Optum

ICD-10-CM Professional for Hospitals

The complete official code set

Codes valid from October 1, 2023 through September 30, 2024

2024

optumcoding.com

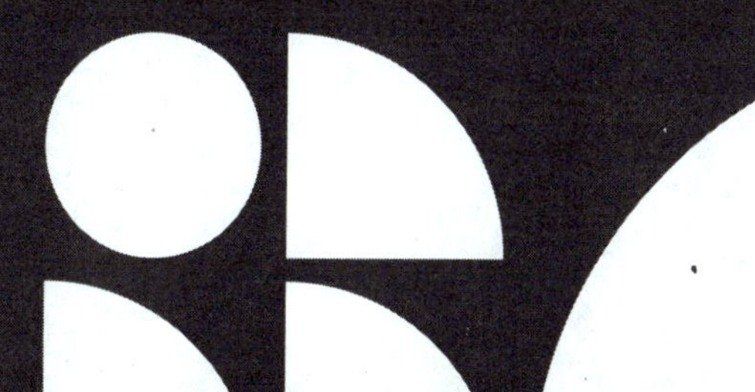

Publisher's Notice

The *ICD-10-CM Professional for Hospitals: The Complete Official Code Set* is designed to be an accurate and authoritative source regarding coding and every reasonable effort has been made to ensure accuracy and completeness of the content. However, Optum makes no guarantee, warranty, or representation that this publication is accurate, complete or without errors. It is understood that Optum is not rendering any legal or other professional services or advice in this publication and that Optum bears no liability for any results or consequences that may arise from the use of this book.

Acknowledgments

Marianne Randall, CPC, *Product Manager*
Anita Schmidt, BS, RHIA, AHIMA-approved ICD-10-CM/PCS Trainer, *Subject Matter Expert*
LaJuana Green, RHIA, CCS, *Subject Matter Expert*
Leanne Patterson, CPC, *Subject Matter Expert*
Jacqueline R. Petersen, MHA, RHIA, CHDA, CPC, *Subject Matter Expert* Laura M. Anderson, RN, BSN, CCDS, *Subject Matter Expert*
Tara Rose, CPC, CPC-I, CPMA, RHIA, CCS-P, *Subject Matter Expert*
Stacy Perry, *Manager, Desktop Publishing*
Tracy Betzler, *Senior Desktop Publishing Specialist*
Hope M. Dunn, *Senior Desktop Publishing Specialist*
Katie Russell, *Desktop Publishing Specialist*
Kate Holden, *Editor*

Our Commitment to Accuracy

Optum is committed to producing accurate and reliable materials.

To report corrections, please email customerassistance@optum.com. You can also reach customer service by calling 1.800.464.3649, option 1.

Made in the USA
ISBN 978-1-62254-883-5

Anita Schmidt, BS, RHIA, AHIMA-approved ICD-10-CM/PCS Trainer

Ms. Schmidt has expertise in ICD-10-CM/PCS, DRG, and CPT with more than 15 years' experience in coding in multiple settings, including inpatient, observation, and same-day surgery. Her experience includes analysis of medical record documentation, assignment of ICD-10-CM and PCS codes, and DRG validation. She has conducted training for ICD-10-CM/PCS and electronic health record. She has also collaborated with clinical documentation specialists to identify documentation needs and potential areas for physician education. Most recently she has been developing content for resource and educational products related to ICD-10-CM, ICD-10-PCS, DRG, and CPT. Ms. Schmidt is an AHIMA-approved ICD-10-CM/PCS trainer and is an active member of the American Health Information Management Association (AHIMA) and the Minnesota Health Information Management Association (MHIMA).

Laura M. Anderson, RN, BSN, CCDS

Ms. Anderson is a Registered Nurse and CDI Specialist/Educator with more than 20 years of experience in the healthcare profession. She obtained her BSN at the University of Minnesota and spent most of her bedside nursing career on Medical-Surgical care units. Her clinical documentation experience began in 2007, covering CDI specialist training, education development, and physician engagement. She has served as a CDI Team Lead and consultant, working with senior leadership to incorporate CDI work into documentation compliance and quality metrics. Ms. Anderson also has a BS degree in Biology (Winthrop University), with research experience in liver cancer and radiation-induced leukemia. She has presented at the state and national levels for the Association of Clinical Documentation Integrity Specialists (ACDIS) and serves as a co-lead for the Minnesota state chapter.

Engagement at every touch point

Optum and Shutterfly Business Solutions are teaming up to give Optum customers new ways to connect with members and patients.

Shutterfly Business Solutions helps health care providers and payers create personalized communications for impactful connections with members and patients. Shutterfly Business Solutions specializes in direct mail, transactional communications, corporate gifting and books for enterprises.

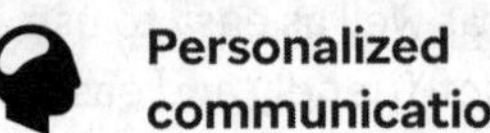

Personalized communications

Simple, automated workflows

Digital printing

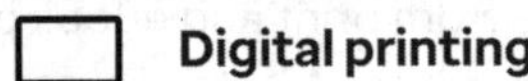

Customized integration

Shutterfly Business Solutions offers:

- **Welcome and engagement campaigns**
  Personalized and branded promotional engagement and targeted offerings, including welcome and reminder, rewards and gifting programs and books
- **Direct mail campaigns**
  Highly personalized and targeted communications, from marketing campaigns, to postcards and announcements, to welcome packets
- **Member and patient communications**
  Automated and compliance-driven mailings including statements, invoices, EOBs, benefit updates or changes
- **Safe, secure and reliable communications that meet regulatory compliance and data privacy standards**

Shutterfly Business Solutions can help you achieve personalized communications and better engagement.

Discover more at:
shutterflybusinesssolutions.com/discover

Contents

How to Use ICD-10-CM Professional for Hospitals 2024

Introduction

ICD-10-CM Professional for Hospitals: The Complete Official Code Set is your definitive coding resource, combining the work of the National Center for Health Statistics (NCHS), Centers for Medicare and Medicaid Services (CMS), American Hospital Association (AHA), and Optum experts to provide the information you need for coding accuracy.

The International Classification of Diseases, 10th Revision, Clinical Modification (ICD-10-CM), is an adaptation of ICD-10, copyrighted by the World Health Organization (WHO). The development and maintenance of this clinical modification (CM) is the responsibility of the NCHS as authorized by WHO. Any new concepts added to ICD-10-CM are based on an established update process through the collaboration of WHO's Update and Revision Committee and the ICD-10-CM Coordination and Maintenance Committee.

In addition to the ICD-10-CM classification, other official government source information has been included in this manual. Depending on the source, updates to information may be annual or quarterly. This manual provides the most current information that was available at the time of publication. For updates to the source documents that may have occurred after this manual was published, please refer to the following:

- **NCHS, International Classification of Diseases, Tenth Revision, Clinical Modification (ICD-10-CM)**

  https://www.cms.gov/medicare/icd-10/2024-icd-10-cm

- **CMS Inpatient Prospective Payment System Proposed Rule and v41 MS-DRG Data Files, FY 2024**

  https://www.cms.gov/medicare/acute-inpatient-pps/fy-2024-ipps-proposed-rule-home-page

  https://www.cms.gov/Medicare/Medicare-Fee-for-Service-Payment/AcuteInpatientPPS/MS-DRG-Classifications-and-Software

- **CMS Risk Adjustment Model, version 24**

  https://www.cms.gov/Medicare/Health-Plans/MedicareAdvtgSpecRateStats/Risk-Adjustors

- **CMS Long-term Care Hospital Prospective Payment System Proposed Rule and Data Files, FY 2024**

  https://www.cms.gov/medicare/medicare-fee-service-payment/longtermcarehospitalpps/ltchpps-regulations-and-notices/cms-1785-p

- **AHA Coding Clinics**

  https://www.codingclinicadvisor.com/

The official NCHS ICD-10-CM classification includes three main sections: the guidelines, the indexes, and the tabular list, all of which make up the bulk of this coding manual. To complement the classification, Optum's coding experts have incorporated Medicare-related coding edits and proprietary features, such as supplementary notations, coding tools, and appendixes, into a comprehensive and easy-to-use reference. This publication is organized as follows:

What's New for 2024

This section provides a high-level overview of the code changes made for FY 2024. The list of codes provided identifies new, revised, and deleted codes. Asterisked codes identify prior midyear changes that were made to the classification, effective April 1, 2023. All changes are based on an official addendum, provided by the NCHS.

Conversion Table

The conversion table was developed by NCHS to help facilitate data retrieval as new codes are added to the ICD-10-CM classification. This table provides a crosswalk from each FY 2024 new code to the equivalent code(s) assigned, prior to October 1, 2023, for that diagnosis or condition. Asterisked codes identify prior midyear additions, effective April 1, 2023. For the full conversion table, refer to the Conversion Table zip file at https://www.cms.gov/medicare/icd-10/2024-icd-10-cm.

10 Steps to Correct Coding

This step-by-step tutorial walks the coder through the process of finding the correct code — from locating the code in the official indexes to verifying the code in the tabular section — while following applicable conventions, guidelines, and instructional notes. Specific examples are provided with detailed explanations of each coding step along with advice for proper sequencing.

Official ICD-10-CM Guidelines for Coding and Reporting

This section provides the full official conventions and guidelines regulating the appropriate assignment and reporting of ICD-10-CM codes. These conventions and guidelines are published by the U.S. Department of Health and Human Services (DHHS) and approved by the cooperating parties (American Health Information Management Association [AHIMA], NCHS, Centers for Disease Control and Prevention [CDC], and the American Hospital Association [AHA]).

Indexes

Index to Diseases and Injuries

The Index to Diseases and Injuries is arranged in alphabetic order by terms specific to a disease, condition, illness, injury, eponym, or abbreviation as well as terms that describe circumstances other than a disease or injury that may require attention from a health care professional.

Neoplasm Table

The Neoplasm Table is arranged in alphabetic order by anatomical site. Codes are then listed in individual columns based upon the histological behavior (malignant, in situ, benign, uncertain, or unspecified) of the neoplasm.

Table of Drugs and Chemicals

The Table of Drugs and Chemicals is arranged in alphabetic order by the specific drug or chemical name. Codes are listed in individual columns based upon the associated intent (poisoning, adverse effect, or underdosing). **Note:** Drugs with an asterisk identify substances added to the table by Optum subject matter experts.

External Causes Index

The External Causes Index is arranged in alphabetic order by main terms that describe the cause, the intent, the place of occurrence, the activity, and the status of the patient at the time the injury occurred or health condition arose.

Index Notations

With

The word "with" or "in" should be interpreted to mean "associated with" or "due to." The classification presumes a causal relationship between the two conditions linked by these terms in the index. These conditions should be coded as related even in the absence of provider documentation explicitly linking them unless the documentation clearly states the conditions are unrelated or when another guideline specifically requires a documented linkage between two conditions (e.g., the sepsis guideline for "acute organ dysfunction that is not clearly associated with the sepsis"). For conditions not specifically linked by these relational terms in the classification or when a guideline requires explicit documentation of a linkage between two conditions, provider documentation must link the conditions to code them as related.

The word "with" in the index is sequenced immediately following the main term, not in alphabetical order.

> **Dermatopolymyositis** M33.9Ø
> with
> myopathy M33.92
> respiratory involvement M33.91
> specified organ involvement NEC M33.99
> amyopathic M33.93

See

When the instruction "see" follows a term in the index, it indicates that another term must be referenced to locate the correct code.

> **Hematoperitoneum** — *see* Hemoperitoneum

See Also

The instructional note "see also" simply provides alternative terms the coder may reference that may be useful in determining the correct code but are not necessary to follow if the main term supplies the appropriate code.

> **Hematinuria** — *see also* Hemaglobinuria
> malarial B5Ø.8

Default Codes

In the index, the default code is the code listed next to the main term and represents the condition most commonly associated with that main term. This code may be assigned when documentation does not support reporting a more specific code. Alternatively, it may provide an unspecified code for the condition.

> **Hemiatrophy** R68.89
> cerebellar G31.9
> face, facial, progressive (Romberg) G51.8
> tongue K14.8

Parentheses

Parentheses in the indexes enclose nonessential modifiers, supplementary words that may be present or absent in the statement of a disease without affecting the code.

> **Pseudomeningocele** (cerebral) (infective) (post-traumatic) G96.198
> postprocedural (spinal) G97.82

Brackets

ICD-10-CM has a coding convention addressing code assignment for manifestations that occur as a result of an underlying condition. This convention requires the underlying condition to be sequenced first, followed by the code or codes for the associated manifestation. In the index, italicized codes in brackets identify manifestation codes.

> **Polyneuropathy** (peripheral) G62.9
> alcoholic G62.1
> amyloid (Portuguese) E85.1 *[G63]*
> transthyretin-related (ATTR) familial E85.1 *[G63]*

Shaded Guides

Exclusive vertical shaded guides in the Index to Diseases and Injuries and External Causes Index help the user easily follow the indent levels for the subentries under a main term. Sequencing rules may apply depending on the level of indent for separate subentries.

> **Hemicrania**
> congenital malformation QØØ.Ø
> continua G44.51
> meaning migraine — *see also* Migraine G43.9Ø9
> paroxysmal G44.Ø39
> chronic G44.Ø49
> intractable G44.Ø41
> not intractable G44.Ø49
> episodic G44.Ø39
> intractable G44.Ø31
> not intractable G44.Ø39
> intractable G44.Ø31
> not intractable G44.Ø39

Following References

The Index to Diseases and Injuries includes "following" references to assist in locating out-of-sequence codes in the tabular list. Out-of-sequence codes contain an alphabetic character (letter) in the third- or fourth-character position. These codes are placed according to the classification rules — according to condition — not according to alphabetic or numeric sequencing rules.

> **Carcinoma** (malignant) — *see also* Neoplasm, by site, malignant
> neuroendocrine — *see also* Tumor, neuroendocrine
> high grade, any site C7A.1 (*following* C75)
> poorly differentiated, any site C7A.1 (*following* C75)

Additional Character Required

The Index to Diseases and Injuries, Neoplasm Table, and External Causes Index provide an icon after certain codes to signify to the user that additional characters are required to make the code valid. The tabular list should be consulted for appropriate character selection.

> **Fall, falling** (accidental) W19 ☑
> building W2Ø.1 ☑

Tabular List of Diseases

ICD-10-CM codes and descriptions are arranged numerically within the tabular list of diseases with 19 separate chapters providing codes associated with a particular body system or nature of injury or disease. There is also a chapter providing codes for external causes of an injury or health conditions, a chapter for codes that address encounters with healthcare facilities for circumstances other than a disease or injury, and finally a chapter for codes that capture special circumstances such as new diseases of uncertain etiology or emergency use codes.

Code and Code Descriptions

ICD-10-CM is an alphanumeric classification system that contains categories, subcategories, and valid codes. The first character is always a letter with any additional characters represented by either a letter or number. A three-character category without further subclassification is equivalent to a valid three-character code. Valid codes may be three, four, five, six, or seven characters in length, with each level of subdivision after a three-character category representing a subcategory. The final level of subdivision is a valid code.

Boldface

Boldface type is used for all codes and descriptions in the tabular list.

Italics

Italicized type is used to identify manifestation codes, those codes that should not be reported as first-listed diagnoses.

Deleted Text

~~Strikethrough~~ on a code and code description indicates a deletion from the classification for the current year.

Key Word

Green font is used throughout the Tabular List of Diseases to differentiate the key words that appear in similar code descriptions in a given category or subcategory. The key word convention is used only in those categories in which there are multiple codes with very similar descriptions with only a few words that differentiate them.

For example, refer to the list of codes below from category H55:

✓4th H55 Nystagmus and other irregular eye movements
✓5th H55.Ø Nystagmus
H55.ØØ Unspecified nystagmus
H55.Ø1 Congenital nystagmus
H55.Ø2 Latent nystagmus
H55.Ø3 Visual deprivation nystagmus
H55.Ø4 Dissociated nystagmus
H55.Ø9 Other forms of nystagmus

The portion of the code description that appears in **green font** in the tabular list helps the coder quickly identify the key terms and the correct code. This convention is especially useful when the codes describe laterality, such as the following codes from subcategory H4Ø.22:

✓6th H4Ø.22 Chronic angle-closure glaucoma
Chronic primary angle closure glaucoma
✓7th H4Ø.221 Chronic angle-closure glaucoma, right eye
✓7th H4Ø.222 Chronic angle-closure glaucoma, left eye
✓7th H4Ø.223 Chronic angle-closure glaucoma, bilateral
✓7th H4Ø.229 Chronic angle-closure glaucoma, unspecified eye

Tabular Notations

Official parenthetical notes as well as Optum's supplementary notations are provided at the chapter, code block, category, subcategory, and individual code level to help the user assign proper codes. The information in the notation can apply to one or more codes depending on where the citation is placed.

Official Notations

Includes Notes

The word INCLUDES appears immediately under certain categories to further define, clarify, or give examples of the content of a code category.

Inclusion Terms

Lists of inclusion terms are included under certain codes. These terms indicate some of the conditions for which that code number may be used. Inclusion terms may be synonyms with the code title, or, in the case of "other specified" codes, the terms may also provide a list of various conditions included within a classification code. The inclusion terms are not exhaustive. The index may provide additional terms that may also be assigned to a given code.

Excludes Notes

ICD-10-CM has two types of excludes notes. Each note has a different definition for use. However, they are similar in that they both indicate that codes excluded from each other are independent of each other.

Excludes 1

An EXCLUDES 1 note is a "pure" excludes. It means "NOT CODED HERE!" An Excludes 1 note indicates mutually exclusive codes: two conditions that cannot be reported together. An Excludes1 note indicates that the code excluded should never be used at the same time as the code above the Excludes1 note. An Excludes1 is used when two conditions cannot occur together, such as a congenital form versus an acquired form of the same condition.

An exception to the Excludes 1 definition is when the two conditions are unrelated to each other. If it is not clear whether the two conditions involving an Excludes 1 note are related or not, query the provider. For example, code F45.8 Other somatoform disorders, has an Excludes 1 note for "sleep related teeth grinding (G47.63)" because "teeth grinding" is an inclusion term under F45.8. Only one of these two codes should be assigned for teeth grinding. However, psychogenic dysmenorrhea is also an inclusion term under F45.8, and a patient could have both this condition and sleep-related teeth grinding. In this case, the two conditions are clearly unrelated to each other, so it would be appropriate to report F45.8 and G47.63 together.

Excludes 2

An EXCLUDES 2 note means "NOT INCLUDED HERE." An Excludes 2 note indicates that although the excluded condition is not part of the condition it is excluded from, a patient may have both conditions at the same time. Therefore, when an Excludes 2 note appears under a code, it may be acceptable to use both the code and the excluded code together if supported by the medical documentation.

Note

The term "NOTE" appears as an icon and precedes the instructional information. These notes function as alerts to highlight coding instructions within the text.

Code First/Use additional code

These instructional notes provide sequencing instruction. They may appear independently of each other or to designate certain etiology/manifestation paired codes. These instructions signal the coder that an additional code should be reported to provide a more complete picture of that diagnosis.

In etiology/manifestation coding, ICD-10-CM requires the underlying condition to be sequenced first, followed by the manifestation. In these situations, codes with "In diseases classified elsewhere" in the code description are never permitted as a first-listed or principal diagnosis code and must be sequenced following the underlying condition code.

Code Also

A "code also" note alerts the coder that more than one code may be required to fully describe the condition. The sequencing depends on the circumstances of the encounter. Factors that may determine sequencing include severity and reason for the encounter.

Revised Text

The revised text ▶◀ "bow ties" alert the user to changes in official notations for the current year. Revised text may include the following:

- A change in a current parenthetical description
- A change in the code(s) associated with a current parenthetical note
- A change in how a current parenthetical note is classified (e.g., an Excludes 1 note that changed to an Excludes 2 note)
- Addition of a new parenthetical note(s) to a code

Deleted Text

~~Strikethrough~~ on official notations indicate a deletion from the classification for the current year.

Optum Notations

AHA Coding Clinic Citations

Coding Clinics are official American Hospital Association (AHA) publications that provide coding advice specific to ICD-10-CM and ICD-10-PCS.

Coding Clinic citations included in this manual are current up to the second quarter of 2023.

These citations identify the year, quarter, and page number of one or more *Coding Clinic* publications that may have coding advice relevant to a particular code or group of codes. With the most current citation listed first, these notations are preceded by the symbol **AHA:** and appear in purple type.

> **I15.1 Hypertension secondary to other renal disorders**
> AHA: 2016, 3Q, 22

Definitions

Definitions explain a specific term, condition, or disease process in layman's terms. These notations are preceded by the symbol **DEF:** and appear in purple type.

> ✓5th **M51.4 Schmorl's nodes**
> **DEF:** Irregular bone defect in the margin of the vertebral body that causes herniation into the end plate of the vertebral body.

Coding Tips

The tips in the tabular list offer coding advice that is not readily available within the ICD-10-CM classification. It may relate official coding guidelines, indexing nuances, or advice from *AHA's Coding Clinic for ICD-10-CM/PCS*. These notations are preceded by the symbol **TIP:** and appear in brown type.

> ✓5th **B97.2 Coronavirus as the cause of diseases classified elsewhere**
> **TIP:** Do not report a code from this subcategory for COVID-19; refer to U07.1.

Icons

Note: The following icons are placed to the left of the code.

Changes to ICD-10-CM codes since the last published edition of this manual are highlighted in two ways:

The following green icons identify new or revised codes effective April 1, 2023:

● **New Code — Midyear**

▲ **Revised Code — Midyear**

The following black icons identify new or revised codes effective October 1, 2023:

● **New Code**

▲ **Revised Code**

✓ **Additional Characters Required**

✓4th This symbol indicates that the code requires a 4th character.

✓5th This symbol indicates that the code requires a 5th character.

✓6th This symbol indicates that the code requires a 6th character.

✓7th This symbol indicates that the code requires a 7th character.

> ✓5th **H60.3 Other infective otitis externa**
> ✓6th **H60.31 Diffuse otitis externa**
> **H60.311 Diffuse otitis externa, right ear**
> **H60.312 Diffuse otitis externa, left ear**
> **H60.313 Diffuse otitis externa, bilateral**
> **H60.319 Diffuse otitis externa, unspecified ear**

✓x7th **Placeholder Alert**

This symbol indicates that the code requires a 7th character following the placeholder "X". Codes with fewer than six characters that require a 7th character must contain placeholder "X" to fill in the empty character(s).

> ✓x7th **T16.1 Foreign body in right ear**

Most icons in this manual, placed at the end of the code description, include official edits from the following sources:

- Inpatient prospective payment system (IPPS)
- CMS HCC risk-adjustment model

In most instances, FY 2024 data from the above sources were not available at the time this book was printed. In an effort to make available the most current source information, Optum has provided a document identifying FY 2024 changes to edit designations for ICD-10-CM codes. Edit changes identified in this document may include:

- Age
- Sex
- Hospital-acquired condition
- Major HIV-related diagnosis
- Major complication/comorbidity
- Complication/comorbidity
- Manifestation
- Unacceptable principal diagnosis
- Questionable principal diagnosis
- Unspecified site
- CMS-HC

This document can be accessed at the following:

https://www.optumcoding.com/ProductUpdates/
Title: "2024 ICD-10-CM Inpatient Edit Changes"
Password: 24FACILITY

Age Edits

N **Newborn Age: 0**
These diagnoses are intended for newborns and neonates and the patient's age must be 0 years.

N47.Ø Adherent prepuce, newborn N♂

P **Pediatric Age: 0-17**
These diagnoses are intended for children and the patient's age must be between 0 and 17 years.

L21.1 Seborrheic infantile dermatitis P

M **Maternity Age: 9-64**
These diagnoses are intended for childbearing patients between the age of 9 and 64 years.

OØ2.9 Abnormal product of conception, unspecified M♀

A **Adult Age: 15-124**
These diagnoses are intended for patients between the age of 15 and 124 years.

> **R54 Age-related physical debility** A
> Frailty
> Old age
> Senescence
> Senile asthenia
> Senile debility
> **EXCLUDES 1** *age-related cognitive decline (R41.81)*
> *sarcopenia (M62.84)*
> *senile psychosis (FØ3)*
> *senility NOS (R41.81)*

Sex Edits

♂ **Male diagnosis only**

Q98.Ø Klinefelter syndrome karyotype 47, XXY ♂

♀ **Female diagnosis only**

N35.12 Postinfective urethral stricture, not elsewhere classified, female ♀

H1-H14 Hospital Acquired Condition (HAC)
These icons identify codes that are high-cost and/or high-volume (CC or MCC) that when assigned as a secondary diagnosis result in assignment of a case to a higher-paying MS-DRG. The condition or diagnosis represented by these codes is considered reasonably preventable through the application of evidence-based guidelines. If the condition is not present on admission (meaning it developed during the hospital admission), the case will not group to the higher-paying MS-DRG based solely upon the reporting of the HAC code. Many of these HACs are conditional and are based on reporting the specific diagnosis code(s) in combination with certain procedure codes.

Note: Hospital-acquired conditions do not impact MS-LTC-DRG assignment.

N15.1 Renal and perinephric abscess MCC H6

CC **CC Condition**
This icon identifies a complication or comorbidity diagnosis that may affect DRG assignment. A complication or comorbidity diagnosis, CC condition, is defined as a significant acute disease, a significant acute manifestation of a chronic disease, an advanced or end-stage chronic disease, or a chronic disease associated with systemic physiological decompensation and debility that have consistently greater impact on hospital resources.

G9Ø.59 Complex regional pain syndrome I of other specified site 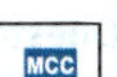

MCC **MCC Condition**
This icon identifies a major complication or comorbidity diagnosis that may affect DRG assignment. An MCC condition meets the same criteria as a CC condition but is associated with a higher acuity level and hospital resource consumption is expected to be higher than that for a CC condition. There are fewer conditions that meet the criteria as an MCC than those for a CC condition.

✓7th **S35.238 Other injury of inferior mesenteric artery** MCC

Note: The assignment of an MS-DRG or MS-LTC-DRG often depends on the presence or absence of a secondary diagnosis code that is designated as an MCC or CC. However, in some instances the MCC or CC designation for that secondary diagnosis code is negated due to its relationship with the principal diagnosis; this is referred to as CC exclusion. The ICD-10 MS-DRG Definitions Manual included with the IPPS final rule provides a list of all principal diagnosis codes that would render ineffective the MCC/CC designation for a particular ICD-10-CM code when used as a secondary diagnosis. Optum has provided this CC exclusion list in an easily searchable data file, which can be accessed at the following:

https://www.optumcoding.com/ProductUpdates/
Title: "2024 ICD-10-CM for Hospitals CC Excludes Data File"
Password: 24FACILITY

UNS **Unspecified Site**
This icon identifies codes that are considered an MCC or CC but lack specificity in regard to their anatomical location. The medical record documentation should be reviewed carefully, to ensure that no other code within the same category or subcategory can be assigned for greater specificity.

G81.ØØ Flaccid hemiplegia affecting unspecified side CC UNS HCC

UPD **Unacceptable Principal Diagnosis**
This icon identifies codes that should not be assigned as principal diagnosis for *inpatient* admissions. Codes with an unacceptable principal diagnosis edit are considered supplementary — describing circumstances that influence an individual's health status or an additional code — identifying conditions that are not specific manifestations but may be due to an underlying cause.

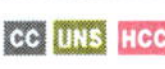 **T48.5X5 Adverse effect of other anti-common-cold drugs** UPD

HIV **HIV-related Condition**
This icon identifies codes that are considered a major HIV-related diagnosis. When the condition is coded in combination with a diagnosis of human immunodeficiency virus (HIV), code B2Ø, the case will move from MS-DRG/MS-LTC-DRG 977 to MS-DRGs/MS-LTC-DRGs 974-976.

G96.9 Disorder of central nervous system, unspecified HIV

 **CMS-HCC Condition**

This icon identifies codes that are included in the CMS-HCC risk-adjustment model.

> **Y62.2 Failure of sterile precautions during kidney dialysis and other perfusion** 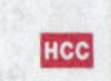

Color Bars

Manifestation Code

Codes defined as manifestation codes appear in italic type, with a blue color bar over the code description. A manifestation cannot be reported as a first-listed code; it is sequenced as a secondary diagnosis with the underlying disease code listed first.

> *G32.89* ***Other specified degenerative disorders of nervous system in diseases classified elsewhere***
> Degenerative encephalopathy in diseases classified elsewhere

Questionable Admission Diagnoses

Questionable admission diagnoses will appear with a yellow color bar over the code description. These codes, although not unacceptable as a PDx, may be considered a "questionable admission" when used as PDx in an acute care hospital.

> **E66.Ø9 Other obesity due to excess calories**

Wrong Procedure Performed Edit

An orange color bar over the code title indicates the Wrong Procedure Performed edit. This edit was created to identify cases in which wrong surgeries occurred. Any claim with a code from Y65.51-Y65.53 will be denied and returned to the provider. A surgical or other invasive procedure is considered to be a wrong procedure if one of the following is true:

- The procedure was performed on the wrong site.
- The procedure was performed on the wrong patient.
- The incorrect procedure was performed on a patient.

> **Y65.51 Performance of wrong procedure (operation) on correct patient**
> Wrong device implanted into correct surgical site
> **EXCLUDES 1** *performance of correct procedure (operation) on wrong side or body part (Y65.53)*

Unspecified Diagnosis

Codes that appear with a gray color bar over the alphanumeric code identify unspecified diagnoses. These codes should be used in limited circumstances, when neither the diagnostic statement nor the documentation provides enough information to assign a more specific diagnosis code. The abbreviation NOS, "not otherwise specified," in the tabular list may be interpreted as "unspecified."

> **GØ3.9 Meningitis, unspecified** MCC
> Arachnoiditis (spinal) NOS

Chapter-Level Notations

Chapter-Specific Guidelines with Coding Examples

Each chapter begins with the Official Guidelines for Coding and Reporting specific to that chapter, where provided. Coding examples specific to inpatient care settings have been provided to illustrate the coding and/or sequencing guidance in these guidelines.

Muscle and Tendon Table

ICD-10-CM categorizes certain muscles and tendons in the upper and lower extremities by their action (e.g., extension or flexion) as well as their anatomical location. The Muscle/Tendon table is provided at the beginning of chapter 13 and chapter 19 to help users when code selection depends on the action of the muscle and/or tendon.

Note: This table is not all-inclusive, and proper code assignment should be based on the provider's documentation.

Illustrations

This section includes illustrations of normal anatomy with ICD-10-CM-specific terminology.

What's New for 2024

Official Updates

A summary of changes to the official ICD-10-CM code set is provided below, identifying changes made for fiscal 2024, effective October 1, 2023, to September 30, 2024. Asterisked codes identify prior midyear changes that were made to the classification, effective April 1, 2023. All code changes were made by the agency charged with maintaining and updating the ICD-10-CM code set, the National Center for Health Statistics (NCHS), a section of the Centers for Disease Control and Prevention (CDC).

437 New Codes

A41.54 B96.83 D13.91 D13.99 D48.110
D48.111 D48.112 D48.113 D48.114 D48.115
D48.116 D48.117 D48.118 D48.119 D48.19
D57.04 D57.214 D57.414 D57.434 D57.454
D57.814 D61.02 D89.84 E20.810 E20.811
E20.812 E20.818 E20.819 E20.89 E74.05
E75.27 E75.28 E79.81 E79.82 E79.89
E88.43 E88.810 E88.811 E88.818 E88.819
E88.A G11.5 G11.6 G20.A1 G20.A2
G20.B1 G20.B2 G20.C G23.3 G31.80
G31.86 G37.81 G37.89 G40.C01 G40.C09
G40.C11 G40.C19 G43.E01 G43.E09 G43.E11
G43.E19 G90.B G93.42 G93.43 G93.44
H36.811 H36.812 H36.813 H36.819 H36.821
H36.822 H36.823 H36.829 H36.89 H50.621
H50.622 H50.629 H50.631 H50.632 H50.639
H50.641 H50.642 H50.649 H50.651 H50.652
H50.659 H50.661 H50.662 H50.669 H50.671
H50.672 H50.679 H50.681 H50.682 H50.689
H57.8A1 H57.8A2 H57.8A3 H57.8A9 I1A.0
I20.81 I20.89 I21.B I24.81 I24.89
I25.85 I47.10 I47.11 I47.19 J15.61
J15.69 J44.81 J44.89 J4A.0 J4A.8
J4A.9 K35.200 K35.201 K35.209 K35.210
K35.211 K35.219 K63.8211 K63.8212 K63.8219
K63.822 K63.829 K68.2 K68.3 K90.821
K90.822 K90.829 K90.83 M80.0B1A M80.0B1D
M80.0B1G M80.0B1K M80.0B1P M80.0B1S M80.0B2A
M80.0B2D M80.0B2G M80.0B2K M80.0B2P M80.0B2S
M80.0B9A M80.0B9D M80.0B9G M80.0B9K M80.0B9P
M80.0B9S M80.8B1A M80.8B1D M80.8B1G M80.8B1K
M80.8B1P M80.8B1S M80.8B2A M80.8B2D M80.8B2G
M80.8B2K M80.8B2P M80.8B2S M80.8B9A M80.8B9D
M80.8B9G M80.8B9K M80.8B9P M80.8B9S N02.B1
N02.B2 N02.B3 N02.B4 N02.B5 N02.B6
N02.B9 N04.20 N04.21 N04.22 N04.29
N06.20 N06.21 N06.22 N06.29 O26.641
O26.642 O26.643 O26.649 O90.41 O90.49
Q44.70 Q44.71 Q44.79 Q75.001 Q75.002
Q75.009 Q75.01 Q75.021 Q75.022 Q75.029
Q75.03 Q75.041 Q75.042 Q75.049 Q75.051
Q75.052 Q75.058 Q75.08 Q87.83 Q87.84
Q87.85 Q93.52 R09.A0 R09.A1 R09.A2
R09.A9 R40.2A R92.30 R92.311 R92.312
R92.313 R92.321 R92.322 R92.323 R92.331
R92.332 R92.333 R92.341 R92.342 R92.343
T56.821A T56.821D T56.821S T56.822A T56.822D
T56.822S T56.823A T56.823D T56.823S T56.824A
T56.824D T56.824S T74.A1XA* T74.A1XD* T74.A1XS*
T74.A2XA* T74.A2XD* T74.A2XS* T76.A1XA* T76.A1XD*
T76.A1XS* T76.A2XA* T76.A2XD* T76.A2XS* W44.8XXA
W44.8XXD W44.8XXS W44.9XXA W44.9XXD W44.9XXS
W44.A0XA W44.A0XD W44.A0XS W44.A1XA W44.A1XD
W44.A1XS W44.A9XA W44.A9XD W44.A9XS W44.B0XA
W44.B0XD W44.B0XS W44.B1XA W44.B1XD W44.B1XS
W44.B2XA W44.B2XD W44.B2XS W44.B3XA W44.B3XD
W44.B3XS W44.B4XA W44.B4XD W44.B4XS W44.B5XA
W44.B5XD W44.B5XS W44.B9XA W44.B9XD W44.B9XS
W44.C0XA W44.C0XD W44.C0XS W44.C1XA W44.C1XD
W44.C1XS W44.C2XA W44.C2XD W44.C2XS W44.D0XA
W44.D0XD W44.D0XS W44.D1XA W44.D1XD W44.D1XS
W44.D2XA W44.D2XD W44.D2XS W44.D3XA W44.D3XD
W44.D3XS W44.D4XA W44.D4XD W44.D4XS W44.D9XA
W44.D9XD W44.D9XS W44.E0XA W44.E0XD W44.E0XS
W44.E1XA W44.E1XD W44.E1XS W44.E2XA W44.E2XD
W44.E2XS W44.E3XA W44.E3XD W44.E3XS W44.E4XA
W44.E4XD W44.E4XS W44.E9XA W44.E9XD W44.E9XS
W44.F0XA W44.F0XD W44.F0XS W44.F1XA W44.F1XD
W44.F1XS W44.F2XA W44.F2XD W44.F2XS W44.F3XA
W44.F3XD W44.F3XS W44.F4XA W44.F4XD W44.F4XS
W44.F9XA W44.F9XD W44.F9XS W44.G0XA W44.G0XD
W44.G0XS W44.G1XA W44.G1XD W44.G1XS W44.G2XA
W44.G2XD W44.G2XS W44.G3XA W44.G3XD W44.G3XS
W44.G9XA W44.G9XD W44.G9XS W44.H0XA W44.H0XD
W44.H0XS W44.H1XA W44.H1XD W44.H1XS W44.H2XA
W44.H2XD W44.H2XS Y07.010* Y07.011* Y07.020*
Y07.021* Y07.030* Y07.031* Y07.040* Y07.041*
Y07.050* Y07.051* Y07.44* Y07.45* Y07.46*
Y07.47* Y07.54* Z02.84 Z05.81 Z05.89
Z16.13 Z22.340 Z22.341 Z22.349 Z22.350
Z22.358 Z22.359 Z29.81 Z29.89 Z55.6*
Z58.81* Z58.89* Z59.10* Z59.11* Z59.12*
Z59.19* Z62.23 Z62.24 Z62.814* Z62.815*
Z62.823 Z62.831 Z62.832 Z62.833 Z62.892
Z83.710 Z83.711 Z83.718 Z83.719 Z91.141*
Z91.148* Z91.151* Z91.158* Z91.413* Z91.414*
Z91.85 Z91.A41 Z91.A48 Z91.A51 Z91.A58
Z91.A91 Z91.A98

14 Revised Codes

Note: Each code is listed with its revised description only.

I25.112	Atherosclerotic heart disease of native coronary artery with refractory angina pectoris
I71.51	Supraceliac aneurysm of the thoracoabdominal aorta, ruptured
I71.52	Paravisceral aneurysm of the thoracoabdominal aorta, ruptured
I71.61	Supraceliac aneurysm of the thoracoabdominal aorta, without rupture
I71.62	Paravisceral aneurysm of the thoracoabdominal aorta, without rupture
N35.812	Other bulbous urethral stricture, male
P19.9	Metabolic acidemia in newborn, unspecified
Q85.81	PTEN hamartoma tumor syndrome
Q87.40	Marfan syndrome, unspecified
Q87.410	Marfan syndrome with aortic dilation
Q87.418	Marfan syndrome with other cardiovascular manifestations
Q87.42	Marfan syndrome with ocular manifestations
Q87.43	Marfan syndrome with skeletal manifestation
Z59.87*	Material hardship due to limited financial resources, not elsewhere classified

Proprietary Updates

The following proprietary features have also been added:

- New definitions that describe, in lay terms, a specific condition or disease process
- New coding tips that provide coding advice beyond the code classification
- Updated *AHA Coding Clinic* references through second quarter 2023

Conversion Table of ICD-10-CM Codes

The FY 2024 (October 1, 2023-September 30, 2024) Conversion Table for new ICD-10-CM codes is provided to assist users in data retrieval. For each new code the table shows its previously assigned code equivalent. Asterisks identify new codes added to the classification April 1, 2023.

Code Assignment Beginning 10/1/2023	Previous Code(s) Assignment
A41.54	A41.59
B96.83	B96.89
D13.91	D13.9
D13.99	D13.9
D48.11Ø	D48.1
D48.111	D48.1
D48.112	D48.1
D48.113	D48.1
D48.114	D48.1
D48.115	D48.1
D48.116	D48.1
D48.117	D48.1
D48.118	D48.1
D48.119	D48.1
D48.19	D48.1
D57.Ø4	D57.Ø9
D57.214	D57.218
D57.414	D57.418
D57.434	D57.438
D57.454	D57.458
D57.814	D57.818
D61.Ø2	D61.Ø9
D89.84	D89.89
E2Ø.81Ø	E2Ø.8
E2Ø.811	E2Ø.8
E2Ø.812	E2Ø.8
E2Ø.818	E2Ø.8
E2Ø.819	E2Ø.8
E2Ø.89	E2Ø.8
E74.Ø5	E74.Ø9
E75.27	E75.29
E75.28	E75.29
E79.81	E79.8
E79.82	E79.8
E79.89	E79.8
E88.43	E88.49
E88.81Ø	E88.81
E88.811	E88.81
E88.818	E88.81
E88.819	E88.81
E88.A	R64
G11.5	G11.8 and E23.Ø and KØØ.Ø
G11.6	G11.8
G2Ø.A1	G2Ø
G2Ø.A2	G2Ø
G2Ø.B1	G2Ø
G2Ø.B2	G2Ø
G2Ø.C	G2Ø
G23.3	G23.8
G31.8Ø	G31.89
G31.86	G31.89
G37.81	G37.8
G37.89	G37.8
G4Ø.CØ1	G4Ø.3Ø1
G4Ø.CØ9	G4Ø.3Ø9
G4Ø.C11	G4Ø.311
G4Ø.C19	G4Ø.319
G43.EØ1	G43.8Ø1
G43.EØ9	G43.8Ø9
G43.E11	G43.811
G43.E19	G43.819
G9Ø.B	G9Ø.8
G93.42	G93.49
G93.43	G93.49
G93.44	G93.49
H36.811	H35.2Ø-H35.23
H36.812	H35.2Ø-H35.23
H36.813	H35.2Ø-H35.23
H36.819	H35.2Ø-H35.23
H36.821	H35.2Ø-H35.23
H36.822	H35.2Ø-H35.23
H36.823	H35.2Ø-H35.23
H36.829	H35.2Ø-H35.23
H36.89	H35.2Ø-H35.23
H5Ø.621	H5Ø.69
H5Ø.622	H5Ø.69
H5Ø.629	H5Ø.69
H5Ø.631	H5Ø.69
H5Ø.632	H5Ø.69
H5Ø.639	H5Ø.69
H5Ø.641	H5Ø.69
H5Ø.642	H5Ø.69
H5Ø.649	H5Ø.69
H5Ø.651	H5Ø.69
H5Ø.652	H5Ø.69
H5Ø.659	H5Ø.69
H5Ø.661	H5Ø.69
H5Ø.662	H5Ø.69
H5Ø.669	H5Ø.69
H5Ø.671	H5Ø.69
H5Ø.672	H5Ø.69
H5Ø.679	H5Ø.69
H5Ø.681	H5Ø.69
H5Ø.682	H5Ø.69
H5Ø.689	H5Ø.69
H57.8A1	H57.89
H57.8A2	H57.89
H57.8A3	H57.89
H57.8A9	H57.89
I1A.Ø	I1Ø-I15.9
I2Ø.81	I2Ø.8
I2Ø.89	I2Ø.8
I21.B	I21.A9
I24.81	I24.8
I24.89	I24.8
I25.85	I25.89
I47.1Ø	I47.1
I47.11	I47.1
I47.19	I47.1
J15.61	J15.6
J15.69	J15.6
J44.81	J42
J44.89	J42
J4A.Ø	J44.Ø-J44.1; J44.9
J4A.8	J44.Ø-J44.1; J44.9
J4A.9	J44.Ø-J44.1; J44.9
K35.2ØØ	K35.2Ø
K35.2Ø1	K35.2Ø
K35.2Ø9	K35.2Ø
K35.21Ø	K35.21
K35.211	K35.21
K35.219	K35.21
K63.8211	K63.89
K63.8212	K63.89
K63.8219	K63.89
K63.822	K63.89
K63.829	K63.89
K68.2	K68.9
K68.3	K68.9
K9Ø.821	K9Ø.89
K9Ø.822	K9Ø.89
K9Ø.829	K9Ø.89
K9Ø.83	K9Ø.89
M8Ø.ØB1A	M8Ø.ØAXA
M8Ø.ØB1D	M8Ø.ØAXD
M8Ø.ØB1G	M8Ø.ØAXG
M8Ø.ØB1K	M8Ø.ØAXK
M8Ø.ØB1P	M8Ø.ØAXP
M8Ø.ØB1S	M8Ø.ØAXS
M8Ø.ØB2A	M8Ø.ØAXA
M8Ø.ØB2D	M8Ø.ØAXD
M8Ø.ØB2G	M8Ø.ØAXG
M8Ø.ØB2K	M8Ø.ØAXK
M8Ø.ØB2P	M8Ø.ØAXP
M8Ø.ØB2S	M8Ø.ØAXS
M8Ø.ØB9A	M8Ø.ØAXA
M8Ø.ØB9D	M8Ø.ØAXD
M8Ø.ØB9G	M8Ø.ØAXG
M8Ø.ØB9K	M8Ø.ØAXK
M8Ø.ØB9P	M8Ø.ØAXP
M8Ø.ØB9S	M8Ø.ØAXS
M8Ø.8B1A	M8Ø.8ØXA
M8Ø.8B1D	M8Ø.8AXD
M8Ø.8B1G	M8Ø.8AXG
M8Ø.8B1K	M8Ø.8AXK
M8Ø.8B1P	M8Ø.8AXP
M8Ø.8B1S	M8Ø.8AXS
M8Ø.8B2A	M8Ø.8ØXA
M8Ø.8B2D	M8Ø.8AXD
M8Ø.8B2G	M8Ø.8AXG
M8Ø.8B2K	M8Ø.8AXK
M8Ø.8B2P	M8Ø.8AXP
M8Ø.8B2S	M8Ø.8AXS
M8Ø.8B9A	M8Ø.8ØXA
M8Ø.8B9D	M8Ø.8AXD
M8Ø.8B9G	M8Ø.8AXG
M8Ø.8B9K	M8Ø.8AXK
M8Ø.8B9P	M8Ø.8AXP
M8Ø.8B9S	M8Ø.8AXS
NØ2.B1	NØ2.Ø-NØ2.1
NØ2.B2	NØ2.1
NØ2.B3	NØ2.2
NØ2.B4	NØ2.2
NØ2.B5	NØ2.3
NØ2.B6	NØ2.5
NØ2.B9	NØ2.8
NØ4.2Ø	NØ4.2
NØ4.21	NØ4.2
NØ4.22	NØ4.2
NØ4.29	NØ4.2
NØ6.2Ø	NØ6.2
NØ6.21	NØ6.2
NØ6.22	NØ6.2
NØ6.29	NØ6.2
O26.641	O26.611
O26.642	O26.612
O26.643	O26.613
O26.649	O26.619
O9Ø.41	O9Ø.4
O9Ø.49	O9Ø.4
Q44.7Ø	Q44.7
Q44.71	Q44.7
Q44.79	Q44.7
Q75.ØØ1	Q75.Ø
Q75.ØØ2	Q75.Ø
Q75.ØØ9	Q75.Ø
Q75.Ø1	Q75.Ø
Q75.Ø21	Q75.Ø
Q75.Ø22	Q75.Ø
Q75.Ø29	Q75.Ø
Q75.Ø3	Q75.Ø
Q75.Ø41	Q75.Ø
Q75.Ø42	Q75.Ø
Q75.Ø49	Q75.Ø
Q75.Ø51	Q75.Ø
Q75.Ø52	Q75.Ø
Q75.Ø58	Q75.Ø
Q75.Ø8	Q75.Ø
Q87.83	Q87.89
Q87.84	Q87.89
Q87.85	Q87.89
Q93.52	Q93.59
RØ9.AØ	RØ9.89
RØ9.A1	RØ9.89
RØ9.A2	RØ9.89
RØ9.A9	RØ9.89
R4Ø.2A	R4Ø.2Ø
R92.3Ø	R92.2
R92.311	R92.2
R92.312	R92.2
R92.313	R92.2
R92.321	R92.2
R92.322	R92.2
R92.323	R92.2
R92.331	R92.2
R92.332	R92.2
R92.333	R92.2
R92.341	R92.2
R92.342	R92.2
R92.343	R92.2
T56.821A	T56.891A
T56.821D	T56.891D
T56.821S	T56.891S
T56.822A	T56.892A
T56.822D	T56.892D
T56.822S	T56.892S
T56.823A	T56.893A
T56.823D	T56.893D
T56.823S	T56.893S
T56.824A	T56.894A
T56.824D	T56.894D
T56.824S	T56.894S
*T74.A1XA	T74.91XA
*T74.A1XD	T74.91XD
*T74.A1XS	T74.91XS
*T74.A2XA	T74.92XA
*T74.A2XD	T74.92XD
*T74.A2XS	T74.92XS
*T76.A1XA	T76.91XA
*T76.A1XD	T76.91XD
*T76.A1XS	T76.91XS
*T76.A2XA	T76.92XA
*T76.A2XD	T76.92XD
*T76.A2XS	T76.92XS
W44.8XXA	Codes in Categories T15-T19
W44.8XXD	Codes in Categories T15-T19
W44.8XXS	Codes in Categories T15-T19
W44.9XXA	Codes in Categories T15-T19
W44.9XXD	Codes in Categories T15-T19
W44.9XXS	Codes in Categories T15-T19
W44.AØXA	Codes in Categories T15-T19
W44.AØXD	Codes in Categories T15-T19
W44.AØXS	Codes in Categories T15-T19
W44.A1XA	Codes in Categories T15-T19
W44.A1XD	Codes in Categories T15-T19

Code Assignment Beginning 10/1/2023	Previous Code(s) Assignment
W44.A1XS	Codes in Categories T15-T19
W44.A9XA	Codes in Categories T15-T19
W44.A9XD	Codes in Categories T15-T19
W44.A9XS	Codes in Categories T15-T19
W44.BØXA	Codes in Categories T15-T19
W44.BØXD	Codes in Categories T15-T19
W44.BØXS	Codes in Categories T15-T19
W44.B1XA	Codes in Categories T15-T19
W44.B1XD	Codes in Categories T15-T19
W44.B1XS	Codes in Categories T15-T19
W44.B2XA	Codes in Categories T15-T19
W44.B2XD	Codes in Categories T15-T19
W44.B2XS	Codes in Categories T15-T19
W44.B3XA	Codes in Categories T15-T19
W44.B3XD	Codes in Categories T15-T19
W44.B3XS	Codes in Categories T15-T19
W44.B4XA	Codes in Categories T15-T19
W44.B4XD	Codes in Categories T15-T19
W44.B4XS	Codes in Categories T15-T19
W44.B5XA	Codes in Categories T15-T19
W44.B5XD	Codes in Categories T15-T19
W44.B5XS	Codes in Categories T15-T19
W44.B9XA	Codes in Categories T15-T19

Code Assignment Beginning 10/1/2023	Previous Code(s) Assignment
W44.B9XD	Codes in Categories T15-T19
W44.B9XS	Codes in Categories T15-T19
W44.CØXA	Codes in Categories T15-T19
W44.CØXD	Codes in Categories T15-T19
W44.CØXS	Codes in Categories T15-T19
W44.C1XA	Codes in Categories T15-T19
W44.C1XD	Codes in Categories T15-T19
W44.C1XS	Codes in Categories T15-T19
W44.C2XA	Codes in Categories T15-T19
W44.C2XD	Codes in Categories T15-T19
W44.C2XS	Codes in Categories T15-T19
W44.DØXA	Codes in Categories T15-T19
W44.DØXD	Codes in Categories T15-T19
W44.DØXS	Codes in Categories T15-T19
W44.D1XA	Codes in Categories T15-T19
W44.D1XD	Codes in Categories T15-T19
W44.D1XS	Codes in Categories T15-T19
W44.D2XA	Codes in Categories T15-T19
W44.D2XD	Codes in Categories T15-T19
W44.D2XS	Codes in Categories T15-T19
W44.D3XA	Codes in Categories T15-T19
W44.D3XD	Codes in Categories T15-T19
W44.D3XS	Codes in Categories T15-T19

Code Assignment Beginning 10/1/2023	Previous Code(s) Assignment
W44.D4XA	Codes in Categories T15-T19
W44.D4XD	Codes in Categories T15-T19
W44.D4XS	Codes in Categories T15-T19
W44.D9XA	Codes in Categories T15-T19
W44.D9XD	Codes in Categories T15-T19
W44.D9XS	Codes in Categories T15-T19
W44.EØXA	Codes in Categories T15-T19
W44.EØXD	Codes in Categories T15-T19
W44.EØXS	Codes in Categories T15-T19
W44.E1XA	Codes in Categories T15-T19
W44.E1XD	Codes in Categories T15-T19
W44.E1XS	Codes in Categories T15-T19
W44.E2XA	Codes in Categories T15-T19
W44.E2XD	Codes in Categories T15-T19
W44.E2XS	Codes in Categories T15-T19
W44.E3XA	Codes in Categories T15-T19
W44.E3XD	Codes in Categories T15-T19
W44.E3XS	Codes in Categories T15-T19
W44.E4XA	Codes in Categories T15-T19
W44.E4XD	Codes in Categories T15-T19
W44.E4XS	Codes in Categories T15-T19
W44.E9XA	Codes in Categories T15-T19
W44.E9XD	Codes in Categories T15-T19

Code Assignment Beginning 10/1/2023	Previous Code(s) Assignment
W44.E9XS	Codes in Categories T15-T19
W44.FØXA	Codes in Categories T15-T19
W44.FØXD	Codes in Categories T15-T19
W44.FØXS	Codes in Categories T15-T19
W44.F1XA	Codes in Categories T15-T19
W44.F1XD	Codes in Categories T15-T19
W44.F1XS	Codes in Categories T15-T19
W44.F2XA	Codes in Categories T15-T19
W44.F2XD	Codes in Categories T15-T19
W44.F2XS	Codes in Categories T15-T19
W44.F3XA	Codes in Categories T15-T19
W44.F3XD	Codes in Categories T15-T19
W44.F3XS	Codes in Categories T15-T19
W44.F4XA	Codes in Categories T15-T19
W44.F4XD	Codes in Categories T15-T19
W44.F4XS	Codes in Categories T15-T19
W44.F9XA	Codes in Categories T15-T19
W44.F9XD	Codes in Categories T15-T19
W44.F9XS	Codes in Categories T15-T19
W44.GØXA	Codes in Categories T15-T19
W44.GØXD	Codes in Categories T15-T19
W44.GØXS	Codes in Categories T15-T19
W44.G1XA	Codes in Categories T15-T19

Code Assignment Beginning 10/1/2023	Previous Code(s) Assignment
W44.G1XD	Codes in Categories T15-T19
W44.G1XS	Codes in Categories T15-T19
W44.G2XA	Codes in Categories T15-T19
W44.G2XD	Codes in Categories T15-T19
W44.G2XS	Codes in Categories T15-T19
W44.G3XA	Codes in Categories T15-T19
W44.G3XD	Codes in Categories T15-T19
W44.G3XS	Codes in Categories T15-T19
W44.G9XA	Codes in Categories T15-T19
W44.G9XD	Codes in Categories T15-T19
W44.G9XS	Codes in Categories T15-T19
W44.HØXA	Codes in Categories T15-T19
W44.HØXD	Codes in Categories T15-T19
W44.HØXS	Codes in Categories T15-T19
W44.H1XA	Codes in Categories T15-T19
W44.H1XD	Codes in Categories T15-T19
W44.H1XS	Codes in Categories T15-T19
W44.H2XA	Codes in Categories T15-T19
W44.H2XD	Codes in Categories T15-T19
W44.H2XS	Codes in Categories T15-T19
*YØ7.Ø1Ø	YØ7.Ø1
*YØ7.Ø11	YØ7.Ø1
*YØ7.Ø2Ø	YØ7.Ø2
*YØ7.Ø21	YØ7.Ø2
*YØ7.Ø3Ø	YØ7.Ø3
*YØ7.Ø31	YØ7.Ø3
*YØ7.Ø4Ø	YØ7.Ø4
*YØ7.Ø41	YØ7.Ø4

Code Assignment Beginning 10/1/2023	Previous Code(s) Assignment
*YØ7.Ø5Ø	YØ7.Ø1-YØ7.Ø4
*YØ7.Ø51	YØ7.Ø1-YØ7.Ø4
*YØ7.44	YØ7.499
*YØ7.45	YØ7.499
*YØ7.46	YØ7.499
*YØ7.47	YØ7.499
*YØ7.54	YØ7.59
ZØ2.84	ZØ2.89
ZØ5.81	ZØ5.8
ZØ5.89	ZØ5.8
Z16.13	Z16.19
Z22.34Ø	Z22.39
Z22.341	Z22.39
Z22.349	Z22.39
Z22.35Ø	Z22.39
Z22.358	Z22.39
Z22.359	Z22.39
Z29.81	Z29.8
Z29.89	Z29.8
*Z55.6	Z55.8
*Z58.81	Z59.89
*Z58.89	Z59.89
*Z59.1Ø	Z59.1
*Z59.11	Z59.1
*Z59.12	Z59.1
*Z59.19	Z59.1
Z62.23	Z62.29
Z62.24	Z62.29
*Z62.814	Z62.819
*Z62.815	Z62.819
Z62.823	Z62.898
Z62.831	Z62.898
Z62.832	Z62.898
Z62.833	Z62.898
Z62.892	Z62.898
Z83.71Ø	Z83.71
Z83.711	Z83.71
Z83.718	Z83.71
Z83.719	Z83.71
*Z91.141	Z91.14
*Z91.148	Z91.14
*Z91.151	Z91.15
*Z91.158	Z91.15
*Z91.413	Z91.419
*Z91.414	Z91.419
Z91.85	Z91.89
Z91.A41	Z91.A4
Z91.A48	Z91.A4
Z91.A51	Z91.A5
Z91.A58	Z91.A5
Z91.A91	Z91.A9
Z91.A98	Z91.A9

10 Steps to Correct Coding

Follow the 10 steps below to correctly code encounters for health care services.

Step 1: Identify the reason for the visit or encounter (i.e., a sign, symptom, diagnosis and/or condition).

The medical record documentation should accurately reflect the patient's condition, using terminology that includes specific diagnoses and symptoms or clearly states the reasons for the encounter.

Choosing the main term that best describes the reason chiefly responsible for the service provided is the most important step in coding. If symptoms are present and documented but a definitive diagnosis has not yet been determined, code the symptoms. *For outpatient cases, do not code conditions that are referred to as "rule out," "suspected," "probable," or "questionable."* Diagnoses often are not established at the time of the initial encounter/visit and may require two or more visits to be established. Code only what is documented in the available outpatient records and only to the highest degree of certainty known at the time of the patient's visit. For inpatient medical records, uncertain diagnoses may be reported if documented at the time of discharge.

Step 2: After selecting the reason for the encounter, consult the alphabetic index.

The most critical rule is to begin code selection in the alphabetic index. Never turn first to the tabular list. The index provides cross-references, essential and nonessential modifiers, and other instructional notations that may not be found in the tabular list.

Step 3: Locate the main term entry.

The alphabetic index lists conditions, which may be expressed as nouns or eponyms, with critical use of adjectives. Some conditions known by several names have multiple main entries. Reasons for encounters may be located under general terms such as admission, encounter, and examination. Other general terms such as history, status (post), or presence (of) can be used to locate other factors influencing health.

Step 4: Scan subterm entries.

Scan the subterm entries, as appropriate, being sure to review continued lines and additional subterms that may appear in the next column or on the next page. Shaded vertical guidelines in the index indicate the indentation level for each subterm in relation to the main terms.

Step 5: Pay close attention to index instructions.

- Parentheses ( ) enclose nonessential modifiers, terms that are supplementary words or explanatory information that may or may not appear in the diagnostic statement and do not affect code selection.
- Brackets [ ] enclose manifestation codes that can be used only as secondary codes to the underlying condition code immediately preceding it. If used, manifestation codes must be reported with the appropriate etiology codes.
- Default codes are listed next to the main term and represent the condition most commonly associated with the main term or the unspecified code for the main term.
- *"See"* cross-references, identified by italicized type and "code by" cross-references indicate that another term *must be referenced* to locate the correct code.
- *"See also"* cross-references, identified by italicized type, provide alternative terms that may be useful to look up but *are not mandatory*.
- "Omit code" cross-references identify instances when a code is not applicable depending on the condition being coded.
- "With" subterms are listed out of alphabetic order and identify a presumed causal relationship between the two conditions they link.
- "Due to" subterms identify a relationship between the two conditions they link.
- "NEC," abbreviation for "not elsewhere classified," follows some main terms or subterms and indicates that there is no specific code for the condition even though the medical documentation may be very specific.
- "NOS," abbreviation for "not otherwise specified," follows some main terms or subterms and is the equivalent of unspecified; NOS signifies that the information in the medical record is insufficient for assigning a more specific code.
- *Following* references help coders locate alphanumeric codes that are out of sequence in the tabular section.
- Check-additional-character symbols flag codes that require additional characters to make the code valid; the characters available to complete the code should be verified in the tabular section.

Step 6: Choose a potential code and locate it in the tabular list.

To prevent coding errors, always use both the alphabetic index (to identify a code) and the tabular list (to verify a code), as the index does not include the important instructional notes found in the tabular list. An added benefit of using the tabular list, which groups like things together, is that while looking at one code in the list, a coder might see a more specific one that would have been missed had the coder relied solely on the alphabetic index. Additionally, many of the codes require a fourth, fifth, sixth, or seventh character to be valid, and many of these characters can be found only in the tabular list.

Step 7: Read all instructional material in the tabular section.

The coder must follow any Includes, Excludes 1 and Excludes 2 notes, and other instructional notes, such as "Code first" and "Use additional code," listed in the tabular list for the chapter, category, subcategory, and subclassification levels of code selection that direct the coder to use a different or additional code. Any codes in the tabular range A00.0–T88.9, Z00–Z99.8, and U00–U85 may be used to identify the diagnostic reason for the encounter. The tabular list encompasses many codes describing disease and injury classifications (e.g., infectious and parasitic diseases, neoplasms, symptoms, nervous and circulatory system, etc.).

Codes that describe symptoms and signs, as opposed to definitive diagnoses, should be reported when an established diagnosis has not been made (confirmed) by the physician. Chapter 18 of the ICD-10-CM code book, "Symptoms, Signs, and Abnormal Clinical and Laboratory Findings, Not Elsewhere Classified" (codes RØØ–R99), contains many, but not all, codes for symptoms.

ICD-10-CM classifies encounters with health care providers for circumstances other than a disease or injury in chapter 21, "Factors Influencing Health Status and Contact with Health Services" (codes ZØØ–Z99). Circumstances other than a disease or injury often are recorded as chiefly responsible for the encounter.

A code is invalid if it does not include the full number of characters (greatest level of specificity) required. Codes in ICD-10-CM can contain from three to seven alphanumeric characters. A three-character code is to be used only if the category is not further subdivided into four-, five-, six-, or seven-character codes. Placeholder character X is used as part of an alphanumeric code to allow for future expansion and as a placeholder for empty characters in a code that requires a seventh character but has no fourth, fifth, or sixth character. Note that certain categories require seventh characters that apply to all codes in that category. Always check the category level for applicable seventh characters for that category.

Step 8: Consult the official ICD-10-CM conventions and guidelines.

The *ICD-10-CM Official Guidelines for Coding and Reporting* govern the use of certain codes. These guidelines provide both general and chapter-specific coding guidance.

Step 9: Confirm and assign the code.

Having reviewed all relevant information concerning the possible code choices, assign the code that most completely describes the condition.

Repeat steps 1 through 9 for all additional documented conditions that meet the following criteria:

- They exist at the time of the visit *AND*
- They require or affect patient care, treatment, or management

Step 10: Sequence codes correctly.

Sequencing is the order in which the codes are listed on the claim. List first the ICD-10-CM code for the diagnosis, condition, problem, or other reason for the encounter/visit that is shown in the medical record to be chiefly responsible for the services provided. List additional codes that describe any coexisting conditions. Follow the official coding guidelines (see the guidelines, section II, "Selection of Principal Diagnosis"; section III, "Reporting Additional Diagnoses"; and section IV, "Diagnostic Coding and Reporting Guidelines for Outpatient Services") on proper sequencing of codes.

Coding Examples

Diagnosis: Anorexia

Step 1: The reason for the encounter was the condition, anorexia.

Step 2: Consult the alphabetic index.

Step 3: Locate the main term "Anorexia."

Step 4: Two possible subterms are available, "hysterical" and "nervosa." Neither is documented in this instance, however, so they cannot be used in code selection.

Step 5: The code listed next to the main term is called the default code selection. Because the two subentries (essential modifiers) do not apply in this instance, the default code (R63.Ø) should be used.

Step 6: Turn to code R63.Ø in the tabular list and read all instructional notes.

Step 7: The Excludes 1 note at code R63.Ø indicates that anorexia nervosa and loss of appetite determined to be of nonorganic origin should be reported with a code from chapter 5. The diagnostic statement does not describe the condition as anorexia nervosa, however, and does not indicate that the anorexia is of a nonorganic origin. There is no further division of the category past the fourth-character subcategory. Therefore, code R63.Ø is at the highest level of specificity.

Step 8: Review of official guideline I.C.18 indicates that a symptom code is appropriate when a more definitive diagnosis is not documented.

Step 9: The default code, R63.Ø Anorexia, is the correct code selection.

Repeat steps 1 through 9 for any concomitant diagnoses.

Step 10: Since anorexia is listed as the chief reason for the health care encounter, the first-listed, or principal, diagnosis is R63.Ø. Note that this is a chapter 18 symptom code but can be assigned for both inpatient and outpatient records since the provider did not establish a more definitive diagnosis, according to sections II.A and IV.D.

Diagnosis: Acute bronchitis

Step 1: The reason for the encounter was the condition, acute bronchitis.

Step 2: Consult the alphabetic index.

Step 3: Locate the main term "Bronchitis."

Step 4: There is a subterm for "acute or subacute." Additional subterms are not included in the diagnostic statement.

Step 5: Nonessential modifiers (with bronchospasm or obstruction) are terms that do not affect code assignment. Since no other subterms indented under "acute" apply here, the code listed next to this subentry—in this case J2Ø.9—should be chosen.

Step 6: Turn to code J2Ø.9 in the tabular list and read all instructional notes.

Step 7: The Includes note under category J2Ø lists alternative terms for acute bronchitis. Note that the list is not exhaustive but is only a representative selection of diagnoses that are included in the subcategory. The Excludes 1 note refers to category J4Ø for bronchitis and tracheobronchitis NOS. There are several conditions in the Excludes 2 notes that, if applicable, can be coded in addition to this code.

Note that the codes included in J2Ø represent acute bronchitis due to various infectious organisms that could be selected if identified in the documentation. In this case, the organism was not identified and there is no further division of the category past the fourth character subcategory. Therefore, code J2Ø.9 is at the highest level of specificity.

Step 8: Review of official guideline I.C.10 provides no additional information affecting the code selected.

Step 9: Assign code J2Ø.9 Acute bronchitis, unspecified.

Repeat steps 1 through 9 for any concomitant diagnoses.

Step 10: In the absence of additional diagnoses that may affect sequencing, code J2Ø.9 should be sequenced as the first-listed, or principal, diagnosis.

Diagnosis: Cerebellar ataxia in myxedema

Step 1: The reason for the encounter was the condition, cerebellar ataxia.

Step 2: Consult the alphabetic index.

Step 3: Locate the main term "Ataxia."

Step 4: Available subterms include "cerebellar (hereditary)," with additional indented subterms for "in" and "myxedema," all essential modifiers that are included in the diagnostic statement. Two codes are provided, EØ3.9 and G13.2, the latter of which is in brackets.

Step 5: Note the nonessential modifier (in parentheses) after the subterm cerebellar includes the term "hereditary." Because it is in parentheses, this term is not required in the diagnostic statement for this subentry to apply. The brackets around G13.2 identify this code as a manifestation of the condition described by code EØ3.9 and indicate that the two must be reported together and sequencing rules apply.

Step 6: Locate codes EØ3.9 and G13.2 in the tabular list, and read all instructional notes.

Step 7: For code EØ3.9, there are no instructional notes in the tabular list at the category EØ3 or code level that indicate that this condition should be coded elsewhere in the classification or that additional codes are required. Without further information from the diagnostic statement, myxedema, not otherwise specified (NOS), is appropriately reported with code EØ3.9 Hypothyroidism, unspecified, according to the inclusion term at this code.

Code G13.2 in the tabular list has an instructional note to "Code first underlying disease," which includes conditions found in category EØ3.-. Based on this note, codes EØ3.9 and G13.2 are to be coded together, with G13.2 listed only as a secondary diagnosis. This correlates with what the alphabetic index indicated. As there is no further division of codes in category G13 beyond the fourth character, G13.2 is at the highest level of specificity.

Step 8: Although there are some general conventions, such as how to interpret brackets in the alphabetic index, no chapter-specific guidelines apply to this coding scenario.

Step 9: Assign codes EØ3.9 Hypothyroidism, unspecified, and G13.2 Systemic atrophy primarily affecting the central nervous system in myxedema.

Repeat steps 1 through 9 for any concomitant diagnoses.

Step 10: Based on the alphabetic index and tabular instructional notations, code EØ3.9 should be sequenced as the first-listed, or principal, diagnosis followed by G13.2 as a secondary diagnosis.

Diagnosis: Decubitus ulcer of right elbow with skin loss and necrosis of subcutaneous tissue

Step 1: The reason for the encounter was the condition, decubitus ulcer.

Step 2: Consult the alphabetic index.

Step 3: Locate the main term "Ulcer."

Step 4: For the subterm "decubitus," there is no code provided or additional subterms indented, but a cross-reference is listed.

Step 5: The italicized cross-reference instructs the coder to "*see* Ulcer, pressure, by site."

Repeat steps 3 through 5 for the cross-reference:

Step 3: Locate the main term "Ulcer."

Step 4: Review the subentries for the subterm "pressure." The next level of indent lists either the site of the ulcer or the specific stage of the ulcer (stage 1–4, unstageable, and unspecified stages). The diagnostic statement provides the site, right elbow, and the extent of tissue damage (skin loss and necrosis of subcutaneous tissue) but does not specifically state that the ulcer is stage 1, stage 2, etc. Nonessential modifiers (in parentheses) at each stage include a description of the typical extent of damage at each stage. For example, stage 1 describes "pre-ulcer skin changes limited to persistent focal edema." Based on the documentation in the record, the coder can correlate the documentation to the nonessential modifiers and choose the specific stage from the index. The coder can also go directly to the body site, choosing the stage of the ulcer after reviewing the code options and instructional notations in the tabular list.

The diagnostic statement indicates that the extent of the damage to the elbow includes skin loss and necrosis of subcutaneous tissue, coinciding with the nonessential modifier next to the subentry "stage 3." The body site of elbow (L89.Ø-) is listed as another level of indent with other body sites.

Step 5: Note that code L89.Ø is followed by a dash and an additional-character-required icon, which indicate that more characters are needed to complete the code. From here, the tabular listing for L89.Ø- can be consulted.

Step 6: Locate code L89.Ø- in the tabular list and read all instructional notes.

Step 7: The tabular listing at category L89 has an Includes note for "decubitus ulcer," which confirms that category L89 is the appropriate category to represent what is documented in the diagnostic statement.

Several Excludes 2 notes are also listed at the category level. Excludes 2 notes represent conditions that can occur concomitantly with the decubitus ulcer and can be coded in addition to code L89, if supported by the documentation.

The subcategory codes under L89.Ø indicate that the fifth character describes laterality. Locate the right elbow at subcategory L89.Ø1. See that an additional sixth character to specify the stage of the ulcer is now needed to complete the code. The stage can be determined either by the specific documentation of the stage (e.g., stage 1, stage 2) or, in this case, a description that matches one of the inclusion terms that follow each stage code. For example, the diagnostic description in this case of "skin loss and necrosis of the subcutaneous tissue" matches the inclusion term under L89.Ø13 Pressure ulcer of right elbow, stage 3. No additional characters are required because code L89.Ø13 is at its highest level of specificity.

Step 8: The official guidelines contain quite a bit of information relating to pressure ulcers in chapter-specific guideline I.C.12 as well as information in general guideline I.B.14. These and any other pertinent guidelines should be reviewed to ensure appropriate code assignment.

Step 9: Assign code L89.Ø13 Pressure ulcer of right elbow, stage 3.

Repeat steps 1 through 9 for any concomitant diagnoses.

Step 10: Since the decubitus ulcer is listed as the chief reason for the health care encounter, the first-listed, or principal, diagnosis is L89.Ø13. However, according to the code first instructional note at the L89 category level, gangrene (I96) would be sequenced before the pressure ulcer if it were documented.

Diagnosis: Emergency department visit for bimalleolar fracture of the right ankle due to trauma

Step 1: The reason for the encounter was the condition, bimalleolar fracture.

Step 2: Consult the alphabetic index.

Step 3: Locate the main term "Fracture." Note that many main terms represent fractures: "Fracture, burst," "Fracture, chronic," "Fracture, insufficiency," "Fracture, nontraumatic NEC," "Fracture, pathological," and "Fracture, traumatic." Since the diagnostic statement specifically states that this fracture was the result of trauma, the main term "Fracture, traumatic" should be used.

Step 4: Subterms that should be referenced are "ankle" and "bimalleolar (displaced)," which lists code S82.84-.

Step 5: A nonessential modifier (in parentheses) next to the term bimalleolar for "displaced" indicates that S82.84- is the default category unless the fracture is specifically identified as "nondisplaced."

Note that code S82.84- is followed by a dash and an additional-character icon, both of which indicate that more characters are required. From here, the tabular list can be consulted.

Step 6: Locate code S82.84- in the tabular list and read all instructional notes.

Step 7: The instructional notes at category S82 indicate that fractures not specified as displaced or nondisplaced default to displaced and that fractures not designated as open or closed default to closed. Additional instructional notes can be found at the category level but none pertain to the current scenario.

Read through the subcategory codes under S82.84, and note that the sixth character specifies displaced or nondisplaced and laterality. Based on the index nonessential modifier (displaced) and the code note at category S82, code selection should identify a displaced fracture of the right side. A displaced bimalleolar fracture of the right lower leg is coded to S82.841.

To complete the code, a seventh character must be assigned to identify the type of encounter (initial, subsequent, or sequela) and whether the fracture is open or closed. Most of the codes in category S82 require a seventh character represented in the list at the category level. However, it is important to note that some subcategories have their own specific set of seventh characters. In this instance, subcategory S82.84- does not have a unique set of seventh characters and the list provided at the category level should be used. Without documentation of the fracture being open, the tabular notation indicates that the default is closed. Character A, representing "initial encounter for closed fracture," listed in the box at the category level is the most appropriate option.

2024 ICD-10-CM Official Guidelines for Coding and Reporting

Narrative changes effective October 1, 2023 appear in **bold** text

Narrative changes effective April 1, 2023 appear in shaded text

Items underlined have been moved within the guidelines since the FY 2023 version

Italics are used to indicate revisions to heading changes

The Centers for Medicare and Medicaid Services (CMS) and the National Center for Health Statistics (NCHS), two departments within the U.S. Federal Government's Department of Health and Human Services (DHHS) provide the following guidelines for coding and reporting using the International Classification of Diseases, 10th Revision, Clinical Modification (ICD-10-CM). These guidelines should be used as a companion document to the official version of the ICD-10-CM as published on the NCHS website. The ICD-10-CM is a morbidity classification published by the United States for classifying diagnoses and reason for visits in all health care settings. The ICD-10-CM is based on the ICD-10, the statistical classification of disease published by the World Health Organization (WHO).

These guidelines have been approved by the four organizations that make up the Cooperating Parties for the ICD-10-CM: the American Hospital Association (AHA), the American Health Information Management Association (AHIMA), CMS, and NCHS.

These guidelines are a set of rules that have been developed to accompany and complement the official conventions and instructions provided within the ICD-10-CM itself. The instructions and conventions of the classification take precedence over guidelines. These guidelines are based on the coding and sequencing instructions in the Tabular List and Alphabetic Index of ICD-10-CM, but provide additional instruction. Adherence to these guidelines when assigning ICD-10-CM diagnosis codes is required under the Health Insurance Portability and Accountability Act (HIPAA). The diagnosis codes (Tabular List and Alphabetic Index) have been adopted under HIPAA for all healthcare settings. A joint effort between the healthcare provider and the coder is essential to achieve complete and accurate documentation, code assignment, and reporting of diagnoses and procedures. These guidelines have been developed to assist both the healthcare provider and the coder in identifying those diagnoses that are to be reported. The importance of consistent, complete documentation in the medical record cannot be overemphasized. Without such documentation accurate coding cannot be achieved. The entire record should be reviewed to determine the specific reason for the encounter and the conditions treated.

The term encounter is used for all settings, including hospital admissions. In the context of these guidelines, the term provider is used throughout the guidelines to mean physician or any qualified health care practitioner who is legally accountable for establishing the patient's diagnosis. Only this set of guidelines, approved by the Cooperating Parties, is official.

The guidelines are organized into sections. Section I includes the structure and conventions of the classification and general guidelines that apply to the entire classification, and chapter-specific guidelines that correspond to the chapters as they are arranged in the classification. Section II includes guidelines for selection of principal diagnosis for non-outpatient settings. Section III includes guidelines for reporting additional diagnoses in non-outpatient settings. Section IV is for outpatient coding and reporting. It is necessary to review all sections of the guidelines to fully understand all of the rules and instructions needed to code properly.

Section I. Conventions, general coding guidelines and chapter specific guidelines

The conventions, general guidelines and chapter-specific guidelines are applicable to all health care settings unless otherwise indicated. The conventions and instructions of the classification take precedence over guidelines.

A. Conventions for the ICD-10-CM

The conventions for the ICD-10-CM are the general rules for use of the classification independent of the guidelines. These conventions are incorporated within the Alphabetic Index and Tabular List of the ICD-10-CM as instructional notes.

1. **The Alphabetic Index and Tabular List**
   The ICD-10-CM is divided into the Alphabetic Index, an alphabetical list of terms and their corresponding code, and the Tabular List, a structured list of codes divided into chapters based on body system or condition. The Alphabetic Index consists of the following parts: the Index of Diseases and Injury, the Index of External Causes of Injury, the Table of Neoplasms and the Table of Drugs and Chemicals.
   See Section I.C.2. Neoplasms
   See Section I.C.19. Adverse effects, poisoning, underdosing and toxic effects
2. **Format and Structure:**
   The ICD-10-CM Tabular List contains categories, subcategories and codes. Characters for categories, subcategories and codes may be either a letter or a number. All categories are 3 characters. A three-character category that has no further subdivision is equivalent to a code. Subcategories are either 4 or 5 characters. Codes may be 3, 4, 5, 6 or 7 characters. That is, each level of subdivision after a category is a subcategory. The final level of subdivision is a code. Codes that have applicable 7th characters are still referred to as codes, not subcategories. A code that has an applicable 7th character is considered invalid without the 7th character.
   The ICD-10-CM uses an indented format for ease in reference.
3. **Use of codes for reporting purposes**
   For reporting purposes only codes are permissible, not categories or subcategories, and any applicable 7th character is required.
4. **Placeholder character**
   The ICD-10-CM utilizes a placeholder character "X". The "X" is used as a placeholder at certain codes to allow for future expansion. An example of this is at the poisoning, adverse effect and underdosing codes, categories T36-T5Ø. Where a placeholder exists, the X must be used in order for the code to be considered a valid code.
5. **7th Characters**
   Certain ICD-10-CM categories have applicable 7th characters. The applicable 7th character is required for all codes within the category, or as the notes in the Tabular List instruct. The 7th character must always be the 7th character in the data field. If a code that requires a 7th character is not 6 characters, a placeholder X must be used to fill in the empty characters.
6. **Abbreviations**
   a. **Alphabetic Index abbreviations**
      NEC "Not elsewhere classifiable"
      This abbreviation in the Alphabetic Index represents "other specified." When a specific code is not available for a condition, the Alphabetic Index directs the coder to the "other specified" code in the Tabular List.
      NOS "Not otherwise specified"
      This abbreviation is the equivalent of unspecified.
   b. **Tabular List abbreviations**
      NEC "Not elsewhere classifiable"
      This abbreviation in the Tabular List represents "other specified". When a specific code is not available for a condition, the Tabular List includes an NEC entry under a code to identify the code as the "other specified" code.
      NOS "Not otherwise specified"
      This abbreviation is the equivalent of unspecified.
7. **Punctuation**
   [ ] Brackets are used in the Tabular List to enclose synonyms, alternative wording or explanatory phrases. Brackets are used in the Alphabetic Index to identify manifestation codes.
   ( ) Parentheses are used in both the Alphabetic Index and Tabular List to enclose supplementary words that may be present or absent in the statement of a disease or procedure without affecting the code number to which it is assigned. The terms within the parentheses are referred to as nonessential modifiers. The nonessential modifiers in the Alphabetic Index to Diseases apply to subterms following a main term except when a nonessential modifier and a subentry are mutually exclusive, the subentry takes precedence. For example, in the ICD-10-CM Alphabetic Index under the main term Enteritis, "acute" is a nonessential modifier and "chronic" is a subentry. In this case, the nonessential modifier "acute" does not apply to the subentry "chronic".
   : Colons are used in the Tabular List after an incomplete term which needs one or more of the modifiers following the colon to make it assignable to a given category.
8. **Use of "and".**
   See Section I.A.14. Use of the term "And"
9. **Other and Unspecified codes**
   a. **"Other" codes**
      Codes titled "other" or "other specified" are for use when the information in the medical record provides detail for which a specific code does not exist. Alphabetic Index entries with NEC in the line designate "other" codes in the Tabular List. These Alphabetic Index entries represent specific disease entities for which no specific code exists, so the term is included within an "other" code.
   b. **"Unspecified" codes**
      Codes titled "unspecified" are for use when the information in the medical record is insufficient to assign a more specific code. For those categories for which an unspecified code is not provided, the "other specified" code may represent both other and unspecified.
      See Section I.B.18. Use of Signs/Symptom/Unspecified Codes
10. **Includes Notes**
    This note appears immediately under a three-character code title to further define, or give examples of, the content of the category.
11. **Inclusion terms**
    List of terms is included under some codes. These terms are the conditions for which that code is to be used. The terms may be synonyms of the code title, or, in the case of "other specified" codes, the terms are a list of the various conditions assigned to that code. The inclusion terms are not necessarily exhaustive. Additional terms found only in the Alphabetic Index may also be assigned to a code.
12. **Excludes Notes**
    The ICD-10-CM has two types of excludes notes. Each type of note has a different definition for use, but they are all similar in that they indicate that codes excluded from each other are independent of each other.
    a. **Excludes1**
       A type 1 Excludes note is a pure excludes note. It means "NOT CODED HERE!" An Excludes1 note indicates that the code excluded should never be used at the same time as the code above the Excludes1 note. An Excludes1 is used when two conditions cannot occur together, such as a congenital form versus an acquired form of the same condition.
       An exception to the Excludes1 definition is the circumstance when the two conditions are unrelated to each other. If it is not clear whether the two conditions involving an Excludes1 note are related or not, query the provider. For example, code F45.8, Other somatoform disorders, has an Excludes1 note for "sleep related teeth grinding (G47.63)," because "teeth grinding" is an inclusion term under F45.8. Only one of these two codes should be assigned for teeth grinding. However psychogenic dysmenorrhea is also an inclusion term under F45.8, and a patient could have both this condition and sleep related teeth grinding. In this case, the two conditions are clearly unrelated to each other, and so it would be appropriate to report F45.8 and G47.63 together.
    b. **Excludes2**
       A type 2 Excludes note represents "Not included here." An excludes2 note indicates that the condition excluded is not part of the condition represented by the code, but a patient may have both conditions at the same time. When an Excludes2 note appears under a code, it is acceptable to use both the code and the excluded code together, when appropriate.
13. **Etiology/manifestation convention ("code first", "use additional code" and "in diseases classified elsewhere" notes)**
    Certain conditions have both an underlying etiology and multiple body system manifestations due to the underlying etiology. For such conditions, the ICD-10-CM has a coding convention that requires the underlying condition be sequenced first, if applicable, followed by the manifestation. Wherever such a combination exists, there is a "use additional code" note at the etiology code, and a "code first" note at the manifestation code. These instructional notes indicate the proper sequencing order of the codes, etiology followed by manifestation.
    In most cases the manifestation codes will have in the code title, "in diseases classified elsewhere." Codes with this title are a component of the etiology/manifestation convention. The code title indicates that it is a manifestation code. "In diseases classified elsewhere" codes are never permitted to be used as first listed or principal diagnosis codes. They must be used in conjunction with an underlying condition code and they must be listed following the underlying condition. See category FØ2, Dementia in other diseases classified elsewhere, for an example of this convention.
    There are manifestation codes that do not have "in diseases classified elsewhere" in the title. For such codes, there is a "use additional code" note at the etiology code and a "code first" note at the manifestation code, and the rules for sequencing apply.

In addition to the notes in the Tabular List, these conditions also have a specific Alphabetic Index entry structure. In the Alphabetic Index both conditions are listed together with the etiology code first followed by the manifestation codes in brackets. The code in brackets is always to be sequenced second.

An example of the etiology/manifestation convention is dementia with Parkinson's disease. In the Alphabetic Index, **a** code **from category** G2Ø is listed first, followed by code FØ2.8Ø or FØ2.81- in brackets. **A** code **from category G2Ø**- represents the underlying etiology, Parkinson's disease, and must be sequenced first, whereas codes FØ2.8Ø and FØ2.81- represent the manifestation of dementia in diseases classified elsewhere, with or without behavioral disturbance.

"Code first" and "Use additional code" notes are also used as sequencing rules in the classification for certain codes that are not part of an etiology/manifestation combination.

See Section I.B.7. Multiple coding for a single condition.

14. **"And"**

The word "and" should be interpreted to mean either "and" or "or" when it appears in a title.

For example, cases of "tuberculosis of bones", "tuberculosis of joints" and "tuberculosis of bones and joints" are classified to subcategory A18.Ø, Tuberculosis of bones and joints.

15. **"With"**

The word "with" or "in" should be interpreted to mean "associated with" or "due to" when it appears in a code title, the Alphabetic Index (either under a main term or subterm), or an instructional note in the Tabular List. The classification presumes a causal relationship between the two conditions linked by these terms in the Alphabetic Index or Tabular List. These conditions should be coded as related even in the absence of provider documentation explicitly linking them, unless the documentation clearly states the conditions are unrelated or when another guideline exists that specifically requires a documented linkage between two conditions (e.g., sepsis guideline for "acute organ dysfunction that is not clearly associated with the sepsis").

For conditions not specifically linked by these relational terms in the classification or when a guideline requires that a linkage between two conditions be explicitly documented, provider documentation must link the conditions in order to code them as related.

The word "with" in the Alphabetic Index is sequenced immediately following the main term or subterm, not in alphabetical order.

16. **"See" and "See Also"**

The "see" instruction following a main term in the Alphabetic Index indicates that another term should be referenced. It is necessary to go to the main term referenced with the "see" note to locate the correct code.

A "see also" instruction following a main term in the Alphabetic Index instructs that there is another main term that may also be referenced that may provide additional Alphabetic Index entries that may be useful. It is not necessary to follow the "see also" note when the original main term provides the necessary code.

17. **"Code also" note**

A "code also" note instructs that two codes may be required to fully describe a condition, but this note does not provide sequencing direction. The sequencing depends on the circumstances of the encounter.

18. **Default codes**

A code listed next to a main term in the ICD-10-CM Alphabetic Index is referred to as a default code. The default code represents that condition that is most commonly associated with the main term or is the unspecified code for the condition. If a condition is documented in a medical record (for example, appendicitis) without any additional information, such as acute or chronic, the default code should be assigned.

19. **Code assignment and Clinical Criteria**

The assignment of a diagnosis code is based on the provider's diagnostic statement that the condition exists. The provider's statement that the patient has a particular condition is sufficient. Code assignment is not based on clinical criteria used by the provider to establish the diagnosis. If there is conflicting medical record documentation, query the provider.

B. General Coding Guidelines

1. **Locating a code in the ICD-10-CM**

To select a code in the classification that corresponds to a diagnosis or reason for visit documented in a medical record, first locate the term in the Alphabetic Index, and then verify the code in the Tabular List. Read and be guided by instructional notations that appear in both the Alphabetic Index and the Tabular List.

It is essential to use both the Alphabetic Index and Tabular List when locating and assigning a code. The Alphabetic Index does not always provide the full code. Selection of the full code, including laterality and any applicable 7th character can only be done in the Tabular List. A dash (-) at the end of an Alphabetic Index entry indicates that additional characters are required. Even if a dash is not included at the Alphabetic Index entry, it is necessary to refer to the Tabular List to verify that no 7th character is required.

2. **Level of Detail in Coding**

Diagnosis codes are to be used and reported at their highest number of characters available and to the highest level of specificity documented in the medical record.

ICD-10-CM diagnosis codes are composed of codes with 3, 4, 5, 6 or 7 characters. Codes with three characters are included in ICD-10-CM as the heading of a category of codes that may be further subdivided by the use of fourth and/or fifth characters and/or sixth characters, which provide greater detail.

A three-character code is to be used only if it is not further subdivided. A code is invalid if it has not been coded to the full number of characters required for that code, including the 7th character, if applicable.

3. **Code or codes from AØØ.Ø through T88.9, ZØØ-Z99.8, UØØ-U85**

The appropriate code or codes from AØØ.Ø through T88.9, ZØØ-Z99.8, and UØØ-U85 must be used to identify diagnoses, symptoms, conditions, problems, complaints or other reason(s) for the encounter/visit.

4. **Signs and symptoms**

Codes that describe symptoms and signs, as opposed to diagnoses, are acceptable for reporting purposes when a related definitive diagnosis has not been established (confirmed) by the provider. Chapter 18 of ICD-10-CM, Symptoms, Signs, and Abnormal Clinical and Laboratory Findings, Not Elsewhere Classified (codes RØØ.Ø-R99) contains many, but not all, codes for symptoms.

See Section I.B.18. Use of Signs/Symptom/Unspecified Codes

5. **Conditions that are an integral part of a disease process**

Signs and symptoms that are associated routinely with a disease process should not be assigned as additional codes, unless otherwise instructed by the classification.

6. **Conditions that are not an integral part of a disease process**

Additional signs and symptoms that may not be associated routinely with a disease process should be coded when present.

7. **Multiple coding for a single condition**

In addition to the etiology/manifestation convention that requires two codes to fully describe a single condition that affects multiple body systems, there are other single conditions that also require more than one code. "Use additional code" notes are found in the Tabular List at codes that are not part of an etiology/manifestation pair where a secondary code is useful to fully describe a condition. The sequencing rule is the same as the etiology/manifestation pair, "use additional code" indicates that a secondary code should be added, if known.

For example, for bacterial infections that are not included in chapter 1, a secondary code from category B95, Streptococcus, Staphylococcus, and Enterococcus, as the cause of diseases classified elsewhere, or B96, Other bacterial agents as the cause of diseases classified elsewhere, may be required to identify the bacterial organism causing the infection. A "use additional code" note will normally be found at the infectious disease code, indicating a need for the organism code to be added as a secondary code.

"Code first" notes are also under certain codes that are not specifically manifestation codes but may be due to an underlying cause. When there is a "code first" note and an underlying condition is present, the underlying condition should be sequenced first, if known.

"Code, if applicable, any causal condition first" notes indicate that this code may be assigned as a principal diagnosis when the causal condition is unknown or not applicable. If a causal condition is known, then the code for that condition should be sequenced as the principal or first-listed diagnosis.

Multiple codes may be needed for sequela, complication codes and obstetric codes to more fully describe a condition. See the specific guidelines for these conditions for further instruction.

8. **Acute and Chronic Conditions**

If the same condition is described as both acute (subacute) and chronic, and separate subentries exist in the Alphabetic Index at the same indentation level, code both and sequence the acute (subacute) code first.

9. **Combination Code**

A combination code is a single code used to classify:

Two diagnoses, or

A diagnosis with an associated secondary process (manifestation)

A diagnosis with an associated complication

Combination codes are identified by referring to subterm entries in the Alphabetic Index and by reading the inclusion and exclusion notes in the Tabular List.

Assign only the combination code when that code fully identifies the diagnostic conditions involved or when the Alphabetic Index so directs. Multiple coding should not be used when the classification provides a combination code that clearly identifies all of the elements documented in the diagnosis. When the combination code lacks necessary specificity in describing the manifestation or complication, an additional code should be used as a secondary code.

10. Sequela (Late Effects)

A sequela is the residual effect (condition produced) after the acute phase of an illness or injury has terminated. There is no time limit on when a sequela code can be used. The residual may be apparent early, such as in cerebral infarction, or it may occur months or years later, such as that due to a previous injury. Examples of sequela include: scar formation resulting from a burn, deviated septum due to a nasal fracture, and infertility due to tubal occlusion from old tuberculosis. Coding of sequela generally requires two codes sequenced in the following order: the condition or nature of the sequela is sequenced first. The sequela code is sequenced second.

An exception to the above guidelines are those instances where the code for the sequela is followed by a manifestation code identified in the Tabular List and title, or the sequela code has been expanded (at the fourth, fifth or sixth character levels) to include the manifestation(s). The code for the acute phase of an illness or injury that led to the sequela is never used with a code for the late effect.

See Section I.C.9. Sequelae of cerebrovascular disease

See Section I.C.15. Sequelae of complication of pregnancy, childbirth and the puerperium

See Section I.C.19. Application of 7th characters for Chapter 19

11. Impending or Threatened Condition

Code any condition described at the time of discharge as "impending" or "threatened" as follows:

If it did occur, code as confirmed diagnosis.

If it did not occur, reference the Alphabetic Index to determine if the condition has a subentry term for "impending" or "threatened" and also reference main term entries for "Impending" and for "Threatened."

If the subterms are listed, assign the given code.

If the subterms are not listed, code the existing underlying condition(s) and not the condition described as impending or threatened.

12. Reporting Same Diagnosis Code More than Once

Each unique ICD-10-CM diagnosis code may be reported only once for an encounter. This applies to bilateral conditions when there are no distinct codes identifying laterality or two different conditions classified to the same ICD-10-CM diagnosis code.

13. Laterality

Some ICD-10-CM codes indicate laterality, specifying whether the condition occurs on the left, right or is bilateral. If no bilateral code is provided and the condition is bilateral, assign separate codes for both the left and right side. If the side is not identified in the medical record, assign the code for the unspecified side.

When a patient has a bilateral condition and each side is treated during separate encounters, assign the "bilateral" code (as the condition still exists on both sides), including for the encounter to treat the first side. For the second encounter for treatment after one side has previously been treated and the condition no longer exists on that side, assign the appropriate unilateral code for the side where the condition still exists (e.g., cataract surgery performed on each eye in separate encounters). The bilateral code would not be assigned for the subsequent encounter, as the patient no longer has the condition in the previously-treated site. If the treatment on the first side did not completely resolve the condition, then the bilateral code would still be appropriate.

When laterality is not documented by the patient's provider, code assignment for the affected side may be based on medical record documentation from other clinicians. If there is conflicting medical record documentation regarding the affected side, the patient's provider should be queried for clarification. Codes for "unspecified" side should rarely be used, such as when the documentation in the record is insufficient to determine the affected side and it is not possible to obtain clarification.

14. Documentation by Clinicians Other than the Patient's Provider

Code assignment is based on the documentation by the patient's provider (i.e., physician or other qualified healthcare practitioner legally accountable for establishing the patient's diagnosis). There are a few exceptions when code assignment may be based on medical record documentation from clinicians who are not the patient's provider (i.e., physician or other qualified healthcare practitioner legally accountable for establishing the patient's diagnosis). In this context, "clinicians" other than the patient's provider refer to healthcare professionals permitted, based on regulatory or accreditation requirements or internal hospital policies, to document in a patient's official medical record.

These exceptions include codes for:

- Body Mass Index (BMI)
- Depth of non-pressure chronic ulcers
- Pressure ulcer stage
- Coma scale
- NIH stroke scale (NIHSS)
- Social determinants of health (SDOH) **classified to Chapter 21**
- Laterality
- Blood alcohol level
- Underimmunization status

This information is typically, or may be, documented by other clinicians involved in the care of the patient (e.g., a dietitian often documents the BMI, a nurse often documents the pressure ulcer stages, and an emergency medical technician often documents the coma scale). However, the associated diagnosis (such as overweight, obesity, acute stroke, pressure ulcer, or a condition classifiable to category F1Ø, Alcohol related disorders) must be documented by the patient's provider. If there is conflicting medical record documentation, either from the same clinician or different clinicians, the patient's provider should be queried for clarification.

The BMI, coma scale, NIHSS, blood alcohol level codes, codes for social determinants of health and underimmunization status should only be reported as secondary diagnoses.

See Section I.C.21.c.17. for additional information regarding coding social determinants of health.

15. Syndromes

Follow the Alphabetic Index guidance when coding syndromes. In the absence of Alphabetic Index guidance, assign codes for the documented manifestations of the syndrome. Additional codes for manifestations that are not an integral part of the disease process may also be assigned when the condition does not have a unique code.

16. Documentation of Complications of Care

Code assignment is based on the provider's documentation of the relationship between the condition and the care or procedure, unless otherwise instructed by the classification. The guideline extends to any complications of care, regardless of the chapter the code is located in. It is important to note that not all conditions that occur during or following medical care or surgery are classified as complications. There must be a cause-and-effect relationship between the care provided and the condition, and the documentation must support that the condition is clinically significant. It is not necessary for the provider to explicitly document the term "complication." For example, if the condition alters the course of the surgery as documented in the operative report, then it would be appropriate to report a complication code. Query the provider for clarification if the documentation is not clear as to the relationship between the condition and the care or procedure.

17. Borderline Diagnosis

If the provider documents a "borderline" diagnosis at the time of discharge, the diagnosis is coded as confirmed, unless the classification provides a specific entry (e.g., borderline diabetes). If a borderline condition has a specific index entry in ICD-10-CM, it should be coded as such. Since borderline conditions are not uncertain diagnoses, no distinction is made between the care setting (inpatient versus outpatient). Whenever the documentation is unclear regarding a borderline condition, coders are encouraged to query for clarification.

18. Use of Sign/Symptom/Unspecified Codes

Sign/symptom and "unspecified" codes have acceptable, even necessary, uses. While specific diagnosis codes should be reported when they are supported by the available medical record documentation and clinical knowledge of the patient's health condition, there are instances when signs/symptoms or unspecified codes are the best choices for accurately reflecting the healthcare encounter. Each healthcare encounter should be coded to the level of certainty known for that encounter.

As stated in the introductory section of these official coding guidelines, a joint effort between the healthcare provider and the coder is essential to achieve complete and accurate documentation, code assignment, and reporting of diagnoses and procedures. The importance of consistent, complete documentation in the medical record cannot be overemphasized. Without such documentation accurate coding cannot be achieved. The entire record should be reviewed to determine the specific reason for the encounter and the conditions treated.

If a definitive diagnosis has not been established by the end of the encounter, it is appropriate to report codes for sign(s) and/or symptom(s) in lieu of a definitive diagnosis. When sufficient clinical information isn't known or available about a particular health condition to assign a more specific code, it is acceptable to report the appropriate "unspecified" code (e.g., a diagnosis of pneumonia has been determined, but not the specific type). Unspecified codes should be reported when they are the codes that most accurately reflect what is known about the patient's condition at the time of that particular encounter. It would be inappropriate to select a specific code that is not supported by the medical record documentation or conduct medically unnecessary diagnostic testing in order to determine a more specific code.

19. Coding for Healthcare Encounters in Hurricane Aftermath

a. Use of External Cause of Morbidity Codes

An external cause of morbidity code should be assigned to identify the cause of the injury(ies) incurred as a result of the hurricane. The use of external cause of morbidity codes is supplemental to the application of ICD-10-CM codes. External cause of morbidity codes are never to be recorded as a principal diagnosis (first-listed in non-inpatient settings). The appropriate injury code should be sequenced before any external cause codes. The external cause of morbidity codes capture how the injury or health condition happened (cause), the intent (unintentional or accidental; or intentional, such as suicide or assault), the place where the event occurred, the activity of the patient at the time of the event, and the person's status (e.g., civilian, military). They should not be assigned for encounters to treat hurricane victims' medical conditions when no injury, adverse effect or poisoning is involved. External cause of morbidity codes should be assigned for each encounter for care and treatment of the injury. External cause of morbidity codes may be assigned in all health care settings. For the purpose of capturing complete and accurate ICD-10-CM data in the aftermath of the hurricane, a healthcare setting should be considered as any location where medical care is provided by licensed healthcare professionals.

b. Sequencing of External Causes of Morbidity Codes

Codes for cataclysmic events, such as a hurricane, take priority over all other external cause codes except child and adult abuse and terrorism and should be sequenced before other external cause of injury codes. Assign as many external cause of morbidity codes as necessary to fully explain each cause. For example, if an injury occurs as a result of a building collapse during the hurricane, external cause codes for both the hurricane and the building collapse should be assigned, with the external causes code for hurricane being sequenced as the first external cause code. For injuries incurred as a direct result of the hurricane, assign the appropriate code(s) for the injuries, followed by the code X37.Ø-, Hurricane (with the appropriate 7th character), and any other applicable external cause of injury codes. Code X37.Ø- also should be assigned when an injury is incurred as a result of flooding caused by a levee breaking related to the hurricane. Code X38.-, Flood (with the appropriate 7th character), should be assigned when an injury is from flooding resulting directly from the storm. Code X36.Ø.-, Collapse of dam or man-made structure, should not be assigned when the cause of the collapse is due to the hurricane. Use of code X36.Ø- is limited to collapses of man-made structures due to earth surface movements, not due to storm surges directly from a hurricane.

c. Other External Causes of Morbidity Code Issues

For injuries that are not a direct result of the hurricane, such as an evacuee that has incurred an injury as a result of a motor vehicle accident, assign the appropriate external cause of morbidity code(s) to describe the cause of the injury, but do not assign code X37.Ø-, Hurricane. If it is not clear whether the injury was a direct result of the hurricane, assume the injury is due to the hurricane and assign code X37.Ø-, Hurricane, as well as any other applicable external cause of morbidity codes. In addition to code X37.Ø-, Hurricane, other possible applicable external cause of morbidity codes include:

X3Ø-, Exposure to excessive natural heat
X31-, Exposure to excessive natural cold
X38-, Flood

d. Use of Z codes

Z codes (other reasons for healthcare encounters) may be assigned as appropriate to further explain the reasons for presenting for healthcare services, including transfers between healthcare facilities, or provide additional information relevant to a patient encounter. The ICD-10-CM Official Guidelines for Coding and Reporting identify which codes maybe assigned as principal or first-listed diagnosis only, secondary diagnosis only, or principal/first-listed or secondary (depending on the circumstances). Possible applicable Z codes include:

Z59.Ø-, Homelessness
Z59.1, Inadequate housing
Z59.5, Extreme poverty
Z75.1, Person awaiting admission to adequate facility elsewhere
Z75.3, Unavailability and inaccessibility of health-care facilities
Z75.4, Unavailability and inaccessibility of other helping agencies
Z76.2, Encounter for health supervision and care of other healthy infant and child
Z99.12, Encounter for respirator [ventilator] dependence during power failure

The external cause of morbidity codes and the Z codes listed above are not an all-inclusive list. Other codes may be applicable to the encounter based upon the documentation. Assign as many codes as necessary to fully explain each healthcare encounter. Since patient history information may be very limited, use any available documentation to assign the appropriate external cause of morbidity and Z codes.

C. Chapter-Specific Coding Guidelines

In addition to general coding guidelines, there are guidelines for specific diagnoses and/or conditions in the classification. Unless otherwise indicated, these guidelines apply to all health care settings. Please refer to Section II for guidelines on the selection of principal diagnosis.

1. Chapter 1: Certain Infectious and Parasitic Diseases (AØØ-B99), UØ7.1, UØ9.9

a. Human Immunodeficiency Virus (HIV) Infections

1) Code only confirmed cases

Code only confirmed cases of HIV infection/illness. This is an exception to the hospital inpatient guideline Section II, H.

In this context, "confirmation" does not require documentation of positive serology or culture for HIV; the provider's diagnostic statement that the patient is HIV positive or has an HIV-related illness is sufficient.

2) Selection and sequencing of HIV codes

(a) Patient admitted for HIV-related condition

If a patient is admitted for an HIV-related condition, the principal diagnosis should be B2Ø, Human immunodeficiency virus [HIV] disease followed by additional diagnosis codes for all reported HIV-related conditions.

An exception to this guideline is if the reason for admission is hemolytic-uremic syndrome associated with HIV disease. Assign code D59.31, Infection- associated hemolytic-uremic syndrome, followed by code B2Ø, Human immunodeficiency virus [HIV] disease.

(b) Patient with HIV disease admitted for unrelated condition

If a patient with HIV disease is admitted for an unrelated condition (such as a traumatic injury), the code for the unrelated condition (e.g., the nature of injury code) should be the principal diagnosis. Other diagnoses would be B2Ø followed by additional diagnosis codes for all reported HIV-related conditions.

(c) Whether the patient is newly diagnosed

Whether the patient is newly diagnosed or has had previous admissions/encounters for HIV conditions is irrelevant to the sequencing decision.

(d) Asymptomatic human immunodeficiency virus

Z21, Asymptomatic human immunodeficiency virus [HIV] infection status, is to be applied when the patient without any documentation of symptoms is listed as being "HIV positive," "known HIV," "HIV test positive," or similar terminology. Do not use this code if the term "AIDS" or "HIV disease" is used or if the patient is treated for any HIV-related illness or is described as having any condition(s) resulting from his/her HIV positive status; use B2Ø in these cases.

(e) Patients with inconclusive HIV serology

Patients with inconclusive HIV serology, but no definitive diagnosis or manifestations of the illness, may be assigned code R75, Inconclusive laboratory evidence of human immunodeficiency virus [HIV].

(f) Previously diagnosed HIV-related illness

Patients with any known prior diagnosis of an HIV-related illness should be coded to B2Ø. Once a patient has developed an HIV-related illness, the patient should always be assigned code B2Ø on every subsequent admission/encounter. Patients previously diagnosed with any HIV illness (B2Ø) should never be assigned to R75 or Z21, Asymptomatic human immunodeficiency virus [HIV] infection status.

(g) HIV Infection in Pregnancy, Childbirth and the Puerperium

During pregnancy, childbirth or the puerperium, a patient admitted (or presenting for a health care encounter) because of an HIV-related illness should receive a principal diagnosis code of O98.7-, Human immunodeficiency [HIV] disease complicating pregnancy, childbirth and the puerperium, followed by B2Ø and the code(s) for the HIV-related illness(es). Codes from Chapter 15 always take sequencing priority.

Patients with asymptomatic HIV infection status admitted (or presenting for a health care encounter) during pregnancy, childbirth, or the puerperium should receive codes of O98.7- and Z21.

(h) Encounters for testing for HIV

If a patient is being seen to determine his/her HIV status, use code Z11.4, Encounter for screening for human immunodeficiency virus [HIV]. Use additional codes for any associated high-risk behavior, if applicable.

If a patient with signs or symptoms is being seen for HIV testing, code the signs and symptoms. An additional counseling code Z71.7, Human immunodeficiency virus [HIV] counseling, may be used if counseling is provided during the encounter for the test.

When a patient returns to be informed of his/her HIV test results and the test result is negative, use code Z71.7, Human immunodeficiency virus [HIV] counseling.

If the results are positive, see previous guidelines and assign codes as appropriate.

(i) HIV managed by antiretroviral medication

If a patient with documented HIV disease, HIV-related illness or AIDS is currently managed on antiretroviral medications, assign code B2Ø, Human immunodeficiency virus [HIV] disease. Code Z79.899, Other long term (current) drug therapy, may be assigned as an additional code to identify the long-term (current) use of antiretroviral medications.

(j) Encounter for HIV Prophylaxis Measures

When a patient is seen for administration of pre-exposure prophylaxis medication for HIV, assign code Z29.81, Encounter for HIV pre-exposure prophylaxis.

Pre-exposure prophylaxis (PrEP) is intended to prevent infection in people who are at risk for getting HIV through sex or injection drug use. Any risk factors for HIV should also be coded.

b. Infectious agents as the cause of diseases classified to other chapters

Certain infections are classified in chapters other than Chapter 1 and no organism is identified as part of the infection code. In these instances, it is necessary to use an additional code from Chapter 1 to identify the organism. A code from category B95, Streptococcus, Staphylococcus, and Enterococcus as the cause of diseases classified to other chapters, B96, Other bacterial agents as the cause of diseases classified to other chapters, or B97, Viral agents as the cause of diseases classified to other chapters, is to be used as an additional code to identify the organism. An instructional note will be found at the infection code advising that an additional organism code is required.

c. Infections resistant to antibiotics

Many bacterial infections are resistant to current antibiotics. It is necessary to identify all infections documented as antibiotic resistant. Assign a code from category Z16, Resistance to antimicrobial drugs, following the infection code only if the infection code does not identify drug resistance.

d. Sepsis, Severe Sepsis, and Septic Shock Infections resistant to antibiotics

1) Coding of Sepsis and Severe Sepsis

(a) Sepsis

For a diagnosis of sepsis, assign the appropriate code for the underlying systemic infection. If the type of infection or causal organism is not further specified, assign code A41.9, Sepsis, unspecified organism.

A code from subcategory R65.2, Severe sepsis, should not be assigned unless severe sepsis or an associated acute organ dysfunction is documented.

(i) Negative or inconclusive blood cultures and sepsis

Negative or inconclusive blood cultures do not preclude a diagnosis of sepsis in patients with clinical evidence of the condition; however, the provider should be queried.

(ii) Urosepsis

The term urosepsis is a nonspecific term. It is not to be considered synonymous with sepsis. It has no default code in the Alphabetic Index. Should a provider use this term, he/she must be queried for clarification.

(iii) Sepsis with organ dysfunction

If a patient has sepsis and associated acute organ dysfunction or multiple organ dysfunction (MOD), follow the instructions for coding severe sepsis.

(iv) Acute organ dysfunction that is not clearly associated with the sepsis

If a patient has sepsis and an acute organ dysfunction, but the medical record documentation indicates that the acute organ dysfunction is related to a medical condition other than the sepsis, do not assign a code from subcategory R65.2, Severe sepsis. An acute organ dysfunction must be associated with the sepsis in order to assign the severe sepsis code. If the documentation is not clear as to whether an acute organ dysfunction is related to the sepsis or another medical condition, query the provider.

(b) Severe sepsis

The coding of severe sepsis requires a minimum of 2 codes: first a code for the underlying systemic infection, followed by a code from subcategory R65.2, Severe sepsis. If the causal organism is not documented, assign code A41.9, Sepsis, unspecified organism, for the infection. Additional code(s) for the associated acute organ dysfunction are also required.

Due to the complex nature of severe sepsis, some cases may require querying the provider prior to assignment of the codes.

2) Septic shock

Septic shock generally refers to circulatory failure associated with severe sepsis, and therefore, it represents a type of acute organ dysfunction.

For cases of septic shock, the code for the systemic infection should be sequenced first, followed by code R65.21, Severe sepsis with septic shock or code T81.12, Postprocedural septic shock.

Any additional codes for the other acute organ dysfunctions should also be assigned. As noted in the sequencing instructions in the Tabular List, the code for septic shock cannot be assigned as a principal diagnosis.

3) Sequencing of severe sepsis

If severe sepsis is present on admission, and meets the definition of principal diagnosis, the underlying systemic infection should be assigned as principal diagnosis followed by the appropriate code from subcategory R65.2 as required by the sequencing rules in the Tabular List. A code from subcategory R65.2 can never be assigned as a principal diagnosis.

When severe sepsis develops during an encounter (it was not present on admission), the underlying systemic infection and the appropriate code from subcategory R65.2 should be assigned as secondary diagnoses.

Severe sepsis may be present on admission, but the diagnosis may not be confirmed until sometime after admission. If the documentation is not clear whether severe sepsis was present on admission, the provider should be queried.

For infection-associated hemolytic-uremic syndrome with severe sepsis, see guideline I.C.1.d.9.

4) Sepsis or severe sepsis with a localized infection

If the reason for admission is sepsis or severe sepsis and a localized infection, such as pneumonia or cellulitis, a code(s) for the underlying systemic infection should be assigned first and the code for the localized infection should be assigned as a secondary diagnosis. If the patient has severe sepsis, a code from subcategory R65.2 should also be assigned as a secondary diagnosis. If the patient is admitted with a localized infection, such as pneumonia, and sepsis/severe sepsis doesn't develop until after admission, the localized infection should be assigned first, followed by the appropriate sepsis/severe sepsis codes.

For hemolytic-uremic syndrome associated with sepsis, see guideline I. C.1.d.9.

5) Sepsis due to a postprocedural infection

(a) Documentation of causal relationship

As with all postprocedural complications, code assignment is based on the provider's documentation of the relationship between the infection and the procedure.

(b) Sepsis due to a postprocedural infection

For **sepsis** following a **postprocedural wound (surgical site) infection**, a code from T81.4**1**, to T81.43, Infection following a procedure, or a code from O86.ØØ to O86.Ø3, Infection of obstetric surgical wound, that identifies the site of the infection should be **sequenced** first, if known. Assign an additional code for sepsis following a procedure (T81.44) or sepsis following an obstetrical procedure (O86.Ø4). Use an additional code to identify the infectious agent. If the patient has severe sepsis, the appropriate code from subcategory R65.2 should also be assigned with the additional code(s) for any acute organ dysfunction.

For infections following infusion, transfusion, therapeutic injection, or immunization, a code from subcategory T8Ø.2, Infections following infusion, transfusion, and therapeutic injection, or code T88.Ø-, Infection following immunization, should be coded first, followed by the code for the specific infection. If the patient has severe sepsis, the appropriate code from subcategory R65.2 should also be assigned, with the additional codes(s) for any acute organ dysfunction.

(c) Postprocedural infection and postprocedural septic shock

If a postprocedural infection has resulted in postprocedural septic shock, assign the codes indicated above for sepsis due to a postprocedural infection, followed by code T81.12-,

Postprocedural septic shock. Do not assign code R65.21, Severe sepsis with septic shock. Additional code(s) should be assigned for any acute organ dysfunction.

6) Sepsis and severe sepsis associated with a noninfectious process (condition)

In some cases, a noninfectious process (condition) such as trauma, may lead to an infection which can result in sepsis or severe sepsis. If sepsis or severe sepsis is documented as associated with a noninfectious condition, such as a burn or serious injury, and this condition meets the definition for principal diagnosis, the code for the noninfectious condition should be sequenced first, followed by the code for the resulting infection. If severe sepsis is present, a code from subcategory R65.2 should also be assigned with any associated organ dysfunction(s) codes. It is not necessary to assign a code from subcategory R65.1, Systemic inflammatory response syndrome (SIRS) of non-infectious origin, for these cases.

If the infection meets the definition of principal diagnosis, it should be sequenced before the non-infectious condition. When both the associated non-infectious condition and the infection meet the definition of principal diagnosis, either may be assigned as principal diagnosis.

Only one code from category R65, Symptoms and signs specifically associated with systemic inflammation and infection, should be assigned. Therefore, when a non-infectious condition leads to an infection resulting in severe sepsis, assign the appropriate code from subcategory R65.2, Severe sepsis. Do not additionally assign a code from subcategory R65.1, Systemic inflammatory response syndrome (SIRS) of non-infectious origin.

See Section I.C.18. SIRS due to non-infectious process

7) Sepsis and septic shock complicating abortion, pregnancy, childbirth, and the puerperium

See Section I.C.15. Sepsis and septic shock complicating abortion, pregnancy, childbirth and the puerperium

8) Newborn sepsis

See Section I.C.16. f. Bacterial sepsis of Newborn

9) Hemolytic-uremic syndrome associated with sepsis

If the reason for admission is hemolytic-uremic syndrome that is associated with sepsis, assign code D59.31, Infection-associated hemolytic-uremic syndrome, as the principal diagnosis. Codes for the underlying systemic infection and any other conditions (such as severe sepsis) should be assigned as secondary diagnoses.

e. Methicillin Resistant Staphylococcus aureus (MRSA) Conditions

1) Selection and sequencing of MRSA codes

(a) Combination codes for MRSA infection

When a patient is diagnosed with an infection that is due to methicillin resistant *Staphylococcus aureus* (MRSA), and that infection has a combination code that includes the causal organism (e.g., sepsis, pneumonia) assign the appropriate combination code for the condition (e.g., code A41.Ø2, Sepsis due to Methicillin resistant Staphylococcus aureus or code J15.212, Pneumonia due to Methicillin resistant Staphylococcus aureus). Do not assign code B95.62, Methicillin resistant Staphylococcus aureus infection as the cause of diseases classified elsewhere, as an additional code, because the combination code includes the type of infection and the MRSA organism. Do not assign a code from subcategory Z16.11, Resistance to penicillins, as an additional diagnosis.

See Section C.1. for instructions on coding and sequencing of sepsis and severe sepsis.

(b) Other codes for MRSA infection

When there is documentation of a current infection (e.g., wound infection, stitch abscess, urinary tract infection) due to MRSA, and that infection does not have a combination code that includes the causal organism, assign the appropriate code to identify the condition along with code B95.62, Methicillin resistant Staphylococcus aureus infection as the cause of diseases classified elsewhere for the MRSA infection. Do not assign a code from subcategory Z16.11, Resistance to penicillins.

(c) Methicillin susceptible Staphylococcus aureus (MSSA) and MRSA colonization

The condition or state of being colonized or carrying MSSA or MRSA is called colonization or carriage, while an individual person is described as being colonized or being a carrier.

Colonization means that MSSA or MSRA is present on or in the body without necessarily causing illness. A positive MRSA colonization test might be documented by the provider as "MRSA screen positive" or "MRSA nasal swab positive".

Assign code Z22.322, Carrier or suspected carrier of Methicillin resistant Staphylococcus aureus, for patients documented as having MRSA colonization. Assign code Z22.321, Carrier or suspected carrier of Methicillin susceptible Staphylococcus aureus, for patients documented as having MSSA colonization. Colonization is not necessarily indicative of a disease process or as the cause of a specific condition the patient may have unless documented as such by the provider.

(d) MRSA colonization and infection

If a patient is documented as having both MRSA colonization and infection during a hospital admission, code Z22.322, Carrier or suspected carrier of Methicillin resistant Staphylococcus aureus, and a code for the MRSA infection may both be assigned.

f. Zika virus infections

1) Code only confirmed cases

Code only a confirmed diagnosis of Zika virus (A92.5, Zika virus disease) as documented by the provider. This is an exception to the hospital inpatient guideline Section II, H. In this context, "confirmation" does not require documentation of the type of test performed; the provider's diagnostic statement that the condition is confirmed is sufficient. This code should be assigned regardless of the stated mode of transmission.

If the provider documents "suspected", "possible" or "probable" Zika, do not assign code A92.5. Assign a code(s) explaining the reason for encounter (such as fever, rash, or joint pain) or Z2Ø.821, Contact with and (suspected) exposure to Zika virus.

g. Coronavirus infections

1) COVID-19 infection (infection due to SARS-CoV-2)

(a) Code only confirmed cases

Code only a confirmed diagnosis of the 2019 novel coronavirus disease (COVID-19) as documented by the provider, or documentation of a positive COVID-19 test result. For a confirmed diagnosis, assign code UØ7.1, COVID-19. This is an exception to the hospital inpatient guideline Section II, H. In this context, "confirmation" does not require documentation of a positive test result for COVID-19; the provider's documentation that the individual has COVID-19 is sufficient.

If the provider documents "suspected," "possible," "probable," or "inconclusive" COVID-19, do not assign code UØ7.1. Instead, code the signs and symptoms reported. See guideline I.C.1.g.1.g.

(b) Sequencing of codes

When COVID-19 meets the definition of principal diagnosis, code UØ7.1, COVID-19, should be sequenced first, followed by the appropriate codes for associated manifestations, except when another guideline requires that certain codes be sequenced first, such as obstetrics, sepsis, or transplant complications.

For a COVID-19 infection that progresses to sepsis, see Section I.C.1.d. Sepsis, Severe Sepsis, and Septic Shock

See Section I.C.15.s. for COVID-19 infection in pregnancy, childbirth, and the puerperium

See Section I.C.16.h. for COVID-19 infection in newborn

For a COVID-19 infection in a lung transplant patient, see Section I.C.19.g.3.a. Transplant complications other than kidney.

(c) Acute respiratory manifestations of COVID-19

When the reason for the encounter/admission is a respiratory manifestation of COVID-19, assign code UØ7.1, COVID-19, as the principal/first-listed diagnosis and assign code(s) for the respiratory manifestation(s) as additional diagnoses.

The following conditions are examples of common respiratory manifestations of COVID-19.

(i) Pneumonia

For a patient with pneumonia confirmed as due to COVID-19, assign codes UØ7.1, COVID-19, and J12.82, Pneumonia due to coronavirus disease 2019.

(ii) Acute bronchitis

For a patient with acute bronchitis confirmed as due to COVID-19, assign codes UØ7.1, and J2Ø.8, Acute bronchitis due to other specified organisms.

Bronchitis not otherwise specified (NOS) due to COVID-19 should be coded using code UØ7.1 and J4Ø, Bronchitis, not specified as acute or chronic.

(iii) **Lower respiratory infection**

If the COVID-19 is documented as being associated with a lower respiratory infection, not otherwise specified (NOS), or an acute respiratory infection, NOS, codes U07.1 and J22, Unspecified acute lower respiratory infection, should be assigned.

If the COVID-19 is documented as being associated with a respiratory infection, NOS, codes U07.1 and J98.8, Other specified respiratory disorders, should be assigned.

(iv) **Acute respiratory distress syndrome**

For acute respiratory distress syndrome (ARDS) due to COVID-19, assign codes U07.1, and J80, Acute respiratory distress syndrome.

(v) **Acute respiratory failure**

For acute respiratory failure due to COVID-19, assign code U07.1, and code J96.0-, Acute respiratory failure.

(d) **Non-respiratory manifestations of COVID-19**

When the reason for the encounter/admission is a non-respiratory manifestation (e.g., viral enteritis) of COVID-19, assign code U07.1, COVID-19, as the principal/first-listed diagnosis and assign code(s) for the manifestation(s) as additional diagnoses.

(e) **Exposure to COVID-19**

For asymptomatic individuals with actual or suspected exposure to COVID-19, assign code Z20.822, Contact with and (suspected) exposure to COVID-19.

For symptomatic individuals with actual or suspected exposure to COVID-19 and the infection has been ruled out, or test results are inconclusive or unknown, assign code Z20.822, Contact with and (suspected) exposure to COVID-19. See guideline I.C.21.c.1, Contact/Exposure, for additional guidance regarding the use of category Z20 codes.

If COVID-19 is confirmed, see guideline I.C.1.g.1.a.

(f) **Screening for COVID-19**

For screening for COVID-19, including preoperative testing, assign code Z11.52, Encounter for screening for COVID-19.

(g) **Signs and symptoms without definitive diagnosis of COVID-19**

For patients presenting with any signs/symptoms associated with COVID-19 (such as fever, etc.) but a definitive diagnosis has not been established, assign the appropriate code(s) for each of the presenting signs and symptoms such as:

- R05.1, Acute cough, or R05.9, Cough, unspecified
- R06.02 Shortness of breath
- R50.9 Fever, unspecified

If a patient with signs/symptoms associated with COVID-19 also has an actual or suspected contact with or exposure to COVID-19, assign Z20.822, Contact with and (suspected) exposure to COVID-19, as an additional code.

(h) **Asymptomatic individuals who test positive for COVID-19**

For asymptomatic individuals who test positive for COVID-19, see guideline I.C.1.g.1.a. Although the individual is asymptomatic, the individual has tested positive and is considered to have the COVID-19 infection.

(i) **Personal history of COVID-19**

For patients with a history of COVID-19, assign code Z86.16, Personal history of COVID-19.

(j) **Follow-up visits after COVID-19 infection has resolved**

For individuals who previously had COVID-19, without residual symptom(s) or condition(s), and are being seen for follow-up evaluation, and COVID-19 test results are negative, assign codes Z09, Encounter for follow-up examination after completed treatment for conditions other than malignant neoplasm, and Z86.16, Personal history of COVID-19.

For follow-up visits for individuals with symptom(s) or condition(s) related to a previous COVID-19 infection, see guideline I.C.1.g.1.m.

See Section I.C.21.c.8, Factors influencing health states and contact with health services, Follow-up

(k) **Encounter for antibody testing**

For an encounter for antibody testing that is not being performed to confirm a current COVID-19 infection, nor is a follow-up test after resolution of COVID-19, assign Z01.84, Encounter for antibody response examination.

Follow the applicable guidelines above if the individual is being tested to confirm a current COVID-19 infection.

For follow-up testing after a COVID-19 infection, see guideline I.C.1.g.1.j.

(l) **Multisystem Inflammatory Syndrome**

For individuals with multisystem inflammatory syndrome (MIS) and COVID-19, assign code U07.1, COVID-19, as the principal/first-listed diagnosis and assign code M35.81, Multisystem inflammatory syndrome, as an additional diagnosis.

If an individual with a history of COVID-19 develops MIS, assign codes M35.81, Multisystem inflammatory syndrome, and U09.9, Post COVID-19 condition, unspecified.

If an individual with a known or suspected exposure to COVID-19, and no current COVID-19 infection or history of COVID-19, develops MIS, assign codes M35.81, Multisystem inflammatory syndrome, and Z20.822, Contact with and (suspected) exposure to COVID-19.

Additional codes should be assigned for any associated complications of MIS.

(m) **Post COVID-19 Condition**

For sequela of COVID-19, or associated symptoms or conditions that develop following a previous COVID-19 infection, assign a code(s) for the specific symptom(s) or condition(s) related to the previous COVID-19 infection, if known, and code U09.9, Post COVID-19 condition, unspecified.

Code U09.9 should not be assigned for manifestations of an active (current) COVID-19 infection.

If a patient has a condition(s) associated with a previous COVID-19 infection and develops a new active (current) COVID-19 infection, code U09.9 may be assigned in conjunction with code U07.1, COVID-19, to identify that the patient also has a condition(s) associated with a previous COVID-19 infection. Code(s) for the specific condition(s) associated with the previous COVID-19 infection and code(s) for manifestation(s) of the new active (current) COVID-19 infection should also be assigned.

(n) **Underimmunization for COVID-19 Status**

Code Z28.310, Unvaccinated for COVID-19, may be assigned when the patient has not received a COVID-19 vaccine of any type. Code Z28.311, Partially vaccinated for COVID-19, may be assigned when the patient has been partially vaccinated for COVID-19 as per the recommendations of the Centers for Disease Control and Prevention (CDC) in place at the time of the encounter. For information, visit the CDC's website https://www.cdc.gov/coronavirus/2019-ncov/vaccines/.

See Section I.B.14. for underimmunization documentation by clinicians other than patient's provider.

2. Chapter 2: Neoplasms (C00-D49)

General Guidelines

Chapter 2 of the ICD-10-CM contains the codes for most benign and all malignant neoplasms. Certain benign neoplasms, such as prostatic adenomas, may be found in the specific body system chapters. To properly code a neoplasm, it is necessary to determine from the record if the neoplasm is benign, in-situ, malignant, or of uncertain histologic behavior. If malignant, any secondary (metastatic) sites should also be determined.

Primary malignant neoplasms overlapping site boundaries

A primary malignant neoplasm that overlaps two or more contiguous (next to each other) sites should be classified to the subcategory/code .8 ('overlapping lesion'), unless the combination is specifically indexed elsewhere. For multiple neoplasms of the same site that are not contiguous such as tumors in different quadrants of the same breast, codes for each site should be assigned.

Malignant neoplasm of ectopic tissue

Malignant neoplasms of ectopic tissue are to be coded to the site of origin mentioned, e.g., ectopic pancreatic malignant neoplasms involving the stomach are coded to malignant neoplasm of pancreas, unspecified (C25.9).

The neoplasm table in the Alphabetic Index should be referenced first. However, if the histological term is documented, that term should be referenced first, rather than going immediately to the Neoplasm Table, in order to determine which column in the Neoplasm Table is appropriate. For example, if the documentation indicates "adenoma," refer to the term in the Alphabetic Index to review the entries under this term and the instructional note to "see also neoplasm, by site, benign." The table provides the proper code based on the type of neoplasm and the site. It is important to select the proper column in the table that corresponds to the type of neoplasm. The Tabular List should then be referenced to verify that the correct code has been selected from the table and that a more specific site code does not exist.

See Section I.C.21. Factors influencing health status and contact with health services, Status, for information regarding Z15.Ø, codes for genetic susceptibility to cancer.

a. Admission/Encounter for treatment of primary site

If the malignancy is chiefly responsible for occasioning the patient admission/encounter and treatment is directed at the primary site, designate the primary malignancy as the principal/first-listed diagnosis.

The only exception to this guideline is if the administration of chemotherapy, immunotherapy or external beam radiation therapy is chiefly responsible for occasioning the admission/encounter. In that case, assign the appropriate Z51.-- code as the first-listed or principal diagnosis, and the underlying diagnosis or problem for which the service is being performed as a secondary diagnosis.

b. Admission/Encounter for treatment of secondary site

When a patient is admitted because of a primary neoplasm with metastasis and treatment is directed toward the secondary site only, the secondary neoplasm is designated as the principal diagnosis even though the primary malignancy is still present.

c. Coding and sequencing of complications

Coding and sequencing of complications associated with the malignancies or with the therapy thereof are subject to the following guidelines:

1) Anemia associated with malignancy

When admission/encounter is for management of an anemia associated with the malignancy, and the treatment is only for anemia, the appropriate code for the malignancy is sequenced as the principal or first-listed diagnosis followed by the appropriate code for the anemia (such as code D63.Ø, Anemia in neoplastic disease).

2) Anemia associated with chemotherapy, immunotherapy and radiation therapy

When the admission/encounter is for management of an anemia associated with an adverse effect of the administration of chemotherapy or immunotherapy and the only treatment is for the anemia, the anemia code is sequenced first followed by the appropriate codes for the neoplasm and the adverse effect (T45.1X5-, Adverse effect of antineoplastic and immunosuppressive drugs).

When the admission/encounter is for management of an anemia associated with an adverse effect of radiotherapy, the anemia code should be sequenced first, followed by the appropriate neoplasm code and code Y84.2, Radiological procedure and radiotherapy as the cause of abnormal reaction of the patient, or of later complication, without mention of misadventure at the time of the procedure.

3) Management of dehydration due to the malignancy

When the admission/encounter is for management of dehydration due to the malignancy and only the dehydration is being treated (intravenous rehydration), the dehydration is sequenced first, followed by the code(s) for the malignancy.

4) Treatment of a complication resulting from a surgical procedure

When the admission/encounter is for treatment of a complication resulting from a surgical procedure, designate the complication as the principal or first-listed diagnosis if treatment is directed at resolving the complication.

d. Primary malignancy previously excised

When a primary malignancy has been previously excised or eradicated from its site and there is no further treatment directed to that site and there is no evidence of any existing primary malignancy at that site, a code from category Z85, Personal history of malignant neoplasm, should be used to indicate the former site of the malignancy. Any mention of extension, invasion, or metastasis to another site is coded as a secondary malignant neoplasm to that site. The secondary site may be the principal or first-listed diagnosis with the Z85 code used as a secondary code.

See section I.C.2.t. Secondary malignant neoplasm of lymphoid tissue.

e. Admissions/Encounters involving chemotherapy, immunotherapy and radiation therapy

1) Episode of care involves surgical removal of neoplasm

When an episode of care involves the surgical removal of a neoplasm, primary or secondary site, followed by adjunct chemotherapy or radiation treatment during the same episode of care, the code for the neoplasm should be assigned as principal or first-listed diagnosis.

2) Patient admission/encounter chiefly for administration of chemotherapy, immunotherapy and radiation therapy

If a patient admission/encounter is **chiefly** for the administration of chemotherapy, immunotherapy or external beam radiation therapy assign code Z51.Ø, Encounter for antineoplastic radiation therapy, or Z51.11, Encounter for antineoplastic chemotherapy, or Z51.12, Encounter for antineoplastic immunotherapy as the first-listed or principal diagnosis. If a patient receives more than one of these therapies during the same admission, more than one of these codes may be assigned, in any sequence.

The malignancy for which the therapy is being administered should be assigned as a secondary diagnosis.

If a patient admission/encounter is for the insertion or implantation of radioactive elements (e.g., brachytherapy) the appropriate code for the malignancy is sequenced as the principal or first-listed diagnosis. Code Z51.Ø should not be assigned.

3) Patient admitted for radiation therapy, chemotherapy or immunotherapy and develops complications

When a patient is admitted for the purpose of external beam radiotherapy, immunotherapy or chemotherapy and develops complications such as uncontrolled nausea and vomiting or dehydration, the principal or first-listed diagnosis is Z51.Ø, Encounter for antineoplastic radiation therapy, or Z51.11, Encounter for antineoplastic chemotherapy, or Z51.12, Encounter for antineoplastic immunotherapy followed by any codes for the complications.

When a patient is admitted for the purpose of insertion or implantation of radioactive elements (e.g., brachytherapy) and develops complications such as uncontrolled nausea and vomiting or dehydration, the principal or first-listed diagnosis is the appropriate code for the malignancy followed by any codes for the complications.

f. Admission/encounter to determine extent of malignancy

When the reason for admission/encounter is to determine the extent of the malignancy, or for a procedure such as paracentesis or thoracentesis, the primary malignancy or appropriate metastatic site is designated as the principal or first-listed diagnosis, even though chemotherapy or radiotherapy is administered.

g. Symptoms, signs, and abnormal findings listed in Chapter 18 associated with neoplasms

Symptoms, signs, and ill-defined conditions listed in Chapter 18 characteristic of, or associated with, an existing primary or secondary site malignancy cannot be used to replace the malignancy as principal or first-listed diagnosis, regardless of the number of admissions or encounters for treatment and care of the neoplasm.

See section I.C.21. Factors influencing health status and contact with health services, Encounter for prophylactic organ removal.

h. Admission/encounter for pain control/management

See Section I.C.6. for information on coding admission/encounter for pain control/management.

i. Malignancy in two or more noncontiguous sites

A patient may have more than one malignant tumor in the same organ. These tumors may represent different primaries or metastatic disease, depending on the site. Should the documentation be unclear, the provider should be queried as to the status of each tumor so that the correct codes can be assigned.

j. Disseminated malignant neoplasm, unspecified

Code C8Ø.Ø, Disseminated malignant neoplasm, unspecified, is for use only in those cases where the patient has advanced metastatic disease and no known primary or secondary sites are specified. It should not be used in place of assigning codes for the primary site and all known secondary sites.

k. Malignant neoplasm without specification of site

Code C8Ø.1, Malignant (primary) neoplasm, unspecified, equates to Cancer, unspecified. This code should only be used when no determination can be made as to the primary site of a malignancy. This code should rarely be used in the inpatient setting.

l. Sequencing of neoplasm codes

1) Encounter for treatment of primary malignancy

If the reason for the encounter is for treatment of a primary malignancy, assign the malignancy as the principal/first-listed diagnosis. The primary site is to be sequenced first, followed by any metastatic sites.

2) Encounter for treatment of secondary malignancy

When an encounter is for a primary malignancy with metastasis and treatment is directed toward the metastatic (secondary) site(s) only, the metastatic site(s) is designated as the principal/first-listed diagnosis. The primary malignancy is coded as an additional code.

3) Malignant neoplasm in a pregnant patient

When a pregnant patient has a malignant neoplasm, a code from subcategory O9A.1-, Malignant neoplasm complicating pregnancy, childbirth, and the puerperium, should be sequenced first, followed by the appropriate code from Chapter 2 to indicate the type of neoplasm.

4) **Encounter for complication associated with a neoplasm**
When an encounter is for management of a complication associated with a neoplasm, such as dehydration, and the treatment is only for the complication, the complication is coded first, followed by the appropriate code(s) for the neoplasm.
The exception to this guideline is anemia. When the admission/encounter is for management of an anemia associated with the malignancy, and the treatment is only for anemia, the appropriate code for the malignancy is sequenced as the principal or first-listed diagnosis followed by code D63.Ø, Anemia in neoplastic disease.

5) **Complication from surgical procedure for treatment of a neoplasm**
When an encounter is for treatment of a complication resulting from a surgical procedure performed for the treatment of the neoplasm, designate the complication as the principal/first-listed diagnosis. See the guideline regarding the coding of a current malignancy versus personal history to determine if the code for the neoplasm should also be assigned.

6) **Pathologic fracture due to a neoplasm**
When an encounter is for a pathological fracture due to a neoplasm, and the focus of treatment is the fracture, a code from subcategory M84.5, Pathological fracture in neoplastic disease, should be sequenced first, followed by the code for the neoplasm.
If the focus of treatment is the neoplasm with an associated pathological fracture, the neoplasm code should be sequenced first, followed by a code from M84.5 for the pathological fracture.

m. **Current malignancy versus personal history of malignancy**
When a primary malignancy has been excised but further treatment, such as an additional surgery for the malignancy, radiation therapy or chemotherapy is directed to that site, the primary malignancy code should be used until treatment is completed.
When a primary malignancy has been previously excised or eradicated from its site, there is no further treatment (of the malignancy) directed to that site, and there is no evidence of any existing primary malignancy at that site, a code from category Z85, Personal history of malignant neoplasm, should be used to indicate the former site of the malignancy.
Codes from subcategories Z85.Ø – Z85.85 should only be assigned for the former site of a primary malignancy, not the site of a secondary malignancy. Code Z85.89 may be assigned for the former site(s) of either a primary or secondary malignancy.
See Section I.C.21. Factors influencing health status and contact with health services, History (of)

n. **Leukemia, Multiple Myeloma, and Malignant Plasma Cell Neoplasms in remission versus personal history**
The categories for leukemia, and category C9Ø, Multiple myeloma and malignant plasma cell neoplasms, have codes indicating whether or not the leukemia has achieved remission. There are also codes Z85.6, Personal history of leukemia, and Z85.79, Personal history of other malignant neoplasms of lymphoid, hematopoietic and related tissues. If the documentation is unclear as to whether the leukemia has achieved remission, the provider should be queried.
See Section I.C.21. Factors influencing health status and contact with health services, History (of)

o. **Aftercare following surgery for neoplasm**
See Section I.C.21. Factors influencing health status and contact with health services, Aftercare

p. **Follow-up care for completed treatment of a malignancy**
See Section I.C.21. Factors influencing health status and contact with health services, Follow-up

q. **Prophylactic organ removal for prevention of malignancy**
See Section I.C. 21, Factors influencing health status and contact with health services, Prophylactic organ removal

r. **Malignant neoplasm associated with transplanted organ**
A malignant neoplasm of a transplanted organ should be coded as a transplant complication. Assign first the appropriate code from category T86.-, Complications of transplanted organs and tissue, followed by code C8Ø.2, Malignant neoplasm associated with transplanted organ. Use an additional code for the specific malignancy.

s. **Breast Implant Associated Anaplastic Large Cell Lymphoma**
Breast implant associated anaplastic large cell lymphoma (BIA-ALCL) is a type of lymphoma that can develop around breast implants. Assign code C84.7A, Anaplastic large cell lymphoma, ALK-negative, breast, for BIA-ALCL. Do not assign a complication code from chapter 19.

t. **Secondary malignant neoplasm of lymphoid tissue**
When a malignant neoplasm of lymphoid tissue metastasizes beyond the lymph nodes, a code from categories C81-C85 with a final character "9" should be assigned identifying "extranodal and solid organ sites" rather than a code for the secondary neoplasm of the affected solid organ. For example, for metastasis of **diffuse large** B-cell lymphoma to the lung, brain and left adrenal gland, assign code C83.39, Diffuse large B-cell lymphoma, extranodal and solid organ sites.

3. **Chapter 3: Disease of the blood and blood-forming organs and certain disorders involving the immune mechanism (D5Ø-D89)**
Reserved for future guideline expansion

4. **Chapter 4: Endocrine, Nutritional, and Metabolic Diseases (EØØ-E89)**

a. **Diabetes mellitus**
The diabetes mellitus codes are combination codes that include the type of diabetes mellitus, the body system affected, and the complications affecting that body system. As many codes within a particular category as are necessary to describe all of the complications of the disease may be used. They should be sequenced based on the reason for a particular encounter. Assign as many codes from categories EØ8 – E13 as needed to identify all of the associated conditions that the patient has.

1) **Type of diabetes**
The age of a patient is not the sole determining factor, though most type 1 diabetics develop the condition before reaching puberty. For this reason, type 1 diabetes mellitus is also referred to as juvenile diabetes.

2) **Type of diabetes mellitus not documented**
If the type of diabetes mellitus is not documented in the medical record the default is E11.-, Type 2 diabetes mellitus.

3) **Diabetes mellitus and the use of insulin, oral hypoglycemics, and injectable non-insulin drugs**
If the documentation in a medical record does not indicate the type of diabetes but does indicate that the patient uses insulin, code E11-, Type 2 diabetes mellitus, should be assigned. Additional code(s) should be assigned from category Z79 to identify the long-term (current) use of insulin, oral hypoglycemic drugs, or injectable non-insulin antidiabetic, as follows:
If the patient is treated with both oral hypoglycemic drugs and insulin, both code Z79.4, Long term (current) use of insulin, and code Z79.84, Long term (current) use of oral hypoglycemic drugs, should be assigned.
If the patient is treated with both insulin and an injectable non-insulin antidiabetic drug, assign codes Z79.4, Long term (current) use of insulin, and Z79.85, Long-term (current) use of injectable non-insulin antidiabetic drugs.
If the patient is treated with both oral hypoglycemic drugs and an injectable non-insulin antidiabetic drug, assign codes Z79.84, Long term (current) use of oral hypoglycemic drugs, and Z79.85, Long-term (current) use of injectable non-insulin antidiabetic drugs.
Code Z79.4 should not be assigned if insulin is given temporarily to bring a type 2 patient's blood sugar under control during an encounter.

4) **Diabetes mellitus in pregnancy and gestational diabetes**
See Section I.C.15. Diabetes mellitus in pregnancy.
See Section I.C.15. Gestational (pregnancy induced) diabetes

5) **Complications due to insulin pump malfunction**

(a) **Underdose of insulin due to insulin pump failure**
An underdose of insulin due to an insulin pump failure should be assigned to a code from subcategory T85.6, Mechanical complication of other specified internal and external prosthetic devices, implants and grafts, that specifies the type of pump malfunction, as the principal or first-listed code, followed by code T38.3X6-, Underdosing of insulin and oral hypoglycemic [antidiabetic] drugs. Additional codes for the type of diabetes mellitus and any associated complications due to the underdosing should also be assigned.

(b) **Overdose of insulin due to insulin pump failure**
The principal or first-listed code for an encounter due to an insulin pump malfunction resulting in an overdose of insulin, should also be T85.6-, Mechanical complication of other specified internal and external prosthetic devices, implants and grafts, followed by code T38.3X1-, Poisoning by insulin and oral hypoglycemic [antidiabetic] drugs, accidental (unintentional).

6) **Secondary diabetes mellitus**
Codes under categories EØ8, Diabetes mellitus due to underlying condition, EØ9, Drug or chemical induced diabetes mellitus, and E13, Other specified diabetes mellitus, identify complications/manifestations associated with secondary diabetes

mellitus. Secondary diabetes is always caused by another condition or event (e.g., cystic fibrosis, malignant neoplasm of pancreas, pancreatectomy, adverse effect of drug, or poisoning).

(a) Secondary diabetes mellitus and the use of insulin, oral hypoglycemic drugs, or injectable non-insulin drugs

For patients with secondary diabetes mellitus who routinely use insulin, oral hypoglycemic drugs, or injectable non-insulin drugs, additional code(s) from category Z79 should be assigned to identify the long-term (current) use of insulin, oral hypoglycemic drugs, or non-injectable non-insulin drugs as follows:

If the patient is treated with both oral hypoglycemic drugs and insulin, both code Z79.4, Long term (current) use of insulin, and code Z79.84, Long term (current) use of oral hypoglycemic drugs, should be assigned.

If the patient is treated with both insulin and an injectable non-insulin antidiabetic drug, assign codes Z79.4, Long-term (current) use of insulin, and Z79.85, Long-term (current) use of injectable non-insulin antidiabetic drugs.

If the patient is treated with both oral hypoglycemic drugs and an injectable non-insulin antidiabetic drug, assign codes Z79.84, Long-term (current) use of oral hypoglycemic drugs, and Z79.85, Long-term (current) use of injectable non-insulin antidiabetic drugs.

Code Z79.4 should not be assigned if insulin is given temporarily to bring a secondary diabetic patient's blood sugar under control during an encounter.

(b) Assigning and sequencing secondary diabetes codes and its causes

The sequencing of the secondary diabetes codes in relationship to codes for the cause of the diabetes is based on the Tabular List instructions for categories EØ8, EØ9 and E13.

(i) Secondary diabetes mellitus due to pancreatectomy

For postpancreatectomy diabetes mellitus (lack of insulin due to the surgical removal of all or part of the pancreas), assign code E89.1, Postprocedural hypoinsulinemia.

Assign a code from category E13 and a code from subcategory Z9Ø.41, Acquired absence of pancreas, as additional codes.

(ii) Secondary diabetes due to drugs

Secondary diabetes may be caused by an adverse effect of correctly administered medications, poisoning or sequela of poisoning.

See section I.C.19.e. for coding of adverse effects and poisoning, and section I.C.20 for external cause code reporting.

5. Chapter 5: Mental, Behavioral and Neurodevelopmental disorders (FØ1-F99)

a. Pain disorders related to psychological factors

Assign code F45.41, for pain that is exclusively related to psychological disorders. As indicated by the Excludes 1 note under category G89, a code from category G89 should not be assigned with code F45.41.

Code F45.42, Pain disorders with related psychological factors, should be used with a code from category G89, Pain, not elsewhere classified, if there is documentation of a psychological component for a patient with acute or chronic pain.

See Section I.C.6. Pain

b. Mental and behavioral disorders due to psychoactive substance use

1) In Remission

Selection of codes describing "in remission" for categories F1Ø-F19, Mental and behavioral disorders due to psychoactive substance use (categories F1Ø-F19 with -.11, -.21, -.91) requires the provider's clinical judgment and are assigned only on the basis of provider documentation (as defined in the Official Guidelines for Coding and Reporting), unless otherwise instructed by the classification.

Mild substance use disorders in early or sustained remission are classified to the appropriate codes for substance abuse in remission, and moderate or severe substance use disorders in early or sustained remission are classified to the appropriate codes for substance dependence in remission.

2) Psychoactive Substance Use, Abuse and Dependence

When the provider documentation refers to use, abuse and dependence of the same substance (e.g. alcohol, opioid, cannabis, etc.), only one code should be assigned to identify the pattern of use based on the following hierarchy:

- If both use and abuse are documented, assign only the code for abuse
- If both abuse and dependence are documented, assign only the code for dependence
- If use, abuse and dependence are all documented, assign only the code for dependence
- If both use and dependence are documented, assign only the code for dependence.

3) Psychoactive Substance Use, Unspecified

As with all other unspecified diagnoses, the codes for unspecified psychoactive substance use (F1Ø.9-, F11.9-, F12.9-, F13.9-, F14.9-, F15.9-, F16.9-, F18.9-, F19.9-) should only be assigned based on provider documentation and when they meet the definition of a reportable diagnosis (see Section III, Reporting Additional Diagnoses). These codes are to be used only when the psychoactive substance use is associated with a substance related disorder (chapter 5 disorders such as sexual dysfunction, sleep disorder, or a mental or behavioral disorder) or medical condition, and such a relationship is documented by the provider.

4) Medical Conditions Due to Psychoactive Substance Use, Abuse and Dependence

Medical conditions due to substance use, abuse, and dependence are not classified as substance-induced disorders. Assign the diagnosis code for the medical condition as directed by the Alphabetical Index along with the appropriate psychoactive substance use, abuse or dependence code. For example, for alcoholic pancreatitis due to alcohol dependence, assign the appropriate code from subcategory K85.2, Alcohol induced acute pancreatitis, and the appropriate code from subcategory F1Ø.2, such as code F1Ø.2Ø, Alcohol dependence, uncomplicated. It would not be appropriate to assign code F1Ø.288, Alcohol dependence with other alcohol-induced disorder.

5) Blood Alcohol Level

A code from category Y9Ø, Evidence of alcohol involvement determined by blood alcohol level, may be assigned when this information is documented and the patient's provider has documented a condition classifiable to category F1Ø, Alcohol related disorders. The blood alcohol level does not need to be documented by the patient's provider in order for it to be coded.

See Section I.B.14. for blood alcohol level documentation by clinicians other than patient's provider.

c. Factitious Disorder

Factitious disorder imposed on self or Munchausen's syndrome is a disorder in which a person falsely reports or causes his or her own physical or psychological signs or symptoms. For patients with documented factitious disorder on self or Munchausen's syndrome, assign the appropriate code from subcategory F68.1-, Factitious disorder imposed on self.

Munchausen's syndrome by proxy (MSBP) is a disorder in which a caregiver (perpetrator) falsely reports or causes an illness or injury in another person (victim) under his or her care, such as a child, an elderly adult, or a person who has a disability. The condition is also referred to as "factitious disorder imposed on another" or "factitious disorder by proxy." The perpetrator, not the victim, receives this diagnosis. Assign code F68.A, Factitious disorder imposed on another, to the perpetrator's record. For the victim of a patient suffering from MSBP, assign the appropriate code from categories T74, Adult and child abuse, neglect and other maltreatment, confirmed, or T76, Adult and child abuse, neglect and other maltreatment, suspected.

See Section I.C.19.f. Adult and child abuse, neglect and other maltreatment

d. Dementia

The ICD-10-CM classifies dementia (categories FØ1, FØ2, and FØ3) on the basis of the etiology and severity (unspecified, mild, moderate or severe). Selection of the appropriate severity level requires the provider's clinical judgment and codes should be assigned only on the basis of provider documentation (as defined in the *Official Guidelines for Coding and Reporting*), unless otherwise instructed by the classification. If the documentation does not provide information about the severity of the dementia, assign the appropriate code for unspecified severity.

If a patient is admitted to an inpatient acute care hospital or other inpatient facility setting with dementia at one severity level and it progresses to a higher severity level, assign one code for the highest severity level reported during the stay.

6. Chapter 6: Diseases of the Nervous System (GØØ-G99)

a. Dominant/nondominant side

Codes from category G81, Hemiplegia and hemiparesis, and subcategories G83.1, Monoplegia of lower limb, G83.2, Monoplegia of upper limb, and G83.3, Monoplegia, unspecified, identify whether the dominant or nondominant side is affected. Should the affected side be documented, but not specified as dominant or nondominant, and the classification system does not indicate a default, code selection is as follows:

- For ambidextrous patients, the default should be dominant.
- If the left side is affected, the default is non-dominant.
- If the right side is affected, the default is dominant.

b. Pain - Category G89

1) General coding information

Codes in category G89, Pain, not elsewhere classified, may be used in conjunction with codes from other categories and chapters to provide more detail about acute or chronic pain and neoplasm-related pain, unless otherwise indicated below.

If the pain is not specified as acute or chronic, post-thoracotomy, postprocedural, or neoplasm-related, do not assign codes from category G89.

A code from category G89 should not be assigned if the underlying (definitive) diagnosis is known, unless the reason for the encounter is pain control/ management and not management of the underlying condition.

When an admission or encounter is for a procedure aimed at treating the underlying condition (e.g., spinal fusion, kyphoplasty), a code for the underlying condition (e.g., vertebral fracture, spinal stenosis) should be assigned as the principal diagnosis. No code from category G89 should be assigned.

(a) Category G89 Codes as Principal or First-Listed Diagnosis

Category G89 codes are acceptable as principal diagnosis or the first-listed code:

- When pain control or pain management is the reason for the admission/encounter (e.g., a patient with displaced intervertebral disc, nerve impingement and severe back pain presents for injection of steroid into the spinal canal). The underlying cause of the pain should be reported as an additional diagnosis, if known.
- When a patient is admitted for the insertion of a neurostimulator for pain control, assign the appropriate pain code as the principal or first-listed diagnosis. When an admission or encounter is for a procedure aimed at treating the underlying condition and a neurostimulator is inserted for pain control during the same admission/encounter, a code for the underlying condition should be assigned as the principal diagnosis and the appropriate pain code should be assigned as a secondary diagnosis.

(b) Use of Category G89 Codes in Conjunction with Site Specific Pain Codes

(i) Assigning Category G89 and Site-Specific Pain Codes

Codes from category G89 may be used in conjunction with codes that identify the site of pain (including codes from chapter 18) if the category G89 code provides additional information. For example, if the code describes the site of the pain, but does not fully describe whether the pain is acute or chronic, then both codes should be assigned.

(ii) Sequencing of Category G89 Codes with Site-Specific Pain Codes

The sequencing of category G89 codes with site-specific pain codes (including chapter 18 codes), is dependent on the circumstances of the encounter/admission as follows:

- If the encounter is for pain control or pain management, assign the code from category G89 followed by the code identifying the specific site of pain (e.g., encounter for pain management for acute neck pain from trauma is assigned code G89.11, Acute pain due to trauma, followed by code M54.2, Cervicalgia, to identify the site of pain).
- If the encounter is for any other reason except pain control or pain management, and a related definitive diagnosis has not been established (confirmed) by the provider, assign the code for the specific site of pain first, followed by the appropriate code from category G89.

2) Pain due to devices, implants and grafts

See Section I.C.19. Pain due to medical devices

3) Postoperative Pain

The provider's documentation should be used to guide the coding of postoperative pain, as well as *Section III. Reporting Additional Diagnoses* and *Section IV. Diagnostic Coding and Reporting in the Outpatient Setting.*

The default for post-thoracotomy and other postoperative pain not specified as acute or chronic is the code for the acute form.

Routine or expected postoperative pain immediately after surgery should not be coded.

(a) Postoperative pain not associated with specific postoperative complication

Postoperative pain not associated with a specific postoperative complication is assigned to the appropriate postoperative pain code in category G89.

(b) Postoperative pain associated with specific postoperative complication

Postoperative pain associated with a specific postoperative complication (such as painful wire sutures) is assigned to the appropriate code(s) found in Chapter 19, Injury, poisoning, and certain other consequences of external causes. If appropriate, use additional code(s) from category G89 to identify acute or chronic pain (G89.18 or G89.28).

4) Chronic pain

Chronic pain is classified to subcategory G89.2. There is no time frame defining when pain becomes chronic pain. The provider's documentation should be used to guide use of these codes.

5) Neoplasm Related Pain

Code G89.3 is assigned to pain documented as being related, associated or due to cancer, primary or secondary malignancy, or tumor. This code is assigned regardless of whether the pain is acute or chronic.

This code may be assigned as the principal or first-listed code when the stated reason for the admission/encounter is documented as pain control/pain management. The underlying neoplasm should be reported as an additional diagnosis.

When the reason for the admission/encounter is management of the neoplasm and the pain associated with the neoplasm is also documented, code G89.3 may be assigned as an additional diagnosis. It is not necessary to assign an additional code for the site of the pain.

See Section I.C.2. for instructions on the sequencing of neoplasms for all other stated reasons for the admission/encounter (except for pain control/pain management).

6) Chronic pain syndrome

Central pain syndrome (G89.Ø) and chronic pain syndrome (G89.4) are different than the term "chronic pain," and therefore codes should only be used when the provider has specifically documented this condition.

See Section I.C.5. Pain disorders related to psychological factors

7. Chapter 7: Diseases of the Eye and Adnexa (HØØ-H59)

a. Glaucoma

1) Assigning Glaucoma Codes

Assign as many codes from category H4Ø, Glaucoma, as needed to identify the type of glaucoma, the affected eye, and the glaucoma stage.

2) Bilateral glaucoma with same type and stage

When a patient has bilateral glaucoma and both eyes are documented as being the same type and stage, and there is a code for bilateral glaucoma, report only the code for the type of glaucoma, bilateral, with the seventh character for the stage.

When a patient has bilateral glaucoma and both eyes are documented as being the same type and stage, and the classification does not provide a code for bilateral glaucoma (i.e. subcategories H4Ø.1Ø, and H4Ø.2Ø) report only one code for the type of glaucoma with the appropriate seventh character for the stage.

3) Bilateral glaucoma stage with different types or stages

When a patient has bilateral glaucoma and each eye is documented as having a different type or stage, and the classification distinguishes laterality, assign the appropriate code for each eye rather than the code for bilateral glaucoma.

When a patient has bilateral glaucoma and each eye is documented as having a different type, and the classification does not distinguish laterality (i.e., subcategories H4Ø.1Ø, and H4Ø.2Ø), assign one code for each type of glaucoma with the appropriate seventh character for the stage.

When a patient has bilateral glaucoma and each eye is documented as having the same type, but different stage, and the classification does not distinguish laterality (i.e., subcategories H4Ø.1Ø and H4Ø.2Ø), assign a code for the type of glaucoma for each eye with the seventh character for the specific glaucoma stage documented for each eye.

4) **Patient admitted with glaucoma and stage evolves during the admission**
If a patient is admitted with glaucoma and the stage progresses during the admission, assign the code for highest stage documented.

5) **Indeterminate stage glaucoma**
Assignment of the seventh character "4" for "indeterminate stage" should be based on the clinical documentation. The seventh character "4" is used for glaucomas whose stage cannot be clinically determined. This seventh character should not be confused with the seventh character "Ø", unspecified, which should be assigned when there is no documentation regarding the stage of the glaucoma.

b. **Blindness**
If "blindness" or "low vision" of both eyes is documented but the visual impairment category is not documented, assign code H54.3, Unqualified visual loss, both eyes. If "blindness" or "low vision" in one eye is documented but the visual impairment category is not documented, assign a code from H54.6-, Unqualified visual loss, one eye. If "blindness" or "visual loss" is documented without any information about whether one or both eyes are affected, assign code H54.7, Unspecified visual loss.

8. **Chapter 8: Diseases of the Ear and Mastoid Process (H6Ø-H95)**
Reserved for future guideline expansion

9. **Chapter 9: Diseases of the Circulatory System (IØØ-I99)**

a. **Hypertension**
The classification presumes a causal relationship between hypertension and heart involvement and between hypertension and kidney involvement, as the two conditions are linked by the term "with" in the Alphabetic Index. These conditions should be coded as related even in the absence of provider documentation explicitly linking them, unless the documentation clearly states the conditions are unrelated.

For hypertension and conditions not specifically linked by relational terms such as "with," "associated with" or "due to" in the classification, provider documentation must link the conditions in order to code them as related.

1) **Hypertension with Heart Disease**
Hypertension with heart conditions classified to I5Ø.- or I51.4- I51.7, I51.89, I51.9, are assigned to a code from category I11, Hypertensive heart disease. Use additional code(s) from category I5Ø, Heart failure, to identify the type(s) of heart failure in those patients with heart failure.

The same heart conditions (I5Ø.-, I51.4-I51.7, I51.89, I51.9) with hypertension are coded separately if the provider has documented they are unrelated to the hypertension. Sequence according to the circumstances of the admission/encounter.

2) **Hypertensive Chronic Kidney Disease**
Assign codes from category I12, Hypertensive chronic kidney disease, when both hypertension and a condition classifiable to category N18, Chronic kidney disease (CKD), are present. CKD should not be coded as hypertensive if the provider indicates the CKD is not related to the hypertension.

The appropriate code from category N18 should be used as a secondary code with a code from category I12 to identify the stage of chronic kidney disease.

See Section I.C.14. Chronic kidney disease.

If a patient has hypertensive chronic kidney disease and acute renal failure, the acute renal failure should also be coded. Sequence according to the circumstances of the admission/encounter.

3) **Hypertensive Heart and Chronic Kidney Disease**
Assign codes from combination category I13, Hypertensive heart and chronic kidney disease, when there is hypertension with both heart and kidney involvement. If heart failure is present, assign an additional code from category I5Ø to identify the type of heart failure.

The appropriate code from category N18, Chronic kidney disease, should be used as a secondary code with a code from category I13 to identify the stage of chronic kidney disease.

See Section I.C.14. Chronic kidney disease.

The codes in category I13, Hypertensive heart and chronic kidney disease, are combination codes that include hypertension, heart disease and chronic kidney disease. The Includes note at I13 specifies that the conditions included at I11 and I12 are included together in I13. If a patient has hypertension, heart disease and chronic kidney disease, then a code from I13 should be used, not individual codes for hypertension, heart disease and chronic kidney disease, or codes from I11 or I12.

For patients with both acute renal failure and chronic kidney disease, the acute renal failure should also be coded. Sequence according to the circumstances of the admission/encounter.

4) **Hypertensive Cerebrovascular Disease**
For hypertensive cerebrovascular disease, first assign the appropriate code from categories I6Ø-I69, followed by the appropriate hypertension code.

5) **Hypertensive Retinopathy**
Subcategory H35.Ø, Background retinopathy and retinal vascular changes, should be used along with a code from categories I1Ø-I15, in the Hypertensive diseases section, to include the systemic hypertension. The sequencing is based on the reason for the encounter.

6) **Hypertension, Secondary**
Secondary hypertension is due to an underlying condition. Two codes are required: one to identify the underlying etiology and one from category I15 to identify the hypertension. Sequencing of codes is determined by the reason for admission/encounter.

7) **Hypertension, Transient**
Assign code RØ3.Ø, Elevated blood pressure reading without diagnosis of hypertension, unless patient has an established diagnosis of hypertension. Assign code O13.-, Gestational [pregnancy-induced] hypertension without significant proteinuria, or O14.-, Pre-eclampsia, for transient hypertension of pregnancy.

8) **Hypertension, Controlled**
This diagnostic statement usually refers to an existing state of hypertension under control by therapy. Assign the appropriate code from categories I1Ø-I15, Hypertensive diseases.

9) **Hypertension, Uncontrolled**
Uncontrolled hypertension may refer to untreated hypertension or hypertension not responding to current therapeutic regimen. In either case, assign the appropriate code from categories I1Ø-I15, Hypertensive diseases.

10) **Hypertensive Crisis**
Assign a code from category I16, Hypertensive crisis, for documented hypertensive urgency, hypertensive emergency or unspecified hypertensive crisis. Code also any identified hypertensive disease (I1Ø-I15). The sequencing is based on the reason for the encounter.

11) **Pulmonary Hypertension**
Pulmonary hypertension is classified to category I27, Other pulmonary heart diseases. For secondary pulmonary hypertension (I27.1, I27.2-), code also any associated conditions or adverse effects of drugs or toxins. The sequencing is based on the reason for the encounter, except for adverse effects of drugs (See Section I.C.19.e.).

*12) **Hypertension, Resistant***
Resistant hypertension refers to blood pressure of a patient with hypertension that remains above goal in spite of the use of antihypertensive medications. Assign code I1A.Ø, Resistant hypertension, as an additional code when apparent treatment resistant hypertension, treatment resistant hypertension, or true resistant hypertension is documented by the provider. A code for the specific type of existing hypertension is sequenced first, if known.

b. **Atherosclerotic Coronary Artery Disease and Angina**
ICD-10-CM has combination codes for atherosclerotic heart disease with angina pectoris. The subcategories for these codes are I25.11, Atherosclerotic heart disease of native coronary artery with angina pectoris and I25.7, Atherosclerosis of coronary artery bypass graft(s) and coronary artery of transplanted heart with angina pectoris.

When using one of these combination codes it is not necessary to use an additional code for angina pectoris. A causal relationship can be assumed in a patient with both atherosclerosis and angina pectoris, unless the documentation indicates the angina is due to something other than the atherosclerosis.

If a patient with coronary artery disease is admitted due to an acute myocardial infarction (AMI), the AMI should be sequenced before the coronary artery disease.

See Section I.C.9. Acute myocardial infarction (AMI)

c. **Intraoperative and Postprocedural Cerebrovascular Accident**
Medical record documentation should clearly specify the cause-and-effect relationship between the medical intervention and the cerebrovascular accident in order to assign a code for intraoperative or postprocedural cerebrovascular accident.

Proper code assignment depends on whether it was an infarction or hemorrhage and whether it occurred intraoperatively or postoperatively. If it was a cerebral hemorrhage, code assignment depends on the type of procedure performed.

d. **Sequelae of Cerebrovascular Disease**

1) **Category I69, Sequelae of Cerebrovascular disease**

Category I69 is used to indicate conditions classifiable to categories I60-I67 as the causes of sequela (neurologic deficits), themselves classified elsewhere. These "late effects" include neurologic deficits that persist after initial onset of conditions classifiable to categories I60-I67. The neurologic deficits caused by cerebrovascular disease may be present from the onset or may arise at any time after the onset of the condition classifiable to categories I60-I67.

Codes from category I69, Sequelae of cerebrovascular disease, that specify hemiplegia, hemiparesis and monoplegia identify whether the dominant or nondominant side is affected. Should the affected side be documented, but not specified as dominant or nondominant, and the classification system does not indicate a default, code selection is as follows:

- For ambidextrous patients, the default should be dominant.
- If the left side is affected, the default is non-dominant.
- If the right side is affected, the default is dominant.

2) **Codes from category I69 with codes from I60-I67**

Codes from category I69 may be assigned on a health care record with codes from I60-I67, if the patient has a current cerebrovascular disease and deficits from an old cerebrovascular disease.

3) **Codes from category I69 and Personal history of transient ischemic attack (TIA) and cerebral infarction (Z86.73)**

Codes from category I69 should not be assigned if the patient does not have neurologic deficits.

See Section I.C.21.4. History (of) for use of personal history codes

e. **Acute myocardial infarction (AMI)**

1) **Type 1 ST elevation myocardial infarction (STEMI) and non-ST elevation myocardial infarction (NSTEMI)**

The ICD-10-CM codes for type 1 acute myocardial infarction (AMI) identify the site, such as anterolateral wall or true posterior wall. Subcategories I21.0-I21.2 and code I21.3 are used for type 1 ST elevation myocardial infarction (STEMI). Code I21.4, Non-ST elevation (NSTEMI) myocardial infarction, is used for type 1 non-ST elevation myocardial infarction (NSTEMI) and nontransmural MIs.

If a type 1 NSTEMI evolves to STEMI, assign the STEMI code. If a type 1 STEMI converts to NSTEMI due to thrombolytic therapy, it is still coded as STEMI.

For encounters occurring while the myocardial infarction is equal to, or less than, four weeks old, including transfers to another acute setting or a postacute setting, and the myocardial infarction meets the definition for "other diagnoses" (see Section III, Reporting Additional Diagnoses), codes from category I21 may continue to be reported. For encounters after the 4-week time frame and the patient is still receiving care related to the myocardial infarction, the appropriate aftercare code should be assigned, rather than a code from category I21. For old or healed myocardial infarctions not requiring further care, code I25.2, Old myocardial infarction, may be assigned.

2) **Acute myocardial infarction, unspecified**

Code I21.9, Acute myocardial infarction, unspecified, is the default for unspecified acute myocardial infarction or unspecified type. If only type 1 STEMI or transmural MI without the site is documented, assign code I21.3, ST elevation (STEMI) myocardial infarction of unspecified site.

3) **AMI documented as nontransmural or subendocardial but site provided**

If an AMI is documented as nontransmural or subendocardial, but the site is provided, it is still coded as a subendocardial AMI.

See Section I.C.21.3. for information on coding status post administration of tPA in a different facility within the last 24 hours.

4) **Subsequent acute myocardial infarction**

A code from category I22, Subsequent ST elevation (STEMI) and non-ST elevation (NSTEMI) myocardial infarction, is to be used when a patient who has suffered a type 1 or unspecified AMI has a new AMI within the 4 week time frame of the initial AMI. A code from category I22 must be used in conjunction with a code from category I21. The sequencing of the I22 and I21 codes depends on the circumstances of the encounter.

Do not assign code I22 for subsequent myocardial infarctions other than type 1 or unspecified. For subsequent type 2 AMI assign only code I21.A1. For subsequent type 4 or type 5 AMI, assign only code I21.A9.

If a subsequent myocardial infarction of one type occurs within 4 weeks of a myocardial infarction of a different type, assign the appropriate codes from category I21 to identify each type. Do not assign a code from I22. Codes from category I22 should only be assigned if both the initial and subsequent myocardial infarctions are type 1 or unspecified.

5) **Other Types of Myocardial Infarction**

The ICD-10-CM provides codes for different types of myocardial infarction. Type 1 myocardial infarctions are assigned to codes I21.0-I21.4.

Type 2 myocardial infarction (myocardial infarction due to demand ischemia or secondary to ischemic imbalance) is assigned to code I21.A1, Myocardial infarction type 2 with the underlying cause coded first. Do not assign code I24.8, Other forms of acute ischemic heart disease, for the demand ischemia. If a type 2 AMI is described as NSTEMI or STEMI, only assign code I21.A1. Codes I21.01-I21.4 should only be assigned for type 1 AMIs.

Acute myocardial infarctions type 3, 4a, 4b, 4c and 5 are assigned to code I21.A9, Other myocardial infarction type.

The "Code also" and "Code first" notes should be followed related to complications, and for coding of postprocedural myocardial infarctions during or following cardiac surgery.

6) ***Myocardial Infarction with Coronary Microvascular Dysfunction***

Coronary microvascular dysfunction (CMD) is a condition that impacts the microvasculature by restricting microvascular flow and increasing microvascular resistance. Code I21.B, Myocardial infarction with coronary microvascular dysfunction, is assigned for myocardial infarction with coronary microvascular disease, myocardial infarction with coronary microvascular dysfunction, and myocardial infarction with non-obstructive coronary arteries (MINOCA) with microvascular disease.

10. **Chapter 10: Diseases of the Respiratory System (J00-J99), U07.0**

a. **Chronic Obstructive Pulmonary Disease [COPD] and Asthma**

1) **Acute exacerbation of chronic obstructive bronchitis and asthma**

The codes in categories J44 and J45 distinguish between uncomplicated cases and those in acute exacerbation. An acute exacerbation is a worsening or a decompensation of a chronic condition. An acute exacerbation is not equivalent to an infection superimposed on a chronic condition, though an exacerbation may be triggered by an infection.

b. **Acute Respiratory Failure**

1) **Acute respiratory failure as principal diagnosis**

A code from subcategory J96.0, Acute respiratory failure, or subcategory J96.2, Acute and chronic respiratory failure, may be assigned as a principal diagnosis when it is the condition established after study to be chiefly responsible for occasioning the admission to the hospital, and the selection is supported by the Alphabetic Index and Tabular List. However, chapter-specific coding guidelines (such as obstetrics, poisoning, HIV, newborn) that provide sequencing direction take precedence.

2) **Acute respiratory failure as secondary diagnosis**

Respiratory failure may be listed as a secondary diagnosis if it occurs after admission, or if it is present on admission, but does not meet the definition of principal diagnosis.

3) **Sequencing of acute respiratory failure and another acute condition**

When a patient is admitted with respiratory failure and another acute condition, (e.g., myocardial infarction, cerebrovascular accident, aspiration pneumonia), the principal diagnosis will not be the same in every situation. This applies whether the other acute condition is a respiratory or nonrespiratory condition. Selection of the principal diagnosis will be dependent on the circumstances of admission. If both the respiratory failure and the other acute condition are equally responsible for occasioning the admission to the hospital, and there are no chapter-specific sequencing rules, the guideline regarding two or more diagnoses that equally meet the definition for principal diagnosis (Section II, C.) may be applied in these situations.

If the documentation is not clear as to whether acute respiratory failure and another condition are equally responsible for occasioning the admission, query the provider for clarification.

c. **Influenza due to certain identified influenza viruses**

Code only confirmed cases of influenza due to certain identified influenza viruses (category J09), and due to other identified influenza virus (category J10). This is an exception to the hospital inpatient guideline Section II, H. (Uncertain Diagnosis).

In this context, "confirmation" does not require documentation of positive laboratory testing specific for avian or other novel influenza A or other identified influenza virus. However, coding should be based on the provider's diagnostic statement that the patient has avian influenza, or other novel influenza A, for category J09, or has another particular identified strain of influenza, such as H1N1 or H3N2, but not identified as novel or variant, for category J1Ø.

If the provider records "suspected" or "possible" or "probable" avian influenza, or novel influenza, or other identified influenza, then the appropriate influenza code from category J11, Influenza due to unidentified influenza virus, should be assigned. A code from category JØ9, Influenza due to certain identified influenza viruses, should not be assigned nor should a code from category J1Ø, Influenza due to other identified influenza virus.

d. Ventilator associated Pneumonia

1) Documentation of Ventilator associated Pneumonia

As with all procedural or postprocedural complications, code assignment is based on the provider's documentation of the relationship between the condition and the procedure.

Code J95.851, Ventilator associated pneumonia, should be assigned only when the provider has documented ventilator associated pneumonia (VAP). An additional code to identify the organism (e.g., Pseudomonas aeruginosa, code B96.5) should also be assigned. Do not assign an additional code from categories J12-J18 to identify the type of pneumonia.

Code J95.851 should not be assigned for cases where the patient has pneumonia and is on a mechanical ventilator and the provider has not specifically stated that the pneumonia is ventilator-associated pneumonia. If the documentation is unclear as to whether the patient has a pneumonia that is a complication attributable to the mechanical ventilator, query the provider.

2) Ventilator associated Pneumonia Develops after Admission

A patient may be admitted with one type of pneumonia (e.g., code J13, Pneumonia due to Streptococcus pneumonia) and subsequently develop VAP. In this instance, the principal diagnosis would be the appropriate code from categories J12-J18 for the pneumonia diagnosed at the time of admission. Code J95.851, Ventilator associated pneumonia, would be assigned as an additional diagnosis when the provider has also documented the presence of ventilator associated pneumonia.

e. Vaping-related disorders

For patients presenting with condition(s) related to vaping, assign code UØ7.Ø, Vaping-related disorder, as the principal diagnosis. For lung injury due to vaping, assign only code UØ7.Ø. Assign additional codes for other manifestations, such as acute respiratory failure (subcategory J96.Ø-) or pneumonitis (code J68.Ø).

Associated respiratory signs and symptoms due to vaping, such as cough, shortness of breath, etc., are not coded separately, when a definitive diagnosis has been established. However, it would be appropriate to code separately any gastrointestinal symptoms, such as diarrhea and abdominal pain.

See Section I.C.1.g.1.c.i. for Pneumonia confirmed as due to COVID-19

11. Chapter 11: Diseases of the Digestive System (KØØ-K95)

Reserved for future guideline expansion

12. Chapter 12: Diseases of the Skin and Subcutaneous Tissue (LØØ-L99)

a. Pressure ulcer stage codes

1) Pressure ulcer stages

Codes in category L89, Pressure ulcer, identify the site and stage of the pressure ulcer.

The ICD-10-CM classifies pressure ulcer stages based on severity, which is designated by stages 1-4, deep tissue pressure injury, unspecified stage, and unstageable.

Assign as many codes from category L89 as needed to identify all the pressure ulcers the patient has, if applicable.

See Section I.B.14. for pressure ulcer stage documentation by clinicians other than patient's provider.

2) Unstageable pressure ulcers

Assignment of the code for unstageable pressure ulcer (L89.--Ø) should be based on the clinical documentation. These codes are used for pressure ulcers whose stage cannot be clinically determined (e.g., the ulcer is covered by eschar or has been treated with a skin or muscle graft). This code should not be confused with the codes for unspecified stage (L89.--9). When there is no documentation regarding the stage of the pressure ulcer, assign the appropriate code for unspecified stage (L89.-- 9).

If during an encounter, the stage of an unstageable pressure ulcer is revealed after debridement, assign only the code for the stage revealed following debridement.

3) Documented pressure ulcer stage

Assignment of the pressure ulcer stage code should be guided by clinical documentation of the stage or documentation of the terms found in the Alphabetic Index. For clinical terms describing the stage that are not found in the Alphabetic Index, and there is no documentation of the stage, the provider should be queried.

4) Patients admitted with pressure ulcers documented as healed

No code is assigned if the documentation states that the pressure ulcer is completely healed at the time of admission.

5) Pressure ulcers documented as healing

Pressure ulcers described as healing should be assigned the appropriate pressure ulcer stage code based on the documentation in the medical record. If the documentation does not provide information about the stage of the healing pressure ulcer, assign the appropriate code for unspecified stage.

If the documentation is unclear as to whether the patient has a current (new) pressure ulcer or if the patient is being treated for a healing pressure ulcer, query the provider.

For ulcers that were present on admission but healed at the time of discharge, assign the code for the site and stage of the pressure ulcer at the time of admission.

6) Patient admitted with pressure ulcer evolving into another stage during the admission

If a patient is admitted to an inpatient hospital with a pressure ulcer at one stage and it progresses to a higher stage, two separate codes should be assigned: one code for the site and stage of the ulcer on admission and a second code for the same ulcer site and the highest stage reported during the stay.

7) Pressure-induced deep tissue damage

For pressure-induced deep tissue damage or deep tissue pressure injury, assign only the appropriate code for pressure-induced deep tissue damage (L89.--6).

b. Non-Pressure Chronic Ulcers

1) Patients admitted with non-pressure ulcers documented as healed

No code is assigned if the documentation states that the non-pressure ulcer is completely healed at the time of admission.

2) Non-pressure ulcers documented as healing

Non-pressure ulcers described as healing should be assigned the appropriate non-pressure ulcer code based on the documentation in the medical record. If the documentation does not provide information about the severity of the healing non-pressure ulcer, assign the appropriate code for unspecified severity.

If the documentation is unclear as to whether the patient has a current (new) non-pressure ulcer or if the patient is being treated for a healing non-pressure ulcer, query the provider.

For ulcers that were present on admission but healed at the time of discharge, assign the code for the site and severity of the non-pressure ulcer at the time of admission.

3) Patient admitted with non-pressure ulcer that progresses to another severity level during the admission

If a patient is admitted to an inpatient hospital with a non-pressure ulcer at one severity level and it progresses to a higher severity level, two separate codes should be assigned: one code for the site and severity level of the ulcer on admission and a second code for the same ulcer site and the highest severity level reported during the stay.

See Section I.B.14. for pressure ulcer stage documentation by clinicians other than patient's provider

13. Chapter 13: Diseases of the Musculoskeletal System and Connective Tissue (MØØ-M99)

a. Site and laterality

Most of the codes within Chapter 13 have site and laterality designations. The site represents the bone, joint or the muscle involved. For some conditions where more than one bone, joint or muscle is usually involved, such as osteoarthritis, there is a "multiple sites" code available. For categories where no multiple site code is provided and more than one bone, joint or muscle is involved, multiple codes should be used to indicate the different sites involved.

1) Bone versus joint

For certain conditions, the bone may be affected at the upper or lower end, (e.g., avascular necrosis of bone, M87, Osteoporosis, M8Ø, M81). Though the portion of the bone affected may be at the joint, the site designation will be the bone, not the joint.

b. Acute traumatic versus chronic or recurrent musculoskeletal conditions

Many musculoskeletal conditions are a result of previous injury or trauma to a site, or are recurrent conditions. Bone, joint or muscle conditions that are the result of a healed injury are usually found in chapter 13. Recurrent bone, joint or muscle conditions are also usually found in chapter 13. Any current, acute injury should be coded to the appropriate injury code from chapter 19. Chronic or recurrent conditions should generally be coded with a code from chapter 13. If it is difficult to determine from the documentation in the record which code is best to describe a condition, query the provider.

c. Coding of Pathologic Fractures

7th character A is for use as long as the patient is receiving active treatment for the fracture. While the patient may be seen by a new or different provider over the course of treatment for a pathological fracture, assignment of the 7th character is based on whether the patient is undergoing active treatment and not whether the provider is seeing the patient for the first time.

7th character D is to be used for encounters after the patient has completed active treatment for the fracture and is receiving routine care for the fracture during the healing or recovery phase. The other 7th characters, listed under each subcategory in the Tabular List, are to be used for subsequent encounters for treatment of problems associated with the healing, such as malunions, nonunions, and sequelae.

Care for complications of surgical treatment for fracture repairs during the healing or recovery phase should be coded with the appropriate complication codes.

See Section I.C.19. Coding of traumatic fractures.

d. Osteoporosis

Osteoporosis is a systemic condition, meaning that all bones of the musculoskeletal system are affected. Therefore, site is not a component of the codes under category M81, Osteoporosis without current pathological fracture. The site codes under category M8Ø, Osteoporosis with current pathological fracture, identify the site of the fracture, not the osteoporosis.

1) Osteoporosis without pathological fracture

Category M81, Osteoporosis without current pathological fracture, is for use for patients with osteoporosis who do not currently have a pathologic fracture due to the osteoporosis, even if they have had a fracture in the past. For patients with a history of osteoporosis fractures, status code Z87.31Ø, Personal history of (healed) osteoporosis fracture, should follow the code from M81.

2) Osteoporosis with current pathological fracture

Category M8Ø, Osteoporosis with current pathological fracture, is for patients who have a current pathologic fracture at the time of an encounter. The codes under M8Ø identify the site of the fracture. A code from category M8Ø, not a traumatic fracture code, should be used for any patient with known osteoporosis who suffers a fracture, even if the patient had a minor fall or trauma, if that fall or trauma would not usually break a normal, healthy bone.

e. Multisystem Inflammatory Syndrome

See Section I.C.1.g.1.l. for Multisystem Inflammatory Syndrome

14. Chapter 14: Diseases of Genitourinary System (NØØ-N99)

a. Chronic kidney disease

1) Stages of chronic kidney disease (CKD)

The ICD-10-CM classifies CKD based on severity. The severity of CKD is designated by stages 1-5. Stage 2, code N18.2, equates to mild CKD; stage 3, codes N18.3Ø-N18.32, equate to moderate CKD; and stage 4, code N18.4, equates to severe CKD. Code N18.6, End stage renal disease (ESRD), is assigned when the provider has documented end-stage renal disease (ESRD).

If both a stage of CKD and ESRD are documented, assign code N18.6 only.

2) Chronic kidney disease and kidney transplant status

Patients who have undergone kidney transplant may still have some form of chronic kidney disease (CKD) because the kidney transplant may not fully restore kidney function. Therefore, the presence of CKD alone does not constitute a transplant complication. Assign the appropriate N18 code for the patient's stage of CKD and code Z94.Ø, Kidney transplant status. If a transplant complication such as failure or rejection or other transplant complication is documented, see section I.C.19.g for information on coding complications of a kidney transplant. If the documentation is unclear as to whether the patient has a complication of the transplant, query the provider.

3) Chronic kidney disease with other conditions

Patients with CKD may also suffer from other serious conditions, most commonly diabetes mellitus and hypertension. The sequencing of the CKD code in relationship to codes for other contributing conditions is based on the conventions in the Tabular List.

See I.C.9. Hypertensive chronic kidney disease.

See I.C.19. Chronic kidney disease and kidney transplant complications.

15. Chapter 15: Pregnancy, Childbirth, and the Puerperium (OØØ-O9A)

a. General Rules for Obstetric Cases

1) Codes from chapter 15 and sequencing priority

Obstetric cases require codes from chapter 15, codes in the range OØØ-O9A, Pregnancy, Childbirth, and the Puerperium. Chapter 15 codes have sequencing priority over codes from other chapters. Additional codes from other chapters may be used in conjunction with chapter 15 codes to further specify conditions. Should the provider document that the pregnancy is incidental to the encounter, then code Z33.1, Pregnant state, incidental, should be used in place of any chapter 15 codes. It is the provider's responsibility to state that the condition being treated is not affecting the pregnancy.

2) Chapter 15 codes used only on the maternal record

Chapter 15 codes are to be used only on the maternal record, never on the record of the newborn.

3) Final character for trimester

The majority of codes in Chapter 15 have a final character indicating the trimester of pregnancy. The timeframes for the trimesters are indicated at the beginning of the chapter. If trimester is not a component of a code, it is because the condition always occurs in a specific trimester, or the concept of trimester of pregnancy is not applicable. Certain codes have characters for only certain trimesters because the condition does not occur in all trimesters, but it may occur in more than just one.

Assignment of the final character for trimester should be based on the provider's documentation of the trimester (or number of weeks) for the current admission/encounter. This applies to the assignment of trimester for pre-existing conditions as well as those that develop during or are due to the pregnancy. The provider's documentation of the number of weeks may be used to assign the appropriate code identifying the trimester.

Whenever delivery occurs during the current admission, and there is an "in childbirth" option for the obstetric complication being coded, the "in childbirth" code should be assigned. When the classification does not provide an obstetric code with an "in childbirth" option, it is appropriate to assign a code describing the current trimester.

4) Selection of trimester for inpatient admissions that encompass more than one trimester

In instances when a patient is admitted to a hospital for complications of pregnancy during one trimester and remains in the hospital into a subsequent trimester, the trimester character for the antepartum complication code should be assigned on the basis of the trimester when the complication developed, not the trimester of the discharge. If the condition developed prior to the current admission/encounter or represents a pre-existing condition, the trimester character for the trimester at the time of the admission/encounter should be assigned.

5) Unspecified trimester

Each category that includes codes for trimester has a code for "unspecified trimester." The "unspecified trimester" code should rarely be used, such as when the documentation in the record is insufficient to determine the trimester and it is not possible to obtain clarification.

6) 7th character for fetus identification

Where applicable, a 7th character is to be assigned for certain categories (O31, O32, O33.3-O33.6, O35, O36, O4Ø, O41, O6Ø.1, O6Ø.2, O64, and O69) to identify the fetus for which the complication code applies.

Assign 7th character "Ø":

- For single gestations
- When the documentation in the record is insufficient to determine the fetus affected and it is not possible to obtain clarification.
- When it is not possible to clinically determine which fetus is affected.

7) Completed weeks of gestation

In ICD-10-CM, "completed" weeks of gestation refers to full weeks. For example, if the provider documents gestation at 39 weeks and 6 days, the code for 39 weeks of gestation should be assigned, as the patient has not yet reached 40 completed weeks.

b. Selection of OB Principal or First-listed Diagnosis

1) Routine outpatient prenatal visits

For routine outpatient prenatal visits when no complications are present, a code from category Z34, Encounter for supervision of normal pregnancy, should be used as the first-listed diagnosis. These codes should not be used in conjunction with chapter 15 codes.

2) Supervision of High-Risk Pregnancy

Codes from category OØ9, Supervision of high-risk pregnancy, are intended for use only during the prenatal period. For complications during the labor or delivery episode as a result of a high-risk pregnancy, assign the applicable complication codes from Chapter 15. If there are no complications during the labor or delivery episode, assign code O8Ø, Encounter for full-term uncomplicated delivery.

For routine prenatal outpatient visits for patients with high-risk pregnancies, a code from category O09, Supervision of high-risk pregnancy, should be used as the first-listed diagnosis. Secondary chapter 15 codes may be used in conjunction with these codes if appropriate.

3) **Episodes when no delivery occurs**
In episodes when no delivery occurs, the principal diagnosis should correspond to the principal complication of the pregnancy which necessitated the encounter. Should more than one complication exist, all of which are treated or monitored, any of the complication codes may be sequenced first.

4) **When a delivery occurs**
When an obstetric patient is admitted and delivers during that admission, the condition that prompted the admission should be sequenced as the principal diagnosis. If multiple conditions prompted the admission, sequence the one most related to the delivery as the principal diagnosis. A code for any complication of the delivery should be assigned as an additional diagnosis. In cases of cesarean delivery, if the patient was admitted with a condition that resulted in the performance of a cesarean procedure, that condition should be selected as the principal diagnosis. If the reason for the admission was unrelated to the condition resulting in the cesarean delivery, the condition related to the reason for the admission should be selected as the principal diagnosis.

5) **Outcome of delivery**
A code from category Z37, Outcome of delivery, should be included on every maternal record when a delivery has occurred. These codes are not to be used on subsequent records or on the newborn record.

c. **Pre-existing conditions versus conditions due to the pregnancy**
Certain categories in Chapter 15 distinguish between conditions of the mother that existed prior to pregnancy (pre-existing) and those that are a direct result of pregnancy. When assigning codes from Chapter 15, it is important to assess if a condition was pre-existing prior to pregnancy or developed during or due to the pregnancy in order to assign the correct code.

Categories that do not distinguish between pre-existing and pregnancy-related conditions may be used for either. It is acceptable to use codes specifically for the puerperium with codes complicating pregnancy and childbirth if a condition arises postpartum during the delivery encounter.

d. **Pre-existing hypertension in pregnancy**
Category O1Ø, Pre-existing hypertension complicating pregnancy, childbirth and the puerperium, includes codes for hypertensive heart and hypertensive chronic kidney disease. When assigning one of the O1Ø codes that includes hypertensive heart disease or hypertensive chronic kidney disease, it is necessary to add a secondary code from the appropriate hypertension category to specify the type of heart failure or chronic kidney disease.

See Section I.C.9. Hypertension.

e. **Fetal Conditions Affecting the Management of the Mother**

1) **Codes from categories O35 and O36**
Codes from categories O35, Maternal care for known or suspected fetal abnormality and damage, and O36, Maternal care for other fetal problems, are assigned only when the fetal condition is actually responsible for modifying the management of the mother, i.e., by requiring diagnostic studies, additional observation, special care, or termination of pregnancy. The fact that the fetal condition exists does not justify assigning a code from this series to the mother's record.

2) **In utero surgery**
In cases when surgery is performed on the fetus, a diagnosis code from category O35, Maternal care for known or suspected fetal abnormality and damage, should be assigned identifying the fetal condition. Assign the appropriate procedure code for the procedure performed.

No code from Chapter 16, the perinatal codes, should be used on the mother's record to identify fetal conditions. Surgery performed in utero on a fetus is still to be coded as an obstetric encounter.

f. **HIV Infection in Pregnancy, Childbirth and the Puerperium**
During pregnancy, childbirth or the puerperium, a patient admitted because of an HIV-related illness should receive a principal diagnosis from subcategory O98.7-, Human immunodeficiency [HIV] disease complicating pregnancy, childbirth and the puerperium, followed by the code(s) for the HIV-related illness(es).

Patients with asymptomatic HIV infection status admitted during pregnancy, childbirth, or the puerperium should receive codes of O98.7- and Z21, Asymptomatic human immunodeficiency virus [HIV] infection status.

g. **Diabetes mellitus in pregnancy**
Diabetes mellitus is a significant complicating factor in pregnancy. Pregnant patients who are diabetic should be assigned a code from category O24, Diabetes mellitus in pregnancy, childbirth, and the puerperium, first, followed by the appropriate diabetes code(s) (EØ8-E13) from Chapter 4.

h. **Long term use of insulin and oral hypoglycemics**
See section I.C.4.a.3 for information on the long-term use of insulin and oral hypoglycemics.

i. **Gestational (pregnancy induced) diabetes**
Gestational (pregnancy induced) diabetes can occur during the second and third trimester of pregnancy in patients who were not diabetic prior to pregnancy. Gestational diabetes can cause complications in the pregnancy similar to those of pre-existing diabetes mellitus. It also puts the patient at greater risk of developing diabetes after the pregnancy.

Codes for gestational diabetes are in subcategory O24.4, Gestational diabetes mellitus. No other code from category O24, Diabetes mellitus in pregnancy, childbirth, and the puerperium, should be used with a code from O24.4.

The codes under subcategory O24.4 include diet controlled, insulin controlled, and controlled by oral hypoglycemic drugs. If a patient with gestational diabetes is treated with both diet and insulin, only the code for insulin-controlled is required. If a patient with gestational diabetes is treated with both diet and oral hypoglycemic medications, only the code for "controlled by oral hypoglycemic drugs" is required. Codes Z79.4, Long-term (current) use of insulin, Z79.84, Long-term (current) use of oral hypoglycemic drugs, and Z79.85, Long-term (current) use of injectable non-insulin antidiabetic drugs, should not be assigned with codes from subcategory O24.4.

An abnormal glucose tolerance in pregnancy is assigned a code from subcategory O99.81, Abnormal glucose complicating pregnancy, childbirth, and the puerperium.

j. **Sepsis and septic shock complicating abortion, pregnancy, childbirth and the puerperium**
When assigning a chapter 15 code for sepsis complicating abortion, pregnancy, childbirth, and the puerperium, a code for the specific type of infection should be assigned as an additional diagnosis. If severe sepsis is present, a code from subcategory R65.2, Severe sepsis, and code(s) for associated organ dysfunction(s) should also be assigned as additional diagnoses.

k. **Puerperal sepsis**
Code O85, Puerperal sepsis, should be assigned with a secondary code to identify the causal organism (e.g., for a bacterial infection, assign a code from category B95-B96, Bacterial infections in conditions classified elsewhere). A code from category A4Ø, Streptococcal sepsis, or A41, Other sepsis, should not be used for puerperal sepsis. If applicable, use additional codes to identify severe sepsis (R65.2-) and any associated acute organ dysfunction.

Code O85 should not be assigned for sepsis following an obstetrical procedure (See Section I.C.1.d.5.b., Sepsis due to a postprocedural infection).

l. **Alcohol, tobacco and drug use during pregnancy, childbirth and the puerperium**

1) **Alcohol use during pregnancy, childbirth and the puerperium**
Codes under subcategory O99.31, Alcohol use complicating pregnancy, childbirth, and the puerperium, should be assigned for any pregnancy case when a patient uses alcohol during the pregnancy or postpartum. A secondary code from category F1Ø, Alcohol related disorders, should also be assigned to identify manifestations of the alcohol use.

2) **Tobacco use during pregnancy, childbirth and the puerperium**
Codes under subcategory O99.33, Smoking (tobacco) complicating pregnancy, childbirth, and the puerperium, should be assigned for any pregnancy case when a patient uses any type of tobacco product during the pregnancy or postpartum.

A secondary code from category F17, Nicotine dependence, should also be assigned to identify the type of nicotine dependence.

3) **Drug use during pregnancy, childbirth and the puerperium**
Codes under subcategory O99.32, Drug use complicating pregnancy, childbirth, and the puerperium, should be assigned for any pregnancy case when a patient uses drugs during the pregnancy or postpartum. This can involve illegal drugs, or inappropriate use or abuse of prescription drugs. Secondary code(s) from categories F11-F16 and F18-F19 should also be assigned to identify manifestations of the drug use.

m. Poisoning, toxic effects, adverse effects and underdosing in a pregnant patient

A code from subcategory O9A.2, Injury, poisoning and certain other consequences of external causes complicating pregnancy, childbirth, and the puerperium, should be sequenced first, followed by the appropriate injury, poisoning, toxic effect, adverse effect or underdosing code, and then the additional code(s) that specifies the condition caused by the poisoning, toxic effect, adverse effect or underdosing.

See Section I.C.19. Adverse effects, poisoning, underdosing and toxic effects.

n. Normal Delivery, Code O8Ø

1) Encounter for full term uncomplicated delivery

Code O8Ø should be assigned when a patient is admitted for a full-term normal delivery and delivers a single, healthy infant without any complications antepartum, during the delivery, or postpartum during the delivery episode. Code O8Ø is always a principal diagnosis. It is not to be used if any other code from chapter 15 is needed to describe a current complication of the antenatal, delivery, or postnatal period. Additional codes from other chapters may be used with code O8Ø if they are not related to or are in any way complicating the pregnancy.

2) Uncomplicated delivery with resolved antepartum complication

Code O8Ø may be used if the patient had a complication at some point during the pregnancy, but the complication is not present at the time of the admission for delivery.

3) Outcome of delivery for O8Ø

Z37.Ø, Single live birth, is the only outcome of delivery code appropriate for use with O8Ø.

o. The Peripartum and Postpartum Periods

1) Peripartum and Postpartum periods

The postpartum period begins immediately after delivery and continues for six weeks following delivery. The peripartum period is defined as the last month of pregnancy to five months postpartum.

2) Peripartum and postpartum complication

A postpartum complication is any complication occurring within the six-week period.

3) Pregnancy-related complications after 6-week period

Chapter 15 codes may also be used to describe pregnancy-related complications after the peripartum or postpartum period if the provider documents that a condition is pregnancy related.

4) Admission for routine postpartum care following delivery outside hospital

When the mother delivers outside the hospital prior to admission and is admitted for routine postpartum care and no complications are noted, code Z39.Ø, Encounter for care and examination of mother immediately after delivery, should be assigned as the principal diagnosis.

5) Pregnancy associated cardiomyopathy

Pregnancy associated cardiomyopathy, code O9Ø.3, is unique in that it may be diagnosed in the third trimester of pregnancy but may continue to progress months after delivery. For this reason, it is referred to as peripartum cardiomyopathy. Code O9Ø.3 is only for use when the cardiomyopathy develops as a result of pregnancy in a patient who did not have pre-existing heart disease.

p. Code O94, Sequelae of complication of pregnancy, childbirth, and the puerperium

1) Code O94

Code O94, Sequelae of complication of pregnancy, childbirth, and the puerperium, is for use in those cases when an initial complication of a pregnancy develops a sequela or sequelae requiring care or treatment at a future date.

2) After the initial postpartum period

This code may be used at any time after the initial postpartum period.

3) Sequencing of Code O94

This code, like all sequela codes, is to be sequenced following the code describing the sequelae of the complication.

q. Termination of Pregnancy and Spontaneous abortions

1) Abortion with Liveborn Fetus

When an attempted termination of pregnancy results in a liveborn fetus, assign code Z33.2, Encounter for elective termination of pregnancy and a code from category Z37, Outcome of Delivery.

2) Retained Products of Conception following an abortion

Subsequent encounters for retained products of conception following a spontaneous abortion or elective termination of pregnancy, without complications are assigned OØ3.4, Incomplete spontaneous abortion without complication, or code OØ7.4, Failed attempted termination of pregnancy without complication. This advice is appropriate even when the patient was discharged previously with a discharge diagnosis of complete abortion. If the patient has a specific complication associated with the spontaneous abortion or elective termination of pregnancy in addition to retained products of conception, assign the appropriate complication code (e.g., OØ3.-, OØ4.-, OØ7.-) instead of code OØ3.4 or OØ7.4.

3) Complications leading to abortion

Codes from Chapter 15 may be used as additional codes to identify any documented complications of the pregnancy in conjunction with codes in categories in OØ4, OØ7 and OØ8.

4) Hemorrhage following elective abortion

For hemorrhage post elective abortion, assign code OØ4.6, Delayed or excessive hemorrhage following (induced) termination of pregnancy. Do not assign code O72.1, Other immediate postpartum hemorrhage, as this code should not be assigned for post abortion conditions.

r. Abuse in a pregnant patient

For suspected or confirmed cases of abuse of a pregnant patient, a code(s) from subcategories O9A.3, Physical abuse complicating pregnancy, childbirth, and the puerperium, O9A.4, Sexual abuse complicating pregnancy, childbirth, and the puerperium, and O9A.5, Psychological abuse complicating pregnancy, childbirth, and the puerperium, should be sequenced first, followed by the appropriate codes (if applicable) to identify any associated current injury due to physical abuse, sexual abuse, and the perpetrator of abuse.

See Section I.C.19. Adult and child abuse, neglect and other maltreatment.

s. COVID-19 infection in pregnancy, childbirth, and the puerperium

During pregnancy, childbirth or the puerperium, when COVID-19 is the reason for admission/encounter , code O98.5-, Other viral diseases complicating pregnancy, childbirth and the puerperium, should be sequenced as the principal/first-listed diagnosis, and code UØ7.1, COVID-19, and the appropriate codes for associated manifestation(s) should be assigned as additional diagnoses. Codes from Chapter 15 always take sequencing priority.

If the reason for admission/encounter is unrelated to COVID-19 but the patient tests positive for COVID-19 during the admission/encounter, the appropriate code for the reason for admission/encounter should be sequenced as the principal/first-listed diagnosis, and codes O98.5- and UØ7.1, as well as the appropriate codes for associated COVID-19 manifestations, should be assigned as additional diagnoses.

16. Chapter 16: Certain Conditions Originating in the Perinatal Period (PØØ-P96)

For coding and reporting purposes the perinatal period is defined as before birth through the 28th day following birth. The following guidelines are provided for reporting purposes.

a. General Perinatal Rules

1) Use of Chapter 16 Codes

Codes in this chapter are never for use on the maternal record. Codes from Chapter 15, the obstetric chapter, are never permitted on the newborn record. Chapter 16 codes may be used throughout the life of the patient if the condition is still present.

2) Principal Diagnosis for Birth Record

When coding the birth episode in a newborn record, assign a code from category Z38, Liveborn infants according to place of birth and type of delivery, as the principal diagnosis. A code from category Z38 is assigned only once, to a newborn at the time of birth. If a newborn is transferred to another institution, a code from category Z38 should not be used at the receiving hospital.

A code from category Z38 is used only on the newborn record, not on the mother's record.

3) Use of Codes from other Chapters with Codes from Chapter 16

Codes from other chapters may be used with codes from chapter 16 if the codes from the other chapters provide more specific detail. Codes for signs and symptoms may be assigned when a definitive diagnosis has not been established. If the reason for the encounter is a perinatal condition, the code from chapter 16 should be sequenced first.

4) Use of Chapter 16 Codes after the Perinatal Period

Should a condition originate in the perinatal period, and continue throughout the life of the patient, the perinatal code should continue to be used regardless of the patient's age.

5) Birth process or community acquired conditions

If a newborn has a condition that may be either due to the birth process or community acquired and the documentation does not indicate which it is, the default is due to the birth process and the code from Chapter 16 should be used. If the condition is community-acquired, a code from Chapter 16 should not be assigned.

For COVID-19 infection in a newborn, see guideline I.C.16.h.

6) Code all clinically significant conditions

All clinically significant conditions noted on routine newborn examination should be coded. A condition is clinically significant if it requires:

- clinical evaluation; or
- therapeutic treatment; or
- diagnostic procedures; or
- extended length of hospital stay; or
- increased nursing care and/or monitoring; or
- has implications for future health care needs

Note: The perinatal guidelines listed above are the same as the general coding guidelines for "additional diagnoses," except for the final point regarding implications for future health care needs. Codes should be assigned for conditions that have been specified by the provider as having implications for future health care needs.

b. Observation and Evaluation of Newborns for Suspected Conditions not Found

1) Use of ZØ5 codes

Assign a code from category ZØ5, Observation and evaluation of newborn for suspected diseases and conditions ruled out, to identify those instances when a healthy newborn is evaluated for a suspected condition/disease that is determined after study not to be present. Do not use a code from category ZØ5 when the patient is documented to have signs or symptoms of a suspected problem; in such cases code the sign or symptom.

2) ZØ5 on other than the birth record

A code from category ZØ5 may also be assigned as a principal or first-listed code for readmissions or encounters when the code from category Z38 code no longer applies. Codes from category ZØ5 are for use only for healthy newborns and infants for which no condition after study is found to be present.

3) ZØ5 on a birth record

A code from category ZØ5 is to be used as a secondary code after the code from category Z38, Liveborn infants according to place of birth and type of delivery.

c. Coding Additional Perinatal Diagnoses

1) Assigning codes for conditions that require treatment

Assign codes for conditions that require treatment or further investigation, prolong the length of stay, or require resource utilization.

2) Codes for conditions specified as having implications for future health care needs

Assign codes for conditions that have been specified by the provider as having implications for future health care needs.

Note: This guideline should not be used for adult patients.

d. Prematurity and Fetal Growth Retardation

Providers utilize different criteria in determining prematurity. A code for prematurity should not be assigned unless it is documented. Assignment of codes in categories PØ5, Disorders of newborn related to slow fetal growth and fetal malnutrition, and PØ7, Disorders of newborn related to short gestation and low birth weight, not elsewhere classified, should be based on the recorded birth weight and estimated gestational age.

When both birth weight and gestational age are available, two codes from category PØ7 should be assigned, with the code for birth weight sequenced before the code for gestational age.

e. Low birth weight and immaturity status

Codes from category PØ7, Disorders of newborn related to short gestation and low birth weight, not elsewhere classified, are for use for a child or adult who was premature or had a low birth weight as a newborn and this is affecting the patient's current health status.

See Section I.C.21. Factors influencing health status and contact with health services, Status.

f. Bacterial Sepsis of Newborn

Category P36, Bacterial sepsis of newborn, includes congenital sepsis. If a perinate is documented as having sepsis without documentation of congenital or community acquired, the default is congenital and a code from category P36 should be assigned. If the P36 code includes the causal organism, an additional code from category B95, Streptococcus, Staphylococcus, and Enterococcus as the cause of diseases classified elsewhere, or B96, Other bacterial agents as the cause of diseases classified elsewhere, should not be assigned. If the P36 code does not include the causal organism, assign an additional code from category B96. If applicable, use additional codes to identify severe sepsis (R65.2-) and any associated acute organ dysfunction.

g. Stillbirth

Code P95, Stillbirth, is only for use in institutions that maintain separate records for stillbirths. No other code should be used with P95. Code P95 should not be used on the mother's record.

h. COVID-19 Infection in Newborn

For a newborn that tests positive for COVID-19, assign code UØ7.1, COVID-19, and the appropriate codes for associated manifestation(s) in neonates/newborns in the absence of documentation indicating a specific type of transmission. For a newborn that tests positive for COVID-19 and the provider documents the condition was contracted in utero or during the birth process, assign codes P35.8, Other congenital viral diseases, and UØ7.1, COVID-19. When coding the birth episode in a newborn record, the appropriate code from category Z38, Liveborn infants according to place of birth and type of delivery, should be assigned as the principal diagnosis.

17. Chapter 17: Congenital malformations, deformations, and chromosomal abnormalities (QØØ-Q99)

Assign an appropriate code(s) from categories QØØ-Q99, Congenital malformations, deformations, and chromosomal abnormalities when a malformation/deformation or chromosomal abnormality is documented. A malformation/deformation/or chromosomal abnormality may be the principal/first-listed diagnosis on a record or a secondary diagnosis.

When a malformation/deformation or chromosomal abnormality does not have a unique code assignment, assign additional code(s) for any manifestations that may be present.

When the code assignment specifically identifies the malformation/deformation or chromosomal abnormality, manifestations that are an inherent component of the anomaly should not be coded separately. Additional codes should be assigned for manifestations that are not an inherent component.

Codes from Chapter 17 may be used throughout the life of the patient. If a congenital malformation or deformity has been corrected, a personal history code should be used to identify the history of the malformation or deformity. Although present at birth, a malformation/deformation/or chromosomal abnormality may not be identified until later in life. Whenever the condition is diagnosed by the provider, it is appropriate to assign a code from codes QØØ-Q99. For the birth admission, the appropriate code from category Z38, Liveborn infants, according to place of birth and type of delivery, should be sequenced as the principal diagnosis, followed by any congenital anomaly codes, QØØ-Q99.

18. Chapter 18: Symptoms, signs, and abnormal clinical and laboratory findings, not elsewhere classified (RØØ-R99)

Chapter 18 includes symptoms, signs, abnormal results of clinical or other investigative procedures, and ill-defined conditions regarding which no diagnosis classifiable elsewhere is recorded. Signs and symptoms that point to a specific diagnosis have been assigned to a category in other chapters of the classification.

a. Use of symptom codes

Codes that describe symptoms and signs are acceptable for reporting purposes when a related definitive diagnosis has not been established (confirmed) by the provider.

b. Use of a symptom code with a definitive diagnosis code

Codes for signs and symptoms may be reported in addition to a related definitive diagnosis when the sign or symptom is not routinely associated with that diagnosis, such as the various signs and symptoms associated with complex syndromes. The definitive diagnosis code should be sequenced before the symptom code.

Signs or symptoms that are associated routinely with a disease process should not be assigned as additional codes, unless otherwise instructed by the classification.

c. Combination codes that include symptoms

ICD-10-CM contains a number of combination codes that identify both the definitive diagnosis and common symptoms of that diagnosis. When using one of these combination codes, an additional code should not be assigned for the symptom.

d. Repeated falls

Code R29.6, Repeated falls, is for use for encounters when a patient has recently fallen and the reason for the fall is being investigated.

Code Z91.81, History of falling, is for use when a patient has fallen in the past and is at risk for future falls. When appropriate, both codes R29.6 and Z91.81 may be assigned together.

e. Coma

Code R40.20, Unspecified coma, **should** be assigned **when the underlying cause of the coma is not known, or the cause is a traumatic brain injury and the coma scale is not documented in the medical record**.

Do not report codes for unspecified coma, individual or total Glasgow coma scale scores for a patient with a medically induced coma or a sedated patient.

1) **Coma Scale**

The coma scale codes (R4Ø.21- to R4Ø.24-) can be used in conjunction with traumatic brain injury codes. These codes **cannot be used with code R4Ø.2A, Nontraumatic coma due to underlying condition. They** are primarily for use by trauma registries, but they may be used in any setting where this information is collected. The coma scale codes should be sequenced after the diagnosis code(s).

These codes, one from each subcategory, are needed to complete the scale. The 7th character indicates when the scale was recorded. The 7th character should match for all three codes.

At a minimum, report the initial score documented on presentation at your facility. This may be a score from the emergency medicine technician (EMT) or in the emergency department. If desired, a facility may choose to capture multiple coma scale scores.

Assign code R4Ø.24-, Glasgow coma scale, total score, when only the total score is documented in the medical record and not the individual score(s).

If multiple coma scores are captured within the first 24 hours after hospital admission, assign only the code for the score at the time of admission. ICD-10-CM does not classify coma scores that are reported after admission but less than 24 hours later.

See Section I.B.14. for coma scale documentation by clinicians other than patient's provider

f. **Functional quadriplegia**

GUIDELINE HAS BEEN DELETED EFFECTIVE OCTOBER 1, 2017

g. **SIRS due to Non-Infectious Process**

The systemic inflammatory response syndrome (SIRS) can develop as a result of certain non-infectious disease processes, such as trauma, malignant neoplasm, or pancreatitis. When SIRS is documented with a noninfectious condition, and no subsequent infection is documented, the code for the underlying condition, such as an injury, should be assigned, followed by code R65.1Ø, Systemic inflammatory response syndrome (SIRS) of non-infectious origin without acute organ dysfunction, or code R65.11, Systemic inflammatory response syndrome (SIRS) of non-infectious origin with acute organ dysfunction. If an associated acute organ dysfunction is documented, the appropriate code(s) for the specific type of organ dysfunction(s) should be assigned in addition to code R65.11. If acute organ dysfunction is documented, but it cannot be determined if the acute organ dysfunction is associated with SIRS or due to another condition (e.g., directly due to the trauma), the provider should be queried.

h. **Death NOS**

Code R99, Ill-defined and unknown cause of mortality, is only for use in the very limited circumstance when a patient who has already died is brought into an emergency department or other healthcare facility and is pronounced dead upon arrival. It does not represent the discharge disposition of death.

i. **NIHSS Stroke Scale**

The NIH stroke scale (NIHSS) codes (R29.7- -) can be used in conjunction with acute stroke codes (**I6Ø–**I63) to identify the patient's neurological status and the severity of the stroke. The stroke scale codes should be sequenced after the acute stroke diagnosis code(s).

At a minimum, report the initial score documented. If desired, a facility may choose to capture multiple stroke scale scores.

See Section I.B.14. for NIHSS stroke scale documentation by clinicians other than patient's provider

19. **Chapter 19: Injury, poisoning, and certain other consequences of external causes (SØØ-T88)**

a. **Application of 7th Characters in Chapter 19**

Most categories in chapter 19 have a 7th character requirement for each applicable code. Most categories in this chapter have three 7th character values (with the exception of fractures): A, initial encounter, D, subsequent encounter and S, sequela. Categories for traumatic fractures have additional 7th character values. While the patient may be seen by a new or different provider over the course of treatment for an injury, assignment of the 7th character is based on whether the patient is undergoing active treatment and not whether the provider is seeing the patient for the first time.

For complication codes, active treatment refers to treatment for the condition described by the code, even though it may be related to an earlier precipitating problem. For example, code T84.5ØXA, Infection and inflammatory reaction due to unspecified internal joint prosthesis, initial encounter, is used when active treatment is provided for the infection, even though the condition relates to the prosthetic device, implant or graft that was placed at a previous encounter.

7th character "A", initial encounter is used for each encounter where the patient is receiving active treatment for the condition.

7th character "D" subsequent encounter is used for encounters after the patient has completed active treatment of the condition and is receiving routine care for the condition during the healing or recovery phase.

The aftercare Z codes should not be used for aftercare for conditions such as injuries or poisonings, where 7th characters are provided to identify subsequent care. For example, for aftercare of an injury, assign the acute injury code with the 7th character "D" (subsequent encounter).

7th character "S", sequela, is for use for complications or conditions that arise as a direct result of a condition, such as scar formation after a burn. The scars are sequelae of the burn. When using 7th character "S", it is necessary to use both the injury code that precipitated the sequela and the code for the sequela itself. The "S" is added only to the injury code, not the sequela code. The 7th character "S" identifies the injury responsible for the sequela. The specific type of sequela (e.g. scar) is sequenced first, followed by the injury code.

See Section I.B.10. Sequelae, (Late Effects)

b. **Coding of Injuries**

When coding injuries, assign separate codes for each injury unless a combination code is provided, in which case the combination code is assigned. Codes from category TØ7, Unspecified multiple injuries should not be assigned in the inpatient setting unless information for a more specific code is not available. Traumatic injury codes (SØØ-T14.9) are not to be used for normal, healing surgical wounds or to identify complications of surgical wounds.

The code for the most serious injury, as determined by the provider and the focus of treatment, is sequenced first.

1) **Superficial injuries**

Superficial injuries such as abrasions or contusions are not coded when associated with more severe injuries of the same site.

2) **Primary injury with damage to nerves/blood vessels**

When a primary injury results in minor damage to peripheral nerves or blood vessels, the primary injury is sequenced first with additional code(s) for injuries to nerves and spinal cord (such as category SØ4), and/or injury to blood vessels (such as category S15). When the primary injury is to the blood vessels or nerves, that injury should be sequenced first.

3) **Iatrogenic injuries**

Injury codes from Chapter 19 should not be assigned for injuries that occur during, or as a result of, a medical intervention. Assign the appropriate complication code(s).

c. **Coding of Traumatic Fractures**

The principles of multiple coding of injuries should be followed in coding fractures. Fractures of specified sites are coded individually by site in accordance with both the provisions within categories SØ2, S12, S22, S32, S42, S49, S52, S59, S62, S72, S79, S82, S89, S92 and the level of detail furnished by medical record content.

A fracture not indicated as open or closed should be coded to closed. A fracture not indicated whether displaced or not displaced should be coded to displaced.

More specific guidelines are as follows:

1) **Initial vs. subsequent encounter for fractures**

Traumatic fractures are coded using the appropriate 7th character for initial encounter (A, B, C) for each encounter where the patient is receiving active treatment for the fracture. The appropriate 7th character for initial encounter should also be assigned for a patient who delayed seeking treatment for the fracture or nonunion.

Fractures are coded using the appropriate 7th character for subsequent care for encounters after the patient has completed active treatment of the fracture and is receiving routine care for the fracture during the healing or recovery phase.

Care for complications of surgical treatment for fracture repairs during the healing or recovery phase should be coded with the appropriate complication codes.

Care of complications of fractures, such as malunion and nonunion, should be reported with the appropriate 7th character for subsequent care with nonunion (K, M, N,) or subsequent care with malunion (P, Q, R).

Malunion/nonunion: The appropriate 7th character for initial encounter should also be assigned for a patient who delayed seeking treatment for the fracture or nonunion.

The open fracture designations in the assignment of the 7th character for fractures of the forearm, femur and lower leg, including ankle are based on the Gustilo open fracture classification. When the Gustilo classification type is not specified for an open fracture, the 7th character for open fracture type I or II should be assigned (B, E, H, M, Q).

A code from category M8Ø, not a traumatic fracture code, should be used for any patient with known osteoporosis who suffers a fracture, even if the patient had a minor fall or trauma, if that fall or trauma would not usually break a normal, healthy bone.

See Section I.C.13. Osteoporosis.

The aftercare Z codes should not be used for aftercare for traumatic fractures. For aftercare of a traumatic fracture, assign the acute fracture code with the appropriate 7th character.

2) **Multiple fractures sequencing**

Multiple fractures are sequenced in accordance with the severity of the fracture.

3) **Physeal fractures**

For physeal fractures, assign only the code identifying the type of physeal fracture. Do not assign a separate code to identify the specific bone that is fractured.

d. **Coding of Burns and Corrosions**

The ICD-10-CM makes a distinction between burns and corrosions. The burn codes are for thermal burns, except sunburns, that come from a heat source, such as a fire or hot appliance. The burn codes are also for burns resulting from electricity and radiation. Corrosions are burns due to chemicals. The guidelines are the same for burns and corrosions.

Current burns (T2Ø-T25) are classified by depth, extent and by agent (X code). Burns are classified by depth as first degree (erythema), second degree (blistering), and third degree (full-thickness involvement). Burns of the eye and internal organs (T26-T28) are classified by site, but not by degree.

1) **Sequencing of burn and related condition codes**

Sequence first the code that reflects the highest degree of burn when more than one burn is present.

a. When the reason for the admission or encounter is for treatment of external multiple burns, sequence first the code that reflects the burn of the highest degree.

b. When a patient has both internal and external burns, the circumstances of admission govern the selection of the principal diagnosis or first-listed diagnosis.

c. When a patient is admitted for burn injuries and other related conditions such as smoke inhalation and/or respiratory failure, the circumstances of admission govern the selection of the principal or first-listed diagnosis.

2) **Burns of the same anatomic site**

Classify burns of the same anatomic site and on the same side but of different degrees to the subcategory identifying the highest degree recorded in the diagnosis (e.g., for second and third degree burns of right thigh, assign only code T24.311-).

3) **Non-healing burns**

Non-healing burns are coded as acute burns.

Necrosis of burned skin should be coded as a non-healed burn.

4) **Infected burn**

For any documented infected burn site, use an additional code for the infection.

5) **Assign separate codes for each burn site**

When coding burns, assign separate codes for each burn site. Category T3Ø, Burn and corrosion, body region unspecified is extremely vague and should rarely be used.

Codes for burns of "multiple sites" should only be assigned when the medical record documentation does not specify the individual sites.

6) **Burns and corrosions classified according to extent of body surface involved**

Assign codes from category T31, Burns classified according to extent of body surface involved, or T32, Corrosions classified according to extent of body surface involved, for acute burns or corrosions when the site of the burn or corrosion is not specified or when there is a need for additional data. It is advisable to use category T31 as additional coding when needed to provide data for evaluating burn mortality, such as that needed by burn units. It is also advisable to use category T31 as an additional code for reporting purposes when there is mention of a third-degree burn involving 20 percent or more of the body surface. Codes from categories T31 and T32 should not be used for sequelae of burns or corrosions.

Categories T31 and T32 are based on the classic "rule of nines" in estimating body surface involved: head and neck are assigned nine percent, each arm nine percent, each leg 18 percent, the anterior trunk 18 percent, posterior trunk 18 percent, and genitalia one percent. Providers may change these percentage assignments where necessary to accommodate infants and children who have proportionately larger heads than adults, and patients who have large buttocks, thighs, or abdomen that involve burns.

7) **Encounters for treatment of sequela of burns**

Encounters for the treatment of the late effects of burns or corrosions (i.e., scars or joint contractures) should be coded with a burn or corrosion code with the 7th character "S" for sequela.

8) **Sequelae with a late effect code and current burn**

When appropriate, both a code for a current burn or corrosion with 7th character "A" or "D" and a burn or corrosion code with 7th character "S" may be assigned on the same record (when both a current burn and sequelae of an old burn exist). Burns and corrosions do not heal at the same rate and a current healing wound may still exist with sequela of a healed burn or corrosion.

See Section I.B.10. Sequela (Late Effects)

9) **Use of an external cause code with burns and corrosions**

An external cause code should be used with burns and corrosions to identify the source and intent of the burn, as well as the place where it occurred.

e. **Adverse Effects, Poisoning, Underdosing and Toxic Effects**

Codes in categories T36-T65 are combination codes that include the substance that was taken as well as the intent. No additional external cause code is required for poisonings, toxic effects, adverse effects and underdosing codes.

1) **Do not code directly from the Table of Drugs**

Do not code directly from the Table of Drugs and Chemicals. Always refer back to the Tabular List.

2) **Use as many codes as necessary to describe**

Use as many codes as necessary to describe completely all drugs, medicinal or biological substances.

3) **If the same code would describe the causative agent**

If the same code would describe the causative agent for more than one adverse reaction, poisoning, toxic effect or underdosing, assign the code only once.

4) **If two or more drugs, medicinal or biological substances**

If two or more drugs, medicinal or biological substances are taken, code each individually unless a combination code is listed in the Table of Drugs and Chemicals.

If multiple unspecified drugs, medicinal or biological substances were taken, assign the appropriate code from subcategory T5Ø.91, Poisoning by, adverse effect of and underdosing of multiple unspecified drugs, medicaments and biological substances.

5) **The occurrence of drug toxicity is classified in ICD-10-CM as follows:**

(a) **Adverse Effect**

When coding an adverse effect of a drug that has been correctly prescribed and properly administered, assign the appropriate code for the nature of the adverse effect followed by the appropriate code for the adverse effect of the drug (T36-T5Ø). The code for the drug should have a 5th or 6th character "5" (for example T36.ØX5-) Examples of the nature of an adverse effect are tachycardia, delirium, gastrointestinal hemorrhaging, vomiting, hypokalemia, hepatitis, renal failure, or respiratory failure.

(b) **Poisoning**

When coding a poisoning or reaction to the improper use of a medication (e.g., overdose, wrong substance given or taken in error, wrong route of administration), first assign the appropriate code from categories T36-T5Ø. The poisoning codes have an associated intent as their 5th or 6th character (accidental, intentional self-harm, assault and undetermined). If the intent of the poisoning is unknown or unspecified, code the intent as accidental intent. The undetermined intent is only for use if the documentation in the record specifies that the intent cannot be determined. Use additional code(s) for all manifestations of poisonings.

If there is also a diagnosis of abuse or dependence of the substance, the abuse or dependence is assigned as an additional code.

Examples of poisoning include:

(i) Error was made in drug prescription

Errors made in drug prescription or in the administration of the drug by provider, nurse, patient, or other person.

(ii) Overdose of a drug intentionally taken

If an overdose of a drug was intentionally taken or administered and resulted in drug toxicity, it would be coded as a poisoning.

(iii) Nonprescribed drug taken with correctly prescribed and properly administered drug

If a nonprescribed drug or medicinal agent was taken in combination with a correctly prescribed and properly administered drug, any drug toxicity or other reaction resulting from the interaction of the two drugs would be classified as a poisoning.

(iv) Interaction of drug(s) and alcohol
When a reaction results from the interaction of a drug(s) and alcohol, this would be classified as poisoning.

See Section I.C.4. if poisoning is the result of insulin pump malfunctions.

For Sequela (Late Effects) see Section I.B.10.

(c) Underdosing

Underdosing refers to taking less of a medication than is prescribed by a provider or a manufacturer's instruction. Discontinuing the use of a prescribed medication on the patient's own initiative (not directed by the patient's provider) is also classified as an underdosing. For underdosing, assign the code from categories T36-T5Ø (fifth or sixth character "6"). Documentation of a change in the patient's condition is not required in order to assign an underdosing code. Documentation that the patient is taking less of a medication than is prescribed or discontinued the prescribed medication is sufficient for code assignment.

Codes for underdosing should never be assigned as principal or first-listed codes. If a patient has a relapse or exacerbation of the medical condition for which the drug is prescribed because of the reduction in dose, then the medical condition itself should be coded.

Noncompliance (Z91.12-, Z91.13-**,** Z91.14- and **Z91.A4-**) or complication of care (Y63.6-Y63.9) codes are to be used with an underdosing code to indicate intent, if known.

(d) Toxic Effects

When a harmful substance is ingested or comes in contact with a person, this is classified as a toxic effect. The toxic effect codes are in categories T51-T65. **When coding a toxic effect, assign the toxic effect code first, followed by codes for all associated manifestations of the toxic effect.**

Toxic effect codes have an associated intent: accidental, intentional self-harm, assault and undetermined.

For Sequela (Late Effects) see Section I.B.10. Sequela

f. Adult and child abuse, neglect and other maltreatment

Sequence first the appropriate code from categories T74, Adult and child abuse, neglect and other maltreatment, confirmed, or T76, Adult and child abuse, neglect and other maltreatment, suspected, for abuse, neglect and other maltreatment, followed by any accompanying mental health or injury code(s).

If the documentation in the medical record states abuse or neglect, it is coded as confirmed (T74.-). It is coded as suspected if it is documented as suspected (T76.-).

For cases of confirmed abuse or neglect an external cause code from the assault section (X92-YØ9) should be added to identify the cause of any physical injuries. A perpetrator code (YØ7) should be added when the perpetrator of the abuse is known. For suspected cases of abuse or neglect, do not report external cause or perpetrator code.

If a suspected case of abuse, neglect or mistreatment is ruled out during an encounter code ZØ4.71, Encounter for examination and observation following alleged physical adult abuse, ruled out, or code ZØ4.72, Encounter for examination and observation following alleged child physical abuse, ruled out, should be used, not a code from T76.

If a suspected case of alleged rape or sexual abuse is ruled out during an encounter code ZØ4.41, Encounter for examination and observation following alleged adult rape or code ZØ4.42, Encounter for examination and observation following alleged child rape, should be used, not a code from T76.

If a suspected case of forced sexual exploitation or forced labor exploitation is ruled out during an encounter, code ZØ4.81, Encounter for examination and observation of victim following forced sexual exploitation, or code ZØ4.82, Encounter for examination and observation of victim following forced labor exploitation, should be used, not a code from T76.

See Section I.C.15. Abuse in a pregnant patient.

g. Complications of care

1) General guidelines for complications of care

(a) Documentation of complications of care

See Section I.B.16. for information on documentation of complications of care.

2) Pain due to medical devices

Pain associated with devices, implants or grafts left in a surgical site (for example painful hip prosthesis) is assigned to the appropriate code(s) found in Chapter 19, Injury, poisoning, and certain other consequences of external causes. Specific codes for pain due to medical devices are found in the T code section of the ICD-10-CM. Use additional code(s) from category G89 to identify acute or chronic pain due to presence of the device, implant or graft (G89.18 or G89.28).

3) Transplant complications

(a) Transplant complications other than kidney

Codes under category T86, Complications of transplanted organs and tissues, are for use for both complications and rejection of transplanted organs. A transplant complication code is only assigned if the complication affects the function of the transplanted organ. Two codes are required to fully describe a transplant complication: the appropriate code from category T86 and a secondary code that identifies the complication.

Pre-existing conditions or conditions that develop after the transplant are not coded as complications unless they affect the function of the transplanted organs.

See I.C.21. for transplant organ removal status

See I.C.2. for malignant neoplasm associated with transplanted organ.

<u>See I.C.1.d.4. for sequencing of sepsis due to infection in transplanted organ</u>

(b) Kidney transplant complications

Patients who have undergone kidney transplant may still have some form of chronic kidney disease (CKD) because the kidney transplant may not fully restore kidney function. Code T86.1- should be assigned for documented complications of a kidney transplant, such as transplant failure or rejection or other transplant complication. Code T86.1- should not be assigned for post kidney transplant patients who have chronic kidney (CKD) unless a transplant complication such as transplant failure or rejection is documented. If the documentation is unclear as to whether the patient has a complication of the transplant, query the provider.

Conditions that affect the function of the transplanted kidney, other than CKD, should be assigned a code from subcategory T86.1, Complications of transplanted organ, Kidney, and a secondary code that identifies the complication.

For patients with CKD following a kidney transplant, but who do not have a complication such as failure or rejection, *see section I.C.14. Chronic kidney disease and kidney transplant status.*

<u>See I.C.1.d.4. for sequencing of sepsis due to infection in transplanted organ</u>

4) Complication codes that include the external cause

As with certain other T codes, some of the complications of care codes have the external cause included in the code. The code includes the nature of the complication as well as the type of procedure that caused the complication. No external cause code indicating the type of procedure is necessary for these codes.

5) Complications of care codes within the body system chapters

Intraoperative and postprocedural complication codes are found within the body system chapters with codes specific to the organs and structures of that body system. These codes should be sequenced first, followed by a code(s) for the specific complication, if applicable.

Complication codes from the body system chapters should be assigned for intraoperative and postprocedural complications (e.g., the appropriate complication code from chapter 9 would be assigned for a vascular intraoperative or postprocedural complication) unless the complication is specifically indexed to a T code in chapter 19.

20. Chapter 20: External Causes of Morbidity (VØØ-Y99)

The external causes of morbidity codes should never be sequenced as the first-listed or principal diagnosis.

External cause codes are intended to provide data for injury research and evaluation of injury prevention strategies. These codes capture how the injury or health condition happened (cause), the intent (unintentional or accidental; or intentional, such as suicide or assault), the place where the event occurred the activity of the patient at the time of the event, and the person's status (e.g., civilian, military).

There is no national requirement for mandatory ICD-10-CM external cause code reporting. Unless a provider is subject to a state-based external cause code reporting mandate or these codes are required by a particular payer, reporting of ICD-10-CM codes in Chapter 20, External Causes of Morbidity, is not required. In the absence of a mandatory reporting requirement, providers are encouraged to voluntarily report external cause codes, as they provide valuable data for injury research and evaluation of injury prevention strategies.

a. General External Cause Coding Guidelines

1) Used with any code in the range of AØØ.Ø-T88.9, ZØØ-Z99

An external cause code may be used with any code in the range of AØØ.Ø-T88.9, ZØØ-Z99, classification that represents a health condition due to an external cause. Though they are most applicable to injuries, they are also valid for use with such things as infections or diseases due to an external source, and other health conditions, such as a heart attack that occurs during strenuous physical activity.

2) External cause code used for length of treatment

Assign the external cause code, with the appropriate 7th character (initial encounter, subsequent encounter or sequela) for each encounter for which the injury or condition is being treated.

Most categories in chapter 20 have a 7th character requirement for each applicable code. Most categories in this chapter have three 7th character values: A, initial encounter, D, subsequent encounter and S, sequela. While the patient may be seen by a new or different provider over the course of treatment for an injury or condition, assignment of the 7th character for external cause should match the 7th character of the code assigned for the associated injury or condition for the encounter.

3) Use the full range of external cause codes

Use the full range of external cause codes to completely describe the cause, the intent, the place of occurrence, and if applicable, the activity of the patient at the time of the event, and the patient's status, for all injuries, and other health conditions due to an external cause.

4) Assign as many external cause codes as necessary

Assign as many external cause codes as necessary to fully explain each cause. If only one external code can be recorded, assign the code most related to the principal diagnosis.

5) The selection of the appropriate external cause code

The selection of the appropriate external cause code is guided by the Alphabetic Index of External Causes and by Inclusion and Exclusion notes in the Tabular List.

6) External cause code can never be a principal diagnosis

An external cause code can never be a principal (first-listed) diagnosis.

7) Combination external cause codes

Certain of the external cause codes are combination codes that identify sequential events that result in an injury, such as a fall which results in striking against an object. The injury may be due to either event or both. The combination external cause code used should correspond to the sequence of events regardless of which caused the most serious injury.

8) No external cause code needed in certain circumstances

No external cause code from Chapter 20 is needed if the external cause and intent are included in a code from another chapter (e.g., T36.ØX1-, Poisoning by penicillins, accidental (unintentional)).

b. Place of Occurrence Guideline

Codes from category Y92, Place of occurrence of the external cause, are secondary codes for use after other external cause codes to identify the location of the patient at the time of injury or other condition.

Generally, a place of occurrence code is assigned only once, at the initial encounter for treatment. However, in the rare instance that a new injury occurs during hospitalization, an additional place of occurrence code may be assigned. No 7th characters are used for Y92.

Do not use place of occurrence code Y92.9 if the place is not stated or is not applicable.

c. Activity Code

Assign a code from category Y93, Activity code, to describe the activity of the patient at the time the injury or other health condition occurred.

An activity code is used only once, at the initial encounter for treatment. Only one code from Y93 should be recorded on a medical record.

The activity codes are not applicable to poisonings, adverse effects, misadventures or sequela.

Do not assign Y93.9, Unspecified activity, if the activity is not stated.

A code from category Y93 is appropriate for use with external cause and intent codes if identifying the activity provides additional information about the event.

d. Place of Occurrence, Activity, and Status Codes Used with other External Cause Code

When applicable, place of occurrence, activity, and external cause status codes are sequenced after the main external cause code(s). Regardless of the number of external cause codes assigned, generally there should be only one place of occurrence code, one activity code, and one external cause status code assigned to an encounter. However, in the rare instance that a new injury occurs during hospitalization, an additional place of occurrence code may be assigned.

e. If the Reporting Format Limits the Number of External Cause Codes

If the reporting format limits the number of external cause codes that can be used in reporting clinical data, report the code for the cause/intent most related to the principal diagnosis. If the format permits capture of additional external cause codes, the cause/intent, including medical misadventures, of the additional events should be reported rather than the codes for place, activity, or external status.

f. Multiple External Cause Coding Guidelines

More than one external cause code is required to fully describe the external cause of an illness or injury. The assignment of external cause codes should be sequenced in the following priority:

If two or more events cause separate injuries, an external cause code should be assigned for each cause. The first-listed external cause code will be selected in the following order:

External codes for child and adult abuse take priority over all other external cause codes.

See Section I.C.19., Child and Adult abuse guidelines.

External cause codes for terrorism events take priority over all other external cause codes except child and adult abuse.

External cause codes for cataclysmic events take priority over all other external cause codes except child and adult abuse and terrorism.

External cause codes for transport accidents take priority over all other external cause codes except cataclysmic events, child and adult abuse and terrorism.

Activity and external cause status codes are assigned following all causal (intent) external cause codes.

The first-listed external cause code should correspond to the cause of the most serious diagnosis due to an assault, accident, or self-harm, following the order of hierarchy listed above.

g. Child and Adult Abuse Guideline

Adult and child abuse, neglect and maltreatment are classified as assault. Any of the assault codes may be used to indicate the external cause of any injury resulting from the confirmed abuse.

For confirmed cases of abuse, neglect and maltreatment, when the perpetrator is known, a code from YØ7, Perpetrator of maltreatment and neglect, should accompany any other assault codes.

See Section I.C.19. Adult and child abuse, neglect and other maltreatment

h. Unknown or Undetermined Intent Guideline

If the intent (accident, self-harm, assault) of the cause of an injury or other condition is unknown or unspecified, code the intent as accidental intent. All transport accident categories assume accidental intent.

1) Use of undetermined intent

External cause codes for events of undetermined intent are only for use if the documentation in the record specifies that the intent cannot be determined.

i. Sequelae (Late Effects) of External Cause Guidelines

1) Sequelae external cause codes

Sequela are reported using the external cause code with the 7th character "S" for sequela. These codes should be used with any report of a late effect or sequela resulting from a previous injury.

See Section I.B.10. Sequela (Late Effects)

2) Sequela external cause code with a related current injury

A sequela external cause code should never be used with a related current nature of injury code.

3) Use of sequela external cause codes for subsequent visits

Use a late effect external cause code for subsequent visits when a late effect of the initial injury is being treated. Do not use a late effect external cause code for subsequent visits for follow-up care (e.g., to assess healing, to receive rehabilitative therapy) of the injury when no late effect of the injury has been documented.

j. Terrorism Guidelines

1) Cause of injury identified by the Federal Government (FBI) as terrorism

When the cause of an injury is identified by the Federal Government (FBI) as terrorism, the first-listed external cause code should be a code from category Y38, Terrorism. The definition of terrorism employed by the FBI is found at the inclusion note at the beginning of category Y38. Use additional code for place of occurrence (Y92.-). More than one Y38 code may be assigned if the injury is the result of more than one mechanism of terrorism.

2) Cause of an injury is suspected to be the result of terrorism

When the cause of an injury is suspected to be the result of terrorism a code from category Y38 should not be assigned. Suspected cases should be classified as assault.

3) **Code Y38.9, Terrorism, secondary effects**
Assign code Y38.9, Terrorism, secondary effects, for conditions occurring subsequent to the terrorist event. This code should not be assigned for conditions that are due to the initial terrorist act.
It is acceptable to assign code Y38.9 with another code from Y38 if there is an injury due to the initial terrorist event and an injury that is a subsequent result of the terrorist event.

k. **External Cause Status**
A code from category Y99, External cause status, should be assigned whenever any other external cause code is assigned for an encounter, including an Activity code, except for the events noted below. Assign a code from category Y99, External cause status, to indicate the work status of the person at the time the event occurred. The status code indicates whether the event occurred during military activity, whether a non-military person was at work, whether an individual including a student or volunteer was involved in a non-work activity at the time of the causal event.
A code from Y99, External cause status, should be assigned, when applicable, with other external cause codes, such as transport accidents and falls. The external cause status codes are not applicable to poisonings, adverse effects, misadventures or late effects.
Do not assign a code from category Y99 if no other external cause codes (cause, activity) are applicable for the encounter.
An external cause status code is used only once, at the initial encounter for treatment. Only one code from Y99 should be recorded on a medical record.
Do not assign code Y99.9, Unspecified external cause status, if the status is not stated.

21. **Chapter 21: Factors influencing health status and contact with health services (Z00-Z99)**
Note: The chapter specific guidelines provide additional information about the use of Z codes for specified encounters.

a. **Use of Z Codes in Any Healthcare Setting**
Z codes are for use in any healthcare setting. Z codes may be used as either a first-listed (principal diagnosis code in the inpatient setting) or secondary code, depending on the circumstances of the encounter. Certain Z codes may only be used as first-listed or principal diagnosis.

b. **Z Codes Indicate a Reason for an Encounter or Provide Additional Information about a Patient Encounter**
Z codes are not procedure codes. A corresponding procedure code must accompany a Z code to describe any procedure performed.

c. **Categories of Z Codes**

1) **Contact/Exposure**
Category Z20 indicates contact with, and suspected exposure to, communicable diseases. These codes are for patients who are suspected to have been exposed to a disease by close personal contact with an infected individual or are in an area where a disease is epidemic.
Category Z77, Other contact with and (suspected) exposures hazardous to health, indicates contact with and suspected exposures hazardous to health.
Contact/exposure codes may be used as a first-listed code to explain an encounter for testing, or, more commonly, as a secondary code to identify a potential risk.

2) **Inoculations and vaccinations**
Code Z23 is for encounters for inoculations and vaccinations. It indicates that a patient is being seen to receive a prophylactic inoculation against a disease. Procedure codes are required to identify the actual administration of the injection and the type(s) of immunizations given. Code Z23 may be used as a secondary code if the inoculation is given as a routine part of preventive health care, such as a well-baby visit.

3) **Status**
Status codes indicate that a patient is either a carrier of a disease or has the sequelae or residual of a past disease or condition. This includes such things as the presence of prosthetic or mechanical devices resulting from past treatment. A status code is informative, because the status may affect the course of treatment and its outcome. A status code is distinct from a history code. The history code indicates that the patient no longer has the condition.
A status code should not be used with a diagnosis code from one of the body system chapters, if the diagnosis code includes the information provided by the status code. For example, code Z94.1, Heart transplant status, should not be used with a code from subcategory T86.2, Complications of heart transplant. The status code does not provide additional information. The complication code indicates that the patient is a heart transplant patient.
For encounters for weaning from a mechanical ventilator, assign a code from subcategory J96.1, Chronic respiratory failure, followed by code Z99.11, Dependence on respirator [ventilator] status.
The status Z codes/categories are:

Z14 Genetic carrier
Genetic carrier status indicates that a person carries a gene, associated with a particular disease, which may be passed to offspring who may develop that disease. The person does not have the disease and is not at risk of developing the disease.

Z15 Genetic susceptibility to disease
Genetic susceptibility indicates that a person has a gene that increases the risk of that person developing the disease.
Codes from category Z15 should not be used as principal or first-listed codes. If the patient has the condition to which he/she is susceptible, and that condition is the reason for the encounter, the code for the current condition should be sequenced first. If the patient is being seen for follow-up after completed treatment for this condition, and the condition no longer exists, a follow-up code should be sequenced first, followed by the appropriate personal history and genetic susceptibility codes. If the purpose of the encounter is genetic counseling associated with procreative management, code Z31.5, Encounter for genetic counseling, should be assigned as the first-listed code, followed by a code from category Z15. Additional codes should be assigned for any applicable family or personal history.

Z16 Resistance to antimicrobial drugs
This code indicates that a patient has a condition that is resistant to antimicrobial drug treatment. Sequence the infection code first.

Z17 Estrogen receptor status

Z18 Retained foreign body fragments

Z19 Hormone sensitivity malignancy status

Z21 Asymptomatic HIV infection status
This code indicates that a patient has tested positive for HIV but has manifested no signs or symptoms of the disease.

Z22 Carrier of infectious disease
Carrier status indicates that a person harbors the specific organisms of a disease without manifest symptoms and is capable of transmitting the infection.

Z28.3 Underimmunization status
See Section I.B.14. for underimmunization documentation by clinicians other than the patient's provider.

Z33.1 Pregnant state, incidental
This code is a secondary code only for use when the pregnancy is in no way complicating the reason for visit. Otherwise, a code from the obstetric chapter is required.

Z66 Do not resuscitate
This code may be used when it is documented by the provider that a patient is on do not resuscitate status at any time during the stay.

Z67 Blood type

Z68 Body mass index (BMI)
BMI codes should only be assigned when there is an associated, reportable diagnosis (such as obesity). Do not assign BMI codes during pregnancy.
See Section I.B.14. for BMI documentation by clinicians other than the patient's provider.

Z74.01 Bed confinement status

Z76.82 Awaiting organ transplant status

Z78 Other specified health status
Code Z78.1, Physical restraint status, may be used when it is documented by the provider that a patient has been put in restraints during the current encounter. Please note that this code should not be reported when it is documented by the provider that a patient is temporarily restrained during a procedure.

Z79 Long-term (current) drug therapy
Codes from this category indicate a patient's continuous use of a prescribed drug (including such things as aspirin therapy) for the long-term treatment of a condition or for prophylactic use. It is not for use for patients who have addictions to drugs. This subcategory is not for use of medications for detoxification or maintenance programs to prevent withdrawal symptoms (e.g., methadone maintenance for opiate dependence). Assign the

appropriate code for the drug use, abuse, or dependence instead.

Assign a code from Z79 if the patient is receiving a medication for an extended period as a prophylactic measure (such as for the prevention of deep vein thrombosis) or as treatment of a chronic condition (such as arthritis) or a disease requiring a lengthy course of treatment (such as cancer). Do not assign a code from category Z79 for medication being administered for a brief period of time to treat an acute illness or injury (such as a course of antibiotics to treat acute bronchitis).

Z88 Allergy status to drugs, medicaments and biological substances
Except: Z88.9, Allergy status to unspecified drugs, medicaments and biological substances status

Z89 Acquired absence of limb

Z90 Acquired absence of organs, not elsewhere classified

Z91.0- Allergy status, other than to drugs and biological substances

Z92.82 Status post administration of tPA (rtPA) in a different facility within the last 24 hours prior to admission to a current facility

Assign code Z92.82, Status post administration of tPA (rtPA) in a different facility within the last 24 hours prior to admission to current facility, as a secondary diagnosis when a patient is received by transfer into a facility and documentation indicates they were administered tissue plasminogen activator (tPA) within the last 24 hours prior to admission to the current facility.

This guideline applies even if the patient is still receiving the tPA at the time they are received into the current facility.

The appropriate code for the condition for which the tPA was administered (such as cerebrovascular disease or myocardial infarction) should be assigned first.

Code Z92.82 is only applicable to the receiving facility record and not to the transferring facility record.

Z93 Artificial opening status

Z94 Transplanted organ and tissue status

Z95 Presence of cardiac and vascular implants and grafts

Z96 Presence of other functional implants

Z97 Presence of other devices

Z98 Other postprocedural states

Assign code Z98.85, Transplanted organ removal status, to indicate that a transplanted organ has been previously removed. This code should not be assigned for the encounter in which the transplanted organ is removed. The complication necessitating removal of the transplant organ should be assigned for that encounter.

See section I.C.19. for information on the coding of organ transplant complications.

Z99 Dependence on enabling machines and devices, not elsewhere classified

Note: Categories Z89-Z90 and Z93-Z99 are for use only if there are no complications or malfunctions of the organ or tissue replaced, the amputation site or the equipment on which the patient is dependent.

4) History (of)

There are two types of history Z codes, personal and family. Personal history codes explain a patient's past medical condition that no longer exists and is not receiving any treatment, but that has the potential for recurrence, and therefore may require continued monitoring.

Family history codes are for use when a patient has a family member(s) who has had a particular disease that causes the patient to be at higher risk of also contracting the disease.

Personal history codes may be used in conjunction with follow-up codes and family history codes may be used in conjunction with screening codes to explain the need for a test or procedure. History codes are also acceptable on any medical record regardless of the reason for visit. A history of an illness, even if no longer present, is important information that may alter the type of treatment ordered.

The reason for the encounter (for example, screening or counseling) should be sequenced first and the appropriate personal and/or family history code(s) should be assigned as additional diagnos(es).

The history Z code categories are:

Z80 Family history of primary malignant neoplasm

Z81 Family history of mental and behavioral disorders

Z82 Family history of certain disabilities and chronic diseases (leading to disablement)

Z83 Family history of other specific disorders

Z84 Family history of other conditions

Z85 Personal history of malignant neoplasm

Z86 Personal history of certain other diseases

Z87 Personal history of other diseases and conditions

Z91.4- Personal history of psychological trauma, not elsewhere classified

Z91.5- Personal history of self-harm

Z91.81 History of falling

Z91.82 Personal history of military deployment

Z91.85 Personal history of military service

Z92 Personal history of medical treatment
Except: Z92.0, Personal history of contraception
Except: Z92.82, Status post administration of tPA (rtPA) in a different facility within the last 24 hours prior to admission to a current facility

5) Screening

Screening is the testing for disease or disease precursors in seemingly well individuals so that early detection and treatment can be provided for those who test positive for the disease (e.g., screening mammogram).

The testing of a person to rule out or confirm a suspected diagnosis because the patient has some sign or symptom is a diagnostic examination, not a screening. In these cases, the sign or symptom is used to explain the reason for the test.

A screening code may be a first-listed code if the reason for the visit is specifically the screening exam. It may also be used as an additional code if the screening is done during an office visit for other health problems. A screening code is not necessary if the screening is inherent to a routine examination, such as a pap smear done during a routine pelvic examination.

Should a condition be discovered during the screening then the code for the condition may be assigned as an additional diagnosis.

The Z code indicates that a screening exam is planned. A procedure code is required to confirm that the screening was performed.

The screening Z codes/categories:

Z11 Encounter for screening for infectious and parasitic diseases

Z12 Encounter for screening for malignant neoplasms

Z13 Encounter for screening for other diseases and disorders
Except: Z13.9, Encounter for screening, unspecified

Z36 Encounter for antenatal screening for mother

6) Observation

There are three observation Z code categories. They are for use in very limited circumstances when a person is being observed for a suspected condition that is ruled out. The observation codes are not for use if an injury or illness or any signs or symptoms related to the suspected condition are present. In such cases the diagnosis/symptom code is used with the corresponding external cause code.

The observation codes are primarily to be used as a principal/first-listed diagnosis. An observation code may be assigned as a secondary diagnosis code when the patient is being observed for a condition that is ruled out and is unrelated to the principal/first-listed diagnosis. Also, when the principal diagnosis is required to be a code from category Z38, Liveborn infants according to place of birth and type of delivery, then a code from category Z05, Encounter for observation and evaluation of newborn for suspected diseases and conditions ruled out, is sequenced after the Z38 code. Additional codes may be used in addition to the observation code, but only if they are unrelated to the suspected condition being observed.

Codes from subcategory Z03.7, Encounter for suspected maternal and fetal conditions ruled out, may either be used as a first-listed or as an additional code assignment depending on the case. They are for use in very limited circumstances on a maternal record when an encounter is for a suspected maternal or fetal condition that is ruled out during that encounter (for example, a maternal or fetal condition may be suspected due to an abnormal test result). These codes should not be used when the condition is confirmed. In those cases, the confirmed condition should be coded. In addition, these codes are not for use if an illness or any signs or symptoms related to the suspected condition or problem are present. In such cases the diagnosis/symptom code is used.

Additional codes may be used in addition to the code from subcategory Z03.7, but only if they are unrelated to the suspected condition being evaluated.

Codes from subcategory Z03.7 may not be used for encounters for antenatal screening of mother. *See Section I.C.21. Screening.*

For encounters for suspected fetal condition that are inconclusive following testing and evaluation, assign the appropriate code from category O35, O36, O40 or O41.

The observation Z code categories:

- Z03 Encounter for medical observation for suspected diseases and conditions ruled out
- Z04 Encounter for examination and observation for other reasons Except: Z04.9, Encounter for examination and observation for unspecified reason
- Z05 Encounter for observation and evaluation of newborn for suspected diseases and conditions ruled out

7) Aftercare

Aftercare visit codes cover situations when the initial treatment of a disease has been performed and the patient requires continued care during the healing or recovery phase, or for the long-term consequences of the disease. The aftercare Z code should not be used if treatment is directed at a current, acute disease. The diagnosis code is to be used in these cases. Exceptions to this rule are codes Z51.0, Encounter for antineoplastic radiation therapy, and codes from subcategory Z51.1, Encounter for antineoplastic chemotherapy and immunotherapy. These codes are to be first listed, followed by the diagnosis code when a patient's encounter is solely to receive radiation therapy, chemotherapy, or immunotherapy for the treatment of a neoplasm. If the reason for the encounter is more than one type of antineoplastic therapy, code Z51.0 and a code from subcategory Z51.1 may be assigned together, in which case one of these codes would be reported as a secondary diagnosis.

The aftercare Z codes should also not be used for aftercare for injuries. For aftercare of an injury, assign the acute injury code with the appropriate 7th character (for subsequent encounter).

The aftercare codes are generally first listed to explain the specific reason for the encounter. An aftercare code may be used as an additional code when some type of aftercare is provided in addition to the reason for admission and no diagnosis code is applicable. An example of this would be the closure of a colostomy during an encounter for treatment of another condition.

Aftercare codes should be used in conjunction with other aftercare codes or diagnosis codes to provide better detail on the specifics of an aftercare encounter visit, unless otherwise directed by the classification. The sequencing of multiple aftercare codes depends on the circumstances of the encounter.

Certain aftercare Z code categories need a secondary diagnosis code to describe the resolving condition or sequelae. For others, the condition is included in the code title.

Additional Z code aftercare category terms include fitting and adjustment, and attention to artificial openings.

Status Z codes may be used with aftercare Z codes to indicate the nature of the aftercare. For example, code Z95.1, Presence of aortocoronary bypass graft, may be used with code Z48.812, Encounter for surgical aftercare following surgery on the circulatory system, to indicate the surgery for which the aftercare is being performed. A status code should not be used when the aftercare code indicates the type of status, such as using Z43.0, Encounter for attention to tracheostomy, with Z93.0, Tracheostomy status.

The aftercare Z category/codes:

- Z42 Encounter for plastic and reconstructive surgery following medical procedure or healed injury
- Z43 Encounter for attention to artificial openings
- Z44 Encounter for fitting and adjustment of external prosthetic device
- Z45 Encounter for adjustment and management of implanted device
- Z46 Encounter for fitting and adjustment of other devices
- Z47 Orthopedic aftercare
- Z48 Encounter for other postprocedural aftercare
- Z49 Encounter for care involving renal dialysis
- Z51 Encounter for other aftercare and medical care

8) Follow-up

The follow-up codes are used to explain continuing surveillance following completed treatment of a disease, condition, or injury. They imply that the condition has been fully treated and no longer exists. They should not be confused with aftercare codes, or injury codes with a 7th character for subsequent encounter, that explain ongoing care of a healing condition or its sequelae. Follow-up codes may be used in conjunction with history codes to provide the full picture of the healed condition and its treatment. The follow-up code is sequenced first, followed by the history code.

A follow-up code may be used to explain multiple visits. Should a condition be found to have recurred on the follow-up visit, then the diagnosis code for the condition should be assigned in place of the follow-up code.

The follow-up Z **codes/categories:**

- Z08 Encounter for follow-up examination after completed treatment for malignant neoplasm
- Z09 Encounter for follow-up examination after completed treatment for conditions other than malignant neoplasm

Codes Z08, Encounter for follow-up examination after completed treatment for malignant neoplasm, and Z09, Encounter for follow up examination after completed treatment for conditions other than malignant neoplasm, may be assigned following any type of completed treatment modality (including both medical and surgical treatments).

- Z39 Encounter for maternal postpartum care and examination

9) Donor

Codes in category Z52, Donors of organs and tissues, are used for living individuals who are donating blood or other body tissue. These codes are for individuals donating for others, as well as for self-donations. They are not used to identify cadaveric donations.

10) Counseling

Counseling Z codes are used when a patient or family member receives assistance in the aftermath of an illness or injury, or when support is required in coping with family or social problems.

The counseling Z codes/categories:

- Z30.0- Encounter for general counseling and advice on contraception
- Z31.5 Encounter for procreative genetic counseling
- Z31.6- Encounter for general counseling and advice on procreation
- Z32.2 Encounter for childbirth instruction
- Z32.3 Encounter for childcare instruction
- Z69 Encounter for mental health services for victim and perpetrator of abuse
- Z70 Counseling related to sexual attitude, behavior and orientation
- Z71 Persons encountering health services for other counseling and medical advice, not elsewhere classified

  Note: Code Z71.84, Encounter for health counseling related to travel, is to be used for health risk and safety counseling for future travel purposes.

  Code Z71.85, Encounter for immunization safety counseling, is to be used for counseling of the patient or caregiver regarding the safety of a vaccine. This code should not be used for the provision of general information regarding risks and potential side effects during routine encounters for the administration of vaccines.

  Code Z71.87, Encounter for pediatric-to-adult transition counseling, should be assigned when pediatric-to-adult transition counseling is the sole reason for the encounter or when this counseling is provided in addition to other services, such as treatment of a chronic condition. If both transition counseling and treatment of a medical condition are provided during the same encounter, the code(s) for the medical condition(s) treated and code Z71.87 should be assigned, with sequencing depending on the circumstances of the encounter.
- Z76.81 Expectant mother prebirth pediatrician visit

11) Encounters for Obstetrical and Reproductive Services

See Section I.C.15. Pregnancy, Childbirth, and the Puerperium, for further instruction on the use of these codes.

Z codes for pregnancy are for use in those circumstances when none of the problems or complications included in the codes from the Obstetrics chapter exist (a routine prenatal visit or postpartum care). Codes in category Z34, Encounter for supervision of normal pregnancy, are always first listed and are not to be used with any other code from the OB chapter.

Codes in category Z3A, Weeks of gestation, may be assigned to provide additional information about the pregnancy. Category Z3A codes should not be assigned for pregnancies with abortive outcomes (categories O00-O08), elective termination of pregnancy (code Z33.2), nor for postpartum conditions, as category Z3A is not applicable to these conditions. The date of the admission should be used to determine weeks of gestation for inpatient admissions that encompass more than one gestational week.

The outcome of delivery, category Z37, should be included on all maternal delivery records. It is always a secondary code.

Codes in category Z37 should not be used on the newborn record.

Z codes for family planning (contraceptive) or procreative management and counseling should be included on an obstetric record either during the pregnancy or the postpartum stage, if applicable.

Z codes/categories for obstetrical and reproductive services:

Z30 Encounter for contraceptive management
Z31 Encounter for procreative management
Z32.2 Encounter for childbirth instruction
Z32.3 Encounter for childcare instruction
Z33 Pregnant state
Z34 Encounter for supervision of normal pregnancy
Z36 Encounter for antenatal screening of mother
Z3A Weeks of gestation
Z37 Outcome of delivery
Z39 Encounter for maternal postpartum care and examination
Z76.81 Expectant mother prebirth pediatrician visit

12) Newborns and Infants

See Section I.C.16. Newborn (Perinatal) Guidelines, for further instruction on the use of these codes.

Newborn Z codes/categories:

Z76.1 Encounter for health supervision and care of foundling
Z00.1- Encounter for routine child health examination
Z38 Liveborn infants according to place of birth and type of delivery

13) Routine and Administrative Examinations

The Z codes allow for the description of encounters for routine examinations, such as, a general check-up, or, examinations for administrative purposes, such as, a pre-employment physical. The codes are not to be used if the examination is for diagnosis of a suspected condition or for treatment purposes. In such cases the diagnosis code is used. During a routine exam, should a diagnosis or condition be discovered, it should be coded as an additional code. Pre-existing and chronic conditions and history codes may also be included as additional codes as long as the examination is for administrative purposes and not focused on any particular condition.

Some of the codes for routine health examinations distinguish between "with" and "without" abnormal findings. Code assignment depends on the information that is known at the time the encounter is being coded. For example, if no abnormal findings were found during the examination, but the encounter is being coded before test results are back, it is acceptable to assign the code for "without abnormal findings." When assigning a code for "with abnormal findings," additional code(s) should be assigned to identify the specific abnormal finding(s).

Pre-operative examination and pre-procedural laboratory examination Z codes are for use only in those situations when a patient is being cleared for a procedure or surgery and no treatment is given.

The Z codes/categories for routine and administrative examinations:

Z00 Encounter for general examination without complaint, suspected or reported diagnosis
Z01 Encounter for other special examination without complaint, suspected or reported diagnosis
Z02 Encounter for administrative examination
Except: Z02.9, Encounter for administrative examinations, unspecified
Z32.0- Encounter for pregnancy test

14) Miscellaneous Z Codes

The miscellaneous Z codes capture a number of other health care encounters that do not fall into one of the other categories. Some of these codes identify the reason for the encounter; others are for use as additional codes that provide useful information on circumstances that may affect a patient's care and treatment.

Prophylactic Organ Removal

For encounters specifically for prophylactic removal of an organ (such as prophylactic removal of breasts due to a genetic susceptibility to cancer or a family history of cancer), the principal or first-listed code should be a code from category Z40, Encounter for prophylactic surgery, followed by the appropriate codes to identify the associated risk factor (such as genetic susceptibility or family history).

If the patient has a malignancy of one site and is having prophylactic removal at another site to prevent either a new primary malignancy or metastatic disease, a code for the malignancy should also be assigned in addition to a code from subcategory Z40.0, Encounter for prophylactic surgery for risk factors related to malignant neoplasms. A Z40.0 code should not be assigned if the patient is having organ removal for treatment of a malignancy, such as the removal of the testes for the treatment of prostate cancer.

Miscellaneous Z codes/categories:

Z28 Immunization not carried out
Except: Z28.3-, Underimmunization status
Z29 Encounter for other prophylactic measures
Z40 Encounter for prophylactic surgery
Z41 Encounter for procedures for purposes other than remedying health state
Except: Z41.9, Encounter for procedure for purposes other than remedying health state, unspecified
Z53 Persons encountering health services for specific procedures and treatment, not carried out
Z72 Problems related to lifestyle
Note: These codes should be assigned only when the documentation specifies that the patient has an associated problem
Z73 Problems related to life management difficulty
Note: These codes should be assigned only when the documentation specifies that the patient has an associated problem.
Z74 Problems related to care provider dependency
Except: Z74.01, Bed confinement status
Z75 Problems related to medical facilities and other health care
Z76.0 Encounter for issue of repeat prescription
Z76.3 Healthy person accompanying sick person
Z76.4 Other boarder to healthcare facility
Z76.5 Malingerer [conscious simulation]
Z91.1- Patient's noncompliance with medical treatment and regimen
Z91.A- Caregiver's noncompliance with patient's medical treatment and regimen
Z91.83 Wandering in diseases classified elsewhere
Z91.84- Oral health risk factors
Z91.89 Other specified personal risk factors, not elsewhere classified

See Section I.B.14. for Z55-Z65 Persons with potential health hazards related to socioeconomic and psychosocial circumstances, documentation by clinicians other than the patient's provider

15) Nonspecific Z Codes

Certain Z codes are so non-specific, or potentially redundant with other codes in the classification, that there can be little justification for their use in the inpatient setting. Their use in the outpatient setting should be limited to those instances when there is no further documentation to permit more precise coding. Otherwise, any sign or symptom or any other reason for visit that is captured in another code should be used.

Nonspecific Z codes/categories:

Z02.9 Encounter for administrative examinations, unspecified
Z04.9 Encounter for examination and observation for unspecified reason
Z13.9 Encounter for screening, unspecified
Z41.9 Encounter for procedure for purposes other than remedying health state, unspecified
Z52.9 Donor of unspecified organ or tissue
Z86.59 Personal history of other mental and behavioral disorders
Z88.9 Allergy status to unspecified drugs, medicaments and biological substances status
Z92.0 Personal history of contraception

16) Z Codes That May Only be Principal/First-Listed Diagnosis

The following Z codes/categories may only be reported as the principal/first-listed diagnosis, except when there are multiple encounters on the same day and the medical records for the encounters are combined:

Z00 Encounter for general examination without complaint, suspected or reported diagnosis
Except: Z00.6
Z01 Encounter for other special examination without complaint, suspected or reported diagnosis
Z02 Encounter for administrative examination
Z04 Encounter for examination and observation for other reasons
Z33.2 Encounter for elective termination of pregnancy
Z31.81 Encounter for male factor infertility in female patient
Z31.83 Encounter for assisted reproductive fertility procedure cycle

Z31.84 Encounter for fertility preservation procedure
Z34 Encounter for supervision of normal pregnancy
Z39 Encounter for maternal postpartum care and examination
Z38 Liveborn infants according to place of birth and type of delivery
Z40 Encounter for prophylactic surgery
Z42 Encounter for plastic and reconstructive surgery following medical procedure or healed injury
Z51.0 Encounter for antineoplastic radiation therapy
Z51.1- Encounter for antineoplastic chemotherapy and immunotherapy
Z52 Donors of organs and tissues
Except: Z52.9, Donor of unspecified organ or tissue
Z76.1 Encounter for health supervision and care of foundling
Z76.2 Encounter for health supervision and care of other healthy infant and child
Z99.12 Encounter for respirator [ventilator] dependence during power failure

17) Social Determinants of Health

Social determinants of health (SDOH) codes describing social problems, conditions, or risk factors that influence a patient's health should be assigned when this information is documented in the patient's medical record. Assign as many SDOH codes as are necessary to describe all of the social problems, conditions, or risk factors documented during the current episode of care. For example, a patient who lives alone may suffer an acute injury temporarily impacting their ability to perform routine activities of daily living. When documented as such, this would support assignment of code Z60.2, Problems related to living alone. However, merely living alone, without documentation of a risk or unmet need for assistance at home, would not support assignment of code Z60.2. Documentation by a clinician (or patient-reported information that is signed off by a clinician) that the patient expressed concerns with access and availability of food would support assignment of code Z59.41, Food insecurity. Similarly, medical record documentation indicating the patient is homeless would support assignment of a code from subcategory Z59.0-, Homelessness.

For social determinants of health **classified to chapter 21**, such as information found in categories Z55-Z65, Persons with potential health hazards related to socioeconomic and psychosocial circumstances, code assignment may be based on medical record documentation from clinicians involved in the care of the patient who are not the patient's provider since this information represents social information, rather than medical diagnoses. For example, coding professionals may utilize documentation of social information from social workers, community health workers, case managers, or nurses, if their documentation is included in the official medical record.

Patient self-reported documentation may be used to assign codes for social determinants of health, as long as the patient self-reported information is signed-off by and incorporated into the medical record by either a clinician or provider.

Social determinants of health codes are located primarily in these Z code categories:

Z55 Problems related to education and literacy
Z56 Problems related to employment and unemployment
Z57 Occupational exposure to risk factors
Z58 Problems related to physical environment
Z59 Problems related to housing and economic circumstances
Z60 Problems related to social environment
Z62 Problems related to upbringing
Z63 Other problems related to primary support group, including family circumstances
Z64 Problems related to certain psychosocial circumstances
Z65 Problems related to other psychosocial circumstances

See Section I.B.14. Documentation by Clinicians Other than the Patient's Provider.

22. Chapter 22: Codes for Special Purposes (U00-U85)

U07.0 Vaping-related disorder (see Section I.C.10.e., Vaping-related disorders)
U07.1 COVID-19 (see Section I.C.1.g.1., COVID-19 infection)
U09.9 Post COVID-19 condition, unspecified (see Section I.C.1.g.1.m.)

Section II. Selection of Principal Diagnosis

The circumstances of inpatient admission always govern the selection of principal diagnosis. The principal diagnosis is defined in the Uniform Hospital Discharge Data Set (UHDDS) as "that condition established after study to be chiefly responsible for occasioning the admission of the patient to the hospital for care."

The UHDDS definitions are used by hospitals to report inpatient data elements in a standardized manner. These data elements and their definitions can be found in the July 31, 1985, Federal Register (Vol. 50, No, 147), pp. 31038-40.

Since that time, the application of the UHDDS definitions has been expanded to include all non-outpatient settings (acute care, short term, long term care and psychiatric hospitals; home health agencies; rehab facilities; nursing homes, etc.). The UHDDS definitions also apply to hospice services (all levels of care).

In determining principal diagnosis, coding conventions in the ICD-10-CM, the Tabular List and Alphabetic Index take precedence over these official coding guidelines.

(See Section I.A., Conventions for the ICD-10-CM)

The importance of consistent, complete documentation in the medical record cannot be overemphasized. Without such documentation the application of all coding guidelines is a difficult, if not impossible, task.

A. Codes for symptoms, signs, and ill-defined conditions

Codes for symptoms, signs, and ill-defined conditions from Chapter 18 are not to be used as principal diagnosis when a related definitive diagnosis has been established.

B. Two or more interrelated conditions, each potentially meeting the definition for principal diagnosis.

When there are two or more interrelated conditions (such as diseases in the same ICD-10-CM chapter or manifestations characteristically associated with a certain disease) potentially meeting the definition of principal diagnosis, either condition may be sequenced first, unless the circumstances of the admission, the therapy provided, the Tabular List, or the Alphabetic Index indicate otherwise.

C. Two or more diagnoses that equally meet the definition for principal diagnosis

In the unusual instance when two or more diagnoses equally meet the criteria for principal diagnosis as determined by the circumstances of admission, diagnostic workup and/or therapy provided, and the Alphabetic Index, Tabular List, or another coding guidelines does not provide sequencing direction, any one of the diagnoses may be sequenced first.

D. Two or more comparative or contrasting conditions

In those rare instances when two or more contrasting or comparative diagnoses are documented as "either/or" (or similar terminology), they are coded as if the diagnoses were confirmed and the diagnoses are sequenced according to the circumstances of the admission. If no further determination can be made as to which diagnosis should be principal, either diagnosis may be sequenced first.

E. A symptom(s) followed by contrasting/comparative diagnoses

GUIDELINE HAS BEEN DELETED EFFECTIVE OCTOBER 1, 2014

F. Original treatment plan not carried out

Sequence as the principal diagnosis the condition, which after study occasioned the admission to the hospital, even though treatment may not have been carried out due to unforeseen circumstances.

G. Complications of surgery and other medical care

When the admission is for treatment of a complication resulting from surgery or other medical care, the complication code is sequenced as the principal diagnosis. If the complication is classified to the T80-T88 series and the code lacks the necessary specificity in describing the complication, an additional code for the specific complication should be assigned.

H. Uncertain Diagnosis

If the diagnosis documented at the time of discharge is qualified as "probable," "suspected," "likely," "questionable," "possible," or "still to be ruled out," "compatible with," "consistent with," or other similar terms indicating uncertainty, code the condition as if it existed or was established. The bases for these guidelines are the diagnostic workup, arrangements for further workup or observation, and initial therapeutic approach that correspond most closely with the established diagnosis.

Note: This guideline is applicable only to inpatient admissions to short-term, acute, long-term care and psychiatric hospitals.

I. Admission from Observation Unit

1. Admission Following Medical Observation

When a patient is admitted to an observation unit for a medical condition, which either worsens or does not improve, and is subsequently admitted as an inpatient of the same hospital for this same medical condition, the principal diagnosis would be the medical condition which led to the hospital admission.

2. Admission Following Post-Operative Observation

When a patient is admitted to an observation unit to monitor a condition (or complication) that develops following outpatient surgery, and then is subsequently admitted as an inpatient of the same hospital, hospitals should apply the Uniform Hospital Discharge Data Set (UHDDS) definition of principal diagnosis as "that condition established after study to be chiefly responsible for occasioning the admission of the patient to the hospital for care."

J. Admission from Outpatient Surgery

When a patient receives surgery in the hospital's outpatient surgery department and is subsequently admitted for continuing inpatient care at the same hospital, the following guidelines should be followed in selecting the principal diagnosis for the inpatient admission:

- If the reason for the inpatient admission is a complication, assign the complication as the principal diagnosis.
- If no complication, or other condition, is documented as the reason for the inpatient admission, assign the reason for the outpatient surgery as the principal diagnosis.
- If the reason for the inpatient admission is another condition unrelated to the surgery, assign the unrelated condition as the principal diagnosis.

K. Admissions/Encounters for Rehabilitation

When the purpose for the admission/encounter is rehabilitation, sequence first the code for the condition for which the service is being performed. For example, for an admission/encounter for rehabilitation for right-sided dominant hemiplegia following a cerebrovascular infarction, report code I69.351, Hemiplegia and hemiparesis following cerebral infarction affecting right dominant side, as the first-listed or principal diagnosis.

If the condition for which the rehabilitation service is being provided is no longer present, report the appropriate aftercare code as the first-listed or principal diagnosis, unless the rehabilitation service is being provided following an injury. For rehabilitation services following active treatment of an injury, assign the injury code with the appropriate seventh character for subsequent encounter as the first-listed or principal diagnosis. For example, if a patient with severe degenerative osteoarthritis of the hip, underwent hip replacement and the current encounter/admission is for rehabilitation, report code Z47.1, Aftercare following joint replacement surgery, as the first-listed or principal diagnosis. If the patient requires rehabilitation post hip replacement for right intertrochanteric femur fracture, report code S72.141D, Displaced intertrochanteric fracture of right femur, subsequent encounter for closed fracture with routine healing, as the first-listed or principal diagnosis.

See Section I.C.21.c.7., Factors influencing health states and contact with health services, Aftercare.

See Section I.C.19.a., for additional information about the use of 7th characters for injury codes.

Section III. Reporting Additional Diagnoses

GENERAL RULES FOR OTHER (ADDITIONAL) DIAGNOSES

For reporting purposes, the definition for "other diagnoses" is interpreted as additional **clinically significant** conditions that affect patient care in terms of requiring:

clinical evaluation; or
therapeutic treatment; or
diagnostic procedures; or
extended length of hospital stay; or
increased nursing care and/or monitoring.

The UHDDS item #11-b defines Other Diagnoses as "all conditions that coexist at the time of admission, that develop subsequently, or that affect the treatment received and/or the length of stay. Diagnoses that relate to an earlier episode which have no bearing on the current hospital stay are to be excluded." UHDDS definitions apply to inpatients in acute care, short-term, long term care and psychiatric hospital setting. The UHDDS definitions are used by acute care short-term hospitals to report inpatient data elements in a standardized manner. These data elements and their definitions can be found in the July 31, 1985, Federal Register (Vol. 50, No, 147), pp. 31038-40.

Since that time, the application of the UHDDS definitions has been expanded to include all non-outpatient settings (acute care, short term, long term care and psychiatric hospitals; home health agencies; rehab facilities; nursing homes, etc.). The UHDDS definitions also apply to hospice services (all levels of care).

The following guidelines are to be applied in designating "other diagnoses" when neither the Alphabetic Index nor the Tabular List in ICD-10-CM provide direction. The listing of the diagnoses in the patient record is the responsibility of the provider.

A. Previous conditions

If the provider has included a diagnosis in the final diagnostic statement, such as the discharge summary or the face sheet, it should ordinarily be coded. Some providers include in the diagnostic statement resolved conditions or diagnoses and status-post procedures from previous admissions that have no bearing on the current stay. Such conditions are not to be reported and are coded only if required by hospital policy.

However, history codes (categories Z80-Z87) may be used as secondary codes if the historical condition or family history has an impact on current care or influences treatment.

B. Abnormal findings

Abnormal findings (laboratory, x-ray, pathologic, and other diagnostic results) are not coded and reported unless the provider indicates their clinical significance. If the findings are outside the normal range and the provider has ordered other tests to evaluate the condition or prescribed treatment, it is appropriate to ask the provider whether the abnormal finding should be added.

Please note: This differs from the coding practices in the outpatient setting for coding encounters for diagnostic tests that have been interpreted by a provider.

C. Uncertain Diagnosis

If the diagnosis documented at the time of discharge is qualified as "probable," "suspected," "likely," "questionable," "possible," or "still to be ruled out," "compatible with," "consistent with," or other similar terms indicating uncertainty, code the condition as if it existed or was established. The bases for these guidelines are the diagnostic workup, arrangements for further workup or observation, and initial therapeutic approach that correspond most closely with the established diagnosis.

Note: This guideline is applicable only to inpatient admissions to short-term, acute, long-term care and psychiatric hospitals.

Section IV. Diagnostic Coding and Reporting Guidelines for Outpatient Services

These coding guidelines for outpatient diagnoses have been approved for use by hospitals/ providers in coding and reporting hospital-based outpatient services and provider-based office visits. Guidelines in Section I, Conventions, general coding guidelines and chapter-specific guidelines, should also be applied for outpatient services and office visits.

Information about the use of certain abbreviations, punctuation, symbols, and other conventions used in the ICD-10-CM Tabular List (code numbers and titles), can be found in Section IA of these guidelines, under "Conventions Used in the Tabular List." Section I.B. contains general guidelines that apply to the entire classification. Section I.C. contains chapter-specific guidelines that correspond to the chapters as they are arranged in the classification. Information about the correct sequence to use in finding a code is also described in Section I.

The terms encounter and visit are often used interchangeably in describing outpatient service contacts and, therefore, appear together in these guidelines without distinguishing one from the other.

Though the conventions and general guidelines apply to all settings, coding guidelines for outpatient and provider reporting of diagnoses will vary in a number of instances from those for inpatient diagnoses, recognizing that:

The Uniform Hospital Discharge Data Set (UHDDS) definition of principal diagnosis does not apply to hospital-based outpatient services and provider-based office visits.

Coding guidelines for inconclusive diagnoses (probable, suspected, rule out, etc.) were developed for inpatient reporting and do not apply to outpatients.

A. Selection of first-listed condition

In the outpatient setting, the term first-listed diagnosis is used in lieu of principal diagnosis.

In determining the first-listed diagnosis the coding conventions of ICD-10-CM, as well as the general and disease specific guidelines take precedence over the outpatient guidelines.

Diagnoses often are not established at the time of the initial encounter/visit. It may take two or more visits before the diagnosis is confirmed.

The most critical rule involves beginning the search for the correct code assignment through the Alphabetic Index. Never begin searching initially in the Tabular List as this will lead to coding errors.

1. Outpatient Surgery

When a patient presents for outpatient surgery (same day surgery), code the reason for the surgery as the first-listed diagnosis (reason for the encounter), even if the surgery is not performed due to a contraindication.

2. Observation Stay

When a patient is admitted for observation for a medical condition, assign a code for the medical condition as the first-listed diagnosis.

When a patient presents for outpatient surgery and develops complications requiring admission to observation, code the reason for the surgery as the first reported diagnosis (reason for the encounter), followed by codes for the complications as secondary diagnoses.

B. Codes from A00.0 through T88.9, Z00-Z99, U00-U85

The appropriate code(s) from A00.0 through T88.9, Z00-Z99 and U00-U85 must be used to identify diagnoses, symptoms, conditions, problems, complaints, or other reason(s) for the encounter/visit.

C. Accurate reporting of ICD-10-CM diagnosis codes

For accurate reporting of ICD-10-CM diagnosis codes, the documentation should describe the patient's condition, using terminology which includes specific diagnoses as well as symptoms, problems, or reasons for the encounter. There are ICD-10-CM codes to describe all of these.

D. Codes that describe symptoms and signs

Codes that describe symptoms and signs, as opposed to diagnoses, are acceptable for reporting purposes when a diagnosis has not been established (confirmed) by the provider. Chapter 18 of ICD-10-CM, Symptoms, Signs, and Abnormal Clinical and Laboratory Findings Not Elsewhere Classified (codes RØØ-R99) contain many, but not all codes for symptoms.

E. Encounters for circumstances other than a disease or injury

ICD-10-CM provides codes to deal with encounters for circumstances other than a disease or injury. The Factors Influencing Health Status and Contact with Health Services codes (ZØØ-Z99) are provided to deal with occasions when circumstances other than a disease or injury are recorded as diagnosis or problems.

See Section I.C.21. Factors influencing health status and contact with health services.

F. Level of Detail in Coding

1. ICD-10-CM codes with 3, 4, 5, 6 or 7 characters

ICD-10-CM is composed of codes with 3, 4, 5, 6 or 7 characters. Codes with three characters are included in ICD-10-CM as the heading of a category of codes that may be further subdivided by the use of fourth, fifth, sixth or seventh characters to provide greater specificity.

2. Use of full number of characters required for a code

A three-character code is to be used only if it is not further subdivided. A code is invalid if it has not been coded to the full number of characters required for that code, including the 7th character, if applicable.

3. Highest level of specificity

Code to the highest level of specificity when supported by the medical record documentation.

G. ICD-10-CM code for the diagnosis, condition, problem, or other reason for encounter/visit

List first the ICD-10-CM code for the diagnosis, condition, problem, or other reason for encounter/visit shown in the medical record to be chiefly responsible for the services provided. List additional codes that describe any coexisting conditions. In some cases, the first-listed diagnosis may be a symptom when a diagnosis has not been established (confirmed) by the provider.

H. Uncertain diagnosis

Do not code diagnoses documented as "probable", "suspected," "questionable," "rule out," "compatible with," "consistent with," or "working diagnosis" or other similar terms indicating uncertainty. Rather, code the condition(s) to the highest degree of certainty for that encounter/visit, such as symptoms, signs, abnormal test results, or other reason for the visit.

Please note: This differs from the coding practices used by short-term, acute care, long-term care and psychiatric hospitals.

I. Chronic diseases

Chronic diseases treated on an ongoing basis may be coded and reported as many times as the patient receives treatment and care for the condition(s)

J. Code all documented conditions that coexist

Code all documented conditions that coexist at the time of the encounter/visit and that require or affect patient care, treatment or management. Do not code conditions that were previously treated and no longer exist. However, history codes (categories Z8Ø-Z87) may be used as secondary codes if the historical condition or family history has an impact on current care or influences treatment.

K. Patients receiving diagnostic services only

For patients receiving diagnostic services only during an encounter/visit, sequence first the diagnosis, condition, problem, or other reason for encounter/visit shown in the medical record to be chiefly responsible for the outpatient services provided during the encounter/visit. Codes for other diagnoses (e.g., chronic conditions) may be sequenced as additional diagnoses.

For encounters for routine laboratory/radiology testing in the absence of any signs, symptoms, or associated diagnosis, assign ZØ1.89, Encounter for other specified special examinations. If routine testing is performed during the same encounter as a test to evaluate a sign, symptom, or diagnosis, it is appropriate to assign both the Z code and the code describing the reason for the non-routine test.

For outpatient encounters for diagnostic tests that have been interpreted by a physician, and the final report is available at the time of coding, code any confirmed or definitive diagnosis(es) documented in the interpretation. Do not code related signs and symptoms as additional diagnoses.

Please note: This differs from the coding practice in the hospital inpatient setting regarding abnormal findings on test results.

L. Patients receiving therapeutic services only

For patients receiving therapeutic services only during an encounter/visit, sequence first the diagnosis, condition, problem, or other reason for encounter/visit shown in the medical record to be chiefly responsible for the outpatient services provided during the encounter/visit. Codes for other diagnoses (e.g., chronic conditions) may be sequenced as additional diagnoses.

The only exception to this rule is that when the primary reason for the admission/encounter is chemotherapy or radiation therapy, the appropriate Z code for the service is listed first, and the diagnosis or problem for which the service is being performed listed second.

M. Patients receiving preoperative evaluations only

For patients receiving preoperative evaluations only, sequence first a code from subcategory ZØ1.81, Encounter for pre-procedural examinations, to describe the pre-op consultations. Assign a code for the condition to describe the reason for the surgery as an additional diagnosis. Code also any findings related to the pre-op evaluation.

N. Ambulatory surgery

For ambulatory surgery, code the diagnosis for which the surgery was performed. If the postoperative diagnosis is known to be different from the preoperative diagnosis at the time the diagnosis is confirmed, select the postoperative diagnosis for coding, since it is the most definitive.

O. Routine outpatient prenatal visits

See Section I.C.15. Routine outpatient prenatal visits.

P. Encounters for general medical examinations with abnormal findings

The subcategories for encounters for general medical examinations, ZØØ.Ø- and encounter for routine child health examination, ZØØ.12-, provide codes for with and without abnormal findings. Should a general medical examination result in an abnormal finding, the code for general medical examination with abnormal finding should be assigned as the first-listed diagnosis. An examination with abnormal findings refers to a condition/diagnosis that is newly identified or a change in severity of a chronic condition (such as uncontrolled hypertension, or an acute exacerbation of chronic obstructive pulmonary disease) during a routine physical examination. A secondary code for the abnormal finding should also be coded.

Q. Encounters for routine health screenings

See Section I.C.21. Factors influencing health status and contact with health services, Screening

Appendix I. Present on Admission Reporting Guidelines

Introduction

These guidelines are to be used as a supplement to the *ICD-10-CM Official Guidelines for Coding and Reporting* to facilitate the assignment of the Present on Admission (POA) indicator for each diagnosis and external cause of injury code reported on claim forms (UB-04 and 837 Institutional).

These guidelines are not intended to replace any guidelines in the main body of the *ICD-10-CM Official Guidelines for Coding and Reporting*. The POA guidelines are not intended to provide guidance on when a condition should be coded, but rather, how to apply the POA indicator to the final set of diagnosis codes that have been assigned in accordance with Sections I, II, and III of the official coding guidelines. Subsequent to the assignment of the ICD-10-CM codes, the POA indicator should then be assigned to those conditions that have been coded.

As stated in the Introduction to the *ICD-10-CM Official Guidelines for Coding and Reporting*, a joint effort between the healthcare provider and the coder is essential to achieve complete and accurate documentation, code assignment, and reporting of diagnoses and procedures. The importance of consistent, complete documentation in the medical record cannot be overemphasized. Medical record documentation from any provider involved in the care and treatment of the patient may be used to support the determination of whether a condition was present on admission or not. In the context of the official coding guidelines, the term "provider" means a physician or any qualified healthcare practitioner who is legally accountable for establishing the patient's diagnosis.

These guidelines are not a substitute for the provider's clinical judgment as to the determination of whether a condition was/was not present on admission. The provider should be queried regarding issues related to the linking of signs/symptoms, timing of test results, and the timing of findings.

Please see the CDC website for the detailed list of ICD-10-CM codes that do not require the use of a POA indicator (https://www.cdc.gov/nchs/icd/icd10cm.htm). The codes and categories on this exempt list are for circumstances regarding the healthcare encounter or factors influencing health status that do not represent a current disease or injury or that describe conditions that are always present on admission.

General Reporting Requirements

All claims involving inpatient admissions to general acute care hospitals or other facilities that are subject to a law or regulation mandating collection of present on admission information.

Present on admission is defined as present at the time the order for inpatient admission occurs -- conditions that develop during an outpatient encounter, including emergency department, observation, or outpatient surgery, are considered as present on admission.

POA indicator is assigned to principal and secondary diagnoses (as defined in Section II of the Official Guidelines for Coding and Reporting) and the external cause of injury codes.

Issues related to inconsistent, missing, conflicting or unclear documentation must still be resolved by the provider.

If a condition would not be coded and reported based on UHDDS definitions and current official coding guidelines, then the POA indicator would not be reported.

Reporting Options

Y – Yes

N – No

U – Unknown

W – Clinically undetermined

Unreported/Not used – (Exempt from POA reporting)

Reporting Definitions

Y = present at the time of inpatient admission

N = not present at the time of inpatient admission

U = documentation is insufficient to determine if condition is present on admission

W = provider is unable to clinically determine whether condition was present on admission or not

Timeframe for POA Identification and Documentation

There is no required timeframe as to when a provider (per the definition of "provider" used in these guidelines) must identify or document a condition to be present on admission. In some clinical situations, it may not be possible for a provider to make a definitive diagnosis (or a condition may not be recognized or reported by the patient) for a period of time after admission. In some cases, it may be several days before the provider arrives at a definitive diagnosis. This does not mean that the condition was not present on admission. Determination of whether the condition was present on admission or not will be based on the applicable POA guideline as identified in this document, or on the provider's best clinical judgment.

If at the time of code assignment the documentation is unclear as to whether a condition was present on admission or not, it is appropriate to query the provider for clarification.

Assigning the POA Indicator

Condition is on the "Exempt from Reporting" list

Leave the "present on admission" field blank if the condition is on the list of ICD-10-CM codes for which this field is not applicable. This is the only circumstance in which the field may be left blank.

POA Explicitly Documented

Assign Y for any condition the provider explicitly documents as being present on admission.

Assign N for any condition the provider explicitly documents as not present at the time of admission.

Conditions diagnosed prior to inpatient admission

Assign "Y" for conditions that were diagnosed prior to admission (example: hypertension, diabetes mellitus, asthma)

Conditions diagnosed during the admission but clearly present before admission

Assign "Y" for conditions diagnosed during the admission that were clearly present but not diagnosed until after admission occurred.

Diagnoses subsequently confirmed after admission are considered present on admission if at the time of admission they are documented as suspected, possible, rule out, differential diagnosis, or constitute an underlying cause of a symptom that is present at the time of admission.

Condition develops during outpatient encounter prior to inpatient admission

Assign Y for any condition that develops during an outpatient encounter prior to a written order for inpatient admission.

Documentation does not indicate whether condition was present on admission

Assign "U" when the medical record documentation is unclear as to whether the condition was present on admission. "U" should not be routinely assigned and used only in very limited circumstances. Coders are encouraged to query the providers when the documentation is unclear.

Documentation states that it cannot be determined whether the condition was or was not present on admission

Assign "W" when the medical record documentation indicates that it cannot be clinically determined whether or not the condition was present on admission.

Chronic condition with acute exacerbation during the admission

If a single code identifies both the chronic condition and the acute exacerbation, see POA guidelines pertaining to codes that contain multiple clinical concepts.

If a single code only identifies the chronic condition and not the acute exacerbation (e.g., acute exacerbation of chronic leukemia), assign "Y."

Conditions documented as possible, probable, suspected, or rule out at the time of discharge

If the final diagnosis contains a possible, probable, suspected, or rule out diagnosis, and this diagnosis was based on signs, symptoms or clinical findings suspected at the time of inpatient admission, assign "Y."

If the final diagnosis contains a possible, probable, suspected, or rule out diagnosis, and this diagnosis was based on signs, symptoms or clinical findings that were not present on admission, assign "N".

Conditions documented as impending or threatened at the time of discharge

If the final diagnosis contains an impending or threatened diagnosis, and this diagnosis is based on symptoms or clinical findings that were present on admission, assign "Y".

If the final diagnosis contains an impending or threatened diagnosis, and this diagnosis is based on symptoms or clinical findings that were not present on admission, assign "N".

Acute and Chronic Conditions

Assign "Y" for acute conditions that are present at time of admission and N for acute conditions that are not present at time of admission.

Assign "Y" for chronic conditions, even though the condition may not be diagnosed until after admission.

If a single code identifies both an acute and chronic condition, see the POA guidelines for codes that contain multiple clinical concepts.

Codes That Contain Multiple Clinical Concepts

Assign "N" if at least one of the clinical concepts included in the code was not present on admission (e.g., COPD with acute exacerbation and the exacerbation was not present on admission; gastric ulcer that does not start bleeding until after admission; asthma patient develops status asthmaticus after admission).

Assign "Y" if all of the clinical concepts included in the code were present on admission (e.g., duodenal ulcer that perforates prior to admission).

For infection codes that include the causal organism, assign "Y" if the infection (or signs of the infection) were present on admission, even though the culture results may not be known until after admission (e.g., patient is admitted with pneumonia and the provider documents Pseudomonas as the causal organism a few days later).

Same Diagnosis Code for Two or More Conditions

When the same ICD-10-CM diagnosis code applies to two or more conditions during the same encounter (e.g. two separate conditions classified to the same ICD-10-CM diagnosis code):

Assign "Y" if all conditions represented by the single ICD-10-CM code were present on admission (e.g. bilateral unspecified age-related cataracts).

Assign "N" if any of the conditions represented by the single ICD-10-CM code was not present on admission (e.g. traumatic secondary and recurrent hemorrhage and seroma is assigned to a single code T79.2, but only one of the conditions was present on admission).

Obstetrical conditions

Whether or not the patient delivers during the current hospitalization does not affect assignment of the POA indicator. The determining factor for POA assignment is whether the pregnancy complication or obstetrical condition described by the code was present at the time of admission or not.

If the pregnancy complication or obstetrical condition was present on admission (e.g., patient admitted in preterm labor), assign "Y".

If the pregnancy complication or obstetrical condition was not present on admission (e.g., 2nd degree laceration during delivery, postpartum hemorrhage that occurred during current hospitalization, fetal distress develops after admission), assign "N".

If the obstetrical code includes more than one diagnosis and any of the diagnoses identified by the code were not present on admission assign "N". (e.g., Category O11, Pre-existing hypertension with pre-eclampsia)

Perinatal conditions

Newborns are not considered to be admitted until after birth. Therefore, any condition present at birth or that developed in utero is considered present at admission and should be assigned "Y". This includes conditions that occur during delivery (e.g., injury during delivery, meconium aspiration, exposure to streptococcus B in the vaginal canal).

Congenital conditions and anomalies

Assign "Y" for congenital conditions and anomalies except for categories QØØ-Q99, Congenital anomalies, which are on the exempt list. Congenital conditions are always considered present on admission.

External cause of injury codes

Assign "Y" for any external cause code representing an external cause of morbidity that occurred prior to inpatient admission (e.g., patient fell out of bed at home, patient fell out of bed in emergency room prior to admission)

Assign "N" for any external cause code representing an external cause of morbidity that occurred during inpatient hospitalization (e.g., patient fell out of hospital bed during hospital stay, patient experienced an adverse reaction to a medication administered after inpatient admission).

ICD-10-CM Index to Diseases and Injuries

A

Aarskog's syndrome Q87.19
Abandonment — *see* Maltreatment
Abasia (-astasia) (hysterical) F44.4
Abderhalden-Kaufmann-Lignac syndrome (cystinosis) E72.Ø4
Abdomen, abdominal — *see also* condition
acute R1Ø.Ø
angina K55.1
muscle deficiency syndrome Q79.4
Abdominalgia — *see* Pain, abdominal
Abduction contracture, hip or other joint — *see* Contraction, joint
Aberrant (congenital) — *see also* Malposition, congenital
adrenal gland Q89.1
artery (peripheral) Q27.8
basilar NEC Q28.1
cerebral Q28.3
coronary Q24.5
digestive system Q27.8
eye Q15.8
lower limb Q27.8
precerebral Q28.1
pulmonary Q25.79
renal Q27.2
retina Q14.1
specified site NEC Q27.8
subclavian Q27.8
upper limb Q27.8
vertebral Q28.1
breast Q83.8
endocrine gland NEC Q89.2
hepatic duct Q44.5
pancreas Q45.3
parathyroid gland Q89.2
pituitary gland Q89.2
sebaceous glands, mucous membrane, mouth, congenital Q38.6
spleen Q89.Ø9
subclavian artery Q27.8
thymus (gland) Q89.2
thyroid gland Q89.2
vein (peripheral) NEC Q27.8
cerebral Q28.3
digestive system Q27.8
lower limb Q27.8
precerebral Q28.1
specified site NEC Q27.8
upper limb Q27.8
Aberration
distantial — *see* Disturbance, visual
mental F99
Abetalipoproteinemia E78.6
Abiotrophy R68.89
Ablatio, ablation
retinae — *see* Detachment, retina
Ablepharia, ablepharon Q1Ø.3
Abnormal, abnormality, abnormalities — *see also* Anomaly
acid-base balance (mixed) E87.4
albumin R77.Ø
alphafetoprotein R77.2
alveolar ridge KØ8.9
anatomical relationship Q89.9
apertures, congenital, diaphragm Q79.1
atrial septal, specified NEC Q21.19
auditory perception H93.29- ☑
diplacusis — *see* Diplacusis
hyperacusis — *see* Hyperacusis
recruitment — *see* Recruitment, auditory
threshold shift — *see* Shift, auditory threshold
autosomes Q99.9
fragile site Q95.5
basal metabolic rate R94.8
biosynthesis, testicular androgen E29.1
bleeding time R79.1
blood amino-acid level R79.83
blood level (of)
cobalt R79.Ø
copper R79.Ø
iron R79.Ø

Abnormal, abnormality, abnormalities — *continued*
blood level — *continued*
lithium R78.89
magnesium R79.Ø
mineral NEC R79.Ø
zinc R79.Ø
blood pressure
elevated RØ3.Ø
low reading (nonspecific) RØ3.1
blood sugar R73.Ø9
blood-gas level R79.81
bowel sounds R19.15
absent R19.11
hyperactive R19.12
brain scan R94.Ø2
breathing RØ6.9
caloric test R94.138
cerebrospinal fluid R83.9
cytology R83.6
drug level R83.2
enzyme level R83.Ø
hormones R83.1
immunology R83.4
microbiology R83.5
nonmedicinal level R83.3
specified type NEC R83.8
chemistry, blood R79.9
C-reactive protein R79.82
drugs — *see* Findings, abnormal, in blood
gas level R79.81
minerals R79.Ø
pancytopenia D61.818
PTT R79.1
specified NEC R79.89
toxins — *see* Findings, abnormal, in blood
chest sounds (friction) (rales) RØ9.89
chromosome, chromosomal Q99.9
with more than three X chromosomes, female Q97.1
analysis result R89.8
bronchial washings R84.8
cerebrospinal fluid R83.8
cervix uteri NEC R87.89
nasal secretions R84.8
nipple discharge R89.8
peritoneal fluid R85.89
pleural fluid R84.8
prostatic secretions R86.8
saliva R85.89
seminal fluid R86.8
sputum R84.8
synovial fluid R89.8
throat scrapings R84.8
vagina R87.89
vulva R87.89
wound secretions R89.8
dicentric replacement Q93.2
ring replacement Q93.2
sex Q99.8
female phenotype Q97.9
specified NEC Q97.8
male phenotype Q98.9
specified NEC Q98.8
structural male Q98.6
specified NEC Q99.8
clinical findings NEC R68.89
coagulation D68.9
newborn, transient P61.6
profile R79.1
time R79.1
communication — *see* Fistula
conjunctiva, vascular H11.41- ☑
coronary artery Q24.5
cortisol-binding globulin E27.8
course, eustachian tube Q17.8
creatinine clearance R94.4
cytology
anus R85.619
atypical squamous cells cannot exclude high grade squamous intraepithelial lesion (ASC-H) R85.611
atypical squamous cells of undetermined significance (ASC-US) R85.61Ø

Abnormal, abnormality, abnormalities — *continued*
cytology — *continued*
anus — *continued*
cytologic evidence of malignancy R85.614
high grade squamous intraepithelial lesion (HGSIL) R85.613
human papillomavirus (HPV) DNA test
high risk positive R85.81
low risk postive R85.82
inadequate smear R85.615
low grade squamous intraepithelial lesion (LGSIL) R85.612
satisfactory anal smear but lacking transformation zone R85.616
specified NEC R85.618
unsatisfactory smear R85.615
female genital organs — *see* Abnormal, Papanicolaou (smear)
dark adaptation curve H53.61
dentofacial NEC — *see* Anomaly, dentofacial
development, developmental Q89.9
central nervous system QØ7.9
diagnostic imaging
abdomen, abdominal region NEC R93.5
biliary tract R93.2
bladder R93.41
breast R92.8
central nervous system NEC R9Ø.89
cerebrovascular NEC R9Ø.89
coronary circulation R93.1
digestive tract NEC R93.3
gastrointestinal (tract) R93.3
genitourinary organs R93.89
head R93.Ø
heart R93.1
intrathoracic organ NEC R93.89
kidney R93.42- ☑
limbs R93.6
liver R93.2
lung (field) R91.8
musculoskeletal system NEC R93.7
renal pelvis R93.41
retroperitoneum R93.5
site specified NEC R93.89
skin and subcutaneous tissue R93.89
skull R93.Ø
testis R93.81- ☑
ureter R93.41
urinary organs specified NEC R93.49
direction, teeth, fully erupted M26.3Ø
ear ossicles, acquired NEC H74.39- ☑
ankylosis — *see* Ankylosis, ear ossicles
discontinuity — *see* Discontinuity, ossicles, ear
partial loss — *see* Loss, ossicles, ear (partial)
Ebstein Q22.5
echocardiogram R93.1
echoencephalogram R9Ø.81
echogram — *see* Abnormal, diagnostic imaging
electrocardiogram [ECG] [EKG] R94.31
electroencephalogram [EEG] R94.Ø1
electrolyte — *see* Imbalance, electrolyte
electromyogram [EMG] R94.131
electro-oculogram [EOG] R94.11Ø
electrophysiological intracardiac studies R94.39
electroretinogram [ERG] R94.111
erythrocytes
congenital, with perinatal jaundice D58.9
feces (color) (contents) (mucus) R19.5
finding — *see* Findings, abnormal, without diagnosis
fluid
amniotic — *see* Abnormal, specimen, specified
cerebrospinal — *see* Abnormal, cerebrospinal fluid
peritoneal — *see* Abnormal, specimen, digestive organs
pleural — *see* Abnormal, specimen, respiratory organs
synovial — *see* Abnormal, specimen, specified
thorax (bronchial washings) (pleural fluid) — *see* Abnormal, specimen, respiratory organs
vaginal — *see* Abnormal, specimen, female genital organs

Abnormal, abnormality, abnormalities — *continued*
- form
  - teeth K00.2
  - uterus — *see* Anomaly, uterus
- function studies
  - auditory R94.120
  - bladder R94.8
  - brain R94.09
  - cardiovascular R94.30
  - ear R94.128
  - endocrine NEC R94.7
  - eye NEC R94.118
  - kidney R94.4
  - liver R94.5
  - nervous system
    - central NEC R94.09
    - peripheral NEC R94.138
  - pancreas R94.8
  - placenta R94.8
  - pulmonary R94.2
  - special senses NEC R94.128
  - spleen R94.8
  - thyroid R94.6
  - vestibular R94.121
- gait — *see* Gait
  - hysterical F44.4
- gastrin secretion E16.4
- globulin R77.1
  - cortisol-binding E27.8
  - thyroid-binding E07.89
- glomerular, minor — *see also* N00-N07 with fourth character .0 N05.0
- glucagon secretion E16.3
- glucose tolerance (test) (non-fasting) R73.09
- gravitational (G) forces or states (effect of) T75.81 ☑
- hair (color) (shaft) L67.9
  - specified NEC L67.8
- hard tissue formation in pulp (dental) K04.3
- head movement R25.0
- heart
  - rate R00.9
    - specified NEC R00.8
  - shadow R93.1
  - sounds NEC R01.2
- hemoglobin (disease) — *see also* Disease, hemoglobin D58.2
  - trait — *see* Trait, hemoglobin, abnormal
- histology NEC R89.7
- immunological findings R89.4
  - in serum R76.9
    - specified NEC R76.8
- increase in appetite R63.2
- involuntary movement — *see* Abnormal, movement, involuntary
- jaw closure M26.51
- karyotype R89.8
- kidney function test R94.4
- knee jerk R29.2
- leukocyte (cell) (differential) NEC D72.9
- liver function test — *see also* Elevated, liver function, test R79.89
- loss of
  - height R29.890
  - weight R63.4
- mammogram NEC R92.8
  - calcification (calculus) R92.1
  - microcalcification R92.0
- Mantoux test R76.11
- movement (disorder) — *see also* Disorder, movement
  - head R25.0
  - involuntary R25.9
    - fasciculation R25.3
    - of head R25.0
    - spasm R25.2
    - specified type NEC R25.8
    - tremor R25.1
- myoglobin (Aberdeen) (Annapolis) R89.7
- neonatal screening P09.9
  - for
    - congenital adrenal hyperplasia P09.2
    - congenital endocrine disease P09.2
    - congenital hematologic disorders P09.3
    - critical congenital heart disease P09.5
    - cystic fibrosis P09.4
    - hemoglobinopathy P09.3
    - hypothyroidism P09.2
    - inborn errors of metabolism P09.1

Abnormal, abnormality, abnormalities — *continued*
- neonatal screening — *continued*
  - for — *continued*
    - neonatal hearing loss P09.6
    - red cell membrane defects P09.3
    - sickle cell P09.3
    - specified NEC P09.8
- oculomotor study R94.113
- palmar creases Q82.8
- Papanicolaou (smear)
  - anus R85.619
    - atypical squamous cells cannot exclude high grade squamous intraepithelial lesion (ASC-H) R85.611
    - atypical squamous cells of undetermined significance (ASC-US) R85.610
    - cytologic evidence of malignancy R85.614
    - high grade squamous intraepithelial lesion (HGSIL) R85.613
    - human papillomavirus (HPV) DNA test
      - high risk positive R85.81
      - low risk postive R85.82
    - inadequate smear R85.615
    - low grade squamous intraepithelial lesion (LGSIL) R85.612
    - satisfactory anal smear but lacking transformation zone R85.616
    - specified NEC R85.618
    - unsatisfactory smear R85.615
  - bronchial washings R84.6
  - cerebrospinal fluid R83.6
  - cervix R87.619
    - atypical squamous cells cannot exclude high grade squamous intraepithelial lesion (ASC-H) R87.611
    - atypical squamous cells of undetermined significance (ASC-US) R87.610
    - cytologic evidence of malignancy R87.614
    - high grade squamous intraepithelial lesion (HGSIL) R87.613
    - inadequate smear R87.615
    - low grade squamous intraepithelial lesion (LGSIL) R87.612
    - non-atypical endometrial cells R87.618
    - satisfactory cervical smear but lacking transformation zone R87.616
    - specified NEC R87.618
    - thin preparaton R87.619
    - unsatisfactory smear R87.615
  - nasal secretions R84.6
  - nipple discharge R89.6
  - peritoneal fluid R85.69
  - pleural fluid R84.6
  - prostatic secretions R86.6
  - saliva R85.69
  - seminal fluid R86.6
  - sites NEC R89.6
  - sputum R84.6
  - synovial fluid R89.6
  - throat scrapings R84.6
  - vagina R87.629
    - atypical squamous cells cannot exclude high grade squamous intraepithelial lesion (ASC-H) R87.621
    - atypical squamous cells of undetermined significance (ASC-US) R87.620
    - cytologic evidence of malignancy R87.624
    - high grade squamous intraepithelial lesion (HGSIL) R87.623
    - inadequate smear R87.625
    - low grade squamous intraepithelial lesion (LGSIL) R87.622
    - specified NEC R87.628
    - thin preparation R87.629
    - unsatisfactory smear R87.625
  - vulva R87.69
  - wound secretions R89.6
- partial thromboplastin time (PTT) R79.1
- pelvis (bony) — *see* Deformity, pelvis
- percussion, chest (tympany) R09.89
- periods (grossly) — *see* Menstruation
- phonocardiogram R94.39
- plantar reflex R29.2
- plasma
  - protein R77.9
    - specified NEC R77.8
  - viscosity R70.1
- pleural (folds) Q34.0

Abnormal, abnormality, abnormalities — *continued*
- posture R29.3
- product of conception O02.9
  - specified type NEC O02.89
- prothrombin time (PT) R79.1
- pulmonary
  - artery, congenital Q25.79
  - function, newborn P28.89
  - test results R94.2
- pulsations in neck R00.2
- pupillary H21.56- ☑
  - function (reaction) (reflex) — *see* Anomaly, pupil, function
- radiological examination — *see* Abnormal, diagnostic imaging
- red blood cell(s) (morphology) (volume) R71.8
- reflex — *see* Reflex
- renal function test R94.4
- response to nerve stimulation R94.130
- retinal correspondence H53.31
- retinal function study R94.111
- rhythm, heart — *see also* Arrhythmia
- saliva — *see* Abnormal, specimen, digestive organs
- scan
  - kidney R94.4
  - liver R93.2
  - thyroid R94.6
- secretion
  - gastrin E16.4
  - glucagon E16.3
- semen, seminal fluid — *see* Abnormal, specimen, male genital organs
- serum level (of)
  - acid phosphatase R74.8
  - alkaline phosphatase R74.8
  - amylase R74.8
  - enzymes R74.9
    - specified NEC R74.8
  - lipase R74.8
  - triacylglycerol lipase R74.8
- shape
  - gravid uterus — *see* Anomaly, uterus
- sinus venosus Q21.16
- size, tooth, teeth K00.2
- spacing, tooth, teeth, fully erupted M26.30
- specimen
  - digestive organs (peritoneal fluid) (saliva) R85.9
    - cytology R85.69
    - drug level R85.2
    - enzyme level R85.0
    - histology R85.7
    - hormones R85.1
    - immunology R85.4
    - microbiology R85.5
    - nonmedicinal level R85.3
    - specified type NEC R85.89
  - female genital organs (secretions) (smears) R87.9
    - cytology R87.69
      - cervix R87.619
        - human papillomavirus (HPV) DNA test
          - high risk positive R87.810
          - low risk positive R87.820
        - inadequate (unsatisfactory) smear R87.615
        - non-atypical endometrial cells R87.618
        - specified NEC R87.618
      - vagina R87.629
        - human papillomavirus (HPV) DNA test
          - high risk positive R87.811
          - low risk positive R87.821
        - inadequate (unsatisfactory) smear R87.625
      - vulva R87.69
    - drug level R87.2
    - enzyme level R87.0
    - histological R87.7
    - hormones R87.1
    - immunology R87.4
    - microbiology R87.5
    - nonmedicinal level R87.3
    - specified type NEC R87.89
  - male genital organs (prostatic secretions) (semen) R86.9
    - cytology R86.6
    - drug level R86.2
    - enzyme level R86.0
    - histological R86.7

Abnormal, abnormality, abnormalities — *continued*
- specimen — *continued*
  - male genital organs — *continued*
    - hormones R86.1
    - immunology R86.4
    - microbiology R86.5
    - nonmedicinal level R86.3
    - specified type NEC R86.8
  - nipple discharge — *see* Abnormal, specimen, specified
  - respiratory organs (bronchial washings) (nasal secretions) (pleural fluid) (sputum) R84.9
    - cytology R84.6
    - drug level R84.2
    - enzyme level R84.0
    - histology R84.7
    - hormones R84.1
    - immunology R84.4
    - microbiology R84.5
    - nonmedicinal level R84.3
    - specified type NEC R84.8
  - specified organ, system and tissue NOS R89.9
    - cytology R89.6
    - drug level R89.2
    - enzyme level R89.0
    - histology R89.7
    - hormones R89.1
    - immunology R89.4
    - microbiology R89.5
    - nonmedicinal level R89.3
    - specified type NEC R89.8
  - synovial fluid — *see* Abnormal, specimen, specified
  - thorax (bronchial washings) (pleural fluids) — *see* Abnormal, specimen, respiratory organs
  - vagina (secretion) (smear) R87.629
  - vulva (secretion) (smear) R87.69
  - wound secretion — *see* Abnormal, specimen, specified
- spermatozoa — *see* Abnormal, specimen, male genital organs
- sputum (amount) (color) (odor) R09.3
- stool (color) (contents) (mucus) R19.5
  - bloody K92.1
  - guaiac positive R19.5
- synchondrosis Q78.8
- thermography — *see also* Abnormal, diagnostic imaging R93.89
- thyroid-binding globulin E07.89
- tooth, teeth (form) (size) K00.2
- toxicology (findings) R78.9
- transport protein E88.09
- tumor marker NEC R97.8
- ultrasound results — *see* Abnormal, diagnostic imaging
- umbilical cord complicating delivery O69.9 ☑
- urination NEC R39.198
- urine (constituents) R82.90
  - bile R82.2
  - cytological examination R82.89
  - drugs R82.5
  - fat R82.0
  - glucose R81
  - heavy metals R82.6
  - hemoglobin R82.3
  - histological examination R82.89
  - ketones R82.4
  - microbiological examination (culture) R82.79
  - myoglobin R82.1
  - positive culture R82.79
  - protein — *see* Proteinuria
  - specified substance NEC R82.998
    - chromoabnormality NEC R82.91
  - substances nonmedical R82.6
- uterine hemorrhage — *see* Hemorrhage, uterus
- vectorcardiogram R94.39
- visually evoked potential (VEP) R94.112
- white blood cells D72.9
  - specified NEC D72.89
- X-ray examination — *see* Abnormal, diagnostic imaging

Abnormity (any organ or part) — *see* Anomaly

Abocclusion M26.29
- hemolytic disease (newborn) P55.1
- incompatibility reaction ABO — *see* Complication(s), transfusion, incompatibility reaction, ABO

Abolition, language R48.8

Aborter, habitual or recurrent — *see* Loss (of), pregnancy, recurrent

Abortion (complete) (spontaneous) O03.9

Abortion — *continued*
- with
  - retained products of conception — *see* Abortion, incomplete
- attempted (elective) (failed) O07.4
  - complicated by O07.30
    - afibrinogenemia O07.1
    - cardiac arrest O07.36
    - chemical damage of pelvic organ(s) O07.34
    - circulatory collapse O07.31
    - cystitis O07.38
    - defibrination syndrome O07.1
    - electrolyte imbalance O07.33
    - embolism (air) (amniotic fluid) (blood clot) (fat) (pulmonary) (septic) (soap) O07.2
    - endometritis O07.0
    - genital tract and pelvic infection O07.0
    - hemolysis O07.1
    - hemorrhage (delayed) (excessive) O07.1
    - infection
      - genital tract or pelvic O07.0
      - urinary tract tract O07.38
    - intravascular coagulation O07.1
    - laceration of pelvic organ(s) O07.34
    - metabolic disorder O07.33
    - oliguria O07.32
    - oophoritis O07.0
    - parametritis O07.0
    - pelvic peritonitis O07.0
    - perforation of pelvic organ(s) O07.34
    - renal failure or shutdown O07.32
    - salpingitis or salpingo-oophoritis O07.0
    - sepsis O07.37
    - shock O07.31
    - specified condition NEC O07.39
    - tubular necrosis (renal) O07.32
    - uremia O07.32
    - urinary tract infection O07.38
    - venous complication NEC O07.35
      - embolism (air) (amniotic fluid) (blood clot) (fat) (pulmonary) (septic) (soap) O07.2
- complicated (by) (following) O03.80
  - afibrinogenemia O03.6
  - cardiac arrest O03.86
  - chemical damage of pelvic organ(s) O03.84
  - circulatory collapse O03.81
  - cystitis O03.88
  - defibrination syndrome O03.6
  - electrolyte imbalance O03.83
  - embolism (air) (amniotic fluid) (blood clot) (fat) (pulmonary) (septic) (soap) O03.7
  - endometritis O03.5
  - genital tract and pelvic infection O03.5
  - hemolysis O03.6
  - hemorrhage (delayed) (excessive) O03.6
  - infection
    - genital tract or pelvic O03.5
    - urinary tract O03.88
  - intravascular coagulation O03.6
  - laceration of pelvic organ(s) O03.84
  - metabolic disorder O03.83
  - oliguria O03.82
  - oophoritis O03.5
  - parametritis O03.5
  - pelvic peritonitis O03.5
  - perforation of pelvic organ(s) O03.84
  - renal failure or shutdown O03.82
  - salpingitis or salpingo-oophoritis O03.5
  - sepsis O03.87
  - shock O03.81
  - specified condition NEC O03.89
  - tubular necrosis (renal) O03.82
  - uremia O03.82
  - urinary tract infection O03.88
  - venous complication NEC O03.85
    - embolism (air) (amniotic fluid) (blood clot) (fat) (pulmonary) (septic) (soap) O03.7
- failed — *see* Abortion, attempted
- habitual or recurrent N96
  - with current abortion — *see* categories O03-O04
  - without current pregnancy N96
  - care in current pregnancy O26.2- ☑
- incomplete (spontaneous) O03.4
  - complicated (by) (following) O03.30
    - afibrinogenemia O03.1
    - cardiac arrest O03.36
    - chemical damage of pelvic organ(s) O03.34
    - circulatory collapse O03.31
    - cystitis O03.38

Abortion — *continued*
- incomplete — *continued*
  - complicated — *continued*
    - defibrination syndrome O03.1
    - electrolyte imbalance O03.33
    - embolism (air) (amniotic fluid) (blood clot) (fat) (pulmonary) (septic) (soap) O03.2
    - endometritis O03.0
    - genital tract and pelvic infection O03.0
    - hemolysis O03.1
    - hemorrhage (delayed) (excessive) O03.1
    - infection
      - genital tract or pelvic O03.0
      - urinary tract O03.38
    - intravascular coagulation O03.1
    - laceration of pelvic organ(s) O03.34
    - metabolic disorder O03.33
    - oliguria O03.32
    - oophoritis O03.0
    - parametritis O03.0
    - pelvic peritonitis O03.0
    - perforation of pelvic organ(s) O03.34
    - renal failure or shutdown O03.32
    - salpingitis or salpingo-oophoritis O03.0
    - sepsis O03.37
    - shock O03.31
    - specified condition NEC O03.39
    - tubular necrosis (renal) O03.32
    - uremia O03.32
    - urinary infection O03.38
    - venous complication NEC O03.35
      - embolism (air) (amniotic fluid) (blood clot) (fat) (pulmonary) (septic) (soap) O03.2
- induced (encounter for) Z33.2
  - complicated by O04.80
    - afibrinogenemia O04.6
    - cardiac arrest O04.86
    - chemical damage of pelvic organ(s) O04.84
    - circulatory collapse O04.81
    - cystitis O04.88
    - defibrination syndrome O04.6
    - electrolyte imbalance O04.83
    - embolism (air) (amniotic fluid) (blood clot) (fat) (pulmonary) (septic) (soap) O04.7
    - endometritis O04.5
    - genital tract and pelvic infection O04.5
    - hemolysis O04.6
    - hemorrhage (delayed) (excessive) O04.6
    - infection
      - genital tract or pelvic O04.5
      - urinary tract O04.88
    - intravascular coagulation O04.6
    - laceration of pelvic organ(s) O04.84
    - metabolic disorder O04.83
    - oliguria O04.82
    - oophoritis O04.5
    - parametritis O04.5
    - pelvic peritonitis O04.5
    - perforation of pelvic organ(s) O04.84
    - renal failure or shutdown O04.82
    - salpingitis or salpingo-oophoritis O04.5
    - sepsis O04.87
    - shock O04.81
    - specified condition NEC O04.89
    - tubular necrosis (renal) O04.82
    - uremia O04.82
    - urinary tract infection O04.88
    - venous complication NEC O04.85
      - embolism (air) (amniotic fluid) (blood clot) (fat) (pulmonary) (septic) (soap) O04.7
- inevitable O03.4
- missed O02.1
- spontaneous — *see* Abortion (complete) (spontaneous)
  - threatened O20.0
- threatened (spontaneous) O20.0
- tubal O00.10- ☑
  - with intrauterine pregnancy O00.11- ☑

Abortus fever A23.1

Aboulomania F60.7

Abrami's disease D59.8

Abramov-Fiedler myocarditis (acute isolated myocarditis) I40.1

Abrasion T14.8 ☑
- abdomen, abdominal (wall) S30.811 ☑
- alveolar process S00.512 ☑
- ankle S90.51- ☑
- antecubital space — *see* Abrasion, elbow
- anus S30.817 ☑

Abrasion — *continued*
- arm (upper) S4Ø.81- ☑
- auditory canal — *see* Abrasion, ear
- auricle — *see* Abrasion, ear
- axilla — *see* Abrasion, arm
- back, lower S3Ø.81Ø ☑
- breast S2Ø.11- ☑
- brow SØØ.81 ☑
- buttock S3Ø.81Ø ☑
- calf — *see* Abrasion, leg
- canthus — *see* Abrasion, eyelid
- cheek SØØ.81 ☑
  - internal SØØ.512 ☑
- chest wall — *see* Abrasion, thorax
- chin SØØ.81 ☑
- clitoris S3Ø.814 ☑
- cornea SØ5.Ø- ☑
- costal region — *see* Abrasion, thorax
- dental KØ3.1
- digit(s)
  - foot — *see* Abrasion, toe
  - hand — *see* Abrasion, finger
- ear SØØ.41- ☑
- elbow S5Ø.31- ☑
- epididymis S3Ø.813 ☑
- epigastric region S3Ø.811 ☑
- epiglottis S1Ø.11 ☑
- esophagus (thoracic) S27.818 ☑
  - cervical S1Ø.11 ☑
- eyebrow — *see* Abrasion, eyelid
- eyelid SØØ.21- ☑
- face SØØ.81 ☑
- finger(s) S6Ø.41- ☑
  - index S6Ø.41- ☑
  - little S6Ø.41- ☑
  - middle S6Ø.41- ☑
  - ring S6Ø.41- ☑
- flank S3Ø.811 ☑
- foot (except toe(s) alone) S9Ø.81- ☑
  - toe — *see* Abrasion, toe
- forearm S5Ø.81- ☑
  - elbow only — *see* Abrasion, elbow
- forehead SØØ.81 ☑
- genital organs, external
  - female S3Ø.816 ☑
  - male S3Ø.815 ☑
- groin S3Ø.811 ☑
- gum SØØ.512 ☑
- hand S6Ø.51- ☑
- head SØØ.91 ☑
  - ear — *see* Abrasion, ear
  - eyelid — *see* Abrasion, eyelid
  - lip SØØ.511 ☑
  - nose SØØ.31 ☑
  - oral cavity SØØ.512 ☑
  - scalp SØØ.Ø1 ☑
  - specified site NEC SØØ.81 ☑
- heel — *see* Abrasion, foot
- hip S7Ø.21- ☑
- inguinal region S3Ø.811 ☑
- interscapular region S2Ø.419 ☑
- jaw SØØ.81 ☑
- knee S8Ø.21- ☑
- labium (majus) (minus) S3Ø.814 ☑
- larynx S1Ø.11 ☑
- leg (lower) S8Ø.81- ☑
  - knee — *see* Abrasion, knee
  - upper — *see* Abrasion, thigh
- lip SØØ.511 ☑
- lower back S3Ø.81Ø ☑
- lumbar region S3Ø.81Ø ☑
- malar region SØØ.81 ☑
- mammary — *see* Abrasion, breast
- mastoid region SØØ.81 ☑
- mouth SØØ.512 ☑
- nail
  - finger — *see* Abrasion, finger
  - toe — *see* Abrasion, toe
- nape S1Ø.81 ☑
- nasal SØØ.31 ☑
- neck S1Ø.91 ☑
  - specified site NEC S1Ø.81 ☑
  - throat S1Ø.11 ☑
- nose SØØ.31 ☑
- occipital region SØØ.Ø1 ☑
- oral cavity SØØ.512 ☑

Abrasion — *continued*
- orbital region — *see* Abrasion, eyelid
- palate SØØ.512 ☑
- palm — *see* Abrasion, hand
- parietal region SØØ.Ø1 ☑
- pelvis S3Ø.81Ø ☑
- penis S3Ø.812 ☑
- perineum
  - female S3Ø.814 ☑
  - male S3Ø.81Ø ☑
- periocular area — *see* Abrasion, eyelid
- phalanges
  - finger — *see* Abrasion, finger
  - toe — *see* Abrasion, toe
- pharynx S1Ø.11 ☑
- pinna — *see* Abrasion, ear
- popliteal space — *see* Abrasion, knee
- prepuce S3Ø.812 ☑
- pubic region S3Ø.81Ø ☑
- pudendum
  - female S3Ø.816 ☑
  - male S3Ø.815 ☑
- sacral region S3Ø.81Ø ☑
- scalp SØØ.Ø1 ☑
- scapular region — *see* Abrasion, shoulder
- scrotum S3Ø.813 ☑
- shin — *see* Abrasion, leg
- shoulder S4Ø.21- ☑
- skin NEC T14.8 ☑
- sternal region S2Ø.319 ☑
- submaxillary region SØØ.81 ☑
- submental region SØØ.81 ☑
- subungual
  - finger(s) — *see* Abrasion, finger
  - toe(s) — *see* Abrasion, toe
- supraclavicular fossa S1Ø.81 ☑
- supraorbital SØØ.81 ☑
- temple SØØ.81 ☑
- temporal region SØØ.81 ☑
- testis S3Ø.813 ☑
- thigh S7Ø.31- ☑
- thorax, thoracic (wall) S2Ø.91 ☑
  - back S2Ø.41- ☑
  - front S2Ø.31- ☑
- throat S1Ø.11 ☑
- thumb S6Ø.31- ☑
- toe(s) (lesser) S9Ø.416 ☑
  - great S9Ø.41- ☑
- tongue SØØ.512 ☑
- tooth, teeth (dentifrice) (habitual) (hard tissues) (occupational) (ritual) (traditional) KØ3.1
- trachea S1Ø.11 ☑
- tunica vaginalis S3Ø.813 ☑
- tympanum, tympanic membrane — *see* Abrasion, ear
- uvula SØØ.512 ☑
- vagina S3Ø.814 ☑
- vocal cords S1Ø.11 ☑
- vulva S3Ø.814 ☑
- wrist S6Ø.81- ☑

Abrism — *see* Poisoning, food, noxious, plant

Abruptio placentae O45.9- ☑
- with
  - afibrinogenemia O45.Ø1- ☑
  - coagulation defect O45.ØØ- ☑
    - specified NEC O45.Ø9- ☑
  - disseminated intravascular coagulation O45.Ø2- ☑
  - hypofibrinogenemia O45.Ø1- ☑
- specified NEC O45.8- ☑

Abruption, placenta — *see* Abruptio placentae

Abscess (connective tissue) (embolic) (fistulous) (infective) (metastatic) (multiple) (pernicious) (pyogenic) (septic) LØ2.91
- with
  - diverticular disease (intestine) K57.8Ø
    - with bleeding K57.81
    - large intestine K57.2Ø
      - with
        - bleeding K57.21
        - small intestine K57.4Ø
          - with bleeding K57.41
    - small intestine K57.ØØ
      - with
        - bleeding K57.Ø1
        - large intestine K57.4Ø
          - with bleeding K57.41

Abscess — *continued*
- with — *continued*
  - lymphangitis — *code by* site under Abscess
- abdomen, abdominal
  - cavity K65.1
  - wall LØ2.211
- abdominopelvic K65.1
- accessory sinus — *see* Sinusitis
- adrenal (capsule) (gland) E27.8
- alveolar KØ4.7
  - with sinus KØ4.6
- amebic AØ6.4
  - brain (and liver or lung abscess) AØ6.6
  - genitourinary tract AØ6.82
  - liver (without mention of brain or lung abscess) AØ6.4
  - lung (and liver) (without mention of brain abscess) AØ6.5
  - specified site NEC AØ6.89
  - spleen AØ6.89
- anerobic A48.Ø
- ankle — *see* Abscess, lower limb
- anorectal K61.2
- antecubital space — *see* Abscess, upper limb
- antrum (chronic) (Highmore) — *see* Sinusitis, maxillary
- anus K61.Ø
- apical (tooth) KØ4.7
  - with sinus (alveolar) KØ4.6
- appendix K35.33
- areola (acute) (chronic) (nonpuerperal) N61.1
  - puerperal, postpartum or gestational — *see* Infection, nipple
- arm (any part) — *see* Abscess, upper limb
- artery (wall) I77.89
- atheromatous I77.2
- auricle, ear — *see* Abscess, ear, external
- axilla (region) LØ2.41- ☑
  - lymph gland or node LØ4.2
- back (any part, except buttock) LØ2.212
- Bartholin's gland N75.1
  - with
    - abortion — *see* Abortion, by type complicated by, sepsis
    - ectopic or molar pregnancy OØ8.Ø
  - following ectopic or molar pregnancy OØ8.Ø
- Bezold's — *see* Mastoiditis, acute
- bilharziasis B65.1
- bladder (wall) — *see* Cystitis, specified type NEC
- bone (subperiosteal) — *see also* Osteomyelitis, specified type NEC
  - accessory sinus (chronic) — *see* Sinusitis
  - chronic or old — *see* Osteomyelitis, chronic
  - jaw (lower) (upper) M27.2
  - mastoid — *see* Mastoiditis, acute, subperiosteal
  - petrous — *see* Petrositis
  - spinal (tuberculous) A18.Ø1
    - nontuberculous — *see* Osteomyelitis, vertebra
- bowel K63.Ø
- brain (any part) (cystic) (otogenic) GØ6.Ø
  - amebic (with abscess of any other site) AØ6.6
  - gonococcal A54.82
  - pheomycotic (chromomycotic) B43.1
  - tuberculous A17.81
- breast (acute) (chronic) (nonpuerperal) N61.1
  - newborn P39.Ø
  - puerperal, postpartum, gestational — *see* Mastitis, obstetric, purulent
- broad ligament N73.2
  - acute N73.Ø
  - chronic N73.1
- Brodie's (localized) (chronic) M86.8X- ☑
- bronchi J98.Ø9
- buccal cavity K12.2
- bulbourethral gland N34.Ø
- bursa M71.ØØ
  - ankle M71.Ø7- ☑
  - elbow M71.Ø2- ☑
  - foot M71.Ø7- ☑
  - hand M71.Ø4- ☑
  - hip M71.Ø5- ☑
  - knee M71.Ø6- ☑
  - multiple sites M71.Ø9
  - pharyngeal J39.1
  - shoulder M71.Ø1- ☑
  - specified site NEC M71.Ø8
  - wrist M71.Ø3- ☑
- buttock LØ2.31
- canthus — *see* Blepharoconjunctivitis

Abscess — *continued*
- penis — *continued*
  - gonococcal (accessory gland) (periurethral) A54.1
- perianal K61.Ø
- periapical KØ4.7
  - with sinus (alveolar) KØ4.6
- periappendicular K35.33
- pericardial I3Ø.1
- pericecal K35.33
- pericemental — *see* Periodontitis, aggressive, localized
- pericholecystic — *see* Cholecystitis, acute
- pericoronal — *see* Periodontitis, aggressive, localized
- peridental — *see* Periodontitis, aggressive, localized
- perimetric — *see also* Disease, pelvis, inflammatory N73.2
- perinephric, perinephritic — *see* Abscess, kidney
- perineum, perineal (superficial) LØ2.215
  - urethra N34.Ø
- periodontal (parietal) — *see* Periodontitis, aggressive, localized
  - apical KØ4.7
- periosteum, periosteal — *see also* Osteomyelitis, specified type NEC
  - with osteomyelitis — *see also* Osteomyelitis, specified type NEC
    - acute — *see* Osteomyelitis, acute
    - chronic — *see* Osteomyelitis, chronic
- peripharyngeal J39.Ø
- peripleuritic J86.9
  - with fistula J86.Ø
- periprostatic N41.2
- perirectal K61.1
- perirenal (tissue) — *see* Abscess, kidney
- perisinuous (nose) — *see* Sinusitis
- peritoneum, peritoneal (perforated) (ruptured) K65.1
  - with appendicitis — *see also* Appendicitis K35.33
  - pelvic
    - female — *see* Peritonitis, pelvic, female
    - male K65.1
  - postoperative T81.43 ☑
  - puerperal, postpartum, childbirth O85
  - tuberculous A18.31
- peritonsillar J36
- perityphlic K35.33
- periureteral N28.89
- periurethral N34.Ø
  - gonococcal (accessory gland) (periurethral) A54.1
- periuterine — *see also* Disease, pelvis, inflammatory N73.2
- perivesical — *see* Cystitis, specified type NEC
- petrous bone — *see* Petrositis
- phagedenic NOS LØ2.91
  - chancroid A57
- pharynx, pharyngeal (lateral) J39.1
- pilonidal LØ5.Ø1
- pituitary (gland) E23.6
- pleura J86.9
  - with fistula J86.Ø
- popliteal — *see* Abscess, lower limb
- postcecal K35.33
- postlaryngeal J38.7
- postnasal J34.Ø
- postoperative (any site) — *see also* Infection, postoperative wound T81.49 ☑
  - retroperitoneal K68.11
- postpharyngeal J39.Ø
- posttonsillar J36
- post-typhoid AØ1.Ø9
- pouch of Douglas — *see* Peritonitis, pelvic, female
- premammary — *see* Abscess, breast
- prepatellar — *see* Abscess, lower limb
- presacral K68.19
- prostate N41.2
  - gonococcal (acute) (chronic) A54.22
- psoas muscle K68.12
- puerperal — *code by* site under Puerperal, abscess
- pulmonary — *see* Abscess, lung
- pulp, pulpal (dental) KØ4.Ø1
  - irreversible KØ4.Ø2
  - reversible KØ4.Ø1
- rectovaginal septum K63.Ø
- rectovesical — *see* Cystitis, specified type NEC
- rectum K61.1
- renal — *see* Abscess, kidney
- retina — *see* Inflammation, chorioretinal
- retrobulbar — *see* Abscess, orbit
- retrocecal K65.1
- retrolaryngeal J38.7

Abscess — *continued*
- retromammary — *see* Abscess, breast
- retroperitoneal NEC K68.19
  - postprocedural K68.11
- retropharyngeal J39.Ø
- retrouterine — *see* Peritonitis, pelvic, female
- retrovesical — *see* Cystitis, specified type NEC
- root, tooth KØ4.7
  - with sinus (alveolar) KØ4.6
- round ligament — *see also* Disease, pelvis, inflammatory N73.2
- rupture (spontaneous) NOS LØ2.91
- sacrum (tuberculous) A18.Ø1
  - nontuberculous M46.28
- salivary (duct) (gland) K11.3
- scalp (any part) LØ2.811
- scapular — *see* Osteomyelitis, specified type NEC
- sclera — *see* Scleritis
- scrofulous (tuberculous) A18.2
- scrotum N49.2
- seminal vesicle N49.Ø
- septal, dental KØ4.7
  - with sinus (alveolar) KØ4.6
- serous — *see* Periostitis
- shoulder (region) — *see* Abscess, upper limb
- sigmoid K63.Ø
- sinus (accessory) (chronic) (nasal) — *see also* Sinusitis
  - intracranial venous (any) GØ6.Ø
- Skene's duct or gland N34.Ø
- skin — *see* Abscess, by site
- specified site NEC LØ2.818
- spermatic cord N49.1
- sphenoidal (sinus) (chronic) J32.3
- spinal cord (any part) (staphylococcal) GØ6.1
  - tuberculous A17.81
- spine (column) (tuberculous) A18.Ø1
  - epidural GØ6.1
  - nontuberculous — *see* Osteomyelitis, vertebra
- spleen D73.3
  - amebic AØ6.89
- stitch T81.41 ☑
  - following an obstetrical procedure O86.Ø1
- subarachnoid GØ6.2
  - brain GØ6.Ø
  - spinal cord GØ6.1
- subareolar — *see* Abscess, breast
- subcecal K35.33
- subcutaneous — *see also* Abscess, by site
  - following procedure T81.41 ☑
    - obstetrical O86.Ø1
  - pheomycotic (chromomycotic) B43.2
- subdiaphragmatic K65.1
- subdural GØ6.2
  - brain GØ6.Ø
    - sequelae GØ9
  - spinal cord GØ6.1
- sub-fascial, following an obstetrical procedure O86.Ø2
- subgaleal LØ2.811
- subhepatic K65.1
- sublingual K12.2
  - gland K11.3
- submammary — *see* Abscess, breast
- submandibular (region) (space) (triangle) K12.2
  - gland K11.3
- submaxillary (region) LØ2.Ø1
  - gland K11.3
- submental LØ2.Ø1
  - gland K11.3
- subperiosteal — *see* Osteomyelitis, specified type NEC
- subphrenic K65.1
  - following an obstetrical procedure O86.Ø3
  - postoperative T81.43 ☑
- suburethral N34.Ø
- sudoriparous L75.8
- supraclavicular (fossa) — *see* Abscess, upper limb
- supralevator K61.5
- suprapelvic, acute N73.Ø
- suprarenal (capsule) (gland) E27.8
- sweat gland L74.8
- tear duct — *see* Inflammation, lacrimal, passages, acute
- temple LØ2.Ø1
- temporal region LØ2.Ø1
- temporosphenoidal GØ6.Ø
- tendon (sheath) M65.ØØ
  - ankle M65.Ø7- ☑
  - foot M65.Ø7- ☑
  - forearm M65.Ø3- ☑
  - hand M65.Ø4- ☑

Abscess — *continued*
- tendon — *continued*
  - lower leg M65.Ø6- ☑
  - pelvic region M65.Ø5- ☑
  - shoulder region M65.Ø1- ☑
  - specified site NEC M65.Ø8
  - thigh M65.Ø5- ☑
  - upper arm M65.Ø2- ☑
- testis N45.4
- thigh — *see* Abscess, lower limb
- thorax J86.9
  - with fistula J86.Ø
- throat J39.1
- thumb — *see also* Abscess, hand
  - nail — *see* Cellulitis, finger
- thymus (gland) E32.1
- thyroid (gland) EØ6.Ø
- toe (any) — *see also* Abscess, foot
  - nail — *see* Cellulitis, toe
- tongue (staphylococcal) K14.Ø
- tonsil(s) (lingual) J36
- tonsillopharyngeal J36
- tooth, teeth (root) KØ4.7
  - with sinus (alveolar) KØ4.6
  - supporting structures NEC — *see* Periodontitis, aggressive, localized
- trachea J39.8
- trunk LØ2.219
  - abdominal wall LØ2.211
  - back LØ2.212
  - chest wall LØ2.213
  - groin LØ2.214
  - perineum LØ2.215
  - umbilicus LØ2.216
- tubal — *see* Salpingitis
- tuberculous — *see* Tuberculosis, abscess
- tubo-ovarian — *see* Salpingo-oophoritis
- tunica vaginalis N49.1
- umbilicus LØ2.216
- upper
  - limb LØ2.41- ☑
  - respiratory J39.8
- urethral (gland) N34.Ø
- urinary N34.Ø
- uterus, uterine (wall) — *see also* Endometritis
  - ligament — *see also* Disease, pelvis, inflammatory N73.2
  - neck — *see* Cervicitis
- uvula K12.2
- vagina (wall) — *see* Vaginitis
- vaginorectal — *see* Vaginitis
- vas deferens N49.1
- vermiform appendix K35.33
- vertebra (column) (tuberculous) A18.Ø1
  - nontuberculous — *see* Osteomyelitis, vertebra
- vesical — *see* Cystitis, specified type NEC
- vesico-uterine pouch — *see* Peritonitis, pelvic, female
- vitreous (humor) — *see* Endophthalmitis, purulent
- vocal cord J38.3
- von Bezold's — *see* Mastoiditis, acute
- vulva N76.4
- vulvovaginal gland N75.1
- web space — *see* Abscess, hand
- wound T81.49 ☑
- wrist — *see* Abscess, upper limb

Absence (of) (organ or part) (complete or partial)
- adrenal (gland) (congenital) Q89.1
  - acquired E89.6
- albumin in blood E88.Ø9
- alimentary tract (congenital) Q45.8
  - upper Q4Ø.8
- alveolar process (acquired) — *see* Anomaly, alveolar
- ankle (acquired) Z89.44- ☑
- anus (congenital) Q42.3
  - with fistula Q42.2
- aorta (congenital) Q25.41
- appendix, congenital Q42.8
- arm (acquired) Z89.2Ø- ☑
  - above elbow Z89.22- ☑
    - congenital (with hand present) — *see* Agenesis, arm, with hand present
      - and hand — *see* Agenesis, forearm, and hand
  - below elbow Z89.21- ☑
    - congenital (with hand present) — *see* Agenesis, arm, with hand present
      - and hand — *see* Agenesis, forearm, and hand
  - congenital — *see* Defect, reduction, upper limb

Absence — *continued*
- arm — *continued*
  - shoulder (following explantation of shoulder joint prosthesis) (joint) (with or without presence of antibiotic-impregnated cement spacer) Z89.23- ☑
    - congenital (with hand present) — *see* Agenesis, arm, with hand present
- artery (congenital) (peripheral) Q27.8
  - brain Q28.3
  - coronary Q24.5
  - pulmonary Q25.79
  - specified NEC Q27.8
  - umbilical Q27.Ø
- atrial septum (congenital) Q21.19
- auditory canal (congenital) (external) Q16.1
- auricle (ear), congenital Q16.Ø
- bile, biliary duct, congenital Q44.5
- bladder (acquired) Z9Ø.6
  - congenital Q64.5
- bowel sounds R19.11
- brain QØØ.Ø
  - part of QØ4.3
- breast(s) (and nipple(s)) (acquired) Z9Ø.1- ☑
  - congenital Q83.8
- broad ligament Q5Ø.6
- bronchus (congenital) Q32.4
- canaliculus lacrimalis, congenital Q1Ø.4
- cerebellum (vermis) QØ4.3
- cervix (acquired) (with uterus) Z9Ø.71Ø
  - with remaining uterus Z9Ø.712
  - congenital Q51.5
- chin, congenital Q18.8
- cilia (congenital) Q1Ø.3
  - acquired — *see* Madarosis
- clitoris (congenital) Q52.6
- coccyx, congenital Q76.49
- cold sense R2Ø.8
- congenital
  - lumen — *see* Atresia
  - organ or site NEC — *see* Agenesis
  - septum — *see* Imperfect, closure
- corpus callosum QØ4.Ø
- cricoid cartilage, congenital Q31.8
- diaphragm (with hernia), congenital Q79.1
- digestive organ(s) or tract, congenital Q45.8
  - acquired NEC Z9Ø.49
  - upper Q4Ø.8
- ductus arteriosus Q28.8
- duodenum (acquired) Z9Ø.49
  - congenital Q41.Ø
- ear, congenital Q16.9
  - acquired H93.8- ☑
  - auricle Q16.Ø
  - external Q16.Ø
  - inner Q16.5
  - lobe, lobule Q17.8
  - middle, except ossicles Q16.4
    - ossicles Q16.3
  - ossicles Q16.3
- ejaculatory duct (congenital) Q55.4
- endocrine gland (congenital) NEC Q89.2
  - acquired E89.89
- epididymis (congenital) Q55.4
  - acquired Z9Ø.79
- epiglottis, congenital Q31.8
- esophagus (congenital) Q39.8
  - acquired (partial) Z9Ø.49
- eustachian tube (congenital) Q16.2
- extremity (acquired) Z89.9
  - congenital Q73.Ø
  - knee (following explantation of knee joint prosthesis) (joint) (with or without presence of antibiotic-impregnated cement spacer) Z89.52- ☑
  - lower (above knee) Z89.619
    - below knee Z89.51- ☑
  - upper — *see* Absence, arm
- eye (acquired) Z9Ø.Ø1
  - congenital Q11.1
  - muscle (congenital) Q1Ø.3
- eyeball (acquired) Z9Ø.Ø1
- eyelid (fold) (congenital) Q1Ø.3
  - acquired Z9Ø.Ø1
- face, specified part NEC Q18.8
- fallopian tube(s) (acquired) Z9Ø.79
  - congenital Q5Ø.6
- family member (causing problem in home) NEC — *see also* Disruption, family Z63.32

Absence — *continued*
- femur, congenital — *see* Defect, reduction, lower limb, longitudinal, femur
- fibrinogen (congenital) D68.2
  - acquired D65
- finger(s) (acquired) Z89.Ø2- ☑
  - congenital — *see* Agenesis, hand
- foot (acquired) Z89.43- ☑
  - congenital — *see* Agenesis, foot
- forearm (acquired) — *see* Absence, arm, below elbow
- gallbladder (acquired) Z9Ø.49
  - congenital Q44.Ø
- gamma globulin in blood D8Ø.1
  - hereditary D8Ø.Ø
- genital organs
  - acquired (female) (male) Z9Ø.79
  - female, congenital Q52.8
    - external Q52.71
    - internal NEC Q52.8
  - male, congenital Q55.8
- genitourinary organs, congenital NEC
  - female Q52.8
  - male Q55.8
- globe (acquired) Z9Ø.Ø1
  - congenital Q11.1
- glottis, congenital Q31.8
- hand and wrist (acquired) Z89.11- ☑
  - congenital — *see* Agenesis, hand
- head, part (acquired) NEC Z9Ø.Ø9
- heat sense R2Ø.8
- hip (following explantation of hip joint prosthesis) (joint) (with or without presence of antibiotic-impregnated cement spacer) Z89.62- ☑
- hymen (congenital) Q52.4
- ileum (acquired) Z9Ø.49
  - congenital Q41.2
- immunoglobulin, isolated NEC D8Ø.3
  - IgA D8Ø.2
  - IgG D8Ø.3
  - IgM D8Ø.4
- incus (acquired) — *see* Loss, ossicles, ear
  - congenital Q16.3
- inner ear, congenital Q16.5
- intestine (acquired) (small) Z9Ø.49
  - congenital Q41.9
    - specified NEC Q41.8
  - large Z9Ø.49
    - congenital Q42.9
      - specified NEC Q42.8
- iris, congenital Q13.1
- jejunum (acquired) Z9Ø.49
  - congenital Q41.1
- joint
  - acquired
    - hip (following explantation of hip joint prosthesis) (with or without presence of antibiotic-impregnated cement spacer) Z89.62- ☑
    - knee (following explantation of knee joint prosthesis) (with or without presence of antibiotic-impregnated cement spacer) Z89.52- ☑
    - shoulder (following explantation of shoulder joint prosthesis) (with or without presence of antibiotic-impregnated cement spacer) Z89.23- ☑
  - congenital NEC Q74.8
- kidney(s) (acquired) Z9Ø.5
  - congenital Q6Ø.2
    - bilateral Q6Ø.1
    - unilateral Q6Ø.Ø
- knee (following explantation of knee joint prosthesis) (joint) (with or without presence of antibiotic-impregnated cement spacer) Z89.52- ☑
- labyrinth, membranous Q16.5
- larynx (congenital) Q31.8
  - acquired Z9Ø.Ø2
- leg (acquired) (above knee) Z89.61- ☑
  - below knee (acquired) Z89.51- ☑
  - congenital — *see* Defect, reduction, lower limb
- lens (acquired) — *see also* Aphakia
  - congenital Q12.3
  - post cataract extraction Z98.4- ☑
- limb (acquired) — *see* Absence, extremity
- lip Q38.6
- liver (congenital) Q44.79
- lung (fissure) (lobe) (bilateral) (unilateral) (congenital) Q33.3
  - acquired (any part) Z9Ø.2

Absence — *continued*
- menstruation — *see* Amenorrhea
- muscle (congenital) (pectoral) Q79.8
  - ocular Q1Ø.3
- neck, part Q18.8
- neutrophil — *see* Agranulocytosis
- nipple(s) (with breast(s)) (acquired) Z9Ø.1- ☑
  - congenital Q83.2
- nose (congenital) Q3Ø.1
  - acquired Z9Ø.Ø9
- organ
  - of Corti, congenital Q16.5
  - or site, congenital NEC Q89.8
    - acquired NEC Z9Ø.89
- osseous meatus (ear) Q16.4
- ovary (acquired)
  - bilateral Z9Ø.722
  - congenital
    - bilateral Q5Ø.Ø2
    - unilateral Q5Ø.Ø1
  - unilateral Z9Ø.721
- oviduct (acquired)
  - bilateral Z9Ø.722
  - congenital Q5Ø.6
  - unilateral Z9Ø.721
- pancreas (congenital) Q45.Ø
  - acquired Z9Ø.41Ø
    - complete Z9Ø.41Ø
    - partial Z9Ø.411
    - total Z9Ø.41Ø
- parathyroid gland (acquired) E89.2
  - congenital Q89.2
- patella, congenital Q74.1
- penis (congenital) Q55.5
  - acquired Z9Ø.79
- pericardium (congenital) Q24.8
- pituitary gland (congenital) Q89.2
  - acquired E89.3
- prostate (acquired) Z9Ø.79
  - congenital Q55.4
- pulmonary valve Q22.Ø
- punctum lacrimale (congenital) Q1Ø.4
- radius, congenital — *see* Defect, reduction, upper limb, longitudinal, radius
- rectum (congenital) Q42.1
  - with fistula Q42.Ø
  - acquired Z9Ø.49
- respiratory organ NOS Q34.9
- rib (acquired) Z9Ø.89
  - congenital Q76.6
- sacrum, congenital Q76.49
- salivary gland(s), congenital Q38.4
- scrotum, congenital Q55.29
- seminal vesicles (congenital) Q55.4
  - acquired Z9Ø.79
- septum
  - atrial (congenital) Q21.19
  - between aorta and pulmonary artery Q21.4
  - ventricular (congenital) Q2Ø.4
- sex chromosome
  - female phenotype Q97.8
  - male phenotype Q98.8
- skull bone (congenital) Q75.8
  - with
    - anencephaly QØØ.Ø
    - encephalocele — *see* Encephalocele
    - hydrocephalus QØ3.9
      - with spina bifida — *see* Spina bifida, by site, with hydrocephalus
    - microcephaly QØ2
- spermatic cord, congenital Q55.4
- spine, congenital Q76.49
- spleen (congenital) Q89.Ø1
  - acquired Z9Ø.81
- sternum, congenital Q76.7
- stomach (acquired) (partial) Z9Ø.3
  - congenital Q4Ø.2
- superior vena cava, congenital Q26.8
- teeth, tooth (congenital) KØØ.Ø
  - acquired (complete) KØ8.1Ø9
    - class I KØ8.1Ø1
    - class II KØ8.1Ø2
    - class III KØ8.1Ø3
    - class IV KØ8.1Ø4
    - due to
      - caries KØ8.139
        - class I KØ8.131
        - class II KØ8.132
        - class III KØ8.133

- **Absence** — *continued*
  - teeth, tooth — *continued*
    - acquired — *continued*
      - due to — *continued*
        - caries — *continued*
          - class IV KØ8.134
        - periodontal disease KØ8.129
          - class I KØ8.121
          - class II KØ8.122
          - class III KØ8.123
          - class IV KØ8.124
        - specified NEC KØ8.199
          - class I KØ8.191
          - class II KØ8.192
          - class III KØ8.193
          - class IV KØ8.194
        - trauma KØ8.119
          - class I KØ8.111
          - class II KØ8.112
          - class III KØ8.113
          - class IV KØ8.114
      - partial KØ8.4Ø9
        - class I KØ8.4Ø1
        - class II KØ8.4Ø2
        - class III KØ8.4Ø3
        - class IV KØ8.4Ø4
        - due to
          - caries KØ8.439
            - class I KØ8.431
            - class II KØ8.432
            - class III KØ8.433
            - class IV KØ8.434
          - periodontal disease KØ8.429
            - class I KØ8.421
            - class II KØ8.422
            - class III KØ8.423
            - class IV KØ8.424
          - specified NEC KØ8.499
            - class I KØ8.491
            - class II KØ8.492
            - class III KØ8.493
            - class IV KØ8.494
          - trauma KØ8.419
            - class I KØ8.411
            - class II KØ8.412
            - class III KØ8.413
            - class IV KØ8.414
  - tendon (congenital) Q79.8
  - testis (congenital) Q55.Ø
    - acquired Z9Ø.79
  - thumb (acquired) Z89.Ø1- ☑
    - congenital — *see* Agenesis, hand
  - thymus gland Q89.2
  - thyroid (gland) (acquired) E89.Ø
    - cartilage, congenital Q31.8
    - congenital EØ3.1
  - toe(s) (acquired) Z89.42- ☑
    - with foot — *see* Absence, foot and ankle
    - congenital — *see* Agenesis, foot
    - great Z89.41- ☑
  - tongue, congenital Q38.3
  - trachea (cartilage), congenital Q32.1
  - transverse aortic arch, congenital Q25.49
  - tricuspid valve Q22.4
  - umbilical artery, congenital Q27.Ø
  - upper arm and forearm with hand present, congenital — *see* Agenesis, arm, with hand present
  - ureter (congenital) Q62.4
    - acquired Z9Ø.6
  - urethra, congenital Q64.5
  - uterus (acquired) Z9Ø.71Ø
    - with cervix Z9Ø.71Ø
    - with remaining cervical stump Z9Ø.711
    - congenital Q51.Ø
  - uvula, congenital Q38.5
  - vagina, congenital Q52.Ø
  - vas deferens (congenital) Q55.4
    - acquired Z9Ø.79
  - vein (peripheral) congenital NEC Q27.8
    - cerebral Q28.3
    - digestive system Q27.8
    - great Q26.8
    - lower limb Q27.8
    - portal Q26.5
    - precerebral Q28.1
    - specified site NEC Q27.8
    - upper limb Q27.8
  - vena cava (inferior) (superior), congenital Q26.8
- **Absence** — *continued*
  - ventricular septum Q2Ø.4
  - vertebra, congenital Q76.49
  - von Willebrand factor, complete (near) — *see also* Disease, von Willebrand D68.Ø3
  - vulva, congenital Q52.71
  - wrist (acquired) Z89.12- ☑
- **Absorbent system disease** I87.8
- **Absorption**
  - carbohydrate, disturbance K9Ø.49
  - chemical — *see* Table of Drugs and Chemicals
    - through placenta (newborn) PØ4.9
      - environmental substance PØ4.6
      - nutritional substance PØ4.5
      - obstetric anesthetic or analgesic drug PØ4.Ø
  - drug NEC — *see* Table of Drugs and Chemicals
    - addictive
      - through placenta (newborn) — *see also* Newborn, affected by, maternal, use of PØ4.4Ø
        - cocaine PØ4.41
        - hallucinogens PØ4.42
        - specified drug NEC PØ4.49
    - medicinal
      - through placenta (newborn) PØ4.19
    - through placenta (newborn) PØ4.19
      - obstetric anesthetic or analgesic drug PØ4.Ø
  - fat, disturbance K9Ø.49
    - pancreatic K9Ø.3
  - noxious substance — *see* Table of Drugs and Chemicals
  - protein, disturbance K9Ø.49
  - starch, disturbance K9Ø.49
  - toxic substance — *see* Table of Drugs and Chemicals
  - uremic — *see* Uremia
- **Abstinence symptoms, syndrome**
  - alcohol F1Ø.239
    - with delirium F1Ø.231
  - cocaine F14.23
  - neonatal P96.1
  - nicotine — *see* Dependence, drug, nicotine, with, withdrawal
  - opioid F11.93
    - with dependence F11.23
  - psychoactive NEC F19.939
    - with
      - delirium F19.931
      - dependence F19.239
        - with
          - delirium F19.231
          - perceptual disturbance F19.232
        - uncomplicated F19.23Ø
      - perceptual disturbance F19.932
    - uncomplicated F19.93Ø
  - sedative F13.939
    - with
      - delirium F13.931
      - dependence F13.239
        - with
          - delirium F13.231
          - perceptual disturbance F13.232
        - uncomplicated F13.23Ø
      - perceptual disturbance F13.932
    - uncomplicated F13.93Ø
  - stimulant NEC F15.93
    - with dependence F15.23
- **Abulia** R68.89
- **Abulomania** F6Ø.7
- **Abuse**
  - adult — *see* Maltreatment, adult
    - as reason for
      - couple seeking advice (including offender) Z63.Ø
  - alcohol (non-dependent) F1Ø.1Ø
    - with
      - anxiety disorder F1Ø.18Ø
      - intoxication F1Ø.129
        - with delirium F1Ø.121
        - uncomplicated F1Ø.12Ø
      - mood disorder F1Ø.14
      - other specified disorder F1Ø.188
      - psychosis F1Ø.159
        - delusions F1Ø.15Ø
        - hallucinations F1Ø.151
      - sexual dysfunction F1Ø.181
      - sleep disorder F1Ø.182
      - unspecified disorder F1Ø.19
      - withdrawal F1Ø.139
        - with
          - perceptual disturbance F1Ø.132
        - delirium F1Ø.131
- **Abuse** — *continued*
  - alcohol — *continued*
    - with — *continued*
      - withdrawal — *continued*
        - uncomplicated F1Ø.13Ø
    - counseling and surveillance Z71.41
    - in remission (early) (sustained) F1Ø.11
  - amphetamine (or related substance) — *see also* Abuse, drug, stimulant NEC
    - stimulant NEC F15.1Ø
      - with
        - anxiety disorder F15.18Ø
        - intoxication F15.129
          - with
            - delirium F15.121
            - perceptual disturbance F15.122
        - withdrawal F15.13
  - analgesics (non-prescribed) (over the counter) F55.8
  - antacids F55.Ø
  - antidepressants — *see* Abuse, drug, psychoactive NEC
  - anxiolytic — *see* Abuse, drug, sedative
  - barbiturates — *see* Abuse, drug, sedative
  - caffeine — *see* Abuse, drug, stimulant NEC
  - cannabis, cannabinoids — *see* Abuse, drug, cannabis
  - child — *see* Maltreatment, child
  - cocaine — *see* Abuse, drug, cocaine
  - drug NEC (non-dependent) F19.1Ø
    - with sleep disorder F19.182
    - amphetamine type — *see* Abuse, drug, stimulant NEC
    - analgesics (non-prescribed) (over the counter) F55.8
    - antacids F55.Ø
    - antidepressants — *see* Abuse, drug, psychoactive NEC
    - anxiolytics — *see* Abuse, drug, sedative
    - barbiturates — *see* Abuse, drug, sedative
    - caffeine — *see* Abuse, drug, stimulant NEC
    - cannabis F12.1Ø
      - with
        - anxiety disorder F12.18Ø
        - intoxication F12.129
          - with
            - delirium F12.121
            - perceptual disturbance F12.122
          - uncomplicated F12.12Ø
        - other specified disorder F12.188
        - psychosis F12.159
          - delusions F12.15Ø
          - hallucinations F12.151
        - unspecified disorder F12.19
        - withdrawal F12.13
      - in remission (early) (sustained) F12.11
    - cocaine F14.1Ø
      - with
        - anxiety disorder F14.18Ø
        - intoxication F14.129
          - with
            - delirium F14.121
            - perceptual disturbance F14.122
          - uncomplicated F14.12Ø
        - mood disorder F14.14
        - other specified disorder F14.188
        - psychosis F14.159
          - delusions F14.15Ø
          - hallucinations F14.151
        - sexual dysfunction F14.181
        - sleep disorder F14.182
        - unspecified disorder F14.19
        - withdrawal F14.13
      - in remission (early) (sustained) F14.11
    - counseling and surveillance Z71.51
    - hallucinogen F16.1Ø
      - with
        - anxiety disorder F16.18Ø
        - flashbacks F16.183
        - intoxication F16.129
          - with
            - delirium F16.121
            - perceptual disturbance F16.122
          - uncomplicated F16.12Ø
        - mood disorder F16.14
        - other specified disorder F16.188
        - perception disorder, persisting F16.183
        - psychosis F16.159
          - delusions F16.15Ø
          - hallucinations F16.151
        - unspecified disorder F16.19
      - in remission (early) (sustained) F16.11

Abuse — *continued*
- drug — *continued*
  - hashish — *see* Abuse, drug, cannabis
  - herbal or folk remedies F55.1
  - hormones F55.3
  - hypnotics — *see* Abuse, drug, sedative
  - in remission (early) (sustained) F19.11
  - inhalant F18.10
    - with
      - anxiety disorder F18.180
      - dementia, persisting F18.17
      - intoxication F18.129
        - with delirium F18.121
        - uncomplicated F18.120
      - mood disorder F18.14
      - other specified disorder F18.188
      - psychosis F18.159
        - delusions F18.150
        - hallucinations F18.151
      - unspecified disorder F18.19
    - in remission (early) (sustained) F18.11
  - laxatives F55.2
  - LSD — *see* Abuse, drug, hallucinogen
  - marihuana — *see* Abuse, drug, cannabis
  - morphine type (opioids) — *see* Abuse, drug, opioid
  - opioid F11.10
    - with
      - intoxication F11.129
        - with
          - delirium F11.121
          - perceptual disturbance F11.122
        - uncomplicated F11.120
      - mood disorder F11.14
      - opioid-associated amnestic syndrome F11.188
      - other specified disorder F11.188
      - psychosis F11.159
        - delusions F11.150
        - hallucinations F11.151
      - sexual dysfunction F11.181
      - sleep disorder F11.182
      - unspecified disorder F11.19
      - withdrawal F11.13
    - in remission (early) (sustained) F11.11
  - PCP (phencyclidine) (or related substance) — *see* Abuse, drug, hallucinogen
  - psychoactive NEC F19.10
    - with
      - amnestic disorder F19.16
      - anxiety disorder F19.180
      - dementia F19.17
      - intoxication F19.129
        - with
          - delirium F19.121
          - perceptual disturbance F19.122
        - uncomplicated F19.120
      - mood disorder F19.14
      - other specified disorder F19.188
      - psychosis F19.159
        - delusions F19.150
        - hallucinations F19.151
      - sexual dysfunction F19.181
      - sleep disorder F19.182
      - unspecified disorder F19.19
      - withdrawal F19.139
        - with
          - perceptual disturbance F19.132
        - delirium F19.131
        - uncomplicated F19.130
  - sedative, hypnotic or anxiolytic F13.10
    - with
      - anxiety disorder F13.180
      - intoxication F13.129
        - with delirium F13.121
        - uncomplicated F13.120
      - mood disorder F13.14
      - other specified disorder F13.188
      - psychosis F13.159
        - delusions F13.150
        - hallucinations F13.151
      - sexual dysfunction F13.181
      - sleep disorder F13.182
      - unspecified disorder F13.19
      - withdrawal F13.139
        - with
          - perceptual disturbance F13.132
        - delirium F13.131
        - uncomplicated F13.130
    - in remission (early) (sustained) F13.11

Abuse — *continued*
- drug — *continued*
  - solvent — *see* Abuse, drug, inhalant
  - steroids F55.3
  - stimulant NEC F15.10
    - with
      - anxiety disorder F15.180
      - intoxication F15.129
        - with
          - delirium F15.121
          - perceptual disturbance F15.122
        - uncomplicated F15.120
      - mood disorder F15.14
      - other specified disorder F15.188
      - psychosis F15.159
        - delusions F15.150
        - hallucinations F15.151
      - sexual dysfunction F15.181
      - sleep disorder F15.182
      - unspecified disorder F15.19
      - withdrawal F15.13
    - in remission (early) (sustained) F15.11
  - tranquilizers — *see* Abuse, drug, sedative
  - vitamins F55.4
- hallucinogens — *see* Abuse, drug, hallucinogen
- hashish — *see* Abuse, drug, cannabis
- herbal or folk remedies F55.1
- hormones F55.3
- hypnotic — *see* Abuse, drug, sedative
- inhalant — *see* Abuse, drug, inhalant
- laxatives F55.2
- LSD — *see* Abuse, drug, hallucinogen
- marihuana — *see* Abuse, drug, cannabis
- morphine type (opioids) — *see* Abuse, drug, opioid
- non-psychoactive substance NEC F55.8
  - antacids F55.0
  - folk remedies F55.1
  - herbal remedies F55.1
  - hormones F55.3
  - laxatives F55.2
  - steroids F55.3
  - vitamins F55.4
- opioids — *see* Abuse, drug, opioid
- PCP (phencyclidine) (or related substance) — *see* Abuse, drug, hallucinogen
- physical (adult) (child) — *see* Maltreatment
- psychoactive substance — *see* Abuse, drug, psychoactive NEC
- psychological (adult) (child) — *see* Maltreatment
- sedative — *see* Abuse, drug, sedative
- sexual — *see* Maltreatment
- solvent — *see* Abuse, drug, inhalant
- steroids F55.3
- vitamins F55.4

Acalculia R48.8
- developmental F81.2

Acanthamebiasis (with) B60.10
- conjunctiva B60.12
- keratoconjunctivitis B60.13
- meningoencephalitis B60.11
- other specified B60.19

Acanthocephaliasis B83.8

Acanthocheilonemiasis B74.4

Acanthocytosis E78.6

Acantholysis L11.9

Acanthosis (acquired) (nigricans) L83
- benign Q82.8
- congenital Q82.8
- seborrheic L82.1
  - inflamed L82.0
- tongue K14.3

Acapnia E87.3

Acarbia E87.29

Acardia, acardius Q89.8

Acardiacus amorphus Q89.8

Acardiotrophia I51.4

Acariasis B88.0
- scabies B86

Acarodermatitis (urticarioides) B88.0

Acarophobia F40.218

Acatalasemia, acatalasia E80.3

Acathisia (drug induced) G25.71

Accelerated atrioventricular conduction I45.6

Accentuation of personality traits (type A) Z73.1

Accessory (congenital)
- adrenal gland Q89.1
- anus Q43.4
- appendix Q43.4

Accessory — *continued*
- atrioventricular conduction I45.6
- auditory ossicles Q16.3
- auricle (ear) Q17.0
- biliary duct or passage Q44.5
- bladder Q64.79
- blood vessels NEC Q27.9
  - coronary Q24.5
- bone NEC Q79.8
- breast tissue, axilla Q83.1
- carpal bones Q74.0
- cecum Q43.4
- chromosome(s) NEC (nonsex) Q92.9
  - with complex rearrangements NEC Q92.5
    - seen only at prometaphase Q92.8
  - 13 — *see* Trisomy, 13
  - 18 — *see* Trisomy, 18
  - 21 — *see* Trisomy, 21
  - partial Q92.9
  - sex
    - female phenotype Q97.8
- coronary artery Q24.5
- cusp(s), heart valve NEC Q24.8
  - pulmonary Q22.3
- cystic duct Q44.5
- digit(s) Q69.9
- ear (auricle) (lobe) Q17.0
- endocrine gland NEC Q89.2
- eye muscle Q10.3
- eyelid Q10.3
- face bone(s) Q75.8
- fallopian tube (fimbria) (ostium) Q50.6
- finger(s) Q69.0
- foreskin N47.8
- frontonasal process Q75.8
- gallbladder Q44.1
- genital organ(s)
  - female Q52.8
    - external Q52.79
    - internal NEC Q52.8
  - male Q55.8
- genitourinary organs NEC Q89.8
  - female Q52.8
  - male Q55.8
- hallux Q69.2
- heart Q24.8
  - valve NEC Q24.8
    - pulmonary Q22.3
- hepatic ducts Q44.5
- hymen Q52.4
- intestine (large) (small) Q43.4
- kidney Q63.0
- lacrimal canal Q10.6
- leaflet, heart valve NEC Q24.8
- ligament, broad Q50.6
- liver Q44.79
  - duct Q44.5
- lobule (ear) Q17.0
- lung (lobe) Q33.1
- muscle Q79.8
- navicular of carpus Q74.0
- nervous system, part NEC Q07.8
- nipple Q83.3
- nose Q30.8
- organ or site not listed — *see* Anomaly, by site
- ovary Q50.31
- oviduct Q50.6
- pancreas Q45.3
- parathyroid gland Q89.2
- parotid gland (and duct) Q38.4
- pituitary gland Q89.2
- preauricular appendage Q17.0
- prepuce N47.8
- renal arteries (multiple) Q27.2
- rib Q76.6
  - cervical Q76.5
- roots (teeth) K00.2
- salivary gland Q38.4
- sesamoid bones Q74.8
  - foot Q74.2
  - hand Q74.0
- skin tags Q82.8
- spleen Q89.09
- sternum Q76.7
- submaxillary gland Q38.4
- tarsal bones Q74.2
- teeth, tooth K00.1
- tendon Q79.8
- thumb Q69.1

- **Accessory** — *continued*
  - thymus gland Q89.2
  - thyroid gland Q89.2
  - toes Q69.2
  - tongue Q38.3
  - tooth, teeth KØØ.1
  - tragus Q17.Ø
  - ureter Q62.5
  - urethra Q64.79
  - urinary organ or tract NEC Q64.8
  - uterus Q51.28
  - vagina Q52.1Ø
  - valve, heart NEC Q24.8
    - pulmonary Q22.3
  - vertebra Q76.49
  - vocal cords Q31.8
  - vulva Q52.79
- **Accident**
  - birth — *see* Birth, injury
  - cardiac — *see* Infarct, myocardium
  - cerebrovascular (ischemic) I63.9
    - aborted I63.9
    - chronic (old) (remote) (imaging) (without sequelae) Z86.73
      - with residual defects — *see* Sequelae, disease, cerebrovascular
    - embolic I63.- ☑
    - hemorrhagic — *see* Hemorrhage, intracranial, intracerebral
    - old (without sequelae) Z86.73
      - with sequelae (of) — *see* Sequelae, infarction, cerebral
    - thrombotic I63.- ☑
  - coronary — *see* Infarct, myocardium
  - craniovascular I63.9
  - vascular, brain I63.9
- **Accidental** — *see* condition
- **Accommodation** (disorder) — *see also* condition
  - hysterical paralysis of F44.89
  - insufficiency of H52.4
  - paresis — *see* Paresis, of accommodation
  - spasm — *see* Spasm, of accommodation
- **Accouchement** — *see* Delivery
- **Accreta placenta** O43.21- ☑
- **Accretio cordis** (nonrheumatic) I31.Ø
- **Accretions, tooth, teeth** KØ3.6
- **Acculturation difficulty** Z6Ø.3
- **Accumulation secretion, prostate** N42.89
- **Acephalia, acephalism, acephalus, acephaly** QØØ.Ø
- **Acephalobrachia monster** Q89.8
- **Acephalochirus monster** Q89.8
- **Acephalogaster** Q89.8
- **Acephalostomus monster** Q89.8
- **Acephalothorax** Q89.8
- **Acerophobia** F4Ø.298
- **Acetonemia** R79.89
  - in Type 1 diabetes E1Ø.1Ø
    - with coma E1Ø.11
- **Acetonuria** R82.4
- **Achalasia** (cardia) (esophagus) K22.Ø
  - congenital Q39.5
  - pylorus Q4Ø.Ø
  - sphincteral NEC K59.89
- **Ache**(s) — *see* Pain
- **Acheilia** Q38.6
- **Achillobursitis** — *see* Tendinitis, Achilles
- **Achillodynia** — *see* Tendinitis, Achilles
- **Achlorhydria, achlorhydric** (neurogenic) K31.83
  - anemia D5Ø.8
  - diarrhea K31.83
  - psychogenic F45.8
  - secondary to vagotomy K91.1
- **Achluophobia** F4Ø.228
- **Acholia** K82.8
- **Acholuric jaundice** (familial) (splenomegalic) — *see also* Spherocytosis
  - acquired D59.8
- **Achondrogenesis** Q77.Ø
- **Achondroplasia** (osteosclerosis congenita) Q77.4
- **Achroma, cutis** L8Ø
- **Achromat** (ism), achromatopsia (acquired) (congenital) H53.51
- **Achromia, congenital** — *see* Albinism
- **Achromia parasitica** B36.Ø
- **Achylia gastrica** K31.89
  - psychogenic F45.8
- **Acid**
  - burn — *see* Corrosion
  - deficiency
    - amide nicotinic E52
    - ascorbic E54
    - folic E53.8
    - nicotinic E52
    - pantothenic E53.8
  - intoxication — *see also* Acidosis E87.29
  - peptic disease K3Ø
  - phosphatase deficiency E83.39
  - stomach K3Ø
    - psychogenic F45.8
- **Acidemia** — *see also* Acidosis E87.2Ø
  - argininosuccinic E72.22
  - isovaleric E71.11Ø
  - metabolic — *see also* Acidosis, metabolic
    - newborn P19.9
      - first noted before onset of labor P19.Ø
      - first noted during labor P19.1
      - noted at birth P19.2
  - methylmalonic E71.12Ø
  - pipecolic E72.3
  - propionic E71.121
- **Acidity, gastric** (high) K3Ø
  - psychogenic F45.8
- **Acidocytopenia** — *see* Agranulocytosis
- **Acidocytosis** D72.1Ø
- **Acidopenia** — *see* Agranulocytosis
- **Acidosis** (lactic) E87.2Ø
  - in Type 1 diabetes E1Ø.1Ø
    - with coma E1Ø.11
  - kidney, tubular N25.89
  - lactic E87.2Ø
    - acute E87.21
    - chronic E87.22
  - metabolic NEC E87.2Ø
    - with respiratory acidosis E87.4
    - acute E87.21
    - chronic E87.22
    - hyperchloremic, of newborn P74.421
    - late, of newborn P74.Ø
  - mixed metabolic and respiratory, newborn P84
  - newborn P84
  - renal (hyperchloremic) (tubular) N25.89
  - respiratory E87.29
    - acute J96.Ø2
    - chronic J96.12
    - complicated by
      - metabolic
        - acidosis E87.4
        - alkalosis E87.4
  - specified NEC E87.29
- **Aciduria**
  - 4-hydroxybutyric E72.81
  - argininosuccinic E72.22
  - gamma-hydroxybutyric E72.81
  - glutaric (type I) E72.3
    - type II E71.313
    - type III E71.5- ☑
  - orotic (congenital) (hereditary) (pyrimidine deficiency) E79.89
    - anemia D53.Ø
- **Acladiosis** (skin) B36.Ø
- **Aclasis, diaphyseal** Q78.6
- **Acleistocardia** Q21.19
- **Aclusion** — *see* Anomaly, dentofacial, malocclusion
- **Acne** L7Ø.9
  - artificialis L7Ø.8
  - atrophica L7Ø.2
  - cachecticorum (Hebra) L7Ø.8
  - conglobata L7Ø.1
  - cystic L7Ø.Ø
  - decalvans L66.2
  - excoriee (des jeunes filles) L7Ø.5
  - frontalis L7Ø.2
  - indurata L7Ø.Ø
  - infantile L7Ø.4
  - keloid L73.Ø
  - lupoid L7Ø.2
  - necrotic, necrotica (miliaris) L7Ø.2
  - neonatal L7Ø.4
  - nodular L7Ø.Ø
  - occupational L7Ø.8
  - picker's L7Ø.5
  - pustular L7Ø.Ø
  - rodens L7Ø.2
  - rosacea L71.9
- **Acne** — *continued*
  - specified NEC L7Ø.8
  - tropica L7Ø.3
  - varioliformis L7Ø.2
  - vulgaris L7Ø.Ø
- **Acnitis** (primary) A18.4
- **Acosta's disease** T7Ø.29 ☑
- **Acoustic** — *see* condition
- **Acousticophobia** F4Ø.298
- **ACPO** (acute colonic pseudo-obstruction) K59.81
- **Acquired** — *see also* condition
  - immunodeficiency syndrome (AIDS) B2Ø
- **Acrania** QØØ.Ø
- **Acroangiodermatitis** I78.9
- **Acroasphyxia, chronic** I73.89
- **Acrobystitis** N47.7
- **Acrocephalopolysyndactyly** Q87.Ø
- **Acrocephalosyndactyly** Q87.Ø
- **Acrocephaly** Q75.ØØ9
- **Acrochondrohyperplasia** — *see* Syndrome, Marfan
- **Acrocyanosis** I73.89
  - newborn P28.2
    - meaning transient blue hands and feet — *omit code*
- **Acrodermatitis** L3Ø.8
  - atrophicans (chronica) L9Ø.4
  - continua (Hallopeau) L4Ø.2
  - enteropathica (hereditary) E83.2
  - Hallopeau's L4Ø.2
  - infantile papular L44.4
  - perstans L4Ø.2
  - pustulosa continua L4Ø.2
  - recalcitrant pustular L4Ø.2
- **Acrodynia** — *see* Poisoning, mercury
- **Acromegaly, acromegalia** E22.Ø
- **Acromelalgia** I73.81
- **Acromicria, acromikria** Q79.8
- **Acronyx** L6Ø.Ø
- **Acropachy, thyroid** — *see* Thyrotoxicosis
- **Acroparesthesia** (simple) (vasomotor) I73.89
- **Acropathy, thyroid** — *see* Thyrotoxicosis
- **Acrophobia** F4Ø.241
- **Acroposthitis** N47.7
- **Acroscleriasis, acroscleroderma, acrosclerosis** — *see* Sclerosis, systemic
- **Acrosphacelus** I96
- **Acrospiroma, eccrine** — *see* Neoplasm, skin, benign
- **Acrostealgia** — *see* Osteochondropathy
- **Acrotrophodynia** — *see* Immersion
- **ACTH ectopic syndrome** E24.3
- **Actinic** — *see* condition
- **Actinobacillosis, actinobacillus** A28.8
  - mallei A24.Ø
  - muris A25.1
- **Actinomyces israelii** (infection) — *see* Actinomycosis
- **Actinomycetoma** (foot) B47.1
- **Actinomycosis, actinomycotic** A42.9
  - with pneumonia A42.Ø
  - abdominal A42.1
  - cervicofacial A42.2
  - cutaneous A42.89
  - gastrointestinal A42.1
  - pulmonary A42.Ø
  - sepsis A42.7
  - specified site NEC A42.89
- **Actinoneuritis** G62.82
- **Action, heart**
  - disorder I49.9
  - irregular I49.9
    - psychogenic F45.8
- **Activated protein C resistance** D68.51
- **Activation**
  - mast cell (disorder) (syndrome) D89.4Ø
    - idiopathic D89.42
    - monoclonal D89.41
    - secondary D89.43
    - specified type NEC D89.49
- **Active** — *see* condition
- **Acute** — *see also* condition
  - abdomen R1Ø.Ø
  - gallbladder — *see* Cholecystitis, acute
- **Acyanotic heart disease** (congenital) Q24.9
- **Acystia** Q64.5
- **Adair-Dighton syndrome** (brittle bones and blue sclera, deafness) Q78.Ø
- **Adamantinoblastoma** — *see* Ameloblastoma
- **Adamantinoma** — *see also* Cyst, calcifying odontogenic
  - long bones C4Ø.9Ø

- **Adenofibroma** — *continued*
  - endometrioid — *continued*
    - borderline malignancy D39.1Ø
    - malignant C56- ☑
  - mucinous
    - specified site — *see* Neoplasm, benign, by site
    - unspecified site D27.9
  - papillary
    - specified site — *see* Neoplasm, benign, by site
    - unspecified site D27.9
  - prostate — *see* Enlargement, enlarged, prostate
  - serous
    - specified site — *see* Neoplasm, benign, by site
    - unspecified site D27.9
  - specified site — *see* Neoplasm, benign, by site
  - unspecified site D27.9
- **Adenofibrosis**
  - breast — *see* Fibroadenosis, breast
  - endometrioid N8Ø.ØØ
- **Adenoiditis** (chronic) J35.Ø2
  - with tonsillitis J35.Ø3
  - acute JØ3.9Ø
    - recurrent JØ3.91
    - specified organism NEC JØ3.8Ø
      - recurrent JØ3.81
    - staphylococcal JØ3.8Ø
      - recurrent JØ3.81
    - streptococcal JØ3.ØØ
      - recurrent JØ3.Ø1
- **Adenoids** — *see* condition
- **Adenolipoma** — *see* Neoplasm, benign, by site
- **Adenolipomatosis, Launois-Bensaude** E88.89
- **Adenolymphoma**
  - specified site — *see* Neoplasm, benign, by site
  - unspecified site D11.9
- **Adenoma** — *see also* Neoplasm, benign, by site
  - acidophil
    - specified site — *see* Neoplasm, benign, by site
    - unspecified site D35.2
  - acidophil-basophil, mixed
    - specified site — *see* Neoplasm, benign, by site
    - unspecified site D35.2
  - adrenal (cortical) D35.ØØ
    - clear cell D35.ØØ
    - compact cell D35.ØØ
    - glomerulosa cell D35.ØØ
    - heavily pigmented variant D35.ØØ
    - mixed cell D35.ØØ
  - alpha-cell
    - pancreas D13.7
    - specified site NEC — *see* Neoplasm, benign, by site
    - unspecified site D13.7
  - alveolar D14.3Ø
  - apocrine
    - breast D24- ☑
    - specified site NEC — *see* Neoplasm, skin, benign, by site
    - unspecified site D23.9
  - basal cell D11.9
  - basophil
    - specified site — *see* Neoplasm, benign, by site
    - unspecified site D35.2
  - basophil-acidophil, mixed
    - specified site — *see* Neoplasm, benign, by site
    - unspecified site D35.2
  - beta-cell
    - pancreas D13.7
    - specified site NEC — *see* Neoplasm, benign, by site
    - unspecified site D13.7
  - bile duct D13.4
    - common D13.5
    - extrahepatic D13.5
    - intrahepatic D13.4
    - specified site NEC — *see* Neoplasm, benign, by site
    - unspecified site D13.4
  - black D35.ØØ
  - bronchial D38.1
    - cylindroid type — *see* Neoplasm, lung, malignant
  - ceruminous D23.2- ☑
  - chief cell D35.1
  - chromophobe
    - specified site — *see* Neoplasm, benign, by site
    - unspecified site D35.2
  - colloid
    - specified site — *see* Neoplasm, benign, by site
    - unspecified site D34
  - eccrine, papillary — *see* Neoplasm, skin, benign
- **Adenoma** — *continued*
  - endocrine, multiple
    - single specified site — *see* Neoplasm, uncertain behavior, by site
    - two or more specified sites D44- ☑
    - unspecified site D44.9
  - endometrioid — *see also* Neoplasm, benign
    - borderline malignancy — *see* Neoplasm, uncertain behavior, by site
  - eosinophil
    - specified site — *see* Neoplasm, benign, by site
    - unspecified site D35.2
  - fetal
    - specified site — *see* Neoplasm, benign, by site
    - unspecified site D34
  - follicular
    - specified site — *see* Neoplasm, benign, by site
    - unspecified site D34
  - hepatocellular D13.4
  - Hurthle cell D34
  - islet cell
    - pancreas D13.7
    - specified site NEC — *see* Neoplasm, benign, by site
    - unspecified site D13.7
  - liver cell D13.4
  - macrofollicular
    - specified site — *see* Neoplasm, benign, by site
    - unspecified site D34
  - malignant, malignum — *see* Neoplasm, malignant, by site
  - microcystic
    - pancreas D13.6
    - specified site NEC — *see* Neoplasm, benign, by site
    - unspecified site D13.6
  - microfollicular
    - specified site — *see* Neoplasm, benign, by site
    - unspecified site D34
  - mucoid cell
    - specified site — *see* Neoplasm, benign, by site
    - unspecified site D35.2
  - multiple endocrine
    - single specified site — *see* Neoplasm, uncertain behavior, by site
    - two or more specified sites D44- ☑
    - unspecified site D44.9
  - nipple D24- ☑
  - papillary — *see also* Neoplasm, benign, by site
    - eccrine — *see* Neoplasm, skin, benign, by site
  - Pick's tubular
    - specified site — *see* Neoplasm, benign, by site
    - unspecified site
      - female D27.9
      - male D29.2Ø
  - pleomorphic
    - carcinoma in — *see* Neoplasm, salivary gland, malignant
      - specified site — *see* Neoplasm, malignant, by site
      - unspecified site CØ8.9
  - polypoid — *see also* Neoplasm, benign
    - adenocarcinoma in — *see* Neoplasm, malignant, by site
    - adenocarcinoma in situ — *see* Neoplasm, in situ, by site
  - prostate — *see* Neoplasm, benign, prostate
  - rete cell D29.2Ø
  - sebaceous — *see* Neoplasm, skin, benign
  - Sertoli cell
    - specified site — *see* Neoplasm, benign, by site
    - unspecified site
      - female D27.9
      - male D29.2Ø
  - skin appendage — *see* Neoplasm, skin, benign
  - sudoriferous gland — *see* Neoplasm, skin, benign
  - sweat gland — *see* Neoplasm, skin, benign
  - testicular
    - specified site — *see* Neoplasm, benign, by site
    - unspecified site
      - female D27.9
      - male D29.2Ø
  - tubular — *see also* Neoplasm, benign, by site
    - adenocarcinoma in — *see* Neoplasm, malignant, by site
    - adenocarcinoma in situ — *see* Neoplasm, in situ, by site
    - Pick's
      - specified site — *see* Neoplasm, benign, by site
- **Adenoma** — *continued*
  - tubular — *see also* Neoplasm, benign, by site — *continued*
    - Pick's — *continued*
      - unspecified site
        - female D27.9
        - male D29.2Ø
  - tubulovillous — *see also* Neoplasm, benign, by site
    - adenocarcinoma in — *see* Neoplasm, malignant, by site
    - adenocarcinoma in situ — *see* Neoplasm, in situ, by site
  - villous — *see* Neoplasm, uncertain behavior, by site
    - adenocarcinoma in — *see* Neoplasm, malignant, by site
    - adenocarcinoma in situ — *see* Neoplasm, in situ, by site
  - water-clear cell D35.1
- **Adenomatosis**
  - endocrine (multiple) E31.2Ø
    - single specified site — *see* Neoplasm, uncertain behavior, by site
  - erosive of nipple D24- ☑
  - pluriendocrine — *see* Adenomatosis, endocrine
  - pulmonary D38.1
    - malignant — *see* Neoplasm, lung, malignant
  - specified site — *see* Neoplasm, benign, by site
  - unspecified site D12.6
- **Adenomatous**
  - goiter (nontoxic) EØ4.9
    - with hyperthyroidism — *see* Hyperthyroidism, with, goiter, nodular
    - toxic — *see* Hyperthyroidism, with, goiter, nodular
- **Adenomyoma** — *see also* Neoplasm, benign, by site
  - prostate — *see* Enlarged, prostate
- **Adenomyometritis** N8Ø.ØØ
- **Adenomyosis** (uterus) N8Ø.Ø3
- **Adenopathy** (lymph gland) R59.9
  - generalized R59.1
  - inguinal R59.Ø
  - localized R59.Ø
  - mediastinal R59.Ø
  - mesentery R59.Ø
  - syphilitic (secondary) A51.49
  - tracheobronchial R59.Ø
    - tuberculous A15.4
      - primary (progressive) A15.7
  - tuberculous — *see also* Tuberculosis, lymph gland
    - tracheobronchial A15.4
      - primary (progressive) A15.7
- **Adenosalpingitis** — *see* Salpingitis
- **Adenosarcoma** — *see* Neoplasm, malignant, by site
- **Adenosclerosis** I88.8
- **Adenosis** (sclerosing) breast — *see* Fibroadenosis, breast
- **Adenovirus, as cause of disease classified elsewhere** B97.Ø
- **Adentia** (complete) (partial) — *see* Absence, teeth
- **Adherent** — *see also* Adhesions
  - labia (minora) N9Ø.89
  - pericardium (nonrheumatic) I31.Ø
    - rheumatic IØ9.2
  - placenta (with hemorrhage) O72.Ø
    - without hemorrhage O73.Ø
  - prepuce, newborn N47.Ø
  - scar (skin) L9Ø.5
  - tendon in scar L9Ø.5
- **Adhesions, adhesive** (postinfective) K66.Ø
  - with intestinal obstruction K56.5Ø
    - complete K56.52
    - incomplete K56.51
    - partial K56.51
  - abdominal (wall) — *see* Adhesions, peritoneum
  - appendix K38.8
  - bile duct (common) (hepatic) K83.8
  - bladder (sphincter) N32.89
  - bowel — *see* Adhesions, peritoneum
  - cardiac I31.Ø
    - rheumatic IØ9.2
  - cecum — *see* Adhesions, peritoneum
  - cervicovaginal N88.1
    - congenital Q52.8
    - postpartal O9Ø.89
      - old N88.1
  - cervix N88.1
  - ciliary body NEC — *see* Adhesions, iris
  - clitoris N9Ø.89
  - colon — *see* Adhesions, peritoneum
  - common duct K83.8

☑ **Additional Character Required — Refer to the Tabular List for Character Selection**

Admission — *continued*
- attention to artificial opening — *continued*
  - specified site NEC Z43.8
    - intestinal tract Z43.4
    - urinary tract Z43.6
  - tracheostomy Z43.Ø
  - ureterostomy Z43.6
  - urethrostomy Z43.6
- breast augmentation or reduction Z41.1
- breast reconstruction following mastectomy Z42.1
- change of
  - dressing (nonsurgical) Z48.ØØ
  - neuropacemaker device (brain) (peripheral nerve) (spinal cord) Z46.2
    - implanted Z45.42
  - surgical dressing Z48.Ø1
- circumcision, ritual or routine (in absence of diagnosis) Z41.2
- clinical research investigation (control) (normal comparison) (participant) ZØØ.6
- contraceptive management Z3Ø.9
- cosmetic surgery NEC Z41.1
- counseling — *see also* Counseling
  - dietary Z71.3
  - gestational carrier Z31.7
  - HIV Z71.7
  - human immunodeficiency virus Z71.7
  - nonattending third party Z71.Ø
  - procreative management NEC Z31.69
- delivery, full-term, uncomplicated O8Ø
  - cesarean, without indication O82
- desensitization to allergens Z51.6
- dietary surveillance and counseling Z71.3
- ear piercing Z41.3
- examination at health care facility (adult) — *see also* Examination ZØØ.ØØ
  - with abnormal findings ZØØ.Ø1
  - clinical research investigation (control) (normal comparison) (participant) ZØØ.6
  - dental ZØ1.2Ø
    - with abnormal findings ZØ1.21
  - donor (potential) ZØØ.5
  - ear ZØ1.1Ø
    - with abnormal findings NEC ZØ1.118
  - eye ZØ1.ØØ
    - with abnormal findings ZØ1.Ø1
    - following failed vision screening ZØ1.Ø2Ø
      - with abnormal findings ZØ1.Ø21
  - general, specified reason NEC ZØØ.8
  - hearing ZØ1.1Ø
    - with abnormal findings NEC ZØ1.118
    - infant or child (over 28 days old) ZØØ.129
      - with abnormal findings ZØØ.121
  - postpartum checkup Z39.2
  - psychiatric (general) ZØØ.8
    - requested by authority ZØ4.6
  - vision ZØ1.ØØ
    - with abnormal findings ZØ1.Ø1
    - following failed vision screening ZØ1.Ø2Ø
      - with abnormal findings ZØ1.Ø21
    - infant or child (over 28 days old) ZØØ.129
      - with abnormal findings ZØØ.121
- fitting (of)
  - artificial
    - arm — *see* Admission, adjustment, artificial, arm
    - eye Z44.2 ☑
    - leg — *see* Admission, adjustment, artificial, leg
  - brain neuropacemaker Z46.2
    - implanted Z45.42
  - breast prosthesis (external) Z44.3 ☑
  - colostomy belt Z46.89
  - contact lenses Z46.Ø
  - cystostomy device Z46.6
  - dental prosthesis Z46.3
  - dentures Z46.3
  - device NEC
    - abdominal Z46.89
    - nervous system Z46.2
      - implanted — *see* Admission, adjustment, device, implanted, nervous system
    - orthodontic Z46.4
    - prosthetic Z44.9
      - breast Z44.3 ☑
      - dental Z46.3
      - eye Z44.2 ☑
    - substitution
      - auditory Z46.2

Admission — *continued*
- fitting — *continued*
  - device — *continued*
    - substitution — *continued*
      - auditory — *continued*
        - implanted — *see* Admission, adjustment, device, implanted, hearing device
      - nervous system Z46.2
        - implanted — *see* Admission, adjustment, device, implanted, nervous system
      - visual Z46.2
        - implanted Z45.31
  - hearing aid Z46.1
  - ileostomy device Z46.89
  - intestinal appliance or device NEC Z46.89
  - neuropacemaker (brain) (peripheral nerve) (spinal cord) Z46.2
    - implanted Z45.42
  - orthodontic device Z46.4
  - orthopedic device (brace) (cast) (shoes) Z46.89
  - prosthesis Z44.9
    - arm — *see* Admission, adjustment, artificial, arm
    - breast Z44.3 ☑
    - dental Z46.3
    - eye Z44.2 ☑
    - leg — *see* Admission, adjustment, artificial, leg
    - specified type NEC Z44.8
  - spectacles Z46.Ø
- follow-up examination ZØ9
- intrauterine device management Z3Ø.431
  - initial prescription Z3Ø.Ø14
- mental health evaluation ZØØ.8
  - requested by authority ZØ4.6
- observation — *see* Observation
- Papanicolaou smear, cervix Z12.4
  - for suspected malignant neoplasm Z12.4
- plastic and reconstructive surgery following medical procedure or healed injury NEC Z42.8
- plastic surgery, cosmetic NEC Z41.1
- postpartum observation
  - immediately after delivery Z39.Ø
  - routine follow-up Z39.2
- poststerilization (for restoration) Z31.Ø
  - aftercare Z31.42
- procreative management Z31.9
- prophylactic (measure) — *see also* Encounter, prophylactic measures
  - organ removal Z4Ø.ØØ
    - breast Z4Ø.Ø1
    - fallopian tube(s) Z4Ø.Ø3
      - with ovary(s) Z4Ø.Ø2
    - ovary(s) Z4Ø.Ø2
    - specified organ NEC Z4Ø.Ø9
    - testes Z4Ø.Ø9
  - vaccination Z23
- psychiatric examination (general) ZØØ.8
  - requested by authority ZØ4.6
- radiation therapy (antineoplastic) Z51.Ø
- reconstructive surgery following medical procedure or healed injury NEC Z42.8
- removal of
  - cystostomy catheter Z43.5
  - drains Z48.Ø3
  - dressing (nonsurgical) Z48.ØØ
  - implantable subdermal contraceptive Z3Ø.46
  - intrauterine contraceptive device Z3Ø.432
  - neuropacemaker (brain) (peripheral nerve) (spinal cord) Z46.2
    - implanted Z45.42
  - staples Z48.Ø2
  - surgical dressing Z48.Ø1
  - sutures Z48.Ø2
  - ureteral stent Z46.6
- respirator [ventilator] use during power failure Z99.12
- restoration of organ continuity (poststerilization) Z31.Ø
  - aftercare Z31.42
- sensitivity test — *see also* Test, skin
  - allergy NEC ZØ1.82
  - Mantoux Z11.1
- tuboplasty following previous sterilization Z31.Ø
  - aftercare Z31.42
- vasoplasty following previous sterilization Z31.Ø
  - aftercare Z31.42
- vision examination ZØ1.ØØ
  - with abnormal findings ZØ1.Ø1
  - following failed vision screening ZØ1.Ø2Ø
    - with abnormal findings ZØ1.Ø21
  - infant or child (over 28 days old) ZØØ.129

Admission — *continued*
- vision examination — *continued*
  - infant or child — *continued*
    - with abnormal findings ZØØ.121
- waiting period for admission to other facility Z75.1

Adnexitis (suppurative) — *see* Salpingo-oophoritis

Adolescent X-linked adrenoleukodystrophy E71.521

Adrenal (gland) — *see* condition

Adrenalism, tuberculous A18.7

Adrenalitis, adrenitis E27.8
- autoimmune E27.1
- meningococcal, hemorrhagic A39.1

Adrenarche, premature E27.Ø

Adrenocortical syndrome — *see* Cushing's, syndrome

Adrenogenital syndrome E25.9
- acquired E25.8
- congenital E25.Ø
- salt loss E25.Ø

Adrenogenitalism, congenital E25.Ø

Adrenoleukodystrophy E71.529
- neonatal E71.511
- X-linked E71.529
  - Addison only phenotype E71.528
  - Addison-Schilder E71.528
  - adolescent E71.521
  - adrenomyeloneuropathy E71.522
  - childhood cerebral E71.52Ø
  - other specified E71.528

Adrenomyeloneuropathy E71.522

Adventitious bursa — *see* Bursopathy, specified type NEC

Adverse effect — *see* Table of Drugs and Chemicals, categories T36-T5Ø, with 6th character 5

Advice — *see* Counseling

Adynamia (episodica) (hereditary) (periodic) G72.3

Aeration lung imperfect, newborn — *see* Atelectasis

Aerobullosis T7Ø.3 ☑

Aerocele — *see* Embolism, air

Aerodermectasia
- subcutaneous (traumatic) T79.7 ☑

Aerodontalgia T7Ø.29 ☑

Aeroembolism T7Ø.3 ☑

Aerogenes capsulatus infection A48.Ø

Aero-otitis media T7Ø.Ø ☑

Aerophagy, aerophagia (psychogenic) F45.8

Aerophobia F4Ø.228

Aerosinusitis T7Ø.1 ☑

Aerotitis T7Ø.Ø ☑

Affection — *see* Disease

Afibrinogenemia — *see also* Defect, coagulation D68.8
- acquired D65
- congenital D68.2
- following ectopic or molar pregnancy OØ8.1
- in abortion — *see* Abortion, by type, complicated by, afibrinogenemia
- puerperal O72.3

African
- sleeping sickness B56.9
- tick fever A68.1
- trypanosomiasis B56.9
  - gambian B56.Ø
  - rhodesian B56.1

Aftercare — *see also* Care Z51.89
- following surgery (for) (on)
  - amputation Z47.81
  - attention to
    - drains Z48.Ø3
    - dressings (nonsurgical) Z48.ØØ
      - surgical Z48.Ø1
    - sutures Z48.Ø2
  - circulatory system Z48.812
  - delayed (planned) wound closure Z48.1
  - digestive system Z48.815
  - explantation of joint prosthesis (staged procedure)
    - hip Z47.32
    - knee Z47.33
    - shoulder Z47.31
  - genitourinary system Z48.816
  - joint replacement Z47.1
  - neoplasm Z48.3
  - nervous system Z48.811
  - oral cavity Z48.814
  - organ transplant
    - bone marrow Z48.29Ø
    - heart Z48.21
    - heart-lung Z48.28Ø
    - kidney Z48.22
    - liver Z48.23

- **Aftercare** — *continued*
  - following surgery — *continued*
    - organ transplant — *continued*
      - lung Z48.24
      - multiple organs NEC Z48.288
      - specified NEC Z48.298
    - orthopedic NEC Z47.89
    - planned wound closure Z48.1
    - removal of internal fixation device Z47.2
    - respiratory system Z48.813
    - scoliosis Z47.82
    - sense organs Z48.81Ø
    - skin and subcutaneous tissue Z48.817
    - specified body system
      - circulatory Z48.812
      - digestive Z48.815
      - genitourinary Z48.816
      - nervous Z48.811
      - oral cavity Z48.814
      - respiratory Z48.813
      - sense organs Z48.81Ø
      - skin and subcutaneous tissue Z48.817
      - teeth Z48.814
    - specified NEC Z48.89
    - spinal Z47.89
    - teeth Z48.814
  - fracture — *code to* fracture with seventh character D
  - involving
    - removal of
      - drains Z48.Ø3
      - dressings (nonsurgical) Z48.ØØ
      - staples Z48.Ø2
      - surgical dressings Z48.Ø1
      - sutures Z48.Ø2
  - neuropacemaker (brain) (peripheral nerve) (spinal cord) Z46.2
    - implanted Z45.42
  - orthopedic NEC Z47.89
  - postprocedural — *see* Aftercare, following surgery
- **After-cataract** — *see* Cataract, secondary
- **Agalactia** (primary) O92.3
  - elective, secondary or therapeutic O92.5
- **Agammaglobulinemia** (acquired (secondary) (nonfamilial) D8Ø.1
  - with
    - immunoglobulin-bearing B-lymphocytes D8Ø.1
    - lymphopenia D81.9
  - autosomal recessive (Swiss type) D8Ø.Ø
  - Bruton's X-linked D8Ø.Ø
  - common variable (CVAgamma) D8Ø.1
  - congenital sex-linked D8Ø.Ø
  - hereditary D8Ø.Ø
  - lymphopenic D81.9
  - Swiss type (autosomal recessive) D8Ø.Ø
  - X-linked (with growth hormone deficiency) (Bruton) D8Ø.Ø
- **Aganglionosis** (bowel) (colon) Q43.1
- **Age** (old) — *see* Senility
- **Agenesis**
  - adrenal (gland) Q89.1
  - alimentary tract (complete) (partial) NEC Q45.8
    - upper Q4Ø.8
  - anus, anal (canal) Q42.3
    - with fistula Q42.2
  - aorta Q25.41
  - appendix Q42.8
  - arm (complete) Q71.Ø- ☑
    - with hand present Q71.1- ☑
  - artery (peripheral) Q27.9
    - brain Q28.3
    - coronary Q24.5
    - pulmonary Q25.79
    - specified NEC Q27.8
    - umbilical Q27.Ø
  - auditory (canal) (external) Q16.1
  - auricle (ear) Q16.Ø
  - bile duct or passage Q44.5
  - bladder Q64.5
  - bone Q79.9
  - brain QØØ.Ø
    - part of QØ4.3
  - breast (with nipple present) Q83.8
    - with absent nipple Q83.Ø
  - bronchus Q32.4
  - canaliculus lacrimalis Q1Ø.4
  - carpus — *see* Agenesis, hand
  - cartilage Q79.9
  - cecum Q42.8
- **Agenesis** — *continued*
  - cerebellum QØ4.3
  - cervix Q51.5
  - chin Q18.8
  - cilia Q1Ø.3
  - circulatory system, part NOS Q28.9
  - clavicle Q74.Ø
  - clitoris Q52.6
  - coccyx Q76.49
  - colon Q42.9
    - specified NEC Q42.8
  - corpus callosum QØ4.Ø
  - cricoid cartilage Q31.8
  - diaphragm (with hernia) Q79.1
  - digestive organ(s) or tract (complete) (partial) NEC Q45.8
    - upper Q4Ø.8
  - ductus arteriosus Q28.8
  - duodenum Q41.Ø
  - ear Q16.9
    - auricle Q16.Ø
    - lobe Q17.8
  - ejaculatory duct Q55.4
  - endocrine (gland) NEC Q89.2
  - epiglottis Q31.8
  - esophagus Q39.8
  - eustachian tube Q16.2
  - eye Q11.1
    - adnexa Q15.8
  - eyelid (fold) Q1Ø.3
  - face
    - bones NEC Q75.8
    - specified part NEC Q18.8
  - fallopian tube Q5Ø.6
  - femur — *see* Defect, reduction, lower limb, longitudinal, femur
  - fibula — *see* Defect, reduction, lower limb, longitudinal, fibula
  - finger (complete) (partial) — *see* Agenesis, hand
  - foot (and toes) (complete) (partial) Q72.3- ☑
  - forearm (with hand present) — *see* Agenesis, arm, with hand present
    - and hand Q71.2- ☑
  - gallbladder Q44.Ø
  - gastric Q4Ø.2
  - genitalia, genital (organ(s))
    - female Q52.8
      - external Q52.71
      - internal NEC Q52.8
    - male Q55.8
  - glottis Q31.8
  - hair Q84.Ø
  - hand (and fingers) (complete) (partial) Q71.3- ☑
  - heart Q24.8
    - valve NEC Q24.8
      - pulmonary Q22.Ø
  - hepatic Q44.79
  - humerus — *see* Defect, reduction, upper limb
  - hymen Q52.4
  - ileum Q41.2
  - incus Q16.3
  - intestine (small) Q41.9
    - large Q42.9
      - specified NEC Q42.8
  - iris (dilator fibers) Q13.1
  - jaw M26.Ø9
  - jejunum Q41.1
  - kidney(s) (partial) Q6Ø.2
    - bilateral Q6Ø.1
    - unilateral Q6Ø.Ø
  - labium (majus) (minus) Q52.71
  - labyrinth, membranous Q16.5
  - lacrimal apparatus Q1Ø.4
  - larynx Q31.8
  - leg (complete) Q72.Ø- ☑
    - with foot present Q72.1- ☑
    - lower leg (with foot present) — *see* Agenesis, leg, with foot present
      - and foot Q72.2- ☑
  - lens Q12.3
  - limb (complete) Q73.Ø
    - lower — *see* Agenesis, leg
    - upper — *see* Agenesis, arm
  - lip Q38.Ø
  - liver Q44.79
  - lung (fissure) (lobe) (bilateral) (unilateral) Q33.3
  - mandible, maxilla M26.Ø9
  - metacarpus — *see* Agenesis, hand
- **Agenesis** — *continued*
  - metatarsus — *see* Agenesis, foot
  - muscle Q79.8
    - eyelid Q1Ø.3
    - ocular Q15.8
  - musculoskeletal system NEC Q79.8
  - nail(s) Q84.3
  - neck, part Q18.8
  - nerve QØ7.8
  - nervous system, part NEC QØ7.8
  - nipple Q83.2
  - nose Q3Ø.1
  - nuclear QØ7.8
  - organ
    - of Corti Q16.5
    - or site not listed — *see* Anomaly, by site
  - osseous meatus (ear) Q16.1
  - ovary
    - bilateral Q5Ø.Ø2
    - unilateral Q5Ø.Ø1
  - oviduct Q5Ø.6
  - pancreas Q45.Ø
  - parathyroid (gland) Q89.2
  - parotid gland(s) Q38.4
  - patella Q74.1
  - pelvic girdle (complete) (partial) Q74.2
  - penis Q55.5
  - pericardium Q24.8
  - pituitary (gland) Q89.2
  - prostate Q55.4
  - punctum lacrimale Q1Ø.4
  - radioulnar — *see* Defect, reduction, upper limb
  - radius — *see* Defect, reduction, upper limb, longitudinal, radius
  - rectum Q42.1
    - with fistula Q42.Ø
  - renal Q6Ø.2
    - bilateral Q6Ø.1
    - unilateral Q6Ø.Ø
  - respiratory organ NEC Q34.8
  - rib Q76.6
  - roof of orbit Q75.8
  - round ligament Q52.8
  - sacrum Q76.49
  - salivary gland Q38.4
  - scapula Q74.Ø
  - scrotum Q55.29
  - seminal vesicles Q55.4
  - septum
    - atrial Q21.19
    - between aorta and pulmonary artery Q21.4
    - ventricular Q2Ø.4
  - shoulder girdle (complete) (partial) Q74.Ø
  - skull (bone) Q75.8
    - with
      - anencephaly QØØ.Ø
      - encephalocele — *see* Encephalocele
      - hydrocephalus QØ3.9
        - with spina bifida — *see* Spina bifida, by site, with hydrocephalus
      - microcephaly QØ2
  - spermatic cord Q55.4
  - spinal cord QØ6.Ø
  - spine Q76.49
  - spleen Q89.Ø1
  - sternum Q76.7
  - stomach Q4Ø.2
  - submaxillary gland(s) (congenital) Q38.4
  - tarsus — *see* Agenesis, foot
  - tendon Q79.8
  - testicle Q55.Ø
  - thymus (gland) Q89.2
  - thyroid (gland) EØ3.1
    - cartilage Q31.8
  - tibia — *see* Defect, reduction, lower limb, longitudinal, tibia
  - tibiofibular — *see* Defect, reduction, lower limb, specified type NEC
  - toe (and foot) (complete) (partial) — *see* Agenesis, foot
  - tongue Q38.3
  - trachea (cartilage) Q32.1
  - ulna — *see* Defect, reduction, upper limb, longitudinal, ulna
  - upper limb — *see* Agenesis, arm
  - ureter Q62.4
  - urethra Q64.5
  - urinary tract NEC Q64.8
  - uterus Q51.Ø

- **Agenesis** — *continued*
  - uvula Q38.5
  - vagina Q52.Ø
  - vas deferens Q55.4
  - vein(s) (peripheral) Q27.9
    - brain Q28.3
    - great NEC Q26.8
    - portal Q26.5
  - vena cava (inferior) (superior) Q26.8
  - vermis of cerebellum QØ4.3
  - vertebra Q76.49
  - vulva Q52.71
- **Ageusia** R43.2
- **Agitated** — *see* condition
- **Agitation** R45.1
- **Aglossia** (congenital) Q38.3
- **Aglossia-adactylia syndrome** Q87.Ø
- **Aglycogenosis** E74.ØØ
- **Agnosia** (body image) (other senses) (tactile) R48.1
  - developmental F88
  - verbal R48.1
    - auditory R48.1
      - developmental F8Ø.2
    - developmental F8Ø.2
  - visual (object) R48.3
- **Agoraphobia** F4Ø.ØØ
  - with panic disorder F4Ø.Ø1
  - without panic disorder F4Ø.Ø2
- **Agrammatism** R48.8
- **Agranulocytopenia** — *see* Agranulocytosis
- **Agranulocytosis** (chronic) (cyclical) (genetic) (infantile) (periodic) (pernicious) — *see also* Neutropenia D7Ø.9
  - congenital D7Ø.Ø
  - cytoreductive cancer chemotherapy sequela D7Ø.1
  - drug-induced D7Ø.2
    - due to cytoreductive cancer chemotherapy D7Ø.1
  - due to infection D7Ø.3
  - secondary D7Ø.4
    - drug-induced D7Ø.2
      - due to cytoreductive cancer chemotherapy D7Ø.1
- **Agraphia** (absolute) R48.8
  - with alexia R48.Ø
  - developmental F81.81
- **Ague** (dumb) — *see* Malaria
- **Agyria** QØ4.3
- **Ahumada-del Castillo syndrome** E23.Ø
- **Aichomophobia** F4Ø.298
- **AIDS** (related complex) B2Ø
- **Ailment heart** — *see* Disease, heart
- **Ailurophobia** F4Ø.218
- **AIN** — *see* Neoplasia, intraepithelial, anal
- **Ainhum** (disease) L94.6
- **AIPHI** (acute idiopathic pulmonary hemorrhage in infants (over 28 days old)) RØ4.81
- **Air**
  - anterior mediastinum J98.2
  - compressed, disease T7Ø.3 ☑
  - conditioner lung or pneumonitis J67.7
  - embolism (artery) (cerebral) (any site) T79.Ø ☑
    - with ectopic or molar pregnancy OØ8.2
    - due to implanted device NEC — *see* Complications, by site and type, specified NEC
    - following
      - abortion — *see* Abortion by type, complicated by, embolism
      - ectopic or molar pregnancy OØ8.2
      - infusion, therapeutic injection or transfusion T8Ø.Ø ☑
    - in pregnancy, childbirth or puerperium — *see* Embolism, obstetric
    - traumatic T79.Ø ☑
  - hunger, psychogenic F45.8
  - rarefied, effects of — *see* Effect, adverse, high altitude
  - sickness T75.3 ☑
- **Airplane sickness** T75.3 ☑
- **Akathisia** (drug-induced) (treatment-induced) G25.71
  - neuroleptic induced (acute) G25.71
  - tardive G25.71
- **Akinesia** R29.898
- **Akinetic mutism** R41.89
- **Akureyri's disease** G93.39
- **Alactasia, congenital** E73.Ø
- **Alagille (-Watson) syndrome** Q44.71
- **Alastrim** BØ3
- **Albers-Schonberg syndrome** Q78.2
- **Albert's syndrome** — *see* Tendinitis, Achilles
- **Albinism, albino** E7Ø.3Ø
  - with hematologic abnormality E7Ø.339
    - Chediak-Higashi syndrome E7Ø.33Ø
    - Hermansky-Pudlak syndrome E7Ø.331
    - other specified E7Ø.338
  - I E7Ø.32Ø
  - II E7Ø.321
  - ocular E7Ø.319
    - autosomal recessive E7Ø.311
    - other specified E7Ø.318
    - X-linked E7Ø.31Ø
  - oculocutaneous E7Ø.329
    - other specified E7Ø.328
    - tyrosinase (ty) negative E7Ø.32Ø
    - tyrosinase (ty) positive E7Ø.321
  - other specified E7Ø.39
- **Albinismus** E7Ø.3Ø
- **Albright** (-McCune)(-Sternberg) syndrome Q78.1
- **Albuminous** — *see* condition
- **Albuminuria, albuminuric** (acute) (chronic) (subacute) — *see also* Proteinuria R8Ø.9
  - complicating pregnancy — *see* Proteinuria, gestational
    - with
      - gestational hypertension — *see* Pre-eclampsia
      - pre-existing hypertension — *see* Hypertension, complicating pregnancy, pre-existing, with, pre-eclampsia
  - gestational — *see* Proteinuria, gestational
    - with
      - gestational hypertension — *see* Pre-eclampsia
      - pre-existing hypertension — *see* Hypertension, complicating pregnancy, pre-existing, with, pre-eclampsia
  - orthostatic R8Ø.2
  - postural R8Ø.2
  - pre-eclamptic — *see* Pre-eclampsia
  - scarlatinal A38.8
- **Albuminurophobia** F4Ø.298
- **Alcaptonuria** E7Ø.29
- **Alcohol, alcoholic, alcohol-induced**
  - addiction (without remission) F1Ø.2Ø
    - with remission F1Ø.21
  - amnestic disorder, persisting F1Ø.96
    - with dependence F1Ø.26
  - anxiety disorder F1Ø.98Ø
  - bipolar and related disorder F1Ø.94
  - brain syndrome, chronic F1Ø.97
    - with dependence F1Ø.27
  - cardiopathy I42.6
  - counseling and surveillance Z71.41
    - family member Z71.42
  - delirium (acute) (tremens) (withdrawal) F1Ø.921
    - with intoxication F1Ø.921
      - in
        - abuse F1Ø.121
        - dependence F1Ø.221
    - abuse F1Ø.131
      - with intoxication F1Ø.121
    - dependence (acute) (tremens) (withdrawal) F1Ø.231
      - with intoxication F1Ø.221
    - use, unspecified F1Ø.931
      - with intoxication F1Ø.921
  - dementia F1Ø.97
    - with dependence F1Ø.27
  - depressive disorder F1Ø.94
  - deterioration F1Ø.97
    - with dependence F1Ø.27
  - hallucinosis (acute) F1Ø.951
    - in
      - abuse F1Ø.151
      - dependence F1Ø.251
  - insanity F1Ø.959
  - intoxication (acute) (without dependence) F1Ø.129
    - with
      - delirium F1Ø.121
      - dependence F1Ø.229
        - with delirium F1Ø.221
        - uncomplicated F1Ø.22Ø
    - uncomplicated F1Ø.12Ø
  - jealousy F1Ø.988
  - Korsakoff's, Korsakov's, Korsakow's F1Ø.26
  - liver K7Ø.9
    - acute — *see* Disease, liver, alcoholic, hepatitis
  - major neurocognitive disorder, amnestic-confabulatory type F1Ø.96
  - major neurocognitive disorder, nonamnestic-confabulatory type F1Ø.97
  - mania (acute) (chronic) F1Ø.959
- **Alcohol, alcoholic, alcohol-induced** — *continued*
  - mild neurocognitive disorder F1Ø.988
  - paranoia, paranoid (type) psychosis F1Ø.95Ø
  - pellagra E52
  - poisoning, accidental (acute) NEC — *see* Table of Drugs and Chemicals, alcohol, poisoning
  - psychosis — *see* Psychosis, alcoholic
  - psychotic disorder F1Ø.959
  - sexual dysfunction F1Ø.981
  - sleep disorder F1Ø.982
  - withdrawal (without convulsions) F1Ø.239
    - with delirium F1Ø.231
- **Alcoholism** (chronic) (without remission) F1Ø.2Ø
  - with
    - psychosis — *see* Psychosis, alcoholic
    - remission F1Ø.21
  - Korsakov's F1Ø.96
    - with dependence F1Ø.26
- **Alder** (-Reilly) **anomaly or syndrome** (leukocyte granulation) D72.Ø
- **Aldosteronism** E26.9
  - familial (type I) E26.Ø2
  - glucocorticoid-remediable E26.Ø2
  - primary (due to (bilateral) adrenal hyperplasia) E26.Ø9
  - primary NEC E26.Ø9
  - secondary E26.1
  - specified NEC E26.89
- **Aldosteronoma** D44.1Ø
- **Aldrich** (-Wiskott) **syndrome** (eczema-thrombocytopenia) D82.Ø
- **Alektorophobia** F4Ø.218
- **Aleppo boil** B55.1
- **Aleukemic** — *see* condition
- **Aleukia**
  - congenital D7Ø.Ø
  - hemorrhagica D61.9
    - congenital D61.Ø9
  - splenica D73.1
- **Alexia** R48.Ø
  - developmental F81.Ø
  - secondary to organic lesion R48.Ø
- **Algoneurodystrophy** M89.ØØ
  - ankle M89.Ø7- ☑
  - foot M89.Ø7- ☑
  - forearm M89.Ø3- ☑
  - hand M89.Ø4- ☑
  - lower leg M89.Ø6- ☑
  - multiple sites M89.Ø- ☑
  - shoulder M89.Ø1- ☑
  - specified site NEC M89.Ø8
  - thigh M89.Ø5- ☑
  - upper arm M89.Ø2- ☑
- **Algophobia** F4Ø.298
- **Alienation, mental** — *see* Psychosis
- **Alkalemia** E87.3
- **Alkalosis** E87.3
  - metabolic E87.3
    - with respiratory acidosis E87.4
    - of newborn P74.41
  - respiratory E87.3
- **Alkaptonuria** E7Ø.29
- **Allen-Masters syndrome** N83.8
- **Allergy, allergic** (reaction) (to) T78.4Ø ☑
  - air-borne substance NEC (rhinitis) J3Ø.89
  - alveolitis (extrinsic) J67.9
    - due to
      - Aspergillus clavatus J67.4
      - Cryptostroma corticale J67.6
      - organisms (fungal, thermophilic actinomycete) growing in ventilation (air conditioning) systems J67.7
    - specified type NEC J67.8
  - anaphylactic reaction or shock T78.2 ☑
  - angioneurotic edema T78.3 ☑
  - animal (dander) (epidermal) (hair) (rhinitis) J3Ø.81
  - bee sting (anaphylactic shock) — *see* Toxicity, venom, arthropod, bee
  - biological — *see* Allergy, drug
  - colitis — *see also* Colitis, allergic K52.29
  - dander (animal) (rhinitis) J3Ø.81
  - dandruff (rhinitis) J3Ø.81
  - dental restorative material (existing) KØ8.55
  - dermatitis — *see* Dermatitis, contact, allergic
  - diathesis — *see* History, allergy
  - drug, medicament & biological (any) (external) (internal) T78.4Ø ☑

☑ **Additional Character Required — Refer to the Tabular List for Character Selection**

- **Allergy, allergic** — *continued*
  - drug, medicament & biological — *continued*
    - correct substance properly administered — *see* Table of Drugs and Chemicals, by drug, adverse effect
    - wrong substance given or taken NEC (by accident) — *see* Table of Drugs and Chemicals, by drug, poisoning
  - due to pollen J30.1
  - dust (house) (stock) (rhinitis) J30.89
    - with asthma — *see* Asthma, allergic extrinsic
  - eczema — *see* Dermatitis, contact, allergic
  - epidermal (animal) (rhinitis) J30.81
  - feathers (rhinitis) J30.89
  - food (any) (ingested) NEC T78.1 ☑
    - anaphylactic shock — *see* Shock, anaphylactic, due to food
    - dermatitis — *see* Dermatitis, due to, food
    - dietary counseling and surveillance Z71.3
    - in contact with skin L23.6
    - rhinitis J30.5
    - status (without reaction) Z91.018
      - beef Z91.014
      - eggs Z91.012
      - lamb Z91.014
      - mammalian meats Z91.014
      - milk products Z91.011
      - peanuts Z91.010
      - pork Z91.014
      - red meats Z91.014
      - seafood Z91.013
      - specified NEC Z91.018
  - gastrointestinal — *see also* specific type of allergic reaction
    - meaning colitis — *see also* Colitis, allergic K52.29
    - meaning gastroenteritis — *see also* Gastroenteritis, allergic K52.29
    - meaning other adverse food reaction not elsewhere classified T78.1 ☑
  - grain J30.1
  - grass (hay fever) (pollen) J30.1
    - asthma — *see* Asthma, allergic extrinsic
  - hair (animal) (rhinitis) J30.81
  - history (of) — *see* History, allergy
  - horse serum — *see* Allergy, serum
  - inhalant (rhinitis) J30.89
    - pollen J30.1
  - kapok (rhinitis) J30.89
  - medicine — *see* Allergy, drug
  - milk protein — *see also* Allergy, food Z91.011
    - anaphylactic reaction T78.07 ☑
    - dermatitis L27.2
    - enterocolitis syndrome K52.21
    - enteropathy K52.22
    - gastroenteritis K52.29
    - gastroesophageal reflux — *see also* Reaction, adverse, food K21.9
      - with esophagitis (without bleeding) K21.00
        - with bleeding K21.01
    - proctocolitis K52.29
  - nasal, seasonal due to pollen J30.1
  - pneumonia J82.89
  - pollen (any) (hay fever) J30.1
    - asthma — *see* Asthma, allergic extrinsic
  - primrose J30.1
  - primula J30.1
  - proctocolitis K52.29
  - purpura D69.0
  - ragweed (hay fever) (pollen) J30.1
    - asthma — *see* Asthma, allergic extrinsic
  - rose (pollen) J30.1
  - seasonal NEC J30.2
  - Senecio jacobae (pollen) J30.1
  - serum — *see also* Reaction, serum T80.69 ☑
    - anaphylactic shock T80.59 ☑
  - shock (anaphylactic) T78.2 ☑
    - due to
      - administration of blood and blood products T80.51 ☑
      - adverse effect of correct medicinal substance properly administered T88.6 ☑
      - immunization T80.52 ☑
      - serum NEC T80.59 ☑
      - vaccination T80.52 ☑
  - specific NEC T78.49 ☑
  - tree (any) (hay fever) (pollen) J30.1
    - asthma — *see* Asthma, allergic extrinsic
  - upper respiratory J30.9

- **Allergy, allergic** — *continued*
  - urticaria L50.0
  - vaccine — *see* Allergy, serum
  - wheat — *see* Allergy, food
- **Allescheriasis** B48.2
- **Alligator skin disease** Q80.9
- **Allocheiria, allochiria** R20.8
- **Almeida's disease** — *see* Paracoccidioidomycosis
- **Alopecia** (hereditaria) (seborrheica) L65.9
  - androgenic L64.9
    - drug-induced L64.0
    - specified NEC L64.8
  - areata L63.9
    - ophiasis L63.2
    - specified NEC L63.8
    - totalis L63.0
    - universalis L63.1
  - cicatricial L66.9
    - specified NEC L66.8
  - circumscripta L63.9
  - congenital, congenitalis Q84.0
  - due to cytotoxic drugs NEC L65.8
  - mucinosa L65.2
  - postinfective NEC L65.8
  - postpartum L65.0
  - premature L64.8
  - specific (syphilitic) A51.32
  - specified NEC L65.8
  - syphilitic (secondary) A51.32
  - totalis (capitis) L63.0
  - universalis (entire body) L63.1
  - X-ray L58.1
- **Alpers' disease** G31.81
- **Alpine sickness** T70.29 ☑
- **Alport syndrome** Q87.81
- **ALTE** (apparent life threatening event) **in newborn and infant** R68.13
- **Alteration** (of), **Altered**
  - awareness
    - transient R40.4
    - unintended under general anesthesia, during procedure T88.53 ☑
  - mental status R41.82
  - pattern of family relationships affecting child Z62.898
  - sensation
    - following
      - cerebrovascular disease I69.998
        - cerebral infarction I69.398
        - intracerebral hemorrhage I69.198
        - nontraumatic intracranial hemorrhage NEC I69.298
        - specified disease NEC I69.898
        - subarachnoid hemorrhage I69.098
- **Alternating** — *see* condition
- **Altitude, high** (effects) — *see* Effect, adverse, high altitude
- **Aluminosis** (of lung) J63.0
- **Alveolitis**
  - allergic (extrinsic) — *see* Pneumonitis, hypersensitivity
  - due to
    - Aspergillus clavatus J67.4
    - Cryptostroma corticale J67.6
  - fibrosing (cryptogenic) (idiopathic) J84.112
  - jaw M27.3
  - sicca dolorosa M27.3
- **Alveolus, alveolar** — *see* condition
- **Alymphocytosis** D72.810
  - thymic (with immunodeficiency) D82.1
- **Alymphoplasia, thymic** D82.1
- **Alzheimer's disease or sclerosis** — *see* Disease, Alzheimer's
- **Amastia** (with nipple present) Q83.8
  - with absent nipple Q83.0
- **Amathophobia** F40.228
- **Amaurosis** (acquired) (congenital) — *see also* Blindness
  - fugax G45.3
  - hysterical F44.6
  - Leber's congenital H35.50
  - uremic — *see* Uremia
- **Amaurotic idiocy** (infantile) (juvenile) (late) E75.4
- **Amaxophobia** F40.248
- **Ambiguous genitalia** Q56.4
- **Amblyopia** (congenital) (ex anopsia) (partial) (suppression) H53.00- ☑
  - anisometropic — *see* Amblyopia, refractive
  - deprivation H53.01- ☑
  - hysterical F44.6
  - nocturnal — *see also* Blindness, night

- **Amblyopia** — *continued*
  - nocturnal — *see also* Blindness, night — *continued*
    - vitamin A deficiency E50.5
  - refractive H53.02- ☑
  - strabismic H53.03- ☑
  - suspect H53.04- ☑
  - tobacco H53.8
  - toxic NEC H53.8
  - uremic — *see* Uremia
- **Ameba, amebic** (histolytica) — *see also* Amebiasis
  - abscess (liver) A06.4
- **Amebiasis** A06.9
  - with abscess — *see* Abscess, amebic
  - acute A06.0
  - chronic (intestine) A06.1
    - with abscess — *see* Abscess, amebic
  - cutaneous A06.7
  - cutis A06.7
  - cystitis A06.81
  - genitourinary tract NEC A06.82
  - hepatic — *see* Abscess, liver, amebic
  - intestine A06.0
  - nondysenteric colitis A06.2
  - skin A06.7
  - specified site NEC A06.89
- **Ameboma** (of intestine) A06.3
- **Amelia** Q73.0
  - lower limb — *see* Agenesis, leg
  - upper limb — *see* Agenesis, arm
- **Ameloblastoma** — *see also* Cyst, calcifying odontogenic
  - long bones C40.9- ☑
    - lower limb C40.2- ☑
    - upper limb C40.0- ☑
  - malignant C41.1
    - jaw (bone) (lower) C41.1
      - upper C41.0
  - tibial C40.2- ☑
- **Amelogenesis imperfecta** K00.5
  - nonhereditaria (segmentalis) K00.4
- **Amenorrhea** N91.2
  - hyperhormonal E28.8
  - primary N91.0
  - secondary N91.1
- **Amentia** — *see* Disability, intellectual
  - Meynert's (nonalcoholic) F04
- **American**
  - leishmaniasis B55.2
  - mountain tick fever A93.2
- **Ametropia** — *see* Disorder, refraction
- **AMH** (asymptomatic microscopic hematuria) R31.21
- **Amianthosis** J61
- **Amimia** R48.8
- **Amino-acid disorder** E72.9
  - anemia D53.0
- **Aminoacidopathy** E72.9
- **Aminoaciduria** E72.9
- **Amnesia** R41.3
  - anterograde R41.1
  - auditory R48.8
  - dissociative F44.0
    - with dissociative fugue F44.1
  - hysterical F44.0
  - postictal in epilepsy — *see* Epilepsy
  - psychogenic F44.0
  - retrograde R41.2
  - transient global G45.4
- **Amnes(t)ic syndrome** (post-traumatic) F04
  - induced by
    - alcohol F10.96
      - with dependence F10.26
    - psychoactive NEC F19.96
      - with
        - abuse F19.16
        - dependence F19.26
    - sedative F13.96
      - with dependence F13.26
- **Amnion, amniotic** — *see* condition
- **Amnionitis** — *see* Pregnancy, complicated by
- **Amok** F68.8
- **Amoral traits** F60.89
- **Amphetamine** (or other stimulant) **-induced**
  - anxiety disorder F15.980
  - bipolar and related disorder F15.94
  - delirium F15.921
  - depressive disorder F15.94
  - obsessive-compulsive and related disorder F15.988
  - psychotic disorder F15.959

Amphetamine (or other stimulant) **-induced** — *continued*
- sexual dysfunction F15.981
- sleep disorder F15.982
- stimulant withdrawal F15.23

Ampulla
- lower esophagus K22.89
- phrenic K22.89

Amputation — *see also* Absence, by site, acquired
- neuroma (postoperative) (traumatic) — *see* Complications, amputation stump, neuroma
- stump (surgical)
  - abnormal, painful, or with complication (late) — *see* Complications, amputation stump
  - healed or old NOS Z89.9
- traumatic (complete) (partial)
  - arm (upper) (complete) S48.91- ☑
    - at
      - elbow S58.Ø1- ☑
        - partial S58.Ø2- ☑
      - shoulder joint (complete) S48.Ø1- ☑
        - partial S48.Ø2- ☑
    - between
      - elbow and wrist (complete) S58.11- ☑
        - partial S58.12- ☑
      - shoulder and elbow (complete) S48.11- ☑
        - partial S48.12- ☑
    - partial S48.92- ☑
  - breast (complete) S28.21- ☑
    - partial S28.22- ☑
  - clitoris (complete) S38.211 ☑
    - partial S38.212 ☑
  - ear (complete) SØ8.11- ☑
    - partial SØ8.12- ☑
  - finger (complete) (metacarpophalangeal) S68.11- ☑
    - index S68.11- ☑
    - little S68.11- ☑
    - middle S68.11- ☑
    - partial S68.12- ☑
      - index S68.12- ☑
      - little S68.12- ☑
      - middle S68.12- ☑
      - ring S68.12- ☑
    - ring S68.11- ☑
    - thumb — *see* Amputation, traumatic, thumb
    - transphalangeal (complete) S68.61- ☑
      - index S68.61- ☑
      - little S68.61- ☑
      - middle S68.61- ☑
      - partial S68.62- ☑
        - index S68.62- ☑
        - little S68.62- ☑
        - middle S68.62- ☑
        - ring S68.62- ☑
      - ring S68.61- ☑
  - foot (complete) S98.91- ☑
    - at ankle level S98.Ø1- ☑
      - partial S98.Ø2- ☑
    - midfoot S98.31- ☑
      - partial S98.32- ☑
    - partial S98.92- ☑
  - forearm (complete) S58.91- ☑
    - at elbow level (complete) S58.Ø1- ☑
      - partial S58.Ø2- ☑
    - between elbow and wrist (complete) S58.11- ☑
      - partial S58.12- ☑
    - partial S58.92- ☑
  - genital organ(s) (external)
    - female (complete) S38.211 ☑
      - partial S38.212 ☑
    - male
      - penis (complete) S38.221 ☑
        - partial S38.222 ☑
      - scrotum (complete) S38.231 ☑
        - partial S38.232 ☑
      - testes (complete) S38.231 ☑
        - partial S38.232 ☑
  - hand (complete) (wrist level) S68.41- ☑
    - finger(s) alone — *see* Amputation, traumatic, finger
    - partial S68.42- ☑
    - thumb alone — *see* Amputation, traumatic, thumb
    - transmetacarpal (complete) S68.71- ☑
      - partial S68.72- ☑

Amputation — *continued*
- traumatic — *continued*
  - head
    - ear — *see* Amputation, traumatic, ear
    - nose (partial) SØ8.812 ☑
      - complete SØ8.811 ☑
    - part SØ8.89 ☑
      - scalp SØ8.Ø ☑
  - hip (and thigh) (complete) S78.91- ☑
    - at hip joint (complete) S78.Ø1- ☑
      - partial S78.Ø2- ☑
    - between hip and knee (complete) S78.11- ☑
      - partial S78.12- ☑
    - partial S78.92- ☑
  - labium (majus) (minus) (complete) S38.21- ☑
    - partial S38.21- ☑
  - leg (lower) S88.91- ☑
    - at knee level S88.Ø1- ☑
      - partial S88.Ø2- ☑
    - between knee and ankle S88.11- ☑
      - partial S88.12- ☑
    - partial S88.92- ☑
  - nose (partial) SØ8.812 ☑
    - complete SØ8.811 ☑
  - penis (complete) S38.221 ☑
    - partial S38.222 ☑
  - scrotum (complete) S38.231 ☑
    - partial S38.232 ☑
  - shoulder — *see* Amputation, traumatic, arm
    - at shoulder joint — *see* Amputation, traumatic, arm, at shoulder joint
  - testes (complete) S38.231 ☑
    - partial S38.232 ☑
  - thigh — *see* Amputation, traumatic, hip
  - thorax, part of S28.1 ☑
    - breast — *see* Amputation, traumatic, breast
  - thumb (complete) (metacarpophalangeal) S68.Ø1- ☑
    - partial S68.Ø2- ☑
    - transphalangeal (complete) S68.51- ☑
      - partial S68.52- ☑
  - toe (lesser) S98.13- ☑
    - great S98.11- ☑
      - partial S98.12- ☑
    - more than one S98.21- ☑
      - partial S98.22- ☑
    - partial S98.14- ☑
  - vulva (complete) S38.211 ☑
    - partial S38.212 ☑

Amputee (bilateral) (old) Z89.9

Amsterdam dwarfism Q87.19

Amusia R48.8
- developmental F8Ø.89

Amyelencephalus, amyelencephaly QØØ.Ø

Amyelia QØ6.Ø

Amygdalitis — *see* Tonsillitis

Amygdalolith J35.8

Amyloid heart (disease) E85.4 *[I43]*

Amyloidosis (generalized) (primary) E85.9
- with lung involvement E85.4 *[J99]*
- familial E85.2
- genetic E85.2
- heart E85.4 *[I43]*
- hemodialysis-associated E85.3
- light chain (AL) E85.81
- liver E85.4 *[K77]*
- localized E85.4
- neuropathic heredofamilial E85.1
- non-neuropathic heredofamilial E85.Ø
- organ limited E85.4
- Portuguese E85.1
- pulmonary E85.4 *[J99]*
- secondary systemic E85.3
- senile systemic (SSA) E85.82
- skin (lichen) (macular) E85.4 *[L99]*
- specified NEC E85.89
- subglottic E85.4 *[J99]*
- wild-type transthyretin-related (ATTR) E85.82

Amylopectinosis (brancher enzyme deficiency) E74.Ø3

Amylophagia — *see* Pica

Amyoplasia congenita Q79.8

Amyotonia M62.89
- congenita G7Ø.2

Amyotrophia, amyotrophy, amyotrophic G71.8
- congenita Q79.8
- diabetic — *see* Diabetes, amyotrophy

Amyotrophia, amyotrophy, amyotrophic — *continued*
- lateral sclerosis G12.21
- neuralgic G54.5
- spinal progressive G12.25

Anacidity, gastric K31.83
- psychogenic F45.8

Anaerosis of newborn P28.89

Analbuminemia E88.Ø9

Analgesia — *see* Anesthesia

Analphalipoproteinemia E78.6

Anaphylactic
- purpura D69.Ø
- shock or reaction — *see* Shock, anaphylactic

Anaphylactoid shock or reaction — *see* Shock, anaphylactic

Anaphylactoid syndrome of pregnancy O88.Ø1- ☑

Anaphylaxis — *see* Shock, anaphylactic

Anaplasia cervix — *see also* Dysplasia, cervix N87.9

Anaplasmosis [A. phagocytophilum] (transfusion transmitted) A79.82
- human A77.49

Anarthria R47.1

Anasarca R6Ø.1
- cardiac — *see* Failure, heart, congestive
- lung J18.2
- newborn P83.2
- nutritional E43
- pulmonary J18.2
- renal NØ4.9

Anastomosis
- aneurysmal — *see* Aneurysm
- arteriovenous ruptured brain I6Ø.8
  - intracerebral I61.8
  - intraparenchymal I61.8
  - intraventricular I61.5
  - subarachnoid I6Ø.8
- intestinal K63.89
  - complicated NEC K91.89
    - involving urinary tract N99.89
- retinal and choroidal vessels (congenital) Q14.8

Anatomical narrow angle H4Ø.Ø3- ☑

Ancylostoma, ancylostomiasis (braziliense) (caninum) (ceylanicum) (duodenale) B76.Ø
- Necator americanus B76.1

Andersen's disease (glycogen storage) E74.Ø9

Anderson-Fabry disease E75.21

Andes disease T7Ø.29 ☑

Andrews' disease (bacterid) LØ8.89

Androblastoma
- benign
  - specified site — *see* Neoplasm, benign, by site
  - unspecified site
    - female D27.9
    - male D29.2Ø
- malignant
  - specified site — *see* Neoplasm, malignant, by site
  - unspecified site
    - female C56.9
    - male C62.9Ø
- specified site — *see* Neoplasm, uncertain behavior, by site
- tubular
  - with lipid storage
    - specified site — *see* Neoplasm, benign, by site
    - unspecified site
      - female D27.9
      - male D29.2Ø
  - specified site — *see* Neoplasm, benign, by site
  - unspecified site
    - female D27.9
    - male D29.2Ø
- unspecified site
  - female D39.1Ø
  - male D4Ø.1Ø

Androgen insensitivity syndrome — *see also* Syndrome, androgen insensitivity E34.5Ø

Androgen resistance syndrome — *see also* Syndrome, androgen insensitivity E34.5Ø

Android pelvis Q74.2
- with disproportion (fetopelvic) O33.3 ☑
  - causing obstructed labor O65.3

Androphobia F4Ø.29Ø

Anectasis, pulmonary (newborn) — *see* Atelectasis

Anemia (essential) (general) (hemoglobin deficiency) (infantile) (primary) (profound) D64.9

Anemia — *continued*
- with (due to) (in)
  - disorder of
    - anaerobic glycolysis D55.29
    - pentose phosphate pathway D55.1
  - koilonychia D5Ø.9
- achlorhydric D5Ø.8
- achrestic D53.1
- Addison (-Biermer) (pernicious) D51.Ø
- agranulocytic — *see* Agranulocytosis
- amino-acid-deficiency D53.Ø
- aplastic D61.9
  - congenital D61.Ø9
  - drug-induced D61.1
  - due to
    - drugs D61.1
    - external agents NEC D61.2
    - infection D61.2
    - radiation D61.2
  - idiopathic D61.3
  - red cell (pure) D6Ø.9
    - chronic D6Ø.Ø
    - congenital D61.Ø1
    - specified type NEC D6Ø.8
    - transient D6Ø.1
  - specified type NEC D61.89
  - toxic D61.2
- aregenerative
  - congenital D61.Ø9
- asiderotic D5Ø.9
- atypical (primary) D64.9
- Baghdad spring D55.Ø
- Balantidium coli AØ7.Ø
- Biermer's (pernicious) D51.Ø
- blood loss (chronic) D5Ø.Ø
  - acute D62
- bothriocephalus B7Ø.Ø *[D63.8]*
- brickmaker's B76.9 *[D63.8]*
- cerebral I67.89
- childhood D58.9
- chlorotic D5Ø.8
- chronic
  - blood loss D5Ø.Ø
  - hemolytic D58.9
    - idiopathic D59.9
  - simple D53.9
- chronica congenita aregenerativa D61.Ø9
- combined system disease NEC D51.Ø *[G32.Ø]*
  - due to dietary vitamin B12 deficiency D51.3 *[G32.Ø]*
- complicating pregnancy, childbirth or puerperium — *see* Pregnancy, complicated by (management affected by), anemia
- congenital P61.4
  - aplastic D61.Ø9
  - due to isoimmunization NOS P55.9
  - dyserythropoietic, dyshematopoietic D64.4
  - following fetal blood loss P61.3
  - Heinz body D58.2
  - hereditary hemolytic NOS D58.9
  - pernicious D51.Ø
  - spherocytic D58.Ø
- Cooley's (erythroblastic) D56.1
- cytogenic D51.Ø
- deficiency D53.9
  - 2, 3 diphosphoglycurate mutase D55.29
  - 2, 3 PG D55.29
  - 6 phosphogluconate dehydrogenase D55.1
  - 6-PGD D55.1
  - amino-acid D53.Ø
  - combined B12 and folate D53.1
  - enzyme D55.9
    - drug-induced (hemolytic) D59.2
    - glucose-6-phosphate dehydrogenase (G6PD) D55.Ø
    - glycolytic D55.29
    - nucleotide metabolism D55.3
    - related to hexose monophosphate (HMP) shunt pathway NEC D55.1
    - specified type NEC D55.8
  - erythrocytic glutathione D55.1
  - folate D52.9
    - dietary D52.Ø
    - drug-induced D52.1
  - folic acid D52.9
    - dietary D52.Ø
    - drug-induced D52.1
  - G SH D55.1
  - G6PD D55.Ø
  - GGS-R D55.1

Anemia — *continued*
- deficiency — *continued*
  - glucose-6-phosphate dehydrogenase D55.Ø
  - glutathione reductase D55.1
  - glyceraldehyde phosphate dehydrogenase D55.29
  - hexokinase D55.29
  - iron D5Ø.9
    - secondary to blood loss (chronic) D5Ø.Ø
  - nutritional D53.9
    - with
      - poor iron absorption D5Ø.8
      - specified deficiency NEC D53.8
  - phosphofructo-aldolase D55.29
  - phosphoglycerate kinase D55.29
  - PK D55.21
  - protein D53.Ø
  - pyruvate kinase D55.21
  - transcobalamin II D51.2
  - triose-phosphate isomerase D55.29
  - vitamin B12 NOS D51.9
    - dietary D51.3
    - due to
      - intrinsic factor deficiency D51.Ø
      - selective vitamin B12 malabsorption with proteinuria D51.1
    - pernicious D51.Ø
    - specified type NEC D51.8
- Diamond-Blackfan (congenital hypoplastic) D61.Ø1
- dibothriocephalus B7Ø.Ø *[D63.8]*
- dimorphic D53.1
- diphasic D53.1
- Diphyllobothrium (Dibothriocephalus) B7Ø.Ø *[D63.8]*
- due to (in) (with)
  - antineoplastic chemotherapy D64.81
  - blood loss (chronic) D5Ø.Ø
    - acute D62
  - chemotherapy, antineoplastic D64.81
  - chronic disease classified elsewhere NEC D63.8
  - chronic kidney disease D63.1
  - deficiency
    - amino-acid D53.Ø
    - copper D53.8
    - folate (folic acid) D52.9
      - dietary D52.Ø
      - drug-induced D52.1
    - molybdenum D53.8
    - protein D53.Ø
    - zinc D53.8
  - dietary vitamin B12 deficiency D51.3
  - disorder of
    - glutathione metabolism D55.1
    - nucleotide metabolism D55.3
  - drug — *see* Anemia, by type — *see also* Table of Drugs and Chemicals
  - end stage renal disease D63.1
  - enzyme disorder D55.9
  - fetal blood loss P61.3
  - fish tapeworm (D.latum) infestation B7Ø.Ø *[D63.8]*
  - hemorrhage (chronic) D5Ø.Ø
    - acute D62
  - impaired absorption D5Ø.9
  - loss of blood (chronic) D5Ø.Ø
    - acute D62
  - myxedema EØ3.9 *[D63.8]*
  - Necator americanus B76.1 *[D63.8]*
  - prematurity P61.2
  - selective vitamin B12 malabsorption with proteinuria D51.1
  - transcobalamin II deficiency D51.2
- Dyke-Young type (secondary) (symptomatic) D59.19
- dyserythropoietic (congenital) D64.4
- dyshematopoietic (congenital) D64.4
- Egyptian B76.9 *[D63.8]*
- elliptocytosis — *see* Elliptocytosis
- enzyme-deficiency, drug-induced D59.2
- epidemic — *see also* Ancylostomiasis B76.9 *[D63.8]*
- erythroblastic
  - familial D56.1
  - newborn — *see also* Disease, hemolytic P55.9
  - of childhood D56.1
- erythrocytic glutathione deficiency D55.1
- erythropoietin-resistant anemia (EPO resistant anemia) D63.1
- Faber's (achlorhydric anemia) D5Ø.9
- factitious (self-induced blood letting) D5Ø.Ø
- familial erythroblastic D56.1
- Fanconi's (congenital pancytopenia) D61.Ø9
- favism D55.Ø

Anemia — *continued*
- fish tapeworm (D. latum) infestation B7Ø.Ø *[D63.8]*
- folate (folic acid) deficiency D52.9
- glucose-6-phosphate dehydrogenase (G6PD) deficiency D55.Ø
- glutathione-reductase deficiency D55.1
- goat's milk D52.Ø
- granulocytic — *see* Agranulocytosis
- Heinz body, congenital D58.2
- hemolytic D58.9
  - acquired D59.9
    - with hemoglobinuria NEC D59.6
    - autoimmune NEC D59.19
    - infectious D59.4
    - specified type NEC D59.8
    - toxic D59.4
  - acute D59.9
    - due to enzyme deficiency specified type NEC D55.8
    - Lederer's D59.19
  - autoimmune D59.1Ø
    - cold D59.12
    - drug-induced D59.Ø
    - mixed D59.13
    - warm D59.11
  - chronic D58.9
    - idiopathic D59.9
  - cold type (primary) (secondary) (symptomatic) D59.12
  - congenital (spherocytic) — *see* Spherocytosis
  - due to
    - cardiac conditions D59.4
    - drugs (nonautoimmune) D59.2
      - autoimmune D59.Ø
    - enzyme disorder D55.9
      - drug-induced D59.2
    - presence of shunt or other internal prosthetic device D59.4
  - familial D58.9
  - hereditary D58.9
    - due to enzyme disorder D55.9
      - specified type NEC D55.8
    - specified type NEC D58.8
  - idiopathic (chronic) D59.9
  - mechanical D59.4
  - microangiopathic D59.4
  - mixed type (primary) (secondary) (symptomatic) D59.13
  - nonautoimmune D59.4
    - drug-induced D59.2
  - nonspherocytic
    - congenital or hereditary NEC D55.8
      - glucose-6-phosphate dehydrogenase deficiency D55.Ø
      - pyruvate kinase deficiency D55.21
      - type
        - I D55.1
        - II D55.29
    - type
      - I D55.1
      - II D55.29
  - primary
    - autoimmune
      - cold type D59.12
      - mixed type D59.13
      - warm type D59.11
  - secondary D59.4
    - autoimmune
      - cold type D59.12
      - mixed type D59.13
      - warm type D59.11
  - specified (hereditary) type NEC D58.8
  - Stransky-Regala type — *see also* Hemoglobinopathy D58.8
  - symptomatic D59.4
    - autoimmune
      - cold type D59.12
      - mixed type D59.13
      - warm type D59.11
  - toxic D59.4
  - warm type (primary) (secondary) (symptomatic) D59.11
- hemorrhagic (chronic) D5Ø.Ø
  - acute D62
- Herrick's D57.1
- hexokinase deficiency D55.29
- hookworm B76.9 *[D63.8]*
- hypochromic (idiopathic) (microcytic) (normoblastic) D5Ø.9

Anemia — *continued*
- hypochromic — *continued*
  - due to blood loss (chronic) D5Ø.Ø
    - acute D62
  - familial sex-linked D64.Ø
  - pyridoxine-responsive D64.3
  - sideroblastic, sex-linked D64.Ø
- hypoplasia, red blood cells D61.9
  - congenital or familial D61.Ø1
- hypoplastic (idiopathic) D61.9
  - congenital or familial (of childhood) D61.Ø1
- hypoproliferative (refractive) D61.9
- idiopathic D64.9
  - aplastic D61.3
  - hemolytic, chronic D59.9
- in (due to) (with)
  - chronic kidney disease D63.1
  - end stage renal disease D63.1
  - failure, kidney (renal) D63.1
  - neoplastic disease — *see also* Neoplasm D63.Ø
- intertropical — *see also* Ancylostomiasis D63.8
- iron deficiency D5Ø.9
  - secondary to blood loss (chronic) D5Ø.Ø
    - acute D62
  - specified type NEC D5Ø.8
- Joseph-Diamond-Blackfan (congenital hypoplastic) D61.Ø1
- Lederer's (hemolytic) D59.19
- leukoerythroblastic D61.82
- macrocytic D53.9
  - nutritional D52.Ø
  - tropical D52.8
- malarial — *see also* Malaria B54 *[D63.8]*
- malignant (progressive) D51.Ø
- malnutrition D53.9
- marsh — *see also* Malaria B54 *[D63.8]*
- Mediterranean (with other hemoglobinopathy) D56.9
- megaloblastic D53.1
  - combined B12 and folate deficiency D53.1
  - hereditary D51.1
  - nutritional D52.Ø
  - orotic aciduria D53.Ø
  - refractory D53.1
  - specified type NEC D53.1
- megalocytic D53.1
- microcytic (hypochromic) D5Ø.9
  - due to blood loss (chronic) D5Ø.Ø
    - acute D62
  - familial D56.8
- microdrepanocytosis D57.4Ø
- microelliptopoikilocytic (Rietti-Greppi- Micheli) D56.9
- miner's B76.9 *[D63.8]*
- myelodysplastic D46.9
- myelofibrosis D75.81
- myelogenous D64.89
- myelopathic D64.89
- myelophthisic D61.82
- myeloproliferative D47.Z9 (*following* D47.4)
- newborn P61.4
  - due to
    - ABO (antibodies, isoimmunization, maternal/fetal incompatibility) P55.1
    - Rh (antibodies, isoimmunization, maternal/fetal incompatibility) P55.Ø
  - following fetal blood loss P61.3
  - posthemorrhagic (fetal) P61.3
- nonspherocytic hemolytic — *see* Anemia, hemolytic, nonspherocytic
- normocytic (infectional) D64.9
  - due to blood loss (chronic) D5Ø.Ø
    - acute D62
  - myelophthisic D61.82
- nutritional (deficiency) D53.9
  - with
    - poor iron absorption D5Ø.8
    - specified deficiency NEC D53.8
  - megaloblastic D52.Ø
- of prematurity P61.2
- orotaciduric (congenital) (hereditary) D53.Ø
- osteosclerotic D64.89
- ovalocytosis (hereditary) — *see* Elliptocytosis
- paludal — *see also* Malaria B54 *[D63.8]*
- pernicious (congenital) (malignant) (progressive) D51.Ø
- pleochromic D64.89
  - of sprue D52.8
- posthemorrhagic (chronic) D5Ø.Ø
  - acute D62
  - newborn P61.3

Anemia — *continued*
- postoperative (postprocedural)
  - due to (acute) blood loss D62
    - chronic blood loss D5Ø.Ø
  - specified NEC D64.89
- postpartum O9Ø.81
- pressure D64.89
- progressive D64.9
  - malignant D51.Ø
  - pernicious D51.Ø
- protein-deficiency D53.Ø
- pseudoleukemica infantum D64.89
- pure red cell D6Ø.9
  - congenital D61.Ø1
- pyridoxine-responsive D64.3
- pyruvate kinase deficiency D55.21
- refractory D46.4
  - with
    - excess of blasts D46.2Ø
      - 1 (RAEB 1) D46.21
      - 2 (RAEB 2) D46.22
      - in transformation (RAEB T) — *see* Leukemia, acute myeloblastic
    - hemochromatosis D46.1
    - sideroblasts (ring) (RARS) D46.1
  - megaloblastic D53.1
  - sideroblastic D46.1
  - sideropenic D5Ø.9
  - without ring sideroblasts, so stated D46.Ø
  - without sideroblasts without excess of blasts D46.Ø
- Rietti-Greppi-Micheli D56.9
- scorbutic D53.2
- secondary to
  - blood loss (chronic) D5Ø.Ø
    - acute D62
  - hemorrhage (chronic) D5Ø.Ø
    - acute D62
- semiplastic D61.89
- sickle-cell — *see* Disease, sickle-cell
- sideroblastic D64.3
  - hereditary D64.Ø
  - hypochromic, sex-linked D64.Ø
  - pyridoxine-responsive NEC D64.3
  - refractory D46.1
  - secondary (due to)
    - disease D64.1
    - drugs and toxins D64.2
  - specified type NEC D64.3
- sideropenic (refractory) D5Ø.9
  - due to blood loss (chronic) D5Ø.Ø
    - acute D62
- simple chronic D53.9
- specified type NEC D64.89
- spherocytic (hereditary) — *see* Spherocytosis
- splenic D64.89
- splenomegalic D64.89
- stomatocytosis D58.8
- syphilitic (acquired) (late) A52.79 *[D63.8]*
- target cell D64.89
- thalassemia D56.9
- thrombocytopenic — *see* Thrombocytopenia
- toxic D61.2
- tropical B76.9 *[D63.8]*
  - macrocytic D52.8
- tuberculous A18.89 *[D63.8]*
- vegan D51.3
- vitamin
  - B12 deficiency (dietary) pernicious D51.Ø
  - B6-responsive D64.3
- von Jaksch's D64.89
- Witts' (achlorhydric anemia) D5Ø.8

Anemophobia F4Ø.228

Anencephalus, anencephaly QØØ.Ø

Anergasia — *see* Psychosis, organic

Anesthesia, anesthetic R2Ø.Ø
- complication or reaction NEC — *see also* Complications, anesthesia T88.59 ☑
  - due to
    - correct substance properly administered — *see* Table of Drugs and Chemicals, by drug, adverse effect
    - overdose or wrong substance given — *see* Table of Drugs and Chemicals, by drug, poisoning
  - unintended awareness under general anesthesia during procedure T88.53 ☑
    - personal history of Z92.84
- cornea H18.81- ☑

Anesthesia, anesthetic — *continued*
- dissociative F44.6
- functional (hysterical) F44.6
- hyperesthetic, thalamic G89.Ø
- hysterical F44.6
- local skin lesion R2Ø.Ø
- sexual (psychogenic) F52.1
- shock (due to) T88.2 ☑
- skin R2Ø.Ø
- testicular N5Ø.9

Anetoderma (maculosum) (of) L9Ø.8
- Jadassohn-Pellizzari L9Ø.2
- Schweniger-Buzzi L9Ø.1

Aneurin deficiency E51.9

Aneurysm (anastomotic) (artery) (cirsoid) (diffuse) (false) (fusiform) (multiple) (saccular) I72.9
- abdominal (aorta) I71.4Ø
  - infrarenal I71.43
    - ruptured I71.33
  - juxtarenal I71.42
    - ruptured I71.32
  - pararenal I71.41
    - ruptured I71.31
  - ruptured I71.3Ø
  - syphilitic A52.Ø1
- aorta, aortic (nonsyphilitic) I71.9
  - abdominal I71.4Ø
    - dissecting — *see* Dissection, aorta, abdominal
    - ruptured I71.3Ø
  - arch I71.22
    - ruptured I71.12
  - arteriosclerotic I71.9
    - ruptured I71.8
  - ascending I71.21
    - ruptured I71.11
  - congenital Q25.43
  - descending I71.9
    - abdominal I71.4Ø
      - ruptured I71.3Ø
    - ruptured I71.8
    - thoracic I71.23
      - ruptured I71.13
  - dissecting — *see* Dissection, aorta
  - root Q25.43
  - ruptured I71.8
  - sinus, congenital Q25.43
  - syphilitic A52.Ø1
  - thoracic I71.2Ø
    - ruptured I71.1Ø
  - thoracoabdominal I71.6Ø
    - paravisceral I71.62
      - ruptured I71.52
    - ruptured I71.5Ø
    - supraceliac I71.61
      - ruptured I71.51
  - thorax, thoracic I71.2Ø
    - arch I71.22
      - ruptured I71.12
    - ascending I71.21
      - ruptured I71.11
    - descending I71.23
      - ruptured I71.13
    - ruptured I71.1Ø
      - arch I71.12
      - ascending I71.11
      - descending I71.13
  - transverse I71.22
    - ruptured I71.12
  - valve (heart) — *see also* Endocarditis, aortic I35.8
- arteriosclerotic I72.9
  - cerebral I67.1
    - ruptured — *see* Hemorrhage, intracranial, subarachnoid
- arteriovenous (congenital) — *see also* Malformation, arteriovenous
  - acquired I77.Ø
    - brain I67.1
      - ruptured — *see* Aneurysm, arteriovenous, brain, ruptured
    - coronary I25.41
    - pulmonary I28.Ø
  - brain Q28.2
    - ruptured I6Ø.8
      - intracerebral I61.8
      - intraparenchymal I61.8
      - intraventricular I61.5
      - subarachnoid I6Ø.8

- **Angiohemophilia** (A) (B) — *see* Disease, von Willebrand
- **Angioid streaks** (choroid) (macula) (retina) H35.33
- **Angiokeratoma** — *see* Neoplasm, skin, benign
  - corporis diffusum E75.21
- **Angioleiomyoma** — *see* Neoplasm, connective tissue, benign
- **Angiolipoma** — *see also* Lipoma
  - infiltrating — *see* Lipoma
- **Angioma** — *see also* Hemangioma, by site
  - capillary I78.1
  - hemorrhagicum hereditaria I78.Ø
  - intra-abdominal D18.Ø3
  - intracranial D18.Ø2
  - malignant — *see* Neoplasm, connective tissue, malignant
  - plexiform D18.ØØ
    - intra-abdominal D18.Ø3
    - intracranial D18.Ø2
    - skin D18.Ø1
    - specified site NEC D18.Ø9
  - senile I78.1
  - serpiginosum L81.7
  - skin D18.Ø1
  - specified site NEC D18.Ø9
  - spider I78.1
  - stellate I78.1
  - venous Q28.3
- **Angiomatosis** Q82.8
  - bacillary A79.89
  - encephalotrigeminal Q85.89
  - hemorrhagic familial I78.Ø
  - hereditary familial I78.Ø
  - liver K76.4
- **Angiomyolipoma** — *see* Lipoma
- **Angiomyoliposarcoma** — *see* Neoplasm, connective tissue, malignant
- **Angiomyoma** — *see* Neoplasm, connective tissue, benign
- **Angiomyosarcoma** — *see* Neoplasm, connective tissue, malignant
- **Angiomyxoma** — *see* Neoplasm, connective tissue, uncertain behavior
- **Angioneurosis** F45.8
- **Angioneurotic edema** (allergic) (any site) (with urticaria) T78.3 ☑
  - hereditary D84.1
- **Angiopathia, angiopathy** I99.9
  - cerebral I67.9
    - amyloid E85.4 *[I68.Ø]*
  - diabetic (peripheral) — *see* Diabetes, angiopathy
  - peripheral I73.9
    - diabetic — *see* Diabetes, angiopathy
    - specified type NEC I73.89
  - retinae syphilitica A52.Ø5
  - retinalis (juvenilis)
    - diabetic — *see* Diabetes, retinopathy
    - proliferative — *see* Retinopathy, proliferative
- **Angiosarcoma** — *see also* Neoplasm, connective tissue, malignant
  - liver C22.3
- **Angiosclerosis** — *see* Arteriosclerosis
- **Angiospasm** (peripheral) (traumatic) (vessel) — *see also* Vasospasm I73.9
  - brachial plexus G54.Ø
  - cerebral G45.9
  - cervical plexus G54.2
  - nerve
    - arm — *see* Mononeuropathy, upper limb
      - axillary G54.Ø
      - median — *see* Lesion, nerve, median
      - ulnar — *see* Lesion, nerve, ulnar
    - axillary G54.Ø
    - leg — *see* Mononeuropathy, lower limb
    - median — *see* Lesion, nerve, median
    - plantar — *see* Lesion, nerve, plantar
    - ulnar — *see* Lesion, nerve, ulnar
- **Angiospastic disease or edema** I73.9
- **Angiostrongyliasis**
  - due to
    - Parastrongylus
      - cantonensis B83.2
      - costaricensis B81.3
  - intestinal B81.3
- **Anguillulosis** — *see* Strongyloidiasis
- **Angulation**
  - cecum — *see* Obstruction, intestine
  - coccyx (acquired) — *see also* subcategory M43.8 ☑
    - congenital NEC Q76.49
- **Angulation** — *continued*
  - femur (acquired) — *see also* Deformity, limb, specified type NEC, thigh
    - congenital Q74.2
  - intestine (large) (small) — *see* Obstruction, intestine
  - sacrum (acquired) — *see also* subcategory M43.8 ☑
    - congenital NEC Q76.49
  - sigmoid (flexure) — *see* Obstruction, intestine
  - spine — *see* Dorsopathy, deforming, specified NEC
  - tibia (acquired) — *see also* Deformity, limb, specified type NEC, lower leg
    - congenital Q74.2
  - ureter N13.5
    - with infection N13.6
  - wrist (acquired) — *see also* Deformity, limb, specified type NEC, forearm
    - congenital Q74.Ø
- **Angulus infectiosus** (lips) K13.Ø
- **Anhedonia** R45.84
  - sexual F52.Ø
- **Anhidrosis** L74.4
- **Anhydration** E86.Ø
- **Anhydremia** E86.Ø
- **Anidrosis** L74.4
- **Aniridia** (congenital) Q13.1
- **Anisakiasis** (infection) (infestation) B81.Ø
- **Anisakis larvae infestation** B81.Ø
- **Aniseikonia** H52.32
- **Anisocoria** (pupil) H57.Ø2
  - congenital Q13.2
- **Anisocytosis** R71.8
- **Anisometropia** (congenital) H52.31
- **Ankle** — *see* condition
- **Ankyloblepharon** (eyelid) (acquired) — *see also* Blepharophimosis
  - filiforme (adnatum) (congenital) Q1Ø.3
  - total Q1Ø.3
- **Ankyloglossia** Q38.1
- **Ankylosis** (fibrous) (osseous) (joint) M24.6Ø
  - ankle M24.67- ☑
  - arthrodesis status Z98.1
  - cricoarytenoid (cartilage) (joint) (larynx) J38.7
  - dental KØ3.5
  - ear ossicles H74.31- ☑
  - elbow M24.62- ☑
  - foot M24.67- ☑
  - hand M24.64- ☑
  - hip M24.65- ☑
  - incostapedial joint (infectional) — *see* Ankylosis, ear ossicles
  - jaw (temporomandibular) M26.61- ☑
  - knee M24.66- ☑
  - lumbosacral (joint) M43.27
  - postoperative (status) Z98.1
  - produced by surgical fusion, status Z98.1
  - sacro-iliac (joint) M43.28
  - shoulder M24.61- ☑
  - specified site NEC M24.69
  - spine (joint) — *see also* Fusion, spine
    - spondylitic — *see* Spondylitis, ankylosing
  - surgical Z98.1
  - temporomandibular M26.61- ☑
  - tooth, teeth (hard tissues) KØ3.5
  - wrist M24.63- ☑
- **Ankylostoma** — *see* Ancylostoma
- **Ankylostomiasis** — *see* Ancylostomiasis
- **Ankylurethria** — *see* Stricture, urethra
- **Annular** — *see also* condition
  - detachment, cervix N88.8
  - organ or site, congenital NEC — *see* Distortion
  - pancreas (congenital) Q45.1
- **Anoctaminopathy** G71.Ø35
- **Anodontia** (complete) (partial) (vera) KØØ.Ø
  - acquired KØ8.1Ø ☑
- **Anomaly, anomalous** (congenital) (unspecified type) Q89.9
  - abdominal wall NEC Q79.59
  - acoustic nerve QØ7.8
  - adrenal (gland) Q89.1
  - Alder (-Reilly) (leukocyte granulation) D72.Ø
  - alimentary tract Q45.9
    - upper Q4Ø.9
  - alveolar M26.7Ø
    - hyperplasia M26.79
      - mandibular M26.72
      - maxillary M26.71
    - hypoplasia M26.79
- **Anomaly, anomalous** — *continued*
  - alveolar — *continued*
    - hypoplasia — *continued*
      - mandibular M26.74
      - maxillary M26.73
    - ridge (process) M26.79
    - specified NEC M26.79
  - ankle (joint) Q74.2
  - anus Q43.9
  - aorta (arch) NEC Q25.4Ø
    - coarctation (preductal) (postductal) Q25.1
  - aortic cusp or valve Q23.9
  - appendix Q43.8
  - apple peel syndrome Q41.1
  - aqueduct of Sylvius QØ3.Ø
    - with spina bifida — *see* Spina bifida, with hydrocephalus
  - arm Q74.Ø
  - arteriovenous NEC
    - coronary Q24.5
    - gastrointestinal Q27.33
      - acquired — *see* Angiodysplasia
  - artery (peripheral) Q27.9
    - basilar NEC Q28.1
    - cerebral Q28.3
    - coronary Q24.5
    - digestive system Q27.8
    - eye Q15.8
    - great Q25.9
      - specified NEC Q25.8
    - lower limb Q27.8
    - peripheral Q27.9
      - specified NEC Q27.8
    - pulmonary NEC Q25.79
    - renal Q27.2
    - retina Q14.1
    - specified site NEC Q27.8
    - subclavian Q27.8
      - origin Q25.48
    - umbilical Q27.Ø
    - upper limb Q27.8
    - vertebral NEC Q28.1
  - aryteno-epiglottic folds Q31.8
  - atrial
    - bands or folds Q2Ø.8
    - septa Q21.1Ø
  - atrioventricular
    - excitation I45.6
    - septum Q21.Ø
  - auditory canal Q17.8
  - auricle
    - ear Q17.8
      - causing impairment of hearing Q16.9
    - heart Q2Ø.8
  - Axenfeld's Q15.Ø
  - back Q89.9
  - band
    - atrial Q2Ø.8
    - heart Q24.8
    - ventricular Q24.8
  - Bartholin's duct Q38.4
  - biliary duct or passage Q44.5
  - bladder Q64.7Ø
    - absence Q64.5
    - diverticulum Q64.6
    - exstrophy Q64.1Ø
      - cloacal Q64.12
      - extroversion Q64.19
      - specified type NEC Q64.19
      - supravesical fissure Q64.11
    - neck obstruction Q64.31
    - specified type NEC Q64.79
  - bone Q79.9
    - arm Q74.Ø
    - face Q75.9
    - leg Q74.2
    - pelvic girdle Q74.2
    - shoulder girdle Q74.Ø
    - skull Q75.9
      - with
        - anencephaly QØØ.Ø
        - encephalocele — *see* Encephalocele
        - hydrocephalus QØ3.9
          - with spina bifida — *see* Spina bifida, by site, with hydrocephalus
        - microcephaly QØ2
  - brain (multiple) QØ4.9
    - vessel Q28.3
  - breast Q83.9

- **Apiphobia** F4Ø.218
- **Aplasia** — *see also* Agenesis
  - abdominal muscle syndrome Q79.4
  - alveolar process (acquired) — *see* Anomaly, alveolar
    - congenital Q38.6
  - aorta (congenital) Q25.41
  - axialis extracorticalis (congenita) E75.29
  - bone marrow (myeloid) D61.9
    - congenital D61.Ø1
  - brain QØØ.Ø
    - part of QØ4.3
  - bronchus Q32.4
  - cementum KØØ.4
  - cerebellum QØ4.3
  - cervix (congenital) Q51.5
  - congenital pure red cell D61.Ø1
  - corpus callosum QØ4.Ø
  - cutis congenita Q84.8
  - erythrocyte congenital D61.Ø1
  - extracortical axial E75.29
  - eye Q11.1
  - fovea centralis (congenital) Q14.1
  - gallbladder, congenital Q44.Ø
  - iris Q13.1
  - labyrinth, membranous Q16.5
  - limb (congenital) Q73.8
    - lower — *see* Defect, reduction, lower limb
    - upper — *see* Agenesis, arm
  - lung, congenital (bilateral) (unilateral) Q33.3
  - pancreas Q45.Ø
  - parathyroid-thymic D82.1
  - Pelizaeus-Merzbacher E75.27
  - penis Q55.5
  - prostate Q55.4
  - red cell (with thymoma) D6Ø.9
    - acquired D6Ø.9
      - due to drugs D6Ø.9
    - adult D6Ø.9
    - chronic D6Ø.Ø
    - congenital D61.Ø1
    - constitutional D61.Ø1
    - due to drugs D6Ø.9
    - hereditary D61.Ø1
    - of infants D61.Ø1
    - primary D61.Ø1
    - pure D61.Ø1
      - due to drugs D6Ø.9
    - specified type NEC D6Ø.8
    - transient D6Ø.1
  - round ligament Q52.8
  - skin Q84.8
  - spermatic cord Q55.4
  - spleen Q89.Ø1
  - testicle Q55.Ø
  - thymic, with immunodeficiency D82.1
  - thyroid (congenital) (with myxedema) EØ3.1
  - uterus Q51.Ø
  - ventral horn cell QØ6.1
- **Apnea, apneic** (of) (spells) RØ6.81
  - newborn P28.4Ø
    - central P28.41
    - mixed P28.43
    - obstructive P28.42
    - sleep
      - primary P28.3Ø
        - central P28.31
        - mixed P28.33
        - obstructive P28.32
        - specified NEC P28.39
    - specified NEC P28.49
  - prematurity P28.49
  - sleep G47.3Ø
    - central (primary) G47.31
      - idiopathic G47.31
      - in conditions classified elsewhere G47.37
    - obstructive (adult) (pediatric) G47.33
      - hypopnea G47.33
    - primary central G47.31
    - specified NEC G47.39
- **Apneumatosis, newborn** P28.Ø
- **Apocrine metaplasia** (breast) — *see* Dysplasia, mammary, specified type NEC
- **Apophysitis** (bone) — *see also* Osteochondropathy
  - calcaneus M92.8
  - juvenile M92.9
- **Apoplectiform convulsions** (cerebral ischemia) I67.82
- **Apoplexia, apoplexy, apoplectic**
  - adrenal A39.1
- **Apoplexia, apoplexy, apoplectic** — *continued*
  - heart (auricle) (ventricle) — *see* Infarct, myocardium
  - heat T67.Ø1 ☑
  - hemorrhagic (stroke) — *see* Hemorrhage, intracranial
  - meninges, hemorrhagic — *see* Hemorrhage, intracranial, subarachnoid
  - uremic N18.9 *[I68.8]*
- **Appearance**
  - bizarre R46.1
  - specified NEC R46.89
  - very low level of personal hygiene R46.Ø
- **Appendage**
  - epididymal (organ of Morgagni) Q55.4
  - intestine (epiploic) Q43.8
  - preauricular Q17.Ø
  - testicular (organ of Morgagni) Q55.29
- **Appendicitis** (pneumococcal) (retrocecal) K37
  - with
    - gangrene K35.891
      - with localized peritonitis K35.31
    - perforation NOS K35.32
    - peritoneal abscess K35.33
    - peritonitis NEC K35.33
      - generalized K35.2Ø9
        - with
          - abscess K35.219
            - with perforation or rupture K35.211
            - following rupture or perforation of appendix NOS K35.211
            - without perforation or rupture K35.21Ø
          - perforation or rupture K35.2Ø1
        - following rupture or perforation of appendix NOS K35.2Ø1
        - without rupture or perforation of appendix K35.2ØØ
      - localized K35.3Ø
        - with
          - gangrene K35.31
          - perforation K35.32
            - and abscess K35.33
      - rupture (with localized peritonitis) K35.32
  - acute (catarrhal) (fulminating) (obstructive) (retrocecal) (suppurative) K35.8Ø
    - with
      - gangrene K35.891
      - peritoneal abscess K35.33
      - peritonitis NEC K35.33
        - generalized K35.2Ø9
          - with
            - abscess K35.219
              - with perforation or rupture K35.211
              - following rupture or perforation of appendix NOS K35.211
              - without perforation or rupture K35.21Ø
            - perforation or rupture K35.2Ø1
          - following rupture or perforation of appendix NOS K35.2Ø1
          - without rupture or perforation of appendix K35.2ØØ
        - localized K35.3Ø
          - with
            - gangrene K35.31
            - perforation K35.32
              - and abscess K35.33
    - specified NEC K35.89Ø
      - with gangrene K35.891
        - with localized peritonitis K35.31
  - amebic AØ6.89
  - chronic (recurrent) K36
  - exacerbation — *see* Appendicitis, with, gangrene
  - gangrenous — *see* Appendicitis, acute
  - healed (obliterative) K36
  - interval K36
  - neurogenic K36
  - obstructive K36
  - recurrent K36
  - relapsing K36
  - ruptured NOS (with localized peritonitis) K35.32
  - subacute (adhesive) K36
  - subsiding K36
  - suppurative — *see* Appendicitis, acute
  - tuberculous A18.32
- **Appendicopathia oxyurica** B8Ø
- **Appendix, appendicular** — *see also* condition
  - epididymis Q55.4
- **Appendix, appendicular** — *continued*
  - Morgagni
    - female Q5Ø.5
    - male (epididymal) Q55.4
      - testicular Q55.29
  - testis Q55.29
- **Appetite**
  - depraved — *see* Pica
  - excessive R63.2
  - lack or loss — *see also* Anorexia R63.Ø
    - nonorganic origin F5Ø.89
    - psychogenic F5Ø.89
  - perverted (hysterical) — *see* Pica
- **Apple peel syndrome** Q41.1
- **Apprehension state** F41.1
- **Apprehensiveness, abnormal** F41.9
- **Approximal wear** KØ3.Ø
- **Apraxia** (classic) (ideational) (ideokinetic) (ideomotor) (motor) (verbal) R48.2
  - following
    - cerebrovascular disease I69.99Ø
      - cerebral infarction I69.39Ø
      - intracerebral hemorrhage I69.19Ø
      - nontraumatic intracranial hemorrhage NEC I69.29Ø
      - specified disease NEC I69.89Ø
      - subarachnoid hemorrhage I69.Ø9Ø
  - oculomotor, congenital H51.8
- **Aptyalism** K11.7
- **Apudoma** — *see* Neoplasm, uncertain behavior, by site
- **Aqueous misdirection** H4Ø.83- ☑
- **Arabicum elephantiasis** — *see* Infestation, filarial
- **Arachnitis** — *see* Meningitis
- **Arachnodactyly** — *see* Syndrome, Marfan
- **Arachnoiditis** (acute) (adhesive) (basal) (brain) (cerebrospinal) — *see* Meningitis
- **Arachnophobia** F4Ø.21Ø
- **Arboencephalitis, Australian** A83.4
- **Arborization block** (heart) I45.5
- **ARC** (AIDS-related complex) B2Ø
- **Arch**
  - aortic Q25.49
  - bovine Q25.49
- **Arches** — *see* condition
- **Arcuate uterus** Q51.81Ø
- **Arcuatus uterus** Q51.81Ø
- **Arcus** (cornea) senilis — *see* Degeneration, cornea, senile
- **Arc-welder's lung** J63.4
- **Areflexia** R29.2
- **Areola** — *see* condition
- **Argentaffinoma** — *see also* Neoplasm, uncertain behavior, by site
  - malignant — *see* Neoplasm, malignant, by site
  - syndrome E34.Ø
- **Argininemia** E72.21
- **Arginosuccinic aciduria** E72.22
- **Argyll Robertson phenomenon, pupil or syndrome** (syphilitic) A52.19
  - atypical H57.Ø9
  - nonsyphilitic H57.Ø9
- **Argyria, argyriasis**
  - conjunctival H11.13- ☑
  - from drug or medicament — *see* Table of Drugs and Chemicals, by substance
- **Argyrosis, conjunctival** H11.13- ☑
- **Arhinencephaly** QØ4.1
- **Ariboflavinosis** E53.Ø
- **Arm** — *see* condition
- **Arnold-Chiari disease, obstruction or syndrome** (type II) QØ7.ØØ
  - with
    - hydrocephalus QØ7.Ø2
      - with spina bifida QØ7.Ø3
    - spina bifida QØ7.Ø1
      - with hydrocephalus QØ7.Ø3
  - type III — *see* Encephalocele
  - type IV QØ4.8
- **Aromatic amino-acid metabolism disorder** E7Ø.9
  - specified NEC E7Ø.89
- **Arousals, confusional** G47.51
- **Arrest, arrested**
  - cardiac I46.9
    - complicating
      - abortion — *see* Abortion, by type, complicated by, cardiac arrest
      - anesthesia (general) (local) or other sedation — *see* Table of Drugs and Chemicals, by drug

- **Arteriosclerosis, arteriosclerotic** — *continued*
  - with — *continued*
    - critical limb ischemia — *continued*
      - bypass graft — *continued*
        - nonbiological graft — *continued*
          - leg — *continued*
            - with
              - gangrene (and intermittent claudication, rest pain, and ulcer) I70.669
              - rest pain (and intermittent claudication) I70.629
            - bilateral I70.623
              - with
                - gangrene (and intermittent claudication, rest pain, and ulcer) I70.663
                - rest pain (intermittent claudication) I70.623
            - left I70.622
              - with
                - gangrene (and intermittent claudication, rest pain, and ulcer) I70.662
                - rest pain (and intermittent claudication) I70.622
                - ulceration (and intermittent claudication and rest pain) I70.649
                  - ankle I70.643
                  - calf I70.642
                  - foot site NEC I70.645
                  - heel I70.644
                  - lower leg NEC I70.648
                  - midfoot I70.644
                  - thigh I70.641
            - right I70.621
              - with
                - gangrene (and intermittent claudication, rest pain, and ulcer) I70.661
                - rest pain (and intermittent claudication) I70.621
                - ulceration (and intermittent claudication and rest pain) I70.639
                  - ankle I70.633
                  - calf I70.632
                  - foot site NEC I70.635
                  - heel I70.634
                  - lower leg NEC I70.638
                  - midfoot I70.634
                  - thigh I70.631
        - specified graft NEC I70.729
          - leg I70.729
            - with
              - gangrene (and intermittent claudication, rest pain, and ulcer) I70.769
              - rest pain (and intermittent claudication) I70.729
            - bilateral I70.723
              - with
                - gangrene (and intermittent claudication, rest pain, and ulcer) I70.763
                - rest pain (and intermittent claudication) I70.723
            - left I70.722
              - with
                - gangrene (and intermittent claudication, rest pain, and ulcer) I70.762
                - rest pain (and intermittent claudication) I70.722
                - ulceration (and intermittent claudication and rest pain) I70.749
                  - ankle I70.743
                  - calf I70.742
                  - foot site NEC I70.745
                  - heel I70.744
                  - lower leg NEC I70.748
                  - midfoot I70.744
                  - thigh I70.741
            - right I70.721

- **Arteriosclerosis, arteriosclerotic** — *continued*
  - with — *continued*
    - critical limb ischemia — *continued*
      - bypass graft — *continued*
        - specified graft — *continued*
          - leg — *continued*
            - right — *continued*
              - with
                - gangrene (and intermittent claudication, rest pain, and ulcer) I70.761
                - rest pain (and intermittent claudication) I70.721
                - ulceration (and intermittent claudication and rest pain) I70.739
                  - ankle I70.733
                  - calf I70.732
                  - foot site NEC I70.735
                  - heel I70.734
                  - lower leg NEC I70.738
                  - midfoot I70.734
                  - thigh I70.731
      - leg I70.229
        - with
          - gangrene (and intermittent claudication, rest pain, and ulcer) I70.269
          - rest pain (and intermittent claudication) I70.229
        - bilateral I70.223
          - with
            - gangrene (and intermittent claudication, rest pain, and ulcer) I70.263
            - rest pain (and intermittent claudication) I70.223
        - left I70.222
          - with
            - gangrene (and intermittent claudication, rest pain, and ulcer) I70.262
            - rest pain (and intermittent claudication) I70.222
            - ulceration (and intermittent claudication and rest pain) I70.249
              - ankle I70.243
              - calf I70.242
              - foot site NEC I70.245
              - heel I70.244
              - lower leg NEC I70.248
              - midfoot I70.244
              - thigh I70.241
        - right I70.221
          - with
            - gangrene (and intermittent claudication, rest pain, and ulcer) I70.261
            - rest pain (and intermittent claudication) I70.221
            - ulceration (and intermittent claudication and rest pain) I70.239
              - ankle I70.233
              - calf I70.232
              - foot site NEC I70.235
              - heel I70.234
              - lower leg NEC I70.238
              - midfoot I70.234
              - thigh I70.231
  - aorta I70.0
  - arteries of extremities — *see* Arteriosclerosis, extremities
    - with
      - chronic limb-threatening ischemia — *see* Arteriosclerosis, with critical limb ischemia
      - critical limb ischemia — *see* Arteriosclerosis, with critical limb ischemia
  - brain I67.2
    - with infarction — *see* Occlusion, artery, brain or cerebral, with infarction
  - bypass graft
    - with
      - chronic limb-threatening ischemia — *see* Arteriosclerosis, with critical limb ischemia
      - critical limb ischemia — *see* Arteriosclerosis, with critical limb ischemia
    - coronary — *see* Arteriosclerosis, coronary, bypass graft

- **Arteriosclerosis, arteriosclerotic** — *continued*
  - bypass graft — *continued*
    - extremities — *see* Arteriosclerosis, extremities, bypass graft
  - cardiac — *see* Disease, heart, ischemic, atherosclerotic
  - cardiopathy — *see* Disease, heart, ischemic, atherosclerotic
  - cardiorenal — *see* Hypertension, cardiorenal
  - cardiovascular — *see* Disease, heart, ischemic, atherosclerotic
  - carotid — *see also* Occlusion, artery, carotid I65.2- ☑
  - central nervous system I67.2
    - with infarction — *see* Occlusion, artery, cerebral or precerebral, with infarction
  - cerebral I67.2
    - with infarction — *see* Occlusion, artery, brain or cerebral, with infarction
  - cerebrovascular I67.2
    - with infarction — *see* Occlusion, artery, brain or cerebral, with infarction
  - coronary (artery) I25.10
    - due to
      - calcified coronary lesion (severely) I25.84
      - lipid rich plaque I25.83
    - bypass graft I25.810
      - with
        - angina pectoris I25.709
          - with documented spasm I25.701
          - refractory I25.702
          - specified type NEC I25.708
          - unstable I25.700
        - ischemic chest pain I25.709
      - autologous artery I25.810
        - with
          - angina pectoris I25.729
            - with documented spasm I25.721
            - refractory I25.722
            - specified type I25.728
            - unstable I25.720
          - ischemic chest pain I25.729
      - autologous vein I25.810
        - with
          - angina pectoris I25.719
            - with documented spasm I25.711
            - refractory I25.712
            - specified type I25.718
            - unstable I25.710
          - ischemic chest pain I25.719
      - nonautologous biological I25.810
        - with
          - angina pectoris I25.739
            - with documented spasm I25.731
            - refractory I25.732
            - specified type I25.738
            - unstable I25.730
          - ischemic chest pain I25.739
      - specified type NEC I25.810
        - with
          - angina pectoris I25.799
            - with documented spasm I25.791
            - refractory I25.792
            - specified type I25.798
            - unstable I25.790
          - ischemic chest pain I25.799
    - native vessel
      - with
        - angina pectoris I25.119
          - with documented spasm I25.111
          - refractory I25.112
          - specified type NEC I25.118
          - unstable I25.110
        - ischemic chest pain I25.119
    - transplanted heart I25.811
      - bypass graft I25.812
        - with
          - angina pectoris I25.769
            - with documented spasm I25.761
            - refractory I25.762
            - specified type I25.768
            - unstable I25.760
          - ischemic chest pain I25.769
      - native coronary artery I25.811
        - with
          - angina pectoris I25.759
            - with documented spasm I25.751
            - refractory I25.752
            - specified type I25.758
            - unstable I25.750

Arthritis, arthritic — *continued*
- epidemic erythema A25.1
- facet joint — *see also* Spondylosis M47.819
- febrile — *see* Fever, rheumatic
- gonococcal A54.42
- gouty (acute) — *see* Gout
- in (due to)
  - acromegaly — *see also* subcategory M14.8- E22.Ø
  - amyloidosis — *see also* subcategory M14.8- E85.4
  - bacterial disease — *see also* subcategory MØ1 A49.9
  - Behcet's syndrome M35.2
  - caisson disease — *see also* subcategory M14.8- T7Ø.3 ☑
  - coliform bacilli (Escherichia coli) — *see* Arthritis, in, pyogenic organism NEC
  - crystals M11.9
    - dicalcium phosphate — *see* Arthritis, in, crystals, specified type NEC
    - hydroxyapatite M11.Ø- ☑
    - pyrophosphate — *see* Arthritis, in, crystals, specified type NEC
    - specified type NEC M11.8Ø
      - ankle M11.87- ☑
      - elbow M11.82- ☑
      - foot joint M11.87- ☑
      - hand joint M11.84- ☑
      - hip M11.85- ☑
      - knee M11.86- ☑
      - multiple sites M11.8- ☑
      - shoulder M11.81- ☑
      - vertebrae M11.88
      - wrist M11.83- ☑
  - dermatoarthritis, lipoid E78.81
  - dracontiasis (dracunculiasis) — *see also* category MØ1 B72
  - endocrine disorder NEC — *see also* subcategory M14.8- E34.9
  - enteritis, infectious NEC — *see also* category MØ1 AØ9
    - specified organism NEC — *see also* category MØ1 AØ8.8
  - erythema
    - multiforme — *see also* subcategory M14.8- L51.9
    - nodosum — *see also* subcategory M14.8- L52
  - gout — *see* Gout
  - helminthiasis NEC — *see also* category MØ1 B83.9
  - hemochromatosis — *see also* subcategory M14.8- E83.118
  - hemoglobinopathy NEC D58.2 *[M36.3]*
  - hemophilia NEC D66 *[M36.2]*
  - Hemophilus influenzae MØØ.8- ☑ *[B96.3]*
  - Henoch (-Schonlein) purpura D69.Ø *[M36.4]*
  - hyperparathyroidism NEC — *see also* subcategory M14.8- E21.3
  - hypersensitivity reaction NEC T78.49 ☑ *[M36.4]*
  - hypogammaglobulinemia — *see also* subcategory M14.8- D8Ø.1
  - hypothyroidism NEC — *see also* subcategory M14.8- EØ3.9
  - infection — *see* Arthritis, pyogenic or pyemic
    - spine — *see* Spondylopathy, infective
  - infectious disease NEC MØ1 ☑
  - leprosy — *see also* category MØ1 A3Ø.9
  - leukemia NEC C95.9- ☑ *[M36.1]*
  - lipoid dermatoarthritis E78.81
  - Lyme disease A69.23
  - Mediterranean fever, familial — *see also* subcategory M14.8- MØ4.1
  - Meningococcus A39.83
  - metabolic disorder NEC — *see also* subcategory M14.8- E88.9
  - multiple myelomatosis C9Ø.Ø- ☑ *[M36.1]*
  - mumps B26.85
  - mycosis NEC — *see also* category MØ1 B49
  - myelomatosis (multiple) C9Ø.Ø- ☑ *[M36.1]*
  - neurological disorder NEC G98.Ø
  - ochronosis — *see also* subcategory M14.8- E7Ø.29
  - O'nyong-nyong — *see also* category MØ1 A92.1
  - parasitic disease NEC — *see also* category MØ1 B89
  - paratyphoid fever — *see also* category MØ1 AØ1.4
  - Pseudomonas — *see* Arthritis, pyogenic, bacterial NEC
  - psoriasis L4Ø.5Ø
  - pyogenic organism NEC — *see* Arthritis, pyogenic, bacterial NEC
  - Reiter's disease — *see* Reiter's disease

Arthritis, arthritic — *continued*
- in — *continued*
  - respiratory disorder NEC — *see also* subcategory M14.8- J98.9
  - reticulosis, malignant — *see also* subcategory M14.8- C86.Ø
  - rubella BØ6.82
  - Salmonella (arizonae) (cholerae-suis) (enteritidis) (typhimurium) AØ2.23
  - sarcoidosis D86.86
  - specified bacteria NEC — *see* Arthritis, pyogenic, bacterial NEC
  - sporotrichosis B42.82
  - syringomyelia G95.Ø
  - thalassemia NEC D56.9 *[M36.3]*
  - tuberculosis — *see* Tuberculosis, arthritis
  - typhoid fever AØ1.Ø4
  - urethritis, Reiter's — *see* Reiter's disease
  - viral disease NEC — *see also* category MØ1 B34.9
- infectious or infective — *see also* Arthritis, pyogenic or pyemic
  - spine — *see* Spondylopathy, infective
- juvenile MØ8.9Ø
  - with systemic onset — *see* Still's disease
  - ankle MØ8.97- ☑
  - elbow MØ8.92- ☑
  - foot joint MØ8.97- ☑
  - hand joint MØ8.94- ☑
  - hip MØ8.95- ☑
  - knee MØ8.96- ☑
  - multiple site MØ8.99
  - pauciarticular MØ8.4Ø
    - ankle MØ8.47- ☑
    - elbow MØ8.42- ☑
    - foot joint MØ8.47- ☑
    - hand joint MØ8.44- ☑
    - hip MØ8.45- ☑
    - knee MØ8.46- ☑
    - shoulder MØ8.41- ☑
    - specified site NEC MØ8.4A
    - vertebrae MØ8.48
    - wrist MØ8.43- ☑
  - psoriatic L4Ø.54
  - rheumatoid — *see* Arthritis, rheumatoid, juvenile
  - shoulder MØ8.91- ☑
  - specified site NEC MØ8.9A
  - specified type NEC MØ8.8Ø
    - ankle MØ8.87- ☑
    - elbow MØ8.82- ☑
    - foot joint MØ8.87- ☑
    - hand joint MØ8.84- ☑
    - hip MØ8.85- ☑
    - knee MØ8.86- ☑
    - multiple site MØ8.89
    - shoulder MØ8.81- ☑
    - specified joint NEC MØ8.88
    - vertebrae MØ8.88
    - wrist MØ8.83- ☑
  - wrist MØ8.93- ☑
- meaning osteoarthritis — *see* Osteoarthritis
- meningococcal A39.83
- menopausal (any site) NEC — *see* Arthritis, specified form NEC
- mutilans (psoriatic) L4Ø.52
- mycotic NEC — *see also* category MØ1 B49
- neuropathic (Charcot) — *see* Arthropathy, neuropathic
  - diabetic — *see* Diabetes, arthropathy, neuropathic
  - nonsyphilitic NEC G98.Ø
  - syringomyelic G95.Ø
- ochronotic — *see also* subcategory M14.8- E7Ø.29
- palindromic (any site) — *see* Rheumatism, palindromic
- pneumococcal MØØ.1Ø
  - ankle MØØ.17- ☑
  - elbow MØØ.12- ☑
  - foot joint — *see* Arthritis, pneumococcal, ankle
  - hand joint MØØ.14- ☑
  - hip MØØ.15- ☑
  - knee MØØ.16- ☑
  - multiple site MØØ.19
  - shoulder MØØ.11- ☑
  - vertebra MØØ.18
  - wrist MØØ.13- ☑
- postdysenteric — *see* Arthropathy, postdysenteric
- postmeningococcal A39.84
- postrheumatic, chronic — *see* Arthropathy, postrheumatic, chronic

Arthritis, arthritic — *continued*
- primary progressive — *see also* Arthritis, specified form NEC
  - spine — *see* Spondylitis, ankylosing
- psoriatic L4Ø.5Ø
- purulent (any site except spine) — *see* Arthritis, pyogenic or pyemic
  - spine — *see* Spondylopathy, infective
- pyogenic or pyemic (any site except spine) MØØ.9
  - bacterial NEC MØØ.8Ø
    - ankle MØØ.87- ☑
    - elbow MØØ.82- ☑
    - foot joint — *see* Arthritis, pyogenic, bacterial NEC, ankle
    - hand joint MØØ.84- ☑
    - hip MØØ.85- ☑
    - knee MØØ.86- ☑
    - multiple site MØØ.89
    - shoulder MØØ.81- ☑
    - vertebra MØØ.88
    - wrist MØØ.83- ☑
  - pneumococcal — *see* Arthritis, pneumococcal
  - spine — *see* Spondylopathy, infective
  - staphylococcal — *see* Arthritis, staphylococcal
  - streptococcal — *see* Arthritis, streptococcal NEC
    - pneumococcal — *see* Arthritis, pneumococcal
- reactive — *see* Reiter's disease
- rheumatic — *see also* Arthritis, rheumatoid
  - acute or subacute — *see* Fever, rheumatic
- rheumatoid MØ6.9
  - with
    - carditis — *see* Rheumatoid, carditis
    - endocarditis — *see* Rheumatoid, carditis
    - heart involvement NEC — *see* Rheumatoid, carditis
    - lung involvement — *see* Rheumatoid, lung
    - myocarditis — *see* Rheumatoid, carditis
    - myopathy — *see* Rheumatoid, myopathy
    - pericarditis — *see* Rheumatoid, carditis
    - polyneuropathy — *see* Rheumatoid, polyneuropathy
    - rheumatoid factor — *see* Arthritis, rheumatoid, seropositive
    - splenoadenomegaly and leukopenia — *see* Felty's syndrome
    - vasculitis — *see* Rheumatoid, vasculitis
    - visceral involvement NEC — *see* Rheumatoid, arthritis, with involvement of organs NEC
  - juvenile (with or without rheumatoid factor) MØ8.ØØ
    - with systemic onset — *see* Still's disease
    - ankle MØ8.Ø7- ☑
    - elbow MØ8.Ø2- ☑
    - foot joint MØ8.Ø7- ☑
    - hand joint MØ8.Ø4- ☑
    - hip MØ8.Ø5- ☑
    - knee MØ8.Ø6- ☑
    - multiple site MØ8.Ø9
    - shoulder MØ8.Ø1- ☑
    - specified site NEC MØ8.ØA
    - vertebra MØ8.Ø8
    - wrist MØ8.Ø3- ☑
  - seronegative MØ6.ØØ
    - ankle MØ6.Ø7- ☑
    - elbow MØ6.Ø2- ☑
    - foot joint MØ6.Ø7- ☑
    - hand joint MØ6.Ø4- ☑
    - hip MØ6.Ø5- ☑
    - knee MØ6.Ø6- ☑
    - multiple site MØ6.Ø9
    - shoulder MØ6.Ø1- ☑
    - specified site NEC MØ6.ØA
    - vertebra MØ6.Ø8
    - wrist MØ6.Ø3- ☑
  - seropositive MØ5.9
    - specified NEC MØ5.8Ø
      - ankle MØ5.87- ☑
      - elbow MØ5.82- ☑
      - foot joint MØ5.87- ☑
      - hand joint MØ5.84- ☑
      - hip MØ5.85- ☑
      - knee MØ5.86- ☑
      - multiple sites MØ5.89
      - shoulder MØ5.81- ☑
      - specified site NEC MØ5.8A
      - vertebra — *see* Spondylitis, ankylosing
      - wrist MØ5.83- ☑
    - without organ involvement MØ5.7Ø

- **Arthritis, arthritic** — *continued*
  - rheumatoid — *continued*
    - seropositive — *continued*
      - without organ involvement — *continued*
        - ankle M05.77- ☑
        - elbow M05.72- ☑
        - foot joint M05.77- ☑
        - hand joint M05.74- ☑
        - hip M05.75- ☑
        - knee M05.76- ☑
        - multiple sites M05.79
        - shoulder M05.71- ☑
        - specified site NEC M05.7A
        - vertebra — *see* Spondylitis, ankylosing
        - wrist M05.73- ☑
    - specified type NEC M06.80
      - ankle M06.87- ☑
      - elbow M06.82- ☑
      - foot joint M06.87- ☑
      - hand joint M06.84- ☑
      - hip M06.85- ☑
      - knee M06.86- ☑
      - multiple site M06.89
      - shoulder M06.81- ☑
      - specified site NEC M06.8A
      - vertebra M06.88
      - wrist M06.83- ☑
    - spine — *see* Spondylitis, ankylosing
  - rubella B06.82
  - scorbutic — *see also* subcategory M14.8- E54
  - senile or senescent — *see* Osteoarthritis
  - septic (any site except spine) — *see* Arthritis, pyogenic or pyemic
    - spine — *see* Spondylopathy, infective
  - serum (nontherapeutic) (therapeutic) — *see* Arthropathy, postimmunization
  - specified form NEC M13.80
    - ankle M13.87- ☑
    - elbow M13.82- ☑
    - foot joint M13.87- ☑
    - hand joint M13.84- ☑
    - hip M13.85- ☑
    - knee M13.86- ☑
    - multiple site M13.89
    - shoulder M13.81- ☑
    - specified joint NEC M13.88
    - wrist M13.83- ☑
  - spine — *see also* Spondylosis
    - infectious or infective NEC — *see* Spondylopathy, infective
    - Marie-Strumpell — *see* Spondylitis, ankylosing
    - pyogenic — *see* Spondylopathy, infective
    - rheumatoid — *see* Spondylitis, ankylosing
    - traumatic (old) — *see* Spondylopathy, traumatic
    - tuberculous A18.01
  - staphylococcal M00.00
    - ankle M00.07- ☑
    - elbow M00.02- ☑
    - foot joint — *see* Arthritis, staphylococcal, ankle
    - hand joint M00.04- ☑
    - hip M00.05- ☑
    - knee M00.06- ☑
    - multiple site M00.09
    - shoulder M00.01- ☑
    - vertebra M00.08
    - wrist M00.03- ☑
  - streptococcal NEC M00.20
    - ankle M00.27- ☑
    - elbow M00.22- ☑
    - foot joint — *see* Arthritis, streptococcal, ankle
    - hand joint M00.24- ☑
    - hip M00.25- ☑
    - knee M00.26- ☑
    - multiple site M00.29
    - shoulder M00.21- ☑
    - vertebra M00.28
    - wrist M00.23- ☑
  - suppurative — *see* Arthritis, pyogenic or pyemic
  - syphilitic (late) A52.16
    - congenital A50.55 *[M12.80]*
  - syphilitica deformans (Charcot) A52.16
  - temporomandibular joint M26.64- ☑
  - toxic of menopause (any site) — *see* Arthritis, specified form NEC
  - transient — *see* Arthropathy, specified form NEC
  - traumatic (chronic) — *see* Arthropathy, traumatic
  - tuberculous A18.02
- **Arthritis, arthritic** — *continued*
  - tuberculous — *continued*
    - spine A18.01
  - uratic — *see* Gout
  - urethritica (Reiter's) — *see* Reiter's disease
  - vertebral — *see* Spondylopathy, inflammatory
  - villous (any site) — *see* Arthropathy, specified form NEC
- **Arthrocele** — *see* Effusion, joint
- **Arthrodesis status** Z98.1
- **Arthrodynia** — *see also* Pain, joint
- **Arthrodysplasia** Q74.9
- **Arthrofibrosis, joint** — *see* Ankylosis
- **Arthrogryposis** (congenital) Q68.8
  - multiplex congenita Q74.3
- **Arthrokatadysis** M24.7
- **Arthropathy** — *see also* Arthritis M12.9
  - Charcot's — *see* Arthropathy, neuropathic
    - diabetic — *see* Diabetes, arthropathy, neuropathic
    - syringomyelic G95.0
  - cricoarytenoid J38.7
  - crystal (-induced) — *see* Arthritis, in, crystals
  - diabetic NEC — *see* Diabetes, arthropathy
  - distal interphalangeal, psoriatic L40.51
  - enteropathic M07.60
    - ankle M07.67- ☑
    - elbow M07.62- ☑
    - foot joint M07.67- ☑
    - hand joint M07.64- ☑
    - hip M07.65- ☑
    - knee M07.66- ☑
    - multiple site M07.69
    - shoulder M07.61- ☑
    - vertebra M07.68
    - wrist M07.63- ☑
  - facet joint — *see also* Spondylosis M47.819
  - following intestinal bypass M02.00
    - ankle M02.07- ☑
    - elbow M02.02- ☑
    - foot joint M02.07- ☑
    - hand joint M02.04- ☑
    - hip M02.05- ☑
    - knee M02.06- ☑
    - multiple site M02.09
    - shoulder M02.01- ☑
    - vertebra M02.08
    - wrist M02.03- ☑
  - gouty — *see also* Gout
    - in (due to)
      - Lesch-Nyhan syndrome E79.1 *[M14.8-]* ☑
      - sickle-cell disorders D57- ☑ *[M14.8-]* ☑
  - hemophilic NEC D66 *[M36.2]*
    - in (due to)
      - hyperparathyroidism NEC E21.3 *[M14.8-]* ☑
      - metabolic disease NOS E88.9 *[M14.8-]* ☑
  - in (due to)
    - acromegaly E22.0 *[M14.8-]* ☑
    - amyloidosis E85.4 *[M14.8-]* ☑
    - blood disorder NOS D75.9 *[M36.3]*
    - diabetes — *see* Diabetes, arthropathy
    - endocrine disease NOS E34.9 *[M14.8-]* ☑
    - erythema
      - multiforme L51.9 *[M14.8-]* ☑
      - nodosum L52 *[M14.8-]* ☑
    - hemochromatosis E83.118 *[M14.8-]* ☑
    - hemoglobinopathy NEC D58.2 *[M36.3]*
    - hemophilia NEC D66 *[M36.2]*
    - Henoch-Schonlein purpura D69.0 *[M36.4]*
    - hyperthyroidism E05.90 *[M14.8-]* ☑
    - hypothyroidism E03.9 *[M14.8-]* ☑
    - infective endocarditis I33.0 *[M12.80]*
    - leukemia NEC C95.9- ☑ *[M36.1]*
    - malignant histiocytosis C96.A *[M36.1]*
    - metabolic disease NOS E88.9 *[M14.8-]* ☑
    - multiple myeloma C90.0- ☑ *[M36.1]*
    - neoplastic disease NOS (*see also* Neoplasm) D49.9 *[M36.1]*
    - nutritional deficiency — *see also* subcategory M14.8- E63.9
    - psoriasis NOS L40.50
    - sarcoidosis D86.86
    - syphilis (late) A52.77
      - congenital A50.55 *[M12.80]*
    - thyrotoxicosis — *see also* subcategory M14.8- E05.90
    - ulcerative colitis K51.90 *[M07.60]*
- **Arthropathy** — *continued*
  - in — *continued*
    - viral hepatitis (postinfectious) NEC B19.9 *[M12.80]*
    - Whipple's disease — *see also* subcategory M14.8- K90.81
  - Jaccoud — *see* Arthropathy, postrheumatic, chronic
  - juvenile — *see* Arthritis, juvenile
    - psoriatic L40.54
  - mutilans (psoriatic) L40.52
  - neuropathic (Charcot) M14.60
    - ankle M14.67- ☑
    - diabetic — *see* Diabetes, arthropathy, neuropathic
    - elbow M14.62- ☑
    - foot joint M14.67- ☑
    - hand joint M14.64- ☑
    - hip M14.65- ☑
    - knee M14.66- ☑
    - multiple site M14.69
    - nonsyphilitic NEC G98.0
    - shoulder M14.61- ☑
    - syringomyelic G95.0
    - vertebra M14.68
    - wrist M14.63- ☑
  - osteopulmonary — *see* Osteoarthropathy, hypertrophic, specified NEC
  - postdysenteric M02.10
    - ankle M02.17- ☑
    - elbow M02.12- ☑
    - foot joint M02.17- ☑
    - hand joint M02.14- ☑
    - hip M02.15- ☑
    - knee M02.16- ☑
    - multiple site M02.19
    - shoulder M02.11- ☑
    - vertebra M02.18
    - wrist M02.13- ☑
  - postimmunization M02.20
    - ankle M02.27- ☑
    - elbow M02.22- ☑
    - foot joint M02.27- ☑
    - hand joint M02.24- ☑
    - hip M02.25- ☑
    - knee M02.26- ☑
    - multiple site M02.29
    - shoulder M02.21- ☑
    - vertebra M02.28
    - wrist M02.23- ☑
  - postinfectious NEC B99 ☑ *[M12.80]*
    - in (due to)
      - enteritis due to Yersinia enterocolitica A04.6 *[M12.80]*
      - syphilis A52.77
      - viral hepatitis NEC B19.9 *[M12.80]*
  - postrheumatic, chronic (Jaccoud) M12.00
    - ankle M12.07- ☑
    - elbow M12.02- ☑
    - foot joint M12.07- ☑
    - hand joint M12.04- ☑
    - hip M12.05- ☑
    - knee M12.06- ☑
    - multiple site M12.09
    - shoulder M12.01- ☑
    - specified joint NEC M12.08
    - vertebrae M12.08
    - wrist M12.03- ☑
  - psoriatic NEC L40.59
    - interphalangeal, distal L40.51
  - reactive M02.9
    - in (due to)
      - infective endocarditis I33.0 *[M02.9]*
    - specified type NEC M02.80
      - ankle M02.87- ☑
      - elbow M02.82- ☑
      - foot joint M02.87- ☑
      - hand joint M02.84- ☑
      - hip M02.85- ☑
      - knee M02.86- ☑
      - multiple site M02.89
      - shoulder M02.81- ☑
      - vertebra M02.88
      - wrist M02.83- ☑
  - specified form NEC M12.80
    - ankle M12.87- ☑
    - elbow M12.82- ☑
    - foot joint M12.87- ☑
    - hand joint M12.84- ☑
    - hip M12.85- ☑

Atrophia — *continued*
- senilis — *continued*
  - dermatological L90.8
    - due to radiation (nonionizing) (solar) L57.8
- unguium L60.3
  - congenita Q84.6

Atrophie blanche (en plaque) (de Milian) L95.0

Atrophoderma, atrophodermia (of) L90.9
- diffusum (idiopathic) L90.4
- maculatum L90.8
  - et striatum L90.8
    - due to syphilis A52.79
  - syphilitic A51.39
- neuriticum L90.8
- Pasini and Pierini L90.3
- pigmentosum Q82.1
- reticulatum symmetricum faciei L66.4
- senile L90.8
  - due to radiation (nonionizing) (solar) L57.8
- vermiculata (cheeks) L66.4

Atrophy, atrophic (of)
- adrenal (capsule) (gland) E27.49
  - primary (autoimmune) E27.1
- alveolar process or ridge (edentulous) K08.20
- anal sphincter (disuse) N81.84
- appendix K38.8
- arteriosclerotic — *see* Arteriosclerosis
- bile duct (common) (hepatic) K83.8
- bladder N32.89
  - neurogenic N31.8
- blanche (en plaque) (of Milian) L95.0
- bone (senile) NEC — *see also* Disorder, bone, specified type NEC
  - due to
    - tabes dorsalis (neurogenic) A52.11
- brain (cortex) (progressive) G31.9
  - frontotemporal circumscribed — *see also* Dementia, in, diseases specified elsewhere G31.01 *[F02.80]*
    - with behavioral disturbance — *see also* Dementia, in, diseases specified elsewhere G31.01 *[F02.81-]* ☑
  - senile NEC G31.1
- breast N64.2
  - obstetric — *see* Disorder, breast, specified type NEC
- buccal cavity K13.79
- cardiac — *see* Degeneration, myocardial
- cartilage (infectional) (joint) — *see* Disorder, cartilage, specified NEC
- cerebellar — *see* Atrophy, brain
- cerebral — *see* Atrophy, brain
- cervix (mucosa) (senile) (uteri) N88.8
  - menopausal N95.8
- Charcot-Marie-Tooth G60.0
- choroid (central) (macular) (myopic) (retina) H31.10- ☑
  - diffuse secondary H31.12- ☑
  - gyrate H31.23
  - senile H31.11- ☑
- ciliary body — *see* Atrophy, iris
- conjunctiva (senile) H11.89
- corpus cavernosum N48.89
- cortical — *see* Atrophy, brain
- cystic duct K82.8
- Dejerine-Thomas G23.8
- disuse NEC — *see* Atrophy, muscle
- Duchenne-Aran G12.21
- ear H93.8- ☑
- edentulous alveolar ridge K08.20
- endometrium (senile) N85.8
  - cervix N88.8
- enteric K63.89
- epididymis N50.89
- eyeball — *see* Disorder, globe, degenerated condition, atrophy
- eyelid (senile) — *see* Disorder, eyelid, degenerative
- facial (skin) L90.9
- fallopian tube (senile) N83.32- ☑
  - with ovary N83.33- ☑
- fascioscapulohumeral (Landouzy- Dejerine) G71.02
- fatty, thymus (gland) E32.8
- gallbladder K82.8
- gastric K29.40
  - with bleeding K29.41
- gastrointestinal K63.89
- glandular I89.8
- globe H44.52- ☑
- gum — *see* Recession, gingival
- hair L67.8

Atrophy, atrophic — *continued*
- heart (brown) — *see* Degeneration, myocardial
- hemifacial Q67.4
  - Romberg G51.8
- infantile E41
  - paralysis, acute — *see* Poliomyelitis, paralytic
- intestine K63.89
- iris (essential) (progressive) H21.26- ☑
  - specified NEC H21.29
- kidney (senile) (terminal) — *see also* Sclerosis, renal N26.1
  - congenital or infantile Q60.5
    - bilateral Q60.4
    - unilateral Q60.3
  - hydronephrotic — *see* Hydronephrosis
- lacrimal gland (primary) H04.14- ☑
  - secondary H04.15- ☑
- Landouzy-Dejerine G71.02
- laryngitis, infective J37.0
- larynx J38.7
- Leber's optic (hereditary) H47.22
- lip K13.0
- liver (yellow) K72.90
  - with coma K72.91
  - acute, subacute K72.00
    - with coma K72.01
  - chronic K72.10
    - with coma K72.11
- lung (senile) J98.4
- macular (dermatological) L90.8
  - syphilitic, skin A51.39
    - striated A52.79
- mandible (edentulous) K08.20
  - minimal K08.21
  - moderate K08.22
  - severe K08.23
- maxilla K08.20
  - minimal K08.24
  - moderate K08.25
  - severe K08.26
- muscle, muscular (diffuse) (general) (idiopathic) (primary) M62.50
  - ankle M62.57- ☑
  - back M62.5A9
    - cervical M62.5A0
    - lumbosacral M62.5A2
    - thoracic M62.5A1
  - Duchenne-Aran G12.21
  - foot M62.57- ☑
  - forearm M62.53- ☑
  - hand M62.54- ☑
  - infantile spinal G12.0
  - lower leg M62.56- ☑
  - multiple sites M62.59
  - myelopathic — *see* Atrophy, muscle, spinal
  - myotonic G71.11
  - neuritic G58.9
  - neuropathic (peroneal) (progressive) G60.0
  - pelvic (disuse) N81.84
  - peroneal G60.0
  - progressive (bulbar) G12.21
    - adult G12.1
    - infantile (spinal) G12.0
    - spinal G12.25
      - adult G12.1
      - infantile G12.0
  - pseudohypertrophic G71.02
  - shoulder region M62.51- ☑
  - specified site NEC M62.58
  - spinal G12.9
    - adult form G12.1
    - Aran-Duchenne G12.21
    - childhood form, type II G12.1
    - distal G12.1
    - hereditary NEC G12.1
    - infantile, type I (Werdnig-Hoffmann) G12.0
    - juvenile form, type III (Kugelberg- Welander) G12.1
    - progressive G12.25
    - scapuloperoneal form G12.1
    - specified NEC G12.8
  - syphilitic A52.78
  - thigh M62.55- ☑
  - upper arm M62.52- ☑
- myocardium — *see* Degeneration, myocardial
- myometrium (senile) N85.8
  - cervix N88.8
- myopathic NEC — *see* Atrophy, muscle

Atrophy, atrophic — *continued*
- myotonia G71.11
- nail L60.3
- nasopharynx J31.1
- nerve — *see also* Disorder, nerve
  - abducens — *see* Strabismus, paralytic, sixth nerve
  - accessory G52.8
  - acoustic or auditory H93.3 ☑
  - cranial G52.9
    - eighth (auditory) H93.3 ☑
    - eleventh (accessory) G52.8
    - fifth (trigeminal) G50.8
    - first (olfactory) G52.0
    - fourth (trochlear) — *see* Strabismus, paralytic, fourth nerve
    - second (optic) H47.20
    - sixth (abducens) — *see* Strabismus, paralytic, sixth nerve
    - tenth (pneumogastric) (vagus) G52.2
    - third (oculomotor) — *see* Strabismus, paralytic, third nerve
    - twelfth (hypoglossal) G52.3
  - hypoglossal G52.3
  - oculomotor — *see* Strabismus, paralytic, third nerve
  - olfactory G52.0
  - optic (papillomacular bundle)
    - syphilitic (late) A52.15
      - congenital A50.44
  - pneumogastric G52.2
  - trigeminal G50.8
  - trochlear — *see* Strabismus, paralytic, fourth nerve
  - vagus (pneumogastric) G52.2
- neurogenic, bone, tabetic A52.11
- nutritional E43
  - with marasmus E41
- old age R54
- olivopontocerebellar G23.8
- optic (nerve) H47.20
  - glaucomatous H47.23- ☑
  - hereditary H47.22
  - primary H47.21- ☑
  - specified type NEC H47.29- ☑
  - syphilitic (late) A52.15
    - congenital A50.44
- orbit H05.31- ☑
- ovary (senile) N83.31- ☑
  - with fallopian tube N83.33- ☑
- oviduct (senile) — *see* Atrophy, fallopian tube
- palsy, diffuse (progressive) G12.22
- pancreas (duct) (senile) K86.89
- parotid gland K11.0
- pelvic muscle N81.84
- penis N48.89
- pharynx J39.2
- pluriglandular E31.8
  - autoimmune E31.0
- polyarthritis M15.9
- prostate N42.89
- pseudohypertrophic (muscle) G71.02
- renal — *see also* Sclerosis, renal N26.1
- retina, retinal (postinfectional) H35.89
- rhinitis J31.0
- salivary gland K11.0
- scar L90.5
- sclerosis, lobar (of brain) — *see also* Dementia, in, diseases specified elsewhere G31.09 *[F02.80]*
  - with behavioral disturbance — *see also* Dementia, in, diseases specified elsewhere G31.09 *[F02.81-]* ☑
- scrotum N50.89
- seminal vesicle N50.89
- senile R54
  - due to radiation (nonionizing) (solar) L57.8
- skin (patches) (spots) L90.9
  - degenerative (senile) L90.8
  - due to radiation (nonionizing) (solar) L57.8
  - senile L90.8
- spermatic cord N50.89
- spinal (acute) (cord) G95.89
  - muscular — *see* Atrophy, muscle, spinal
  - paralysis G12.20
    - acute — *see* Poliomyelitis, paralytic
    - meaning progressive muscular atrophy G12.25
- spine (column) — *see* Spondylopathy, specified NEC
- spleen (senile) D73.0
- stomach K29.40
  - with bleeding K29.41
- striate (skin) L90.6

- **Atrophy, atrophic** — *continued*
  - striate — *continued*
    - syphilitic A52.79
  - subcutaneous L9Ø.9
  - sublingual gland K11.Ø
  - submandibular gland K11.Ø
  - submaxillary gland K11.Ø
  - Sudeck's — *see* Algoneurodystrophy
  - suprarenal (capsule) (gland) E27.49
    - primary E27.1
  - systemic affecting central nervous system
    - in
      - myxedema EØ3.9 *[G13.2]*
      - neoplastic disease — *see also* Neoplasm D49.9 *[G13.1]*
      - specified disease NEC G13.8
  - tarso-orbital fascia, congenital Q1Ø.3
  - testis N5Ø.Ø
  - thenar, partial — *see* Syndrome, carpal tunnel
  - thymus (fatty) E32.8
  - thyroid (gland) (acquired) EØ3.4
    - with cretinism EØ3.1
    - congenital (with myxedema) EØ3.1
  - tongue (senile) K14.8
    - papillae K14.4
  - trachea J39.8
  - tunica vaginalis N5Ø.89
  - turbinate J34.89
  - tympanic membrane (nonflaccid) H73.82- ☑
    - flaccid H73.81- ☑
  - upper respiratory tract J39.8
  - uterus, uterine (senile) N85.8
    - cervix N88.8
    - due to radiation (intended effect) N85.8
      - adverse effect or misadventure N99.89
  - vagina (senile) N95.2
  - vas deferens N5Ø.89
  - vascular I99.8
  - vertebra (senile) — *see* Spondylopathy, specified NEC
  - vulva (senile) N9Ø.5
  - Werdnig-Hoffmann G12.Ø
  - yellow — *see* Failure, hepatic
- **Attack, attacks**
  - with alteration of consciousness (with automatisms) — *see* Epilepsy, localization-related, symptomatic, with complex partial seizures
  - Adams-Stokes I45.9
  - akinetic — *see* Epilepsy, generalized, specified NEC
  - angina — *see* Angina
  - atonic — *see* Epilepsy, generalized, specified NEC
  - benign shuddering G25.83
  - cataleptic — *see* Catalepsy
  - coronary — *see* Infarct, myocardium
  - cyanotic, newborn P28.2
  - drop NEC R55
  - epileptic — *see* Epilepsy
  - heart — *see* infarct, myocardium
  - hysterical F44.9
  - jacksonian — *see* Epilepsy, localization-related, symptomatic, with simple partial seizures
  - myocardium, myocardial — *see* Infarct, myocardium
  - myoclonic — *see* Epilepsy, generalized, specified NEC
  - panic F41.Ø
  - psychomotor — *see* Epilepsy, localization-related, symptomatic, with complex partial seizures
  - salaam — *see* Epilepsy, spasms
  - schizophreniform, brief F23
  - shuddering, benign G25.83
  - Stokes-Adams I45.9
  - syncope R55
  - transient ischemic (TIA) G45.9
    - specified NEC G45.8
  - unconsciousness R55
    - hysterical F44.89
  - vasomotor R55
  - vasovagal (paroxysmal) (idiopathic) R55
  - without alteration of consciousness — *see* Epilepsy, localization-related, symptomatic, with simple partial seizures
- **Attention** (to)
  - artificial
    - opening (of) Z43.9
      - digestive tract NEC Z43.4
        - colon Z43.3
        - ilium Z43.2
        - stomach Z43.1
      - specified NEC Z43.8
      - trachea Z43.Ø
- **Attention** — *continued*
  - artificial — *continued*
    - opening — *continued*
      - urinary tract NEC Z43.6
        - cystostomy Z43.5
        - nephrostomy Z43.6
        - ureterostomy Z43.6
        - urethrostomy Z43.6
      - vagina Z43.7
  - colostomy Z43.3
  - cystostomy Z43.5
  - deficit disorder or syndrome F98.8
    - with hyperactivity — *see* Disorder, attention-deficit hyperactivity
  - gastrostomy Z43.1
  - ileostomy Z43.2
  - jejunostomy Z43.4
  - nephrostomy Z43.6
  - surgical dressings Z48.Ø1
  - sutures Z48.Ø2
  - tracheostomy Z43.Ø
  - ureterostomy Z43.6
  - urethrostomy Z43.6
- **Attrition**
  - gum — *see* Recession, gingival
  - tooth, teeth (excessive) (hard tissues) KØ3.Ø
- **Atypical, atypism** — *see also* condition
  - cells (on cytolgocial smear) (endocervical) (endometrial) (glandular)
    - cervix R87.619
    - vagina R87.629
  - cervical N87.9
  - endometrium N85.9
    - hyperplasia N85.ØØ
  - parenting situation Z62.9
- **Auditory** — *see* condition
- **Aujeszky's disease** B33.8
- **Aurantiasis, cutis** E67.1
- **Auricle, auricular** — *see also* condition
  - cervical Q18.2
- **Auriculotemporal syndrome** G5Ø.8
- **Austin Flint murmur** (aortic insufficiency) I35.1
- **Australian**
  - Q fever A78
  - X disease A83.4
- **Autism, autistic** (childhood) (infantile) F84.Ø
  - atypical F84.9
  - spectrum disorder F84.Ø
- **Autodigestion** R68.89
- **Autoerythrocyte sensitization** (syndrome) D69.2
- **Autographism** L5Ø.3
- **Autoimmune**
  - disease (systemic) M35.9
  - inhibitors to clotting factors D68.311
  - lymphoproliferative syndrome [ALPS] D89.82
  - thyroiditis EØ6.3
- **Autointoxication** R68.89
- **Automatism** G93.89
  - with temporal sclerosis G93.81
  - epileptic — *see* Epilepsy, localization-related, symptomatic, with complex partial seizures
  - paroxysmal, idiopathic — *see* Epilepsy, localization-related, symptomatic, with complex partial seizures
- **Autonomic, autonomous**
  - bladder (neurogenic) N31.2
  - hysteria seizure F44.5
- **Autosensitivity, erythrocyte** D69.2
- **Autosensitization, cutaneous** L3Ø.2
- **Autosome** — *see* condition by chromosome involved
- **Autotopagnosia** R48.1
- **Autotoxemia** R68.89
- **Autumn** — *see* condition
- **Avellis' syndrome** G46.8
- **Aversion**
  - oral R63.39
    - newborn P92.- ☑
    - nonorganic origin F98.2 ☑
  - sexual F52.1
- **Aviator's**
  - disease or sickness — *see* Effect, adverse, high altitude
  - ear T7Ø.Ø ☑
- **Avitaminosis** (multiple) — *see also* Deficiency, vitamin E56.9
  - B E53.9
    - with
      - beriberi E51.11
      - pellagra E52
- **Avitaminosis** — *continued*
  - B2 E53.Ø
  - B6 E53.1
  - B12 E53.8
  - D E55.9
    - with rickets E55.Ø
  - G E53.Ø
  - K E56.1
  - nicotinic acid E52
- **AVNRT** (atrioventricular nodal re-entrant tachycardia) I47.19
- **AVRT** (atrioventricular nodal re-entrant tachycardia) I47.19
- **Avulsion** (traumatic)
  - blood vessel — *see* Injury, blood vessel
  - bone — *see* Fracture, by site
  - cartilage — *see also* Dislocation, by site
    - symphyseal (inner), complicating delivery O71.6
  - external site other than limb — *see* Wound, open, by site
  - eye SØ5.7- ☑
  - head (intracranial)
    - external site NEC SØ8.89 ☑
    - scalp SØ8.Ø ☑
  - internal organ or site — *see* Injury, by site
  - joint — *see also* Dislocation, by site
    - capsule — *see* Sprain, by site
  - kidney S37.Ø6- ☑
  - ligament — *see* Sprain, by site
  - limb — *see also* Amputation, traumatic, by site
    - skin and subcutaneous tissue — *see* Wound, open, by site
  - muscle — *see* Injury, muscle
  - nerve (root) — *see* Injury, nerve
  - scalp SØ8.Ø ☑
  - skin and subcutaneous tissue — *see* Wound, open, by site
  - spleen S36.Ø32 ☑
  - symphyseal cartilage (inner), complicating delivery O71.6
  - tendon — *see* Injury, muscle
  - tooth SØ3.2 ☑
- **Awareness of heart beat** RØØ.2
- **Axenfeld's**
  - anomaly or syndrome Q15.Ø
  - degeneration (calcareous) Q13.4
- **Axilla, axillary** — *see also* condition
  - breast Q83.1
- **Axonotmesis** — *see* Injury, nerve
- **Ayerza's disease or syndrome** (pulmonary artery sclerosis with pulmonary hypertension) I27.Ø
- **Azoospermia** (organic) N46.Ø1
  - due to
    - drug therapy N46.Ø21
    - efferent duct obstruction N46.Ø23
    - infection N46.Ø22
    - radiation N46.Ø24
    - specified cause NEC N46.Ø29
    - systemic disease N46.Ø25
- **Azotemia** R79.89
  - meaning uremia N19
- **Aztec ear** Q17.3
- **Azygos**
  - continuation inferior vena cava Q26.8
  - lobe (lung) Q33.1

B

- **Baastrup's disease** — *see* Kissing spine
- **Babesiosis** B6Ø.ØØ
  - due to
    - Babesia
      - divergens B6Ø.Ø3
      - duncani B6Ø.Ø2
      - KO-1 B6Ø.Ø9
      - microti B6Ø.Ø1
      - MO-1 B6Ø.Ø3
      - species
        - unspecified B6Ø.ØØ
      - venatorum B6Ø.Ø9
    - specified NEC B6Ø.Ø9
- **Babington's disease** (familial hemorrhagic telangiectasia) I78.Ø
- **Babinski's syndrome** A52.79
- **Baby**
  - crying constantly R68.11
  - floppy (syndrome) P94.2
- **Bacillary** — *see* condition

- **Bacilluria** R82.71
- **Bacillus** — *see also* Infection, bacillus
  - abortus infection A23.1
  - anthracis infection A22.9
  - coli infection — *see also* Escherichia coli B96.2Ø
  - Flexner's AØ3.1
  - mallei infection A24.Ø
  - Shiga's AØ3.Ø
  - suipestifer infection — *see* Infection, salmonella
- **Back** — *see* condition
- **Backache** (postural) M54.9
  - sacroiliac M53.3
  - specified NEC M54.89
- **Backflow** — *see* Reflux
- **Backward reading** (dyslexia) F81.Ø
- **Bacteremia** R78.81
  - with sepsis — *see* Sepsis
- **Bactericholia** — *see* Cholecystitis, acute
- **Bacterid, bacteride** (pustular) L4Ø.3
- **Bacterium, bacteria, bacterial**
  - agent NEC, as cause of disease classified elsewhere B96.89
  - in blood — *see* Bacteremia
  - in urine — *see* Bacteriuria
- **Bacteriuria, bacteruria** R82.71
  - asymptomatic R82.71
- **Bacteroides**
  - fragilis, as cause of disease classified elsewhere B96.6
- **Bad**
  - heart — *see* Disease, heart
  - trip
    - due to drug abuse — *see* Abuse, drug, hallucinogen
    - due to drug dependence — *see* Dependence, drug, hallucinogen
- **Baelz's disease** (cheilitis glandularis apostematosa) K13.Ø
- **Baerensprung's disease** (eczema marginatum) B35.6
- **Bagasse disease or pneumonitis** J67.1
- **Bagassosis** J67.1
- **Baker's cyst** — *see* Cyst, Baker's
- **Bakwin-Krida syndrome** (metaphyseal dysplasia) Q78.5
- **Balancing side interference** M26.56
- **Balanitis** (circinata) (erosiva) (gangrenosa) (phagedenic) (vulgaris) N48.1
  - amebic AØ6.82
  - candidal B37.42
  - due to Haemophilus ducreyi A57
  - gonococcal (acute) (chronic) A54.23
  - xerotica obliterans N48.Ø
- **Balanoposthitis** N47.6
  - gonococcal (acute) (chronic) A54.23
  - ulcerative (specific) A63.8
- **Balanorrhagia** — *see* Balanitis
- **Balantidiasis, balantidiosis** AØ7.Ø
- **Bald tongue** K14.4
- **Baldness** — *see also* Alopecia
  - male-pattern — *see* Alopecia, androgenic
- **Balkan grippe** A78
- **Balloon disease** — *see* Effect, adverse, high altitude
- **Balo's disease** (concentric sclerosis) G37.5
- **Bamberger-Marie disease** — *see* Osteoarthropathy, hypertrophic, specified type NEC
- **Bancroft's filariasis** B74.Ø
- **Band**(s)
  - adhesive — *see* Adhesions, peritoneum
  - anomalous or congenital — *see also* Anomaly, by site
    - heart (atrial) (ventricular) Q24.8
    - intestine Q43.3
    - omentum Q43.3
  - cervix N88.1
  - constricting, congenital Q79.8
  - gallbladder (congenital) Q44.1
  - intestinal (adhesive) — *see* Adhesions, peritoneum
  - obstructive
    - intestine K56.5Ø
      - complete K56.52
      - incomplete K56.51
      - partial K56.51
    - peritoneum K56.5Ø
      - complete K56.52
      - incomplete K56.51
      - partial K56.51
  - periappendiceal, congenital Q43.3
  - peritoneal (adhesive) — *see* Adhesions, peritoneum
  - uterus N73.6
    - internal N85.6
  - vagina N89.5
- **Bandemia** D72.825
- **Bandl's ring** (contraction), complicating delivery O62.4
- **Bangkok hemorrhagic fever** A91
- **Bang's disease** (brucella abortus) A23.1
- **Bankruptcy** (anxiety concerning) Z59.86
- **Bannister's disease** T78.3 ☑
  - hereditary D84.1
- **Banti's disease or syndrome** (with cirrhosis) (with portal hypertension) K76.6
- **Bar, median, prostate** — *see* Enlargement, enlarged, prostate
- **Barcoo disease or rot** — *see* Ulcer, skin
- **Barlow's disease** E54
- **Barodontalgia** T7Ø.29 ☑
- **Baron Munchausen syndrome** — *see* Disorder, factitious
- **Barosinusitis** T7Ø.1 ☑
- **Barotitis** T7Ø.Ø ☑
- **Barotrauma** T7Ø.29 ☑
  - odontalgia T7Ø.29 ☑
  - otitic T7Ø.Ø ☑
  - sinus T7Ø.1 ☑
- **Barraquer** (-Simons) **disease or syndrome** (progressive lipodystrophy) E88.1
- **Barre-Guillain disease or syndrome** G61.Ø
- **Barrel chest** M95.4
- **Barre-Lieou syndrome** (posterior cervical sympathetic) M53.Ø
- **Barrett's**
  - disease — *see* Barrett's, esophagus
  - esophagus K22.7Ø
    - with dysplasia K22.719
      - high grade K22.711
      - low grade K22.71Ø
    - without dysplasia K22.7Ø
  - syndrome — *see* Barrett's, esophagus
  - ulcer K22.1Ø
    - with bleeding K22.11
    - without bleeding K22.1Ø
- **Barsony** (-Polgar) (-Teschendorf) **syndrome** (corkscrew esophagus) K22.4
- **Barth syndrome** E78.71
- **Bartholinitis** (suppurating) N75.8
  - gonococcal (acute) (chronic) (with abscess) A54.1
- **Bartonellosis** A44.9
  - cutaneous A44.1
  - mucocutaneous A44.1
  - specified NEC A44.8
  - systemic A44.Ø
- **Barton's fracture** S52.56- ☑
- **Bartter's syndrome** E26.81
- **Basal** — *see* condition
- **Basan's** (hidrotic) ectodermal dysplasia Q82.4
- **Baseball finger** — *see* Dislocation, finger
- **Basedow's disease** (exophthalmic goiter) — *see* Hyperthyroidism, with, goiter
- **Basic** — *see* condition
- **Basilar** — *see* condition
- **Bason's** (hidrotic) ectodermal dysplasia Q82.4
- **Basopenia** — *see* Agranulocytosis
- **Basophilia** D72.824
- **Basophilism** (cortico-adrenal) (Cushing's) (pituitary) E24.Ø
- **Bassen-Kornzweig disease or syndrome** E78.6
- **Bat ear** Q17.5
- **Bateman's**
  - disease BØ8.1
  - purpura (senile) D69.2
- **Bathing cramp** T75.1 ☑
- **Bathophobia** F4Ø.248
- **Batten** (-Mayou) **disease** E75.4
  - retina E75.4 *[H36.89]*
- **Batten-Steinert syndrome** G71.11
- **Battered** — *see* Maltreatment
- **Battey Mycobacterium infection** A31.Ø
- **Battle exhaustion** F43.Ø
- **Battledore placenta** O43.19- ☑
- **Baumgarten-Cruveilhier cirrhosis, disease or syndrome** K74.69
- **Bauxite fibrosis** (of lung) J63.1
- **Bayle's disease** (general paresis) A52.17
- **Bazin's disease** (primary) (tuberculous) A18.4
- **Beach ear** — *see* Swimmer's, ear
- **Beaded hair** (congenital) Q84.1
- **Beal conjunctivitis or syndrome** B3Ø.2
- **Beard's disease** (neurasthenia) F48.8
- **Beat**(s)
  - atrial, premature I49.1
  - ectopic I49.49
- **Beat**(s) — *continued*
  - elbow — *see* Bursitis, elbow
  - escaped, heart I49.49
  - hand — *see* Bursitis, hand
  - knee — *see* Bursitis, knee
  - premature I49.4Ø
    - atrial I49.1
    - auricular I49.1
    - supraventricular I49.1
- **Beau's**
  - disease or syndrome — *see* Degeneration, myocardial
  - lines (transverse furrows on fingernails) L6Ø.4
- **Bechterev's syndrome** — *see* Spondylitis, ankylosing
- **Becker's**
  - cardiomyopathy I42.8
  - disease
    - idiopathic mural endomyocardial disease I42.3
    - myotonia congenita, recessive form G71.12
  - dystrophy G71.Ø1
  - pigmented hairy nevus D22.5
- **Beck's syndrome** (anterior spinal artery occlusion) I65.8
- **Beckwith-Wiedemann syndrome** Q87.3
- **Bed confinement status** Z74.Ø1
- **Bed sore** — *see* Ulcer, pressure, by site
- **Bedbug bite**(s) — *see* Bite(s), by site, superficial, insect
- **Bedclothes, asphyxiation or suffocation by** — *see* Asphyxia, traumatic, due to, mechanical, trapped
- **Bednar's**
  - aphthae K12.Ø
  - tumor — *see* Neoplasm, malignant, by site
- **Bedridden** Z74.Ø1
- **Bed-sharing, infant** Z72.823
- **Bedsore** — *see* Ulcer, pressure, by site
- **Bedwetting** — *see* Enuresis
- **Bee sting** (with allergic or anaphylactic shock) — *see* Toxicity, venom, arthropod, bee
- **Beer drinker's heart** (disease) I42.6
- **Begbie's disease** (exophthalmic goiter) — *see* Hyperthyroidism, with, goiter
- **Behavior**
  - antisocial
    - adult Z72.811
    - child or adolescent Z72.81Ø
  - disorder, disturbance — *see* Disorder, conduct
  - disruptive — *see* Disorder, conduct
  - drug seeking Z76.5
  - inexplicable R46.2
  - marked evasiveness R46.5
  - obsessive-compulsive R46.81
  - overactivity R46.3
  - poor responsiveness R46.4
  - self-damaging (life-style) Z72.89
  - sleep-incompatible Z72.821
  - slowness R46.4
  - specified NEC R46.89
  - strange (and inexplicable) R46.2
  - suspiciousness R46.5
  - type A pattern Z73.1
  - undue concern or preoccupation with stressful events R46.6
  - verbosity and circumstantial detail obscuring reason for contact R46.7
- **Behcet's disease or syndrome** M35.2
- **Behr's disease** — *see* Degeneration, macula
- **Beigel's disease or morbus** (white piedra) B36.2
- **Bejel** A65
- **Bekhterev's syndrome** — *see* Spondylitis, ankylosing
- **Belching** — *see* Eructation
- **Bell's**
  - mania F3Ø.8
  - palsy, paralysis G51.Ø
    - infant or newborn P11.3
  - spasm G51.3- ☑
- **Bence Jones albuminuria or proteinuria NEC** R8Ø.3
- **Bends** T7Ø.3 ☑
- **Benedikt's paralysis or syndrome** G46.3
- **Benign** — *see also* condition
  - prostatic hyperplasia — *see* Hyperplasia, prostate
- **Bennett's fracture** (displaced) S62.21- ☑
- **Benson's disease** — *see* Deposit, crystalline
- **Bent**
  - back (hysterical) F44.4
  - nose M95.Ø
    - congenital Q67.4
- **Bereavement** (uncomplicated) Z63.4
- **Bergeron's disease** (hysterical chorea) F44.4
- **Berger's disease** — *see* Nephropathy, IgA

Bite(s) — *continued*
- digit(s)
  - hand — *see* Bite, finger
  - toe — *see* Bite, toe
- ear (canal) (external) SØ1.35- ☑
  - superficial NEC SØØ.47- ☑
    - insect SØØ.46- ☑
- elbow S51.Ø5- ☑
  - superficial NEC S5Ø.37- ☑
    - insect S5Ø.36- ☑
- epididymis — *see* Bite, testis
- epigastric region — *see* Bite, abdomen
- epiglottis — *see* Bite, neck, specified site NEC
- esophagus, cervical S11.25 ☑
  - superficial NEC S1Ø.17 ☑
    - insect S1Ø.16 ☑
- eyebrow — *see* Bite, eyelid
- eyelid SØ1.15- ☑
  - superficial NEC SØØ.27- ☑
    - insect SØØ.26- ☑
- face NEC — *see* Bite, head, specified site NEC
- finger(s) S61.259 ☑
  - with
    - damage to nail S61.359 ☑
  - index S61.258 ☑
    - with
      - damage to nail S61.358 ☑
    - left S61.251 ☑
      - with
        - damage to nail S61.351 ☑
    - right S61.25Ø ☑
      - with
        - damage to nail S61.35Ø ☑
    - superficial NEC S6Ø.478 ☑
      - insect S6Ø.46- ☑
  - little S61.25- ☑
    - with
      - damage to nail S61.35- ☑
    - superficial NEC S6Ø.47- ☑
      - insect S6Ø.46- ☑
  - middle S61.25- ☑
    - with
      - damage to nail S61.35- ☑
    - superficial NEC S6Ø.47- ☑
      - insect S6Ø.46- ☑
  - ring S61.25- ☑
    - with
      - damage to nail S61.35- ☑
    - superficial NEC S6Ø.47- ☑
      - insect S6Ø.46- ☑
  - superficial NEC S6Ø.479 ☑
    - insect S6Ø.469 ☑
  - thumb — *see* Bite, thumb
- flank — *see* Bite, abdomen, wall
- flea — *see* Bite, by site, superficial, insect
- foot (except toe(s) alone) S91.35- ☑
  - superficial NEC S9Ø.87- ☑
    - insect S9Ø.86- ☑
  - toe — *see* Bite, toe
- forearm S51.85- ☑
  - elbow only — *see* Bite, elbow
  - superficial NEC S5Ø.87- ☑
    - insect S5Ø.86- ☑
- forehead — *see* Bite, head, specified site NEC
- genital organs, external
  - female S31.552 ☑
    - superficial NEC S3Ø.876 ☑
      - insect S3Ø.866 ☑
    - vagina and vulva — *see* Bite, vulva
  - male S31.551 ☑
    - penis — *see* Bite, penis
    - scrotum — *see* Bite, scrotum
    - superficial NEC S3Ø.875 ☑
      - insect S3Ø.865 ☑
    - testes — *see* Bite, testis
- groin — *see* Bite, abdomen, wall
- gum — *see* Bite, oral cavity
- hand S61.45- ☑
  - finger — *see* Bite, finger
  - superficial NEC S6Ø.57- ☑
    - insect S6Ø.56- ☑
  - thumb — *see* Bite, thumb
- head SØ1.95 ☑
  - cheek — *see* Bite, cheek
  - ear — *see* Bite, ear
  - eyelid — *see* Bite, eyelid

Bite(s) — *continued*
- head — *continued*
  - lip — *see* Bite, lip
  - nose — *see* Bite, nose
  - oral cavity — *see* Bite, oral cavity
  - scalp — *see* Bite, scalp
  - specified site NEC SØ1.85 ☑
    - superficial NEC SØØ.87 ☑
      - insect SØØ.86 ☑
  - superficial NEC SØØ.97 ☑
    - insect SØØ.96 ☑
  - temporomandibular area — *see* Bite, cheek
- heel — *see* Bite, foot
- hip S71.Ø5- ☑
  - superficial NEC S7Ø.27- ☑
    - insect S7Ø.26- ☑
- hymen S31.45 ☑
- hypochondrium — *see* Bite, abdomen, wall
- hypogastric region — *see* Bite, abdomen, wall
- inguinal region — *see* Bite, abdomen, wall
- insect — *see* Bite, by site, superficial, insect
- instep — *see* Bite, foot
- interscapular region — *see* Bite, thorax, back
- jaw — *see* Bite, head, specified site NEC
- knee S81.Ø5- ☑
  - superficial NEC S8Ø.27- ☑
    - insect S8Ø.26- ☑
- labium (majus) (minus) — *see* Bite, vulva
- lacrimal duct — *see* Bite, eyelid
- larynx S11.Ø15 ☑
  - superficial NEC S1Ø.17 ☑
    - insect S1Ø.16 ☑
- leg (lower) S81.85- ☑
  - ankle — *see* Bite, ankle
  - foot — *see* Bite, foot
  - knee — *see* Bite, knee
  - superficial NEC S8Ø.87- ☑
    - insect S8Ø.86- ☑
  - toe — *see* Bite, toe
  - upper — *see* Bite, thigh
- lip SØ1.551 ☑
  - superficial NEC SØØ.571 ☑
    - insect SØØ.561 ☑
- lizard (venomous) — *see* Venom, bite, reptile
- loin — *see* Bite, abdomen, wall
- lower back — *see* Bite, back, lower
- lumbar region — *see* Bite, back, lower
- malar region — *see* Bite, head, specified site NEC
- mammary — *see* Bite, breast
- marine animals (venomous) — *see* Toxicity, venom, marine animal
- mastoid region — *see* Bite, head, specified site NEC
- mouth — *see* Bite, oral cavity
- nail
  - finger — *see* Bite, finger
  - toe — *see* Bite, toe
- nape — *see* Bite, neck, specified site NEC
- nasal (septum) (sinus) — *see* Bite, nose
- nasopharynx — *see* Bite, head, specified site NEC
- neck S11.95 ☑
  - involving
    - cervical esophagus — *see* Bite, esophagus, cervical
    - larynx — *see* Bite, larynx
    - pharynx — *see* Bite, pharynx
    - thyroid gland S11.15 ☑
    - trachea — *see* Bite, trachea
  - specified site NEC S11.85 ☑
    - superficial NEC S1Ø.87 ☑
      - insect S1Ø.86 ☑
  - superficial NEC S1Ø.97 ☑
    - insect S1Ø.96 ☑
  - throat S11.85 ☑
    - superficial NEC S1Ø.17 ☑
      - insect S1Ø.16 ☑
- nose (septum) (sinus) SØ1.25 ☑
  - superficial NEC SØØ.37 ☑
    - insect SØØ.36 ☑
- occipital region — *see* Bite, scalp
- oral cavity SØ1.552 ☑
  - superficial NEC SØØ.572 ☑
    - insect SØØ.562 ☑
- orbital region — *see* Bite, eyelid
- palate — *see* Bite, oral cavity
- palm — *see* Bite, hand
- parietal region — *see* Bite, scalp

Bite(s) — *continued*
- pelvis S31.Ø5Ø ☑
  - with penetration into retroperitoneal space S31.Ø51 ☑
  - superficial NEC S3Ø.87Ø ☑
    - insect S3Ø.86Ø ☑
- penis S31.25 ☑
  - superficial NEC S3Ø.872 ☑
    - insect S3Ø.862 ☑
- perineum
  - female — *see* Bite, vulva
  - male — *see* Bite, pelvis
- periocular area (with or without lacrimal passages) — *see* Bite, eyelid
- phalanges
  - finger — *see* Bite, finger
  - toe — *see* Bite, toe
- pharynx S11.25 ☑
  - superficial NEC S1Ø.17 ☑
    - insect S1Ø.16 ☑
- pinna — *see* Bite, ear
- poisonous — *see* Venom
- popliteal space — *see* Bite, knee
- prepuce — *see* Bite, penis
- pubic region — *see* Bite, abdomen, wall
- rectovaginal septum — *see* Bite, vulva
- red bug B88.Ø
- reptile NEC — *see also* Venom, bite, reptile
  - nonvenomous — *see* Bite, by site
  - snake — *see* Venom, bite, snake
- sacral region — *see* Bite, back, lower
- sacroiliac region — *see* Bite, back, lower
- salivary gland — *see* Bite, oral cavity
- scalp SØ1.Ø5 ☑
  - superficial NEC SØØ.Ø7 ☑
    - insect SØØ.Ø6 ☑
- scapular region — *see* Bite, shoulder
- scrotum S31.35 ☑
  - superficial NEC S3Ø.873 ☑
    - insect S3Ø.863 ☑
- sea-snake (venomous) — *see* Toxicity, venom, snake, sea snake
- shin — *see* Bite, leg
- shoulder S41.Ø5- ☑
  - superficial NEC S4Ø.27- ☑
    - insect S4Ø.26- ☑
- snake — *see also* Venom, bite, snake
  - nonvenomous — *see* Bite, by site
- spermatic cord — *see* Bite, testis
- spider (venomous) — *see* Toxicity, venom, spider
  - nonvenomous — *see* Bite, by site, superficial, insect
- sternal region — *see* Bite, thorax, front
- submaxillary region — *see* Bite, head, specified site NEC
- submental region — *see* Bite, head, specified site NEC
- subungual
  - finger(s) — *see* Bite, finger
  - toe — *see* Bite, toe
- superficial — *see* Bite, by site, superficial
- supraclavicular fossa S11.85 ☑
- supraorbital — *see* Bite, head, specified site NEC
- temple, temporal region — *see* Bite, head, specified site NEC
- temporomandibular area — *see* Bite, cheek
- testis S31.35 ☑
  - superficial NEC S3Ø.873 ☑
    - insect S3Ø.863 ☑
- thigh S71.15- ☑
  - superficial NEC S7Ø.37- ☑
    - insect S7Ø.36- ☑
- thorax, thoracic (wall) S21.95 ☑
  - back S21.25- ☑
    - with penetration into thoracic cavity S21.45- ☑
  - breast — *see* Bite, breast
  - front S21.15- ☑
    - with penetration into thoracic cavity S21.35- ☑
  - superficial NEC S2Ø.97 ☑
    - back S2Ø.47- ☑
    - front S2Ø.37- ☑
    - insect S2Ø.96 ☑
      - back S2Ø.46- ☑
      - front S2Ø.36- ☑
- throat — *see* Bite, neck, throat
- thumb S61.Ø5- ☑
  - with
    - damage to nail S61.15- ☑

- **Bite**(s) — *continued*
  - thumb — *continued*
    - superficial NEC S60.37- ☑
      - insect S60.36- ☑
  - thyroid S11.15 ☑
    - superficial NEC S10.87 ☑
      - insect S10.86 ☑
  - toe(s) S91.15- ☑
    - with
      - damage to nail S91.25- ☑
    - great S91.15- ☑
      - with
        - damage to nail S91.25- ☑
    - lesser S91.15- ☑
      - with
        - damage to nail S91.25- ☑
    - superficial NEC S90.47- ☑
      - great S90.47- ☑
      - insect S90.46- ☑
        - great S90.46- ☑
  - tongue S01.552 ☑
  - trachea S11.025 ☑
    - superficial NEC S10.17 ☑
      - insect S10.16 ☑
  - tunica vaginalis — *see* Bite, testis
  - tympanum, tympanic membrane — *see* Bite, ear
  - umbilical region S31.155 ☑
  - uvula — *see* Bite, oral cavity
  - vagina — *see* Bite, vulva
  - venomous — *see* Venom
  - vocal cords S11.035 ☑
    - superficial NEC S10.17 ☑
      - insect S10.16 ☑
  - vulva S31.45 ☑
    - superficial NEC S30.874 ☑
      - insect S30.864 ☑
  - wrist S61.55- ☑
    - superficial NEC S60.87- ☑
      - insect S60.86- ☑
- **Biting, cheek or lip** K13.1
- **Biventricular failure** (heart) I50.82
- **Bjorck** (-Thorson) **syndrome** (malignant carcinoid) E34.0
- **Black**
  - death A20.9
  - eye S00.1- ☑
  - hairy tongue K14.3
  - heel (foot) S90.3- ☑
  - lung (disease) J60
  - palm (hand) S60.22- ☑
- **Blackfan-Diamond anemia or syndrome** (congenital hypoplastic anemia) D61.01
- **Blackhead** L70.0
- **Blackout** R55
- **Bladder** — *see* condition
- **Blast** (air) (hydraulic) (immersion) (underwater)
  - blindness S05.8X- ☑
  - injury
    - abdomen or thorax — *see* Injury, by site
    - ear (acoustic nerve trauma) — *see* Injury, nerve, acoustic, specified type NEC
    - syndrome NEC T70.8 ☑
- **Blastoma** — *see* Neoplasm, malignant, by site
  - pulmonary — *see* Neoplasm, lung, malignant
- **Blastomycosis, blastomycotic** B40.9
  - Brazilian — *see* Paracoccidioidomycosis
  - cutaneous B40.3
  - disseminated B40.7
  - European — *see* Cryptococcosis
  - generalized B40.7
  - keloidal B48.0
  - North American B40.9
  - primary pulmonary B40.0
  - pulmonary B40.2
    - acute B40.0
    - chronic B40.1
  - skin B40.3
  - South American — *see* Paracoccidioidomycosis
  - specified NEC B40.89
- **Bleb**(s) R23.8
  - emphysematous (lung) (solitary) J43.9
  - endophthalmitis H59.43
  - filtering (vitreous), after glaucoma surgery Z98.83
  - inflammed (infected), postprocedural H59.40
    - stage 1 H59.41
    - stage 2 H59.42
    - stage 3 H59.43
  - lung (ruptured) J43.9
- **Bleb**(s) — *continued*
  - lung — *continued*
    - congenital — *see* Atelectasis
    - newborn P25.8
  - subpleural (emphysematous) J43.9
- **Blebitis, postprocedural** H59.40
  - stage 1 H59.41
  - stage 2 H59.42
  - stage 3 H59.43
- **Bleeder** (familial) (hereditary) — *see* Hemophilia
- **Bleeding** — *see also* Hemorrhage
  - anal K62.5
  - anovulatory N97.0
  - atonic, following delivery O72.1
  - capillary I78.8
    - puerperal O72.2
  - contact (postcoital) N93.0
  - due to uterine subinvolution N85.3
  - ear — *see* Otorrhagia
  - excessive, associated with menopausal onset N92.4
  - familial — *see* Defect, coagulation
  - following intercourse N93.0
  - gastrointestinal K92.2
  - hemorrhoids — *see* Hemorrhoids
  - intermenstrual (regular) N92.3
    - irregular N92.1
  - intraoperative — *see* Complication, intraoperative, hemorrhage
  - irregular N92.6
  - menopausal N92.4
  - newborn, intraventricular — *see* Newborn, affected by, hemorrhage, intraventricular
  - nipple N64.59
  - nose R04.0
  - ovulation N92.3
  - perimenopausal N92.4
  - postclimacteric N95.0
  - postcoital N93.0
  - postmenopausal N95.0
  - postoperative — *see* Complication, postprocedural, hemorrhage
  - preclimacteric N92.4
  - pre-pubertal vaginal N93.1
  - puberty (excessive, with onset of menstrual periods) N92.2
  - rectum, rectal K62.5
    - newborn P54.2
  - tendencies — *see* Defect, coagulation
  - throat R04.1
  - tooth socket (post-extraction) K91.840
  - umbilical stump P51.9
  - uterus, uterine NEC N93.9
    - climacteric N92.4
    - dysfunctional or functional N93.8
    - menopausal N92.4
    - preclimacteric or premenopausal N92.4
    - unrelated to menstrual cycle N93.9
  - vagina, vaginal (abnormal) N93.9
    - dysfunctional or functional N93.8
    - newborn P54.6
    - pre-pubertal N93.1
  - vicarious N94.89
- **Blennorrhagia, blennorrhagic** — *see* Gonorrhea
- **Blennorrhea** (acute) (chronic) — *see also* Gonorrhea
  - inclusion (neonatal) (newborn) P39.1
  - lower genitourinary tract (gonococcal) A54.00
  - neonatorum (gonococcal ophthalmia) A54.31
- **Blepharelosis** — *see* Entropion
- **Blepharitis** (angularis) (ciliaris) (eyelid) (marginal) (nonulcerative) H01.009
  - herpes zoster B02.39
  - left H01.006
    - lower H01.005
    - upper H01.004
    - upper and lower H01.00B
  - right H01.003
    - lower H01.002
    - upper H01.001
    - upper and lower H01.00A
  - squamous H01.029
    - left H01.026
      - lower H01.025
      - upper H01.024
      - upper and lower H01.02B
    - right H01.023
      - lower H01.022
      - upper H01.021
      - upper and lower H01.02A
- **Blepharitis** — *continued*
  - ulcerative H01.019
    - left H01.016
      - lower H01.015
      - upper H01.014
      - upper and lower H01.01B
    - right H01.013
      - lower H01.012
      - upper H01.011
      - upper and lower H01.01A
- **Blepharochalasis** H02.30
  - congenital Q10.0
  - left H02.36
    - lower H02.35
    - upper H02.34
  - right H02.33
    - lower H02.32
    - upper H02.31
- **Blepharoclonus** H02.59
- **Blepharoconjunctivitis** H10.50- ☑
  - angular H10.52- ☑
  - contact H10.53- ☑
  - ligneous H10.51- ☑
- **Blepharophimosis** (eyelid) H02.529
  - congenital Q10.3
  - left H02.526
    - lower H02.525
    - upper H02.524
  - right H02.523
    - lower H02.522
    - upper H02.521
- **Blepharoptosis** H02.40- ☑
  - congenital Q10.0
  - mechanical H02.41- ☑
  - myogenic H02.42- ☑
  - neurogenic H02.43- ☑
  - paralytic H02.43- ☑
- **Blepharopyorrhea, gonococcal** A54.39
- **Blepharospasm** G24.5
  - drug induced G24.01
- **Blighted ovum** O02.0
- **Blind** — *see also* Blindness
  - bronchus (congenital) Q32.4
  - loop syndrome K90.2
    - congenital Q43.8
  - sac, fallopian tube (congenital) Q50.6
  - spot, enlarged — *see* Defect, visual field, localized, scotoma, blind spot area
  - tract or tube, congenital NEC — *see* Atresia, by site
- **Blindness** (acquired) (congenital) (both eyes) H54.0X- ☑
  - blast S05.8X- ☑
  - color — *see* Deficiency, color vision
  - concussion S05.8X- ☑
  - cortical H47.619
    - left brain H47.612
    - right brain H47.611
  - day H53.11
  - due to injury (current episode) S05.9- ☑
    - sequelae — *code to* injury with seventh character S
  - eclipse (total) — *see* Retinopathy, solar
  - emotional (hysterical) F44.6
  - face H53.16
  - hysterical F44.6
  - legal (both eyes) (USA definition) H54.8
  - mind R48.8
  - night H53.60
    - abnormal dark adaptation curve H53.61
    - acquired H53.62
    - congenital H53.63
    - specified type NEC H53.69
    - vitamin A deficiency E50.5
  - one eye (other eye normal) H54.40
    - left (normal vision on right) H54.42- ☑
      - low vision on right H54.12- ☑
    - low vision, other eye H54.10
    - right (normal vision on left) H54.41- ☑
      - low vision on left H54.11- ☑
  - psychic R48.8
  - river B73.01
  - snow — *see* Photokeratitis
  - sun, solar — *see* Retinopathy, solar
  - transient — *see* Disturbance, vision, subjective, loss, transient
  - traumatic (current episode) S05.9- ☑
  - word (developmental) F81.0
    - acquired R48.0
    - secondary to organic lesion R48.0

- **Blister** (nonthermal)
  - abdominal wall S3Ø.821 ☑
  - alveolar process SØØ.522 ☑
  - ankle S9Ø.52- ☑
  - antecubital space — *see* Blister, elbow
  - anus S3Ø.827 ☑
  - arm (upper) S4Ø.82- ☑
  - auditory canal — *see* Blister, ear
  - auricle — *see* Blister, ear
  - axilla — *see* Blister, arm
  - back, lower S3Ø.82Ø ☑
  - beetle dermatitis L24.89
  - breast S2Ø.12- ☑
  - brow SØØ.82 ☑
  - calf — *see* Blister, leg
  - canthus — *see* Blister, eyelid
  - cheek SØØ.82 ☑
    - internal SØØ.522 ☑
  - chest wall — *see* Blister, thorax
  - chin SØØ.82 ☑
  - costal region — *see* Blister, thorax
  - digit(s)
    - foot — *see* Blister, toe
    - hand — *see* Blister, finger
  - due to burn — *see* Burn, by site, second degree
  - ear SØØ.42- ☑
  - elbow S5Ø.32- ☑
  - epiglottis S1Ø.12 ☑
  - esophagus, cervical S1Ø.12 ☑
  - eyebrow — *see* Blister, eyelid
  - eyelid SØØ.22- ☑
  - face SØØ.82 ☑
  - fever BØØ.1
  - finger(s) S6Ø.429 ☑
    - index S6Ø.42- ☑
    - little S6Ø.42- ☑
    - middle S6Ø.42- ☑
    - ring S6Ø.42- ☑
  - foot (except toe(s) alone) S9Ø.82- ☑
    - toe — *see* Blister, toe
  - forearm S5Ø.82- ☑
    - elbow only — *see* Blister, elbow
  - forehead SØØ.82 ☑
  - fracture — *omit code*
  - genital organ
    - female S3Ø.826 ☑
    - male S3Ø.825 ☑
  - gum SØØ.522 ☑
  - hand S6Ø.52- ☑
  - head SØØ.92 ☑
    - ear — *see* Blister, ear
    - eyelid — *see* Blister, eyelid
    - lip SØØ.521 ☑
    - nose SØØ.32 ☑
    - oral cavity SØØ.522 ☑
    - scalp SØØ.Ø2 ☑
    - specified site NEC SØØ.82 ☑
  - heel — *see* Blister, foot
  - hip S7Ø.22- ☑
  - interscapular region S2Ø.429 ☑
  - jaw SØØ.82 ☑
  - knee S8Ø.22- ☑
  - larynx S1Ø.12 ☑
  - leg (lower) S8Ø.82- ☑
    - knee — *see* Blister, knee
    - upper — *see* Blister, thigh
  - lip SØØ.521 ☑
  - malar region SØØ.82 ☑
  - mammary — *see* Blister, breast
  - mastoid region SØØ.82 ☑
  - mouth SØØ.522 ☑
  - multiple, skin, nontraumatic R23.8
  - nail
    - finger — *see* Blister, finger
    - toe — *see* Blister, toe
  - nasal SØØ.32 ☑
  - neck S1Ø.92 ☑
    - specified site NEC S1Ø.82 ☑
    - throat S1Ø.12 ☑
  - nose SØØ.32 ☑
  - occipital region SØØ.Ø2 ☑
  - oral cavity SØØ.522 ☑
  - orbital region — *see* Blister, eyelid
  - palate SØØ.522 ☑
  - palm — *see* Blister, hand
  - parietal region SØØ.Ø2 ☑

- **Blister** — *continued*
  - pelvis S3Ø.82Ø ☑
  - penis S3Ø.822 ☑
  - periocular area — *see* Blister, eyelid
  - phalanges
    - finger — *see* Blister, finger
    - toe — *see* Blister, toe
  - pharynx S1Ø.12 ☑
  - pinna — *see* Blister, ear
  - popliteal space — *see* Blister, knee
  - scalp SØØ.Ø2 ☑
  - scapular region — *see* Blister, shoulder
  - scrotum S3Ø.823 ☑
  - shin — *see* Blister, leg
  - shoulder S4Ø.22- ☑
  - sternal region S2Ø.329 ☑
  - submaxillary region SØØ.82 ☑
  - submental region SØØ.82 ☑
  - subungual
    - finger(s) — *see* Blister, finger
    - toe(s) — *see* Blister, toe
  - supraclavicular fossa S1Ø.82 ☑
  - supraorbital SØØ.82 ☑
  - temple SØØ.82 ☑
  - temporal region SØØ.82 ☑
  - testis S3Ø.823 ☑
  - thermal — *see* Burn, by site, second degree
  - thigh S7Ø.32- ☑
  - thorax, thoracic (wall) S2Ø.92 ☑
    - back S2Ø.42- ☑
    - front S2Ø.32- ☑
  - throat S1Ø.12 ☑
  - thumb S6Ø.32- ☑
  - toe(s) S9Ø.42- ☑
    - great S9Ø.42- ☑
  - tongue SØØ.522 ☑
  - trachea S1Ø.12 ☑
  - tympanum, tympanic membrane — *see* Blister, ear
  - upper arm — *see* Blister, arm (upper)
  - uvula SØØ.522 ☑
  - vagina S3Ø.824 ☑
  - vocal cords S1Ø.12 ☑
  - vulva S3Ø.824 ☑
  - wrist S6Ø.82- ☑
- **Bloating** R14.Ø
- **Bloch-Sulzberger disease or syndrome** Q82.3
- **Block, blocked**
  - alveolocapillary J84.1Ø
  - arborization (heart) I45.5
  - arrhythmic I45.9
  - atrioventricular (incomplete) (partial) I44.3Ø
    - with atrioventricular dissociation I44.2
    - complete I44.2
      - congenital Q24.6
    - congenital Q24.6
    - first degree I44.Ø
    - second degree (types I and II) I44.1
    - specified NEC I44.39
    - third degree I44.2
    - types I and II I44.1
  - auriculoventricular — *see* Block, atrioventricular
  - bifascicular (cardiac) I45.2
  - bundle-branch (complete) (false) (incomplete) I45.4
    - bilateral I45.2
    - left I44.7
      - with right bundle branch block I45.2
      - hemiblock I44.6Ø
        - anterior I44.4
        - posterior I44.5
      - incomplete I44.7
        - with right bundle branch block I45.2
    - right I45.1Ø
      - with
        - left bundle branch block I45.2
        - left fascicular block I45.2
      - specified NEC I45.19
    - Wilson's type I45.19
  - cardiac I45.9
  - conduction I45.9
    - complete I44.2
  - fascicular (left) I44.6Ø
    - anterior I44.4
    - posterior I44.5
    - right I45.Ø
    - specified NEC I44.69
  - foramen Magendie (acquired) G91.1
    - congenital QØ3.1

- **Block, blocked** — *continued*
  - foramen Magendie — *continued*
    - congenital — *continued*
      - with spina bifida — *see* Spina bifida, by site, with hydrocephalus
  - heart I45.9
    - bundle branch I45.4
      - bilateral I45.2
    - complete (atrioventricular) I44.2
    - congenital Q24.6
    - first degree (atrioventricular) I44.Ø
    - second degree (atrioventricular) I44.1
    - specified type NEC I45.5
    - third degree (atrioventricular) I44.2
  - hepatic vein I82.Ø
  - intraventricular (nonspecific) I45.4
    - bundle branch
      - bilateral I45.2
  - kidney N28.9
    - postcystoscopic or postprocedural N99.Ø
  - Mobitz (types I and II) I44.1
  - myocardial — *see* Block, heart
  - nodal I45.5
  - organ or site, congenital NEC — *see* Atresia, by site
  - portal (vein) I81
  - second degree (types I and II) I44.1
  - sinoatrial I45.5
  - sinoauricular I45.5
  - third degree I44.2
  - trifascicular I45.3
  - tubal N97.1
  - vein NOS I82.9Ø
  - Wenckebach (types I and II) I44.1
- **Blockage** — *see* Obstruction
- **Blocq's disease** F44.4
- **Blood**
  - constituents, abnormal R78.9
  - disease D75.9
  - donor — *see* Donor, blood
  - dyscrasia D75.9
    - with
      - abortion — *see* Abortion, by type, complicated by, hemorrhage
      - ectopic pregnancy OØ8.1
      - molar pregnancy OØ8.1
    - following ectopic or molar pregnancy OØ8.1
    - newborn P61.9
    - puerperal, postpartum O72.3
  - flukes NEC — *see* Schistosomiasis
  - in
    - feces K92.1
      - occult R19.5
    - urine — *see* Hematuria
  - mole OØ2.Ø
  - occult in feces R19.5
  - pressure
    - decreased, due to shock following injury T79.4 ☑
    - examination only ZØ1.3Ø
    - fluctuating I99.8
    - high — *see* Hypertension
      - borderline RØ3.Ø
      - incidental reading, without diagnosis of hypertension RØ3.Ø
    - low — *see also* Hypotension
      - incidental reading, without diagnosis of hypotension RØ3.1
  - spitting — *see* Hemoptysis
  - staining cornea — *see* Pigmentation, cornea, stromal
  - transfusion
    - reaction or complication — *see* Complications, transfusion
  - type
    - A (Rh positive) Z67.1Ø
      - Rh negative Z67.11
    - AB (Rh positive) Z67.3Ø
      - Rh negative Z67.31
    - B (Rh positive) Z67.2Ø
      - Rh negative Z67.21
    - O (Rh positive) Z67.4Ø
      - Rh negative Z67.41
    - Rh (positive) Z67.9Ø
      - negative Z67.91
  - vessel rupture — *see* Hemorrhage
  - vomiting — *see* Hematemesis
- **Blood-forming organs, disease** D75.9
- **Bloodgood's disease** — *see* Mastopathy, cystic
- **Bloom** (-Machacek)(-Torre) **syndrome** Q82.8
- **Blount disease or osteochondrosis** M92.51- ☑

Blue
- baby Q24.9
- diaper syndrome E72.Ø9
- dome cyst (breast) — *see* Cyst, breast
- dot cataract Q12.Ø
- nevus D22.9
- sclera Q13.5
  - with fragility of bone and deafness Q78.Ø
- toe syndrome I75.Ø2- ☑

Blueness — *see* Cyanosis

Blues, postpartal O9Ø.6
- baby O9Ø.6

Blurring, visual H53.8

Blushing (abnormal) (excessive) R23.2

BMI — *see* Body, mass index

Boarder, hospital NEC Z76.4
- accompanying sick person Z76.3
- healthy infant or child Z76.2
  - foundling Z76.1

Bockhart's impetigo LØ1.Ø2

Bodechtel-Guttman disease (subacute sclerosing panencephalitis) A81.1

Boder-Sedgwick syndrome (ataxia-telangiectasia) G11.3

Body, bodies
- Aschoff's — *see* Myocarditis, rheumatic
- asteroid, vitreous — *see* Deposit, crystalline
- cytoid (retina) — *see* Occlusion, artery, retina
- drusen (degenerative) (macula) (retinal) — *see also* Degeneration, macula, drusen
  - optic disc — *see* Drusen, optic disc
- foreign — *see* Foreign body
- loose
  - joint, except knee — *see* Loose, body, joint
    - knee M23.4- ☑
  - sheath, tendon — *see* Disorder, tendon, specified type NEC
- mass index (BMI)
  - adult
    - 19.9 or less Z68.1
    - 2Ø.Ø-2Ø.9 Z68.2Ø
    - 21.Ø-21.9 Z68.21
    - 22.Ø-22.9 Z68.22
    - 23.Ø-23.9 Z68.23
    - 24.Ø-24.9 Z68.24
    - 25.Ø-25.9 Z68.25
    - 26.Ø-26.9 Z68.26
    - 27.Ø-27.9 Z68.27
    - 28.Ø-28.9 Z68.28
    - 29.Ø-29.9 Z68.29
    - 3Ø.Ø-3Ø.9 Z68.3Ø
    - 31.Ø-31.9 Z68.31
    - 32.Ø-32.9 Z68.32
    - 33.Ø-33.9 Z68.33
    - 34.Ø-34.9 Z68.34
    - 35.Ø-35.9 Z68.35
    - 36.Ø-36.9 Z68.36
    - 37.Ø-37.9 Z68.37
    - 38.Ø-38.9 Z68.38
    - 39.Ø-39.9 Z68.39
    - 4Ø.Ø-44.9 Z68.41
    - 45.Ø-49.9 Z68.42
    - 5Ø.Ø-59.9 Z68.43
    - 6Ø.Ø-69.9 Z68.44
    - 7Ø and over Z68.45
  - pediatric
    - 5th percentile to less than 85th percentile for age Z68.52
    - 85th percentile to less than 95th percentile for age Z68.53
    - greater than or equal to ninety-fifth percentile for age Z68.54
    - less than fifth percentile for age Z68.51
- Mooser's A75.2
- rice — *see also* Loose, body, joint
  - knee M23.4- ☑
- rocking F98.4

Boeck's
- disease or sarcoid — *see* Sarcoidosis
- lupoid (miliary) D86.3

Boerhaave's syndrome (spontaneous esophageal rupture) K22.3

Boggy
- cervix N88.8
- uterus N85.8

Boil — *see also* Furuncle, by site
- Aleppo B55.1
- Baghdad B55.1
- Delhi B55.1

Boil — *continued*
- lacrimal
  - gland — *see* Dacryoadenitis
  - passages (duct) (sac) — *see* Inflammation, lacrimal, passages, acute
- Natal B55.1
- orbit, orbital — *see* Abscess, orbit
- tropical B55.1

Bold hives — *see* Urticaria

Bombé, iris — *see* Membrane, pupillary

Bone — *see* condition

Bonnevie-Ullrich syndrome — *see also* Turner's syndrome Q87.19

Bonnier's syndrome H81.8 ☑

Bonvale dam fever T73.3 ☑

Bony block of joint — *see* Ankylosis

BOOP (bronchiolitis obliterans organized pneumonia) J84.89

Borderline
- diabetes mellitus R73.Ø3
- hypertension RØ3.Ø
- osteopenia M85.8- ☑
- pelvis, with obstruction during labor O65.1
- personality F6Ø.3

Borna disease A83.9

Bornholm disease B33.Ø

Boston exanthem A88.Ø

Botalli, ductus (patent) (persistent) Q25.Ø

Bothriocephalus latus infestation B7Ø.Ø

Botulism (foodborne intoxication) AØ5.1
- infant A48.51
- non-foodborne A48.52
- wound A48.52

Bouba — *see* Yaws

Bouchard's nodes (with arthropathy) M15.2

Bouffée délirante F23

Bouillaud's disease or syndrome (rheumatic heart disease) IØ1.9

Bourneville's disease Q85.1

Boutonniere deformity (finger) — *see* Deformity, finger, boutonniere

Bouveret (-Hoffmann) **syndrome** (paroxysmal tachycardia) I47.9

Bovine heart — *see* Hypertrophy, cardiac

Bowel — *see* condition

Bowen's
- dermatosis (precancerous) — *see* Neoplasm, skin, in situ
- disease — *see* Neoplasm, skin, in situ
- epithelioma — *see* Neoplasm, skin, in situ
- type
  - epidermoid carcinoma-in-situ — *see* Neoplasm, skin, in situ
  - intraepidermal squamous cell carcinoma — *see* Neoplasm, skin, in situ

Bowing
- femur — *see also* Deformity, limb, specified type NEC, thigh
  - congenital Q68.3
- fibula — *see also* Deformity, limb, specified type NEC, lower leg
  - congenital Q68.4
- forearm — *see* Deformity, limb, specified type NEC, forearm
- leg(s), long bones, congenital Q68.5
- radius — *see* Deformity, limb, specified type NEC, forearm
- tibia — *see also* Deformity, limb, specified type NEC, lower leg
  - congenital Q68.4

Bowleg(s) (acquired) M21.16- ☑
- congenital Q68.5
- rachitic E64.3

Boyd's dysentery AØ3.2

Brachial — *see* condition

Brachycardia RØØ.1

Brachycephaly, non-deformational Q75.Ø22

Bradley's disease AØ8.19

Bradyarrhythmia, cardiac I49.8

Bradycardia (sinoatrial) (sinus) (vagal) RØØ.1
- neonatal P29.12
- reflex G9Ø.Ø9
- tachycardia syndrome I49.5

Bradykinesia R25.8

Bradypnea RØ6.89

Bradytachycardia I49.5

Brailsford's disease or osteochondrosis — *see* Osteochondrosis, juvenile, radius

Brain — *see also* condition
- death G93.82
- syndrome — *see* Syndrome, brain

Branched-chain amino-acid disorder E71.2

Branchial — *see* condition
- cartilage, congenital Q18.2

Branchiogenic remnant (in neck) Q18.Ø

Brandt's syndrome (acrodermatitis enteropathica) E83.2

Brash (water) R12

Bravais-jacksonian epilepsy — *see* Epilepsy, localization-related, symptomatic, with simple partial seizures

Braxton Hicks contractions — *see* False, labor

Brazilian leishmaniasis B55.2

BRBPR K62.5

Break, retina (without detachment) H33.3Ø- ☑
- with retinal detachment — *see* Detachment, retina
- horseshoe tear H33.31- ☑
- multiple H33.33- ☑
- round hole H33.32- ☑

Breakdown
- device, graft or implant — *see also* Complications, by site and type, mechanical T85.618 ☑
  - arterial graft NEC — *see* Complication, cardiovascular device, mechanical, vascular
  - breast (implant) T85.41 ☑
  - catheter NEC T85.618 ☑
    - cystostomy T83.Ø1Ø ☑
    - dialysis (renal) T82.41 ☑
      - intraperitoneal T85.611 ☑
    - Hopkins T83.Ø18 ☑
    - ileostomy T83.Ø18 ☑
    - infusion NEC T82.514 ☑
      - cranial T85.61Ø- ☑
      - epidural T85.61Ø ☑
      - intrathecal T85.61Ø ☑
      - spinal T85.61Ø ☑
      - subarachnoid T85.61Ø ☑
      - subdural T85.61Ø ☑
    - nephrostomy T83.Ø12 ☑
    - urethral indwelling T83.Ø11 ☑
    - urinary NEC T83.Ø18 ☑
    - urostomy T83.Ø18 ☑
  - electronic (electrode) (pulse generator) (stimulator)
    - bone T84.31Ø ☑
    - cardiac T82.119 ☑
      - electrode T82.11Ø ☑
      - pulse generator T82.111 ☑
      - specified type NEC T82.118 ☑
    - nervous system — *see* Complication, prosthetic device, mechanical, electronic nervous system stimulator
    - urinary — *see* Complication, genitourinary, device, urinary, mechanical
  - fixation, internal (orthopedic) NEC — *see* Complication, fixation device, mechanical
  - gastrointestinal — *see* Complications, prosthetic device, mechanical, gastrointestinal device
  - genital NEC T83.418 ☑
    - intrauterine contraceptive device T83.31 ☑
    - penile prosthesis (cylinder) (implanted) (pump) (resevoir) T83.41Ø ☑
    - testicular prosthesis T83.411 ☑
  - heart NEC — *see* Complication, cardiovascular device, mechanical
  - intrathecal infusion pump T85.615 ☑
  - joint prosthesis — *see* Complications, joint prosthesis, internal, mechanical, by site
  - nervous system, specified device NEC T85.615 ☑
  - ocular NEC — *see* Complications, prosthetic device, mechanical, ocular device
  - orthopedic NEC — *see* Complication, orthopedic, device, mechanical
  - specified NEC T85.618 ☑
  - subcutaneous device pocket
    - nervous system prosthetic device, implant, or graft T85.89Ø ☑
    - other internal prosthetic device, implant, or graft T85.898 ☑
  - sutures, permanent T85.612 ☑
    - used in bone repair — *see* Complications, fixation device, internal (orthopedic), mechanical
  - urinary NEC T83.118 ☑
    - graft T83.21 ☑

Bronchitis — *continued*
- suppurative (chronic) J41.1
  - acute or subacute — *see* Bronchitis, acute
- tuberculous A15.5
- under I5 years of age — *see* Bronchitis, acute
  - chronic — *see* Bronchitis, chronic
- viral NEC, acute or subacute — *see also* Bronchitis, acute J2Ø.8

Bronchoalveolitis J18.Ø
Bronchoaspergillosis B44.1
Bronchocele meaning goiter EØ4.Ø
Broncholithiasis J98.Ø9
- tuberculous NEC A15.5

Bronchomalacia J98.Ø9
- congenital Q32.2

Bronchomycosis NOS B49 *[J99]*
- candidal B37.1

Bronchopleuropneumonia — *see* Pneumonia, broncho
Bronchopneumonia — *see* Pneumonia, broncho
Bronchopneumonitis — *see* Pneumonia, broncho
Bronchopulmonary — *see* condition
Bronchopulmonitis — *see* Pneumonia, broncho
Bronchorrhagia (see Hemoptysis)
Bronchorrhea J98.Ø9
- acute J2Ø.9
- chronic (infective) (purulent) J42

Bronchospasm (acute) J98.Ø1
- with
  - bronchiolitis, acute J21.9
  - bronchitis, acute (conditions in J2Ø) — *see* Bronchitis, acute
- due to external agent — *see* condition, respiratory, acute, due to
- exercise induced J45.99Ø

Bronchospirochetosis A69.8
- Castellani A69.8

Bronchostenosis J98.Ø9
Bronchus — *see* condition
Brontophobia F4Ø.22Ø
Bronze baby syndrome P83.88
Brooke's tumor — *see* Neoplasm, skin, benign
Brown enamel of teeth (hereditary) KØØ.5
Brown's sheath syndrome H5Ø.61- ☑
Brown-Sequard disease, paralysis or syndrome G83.81
Bruce sepsis A23.Ø
Brucellosis (infection) A23.9
- abortus A23.1
- canis A23.3
- dermatitis A23.9
- melitensis A23.Ø
- mixed A23.8
- sepsis A23.9
  - melitensis A23.Ø
  - specified NEC A23.8
- suis A23.2

Bruck-de Lange disease Q87.19
Bruck's disease — *see* Deformity, limb
BRUE (brief resolved unexplained event) R68.13
Brugsch's syndrome Q82.8
Bruise (skin surface intact) — *see also* Contusion
- with
  - open wound — *see* Wound, open
- internal organ — *see* Injury, by site
- newborn P54.5
- scalp, due to birth injury, newborn P12.3
- umbilical cord O69.5 ☑

Bruit (arterial) RØ9.89
- cardiac RØ1.1

Brush burn — *see* Abrasion, by site
Bruton's X-linked agammaglobulinemia D8Ø.Ø
Bruxism
- psychogenic F45.8
- sleep related G47.63

Bubbly lung syndrome P27.Ø
Bubo I88.8
- blennorrhagic (gonococcal) A54.89
- chancroidal A57
- climatic A55
- due to Haemophilus ducreyi A57
- gonococcal A54.89
- indolent (nonspecific) I88.8
- inguinal (nonspecific) I88.8
  - chancroidal A57
  - climatic A55
  - due to H. ducreyi A57
  - infective I88.8

Bubo — *continued*
- scrofulous (tuberculous) A18.2
- soft chancre A57
- suppurating — *see* Lymphadenitis, acute
- syphilitic (primary) A51.Ø
  - congenital A5Ø.Ø7
- tropical A55
- virulent (chancroidal) A57

Bubonic plague A2Ø.Ø
Bubonocele — *see* Hernia, inguinal
Buccal — *see* condition
Buchanan's disease or osteochondrosis M91.Ø
Buchem's syndrome (hyperostosis corticalis) M85.2
Bucket-handle fracture or tear (semilunar cartilage) — *see* Tear, meniscus
Budd-Chiari syndrome (hepatic vein thrombosis) I82.Ø
Budgerigar fancier's disease or lung J67.2
Buds
- breast E3Ø.1
  - in newborn P96.89

Buerger's disease (thromboangiitis obliterans) I73.1
Bulbar — *see* condition
Bulbus cordis (left ventricle) (persistent) Q21.8
Bulimia (nervosa) F5Ø.2
- atypical F5Ø.9
- normal weight F5Ø.9

Bulky
- stools R19.5
- uterus N85.2

Bulla (e) R23.8
- lung (emphysematous) (solitary) J43.9
  - newborn P25.8

Bullet wound — *see also* Puncture
- fracture — *code as* Fracture, by site
- internal organ — *see* Injury, by site

Bundle
- branch block (complete) (false) (incomplete) — *see* Block, bundle-branch
- of His — *see* condition

Bunion M21.61- ☑
- tailor's M21.62- ☑

Bunionette M21.62- ☑
Buphthalmia, buphthalmos (congenital) Q15.Ø
Burdwan fever B55.Ø
Burger-Grutz disease or syndrome E78.3
Buried
- penis (congenital) Q55.64
  - acquired N48.83
- roots KØ8.3

Burke's syndrome K86.89
Burkholderia
- cepacia A49.8
- mallei A24.Ø
- pseudomallei — *see* Melioidosis

Burkitt
- cell leukemia C91.Ø- ☑
- lymphoma (malignant) C83.7- ☑
  - small noncleaved, diffuse C83.7- ☑
  - spleen C83.77
  - undifferentiated C83.7- ☑
- tumor C83.7- ☑
- type
  - acute lymphoblastic leukemia C91.Ø- ☑
  - undifferentiated C83.7- ☑

Burn (electricity) (flame) (hot gas, liquid or hot object) (radiation) (steam) (thermal) T3Ø.Ø
- abdomen, abdominal (muscle) (wall) T21.Ø2 ☑
  - first degree T21.12 ☑
  - second degree T21.22 ☑
  - third degree T21.32 ☑
- above elbow T22.Ø39 ☑
  - first degree T22.139 ☑
  - left T22.Ø32 ☑
    - first degree T22.132 ☑
    - second degree T22.232 ☑
    - third degree T22.332 ☑
  - right T22.Ø31 ☑
    - first degree T22.131 ☑
    - second degree T22.231 ☑
    - third degree T22.331 ☑
  - second degree T22.239 ☑
  - third degree T22.339 ☑
- acid (caustic) (external) (internal) — *see* Corrosion, by site
- alimentary tract NEC T28.2 ☑
  - esophagus T28.1 ☑
  - mouth T28.Ø ☑

Burn — *continued*
- alimentary tract — *continued*
  - pharynx T28.Ø ☑
- alkaline (caustic) (external) (internal) — *see* Corrosion, by site
- ankle T25.Ø19 ☑
  - first degree T25.119 ☑
  - left T25.Ø12 ☑
    - first degree T25.112 ☑
    - second degree T25.212 ☑
    - third degree T25.312 ☑
  - multiple with foot — *see* Burn, lower, limb, multiple, ankle and foot
  - right T25.Ø11 ☑
    - first degree T25.111 ☑
    - second degree T25.211 ☑
    - third degree T25.311 ☑
  - second degree T25.219 ☑
  - third degree T25.319 ☑
- anus — *see* Burn, buttock
- arm (lower) (upper) — *see* Burn, upper, limb
- axilla T22.Ø49 ☑
  - first degree T22.149 ☑
  - left T22.Ø42 ☑
    - first degree T22.142 ☑
    - second degree T22.242 ☑
    - third degree T22.342 ☑
  - right T22.Ø41 ☑
    - first degree T22.141 ☑
    - second degree T22.241 ☑
    - third degree T22.341 ☑
  - second degree T22.249 ☑
  - third degree T22.349 ☑
- back (lower) T21.Ø4 ☑
  - first degree T21.14 ☑
  - second degree T21.24 ☑
  - third degree T21.34 ☑
  - upper T21.Ø3 ☑
    - first degree T21.13 ☑
    - second degree T21.23 ☑
    - third degree T21.33 ☑
- blisters — *code as* Burn, second degree, by site
- breast(s) — *see* Burn, chest wall
- buttock(s) T21.Ø5 ☑
  - first degree T21.15 ☑
  - second degree T21.25 ☑
  - third degree T21.35 ☑
- calf T24.Ø39 ☑
  - first degree T24.139 ☑
  - left T24.Ø32 ☑
    - first degree T24.132 ☑
    - second degree T24.232 ☑
    - third degree T24.332 ☑
  - right T24.Ø31 ☑
    - first degree T24.131 ☑
    - second degree T24.231 ☑
    - third degree T24.331 ☑
  - second degree T24.239 ☑
  - third degree T24.339 ☑
- canthus (eye) — *see* Burn, eyelid
- caustic acid or alkaline — *see* Corrosion, by site
- cervix T28.3 ☑
- cheek T2Ø.Ø6 ☑
  - first degree T2Ø.16 ☑
  - second degree T2Ø.26 ☑
  - third degree T2Ø.36 ☑
- chemical (acids) (alkalines) (caustics) (external) (internal) — *see* Corrosion, by site
- chest wall T21.Ø1 ☑
  - first degree T21.11 ☑
  - second degree T21.21 ☑
  - third degree T21.31 ☑
- chin T2Ø.Ø3 ☑
  - first degree T2Ø.13 ☑
  - second degree T2Ø.23 ☑
  - third degree T2Ø.33 ☑
- colon T28.2 ☑
- conjunctiva (and cornea) — *see* Burn, cornea
- cornea (and conjunctiva) T26.1- ☑
  - chemical — *see* Corrosion, cornea
- corrosion (external) (internal) — *see* Corrosion, by site
- deep necrosis of underlying tissue — *code as* Burn, third degree, by site
- dorsum of hand T23.Ø69 ☑
  - first degree T23.169 ☑
  - left T23.Ø62 ☑

- **Burn** — *continued*
  - dorsum of hand — *continued*
    - left — *continued*
      - first degree T23.162 ☑
      - second degree T23.262 ☑
      - third degree T23.362 ☑
    - right T23.061 ☑
      - first degree T23.161 ☑
      - second degree T23.261 ☑
      - third degree T23.361 ☑
    - second degree T23.269 ☑
    - third degree T23.369 ☑
  - due to ingested chemical agent — *see* Corrosion, by site
  - ear (auricle) (external) (canal) T20.01 ☑
    - first degree T20.11 ☑
    - second degree T20.21 ☑
    - third degree T20.31 ☑
  - elbow T22.029 ☑
    - first degree T22.129 ☑
    - left T22.022 ☑
      - first degree T22.122 ☑
      - second degree T22.222 ☑
      - third degree T22.322 ☑
    - right T22.021 ☑
      - first degree T22.121 ☑
      - second degree T22.221 ☑
      - third degree T22.321 ☑
    - second degree T22.229 ☑
    - third degree T22.329 ☑
  - epidermal loss — *code as* Burn, second degree, by site
  - erythema, erythematous — *code as* Burn, first degree, by site
  - esophagus T28.1 ☑
  - extent (percentage of body surface)
    - less than 10 percent T31.0
    - 10-19 percent T31.10
      - with 0-9 percent third degree burns T31.10
      - with 10-19 percent third degree burns T31.11
    - 20-29 percent T31.20
      - with 0-9 percent third degree burns T31.20
      - with 10-19 percent third degree burns T31.21
      - with 20-29 percent third degree burns T31.22
    - 30-39 percent T31.30
      - with 0-9 percent third degree burns T31.30
      - with 10-19 percent third degree burns T31.31
      - with 20-29 percent third degree burns T31.32
      - with 30-39 percent third degree burns T31.33
    - 40-49 percent T31.40
      - with 0-9 percent third degree burns T31.40
      - with 10-19 percent third degree burns T31.41
      - with 20-29 percent third degree burns T31.42
      - with 30-39 percent third degree burns T31.43
      - with 40-49 percent third degree burns T31.44
    - 50-59 percent T31.50
      - with 0-9 percent third degree burns T31.50
      - with 10-19 percent third degree burns T31.51
      - with 20-29 percent third degree burns T31.52
      - with 30-39 percent third degree burns T31.53
      - with 40-49 percent third degree burns T31.54
      - with 50-59 percent third degree burns T31.55
    - 60-69 percent T31.60
      - with 0-9 percent third degree burns T31.60
      - with 10-19 percent third degree burns T31.61
      - with 20-29 percent third degree burns T31.62
      - with 30-39 percent third degree burns T31.63
      - with 40-49 percent third degree burns T31.64
      - with 50-59 percent third degree burns T31.65
      - with 60-69 percent third degree burns T31.66
    - 70-79 percent T31.70
      - with 0-9 percent third degree burns T31.70
      - with 10-19 percent third degree burns T31.71
      - with 20-29 percent third degree burns T31.72
      - with 30-39 percent third degree burns T31.73
      - with 40-49 percent third degree burns T31.74
      - with 50-59 percent third degree burns T31.75
      - with 60-69 percent third degree burns T31.76
      - with 70-79 percent third degree burns T31.77
    - 80-89 percent T31.80
      - with 0-9 percent third degree burns T31.80
      - with 10-19 percent third degree burns T31.81
      - with 20-29 percent third degree burns T31.82
      - with 30-39 percent third degree burns T31.83
      - with 40-49 percent third degree burns T31.84
      - with 50-59 percent third degree burns T31.85
      - with 60-69 percent third degree burns T31.86
      - with 70-79 percent third degree burns T31.87
      - with 80-89 percent third degree burns T31.88

- **Burn** — *continued*
  - extent — *continued*
    - 90 percent or more T31.90
      - with 0-9 percent third degree burns T31.90
      - with 10-19 percent third degree burns T31.91
      - with 20-29 percent third degree burns T31.92
      - with 30-39 percent third degree burns T31.93
      - with 40-49 percent third degree burns T31.94
      - with 50-59 percent third degree burns T31.95
      - with 60-69 percent third degree burns T31.96
      - with 70-79 percent third degree burns T31.97
      - with 80-89 percent third degree burns T31.98
      - with 90 percent or more third degree burns T31.99
  - extremity — *see* Burn, limb
  - eye(s) and adnexa T26.4- ☑
    - with resulting rupture and destruction of eyeball T26.2- ☑
    - conjunctival sac — *see* Burn, cornea
    - cornea — *see* Burn, cornea
    - lid — *see* Burn, eyelid
    - periocular area — *see* Burn, eyelid
    - specified site NEC T26.3- ☑
  - eyeball — *see* Burn, eye
  - eyelid(s) T26.0- ☑
    - chemical — *see* Corrosion, eyelid
  - face — *see* Burn, head
  - finger T23.029 ☑
    - first degree T23.129 ☑
    - left T23.022 ☑
      - first degree T23.122 ☑
      - second degree T23.222 ☑
      - third degree T23.322 ☑
    - multiple sites (without thumb) T23.039 ☑
      - with thumb T23.049 ☑
        - first degree T23.149 ☑
        - left T23.042 ☑
          - first degree T23.142 ☑
          - second degree T23.242 ☑
          - third degree T23.342 ☑
        - right T23.041 ☑
          - first degree T23.141 ☑
          - second degree T23.241 ☑
          - third degree T23.341 ☑
        - second degree T23.249 ☑
        - third degree T23.349 ☑
      - first degree T23.139 ☑
      - left T23.032 ☑
        - first degree T23.132 ☑
        - second degree T23.232 ☑
        - third degree T23.332 ☑
      - right T23.031 ☑
        - first degree T23.131 ☑
        - second degree T23.231 ☑
        - third degree T23.331 ☑
      - second degree T23.239 ☑
      - third degree T23.339 ☑
    - right T23.021 ☑
      - first degree T23.121 ☑
      - second degree T23.221 ☑
      - third degree T23.321 ☑
    - second degree T23.229 ☑
    - third degree T23.329 ☑
  - flank — *see* Burn, abdominal wall
  - foot T25.029 ☑
    - first degree T25.129 ☑
    - left T25.022 ☑
      - first degree T25.122 ☑
      - second degree T25.222 ☑
      - third degree T25.322 ☑
    - multiple with ankle — *see* Burn, lower, limb, multiple, ankle and foot
    - right T25.021 ☑
      - first degree T25.121 ☑
      - second degree T25.221 ☑
      - third degree T25.321 ☑
    - second degree T25.229 ☑
    - third degree T25.329 ☑
  - forearm T22.019 ☑
    - first degree T22.119 ☑
    - left T22.012 ☑
      - first degree T22.112 ☑
      - second degree T22.212 ☑
      - third degree T22.312 ☑
    - right T22.011 ☑
      - first degree T22.111 ☑

- **Burn** — *continued*
  - forearm — *continued*
    - right — *continued*
      - second degree T22.211 ☑
      - third degree T22.311 ☑
    - second degree T22.219 ☑
    - third degree T22.319 ☑
  - forehead T20.06 ☑
    - first degree T20.16 ☑
    - second degree T20.26 ☑
    - third degree T20.36 ☑
  - fourth degree — *code as* Burn, third degree, by site
  - friction — *see* Burn, by site
  - from swallowing caustic or corrosive substance NEC — *see* Corrosion, by site
  - full thickness skin loss — *code as* Burn, third degree, by site
  - gastrointestinal tract NEC T28.2 ☑
    - from swallowing caustic or corrosive substance T28.7 ☑
  - genital organs
    - external
      - female T21.07 ☑
        - first degree T21.17 ☑
        - second degree T21.27 ☑
        - third degree T21.37 ☑
      - male T21.06 ☑
        - first degree T21.16 ☑
        - second degree T21.26 ☑
        - third degree T21.36 ☑
    - internal T28.3 ☑
      - from caustic or corrosive substance T28.8 ☑
  - groin — *see* Burn, abdominal wall
  - hand(s) T23.009 ☑
    - back — *see* Burn, dorsum of hand
    - finger — *see* Burn, finger
    - first degree T23.109 ☑
    - left T23.002 ☑
      - first degree T23.102 ☑
      - second degree T23.202 ☑
      - third degree T23.302 ☑
    - multiple sites with wrist T23.099 ☑
      - first degree T23.199 ☑
      - left T23.092 ☑
        - first degree T23.192 ☑
        - second degree T23.292 ☑
        - third degree T23.392 ☑
      - right T23.091 ☑
        - first degree T23.191 ☑
        - second degree T23.291 ☑
        - third degree T23.391 ☑
      - second degree T23.299 ☑
      - third degree T23.399 ☑
    - palm — *see* Burn, palm
    - right T23.001 ☑
      - first degree T23.101 ☑
      - second degree T23.201 ☑
      - third degree T23.301 ☑
    - second degree T23.209 ☑
    - third degree T23.309 ☑
    - thumb — *see* Burn, thumb
  - head (and face) (and neck) T20.00 ☑
    - cheek — *see* Burn, cheek
    - chin — *see* Burn, chin
    - ear — *see* Burn, ear
    - eye(s) only — *see* Burn, eye
    - first degree T20.10 ☑
    - forehead — *see* Burn, forehead
    - lip — *see* Burn, lip
    - multiple sites T20.09 ☑
      - first degree T20.19 ☑
      - second degree T20.29 ☑
      - third degree T20.39 ☑
    - neck — *see* Burn, neck
    - nose — *see* Burn, nose
    - scalp — *see* Burn, scalp
    - second degree T20.20 ☑
    - third degree T20.30 ☑
  - hip(s) — *see* Burn, thigh
  - inhalation — *see* Burn, respiratory tract
    - caustic or corrosive substance (fumes) — *see* Corrosion, respiratory tract
  - internal organ(s) T28.40 ☑
    - alimentary tract T28.2 ☑
      - esophagus T28.1 ☑
    - eardrum T28.41 ☑

- **Burn** — *continued*
  - internal organ(s) — *continued*
    - esophagus T28.1 ☑
    - from caustic or corrosive substance (swallowing) NEC — *see* Corrosion, by site
    - genitourinary T28.3 ☑
    - mouth T28.0 ☑
    - pharynx T28.0 ☑
    - respiratory tract — *see* Burn, respiratory tract
    - specified organ NEC T28.49 ☑
  - interscapular region — *see* Burn, back, upper
  - intestine (large) (small) T28.2 ☑
  - knee T24.029 ☑
    - first degree T24.129 ☑
    - left T24.022 ☑
      - first degree T24.122 ☑
      - second degree T24.222 ☑
      - third degree T24.322 ☑
    - right T24.021 ☑
      - first degree T24.121 ☑
      - second degree T24.221 ☑
      - third degree T24.321 ☑
    - second degree T24.229 ☑
    - third degree T24.329 ☑
  - labium (majus) (minus) — *see* Burn, genital organs, external, female
  - lacrimal apparatus, duct, gland or sac — *see* Burn, eye, specified site NEC
  - larynx T27.0 ☑
    - with lung T27.1 ☑
  - leg(s) (lower) (upper) — *see* Burn, lower, limb
  - lightning — *see* Burn, by site
  - limb(s)
    - lower (except ankle or foot alone) — *see* Burn, lower, limb
    - upper — *see* Burn, upper limb
  - lip(s) T20.02 ☑
    - first degree T20.12 ☑
    - second degree T20.22 ☑
    - third degree T20.32 ☑
  - lower
    - back — *see* Burn, back
    - limb T24.009 ☑
      - ankle — *see* Burn, ankle
      - calf — *see* Burn, calf
      - first degree T24.109 ☑
      - foot — *see* Burn, foot
      - hip — *see* Burn, thigh
      - knee — *see* Burn, knee
      - left T24.002 ☑
        - first degree T24.102 ☑
        - second degree T24.202 ☑
        - third degree T24.302 ☑
      - multiple sites, except ankle and foot T24.099 ☑
        - ankle and foot T25.099 ☑
          - first degree T25.199 ☑
          - left T25.092 ☑
            - first degree T25.192 ☑
            - second degree T25.292 ☑
            - third degree T25.392 ☑
          - right T25.091 ☑
            - first degree T25.191 ☑
            - second degree T25.291 ☑
            - third degree T25.391 ☑
          - second degree T25.299 ☑
          - third degree T25.399 ☑
        - first degree T24.199 ☑
        - left T24.092 ☑
          - first degree T24.192 ☑
          - second degree T24.292 ☑
          - third degree T24.392 ☑
        - right T24.091 ☑
          - first degree T24.191 ☑
          - second degree T24.291 ☑
          - third degree T24.391 ☑
        - second degree T24.299 ☑
        - third degree T24.399 ☑
      - right T24.001 ☑
        - first degree T24.101 ☑
        - second degree T24.201 ☑
        - third degree T24.301 ☑
      - second degree T24.209 ☑
      - thigh — *see* Burn, thigh
      - third degree T24.309 ☑
      - toe — *see* Burn, toe
  - lung (with larynx and trachea) T27.1 ☑

- **Burn** — *continued*
  - mouth T28.0 ☑
  - neck T20.07 ☑
    - first degree T20.17 ☑
    - second degree T20.27 ☑
    - third degree T20.37 ☑
  - nose (septum) T20.04 ☑
    - first degree T20.14 ☑
    - second degree T20.24 ☑
    - third degree T20.34 ☑
  - ocular adnexa — *see* Burn, eye
  - orbit region — *see* Burn, eyelid
  - palm T23.059 ☑
    - first degree T23.159 ☑
    - left T23.052 ☑
      - first degree T23.152 ☑
      - second degree T23.252 ☑
      - third degree T23.352 ☑
    - right T23.051 ☑
      - first degree T23.151 ☑
      - second degree T23.251 ☑
      - third degree T23.351 ☑
    - second degree T23.259 ☑
    - third degree T23.359 ☑
  - partial thickness — *code as* Burn, by site, second degree
  - pelvis — *see* Burn, trunk
  - penis — *see* Burn, genital organs, external, male
  - perineum
    - female — *see* Burn, genital organs, external, female
    - male — *see* Burn, genital organs, external, male
  - periocular area — *see* Burn, eyelid
  - pharynx T28.0 ☑
  - rectum T28.2 ☑
  - respiratory tract T27.3 ☑
    - larynx — *see* Burn, larynx
    - specified part NEC T27.2 ☑
    - trachea — *see* Burn, trachea
  - sac, lacrimal — *see* Burn, eye, specified site NEC
  - scalp T20.05 ☑
    - first degree T20.15 ☑
    - second degree T20.25 ☑
    - third degree T20.35 ☑
  - scapular region T22.069 ☑
    - first degree T22.169 ☑
    - left T22.062 ☑
      - first degree T22.162 ☑
      - second degree T22.262 ☑
      - third degree T22.362 ☑
    - right T22.061 ☑
      - first degree T22.161 ☑
      - second degree T22.261 ☑
      - third degree T22.361 ☑
    - second degree T22.269 ☑
    - third degree T22.369 ☑
  - sclera — *see* Burn, eye, specified site NEC
  - scrotum — *see* Burn, genital organs, external, male
  - shoulder T22.059 ☑
    - first degree T22.159 ☑
    - left T22.052 ☑
      - first degree T22.152 ☑
      - second degree T22.252 ☑
      - third degree T22.352 ☑
    - right T22.051 ☑
      - first degree T22.151 ☑
      - second degree T22.251 ☑
      - third degree T22.351 ☑
    - second degree T22.259 ☑
    - third degree T22.359 ☑
  - stomach T28.2 ☑
  - temple — *see* Burn, head
  - testis — *see* Burn, genital organs, external, male
  - thigh T24.019 ☑
    - first degree T24.119 ☑
    - left T24.012 ☑
      - first degree T24.112 ☑
      - second degree T24.212 ☑
      - third degree T24.312 ☑
    - right T24.011 ☑
      - first degree T24.111 ☑
      - second degree T24.211 ☑
      - third degree T24.311 ☑
    - second degree T24.219 ☑
    - third degree T24.319 ☑
  - thorax (external) — *see* Burn, trunk
  - throat (meaning pharynx) T28.0 ☑
  - thumb(s) T23.019 ☑

- **Burn** — *continued*
  - thumb(s) — *continued*
    - first degree T23.119 ☑
    - left T23.012 ☑
      - first degree T23.112 ☑
      - second degree T23.212 ☑
      - third degree T23.312 ☑
    - multiple sites with fingers T23.049 ☑
      - first degree T23.149 ☑
      - left T23.042 ☑
        - first degree T23.142 ☑
        - second degree T23.242 ☑
        - third degree T23.342 ☑
      - right T23.041 ☑
        - first degree T23.141 ☑
        - second degree T23.241 ☑
        - third degree T23.341 ☑
      - second degree T23.249 ☑
      - third degree T23.349 ☑
    - right T23.011 ☑
      - first degree T23.111 ☑
      - second degree T23.211 ☑
      - third degree T23.311 ☑
    - second degree T23.219 ☑
    - third degree T23.319 ☑
  - toe T25.039 ☑
    - first degree T25.139 ☑
    - left T25.032 ☑
      - first degree T25.132 ☑
      - second degree T25.232 ☑
      - third degree T25.332 ☑
    - right T25.031 ☑
      - first degree T25.131 ☑
      - second degree T25.231 ☑
      - third degree T25.331 ☑
    - second degree T25.239 ☑
    - third degree T25.339 ☑
  - tongue T28.0 ☑
  - tonsil(s) T28.0 ☑
  - trachea T27.0 ☑
    - with lung T27.1 ☑
  - trunk T21.00 ☑
    - abdominal wall — *see* Burn, abdominal wall
    - anus — *see* Burn, buttock
    - axilla — *see* Burn, upper limb
    - back — *see* Burn, back
    - breast — *see* Burn, chest wall
    - buttock — *see* Burn, buttock
    - chest wall — *see* Burn, chest wall
    - first degree T21.10 ☑
    - flank — *see* Burn, abdominal wall
    - genital
      - female — *see* Burn, genital organs, external, female
      - male — *see* Burn, genital organs, external, male
    - groin — *see* Burn, abdominal wall
    - interscapular region — *see* Burn, back, upper
    - labia — *see* Burn, genital organs, external, female
    - lower back — *see* Burn, back
    - penis — *see* Burn, genital organs, external, male
    - perineum
      - female — *see* Burn, genital organs, external, female
      - male — *see* Burn, genital organs, external, male
    - scapula region — *see* Burn, scapular region
    - scrotum — *see* Burn, genital organs, external, male
    - second degree T21.20 ☑
    - specified site NEC T21.09 ☑
      - first degree T21.19 ☑
      - second degree T21.29 ☑
      - third degree T21.39 ☑
    - testes — *see* Burn, genital organs, external, male
    - third degree T21.30 ☑
    - upper back — *see* Burn, back, upper
    - vulva — *see* Burn, genital organs, external, female
  - unspecified site with extent of body surface involved specified
    - less than 10 percent T31.0
    - 10-19 percent (0-9 percent third degree) T31.10
      - with 10-19 percent third degree T31.11
    - 20-29 percent (0-9 percent third degree) T31.20
      - with
        - 10-19 percent third degree T31.21
        - 20-29 percent third degree T31.22
    - 30-39 percent (0-9 percent third degree) T31.30

- **Burn** — *continued*
  - unspecified site with extent of body surface involved specified — *continued*
    - 30-39 percent — *continued*
      - with
        - 10-19 percent third degree T31.31
        - 20-29 percent third degree T31.32
        - 30-39 percent third degree T31.33
    - 40-49 percent (0-9 percent third degree) T31.40
      - with
        - 10-19 percent third degree T31.41
        - 20-29 percent third degree T31.42
        - 30-39 percent third degree T31.43
        - 40-49 percent third degree T31.44
    - 50-59 percent (0-9 percent third degree) T31.50
      - with
        - 10-19 percent third degree T31.51
        - 20-29 percent third degree T31.52
        - 30-39 percent third degree T31.53
        - 40-49 percent third degree T31.54
        - 50-59 percent third degree T31.55
    - 60-69 percent (0-9 percent third degree) T31.60
      - with
        - 10-19 percent third degree T31.61
        - 20-29 percent third degree T31.62
        - 30-39 percent third degree T31.63
        - 40-49 percent third degree T31.64
        - 50-59 percent third degree T31.65
        - 60-69 percent third degree T31.66
    - 70-79 percent (0-9 percent third degree) T31.70
      - with
        - 10-19 percent third degree T31.71
        - 20-29 percent third degree T31.72
        - 30-39 percent third degree T31.73
        - 40-49 percent third degree T31.74
        - 50-59 percent third degree T31.75
        - 60-69 percent third degree T31.76
        - 70-79 percent third degree T31.77
    - 80-89 percent (0-9 percent third degree) T31.80
      - with
        - 10-19 percent third degree T31.81
        - 20-29 percent third degree T31.82
        - 30-39 percent third degree T31.83
        - 40-49 percent third degree T31.84
        - 50-59 percent third degree T31.85
        - 60-69 percent third degree T31.86
        - 70-79 percent third degree T31.87
        - 80-89 percent third degree T31.88
    - 90 percent or more (0-9 percent third degree) T31.90
      - with
        - 10-19 percent third degree T31.91
        - 20-29 percent third degree T31.92
        - 30-39 percent third degree T31.93
        - 40-49 percent third degree T31.94
        - 50-59 percent third degree T31.95
        - 60-69 percent third degree T31.96
        - 70-79 percent third degree T31.97
        - 80-89 percent third degree T31.98
        - 90-99 percent third degree T31.99
  - upper limb T22.00 ☑
    - above elbow — *see* Burn, above elbow
    - axilla — *see* Burn, axilla
    - elbow — *see* Burn, elbow
    - first degree T22.10 ☑
    - forearm — *see* Burn, forearm
    - hand — *see* Burn, hand
    - interscapular region — *see* Burn, back, upper
    - multiple sites T22.099 ☑
      - first degree T22.199 ☑
      - left T22.092 ☑
        - first degree T22.192 ☑
        - second degree T22.292 ☑
        - third degree T22.392 ☑
      - right T22.091 ☑
        - first degree T22.191 ☑
        - second degree T22.291 ☑
        - third degree T22.391 ☑
      - second degree T22.299 ☑
      - third degree T22.399 ☑
    - scapular region — *see* Burn, scapular region
    - second degree T22.20 ☑
    - shoulder — *see* Burn, shoulder
    - third degree T22.30 ☑
    - wrist — *see* Burn, wrist
  - uterus T28.3 ☑
  - vagina T28.3 ☑
  - vulva — *see* Burn, genital organs, external, female
  - wrist T23.079 ☑

- **Burn** — *continued*
  - wrist — *continued*
    - first degree T23.179 ☑
    - left T23.072 ☑
      - first degree T23.172 ☑
      - second degree T23.272 ☑
      - third degree T23.372 ☑
    - multiple sites with hand T23.099 ☑
      - first degree T23.199 ☑
      - left T23.092 ☑
        - first degree T23.192 ☑
        - second degree T23.292 ☑
        - third degree T23.392 ☑
      - right T23.091 ☑
        - first degree T23.191 ☑
        - second degree T23.291 ☑
        - third degree T23.391 ☑
      - second degree T23.299 ☑
      - third degree T23.399 ☑
    - right T23.071 ☑
      - first degree T23.171 ☑
      - second degree T23.271 ☑
      - third degree T23.371 ☑
    - second degree T23.279 ☑
    - third degree T23.379 ☑
- **Burnett's syndrome** E83.52
- **Burning**
  - feet syndrome E53.9
  - sensation R20.8
  - tongue K14.6
- **Burn-out** (state) Z73.0
- **Burns' disease or osteochondrosis** — *see* Osteochondrosis, juvenile, ulna
- **Bursa** — *see* condition
- **Bursitis** M71.9
  - Achilles — *see* Tendinitis, Achilles
  - adhesive — *see* Bursitis, specified NEC
  - ankle — *see* Enthesopathy, lower limb, ankle, specified type NEC
  - calcaneal — *see* Enthesopathy, foot, specified type NEC
  - collateral ligament, tibial — *see* Bursitis, tibial collateral
  - due to use, overuse, pressure — *see also* Disorder, soft tissue, due to use, specified type NEC
    - specified NEC — *see* Disorder, soft tissue, due to use, specified NEC
  - Duplay's M75.0 ☑
  - elbow NEC M70.3- ☑
    - olecranon M70.2- ☑
  - finger — *see* Disorder, soft tissue, due to use, specified type NEC, hand
  - foot — *see* Enthesopathy, foot, specified type NEC
  - gonococcal A54.49
  - gouty — *see* Gout
  - hand M70.1- ☑
  - hip NEC M70.7- ☑
    - trochanteric M70.6- ☑
  - infective NEC M71.10
    - abscess — *see* Abscess, bursa
    - ankle M71.17- ☑
    - elbow M71.12- ☑
    - foot M71.17- ☑
    - hand M71.14- ☑
    - hip M71.15- ☑
    - knee M71.16- ☑
    - multiple sites M71.19
    - shoulder M71.11- ☑
    - specified site NEC M71.18
    - wrist M71.13- ☑
  - ischial — *see* Bursitis, hip
  - knee NEC M70.5- ☑
    - prepatellar M70.4- ☑
  - occupational NEC — *see also* Disorder, soft tissue, due to use
  - olecranon — *see* Bursitis, elbow, olecranon
  - pharyngeal J39.1
  - popliteal — *see* Bursitis, knee
  - prepatellar M70.4- ☑
  - radiohumeral M70.3- ☑
  - rheumatoid M06.20
    - ankle M06.27- ☑
    - elbow M06.22- ☑
    - foot joint M06.27- ☑
    - hand joint M06.24- ☑
    - hip M06.25- ☑
    - knee M06.26- ☑
    - multiple site M06.29

- **Bursitis** — *continued*
  - rheumatoid — *continued*
    - shoulder M06.21- ☑
    - vertebra M06.28
    - wrist M06.23- ☑
  - scapulohumeral — *see* Bursitis, shoulder
  - semimembranous muscle (knee) — *see* Bursitis, knee
  - shoulder M75.5- ☑
    - adhesive — *see* Capsulitis, adhesive
  - specified NEC M71.50
    - ankle M71.57- ☑
    - due to use, overuse or pressure — *see* Disorder, soft tissue, due to, use
    - elbow M71.52- ☑
    - foot M71.57- ☑
    - hand M71.54- ☑
    - hip M71.55- ☑
    - knee M71.56- ☑
    - shoulder — *see* Bursitis, shoulder
    - specified site NEC M71.58
    - tibial collateral M76.4- ☑
    - wrist M71.53- ☑
  - subacromial — *see* Bursitis, shoulder
  - subcoracoid — *see* Bursitis, shoulder
  - subdeltoid — *see* Bursitis, shoulder
  - syphilitic A52.78
  - Thornwaldt, Tornwaldt J39.2
  - tibial collateral M76.4- ☑
  - toe — *see* Enthesopathy, foot, specified type NEC
  - trochanteric (area) — *see* Bursitis, hip, trochanteric
  - wrist — *see* Bursitis, hand
- **Bursopathy** M71.9
  - specified type NEC M71.80
    - ankle M71.87- ☑
    - elbow M71.82- ☑
    - foot M71.87- ☑
    - hand M71.84- ☑
    - hip M71.85- ☑
    - knee M71.86- ☑
    - multiple sites M71.89
    - shoulder M71.81- ☑
    - specified site NEC M71.88
    - wrist M71.83- ☑
- **Burst stitches or sutures** (complication of surgery) T81.31 ☑
  - external operation wound T81.31 ☑
  - internal operation wound T81.32 ☑
- **Buruli ulcer** A31.1
- **Bury's disease** L95.1
- **Buschke's**
  - disease — *see* Cryptococcosis by site
  - scleredema — *see* Sclerosis, systemic
- **Busse-Buschke disease** — *see* Cryptococcosis by site
- **Buttock** — *see* condition
- **Button**
  - Biskra B55.1
  - Delhi B55.1
  - oriental B55.1
- **Buttonhole deformity** (finger) — *see* Deformity, finger, boutonniere
- **Bwamba fever** A92.8
- **Byssinosis** J66.0
- **Bywaters' syndrome** T79.5 ☑

C

- **Cachexia** E43
  - cancerous R64
  - cardiac — *see* Disease, heart
  - dehydration E86.0
  - due to
    - malnutrition R64
    - underlying condition E88.A
  - exophthalmic — *see* Hyperthyroidism
  - heart — *see* Disease, heart
  - hypophyseal E23.0
  - hypopituitary E23.0
  - lead — *see* Poisoning, lead
  - malignant R64
  - marsh — *see* Malaria
  - nervous F48.8
  - old age R54
  - paludal — *see* Malaria
  - pituitary E23.0
  - pulmonary R64
  - renal N28.9
  - saturnine — *see* Poisoning, lead

Cachexia — *continued*
  senile R54
  Simmonds' E23.Ø
  splenica D73.Ø
  strumipriva EØ3.4
  tuberculous NEC — *see* Tuberculosis
CADASIL (cerebral autosomal dominant arteriopathy with subcortical infarcts and leukoencephalopathy) I67.85Ø
Cafe, au lait spots L81.3
Caffeine-induced
  anxiety disorder F15.98Ø
  sleep disorder F15.982
Caffey's syndrome Q78.8
Caisson disease T7Ø.3 ☑
Cake kidney Q63.1
Caked breast (puerperal, postpartum) O92.79
Calabar swelling B74.3
Calcaneal spur — *see* Spur, bone, calcaneal
Calcaneo-apophysitis M92.8
Calcareous — *see* condition
Calcicosis J62.8
Calciferol (vitamin D) deficiency E55.9
  with rickets E55.Ø
Calcification
  adrenal (capsule) (gland) E27.49
    tuberculous B9Ø.8 *[E35]*
  aorta I7Ø.Ø
  artery (annular) — *see* Arteriosclerosis
  auricle (ear) — *see* Disorder, pinna, specified type NEC
  basal ganglia G23.8
  bladder N32.89
    due to Schistosoma hematobium B65.Ø
  brain (cortex) — *see* Calcification, cerebral
  bronchus J98.Ø9
  bursa M71.4Ø
    ankle M71.47- ☑
    elbow M71.42- ☑
    foot M71.47- ☑
    hand M71.44- ☑
    hip M71.45- ☑
    knee M71.46- ☑
    multiple sites M71.49
    shoulder M75.3- ☑
    specified site NEC M71.48
    wrist M71.43- ☑
  cardiac — *see* Degeneration, myocardial
  cerebral (cortex) G93.89
    artery I67.2
  cervix (uteri) N88.8
  choroid plexus G93.89
  conjunctiva — *see* Concretion, conjunctiva
  corpora cavernosa (penis) N48.89
  cortex (brain) — *see* Calcification, cerebral
  dental pulp (nodular) KØ4.2
  dentinal papilla KØØ.4
  fallopian tube N83.8
  falx cerebri G96.198
  gallbladder K82.8
  general E83.59
  heart — *see also* Degeneration, myocardial
    valve — *see also* Endocarditis
      mitral — *see* Calcification, mitral
  idiopathic infantile arterial (IIAC) Q28.8
  intervertebral cartilage or disc (postinfective) — *see* Disorder, disc, specified NEC
  intracranial — *see* Calcification, cerebral
  joint — *see* Disorder, joint, specified type NEC
  kidney N28.89
    tuberculous N29 *[B9Ø.1]*
  larynx (senile) J38.7
  lens — *see* Cataract, specified NEC
  lung (active) (postinfectional) J98.4
    tuberculous B9Ø.9
  lymph gland or node (postinfectional) I89.8
    tuberculous — *see also* Tuberculosis, lymph gland B9Ø.8
  mammographic R92.1
  massive (paraplegic) — *see* Myositis, ossificans, in, quadriplegia
  medial — *see* Arteriosclerosis, extremities
  meninges (cerebral) (spinal) G96.198
  metastatic E83.59
  mitral (valve)
    annular I34.81
      nonrheumatic I34.81
      rheumatic IØ5.8

Calcification — *continued*
  mitral — *continued*
    annulus I34.81
      nonrheumatic I34.81
      rheumatic IØ5.8
  Monckeberg's — *see* Arteriosclerosis, extremities
  muscle M61.9
    due to burns — *see* Myositis, ossificans, in, burns
    paralytic — *see* Myositis, ossificans, in, quadriplegia
    specified type NEC M61.4Ø
      ankle M61.47- ☑
      foot M61.47- ☑
      forearm M61.43- ☑
      hand M61.44- ☑
      lower leg M61.46- ☑
      multiple sites M61.49
      pelvic region M61.45- ☑
      shoulder region M61.41- ☑
      specified site NEC M61.48
      thigh M61.45- ☑
      upper arm M61.42- ☑
  myocardium, myocardial — *see* Degeneration, myocardial
  ovary N83.8
  pancreas K86.89
  penis N48.89
  periarticular — *see* Disorder, joint, specified type NEC
  pericardium — *see also* Pericarditis I31.1
  pineal gland E34.8
  pleura J94.8
    postinfectional J94.8
    tuberculous NEC B9Ø.9
  pulpal (dental) (nodular) KØ4.2
  sclera H15.89
  spleen D73.89
  subcutaneous L94.2
  suprarenal (capsule) (gland) E27.49
  tendon (sheath) — *see also* Tenosynovitis, specified type NEC
    with bursitis, synovitis or tenosynovitis — *see* Tendinitis, calcific
  trachea J39.8
  ureter N28.89
  uterus N85.8
  vitreous — *see* Deposit, crystalline
Calcified — *see* Calcification
Calcinosis (interstitial) (tumoral) (universalis) E83.59
  with Raynaud's phenomenon, esophageal dysfunction, sclerodactyly, telangiectasia (CREST syndrome) M34.1
  circumscripta (skin) L94.2
  cutis L94.2
Calciphylaxis — *see also* Calcification, by site E83.59
Calcium
  deposits — *see* Calcification, by site
  metabolism disorder E83.5Ø
  salts or soaps in vitreous — *see* Deposit, crystalline
Calciuria R82.994
Calculi — *see* Calculus
Calculosis, intrahepatic — *see* Calculus, bile duct
Calculus, calculi, calculous
  ampulla of Vater — *see* Calculus, bile duct
  anuria (impacted) (recurrent) — *see also* Calculus, urinary N2Ø.9
  appendix K38.1
  bile duct (common) (hepatic) K8Ø.5Ø
    with
      calculus of gallbladder — *see* Calculus, gallbladder and bile duct
      cholangitis K8Ø.3Ø
        with
          cholecystitis — *see* Calculus, bile duct, with cholecystitis
          obstruction K8Ø.31
        acute K8Ø.32
          with
            chronic cholangitis K8Ø.36
              with obstruction K8Ø.37
            obstruction K8Ø.33
        chronic K8Ø.34
          with
            acute cholangitis K8Ø.36
              with obstruction K8Ø.37
            obstruction K8Ø.35
      cholecystitis (with cholangitis) K8Ø.4Ø
        with obstruction K8Ø.41
        acute K8Ø.42

Calculus, calculi, calculous — *continued*
  bile duct — *continued*
    with — *continued*
      cholecystitis — *continued*
        acute — *continued*
          with
            chronic cholecystitis K8Ø.46
              with obstruction K8Ø.47
            obstruction K8Ø.43
        chronic K8Ø.44
          with
            acute cholecystitis K8Ø.46
              with obstruction K8Ø.47
            obstruction K8Ø.45
  biliary — *see also* Calculus, gallbladder
    specified NEC K8Ø.8Ø
      with obstruction K8Ø.81
  bilirubin, multiple — *see* Calculus, gallbladder
  bladder (encysted) (impacted) (urinary) (diverticulum) N21.Ø
  bronchus J98.Ø9
  calyx (kidney) (renal) — *see* Calculus, kidney
  cholesterol (pure) (solitary) — *see* Calculus, gallbladder
  common duct (bile) — *see* Calculus, bile duct
  conjunctiva — *see* Concretion, conjunctiva
  cystic N21.Ø
    duct — *see* Calculus, gallbladder
  dental (subgingival) (supragingival) KØ3.6
  diverticulum
    bladder N21.Ø
    kidney N2Ø.Ø
  epididymis N5Ø.89
  gallbladder K8Ø.2Ø
    with
      bile duct calculus — *see* Calculus, gallbladder and bile duct
      cholecystitis K8Ø.1Ø
        with obstruction K8Ø.11
        acute K8Ø.ØØ
          with
            chronic cholecystitis K8Ø.12
              with obstruction K8Ø.13
            obstruction K8Ø.Ø1
        chronic K8Ø.1Ø
          with
            acute cholecystitis K8Ø.12
              with obstruction K8Ø.13
            obstruction K8Ø.11
        specified NEC K8Ø.18
          with obstruction K8Ø.19
      obstruction K8Ø.21
  gallbladder and bile duct K8Ø.7Ø
    with
      cholecystitis K8Ø.6Ø
        with obstruction K8Ø.61
        acute K8Ø.62
          with
            chronic cholecystitis K8Ø.66
              with obstruction K8Ø.67
            obstruction K8Ø.63
        chronic K8Ø.64
          with
            acute cholecystitis K8Ø.66
              with obstruction K8Ø.67
            obstruction K8Ø.65
      obstruction K8Ø.71
  hepatic (duct) — *see* Calculus, bile duct
  ileal conduit N21.8
  intestinal (impaction) (obstruction) K56.49
  kidney (impacted) (multiple) (pelvis) (recurrent) (staghorn) N2Ø.Ø
    with calculus, ureter N2Ø.2
    congenital Q63.8
  lacrimal passages — *see* Dacryolith
  liver (impacted) — *see* Calculus, bile duct
  lung J98.4
  mammographic R92.1
  nephritic (impacted) (recurrent) — *see* Calculus, kidney
  nose J34.89
  pancreas (duct) K86.89
  parotid duct or gland K11.5
  pelvis, encysted — *see* Calculus, kidney
  prostate N42.Ø
  pulmonary J98.4
  pyelitis (impacted) (recurrent) N2Ø.Ø
    with hydronephrosis N13.6
  pyelonephritis (impacted) (recurrent) — *see* category N2Ø ☑

- **Calculus, calculi, calculous** — *continued*
  - pyelonephritis — *see* category — *continued*
    - with hydronephrosis N13.6
  - renal (impacted) (recurrent) — *see* Calculus, kidney
  - salivary (duct) (gland) K11.5
  - seminal vesicle N5Ø.89
  - staghorn — *see* Calculus, kidney
  - Stensen's duct K11.5
  - stomach K31.89
  - sublingual duct or gland K11.5
    - congenital Q38.4
  - submandibular duct, gland or region K11.5
  - submaxillary duct, gland or region K11.5
  - suburethral N21.8
  - tonsil J35.8
  - tooth, teeth (subgingival) (supragingival) KØ3.6
  - tunica vaginalis N5Ø.89
  - ureter (impacted) (recurrent) N2Ø.1
    - with calculus, kidney N2Ø.2
      - with hydronephrosis N13.2
        - with infection N13.6
  - ureteropelvic junction N2Ø.1
  - urethra (impacted) N21.1
  - urinary (duct) (impacted) (passage) (tract) N2Ø.9
    - with hydronephrosis N13.2
      - with infection N13.6
    - in (due to)
    - lower N21.9
      - specified NEC N21.8
  - vagina N89.8
  - vesical (impacted) N21.Ø
  - Wharton's duct K11.5
  - xanthine E79.82 *[N22]*
- **Calicectasis** N28.89
- **Caliectasis** N28.89
- **California**
  - disease B38.9
  - encephalitis A83.5
- **Caligo cornea** — *see* Opacity, cornea, central
- **Callositas, callosity** (infected) L84
- **Callus** (infected) L84
  - bone — *see* Osteophyte
    - excessive, following fracture — *code as* Sequelae of fracture
- **CALME** (childhood asymmetric labium majus enlargement) N9Ø.61
- **Calorie deficiency or malnutrition** — *see also* Malnutrition E46
- **Calpainopathy** (primary) G71.Ø32
  - autosomal dominant G71.Ø31
  - autosomal recessive G71.Ø32
- **Calve-Perthes disease** — *see* Legg-Calve-Perthes disease
- **Calve's disease** — *see* Osteochondrosis, juvenile, spine
- **Calvities** — *see* Alopecia, androgenic
- **Cameroon fever** — *see* Malaria
- **Camptocormia** (hysterical) F44.4
- **Camurati-Engelmann syndrome** Q78.3
- **Canal** — *see also* condition
  - atrioventricular Q21.2Ø
    - common Q21.23
    - incomplete Q21.21
    - intermediate Q21.22
    - partial Q21.21
    - transitional Q21.22
- **Canaliculitis** (lacrimal) (acute) (subacute) HØ4.33- ☑
  - Actinomyces A42.89
  - chronic HØ4.42- ☑
- **Canavan disease** E75.28
- **Canceled procedure** (surgical) Z53.9
  - because of
    - contraindication Z53.Ø9
      - smoking Z53.Ø1
    - left against medical advice (AMA) Z53.29
    - patient's decision Z53.2Ø
      - for reasons of belief or group pressure Z53.1
      - specified reason NEC Z53.29
    - specified reason NEC Z53.8
- **Cancer** — *see also* Neoplasm, by site, malignant
  - bile duct type liver C22.1
  - blood — *see* Leukemia
  - breast — *see also* Neoplasm, breast, malignant C5Ø.91- ☑
  - hepatocellular C22.Ø
  - lung — *see also* Neoplasm, lung, malignant C34.9Ø
  - ovarian — *see also* Neoplasm ovary, malignant C56.9
  - unspecified site (primary) C8Ø.1
- **Cancer** (o) **phobia** F45.29
- **Cancerous** — *see* Neoplasm, malignant, by site
- **Cancrum oris** A69.Ø
- **Candidiasis, candidal** B37.9
  - balanitis B37.42
  - bronchitis B37.1
  - cheilitis B37.83
  - congenital P37.5
  - cystitis B37.41
  - disseminated B37.7
  - endocarditis B37.6
  - enteritis B37.82
  - esophagitis B37.81
  - intertrigo B37.2
  - lung B37.1
  - meningitis B37.5
  - mouth B37.Ø
  - nails B37.2
  - neonatal P37.5
  - onychia B37.2
  - oral B37.Ø
  - osteomyelitis B37.89
  - otitis externa B37.84
  - paronychia B37.2
  - perionyxis B37.2
  - pneumonia B37.1
  - proctitis B37.82
  - pulmonary B37.1
  - pyelonephritis B37.49
  - sepsis B37.7
  - skin B37.2
  - specified site NEC B37.89
  - stomatitis B37.Ø
  - systemic B37.7
  - urethritis B37.41
  - urogenital site NEC B37.49
  - vagina (acute) B37.31
    - chronic (recurrent) B37.32
  - vulva (acute) B37.31
    - chronic (recurrent) B37.32
  - vulvovaginitis (acute) B37.31
    - chronic (recurrent) B37.32
- **Candidid** L3Ø.2
- **Candidosis** — *see* Candidiasis
- **Candiru infection or infestation** B88.8
- **Canities** (premature) L67.1
  - congenital Q84.2
- **Canker** (mouth) (sore) K12.Ø
  - rash A38.9
- **Cannabinosis** J66.2
- **Cannabis induced**
  - anxiety disorder F12.98Ø
  - psychotic disorder F12.959
  - sleep disorder F12.988
- **Canton fever** A75.9
- **Cantrell's syndrome** Q87.89
- **Capillariasis** (intestinal) B81.1
  - hepatic B83.8
- **Capillary** — *see* condition
- **Caplan's syndrome** — *see* Rheumatoid, lung
- **Capsule** — *see* condition
- **Capsulitis** (joint) — *see also* Enthesopathy
  - adhesive (shoulder) M75.Ø- ☑
  - hepatic K65.8
  - labyrinthine — *see* Otosclerosis, specified NEC
  - thyroid EØ6.9
- **Caput**
  - crepitus Q75.8
  - medusae I86.8
  - succedaneum P12.81
- **Car sickness** T75.3 ☑
- **Carapata** (disease) A68.Ø
- **Carate** — *see* Pinta
- **Carbon lung** J6Ø
- **Carbuncle** LØ2.93
  - abdominal wall LØ2.231
  - anus K61.Ø
  - auditory canal, external — *see* Abscess, ear, external
  - auricle ear — *see* Abscess, ear, external
  - axilla LØ2.43- ☑
  - back (any part) LØ2.232
  - breast N61.1
  - buttock LØ2.33
  - cheek (external) LØ2.Ø3
  - chest wall LØ2.233
  - chin LØ2.Ø3
  - corpus cavernosum N48.21
  - ear (any part) (external) (middle) — *see* Abscess, ear, external
- **Carbuncle** — *continued*
  - external auditory canal — *see* Abscess, ear, external
  - eyelid — *see* Abscess, eyelid
  - face NEC LØ2.Ø3
  - femoral (region) — *see* Carbuncle, lower limb
  - finger — *see* Carbuncle, hand
  - flank LØ2.231
  - foot LØ2.63- ☑
  - forehead LØ2.Ø3
  - genital — *see* Abscess, genital
  - gluteal (region) LØ2.33
  - groin LØ2.234
  - hand LØ2.53- ☑
  - head NEC LØ2.831
  - heel — *see* Carbuncle, foot
  - hip — *see* Carbuncle, lower limb
  - kidney — *see* Abscess, kidney
  - knee — *see* Carbuncle, lower limb
  - labium (majus) (minus) N76.4
  - lacrimal
    - gland — *see* Dacryoadenitis
    - passages (duct) (sac) — *see* Inflammation, lacrimal, passages, acute
  - leg — *see* Carbuncle, lower limb
  - lower limb LØ2.43- ☑
  - malignant A22.Ø
  - navel LØ2.236
  - neck LØ2.13
  - nose (external) (septum) J34.Ø
  - orbit, orbital — *see* Abscess, orbit
  - palmar (space) — *see* Carbuncle, hand
  - partes posteriores LØ2.33
  - pectoral region LØ2.233
  - penis N48.21
  - perineum LØ2.235
  - pinna — *see* Abscess, ear, external
  - popliteal — *see* Carbuncle, lower limb
  - scalp LØ2.831
  - seminal vesicle N49.Ø
  - shoulder — *see* Carbuncle, upper limb
  - specified site NEC LØ2.838
  - temple (region) LØ2.Ø3
  - thumb — *see* Carbuncle, hand
  - toe — *see* Carbuncle, foot
  - trunk LØ2.239
    - abdominal wall LØ2.231
    - back LØ2.232
    - chest wall LØ2.233
    - groin LØ2.234
    - perineum LØ2.235
    - umbilicus LØ2.236
  - umbilicus LØ2.236
  - upper limb LØ2.43- ☑
  - urethra N34.Ø
  - vulva N76.4
- **Carbunculus** — *see* Carbuncle
- **Carcinoid** (tumor) — *see* Tumor, carcinoid
- **Carcinoidosis** E34.Ø
- **Carcinoma** (malignant) — *see also* Neoplasm, by site, malignant
  - acidophil
    - specified site — *see* Neoplasm, malignant, by site
    - unspecified site C75.1
  - acidophil-basophil, mixed
    - specified site — *see* Neoplasm, malignant, by site
    - unspecified site C75.1
  - adnexal (skin) — *see* Neoplasm, skin, malignant
  - adrenal cortical C74.Ø- ☑
  - alveolar — *see* Neoplasm, lung, malignant
    - cell — *see* Neoplasm, lung, malignant
  - ameloblastic C41.1
    - upper jaw (bone) C41.Ø
  - apocrine
    - breast — *see* Neoplasm, breast, malignant
    - specified site NEC — *see* Neoplasm, skin, malignant
    - unspecified site C44.99
  - basal cell (pigmented) (*see also* Neoplasm, skin, malignant) C44.91
    - fibro-epithelial — *see* Neoplasm, skin, malignant
    - morphea — *see* Neoplasm, skin, malignant
    - multicentric — *see* Neoplasm, skin, malignant
  - basaloid
  - basal-squamous cell, mixed — *see* Neoplasm, skin, malignant
  - basophil
    - specified site — *see* Neoplasm, malignant, by site
    - unspecified site C75.1

- **Caries** — *continued*
  - dental — *continued*
    - coronal surface
      - chewing surface
        - limited to enamel K02.51
        - penetrating into dentin K02.52
        - penetrating into pulp K02.53
      - pit and fissure surface
        - limited to enamel K02.51
        - penetrating into dentin K02.52
        - penetrating into pulp K02.53
      - smooth surface
        - limited to enamel K02.61
        - penetrating into dentin K02.62
        - penetrating into pulp K02.63
    - pit and fissure surface
      - limited to enamel K02.51
      - penetrating into dentin K02.52
      - penetrating into pulp K02.53
    - primary, cervical origin K02.52
    - root K02.7
    - smooth surface
      - limited to enamel K02.61
      - penetrating into dentin K02.62
      - penetrating into pulp K02.63
  - external meatus — *see* Disorder, ear, external, specified type NEC
  - hip (tuberculous) A18.02
  - initial (tooth)
    - chewing surface K02.51
    - pit and fissure surface K02.51
    - smooth surface K02.61
  - knee (tuberculous) A18.02
  - labyrinth H83.8 ☑
  - limb NEC (tuberculous) A18.03
  - mastoid process (chronic) — *see* Mastoiditis, chronic
    - tuberculous A18.03
  - middle ear H74.8 ☑
  - nose (tuberculous) A18.03
  - orbit (tuberculous) A18.03
  - ossicles, ear — *see* Abnormal, ear ossicles
  - petrous bone — *see* Petrositis
  - root (dental) (tooth) K02.7
  - sacrum (tuberculous) A18.01
  - spine, spinal (column) (tuberculous) A18.01
  - syphilitic A52.77
    - congenital (early) A50.02 *[M90.80]*
  - tooth, teeth — *see* Caries, dental
  - tuberculous A18.03
  - vertebra (column) (tuberculous) A18.01
- **Carious teeth** — *see* Caries, dental
- **Carneous mole** O02.0
- **Carnitine insufficiency** E71.40
- **Carotenemia** (dietary) E67.1
- **Carotenosis** (cutis) (skin) E67.1
- **Carotid body or sinus syndrome** G90.01
- **Carotidynia** G90.01
- **Carpal tunnel syndrome** — *see* Syndrome, carpal tunnel
- **Carpenter's syndrome** Q87.0
- **Carpopedal spasm** — *see* Tetany
- **Carr-Barr-Plunkett syndrome** Q97.1
- **Carrier** (suspected) of
  - Acinetobacter baumannii Z22.349
    - carbapenem-resistant Z22.340
    - carbapenem-sensitive Z22.341
  - amebiasis Z22.1
  - bacterial disease NEC Z22.39
    - diphtheria Z22.2
    - intestinal infectious NEC Z22.1
      - typhoid Z22.0
    - meningococcal Z22.31
    - sexually transmitted Z22.4
    - specified NEC Z22.39
    - staphylococcal (Methicillin susceptible) Z22.321
      - Methicillin resistant Z22.322
    - streptococcal Z22.338
      - group B Z22.330
        - complicating pregnancy or delivery O99.82- ☑
    - typhoid Z22.0
  - cholera Z22.1
  - diphtheria Z22.2
  - E. coli (Escherichia coli) Z22.35- ☑
  - Enterobacterales Z22.359
    - carbapenem-resistant Z22.350
    - carbapenem-sensitive Z22.358
    - Enterobacterales, specified type NEC Z22.358
    - ESBL-producing Z22.358
- **Carrier** of — *continued*
  - Enterobacterales — *continued*
    - extended-spectrum beta-lactamase producing Z22.358
  - gastrointestinal pathogens NEC Z22.1
  - genetic Z14.8
    - cystic fibrosis Z14.1
    - hemophilia A (asymptomatic) Z14.01
      - symptomatic Z14.02
  - gestational, pregnant Z33.1
  - gonorrhea Z22.4
  - HAA (hepatitis Australian-antigen) B18.8
  - HB (c)(s)-AG B18.1
  - hepatitis (viral) B18.9
    - Australia-antigen (HAA) B18.8
    - B surface antigen (HBsAg) B18.1
      - with acute delta- (super)infection B17.0
    - C B18.2
    - specified NEC B18.8
  - human T-cell lymphotropic virus type-1 (HTLV-1) infection Z22.6
  - infectious organism Z22.9
    - specified NEC Z22.8
  - K. pneumoniae (Klebsiella pneumoniae) Z22.35- ☑
  - meningococci Z22.31
  - Salmonella typhosa Z22.0
  - serum hepatitis — *see* Carrier, hepatitis
  - staphylococci (Methicillin susceptible) Z22.321
    - Methicillin resistant Z22.322
  - streptococci Z22.338
    - group B Z22.330
      - complicating pregnancy or delivery O99.82- ☑
  - syphilis Z22.4
  - typhoid Z22.0
  - venereal disease NEC Z22.4
- **Carrion's disease** A44.0
- **Carter's relapsing fever** (Asiatic) A68.1
- **Cartilage** — *see* condition
- **Caruncle** (inflamed)
  - conjunctiva (acute) — *see* Conjunctivitis, acute
  - labium (majus) (minus) N90.89
  - lacrimal — *see* Inflammation, lacrimal, passages
  - myrtiform N89.8
  - urethral (benign) N36.2
- **Cascade stomach** K31.2
- **Caseation lymphatic gland** (tuberculous) A18.2
- **Cassidy** (-Scholte) syndrome (malignant carcinoid) E34.0
- **Castellani's disease** A69.8
- **Castration, traumatic, male** S38.231 ☑
- **Casts in urine** R82.998
- **Cat**
  - cry syndrome Q93.4
  - ear Q17.3
  - eye syndrome Q92.8
- **Catabolism, senile** R54
- **Catalepsy** (hysterical) F44.2
  - schizophrenic F20.2
- **Cataplexy** (idiopathic) — *see* Narcolepsy
- **Cataract** (cortical) (immature) (incipient) H26.9
  - with
    - neovascularization — *see* Cataract, complicated
  - age-related — *see* Cataract, senile
  - anterior
    - and posterior axial embryonal Q12.0
    - pyramidal Q12.0
  - associated with
    - galactosemia E74.21 *[H28]*
    - myotonic disorders G71.19 *[H28]*
  - blue Q12.0
  - central Q12.0
  - cerulean Q12.0
  - complicated H26.20
    - with
      - neovascularization H26.21- ☑
      - ocular disorder H26.22- ☑
    - glaucomatous flecks H26.23- ☑
  - congenital Q12.0
  - coraliform Q12.0
  - coronary Q12.0
  - crystalline Q12.0
  - diabetic — *see* Diabetes, cataract
  - drug-induced H26.3- ☑
  - due to
    - ocular disorder — *see* Cataract, complicated
    - radiation H26.8
  - electric H26.8
  - extraction status Z98.4- ☑
  - glass-blower's H26.8
- **Cataract** — *continued*
  - heat ray H26.8
  - heterochromic — *see* Cataract, complicated
  - hypermature — *see* Cataract, senile, morgagnian type
  - in (due to)
    - chronic iridocyclitis — *see* Cataract, complicated
    - diabetes — *see* Diabetes, cataract
    - endocrine disease E34.9 *[H28]*
    - eye disease — *see* Cataract, complicated
    - hypoparathyroidism E20.9 *[H28]*
    - malnutrition-dehydration E46 *[H28]*
    - metabolic disease E88.9 *[H28]*
    - myotonic disorders G71.19 *[H28]*
    - nutritional disease E63.9 *[H28]*
  - infantile — *see* Cataract, presenile
  - irradiational — *see* Cataract, specified NEC
  - juvenile — *see* Cataract, presenile
  - malnutrition-dehydration E46 *[H28]*
  - morgagnian — *see* Cataract, senile, morgagnian type
  - myotonic G71.19 *[H28]*
  - myxedema E03.9 *[H28]*
  - nuclear
    - embryonal Q12.0
    - sclerosis — *see* Cataract, senile, nuclear
  - presenile H26.00- ☑
    - combined forms H26.06- ☑
    - cortical H26.01- ☑
    - lamellar — *see* Cataract, presenile, cortical
    - nuclear H26.03- ☑
    - specified NEC H26.09
    - subcapsular polar (anterior) H26.04- ☑
      - posterior H26.05- ☑
    - zonular — *see* Cataract, presenile, cortical
  - secondary H26.40
    - Soemmering's ring H26.41- ☑
    - specified NEC H26.49- ☑
    - to eye disease — *see* Cataract, complicated
  - senile H25.9
    - brunescens — *see* Cataract, senile, nuclear
    - combined forms H25.81- ☑
    - coronary — *see* Cataract, senile, incipient
    - cortical H25.01- ☑
    - hypermature — *see* Cataract, senile, morgagnian type
    - incipient (mature) (total) H25.09- ☑
      - cortical — *see* Cataract, senile, cortical
      - subcapsular — *see* Cataract, senile, subcapsular
    - morgagnian type (hypermature) H25.2- ☑
    - nuclear (sclerosis) H25.1- ☑
    - polar subcapsular (anterior) (posterior) — *see* Cataract, senile, incipient
    - punctate — *see* Cataract, senile, incipient
    - specified NEC H25.89
    - subcapsular polar (anterior) H25.03- ☑
      - posterior H25.04- ☑
  - snowflake — *see* Diabetes, cataract
  - specified NEC H26.8
  - toxic — *see* Cataract, drug-induced
  - traumatic H26.10- ☑
    - localized H26.11- ☑
    - partially resolved H26.12- ☑
    - total H26.13- ☑
  - zonular (perinuclear) Q12.0
- **Cataracta** — *see also* Cataract
  - brunescens — *see* Cataract, senile, nuclear
  - centralis pulverulenta Q12.0
  - cerulea Q12.0
  - complicata — *see* Cataract, complicated
  - congenita Q12.0
  - coralliformis Q12.0
  - coronaria Q12.0
  - diabetic — *see* Diabetes, cataract
  - membranacea
    - accreta — *see* Cataract, secondary
    - congenita Q12.0
  - nigra — *see* Cataract, senile, nuclear
  - sunflower — *see* Cataract, complicated
- **Catarrh, catarrhal** (acute) (febrile) (infectious) (inflammation) — *see also* condition J00
  - bronchial — *see* Bronchitis
  - chest — *see* Bronchitis
  - chronic J31.0
  - due to congenital syphilis A50.03
  - enteric — *see* Enteritis
  - eustachian H68.009
  - fauces — *see* Pharyngitis
  - gastrointestinal — *see* Enteritis

Catarrh, catarrhal — *continued*
gingivitis KØ5.ØØ
nonplaque induced KØ5.Ø1
plaque induced KØ5.ØØ
hay — *see* Fever, hay
intestinal — *see* Enteritis
larynx, chronic J37.Ø
liver B15.9
with hepatic coma B15.Ø
lung — *see* Bronchitis
middle ear, chronic — *see* Otitis, media, nonsuppurative, chronic, serous
mouth K12.1
nasal (chronic) — *see* Rhinitis
nasobronchial J31.1
nasopharyngeal (chronic) J31.1
acute JØØ
pulmonary — *see* Bronchitis
spring (eye) (vernal) — *see* Conjunctivitis, acute, atopic
summer (hay) — *see* Fever, hay
throat J31.2
tubotympanal — *see also* Otitis, media, nonsuppurative
chronic — *see* Otitis, media, nonsuppurative, chronic, serous
Catatonia (schizophrenic) F2Ø.2
Catatonic
disorder due to known physiologic condition FØ6.1
schizophrenia F2Ø.2
stupor R4Ø.1
Cat-scratch — *see also* Abrasion
disease or fever A28.1
Cauda equina — *see* condition
Cauliflower ear M95.1- ☑
Causalgia (upper limb) G56.4- ☑
lower limb G57.7- ☑
Cause
external, general effects T75.89 ☑
Caustic burn — *see* Corrosion, by site
Cavare's disease (familial periodic paralysis) G72.3
Cave-in, injury
crushing (severe) — *see* Crush
suffocation — *see* Asphyxia, traumatic, due to low oxygen, due to cave-in
Cavernitis (penis) N48.29
Cavernositis N48.29
Cavernous — *see* condition
Cavitation of lung — *see also* Tuberculosis, pulmonary
nontuberculous J98.4
Cavities, dental — *see* Caries, dental
Cavity
lung — *see* Cavitation of lung
optic papilla Q14.2
pulmonary — *see* Cavitation of lung
Cavovarus foot, congenital Q66.1- ☑
Cavus foot (congenital) Q66.7- ☑
acquired — *see* Deformity, limb, foot, specified NEC
Cazenave's disease L1Ø.2
CDKL5 (Cyclin-Dependent Kinase-Like 5 Deficiency Disorder) G4Ø.42
Cecitis K52.9
with perforation, peritonitis, or rupture K65.8
Cecoureterocele Q62.32
Cecum — *see* condition
Celiac
artery compression syndrome I77.4
disease (with steatorrhea) K9Ø.Ø
infantilism K9Ø.Ø
Cell(s), **cellular** — *see also* condition
in urine R82.998
Cellulitis (diffuse) (phlegmonous) (septic) (suppurative) LØ3.9Ø
abdominal wall LØ3.311
anaerobic A48.Ø
ankle — *see* Cellulitis, lower limb
anus K61.Ø
arm — *see* Cellulitis, upper limb
auricle (ear) — *see* Cellulitis, ear
axilla LØ3.11- ☑
back (any part) LØ3.312
breast (acute) (nonpuerperal) (subacute) N61.Ø
nipple N61.Ø
broad ligament
acute N73.Ø
buttock LØ3.317
cervical (meaning neck) LØ3.221
cervix (uteri) — *see* Cervicitis
cheek (external) LØ3.211

Cellulitis — *continued*
cheek — *continued*
internal K12.2
chest wall LØ3.313
chronic LØ3.9Ø
clostridial A48.Ø
corpus cavernosum N48.22
digit
finger — *see* Cellulitis, finger
toe — *see* Cellulitis, toe
Douglas' cul-de-sac or pouch
acute N73.Ø
drainage site (following operation) T81.49 ☑
ear (external) H6Ø.1- ☑
eosinophilic (granulomatous) L98.3
erysipelatous — *see* Erysipelas
external auditory canal — *see* Cellulitis, ear
eyelid — *see* Abscess, eyelid
face NEC LØ3.211
finger (intrathecal) (periosteal) (subcutaneous) (subcuticular) LØ3.Ø1- ☑
foot — *see* Cellulitis, lower limb
gangrenous — *see* Gangrene
genital organ NEC
female (external) N76.4
male N49.9
multiple sites N49.8
specified NEC N49.8
gluteal (region) LØ3.317
gonococcal A54.89
groin LØ3.314
hand — *see* Cellulitis, upper limb
head NEC LØ3.811
face (any part, except ear, eye and nose) LØ3.211
heel — *see* Cellulitis, lower limb
hip — *see* Cellulitis, lower limb
jaw (region) LØ3.211
knee — *see* Cellulitis, lower limb
labium (majus) (minus) — *see* Vulvitis
lacrimal passages — *see* Inflammation, lacrimal, passages
larynx J38.7
leg — *see* Cellulitis, lower limb
lip K13.Ø
lower limb LØ3.11- ☑
toe — *see* Cellulitis, toe
mouth (floor) K12.2
multiple sites, so stated LØ3.9Ø
nasopharynx J39.1
navel LØ3.316
newborn P38.9
with mild hemorrhage P38.1
without hemorrhage P38.9
neck (region) LØ3.221
nipple (acute) (nonpuerperal) (subacute) N61.Ø
nose (septum) (external) J34.Ø
orbit, orbital HØ5.Ø1- ☑
palate (soft) K12.2
pectoral (region) LØ3.313
pelvis, pelvic (chronic)
female — *see also* Disease, pelvis, inflammatory N73.2
acute N73.Ø
following ectopic or molar pregnancy OØ8.Ø
male K65.Ø
penis N48.22
perineal, perineum LØ3.315
periorbital LØ3.213
perirectal K61.1
peritonsillar J36
periurethral N34.Ø
periuterine — *see also* Disease, pelvis, inflammatory N73.2
acute N73.Ø
pharynx J39.1
preseptal LØ3.213
rectum K61.1
retroperitoneal K68.9
round ligament
acute N73.Ø
scalp (any part) LØ3.811
scrotum N49.2
seminal vesicle N49.Ø
shoulder — *see* Cellulitis, upper limb
specified site NEC LØ3.818
submandibular (region) (space) (triangle) K12.2
gland K11.3
submaxillary (region) K12.2

Cellulitis — *continued*
submaxillary — *continued*
gland K11.3
thigh — *see* Cellulitis, lower limb
thumb (intrathecal) (periosteal) (subcutaneous) (subcuticular) — *see* Cellulitis, finger
toe (intrathecal) (periosteal) (subcutaneous) (subcuticular) LØ3.Ø3- ☑
tonsil J36
trunk LØ3.319
abdominal wall LØ3.311
back (any part) LØ3.312
buttock LØ3.317
chest wall LØ3.313
groin LØ3.314
perineal, perineum LØ3.315
umbilicus LØ3.316
tuberculous (primary) A18.4
umbilicus LØ3.316
upper limb LØ3.11- ☑
axilla — *see* Cellulitis, axilla
finger — *see* Cellulitis, finger
thumb — *see* Cellulitis, finger
vaccinal T88.Ø ☑
vocal cord J38.3
vulva — *see* Vulvitis
wrist — *see* Cellulitis, upper limb
Cementoblastoma, benign — *see* Cyst, calcifying odontogenic
Cementoma — *see* Cyst, calcifying odontogenic
Cementoperiostitis — *see* Periodontitis
Cementosis KØ3.4
Central auditory processing disorder H93.25
Central pain syndrome G89.Ø
Cephalematocele, cephal(o)hematocele
newborn P52.8
birth injury P1Ø.8
traumatic — *see* Hematoma, brain
Cephalematoma, cephalhematoma (calcified)
newborn (birth injury) P12.Ø
traumatic — *see* Hematoma, brain
Cephalgia, cephalalgia — *see also* Headache
histamine G44.ØØ9
intractable G44.ØØ1
not intractable G44.ØØ9
trigeminal autonomic (TAC) NEC G44.Ø99
intractable G44.Ø91
not intractable G44.Ø99
Cephalic — *see* condition
Cephalitis — *see* Encephalitis
Cephalocele — *see* Encephalocele
Cephalomenia N94.89
Cephalopelvic — *see* condition
Cerclage (with cervical incompetence) in pregnancy — *see* Incompetence, cervix, in pregnancy
Cerebellitis — *see* Encephalitis
Cerebellum, cerebellar — *see* condition
Cerebral — *see* condition
Cerebritis — *see* Encephalitis
Cerebro-hepato-renal syndrome Q87.89
Cerebromalacia — *see* Softening, brain
sequelae of cerebrovascular disease I69.398
Cerebroside lipidosis E75.22
Cerebrospasticity (congenital) G8Ø.1
Cerebrospinal — *see* condition
Cerebrum — *see* condition
Ceroid-lipofuscinosis, neuronal E75.4
Cerumen (accumulation) (impacted) H61.2- ☑
Cervical — *see also* condition
auricle Q18.2
dysplasia in pregnancy — *see* Abnormal, cervix, in pregnancy or childbirth
erosion in pregnancy — *see* Abnormal, cervix, in pregnancy or childbirth
fibrosis in pregnancy — *see* Abnormal, cervix, in pregnancy or childbirth
fusion syndrome Q76.1
rib Q76.5
shortening (complicating pregnancy) O26.87- ☑
Cervicalgia M54.2
Cervicitis (acute) (atrophic) (chronic) (nonvenereal) (senile) (subacute) (with ulceration) N72
with
abortion — *see* Abortion, by type complicated by genital tract and pelvic infection
ectopic pregnancy OØ8.Ø
molar pregnancy OØ8.Ø

Chlamydia, chlamydial — *continued*
- endometritis A56.11
- epididymitis A56.19
- female
  - pelvic inflammatory disease A56.11
  - pelviperitonitis A56.11
- orchitis A56.19
- peritonitis A74.81
- pharyngitis A56.4
- proctitis A56.3
- psittaci (infection) A7Ø
- salpingitis A56.11
- sexually-transmitted infection NEC A56.8
- specified NEC A74.89
- urethritis A56.Ø1
- vulvovaginitis A56.Ø2

Chlamydiosis — *see* Chlamydia

Chloasma (skin) (idiopathic) (symptomatic) L81.1
- eyelid HØ2.719
  - hyperthyroid EØ5.9Ø *[HØ2.719]*
    - with thyroid storm EØ5.91 *[HØ2.719]*
  - left HØ2.716
    - lower HØ2.715
    - upper HØ2.714
  - right HØ2.713
    - lower HØ2.712
    - upper HØ2.711

Chloroma C92.3- ☑

Chlorosis D5Ø.9
- Egyptian B76.9 *[D63.8]*
- miner's B76.9 *[D63.8]*

Chlorotic anemia D5Ø.8

Chocolate cyst (ovary) N8Ø.1Ø- ☑

Choked
- disc or disk — *see* Papilledema
- on food, phlegm, or vomitus NOS — *see* Foreign body, by site
- while vomiting NOS — *see* Foreign body, by site

Chokes (resulting from bends) T7Ø.3 ☑

Choking sensation RØ9.89

Cholangiectasis K83.8

Cholangiocarcinoma
- with hepatocellular carcinoma, combined C22.Ø
- liver C22.1
- specified site NEC — *see* Neoplasm, malignant, by site
- unspecified site C22.1

Cholangiohepatitis K83.8
- due to fluke infestation B66.1

Cholangiohepatoma C22.Ø

Cholangiolitis (acute) (chronic) (extrahepatic) (gangrenous) (intrahepatic) K83.Ø9
- paratyphoidal — *see* Fever, paratyphoid
- typhoidal AØ1.Ø9

Cholangioma D13.4
- malignant — *see* Cholangiocarcinoma

Cholangitis (ascending) (recurrent) (secondary) (stenosing) (suppurative) K83.Ø9
- with calculus, bile duct — *see* Calculus, bile duct, with cholangitis
- chronic nonsuppurative destructive K74.3
- primary K83.Ø9
  - sclerosing K83.Ø1
- sclerosing K83.Ø9

Cholecystectasia K82.8

Cholecystitis K81.9
- with
  - calculus, stones in
    - bile duct (common) (hepatic) — *see* Calculus, bile duct, with cholecystitis
    - cystic duct — *see* Calculus, gallbladder, with cholecystitis
    - gallbladder — *see* Calculus, gallbladder, with cholecystitis
  - choledocholithiasis — *see* Calculus, bile duct, with cholecystitis
  - cholelithiasis — *see* Calculus, gallbladder, with cholecystitis
  - gangrene of gallbladder K82.A1
  - perforation of gallbladder K82.A2
- acute (emphysematous) (gangrenous) (suppurative) K81.Ø
  - with
    - calculus, stones in
      - cystic duct — *see* Calculus, gallbladder, with cholecystitis, acute
      - gallbladder — *see* Calculus, gallbladder, with cholecystitis, acute

Cholecystitis — *continued*
- acute — *continued*
  - with — *continued*
    - choledocholithiasis — *see* Calculus, bile duct, with cholecystitis, acute
    - cholelithiasis — *see* Calculus, gallbladder, with cholecystitis, acute
    - chronic cholecystitis K81.2
      - with gallbladder calculus K8Ø.12
        - with obstruction K8Ø.13
- chronic K81.1
  - with acute cholecystitis K81.2
    - with gallbladder calculus K8Ø.12
      - with obstruction K8Ø.13
- emphysematous (acute) — *see* Cholecystitis, acute
- gangrenous — *see* Cholecystitis, acute
- paratyphoidal, current AØ1.4
- suppurative — *see* Cholecystitis, acute
- typhoidal AØ1.Ø9

Cholecystolithiasis — *see* Calculus, gallbladder

Choledochitis (suppurative) K83.Ø9

Choledocholith — *see* Calculus, bile duct

Choledocholithiasis (common duct) (hepatic duct) — *see* Calculus, bile duct
- cystic — *see* Calculus, gallbladder
- typhoidal AØ1.Ø9

Cholelithiasis (cystic duct) (gallbladder) (impacted) (multiple) — *see* Calculus, gallbladder
- bile duct (common) (hepatic) — *see* Calculus, bile duct
- hepatic duct — *see* Calculus, bile duct
- specified NEC K8Ø.8Ø
  - with obstruction K8Ø.81

Cholemia — *see also* Jaundice
- familial (simple) (congenital) E8Ø.4
- Gilbert's E8Ø.4

Choleperitoneum, choleperitonitis K65.3

Cholera (Asiatic) (epidemic) (malignant) AØØ.9
- antimonial — *see* Poisoning, antimony
- classical AØØ.Ø
- due to Vibrio cholerae Ø1 AØØ.9
  - biovar cholerae AØØ.Ø
  - biovar eltor AØØ.1
  - el tor AØØ.1
- el tor AØØ.1

Cholerine — *see* Cholera

Cholestasis NEC K83.1
- with hepatocyte injury K71.Ø
- due to total parenteral nutrition (TPN) K76.89
- pure K71.Ø

Cholesteatoma (ear) (middle) (with reaction) H71.9- ☑
- attic H71.Ø- ☑
- external ear (canal) H6Ø.4- ☑
- mastoid H71.2- ☑
- postmastoidectomy cavity (recurrent) — *see* Complications, postmastoidectomy, recurrent cholesteatoma
- recurrent (postmastoidectomy) — *see* Complications, postmastoidectomy, recurrent cholesteatoma
- tympanum H71.1- ☑

Cholesteatosis, diffuse H71.3- ☑

Cholesteremia E78.ØØ

Cholesterin in vitreous — *see* Deposit, crystalline

Cholesterol
- deposit
  - retina H35.89
  - vitreous — *see* Deposit, crystalline
- elevated (high) E78.ØØ
  - with elevated (high) triglycerides E78.2
  - screening for Z13.22Ø
- imbibition of gallbladder K82.4

Cholesterolemia (essential) (pure) E78.ØØ
- familial E78.Ø1
- hereditary E78.Ø1

Cholesterolosis, cholesterosis (gallbladder) K82.4
- cerebrotendinous E75.5

Cholocolic fistula K82.3

Choluria R82.2

Chondritis M94.8X9
- aurical H61.Ø3- ☑
- costal (Tietze's) M94.Ø
- external ear H61.Ø3- ☑
- patella, posttraumatic — *see* Chondromalacia, patella
- pinna H61.Ø3- ☑
- purulent M94.8X- ☑
- tuberculous NEC A18.Ø2
  - intervertebral A18.Ø1

Chondroblastoma — *see also* Neoplasm, bone, benign

Chondroblastoma — *continued*
- malignant — *see* Neoplasm, bone, malignant

Chondrocalcinosis M11.2Ø
- ankle M11.27- ☑
- elbow M11.22- ☑
- familial M11.1Ø
  - ankle M11.17- ☑
  - elbow M11.12- ☑
  - foot joint M11.17- ☑
  - hand joint M11.14- ☑
  - hip M11.15- ☑
  - knee M11.16- ☑
  - multiple site M11.19
  - shoulder M11.11- ☑
  - vertebrae M11.18
  - wrist M11.13- ☑
- foot joint M11.27- ☑
- hand joint M11.24- ☑
- hip M11.25- ☑
- knee M11.26- ☑
- multiple site M11.29
- shoulder M11.21- ☑
- specified type NEC M11.2Ø
  - ankle M11.27- ☑
  - elbow M11.22- ☑
  - foot joint M11.27- ☑
  - hand joint M11.24- ☑
  - hip M11.25- ☑
  - knee M11.26- ☑
  - multiple site M11.29
  - shoulder M11.21- ☑
  - vertebrae M11.28
  - wrist M11.23- ☑
- vertebrae M11.28
- wrist M11.23- ☑

Chondrodermatitis nodularis helicis or anthelicis — *see* Perichondritis, ear

Chondrodysplasia Q78.9
- with hemangioma Q78.4
- calcificans congenita Q77.3
- fetalis Q77.4
- metaphyseal (Jansen's) (McKusick's) (Schmid's) Q78.8
- punctata Q77.3

Chondrodystrophy, chondrodystrophia (familial) (fetalis) (hypoplastic) Q78.9
- calcificans congenita Q77.3
- myotonic (congenital) G71.13
- punctata Q77.3

Chondroectodermal dysplasia Q77.6

Chondrogenesis imperfecta Q77.4

Chondrolysis M94.35- ☑

Chondroma — *see also* Neoplasm, cartilage, benign
- juxtacortical — *see* Neoplasm, bone, benign
- periosteal — *see* Neoplasm, bone, benign

Chondromalacia (systemic) M94.2Ø
- acromioclavicular joint M94.21- ☑
- ankle M94.27- ☑
- elbow M94.22- ☑
- foot joint M94.27- ☑
- glenohumeral joint M94.21- ☑
- hand joint M94.24- ☑
- hip M94.25- ☑
- knee M94.26- ☑
  - patella M22.4- ☑
- multiple sites M94.29
- patella M22.4- ☑
- rib M94.28
- sacroiliac joint M94.259
- shoulder M94.21- ☑
- sternoclavicular joint M94.21- ☑
- vertebral joint M94.28
- wrist M94.23- ☑

Chondromatosis — *see also* Neoplasm, cartilage, uncertain behavior
- internal Q78.4

Chondromyxosarcoma — *see* Neoplasm, cartilage, malignant

Chondro-osteodysplasia (Morquio-Brailsford type) E76.219

Chondro-osteodystrophy E76.29

Chondro-osteoma — *see* Neoplasm, bone, benign

Chondropathia tuberosa M94.Ø

Chondrosarcoma — *see* Neoplasm, cartilage, malignant
- juxtacortical — *see* Neoplasm, bone, malignant
- mesenchymal — *see* Neoplasm, connective tissue, malignant
- myxoid — *see* Neoplasm, cartilage, malignant

Cirrhosis, cirrhotic — *continued*
nutritional — *continued*
alcoholic K7Ø.3Ø
with ascites K7Ø.31
obstructive — *see* Cirrhosis, biliary
ovarian N83.8
pancreas (duct) K86.89
pigmentary E83.11Ø
portal K74.69
alcoholic K7Ø.3Ø
with ascites K7Ø.31
postnecrotic K74.69
alcoholic K7Ø.3Ø
with ascites K7Ø.31
pulmonary J84.1Ø
renal — *see* Sclerosis, renal
spleen D73.2
stasis K76.1
Todd's K74.3
unilobar K74.3
xanthomatous (biliary) K74.5
due to xanthomatosis (familial) (metabolic) (primary) E78.2
Cistern, subarachnoid R93.Ø
Citrullinemia E72.23
Citrullinuria E72.23
Civatte's disease or poikiloderma L57.3
CLAD — *see* Dysfunction, chronic, lung allograft
Clam digger's itch B65.3
Clammy skin R23.1
Clap — *see* Gonorrhea
Clarke-Hadfield syndrome (pancreatic infantilism) K86.89
Clark's paralysis G8Ø.9
Clastothrix L67.8
Claude Bernard-Horner syndrome G9Ø.2
traumatic — *see* Injury, nerve, cervical sympathetic
Claude's disease or syndrome G46.3
Claudicatio venosa intermittens I87.8
Claudication (intermittent) I73.9
cerebral (artery) G45.9
spinal cord (arteriosclerotic) G95.19
syphilitic A52.Ø9
venous (axillary) I87.8
Claustrophobia F4Ø.24Ø
Clavus (infected) L84
Clawfoot (congenital) Q66.89
acquired — *see* Deformity, limb, clawfoot
Clawhand (acquired) — *see also* Deformity, limb, clawhand
congenital Q68.1
Clawtoe (congenital) Q66.89
acquired — *see* Deformity, toe, specified NEC
Clay eating — *see* Pica
Cleansing of artificial opening — *see* Attention to, artificial, opening
Cleft (congenital) — *see also* Imperfect, closure
alveolar process M26.79
branchial (persistent) Q18.2
cyst Q18.Ø
fistula Q18.Ø
sinus Q18.Ø
cricoid cartilage, posterior Q31.8
cyst Q18.Ø
fistula Q18.Ø
sinus Q18.Ø
foot Q72.7 ☑
hand Q71.6 ☑
lip (unilateral) Q36.9
with cleft palate Q37.9
hard Q37.1
with soft Q37.5
soft Q37.3
with hard Q37.5
bilateral Q36.Ø
with cleft palate Q37.8
hard Q37.Ø
with soft Q37.4
soft Q37.2
with hard Q37.4
median Q36.1
nose Q3Ø.2
palate Q35.9
with cleft lip (unilateral) Q37.9
bilateral Q37.8
hard Q35.1
with
cleft lip (unilateral) Q37.1

Cleft — *continued*
palate — *continued*
hard — *continued*
with — *continued*
cleft lip — *continued*
bilateral Q37.Ø
soft Q35.5
with cleft lip (unilateral) Q37.5
bilateral Q37.4
medial Q35.5
soft Q35.3
with
cleft lip (unilateral) Q37.3
bilateral Q37.2
hard Q35.5
with cleft lip (unilateral) Q37.5
bilateral Q37.4
penis Q55.69
scrotum Q55.29
thyroid cartilage Q31.8
uvula Q35.7
Cleidocranial dysostosis Q74.Ø
Cleptomania F63.2
Clicking hip (newborn) R29.4
Climacteric (female) — *see also* Menopause
arthritis (any site) NEC — *see* Arthritis, specified form NEC
depression (single episode) F32.89
recurrent episode F33.8
male (symptoms) (syndrome) NEC N5Ø.89
melancholia (single episode) F32.89
recurrent episode F33.8
paranoid state F22
polyarthritis NEC — *see* Arthritis, specified form NEC
symptoms (female) N95.1
Clinical research investigation (clinical trial) (control subject) (normal comparison) (participant) ZØØ.6
Clitoris — *see* condition
Cloaca (persistent) Q43.7
Clonorchiasis, clonorchis infection (liver) B66.1
Clonus R25.8
Closed bite M26.29
Clostridium (C.) **perfringens, as cause of disease classified elsewhere** B96.7
Closure
congenital, nose Q3Ø.Ø
cranial sutures, premature Q75.ØØ9
defective or imperfect NEC — *see* Imperfect, closure
fistula, delayed — *see* Fistula
foramen ovale, imperfect Q21.12
hymen N89.6
interauricular septum, defective Q21.19
interventricular septum, defective Q21.Ø
lacrimal duct — *see also* Stenosis, lacrimal, duct
congenital Q1Ø.5
nose (congenital) Q3Ø.Ø
acquired M95.Ø
of artificial opening — *see* Attention to, artificial, opening
vagina N89.5
valve — *see* Endocarditis
vulva N9Ø.5
Clot (blood) — *see also* Embolism
artery (obstruction) (occlusion) — *see* Embolism
bladder N32.89
brain (intradural or extradural) — *see* Occlusion, artery, cerebral
circulation I74.9
heart — *see also* Infarct, myocardium
not resulting in infarction I51.3
vein — *see* Thrombosis
Clouded state R4Ø.1
epileptic — *see* Epilepsy, specified NEC
paroxysmal — *see* Epilepsy, specified NEC
Cloudy antrum, antra J32.Ø
Clouston's (hidrotic) **ectodermal dysplasia** Q82.4
Cloverleaf skull Q75.Ø51
Clubbed nail pachydermoperiostosis M89.4Ø *[L62]*
Clubbing of finger(s) (nails) R68.3
Clubfinger R68.3
congenital Q68.1
Clubfoot (congenital) Q66.89
acquired — *see* Deformity, limb, clubfoot
equinovarus Q66.Ø- ☑
paralytic — *see* Deformity, limb, clubfoot
Clubhand (congenital) (radial) Q71.4- ☑
acquired — *see* Deformity, limb, clubhand

Clubnail R68.3
congenital Q84.6
Clump, kidney Q63.1
Clumsiness, clumsy child syndrome F82
Cluttering F8Ø.81
Clutton's joints A5Ø.51 *[M12.8Ø]*
Coagulation, intravascular (diffuse) (disseminated) — *see also* Defibrination syndrome
complicating abortion — *see* Abortion, by type, complicated by, intravascular coagulation
COVID-19 associated — *see also* COVID-19 D65
following ectopic or molar pregnancy OØ8.1
Coagulopathy — *see also* Defect, coagulation
consumption D65
intravascular D65
newborn P6Ø
Coalition
calcaneo-scaphoid Q66.89
tarsal Q66.89
Coalminer's
elbow — *see* Bursitis, elbow, olecranon
lung or pneumoconiosis J6Ø
Coalworker's lung or pneumoconiosis J6Ø
Coarctation
aorta (preductal) (postductal) Q25.1
pulmonary artery Q25.71
Coated tongue K14.3
Coats' disease (exudative retinopathy) — *see* Retinopathy, exudative
Cocaine-induced
anxiety disorder F14.98Ø
bipolar and related disorder F14.94
depressive disorder F14.94
obsessive-compulsive and related disorder F14.988
psychotic disorder F14.959
sexual dysfunction F14.981
sleep disorder F14.982
Cocainism — *see* Disorder, cocaine use
Coccidioidomycosis B38.9
cutaneous B38.3
disseminated B38.7
generalized B38.7
meninges B38.4
prostate B38.81
pulmonary B38.2
acute B38.Ø
chronic B38.1
skin B38.3
specified NEC B38.89
Coccidioidosis — *see* Coccidioidomycosis
Coccidiosis (intestinal) AØ7.3
Coccydynia, coccygodynia M53.3
Coccyx — *see* condition
Cochin-China diarrhea K9Ø.1
Cockayne's syndrome Q87.19
Cocked up toe — *see* Deformity, toe, specified NEC
Cock's peculiar tumor L72.3
Codman's tumor — *see* Neoplasm, bone, benign
Coenurosis B71.8
Coffee-worker's lung J67.8
Cogan's syndrome H16.32- ☑
oculomotor apraxia H51.8
Coitus, painful (female) N94.1Ø
male N53.12
psychogenic F52.6
Cold JØØ
with influenza, flu, or grippe — *see* Influenza, with, respiratory manifestations NEC
agglutinin disease or hemoglobinuria (chronic) D59.12
bronchial — *see* Bronchitis
chest — *see* Bronchitis
common (head) JØØ
effects of T69.9 ☑
specified effect NEC T69.8 ☑
excessive, effects of T69.9 ☑
specified effect NEC T69.8 ☑
exhaustion from T69.8 ☑
exposure to T69.9 ☑
specified effect NEC T69.8 ☑
head JØØ
injury syndrome (newborn) P8Ø.Ø
on lung — *see* Bronchitis
rose J3Ø.1
sensitivity, auto-immune D59.12
symptoms JØØ
virus JØØ
Coldsore BØØ.1

- **Colibacillosis** A49.8
  - as the cause of other disease — *see also* Escherichia coli B96.20
  - generalized — *see also* Sepsis, Escherichia coli A41.51
- **Colic** (bilious) (infantile) (intestinal) (recurrent) (spasmodic) R10.83
  - abdomen R10.83
    - psychogenic F45.8
  - appendix, appendicular K38.8
  - bile duct — *see* Calculus, bile duct
  - biliary — *see* Calculus, bile duct
  - common duct — *see* Calculus, bile duct
  - cystic duct — *see* Calculus, gallbladder
  - Devonshire NEC — *see* Poisoning, lead
  - gallbladder — *see* Calculus, gallbladder
  - gallstone — *see* Calculus, gallbladder
    - gallbladder or cystic duct — *see* Calculus, gallbladder
  - hepatic (duct) — *see* Calculus, bile duct
  - hysterical F45.8
  - kidney N23
  - lead NEC — *see* Poisoning, lead
  - mucous K58.9
    - with diarrhea K58.0
    - psychogenic F54
  - nephritic N23
  - painter's NEC — *see* Poisoning, lead
  - pancreas K86.89
  - psychogenic F45.8
  - renal N23
  - saturnine NEC — *see* Poisoning, lead
  - ureter N23
  - urethral N36.8
    - due to calculus N21.1
  - uterus NEC N94.89
    - menstrual — *see* Dysmenorrhea
  - worm NOS B83.9
- **Colicystitis** — *see* Cystitis
- **Colitis** (acute) (catarrhal) (chronic) (noninfective) (hemorrhagic) — *see also* Enteritis K52.9
  - allergic K52.29
    - with
      - food protein-induced enterocolitis syndrome K52.21
      - proctocolitis K52.29
  - amebic (acute) — *see also* Amebiasis A06.0
    - nondysenteric A06.2
  - anthrax A22.2
  - bacillary — *see* Infection, Shigella
  - balantidial A07.0
  - Clostridium difficile
    - not specified as recurrent A04.72
    - recurrent A04.71
  - coccidial A07.3
  - collagenous K52.831
  - cystica superficialis K52.89
  - dietary counseling and surveillance (for) Z71.3
  - dietetic — *see also* Colitis, allergic K52.29
  - drug-induced K52.1
  - due to radiation K52.0
  - eosinophilic K52.82
  - food hypersensitivity — *see also* Colitis, allergic K52.29
  - giardial A07.1
  - granulomatous — *see* Enteritis, regional, large intestine
  - indeterminate, so stated K52.3
  - infectious — *see* Enteritis, infectious
  - ischemic K55.9
    - acute (subacute) — *see also* Ischemia, intestine, acute K55.039
    - chronic K55.1
    - due to mesenteric artery insufficiency K55.1
    - fulminant (acute) — *see also* Ischemia, intestine, acute K55.039
  - left sided K51.50
    - with
      - abscess K51.514
      - complication K51.519
        - specified NEC K51.518
      - fistula K51.513
      - obstruction K51.512
      - rectal bleeding K51.511
  - lymphocytic K52.832
  - membranous
    - psychogenic F54
  - microscopic K52.839
    - specified NEC K52.838
  - mucous — *see* Syndrome, irritable, bowel
    - psychogenic F54

Colitis — *continued*

  - noninfective K52.9
    - specified NEC K52.89
  - polyposa — *see* Polyp, colon, inflammatory
  - protozoal A07.9
  - pseudomembranous
    - not specified as recurrent A04.72
    - recurrent A04.71
  - pseudomucinous — *see* Syndrome, irritable, bowel
  - regional — *see* Enteritis, regional, large intestine
    - infectious A09
  - segmental — *see* Enteritis, regional, large intestine
  - septic — *see* Enteritis, infectious
  - spastic K58.9
    - with diarrhea K58.0
    - psychogenic F54
  - staphylococcal A04.8
    - foodborne A05.0
  - subacute ischemic — *see also* Ischemia, intestine, acute K55.039
  - thromboulcerative — *see also* Ischemia, intestine, acute K55.039
  - toxic NEC K52.1
    - due to Clostridium difficile
      - not specified as recurrent A04.72
      - recurrent A04.71
  - transmural — *see* Enteritis, regional, large intestine
  - trichomonal A07.8
  - tuberculous (ulcerative) A18.32
  - ulcerative (chronic) K51.90
    - with
      - complication K51.919
        - abscess K51.914
        - fistula K51.913
        - obstruction K51.912
        - rectal bleeding K51.911
        - specified complication NEC K51.918
    - enterocolitis — *see* Enterocolitis, ulcerative
    - ileocolitis — *see* Ileocolitis, ulcerative
    - mucosal proctocolitis — *see* Proctocolitis, mucosal
    - proctitis — *see* Proctitis, ulcerative
    - pseudopolyposis — *see* Polyp, colon, inflammatory
    - psychogenic F54
    - rectosigmoiditis — *see* Rectosigmoiditis, ulcerative
    - specified type NEC K51.80
      - with
        - complication K51.819
          - abscess K51.814
          - fistula K51.813
          - obstruction K51.812
          - rectal bleeding K51.811
          - specified complication NEC K51.818
- **Collagenosis, collagen disease** (nonvascular) (vascular) M35.9
  - cardiovascular I42.8
  - reactive perforating L87.1
  - specified NEC M35.89
- **Collapse** R55
  - adrenal E27.2
  - cardiorespiratory R57.0
  - cardiovascular R57.0
    - newborn P29.89
  - circulatory (peripheral) R57.9
    - during or after labor and delivery O75.1
    - following ectopic or molar pregnancy O08.3
    - newborn P29.89
  - during or
    - after labor and delivery O75.1
    - resulting from a procedure, not elsewhere classified T81.10 ☑
  - external ear canal — *see* Stenosis, external ear canal
  - general R55
  - heart — *see* Disease, heart
  - heat T67.1 ☑
  - hysterical F44.89
  - labyrinth, membranous (congenital) Q16.5
  - lung (massive) — *see also* Atelectasis J98.19
    - pressure due to anesthesia (general) (local) or other sedation T88.2 ☑
      - during labor and delivery O74.1
      - in pregnancy O29.02- ☑
      - postpartum, puerperal O89.09
  - myocardial — *see* Disease, heart
  - nervous F48.8
  - neurocirculatory F45.8
  - nose M95.0
  - postoperative T81.10 ☑
  - pulmonary — *see also* Atelectasis J98.19

Collapse — *continued*

  - pulmonary — *see also* Atelectasis — *continued*
    - newborn — *see* Atelectasis
  - trachea J39.8
  - tracheobronchial J98.09
  - valvular — *see* Endocarditis
  - vascular (peripheral) R57.9
    - during or after labor and delivery O75.1
    - following ectopic or molar pregnancy O08.3
    - newborn P29.89
  - vertebra M48.50- ☑
    - cervical region M48.52- ☑
    - cervicothoracic region M48.53- ☑
    - in (due to)
      - neoplasm (metastasis) M84.58- ☑
      - osteoporosis — *see also* Osteoporosis M80.88 ☑
        - cervical region M80.88 ☑
        - cervicothoracic region M80.88 ☑
        - lumbar region M80.88 ☑
        - lumbosacral region M80.88 ☑
        - multiple sites M80.88 ☑
        - occipito-atlanto-axial region M80.88 ☑
        - sacrococcygeal region M80.88 ☑
        - thoracic region M80.88 ☑
        - thoracolumbar region M80.88 ☑
      - specified disease NEC M48.50- ☑
        - cervical region M48.52- ☑
        - cervicothoracic region M48.53- ☑
        - lumbar region M48.56- ☑
        - lumbosacral region M48.57- ☑
        - occipito-atlanto-axial region M48.51- ☑
        - sacrococcygeal region M48.58- ☑
        - thoracic region M48.54- ☑
        - thoracolumbar region M48.55- ☑
    - lumbar region M48.56- ☑
    - lumbosacral region M48.57- ☑
    - occipito-atlanto-axial region M48.51- ☑
    - sacrococcygeal region M48.58- ☑
    - thoracic region M48.54- ☑
    - thoracolumbar region M48.55- ☑
- **Collateral** — *see also* condition
  - circulation (venous) I87.8
  - dilation, veins I87.8
- **Colles' fracture** S52.53- ☑
- **Collet** (-Sicard) syndrome G52.7
- **Collier's asthma or lung** J60
- **Collodion baby** Q80.2
- **Colloid nodule** (of thyroid) (cystic) E04.1
- **Coloboma** (iris) Q13.0
  - eyelid Q10.3
  - fundus Q14.8
  - lens Q12.2
  - optic disc (congenital) Q14.2
    - acquired H47.31- ☑
- **Coloenteritis** — *see* Enteritis
- **Colon** — *see* condition
- **Colonization**
  - MRSA (Methicillin resistant Staphylococcus aureus) Z22.322
  - MSSA (Methicillin susceptible Staphylococcus aureus) Z22.321
  - status — *see* Carrier (suspected) of
- **Coloptosis** K63.4
- **Color blindness** — *see* Deficiency, color vision
- **Colostomy**
  - attention to Z43.3
  - fitting or adjustment Z46.89
  - malfunctioning K94.03
  - status Z93.3
- **Colpitis** (acute) — *see* Vaginitis
- **Colpocele** N81.5
- **Colpocystitis** — *see* Vaginitis
- **Colpospasm** N94.2
- **Column, spinal, vertebral** — *see* condition
- **Coma** R40.20
  - with
    - motor response (none) R40.231 ☑
      - abnormal extensor posturing to pain or noxious stimuli (< 2 years of age) R40.232 ☑
      - abnormal flexure posturing to pain or noxious stimuli (0-5 years of age) R40.233 ☑
      - extensor posturing to pain or noxious stimuli (2-5 years of age) R40.232 ☑
      - flexion/decorticate posturing (< 2 years of age) R40.233 ☑
      - localizes pain (2-5 years of age) R40.235 ☑

- **Coma** — *continued*
  - with — *continued*
    - motor response — *continued*
      - normal or spontaneous movement (< 2 years of age) R4Ø.236 ☑
      - obeys commands (2-5 years of age) R4Ø.236 ☑
      - score of
        - 1 R4Ø.231 ☑
        - 2 R4Ø.232 ☑
        - 3 R4Ø.233 ☑
        - 4 R4Ø.234 ☑
        - 5 R4Ø.235 ☑
        - 6 R4Ø.236 ☑
      - withdraws from pain or noxious stimuli (Ø-5 years of age) R4Ø.234 ☑
      - withdraws to touch (< 2 years of age) R4Ø.235 ☑
    - opening of eyes (never) R4Ø.211 ☑
      - in response to
        - pain R4Ø.212 ☑
        - sound R4Ø.213 ☑
      - score of
        - 1 R4Ø.211 ☑
        - 2 R4Ø.212 ☑
        - 3 R4Ø.213 ☑
        - 4 R4Ø.214 ☑
      - spontaneous R4Ø.214 ☑
    - verbal response (none) R4Ø.221 ☑
      - confused conversation R4Ø.224 ☑
      - cooing or babbling or crying appropriately (<2 years of age) R4Ø.225 ☑
      - inappropriate crying or screaming (< 2 years of age) R4Ø.223 ☑
      - inappropriate words (2-5 years of age) R4Ø.224 ☑
      - inappropriate words R4Ø.223 ☑
      - incomprehensible sounds (2-5 years of age) R4Ø.222 ☑
      - incomprehensible words R4Ø.222 ☑
      - irritable cries (< 2 years of age) R4Ø.224 ☑
      - moans/grunts to pain; restless (< 2 years old) R4Ø.222 ☑
      - oriented R4Ø.225 ☑
      - score of
        - 1 R4Ø.221 ☑
        - 2 R4Ø.222 ☑
        - 3 R4Ø.223 ☑
        - 4 R4Ø.224 ☑
        - 5 R4Ø.225 ☑
      - screaming (2-5 years of age) R4Ø.223 ☑
      - uses appropriate words (2-5 years of age) R4Ø.225 ☑
  - eclamptic — *see* Eclampsia
  - epileptic — *see* Epilepsy
  - Glasgow, scale score — *see* Glasgow coma scale
  - hepatic — *see* Failure, hepatic, by type, with coma
  - hyperglycemic (diabetic) — *see* Diabetes, by type, with hyperosmolarity, with coma
  - hyperosmolar (diabetic) — *see* Diabetes, by type, with hyperosmolarity, with coma
  - hypoglycemic (diabetic) — *see* Diabetes, by type, with hypoglycemia, with coma
    - nondiabetic E15
  - in diabetes — *see* Diabetes, coma
  - insulin-induced — *see* Coma, hypoglycemic
  - ketoacidotic (diabetic) — *see* Diabetes, by type, with ketoacidosis, with coma
  - myxedematous EØ3.5
  - newborn P91.5
  - nontraumatic, due to underlying condition R4Ø.2A
  - persistent vegetative state R4Ø.3
  - secondary R4Ø.2A
  - specified NEC, without documented Glasgow coma scale score, or with partial Glasgow coma scale score reported R4Ø.244 ☑
- **Comatose** — *see* Coma
- **Combat fatigue** F43.Ø
- **Combined** — *see* condition
- **Comedo, comedones** (giant) L7Ø.Ø
- **Comedocarcinoma** — *see also* Neoplasm, breast, malignant
  - noninfiltrating
    - breast DØ5.8- ☑
    - specified site — *see* Neoplasm, in situ, by site
    - unspecified site DØ5.8- ☑
- **Comedomastitis** — *see* Ectasia, mammary duct
- **Comminuted fracture** — *code as* Fracture, closed
- **Common**
  - arterial trunk Q2Ø.Ø
  - atrioventricular canal Q21.23
  - atrium Q21.19
  - cold (head) JØØ
  - truncus (arteriosus) Q2Ø.Ø
  - variable immunodeficiency — *see* Immunodeficiency, common variable
  - ventricle Q2Ø.4
- **Commotio, commotion** (current)
  - brain — *see* Injury, intracranial, concussion
  - cerebri — *see* Injury, intracranial, concussion
  - retinae SØ5.8X- ☑
  - spinal cord — *see* Injury, spinal cord, by region
  - spinalis — *see* Injury, spinal cord, by region
- **Communication**
  - between
    - base of aorta and pulmonary artery Q21.4
    - left ventricle and right atrium Q2Ø.5
    - pericardial sac and pleural sac Q34.8
    - pulmonary artery and pulmonary vein, congenital Q25.72
  - congenital between uterus and digestive or urinary tract Q51.7
- **Compartment syndrome** (deep) (posterior) (traumatic) T79.AØ ☑ (*following* T79.7)
  - abdomen T79.A3 ☑ (*following* T79.7)
  - lower extremity (hip, buttock, thigh, leg, foot, toes) T79.A2 ☑ (*following* T79.7)
  - nontraumatic
    - abdomen M79.A3 (*following* M79.7)
    - lower extremity (hip, buttock, thigh, leg, foot, toes) M79.A2- ☑ (*following* M79.7)
    - specified site NEC M79.A9 (*following* M79.7)
    - upper extremity (shoulder, arm, forearm, wrist, hand, fingers) M79.A1- ☑ (*following* M79.7)
  - specified site NEC T79.A9 ☑ (*following* T79.7)
  - upper extremity (shoulder, arm, forearm, wrist, hand, fingers) T79.A1- ☑ (*following* T79.7)
- **Compensation**
  - failure — *see* Disease, heart
  - neurosis, psychoneurosis — *see* Disorder, factitious
- **Complaint** — *see also* Disease
  - bowel, functional K59.9
    - psychogenic F45.8
  - intestine, functional K59.9
    - psychogenic F45.8
  - kidney — *see* Disease, renal
  - miners' J6Ø
- **Complete** — *see* condition
- **Complex**
  - Addison-Schilder E71.528
  - cardiorenal — *see* Hypertension, cardiorenal
  - Costen's M26.69
  - disseminated mycobacterium avium- intracellulare (DMAC) A31.2
  - Eisenmenger's (ventricular septal defect) I27.83
  - hypersexual F52.8
  - jumped process, spine — *see* Dislocation, vertebra
  - primary, tuberculous A15.7
  - Schilder-Addison E71.528
  - subluxation (vertebral) M99.19
    - abdomen M99.19
    - acromioclavicular M99.17
    - cervical region M99.11
    - cervicothoracic M99.11
    - costochondral M99.18
    - costovertebral M99.18
    - head region M99.1Ø
    - hip M99.15
    - lower extremity M99.16
    - lumbar region M99.13
    - lumbosacral M99.13
    - occipitocervical M99.1Ø
    - pelvic region M99.15
    - pubic M99.15
    - rib cage M99.18
    - sacral region M99.14
    - sacrococcygeal M99.14
    - sacroiliac M99.14
    - specified NEC M99.19
    - sternochondral M99.18
    - sternoclavicular M99.17
    - thoracic region M99.12
    - thoracolumbar M99.12
    - upper extremity M99.17
- **Complex** — *continued*
  - Taussig-Bing (transposition, aorta and overriding pulmonary artery) Q2Ø.1
- **Complication**(s) (from) (of)
  - accidental puncture or laceration during a procedure (of) — *see* Complications, intraoperative (intraprocedural), puncture or laceration
  - amputation stump (surgical) (late) NEC T87.9
    - dehiscence T87.81
    - infection or inflammation T87.4Ø
      - lower limb T87.4- ☑
      - upper limb T87.4- ☑
    - necrosis T87.5Ø
      - lower limb T87.5- ☑
      - upper limb T87.5- ☑
    - neuroma T87.3Ø
      - lower limb T87.3- ☑
      - upper limb T87.3- ☑
    - specified type NEC T87.89
  - anastomosis (and bypass) — *see also* Complications, prosthetic device or implant
    - intestinal (internal) NEC K91.89
      - involving urinary tract N99.89
    - urinary tract (involving intestinal tract) N99.89
    - vascular — *see* Complications, cardiovascular device or implant
  - anesthesia, anesthetic — *see also* Anesthesia, complication T88.59 ☑
    - brain, postpartum, puerperal O89.2
    - cardiac
      - in
        - labor and delivery O74.2
        - pregnancy O29.19- ☑
      - postpartum, puerperal O89.1
    - central nervous system
      - in
        - labor and delivery O74.3
        - pregnancy O29.29- ☑
      - postpartum, puerperal O89.2
    - difficult or failed intubation T88.4 ☑
      - in pregnancy O29.6- ☑
    - failed sedation (conscious) (moderate) during procedure T88.52 ☑
    - general, unintended awareness during procedure T88.53 ☑
    - hyperthermia, malignant T88.3 ☑
    - hypothermia T88.51 ☑
    - intubation failure T88.4 ☑
    - malignant hyperthermia T88.3 ☑
    - pulmonary
      - in
        - labor and delivery O74.1
        - pregnancy NEC O29.Ø9- ☑
      - postpartum, puerperal O89.Ø9
    - shock T88.2 ☑
    - spinal and epidural
      - in
        - labor and delivery NEC O74.6
          - headache O74.5
        - pregnancy NEC O29.5X- ☑
      - postpartum, puerperal NEC O89.5
        - headache O89.4
    - unintended awareness under general anesthesia during procedure T88.53 ☑
  - anti-reflux device — *see* Complications, esophageal anti-reflux device
  - aortic (bifurcation) graft — *see* Complications, graft, vascular
  - aortocoronary (bypass) graft — *see* Complications, coronary artery (bypass) graft
  - aortofemoral (bypass) graft — *see* Complications, extremity artery (bypass) graft
  - arteriovenous
    - fistula, surgically created T82.9 ☑
      - embolism T82.818 ☑
      - fibrosis T82.828 ☑
      - hemorrhage T82.838 ☑
      - infection or inflammation T82.7 ☑
      - mechanical
        - breakdown T82.51Ø ☑
        - displacement T82.52Ø ☑
        - leakage T82.53Ø ☑
        - malposition T82.52Ø ☑
        - obstruction T82.59Ø ☑
        - perforation T82.59Ø ☑
        - protrusion T82.59Ø ☑
      - pain T82.848 ☑

- **Complication**(s) — *continued*
  - arteriovenous — *continued*
    - fistula, surgically created — *continued*
      - specified type NEC T82.898 ☑
      - stenosis T82.858 ☑
      - thrombosis T82.868 ☑
    - shunt, surgically created T82.9 ☑
      - embolism T82.818 ☑
      - fibrosis T82.828 ☑
      - hemorrhage T82.838 ☑
      - infection or inflammation T82.7 ☑
      - mechanical
        - breakdown T82.511 ☑
        - displacement T82.521 ☑
        - leakage T82.531 ☑
        - malposition T82.521 ☑
        - obstruction T82.591 ☑
        - perforation T82.591 ☑
        - protrusion T82.591 ☑
      - pain T82.848 ☑
      - specified type NEC T82.898 ☑
      - stenosis T82.858 ☑
      - thrombosis T82.868 ☑
  - arthroplasty — *see* Complications, joint prosthesis
  - artificial
    - fertilization or insemination N98.9
      - attempted introduction (of)
        - embryo in embryo transfer N98.3
        - ovum following in vitro fertilization N98.2
      - hyperstimulation of ovaries N98.1
      - infection N98.0
      - specified NEC N98.8
    - heart T82.9 ☑
      - embolism T82.817 ☑
      - fibrosis T82.827 ☑
      - hemorrhage T82.837 ☑
      - infection or inflammation T82.7 ☑
      - mechanical
        - breakdown T82.512 ☑
        - displacement T82.522 ☑
        - leakage T82.532 ☑
        - malposition T82.522 ☑
        - obstruction T82.592 ☑
        - perforation T82.592 ☑
        - protrusion T82.592 ☑
      - pain T82.847 ☑
      - specified type NEC T82.897 ☑
      - stenosis T82.857 ☑
      - thrombosis T82.867 ☑
    - opening
      - cecostomy — *see* Complications, colostomy
      - colostomy — *see* Complications, colostomy
      - cystostomy — *see* Complications, cystostomy
      - enterostomy — *see* Complications, enterostomy
      - gastrostomy — *see* Complications, gastrostomy
      - ileostomy — *see* Complications, enterostomy
      - jejunostomy — *see* Complications, enterostomy
      - nephrostomy — *see* Complications, stoma, urinary tract
      - tracheostomy — *see* Complications, tracheostomy
      - ureterostomy — *see* Complications, stoma, urinary tract
      - urethrostomy — *see* Complications, stoma, urinary tract
  - balloon implant or device
    - gastrointestinal T85.9 ☑
      - embolism T85.818 ☑
      - fibrosis T85.828 ☑
      - hemorrhage T85.838 ☑
      - infection and inflammation T85.79 ☑
      - pain T85.848 ☑
      - specified type NEC T85.898 ☑
      - stenosis T85.858 ☑
      - thrombosis T85.868 ☑
    - vascular (counterpulsation) T82.9 ☑
      - embolism T82.818 ☑
      - fibrosis T82.828 ☑
      - hemorrhage T82.838 ☑
      - infection or inflammation T82.7 ☑
      - mechanical
        - breakdown T82.513 ☑
        - displacement T82.523 ☑
        - leakage T82.533 ☑
        - malposition T82.523 ☑
        - obstruction T82.593 ☑

- **Complication**(s) — *continued*
  - balloon implant or device — *continued*
    - vascular — *continued*
      - mechanical — *continued*
        - perforation T82.593 ☑
        - protrusion T82.593 ☑
      - pain T82.848 ☑
      - specified type NEC T82.898 ☑
      - stenosis T82.858 ☑
      - thrombosis T82.868 ☑
  - bariatric procedure
    - gastric band procedure K95.09
      - infection K95.01
    - specified procedure NEC K95.89
      - infection K95.81
  - bile duct implant (prosthetic) T85.9 ☑
    - embolism T85.818 ☑
    - fibrosis T85.828 ☑
    - hemorrhage T85.838 ☑
    - infection and inflammation T85.79 ☑
    - mechanical
      - breakdown T85.510 ☑
      - displacement T85.520 ☑
      - malfunction T85.510 ☑
      - malposition T85.520 ☑
      - obstruction T85.590 ☑
      - perforation T85.590 ☑
      - protrusion T85.590 ☑
      - specified NEC T85.590 ☑
    - pain T85.848 ☑
    - specified type NEC T85.898 ☑
    - stenosis T85.858 ☑
    - thrombosis T85.868 ☑
  - bladder device (auxiliary) — *see* Complications, genitourinary, device or implant, urinary system
  - bleeding (postoperative) — *see* Complication, postoperative, hemorrhage
    - intraoperative — *see* Complication, intraoperative, hemorrhage
  - blood vessel graft — *see* Complications, graft, vascular
  - bone
    - device NEC T84.9 ☑
      - embolism T84.81 ☑
      - fibrosis T84.82 ☑
      - hemorrhage T84.83 ☑
      - infection or inflammation T84.7 ☑
      - mechanical
        - breakdown T84.318 ☑
        - displacement T84.328 ☑
        - malposition T84.328 ☑
        - obstruction T84.398 ☑
        - perforation T84.398 ☑
        - protrusion T84.398 ☑
      - pain T84.84 ☑
      - specified type NEC T84.89 ☑
      - stenosis T84.85 ☑
      - thrombosis T84.86 ☑
    - graft — *see* Complications, graft, bone
    - growth stimulator (electrode) — *see* Complications, electronic stimulator device, bone
    - marrow transplant — *see* Complications, transplant, bone, marrow
  - brain neurostimulator (electrode) — *see* Complications, electronic stimulator device, brain
  - breast implant (prosthetic) T85.9 ☑
    - capsular contracture T85.44 ☑
    - embolism T85.818 ☑
    - fibrosis T85.828 ☑
    - hemorrhage T85.838 ☑
    - infection and inflammation T85.79 ☑
    - mechanical
      - breakdown T85.41 ☑
      - displacement T85.42 ☑
      - leakage T85.43 ☑
      - malposition T85.42 ☑
      - obstruction T85.49 ☑
      - perforation T85.49 ☑
      - protrusion T85.49 ☑
      - specified NEC T85.49 ☑
    - pain T85.848 ☑
    - specified type NEC T85.898 ☑
    - stenosis T85.858 ☑
    - thrombosis T85.868 ☑
  - bypass — *see also* Complications, prosthetic device or implant

- **Complication**(s) — *continued*
  - bypass — *see also* Complications, prosthetic device or implant — *continued*
    - aortocoronary — *see* Complications, coronary artery (bypass) graft
    - arterial — *see also* Complications, graft, vascular
      - extremity — *see* Complications, extremity artery (bypass) graft
  - cardiac — *see also* Disease, heart
    - device, implant or graft T82.9 ☑
      - embolism T82.817 ☑
      - fibrosis T82.827 ☑
      - hemorrhage T82.837 ☑
      - infection or inflammation T82.7 ☑
        - valve prosthesis T82.6 ☑
      - mechanical
        - breakdown T82.519 ☑
          - specified device NEC T82.518 ☑
        - displacement T82.529 ☑
          - specified device NEC T82.528 ☑
        - leakage T82.539 ☑
          - specified device NEC T82.538 ☑
        - malposition T82.529 ☑
          - specified device NEC T82.528 ☑
        - obstruction T82.599 ☑
          - specified device NEC T82.598 ☑
        - perforation T82.599 ☑
          - specified device NEC T82.598 ☑
        - protrusion T82.599 ☑
          - specified device NEC T82.598 ☑
      - pain T82.847 ☑
      - specified type NEC T82.897 ☑
      - stenosis T82.857 ☑
      - thrombosis T82.867 ☑
  - cardiovascular device, graft or implant T82.9 ☑
    - aortic graft — *see* Complications, graft, vascular
    - arteriovenous
      - fistula, artificial — *see* Complication, arteriovenous, fistula, surgically created
      - shunt — *see* Complication, arteriovenous, shunt, surgically created
    - artificial heart — *see* Complication, artificial, heart
    - balloon (counterpulsation) device — *see* Complication, balloon implant, vascular
    - carotid artery graft — *see* Complications, graft, vascular
    - coronary bypass graft — *see* Complication, coronary artery (bypass) graft
    - dialysis catheter (vascular) — *see* Complication, catheter, dialysis
    - electronic T82.9 ☑
      - electrode T82.9 ☑
        - embolism T82.817 ☑
        - fibrosis T82.827 ☑
        - hemorrhage T82.837 ☑
        - infection T82.7 ☑
        - mechanical
          - breakdown T82.110 ☑
          - displacement T82.120 ☑
          - leakage T82.190 ☑
          - obstruction T82.190 ☑
          - perforation T82.190 ☑
          - protrusion T82.190 ☑
          - specified type NEC T82.190 ☑
        - pain T82.847 ☑
        - specified NEC T82.897 ☑
        - stenosis T82.857 ☑
        - thrombosis T82.867 ☑
      - embolism T82.817 ☑
      - fibrosis T82.827 ☑
      - hemorrhage T82.837 ☑
      - infection T82.7 ☑
      - mechanical
        - breakdown T82.119 ☑
        - displacement T82.129 ☑
        - leakage T82.199 ☑
        - obstruction T82.199 ☑
        - perforation T82.199 ☑
        - protrusion T82.199 ☑
        - specified type NEC T82.199 ☑
      - pain T82.847 ☑
      - pulse generator T82.9 ☑
        - embolism T82.817 ☑
        - fibrosis T82.827 ☑
        - hemorrhage T82.837 ☑
        - infection T82.7 ☑

Complication(s) — *continued*
- cardiovascular device, graft or implant — *continued*
  - electronic — *continued*
    - pulse generator — *continued*
      - mechanical
        - breakdown T82.111 ☑
        - displacement T82.121 ☑
        - leakage T82.191 ☑
        - obstruction T82.191 ☑
        - perforation T82.191 ☑
        - protrusion T82.191 ☑
        - specified type NEC T82.191 ☑
      - pain T82.847 ☑
      - specified NEC T82.897 ☑
      - stenosis T82.857 ☑
      - thrombosis T82.867 ☑
    - specified condition NEC T82.897 ☑
    - specified device NEC T82.9 ☑
      - embolism T82.817 ☑
      - fibrosis T82.827 ☑
      - hemorrhage T82.837 ☑
      - infection T82.7 ☑
      - mechanical
        - breakdown T82.118 ☑
        - displacement T82.128 ☑
        - leakage T82.198 ☑
        - obstruction T82.198 ☑
        - perforation T82.198 ☑
        - protrusion T82.198 ☑
        - specified type NEC T82.198 ☑
      - pain T82.847 ☑
      - specified NEC T82.897 ☑
      - stenosis T82.857 ☑
      - thrombosis T82.867 ☑
    - stenosis T82.857 ☑
    - thrombosis T82.867 ☑
  - extremity artery graft — *see* Complication, extremity artery (bypass) graft
  - femoral artery graft — *see* Complication, extremity artery (bypass) graft
  - heart
    - transplant — *see* Complication, transplant, heart
    - valve — *see* Complication, prosthetic device, heart valve
      - graft — *see* Complication, heart, valve, graft
  - heart-lung transplant — *see* Complication, transplant, heart, with lung
  - infection or inflammation T82.7 ☑
  - umbrella device — *see* Complication, umbrella device, vascular
  - vascular graft (or anastomosis) — *see* Complication, graft, vascular
- carotid artery (bypass) graft — *see* Complications, graft, vascular
- catheter (device) NEC — *see also* Complications, prosthetic device or implant
  - cranial infusion
    - infection and inflammation T85.735 ☑
    - mechanical
      - breakdown T85.61Ø ☑
      - displacement T85.62Ø ☑
      - leakage T85.63Ø ☑
      - malfunction T85.69Ø ☑
      - malposition T85.62Ø ☑
      - obstruction T85.69Ø ☑
      - perforation T85.69Ø ☑
      - protrusion T85.69Ø ☑
      - specified NEC T85.69Ø ☑
  - cystostomy T83.9 ☑
    - embolism T83.81 ☑
    - fibrosis T83.82 ☑
    - hemorrhage T83.83 ☑
    - infection and inflammation T83.51Ø ☑
    - mechanical
      - breakdown T83.Ø1Ø ☑
      - displacement T83.Ø2Ø ☑
      - leakage T83.Ø3Ø ☑
      - malposition T83.Ø2Ø ☑
      - obstruction T83.Ø9Ø ☑
      - perforation T83.Ø9Ø ☑
      - protrusion T83.Ø9Ø ☑
      - specified NEC T83.Ø9Ø ☑
    - pain T83.84 ☑
    - specified type NEC T83.89 ☑
    - stenosis T83.85 ☑
    - thrombosis T83.86 ☑

Complication(s) — *continued*
- catheter — *see also* Complications, prosthetic device or implant — *continued*
  - dialysis (vascular) T82.9 ☑
    - embolism T82.818 ☑
    - fibrosis T82.828 ☑
    - hemorrhage T82.838 ☑
    - infection and inflammation T82.7 ☑
    - intraperitoneal — *see* Complications, catheter, intraperitoneal
    - mechanical
      - breakdown T82.41 ☑
      - displacement T82.42 ☑
      - leakage T82.43 ☑
      - malposition T82.42 ☑
      - obstruction T82.49 ☑
      - perforation T82.49 ☑
      - protrusion T82.49 ☑
    - pain T82.848 ☑
    - specified type NEC T82.898 ☑
    - stenosis T82.858 ☑
    - thrombosis T82.868 ☑
  - epidural infusion T85.9 ☑
    - embolism T85.81Ø ☑
    - fibrosis T85.82Ø ☑
    - hemorrhage T85.83Ø ☑
    - infection and inflammation T85.735 ☑
    - mechanical
      - breakdown T85.61Ø ☑
      - displacement T85.62Ø ☑
      - leakage T85.63Ø ☑
      - malfunction T85.69Ø ☑
      - malposition T85.62Ø ☑
      - obstruction T85.69Ø ☑
      - perforation T85.69Ø ☑
      - protrusion T85.69Ø ☑
      - specified NEC T85.69Ø ☑
    - pain T85.84Ø ☑
    - specified type NEC T85.89Ø ☑
    - stenosis T85.85Ø ☑
    - thrombosis T85.86Ø ☑
  - intraperitoneal dialysis T85.9 ☑
    - embolism T85.818 ☑
    - fibrosis T85.828 ☑
    - hemorrhage T85.838 ☑
    - infection and inflammation T85.71 ☑
    - mechanical
      - breakdown T85.611 ☑
      - displacement T85.621 ☑
      - leakage T85.631 ☑
      - malfunction T85.611 ☑
      - malposition T85.621 ☑
      - obstruction T85.691 ☑
      - perforation T85.691 ☑
      - protrusion T85.691 ☑
      - specified NEC T85.691 ☑
    - pain T85.848 ☑
    - specified type NEC T85.898 ☑
    - stenosis T85.858 ☑
    - thrombosis T85.868 ☑
  - intrathecal infusion
    - infection and inflammation T85.735 ☑
    - mechanical
      - breakdown T85.61Ø ☑
      - displacement T85.62Ø ☑
      - leakage T85.63Ø ☑
      - malfunction T85.69Ø ☑
      - malposition T85.62Ø ☑
      - obstruction T85.69Ø ☑
      - perforation T85.69Ø ☑
      - protrusion T85.69Ø ☑
      - specified NEC T85.69Ø ☑
  - intravenous infusion T82.9 ☑
    - embolism T82.818 ☑
    - fibrosis T82.828 ☑
    - hemorrhage T82.838 ☑
    - infection or inflammation T82.7 ☑
    - mechanical
      - breakdown T82.514 ☑
      - displacement T82.524 ☑
      - leakage T82.534 ☑
      - malposition T82.524 ☑
      - obstruction T82.594 ☑
      - perforation T82.594 ☑
      - protrusion T82.594 ☑
    - pain T82.848 ☑

Complication(s) — *continued*
- catheter — *see also* Complications, prosthetic device or implant — *continued*
  - intravenous infusion — *continued*
    - specified type NEC T82.898 ☑
    - stenosis T82.858 ☑
    - thrombosis T82.868 ☑
  - spinal infusion
    - infection and inflammation T85.735 ☑
    - mechanical
      - breakdown T85.61Ø ☑
      - displacement T85.62Ø ☑
      - leakage T85.63Ø ☑
      - malfunction T85.69Ø ☑
      - malposition T85.62Ø ☑
      - obstruction T85.69Ø ☑
      - perforation T85.69Ø ☑
      - protrusion T85.69Ø ☑
      - specified NEC T85.69Ø ☑
  - subarachnoid infusion
    - infection and inflammation T85.735 ☑
    - mechanical
      - breakdown T85.61Ø ☑
      - displacement T85.62Ø ☑
      - leakage T85.63Ø ☑
      - malfunction T85.69Ø ☑
      - malposition T85.62Ø ☑
      - obstruction T85.69Ø ☑
      - perforation T85.69Ø ☑
      - protrusion T85.69Ø ☑
      - specified NEC T85.69Ø ☑
  - subdural infusion T85.9 ☑
    - embolism T85.81Ø ☑
    - fibrosis T85.82Ø ☑
    - hemorrhage T85.83Ø ☑
    - infection and inflammation T85.735 ☑
    - mechanical
      - breakdown T85.61Ø ☑
      - displacement T85.62Ø ☑
      - leakage T85.63Ø ☑
      - malfunction T85.69Ø ☑
      - malposition T85.62Ø ☑
      - obstruction T85.69Ø ☑
      - perforation T85.69Ø ☑
      - protrusion T85.69Ø ☑
      - specified NEC T85.69Ø ☑
    - pain T85.84Ø ☑
    - specified type NEC T85.89Ø ☑
    - stenosis T85.85Ø ☑
    - thrombosis T85.86Ø ☑
  - urethral T83.9 ☑
    - displacement T83.Ø28 ☑
    - embolism T83.81 ☑
    - fibrosis T83.82 ☑
    - hemorrhage T83.83 ☑
    - indwelling
      - breakdown T83.Ø11 ☑
      - displacement T83.Ø21 ☑
      - infection and inflammation T83.511 ☑
      - leakage T83.Ø31 ☑
      - specified complication NEC T83.Ø91 ☑
    - infection and inflammation T83.511 ☑
    - leakage T83.Ø38 ☑
    - malposition T83.Ø28 ☑
    - mechanical
      - breakdown T83.Ø11 ☑
    - obstruction (mechanical) T83.Ø91 ☑
    - pain T83.84 ☑
    - perforation T83.Ø91 ☑
    - protrusion T83.Ø91 ☑
    - specified type NEC T83.Ø91 ☑
    - stenosis T83.85 ☑
    - thrombosis T83.86 ☑
  - urinary NEC
    - breakdown T83.Ø18 ☑
    - displacement T83.Ø28 ☑
    - infection and inflammation T83.518 ☑
    - leakage T83.Ø38 ☑
    - specified complication NEC T83.Ø98 ☑
- cecostomy (stoma) — *see* Complications, colostomy
- cesarean delivery wound NEC O9Ø.89
  - disruption O9Ø.Ø
  - hematoma O9Ø.2
  - infection (following delivery) O86.ØØ
- chemotherapy (antineoplastic) NEC T88.7 ☑

- **Complication**(s) — *continued*
  - gastrostomy — *continued*
    - specified complication NEC K94.29
  - genitourinary
    - device or implant T83.9 ☑
      - genital tract T83.9 ☑
        - infection or inflammation T83.69 ☑
        - intrauterine contraceptive device — *see* Complications, intrauterine, contraceptive device
        - mechanical — *see* Complications, by device, mechanical
        - mesh — *see* Complications, prosthetic device or implant, mesh
        - penile prosthesis — *see* Complications, prosthetic device, penile
        - specified type NEC T83.89 ☑
          - embolism T83.81 ☑
          - fibrosis T83.82 ☑
          - hemorrhage T83.83 ☑
          - pain T83.84 ☑
          - specified complication NEC T83.89 ☑
          - stenosis T83.85 ☑
          - thrombosis T83.86 ☑
        - vaginal mesh — *see* Complications, prosthetic device or implant, mesh
      - urinary system T83.9 ☑
        - cystostomy catheter — *see* Complication, catheter, cystostomy
        - electronic stimulator — *see* Complications, electronic stimulator device, urinary
        - indwelling urethral catheter — *see* Complications, catheter, urethral, indwelling
        - infection or inflammation T83.598 ☑
          - indwelling urethral catheter T83.511 ☑
        - kidney transplant — *see* Complication, transplant, kidney
        - organ graft — *see* Complication, graft, urinary organ
        - specified type NEC T83.89 ☑
          - embolism T83.81 ☑
          - fibrosis T83.82 ☑
          - hemorrhage T83.83 ☑
          - mechanical T83.198 ☑
            - breakdown T83.118 ☑
            - displacement T83.128 ☑
            - malfunction T83.118 ☑
            - malposition T83.128 ☑
            - obstruction T83.198 ☑
            - perforation T83.198 ☑
            - protrusion T83.198 ☑
            - specified NEC T83.198 ☑
        - sphincter implant — *see* Complications, implant, urinary sphincter
        - sphincter, implanted T83.191 ☑
        - stent (ileal conduit) (nephroureteral) T83.193 ☑
          - pain T83.84 ☑
          - specified complication NEC T83.89 ☑
          - stenosis T83.85 ☑
          - thrombosis T83.86 ☑
          - ureteral indwelling T83.192 ☑
    - postprocedural
      - pelvic peritoneal adhesions N99.4
      - renal failure N99.Ø
      - specified NEC N99.89
      - stoma — *see* Complications, stoma, urinary tract
      - urethral stricture — *see* Stricture, urethra, postprocedural
      - vaginal
        - adhesions N99.2
        - vault prolapse N99.3
  - graft (bypass) (patch) — *see also* Complications, prosthetic device or implant
    - aorta — *see* Complications, graft, vascular
    - arterial — *see* Complication, graft, vascular
    - bone T86.839
      - failure T86.831
      - infection T86.832
      - mechanical T84.318 ☑
        - breakdown T84.318 ☑
        - displacement T84.328 ☑
        - protrusion T84.398 ☑
        - specified type NEC T84.398 ☑
      - rejection T86.83Ø
      - specified type NEC T86.838
    - carotid artery — *see* Complications, graft, vascular

- **Complication**(s) — *continued*
  - graft — *see also* Complications, prosthetic device or implant — *continued*
    - cornea T86.849- ☑
      - failure T86.841- ☑
      - infection T86.842- ☑
      - mechanical T85.398 ☑
        - breakdown T85.318 ☑
        - displacement T85.328 ☑
        - protrusion T85.398 ☑
        - specified type NEC T85.398 ☑
      - rejection T86.84Ø- ☑
      - retroprosthetic membrane T85.398 ☑
      - specified type NEC T86.848- ☑
    - femoral artery (bypass) — *see* Complication, extremity artery (bypass) graft
    - genital organ or tract — *see* Complications, genitourinary, device or implant, genital tract
    - muscle T84.9 ☑
      - breakdown T84.41Ø ☑
      - displacement T84.42Ø ☑
      - embolism T84.81 ☑
      - fibrosis T84.82 ☑
      - hemorrhage T84.83 ☑
      - infection and inflammation T84.7 ☑
      - mechanical NEC T84.49Ø ☑
      - pain T84.84 ☑
      - specified type NEC T84.89 ☑
      - stenosis T84.85 ☑
      - thrombosis T84.86 ☑
    - nerve — *see* Complication, prosthetic device or implant, specified NEC
    - skin — *see* Complications, prosthetic device or implant, skin graft
    - tendon T84.9 ☑
      - breakdown T84.41Ø ☑
      - displacement T84.42Ø ☑
      - embolism T84.81 ☑
      - fibrosis T84.82 ☑
      - hemorrhage T84.83 ☑
      - infection and inflammation T84.7 ☑
      - mechanical NEC T84.49Ø ☑
      - pain T84.84 ☑
      - specified type NEC T84.89 ☑
      - stenosis T84.85 ☑
      - thrombosis T84.86 ☑
    - urinary organ T83.9 ☑
      - embolism T83.81 ☑
      - fibrosis T83.82 ☑
      - hemorrhage T83.83 ☑
      - infection and inflammation T83.598 ☑
        - indwelling urethral catheter T83.511 ☑
      - mechanical
        - breakdown T83.21 ☑
        - displacement T83.22 ☑
        - erosion T83.24 ☑
        - exposure T83.25 ☑
        - leakage T83.23 ☑
        - malposition T83.22 ☑
        - obstruction T83.29 ☑
        - perforation T83.29 ☑
        - protrusion T83.29 ☑
        - specified NEC T83.29 ☑
      - pain T83.84 ☑
      - specified type NEC T83.89 ☑
      - stenosis T83.85 ☑
      - thrombosis T83.86 ☑
    - vascular T82.9 ☑
      - embolism T82.818 ☑
      - femoral artery — *see* Complication, extremity artery (bypass) graft
      - fibrosis T82.828 ☑
      - hemorrhage T82.838 ☑
      - mechanical
        - breakdown T82.319 ☑
          - aorta (bifurcation) T82.31Ø ☑
          - carotid artery T82.311 ☑
          - specified vessel NEC T82.318 ☑
        - displacement T82.329 ☑
          - aorta (bifurcation) T82.32Ø ☑
          - carotid artery T82.321 ☑
          - specified vessel NEC T82.328 ☑
        - leakage T82.339 ☑
          - aorta (bifurcation) T82.33Ø ☑
          - carotid artery T82.331 ☑
          - specified vessel NEC T82.338 ☑

- **Complication**(s) — *continued*
  - graft — *see also* Complications, prosthetic device or implant — *continued*
    - vascular — *continued*
      - mechanical — *continued*
        - malposition T82.329 ☑
          - aorta (bifurcation) T82.32Ø ☑
          - carotid artery T82.321 ☑
          - specified vessel NEC T82.328 ☑
        - obstruction T82.399 ☑
          - aorta (bifurcation) T82.39Ø ☑
          - carotid artery T82.391 ☑
          - specified vessel NEC T82.398 ☑
        - perforation T82.399 ☑
          - aorta (bifurcation) T82.39Ø ☑
          - carotid artery T82.391 ☑
          - specified vessel NEC T82.398 ☑
        - protrusion T82.399 ☑
          - aorta (bifurcation) T82.39Ø ☑
          - carotid artery T82.391 ☑
          - specified vessel NEC T82.398 ☑
      - pain T82.848 ☑
      - specified complication NEC T82.898 ☑
      - stenosis T82.858 ☑
      - thrombosis T82.868 ☑
  - heart I51.9
    - assist device
      - infection and inflammation T82.7 ☑
    - following acute myocardial infarction — *see* Complications, following, acute myocardial infarction
    - postoperative — *see* Complications, circulatory system
    - transplant — *see* Complication, transplant, heart
      - and lung(s) — *see* Complications, transplant, heart, with lung
    - valve
      - graft (biological) T82.9 ☑
        - embolism T82.817 ☑
        - fibrosis T82.827 ☑
        - hemorrhage T82.837 ☑
        - infection and inflammation T82.7 ☑
        - mechanical T82.228 ☑
          - breakdown T82.221 ☑
          - displacement T82.222 ☑
          - leakage T82.223 ☑
          - malposition T82.222 ☑
          - obstruction T82.228 ☑
          - perforation T82.228 ☑
          - protrusion T82.228 ☑
        - pain T82.847 ☑
        - specified type NEC T82.897 ☑
        - stenosis T82.857 ☑
        - thrombosis T82.867 ☑
      - prosthesis T82.9 ☑
        - embolism T82.817 ☑
        - fibrosis T82.827 ☑
        - hemorrhage T82.837 ☑
        - infection or inflammation T82.6 ☑
        - mechanical T82.Ø9 ☑
          - breakdown T82.Ø1 ☑
          - displacement T82.Ø2 ☑
          - leakage T82.Ø3 ☑
          - malposition T82.Ø2 ☑
          - obstruction T82.Ø9 ☑
          - perforation T82.Ø9 ☑
          - protrusion T82.Ø9 ☑
        - pain T82.847 ☑
        - specified type NEC T82.897 ☑
          - mechanical T82.Ø9 ☑
        - stenosis T82.857 ☑
        - thrombosis T82.867 ☑
  - hematoma
    - intraoperative — *see* Complication, intraoperative, hemorrhage
    - postprocedural — *see* Complication, postprocedural, hematoma
  - hemodialysis — *see* Complications, dialysis
  - hemorrhage
    - intraoperative — *see* Complication, intraoperative, hemorrhage
    - postprocedural — *see* Complication, postprocedural, hemorrhage
  - IEC (immune effector cellular) therapy T8Ø.82 ☑
  - ileostomy (stoma) — *see* Complications, enterostomy
  - immune effector cellular (IEC) therapy T8Ø.82 ☑

Complication(s) — *continued*
- immunization (procedure) — *see* Complications, vaccination
- implant — *see also* Complications, by site and type
  - urinary sphincter T83.9 ☑
    - embolism T83.81 ☑
    - fibrosis T83.82 ☑
    - hemorrhage T83.83 ☑
    - infection and inflammation T83.591 ☑
    - mechanical
      - breakdown T83.111 ☑
      - displacement T83.121 ☑
      - leakage T83.191 ☑
      - malposition T83.121 ☑
      - obstruction T83.191 ☑
      - perforation T83.191 ☑
      - protrusion T83.191 ☑
      - specified NEC T83.191 ☑
    - pain T83.84 ☑
    - specified type NEC T83.89 ☑
    - stenosis T83.85 ☑
    - thrombosis T83.86 ☑
- infusion (procedure) T8Ø.9Ø ☑
  - air embolism T8Ø.Ø ☑
  - blood — *see* Complications, transfusion
  - catheter — *see* Complications, catheter
  - infection T8Ø.29 ☑
  - pump — *see* Complications, cardiovascular, device or implant
  - sepsis T8Ø.29 ☑
  - serum reaction — *see also* Reaction, serum T8Ø.69 ☑
    - anaphylactic shock — *see also* Shock, anaphylactic T8Ø.59 ☑
  - specified type NEC T8Ø.89 ☑
- inhalation therapy NEC T81.81 ☑
- injection (procedure) T8Ø.9Ø ☑
  - drug reaction — *see* Reaction, drug
  - infection T8Ø.29 ☑
  - sepsis T8Ø.29 ☑
  - serum (prophylactic) (therapeutic) — *see* Complications, vaccination
  - specified type NEC T8Ø.89 ☑
  - vaccine (any) — *see* Complications, vaccination
- inoculation (any) — *see* Complications, vaccination
- insulin pump
  - infection and inflammation T85.72 ☑
  - mechanical
    - breakdown T85.614 ☑
    - displacement T85.624 ☑
    - leakage T85.633 ☑
    - malposition T85.624 ☑
    - obstruction T85.694 ☑
    - perforation T85.694 ☑
    - protrusion T85.694 ☑
    - specified NEC T85.694 ☑
- intestinal pouch NEC K91.858
- intraocular lens (prosthetic) T85.9 ☑
  - embolism T85.818 ☑
  - fibrosis T85.828 ☑
  - hemorrhage T85.838 ☑
  - infection and inflammation T85.79 ☑
  - mechanical
    - breakdown T85.21 ☑
    - displacement T85.22 ☑
    - malposition T85.22 ☑
    - obstruction T85.29 ☑
    - perforation T85.29 ☑
    - protrusion T85.29 ☑
    - specified NEC T85.29 ☑
  - pain T85.848 ☑
  - specified type NEC T85.898 ☑
  - stenosis T85.858 ☑
  - thrombosis T85.868 ☑
- intraoperative (intraprocedural)
  - cardiac arrest — *see also* Infarct, myocardium, associated with revascularization procedure
    - during cardiac surgery I97.71Ø
    - during other surgery I97.711
  - cardiac functional disturbance NEC — *see also* Infarct, myocardium, associated with revascularization procedure
    - during cardiac surgery I97.79Ø
    - during other surgery I97.791

Complication(s) — *continued*
- intraoperative — *continued*
  - hemorrhage (hematoma) (of)
    - circulatory system organ or structure
      - during cardiac bypass I97.411
      - during cardiac catheterization I97.41Ø
      - during other circulatory system procedure I97.418
      - during other procedure I97.42
    - digestive system organ
      - during procedure on digestive system K91.61
      - during procedure on other organ K91.62
    - ear
      - during procedure on ear and mastoid process H95.21
      - during procedure on other organ H95.22
    - endocrine system organ or structure
      - during procedure on endocrine system organ or structure E36.Ø1
      - during procedure on other organ E36.Ø2
    - eye and adnexa
      - during ophthalmic procedure H59.11- ☑
      - during other procedure H59.12- ☑
    - genitourinary organ or structure
      - during procedure on genitourinary organ or structure N99.61
      - during procedure on other organ N99.62
    - mastoid process
      - during procedure on ear and mastoid process H95.21
      - during procedure on other organ H95.22
    - musculoskeletal structure
      - during musculoskeletal surgery M96.81Ø
      - during non-orthopedic surgery M96.811
      - during orthopedic surgery M96.81Ø
    - nervous system
      - during a nervous system procedure G97.31
      - during other procedure G97.32
    - respiratory system
      - during other procedure J95.62
      - during procedure on respiratory system organ or structure J95.61
    - skin and subcutaneous tissue
      - during a dermatologic procedure L76.Ø1
      - during a procedure on other organ L76.Ø2
    - spleen
      - during a procedure on other organ D78.Ø2
      - during a procedure on the spleen D78.Ø1
  - puncture or laceration (accidental) (unintentional) (of)
    - brain
      - during a nervous system procedure G97.48
      - during other procedure G97.49
    - circulatory system organ or structure
      - during circulatory system procedure I97.51
      - during other procedure I97.52
    - digestive system
      - during procedure on digestive system K91.71
      - during procedure on other organ K91.72
    - ear
      - during procedure on ear and mastoid process H95.31
      - during procedure on other organ H95.32
    - endocrine system organ or structure
      - during procedure on endocrine system organ or structure E36.11
      - during procedure on other organ E36.12
    - eye and adnexa
      - during ophthalmic procedure H59.21- ☑
      - during other procedure H59.22- ☑
    - genitourinary organ or structure
      - during procedure on genitourinary organ or structure N99.71
      - during procedure on other organ N99.72
    - mastoid process
      - during procedure on ear and mastoid process H95.31
      - during procedure on other organ H95.32
    - musculoskeletal structure
      - during musculoskeletal surgery M96.82Ø
      - during non-orthopedic surgery M96.821
      - during orthopedic surgery M96.82Ø
    - nervous system
      - during a nervous system procedure G97.48
      - during other procedure G97.49
    - respiratory system
      - during other procedure J95.72
      - during procedure on respiratory system organ or structure J95.71

Complication(s) — *continued*
- intraoperative — *continued*
  - puncture or laceration — *continued*
    - skin and subcutaneous tissue
      - during a dermatologic procedure L76.11
      - during a procedure on other organ L76.12
    - spleen
      - during a procedure on other organ D78.12
      - during a procedure on the spleen D78.11
  - specified NEC
    - circulatory system I97.88
    - digestive system K91.81
    - ear H95.88
    - endocrine system E36.8
    - eye and adnexa H59.88
    - genitourinary system N99.81
    - mastoid process H95.88
    - musculoskeletal structure M96.89
    - nervous system G97.81
    - respiratory system J95.88
    - skin and subcutaneous tissue L76.81
    - spleen D78.81
- intraperitoneal catheter (dialysis) (infusion) — *see* Complication(s), catheter, intraperitoneal dialysis
- intrathecal infusion pump
  - infection and inflammation T85.738 ☑
  - mechanical
    - breakdown T85.615 ☑
    - displacement T85.625 ☑
    - leakage T85.635 ☑
    - malfunction T85.695 ☑
    - malposition T85.625 ☑
    - obstruction T85.695 ☑
    - perforation T85.695 ☑
    - protrusion T85.695 ☑
    - specified NEC T85.695 ☑
- intrauterine
  - contraceptive device
    - embolism T83.81 ☑
    - fibrosis T83.82 ☑
    - hemorrhage T83.83 ☑
    - infection and inflammation T83.69 ☑
    - mechanical
      - breakdown T83.31 ☑
      - displacement T83.32 ☑
      - malposition T83.32 ☑
      - obstruction T83.39 ☑
      - perforation T83.39 ☑
      - protrusion T83.39 ☑
      - specified NEC T83.39 ☑
    - pain T83.84 ☑
    - specified type NEC T83.89 ☑
    - stenosis T83.85 ☑
    - thrombosis T83.86 ☑
  - procedure (fetal), to newborn P96.5
- jejunostomy (stoma) — *see* Complications, enterostomy
- joint prosthesis, internal T84.9 ☑
  - breakage (fracture) T84.Ø1- ☑
  - dislocation T84.Ø2- ☑
  - fracture T84.Ø1- ☑
  - infection or inflammation T84.5Ø ☑
    - hip T84.5- ☑
    - knee T84.5- ☑
    - specified joint NEC T84.59 ☑
  - instability T84.Ø2- ☑
  - malposition — *see* Complications, joint prosthesis, mechanical, displacement
  - mechanical
    - breakage, broken T84.Ø1- ☑
    - dislocation T84.Ø2- ☑
    - displacement T84.Ø2- ☑
    - fracture T84.Ø1- ☑
    - instability T84.Ø2- ☑
    - leakage — *see* Complications, joint prosthesis, mechanical, specified NEC
    - loosening T84.Ø39 ☑
      - hip T84.Ø3- ☑
      - knee T84.Ø3- ☑
      - specified joint NEC T84.Ø38 ☑
    - obstruction — *see* Complications, joint prosthesis, mechanical, specified NEC
    - perforation — *see* Complications, joint prosthesis, mechanical, specified NEC
    - osteolysis T84.Ø59 ☑
      - hip T84.Ø5- ☑
      - knee T84.Ø5- ☑

- **Complication**(s) — *continued*
  - joint prosthesis, internal — *continued*
    - mechanical — *continued*
      - perforation — *see* Complications, joint prosthesis, mechanical, specified — *continued*
        - osteolysis — *continued*
          - other specified joint T84.Ø58 ☑
      - periprosthetic osteolysis, by site T84.Ø5- ☑
      - protrusion — *see* Complications, joint prosthesis, mechanical, specified NEC
      - specified complication NEC T84.Ø99 ☑
        - hip T84.Ø9- ☑
        - knee T84.Ø9- ☑
        - other specified joint T84.Ø98 ☑
      - subluxation T84.Ø2- ☑
      - wear of articular bearing surface T84.Ø69 ☑
        - hip T84.Ø6- ☑
        - knee T84.Ø6- ☑
        - other specified joint T84.Ø68 ☑
    - specified joint NEC T84.89 ☑
      - embolism T84.81 ☑
      - fibrosis T84.82 ☑
      - hemorrhage T84.83 ☑
      - pain T84.84 ☑
      - specified complication NEC T84.89 ☑
      - stenosis T84.85 ☑
      - thrombosis T84.86 ☑
    - subluxation T84.Ø2- ☑
  - kidney transplant — *see* Complications, transplant, kidney
  - labor O75.9
    - specified NEC O75.89
  - liver transplant (immune or nonimmune) — *see* Complications, transplant, liver
  - lumbar puncture G97.1
    - cerebrospinal fluid leak G97.Ø
    - headache or reaction G97.1
  - lung transplant — *see* Complications, transplant, lung
    - and heart — *see* Complications, transplant, lung, with heart
  - male genital N5Ø.9
    - device, implant or graft — *see* Complications, genitourinary, device or implant, genital tract
    - postprocedural or postoperative — *see* Complications, genitourinary, postprocedural
    - specified NEC N99.89
  - mastoid (process) procedure
    - intraoperative H95.88
      - hematoma — *see* Complications, intraoperative, hemorrhage (hematoma) (of), mastoid process
      - hemorrhage — *see* Complications, intraoperative, hemorrhage (hematoma) (of), mastoid process
      - laceration — *see* Complications, intraoperative, puncture or laceration, mastoid process
      - specified NEC H95.88
    - postmastoidectomy — *see* Complications, postmastoidectomy
    - postoperative H95.89
      - external ear canal stenosis H95.81 ☑
      - hematoma — *see* Complications, postprocedural, hematoma (of), mastoid process
      - hemorrhage — *see* Complications, postprocedural, hemorrhage (of), mastoid process
      - postmastoidectomy — *see* Complications, postmastoidectomy
      - seroma — *see* Complications, postprocedural, seroma (of), mastoid process
      - specified NEC H95.89
  - mastoidectomy cavity — *see* Complications, postmastoidectomy
  - mechanical — *see* Complications, by site and type, mechanical
  - medical procedures — *see also* Complication(s), intraoperative T88.9 ☑
  - metabolic E88.9
    - postoperative E89.89
      - specified NEC E89.89
  - molar pregnancy NOS OØ8.9
    - damage to pelvic organs OØ8.6
    - embolism OØ8.2
    - genital infection OØ8.Ø
    - hemorrhage (delayed) (excessive) OØ8.1
    - metabolic disorder OØ8.5
    - renal failure OØ8.4
    - shock OØ8.3

- **Complication**(s) — *continued*
  - molar pregnancy — *continued*
    - specified type NEC OØ8.Ø
    - venous complication NEC OØ8.7
  - musculoskeletal system — *see also* Complication, intraoperative (intraprocedural), by site
    - device, implant or graft NEC — *see* Complications, orthopedic, device or implant
    - internal fixation (nail) (plate) (rod) — *see* Complications, fixation device, internal
    - joint prosthesis — *see* Complications, joint prosthesis
    - post radiation M96.89
      - kyphosis M96.2
      - scoliosis M96.5
      - specified complication NEC M96.89
    - postoperative (postprocedural) M96.89
      - with osteoporosis — *see* Osteoporosis
      - fracture following insertion of device — *see* Fracture, following insertion of orthopedic implant, joint prosthesis or bone plate
      - joint instability after prosthesis removal M96.89
      - lordosis M96.4
      - postlaminectomy syndrome NEC M96.1
        - kyphosis M96.3
      - pseudarthrosis M96.Ø
      - specified complication NEC M96.89
  - nephrostomy (stoma) — *see* Complications, stoma, urinary tract, external NEC
  - nervous system G98.8
    - central G96.9
    - device, implant or graft — *see also* Complication, prosthetic device or implant, specified NEC
      - electronic stimulator (electrode(s)) — *see* Complications, electronic stimulator device
      - specified NEC
        - infection and inflammation T85.738 ☑
        - mechanical T85.695 ☑
          - breakdown T85.615 ☑
          - displacement T85.625 ☑
          - leakage T85.635 ☑
          - malfunction T85.695 ☑
          - malposition T85.625 ☑
          - obstruction T85.695 ☑
          - perforation T85.695 ☑
          - protrusion T85.695 ☑
          - specified NEC T85.695 ☑
      - ventricular shunt — *see* Complications, ventricular shunt
    - electronic stimulator (electrode(s)) — *see* Complications, electronic stimulator device
    - postprocedural G97.82
      - intracranial hypotension G97.2
      - specified NEC G97.82
      - spinal fluid leak G97.Ø
  - newborn, due to intrauterine (fetal) procedure P96.5
  - nonabsorbable (permanent) sutures — *see* Complication, sutures, permanent
  - obstetric O75.9
    - procedure (instrumental) (manual) (surgical) specified NEC O75.4
    - specified NEC O75.89
    - surgical wound NEC O9Ø.89
      - hematoma O9Ø.2
      - infection O86.ØØ
  - ocular lens implant — *see* Complications, intraocular lens
  - ophthalmologic
    - postprocedural bleb — *see* Blebitis
  - orbital prosthesis T85.9 ☑
    - embolism T85.818 ☑
    - fibrosis T85.828 ☑
    - hemorrhage T85.838 ☑
    - infection and inflammation T85.79 ☑
    - mechanical
      - breakdown T85.31- ☑
      - displacement T85.32- ☑
      - malposition T85.32- ☑
      - obstruction T85.39- ☑
      - perforation T85.39- ☑
      - protrusion T85.39- ☑
      - specified NEC T85.39- ☑
    - pain T85.848 ☑
    - specified type NEC T85.898 ☑
    - stenosis T85.858 ☑
    - thrombosis T85.868 ☑

- **Complication**(s) — *continued*
  - organ or tissue transplant (partial) (total) — *see* Complications, transplant
  - orthopedic — *see also* Disorder, soft tissue
    - device or implant T84.9 ☑
      - bone
        - device or implant — *see* Complication, bone, device NEC
        - graft — *see* Complication, graft, bone
      - breakdown T84.418 ☑
      - displacement T84.428 ☑
      - electronic bone stimulator — *see* Complications, electronic stimulator device, bone
      - embolism T84.81 ☑
      - fibrosis T84.82 ☑
      - fixation device — *see* Complication, fixation device, internal
      - hemorrhage T84.83 ☑
      - infection or inflammation T84.7 ☑
      - joint prosthesis — *see* Complication, joint prosthesis, internal
      - malfunction T84.418 ☑
      - malposition T84.428 ☑
      - mechanical NEC T84.498 ☑
      - muscle graft — *see* Complications, graft, muscle
      - obstruction T84.498 ☑
      - pain T84.84 ☑
      - perforation T84.498 ☑
      - protrusion T84.498 ☑
      - specified complication NEC T84.89 ☑
      - stenosis T84.85 ☑
      - tendon graft — *see* Complications, graft, tendon
      - thrombosis T84.86 ☑
    - fracture (following insertion of device) — *see* Fracture, following insertion of orthopedic implant, joint prosthesis or bone plate
    - postprocedural M96.89
      - fracture — *see* Fracture, following insertion of orthopedic implant, joint prosthesis or bone plate
      - postlaminectomy syndrome NEC M96.1
        - kyphosis M96.3
        - lordosis M96.4
      - postradiation
        - kyphosis M96.2
        - scoliosis M96.5
      - pseudarthrosis post-fusion M96.Ø
      - specified type NEC M96.89
  - pacemaker (cardiac) — *see* Complications, cardiovascular device or implant, electronic
  - pancreas transplant — *see* Complications, transplant, pancreas
  - penile prosthesis (implant) — *see* Complications, prosthetic device, penile
  - perfusion NEC T8Ø.9Ø ☑
  - perineal repair (obstetrical) NEC O9Ø.89
    - disruption O9Ø.1
    - hematoma O9Ø.2
    - infection (following delivery) O86.Ø9
  - phototherapy T88.9 ☑
    - specified NEC T88.8 ☑
  - postmastoidectomy NEC H95.19- ☑
    - cyst, mucosal H95.13- ☑
    - granulation H95.12- ☑
    - inflammation, chronic H95.11- ☑
    - recurrent cholesteatoma H95.Ø- ☑
  - postoperative — *see* Complications, postprocedural
    - circulatory — *see* Complications, circulatory system
    - ear — *see* Complications, ear
    - endocrine — *see* Complications, endocrine
    - eye — *see* Complications, eye
    - lumbar puncture G97.1
      - cerebrospinal fluid leak G97.Ø
    - nervous system (central) (peripheral) — *see* Complications, nervous system
    - respiratory system — *see* Complications, respiratory system
  - postprocedural — *see also* Complications, surgical procedure
    - cardiac arrest — *see also* Infarct, myocardium, associated with revascularization procedure
      - following cardiac surgery I97.12Ø
      - following other surgery I97.121
    - cardiac functional disturbance NEC — *see also* Infarct, myocardium, associated with revascularization procedure
      - following cardiac surgery I97.19Ø

- **Complication**(s) — *continued*
  - postprocedural — *see also* Complications, surgical procedure — *continued*
    - cardiac functional disturbance — *see also* Infarct, myocardium, associated with revascularization procedure — *continued*
      - following other surgery I97.191
    - cardiac insufficiency
      - following cardiac surgery I97.110
      - following other surgery I97.111
    - chorioretinal scars following retinal surgery H59.81- ☑
    - following cataract surgery
      - cataract (lens) fragments H59.02- ☑
      - cystoid macular edema H59.03- ☑
      - specified NEC H59.09- ☑
      - vitreous (touch) syndrome H59.01- ☑
    - heart failure
      - following cardiac surgery I97.130
      - following other surgery I97.131
    - hematoma (of)
      - circulatory system organ or structure
        - following cardiac bypass I97.631
        - following cardiac catheterization I97.630
        - following other circulatory system procedure I97.638
        - following other procedure I97.621
      - digestive system
        - following procedure on digestive system K91.870
        - following procedure on other organ K91.871
      - ear
        - following other procedure H95.52
        - following procedure on ear and mastoid process H95.51
      - endocrine system
        - following endocrine system procedure E89.820
        - following other procedure E89.821
      - eye and adnexa
        - following ophthalmic procedure H59.33- ☑
        - following other procedure H59.34- ☑
      - genitourinary organ or structure
        - following procedure on genitourinary organ or structure N99.840
        - following procedure on other organ N99.841
      - mastoid process
        - following other procedure H95.52
        - following procedure on ear and mastoid process H95.51
      - musculoskeletal structure
        - following musculoskeletal surgery M96.840
        - following non-orthopedic surgery M96.841
        - following orthopedic surgery M96.840
      - nervous system
        - following nervous system procedure G97.61
        - following other procedure G97.62
      - respiratory system
        - following other procedure J95.861
        - following procedure on respiratory system organ or structure J95.860
      - skin and subcutaneous tissue
        - following dermatologic procedure L76.31
        - following procedure on other organ L76.32
      - spleen
        - following procedure on other organ D78.32
        - following procedure on the spleen D78.31
    - hemorrhage (of)
      - circulatory system organ or structure
        - following cardiac bypass I97.611
        - following cardiac catheterization I97.610
        - following other circulatory system procedure I97.618
        - following other procedure I97.620
      - digestive system
        - following procedure on digestive system K91.840
        - following procedure on other organ K91.841
      - ear
        - following other procedure H95.42
        - following procedure on ear and mastoid process H95.41
      - endocrine system
        - following endocrine system procedure E89.810
        - following other procedure E89.811
      - eye and adnexa
        - following ophthalmic procedure H59.31- ☑

- **Complication**(s) — *continued*
  - postprocedural — *see also* Complications, surgical procedure — *continued*
    - hemorrhage — *continued*
      - eye and adnexa — *continued*
        - following other procedure H59.32- ☑
      - genitourinary organ or structure
        - following procedure on genitourinary organ or structure N99.820
        - following procedure on other organ N99.821
      - mastoid process
        - following other procedure H95.42
        - following procedure on ear and mastoid process H95.41
      - musculoskeletal structure
        - following musculoskeletal surgery M96.830
        - following non-orthopedic surgery M96.831
        - following orthopedic surgery M96.830
      - nervous system
        - following nervous system procedure G97.51
        - following other procedure G97.52
      - respiratory system
        - following a respiratory system procedure J95.830
        - following other procedure J95.831
      - skin and subcutaneous tissue
        - following a procedure on other organ L76.22
        - following dermatologic procedure L76.21
      - spleen
        - following procedure on other organ D78.22
        - following procedure on the spleen D78.21
    - seroma (of)
      - circulatory system organ or structure
        - following cardiac bypass I97.641
        - following cardiac catheterization I97.640
        - following other circulatory system procedure I97.648
        - following other procedure I97.622
      - digestive system
        - following procedure on digestive system K91.872
        - following procedure on other organ K91.873
      - ear
        - following other procedure H95.54
        - following procedure on ear and mastoid process H95.53
      - endocrine system
        - following endocrine system procedure E89.822
        - following other procedure E89.823
      - eye and adnexa
        - following ophthalmic procedure H59.35- ☑
        - following other procedure H59.36- ☑
      - genitourinary organ or structure
        - following procedure on genitourinary organ or structure N99.842
        - following procedure on other organ N99.843
      - mastoid process
        - following other procedure H95.54
        - following procedure on ear and mastoid process H95.53
      - musculoskeletal structure
        - following musculoskeletal surgery M96.842
        - following non-orthopedic surgery M96.843
        - following orthopedic surgery M96.842
      - nervous system
        - following nervous system procedure G97.63
        - following other procedure G97.64
      - respiratory system
        - following other procedure J95.863
        - following procedure on respiratory system organ or structure J95.862
      - skin and subcutaneous tissue
        - following dermatologic procedure L76.33
        - following procedure on other organ L76.34
      - spleen
        - following procedure on other organ D78.34
        - following procedure on the spleen D78.33
    - specified NEC
      - circulatory system I97.89
      - digestive K91.89
      - ear H95.89
      - endocrine E89.89
      - eye and adnexa H59.89
      - genitourinary N99.89
      - mastoid process H95.89
      - metabolic E89.89
      - musculoskeletal structure M96.89
      - nervous system G97.82

- **Complication**(s) — *continued*
  - postprocedural — *see also* Complications, surgical procedure — *continued*
    - specified — *continued*
      - respiratory system J95.89
      - skin and subcutaneous tissue L76.82
      - spleen D78.89
  - pregnancy NEC — *see* Pregnancy, complicated by
  - prosthetic device or implant T85.9 ☑
    - bile duct — *see* Complications, bile duct implant
    - breast — *see* Complications, breast implant
    - bulking agent
      - ureteral
        - erosion T83.714 ☑
        - exposure T83.724 ☑
      - urethral
        - erosion T83.713 ☑
        - exposure T83.723 ☑
    - cardiac and vascular NEC — *see* Complications, cardiovascular device or implant
    - corneal transplant — *see* Complications, graft, cornea
    - electronic nervous system stimulator — *see* Complications, electronic stimulator device
    - epidural infusion catheter — *see* Complications, catheter, epidural
    - esophageal anti-reflux device — *see* Complications, esophageal anti-reflux device
    - genital organ or tract — *see* Complications, genitourinary, device or implant, genital tract
      - specified NEC T83.79- ☑
    - heart valve — *see* Complications, heart, valve, prosthesis
    - infection or inflammation T85.79 ☑
      - intestine transplant T86.852
      - liver transplant T86.43
      - lung transplant T86.812
      - pancreas transplant T86.892
      - skin graft T86.822
    - intraocular lens — *see* Complications, intraocular lens
    - intraperitoneal (dialysis) catheter — *see* Complication(s), catheter, intraperitoneal dialysis
    - joint — *see* Complications, joint prosthesis, internal
    - mechanical NEC T85.698 ☑
      - dialysis catheter (vascular) — *see also* Complication, catheter, dialysis, mechanical
        - peritoneal — *see* Complication(s), catheter, intraperitoneal dialysis
      - gastrointestinal device T85.598 ☑
      - ocular device T85.398 ☑
      - subdural (infusion) catheter T85.690 ☑
      - suture, permanent T85.692 ☑
        - that for bone repair — *see* Complications, fixation device, internal (orthopedic), mechanical
      - ventricular shunt
        - breakdown T85.01 ☑
        - displacement T85.02 ☑
        - leakage T85.03 ☑
        - malposition T85.02 ☑
        - obstruction T85.09 ☑
        - perforation T85.09 ☑
        - protrusion T85.09 ☑
        - specified NEC T85.09 ☑
    - mesh
      - erosion (to surrounding organ or tissue) T83.718 ☑
        - urethral (into pelvic floor muscles) T83.712 ☑
        - vaginal (into pelvic floor muscles) T83.711 ☑
      - exposure (into surrounding organ or tissue) T83.728 ☑
        - urethral (through urethral wall) T83.722 ☑
        - vaginal (into vagina) (through vaginal wall) T83.721 ☑
    - orbital — *see* Complications, orbital prosthesis
    - penile T83.9 ☑
      - embolism T83.81 ☑
      - fibrosis T83.82 ☑
      - hemorrhage T83.83 ☑
      - infection and inflammation T83.61 ☑
      - mechanical
        - breakdown T83.410 ☑
        - displacement T83.420 ☑
        - leakage T83.490 ☑
        - malposition T83.420 ☑
        - obstruction T83.490 ☑

- **Complication**(s) — *continued*
  - surgical procedure — *continued*
    - hyperglycemia (postpancreatectomy) E89.1
    - hypoinsulinemia (postpancreatectomy) E89.1
    - hypoparathyroidism (postparathyroidectomy) E89.2
    - hypopituitarism (posthypophysectomy) E89.3
    - hypothyroidism (post-thyroidectomy) E89.0
    - intestinal obstruction — *see also* Obstruction, intestine, postoperative K91.30
    - intracranial hypotension following ventricular shunting (ventriculostomy) G97.2
    - lymphedema I97.89
      - postmastectomy I97.2
    - malabsorption (postsurgical) NEC K91.2
      - osteoporosis — *see* Osteoporosis, postsurgical malabsorption
    - mastoidectomy cavity NEC — *see* Complications, postmastoidectomy
    - metabolic E89.89
      - specified NEC E89.89
    - musculoskeletal — *see* Complications, musculoskeletal system
    - nervous system (central) (peripheral) — *see* Complications, nervous system
    - ovarian failure E89.40
      - asymptomatic E89.40
      - symptomatic E89.41
    - peripheral vascular — *see* Complications, surgical procedure, vascular
    - postcardiotomy syndrome I97.0
    - postcholecystectomy syndrome K91.5
    - postcommissurotomy syndrome I97.0
    - postgastrectomy dumping syndrome K91.1
    - postlaminectomy syndrome NEC M96.1
      - kyphosis M96.3
    - postmastectomy lymphedema syndrome I97.2
    - postmastoidectomy cholesteatoma — *see* Complications, postmastoidectomy, recurrent cholesteatoma
    - postvagotomy syndrome K91.1
    - postvalvulotomy syndrome I97.0
    - pulmonary insufficiency (acute) J95.2
      - chronic J95.3
      - following thoracic surgery J95.1
    - reattached body part — *see* Complications, reattached
    - respiratory — *see* Complications, respiratory system
    - shock (hypovolemic) T81.19 ☑
    - spleen (postoperative) D78.89
      - intraoperative D78.81
    - stitch abscess T81.41 ☑
    - subglottic stenosis (postsurgical) J95.5
    - testicular hypofunction E89.5
    - transplant — *see* Complications, organ or tissue transplant
    - urinary NEC N99.89
    - vaginal vault prolapse (posthysterectomy) N99.3
    - vascular (peripheral)
      - artery T81.719 ☑
        - mesenteric T81.710 ☑
        - renal T81.711 ☑
        - specified NEC T81.718 ☑
      - vein T81.72 ☑
    - wound infection T81.49 ☑
  - suture, permanent (wire) NEC T85.9 ☑
    - with repair of bone — *see* Complications, fixation device, internal
    - embolism T85.818 ☑
    - fibrosis T85.828 ☑
    - hemorrhage T85.838 ☑
    - infection and inflammation T85.79 ☑
    - mechanical
      - breakdown T85.612 ☑
      - displacement T85.622 ☑
      - malfunction T85.612 ☑
      - malposition T85.622 ☑
      - obstruction T85.692 ☑
      - perforation T85.692 ☑
      - protrusion T85.692 ☑
      - specified NEC T85.692 ☑
    - pain T85.848 ☑
    - specified type NEC T85.898 ☑
    - stenosis T85.858 ☑
    - thrombosis T85.868 ☑
  - tracheostomy J95.00
    - granuloma J95.09
    - hemorrhage J95.01

- **Complication**(s) — *continued*
  - tracheostomy — *continued*
    - infection J95.02
    - malfunction J95.03
    - mechanical J95.03
    - obstruction J95.03
    - specified type NEC J95.09
    - tracheo-esophageal fistula J95.04
  - transfusion (blood) (lymphocytes) (plasma) T80.92 ☑
    - air emblism T80.0 ☑
    - circulatory overload E87.71
    - febrile nonhemolytic transfusion reaction R50.84
    - hemochromatosis E83.111
    - hemolysis T80.89 ☑
    - hemolytic reaction (antigen unspecified) T80.919 ☑
    - incompatibility reaction (antigen unspecified) T80.919 ☑
      - ABO T80.30 ☑
        - delayed serologic (DSTR) T80.39 ☑
        - hemolytic transfusion reaction (HTR) (unspecified time after transfusion) T80.319 ☑
          - acute (AHTR) (less than 24 hours after transfusion) T80.310 ☑
          - delayed (DHTR) (24 hours or more after transfusion) T80.311 ☑
        - specified NEC T80.39 ☑
      - acute (antigen unspecified) T80.910 ☑
      - delayed (antigen unspecified) T80.911 ☑
      - delayed serologic (DSTR) T80.89 ☑
      - non-ABO (minor antigens (Duffy) (K) (Kell) (Kidd) (Lewis) (M) (N) (P) (S)) T80.A0 ☑ (*following* T80.4)
        - delayed serologic (DSTR) T80.A9 ☑ (*following* T80.4)
        - hemolytic transfusion reaction (HTR) (unspecified time after transfusion) T80.A19 ☑ (*following* T80.4)
          - acute (AHTR) (less than 24 hours after transfusion) T80.A10 ☑ (*following* T80.4)
          - delayed (DHTR) (24 hours or more after transfusion) T80.A11 ☑ (*following* T80.4)
        - specified NEC T80.A9 ☑ (*following* T80.4)
      - Rh (antigens (C) (c) (D) (E) (e)) (factor) T80.40 ☑
        - delayed serologic (DSTR) T80.49 ☑
        - hemolytic transfusion reaction (HTR) (unspecified time after transfusion) T80.419 ☑
          - acute (AHTR) (less than 24 hours after transfusion) T80.410 ☑
          - delayed (DHTR) (24 hours or more after transfusion) T80.411 ☑
        - specified NEC T80.49 ☑
    - infection T80.29 ☑
      - acute T80.22- ☑
    - reaction NEC T80.89 ☑
    - sepsis T80.29 ☑
    - shock T80.89 ☑
  - transplant T86.90
    - bone T86.839
      - failure T86.831
      - infection T86.832
      - rejection T86.830
      - specified type NEC T86.838
    - bone marrow T86.00
      - failure T86.02
      - infection T86.03
      - rejection T86.01
      - specified type NEC T86.09
    - cornea T86.849- ☑
      - failure T86.841- ☑
      - infection T86.842- ☑
      - rejection T86.840- ☑
      - specified type NEC T86.848- ☑
    - failure T86.92
    - heart T86.20
      - with lung T86.30
      - cardiac allograft vasculopathy T86.290
        - failure T86.32
        - infection T86.33
        - rejection T86.31
        - specified type NEC T86.39
      - failure T86.22
      - infection T86.23
      - rejection T86.21
      - specified type NEC T86.298
    - infection T86.93

- **Complication**(s) — *continued*
  - transplant — *continued*
    - intestine T86.859
      - failure T86.851
      - infection T86.852
      - rejection T86.850
      - specified type NEC T86.858
    - kidney T86.10
      - failure T86.12
      - infection T86.13
      - rejection T86.11
      - specified type NEC T86.19
    - liver T86.40
      - failure T86.42
      - infection T86.43
      - rejection T86.41
      - specified type NEC T86.49
    - lung T86.819
      - with heart T86.30
        - failure T86.32
        - infection T86.33
        - rejection T86.31
        - specified type NEC T86.39
      - failure T86.811
      - infection T86.812
      - rejection T86.810
      - specified type NEC T86.818
    - malignant neoplasm C80.2
    - pancreas T86.899
      - failure T86.891
      - infection T86.892
      - rejection T86.890
      - specified type NEC T86.898
    - peripheral blood stem cells T86.5
    - post-transplant lymphoproliferative disorder (PTLD) D47.Z1 (*following* D47.4)
    - rejection T86.91
    - skin T86.829
      - failure T86.821
      - infection T86.822
      - rejection T86.820
      - specified type NEC T86.828
    - specified
      - tissue T86.899
        - failure T86.891
        - infection T86.892
        - rejection T86.890
        - specified type NEC T86.898
      - type NEC T86.99
    - stem cell (from peripheral blood) (from umbilical cord) T86.5
    - umbilical cord stem cells T86.5
  - trauma (early) T79.9 ☑
    - specified NEC T79.8 ☑
  - ultrasound therapy NEC T88.9 ☑
  - umbilical cord NEC
    - complicating delivery O69.9 ☑
      - specified NEC O69.89 ☑
  - umbrella device, vascular T82.9 ☑
    - embolism T82.818 ☑
    - fibrosis T82.828 ☑
    - hemorrhage T82.838 ☑
    - infection or inflammation T82.7 ☑
    - mechanical
      - breakdown T82.515 ☑
      - displacement T82.525 ☑
      - leakage T82.535 ☑
      - malposition T82.525 ☑
      - obstruction T82.595 ☑
      - perforation T82.595 ☑
      - protrusion T82.595 ☑
    - pain T82.848 ☑
    - specified type NEC T82.898 ☑
    - stenosis T82.858 ☑
    - thrombosis T82.868 ☑
  - urethral catheter — *see* Complications, catheter, urethral, indwelling
  - vaccination T88.1 ☑
    - anaphylaxis NEC T80.52 ☑
    - arthropathy — *see* Arthropathy, postimmunization
    - cellulitis T88.0 ☑
    - encephalitis or encephalomyelitis G04.02
    - infection (general) (local) NEC T88.0 ☑
    - meningitis G03.8
    - myelitis G04.02
    - protein sickness T80.62 ☑
    - rash T88.1 ☑
    - reaction (allergic) T88.1 ☑

- **Complication**(s) — *continued*
  - vaccination — *continued*
    - reaction — *continued*
      - serum T80.62 ☑
    - sepsis T88.0 ☑
    - serum intoxication, sickness, rash, or other serum reaction NEC T80.62 ☑
      - anaphylactic shock T80.52 ☑
    - shock (allergic) (anaphylactic) T80.52 ☑
    - vaccinia (generalized) (localized) T88.1 ☑
  - vas deferens device or implant — *see* Complications, genitourinary, device or implant, genital tract
  - vascular I99.9
    - device or implant T82.9 ☑
      - embolism T82.818 ☑
      - fibrosis T82.828 ☑
      - hemorrhage T82.838 ☑
      - infection or inflammation T82.7 ☑
      - mechanical
        - breakdown T82.519 ☑
          - specified device NEC T82.518 ☑
        - displacement T82.529 ☑
          - specified device NEC T82.528 ☑
        - leakage T82.539 ☑
          - specified device NEC T82.538 ☑
        - malposition T82.529 ☑
          - specified device NEC T82.528 ☑
        - obstruction T82.599 ☑
          - specified device NEC T82.598 ☑
        - perforation T82.599 ☑
          - specified device NEC T82.598 ☑
        - protrusion T82.599 ☑
          - specified device NEC T82.598 ☑
      - pain T82.848 ☑
      - specified type NEC T82.898 ☑
      - stenosis T82.858 ☑
      - thrombosis T82.868 ☑
    - dialysis catheter — *see* Complication, catheter, dialysis
    - following infusion, therapeutic injection or transfusion T80.1 ☑
    - graft T82.9 ☑
      - embolism T82.818 ☑
      - fibrosis T82.828 ☑
      - hemorrhage T82.838 ☑
      - mechanical
        - breakdown T82.319 ☑
          - aorta (bifurcation) T82.310 ☑
          - carotid artery T82.311 ☑
          - specified vessel NEC T82.318 ☑
        - displacement T82.329 ☑
          - aorta (bifurcation) T82.320 ☑
          - carotid artery T82.321 ☑
          - specified vessel NEC T82.328 ☑
        - leakage T82.339 ☑
          - aorta (bifurcation) T82.330 ☑
          - carotid artery T82.331 ☑
          - femoral artery T82.332 ☑
          - specified vessel NEC T82.338 ☑
        - malposition T82.329 ☑
          - aorta (bifurcation) T82.320 ☑
          - carotid artery T82.321 ☑
          - specified vessel NEC T82.328 ☑
        - obstruction T82.399 ☑
          - aorta (bifurcation) T82.390 ☑
          - carotid artery T82.391 ☑
          - specified vessel NEC T82.398 ☑
        - perforation T82.399 ☑
          - aorta (bifurcation) T82.390 ☑
          - carotid artery T82.391 ☑
          - specified vessel NEC T82.398 ☑
        - protrusion T82.399 ☑
          - aorta (bifurcation) T82.390 ☑
          - carotid artery T82.391 ☑
          - specified vessel NEC T82.398 ☑
      - pain T82.848 ☑
      - specified complication NEC T82.898 ☑
      - stenosis T82.858 ☑
      - thrombosis T82.868 ☑
    - postoperative — *see* Complications, postoperative, circulatory
  - vena cava device (filter) (sieve) (umbrella) — *see* Complications, umbrella device, vascular
  - ventilation therapy NEC T81.81 ☑
  - ventilator
    - mechanical J95.850

- **Complication**(s) — *continued*
  - ventilator — *continued*
    - mechanical — *continued*
      - specified NEC J95.859
  - ventricular (communicating) shunt (device) T85.9 ☑
    - embolism T85.810 ☑
    - fibrosis T85.820 ☑
    - hemorrhage T85.830 ☑
    - infection and inflammation T85.730 ☑
    - mechanical
      - breakdown T85.01 ☑
      - displacement T85.02 ☑
      - leakage T85.03 ☑
      - malposition T85.02 ☑
      - obstruction T85.09 ☑
      - perforation T85.09 ☑
      - protrusion T85.09 ☑
      - specified NEC T85.09 ☑
    - pain T85.840 ☑
    - specified type NEC T85.890 ☑
    - stenosis T85.850 ☑
    - thrombosis T85.860 ☑
  - wire suture, permanent (implanted) — *see* Complications, suture, permanent
- **Compressed air disease** T70.3 ☑
- **Compression**
  - with injury — *code by* Nature of injury
  - artery I77.1
    - celiac, syndrome I77.4
  - brachial plexus G54.0
  - brain (stem) G93.5
    - due to
      - contusion (diffuse) — *see also* Injury, intracranial, diffuse S06.A0 ☑
        - with herniation S06.A1 ☑
        - focal — *see also* Injury, intracranial, focal S06.A0 ☑
          - with herniation S06.A1 ☑
      - injury NEC — *see also* Injury, intracranial, diffuse S06.A0 ☑
    - nontraumatic G93.5
    - traumatic — *see also* Injury, intracranial, diffuse S06.A0 ☑
      - with herniation S06.A1 ☑
  - bronchus J98.09
  - cauda equina G83.4
  - celiac (artery) (axis) I77.4
  - cerebral — *see* Compression, brain
  - cervical plexus G54.2
  - cord
    - spinal — *see* Compression, spinal
    - umbilical — *see* Compression, umbilical cord
  - cranial nerve G52.9
    - eighth H93.3 ☑
    - eleventh G52.8
    - fifth G50.8
    - first G52.0
    - fourth — *see* Strabismus, paralytic, fourth nerve
    - ninth G52.1
    - second — *see* Disorder, nerve, optic
    - seventh G51.8
    - sixth — *see* Strabismus, paralytic, sixth nerve
    - tenth G52.2
    - third — *see* Strabismus, paralytic, third nerve
    - twelfth G52.3
  - diver's squeeze T70.3 ☑
  - during birth (newborn) P15.9
  - esophagus K22.2
  - eustachian tube — *see* Obstruction, eustachian tube, cartilagenous
  - facies Q67.1
  - fracture
    - nontraumatic NOS — *see* Collapse, vertebra
    - pathological — *see* Fracture, pathological
    - traumatic — *see* Fracture, traumatic
  - heart — *see* Disease, heart
  - intestine — *see* Obstruction, intestine
  - laryngeal nerve, recurrent G52.2
    - with paralysis of vocal cords and larynx J38.00
      - bilateral J38.02
      - unilateral J38.01
  - lumbosacral plexus G54.1
  - lung J98.4
  - lymphatic vessel I89.0
  - medulla — *see* Compression, brain
  - nerve — *see also* Disorder, nerve G58.9
    - arm NEC — *see* Mononeuropathy, upper limb

- **Compression** — *continued*
  - nerve — *see also* Disorder, nerve — *continued*
    - axillary G54.0
    - cranial — *see* Compression, cranial nerve
    - leg NEC — *see* Mononeuropathy, lower limb
    - median (in carpal tunnel) — *see* Syndrome, carpal tunnel
    - optic — *see* Disorder, nerve, optic
    - plantar — *see* Lesion, nerve, plantar
    - posterior tibial (in tarsal tunnel) — *see* Syndrome, tarsal tunnel
    - root or plexus NOS (in) G54.9
      - intervertebral disc disorder NEC — *see* Disorder, disc, with, radiculopathy
        - with myelopathy — *see* Disorder, disc, with, myelopathy
      - neoplastic disease — *see also* Neoplasm D49.9 *[G55]*
      - spondylosis — *see* Spondylosis, with radiculopathy
    - sciatic (acute) — *see* Lesion, nerve, sciatic
    - sympathetic G90.8
    - traumatic — *see* Injury, nerve
    - ulnar — *see* Lesion, nerve, ulnar
    - upper extremity NEC — *see* Mononeuropathy, upper limb
  - spinal (cord) G95.20
    - by displacement of intervertebral disc NEC — *see also* Disorder, disc, with, myelopathy
    - nerve root NOS G54.9
      - due to displacement of intervertebral disc NEC — *see* Disorder, disc, with, radiculopathy
        - with myelopathy — *see* Disorder, disc, with, myelopathy
    - specified NEC G95.29
    - spondylogenic (cervical) (lumbar, lumbosacral) (thoracic) — *see* Spondylosis, with myelopathy NEC
      - anterior — *see* Syndrome, anterior, spinal artery, compression
    - traumatic — *see* Injury, spinal cord, by region
  - subcostal nerve (syndrome) — *see* Mononeuropathy, upper limb, specified NEC
  - sympathetic nerve NEC G90.8
  - syndrome T79.5 ☑
  - trachea J39.8
  - ulnar nerve (by scar tissue) — *see* Lesion, nerve, ulnar
  - umbilical cord
    - complicating delivery O69.2 ☑
      - cord around neck O69.1 ☑
      - prolapse O69.0 ☑
      - specified NEC O69.2 ☑
  - ureter N13.5
  - vein I87.1
  - vena cava (inferior) (superior) I87.1
- **Compulsion, compulsive**
  - gambling F63.0
  - neurosis F42.8
  - personality F60.5
  - states F42.8
  - swearing F42.8
    - in Gilles de la Tourette's syndrome F95.2
  - tics and spasms F95.9
- **Concato's disease** (pericardial polyserositis) A19.9
  - nontubercular I31.1
  - pleural — *see* Pleurisy, with effusion
- **Concavity chest wall** M95.4
- **Concealed penis** Q55.64
- **Concern** (normal) **about sick person in family** Z63.6
- **Concrescence** (teeth) K00.2
- **Concretio cordis** I31.1
  - rheumatic I09.2
- **Concretion** — *see also* Calculus
  - appendicular K38.1
  - canaliculus — *see* Dacryolith
  - clitoris N90.89
  - conjunctiva H11.12- ☑
  - eyelid — *see* Disorder, eyelid, specified type NEC
  - lacrimal passages — *see* Dacryolith
  - prepuce (male) N47.8
  - salivary gland (any) K11.5
  - seminal vesicle N50.89
  - tonsil J35.8
- **Concussion** (brain) (cerebral) (current) S06.0X9 ☑
  - with
    - loss of consciousness
      - 30 minutes or less S06.0X1 ☑

Contraception, contraceptive — *continued*
- initial prescription — *continued*
  - transdermal patch hormonal Z3Ø.Ø16
  - vaginal ring hormonal Z3Ø.Ø15
- maintenance Z3Ø.4Ø
  - barrier Z3Ø.49
  - diaphragm Z3Ø.49
  - examination Z3Ø.8
  - injectable Z3Ø.42
  - intrauterine device Z3Ø.431
  - pills Z3Ø.41
  - specified type NEC Z3Ø.49
  - subdermal implantable Z3Ø.46
  - transdermal patch hormonal Z3Ø.45
  - vaginal ring hormonal Z3Ø.44
- management Z3Ø.9
  - specified NEC Z3Ø.8
- postcoital (emergency) Z3Ø.Ø12
- prescription Z3Ø.Ø19
  - repeat Z3Ø.4Ø
- sterilization Z3Ø.2
- surveillance (drug) — *see* Contraception, maintenance

Contraction(s), contracture, contracted
- Achilles tendon — *see also* Short, tendon, Achilles
  - congenital Q66.89
- amputation stump (surgical) (flexion) (late) (next proximal joint) T87.89
- anus K59.89
- bile duct (common) (hepatic) K83.8
- bladder N32.89
  - neck or sphincter N32.Ø
- bowel, cecum, colon or intestine, any part — *see* Obstruction, intestine
- Braxton Hicks — *see* False, labor
- breast implant, capsular T85.44 ☑
- bronchial J98.Ø9
- burn (old) — *see* Cicatrix
- cervix — *see* Stricture, cervix
- cicatricial — *see* Cicatrix
- conjunctiva, trachomatous, active A71.1
  - sequelae (late effect) B94.Ø
- Dupuytren's M72.Ø
- eyelid — *see* Disorder, eyelid function
- fascia (lata) (postural) M72.8
  - Dupuytren's M72.Ø
  - palmar M72.Ø
  - plantar M72.2
- finger NEC — *see also* Deformity, finger
  - congenital Q68.1
  - joint — *see* Contraction, joint, hand
- flaccid — *see* Contraction, paralytic
- gallbladder K82.Ø
- heart valve — *see* Endocarditis
- hip — *see* Contraction, joint, hip
- hourglass
  - bladder N32.89
    - congenital Q64.79
  - gallbladder K82.Ø
    - congenital Q44.1
  - stomach K31.89
    - congenital Q4Ø.2
    - psychogenic F45.8
  - uterus (complicating delivery) O62.4
- hysterical F44.4
- internal os — *see* Stricture, cervix
- joint (abduction) (acquired) (adduction) (flexion) (rotation) M24.5Ø
  - ankle M24.57- ☑
  - congenital NEC Q68.8
    - hip Q65.89
  - elbow M24.52- ☑
  - foot joint M24.57- ☑
  - hand joint M24.54- ☑
  - hip M24.55- ☑
    - congenital Q65.89
  - hysterical F44.4
  - knee M24.56- ☑
  - shoulder M24.51- ☑
  - specified site NEC M24.59
  - wrist M24.53- ☑
- kidney (granular) (secondary) N26.9
  - congenital Q63.8
  - hydronephritic — *see* Hydronephrosis
  - Page N26.2
  - pyelonephritic — *see* Pyelitis, chronic
  - tuberculous A18.11
- ligament — *see also* Disorder, ligament
  - congenital Q79.8
- muscle (postinfective) (postural) NEC M62.4Ø
  - with contracture of joint — *see* Contraction, joint
  - ankle M62.47- ☑
  - congenital Q79.8
    - sternocleidomastoid Q68.Ø
  - extraocular — *see* Strabismus
  - eye (extrinsic) — *see* Strabismus
  - foot M62.47- ☑
  - forearm M62.43- ☑
  - hand M62.44- ☑
  - hysterical F44.4
  - ischemic (Volkmann's) T79.6 ☑
  - lower leg M62.46- ☑
  - multiple sites M62.49
  - pelvic region M62.45- ☑
  - posttraumatic — *see* Strabismus, paralytic
  - psychogenic F45.8
    - conversion reaction F44.4
  - shoulder region M62.41- ☑
  - specified site NEC M62.48
  - thigh M62.45- ☑
  - upper arm M62.42- ☑
- neck — *see* Torticollis
- ocular muscle — *see* Strabismus
- organ or site, congenital NEC — *see* Atresia, by site
- outlet (pelvis) — *see* Contraction, pelvis
- palmar fascia M72.Ø
- paralytic
  - joint — *see* Contraction, joint
  - muscle — *see also* Contraction, muscle NEC
    - ocular — *see* Strabismus, paralytic
- pelvis (acquired) (general) M95.5
  - with disproportion (fetopelvic) O33.1
    - causing obstructed labor O65.1
    - inlet O33.2
    - mid-cavity O33.3 ☑
    - outlet O33.3 ☑
- plantar fascia M72.2
- premature
  - atrium I49.1
  - auriculoventricular I49.49
  - heart I49.49
  - junctional I49.2
  - supraventricular I49.1
  - ventricular I49.3
- prostate N42.89
- pylorus NEC — *see also* Pylorospasm
  - psychogenic F45.8
- rectum, rectal (sphincter) K59.89
- ring (Bandl's) (complicating delivery) O62.4
- scar — *see* Cicatrix
- spine — *see* Dorsopathy, deforming
- sternocleidomastoid (muscle), congenital Q68.Ø
- stomach K31.89
  - hourglass K31.89
    - congenital Q4Ø.2
    - psychogenic F45.8
  - psychogenic F45.8
- tendon (sheath) M62.4Ø
  - with contracture of joint — *see* Contraction, joint
  - Achilles — *see* Short, tendon, Achilles
  - ankle M62.47- ☑
    - Achilles — *see* Short, tendon, Achilles
  - foot M62.47- ☑
  - forearm M62.43- ☑
  - hand M62.44- ☑
  - lower leg M62.46- ☑
  - multiple sites M62.49
  - neck M62.48
  - pelvic region M62.45- ☑
  - shoulder region M62.41- ☑
  - specified site NEC M62.48
  - thigh M62.45- ☑
  - thorax M62.48
  - trunk M62.48
  - upper arm M62.42- ☑
- toe — *see* Deformity, toe, specified NEC
- ureterovesical orifice (postinfectional) N13.5
  - with infection N13.6
- urethra — *see also* Stricture, urethra
  - orifice N32.Ø
- uterus N85.8
  - abnormal NEC O62.9
  - clonic (complicating delivery) O62.4
  - dyscoordinate (complicating delivery) O62.4

Contraction(s), contracture, contracted — *continued*
- uterus — *continued*
  - hourglass (complicating delivery) O62.4
  - hypertonic O62.4
  - hypotonic NEC O62.2
  - inadequate
    - primary O62.Ø
    - secondary O62.1
  - incoordinate (complicating delivery) O62.4
  - poor O62.2
  - tetanic (complicating delivery) O62.4
- vagina (outlet) N89.5
- vesical N32.89
  - neck or urethral orifice N32.Ø
- visual field — *see* Defect, visual field, generalized
- Volkmann's (ischemic) T79.6 ☑

Contusion (skin surface intact) T14.8 ☑
- abdomen, abdominal (muscle) (wall) S3Ø.1 ☑
- adnexa, eye NEC SØ5.8X- ☑
- adrenal gland S37.812 ☑
- alveolar process SØØ.532 ☑
- ankle S9Ø.Ø- ☑
- antecubital space — *see* Contusion, forearm
- anus S3Ø.3 ☑
- arm (upper) S4Ø.Ø2- ☑
  - lower (with elbow) — *see* Contusion, forearm
- auditory canal — *see* Contusion, ear
- auricle — *see* Contusion, ear
- axilla — *see* Contusion, arm, upper
- back — *see also* Contusion, thorax, back
  - lower S3Ø.Ø ☑
- bile duct S36.13 ☑
- bladder S37.22 ☑
- bone NEC T14.8 ☑
- brain (diffuse) — *see* Injury, intracranial, diffuse
  - focal — *see* Injury, intracranial, focal
- brainstem SØ6.38- ☑
- breast S2Ø.Ø- ☑
- broad ligament S37.892 ☑
- brow SØØ.83 ☑
- buttock S3Ø.Ø ☑
- canthus, eye SØØ.1- ☑
- cauda equina S34.3 ☑
- cerebellar, traumatic SØ6.37- ☑
- cerebral SØ6.33- ☑
  - left side SØ6.32- ☑
  - right side SØ6.31- ☑
- cheek SØØ.83 ☑
  - internal SØØ.532 ☑
- chest (wall) — *see* Contusion, thorax
- chin SØØ.83 ☑
- clitoris S3Ø.23 ☑
- colon — *see* Injury, intestine, large, contusion
- common bile duct S36.13 ☑
- conjunctiva SØ5.1- ☑
  - with foreign body (in conjunctival sac) — *see* Foreign body, conjunctival sac
- conus medullaris (spine) S34.139 ☑
- cornea — *see* Contusion, eyeball
  - with foreign body — *see* Foreign body, cornea
- corpus cavernosum S3Ø.21 ☑
- cortex (brain) (cerebral) — *see* Injury, intracranial, diffuse
  - focal — *see* Injury, intracranial, focal
- costal region — *see* Contusion, thorax
- cystic duct S36.13 ☑
- diaphragm S27.8Ø2 ☑
- duodenum S36.42Ø ☑
- ear SØØ.43- ☑
- elbow S5Ø.Ø- ☑
  - with forearm — *see* Contusion, forearm
- epididymis S3Ø.22 ☑
- epigastric region S3Ø.1 ☑
- epiglottis S1Ø.Ø ☑
- esophagus (thoracic) S27.812 ☑
  - cervical S1Ø.Ø ☑
- eyeball SØ5.1- ☑
- eyebrow SØØ.1- ☑
- eyelid (and periocular area) SØØ.1- ☑
- face NEC SØØ.83 ☑
- fallopian tube S37.529 ☑
  - bilateral S37.522 ☑
  - unilateral S37.521 ☑
- femoral triangle S3Ø.1 ☑
- finger(s) S6Ø.ØØ ☑

- **Cor** — *continued*
  - pulmonale — *continued*
    - chronic I27.81
      - with chronic pulmonary embolism I27.82
  - triatriatum, triatrium Q24.2
  - triloculare Q20.8
    - biatrium Q20.4
    - biventriculare Q21.19
- **Corbus' disease** (gangrenous balanitis) N48.1
- **Cord** — *see also* condition
  - around neck
    - complicating delivery O69.81 ☑
      - with compression O69.1 ☑
  - bladder G95.89
    - tabetic A52.19
- **Cordis ectopia** Q24.8
- **Corditis** (spermatic) N49.1
- **Corectopia** Q13.2
- **Cori's disease** (glycogen storage) E74.03
- **Corkhandler's disease or lung** J67.3
- **Corkscrew esophagus** K22.4
- **Corkworker's disease or lung** J67.3
- **Corn** (infected) L84
- **Cornea** — *see also* condition
  - donor Z52.5
  - plana Q13.4
- **Cornelia de Lange syndrome** Q87.19
- **Cornu cutaneum** L85.8
- **Cornual gestation or pregnancy** O00.80
  - with intrauterine pregnancy O00.81
- **Coronary** (artery) — *see* condition
- **Coronavirus** (infection)
  - 2019 — *see also* COVID-19 U07.1
  - as cause of diseases classified elsewhere B97.29
  - coronavirus-19 — *see also* COVID-19 U07.1
  - COVID-19 — *see also* COVID-19 U07.1
  - SARS-associated B97.21
- **Corpora** — *see also* condition
  - amylacea, prostate N42.89
  - cavernosa — *see* condition
- **Corpulence** — *see* Obesity
- **Corpus** — *see* condition
- **Corrected transposition** Q20.5
- **Corrosion** (injury) (acid) (caustic) (chemical) (lime) (external) (internal) T30.4
  - abdomen, abdominal (muscle) (wall) T21.42 ☑
    - first degree T21.52 ☑
    - second degree T21.62 ☑
    - third degree T21.72 ☑
  - above elbow T22.439 ☑
    - first degree T22.539 ☑
    - left T22.432 ☑
      - first degree T22.532 ☑
      - second degree T22.632 ☑
      - third degree T22.732 ☑
    - right T22.431 ☑
      - first degree T22.531 ☑
      - second degree T22.631 ☑
      - third degree T22.731 ☑
    - second degree T22.639 ☑
    - third degree T22.739 ☑
  - alimentary tract NEC T28.7 ☑
  - ankle T25.419 ☑
    - first degree T25.519 ☑
    - left T25.412 ☑
      - first degree T25.512 ☑
      - second degree T25.612 ☑
      - third degree T25.712 ☑
    - multiple with foot — *see* Corrosion, lower, limb, multiple, ankle and foot
    - right T25.411 ☑
      - first degree T25.511 ☑
      - second degree T25.611 ☑
      - third degree T25.711 ☑
    - second degree T25.619 ☑
    - third degree T25.719 ☑
  - anus — *see* Corrosion, buttock
  - arm(s) (meaning upper limb(s)) — *see* Corrosion, upper limb
  - axilla T22.449 ☑
    - first degree T22.549 ☑
    - left T22.442 ☑
      - first degree T22.542 ☑
      - second degree T22.642 ☑
      - third degree T22.742 ☑
    - right T22.441 ☑

- **Corrosion** — *continued*
  - axilla — *continued*
    - right — *continued*
      - first degree T22.541 ☑
      - second degree T22.641 ☑
      - third degree T22.741 ☑
    - second degree T22.649 ☑
    - third degree T22.749 ☑
  - back (lower) T21.44 ☑
    - first degree T21.54 ☑
    - second degree T21.64 ☑
    - third degree T21.74 ☑
    - upper T21.43 ☑
      - first degree T21.53 ☑
      - second degree T21.63 ☑
      - third degree T21.73 ☑
  - blisters — *code as* Corrosion, second degree, by site
  - breast(s) — *see* Corrosion, chest wall
  - buttock(s) T21.45 ☑
    - first degree T21.55 ☑
    - second degree T21.65 ☑
    - third degree T21.75 ☑
  - calf T24.439 ☑
    - first degree T24.539 ☑
    - left T24.432 ☑
      - first degree T24.532 ☑
      - second degree T24.632 ☑
      - third degree T24.732 ☑
    - right T24.431 ☑
      - first degree T24.531 ☑
      - second degree T24.631 ☑
      - third degree T24.731 ☑
    - second degree T24.639 ☑
    - third degree T24.739 ☑
  - canthus (eye) — *see* Corrosion, eyelid
  - cervix T28.8 ☑
  - cheek T20.46 ☑
    - first degree T20.56 ☑
    - second degree T20.66 ☑
    - third degree T20.76 ☑
  - chest wall T21.41 ☑
    - first degree T21.51 ☑
    - second degree T21.61 ☑
    - third degree T21.71 ☑
  - chin T20.43 ☑
    - first degree T20.53 ☑
    - second degree T20.63 ☑
    - third degree T20.73 ☑
  - colon T28.7 ☑
  - conjunctiva (and cornea) — *see* Corrosion, cornea
  - cornea (and conjunctiva) T26.6- ☑
  - deep necrosis of underlying tissue — *code as* Corrosion, third degree, by site
  - dorsum of hand T23.469 ☑
    - first degree T23.569 ☑
    - left T23.462 ☑
      - first degree T23.562 ☑
      - second degree T23.662 ☑
      - third degree T23.762 ☑
    - right T23.461 ☑
      - first degree T23.561 ☑
      - second degree T23.661 ☑
      - third degree T23.761 ☑
    - second degree T23.669 ☑
    - third degree T23.769 ☑
  - ear (auricle) (external) (canal) T20.41 ☑
    - drum T28.91 ☑
    - first degree T20.51 ☑
    - second degree T20.61 ☑
    - third degree T20.71 ☑
  - elbow T22.429 ☑
    - first degree T22.529 ☑
    - left T22.422 ☑
      - first degree T22.522 ☑
      - second degree T22.622 ☑
      - third degree T22.722 ☑
    - right T22.421 ☑
      - first degree T22.521 ☑
      - second degree T22.621 ☑
      - third degree T22.721 ☑
    - second degree T22.629 ☑
    - third degree T22.729 ☑
  - entire body — *see* Corrosion, multiple body regions
  - epidermal loss — *code as* Corrosion, second degree, by site
  - epiglottis T27.4 ☑

- **Corrosion** — *continued*
  - erythema, erythematous — *code as* Corrosion, first degree, by site
  - esophagus T28.6 ☑
  - extent (percentage of body surface)
    - less than 10 percent T32.0
    - 10-19 percent (0-9 percent third degree) T32.10
      - with 10-19 percent third degree T32.11
    - 20-29 percent (0-9 percent third degree) T32.20
      - with
        - 10-19 percent third degree T32.21
        - 20-29 percent third degree T32.22
    - 30-39 percent (0-9 percent third degree) T32.30
      - with
        - 10-19 percent third degree T32.31
        - 20-29 percent third degree T32.32
        - 30-39 percent third degree T32.33
    - 40-49 percent (0-9 percent third degree) T32.40
      - with
        - 10-19 percent third degree T32.41
        - 20-29 percent third degree T32.42
        - 30-39 percent third degree T32.43
        - 40-49 percent third degree T32.44
    - 50-59 percent (0-9 percent third degree) T32.50
      - with
        - 10-19 percent third degree T32.51
        - 20-29 percent third degree T32.52
        - 30-39 percent third degree T32.53
        - 40-49 percent third degree T32.54
        - 50-59 percent third degree T32.55
    - 60-69 percent (0-9 percent third degree) T32.60
      - with
        - 10-19 percent third degree T32.61
        - 20-29 percent third degree T32.62
        - 30-39 percent third degree T32.63
        - 40-49 percent third degree T32.64
        - 50-59 percent third degree T32.65
        - 60-69 percent third degree T32.66
    - 70-79 percent (0-9 percent third degree) T32.70
      - with
        - 10-19 percent third degree T32.71
        - 20-29 percent third degree T32.72
        - 30-39 percent third degree T32.73
        - 40-49 percent third degree T32.74
        - 50-59 percent third degree T32.75
        - 60-69 percent third degree T32.76
        - 70-79 percent third degree T32.77
    - 80-89 percent (0-9 percent third degree) T32.80
      - with
        - 10-19 percent third degree T32.81
        - 20-29 percent third degree T32.82
        - 30-39 percent third degree T32.83
        - 40-49 percent third degree T32.84
        - 50-59 percent third degree T32.85
        - 60-69 percent third degree T32.86
        - 70-79 percent third degree T32.87
        - 80-89 percent third degree T32.88
    - 90 percent or more (0-9 percent third degree) T32.90
      - with
        - 10-19 percent third degree T32.91
        - 20-29 percent third degree T32.92
        - 30-39 percent third degree T32.93
        - 40-49 percent third degree T32.94
        - 50-59 percent third degree T32.95
        - 60-69 percent third degree T32.96
        - 70-79 percent third degree T32.97
        - 80-89 percent third degree T32.98
        - 90-99 percent third degree T32.99
  - extremity — *see* Corrosion, limb
  - eye(s) and adnexa T26.9- ☑
    - with resulting rupture and destruction of eyeball T26.7- ☑
    - conjunctival sac — *see* Corrosion, cornea
    - cornea — *see* Corrosion, cornea
    - lid — *see* Corrosion, eyelid
    - periocular area — *see* Corrosion eyelid
    - specified site NEC T26.8- ☑
  - eyeball — *see* Corrosion, eye
  - eyelid(s) T26.5- ☑
  - face — *see* Corrosion, head
  - finger T23.429 ☑
    - first degree T23.529 ☑
    - left T23.422 ☑
      - first degree T23.522 ☑
      - second degree T23.622 ☑
      - third degree T23.722 ☑
    - multiple sites (without thumb) T23.439 ☑
      - with thumb T23.449 ☑

Corrosion — *continued*
- finger — *continued*
  - multiple sites — *continued*
    - with thumb — *continued*
      - first degree T23.549 ☑
      - left T23.442 ☑
        - first degree T23.542 ☑
        - second degree T23.642 ☑
        - third degree T23.742 ☑
      - right T23.441 ☑
        - first degree T23.541 ☑
        - second degree T23.641 ☑
        - third degree T23.741 ☑
      - second degree T23.649 ☑
      - third degree T23.749 ☑
    - first degree T23.539 ☑
    - left T23.432 ☑
      - first degree T23.532 ☑
      - second degree T23.632 ☑
      - third degree T23.732 ☑
    - right T23.431 ☑
      - first degree T23.531 ☑
      - second degree T23.631 ☑
      - third degree T23.731 ☑
    - second degree T23.639 ☑
    - third degree T23.739 ☑
  - right T23.421 ☑
    - first degree T23.521 ☑
    - second degree T23.621 ☑
    - third degree T23.721 ☑
  - second degree T23.629 ☑
  - third degree T23.729 ☑
- flank — *see* Corrosion, abdomen
- foot T25.429 ☑
  - first degree T25.529 ☑
  - left T25.422 ☑
    - first degree T25.522 ☑
    - second degree T25.622 ☑
    - third degree T25.722 ☑
  - multiple with ankle — *see* Corrosion, lower, limb, multiple, ankle and foot
  - right T25.421 ☑
    - first degree T25.521 ☑
    - second degree T25.621 ☑
    - third degree T25.721 ☑
  - second degree T25.629 ☑
  - third degree T25.729 ☑
- forearm T22.419 ☑
  - first degree T22.519 ☑
  - left T22.412 ☑
    - first degree T22.512 ☑
    - second degree T22.612 ☑
    - third degree T22.712 ☑
  - right T22.411 ☑
    - first degree T22.511 ☑
    - second degree T22.611 ☑
    - third degree T22.711 ☑
  - second degree T22.619 ☑
  - third degree T22.719 ☑
- forehead T20.46 ☑
  - first degree T20.56 ☑
  - second degree T20.66 ☑
  - third degree T20.76 ☑
- fourth degree — *code as* Corrosion, third degree, by site
- full thickness skin loss — *code as* Corrosion, third degree, by site
- gastrointestinal tract NEC T28.7 ☑
- genital organs
  - external
    - female T21.47 ☑
      - first degree T21.57 ☑
      - second degree T21.67 ☑
      - third degree T21.77 ☑
    - male T21.46 ☑
      - first degree T21.56 ☑
      - second degree T21.66 ☑
      - third degree T21.76 ☑
  - internal T28.8 ☑
- groin — *see* Corrosion, abdominal wall
- hand(s) T23.409 ☑
  - back — *see* Corrosion, dorsum of hand
  - finger — *see* Corrosion, finger
  - first degree T23.509 ☑
  - left T23.402 ☑
    - first degree T23.502 ☑

Corrosion — *continued*
- hand(s) — *continued*
  - left — *continued*
    - second degree T23.602 ☑
    - third degree T23.702 ☑
  - multiple sites with wrist T23.499 ☑
    - first degree T23.599 ☑
    - left T23.492 ☑
      - first degree T23.592 ☑
      - second degree T23.692 ☑
      - third degree T23.792 ☑
    - right T23.491 ☑
      - first degree T23.591 ☑
      - second degree T23.691 ☑
      - third degree T23.791 ☑
    - second degree T23.699 ☑
    - third degree T23.799 ☑
  - palm — *see* Corrosion, palm
  - right T23.401 ☑
    - first degree T23.501 ☑
    - second degree T23.601 ☑
    - third degree T23.701 ☑
  - second degree T23.609 ☑
  - third degree T23.709 ☑
  - thumb — *see* Corrosion, thumb
- head (and face) (and neck) T20.40 ☑
  - cheek — *see* Corrosion, cheek
  - chin — *see* Corrosion, chin
  - ear — *see* Corrosion, ear
  - eye(s) only — *see* Corrosion, eye
  - first degree T20.50 ☑
  - forehead — *see* Corrosion, forehead
  - lip — *see* Corrosion, lip
  - multiple sites T20.49 ☑
    - first degree T20.59 ☑
    - second degree T20.69 ☑
    - third degree T20.79 ☑
  - neck — *see* Corrosion, neck
  - nose — *see* Corrosion, nose
  - scalp — *see* Corrosion, scalp
  - second degree T20.60 ☑
  - third degree T20.70 ☑
- hip(s) — *see* Corrosion, lower, limb
- inhalation — *see* Corrosion, respiratory tract
- internal organ(s) — *see also* Corrosion, by site T28.90 ☑
  - alimentary tract T28.7 ☑
    - esophagus T28.6 ☑
  - esophagus T28.6 ☑
  - genitourinary T28.8 ☑
  - mouth T28.5 ☑
  - pharynx T28.5 ☑
  - specified organ NEC T28.99 ☑
- interscapular region — *see* Corrosion, back, upper
- intestine (large) (small) T28.7 ☑
- knee T24.429 ☑
  - first degree T24.529 ☑
  - left T24.422 ☑
    - first degree T24.522 ☑
    - second degree T24.622 ☑
    - third degree T24.722 ☑
  - right T24.421 ☑
    - first degree T24.521 ☑
    - second degree T24.621 ☑
    - third degree T24.721 ☑
  - second degree T24.629 ☑
  - third degree T24.729 ☑
- labium (majus) (minus) — *see* Corrosion, genital organs, external, female
- lacrimal apparatus, duct, gland or sac — *see* Corrosion, eye, specified site NEC
- larynx T27.4 ☑
  - with lung T27.5 ☑
- leg(s) (meaning lower limb(s)) — *see* Corrosion, lower limb
- limb(s)
  - lower — *see* Corrosion, lower, limb
  - upper — *see* Corrosion, upper limb
- lip(s) T20.42 ☑
  - first degree T20.52 ☑
  - second degree T20.62 ☑
  - third degree T20.72 ☑
- lower
  - back — *see* Corrosion, back
  - limb T24.409 ☑
    - ankle — *see* Corrosion, ankle

Corrosion — *continued*
- lower — *continued*
  - limb — *continued*
    - calf — *see* Corrosion, calf
    - first degree T24.509 ☑
    - foot — *see* Corrosion, foot
    - knee — *see* Corrosion, knee
    - left T24.402 ☑
      - first degree T24.502 ☑
      - second degree T24.602 ☑
      - third degree T24.702 ☑
    - multiple sites, except ankle and foot T24.499 ☑
      - ankle and foot T25.499 ☑
        - first degree T25.599 ☑
        - left T25.492 ☑
          - first degree T25.592 ☑
          - second degree T25.692 ☑
          - third degree T25.792 ☑
        - right T25.491 ☑
          - first degree T25.591 ☑
          - second degree T25.691 ☑
          - third degree T25.791 ☑
        - second degree T25.699 ☑
        - third degree T25.799 ☑
      - first degree T24.599 ☑
      - left T24.492 ☑
        - first degree T24.592 ☑
        - second degree T24.692 ☑
        - third degree T24.792 ☑
      - right T24.491 ☑
        - first degree T24.591 ☑
        - second degree T24.691 ☑
        - third degree T24.791 ☑
      - second degree T24.699 ☑
      - third degree T24.799 ☑
    - right T24.401 ☑
      - first degree T24.501 ☑
      - second degree T24.601 ☑
      - third degree T24.701 ☑
    - second degree T24.609 ☑
    - thigh — *see* Corrosion, thigh
    - third degree T24.709 ☑
- lung (with larynx and trachea) T27.5 ☑
- mouth T28.5 ☑
- neck T20.47 ☑
  - first degree T20.57 ☑
  - second degree T20.67 ☑
  - third degree T20.77 ☑
- nose (septum) T20.44 ☑
  - first degree T20.54 ☑
  - second degree T20.64 ☑
  - third degree T20.74 ☑
- ocular adnexa — *see* Corrosion, eye
- orbit region — *see* Corrosion, eyelid
- palm T23.459 ☑
  - first degree T23.559 ☑
  - left T23.452 ☑
    - first degree T23.552 ☑
    - second degree T23.652 ☑
    - third degree T23.752 ☑
  - right T23.451 ☑
    - first degree T23.551 ☑
    - second degree T23.651 ☑
    - third degree T23.751 ☑
  - second degree T23.659 ☑
  - third degree T23.759 ☑
- partial thickness — *code as* Corrosion, unspecified degree, by site
- pelvis — *see* Corrosion, trunk
- penis — *see* Corrosion, genital organs, external, male
- perineum
  - female — *see* Corrosion, genital organs, external, female
  - male — *see* Corrosion, genital organs, external, male
- periocular area — *see* Corrosion, eyelid
- pharynx T28.5 ☑
- rectum T28.7 ☑
- respiratory tract T27.7 ☑
  - larynx — *see* Corrosion, larynx
  - specified part NEC T27.6 ☑
  - trachea — *see* Corrosion, larynx
- sac, lacrimal — *see* Corrosion, eye, specified site NEC
- scalp T20.45 ☑
  - first degree T20.55 ☑
  - second degree T20.65 ☑
  - third degree T20.75 ☑

Corrosion — *continued*
- scapular region T22.469 ☑
  - first degree T22.569 ☑
  - left T22.462 ☑
    - first degree T22.562 ☑
    - second degree T22.662 ☑
    - third degree T22.762 ☑
  - right T22.461 ☑
    - first degree T22.561 ☑
    - second degree T22.661 ☑
    - third degree T22.761 ☑
  - second degree T22.669 ☑
  - third degree T22.769 ☑
- sclera — *see* Corrosion, eye, specified site NEC
- scrotum — *see* Corrosion, genital organs, external, male
- shoulder T22.459 ☑
  - first degree T22.559 ☑
  - left T22.452 ☑
    - first degree T22.552 ☑
    - second degree T22.652 ☑
    - third degree T22.752 ☑
  - right T22.451 ☑
    - first degree T22.551 ☑
    - second degree T22.651 ☑
    - third degree T22.751 ☑
  - second degree T22.659 ☑
  - third degree T22.759 ☑
- stomach T28.7 ☑
- temple — *see* Corrosion, head
- testis — *see* Corrosion, genital organs, external, male
- thigh T24.419 ☑
  - first degree T24.519 ☑
  - left T24.412 ☑
    - first degree T24.512 ☑
    - second degree T24.612 ☑
    - third degree T24.712 ☑
  - right T24.411 ☑
    - first degree T24.511 ☑
    - second degree T24.611 ☑
    - third degree T24.711 ☑
  - second degree T24.619 ☑
  - third degree T24.719 ☑
- thorax (external) — *see* Corrosion, trunk
- throat (meaning pharynx) T28.5 ☑
- thumb(s) T23.419 ☑
  - first degree T23.519 ☑
  - left T23.412 ☑
    - first degree T23.512 ☑
    - second degree T23.612 ☑
    - third degree T23.712 ☑
  - multiple sites with fingers T23.449 ☑
    - first degree T23.549 ☑
    - left T23.442 ☑
      - first degree T23.542 ☑
      - second degree T23.642 ☑
      - third degree T23.742 ☑
    - right T23.441 ☑
      - first degree T23.541 ☑
      - second degree T23.641 ☑
      - third degree T23.741 ☑
    - second degree T23.649 ☑
    - third degree T23.749 ☑
  - right T23.411 ☑
    - first degree T23.511 ☑
    - second degree T23.611 ☑
    - third degree T23.711 ☑
  - second degree T23.619 ☑
  - third degree T23.719 ☑
- toe T25.439 ☑
  - first degree T25.539 ☑
  - left T25.432 ☑
    - first degree T25.532 ☑
    - second degree T25.632 ☑
    - third degree T25.732 ☑
  - right T25.431 ☑
    - first degree T25.531 ☑
    - second degree T25.631 ☑
    - third degree T25.731 ☑
  - second degree T25.639 ☑
  - third degree T25.739 ☑
- tongue T28.5 ☑
- tonsil(s) T28.5 ☑
- total body — *see* Corrosion, multiple body regions
- trachea T27.4 ☑

Corrosion — *continued*
- trachea — *continued*
  - with lung T27.5 ☑
- trunk T21.40 ☑
  - abdominal wall — *see* Corrosion, abdominal wall
  - anus — *see* Corrosion, buttock
  - axilla — *see* Corrosion, upper limb
  - back — *see* Corrosion, back
  - breast — *see* Corrosion, chest wall
  - buttock — *see* Corrosion, buttock
  - chest wall — *see* Corrosion, chest wall
  - first degree T21.50 ☑
  - flank — *see* Corrosion, abdominal wall
  - genital
    - female — *see* Corrosion, genital organs, external, female
    - male — *see* Corrosion, genital organs, external, male
  - groin — *see* Corrosion, abdominal wall
  - interscapular region — *see* Corrosion, back, upper
  - labia — *see* Corrosion, genital organs, external, female
  - lower back — *see* Corrosion, back
  - penis — *see* Corrosion, genital organs, external, male
  - perineum
    - female — *see* Corrosion, genital organs, external, female
    - male — *see* Corrosion, genital organs, external, male
  - scapular region — *see* Corrosion, upper limb
  - scrotum — *see* Corrosion, genital organs, external, male
  - second degree T21.60 ☑
  - shoulder — *see* Corrosion, upper limb
  - specified site NEC T21.49 ☑
    - first degree T21.59 ☑
    - second degree T21.69 ☑
    - third degree T21.79 ☑
  - testes — *see* Corrosion, genital organs, external, male
  - third degree T21.70 ☑
  - upper back — *see* Corrosion, back, upper
  - vagina T28.8 ☑
  - vulva — *see* Corrosion, genital organs, external, female
- unspecified site with extent of body surface involved specified
  - less than 10 percent T32.0
  - 10-19 percent (0-9 percent third degree) T32.10
    - with 10-19 percent third degree T32.11
  - 20-29 percent (0-9 percent third degree) T32.20
    - with
      - 10-19 percent third degree T32.21
      - 20-29 percent third degree T32.22
  - 30-39 percent (0-9 percent third degree) T32.30
    - with
      - 10-19 percent third degree T32.31
      - 20-29 percent third degree T32.32
      - 30-39 percent third degree T32.33
  - 40-49 percent (0-9 percent third degree) T32.40
    - with
      - 10-19 percent third degree T32.41
      - 20-29 percent third degree T32.42
      - 30-39 percent third degree T32.43
      - 40-49 percent third degree T32.44
  - 50-59 percent (0-9 percent third degree) T32.50
    - with
      - 10-19 percent third degree T32.51
      - 20-29 percent third degree T32.52
      - 30-39 percent third degree T32.53
      - 40-49 percent third degree T32.54
      - 50-59 percent third degree T32.55
  - 60-69 percent (0-9 percent third degree) T32.60
    - with
      - 10-19 percent third degree T32.61
      - 20-29 percent third degree T32.62
      - 30-39 percent third degree T32.63
      - 40-49 percent third degree T32.64
      - 50-59 percent third degree T32.65
      - 60-69 percent third degree T32.66
  - 70-79 percent (0-9 percent third degree) T32.70
    - with
      - 10-19 percent third degree T32.71
      - 20-29 percent third degree T32.72
      - 30-39 percent third degree T32.73
      - 40-49 percent third degree T32.74
      - 50-59 percent third degree T32.75

Corrosion — *continued*
- unspecified site with extent of body surface involved specified — *continued*
  - 70-79 percent — *continued*
    - with — *continued*
      - 60-69 percent third degree T32.76
      - 70-79 percent third degree T32.77
  - 80-89 percent (0-9 percent third degree) T32.80
    - with
      - 10-19 percent third degree T32.81
      - 20-29 percent third degree T32.82
      - 30-39 percent third degree T32.83
      - 40-49 percent third degree T32.84
      - 50-59 percent third degree T32.85
      - 60-69 percent third degree T32.86
      - 70-79 percent third degree T32.87
      - 80-89 percent third degree T32.88
  - 90 percent or more (0-9 percent third degree) T32.90
    - with
      - 10-19 percent third degree T32.91
      - 20-29 percent third degree T32.92
      - 30-39 percent third degree T32.93
      - 40-49 percent third degree T32.94
      - 50-59 percent third degree T32.95
      - 60-69 percent third degree T32.96
      - 70-79 percent third degree T32.97
      - 80-89 percent third degree T32.98
      - 90-99 percent third degree T32.99
- upper limb (axilla) (scapular region) T22.40 ☑
  - above elbow — *see* Corrosion, above elbow
  - axilla — *see* Corrosion, axilla
  - elbow — *see* Corrosion, elbow
  - first degree T22.50 ☑
  - forearm — *see* Corrosion, forearm
  - hand — *see* Corrosion, hand
  - interscapular region — *see* Corrosion, back, upper
  - multiple sites T22.499 ☑
    - first degree T22.599 ☑
    - left T22.492 ☑
      - first degree T22.592 ☑
      - second degree T22.692 ☑
      - third degree T22.792 ☑
    - right T22.491 ☑
      - first degree T22.591 ☑
      - second degree T22.691 ☑
      - third degree T22.791 ☑
    - second degree T22.699 ☑
    - third degree T22.799 ☑
  - scapular region — *see* Corrosion, scapular region
  - second degree T22.60 ☑
  - shoulder — *see* Corrosion, shoulder
  - third degree T22.70 ☑
  - wrist — *see* Corrosion, hand
- uterus T28.8 ☑
- vagina T28.8 ☑
- vulva — *see* Corrosion, genital organs, external, female
- wrist T23.479 ☑
  - first degree T23.579 ☑
  - left T23.472 ☑
    - first degree T23.572 ☑
    - second degree T23.672 ☑
    - third degree T23.772 ☑
  - multiple sites with hand T23.499 ☑
    - first degree T23.599 ☑
    - left T23.492 ☑
      - first degree T23.592 ☑
      - second degree T23.692 ☑
      - third degree T23.792 ☑
    - right T23.491 ☑
      - first degree T23.591 ☑
      - second degree T23.691 ☑
      - third degree T23.791 ☑
    - second degree T23.699 ☑
    - third degree T23.799 ☑
  - right T23.471 ☑
    - first degree T23.571 ☑
    - second degree T23.671 ☑
    - third degree T23.771 ☑
  - second degree T23.679 ☑
  - third degree T23.779 ☑

Corrosive burn — *see* Corrosion

Corsican fever — *see* Malaria

Cortical — *see* condition

Cortico-adrenal — *see* condition

Coryza (acute) J00
- with grippe or influenza — *see* Influenza, with, respiratory manifestations NEC

Coryza — *continued*
  syphilitic
    congenital (chronic) A5Ø.Ø5
Co-sleeping, child-caregiver Z72.823
Costen's syndrome or complex M26.69
Costiveness — *see* Constipation
Costochondritis M94.Ø
Cot death R99
Cotard's syndrome F22
Cotia virus BØ8.8
Cotton wool spots (retinal) H35.81
Cotungo's disease — *see* Sciatica
Cough (affected) (epidemic) (nervous) RØ5.9
  with hemorrhage — *see* Hemoptysis
  acute RØ5.1
  bronchial RØ5.8
    with grippe or influenza — *see* Influenza, with, respiratory manifestations NEC
  chronic RØ5.3
  functional F45.8
  hysterical F45.8
  laryngeal, spasmodic RØ5.8
  paroxysmal, due to Bordetella pertussis (without pneumonia) A37.ØØ
    with pneumonia A37.Ø1
  persistent RØ5.3
  psychogenic F45.8
  refractory RØ5.3
  smokers' J41.Ø
  specified NEC RØ5.8
  subacute RØ5.2
  syncope RØ5.4
  tea taster's B49
  unexplained RØ5.3
Counseling (for) Z71.9
  abuse NEC
    perpetrator Z69.82
    victim Z69.81
  alcohol abuser Z71.41
    family Z71.42
  child abuse
    nonparental
      perpetrator Z69.Ø21
      victim Z69.Ø2Ø
    parental
      perpetrator Z69.Ø11
      victim Z69.Ø1Ø
  consanguinity Z71.89
  contraceptive Z3Ø.Ø9
  dietary Z71.3
  drug abuser Z71.51
    family member Z71.52
  exercise Z71.82
  family Z71.89
  fertility preservation (prior to cancer therapy) (prior to removal of gonads) Z31.62
  for non-attending third party Z71.Ø
    related to sexual behavior or orientation Z7Ø.2
  genetic
    nonprocreative Z71.83
    procreative NEC Z31.5
  gestational carrier Z31.7
  health (advice) (education) (instruction) — *see* Counseling, medical
    risk for travel (international) Z71.84
  human immunodeficiency virus (HIV) Z71.7
  immunization safety Z71.85
  impotence Z7Ø.1
  insulin pump use Z46.81
  medical (for) Z71.9
    boarding school resident Z59.3
    consanguinity Z71.89
    feared complaint and no disease found Z71.1
    human immunodeficiency virus (HIV) Z71.7
    institutional resident Z59.3
    on behalf of another Z71.Ø
      related to sexual behavior or orientation Z7Ø.2
    person living alone — *see also* Consultation, specified reason NEC Z6Ø.2
    specified reason NEC Z71.89
  natural family planning
    procreative Z31.61
    to avoid pregnancy Z3Ø.Ø2
  pediatric-to-adult transition Z71.87
  perpetrator (of)
    abuse NEC Z69.82
    child abuse
      non-parental Z69.Ø21

Counseling — *continued*
  perpetrator — *continued*
    child abuse — *continued*
      parental Z69.Ø11
    rape NEC Z69.82
    spousal abuse Z69.12
  procreative NEC Z31.69
    fertility preservation (prior to cancer therapy) (prior to removal of gonads) Z31.62
    using natural family planning Z31.61
  promiscuity Z7Ø.1
  rape victim Z69.81
  religious Z71.81
  safety for travel (international) Z71.84
  sex, sexual (related to) Z7Ø.9
    attitude(s) Z7Ø.Ø
    behavior or orientation Z7Ø.1
    combined concerns Z7Ø.3
    non-responsiveness Z7Ø.1
    on behalf of third party Z7Ø.2
    specified reason NEC Z7Ø.8
  socioeconomic factors Z71.88
  specified reason NEC Z71.89
  spiritual Z71.81
  spousal abuse (perpetrator) Z69.12
    victim Z69.11
  substance abuse Z71.89
    alcohol Z71.41
    drug Z71.51
    tobacco Z71.6
  tobacco use Z71.6
  travel (international) Z71.84
  use (of)
    insulin pump Z46.81
  vaccine product safety Z71.85
  victim (of)
    abuse Z69.81
    child abuse
      by parent Z69.Ø1Ø
      non-parental Z69.Ø2Ø
    rape NEC Z69.81
Coupled rhythm RØØ.8
Couvelaire syndrome or uterus (complicating delivery) O45.8X- ☑
COVID-19 UØ7.1
  condition post UØ9.9
  contact (with) Z2Ø.822
  exposure (to) Z2Ø.822
  history of (personal) Z86.16
  long (haul) UØ9.9
  partially vaccinated (for) Z28.311
  pneumonia J12.82
  screening Z11.52
  sequelae (post acute) UØ9.9
  unvaccinated (for) Z28.31Ø
Cowperitis — *see* Urethritis
Cowper's gland — *see* condition
Cowpox BØ8.Ø1Ø
  due to vaccination T88.1 ☑
Coxa
  magna M91.4- ☑
  plana M91.2- ☑
  valga (acquired) — *see also* Deformity, limb, specified type NEC, thigh
    congenital Q65.81
    sequelae (late effect) of rickets E64.3
  vara (acquired) — *see also* Deformity, limb, specified type NEC, thigh
    congenital Q65.82
    sequelae (late effect) of rickets E64.3
Coxalgia, coxalgic (nontuberculous) — *see also* Pain, joint, hip
  tuberculous A18.Ø2
Coxitis — *see* Monoarthritis, hip
Coxsackie (virus) (infection) B34.1
  as cause of disease classified elsewhere B97.11
  carditis B33.2Ø
  central nervous system NEC A88.8
  endocarditis B33.21
  enteritis AØ8.39
  meningitis (aseptic) A87.Ø
  myocarditis B33.22
  pericarditis B33.23
  pharyngitis BØ8.5
  pleurodynia B33.Ø
  specific disease NEC B33.8
Crabs, meaning pubic lice B85.3
Crack baby PØ4.41

Cracked nipple N64.Ø
  associated with
    lactation O92.13
    pregnancy O92.11- ☑
    puerperium O92.12
Cracked tooth KØ3.81
Cradle cap L21.Ø
Craft neurosis F48.8
Cramp(s) R25.2
  abdominal — *see* Pain, abdominal
  bathing T75.1 ☑
  colic R1Ø.83
    psychogenic F45.8
  due to immersion T75.1 ☑
  fireman T67.2 ☑
  heat T67.2 ☑
  immersion T75.1 ☑
  intestinal — *see* Pain, abdominal
    psychogenic F45.8
  leg, sleep related G47.62
  limb (lower) (upper) NEC R25.2
    sleep related G47.62
  linotypist's F48.8
    organic G25.89
  muscle (limb) (general) R25.2
    due to immersion T75.1 ☑
    psychogenic F45.8
  occupational (hand) F48.8
    organic G25.89
  salt-depletion E87.1
  sleep related, leg G47.62
  stoker's T67.2 ☑
  swimmer's T75.1 ☑
  telegrapher's F48.8
    organic G25.89
  typist's F48.8
    organic G25.89
  uterus N94.89
    menstrual — *see* Dysmenorrhea
  writer's F48.8
    organic G25.89
Cranial — *see* condition
Craniocleidodysostosis Q74.Ø
Craniofenestria (skull) Q75.8
Craniolacunia (skull) Q75.8
Craniopagus Q89.4
Craniopathy, metabolic M85.2
Craniopharyngeal — *see* condition
Craniopharyngioma D44.4
Craniorachischisis (totalis) QØØ.1
Cranioschisis Q75.8
Craniostenosis Q75.ØØ9
Craniosynostosis Q75.ØØ9
  bilateral Q75.ØØ2
  coronal Q75.Ø29
    bilateral Q75.Ø22
    unilateral Q75.Ø21
  lambdoid Q75.Ø49
    bilateral Q75.Ø42
    unilateral Q75.Ø41
  metopic Q75.Ø3
  multi-suture, specified NEC Q75.Ø58
  sagittal Q75.Ø1
  single-suture, specified NEC Q75.Ø8
  unilateral Q75.ØØ1
Craniotabes (cause unknown) M83.8
  neonatal P96.3
  rachitic E64.3
  syphilitic A5Ø.56
Cranium — *see* condition
Craw-craw — *see* Onchocerciasis
Creaking joint — *see* Derangement, joint, specified type NEC
Creeping
  eruption B76.9
  palsy or paralysis G12.22
Crenated tongue K14.8
Creotoxism AØ5.9
Crepitus
  caput Q75.8
  joint — *see* Derangement, joint, specified type NEC
Crescent or conus choroid, congenital Q14.3
CREST syndrome M34.1
Cretin, cretinism (congenital) (endemic) (nongoitrous) (sporadic) EØØ.9
  pelvis
    with disproportion (fetopelvic) O33.Ø

- **Cretin, cretinism** — *continued*
  - pelvis — *continued*
    - with disproportion — *continued*
      - causing obstructed labor O65.Ø
  - type
    - hypothyroid EØØ.1
    - mixed EØØ.2
    - myxedematous EØØ.1
    - neurological EØØ.Ø
- **Creutzfeldt-Jakob disease or syndrome** (with dementia) A81.ØØ
  - familial A81.Ø9
  - iatrogenic A81.Ø9
  - specified NEC A81.Ø9
  - sporadic A81.Ø9
  - variant (vCJD) A81.Ø1
- **Crib death** R99
- **Cribriform hymen** Q52.3
- **Cri-du-chat syndrome** Q93.4
- **Crigler-Najjar disease or syndrome** E8Ø.5
- **Crime, victim of** Z65.4
- **Crimean hemorrhagic fever** A98.Ø
- **Criminalism** F6Ø.2
- **Crisis**
  - abdomen R1Ø.Ø
  - acute reaction F43.Ø
  - addisonian E27.2
  - adrenal (cortical) E27.2
  - celiac K9Ø.Ø
  - Dietl's N13.8
  - emotional — *see also* Disorder, adjustment
    - acute reaction to stress F43.Ø
    - specific to childhood and adolescence F93.8
  - glaucomatocyclitic — *see* Glaucoma, secondary, inflammation
  - heart — *see* Failure, heart
  - nitritoid I95.2
    - correct substance properly administered — *see* Table of Drugs and Chemicals, by drug, adverse effect
    - overdose or wrong substance given or taken — *see* Table of Drugs and Chemicals, by drug, poisoning
  - oculogyric H51.8
    - psychogenic F45.8
  - Pel's (tabetic) A52.11
  - psychosexual identity F64.2
  - renal N28.Ø
  - sickle-cell — *see also* Disease, sickle-cell, by type, with crisis D57.ØØ
    - with
      - acute chest syndrome D57.Ø1
      - cerebral vascular involvement D57.Ø3
      - complication specified NEC D57.Ø9
      - pain (vaso-occlusive) D57.ØØ
      - splenic sequestration D57.Ø2
  - state (acute reaction) F43.Ø
  - tabetic A52.11
  - thyroid — *see* Thyrotoxicosis with thyroid storm
  - thyrotoxic — *see* Thyrotoxicosis with thyroid storm
- **Crocq's disease** (acrocyanosis) I73.89
- **Crohn's disease** — *see* Enteritis, regional
- **Crooked septum, nasal** J34.2
- **Cross syndrome** E7Ø.328
- **Crossbite** (anterior) (posterior) M26.24
- **Cross-eye** — *see* Strabismus, convergent concomitant
- **Croup, croupous** (catarrhal) (infectious) (inflammatory) (nondiphtheritic) JØ5.Ø
  - bronchial J2Ø.9
  - diphtheritic A36.2
  - false J38.5
  - spasmodic J38.5
    - diphtheritic A36.2
  - stridulous J38.5
    - diphtheritic A36.2
- **Crouzon's disease** Q75.1
- **Crowding, tooth, teeth, fully erupted** M26.31
- **CRST syndrome** M34.1
- **Cruchet's disease** A85.8
- **Cruelty in children** — *see also* Disorder, conduct
- **Crural ulcer** — *see* Ulcer, lower limb
- **Crush, crushed, crushing** T14.8 ☑
  - abdomen S38.1 ☑
  - ankle S97.Ø- ☑
  - arm (upper) (and shoulder) S47.- ☑
  - axilla — *see* Crush, arm
  - back, lower S38.1 ☑
- **Crush, crushed, crushing** — *continued*
  - buttock S38.1 ☑
  - cheek SØ7.Ø ☑
  - chest S28.Ø ☑
  - cranium SØ7.1 ☑
  - ear SØ7.Ø ☑
  - elbow S57.Ø- ☑
  - extremity
    - lower
      - ankle — *see* Crush, ankle
      - below knee — *see* Crush, leg
      - foot — *see* Crush, foot
      - hip — *see* Crush, hip
      - knee — *see* Crush, knee
      - thigh — *see* Crush, thigh
      - toe — *see* Crush, toe
    - upper
      - below elbow S67.9- ☑
      - elbow — *see* Crush, elbow
      - finger — *see* Crush, finger
      - forearm — *see* Crush, forearm
      - hand — *see* Crush, hand
      - thumb — *see* Crush, thumb
      - upper arm — *see* Crush, arm
      - wrist — *see* Crush, wrist
  - face SØ7.Ø ☑
  - finger(s) S67.1- ☑
    - with hand (and wrist) — *see* Crush, hand, specified site NEC
    - index S67.19- ☑
    - little S67.19- ☑
    - middle S67.19- ☑
    - ring S67.19- ☑
    - thumb — *see* Crush, thumb
  - foot S97.8- ☑
    - toe — *see* Crush, toe
  - forearm S57.8- ☑
  - genitalia, external
    - female S38.ØØ2 ☑
      - vagina S38.Ø3 ☑
      - vulva S38.Ø3 ☑
    - male S38.ØØ1 ☑
      - penis S38.Ø1 ☑
      - scrotum S38.Ø2 ☑
      - testis S38.Ø2 ☑
  - hand (except fingers alone) S67.2- ☑
    - with wrist S67.4- ☑
  - head SØ7.9 ☑
    - specified NEC SØ7.8 ☑
  - heel — *see* Crush, foot
  - hip S77.Ø- ☑
    - with thigh S77.2- ☑
  - internal organ (abdomen, chest, or pelvis) NEC T14.8 ☑
  - knee S87.Ø- ☑
  - labium (majus) (minus) S38.Ø3 ☑
  - larynx S17.Ø ☑
  - leg (lower) S87.8- ☑
    - knee — *see* Crush, knee
  - lip SØ7.Ø ☑
  - lower
    - back S38.1 ☑
    - leg — *see* Crush, leg
  - neck S17.9 ☑
  - nerve — *see* Injury, nerve
  - nose SØ7.Ø ☑
  - pelvis S38.1 ☑
  - penis S38.Ø1 ☑
  - scalp SØ7.8 ☑
  - scapular region — *see* Crush, arm
  - scrotum S38.Ø2 ☑
  - severe, unspecified site T14.8 ☑
  - shoulder (and upper arm) — *see* Crush, arm
  - skull SØ7.1 ☑
  - syndrome (complication of trauma) T79.5 ☑
  - testis S38.Ø2 ☑
  - thigh S77.1- ☑
    - with hip S77.2- ☑
  - throat S17.8 ☑
  - thumb S67.Ø- ☑
    - with hand (and wrist) — *see* Crush, hand, specified site NEC
  - toe(s) S97.1Ø- ☑
    - great S97.11- ☑
    - lesser S97.12- ☑
  - trachea S17.Ø ☑
  - vagina S38.Ø3 ☑
- **Crush, crushed, crushing** — *continued*
  - vulva S38.Ø3 ☑
  - wrist S67.3- ☑
    - with hand S67.4- ☑
- **Crusta lactea** L21.Ø
- **Crusts** R23.4
- **Crutch paralysis** — *see* Injury, brachial plexus
- **Cruveilhier-Baumgarten cirrhosis, disease or syndrome** K74.69
- **Cruveilhier's atrophy or disease** G12.8
- **Crying** (constant) (continuous) (excessive)
  - child, adolescent, or adult R45.83
  - infant (baby) (newborn) R68.11
- **Cryofibrinogenemia** D89.2
- **Cryoglobulinemia** (essential) (idiopathic) (mixed) (primary) (purpura) (secondary) (vasculitis) D89.1
  - with lung involvement D89.1 *[J99]*
- **Cryptitis** (anal) (rectal) K62.89
- **Cryptococcosis, cryptococcus** (infection) (neoformans) B45.9
  - bone B45.3
  - cerebral B45.1
  - cutaneous B45.2
  - disseminated B45.7
  - generalized B45.7
  - meningitis B45.1
  - meningocerebralis B45.1
  - osseous B45.3
  - pulmonary B45.Ø
  - skin B45.2
  - specified NEC B45.8
- **Cryptopapillitis** (anus) K62.89
- **Cryptophthalmos** Q11.2
  - syndrome Q87.Ø
- **Cryptorchid, cryptorchism, cryptorchidism** Q53.9
  - bilateral Q53.2Ø
    - abdominal Q53.211
    - perineal Q53.22
  - unilateral Q53.1Ø
    - abdominal Q53.111
    - perineal Q53.12
- **Cryptosporidiosis** AØ7.2
  - hepatobiliary B88.8
  - respiratory B88.8
- **Cryptostromosis** J67.6
- **Crystalluria** R82.998
- **Cubitus**
  - congenital Q68.8
  - valgus (acquired) M21.Ø- ☑
    - congenital Q68.8
    - sequelae (late effect) of rickets E64.3
  - varus (acquired) M21.1- ☑
    - congenital Q68.8
    - sequelae (late effect) of rickets E64.3
- **Cultural deprivation or shock** Z6Ø.3
- **Curling esophagus** K22.4
- **Curling's ulcer** — *see* Ulcer, peptic, acute
- **Curschmann** (-Batten) (-Steinert) **disease or syndrome** G71.11
- **Curse, Ondine's** — *see* Apnea, sleep
- **Curvature**
  - organ or site, congenital NEC — *see* Distortion
  - penis (lateral) Q55.61
  - Pott's (spinal) A18.Ø1
  - radius, idiopathic, progressive (congenital) Q74.Ø
  - spine (acquired) (angular) (idiopathic) (incorrect) (postural) — *see* Dorsopathy, deforming
    - congenital Q67.5
    - due to or associated with
      - Charcot-Marie-Tooth disease — *see also* subcategory M49.8 G6Ø.Ø
      - osteitis
        - deformans M88.88
        - fibrosa cystica — *see also* subcategory M49.8 E21.Ø
      - tuberculosis (Pott's curvature) A18.Ø1
    - sequelae (late effect) of rickets E64.3
    - tuberculous A18.Ø1
- **Cushingoid due to steroid therapy** E24.2
  - correct substance properly administered — *see* Table of Drugs and Chemicals, by drug, adverse effect
  - overdose or wrong substance given or taken — *see* Table of Drugs and Chemicals, by drug, poisoning
- **Cushing's**
  - syndrome or disease E24.9
    - drug-induced E24.2
    - iatrogenic E24.2

- **Cushing's** — *continued*
  - syndrome or disease — *continued*
    - pituitary-dependent E24.Ø
    - specified NEC E24.8
  - ulcer — *see* Ulcer, peptic, acute
- **Cusp, Carabelli** — *omit code*
- **Cut** (external) — *see also* Laceration
  - muscle — *see* Injury, muscle
- **Cutaneous** — *see also* condition
  - hemorrhage R23.3
  - larva migrans B76.9
- **Cutis** — *see also* condition
  - hyperelastica Q82.8
    - acquired L57.4
  - laxa (hyperelastica) — *see* Dermatolysis
  - marmorata R23.8
  - osteosis L94.2
  - pendula — *see* Dermatolysis
  - rhomboidalis nuchae L57.2
  - verticis gyrata Q82.8
    - acquired L91.8
- **Cyanosis** R23.Ø
  - due to
    - patent foramen botalli Q21.12
    - persistent foramen ovale Q21.12
  - enterogenous D74.8
  - paroxysmal digital — *see* Raynaud's disease
    - with gangrene I73.Ø1
  - retina, retinal H35.89
- **Cyanotic heart disease** I24.9
  - congenital Q24.9
- **Cycle**
  - anovulatory N97.Ø
  - menstrual, irregular N92.6
- **Cyclencephaly** QØ4.9
- **Cyclical vomiting, in migraine** — *see also* Vomiting, cyclical G43.AØ (*following* G43.7)
  - psychogenic F5Ø.89
- **Cyclitis** — *see also* Iridocyclitis H2Ø.9
  - chronic — *see* Iridocyclitis, chronic
  - Fuchs' heterochromic H2Ø.81- ☑
  - granulomatous — *see* Iridocyclitis, chronic
  - lens-induced — *see* Iridocyclitis, lens-induced
  - posterior H3Ø.2- ☑
- **Cycloid personality** F34.Ø
- **Cyclophoria** H5Ø.54
- **Cyclopia, cyclops** Q87.Ø
- **Cyclopism** Q87.Ø
- **Cyclosporiasis** AØ7.4
- **Cyclothymia** F34.Ø
- **Cyclothymic personality** F34.Ø
- **Cyclotropia** H5Ø.41- ☑
- **Cylindroma** — *see also* Neoplasm, malignant, by site
  - eccrine dermal — *see* Neoplasm, skin, benign
  - skin — *see* Neoplasm, skin, benign
- **Cylindruria** R82.998
- **Cynanche**
  - diphtheritic A36.2
  - tonsillaris J36
- **Cynophobia** F4Ø.218
- **Cynorexia** R63.2
- **Cyphosis** — *see* Kyphosis
- **Cyprus fever** — *see* Brucellosis
- **Cyst** (colloid) (mucous) (simple) (retention)
  - adenoid (infected) J35.8
  - adrenal gland E27.8
    - congenital Q89.1
  - air, lung J98.4
  - allantoic Q64.4
  - alveolar process (jaw bone) M27.4Ø
  - amnion, amniotic O41.8X- ☑
  - aneurysmal M27.49
  - anterior
    - chamber (eye) — *see* Cyst, iris
    - nasopalatine KØ9.1
  - antrum J34.1
  - anus K62.89
  - apical (tooth) (periodontal) KØ4.8
  - appendix K38.8
  - arachnoid, brain (acquired) G93.Ø
    - congenital QØ4.6
  - arytenoid J38.7
  - Baker's M71.2- ☑
    - ruptured M66.Ø
    - tuberculous A18.Ø2
  - Bartholin's gland N75.Ø
  - bile duct (common) (hepatic) K83.5

- **Cyst** — *continued*
  - bladder (multiple) (trigone) N32.89
  - blue dome (breast) — *see* Cyst, breast
  - bone (local) NEC M85.6Ø
    - aneurysmal M85.5Ø
      - ankle M85.57- ☑
      - foot M85.57- ☑
      - forearm M85.53- ☑
      - hand M85.54- ☑
      - jaw M27.49
      - lower leg M85.56- ☑
      - multiple site M85.59
      - neck M85.58
      - rib M85.58
      - shoulder M85.51- ☑
      - skull M85.58
      - specified site NEC M85.58
      - thigh M85.55- ☑
      - toe M85.57- ☑
      - upper arm M85.52- ☑
      - vertebra M85.58
    - solitary M85.4Ø
      - ankle M85.47- ☑
      - fibula M85.46- ☑
      - foot M85.47- ☑
      - hand M85.44- ☑
      - humerus M85.42- ☑
      - jaw M27.49
      - neck M85.48
      - pelvis M85.45- ☑
      - radius M85.43- ☑
      - rib M85.48
      - shoulder M85.41- ☑
      - skull M85.48
      - specified site NEC M85.48
      - tibia M85.46- ☑
      - toe M85.47- ☑
      - ulna M85.43- ☑
      - vertebra M85.48
    - specified type NEC M85.6Ø
      - ankle M85.67- ☑
      - foot M85.67- ☑
      - forearm M85.63- ☑
      - hand M85.64- ☑
      - jaw M27.4Ø
        - developmental (nonodontogenic) KØ9.1
          - odontogenic KØ9.Ø
        - latent M27.Ø
      - lower leg M85.66- ☑
      - multiple site M85.69
      - neck M85.68
      - rib M85.68
      - shoulder M85.61- ☑
      - skull M85.68
      - specified site NEC M85.68
      - thigh M85.65- ☑
      - toe M85.67- ☑
      - upper arm M85.62- ☑
      - vertebra M85.68
  - brain (acquired) G93.Ø
    - congenital QØ4.6
    - hydatid B67.99 *[G94]*
    - third ventricle (colloid), congenital QØ4.6
  - branchial (cleft) Q18.Ø
  - branchiogenic Q18.Ø
  - breast (benign) (blue dome) (pedunculated) (solitary) N6Ø.Ø- ☑
    - involution — *see* Dysplasia, mammary, specified type NEC
    - sebaceous — *see* Dysplasia, mammary, specified type NEC
  - broad ligament (benign) N83.8
  - bronchogenic (mediastinal) (sequestration) J98.4
    - congenital Q33.Ø
  - buccal KØ9.8
  - bulbourethral gland N36.8
  - bursa, bursal NEC M71.3Ø
    - with rupture — *see* Rupture, synovium
    - ankle M71.37- ☑
    - elbow M71.32- ☑
    - foot M71.37- ☑
    - hand M71.34- ☑
    - hip M71.35- ☑
    - multiple sites M71.39
    - pharyngeal J39.2
    - popliteal space — *see* Cyst, Baker's
    - shoulder M71.31- ☑

- **Cyst** — *continued*
  - bursa, bursal — *continued*
    - specified site NEC M71.38
    - wrist M71.33- ☑
  - calcifying odontogenic D16.5
    - upper jaw (bone) (maxilla) D16.4
  - canal of Nuck (female) N94.89
    - congenital Q52.4
  - canthus — *see* Cyst, conjunctiva
  - carcinomatous — *see* Neoplasm, malignant, by site
  - cauda equina G95.89
  - cavum septi pellucidi — *see* Cyst, brain
  - celomic (pericardium) Q24.8
  - cerebellopontine (angle) — *see* Cyst, brain
  - cerebellum — *see* Cyst, brain
  - cerebral — *see* Cyst, brain
  - cervical lateral Q18.Ø
  - cervix NEC N88.8
    - embryonic Q51.6
    - nabothian N88.8
  - chiasmal optic NEC — *see* Disorder, optic, chiasm
  - chocolate (ovary) N8Ø.1Ø- ☑
  - choledochus, congenital Q44.4
  - chorion O41.8X- ☑
  - choroid plexus G93.Ø
    - congenital QØ4.6
  - ciliary body — *see* Cyst, iris
  - clitoris N9Ø.7
  - colon K63.89
  - common (bile) duct K83.5
  - congenital NEC Q89.8
    - adrenal gland Q89.1
    - epiglottis Q31.8
    - esophagus Q39.8
    - fallopian tube Q5Ø.4
    - kidney Q61.ØØ
      - more than one (multiple) Q61.Ø2
        - specified as polycystic Q61.3
          - adult type Q61.2
          - infantile type NEC Q61.19
            - collecting duct dilation Q61.11
      - solitary Q61.Ø1
    - larynx Q31.8
    - liver Q44.6
    - lung Q33.Ø
    - mediastinum Q34.1
    - ovary Q5Ø.1
    - oviduct Q5Ø.4
    - periurethral (tissue) Q64.79
    - prepuce Q55.69
    - salivary gland (any) Q38.4
    - sublingual Q38.6
    - submaxillary gland Q38.6
    - thymus (gland) Q89.2
    - tongue Q38.3
    - ureterovesical orifice Q62.8
    - vulva Q52.79
  - conjunctiva H11.44- ☑
  - cornea H18.89- ☑
  - corpora quadrigemina G93.Ø
  - corpus
    - albicans N83.29- ☑
    - luteum (hemorrhagic) (ruptured) N83.1- ☑
  - Cowper's gland (benign) (infected) N36.8
  - cranial meninges G93.Ø
  - craniobuccal pouch E23.6
  - craniopharyngeal pouch E23.6
  - cystic duct K82.8
  - Cysticercus — *see* Cysticercosis
  - Dandy-Walker QØ3.1
    - with spina bifida — *see* Spina bifida
  - dental (root) KØ4.8
    - developmental KØ9.Ø
    - eruption KØ9.Ø
    - primordial KØ9.Ø
  - dentigerous (mandible) (maxilla) KØ9.Ø
  - dermoid — *see* Neoplasm, benign, by site
    - with malignant transformation C56.- ☑
    - implantation
      - external area or site (skin) NEC L72.Ø
      - iris — *see* Cyst, iris, implantation
      - vagina N89.8
      - vulva N9Ø.7
    - mouth KØ9.8
    - oral soft tissue KØ9.8
    - sacrococcygeal — *see* Cyst, pilonidal
  - developmental KØ9.1
    - odontogenic KØ9.Ø

- **Cyst** — *continued*
  - developmental — *continued*
    - oral region (nonodontogenic) KØ9.1
    - ovary, ovarian Q5Ø.1
  - dura (cerebral) G93.Ø
    - spinal G96.198
  - ear (external) Q18.1
  - echinococcal — *see* Echinococcus
  - embryonic
    - cervix uteri Q51.6
    - fallopian tube Q5Ø.4
    - vagina Q52.4
  - endometrium, endometrial (uterus) N85.8
    - ectopic — *see* Endometriosis
  - enterogenous Q43.8
  - epidermal, epidermoid (inclusion) (*see also* Cyst, skin) L72.Ø
    - mouth KØ9.8
    - oral soft tissue KØ9.8
  - epididymis N5Ø.3
  - epiglottis J38.7
  - epiphysis cerebri E34.8
  - epithelial (inclusion) L72.Ø
  - epoophoron Q5Ø.5
  - eruption KØ9.Ø
  - esophagus K22.89
  - ethmoid sinus J34.1
  - external female genital organs NEC N9Ø.7
  - eyelid (sebaceous) HØ2.829
    - infected — *see* Hordeolum
    - left HØ2.826
      - lower HØ2.825
      - upper HØ2.824
    - right HØ2.823
      - lower HØ2.822
      - upper HØ2.821
  - eye NEC H57.89
    - congenital Q15.8
  - fallopian tube N83.8
    - congenital Q5Ø.4
  - fimbrial (twisted) Q5Ø.4
  - fissural (oral region) KØ9.1
  - follicle (graafian) (hemorrhagic) N83.Ø- ☑
    - nabothian N88.8
  - follicular (atretic) (hemorrhagic) (ovarian) N83.Ø- ☑
    - dentigerous KØ9.Ø
    - odontogenic KØ9.Ø
    - skin L72.9
      - specified NEC L72.8
  - frontal sinus J34.1
  - gallbladder K82.8
  - ganglion — *see* Ganglion
  - Gartner's duct Q52.4
  - gingiva KØ9.Ø
  - gland of Moll — *see* Cyst, eyelid
  - globulomaxillary KØ9.1
  - graafian follicle (hemorrhagic) N83.Ø- ☑
  - granulosal lutein (hemorrhagic) N83.1- ☑
  - hemangiomatous D18.ØØ
    - intra-abdominal D18.Ø3
    - intracranial D18.Ø2
    - skin D18.Ø1
    - specified site NEC D18.Ø9
  - hemorrhagic M27.49
  - hydatid — *see also* Echinococcus B67.9Ø
    - brain B67.99 *[G94]*
    - liver — *see also* Cyst, liver, hydatid B67.8
    - lung NEC B67.99 *[J99]*
    - Morgagni
      - female Q5Ø.5
      - male (epididymal) Q55.4
        - testicular Q55.29
    - specified site NEC B67.99
  - hymen N89.8
    - embryonic Q52.4
  - hypopharynx J39.2
  - hypophysis, hypophyseal (duct) (recurrent) E23.6
    - cerebri E23.6
  - implantation (dermoid)
    - external area or site (skin) NEC L72.Ø
    - iris — *see* Cyst, iris, implantation
    - vagina N89.8
    - vulva N9Ø.7
  - incisive canal KØ9.1
  - inclusion (epidermal) (epithelial) (epidermoid) (squamous) L72.Ø
    - not of skin — *code under* Cyst, by site
  - intestine (large) (small) K63.89

- **Cyst** — *continued*
  - intracranial — *see* Cyst, brain
  - intraligamentous — *see also* Disorder, ligament
    - knee — *see* Derangement, knee
  - intrasellar E23.6
  - iris H21.3Ø9
    - exudative H21.31- ☑
    - idiopathic H21.3Ø- ☑
    - implantation H21.32- ☑
    - parasitic H21.33- ☑
    - pars plana (primary) H21.34- ☑
      - exudative H21.35- ☑
  - jaw (bone) M27.4Ø
    - aneurysmal M27.49
    - developmental (odontogenic) KØ9.Ø
    - fissural KØ9.1
    - hemorrhagic M27.49
    - traumatic M27.49
  - joint NEC — *see* Disorder, joint, specified type NEC
  - kidney N28.1
    - acquired N28.1
    - calyceal — *see* Hydronephrosis
    - congenital Q61.ØØ
    - more than one (multiple) Q61.Ø2
      - specified as polycystic Q61.3
        - adult type (autosomal dominant) Q61.2
        - infantile type (autosomal recessive) NEC Q61.19
          - collecting duct dilation Q61.11
    - pyelogenic — *see* Hydronephrosis
    - simple N28.1
    - solitary (single) N28.1
      - acquired N28.1
      - congenital Q61.Ø1
  - labium (majus) (minus) N9Ø.7
    - sebaceous N9Ø.7
  - lacrimal — *see also* Disorder, lacrimal system, specified NEC
    - gland HØ4.13- ☑
    - passages or sac — *see* Disorder, lacrimal system, specified NEC
  - larynx J38.7
  - lateral periodontal KØ9.Ø
  - lens H27.8
    - congenital Q12.8
  - lip (gland) K13.Ø
  - liver (idiopathic) (simple) K76.89
    - congenital Q44.6
    - hydatid B67.8
      - granulosus B67.Ø
      - multilocularis B67.5
  - lung J98.4
    - congenital Q33.Ø
    - giant bullous J43.9
  - lutein N83.1- ☑
  - lymphangiomatous D18.1
  - lymphoepithelial, oral soft tissue KØ9.8
  - macula — *see* Degeneration, macula, hole
  - malignant — *see* Neoplasm, malignant, by site
  - mammary gland — *see* Cyst, breast
  - mandible M27.4Ø
    - dentigerous KØ9.Ø
    - radicular KØ4.8
  - maxilla M27.4Ø
    - dentigerous KØ9.Ø
    - radicular KØ4.8
  - medial, face and neck Q18.8
  - median
    - anterior maxillary KØ9.1
    - palatal KØ9.1
  - mediastinum, congenital Q34.1
  - meibomian (gland) — *see* Chalazion
    - infected — *see* Hordeolum
  - membrane, brain G93.Ø
  - meninges (cerebral) G93.Ø
    - spinal G96.198
  - meniscus, knee — *see* Derangement, knee, meniscus, cystic
  - mesentery, mesenteric K66.8
    - chyle I89.8
  - mesonephric duct
    - female Q5Ø.5
    - male Q55.4
  - milk N64.89
  - Morgagni (hydatid)
    - female Q5Ø.5
    - male (epididymal) Q55.4
      - testicular Q55.29

- **Cyst** — *continued*
  - mouth KØ9.8
  - Mullerian duct Q5Ø.4
    - appendix testis Q55.29
    - cervix Q51.6
    - fallopian tube Q5Ø.4
    - female Q5Ø.4
    - male Q55.29
    - prostatic utricle Q55.4
    - vagina (embryonal) Q52.4
  - multilocular (ovary) D39.1Ø
    - benign — *see* Neoplasm, benign, by site
  - myometrium N85.8
  - nabothian (follicle) (ruptured) N88.8
  - nasoalveolar KØ9.1
  - nasolabial KØ9.1
  - nasopalatine (anterior) (duct) KØ9.1
  - nasopharynx J39.2
  - neoplastic — *see* Neoplasm, uncertain behavior, by site
    - benign — *see* Neoplasm, benign, by site
  - nerve root
    - cervical G96.191
    - lumbar G96.191
    - sacral G96.191
    - thoracic G96.191
  - nervous system NEC G96.89
  - neuroenteric (congenital) QØ6.8
  - nipple — *see* Cyst, breast
  - nose (turbinates) J34.1
    - sinus J34.1
  - odontogenic, developmental KØ9.Ø
  - omentum (lesser) K66.8
    - congenital Q45.8
  - ora serrata — *see* Cyst, retina, ora serrata
  - oral
    - region KØ9.9
      - developmental (nonodontogenic) KØ9.1
      - specified NEC KØ9.8
    - soft tissue KØ9.9
      - specified NEC KØ9.8
  - orbit HØ5.81- ☑
  - ovary, ovarian (twisted) N83.2Ø- ☑
    - adherent N83.2Ø- ☑
    - chocolate N8Ø.1Ø- ☑
    - corpus
      - albicans N83.29- ☑
      - luteum (hemorrhagic) N83.1- ☑
    - dermoid D27.9
    - developmental Q5Ø.1
    - due to failure of involution NEC N83.2Ø- ☑
    - endometrial N8Ø.1Ø- ☑
    - follicular (graafian) (hemorrhagic) N83.Ø- ☑
    - hemorrhagic N83.2Ø- ☑
    - in pregnancy or childbirth O34.8- ☑
      - with obstructed labor O65.5
    - multilocular D39.1Ø
    - pseudomucinous D27.9
    - retention N83.29- ☑
    - serous N83.2Ø- ☑
    - specified NEC N83.29- ☑
    - theca lutein (hemorrhagic) N83.1- ☑
    - tuberculous A18.18
  - oviduct N83.8
  - palate (median) (fissural) KØ9.1
  - palatine papilla (jaw) KØ9.1
  - pancreas, pancreatic (hemorrhagic) (true) K86.2
    - congenital Q45.2
    - false K86.3
  - paralabral
    - hip M24.85- ☑
    - shoulder S43.43- ☑
  - paramesonephric duct Q5Ø.4
    - female Q5Ø.4
    - male Q55.29
  - paranephric N28.1
  - paraphysis, cerebri, congenital QØ4.6
  - parasitic B89
  - parathyroid (gland) E21.4
  - paratubal N83.8
  - paraurethral duct N36.8
  - paroophoron Q5Ø.5
  - parotid gland K11.6
  - parovarian Q5Ø.5
  - pelvis, female N94.89
    - in pregnancy or childbirth O34.8- ☑
      - causing obstructed labor O65.5
  - penis (sebaceous) N48.89

☑ **Additional Character Required — Refer to the Tabular List for Character Selection**

D

- **Da Costa's syndrome** F45.8
- **Daae** (-Finsen) **disease** (epidemic pleurodynia) B33.Ø
- **Dabney's grip** B33.Ø
- **Dacryoadenitis, dacryadenitis** HØ4.ØØ- ☑
  - acute HØ4.Ø1- ☑
  - chronic HØ4.Ø2- ☑
- **Dacryocystitis** HØ4.3Ø- ☑
  - acute HØ4.32- ☑
  - chronic HØ4.41- ☑
  - neonatal P39.1
  - phlegmonous HØ4.31- ☑
  - syphilitic A52.71
    - congenital (early) A5Ø.Ø1
  - trachomatous, active A71.1
    - sequelae (late effect) B94.Ø
- **Dacryocystoblenorrhea** — *see* Inflammation, lacrimal, passages, chronic
- **Dacryocystocele** — *see* Disorder, lacrimal system, changes
- **Dacryolith, dacryolithiasis** HØ4.51- ☑
- **Dacryoma** — *see* Disorder, lacrimal system, changes
- **Dacryopericystitis** — *see* Dacryocystitis
- **Dacryops** HØ4.11- ☑
- **Dacryostenosis** — *see also* Stenosis, lacrimal
  - congenital Q1Ø.5
- **Dactylitis**
  - bone — *see* Osteomyelitis
  - sickle-cell D57.ØØ
    - Hb C D57.219
    - Hb SS D57.ØØ
    - specified NEC D57.819
  - skin LØ8.9
  - syphilitic A52.77
  - tuberculous A18.Ø3
- **Dactylolysis spontanea** (ainhum) L94.6
- **Dactylosymphysis** Q7Ø.9
  - fingers — *see* Syndactylism, complex, fingers
  - toes — *see* Syndactylism, complex, toes
- **Damage**
  - arteriosclerotic — *see* Arteriosclerosis
  - brain (nontraumatic) G93.9
    - anoxic, hypoxic G93.1
      - resulting from a procedure G97.82
    - child NEC G8Ø.9
    - due to birth injury P11.2
  - cardiorenal (vascular) — *see* Hypertension, cardiorenal
  - cerebral NEC — *see* Damage, brain
  - coccyx, complicating delivery O71.6
  - coronary — *see* Disease, heart, ischemic
  - deep tissue, pressure-induced — *see also* L89 with final character .6
  - eye, birth injury P15.3
  - liver (nontraumatic) K76.9
    - alcoholic K7Ø.9
    - due to drugs — *see* Disease, liver, toxic
    - toxic — *see* Disease, liver, toxic
  - lung
    - dabbing (related) UØ7.Ø
    - electronic cigarette (related) UØ7.Ø
    - vaping (associated) (device) (product) (use) UØ7.Ø
  - medication T88.7 ☑
  - organ
    - dabbing (related) UØ7.Ø
    - electronic cigarette (related) UØ7.Ø
    - vaping (associated) (device) (product) (use) UØ7.Ø
  - pelvic
    - joint or ligament, during delivery O71.6
    - organ NEC
      - during delivery O71.5
      - following ectopic or molar pregnancy OØ8.6
  - renal — *see* Disease, renal
  - subendocardium, subendocardial — *see* Degeneration, myocardial
  - vascular I99.9
- **Dana-Putnam syndrome** (subacute combined sclerosis with pernicious anemia) — *see* Degeneration, combined
- **Danbolt** (-Cross) **syndrome** (acrodermatitis enteropathica) E83.2
- **Dandruff** L21.Ø
- **Dandy-Walker syndrome** QØ3.1
  - with spina bifida — *see* Spina bifida
- **Danlos' syndrome** — *see also* Syndrome, Ehlers-Danlos Q79.6Ø
- **Darier** (-White) **disease** (congenital) Q82.8
  - meaning erythema annulare centrifugum L53.1
- **Darier-Roussy sarcoid** D86.3
- **Darling's disease or histoplasmosis** B39.4
- **Darwin's tubercle** Q17.8
- **Dawson's** (inclusion body) **encephalitis** A81.1
- **De Beurmann** (-Gougerot) **disease** B42.1
- **De la Tourette's syndrome** F95.2
- **De Lange's syndrome** Q87.19
- **De Morgan's spots** (senile angiomas) I78.1
- **De Quervain's**
  - disease (tendon sheath) M65.4
  - syndrome E34.51
  - thyroiditis (subacute granulomatous thyroiditis) EØ6.1
- **De Toni-Fanconi** (-Debre) **syndrome** E72.Ø9
  - with cystinosis E72.Ø4
- **Dead**
  - fetus, retained (mother) O36.4 ☑
    - early pregnancy OØ2.1
  - labyrinth H83.2 ☑
  - ovum, retained OØ2.Ø
- **Deaf nonspeaking NEC** H91.3
- **Deafmutism** (acquired) (congenital) NEC H91.3
  - hysterical F44.6
  - syphilitic, congenital — *see also* subcategory H94.8 A5Ø.Ø9
- **Deafness** (acquired) (complete) (hereditary) (partial) H91.9- ☑
  - with blue sclera and fragility of bone Q78.Ø
  - auditory fatigue — *see* Deafness, specified type NEC
  - aviation T7Ø.Ø ☑
    - nerve injury — *see* Injury, nerve, acoustic, specified type NEC
  - boilermaker's H83.3 ☑
  - central — *see* Deafness, sensorineural
  - conductive H9Ø.2
    - and sensorineural
      - mixed H9Ø.8
        - bilateral H9Ø.6
    - bilateral H9Ø.Ø
    - unilateral H9Ø.1- ☑
      - with restricted hearing on the contralateral side H9Ø.A- ☑
  - congenital H9Ø.5
    - with blue sclera and fragility of bone Q78.Ø
  - due to toxic agents — *see* Deafness, ototoxic
  - emotional (hysterical) F44.6
  - functional (hysterical) F44.6
  - high frequency H91.9- ☑
  - hysterical F44.6
  - low frequency H91.9- ☑
  - mental R48.8
  - mixed conductive and sensorineural H9Ø.8
    - bilateral H9Ø.6
    - unilateral H9Ø.7- ☑
  - nerve — *see* Deafness, sensorineural
  - neural — *see* Deafness, sensorineural
  - noise-induced — *see also* subcategory H83.3 ☑
    - nerve injury — *see* Injury, nerve, acoustic, specified type NEC
  - nonspeaking H91.3
  - ototoxic H91.Ø ☑
  - perceptive — *see* Deafness, sensorineural
  - psychogenic (hysterical) F44.6
  - sensorineural H9Ø.5
    - and conductive
      - bilateral H9Ø.6
      - mixed H9Ø.8
        - bilateral H9Ø.6
    - bilateral H9Ø.3
    - unilateral H9Ø.4- ☑
      - with restricted hearing on the contralateral side H9Ø.A- ☑
  - sensory — *see* Deafness, sensorineural
  - specified type NEC H91.8 ☑
  - sudden (idiopathic) H91.2- ☑
  - syphilitic A52.15
  - transient ischemic H93.Ø1- ☑
  - traumatic — *see* Injury, nerve, acoustic, specified type NEC
  - word (developmental) H93.25
- **Death** (cause unknown) (of) (unexplained) (unspecified cause) R99
  - brain G93.82
  - cardiac (sudden) (with successful resuscitation) — *see* Arrest, cardiac
    - family history of Z82.41
- **Death** — *continued*
  - cardiac — *see* Arrest, cardiac — *continued*
    - personal history of Z86.74
  - family member (assumed) Z63.4
- **Debility** (chronic) (general) (nervous) R53.81
  - congenital or neonatal NOS P96.9
  - nervous R53.81
  - old age R54
  - senile R54
- **Debove's disease** (splenomegaly) R16.1
- **Debt, burdensome** Z59.86
- **Decalcification**
  - bone — *see* Osteoporosis
  - teeth KØ3.89
- **Decapsulation, kidney** N28.89
- **Decay**
  - dental — *see* Caries, dental
  - senile R54
  - tooth, teeth — *see* Caries, dental
- **Deciduitis** (acute)
  - following ectopic or molar pregnancy OØ8.Ø
- **Decline** (general) — *see* Debility
  - cognitive, age-associated R41.81
- **Decompensation**
  - cardiac (acute) (chronic) — *see* Disease, heart
  - cardiovascular — *see* Disease, cardiovascular
  - heart — *see* Disease, heart
  - hepatic — *see* Failure, hepatic
  - myocardial (acute) (chronic) — *see* Disease, heart
  - respiratory J98.8
- **Decompression sickness** T7Ø.3 ☑
- **Decrease** (d)
  - absolute neutrophile count — *see* Neutropenia
  - blood
    - platelets — *see* Thrombocytopenia
    - pressure RØ3.1
      - due to shock following
        - injury T79.4 ☑
        - operation T81.19 ☑
  - estrogen E28.39
    - postablative E89.4Ø
      - asymptomatic E89.4Ø
      - symptomatic E89.41
  - fragility of erythrocytes D58.8
  - function
    - lipase (pancreatic) K9Ø.3
    - ovary in hypopituitarism E23.Ø
    - parenchyma of pancreas K86.89
    - pituitary (gland) (anterior) (lobe) E23.Ø
      - posterior (lobe) E23.Ø
  - functional activity R68.89
  - glucose R73.Ø9
  - hematocrit R71.Ø
  - hemoglobin R71.Ø
  - leukocytes D72.819
    - specified NEC D72.818
  - libido R68.82
  - lymphocytes D72.81Ø
  - platelets D69.6
  - respiration, due to shock following injury T79.4 ☑
  - sexual desire R68.82
  - tear secretion NEC — *see* Syndrome, dry eye
  - tolerance
    - fat K9Ø.49
    - glucose R73.Ø9
    - pancreatic K9Ø.3
    - salt and water E87.8
  - vision NEC H54.7
  - white blood cell count D72.819
    - specified NEC D72.818
- **Decubitus** (ulcer) — *see* Ulcer, pressure, by site
  - cervix N86
- **Deepening acetabulum** — *see* Derangement, joint, specified type NEC, hip
- **Defect, defective** Q89.9
  - 3-beta-hydroxysteroid dehydrogenase E25.Ø
  - 11-hydroxylase E25.Ø
  - 21-hydroxylase E25.Ø
  - abdominal wall, congenital Q79.59
  - antibody immunodeficiency D8Ø.9
  - aorticopulmonary septum Q21.4
  - atrial septal Q21.1Ø
    - coronary sinus Q21.13
    - following acute myocardial infarction (current complication) I23.1
    - ostium primum type (type I) Q21.2Ø

Deficiency, deficient — *continued*
- kappa-light chain D8Ø.8
- labile factor (congenital) (hereditary) D68.2
  - acquired D68.4
- lacrimal fluid (acquired) — *see also* Syndrome, dry eye
  - congenital Q1Ø.6
- lactase
  - congenital E73.Ø
  - secondary E73.1
- Laki-Lorand factor D68.2
- LCAD (long chain acyl CoA dehydrogenase deficiency) E71.31Ø
- lecithin cholesterol acyltransferase E78.6
- lipocaic K86.89
- lipoprotein (familial) (high density) E78.6
- liver phosphorylase E74.Ø9
- lysosomal alpha-1, 4 glucosidase E74.Ø2
- lysosome-associated membrane protein 2 [LAMP2] E74.Ø5
- magnesium E61.2
- major histocompatibility complex
  - class I D81.6
  - class II D81.7
- manganese E61.3
- MCAD (medium chain acyl CoA dehydrogenase deficiency) E71.311
- menadione (vitamin K) E56.1
  - newborn P53
- mental (familial) (hereditary) — *see* Disability, intellectual
- methylenetetrahydrofolate reductase (MTHFR) E72.12
- mevalonate kinase MØ4.1
- mineralocorticoid E27.49
  - with glucocorticoid E27.49
- mineral NEC E61.8
- molybdenum (nutritional) E61.5
- moral F6Ø.2
- multiple nutrient elements E61.7
- multiple sulfatase (MSD) E75.26
- muscle
  - carnitine (palmityltransferase) E71.314
  - phosphofructokinase E74.Ø9
- myoadenylate deaminase E79.2
- myocardial — *see* Insufficiency, myocardial
- myophosphorylase E74.Ø4
- NADH diaphorase or reductase (congenital) D74.Ø
- NADH-methemoglobin reductase (congenital) D74.Ø
- natrium E87.1
- niacin (amide) (-tryptophan) E52
- nicotinamide E52
- nicotinic acid E52
- number of teeth — *see* Anodontia
- nutrient element E61.9
  - multiple E61.7
  - specified NEC E61.8
- nutrition, nutritional — *see also* Nutrition deficient E63.9
  - sequelae — *see* Sequelae, nutritional deficiency
  - specified NEC E63.8
- of interleukin 1 receptor antagonist [DIRA] MØ4.8
- ornithine transcarbamylase E72.4
- ovarian E28.39
- oxygen — *see* Anoxia
- pantothenic acid E53.8
- parathyroid (gland) E2Ø.9
- perineum (female) N81.89
- phenylalanine hydroxylase E7Ø.1
- phosphoenolpyruvate carboxykinase E74.4
- phosphofructokinase E74.19
- phosphomannomutuse E74.818
- phosphomannose isomerase E74.818
- phosphomannosyl mutase E74.818
- phosphorylase kinase, liver E74.Ø9
- pituitary hormone (isolated) E23.Ø
- plasma thromboplastin
  - antecedent (PTA) D68.1
  - component (PTC) D67
- plasminogen (type 1) (type 2) E88.Ø2
- platelet NEC D69.1
  - constitutional — *see* Disease, von Willebrand
- polyglandular E31.8
  - autoimmune E31.Ø
- potassium (K) E87.6
- prepuce N47.3
- proaccelerin (congenital) (hereditary) D68.2
  - acquired D68.4
- proconvertin factor (congenital) (hereditary) D68.2
  - acquired D68.4

Deficiency, deficient — *continued*
- protein — *see also* Malnutrition E46
  - anemia D53.Ø
  - C D68.59
  - S D68.59
- prothrombin (congenital) (hereditary) D68.2
  - acquired D68.4
- Prower factor D68.2
- pseudocholinesterase E88.Ø9
- PTA (plasma thromboplastin antecedent) D68.1
- PTC (plasma thromboplastin component) D67
- purine nucleoside phosphorylase (PNP) D81.5
- pyracin (alpha) (beta) E53.1
- pyridoxal E53.1
- pyridoxamine E53.1
- pyridoxine (derivatives) E53.1
- pyruvate
  - carboxylase E74.4
  - dehydrogenase E74.4
- riboflavin (vitamin B2) E53.Ø
- salt E87.1
- SCAD (short chain acyl CoA dehydrogenase deficiency) E71.312
- secretion
  - ovary E28.39
  - salivary gland (any) K11.7
  - urine R34
- selenium (dietary) E59
- serum antitrypsin, familial E88.Ø1
- short stature homeobox gene (SHOX)
  - with
    - dyschondrosteosis Q78.8
    - short stature (idiopathic) E34.328
    - Turner's syndrome Q96.9
- sodium (Na) E87.1
- SPCA (factor VII) D68.2
- sphincter, intrinsic N36.42
  - with urethral hypermobility N36.43
- stable factor (congenital) (hereditary) D68.2
  - acquired D68.4
- Stuart-Prower (factor X) D68.2
- succinic semialdehyde dehydrogenase E72.81
- sucrase E74.39
- sulfatase E75.26
- sulfite oxidase E72.19
- thiamin, thiaminic (chloride) E51.9
  - beriberi (dry) E51.11
    - wet E51.12
- thrombokinase D68.2
  - newborn P53
- thyroid (gland) — *see* Hypothyroidism
- tocopherol E56.Ø
- tooth bud KØØ.Ø
- transcobalamine II (anemia) D51.2
- vanadium E61.6
- vascular I99.9
- vasopressin E23.2
- vertical ridge KØ6.8
- viosterol — *see* Deficiency, calciferol
- vitamin (multiple) NOS E56.9
  - A E5Ø.9
    - with
      - Bitot's spot (corneal) E5Ø.1
      - follicular keratosis E5Ø.8
      - keratomalacia E5Ø.4
      - manifestations NEC E5Ø.8
      - night blindness E5Ø.5
      - scar of cornea, xerophthalmic E5Ø.6
      - xeroderma E5Ø.8
      - xerophthalmia E5Ø.7
      - xerosis
        - conjunctival E5Ø.Ø
          - and Bitot's spot E5Ø.1
        - cornea E5Ø.2
          - and ulceration E5Ø.3
    - sequelae E64.1
  - B (complex) NOS E53.9
    - with
      - beriberi (dry) E51.11
        - wet E51.12
      - pellagra E52
  - B1 NOS E51.9
    - beriberi (dry) E51.11
      - with circulatory system manifestations E51.11
      - wet E51.12
  - B12 E53.8
  - B2 (riboflavin) E53.Ø
  - B6 E53.1
  - C E54

Deficiency, deficient — *continued*
- vitamin — *continued*
  - C — *continued*
    - sequelae E64.2
  - D E55.9
    - with
      - adult osteomalacia M83.8
      - rickets — *see* Rickets
    - 25-hydroxylase E83.32
  - E E56.Ø
  - folic acid E53.8
  - G E53.Ø
  - group B E53.9
    - specified NEC E53.8
  - H (biotin) E53.8
  - K E56.1
    - of newborn P53
  - nicotinic E52
  - P E56.8
  - PP (pellagra-preventing) E52
  - specified NEC E56.8
  - thiamin E51.9
    - beriberi — *see* Beriberi
- VLCAD (very long chain acyl CoA dehydrogenase deficiency) E71.31Ø
- von Willebrand factor
  - partial quantitative — *see also* Disease, von Willebrand D68.Ø1
  - total quantitative — *see also* Disease, von Willebrand D68.Ø3
- zinc, dietary E6Ø

Deficit — *see also* Deficiency
- attention and concentration R41.84Ø
  - disorder — *see* Attention, deficit
  - following
    - cerebral infarction I69.31Ø
    - cerebrovascular disease I69.91Ø
      - specified disease NEC I69.81Ø
    - nontraumatic
      - intracerebral hemorrhage I69.11Ø
      - specified intracranial hemorrhage NEC I69.21Ø
      - subarachnoid hemorrhage I69.Ø1Ø
- cognitive
  - communication R41.841
  - emotional
    - following
      - cerebral infarction I69.315
      - cerebrovascular disease I69.915
        - specified disease NEC I69.815
      - nontraumatic
        - intracerebral hemorrhage I69.115
        - specified intracranial hemorrhage NEC I69.215
        - subarachnoid hemorrhage I69.Ø15
  - following
    - cerebral infarction I69.319
    - cerebrovascular disease I69.919
      - specified disease NEC I69.819
    - nontraumatic
      - intracerebral hemorrhage I69.119
      - specified intracranial hemorrhage NEC I69.219
      - subarachnoid hemorrhage I69.Ø19
  - social
    - following
      - cerebral infarction I69.315
      - cerebrovascular disease I69.915
        - specified disease NEC I69.815
      - nontraumatic
        - intracerebral hemorrhage I69.115
        - specified intracranial hemorrhage NEC I69.215
        - subarachnoid hemorrhage I69.Ø15
- cognitive NEC R41.89
  - following
    - cerebral infarction I69.318
    - cerebrovascular disease I69.918
      - specified disease NEC I69.818
    - nontraumatic
      - intracerebral hemorrhage I69.118
      - specified intracranial hemorrhage NEC I69.218
      - subarachnoid hemorrhage I69.Ø18
- concentration R41.84Ø
- executive function R41.844
  - following
    - cerebral infarction I69.314
    - cerebrovascular disease I69.914
      - specified disease NEC I69.814
    - nontraumatic
      - intracerebral hemorrhage I69.114

- **Deformity** — *continued*
  - head — *continued*
    - congenital Q75.8
  - heart (congenital) Q24.9
    - septum Q21.9
      - auricular — *see also* Defect, atrial septal Q21.1Ø
      - ventricular Q21.Ø
    - valve (congenital) NEC Q24.8
      - acquired — *see* Endocarditis
  - heel (acquired) — *see* Deformity, foot
  - hepatic duct (congenital) Q44.5
    - acquired K83.8
  - hip (joint) (acquired) (*see also* Deformity, limb, thigh)
    - congenital Q65.9
    - due to (previous) juvenile osteochondrosis — *see* Coxa, plana
    - flexion — *see* Contraction, joint, hip
  - hourglass — *see* Contraction, hourglass
  - humerus (acquired) M21.82- ☑
    - congenital Q74.Ø
  - hypophyseal (congenital) Q89.2
  - ileocecal (coil) (valve) (acquired) K63.89
    - congenital Q43.9
  - ileum (congenital) Q43.9
    - acquired K63.89
  - ilium (acquired) M95.5
    - congenital Q74.2
  - integument (congenital) Q84.9
  - intervertebral cartilage or disc (acquired) — *see* Disorder, disc, specified NEC
  - intestine (large) (small) (congenital) NOS Q43.9
    - acquired K63.89
  - intrinsic minus or plus (hand) — *see* Deformity, limb, specified type NEC, forearm
  - iris (acquired) H21.89
    - congenital Q13.2
  - ischium (acquired) M95.5
    - congenital Q74.2
  - jaw (acquired) (congenital) M26.9
  - joint (acquired) NEC M21.9Ø
    - congenital Q68.8
    - elbow M21.92- ☑
    - hand M21.94- ☑
    - hip M21.95- ☑
    - knee M21.96- ☑
    - shoulder M21.92- ☑
    - wrist M21.93- ☑
  - kidney(s) (calyx) (pelvis) (congenital) Q63.9
    - acquired N28.89
    - artery (congenital) Q27.2
      - acquired I77.89
  - Klippel-Feil (brevicollis) Q76.1
  - knee (acquired) NEC — *see also* Deformity, limb, lower leg
    - congenital Q68.2
  - labium (majus) (minus) (congenital) Q52.79
    - acquired N9Ø.89
  - lacrimal passages or duct (congenital) NEC Q1Ø.6
    - acquired — *see* Disorder, lacrimal system, changes
  - larynx (muscle) (congenital) Q31.8
    - acquired J38.7
    - web (glottic) Q31.Ø
  - leg (upper) (acquired) NEC — *see also* Deformity, limb, thigh
    - congenital Q68.8
    - lower leg — *see* Deformity, limb, lower leg
  - lens (acquired) H27.8
    - congenital Q12.9
  - lid (fold) (acquired) — *see also* Disorder, eyelid, specified type NEC
    - congenital Q1Ø.3
  - ligament (acquired) — *see* Disorder, ligament
    - congenital Q79.9
  - limb (acquired) M21.9Ø
    - clawfoot M21.53- ☑
    - clawhand M21.51- ☑
      - congenital Q68.1
    - clubfoot M21.54- ☑
    - clubhand M21.52- ☑
    - congenital, except reduction deformity Q74.9
    - flat foot M21.4- ☑
    - flexion M21.2Ø
      - ankle M21.27- ☑
      - elbow M21.22- ☑
      - finger M21.24- ☑
      - hip M21.25- ☑
      - knee M21.26- ☑
      - shoulder M21.21- ☑

- **Deformity** — *continued*
  - limb — *continued*
    - flexion — *continued*
      - toe M21.27- ☑
      - wrist M21.23- ☑
    - foot
      - claw — *see* Deformity, limb, clawfoot
      - club — *see* Deformity, limb, clubfoot
      - drop M21.37- ☑
      - flat — *see* Deformity, limb, flat foot
      - specified NEC M21.6X- ☑
    - forearm M21.93- ☑
    - hand M21.94- ☑
    - lower leg M21.96- ☑
    - specified type NEC M21.8Ø
      - forearm M21.83- ☑
      - lower leg M21.86- ☑
      - thigh M21.85- ☑
      - upper arm M21.82- ☑
    - thigh M21.95- ☑
    - unequal length M21.7Ø
      - short site is
        - femur M21.75- ☑
        - fibula M21.76- ☑
        - humerus M21.72- ☑
        - radius M21.73- ☑
        - tibia M21.76- ☑
        - ulna M21.73- ☑
    - upper arm M21.92- ☑
    - valgus — *see* Deformity, valgus
    - varus — *see* Deformity, varus
    - wrist drop M21.33- ☑
  - lip (acquired) NEC K13.Ø
    - congenital Q38.Ø
  - liver (congenital) Q44.7Ø
    - acquired K76.89
  - lumbosacral (congenital) (joint) (region) Q76.49
    - acquired — *see* subcategory M43.8 ☑
    - kyphosis — *see* Kyphosis, congenital
    - lordosis — *see* Lordosis, congenital
  - lung (congenital) Q33.9
    - acquired J98.4
  - lymphatic system, congenital Q89.9
  - Madelung's (radius) Q74.Ø
  - mandible (acquired) (congenital) M26.9
  - maxilla (acquired) (congenital) M26.9
  - meninges or membrane (congenital) QØ7.9
    - cerebral QØ4.8
      - acquired G96.198
    - spinal cord (congenital) QØ6.- ☑
      - acquired G96.198
  - metacarpus (acquired) — *see* Deformity, limb, forearm
    - congenital Q74.Ø
  - metatarsus (acquired) — *see* Deformity, foot
    - congenital Q66.9- ☑
  - middle ear (congenital) Q16.4
    - ossicles Q16.3
  - mitral (leaflets) (valve) IØ5.8
    - parachute Q23.2
    - stenosis, congenital Q23.2
  - mouth (acquired) K13.79
    - congenital Q38.6
  - multiple, congenital NEC Q89.7
  - muscle (acquired) M62.89
    - congenital Q79.9
      - sternocleidomastoid Q68.Ø
  - musculoskeletal system (acquired) M95.9
    - congenital Q79.9
    - specified NEC M95.8
  - nail (acquired) L6Ø.8
    - congenital Q84.6
  - nasal — *see* Deformity, nose
  - neck (acquired) M95.3
    - congenital Q18.9
      - sternocleidomastoid Q68.Ø
  - nervous system (congenital) QØ7.9
  - nipple (congenital) Q83.9
    - acquired N64.89
  - nose (acquired) (cartilage) M95.Ø
    - bone (turbinate) M95.Ø
    - congenital Q3Ø.9
      - bent or squashed Q67.4
    - saddle M95.Ø
      - syphilitic A5Ø.57
    - septum (acquired) J34.2
      - congenital Q3Ø.8
    - sinus (wall) (congenital) Q3Ø.8

- **Deformity** — *continued*
  - nose — *continued*
    - sinus — *continued*
      - acquired M95.Ø
    - syphilitic (congenital) A5Ø.57
      - late A52.73
  - ocular muscle (congenital) Q1Ø.3
    - acquired — *see* Strabismus, mechanical
  - opticociliary vessels (congenital) Q13.2
  - orbit (eye) (acquired) HØ5.3Ø
    - atrophy — *see* Atrophy, orbit
    - congenital Q1Ø.7
    - due to
      - bone disease NEC HØ5.32- ☑
      - trauma or surgery HØ5.33- ☑
    - enlargement — *see* Enlargement, orbit
    - exostosis — *see* Exostosis, orbit
  - organ of Corti (congenital) Q16.5
  - ovary (congenital) Q5Ø.39
    - acquired N83.8
  - oviduct, acquired N83.8
  - palate (congenital) Q38.5
    - acquired M27.8
    - cleft (congenital) — *see* Cleft, palate
  - pancreas (congenital) Q45.3
    - acquired K86.89
  - parathyroid (gland) Q89.2
  - parotid (gland) (congenital) Q38.4
    - acquired K11.8
  - patella (acquired) — *see* Disorder, patella, specified NEC
  - pelvis, pelvic (acquired) (bony) M95.5
    - with disproportion (fetopelvic) O33.Ø
      - causing obstructed labor O65.Ø
    - congenital Q74.2
    - rachitic sequelae (late effect) E64.3
  - penis (glans) (congenital) Q55.69
    - acquired N48.89
  - pericardium (congenital) Q24.8
    - acquired — *see* Pericarditis
  - pharynx (congenital) Q38.8
    - acquired J39.2
  - pinna, acquired — *see also* Disorder, pinna, deformity
    - congenital Q17.9
  - pituitary (congenital) Q89.2
  - posture — *see* Dorsopathy, deforming
  - prepuce (congenital) Q55.69
    - acquired N47.8
  - prostate (congenital) Q55.4
    - acquired N42.89
  - pupil (congenital) Q13.2
    - acquired — *see* Abnormality, pupillary
  - pylorus (congenital) Q4Ø.3
    - acquired K31.89
  - rachitic (acquired), old or healed E64.3
  - radius (acquired) — *see also* Deformity, limb, forearm
    - congenital Q68.8
  - rectum (congenital) Q43.9
    - acquired K62.89
  - reduction (extremity) (limb), congenital — *see also* condition and site Q73.8
    - brain QØ4.3
    - lower — *see* Defect, reduction, lower limb
    - upper — *see* Defect, reduction, upper limb
  - renal — *see* Deformity, kidney
  - respiratory system (congenital) Q34.9
  - rib (acquired) M95.4
    - congenital Q76.6
      - cervical Q76.5
  - rotation (joint) (acquired) — *see* Deformity, limb, specified site NEC
    - congenital Q74.9
    - hip — *see* Deformity, limb, specified type NEC, thigh
      - congenital Q65.89
  - sacroiliac joint (congenital) — *see* subcategory Q74.2
    - acquired — *see* subcategory M43.8 ☑
  - sacrum (acquired) — *see* subcategory M43.8 ☑
  - saddle
    - back — *see* Lordosis
    - nose M95.Ø
      - syphilitic A5Ø.57
  - salivary gland or duct (congenital) Q38.4
    - acquired K11.8
  - scapula (acquired) M95.8
    - congenital Q68.8
  - scrotum (congenital) — *see also* Malformation, testis and scrotum
    - acquired N5Ø.89

- **Delay, delayed** — *continued*
  - development — *continued*
    - speech — *continued*
      - due to hearing loss F8Ø.4
    - spelling F81.81
  - ejaculation F52.32
  - gastric emptying K3Ø
  - menarche E3Ø.Ø
  - menstruation (cause unknown) N91.Ø
  - milestone R62.Ø
  - passage of meconium (newborn) P76.Ø
  - primary respiration P28.9
  - puberty (constitutional) E3Ø.Ø
  - separation of umbilical cord P96.82
  - sexual maturation, female E3Ø.Ø
  - sleep phase syndrome G47.21
  - union, fracture — *see* Fracture, by site
  - vaccination Z28.9
- **Deletion**(s)
  - autosome Q93.9
    - identified by fluorescence in situ hybridization (FISH) Q93.89
    - identified by in situ hybridization (ISH) Q93.89
  - chromosome
    - with complex rearrangements NEC Q93.7
    - part of NEC Q93.59
    - seen only at prometaphase Q93.89
    - short arm
      - 22q11.2 Q93.81
      - 4 Q93.3
      - 5p Q93.4
    - specified NEC Q93.89
  - long arm chromosome 18 or 21 Q93.89
    - with complex rearrangements NEC Q93.7
  - microdeletions NEC Q93.88
- **Delhi boil or button** B55.1
- **Delinquency** (juvenile) (neurotic) F91.8
  - group Z72.81Ø
- **Delinquent immunization status** Z28.39
  - COVID-19 Z28.31- ☑
- **Delirium, delirious** (acute or subacute) (not alcohol- or drug-induced) (with dementia) R41.Ø
  - alcoholic (acute) (tremens) (withdrawal) F1Ø.921
    - with intoxication F1Ø.921
      - in
        - abuse F1Ø.121
        - dependence F1Ø.221
  - due to (secondary to)
    - alcohol
      - intoxication F1Ø.921
        - in
          - abuse F1Ø.121
          - dependence F1Ø.221
      - withdrawal F1Ø.231
    - amphetamine intoxication F15.921
      - in
        - abuse F15.121
        - dependence F15.221
    - anxiolytic
      - intoxication F13.921
        - in
          - abuse F13.121
          - dependence F13.221
      - withdrawal F13.231
    - cannabis intoxication (acute) F12.921
      - in
        - abuse F12.121
        - dependence F12.221
    - cocaine intoxication (acute) F14.921
      - in
        - abuse F14.121
        - dependence F14.221
    - general medical condition FØ5
    - hallucinogen intoxication F16.921
      - in
        - abuse F16.121
        - dependence F16.221
    - hypnotic
      - intoxication F13.921
        - in
          - abuse F13.121
          - dependence F13.221
      - withdrawal F13.231
    - inhalant intoxication (acute) F18.921
      - in
        - abuse F18.121
        - dependence F18.221
    - multiple etiologies FØ5

- **Delirium, delirious** — *continued*
  - due to — *continued*
    - opioid intoxication (acute) F11.921
      - in
        - abuse F11.121
        - dependence F11.221
    - other (or unknown) substance F19.921
    - phencyclidine intoxication (acute) F16.921
      - in
        - abuse F16.121
        - dependence F16.221
    - psychoactive substance NEC intoxication (acute) F19.921
      - in
        - abuse F19.121
        - dependence F19.221
    - sedative
      - intoxication F13.921
        - in
          - abuse F13.121
          - dependence F13.221
      - withdrawal F13.231
    - unknown etiology R41.Ø
  - exhaustion F43.Ø
  - hysterical F44.89
  - postprocedural (postoperative) FØ5
  - puerperal FØ5
  - thyroid — *see* Thyrotoxicosis with thyroid storm
  - traumatic — *see* Injury, intracranial
  - tremens (alcohol-induced) F1Ø.231
    - sedative-induced F13.231
- **Delivery** (childbirth) (labor)
  - arrested active phase O62.1
  - cesarean (for)
    - abnormal
      - pelvis (bony) (deformity) (major) NEC with disproportion (fetopelvic) O33.Ø
        - with obstructed labor O65.Ø
      - presentation or position O32.9 ☑
    - abruptio placentae — *see also* Abruptio placentae O45.9- ☑
    - acromion presentation O32.2 ☑
    - atony, uterus O62.2
    - breech presentation O32.1 ☑
      - incomplete O32.8 ☑
    - brow presentation O32.3 ☑
    - cephalopelvic disproportion O33.9
    - cerclage O34.3- ☑
    - chin presentation O32.3 ☑
    - cicatrix of cervix O34.4- ☑
    - contracted pelvis (general)
      - inlet O33.2
      - outlet O33.3 ☑
    - cord presentation or prolapse O69.Ø ☑
    - cystocele O34.8- ☑
    - deformity (acquired) (congenital)
      - pelvic organs or tissues NEC O34.8- ☑
      - pelvis (bony) NEC O33.Ø
    - disproportion NOS O33.9
    - eclampsia — *see* Eclampsia
    - face presentation O32.3 ☑
    - failed
      - forceps O66.5
      - induction of labor O61.9
        - instrumental O61.1
        - mechanical O61.1
        - medical O61.Ø
        - specified NEC O61.8
        - surgical O61.1
      - trial of labor NOS O66.4Ø
        - following previous cesarean delivery O66.41
      - vacuum extraction O66.5
      - ventouse O66.5
    - fetal-maternal hemorrhage O43.Ø1- ☑
    - hemorrhage (intrapartum) O67.9
      - with coagulation defect O67.Ø
      - specified cause NEC O67.8
    - high head at term O32.4 ☑
    - hydrocephalic fetus O33.6 ☑
    - incarceration of uterus O34.51- ☑
    - incoordinate uterine action O62.4
    - increased size, fetus O33.5 ☑
    - inertia, uterus O62.2
      - primary O62.Ø
      - secondary O62.1
    - isthmocele O34.22
    - lateroversion, uterus O34.59- ☑
    - mal lie O32.9 ☑

- **Delivery** — *continued*
  - cesarean — *continued*
    - malposition
      - fetus O32.9 ☑
      - pelvic organs or tissues NEC O34.8- ☑
      - uterus NEC O34.59- ☑
    - malpresentation NOS O32.9 ☑
    - oblique presentation O32.2 ☑
    - occurring after 37 completed weeks of gestation but before 39 completed weeks gestation due to (spontaneous) onset of labor O75.82
    - oversize fetus O33.5 ☑
    - pelvic tumor NEC O34.8- ☑
    - placenta previa O44.Ø- ☑
      - complete O44.Ø- ☑
        - with hemorrhage O44.1- ☑
    - placental insufficiency O36.51- ☑
    - planned, occurring after 37 completed weeks of gestation but before 39 completed weeks gestation due to (spontaneous) onset of labor O75.82
    - polyp, cervix O34.4- ☑
      - causing obstructed labor O65.5
    - poor dilatation, cervix O62.Ø
    - pre-eclampsia O14.94
      - mild O14.Ø4
      - moderate O14.Ø4
      - severe O14.14
        - with hemolysis, elevated liver enzymes and low platelet count (HELLP) O14.24
    - previous
      - cesarean delivery O34.219
        - classical (vertical) scar O34.212
        - isthmocele O34.22
        - low transverse scar O34.211
        - mid-transverse T incision O34.218
        - scar
          - defect (isthmocele) O34.22
          - specified type NEC O34.218
      - surgery (to)
        - cervix O34.4- ☑
        - gynecological NEC O34.8- ☑
        - rectum O34.7- ☑
        - uterus O34.29
        - vagina O34.6- ☑
    - prolapse
      - arm or hand O32.2 ☑
      - uterus O34.52- ☑
    - prolonged labor NOS O63.9
    - rectocele O34.8- ☑
    - retroversion
      - uterus O34.53- ☑
    - rigid
      - cervix O34.4- ☑
      - pelvic floor O34.8- ☑
      - perineum O34.7- ☑
      - vagina O34.6- ☑
      - vulva O34.7- ☑
    - sacculation, pregnant uterus O34.59- ☑
    - scar(s)
      - cervix O34.4- ☑
      - cesarean delivery O34.219
        - classical (vertical) O34.212
        - isthmocele O34.22
        - low transverse O34.211
        - mid-transverse T incision O34.218
        - scar
          - defect (isthmocele) O34.22
          - specified type NEC O34.218
      - defect (isthmocele) O34.22
      - transmural uterine O34.29
      - uterus O34.29
    - Shirodkar suture in situ O34.3- ☑
    - shoulder presentation O32.2 ☑
    - stenosis or stricture, cervix O34.4- ☑
    - streptococcus group B (GBS) carrier state O99.824
    - transmural uterine scar O34.29
    - transverse presentation or lie O32.2 ☑
    - tumor, pelvic organs or tissues NEC O34.8- ☑
      - cervix O34.4- ☑
    - umbilical cord presentation or prolapse O69.Ø ☑
    - without indication O82
  - completely normal case O8Ø
  - complicated O75.9
    - by
      - abnormal, abnormality (of)
        - forces of labor O62.9

- **Delivery** — *continued*
  - complicated — *continued*
    - by — *continued*
      - malposition, malpresentation — *continued*
        - without obstruction — *see also* Delivery, complicated by, obstruction — *continued*
          - specified NEC O32.8 ☑
          - transverse O32.2 ☑
          - unstable lie O32.Ø ☑
      - meconium in amniotic fluid O77.Ø
      - mental disorder NEC O99.344
      - metrorrhexis — *see* Delivery, complicated by, rupture, uterus
      - nervous system disorder O99.354
      - obesity (pre-existing) O99.214
      - obesity surgery status O99.844
      - obstetric trauma O71.9
        - specified NEC O71.89
      - obstructed labor
        - due to
          - breech (complete) (frank) presentation O64.1 ☑
            - incomplete O64.8 ☑
          - brow presentation O64.3 ☑
          - buttock presentation O64.1 ☑
          - chin presentation O64.2 ☑
          - compound presentation O64.5 ☑
          - contracted pelvis O65.1
          - deep transverse arrest O64.Ø ☑
          - deformed pelvis O65.Ø
          - dystocia (fetal) O66.9
            - due to
              - conjoined twins O66.3
              - fetal
                - abnormality NEC O66.3
                - ascites O66.3
                - hydrops O66.3
                - meningomyelocele O66.3
                - sacral teratoma O66.3
                - tumor O66.3
              - hydrocephalic fetus O66.3
            - shoulder O66.Ø
          - face presentation O64.2 ☑
          - fetopelvic disproportion O65.4
          - footling presentation O64.8 ☑
          - impacted shoulders O66.Ø
          - incomplete rotation of fetal head O64.Ø ☑
          - large fetus O66.2
          - locked twins O66.1
          - malposition O64.9 ☑
            - specified NEC O64.8 ☑
          - malpresentation O64.9 ☑
            - specified NEC O64.8 ☑
          - multiple fetuses NEC O66.6
          - pelvic
            - abnormality (maternal) O65.9
              - organ O65.5
              - specified NEC O65.8
            - contraction
              - inlet O65.2
              - mid-cavity O65.3
              - outlet O65.3
          - persistent (position)
            - occipitoiliac O64.Ø ☑
            - occipitoposterior O64.Ø ☑
            - occipitosacral O64.Ø ☑
            - occipitotransverse O64.Ø ☑
          - prolapsed arm O64.4 ☑
          - shoulder presentation O64.4 ☑
        - specified NEC O66.8
      - pathological retraction ring, uterus O62.4
      - penetration, pregnant uterus by instrument O71.1
      - perforation — *see* Delivery, complicated by, laceration
      - placenta, placental
        - ablatio — *see also* Abruptio placentae O45.9- ☑
        - abnormality O43.9- ☑
          - specified NEC O43.89- ☑
        - abruptio — *see also* Abruptio placentae O45.9- ☑
        - accreta O43.21- ☑
        - adherent (with hemorrhage) O72.Ø
          - without hemorrhage O73.Ø

- **Delivery** — *continued*
  - complicated — *continued*
    - by — *continued*
      - placenta, placental — *continued*
        - detachment (premature) — *see also* Abruptio placentae O45.9- ☑
        - disorder O43.9- ☑
          - specified NEC O43.89- ☑
        - hemorrhage NEC O67.8
        - increta O43.22- ☑
        - low (implantation) (lying) O44.4- ☑
          - with hemorrhage O44.5- ☑
        - malformation O43.1Ø- ☑
        - malposition O44.Ø- ☑
          - without hemorrhage O44.1- ☑
        - percreta O43.23- ☑
        - previa (central) (complete) (lateral) (total) O44.Ø- ☑
          - with hemorrhage O44.1- ☑
          - marginal O44.2- ☑
            - with hemorrhage O44.3- ☑
          - partial O44.2- ☑
            - with hemorrhage O44.3- ☑
        - retained (with hemorrhage) O72.Ø
          - without hemorrhage O73.Ø
        - separation (premature) O45.9- ☑
          - specified NEC O45.8X- ☑
        - vicious insertion O44.1- ☑
      - precipitate labor O62.3
      - premature rupture, membranes — *see also* Pregnancy, complicated by, premature rupture of membranes O42.9Ø
      - prolapse
        - arm or hand O32.2 ☑
        - cord (umbilical) O69.Ø ☑
        - foot or leg O32.8 ☑
        - uterus O34.52- ☑
      - prolonged labor O63.9
        - first stage O63.Ø
        - second stage O63.1
      - protozoal disease (maternal) O98.62
      - respiratory disease NEC O99.52
      - retained membranes or portions of placenta O72.2
        - without hemorrhage O73.1
      - retarded birth O63.9
      - retention of secundines (with hemorrhage) O72.Ø
        - without hemorrhage O73.Ø
        - partial O72.2
          - without hemorrhage O73.1
      - rupture
        - bladder (urinary) O71.5
        - cervix O71.3
        - pelvic organ NEC O71.5
        - urethra O71.5
        - uterus (during or after labor) O71.1
          - before labor O71.Ø- ☑
      - separation, pubic bone (symphysis pubis) O71.6
      - shock O75.1
      - shoulder presentation O64.4 ☑
      - skin disorder NEC O99.72
      - spasm, cervix O62.4
      - stenosis or stricture, cervix O65.5
      - streptococcus group B (GBS) carrier state O99.824
      - subluxation of symphysis (pubis) O26.72
      - syphilis (maternal) O98.12
      - tear — *see* Delivery, complicated by, laceration
      - tetanic uterus O62.4
      - trauma (obstetrical) — *see also* Delivery, complicated, by, damage to O71.9
        - non-obstetric O9A.22 (*following* O99)
        - periurethral O71.82
        - specified NEC O71.89
      - tuberculosis (maternal) O98.Ø2
      - tumor, pelvic organs or tissues NEC O65.5
      - umbilical cord around neck
        - with compression O69.1 ☑
        - without compression O69.81 ☑
      - uterine inertia O62.2
        - during latent phase of labor O62.Ø
        - primary O62.Ø
        - secondary O62.1
      - vasa previa O69.4 ☑
      - velamentous insertion of cord O43.12- ☑
    - specified complication NEC O75.89
  - delayed NOS O63.9

- **Delivery** — *continued*
  - delayed — *continued*
    - following rupture of membranes
      - artificial O75.5
    - second twin, triplet, etc. O63.2
  - forceps, low following failed vacuum extraction O66.5
  - missed (at or near term) O36.4 ☑
  - normal O8Ø
  - obstructed — *see* Delivery, complicated by, obstructed labor
  - precipitate O62.3
  - preterm — *see also* Pregnancy, complicated by, preterm labor O6Ø.1Ø ☑
  - spontaneous O8Ø
  - term pregnancy NOS O8Ø
  - uncomplicated O8Ø
  - vaginal, following previous cesarean delivery O34.219
    - classical (vertical) scar O34.212
    - low transverse scar O34.211
    - mid-transverse T incision O34.218
    - scar
      - defect (isthmocele) O34.22
      - specified type NEC O34.218
- **Delusions** (paranoid) — *see* Disorder, delusional
- **Dementia** (degenerative (primary)) (old age) (persisting) (unspecified severity) (without behavioral disturbance, psychotic disturbance, mood disturbance, and anxiety) FØ3.9Ø
  - with
    - aberrant motor behavior (exit-seeking) (pacing) (restlessness) (rocking) FØ3.911
    - agitation FØ3.911
    - anxiety FØ3.94
    - behavioral disturbances (sexual disinhibition) (sleep disturbance) (social disinhibition) FØ3.918
      - specified NEC FØ3.918
    - Lewy bodies — *see also* Dementia, in, diseases specified elsewhere G31.83 *[FØ2.8Ø]*
      - with behavioral disturbance — *see also* Dementia, in, diseases specified elsewhere G31.83 *[FØ2.81-]* ☑
    - mood disturbance (anhedonia) (apathy) (depression) FØ3.93
    - Parkinsonism — *see also* Dementia, in, diseases specified elsewhere G2Ø.C *[FØ2.8Ø]*
      - with behavioral disturbance — *see also* Dementia, in, diseases specified elsewhere G2Ø.C *[FØ2.81-]* ☑
    - Parkinson's disease — *see also* Dementia, in, diseases specified elsewhere G2Ø.A1 *[FØ2.8Ø]*
      - with behavioral disturbance — *see also* Dementia, in, diseases specified elsewhere G2Ø.A1 *[FØ2.81-]* ☑
    - psychotic disturbance (delusional state) (hallucinations) (paranoia) (suspiciousness) FØ3.92
    - verbal or physical behaviors (anger) (aggression) (combativeness) (profanity) (shouting) (threatening) (violence) FØ3.911
  - alcoholic F1Ø.97
    - with dependence F1Ø.27
  - Alzheimer's type — *see* Disease, Alzheimer's
  - arteriosclerotic — *see* Dementia, vascular
  - atypical, Alzheimer's type — *see* Disease, Alzheimer's, specified NEC
  - congenital — *see* Disability, intellectual
  - frontal (lobe) — *see also* Dementia, in, diseases specified elsewhere G31.Ø9 *[FØ2.8Ø]*
    - with behavioral disturbance — *see also* Dementia, in, diseases specified elsewhere G31.Ø9 *[FØ2.81-]* ☑
  - frontotemporal G31.Ø9 *[FØ2.8Ø]*
    - with behavioral disturbance G31.Ø9 *[FØ2.81]* ☑
    - specified NEC — *see also* Dementia, in, diseases specified elsewhere G31.Ø9 *[FØ2.8Ø]*
      - with behavioral disturbance — *see also* Dementia, in, diseases specified elsewhere G31.Ø9 *[FØ2.81-]* ☑
  - in (due to)
    - alcohol F1Ø.97
      - with dependence F1Ø.27
    - Alzheimer's disease — *see* Disease, Alzheimer's
    - arteriosclerotic brain disease — *see* Dementia, vascular
    - cerebral lipidoses — *see also* Dementia, in, diseases specified elsewhere E75.- ☑ *[FØ2.8Ø]*

Dementia — *continued*
- praecox — *see* Schizophrenia
- presenile F03 ☑
  - Alzheimer's type — *see* Disease, Alzheimer's, early onset
- primary degenerative F03 ☑
- progressive, syphilitic A52.17
- senile F03 ☑
  - with acute confusional state F05
  - Alzheimer's type — *see* Disease, Alzheimer's, late onset
  - depressed or paranoid type F03 ☑
- severe F03.C0
  - with
    - aberrant motor behavior (exit-seeking) (pacing) (restlessness) (rocking) F03.C11
    - agitation F03.C11
    - anxiety F03.C4
    - behavioral disturbances (sexual disinhibition) (sleep disturbance) (social disinhibition) F03.C18
      - specified NEC F03.C18
    - mood disturbance (anhedonia) (apathy) (depression) F03.C3
    - psychotic disturbance (delusional state) (hallucinations) (paranoia) (suspiciousness) F03.C2
    - verbal or physical behaviors (anger) (aggression) (combativeness) (profanity) (shouting) (threatening) (violence) F03.C11
- vascular (acute onset) (mixed) (multi-infarct) (subcortical) (unspecified severity) (without behavioral disturbance, psychotic disturbance, mood disturbance, and anxiety) F01.50
  - with
    - aberrant motor behavior (exit-seeking) (pacing) (restlessness) (rocking) F01.511
    - agitation F01.511
    - anxiety F01.54
    - behavioral disturbances (sleep disturbance) (sexual disinhibition) (social disinhibition) F01.518
      - specified NEC F01.518
    - mood disturbance (anhedonia) (apathy) (depression) F01.53
    - psychotic disturbance (delusional state) (hallucinations) (paranoia) (suspiciousness) F01.52
    - verbal or physical behaviors (anger) (aggression) (combativeness) (profanity) (shouting) (threatening) (violence) F01.511
  - mild F01.A0
    - with
      - aberrant motor behavior (exit-seeking) (pacing) (restlessness) (rocking) F01.A11
      - agitation F01.A11
      - anxiety F01.A4
      - behavioral disturbances (sleep disturbance) (sexual disinhibition) (social disinhibition) F01.A18
        - specified NEC F01.A18
      - mood disturbance (anhedonia) (apathy) (depression) F01.A3
      - psychotic disturbance (delusional state) (hallucinations) (paranoia) (suspiciousness) F01.A2
      - verbal or physical behaviors (anger) (aggression) (combativeness) (profanity) (shouting) (threatening) (violence) F01.A11
  - moderate F01.B0
    - with
      - aberrant motor behavior (exit-seeking) (pacing) (restlessness) (rocking) F01.B11
      - agitation F01.B11
      - anxiety F01.B4
      - behavioral disturbances (sleep disturbance) (sexual disinhibition) (social disinhibition) F01.B18
        - specified NEC F01.B18
      - mood disturbance (anhedonia) (apathy) (depression) F01.B3
      - psychotic disturbance (delusional state) (hallucinations) (paranoia) (suspiciousness) F01.B2
      - verbal or physical behaviors (anger) (aggression) (combativeness) (profanity) (shouting) (threatening) (violence) F01.B11
  - severe F01.C0

Dementia — *continued*
- vascular — *continued*
  - severe — *continued*
    - with
      - aberrant motor behavior (exit-seeking) (pacing) (restlessness) (rocking) F01.C11
      - agitation F01.C11
      - anxiety F01.C4
      - behavioral disturbances (sleep disturbance) (sexual disinhibition) (social disinhibition) F01.C18
        - specified NEC F01.C18
      - mood disturbance (anhedonia) (apathy) (depression) F01.C3
      - psychotic disturbance (delusional state) (hallucinations) (paranoia) (suspiciousness) F01.C2
      - verbal or physical behaviors (anger) (aggression) (combativeness) (profanity) (shouting) (threatening) (violence) F01.C11

Demineralization, bone — *see* Osteoporosis

Demodex folliculorum (infestation) B88.0

Demophobia F40.248

Demoralization R45.3

Demyelination, demyelinization
- central nervous system G37.9
  - specified NEC G37.89
- corpus callosum (central) G37.1
- disseminated, acute G36.9
  - specified NEC G36.8
- global G35
- in optic neuritis G36.0

Dengue (classical) (fever) A90
- hemorrhagic A91
- sandfly A93.1

Dennie-Marfan syphilitic syndrome A50.45

Dens evaginatus, in dente or invaginatus K00.2

Dense breasts — *see also* Density, breast R92.30

Density
- breast R92.30
  - mammographic
    - extreme R92.34- ☑
    - fatty tissue R92.31- ☑
    - fibroglandular R92.32- ☑
    - heterogeneous R92.33- ☑
- increased, bone (disseminated) (generalized) (spotted) — *see* Disorder, bone, density and structure, specified type NEC
- low R92.30
- lung (nodular) J98.4

Dental — *see also* condition
- examination Z01.20
  - with abnormal findings Z01.21
- restoration
  - aesthetically inadequate or displeasing K08.56
  - defective K08.50
    - specified NEC K08.59
  - failure of marginal integrity K08.51
  - failure of periodontal anatomical integrity K08.54

Dentia praecox K00.6

Denticles (pulp) K04.2

Dentigerous cyst K09.0

Dentin
- irregular (in pulp) K04.3
- opalescent K00.5
- secondary (in pulp) K04.3
- sensitive K03.89

Dentinogenesis imperfecta K00.5

Dentinoma — *see* Cyst, calcifying odontogenic

Dentition (syndrome) K00.7
- delayed K00.6
- difficult K00.7
- precocious K00.6
- premature K00.6
- retarded K00.6

Dependence (on) (syndrome) F19.20
- with remission F19.21
- alcohol (ethyl) (methyl) (without remission) F10.20
  - with
    - amnestic disorder, persisting F10.26
    - anxiety disorder F10.280
    - dementia, persisting F10.27
    - intoxication F10.229
      - with delirium F10.221
      - uncomplicated F10.220
    - mood disorder F10.24
    - psychotic disorder F10.259

Dependence — *continued*
- alcohol — *continued*
  - with — *continued*
    - psychotic disorder — *continued*
      - with
        - delusions F10.250
        - hallucinations F10.251
    - remission F10.21
    - sexual dysfunction F10.281
    - sleep disorder F10.282
    - specified disorder NEC F10.288
    - withdrawal F10.239
      - with
        - delirium F10.231
        - perceptual disturbance F10.232
      - uncomplicated F10.230
  - counseling and surveillance Z71.41
  - in remission F10.21
- amobarbital — *see* Dependence, drug, sedative
- amphetamine(s) (type) — *see* Dependence, drug, stimulant NEC
- amytal (sodium) — *see* Dependence, drug, sedative
- analgesic NEC F55.8
- anesthetic (agent) (gas) (general) (local) NEC — *see* Dependence, drug, psychoactive NEC
- anxiolytic NEC — *see* Dependence, drug, sedative
- barbital(s) — *see* Dependence, drug, sedative
- barbiturate(s) (compounds) (drugs classifiable to T42) — *see* Dependence, drug, sedative
- benzedrine — *see* Dependence, drug, stimulant NEC
- bhang — *see* Dependence, drug, cannabis
- bromide(s) NEC — *see* Dependence, drug, sedative
- caffeine — *see* Dependence, drug, stimulant NEC
- cannabis (sativa) (indica) (resin) (derivatives) (type) — *see* Dependence, drug, cannabis
- chloral (betaine) (hydrate) — *see* Dependence, drug, sedative
- chlordiazepoxide — *see* Dependence, drug, sedative
- coca (leaf) (derivatives) — *see* Dependence, drug, cocaine
- cocaine — *see* Dependence, drug, cocaine
- codeine — *see* Dependence, drug, opioid
- combinations of drugs F19.20
- dagga — *see* Dependence, drug, cannabis
- demerol — *see* Dependence, drug, opioid
- dexamphetamine — *see* Dependence, drug, stimulant NEC
- dexedrine — *see* Dependence, drug, stimulant NEC
- dextromethorphan — *see* Dependence, drug, opioid
- dextromoramide — *see* Dependence, drug, opioid
- dextro-nor-pseudo-ephedrine — *see* Dependence, drug, stimulant NEC
- dextrorphan — *see* Dependence, drug, opioid
- diazepam — *see* Dependence, drug, sedative
- dilaudid — *see* Dependence, drug, opioid
- D-lysergic acid diethylamide — *see* Dependence, drug, hallucinogen
- drug NEC F19.20
  - with sleep disorder F19.282
  - cannabis F12.20
    - with
      - anxiety disorder F12.280
      - intoxication F12.229
        - with
          - delirium F12.221
          - perceptual disturbance F12.222
        - uncomplicated F12.220
      - other specified disorder F12.288
      - psychosis F12.259
        - delusions F12.250
        - hallucinations F12.251
      - unspecified disorder F12.29
      - withdrawal F12.23
    - in remission F12.21
  - cocaine F14.20
    - with
      - anxiety disorder F14.280
      - intoxication F14.229
        - with
          - delirium F14.221
          - perceptual disturbance F14.222
        - uncomplicated F14.220
      - mood disorder F14.24
      - other specified disorder F14.288
      - psychosis F14.259
        - delusions F14.250
        - hallucinations F14.251
      - sexual dysfunction F14.281

- **Dependence** — *continued*
  - drug — *continued*
    - cocaine — *continued*
      - with — *continued*
        - sleep disorder F14.282
        - unspecified disorder F14.29
        - withdrawal F14.23
      - in remission F14.21
      - withdrawal symptoms in newborn P96.1
    - counseling and surveillance Z71.51
    - hallucinogen F16.20
      - with
        - anxiety disorder F16.280
        - flashbacks F16.283
        - intoxication F16.229
          - with delirium F16.221
          - uncomplicated F16.220
        - mood disorder F16.24
        - other specified disorder F16.288
        - perception disorder, persisting F16.283
        - psychosis F16.259
          - delusions F16.250
          - hallucinations F16.251
        - unspecified disorder F16.29
      - in remission F16.21
    - in remission F19.21
    - inhalant F18.20
      - with
        - anxiety disorder F18.280
        - dementia, persisting F18.27
        - intoxication F18.229
          - with delirium F18.221
          - uncomplicated F18.220
        - mood disorder F18.24
        - other specified disorder F18.288
        - psychosis F18.259
          - delusions F18.250
          - hallucinations F18.251
        - unspecified disorder F18.29
      - in remission F18.21
    - nicotine F17.200
      - with disorder F17.209
        - in remission F17.201
        - specified disorder NEC F17.208
        - withdrawal F17.203
      - chewing tobacco F17.220
        - with disorder F17.229
          - in remission F17.221
          - specified disorder NEC F17.228
          - withdrawal F17.223
      - cigarettes F17.210
        - with disorder F17.219
          - in remission F17.211
          - specified disorder NEC F17.218
          - withdrawal F17.213
      - specified product NEC F17.290
        - with disorder F17.299
          - remission F17.291
          - specified disorder NEC F17.298
          - withdrawal F17.293
    - opioid F11.20
      - with
        - intoxication F11.229
          - with
            - delirium F11.221
            - perceptual disturbance F11.222
          - uncomplicated F11.220
        - mood disorder F11.24
        - opioid-associated amnestic syndrome F11.288
        - other specified disorder F11.288
        - psychosis F11.259
          - delusions F11.250
          - hallucinations F11.251
        - sexual dysfunction F11.281
        - sleep disorder F11.282
        - unspecified disorder F11.29
        - withdrawal F11.23
      - in remission F11.21
    - psychoactive NEC F19.20
      - with
        - amnestic disorder F19.26
        - anxiety disorder F19.280
        - dementia F19.27
        - intoxication F19.229
          - with
            - delirium F19.221
            - perceptual disturbance F19.222
          - uncomplicated F19.220
        - mood disorder F19.24

- **Dependence** — *continued*
  - drug — *continued*
    - psychoactive — *continued*
      - with — *continued*
        - other specified disorder F19.288
        - psychosis F19.259
          - delusions F19.250
          - hallucinations F19.251
        - sexual dysfunction F19.281
        - sleep disorder F19.282
        - unspecified disorder F19.29
        - withdrawal F19.239
          - with
            - delirium F19.231
            - perceptual disturbance F19.232
          - uncomplicated F19.230
      - in remission F19.21
    - sedative, hypnotic or anxiolytic F13.20
      - with
        - amnestic disorder F13.26
        - anxiety disorder F13.280
        - dementia, persisting F13.27
        - intoxication F13.229
          - with delirium F13.221
          - uncomplicated F13.220
        - mood disorder F13.24
        - other specified disorder F13.288
        - psychosis F13.259
          - delusions F13.250
          - hallucinations F13.251
        - sexual dysfunction F13.281
        - sleep disorder F13.282
        - unspecified disorder F13.29
        - withdrawal F13.239
          - with
            - delirium F13.231
            - perceptual disturbance F13.232
          - uncomplicated F13.230
      - in remission F13.21
    - stimulant NEC F15.20
      - with
        - anxiety disorder F15.280
        - intoxication F15.229
          - with
            - delirium F15.221
            - perceptual disturbance F15.222
          - uncomplicated F15.220
        - mood disorder F15.24
        - other specified disorder F15.288
        - psychosis F15.259
          - delusions F15.250
          - hallucinations F15.251
        - sexual dysfunction F15.281
        - sleep disorder F15.282
        - unspecified disorder F15.29
        - withdrawal F15.23
      - in remission F15.21
  - ethyl
    - alcohol (without remission) F10.20
      - with remission F10.21
    - bromide — *see* Dependence, drug, sedative
    - carbamate F19.20
    - chloride F19.20
    - morphine — *see* Dependence, drug, opioid
  - ganja — *see* Dependence, drug, cannabis
  - glue (airplane) (sniffing) — *see* Dependence, drug, inhalant
  - glutethimide — *see* Dependence, drug, sedative
  - hallucinogenics — *see* Dependence, drug, hallucinogen
  - hashish — *see* Dependence, drug, cannabis
  - hemp — *see* Dependence, drug, cannabis
  - heroin (salt) (any) — *see* Dependence, drug, opioid
  - hypnotic NEC — *see* Dependence, drug, sedative
  - Indian hemp — *see* Dependence, drug, cannabis
  - inhalants — *see* Dependence, drug, inhalant
  - khat — *see* Dependence, drug, stimulant NEC
  - laudanum — *see* Dependence, drug, opioid
  - LSD (-25) (derivatives) — *see* Dependence, drug, hallucinogen
  - luminal — *see* Dependence, drug, sedative
  - lysergic acid — *see* Dependence, drug, hallucinogen
  - maconha — *see* Dependence, drug, cannabis
  - marihuana — *see* Dependence, drug, cannabis
  - meprobamate — *see* Dependence, drug, sedative
  - mescaline — *see* Dependence, drug, hallucinogen
  - methadone — *see* Dependence, drug, opioid
  - methamphetamine(s) — *see* Dependence, drug, stimulant NEC

- **Dependence** — *continued*
  - methaqualone — *see* Dependence, drug, sedative
  - methyl
    - alcohol (without remission) F10.20
      - with remission F10.21
    - bromide — *see* Dependence, drug, sedative
    - morphine — *see* Dependence, drug, opioid
    - phenidate — *see* Dependence, drug, stimulant NEC
    - sulfonal — *see* Dependence, drug, sedative
  - morphine (sulfate) (sulfite) (type) — *see* Dependence, drug, opioid
  - narcotic (drug) NEC — *see* Dependence, drug, opioid
  - nembutal — *see* Dependence, drug, sedative
  - neraval — *see* Dependence, drug, sedative
  - neravan — *see* Dependence, drug, sedative
  - neurobarb — *see* Dependence, drug, sedative
  - nicotine — *see* Dependence, drug, nicotine
  - nitrous oxide F19.20
  - nonbarbiturate sedatives and tranquilizers with similar effect — *see* Dependence, drug, sedative
  - on
    - artificial heart (fully implantable) (mechanical) Z95.812
    - aspirator Z99.0
    - care provider (because of) Z74.9
      - impaired mobility Z74.09
      - need for
        - assistance with personal care Z74.1
        - continuous supervision Z74.3
      - no other household member able to render care Z74.2
      - specified reason NEC Z74.8
    - machine Z99.89
      - enabling NEC Z99.89
      - specified type NEC Z99.89
    - renal dialysis (hemodialysis) (peritoneal) Z99.2
    - respirator Z99.11
    - ventilator Z99.11
    - wheelchair Z99.3
  - opiate — *see* Dependence, drug, opioid
  - opioids — *see* Dependence, drug, opioid
  - opium (alkaloids) (derivatives) (tincture) — *see* Dependence, drug, opioid
  - oxygen (long-term) (supplemental) Z99.81
  - paraldehyde — *see* Dependence, drug, sedative
  - paregoric — *see* Dependence, drug, opioid
  - PCP (phencyclidine) (or related substance) — *see* Dependence, drug, hallucinogen
  - pentobarbital — *see* Dependence, drug, sedative
  - pentobarbitone (sodium) — *see* Dependence, drug, sedative
  - pentothal — *see* Dependence, drug, sedative
  - peyote — *see* Dependence, drug, hallucinogen
  - phencyclidine (PCP) (or related substance) — *see* Dependence, drug, hallucinogen
  - phenmetrazine — *see* Dependence, drug, stimulant NEC
  - phenobarbital — *see* Dependence, drug, sedative
  - polysubstance F19.20
  - psilocibin, psilocin, psilocyn, psilocyline — *see* Dependence, drug, hallucinogen
  - psychostimulant NEC — *see* Dependence, drug, stimulant NEC
  - secobarbital — *see* Dependence, drug, sedative
  - seconal — *see* Dependence, drug, sedative
  - sedative NEC — *see* Dependence, drug, sedative
  - specified drug NEC — *see* Dependence, drug
  - stimulant NEC — *see* Dependence, drug, stimulant NEC
  - substance NEC — *see* Dependence, drug
  - supplemental oxygen Z99.81
  - tobacco — *see* Dependence, drug, nicotine
    - counseling and surveillance Z71.6
  - tranquilizer NEC — *see* Dependence, drug, sedative
  - vitamin B6 E53.1
  - volatile solvents — *see* Dependence, drug, inhalant
- **Dependency**
  - care-provider Z74.9
  - passive F60.7
  - reactions (persistent) F60.7
- **Depersonalization** (in neurotic state) (neurotic) (syndrome) F48.1
- **Depletion**
  - extracellular fluid E86.9
  - plasma E86.1
  - potassium E87.6
    - nephropathy N25.89
  - salt or sodium E87.1

- **Dermatitis** — *continued*
  - contact — *continued*
    - allergic — *continued*
      - due to — *continued*
        - cosmetics L23.2
        - dander (cat) (dog) L23.81
        - drugs in contact with skin L23.3
        - dyes L23.4
        - food in contact with skin L23.6
        - hair (cat) (dog) L23.81
        - insecticide L23.5
        - metals L23.Ø
        - nickel L23.Ø
        - plants, non-food L23.7
        - plastic L23.5
        - rubber L23.5
        - specified agent NEC L23.89
    - due to
      - cement L25.3
      - chemical products NEC L25.3
      - cosmetics L25.Ø
      - dander (cat) (dog) L23.81
      - drugs in contact with skin L25.1
      - dyes L25.2
      - food in contact with skin L25.4
      - hair (cat) (dog) L23.81
      - plants, non-food L25.5
      - specified agent NEC L25.8
    - irritant L24.9
      - due to
        - body fluids L24.AØ
          - feces L24.A2
          - incontinence (dual) (fecal) (urinary) L24.A2
          - saliva L24.A1
          - specified NEC L24.A9
          - urine L24.A2
          - wound exudate L24.A9
        - cement L24.5
        - chemical products NEC L24.5
        - cosmetics L24.3
        - detergents L24.Ø
        - drugs in contact with skin L24.4
        - exudate L24.A9
        - food in contact with skin L24.6
        - friction L24.AØ
        - oils and greases L24.1
        - plants, non-food L24.7
        - solvents L24.2
        - specified agent NEC L24.89
      - related to
        - colostomy L24.B3
        - endotracheal tube L24.A9
        - enterocutaneous fistula L24.B3
        - gastrostomy L24.B1
        - ileostomy L24.B3
        - jejunostomy L24.B1
        - saliva or spit fistula L24.B1
        - stoma or fistula L24.BØ
          - digestive L24.B1
          - fecal or urinary L24.B3
          - respiratory L24.B2
        - tracheostomy L24.B2
  - contusiformis L52
  - desquamative L3Ø.8
  - diabetic — *see* EØ8-E13 with .62Ø
  - diaper L22
  - diphtheritica A36.3
  - dry skin L85.3
  - due to
    - acetone (contact) (irritant) L24.2
    - acids (contact) (irritant) L24.5
    - adhesive(s) (allergic) (contact) (plaster) L23.1
      - irritant L24.5
    - alcohol (irritant) (skin contact) (substances in category T51) L24.2
      - taken internally L27.8
    - alkalis (contact) (irritant) L24.5
    - arsenic (ingested) L27.8
    - carbon disulfide (contact) (irritant) L24.2
    - caustics (contact) (irritant) L24.5
    - cement (contact) L25.3
    - cereal (ingested) L27.2
    - chemical(s) NEC L25.3
      - taken internally L27.8
    - chlorocompounds L24.2
    - chromium (contact) (irritant) L24.81
    - coffee (ingested) L27.2
    - cold weather L3Ø.8

- **Dermatitis** — *continued*
  - due to — *continued*
    - cosmetics (contact) L25.Ø
      - allergic L23.2
      - irritant L24.3
    - cyclohexanes L24.2
    - dander (cat) (dog) L23.81
    - Demodex species B88.Ø
    - Dermanyssus gallinae B88.Ø
    - detergents (contact) (irritant) L24.Ø
    - dichromate L24.81
    - drugs and medicaments (generalized) (internal use) L27.Ø
      - external — *see* Dermatitis, due to, drugs, in contact with skin
      - in contact with skin L25.1
        - allergic L23.3
        - irritant L24.4
      - localized skin eruption L27.1
      - specified substance — *see* Table of Drugs and Chemicals
    - dyes (contact) L25.2
      - allergic L23.4
      - irritant L24.89
    - epidermophytosis — *see* Dermatophytosis
    - esters L24.2
    - external irritant NEC L24.9
    - exudate (wound fluids) L24.A9
    - fish (ingested) L27.2
    - flour (ingested) L27.2
    - food (ingested) L27.2
      - in contact with skin L25.4
    - fruit (ingested) L27.2
    - furs (allergic) (contact) L23.81
    - glues — *see* Dermatitis, due to, adhesives
    - glycols L24.2
    - greases NEC (contact) (irritant) L24.1
    - hair (cat) (dog) L23.81
    - hot
      - objects and materials — *see* Burn
      - weather or places L59.Ø
    - hydrocarbons L24.2
    - infrared rays L59.8
    - ingestion, ingested substance L27.9
      - chemical NEC L27.8
      - drugs and medicaments — *see* Dermatitis, due to, drugs
      - food L27.2
      - specified NEC L27.8
    - insecticide in contact with skin L24.5
    - internal agent L27.9
      - drugs and medicaments (generalized) — *see* Dermatitis, due to, drugs
      - food L27.2
    - irradiation — *see* Dermatitis, due to, radioactive substance
    - ketones L24.2
    - lacquer tree (allergic) (contact) L23.7
    - light (sun) NEC L57.8
      - acute L56.8
      - other L59.8
    - Liponyssoides sanguineus B88.Ø
    - low temperature L3Ø.8
    - meat (ingested) L27.2
    - metals, metal salts (contact) (irritant) L24.81
    - milk (ingested) L27.2
    - nickel (contact) (irritant) L24.81
    - nylon (contact) (irritant) L24.5
    - oils NEC (contact) (irritant) L24.1
    - paint solvent (contact) (irritant) L24.2
    - petroleum products (contact) (irritant) (substances in T52.Ø) L24.2
    - plants NEC (contact) L25.5
      - allergic L23.7
      - irritant L24.7
    - plasters (adhesive) (any) (allergic) (contact) L23.1
      - irritant L24.5
    - plastic (contact) L25.3
    - preservatives (contact) — *see* Dermatitis, due to, chemical, in contact with skin
    - primrose (allergic) (contact) L23.7
    - primula (allergic) (contact) L23.7
    - radiation L59.8
      - nonionizing (chronic exposure) L57.8
      - sun NEC L57.8
        - acute L56.8
    - radioactive substance L58.9
      - acute L58.Ø

- **Dermatitis** — *continued*
  - due to — *continued*
    - radioactive substance — *continued*
      - chronic L58.1
    - radium L58.9
      - acute L58.Ø
      - chronic L58.1
    - ragweed (allergic) (contact) L23.7
    - Rhus (allergic) (contact) (diversiloba) (radicans) (toxicodendron) (venenata) (verniciflua) L23.7
    - rubber (contact) L24.5
    - Senecio jacobaea (allergic) (contact) L23.7
    - solvents (contact) (irritant) (substances in category T52) L24.2
    - specified agent NEC (contact) L25.8
      - allergic L23.89
      - irritant L24.89
    - sunshine NEC L57.8
      - acute L56.8
    - tetrachlorethylene (contact) (irritant) L24.2
    - toluene (contact) (irritant) L24.2
    - turpentine (contact) L24.2
    - ultraviolet rays (sun NEC) (chronic exposure) L57.8
      - acute L56.8
    - vaccine or vaccination L27.Ø
      - specified substance — *see* Table of Drugs and Chemicals
    - varicose veins — *see* Varix, leg, with, inflammation
    - X-rays L58.9
      - acute L58.Ø
      - chronic L58.1
  - dyshydrotic L3Ø.1
  - dysmenorrheica N94.6
  - escharotica — *see* Burn
  - exfoliative, exfoliativa (generalized) L26
    - neonatorum LØØ
  - eyelid — *see also* Dermatosis, eyelid HØ1.9
    - allergic HØ1.119
      - left HØ1.116
        - lower HØ1.115
        - upper HØ1.114
      - right HØ1.113
        - lower HØ1.112
        - upper HØ1.111
    - contact — *see* Dermatitis, eyelid, allergic
    - due to
      - Demodex species B88.Ø
      - herpes (zoster) BØ2.39
        - simplex BØØ.59
    - eczematous HØ1.139
      - left HØ1.136
        - lower HØ1.135
        - upper HØ1.134
      - right HØ1.133
        - lower HØ1.132
        - upper HØ1.131
    - specified NEC HØ1.8
  - facta, factitia, factitial L98.1
    - psychogenic F54
  - flexural NEC L2Ø.82
  - friction L3Ø.4
  - fungus B36.9
    - specified type NEC B36.8
  - gangrenosa, gangrenous infantum LØ8.Ø
  - harvest mite B88.Ø
  - heat L59.Ø
  - herpesviral, vesicular (ear) (lip) BØØ.1
  - herpetiformis (bullous) (erythematous) (pustular) (vesicular) L13.Ø
    - juvenile L12.2
    - senile L12.Ø
  - hiemalis L3Ø.8
  - hypostatic, hypostatica — *see* Varix, leg, with, inflammation
  - infectious eczematoid L3Ø.3
  - infective L3Ø.3
  - irritant — *see* Dermatitis, contact, irritant
  - Jacquet's (diaper dermatitis) L22
  - Leptus B88.Ø
  - lichenified NEC L28.Ø
  - medicamentosa (generalized) (internal use) — *see* Dermatitis, due to drugs
  - mite B88.Ø
  - multiformis L13.Ø
    - juvenile L12.2
  - napkin L22
  - neurotica L13.Ø
  - nummular L3Ø.Ø

Dermatitis — *continued*
- papillaris capillitii L73.Ø
- pellagrous E52
- perioral L71.Ø
- photocontact L56.2
- polymorpha dolorosa L13.Ø
- pruriginosa L13.Ø
- pruritic NEC L3Ø.8
- psychogenic F54
- purulent LØ8.Ø
- pustular
  - contagious BØ8.Ø2
  - subcorneal L13.1
- pyococcal LØ8.Ø
- pyogenica LØ8.Ø
- repens L4Ø.2
- Ritter's (exfoliativa) LØØ
- Schamberg's L81.7
- schistosome B65.3
- seasonal bullous L3Ø.8
- seborrheic L21.9
  - infantile L21.1
  - specified NEC L21.8
- sensitization NOS L23.9
- septic LØ8.Ø
- solare L57.8
- specified NEC L3Ø.8
- stasis I87.2
  - with
    - varicose ulcer — *see* Varix, leg, with ulcer, with inflammation
    - varicose veins — *see* Varix, leg, with, inflammation
  - due to postthrombotic syndrome — *see* Syndrome, postthrombotic
- suppurative LØ8.Ø
- traumatic NEC L3Ø.4
- trophoneurotica L13.Ø
- ultraviolet (sun) (chronic exposure) L57.8
  - acute L56.8
- varicose — *see* Varix, leg, with, inflammation
- vegetans L1Ø.1
- verrucosa B43.Ø
- vesicular, herpesviral BØØ.1

Dermatoarthritis, lipoid E78.81

Dermatochalasis, eyelid HØ2.839
- left HØ2.836
  - lower HØ2.835
  - upper HØ2.834
- right HØ2.833
  - lower HØ2.832
  - upper HØ2.831

Dermatofibroma (lenticulare) — *see* Neoplasm, skin, benign
- protuberans — *see* Neoplasm, skin, uncertain behavior

Dermatofibrosarcoma (pigmented) (protuberans) — *see* Neoplasm, skin, malignant

Dermatographia L5Ø.3

Dermatolysis (exfoliativa) (congenital) Q82.8
- acquired L57.4
- eyelids — *see* Blepharochalasis
- palpebrarum — *see* Blepharochalasis
- senile L57.4

Dermatomegaly NEC Q82.8

Dermatomucosomyositis — *see also* Dermatomyositis M33.1Ø
- with
  - myopathy M33.12
  - respiratory involvement M33.11
  - specified organ involvement NEC M33.19

Dermatomycosis B36.9
- furfuracea B36.Ø
- specified type NEC B36.8

Dermatomyositis (acute) (chronic) — *see also* Dermatopolymyositis
- adult — *see also* Dermatomyositis, specified NEC M33.1Ø
- in (due to) neoplastic disease — *see also* Neoplasm D49.9 *[M36.Ø]*
- juvenile M33.ØØ
  - with
    - myopathy M33.Ø2
    - respiratory involvement M33.Ø1
    - specified organ involvement NEC M33.Ø9
  - amyopathic M33.Ø3
  - without myopathy M33.Ø3
- specified NEC M33.1Ø

Dermatomyositis — *continued*
- specified — *continued*
  - with
    - myopathy M33.12
    - respiratory involvement M33.11
    - specified organ involvement NEC M33.19
  - amyopathic M33.13
  - without myopathy M33.13

Dermatoneuritis of children — *see* Poisoning, mercury

Dermatophilosis A48.8

Dermatophytid L3Ø.2

Dermatophytide — *see* Dermatophytosis

Dermatophytosis (epidermophyton) (infection) (Microsporum) (tinea) (Trichophyton) B35.9
- beard B35.Ø
- body B35.4
- capitis B35.Ø
- corporis B35.4
- deep-seated B35.8
- disseminated B35.8
- foot B35.3
- granulomatous B35.8
- groin B35.6
- hand B35.2
- nail B35.1
- perianal (area) B35.6
- scalp B35.Ø
- specified NEC B35.8

Dermatopolymyositis M33.9Ø
- with
  - myopathy M33.92
  - respiratory involvement M33.91
  - specified organ involvement NEC M33.99
- amyopathic M33.93
- in neoplastic disease — *see also* Neoplasm D49.9 *[M36.Ø]*
- juvenile M33.ØØ
  - with
    - myopathy M33.Ø2
    - respiratory involvement M33.Ø1
    - specified organ involvement NEC M33.Ø9
  - amyopathic M33.Ø3
  - without myopathy M33.Ø3
- specified NEC M33.1Ø
  - amyopathic M33.13
  - myopathy M33.12
  - respiratory involvement M33.11
  - specified organ involvement NEC M33.19
  - without myopathy M33.13
- without myopathy M33.93

Dermatopolyneuritis — *see* Poisoning, mercury

Dermatorrhexis — *see also* Syndrome, Ehlers-Danlos Q79.6Ø
- acquired L57.4

Dermatosclerosis — *see also* Scleroderma
- localized L94.Ø

Dermatosis L98.9
- Andrews' LØ8.89
- Bowen's — *see* Neoplasm, skin, in situ
- bullous L13.9
  - specified NEC L13.8
- exfoliativa L26
- eyelid (noninfectious) — *see also* Dermatitis, eyelid HØ1.9
  - discoid lupus erythematosus — *see* Lupus, erythematosus, eyelid
  - xeroderma — *see* Xeroderma, acquired, eyelid
- factitial L98.1
- febrile neutrophilic L98.2
- gonococcal A54.89
- herpetiformis L13.Ø
  - juvenile L12.2
- linear IgA L13.8
- menstrual NEC L98.8
- neutrophilic, febrile L98.2
- occupational — *see* Dermatitis, contact
- papulosa nigra L82.1
- pigmentary L81.9
  - progressive L81.7
  - Schamberg's L81.7
- psychogenic F54
- purpuric, pigmented L81.7
- pustular, subcorneal L13.1
- transient acantholytic L11.1

Dermographia, dermographism L5Ø.3

Dermoid (cyst) — *see also* Neoplasm, benign, by site
- with malignant transformation C56- ☑
- due to radiation (nonionizing) L57.8

Dermopathy
- infiltrative with thyrotoxicosis — *see* Thyrotoxicosis
- nephrogenic fibrosing L9Ø.8

Dermophytosis — *see* Dermatophytosis

Descemetocele H18.73- ☑

Descemet's membrane — *see* condition

Descending — *see* condition

Descensus uteri — *see* Prolapse, uterus

Desert
- rheumatism B38.Ø
- sore — *see* Ulcer, skin

Desertion (newborn) — *see* Maltreatment

Desmoid (extra-abdominal) (tumor) — *see* Neoplasm, connective tissue, uncertain behavior
- abdominal wall D48.113
- back D48.117
- buttock D48.116
- chest wall D48.111
- extremity
  - lower D48.116
  - upper D48.115
- head and neck D48.11Ø
- intraabdominal D48.114
- intrathoracic D48.112
- pelvic cavity D48.114
- pelvic girdle D48.116
- peritoneal D48.114
- retroperitoneal D48.114
- shoulder girdle D48.115
- site unspecified D48.119
- specified site NEC D48.118

Despondency F32.A

Desquamation, skin R23.4

Destruction, destructive — *see also* Damage
- articular facet — *see also* Derangement, joint, specified type NEC
  - knee M23.8X- ☑
  - vertebra — *see* Spondylosis
- bone — *see also* Disorder, bone, specified type NEC
  - syphilitic A52.77
- joint — *see also* Derangement, joint, specified type NEC
  - sacroiliac M53.3
- rectal sphincter K62.89
- septum (nasal) J34.89
- tuberculous NEC — *see* Tuberculosis
- tympanum, tympanic membrane (nontraumatic) — *see* Disorder, tympanic membrane, specified NEC
- vertebral disc — *see* Degeneration, intervertebral disc

Destructiveness — *see also* Disorder, conduct
- adjustment reaction — *see* Disorder, adjustment

Desultory labor O62.2

Detachment
- cartilage — *see* Sprain
- cervix, annular N88.8
  - complicating delivery O71.3
- choroid (old) (postinfectional) (simple) (spontaneous) H31.4Ø- ☑
  - hemorrhagic H31.41- ☑
  - serous H31.42- ☑
- ligament — *see* Sprain
- meniscus (knee) — *see also* Derangement, knee, meniscus, specified NEC
  - current injury — *see* Tear, meniscus
  - due to old tear or injury — *see* Derangement, knee, meniscus, due to old tear
- retina (without retinal break) (serous) H33.2- ☑
  - with retinal:
    - break H33.ØØ- ☑
      - giant H33.Ø3- ☑
      - multiple H33.Ø2- ☑
      - single H33.Ø1- ☑
    - dialysis H33.Ø4- ☑
  - pigment epithelium — *see* Degeneration, retina, separation of layers, pigment epithelium detachment
  - rhegmatogenous — *see* Detachment, retina, with retinal, break
  - specified NEC H33.8
  - total H33.Ø5- ☑
  - traction H33.4- ☑
- vitreous (body) H43.81 ☑

Detergent asthma J69.8

Deterioration
- epileptic FØ6.8
- general physical R53.81
- heart, cardiac — *see* Degeneration, myocardial

Deterioration — *continued*
- mental — *see* Psychosis
- myocardial, myocardium — *see* Degeneration, myocardial
- senile (simple) R54

Deuteranomaly (anomalous trichromat) H53.53

Deuteranopia (complete) (incomplete) H53.53

Development
- abnormal, bone Q79.9
- arrested R62.5Ø
  - bone — *see* Arrest, development or growth, bone
  - child R62.5Ø
  - due to malnutrition E45
- defective, congenital — *see also* Anomaly, by site
  - cauda equina QØ6.3
  - left ventricle Q24.8
    - in hypoplastic left heart syndrome Q23.4
  - valve Q24.8
    - pulmonary Q22.3
- delayed — *see also* Delay, development R62.5Ø
  - arithmetical skills F81.2
  - language (skills) (expressive) F8Ø.1
  - learning skill F81.9
  - mixed skills F88
  - motor coordination F82
  - reading F81.Ø
  - specified learning skill NEC F81.89
  - speech F8Ø.9
  - spelling F81.81
  - written expression F81.81
- imperfect, congenital — *see also* Anomaly, by site
  - heart Q24.9
  - lungs Q33.6
- incomplete
  - bronchial tree Q32.4
  - organ or site not listed — *see* Hypoplasia, by site
  - respiratory system Q34.9
- sexual, precocious NEC E3Ø.1
- tardy, mental — *see also* Disability, intellectual F79

Developmental — *see* condition
- testing, infant or child — *see* Examination, child

Devergie's disease (pityriasis rubra pilaris) L44.Ø

Deviation (in)
- conjugate palsy (eye) (spastic) H51.Ø
- esophagus (acquired) K22.89
- eye, skew H51.8
- midline (jaw) (teeth) (dental arch) M26.29
  - specified site NEC — *see* Malposition
- nasal septum J34.2
  - congenital Q67.4
- opening and closing of the mandible M26.53
- organ or site, congenital NEC — *see* Malposition, congenital
- septum (nasal) (acquired) J34.2
  - congenital Q67.4
- sexual F65.9
  - bestiality F65.89
  - erotomania F52.8
  - exhibitionism F65.2
  - fetishism, fetishistic F65.Ø
    - transvestism F65.1
  - frotteurism F65.81
  - masochism F65.51
  - multiple F65.89
  - necrophilia F65.89
  - nymphomania F52.8
  - pederosis F65.4
  - pedophilia F65.4
  - sadism, sadomasochism F65.52
  - satyriasis F52.8
  - specified type NEC F65.89
  - transvestism F64.1
  - voyeurism F65.3
- teeth, midline M26.29
- trachea J39.8
- ureter, congenital Q62.61

Device
- cerebral ventricle (communicating) in situ Z98.2
- contraceptive — *see* Contraceptive, device
- drainage, cerebrospinal fluid, in situ Z98.2

Devic's disease G36.Ø

Devil's
- grip B33.Ø
- pinches (purpura simplex) D69.2

Devitalized tooth KØ4.99

Devonshire colic — *see* Poisoning, lead

Dextraposition, aorta Q2Ø.3
- in tetralogy of Fallot Q21.3

Dextrinosis, limit (debrancher enzyme deficiency) E74.Ø3

Dextrocardia (true) Q24.Ø
- with
  - complete transposition of viscera Q89.3
  - situs inversus Q89.3

Dextrotransposition, aorta Q2Ø.3

d-glycericacidemia E72.59

Dhat syndrome F48.8

Dhobi itch B35.6

Di George's syndrome D82.1

Di Guglielmo's disease C94.Ø- ☑

Diabetes, diabetic (mellitus) (sugar) E11.9
- with
  - amyotrophy E11.44
  - arthropathy NEC E11.618
  - autonomic (poly)neuropathy E11.43
  - cataract E11.36
  - Charcot's joints E11.61Ø
  - chronic kidney disease E11.22
  - circulatory complication NEC E11.59
  - coma due to
    - hyperosmolarity E11.Ø1
    - hypoglycemia E11.641
    - ketoacidosis E11.11
  - complication E11.8
    - specified NEC E11.69
  - dermatitis E11.62Ø
  - foot ulcer E11.621
  - gangrene E11.52
  - gastroparalysis E11.43
  - gastroparesis E11.43
  - glomerulonephrosis, intracapillary E11.21
  - glomerulosclerosis, intercapillary E11.21
  - hyperglycemia E11.65
  - hyperosmolarity E11.ØØ
    - with coma E11.Ø1
  - hypoglycemia E11.649
    - with coma E11.641
  - ketoacidosis E11.1Ø
    - with coma E11.11
  - kidney complications NEC E11.29
  - Kimmelstiel-Wilson disease E11.21
  - loss of protective sensation (LOPS) — *see* Diabetes, by type, with neuropathy
  - mononeuropathy E11.41
  - myasthenia E11.44
  - necrobiosis lipoidica E11.62Ø
  - nephropathy E11.21
  - neuralgia E11.42
  - neurologic complication NEC E11.49
  - neuropathic arthropathy E11.61Ø
  - neuropathy E11.4Ø
  - ophthalmic complication NEC E11.39
  - oral complication NEC E11.638
  - osteomyelitis E11.69
  - periodontal disease E11.63Ø
  - peripheral angiopathy E11.51
    - with gangrene E11.52
  - polyneuropathy E11.42
  - renal complication NEC E11.29
  - renal tubular degeneration E11.29
  - retinopathy E11.319
    - with macular edema E11.311
      - resolved following treatment E11.37- ☑
    - nonproliferative E11.329 ☑
      - with macular edema E11.321 ☑
      - mild E11.329 ☑
        - with macular edema E11.321 ☑
      - moderate E11.339 ☑
        - with macular edema E11.331 ☑
      - severe E11.349 ☑
        - with macular edema E11.341 ☑
    - proliferative E11.359 ☑
      - with
        - combined traction retinal detachment and rhegmatogenous retinal detachment E11.354 ☑
        - macular edema E11.351 ☑
        - stable proliferative diabetic retinopathy E11.355 ☑
        - traction retinal detachment involving the macula E11.352 ☑
        - traction retinal detachment not involving the macula E11.353 ☑
  - skin complication NEC E11.628
  - skin ulcer NEC E11.622
- brittle — *see* Diabetes, type 1
- bronzed E83.11Ø

Diabetes, diabetic — *continued*
- complicating pregnancy — *see* Pregnancy, complicated by, diabetes
- dietary counseling and surveillance Z71.3
- due to
  - autoimmune process — *see* Diabetes, type 1
  - immune mediated pancreatic islet beta-cell destruction — *see* Diabetes, type 1
  - pancreatectomy — *see* Diabetes, specified type NEC
- due to drug or chemical EØ9.9
  - with
    - amyotrophy EØ9.44
    - arthropathy NEC EØ9.618
    - autonomic (poly)neuropathy EØ9.43
    - cataract EØ9.36
    - Charcot's joints EØ9.61Ø
    - chronic kidney disease EØ9.22
    - circulatory complication NEC EØ9.59
    - complication EØ9.8
      - specified NEC EØ9.69
    - dermatitis EØ9.62Ø
    - foot ulcer EØ9.621
    - gangrene EØ9.52
    - gastroparalysis EØ9.43
    - gastroparesis EØ9.43
    - glomerulonephrosis, intracapillary EØ9.21
    - glomerulosclerosis, intercapillary EØ9.21
    - hyperglycemia EØ9.65
    - hyperosmolarity EØ9.ØØ
      - with coma EØ9.Ø1
    - hypoglycemia EØ9.649
      - with coma EØ9.641
    - ketoacidosis EØ9.1Ø
      - with coma EØ9.11
    - kidney complications NEC EØ9.29
    - Kimmelstiel-Wilson disease EØ9.21
    - mononeuropathy EØ9.41
    - myasthenia EØ9.44
    - necrobiosis lipoidica EØ9.62Ø
    - nephropathy EØ9.21
    - neuralgia EØ9.42
    - neurologic complication NEC EØ9.49
    - neuropathic arthropathy EØ9.61Ø
    - neuropathy EØ9.4Ø
    - ophthalmic complication NEC EØ9.39
    - oral complication NEC EØ9.638
    - periodontal disease EØ9.63Ø
    - peripheral angiopathy EØ9.51
      - with gangrene EØ9.52
    - polyneuropathy EØ9.42
    - renal complication NEC EØ9.29
    - renal tubular degeneration EØ9.29
    - retinopathy EØ9.319
      - with macular edema EØ9.311
        - resolved following treatment EØ9.37 ☑
      - nonproliferative EØ9.329 ☑
        - with macular edema EØ9.321 ☑
        - mild EØ9.329 ☑
          - with macular edema EØ9.321 ☑
        - moderate EØ9.339 ☑
          - with macular edema EØ9.331 ☑
        - severe EØ9.349 ☑
          - with macular edema EØ9.341 ☑
      - proliferative EØ9.359 ☑
        - with
          - combined traction retinal detachment and rhegmatogenous retinal detachment EØ9.354 ☑
          - macular edema EØ9.351 ☑
          - stable proliferative diabetic retinopathy EØ9.355 ☑
          - traction retinal detachment involving the macula EØ9.352 ☑
          - traction retinal detachment not involving the macula EØ9.353 ☑
    - skin complication NEC EØ9.628
    - skin ulcer NEC EØ9.622
- due to underlying condition EØ8.9
  - with
    - amyotrophy EØ8.44
    - arthropathy NEC EØ8.618
    - autonomic (poly)neuropathy EØ8.43
    - cataract EØ8.36
    - Charcot's joints EØ8.61Ø
    - chronic kidney disease EØ8.22
    - circulatory complication NEC EØ8.59
    - complication EØ8.8
      - specified NEC EØ8.69

- **Diabetes, diabetic** — *continued*
  - due to underlying condition — *continued*
    - with — *continued*
      - dermatitis E08.620
      - foot ulcer E08.621
      - gangrene E08.52
      - gastroparalysis E08.43
      - gastroparesis E08.43
      - glomerulonephrosis, intracapillary E08.21
      - glomerulosclerosis, intercapillary E08.21
      - hyperglycemia E08.65
      - hyperosmolarity E08.00
        - with coma E08.01
      - hypoglycemia E08.649
        - with coma E08.641
      - ketoacidosis E08.10
        - with coma E08.11
      - kidney complications NEC E08.29
      - Kimmelstiel-WIlson disease E08.21
      - mononeuropathy E08.41
      - myasthenia E08.44
      - necrobiosis lipoidica E08.620
      - nephropathy E08.21
      - neuralgia E08.42
      - neurologic complication NEC E08.49
      - neuropathic arthropathy E08.610
      - neuropathy E08.40
      - ophthalmic complication NEC E08.39
      - oral complication NEC E08.638
      - periodontal disease E08.630
      - peripheral angiopathy E08.51
        - with gangrene E08.52
      - polyneuropathy E08.42
      - renal complication NEC E08.29
      - renal tubular degeneration E08.29
      - retinopathy E08.319
        - with macular edema E08.311
        - resolved following treatment E08.37 ☑
        - nonproliferative E08.329 ☑
          - with macular edema E08.321 ☑
          - mild E08.329 ☑
            - with macular edema E08.321 ☑
          - moderate E08.339 ☑
            - with macular edema E08.331 ☑
          - severe E08.349 ☑
            - with macular edema E08.341 ☑
        - proliferative E08.359 ☑
          - with
            - combined traction retinal detachment and rhegmatogenous retinal detachment E08.354 ☑
            - macular edema E08.351 ☑
            - stable proliferative diabetic retinopathy E08.355 ☑
            - traction retinal detachment involving the macula E08.352 ☑
            - traction retinal detachment not involving the macula E08.353 ☑
      - skin complication NEC E08.628
      - skin ulcer NEC E08.622
  - gestational (in pregnancy) O24.419
    - affecting newborn P70.0
    - diet controlled O24.410
    - in childbirth O24.429
      - diet controlled O24.420
      - insulin (and diet) controlled O24.424
      - oral drug controlled (antidiabetic) (hypoglycemic) O24.425
    - insulin (and diet) controlled O24.414
    - oral drug controlled (antidiabetic) (hypoglycemic) O24.415
    - puerperal O24.439
      - diet controlled O24.430
      - insulin (and diet) controlled O24.434
      - oral drug controlled (antidiabetic) (hypoglycemic) O24.435
  - hepatogenous E13.9
  - idiopathic — *see* Diabetes, type 1
  - inadequately controlled — *see* Diabetes, by type, with hyperglycemia
  - insipidus E23.2
    - nephrogenic N25.1
    - pituitary E23.2
    - vasopressin resistant N25.1
  - insulin dependent — *code to* type of diabetes
  - juvenile-onset — *see* Diabetes, type 1
  - ketosis-prone — *see* Diabetes, type 1
  - latent R73.03

- **Diabetes, diabetic** — *continued*
  - neonatal (transient) P70.2
  - non-insulin dependent — *code to* type of diabetes
  - out of control — *see* Diabetes, by type, with hyperglycemia
  - phosphate E83.39
  - poorly controlled — *see* Diabetes, by type, with hyperglycemia
  - postpancreatectomy — *see* Diabetes, specified type NEC
  - postprocedural — *see* Diabetes, specified type NEC
  - retina, hemorrhage E13.39
  - secondary diabetes mellitus NEC — *see* Diabetes, specified type NEC
  - specified type NEC E13.9
    - with
      - amyotrophy E13.44
      - arthropathy NEC E13.618
      - autonomic (poly)neuropathy E13.43
      - cataract E13.36
      - Charcot's joints E13.610
      - chronic kidney disease E13.22
      - circulatory complication NEC E13.59
      - complication E13.8
        - specified NEC E13.69
      - dermatitis E13.620
      - foot ulcer E13.621
      - gangrene E13.52
      - gastroparalysis E13.43
      - gastroparesis E13.43
      - glomerulonephrosis, intracapillary E13.21
      - glomerulosclerosis, intercapillary E13.21
      - hyperglycemia E13.65
      - hyperosmolarity E13.00
        - with coma E13.01
      - hypoglycemia E13.649
        - with coma E13.641
      - ketoacidosis E13.10
        - with coma E13.11
      - kidney complications NEC E13.29
      - Kimmelstiel-Wilson disease E13.21
      - mononeuropathy E13.41
      - myasthenia E13.44
      - necrobiosis lipoidica E13.620
      - nephropathy E13.21
      - neuralgia E13.42
      - neurologic complication NEC E13.49
      - neuropathic arthropathy E13.610
      - neuropathy E13.40
      - ophthalmic complication NEC E13.39
      - oral complication NEC E13.638
      - periodontal disease E13.630
      - peripheral angiopathy E13.51
        - with gangrene E13.52
      - polyneuropathy E13.42
      - renal complication NEC E13.29
      - renal tubular degeneration E13.29
      - retinopathy E13.319
        - with macular edema E13.311
        - resolved following treatment E13.37 ☑
        - nonproliferative E13.329 ☑
          - with macular edema E13.321 ☑
          - mild E13.329 ☑
            - with macular edema E13.321 ☑
          - moderate E13.339 ☑
            - with macular edema E13.331 ☑
          - severe E13.349 ☑
            - with macular edema E13.341 ☑
        - proliferative E13.359 ☑
          - with
            - combined traction retinal detachment and rhegmatogenous retinal detachment E13.354 ☑
            - macular edema E13.351 ☑
            - stable proliferative diabetic retinopathy E13.355 ☑
            - traction retinal detachment involving the macula E13.352 ☑
            - traction retinal detachment not involving the macula E13.353 ☑
      - skin complication NEC E13.628
      - skin ulcer NEC E13.622
  - steroid-induced — *see* Diabetes, due to, drug or chemical
  - type 1 E10.9
    - with
      - amyotrophy E10.44
      - arthropathy NEC E10.618

- **Diabetes, diabetic** — *continued*
  - type 1 — *continued*
    - with — *continued*
      - autonomic (poly)neuropathy E10.43
      - cataract E10.36
      - Charcot's joints E10.610
      - chronic kidney disease E10.22
      - circulatory complication NEC E10.59
      - coma due to
        - hypoglycemia E10.641
        - ketoacidosis E10.11
      - complication E10.8
        - specified NEC E10.69
      - dermatitis E10.620
      - foot ulcer E10.621
      - gangrene E10.52
      - gastroparalysis E10.43
      - gastroparesis E10.43
      - glomerulonephrosis, intracapillary E10.21
      - glomerulosclerosis, intercapillary E10.21
      - hyperglycemia E10.65
      - hypoglycemia E10.649
        - with coma E10.641
      - ketoacidosis E10.10
        - with coma E10.11
      - kidney complications NEC E10.29
      - Kimmelstiel-Wilson disease E10.21
      - mononeuropathy E10.41
      - myasthenia E10.44
      - necrobiosis lipoidica E10.620
      - nephropathy E10.21
      - neuralgia E10.42
      - neurologic complication NEC E10.49
      - neuropathic arthropathy E10.610
      - neuropathy E10.40
      - ophthalmic complication NEC E10.39
      - oral complication NEC E10.638
      - osteomyelitis E10.69
      - periodontal disease E10.630
      - peripheral angiopathy E10.51
        - with gangrene E10.52
      - polyneuropathy E10.42
      - renal complication NEC E10.29
      - renal tubular degeneration E10.29
      - retinopathy E10.319
        - with macular edema E10.311
        - resolved following treatment E10.37 ☑
        - nonproliferative E10.329 ☑
          - with macular edema E10.321 ☑
          - mild E10.329 ☑
            - with macular edema E10.321 ☑
          - moderate E10.339 ☑
            - with macular edema E10.331 ☑
          - severe E10.349 ☑
            - with macular edema E10.341 ☑
        - proliferative E10.359 ☑
          - with
            - combined traction retinal detachment and rhegmatogenous retinal detachment E10.354 ☑
            - macular edema E10.351 ☑
            - stable proliferative diabetic retinopathy E10.355 ☑
            - traction retinal detachment involving the macula E10.352 ☑
            - traction retinal detachment not involving the macula E10.353 ☑
      - skin complication NEC E10.628
      - skin ulcer NEC E10.622
  - type 2 E11.9
    - with
      - amyotrophy E11.44
      - arthropathy NEC E11.618
      - autonomic (poly)neuropathy E11.43
      - cataract E11.36
      - Charcot's joints E11.610
      - chronic kidney disease E11.22
      - circulatory complication NEC E11.59
      - coma due to
        - hyperosmolarity E11.01
        - hypoglycemia E11.641
        - ketoacidosis E11.1- ☑
      - complication E11.8
        - specified NEC E11.69
      - dermatitis E11.620
      - foot ulcer E11.621
      - gangrene E11.52
      - gastroparalysis E11.43

- **Diabetes, diabetic** — *continued*
  - type 2 — *continued*
    - with — *continued*
      - gastroparesis E11.43
      - glomerulonephrosis, intracapillary E11.21
      - glomerulosclerosis, intercapillary E11.21
      - hyperglycemia E11.65
      - hyperosmolarity E11.ØØ
        - with coma E11.Ø1
      - hypoglycemia E11.649
        - with coma E11.641
      - ketoacidosis E11.1Ø
        - with coma E11.11
      - kidney complications NEC E11.29
      - Kimmelstiel-Wilson disease E11.21
      - mononeuropathy E11.41
      - myasthenia E11.44
      - necrobiosis lipoidica E11.62Ø
      - nephropathy E11.21
      - neuralgia E11.42
      - neurologic complication NEC E11.49
      - neuropathic arthropathy E11.61Ø
      - neuropathy E11.4Ø
      - ophthalmic complication NEC E11.39
      - oral complication NEC E11.638
      - osteomyelitis E11.69
      - periodontal disease E11.63Ø
      - peripheral angiopathy E11.51
        - with gangrene E11.52
      - polyneuropathy E11.42
      - renal complication NEC E11.29
      - renal tubular degeneration E11.29
      - retinopathy E11.319
        - with macular edema E11.311
        - resolved following treatment E11.37 ☑
        - nonproliferative E11.329 ☑
          - with macular edema E11.321 ☑
          - mild E11.329 ☑
            - with macular edema E11.321 ☑
          - moderate E11.339 ☑
            - with macular edema E11.331 ☑
          - severe E11.349 ☑
            - with macular edema E11.341 ☑
        - proliferative E11.359 ☑
          - with
            - combined traction retinal detachment and rhegmatogenous retinal detachment E11.354 ☑
            - macular edema E11.351 ☑
            - stable proliferative diabetic retinopathy E11.355 ☑
            - traction retinal detachment involving the macula E11.352 ☑
            - traction retinal detachment not involving the macula E11.353 ☑
      - skin complication NEC E11.628
      - skin ulcer NEC E11.622
  - uncontrolled
    - meaning
      - hyperglycemia — *see* Diabetes, by type, with, hyperglycemia
      - hypoglycemia — *see* Diabetes, by type, with, hypoglycemia
- **Diacyclothrombopathia** D69.1
- **Diagnosis deferred** R69
- **Dialysis** (intermittent) (treatment)
  - noncompliance (with) Z91.158
    - due to financial hardship Z91.151
  - renal (hemodialysis) (peritoneal), status Z99.2
  - retina, retinal — *see* Detachment, retina, with retinal, dialysis
- **Diamond-Blackfan anemia** (congenital hypoplastic) D61.Ø1
- **Diamond-Gardener syndrome** (autoerythrocyte sensitization) D69.2
- **Diaper rash** L22
- **Diaphoresis** (excessive) R61
- **Diaphragm** — *see* condition
- **Diaphragmalgia** RØ7.1
- **Diaphragmatitis, diaphragmitis** J98.6
- **Diaphysial aclasis** Q78.6
- **Diaphysitis** — *see* Osteomyelitis, specified type NEC
- **Diarrhea, diarrheal** (disease) (infantile) (inflammatory) R19.7
  - achlorhydric K31.83
  - allergic K52.29
    - due to
      - colitis — *see* Colitis, allergic
      - enteritis — *see* Enteritis, allergic
  - amebic — *see also* Amebiasis AØ6.Ø
    - with abscess — *see* Abscess, amebic
    - acute AØ6.Ø
    - chronic AØ6.1
    - nondysenteric AØ6.2
  - bacillary — *see* Dysentery, bacillary
  - balantidial AØ7.Ø
  - cachectic NEC K52.89
  - Chilomastix AØ7.8
  - choleriformis AØØ.1
  - chronic (noninfectious) K52.9
  - coccidial AØ7.3
  - Cochin-China K9Ø.1
    - strongyloidiasis B78.Ø
  - Dientamoeba AØ7.8
  - dietetic — *see also* Diarrhea, allergic K52.29
  - drug-induced K52.1
  - due to
    - bacteria AØ4.9
      - specified NEC AØ4.8
    - Campylobacter AØ4.5
    - Capillaria philippinensis B81.1
    - Clostridium difficile
      - not specified as recurrent AØ4.72
      - recurrent AØ4.71
    - Clostridium perfringens (C) (F) AØ4.8
    - Cryptosporidium AØ7.2
    - drugs K52.1
    - Escherichia coli AØ4.4
      - enteroaggregative AØ4.4
      - enterohemorrhagic AØ4.3
      - enteroinvasive AØ4.2
      - enteropathogenic AØ4.Ø
      - enterotoxigenic AØ4.1
      - specified NEC AØ4.4
    - food hypersensitivity — *see also* Diarrhea, allergic K52.29
    - Necator americanus B76.1
    - S. japonicum B65.2
    - specified organism NEC AØ8.8
      - bacterial AØ4.8
      - viral AØ8.39
    - Staphylococcus AØ4.8
    - Trichuris trichiuria B79
    - virus — *see* Enteritis, viral
    - Yersinia enterocolitica AØ4.6
  - dysenteric AØ9
  - endemic AØ9
  - epidemic AØ9
  - flagellate AØ7.9
  - Flexner's (ulcerative) AØ3.1
  - functional K59.1
    - following gastrointestinal surgery K91.89
    - psychogenic F45.8
  - Giardia lamblia AØ7.1
  - giardial AØ7.1
  - hill K9Ø.1
  - infectious AØ9
  - malarial — *see* Malaria
  - mite B88.Ø
  - mycotic NEC B49
  - neonatal (noninfectious) P78.3
  - nervous F45.8
  - neurogenic K59.1
  - noninfectious K52.9
  - postgastrectomy K91.1
  - postvagotomy K91.1
  - protozoal AØ7.9
    - specified NEC AØ7.8
  - psychogenic F45.8
  - specified
    - bacterium NEC AØ4.8
    - virus NEC AØ8.39
  - strongyloidiasis B78.Ø
  - toxic K52.1
  - trichomonal AØ7.8
  - tropical K9Ø.1
  - tuberculous A18.32
  - viral — *see* Enteritis, viral
- **Diastasis**
  - cranial bones M84.88
    - congenital NEC Q75.8
  - joint (traumatic) — *see* Dislocation
  - muscle M62.ØØ
    - ankle M62.Ø7- ☑
    - congenital Q79.8
    - foot M62.Ø7- ☑
    - forearm M62.Ø3- ☑
    - hand M62.Ø4- ☑
    - lower leg M62.Ø6- ☑
    - pelvic region M62.Ø5- ☑
    - shoulder region M62.Ø1- ☑
    - specified site NEC M62.Ø8
    - thigh M62.Ø5- ☑
    - upper arm M62.Ø2- ☑
  - recti (abdomen)
    - complicating delivery O71.89
    - congenital Q79.59
- **Diastema, tooth, teeth, fully erupted** M26.32
- **Diastematomyelia** QØ6.2
- **Diataxia, cerebral** G8Ø.4
- **Diathesis**
  - allergic — *see* History, allergy
  - bleeding (familial) D69.9
  - cystine (familial) E72.ØØ
  - gouty — *see* Gout
  - hemorrhagic (familial) D69.9
    - newborn NEC P53
  - spasmophilic R29.Ø
- **Diaz's disease or osteochondrosis** (juvenile) (talus) — *see* Osteochondrosis, juvenile, tarsus
- **Dibothriocephalus, dibothriocephaliasis** (latus) (infection) (infestation) B7Ø.Ø
  - larval B7Ø.1
- **Dicephalus, dicephaly** Q89.4
- **Dichotomy, teeth** KØØ.2
- **Dichromat, dichromatopsia** (congenital) — *see* Deficiency, color vision
- **Dichuchwa** A65
- **Dicroceliasis** B66.2
- **Didelphia, didelphys** — *see* Double uterus
- **Didymytis** N45.1
  - with orchitis N45.3
- **Dietary**
  - inadequacy or deficiency E63.9
  - surveillance and counseling Z71.3
- **Dietl's crisis** N13.8
- **Dieulafoy lesion** (hemorrhagic)
  - duodenum K31.82
  - esophagus K22.89
  - intestine (colon) K63.81
  - stomach K31.82
- **Difficult, difficulty** (in)
  - acculturation Z6Ø.3
  - feeding R63.3Ø
    - elderly R63.39
    - infant NOS R63.39
    - newborn P92.9
      - breast P92.5
      - specified NEC P92.8
    - nonorganic (infant or child) F98.29
    - specified NEC R63.39
  - intubation, in anesthesia T88.4 ☑
  - mechanical, gastroduodenal stoma K91.89
    - causing obstruction — *see also* Obstruction, intestine, postoperative K91.3Ø
  - micturition
    - need to immediately re-void R39.191
    - position dependent R39.192
    - specified NEC R39.198
  - reading (developmental) F81.Ø
    - secondary to emotional disorders F93.9
  - spelling (specific) F81.81
    - with reading disorder F81.89
    - due to inadequate teaching Z55.8
  - swallowing — *see* Dysphagia
  - understanding
    - health related information Z55.6
    - medication instructions Z55.6
  - walking R26.2
  - work
    - conditions NEC Z56.5
    - schedule Z56.3
- **Diffuse** — *see* condition
- **Digestive** — *see* condition
- **Dihydropyrimidine dehydrogenase disease** (DPD) E88.89
- **Diktyoma** — *see* Neoplasm, malignant, by site
- **Dilaceration, tooth** KØØ.4

Dilatation
- anus K59.89
  - venule — *see* Hemorrhoids
- aorta (focal) (general) — *see* Ectasia, aorta
  - with aneuysm — *see* Aneurysm, aorta
  - congenital Q25.44
- artery — *see* Aneurysm
- bladder (sphincter) N32.89
  - congenital Q64.79
- blood vessel I99.8
- bronchial J47.9
  - with
    - exacerbation (acute) J47.1
    - lower respiratory infection J47.Ø
- calyx N28.89
  - due to obstruction — *see* Hydronephrosis
- capillaries I78.8
- cardiac (acute) (chronic) — *see also* Hypertrophy, cardiac
  - congenital Q24.8
    - valve NEC Q24.8
      - pulmonary Q22.3
  - valve — *see* Endocarditis
- cavum septi pellucidi QØ6.8
- cervix (uteri) — *see also* Incompetency, cervix
  - incomplete, poor, slow complicating delivery O62.Ø
- colon K59.39
  - congenital Q43.1
  - psychogenic F45.8
  - toxic K59.31
- common duct (acquired) K83.8
  - congenital Q44.5
- cystic duct (acquired) K82.8
  - congenital Q44.5
- duct, mammary — *see* Ectasia, mammary duct
- duodenum K59.89
- esophagus K22.89
  - congenital Q39.5
  - due to achalasia K22.Ø
- eustachian tube, congenital Q17.8
- gallbladder K82.8
- gastric — *see* Dilatation, stomach
- heart (acute) (chronic) — *see also* Hypertrophy, cardiac
  - congenital Q24.8
  - valve — *see* Endocarditis
- ileum K59.89
  - psychogenic F45.8
- jejunum K59.89
  - psychogenic F45.8
- kidney (calyx) (collecting structures) (cystic) (parenchyma) (pelvis) (idiopathic) N28.89
  - due to obstruction — *see* Hydronephrosis
- lacrimal passages or duct — *see* Disorder, lacrimal system, changes
- lymphatic vessel I89.Ø
- mammary duct — *see* Ectasia, mammary duct
- Meckel's diverticulum (congenital) Q43.Ø
  - malignant — *see* Table of Neoplasms, small intestine, malignant
- myocardium (acute) (chronic) — *see* Hypertrophy, cardiac
- organ or site, congenital NEC — *see* Distortion
- pancreatic duct K86.89
- pericardium — *see* Pericarditis
- pharynx J39.2
- prostate N42.89
- pulmonary
  - artery (idiopathic) I28.8
  - valve, congenital Q22.3
- pupil H57.Ø4
- rectum K59.39
- saccule, congenital Q16.5
- salivary gland (duct) K11.8
- sphincter ani K62.89
- stomach K31.89
  - acute K31.Ø
  - psychogenic F45.8
- submaxillary duct K11.8
- trachea, congenital Q32.1
- ureter (idiopathic) N28.82
  - congenital Q62.2
  - due to obstruction N13.4
- urethra (acquired) N36.8
- vasomotor I73.9
- vein I86.8
- ventricular, ventricle (acute) (chronic) — *see also* Hypertrophy, cardiac
  - cerebral, congenital QØ4.8
- venule NEC I86.8
- vesical orifice N32.89

Dilated, dilation — *see* Dilatation

Diminished, diminution
- hearing (acuity) — *see* Deafness
- sense or sensation (cold) (heat) (tactile) (vibratory) R2Ø.8
- vision NEC H54.7
- vital capacity R94.2

Diminuta taenia B71.Ø

Dimitri-Sturge-Weber disease Q85.89

Dimple
- congenital sacral Q82.6
- parasacral Q82.6
- pilonidal or postanal — *see* Cyst, pilonidal

Dioctophyme renalis (infection) (infestation) B83.8

Dipetalonemiasis B74.4

Diphallus Q55.69

Diphtheria, diphtheritic (gangrenous) (hemorrhagic) A36.9
- carrier (suspected) Z22.2
- cutaneous A36.3
- faucial A36.Ø
- infection of wound A36.3
- laryngeal A36.2
- myocarditis A36.81
- nasal, anterior A36.89
- nasopharyngeal A36.1
- neurological complication A36.89
- pharyngeal A36.Ø
- specified site NEC A36.89
- tonsillar A36.Ø

Diphyllobothriasis (intestine) B7Ø.Ø
- larval B7Ø.1

Diplacusis H93.22- ☑

Diplegia (upper limbs) G83.Ø
- congenital (cerebral) G8Ø.8
- facial G51.Ø
- lower limbs G82.2Ø
- spastic G8Ø.1

Diplococcus, diplococcal — *see* condition

Diplopia H53.2

Dipsomania F1Ø.2Ø
- with
  - psychosis — *see* Psychosis, alcoholic
  - remission F1Ø.21

Dipylidiasis B71.1

DIRA (deficiency of interleukin 1 receptor antagonist) MØ4.8

Direction, teeth, abnormal, fully erupted M26.3Ø

Dirofilariasis B74.8

Dirt-eating child F98.3

Disability, disabilities
- heart — *see* Disease, heart
- intellectual F79
  - with
    - autistic features F84.9
    - pathogenic CHAMP1 (genetic) (variant) F78.A9
    - pathogenic HNRNPH2 (genetic) (variant) F78.A9
    - pathogenic SATB2 (genetic) (variant) F78.A9
    - pathogenic SETBP1 (genetic) (variant) F78.A9
    - pathogenic STXBP1 (genetic) (variant) F78.A9
    - pathogenic SYNGAP1 (genetic) (variant) F78.A1
  - autosomal dominant F78.A9
  - autosomal recessive F78.A9
  - genetic related F78.A9
    - with
      - pathogenic CHAMP1 (variant) F78.A9
      - pathogenic HNRNPH2 (variant) F78.A9
      - pathogenic SATB2 (variant) F78.A9
      - pathogenic SETBP1 (variant) F78.A9
      - pathogenic STXBP1 (variant) F78.A9
      - pathogenic SYNGAP1 (variant) F78.A1
    - specified NEC F78.A9
    - SYNGAP1-related F78.A1
  - in
    - autosomal dominant mental retardation F78.A9
    - autosomal recessive mental retardation F78.A9
    - SATB2-associated syndrome F78.A9
    - SETBP1 disorder F78.A9
    - STXBP1 encephalopathy with epilepsy — *see also* Encephalopathy; and — *see also* Epilepsy
    - X-linked mental retardation (syndromic) (Bain type) F78.A9
  - mild (I.Q. 5Ø-69) F7Ø
  - moderate (I.Q. 35-49) F71
  - profound (I.Q. under 2Ø) F73
  - severe (I.Q. 2Ø-34) F72
  - specified level NEC F78.A9
  - SYNGAP1-related F78.A1
  - X-linked (syndromic) (Bain type) F78.A9
- knowledge acquisition F81.9
- learning F81.9
- limiting activities Z73.6
- spelling, specific F81.81

Disappearance of family member Z63.4

Disarticulation — *see* Amputation
- meaning traumatic amputation — *see* Amputation, traumatic

Discharge (from)
- abnormal finding in — *see* Abnormal, specimen
- breast (female) (male) N64.52
- diencephalic autonomic idiopathic — *see* Epilepsy, specified NEC
- ear — *see also* Otorrhea
  - blood — *see* Otorrhagia
- excessive urine R35.89
- nipple N64.52
- penile R36.9
- postnasal RØ9.82
- prison, anxiety concerning Z65.2
- urethral R36.9
  - without blood R36.Ø
  - hematospermia R36.1
- vaginal N89.8

Discitis, diskitis M46.4Ø
- cervical region M46.42
- cervicothoracic region M46.43
- lumbar region M46.46
- lumbosacral region M46.47
- multiple sites M46.49
- occipito-atlanto-axial region M46.41
- pyogenic — *see* Infection, intervertebral disc, pyogenic
- sacrococcygeal region M46.48
- thoracic region M46.44
- thoracolumbar region M46.45

Discoid
- meniscus (congenital) Q68.6
- semilunar cartilage (congenital) — *see* Derangement, knee, meniscus, specified NEC

Discoloration
- nails L6Ø.8
- teeth (posteruptive) KØ3.7
  - during formation KØØ.8

Discomfort
- chest RØ7.89
- visual H53.14- ☑

Discontinuity, ossicles, ear H74.2- ☑

Discord (with)
- boss Z56.4
- classmates Z55.4
- counselor Z64.4
- employer Z56.4
- family Z63.8
- fellow employees Z56.4
- in-laws Z63.1
- landlord Z59.2
- lodgers Z59.2
- neighbors Z59.2
- probation officer Z64.4
- social worker Z64.4
- teachers Z55.4
- workmates Z56.4

Discordant connection
- atrioventricular (congenital) Q2Ø.5
- ventriculoarterial Q2Ø.3

Discrepancy
- centric occlusion maximum intercuspation M26.55
- leg length (acquired) — *see* Deformity, limb, unequal length
  - congenital — *see* Defect, reduction, lower limb
- uterine size date O26.84- ☑

Discrimination
- ethnic Z6Ø.5
- political Z6Ø.5
- racial Z6Ø.5
- religious Z6Ø.5
- sex Z6Ø.5

Disease, diseased — *see also* Syndrome
- absorbent system I87.8
- acid-peptic K3Ø
- Acosta's T7Ø.29 ☑

Disease, diseased — *continued*
- Castellani's A69.8
- Castleman (unicentric) (multicentric) D47.Z2
  - HHV-8-associated — *see also* Herpesvirus, human, 8 D47.Z2
- cat-scratch A28.1
- Cavare's (familial periodic paralysis) G72.3
- cecum K63.9
- celiac (adult) (infantile) (with steatorrhea) K9Ø.Ø
- cellular tissue L98.9
- central core G71.29
- cerebellar, cerebellum — *see* Disease, brain
- cerebral — *see also* Disease, brain
  - degenerative — *see* Degeneration, brain
- cerebrospinal G96.9
- cerebrovascular I67.9
  - acute I67.89
    - embolic I63.4- ☑
    - thrombotic I63.3- ☑
  - arteriosclerotic I67.2
  - hereditary NEC I67.858
  - specified NEC I67.89
- cervix (uteri) (noninflammatory) N88.9
  - inflammatory — *see* Cervicitis
  - specified NEC N88.8
- Chabert's A22.9
- Chandler's (osteochondritis dissecans, hip) — *see* Osteochondritis, dissecans, hip
- Charlouis — *see* Yaws
- Chediak-Steinbrinck (-Higashi) (congenital gigantism of peroxidase granules) E7Ø.33Ø
- chest J98.9
- Chiari's (hepatic vein thrombosis) I82.Ø
- Chicago B4Ø.9
- Chignon B36.8
- chigo, chigoe B88.1
- childhood granulomatous D71
- Chinese liver fluke B66.1
- chlamydial A74.9
  - specified NEC A74.89
- cholecystic K82.9
- choroid H31.9
  - specified NEC H31.8
- Christmas D67
- chronic bullous of childhood L12.2
- chylomicron retention E78.3
- ciliary body H21.9
  - specified NEC H21.89
- circulatory (system) NEC I99.8
  - newborn P29.9
  - syphilitic A52.ØØ
    - congenital A5Ø.54
- coagulation factor deficiency (congenital) — *see* Defect, coagulation
- coccidioidal — *see* Coccidioidomycosis
- cold
  - agglutinin or hemoglobinuria D59.12
    - paroxysmal D59.6
  - hemagglutinin (chronic) D59.12
- collagen NOS (nonvascular) (vascular) M35.9
  - specified NEC M35.89
- colon K63.9
  - functional K59.9
    - congenital Q43.2
  - ischemic — *see also* Ischemia, intestine, acute K55.Ø39
- colonic inflammatory bowel, unclassified (IBDU) K52.3
- combined system — *see* Degeneration, combined
- compressed air T7Ø.3 ☑
- Concato's (pericardial polyserositis) A19.9
  - nontubercular I31.1
  - pleural — *see* Pleurisy, with effusion
- conjunctiva H11.9
  - chlamydial A74.Ø
  - specified NEC H11.89
  - viral B3Ø.9
    - specified NEC B3Ø.8
- connective tissue, systemic (diffuse) M35.9
  - in (due to)
    - hypogammaglobulinemia D8Ø.1 *[M36.8]*
    - ochronosis E7Ø.29 *[M36.8]*
  - specified NEC M35.89
- Conor and Bruch's (boutonneuse fever) A77.1
- Cooper's — *see* Mastopathy, cystic
- Cori's (glycogenosis III) E74.Ø3
- corkhandler's or corkworker's J67.3
- cornea H18.9
  - specified NEC H18.89- ☑
- coronary (artery) — *see* Disease, heart, ischemic, atherosclerotic
  - congenital Q24.5
  - microvascular
    - with
      - angina pectoris I2Ø.81
      - myocardial infarction I21.B
    - acute I24.81
    - chronic I25.85
  - ostial, syphilitic (aortic) (mitral) (pulmonary) A52.Ø3
- corpus cavernosum N48.9
  - specified NEC N48.89
- Cotugno's — *see* Sciatica
- COVID-19 UØ7.1
- coxsackie (virus) NEC B34.1
- cranial nerve NOS G52.9
- Creutzfeldt-Jakob — *see* Creutzfeldt-Jakob disease or syndrome
- Crocq's (acrocyanosis) I73.89
- Crohn's — *see* Enteritis, regional
- Curschmann G71.11
- cystic
  - breast (chronic) — *see* Mastopathy, cystic
  - kidney, congenital Q61.9
  - liver, congenital Q44.6
  - lung J98.4
    - congenital Q33.Ø
- cytomegalic inclusion (generalized) B25.9
  - with pneumonia B25.Ø
  - congenital P35.1
- cytomegaloviral B25.9
  - specified NEC B25.8
- Czerny's (periodic hydrarthrosis of the knee) — *see* Effusion, joint, knee
- Daae (-Finsen) (epidemic pleurodynia) B33.Ø
- Danon E74.Ø5
- Darling's — *see* Histoplasmosis capsulati
- de Quervain's (tendon sheath) M65.4
  - thyroid (subacute granulomatous thyroiditis) EØ6.1
- Debove's (splenomegaly) R16.1
- deer fly — *see* Tularemia
- Degos' I77.89
- demyelinating, demyelinizating (nervous system) G37.9
  - multiple sclerosis G35
  - specified NEC G37.89
- dense deposit — *see also* NØØ-NØ7 with fourth character .6 NØ5.6
- deposition, hydroxyapatite — *see* Disease, hydroxyapatite deposition
- Devergie's (pityriasis rubra pilaris) L44.Ø
- Devic's G36.Ø
- diaphorase deficiency D74.Ø
- diaphragm J98.6
- diarrheal, infectious NEC AØ9
- digestive system K92.9
  - specified NEC K92.89
- disc, degenerative — *see* Degeneration, intervertebral disc
- discogenic — *see also* Displacement, intervertebral disc NEC
  - with myelopathy — *see* Disorder, disc, with, myelopathy
- diverticular — *see* Diverticula
- Dubois (thymus) A5Ø.59 *[E35]*
- Duchenne-Griesinger G71.Ø1
- Duchenne's
  - muscular dystrophy G71.Ø1
  - pseudohypertrophy, muscles G71.Ø1
- ductless glands E34.9
- Duhring's (dermatitis herpetiformis) L13.Ø
- duodenum K31.9
  - specified NEC K31.89
- Dupre's (meningism) R29.1
- Dupuytren's (muscle contracture) M72.Ø
- Durand-Nicholas-Favre (climatic bubo) A55
- Duroziez's (congenital mitral stenosis) Q23.2
- ear — *see* Disorder, ear
- Eberth's — *see* Fever, typhoid
- Ebola (virus) A98.4
- Ebstein's heart Q22.5
- Echinococcus — *see* Echinococcus
- echovirus NEC B34.1
- Eddowes' (brittle bones and blue sclera) Q78.Ø
- edentulous (alveolar) ridge KØ6.9
  - specified NEC KØ6.8
- Edsall's T67.2 ☑
- Eichstedt's (pityriasis versicolor) B36.Ø
- Eisenmenger's (irreversible) I27.83
- Ellis-van Creveld (chondroectodermal dysplasia) Q77.6
- end stage renal (ESRD) N18.6
  - due to hypertension I12.Ø
- endocrine glands or system NEC E34.9
- endomyocardial (eosinophilic) I42.3
- English (rickets) E55.Ø
- enteroviral, enterovirus NEC B34.1
  - central nervous system NEC A88.8
- epidemic B99.9
  - specified NEC B99.8
- epididymis N5Ø.9
- Erb (-Landouzy) G71.Ø2
- Erdheim-Chester (ECD) E88.89
- esophagus K22.9
  - functional K22.4
  - psychogenic F45.8
  - specified NEC K22.89
- Eulenburg's (congenital paramyotonia) G71.19
- eustachian tube — *see* Disorder, eustachian tube
- external
  - auditory canal — *see* Disorder, ear, external
  - ear — *see* Disorder, ear, external
- extrapyramidal G25.9
  - specified NEC G25.89
- eye H57.9
  - anterior chamber H21.9
  - inflammatory NEC H57.89
  - muscle (external) — *see* Strabismus
  - specified NEC H57.89
  - syphilitic — *see* Oculopathy, syphilitic
- eyeball H44.9
  - specified NEC H44.89
- eyelid — *see* Disorder, eyelid
  - specified NEC — *see* Disorder, eyelid, specified type NEC
- eyeworm of Africa B74.3
- facial nerve (seventh) G51.9
  - newborn (birth injury) P11.3
- Fahr (of brain) G23.8
- Fahr Volhard (of kidney) I12.- ☑
- fallopian tube (noninflammatory) N83.9
  - inflammatory — *see* Salpingo-oophoritis
  - specified NEC N83.8
- familial periodic paralysis G72.3
- Fanconi's (congenital pancytopenia) D61.Ø9
- fascia NEC — *see also* Disorder, muscle
  - inflammatory — *see* Myositis
  - specified NEC M62.89
- Fauchard's (periodontitis) — *see* Periodontitis
- Favre-Durand-Nicolas (climatic bubo) A55
- Fede's K14.Ø
- Feer's — *see* Poisoning, mercury
- female pelvic inflammatory — *see also* Disease, pelvis, inflammatory N73.9
  - syphilitic (secondary) A51.42
  - tuberculous A18.17
- Fernels' (aortic aneurysm) I71.9
- fibrocaseous of lung — *see* Tuberculosis, pulmonary
- fibrocystic — *see* Fibrocystic disease
- Fiedler's (leptospiral jaundice) A27.Ø
- fifth BØ8.3
- file-cutter's — *see* Poisoning, lead
- fish-skin Q8Ø.9
  - acquired L85.Ø
- Flajani (-Basedow) (exophthalmic goiter) — *see* Hyperthyroidism, with, goiter (diffuse)
- flax-dresser's J66.1
- fluke — *see* Infestation, fluke
- foot and mouth BØ8.8
- foot process NØ4.9
- Forbes' (glycogenosis III) E74.Ø3
- Fordyce-Fox (apocrine miliaria) L75.2
- Fordyce's (ectopic sebaceous glands) (mouth) Q38.6
- Forestier's (rhizomelic pseudopolyarthritis) M35.3
  - meaning ankylosing hyperostosis — *see* Hyperostosis, ankylosing
- Fothergill's
  - neuralgia — *see* Neuralgia, trigeminal
  - scarlatina anginosa A38.9
- Fournier (gangrene) N49.3
  - female N76.82
  - vagina and vulva N76.82
- fourth BØ8.8
- Fox (-Fordyce) (apocrine miliaria) L75.2
- Francis' — *see* Tularemia
- Franklin C88.2

- **Disease, diseased** — *continued*
  - hemoglobin or Hb — *continued*
    - SE D57.8- ☑
    - spherocytosis D58.0
    - unstable, hemolytic D58.2
  - hemolytic (newborn) P55.9
    - autoimmune D59.10
      - cold type (primary) (secondary) (symptomatic) D59.12
      - mixed type (primary) (secondary) (symptomatic) D59.13
      - warm type (primary) (secondary) (symptomatic) D59.11
    - drug-induced D59.0
    - due to or with
      - incompatibility
        - ABO (blood group) P55.1
        - blood (group) (Duffy) (K) (Kell) (Kidd) (Lewis) (M) (S) NEC P55.8
        - Rh (blood group) (factor) P55.0
      - Rh negative mother P55.0
    - specified type NEC P55.8
    - unstable hemoglobin D58.2
  - hemorrhagic D69.9
    - newborn P53
  - Henoch (-Schonlein) (purpura nervosa) D69.0
  - hepatic — *see* Disease, liver
  - hepatolenticular E83.01
  - heredodegenerative NEC
    - spinal cord G95.89
  - herpesviral, disseminated B00.7
  - Hers' (glycogenosis VI) E74.09
  - Herter (-Gee) (-Heubner) (nontropical sprue) K90.0
  - Heubner-Herter (nontropical sprue) K90.0
  - high fetal gene or hemoglobin thalassemia D56.9
  - Hildenbrand's — *see* Typhus
  - hip (joint) M25.9
    - congenital Q65.89
    - suppurative M00.9
    - tuberculous A18.02
  - His (-Werner) (trench fever) A79.0
  - Hodgson's — *see also* Aneurysm, aorta, thorax I71.20
    - ruptured — *see also* Aneurysm, aorta, thorax, ruptured I71.10
  - Holla — *see* Spherocytosis
  - hookworm B76.9
    - specified NEC B76.8
  - host-versus-graft D89.813
    - acute D89.810
    - acute on chronic D89.812
    - chronic D89.811
  - human immunodeficiency virus (HIV) B20
  - Huntington's G10
    - with dementia — *see also* Dementia, in, diseases specified elsewhere G10 *[F02.80]*
  - Hunt's (herpetic geniculate ganglionitis) (neuralgia) B02.21
    - dyssynergia cerebellaris myoclonica G11.19
  - Hutchinson's (cheiropompholyx) — *see* Hutchinson's disease
  - hyaline (diffuse) (generalized)
    - membrane (lung) (newborn) P22.0
      - adult J80
  - hydatid — *see* Echinococcus
  - hydroxyapatite deposition M11.00
    - ankle M11.07- ☑
    - elbow M11.02- ☑
    - foot joint M11.07- ☑
    - hand joint M11.04- ☑
    - hip M11.05- ☑
    - knee M11.06- ☑
    - multiple site M11.09
    - shoulder M11.01- ☑
    - vertebra M11.08
    - wrist M11.03- ☑
  - hyperkinetic — *see* Hyperkinesia
  - hypertensive — *see* Hypertension
  - hypophysis E23.7
  - Iceland G93.39
  - I-cell E77.0
  - IgG4-related D89.84
  - immune D89.9
  - immunoglobulin G4-related D89.84
  - immunoproliferative (malignant) C88.9
    - small intestinal C88.3
    - specified NEC C88.8
  - inclusion B25.9
    - salivary gland B25.9

- **Disease, diseased** — *continued*
  - infectious, infective B99.9
    - congenital P37.9
      - specified NEC P37.8
      - viral P35.9
        - specified type NEC P35.8
    - specified NEC B99.8
  - inflammatory
    - penis N48.29
      - abscess N48.21
      - cellulitis N48.22
    - prepuce N47.7
      - balanoposthitis N47.6
    - tubo-ovarian — *see* Salpingo-oophoritis
  - intervertebral disc — *see also* Disorder, disc
    - with myelopathy — *see* Disorder, disc, with, myelopathy
    - cervical, cervicothoracic — *see* Disorder, disc, cervical
      - with
        - myelopathy — *see* Disorder, disc, cervical, with myelopathy
        - neuritis, radiculitis or radiculopathy — *see* Disorder, disc, cervical, with neuritis
        - specified NEC — *see* Disorder, disc, cervical, specified type NEC
    - lumbar (with)
      - myelopathy M51.06
      - neuritis, radiculitis, radiculopathy or sciatica M51.16
      - specified NEC M51.86
    - lumbosacral (with)
      - neuritis, radiculitis, radiculopathy or sciatica M51.17
      - specified NEC M51.87
    - specified NEC — *see* Disorder, disc, specified NEC
    - thoracic (with)
      - myelopathy M51.04
      - neuritis, radiculitis or radiculopathy M51.14
      - specified NEC M51.84
    - thoracolumbar (with)
      - myelopathy M51.05
      - neuritis, radiculitis or radiculopathy M51.15
      - specified NEC M51.85
  - intestine K63.9
    - functional K59.9
      - psychogenic F45.8
      - specified NEC K59.89
    - organic K63.9
    - protozoal A07.9
    - specified NEC K63.89
  - iris H21.9
    - specified NEC H21.89
  - iron metabolism or storage E83.10
  - island (scrub typhus) A75.3
  - itai-itai — *see* Poisoning, cadmium
  - Jakob-Creutzfeldt — *see* Creutzfeldt-Jakob disease or syndrome
  - jaw M27.9
    - fibrocystic M27.49
    - specified NEC M27.8
  - jigger B88.1
  - joint — *see also* Disorder, joint
    - Charcot's — *see* Arthropathy, neuropathic (Charcot)
    - degenerative — *see* Osteoarthritis
      - multiple M15.9
      - spine — *see* Spondylosis
    - facet joint — *see also* Spondylosis M47.819
    - hypertrophic — *see* Osteoarthritis
    - sacroiliac M53.3
    - specified NEC — *see* Disorder, joint, specified type NEC
    - spine NEC — *see* Dorsopathy
    - suppurative — *see* Arthritis, pyogenic or pyemic
  - Jourdain's (acute gingivitis) K05.00
    - nonplaque induced K05.01
    - plaque induced K05.00
  - Kaschin-Beck (endemic polyarthritis) M12.10
    - ankle M12.17- ☑
    - elbow M12.12- ☑
    - foot joint M12.17- ☑
    - hand joint M12.14- ☑
    - hip M12.15- ☑
    - knee M12.16- ☑
    - multiple site M12.19
    - shoulder M12.11- ☑
    - vertebra M12.18
    - wrist M12.13- ☑

- **Disease, diseased** — *continued*
  - Katayama B65.2
  - Kedani (scrub typhus) A75.3
  - Keshan E59
  - kidney (functional) (pelvis) N28.9
    - chronic N18.9
      - hypertensive — *see* Hypertension, kidney
      - stage 1 N18.1
      - stage 2 (mild) N18.2
      - stage 3 (moderate) N18.30
      - stage 3a N18.31
      - stage 3b N18.32
      - stage 4 (severe) N18.4
      - stage 5 N18.5
    - complicating pregnancy — *see* Pregnancy, complicated by, renal disease
    - cystic (congenital) Q61.9
    - fibrocystic (congenital) Q61.8
    - hypertensive — *see* Hypertension, kidney
    - in (due to)
      - schistosomiasis (bilharziasis) B65.9 *[N29]*
    - multicystic Q61.4
    - polycystic Q61.3
      - adult type Q61.2
      - childhood type NEC Q61.19
        - collecting duct dilatation Q61.11
  - Kimmelstiel (-Wilson) (intercapillary polycystic (congenital) glomerulosclerosis) — *see* E08-E13 with .21
  - Kinnier Wilson's (hepatolenticular degeneration) E83.01
  - kissing — *see* Mononucleosis, infectious
  - Klebs' — *see also* Glomerulonephritis N05- ☑
  - Klippel-Feil (brevicollis) Q76.1
  - Kohler-Pellegrini-Stieda (calcification, knee joint) — *see* Bursitis, tibial collateral
  - Kok Q89.8
  - Konig's (osteochondritis dissecans) — *see* Osteochondritis, dissecans
  - Korsakoff's (nonalcoholic) F04
    - alcoholic F10.96
      - with dependence F10.26
  - Kostmann's (infantile genetic agranulocytosis) D70.0
  - kuru A81.81
  - Kyasanur Forest A98.2
  - labyrinth, ear — *see* Disorder, ear, inner
  - lacrimal system — *see* Disorder, lacrimal system
  - Lafora body — *see also* Epilepsy, progressive, Lafora G40.C09
  - Lancereaux-Mathieu (leptospiral jaundice) A27.0
  - Landry's G61.0
  - Larrey-Weil (leptospiral jaundice) A27.0
  - larynx J38.7
  - legionnaires' A48.1
    - nonpneumonic A48.2
  - Lenegre's I44.2
  - lens H27.9
    - specified NEC H27.8
  - Lev's (acquired complete heart block) I44.2
  - Lewy body (dementia) — *see also* Dementia, in, diseases specified elsewhere G31.83 *[F02.80]*
    - with behavioral disturbance — *see also* Dementia, in, diseases specified elsewhere G31.83 *[F02.81-]* ☑
  - Lichtheim's (subacute combined sclerosis with pernicious anemia) D51.0
  - Lightwood's (renal tubular acidosis) N25.89
  - Lignac's (cystinosis) E72.04
  - lip K13.0
  - lipid-storage E75.6
    - specified NEC E75.5
  - Lipschutz's N76.6
  - liver (chronic) (organic) K76.9
    - alcoholic (chronic) K70.9
      - acute — *see* Disease, liver, alcoholic, hepatitis
      - cirrhosis K70.30
        - with ascites K70.31
      - failure K70.40
        - with coma K70.41
      - fatty liver K70.0
      - fibrosis K70.2
      - hepatitis K70.10
        - with ascites K70.11
      - sclerosis K70.2
    - cystic, congenital Q44.6
    - drug-induced (idiosyncratic) (toxic) (predictable) (unpredictable) — *see* Disease, liver, toxic
    - end stage K72.1- ☑
      - due to hepatitis — *see* Hepatitis
      - with coma K72.11

- **Disease, diseased** — *continued*
  - liver — *continued*
    - fatty, nonalcoholic (NAFLD) K76.Ø
      - alcoholic K7Ø.Ø
    - fibrocystic (congenital) Q44.6
    - fluke
      - Chinese B66.1
      - oriental B66.1
      - sheep B66.3
    - gestational alloimmune (GALD) P78.84
    - glycogen storage E74.Ø9 *[K77]*
    - in (due to)
      - schistosomiasis (bilharziasis) B65.9 *[K77]*
    - inflammatory K75.9
      - alcoholic K7Ø.1 ☑
      - specified NEC K75.89
    - polycystic (congenital) Q44.6
    - toxic K71.9
      - with
        - cholestasis K71.Ø
        - cirrhosis (liver) K71.7
        - fibrosis (liver) K71.7
        - focal nodular hyperplasia K71.8
        - hepatic granuloma K71.8
        - hepatic necrosis K71.1Ø
          - with coma K71.11
        - hepatitis NEC K71.6
          - acute K71.2
          - chronic
            - active K71.5Ø
              - with ascites K71.51
            - lobular K71.4
            - persistent K71.3
          - lupoid K71.5Ø
            - with ascites K71.51
        - peliosis hepatis K71.8
        - veno-occlusive disease (VOD) of liver K71.8
    - veno-occlusive K76.5
  - Lobo's (keloid blastomycosis) B48.Ø
  - Lobstein's (brittle bones and blue sclera) Q78.Ø
  - Ludwig's (submaxillary cellulitis) K12.2
  - lumbosacral region M53.87
  - lung J98.4
    - black J6Ø
    - congenital Q33.9
    - cystic J98.4
      - congenital Q33.Ø
    - dabbing (related) UØ7.Ø
    - electronic cigarette (related) UØ7.Ø
    - fibroid (chronic) — *see* Fibrosis, lung
    - fluke B66.4
      - oriental B66.4
    - in
      - amyloidosis E85.4 *[J99]*
      - sarcoidosis D86.Ø
      - Sjogren's syndrome M35.Ø2
      - systemic
        - lupus erythematosus M32.13
        - sclerosis M34.81
    - interstitial J84.9
      - with progressive fibrotic phenotype, in diseases classified elsewhere J84.17Ø
      - drug-induced — *see* Disorder, lung, interstitial, drug-induced
      - of childhood, specified NEC J84.848
        - drug-induced — *see* Disorder, lung, interstitial, drug-induced
      - respiratory bronchiolitis J84.115
      - specified NEC J84.89
    - obstructive (chronic) J44.9
      - with
        - acute
          - bronchitis J44.Ø
          - exacerbation NEC J44.1
          - lower respiratory infection J44.Ø
        - alveolitis, allergic J67.9
        - asthma J44.9
        - bronchiectasis J47.9
          - with
            - exacerbation (acute) J47.1
            - lower respiratory infection J47.Ø
        - bronchitis J44.89
          - with
            - exacerbation (acute) J44.1
            - lower respiratory infection J44.Ø
        - emphysema J43.9
        - hypersensitivity pneumonitis J67.9
      - decompensated J44.1

- **Disease, diseased** — *continued*
  - lung — *continued*
    - obstructive — *continued*
      - decompensated — *continued*
        - with
          - exacerbation (acute) J44.1
    - polycystic J98.4
      - congenital Q33.Ø
    - rheumatoid (diffuse) (interstitial) — *see* Rheumatoid, lung
    - vaping (associated) (device) (product) (use) UØ7.Ø
  - Lutembacher's (atrial septal defect with mitral stenosis) Q21.19
  - Lyme A69.2Ø
  - lymphatic (gland) (system) (channel) (vessel) I89.9
  - lymphoproliferative D47.9
    - specified NEC D47.Z9 (*following* D47.4)
    - T-gamma D47.Z9 (*following* D47.4)
    - X-linked D82.3
  - Magitot's M27.2
  - malarial — *see* Malaria
  - malignant — *see also* Neoplasm, malignant, by site
  - Manson's B65.1
  - maple bark J67.6
  - maple-syrup-urine E71.Ø
  - Marburg (virus) A98.3
  - Marion's (bladder neck obstruction) N32.Ø
  - Marsh's (exophthalmic goiter) — *see* Hyperthyroidism, with, goiter (diffuse)
  - mastoid (process) — *see* Disorder, ear, middle
  - Mathieu's (leptospiral jaundice) A27.Ø
  - Maxcy's A75.2
  - McArdle (-Schmid-Pearson) (glycogenosis V) E74.Ø4
  - mediastinum J98.59
  - medullary center (idiopathic) (respiratory) G93.89
  - Meige's (chronic hereditary edema) Q82.Ø
  - meningococcal — *see* Infection, meningococcal
  - mental F99
    - organic FØ9
  - mesenchymal M35.9
  - mesenteric embolic — *see also* Ischemia, intestine, acute K55.Ø39
  - metabolic, metabolism E88.9
    - bilirubin E8Ø.7
  - metal-polisher's J62.8
  - metastatic — *see also* Neoplasm, secondary, by site C79.9
  - microvascular - code to condition
  - microvillus
    - atrophy Q43.8
    - inclusion (MVD) Q43.8
  - middle ear — *see* Disorder, ear, middle
  - Mikulicz' (dryness of mouth, absent or decreased lacrimation) K11.8
  - Milroy's (chronic hereditary edema) Q82.Ø
  - Minamata — *see* Poisoning, mercury
  - minicore G71.29
  - Minor's G95.19
  - Minot's (hemorrhagic disease, newborn) P53
  - Minot-von Willebrand-Jurgens (angiohemophilia) — *see* Disease, von Willebrand
  - Mitchell's (erythromelalgia) I73.81
  - mitral (valve) IØ5.9
    - nonrheumatic I34.9
  - mixed connective tissue M35.1
  - MOG antibody G37.81
  - moldy hay J67.Ø
  - Monge's T7Ø.29 ☑
  - Morgagni-Adams-Stokes (syncope with heart block) I45.9
  - Morgagni's (syndrome) (hyperostosis frontalis interna) M85.2
  - Morton's (with metatarsalgia) — *see* Lesion, nerve, plantar
  - Morvan's G6Ø.8
  - motor neuron (bulbar) (mixed type) (spinal) G12.2Ø
    - amyotrophic lateral sclerosis G12.21
    - familial G12.24
    - progressive bulbar palsy G12.22
    - specified NEC G12.29
  - moyamoya I67.5
  - mu heavy chain disease C88.2
  - multicore G71.29
  - multiminicore G71.29
  - muscle — *see also* Disorder, muscle
    - inflammatory — *see* Myositis
    - ocular (external) — *see* Strabismus

- **Disease, diseased** — *continued*
  - musculoskeletal system, soft tissue — *see also* Disorder, soft tissue
    - specified NEC — *see* Disorder, soft tissue, specified type NEC
  - mushroom workers' J67.5
  - mycotic B49
  - myelin oligodendrocyte glycoprotein antibody G37.81
  - myelodysplastic — *see also* Syndrome, myelodysplasia C94.6
  - myelodysplastic/myeloproliferative neoplasm, unclassifiable C94.6
  - myeloproliferative D47.1
    - chronic D47.1
    - not classified C94.6
    - specified NEC C94.6
    - unclassifiable C94.6
  - myocardium, myocardial — *see also* Degeneration, myocardial I51.5
    - primary (idiopathic) I42.9
  - myoneural G7Ø.9
  - Naegeli's D69.1
  - nails L6Ø.9
    - specified NEC L6Ø.8
  - Nairobi (sheep virus) A93.8
  - nasal J34.9
  - nemaline body G71.21
  - nerve — *see* Disorder, nerve
  - nervous system G98.8
    - autonomic G9Ø.9
    - central G96.9
      - specified NEC G96.89
    - congenital QØ7.9
    - parasympathetic G9Ø.9
    - specified NEC G98.8
    - sympathetic G9Ø.9
    - vegetative G9Ø.9
  - neuromuscular system G7Ø.9
  - Newcastle B3Ø.8
  - Nicolas (-Durand)-Favre (climatic bubo) A55
  - nipple N64.9
    - Paget's C5Ø.Ø1- ☑
      - female C5Ø.Ø1- ☑
      - male C5Ø.Ø2- ☑
  - Nishimoto (-Takeuchi) I67.5
  - nonarthropod-borne NOS (viral) B34.9
    - enterovirus NEC B34.1
  - nonautoimmune hemolytic D59.4
    - drug-induced D59.2
  - Nonne-Milroy-Meige (chronic hereditary edema) Q82.Ø
  - nose J34.9
  - nucleus pulposus — *see* Disorder, disc
  - nutritional E63.9
  - oast-house-urine E72.19
    - ocular
      - herpesviral BØØ.5Ø
      - zoster BØ2.3Ø
  - obliterative vascular I77.1
  - Ohara's — *see* Tularemia
  - Opitz's (congestive splenomegaly) D73.2
  - Oppenheim-Urbach (necrobiosis lipoidica diabeticorum) — *see* EØ8-E13 with .62Ø
  - optic nerve NEC — *see* Disorder, nerve, optic
  - orbit — *see* Disorder, orbit
  - organ
    - dabbing (related) UØ7.Ø
    - electronic cigarette (related) UØ7.Ø
    - vaping (associated) (device) (product) (use) UØ7.Ø
  - Oriental liver fluke B66.1
  - Oriental lung fluke B66.4
  - Ormond's N13.5
  - Oropouche virus A93.Ø
  - Osler-Rendu (familial hemorrhagic telangiectasia) I78.Ø
  - osteofibrocystic E21.Ø
  - Otto's M24.7
  - outer ear — *see* Disorder, ear, external
  - ovary (noninflammatory) N83.9
    - cystic N83.2Ø- ☑
    - inflammatory — *see* Salpingo-oophoritis
    - polycystic E28.2
    - specified NEC N83.8
  - Owren's (congenital) — *see* Defect, coagulation
  - p11Ød-activating mutation causing senescent T cells, lymphadenopathy, and immunodeficiency [PASLI] D81.82
  - pancreas K86.9
    - cystic K86.2
    - fibrocystic E84.9

Disease, diseased — *continued*
- pancreas — *continued*
  - specified NEC K86.89
- panvalvular IØ8.9
  - specified NEC IØ8.8
- parametrium (noninflammatory) N83.9
- parasitic B89
  - cerebral NEC B71.9 *[G94]*
  - intestinal NOS B82.9
  - mouth B37.Ø
  - skin NOS B88.9
  - specified type — *see* Infestation
  - tongue B37.Ø
- parathyroid (gland) E21.5
  - specified NEC E21.4
- Parkinson's G2Ø.A1
  - with dyskinesia
    - with
      - fluctuations G2Ø.B2
      - OFF episodes G2Ø.B2
    - without mention of
      - fluctuations G2Ø.B1
      - OFF episodes G2Ø.B1
  - without dyskinesia
    - with
      - fluctuations G2Ø.A2
      - OFF episodes G2Ø.A2
    - without mention of
      - fluctuations G2Ø.A1
      - OFF episodes G2Ø.A1
- parodontal KØ5.6
- Parrot's (syphilitic osteochondritis) A5Ø.Ø2
- Parry's (exophthalmic goiter) — *see* Hyperthyroidism, with, goiter (diffuse)
- Parson's (exophthalmic goiter) — *see* Hyperthyroidism, with, goiter (diffuse)
- Paxton's (white piedra) B36.2
- pearl-worker's — *see* Osteomyelitis, specified type NEC
- Pellegrini-Stieda (calcification, knee joint) — *see* Bursitis, tibial collateral
- pelvis, pelvic
  - female NOS N94.9
    - specified NEC N94.89
  - gonococcal (acute) (chronic) A54.24
  - inflammatory (female) N73.9
    - acute N73.Ø
    - chlamydial A56.11
    - chronic N73.1
    - specified NEC N73.8
    - syphilitic (secondary) A51.42
      - late A52.76
    - tuberculous A18.17
  - organ, female N94.9
  - peritoneum, female NEC N94.89
- penis N48.9
  - inflammatory N48.29
    - abscess N48.21
    - cellulitis N48.22
  - specified NEC N48.89
- periapical tissues NOS KØ4.9Ø
- periodontal KØ5.6
  - specified NEC KØ5.5
- periosteum — *see* Disorder, bone, specified type NEC
- peripheral
  - arterial I73.9
  - autonomic nervous system G9Ø.9
  - nerves — *see* Polyneuropathy
  - vascular NOS I73.9
    - in diabetes mellitus — *see* Diabetes, by type, with peripheral angiopathy
- peritoneum K66.9
  - pelvic, female NEC N94.89
  - specified NEC K66.8
- persistent mucosal (middle ear) H66.2Ø
  - left H66.22
    - with right H66.23
  - right H66.21
    - with left H66.23
- Petit's — *see* Hernia, abdomen, specified site NEC
- pharynx J39.2
  - specified NEC J39.2
- Phocas' — *see* Mastopathy, cystic
- photochromogenic (acid-fast bacilli) (pulmonary) A31.Ø
  - nonpulmonary A31.9
- Pick's — *see also* Dementia, in, diseases specified elsewhere G31.Ø1 *[FØ2.8Ø]*

Disease, diseased — *continued*
- Pick's — *see also* Dementia, in, diseases specified elsewhere — *continued*
  - with behavioral disturbance — *see also* Dementia, in, diseases specified elsewhere G31.Ø1 *[FØ2.81-]* ☑
  - brain G31.Ø1 *[FØ2.8Ø]*
    - with behavioral disturbance — *see also* Dementia, in, diseases specified elsewhere G31.Ø1 *[FØ2.81-]* ☑
  - of pericardium (pericardial pseudocirrhosis of liver) I31.1
- pigeon fancier's J67.2
- pineal gland E34.8
- pink — *see* Poisoning, mercury
- Pinkus' (lichen nitidus) L44.1
- pinworm B8Ø
- Piry virus A93.8
- pituitary (gland) E23.7
- pituitary-snuff-taker's J67.8
- pleura (cavity) J94.9
  - specified NEC J94.8
- pneumatic drill (hammer) T75.21 ☑
- Pollitzer's (hidradenitis suppurativa) L73.2
- polycystic
  - kidney or renal Q61.3
    - adult type Q61.2
    - childhood type NEC Q61.19
      - collecting duct dilatation Q61.11
  - liver or hepatic Q44.6
  - lung or pulmonary J98.4
    - congenital Q33.Ø
  - ovary, ovaries E28.2
  - spleen Q89.Ø9
- polyethylene T84.Ø5- ☑
- Pompe's (glycogenosis II) E74.Ø2
- Posadas-Wernicke B38.9
- Potain's (pulmonary edema) — *see* Edema, lung
- prepuce N47.8
  - inflammatory N47.7
    - balanoposthitis N47.6
- Pringle's (tuberous sclerosis) Q85.1
- prion, central nervous system A81.9
  - specified NEC A81.89
- prostate N42.9
  - specified NEC N42.89
- protozoal B64
  - acanthamebiasis — *see* Acanthamebiasis
  - African trypanosomiasis — *see* African trypanosomiasis
  - babesiosis — *see also* Babesiosis B6Ø.ØØ
  - Chagas disease — *see* Chagas disease
  - intestine, intestinal AØ7.9
  - leishmaniasis — *see* Leishmaniasis
  - malaria — *see* Malaria
  - naegleriasis B6Ø.2
  - pneumocystosis B59
  - specified organism NEC B6Ø.8
  - toxoplasmosis — *see* Toxoplasmosis
- pseudo-Hurler's E77.Ø
- psychiatric F99
- psychotic — *see* Psychosis
- Puente's (simple glandular cheilitis) K13.Ø
- puerperal — *see also* Puerperal O9Ø.89
- pulmonary — *see also* Disease, lung
  - artery I28.9
  - chronic obstructive J44.9
    - with
      - acute bronchitis J44.Ø
      - exacerbation (acute) J44.1
      - lower respiratory infection (acute) J44.Ø
    - decompensated J44.1
      - with
        - exacerbation (acute) J44.1
  - heart I27.9
    - specified NEC I27.89
  - hypertensive (vascular) — *see also* Hypertension, pulmonary I27.2Ø
    - NEC I27.2 ☑
    - primary (idiopathic) I27.Ø
  - valve I37.9
    - rheumatic IØ9.89
- pulp (dental) NOS KØ4.9Ø
- pulseless M31.4
- Putnam's (subacute combined sclerosis with pernicious anemia) D51.Ø
- Pyle (-Cohn) (metaphyseal dysplasia) Q78.5
- ragpicker's or ragsorter's A22.1

Disease, diseased — *continued*
- Raynaud's — *see* Raynaud's disease
- reactive airway — *see* Asthma
- Reclus' (cystic) — *see* Mastopathy, cystic
- rectum K62.9
  - specified NEC K62.89
- Refsum's (heredopathia atactica polyneuritiformis) G6Ø.1
- renal (functional) (pelvis) — *see also* Disease, kidney N28.9
  - with
    - edema — *see* Nephrosis
    - glomerular lesion — *see* Glomerulonephritis
      - with edema — *see* Nephrosis
    - interstitial nephritis N12
  - acute N28.9
  - chronic — *see also* Disease, kidney, chronic N18.9
  - cystic, congenital Q61.9
  - diabetic — *see* EØ8-E13 with .22
  - end-stage (failure) N18.6
    - due to hypertension I12.Ø
  - fibrocystic (congenital) Q61.8
  - hypertensive — *see* Hypertension, kidney
  - lupus M32.14
  - phosphate-losing (tubular) N25.Ø
  - polycystic (congenital) Q61.3
    - adult type Q61.2
    - childhood type NEC Q61.19
      - collecting duct dilatation Q61.11
  - rapidly progressive NØ1.9
  - subacute NØ1.9
- Rendu-Osler-Weber (familial hemorrhagic telangiectasia) I78.Ø
- renovascular (arteriosclerotic) — *see* Hypertension, kidney
- respiratory (tract) J98.9
  - acute or subacute NOS JØ6.9
    - due to
      - chemicals, gases, fumes or vapors (inhalation) J68.3
      - external agent J7Ø.9
        - specified NEC J7Ø.8
      - radiation J7Ø.Ø
      - smoke inhalation J7Ø.5
    - noninfectious J39.8
  - chronic NOS J98.9
    - due to
      - chemicals, gases, fumes or vapors J68.4
      - external agent J7Ø.9
        - specified NEC J7Ø.8
      - radiation J7Ø.1
    - newborn P27.9
      - specified NEC P27.8
  - due to
    - chemicals, gases, fumes or vapors J68.9
      - acute or subacute NEC J68.3
      - chronic J68.4
    - external agent J7Ø.9
      - specified NEC J7Ø.8
  - newborn P28.9
    - specified type NEC P28.89
  - upper J39.9
    - acute or subacute JØ6.9
    - noninfectious NEC J39.8
    - specified NEC J39.8
    - streptococcal JØ6.9
- retina, retinal H35.9
  - Batten's or Batten-Mayou E75.4 *[H36.89]*
  - specified NEC H35.89
- rheumatoid — *see* Arthritis, rheumatoid
- rickettsial NOS A79.9
  - specified type NEC A79.89
- Riga (-Fede) (cachectic aphthae) K14.Ø
- Riggs' (compound periodontitis) — *see* Periodontitis
- Ritter's LØØ
- Rivalta's (cervicofacial actinomycosis) A42.2
- Robles' (onchocerciasis) B73.Ø1
- rod body G71.21
- Roger's (congenital interventricular septal defect) Q21.Ø
- Rosenthal's (factor XI deficiency) D68.1
- Ross River B33.1
- Rossbach's (hyperchlorhydria) K31.89
  - psychogenic F45.8
- Rotes Querol — *see* Hyperostosis, ankylosing
- Roth (-Bernhardt) — *see* Mononeuropathy, lower limb, meralgia paresthetica
- Runeberg's (progressive pernicious anemia) D51.Ø
- sacroiliac NEC M53.3

Index

Disease, diseased — Disease, diseased

- **Disease, diseased** — *continued*
  - salivary gland or duct K11.9
    - inclusion B25.9
    - specified NEC K11.8
    - virus B25.9
  - sandworm B76.9
  - Schimmelbusch's — *see* Mastopathy, cystic
  - Schmorl's — *see* Schmorl's disease or nodes
  - Schonlein (-Henoch) (purpura rheumatica) D69.Ø
  - Schottmuller's — *see* Fever, paratyphoid
  - Schultz's (agranulocytosis) — *see* Agranulocytosis
  - Schwalbe-Ziehen-Oppenheim G24.1
  - Schwartz-Jampel G71.13
  - sclera H15.9
    - specified NEC H15.89
  - scrofulous (tuberculous) A18.2
  - scrotum N5Ø.9
  - sebaceous glands L73.9
  - semilunar cartilage, cystic — *see also* Derangement, knee, meniscus, cystic
  - seminal vesicle N5Ø.9
  - serum NEC — *see also* Reaction, serum T8Ø.69 ☑
  - sexually transmitted A64
    - anogenital
      - herpesviral infection — *see* Herpes, anogenital
      - warts A63.Ø
    - chancroid A57
    - chlamydial infection — *see* Chlamydia
    - gonorrhea — *see* Gonorrhea
    - granuloma inguinale A58
    - specified organism NEC A63.8
    - syphilis — *see* Syphilis
    - trichomoniasis — *see* Trichomoniasis
  - Sezary C84.1- ☑
  - shimamushi (scrub typhus) A75.3
  - shipyard B3Ø.Ø
  - sickle-cell D57.1
    - with
      - acute chest syndrome D57.Ø1
      - cerebral vascular involvement D57.Ø3
      - crisis (painful) D57.ØØ
        - with
          - complication specified NEC D57.Ø9
          - dactylitis D57.Ø4
      - dactylitis D57.Ø4
      - pain (vaso-occlusive) D57.ØØ
      - priapism D57.Ø9
      - splenic sequestration D57.Ø2
    - elliptocytosis D57.8- ☑
    - Hb-C D57.2Ø
      - with
        - acute chest syndrome D57.211
        - cerebral vascular involvement D57.213
        - crisis D57.219
          - with
            - dactylitis D57.214
            - specified complication NEC D57.218
        - dactylitis D57.214
        - pain (vaso-occlusive) D57.219
        - priapism D57.218
        - splenic sequestration D57.212
      - without crisis D57.2Ø
    - Hb-SD D57.8Ø
      - with
        - acute chest syndrome D57.811
        - cerebral vascular involvement D57.813
        - crisis D57.819
          - with
            - complication specified NEC D57.818
            - dactylitis D57.814
        - dactylitis D57.814
        - pain (vaso-occlusive) D57.819
        - splenic sequestration D57.812
      - without crisis D57.8Ø
    - Hb-SE D57.8Ø
      - with
        - acute chest syndrome D57.811
        - cerebral vascular involvement D57.813
        - crisis D57.819
          - with
            - complication specified NEC D57.818
            - dactylitis D57.814
        - dactylitis D57.814
        - pain (vaso-occlusive) D57.819
        - splenic sequestration D57.812
      - without crisis D57.8Ø
    - specified NEC D57.8Ø

- **Disease, diseased** — *continued*
  - sickle-cell — *continued*
    - specified — *continued*
      - with
        - acute chest syndrome D57.811
        - cerebral vascular involvement D57.813
        - crisis D57.819
          - with
            - complication specified NEC D57.818
            - dactylitis D57.814
        - dactylitis D57.814
        - pain (vaso-occlusive) D57.819
        - splenic sequestration D57.812
      - without crisis D57.8Ø
    - spherocytosis D57.8Ø
      - with
        - acute chest syndrome D57.811
        - cerebral vascular involvement D57.813
        - crisis D57.819
          - with complication specified NEC D57.818
        - pain (vaso-occlusive) D57.819
        - splenic sequestration D57.812
      - without crisis D57.8Ø
    - thalassemia D57.4Ø
      - with
        - acute chest syndrome D57.411
          - with dactylitis D57.414
          - with specified complication NEC D57.418
        - cerebral vascular involvement D57.413
        - crisis (painful) D57.419
          - with specified complication NEC D57.418
        - dactylitis D57.414
        - pain (vaso-occlusive) D57.419
        - splenic sequestration D57.412
      - beta plus D57.44
        - with
          - acute chest syndrome D57.451
            - with dactylitis D57.454
          - cerebral vascular involvement D57.453
          - crisis D57.459
            - with specified complication NEC D57.458
          - dactylitis D57.454
          - pain (vaso-occlusive) D57.459
          - splenic sequestration D57.452
        - without crisis D57.44
      - beta zero D57.42
        - with
          - acute chest syndrome D57.431
            - with dactylitis D57.434
          - cerebral vascular involvement D57.433
          - crisis D57.439
            - with specified complication NEC D57.438
          - dactylitis D57.434
          - pain (vaso-occlusive) D57.439
          - splenic sequestration D57.432
        - without crisis D57.42
  - silo-filler's J68.8
    - bronchitis J68.Ø
    - pneumonitis J68.Ø
    - pulmonary edema J68.1
  - simian B BØØ.4
  - Simons' (progressive lipodystrophy) E88.1
  - sin nombre virus B33.4
  - sinus — *see* Sinusitis
  - Sirkari's B55.Ø
  - sixth BØ8.2Ø
    - due to human herpesvirus 6 BØ8.21
    - due to human herpesvirus 7 BØ8.22
  - skin L98.9
    - due to metabolic disorder NEC E88.9 *[L99]*
    - specified NEC L98.8
  - slim (HIV) B2Ø
  - small vessel I73.9
  - Sneddon-Wilkinson (subcorneal pustular dermatosis) L13.1
  - South African creeping B88.Ø
  - spinal (cord) G95.9
    - congenital QØ6.9
    - specified NEC G95.89
  - spine — *see also* Spondylopathy
    - joint — *see* Dorsopathy
    - tuberculous A18.Ø1
  - spinocerebellar (hereditary) G11.9
    - specified NEC G11.8
  - spleen D73.9
    - amyloid E85.4 *[D77]*
    - organic D73.9

- **Disease, diseased** — *continued*
  - spleen — *continued*
    - polycystic Q89.Ø9
    - postinfectional D73.89
  - sponge-diver's — *see* Toxicity, venom, marine animal, sea anemone
  - Startle Q89.8
  - Steinert's G71.11
  - Sticker's (erythema infectiosum) BØ8.3
  - Stieda's (calcification, knee joint) — *see* Bursitis, tibial collateral
  - Stokes' (exophthalmic goiter) — *see* Hyperthyroidism, with, goiter (diffuse)
  - Stokes-Adams (syncope with heart block) I45.9
  - stomach K31.9
    - functional, psychogenic F45.8
    - specified NEC K31.89
  - stonemason's J62.8
  - storage
    - glycogen — *see* Disease, glycogen storage
    - mucopolysaccharide — *see* Mucopolysaccharidosis
  - striatopallidal system NEC G25.89
  - Stuart-Prower (congenital factor X deficiency) D68.2
  - Stuart's (congenital factor X deficiency) D68.2
  - subcutaneous tissue — *see* Disease, skin
  - supporting structures of teeth KØ8.9
    - specified NEC KØ8.89
  - suprarenal (capsule) (gland) E27.9
    - hyperfunction E27.Ø
    - specified NEC E27.8
  - sweat glands L74.9
    - specified NEC L74.8
  - Sweeley-Klionsky E75.21
  - Swift (-Feer) — *see* Poisoning, mercury
  - swimming-pool granuloma A31.1
  - Sylvest's (epidemic pleurodynia) B33.Ø
  - sympathetic nervous system G9Ø.9
  - synovium — *see* Disorder, synovium
  - syphilitic — *see* Syphilis
  - systemic tissue mast cell D47.Ø2
  - tanapox (virus) BØ8.71
  - Tangier E78.6
  - Tarral-Besnier (pityriasis rubra pilaris) L44.Ø
  - Tauri's E74.Ø9
  - tear duct — *see* Disorder, lacrimal system
  - tendon, tendinous — *see also* Disorder, tendon
    - nodular — *see* Trigger finger
  - terminal vessel I73.9
  - testis N5Ø.9
  - thalassemia Hb-S — *see* Disease, sickle-cell, thalassemia
  - Thaysen-Gee (nontropical sprue) K9Ø.Ø
  - Thomsen G71.12
  - throat J39.2
    - septic JØ2.Ø
  - thromboembolic — *see* Embolism
  - thymus (gland) E32.9
    - specified NEC E32.8
  - thyroid (gland) EØ7.9
    - heart — *see also* Hyperthyroidism EØ5.9Ø *[I43]*
      - with thyroid storm EØ5.91 *[I43]*
    - specified NEC EØ7.89
  - Tietze's M94.Ø
  - tongue K14.9
    - specified NEC K14.8
  - tonsils, tonsillar (and adenoids) J35.9
  - tooth, teeth KØ8.9
    - hard tissues KØ3.9
      - specified NEC KØ3.89
    - pulp NEC KØ4.99
    - specified NEC KØ8.89
  - Tourette's F95.2
  - trachea NEC J39.8
  - tricuspid IØ7.9
    - nonrheumatic I36.9
  - triglyceride-storage E75.5
  - trophoblastic — *see* Mole, hydatidiform
  - tsutsugamushi A75.3
  - tube (fallopian) (noninflammatory) N83.9
    - inflammatory — *see* Salpingitis
    - specified NEC N83.8
  - tuberculous NEC — *see* Tuberculosis
  - tubo-ovarian (noninflammatory) N83.9
    - inflammatory — *see* Salpingo-oophoritis
    - specified NEC N83.8
  - tubotympanic, chronic — *see* Otitis, media, suppurative, chronic, tubotympanic
  - tubulo-interstitial N15.9
    - specified NEC N15.8

- **Disease, diseased** — *continued*
  - tympanum — *see* Disorder, tympanic membrane
  - Uhl's Q24.8
  - Underwood's (sclerema neonatorum) P83.Ø
  - Unverricht (-Lundborg) — *see* Epilepsy, generalized, idiopathic
  - Urbach-Oppenheim (necrobiosis lipoidica diabeticorum) — *see* EØ8-E13 with .62Ø
  - ureter N28.9
    - in (due to)
      - schistosomiasis (bilharziasis) B65.Ø *[N29]*
  - urethra N36.9
    - specified NEC N36.8
  - urinary (tract) N39.9
    - bladder N32.9
      - specified NEC N32.89
    - specified NEC N39.8
  - uterus (noninflammatory) N85.9
    - infective — *see* Endometritis
    - inflammatory — *see* Endometritis
    - specified NEC N85.8
  - uveal tract (anterior) H21.9
    - posterior H31.9
  - vagabond's B85.1
  - vagina, vaginal (noninflammatory) N89.9
    - inflammatory NEC N76.89
    - specified NEC N89.8
  - valve, valvular I38
    - multiple IØ8.9
      - specified NEC IØ8.8
  - van Creveld-von Gierke (glycogenosis I) E74.Ø1
  - vas deferens N5Ø.9
  - vascular I99.9
    - arteriosclerotic — *see* Arteriosclerosis
    - ciliary body NEC — *see* Disorder, iris, vascular
    - hypertensive — *see* Hypertension
    - iris NEC — *see* Disorder, iris, vascular
    - obliterative I77.1
      - peripheral I73.9
    - occlusive I99.8
    - peripheral (occlusive) I73.9
      - in diabetes mellitus — *see* EØ8-E13 with .51
  - vasomotor I73.9
  - vasospastic I73.9
  - vein I87.9
  - venereal — *see also* Disease, sexually transmitted A64
    - chlamydial NEC A56.8
      - anus A56.3
      - genitourinary NOS A56.2
      - pharynx A56.4
      - rectum A56.3
    - fifth A55
    - sixth A55
    - specified nature or type NEC A63.8
  - vertebra, vertebral — *see also* Spondylopathy
    - disc — *see* Disorder, disc
  - vibration — *see* Vibration, adverse effects
  - viral, virus — *see also* Disease, by type of virus B34.9
    - arbovirus NOS A94
    - arthropod-borne NOS A94
    - congenital P35.9
      - specified NEC P35.8
    - Hanta (with renal manifestations) (Dobrava) (Puumala) (Seoul) A98.5
      - with pulmonary manifestations (Andes) (Bayou) (Bermejo) (Black Creek Canal) (Choclo) (Juquitiba) (Laguna negra) (Lechiguanas) (New York) (Oran) (Sin nombre) B33.4
    - Hantaan (Korean hemorrhagic fever) A98.5
    - human immunodeficiency (HIV) B2Ø
    - Kunjin A83.4
    - nonarthropod-borne NOS B34.9
    - Powassan A84.81
    - Rocio (encephalitis) A83.6
    - Sin nombre (Hantavirus) (cardio)-pulmonary syndrome) B33.4
    - Tahyna B33.8
    - vesicular stomatitis A93.8
  - vitreous H43.9
    - specified NEC H43.89
  - vocal cord J38.3
  - Volkmann's, acquired T79.6 ☑
  - von Eulenburg's (congenital paramyotonia) G71.19
  - von Gierke's (glycogenosis I) E74.Ø1
  - von Graefe's — *see* Strabismus, paralytic, ophthalmoplegia, progressive
  - von Willebrand (-Jurgens) (angiohemophilia) D68.ØØ
    - acquired D68.Ø4

- **Disease, diseased** — *continued*
  - von Willebrand — *continued*
    - platelet-type D68.Ø9
    - pseudo D68.Ø9
    - specified NEC D68.Ø9
    - type 1 D68.Ø1
    - type 1C D68.Ø1
    - type 2 D68.Ø29
      - type 2A D68.Ø2Ø
      - type 2B D68.Ø21
      - type 2M D68.Ø22
      - type 2N D68.Ø23
    - type 3 D68.Ø3
  - Vrolik's (osteogenesis imperfecta) Q78.Ø
  - vulva (noninflammatory) N9Ø.9
    - inflammatory NEC N76.89
    - specified NEC N9Ø.89
  - Wallgren's (obstruction of splenic vein with collateral circulation) I87.8
  - Wassilieff's (leptospiral jaundice) A27.Ø
  - wasting NEC E88.A
    - due to
      - malnutrition E43
        - with marasmus E41
      - underlying condition E88.A
      - with marasmus E41
  - Waterhouse-Friderichsen A39.1
  - Wegner's (syphilitic osteochondritis) A5Ø.Ø2
  - Weil's (leptospiral jaundice of lung) A27.Ø
  - Weir Mitchell's (erythromelalgia) I73.81
  - Werdnig-Hoffmann G12.Ø
  - Wermer's E31.21
  - Werner-His (trench fever) A79.Ø
  - Werner-Schultz (neutropenic splenomegaly) D73.81
  - Wernicke-Posadas B38.9
  - whipworm B79
  - white blood cells D72.9
    - specified NEC D72.89
  - white matter R9Ø.82
  - white-spot, meaning lichen sclerosus et atrophicus L9Ø.Ø
    - penis N48.Ø
    - vulva N9Ø.4
  - Wilkie's K55.1
  - Wilkinson-Sneddon (subcorneal pustular dermatosis) L13.1
  - Willis' — *see* Diabetes
  - Wilson's (hepatolenticular degeneration) E83.Ø1
  - woolsorter's A22.1
  - yaba monkey tumor BØ8.72
  - yaba pox (virus) BØ8.72
  - Zika virus A92.5
    - congenital P35.4
  - zoonotic, bacterial A28.9
    - specified type NEC A28.8
- **Disfigurement** (due to scar) L9Ø.5
- **Disgerminoma** — *see* Dysgerminoma
- **DISH** (diffuse idiopathic skeletal hyperostosis) — *see* Hyperostosis, ankylosing
- **Disinsertion, retina** — *see* Detachment, retina
- **Dislocatable hip, congenital** Q65.6
- **Dislocation** (articular)
  - with fracture — *see* Fracture
  - acromioclavicular (joint) S43.1Ø- ☑
    - with displacement
      - 1ØØ%-2ØØ% S43.12- ☑
      - more than 2ØØ% S43.13- ☑
    - inferior S43.14- ☑
    - posterior S43.15- ☑
  - ankle S93.Ø- ☑
  - astragalus — *see* Dislocation, ankle
  - atlantoaxial S13.121 ☑
  - atlantooccipital S13.111 ☑
  - atloidooccipital S13.111 ☑
  - breast bone S23.29 ☑
  - capsule, joint — *code by* site under Dislocation
  - carpal (bone) — *see* Dislocation, wrist
  - carpometacarpal (joint) NEC S63.Ø5- ☑
    - thumb S63.Ø4- ☑
  - cartilage (joint) — *code by* site under Dislocation
  - cervical spine (vertebra) — *see* Dislocation, vertebra, cervical
  - chronic — *see* Dislocation, recurrent
  - clavicle — *see* Dislocation, acromioclavicular joint
  - coccyx S33.2 ☑
  - congenital NEC Q68.8
  - coracoid — *see* Dislocation, shoulder
  - costal cartilage S23.29 ☑

- **Dislocation** — *continued*
  - costochondral S23.29 ☑
  - cricoarytenoid articulation S13.29 ☑
  - cricothyroid articulation S13.29 ☑
  - dorsal vertebra — *see* Dislocation, vertebra, thoracic
  - ear ossicle — *see* Discontinuity, ossicles, ear
  - elbow S53.1Ø- ☑
    - congenital Q68.8
    - pathological — *see* Dislocation, pathological NEC, elbow
    - radial head alone — *see* Dislocation, radial head
    - recurrent — *see* Dislocation, recurrent, elbow
    - traumatic S53.1Ø- ☑
      - anterior S53.11- ☑
      - lateral S53.14- ☑
      - medial S53.13- ☑
      - posterior S53.12- ☑
      - specified type NEC S53.19- ☑
  - eye, nontraumatic — *see* Luxation, globe
  - eyeball, nontraumatic — *see* Luxation, globe
  - femur
    - distal end — *see* Dislocation, knee
    - proximal end — *see* Dislocation, hip
  - fibula
    - distal end — *see* Dislocation, ankle
    - proximal end — *see* Dislocation, knee
  - finger S63.25- ☑
    - index S63.25- ☑
    - interphalangeal S63.27- ☑
      - distal S63.29- ☑
        - index S63.29- ☑
        - little S63.29- ☑
        - middle S63.29- ☑
        - ring S63.29- ☑
      - index S63.27- ☑
      - little S63.27- ☑
      - middle S63.27- ☑
      - proximal S63.28- ☑
        - index S63.28- ☑
        - little S63.28- ☑
        - middle S63.28- ☑
        - ring S63.28- ☑
      - ring S63.27- ☑
    - little S63.25- ☑
    - metacarpophalangeal S63.26- ☑
      - index S63.26- ☑
      - little S63.26- ☑
      - middle S63.26- ☑
      - ring S63.26- ☑
    - middle S63.25- ☑
    - recurrent — *see* Dislocation, recurrent, finger
    - ring S63.25- ☑
    - thumb — *see* Dislocation, thumb
  - foot S93.3Ø- ☑
    - recurrent — *see* Dislocation, recurrent, foot
    - specified site NEC S93.33- ☑
    - tarsal joint S93.31- ☑
    - tarsometatarsal joint S93.32- ☑
    - toe — *see* Dislocation, toe
  - fracture — *see* Fracture
  - glenohumeral (joint) — *see* Dislocation, shoulder
  - glenoid — *see* Dislocation, shoulder
  - habitual — *see* Dislocation, recurrent
  - hip S73.ØØ- ☑
    - anterior S73.Ø3- ☑
      - obturator S73.Ø2- ☑
    - central S73.Ø4- ☑
    - congenital (total) Q65.2
      - bilateral Q65.1
      - partial Q65.5
        - bilateral Q65.4
        - unilateral Q65.3- ☑
      - unilateral Q65.Ø- ☑
    - developmental M24.85- ☑
    - pathological — *see* Dislocation, pathological NEC, hip
    - posterior S73.Ø1- ☑
    - recurrent — *see* Dislocation, recurrent, hip
  - humerus, proximal end — *see* Dislocation, shoulder
  - incomplete — *see* Subluxation, by site
  - incus — *see* Discontinuity, ossicles, ear
  - infracoracoid — *see* Dislocation, shoulder
  - innominate (pubic junction) (sacral junction) S33.39 ☑
    - acetabulum — *see* Dislocation, hip
  - interphalangeal (joint(s))
    - finger S63.279 ☑

- **Dislocation** — *continued*
  - wrist — *continued*
    - distal radioulnar joint — *see* Dislocation, radioulnar (joint), distal
    - metacarpal bone, proximal — *see* Dislocation, metacarpal (bone), proximal end
    - midcarpal — *see* Dislocation, midcarpal (joint)
    - radiocarpal joint — *see* Dislocation, radiocarpal (joint)
    - recurrent — *see* Dislocation, recurrent, wrist
    - specified site NEC S63.09- ☑
    - ulna — *see* Dislocation, ulna, distal end
  - xiphoid cartilage S23.29 ☑
- **Disorder** (of) — *see also* Disease
  - acantholytic L11.9
    - specified NEC L11.8
  - acute
    - psychotic — *see* Psychosis, acute
    - stress F43.0
  - adjustment (grief) F43.20
    - with
      - anxiety F43.22
        - with depressed mood F43.23
      - conduct disturbance F43.24
        - with emotional disturbance F43.25
      - depressed mood F43.21
        - with anxiety F43.23
      - other specified symptom F43.29
  - adrenal (capsule) (gland) (medullary) E27.9
    - specified NEC E27.8
  - adrenogenital — *see also* Adrenogenital syndrome E25.9
    - drug-induced E25.8
    - iatrogenic E25.8
    - idiopathic E25.8
  - adult personality (and behavior) F69
    - specified NEC F68.8
  - affective (mood) — *see* Disorder, mood
  - aggressive, unsocialized F91.1
  - alcohol use
    - mild F10.10
      - with
        - alcohol intoxication F10.129
          - delirium F10.121
        - alcohol-induced
          - anxiety disorder F10.180
          - bipolar and related disorder F10.14
          - depressive disorder F10.14
          - psychotic disorder F10.159
          - sexual dysfunction F10.181
          - sleep disorder F10.182
      - in remission (early) (sustained) F10.11
    - moderate or severe F10.20
      - with
        - alcohol intoxication F10.229
          - delirium F10.221
        - alcohol-induced
          - anxiety disorder F10.280
          - bipolar and related disorder F10.24
          - depressive disorder F10.24
          - major neurocognitive disorder, amnestic-confabulatory type F10.26
          - major neurocognitive disorder, non-amnestic-confabulatory type F10.27
          - mild neurocognitive disorder F10.288
          - psychotic disorder F10.259
          - sexual dysfunction F10.281
          - sleep disorder F10.282
      - in remission (early) (sustained) F10.21
  - alcohol-related F10.99
    - with
      - amnestic disorder, persisting F10.96
      - anxiety disorder F10.980
      - dementia, persisting F10.97
      - intoxication F10.929
        - with delirium F10.921
        - uncomplicated F10.920
      - mood disorder F10.94
      - other specified F10.988
      - psychotic disorder F10.959
        - with
          - delusions F10.950
          - hallucinations F10.951
      - sexual dysfunction F10.981
      - sleep disorder F10.982
  - allergic — *see* Allergy
  - alveolar NEC J84.09

- **Disorder** — *continued*
  - amino-acid
    - cystathioninuria E72.19
    - cystinosis E72.04
    - cystinuria E72.01
    - glycinuria E72.09
    - homocystinuria E72.11
    - metabolism — *see* Disturbance, metabolism, amino-acid
      - specified NEC E72.89
    - neonatal, transitory P74.8
    - renal transport NEC E72.09
    - transport NEC E72.09
  - amnesic, amnestic
    - alcohol-induced F10.96
      - with dependence F10.26
    - due to (secondary to) general medical condition F04
    - psychoactive NEC-induced F19.96
      - with
        - abuse F19.16
        - dependence F19.26
    - sedative, hypnotic or anxiolytic-induced F13.96
      - with dependence F13.26
  - amphetamine (or other stimulant) use
    - mild
      - with
        - amphetamine, cocaine, or other stimulant intoxication
          - with perceptual disturbances F15.122
          - without perceptual disturbances F15.129
        - amphetamine (or other stimulant) -induced
          - anxiety disorder F15.180
          - bipolar and related disorder F15.14
          - depressive disorder F15.14
          - obsessive-compulsive and related disorder F15.188
          - psychotic disorder F15.159
          - sexual dysfunction F15.181
        - intoxication delirium F15.121
    - moderate or severe
      - with
        - amphetamine, cocaine, or other stimulant intoxication
          - with perceptual disturbances F15.222
          - without perceptual disturbances F15.229
        - amphetamine (or other stimulant) -induced
          - anxiety disorder F15.280
          - bipolar and related disorder F15.24
          - depressive disorder F15.24
          - obsessive-compulsive and related disorder F15.288
          - psychotic disorder F15.259
          - sexual dysfunction F15.281
        - intoxication delirium F15.221
  - amphetamine-type substance use
    - mild F15.10
      - in remission (early) (sustained) F15.11
    - moderate F15.20
      - in remission (early) (sustained) F15.21
    - severe F15.20
      - in remission (early) (sustained) F15.21
  - anaerobic glycolysis with anemia D55.29
  - anxiety F41.9
    - due to (secondary to)
      - alcohol F10.980
        - in
          - abuse F10.180
          - dependence F10.280
      - amphetamine F15.980
        - in
          - abuse F15.180
          - dependence F15.280
      - anxiolytic F13.980
        - in
          - abuse F13.180
          - dependence F13.280
      - caffeine F15.980
        - in
          - abuse F15.180
          - dependence F15.280
      - cannabis F12.980
        - in
          - abuse F12.180
          - dependence F12.280
      - cocaine F14.980
        - in
          - abuse F14.180
          - dependence F14.180
      - general medical condition F06.4

- **Disorder** — *continued*
  - anxiety — *continued*
    - due to — *continued*
      - hallucinogen F16.980
        - in
          - abuse F16.180
          - dependence F16.280
      - hypnotic F13.980
        - in
          - abuse F13.180
          - dependence F13.280
      - inhalant F18.980
        - in
          - abuse F18.180
          - dependence F18.280
      - phencyclidine F16.980
        - in
          - abuse F16.180
          - dependence F16.280
      - psychoactive substance NEC F19.980
        - in
          - abuse F19.180
          - dependence F19.280
      - sedative F13.980
        - in
          - abuse F13.180
          - dependence F13.280
      - volatile solvents F18.980
        - in
          - abuse F18.180
          - dependence F18.280
    - generalized F41.1
    - illness F45.21
    - mixed
      - with depression (mild) F41.8
      - specified NEC F41.3
    - organic F06.4
    - phobic F40.9
      - of childhood F40.8
    - specified NEC F41.8
  - aortic valve — *see* Endocarditis, aortic
  - aromatic amino-acid metabolism E70.9
    - specified NEC E70.89
  - arteriole NEC I77.89
  - artery NEC I77.89
  - articulation — *see* Disorder, joint
  - attachment (childhood)
    - disinhibited F94.2
    - reactive F94.1
  - attention-deficit hyperactivity (adolescent) (adult) (child) F90.9
    - combined
      - presentation F90.2
      - type F90.2
    - hyperactive
      - impulsive presentation F90.1
      - type F90.1
    - inattentive
      - presentation F90.0
      - type F90.0
    - specified type NEC F90.8
  - attention-deficit without hyperactivity (adolescent) (adult) (child) F98.8
  - auditory processing (central) H93.25
  - autism spectrum F84.0
  - autistic F84.0
  - autoimmune D89.89
  - autonomic nervous system G90.9
    - specified NEC G90.8
  - avoidant
    - child or adolescent F40.10
    - restrictive food intake F50.82
  - balance
    - acid-base E87.8
      - mixed E87.4
    - electrolyte E87.8
    - fluid NEC E87.8
  - behavioral (disruptive) — *see* Disorder, conduct
  - bereavement, persistent complex F43.81
  - beta-amino-acid metabolism E72.89
  - bile acid and cholesterol metabolism E78.70
    - Barth syndrome E78.71
    - other specified E78.79
    - Smith-Lemli-Opitz syndrome E78.72
  - bilirubin excretion E80.6
  - binge eating F50.81
  - binocular
    - movement H51.9

- **Disorder** — *continued*
  - binocular — *continued*
    - movement — *continued*
      - convergence
        - excess H51.12
        - insufficiency H51.11
      - internuclear ophthalmoplegia — *see* Ophthalmoplegia, internuclear
      - palsy of conjugate gaze H51.Ø
      - specified type NEC H51.8
    - vision NEC — *see* Disorder, vision, binocular
  - bipolar (I) seasonal) (type I) F31.9
    - and related due to a known physiological condition
      - with
        - manic features FØ6.33
        - manic- or hypomanic-like episodes FØ6.33
        - mixed features FØ6.34
    - current (or most recent) episode
      - depressed F31.9
        - with psychotic features F31.5
        - without psychotic features F31.3Ø
          - mild F31.31
          - moderate F31.32
          - severe (without psychotic features) F31.4
            - with psychotic features F31.5
      - hypomanic F31.Ø
      - manic F31.9
        - with psychotic features F31.2
        - without psychotic features F31.1Ø
          - mild F31.11
          - moderate F31.12
          - severe (without psychotic features) F31.13
            - with psychotic features F31.2
      - mixed F31.6Ø
        - mild F31.61
        - moderate F31.62
        - severe (without psychotic features) F31.63
          - with psychotic features F31.64
      - severe depression (without psychotic features) F31.4
        - with psychotic features F31.5
    - II (type 2) F31.81
    - in remission (currently) F31.7Ø
      - in full remission
        - most recent episode
          - depressed F31.76
          - hypomanic F31.72
          - manic F31.74
          - mixed F31.78
      - in partial remission
        - most recent episode
          - depressed F31.75
          - hypomanic F31.71
          - manic F31.73
          - mixed F31.77
    - organic FØ6.3Ø
    - single manic episode F3Ø.9
      - mild F3Ø.11
      - moderate F3Ø.12
      - severe (without psychotic symptoms) F3Ø.13
        - with psychotic symptoms F3Ø.2
    - specified NEC F31.89
  - bladder N32.9
    - functional NEC N31.9
    - in schistosomiasis B65.Ø *[N33]*
    - specified NEC N32.89
  - bleeding D68.9
  - blood D75.9
    - in congenital early syphilis A5Ø.Ø9 *[D77]*
  - body dysmorphic F45.22
  - bone M89.9
    - continuity M84.9
      - specified type NEC M84.8Ø
        - ankle M84.87- ☑
        - fibula M84.86- ☑
        - foot M84.87- ☑
        - hand M84.84- ☑
        - humerus M84.82- ☑
        - neck M84.88
        - pelvis M84.859
        - radius M84.83- ☑
        - rib M84.88
        - shoulder M84.81- ☑
        - skull M84.88
        - thigh M84.85- ☑
        - tibia M84.86- ☑
        - ulna M84.83- ☑

- **Disorder** — *continued*
  - bone — *continued*
    - continuity — *continued*
      - specified type — *continued*
        - vertebra M84.88
    - density and structure M85.9
      - cyst — *see also* Cyst, bone, specified type NEC
        - aneurysmal — *see* Cyst, bone, aneurysmal
        - solitary — *see* Cyst, bone, solitary
      - diffuse idiopathic skeletal hyperostosis — *see* Hyperostosis, ankylosing
      - fibrous dysplasia (monostotic) — *see* Dysplasia, fibrous, bone
      - fluorosis — *see* Fluorosis, skeletal
      - hyperostosis of skull M85.2
      - osteitis condensans — *see* Osteitis, condensans
      - specified type NEC M85.8- ☑
        - ankle M85.87- ☑
        - foot M85.87- ☑
        - forearm M85.83- ☑
        - hand M85.84- ☑
        - lower leg M85.86- ☑
        - multiple sites M85.89
        - neck M85.88
        - rib M85.88
        - shoulder M85.81- ☑
        - skull M85.88
        - thigh M85.85- ☑
        - upper arm M85.82- ☑
        - vertebra M85.88
    - development and growth NEC M89.2Ø
      - carpus M89.24- ☑
      - clavicle M89.21- ☑
      - femur M89.25- ☑
      - fibula M89.26- ☑
      - finger M89.24- ☑
      - humerus M89.22- ☑
      - ilium M89.28
      - ischium M89.28
      - metacarpus M89.24- ☑
      - metatarsus M89.27- ☑
      - multiple sites M89.29
      - neck M89.28
      - radius M89.23- ☑
      - rib M89.28
      - scapula M89.21- ☑
      - skull M89.28
      - tarsus M89.27- ☑
      - tibia M89.26- ☑
      - toe M89.27- ☑
      - ulna M89.23- ☑
      - vertebra M89.28
    - specified type NEC M89.8X- ☑
  - brachial plexus G54.Ø
  - branched-chain amino-acid metabolism E71.2
    - specified NEC E71.19
  - breast N64.9
    - agalactia — *see* Agalactia
    - associated with
      - lactation O92.7Ø
        - specified NEC O92.79
      - pregnancy O92.2Ø
        - specified NEC O92.29
      - puerperium O92.2Ø
        - specified NEC O92.29
    - cracked nipple — *see* Cracked nipple
    - galactorrhea — *see* Galactorrhea
    - hypogalactia O92.4
    - lactation disorder NEC O92.79
    - mastitis — *see* Mastitis
    - nipple infection — *see* Infection, nipple
    - retracted nipple — *see* Retraction, nipple
    - specified type NEC N64.89
  - Briquet's F45.Ø
  - bullous, in diseases classified elsewhere L14
  - caffeine use
    - mild
      - with
        - caffeine-induced
          - anxiety disorder F15.18Ø
          - sleep disorder F15.182
    - moderate or severe
      - with
        - caffeine-induced
          - anxiety disorder F15.28Ø
          - sleep disorder F15.282

- **Disorder** — *continued*
  - cannabis use
    - mild F12.1Ø
      - with
        - cannabis intoxication delirium F12.121
          - with perceptual disturbances F12.122
          - without perceptual disturbances F12.129
        - cannabis-induced
          - anxiety disorder F12.18Ø
          - psychotic disorder F12.159
          - sleep disorder F12.188
      - in remission (early) (sustained) F12.11
    - moderate or severe F12.2Ø
      - with
        - cannabis intoxication
          - with perceptual disturbances F12.222
          - without perceptual disturbances F12.229
        - cannabis-induced
          - anxiety disorder F12.28Ø
          - psychotic disorder F12.259
          - sleep disorder F12.288
        - delirium F12.221
      - in remission (early) (sustained) F12.21
  - carbohydrate
    - absorption, intestinal NEC E74.39
    - metabolism (congenital) E74.9
      - specified NEC E74.89
  - cardiac, functional I51.89
  - carnitine metabolism E71.4Ø
  - cartilage M94.9
    - articular NEC — *see* Derangement, joint, articular cartilage
      - chondrocalcinosis — *see* Chondrocalcinosis
    - specified type NEC M94.8X- ☑
      - articular — *see* Derangement, joint, articular cartilage
      - multiple sites M94.8XØ
  - catatonia (due to known physiological condition) (with another mental disorder) FØ6.1
  - catatonic
    - due to (secondary to) known physiological condition FØ6.1
    - organic FØ6.1
  - central auditory processing H93.25
  - cervical
    - region NEC M53.82
    - root (nerve) NEC G54.2
  - character NOS F6Ø.9
  - childhood disintegrative NEC F84.3
  - cholesterol and bile acid metabolism E78.7Ø
    - Barth syndrome E78.71
    - other specified E78.79
    - Smith-Lemli-Opitz syndrome E78.72
  - choroid H31.9
    - atrophy — *see* Atrophy, choroid
    - degeneration — *see* Degeneration, choroid
    - detachment — *see* Detachment, choroid
    - dystrophy — *see* Dystrophy, choroid
    - hemorrhage — *see* Hemorrhage, choroid
    - rupture — *see* Rupture, choroid
    - scar — *see* Scar, chorioretinal
    - solar retinopathy — *see* Retinopathy, solar
    - specified type NEC H31.8
  - ciliary body — *see* Disorder, iris
    - degeneration — *see* Degeneration, ciliary body
  - coagulation (factor) — *see also* Defect, coagulation D68.9
    - newborn, transient P61.6
  - cocaine use
    - mild F14.1Ø
      - with
        - amphetamine, cocaine, or other stimulant intoxication
          - with perceptual disturbances F14.122
          - without perceptual disturbances F14.129
        - cocaine intoxication delirium F14.121
        - cocaine-induced
          - anxiety disorder F14.18Ø
          - bipolar and related disorder F14.14
          - depressive disorder F14.14
          - obsessive-compulsive and related disorder F14.188
          - psychotic disorder F14.159
          - sexual dysfunction F14.181
          - sleep disorder F14.182
      - in remission (early) (sustained) F14.11
    - moderate or severe F14.2Ø

- **Disorder** — *continued*
  - cocaine use — *continued*
    - moderate or severe — *continued*
      - with
        - amphetamine, cocaine, or other stimulant intoxication
          - with perceptual disturbances F14.222
          - without perceptual disturbances F14.229
        - cocaine intoxication delirium F14.221
        - cocaine-induced
          - anxiety disorder F14.280
          - bipolar and related disorder F14.24
          - depressive disorder F14.24
          - obsessive-compulsive and related disorder F14.288
          - psychotic disorder F14.259
          - sexual dysfunction F14.281
          - sleep disorder F14.282
      - in remission (early) (sustained) F14.21
  - coccyx NEC M53.3
  - cognitive F09
    - due to (secondary to) general medical condition F09
    - persisting R41.89
      - due to
        - alcohol F10.97
          - with dependence F10.27
        - anxiolytics F13.97
          - with dependence F13.27
        - hypnotics F13.97
          - with dependence F13.27
        - sedatives F13.97
          - with dependence F13.27
        - specified substance NEC F19.97
          - with
            - abuse F19.17
            - dependence F19.27
  - communication F80.9
    - social pragmatic F80.82
  - conduct (childhood) F91.9
    - adjustment reaction — *see* Disorder, adjustment
    - adolescent onset type F91.2
    - childhood onset type F91.1
    - compulsive F63.9
    - confined to family context F91.0
    - depressive F91.8
    - group type F91.2
    - hyperkinetic — *see* Disorder, attention-deficit hyperactivity
    - oppositional defiance F91.3
    - socialized F91.2
    - solitary aggressive type F91.1
    - specified NEC F91.8
    - unsocialized (aggressive) F91.1
  - conduction, heart I45.9
  - congenital glycosylation (CDG) E74.89
  - conjunctiva H11.9
    - infection — *see* Conjunctivitis
  - connective tissue, localized L94.9
    - specified NEC L94.8
  - conversion (functional neurological symptom disorder)
    - with
      - abnormal movement F44.4
      - anesthesia or sensory loss F44.6
      - attacks or seizures F44.5
      - mixed symptoms F44.7
      - special sensory symptoms F44.6
      - speech symptoms F44.4
      - swallowing symptoms F44.4
      - weakness or paralysis F44.4
  - convulsive (secondary) — *see* Convulsions
  - cornea H18.9
    - deformity — *see* Deformity, cornea
    - degeneration — *see* Degeneration, cornea
    - deposits — *see* Deposit, cornea
    - due to contact lens H18.82- ☑
      - specified as edema — *see* Edema, cornea
    - edema — *see* Edema, cornea
    - keratitis — *see* Keratitis
    - keratoconjunctivitis — *see* Keratoconjunctivitis
    - membrane change — *see* Change, corneal membrane
    - neovascularization — *see* Neovascularization, cornea
    - scar — *see* Opacity, cornea
    - specified type NEC H18.89- ☑
    - ulcer — *see* Ulcer, cornea
  - corpus cavernosum N48.9
  - cranial nerve — *see* Disorder, nerve, cranial

- **Disorder** — *continued*
  - Cyclin-Dependent Kinase-Like 5 Deficiency (CDKL5) G40.42
  - cyclothymic F34.0
  - defiant oppositional F91.3
  - delusional (persistent) (systematized) F22
    - induced F24
  - depersonalization F48.1
  - depressive F32.A
    - due to known physiological condition
      - with
        - depressive features F06.31
        - major depressive-like episode F06.32
        - mixed features F06.34
    - major F32.9
      - with psychotic symptoms F32.3
      - in remission (full) F32.5
        - partial F32.4
      - recurrent F33.9
        - with psychotic features F33.3
      - single episode F32.9
        - mild F32.0
        - moderate F32.1
        - severe (without psychotic symptoms) F32.2
          - with psychotic symptoms F32.3
    - organic F06.31
    - persistent F34.1
    - recurrent F33.9
      - current episode
        - mild F33.0
        - moderate F33.1
        - severe (without psychotic symptoms) F33.2
          - with psychotic symptoms F33.3
      - in remission F33.40
        - full F33.42
        - partial F33.41
      - specified NEC F33.8
    - single episode — *see* Episode, depressive
    - specified NEC F32.89
  - developmental F89
    - arithmetical skills F81.2
    - coordination (motor) F82
    - expressive writing F81.81
    - language F80.9
      - expressive F80.1
      - mixed receptive and expressive F80.2
      - receptive type F80.2
      - specified NEC F80.89
    - learning F81.9
      - arithmetical F81.2
      - reading F81.0
    - mixed F88
    - motor coordination or function F82
    - pervasive F84.9
      - specified NEC F84.8
    - phonological F80.0
    - reading F81.0
    - scholastic skills — *see also* Disorder, learning
      - mixed F81.89
    - specified NEC F88
    - speech F80.9
      - articulation F80.0
      - specified NEC F80.89
    - written expression F81.81
  - diaphragm J98.6
  - digestive (system) K92.9
    - newborn P78.9
      - specified NEC P78.89
    - postprocedural — *see* Complication, gastrointestinal
    - psychogenic F45.8
  - disc (intervertebral) M51.9
    - with
      - myelopathy
        - cervical region M50.00
        - cervicothoracic region M50.03
        - high cervical region M50.01
        - lumbar region M51.06
        - mid-cervical region M50.020
        - sacrococcygeal region M53.3
        - thoracic region M51.04
        - thoracolumbar region M51.05
      - radiculopathy
        - cervical region M50.10
        - cervicothoracic region M50.13
        - high cervical region M50.11
        - lumbar region M51.16
        - lumbosacral region M51.17
        - mid-cervical region M50.120
        - sacrococcygeal region M53.3

- **Disorder** — *continued*
  - disc — *continued*
    - with — *continued*
      - radiculopathy — *continued*
        - thoracic region M51.14
        - thoracolumbar region M51.15
    - cervical M50.90
      - with
        - myelopathy M50.00
          - C2-C3 M50.01
          - C3-C4 M50.01
          - C4-C5 M50.021
          - C5-C6 M50.022
          - C6-C7 M50.023
          - C7-T1 M50.03
          - cervicothoracic region M50.03
          - high cervical region M50.01
          - mid-cervical region M50.020
        - neuritis, radiculitis or radiculopathy M50.10
          - C2-C3 M50.11
          - C3-C4 M50.11
          - C4-C5 M50.121
          - C5-C6 M50.122
          - C6-C7 M50.123
          - C7-T1 M50.13
          - cervicothoracic region M50.13
          - high cervical region M50.11
          - mid-cervical region M50.120
      - C2-C3 M50.91
      - C3-C4 M50.91
      - C4-C5 M50.921
      - C5-C6 M50.922
      - C6-C7 M50.923
      - C7-T1 M50.93
      - cervicothoracic region M50.93
      - degeneration M50.30
        - C2-C3 M50.31
        - C3-C4 M50.31
        - C4-C5 M50.321
        - C5-C6 M50.322
        - C6-C7 M50.323
        - C7-T1 M50.33
        - cervicothoracic region M50.33
        - high cervical region M50.31
        - mid-cervical region M50.320
      - displacement M50.20
        - C2-C3 M50.21
        - C3-C4 M50.21
        - C4-C5 M50.221
        - C5-C6 M50.222
        - C6-C7 M50.223
        - C7-T1 M50.23
        - cervicothoracic region M50.23
        - high cervical region M50.21
        - mid-cervical region M50.220
      - high cervical region M50.91
      - mid-cervical region M50.920
      - specified type NEC M50.80
        - C2-C3 M50.81
        - C3-C4 M50.81
        - C4-C5 M50.821
        - C5-C6 M50.822
        - C6-C7 M50.823
        - C7-T1 M50.83
        - cervicothoracic region M50.83
        - high cervical region M50.81
        - mid-cervical region M50.820
    - specified NEC
      - lumbar region M51.86
      - lumbosacral region M51.87
      - sacrococcygeal region M53.3
      - thoracic region M51.84
      - thoracolumbar region M51.85
  - disinhibited attachment (childhood) F94.2
  - disintegrative, childhood NEC F84.3
  - disruptive F91.9
    - mood dysregulation F34.81
    - specified NEC F91.8
  - disruptive behavior — *see* Disorder, conduct
  - dissocial personality F60.2
  - dissociative F44.9
    - affecting
      - motor function F44.4
        - and sensation F44.7
      - sensation F44.6
        - and motor function F44.7
    - brief reactive F43.0
    - due to (secondary to) general medical condition F06.8

Disorder — *continued*
- dissociative — *continued*
  - mixed F44.7
  - organic FØ6.8
  - other specified NEC F44.89
- double heterozygous sickling — *see* Disease, sickle-cell
- dream anxiety F51.5
- drug induced hemorrhagic D68.32
- drug related F19.99
  - abuse — *see* Abuse, drug
  - dependence — *see* Dependence, drug
- dysmorphic body F45.22
- dysthymic F34.1
- ear H93.9- ☑
  - bleeding — *see* Otorrhagia
  - deafness — *see* Deafness
  - degenerative H93.Ø9- ☑
  - discharge — *see* Otorrhea
  - external H61.9- ☑
    - auditory canal stenosis — *see* Stenosis, external ear canal
    - exostosis — *see* Exostosis, external ear canal
    - impacted cerumen — *see* Impaction, cerumen
    - otitis — *see* Otitis, externa
    - perichondritis — *see* Perichondritis, ear
    - pinna — *see* Disorder, pinna
    - specified type NEC H61.89- ☑
  - inner H83.9- ☑
    - vestibular dysfunction — *see* Disorder, vestibular function
  - middle H74.9- ☑
    - adhesive H74.1- ☑
    - ossicle — *see* Abnormal, ear ossicles
    - polyp — *see* Polyp, ear (middle)
    - specified NEC, in diseases classified elsewhere H75.8- ☑
  - postprocedural — *see* Complications, ear, procedure
  - specified NEC, in diseases classified elsewhere H94.8- ☑
- eating (adult) (psychogenic) F5Ø.9
  - anorexia — *see* Anorexia
  - binge F5Ø.81
  - bulimia F5Ø.2
  - child F98.29
    - pica F98.3
    - rumination disorder F98.21
  - pica F5Ø.89
    - childhood F98.3
  - specified NEC F5Ø.89
- electrolyte (balance) NEC E87.8
  - with
    - abortion — *see* Abortion by type complicated by specified condition NEC
    - ectopic pregnancy OØ8.5
    - molar pregnancy OØ8.5
  - acidosis (lactic) (metabolic) E87.2Ø
    - acute E87.21
    - chronic E87.22
    - respiratory E87.29
    - specified NEC E87.29
  - alkalosis (metabolic) (respiratory) E87.3
- elimination, transepidermal L87.9
  - specified NEC L87.8
- emotional (persistent) F34.9
  - of childhood F93.9
    - specified NEC F93.8
- endocrine E34.9
  - postprocedural E89.89
    - specified NEC E89.89
- erectile (male) (organic) — *see also* Dysfunction, sexual, male, erectile N52.9
  - nonorganic F52.21
- erythematous — *see* Erythema
- esophagus K22.9
  - functional K22.4
  - psychogenic F45.8
- eustachian tube H69.9- ☑
  - infection — *see* Salpingitis, eustachian
  - obstruction — *see* Obstruction, eustachian tube
  - patulous — *see* Patulous, eustachian tube
  - specified NEC H69.8- ☑
- exhibitionistic F65.2
- extrapyramidal G25.9
  - in deseases classified elsewhere — *see* category G26
  - specified type NEC G25.89
- eye H57.9

Disorder — *continued*
- eye — *continued*
  - postprocedural — *see* Complication, postprocedural, eye
- eyelid HØ2.9
  - cyst — *see* Cyst, eyelid
  - degenerative HØ2.7Ø
    - chloasma — *see* Chloasma, eyelid
    - madarosis — *see* Madarosis
    - specified type NEC HØ2.79
    - vitiligo — *see* Vitiligo, eyelid
    - xanthelasma — *see* Xanthelasma
  - dermatochalasis — *see* Dermatochalasis
  - edema — *see* Edema, eyelid
  - elephantiasis — *see* Elephantiasis, eyelid
  - foreign body, retained — *see* Foreign body, retained, eyelid
  - function HØ2.59
    - abnormal innervation syndrome — *see* Syndrome, abnormal innervation
    - blepharochalasis — *see* Blepharochalasis
    - blepharoclonus — *see* Blepharoclonus
    - blepharophimosis — *see* Blepharophimosis
    - blepharoptosis — *see* Blepharoptosis
    - lagophthalmos — *see* Lagophthalmos
    - lid retraction — *see* Retraction, lid
  - hypertrichosis — *see* Hypertrichosis, eyelid
  - specified type NEC HØ2.89
  - vascular HØ2.879
    - left HØ2.876
      - lower HØ2.875
      - upper HØ2.874
    - right HØ2.873
      - lower HØ2.872
      - upper HØ2.871
- factitious
  - by proxy F68.A
  - imposed on another F68.A
  - imposed on self F68.1Ø
    - with predominantly
      - psychological symptoms F68.11
        - with physical symptoms F68.13
      - physical symptoms F68.12
        - with psychological symptoms F68.13
- factor, coagulation — *see* Defect, coagulation
- fatty acid
  - metabolism E71.3Ø
    - specified NEC E71.39
  - oxidation
    - LCAD E71.31Ø
    - MCAD E71.311
    - SCAD E71.312
    - specified deficiency NEC E71.318
- feeding (infant or child) — *see also* Disorder, eating R63.3Ø
  - or eating disorder F5Ø.9
  - pediatric
    - acute R63.31
    - chronic R63.32
  - specified NEC F5Ø.9
- feigned (with obvious motivation) Z76.5
  - without obvious motivation — *see* Disorder, factitious
- female
  - hypoactive sexual desire F52.Ø
  - orgasmic F52.31
  - sexual interest/arousal F52.22
- fetishistic F65.Ø
- fibroblastic M72.9
  - specified NEC M72.8
- fluency
  - adult onset F98.5
  - childhood onset F8Ø.81
  - following
    - cerebral infarction I69.323
    - cerebrovascular disease I69.923
      - specified disease NEC I69.823
    - intracerebral hemorrhage I69.123
    - nontraumatic intracranial hemorrhage NEC I69.223
    - subarachnoid hemorrhage I69.Ø23
  - in conditions classified elsewhere R47.82
- fluid balance E87.8
- follicular (skin) L73.9
  - specified NEC L73.8
- frotteuristic F65.81
- fructose metabolism E74.1Ø
  - essential fructosuria E74.11

Disorder — *continued*
- fructose metabolism — *continued*
  - fructokinase deficiency E74.11
  - fructose-1, 6-diphosphatase deficiency E74.19
  - hereditary fructose intolerance E74.12
  - other specified E74.19
- functional polymorphonuclear neutrophils D71
- gallbladder, biliary tract and pancreas in diseases classified elsewhere K87
- gambling F63.Ø
- gamma aminobutyric acid (GABA) metabolism E72.81
- gamma-glutamyl cycle E72.89
- gastric (functional) K31.9
  - motility K3Ø
  - psychogenic F45.8
  - secretion K3Ø
- gastrointestinal (functional) NOS K92.9
  - newborn P78.9
  - psychogenic F45.8
- gender incongruence F64.9
  - in adolescents and adults F64.Ø
  - of childhood F64.2
- gender-identity or -role F64.9
  - childhood F64.2
  - effect on relationship F66
  - of adolescence or adulthood F64.Ø
    - nontranssexual F64.8
  - specified NEC F64.8
  - uncertainty F66
- genito-pelvic pain penetration F52.6
- genitourinary system
  - female N94.9
  - male N5Ø.9
  - psychogenic F45.8
- globe H44.9
  - degenerated condition H44.5Ø
    - absolute glaucoma H44.51- ☑
    - atrophy H44.52- ☑
    - leucocoria H44.53- ☑
  - degenerative H44.3Ø
    - chalcosis H44.31- ☑
    - myopia — *see also* Myopia, degenerative H44.2- ☑
    - siderosis H44.32- ☑
    - specified type NEC H44.39- ☑
  - endophthalmitis — *see* Endophthalmitis
  - foreign body, retained — *see* Foreign body, intraocular, old, retained
  - hemophthalmos — *see* Hemophthalmos
  - hypotony H44.4Ø
    - due to
      - ocular fistula H44.42- ☑
      - specified disorder NEC H44.43- ☑
    - flat anterior chamber H44.41- ☑
    - primary H44.44- ☑
  - luxation — *see* Luxation, globe
  - specified type NEC H44.89
- glomerular (in) NØ5.9
  - amyloidosis E85.4 *[NØ8]*
  - cryoglobulinemia D89.1 *[NØ8]*
  - disseminated intravascular coagulation D65 *[NØ8]*
  - Fabry's disease E75.21 *[NØ8]*
  - familial lecithin cholesterol acyltransferase deficiency E78.6 *[NØ8]*
  - Goodpasture's syndrome M31.Ø
  - hemolytic-uremic syndrome — *see* Syndrome, hemolytic-uremic
  - Henoch (-Schonlein) purpura D69.Ø *[NØ8]*
  - malariae malaria B52.Ø
  - microscopic polyangiitis M31.7 *[NØ8]*
  - multiple myeloma C9Ø.Ø- ☑ *[NØ8]*
  - mumps B26.83
  - schistosomiasis B65.9 *[NØ8]*
  - sepsis NEC A41.- ☑ *[NØ8]*
    - streptococcal A4Ø.- ☑ *[NØ8]*
  - sickle-cell disorders D57.- ☑ *[NØ8]*
  - strongyloidiasis B78.9 *[NØ8]*
  - subacute bacterial endocarditis I33.Ø *[NØ8]*
  - syphilis A52.75
  - systemic lupus erythematosus M32.14
  - thrombotic thrombocytopenic purpura M31.19 *[NØ8]*
  - Waldenstrom macroglobulinemia C88.Ø *[NØ8]*
  - Wegener's granulomatosis M31.31
- gluconeogenesis E74.4
- glucosaminoglycan metabolism — *see* Disorder, metabolism, glucosaminoglycan
- glucose transport E74.819

- **Disorder** — *continued*
  - male
    - erectile (organic) — *see also* Dysfunction, sexual, male, erectile N52.9
      - nonorganic F52.21
    - hypoactive sexual desire F52.0
    - orgasmic F52.32
  - manic F30.9
    - organic F06.33
  - mast cell activation — *see* Activation, mast cell
  - mastoid — *see also* Disorder, ear, middle
    - postprocedural — *see* Complications, ear, procedure
  - meninges, specified type NEC G96.198
  - meniscus — *see* Derangement, knee, meniscus
  - menopausal N95.9
    - specified NEC N95.8
  - menstrual N92.6
    - psychogenic F45.8
    - specified NEC N92.5
  - mental (or behavioral) (nonpsychotic) F99
    - due to (secondary to)
      - amphetamine
        - due to drug abuse — *see* Abuse, drug, stimulant
        - due to drug dependence — *see* Dependence, drug, stimulant
      - brain disease, damage and dysfunction F09
      - caffeine use
        - due to drug abuse — *see* Abuse, drug, stimulant
        - due to drug dependence — *see* Dependence, drug, stimulant
      - cannabis use
        - due to drug abuse — *see* Abuse, drug, cannabis
        - due to drug dependence — *see* Dependence, drug, cannabis
      - general medical condition F09
      - sedative or hypnotic use
        - due to drug abuse — *see* Abuse, drug, sedative
        - due to drug dependence — *see* Dependence, drug, sedative
      - tobacco (nicotine) use — *see* Dependence, drug, nicotine
    - following organic brain damage F07.9
      - frontal lobe syndrome F07.0
      - personality change F07.0
      - postconcussional syndrome F07.81
      - specified NEC F07.89
    - infancy, childhood or adolescence F98.9
    - neurotic — *see* Neurosis
    - organic or symptomatic F09
    - presenile, psychotic F03 ☑
    - problem NEC
    - psychoneurotic — *see* Neurosis
    - psychotic — *see* Psychosis
    - puerperal F53.0
    - senile, psychotic NEC F03 ☑
  - metabolic, amino acid, transitory, newborn P74.8
  - metabolism NOS E88.9
    - amino-acid E72.9
      - aromatic E70.9
        - albinism — *see* Albinism
        - histidine E70.40
          - histidinemia E70.41
          - other specified E70.49
        - hyperphenylalaninemia E70.1
          - classical phenylketonuria E70.0
        - other specified E70.89
        - tryptophan E70.5
        - tyrosine E70.20
          - hypertyrosinemia E70.21
          - other specified E70.29
      - branched chain E71.2
        - 3-methylglutaconic aciduria E71.111
        - hyperleucine-isoleucinemia E71.19
        - hypervalinemia E71.19
        - isovaleric acidemia E71.110
        - maple syrup urine disease E71.0
        - methylmalonic acidemia E71.120
        - organic aciduria NEC E71.118
        - other specified E71.19
        - proprionate NEC E71.128
        - proprionic acidemia E71.121
      - glycine E72.50
        - d-glycericacidemia E72.59
        - hyperhydroxyprolinemia E72.59

- **Disorder** — *continued*
  - metabolism — *continued*
    - amino-acid — *continued*
      - glycine — *continued*
        - hyperoxaluria R82.992
          - primary E72.53
        - hyperprolinemia E72.59
        - non-ketotic hyperglycinemia E72.51
        - other specified E72.59
        - sarcosinemia E72.59
        - trimethylaminuria E72.52
      - hydroxylysine E72.3
      - lysine E72.3
      - ornithine E72.4
      - other specified E72.89
        - beta-amino acid E72.89
        - gamma-glutamyl cycle E72.89
      - straight-chain E72.89
      - sulfur-bearing E72.10
        - homocystinuria E72.11
        - methylenetetrahydrofolate reductase deficiency E72.12
        - other specified E72.19
    - bile acid and cholesterol metabolism E78.70
    - bilirubin E80.7
      - specified NEC E80.6
    - calcium E83.50
      - hypercalcemia E83.52
      - hypocalcemia E83.51
      - other specified E83.59
    - carbohydrate E74.9
      - specified NEC E74.89
    - cholesterol and bile acid metabolism E78.70
    - congenital E88.9
    - copper E83.00
      - specified type NEC E83.09
      - Wilson's disease E83.01
    - cystinuria E72.01
    - fructose E74.10
    - galactose E74.20
    - glucosaminoglycan E76.9
      - mucopolysaccharidosis — *see* Mucopolysaccharidosis
      - specified NEC E76.8
    - glutamine E72.89
    - glycine E72.50
    - glycogen storage (hepatorenal) E74.09
    - glycoprotein E77.9
      - specified NEC E77.8
    - glycosaminoglycan E76.9
      - specified NEC E76.8
    - in labor and delivery O75.89
    - iron E83.10
    - isoleucine E71.19
    - leucine E71.19
    - lipoid E78.9
    - lipoprotein E78.9
      - specified NEC E78.89
    - magnesium E83.40
      - hypermagnesemia E83.41
      - hypomagnesemia E83.42
      - other specified E83.49
    - mineral E83.9
      - specified NEC E83.89
    - mitochondrial E88.40
      - MELAS syndrome E88.41
      - MERRF syndrome (myoclonic epilepsy associated with ragged-red fibers) E88.42
      - other specified E88.49
      - tRNA synthetases E88.43
    - ornithine E72.4
    - phosphatases E83.30
    - phosphorus E83.30
      - acid phosphatase deficiency E83.39
      - hypophosphatasia E83.39
      - hypophosphatemia E83.39
        - familial E83.31
      - other specified E83.39
      - pseudovitamin D deficiency E83.32
    - plasma protein NEC E88.09
    - porphyrin — *see* Porphyria
    - postprocedural E89.89
      - specified NEC E89.89
    - purine E79.9
      - specified NEC E79.89
    - pyrimidine E79.9
      - specified NEC E79.89
    - pyruvate E74.4
    - serine E72.89

- **Disorder** — *continued*
  - metabolism — *continued*
    - sodium E87.8
    - specified NEC E88.89
    - threonine E72.89
    - valine E71.19
    - zinc E83.2
  - methylmalonic acidemia E71.120
  - micturition NEC — *see also* Difficulty, micturition R39.198
    - feeling of incomplete emptying R39.14
    - hesitancy R39.11
    - poor stream R39.12
    - psychogenic F45.8
    - split stream R39.13
    - straining R39.16
    - urgency R39.15
  - mild neurocognitive G31.84
    - due to known physiological condition (without behavioral disturbance) F06.70
      - with behavioral disturbance F06.71
  - mitochondrial metabolism E88.40
  - mitral (valve) — *see* Endocarditis, mitral
  - mixed
    - anxiety and depressive F41.8
    - of scholastic skills (developmental) F81.89
    - receptive expressive language F80.2
  - mood F39
    - bipolar — *see* Disorder, bipolar
    - depressive — *see* Disorder, depressive
    - due to (secondary to)
      - alcohol F10.94
      - amphetamine F15.94
        - in
          - abuse F15.14
          - dependence F15.24
      - anxiolytic F13.94
        - in
          - abuse F13.14
          - dependence F13.24
      - cocaine F14.94
        - in
          - abuse F14.14
          - dependence F14.24
      - general medical condition F06.30
      - hallucinogen F16.94
        - in
          - abuse F16.14
          - dependence F16.24
      - hypnotic F13.94
        - in
          - abuse F13.14
          - dependence F13.24
      - inhalant F18.94
        - in
          - abuse F18.14
          - dependence F18.24
      - opioid F11.94
        - in
          - abuse F11.14
          - dependence F11.24
      - phencyclidine (PCP) F16.94
        - in
          - abuse F16.14
          - dependence F16.24
      - physiological condition F06.30
        - with
          - depressive features F06.31
          - major depressive-like episode F06.32
          - manic features F06.33
          - mixed features F06.34
      - psychoactive substance NEC F19.94
        - in
          - abuse F19.14
          - dependence F19.24
      - sedative F13.94
        - in
          - abuse F13.14
          - dependence F13.24
      - volatile solvents F18.94
        - in
          - abuse F18.14
          - dependence F18.24
    - manic episode F30.9
      - with psychotic symptoms F30.2
      - in remission (full) F30.4
        - partial F30.3
      - specified type NEC F30.8
      - without psychotic symptoms F30.10

- **Disorder** — *continued*
  - mood — *continued*
    - manic episode — *continued*
      - without psychotic symptoms — *continued*
        - mild F3Ø.11
        - moderate F3Ø.12
        - severe F3Ø.13
    - organic FØ6.3Ø
      - right hemisphere FØ7.89
    - persistent F34.9
      - cyclothymia F34.Ø
      - dysthymia F34.1
      - specified type NEC F34.89
    - recurrent F39
    - right hemisphere organic FØ7.89
  - movement G25.9
    - drug-induced G25.7Ø
      - akathisia G25.71
      - specified NEC G25.79
    - hysterical F44.4
    - in diseases classified elsewhere — *see* category G26
    - periodic limb G47.61
      - sleep related G47.61
    - sleep related NEC G47.69
    - specified NEC G25.89
    - stereotyped F98.4
    - treatment-induced G25.9
  - multiple personality F44.81
  - muscle M62.9
    - attachment, spine — *see* Enthesopathy, spinal
    - in trichinellosis — *see* Trichinellosis, with muscle disorder
    - psychogenic F45.8
    - specified type NEC M62.89
    - tone, newborn P94.9
      - specified NEC P94.8
  - muscular
    - attachments — *see also* Enthesopathy
      - spine — *see* Enthesopathy, spinal
    - urethra N36.44
  - musculoskeletal system, soft tissue — *see* Disorder, soft tissue
    - postprocedural M96.89
    - psychogenic F45.8
  - myoneural G7Ø.9
    - due to lead G7Ø.1
    - specified NEC G7Ø.89
    - toxic G7Ø.1
  - myotonic NEC G71.19
  - nail, in diseases classified elsewhere L62
  - neck region NEC — *see* Dorsopathy, specified NEC
  - neonatal onset multisystemic inflammatory (NOMID) MØ4.2
  - nerve G58.9
    - abducent NEC — *see* Strabismus, paralytic, sixth nerve
    - accessory G52.8
    - acoustic — *see* subcategory H93.3 ☑
    - auditory — *see* subcategory H93.3 ☑
    - auriculotemporal G5Ø.8
    - axillary G54.Ø
    - cerebral — *see* Disorder, nerve, cranial
    - cranial G52.9
      - eighth — *see* subcategory H93.3 ☑
      - eleventh G52.8
      - fifth G5Ø.9
      - first G52.Ø
      - fourth NEC — *see* Strabismus, paralytic, fourth nerve
      - multiple G52.7
      - ninth G52.1
      - second NEC — *see* Disorder, nerve, optic
      - seventh NEC G51.8
      - sixth NEC — *see* Strabismus, paralytic, sixth nerve
      - specified NEC G52.8
      - tenth G52.2
      - third NEC — *see* Strabismus, paralytic, third nerve
      - twelfth G52.3
    - entrapment — *see* Neuropathy, entrapment
    - facial G51.9
      - specified NEC G51.8
    - femoral — *see* Lesion, nerve, femoral
    - glossopharyngeal NEC G52.1
    - hypoglossal G52.3
    - intercostal G58.Ø
    - lateral
      - cutaneous of thigh — *see* Mononeuropathy, lower limb, meralgia paresthetica

- **Disorder** — *continued*
  - nerve — *continued*
    - lateral — *continued*
      - popliteal — *see* Lesion, nerve, popliteal
    - lower limb — *see* Mononeuropathy, lower limb
    - medial popliteal — *see* Lesion, nerve, popliteal, medial
    - median NEC — *see* Lesion, nerve, median
    - multiple G58.7
    - oculomotor NEC — *see* Strabismus, paralytic, third nerve
    - olfactory G52.Ø
    - optic NEC H47.Ø9- ☑
      - hemorrhage into sheath — *see* Hemorrhage, optic nerve
      - ischemic H47.Ø1- ☑
    - peroneal — *see* Lesion, nerve, popliteal
    - phrenic G58.8
    - plantar — *see* Lesion, nerve, plantar
    - pneumogastric G52.2
    - posterior tibial — *see* Syndrome, tarsal tunnel
    - radial — *see* Lesion, nerve, radial
    - recurrent laryngeal G52.2
    - root G54.9
      - cervical G54.2
      - lumbosacral G54.1
      - specified NEC G54.8
      - thoracic G54.3
    - sciatic NEC — *see* Lesion, nerve, sciatic
    - specified NEC G58.8
      - lower limb — *see* Mononeuropathy, lower limb, specified NEC
      - upper limb — *see* Mononeuropathy, upper limb, specified NEC
    - sympathetic G9Ø.9
    - tibial — *see* Lesion, nerve, popliteal, medial
    - trigeminal G5Ø.9
      - specified NEC G5Ø.8
    - trochlear NEC — *see* Strabismus, paralytic, fourth nerve
    - ulnar — *see* Lesion, nerve, ulnar
    - upper limb — *see* Mononeuropathy, upper limb
    - vagus G52.2
  - nervous system G98.8
    - autonomic (peripheral) G9Ø.9
      - specified NEC G9Ø.8
    - central G96.9
      - specified NEC G96.89
    - parasympathetic G9Ø.9
    - specified NEC G98.8
    - sympathetic G9Ø.9
    - vegetative G9Ø.9
  - neurocognitive R41.9
    - with Lewy bodies — *see also* Dementia, in, diseases specified elsewhere G31.83 *[FØ2.-]* ☑
    - frontotemporal, specified NEC — *see also* Dementia, in, diseases specified elsewhere G31.Ø9 *[FØ2.-]* ☑
    - major — *see also* Dementia FØ3.- ☑
      - due to vascular disease — *see* Dementia, vascular
        - mild — *see* Dementia, vascular, mild
        - moderate — *see* Dementia, vascular, moderate
        - severe — *see* Dementia, vascular, severe
      - in (due to) (other diseases classified elsewhere) — *see also* Dementia, in (due to) FØ2.8Ø
        - with
          - aggressive behavior — *see also* Dementia, in (due to) FØ2.81- ☑
          - combative behavior — *see also* Dementia, in (due to) FØ2.81- ☑
          - violent behavior — *see also* Dementia, in (due to) FØ2.81- ☑
    - mild (of uncertain or unknown etiology) — *see also* Disorder, mild neurocognitive G31.84
  - neurodevelopmental F89
    - specified NEC F88
  - neurohypophysis NEC E23.3
  - neurological NEC R29.818
  - neuromuscular G7Ø.9
    - hereditary NEC G71.9
    - specified NEC G7Ø.89
    - toxic G7Ø.1
  - neurotic F48.9
    - specified NEC F48.8
  - neutrophil, polymorphonuclear D71
  - nicotine use — *see* Dependence, drug, nicotine

- **Disorder** — *continued*
  - nightmare F51.5
  - non-rapid eye movement sleep arousal
    - sleep terror type F51.4
    - sleepwalking type F51.3
  - nose J34.9
    - specified NEC J34.89
  - obsessive-compulsive F42.9
    - and related disorder due to a known physiological condition FØ6.8
  - odontogenesis NOS KØØ.9
  - opioid use
    - with
      - opioid-induced psychotic disorder F11.959
        - with
          - delusions F11.95Ø
          - hallucinations F11.951
    - due to drug abuse — *see* Abuse, drug, opioid
    - due to drug dependence — *see* Dependence, drug, opioid
    - mild F11.1Ø
      - with
        - opioid-induced
          - anxiety disorder F11.188
          - depressive disorder F11.14
          - sexual dysfunction F11.181
        - opioid intoxication
          - with perceptual disturbances F11.122
          - delirium F11.121
          - without perceptual disturbances F11.129
      - in remission (early) (sustained) F11.11
    - moderate or severe F11.2Ø
      - with
        - opioid-induced
          - anxiety disorder F11.288
          - anxiety disorder F11.988
          - depressive disorder F11.24
          - depressive disorder F11.94
          - sexual dysfunction F11.281
          - sexual dysfunction F11.981
        - opioid intoxication
          - with perceptual disturbances F11.222
          - delirium F11.221
          - without perceptual disturbances F11.229
      - in remission (early) (sustained) F11.21
  - oppositional defiant F91.3
  - optic
    - chiasm H47.49
      - due to
        - inflammatory disorder H47.41
        - neoplasm H47.42
        - vascular disorder H47.43
    - disc H47.39- ☑
      - coloboma — *see* Coloboma, optic disc
      - drusen — *see* Drusen, optic disc
      - pseudopapilledema — *see* Pseudopapilledema
    - radiations — *see* Disorder, visual, pathway
    - tracts — *see* Disorder, visual, pathway
  - orbit HØ5.9
    - cyst — *see* Cyst, orbit
    - deformity — *see* Deformity, orbit
    - edema — *see* Edema, orbit
    - enophthalmos — *see* Enophthalmos
    - exophthalmos — *see* Exophthalmos
    - hemorrhage — *see* Hemorrhage, orbit
    - inflammation — *see* Inflammation, orbit
    - myopathy — *see* Myopathy, extraocular muscles
    - retained foreign body — *see* Foreign body, orbit, old
    - specified type NEC HØ5.89
  - organic
    - anxiety FØ6.4
    - catatonic FØ6.1
    - delusional FØ6.2
    - dissociative FØ6.8
    - emotionally labile (asthenic) FØ6.8
    - mood (affective) FØ6.3Ø
    - schizophrenia-like FØ6.2
  - orgasmic (female) F52.31
    - male F52.32
  - ornithine metabolism E72.4
  - overanxious F41.1
    - of childhood F93.8
  - pain
    - with related psychological factors F45.42
    - exclusively related to psychological factors F45.41
    - genito-pelvic penetration disorder F52.6
  - pancreatic internal secretion E16.9

- **Disorder** — *continued*
  - pancreatic internal secretion — *continued*
    - specified NEC E16.8
  - panic F41.Ø
    - with agoraphobia F4Ø.Ø1
  - papulosquamous L44.9
    - in diseases classified elsewhere L45
    - specified NEC L44.8
  - paranoid F22
    - induced F24
    - shared F24
  - paraphilic F65.9
    - specified NEC F65.89
  - parathyroid (gland) E21.5
    - specified NEC E21.4
  - parietoalveolar NEC J84.Ø9
  - paroxysmal, mixed R56.9
  - patella M22.9- ☑
    - chondromalacia — *see* Chondromalacia, patella
    - derangement NEC M22.3X- ☑
    - recurrent
      - dislocation — *see* Dislocation, patella, recurrent
      - subluxation — *see* Dislocation, patella, recurrent, incomplete
    - specified NEC M22.8X- ☑
  - patellofemoral M22.2X- ☑
  - pedophilic F65.4
  - pentose phosphate pathway with anemia D55.1
  - perception, due to hallucinogens F16.983
    - in
      - abuse F16.183
      - dependence F16.283
  - peripheral nervous system NEC G64
  - peroxisomal E71.5Ø
    - biogenesis
      - neonatal adrenoleukodystrophy E71.511
      - specified disorder NEC E71.518
      - Zellweger syndrome E71.51Ø
    - rhizomelic chondrodysplasia punctata E71.54Ø
    - specified form NEC E71.548
      - group 1 E71.518
      - group 2 E71.53
      - group 3 E71.542
    - X-linked adrenoleukodystrophy E71.529
      - adolescent E71.521
      - adrenomyeloneuropathy E71.522
      - childhood E71.52Ø
      - specified form NEC E71.528
    - Zellweger-like syndrome E71.541
  - persistent
    - (somatoform) pain F45.41
    - affective (mood) F34.9
  - personality — *see also* Personality F6Ø.9
    - affective F34.Ø
    - aggressive F6Ø.3
    - amoral F6Ø.2
    - anankastic F6Ø.5
    - antisocial F6Ø.2
    - anxious F6Ø.6
    - asocial F6Ø.2
    - asthenic F6Ø.7
    - avoidant F6Ø.6
    - borderline F6Ø.3
    - change (secondary) due to general medical condition FØ7.Ø
    - compulsive F6Ø.5
    - cyclothymic F34.Ø
    - dependent (passive) F6Ø.7
    - depressive F34.1
    - dissocial F6Ø.2
    - emotional instability F6Ø.3
    - expansive paranoid F6Ø.Ø
    - explosive F6Ø.3
    - following organic brain damage FØ7.9
    - histrionic F6Ø.4
    - hyperthymic F34.Ø
    - hypothymic F34.1
    - hysterical F6Ø.4
    - immature F6Ø.89
    - inadequate F6Ø.7
    - labile F6Ø.3
    - mixed (nonspecific) F6Ø.89
    - moral deficiency F6Ø.2
    - narcissistic F6Ø.81
    - negativistic F6Ø.89
    - obsessional F6Ø.5
    - obsessive (-compulsive) F6Ø.5
    - organic FØ7.9

- **Disorder** — *continued*
  - personality — *see also* Personality — *continued*
    - overconscientious F6Ø.5
    - paranoid F6Ø.Ø
    - passive (-dependent) F6Ø.7
    - passive-aggressive F6Ø.89
    - pathological NEC F6Ø.9
    - pseudosocial F6Ø.2
    - psychopathic F6Ø.2
    - schizoid F6Ø.1
    - schizotypal F21
    - self-defeating F6Ø.7
    - specified NEC F6Ø.89
    - type A F6Ø.5
    - unstable (emotional) F6Ø.3
  - pervasive, developmental F84.9
  - phencyclidine use
    - mild F16.1Ø
      - with
        - phencyclidine intoxication F16.129
        - phencyclidine intoxication delirium F16.121
        - phencyclidine-induced
          - anxiety disorder F16.18Ø
          - bipolar and related disorder F16.14
          - depressive disorder F16.14
          - psychotic disorder F16.159
      - in remission (early) (sustained) F16.11
    - moderate or severe F16.2Ø
      - with
        - phencyclidine intoxication F16.229
        - phencyclidine intoxication delirium F16.221
        - phencyclidine-induced
          - anxiety disorder F16.28Ø
          - bipolar and related disorder F16.14
          - depressive disorder F16.24
          - psychotic disorder F16.259
      - in remission (early) (sustained) F16.21
  - phobic anxiety, childhood F4Ø.8
  - phosphate-losing tubular N25.Ø
  - pigmentation L81.9
    - choroid, congenital Q14.3
    - diminished melanin formation L81.6
    - iron L81.8
    - specified NEC L81.8
  - pinna (noninfective) H61.1Ø- ☑
    - deformity, acquired H61.11- ☑
    - hematoma H61.12- ☑
    - perichondritis — *see* Perichondritis, ear
    - specified type NEC H61.19- ☑
  - pituitary gland E23.7
    - iatrogenic (postprocedural) E89.3
    - specified NEC E23.6
  - platelet-activating anti-PF4, specified NEC D75.84
  - platelets D69.1
  - plexus G54.9
    - specified NEC G54.8
  - polymorphonuclear neutrophils D71
  - porphyrin metabolism — *see* Porphyria
  - postconcussional FØ7.81
  - posthallucinogen perception F16.983
    - in
      - abuse F16.183
      - dependence F16.283
  - postmenopausal N95.9
    - specified NEC N95.8
  - postprocedural (postoperative) — *see* Complications, postprocedural
  - post-transplant lymphoproliferative D47.Z1 (*following* D47.4)
  - post-traumatic stress (PTSD) F43.1Ø
    - acute F43.11
    - chronic F43.12
  - premenstrual dysphoric (PMDD) F32.81
  - prepuce N47.8
  - propionic acidemia E71.121
  - prostate N42.9
    - specified NEC N42.89
  - psychogenic NOS — *see also* condition F45.9
    - anxiety F41.8
    - appetite F5Ø.9
    - asthenic F48.8
    - cardiovascular (system) F45.8
    - compulsive F42.8
    - cutaneous F54
    - depressive F32.9
    - digestive (system) F45.8
    - dysmenorrheic F45.8
    - dyspneic F45.8

- **Disorder** — *continued*
  - psychogenic — *see also* condition — *continued*
    - endocrine (system) F54
    - eye NEC F45.8
    - feeding — *see* Disorder, eating
    - functional NEC F45.8
    - gastric F45.8
    - gastrointestinal (system) F45.8
    - genitourinary (system) F45.8
    - heart (function) (rhythm) F45.8
    - hyperventilatory F45.8
    - hypochondriacal — *see* Disorder, hypochondriacal
    - intestinal F45.8
    - joint F45.8
    - learning F81.9
    - limb F45.8
    - lymphatic (system) F45.8
    - menstrual F45.8
    - micturition F45.8
    - monoplegic NEC F44.4
    - motor F44.4
    - muscle F45.8
    - musculoskeletal F45.8
    - neurocirculatory F45.8
    - obsessive F42.8
    - occupational F48.8
    - organ or part of body NEC F45.8
    - paralytic NEC F44.4
    - phobic F4Ø.9
    - physical NEC F45.8
    - rectal F45.8
    - respiratory (system) F45.8
    - rheumatic F45.8
    - sexual (function) F52.9
    - skin (allergic) (eczematous) F54
    - sleep F51.9
    - specified part of body NEC F45.8
    - stomach F45.8
  - psychological F99
    - associated with
      - disease classified elsewhere F54
      - sexual
        - development F66
        - relationship F66
      - uncertainty about gender identity F64.9
  - psychomotor NEC F44.4
    - hysterical F44.4
  - psychoneurotic — *see also* Neurosis
    - mixed NEC F48.8
  - psychophysiologic — *see* Disorder, somatoform
  - psychosexual F65.9
    - development F66
    - identity of childhood F64.2
  - psychosomatic NOS — *see* Disorder, somatoform
    - multiple F45.Ø
    - undifferentiated F45.1
  - psychotic — *see* Psychosis
    - transient (acute) F23
  - puberty E3Ø.9
    - specified NEC E3Ø.8
  - pulmonary (valve) — *see* Endocarditis, pulmonary
  - purine metabolism E79.9
  - pyrimidine metabolism E79.9
  - pyruvate metabolism E74.4
  - reactive attachment (childhood) F94.1
  - reading R48.Ø
    - developmental (specific) F81.Ø
  - receptive language F8Ø.2
  - receptor, hormonal, peripheral — *see also* Syndrome, androgen insensitivity E34.5Ø
  - recurrent brief depressive F33.8
  - reflex R29.2
  - refraction H52.7
    - aniseikonia H52.32
    - anisometropia H52.31
    - astigmatism — *see* Astigmatism
    - hypermetropia — *see* Hypermetropia
    - myopia — *see* Myopia
    - presbyopia H52.4
    - specified NEC H52.6
  - relationship F68.8
    - due to sexual orientation F66
  - REM sleep behavior G47.52
  - renal function, impaired (tubular) N25.9
  - resonance R49.9
    - specified NEC R49.8
  - respiratory function, impaired — *see also* Failure, respiration

- **Disorder** — *continued*
  - respiratory function, impaired — *see also* Failure, respiration — *continued*
    - postprocedural — *see* Complication, postoperative, respiratory system
    - psychogenic F45.8
  - retina H35.9
    - angioid streaks H35.33
    - changes in vascular appearance H35.01- ☑
    - degeneration — *see* Degeneration, retina
    - dystrophy (hereditary) — *see* Dystrophy, retina
    - edema H35.81
    - hemorrhage — *see* Hemorrhage, retina
    - ischemia H35.82
    - macular degeneration — *see* Degeneration, macula
    - microaneurysms H35.04- ☑
    - microvascular abnormality NEC H35.09
    - neovascularization — *see* Neovascularization, retina
    - retinopathy — *see* Retinopathy
    - separation of layers H35.70
      - central serous chorioretinopathy H35.71- ☑
      - pigment epithelium detachment (serous) H35.72- ☑
        - hemorrhagic H35.73- ☑
    - specified type NEC H35.89
    - telangiectasis — *see* Telangiectasis, retina
    - vasculitis — *see* Vasculitis, retina
  - retroperitoneal K68.9
  - right hemisphere organic affective F07.89
  - rumination (infant or child) F98.21
  - sacrum, sacrococcygeal NEC M53.3
  - schizoaffective F25.9
    - bipolar type F25.0
    - depressive type F25.1
    - manic type F25.0
    - mixed type F25.0
    - specified NEC F25.8
  - schizoid of childhood F84.5
  - schizophrenia spectrum and other psychotic disorder F29
    - specified NEC F28
  - schizophreniform F20.81
    - brief F23
  - schizotypal (personality) F21
  - seasonal affective, recurrent episodes F33.- ☑
  - secretion, thyrocalcitonin E07.0
  - sedative, hypnotic, or anxiolytic use
    - mild F13.10
      - with
        - sedative, hypnotic, or anxiolytic intoxication F13.129
        - sedative, hypnotic, or anxiolytic intoxication delirium F13.121
        - sedative, hypnotic, or anxiolytic-induced
          - anxiety disorder F13.180
          - bipolar and related disorder F13.14
          - depressive disorder F13.14
          - psychotic disorder F13.159
          - sexual dysfunction F13.181
      - in remission (early) (sustained) F13.11
    - moderate or severe F13.20
      - with
        - sedative, hypnotic, or anxiolytic intoxication F13.229
        - sedative, hypnotic, or anxiolytic intoxication delirium F13.221
        - sedative, hypnotic, or anxiolytic-induced
          - anxiety disorder F13.280
          - bipolar and related disorder F13.24
          - depressive disorder F13.24
          - major neurocognitive disorder F13.27
          - mild neurocognitive disorder F13.288
          - psychotic disorder F13.259
          - sexual dysfunction F13.281
      - in remission (early) (sustained) F13.21
  - seizure — *see also* Epilepsy G40.909
    - intractable G40.919
      - with status epilepticus G40.911
  - semantic pragmatic F80.89
    - with autism F84.0
  - sense of smell R43.1
    - psychogenic F45.8
  - separation anxiety, of childhood F93.0
  - sexual
    - aversion F52.1
    - function, psychogenic F52.9
    - interest/arousal, female F52.22
    - masochism F65.51

- **Disorder** — *continued*
  - sexual — *continued*
    - maturation F66
    - nonorganic F52.9
    - preference — *see also* Deviation, sexual F65.9
      - fetishistic transvestism F65.1
    - relationship F66
    - sadism F65.52
  - shyness, of childhood and adolescence F40.10
  - sibling rivalry F93.8
  - sickle-cell (sickling) (homozygous) — *see* Disease, sickle-cell
    - heterozygous D57.3
    - specified type NEC D57.8- ☑
    - trait D57.3
  - sinus (nasal) J34.9
    - specified NEC J34.89
  - skin L98.9
    - atrophic L90.9
      - specified NEC L90.8
    - granulomatous L92.9
      - specified NEC L92.8
    - hypertrophic L91.9
      - specified NEC L91.8
    - infiltrative NEC L98.6
    - newborn P83.9
      - specified NEC P83.88
    - picking F42.4
    - psychogenic (allergic) (eczematous) F54
  - sleep G47.9
    - breathing-related — *see* Apnea, sleep
    - circadian rhythm G47.20
      - advance sleep phase type G47.22
      - delayed sleep phase type G47.21
      - due to
        - alcohol
          - abuse F10.182
          - dependence F10.282
          - use F10.982
        - amphetamines
          - abuse F15.182
          - dependence F15.282
          - use F15.982
        - caffeine
          - abuse F15.182
          - dependence F15.282
          - use F15.982
        - cocaine
          - abuse F14.182
          - dependence F14.282
          - use F14.982
        - drug NEC
          - abuse F19.182
          - dependence F19.282
          - use F19.982
        - opioid
          - abuse F11.182
          - dependence F11.282
          - use F11.982
        - psychoactive substance NEC
          - abuse F19.182
          - dependence F19.282
          - use F19.982
        - sedative, hypnotic, or anxiolytic
          - abuse F13.182
          - dependence F13.282
          - use F13.982
        - stimulant NEC
          - abuse F15.182
          - dependence F15.282
          - use F15.982
      - free running type G47.24
      - in conditions classified elsewhere G47.27
      - irregular sleep wake type G47.23
      - jet lag type G47.25
      - non-24-hour sleep-wake type G47.24
      - shift work type G47.26
      - specified NEC G47.29
    - due to
      - alcohol
        - abuse F10.182
        - dependence F10.282
        - use F10.982
      - amphetamine
        - abuse F15.182
        - dependence F15.282
        - use F15.982
      - anxiolytic
        - abuse F13.182

- **Disorder** — *continued*
  - sleep — *continued*
    - due to — *continued*
      - anxiolytic — *continued*
        - dependence F13.282
        - use F13.982
      - caffeine
        - abuse F15.182
        - dependence F15.282
        - use F15.982
      - cocaine
        - abuse F14.182
        - dependence F14.282
        - use F14.982
      - drug NEC
        - abuse F19.182
        - dependence F19.282
        - use F19.982
      - hypnotic
        - abuse F13.182
        - dependence F13.282
        - use F13.982
      - opioid
        - abuse F11.182
        - dependence F11.282
        - use F11.982
      - psychoactive substance NEC
        - abuse F19.182
        - dependence F19.282
        - use F19.982
      - sedative
        - abuse F13.182
        - dependence F13.282
        - use F13.982
      - stimulant NEC
        - abuse F15.182
        - dependence F15.282
        - use F15.982
    - emotional F51.9
    - excessive somnolence — *see* Hypersomnia
    - hypersomnia type — *see* Hypersomnia
    - initiating or maintaining — *see* Insomnia
    - nightmares F51.5
    - nonorganic F51.9
      - specified NEC F51.8
    - parasomnia type G47.50
    - specified NEC G47.8
    - terrors F51.4
    - walking F51.3
  - sleep-wake pattern or schedule — *see also* Disorder, sleep, circadian rhythm G47.9
    - specified NEC G47.8
  - social
    - anxiety (of childhood) F40.10
      - generalized F40.11
    - functioning in childhood F94.9
      - specified NEC F94.8
    - pragmatic F80.82
  - soft tissue M79.9
    - ankle M79.9
    - due to use, overuse and pressure M70.90
      - ankle M70.97- ☑
      - bursitis — *see* Bursitis
      - foot M70.97- ☑
      - forearm M70.93- ☑
      - hand M70.94- ☑
      - lower leg M70.96- ☑
      - multiple sites M70.99
      - pelvic region M70.95- ☑
      - shoulder region M70.91- ☑
      - specified site NEC M70.98
      - specified type NEC M70.80
        - ankle M70.87- ☑
        - foot M70.87- ☑
        - forearm M70.83- ☑
        - hand M70.84- ☑
        - lower leg M70.86- ☑
        - multiple sites M70.89
        - pelvic region M70.85- ☑
        - shoulder region M70.81- ☑
        - specified site NEC M70.88
        - thigh M70.85- ☑
        - upper arm M70.82- ☑
      - thigh M70.95- ☑
      - upper arm M70.92- ☑
    - foot M79.9
    - forearm M79.9
    - hand M79.9

- **Disorder** — *continued*
  - voice — *continued*
    - specified type NEC R49.8
  - volatile solvent use
    - due to drug abuse — *see* Abuse, drug, inhalant
    - due to drug dependence — *see* Dependence, drug, inhalant
  - voyeuristic F65.3
  - white blood cells D72.9
    - specified NEC D72.89
  - withdrawing, child or adolescent F4Ø.1Ø
- **Disorientation** R41.Ø
- **Displacement, displaced**
  - acquired traumatic of bone, cartilage, joint, tendon NEC — *see* Dislocation
  - adrenal gland (congenital) Q89.1
  - appendix, retrocecal (congenital) Q43.8
  - auricle (congenital) Q17.4
  - bladder (acquired) N32.89
    - congenital Q64.19
  - brachial plexus (congenital) QØ7.8
  - brain stem, caudal (congenital) QØ4.8
  - canaliculus (lacrimalis), congenital Q1Ø.6
  - cardia through esophageal hiatus (congenital) Q4Ø.1
  - cerebellum, caudal (congenital) QØ4.8
  - cervix — *see* Malposition, uterus
  - colon (congenital) Q43.3
  - device, implant or graft — *see also* Complications, by site and type, mechanical T85.628 ☑
    - arterial graft NEC — *see* Complication, cardiovascular device, mechanical, vascular
    - breast (implant) T85.42 ☑
    - catheter NEC T85.628 ☑
      - dialysis (renal) T82.42 ☑
        - intraperitoneal T85.621 ☑
      - infusion NEC T82.524 ☑
        - spinal (epidural) (subdural) T85.62Ø ☑
      - urinary
        - cystostomy T83.Ø2Ø ☑
        - Hopkins T83.Ø28 ☑
        - ileostomy T83.Ø28 ☑
        - indwelling T83.Ø21 ☑
        - nephrostomy T83.Ø22 ☑
        - specified NEC T83.Ø28 ☑
        - urostomy T83.Ø28 ☑
    - electronic (electrode) (pulse generator) (stimulator) — *see* Complication, electronic stimulator
    - fixation, internal (orthopedic) NEC — *see* Complication, fixation device, mechanical
    - gastrointestinal — *see* Complications, prosthetic device, mechanical, gastrointestinal device
    - genital NEC T83.428 ☑
      - intrauterine contraceptive device (string) T83.32 ☑
      - penile prosthesis (cylinder) (implanted) (pump) (reservoir) T83.42Ø ☑
      - testicular prosthesis T83.421 ☑
    - heart NEC — *see* Complication, cardiovascular device, mechanical
    - joint prosthesis — *see* Complications, joint prosthesis, mechanical
    - ocular — *see* Complications, prosthetic device, mechanical, ocular device
    - orthopedic NEC — *see* Complication, orthopedic, device or graft, mechanical
    - specified NEC T85.628 ☑
    - urinary NEC T83.128 ☑
      - graft T83.22 ☑
      - sphincter, implanted T83.121 ☑
      - stent (ileal conduit) (nephroureteral) T83.123 ☑
        - ureteral indwelling T83.122 ☑
    - vascular NEC — *see* Complication, cardiovascular device, mechanical
    - ventricular intracranial shunt T85.Ø2 ☑
  - electronic stimulator
    - bone T84.32Ø ☑
    - cardiac — *see* Complications, cardiac device, electronic
    - nervous system — *see* Complication, prosthetic device, mechanical, electronic nervous system stimulator
    - urinary — *see* Complications, electronic stimulator, urinary
  - esophageal mucosa into cardia of stomach, congenital Q39.8
  - esophagus (acquired) K22.89
    - congenital Q39.8
- **Displacement, displaced** — *continued*
  - eyeball (acquired) (lateral) (old) — *see* Displacement, globe
    - congenital Q15.8
    - current — *see* Avulsion, eye
  - fallopian tube (acquired) N83.4- ☑
    - congenital Q5Ø.6
    - opening (congenital) Q5Ø.6
  - gallbladder (congenital) Q44.1
  - gastric mucosa (congenital) Q4Ø.2
  - globe (acquired) (old) (lateral) HØ5.21- ☑
    - current — *see* Avulsion, eye
  - heart (congenital) Q24.8
    - acquired I51.89
  - hymen (upward) (congenital) Q52.4
  - intervertebral disc NEC
    - with myelopathy — *see* Disorder, disc, with, myelopathy
    - cervical, cervicothoracic (with) M5Ø.2Ø
      - myelopathy — *see* Disorder, disc, cervical, with myelopathy
      - neuritis, radiculitis or radiculopathy — *see* Disorder, disc, cervical, with neuritis
    - due to trauma — *see* Dislocation, vertebra
    - lumbar region M51.26
      - with
        - myelopathy M51.Ø6
        - neuritis, radiculitis, radiculopathy or sciatica M51.16
    - lumbosacral region M51.27
      - with
        - neuritis, radiculitis, radiculopathy or sciatica M51.17
    - sacrococcygeal region M53.3
    - thoracic region M51.24
      - with
        - myelopathy M51.Ø4
        - neuritis, radiculitis, radiculopathy M51.14
    - thoracolumbar region M51.25
      - with
        - myelopathy M51.Ø5
        - neuritis, radiculitis, radiculopathy M51.15
  - intrauterine device (string) T83.32 ☑
  - kidney (acquired) N28.83
    - congenital Q63.2
  - lachrymal, lacrimal apparatus or duct (congenital) Q1Ø.6
  - lens, congenital Q12.1
  - macula (congenital) Q14.1
  - Meckel's diverticulum Q43.Ø
    - malignant — *see* Table of Neoplasms, small intestine, malignant
  - nail (congenital) Q84.6
    - acquired L6Ø.8
  - opening of Wharton's duct in mouth Q38.4
  - organ or site, congenital NEC — *see* Malposition, congenital
  - ovary (acquired) N83.4- ☑
    - congenital Q5Ø.39
    - free in peritoneal cavity (congenital) Q5Ø.39
    - into hernial sac N83.4- ☑
  - oviduct (acquired) N83.4- ☑
    - congenital Q5Ø.6
  - parathyroid (gland) E21.4
  - parotid gland (congenital) Q38.4
  - punctum lacrimale (congenital) Q1Ø.6
  - sacro-iliac (joint) (congenital) Q74.2
    - current injury S33.2 ☑
    - old — *see* subcategory M53.2 ☑
  - salivary gland (any) (congenital) Q38.4
  - spleen (congenital) Q89.Ø9
  - stomach, congenital Q4Ø.2
  - sublingual duct Q38.4
  - tongue (downward) (congenital) Q38.3
  - tooth, teeth, fully erupted M26.3Ø
    - horizontal M26.33
    - vertical M26.34
  - trachea (congenital) Q32.1
  - ureter or ureteric opening or orifice (congenital) Q62.62
  - uterine opening of oviducts or fallopian tubes Q5Ø.6
  - uterus, uterine — *see* Malposition, uterus
  - ventricular septum Q21.Ø
    - with rudimentary ventricle Q2Ø.4
- **Disproportion**
  - between native and reconstructed breast N65.1
  - fiber-type G71.2Ø
    - congenital G71.29
- **Disruptio uteri** — *see* Rupture, uterus
- **Disruption** (of)
  - ciliary body NEC H21.89
  - closure of
    - cornea T81.31 ☑
    - craniotomy T81.32 ☑
    - fascia (muscular) (superficial) T81.32 ☑
    - internal organ or tissue T81.32 ☑
    - laceration (external) (internal) T81.33 ☑
    - ligament T81.32 ☑
    - mucosa T81.31 ☑
    - muscle or muscle flap T81.32 ☑
    - ribs or rib cage T81.32 ☑
    - skin and subcutaneous tissue (full-thickness) (superficial) T81.31 ☑
    - skull T81:32 ☑
    - sternum (sternotomy) T81.32 ☑
    - tendon T81.32 ☑
    - traumatic laceration (external) (internal) T81.33 ☑
  - family Z63.8
    - due to
      - absence of family member due to military deployment Z63.31
      - absence of family member NEC Z63.32
      - alcoholism and drug addiction in family Z63.72
      - bereavement Z63.4
      - death (assumed) or disappearance of family member Z63.4
      - divorce or separation Z63.5
      - drug addiction in family Z63.72
      - return of family member from military deployment (current or past conflict) Z63.71
      - stressful life events NEC Z63.79
  - iris NEC H21.89
  - ligament(s) — *see also* Sprain
    - knee
      - current injury — *see* Dislocation, knee
      - old (chronic) — *see* Derangement, knee, instability
      - spontaneous NEC — *see* Derangement, knee, disruption ligament
  - ossicular chain — *see* Discontinuity, ossicles, ear
  - pelvic ring (stable) S32.81Ø ☑
    - unstable S32.811 ☑
  - traumatic injury wound repair T81.33 ☑
  - wound T81.3Ø ☑
    - episiotomy O9Ø.1
    - operation T81.31 ☑
      - cesarean O9Ø.Ø
      - external operation wound (superficial) T81.31 ☑
      - internal operation wound (deep) T81.32 ☑
    - perineal (obstetric) O9Ø.1
    - traumatic injury repair T81.33 ☑
- **Dissatisfaction with**
  - employment Z56.9
  - school environment Z55.4
- **Dissecting** — *see* condition
- **Dissection**
  - aorta I71.ØØ
    - abdominal I71.Ø2
    - thoracic I71.Ø19
      - aortic arch I71.Ø11
      - ascending aorta I71.Ø1Ø
      - descending thoracic aorta I71.Ø12
    - thoracoabdominal I71.Ø3
  - artery I77.7Ø
    - basilar (trunk) I77.75
    - carotid I77.71
    - cerebral (nonruptured) I67.Ø
      - ruptured — *see* Hemorrhage, intracranial, subarachnoid
    - coronary I25.42
    - extremity
      - lower I77.77
      - upper I77.76
    - iliac I77.72
    - precerebral
      - congenital (nonruptured) Q28.1
      - specified site NEC I77.75
    - renal I77.73
    - specified NEC I77.79
    - vertebral I77.74
  - precerebral artery, congenital (nonruptured) Q28.1
    - Heartland A93.8
  - traumatic — *see* Wound, open, by site
  - vascular I99.8
  - wound — *see* Wound, open
- **Disseminated** — *see* condition

Division
- cervix uteri (acquired) N88.8
- glans penis Q55.69
- labia minora (congenital) Q52.79
- ligament (partial or complete) (current) — *see also* Sprain
  - with open wound — *see* Wound, open
- muscle (partial or complete) (current) — *see also* Injury, muscle
  - with open wound — *see* Wound, open
- nerve (traumatic) — *see* Injury, nerve
- spinal cord — *see* Injury, spinal cord, by region
- vein I87.8

Divorce, causing family disruption Z63.5

Dix-Hallpike neurolabyrinthitis — *see* Neuronitis, vestibular

Dizziness R42
- hysterical F44.89
- psychogenic F45.8

DMAC (disseminated mycobacterium avium-intracellulare complex) A31.2

DNR (do not resuscitate) Z66

Doan-Wiseman syndrome (primary splenic neutropenia) — *see* Agranulocytosis

Doehle-Heller aortitis A52.02

Dog bite — *see* Bite

Dohle body panmyelopathic syndrome D72.0

Dolichocephaly Q67.2
- non-deformational Q75.01

Dolichocolon Q43.8

Dolichostenomelia — *see* Syndrome, Marfan

Donohue's syndrome E34.8

Donor (organ or tissue) Z52.9
- blood (whole) Z52.000
  - autologous Z52.010
  - specified component (lymphocytes) (platelets) NEC Z52.008
    - autologous Z52.018
    - specified donor NEC Z52.098
  - specified donor NEC Z52.090
  - stem cells Z52.001
    - autologous Z52.011
    - specified donor NEC Z52.091
- bone Z52.20
  - autologous Z52.21
  - marrow Z52.3
  - specified type NEC Z52.29
- cornea Z52.5
- egg (Oocyte) Z52.819
  - age 35 and over Z52.812
    - anonymous recipient Z52.812
    - designated recipient Z52.813
  - under age 35 Z52.810
    - anonymous recipient Z52.810
    - designated recipient Z52.811
- kidney Z52.4
- liver Z52.6
- lung Z52.89
- lymphocyte — *see* Donor, blood, specified components NEC
- Oocyte — *see* Donor, egg
- platelets Z52.008
- potential, examination of Z00.5
- semen Z52.89
- skin Z52.10
  - autologous Z52.11
  - specified type NEC Z52.19
- specified organ or tissue NEC Z52.89
- sperm Z52.89

Donovanosis A58

Dorsalgia M54.9
- psychogenic F45.41
- specified NEC M54.89

Dorsopathy M53.9
- deforming M43.9
  - specified NEC — *see* subcategory M43.8 ☑
- specified NEC M53.80
  - cervical region M53.82
  - cervicothoracic region M53.83
  - lumbar region M53.86
  - lumbosacral region M53.87
  - occipito-atlanto-axial region M53.81
  - sacrococcygeal region M53.88
  - thoracic region M53.84
  - thoracolumbar region M53.85

Double
- albumin E88.09
- aortic arch Q25.45

Double — *continued*
- auditory canal Q17.8
- auricle (heart) Q20.8
- bladder Q64.79
- cervix Q51.820
  - with doubling of uterus (and vagina) Q51.10
    - with obstruction Q51.11
- inlet ventricle Q20.4
- kidney with double pelvis (renal) Q63.0
- meatus urinarius Q64.75
- monster Q89.4
- outlet
  - left ventricle Q20.2
  - right ventricle Q20.1
- pelvis (renal) with double ureter Q62.5
- tongue Q38.3
- ureter (one or both sides) Q62.5
  - with double pelvis (renal) Q62.5
- urethra Q64.74
- urinary meatus Q64.75
- uterus Q51.28
  - with
    - doubling of cervix (and vagina) Q51.10
      - with obstruction Q51.11
  - complete Q51.21
  - in pregnancy or childbirth O34.0- ☑
    - causing obstructed labor O65.5
  - partial Q51.22
  - specified NEC Q51.28
- vagina Q52.10
  - with doubling of uterus (and cervix) Q51.10
    - with obstruction Q51.11
- vision H53.2
- vulva Q52.79

Doubled up Z59.01

Douglas' pouch, cul-de-sac — *see* condition

Down syndrome Q90.9
- meiotic nondisjunction Q90.0
- mitotic nondisjunction Q90.1
- mosaicism Q90.1
- translocation Q90.2

DPD (dihydropyrimidine dehydrogenase deficiency) E88.89

Dracontiasis B72

Dracunculiasis, dracunculosis B72

Dream state, hysterical F44.89

Drepanocytic anemia — *see* Disease, sickle-cell

Dresbach's syndrome (elliptocytosis) D58.1

Dreschlera (hawaiiensis) (infection) B43.8

Dressler's syndrome I24.1

Drift, ulnar — *see* Deformity, limb, specified type NEC, forearm

Drinking (alcohol)
- excessive, to excess NEC (without dependence) F10.10
  - habitual (continual) (without remission) F10.20
    - with remission F10.21

Drip, postnasal (chronic) R09.82
- due to
  - allergic rhinitis — *see* Rhinitis, allergic
  - common cold J00
  - gastroesophageal reflux — *see* Reflux, gastroesophageal
  - nasopharyngitis — *see* Nasopharyngitis
  - other known condition — *code to* condition
  - sinusitis — *see* Sinusitis

Droop
- facial R29.810
  - cerebrovascular disease I69.992
    - cerebral infarction I69.392
    - intracerebral hemorrhage I69.192
    - nontraumatic intracranial hemorrhage NEC I69.292
    - specified disease NEC I69.892
    - subarachnoid hemorrhage I69.092

Drop (in)
- attack NEC R55
- finger — *see* Deformity, finger
- foot — *see* Deformity, limb, foot, drop
- hematocrit (precipitous) R71.0
- hemoglobin R71.0
- toe — *see* Deformity, toe, specified NEC
- wrist — *see* Deformity, limb, wrist drop

Dropped heart beats I45.9

Dropsy, dropsical — *see also* Hydrops
- abdomen R18.8
- brain — *see* Hydrocephalus
- cardiac, heart — *see* Failure, heart, congestive
- gangrenous — *see* Gangrene

Dropsy, dropsical — *continued*
- heart — *see* Failure, heart, congestive
- kidney — *see* Nephrosis
- lung — *see* Edema, lung
- newborn due to isoimmunization P56.0
- pericardium — *see* Pericarditis

Drowned, drowning (near) T75.1 ☑

Drowsiness R40.0

Drug
- abuse counseling and surveillance Z71.51
- addiction — *see* Dependence
- dependence — *see* Dependence
- habit — *see* Dependence
- harmful use — *see* Abuse, drug
- induced fever R50.2
- overdose — *see* Table of Drugs and Chemicals, by drug, poisoning
- poisoning — *see* Table of Drugs and Chemicals, by drug, poisoning
- resistant organism infection — *see also* Resistant, organism, to, drug Z16.30
- therapy
  - long term (current) (prophylactic) — *see* Therapy, drug long-term (current) (prophylactic)
  - short term — *omit code*
- wrong substance given or taken in error — *see* Table of Drugs and Chemicals, by drug, poisoning

Drunkenness (without dependence) F10.129
- acute in alcoholism F10.229
- chronic (without remission) F10.20
  - with remission F10.21
- pathological (without dependence) F10.129
  - with dependence F10.229
- sleep F51.9

Drusen
- macula (degenerative) (retina) — *see* Degeneration, macula, drusen
- optic disc H47.32- ☑

Dry, dryness — *see also* condition
- larynx J38.7
- mouth R68.2
  - due to dehydration E86.0
- nose J34.89
- socket (teeth) M27.3
- throat J39.2

DSAP L56.5

Duane's syndrome H50.81- ☑

Dubin-Johnson disease or syndrome E80.6

Dubois' disease (thymus gland) A50.59 *[E35]*

Dubowitz' syndrome Q87.19

Duchenne-Aran muscular atrophy G12.21

Duchenne-Griesinger disease G71.01

Duchenne's
- disease or syndrome
  - motor neuron disease G12.22
  - muscular dystrophy G71.01
- locomotor ataxia (syphilitic) A52.11
- paralysis
  - birth injury P14.0
  - due to or associated with
    - motor neuron disease G12.22
    - muscular dystrophy G71.01

Ducrey's chancre A57

Duct, ductus — *see* condition

Duhring's disease (dermatitis herpetiformis) L13.0

Dullness, cardiac (decreased) (increased) R01.2

Dumb ague — *see* Malaria

Dumbness — *see* Aphasia

Dumdum fever B55.0

Dumping syndrome (postgastrectomy) K91.1

Duodenitis (nonspecific) (peptic) K29.80
- with bleeding K29.81
- erosive — *see* Ulcer, duodenum

Duodenocholangitis — *see* Cholangitis

Duodenum, duodenal — *see* condition

Duplay's bursitis or periarthritis M75.0 ☑

Duplication, duplex — *see also* Accessory
- alimentary tract Q45.8
- anus Q43.4
- appendix (and cecum) Q43.4
- biliary duct (any) Q44.5
- bladder Q64.79
- cecum (and appendix) Q43.4
- cervix Q51.820
- chromosome NEC — *see also* Trisomy
  - with complex rearrangements NEC Q92.5
  - seen only at prometaphase Q92.8

☑ **Additional Character Required — Refer to the Tabular List for Character Selection**

- **Ectropion** — *continued*
  - eyelid — *continued*
    - paralytic — *continued*
      - right — *continued*
        - upper HØ2.151
    - right HØ2.1Ø3
      - lower HØ2.1Ø2
      - upper HØ2.1Ø1
    - senile HØ2.139
      - left HØ2.136
        - lower HØ2.135
        - upper HØ2.134
      - right HØ2.133
        - lower HØ2.132
        - upper HØ2.131
    - spastic HØ2.149
      - left HØ2.146
        - lower HØ2.145
        - upper HØ2.144
      - right HØ2.143
        - lower HØ2.142
        - upper HØ2.141
  - iris H21.89
  - lip (acquired) K13.Ø
    - congenital Q38.Ø
  - urethra N36.8
  - uvea H21.89
- **Eczema** (acute) (chronic) (erythematous) (fissum) (rubrum) (squamous) — *see also* Dermatitis L3Ø.9
  - contact — *see* Dermatitis, contact
  - dyshydrotic L3Ø.1
  - external ear — *see* Otitis, externa, acute, eczematoid
  - flexural L2Ø.82
  - herpeticum BØØ.Ø
  - hypertrophicum L28.Ø
  - hypostatic — *see* Varix, leg, with, inflammation
  - impetiginous LØ1.1
  - infantile (due to any substance) L2Ø.83
    - intertriginous L21.1
    - seborrheic L21.1
  - intertriginous NEC L3Ø.4
    - infantile L21.1
  - intrinsic (allergic) L2Ø.84
  - lichenified NEC L28.Ø
  - marginatum (hebrae) B35.6
  - pustular L3Ø.3
  - stasis I87.2
    - with varicose veins — *see* Varix, leg, with, inflammation
  - vaccination, vaccinatum T88.1 ☑
  - varicose — *see* Varix, leg, with, inflammation
- **Eczematid** L3Ø.2
- **Eddowes** (-Spurway) **syndrome** Q78.Ø
- **Edema, edematous** (infectious) (pitting) (toxic) R6Ø.9
  - with nephritis — *see* Nephrosis
  - allergic T78.3 ☑
  - amputation stump (surgical) (sequelae (late effect)) T87.89
  - angioneurotic (allergic) (any site) (with urticaria) T78.3 ☑
    - hereditary D84.1
  - angiospastic I73.9
  - Berlin's (traumatic) SØ5.8X- ☑
  - brain (cytotoxic) (vasogenic) G93.6
    - due to birth injury P11.Ø
    - newborn (anoxia or hypoxia) P52.4
      - birth injury P11.Ø
    - traumatic — *see* Injury, intracranial, cerebral edema
  - cardiac — *see* Failure, heart, congestive
  - cardiovascular — *see* Failure, heart, congestive
  - cerebral — *see* Edema, brain
  - cerebrospinal — *see* Edema, brain
  - cervix (uteri) (acute) N88.8
    - puerperal, postpartum O9Ø.89
  - chronic hereditary Q82.Ø
  - circumscribed, acute T78.3 ☑
    - hereditary D84.1
  - conjunctiva H11.42- ☑
  - cornea H18.2- ☑
    - idiopathic H18.22- ☑
    - secondary H18.23- ☑
      - due to contact lens H18.21- ☑
  - due to
    - lymphatic obstruction I89.Ø
    - salt retention E87.Ø
  - epiglottis — *see* Edema, glottis
  - essential, acute T78.3 ☑
    - hereditary D84.1

- **Edema, edematous** — *continued*
  - extremities, lower — *see* Edema, legs
  - eyelid NEC HØ2.849
    - left HØ2.846
      - lower HØ2.845
      - upper HØ2.844
    - right HØ2.843
      - lower HØ2.842
      - upper HØ2.841
  - familial, hereditary Q82.Ø
  - famine — *see* Malnutrition, severe
  - generalized R6Ø.1
  - glottis, glottic, glottidis (obstructive) (passive) J38.4
    - allergic T78.3 ☑
      - hereditary D84.1
  - heart — *see* Failure, heart, congestive
  - heat T67.7 ☑
  - hereditary Q82.Ø
  - inanition — *see* Malnutrition, severe
  - intracranial G93.6
  - iris H21.89
  - joint — *see* Effusion, joint
  - larynx — *see* Edema, glottis
  - legs R6Ø.Ø
    - due to venous obstruction I87.1
    - hereditary Q82.Ø
  - localized R6Ø.Ø
    - due to venous obstruction I87.1
  - lower limbs — *see* Edema, legs
  - lung J81.1
    - with heart condition or failure — *see* Failure, ventricular, left
      - newborn P29.Ø
    - acute J81.Ø
    - chemical (acute) J68.1
      - chronic J68.1
    - chronic J81.1
      - due to
        - chemicals, gases, fumes or vapors (inhalation) J68.1
        - external agent J7Ø.9
          - specified NEC J7Ø.8
        - radiation J7Ø.1
    - due to
      - chemicals, fumes or vapors (inhalation) J68.1
      - external agent J7Ø.9
        - specified NEC J7Ø.8
      - high altitude T7Ø.29 ☑
      - near drowning T75.1 ☑
      - radiation J7Ø.Ø
    - meaning failure, left ventricle I5Ø.1
  - lymphatic I89.Ø
    - due to mastectomy I97.2
  - macula H35.81
    - cystoid, following cataract surgery — *see* Complications, postprocedural, following cataract surgery
    - diabetic — *see* Diabetes, by type, with, retinopathy, with macular edema
  - malignant — *see* Gangrene, gas
  - Milroy's Q82.Ø
  - nasopharynx J39.2
  - newborn P83.3Ø
    - hydrops fetalis — *see* Hydrops, fetalis
    - specified NEC P83.39
  - nutritional — *see also* Malnutrition, severe
    - with dyspigmentation, skin and hair E4Ø
  - optic disc or nerve — *see* Papilledema
  - orbit HØ5.22- ☑
  - pancreas K86.89
  - papilla, optic — *see* Papilledema
  - penis N48.89
  - periodic T78.3 ☑
    - hereditary D84.1
  - pharynx J39.2
  - pulmonary — *see* Edema, lung
  - Quincke's T78.3 ☑
    - hereditary D84.1
  - renal — *see* Nephrosis
  - retina H35.81
    - diabetic — *see* Diabetes, by type, with, retinopathy, with macular edema
  - salt E87.Ø
  - scrotum N5Ø.89
  - seminal vesicle N5Ø.89
  - spermatic cord N5Ø.89
  - spinal (cord) (vascular) (nontraumatic) G95.19
  - starvation — *see* Malnutrition, severe

- **Edema, edematous** — *continued*
  - stasis — *see* Hypertension, venous, (chronic)
  - subglottic — *see* Edema, glottis
  - supraglottic — *see* Edema, glottis
  - testis N44.8
  - tunica vaginalis N5Ø.89
  - vas deferens N5Ø.89
  - vulva (acute) N9Ø.89
- **Edentulism** — *see* Absence, teeth, acquired
- **Edsall's disease** T67.2 ☑
- **Educational handicap** Z55.9
  - less than a high school diploma Z55.5
  - no general equivalence degree (GED) Z55.5
  - specified NEC Z55.8
- **Edward's syndrome** — *see* Trisomy, 18
- **Effect**(s) (of) (from) — *see* Effect, adverse NEC
- **Effect, adverse**
  - abnormal gravitational (G) forces or states T75.81 ☑
  - abuse — *see* Maltreatment
  - air pressure T7Ø.9 ☑
    - specified NEC T7Ø.8 ☑
  - altitude (high) — *see* Effect, adverse, high altitude
  - anesthesia — *see also* Anesthesia T88.59 ☑
    - in labor and delivery O74.9
    - local, toxic
      - in labor and delivery O74.4
      - in pregnancy NEC O29.3- ☑
      - postpartum, puerperal O89.3
    - postpartum, puerperal O89.9
    - specified NEC T88.59 ☑
      - in labor and delivery O74.8
      - postpartum, puerperal O89.8
    - spinal and epidural T88.59 ☑
      - headache T88.59 ☑
        - in labor and delivery O74.5
        - postpartum, puerperal O89.4
      - specified NEC
        - in labor and delivery O74.6
        - postpartum, puerperal O89.5
  - antitoxin — *see* Complications, vaccination
  - atmospheric pressure T7Ø.9 ☑
    - due to explosion T7Ø.8 ☑
    - high T7Ø.3 ☑
    - low — *see* Effect, adverse, high altitude
    - specified effect NEC T7Ø.8 ☑
  - biological, correct substance properly administered — *see* Effect, adverse, drug
  - blood (derivatives) (serum) (transfusion) — *see* Complications, transfusion
  - chemical substance — *see* Table of Drugs and Chemicals
  - cold (temperature) (weather) T69.9 ☑
    - chilblains T69.1 ☑
    - frostbite — *see* Frostbite
    - specified effect NEC T69.8 ☑
  - drugs and medicaments T88.7 ☑
    - specified drug — *see* Table of Drugs and Chemicals, by drug, adverse effect
    - specified effect — *code to* condition
  - electric current, electricity (shock) T75.4 ☑
    - burn — *see* Burn
  - exertion (excessive) T73.3 ☑
  - exposure — *see* Exposure
  - external cause NEC T75.89 ☑
  - foodstuffs T78.1 ☑
    - allergic reaction — *see* Allergy, food
      - causing anaphylaxis — *see* Shock, anaphylactic, due to food
    - noxious — *see* Poisoning, food, noxious
  - gases, fumes, or vapors T59.9- ☑
    - specified agent — *see* Table of Drugs and Chemicals
  - glue (airplane) sniffing
    - due to drug abuse — *see* Abuse, drug, inhalant
    - due to drug dependence — *see* Dependence, drug, inhalant
  - heat — *see* Heat
  - high altitude NEC T7Ø.29 ☑
    - anoxia T7Ø.29 ☑
    - on
      - ears T7Ø.Ø ☑
      - sinuses T7Ø.1 ☑
    - polycythemia D75.1
  - high pressure fluids T7Ø.4 ☑
  - hot weather — *see* Heat
  - hunger T73.Ø ☑
  - immersion, foot — *see* Immersion
  - immunization — *see* Complications, vaccination

- **Effect, adverse** — *continued*
  - immunological agents — *see* Complications, vaccination
  - infrared (radiation) (rays) NOS T66 ☑
    - dermatitis or eczema L59.8
  - infusion — *see* Complications, infusion
  - lack of care of infants — *see* Maltreatment, child
  - lightning — *see* Lightning
  - medical care T88.9 ☑
    - specified NEC T88.8 ☑
  - medicinal substance, correct, properly administered — *see* Effect, adverse, drug
  - motion T75.3 ☑
  - noise, on inner ear — *see* subcategory H83.3 ☑
  - overheated places — *see* Heat
  - psychosocial, of work environment Z56.5
  - radiation (diagnostic) (infrared) (natural source) (therapeutic) (ultraviolet) (X-ray) NOS T66 ☑
    - dermatitis or eczema — *see* Dermatitis, due to, radiation
    - fibrosis of lung J7Ø.1
    - pneumonitis J7Ø.Ø
    - pulmonary manifestations
      - acute J7Ø.Ø
      - chronic J7Ø.1
    - skin L59.9
  - radioactive substance NOS
    - dermatitis or eczema — *see* Radiodermatitis
  - reduced temperature T69.9 ☑
    - immersion foot or hand — *see* Immersion
    - specified effect NEC T69.8 ☑
  - serum NEC — *see also* Reaction, serum T8Ø.69 ☑
  - specified NEC T78.8 ☑
    - external cause NEC T75.89 ☑
  - strangulation — *see* Asphyxia, traumatic
  - submersion T75.1 ☑
  - thirst T73.1 ☑
  - toxic — *see* Toxicity
  - transfusion — *see* Complications, transfusion
  - ultraviolet (radiation) (rays) NOS T66 ☑
    - burn — *see* Burn
    - dermatitis or eczema — *see* Dermatitis, due to, ultraviolet rays
      - acute L56.8
  - vaccine (any) — *see* Complications, vaccination
  - vibration — *see* Vibration, adverse effects
  - water pressure NEC T7Ø.9 ☑
    - specified NEC T7Ø.8 ☑
  - weightlessness T75.82 ☑
  - whole blood — *see* Complications, transfusion
  - work environment Z56.5
- **Effects, late** — *see* Sequelae
- **Effluvium**
  - anagen L65.1
  - telogen L65.Ø
- **Effort syndrome** (psychogenic) F45.8
- **Effusion**
  - amniotic fluid — *see* Pregnancy, complicated by, premature rupture of membranes
  - brain (serous) G93.6
  - bronchial — *see* Bronchitis
  - cerebral G93.6
  - cerebrospinal — *see also* Meningitis
    - vessel G93.6
  - chest — *see* Effusion, pleura
  - chylous, chyliform (pleura) J94.Ø
  - intracranial G93.6
  - joint M25.4Ø
    - ankle M25.47- ☑
    - elbow M25.42- ☑
    - foot joint M25.47- ☑
    - hand joint M25.44- ☑
    - hip M25.45- ☑
    - knee M25.46- ☑
    - shoulder M25.41- ☑
    - specified joint NEC M25.48
    - wrist M25.43- ☑
  - malignant pleural J91.Ø
  - meninges — *see* Meningitis
  - pericardium, pericardial (noninflammatory) I31.39
    - acute — *see* Pericarditis, acute
    - malignant, in disease classified elsewhere I31.31
    - specified type, NEC I31.39
  - peritoneal (chronic) R18.8
  - pleura, pleurisy, pleuritic, pleuropericardial J9Ø
    - chylous, chyliform J94.Ø
    - due to systemic lupus erythematosis M32.13
- **Effusion** — *continued*
  - pleura, pleurisy, pleuritic, pleuropericardial — *continued*
    - in conditions classified elsewhere J91.8
    - influenzal — *see* Influenza, with, respiratory manifestations NEC
    - malignant J91.Ø
    - newborn P28.89
    - tuberculous NEC A15.6
      - primary (progressive) A15.7
  - spinal — *see* Meningitis
  - thorax, thoracic — *see* Effusion, pleura
- **Egg shell nails** L6Ø.3
  - congenital Q84.6
- **EGPA** (eosinophilic granulomatosis with polyangiitis) M3Ø.1
- **Egyptian splenomegaly** B65.1
- **Ehlers-Danlos syndrome** — *see also* Syndrome, Ehlers-Danlos Q79.6Ø
- **Ehrlichiosis** A77.4Ø
  - due to
    - E. chafeensis A77.41
    - E. ewingii A77.49
    - E. muris euclairensis A77.49
    - E. sennetsu A79.81
    - specified organism NEC A77.49
- **Eichstedt's disease** B36.Ø
- **Eisenmenger's**
  - complex or syndrome I27.83
  - defect Q21.8
- **Ejaculation**
  - delayed F52.32
  - painful N53.12
  - premature F52.4
  - retarded N53.11
  - retrograde N53.14
  - semen, painful N53.12
    - psychogenic F52.6
- **Ekbom's syndrome** (restless legs) G25.81
- **Ekman's syndrome** (brittle bones and blue sclera) Q78.Ø
- **Elastic skin** Q82.8
  - acquired L57.4
- **Elastofibroma** — *see* Neoplasm, connective tissue, benign
- **Elastoma** (juvenile) Q82.8
  - Miescher's L87.2
- **Elastomyofibrosis** I42.4
- **Elastosis**
  - actinic, solar L57.8
  - atrophicans (senile) L57.4
  - perforans serpiginosa L87.2
  - senilis L57.4
- **Elbow** — *see* condition
- **Electric current, electricity, effects** (concussion) (fatal) (nonfatal) (shock) T75.4 ☑
  - burn — *see* Burn
- **Electric feet syndrome** E53.8
- **Electrocution** T75.4 ☑
  - from electroshock gun (taser) T75.4 ☑
- **Electrolyte imbalance** E87.8
  - with
    - abortion — *see* Abortion by type, complicated by, electrolyte imbalance
    - ectopic pregnancy OØ8.5
    - molar pregnancy OØ8.5
- **Elephantiasis** (nonfilarial) I89.Ø
  - arabicum — *see* Infestation, filarial
  - bancroftian B74.Ø
  - congenital (any site) (hereditary) Q82.Ø
  - due to
    - Brugia (malayi) B74.1
      - timori B74.2
    - mastectomy I97.2
    - Wuchereria (bancrofti) B74.Ø
  - eyelid HØ2.859
    - left HØ2.856
      - lower HØ2.855
      - upper HØ2.854
    - right HØ2.853
      - lower HØ2.852
      - upper HØ2.851
  - filarial, filariensis — *see* Infestation, filarial
  - glandular I89.Ø
  - graecorum A3Ø.9
  - lymphangiectatic I89.Ø
  - lymphatic vessel I89.Ø
    - due to mastectomy I97.2
  - scrotum (nonfilarial) I89.Ø
- **Elephantiasis** — *continued*
  - streptococcal I89.Ø
  - surgical I97.89
    - postmastectomy I97.2
  - telangiectodes I89.Ø
  - vulva (nonfilarial) N9Ø.89
- **Elevated, elevation**
  - alanine transaminase (ALT) R74.Ø1
  - ALT (alanine transaminase) R74.Ø1
  - antibody titer R76.Ø
  - aspartate transaminase (AST) R74.Ø1
  - AST (aspartate transaminase) R74.Ø1
  - basal metabolic rate R94.8
  - blood pressure — *see also* Hypertension
    - reading (incidental) (isolated) (nonspecific), no diagnosis of hypertension RØ3.Ø
  - blood sugar R73.9
  - body temperature (of unknown origin) R5Ø.9
  - cancer antigen 125 [CA 125] R97.1
  - carcinoembryonic antigen [CEA] R97.Ø
  - cholesterol E78.ØØ
    - with high triglycerides E78.2
  - conjugate, eye H51.Ø
  - C-reactive protein (CRP) R79.82
  - diaphragm, congenital Q79.1
  - erythrocyte sedimentation rate R7Ø.Ø
  - fasting glucose R73.Ø1
  - fasting triglycerides E78.1
  - finding on laboratory examination — *see* Findings, abnormal, inconclusive, without diagnosis, by type of exam
  - GFR (glomerular filtration rate) — *see* Findings, abnormal, inconclusive, without diagnosis, by type of exam
  - glucose tolerance (oral) R73.Ø2
  - immunoglobulin level R76.8
  - indoleacetic acid R82.5
  - lactic acid dehydrogenase (LDH) level R74.Ø2
  - leukocytes D72.829
  - lipoprotein a (Lp(a)) level E78.41
  - liver function
    - study R94.5
    - test R79.89
      - alkaline phosphatase R74.8
      - aminotransferase R74.Ø1
      - bilirubin R17
      - hepatic enzyme R74.8
      - lactate dehydrogenase R74.Ø2
  - Lp(a) (lipoprotein(a)) E78.41
  - lymphocytes D72.82Ø
  - prostate specific antigen [PSA] R97.2Ø
  - Rh titer — *see* Complication(s), transfusion, incompatibility reaction, Rh (factor)
  - scapula, congenital Q74.Ø
  - sedimentation rate R7Ø.Ø
  - SGOT R74.Ø1
  - SGPT R74.Ø1
  - transaminase level R74.Ø1
  - triglycerides E78.1
    - with high cholesterol E78.2
  - troponin R79.89
  - tumor associated antigens [TAA] NEC R97.8
  - tumor specific antigens [TSA] NEC R97.8
  - urine level of
    - 17-ketosteroids R82.5
    - catecholamine R82.5
    - indoleacetic acid R82.5
    - steroids R82.5
    - vanillylmandelic acid (VMA) R82.5
  - venous pressure I87.8
  - white blood cell count D72.829
    - specified NEC D72.828
- **Elliptocytosis** (congenital) (hereditary) D58.1
  - Hb C (disease) D58.1
  - hemoglobin disease D58.1
  - sickle-cell (disease) D57.8- ☑
    - trait D57.3
- **Ellison-Zollinger syndrome** E16.4
- **Ellis-van Creveld syndrome** (chondroectodermal dysplasia) Q77.6
- **Elongated, elongation** (congenital) — *see also* Distortion
  - bone Q79.9
  - cervix (uteri) Q51.828
    - acquired N88.4
    - hypertrophic N88.4
  - colon Q43.8
  - common bile duct Q44.5

- **Embolism** — *continued*
  - spleen, splenic (artery) I74.8
  - upper extremity I74.2
  - vein (acute) I82.9Ø
    - antecubital I82.61- ☑
      - chronic I82.71- ☑
    - axillary I82.A1- ☑ (*following* I82.7)
      - chronic I82.A2- ☑ (*following* I82.7)
    - basilic I82.61- ☑
      - chronic I82.71- ☑
    - brachial I82.62- ☑
      - chronic I82.72- ☑
    - brachiocephalic (innominate) I82.29Ø
      - chronic I82.291
    - calf, muscle I82.46- ☑
      - chronic I82.56- ☑
    - cephalic I82.61- ☑
      - chronic I82.71- ☑
    - chronic I82.91
    - deep (DVT) I82.4Ø- ☑
      - calf I82.4Z- ☑
        - chronic I82.5Z- ☑
      - lower leg I82.4Z- ☑
        - chronic I82.5Z- ☑
      - thigh I82.4Y- ☑
        - chronic I82.5Y- ☑
      - upper leg I82.4Y ☑
        - chronic I82.5Y-
    - femoral I82.41- ☑
      - chronic I82.51- ☑
    - gastrocnemial I82.46- ☑
      - chronic I82.56- ☑
    - iliac (iliofemoral) I82.42- ☑
      - chronic I82.52- ☑
    - innominate I82.29Ø
      - chronic I82.291
    - internal jugular I82.C1- ☑ (*following* I82.7)
      - chronic I82.C2- ☑ (*following* I82.7)
    - lower extremity
      - deep I82.4Ø- ☑
        - chronic I82.5Ø- ☑
        - specified NEC I82.49- ☑
          - chronic NEC I82.59- ☑
      - distal
        - deep I82.4Z- ☑
      - proximal
        - deep I82.4Y- ☑
          - chronic I82.5Y- ☑
      - superficial I82.81- ☑
    - peroneal I82.45- ☑
      - chronic I82.55- ☑
    - popliteal I82.43- ☑
      - chronic I82.53- ☑
    - radial I82.62- ☑
      - chronic I82.72- ☑
    - renal I82.3
    - saphenous (greater) (lesser) I82.81- ☑
    - soleal I82.46- ☑
      - chronic I82.56- ☑
    - specified NEC I82.89Ø
      - chronic NEC I82.891
    - subclavian I82.B1- ☑ (*following* I82.7)
      - chronic I82.B2- ☑ (*following* I82.7)
    - thoracic NEC I82.29Ø
      - chronic I82.291
    - tibial I82.44- ☑
      - chronic I82.54- ☑
    - ulnar I82.62- ☑
      - chronic I82.72- ☑
    - upper extremity I82.6Ø- ☑
      - chronic I82.7Ø- ☑
      - deep I82.62- ☑
        - chronic I82.72- ☑
      - superficial I82.61- ☑
        - chronic I82.71- ☑
    - vena cava
      - inferior (acute) I82.22Ø
        - chronic I82.221
      - superior (acute) I82.21Ø
        - chronic I82.211
    - venous sinus GØ8
    - vessels of brain — *see* Occlusion, artery, cerebral
- **Embolus** — *see* Embolism
- **Embryoma** — *see also* Neoplasm, uncertain behavior, by site
  - benign — *see* Neoplasm, benign, by site
- **Embryoma** — *continued*
  - kidney C64.- ☑
  - liver C22.Ø
  - malignant — *see also* Neoplasm, malignant, by site
    - kidney C64.- ☑
    - liver C22.Ø
    - testis C62.9- ☑
      - descended (scrotal) C62.1- ☑
      - undescended C62.Ø- ☑
  - testis C62.9- ☑
    - descended (scrotal) C62.1- ☑
    - undescended C62.Ø- ☑
- **Embryonic**
  - circulation Q28.9
  - heart Q28.9
  - vas deferens Q55.4
- **Embryopathia NOS** Q89.9
- **Embryotoxon** Q13.4
- **Emesis** — *see* Vomiting
- **Emotional lability** R45.86
- **Emotionality, pathological** F6Ø.3
- **Emotogenic disease** — *see* Disorder, psychogenic
- **Emphysema** (atrophic) (bullous) (chronic) (interlobular) (lung) (obstructive) (pulmonary) (senile) (vesicular) J43.9
  - cellular tissue (traumatic) T79.7 ☑
    - surgical T81.82 ☑
  - centrilobular J43.2
  - compensatory J98.3
  - congenital (interstitial) P25.Ø
  - conjunctiva H11.89
  - connective tissue (traumatic) T79.7 ☑
    - surgical T81.82 ☑
  - due to chemicals, gases, fumes or vapors — *see also* Disease, respiratory, chronic, due to chemicals, gases, fumes or vapors J43- ☑
  - eyelid(s) — *see* Disorder, eyelid, specified type NEC
    - surgical T81.82 ☑
    - traumatic T79.7 ☑
  - interstitial J98.2
    - congenital P25.Ø
    - perinatal period P25.Ø
  - laminated tissue T79.7 ☑
    - surgical T81.82 ☑
  - mediastinal J98.2
    - newborn P25.2
  - orbit, orbital — *see* Disorder, orbit, specified type NEC
  - panacinar J43.1
  - panlobular J43.1
  - specified NEC J43.8
  - subcutaneous (traumatic) T79.7 ☑
    - nontraumatic J98.2
    - postprocedural T81.82 ☑
    - surgical T81.82 ☑
  - surgical T81.82 ☑
  - thymus (gland) (congenital) E32.8
  - traumatic (subcutaneous) T79.7 ☑
  - unilateral J43.Ø
- **Empty nest syndrome** Z6Ø.Ø
- **Empyema** (acute) (chest) (double) (pleura) (supradiaphragmatic) (thorax) J86.9
  - with fistula J86.Ø
  - accessory sinus (chronic) — *see* Sinusitis
  - antrum (chronic) — *see* Sinusitis, maxillary
  - brain (any part) — *see* Abscess, brain
  - ethmoidal (chronic) (sinus) — *see* Sinusitis, ethmoidal
  - extradural — *see* Abscess, extradural
  - frontal (chronic) (sinus) — *see* Sinusitis, frontal
  - gallbladder K81.Ø
  - mastoid (process) (acute) — *see* Mastoiditis, acute
  - maxilla, maxillary M27.2
    - sinus (chronic) — *see* Sinusitis, maxillary
  - nasal sinus (chronic) — *see* Sinusitis
  - sinus (accessory) (chronic) (nasal) — *see* Sinusitis
  - sphenoidal (sinus) (chronic) — *see* Sinusitis, sphenoidal
  - subarachnoid — *see* Abscess, extradural
  - subdural — *see* Abscess, subdural
  - tuberculous A15.6
  - ureter — *see* Ureteritis
  - ventricular — *see* Abscess, brain
- **En coup de sabre lesion** L94.1
- **Enamel pearls** KØØ.2
- **Enameloma** KØØ.2
- **Enanthema, viral** BØ9
- **Encephalitis** (chronic) (hemorrhagic) (idiopathic) (nonepidemic) (spurious) (subacute) GØ4.9Ø
  - acute — *see also* Encephalitis, viral A86
- **Encephalitis** — *continued*
  - acute — *see also* Encephalitis, viral — *continued*
    - disseminated GØ4.ØØ
      - infectious GØ4.Ø1
      - noninfectious GØ4.81
      - postimmunization (postvaccination) GØ4.Ø2
      - postinfectious GØ4.Ø1
    - inclusion body A85.8
    - necrotizing hemorrhagic GØ4.3Ø
      - postimmunization GØ4.32
      - postinfectious GØ4.31
      - specified NEC GØ4.39
  - arboviral, arbovirus NEC A85.2
  - arthropod-borne NEC (viral) A85.2
  - Australian A83.4
  - California (virus) A83.5
  - Central European (tick-borne) A84.1
  - Czechoslovakian A84.1
  - Dawson's (inclusion body) A81.1
  - diffuse sclerosing A81.1
  - disseminated, acute GØ4.ØØ
  - due to
    - cat scratch disease A28.1
    - human immunodeficiency virus (HIV) disease B2Ø *[GØ5.3]*
    - malaria — *see* Malaria
    - rickettsiosis — *see* Rickettsiosis
    - smallpox inoculation GØ4.Ø2
    - typhus — *see* Typhus
  - Eastern equine A83.2
  - endemic (viral) A86
  - epidemic NEC (viral) A86
  - equine (acute) (infectious) (viral) A83.9
    - Eastern A83.2
    - Venezuelan A92.2
    - Western A83.1
  - Far Eastern (tick-borne) A84.Ø
  - following vaccination or other immunization procedure GØ4.Ø2
  - herpes zoster BØ2.Ø
  - herpesviral BØØ.4
    - due to herpesvirus 6 B1Ø.Ø1
    - due to herpesvirus 7 B1Ø.Ø9
    - specified NEC B1Ø.Ø9
  - Ilheus (virus) A83.8
  - in (due to)
    - actinomycosis A42.82
    - adenovirus A85.1
    - African trypanosomiasis B56.9 *[GØ5.3]*
    - Chagas' disease (chronic) B57.42
    - cytomegalovirus B25.8
    - enterovirus A85.Ø
    - herpes (simplex) virus BØØ.4
      - due to herpesvirus 6 B1Ø.Ø1
      - due to herpesvirus 7 B1Ø.Ø9
      - specified NEC B1Ø.Ø9
    - infectious disease NEC B99 ☑ *[GØ5.3]*
    - influenza — *see* Influenza, with, encephalopathy
    - listeriosis A32.12
    - measles BØ5.Ø
    - mumps B26.2
    - naegleriasis B6Ø.2
    - parasitic disease NEC B89 *[GØ5.3]*
    - poliovirus A8Ø.9 *[GØ5.3]*
    - rubella BØ6.Ø1
    - syphilis
      - congenital A5Ø.42
      - late A52.14
    - systemic lupus erythematosus M32.19 *[GØ5.3]*
    - toxoplasmosis (acquired) B58.2
      - congenital P37.1
    - tuberculosis A17.82
    - zoster BØ2.Ø
  - inclusion body A81.1
  - infectious (acute) (virus) NEC A86
  - Japanese (B type) A83.Ø
  - La Crosse A83.5
  - lead — *see* Poisoning, lead
  - lethargica (acute) (infectious) A85.8
  - louping ill A84.89
  - lupus erythematosus, systemic M32.19 *[GØ5.3]*
  - lymphatica A87.2
  - Mengo A85.8
  - meningococcal A39.81
  - Murray Valley A83.4
  - otitic NEC H66.4Ø *[GØ5.3]*
  - parasitic NOS B71.9
  - periaxial G37.Ø

Encephalitis — *continued*
- periaxialis (concentrica) (diffuse) G37.5
- postchickenpox B01.11
- postexanthematous NEC B09
- postimmunization G04.02
- postinfectious NEC G04.01
- postmeasles B05.0
- postvaccinal G04.02
- postvaricella B01.11
- postviral NEC A86
- Powassan A84.81
- Rasmussen G04.81
- Rio Bravo A85.8
- Russian
  - autumnal A83.0
  - spring-summer (taiga) A84.0
- saturnine — *see* Poisoning, lead
- specified NEC G04.81
- St. Louis A83.3
- subacute sclerosing A81.1
- summer A83.0
- suppurative G04.81
- tick-borne A84.9
- Torula, torular (cryptococcal) B45.1
- toxic NEC G92.8
- trichinosis B75 *[G05.3]*
- type
  - B A83.0
  - C A83.3
- van Bogaert's A81.1
- Venezuelan equine A92.2
- Vienna A85.8
- viral, virus A86
  - arthropod-borne NEC A85.2
    - mosquito-borne A83.9
      - Australian X disease A83.4
      - California virus A83.5
      - Eastern equine A83.2
      - Japanese (B type) A83.0
      - Murray Valley A83.4
      - specified NEC A83.8
      - St. Louis A83.3
      - type B A83.0
      - type C A83.3
      - Western equine A83.1
    - tick-borne A84.9
      - biundulant A84.1
      - central European A84.1
      - Czechoslovakian A84.1
      - diphasic meningoencephalitis A84.1
      - Far Eastern A84.0
      - Russian spring-summer (taiga) A84.0
      - specified NEC A84.89
  - specified type NEC A85.8
  - tick-borne, specified NEC A84.89
- Western equine A83.1

Encephalocele Q01.9
- frontal Q01.0
- nasofrontal Q01.1
- occipital Q01.2
- specified NEC Q01.8

Encephalocystocele — *see* Encephalocele

Encephaloduroarteriomyosynangiosis (EDAMS) I67.5

Encephalomalacia (brain) (cerebellar) (cerebral) — *see* Softening, brain

Encephalomeningitis — *see* Meningoencephalitis

Encephalomeningocele — *see* Encephalocele

Encephalomeningomyelitis — *see* Meningoencephalitis

Encephalomyelitis — *see also* Encephalitis G04.90
- acute disseminated G04.00
  - infectious G04.01
  - noninfectious G04.81
  - postimmunization G04.02
  - postinfectious G04.01
- acute necrotizing hemorrhagic G04.30
  - postimmunization G04.32
  - postinfectious G04.31
  - specified NEC G04.39
- equine A83.9
  - Eastern A83.2
  - Venezuelan A92.2
  - Western A83.1
- in diseases classified elsewhere G05.3
- myalgic G93.32
  - chronic fatigue syndrome [ME/CFS] G93.32
- postchickenpox B01.11
- postinfectious NEC G04.01
- postmeasles B05.0

Encephalomyelitis — *continued*
- postvaccinal G04.02
- postvaricella B01.11
- rubella B06.01
- specified NEC G04.81
- Venezuelan equine A92.2

Encephalomyelocele — *see* Encephalocele

Encephalomyelomeningitis — *see* Meningoencephalitis

Encephalomyelopathy G96.9

Encephalomyeloradiculitis (acute) G61.0

Encephalomyeloradiculoneuritis (acute) (Guillain-Barre) G61.0

Encephalomyeloradiculopathy G96.9

Encephalopathia hyperbilirubinemica, newborn P57.9
- due to isoimmunization (conditions in P55) P57.0

Encephalopathy (acute) G93.40
- acute necrotizing hemorrhagic G04.30
  - postimmunization G04.32
  - postinfectious G04.31
  - specified NEC G04.39
- alcoholic G31.2
- anoxic — *see* Damage, brain, anoxic
- arteriosclerotic I67.2
- centrolobar progressive (Schilder) G37.0
- congenital Q07.9
- degenerative, in specified disease NEC G32.89
- demyelinating callosal G37.1
- due to
  - drugs — *see also* Table of Drugs and Chemicals G92.8
- hepatic (without coma) K76.82
- hyperbilirubinemic, newborn P57.9
  - due to isoimmunization (conditions in P55) P57.0
- hypertensive I67.4
- hypoglycemic E16.2
- hypoxic — *see* Damage, brain, anoxic
- hypoxic ischemic P91.60
  - mild P91.61
  - moderate P91.62
  - severe P91.63
- in (due to) (with)
  - birth injury P11.1
  - hyperinsulinism E16.1 *[G94]*
  - influenza — *see* Influenza, with, encephalopathy
  - lack of vitamin — *see also* Deficiency, vitamin E56.9 *[G32.89]*
  - neoplastic disease — *see also* Neoplasm D49.9 *[G13.1]*
  - serum — *see also* Reaction, serum T80.69 ☑
  - syphilis A52.17
  - trauma (postconcussional) F07.81
    - current injury — *see* Injury, intracranial
  - vaccination G04.02
- lead — *see* Poisoning, lead
- metabolic G93.41
  - drug induced G92.8
  - toxic G92.8
- myoclonic, early, symptomatic — *see* Epilepsy, generalized, specified NEC
- necrotizing, subacute (Leigh) G31.82
- neonatal P91.819
  - in diseases classified elsewhere P91.811
- pellagrous E52 *[G32.89]*
- portal-systemic K76.82
- postcontusional F07.81
  - current injury — *see* Injury, intracranial, diffuse
- posthypoglycemic (coma) E16.1 *[G94]*
- postradiation G93.89
- saturnine — *see* Poisoning, lead
- septic G93.41
- specified NEC G93.49
- spongioform, subacute (viral) A81.09
- toxic G92.9
  - metabolic G92.8
- traumatic (postconcussional) F07.81
  - current injury — *see* Injury, intracranial
- vitamin B deficiency NEC E53.9 *[G32.89]*
  - vitamin B1 E51.2
- Wernicke's E51.2

Encephalorrhagia — *see* Hemorrhage, intracranial, intracerebral

Encephalosis, posttraumatic F07.81

Enchondroma — *see also* Neoplasm, bone, benign

Enchondromatosis (cartilaginous) (multiple) Q78.4

Encopresis R15.9
- functional F98.1
- nonorganic origin F98.1

Encopresis — *continued*
- psychogenic F98.1

Encounter (with health service) (for) Z76.89
- adjustment and management (of)
  - breast implant Z45.81 ☑
  - implanted device NEC Z45.89
  - myringotomy device (stent) (tube) Z45.82
  - neurostimulator (brain) (gastric) (peripheral nerve) (sacral nerve) (spinal cord) (vagus nerve) Z45.42
- administrative purpose only Z02.9
  - examination for
    - adoption Z02.82
    - armed forces Z02.3
    - child welfare Z02.84
    - disability determination Z02.71
    - driving license Z02.4
    - employment Z02.1
    - insurance Z02.6
    - medical certificate NEC Z02.79
    - paternity testing Z02.81
    - residential institution admission Z02.2
    - school admission Z02.0
    - sports Z02.5
  - specified reason NEC Z02.89
- aftercare — *see* Aftercare
- antenatal screening Z36.9
  - cervical length Z36.86
  - chromosomal anomalies Z36.0
  - congenital cardiac abnormalities Z36.83
  - elevated maternal serum alphafetoprotein Z36.1
  - fetal growth retardation Z36.4
  - fetal lung maturity Z36.84
  - fetal macrosomia Z36.88
  - hydrops fetalis Z36.81
  - intrauterine growth restriction (IUGR) /small-for-dates Z36.4
  - isoimmunization Z36.5
  - large-for-dates Z36.88
  - malformations Z36.3
  - non-visualized anatomy on a previous scan Z36.2
  - nuchal translucency Z36.82
  - raised alphafetoprotein level Z36.1
  - risk of pre-term labor Z36.86
  - specified follow-up NEC Z36.2
  - specified genetic defects NEC Z36.8A
  - specified type NEC Z36.89
  - Streptococcus B Z36.85
  - suspected anomaly Z36.3
  - uncertain dates Z36.87
- assisted reproductive fertility procedure cycle Z31.83
- blood typing Z01.83
  - Rh typing Z01.83
- breast augmentation or reduction Z41.1
- breast implant exchange (different material) (different size) Z45.81 ☑
- breast reconstruction following mastectomy Z42.1
- check-up — *see* Examination
- chemotherapy for neoplasm Z51.11
- child welfare screening exam Z02.84
- colonoscopy, screening Z12.11
- counseling — *see* Counseling
- delivery, full-term, uncomplicated O80
  - cesarean, without indication O82
- desensitization to allergens Z51.6
- ear piercing Z41.3
- examination — *see* Examination
- expectant parent(s) (adoptive) pre-birth pediatrician visit Z76.81
- fertility preservation procedure (prior to cancer therapy) (prior to removal of gonads) Z31.84
- fitting (of) — *see* Fitting (and adjustment) (of)
- genetic
  - counseling
    - nonprocreative Z71.83
    - procreative Z31.5
  - testing — *see* Test, genetic
- hearing conservation and treatment Z01.12
- HIV
  - pre-exposure prophylaxis Z29.81
  - PrEP Z29.81
- immunotherapy for neoplasm Z51.12
- in vitro fertilization cycle Z31.83
- instruction (in)
  - child care (postpartal) (prenatal) Z32.3
  - childbirth Z32.2
  - natural family planning
    - procreative Z31.61

- **Encounter** — *continued*
  - instruction — *continued*
    - natural family planning — *continued*
      - to avoid pregnancy Z3Ø.Ø2
  - insulin pump titration Z46.81
  - joint prosthesis insertion following prior explantation of joint prosthesis (staged procedure)
    - hip Z47.32
    - knee Z47.33
    - shoulder Z47.31
  - laboratory (as part of a general medical examination) ZØØ.ØØ
    - with abnormal findings ZØØ.Ø1
  - mental health services (for)
    - abuse NEC
      - perpetrator Z69.82
      - victim Z69.81
    - child abuse
      - nonparental
        - perpetrator Z69.Ø21
        - victim Z69.Ø2Ø
      - parental
        - perpetrator Z69.Ø11
        - victim Z69.Ø1Ø
    - child neglect
      - nonparental
        - perpetrator Z69.Ø21
        - victim Z69.Ø2Ø
      - parental
        - perpetrator Z69.Ø11
        - victim Z69.Ø1Ø
    - child psychological abuse
      - nonparental
        - perpetrator Z69.Ø21
        - victim Z69.Ø2Ø
      - parental
        - perpetrator Z69.Ø11
        - victim Z69.Ø1Ø
    - child sexual abuse
      - nonparental
        - perpetrator Z69.Ø21
        - victim Z69.Ø2Ø
      - parental
        - perpetrator Z69.Ø11
        - victim Z69.Ø1Ø
    - non-spousal adult abuse
      - perpetrator Z69.82
      - victim Z69.81
    - spousal or partner
      - abuse
        - perpetrator Z69.12
        - victim Z69.11
      - neglect
        - perpetrator Z69.12
        - victim Z69.11
      - psychological abuse
        - perpetrator Z69.12
        - victim Z69.11
      - violence
        - perpetrator (physical) (sexual) Z69.12
        - victim (physical) Z69.11
          - sexual Z69.81
  - observation (for) (ruled out)
    - alarm, without findings
      - apnea ZØ3.83
      - bradycardia ZØ3.83
      - oximeter ZØ3.83
    - condition suspected related to home physiologic monitoring device ZØ3.83
      - newborn ZØ5.81
        - apnea alarm ZØ5.81
        - bradycardia alarm ZØ5.81
        - malfunction of home cardiorespiratory monitor ZØ5.81
        - non-specific findings home physiologic monitoring device ZØ5.81
        - pulse oximeter alarm without findings ZØ5.81
    - exposure to (suspected)
      - anthrax ZØ3.81Ø
      - biological agent NEC ZØ3.818
    - malfunction of home cardiorespiratory monitor ZØ3.83
    - non-specific findings home physiologic monitoring device ZØ3.83
  - pediatrician visit, by expectant parent(s) (adoptive) Z76.81
  - placental sample (taken vaginally) — *see also* Encounter, antenatal screening Z36.9

- **Encounter** — *continued*
  - plastic and reconstructive surgery following medical procedure or healed injury NEC Z42.8
  - postoperative — *see* Aftercare
  - pregnancy
    - supervision of — *see* Pregnancy, supervision of
    - test Z32.ØØ
      - result negative Z32.Ø2
      - result positive Z32.Ø1
  - procreative management and counseling for gestational carrier Z31.7
  - prophylactic measures Z29.9
    - antivenin Z29.12
    - fluoride administration Z29.3
    - HIV pre-exposure Z29.81
    - immunotherapy for respiratory syncytial virus (RSV) Z29.11
    - rabies immune globin Z29.14
    - Rho (D) immune globulin Z29.13
    - specified NEC Z29.89
  - radiation therapy (antineoplastic) Z51.Ø
  - radiological (as part of a general medical examination) ZØØ.ØØ
    - with abnormal findings ZØØ.Ø1
  - reconstructive surgery following medical procedure or healed injury NEC Z42.8
  - removal (of) — *see also* Removal
    - artificial
      - arm Z44.ØØ- ☑
        - complete Z44.Ø1- ☑
        - partial Z44.Ø2- ☑
      - eye Z44.2- ☑
      - leg Z44.1Ø- ☑
        - complete Z44.11- ☑
        - partial Z44.12- ☑
    - breast implant Z45.81 ☑
      - tissue expander (with or without synchronous insertion of permanent implant) Z45.81 ☑
    - device Z46.9
      - specified NEC Z46.89
    - external
      - fixation device — *code to* fracture with seventh character D
      - prosthesis, prosthetic device Z44.9
        - breast Z44.3- ☑
        - specified NEC Z44.8
    - implanted device NEC Z45.89
    - insulin pump Z46.81
    - internal fixation device Z47.2
    - myringotomy device (stent) (tube) Z45.82
    - nervous system device NEC Z46.2
      - brain neuropacemaker Z46.2
      - visual substitution device Z46.2
        - implanted Z45.31
    - non-vascular catheter Z46.82
    - orthodontic device Z46.4
    - stent
      - ureteral Z46.6
    - urinary device Z46.6
  - repeat cervical smear to confirm findings of recent normal smear following initial abnormal smear ZØ1.42
  - respirator [ventilator] use during power failure Z99.12
  - Rh typing ZØ1.83
  - screening — *see* Screening
  - specified NEC Z76.89
  - sterilization Z3Ø.2
  - suspected condition, ruled out
    - amniotic cavity and membrane ZØ3.71
    - cervical shortening ZØ3.75
    - fetal anomaly ZØ3.73
    - fetal growth ZØ3.74
    - maternal and fetal conditions NEC ZØ3.79
    - oligohydramnios ZØ3.71
    - placental problem ZØ3.72
    - polyhydramnios ZØ3.71
  - suspected exposure (to), ruled out
    - anthrax ZØ3.81Ø
    - biological agents NEC ZØ3.818
  - termination of pregnancy, elective Z33.2
  - testing — *see* Test
  - therapeutic drug level monitoring Z51.81
  - titration, insulin pump Z46.81
  - to determine fetal viability of pregnancy O36.8Ø ☑
  - training
    - insulin pump Z46.81
  - X-ray of chest (as part of a general medical examination) ZØØ.ØØ

- **Encounter** — *continued*
  - X-ray of chest — *continued*
    - with abnormal findings ZØØ.Ø1
- **Encystment** — *see* Cyst
- **Endarteritis** (bacterial, subacute) (infective) I77.6
  - brain I67.7
  - cerebral or cerebrospinal I67.7
  - deformans — *see* Arteriosclerosis
  - embolic — *see* Embolism
  - obliterans — *see also* Arteriosclerosis
    - pulmonary I28.8
  - pulmonary I28.8
  - retina — *see* Vasculitis, retina
  - senile — *see* Arteriosclerosis
  - syphilitic A52.Ø9
    - brain or cerebral A52.Ø4
    - congenital A5Ø.54 *[I79.8]*
  - tuberculous A18.89
- **Endemic** — *see* condition
- **Endocarditis** (chronic) (marantic) (nonbacterial) (thrombotic) (valvular) I38
  - with rheumatic fever (conditions in IØØ)
    - active — *see* Endocarditis, acute, rheumatic
    - inactive or quiescent (with chorea) IØ9.1
  - acute or subacute I33.9
    - infective I33.Ø
    - rheumatic (aortic) (mitral) (pulmonary) (tricuspid) IØ1.1
      - with chorea (acute) (rheumatic) (Sydenham's) IØ2.Ø
  - aortic (heart) (nonrheumatic) (valve) I35.8
    - with
      - mitral disease IØ8.Ø
        - with tricuspid (valve) disease IØ8.3
        - active or acute IØ1.1
          - with chorea (acute) (rheumatic) (Sydenham's) IØ2.Ø
      - rheumatic fever (conditions in IØØ)
        - active — *see* Endocarditis, acute, rheumatic
        - inactive or quiescent (with chorea) IØ6.9
      - tricuspid (valve) disease IØ8.2
        - with mitral (valve) disease IØ8.3
    - acute or subacute I33.9
    - arteriosclerotic I35.8
    - rheumatic IØ6.9
      - with mitral disease IØ8.Ø
        - with tricuspid (valve) disease IØ8.3
        - active or acute IØ1.1
          - with chorea (acute) (rheumatic) (Sydenham's) IØ2.Ø
      - active or acute IØ1.1
        - with chorea (acute) (rheumatic) (Sydenham's) IØ2.Ø
      - specified NEC IØ6.8
    - specified cause NEC I35.8
    - syphilitic A52.Ø3
  - arteriosclerotic I38
  - atypical verrucous (Libman-Sacks) M32.11
  - bacterial (acute) (any valve) (subacute) I33.Ø
  - candidal B37.6
  - congenital Q24.8
  - constrictive I33.Ø
  - Coxiella burnetii A78 *[I39]*
  - Coxsackie B33.21
  - due to
    - prosthetic cardiac valve T82.6 ☑
    - Q fever A78 *[I39]*
    - Serratia marcescens I33.Ø
    - typhoid (fever) AØ1.Ø2
  - gonococcal A54.83
  - infectious or infective (acute) (any valve) (subacute) I33.Ø
  - lenta (acute) (any valve) (subacute) I33.Ø
  - Libman-Sacks M32.11
  - listerial A32.82
  - Loffler's I42.3
  - malignant (acute) (any valve) (subacute) I33.Ø
  - meningococcal A39.51
  - mitral (chronic) (double) (fibroid) (heart) (inactive) (valve) (with chorea) IØ5.9
    - with
      - aortic (valve) disease IØ8.Ø
        - with tricuspid (valve) disease IØ8.3
        - active or acute IØ1.1
          - with chorea (acute) (rheumatic) (Sydenham's) IØ2.Ø
      - rheumatic fever (conditions in IØØ)
        - active — *see* Endocarditis, acute, rheumatic

- **Endocarditis** — *continued*
  - mitral — *continued*
    - with — *continued*
      - rheumatic fever — *continued*
        - inactive or quiescent (with chorea) I05.9
      - tricuspid (valve) disease I08.1
        - with aortic (valve) disease I08.3
    - active or acute I01.1
      - with chorea (acute) (rheumatic) (Sydenham's) I02.0
      - bacterial I33.0
    - arteriosclerotic I34.89
    - nonrheumatic I34.89
      - acute or subacute I33.9
    - specified NEC I05.8
  - monilial B37.6
  - multiple valves I08.9
    - specified disorders I08.8
  - mycotic (acute) (any valve) (subacute) I33.0
  - pneumococcal (acute) (any valve) (subacute) I33.0
  - pulmonary (chronic) (heart) (valve) I37.8
    - with rheumatic fever (conditions in I00)
      - active — *see* Endocarditis, acute, rheumatic
      - inactive or quiescent (with chorea) I09.89
        - with aortic, mitral or tricuspid disease I08.8
    - acute or subacute I33.9
      - rheumatic I01.1
        - with chorea (acute) (rheumatic) (Sydenham's) I02.0
    - arteriosclerotic I37.8
    - congenital Q22.2
    - rheumatic (chronic) (inactive) (with chorea) I09.89
      - active or acute I01.1
        - with chorea (acute) (rheumatic) (Sydenham's) I02.0
    - syphilitic A52.03
  - purulent (acute) (any valve) (subacute) I33.0
  - Q fever A78 *[I39]*
  - rheumatic (chronic) (inactive) (with chorea) I09.1
    - active or acute (aortic) (mitral) (pulmonary) (tricuspid) I01.1
      - with chorea (acute) (rheumatic) (Sydenham's) I02.0
  - rheumatoid — *see* Rheumatoid, carditis
  - septic (acute) (any valve) (subacute) I33.0
  - streptococcal (acute) (any valve) (subacute) I33.0
  - subacute — *see* Endocarditis, acute
  - suppurative (acute) (any valve) (subacute) I33.0
  - syphilitic A52.03
  - toxic I33.9
  - tricuspid (chronic) (heart) (inactive) (rheumatic) (valve) (with chorea) I07.9
    - with
      - aortic (valve) disease I08.2
        - mitral (valve) disease I08.3
      - mitral (valve) disease I08.1
        - aortic (valve) disease I08.3
      - rheumatic fever (conditions in I00)
        - active — *see* Endocarditis, acute, rheumatic
        - inactive or quiescent (with chorea) I07.8
    - active or acute I01.1
      - with chorea (acute) (rheumatic) (Sydenham's) I02.0
    - arteriosclerotic I36.8
    - nonrheumatic I36.8
      - acute or subacute I33.9
    - specified cause, except rheumatic I36.8
  - tuberculous — *see* Tuberculosis, endocarditis
  - typhoid A01.02
  - ulcerative (acute) (any valve) (subacute) I33.0
  - vegetative (acute) (any valve) (subacute) I33.0
  - verrucous (atypical) (nonbacterial) (nonrheumatic) M32.11
- **Endocardium, endocardial** — *see also* condition
  - cushion defect Q21.20
- **Endocervicitis** — *see also* Cervicitis
  - due to intrauterine (contraceptive) device T83.69 ☑
  - hyperplastic N72
- **Endocrine** — *see* condition
- **Endocrinopathy, pluriglandular** E31.9
- **Endodontic**
  - overfill M27.52
  - underfill M27.53
- **Endodontitis** K04.01
  - irreversible K04.02
  - reversible K04.01
- **Endomastoiditis** — *see* Mastoiditis
- **Endometrioma** N80.12- ☑
- **Endometriosis** N80.9
  - abdomen, abdominal N80.C0
    - specified site, NEC N80.C9
    - wall N80.C19
      - fascia and muscular layers N80.C11
      - subcutaneous tissue N80.C10
      - unspecified depth N80.C19
  - appendix N80.549
    - deep N80.542
    - superficial N80.541
  - bladder (unspecified depth) N80.A0
    - deep N80.A2
    - superficial N80.A1
  - bowel N80.50
  - broad ligament N80.3C ☑
  - cardiothoracic space N80.B6
  - cecum N80.539
    - deep N80.532
    - superficial N80.531
  - cervix N80.0- ☑
  - colon N80.559
    - descending N80.559
      - deep N80.552
      - superficial N80.551
    - sigmoid N80.529
      - deep N80.522
      - superficial N80.521
    - transverse N80.559
      - deep N80.552
      - superficial N80.551
  - cul-de-sac (Douglas')
    - anterior (unspecified depth) N80.319
      - deep N80.312
      - superficial N80.311
    - posterior (unspecified depth) N80.329
      - deep N80.322
      - superficial N80.321
  - deep
    - involving muscular wall of fallopian tube N80.22 ☑
    - retrocervical N80.02
  - diaphragm N80.B39
    - deep N80.B32
    - superficial N80.B31
    - unspecified depth N80.B39
  - exocervix N80.01
  - extra-pelvic abdominal peritoneum N80.C4
  - fallopian tube (unspecified depth) N80.20- ☑
    - deep N80.22- ☑
    - superficial N80.21- ☑
  - female genital organ NEC N80.8
  - gallbladder N80.8
  - in scar of skin N80.6
  - inguinal canal N80.C3
  - internal N80.02
  - intestine N80.50
    - small N80.569
      - deep (multifocal) N80.562
      - superficial N80.561
  - lung N80.B2
  - mediastinal space N80.B5
  - myometrium N80.03
  - nerve
    - femoral N80.D6
    - obturator N80.D3
    - pelvic N80.D0
      - splanchnic N80.D1
    - pudendal N80.D5
    - retroperitoneum, NEC N80.D9
    - sacral splanchnic N80.D1
    - sciatic N80.D4
    - specified, NEC N80.D9
  - ovary (unspecified depth) N80.10- ☑
    - deep N80.12- ☑
    - superficial N80.11- ☑
  - parametrium N80.399
  - pelvic
    - brim N80.38- ☑
      - deep N80.37- ☑
      - superficial N80.36- ☑
    - peritoneum N80.30
      - specified sites, NEC N80.399
        - deep N80.392
        - superficial N80.391
    - sidewall N80.35- ☑
      - deep N80.34- ☑
      - superficial N80.33- ☑
  - pericardial space N80.B4
  - peritoneal (pelvic) N80.30
- **Endometriosis** — *continued*
  - pleura N80.B1
  - rectovaginal septum N80.40
    - with involvement of vagina N80.42
    - without involvement of vagina N80.41
  - rectum N80.519
    - deep (multifocal) N80.512
    - superficial N80.511
  - retroperitoneum N80.30
  - round ligament N80.3C9
  - sacral nerve roots N80.D2
  - skin (scar) N80.6
  - specified site NEC N80.8
  - stromal D39.0
  - thorax N80.B- ☑
  - umbilicus N80.C2
  - ureter N80.A69
    - deep N80.A5- ☑
    - extrinsic N80.A4- ☑
    - intrinsic N80.A5- ☑
    - superficial N80.A4- ☑
    - unspecified depth N80.A6- ☑
  - uterosacral ligament(s) N80.3C- ☑
    - deep N80.3B- ☑
    - superficial N80.3A- ☑
  - uterus N80.00
    - deep N80.02
    - internal N80.02
    - superficial N80.01
  - vagina N80.42
  - vulva N80.8
- **Endometritis** (decidual) (nonspecific) (purulent) (senile) (atrophic) (suppurative) N71.9
  - with ectopic pregnancy O08.0
  - acute N71.0
  - blenorrhagic (gonococcal) (acute) (chronic) A54.24
  - cervix, cervical (with erosion or ectropion) — *see also* Cervicitis
    - hyperplastic N72
  - chlamydial A56.11
  - chronic N71.1
  - following
    - abortion — *see* Abortion by type complicated by genital infection
    - ectopic or molar pregnancy O08.0
  - gonococcal, gonorrheal (acute) (chronic) A54.24
  - hyperplastic — *see also* Hyperplasia, endometrial N85.00
    - cervix N72
  - puerperal, postpartum, childbirth O86.12
  - subacute N71.0
  - tuberculous A18.17
- **Endometrium** — *see* condition
- **Endomyocardiopathy, South African** I42.3
- **Endomyocarditis** — *see* Endocarditis
- **Endomyofibrosis** I42.3
- **Endomyometritis** — *see* Endometritis
- **Endopericarditis** — *see* Endocarditis
- **Endoperineuritis** — *see* Disorder, nerve
- **Endophlebitis** — *see* Phlebitis
- **Endophthalmia** — *see* Endophthalmitis, purulent
- **Endophthalmitis** (acute) (infective) (metastatic) (subacute) H44.009
  - bleb associated — *see also* Bleb, inflamed (infected), postprocedural H59.4 ☑
  - gonorrheal A54.39
  - in (due to)
    - cysticercosis B69.1
    - onchocerciasis B73.01
    - toxocariasis B83.0
  - panuveitis — *see* Panuveitis
  - parasitic H44.12- ☑
  - purulent H44.00- ☑
    - panophthalmitis — *see* Panophthalmitis
    - vitreous abscess H44.02- ☑
  - specified NEC H44.19
  - sympathetic — *see* Uveitis, sympathetic
- **Endosalpingioma** D28.2
- **Endosalpingiosis** N94.89
- **Endosteitis** — *see* Osteomyelitis
- **Endothelioma, bone** — *see* Neoplasm, bone, malignant
- **Endotheliosis** (hemorrhagic infectional) D69.8
- **Endotoxemia** — code to condition
- **Endotrachelitis** — *see* Cervicitis
- **Engelmann** (-Camurati) **syndrome** Q78.3
- **English disease** — *see* Rickets
- **Engman's disease** L30.3

Enterocolitis — *continued*
- granulomatous — *see* Enteritis, regional
- hemorrhagic (acute) — *see also* Ischemia, intestine, acute K55.059
  - chronic K55.1
- infectious NEC A09
- ischemic K55.9
- necrotizing K55.30
  - with
    - perforation K55.33
    - pneumatosis K55.32
      - and perforation K55.33
  - due to Clostridium difficile
    - not specified as recurrent A04.72
    - recurrent A04.71
  - in non-newborn K55.30
    - stage 1 (without pneumatosis, without perforation) K55.31
    - stage 2 (with pneumatosis, without perforation) K55.32
    - stage 3 (with pneumatosis, with perforation) K55.33
  - in newborn P77.9
    - stage 1 (without pneumatosis, without perforation) P77.1
    - stage 2 (with pneumatosis, without perforation) P77.2
    - stage 3 (with pneumatosis, with perforation) P77.3
  - without pneumatosis or perforation K55.31
- noninfectious K52.9
  - newborn — *see* Enterocolitis, necrotizing, in newborn
- pseudomembranous (newborn)
  - not specified as recurrent A04.72
  - recurrent A04.71
- radiation K52.0
  - newborn — *see* Enterocolitis, necrotizing, in newborn
- ulcerative (chronic) — *see* Pancolitis, ulcerative (chronic)

Enterogastritis — *see* Enteritis

Enteropathy K63.9
- celiac-gluten-sensitive K90.0
  - non-celiac K90.41
- food protein-induced K52.22
- hemorrhagic, terminal — *see also* Ischemia, intestine, acute K55.059
- protein-losing K90.49

Enteroperitonitis — *see* Peritonitis

Enteroptosis K63.4

Enterorrhagia K92.2

Enterospasm — *see also* Syndrome, irritable, bowel
- psychogenic F45.8

Enterostenosis — *see also* Obstruction, intestine, specified NEC K56.699

Enterostomy
- complication — *see* Complication, enterostomy
- status Z93.4

Enterovirus, as cause of disease classified elsewhere B97.10
- coxsackievirus B97.11
- echovirus B97.12
- other specified B97.19

Enthesopathy (peripheral) M77.9
- Achilles tendinitis — *see* Tendinitis, Achilles
- ankle and tarsus M77.5- ☑
  - specified type NEC — *see* Enthesopathy, foot, specified type NEC
- anterior tibial syndrome M76.81- ☑
- calcaneal spur — *see* Spur, bone, calcaneal
- elbow region M77.8
  - lateral epicondylitis — *see* Epicondylitis, lateral
  - medial epicondylitis — *see* Epicondylitis, medial
- foot NEC M77.8
  - metatarsalgia — *see* Metatarsalgia
  - specified type NEC M77.5- ☑
- forearm M77.8
- gluteal tendinitis — *see* Tendinitis, gluteal
- hand M77.8
- hip — *see* Enthesopathy, lower limb, specified type NEC
- iliac crest spur — *see* Spur, bone, iliac crest
- iliotibial band syndrome — *see* Syndrome, iliotibial band
- knee — *see* Enthesopathy, lower limb, lower leg, specified type NEC
- lateral epicondylitis — *see* Epicondylitis, lateral

Enthesopathy — *continued*
- lower limb (excluding foot) M76.9
  - Achilles tendinitis — *see* Tendinitis, Achilles
  - ankle and tarsus M77.5- ☑
    - specified type NEC — *see* Enthesopathy, foot, specified type NEC
  - anterior tibial syndrome M76.81- ☑
  - gluteal tendinitis — *see* Tendinitis, gluteal
  - iliac crest spur — *see* Spur, bone, iliac crest
  - iliotibial band syndrome — *see* Syndrome, iliotibial band
  - patellar tendinitis — *see* Tendinitis, patellar
  - pelvic region — *see* Enthesopathy, lower limb, specified type NEC
  - peroneal tendinitis — *see* Tendinitis, peroneal
  - posterior tibial syndrome M76.82- ☑
  - psoas tendinitis — *see* Tendinitis, psoas
  - specified type NEC M76.89- ☑
  - tibial collateral bursitis — *see* Bursitis, tibial collateral
- medial epicondylitis — *see* Epicondylitis, medial
- metatarsalgia — *see* Metatarsalgia
- multiple sites M77.8
- patellar tendinitis — *see* Tendinitis, patellar
- pelvis M77.8
- periarthritis of wrist — *see* Periarthritis, wrist
- peroneal tendinitis — *see* Tendinitis, peroneal
- posterior tibial syndrome M76.82- ☑
- psoas tendinitis — *see* Tendinitis, psoas
- shoulder M77.8
- shoulder region — *see* Lesion, shoulder
- specified type NEC M77.8
- spinal M46.00
  - cervical region M46.02
  - cervicothoracic region M46.03
  - lumbar region M46.06
  - lumbosacral region M46.07
  - multiple sites M46.09
  - occipito-atlanto-axial region M46.01
  - sacrococcygeal region M46.08
  - thoracic region M46.04
  - thoracolumbar region M46.05
- tibial collateral bursitis — *see* Bursitis, tibial collateral
- upper arm M77.8
- wrist and carpus NEC M77.8
  - calcaneal spur — *see* Spur, bone, calcaneal
  - periarthritis of wrist — *see* Periarthritis, wrist

Entomophobia F40.218

Entomophthoromycosis B46.8

Entrance, air into vein — *see* Embolism, air

Entrapment
- muscle
  - eye
    - extraocular H50.68- ☑
    - oblique
      - inferior H50.62- ☑
      - superior H50.66- ☑
    - rectus
      - inferior H50.63- ☑
      - lateral H50.64- ☑
      - medial H50.65- ☑
      - superior H50.67- ☑
- nerve — *see* Neuropathy, entrapment

Entropion (eyelid) (paralytic) H02.009
- cicatricial H02.019
  - left H02.016
    - lower H02.015
    - upper H02.014
  - right H02.013
    - lower H02.012
    - upper H02.011
- congenital Q10.2
- left H02.006
  - lower H02.005
  - upper H02.004
- mechanical H02.029
  - left H02.026
    - lower H02.025
    - upper H02.024
  - right H02.023
    - lower H02.022
    - upper H02.021
- right H02.003
  - lower H02.002
  - upper H02.001
- senile H02.039
  - left H02.036

Entropion — *continued*
- senile — *continued*
  - left — *continued*
    - lower H02.035
    - upper H02.034
  - right H02.033
    - lower H02.032
    - upper H02.031
- spastic H02.049
  - left H02.046
    - lower H02.045
    - upper H02.044
  - right H02.043
    - lower H02.042
    - upper H02.041

Enucleated eye (traumatic, current) S05.7- ☑

Enuresis R32
- functional F98.0
- habit disturbance F98.0
- nocturnal N39.44
  - psychogenic F98.0
- nonorganic origin F98.0
- psychogenic F98.0

Eosinopenia — *see* Agranulocytosis

Eosinophilia (allergic) (idiopathic) (secondary) D72.10
- with
  - angiolymphoid hyperplasia (ALHE) D18.01
- familial D72.19
- hereditary D72.19
- in disease classified elsewhere D72.18
- infiltrative — *see* Eosinophilia, pulmonary
- Loffler's J82.89
- peritoneal — *see* Peritonitis, eosinophilic
- pulmonary NEC J82.89
  - acute J82.82
  - asthmatic J82.83
  - chronic J82.81
- specified NEC D72.19
- tropical (pulmonary) J82.89

Eosinophilia-myalgia syndrome M35.89

Ependymitis (acute) (cerebral) (chronic) (granular) — *see* Encephalomyelitis

Ependymoblastoma
- specified site — *see* Neoplasm, malignant, by site
- unspecified site C71.9

Ependymoma (epithelial) (malignant)
- anaplastic
  - specified site — *see* Neoplasm, malignant, by site
  - unspecified site C71.9
- benign
  - specified site — *see* Neoplasm, benign, by site
  - unspecified site D33.2
- myxopapillary D43.2
  - specified site — *see* Neoplasm, uncertain behavior, by site
  - unspecified site D43.2
- papillary D43.2
  - specified site — *see* Neoplasm, uncertain behavior, by site
  - unspecified site D43.2
- specified site — *see* Neoplasm, malignant, by site
- unspecified site C71.9

Ependymopathy G93.89

Ephelis, ephelides L81.2

Epiblepharon (congenital) Q10.3

Epicanthus, epicanthic fold (eyelid) (congenital) Q10.3

Epicondylitis (elbow)
- lateral M77.1- ☑
- medial M77.0- ☑

Epicystitis — *see* Cystitis

Epidemic — *see* condition

Epidermidalization, cervix — *see* Dysplasia, cervix

Epidermis, epidermal — *see* condition

Epidermodysplasia verruciformis B07.8

Epidermolysis
- bullosa (congenital) Q81.9
  - acquired L12.30
    - drug-induced L12.31
    - specified cause NEC L12.35
  - dystrophica Q81.2
  - letalis Q81.1
  - simplex Q81.0
  - specified NEC Q81.8
- necroticans combustiformis L51.2
  - due to drug — *see* Table of Drugs and Chemicals, by drug

Epidermophytid — *see* Dermatophytosis

Epidermophytosis (infected) — *see* Dermatophytosis

- **Epididymis** — *see* condition
- **Epididymitis** (acute) (nonvenereal) (recurrent) (residual) N45.1
  - with orchitis N45.3
  - blennorrhagic (gonococcal) A54.23
  - caseous (tuberculous) A18.15
  - chlamydial A56.19
  - filarial — *see also* Infestation, filarial B74.9 *[N51]*
  - gonococcal A54.23
  - syphilitic A52.76
  - tuberculous A18.15
- **Epididymo-orchitis** — *see also* Epididymitis N45.3
- **Epidural** — *see* condition
- **Epigastrium, epigastric** — *see* condition
- **Epigastrocele** — *see* Hernia, ventral
- **Epiglottis** — *see* condition
- **Epiglottitis, epiglottiditis** (acute) J05.10
  - with obstruction J05.11
  - chronic J37.0
- **Epignathus** Q89.4
- **Epilepsia partialis continua** — *see also* Kozhevnikof's epilepsy G40.1- ☑
- **Epilepsy, epileptic, epilepsia** (attack) (cerebral) (convulsion) (fit) (seizure) G40.909

> *Note: the following terms are to be considered equivalent to intractable: pharmacoresistant (pharmacologically resistant), treatment resistant, refractory (medically) and poorly controlled*

  - with
    - complex partial seizures — *see* Epilepsy, localization-related, symptomatic, with complex partial seizures
    - grand mal seizures on awakening — *see* Epilepsy, generalized, specified NEC
    - myoclonic absences — *see* Epilepsy, generalized, specified NEC
    - myoclonic-astatic seizures — *see* Epilepsy, generalized, specified NEC
    - simple partial seizures — *see* Epilepsy, localization-related, symptomatic, with simple partial seizures
  - akinetic — *see* Epilepsy, generalized, specified NEC
  - benign childhood with centrotemporal EEG spikes — *see* Epilepsy, localization-related, idiopathic
  - benign myoclonic in infancy G40.80- ☑
  - Bravais-jacksonian — *see* Epilepsy, localization-related, symptomatic, with simple partial seizures
  - childhood
    - with occipital EEG paroxysms — *see* Epilepsy, localization-related, idiopathic
    - absence G40.A09 (*following* G40.3)
      - intractable G40.A19 (*following* G40.3)
        - with status epilepticus G40.A11 (*following* G40.3)
        - without status epilepticus G40.A19 (*following* G40.3)
      - not intractable G40.A09 (*following* G40.3)
        - with status epilepticus G40.A01 (*following* G40.3)
        - without status epilepticus G40.A09 (*following* G40.3)
  - climacteric — *see* Epilepsy, specified NEC
  - cysticercosis B69.0
  - deterioration (mental) F06.8
  - due to syphilis A52.19
  - focal — *see* Epilepsy, localization-related, symptomatic, with simple partial seizures
  - generalized
    - idiopathic G40.309
      - intractable G40.319
        - with status epilepticus G40.311
        - without status epilepticus G40.319
      - not intractable G40.309
        - with status epilepticus G40.301
        - without status epilepticus G40.309
    - specified NEC G40.409
      - intractable G40.419
        - with status epilepticus G40.411
        - without status epilepticus G40.419
      - not intractable G40.409
        - with status epilepticus G40.401
        - without status epilepticus G40.409
  - impulsive petit mal — *see* Epilepsy, juvenile myoclonic
  - intractable G40.919
    - with status epilepticus G40.911
    - without status epilepticus G40.919
  - juvenile absence G40.A09 (*following* G40.3)

Epilepsy, epileptic, epilepsia — *continued*

  - juvenile absence — *continued*
    - intractable G40.A19 (*following* G40.3)
      - with status epilepticus G40.A11 (*following* G40.3)
      - without status epilepticus G40.A19 (*following* G40.3)
    - not intractable G40.A09 (*following* G40.3)
      - with status epilepticus G40.A01 (*following* G40.3)
      - without status epilepticus G40.A09 (*following* G40.3)
  - juvenile myoclonic G40.B09 (*following* G40.3)
    - intractable G40.B19 (*following* G40.3)
      - with status epilepticus G40.B11 (*following* G40.3)
      - without status epilepticus G40.B19 (*following* G40.3)
    - not intractable G40.B09 (*following* G40.3)
      - with status epilepticus G40.B01 (*following* G40.3)
      - without status epilepticus G40.B09 (*following* G40.3)
  - Lafora progressive myoclonus — *see also* Epilepsy, progressive, Lafora G40.C09
  - localization-related (focal) (partial)
    - idiopathic G40.009
      - with seizures of localized onset G40.009
        - intractable G40.019
          - with status epilepticus G40.011
          - without status epilepticus G40.019
        - not intractable G40.009
          - with status epilepticus G40.001
          - without status epilepticus G40.009
    - symptomatic
      - with complex partial seizures G40.209
        - intractable G40.219
          - with status epilepticus G40.211
          - without status epilepticus G40.219
        - not intractable G40.209
          - with status epilepticus G40.201
          - without status epilepticus G40.209
      - with simple partial seizures G40.109
        - intractable G40.119
          - with status epilepticus G40.111
          - without status epilepticus G40.119
        - not intractable G40.109
          - with status epilepticus G40.101
          - without status epilepticus G40.109
  - myoclonus, myoclonic — *see also* Epilepsy, generalized, specified NEC
    - progressive — *see also* Epilepsy, generalized, idiopathic
      - Lafora G40.C09
        - intractable G40.C19
          - with status epilepticus G40.C11
          - without status epilepticus G40.C19
        - not intractable G40.C09
          - with status epilepticus G40.C01
          - without status epilepticus G40.C09
      - type 1 — *see* Epilepsy, generalized, idiopathic
      - type 2 — *see* Epilepsy, myoclonus, progressive, Lafora
    - severe, in infancy (SMEI) G40.83- ☑
  - not intractable G40.909
    - with status epilepticus G40.901
    - without status epilepticus G40.909
  - on awakening — *see* Epilepsy, generalized, specified NEC
  - parasitic NOS B71.9 *[G94]*
  - partial — *see* Epilepsy, localization-related, symptomatic, with simple partial seizures
  - partialis continua — *see also* Kozhevnikof's epilepsy G40.1- ☑
  - peripheral — *see* Epilepsy, specified NEC
  - polymorphic, in infancy (PMEI) G40.83- ☑
  - procursiva — *see* Epilepsy, localization-related, symptomatic, with simple partial seizures
  - progressive (familial) myoclonic — *see* Epilepsy, myoclonus, progressive
    - Lafora — *see also* Epilepsy, progressive, Lafora G40.C09
  - reflex — *see* Epilepsy, specified NEC
  - related to
    - alcohol G40.509
      - not intractable G40.509
        - with status epilepticus G40.501
        - without status epliepticus G40.509
    - drugs G40.509
      - not intractable G40.509
        - with status epilepticus G40.501
        - without status epliepticus G40.509

Epilepsy, epileptic, epilepsia — *continued*

  - related to — *continued*
    - external causes G40.509
      - not intractable G40.509
        - with status epilepticus G40.501
        - without status epliepticus G40.509
    - hormonal changes G40.509
      - not intractable G40.509
        - with status epilepticus G40.501
        - without status epliepticus G40.509
    - sleep deprivation G40.509
      - not intractable G40.509
        - with status epilepticus G40.501
        - without status epliepticus G40.509
    - stress G40.509
      - not intractable G40.509
        - with status epilepticus G40.501
        - without status epliepticus G40.509
  - somatomotor — *see* Epilepsy, localization-related, symptomatic, with simple partial seizures
  - somatosensory — *see* Epilepsy, localization-related, symptomatic, with simple partial seizures
  - spasms G40.822
    - intractable G40.824
      - with status epilepticus G40.823
      - without status epilepticus G40.824
    - not intractable G40.822
      - with status epilepticus G40.821
      - without status epilepticus G40.822
  - specified NEC G40.802
    - intractable G40.804
      - with status epilepticus G40.803
      - without status epilepticus G40.804
    - not intractable G40.802
      - with status epilepticus G40.801
      - without status epilepticus G40.802
  - syndromes
    - generalized
      - idiopathic G40.309
        - intractable G40.319
          - with status epilepticus G40.311
          - without status epilepticus G40.319
        - not intractable G40.309
          - with status epilepticus G40.301
          - without status epilepticus G40.309
      - specified NEC G40.409
        - intractable G40.419
          - with status epilepticus G40.411
          - without status epilepticus G40.419
        - not intractable G40.409
          - with status epilepticus G40.401
          - without status epilepticus G40.409
    - localization-related (focal) (partial)
      - idiopathic G40.009
        - with seizures of localized onset G40.009
          - intractable G40.019
            - with status epilepticus G40.011
            - without status epilepticus G40.019
          - not intractable G40.009
            - with status epilepticus G40.001
            - without status epilepticus G40.009
      - symptomatic
        - with complex partial seizures G40.209
          - intractable G40.219
            - with status epilepticus G40.211
            - without status epilepticus G40.219
          - not intractable G40.209
            - with status epilepticus G40.201
            - without status epilepticus G40.209
        - with simple partial seizures G40.109
          - intractable G40.119
            - with status epilepticus G40.111
            - without status epilepticus G40.119
          - not intractable G40.109
            - with status epilepticus G40.101
            - without status epilepticus G40.109
    - specified NEC G40.802
      - intractable G40.804
        - with status epilepticus G40.803
        - without status epilepticus G40.804
      - not intractable G40.802
        - with status epilepticus G40.801
        - without status epilepticus G40.802
  - tonic (-clonic) — *see* Epilepsy, generalized, specified NEC
  - twilight F05
  - uncinate (gyrus) — *see* Epilepsy, localization-related, symptomatic, with complex partial seizures

- **Erythrocytosis** (megalosplenic) (secondary) D75.1
  - familial D75.Ø
  - oval, hereditary — *see* Elliptocytosis
  - secondary D75.1
  - stress D75.1
- **Erythroderma** (secondary) — *see also* Erythema L53.9
  - bullous ichthyosiform, congenital Q8Ø.3
  - desquamativum L21.1
  - ichthyosiform, congenital (bullous) Q8Ø.3
  - neonatorum P83.88
  - psoriaticum L4Ø.8
- **Erythrodysesthesia, palmar plantar** (PPE) L27.1
- **Erythrogenesis imperfecta** D61.Ø9
- **Erythroleukemia** C94.Ø- ☑
- **Erythromelalgia** I73.81
- **Erythrophagocytosis** D75.89
- **Erythrophobia** F4Ø.298
- **Erythroplakia, oral epithelium, and tongue** K13.29
- **Erythroplasia** (Queyrat) DØ7.4
  - specified site — *see* Neoplasm, skin, in situ
  - unspecified site DØ7.4
- **Escherichia coli** (E. coli), **as cause of disease classified elsewhere** B96.2Ø
  - non-O157 Shiga toxin-producing (with known O group) B96.22
  - non-Shiga toxin-producing B96.29
  - O157 B96.21
  - O157 with confirmation of Shiga toxin when H antigen is unknown, or is not H7 B96.21
  - O157:H- (nonmotile) with confirmation of Shiga toxin B96.21
  - O157:H7 with or without confirmation of Shiga toxin-production B96.21
    - specified NEC B96.22
  - Shiga toxin-producing (with unspecified O group) (STEC) B96.23
  - specified NEC B96.29
- **Esophagismus** K22.4
- **Esophagitis** (acute) (alkaline) (chemical) (chronic) (infectional) (necrotic) (peptic) (postoperative) (without bleeding) K2Ø.9Ø
  - with bleeding K2Ø.91
  - candidal B37.81
  - due to gastrointestinal reflux disease (without bleeding) K21.ØØ
    - with bleeding K21.Ø1
  - eosinophilic K2Ø.Ø
  - reflux K21.ØØ
    - with bleeding K21.Ø1
  - specified NEC (without bleeding) K2Ø.8Ø
    - with bleeding K2Ø.81
  - tuberculous A18.83
  - ulcerative K22.1Ø
    - with bleeding K22.11
- **Esophagocele** K22.5
- **Esophagomalacia** K22.89
- **Esophagospasm** K22.4
- **Esophagostenosis** K22.2
- **Esophagostomiasis** B81.8
- **Esophagotracheal** — *see* condition
- **Esophagus** — *see* condition
- **Esophoria** H5Ø.51
  - convergence, excess H51.12
  - divergence, insufficiency H51.8
- **Esotropia** — *see* Strabismus, convergent concomitant
- **Espundia** B55.2
- **Essential** — *see* condition
- **Esthesioneuroblastoma** C3Ø.Ø
- **Esthesioneurocytoma** C3Ø.Ø
- **Esthesioneuroepithelioma** C3Ø.Ø
- **Esthiomene** A55
- **Estivo-autumnal malaria** (fever) B5Ø.9
- **Estrangement** (marital) Z63.5
  - parent-child NEC Z62.89Ø
- **Estriasis** — *see* Myiasis
- **Ethanolism** — *see* Alcoholism
- **Etherism** — *see* Dependence, drug, inhalant
- **Ethmoid, ethmoidal** — *see* condition
- **Ethmoiditis** (chronic) (nonpurulent) (purulent) — *see also* Sinusitis, ethmoidal
  - influenzal — *see* Influenza, with, respiratory manifestations NEC
  - Woakes' J33.1
- **Ethylism** — *see* Alcoholism
- **Eulenburg's disease** (congenital paramyotonia) G71.19
- **Eumycetoma** B47.Ø
- **Eunuchoidism** E29.1
- **Eunuchoidism** — *continued*
  - hypogonadotropic E23.Ø
- **European blastomycosis** — *see* Cryptococcosis
- **Eustachian** — *see* condition
- **Evaluation** (for) (of)
  - development state
    - adolescent ZØØ.3
    - period of
      - delayed growth in childhood ZØØ.7Ø
        - with abnormal findings ZØØ.71
      - rapid growth in childhood ZØØ.2
    - puberty ZØØ.3
  - growth and developmental state (period of rapid growth) ZØØ.2
    - delayed growth ZØØ.7Ø
      - with abnormal findings ZØØ.71
  - mental health (status) ZØØ.8
    - requested by authority ZØ4.6
  - period of
    - delayed growth in childhood ZØØ.7Ø
      - with abnormal findings ZØØ.71
    - rapid growth in childhood ZØØ.2
  - suspected condition — *see* Observation
- **Evans syndrome** D69.41
- **Event**
  - apparent life threatening in newborn and infant (ALTE) R68.13
  - brief resolved unexplained event (BRUE) R68.13
- **Eventration** — *see also* Hernia, ventral
  - colon into chest — *see* Hernia, diaphragm
  - diaphragm (congenital) Q79.1
- **Eversion**
  - bladder N32.89
  - cervix (uteri) N86
    - with cervicitis N72
  - foot NEC — *see also* Deformity, valgus, ankle
    - congenital Q66.6
  - punctum lacrimale (postinfectional) (senile) HØ4.52- ☑
  - ureter (meatus) N28.89
  - urethra (meatus) N36.8
  - uterus N81.4
- **Evidence**
  - cytologic
    - of malignancy on anal smear R85.614
    - of malignancy on cervical smear R87.614
    - of malignancy on vaginal smear R87.624
- **Evisceration**
  - birth injury P15.8
  - traumatic NEC
    - eye — *see* Enucleated eye
- **Evulsion** — *see* Avulsion
- **Ewing's sarcoma or tumor** — *see* Neoplasm, bone, malignant
- **Examination** (for) (following) (general) (of) (routine) ZØØ.ØØ
  - with abnormal findings ZØØ.Ø1
  - abuse, physical (alleged), ruled out
    - adult ZØ4.71
    - child ZØ4.72
  - adolescent (development state) ZØØ.3
  - alleged rape or sexual assault (victim), ruled out
    - adult ZØ4.41
    - child ZØ4.42
  - allergy ZØ1.82
  - annual (adult) (periodic) (physical) ZØØ.ØØ
    - with abnormal findings ZØØ.Ø1
    - gynecological ZØ1.419
      - with abnormal findings ZØ1.411
  - antibody response ZØ1.84
  - blood — *see* Examination, laboratory
  - blood pressure ZØ1.3Ø
    - with abnormal findings ZØ1.31
  - cancer staging — *see* Neoplasm, malignant, by site
  - cervical Papanicolaou smear Z12.4
    - as part of routine gynecological examination ZØ1.419
      - with abnormal findings ZØ1.411
  - child (over 28 days old) ZØØ.129
    - with abnormal findings ZØØ.121
    - under 28 days old — *see* Newborn, examination
  - clinical research control or normal comparison (control) (participant) ZØØ.6
  - contraceptive (drug) maintenance (routine) Z3Ø.8
    - device (intrauterine) Z3Ø.431
  - dental ZØ1.2Ø
    - with abnormal findings ZØ1.21
  - developmental — *see* Examination, child
  - donor (potential) ZØØ.5
- **Examination** — *continued*
  - ear ZØ1.1Ø
    - with abnormal findings NEC ZØ1.118
  - eye ZØ1.ØØ
    - with abnormal findings ZØ1.Ø1
    - following failed vision screening ZØ1.Ø2Ø
      - with abnormal findings ZØ1.Ø21
  - follow-up (routine) (following) ZØ9
    - chemotherapy NEC ZØ9
      - malignant neoplasm ZØ8
    - fracture ZØ9
    - malignant neoplasm ZØ8
    - postpartum Z39.2
    - psychotherapy ZØ9
    - radiotherapy NEC ZØ9
      - malignant neoplasm ZØ8
    - surgery NEC ZØ9
      - malignant neoplasm ZØ8
  - following
    - accident NEC ZØ4.3
      - transport ZØ4.1
      - work ZØ4.2
    - assault, alleged, ruled out
      - adult ZØ4.71
      - child ZØ4.72
    - motor vehicle accident ZØ4.1
    - treatment (for) ZØ9
      - combined NEC ZØ9
        - fracture ZØ9
        - malignant neoplasm ZØ8
      - malignant neoplasm ZØ8
      - mental disorder ZØ9
      - specified condition NEC ZØ9
  - forced sexual exploitation ZØ4.81
  - forced labor exploitation ZØ4.82
  - gynecological ZØ1.419
    - with abnormal findings ZØ1.411
    - for contraceptive maintenance Z3Ø.8
  - health — *see* Examination, medical
  - hearing ZØ1.1Ø
    - with abnormal findings NEC ZØ1.118
    - following failed hearing screening ZØ1.11Ø
    - infant or child (over 28 days old) ZØØ.129
      - with abnormal findings ZØØ.121
  - immunity status testing ZØ1.84
  - laboratory (as part of a general medical examination) ZØØ.ØØ
    - with abnormal findings ZØØ.Ø1
    - preprocedural ZØ1.812
  - lactating mother Z39.1
  - medical (adult) (for) (of) ZØØ.ØØ
    - with abnormal findings ZØØ.Ø1
    - administrative purpose only ZØ2.9
      - specified NEC ZØ2.89
    - admission to
      - armed forces ZØ2.3
      - old age home ZØ2.2
      - prison ZØ2.89
      - residential institution ZØ2.2
      - school ZØ2.Ø
        - following illness or medical treatment ZØ2.Ø
      - summer camp ZØ2.89
    - adoption ZØ2.82
    - blood alcohol or drug level ZØ2.83
    - camp (summer) ZØ2.89
    - clinical research, normal subject (control) (participant) ZØØ.6
    - control subject in clinical research (normal comparison) (participant) ZØØ.6
    - donor (potential) ZØØ.5
    - driving license ZØ2.4
    - general (adult) ZØØ.ØØ
      - with abnormal findings ZØØ.Ø1
    - immigration ZØ2.89
    - insurance purposes ZØ2.6
    - marriage ZØ2.89
    - medicolegal reasons NEC ZØ4.89
    - naturalization ZØ2.89
    - participation in sport ZØ2.5
    - paternity testing ZØ2.81
    - population survey ZØØ.8
    - pre-employment ZØ2.1
    - pre-operative — *see* Examination, pre-procedural
    - pre-procedural
      - cardiovascular ZØ1.81Ø
      - respiratory ZØ1.811
      - specified NEC ZØ1.818
    - preschool children
      - for admission to school ZØ2.Ø

Examination — *continued*
- medical — *continued*
  - prisoners
    - for entrance into prison Z02.89
  - recruitment for armed forces Z02.3
  - specified NEC Z00.8
  - sport competition Z02.5
- medicolegal reason NEC Z04.89
  - following
    - forced sexual exploitation Z04.81
    - forced labor exploitation Z04.82
- newborn — *see* Newborn, examination
- pelvic (annual) (periodic) Z01.419
  - with abnormal findings Z01.411
- period of rapid growth in childhood Z00.2
- periodic (adult) (annual) (routine) Z00.00
  - with abnormal findings Z00.01
- physical (adult) — *see also* Examination, medical Z00.00
  - sports Z02.5
- postpartum
  - immediately after delivery Z39.0
  - routine follow-up Z39.2
- pre-chemotherapy (antineoplastic) Z01.818
- prenatal (normal pregnancy) — *see also* Pregnancy, normal Z34.9- ☑
- pre-procedural (pre-operative)
  - cardiovascular Z01.810
  - laboratory Z01.812
  - respiratory Z01.811
  - specified NEC Z01.818
- prior to chemotherapy (antineoplastic) Z01.818
- psychiatric NEC Z00.8
  - follow-up not needing further care Z09
  - requested by authority Z04.6
- radiological (as part of a general medical examination) Z00.00
  - with abnormal findings Z00.01
- repeat cervical smear to confirm findings of recent normal smear following initial abnormal smear Z01.42
- skin (hypersensitivity) Z01.82
- special — *see also* Examination, by type Z01.89
  - specified type NEC Z01.89
- specified type or reason NEC Z04.89
- teeth Z01.20
  - with abnormal findings Z01.21
- urine — *see* Examination, laboratory
- vision Z01.00
  - with abnormal findings Z01.01
  - following failed vision screening Z01.020
    - with abnormal findings Z01.021
  - infant or child (over 28 days old) Z00.129
    - with abnormal findings Z00.121

Exanthem, exanthema — *see also* Rash
- with enteroviral vesicular stomatitis B08.4
- Boston A88.0
- epidemic with meningitis A88.0 *[G02]*
- subitum B08.20
  - due to human herpesvirus 6 B08.21
  - due to human herpesvirus 7 B08.22
- viral, virus B09
  - specified type NEC B08.8

Excess, excessive, excessively
- alcohol level in blood R78.0
- androgen (ovarian) E28.1
- attrition, tooth, teeth K03.0
- carotene, carotin (dietary) E67.1
- cold, effects of T69.9 ☑
  - specified effect NEC T69.8 ☑
- convergence H51.12
- crying
  - in child, adolescent, or adult R45.83
  - in infant R68.11
- development, breast N62
- divergence H51.8
- drinking (alcohol) NEC (without dependence) F10.10
  - habitual (continual) (without remission) F10.20
- eating R63.2
- estrogen E28.0
- fat — *see also* Obesity
  - in heart — *see* Degeneration, myocardial
  - localized E65
- foreskin N47.8
- gas R14.0
- glucagon E16.3
- heat — *see* Heat
- intermaxillary vertical dimension of fully erupted teeth M26.37

Excess, excessive, excessively — *continued*
- interocclusal distance of fully erupted teeth M26.37
- kalium E87.5
- large
  - colon K59.39
    - congenital Q43.8
  - infant P08.0
  - organ or site, congenital NEC — *see* Anomaly, by site
- long
  - organ or site, congenital NEC — *see* Anomaly, by site
- menstruation (with regular cycle) N92.0
  - with irregular cycle N92.1
- napping Z72.821
- natrium E87.0
- number of teeth K00.1
- nutrient (dietary) NEC R63.2
- potassium (K) E87.5
- salivation K11.7
- secretion — *see also* Hypersecretion
  - milk O92.6
  - sputum R09.3
  - sweat R61
- sexual drive F52.8
- short
  - organ or site, congenital NEC — *see* Anomaly, by site
  - umbilical cord in labor or delivery O69.3 ☑
- skin L98.7
  - and subcutaneous tissue L98.7
  - eyelid (acquired) — *see* Blepharochalasis
    - congenital Q10.3
- sodium (Na) E87.0
- spacing of fully erupted teeth M26.32
- sputum R09.3
- sweating R61
- thirst R63.1
  - due to deprivation of water T73.1 ☑
- transportation time Z59.82
- tuberosity of jaw M26.07
- vitamin
  - A (dietary) E67.0
    - administered as drug (prolonged intake) — *see* Table of Drugs and Chemicals, vitamins, adverse effect
    - overdose or wrong substance given or taken — *see* Table of Drugs and Chemicals, vitamins, poisoning
  - D (dietary) E67.3
    - administered as drug (prolonged intake) — *see* Table of Drugs and Chemicals, vitamins, adverse effect
    - overdose or wrong substance given or taken — *see* Table of Drugs and Chemicals, vitamins, poisoning
- weight
  - gain R63.5
  - loss R63.4

Excitability, abnormal, under minor stress (personality disorder) F60.3

Excitation
- anomalous atrioventricular I45.6
- psychogenic F30.8
- reactive (from emotional stress, psychological trauma) F30.8

Excitement
- hypomanic F30.8
- manic F30.9
- mental, reactive (from emotional stress, psychological trauma) F30.8
- state, reactive (from emotional stress, psychological trauma) F30.8

Excoriation (traumatic) — *see also* Abrasion
- neurotic L98.1
- skin picking disorder F42.4

Exfoliation
- due to erythematous conditions according to extent of body surface involved L49.0
  - 10-19 percent of body surface L49.1
  - 20-29 percent of body surface L49.2
  - 30-39 percent of body surface L49.3
  - 40-49 percent of body surface L49.4
  - 50-59 percent of body surface L49.5
  - 60-69 percent of body surface L49.6
  - 70-79 percent of body surface L49.7
  - 80-89 percent of body surface L49.8
  - 90-99 percent of body surface L49.9

Exfoliation — *continued*
- due to erythematous conditions according to extent of body surface involved — *continued*
  - less than 10 percent of body surface L49.0
- teeth, due to systemic causes K08.0

Exfoliative — *see* condition

Exhaustion, exhaustive (physical NEC) R53.83
- battle F43.0
- cardiac — *see* Failure, heart
- delirium F43.0
- due to
  - cold T69.8 ☑
  - excessive exertion T73.3 ☑
  - exposure T73.2 ☑
  - neurasthenia F48.8
- heart — *see* Failure, heart
- heat — *see also* Heat, exhaustion T67.5 ☑
  - due to
    - salt depletion T67.4 ☑
    - water depletion T67.3 ☑
- maternal, complicating delivery O75.81
- mental F48.8
- myocardium, myocardial — *see* Failure, heart
- nervous F48.8
- old age R54
- psychogenic F48.8
- psychosis F43.0
- senile R54
- vital NEC Z73.0

Exhibitionism F65.2

Exocervicitis — *see* Cervicitis

Exomphalos Q79.2
- meaning hernia — *see* Hernia, umbilicus

Exophoria H50.52
- convergence, insufficiency H51.11
- divergence, excess H51.8

Exophthalmos H05.2- ☑
- congenital Q15.8
- constant NEC H05.24- ☑
- displacement, globe — *see* Displacement, globe
- due to thyrotoxicosis (hyperthyroidism) — *see* Hyperthyroidism, with, goiter (diffuse)
- dysthyroid — *see* Hyperthyroidism, with, goiter (diffuse)
- goiter — *see* Hyperthyroidism, with, goiter (diffuse)
- intermittent NEC H05.25- ☑
- malignant — *see* Hyperthyroidism, with, goiter (diffuse)
- orbital
  - edema — *see* Edema, orbit
  - hemorrhage — *see* Hemorrhage, orbit
- pulsating NEC H05.26- ☑
- thyrotoxic, thyrotropic — *see* Hyperthyroidism, with, goiter (diffuse)

Exostosis — *see also* Disorder, bone
- cartilaginous — *see* Neoplasm, bone, benign
- congenital (multiple) Q78.6
- external ear canal H61.81- ☑
- gonococcal A54.49
- jaw (bone) M27.8
- multiple, congenital Q78.6
- orbit H05.35- ☑
- osteocartilaginous — *see* Neoplasm, bone, benign
- syphilitic A52.77

Exotropia — *see* Strabismus, divergent concomitant

Explanation of
- investigation finding Z71.2
- medication Z71.89

Exploitation
- labor
  - confirmed
    - adult forced T74.61 ☑
    - child forced T74.62 ☑
  - suspected
    - adult forced T76.61 ☑
    - child forced T76.62 ☑
- sexual
  - confirmed
    - adult forced T74.51 ☑
    - child T74.52 ☑
  - suspected
    - adult forced T76.51 ☑
    - child T76.52 ☑

Exposure (to) — *see also* Contact, with T75.89 ☑
- acariasis Z20.7
- AIDS virus Z20.6
- air pollution Z77.110
- algae and algae toxins Z77.121

- **Exposure** — *continued*
  - algae bloom Z77.121
  - anthrax Z20.810
  - aromatic amines Z77.020
  - aromatic (hazardous) compounds NEC Z77.028
  - aromatic dyes NOS Z77.028
  - arsenic Z77.010
  - asbestos Z77.090
  - bacterial disease NEC Z20.818
  - benzene Z77.021
  - blue-green algae bloom Z77.121
  - body fluids (potentially hazardous) Z77.21
  - brown tide Z77.121
  - chemicals (chiefly nonmedicinal) (hazardous) NEC Z77.098
  - cholera Z20.09
  - chromium compounds Z77.018
  - cold, effects of T69.9 ☑
    - specified effect NEC T69.8 ☑
  - communicable disease Z20.9
    - bacterial NEC Z20.818
    - specified NEC Z20.89
    - viral NEC Z20.828
    - Zika virus Z20.821
  - coronavirus (disease) (novel) 2019 Z20.822
  - COVID-19 Z20.822
  - cyanobacteria bloom Z77.121
  - disaster Z65.5
  - discrimination Z60.5
  - dyes Z77.098
  - effects of T73.9 ☑
  - environmental tobacco smoke (acute) (chronic) Z77.22
  - Escherichia coli (E. coli) Z20.01
  - exhaustion due to T73.2 ☑
  - fiberglass — *see* Table of Drugs and Chemicals, fiberglass
  - German measles Z20.4
  - gonorrhea Z20.2
  - hazardous metals NEC Z77.018
  - hazardous substances NEC Z77.29
  - hazards in the physical environment NEC Z77.128
  - hazards to health NEC Z77.9
  - human immunodeficiency virus (HIV) Z20.6
  - human T-lymphotropic virus type-1 (HTLV-1) Z20.89
  - implanted
    - mesh — *see* Complications, prosthetic device or implant, mesh
    - prosthetic materials NEC — *see* Complications, prosthetic materials NEC
  - infestation (parasitic) NEC Z20.7
  - intestinal infectious disease NEC Z20.09
    - Escherichia coli (E. coli) Z20.01
  - lead Z77.011
  - meningococcus Z20.811
  - mold (toxic) Z77.120
  - nickel dust Z77.018
  - noise Z77.122
  - occupational
    - air contaminants NEC Z57.39
    - dust Z57.2
    - environmental tobacco smoke Z57.31
    - extreme temperature Z57.6
    - noise Z57.0
    - radiation Z57.1
    - risk factors Z57.9
      - specified NEC Z57.8
    - toxic agents (gases) (liquids) (solids) (vapors) in agriculture Z57.4
    - toxic agents (gases) (liquids) (solids) (vapors) in industry NEC Z57.5
    - vibration Z57.7
  - parasitic disease NEC Z20.7
  - pediculosis Z20.7
  - persecution Z60.5
  - pfiesteria piscicida Z77.121
  - poliomyelitis Z20.89
  - pollution
    - air Z77.110
    - environmental NEC Z77.118
    - soil Z77.112
    - water Z77.111
  - polycyclic aromatic hydrocarbons Z77.028
  - prenatal (drugs) (toxic chemicals) — *see* Newborn, affected by, noxious substances transmitted via placenta or breast milk
  - rabies Z20.3
  - radiation, naturally occurring NEC Z77.123
  - radon Z77.123

- **Exposure** — *continued*
  - red tide (Florida) Z77.121
  - rubella Z20.4
  - SARS-CoV-2 Z20.822
  - second hand tobacco smoke (acute) (chronic) Z77.22
    - in the perinatal period P96.81
  - sexually-transmitted disease Z20.2
  - smallpox (laboratory) Z20.89
  - syphilis Z20.2
  - terrorism Z65.4
  - torture Z65.4
  - tuberculosis Z20.1
  - uranium Z77.012
  - varicella Z20.820
  - venereal disease Z20.2
  - viral disease NEC Z20.828
  - war Z65.5
  - water pollution Z77.111
  - Zika virus Z20.821
- **Exsanguination** — *see* Hemorrhage
- **Exstrophy**
  - abdominal contents Q45.8
  - bladder Q64.10
    - cloacal Q64.12
    - specified type NEC Q64.19
    - supravesical fissure Q64.11
- **Extensive** — *see* condition
- **Extra** — *see also* Accessory
  - marker chromosomes (normal individual) Q92.61
    - in abnormal individual Q92.62
  - rib Q76.6
    - cervical Q76.5
- **Extrasystoles** (supraventricular) I49.49
  - atrial I49.1
  - auricular I49.1
  - junctional I49.2
  - ventricular I49.3
- **Extrauterine gestation or pregnancy** — *see* Pregnancy, by site
- **Extravasation**
  - blood R58
  - chyle into mesentery I89.8
  - pelvicalyceal N13.8
  - pyelosinus N13.8
  - urine (from ureter) R39.0
  - vesicant agent
    - antineoplastic chemotherapy T80.810 ☑
    - other agent NEC T80.818 ☑
- **Extremity** — *see* condition, limb
- **Extrophy** — *see* Exstrophy
- **Extroversion**
  - bladder Q64.19
  - uterus N81.4
    - complicating delivery O71.2
    - postpartal (old) N81.4
- **Extruded tooth** (teeth) M26.34
- **Extrusion**
  - breast implant (prosthetic) T85.42 ☑
  - eye implant (globe) (ball) T85.328 ☑
  - intervertebral disc — *see* Displacement, intervertebral disc
  - ocular lens implant (prosthetic) — *see* Complications, intraocular lens
  - vitreous — *see* Prolapse, vitreous
- **Exudate**
  - causing irritant dermatitis L24.A9
  - pleural — *see* Effusion, pleura
  - retina H35.89
  - wound fluids causing irritant dermatitis L24.A9
- **Exudative** — *see* condition
- **Eye, eyeball, eyelid** — *see* condition
- **Eyestrain** — *see* Disturbance, vision, subjective
- **Eyeworm disease of Africa** B74.3

F

- **Faber's syndrome** (achlorhydric anemia) D50.9
- **Fabry (-Anderson) disease** E75.21
- **Facet syndrome** M47.89- ☑
- **Faciocephalalgia, autonomic** — *see also* Neuropathy, peripheral, autonomic G90.09
- **Factor**(s)
  - psychic, associated with diseases classified elsewhere F54
  - psychological
    - affecting physical conditions F54
    - or behavioral
      - affecting general medical condition F54

- **Factor**(s) — *continued*
  - psychological — *continued*
    - or behavioral — *continued*
      - associated with disorders or diseases classified elsewhere F54
- **Fahr disease** (of brain) G23.8
- **Fahr Volhard disease** (of kidney) I12.- ☑
- **Failure, failed**
  - abortion — *see* Abortion, attempted
  - aortic (valve) I35.8
    - rheumatic I06.8
  - attempted abortion — *see* Abortion, attempted
  - biventricular I50.82
    - due to left heart failure I50.814
  - bone marrow — *see* Anemia, aplastic
  - cardiac — *see* Failure, heart
  - cardiorenal (chronic) — *see also* Failure, renal, and Failure, heart I50.9
    - hypertensive I13.2
  - cardiorespiratory — *see also* Failure, heart R09.2
  - cardiovascular (chronic) — *see* Failure, heart
  - cerebrovascular I67.9
  - cervical dilatation in labor O62.0
  - circulation, circulatory (peripheral) R57.9
    - newborn P29.89
  - compensation — *see* Disease, heart
  - compliance with medical treatment or regimen — *see* Noncompliance
  - congestive — *see* Failure, heart, congestive
  - dental implant (endosseous) M27.69
    - due to
      - failure of dental prosthesis M27.63
      - lack of attached gingiva M27.62
      - occlusal trauma (poor prosthetic design) M27.62
      - parafunctional habits M27.62
      - periodontal infection (peri-implantitis) M27.62
      - poor oral hygiene M27.62
    - osseointegration M27.61
      - due to
        - complications of systemic disease M27.61
        - poor bone quality M27.61
      - iatrogenic M27.61
    - post-osseointegration
      - biological M27.62
      - due to complications of systemic disease M27.62
      - iatrogenic M27.62
      - mechanical M27.63
    - pre-integration M27.61
    - pre-osseointegration M27.61
    - specified NEC M27.69
  - descent of head (at term) of pregnancy (mother) O32.4 ☑
  - endosseous dental implant — *see* Failure, dental implant
  - engagement of head (term of pregnancy) (mother) O32.4 ☑
  - erection (penile) — *see also* Dysfunction, sexual, male, erectile N52.9
    - nonorganic F52.21
  - examination(s), anxiety concerning Z55.2
  - expansion terminal respiratory units (newborn) (primary) P28.0
  - forceps NOS (with subsequent cesarean delivery) O66.5
  - gain weight (child over 28 days old) R62.51
    - adult R62.7
    - newborn P92.6
  - genital response (male) F52.21
    - female F52.22
  - heart (acute) (senile) (sudden) I50.9
    - with
      - acute pulmonary edema — *see* Failure, ventricular, left
      - decompensation I50.9
        - with
          - normal ejection fraction I50.33
          - preserved ejection fraction I50.33
          - reduced ejection fraction I50.23
            - with diastolic dysfunction I50.43
        - combined systolic and diastolic I50.43
        - diastolic I50.33
        - right I50.813
        - systolic I50.23
      - dilatation — *see* Disease, heart
      - hypertension — *see* Hypertension, heart
      - normal ejection fraction — *see* Failure, heart, diastolic
      - preserved ejection fraction — *see* Failure, heart, diastolic

- **Failure, failed** — *continued*
  - heart — *continued*
    - with — *continued*
      - reduced ejection fraction — *see* Failure, heart, systolic
    - arteriosclerotic I7Ø.9Ø
    - biventricular I5Ø.82
      - due to left heart failure I5Ø.814
    - combined left-right sided I5Ø.82
      - due to left heart failure I5Ø.814
    - compensated — *see also* Failure, heart, by type as diastolic or systolic, chronic I5Ø.9
    - complicating
      - anesthesia (general) (local) or other sedation
        - in labor and delivery O74.2
        - in pregnancy O29.12- ☑
        - postpartum, puerperal O89.1
      - delivery (cesarean) (instrumental) O75.4
    - congestive I5Ø.9
      - with rheumatic fever (conditions in IØØ)
        - active IØ1.8
        - inactive or quiescent (with chorea) IØ9.81
      - newborn P29.Ø
      - rheumatic (chronic) (inactive) (with chorea) IØ9.81
        - active or acute IØ1.8
          - with chorea IØ2.Ø
    - decompensated — *see also* Failure, heart, by type as diastolic or systolic, acute and chronic I5Ø.9
    - degenerative — *see* Degeneration, myocardial
    - diastolic (congestive) (left ventricular) I5Ø.3Ø
      - acute (congestive) I5Ø.31
        - and (on) chronic (congestive) I5Ø.33
      - chronic (congestive) I5Ø.32
        - and (on) acute (congestive) I5Ø.33
      - combined with systolic (congestive) I5Ø.4Ø
        - acute (congestive) I5Ø.41
          - and (on) chronic (congestive) I5Ø.43
        - chronic (congestive) I5Ø.42
          - and (on) acute (congestive) I5Ø.43
    - due to presence of cardiac prosthesis I97.13- ☑
    - end stage — *see also* Failure, heart, by type as diastolic or systolic, chronic I5Ø.84
    - following cardiac surgery I97.13- ☑
    - high output NOS I5Ø.83
    - hypertensive — *see* Hypertension, heart
    - left (ventricular) — *see also* Failure, ventricular, left
      - combined diastolic and systolic — *see* Failure, heart, diastolic, combined with systolic
      - diastolic — *see* Failure, heart, diastolic
      - systolic — *see* Failure, heart, systolic
    - low output (syndrome) NOS I5Ø.9
    - newborn P29.Ø
    - organic — *see* Disease, heart
    - peripartum O9Ø.3
    - postprocedural I97.13- ☑
    - rheumatic (chronic) (inactive) IØ9.9
    - right (isolated) (ventricular) I5Ø.81Ø
      - acute I5Ø.811
        - and (on) chronic I5Ø.813
      - chronic I5Ø.812
        - and acute I5Ø.813
      - secondary to left heart failure I5Ø.814
    - specified NEC I5Ø.89

> *Note: heart failure stages A, B, C, and D are based on the American College of Cardiology and American Heart Association stages of heart failure, which complement and should not be confused with the New York Heart Association Classification of Heart Failure, into Class I, Class II, Class III, and Class IV*

-
  -
    - stage A Z91.89
    - stage B — *see also* Failure, heart, by type as diastolic or systolic I5Ø.9
    - stage C — *see also* Failure, heart, by type as diastolic or systolic I5Ø.9
    - stage D — *see also* Failure, heart, by type as diastolic or systolic, chronic I5Ø.84
    - systolic (congestive) (left ventricular) I5Ø.2Ø
      - acute (congestive) I5Ø.21
        - and (on) chronic (congestive) I5Ø.23
      - chronic (congestive) I5Ø.22
        - and (on) acute (congestive) I5Ø.23
      - combined with diastolic (congestive) I5Ø.4Ø
        - acute (congestive) I5Ø.41
          - and (on) chronic (congestive) I5Ø.43
        - chronic (congestive) I5Ø.42
          - and (on) acute (congestive) I5Ø.43

- **Failure, failed** — *continued*
  - heart — *continued*
    - thyrotoxic — *see also* Thyrotoxicosis EØ5.9Ø *[I43]*
      - with
        - high output — *see also* Thyrotoxicosis I5Ø.83
        - thyroid storm EØ5.91 *[I43]*
          - high output — *see also* Thyrotoxicosis I5Ø.83
    - valvular — *see* Endocarditis
  - hepatic K72.9Ø
    - with coma K72.91
    - acute or subacute K72.1Ø
      - with coma K72.Ø1
      - due to drugs K71.1Ø
        - with coma K71.11
    - alcoholic (acute) (chronic) (subacute) K7Ø.4Ø
      - with coma K7Ø.41
    - chronic K72.1Ø
      - with coma K72.11
      - due to drugs (acute) (subacute) (chronic) K71.1Ø
        - with coma K71.11
    - due to drugs (acute) (subacute) (chronic) K71.1Ø
      - with coma K71.11
    - end stage K72.1Ø
      - with coma K72.11
    - postprocedural K91.82
  - hepatorenal K76.7
  - induction (of labor) O61.9
    - abortion — *see* Abortion, attempted
    - by
      - oxytocic drugs O61.Ø
      - prostaglandins O61.Ø
    - instrumental O61.1
    - mechanical O61.1
    - medical O61.Ø
    - specified NEC O61.8
    - surgical O61.1
  - intestinal failure K9Ø.83
  - intubation during anesthesia T88.4 ☑
    - in pregnancy O29.6- ☑
    - labor and delivery O74.7
    - postpartum, puerperal O89.6
  - involution, thymus (gland) E32.Ø
  - kidney — *see also* Disease, kidney, chronic N19
    - acute — *see also* Failure, renal, acute N17.9
  - lactation (complete) O92.3
    - partial O92.4
  - Leydig's cell, adult E29.1
  - liver — *see* Failure, hepatic
  - menstruation at puberty N91.Ø
  - mitral IØ5.8
  - myocardial, myocardium — *see also* Failure, heart I5Ø.9
    - chronic — *see also* Failure, heart, congestive I5Ø.9
    - congestive — *see also* Failure, heart, congestive I5Ø.9
  - newborn screening — *see* Abnormal, neonatal screening
    - neonatal congenital heart disease PØ9.5
  - orgasm (female) (psychogenic) F52.31
    - male F52.32
  - ovarian (primary) E28.39
    - iatrogenic E89.4Ø
      - asymptomatic E89.4Ø
      - symptomatic E89.41
    - postprocedural (postablative) (postirradiation) (postsurgical) E89.4Ø
      - asymptomatic E89.4Ø
      - symptomatic E89.41
  - ovulation causing infertility N97.Ø
  - polyglandular, autoimmune E31.Ø
  - prosthetic joint implant — *see* Complications, joint prosthesis, mechanical, breakdown, by site
  - renal N19
    - with
      - tubular necrosis (acute) N17.Ø
    - acute N17.9
      - with
        - cortical necrosis N17.1
        - medullary necrosis N17.2
        - tubular necrosis N17.Ø
      - specified NEC N17.8
    - chronic N18.9
      - hypertensive — *see* Hypertension, kidney
    - congenital P96.Ø
    - end stage (chronic) N18.6
      - due to hypertension I12.Ø

- **Failure, failed** — *continued*
  - renal — *continued*
    - following
      - abortion — *see* Abortion by type complicated by specified condition NEC
      - crushing T79.5 ☑
      - ectopic or molar pregnancy OØ8.4
      - labor and delivery (acute) O9Ø.49
    - hypertensive — *see* Hypertension, kidney
    - postprocedural N99.Ø
  - respiration, respiratory J96.9Ø
    - with
      - hypercapnia J96.92
      - hypercarbia J96.92
      - hypoxia J96.91
    - acute J96.ØØ
      - with
        - hypercapnia J96.Ø2
        - hypercarbia J96.Ø2
        - hypoxia J96.Ø1
    - center G93.89
    - acute and (on) chronic J96.2Ø
      - with
        - hypercapnia J96.22
        - hypercarbia J96.22
        - hypoxia J96.21
    - chronic J96.1Ø
      - with
        - hypercapnia J96.12
        - hypercarbia J96.12
        - hypoxia J96.11
    - newborn P28.5
    - postprocedural (acute) J95.821
      - acute and chronic J95.822
  - rotation
    - cecum Q43.3
    - colon Q43.3
    - intestine Q43.3
    - kidney Q63.2
  - sedation (conscious) (moderate) during procedure T88.52 ☑
    - history of Z92.83
  - segmentation — *see also* Fusion
    - fingers — *see* Syndactylism, complex, fingers
    - vertebra Q76.49
      - with scoliosis Q76.3
  - seminiferous tubule, adult E29.1
  - senile (general) R54
  - sexual arousal (male) F52.21
    - female F52.22
  - testicular endocrine function E29.1
  - to thrive (child over 28 days old) R62.51
    - adult R62.7
    - newborn P92.6
  - transplant T86.92
    - bone T86.831
      - marrow T86.Ø2
    - cornea T86.841- ☑
    - heart T86.22
      - with lung(s) T86.32
    - intestine T86.851
    - kidney T86.12
    - liver T86.42
    - lung(s) T86.811
      - with heart T86.32
    - pancreas T86.891
    - skin (allograft) (autograft) T86.821
    - specified organ or tissue NEC T86.891
    - stem cell (peripheral blood) (umbilical cord) T86.5
  - trial of labor (with subsequent cesarean delivery) O66.4Ø
    - following previous cesarean delivery O66.41
  - tubal ligation N99.89
  - urinary — *see* Disease, kidney, chronic
  - vacuum extraction NOS (with subsequent cesarean delivery) O66.5
  - vasectomy N99.89
  - ventouse NOS (with subsequent cesarean delivery) O66.5
  - ventricular — *see also* Failure, heart I5Ø.9
    - left — *see also* Failure, heart, left I5Ø.1
      - with rheumatic fever (conditions in IØØ)
        - active IØ1.8
          - with chorea IØ2.Ø
        - inactive or quiescent (with chorea) IØ9.81
      - rheumatic (chronic) (inactive) (with chorea) IØ9.81
        - active or acute IØ1.8

- **Failure, failed** — *continued*
  - ventricular — *see also* Failure, heart — *continued*
    - left — *see also* Failure, heart, left — *continued*
      - rheumatic — *continued*
        - active or acute — *continued*
          - with chorea IØ2.Ø
    - right — *see* Failure, heart, right
  - vital centers, newborn P91.88
- **Fainting** (fit) R55
- **Fallen arches** — *see* Deformity, limb, flat foot
- **Falling, falls** (repeated) R29.6
  - any organ or part — *see* Prolapse
- **Fallopian**
  - insufflation Z31.41
  - tube — *see* condition
- **Fallot's**
  - pentalogy Q21.8
  - tetrad or tetralogy Q21.3
  - triad or trilogy Q22.3
- **False** — *see also* condition
  - croup J38.5
  - joint — *see* Nonunion, fracture
  - labor (pains) O47.9
    - at or after 37 completed weeks of gestation O47.1
    - before 37 completed weeks of gestation O47.Ø- ☑
  - passage, urethra (prostatic) N36.5
  - pregnancy F45.8
- **Family, familial** — *see also* condition
  - disruption Z63.8
    - involving divorce or separation Z63.5
  - Li-Fraumeni (syndrome) Z15.Ø1
  - planning advice Z3Ø.Ø9
  - problem Z63.9
    - specified NEC Z63.8
  - retinoblastoma C69.2- ☑
- **Famine** (effects of) T73.Ø ☑
  - edema — *see* Malnutrition, severe
- **Fanconi** (-de Toni)(-Debre) **syndrome** E72.Ø9
  - with cystinosis E72.Ø4
- **Fanconi's anemia** (congenital pancytopenia) D61.Ø9
- **Farber's disease or syndrome** E75.29
- **Farcy** A24.Ø
- **Farmer's**
  - lung J67.Ø
  - skin L57.8
- **Farsightedness** — *see* Hypermetropia
- **Fascia** — *see* condition
- **Fasciculation** R25.3
- **Fasciitis** M72.9
  - diffuse (eosinophilic) M35.4
  - infective M72.8
    - necrotizing M72.6
  - necrotizing M72.6
  - nodular M72.4
  - perirenal (with ureteral obstruction) N13.5
    - with infection N13.6
  - plantar M72.2
  - specified NEC M72.8
  - traumatic (old) M72.8
    - current — *code by* site under Sprain
- **Fascioliasis** B66.3
- **Fasciolopsis, fasciolopsiasis** (intestinal) B66.5
- **Fascioscapulohumeral myopathy** G71.Ø2
- **Fast pulse** RØØ.Ø
- **Fat**
  - embolism — *see* Embolism, fat
  - excessive — *see also* Obesity
    - in heart — *see* Degeneration, myocardial
  - in stool R19.5
  - localized (pad) E65
    - heart — *see* Degeneration, myocardial
    - knee M79.4
    - retropatellar M79.4
  - necrosis
    - breast N64.1
    - mesentery K65.4
    - omentum K65.4
  - pad E65
    - knee M79.4
- **Fatigue** R53.83
  - auditory deafness — *see* Deafness
  - chronic R53.82
  - combat F43.Ø
  - general R53.83
    - psychogenic F48.8
  - heat (transient) T67.6 ☑
  - muscle M62.89
- **Fatigue** — *continued*
  - myocardium — *see* Failure, heart
  - neoplasm-related R53.Ø
  - nervous, neurosis F48.8
  - operational F48.8
  - psychogenic (general) F48.8
  - senile R54
  - voice R49.8
- **Fatness** — *see* Obesity
- **Fatty** — *see also* condition
  - apron E65
  - degeneration — *see* Degeneration, fatty
  - heart (enlarged) — *see* Degeneration, myocardial
  - liver NEC K76.Ø
    - alcoholic K7Ø.Ø
    - nonalcoholic K76.Ø
  - necrosis — *see* Degeneration, fatty
- **Fauces** — *see* condition
- **Fauchard's disease** (periodontitis) — *see* Periodontitis
- **Faucitis** JØ2.9
- **Favism** (anemia) D55.Ø
- **Favus** — *see* Dermatophytosis
- **Fazio-Londe disease or syndrome** G12.1
- **Fear complex or reaction** F4Ø.9
- **Fear of** — *see* Phobia
- **Feared complaint unfounded** Z71.1
- **Febris, febrile** — *see also* Fever
  - flava — *see also* Fever, yellow A95.9
  - melitensis A23.Ø
  - pestis — *see* Plague
  - recurrens — *see* Fever, relapsing
  - rubra A38.9
- **Fecal**
  - incontinence R15.9
  - smearing R15.1
  - soiling R15.1
  - urgency R15.2
- **Fecalith** (impaction) K56.41
  - appendix K38.1
  - congenital P76.8
- **Fede's disease** K14.Ø
- **Feeble rapid pulse due to shock following injury** T79.4 ☑
- **Feeble-minded** F7Ø
- **Feeding**
  - difficulties R63.3Ø
  - problem (elderly) (infant) R63.39
    - newborn P92.9
      - specified NEC P92.8
    - nonorganic (adult) — *see* Disorder, eating
- **Feeling** (of)
  - foreign body in throat RØ9.89
- **Feer's disease** — *see* Poisoning, mercury
- **Feet** — *see* condition
- **Feigned illness** Z76.5
- **Feil-Klippel syndrome** (brevicollis) Q76.1
- **Feinmesser's** (hidrotic) **ectodermal dysplasia** Q82.4
- **Felinophobia** F4Ø.218
- **Felon** — *see also* Cellulitis, digit
  - with lymphangitis — *see* Lymphangitis, acute, digit
- **Felty's syndrome** MØ5.ØØ
  - ankle MØ5.Ø7- ☑
  - elbow MØ5.Ø2- ☑
  - foot joint MØ5.Ø7- ☑
  - hand joint MØ5.Ø4- ☑
  - hip MØ5.Ø5- ☑
  - knee MØ5.Ø6- ☑
  - multiple site MØ5.Ø9
  - shoulder MØ5.Ø1- ☑
  - vertebra — *see* Spondylitis, ankylosing
  - wrist MØ5.Ø3- ☑
- **Female genital cutting status** — *see* Female genital mutilation status (FGM)
- **Female genital mutilation status** (FGM) N9Ø.81Ø
  - specified NEC N9Ø.818
  - type I (clitorectomy status) N9Ø.811
  - type II (clitorectomy with excision of labia minora status) N9Ø.812
  - type III (infibulation status) N9Ø.813
  - type IV N9Ø.818
- **Femur, femoral** — *see* condition
- **Fenestration, fenestrated** — *see also* Imperfect, closure
  - aortico-pulmonary Q21.4
  - atrial septum Q21.11
  - cusps, heart valve NEC Q24.8
    - pulmonary Q22.3
  - pulmonic cusps Q22.3
- **Fernell's disease** (aortic aneurysm) I71.9
- **Fertile eunuch syndrome** E23.Ø
- **Fetid**
  - breath R19.6
  - sweat L75.Ø
- **Fetishism** F65.Ø
  - transvestic F65.1
- **Fetus, fetal** — *see also* condition
  - alcohol syndrome (dysmorphic) Q86.Ø
  - compressus O31.Ø- ☑
  - hydantoin syndrome Q86.1
  - lung tissue P28.Ø
  - papyraceous O31.Ø- ☑
- **Fever** (inanition) (of unknown origin) (persistent) (with chills) (with rigor) R5Ø.9
  - abortus A23.1
  - Aden (dengue) A9Ø
  - African tick bite A77.8
  - African tick-borne A68.1
  - American
    - mountain (tick) A93.2
    - spotted A77.Ø
  - aphthous BØ8.8
  - arbovirus, arboviral A94
    - hemorrhagic A94
    - specified NEC A93.8
  - Argentinian hemorrhagic A96.Ø
  - Assam B55.Ø
  - Australian Q A78
  - Bangkok hemorrhagic A91
  - Barmah forest A92.8
  - Bartonella A44.Ø
  - bilious, hemoglobinuric B5Ø.8
  - blackwater B5Ø.8
  - blister BØØ.1
  - Bolivian hemorrhagic A96.1
  - Bonvale dam T73.3 ☑
  - boutonneuse A77.1
  - brain — *see* Encephalitis
  - Brazilian purpuric A48.4
  - breakbone A9Ø
  - Bullis A77.Ø
  - Bunyamwera A92.8
  - Burdwan B55.Ø
  - Bwamba A92.8
  - Cameroon — *see* Malaria
  - Canton A75.9
  - catarrhal (acute) JØØ
    - chronic J31.Ø
  - cat-scratch A28.1
  - Central Asian hemorrhagic A98.Ø
  - cerebral — *see* Encephalitis
  - cerebrospinal meningococcal A39.Ø
  - Chagres B5Ø.9
  - Chandipura A92.8
  - Changuinola A93.1
  - Charcot's (biliary) (hepatic) (intermittent) — *see* Calculus, bile duct
  - Chikungunya (viral) (hemorrhagic) A92.Ø
  - Chitral A93.1
  - Colombo — *see* Fever, paratyphoid
  - Colorado tick (virus) A93.2
  - congestive (remittent) — *see* Malaria
  - Congo virus A98.Ø
  - continued malarial B5Ø.9
  - Corsican — *see* Malaria
  - Crimean-Congo hemorrhagic A98.Ø
  - Cyprus — *see* Brucellosis
  - dandy A9Ø
  - deer fly — *see* Tularemia
  - dengue (virus) A9Ø
    - hemorrhagic A91
    - sandfly A93.1
  - desert B38.Ø
  - drug induced R5Ø.2
  - due to
    - conditions classified elsewhere R5Ø.81
    - heat T67.Ø1 ☑
  - enteric AØ1.ØØ
  - enteroviral exanthematous (Boston exanthem) A88.Ø
  - ephemeral (of unknown origin) R5Ø.9
  - epidemic hemorrhagic A98.5
  - erysipelatous — *see* Erysipelas
  - estivo-autumnal (malarial) B5Ø.9
  - famine A75.Ø
  - five day A79.Ø
  - following delivery O86.4
  - Fort Bragg A27.89

- **Fibrosis, fibrotic** — *continued*
  - lung — *continued*
    - with — *continued*
      - silicosis J62.8
    - capillary J84.1Ø
    - congenital P27.8
    - diffuse (idiopathic) J84.1Ø
      - chemicals, gases, fumes or vapors (inhalation) — *see also* Disease, respiratory, chronic, due to chemicals, gases, fumes or vapors J84.1Ø
      - interstitial J84.1Ø
        - acute J84.114
      - talc J62.Ø
    - following radiation J7Ø.1
    - idiopathic J84.112
    - postinflammatory J84.1Ø
    - silicotic J62.8
    - tuberculous — *see* Tuberculosis, pulmonary
  - lymphatic gland I89.8
  - median bar — *see* Hyperplasia, prostate
  - mediastinum (idiopathic) J98.59
  - meninges G96.198
  - myocardium, myocardial — *see* Myocarditis
  - ovary N83.8
  - oviduct N83.8
  - pancreas K86.89
  - penis NEC N48.6
  - pericardium I31.Ø
  - perineum, in pregnancy or childbirth O34.7- ☑
    - causing obstructed labor O65.5
  - pleura J94.1
  - popliteal fat pad M79.4
  - prostate (chronic) — *see* Hyperplasia, prostate
  - pulmonary — *see also* Fibrosis, lung J84.1Ø
    - congenital P27.8
    - idiopathic J84.112
  - rectal sphincter K62.89
  - retroperitoneal K68.2
    - with infection N13.6
    - idiopathic (with ureteral obstruction) N13.5
  - sclerosing mesenteric (idiopathic) K65.4
  - scrotum N5Ø.89
  - seminal vesicle N5Ø.89
  - senile R54
  - skin L9Ø.5
  - spermatic cord N5Ø.89
  - spleen D73.89
    - in schistosomiasis (bilharziasis) B65.9 *[D77]*
  - subepidermal nodular — *see* Neoplasm, skin, benign
  - submucous (oral) (tongue) K13.5
  - testis N44.8
    - chronic, due to syphilis A52.76
  - thymus (gland) E32.8
  - tongue, submucous K13.5
  - tunica vaginalis N5Ø.89
  - uterus (non-neoplastic) N85.8
  - vagina N89.8
  - valve, heart — *see* Endocarditis
  - vas deferens N5Ø.89
  - vein I87.8
- **Fibrositis** (periarticular) M79.7
  - nodular, chronic (Jaccoud's) (rheumatoid) — *see* Arthropathy, postrheumatic, chronic
- **Fibrothorax** J94.1
- **Fibrotic** — *see* Fibrosis
- **Fibrous** — *see* condition
- **Fibroxanthoma** — *see also* Neoplasm, connective tissue, benign
  - atypical — *see* Neoplasm, connective tissue, uncertain behavior
  - malignant — *see* Neoplasm, connective tissue, malignant
- **Fibroxanthosarcoma** — *see* Neoplasm, connective tissue, malignant
- **Fiedler's**
  - disease (icterohemorrhagic leptospirosis) A27.Ø
  - myocarditis (acute) I4Ø.1
- **Fifth disease** BØ8.3
  - venereal A55
- **Filaria, filarial, filariasis** — *see* Infestation, filarial
- **Filatov's disease** — *see* Mononucleosis, infectious
- **File-cutter's disease** — *see* Poisoning, lead
- **Filling defect**
  - biliary tract R93.2
  - bladder R93.41
  - duodenum R93.3
  - gallbladder R93.2
  - gastrointestinal tract R93.3
  - intestine R93.3
  - kidney R93.42- ☑
  - stomach R93.3
  - ureter R93.41
  - urinary organs, specified NEC R93.49
- **Fimbrial cyst** Q5Ø.4
- **Financial problem affecting care NOS** Z59.9
  - bankruptcy Z59.89
  - foreclosure on loan Z59.89
    - home loan Z59.81- ☑
  - strain Z59.86
- **Findings, abnormal, inconclusive, without diagnosis** — *see also* Abnormal
  - 17-ketosteroids, elevated R82.5
  - acetonuria R82.4
  - alcohol in blood R78.Ø
  - anisocytosis R71.8
  - antenatal screening of mother O28.9
    - biochemical O28.1
    - chromosomal O28.5
    - cytological O28.2
    - genetic O28.5
    - hematological O28.Ø
    - radiological O28.4
    - specified NEC O28.8
    - ultrasonic O28.3
  - antibody titer, elevated R76.Ø
  - anticardiolipin antibody R76.Ø
  - antiphosphatidylglycerol antibody R76.Ø
  - antiphosphatidylinositol antibody R76.Ø
  - antiphosphatidylserine antibody R76.Ø
  - antiphospholipid antibody R76.Ø
  - bacteriuria R82.71
  - bicarbonate E87.8
  - bile in urine R82.2
  - blood sugar R73.Ø9
    - high R73.9
    - low (transient) E16.2
  - body fluid or substance, specified NEC R88.8
  - casts, urine R82.998
  - catecholamines R82.5
  - cells, urine R82.998
  - chloride E87.8
  - cholesterol E78.9
    - high E78.ØØ
      - with high triglycerides E78.2
  - chyluria R82.Ø
  - cloudy
    - dialysis effluent R88.Ø
    - urine R82.9Ø
  - creatinine clearance R94.4
  - crystals, urine R82.998
  - culture
    - blood R78.81
    - positive — *see* Positive, culture
  - echocardiogram R93.1
  - electrolyte level, urinary R82.998
  - function study NEC R94.8
    - bladder R94.8
    - endocrine NEC R94.7
      - thyroid R94.6
    - kidney R94.4
    - liver R94.5
    - pancreas R94.8
    - placenta R94.8
    - pulmonary R94.2
    - spleen R94.8
  - gallbladder, nonvisualization R93.2
  - glucose (tolerance test) (non-fasting) R73.Ø9
  - glycosuria R81
  - heart
    - shadow R93.1
    - sounds RØ1.2
  - hematinuria R82.3
  - hematocrit drop (precipitous) R71.Ø
  - hemoglobinuria R82.3
  - human papillomavirus (HPV) DNA test positive
    - cervix
      - high risk R87.81Ø
      - low risk R87.82Ø
    - vagina
      - high risk R87.811
      - low risk R87.821
  - in blood (of substance not normally found in blood) R78.9
    - addictive drug NEC R78.4
    - alcohol (excessive level) R78.Ø
    - cocaine R78.2
    - hallucinogen R78.3
    - heavy metals (abnormal level) R78.79
    - lead R78.71
    - lithium (abnormal level) R78.89
    - opiate drug R78.1
    - psychotropic drug R78.5
    - specified substance NEC R78.89
    - steroid agent R78.6
  - indoleacetic acid, elevated R82.5
  - ketonuria R82.4
  - lactic acid dehydrogenase (LDH) R74.Ø2
  - liver function test — *see also* Elevated, liver function, test R79.89
  - mammogram NEC R92.8
    - calcification (calculus) R92.1
    - inconclusive result R92.2
    - microcalcification R92.Ø
  - mediastinal shift R93.89
  - melanin, urine R82.998
  - myoglobinuria R82.1
  - neonatal screening — *see* Abnormal, neonatal screening
  - newborn screens, state mandated — *see* Abnormal, neonatal screening
  - nonvisualization of gallbladder R93.2
  - odor of urine NOS R82.9Ø
  - Papanicolaou cervix R87.619
    - non-atypical endometrial cells R87.618
  - pneumoencephalogram R93.Ø
  - poikilocytosis R71.8
  - potassium (deficiency) E87.6
    - excess E87.5
  - PPD R76.11
  - radiologic (X-ray) R93.89
    - abdomen R93.5
    - biliary tract R93.2
    - breast R92.8
    - gastrointestinal tract R93.3
    - genitourinary organs R93.89
    - head R93.Ø
    - inconclusive due to excess body fat of patient R93.9
    - intrathoracic organs NEC R93.1
    - musculoskeletal
      - limbs R93.6
      - other than limb R93.7
    - placenta R93.89
    - retroperitoneum R93.5
    - skin R93.89
    - skull R93.Ø
    - subcutaneous tissue R93.89
    - testis R93.81- ☑
  - red blood cell (count) (morphology) (sickling) (volume) R71.8
  - scan NEC R94.8
    - bladder R94.8
    - bone R94.8
    - kidney R94.4
    - liver R93.2
    - lung R94.2
    - pancreas R94.8
    - placental R94.8
    - spleen R94.8
    - thyroid R94.6
  - sedimentation rate, elevated R7Ø.Ø
  - SGOT R74.Ø1
  - SGPT R74.Ø1
  - sodium (deficiency) E87.1
    - excess E87.Ø
  - specified body fluid NEC R88.8
  - stress test R94.39
  - testis R93.81- ☑
  - thyroid (function) (metabolic rate) (scan) (uptake) R94.6
  - transaminase (level) R74.Ø1
  - triglycerides E78.9
    - high E78.1
      - with high cholesterol E78.2
  - tuberculin skin test (without active tuberculosis) R76.11
  - urine R82.9Ø
    - acetone R82.4
    - bacteria R82.71
    - bile R82.2
    - casts or cells R82.998
    - chyle R82.Ø
    - culture positive R82.79

- **Findings, abnormal, inconclusive, without diagnosis** — *continued*
  - urine — *continued*
    - glucose R81
    - hemoglobin R82.3
    - ketone R82.4
    - sugar R81
  - vanillylmandelic acid (VMA), elevated R82.5
  - vectorcardiogram (VCG) R94.39
  - ventriculogram R93.Ø
  - white blood cell (count) (differential) (morphology) D72.9
  - xerography R92.8
- **Finger** — *see* condition
- **Fire, Saint Anthony's** — *see* Erysipelas
- **Fire-setting**
  - pathological (compulsive) F63.1
- **Fish hook stomach** K31.89
- **Fishmeal-worker's lung** J67.8
- **Fissure, fissured**
  - anus, anal K6Ø.2
    - acute K6Ø.Ø
    - chronic K6Ø.1
    - congenital Q43.8
  - ear, lobule, congenital Q17.8
  - epiglottis (congenital) Q31.8
  - larynx J38.7
    - congenital Q31.8
  - lip K13.Ø
    - congenital — *see* Cleft, lip
  - nipple N64.Ø
    - associated with
      - lactation O92.13
      - pregnancy O92.11- ☑
      - puerperium O92.12
  - nose Q3Ø.2
  - palate (congenital) — *see* Cleft, palate
  - skin R23.4
  - spine (congenital) — *see also* Spina bifida
    - with hydrocephalus — *see* Spina bifida, by site, with hydrocephalus
  - tongue (acquired) K14.5
    - congenital Q38.3
- **Fistula** (cutaneous) L98.8
  - abdomen (wall) K63.2
    - bladder N32.2
    - intestine NEC K63.2
    - ureter N28.89
    - uterus N82.5
  - abdominorectal K63.2
  - abdominosigmoidal K63.2
  - abdominothoracic J86.Ø
  - abdominouterine N82.5
    - congenital Q51.7
  - abdominovesical N32.2
  - accessory sinuses — *see* Sinusitis
  - actinomycotic — *see* Actinomycosis
  - alveolar antrum — *see* Sinusitis, maxillary
  - alveolar process KØ4.6
  - anorectal K6Ø.5
  - antrobuccal — *see* Sinusitis, maxillary
  - antrum — *see* Sinusitis, maxillary
  - anus, anal (recurrent) (infectional) K6Ø.3
    - congenital Q43.6
      - with absence, atresia and stenosis Q42.2
    - tuberculous A18.32
  - aorta-duodenal I77.2
  - appendix, appendicular K38.3
  - arteriovenous (acquired) (nonruptured) I77.Ø
    - brain I67.1
      - congenital Q28.2
        - ruptured — *see* Fistula, arteriovenous, brain, ruptured
      - ruptured I6Ø.8
        - intracerebral I61.8
        - intraparenchymal I61.8
        - intraventricular I61.5
        - subarachnoid I6Ø.8
    - cerebral — *see* Fistula, arteriovenous, brain
    - congenital (peripheral) — *see also* Malformation, arteriovenous
      - brain Q28.2
        - ruptured — *see* Fistula, arteriovenous, brain, ruptured
      - coronary Q24.5
      - pulmonary Q25.72
    - coronary I25.41
      - congenital Q24.5

- **Fistula** — *continued*
  - arteriovenous — *continued*
    - pulmonary I28.Ø
      - congenital Q25.72
    - surgically created (for dialysis) Z99.2
      - complication — *see* Complication, arteriovenous, fistula, surgically created
    - traumatic — *see* Injury, blood vessel
  - artery I77.2
  - aural (mastoid) — *see* Mastoiditis, chronic
  - auricle — *see also* Disorder, pinna, specified type NEC
    - congenital Q18.1
  - Bartholin's gland N82.8
  - bile duct (common) (hepatic) K83.3
    - with calculus, stones — *see also* Calculus, bile duct K83.3
  - biliary (tract) — *see* Fistula, bile duct
  - bladder (sphincter) NEC — *see also* Fistula, vesico- N32.2
    - into seminal vesicle N32.2
  - bone — *see also* Disorder, bone, specified type NEC
    - with osteomyelitis, chronic — *see* Osteomyelitis, chronic, with draining sinus
  - brain G93.89
    - arteriovenous (acquired) — *see also* Fistula, arteriovenous, brain I67.1
      - congenital Q28.2
  - branchial (cleft) Q18.Ø
  - branchiogenous Q18.Ø
  - breast N61.Ø
    - puerperal, postpartum or gestational, due to mastitis (purulent) — *see* Mastitis, obstetric, purulent
  - bronchial J86.Ø
  - bronchocutaneous, bronchomediastinal, bronchopleural, bronchopleuromediastinal (infective) J86.Ø
    - tuberculous NEC A15.5
  - bronchoesophageal J86.Ø
    - congenital Q39.2
      - with atresia of esophagus Q39.1
  - bronchovisceral J86.Ø
  - buccal cavity (infective) K12.2
  - cecosigmoidal K63.2
  - cecum K63.2
  - cerebrospinal (fluid) G96.Ø8
  - cervical, lateral Q18.1
  - cervicoaural Q18.1
  - cervicosigmoidal N82.4
  - cervicovesical N82.1
  - cervix N82.8
  - chest (wall) J86.Ø
  - cholecystenteric — *see* Fistula, gallbladder
  - cholecystocolic — *see* Fistula, gallbladder
  - cholecystocolonic — *see* Fistula, gallbladder
  - cholecystoduodenal — *see* Fistula, gallbladder
  - cholecystogastric — *see* Fistula, gallbladder
  - cholecystointestinal — *see* Fistula, gallbladder
  - choledochoduodenal — *see* Fistula, bile duct
  - cholocolic K82.3
  - coccyx — *see* Sinus, pilonidal
  - colon K63.2
  - colostomy K94.Ø9
  - colovesical N32.1
  - common duct — *see* Fistula, bile duct
  - congenital, site not listed — *see* Anomaly, by site
  - coronary, arteriovenous I25.41
    - congenital Q24.5
  - costal region J86.Ø
  - cul-de-sac, Douglas' N82.8
  - cystic duct — *see also* Fistula, gallbladder
    - congenital Q44.5
  - dental KØ4.6
  - diaphragm J86.Ø
  - duodenum K31.6
  - ear (external) (canal) — *see* Disorder, ear, external, specified type NEC
  - enterocolic K63.2
  - enterocutaneous K63.2
  - enterouterine N82.4
    - congenital Q51.7
  - enterovaginal N82.4
    - congenital Q52.2
    - large intestine N82.3
    - small intestine N82.2
  - enterovesical N32.1
  - epididymis N5Ø.89
    - tuberculous A18.15
  - esophagobronchial J86.Ø
    - congenital Q39.2

- **Fistula** — *continued*
  - esophagobronchial — *continued*
    - congenital — *continued*
      - with atresia of esophagus Q39.1
  - esophagocutaneous K22.89
  - esophagopleural-cutaneous J86.Ø
  - esophagotracheal J86.Ø
    - congenital Q39.2
      - with atresia of esophagus Q39.1
  - esophagus K22.89
    - congenital Q39.2
      - with atresia of esophagus Q39.1
  - ethmoid — *see* Sinusitis, ethmoidal
  - eyeball (cornea) (sclera) — *see* Disorder, globe, hypotony
  - eyelid HØ1.8
  - fallopian tube, external N82.5
  - fecal K63.2
    - congenital Q43.6
  - from periapical abscess KØ4.6
  - frontal sinus — *see* Sinusitis, frontal
  - gallbladder K82.3
    - with calculus, cholelithiasis, stones — *see* Calculus, gallbladder
  - gastric K31.6
  - gastrocolic K31.6
    - congenital Q4Ø.2
    - tuberculous A18.32
  - gastroenterocolic K31.6
  - gastroesophageal K31.6
  - gastrojejunal K31.6
  - gastrojejunocolic K31.6
  - genital tract (female) N82.9
    - specified NEC N82.8
    - to intestine NEC N82.4
    - to skin N82.5
  - hepatic artery-portal vein, congenital Q26.6
  - hepatopleural J86.Ø
  - hepatopulmonary J86.Ø
  - ileorectal or ileosigmoidal K63.2
  - ileovaginal N82.2
  - ileovesical N32.1
  - ileum K63.2
  - in ano K6Ø.3
    - tuberculous A18.32
  - inner ear (labyrinth) — *see* subcategory H83.1 ☑
  - intestine NEC K63.2
  - intestinocolonic (abdominal) K63.2
  - intestinoureteral N28.89
  - intestinouterine N82.4
  - intestinovaginal N82.4
    - large intestine N82.3
    - small intestine N82.2
  - intestinovesical N32.1
  - ischiorectal (fossa) K61.39
  - jejunum K63.2
  - joint M25.1Ø
    - ankle M25.17- ☑
    - elbow M25.12- ☑
    - foot joint M25.17- ☑
    - hand joint M25.14- ☑
    - hip M25.15- ☑
    - knee M25.16- ☑
    - shoulder M25.11- ☑
    - specified joint NEC M25.18
    - tuberculous — *see* Tuberculosis, joint
    - vertebrae M25.18
    - wrist M25.13- ☑
  - kidney N28.89
  - labium (majus) (minus) N82.8
  - labyrinth — *see* subcategory H83.1 ☑
  - lacrimal (gland) (sac) HØ4.61- ☑
  - lacrimonasal duct — *see* Fistula, lacrimal
  - laryngotracheal, congenital Q34.8
  - larynx J38.7
  - lip K13.Ø
    - congenital Q38.Ø
  - lumbar, tuberculous A18.Ø1
  - lung J86.Ø
  - lymphatic I89.8
  - mammary (gland) N61.Ø
  - mastoid (process) (region) — *see* Mastoiditis, chronic
  - maxillary J32.Ø
  - medial, face and neck Q18.8
  - mediastinal J86.Ø
  - mediastinobronchial J86.Ø
  - mediastinocutaneous J86.Ø
  - middle ear — *see* subcategory H74.8 ☑

- **Fixation** — *continued*
  - vocal cord J38.3
- **Flabby ridge** K06.8
- **Flaccid** — *see also* condition
  - palate, congenital Q38.5
- **Flail**
  - chest S22.5 ☑
    - associated with chest compression and cardiopulmonary resuscitation M96.A4
    - newborn (birth injury) P13.8
  - joint (paralytic) M25.20
    - ankle M25.27- ☑
    - elbow M25.22- ☑
    - foot joint M25.27- ☑
    - hand joint M25.24- ☑
    - hip M25.25- ☑
    - knee M25.26- ☑
    - shoulder M25.21- ☑
    - specified joint NEC M25.28
    - wrist M25.23- ☑
- **Flajani's disease** — *see* Hyperthyroidism, with, goiter (diffuse)
- **Flap, liver** K71.3
- **Flashbacks** (residual to hallucinogen use) F16.283
- **Flat**
  - affect R45.89
  - chamber (eye) — *see* Disorder, globe, hypotony, flat anterior chamber
  - chest, congenital Q67.8
  - foot (acquired) (fixed type) (painful) (postural) — *see also* Deformity, limb, flat foot
    - congenital (rigid) (spastic (everted)) Q66.5- ☑
    - rachitic sequelae (late effect) E64.3
  - organ or site, congenital NEC — *see* Anomaly, by site
  - pelvis M95.5
    - with disproportion (fetopelvic) O33.0
      - causing obstructed labor O65.0
    - congenital Q74.2
- **Flatau-Schilder disease** G37.0
- **Flatback syndrome** M40.30
  - lumbar region M40.36
  - lumbosacral region M40.37
  - thoracolumbar region M40.35
- **Flattening**
  - head, femur M89.8X5
  - hip — *see* Coxa, plana
  - lip (congenital) Q18.8
  - nose (congenital) Q67.4
    - acquired M95.0
- **Flatulence** R14.3
  - psychogenic F45.8
- **Flatus** R14.3
  - vaginalis N89.8
- **Flax-dresser's disease** J66.1
- **Flea bite** — *see* Injury, bite, by site, superficial, insect
- **Flecks, glaucomatous** (subcapsular) — *see* Cataract, complicated
- **Fleischer** (-Kayser) **ring** (cornea) H18.04- ☑
- **Fleshy mole** O02.0
- **Flexibilitas cerea** — *see* Catalepsy
- **Flexion**
  - amputation stump (surgical) T87.89
  - cervix — *see* Malposition, uterus
  - contracture, joint — *see* Contraction, joint
  - deformity, joint — *see also* Deformity, limb, flexion M21.20
    - hip, congenital Q65.89
  - uterus — *see also* Malposition, uterus
    - lateral — *see* Lateroversion, uterus
- **Flexner-Boyd dysentery** A03.2
- **Flexner's dysentery** A03.1
- **Flexure** — *see* Flexion
- **Flint murmur** (aortic insufficiency) I35.1
- **Floater, vitreous** — *see* Opacity, vitreous
- **Floating**
  - cartilage (joint) — *see also* Loose, body, joint
    - knee — *see* Derangement, knee, loose body
  - gallbladder, congenital Q44.1
  - kidney N28.89
    - congenital Q63.8
  - spleen D73.89
- **Flooding** N92.0
- **Floor** — *see* condition
- **Floppy**
  - baby syndrome (nonspecific) P94.2
  - iris syndrome (intraoperative) (IFIS) H21.81
  - nonrheumatic mitral valve syndrome I34.1
- **Flu** — *see also* Influenza
  - avian — *see also* Influenza, due to, identified novel influenza A virus J09.X2
  - bird — *see also* Influenza, due to, identified novel influenza A virus J09.X2
  - intestinal NEC A08.4
  - swine (viruses that normally cause infections in pigs) — *see also* Influenza, due to, identified novel influenza A virus J09.X2
- **Fluctuating blood pressure** I99.8
- **Fluid**
  - abdomen R18.8
  - chest J94.8
  - heart — *see* Failure, heart, congestive
  - joint — *see* Effusion, joint
  - loss (acute) E86.9
  - lung — *see* Edema, lung
  - overload E87.70
    - specified NEC E87.79
  - peritoneal cavity R18.8
  - pleural cavity J94.8
  - retention R60.9
- **Flukes NEC** — *see also* Infestation, fluke
  - blood NEC — *see* Schistosomiasis
  - liver B66.3
- **Fluor** (vaginalis) N89.8
  - trichomonal or due to Trichomonas (vaginalis) A59.00
- **Fluorosis**
  - dental K00.3
  - skeletal M85.10
    - ankle M85.17- ☑
    - foot M85.17- ☑
    - forearm M85.13- ☑
    - hand M85.14- ☑
    - lower leg M85.16- ☑
    - multiple site M85.19
    - neck M85.18
    - rib M85.18
    - shoulder M85.11- ☑
    - skull M85.18
    - specified site NEC M85.18
    - thigh M85.15- ☑
    - toe M85.17- ☑
    - upper arm M85.12- ☑
    - vertebra M85.18
- **Flush syndrome** E34.0
- **Flushing** R23.2
  - menopausal N95.1
- **Flutter**
  - atrial or auricular I48.92
    - atypical I48.4
    - type I I48.3
    - type II I48.4
    - typical I48.3
  - heart I49.8
    - atrial or auricular I48.92
      - atypical I48.4
      - type I I48.3
      - type II I48.4
      - typical I48.3
    - ventricular I49.02
  - ventricular I49.02
- **FNHTR** (febrile nonhemolytic transfusion reaction) R50.84
- **Fochier's abscess** — *code by* site under Abscess
- **Focus, Assmann's** — *see* Tuberculosis, pulmonary
- **Fogo selvagem** L10.3
- **Foix-Alajouanine syndrome** G95.19
- **Fold, folds** (anomalous) — *see also* Anomaly, by site
  - Descemet's membrane — *see* Change, corneal membrane, Descemet's, fold
  - epicanthic Q10.3
  - heart Q24.8
- **Folie a deux** F24
- **Follicle**
  - cervix (nabothian) (ruptured) N88.8
  - graafian, ruptured, with hemorrhage N83.0- ☑
  - nabothian N88.8
- **Follicular** — *see* condition
- **Folliculitis** (superficial) L73.9
  - abscedens et suffodiens L66.3
  - cyst N83.0- ☑
  - decalvans L66.2
  - deep — *see* Furuncle, by site
  - gonococcal (acute) (chronic) A54.01
  - keloid, keloidalis L73.0
  - pustular L01.02
  - ulerythematosa reticulata L66.4
- **Folliculome lipidique**
  - specified site — *see* Neoplasm, benign, by site
  - unspecified site
    - female D27.9
    - male D29.20
- **Følling's disease** E70.0
- **Follow-up** — *see* Examination, follow-up
- **Fong's syndrome** (hereditary osteo-onychodysplasia) Q87.2
- **Food**
  - allergy L27.2
  - asphyxia (from aspiration or inhalation) — *see* Foreign body, by site
  - choked on — *see* Foreign body, by site
  - deprivation T73.0 ☑
    - specified kind of food NEC E63.8
  - insecurity Z59.41
  - intoxication — *see* Poisoning, food
  - lack of T73.0 ☑
  - poisoning — *see* Poisoning, food
  - rejection NEC — *see* Disorder, eating
  - strangulation or suffocation — *see* Foreign body, by site
  - toxemia — *see* Poisoning, food
- **Foot** — *see* condition
- **Foramen ovale** (nonclosure) (patent) (persistent) Q21.12
- **Forbes' glycogen storage disease** E74.03
- **Fordyce-Fox disease** L75.2
- **Fordyce's disease** (mouth) Q38.6
- **Forearm** — *see* condition
- **Foreclosure on loan** Z59.89
- **Foreign body**
  - with
    - laceration — *see* Laceration, by site, with foreign body
    - puncture wound — *see* Puncture, by site, with foreign body
  - accidentally left following a procedure T81.509 ☑
    - aspiration T81.506 ☑
      - resulting in
        - adhesions T81.516 ☑
        - obstruction T81.526 ☑
        - perforation T81.536 ☑
        - specified complication NEC T81.596 ☑
    - cardiac catheterization T81.505 ☑
      - resulting in
        - acute reaction T81.60 ☑
          - aseptic peritonitis T81.61 ☑
          - specified NEC T81.69 ☑
        - adhesions T81.515 ☑
        - obstruction T81.525 ☑
        - perforation T81.535 ☑
        - specified complication NEC T81.595 ☑
    - causing
      - acute reaction T81.60 ☑
        - aseptic peritonitis T81.61 ☑
        - specified complication NEC T81.69 ☑
      - adhesions T81.519 ☑
      - aseptic peritonitis T81.61 ☑
      - obstruction T81.529 ☑
      - perforation T81.539 ☑
      - specified complication NEC T81.599 ☑
    - endoscopy T81.504 ☑
      - resulting in
        - adhesions T81.514 ☑
        - obstruction T81.524 ☑
        - perforation T81.534 ☑
        - specified complication NEC T81.594 ☑
    - immunization T81.503 ☑
      - resulting in
        - adhesions T81.513 ☑
        - obstruction T81.523 ☑
        - perforation T81.533 ☑
        - specified complication NEC T81.593 ☑
    - infusion T81.501 ☑
      - resulting in
        - adhesions T81.511 ☑
        - obstruction T81.521 ☑
        - perforation T81.531 ☑
        - specified complication NEC T81.591 ☑
    - injection T81.503 ☑
      - resulting in
        - adhesions T81.513 ☑
        - obstruction T81.523 ☑
        - perforation T81.533 ☑
        - specified complication NEC T81.593 ☑

- **Foreign body** — *continued*
  - pharynx — *continued*
    - causing
      - asphyxiation T17.2ØØ ☑
        - food (bone) (seed) T17.22Ø ☑
        - gastric contents (vomitus) T17.21Ø ☑
        - specified type NEC T17.29Ø ☑
      - injury NEC T17.2Ø8 ☑
        - food (bone) (seed) T17.228 ☑
        - gastric contents (vomitus) T17.218 ☑
        - specified type NEC T17.298 ☑
  - respiratory tract T17.9Ø8 ☑
    - bronchioles — *see* Foreign body, respiratory tract, specified site NEC
    - bronchus — *see* Foreign body, bronchus
    - causing
      - asphyxiation T17.9ØØ ☑
        - food (bone) (seed) T17.92Ø ☑
        - gastric contents (vomitus) T17.91Ø ☑
        - specified type NEC T17.99Ø ☑
      - injury NEC T17.9Ø8 ☑
        - food (bone) (seed) T17.928 ☑
        - gastric contents (vomitus) T17.918 ☑
        - specified type NEC T17.998 ☑
    - larynx — *see* Foreign body, larynx
    - lung — *see* Foreign body, respiratory tract, specified site NEC
    - multiple parts — *see* Foreign body, respiratory tract, specified site NEC
    - nasal sinus T17.Ø ☑
    - nasopharynx — *see* Foreign body, pharynx
    - nose T17.1 ☑
    - nostril T17.1 ☑
    - pharynx — *see* Foreign body, pharynx
    - specified site NEC T17.8Ø8 ☑
      - causing
        - asphyxiation T17.8ØØ ☑
          - food (bone) (seed) T17.82Ø ☑
          - gastric contents (vomitus) T17.81Ø ☑
          - specified type NEC T17.89Ø ☑
        - injury NEC T17.8Ø8 ☑
          - food (bone) (seed) T17.828 ☑
          - gastric contents (vomitus) T17.818 ☑
          - specified type NEC T17.898 ☑
    - throat — *see* Foreign body, pharynx
    - trachea — *see* Foreign body, trachea
  - retained (old) (nonmagnetic) (in)
    - anterior chamber (eye) — *see* Foreign body, intraocular, old, retained, anterior chamber
      - magnetic — *see* Foreign body, intraocular, old, retained, magnetic, anterior chamber
    - ciliary body — *see* Foreign body, intraocular, old, retained, ciliary body
      - magnetic — *see* Foreign body, intraocular, old, retained, magnetic, ciliary body
    - eyelid HØ2.819
      - left HØ2.816
        - lower HØ2.815
        - upper HØ2.814
      - right HØ2.813
        - lower HØ2.812
        - upper HØ2.811
    - fragments — *see* Retained, foreign body fragments (type of)
    - globe — *see* Foreign body, intraocular, old, retained
      - magnetic — *see* Foreign body, intraocular, old, retained, magnetic
    - intraocular — *see* Foreign body, intraocular, old, retained
      - magnetic — *see* Foreign body, intraocular, old, retained, magnetic
    - iris — *see* Foreign body, intraocular, old, retained, iris
      - magnetic — *see* Foreign body, intraocular, old, retained, magnetic, iris
    - lens — *see* Foreign body, intraocular, old, retained, lens
      - magnetic — *see* Foreign body, intraocular, old, retained, magnetic, lens
    - muscle — *see* Foreign body, retained, soft tissue
    - orbit — *see* Foreign body, orbit, old
    - posterior wall of globe — *see* Foreign body, intraocular, old, retained, posterior wall
      - magnetic — *see* Foreign body, intraocular, old, retained, magnetic, posterior wall
    - retrobulbar — *see* Foreign body, orbit, old, retrobulbar

- **Foreign body** — *continued*
  - retained — *continued*
    - soft tissue M79.5
    - vitreous — *see* Foreign body, intraocular, old, retained, vitreous body
      - magnetic — *see* Foreign body, intraocular, old, retained, magnetic, vitreous body
  - retina SØ5.5- ☑
  - sensation — *see* Sensation, foreign body
  - superficial, without open wound
    - abdomen, abdominal (wall) S3Ø.851 ☑
    - alveolar process SØØ.552 ☑
    - ankle S9Ø.55- ☑
    - antecubital space — *see* Foreign body, superficial, forearm
    - anus S3Ø.857 ☑
    - arm (upper) S4Ø.85- ☑
    - auditory canal — *see* Foreign body, superficial, ear
    - auricle — *see* Foreign body, superficial, ear
    - axilla — *see* Foreign body, superficial, arm
    - back, lower S3Ø.85Ø ☑
    - breast S2Ø.15- ☑
    - brow SØØ.85 ☑
    - buttock S3Ø.85Ø ☑
    - calf — *see* Foreign body, superficial, leg
    - canthus — *see* Foreign body, superficial, eyelid
    - cheek SØØ.85 ☑
      - internal SØØ.552 ☑
    - chest wall — *see* Foreign body, superficial, thorax
    - chin SØØ.85 ☑
    - clitoris S3Ø.854 ☑
    - costal region — *see* Foreign body, superficial, thorax
    - digit(s)
      - foot — *see* Foreign body, superficial, toe
      - hand — *see* Foreign body, superficial, finger
    - ear SØØ.45- ☑
    - elbow S5Ø.35- ☑
    - epididymis S3Ø.853 ☑
    - epigastric region S3Ø.851 ☑
    - epiglottis S1Ø.15 ☑
    - esophagus, cervical S1Ø.15 ☑
    - eyebrow — *see* Foreign body, superficial, eyelid
    - eyelid SØØ.25- ☑
    - face SØØ.85 ☑
    - finger(s) S6Ø.459 ☑
      - index S6Ø.45- ☑
      - little S6Ø.45- ☑
      - middle S6Ø.45- ☑
      - ring S6Ø.45- ☑
    - flank S3Ø.851 ☑
    - foot (except toe(s) alone) S9Ø.85- ☑
      - toe — *see* Foreign body, superficial, toe
    - forearm S5Ø.85- ☑
      - elbow only — *see* Foreign body, superficial, elbow
    - forehead SØØ.85 ☑
    - genital organs, external
      - female S3Ø.856 ☑
      - male S3Ø.855 ☑
    - groin S3Ø.851 ☑
    - gum SØØ.552 ☑
    - hand S6Ø.55- ☑
    - head SØØ.95 ☑
      - ear — *see* Foreign body, superficial, ear
      - eyelid — *see* Foreign body, superficial, eyelid
      - lip SØØ.551 ☑
      - nose SØØ.35 ☑
      - oral cavity SØØ.552 ☑
      - scalp SØØ.Ø5 ☑
      - specified site NEC SØØ.85 ☑
    - heel — *see* Foreign body, superficial, foot
    - hip S7Ø.25- ☑
    - inguinal region S3Ø.851 ☑
    - interscapular region S2Ø.459 ☑
    - jaw SØØ.85 ☑
    - knee S8Ø.25- ☑
    - labium (majus) (minus) S3Ø.854 ☑
    - larynx S1Ø.15 ☑
    - leg (lower) S8Ø.85- ☑
      - knee — *see* Foreign body, superficial, knee
      - upper — *see* Foreign body, superficial, thigh
    - lip SØØ.551 ☑
    - lower back S3Ø.85Ø ☑
    - lumbar region S3Ø.85Ø ☑
    - malar region SØØ.85 ☑
    - mammary — *see* Foreign body, superficial, breast

- **Foreign body** — *continued*
  - superficial, without open wound — *continued*
    - mastoid region SØØ.85 ☑
    - mouth SØØ.552 ☑
    - nail
      - finger — *see* Foreign body, superficial, finger
      - toe — *see* Foreign body, superficial, toe
    - nape S1Ø.85 ☑
    - nasal SØØ.35 ☑
    - neck S1Ø.95 ☑
      - specified site NEC S1Ø.85 ☑
      - throat S1Ø.15 ☑
    - nose SØØ.35 ☑
    - occipital region SØØ.Ø5 ☑
    - oral cavity SØØ.552 ☑
    - orbital region — *see* Foreign body, superficial, eyelid
    - palate SØØ.552 ☑
    - palm — *see* Foreign body, superficial, hand
    - parietal region SØØ.Ø5 ☑
    - pelvis S3Ø.85Ø ☑
    - penis S3Ø.852 ☑
    - perineum
      - female S3Ø.854 ☑
      - male S3Ø.85Ø ☑
    - periocular area — *see* Foreign body, superficial, eyelid
    - phalanges
      - finger — *see* Foreign body, superficial, finger
      - toe — *see* Foreign body, superficial, toe
    - pharynx S1Ø.15 ☑
    - pinna — *see* Foreign body, superficial, ear
    - popliteal space — *see* Foreign body, superficial, knee
    - prepuce S3Ø.852 ☑
    - pubic region S3Ø.85Ø ☑
    - pudendum
      - female S3Ø.856 ☑
      - male S3Ø.855 ☑
    - sacral region S3Ø.85Ø ☑
    - scalp SØØ.Ø5 ☑
    - scapular region — *see* Foreign body, superficial, shoulder
    - scrotum S3Ø.853 ☑
    - shin — *see* Foreign body, superficial, leg
    - shoulder S4Ø.25- ☑
    - sternal region S2Ø.359 ☑
    - submaxillary region SØØ.85 ☑
    - submental region SØØ.85 ☑
    - subungual
      - finger(s) — *see* Foreign body, superficial, finger
      - toe(s) — *see* Foreign body, superficial, toe
    - supraclavicular fossa S1Ø.85 ☑
    - supraorbital SØØ.85 ☑
    - temple SØØ.85 ☑
    - temporal region SØØ.85 ☑
    - testis S3Ø.853 ☑
    - thigh S7Ø.35- ☑
    - thorax, thoracic (wall) S2Ø.95 ☑
      - back S2Ø.45- ☑
      - front S2Ø.35- ☑
    - throat S1Ø.15 ☑
    - thumb S6Ø.35- ☑
    - toe(s) (lesser) S9Ø.456 ☑
      - great S9Ø.45- ☑
    - tongue SØØ.552 ☑
    - trachea S1Ø.15 ☑
    - tunica vaginalis S3Ø.853 ☑
    - tympanum, tympanic membrane — *see* Foreign body, superficial, ear
    - uvula SØØ.552 ☑
    - vagina S3Ø.854 ☑
    - vocal cords S1Ø.15 ☑
    - vulva S3Ø.854 ☑
    - wrist S6Ø.85- ☑
  - swallowed T18.9 ☑
  - trachea T17.4Ø8 ☑
    - causing
      - asphyxiation T17.4ØØ ☑
        - food (bone) (seed) T17.42Ø ☑
        - gastric contents (vomitus) T17.41Ø ☑
        - specified type NEC T17.49Ø ☑
      - injury NEC T17.4Ø8 ☑
        - food (bone) (seed) T17.428 ☑
        - gastric contents (vomitus) T17.418 ☑
        - specified type NEC T17.498 ☑

- **Fracture, traumatic** — *continued*
  - carpal bone(s) — *continued*
    - navicular — *continued*
      - middle third (displaced) S62.Ø2- ☑
        - nondisplaced S62.Ø2- ☑
      - proximal third (displaced) S62.Ø3- ☑
        - nondisplaced S62.Ø3- ☑
      - volar tuberosity — *see* Fracture, carpal bones, navicular, distal pole
    - os magnum — *see* Fracture, carpal bones, capitate
    - pisiform (displaced) S62.16- ☑
      - nondisplaced S62.16- ☑
    - semilunar — *see* Fracture, carpal bones, lunate
    - smaller multangular — *see* Fracture, carpal bones, trapezoid
    - trapezium (displaced) S62.17- ☑
      - nondisplaced S62.17- ☑
    - trapezoid (displaced) S62.18- ☑
      - nondisplaced S62.18- ☑
    - triquetrum (displaced) S62.11- ☑
      - nondisplaced S62.11- ☑
    - unciform — *see* Fracture, carpal bones, hamate
  - cervical — *see* Fracture, vertebra, cervical
  - clavicle S42.ØØ- ☑
    - acromial end (displaced) S42.Ø3- ☑
      - nondisplaced S42.Ø3- ☑
    - birth injury P13.4
    - lateral end — *see* Fracture, clavicle, acromial end
    - shaft (displaced) S42.Ø2- ☑
      - nondisplaced S42.Ø2- ☑
    - sternal end (anterior) (displaced) S42.Ø1- ☑
      - nondisplaced S42.Ø1- ☑
      - posterior S42.Ø1- ☑
  - coccyx S32.2 ☑
  - collapsed — *see* Collapse, vertebra
  - collar bone — *see* Fracture, clavicle
  - Colles' — *see* Colles' fracture
  - coronoid process — *see* Fracture, ulna, upper end, coronoid process
  - corpus cavernosum penis S39.84Ø ☑
  - costochondral cartilage S23.41 ☑
  - costochondral, costosternal junction — *see* Fracture, rib
  - cranium — *see* Fracture, skull
  - cricoid cartilage S12.8 ☑
  - cuboid (ankle) — *see* Fracture, tarsal, cuboid
  - cuneiform
    - foot — *see* Fracture, tarsal, cuneiform
    - wrist — *see* Fracture, carpal, triquetrum
  - delayed union — *see* Delay, union, fracture
  - dental restorative material KØ8.539
    - with loss of material KØ8.531
    - without loss of material KØ8.53Ø
  - due to
    - birth injury — *see* Birth, injury, fracture
    - osteoporosis — *see* Osteoporosis, with fracture
  - Dupuytren's — *see* Fracture, ankle, lateral malleolus
  - elbow S42.4Ø- ☑
  - ethmoid (bone) (sinus) — *see* Fracture, skull, base
  - face bone SØ2.92 ☑
  - fatigue — *see also* Fracture, stress
    - vertebra M48.4Ø ☑
      - cervical region M48.42 ☑
      - cervicothoracic region M48.43 ☑
      - lumbar region M48.46 ☑
      - lumbosacral region M48.47 ☑
      - occipito-atlanto-axial region M48.41 ☑
      - sacrococcygeal region M48.48 ☑
      - thoracic region M48.44 ☑
      - thoracolumbar region M48.45 ☑
  - femur, femoral S72.9- ☑
    - basicervical (basal) S72.Ø ☑
    - birth injury P13.2
    - capital epiphyseal S79.Ø1- ☑
    - condyles, epicondyles — *see* Fracture, femur, lower end
    - distal end — *see* Fracture, femur, lower end
    - epiphysis
      - head — *see* Fracture, femur, upper end, epiphysis
      - lower — *see* Fracture, femur, lower end, epiphysis
      - upper — *see* Fracture, femur, upper end, epiphysis
    - following insertion of implant, prosthesis or plate M96.66- ☑
    - head — *see* Fracture, femur, upper end, head

- **Fracture, traumatic** — *continued*
  - femur, femoral — *continued*
    - intertrochanteric — *see* Fracture, femur, trochanteric
    - intratrochanteric — *see* Fracture, femur, trochanteric
    - lower end S72.4Ø- ☑
      - condyle (displaced) S72.41- ☑
        - lateral (displaced) S72.42- ☑
          - nondisplaced S72.42- ☑
        - medial (displaced) S72.43- ☑
          - nondisplaced S72.43- ☑
        - nondisplaced S72.41- ☑
      - epiphysis (displaced) S72.44- ☑
        - nondisplaced S72.44- ☑
      - physeal S79.1Ø- ☑
        - Salter-Harris
          - Type I S79.11- ☑
          - Type II S79.12- ☑
          - Type III S79.13- ☑
          - Type IV S79.14- ☑
        - specified NEC S79.19- ☑
      - specified NEC S72.49- ☑
      - supracondylar (displaced) S72.45- ☑
        - with intracondylar extension (displaced) S72.46- ☑
          - nondisplaced S72.46- ☑
        - nondisplaced S72.45- ☑
      - torus S72.47- ☑
    - neck — *see* Fracture, femur, upper end, neck
    - pertrochanteric — *see* Fracture, femur, trochanteric
    - shaft (lower third) (middle third) (upper third) S72.3Ø- ☑
      - comminuted (displaced) S72.35- ☑
        - nondisplaced S72.35- ☑
      - oblique (displaced) S72.33- ☑
        - nondisplaced S72.33- ☑
      - segmental (displaced) S72.36- ☑
        - nondisplaced S72.36- ☑
      - specified NEC S72.39- ☑
      - spiral (displaced) S72.34- ☑
        - nondisplaced S72.34- ☑
      - transverse (displaced) S72.32- ☑
        - nondisplaced S72.32- ☑
    - specified site NEC — *see* subcategory S72.8 ☑
    - subcapital (displaced) S72.Ø1- ☑
    - subtrochanteric (region) (section) (displaced) S72.2- ☑
      - nondisplaced S72.2- ☑
    - transcervical — *see* Fracture, femur, midcervical
    - transtrochanteric — *see* Fracture, femur, trochanteric
    - trochanteric S72.1Ø- ☑
      - apophyseal (displaced) S72.13- ☑
        - nondisplaced S72.13- ☑
      - greater trochanter (displaced) S72.11- ☑
        - nondisplaced S72.11- ☑
      - intertrochanteric (displaced) S72.14- ☑
        - nondisplaced S72.14- ☑
      - lesser trochanter (displaced) S72.12- ☑
        - nondisplaced S72.12- ☑
    - upper end S72.ØØ- ☑
      - apophyseal (displaced) S72.13- ☑
        - nondisplaced S72.13- ☑
      - cervicotrochanteric — *see* Fracture, femur, upper end, neck, base
      - epiphysis (displaced) S72.Ø2- ☑
        - nondisplaced S72.Ø2- ☑
      - head S72.Ø5- ☑
        - articular (displaced) S72.Ø6- ☑
          - nondisplaced S72.Ø6- ☑
        - specified NEC S72.Ø9- ☑
      - intertrochanteric (displaced) S72.14- ☑
        - nondisplaced S72.14- ☑
      - intracapsular S72.Ø1- ☑
      - midcervical (displaced) S72.Ø3- ☑
        - nondisplaced S72.Ø3- ☑
      - neck S72.ØØ- ☑
        - base (displaced) S72.Ø4- ☑
          - nondisplaced S72.Ø4- ☑
        - specified NEC S72.Ø9- ☑
      - pertrochanteric — *see* Fracture, femur, upper end, trochanteric
      - physeal S79.ØØ- ☑
        - Salter-Harris type I S79.Ø1- ☑
        - specified NEC S79.Ø9- ☑

- **Fracture, traumatic** — *continued*
  - femur, femoral — *continued*
    - upper end — *continued*
      - subcapital (displaced) S72.Ø1- ☑
      - subtrochanteric (displaced) S72.2- ☑
        - nondisplaced S72.2- ☑
      - transcervical — *see* Fracture, femur, upper end, midcervical
      - trochanteric S72.1Ø- ☑
        - greater (displaced) S72.11- ☑
          - nondisplaced S72.11- ☑
        - lesser (displaced) S72.12- ☑
          - nondisplaced S72.12- ☑
  - fibula (shaft) (styloid) S82.4Ø- ☑
    - comminuted (displaced) S82.45- ☑
      - nondisplaced S82.45- ☑
    - following insertion of implant, prosthesis or plate M96.67- ☑
    - involving ankle or malleolus — *see* Fracture, fibula, lateral malleolus
    - lateral malleolus (displaced) S82.6- ☑
      - nondisplaced S82.6- ☑
    - lower end
      - physeal S89.3Ø- ☑
        - Salter-Harris
          - Type I S89.31- ☑
          - Type II S89.32- ☑
        - specified NEC S89.39- ☑
      - specified NEC S82.83- ☑
      - torus S82.82- ☑
    - oblique (displaced) S82.43- ☑
      - nondisplaced S82.43- ☑
    - segmental (displaced) S82.46- ☑
      - nondisplaced S82.46- ☑
    - specified NEC S82.49- ☑
    - spiral (displaced) S82.44- ☑
      - nondisplaced S82.44- ☑
    - transverse (displaced) S82.42- ☑
      - nondisplaced S82.42- ☑
    - upper end
      - physeal S89.2Ø- ☑
        - Salter-Harris
          - Type I S89.21- ☑
          - Type II S89.22- ☑
        - specified NEC S89.29- ☑
      - specified NEC S82.83- ☑
      - torus S82.81- ☑
  - finger (except thumb) S62.6Ø- ☑
    - distal phalanx (displaced) S62.63- ☑
      - nondisplaced S62.66- ☑
    - index S62.6Ø- ☑
      - distal phalanx (displaced) S62.63- ☑
        - nondisplaced S62.66- ☑
      - middle phalanx (displaced) S62.62- ☑
        - nondisplaced S62.65- ☑
      - proximal phalanx (displaced) S62.61- ☑
        - nondisplaced S62.64- ☑
    - little S62.6Ø- ☑
      - distal phalanx (displaced) S62.63- ☑
        - nondisplaced S62.66- ☑
      - middle phalanx (displaced) S62.62- ☑
        - nondisplaced S62.65- ☑
      - proximal phalanx (displaced) S62.61- ☑
        - nondisplaced S62.64- ☑
    - middle S62.6Ø- ☑
      - distal phalanx (displaced) S62.63- ☑
        - nondisplaced S62.66- ☑
      - middle phalanx (displaced) S62.62- ☑
        - nondisplaced S62.65- ☑
      - proximal phalanx (displaced) S62.61- ☑
        - nondisplaced S62.64- ☑
    - middle phalanx (displaced) S62.62- ☑
      - nondisplaced S62.65- ☑
    - proximal phalanx (displaced) S62.61- ☑
      - nondisplaced S62.64- ☑
    - ring S62.6Ø- ☑
      - distal phalanx (displaced) S62.63- ☑
        - nondisplaced S62.66- ☑
      - middle phalanx (displaced) S62.62- ☑
        - nondisplaced S62.65- ☑
      - proximal phalanx (displaced) S62.61- ☑
        - nondisplaced S62.64- ☑
    - thumb — *see* Fracture, thumb
  - following insertion (intraoperative) (postoperative) of orthopedic implant, joint prosthesis or bone plate M96.69

Fracture, traumatic — *continued*
- following insertion of orthopedic implant, joint prosthesis or bone plate — *continued*
  - femur M96.66- ☑
  - fibula M96.67- ☑
  - humerus M96.62- ☑
  - pelvis M96.65
  - radius M96.63- ☑
  - specified bone NEC M96.69
  - tibia M96.67- ☑
  - ulna M96.63- ☑
- foot S92.9Ø- ☑
  - astragalus — *see* Fracture, tarsal, talus
  - calcaneus — *see* Fracture, tarsal, calcaneus
  - cuboid — *see* Fracture, tarsal, cuboid
  - cuneiform — *see* Fracture, tarsal, cuneiform
  - metatarsal — *see* Fracture, metatarsal
  - navicular — *see* Fracture, tarsal, navicular
  - sesamoid S92.81- ☑
  - specified NEC S92.81- ☑
  - talus — *see* Fracture, tarsal, talus
  - tarsal — *see* Fracture, tarsal
  - toe — *see* Fracture, toe
- forearm S52.9- ☑
  - radius — *see* Fracture, radius
  - ulna — *see* Fracture, ulna
- fossa (anterior) (middle) (posterior) SØ2.19 ☑
- fragility — *see* Fracture, pathological, due to osteoporosis
- frontal (bone) (skull) SØ2.Ø ☑
  - sinus SØ2.19 ☑
- glenoid (cavity) (scapula) — *see* Fracture, scapula, glenoid cavity
- greenstick — *see* Fracture, by site
- hallux — *see* Fracture, toe, great
- hand S62.9- ☑
  - carpal — *see* Fracture, carpal bone
  - finger (except thumb) — *see* Fracture, finger
  - metacarpal — *see* Fracture, metacarpal
  - navicular (scaphoid) (hand) — *see* Fracture, carpal bone, navicular
  - thumb — *see* Fracture, thumb
- healed or old
  - with complications — *code by* Nature of the complication
- heel bone — *see* Fracture, tarsal, calcaneus
- Hill-Sachs S42.29- ☑
- hip — *see* Fracture, femur, neck
- humerus S42.3Ø- ☑
  - anatomical neck — *see* Fracture, humerus, upper end
  - articular process — *see* Fracture, humerus, lower end
  - capitellum — *see* Fracture, humerus, lower end, condyle, lateral
  - distal end — *see* Fracture, humerus, lower end
  - epiphysis
    - lower — *see* Fracture, humerus, lower end, physeal
    - upper — *see* Fracture, humerus, upper end, physeal
  - external condyle — *see* Fracture, humerus, lower end, condyle, lateral
  - following insertion of implant, prosthesis or plate M96.62- ☑
  - great tuberosity — *see* Fracture, humerus, upper end, greater tuberosity
  - intercondylar — *see* Fracture, humerus, lower end
  - internal epicondyle — *see* Fracture, humerus, lower end, epicondyle, medial
  - lesser tuberosity — *see* Fracture, humerus, upper end, lesser tuberosity
  - lower end S42.4Ø- ☑
    - condyle
      - lateral (displaced) S42.45- ☑
        - nondisplaced S42.45- ☑
      - medial (displaced) S42.46- ☑
        - nondisplaced S42.46- ☑
    - epicondyle
      - lateral (displaced) S42.43- ☑
        - nondisplaced S42.43- ☑
      - medial (displaced) S42.44- ☑
        - incarcerated S42.44- ☑
        - nondisplaced S42.44- ☑
    - physeal S49.1Ø- ☑
      - Salter-Harris
        - Type I S49.11- ☑

Fracture, traumatic — *continued*
- humerus — *continued*
  - lower end — *continued*
    - physeal — *continued*
      - Salter-Harris — *continued*
        - Type II S49.12- ☑
        - Type III S49.13- ☑
        - Type IV S49.14- ☑
      - specified NEC S49.19- ☑
    - specified NEC (displaced) S42.49- ☑
      - nondisplaced S42.49- ☑
    - supracondylar (simple) (displaced) S42.41- ☑
      - with intercondylar fracture — *see* Fracture, humerus, lower end
      - comminuted (displaced) S42.42- ☑
        - nondisplaced S42.42- ☑
      - nondisplaced S42.41- ☑
    - torus S42.48- ☑
    - transcondylar (displaced) S42.47- ☑
      - nondisplaced S42.47- ☑
  - proximal end — *see* Fracture, humerus, upper end
  - shaft S42.3Ø- ☑
    - comminuted (displaced) S42.35- ☑
      - nondisplaced S42.35- ☑
    - greenstick S42.31- ☑
    - oblique (displaced) S42.33- ☑
      - nondisplaced S42.33- ☑
    - segmental (displaced) S42.36- ☑
      - nondisplaced S42.36- ☑
    - specified NEC S42.39- ☑
    - spiral (displaced) S42.34- ☑
      - nondisplaced S42.34- ☑
    - transverse (displaced) S42.32- ☑
      - nondisplaced S42.32- ☑
  - supracondylar — *see* Fracture, humerus, lower end
  - surgical neck — *see* Fracture, humerus, upper end, surgical neck
  - trochlea — *see* Fracture, humerus, lower end, condyle, medial
  - tuberosity — *see* Fracture, humerus, upper end
  - upper end S42.2Ø- ☑
    - anatomical neck — *see* Fracture, humerus, upper end, specified NEC
    - articular head — *see* Fracture, humerus, upper end, specified NEC
    - epiphysis — *see* Fracture, humerus, upper end, physeal
    - greater tuberosity (displaced) S42.25- ☑
      - nondisplaced S42.25- ☑
    - lesser tuberosity (displaced) S42.26- ☑
      - nondisplaced S42.26- ☑
    - physeal S49.ØØ- ☑
      - Salter-Harris
        - Type I S49.Ø1- ☑
        - Type II S49.Ø2- ☑
        - Type III S49.Ø3- ☑
        - Type IV S49.Ø4- ☑
      - specified NEC S49.Ø9- ☑
    - specified NEC (displaced) S42.29- ☑
      - nondisplaced S42.29- ☑
    - surgical neck (displaced) S42.21- ☑
      - four-part S42.24- ☑
      - nondisplaced S42.21- ☑
      - three-part S42.23- ☑
      - two-part (displaced) S42.22- ☑
        - nondisplaced S42.22- ☑
    - torus S42.27- ☑
    - transepiphyseal — *see* Fracture, humerus, upper end, physeal
- hyoid bone S12.8 ☑
- ilium S32.3Ø- ☑
  - with disruption of pelvic ring — *see* Disruption, pelvic ring
  - avulsion (displaced) S32.31- ☑
    - nondisplaced S32.31- ☑
  - specified NEC S32.39- ☑
- impaction, impacted — *code as* Fracture, by site
- innominate bone — *see* Fracture, ilium
- instep — *see* Fracture, foot
- ischium S32.6Ø- ☑
  - with disruption of pelvic ring — *see* Disruption, pelvic ring
  - avulsion (displaced) S32.61- ☑
    - nondisplaced S32.61- ☑
  - specified NEC S32.69- ☑
- jaw (bone) (lower) — *see* Fracture, mandible

Fracture, traumatic — *continued*
- jaw — *see* Fracture, mandible — *continued*
  - upper — *see* Fracture, maxilla
- joint prosthesis — *see* Complications, joint prosthesis, mechanical, breakdown, by site
  - periprosthetic — *see* Fracture, traumatic, periprosthetic
- knee cap — *see* Fracture, patella
- larynx S12.8 ☑
- late effects — *see* Sequelae, fracture
- leg (lower) S82.9- ☑
  - ankle — *see* Fracture, ankle
  - femur — *see* Fracture, femur
  - fibula — *see* Fracture, fibula
  - malleolus — *see* Fracture, ankle
  - patella — *see* Fracture, patella
  - specified site NEC S82.89- ☑
  - tibia — *see* Fracture, tibia
- lumbar spine — *see* Fracture, vertebra, lumbar
- lumbosacral spine S32.9 ☑
- Maisonneuve's (displaced) S82.86- ☑
  - nondisplaced S82.86- ☑
- malar bone — *see also* Fracture, maxilla SØ2.4ØØ ☑
  - left side SØ2.4ØB ☑
  - right side SØ2.4ØA ☑
- malleolus — *see* Fracture, ankle
- malunion — *see* Fracture, by site
- mandible (lower jaw (bone)) SØ2.6Ø9 ☑
  - alveolus SØ2.67- ☑
  - angle (of jaw) SØ2.65- ☑
  - body, unspecified SØ2.6ØØ ☑
    - left side SØ2.6Ø2 ☑
    - right side SØ2.6Ø1 ☑
  - condylar process SØ2.61- ☑
  - coronoid process SØ2.63- ☑
  - ramus, unspecified SØ2.64- ☑
  - specified site NEC SØ2.69 ☑
  - subcondylar process SØ2.62- ☑
  - symphysis SØ2.66 ☑
- manubrium (sterni) S22.21 ☑
  - dissociation from sternum S22.23 ☑
- march — *see* Fracture, traumatic, stress, by site
- maxilla, maxillary (bone) (sinus) (superior) (upper jaw) SØ2.4Ø1 ☑
  - alveolus SØ2.42 ☑
  - inferior — *see* Fracture, mandible
  - LeFort I SØ2.411 ☑
  - LeFort II SØ2.412 ☑
  - LeFort III SØ2.413 ☑
  - left side SØ2.4ØD ☑
  - right side SØ2.4ØC ☑
- metacarpal S62.3Ø9 ☑
  - base (displaced) S62.319 ☑
    - nondisplaced S62.349 ☑
  - fifth S62.3Ø- ☑
    - base (displaced) S62.31- ☑
      - nondisplaced S62.34- ☑
    - neck (displaced) S62.33- ☑
      - nondisplaced S62.36- ☑
    - shaft (displaced) S62.32- ☑
      - nondisplaced S62.35- ☑
    - specified NEC S62.398 ☑
  - first S62.2Ø- ☑
    - base NEC (displaced) S62.23- ☑
      - nondisplaced S62.23- ☑
    - Bennett's — *see* Bennett's fracture
    - neck (displaced) S62.25- ☑
      - nondisplaced S62.25- ☑
    - shaft (displaced) S62.24- ☑
      - nondisplaced S62.24- ☑
    - specified NEC S62.29- ☑
  - fourth S62.3Ø- ☑
    - base (displaced) S62.31- ☑
      - nondisplaced S62.34- ☑
    - neck (displaced) S62.33- ☑
      - nondisplaced S62.36- ☑
    - shaft (displaced) S62.32- ☑
      - nondisplaced S62.35- ☑
    - specified NEC S62.39- ☑
  - neck (displaced) S62.33- ☑
    - nondisplaced S62.36- ☑
  - Rolando's — *see* Rolando's fracture
  - second S62.3Ø- ☑
    - base (displaced) S62.31- ☑
      - nondisplaced S62.34- ☑
    - neck (displaced) S62.33- ☑

☑ **Additional Character Required — Refer to the Tabular List for Character Selection**

- **Fracture, traumatic** — *continued*
  - tibia — *continued*
    - lower end — *continued*
      - physeal — *continued*
        - Salter-Harris
          - Type I S89.11- ☑
          - Type II S89.12- ☑
          - Type III S89.13- ☑
          - Type IV S89.14- ☑
        - specified NEC S89.19- ☑
      - pilon (displaced) S82.87- ☑
        - nondisplaced S82.87- ☑
      - specified NEC S82.39- ☑
      - torus S82.31- ☑
    - malleolus — *see* Fracture, ankle, medial malleolus
    - oblique (displaced) S82.23- ☑
      - nondisplaced S82.23- ☑
    - pilon — *see* Fracture, tibia, lower end, pilon
    - proximal end — *see* Fracture, tibia, upper end
    - segmental (displaced) S82.26- ☑
      - nondisplaced S82.26- ☑
    - specified NEC S82.29- ☑
    - spine — *see* Fracture, tibia, upper end, spine
    - spiral (displaced) S82.24- ☑
      - nondisplaced S82.24- ☑
    - transverse (displaced) S82.22- ☑
      - nondisplaced S82.22- ☑
    - tuberosity — *see* Fracture, tibia, upper end, tuberosity
    - upper end S82.10- ☑
      - bicondylar (displaced) S82.14- ☑
        - nondisplaced S82.14- ☑
      - lateral condyle (displaced) S82.12- ☑
        - nondisplaced S82.12- ☑
      - medial condyle (displaced) S82.13- ☑
        - nondisplaced S82.13- ☑
      - physeal S89.00- ☑
        - Salter-Harris
          - Type I S89.01- ☑
          - Type II S89.02- ☑
          - Type III S89.03- ☑
          - Type IV S89.04- ☑
        - specified NEC S89.09- ☑
      - plateau — *see* Fracture, tibia, upper end, bicondylar
      - specified NEC S82.19- ☑
      - spine (displaced) S82.11- ☑
        - nondisplaced S82.11- ☑
      - torus S82.16- ☑
      - tuberosity (displaced) S82.15- ☑
        - nondisplaced S82.15- ☑
  - toe S92.91- ☑
    - great (displaced) S92.40- ☑
      - distal phalanx (displaced) S92.42- ☑
        - nondisplaced S92.42- ☑
      - nondisplaced S92.40- ☑
      - proximal phalanx (displaced) S92.41- ☑
        - nondisplaced S92.41- ☑
      - specified NEC S92.49- ☑
    - lesser (displaced) S92.50- ☑
      - distal phalanx (displaced) S92.53- ☑
        - nondisplaced S92.53- ☑
      - middle phalanx (displaced) S92.52- ☑
        - nondisplaced S92.52- ☑
      - nondisplaced S92.50- ☑
      - proximal phalanx (displaced) S92.51- ☑
        - nondisplaced S92.51- ☑
      - specified NEC S92.59- ☑
    - physeal
      - phalanx S99.20- ☑
        - Salter-Harris
          - Type I S99.21- ☑
          - Type II S99.22- ☑
          - Type III S99.23- ☑
          - Type IV S99.24- ☑
        - specified NEC S99.29- ☑
  - tooth (root) S02.5 ☑
  - trachea (cartilage) S12.8 ☑
  - transverse process — *see* Fracture, vertebra
  - trapezium or trapezoid bone — *see* Fracture, carpal
  - trimalleolar — *see* Fracture, ankle, trimalleolar
  - triquetrum (cuneiform of carpus) — *see* Fracture, carpal, triquetrum
  - trochanter — *see* Fracture, femur, trochanteric
  - tuberosity (external) — *see* Fracture, traumatic, by site
  - ulna (shaft) S52.20- ☑

- **Fracture, traumatic** — *continued*
  - ulna — *continued*
    - bent bone S52.28- ☑
    - coronoid process — *see* Fracture, ulna, upper end, coronoid process
    - distal end — *see* Fracture, ulna, lower end
    - following insertion of implant, prosthesis or plate M96.63- ☑
    - head S52.60- ☑
    - lower end S52.60- ☑
      - physeal S59.00- ☑
        - Salter-Harris
          - Type I S59.01- ☑
          - Type II S59.02- ☑
          - Type III S59.03- ☑
          - Type IV S59.04- ☑
        - specified NEC S59.09- ☑
      - specified NEC S52.69- ☑
      - styloid process (displaced) S52.61- ☑
        - nondisplaced S52.61- ☑
      - torus S52.62- ☑
    - proximal end — *see* Fracture, ulna, upper end
    - shaft S52.20- ☑
      - comminuted (displaced) S52.25- ☑
        - nondisplaced S52.25- ☑
      - greenstick S52.21- ☑
      - Monteggia's — *see* Monteggia's fracture
      - oblique (displaced) S52.23- ☑
        - nondisplaced S52.23- ☑
      - segmental (displaced) S52.26- ☑
        - nondisplaced S52.26- ☑
      - specified NEC S52.29- ☑
      - spiral (displaced) S52.24- ☑
        - nondisplaced S52.24- ☑
      - transverse (displaced) S52.22- ☑
        - nondisplaced S52.22- ☑
    - upper end S52.00- ☑
      - coronoid process (displaced) S52.04- ☑
        - nondisplaced S52.04- ☑
      - olecranon process (displaced) S52.02- ☑
        - with intraarticular extension S52.03- ☑
        - nondisplaced S52.02- ☑
          - with intraarticular extension S52.03- ☑
      - specified NEC S52.09- ☑
      - torus S52.01- ☑
  - unciform — *see* Fracture, carpal, hamate
  - vault of skull S02.0 ☑
  - vertebra, vertebral (arch) (body) (column) (neural arch) (pedicle) (spinous process) (transverse process)
    - atlas — *see* Fracture, neck, cervical vertebra, first
    - axis — *see* Fracture, neck, cervical vertebra, second
    - cervical (teardrop) S12.9 ☑
      - axis — *see* Fracture, neck, cervical vertebra, second
      - first (atlas) — *see* Fracture, neck, cervical vertebra, first
      - second (axis) — *see* Fracture, neck, cervical vertebra, second
    - chronic M84.48 ☑
    - coccyx S32.2 ☑
    - dorsal — *see* Fracture, thorax, vertebra
    - lumbar S32.009 ☑
      - burst (stable) S32.001 ☑
        - unstable S32.002 ☑
      - fifth S32.059 ☑
        - burst (stable) S32.051 ☑
          - unstable S32.052 ☑
        - specified type NEC S32.058 ☑
        - wedge compression S32.050 ☑
      - first S32.019 ☑
        - burst (stable) S32.011 ☑
          - unstable S32.012 ☑
        - specified type NEC S32.018 ☑
        - wedge compression S32.010 ☑
      - fourth S32.049 ☑
        - burst (stable) S32.041 ☑
          - unstable S32.042 ☑
        - specified type NEC S32.048 ☑
        - wedge compression S32.040 ☑
      - second S32.029 ☑
        - burst (stable) S32.021 ☑
          - unstable S32.022 ☑
        - specified type NEC S32.028 ☑
        - wedge compression S32.020 ☑
      - specified type NEC S32.008 ☑
      - third S32.039 ☑

- **Fracture, traumatic** — *continued*
  - vertebra, vertebral — *continued*
    - lumbar — *continued*
      - third — *continued*
        - burst (stable) S32.031 ☑
          - unstable S32.032 ☑
        - specified type NEC S32.038 ☑
        - wedge compression S32.030 ☑
      - wedge compression S32.000 ☑
    - metastatic — *see* Collapse, vertebra, in, specified disease NEC — *see also* Neoplasm
    - newborn (birth injury) P11.5
    - sacrum S32.10 ☑
      - specified NEC S32.19 ☑
      - Type
        - 1 S32.14 ☑
        - 2 S32.15 ☑
        - 3 S32.16 ☑
        - 4 S32.17 ☑
      - Zone
        - I S32.119 ☑
          - displaced (minimally) S32.111 ☑
            - severely S32.112 ☑
          - nondisplaced S32.110 ☑
        - II S32.129 ☑
          - displaced (minimally) S32.121 ☑
            - severely S32.122 ☑
          - nondisplaced S32.120 ☑
        - III S32.139 ☑
          - displaced (minimally) S32.131 ☑
            - severely S32.132 ☑
          - nondisplaced S32.130 ☑
    - thoracic — *see* Fracture, thorax, vertebra
  - vertex S02.0 ☑
  - vomer (bone) S02.2 ☑
  - wrist S62.10- ☑
    - carpal — *see* Fracture, carpal bone
    - navicular (scaphoid) (hand) — *see* Fracture, carpal, navicular
  - xiphisternum, xiphoid (process) S22.24 ☑
    - associated with chest compression and cardiopulmonary resuscitation M96.A1
  - zygoma S02.402 ☑
    - left side S02.40F ☑
    - right side S02.40E ☑
- **Fragile, fragility**
  - autosomal site Q95.5
  - bone, congenital (with blue sclera) Q78.0
  - capillary (hereditary) D69.8
  - hair L67.8
  - nails L60.3
  - non-sex chromosome site Q95.5
  - X chromosome Q99.2
- **Fragilitas**
  - crinium L67.8
  - ossium (with blue sclerae) (hereditary) Q78.0
  - unguium L60.3
    - congenital Q84.6
- **Fragments, cataract** (lens), **following cataract surgery** H59.02- ☑
  - retained foreign body — *see* Retained, foreign body fragments (type of)
- **Frailty** (frail) R54
  - mental R41.81
- **Frambesia, frambesial** (tropica) — *see also* Yaws
  - initial lesion or ulcer A66.0
  - primary A66.0
- **Frambeside**
  - gummatous A66.4
  - of early yaws A66.2
- **Frambesioma** A66.1
- **Franceschetti-Klein** (-Wildervanck) **disease or syndrome** Q75.4
- **Francis' disease** — *see* Tularemia
- **Franklin disease** C88.2
- **Frank's essential thrombocytopenia** D69.3
- **Fraser's syndrome** Q87.0
- **Freckle**(s) L81.2
  - malignant melanoma in — *see* Melanoma
  - melanotic (Hutchinson's) — *see* Melanoma, in situ
  - retinal D49.81
- **Frederickson's hyperlipoproteinemia, type**
  - I and V E78.3
  - IIA E78.00
  - IIB and III E78.2
  - IV E78.1
- **Freeman Sheldon syndrome** Q87.0

- **Freezing** — *see also* Effect, adverse, cold T69.9 ☑
- **Freiberg's disease** (infraction of metatarsal head or osteochondrosis) — *see* Osteochondrosis, juvenile, metatarsus
- **Frei's disease** A55
- **Fremitus, friction, cardiac** RØ1.2
- **Frenum, frenulum**
  - external os Q51.828
  - tongue (shortening) (congenital) Q38.1
- **Frequency micturition** (nocturnal) R35.Ø
  - psychogenic F45.8
- **Frey's syndrome**
  - auriculotemporal G5Ø.8
  - hyperhidrosis L74.52
- **Friction**
  - burn — *see* Burn, by site
  - fremitus, cardiac RØ1.2
  - precordial RØ1.2
  - sounds, chest RØ9.89
- **Friderichsen-Waterhouse syndrome or disease** A39.1
- **Friedlander's B** (bacillus) **NEC** — *see also* condition A49.8
- **Friedreich's**
  - ataxia G11.11
  - combined systemic disease G11.11
  - facial hemihypertrophy Q67.4
  - sclerosis (cerebellum) (spinal cord) G11.11
- **Frigidity** F52.22
- **Frohlich's syndrome** E23.6
- **Frontal** — *see also* condition
  - lobe syndrome FØ7.Ø
- **Frostbite** (superficial) T33.9Ø ☑
  - with
    - partial thickness skin loss — *see* Frostbite (superficial), by site
    - tissue necrosis T34.9Ø ☑
  - abdominal wall T33.3 ☑
    - with tissue necrosis T34.3 ☑
  - ankle T33.81- ☑
    - with tissue necrosis T34.81- ☑
  - arm T33.4- ☑
    - with tissue necrosis T34.4- ☑
    - finger(s) — *see* Frostbite, finger
    - hand — *see* Frostbite, hand
    - wrist — *see* Frostbite, wrist
  - ear T33.Ø1- ☑
    - with tissue necrosis T34.Ø1- ☑
  - face T33.Ø9 ☑
    - with tissue necrosis T34.Ø9 ☑
  - finger T33.53- ☑
    - with tissue necrosis T34.53- ☑
  - foot T33.82- ☑
    - with tissue necrosis T34.82- ☑
  - hand T33.52- ☑
    - with tissue necrosis T34.52- ☑
  - head T33.Ø9 ☑
    - with tissue necrosis T34.Ø9 ☑
    - ear — *see* Frostbite, ear
    - nose — *see* Frostbite, nose
  - hip (and thigh) T33.6- ☑
    - with tissue necrosis T34.6- ☑
  - knee T33.7- ☑
    - with tissue necrosis T34.7- ☑
  - leg T33.9- ☑
    - with tissue necrosis T34.9- ☑
    - ankle — *see* Frostbite, ankle
    - foot — *see* Frostbite, foot
    - knee — *see* Frostbite, knee
    - lower T33.7- ☑
      - with tissue necrosis T34.7- ☑
    - thigh — *see* Frostbite, hip
    - toe — *see* Frostbite, toe
  - limb
    - lower T33.99 ☑
      - with tissue necrosis T34.99 ☑
    - upper — *see* Frostbite, arm
  - neck T33.1 ☑
    - with tissue necrosis T34.1 ☑
  - nose T33.Ø2 ☑
    - with tissue necrosis T34.Ø2 ☑
  - pelvis T33.3 ☑
    - with tissue necrosis T34.3 ☑
  - specified site NEC T33.99 ☑
    - with tissue necrosis T34.99 ☑
  - thigh — *see* Frostbite, hip
  - thorax T33.2 ☑
    - with tissue necrosis T34.2 ☑
- **Frostbite** — *continued*
  - toes T33.83- ☑
    - with tissue necrosis T34.83- ☑
  - trunk T33.99 ☑
    - with tissue necrosis T34.99 ☑
  - wrist T33.51- ☑
    - with tissue necrosis T34.51- ☑
- **Frotteurism** F65.81
- **Frozen** — *see also* Effect, adverse, cold T69.9 ☑
  - pelvis (female) N94.89
    - male K66.8
  - shoulder — *see* Capsulitis, adhesive
- **Fructokinase deficiency** E74.11
- **Fructose 1,6 diphosphatase deficiency** E74.19
- **Fructosemia** (benign) (essential) E74.12
- **Fructosuria** (benign) (essential) E74.11
- **Fuchs'**
  - black spot (myopic) — *see also* Myopia, degenerative H44.2- ☑
  - dystrophy (corneal endothelium) H18.51- ☑
  - heterochromic cyclitis — *see* Cyclitis, Fuchs' heterochromic
- **Fucosidosis** E77.1
- **Fugue** R68.89
  - dissociative F44.1
  - hysterical (dissociative) F44.1
  - postictal in epilepsy — *see* Epilepsy
  - reaction to exceptional stress (transient) F43.Ø
- **Fulminant, fulminating** — *see* condition
- **Functional** — *see also* condition
  - bleeding (uterus) N93.8
- **Functioning, intellectual, borderline** R41.83
- **Fundus** — *see* condition
- **Fungemia NOS** B49
- **Fungus, fungous**
  - cerebral G93.89
  - disease NOS B49
  - infection — *see* Infection, fungus
- **Funiculitis** (acute) (chronic) (endemic) N49.1
  - gonococcal (acute) (chronic) A54.23
  - tuberculous A18.15
- **Funnel**
  - breast (acquired) M95.4
    - congenital Q67.6
    - sequelae (late effect) of rickets E64.3
  - chest (acquired) M95.4
    - congenital Q67.6
    - sequelae (late effect) of rickets E64.3
  - pelvis (acquired) M95.5
    - with disproportion (fetopelvic) O33.3 ☑
      - causing obstructed labor O65.3
    - congenital Q74.2
- **FUO** (fever of unknown origin) R5Ø.9
- **Furfur** L21.Ø
  - microsporon B36.Ø
- **Furrier's lung** J67.8
- **Furrowed** K14.5
  - nail(s) (transverse) L6Ø.4
    - congenital Q84.6
  - tongue K14.5
    - congenital Q38.3
- **Furuncle** LØ2.92
  - abdominal wall LØ2.221
  - ankle — *see* Furuncle, lower limb
  - antecubital space — *see* Furuncle, upper limb
  - anus K61.Ø
  - arm — *see* Furuncle, upper limb
  - auditory canal, external — *see* Abscess, ear, external
  - auricle (ear) — *see* Abscess, ear, external
  - axilla (region) LØ2.42- ☑
  - back (any part) LØ2.222
  - breast N61.1
  - buttock LØ2.32
  - cheek (external) LØ2.Ø2
  - chest wall LØ2.223
  - chin LØ2.Ø2
  - corpus cavernosum N48.21
  - ear, external — *see* Abscess, ear, external
  - external auditory canal — *see* Abscess, ear, external
  - eyelid — *see* Abscess, eyelid
  - face LØ2.Ø2
  - femoral (region) — *see* Furuncle, lower limb
  - finger — *see* Furuncle, hand
  - flank LØ2.221
  - foot LØ2.62- ☑
  - forehead LØ2.Ø2
  - gluteal (region) LØ2.32
- **Furuncle** — *continued*
  - groin LØ2.224
  - hand LØ2.52- ☑
  - head LØ2.821
    - face LØ2.Ø2
  - hip — *see* Furuncle, lower limb
  - kidney — *see* Abscess, kidney
  - knee — *see* Furuncle, lower limb
  - labium (majus) (minus) N76.4
  - lacrimal
    - gland — *see* Dacryoadenitis
    - passages (duct) (sac) — *see* Inflammation, lacrimal, passages, acute
  - leg (any part) — *see* Furuncle, lower limb
  - lower limb LØ2.42- ☑
  - malignant A22.Ø
  - mouth K12.2
  - navel LØ2.226
  - neck LØ2.12
  - nose J34.Ø
  - orbit, orbital — *see* Abscess, orbit
  - palmar (space) — *see* Furuncle, hand
  - partes posteriores LØ2.32
  - pectoral region LØ2.223
  - penis N48.21
  - perineum LØ2.225
  - pinna — *see* Abscess, ear, external
  - popliteal — *see* Furuncle, lower limb
  - prepatellar — *see* Furuncle, lower limb
  - scalp LØ2.821
  - seminal vesicle N49.Ø
  - shoulder — *see* Furuncle, upper limb
  - specified site NEC LØ2.828
  - submandibular K12.2
  - temple (region) LØ2.Ø2
  - thumb — *see* Furuncle, hand
  - toe — *see* Furuncle, foot
  - trunk LØ2.229
    - abdominal wall LØ2.221
    - back LØ2.222
    - chest wall LØ2.223
    - groin LØ2.224
    - perineum LØ2.225
    - umbilicus LØ2.226
  - umbilicus LØ2.226
  - upper limb LØ2.42- ☑
  - vulva N76.4
- **Furunculosis** — *see* Furuncle
- **Fused** — *see* Fusion, fused
- **Fusion, fused** (congenital)
  - astragaloscaphoid Q74.2
  - atria Q21.19
  - auditory canal Q16.1
  - auricles, heart Q21.19
  - binocular with defective stereopsis H53.32
  - bone Q79.8
  - cervical spine M43.22
  - choanal Q3Ø.Ø
  - commissure, mitral valve Q23.2
  - cusps, heart valve NEC Q24.8
    - mitral Q23.2
    - pulmonary Q22.1
    - tricuspid Q22.4
  - ear ossicles Q16.3
  - fingers Q7Ø.Ø ☑
  - hymen Q52.3
  - joint (acquired) — *see also* Ankylosis
    - congenital Q74.8
  - kidneys (incomplete) Q63.1
  - labium (majus) (minus) Q52.5
  - larynx and trachea Q34.8
  - limb, congenital Q74.8
    - lower Q74.2
    - upper Q74.Ø
  - lobes, lung Q33.8
  - lumbosacral (acquired) M43.27
    - arthrodesis status Z98.1
    - congenital Q76.49
    - postprocedural status Z98.1
  - nares, nose, nasal, nostril(s) Q3Ø.Ø
  - organ or site not listed — *see* Anomaly, by site
  - ossicles Q79.9
    - auditory Q16.3
  - pulmonic cusps Q22.1
  - ribs Q76.6
  - sacroiliac (joint) (acquired) M43.28
    - arthrodesis status Z98.1
    - congenital Q74.2

☑ **Additional Character Required — Refer to the Tabular List for Character Selection**

G

- **Gastritis** — *continued*
  - specified NEC K29.6Ø
    - with bleeding K29.61
  - superficial chronic K29.3Ø
    - with bleeding K29.31
  - tuberculous A18.83
  - viral NEC AØ8.4
- **Gastrocarcinoma** — *see* Neoplasm, malignant, stomach
- **Gastrocolic** — *see* condition
- **Gastrodisciasis, gastrodiscoidiasis** B66.8
- **Gastroduodenitis** K29.9Ø
  - with bleeding K29.91
  - virus, viral AØ8.4
    - specified type NEC AØ8.39
- **Gastrodynia** — *see* Pain, abdominal
- **Gastroenteritis** (acute) (chronic) (noninfectious) — *see also* Enteritis K52.9
  - allergic K52.29
    - with
      - eosinophilic gastritis or gastroenteritis K52.81
      - food protein-induced enterocolitis syndrome K52.21
      - food protein-induced enteropathy K52.22
  - dietetic — *see also* Gastroenteritis, allergic K52.29
  - drug-induced K52.1
  - due to
    - Cryptosporidium AØ7.2
    - drugs K52.1
    - food poisoning — *see* Intoxication, foodborne
    - radiation K52.Ø
  - eosinophilic K52.81
  - epidemic (infectious) AØ9
  - food hypersensitivity — *see also* Gastroenteritis, allergic K52.29
  - infectious — *see* Enteritis, infectious
  - influenzal — *see* Influenza, with gastroenteritis
  - noninfectious K52.9
    - specified NEC K52.89
  - rotaviral AØ8.Ø
  - Salmonella AØ2.Ø
  - toxic K52.1
  - viral NEC AØ8.4
    - acute infectious AØ8.39
      - type Norwalk AØ8.11
    - infantile (acute) AØ8.39
    - Norwalk agent AØ8.11
    - rotaviral AØ8.Ø
    - severe of infants AØ8.39
    - specified type NEC AØ8.39
- **Gastroenteropathy** — *see also* Gastroenteritis K52.9
  - acute, due to Norovirus AØ8.11
  - acute, due to Norwalk agent AØ8.11
  - infectious AØ9
- **Gastroenteroptosis** K63.4
- **Gastroesophageal laceration- hemorrhage syndrome** K22.6
- **Gastrointestinal** — *see* condition
- **Gastrojejunal** — *see* condition
- **Gastrojejunitis** — *see also* Enteritis K52.9
- **Gastrojejunocolic** — *see* condition
- **Gastroliths** K31.89
- **Gastromalacia** K31.89
- **Gastroparalysis** K31.84
  - diabetic — *see* Diabetes, gastroparalysis
- **Gastroparesis** K31.84
  - diabetic — *see* Diabetes, by type, with gastroparesis
- **Gastropathy** K31.9
  - congestive portal — *see also* Hypertension, portal K31.89
  - erythematous K29.7Ø
  - exudative K9Ø.89
  - portal hypertensive — *see also* Hypertension, portal K31.89
  - specified NEC K31.89
- **Gastroptosis** K31.89
- **Gastrorrhagia** K92.2
  - psychogenic F45.8
- **Gastroschisis** (congenital) Q79.3
- **Gastrospasm** (neurogenic) (reflex) K31.89
  - neurotic F45.8
  - psychogenic F45.8
- **Gastrostaxis** — *see* Gastritis, with bleeding
- **Gastrostenosis** K31.89
- **Gastrostomy**
  - attention to Z43.1
  - status Z93.1
- **Gastrosuccorrhea** (continuous) (intermittent) K31.89
  - neurotic F45.8
- **Gastrosuccorrhea** — *continued*
  - psychogenic F45.8
- **Gatophobia** F4Ø.218
- **Gaucher's disease or splenomegaly** (adult) (infantile) E75.22
- **Gee** (-Herter)(-Thaysen) **disease** (nontropical sprue) K9Ø.Ø
- **Gelineau's syndrome** G47.419
  - with cataplexy G47.411
- **Gemination, tooth, teeth** KØØ.2
- **Gemistocytoma**
  - specified site — *see* Neoplasm, malignant, by site
  - unspecified site C71.9
- **General, generalized** — *see* condition
- **Genetic**
  - carrier (status)
    - cystic fibrosis Z14.1
    - hemophilia A (asymptomatic) Z14.Ø1
      - symptomatic Z14.Ø2
    - specified NEC Z14.8
  - susceptibility to disease NEC Z15.89
    - malignant neoplasm Z15.Ø9
      - breast Z15.Ø1
      - endometrium Z15.Ø4
      - ovary Z15.Ø2
      - prostate Z15.Ø3
      - specified NEC Z15.Ø9
    - multiple endocrine neoplasia Z15.81
- **Genital** — *see* condition
- **Genito-anorectal syndrome** A55
- **Genitourinary system** — *see* condition
- **Genu**
  - congenital Q74.1
  - extrorsum (acquired) — *see also* Deformity, varus, knee
    - congenital Q74.1
    - sequelae (late effect) of rickets E64.3
  - introrsum (acquired) — *see also* Deformity, valgus, knee
    - congenital Q74.1
    - sequelae (late effect) of rickets E64.3
  - rachitic (old) E64.3
  - recurvatum (acquired) — *see also* Deformity, limb, specified type NEC, lower leg
    - congenital Q68.2
    - sequelae (late effect) of rickets E64.3
  - valgum (acquired) (knock-knee) M21.Ø6- ☑
    - congenital Q74.1
    - sequelae (late effect) of rickets E64.3
  - varum (acquired) (bowleg) M21.16- ☑
    - congenital Q74.1
    - sequelae (late effect) of rickets E64.3
- **Geographic tongue** K14.1
- **Geophagia** — *see* Pica
- **Geotrichosis** B48.3
  - stomatitis B48.3
- **Gephyrophobia** F4Ø.242
- **Gerbode defect** Q21.Ø
- **GERD** (gastroesophageal reflux disease) K21.9
- **Gerhardt's**
  - disease (erythromelalgia) I73.81
  - syndrome (vocal cord paralysis) J38.ØØ
    - bilateral J38.Ø2
    - unilateral J38.Ø1
- **German measles** — *see also* Rubella
  - exposure to Z2Ø.4
- **Germinoblastoma** (diffuse) C85.9- ☑
  - follicular C82.9- ☑
- **Germinoma** — *see* Neoplasm, malignant, by site
- **Gerontoxon** — *see* Degeneration, cornea, senile
- **Gerstmann's syndrome** R48.8
  - developmental F81.2
- **Gerstmann-Straussler-Scheinker syndrome** (GSS) A81.82
- **Gestation** (period) — *see also* Pregnancy
  - ectopic — *see* Pregnancy, by site
  - multiple O3Ø.9- ☑
    - greater than quadruplets — *see* Pregnancy, multiple (gestation), specified NEC
    - specified NEC — *see* Pregnancy, multiple (gestation), specified NEC
- **Gestational**
  - mammary abscess O91.11- ☑
  - purulent mastitis O91.11- ☑
  - subareolar abscess O91.11- ☑
- **Ghon tubercle, primary infection** A15.7
- **Ghost**
  - teeth KØØ.4
  - vessels (cornea) H16.41- ☑
- **Ghoul hand** A66.3
- **Gianotti-Crosti disease** L44.4
- **Giant**
  - cell
    - epulis KØ6.8
    - peripheral granuloma KØ6.8
  - esophagus, congenital Q39.5
  - kidney, congenital Q63.3
  - urticaria T78.3 ☑
    - hereditary D84.1
- **Giardiasis** AØ7.1
- **Gibert's disease or pityriasis** L42
- **Giddiness** R42
  - hysterical F44.89
  - psychogenic F45.8
- **Gierke's disease** (glycogenosis I) E74.Ø1
- **Gigantism** (cerebral) (hypophyseal) (pituitary) E22.Ø
  - constitutional E34.4
- **Gilbert's disease or syndrome** E8Ø.4
- **Gilchrist's disease** B4Ø.9
- **Gilford-Hutchinson disease** E34.8
- **Gilles de la Tourette's disease or syndrome** (motor-verbal tic) F95.2
- **Gingivitis** KØ5.1Ø
  - acute (catarrhal) KØ5.ØØ
    - necrotizing A69.1
    - nonplaque induced KØ5.Ø1
    - plaque induced KØ5.ØØ
  - chronic (desquamative) (hyperplastic) (simple marginal) (pregnancy associated) (ulcerative) KØ5.1Ø
    - nonplaque induced KØ5.11
    - plaque induced KØ5.1Ø
  - expulsiva — *see* Periodontitis
  - necrotizing ulcerative (acute) A69.1
  - pellagrous E52
    - acute necrotizing A69.1
  - Vincent's A69.1
- **Gingivoglossitis** K14.Ø
- **Gingivopericementitis** — *see* Periodontitis
- **Gingivosis** — *see* Gingivitis, chronic
- **Gingivostomatitis** KØ5.1Ø
  - herpesviral BØØ.2
  - necrotizing ulcerative (acute) A69.1
- **Gland, glandular** — *see* condition
- **Glanders** A24.Ø
- **Glanzmann** (-Naegeli) **disease or thrombasthenia** D69.1
- **Glasgow coma scale**
  - total score
    - 3-8 R4Ø.243 ☑
    - 9-12 R4Ø.242 ☑
    - 13-15 R4Ø.241 ☑
- **Glass-blower's disease** (cataract) — *see* Cataract, specified NEC
- **Glaucoma** H4Ø.9
  - with
    - increased episcleral venous pressure H4Ø.81- ☑
    - pseudoexfoliation of lens — *see* Glaucoma, open angle, primary, capsular
  - absolute H44.51- ☑
  - angle-closure (primary) H4Ø.2Ø- ☑
    - acute (attack) (crisis) H4Ø.21- ☑
    - chronic H4Ø.22- ☑
    - intermittent H4Ø.23- ☑
    - residual stage H4Ø.24- ☑
  - borderline H4Ø.ØØ- ☑
  - capsular (with pseudoexfoliation of lens) — *see* Glaucoma, open angle, primary, capsular
  - childhood Q15.Ø
  - closed angle — *see* Glaucoma, angle-closure
  - congenital Q15.Ø
  - corticosteroid-induced — *see* Glaucoma, secondary, drugs
  - hypersecretion H4Ø.82- ☑
  - in (due to)
    - amyloidosis E85.4 *[H42]*
    - aniridia Q13.1 *[H42]*
    - concussion of globe — *see* Glaucoma, secondary, trauma
    - dislocation of lens — *see* Glaucoma, secondary
    - disorder of lens NEC — *see* Glaucoma, secondary
    - drugs — *see* Glaucoma, secondary, drugs
    - endocrine disease NOS E34.9 *[H42]*
    - eye
      - inflammation — *see* Glaucoma, secondary, inflammation
      - trauma — *see* Glaucoma, secondary, trauma

- **Glaucoma** — *continued*
  - in — *continued*
    - hypermature cataract — *see* Glaucoma, secondary
    - iridocyclitis — *see* Glaucoma, secondary, inflammation
    - lens disorder — *see* Glaucoma, secondary
    - Lowe's syndrome E72.Ø3 *[H42]*
    - metabolic disease NOS E88.9 *[H42]*
    - ocular disorders NEC — *see* Glaucoma, secondary
    - onchocerciasis B73.Ø2
    - pupillary block — *see* Glaucoma, secondary
    - retinal vein occlusion — *see* Glaucoma, secondary
    - Rieger's anomaly Q13.81 *[H42]*
    - rubeosis of iris — *see* Glaucoma, secondary
    - tumor of globe — *see* Glaucoma, secondary
  - infantile Q15.Ø
  - low tension — *see* Glaucoma, open angle, primary, low-tension
  - malignant H4Ø.83- ☑
  - narrow angle — *see* Glaucoma, angle-closure
  - newborn Q15.Ø
  - noncongestive (chronic) — *see* Glaucoma, open angle
  - nonobstructive — *see* Glaucoma, open angle
  - obstructive — *see also* Glaucoma, angle-closure
    - due to lens changes — *see* Glaucoma, secondary
  - open angle H4Ø.1Ø- ☑
    - primary H4Ø.11- ☑
      - capsular (with pseudoexfoliation of lens) H4Ø.14- ☑
      - low-tension H4Ø.12- ☑
      - pigmentary H4Ø.13- ☑
      - residual stage H4Ø.15- ☑
  - phacolytic — *see* Glaucoma, secondary
  - pigmentary — *see* Glaucoma, open angle, primary, pigmentary
  - postinfectious — *see* Glaucoma, secondary, inflammation
  - secondary (to) H4Ø.5- ☑
    - drugs H4Ø.6- ☑
    - inflammation H4Ø.4- ☑
    - trauma H4Ø.3- ☑
  - simple (chronic) H4Ø.11- ☑
  - simplex H4Ø.11- ☑
  - specified type NEC H4Ø.89
  - suspect H4Ø.ØØ- ☑
  - syphilitic A52.71
  - traumatic — *see also* Glaucoma, secondary, trauma
    - newborn (birth injury) P15.3
  - tuberculous A18.59
- **Glaucomatous flecks** (subcapsular) — *see* Cataract, complicated
- **Glazed tongue** K14.4
- **Gleet** (gonococcal) A54.Ø1
- **Glenard's disease** K63.4
- **Glioblastoma** (multiforme)
  - with sarcomatous component
    - specified site — *see* Neoplasm, malignant, by site
    - unspecified site C71.9
  - giant cell
    - specified site — *see* Neoplasm, malignant, by site
    - unspecified site C71.9
  - specified site — *see* Neoplasm, malignant, by site
  - unspecified site C71.9
- **Glioma** (malignant)
  - astrocytic
    - specified site — *see* Neoplasm, malignant, by site
    - unspecified site C71.9
  - mixed
    - specified site — *see* Neoplasm, malignant, by site
    - unspecified site C71.9
  - nose Q3Ø.8
  - specified site NEC — *see* Neoplasm, malignant, by site
  - subependymal D43.2
    - specified site — *see* Neoplasm, uncertain behavior, by site
    - unspecified site D43.2
  - unspecified site C71.9
- **Gliomatosis cerebri** C71.Ø
- **Glioneuroma** — *see* Neoplasm, uncertain behavior, by site
- **Gliosarcoma**
  - specified site — *see* Neoplasm, malignant, by site
  - unspecified site C71.9
- **Gliosis** (cerebral) G93.89
  - spinal G95.89
- **Glisson's disease** — *see* Rickets
- **Globinuria** R82.3
- **Globus** (hystericus) F45.8
- **Glomangioma** D18.ØØ
  - intra-abdominal D18.Ø3
  - intracranial D18.Ø2
  - skin D18.Ø1
  - specified site NEC D18.Ø9
- **Glomangiomyoma** D18.ØØ
  - intra-abdominal D18.Ø3
  - intracranial D18.Ø2
  - skin D18.Ø1
  - specified site NEC D18.Ø9
- **Glomangiosarcoma** — *see* Neoplasm, connective tissue, malignant
- **Glomerular**
  - disease in syphilis A52.75
  - nephritis — *see* Glomerulonephritis
- **Glomerulitis** — *see* Glomerulonephritis
- **Glomerulonephritis** — *see also* Nephritis NØ5.9
  - with
    - C3
      - glomerulonephritis NØ5.A
      - glomerulopathy NØ5.A
        - with dense deposit disease NØ5.6
    - edema — *see* Nephrosis
    - minimal change NØ5.Ø
    - minor glomerular abnormality NØ5.Ø
  - acute NØØ.9
  - chronic NØ3.9
  - crescentic (diffuse) NEC — *see also* NØØ-NØ7 with fourth character .7 NØ5.7
  - dense deposit — *see also* NØØ-NØ7 with fourth character .6 NØ5.6
  - diffuse
    - crescentic — *see also* NØØ-NØ7 with fourth character .7 NØ5.7
    - endocapillary proliferative — *see also* NØØ-NØ7 with fourth character .4 NØ5.4
    - membranous — *see also* NØØ-NØ7 with fourth character .2 NØ5.2
    - mesangial proliferative — *see also* NØØ-NØ7 with fourth character .3 NØ5.3
    - mesangiocapillary — *see also* NØØ-NØ7 with fourth character .5 NØ5.5
    - sclerosing N18.9
  - endocapillary proliferative (diffuse) NEC — *see also* NØØ-NØ7 with fourth character .4 NØ5.4
  - extracapillary NEC — *see also* NØØ-NØ7 with fourth character .7 NØ5.7
  - focal (and segmental) — *see also* NØØ-NØ7 with fourth character .1 NØ5.1
  - hypocomplementemic — *see* Glomerulonephritis, membranoproliferative
  - IgA — *see* Nephropathy, IgA
  - immune complex (circulating) NEC NØ5.8
  - in (due to)
    - amyloidosis E85.4 *[NØ8]*
    - bilharziasis B65.9 *[NØ8]*
    - cryoglobulinemia D89.1 *[NØ8]*
    - defibrination syndrome D65 *[NØ8]*
    - diabetes mellitus — *see* Diabetes, glomerulosclerosis
    - disseminated intravascular coagulation D65 *[NØ8]*
    - Fabry (-Anderson) disease E75.21 *[NØ8]*
    - Goodpasture's syndrome M31.Ø
    - hemolytic-uremic syndrome — *see* Syndrome, hemolytic-uremic
    - Henoch (-Schonlein) purpura D69.Ø *[NØ8]*
    - lecithin cholesterol acyltransferase deficiency E78.6 *[NØ8]*
    - microscopic polyangiitis M31.7 *[NØ8]*
    - multiple myeloma C9Ø.Ø- ☑ *[NØ8]*
    - Plasmodium malariae B52.Ø
    - schistosomiasis B65.9 *[NØ8]*
    - sepsis A41.9 *[NØ8]*
      - streptococcal A4Ø- ☑ *[NØ8]*
    - sickle-cell disorders D57.- ☑ *[NØ8]*
    - strongyloidiasis B78.9 *[NØ8]*
    - subacute bacterial endocarditis I33.Ø *[NØ8]*
    - syphilis (late) congenital A5Ø.59 *[NØ8]*
    - systemic lupus erythematosus M32.14
    - thrombotic thrombocytopenic purpura M31.19 *[NØ8]*
    - typhoid fever AØ1.Ø9
    - Waldenstrom macroglobulinemia C88.Ø *[NØ8]*
    - Wegener's granulomatosis M31.31
  - latent or quiescent NØ3.9
- **Glomerulonephritis** — *continued*
  - lobular, lobulonodular — *see* Glomerulonephritis, membranoproliferative
  - membranoproliferative (diffuse)(type 1 or 3) — *see also* NØØ-NØ7 with fourth character .5 NØ5.5
    - dense deposit (type 2) NEC — *see also* NØØ-NØ7 with fourth character .6 NØ5.6
  - membranous (diffuse) NEC — *see also* NØØ-NØ7 with fourth character .2 NØ5.2
  - mesangial
    - IgA/IgG — *see* Nephropathy, IgA
    - proliferative (diffuse) NEC — *see also* NØØ-NØ7 with fourth character .3 NØ5.3
  - mesangiocapillary (diffuse) NEC — *see also* NØØ-NØ7 with fourth character .5 NØ5.5
  - necrotic, necrotizing NEC — *see also* NØØ- NØ7 with fourth character .8 NØ5.8
  - nodular — *see* Glomerulonephritis, membranoproliferative
  - poststreptococcal NEC NØ5.9
    - acute NØØ.9
    - chronic NØ3.9
    - rapidly progressive NØ1.9
  - proliferative NEC — *see also* NØØ-NØ7 with fourth character .8 NØ5.8
    - diffuse (lupus) M32.14
  - rapidly progressive NØ1.9
  - sclerosing, diffuse N18.9
  - specified pathology NEC — *see also* NØØ- NØ7 with fourth character .8 NØ5.8
  - subacute NØ1.9
- **Glomerulopathy** — *see* Glomerulonephritis
- **Glomerulosclerosis** — *see also* Sclerosis, renal
  - intercapillary (nodular) (with diabetes) — *see* Diabetes, glomerulosclerosis
  - intracapillary — *see* Diabetes, glomerulosclerosis
- **Glossagra** K14.6
- **Glossalgia** K14.6
- **Glossitis** (chronic superficial) (gangrenous) (Moeller's) K14.Ø
  - areata exfoliativa K14.1
  - atrophic K14.4
  - benign migratory K14.1
  - cortical superficial, sclerotic K14.Ø
  - Hunter's D51.Ø
  - interstitial, sclerous K14.Ø
  - median rhomboid K14.2
  - pellagrous E52
  - superficial, chronic K14.Ø
- **Glossocele** K14.8
- **Glossodynia** K14.6
  - exfoliativa K14.4
- **Glossoncus** K14.8
- **Glossopathy** K14.9
- **Glossophytia** K14.3
- **Glossoplegia** K14.8
- **Glossoptosis** K14.8
- **Glossopyrosis** K14.6
- **Glossotrichia** K14.3
- **Glossy skin** L9Ø.8
- **Glottis** — *see* condition
- **Glottitis** — *see also* Laryngitis JØ4.Ø
- **Glucagonoma**
  - pancreas
    - benign D13.7
    - malignant C25.4
    - uncertain behavior D37.8
  - specified site NEC
    - benign — *see* Neoplasm, benign, by site
    - malignant — *see* Neoplasm, malignant, by site
    - uncertain behavior — *see* Neoplasm, uncertain behavior, by site
  - unspecified site
    - benign D13.7
    - malignant C25.4
    - uncertain behavior D37.8
- **Glucoglycinuria** E72.51
- **Glucose-galactose malabsorption** E74.39
- **Glue**
  - ear — *see* Otitis, media, nonsuppurative, chronic, mucoid
  - sniffing (airplane) — *see* Abuse, drug, inhalant
    - dependence — *see* Dependence, drug, inhalant
- **GLUT1 deficiency syndrome 1, infantile onset** E74.81Ø
- **GLUT1 deficiency syndrome 2, childhood onset** E74.81Ø
- **Glutaric aciduria** E72.3

Glycinemia E72.51
Glycinuria (renal) (with ketosis) E72.Ø9
Glycogen
  infiltration — *see* Disease, glycogen storage
  storage disease — *see* Disease, glycogen storage
Glycogenosis (diffuse) (generalized) — *see also* Disease, glycogen storage
  cardiac E74.Ø2 *[I43]*
  diabetic, secondary — *see* Diabetes, glycogenosis, secondary
  pulmonary interstitial J84.842
Glycopenia E16.2
Glycosuria R81
  renal E74.818
Gnathostoma spinigerum (infection) (infestation), **gnathostomiasis** (wandering swelling) B83.1
Goiter (plunging) (substernal) EØ4.9
  with
    hyperthyroidism (recurrent) — *see* Hyperthyroidism, with, goiter
    thyrotoxicosis — *see* Hyperthyroidism, with, goiter
  adenomatous — *see* Goiter, nodular
  cancerous C73
  congenital (nontoxic) EØ3.Ø
    diffuse EØ3.Ø
    parenchymatous EØ3.Ø
    transitory, with normal functioning P72.Ø
  cystic EØ4.2
    due to iodine-deficiency EØ1.1
  due to
    enzyme defect in synthesis of thyroid hormone EØ7.1
    iodine-deficiency (endemic) EØ1.2
  dyshormonogenetic (familial) EØ7.1
  endemic (iodine-deficiency) EØ1.2
    diffuse EØ1.Ø
    multinodular EØ1.1
  exophthalmic — *see* Hyperthyroidism, with, goiter
  iodine-deficiency (endemic) EØ1.2
    diffuse EØ1.Ø
    multinodular EØ1.1
    nodular EØ1.1
  lingual Q89.2
  lymphadenoid EØ6.3
  malignant C73
  multinodular (cystic) (nontoxic) EØ4.2
    toxic or with hyperthyroidism EØ5.2Ø
      with thyroid storm EØ5.21
  neonatal NEC P72.Ø
  nodular (nontoxic) (due to) EØ4.9
    with
      hyperthyroidism EØ5.2Ø
        with thyroid storm EØ5.21
      thyrotoxicosis EØ5.2Ø
        with thyroid storm EØ5.21
    endemic EØ1.1
    iodine-deficiency EØ1.1
    sporadic EØ4.9
    toxic EØ5.2Ø
      with thyroid storm EØ5.21
  nontoxic EØ4.9
    diffuse (colloid) EØ4.Ø
    multinodular EØ4.2
    simple EØ4.Ø
    specified NEC EØ4.8
    uninodular EØ4.1
  simple EØ4.Ø
  toxic — *see* Hyperthyroidism, with, goiter
  uninodular (nontoxic) EØ4.1
    toxic or with hyperthyroidism EØ5.1Ø
      with thyroid storm EØ5.11
Goiter-deafness syndrome EØ7.1
Goldberg syndrome Q89.8
Goldberg-Maxwell syndrome E34.51
Goldblatt's hypertension or kidney I7Ø.1
Goldenhar (-Gorlin) **syndrome** Q87.Ø
Goldflam-Erb disease or syndrome G7Ø.ØØ
  with exacerbation (acute) G7Ø.Ø1
  in crisis G7Ø.Ø1
Goldscheider's disease Q81.8
Goldstein's disease (familial hemorrhagic telangiectasia) I78.Ø
Golfer's elbow — *see* Epicondylitis, medial
Gonadoblastoma
  specified site — *see* Neoplasm, uncertain behavior, by site
  unspecified site
    female D39.1Ø
Gonadoblastoma — *continued*
  unspecified site — *continued*
    male D4Ø.1Ø
Gonecystitis — *see* Vesiculitis
Gongylonemiasis B83.8
Goniosynechiae — *see* Adhesions, iris, goniosynechiae
Gonococcemia A54.86
Gonococcus, gonococcal (disease) (infection) — *see also* condition A54.9
  anus A54.6
  bursa, bursitis A54.49
  conjunctiva, conjunctivitis (neonatorum) A54.31
  endocardium A54.83
  eye A54.3Ø
    conjunctivitis A54.31
    iridocyclitis A54.32
    keratitis A54.33
    newborn A54.31
    other specified A54.39
  fallopian tubes (acute) (chronic) A54.24
  genitourinary (organ) (system) (tract) (acute)
    lower A54.ØØ
      with abscess (accessory gland) (periurethral) A54.1
    upper — *see also* condition A54.29
  heart A54.83
  iridocyclitis A54.32
  joint A54.42
  lymphatic (gland) (node) A54.89
  meninges, meningitis A54.81
  musculoskeletal A54.4Ø
    arthritis A54.42
    osteomyelitis A54.43
    other specified A54.49
    spondylopathy A54.41
  pelviperitonitis A54.24
  pelvis (acute) (chronic) A54.24
  pharynx A54.5
  proctitis A54.6
  pyosalpinx (acute) (chronic) A54.24
  rectum A54.6
  skin A54.89
  specified site NEC A54.89
  tendon sheath A54.49
  throat A54.5
  urethra (acute) (chronic) A54.Ø1
    with abscess (accessory gland) (periurethral) A54.1
  vulva (acute) (chronic) A54.Ø2
Gonocytoma
  specified site — *see* Neoplasm, uncertain behavior, by site
  unspecified site
    female D39.1Ø
    male D4Ø.1Ø
Gonorrhea (acute) (chronic) A54.9
  Bartholin's gland (acute) (chronic) (purulent) A54.Ø2
    with abscess (accessory gland) (periurethral) A54.1
  bladder A54.Ø1
  cervix A54.Ø3
  conjunctiva, conjunctivitis (neonatorum) A54.31
  contact Z2Ø.2
  Cowper's gland (with abscess) A54.1
  exposure to Z2Ø.2
  fallopian tube (acute) (chronic) A54.24
  kidney (acute) (chronic) A54.21
  lower genitourinary tract A54.ØØ
    with abscess (accessory gland) (periurethral) A54.1
  ovary (acute) (chronic) A54.24
  pelvis (acute) (chronic) A54.24
    female pelvic inflammatory disease A54.24
  penis A54.Ø9
  prostate (acute) (chronic) A54.22
  seminal vesicle (acute) (chronic) A54.23
  specified site not listed — *see also* Gonococcus A54.89
  spermatic cord (acute) (chronic) A54.23
  urethra A54.Ø1
    with abscess (accessory gland) (periurethral) A54.1
  vagina A54.Ø2
  vas deferens (acute) (chronic) A54.23
  vulva A54.Ø2
Goodall's disease AØ8.19
Goodpasture's syndrome M31.Ø
Gopalan's syndrome (burning feet) E53.Ø
Gorlin-Chaudry-Moss syndrome Q87.Ø
Gottron's papules L94.4
Gougerot-Blum syndrome (pigmented purpuric lichenoid dermatitis) L81.7
Gougerot-Carteaud disease or syndrome (confluent reticulate papillomatosis) L83
Gougerot's syndrome (trisymptomatic) L81.7
Gouley's syndrome (constrictive pericarditis) I31.1
Goundou A66.6
Gout, chronic — *see also* Gout, gouty M1A.9 ☑ *(following MØ8)*
  drug-induced M1A.2Ø ☑ *(following MØ8)*
    ankle M1A.27- ☑ *(following MØ8)*
    elbow M1A.22- ☑ *(following MØ8)*
    foot joint M1A.27- ☑ *(following MØ8)*
    hand joint M1A.24- ☑ *(following MØ8)*
    hip M1A.25- ☑ *(following MØ8)*
    knee M1A.26- ☑ *(following MØ8)*
    multiple site M1A.29- ☑ *(following MØ8)*
    shoulder M1A.21- ☑ *(following MØ8)*
    vertebrae M1A.28 ☑ *(following MØ8)*
    wrist M1A.23- ☑ *(following MØ8)*
  idiopathic M1A.ØØ ☑ *(following MØ8)*
    ankle M1A.Ø7- ☑ *(following MØ8)*
    elbow M1A.Ø2- ☑ *(following MØ8)*
    foot joint M1A.Ø7- ☑ *(following MØ8)*
    hand joint M1A.Ø4- ☑ *(following MØ8)*
    hip M1A.Ø5- ☑ *(following MØ8)*
    knee M1A.Ø6- ☑ *(following MØ8)*
    multiple site M1A.Ø9 ☑ *(following MØ8)*
    shoulder M1A.Ø1- ☑ *(following MØ8)*
    vertebrae M1A.Ø8 ☑ *(following MØ8)*
    wrist M1A.Ø3- ☑ *(following MØ8)*
  in (due to) renal impairment M1A.3Ø ☑ *(following MØ8)*
    ankle M1A.37- ☑ *(following MØ8)*
    elbow M1A.32- ☑ *(following MØ8)*
    foot joint M1A.37- ☑ *(following MØ8)*
    hand joint M1A.34- ☑ *(following MØ8)*
    hip M1A.35- ☑ *(following MØ8)*
    knee M1A.36- ☑ *(following MØ8)*
    multiple site M1A.39 ☑ *(following MØ8)*
    shoulder M1A.31- ☑ *(following MØ8)*
    vertebrae M1A.38 ☑ *(following MØ8)*
    wrist M1A.33- ☑ *(following MØ8)*
  lead-induced M1A.1Ø ☑ *(following MØ8)*
    ankle M1A.17- ☑ *(following MØ8)*
    elbow M1A.12- ☑ *(following MØ8)*
    foot joint M1A.17- ☑ *(following MØ8)*
    hand joint M1A.14- ☑ *(following MØ8)*
    hip M1A.15- ☑ *(following MØ8)*
    knee M1A.16- ☑ *(following MØ8)*
    multiple site M1A.19 ☑ *(following MØ8)*
    shoulder M1A.11- ☑ *(following MØ8)*
    vertebrae M1A.18 ☑ *(following MØ8)*
    wrist M1A.13- ☑ *(following MØ8)*
  primary — *see* Gout, chronic, idiopathic
  saturnine — *see* Gout, chronic, lead-induced
  secondary NEC M1A.4Ø ☑ *(following MØ8)*
    ankle M1A.47- ☑ *(following MØ8)*
    elbow M1A.42- ☑ *(following MØ8)*
    foot joint M1A.47- ☑ *(following MØ8)*
    hand joint M1A.44- ☑ *(following MØ8)*
    hip M1A.45- ☑ *(following MØ8)*
    knee M1A.46- ☑ *(following MØ8)*
    multiple site M1A.49 ☑ *(following MØ8)*
    shoulder M1A.41- ☑ *(following MØ8)*
    vertebrae M1A.48 ☑ *(following MØ8)*
    wrist M1A.43- ☑ *(following MØ8)*
  syphilitic — *see also* subcategory M14.8- A52.77
  tophi M1A.9 ☑ *(following MØ8)*
Gout, gouty (acute) (attack) (flare) — *see also* Gout, chronic M1Ø.9
  drug-induced M1Ø.2Ø
    ankle M1Ø.27- ☑
    elbow M1Ø.22- ☑
    foot joint M1Ø.27- ☑
    hand joint M1Ø.24- ☑
    hip M1Ø.25- ☑
    knee M1Ø.26- ☑
    multiple site M1Ø.29
    shoulder M1Ø.21- ☑
    vertebrae M1Ø.28
    wrist M1Ø.23- ☑
  idiopathic M1Ø.ØØ
    ankle M1Ø.Ø7- ☑
    elbow M1Ø.Ø2- ☑
    foot joint M1Ø.Ø7- ☑
    hand joint M1Ø.Ø4- ☑
    hip M1Ø.Ø5- ☑
    knee M1Ø.Ø6- ☑

- **Gout, gouty** — *continued*
  - idiopathic — *continued*
    - multiple site M1Ø.Ø9
    - shoulder M1Ø.Ø1- ☑
    - vertebrae M1Ø.Ø8
    - wrist M1Ø.Ø3- ☑
  - in (due to) renal impairment M1Ø.3Ø
    - ankle M1Ø.37- ☑
    - elbow M1Ø.32- ☑
    - foot joint M1Ø.37- ☑
    - hand joint M1Ø.34- ☑
    - hip M1Ø.35- ☑
    - knee M1Ø.36- ☑
    - multiple site M1Ø.39
    - shoulder M1Ø.31- ☑
    - vertebrae M1Ø.38
    - wrist M1Ø.33- ☑
  - lead-induced M1Ø.1Ø
    - ankle M1Ø.17- ☑
    - elbow M1Ø.12- ☑
    - foot joint M1Ø.17- ☑
    - hand joint M1Ø.14- ☑
    - hip M1Ø.15- ☑
    - knee M1Ø.16- ☑
    - multiple site M1Ø.19
    - shoulder M1Ø.11- ☑
    - vertebrae M1Ø.18
    - wrist M1Ø.13- ☑
  - primary — *see* Gout, idiopathic
  - saturnine — *see* Gout, lead-induced
  - secondary NEC M1Ø.4Ø
    - ankle M1Ø.47- ☑
    - elbow M1Ø.42- ☑
    - foot joint M1Ø.47- ☑
    - hand joint M1Ø.44- ☑
    - hip M1Ø.45- ☑
    - knee M1Ø.46- ☑
    - multiple site M1Ø.49
    - shoulder M1Ø.41- ☑
    - vertebrae M1Ø.48
    - wrist M1Ø.43- ☑
  - syphilitic — *see also* subcategory M14.8- A52.77
  - tophi — *see* Gout, chronic
- **Gower's**
  - muscular dystrophy G71.Ø1
  - syndrome (vasovagal attack) R55
- **Gradenigo's syndrome** — *see* Otitis, media, suppurative, acute
- **Graefe's disease** — *see* Strabismus, paralytic, ophthalmoplegia, progressive
- **Graft-versus-host disease** D89.813
  - acute D89.81Ø
  - acute on chronic D89.812
  - chronic D89.811
- **Grain mite** (itch) B88.Ø
- **Grainhandler's disease or lung** J67.8
- **Grand mal** — *see* Epilepsy, generalized, specified NEC
- **Grand multipara status only** (not pregnant) Z64.1
  - pregnant — *see* Pregnancy, complicated by, grand multiparity
- **Granite worker's lung** J62.8
- **Granular** — *see also* condition
  - inflammation, pharynx J31.2
  - kidney (contracting) — *see* Sclerosis, renal
  - liver K74.69
- **Granulation tissue** (abnormal) (excessive) L92.9
  - postmastoidectomy cavity — *see* Complications, postmastoidectomy, granulation
- **Granulocytopenia** (primary) (malignant) — *see* Agranulocytosis
- **Granuloma** L92.9
  - abdomen K66.8
    - from residual foreign body L92.3
    - pyogenicum L98.Ø
  - actinic L57.5
  - annulare (perforating) L92.Ø
  - apical KØ4.5
  - aural — *see* Otitis, externa, specified NEC
  - beryllium (skin) L92.3
  - bone
    - eosinophilic C96.6
    - from residual foreign body — *see* Osteomyelitis, specified type NEC
    - lung C96.6
  - brain (any site) GØ6.Ø
    - schistosomiasis B65.9 *[GØ7]*
  - canaliculus lacrimalis — *see* Granuloma, lacrimal

- **Granuloma** — *continued*
  - candidal (cutaneous) B37.2
  - cerebral (any site) GØ6.Ø
  - coccidioidal (primary) (progressive) B38.7
    - lung B38.1
    - meninges B38.4
  - colon K63.89
  - conjunctiva H11.22- ☑
  - dental KØ4.5
  - ear, middle — *see* Cholesteatoma
  - eosinophilic C96.6
    - bone C96.6
    - lung C96.6
    - oral mucosa K13.4
    - skin L92.2
  - eyelid HØ1.8
  - facial (e) L92.2
  - foreign body (in soft tissue) NEC M6Ø.2Ø
    - ankle M6Ø.27- ☑
    - foot M6Ø.27- ☑
    - forearm M6Ø.23- ☑
    - hand M6Ø.24- ☑
    - in operation wound — *see* Foreign body, accidentally left during a procedure
    - lower leg M6Ø.26- ☑
    - pelvic region M6Ø.25- ☑
    - shoulder region M6Ø.21- ☑
    - skin L92.3
    - specified site NEC M6Ø.28
    - subcutaneous tissue L92.3
    - thigh M6Ø.25- ☑
    - upper arm M6Ø.22- ☑
  - gangraenescens M31.2
  - genito-inguinale A58
  - giant cell (central) (reparative) (jaw) M27.1
    - gingiva (peripheral) KØ6.8
  - gland (lymph) I88.8
  - hepatic NEC K75.3
    - in (due to)
      - berylliosis J63.2 *[K77]*
      - sarcoidosis D86.89
  - Hodgkin C81.9- ☑
  - ileum K63.89
  - infectious B99.9
    - specified NEC B99.8
  - inguinale (Donovan) (venereal) A58
  - intestine NEC K63.89
  - intracranial (any site) GØ6.Ø
  - intraspinal (any part) GØ6.1
  - iridocyclitis — *see* Iridocyclitis, chronic
  - jaw (bone) (central) M27.1
    - reparative giant cell M27.1
  - kidney — *see also* Infection, kidney N15.8
  - lacrimal HØ4.81- ☑
  - larynx J38.7
  - lethal midline (faciale(e)) M31.2
  - liver NEC — *see* Granuloma, hepatic
  - lung (infectious) — *see also* Fibrosis, lung
    - coccidioidal B38.1
    - eosinophilic C96.6
  - Majocchi's B35.8
  - malignant (facial(e)) M31.2
  - mandible (central) M27.1
  - midline (lethal) M31.2
  - monilial (cutaneous) B37.2
  - nasal sinus — *see* Sinusitis
  - operation wound T81.89 ☑
    - foreign body — *see* Foreign body, accidentally left during a procedure
    - stitch T81.89 ☑
    - talc — *see* Foreign body, accidentally left during a procedure
  - oral mucosa K13.4
  - orbit, orbital HØ5.11- ☑
  - paracoccidioidal B41.8
  - penis, venereal A58
  - periapical KØ4.5
  - peritoneum K66.8
    - due to ova of helminths NOS — *see also* Helminthiasis B83.9 *[K67]*
  - postmastoidectomy cavity — *see* Complications, postmastoidectomy, recurrent cholesteatoma
  - prostate N42.89
  - pudendi (ulcerating) A58
  - pulp, internal (tooth) KØ3.3
  - pyogenic, pyogenicum (of) (skin) L98.Ø
    - gingiva KØ6.8
    - maxillary alveolar ridge KØ4.5

- **Granuloma** — *continued*
  - pyogenic, pyogenicum — *continued*
    - oral mucosa K13.4
  - rectum K62.89
  - reticulohistiocytic D76.3
  - rubrum nasi L74.8
  - Schistosoma — *see* Schistosomiasis
  - septic (skin) L98.Ø
  - silica (skin) L92.3
  - sinus (accessory) (infective) (nasal) — *see* Sinusitis
  - skin L92.9
    - from residual foreign body L92.3
    - pyogenicum L98.Ø
  - spine
    - syphilitic (epidural) A52.19
    - tuberculous A18.Ø1
  - stitch (postoperative) T81.89 ☑
  - suppurative (skin) L98.Ø
  - swimming pool A31.1
  - talc — *see also* Granuloma, foreign body
    - in operation wound — *see* Foreign body, accidentally left during a procedure
  - telangiectaticum (skin) L98.Ø
  - tracheostomy J95.Ø9
  - trichophyticum B35.8
  - tropicum A66.4
  - umbilical P83.81
  - umbilicus P83.81
  - urethra N36.8
  - uveitis — *see* Iridocyclitis, chronic
  - vagina A58
  - venereum A58
  - vocal cord J38.3
- **Granulomatosis** L92.9
  - with polyangiitis M31.3- ☑
  - eosinophilic, with polyangiitis [EGPA] M3Ø.1
  - lymphoid C83.8- ☑
  - miliary (listerial) A32.89
  - necrotizing, respiratory M31.3Ø
  - progressive septic D71
  - specified NEC L92.8
  - Wegener's M31.3Ø
    - with renal involvement M31.31
- **Granulomatous tissue** (abnormal) (excessive) L92.9
- **Granulosis rubra nasi** L74.8
- **Graphite fibrosis** (of lung) J63.3
- **Graphospasm** F48.8
  - organic G25.89
- **Grating scapula** M89.8X1
- **Gravel** (urinary) — *see* Calculus, urinary
- **Graves' disease** — *see* Hyperthyroidism, with, goiter
- **Gravis** — *see* condition
- **Grawitz tumor** C64.- ☑
- **Gray syndrome** (newborn) P93.Ø
- **Grayness, hair** (premature) L67.1
  - congenital Q84.2
- **Green sickness** D5Ø.8
- **Greenfield's disease**
  - meaning
    - concentric sclerosis (encephalitis periaxialis concentrica) G37.5
    - metachromatic leukodystrophy E75.25
- **Greenstick fracture** — *code as* Fracture, by site
- **Grey syndrome** (newborn) P93.Ø
- **Grief** F43.21
  - complicated F34.81
  - prolonged F43.81
  - reaction — *see also* Disorder, adjustment F43.2Ø
- **Griesinger's disease** B76.Ø
- **Grinder's lung or pneumoconiosis** J62.8
- **Grinding, teeth**
  - psychogenic F45.8
  - sleep related G47.63
- **Grip**
  - Dabney's B33.Ø
  - devil's B33.Ø
- **Grippe, grippal** — *see also* Influenza
  - Balkan A78
  - summer, of Italy A93.1
- **Grisel's disease** M43.6
- **Groin** — *see* condition
- **Grooved tongue** K14.5
- **Ground itch** B76.9
- **Grover's disease or syndrome** L11.1
- **Growing pains, children** R29.898
- **Growth** (fungoid) (neoplastic) (new) — *see also* Neoplasm
  - adenoid (vegetative) J35.8

- **Hematemesis** — *continued*
  - with ulcer — *code by site under* Ulcer, with hemorrhage K27.4
  - newborn, neonatal P54.Ø
    - due to swallowed maternal blood P78.2
- **Hematidrosis** L74.8
- **Hematinuria** — *see also* Hemoglobinuria
  - malarial B5Ø.8
- **Hematobilia** K83.8
- **Hematocele**
  - female NEC N94.89
    - with ectopic pregnancy OØØ.9Ø
      - with intrauterine pregnancy OØØ.91
    - ovary N83.8
  - male N5Ø.1
- **Hematochezia** — *see also* Melena K92.1
- **Hematochyluria** — *see also* Infestation, filarial
  - schistosomiasis (bilharziasis) B65.Ø
- **Hematocolpos** (with hematometra or hematosalpinx) N89.7
- **Hematocornea** — *see* Pigmentation, cornea, stromal
- **Hematogenous** — *see* condition
- **Hematoma** (traumatic) (skin surface intact) — *see also* Contusion
  - with
    - injury of internal organs — *see* Injury, by site
    - open wound — *see* Wound, open
  - amputation stump (surgical) (late) T87.89
  - aorta, dissecting I71.ØØ
    - abdominal I71.Ø2
    - thoracic — *see also* Dissection, aorta, thoracic I71.Ø19
    - thoracoabdominal I71.Ø3
  - aortic intramural — *see* Dissection, aorta
  - arterial (complicating trauma) — *see* Injury, blood vessel, by site
  - auricle — *see* Contusion, ear
    - nontraumatic — *see* Disorder, pinna, hematoma
  - birth injury NEC P15.8
  - brain (traumatic)
    - with
      - cerebral laceration or contusion (diffuse) — *see* Injury, intracranial, diffuse
        - focal — *see* Injury, intracranial, focal
    - cerebellar, traumatic SØ6.37- ☑
    - intracerebral, traumatic — *see* Injury, intracranial, intracerebral hemorrhage
    - newborn NEC P52.4
      - birth injury P1Ø.1
    - nontraumatic — *see* Hemorrhage, intracranial
    - subarachnoid, arachnoid, traumatic — *see* Injury, intracranial, subarachnoid hemorrhage
    - subdural, traumatic — *see* Injury, intracranial, subdural hemorrhage
  - breast (nontraumatic) N64.89
  - broad ligament (nontraumatic) N83.7
    - traumatic S37.892 ☑
  - cerebellar, traumatic SØ6.37- ☑
  - cerebral — *see* Hematoma, brain
  - cerebrum SØ6.36- ☑
    - left SØ6.35- ☑
    - right SØ6.34- ☑
  - cesarean delivery wound O9Ø.2
  - complicating delivery (perineal) (pelvic) (vagina) (vulva) O71.7
  - corpus cavernosum (nontraumatic) N48.89
  - epididymis (nontraumatic) N5Ø.1
  - epidural (traumatic) — *see* Injury, intracranial, epidural hemorrhage
    - spinal — *see* Injury, spinal cord, by region
  - episiotomy O9Ø.2
  - face, birth injury P15.4
  - genital organ NEC (nontraumatic)
    - female (nonobstetric) N94.89
      - traumatic S3Ø.2Ø2 ☑
    - male N5Ø.1
      - traumatic S3Ø.2Ø1 ☑
  - internal organs — *see* Injury, by site
  - intracerebral, traumatic — *see* Injury, intracranial, intracerebral hemorrhage
  - intraoperative — *see* Complications, intraoperative, hemorrhage
  - labia (nontraumatic) (nonobstetric) N9Ø.89
  - liver (subcapsular) (nontraumatic) K76.89
    - birth injury P15.Ø
  - mediastinum — *see* Injury, intrathoracic
  - mesosalpinx (nontraumatic) N83.7
- **Hematoma** — *continued*
  - mesosalpinx — *continued*
    - traumatic S37.898 ☑
  - muscle — code by site under Contusion
  - nontraumatic
    - muscle M79.81
    - soft tissue M79.81
  - obstetrical surgical wound O9Ø.2
  - orbit, orbital (nontraumatic) — *see also* Hemorrhage, orbit
    - traumatic — *see* Contusion, orbit
  - pelvis (female) (nontraumatic) (nonobstetric) N94.89
    - obstetric O71.7
    - traumatic — *see* Injury, by site
  - penis (nontraumatic) N48.89
    - birth injury P15.5
  - perianal (nontraumatic) K64.5
  - perineal S3Ø.23 ☑
    - complicating delivery O71.7
  - perirenal — *see* Injury, kidney
  - peritoneal K66.1
  - pinna — *see* Contusion, ear
    - nontraumatic — *see* Disorder, pinna, hematoma
  - placenta O43.89- ☑
  - postoperative (postprocedural) — *see* Complication, postprocedural, hematoma
  - retroperitoneal (nontraumatic) K68.3
    - traumatic S36.892 ☑
  - scrotum, superficial S3Ø.22 ☑
    - birth injury P15.5
  - seminal vesicle (nontraumatic) N5Ø.1
    - traumatic S37.892 ☑
  - spermatic cord (traumatic) S37.892 ☑
    - nontraumatic N5Ø.1
  - spinal (cord) (meninges) — *see also* Injury, spinal cord, by region
    - newborn (birth injury) P11.5
  - spleen D73.5
    - intraoperative — *see* Complications, intraoperative, hemorrhage, spleen
    - postprocedural (postoperative) — *see* Complications, postprocedural, hemorrhage, spleen
  - sternocleidomastoid, birth injury P15.2
  - sternomastoid, birth injury P15.2
  - subarachnoid (traumatic) — *see* Injury, intracranial, subarachnoid hemorrhage
    - newborn (nontraumatic) P52.5
      - due to birth injury P1Ø.3
    - nontraumatic — *see* Hemorrhage, intracranial, subarachnoid
  - subdural (traumatic) — *see* Injury, intracranial, subdural hemorrhage
    - newborn (localized) P52.8
      - birth injury P1Ø.Ø
    - nontraumatic — *see* Hemorrhage, intracranial, subdural
  - superficial, newborn P54.5
  - testis (nontraumatic) N5Ø.1
    - birth injury P15.5
  - tunica vaginalis (nontraumatic) N5Ø.1
  - umbilical cord, complicating delivery O69.5 ☑
  - uterine ligament (broad) (nontraumatic) N83.7
    - traumatic S37.892 ☑
  - vagina (ruptured) (nontraumatic) N89.8
    - complicating delivery O71.7
  - vas deferens (nontraumatic) N5Ø.1
    - traumatic S37.892 ☑
  - vitreous — *see* Hemorrhage, vitreous
  - vulva (nontraumatic) (nonobstetric) N9Ø.89
    - complicating delivery O71.7
    - newborn (birth injury) P15.5
- **Hematometra** N85.7
  - with hematocolpos N89.7
- **Hematomyelia** (central) G95.19
  - newborn (birth injury) P11.5
  - traumatic T14.8 ☑
- **Hematomyelitis** GØ4.9Ø
- **Hematoperitoneum** — *see* Hemoperitoneum
- **Hematophobia** F4Ø.23Ø
- **Hematopneumothorax** (see Hemothorax)
- **Hematopoiesis, cyclic** D7Ø.4
- **Hematoporphyria** — *see* Porphyria
- **Hematorachis, hematorrhachis** G95.19
  - newborn (birth injury) P11.5
- **Hematosalpinx** N83.6
  - with
    - hematocolpos N89.7
    - hematometra N85.7
- **Hematosalpinx** — *continued*
  - with — *continued*
    - hematometra — *continued*
      - with hematocolpos N89.7
  - infectional — *see* Salpingitis
- **Hematospermia** R36.1
- **Hematothorax** (see Hemothorax)
- **Hematuria** R31.9
  - benign (familial) (of childhood) — *see also* Hematuria, idiopathic
    - essential microscopic R31.1
  - due to sulphonamide, sulfonamide — *see* Table of Drugs and Chemicals, by drug
  - endemic — *see also* Schistosomiasis B65.Ø
  - gross R31.Ø
  - idiopathic NØ2.9
    - with glomerular lesion
      - C3
        - glomerulonephritis NØ2.A
        - glomerulopathy NØ2.A
          - with dense deposit disease NØ2.6
      - crescentic (diffuse) glomerulonephritis NØ2.7
      - dense deposit disease NØ2.6
      - endocapillary proliferative glomerulonephritis NØ2.4
      - focal and segmental hyalinosis or sclerosis NØ2.1
      - membranoproliferative (diffuse) NØ2.5
      - membranous (diffuse) NØ2.2
      - mesangial proliferative (diffuse) NØ2.3
      - mesangiocapillary (diffuse) NØ2.5
      - minor abnormality NØ2.Ø
      - proliferative NEC NØ2.8
      - specified pathology NEC NØ2.8
  - intermittent — *see* Hematuria, idiopathic
  - malarial B5Ø.8
  - microscopic NEC (with symptoms) R31.29
    - asymptomatic R31.21
    - benign essential R31.1
  - paroxysmal — *see also* Hematuria, idiopathic
    - nocturnal D59.5
  - persistent — *see* Hematuria, idiopathic
  - recurrent — *see* Hematuria, idiopathic
  - tropical — *see also* Schistosomiasis B65.Ø
  - tuberculous A18.13
- **Hemeralopia** (day blindness) H53.11
  - vitamin A deficiency E5Ø.5
- **Hemi-akinesia** R41.4
- **Hemianalgesia** R2Ø.Ø
- **Hemianencephaly** QØØ.Ø
- **Hemianesthesia** R2Ø.Ø
- **Hemianopia, hemianopsia** (heteronymous) H53.47
  - homonymous H53.46- ☑
  - syphilitic A52.71
- **Hemiathetosis** R25.8
- **Hemiatrophy** R68.89
  - cerebellar G31.9
  - face, facial, progressive (Romberg) G51.8
  - tongue K14.8
- **Hemiballism** (us) G25.5
- **Hemicardia** Q24.8
- **Hemicephalus, hemicephaly** QØØ.Ø
- **Hemichorea** G25.5
- **Hemicolitis, left** — *see* Colitis, left sided
- **Hemicrania**
  - congenital malformation QØØ.Ø
  - continua G44.51
  - meaning migraine — *see also* Migraine G43.9Ø9
  - paroxysmal G44.Ø39
    - chronic G44.Ø49
      - intractable G44.Ø41
      - not intractable G44.Ø49
    - episodic G44.Ø39
      - intractable G44.Ø31
      - not intractable G44.Ø39
    - intractable G44.Ø31
    - not intractable G44.Ø39
- **Hemidystrophy** — *see* Hemiatrophy
- **Hemiectromelia** Q73.8
- **Hemihypalgesia** R2Ø.8
- **Hemihypesthesia** R2Ø.1
- **Hemi-inattention** R41.4
- **Hemimegalencephaly** QØ4.5
- **Hemimelia** Q73.8
  - lower limb — *see* Defect, reduction, lower limb, specified type NEC
  - upper limb — *see* Defect, reduction, upper limb, specified type NEC
- **Hemiparalysis** — *see* Hemiplegia

- **Hemorrhage, hemorrhagic** — *continued*
  - due to or associated with — *continued*
    - device, implant or graft — *see also* Complications, by site and type, specified — *continued*
      - gastrointestinal (bile duct) (esophagus) T85.838 ☑
      - genital NEC T83.83 ☑
      - heart NEC T82.837 ☑
      - joint prosthesis T84.83 ☑
      - ocular (corneal graft) (orbital implant) NEC T85.838 ☑
      - orthopedic NEC T84.83 ☑
        - bone graft T86.838
      - specified NEC T85.838 ☑
      - urinary NEC T83.83 ☑
      - vascular NEC T82.838 ☑
      - ventricular intracranial shunt T85.83Ø ☑
  - duodenum, duodenal K92.2
    - ulcer — *see* Ulcer, duodenum, with hemorrhage
  - dura mater — *see* Hemorrhage, intracranial, subdural
  - endotracheal — *see* Hemorrhage, lung
  - epicranial subaponeurotic (massive), birth injury P12.2
  - epidural (traumatic) — *see also* Injury, intracranial, epidural hemorrhage
    - nontraumatic I62.1
  - esophagus K22.89
    - varix I85.Ø1
      - secondary I85.11
  - excessive, following ectopic gestation (subsequent episode) OØ8.1
  - extradural (traumatic) — *see* Injury, intracranial, epidural hemorrhage
    - birth injury P1Ø.8
    - newborn (anoxic) (nontraumatic) P52.8
    - nontraumatic I62.1
  - eye NEC H57.89
    - fundus — *see* Hemorrhage, retina
    - lid — *see* Disorder, eyelid, specified type NEC
  - fallopian tube N83.6
  - fibrinogenolysis — *see* Fibrinolysis
  - fibrinolytic (acquired) — *see* Fibrinolysis
  - from
    - ear (nontraumatic) — *see* Otorrhagia
    - tracheostomy stoma J95.Ø1
  - fundus, eye — *see* Hemorrhage, retina
  - funis — *see* Hemorrhage, umbilicus, cord
  - gastric — *see* Hemorrhage, stomach
  - gastroenteric K92.2
    - newborn P54.3
  - gastrointestinal (tract) K92.2
    - newborn P54.3
  - genital organ, male N5Ø.1
  - genitourinary (tract) NOS R31.9
  - gingiva KØ6.8
  - globe (eye) — *see* Hemophthalmos
  - graafian follicle cyst (ruptured) N83.Ø- ☑
  - gum KØ6.8
  - heart I51.89
  - hypopharyngeal (throat) RØ4.1
  - intermenstrual (regular) N92.3
    - irregular N92.1
  - internal (organs) NEC R58
    - capsule I61.Ø
    - ear — *see* subcategory H83.8 ☑
    - newborn P54.8
  - intestine K92.2
    - newborn P54.3
  - intra-abdominal R58
  - intra-alveolar (lung), newborn P26.8
  - intracerebral (nontraumatic) — *see* Hemorrhage, intracranial, intracerebral
  - intracranial (nontraumatic) I62.9
    - birth injury P1Ø.9
    - epidural, nontraumatic I62.1
    - extradural, nontraumatic I62.1
    - intracerebral (nontraumatic) (in) I61.9
      - brain stem I61.3
      - cerebellum I61.4
      - hemisphere I61.2
        - cortical (superficial) I61.1
        - subcortical (deep) I61.Ø
      - intraoperative
        - during a nervous system procedure G97.31
        - during other procedure G97.32
      - intraventricular I61.5
      - multiple localized I61.6
      - newborn P52.4
        - birth injury P1Ø.1

- **Hemorrhage, hemorrhagic** — *continued*
  - intracranial — *continued*
    - intracerebral — *continued*
      - postprocedural
        - following a nervous system procedure G97.51
        - following other procedure G97.52
      - specified NEC I61.8
      - superficial I61.1
      - traumatic (diffuse) — *see* Injury, intracranial, diffuse
        - focal — *see* Injury, intracranial, focal
    - newborn P52.9
      - specified NEC P52.8
    - subarachnoid (nontraumatic) (from) I6Ø.9
      - intracranial (cerebral) artery I6Ø.7
        - anterior communicating I6Ø.2
        - basilar I6Ø.4
        - carotid siphon and bifurcation I6Ø.Ø- ☑
        - communicating I6Ø.7
          - anterior I6Ø.2
          - posterior I6Ø.3- ☑
        - middle cerebral I6Ø.1- ☑
        - posterior communicating I6Ø.3- ☑
        - specified artery NEC I6Ø.6
        - vertebral I6Ø.5- ☑
      - newborn P52.5
        - birth injury P1Ø.3
      - specified NEC I6Ø.8
      - traumatic SØ6.6X- ☑
    - subdural (nontraumatic) I62.ØØ
      - acute I62.Ø1
      - birth injury P1Ø.Ø
      - chronic I62.Ø3
      - newborn (anoxic) (hypoxic) P52.8
        - birth injury P1Ø.Ø
      - spinal G95.19
      - subacute I62.Ø2
      - traumatic — *see* Injury, intracranial, subdural hemorrhage
    - traumatic — *see* Injury, intracranial, focal brain injury
  - intramedullary NEC G95.19
  - intraocular — *see* Hemophthalmos
  - intraoperative, intraprocedural — *see* Complication, hemorrhage (hematoma), intraoperative (intraprocedural), by site
  - intrapartum — *see* Hemorrhage, complicating, delivery
  - intrapelvic
    - female N94.89
    - male K66.1
  - intraperitoneal K66.1
  - intrapontine I61.3
  - intraprocedural — *see* Complication, hemorrhage (hematoma), intraoperative (intraprocedural), by site
  - intrauterine N85.7
    - complicating delivery — *see also* Hemorrhage, complicating, delivery O67.9
    - postpartum — *see* Hemorrhage, postpartum
  - intraventricular I61.5
    - newborn (nontraumatic) — *see also* Newborn, affected by, hemorrhage P52.3
      - due to birth injury P1Ø.2
      - grade
        - 1 P52.Ø
        - 2 P52.1
        - 3 P52.21
        - 4 P52.22
  - intravesical N32.89
  - iris (postinfectional) (postinflammatory) (toxic) — *see* Hyphema
  - joint (nontraumatic) — *see* Hemarthrosis
  - kidney N28.89
  - knee (joint) (nontraumatic) — *see* Hemarthrosis, knee
  - labyrinth — *see* subcategory H83.8 ☑
  - lenticular striate artery I61.Ø
  - ligature, vessel — *see* Hemorrhage, postoperative
  - liver K76.89
  - lung RØ4.89
    - newborn P26.9
      - massive P26.1
      - specified NEC P26.8
    - tuberculous — *see* Tuberculosis, pulmonary
  - massive umbilical, newborn P51.Ø
  - mediastinum — *see* Hemorrhage, lung
  - medulla I61.3
  - membrane (brain) I6Ø.8
    - spinal cord — *see* Hemorrhage, spinal cord

- **Hemorrhage, hemorrhagic** — *continued*
  - meninges, meningeal (brain) (middle) I6Ø.8
    - spinal cord — *see* Hemorrhage, spinal cord
  - mesentery K66.1
  - metritis — *see* Endometritis
  - mouth K13.79
  - mucous membrane NEC R58
    - newborn P54.8
  - muscle M62.89
  - nail (subungual) L6Ø.8
  - nasal turbinate RØ4.Ø
    - newborn P54.8
  - navel, newborn P51.9
  - newborn P54.9
    - specified NEC P54.8
  - nipple N64.59
  - nose RØ4.Ø
    - newborn P54.8
  - omentum K66.1
  - optic nerve (sheath) H47.Ø2- ☑
  - orbit, orbital HØ5.23- ☑
  - ovary NEC N83.8
  - oviduct N83.6
  - pancreas K86.89
  - parathyroid (gland) (spontaneous) E21.4
  - parturition — *see* Hemorrhage, complicating, delivery
  - penis N48.89
  - pericardium, pericarditis I31.2
  - peritoneum, peritoneal K66.1
  - peritonsillar tissue J35.8
    - due to infection J36
  - petechial R23.3
    - due to autosensitivity, erythrocyte D69.2
  - pituitary (gland) E23.6
  - pleura — *see* Hemorrhage, lung
  - polioencephalitis, superior E51.2
  - polymyositis — *see* Polymyositis
  - pons, pontine I61.3
  - posterior fossa (nontraumatic) I61.8
    - newborn P52.6
  - postmenopausal N95.Ø
  - postnasal RØ4.Ø
  - postoperative — *see* Complications, postprocedural, hemorrhage, by site
  - postpartum NEC (following delivery of placenta) O72.1
    - delayed or secondary O72.2
    - retained placenta O72.Ø
    - third stage O72.Ø
  - pregnancy — *see* Hemorrhage, antepartum
  - preretinal — *see* Hemorrhage, retina
  - prostate N42.1
  - puerperal — *see* Hemorrhage, postpartum
    - delayed or secondary O72.2
  - pulmonary RØ4.89
    - newborn P26.9
      - massive P26.1
      - specified NEC P26.8
    - tuberculous — *see* Tuberculosis, pulmonary
  - purpura (primary) D69.3
  - rectum (sphincter) K62.5
    - newborn P54.2
  - recurring, following initial hemorrhage at time of injury T79.2 ☑
  - renal N28.89
  - respiratory passage or tract RØ4.9
    - specified NEC RØ4.89
  - retina, retinal (vessels) H35.6- ☑
    - diabetic — *see* Microaneurysm, retinal, diabetic
  - retroperitoneal K68.3
  - scalp R58
  - scrotum N5Ø.1
  - secondary (nontraumatic) R58
    - following initial hemorrhage at time of injury T79.2 ☑
  - seminal vesicle N5Ø.1
  - skin R23.3
    - newborn P54.5
  - slipped umbilical ligature P51.8
  - spermatic cord N5Ø.1
  - spinal (cord) G95.19
    - newborn (birth injury) P11.5
  - spleen D73.5
    - intraoperative — *see* Complications, intraoperative, hemorrhage, spleen
    - postprocedural — *see* Complications, postprocedural, hemorrhage, spleen
  - stomach K92.2
    - newborn P54.3

- **Hepatosis** K76.89
- **Hepatosplenomegaly** R16.2
  - hyperlipemic (Burger-Grutz type) E78.3 *[K77]*
- **Hereditary** — *see* condition
- **Hereditary alpha tryptasemia** (syndrome) D89.44
- **Heredodegeneration, macular** — *see* Dystrophy, retina
- **Heredopathia atactica polyneuritiformis** G60.1
- **Heredosyphilis** — *see* Syphilis, congenital
- **Herlitz' syndrome** Q81.1
- **Hermansky-Pudlak syndrome** E70.331
- **Hermaphrodite, hermaphroditism** (true) Q56.0
  - 46,XX with streak gonads Q99.1
  - 46,XX/46,XY Q99.0
  - 46,XY with streak gonads Q99.1
  - chimera 46,XX/46,XY Q99.0
- **Hernia, hernial** (acquired) (recurrent) K46.9
  - with
    - gangrene — *see* Hernia, by site, with, gangrene
    - incarceration — *see* Hernia, by site, with, obstruction
    - irreducible — *see* Hernia, by site, with, obstruction
    - obstruction — *see* Hernia, by site, with, obstruction
    - strangulation — *see* Hernia, by site, with, obstruction
  - abdomen, abdominal K46.9
    - with
      - gangrene (and obstruction) K46.1
      - obstruction K46.0
    - femoral — *see* Hernia, femoral
    - incisional — *see* Hernia, incisional
    - inguinal — *see* Hernia, inguinal
    - specified site NEC K45.8
      - with
        - gangrene (and obstruction) K45.1
        - obstruction K45.0
    - umbilical — *see* Hernia, umbilical
    - wall — *see* Hernia, ventral
  - appendix — *see* Hernia, abdomen
  - bladder (mucosa) (sphincter)
    - congenital (female) (male) Q79.51
    - female — *see* Cystocele
    - male N32.89
  - brain, congenital — *see* Encephalocele
  - cartilage, vertebra — *see* Displacement, intervertebral disc
  - cerebral, congenital — *see also* Encephalocele
    - endaural Q01.8
  - ciliary body (traumatic) S05.2- ☑
  - colon — *see* Hernia, abdomen
  - Cooper's — *see* Hernia, abdomen, specified site NEC
  - crural — *see* Hernia, femoral
  - diaphragm, diaphragmatic K44.9
    - with
      - gangrene (and obstruction) K44.1
      - obstruction K44.0
    - congenital Q79.0
  - direct (inguinal) — *see* Hernia, inguinal
  - diverticulum, intestine — *see* Hernia, abdomen
  - double (inguinal) — *see* Hernia, inguinal, bilateral
  - due to adhesions (with obstruction) K56.50
  - epigastric — *see also* Hernia, ventral K43.9
  - esophageal hiatus — *see* Hernia, hiatal
  - external (inguinal) — *see* Hernia, inguinal
  - fallopian tube N83.4- ☑
  - fascia M62.89
  - femoral K41.90
    - with
      - gangrene (and obstruction) K41.40
        - not specified as recurrent K41.40
        - recurrent K41.41
      - obstruction K41.30
        - not specified as recurrent K41.30
        - recurrent K41.31
    - not specified as recurrent K41.90
    - recurrent K41.91
    - bilateral K41.20
      - with
        - gangrene (and obstruction) K41.10
          - not specified as recurrent K41.10
          - recurrent K41.11
        - obstruction K41.00
          - not specified as recurrent K41.00
          - recurrent K41.01
      - not specified as recurrent K41.20
      - recurrent K41.21
    - unilateral K41.90
      - with
        - gangrene (and obstruction) K41.40
          - not specified as recurrent K41.40

- **Hernia, hernial** — *continued*
  - femoral — *continued*
    - unilateral — *continued*
      - with — *continued*
        - gangrene — *continued*
          - recurrent K41.41
        - obstruction K41.30
          - not specified as recurrent K41.30
          - recurrent K41.31
      - not specified as recurrent K41.90
      - recurrent K41.91
  - foramen magnum G93.5
    - congenital Q01.8
  - funicular (umbilical) — *see also* Hernia, umbilicus
    - spermatic (cord) — *see* Hernia, inguinal
  - gastrointestinal tract — *see* Hernia, abdomen
  - Hesselbach's — *see* Hernia, femoral, specified site NEC
  - hiatal (esophageal) (sliding) K44.9
    - with
      - gangrene (and obstruction) K44.1
      - obstruction K44.0
    - congenital Q40.1
  - hypogastric — *see* Hernia, ventral
  - incarcerated — *see also* Hernia, by site, with obstruction
    - with gangrene — *see* Hernia, by site, with gangrene
  - incisional K43.2
    - with
      - gangrene (and obstruction) K43.1
      - obstruction K43.0
  - indirect (inguinal) — *see* Hernia, inguinal
  - inguinal (direct) (external) (funicular) (indirect) (internal) (oblique) (scrotal) (sliding) K40.90
    - with
      - gangrene (and obstruction) K40.40
        - not specified as recurrent K40.40
        - recurrent K40.41
      - obstruction K40.30
        - not specified as recurrent K40.30
        - recurrent K40.31
    - not specified as recurrent K40.90
    - recurrent K40.91
    - bilateral K40.20
      - with
        - gangrene (and obstruction) K40.10
          - not specified as recurrent K40.10
          - recurrent K40.11
        - obstruction K40.00
          - not specified as recurrent K40.00
          - recurrent K40.01
      - not specified as recurrent K40.20
      - recurrent K40.21
    - unilateral K40.90
      - with
        - gangrene (and obstruction) K40.40
          - not specified as recurrent K40.40
          - recurrent K40.41
        - obstruction K40.30
          - not specified as recurrent K40.30
          - recurrent K40.31
      - not specified as recurrent K40.90
      - recurrent K40.91
  - internal — *see also* Hernia, abdomen
    - inguinal — *see* Hernia, inguinal
  - interstitial — *see* Hernia, abdomen
  - intervertebral cartilage or disc — *see* Displacement, intervertebral disc
  - intestine, intestinal — *see* Hernia, by site
  - intra-abdominal — *see* Hernia, abdomen
  - iris (traumatic) S05.2- ☑
  - irreducible — *see also* Hernia, by site, with obstruction
    - with gangrene — *see* Hernia, by site, with gangrene
  - ischiatic — *see* Hernia, abdomen, specified site NEC
  - ischiorectal — *see* Hernia, abdomen, specified site NEC
  - lens (traumatic) S05.2- ☑
  - linea (alba) (semilunaris) — *see* Hernia, ventral
  - Littre's — *see* Hernia, abdomen
  - lumbar — *see* Hernia, abdomen, specified site NEC
  - lung (subcutaneous) J98.4
  - mediastinum J98.59
  - mesenteric (internal) — *see* Hernia, abdomen
  - midline — *see* Hernia, ventral
  - muscle (sheath) M62.89
  - nucleus pulposus — *see* Displacement, intervertebral disc
  - oblique (inguinal) — *see* Hernia, inguinal
  - obstructive — *see also* Hernia, by site, with obstruction
    - with gangrene — *see* Hernia, by site, with gangrene

- **Hernia, hernial** — *continued*
  - obturator — *see* Hernia, abdomen, specified site NEC
  - omental — *see* Hernia, abdomen
  - ovary N83.4- ☑
  - oviduct N83.4- ☑
  - paraesophageal — *see also* Hernia, diaphragm
    - congenital Q40.1
  - parastomal K43.5
    - with
      - gangrene (and obstruction) K43.4
      - obstruction K43.3
  - paraumbilical — *see* Hernia, umbilicus
  - perineal — *see* Hernia, abdomen, specified site NEC
  - Petit's — *see* Hernia, abdomen, specified site NEC
  - postoperative — *see* Hernia, incisional
  - pregnant uterus — *see* Abnormal, uterus in pregnancy or childbirth
  - prevesical N32.89
  - properitoneal — *see* Hernia, abdomen, specified site NEC
  - pudendal — *see* Hernia, abdomen, specified site NEC
  - rectovaginal N81.6
  - retroperitoneal — *see* Hernia, abdomen, specified site NEC
  - Richter's — *see* Hernia, abdomen, with obstruction
  - Rieux's, Riex's — *see* Hernia, abdomen, specified site NEC
  - sac condition (adhesion) (dropsy) (inflammation) (laceration) (suppuration) — *code by site under* Hernia
  - sciatic — *see* Hernia, abdomen, specified site NEC
  - scrotum, scrotal — *see* Hernia, inguinal
  - sliding (inguinal) — *see also* Hernia, inguinal
    - hiatus — *see* Hernia, hiatal
  - spigelian — *see* Hernia, ventral
  - spinal — *see* Spina bifida
  - strangulated — *see also* Hernia, by site, with obstruction
    - with gangrene — *see* Hernia, by site, with gangrene
  - subxiphoid — *see* Hernia, ventral
  - supra-umbilicus — *see* Hernia, ventral
  - tendon — *see* Disorder, tendon, specified type NEC
  - Treitz's (fossa) — *see* Hernia, abdomen, specified site NEC
  - tunica vaginalis Q55.29
  - umbilicus, umbilical K42.9
    - with
      - gangrene (and obstruction) K42.1
      - obstruction K42.0
  - ureter N28.89
  - urethra, congenital Q64.79
  - urinary meatus, congenital Q64.79
  - uterus N81.4
    - pregnant — *see* Abnormal, uterus in pregnancy or childbirth
  - vaginal (anterior) (wall) — *see* Cystocele
  - Velpeau's — *see* Hernia, femoral
  - ventral K43.9
    - with
      - gangrene (and obstruction) K43.7
      - obstruction K43.6
    - incisional K43.2
      - with
        - gangrene (and obstruction) K43.1
        - obstruction K43.0
    - recurrent — *see* Hernia, incisional
    - specified NEC K43.9
      - with
        - gangrene (and obstruction) K43.7
        - obstruction K43.6
  - vesical
    - congenital (female) (male) Q79.51
    - female — *see* Cystocele
    - male N32.89
  - vitreous (into wound) S05.2- ☑
    - into anterior chamber — *see* Prolapse, vitreous
- **Herniation** — *see also* Hernia
  - brain (stem) G93.5
    - nontraumatic G93.5
    - traumatic S06.A1 ☑
      - cerebellar S06.A1 ☑
      - subfalcine (cingulate) S06.A1 ☑
      - tonsillar S06.A1 ☑
      - transtentorial (central) (upward cerebellar) S06.A1 ☑
      - uncal S06.A1 ☑
  - cerebral G93.5

- **History** — *continued*
  - personal — *see also* History, family — *continued*
    - disease or disorder — *continued*
      - infectious — *continued*
        - malaria Z86.13
        - Methicillin resistant Staphylococcus aureus (MRSA) Z86.14
        - poliomyelitis Z86.12
        - SARS-CoV-2 Z86.16
        - specified NEC Z86.19
        - tuberculosis Z86.11
      - mental NEC Z86.59
      - metabolic Z86.39
        - diabetic foot ulcer Z86.31
        - gestational diabetes Z86.32
        - specified type NEC Z86.39
      - musculoskeletal NEC Z87.39
      - nervous system Z86.69
      - nutritional Z86.39
      - parasitic Z86.19
      - respiratory system NEC Z87.09
      - sense organs Z86.69
      - skin Z87.2
      - specified site or type NEC Z87.898
      - subcutaneous tissue Z87.2
      - trophoblastic Z87.59
      - urinary system NEC Z87.448
    - drug dependence — *see* Dependence, drug, by type, in remission
    - drug therapy
      - antineoplastic chemotherapy Z92.21
      - estrogen Z92.23
      - immunosuppression Z92.25
      - inhaled steroids Z92.240
      - monoclonal drug Z92.22
      - specified NEC Z92.29
      - steroid Z92.241
      - systemic steroids Z92.241
    - dysplasia
      - cervical (mild) (moderate) Z87.410
        - severe (grade III) Z86.001
      - prostatic Z87.430
      - vaginal (mild) (moderate) Z87.411
        - severe (grade III) Z86.002
      - vulvar (mild) (moderate) Z87.412
        - severe (grade III) Z86.002
    - embolism (venous) Z86.718
      - pulmonary Z86.711
    - encephalitis Z86.61
    - estrogen therapy Z92.23
    - extracorporeal membrane oxygenation (ECMO) Z92.81
    - failed conscious sedation Z92.83
    - failed moderate sedation Z92.83
    - fall, falling Z91.81
    - forced labor or sexual exploitation Z91.42
      - in childhood Z62.813
    - fracture (healed)
      - fatigue Z87.312
      - fragility Z87.310
      - osteoporosis Z87.310
      - pathological NEC Z87.311
      - stress Z87.312
      - traumatic Z87.81
    - gene therapy Z92.86
    - gestational diabetes Z86.32
    - hepatitis
      - B Z86.19
      - C Z86.19
    - Hodgkin disease Z85.71
    - hyperthermia, malignant Z88.4
    - hypospadias (corrected) Z87.710
    - hysterectomy Z90.710
    - immunosuppression therapy Z92.25
    - in situ neoplasm
      - breast Z86.000
      - cervix uteri Z86.001
      - digestive organs, specified NEC Z86.004
      - esophagus Z86.003
      - genital organs, specified NEC Z86.002
      - melanoma Z86.006
      - middle ear Z86.005
      - oral cavity Z86.003
      - respiratory system Z86.005
      - skin Z86.007
      - specified NEC Z86.008
      - stomach Z86.003
    - in utero procedure during pregnancy Z98.870
    - in utero procedure while a fetus Z98.871

- **History** — *continued*
  - personal — *see also* History, family — *continued*
    - infection NEC Z86.19
      - central nervous system Z86.61
      - coronavirus (disease) (novel) 2019 Z86.16
      - COVID-19 Z86.16
      - latent tuberculosis Z86.15
      - Methicillin resistant Staphylococcus aureus (MRSA) Z86.14
      - SARS-CoV-2 Z86.16
      - urinary (recurrent) (tract) Z87.440
    - injury NEC Z87.828
    - irradiation Z92.3
    - kidney stones Z87.442
    - latent tuberculosis infection Z86.15
    - leukemia Z85.6
    - lymphoma (non-Hodgkin) Z85.72
    - malignant melanoma (skin) Z85.820
    - malignant neoplasm (of) Z85.9
      - accessory sinuses Z85.22
      - anus NEC Z85.048
        - carcinoid Z85.040
      - bladder Z85.51
      - bone Z85.830
      - brain Z85.841
      - breast Z85.3
      - bronchus NEC Z85.118
        - carcinoid Z85.110
      - carcinoid — *see* History, personal (of), malignant neoplasm, by site, carcinoid
      - cervix Z85.41
      - colon NEC Z85.038
        - carcinoid Z85.030
      - digestive organ Z85.00
        - specified NEC Z85.09
      - endocrine gland NEC Z85.858
      - epididymis Z85.48
      - esophagus Z85.01
      - eye Z85.840
      - gastrointestinal tract — *see* History, malignant neoplasm, digestive organ
      - genital organ
        - female Z85.40
          - specified NEC Z85.44
        - male Z85.45
          - specified NEC Z85.49
      - hematopoietic NEC Z85.79
      - intrathoracic organ Z85.20
      - kidney NEC Z85.528
        - carcinoid Z85.520
      - large intestine NEC Z85.038
        - carcinoid Z85.030
      - larynx Z85.21
      - liver Z85.05
      - lung NEC Z85.118
        - carcinoid Z85.110
      - mediastinum Z85.29
      - Merkel cell Z85.821
      - middle ear Z85.22
      - nasal cavities Z85.22
      - nervous system NEC Z85.848
      - oral cavity Z85.819
        - specified site NEC Z85.818
      - ovary Z85.43
      - pancreas Z85.07
      - pelvis Z85.53
      - pharynx Z85.819
        - specified site NEC Z85.818
      - pleura Z85.29
      - prostate Z85.46
      - rectosigmoid junction NEC Z85.048
        - carcinoid Z85.040
      - rectum NEC Z85.048
        - carcinoid Z85.040
      - respiratory organ Z85.20
      - sinuses, accessory Z85.22
      - skin NEC Z85.828
        - melanoma Z85.820
        - Merkel cell Z85.821
      - small intestine NEC Z85.068
        - carcinoid Z85.060
      - soft tissue Z85.831
      - specified site NEC Z85.89
      - stomach NEC Z85.028
        - carcinoid Z85.020
      - testis Z85.47
      - thymus NEC Z85.238
        - carcinoid Z85.230
      - thyroid Z85.850

- **History** — *continued*
  - personal — *see also* History, family — *continued*
    - malignant neoplasm — *continued*
      - tongue Z85.810
      - trachea Z85.12
      - urinary organ or tract Z85.50
        - specified NEC Z85.59
      - uterus Z85.42
    - maltreatment Z91.89
    - medical treatment NEC Z92.89
    - melanoma Z85.820
      - in situ Z86.006
      - malignant (skin) Z85.820
    - meningitis Z86.61
    - mental disorder Z86.59
    - Merkel cell carcinoma (skin) Z85.821
    - Methicillin resistant Staphylococcus aureus (MRSA) Z86.14
    - military deployment Z91.82
    - military service Z91.85
    - military war, peacekeeping and humanitarian deployment (current or past conflict) Z91.82
    - myocardial infarction (old) I25.2
    - necrotizing enterocolitis of newborn (corrected) Z87.61
    - neglect (in)
      - adult Z91.412
      - childhood Z62.812
    - neoplasia
      - anal intraepithelial, III [AIN III] Z86.004
      - high-grade prostatic intraepithelial, III [HGPIN III] Z86.002
      - vaginal intraepithelial, III [VAIN III] Z86.002
      - vulvar intraepithelial, III [VIN III] Z86.002
    - neoplasm
      - benign Z86.018
        - brain Z86.011
        - colon polyp Z86.010
      - in situ
        - breast Z86.000
        - cervix uteri Z86.001
        - digestive organs, specified NEC Z86.004
        - esophagus Z86.003
        - genital organs, specified NEC Z86.002
        - melanoma Z86.006
        - middle ear Z86.005
        - oral cavity Z86.003
        - respiratory system Z86.005
        - skin Z86.007
        - specified NEC Z86.008
        - stomach Z86.003
      - malignant — *see* History of, malignant neoplasm
      - uncertain behavior Z86.03
    - nephrotic syndrome Z87.441
    - nicotine dependence Z87.891
    - noncompliance with medical treatment or regimen — *see* Noncompliance
    - nutritional deficiency Z86.39
    - obstetric complications Z87.59
      - childbirth Z87.59
      - pregnancy Z87.59
      - pre-term labor Z87.51
      - puerperium Z87.59
    - osteoporosis fractures Z87.31 ☑
    - parasuicide (attempt) Z91.51
    - physical trauma NEC Z87.828
      - self-harm or suicide attempt Z91.51
    - pneumonia (recurrent) Z87.01
    - poisoning NEC Z91.89
      - self-harm or suicide attempt Z91.51
    - poor personal hygiene Z91.89
    - preterm labor Z87.51
    - procedure during pregnancy Z98.870
    - procedure while a fetus Z98.871
    - prolonged reversible ischemic neurologic deficit (PRIND) Z86.73
    - prostatic dysplasia Z87.430
    - psychological
      - abuse
        - adult Z91.411
        - child Z62.811
      - trauma, specified NEC Z91.49
    - radiation therapy Z92.3
    - removal
      - implant
        - breast Z98.86
    - renal calculi Z87.442
    - respiratory condition NEC Z87.09
    - retained foreign body fully removed Z87.821

- **History** — *continued*
  - personal — *see also* History, family — *continued*
    - risk factors NEC Z91.89
    - SARS-CoV-2 infection Z86.16
    - self-harm
      - nonsuicidal Z91.52
      - suicidal Z91.51
    - self-inflicted injury without suicidal intent Z91.52
    - self-injury
      - nonsuicidal Z91.52
    - self-mutilation Z91.52
    - self-poisoning attempt Z91.51
    - sex reassignment Z87.89Ø
    - sleep-wake cycle problem Z72.821
    - specified NEC Z87.898
    - steroid therapy (systemic) Z92.241
      - inhaled Z92.24Ø
    - stroke without residual deficits Z86.73
    - substance abuse NEC F1Ø-F19
    - sudden cardiac arrest Z86.74
    - sudden cardiac death successfully resuscitated Z86.74
    - suicidal behavior Z91.51
    - suicide attempt Z91.51
    - surgery NEC Z98.89Ø
      - with uterine scar Z98.891
      - sex reassignment Z87.89Ø
      - transplant — *see* Transplant
    - thrombophlebitis Z86.72
    - thrombosis (venous) Z86.718
      - pulmonary Z86.711
    - tobacco dependence Z87.891
    - tracheoesophageal
      - atresia Z87.731
      - fistula Z87.731
    - transient ischemic attack (TIA) without residual deficits Z86.73
    - trauma (physical) NEC Z87.828
      - psychological NEC Z91.49
      - self-harm Z91.51
    - traumatic brain injury Z87.82Ø
    - tuberculosis, latent infection Z86.15
    - unhealthy sleep-wake cycle Z72.821
    - unintended awareness under general anesthesia Z92.84
    - urinary calculi Z87.442
    - urinary (recurrent) (tract) infection(s) Z87.44Ø
    - uterine scar from previous surgery Z98.891
    - vaginal dysplasia Z87.411
    - venous thrombosis or embolism Z86.718
      - pulmonary Z86.711
    - vulvar dysplasia Z87.412
- **His-Werner disease** A79.Ø
- **HIV** — *see also* Human, immunodeficiency virus B2Ø
  - laboratory evidence (nonconclusive) R75
  - nonconclusive test (in infants) R75
  - positive, seropositive Z21
- **Hives** (bold) — *see* Urticaria
- **Hoarseness** R49.Ø
- **Hobo** Z59.ØØ
- **Hodgkin disease** — *see* Lymphoma, Hodgkin
- **Hodgson's** — *see also* Aneurysm, aorta, thorax I71.2Ø
  - ruptured — *see also* Aneurysm, aorta, thorax, ruptured I71.1Ø
- **Hoffa-Kastert disease** E88.89
- **Hoffa's disease** E88.89
- **Hoffmann-Bouveret syndrome** I47.9
- **Hoffmann's syndrome** EØ3.9 *[G73.7]*
- **Hole** (round)
  - macula H35.34- ☑
  - retina (without detachment) — *see* Break, retina, round hole
    - with detachment — *see* Detachment, retina, with retinal, break
- **Holiday relief care** Z75.5
- **Hollenhorst's plaque** — *see* Occlusion, artery, retina
- **Hollow foot** (congenital) Q66.7- ☑
  - acquired — *see* Deformity, limb, foot, specified NEC
- **Holoprosencephaly** QØ4.2
- **Holt-Oram syndrome** Q87.2
- **Homelessness** Z59.ØØ
  - sheltered Z59.Ø1
  - unsheltered Z59.Ø2
- **Homesickness** — *see* Disorder, adjustment
- **Homocysteinemia** R79.83
- **Homocystinemia** R79.83
- **Homocystinuria** E72.11
- **Homogentisate 1,2-dioxygenase deficiency** E7Ø.29
- **Homologous serum hepatitis** (prophylactic) (therapeutic) — *see* Hepatitis, viral, type B
- **Honeycomb lung** J98.4
  - congenital Q33.Ø
- **Hooded**
  - clitoris Q52.6
  - penis Q55.69
- **Hookworm** (disease) (infection) (infestation) B76.9
  - with anemia B76.9 *[D63.8]*
  - specified NEC B76.8
- **Hordeolum** (eyelid) (externum) (recurrent) HØØ.Ø19
  - internum HØØ.Ø29
    - left HØØ.Ø26
      - lower HØØ.Ø25
      - upper HØØ.Ø24
    - right HØØ.Ø23
      - lower HØØ.Ø22
      - upper HØØ.Ø21
  - left HØØ.Ø16
    - lower HØØ.Ø15
    - upper HØØ.Ø14
  - right HØØ.Ø13
    - lower HØØ.Ø12
    - upper HØØ.Ø11
- **Horn**
  - cutaneous L85.8
  - nail L6Ø.2
    - congenital Q84.6
- **Horner** (-Claude Bernard) **syndrome** G9Ø.2
  - traumatic — *see* Injury, nerve, cervical sympathetic
- **Horseshoe kidney** (congenital) Q63.1
- **Horton's headache or neuralgia** G44.Ø99
  - intractable G44.Ø91
  - not intractable G44.Ø99
- **Hospital hopper syndrome** — *see* Disorder, factitious
- **Hospitalism in children** — *see* Disorder, adjustment
- **Hostility** R45.5
  - towards child Z62.3
- **Hot flashes**
  - menopausal N95.1
- **Hourglass** (contracture) — *see also* Contraction, hourglass
  - stomach K31.89
    - congenital Q4Ø.2
    - stricture K31.2
- **Household, housing circumstance affecting care** Z59.9
  - specified NEC Z59.89
- **Housemaid's knee** — *see* Bursitis, prepatellar
- **HSCT-TMA** (hematopoietic stem cell transplantation-associated thrombotic microangiopathy) M31.11
- **Hudson** (-Stahli) **line** (cornea) — *see* Pigmentation, cornea, anterior
- **Human**
  - bite (open wound) — *see also* Bite
    - intact skin surface — *see* Bite, superficial
  - herpesvirus — *see* Herpes
  - immunodeficiency virus (HIV) disease (infection) B2Ø
    - asymptomatic status Z21
    - contact Z2Ø.6
    - counseling Z71.7
    - dementia — *see also* Dementia, in, diseases specified elsewhere B2Ø *[FØ2.8Ø]*
      - with behavioral disturbance — *see also* Dementia, in, diseases specified elsewhere B2Ø *[FØ2.81-]* ☑
    - exposure to Z2Ø.6
    - laboratory evidence R75
    - type-2 (HIV 2) as cause of disease classified elsewhere B97.35
  - papillomavirus (HPV)
    - DNA test positive
      - high risk
        - cervix R87.81Ø
        - vagina R87.811
      - low risk
        - cervix R87.82Ø
        - vagina R87.821
    - screening for Z11.51
  - T-cell lymphotropic virus
    - type-1 (HTLV-I) infection B33.3
      - as cause of disease classified elsewhere B97.33
      - carrier Z22.6
    - type-2 (HTLV-II) as cause of disease classified elsewhere B97.34
- **Humidifier lung or pneumonitis** J67.7
- **Humiliation** (experience) **in childhood** Z62.898
- **Humpback** (acquired) — *see* Kyphosis
- **Hunchback** (acquired) — *see* Kyphosis
- **Hunger** T73.Ø ☑
  - air, psychogenic F45.8
- **Hungry bone syndrome** E83.81
- **Hunner's ulcer** — *see* Cystitis, chronic, interstitial
- **Hunter's**
  - glossitis D51.Ø
  - syndrome E76.1
- **Huntington's disease or chorea** G1Ø
  - with dementia — *see also* Dementia, in, diseases specified elsewhere G1Ø *[FØ2.8Ø]*
    - with behavioral disturbance — *see also* Dementia, in, diseases specified elsewhere G1Ø *[FØ2.81-]* ☑
- **Hunt's**
  - disease or syndrome (herpetic geniculate ganglionitis) BØ2.21
    - dyssynergia cerebellaris myoclonica G11.19
  - neuralgia BØ2.21
- **Hurler** (-Scheie) **disease or syndrome** E76.Ø2
- **Hurst's disease** G36.1
- **Hurthle cell**
  - adenocarcinoma C73
  - adenoma D34
  - carcinoma C73
  - tumor D34
- **Hutchinson-Boeck disease or syndrome** — *see* Sarcoidosis
- **Hutchinson-Gilford disease or syndrome** E34.8
- **Hutchinson's**
  - disease, meaning
    - angioma serpiginosum L81.7
    - pompholyx (cheiropompholyx) L3Ø.1
    - prurigo estivalis L56.4
    - summer eruption or summer prurigo L56.4
  - melanotic freckle — *see* Melanoma, in situ
    - malignant melanoma in — *see* Melanoma
  - teeth or incisors (congenital syphilis) A5Ø.52
  - triad (congenital syphilis) A5Ø.53
- **Hyalin plaque, sclera, senile** H15.89
- **Hyaline membrane** (disease) (lung) (pulmonary) (newborn) P22.Ø
- **Hyalinosis**
  - cutis (et mucosae) E78.89
  - focal and segmental (glomerular) — *see also* NØØ-NØ7 with fourth character .1 NØ5.1
- **Hyalitis, hyalosis, asteroid** — *see also* Deposit, crystalline
  - syphilitic (late) A52.71
- **Hydatid**
  - cyst or tumor — *see* Echinococcus
  - mole — *see* Hydatidiform mole
  - Morgagni
    - female Q5Ø.5
    - male (epididymal) Q55.4
      - testicular Q55.29
- **Hydatidiform mole** (benign) (complicating pregnancy) (delivered) (undelivered) OØ1.9
  - classical OØ1.Ø
  - complete OØ1.Ø
  - incomplete OØ1.1
  - invasive D39.2
  - malignant D39.2
  - partial OØ1.1
- **Hydatidosis** — *see* Echinococcus
- **Hydradenitis** (axillaris) (suppurative) L73.2
- **Hydradenoma** — *see* Hidradenoma
- **Hydramnios** O4Ø.- ☑
- **Hydrancephaly, hydranencephaly** QØ4.3
  - with spina bifida — *see* Spina bifida, with hydrocephalus
- **Hydrargyrism NEC** — *see* Poisoning, mercury
- **Hydrarthrosis** — *see also* Effusion, joint
  - gonococcal A54.42
  - intermittent M12.4Ø
    - ankle M12.47- ☑
    - elbow M12.42- ☑
    - foot joint M12.47- ☑
    - hand joint M12.44- ☑
    - hip M12.45- ☑
    - knee M12.46- ☑
    - multiple site M12.49
    - shoulder M12.41- ☑
    - specified joint NEC M12.48
    - wrist M12.43- ☑
  - of yaws (early) (late) — *see also* subcategory M14.8- A66.6

Hyperplasia, hyperplastic — *continued*
- endometrium, endometrial (adenomatous) (cystic) (glandular) (glandular-cystic) (polypoid) N85.ØØ
  - with atypia N85.Ø2
  - benign N85.Ø1
  - cervix — *see* Dysplasia, cervix
  - complex (without atypia) N85.Ø1
  - simple (without atypia) N85.Ø1
- epithelial L85.9
  - focal, oral, including tongue K13.29
  - nipple N62
  - skin L85.9
  - tongue K13.29
  - vaginal wall N89.3
- erythroid D75.89
- fibromuscular of artery (carotid) (renal) I77.3
- genital
  - female NEC N94.89
  - male N5Ø.89
- gingiva KØ6.1
- glandularis cystica uteri (interstitialis) — *see also* Hyperplasia, endometrial N85.ØØ
- gum KØ6.1
- hymen, congenital Q52.4
- irritative, edentulous (alveolar) KØ6.2
- jaw M26.Ø9
  - alveolar M26.79
  - lower M26.Ø3
    - alveolar M26.72
  - upper M26.Ø1
    - alveolar M26.71
- kidney (congenital) Q63.3
- labia N9Ø.69
  - epithelial N9Ø.3
- liver (congenital) Q44.79
  - nodular, focal K76.89
- lymph gland or node R59.9
- mandible, mandibular M26.Ø3
  - alveolar M26.72
  - unilateral condylar M27.8
- maxilla, maxillary M26.Ø1
  - alveolar M26.71
- myometrium, myometrial N85.2
- neuroendocrine cell, of infancy J84.841
- nose
  - lymphoid J34.89
  - polypoid J33.9
- oral mucosa (irritative) K13.6
- organ or site, congenital NEC — *see* Anomaly, by site
- ovary N83.8
- palate, papillary (irritative) K13.6
- pancreatic islet cells E16.9
  - alpha E16.8
    - with excess
      - gastrin E16.4
      - glucagon E16.3
  - beta E16.1
- parathyroid (gland) E21.Ø
- pharynx (lymphoid) J39.2
- prostate (adenofibromatous) N4Ø.Ø
  - with lower urinary tract symptoms (LUTS) N4Ø.1
    - nodular N4Ø.3
  - nodular N4Ø.2
    - with lower urinary tract symptoms (LUTS) N4Ø.3
  - without lower urinary tract symtpoms (LUTS) N4Ø.Ø
    - nodular N4Ø.2
- renal artery I77.89
- reticulo-endothelial (cell) D75.89
- salivary gland (any) K11.1
- Schimmelbusch's — *see* Mastopathy, cystic
- suprarenal capsule (gland) E27.8
- thymus (gland) (persistent) E32.Ø
- thyroid (gland) — *see* Goiter
- tonsils (faucial) (infective) (lingual) (lymphoid) J35.1
  - with adenoids J35.3
- unilateral condylar M27.8
- uterus, uterine N85.2
  - endometrium (glandular) — *see also* Hyperplasia, endometrial N85.ØØ
- vulva N9Ø.69
  - epithelial N9Ø.3

Hyperpnea — *see* Hyperventilation

Hyperpotassemia E87.5

Hyperprebetalipoproteinemia (familial) E78.1

Hyperprolactinemia E22.1

Hyperprolinemia (type I) (type II) E72.59

Hyperproteinemia E88.Ø9

Hyperprothrombinemia, causing coagulation factor deficiency D68.4

Hyperpyrexia R5Ø.9
- heat (effects) T67.Ø1 ☑
- malignant, due to anesthetic T88.3 ☑
- rheumatic — *see* Fever, rheumatic
- unknown origin R5Ø.9

Hyper-reflexia R29.2

Hypersalivation K11.7

Hypersecretion
- ACTH (not associated with Cushing's syndrome) E27.Ø
  - pituitary E24.Ø
- adrenaline E27.5
- adrenomedullary E27.5
- androgen (testicular) E29.Ø
  - ovarian (drug-induced) (iatrogenic) E28.1
- calcitonin EØ7.Ø
- catecholamine E27.5
- corticoadrenal E24.9
- cortisol E24.9
- epinephrine E27.5
- estrogen E28.Ø
- gastric K31.89
  - psychogenic F45.8
- gastrin E16.4
- glucagon E16.3
- hormone(s)
  - ACTH (not associated with Cushing's syndrome) E27.Ø
    - pituitary E24.Ø
  - antidiuretic E22.2
  - growth E22.Ø
  - intestinal NEC E34.1
  - ovarian androgen E28.1
  - pituitary E22.9
  - testicular E29.Ø
  - thyroid stimulating EØ5.8Ø
    - with thyroid storm EØ5.81
- insulin — *see* Hyperinsulinism
- lacrimal glands — *see* Epiphora
- medulloadrenal E27.5
- milk O92.6
- ovarian androgens E28.1
- salivary gland (any) K11.7
- thyrocalcitonin EØ7.Ø
- upper respiratory J39.8

Hypersegmentation, leukocytic, hereditary D72.Ø

Hypersensitive, hypersensitiveness, hypersensitivity — *see also* Allergy
- carotid sinus G9Ø.Ø1
- colon — *see* Irritable, colon
- drug T88.7 ☑
- gastrointestinal K52.29
  - immediate K52.29
  - psychogenic F45.8
- labyrinth — *see* subcategory H83.2 ☑
- pain R2Ø.8
- pneumonitis — *see* Pneumonitis, allergic
- reaction T78.4Ø ☑
  - upper respiratory tract NEC J39.3

Hypersomnia (organic) G47.1Ø
- due to
  - alcohol
    - abuse F1Ø.182
    - dependence F1Ø.282
    - use F1Ø.982
  - amphetamines
    - abuse F15.182
    - dependence F15.282
    - use F15.982
  - caffeine
    - abuse F15.182
    - dependence F15.282
    - use F15.982
  - cocaine
    - abuse F14.182
    - dependence F14.282
    - use F14.982
  - drug NEC
    - abuse F19.182
    - dependence F19.282
    - use F19.982
  - medical condition G47.14
  - mental disorder F51.13
  - opioid
    - abuse F11.182
    - dependence F11.282
    - use F11.982

Hypersomnia — *continued*
- due to — *continued*
  - psychoactive substance NEC
    - abuse F19.182
    - dependence F19.282
    - use F19.982
  - sedative, hypnotic, or anxiolytic
    - abuse F13.182
    - dependence F13.282
    - use F13.982
  - stimulant NEC
    - abuse F15.182
    - dependence F15.282
    - use F15.982
- idiopathic G47.11
  - with long sleep time G47.11
  - without long sleep time G47.12
- menstrual related G47.13
- nonorganic origin F51.11
  - specified NEC F51.19
- not due to a substance or known physiological condition F51.11
  - specified NEC F51.19
- primary F51.11
- recurrent G47.13
- specified NEC G47.19

Hypersplenia, hypersplenism D73.1

Hyperstimulation, ovaries (associated with induced ovulation) N98.1

Hypersusceptibility — *see* Allergy

Hypertelorism (ocular) (orbital) Q75.2

Hypertension, hypertensive (accelerated) (benign) (essential) (idiopathic) (malignant) (systemic) I1Ø
- with
  - heart failure (congestive) I11.Ø
  - heart involvement (conditions in I5Ø.- or I51.4-I51.7, I51.89, I51.9, due to hypertension) — *see* Hypertension, heart
  - kidney involvement — *see* Hypertension, kidney
- benign, intracranial G93.2
- borderline RØ3.Ø
- cardiorenal (disease) I13.1Ø
  - with heart failure I13.Ø
    - with stage 1 through stage 4 chronic kidney disease I13.Ø
    - with stage 5 or end stage renal disease I13.2
  - without heart failure I13.1Ø
    - with stage 1 through stage 4 chronic kidney disease I13.1Ø
    - with stage 5 or end stage renal disease I13.11
- cardiovascular
  - disease (arteriosclerotic) (sclerotic) — *see* Hypertension, heart
  - renal (disease) — *see* Hypertension, cardiorenal
- chronic venous — *see* Hypertension, venous (chronic)
- complicating
  - childbirth (labor) O16.4
    - pre-existing O1Ø.92
      - with
        - heart disease O1Ø.12
          - with renal disease O1Ø.32
        - pre-eclampsia O11.4
        - renal disease O1Ø.22
          - with heart disease O1Ø.32
      - essential O1Ø.Ø2
      - secondary O1Ø.42
  - pregnancy O16.- ☑
    - with edema — *see also* Pre-eclampsia O14.9- ☑
    - gestational (pregnancy induced) (without proteinuria) O13.- ☑
      - with proteinuria O14.9- ☑
        - mild pre-eclampsia O14.Ø- ☑
        - moderate pre-eclampsia O14.Ø- ☑
        - severe pre-eclampsia O14.1- ☑
          - with hemolysis, elevated liver enzymes and low platelet count (HELLP) O14.2- ☑
    - pre-existing O1Ø.91- ☑
      - with
        - heart disease O1Ø.11- ☑
          - with renal disease O1Ø.31- ☑
        - pre-eclampsia — *see* category O11
        - renal disease O1Ø.21- ☑
          - with heart disease O1Ø.31- ☑
      - essential O1Ø.Ø1- ☑
      - secondary O1Ø.41- ☑
    - transient O13- ☑
  - puerperium, pre-existing O16.5

- **Hypomenorrhea** — *see* Oligomenorrhea
- **Hypometabolism** R63.8
- **Hypomotility**
  - gastrointestinal (tract) K31.89
    - psychogenic F45.8
  - intestine K59.89
    - psychogenic F45.8
  - stomach K31.89
    - psychogenic F45.8
- **Hypomyelination - hypogonadotropic hypogonadism - hypodontia** G11.5
- **Hypomyelination with atrophy of the basal ganglia and cerebellum** (H-ABC) G23.3
- **Hyponasality** R49.22
- **Hyponatremia** E87.1
- **Hypo-osmolality** E87.1
- **Hypo-ovarianism, hypo-ovarism** E28.39
- **Hypoparathyroidism** E2Ø.9
  - autoimmune E2Ø.812
  - due to impaired parathyroid hormone secretion, unspecified E2Ø.819
  - familial E2Ø.89
    - isolated E2Ø.818
  - idiopathic E2Ø.Ø
  - neonatal, transitory P71.4
  - postprocedural E89.2
  - secondary, in diseases classified elsewhere E2Ø.811
  - specified NEC E2Ø.89
    - due to impaired parathyroid hormone secretion E2Ø.818
- **Hypoperfusion** (in)
  - newborn P96.89
- **Hypopharyngitis** — *see* Laryngopharyngitis
- **Hypophoria** H5Ø.53
- **Hypophosphatemia, hypophosphatasia** (acquired) (congenital) (renal) E83.39
  - familial E83.31
- **Hypophyseal, hypophysis** — *see also* condition
  - dwarfism E23.Ø
  - gigantism E22.Ø
- **Hypopiesis** — *see* Hypotension
- **Hypopinealism** E34.8
- **Hypopituitarism** (juvenile) E23.Ø
  - drug-induced E23.1
  - due to
    - hypophysectomy E89.3
    - radiotherapy E89.3
  - iatrogenic NEC E23.1
  - postirradiation E89.3
  - postpartum O99.285
  - postprocedural E89.3
- **Hypoplasia, hypoplastic**
  - adrenal (gland), congenital Q89.1
  - alimentary tract, congenital Q45.8
    - upper Q4Ø.8
  - anus, anal (canal) Q42.3
    - with fistula Q42.2
  - aorta, aortic Q25.42
    - ascending, in hypoplastic left heart syndrome Q23.4
    - valve Q23.1
      - in hypoplastic left heart syndrome Q23.4
  - areola, congenital Q83.8
  - arm (congenital) — *see* Defect, reduction, upper limb
  - artery (peripheral) Q27.8
    - brain (congenital) Q28.3
    - coronary Q24.5
    - digestive system Q27.8
    - lower limb Q27.8
    - pulmonary Q25.79
      - functional, unilateral J43.Ø
    - retinal (congenital) Q14.1
    - specified site NEC Q27.8
    - umbilical Q27.Ø
    - upper limb Q27.8
  - auditory canal Q17.8
    - causing impairment of hearing Q16.9
  - biliary duct or passage Q44.5
  - bone NOS Q79.9
    - face Q75.8
    - marrow D61.9
      - megakaryocytic D69.49
    - skull — *see* Hypoplasia, skull
  - brain QØ2
    - gyri QØ4.3
    - part of QØ4.3
  - breast (areola) N64.82
  - bronchus Q32.4
  - cardiac Q24.8

- **Hypoplasia, hypoplastic** — *continued*
  - carpus — *see* Defect, reduction, upper limb, specified type NEC
  - cartilage hair Q78.8
  - cecum Q42.8
  - cementum KØØ.4
  - cephalic QØ2
  - cerebellum QØ4.3
  - cervix (uteri), congenital Q51.821
  - clavicle (congenital) Q74.Ø
  - coccyx Q76.49
  - colon Q42.9
    - specified NEC Q42.8
  - corpus callosum QØ4.Ø
  - cricoid cartilage Q31.2
  - digestive organ(s) or tract NEC Q45.8
    - upper (congenital) Q4Ø.8
  - ear (auricle) (lobe) Q17.2
    - middle Q16.4
  - enamel of teeth (neonatal) (postnatal) (prenatal) KØØ.4
  - endocrine (gland) NEC Q89.2
  - endometrium N85.8
  - epididymis (congenital) Q55.4
  - epiglottis Q31.2
  - erythroid, congenital D61.Ø1
  - esophagus (congenital) Q39.8
  - eustachian tube Q17.8
  - eye Q11.2
  - eyelid (congenital) Q1Ø.3
  - face Q18.8
    - bone(s) Q75.8
  - femur (congenital) — *see* Defect, reduction, lower limb, specified type NEC
  - fibula (congenital) — *see* Defect, reduction, lower limb, specified type NEC
  - finger (congenital) — *see* Defect, reduction, upper limb, specified type NEC
  - focal dermal Q82.8
  - foot — *see* Defect, reduction, lower limb, specified type NEC
  - gallbladder Q44.Ø
  - genitalia, genital organ(s)
    - female, congenital Q52.8
      - external Q52.79
      - internal NEC Q52.8
    - in adiposogenital dystrophy E23.6
  - glottis Q31.2
  - hair Q84.2
  - hand (congenital) — *see* Defect, reduction, upper limb, specified type NEC
  - heart Q24.8
  - humerus (congenital) — *see* Defect, reduction, upper limb, specified type NEC
  - intestine (small) Q41.9
    - large Q42.9
      - specified NEC Q42.8
  - jaw M26.Ø9
    - alveolar M26.79
    - lower M26.Ø4
      - alveolar M26.74
    - upper M26.Ø2
      - alveolar M26.73
  - kidney(s) Q6Ø.5
    - bilateral Q6Ø.4
    - unilateral Q6Ø.3
  - labium (majus) (minus), congenital Q52.79
  - larynx Q31.2
  - left heart syndrome Q23.4
  - leg (congenital) — *see* Defect, reduction, lower limb
  - limb Q73.8
    - lower (congenital) — *see* Defect, reduction, lower limb
    - upper (congenital) — *see* Defect, reduction, upper limb
  - liver Q44.79
  - lung (lobe) (not associated with short gestation) Q33.6
    - associated with immaturity, low birth weight, prematurity, or short gestation P28.Ø
  - mammary (areola), congenital Q83.8
  - mandible, mandibular M26.Ø4
    - alveolar M26.74
    - unilateral condylar M27.8
  - maxillary M26.Ø2
    - alveolar M26.73
  - medullary D61.9
  - megakaryocytic D69.49
  - metacarpus — *see* Defect, reduction, upper limb, specified type NEC

- **Hypoplasia, hypoplastic** — *continued*
  - metatarsus — *see* Defect, reduction, lower limb, specified type NEC
  - muscle Q79.8
  - nail(s) Q84.6
  - nose, nasal Q3Ø.1
  - optic nerve H47.Ø3- ☑
  - osseous meatus (ear) Q17.8
  - ovary, congenital Q5Ø.39
  - pancreas Q45.Ø
  - parathyroid (gland) Q89.2
  - parotid gland Q38.4
  - patella Q74.1
  - pelvis, pelvic girdle Q74.2
  - penis (congenital) Q55.62
  - peripheral vascular system Q27.8
    - digestive system Q27.8
    - lower limb Q27.8
    - specified site NEC Q27.8
    - upper limb Q27.8
  - pituitary (gland) (congenital) Q89.2
  - pulmonary (not associated with short gestation) Q33.6
    - artery, functional J43.Ø
    - associated with short gestation P28.Ø
  - radioulnar — *see* Defect, reduction, upper limb, specified type NEC
  - radius — *see* Defect, reduction, upper limb
  - rectum Q42.1
    - with fistula Q42.Ø
  - respiratory system NEC Q34.8
  - rib Q76.6
  - right heart syndrome Q22.6
  - sacrum Q76.49
  - scapula Q74.Ø
  - scrotum Q55.1
  - shoulder girdle Q74.Ø
  - skin Q82.8
  - skull (bone) Q75.8
    - with
      - anencephaly QØØ.Ø
      - encephalocele — *see* Encephalocele
      - hydrocephalus QØ3.9
        - with spina bifida — *see* Spina bifida, by site, with hydrocephalus
      - microcephaly QØ2
  - spinal (cord) (ventral horn cell) QØ6.1
  - spine Q76.49
  - sternum Q76.7
  - tarsus — *see* Defect, reduction, lower limb, specified type NEC
  - testis Q55.1
  - thymic, with immunodeficiency D82.1
  - thymus (gland) Q89.2
    - with immunodeficiency D82.1
  - thyroid (gland) EØ3.1
    - cartilage Q31.2
  - tibiofibular (congenital) — *see* Defect, reduction, lower limb, specified type NEC
  - toe — *see* Defect, reduction, lower limb, specified type NEC
  - tongue Q38.3
  - Turner's KØØ.4
  - ulna (congenital) — *see* Defect, reduction, upper limb
  - umbilical artery Q27.Ø
  - unilateral condylar M27.8
  - ureter Q62.8
  - uterus, congenital Q51.811
  - vagina Q52.4
  - vascular NEC peripheral Q27.8
    - brain Q28.3
    - digestive system Q27.8
    - lower limb Q27.8
    - specified site NEC Q27.8
    - upper limb Q27.8
  - vein(s) (peripheral) Q27.8
    - brain Q28.3
    - digestive system Q27.8
    - great Q26.8
    - lower limb Q27.8
    - specified site NEC Q27.8
    - upper limb Q27.8
  - vena cava (inferior) (superior) Q26.8
  - vertebra Q76.49
  - vulva, congenital Q52.79
  - zonule (ciliary) Q12.8
- **Hypoplasminogenemia** E88.Ø2
- **Hypopnea, obstructive sleep apnea** G47.33
- **Hypopotassemia** E87.6

- **Hypoproconvertinemia, congenital** (hereditary) D68.2
- **Hypoproteinemia** E77.8
- **Hypoprothrombinemia** (congenital) (hereditary) (idiopathic) D68.2
  - acquired D68.4
  - newborn, transient P61.6
- **Hypoptyalism** K11.7
- **Hypopyon** (eye) (anterior chamber) — *see* Iridocyclitis, acute, hypopyon
- **Hypopyrexia** R68.Ø
- **Hyporeflexia** R29.2
- **Hyposecretion**
  - ACTH E23.Ø
  - antidiuretic hormone E23.2
  - ovary E28.39
  - salivary gland (any) K11.7
  - vasopressin E23.2
- **Hyposegmentation, leukocytic, hereditary** D72.Ø
- **Hyposiderinemia** D5Ø.9
- **Hypospadias** Q54.9
  - balanic Q54.Ø
  - coronal Q54.Ø
  - glandular Q54.Ø
  - penile Q54.1
  - penoscrotal Q54.2
  - perineal Q54.3
  - specified NEC Q54.8
- **Hypospermatogenesis** — *see* Oligospermia
- **Hyposplenism** D73.Ø
- **Hypostasis pulmonary, passive** — *see* Edema, lung
- **Hypostatic** — *see* condition
- **Hyposthenuria** N28.89
- **Hypotension** (arterial) (constitutional) I95.9
  - chronic I95.89
  - due to (of) hemodialysis I95.3
  - drug-induced I95.2
  - iatrogenic I95.89
  - idiopathic (permanent) I95.Ø
  - intracranial G96.81Ø
    - following
      - lumbar cerebrospinal fluid shunting G97.83
      - specified procedure NEC G97.84
      - ventricular shunting (ventriculostomy) G97.2
    - specified NEC G96.819
    - spontaneous G96.811
  - intra-dialytic I95.3
  - maternal, syndrome (following labor and delivery) O26.5- ☑
  - neurogenic, orthostatic G9Ø.3
  - orthostatic (chronic) I95.1
    - due to drugs I95.2
    - neurogenic G9Ø.3
  - postoperative I95.81
  - postural I95.1
  - specified NEC I95.89
- **Hypothermia** (accidental) T68 ☑
  - due to anesthesia, anesthetic T88.51 ☑
  - low environmental temperature T68 ☑
  - neonatal P8Ø.9
    - environmental (mild) NEC P8Ø.8
    - mild P8Ø.8
    - severe (chronic) (cold injury syndrome) P8Ø.Ø
    - specified NEC P8Ø.8
  - not associated with low environmental temperature R68.Ø
- **Hypothyroidism** (acquired) EØ3.9
  - autoimmune — *see* Thyroiditis, autoimmune
  - congenital (without goiter) EØ3.1
    - with goiter (diffuse) EØ3.Ø
  - due to
    - exogenous substance NEC EØ3.2
    - iodine-deficiency, acquired EØ1.8
      - subclinical EØ2
    - irradiation therapy E89.Ø
    - medicament NEC EØ3.2
    - P-aminosalicylic acid (PAS) EØ3.2
    - phenylbutazone EØ3.2
    - resorcinol EØ3.2
    - sulfonamide EØ3.2
    - surgery E89.Ø
    - thiourea group drugs EØ3.2
  - iatrogenic NEC EØ3.2
  - iodine-deficiency (acquired) EØ1.8
    - congenital — *see* Syndrome, iodine- deficiency, congenital
    - subclinical EØ2
  - neonatal, transitory P72.2
  - postinfectious EØ3.3
- **Hypothyroidism** — *continued*
  - postirradiation E89.Ø
  - postprocedural E89.Ø
  - postsurgical E89.Ø
  - specified NEC EØ3.8
  - subclinical, iodine-deficiency related EØ2
- **Hypotonia, hypotonicity, hypotony**
  - bladder N31.2
  - congenital (benign) P94.2
  - eye — *see* Disorder, globe, hypotony
- **Hypotrichosis** — *see* Alopecia
- **Hypotropia** H5Ø.2- ☑
- **Hypoventilation** RØ6.89
  - congenital central alveolar G47.35
  - sleep related
    - idiopathic nonobstructive alveolar G47.34
    - in conditions classified elsewhere G47.36
- **Hypovitaminosis** — *see* Deficiency, vitamin
- **Hypovolemia** E86.1
  - surgical shock T81.19 ☑
  - traumatic (shock) T79.4 ☑
- **Hypoxemia** RØ9.Ø2
  - newborn P84
  - sleep related, in conditions classified elsewhere G47.36
- **Hypoxia** — *see also* Anoxia RØ9.Ø2
  - cerebral, during a procedure NEC G97.81
    - postprocedural NEC G97.82
  - intrauterine P84
  - myocardial — *see* Insufficiency, coronary
  - newborn P84
  - sleep-related G47.34
- **Hypsarhythmia** — *see* Epilepsy, generalized, specified NEC
- **Hysteralgia, pregnant uterus** O26.89- ☑
- **Hysteria, hysterical** (conversion) (dissociative state) F44.9
  - anxiety F41.8
  - convulsions F44.5
  - psychosis, acute F44.9
- **Hysteroepilepsy** F44.5

I

- **IBDU** (colonic inflammatory bowel dissease unclassified) K52.3
- **ICANS** (immune effector cell-associated neurotoxicity syndrome) — *see* Syndrome, immune effector cell-associated neurotoxicity
- **Ichthyoparasitism due to Vandellia cirrhosa** B88.8
- **Ichthyosis** (congenital) Q8Ø.9
  - acquired L85.Ø
  - fetalis Q8Ø.4
  - hystrix Q8Ø.8
  - lamellar Q8Ø.2
  - lingual K13.29
  - palmaris and plantaris Q82.8
  - simplex Q8Ø.Ø
  - vera Q8Ø.8
  - vulgaris Q8Ø.Ø
  - X-linked Q8Ø.1
- **Ichthyotoxism** — *see* Poisoning, fish
  - bacterial — *see* Intoxication, foodborne
- **Icteroanemia, hemolytic** (acquired) D59.9
  - congenital — *see* Spherocytosis
- **Icterus** — *see also* Jaundice
  - conjunctiva R17
  - gravis, newborn P55.Ø
  - hematogenous (acquired) D59.9
  - hemolytic (acquired) D59.9
    - congenital — *see* Spherocytosis
  - hemorrhagic (acute) (leptospiral) (spirochetal) A27.Ø
    - newborn P53
  - infectious B15.9
    - with hepatic coma B15.Ø
    - leptospiral A27.Ø
    - spirochetal A27.Ø
  - neonatorum — *see* Jaundice, newborn
  - newborn P59.9
  - spirochetal A27.Ø
- **Ictus solaris, solis** T67.Ø1 ☑
- **Id reaction** (due to bacteria) L3Ø.2
- **Ideation**
  - homicidal R45.85Ø
  - suicidal R45.851
- **Identity disorder** (child) F64.9
  - gender role F64.2
  - psychosexual F64.2
- **Idioglossia** F8Ø.Ø
- **Idiopathic** — *see* condition
- **Idiot, idiocy** (congenital) F73
  - amaurotic (Bielschowsky(-Jansky)) (family) (infantile (late)) (juvenile (late)) (Vogt-Spielmeyer) E75.4
  - microcephalic QØ2
- **IgE asthma** J45.9Ø9
- **IIAC** (idiopathic infantile arterial calcification) Q28.8
- **Ileitis** (chronic) (noninfectious) — *see also* Enteritis K52.9
  - backwash — *see* Pancolitis, ulcerative (chronic)
  - infectious AØ9
  - regional (ulcerative) — *see* Enteritis, regional, small intestine
  - segmental — *see* Enteritis, regional
  - terminal (ulcerative) — *see* Enteritis, regional, small intestine
- **Ileocolitis** — *see also* Enteritis K52.9
  - infectious AØ9
  - regional — *see* Enteritis, regional
  - ulcerative K51.Ø- ☑
- **Ileostomy**
  - attention to Z43.2
  - malfunctioning K94.13
  - status Z93.2
    - with complication — *see* Complications, enterostomy
- **Ileotyphus** — *see* Typhoid
- **Ileum** — *see* condition
- **Ileus** (bowel) (colon) (inhibitory) (intestine) K56.7
  - adynamic K56.Ø
  - due to gallstone (in intestine) K56.3
  - duodenal (chronic) K31.5
  - gallstone K56.3
  - mechanical NEC — *see also* Obstruction, intestine, specified NEC K56.699
  - meconium P76.Ø
    - in cystic fibrosis E84.11
    - meaning meconium plug (without cystic fibrosis) P76.Ø
  - myxedema K59.89
  - neurogenic K56.Ø
    - Hirschsprung's disease or megacolon Q43.1
  - newborn
    - due to meconium P76.Ø
      - in cystic fibrosis E84.11
      - meaning meconium plug (without cystic fibrosis) P76.Ø
    - transitory P76.1
  - obstructive — *see also* Obstruction, intestine, specified NEC K56.699
  - paralytic K56.Ø
  - postoperative K91.89
- **Iliac** — *see* condition
- **Iliotibial band syndrome** M76.3- ☑
- **Illiteracy** Z55.Ø
  - health Z55.6
- **Illness** — *see also* Disease R69
  - manic-depressive — *see* Disorder, bipolar
- **Imbalance** R26.89
  - autonomic G9Ø.8
  - constituents of food intake E63.1
  - electrolyte E87.8
    - with
      - abortion — *see* Abortion by type, complicated by, electrolyte imbalance
      - molar pregnancy OØ8.5
    - due to hyperemesis gravidarum O21.1
    - following ectopic or molar pregnancy OØ8.5
    - neonatal, transitory NEC P74.49
      - potassium
        - hyperkalemia P74.31
        - hypokalemia P74.32
      - sodium
        - hypernatremia P74.21
        - hyponatremia P74.22
  - endocrine E34.9
  - eye muscle NOS H5Ø.9
  - hormone E34.9
  - hysterical F44.4
  - labyrinth — *see* subcategory H83.2 ☑
  - posture R29.3
  - protein-energy — *see* Malnutrition
  - sympathetic G9Ø.8
- **Imbecile, imbecility** (I.Q. 35-49) F71
- **Imbedding, intrauterine device** T83.39 ☑
- **Imbibition, cholesterol** (gallbladder) K82.4
- **Imbrication, teeth,, fully erupted** M26.3Ø
- **Imerslund** (-Gräsbeck) **syndrome** D51.1

- **Immature** — *see also* Immaturity
  - birth (less than 37 completed weeks) — *see* Preterm, newborn
    - extremely (less than 28 completed weeks) — *see* Immaturity, extreme
  - personality F6Ø.89
- **Immaturity** (less than 37 completed weeks) — *see also* Preterm, newborn
  - extreme of newborn (less than 28 completed weeks of gestation) (less than 196 completed days of gestation) (unspecified weeks of gestation) PØ7.2Ø
    - gestational age
      - 23 completed weeks (23 weeks, Ø days through 23 weeks, 6 days) PØ7.22
      - 24 completed weeks (24 weeks, Ø days through 24 weeks, 6 days) PØ7.23
      - 25 completed weeks (25 weeks, Ø days through 25 weeks, 6 days) PØ7.24
      - 26 completed weeks (26 weeks, Ø days through 26 weeks, 6 days) PØ7.25
      - 27 completed weeks (27 weeks, Ø days through 27 weeks, 6 days) PØ7.26
      - less than 23 completed weeks PØ7.21
  - fetus or infant light-for-dates — *see* Light-for-dates
  - lung, newborn P28.Ø
  - organ or site NEC — *see* Hypoplasia
  - pulmonary, newborn P28.Ø
  - reaction F6Ø.89
  - sexual (female) (male), after puberty E3Ø.Ø
- **Immersion** T75.1 ☑
  - foot T69.Ø2- ☑
  - hand T69.Ø1- ☑
- **Immobile, immobility**
  - complete, due to severe physical disability or frailty R53.2
  - intestine K59.89
  - syndrome (paraplegic) M62.3
- **Immune reconstitution** (inflammatory) syndrome [IRIS] D89.3
- **Immunization** — *see also* Vaccination
  - ABO — *see* Incompatibility, ABO
    - in newborn P55.1
  - appropriate for age
    - child (over 28 days old) ZØØ.129
      - with abnormal findings ZØØ.121
  - complication — *see* Complications, vaccination
  - encounter for Z23
  - not done (not carried out) — *see also* Underimmunization status Z28.9
    - because (of)
      - acute illness of patient Z28.Ø1
      - allergy to vaccine (or component) Z28.Ø4
      - caregiver refusal Z28.82
      - chronic illness of patient Z28.Ø2
      - contraindication NEC Z28.Ø9
      - delay in delivery of vaccine Z28.83
      - group pressure Z28.1
      - guardian refusal Z28.82
      - immune compromised state of patient Z28.Ø3
      - lack of availability of vaccine Z28.83
      - manufacturer delay of vaccine Z28.83
      - parent refusal Z28.82
      - patient had disease being vaccinated against Z28.81
      - patient refusal Z28.21
      - patient's belief Z28.1
      - religious beliefs of patient Z28.1
      - specified reason NEC Z28.89
        - of patient Z28.29
      - unavailability of vaccine Z28.83
      - unspecified patient reason Z28.2Ø
  - partial — *see also* Underimmunization status
    - for COVID-19 Z28.311
  - Rh factor
    - affecting management of pregnancy NEC O36.Ø9- ☑
      - anti-D antibody O36.Ø1- ☑
    - from transfusion — *see* Complication(s), transfusion, incompatibility reaction, Rh (factor)
- **Immunocompromised NOS** D84.9
- **Immunocytoma** C83.Ø- ☑
- **Immunodeficiency** D84.9
  - with
    - adenosine-deaminase deficiency — *see also* Deficiency, adenosine deaminase D81.3Ø
    - antibody defects D8Ø.9
      - specified type NEC D8Ø.8
    - hyperimmunoglobulinemia D8Ø.6

- **Immunodeficiency** — *continued*
  - with — *continued*
    - increased immunoglobulin M (IgM) D8Ø.5
    - major defect D82.9
      - specified type NEC D82.8
    - partial albinism D82.8
    - short-limbed stature D82.2
    - thrombocytopenia and eczema D82.Ø
  - antibody with
    - hyperimmunoglobulinemia D8Ø.6
    - near-normal immunoglobulins D8Ø.6
  - autosomal recessive, Swiss type D8Ø.Ø
  - combined D81.9
    - biotin-dependent carboxylase D81.819
      - biotinidase D81.81Ø
      - holocarboxylase synthetase D81.818
      - specified type NEC D81.818
    - severe (SCID) D81.9
      - with
        - low or normal B-cell numbers D81.2
        - low T- and B-cell numbers D81.1
        - reticular dysgenesis D81.Ø
    - specified type NEC D81.89
  - common variable D83.9
    - with
      - abnormalities of B-cell numbers and function D83.Ø
      - autoantibodies to B- or T-cells D83.2
      - immunoregulatory T-cell disorders D83.1
    - specified type NEC D83.8
  - due to
    - conditions classified elsewhere D84.81
    - drugs D84.821
    - external causes D84.822
    - medication (current or past) D84.821
  - following hereditary defective response to Epstein-Barr virus (EBV) D82.3
  - selective, immunoglobulin
    - A (IgA) D8Ø.2
    - G (IgG) (subclasses) D8Ø.3
    - M (IgM) D8Ø.4
  - severe combined (SCID) D81.9
    - due to adenosine deaminase deficiency D81.31
  - specified type NEC D84.89
  - X-linked, with increased IgM D8Ø.5
- **Immunodeficient NOS** D84.9
- **Immunosuppressed NOS** D84.9
- **Immunotherapy** (encounter for)
  - antineoplastic Z51.12
- **Impaction, impacted**
  - bowel, colon, rectum — *see also* Impaction, fecal K56.49
    - by gallstone K56.3
  - calculus — *see* Calculus
  - cerumen (ear) (external) H61.2- ☑
  - cuspid — *see* Impaction, tooth
  - dental (same or adjacent tooth) KØ1.1
  - fecal, feces K56.41
  - fracture — *see* Fracture, by site
  - gallbladder — *see* Calculus, gallbladder
  - gallstone(s) — *see* Calculus, gallbladder
    - bile duct (common) (hepatic) — *see* Calculus, bile duct
    - cystic duct — *see* Calculus, gallbladder
    - in intestine, with obstruction (any part) K56.3
  - intestine (calculous) NEC — *see also* Impaction, fecal K56.49
    - gallstone, with ileus K56.3
  - intrauterine device (IUD) T83.39 ☑
  - molar — *see* Impaction, tooth
  - shoulder, causing obstructed labor O66.Ø
  - tooth, teeth KØ1.1
  - turbinate J34.89
- **Impaired, impairment** (function)
  - auditory discrimination — *see* Abnormal, auditory perception
  - cognitive, mild, of uncertain or unknown etiology G31.84
  - dual sensory Z73.82
  - fasting glucose R73.Ø1
  - glucose tolerance (oral) R73.Ø2
  - hearing — *see* Deafness
  - heart — *see* Disease, heart
  - kidney N28.9
    - disorder resulting from N25.9
      - specified NEC N25.89
  - liver K72.9Ø
    - with coma K72.91

- **Impaired, impairment** — *continued*
  - mastication KØ8.89
  - mild cognitive G31.84
    - of uncertain or unknown etiology G31.84
  - mild neurocognitive
    - due to known physiological condition (without behavioral disturbance) FØ6.7Ø
      - with behavioral disturbance FØ6.71
  - mobility
    - ear ossicles — *see* Ankylosis, ear ossicles
    - requiring care provider Z74.Ø9
  - myocardium, myocardial — *see* Insufficiency, myocardial
  - rectal sphincter R19.8
  - renal (acute) (chronic) N28.9
    - disorder resulting from N25.9
      - specified NEC N25.89
  - vision NEC H54.7
    - both eyes H54.3
- **Impediment, speech** — *see also* Disorder, speech R47.9
  - psychogenic (childhood) F98.8
  - slurring R47.81
  - specified NEC R47.89
- **Impending**
  - coronary syndrome I2Ø.Ø
  - delirium tremens F1Ø.239
  - myocardial infarction I2Ø.Ø
- **Imperception auditory** (acquired) — *see also* Deafness
  - congenital H93.25
- **Imperfect**
  - aeration, lung (newborn) NEC — *see* Atelectasis
  - closure (congenital)
    - alimentary tract NEC Q45.8
      - lower Q43.8
      - upper Q4Ø.8
    - atrioventricular ostium Q21.2Ø
    - atrium (secundum) Q21.11
    - branchial cleft NOS Q18.2
      - cyst Q18.Ø
      - fistula Q18.Ø
      - sinus Q18.Ø
    - choroid Q14.3
    - cricoid cartilage Q31.8
    - cusps, heart valve NEC Q24.8
      - pulmonary Q22.3
    - ductus
      - arteriosus Q25.Ø
      - Botalli Q25.Ø
    - ear drum (causing impairment of hearing) Q16.4
    - esophagus with communication to bronchus or trachea Q39.1
    - eyelid Q1Ø.3
    - foramen
      - botalli Q21.12
      - ovale Q21.12
    - genitalia, genital organ(s) or system
      - female Q52.8
        - external Q52.79
        - internal NEC Q52.8
      - male Q55.8
    - glottis Q31.8
    - interatrial ostium or septum Q21.19
    - interauricular ostium or septum Q21.19
    - interventricular ostium or septum Q21.Ø
    - larynx Q31.8
    - lip — *see* Cleft, lip
    - nasal septum Q3Ø.3
    - nose Q3Ø.2
    - omphalomesenteric duct Q43.Ø
    - optic nerve entry Q14.2
    - organ or site not listed — *see* Anomaly, by site
    - ostium
      - interatrial Q21.19
      - interauricular Q21.19
      - interventricular Q21.Ø
    - palate — *see* Cleft, palate
    - preauricular sinus Q18.1
    - retina Q14.1
    - roof of orbit Q75.8
    - sclera Q13.5
    - septum
      - aorticopulmonary Q21.4
      - atrial (secundum) Q21.19
      - between aorta and pulmonary artery Q21.4
      - heart Q21.9
      - interatrial (secundum) Q21.19
      - interauricular (secundum) Q21.19
      - interventricular Q21.Ø

- **Imperfect** — *continued*
  - closure — *continued*
    - septum — *continued*
      - interventricular — *continued*
        - in tetralogy of Fallot Q21.3
      - nasal Q3Ø.3
      - ventricular Q21.Ø
        - with pulmonary stenosis or atresia, dextraposition of aorta, and hypertrophy of right ventricle Q21.3
        - in tetralogy of Fallot Q21.3
    - skull Q75.ØØ9
      - with
        - anencephaly QØØ.Ø
        - encephalocele — *see* Encephalocele
        - hydrocephalus QØ3.9
          - with spina bifida — *see* Spina bifida, by site, with hydrocephalus
        - microcephaly QØ2
    - spine (with meningocele) — *see* Spina bifida
    - trachea Q32.1
    - tympanic membrane (causing impairment of hearing) Q16.4
    - uterus Q51.818
    - vitelline duct Q43.Ø
  - erection — *see* Dysfunction, sexual, male, erectile
  - fusion — *see* Imperfect, closure
  - inflation, lung (newborn) — *see* Atelectasis
  - posture R29.3
  - rotation, intestine Q43.3
  - septum, ventricular Q21.Ø
- **Imperfectly descended testis** — *see* Cryptorchid
- **Imperforate** (congenital) — *see also* Atresia
  - anus Q42.3
    - with fistula Q42.2
  - cervix (uteri) Q51.828
  - esophagus Q39.Ø
    - with tracheoesophageal fistula Q39.1
  - hymen Q52.3
  - jejunum Q41.1
  - pharynx Q38.8
  - rectum Q42.1
    - with fistula Q42.Ø
  - urethra Q64.39
  - vagina Q52.4
- **Impervious** (congenital) — *see also* Atresia
  - anus Q42.3
    - with fistula Q42.2
  - bile duct Q44.2
  - esophagus Q39.Ø
    - with tracheoesophageal fistula Q39.1
  - intestine (small) Q41.9
    - large Q42.9
      - specified NEC Q42.8
  - rectum Q42.1
    - with fistula Q42.Ø
  - ureter — *see* Atresia, ureter
  - urethra Q64.39
- **Impetiginization of dermatoses** LØ1.1
- **Impetigo** (any organism) (any site) (circinate) (contagiosa) (simplex) (vulgaris) LØ1.ØØ
  - Bockhart's LØ1.Ø2
  - bullous, bullosa LØ1.Ø3
  - external ear LØ1.ØØ *[H62.4Ø]*
  - follicularis LØ1.Ø2
  - furfuracea L3Ø.5
  - herpetiformis L4Ø.1
    - nonobstetrical L4Ø.1
  - neonatorum LØ1.Ø3
  - nonbullous LØ1.Ø1
  - specified type NEC LØ1.Ø9
  - ulcerative LØ1.Ø9
- **Impingement** (on teeth)
  - joint — *see* Disorder, joint, specified type NEC
  - soft tissue
    - anterior M26.81
    - posterior M26.82
- **Implant, endometrial** N8Ø.9
- **Implantation**
  - anomalous — *see* Anomaly, by site
    - ureter Q62.63
  - cyst
    - external area or site (skin) NEC L72.Ø
    - iris — *see* Cyst, iris, implantation
    - vagina N89.8
    - vulva N9Ø.7
  - dermoid (cyst) — *see* Implantation, cyst
- **Impotence** (sexual) N52.9
- **Impotence** — *continued*
  - counseling Z7Ø.1
  - organic origin — *see also* Dysfunction, sexual, male, erectile N52.9
  - psychogenic F52.21
- **Impression, basilar** Q75.8
- **Imprisonment, anxiety concerning** Z65.1
- **Improper care** (child) (newborn) — *see* Maltreatment
- **Improperly tied umbilical cord** (causing hemorrhage) P51.8
- **Impulsiveness** (impulsive) R45.87
- **Inability to**
  - comply with dietary regimen Z91.118
  - swallow — *see* Aphagia
- **Inaccessible, inaccessibility**
  - health care NEC Z75.3
    - due to
      - waiting period Z75.2
        - for admission to facility elsewhere Z75.1
  - other helping agencies Z75.4
  - transportation Z59.82
- **Inactive** — *see* condition
- **Inadequate, inadequacy**
  - aesthetics of dental restoration KØ8.56
  - biologic, constitutional, functional, or social F6Ø.7
  - development
    - child R62.5Ø
    - genitalia
      - after puberty NEC E3Ø.Ø
      - congenital
        - female Q52.8
          - external Q52.79
          - internal Q52.8
        - male Q55.8
    - lungs Q33.6
      - associated with short gestation P28.Ø
    - organ or site not listed — *see* Anomaly, by site
  - diet (causing nutritional deficiency) E63.9
  - drinking-water supply Z58.6
  - eating habits Z72.4
  - environment, household Z59.11
  - family support Z63.8
  - food (supply) NEC Z59.48
    - hunger effects T73.Ø ☑
  - functional F6Ø.7
  - household care, due to
    - family member
      - handicapped or ill Z74.2
      - on vacation Z75.5
      - temporarily away from home Z74.2
    - technical defects in home Z59.19
    - temporary absence from home of person rendering care Z74.2
  - housing Z59.1Ø
    - environmental temperature Z59.11
    - heating Z59.11
    - space Z59.19
    - specified NEC Z59.19
    - utilities Z59.12
  - income (financial) Z59.6
  - intrafamilial communication Z63.8
  - material resources due to limited financial resources, specified NEC Z59.87
  - mental — *see* Disability, intellectual
  - parental supervision or control of child Z62.Ø
  - personality F6Ø.7
  - pulmonary
    - function RØ6.89
      - newborn P28.5
    - ventilation, newborn P28.5
  - sample of cytologic smear
    - anus R85.615
    - cervix R87.615
    - vagina R87.625
  - social F6Ø.7
    - insurance Z59.7
    - skills NEC Z73.4
    - social support Z6Ø.8
  - supervision of child by parent Z62.Ø
  - teaching affecting education Z55.8
  - transportation Z59.82
  - welfare support Z59.7
- **Inanition** R64
  - with edema — *see* Malnutrition, severe
  - due to
    - deprivation of food T73.Ø ☑
    - malnutrition — *see* Malnutrition
  - fever R5Ø.9
- **Inappropriate**
  - change in quantitative human chorionic gonadotropin (hCG) in early pregnancy OØ2.81
  - diet or eating habits Z72.4
  - level of quantitative human chorionic gonadotropin (hCG) for gestational age in early pregnancy OØ2.81
  - secretion
    - antidiuretic hormone (ADH) (excessive) E22.2
      - deficiency E23.2
    - pituitary (posterior) E22.2
  - sinus tachycardia, so stated (IST) I47.11
- **Inattention at or after birth** — *see* Neglect
- **Incarceration, incarcerated**
  - enterocele K46.Ø
    - gangrenous K46.1
  - epiplocele K46.Ø
    - gangrenous K46.1
  - exomphalos K42.Ø
    - gangrenous K42.1
  - hernia — *see also* Hernia, by site, with obstruction
    - with gangrene — *see* Hernia, by site, with gangrene
  - iris, in wound — *see* Injury, eye, laceration, with prolapse
  - lens, in wound — *see* Injury, eye, laceration, with prolapse
  - omphalocele K42.Ø
  - prison, anxiety concerning Z65.1
  - rupture — *see* Hernia, by site
  - sarcoepiplocele K46.Ø
    - gangrenous K46.1
  - sarcoepiplomphalocele K42.Ø
    - with gangrene K42.1
  - uterus N85.8
    - gravid O34.51- ☑
      - causing obstructed labor O65.5
- **Incised wound**
  - external — *see* Laceration
  - internal organs — *see* Injury, by site
- **Incision, incisional**
  - hernia K43.2
    - with
      - gangrene (and obstruction) K43.1
      - obstruction K43.Ø
  - surgical, complication — *see* Complications, surgical procedure
  - traumatic
    - external — *see* Laceration
    - internal organs — *see* Injury, by site
- **Inclusion**
  - azurophilic leukocytic D72.Ø
  - blennorrhea (neonatal) (newborn) P39.1
  - gallbladder in liver (congenital) Q44.1
- **Incompatibility**
  - ABO
    - affecting management of pregnancy O36.11- ☑
      - anti-A sensitization O36.11- ☑
      - anti-B sensitization O36.19- ☑
      - specified NEC O36.19- ☑
    - infusion or transfusion reaction — *see* Complication(s), transfusion, incompatibility reaction, ABO
    - newborn P55.1
  - blood (group) (Duffy) (K) (Kell) (Kidd) (Lewis) (M) (S) NEC
    - affecting management of pregnancy O36.11- ☑
      - anti-A sensitization O36.11- ☑
      - anti-B sensitization O36.19- ☑
    - infusion or transfusion reaction T8Ø.89 ☑
    - newborn P55.8
  - divorce or estrangement Z63.5
  - Rh (blood group) (factor) Z31.82
    - affecting management of pregnancy NEC O36.Ø9- ☑
      - anti-D antibody O36.Ø1- ☑
    - infusion or transfusion reaction — *see* Complication(s), transfusion, incompatibility reaction, Rh (factor)
    - newborn P55.Ø
  - rhesus — *see* Incompatibility, Rh
- **Incompetency, incompetent, incompetence**
  - annular
    - aortic (valve) — *see* Insufficiency, aortic
    - mitral (valve) I34.Ø
    - pulmonary valve (heart) I37.1
  - aortic (valve) — *see* Insufficiency, aortic
  - cardiac valve — *see* Endocarditis
  - cervix, cervical (os) N88.3
    - in pregnancy O34.3- ☑

- **Incompetency, incompetent, incompetence** — *continued*
  - chronotropic I45.89
    - with
      - autonomic dysfunction G9Ø.8
      - ischemic heart disease I25.89
      - left ventricular dysfunction I51.89
      - sinus node dysfunction I49.8
  - esophagogastric (junction) (sphincter) K22.Ø
  - mitral (valve) — *see* Insufficiency, mitral
  - pelvic fundus N81.89
  - pubocervical tissue N81.82
  - pulmonary valve (heart) I37.1
    - congenital Q22.3
  - rectovaginal tissue N81.83
  - tricuspid (annular) (valve) — *see* Insufficiency, tricuspid
  - valvular — *see* Endocarditis
    - congenital Q24.8
  - vein, venous (saphenous) (varicose) — *see* Varix, leg
- **Incomplete** — *see also* condition
  - atrioventricular
    - canal Q21.21
    - septal defect Q21.21
  - bladder, emptying R33.9
  - defecation R15.Ø
  - endocardial cushion defect Q21.21
  - expansion lungs (newborn) NEC — *see* Atelectasis
  - rotation, intestine Q43.3
- **Inconclusive**
  - diagnostic imaging due to excess body fat of patient R93.9
  - findings on diagnostic imaging of breast NEC R92.8
    - mammogram R92.2
- **Incontinence** R32
  - anal sphincter R15.9
  - coital N39.491
  - feces R15.9
    - nonorganic origin F98.1
  - insensible (urinary) N39.42
  - overflow N39.49Ø
  - postural (urinary) N39.492
  - psychogenic F45.8
  - rectal R15.9
  - reflex N39.498
  - stress (female) (male) N39.3
    - and urge N39.46
  - urethral sphincter R32
  - urge N39.41
    - and stress (female) (male) N39.46
  - urine (urinary) R32
    - continuous N39.45
    - due to cognitive impairment, or severe physical disability or immobility R39.81
    - functional R39.81
    - insensible N39.42
    - mixed (stress and urge) N39.46
    - nocturnal N39.44
    - nonorganic origin F98.Ø
    - overflow N39.49Ø
    - post dribbling N39.43
    - postural N39.492
    - reflex N39.498
    - specified NEC N39.498
    - stress (female) (male) N39.3
      - and urge N39.46
    - total N39.498
    - unaware N39.42
    - urge N39.41
      - and stress (female) (male) N39.46
- **Incontinentia pigmenti** Q82.3
- **Incoordinate, incoordination**
  - esophageal-pharyngeal (newborn) — *see* Dysphagia
  - muscular R27.8
  - uterus (action) (contractions) (complicating delivery) O62.4
- **Increase, increased**
  - abnormal, in development R63.8
  - androgens (ovarian) E28.1
  - anticoagulants (antithrombin) (anti-VIIIa) (anti-IXa) (anti-Xa) (anti-XIa) — *see* Circulating anticoagulants
  - cold sense R2Ø.8
  - estrogen E28.Ø
  - function
    - adrenal
      - cortex — *see* Cushing's, syndrome
      - medulla E27.5
    - pituitary (gland) (anterior) (lobe) E22.9
- **Increase, increased** — *continued*
  - function — *continued*
    - pituitary — *continued*
      - posterior E22.2
  - heat sense R2Ø.8
  - intracranial pressure (benign) G93.2
  - permeability, capillaries I78.8
  - pressure, intracranial G93.2
  - secretion
    - gastrin E16.4
    - glucagon E16.3
    - pancreas, endocrine E16.9
      - growth hormone-releasing hormone E16.8
      - pancreatic polypeptide E16.8
      - somatostatin E16.8
      - vasoactive-intestinal polypeptide E16.8
  - sphericity, lens Q12.4
  - splenic activity D73.1
  - venous pressure I87.8
    - portal K76.6
- **Increta placenta** O43.22- ☑
- **Incrustation, cornea, foreign body** (lead)(zinc) — *see* Foreign body, cornea
- **Incyclophoria** H5Ø.54
- **Incyclotropia** — *see* Cyclotropia
- **Indeterminate sex** Q56.4
- **India rubber skin** Q82.8
- **Indigestion** (acid) (bilious) (functional) K3Ø
  - catarrhal K31.89
  - due to decomposed food NOS AØ5.9
  - nervous F45.8
  - psychogenic F45.8
- **Indirect** — *see* condition
- **Induratio penis plastica** N48.6
- **Induration, indurated**
  - brain G93.89
  - breast (fibrous) N64.51
    - puerperal, postpartum O92.29
  - broad ligament N83.8
  - chancre
    - anus A51.1
    - congenital A5Ø.Ø7
    - extragenital NEC A51.2
  - corpora cavernosa (penis) (plastic) N48.6
  - liver (chronic) K76.89
  - lung (black) (chronic) (fibroid) — *see also* Fibrosis, lung J84.1Ø
    - essential brown J84.Ø3
  - penile (plastic) N48.6
  - phlebitic — *see* Phlebitis
  - skin R23.4
- **Inebriety** (without dependence) — *see* Alcohol, intoxication
- **Inefficiency, kidney** N28.9
- **Inelasticity, skin** R23.4
- **Inequality, leg** (length) (acquired) — *see also* Deformity, limb, unequal length
  - congenital — *see* Defect, reduction, lower limb
  - lower leg — *see* Deformity, limb, unequal length
- **Inertia**
  - bladder (neurogenic) N31.2
  - stomach K31.89
    - psychogenic F45.8
  - uterus, uterine during labor O62.2
    - during latent phase of labor O62.Ø
    - primary O62.Ø
    - secondary O62.1
  - vesical (neurogenic) N31.2
- **Infancy, infantile, infantilism** — *see also* condition
  - celiac K9Ø.Ø
  - genitalia, genitals (after puberty) E3Ø.Ø
  - Herter's (nontropical sprue) K9Ø.Ø
  - intestinal K9Ø.Ø
  - Lorain E23.Ø
  - pancreatic K86.89
  - pelvis M95.5
    - with disproportion (fetopelvic) O33.1
      - causing obstructed labor O65.1
  - pituitary E23.Ø
  - renal N25.Ø
  - uterus — *see* Infantile, genitalia
- **Infant**(s) — *see also* Infancy
  - excessive crying R68.11
  - irritable child R68.12
  - lack of care — *see* Neglect
  - liveborn (singleton) Z38.2
    - born in hospital Z38.ØØ
      - by cesarean Z38.Ø1
- **Infant(s)** — *continued*
  - liveborn — *continued*
    - born outside hospital Z38.1
    - multiple NEC Z38.8
      - born in hospital Z38.68
        - by cesarean Z38.69
      - born outside hospital Z38.7
    - quadruplet Z38.8
      - born in hospital Z38.63
        - by cesarean Z38.64
      - born outside hospital Z38.7
    - quintuplet Z38.8
      - born in hospital Z38.65
        - by cesarean Z38.66
      - born outside hospital Z38.7
    - triplet Z38.8
      - born in hospital Z38.61
        - by cesarean Z38.62
      - born outside hospital Z38.7
    - twin Z38.5
      - born in hospital Z38.3Ø
        - by cesarean Z38.31
      - born outside hospital Z38.4
  - of diabetic mother (syndrome of) P7Ø.1
    - gestational diabetes P7Ø.Ø
- **Infantile** — *see also* condition
  - genitalia, genitals E3Ø.Ø
  - os, uterine E3Ø.Ø
  - penis E3Ø.Ø
  - testis E29.1
  - uterus E3Ø.Ø
- **Infantilism** — *see* Infancy
- **Infarct, infarction**
  - adrenal (capsule) (gland) E27.49
  - appendices epiploicae — *see also* Infarct, intestine K55.Ø69
  - bowel — *see also* Infarct, intestine K55.Ø69
  - brain (stem) — *see* Infarct, cerebral
  - breast N64.89
  - brewer's (kidney) N28.Ø
  - cardiac — *see* Infarct, myocardium
  - cerebellar — *see* Infarct, cerebral
  - cerebral (acute) — *see also* Occlusion, artery cerebral or precerebral, with infarction I63.9-
    - aborted I63.9
    - chronic (imaging) (old) (remote) (without sequelae) Z86.73
      - with residual defects — *see* Sequelae, disease, cerebrovascular
    - cortical I63.9
    - due to
      - cerebral venous thrombosis, nonpyogenic I63.6
      - embolism
        - cerebral arteries I63.4- ☑
        - precerebral arteries I63.1- ☑
      - occlusion NEC
        - cerebral arteries I63.5- ☑
        - precerebral arteries I63.2- ☑
        - small artery I63.81
      - stenosis NEC
        - cerebral arteries I63.5- ☑
        - precerebral arteries I63.2- ☑
        - small artery I63.81
      - thrombosis
        - cerebral artery I63.3- ☑
        - precerebral artery I63.Ø- ☑
    - intraoperative
      - during cardiac surgery I97.81Ø
      - during other surgery I97.811
    - neonatal P91.82- ☑
    - perinatal (arterial ischemic) P91.82- ☑
    - postprocedural
      - following cardiac surgery I97.82Ø
      - following other surgery I97.821
    - specified NEC I63.89
  - colon (acute) (agnogenic) (embolic) (hemorrhagic) (nonocclusive) (nonthrombotic) (occlusive) (segmental) (thrombotic) (with gangrene) — *see also* Infarct, intestine K55.Ø49
  - coronary artery — *see* Infarct, myocardium
  - embolic — *see* Embolism
  - fallopian tube N83.8
  - gallbladder K82.8
  - heart — *see* Infarct, myocardium
  - hepatic K76.3
  - hypophysis (anterior lobe) E23.6
  - impending (myocardium) I2Ø.Ø

Infection, infected, infective — *continued*
- due to or resulting from — *continued*
  - device, implant or graft — *see also* Complications, by site and type, infection or inflammation — *continued*
    - electronic — *continued*
      - urinary (indwelling) T83.51 ☑
    - fixation, internal (orthopedic) NEC — *see* Complication, fixation device, infection
    - gastrointestinal (bile duct) (esophagus) T85.79 ☑
      - neurostimulator electrode (lead) T85.732 ☑
    - genital NEC T83.69 ☑
    - heart NEC T82.7 ☑
      - valve (prosthesis) T82.6 ☑
        - graft T82.7 ☑
    - joint prosthesis — *see* Complication, joint prosthesis, infection
    - ocular (corneal graft) (orbital implant) NEC T85.79 ☑
    - orthopedic NEC T84.7 ☑
    - penile (cylinder) (pump) (resevoir) T83.61 ☑
    - specified NEC T85.79 ☑
    - testicular T83.62 ☑
    - urinary NEC T83.598 ☑
      - ileal conduit stent T83.593 ☑
      - implanted neurostimulation T83.59Ø ☑
      - implanted sphincter T83.591 ☑
      - indwelling ureteral stent T83.592 ☑
      - nephroureteral stent T83.593 ☑
      - specified stent NEC T83.593 ☑
    - vascular NEC T82.7 ☑
    - ventricular intracranial (communicating) shunt T85.73Ø ☑
  - Hickman catheter T8Ø.219 ☑
    - bloodstream T8Ø.211 ☑
    - localized T8Ø.212 ☑
    - specified NEC T8Ø.218 ☑
  - immunization or vaccination T88.Ø ☑
  - infusion, injection or transfusion NEC T8Ø.29 ☑
  - injury NEC — *code by* site under Wound, open
  - peripherally inserted central catheter (PICC) T8Ø.219 ☑
    - bloodstream T8Ø.211 ☑
    - localized T8Ø.212 ☑
    - specified NEC T8Ø.218 ☑
  - portacath (port-a-cath) T8Ø.219 ☑
    - bloodstream T8Ø.211 ☑
    - localized T8Ø.212 ☑
    - specified NEC T8Ø.218 ☑
  - protozoa of the order Piroplasmida NEC B6Ø.Ø9
  - pulmonary artery catheter — *see* Infection, due to or resulting from, central venous catheter
  - surgery T81.4Ø ☑
  - Swan Ganz catheter — *see* Infection, due to or resulting from, central venous catheter
  - triple lumen catheter T8Ø.219 ☑
    - bloodstream T8Ø.211 ☑
    - localized T8Ø.212 ☑
    - specified NEC T8Ø.218 ☑
  - umbilical venous catheter T8Ø.219 ☑
    - bloodstream T8Ø.211 ☑
    - localized T8Ø.212 ☑
    - specified NEC T8Ø.218 ☑
- during labor NEC O75.3
- ear (middle) — *see also* Otitis media
  - external — *see* Otitis, externa, infective
  - inner — *see* subcategory H83.Ø ☑
- Eberthella typhosa AØ1.ØØ
- Echinococcus — *see* Echinococcus
- echovirus
  - as cause of disease classified elsewhere B97.12
  - unspecified nature or site B34.1
- endocardium I33.Ø
- endocervix — *see* Cervicitis
- Entamoeba — *see* Amebiasis
- enteric — *see* Enteritis, infectious
- Enterobacter sakazakii B96.89
- Enterobius vermicularis B8Ø
- enterostomy K94.12
- enterovirus B34.1
  - as cause of disease classified elsewhere B97.1Ø
    - coxsackievirus B97.11
    - echovirus B97.12
    - specified NEC B97.19
- Entomophthora B46.8
- Epidermophyton — *see* Dermatophytosis

Infection, infected, infective — *continued*
- epididymis — *see* Epididymitis
- episiotomy (puerperal) O86.Ø9
- Erysipelothrix (insidiosa) (rhusiopathiae) — *see* Erysipeloid
- erythema infectiosum BØ8.3
- Escherichia (E.) coli NEC A49.8
  - as cause of disease classified elsewhere — *see also* Escherichia coli B96.2Ø
  - congenital P39.8
    - sepsis P36.4
  - generalized A41.51
  - intestinal — *see* Enteritis, infectious, due to, Escherichia coli
- ethmoidal (chronic) (sinus) — *see* Sinusitis, ethmoidal
- eustachian tube (ear) — *see* Salpingitis, eustachian
- external auditory canal (meatus) NEC — *see* Otitis, externa, infective
- eye (purulent) — *see* Endophthalmitis, purulent
- eyelid — *see* Inflammation, eyelid
- fallopian tube — *see* Salpingo-oophoritis
- Fasciola (gigantica) (hepatica) (indica) B66.3
- Fasciolopsis (buski) B66.5
- filarial — *see* Infestation, filarial
- finger (skin) LØ8.9
  - nail LØ3.Ø1- ☑
    - fungus B35.1
- fish tapeworm B7Ø.Ø
  - larval B7Ø.1
- flagellate, intestinal AØ7.9
- fluke — *see* Infestation, fluke
- focal
  - teeth (pulpal origin) KØ4.7
  - tonsils J35.Ø1
- Fonsecaea (compactum) (pedrosoi) B43.Ø
- food — *see* Intoxication, foodborne
- foot (skin) LØ8.9
  - dermatophytic fungus B35.3
- Francisella tularensis — *see* Tularemia
- frontal (sinus) (chronic) — *see* Sinusitis, frontal
- fungus NOS B49
  - beard B35.Ø
  - dermatophytic — *see* Dermatophytosis
  - foot B35.3
  - groin B35.6
  - hand B35.2
  - nail B35.1
  - pathogenic to compromised host only B48.8
  - perianal (area) B35.6
  - scalp B35.Ø
  - skin B36.9
    - foot B35.3
    - hand B35.2
    - toenails B35.1
- Fusarium B48.8
- gallbladder — *see* Cholecystitis
- gas bacillus — *see* Gangrene, gas
- gastrointestinal — *see* Enteritis, infectious
- generalized NEC — *see* Sepsis
- generator pocket, implanted electronic neurostimulator T85.734 ☑
- genital organ or tract
  - female — *see* Disease, pelvis, inflammatory
  - male N49.9
    - multiple sites N49.8
    - specified NEC N49.8
- Ghon tubercle, primary A15.7
- Giardia lamblia AØ7.1
- gingiva (chronic) KØ5.1Ø
  - acute KØ5.ØØ
    - nonplaque induced KØ5.Ø1
    - plaque induced KØ5.ØØ
  - nonplaque induced KØ5.11
  - plaque induced KØ5.1Ø
- glanders A24.Ø
- glenosporopsis B48.Ø
- Gnathostoma (spinigerum) B83.1
- Gongylonema B83.8
- gonococcal — *see* Gonococcus
- gram-negative bacilli NOS A49.9
- guinea worm B72
- gum (chronic) KØ5.1Ø
  - acute KØ5.ØØ
    - nonplaque induced KØ5.Ø1
    - plaque induced KØ5.ØØ
  - nonplaque induced KØ5.11
  - plaque induced KØ5.1Ø
- Haemophilus — *see* Infection, Hemophilus

Infection, infected, infective — *continued*
- heart — *see* Carditis
- Helicobacter pylori AØ4.8
  - as cause of disease classified elsewhere B96.81
- helminths B83.9
  - intestinal B82.Ø
    - mixed (types classifiable to more than one of the titles B65.Ø-B81.3 and B81.8) B81.4
    - specified type NEC B81.8
  - specified type NEC B83.8
- Hemophilus
  - aegyptius, systemic A48.4
  - ducrey (any location) A57
  - generalized A41.3
  - influenzae NEC A49.2
    - as cause of disease classified elsewhere B96.3
- herpes (simplex) — *see also* Herpes
  - congenital P35.2
  - disseminated BØØ.7
  - zoster BØ2.9
- herpesvirus, herpesviral — *see* Herpes
- Heterophyes (heterophyes) B66.8
- hip (joint) NEC MØØ.9
  - due to internal joint prosthesis
    - left T84.52 ☑
    - right T84.51 ☑
  - skin NEC LØ8.9
- Histoplasma — *see* Histoplasmosis
  - American B39.4
  - capsulatum B39.4
- hookworm B76.9
- human
  - papilloma virus A63.Ø
  - T-cell lymphotropic virus type-1 (HTLV-1) B33.3
- hydrocele N43.Ø
- Hymenolepis B71.Ø
- hypopharynx — *see* Pharyngitis
- inguinal (lymph) glands LØ4.1
  - due to soft chancre A57
- intervertebral disc, pyogenic M46.3Ø
  - cervical region M46.32
  - cervicothoracic region M46.33
  - lumbar region M46.36
  - lumbosacral region M46.37
  - multiple sites M46.39
  - occipito-atlanto-axial region M46.31
  - sacrococcygeal region M46.38
  - thoracic region M46.34
  - thoracolumbar region M46.35
- intestine, intestinal — *see* Enteritis, infectious
  - specified NEC AØ8.8
- intra-amniotic affecting newborn NEC P39.2
- intrauterine inflammation O41.12- ☑
- Isospora belli or hominis AØ7.3
- Japanese B encephalitis A83.Ø
- jaw (bone) (lower) (upper) M27.2
- joint NEC MØØ.9
  - due to internal joint prosthesis T84.5Ø ☑
- kidney (cortex) (hematogenous) N15.9
  - with calculus N2Ø.Ø
    - with hydronephrosis N13.6
  - following ectopic gestation OØ8.83
  - pelvis and ureter (cystic) N28.85
  - puerperal (postpartum) O86.21
  - specified NEC N15.8
- Klebsiella (K.) pneumoniae NEC A49.8
  - as cause of disease classified elsewhere B96.1
- knee (joint) NEC MØØ.9
  - joint MØØ.9
  - due to internal joint prosthesis
    - left T84.54 ☑
    - right T84.53 ☑
  - skin LØ8.9
- Koch's — *see* Tuberculosis
- labia (majora) (minora) (acute) — *see* Vulvitis
- lacrimal
  - gland — *see* Dacryoadenitis
  - passages (duct) (sac) — *see* Inflammation, lacrimal, passages
- lancet fluke B66.2
- larynx NEC J38.7
- leg (skin) NOS LØ8.9
- Legionella pneumophila A48.1
  - nonpneumonic A48.2
- Leishmania — *see also* Leishmaniasis
  - aethiopica B55.1
  - braziliensis B55.2
  - chagasi B55.Ø

Infection, infected, infective — *continued*
- respiratory — *continued*
  - upper (acute) NOS JØ6.9
    - chronic J39.8
    - streptococcal JØ6.9
    - viral NOS JØ6.9
      - due to respiratory syncytial virus (RSV) JØ6.9 *[B97.4]*
- resulting from
  - presence of internal prosthesis, implant, graft — *see* Complications, by site and type, infection
- retortamoniasis AØ7.8
- retroperitoneal NEC K68.9
- retrovirus B33.3
  - as cause of disease classified elsewhere B97.3Ø
    - human
      - immunodeficiency, type 2 (HIV 2) B97.35
      - T-cell lymphotropic
        - type I (HTLV-I) B97.33
        - type II (HTLV-II) B97.34
    - lentivirus B97.31
    - oncovirus B97.32
    - specified NEC B97.39
- Rhinosporidium (seeberi) B48.1
- rhinovirus
  - as cause of disease classified elsewhere B97.89
  - unspecified nature or site B34.8
- Rhizopus — *see* Mucormycosis
- rickettsial NOS A79.9
- roundworm (large) NEC B82.Ø
  - Ascariasis — *see also* Ascariasis B77.9
- rubella — *see* Rubella
- Saccharomyces — *see* Candidiasis
- salivary duct or gland (any) — *see* Sialoadenitis
- Salmonella (aertrycke) (arizonae) (callinarum) (choleraesuis) (enteritidis) (suipestifer) (typhimurium) AØ2.9
  - with
    - (gastro)enteritis AØ2.Ø
    - sepsis AØ2.1
    - specified manifestation NEC AØ2.8
  - due to food (poisoning) AØ2.9
  - hirschfeldii AØ1.3
  - localized AØ2.2Ø
    - arthritis AØ2.23
    - meningitis AØ2.21
    - osteomyelitis AØ2.24
    - pneumonia AØ2.22
    - pyelonephritis AØ2.25
    - specified NEC AØ2.29
  - paratyphi AØ1.4
    - A AØ1.1
    - B AØ1.2
    - C AØ1.3
  - schottmuelleri AØ1.2
  - typhi, typhosa — *see* Typhoid
- Sarcocystis AØ7.8
- SARS-CoV-2 — *see* Infection, COVID-19
- scabies B86
- Schistosoma — *see* Infestation, Schistosoma
- scrotum (acute) NEC N49.2
- seminal vesicle — *see* Vesiculitis
- septic
  - localized, skin — *see* Abscess
- Serratia NEC A49.8
  - as cause of disease classified elsewhere B96.89
  - generalized A41.53
- sheep liver fluke B66.3
- Shigella AØ3.9
  - boydii AØ3.2
  - dysenteriae AØ3.Ø
  - flexneri AØ3.1
  - group
    - A AØ3.Ø
    - B AØ3.1
    - C AØ3.2
    - D AØ3.3
  - Schmitz (-Stutzer) AØ3.Ø
  - schmitzii AØ3.Ø
  - shigae AØ3.Ø
  - sonnei AØ3.3
  - specified NEC AØ3.8
- shoulder (joint) NEC MØØ.9
  - due to internal joint prosthesis T84.59 ☑
  - skin NEC LØ8.9
- sinus (accessory) (chronic) (nasal) — *see also* Sinusitis
  - pilonidal — *see* Sinus, pilonidal
  - skin NEC LØ8.89

Infection, infected, infective — *continued*
- Skene's duct or gland — *see* Urethritis
- skin (local) (staphylococcal) (streptococcal) LØ8.9
  - abscess — *code by* site under Abscess
  - cellulitis — *code by* site under Cellulitis
  - due to fungus B36.9
    - specified type NEC B36.8
  - mycotic B36.9
    - specified type NEC B36.8
  - newborn P39.4
  - ulcer — *see* Ulcer, skin
- slow virus A81.9
  - specified NEC A81.89
- Sparganum (mansoni) (proliferum) (baxteri) B7Ø.1
- specific — *see also* Syphilis
  - to perinatal period — *see* Infection, congenital
- specified NEC B99.8
- spermatic cord NEC N49.1
- sphenoidal (sinus) — *see* Sinusitis, sphenoidal
- spinal cord NOS — *see also* Myelitis GØ4.91
  - abscess GØ6.1
  - meninges — *see* Meningitis
  - streptococcal GØ4.89
- Spirillum A25.Ø
- spirochetal NOS A69.9
  - lung A69.8
  - specified NEC A69.8
- Spirometra larvae B7Ø.1
- spleen D73.89
- Sporotrichum, Sporothrix (schenckii) — *see* Sporotrichosis
- staphylococcal, unspecified site
  - as cause of disease classified elsewhere B95.8
    - aureus (methicillin susceptible) (MSSA) B95.61
      - methicillin resistant (MRSA) B95.62
    - specified NEC B95.7
  - aureus (methicillin susceptible) (MSSA) A49.Ø1
    - methicillin resistant (MRSA) A49.Ø2
  - food poisoning AØ5.Ø
  - generalized (purulent) A41.2
  - pneumonia — *see* Pneumonia, staphylococcal
- Stellantchasmus falcatus B66.8
- streptobacillus moniliformis A25.1
- streptococcal NEC A49.1
  - as cause of disease classified elsewhere B95.5
  - B genitourinary complicating
    - childbirth O98.82
    - pregnancy O98.81- ☑
    - puerperium O98.83
  - congenital
    - sepsis P36.1Ø
      - group B P36.Ø
      - specified NEC P36.19
  - generalized (purulent) A4Ø.9
- Streptomyces B47.1
- Strongyloides (stercoralis) — *see* Strongyloidiasis
- stump (amputation) (surgical) — *see* Complication, amputation stump, infection
- subcutaneous tissue, local LØ8.9
- suipestifer — *see* Infection, salmonella
- swimming pool bacillus A31.1
- Taenia — *see* Infestation, Taenia
- Taeniarhynchus saginatus B68.1
- tapeworm — *see* Infestation, tapeworm
- tendon (sheath) — *see* Tenosynovitis, infective NEC
- Ternidens diminutus B81.8
- testis — *see* Orchitis
- threadworm B8Ø
- throat — *see* Pharyngitis
- thyroglossal duct K14.8
- toe (skin) LØ8.9
  - cellulitis LØ3.Ø3- ☑
    - fungus B35.1
  - nail LØ3.Ø3- ☑
    - fungus B35.1
- tongue NEC K14.Ø
  - parasitic B37.Ø
- tonsil (and adenoid) (faucial) (lingual) (pharyngeal) — *see* Tonsillitis
- tooth, teeth KØ4.7
  - periapical KØ4.7
  - peridental, periodontal KØ5.2Ø
    - generalized — *see* Periodontitis, aggressive, generalized
    - localized — *see* Periodontitis, aggressive, localized
  - pulp KØ4.Ø1
    - irreversible KØ4.Ø2

Infection, infected, infective — *continued*
- tooth, teeth — *continued*
  - pulp — *continued*
    - reversible KØ4.Ø1
  - socket M27.3
- TORCH — *see* Infection, congenital
  - without active infection PØØ.2
- Torula histolytica — *see* Cryptococcosis
- Toxocara (canis) (cati) (felis) B83.Ø
- Toxoplasma gondii — *see* Toxoplasma
- trachea, chronic J42
- trematode NEC — *see* Infestation, fluke
- trench fever A79.Ø
- Treponema pallidum — *see* Syphilis
- Trichinella (spiralis) B75
- Trichomonas A59.9
  - cervix A59.Ø9
  - intestine AØ7.8
  - prostate A59.Ø2
  - specified site NEC A59.8
  - urethra A59.Ø3
  - urogenitalis A59.ØØ
  - vagina A59.Ø1
  - vulva A59.Ø1
- Trichophyton, trichophytic — *see* Dermatophytosis
- Trichosporon (beigelii) cutaneum B36.2
- Trichostrongylus B81.2
- Trichuris (trichiura) B79
- Trombicula (irritans) B88.Ø
- Trypanosoma
  - brucei
    - gambiense B56.Ø
    - rhodesiense B56.1
  - cruzi — *see* Chagas' disease
- tubal — *see* Salpingo-oophoritis
- tuberculous
  - latent (LTBI) Z22.7
  - NEC — *see* Tuberculosis
- tubo-ovarian — *see* Salpingo-oophoritis
- tunica vaginalis N49.1
- tunnel T8Ø.212 ☑
- tympanic membrane NEC — *see* Myringitis
- typhoid (abortive) (ambulant) (bacillus) — *see* Typhoid
- typhus A75.9
  - flea-borne A75.2
  - mite-borne A75.3
  - recrudescent A75.1
  - tick-borne A77.9
    - African A77.1
    - North Asian A77.2
- umbilicus LØ8.82
- ureter — *see* Ureteritis
- urethra — *see* Urethritis
- urinary (tract) N39.Ø
  - bladder — *see* Cystitis
  - complicating
    - pregnancy O23.4- ☑
      - specified type NEC O23.3- ☑
  - kidney — *see* Infection, kidney
  - newborn P39.3
  - puerperal (postpartum) O86.2Ø
  - tuberculous A18.13
  - urethra — *see* Urethritis
- uterus, uterine — *see* Endometritis
- vaccination T88.Ø ☑
- vaccinia not from vaccination BØ8.Ø11
- vagina (acute) — *see* Vaginitis
- varicella BØ1.9
- varicose veins — *see* Varix
- vas deferens NEC N49.1
- vesical — *see* Cystitis
- Vibrio
  - cholerae AØØ.Ø
    - El Tor AØØ.1
  - parahaemolyticus (food poisoning) AØ5.3
  - vulnificus
    - as cause of disease classified elsewhere B96.82
    - foodborne intoxication AØ5.5
- Vincent's (gum) (mouth) (tonsil) A69.1
- virus, viral NOS B34.9
  - adenovirus
    - as cause of disease classified elsewhere B97.Ø
    - unspecified nature or site B34.Ø
  - arborvirus, arbovirus arthropod-borne A94
  - as cause of disease classified elsewhere B97.89
    - adenovirus B97.Ø
    - coronavirus B97.29
      - SARS-associated B97.21

Infection, infected, infective — Infection, infected, infective

- **Infestation** — *continued*
  - helminth — *continued*
    - gnathostomiasis B83.1
    - hirudiniasis, internal B83.4
    - intestinal B82.Ø
      - angiostrongyliasis B81.3
      - anisakiasis B81.Ø
      - ascariasis — *see* Ascariasis
      - capillariasis B81.1
      - cysticercosis — *see* Cysticercosis
      - diphyllobothriasis — *see* Infestation, diphyllobothriasis
      - dracunculiasis B72
      - echinococcus — *see* Echinococcosis
      - enterobiasis B8Ø
      - filariasis — *see* Infestation, filarial
      - fluke — *see* Infestation, fluke
      - hookworm — *see* Infestation, hookworm
      - mixed (types classifiable to more than one of the titles B65.Ø-B81.3 and B81.8) B81.4
      - onchocerciasis — *see* Onchocerciasis
      - schistosomiasis — *see* Infestation, schistosoma
      - specified
        - cestode NEC — *see* Infestation, cestode
        - type NEC B81.8
      - strongyloidiasis — *see* Strongyloidiasis
      - taenia — *see* Infestation, taenia
      - trichinellosis B75
      - trichostrongyliasis B81.2
      - trichuriasis B79
    - specified type NEC B83.8
    - syngamiasis B83.3
    - visceral larva migrans B83.Ø
  - Heterophyes (heterophyes) B66.8
  - hookworm B76.9
    - ancylostomiasis B76.Ø
    - necatoriasis B76.1
    - specified type NEC B76.8
  - Hymenolepis (diminuta) (nana) B71.Ø
  - intestinal NEC B82.9
  - leeches (aquatic) (land) — *see* Hirudiniasis
  - Leishmania — *see* Leishmaniasis
  - lice, louse — *see* Infestation, Pediculus
  - Linguatula B88.8
  - Liponyssoides sanguineus B88.Ø
  - Loa loa B74.3
    - conjunctival B74.3
    - eyelid B74.3
  - louse — *see* Infestation, Pediculus
  - maggots — *see* Myiasis
  - Mansonella (ozzardi) (perstans) (streptocerca) B74.4
  - Medina (worm) B72
  - Metagonimus (yokogawai) B66.8
  - microfilaria streptocerca — *see* Onchocerciasis
    - eye B73.ØØ
    - eyelid B73.Ø9
  - mites B88.9
    - scabic B86
  - Monilia (albicans) — *see* Candidiasis
  - mouth B37.Ø
  - Necator americanus B76.1
  - nematode NEC (intestinal) B82.Ø
    - Ancylostoma B76.Ø
    - conjunctiva NEC B83.9
    - Enterobius vermicularis B8Ø
    - Gnathostoma spinigerum B83.1
    - physaloptera B8Ø
    - specified NEC B81.8
    - trichostrongylus B81.2
    - trichuris (trichuria) B79
  - Oesophagostomum (apiostomum) B81.8
  - Oestrus ovis — *see also* Myiasis B87.9
  - Onchocerca (volvulus) — *see* Onchocerciasis
  - Opisthorchis (felineus) (viverrini) B66.Ø
  - orbit, parasitic NOS B89
  - Oxyuris vermicularis B8Ø
  - Paragonimus (westermani) B66.4
  - parasite, parasitic B89
    - eyelid B89
    - intestinal NOS B82.9
    - mouth B37.Ø
    - skin B88.9
    - tongue B37.Ø
  - Parastrongylus
    - cantonensis B83.2
    - costaricensis B81.3
  - Pediculus B85.2
    - body B85.1
    - capitis (humanus) (any site) B85.Ø
    - corporis (humanus) (any site) B85.1
    - head B85.Ø
    - mixed (classifiable to more than one of the titles B85.Ø - B85.3) B85.4
    - pubis (any site) B85.3
  - Pentastoma B88.8
  - pest Z59.19
  - Phthirus (pubis) (any site) B85.3
    - with any infestation classifiable to B85.Ø - B85.2 B85.4
  - pinworm B8Ø
  - pork tapeworm (adult) B68.Ø
  - protozoal NEC B64
    - intestinal AØ7.9
      - specified NEC AØ7.8
    - specified NEC B6Ø.8
  - pubic, louse B85.3
  - rat tapeworm B71.Ø
  - red bug B88.Ø
  - roundworm (large) NEC B82.Ø
    - Ascariasis — *see also* Ascariasis B77.9
  - sandflea B88.1
  - Sarcoptes scabiei B86
  - scabies B86
  - Schistosoma B65.9
    - bovis B65.8
    - cercariae B65.3
    - haematobium B65.Ø
    - intercalatum B65.8
    - japonicum B65.2
    - mansoni B65.1
    - mattheei B65.8
    - mekongi B65.8
    - specified type NEC B65.8
    - spindale B65.8
  - screw worms — *see* Myiasis
  - skin NOS B88.9
  - Sparganum (mansoni) (proliferum) (baxteri) B7Ø.1
    - larval B7Ø.1
  - specified type NEC B88.8
  - Spirometra larvae B7Ø.1
  - Stellantchasmus falcatus B66.8
  - Strongyloides stercoralis — *see* Strongyloidiasis
  - Taenia B68.9
    - diminuta B71.Ø
    - echinococcus — *see* Echinococcus
    - mediocanellata B68.1
    - nana B71.Ø
    - saginata B68.1
    - solium (intestinal form) B68.Ø
      - larval form — *see* Cysticercosis
  - Taeniarhynchus saginatus B68.1
  - tapeworm B71.9
    - beef B68.1
    - broad B7Ø.Ø
      - larval B7Ø.1
    - dog B67.4
    - dwarf B71.Ø
    - fish B7Ø.Ø
      - larval B7Ø.1
    - pork B68.Ø
    - rat B71.Ø
  - Ternidens diminutus B81.8
  - Tetranychus molestissimus B88.Ø
  - threadworm B8Ø
  - tongue B37.Ø
  - Toxocara (canis) (cati) (felis) B83.Ø
  - trematode(s) NEC — *see* Infestation, fluke
  - Trichinella (spiralis) B75
  - Trichocephalus B79
  - Trichomonas — *see* Trichomoniasis
  - Trichostrongylus B81.2
  - Trichuris (trichiura) B79
  - Trombicula (irritans) B88.Ø
  - Tunga penetrans B88.1
  - Uncinaria americana B76.1
  - Vandellia cirrhosa B88.8
  - whipworm B79
  - worms B83.9
    - intestinal B82.Ø
  - Wuchereria (bancrofti) B74.Ø
- **Infiltrate, infiltration**
  - amyloid (generalized) (localized) — *see* Amyloidosis
  - calcareous NEC R89.7
    - localized — *see* Degeneration, by site
  - calcium salt R89.7
  - cardiac
    - fatty — *see* Degeneration, myocardial
    - glycogenic E74.Ø2 *[I43]*
  - corneal — *see* Edema, cornea
  - eyelid — *see* Inflammation, eyelid
  - glycogen, glycogenic — *see* Disease, glycogen storage
  - heart, cardiac
    - fatty — *see* Degeneration, myocardial
    - glycogenic E74.Ø2 *[I43]*
  - inflammatory in vitreous H43.89
  - kidney N28.89
  - leukemic — *see* Leukemia
  - liver K76.89
    - fatty — *see* Fatty, liver NEC
    - glycogen — *see also* Disease, glycogen storage E74.Ø3 *[K77]*
  - lung R91.8
    - eosinophilic — *see* Eosinophilia, pulmonary
  - lymphatic — *see also* Leukemia, lymphatic C91.9- ☑
    - gland I88.9
  - muscle, fatty M62.89
  - myocardium, myocardial
    - fatty — *see* Degeneration, myocardial
    - glycogenic E74.Ø2 *[I43]*
  - on chest x-ray R91.8
  - pulmonary R91.8
    - with eosinophilia — *see* Eosinophilia, pulmonary
  - skin (lymphocytic) L98.6
  - thymus (gland) (fatty) E32.8
  - urine R39.Ø
  - vesicant agent
    - antineoplastic chemotherapy T8Ø.81Ø ☑
    - other agent NEC T8Ø.818 ☑
  - vitreous body H43.89
- **Infirmity** R68.89
  - senile R54
- **Inflammation, inflamed, inflammatory** (with exudation)
  - abducent (nerve) — *see* Strabismus, paralytic, sixth nerve
  - accessory sinus (chronic) — *see* Sinusitis
  - adrenal (gland) E27.8
  - alveoli, teeth M27.3
    - scorbutic E54
  - anal canal, anus K62.89
  - antrum (chronic) — *see* Sinusitis, maxillary
  - appendix — *see* Appendicitis
  - arachnoid — *see* Meningitis
  - areola N61.Ø
    - puerperal, postpartum or gestational — *see* Infection, nipple
  - areolar tissue NOS LØ8.9
  - artery — *see* Arteritis
  - auditory meatus (external) — *see* Otitis, externa
  - Bartholin's gland N75.8
  - bile duct (common) (hepatic) or passage — *see* Cholangitis
  - bladder — *see* Cystitis
  - bone — *see* Osteomyelitis
  - brain — *see also* Encephalitis
    - membrane — *see* Meningitis
  - breast N61.Ø
    - puerperal, postpartum, gestational — *see* Mastitis, obstetric
  - broad ligament — *see* Disease, pelvis, inflammatory
  - bronchi — *see* Bronchitis
  - catarrhal JØØ
  - cecum — *see* Appendicitis
  - cerebral — *see also* Encephalitis
    - membrane — *see* Meningitis
  - cerebrospinal
    - meningococcal A39.Ø
  - cervix (uteri) — *see* Cervicitis
  - chest J98.8
  - chorioretinal H3Ø.9- ☑
    - cyclitis — *see* Cyclitis
    - disseminated H3Ø.1Ø- ☑
      - generalized H3Ø.13- ☑
      - peripheral H3Ø.12- ☑
      - posterior pole H3Ø.11- ☑
    - epitheliopathy — *see* Epitheliopathy
    - focal H3Ø.ØØ- ☑
      - juxtapapillary H3Ø.Ø1- ☑
      - macular H3Ø.Ø4- ☑

- **Inflammation, inflamed, inflammatory** — *continued*
  - chorioretinal — *continued*
    - focal — *continued*
      - paramacular — *see* Inflammation, chorioretinal, focal, macular
      - peripheral H3Ø.Ø3- ☑
      - posterior pole H3Ø.Ø2- ☑
    - specified type NEC H3Ø.89- ☑
  - choroid — *see* Inflammation, chorioretinal
  - chronic, postmastoidectomy cavity — *see* Complications, postmastoidectomy, inflammation
  - colon — *see* Enteritis
  - connective tissue (diffuse) NEC — *see* Disorder, soft tissue, specified type NEC
  - cornea — *see* Keratitis
  - corpora cavernosa N48.29
  - cranial nerve — *see* Disorder, nerve, cranial
  - Douglas' cul-de-sac or pouch (chronic) N73.Ø
  - due to device, implant or graft — *see also* Complications, by site and type, infection or inflammation
    - arterial graft T82.7 ☑
    - breast (implant) T85.79 ☑
    - catheter T85.79 ☑
      - dialysis (renal) T82.7 ☑
        - intraperitoneal T85.71 ☑
      - infusion T82.7 ☑
        - cranial T85.735 ☑
        - intrathecal T85.735 ☑
        - spinal (epidural) (subdural) T85.735 ☑
        - subarachnoid T85.735 ☑
      - urinary T83.518 ☑
        - cystostomy T83.51Ø ☑
        - Hopkins T83.518 ☑
        - ileostomy T83.518 ☑
        - nephrostomy T83.512 ☑
        - specified NEC T83.518 ☑
        - urethral indwelling T83.511 ☑
        - urostomy T83.518 ☑
    - electronic (electrode) (pulse generator) (stimulator)
      - bone T84.7 ☑
      - cardiac T82.7 ☑
      - nervous system T85.738 ☑
        - brain T85.731 ☑
        - cranial nerve T85.732 ☑
        - gastric nerve T85.732 ☑
        - neurostimulator generator T85.734 ☑
        - peripheral nerve T85.732 ☑
        - sacral nerve T85.732 ☑
        - spinal cord T85.733 ☑
        - vagal nerve T85.732 ☑
      - urinary T83.59Ø ☑
    - fixation, internal (orthopedic) NEC — *see* Complication, fixation device, infection
    - gastrointestinal (bile duct) (esophagus) T85.79 ☑
      - neurostimulator electrode (lead) T85.732 ☑
    - genital NEC T83.69 ☑
    - heart NEC T82.7 ☑
      - valve (prosthesis) T82.6 ☑
        - graft T82.7 ☑
    - joint prosthesis — *see* Complication, joint prosthesis, infection
    - ocular (corneal graft) (orbital implant) NEC T85.79 ☑
    - orthopedic NEC T84.7 ☑
    - penile (cylinder) (pump) (resevoir) T83.61 ☑
    - specified NEC T85.79 ☑
    - testicular T83.62 ☑
    - urinary NEC T83.598 ☑
      - ileal conduit stent T83.593 ☑
      - implanted neurostimulation T83.59Ø ☑
      - implanted sphincter T83.591 ☑
      - indwelling ureteral stent T83.592 ☑
      - nephroureteral stent T83.593 ☑
      - specified stent NEC T83.593 ☑
    - vascular NEC T82.7 ☑
    - ventricular intracranial (communicating) shunt T85.73Ø ☑
  - duodenum K29.8Ø
    - with bleeding K29.81
  - dura mater — *see* Meningitis
  - ear (middle) — *see also* Otitis, media
    - external — *see* Otitis, externa
    - inner — *see* subcategory H83.Ø ☑
  - epididymis — *see* Epididymitis
  - esophagus — *see* Esophagitis
  - ethmoidal (sinus) (chronic) — *see* Sinusitis, ethmoidal

- **Inflammation, inflamed, inflammatory** — *continued*
  - eustachian tube (catarrhal) — *see* Salpingitis, eustachian
  - eyelid HØ1.9
    - abscess — *see* Abscess, eyelid
    - blepharitis — *see* Blepharitis
    - chalazion — *see* Chalazion
    - dermatosis (noninfectious) — *see* Dermatosis, eyelid
    - hordeolum — *see* Hordeolum
    - specified NEC HØ1.8
  - fallopian tube — *see* Salpingo-oophoritis
  - fascia — *see* Myositis
  - follicular, pharynx J31.2
  - frontal (sinus) (chronic) — *see* Sinusitis, frontal
  - gallbladder — *see* Cholecystitis
  - gastric — *see* Gastritis
  - gastrointestinal — *see* Enteritis
  - genital organ (internal) (diffuse)
    - female — *see* Disease, pelvis, inflammatory
    - male N49.9
      - multiple sites N49.8
      - specified NEC N49.8
  - gland (lymph) — *see* Lymphadenitis
  - glottis — *see* Laryngitis
  - granular, pharynx J31.2
  - gum KØ5.1Ø
    - nonplaque induced KØ5.11
    - plaque induced KØ5.1Ø
  - heart — *see* Carditis
  - hepatic duct — *see* Cholangitis
  - ileoanal (internal) pouch K91.85Ø
  - ileum — *see also* Enteritis
    - regional or terminal — *see* Enteritis, regional
  - intestinal pouch K91.85Ø
  - intestine (any part) — *see* Enteritis
  - jaw (acute) (bone) (chronic) (lower) (suppurative) (upper) M27.2
  - joint NEC — *see* Arthritis
    - sacroiliac M46.1
  - kidney — *see* Nephritis
  - knee (joint) M13.169
    - tuberculous A18.Ø2
  - labium (majus) (minus) — *see* Vulvitis
  - lacrimal
    - gland — *see* Dacryoadenitis
    - passages (duct) (sac) — *see also* Dacryocystitis
      - canaliculitis — *see* Canaliculitis, lacrimal
  - larynx — *see* Laryngitis
  - leg NOS LØ8.9
  - lip K13.Ø
  - liver (capsule) — *see also* Hepatitis
    - chronic K73.9
    - suppurative K75.Ø
  - lung (acute) — *see also* Pneumonia
    - chronic J98.4
  - lymph gland or node — *see* Lymphadenitis
  - lymphatic vessel — *see* Lymphangitis
  - maxilla, maxillary M27.2
    - sinus (chronic) — *see* Sinusitis, maxillary
  - membranes of brain or spinal cord — *see* Meningitis
  - meninges — *see* Meningitis
  - mouth K12.1
  - muscle — *see* Myositis
  - myocardium — *see* Myocarditis
  - nasal sinus (chronic) — *see* Sinusitis
  - nasopharynx — *see* Nasopharyngitis
  - navel LØ8.82
  - nerve NEC — *see* Neuritis
  - nipple N61.Ø
    - puerperal, postpartum or gestational — *see* Infection, nipple
  - nose — *see* Rhinitis
  - oculomotor (nerve) — *see* Strabismus, paralytic, third nerve
  - optic nerve — *see* Neuritis, optic
  - orbit (chronic) HØ5.1Ø
    - acute HØ5.ØØ
      - abscess — *see* Abscess, orbit
      - cellulitis — *see* Cellulitis, orbit
      - osteomyelitis — *see* Osteomyelitis, orbit
      - periostitis — *see* Periostitis, orbital
      - tenonitis — *see* Tenonitis, eye
    - granuloma — *see* Granuloma, orbit
    - myositis — *see* Myositis, orbital
  - ovary — *see* Salpingo-oophoritis
  - oviduct — *see* Salpingo-oophoritis

- **Inflammation, inflamed, inflammatory** — *continued*
  - pancreas (acute) — *see* Pancreatitis
  - parametrium N73.Ø
  - parotid region LØ8.9
  - pelvis, female — *see* Disease, pelvis, inflammatory
  - penis (corpora cavernosa) N48.29
  - perianal K62.89
  - pericardium — *see* Pericarditis
  - perineum (female) (male) LØ8.9
  - perirectal K62.89
  - peritoneum — *see* Peritonitis
  - periuterine — *see* Disease, pelvis, inflammatory
  - perivesical — *see* Cystitis
  - petrous bone (acute) (chronic) — *see* Petrositis
  - pharynx (acute) — *see* Pharyngitis
  - pia mater — *see* Meningitis
  - pleura — *see* Pleurisy
  - polyp, colon — *see also* Polyp, colon, inflammatory K51.4Ø
  - prostate — *see also* Prostatitis
    - specified type NEC N41.8
  - rectosigmoid — *see* Rectosigmoiditis
  - rectum — *see also* Proctitis K62.89
  - respiratory, upper — *see also* Infection, respiratory, upper JØ6.9
    - acute, due to radiation J7Ø.Ø
    - chronic, due to external agent — *see* condition, respiratory, chronic, due to
    - due to
      - chemicals, gases, fumes or vapors (inhalation) J68.2
      - radiation J7Ø.1
  - retina — *see* Chorioretinitis
  - retrocecal — *see* Appendicitis
  - retroperitoneal — *see* Peritonitis
  - salivary duct or gland (any) (suppurative) — *see* Sialoadenitis
  - scorbutic, alveoli, teeth E54
  - scrotum N49.2
  - seminal vesicle — *see* Vesiculitis
  - sigmoid — *see* Enteritis
  - sinus — *see* Sinusitis
  - Skene's duct or gland — *see* Urethritis
  - skin LØ8.9
  - spermatic cord N49.1
  - sphenoidal (sinus) — *see* Sinusitis, sphenoidal
  - spinal
    - cord — *see* Encephalitis
    - membrane — *see* Meningitis
    - nerve — *see* Disorder, nerve
  - spine — *see* Spondylopathy, inflammatory
  - spleen (capsule) D73.89
  - stomach — *see* Gastritis
  - subcutaneous tissue LØ8.9
  - suprarenal (gland) E27.8
  - synovial — *see* Tenosynovitis
  - tendon (sheath) NEC — *see* Tenosynovitis
  - testis — *see* Orchitis
  - throat (acute) — *see* Pharyngitis
  - thymus (gland) E32.8
  - thyroid (gland) — *see* Thyroiditis
  - tongue K14.Ø
  - tonsil — *see* Tonsillitis
  - trachea — *see* Tracheitis
  - trochlear (nerve) — *see* Strabismus, paralytic, fourth nerve
  - tubal — *see* Salpingo-oophoritis
  - tuberculous NEC — *see* Tuberculosis
  - tubo-ovarian — *see* Salpingo-oophoritis
  - tunica vaginalis N49.1
  - tympanic membrane — *see* Tympanitis
  - umbilicus, umbilical LØ8.82
  - uterine ligament — *see* Disease, pelvis, inflammatory
  - uterus (catarrhal) — *see* Endometritis
  - uveal tract (anterior) NOS — *see also* Iridocyclitis
    - posterior — *see* Chorioretinitis
  - vagina — *see* Vaginitis
  - vas deferens N49.1
  - vein — *see also* Phlebitis
    - intracranial or intraspinal (septic) GØ8
    - thrombotic I8Ø.9
      - leg — *see* Phlebitis, leg
      - lower extremity — *see* Phlebitis, leg
  - vocal cord J38.3
  - vulva — *see* Vulvitis
  - Wharton's duct (suppurative) — *see* Sialoadenitis

Index

Inflation, lung, imperfect — Injury

- **Injury** — *continued*
  - intra-abdominal — *continued*
    - adrenal gland — *see* Injury, adrenal gland
    - bladder — *see* Injury, bladder
    - colon — *see* Injury, intestine, large
    - contusion S36.92 ☑
    - fallopian tube — *see* Injury, fallopian tube
    - gallbladder — *see* Injury, gallbladder
    - intestine — *see* Injury, intestine
    - kidney — *see* Injury, kidney
    - laceration S36.93 ☑
    - liver — *see* Injury, liver
    - ovary — *see* Injury, ovary
    - pancreas — *see* Injury, pancreas
    - pelvic NOS S37.90 ☑
    - peritoneum — *see* Injury, intra-abdominal, specified, site NEC
    - prostate — *see* Injury, prostate
    - rectum — *see* Injury, intestine, large, rectum
    - retroperitoneum — *see* Injury, intra-abdominal, specified, site NEC
    - seminal vesicle — *see* Injury, pelvis, organ, specified site NEC
    - small intestine — *see* Injury, intestine, small
    - specified
      - pelvic S37.90 ☑
        - specified
          - site NEC S37.899 ☑
            - specified type NEC S37.898 ☑
          - type NEC S37.99 ☑
      - site NEC S36.899 ☑
        - contusion S36.892 ☑
        - laceration S36.893 ☑
        - specified type NEC S36.898 ☑
      - type NEC S36.99 ☑
    - spleen — *see* Injury, spleen
    - stomach — *see* Injury, stomach
    - ureter — *see* Injury, ureter
    - urethra — *see* Injury, urethra
    - uterus — *see* Injury, uterus
    - vas deferens — *see* Injury, pelvis, organ, specified site NEC
  - intracranial (traumatic) — *see also* if applicable, Compression, brain, traumatic S06.9- ☑
    - cerebellar hemorrhage, traumatic — *see* Injury, intracranial, focal
    - cerebral edema, traumatic S06.1X- ☑
      - diffuse S06.1X- ☑
      - focal S06.1X- ☑
    - diffuse (axonal) S06.2X- ☑
    - epidural hemorrhage (traumatic) S06.4X- ☑
    - focal brain injury S06.30- ☑
      - contusion — *see* Contusion, cerebral
      - laceration — *see* Laceration, cerebral
    - intracerebral hemorrhage, traumatic S06.36- ☑
      - left side S06.35- ☑
      - right side S06.34- ☑
    - specified NEC S06.89- ☑
    - subarachnoid hemorrhage, traumatic S06.6X- ☑
    - subdural hemorrhage, traumatic S06.5X- ☑
  - intraocular — *see* Injury, eyeball, penetrating
  - intrathoracic S27.9 ☑
    - bronchus S27.409 ☑
      - bilateral S27.402 ☑
      - blast injury (primary) S27.419 ☑
        - bilateral S27.412 ☑
        - secondary — *see* Injury, intrathoracic, bronchus, specified type NEC
        - unilateral S27.411 ☑
      - contusion S27.429 ☑
        - bilateral S27.422 ☑
        - unilateral S27.421 ☑
      - laceration S27.439 ☑
        - bilateral S27.432 ☑
        - unilateral S27.431 ☑
      - specified type NEC S27.499 ☑
        - bilateral S27.492 ☑
        - unilateral S27.491 ☑
      - unilateral S27.401 ☑
    - diaphragm S27.809 ☑
      - contusion S27.802 ☑
      - laceration S27.803 ☑
      - specified type NEC S27.808 ☑
    - esophagus (thoracic) S27.819 ☑
      - contusion S27.812 ☑
      - laceration S27.813 ☑

- **Injury** — *continued*
  - intrathoracic — *continued*
    - esophagus — *continued*
      - specified type NEC S27.818 ☑
    - heart — *see* Injury, heart
    - hemopneumothorax S27.2 ☑
    - hemothorax S27.1 ☑
    - lung S27.309 ☑
      - aspiration J69.0
      - bilateral S27.302 ☑
      - blast injury (primary) S27.319 ☑
        - bilateral S27.312 ☑
        - secondary — *see* Injury, intrathoracic, lung, specified type NEC
        - unilateral S27.311 ☑
      - contusion S27.329 ☑
        - bilateral S27.322 ☑
        - unilateral S27.321 ☑
      - laceration S27.339 ☑
        - bilateral S27.332 ☑
        - unilateral S27.331 ☑
      - specified type NEC S27.399 ☑
        - bilateral S27.392 ☑
        - unilateral S27.391 ☑
      - unilateral S27.301 ☑
    - pleura S27.60 ☑
      - laceration S27.63 ☑
      - specified type NEC S27.69 ☑
    - pneumothorax S27.0 ☑
    - specified organ NEC S27.899 ☑
      - contusion S27.892 ☑
      - laceration S27.893 ☑
      - specified type NEC S27.898 ☑
    - thoracic duct — *see* Injury, intrathoracic, specified organ NEC
    - thymus gland — *see* Injury, intrathoracic, specified organ NEC
    - trachea, thoracic S27.50 ☑
      - blast (primary) S27.51 ☑
      - contusion S27.52 ☑
      - laceration S27.53 ☑
      - specified type NEC S27.59 ☑
  - iris — *see* Injury, eye, specified site NEC
    - penetrating — *see* Injury, eyeball, penetrating
  - jaw S09.93 ☑
  - jejunum — *see* Injury, intestine, small
  - joint NOS T14.8 ☑
    - old or residual — *see* Disorder, joint, specified type NEC
  - kidney S37.00- ☑
    - acute (nontraumatic) N17.9
    - contusion — *see* Contusion, kidney
    - laceration — *see* Laceration, kidney
    - specified NEC S37.09- ☑
  - knee S89.9- ☑
    - contusion — *see* Contusion, knee
    - dislocation — *see* Dislocation, knee
    - meniscus (lateral) (medial) — *see* Sprain, knee, specified site NEC
      - old injury or tear — *see* Derangement, knee, meniscus, due to old injury
    - open — *see* Wound, open, knee
    - specified NEC S89.8- ☑
    - sprain — *see* Sprain, knee
    - superficial — *see* Injury, superficial, knee
  - labium (majus) (minus) S39.94 ☑
  - labyrinth, ear S09.30- ☑
  - lacrimal apparatus, duct, gland, or sac — *see* Injury, eye, specified site NEC
  - larynx NEC S19.81 ☑
  - leg (lower) S89.9- ☑
    - blood vessel — *see* Injury, blood vessel, leg
    - contusion — *see* Contusion, leg
    - fracture — *see* Fracture, leg
    - muscle — *see* Injury, muscle, leg
    - nerve — *see* Injury, nerve, leg
    - open — *see* Wound, open, leg
    - specified NEC S89.8- ☑
    - superficial — *see* Injury, superficial, leg
  - lens, eye — *see* Injury, eye, specified site NEC
    - penetrating — *see* Injury, eyeball, penetrating
  - limb NEC T14.8 ☑
  - lip S09.93 ☑
  - liver S36.119 ☑
    - contusion S36.112 ☑
    - laceration S36.113 ☑

- **Injury** — *continued*
  - liver — *continued*
    - laceration — *continued*
      - major (stellate) S36.116 ☑
      - minor S36.114 ☑
      - moderate S36.115 ☑
    - specified NEC S36.118 ☑
  - lower back S39.92 ☑
    - specified NEC S39.82 ☑
  - lumbar, lumbosacral (region) S39.92 ☑
    - plexus — *see* Injury, lumbosacral plexus
  - lumbosacral plexus S34.4 ☑
  - lung — *see also* Injury, intrathoracic, lung
    - aspiration J69.0
    - dabbing (related) U07.0
    - electronic cigarette (related) U07.0
    - EVALI - [e-cigarette, or vaping, product use associated] U07.0
    - transfusion-related (TRALI) J95.84
    - vaping (associated) (device) (product) (use) U07.0
  - lymphatic thoracic duct — *see* Injury, intrathoracic, specified organ NEC
  - malar region S09.93 ☑
  - mastoid region S09.90 ☑
  - maxilla S09.93 ☑
  - mediastinum — *see* Injury, intrathoracic, specified organ NEC
  - membrane, brain — *see* Injury, intracranial
  - meningeal artery — *see* Injury, intracranial, subdural hemorrhage
  - meninges (cerebral) — *see* Injury, intracranial
  - mesenteric
    - artery
      - branch S35.299 ☑
        - laceration (minor) (superficial) S35.291 ☑
          - major S35.292 ☑
        - specified NEC S35.298 ☑
      - inferior S35.239 ☑
        - laceration (minor) (superficial) S35.231 ☑
          - major S35.232 ☑
        - specified NEC S35.238 ☑
      - superior S35.229 ☑
        - laceration (minor) (superficial) S35.221 ☑
          - major S35.222 ☑
        - specified NEC S35.228 ☑
    - plexus (inferior) (superior) — *see* Injury, nerve, lumbosacral, sympathetic
    - vein
      - inferior S35.349 ☑
        - laceration S35.341 ☑
        - specified NEC S35.348 ☑
      - superior S35.339 ☑
        - laceration S35.331 ☑
        - specified NEC S35.338 ☑
  - mesentery — *see* Injury, intra-abdominal, specified site NEC
  - mesosalpinx — *see* Injury, pelvic organ, specified site NEC
  - middle ear S09.30- ☑
  - midthoracic region NOS S29.9 ☑
  - mouth S09.93 ☑
  - multiple NOS T07 ☑
  - muscle (and fascia) (and tendon)
    - abdomen S39.001 ☑
      - laceration S39.021 ☑
      - specified type NEC S39.091 ☑
      - strain S39.011 ☑
    - abductor
      - thumb, forearm level — *see* Injury, muscle, thumb, abductor
    - adductor
      - thigh S76.20- ☑
        - laceration S76.22- ☑
        - specified type NEC S76.29- ☑
        - strain S76.21- ☑
    - ankle — *see* Injury, muscle, foot
    - anterior muscle group, at leg level (lower) S86.20- ☑
      - laceration S86.22- ☑
      - specified type NEC S86.29- ☑
      - strain S86.21- ☑
    - arm (upper) — *see* Injury, muscle, shoulder
    - biceps (parts NEC) S46.20- ☑
      - laceration S46.22- ☑
      - long head S46.10- ☑
        - laceration S46.12- ☑
        - specified type NEC S46.19- ☑

Index

Injury — Injury

Injury — *continued*
  nerve — *continued*
    pelvis — *see* Injury, nerve, abdomen, specified site NEC
      peripheral — *see* Injury, nerve, abdomen, peripheral
    peripheral NEC T14.8 ☑
      abdomen — *see* Injury, nerve, abdomen, peripheral
      lower back — *see* Injury, nerve, abdomen, peripheral
      neck — *see* Injury, nerve, neck, peripheral
      pelvis — *see* Injury, nerve, abdomen, peripheral
      specified NEC T14.8 ☑
    peroneal (lower leg level) S84.1- ☑
      foot S94.2- ☑
    plexus
      brachial — *see* Injury, brachial plexus
      celiac, coeliac — *see* Injury, nerve, lumbosacral, sympathetic
      mesenteric, inferior — *see* Injury, nerve, lumbosacral, sympathetic
      sacral — *see* Injury, lumbosacral plexus
      spinal
        brachial — *see* Injury, brachial plexus
        lumbosacral — *see* Injury, lumbosacral plexus
    pneumogastric — *see* Injury, nerve, vagus
    radial (forearm level) S54.2- ☑
      hand (level) S64.2- ☑
      upper arm (level) S44.2- ☑
      wrist (level) — *see* Injury, nerve, radial, hand
    root — *see* Injury, nerve, spinal, root
    sacral plexus — *see* Injury, lumbosacral plexus
    sacral spinal — *see* Injury, spinal, sacral
      peripheral S34.6 ☑
      root S34.22 ☑
      sympathetic S34.5 ☑
    sciatic (hip level) (thigh level) S74.Ø- ☑
    second cranial (optic) — *see* Injury, nerve, optic
    seventh cranial (facial) — *see* Injury, nerve, facial
    shoulder — *see* Injury, nerve, arm
    sixth cranial (abducent) — *see* Injury, nerve, abducens
    spinal
      plexus — *see* Injury, nerve, plexus, spinal
      root
        cervical S14.2 ☑
        dorsal S24.2 ☑
        lumbar S34.21 ☑
        sacral S34.22 ☑
        thoracic — *see* Injury, nerve, spinal, root, dorsal
    splanchnic — *see* Injury, nerve, lumbosacral, sympathetic
    sympathetic NEC — *see* Injury, nerve, lumbosacral, sympathetic
      cervical — *see* Injury, nerve, cervical sympathetic
    tenth cranial (pneumogastric or vagus) — *see* Injury, nerve, vagus
    thigh (level) — *see* Injury, nerve, hip
      cutaneous sensory — *see* Injury, nerve, cutaneous sensory, hip
      femoral — *see* Injury, nerve, femoral
      sciatic — *see* Injury, nerve, sciatic
      specified NEC — *see* Injury, nerve, hip
    third cranial (oculomotor) — *see* Injury, nerve, oculomotor
    thorax S24.9 ☑
      peripheral S24.3 ☑
      specified site NEC S24.8 ☑
      sympathetic S24.4 ☑
    thumb, digital — *see* Injury, nerve, digital, thumb
    tibial (lower leg level) (posterior) S84.Ø- ☑
    toe — *see* Injury, nerve, ankle
    trigeminal SØ4.3- ☑
      contusion SØ4.3- ☑
      laceration SØ4.3- ☑
      specified type NEC SØ4.3- ☑
    trochlear SØ4.2- ☑
      contusion SØ4.2- ☑
      laceration SØ4.2- ☑
      specified type NEC SØ4.2- ☑
    twelfth cranial (hypoglossal) — *see* Injury, nerve, hypoglossal
    ulnar (forearm level) S54.Ø- ☑
      arm (upper) (level) S44.Ø- ☑

Injury — *continued*
  nerve — *continued*
    ulnar — *continued*
      hand (level) S64.Ø- ☑
      wrist (level) — *see* Injury, nerve, ulnar, hand
    vagus SØ4.89- ☑
      specified type NEC SØ4.89- ☑
    wrist (level) — *see* Injury, nerve, hand
  ninth cranial nerve (glossopharyngeal) — *see* Injury, nerve, glossopharyngeal
  nose (septum) SØ9.92 ☑
  obstetrical O71.9
    specified NEC O71.89
  occipital (region) (scalp) SØ9.9Ø ☑
    lobe — *see* Injury, intracranial
  optic chiasm SØ4.Ø2 ☑
  optic radiation SØ4.Ø3- ☑
  optic tract and pathways SØ4.Ø3- ☑
  orbit, orbital (region) — *see* Injury, eye
    penetrating (with foreign body) — *see* Injury, eye, orbit, penetrating
    specified NEC — *see* Injury, eye, specified site NEC
  ovary, ovarian S37.4Ø9 ☑
    bilateral S37.4Ø2 ☑
      contusion S37.422 ☑
      laceration S37.432 ☑
      specified type NEC S37.492 ☑
    blood vessel — *see* Injury, blood vessel, ovarian
    contusion S37.429 ☑
      bilateral S37.422 ☑
      unilateral S37.421 ☑
    laceration S37.439 ☑
      bilateral S37.432 ☑
      unilateral S37.431 ☑
    specified type NEC S37.499 ☑
      bilateral S37.492 ☑
      unilateral S37.491 ☑
    unilateral S37.4Ø1 ☑
      contusion S37.421 ☑
      laceration S37.431 ☑
      specified type NEC S37.491 ☑
  palate (hard) (soft) SØ9.93 ☑
  pancreas S36.2Ø9 ☑
    body S36.2Ø1 ☑
      contusion S36.221 ☑
      laceration S36.231 ☑
        major S36.261 ☑
        minor S36.241 ☑
        moderate S36.251 ☑
      specified type NEC S36.291 ☑
    contusion S36.229 ☑
    head S36.2ØØ ☑
      contusion S36.22Ø ☑
      laceration S36.23Ø ☑
        major S36.26Ø ☑
        minor S36.24Ø ☑
        moderate S36.25Ø ☑
      specified type NEC S36.29Ø ☑
    laceration S36.239 ☑
      major S36.269 ☑
      minor S36.249 ☑
      moderate S36.259 ☑
    specified type NEC S36.299 ☑
    tail S36.2Ø2 ☑
      contusion S36.222 ☑
      laceration S36.232 ☑
        major S36.262 ☑
        minor S36.242 ☑
        moderate S36.252 ☑
      specified type NEC S36.292 ☑
  parietal (region) (scalp) SØ9.9Ø ☑
    lobe — *see* Injury, intracranial
  patellar ligament (tendon) S76.1Ø- ☑
    laceration S76.12- ☑
    specified NEC S76.19- ☑
    strain S76.11- ☑
  pelvis, pelvic (floor) S39.93 ☑
    complicating delivery O7Ø.1
    joint or ligament, complicating delivery O71.6
    organ S37.9Ø ☑
      with ectopic or molar pregnancy OØ8.6
      complication of abortion — *see* Abortion
      contusion S37.92 ☑
      following ectopic or molar pregnancy OØ8.6
      laceration S37.93 ☑
      obstetrical trauma NEC O71.5

Injury — *continued*
  pelvis, pelvic — *continued*
    organ — *continued*
      specified
        site NEC S37.899 ☑
          contusion S37.892 ☑
          laceration S37.893 ☑
          specified type NEC S37.898 ☑
        type NEC S37.99 ☑
    specified NEC S39.83 ☑
  penis S39.94 ☑
  perineum S39.94 ☑
  peritoneum S36.81 ☑
    laceration S36.893 ☑
  periurethral tissue — *see* Injury, urethra
    complicating delivery O71.82
  phalanges
    foot — *see* Injury, foot
    hand — *see* Injury, hand
  pharynx NEC S19.85 ☑
  pleura — *see* Injury, intrathoracic, pleura
  plexus
    brachial — *see* Injury, brachial plexus
    cardiac — *see* Injury, nerve, thorax, sympathetic
    celiac, coeliac — *see* Injury, nerve, lumbosacral, sympathetic
    esophageal — *see* Injury, nerve, thorax, sympathetic
    hypogastric — *see* Injury, nerve, lumbosacral, sympathetic
    lumbar, lumbosacral — *see* Injury, lumbosacral plexus
    mesenteric — *see* Injury, nerve, lumbosacral, sympathetic
    pulmonary — *see* Injury, nerve, thorax, sympathetic
  postcardiac surgery (syndrome) I97.Ø
  prepuce S39.94 ☑
  pressure
    injury — *see* Ulcer, pressure, by site
  prostate S37.829 ☑
    contusion S37.822 ☑
    laceration S37.823 ☑
    specified type NEC S37.828 ☑
  pubic region S39.94 ☑
  pudendum S39.94 ☑
  pulmonary plexus — *see* Injury, nerve, thorax, sympathetic
  rectovaginal septum NEC S39.83 ☑
  rectum — *see* Injury, intestine, large, rectum
  retina — *see* Injury, eye, specified site NEC
    penetrating — *see* Injury, eyeball, penetrating
  retroperitoneal — *see* Injury, intra-abdominal, specified site NEC
  rotator cuff (muscle(s)) (tendon(s)) S46.ØØ- ☑
    laceration S46.Ø2- ☑
    specified type NEC S46.Ø9- ☑
    strain S46.Ø1- ☑
  round ligament — *see* Injury, pelvic organ, specified site NEC
  sacral plexus — *see* Injury, lumbosacral plexus
  salivary duct or gland SØ9.93 ☑
  scalp SØ9.9Ø ☑
    newborn (birth injury) P12.9
      due to monitoring (electrode) (sampling incision) P12.4
      specified NEC P12.89
        caput succedaneum P12.81
  scapular region — *see* Injury, shoulder
  sclera — *see* Injury, eye, specified site NEC
    penetrating — *see* Injury, eyeball, penetrating
  scrotum S39.94 ☑
  second cranial nerve (optic) — *see* Injury, nerve, optic
  self-inflicted, without suicidal intent R45.88
  seminal vesicle — *see* Injury, pelvic organ, specified site NEC
  seventh cranial nerve (facial) — *see* Injury, nerve, facial
  shoulder S49.9- ☑
    blood vessel — *see* Injury, blood vessel, arm
    contusion — *see* Contusion, shoulder
    dislocation — *see* Dislocation, shoulder
    fracture — *see* Fracture, shoulder
    muscle — *see* Injury, muscle, shoulder
    nerve — *see* Injury, nerve, shoulder
    open — *see* Wound, open, shoulder
    specified type NEC S49.8- ☑
    sprain — *see* Sprain, shoulder girdle
    superficial — *see* Injury, superficial, shoulder

Injury — *continued*
  superficial — *continued*
    toe(s) — *continued*
      external constriction — *see* Constriction, external, toe
      foreign body — *see* Foreign body, superficial, toe
      great S9Ø.93- ☑
    tongue — *see* Injury, superficial, oral cavity
    tooth, teeth — *see* Injury, superficial, oral cavity
    trachea S1Ø.1Ø ☑
    tunica vaginalis S3Ø.94 ☑
    tympanum, tympanic membrane — *see* Injury, superficial, ear
    uvula — *see* Injury, superficial, oral cavity
    vagina S3Ø.95 ☑
    vocal cords — *see* Injury, superficial, throat
    vulva S3Ø.95 ☑
    wrist S6Ø.91- ☑
  supraclavicular region — *see* Injury, neck
  supraorbital SØ9.93 ☑
  suprarenal gland (multiple) — *see* Injury, adrenal
  surgical complication (external or internal site) — *see* Laceration, accidental complicating surgery
  temple SØ9.9Ø ☑
  temporal region SØ9.9Ø ☑
  tendon — *see also* Injury, muscle, by site
    abdomen — *see* Injury, muscle, abdomen
    Achilles — *see* Injury, Achilles tendon
    lower back — *see* Injury, muscle, lower back
    pelvic organs — *see* Injury, muscle, pelvis
  tenth cranial nerve (pneumogastric or vagus) — *see* Injury, nerve, vagus
  testis S39.94 ☑
  thigh S79.92- ☑
    blood vessel — *see* Injury, blood vessel, hip
    contusion — *see* Contusion, thigh
    fracture — *see* Fracture, femur
    muscle — *see* Injury, muscle, thigh
    nerve — *see* Injury, nerve, thigh
    open — *see* Wound, open, thigh
    specified NEC S79.82- ☑
    superficial — *see* Injury, superficial, thigh
  third cranial nerve (oculomotor) — *see* Injury, nerve, oculomotor
  thorax, thoracic S29.9 ☑
    blood vessel — *see* Injury, blood vessel, thorax
    cavity — *see* Injury, intrathoracic
    dislocation — *see* Dislocation, thorax
    external (wall) S29.9 ☑
      contusion — *see* Contusion, thorax
      nerve — *see* Injury, nerve, thorax
      open — *see* Wound, open, thorax
      specified NEC S29.8 ☑
      sprain — *see* Sprain, thorax
      superficial — *see* Injury, superficial, thorax
    fracture — *see* Fracture, thorax
    internal — *see* Injury, intrathoracic
    intrathoracic organ — *see* Injury, intrathoracic
    sympathetic ganglion — *see* Injury, nerve, thorax, sympathetic
  throat — *see also* Injury, neck S19.9 ☑
  thumb S69.9- ☑
    blood vessel — *see* Injury, blood vessel, thumb
    contusion — *see* Contusion, thumb
    dislocation — *see* Dislocation, thumb
    fracture — *see* Fracture, thumb
    muscle — *see* Injury, muscle, thumb
    nerve — *see* Injury, nerve, digital, thumb
    open — *see* Wound, open, thumb
    specified NEC S69.8- ☑
    sprain — *see* Sprain, thumb
    superficial — *see* Injury, superficial, thumb
  thymus (gland) — *see* Injury, intrathoracic, specified organ NEC
  thyroid (gland) NEC S19.84 ☑
  toe S99.92- ☑
    contusion — *see* Contusion, toe
    dislocation — *see* Dislocation, toe
    fracture — *see* Fracture, toe
    muscle — *see* Injury, muscle, toe
    open — *see* Wound, open, toe
    specified type NEC S99.82- ☑
    sprain — *see* Sprain, toe
    superficial — *see* Injury, superficial, toe
  tongue SØ9.93 ☑

Injury — *continued*
  tonsil SØ9.93 ☑
  tooth SØ9.93 ☑
  trachea (cervical) NEC S19.82 ☑
    thoracic — *see* Injury, intrathoracic, trachea, thoracic
  transfusion-related acute lung (TRALI) J95.84
  tunica vaginalis S39.94 ☑
  twelfth cranial nerve (hypoglossal) — *see* Injury, nerve, hypoglossal
  ureter S37.1Ø ☑
    contusion S37.12 ☑
    laceration S37.13 ☑
    specified type NEC S37.19 ☑
  urethra (sphincter) S37.3Ø ☑
    at delivery O71.5
    contusion S37.32 ☑
    laceration S37.33 ☑
    specified type NEC S37.39 ☑
  urinary organ S37.9Ø ☑
    contusion S37.92 ☑
    laceration S37.93 ☑
    specified
      site NEC S37.899 ☑
        contusion S37.892 ☑
        laceration S37.893 ☑
        specified type NEC S37.898 ☑
      type NEC S37.99 ☑
  uterus, uterine S37.6Ø ☑
    with ectopic or molar pregnancy OØ8.6
    blood vessel — *see* Injury, blood vessel, iliac
    contusion S37.62 ☑
    laceration S37.63 ☑
      cervix at delivery O71.3
    rupture associated with obstetrics — *see* Rupture, uterus
    specified type NEC S37.69 ☑
  uvula SØ9.93 ☑
  vagina S39.93 ☑
    abrasion S3Ø.814 ☑
    bite S31.45 ☑
      insect S3Ø.864 ☑
      superficial NEC S3Ø.874 ☑
    contusion S3Ø.23 ☑
    crush S38.Ø3 ☑
    during delivery — *see* Laceration, vagina, during delivery
    external constriction S3Ø.844 ☑
    insect bite S3Ø.864 ☑
    laceration S31.41 ☑
      with foreign body S31.42 ☑
    open wound S31.4Ø ☑
    puncture S31.43 ☑
      with foreign body S31.44 ☑
    superficial S3Ø.95 ☑
      foreign body S3Ø.854 ☑
  vas deferens — *see* Injury, pelvic organ, specified site NEC
  vascular NEC T14.8 ☑
  vein — *see* Injury, blood vessel
  vena cava (superior) S25.2Ø ☑
    inferior S35.1Ø ☑
      laceration (minor) (superficial) S35.11 ☑
        major S35.12 ☑
      specified type NEC S35.19 ☑
    laceration (minor) (superficial) S25.21 ☑
      major S25.22 ☑
    specified type NEC S25.29 ☑
  vesical (sphincter) — *see* Injury, bladder
  visual cortex SØ4.Ø4- ☑
  vitreous (humor) SØ5.9Ø ☑
    specified NEC SØ5.8X- ☑
  vocal cord NEC S19.83 ☑
  vulva S39.94 ☑
    abrasion S3Ø.814 ☑
    bite S31.45 ☑
      insect S3Ø.864 ☑
      superficial NEC S3Ø.874 ☑
    contusion S3Ø.23 ☑
    crush S38.Ø3 ☑
    during delivery — *see* Laceration, perineum, female, during delivery
    external constriction S3Ø.844 ☑
    insect bite S3Ø.864 ☑
    laceration S31.41 ☑
      with foreign body S31.42 ☑
    open wound S31.4Ø ☑

Injury — *continued*
  vulva — *continued*
    puncture S31.43 ☑
      with foreign body S31.44 ☑
    superficial S3Ø.95 ☑
      foreign body S3Ø.854 ☑
  whiplash (cervical spine) S13.4 ☑
  wrist S69.9- ☑
    blood vessel — *see* Injury, blood vessel, hand
    contusion — *see* Contusion, wrist
    dislocation — *see* Dislocation, wrist
    fracture — *see* Fracture, wrist
    muscle — *see* Injury, muscle, hand
    nerve — *see* Injury, nerve, hand
    open — *see* Wound, open, wrist
    specified NEC S69.8- ☑
    sprain — *see* Sprain, wrist
    superficial — *see* Injury, superficial, wrist

Inoculation — *see also* Vaccination
  complication or reaction — *see* Complications, vaccination

Insanity, insane — *see also* Psychosis
  adolescent — *see* Schizophrenia
  confusional F28
    acute or subacute FØ5
  delusional F22
  senile FØ3 ☑

Insect
  bite — *see* Bite, by site, superficial, insect
  venomous, poisoning NEC (by) — *see* Venom, arthropod

Insecurity
  financial Z59.86
  food Z59.41
  transportation Z59.82

Insensitivity
  adrenocorticotropin hormone (ACTH) E27.49
  androgen E34.5Ø
    complete E34.51
    partial E34.52

Insertion
  cord (umbilical) lateral or velamentous O43.12- ☑
  intrauterine contraceptive device (encounter for) — *see* Intrauterine contraceptive device

Insolation (sunstroke) T67.Ø1 ☑

Insomnia (organic) G47.ØØ
  adjustment F51.Ø2
  adjustment disorder F51.Ø2
  behavioral, of childhood Z73.819
    combined type Z73.812
    limit setting type Z73.811
    sleep-onset association type Z73.81Ø
  childhood Z73.819
  chronic F51.Ø4
    somatized tension F51.Ø4
  conditioned F51.Ø4
  due to
    alcohol
      abuse F1Ø.182
      dependence F1Ø.282
      use F1Ø.982
    amphetamines
      abuse F15.182
      dependence F15.282
      use F15.982
    anxiety disorder F51.Ø5
    caffeine
      abuse F15.182
      dependence F15.282
      use F15.982
    cocaine
      abuse F14.182
      dependence F14.282
      use F14.982
    depression F51.Ø5
    drug NEC
      abuse F19.182
      dependence F19.282
      use F19.982
    medical condition G47.Ø1
    mental disorder NEC F51.Ø5
    opioid
      abuse F11.182
      dependence F11.282
      use F11.982
    psychoactive substance NEC
      abuse F19.182
      dependence F19.182

- **Insomnia** — *continued*
  - due to — *continued*
    - psychoactive substance — *continued*
      - use F19.982
    - sedative, hypnotic, or anxiolytic
      - abuse F13.182
      - dependence F13.282
      - use F13.982
    - stimulant NEC
      - abuse F15.182
      - dependence F15.282
      - use F15.982
  - fatal familial (FFI) A81.83
  - idiopathic F51.Ø1
  - learned F51.3
  - nonorganic origin F51.Ø1
  - not due to a substance or known physiological condition F51.Ø1
    - specified NEC F51.Ø9
  - paradoxical F51.Ø3
  - primary F51.Ø1
  - psychiatric F51.Ø5
  - psychophysiologic F51.Ø4
  - related to psychopathology F51.Ø5
  - short-term F51.Ø2
  - specified NEC G47.Ø9
  - stress-related F51.Ø2
  - transient F51.Ø2
  - without objective findings F51.Ø2
- **Inspiration**
  - food or foreign body — *see* Foreign body, by site
  - mucus — *see* Asphyxia, mucus
- **Inspissated bile syndrome** (newborn) P59.1
- **Instability**
  - emotional (excessive) F6Ø.3
  - housing
    - housed Z59.819
      - with risk of homelessness Z59.811
      - homelessness in past 12 months Z59.812
  - joint (post-traumatic) M25.3Ø
    - ankle M25.37- ☑
    - due to old ligament injury — *see* Disorder, ligament
    - elbow M25.32- ☑
    - flail — *see* Flail, joint
    - foot M25.37- ☑
    - hand M25.34- ☑
    - hip M25.35- ☑
    - knee M25.36- ☑
    - lumbosacral — *see* subcategory M53.2 ☑
    - prosthesis — *see* Complications, joint prosthesis, mechanical, displacement, by site
    - sacroiliac — *see* subcategory M53.2 ☑
    - secondary to
      - old ligament injury — *see* Disorder, ligament
      - removal of joint prosthesis M96.89
    - shoulder (region) M25.31- ☑
    - specified site NEC M25.39
    - spine — *see* subcategory M53.2 ☑
    - wrist M25.33- ☑
  - knee (chronic) M23.5- ☑
  - lumbosacral — *see* subcategory M53.2 ☑
  - nervous F48.8
  - personality (emotional) F6Ø.3
  - spine — *see* Instability, joint, spine
  - vasomotor R55
- **Institutional syndrome** (childhood) F94.2
- **Institutionalization, affecting child** Z62.22
  - disinhibited attachment F94.2
- **Insufficiency, insufficient**
  - accommodation, old age H52.4
  - adrenal (gland) E27.4Ø
    - primary E27.1
  - adrenocortical E27.4Ø
    - drug-induced E27.3
    - iatrogenic E27.3
    - primary E27.1
  - anatomic crown height KØ8.89
  - anterior (occlusal) guidance M26.54
  - anus K62.89
  - aortic (valve) I35.1
    - with
      - mitral (valve) disease IØ8.Ø
        - with tricuspid (valve) disease IØ8.3
      - stenosis I35.2
      - tricuspid (valve) disease IØ8.2
        - with mitral (valve) disease IØ8.3
    - congenital Q23.1
    - rheumatic IØ6.1

- **Insufficiency, insufficient** — *continued*
  - aortic — *continued*
    - rheumatic — *continued*
      - with
        - mitral (valve) disease IØ8.Ø
          - with tricuspid (valve) disease IØ8.3
        - stenosis IØ6.2
          - with mitral (valve) disease IØ8.Ø
            - with tricuspid (valve) disease IØ8.3
        - tricuspid (valve) disease IØ8.2
          - with mitral (valve) disease IØ8.3
    - specified cause NEC I35.1
    - syphilitic A52.Ø3
  - arterial I77.1
    - basilar G45.Ø
    - carotid (hemispheric) G45.1
    - cerebral I67.81
    - coronary (acute or subacute) I24.89
    - mesenteric K55.1
    - peripheral I73.9
    - precerebral (multiple) (bilateral) G45.2
    - vertebral G45.Ø
  - arteriovenous I99.8
  - biliary K83.8
  - cardiac — *see also* Insufficiency, myocardial
    - due to presence of (cardiac) prosthesis I97.11- ☑
    - postprocedural I97.11- ☑
  - cardiorenal, hypertensive I13.2
  - cardiovascular — *see* Disease, cardiovascular
  - cerebrovascular (acute) I67.81
    - with transient focal neurological signs and symptoms G45.8
  - circulatory NEC I99.8
    - newborn P29.89
  - clinical crown length KØ8.89
  - convergence H51.11
  - coronary (acute or subacute) I24.89
    - chronic or with a stated duration of over 4 weeks I25.89
  - corticoadrenal E27.4Ø
    - primary E27.1
  - dietary E63.9
  - divergence H51.8
  - food T73.Ø ☑
  - gastroesophageal K22.89
  - gonadal
    - ovary E28.39
    - testis E29.1
  - heart — *see also* Insufficiency, myocardial
    - newborn P29.Ø
    - valve — *see* Endocarditis
  - hepatic — *see* Failure, hepatic
  - idiopathic autonomic G9Ø.Ø9
  - interocclusal distance of fully erupted teeth (ridge) M26.36
  - kidney N28.9
    - acute N28.9
    - chronic N18.9
  - lacrimal (secretion) HØ4.12- ☑
    - passages — *see* Stenosis, lacrimal
  - liver — *see* Failure, hepatic
  - lung — *see* Insufficiency, pulmonary
  - mental (congenital) — *see* Disability, intellectual
  - mesenteric K55.1
  - mitral (valve) I34.Ø
    - with
      - aortic valve disease IØ8.Ø
        - with tricuspid (valve) disease IØ8.3
      - obstruction or stenosis IØ5.2
        - with aortic valve disease IØ8.Ø
      - tricuspid (valve) disease IØ8.1
        - with aortic (valve) disease IØ8.3
    - congenital Q23.3
    - rheumatic IØ5.1
      - with
        - aortic valve disease IØ8.Ø
          - with tricuspid (valve) disease IØ8.3
        - obstruction or stenosis IØ5.2
          - with aortic valve disease IØ8.Ø
            - with tricuspid (valve) disease IØ8.3
        - tricuspid (valve) disease IØ8.1
          - with aortic (valve) disease IØ8.3
      - active or acute IØ1.1
        - with chorea, rheumatic (Sydenham's) IØ2.Ø
    - specified cause, except rheumatic I34.Ø
  - muscle — *see also* Disease, muscle
    - heart — *see* Insufficiency, myocardial
    - ocular NEC H5Ø.9

- **Insufficiency, insufficient** — *continued*
  - myocardial, myocardium (with arteriosclerosis) — *see also* Failure, heart I5Ø.9
    - with
      - rheumatic fever (conditions in IØØ) IØ9.Ø
        - active, acute or subacute IØ1.2
          - with chorea IØ2.Ø
        - inactive or quiescent (with chorea) IØ9.Ø
    - congenital Q24.8
    - hypertensive — *see* Hypertension, heart
    - newborn P29.Ø
    - rheumatic IØ9.Ø
      - active, acute, or subacute IØ1.2
    - syphilitic A52.Ø6
  - nourishment — *see also* Nutrition deficient T73.Ø ☑
  - pancreatic K86.89
    - exocrine K86.81
  - parathyroid (gland) E2Ø.9
  - peripheral vascular (arterial) I73.9
  - pituitary E23.Ø
  - placental (mother) O36.51- ☑
  - platelets D69.6
  - prenatal care affecting management of pregnancy OØ9.3- ☑
  - progressive pluriglandular E31.Ø
  - pulmonary J98.4
    - acute, following surgery (nonthoracic) J95.2
      - thoracic J95.1
    - chronic, following surgery J95.3
    - following
      - shock J98.4
      - trauma J98.4
    - newborn P28.89
    - valve I37.1
      - with stenosis I37.2
      - congenital Q22.2
      - rheumatic IØ9.89
        - with aortic, mitral or tricuspid (valve) disease IØ8.8
  - pyloric K31.89
  - renal (acute) N28.9
    - chronic N18.9
  - respiratory RØ6.89
    - newborn P28.5
  - rotation — *see* Malrotation
  - sleep syndrome F51.12
  - social insurance Z59.7
  - suprarenal E27.4Ø
    - primary E27.1
  - tarso-orbital fascia, congenital Q1Ø.3
  - testis E29.1
  - thyroid (gland) (acquired) EØ3.9
    - congenital EØ3.1
  - tricuspid (valve) (rheumatic) IØ7.1
    - with
      - aortic (valve) disease IØ8.2
        - with mitral (valve) disease IØ8.3
      - mitral (valve) disease IØ8.1
        - with aortic (valve) disease IØ8.3
      - obstruction or stenosis IØ7.2
        - with aortic (valve) disease IØ8.2
          - with mitral (valve) disease IØ8.3
    - congenital Q22.8
    - nonrheumatic I36.1
      - with stenosis I36.2
  - urethral sphincter R32
  - valve, valvular (heart) I38
    - aortic — *see* Insufficiency, aortic (valve)
    - congenital Q24.8
    - mitral — *see* Insufficiency, mitral (valve)
    - pulmonary — *see* Insufficiency, pulmonary, valve
    - tricuspid — *see* Insufficiency, tricuspid (valve)
  - vascular I99.8
    - intestine K55.9
      - acute — *see also* Ischemia, intestine, acute K55.Ø59
    - mesenteric K55.1
    - peripheral I73.9
    - renal — *see* Hypertension, kidney
  - velopharyngeal
    - acquired K13.79
    - congenital Q38.8
  - venous (chronic) (peripheral) I87.2
  - ventricular — *see* Insufficiency, myocardial
  - welfare support Z59.7
- **Insufflation, fallopian** Z31.41
- **Insular** — *see* condition

Insulinoma
- pancreas
  - benign D13.7
  - malignant C25.4
  - uncertain behavior D37.8
- specified site
  - benign — *see* Neoplasm, by site, benign
  - malignant — *see* Neoplasm, by site, malignant
  - uncertain behavior — *see* Neoplasm, by site, uncertain behavior
- unspecified site
  - benign D13.7
  - malignant C25.4
  - uncertain behavior D37.8

Insuloma — *see* Insulinoma

Interference
- balancing side M26.56
- non-working side M26.56

Intermenstrual — *see* condition

Intermittent — *see* condition

Internal — *see* condition

Interrogation
- cardiac defibrillator (automatic) (implantable) Z45.Ø2
- cardiac pacemaker Z45.Ø18
- cardiac (event) (loop) recorder Z45.Ø9
- infusion pump (implanted) (intrathecal) Z45.1
- neurostimulator Z46.2

Interruption
- aortic arch Q25.21
- bundle of His I44.3Ø
- phase-shift, sleep cycle — *see* Disorder, sleep, circadian rhythm
- sleep phase-shift, or 24 hour sleep-wake cycle — *see* Disorder, sleep, circadian rhythm

Interstitial — *see* condition

Intertrigo L3Ø.4
- labialis K13.Ø

Intervertebral disc — *see* condition

Intestine, intestinal — *see* condition

Intolerance
- carbohydrate K9Ø.49
- disaccharide, hereditary E73.Ø
- fat NEC K9Ø.49
  - pancreatic K9Ø.3
- food K9Ø.49
  - dietary counseling and surveillance Z71.3
- fructose E74.1Ø
  - hereditary E74.12
- glucose (-galactose) E74.39
- gluten K9Ø.41
- lactose E73.9
  - specified NEC E73.8
- lysine E72.3
- milk NEC K9Ø.49
  - lactose E73.9
- orthostatic, chronic G9Ø.A
- protein K9Ø.49
- starch NEC K9Ø.49
- sucrose (-isomaltose) E74.31

Intoxicated NEC (without dependence) — *see* Alcohol, intoxication

Intoxication
- acid — *see also* Acidosis E87.29
- alcoholic (acute) (without dependence) — *see* Alcohol, intoxication
- alimentary canal K52.1
- amphetamine (without dependence) — *see also* Abuse, drug, stimulant, with intoxication
  - with dependence — *see* Dependence, drug, stimulant, with intoxication
  - stimulant NEC F15.1Ø
    - with
      - anxiety disorder F15.18Ø
      - intoxication F15.129
        - with
          - delirium F15.121
          - perceptual disturbance F15.122
- anxiolytic (acute) (without dependence) — *see* Abuse, drug, sedative, with intoxication
  - with dependence — *see* Dependence, drug, sedative, with intoxication
- caffeine F15.929
  - with dependence — *see* Dependence, drug, stimulant, with intoxication
- cannabinoids (acute) (without dependence) — *see* Use, cannabis, with intoxication
  - with
    - abuse — *see* Abuse, drug, cannabis, with intoxication
    - dependence — *see* Dependence, drug, cannabis, with intoxication
- chemical — *see* Table of Drugs and Chemicals
  - via placenta or breast milk — *see* - Absorption, chemical, through placenta
- cocaine (acute) (without dependence) — *see* Abuse, drug, cocaine, with intoxication
  - with dependence — *see* Dependence, drug, cocaine, with intoxication
- drug
  - acute (without dependence) — *see* Abuse, drug, by type with intoxication
    - with dependence — *see* Dependence, drug, by type with intoxication
  - addictive
    - via placenta or breast milk — *see* Absorption, drug, addictive, through placenta
  - newborn P93.8
    - gray baby syndrome P93.Ø
  - overdose or wrong substance given or taken — *see* Table of Drugs and Chemicals, by drug, poisoning
- enteric K52.1
- foodborne AØ5.9
  - bacterial AØ5.9
  - classical (Clostridium botulinum) AØ5.1
  - due to
    - Bacillus cereus AØ5.4
    - bacterium AØ5.9
      - specified NEC AØ5.8
    - Clostridium
      - botulinum AØ5.1
      - perfringens AØ5.2
      - welchii AØ5.2
    - Salmonella AØ2.9
      - with
        - (gastro)enteritis AØ2.Ø
        - localized infection(s) AØ2.2Ø
          - arthritis AØ2.23
          - meningitis AØ2.21
          - osteomyelitis AØ2.24
          - pneumonia AØ2.22
          - pyelonephritis AØ2.25
          - specified NEC AØ2.29
        - sepsis AØ2.1
        - specified manifestation NEC AØ2.8
    - Staphylococcus AØ5.Ø
    - Vibrio
      - parahaemolyticus AØ5.3
      - vulnificus AØ5.5
  - enterotoxin, staphylococcal AØ5.Ø
  - noxious — *see* Poisoning, food, noxious
- gastrointestinal K52.1
- hallucinogenic (without dependence) — *see* Abuse, drug, hallucinogen, with intoxication
  - with dependence — *see* Dependence, drug, hallucinogen, with intoxication
- hepatocerebral intoxication K76.82
- hypnotic (acute) (without dependence) — *see* Abuse, drug, sedative, with intoxication
  - with dependence — *see* Dependence, drug, sedative, with intoxication
- inhalant (acute) (without dependence) — *see* Abuse, drug, inhalant, with intoxication
  - with dependence — *see* Dependence, drug, inhalant, with intoxication
- meaning
  - inebriation — *see* category F1Ø ☑
  - poisoning — *see* Table of Drugs and Chemicals
- methyl alcohol (acute) (without dependence) — *see* Alcohol, intoxication
- opioid (acute) (without dependence) — *see* Abuse, drug, opioid, with intoxication
  - with dependence — *see* Dependence, drug, opioid, with intoxication
- pathologic NEC (without dependence) — *see* Alcohol, intoxication
- phencyclidine (without dependence) — *see* Abuse, drug, hallucinogen, with intoxication
  - with dependence — *see* Dependence, drug, hallucinogen, with intoxication
- potassium (K) E87.5
- psychoactive substance NEC (without dependence) — *see* Abuse, drug, psychoactive NEC, with intoxication
  - with dependence — *see* Dependence, drug, psychoactive NEC, with intoxication
- sedative (acute) (without dependence) — *see* Abuse, drug, sedative, with intoxication
  - with dependence — *see* Dependence, drug, sedative, with intoxication
- serum — *see also* Reaction, serum T8Ø.69 ☑
- uremic — *see* Uremia
- volatile solvents (acute) (without dependence) — *see* Abuse, drug, inhalant, with intoxication
  - with dependence — *see* Dependence, drug, inhalant, with intoxication
- water E87.79

Intraabdominal testis, testes
- bilateral Q53.211
- unilateral Q53.111

Intracranial — *see* condition

Intrahepatic gallbladder Q44.1

Intraligamentous — *see* condition

Intrathoracic — *see also* condition
- kidney Q63.2

Intrauterine contraceptive device
- checking Z3Ø.431
- in situ Z97.5
- insertion Z3Ø.43Ø
  - immediately following removal Z3Ø.433
- management Z3Ø.431
- reinsertion Z3Ø.433
- removal Z3Ø.432
- replacement Z3Ø.433
- retention in pregnancy O26.3- ☑

Intraventricular — *see* condition

Intrinsic deformity — *see* Deformity

Intubation, difficult or failed T88.4 ☑

Intumescence, lens (eye) (cataract) — *see* Cataract

Intussusception (bowel) (colon) (enteric) (ileocecal) (ileocolic) (intestine) (rectum) K56.1
- appendix K38.8
- congenital Q43.8
- ureter (with obstruction) N13.5

Invagination (bowel, colon, intestine or rectum) K56.1

Inversion
- albumin-globulin (A-G) ratio E88.Ø9
- bladder N32.89
- cecum — *see* Intussusception
- cervix N88.8
- chromosome in normal individual Q95.1
- circadian rhythm — *see* Disorder, sleep, circadian rhythm
- nipple N64.59
  - congenital Q83.8
  - gestational — *see* Retraction, nipple
  - puerperal, postpartum — *see* Retraction, nipple
- nyctohemeral rhythm — *see* Disorder, sleep, circadian rhythm
- optic papilla Q14.2
- organ or site, congenital NEC — *see* Anomaly, by site
- sleep rhythm — *see* Disorder, sleep, circadian rhythm
- testis (congenital) Q55.29
- uterus (chronic) (postinfectional) (postpartal, old) N85.5
  - postpartum O71.2
- vagina (posthysterectomy) N99.3
- ventricular Q2Ø.5

Investigation — *see also* Examination ZØ4.9
- clinical research subject (control) (normal comparison) (participant) ZØØ.6

Involuntary movement, abnormal R25.9

Involution, involutional — *see also* condition
- breast, cystic — *see* Dysplasia, mammary, specified type NEC
- depression (single episode) F32.89
  - recurrent episode F33.9
- melancholia (single episode) F32.89
  - recurrent episode F33.8
- ovary, senile — *see* Atrophy, ovary
- thymus failure E32.8

I.Q.
- 2Ø-34 F72
- 35-49 F71
- 5Ø-69 F7Ø
- under 2Ø F73

IRDS (type I) P22.Ø
- type II P22.1

Irideremia Q13.1

- **Issue of** — *continued*
  - repeat prescription (appliance) (glasses) (medicinal substance, medicament, medicine) Z76.Ø
    - contraception — *see* Contraception
- **IST** (inappropriate sinus tachycardia, so stated) I47.11
- **Itch, itching** — *see also* Pruritus
  - baker's L23.6
  - barber's B35.Ø
  - bricklayer's L24.5
  - cheese B88.Ø
  - clam digger's B65.3
  - coolie B76.9
  - copra B88.Ø
  - dew B76.9
  - dhobi B35.6
  - filarial — *see* Infestation, filarial
  - grain B88.Ø
  - grocer's B88.Ø
  - ground B76.9
  - harvest B88.Ø
  - jock B35.6
  - Malabar B35.5
    - beard B35.Ø
    - foot B35.3
    - scalp B35.Ø
  - meaning scabies B86
  - Norwegian B86
  - perianal L29.Ø
  - poultrymen's B88.Ø
  - sarcoptic B86
  - scabies B86
  - scrub B88.Ø
  - straw B88.Ø
  - swimmer's B65.3
  - water B76.9
  - winter L29.8
- **Ivemark's syndrome** (asplenia with congenital heart disease) Q89.Ø1
- **Ivory bones** Q78.2
- **Ixodiasis NEC** B88.8

J

- **Jaccoud's syndrome** — *see* Arthropathy, postrheumatic, chronic
- **Jackson's**
  - membrane Q43.3
  - paralysis or syndrome G83.89
  - veil Q43.3
- **Jacquet's dermatitis** (diaper dermatitis) L22
- **Jadassohn-Pellizari's disease or anetoderma** L9Ø.2
- **Jadassohn's**
  - blue nevus — *see* Nevus
  - intraepidermal epithelioma — *see* Neoplasm, skin, benign
- **Jaffe-Lichtenstein** (-Uehlinger) **syndrome** — *see* Dysplasia, fibrous, bone NEC
- **Jakob-Creutzfeldt disease or syndrome** — *see* Creutzfeldt-Jakob disease or syndrome
- **Jaksch-Luzet disease** D64.89
- **Jamaican**
  - neuropathy G92.8
  - paraplegic tropical ataxic-spastic syndrome G92.8
- **Janet's disease** F48.8
- **Janiceps** Q89.4
- **Jansky-Bielschowsky amaurotic idiocy** E75.4
- **Japanese**
  - B-type encephalitis A83.Ø
  - river fever A75.3
- **Jaundice** (yellow) R17
  - acholuric (familial) (splenomegalic) — *see also* Spherocytosis
    - acquired D59.8
  - breast-milk (inhibitor) P59.3
  - catarrhal (acute) B15.9
    - with hepatic coma B15.Ø
  - cholestatic (benign) R17
  - due to or associated with
    - delayed conjugation P59.8
      - associated with (due to) preterm delivery P59.Ø
    - preterm delivery P59.Ø
  - epidemic (catarrhal) B15.9
    - with hepatic coma B15.Ø
    - leptospiral A27.Ø
    - spirochetal A27.Ø
  - familial nonhemolytic (congenital) (Gilbert) E8Ø.4
    - Crigler-Najjar E8Ø.5
  - febrile (acute) B15.9
- **Jaundice** — *continued*
  - febrile — *continued*
    - with hepatic coma B15.Ø
    - leptospiral A27.Ø
    - spirochetal A27.Ø
  - hematogenous D59.9
  - hemolytic (acquired) D59.9
    - congenital — *see* Spherocytosis
  - hemorrhagic (acute) (leptospiral) (spirochetal) A27.Ø
  - infectious (acute) (subacute) B15.9
    - with hepatic coma B15.Ø
    - leptospiral A27.Ø
    - spirochetal A27.Ø
  - leptospiral (hemorrhagic) A27.Ø
  - malignant (without coma) K72.9Ø
    - with coma K72.91
  - neonatal — *see* Jaundice, newborn
  - newborn P59.9
    - due to or associated with
      - ABO
        - antibodies P55.1
        - incompatibility, maternal/fetal P55.1
        - isoimmunization P55.1
      - absence or deficiency of enzyme system for bilirubin conjugation (congenital) P59.8
      - bleeding P58.1
      - breast milk inhibitors to conjugation P59.3
        - associated with preterm delivery P59.Ø
      - bruising P58.Ø
      - Crigler-Najjar syndrome E8Ø.5
      - delayed conjugation P59.8
        - associated with preterm delivery P59.Ø
      - drugs or toxins
        - given to newborn P58.42
        - transmitted from mother P58.41
      - excessive hemolysis P58.9
        - due to
          - bleeding P58.1
          - bruising P58.Ø
          - drugs or toxins
            - given to newborn P58.42
            - transmitted from mother P58.41
          - infection P58.2
          - polycythemia P58.3
          - swallowed maternal blood P58.5
        - specified type NEC P58.8
      - galactosemia E74.21
      - Gilbert syndrome E8Ø.4
      - hemolytic disease P55.9
        - ABO isoimmunization P55.1
        - Rh isoimmunization P55.Ø
        - specified NEC P55.8
      - hepatocellular damage P59.2Ø
        - specified NEC P59.29
      - hereditary hemolytic anemia P58.8
      - hypothyroidism, congenital EØ3.1
      - incompatibility, maternal/fetal NOS P55.9
      - infection P58.2
      - inspissated bile syndrome P59.1
      - isoimmunization NOS P55.9
      - mucoviscidosis E84.9
      - polycythemia P58.3
      - preterm delivery P59.Ø
      - Rh
        - antibodies P55.Ø
        - incompatibility, maternal/fetal P55.Ø
        - isoimmunization P55.Ø
      - specified cause NEC P59.8
      - swallowed maternal blood P58.5
    - spherocytosis (congenital) D58.Ø
  - nonhemolytic congenital familial (Gilbert) E8Ø.4
  - nuclear, newborn — *see also* Kernicterus of newborn P57.9
  - obstructive — *see also* Obstruction, bile duct K83.1
  - post-immunization — *see* Hepatitis, viral, type, B
  - post-transfusion — *see* Hepatitis, viral, type, B
  - regurgitation — *see also* Obstruction, bile duct K83.1
  - serum (homologous) (prophylactic) (therapeutic) — *see* Hepatitis, viral, type, B
  - spirochetal (hemorrhagic) A27.Ø
  - symptomatic R17
    - newborn P59.9
- **Jaw** — *see* condition
- **Jaw-winking phenomenon or syndrome** QØ7.8
- **Jealousy**
  - alcoholic F1Ø.988
  - childhood F93.8
  - sibling F93.8
- **Jejunitis** — *see* Enteritis
- **Jejunostomy status** Z93.4
- **Jejunum, jejunal** — *see* condition
- **Jensen's disease** — *see* Inflammation, chorioretinal, focal, juxtapapillary
- **Jerks, myoclonic** G25.3
- **Jervell-Lange-Nielsen syndrome** I45.81
- **Jeune's disease** Q77.2
- **Jigger disease** B88.1
- **Job's syndrome** (chronic granulomatous disease) D71
- **Joint** — *see also* condition
  - mice — *see* Loose, body, joint
    - knee M23.4- ☑
- **Jordan's anomaly or syndrome** D72.Ø
- **Joseph-Diamond-Blackfan anemia** (congenital hypoplastic) D61.Ø1
- **Jungle yellow fever** A95.Ø
- **Jüngling's disease** — *see* Sarcoidosis
- **Juvenile** — *see* condition

K

- **Kahler's disease** C9Ø.Ø- ☑
- **Kakke** E51.11
- **Kala-azar** B55.Ø
- **Kallmann's syndrome** E23.Ø
- **Kanner's syndrome** (autism) — *see* Psychosis, childhood
- **Kaposi's**
  - dermatosis (xeroderma pigmentosum) Q82.1
  - lichen ruber L44.Ø
    - acuminatus L44.Ø
  - sarcoma
    - colon C46.4
    - connective tissue C46.1
    - gastrointestinal organ C46.4
    - lung C46.5- ☑
    - lymph node (multiple) C46.3
    - palate (hard) (soft) C46.2
    - rectum C46.4
    - skin (multiple sites) C46.Ø
    - specified site NEC C46.7
    - stomach C46.4
    - unspecified site C46.9
  - varicelliform eruption BØØ.Ø
    - vaccinia T88.1 ☑
- **Kartagener's syndrome or triad** (sinusitis, bronchiectasis, situs inversus) Q89.3
- **Karyotype**
  - with abnormality except iso (Xq) Q96.2
  - 45,X Q96.Ø
  - 46,X
    - iso (Xq) Q96.1
  - 46,XX Q98.3
    - with streak gonads Q5Ø.32
    - hermaphrodite (true) Q99.1
    - male Q98.3
  - 46,XY
    - with streak gonads Q56.1
    - female Q97.3
    - hermaphrodite (true) Q99.1
  - 47,XXX Q97.Ø
  - 47,XXY Q98.Ø
  - 47,XYY Q98.5
- **Kaschin-Beck disease** — *see* Disease, Kaschin-Beck
- **Katayama's disease or fever** B65.2
- **Kawasaki's syndrome** M3Ø.3
- **Kayser-Fleischer ring** (cornea) (pseudosclerosis) H18.Ø4- ☑
- **Kaznelson's syndrome** (congenital hypoplastic anemia) D61.Ø1
- **Kearns-Sayre syndrome** H49.81- ☑
- **Kedani fever** A75.3
- **Kelis** L91.Ø
- **Kelly** (-Patterson) **syndrome** (sideropenic dysphagia) D5Ø.1
- **Keloid, cheloid** L91.Ø
  - acne L73.Ø
  - Addison's L94.Ø
  - cornea — *see* Opacity, cornea
  - Hawkin's L91.Ø
  - scar L91.Ø
- **Keloma** L91.Ø
- **Kenya fever** A77.1
- **Keratectasia** — *see also* Ectasia, cornea
  - congenital Q13.4
- **Keratinization of alveolar ridge mucosa**
  - excessive K13.23

Keratinization of alveolar ridge mucosa — *continued*
  minimal K13.22
Keratinized residual ridge mucosa
  excessive K13.23
  minimal K13.22
Keratitis (nodular) (nonulcerative) (simple) (zonular) H16.9
  with ulceration (central) (marginal) (perforated) (ring) — *see* Ulcer, cornea
  actinic — *see* Photokeratitis
  arborescens (herpes simplex) BØØ.52
  areolar H16.11- ☑
  bullosa H16.8
  deep H16.3Ø9
    specified type NEC H16.399
  dendritic (a) (herpes simplex) BØØ.52
  disciform (is) (herpes simplex) BØØ.52
    varicella BØ1.81
  filamentary H16.12- ☑
  gonococcal (congenital or prenatal) A54.33
  herpes, herpetic (simplex) BØØ.52
    zoster BØ2.33
  in (due to)
    acanthamebiasis B6Ø.13
    adenovirus B3Ø.Ø
    exanthema — *see also* Exanthem BØ9
    herpes (simplex) virus BØØ.52
    measles BØ5.81
    syphilis A5Ø.31
    tuberculosis A18.52
    zoster BØ2.33
  interstitial (nonsyphilitic) H16.3Ø- ☑
    diffuse H16.32- ☑
    herpes, herpetic (simplex) BØØ.52
      zoster BØ2.33
    sclerosing H16.33- ☑
    specified type NEC H16.39- ☑
    syphilitic (congenital) (late) A5Ø.31
    tuberculous A18.52
  macular H16.11- ☑
  nummular H16.11- ☑
  oyster shuckers' H16.8
  parenchymatous — *see* Keratitis, interstitial
  petrificans H16.8
  postmeasles BØ5.81
  punctata
    leprosa A3Ø.9 *[H16.14-]* ☑
    syphilitic (profunda) A5Ø.31
  punctate H16.14- ☑
  purulent H16.8
  rosacea L71.8
  sclerosing H16.33- ☑
  specified type NEC H16.8
  stellate H16.11- ☑
  striate H16.11- ☑
  superficial H16.1Ø- ☑
    with conjunctivitis — *see* Keratoconjunctivitis
    due to light — *see* Photokeratitis
  suppurative H16.8
  syphilitic (congenital) (prenatal) A5Ø.31
  trachomatous A71.1
    sequelae B94.Ø
  tuberculous A18.52
  vesicular H16.8
  xerotic — *see also* Keratomalacia H16.8
    vitamin A deficiency E5Ø.4
Keratoacanthoma L85.8
Keratocele — *see* Descemetocele
Keratoconjunctivitis H16.2Ø- ☑
  Acanthamoeba B6Ø.13
  adenoviral B3Ø.Ø
  epidemic B3Ø.Ø
  exposure H16.21- ☑
  herpes, herpetic (simplex) BØØ.52
    zoster BØ2.33
  in exanthema — *see also* Exanthem BØ9
  infectious B3Ø.Ø
  lagophthalmic — *see* Keratoconjunctivitis, specified type NEC
  neurotrophic H16.23- ☑
  phlyctenular H16.25- ☑
  postmeasles BØ5.81
  shipyard B3Ø.Ø
  sicca (Sjogren's) M35.Ø- ☑
    not Sjogren's H16.22- ☑
  specified type NEC H16.29- ☑

Keratoconjunctivitis — *continued*
  tuberculous (phlyctenular) A18.52
  vernal H16.26- ☑
Keratoconus H18.6Ø- ☑
  congenital Q13.4
  stable H18.61- ☑
  unstable H18.62- ☑
Keratocyst (dental) (odontogenic) — *see* Cyst, calcifying odontogenic
Keratoderma, keratodermia (congenital) (palmaris et plantaris) (symmetrical) Q82.8
  acquired L85.1
    in diseases classified elsewhere L86
  climactericum L85.1
  gonococcal A54.89
  gonorrheal A54.89
  punctata L85.2
  Reiter's — *see* Reiter's disease
Keratodermatocele — *see* Descemetocele
Keratoglobus H18.79 ☑
  congenital Q15.8
    with glaucoma Q15.Ø
Keratohemia — *see* Pigmentation, cornea, stromal
Keratoiritis — *see also* Iridocyclitis
  syphilitic A5Ø.39
  tuberculous A18.54
Keratoma L57.Ø
  palmaris and plantaris hereditarium Q82.8
  senile L57.Ø
Keratomalacia H18.44- ☑
  vitamin A deficiency E5Ø.4
Keratomegaly Q13.4
Keratomycosis B49
  nigrans, nigricans (palmaris) B36.1
Keratopathy H18.9
  band H18.42- ☑
  bullous (aphakic), following cataract surgery H59.Ø1- ☑
  bullous H18.1- ☑
Keratoscleritis, tuberculous A18.52
Keratosis L57.Ø
  actinic L57.Ø
  arsenical L85.8
  congenital, specified NEC Q8Ø.8
  female genital NEC N94.89
  follicularis Q82.8
    acquired L11.Ø
    congenita Q82.8
    et parafollicularis in cutem penetrans L87.Ø
    spinulosa (decalvans) Q82.8
    vitamin A deficiency E5Ø.8
  gonococcal A54.89
  lichenoid L82.Ø
  male genital (external) N5Ø.89
  nigricans L83
  obturans, external ear (canal) — *see* Cholesteatoma, external ear
  palmaris et plantaris (inherited) (symmetrical) Q82.8
    acquired L85.1
  penile N48.89
  pharynx J39.2
  pilaris, acquired L85.8
  punctata (palmaris et plantaris) L85.2
  scrotal N5Ø.89
  seborrheic L82.1
    inflamed L82.Ø
  senile L57.Ø
  solar L57.Ø
  tonsillaris J35.8
  vagina N89.4
  vegetans Q82.8
  vitamin A deficiency E5Ø.8
  vocal cord J38.3
Kerato-uveitis — *see* Iridocyclitis
Kerion (celsi) B35.Ø
Kernicterus of newborn (not due to isoimmunization) P57.9
  due to isoimmunization (conditions in P55.Ø-P55.9) P57.Ø
  specified type NEC P57.8
Kerunoparalysis T75.Ø9 ☑
Keshan disease E59
Ketoacidosis E87.29
  diabetic — *see* Diabetes, by type, with ketoacidosis
Ketonuria R82.4
Ketosis NEC E88.89
  diabetic — *see* Diabetes, by type, with ketoacidosis
Kew Garden fever A79.1
Kidney — *see* condition

Kienbock's disease — *see also* Osteochondrosis, juvenile, hand, carpal lunate
  adult M93.1
Kimmelstiel (-Wilson) **disease** — *see* Diabetes, Kimmelstiel (-Wilson) disease
Kink, kinking
  artery I77.1
  hair (acquired) L67.8
  ileum or intestine — *see* Obstruction, intestine
  Lane's — *see* Obstruction, intestine
  organ or site, congenital NEC — *see* Anomaly, by site
  ureter (pelvic junction) N13.5
    with
      hydronephrosis N13.1
        with infection N13.6
      pyelonephritis (chronic) N11.1
    congenital Q62.39
  vein(s) I87.8
    caval I87.1
    peripheral I87.1
Kinnier Wilson's disease (hepatolenticular degeneration) E83.Ø1
Kissing spine M48.2Ø
  cervical region M48.22
  cervicothoracic region M48.23
  lumbar region M48.26
  lumbosacral region M48.27
  occipito-atlanto-axial region M48.21
  thoracic region M48.24
  thoracolumbar region M48.25
Klatskin's tumor C22.1
Klauder's disease A26.8
Klebs' disease — *see also* Glomerulonephritis NØ5- ☑
Klebsiella (K.) **pneumoniae, as cause of disease classified elsewhere** B96.1
Kleeblattschaedel skull Q75.Ø51
Klein (e)-**Levin syndrome** G47.13
Kleptomania F63.2
Klinefelter's syndrome Q98.4
  karyotype 47,XXY Q98.Ø
  male with more than two X chromosomes Q98.1
Klippel-Feil deficiency, disease, or syndrome (brevicollis) Q76.1
Klippel's disease I67.2
Klippel-Trenaunay (-Weber) **syndrome** Q87.2
Klumpke (-Dejerine) **palsy, paralysis** (birth) (newborn) P14.1
Knee — *see* condition
Knock knee (acquired) M21.Ø6- ☑
  congenital Q74.1
Knot(s)
  intestinal, syndrome (volvulus) K56.2
  surfer S89.8- ☑
  umbilical cord (true) O69.2 ☑
Knotting (of)
  hair L67.8
  intestine K56.2
Knuckle pad (Garrod's) M72.1
Koch's
  infection — *see* Tuberculosis
  relapsing fever A68.9
Koch-Weeks' conjunctivitis — *see* Conjunctivitis, acute, mucopurulent
Koebner's syndrome Q81.8
Koenig's disease (osteochondritis dissecans) — *see* Osteochondritis, dissecans
Kohler-Pellegrini-Steida disease or syndrome (calcification, knee joint) — *see* Bursitis, tibial collateral
Kohler's disease
  patellar — *see* Osteochondrosis, juvenile, patella
  tarsal navicular — *see* Osteochondrosis, juvenile, tarsus
Koilonychia L6Ø.3
  congenital Q84.6
Kojevnikov's, epilepsy — *see* Kozhevnikof's epilepsy
Koplik's spots BØ5.9
Kopp's asthma E32.8
Korsakoff's (Wernicke) **disease, psychosis or syndrome** (alcoholic) F1Ø.96
  with dependence F1Ø.26
  drug-induced
    due to drug abuse — *see* Abuse, drug, by type, with amnestic disorder
    due to drug dependence — *see* Dependence, drug, by type, with amnestic disorder
  nonalcoholic FØ4
Korsakov's disease, psychosis or syndrome — *see* Korsakoff's disease

- **Korsakow's disease, psychosis or syndrome** — *see* Korsakoff's disease
- **Kostmann's disease or syndrome** (infantile genetic agranulocytosis) — *see* Agranulocytosis
- **Kozhevnikof's epilepsy** G40.109
  - intractable G40.119
    - with status epilepticus G40.111
    - without status epilepticus G40.119
  - not intractable G40.109
    - with status epilepticus G40.101
    - without status epilepticus G40.109
- **Krabbe's**
  - disease E75.23
  - syndrome, congenital muscle hypoplasia Q79.8
- **Kraepelin-Morel disease** — *see* Schizophrenia
- **Kraft-Weber-Dimitri disease** Q85.89
- **Kraurosis**
  - ani K62.89
  - penis N48.0
  - vagina N89.8
  - vulva N90.4
- **Kreotoxism** A05.9
- **Krukenberg's**
  - spindle — *see* Pigmentation, cornea, posterior
  - tumor C79.6- ☑
- **Kufs' disease** E75.4
- **Kugelberg-Welander disease** G12.1
- **Kuhnt-Junius degeneration** — *see also* Degeneration, macula H35.32- ☑
- **Kummell's disease or spondylitis** — *see* Spondylopathy, traumatic
- **Kupffer cell sarcoma** C22.3
- **Kuru** A81.81
- **Kussmaul's**
  - disease M30.0
  - respiration E87.29
    - in diabetic acidosis — *see* Diabetes, by type, with ketoacidosis
- **Kwashiorkor** E40
  - marasmic, marasmus type E42
- **Kyasanur Forest disease** A98.2
- **Kyphoscoliosis, kyphoscoliotic** (acquired) — *see also* Scoliosis M41.9
  - congenital Q67.5
  - heart (disease) I27.1
  - sequelae of rickets E64.3
  - tuberculous A18.01
- **Kyphosis, kyphotic** (acquired) M40.209
  - cervical region M40.202
  - cervicothoracic region M40.203
  - congenital Q76.419
    - cervical region Q76.412
    - cervicothoracic region Q76.413
    - occipito-atlanto-axial region Q76.411
    - thoracic region Q76.414
    - thoracolumbar region Q76.415
  - Morquio-Brailsford type (spinal) — *see also* subcategory M49.8 E76.219
  - postlaminectomy M96.3
  - postradiation therapy M96.2
  - postural (adolescent) M40.00
    - cervicothoracic region M40.03
    - thoracic region M40.04
    - thoracolumbar region M40.05
  - secondary NEC M40.10
    - cervical region M40.12
    - cervicothoracic region M40.13
    - thoracic region M40.14
    - thoracolumbar region M40.15
  - sequelae of rickets E64.3
  - specified type NEC M40.299
    - cervical region M40.292
    - cervicothoracic region M40.293
    - thoracic region M40.294
    - thoracolumbar region M40.295
  - syphilitic, congenital A50.56
  - thoracic region M40.204
  - thoracolumbar region M40.205
  - tuberculous A18.01
- **Kyrle disease** L87.0

L

- **Labia, labium** — *see* condition
- **Labile**
  - blood pressure R09.89
  - vasomotor system I73.9
- **Labioglossal paralysis** G12.29
- **Labium leporinum** — *see* Cleft, lip
- **Labor** — *see* Delivery
- **Labored breathing** — *see* Hyperventilation
- **Labyrinthitis** (circumscribed) (destructive) (diffuse) (inner ear) (latent) (purulent) (suppurative) — *see also* subcategory H83.0 ☑
  - syphilitic A52.79
- **Laceration**
  - with abortion — *see* Abortion, by type, complicated by laceration of pelvic organs
  - abdomen, abdominal
    - wall S31.119 ☑
      - with
        - foreign body S31.129 ☑
        - penetration into peritoneal cavity S31.619 ☑
          - with foreign body S31.629 ☑
      - epigastric region S31.112 ☑
        - with
          - foreign body S31.122 ☑
          - penetration into peritoneal cavity S31.612 ☑
            - with foreign body S31.622 ☑
      - left
        - lower quadrant S31.114 ☑
          - with
            - foreign body S31.124 ☑
            - penetration into peritoneal cavity S31.614 ☑
              - with foreign body S31.624 ☑
        - upper quadrant S31.111 ☑
          - with
            - foreign body S31.121 ☑
            - penetration into peritoneal cavity S31.611 ☑
              - with foreign body S31.621 ☑
      - periumbilic region S31.115 ☑
        - with
          - foreign body S31.125 ☑
          - penetration into peritoneal cavity S31.615 ☑
            - with foreign body S31.625 ☑
      - right
        - lower quadrant S31.113 ☑
          - with
            - foreign body S31.123 ☑
            - penetration into peritoneal cavity S31.613 ☑
              - with foreign body S31.623 ☑
        - upper quadrant S31.110 ☑
          - with
            - foreign body S31.120 ☑
            - penetration into peritoneal cavity S31.610 ☑
              - with foreign body S31.620 ☑
  - accidental, complicating surgery — *see* Complications, surgical, accidental puncture or laceration
  - Achilles tendon S86.02- ☑
  - adrenal gland S37.813 ☑
  - alveolar (process) — *see* Laceration, oral cavity
  - ankle S91.01- ☑
    - with
      - foreign body S91.02- ☑
  - antecubital space — *see* Laceration, elbow
  - anus (sphincter) S31.831 ☑
    - with
      - ectopic or molar pregnancy O08.6
      - foreign body S31.832 ☑
    - complicating delivery — *see* Delivery, complicated, by, laceration, anus (sphincter)
    - following ectopic or molar pregnancy O08.6
    - nontraumatic, nonpuerperal — *see* Fissure, anus
  - arm (upper) S41.11- ☑
    - with foreign body S41.12- ☑
    - lower — *see* Laceration, forearm
  - auditory canal (external) (meatus) — *see* Laceration, ear
  - auricle, ear — *see* Laceration, ear
  - axilla — *see* Laceration, arm
  - back — *see also* Laceration, thorax, back
    - lower S31.010 ☑
      - with
        - foreign body S31.020 ☑
          - with penetration into retroperitoneal space S31.021 ☑
        - penetration into retroperitoneal space S31.011 ☑
  - bile duct S36.13 ☑

- **Laceration** — *continued*
  - bladder S37.23 ☑
    - with ectopic or molar pregnancy O08.6
    - following ectopic or molar pregnancy O08.6
    - obstetrical trauma O71.5
  - blood vessel — *see* Injury, blood vessel
  - bowel — *see also* Laceration, intestine
    - with ectopic or molar pregnancy O08.6
    - complicating abortion — *see* Abortion, by type, complicated by, specified condition NEC
    - following ectopic or molar pregnancy O08.6
    - obstetrical trauma O71.5
  - brain (any part) (cortex) (diffuse) (membrane) — *see also* Injury, intracranial, diffuse
    - during birth P10.8
      - with hemorrhage P10.1
    - focal — *see* Injury, intracranial, focal brain injury
  - brainstem S06.38- ☑
  - breast S21.01- ☑
    - with foreign body S21.02- ☑
  - broad ligament S37.893 ☑
    - with ectopic or molar pregnancy O08.6
    - following ectopic or molar pregnancy O08.6
    - laceration syndrome N83.8
    - obstetrical trauma O71.6
    - syndrome (laceration) N83.8
  - buttock S31.801 ☑
    - with foreign body S31.802 ☑
    - left S31.821 ☑
      - with foreign body S31.822 ☑
    - right S31.811 ☑
      - with foreign body S31.812 ☑
  - calf — *see* Laceration, leg
  - canaliculus lacrimalis — *see* Laceration, eyelid
  - canthus, eye — *see* Laceration, eyelid
  - capsule, joint — *see* Sprain
  - causing eversion of cervix uteri (old) N86
  - central (perineal), complicating delivery O70.9
  - cerebellum, traumatic S06.37- ☑
  - cerebral S06.33- ☑
    - during birth P10.8
      - with hemorrhage P10.1
    - left side S06.32- ☑
    - right side S06.31- ☑
  - cervix (uteri)
    - with ectopic or molar pregnancy O08.6
    - following ectopic or molar pregnancy O08.6
    - nonpuerperal, nontraumatic N88.1
    - obstetrical trauma (current) O71.3
    - old (postpartal) N88.1
    - traumatic S37.63 ☑
  - cheek (external) S01.41- ☑
    - with foreign body S01.42- ☑
    - internal — *see* Laceration, oral cavity
  - chest wall — *see* Laceration, thorax
  - chin — *see* Laceration, head, specified site NEC
  - chordae tendinae NEC I51.1
    - concurrent with acute myocardial infarction — *see* Infarct, myocardium
    - following acute myocardial infarction (current complication) I23.4
  - clitoris — *see* Laceration, vulva
  - colon — *see* Laceration, intestine, large, colon
  - common bile duct S36.13 ☑
  - cortex (cerebral) — *see* Injury, intracranial, diffuse
  - costal region — *see* Laceration, thorax
  - cystic duct S36.13 ☑
  - diaphragm S27.803 ☑
  - digit(s)
    - foot — *see* Laceration, toe
    - hand — *see* Laceration, finger
  - duodenum S36.430 ☑
  - ear (canal) (external) S01.31- ☑
    - with foreign body S01.32- ☑
    - drum S09.2- ☑
  - elbow S51.01- ☑
    - with
      - foreign body S51.02- ☑
  - epididymis — *see* Laceration, testis
  - epigastric region — *see* Laceration, abdomen, wall, epigastric region
  - esophagus K22.89
    - traumatic
      - cervical S11.21 ☑
        - with foreign body S11.22 ☑
      - thoracic S27.813 ☑
  - eye (ball) S05.3- ☑

- **Laceration** — *continued*
  - eye — *continued*
    - with prolapse or loss of intraocular tissue SØ5.2- ☑
    - penetrating SØ5.6- ☑
  - eyebrow — *see* Laceration, eyelid
  - eyelid SØ1.11- ☑
    - with foreign body SØ1.12- ☑
  - face NEC — *see* Laceration, head, specified site NEC
  - fallopian tube S37.539 ☑
    - bilateral S37.532 ☑
    - unilateral S37.531 ☑
  - finger(s) S61.219 ☑
    - with
      - damage to nail S61.319 ☑
        - with
          - foreign body S61.329 ☑
      - foreign body S61.229 ☑
    - index S61.218 ☑
      - with
        - damage to nail S61.318 ☑
          - with
            - foreign body S61.328 ☑
        - foreign body S61.228 ☑
      - left S61.211 ☑
        - with
          - damage to nail S61.311 ☑
            - with
              - foreign body S61.321 ☑
          - foreign body S61.221 ☑
      - right S61.21Ø ☑
        - with
          - damage to nail S61.31Ø ☑
            - with
              - foreign body S61.32Ø ☑
          - foreign body S61.22Ø ☑
    - little S61.218 ☑
      - with
        - damage to nail S61.318 ☑
          - with
            - foreign body S61.328 ☑
        - foreign body S61.228 ☑
      - left S61.217 ☑
        - with
          - damage to nail S61.317 ☑
            - with
              - foreign body S61.327 ☑
          - foreign body S61.227 ☑
      - right S61.216 ☑
        - with
          - damage to nail S61.316 ☑
            - with
              - foreign body S61.326 ☑
          - foreign body S61.226 ☑
    - middle S61.218 ☑
      - with
        - damage to nail S61.318 ☑
          - with
            - foreign body S61.328 ☑
        - foreign body S61.228 ☑
      - left S61.213 ☑
        - with
          - damage to nail S61.313 ☑
            - with
              - foreign body S61.323 ☑
          - foreign body S61.223 ☑
      - right S61.212 ☑
        - with
          - damage to nail S61.312 ☑
            - with
              - foreign body S61.322 ☑
          - foreign body S61.222 ☑
    - ring S61.218 ☑
      - with
        - damage to nail S61.318 ☑
          - with
            - foreign body S61.328 ☑
        - foreign body S61.228 ☑
      - left S61.215 ☑
        - with
          - damage to nail S61.315 ☑
            - with
              - foreign body S61.325 ☑
          - foreign body S61.225 ☑
      - right S61.214 ☑
        - with
          - damage to nail S61.314 ☑

- **Laceration** — *continued*
  - finger(s) — *continued*
    - ring — *continued*
      - right — *continued*
        - with — *continued*
          - damage to nail — *continued*
            - with
              - foreign body S61.324 ☑
          - foreign body S61.224 ☑
  - flank S31.119 ☑
    - with foreign body S31.129 ☑
  - foot (except toe(s) alone) S91.319 ☑
    - with foreign body S91.329 ☑
    - left S91.312 ☑
      - with foreign body S91.322 ☑
    - right S91.311 ☑
      - with foreign body S91.321 ☑
    - toe — *see* Laceration, toe
  - forearm S51.819 ☑
    - with
      - foreign body S51.829 ☑
    - elbow only — *see* Laceration, elbow
    - left S51.812 ☑
      - with
        - foreign body S51.822 ☑
    - right S51.811 ☑
      - with
        - foreign body S51.821 ☑
  - forehead SØ1.81 ☑
    - with foreign body SØ1.82 ☑
  - fourchette O7Ø.Ø
    - with ectopic or molar pregnancy OØ8.6
    - complicating delivery O7Ø.Ø
    - following ectopic or molar pregnancy OØ8.6
  - gallbladder S36.123 ☑
  - genital organs, external
    - female S31.512 ☑
      - with foreign body S31.522 ☑
      - vagina — *see* Laceration, vagina
      - vulva — *see* Laceration, vulva
    - male S31.511 ☑
      - with foreign body S31.521 ☑
      - penis — *see* Laceration, penis
      - scrotum — *see* Laceration, scrotum
      - testis — *see* Laceration, testis
  - groin — *see* Laceration, abdomen, wall
  - gum — *see* Laceration, oral cavity
  - hand S61.419 ☑
    - with
      - foreign body S61.429 ☑
    - finger — *see* Laceration, finger
    - left S61.412 ☑
      - with
        - foreign body S61.422 ☑
    - right S61.411 ☑
      - with
        - foreign body S61.421 ☑
    - thumb — *see* Laceration, thumb
  - head SØ1.91 ☑
    - with foreign body SØ1.92 ☑
    - cheek — *see* Laceration, cheek
    - ear — *see* Laceration, ear
    - eyelid — *see* Laceration, eyelid
    - lip — *see* Laceration, lip
    - nose — *see* Laceration, nose
    - oral cavity — *see* Laceration, oral cavity
    - scalp SØ1.Ø1 ☑
      - with foreign body SØ1.Ø2 ☑
    - specified site NEC SØ1.81 ☑
      - with foreign body SØ1.82 ☑
    - temporomandibular area — *see* Laceration, cheek
  - heart — *see* Injury, heart, laceration
  - heel — *see* Laceration, foot
  - hepatic duct S36.13 ☑
  - hip S71.Ø19 ☑
    - with foreign body S71.Ø29 ☑
    - left S71.Ø12 ☑
      - with foreign body S71.Ø22 ☑
    - right S71.Ø11 ☑
      - with foreign body S71.Ø21 ☑
  - hymen — *see* Laceration, vagina
  - hypochondrium — *see* Laceration, abdomen, wall
  - hypogastric region — *see* Laceration, abdomen, wall
  - ileum S36.438 ☑
  - inguinal region — *see* Laceration, abdomen, wall
  - instep — *see* Laceration, foot

- **Laceration** — *continued*
  - internal organ — *see* Injury, by site
  - interscapular region — *see* Laceration, thorax, back
  - intestine
    - large
      - colon S36.539 ☑
        - ascending S36.53Ø ☑
        - descending S36.532 ☑
        - sigmoid S36.533 ☑
        - specified site NEC S36.538 ☑
      - rectum S36.63 ☑
        - transverse S36.531 ☑
    - small S36.439 ☑
      - duodenum S36.43Ø ☑
      - specified site NEC S36.438 ☑
  - intra-abdominal organ S36.93 ☑
    - intestine — *see* Laceration, intestine
    - liver — *see* Laceration, liver
    - pancreas — *see* Laceration, pancreas
    - peritoneum S36.81 ☑
    - specified site NEC S36.893 ☑
    - spleen — *see* Laceration, spleen
    - stomach — *see* Laceration, stomach
  - intracranial NEC — *see also* Injury, intracranial, diffuse
    - birth injury P1Ø.9
  - jaw — *see* Laceration, head, specified site NEC
  - jejunum S36.438 ☑
  - joint capsule — *see* Sprain, by site
  - kidney S37.Ø3- ☑
    - major (greater than 3 cm) (massive) (stellate) S37.Ø6- ☑
    - minor (less than 1 cm) S37.Ø4- ☑
    - moderate (1 to 3 cm) S37.Ø5- ☑
      - multiple S37.Ø6- ☑
  - knee S81.Ø1- ☑
    - with foreign body S81.Ø2- ☑
  - labium (majus) (minus) — *see* Laceration, vulva
  - lacrimal duct — *see* Laceration, eyelid
  - large intestine — *see* Laceration, intestine, large
  - larynx S11.Ø11 ☑
    - with foreign body S11.Ø12 ☑
  - leg (lower) S81.819 ☑
    - with foreign body S81.829 ☑
    - foot — *see* Laceration, foot
    - knee — *see* Laceration, knee
    - left S81.812 ☑
      - with foreign body S81.822 ☑
    - right S81.811 ☑
      - with foreign body S81.821 ☑
    - upper — *see* Laceration, thigh
  - ligament — *see* Sprain
  - lip SØ1.511 ☑
    - with foreign body SØ1.521 ☑
  - liver S36.113 ☑
    - major (stellate) S36.116 ☑
    - minor S36.114 ☑
    - moderate S36.115 ☑
  - loin — *see* Laceration, abdomen, wall
  - lower back — *see* Laceration, back, lower
  - lumbar region — *see* Laceration, back, lower
  - lung S27.339 ☑
    - bilateral S27.332 ☑
    - unilateral S27.331 ☑
  - malar region — *see* Laceration, head, specified site NEC
  - mammary — *see* Laceration, breast
  - mastoid region — *see* Laceration, head, specified site NEC
  - meninges — *see* Injury, intracranial, diffuse
  - meniscus — *see* Tear, meniscus
  - mesentery S36.893 ☑
  - mesosalpinx S37.893 ☑
  - mouth — *see* Laceration, oral cavity
  - muscle — *see* Injury, muscle, by site, laceration
  - nail
    - finger — *see* Laceration, finger, with damage to nail
    - toe — *see* Laceration, toe, with damage to nail
  - nasal (septum) (sinus) — *see* Laceration, nose
  - nasopharynx — *see* Laceration, head, specified site NEC
  - neck S11.91 ☑
    - with foreign body S11.92 ☑
    - involving
      - cervical esophagus S11.21 ☑
        - with foreign body S11.22 ☑
      - larynx — *see* Laceration, larynx
      - pharynx — *see* Laceration, pharynx

- **Laceration** — *continued*
  - neck — *continued*
    - involving — *continued*
      - thyroid gland — *see* Laceration, thyroid gland
      - trachea — *see* Laceration, trachea
    - specified site NEC S11.81 ☑
      - with foreign body S11.82 ☑
  - nerve — *see* Injury, nerve
  - nose (septum) (sinus) SØ1.21 ☑
    - with foreign body SØ1.22 ☑
  - ocular NOS SØ5.3- ☑
    - adnexa NOS SØ1.11- ☑
  - oral cavity SØ1.512 ☑
    - with foreign body SØ1.522 ☑
  - orbit (eye) — *see* Wound, open, ocular, orbit
  - ovary S37.439 ☑
    - bilateral S37.432 ☑
    - unilateral S37.431 ☑
  - palate — *see* Laceration, oral cavity
  - palm — *see* Laceration, hand
  - pancreas S36.239 ☑
  - pelvic S31.Ø1Ø ☑
    - with
      - foreign body S31.Ø2Ø ☑
        - penetration into retroperitoneal cavity S31.Ø21 ☑
      - penetration into retroperitoneal cavity S31.Ø11 ☑
    - floor — *see also* Laceration, back, lower
      - with ectopic or molar pregnancy OØ8.6
      - complicating delivery O7Ø.1
      - following ectopic or molar pregnancy OØ8.6
      - old (postpartal) N81.89
    - organ S37.93 ☑
  - penis S31.21 ☑
    - with foreign body S31.22 ☑
  - perineum
    - female S31.41 ☑
      - with
        - ectopic or molar pregnancy OØ8.6
        - foreign body S31.42 ☑
      - during delivery O7Ø.9
        - first degree O7Ø.Ø
        - fourth degree O7Ø.3
        - second degree O7Ø.1
        - third degree — *see also* Delivery, complicated, by, laceration, perineum, third degree O7Ø.2Ø
      - old (postpartal) N81.89
      - postpartal N81.89
      - secondary (postpartal) O9Ø.1
    - male S31.119 ☑
      - with foreign body S31.129 ☑
  - periocular area (with or without lacrimal passages) — *see* Laceration, eyelid
  - peritoneum S36.893 ☑
  - periumbilic region — *see* Laceration, abdomen, wall, periumbilic
  - periurethral tissue — *see* Laceration, urethra
  - phalanges
    - finger — *see* Laceration, finger
    - toe — *see* Laceration, toe
  - pharynx S11.21 ☑
    - with foreign body S11.22 ☑
  - pinna — *see* Laceration, ear
  - popliteal space — *see* Laceration, knee
  - prepuce — *see* Laceration, penis
  - prostate S37.823 ☑
  - pubic region S31.119 ☑
    - with foreign body S31.129 ☑
  - pudendum — *see* Laceration, genital organs, external
  - rectovaginal septum — *see* Laceration, vagina
  - rectum S36.63 ☑
  - retroperitoneum S36.893 ☑
  - round ligament S37.893 ☑
  - sacral region — *see* Laceration, back, lower
  - sacroiliac region — *see* Laceration, back, lower
  - salivary gland — *see* Laceration, oral cavity
  - scalp SØ1.Ø1 ☑
    - with foreign body SØ1.Ø2 ☑
  - scapular region — *see* Laceration, shoulder
  - scrotum S31.31 ☑
    - with foreign body S31.32 ☑
  - seminal vesicle S37.893 ☑
  - shin — *see* Laceration, leg
  - shoulder S41.Ø19 ☑

- **Laceration** — *continued*
  - shoulder — *continued*
    - with foreign body S41.Ø29 ☑
    - left S41.Ø12 ☑
      - with foreign body S41.Ø22 ☑
    - right S41.Ø11 ☑
      - with foreign body S41.Ø21 ☑
  - small intestine — *see* Laceration, intestine, small
  - spermatic cord — *see* Laceration, testis
  - spinal cord (meninges) — *see also* Injury, spinal cord, by region
    - due to injury at birth P11.5
    - newborn (birth injury) P11.5
  - spleen S36.Ø39 ☑
    - major (massive) (stellate) S36.Ø32 ☑
    - moderate S36.Ø31 ☑
    - superficial (minor) S36.Ø3Ø ☑
  - sternal region — *see* Laceration, thorax, front
  - stomach S36.33 ☑
  - submaxillary region — *see* Laceration, head, specified site NEC
  - submental region — *see* Laceration, head, specified site NEC
  - subungual
    - finger(s) — *see* Laceration, finger, with damage to nail
    - toe(s) — *see* Laceration, toe, with damage to nail
  - suprarenal gland — *see* Laceration, adrenal gland
  - temple, temporal region — *see* Laceration, head, specified site NEC
  - temporomandibular area — *see* Laceration, cheek
  - tendon — *see* Injury, muscle, by site, laceration
    - Achilles S86.Ø2- ☑
  - tentorium cerebelli — *see* Injury, intracranial, diffuse
  - testis S31.31 ☑
    - with foreign body S31.32 ☑
  - thigh S71.11- ☑
    - with foreign body S71.12- ☑
  - thorax, thoracic (wall) S21.91 ☑
    - with foreign body S21.92 ☑
      - back S21.22- ☑
        - with penetration into thoracic cavity S21.42- ☑
      - front S21.12- ☑
        - with penetration into thoracic cavity S21.32- ☑
    - back S21.21- ☑
      - with
        - foreign body S21.22- ☑
          - with penetration into thoracic cavity S21.42- ☑
        - penetration into thoracic cavity S21.41- ☑
    - breast — *see* Laceration, breast
    - front S21.11- ☑
      - with
        - foreign body S21.12- ☑
          - with penetration into thoracic cavity S21.32- ☑
        - penetration into thoracic cavity S21.31- ☑
  - thumb S61.Ø19 ☑
    - with
      - damage to nail S61.119 ☑
        - with
          - foreign body S61.129 ☑
      - foreign body S61.Ø29 ☑
    - left S61.Ø12 ☑
      - with
        - damage to nail S61.112 ☑
          - with
            - foreign body S61.122 ☑
        - foreign body S61.Ø22 ☑
    - right S61.Ø11 ☑
      - with
        - damage to nail S61.111 ☑
          - with
            - foreign body S61.121 ☑
        - foreign body S61.Ø21 ☑
  - thyroid gland S11.11 ☑
    - with foreign body S11.12 ☑
  - toe(s) S91.119 ☑
    - with
      - damage to nail S91.219 ☑
        - with
          - foreign body S91.229 ☑
      - foreign body S91.129 ☑
    - great S91.113 ☑

- **Laceration** — *continued*
  - toe(s) — *continued*
    - great — *continued*
      - with
        - damage to nail S91.213 ☑
          - with
            - foreign body S91.223 ☑
        - foreign body S91.123 ☑
      - left S91.112 ☑
        - with
          - damage to nail S91.212 ☑
            - with
              - foreign body S91.222 ☑
          - foreign body S91.122 ☑
      - right S91.111 ☑
        - with
          - damage to nail S91.211 ☑
            - with
              - foreign body S91.221 ☑
          - foreign body S91.121 ☑
    - lesser S91.116 ☑
      - with
        - damage to nail S91.216 ☑
          - with
            - foreign body S91.226 ☑
        - foreign body S91.126 ☑
      - left S91.115 ☑
        - with
          - damage to nail S91.215 ☑
            - with
              - foreign body S91.225 ☑
          - foreign body S91.125 ☑
      - right S91.114 ☑
        - with
          - damage to nail S91.214 ☑
            - with
              - foreign body S91.224 ☑
          - foreign body S91.124 ☑
  - tongue — *see* Laceration, oral cavity
  - trachea S11.Ø21 ☑
    - with foreign body S11.Ø22 ☑
  - tunica vaginalis — *see* Laceration, testis
  - tympanum, tympanic membrane — *see* Laceration, ear, drum
  - umbilical region S31.115 ☑
    - with foreign body S31.125 ☑
  - ureter S37.13 ☑
  - urethra S37.33 ☑
    - with or following ectopic or molar pregnancy OØ8.6
    - obstetrical trauma O71.5
  - urinary organ NEC S37.893 ☑
  - uterus S37.63 ☑
    - with ectopic or molar pregnancy OØ8.6
    - following ectopic or molar pregnancy OØ8.6
    - nonpuerperal, nontraumatic N85.8
    - obstetrical trauma NEC O71.81
    - old (postpartal) N85.8
  - uvula — *see* Laceration, oral cavity
  - vagina S31.41 ☑
    - with
      - ectopic or molar pregnancy OØ8.6
      - foreign body S31.42 ☑
    - during delivery O71.4
      - with perineal laceration — *see* Laceration, perineum, female, during delivery
    - following ectopic or molar pregnancy OØ8.6
    - nonpuerperal, nontraumatic N89.8
    - old (postpartal) N89.8
  - vas deferens S37.893 ☑
  - vesical — *see* Laceration, bladder
  - vocal cords S11.Ø31 ☑
    - with foreign body S11.Ø32 ☑
  - vulva S31.41 ☑
    - with
      - ectopic or molar pregnancy OØ8.6
      - foreign body S31.42 ☑
    - complicating delivery O7Ø.Ø
    - following ectopic or molar pregnancy OØ8.6
    - nonpuerperal, nontraumatic N9Ø.89
    - old (postpartal) N9Ø.89
  - wrist S61.519 ☑
    - with
      - foreign body S61.529 ☑
    - left S61.512 ☑
      - with
        - foreign body S61.522 ☑
    - right S61.511 ☑

- **Laceration** — *continued*
  - wrist — *continued*
    - right — *continued*
      - with
        - foreign body S61.521 ☑
- **Lack of**
  - achievement in school Z55.3
  - adequate
    - food Z59.48
    - intermaxillary vertical dimension of fully erupted teeth M26.36
    - sleep Z72.82Ø
  - air conditioning Z59.11
  - appetite (see Anorexia) R63.Ø
  - awareness R41.9
  - basic services in physical environment Z58.81
  - care
    - in home Z74.2
    - of infant (at or after birth) T76.Ø2 ☑
      - confirmed T74.Ø2 ☑
  - cognitive functions R41.9
  - coordination R27.9
    - ataxia R27.Ø
    - specified type NEC R27.8
  - development (physiological) R62.5Ø
    - failure to thrive (child over 28 days old) R62.51
      - adult R62.7
      - newborn P92.6
    - short stature R62.52
    - specified type NEC R62.59
  - electricity services Z59.12
  - emotional support Z6Ø.8
  - energy R53.83
  - financial resources Z59.6
  - food Z59.48
  - gas services Z59.12
  - growth R62.52
  - heating Z59.11
  - housing (permanent) (temporary) Z59.ØØ
    - adequate Z59.1Ø
  - learning experiences in childhood Z62.898
  - leisure time (affecting life-style) Z73.2
  - material resources due to limited financial resources, specified NEC Z59.87
  - memory — *see also* Amnesia
    - mild, following organic brain damage FØ6.8
  - oil services Z59.12
  - ovulation N97.Ø
  - parental supervision or control of child Z62.Ø
  - person able to render necessary care Z74.2
  - physical exercise Z72.3
  - play experience in childhood Z62.898
  - posterior occlusal support M26.57
  - relaxation (affecting life-style) Z73.2
  - safe drinking water Z58.6
  - sexual
    - desire F52.Ø
    - enjoyment F52.1
  - shelter Z59.Ø2
  - sleep (adequate) Z72.82Ø
  - supervision of child by parent Z62.Ø
  - support, posterior occlusal M26.57
  - transportation Z59.82
  - water T73.1 ☑
    - safe drinking Z58.6
    - services Z59.12
- **Lacrimal** — *see* condition
- **Lacrimation, abnormal** — *see* Epiphora
- **Lacrimonasal duct** — *see* condition
- **Lactate, elevated** — *see* Acidosis, lactic
- **Lactation, lactating** (breast) (puerperal, postpartum)
  - associated
    - cracked nipple O92.13
    - retracted nipple O92.Ø3
  - defective O92.4
  - disorder NEC O92.79
  - excessive O92.6
  - failed (complete) O92.3
    - partial O92.4
  - mastitis NEC — *see* Mastitis, obstetric
  - mother (care and/or examination) Z39.1
  - nonpuerperal N64.3
- **Lacticemia, excessive** — *see also* Acidosis E87.2Ø
- **Lacunar skull** Q75.8
- **Laennec's cirrhosis** K7Ø.3Ø
  - with ascites K7Ø.31
  - nonalcoholic K74.69
- **Lafora disease** — *see also* Epilepsy, progressive, Lafora G4Ø.CØ9
- **Lag, lid** (nervous) — *see* Retraction, lid
- **Lagophthalmos** (eyelid) (nervous) HØ2.2Ø9
  - bilateral, upper and lower eyelids HØ2.2ØC
  - cicatricial HØ2.219
    - bilateral, upper and lower eyelids HØ2.21C
    - left HØ2.216
      - lower HØ2.215
      - upper HØ2.214
      - upper and lower eyelids HØ2.21B
    - right HØ2.213
      - lower HØ2.212
      - upper HØ2.211
      - upper and lower eyelids HØ2.21A
  - keratoconjunctivitis — *see* Keratoconjunctivitis
  - left HØ2.2Ø6
    - lower HØ2.2Ø5
    - upper HØ2.2Ø4
    - upper and lower eyelids HØ2.2ØB
  - mechanical HØ2.229
    - bilateral, upper and lower eyelids HØ2.22C
    - left HØ2.226
      - lower HØ2.225
      - upper HØ2.224
      - upper and lower eyelids HØ2.22B
    - right HØ2.223
      - lower HØ2.222
      - upper HØ2.221
      - upper and lower eyelids HØ2.22A
  - paralytic HØ2.239
    - bilateral, upper and lower eyelids HØ2.23C
    - left HØ2.236
      - lower HØ2.235
      - upper HØ2.234
      - upper and lower eyelids HØ2.23B
    - right HØ2.233
      - lower HØ2.232
      - upper HØ2.231
      - upper and lower eyelids HØ2.23A
  - right HØ2.2Ø3
    - lower HØ2.2Ø2
    - upper HØ2.2Ø1
    - upper and lower eyelids HØ2.2ØA
- **Laki-Lorand factor deficiency** — *see* Defect, coagulation, specified type NEC
- **Lalling** F8Ø.Ø
- **Lambert-Eaton syndrome** — *see* Syndrome, Lambert-Eaton
- **Lambliasis, lambliosis** AØ7.1
- **Landau-Kleffner syndrome** — *see* Epilepsy, specified NEC
- **Landouzy-Dejerine dystrophy or facioscapulohumeral atrophy** G71.Ø2
- **Landouzy's disease** (icterohemorrhagic leptospirosis) A27.Ø
- **Landry-Guillain-Barre, syndrome or paralysis** G61.Ø
- **Landry's disease or paralysis** G61.Ø
- **Lane's**
  - band Q43.3
  - kink — *see* Obstruction, intestine
  - syndrome K9Ø.2
- **Langdon Down syndrome** — *see* Trisomy, 21
- **Lapsed immunization schedule status** Z28.39
- **Large**
  - baby (regardless of gestational age) (4ØØØg to 4499g) PØ8.1
  - ear, congenital Q17.1
  - physiological cup Q14.2
  - stature R68.89
- **Large-for-dates NEC** (infant) (4ØØØg to 4499g) PØ8.1
  - affecting management of pregnancy O36.6- ☑
  - exceptionally (45ØØg or more) PØ8.Ø
- **Larsen-Johansson disease orosteochondrosis** — *see* Osteochondrosis, juvenile, patella
- **Larsen's syndrome** (flattened facies and multiple congenital dislocations) Q74.8
- **Larva migrans**
  - cutaneous B76.9
    - Ancylostoma B76.Ø
  - visceral B83.Ø
- **Laryngeal** — *see* condition
- **Laryngismus** (stridulus) J38.5
  - congenital P28.89
  - diphtheritic A36.2
- **Laryngitis** (acute) (edematous) (fibrinous) (infective) (infiltrative) (malignant) (membranous) (phlegmonous) (pneumococcal) (pseudomembranous) (septic) (subglottic) (suppurative) (ulcerative) JØ4.Ø
  - with
    - influenza, flu, or grippe — *see* Influenza, with, laryngitis
    - tracheitis (acute) — *see* Laryngotracheitis
  - atrophic J37.Ø
  - catarrhal J37.Ø
  - chronic J37.Ø
    - with tracheitis (chronic) J37.1
  - diphtheritic A36.2
  - due to external agent — *see* Inflammation, respiratory, upper, due to
  - H. influenzae JØ4.Ø
  - Hemophilus influenzae JØ4.Ø
  - hypertrophic J37.Ø
  - influenzal — *see* Influenza, with, respiratory manifestations NEC
  - obstructive JØ5.Ø
  - sicca J37.Ø
  - spasmodic JØ5.Ø
    - acute JØ4.Ø
  - streptococcal JØ4.Ø
  - stridulous JØ5.Ø
  - syphilitic (late) A52.73
    - congenital A5Ø.59 *[J99]*
      - early A5Ø.Ø3 *[J99]*
  - tuberculous A15.5
  - Vincent's A69.1
- **Laryngocele** (congenital) (ventricular) Q31.3
- **Laryngofissure** J38.7
  - congenital Q31.8
- **Laryngomalacia** (congenital) Q31.5
- **Laryngopharyngitis** (acute) JØ6.Ø
  - chronic J37.Ø
  - due to external agent — *see* Inflammation, respiratory, upper, due to
- **Laryngoplegia** J38.ØØ
  - bilateral J38.Ø2
  - unilateral J38.Ø1
- **Laryngoptosis** J38.7
- **Laryngospasm** J38.5
- **Laryngostenosis** J38.6
- **Laryngotracheitis** (acute) (Infectional) (infective) (viral) JØ4.2
  - atrophic J37.1
  - catarrhal J37.1
  - chronic J37.1
  - diphtheritic A36.2
  - due to external agent — *see* Inflammation, respiratory, upper, due to
  - Hemophilus influenzae JØ4.2
  - hypertrophic J37.1
  - influenzal — *see* Influenza, with, respiratory manifestations NEC
  - pachydermic J38.7
  - sicca J37.1
  - spasmodic J38.5
    - acute JØ5.Ø
  - streptococcal JØ4.2
  - stridulous J38.5
  - syphilitic (late) A52.73
    - congenital A5Ø.59 *[J99]*
      - early A5Ø.Ø3 *[J99]*
  - tuberculous A15.5
  - Vincent's A69.1
- **Laryngotracheobronchitis** — *see* Bronchitis
- **Larynx, laryngeal** — *see* condition
- **Lassa fever** A96.2
- **Lassitude** — *see* Weakness
- **Late**
  - talker R62.Ø
  - walker R62.Ø
- **Late effect**(s) — *see* Sequelae
- **Latent** — *see* condition
- **Laterocession** — *see* Lateroversion
- **Lateroflexion** — *see* Lateroversion
- **Lateroversion**
  - cervix — *see* Lateroversion, uterus
  - uterus, uterine (cervix) (postinfectional) (postpartal, old) N85.4
    - congenital Q51.818
    - in pregnancy or childbirth O34.59- ☑
- **Lathyrism** — *see* Poisoning, food, noxious, plant
- **Launois' syndrome** (pituitary gigantism) E22.Ø
- **Launois-Bensaude adenolipomatosis** E88.89

Laurence-Moon syndrome Q87.84
Lax, laxity — *see also* Relaxation
- ligament (ous) — *see also* Disorder, ligament
  - familial M35.7
  - knee — *see* Derangement, knee
- skin (acquired) L57.4
  - congenital Q82.8

Laxative habit F55.2
Lazy leukocyte syndrome D7Ø.8
Lead miner's lung J63.6
Leak, leakage
- air NEC J93.82
  - postprocedural J95.812
- amniotic fluid — *see* Rupture, membranes, premature
- blood (microscopic), fetal, into maternal circulation affecting management of pregnancy — *see* Pregnancy, complicated by
- cerebrospinal fluid G96.ØØ
  - cranial
    - postoperative G96.Ø8
    - specified NEC G96.Ø8
    - spontaneous G96.Ø1
    - traumatic G96.Ø8
  - from spinal (lumbar) puncture G97.Ø
  - spinal
    - postoperative G96.Ø9
    - post-traumatic G96.Ø9
    - specified NEC G96.Ø9
    - spontaneous G96.Ø2
  - spontaneous
    - from
      - skull base G96.Ø1
      - spine G96.Ø2
- CSF — *see* Leak, cerebrospinal fluid
- device, implant or graft — *see also* Complications, by site and type, mechanical
  - arterial graft NEC — *see* Complication, vascular, graft, mechanical, leakage T82.838 ☑
  - breast (implant) T85.43 ☑
  - catheter NEC T85.638 ☑
    - dialysis (renal) T82.43 ☑
      - intraperitoneal T85.631 ☑
    - infusion NEC T82.534 ☑
      - spinal (epidural) (subdural) T85.63Ø ☑
    - urinary T83.Ø38 ☑
      - cystostomy T83.Ø3Ø ☑
      - Hopkins T83.Ø38 ☑
      - ileostomy T83.Ø38 ☑
      - indwelling T83.Ø31 ☑
      - nephrostomy T83.Ø32 ☑
      - specified T83.Ø38 ☑
      - urostomy T83.Ø38 ☑
  - gastrointestinal — *see* Complications, prosthetic device, mechanical, gastrointestinal device
  - genital NEC T83.498 ☑
    - penile prosthesis (cylinder) (implanted) (pump) (reservoir) T83.49Ø ☑
    - testicular prosthesis T83.491 ☑
  - heart NEC — *see* Complication, cardiovascular device, mechanical
  - joint prosthesis — *see* Complications, joint prosthesis, mechanical, specified NEC, by site
  - ocular NEC — *see* Complications, prosthetic device, mechanical, ocular device
  - orthopedic NEC — *see* Complication, orthopedic, device, mechanical
  - persistent air J93.82
  - specified NEC T85.638 ☑
  - urinary NEC — *see also* Complication, genitourinary, device, urinary, mechanical
    - graft T83.23 ☑
  - vascular NEC — *see* Complication, cardiovascular device, mechanical
  - ventricular intracranial shunt T85.Ø3 ☑
- urine — *see* Incontinence

Leaky heart — *see* Endocarditis
Learning defect (specific) F81.9
Leather bottle stomach C16.9
Leber's
- congenital amaurosis H35.5Ø
- optic atrophy (hereditary) H47.22

Lederer's anemia D59.19
Leeches (external) — *see* Hirudiniasis
Leg — *see* condition
Legg (-Calve)-**Perthes disease, syndrome or osteochondrosis** M91.1- ☑
Legionellosis A48.1
- nonpneumonic A48.2

Legionnaires'
- disease A48.1
  - nonpneumonic A48.2
- pneumonia A48.1

Leigh's disease G31.82
Leiner's disease L21.1
Leiofibromyoma — *see* Leiomyoma
Leiomyoblastoma — *see* Neoplasm, connective tissue, benign
Leiomyofibroma — *see also* Neoplasm, connective tissue, benign
- uterus (cervix) (corpus) D25.9

Leiomyoma — *see also* Neoplasm, connective tissue, benign
- bizarre — *see* Neoplasm, connective tissue, benign
- cellular — *see* Neoplasm, connective tissue, benign
- epithelioid — *see* Neoplasm, connective tissue, benign
- uterus (cervix) (corpus) D25.9
  - intramural D25.1
  - submucous D25.Ø
  - subserosal D25.2
- vascular — *see* Neoplasm, connective tissue, benign

Leiomyoma, leiomyomatosis (intravascular) — *see* Neoplasm, connective tissue, uncertain behavior
Leiomyosarcoma — *see also* Neoplasm, connective tissue, malignant
- epithelioid — *see* Neoplasm, connective tissue, malignant
- myxoid — *see* Neoplasm, connective tissue, malignant

Leishmaniasis B55.9
- American (mucocutaneous) B55.2
  - cutaneous B55.1
- Asian Desert B55.1
- Brazilian B55.2
- cutaneous (any type) B55.1
- dermal — *see also* Leishmaniasis, cutaneous
  - post-kala-azar B55.Ø
- eyelid B55.1
- infantile B55.Ø
- Mediterranean B55.Ø
- mucocutaneous (American) (New World) B55.2
- naso-oral B55.2
- nasopharyngeal B55.2
- old world B55.1
- tegumentaria diffusa B55.1
- visceral B55.Ø

Leishmanoid, dermal — *see also* Leishmaniasis, cutaneous
- post-kala-azar B55.Ø

Lenegre's disease I44.2
Lengthening, leg — *see* Deformity, limb, unequal length
Lennert's lymphoma — *see* Lymphoma, Lennert's
Lennox-Gastaut syndrome G4Ø.812
- intractable G4Ø.814
  - with status epilepticus G4Ø.813
  - without status epilepticus G4Ø.814
- not intractable G4Ø.812
  - with status epilepticus G4Ø.811
  - without status epilepticus G4Ø.812

Lens — *see* condition
Lenticonus (anterior) (posterior) (congenital) Q12.8
Lenticular degeneration, progressive E83.Ø1
Lentiglobus (posterior) (congenital) Q12.8
Lentigo (congenital) L81.4
- maligna — *see also* Melanoma, in situ
  - melanoma — *see* Melanoma

Lentivirus, as cause of disease classified elsewhere B97.31
Leontiasis
- ossium M85.2
- syphilitic (late) A52.78
  - congenital A5Ø.59

Lepothrix A48.8
Lepra — *see* Leprosy
Leprechaunism E34.8
Leprosy A3Ø.- ☑
- with muscle disorder A3Ø.9 *[M63.8Ø]*
  - ankle A3Ø.9 *[M63.87-]* ☑
  - foot A3Ø.9 *[M63.87-]* ☑
  - forearm A3Ø.9 *[M63.83-]* ☑
  - hand A3Ø.9 *[M63.84-]* ☑
  - lower leg A3Ø.9 *[M63.86-]* ☑
  - multiple sites A3Ø.9 *[M63.89]*
  - pelvic region A3Ø.9 *[M63.85-]* ☑
  - shoulder region A3Ø.9 *[M63.81-]* ☑
  - specified site NEC A3Ø.9 *[M63.88]*
  - thigh A3Ø.9 *[M63.85-]* ☑
  - upper arm A3Ø.9 *[M63.82-]* ☑
- anesthetic A3Ø.9
- BB A3Ø.3
- BL A3Ø.4
- borderline (infiltrated) (neuritic) A3Ø.3
  - lepromatous A3Ø.4
  - tuberculoid A3Ø.2
- BT A3Ø.2
- dimorphous (infiltrated) (neuritic) A3Ø.3
- I A3Ø.Ø
- indeterminate (macular) (neuritic) A3Ø.Ø
- lepromatous (diffuse) (infiltrated) (macular) (neuritic) (nodular) A3Ø.5
- LL A3Ø.5
- macular (early) (neuritic) (simple) A3Ø.9
- maculoanesthetic A3Ø.9
- mixed A3Ø.3
- neural A3Ø.9
- nodular A3Ø.5
- primary neuritic A3Ø.3
- specified type NEC A3Ø.8
- TT A3Ø.1
- tuberculoid (major) (minor) A3Ø.1

Leptocytosis, hereditary D56.9
Leptomeningitis (chronic) (circumscribed) (hemorrhagic) (nonsuppurative) — *see* Meningitis
Leptomeningopathy G96.198
Leptospiral — *see* condition
Leptospirochetal — *see* condition
Leptospirosis A27.9
- canicola A27.89
- due to Leptospira interrogans serovar icterohaemorrhagiae A27.Ø
- icterohemorrhagica A27.Ø
- pomona A27.89
- Weil's disease A27.Ø

Leptus dermatitis B88.Ø
Leriche's syndrome (aortic bifurcation occlusion) I74.Ø9
Leri's pleonosteosis Q78.8
Leri-Weill syndrome Q77.8
Lermoyez' syndrome — *see* Vertigo, peripheral NEC
Lesch-Nyhan syndrome E79.1
Leser-Trélat disease L82.1
- inflamed L82.Ø

Lesion(s) (nontraumatic)
- abducens nerve — *see* Strabismus, paralytic, sixth nerve
- alveolar process KØ8.9
- angiocentric immunoproliferative D47.Z9 (*following* D47.4)
- anorectal K62.9
- aortic (valve) I35.9
- auditory nerve — *see* subcategory H93.3 ☑
- basal ganglion G25.9
- bile duct — *see* Disease, bile duct
- biomechanical M99.9
  - specified type NEC M99.89
    - abdomen M99.89
    - acromioclavicular M99.87
    - cervical region M99.81
    - cervicothoracic M99.81
    - costochondral M99.88
    - costovertebral M99.88
    - head region M99.8Ø
    - hip M99.85
    - lower extremity M99.86
    - lumbar region M99.83
    - lumbosacral M99.83
    - occipitocervical M99.8Ø
    - pelvic region M99.85
    - pubic M99.85
    - rib cage M99.88
    - sacral region M99.84
    - sacrococcygeal M99.84
    - sacroiliac M99.84
    - specified NEC M99.89
    - sternochondral M99.88
    - sternoclavicular M99.87
    - thoracic region M99.82
    - thoracolumbar M99.82
    - upper extremity M99.87
- bladder N32.9
- bone — *see* Disorder, bone
- brachial plexus G54.Ø
- brain G93.9

- **Lipochondrodystrophy** E76.Ø1
- **Lipochrome histiocytosis** (familial) D71
- **Lipodermatosclerosis** — *see also* Insufficiency, venous M79.3
  - with
    - varicose veins — *see* Varix, leg, with, inflammation
      - ulcerated — *see* Varix, leg, with, ulcer, with inflammation by site
  - ulcerated — *see* Ulcer, by site
- **Lipodystrophia progressiva** E88.1
- **Lipodystrophy** (progressive) E88.1
  - insulin E88.1
  - intestinal K9Ø.81
  - mesenteric K65.4
- **Lipofibroma** — *see* Lipoma
- **Lipofuscinosis, neuronal** (with ceroidosis) E75.4
- **Lipogranuloma, sclerosing** L92.8
- **Lipogranulomatosis** E78.89
- **Lipoid** — *see also* condition
  - histiocytosis D76.3
    - essential E75.29
  - nephrosis NØ4.9
  - proteinosis of Urbach E78.89
- **Lipoidemia** — *see* Hyperlipidemia
- **Lipoidosis** — *see* Lipidosis
- **Lipoma** D17.9
  - fetal D17.9
    - fat cell D17.9
  - infiltrating D17.9
  - intramuscular D17.9
  - pleomorphic D17.9
  - site classification
    - arms (skin) (subcutaneous) D17.2- ☑
    - connective tissue D17.3Ø
      - intra-abdominal D17.5
      - intrathoracic D17.4
      - peritoneum D17.79
      - retroperitoneum D17.79
      - specified site NEC D17.39
      - spermatic cord D17.6
    - face (skin) (subcutaneous) D17.Ø
    - genitourinary organ NEC D17.72
    - head (skin) (subcutaneous) D17.Ø
    - intra-abdominal D17.5
    - intrathoracic D17.4
    - kidney D17.71
    - legs (skin) (subcutaneous) D17.2- ☑
    - neck (skin) (subcutaneous) D17.Ø
    - peritoneum D17.79
    - retroperitoneum D17.79
    - skin D17.3Ø
      - specified site NEC D17.39
    - specified site NEC D17.79
    - spermatic cord D17.6
    - subcutaneous D17.3Ø
      - specified site NEC D17.39
    - trunk (skin) (subcutaneous) D17.1
    - unspecified D17.9
  - spindle cell D17.9
- **Lipomatosis** E88.2
  - dolorosa (Dercum) E88.2
  - fetal — *see* Lipoma
  - Launois-Bensaude E88.89
- **Lipomyoma** — *see* Lipoma
- **Lipomyxoma** — *see* Lipoma
- **Lipomyxosarcoma** — *see* Neoplasm, connective tissue, malignant
- **Lipoprotein metabolism disorder** E78.9
- **Lipoproteinemia** E78.5
  - broad-beta E78.2
  - floating-beta E78.2
  - hyper-pre-beta E78.1
- **Liposarcoma** — *see also* Neoplasm, connective tissue, malignant
  - dedifferentiated — *see* Neoplasm, connective tissue, malignant
  - differentiated type — *see* Neoplasm, connective tissue, malignant
  - embryonal — *see* Neoplasm, connective tissue, malignant
  - mixed type — *see* Neoplasm, connective tissue, malignant
  - myxoid — *see* Neoplasm, connective tissue, malignant
  - pleomorphic — *see* Neoplasm, connective tissue, malignant
  - round cell — *see* Neoplasm, connective tissue, malignant
- **Liposarcoma** — *continued*
  - well differentiated type — *see* Neoplasm, connective tissue, malignant
- **Liposynovitis prepatellaris** E88.89
- **Lipping, cervix** N86
- **Lipschütz disease or ulcer** N76.6
- **Lipuria** R82.Ø
  - schistosomiasis (bilharziasis) B65.Ø
- **Lisping** F8Ø.Ø
- **Lissauer's paralysis** A52.17
- **Lissencephalia, lissencephaly** QØ4.3
- **Listeriosis, listerellosis** A32.9
  - congenital (disseminated) P37.2
  - cutaneous A32.Ø
  - neonatal, newborn (disseminated) P37.2
  - oculoglandular A32.81
  - specified NEC A32.89
- **Lithemia** E79.Ø
- **Lithiasis** — *see* Calculus
- **Lithosis** J62.8
- **Lithuria** R82.998
- **Litigation, anxiety concerning** Z65.3
- **Little leaguer's elbow** — *see* Epicondylitis, medial
- **Little's disease** G8Ø.9
- **Littre's**
  - gland — *see* condition
  - hernia — *see* Hernia, abdomen
- **Littritis** — *see* Urethritis
- **Livedo** (annularis) (racemosa) (reticularis) R23.1
- **Liver** — *see* condition
- **Living alone** (problems with) Z6Ø.2
  - with handicapped person Z74.2
- **Living in a shelter** (motel) (scattered site housing) (temporary or transitional living situation) Z59.Ø1
- **Lloyd's syndrome** — *see* Adenomatosis, endocrine
- **Loa loa, loaiasis, loasis** B74.3
- **Lobar** — *see* condition
- **Lobomycosis** B48.Ø
- **Lobo's disease** B48.Ø
- **Lobotomy syndrome** FØ7.Ø
- **Lobstein** (-Ekman) **disease or syndrome** Q78.Ø
- **Lobster-claw hand** Q71.6- ☑
- **Lobulation** (congenital) — *see also* Anomaly, by site
  - kidney, Q63.1
  - liver, abnormal Q44.79
  - spleen Q89.Ø9
- **Lobule, lobular** — *see* condition
- **Local, localized** — *see* condition
- **Locked twins causing obstructed labor** O66.1
- **Locked-in state** G83.5
- **Locking**
  - joint — *see* Derangement, joint, specified type NEC
    - knee — *see* Derangement, knee
- **Lockjaw** — *see* Tetanus
- **Loffler's**
  - endocarditis I42.3
  - eosinophilia J82.89
  - pneumonia J82.89
  - syndrome (eosinophilic pneumonitis) J82.89
- **Loiasis** (with conjunctival infestation) (eyelid) B74.3
- **Lone Star fever** A77.Ø
- **Loneliness** R45.89
- **Long**
  - COVID (-19) — *see also* COVID-19 UØ9.9
  - labor O63.9
    - first stage O63.Ø
    - second stage O63.1
  - QT syndrome I45.81
- **Longitudinal stripes or grooves, nails** L6Ø.8
  - congenital Q84.6
- **Long-term** (current) (prophylactic) **drug therapy** (use of)
  - 5-fluorouracil Z79.631
  - 6-mercaptopurine Z79.631
  - adalimumab Z79.62Ø
  - agents affecting estrogen receptors and estrogen levels NEC Z79.818
  - alkylating agent Z79.63Ø
  - anastrozole (Arimidex) Z79.811
  - antibiotics Z79.2
    - short-term use — *omit code*
  - anticoagulants Z79.Ø1
  - antidiabetic drugs, injectable, non-insulin Z79.85
  - anti-inflammatory, non-steroidal (NSAID) Z79.1
  - antimetabolite agent Z79.631
  - antiplatelet Z79.Ø2
  - antithrombotics Z79.Ø2
- **Long-term** (current) (prophylactic) **drug therapy** — *continued*
  - antitumor antibiotic Z79.632
  - apremilast Z79.61
  - aromatase inhibitors Z79.811
  - aspirin Z79.82
  - azathioprine Z79.624
  - birth control pill or patch Z79.3
  - bisphosphonates Z79.83
  - bleomycin Z79.632
  - calcineurin inhibitor Z79.621
  - chlorambucil Z79.63Ø
  - cisplatin Z79.63Ø
  - contraceptive, oral Z79.3
  - cyclophosphamide Z79.63Ø
  - cyclosporine Z79.621
  - cytarabine Z79.631
  - doxorubicin Z79.632
  - drug, specified NEC Z79.899
  - estrogen receptor downregulators Z79.818
  - etanercept Z79.62Ø
  - etoposide Z79.634
  - Evista Z79.81Ø
  - exemestane (Aromasin) Z79.811
  - Fareston Z79.81Ø
  - fulvestrant (Faslodex) Z79.818
  - gonadotropin-releasing hormone (GnRH) agonist Z79.818
  - goserelin acetate (Zoladex) Z79.818
  - hormone replacement Z79.89Ø
  - hydroxyurea Z79.64
  - immunomodulators, unspecified Z79.6Ø
    - specified NEC Z79.69
  - immunomodulatory imide drug Z79.61
  - immunosuppressants, unspecified Z79.6Ø
    - specified NEC Z79.69
  - immunosuppressive biologic Z79.62Ø
  - infliximab Z79.62Ø
  - inhibitors of nucleotide synthesis Z79.624
  - insulin Z79.4
  - irinotecan Z79.634
  - Janus kinase inhibitor Z79.622
  - lenalidomide Z79.61
  - letrozole (Femara) Z79.811
  - leuprolide acetate (leuprorelin) (Lupron) Z79.818
  - mammalian target of rapamycin (mTOR) inhibitor Z79.623
  - megestrol acetate (Megace) Z79.818
  - methadone for pain management Z79.891
  - mitomycin C Z79.632
  - mitotic inhibitor Z79.633
  - monoclonal antibodies Z79.62Ø
  - myelosuppressive agent Z79.64
  - Nolvadex Z79.81Ø
  - non-insulin antidiabetic drug, injectable Z79.899
  - non-steroidal anti-inflammatories (NSAID) Z79.1
  - omycophenolate Z79.624
  - opiate analgesic Z79.891
  - oral
    - antidiabetic Z79.84
    - contraceptive Z79.3
    - hypoglycemic Z79.84
  - paclitaxel Z79.633
  - plant alkaloids Z79.633
  - pomalidomide Z79.61
  - purine synthesis (IMDH) inhibitors Z79.624
  - raloxifene (Evista) Z79.81Ø
  - selective estrogen receptor modulators (SERMs) Z79.81Ø
  - sirolimus Z79.623
  - steroids
    - inhaled Z79.51
    - systemic Z79.52
  - tacrolimus Z79.621
  - tamoxifen (Nolvadex) Z79.81Ø
  - tofacitinib Z79.622
  - topoisomerase inhibitor Z79.634
  - topotecan Z79.634
  - toremifene (Fareston) Z79.81Ø
  - vinblastine Z79.633
  - vincristine Z79.633
- **Loop**
  - intestine — *see* Volvulus
  - vascular on papilla (optic) Q14.2
- **Loose** — *see also* condition
  - body
    - joint M24.ØØ
      - ankle M24.Ø7- ☑
      - elbow M24.Ø2- ☑

Loose — *continued*
- body — *continued*
  - joint — *continued*
    - hand M24.Ø4- ☑
    - hip M24.Ø5- ☑
    - knee M23.4- ☑
    - shoulder (region) M24.Ø1- ☑
    - specified site NEC M24.Ø8
    - temporomandibular M24.Ø8
    - toe M24.Ø7- ☑
    - vertebra M24.Ø8
    - wrist M24.Ø3- ☑
  - knee M23.4- ☑
  - sheath, tendon — *see* Disorder, tendon, specified type NEC
- cartilage — *see* Loose, body, joint
- skin and subcutaneous tissue (following bariatric surgery weight loss) (following dietary weight loss) L98.7
- tooth, teeth KØ8.89

Loosening
- aseptic
  - joint prosthesis — *see* Complications, joint prosthesis, mechanical, loosening, by site
- epiphysis — *see* Osteochondropathy
- mechanical
  - joint prosthesis — *see* Complications, joint prosthesis, mechanical, loosening, by site

Looser-Milkman (-Debray) **syndrome** M83.8

Lop ear (deformity) Q17.3

Lorain (-Levi) **short stature syndrome** E23.Ø

Lordosis M4Ø.5Ø
- acquired — *see* Lordosis, specified type NEC
- congenital Q76.429
  - lumbar region Q76.426
  - lumbosacral region Q76.427
  - sacral region Q76.428
  - sacrococcygeal region Q76.428
  - thoracolumbar region Q76.425
- lumbar region M4Ø.56
- lumbosacral region M4Ø.57
- postsurgical M96.4
- postural — *see* Lordosis, specified type NEC
- rachitic (late effect) (sequelae) E64.3
- sequelae of rickets E64.3
- specified type NEC M4Ø.4Ø
  - lumbar region M4Ø.46
  - lumbosacral region M4Ø.47
  - thoracolumbar region M4Ø.45
- thoracolumbar region M4Ø.55
- tuberculous A18.Ø1

Loss (of)
- appetite — *see also* Anorexia R63.Ø
  - hysterical F5Ø.89
  - nonorganic origin F5Ø.89
  - psychogenic F5Ø.89
- blood — *see* Hemorrhage
- bone — *see* Loss, substance of, bone
- consciousness, transient R55
  - traumatic — *see* Injury, intracranial
- control, sphincter, rectum R15.9
  - nonorganic origin F98.1
- elasticity, skin R23.4
- family (member) in childhood Z62.898
- fluid (acute) E86.9
- function of labyrinth — *see* subcategory H83.2 ☑
- hair, nonscarring — *see* Alopecia
- hearing — *see also* Deafness
  - central NOS H9Ø.5
  - conductive H9Ø.2
    - bilateral H9Ø.Ø
    - unilateral
      - with
        - restricted hearing on the contralateral side H9Ø.A1- ☑
        - unrestricted hearing on the contralateral side H9Ø.1- ☑
  - mixed conductive and sensorineural hearing loss H9Ø.8
    - bilateral H9Ø.6
    - unilateral
      - with
        - restricted hearing on the contralateral side H9Ø.A3- ☑
        - unrestricted hearing on the contralateral side H9Ø.7- ☑
  - neural NOS H9Ø.5
  - perceptive NOS H9Ø.5

Loss — *continued*
- hearing — *see also* Deafness — *continued*
  - sensorineural NOS H9Ø.5
    - bilateral H9Ø.3
    - unilateral
      - with
        - restricted hearing onthe contralateral side H9Ø.A2- ☑
        - unrestricted hearing on the contralateral side H9Ø.4- ☑
  - sensory NOS H9Ø.5
- height R29.89Ø
- limb or member, traumatic, current — *see* Amputation, traumatic
- love relationship in childhood Z62.898
- memory — *see also* Amnesia
  - mild, following organic brain damage FØ6.8
- mind — *see* Psychosis
- occlusal vertical dimension of fully erupted teeth M26.37
- organ or part — *see* Absence, by site, acquired
- ossicles, ear (partial) H74.32- ☑
- parent in childhood Z63.4
- pregnancy, recurrent N96
  - care in current pregnancy O26.2- ☑
  - without current pregnancy N96
- recurrent pregnancy — *see* Loss, pregnancy, recurrent
- self-esteem, in childhood Z62.898
- sense of
  - smell — *see* Disturbance, sensation, smell
  - taste — *see* Disturbance, sensation, taste
  - touch R2Ø.8
- sensory R44.9
  - dissociative F44.6
- sexual desire F52.Ø
- sight (acquired) (complete) (congenital) — *see* Blindness
- substance of
  - bone — *see* Disorder, bone, density and structure, specified NEC
    - horizontal alveolar KØ6.3
  - cartilage — *see* Disorder, cartilage, specified type NEC
    - auricle (ear) — *see* Disorder, pinna, specified type NEC
  - vitreous (humor) H15.89
- tooth, teeth — *see* Absence, teeth, acquired
- vision, visual H54.7
  - both eyes H54.3
  - one eye H54.6Ø
    - left (normal vision on right) H54.62
    - right (normal vision on left) H54.61
  - specified as blindness — *see* Blindness
  - subjective
    - sudden H53.13- ☑
    - transient H53.12- ☑
- vitreous — *see* Prolapse, vitreous
- voice — *see* Aphonia
- weight (abnormal) (cause unknown) R63.4

Louis-Bar syndrome (ataxia-telangiectasia) G11.3

Louping ill (encephalitis) A84.89

Louse, lousiness — *see* Lice

Low
- achiever, school Z55.3
- back syndrome M54.5Ø
- basal metabolic rate R94.8
- birthweight (2499 grams or less) PØ7.1Ø
  - with weight of
    - 1ØØØ-1249 grams PØ7.14
    - 125Ø-1499 grams PØ7.15
    - 15ØØ-1749 grams PØ7.16
    - 175Ø-1999 grams PØ7.17
    - 2ØØØ-2499 grams PØ7.18
  - extreme (999 grams or less) PØ7.ØØ
    - with weight of
      - 499 grams or less PØ7.Ø1
      - 5ØØ-749 grams PØ7.Ø2
      - 75Ø-999 grams PØ7.Ø3
  - for gestational age — *see* Light for dates
- blood pressure — *see also* Hypotension
  - reading (incidental) (isolated) (nonspecific) RØ3.1
- cardiac reserve — *see* Disease, heart
- function — *see also* Hypofunction
  - kidney N28.9
- hematocrit D64.9
- hemoglobin D64.9
- income Z59.6
- level of literacy Z55.Ø

Low — *continued*
- lying
  - kidney N28.89
  - organ or site, congenital — *see* Malposition, congenital
- output syndrome (cardiac) — *see* Failure, heart
- platelets (blood) — *see* Thrombocytopenia
- reserve, kidney N28.89
- salt syndrome E87.1
- self esteem R45.81
- set ears Q17.4
- vision H54.2X- ☑
  - one eye (other eye normal) H54.5Ø
    - left (normal vision on right)
      - category 1 H54.52A1
      - category 2 H54.52A2
    - other eye blind — *see* Blindness
    - right (normal vision on left)
      - category 1 H54.511A
      - category 2 H54.512A
- von Willebrand factor R79.1

Low-density-lipoprotein-type (LDL) **hyperlipoproteinemia** E78.ØØ

Lowe's syndrome E72.Ø3

Lown-Ganong-Levine syndrome I45.6

LSD reaction (acute) (without dependence) F16.9Ø
- with dependence F16.2Ø

L-shaped kidney Q63.8

LTBI (latent tuberculosis infection) Z22.7

Ludwig's angina or disease K12.2

Lues (venerea), **luetic** — *see* Syphilis

Luetscher's syndrome (dehydration) E86.Ø

Lumbago, lumbalgia M54.5Ø
- with sciatica M54.4- ☑
  - due to intervertebral disc disorder M51.17
- due to displacement, intervertebral disc M51.27
  - with sciatica M51.17

Lumbar — *see* condition

Lumbarization, vertebra, congenital Q76.49

Lumbermen's itch B88.Ø

Lump — *see also* Mass
- breast N63.Ø
  - axillary tail
    - left N63.32
    - right N63.31
  - left
    - lower inner quadrant N63.24
    - lower outer quadrant N63.23
    - overlapping quadrants N63.25
    - unspecified quadrant N63.2Ø
    - upper inner quadrant N63.22
    - upper outer quadrant N63.21
  - right
    - lower inner quadrant N63.14
    - lower outer quadrant N63.13
    - overlapping quadrants N63.15
    - unspecified quadrant N63.1Ø
    - upper inner quadrant N63.12
    - upper outer quadrant N63.11
  - subareolar
    - left N63.42
    - right N63.41

Lunacy — *see* Psychosis

Lung — *see* condition

Lupoid (miliary) **of Boeck** D86.3

Lupus
- anticoagulant D68.62
  - with
    - hemorrhagic disorder D68.312
    - hypercoagulable state D68.62
  - finding without diagnosis R76.Ø
- discoid (local) L93.Ø
- erythematosus (discoid) (local) L93.Ø
  - disseminated — *see* Lupus, erythematosus, systemic
  - eyelid HØ1.129
    - left HØ1.126
      - lower HØ1.125
      - upper HØ1.124
    - right HØ1.123
      - lower HØ1.122
      - upper HØ1.121
  - profundus L93.2
  - specified NEC L93.2
  - subacute cutaneous L93.1
  - systemic M32.9
    - with organ or system involvement M32.1Ø
      - endocarditis M32.11
      - lung M32.13

- **Lupus** — *continued*
  - erythematosus — *continued*
    - systemic — *continued*
      - with organ or system involvement — *continued*
        - pericarditis M32.12
        - renal (glomerular) M32.14
          - tubulo-interstitial M32.15
        - specified organ or system NEC M32.19
      - drug-induced M32.Ø
      - inhibitor (presence of) D68.62
        - with
          - hemorrhagic disorder D68.312
          - hypercoagulable state D68.62
        - finding without diagnosis R76.Ø
      - specified NEC M32.8
  - exedens A18.4
  - hydralazine M32.Ø
    - correct substance properly administered — *see* Table of Drugs and Chemicals, by drug, adverse effect
    - overdose or wrong substance given or taken — *see* Table of Drugs and Chemicals, by drug, poisoning
  - nephritis (chronic) M32.14
  - nontuberculous, not disseminated L93.Ø
  - panniculitis L93.2
  - pernio (Besnier) D86.3
  - systemic — *see* Lupus, erythematosus, systemic
  - tuberculous A18.4
    - eyelid A18.4
  - vulgaris A18.4
    - eyelid A18.4
- **Luteinoma** D27.- ☑
- **Lutembacher's disease or syndrome** (atrial septal defect with mitral stenosis) Q21.19
- **Luteoma** D27.- ☑
- **Lutz** (-Splendore-de Almeida) **disease** — *see* Paracoccidioidomycosis
- **Luxation** — *see also* Dislocation
  - eyeball (nontraumatic) — *see* Luxation, globe
    - birth injury P15.3
  - globe, nontraumatic H44.82- ☑
  - lacrimal gland — *see* Dislocation, lacrimal gland
  - lens (old) (partial) (spontaneous)
    - congenital Q12.1
      - syphilitic A5Ø.39
- **Lycanthropy** F22
- **Lyell's syndrome** L51.2
  - due to drug L51.2
    - correct substance properly administered — *see* Table of Drugs and Chemicals, by drug, adverse effect
    - overdose or wrong substance given or taken — *see* Table of Drugs and Chemicals, by drug, poisoning
- **Lyme disease** A69.2Ø
- **Lymph**
  - gland or node — *see* condition
  - scrotum — *see* Infestation, filarial
- **Lymphadenitis** I88.9
  - with ectopic or molar pregnancy OØ8.Ø
  - acute LØ4.9
    - axilla LØ4.2
    - face LØ4.Ø
    - head LØ4.Ø
    - hip LØ4.3
    - limb
      - lower LØ4.3
      - upper LØ4.2
    - neck LØ4.Ø
    - shoulder LØ4.2
    - specified site NEC LØ4.8
    - trunk LØ4.1
  - anthracosis (occupational) J6Ø
  - any site, except mesenteric I88.9
    - chronic I88.1
    - subacute I88.1
  - breast
    - gestational — *see* Mastitis, obstetric
    - puerperal, postpartum (nonpurulent) O91.22
  - chancroidal (congenital) A57
  - chronic I88.1
    - mesenteric I88.Ø
  - due to
    - Brugia (malayi) B74.1
      - timori B74.2
    - chlamydial lymphogranuloma A55
- **Lymphadenitis** — *continued*
  - due to — *continued*
    - diphtheria (toxin) A36.89
    - lymphogranuloma venereum A55
    - Wuchereria bancrofti B74.Ø
  - following ectopic or molar pregnancy OØ8.Ø
  - gonorrheal A54.89
  - infective — *see* Lymphadenitis, acute
  - mesenteric (acute) (chronic) (nonspecific) (subacute) I88.Ø
    - due to Salmonella typhi AØ1.Ø9
    - tuberculous A18.39
  - mycobacterial A31.8
  - purulent — *see* Lymphadenitis, acute
  - pyogenic — *see* Lymphadenitis, acute
  - regional, nonbacterial I88.8
  - septic — *see* Lymphadenitis, acute
  - subacute, unspecified site I88.1
  - suppurative — *see* Lymphadenitis, acute
  - syphilitic (early) (secondary) A51.49
    - late A52.79
  - tuberculous — *see* Tuberculosis, lymph gland
  - venereal (chlamydial) A55
- **Lymphadenoid goiter** EØ6.3
- **Lymphadenopathy** (generalized) R59.1
  - angioimmunoblastic, with dysproteinemia (AILD) C86.5
  - due to toxoplasmosis (acquired) B58.89
    - congenital (acute) (subacute) (chronic) P37.1
  - localized R59.Ø
  - syphilitic (early) (secondary) A51.49
- **Lymphadenosis** R59.1
- **Lymphangiectasis** I89.Ø
  - conjunctiva H11.89
  - postinfectional I89.Ø
  - scrotum I89.Ø
- **Lymphangiectatic elephantiasis, nonfilarial** I89.Ø
- **Lymphangioendothelioma** D18.1
  - malignant — *see* Neoplasm, connective tissue, malignant
- **Lymphangioleiomyomatosis** J84.81
- **Lymphangioma** D18.1
  - capillary D18.1
  - cavernous D18.1
  - cystic D18.1
  - malignant — *see* Neoplasm, connective tissue, malignant
- **Lymphangiomyoma** D18.1
- **Lymphangiomyomatosis** J84.81
- **Lymphangiosarcoma** — *see* Neoplasm, connective tissue, malignant
- **Lymphangitis** I89.1
  - with
    - abscess — *code by* site under Abscess
    - cellulitis — *code by* site under Cellulitis
    - ectopic or molar pregnancy OØ8.Ø
  - acute LØ3.91
    - abdominal wall LØ3.321
    - ankle — *see* Lymphangitis, acute, lower limb
    - arm — *see* Lymphangitis, acute, upper limb
    - auricle (ear) — *see* Lymphangitis, acute, ear
    - axilla LØ3.12- ☑
    - back (any part) LØ3.322
    - buttock LØ3.327
    - cervical (meaning neck) LØ3.222
    - cheek (external) LØ3.212
    - chest wall LØ3.323
    - digit
      - finger — *see* Lymphangitis, acute, finger
      - toe — *see* Lymphangitis, acute, toe
    - ear (external) H6Ø.1- ☑
    - external auditory canal — *see* Lymphangitis, acute, ear
    - eyelid — *see* Abscess, eyelid
    - face NEC LØ3.212
    - finger (intrathecal) (periosteal) (subcutaneous) (subcuticular) LØ3.Ø2- ☑
    - foot — *see* Lymphangitis, acute, lower limb
    - gluteal (region) LØ3.327
    - groin LØ3.324
    - hand — *see* Lymphangitis, acute, upper limb
    - head NEC LØ3.891
      - face (any part, except ear, eye and nose) LØ3.212
    - heel — *see* Lymphangitis, acute, lower limb
    - hip — *see* Lymphangitis, acute, lower limb
    - jaw (region) LØ3.212
    - knee — *see* Lymphangitis, acute, lower limb
    - leg — *see* Lymphangitis, acute, lower limb
- **Lymphangitis** — *continued*
  - acute — *continued*
    - lower limb LØ3.12- ☑
      - toe — *see* Lymphangitis, acute, toe
    - navel LØ3.326
    - neck (region) LØ3.222
    - orbit, orbital — *see* Cellulitis, orbit
    - pectoral (region) LØ3.323
    - perineal, perineum LØ3.325
    - scalp (any part) LØ3.891
    - shoulder — *see* Lymphangitis, acute, upper limb
    - specified site NEC LØ3.898
    - thigh — *see* Lymphangitis, acute, lower limb
    - thumb (intrathecal) (periosteal) (subcutaneous) (subcuticular) — *see* Lymphangitis, acute, finger
    - toe (intrathecal) (periosteal) (subcutaneous) (subcuticular) LØ3.Ø4- ☑
    - trunk LØ3.329
      - abdominal wall LØ3.321
      - back (any part) LØ3.322
      - buttock LØ3.327
      - chest wall LØ3.323
      - groin LØ3.324
      - perineal, perineum LØ3.325
      - umbilicus LØ3.326
    - umbilicus LØ3.326
    - upper limb LØ3.12- ☑
      - axilla — *see* Lymphangitis, acute, axilla
      - finger — *see* Lymphangitis, acute, finger
      - thumb — *see* Lymphangitis, acute, finger
    - wrist — *see* Lymphangitis, acute, upper limb
  - breast
    - gestational — *see* Mastitis, obstetric
  - chancroidal A57
  - chronic (any site) I89.1
  - due to
    - Brugia (malayi) B74.1
      - timori B74.2
    - Wuchereria bancrofti B74.Ø
  - following ectopic or molar pregnancy OØ8.89
  - penis
    - acute N48.29
    - gonococcal (acute) (chronic) A54.Ø9
  - puerperal, postpartum, childbirth O86.89
  - strumous, tuberculous A18.2
  - subacute (any site) I89.1
  - tuberculous — *see* Tuberculosis, lymph gland
- **Lymphatic** (vessel) — *see* condition
- **Lymphatism** E32.8
- **Lymphectasia** I89.Ø
- **Lymphedema** (acquired) — *see also* Elephantiasis
  - congenital Q82.Ø
  - hereditary (chronic) (idiopathic) Q82.Ø
  - postmastectomy I97.2
  - praecox I89.Ø
  - secondary I89.Ø
  - surgical NEC I97.89
    - postmastectomy (syndrome) I97.2
- **Lymphoblastic** — *see* condition
- **Lymphoblastoma** (diffuse) — *see* Lymphoma, lymphoblastic (diffuse)
  - giant follicular — *see* Lymphoma, lymphoblastic (diffuse)
  - macrofollicular — *see* Lymphoma, lymphoblastic (diffuse)
- **Lymphocele** I89.8
- **Lymphocytic**
  - chorioencephalitis (acute) (serous) A87.2
  - choriomeningitis (acute) (serous) A87.2
  - meningoencephalitis A87.2
- **Lymphocytoma, benign cutis** L98.8
- **Lymphocytopenia** D72.81Ø
- **Lymphocytosis** (symptomatic) D72.82Ø
  - infectious (acute) B33.8
- **Lymphoepithelioma** — *see* Neoplasm, malignant, by site
- **Lymphogranuloma** (malignant) — *see also* Lymphoma, Hodgkin
  - chlamydial A55
  - inguinale A55
  - venereum (any site) (chlamydial) (with stricture of rectum) A55
- **Lymphogranulomatosis** (malignant) — *see also* Lymphoma, Hodgkin
  - benign (Boeck's sarcoid) (Schaumann's) D86.1
- **Lymphohistiocytosis, hemophagocytic** (familial) D76.1
- **Lymphoid** — *see* condition

- **Lymphoma** (of) (malignant) C85.9Ø
  - adult T-cell (HTLV-1-associated) (acute variant) (chronic variant) (lymphomatoid variant) (smouldering variant) C91.5- ☑
  - anaplastic large cell
    - ALK-negative C84.7- ☑
    - ALK-positive C84.6- ☑
    - breast implant associated (BIA-ALCL) C84.7A
    - CD3Ø-positive C84.6- ☑
    - primary cutaneous C86.6
  - angioimmunoblastic T-cell C86.5
  - BALT C88.4
  - B-cell C85.1- ☑
  - blastic NK-cell C86.4
  - blastic plasmacytoid dendritic cell neoplasm (BPDCN) C86.4
  - B-precursor C83.5- ☑
  - bronchial-associated lymphoid tissue [BALT-lymphoma] C88.4
  - Burkitt (atypical) C83.7- ☑
  - Burkitt-like C83.7- ☑
  - centrocytic C83.1- ☑
  - cutaneous follicle center C82.6- ☑
  - cutaneous T-cell C84.A- ☑ (*following* C84.7)
  - diffuse follicle center C82.5- ☑
  - diffuse large cell C83.3- ☑
    - anaplastic C83.3- ☑
    - B-cell C83.3- ☑
    - CD3Ø-positive C83.3- ☑
    - centroblastic C83.3- ☑
    - immunoblastic C83.3- ☑
    - plasmablastic C83.3- ☑
    - subtype not specified C83.3- ☑
    - T-cell rich C83.3- ☑
  - enteropathy-type (associated) (intestinal) T-cell C86.2
  - extranodal marginal zone B-cell lymphoma of mucosa-associated lymphoid tissue [MALT-lymphoma] C88.4
  - extranodal NK/T-cell, nasal type C86.Ø
  - follicular C82.9- ☑
    - grade
      - I C82.Ø- ☑
      - II C82.1- ☑
      - III C82.2- ☑
      - IIIa C82.3- ☑
      - IIIb C82.4- ☑
    - specified NEC C82.8- ☑
  - hepatosplenic T-cell (alpha-beta) (gamma-delta) C86.1
  - histiocytic C85.9- ☑
    - true C96.A (*following* C96.6)
  - Hodgkin C81.9- ☑
    - lymphocyte depleted (classical) C81.3- ☑
    - lymphocyte-rich (classical) C81.4- ☑
    - mixed cellularity (classical) C81.2- ☑
    - nodular
      - lymphocyte predominant C81.Ø- ☑
      - sclerosis (classical) C81.1- ☑
    - nodular sclerosis (classical) C81.1- ☑
    - specified NEC (classical) C81.7- ☑
  - intravascular large B-cell C83.8- ☑
  - Lennert's C84.4- ☑
  - lymphoblastic (diffuse) C83.5- ☑
  - lymphoblastic B-cell C83.5- ☑
  - lymphoblastic T-cell C83.5- ☑
  - lymphoepithelioid C84.4- ☑
  - lymphoplasmacytic C83.Ø- ☑
    - with IgM-production C88.Ø
  - MALT C88.4
  - mantle cell C83.1- ☑
  - mature T-cell NEC C84.4- ☑
  - mature T/NK-cell C84.9- ☑
    - specified NEC C84.Z- ☑ (*following* C84.7)
  - mediastinal (thymic) large B-cell C85.2- ☑
  - Mediterranean C88.3
  - mucosa-associated lymphoid tissue [MALT-lymphoma] C88.4
  - NK/T cell C84.9- ☑
  - nodal marginal zone C83.Ø- ☑
  - non-follicular (diffuse) C83.9- ☑
    - specified NEC C83.8- ☑
  - non-Hodgkin — *see also* Lymphoma, by type C85.9- ☑
    - specified NEC C85.8- ☑
  - non-leukemic variant of B-CLL C83.Ø- ☑
  - peripheral T-cell NEC C84.4- ☑
  - primary cutaneous
    - anaplastic large cell C86.6
    - CD3Ø-positive large T-cell C86.6
  - primary effusion B-cell C83.8- ☑
  - SALT C88.4
  - skin-associated lymphoid tissue [SALT-lymphoma] C88.4
  - small cell B-cell C83.Ø- ☑
  - splenic marginal zone C83.Ø- ☑
  - subcutaneous panniculitis-like T-cell C86.3
  - T-precursor C83.5- ☑
  - true histiocytic C96.A (*following* C96.6)
- **Lymphomatosis** — *see* Lymphoma
- **Lymphopathia venereum, veneris** A55
- **Lymphopenia** D72.81Ø
- **Lymphoplasmacytic leukemia** — *see* Leukemia, chronic lymphocytic, B-cell type
- **Lymphoproliferation, X-linked disease** D82.3
- **Lymphoreticulosis, benign** (of inoculation) A28.1
- **Lymphorrhea** I89.8
- **Lymphosarcoma** (diffuse) — *see also* Lymphoma C85.9- ☑
- **Lymphostasis** I89.8
- **Lypemania** — *see* Melancholia
- **Lysine and hydroxylysine metabolism disorder** E72.3
- **Lyssa** — *see* Rabies

M

- **Macacus ear** Q17.3
- **Maceration, wet feet, tropical** (syndrome) T69.Ø2- ☑
- **MacLeod's syndrome** J43.Ø
- **Macrocephalia, macrocephaly** Q75.3
- **Macrocheilia, macrochilia** (congenital) Q18.6
- **Macrocolon** — *see also* Megacolon Q43.1
- **Macrocornea** Q15.8
  - with glaucoma Q15.Ø
- **Macrocytic** — *see* condition
- **Macrocytosis** D75.89
- **Macrodactylia, macrodactylism** (fingers) (thumbs) Q74.Ø
  - toes Q74.2
- **Macrodontia** KØØ.2
- **Macrogenia** M26.Ø5
- **Macrogenitosomia** (adrenal) (male) (praecox) E25.9
  - congenital E25.Ø
- **Macroglobulinemia** (idiopathic) (primary) C88.Ø
  - monoclonal (essential) D47.2
  - Waldenstrom C88.Ø
- **Macroglossia** (congenital) Q38.2
  - acquired K14.8
- **Macrognathia, macrognathism** (congenital) (mandibular) (maxillary) M26.Ø9
- **Macrogyria** (congenital) QØ4.8
- **Macrohydrocephalus** — *see* Hydrocephalus
- **Macromastia** — *see* Hypertrophy, breast
- **Macrophthalmos** Q11.3
  - in congenital glaucoma Q15.Ø
- **Macropsia** H53.15
- **Macrosigmoid** K59.39
  - congenital Q43.2
- **Macrospondylitis , acromegalic** E22.Ø
- **Macrostomia** (congenital) Q18.4
- **Macrotia** (external ear) (congenital) Q17.1
- **Macula**
  - cornea, corneal — *see* Opacity, cornea
  - degeneration (atrophic) (exudative) (senile) — *see also* Degeneration, macula
    - hereditary — *see* Dystrophy, retina
- **Maculae ceruleae** B85.1
- **Maculopathy, toxic** — *see* Degeneration, macula, toxic
- **Madarosis** (eyelid) HØ2.729
  - left HØ2.726
    - lower HØ2.725
    - upper HØ2.724
  - right HØ2.723
    - lower HØ2.722
    - upper HØ2.721
- **Madelung's**
  - deformity (radius) Q74.Ø
  - disease
    - radial deformity Q74.Ø
    - symmetrical lipomas, neck E88.89
- **Madness** — *see* Psychosis
- **Madura**
  - foot B47.9
    - actinomycotic B47.1
    - mycotic B47.Ø
- **Maduromycosis** B47.Ø
- **Maffucci's syndrome** Q78.4
- **Magnesium metabolism disorder** — *see* Disorder, metabolism, magnesium
- **Main en griffe** (acquired) — *see also* Deformity, limb, clawhand
  - congenital Q68.1
- **Maintenance** (encounter for)
  - antineoplastic chemotherapy Z51.11
  - antineoplastic radiation therapy Z51.Ø
  - methadone F11.2Ø
- **Majocchi's**
  - disease L81.7
  - granuloma B35.8
- **Major** — *see* condition
- **Mal de los pintos** — *see* Pinta
- **Mal de mer** T75.3 ☑
- **Malabar itch** (any site) B35.5
- **Malabsorption** K9Ø.9
  - calcium K9Ø.89
  - carbohydrate K9Ø.49
  - disaccharide E73.9
  - fat K9Ø.49
  - galactose E74.2Ø
  - glucose (-galactose) E74.39
  - intestinal K9Ø.9
    - specified NEC K9Ø.89
  - isomaltose E74.31
  - lactose E73.9
  - methionine E72.19
  - monosaccharide E74.39
  - postgastrectomy K91.2
  - postsurgical K91.2
  - protein K9Ø.49
  - starch K9Ø.49
  - sucrose E74.39
  - syndrome K9Ø.9
    - postsurgical K91.2
- **Malacia, bone** (adult) M83.9
  - juvenile — *see* Rickets
- **Malacoplakia**
  - bladder N32.89
  - pelvis (kidney) N28.89
  - ureter N28.89
  - urethra N36.8
- **Malacosteon, juvenile** — *see* Rickets
- **Maladaptation** — *see* Maladjustment
- **Maladie de Roger** Q21.Ø
- **Maladjustment**
  - conjugal Z63.Ø
    - involving divorce or estrangement Z63.5
  - educational Z55.4
  - family Z63.9
  - marital Z63.Ø
    - involving divorce or estrangement Z63.5
  - occupational NEC Z56.89
  - simple, adult — *see* Disorder, adjustment
  - situational — *see* Disorder, adjustment
  - social Z6Ø.9
    - due to
      - acculturation difficulty Z6Ø.3
      - discrimination and persecution (perceived) Z6Ø.5
      - exclusion and isolation Z6Ø.4
      - life-cycle (phase of life) transition Z6Ø.Ø
      - rejection Z6Ø.4
      - specified reason NEC Z6Ø.8
- **Malaise** R53.81
- **Malakoplakia** — *see* Malacoplakia
- **Malaria, malarial** (fever) B54
  - with
    - blackwater fever B5Ø.8
      - hemoglobinuric (bilious) B5Ø.8
    - hemoglobinuria B5Ø.8
  - accidentally induced (therapeutically) — *code by* type under Malaria
  - algid B5Ø.9
  - cerebral B5Ø.Ø *[G94]*
  - clinically diagnosed (without parasitological confirmation) B54
  - congenital NEC P37.4
    - falciparum P37.3
  - congestion, congestive B54
  - continued (fever) B5Ø.9
  - estivo-autumnal B5Ø.9
  - falciparum B5Ø.9

- **Malposition** — *continued*
  - congenital — *continued*
    - intestine (large) (small) Q43.8
      - with anomalous adhesions, fixation or malrotation Q43.3
    - joint NEC Q68.8
    - kidney Q63.2
    - larynx Q31.8
    - limb Q68.8
      - lower Q68.8
      - upper Q68.8
    - liver Q44.79
    - lung (lobe) Q33.8
    - nail(s) Q84.6
    - nerve QØ7.8
    - nervous system NEC QØ7.8
    - nose, nasal (septum) Q3Ø.8
    - organ or site not listed — *see* Anomaly, by site
    - ovary Q5Ø.39
    - pancreas Q45.3
    - parathyroid (gland) Q89.2
    - patella Q74.1
    - peripheral vascular system Q27.8
    - pituitary (gland) Q89.2
    - respiratory organ or system NEC Q34.8
    - rib (cage) Q76.6
      - supernumerary in cervical region Q76.5
    - scapula Q74.Ø
    - shoulder Q74.Ø
    - spinal cord QØ6.8
    - spleen Q89.Ø9
    - sternum NEC Q76.7
    - stomach Q4Ø.2
    - symphysis pubis Q74.2
    - thymus (gland) Q89.2
    - thyroid (gland) (tissue) Q89.2
      - cartilage Q31.8
    - toe(s) Q66.9- ☑
      - supernumerary Q69.2
    - tongue Q38.3
    - trachea Q32.1
    - ureter Q62.6Ø
      - deviation Q62.61
      - displacement Q62.62
      - ectopia Q62.63
      - specified type NEC Q62.69
    - uterus Q51.818
    - vein(s) (peripheral) Q27.8
      - great Q26.8
    - vena cava (inferior) (superior) Q26.8
  - device, implant or graft — *see also* Complications, by site and type, mechanical T85.628 ☑
    - arterial graft NEC — *see* Complication, cardiovascular device, mechanical, vascular
    - breast (implant) T85.42 ☑
    - catheter NEC T85.628 ☑
      - cystostomy T83.Ø2Ø ☑
      - dialysis (renal) T82.42 ☑
        - intraperitoneal T85.621 ☑
      - infusion NEC T82.524 ☑
        - spinal (epidural) (subdural) T85.62Ø ☑
      - urinary — *see* also Displacement, device, catheter, urinary T83.Ø28 ☑
    - electronic (electrode) (pulse generator) (stimulator)
      - bone T84.32Ø ☑
      - cardiac T82.129 ☑
        - electrode T82.12Ø ☑
        - pulse generator T82.121 ☑
        - specified type NEC T82.128 ☑
      - nervous system — *see* Complication, prosthetic device, mechanical, electronic nervous system stimulator
      - urinary — *see* Complication, genitourinary, device, urinary, mechanical
    - fixation, internal (orthopedic) NEC — *see* Complication, fixation device, mechanical
    - gastrointestinal — *see* Complications, prosthetic device, mechanical, gastrointestinal device
    - genital NEC T83.428 ☑
      - intrauterine contraceptive device (string) T83.32 ☑
      - penile prosthesis (cylinder) (implanted) (pump) (reservoir) T83.42Ø ☑
      - testicular prosthesis T83.421 ☑
    - heart NEC — *see* Complication, cardiovascular device, mechanical
    - joint prosthesis — *see* Complication, joint prosthesis, mechanical

- **Malposition** — *continued*
  - device, implant or graft — *see also* Complications, by site and type, mechanical — *continued*
    - ocular NEC — *see* Complications, prosthetic device, mechanical, ocular device
    - orthopedic NEC — *see* Complication, orthopedic, device, mechanical
    - specified NEC T85.628 ☑
    - urinary NEC — *see also* Complication, genitourinary, device, urinary, mechanical
      - graft T83.22 ☑
    - vascular NEC — *see* Complication, cardiovascular device, mechanical
    - ventricular intracranial shunt T85.Ø2 ☑
  - fetus — *see* Pregnancy, complicated by (management affected by), presentation, fetal
  - gallbladder K82.8
  - gastrointestinal tract, congenital Q45.8
  - heart, congenital NEC Q24.8
  - joint prosthesis — *see* Complications, joint prosthesis, mechanical, displacement, by site
  - stomach K31.89
    - congenital Q4Ø.2
  - tooth, teeth, fully erupted M26.3Ø
  - uterus (acute) (acquired) (adherent) (asymptomatic) (postinfectional) (postpartal, old) N85.4
    - anteflexion or anteversion N85.4
      - congenital Q51.818
    - flexion N85.4
      - lateral — *see* Lateroversion, uterus
    - inversion N85.5
    - lateral (flexion) (version) — *see* Lateroversion, uterus
      - in pregnancy or childbirth — *see* subcategory O34.5 ☑
    - retroflexion or retroversion — *see* Retroversion, uterus
- **Malposture** R29.3
- **Malrotation**
  - cecum Q43.3
  - colon Q43.3
  - intestine Q43.3
  - kidney Q63.2
- **Malta fever** — *see* Brucellosis
- **Maltreatment**
  - adult
    - abandonment
      - confirmed T74.Ø1 ☑
      - suspected T76.Ø1 ☑
    - bullying
      - confirmed T74.31 ☑
      - suspected T76.31 ☑
    - confirmed T74.91 ☑
    - financial
      - confirmed T74.A1 ☑
      - suspected T76.A1 ☑
    - history of Z91.419
    - intimidation (through social media)
      - confirmed T74.31 ☑
      - suspected T76.31 ☑
    - neglect
      - confirmed T74.Ø1 ☑
      - suspected T76.Ø1 ☑
    - physical abuse
      - confirmed T74.11 ☑
      - suspected T76.11 ☑
    - psychological abuse
      - confirmed T74.31 ☑
      - history of Z91.411
      - suspected T76.31 ☑
    - sexual abuse
      - confirmed T74.21 ☑
      - suspected T76.21 ☑
    - suspected T76.91 ☑
    - threatened abuse (harm) (physical violence) (sexual abuse)
      - confirmed T74.31 ☑
      - suspected T76.31 ☑
  - child
    - abandonment
      - confirmed T74.Ø2 ☑
      - suspected T76.Ø2 ☑
    - bullying
      - confirmed T74.32 ☑
      - suspected T76.32 ☑
    - confirmed T74.92 ☑
    - financial
      - confirmed T74.A2 ☑

- **Maltreatment** — *continued*
  - child — *continued*
    - financial — *continued*
      - suspected T76.A2 ☑
    - history of — *see* History, personal (of), abuse
    - intimidation (through social media)
      - confirmed T74.32 ☑
      - suspected T76.32 ☑
    - neglect
      - confirmed T74.Ø2 ☑
      - history of — *see* History, personal (of), abuse
      - suspected T76.Ø2 ☑
    - physical abuse
      - confirmed T74.12 ☑
      - history of — *see* History, personal (of), abuse
      - suspected T76.12 ☑
    - psychological abuse
      - confirmed T74.32 ☑
      - history of — *see* History, personal (of), abuse
      - suspected T76.32 ☑
    - sexual abuse
      - confirmed T74.22 ☑
      - history of — *see* History, personal (of), abuse
      - suspected T76.22 ☑
    - suspected T76.92 ☑
    - threatened abuse (harm) (physical violence) (sexual abuse)
      - confirmed T74.32 ☑
      - suspected T76.32 ☑
  - personal history of Z91.89
- **Maltworker's lung** J67.4
- **Malunion, fracture** — *see* Fracture, by site
- **Mammillitis** N61.Ø
  - puerperal, postpartum O91.Ø2
- **Mammitis** — *see* Mastitis
- **Mammogram** (examination) Z12.39
  - routine Z12.31
- **Mammoplasia** N62
- **Management** (of)
  - bone conduction hearing device (implanted) Z45.32Ø
  - cardiac pacemaker NEC Z45.Ø18
  - cerebrospinal fluid drainage device Z45.41
  - cochlear device (implanted) Z45.321
  - contraceptive Z3Ø.9
    - specified NEC Z3Ø.8
  - implanted device Z45.9
    - specified NEC Z45.89
  - infusion pump Z45.1
  - procreative Z31.9
    - male factor infertility in female Z31.81
    - specified NEC Z31.89
  - prosthesis (external) — *see also* Fitting Z44.9
    - implanted Z45.9
      - specified NEC Z45.89
  - renal dialysis catheter Z49.Ø1
  - vascular access device Z45.2
- **Mangled** — *see* specified injury by site
- **Mania** (monopolar) — *see also* Disorder, mood, manic episode
  - with psychotic symptoms F3Ø.2
  - without psychotic symptoms F3Ø.1Ø
    - mild F3Ø.11
    - moderate F3Ø.12
    - severe F3Ø.13
  - Bell's F3Ø.8
  - chronic (recurrent) F31.89
  - hysterical F44.89
  - puerperal F3Ø.8
  - recurrent F31.89
- **Manic depression** F31.9
- **Manic-depressive insanity, psychosis, or syndrome** — *see* Disorder, bipolar
- **Mannosidosis** E77.1
- **Mansonelliasis, mansonellosis** B74.4
- **Manson's**
  - disease B65.1
  - schistosomiasis B65.1
- **Manual** — *see* condition
- **Maple-bark-stripper's lung** (disease) J67.6
- **Maple-syrup-urine disease** E71.Ø
- **Marable's syndrome** (celiac artery compression) I77.4
- **Marasmus** E41
  - due to malnutrition E41
  - intestinal E41
  - nutritional E41
  - senile R54
  - tuberculous NEC — *see* Tuberculosis

- **Melanosarcoma** — *continued*
  - epithelioid cell — *see* Melanoma
- **Melanosis** L81.4
  - addisonian E27.1
    - tuberculous A18.7
  - adrenal E27.1
  - colon K63.89
  - conjunctiva — *see* Pigmentation, conjunctiva
    - congenital Q13.89
  - cornea (presenile) (senile) — *see also* Pigmentation, cornea
    - congenital Q13.4
  - eye NEC H57.89
    - congenital Q15.8
  - lenticularis progressiva Q82.1
  - liver K76.89
  - precancerous — *see also* Melanoma, in situ
    - malignant melanoma in — *see* Melanoma
  - Riehl's L81.4
  - sclera H15.89
    - congenital Q13.89
  - suprarenal E27.1
  - tar L81.4
  - toxic L81.4
- **Melanuria** R82.998
- **MELAS syndrome** E88.41
- **Melasma** L81.1
  - adrenal (gland) E27.1
  - suprarenal (gland) E27.1
- **Melena** K92.1
  - with ulcer — *code by* site under Ulcer, with hemorrhage K27.4
  - due to swallowed maternal blood P78.2
  - newborn, neonatal P54.1
    - due to swallowed maternal blood P78.2
- **Meleney's**
  - gangrene (cutaneous) — *see* Ulcer, skin
  - ulcer (chronic undermining) — *see* Ulcer, skin
- **Melioidosis** A24.9
  - acute A24.1
  - chronic A24.2
  - fulminating A24.1
  - pneumonia A24.1
  - pulmonary (chronic) A24.2
    - acute A24.1
    - subacute A24.2
  - sepsis A24.1
  - specified NEC A24.3
  - subacute A24.2
- **Melitensis, febris** A23.Ø
- **Melkersson** (-Rosenthal) **syndrome** G51.2
- **Mellitus, diabetes** — *see* Diabetes
- **Melorheostosis** (bone) — *see* Disorder, bone, density and structure, specified NEC
- **Meloschisis** Q18.4
- **Melotia** Q17.4
- **Membrana**
  - capsularis lentis posterior Q13.89
  - epipapillaris Q14.2
- **Membranacea placenta** O43.19- ☑
- **Membranaceous uterus** N85.8
- **Membrane**(s), membranous — *see also* condition
  - cyclitic — *see* Membrane, pupillary
  - folds, congenital — *see* Web
  - Jackson's Q43.3
  - over face of newborn P28.9
  - premature rupture — *see* Rupture, membranes, premature
  - pupillary H21.4- ☑
    - persistent Q13.89
  - retained (with hemorrhage) (complicating delivery) O72.2
    - without hemorrhage O73.1
  - secondary cataract — *see* Cataract, secondary
  - unruptured (causing asphyxia) — *see* Asphyxia, newborn
  - vitreous — *see* Opacity, vitreous, membranes and strands
- **Membranitis** — *see* Chorioamnionitis
- **Memory disturbance, lack or loss** — *see also* Amnesia
  - mild, following organic brain damage F06.8
- **Menadione deficiency** E56.1
- **Menarche**
  - delayed E30.Ø
  - precocious E30.1
- **Mendacity, pathologic** F60.2
- **Mendelson's syndrome** (due to anesthesia) J95.4
  - in labor and delivery O74.Ø
- **Mendelson's syndrome** — *continued*
  - in pregnancy O29.Ø1- ☑
  - obstetric O74.Ø
  - postpartum, puerperal O89.Ø1
- **Menetrier's disease or syndrome** K29.6Ø
  - with bleeding K29.61
- **Meniere's disease, syndrome or vertigo** H81.Ø- ☑
- **Meninges, meningeal** — *see* condition
- **Meningioma** — *see also* Neoplasm, meninges, benign
  - angioblastic — *see* Neoplasm, meninges, benign
  - angiomatous — *see* Neoplasm, meninges, benign
  - atypical — *see* Neoplasm, meninges, uncertain behavior
  - endotheliomatous — *see* Neoplasm, meninges, benign
  - fibroblastic — *see* Neoplasm, meninges, benign
  - fibrous — *see* Neoplasm, meninges, benign
  - hemangioblastic — *see* Neoplasm, meninges, benign
  - hemangiopericytic — *see* Neoplasm, meninges, benign
  - malignant — *see* Neoplasm, meninges, malignant
  - meningiothelial — *see* Neoplasm, meninges, benign
  - meningotheliomatous — *see* Neoplasm, meninges, benign
  - mixed — *see* Neoplasm, meninges, benign
  - multiple — *see* Neoplasm, meninges, uncertain behavior
  - papillary — *see* Neoplasm, meninges, uncertain behavior
  - psammomatous — *see* Neoplasm, meninges, benign
  - syncytial — *see* Neoplasm, meninges, benign
  - transitional — *see* Neoplasm, meninges, benign
- **Meningiomatosis** (diffuse) — *see* Neoplasm, meninges, uncertain behavior
- **Meningism** — *see* Meningismus
- **Meningismus** (infectional) (pneumococcal) R29.1
  - due to serum or vaccine R29.1
  - influenzal — *see* Influenza, with, manifestations NEC
- **Meningitis** (basal) (basic) (brain) (cerebral) (cervical) (congestive) (diffuse) (hemorrhagic) (infantile) (membranous) (metastatic) (nonspecific) (pontine) (progressive) (simple) (spinal) (subacute) (sympathetic) (toxic) G03.9
  - abacterial G03.Ø
  - actinomycotic A42.81
  - adenoviral A87.1
  - arbovirus A87.8
  - aseptic (acute) G03.Ø
  - bacterial G0Ø.9
    - Escherichia coli (E. coli) GØØ.8
    - Friedlander (bacillus) GØØ.8
    - gram-negative GØØ.9
    - H. influenzae GØØ.Ø
    - Klebsiella GØØ.8
    - pneumococcal GØØ.1
    - specified organism NEC GØØ.8
    - staphylococcal GØØ.3
    - streptococcal (acute) GØØ.2
  - benign recurrent (Mollaret) GØ3.2
  - candidal B37.5
  - caseous (tuberculous) A17.Ø
  - cerebrospinal A39.Ø
  - chronic NEC GØ3.1
  - clear cerebrospinal fluid NEC GØ3.Ø
  - coxsackievirus A87.Ø
  - cryptococcal B45.1
  - diplococcal (gram positive) A39.Ø
  - echovirus A87.Ø
  - enteroviral A87.Ø
  - eosinophilic B83.2
  - epidemic NEC A39.Ø
  - Escherichia coli (E. coli) GØØ.8
  - fibrinopurulent GØØ.9
    - specified organism NEC GØØ.8
  - Friedlander (bacillus) GØØ.8
  - gonococcal A54.81
  - gram-negative cocci GØØ.9
  - gram-positive cocci GØØ.9
  - H. influenzae GØØ.Ø
  - Haemophilus (influenzae) GØØ.Ø
  - in (due to)
    - adenovirus A87.1
    - African trypanosomiasis B56.9 *[GØ2]*
    - anthrax A22.8
    - bacterial disease NEC A48.8 *[GØ1]*
    - Chagas' disease (chronic) B57.41
    - chickenpox BØ1.Ø
    - coccidioidomycosis B38.4
    - Diplococcus pneumoniae GØØ.1
    - enterovirus A87.Ø
- **Meningitis** — *continued*
  - in — *continued*
    - herpes (simplex) virus BØØ.3
      - zoster BØ2.1
    - infectious mononucleosis B27.92
    - leptospirosis A27.81
    - Listeria monocytogenes A32.11
    - Lyme disease A69.21
    - measles BØ5.1
    - mumps (virus) B26.1
    - neurosyphilis (late) A52.13
    - parasitic disease NEC B89 *[GØ2]*
    - poliovirus A8Ø.9 *[GØ2]*
    - preventive immunization, inoculation or vaccination GØ3.8
    - rubella BØ6.Ø2
    - Salmonella infection AØ2.21
    - specified cause NEC GØ3.8
    - Streptococcal pneumoniae GØØ.1
    - typhoid fever AØ1.Ø1
    - varicella BØ1.Ø
    - viral disease NEC A87.8
    - whooping cough A37.9Ø
    - zoster BØ2.1
  - infectious GØØ.9
  - influenzal (H. influenzae) GØØ.Ø
  - Klebsiella GØØ.8
  - leptospiral (aseptic) A27.81
  - lymphocytic (acute) (benign) (serous) A87.2
  - meningococcal A39.Ø
  - Mima polymorpha GØØ.8
  - Mollaret (benign recurrent) GØ3.2
  - monilial B37.5
  - mycotic NEC B49 *[GØ2]*
  - Neisseria A39.Ø
  - nonbacterial GØ3.Ø
  - nonpyogenic NEC GØ3.Ø
  - ossificans G96.198
  - pneumococcal streptococcus pneumoniae GØØ.1
  - poliovirus A8Ø.9 *[GØ2]*
  - postmeasles BØ5.1
  - purulent GØØ.9
    - specified organism NEC GØØ.8
  - pyogenic GØØ.9
    - specified organism NEC GØØ.8
  - Salmonella (arizonae) (Cholerae-Suis) (enteritidis) (typhimurium) AØ2.21
  - septic GØØ.9
    - specified organism NEC GØØ.8
  - serosa circumscripta NEC GØ3.Ø
  - serous NEC G93.2
  - specified organism NEC GØØ.8
  - sporotrichosis B42.81
  - staphylococcal GØØ.3
  - sterile GØ3.Ø
  - Streptococcal (acute) GØØ.2
    - pneumoniae GØØ.1
  - suppurative GØØ.9
    - specified organism NEC GØØ.8
  - syphilitic (late) (tertiary) A52.13
    - acute A51.41
    - congenital A5Ø.41
    - secondary A51.41
  - Torula histolytica (cryptococcal) B45.1
  - traumatic (complication of injury) T79.8 ☑
  - tuberculous A17.Ø
  - typhoid AØ1.Ø1
  - viral NEC A87.9
  - Yersinia pestis A2Ø.3
- **Meningocele** (spinal) — *see also* Spina bifida
  - with hydrocephalus — *see* Spina bifida, by site, with hydrocephalus
  - acquired (traumatic) G96.198
  - cerebral — *see* Encephalocele
- **Meningocerebritis** — *see* Meningoencephalitis
- **Meningococcemia** A39.4
  - acute A39.2
  - chronic A39.3
- **Meningococcus, meningococcal** — *see also* condition A39.9
  - adrenalitis, hemorrhagic A39.1
  - carrier (suspected) of Z22.31
  - meningitis (cerebrospinal) A39.Ø
- **Meningoencephalitis** — *see also* Encephalitis GØ4.9Ø
  - acute NEC — *see also* Encephalitis, viral A86
  - bacterial NEC GØ4.2
  - California A83.5
  - diphasic A84.1

Index

Melanosarcoma — Meningoencephalitis

- **Meningoencephalitis** — *continued*
  - eosinophilic B83.2
  - epidemic A39.81
  - herpesviral, herpetic BØØ.4
    - due to herpesvirus 6 B1Ø.Ø1
    - due to herpesvirus 7 B1Ø.Ø9
    - specified NEC B1Ø.Ø9
  - in (due to)
    - blastomycosis NEC B4Ø.81
    - diseases classified elsewhere GØ5.3
    - free-living amebae B6Ø.2
    - H. influenzae GØØ.Ø
    - Hemophilus influenzae (H .influenzae) GØØ.Ø
    - herpes BØØ.4
      - due to herpesvirus 6 B1Ø.Ø1
      - due to herpesvirus 7 B1Ø.Ø9
      - specified NEC B1Ø.Ø9
    - Lyme disease A69.22
    - mercury — *see* subcategory T56.1 ☑
    - mumps B26.2
    - Naegleria (amebae) (organisms) (fowleri) B6Ø.2
    - Parastrongylus cantonensis B83.2
    - toxoplasmosis (acquired) B58.2
      - congenital P37.1
  - infectious (acute) (viral) A86
  - influenzal (H. influenzae) GØØ.Ø
  - Listeria monocytogenes A32.12
  - lymphocytic (serous) A87.2
  - mumps B26.2
  - parasitic NEC B89 *[GØ5.3]*
  - pneumococcal GØ4.2
  - primary amebic B6Ø.2
  - specific (syphilitic) A52.14
  - specified organism NEC GØ4.81
  - staphylococcal GØ4.2
  - streptococcal GØ4.2
  - syphilitic A52.14
  - toxic NEC G92.8
    - due to mercury — *see* subcategory T56.1 ☑
  - tuberculous A17.82
  - virus NEC A86
- **Meningoencephalocele** — *see also* Encephalocele
  - syphilitic A52.19
    - congenital A5Ø.49
- **Meningoencephalomyelitis** — *see also* Meningoencephalitis
  - acute NEC (viral) A86
    - disseminated GØ4.ØØ
      - postimmunization or postvaccination GØ4.Ø2
      - postinfectious GØ4.Ø1
  - due to
    - actinomycosis A42.82
    - Torula B45.1
    - Toxoplasma or toxoplasmosis (acquired) B58.2
      - congenital P37.1
  - postimmunization or postvaccination GØ4.Ø2
- **Meningoencephalomyelopathy** G96.9
- **Meningoencephalopathy** G96.9
- **Meningomyelitis** — *see also* Meningoencephalitis
  - bacterial NEC GØ4.2
  - blastomycotic NEC B4Ø.81
  - cryptococcal B45.1
  - in diseases classified elsewhere GØ5.4
  - meningococcal A39.81
  - syphilitic A52.14
  - tuberculous A17.82
- **Meningomyelocele** — *see also* Spina bifida
  - syphilitic A52.19
- **Meningomyeloneuritis** — *see* Meningoencephalitis
- **Meningoradiculitis** — *see* Meningitis
- **Meningovascular** — *see* condition
- **Menkes' disease or syndrome** E83.Ø9
  - meaning maple-syrup-urine disease E71.Ø
- **Menometrorrhagia** N92.1
- **Menopause, menopausal** (asymptomatic) (state) Z78.Ø
  - arthritis (any site) NEC — *see* Arthritis, specified form NEC
  - bleeding N92.4
  - depression (single episode) F32.89
    - agitated (single episode) F32.2
      - recurrent episode F33.9
    - psychotic (single episode) F32.89
      - recurrent episode F33.9
    - recurrent episode F33.8
  - melancholia (single episode) F32.89
    - recurrent episode F33.8
  - paranoid state F22
- **Menopause, menopausal** — *continued*
  - postirradiation (postprocedural)
    - asymptomatic E89.4Ø
    - symptomatic E89.41
  - premature E28.319
    - asymptomatic E28.319
      - postirradiation E89.4Ø
      - postsurgical E89.4Ø
    - symptomatic E28.31Ø
      - postirradiation E89.41
      - postsurgical E89.41
  - psychosis NEC F28
  - symptomatic N95.1
  - toxic polyarthritis NEC — *see* Arthritis, specified form NEC
- **Menorrhagia** (primary) N92.Ø
  - climacteric N92.4
    - menopausal N92.4
  - menopausal N92.4
  - perimenopausal N92.4
  - postclimacteric N95.Ø
  - postmenopausal N95.Ø
  - preclimacteric or premenopausal N92.4
  - pubertal (menses retained) N92.2
- **Menostaxis** N92.Ø
- **Menses, retention** N94.89
- **Menstrual** — *see* Menstruation
- **Menstruation**
  - absent — *see* Amenorrhea
  - anovulatory N97.Ø
  - cycle, irregular N92.6
  - delayed N91.Ø
  - disorder N93.9
    - psychogenic F45.8
  - during pregnancy O2Ø.8
  - excessive (with regular cycle) N92.Ø
    - with irregular cycle N92.1
    - at puberty N92.2
  - frequent N92.Ø
  - infrequent — *see* Oligomenorrhea
  - irregular N92.6
    - specified NEC N92.5
  - latent N92.5
  - membranous N92.5
  - painful — *see also* Dysmenorrhea N94.6
    - primary N94.4
    - psychogenic F45.8
    - secondary N94.5
  - passage of clots N92.Ø
  - precocious E3Ø.1
  - protracted N92.5
  - rare — *see* Oligomenorrhea
  - retained N94.89
  - retrograde N92.5
  - scanty — *see* Oligomenorrhea
  - suppression N94.89
  - vicarious (nasal) N94.89
- **Mental** — *see also* condition
  - deficiency — *see* Disability, intellectual
  - deterioration — *see* Psychosis
  - disorder — *see* Disorder, mental
  - exhaustion F48.8
  - insufficiency (congenital) — *see* Disability, intellectual
  - observation without need for further medical care ZØ3.89
  - retardation — *see* Disability, intellectual
  - subnormality — *see* Disability, intellectuall
  - upset — *see* Disorder, mental
- **Meralgia paresthetica** G57.1- ☑
- **Mercurial** — *see* condition
- **Mercurialism** — *see* subcategory T56.1 ☑
- **Merkel cell tumor** — *see* Carcinoma, Merkel cell
- **Merocele** — *see* Hernia, femoral
- **Meromelia**
  - lower limb — *see* Defect, reduction, lower limb
    - intercalary
      - femur — *see* Defect, reduction, lower limb, specified type NEC
        - tibiofibular (complete) (incomplete) — *see* Defect, reduction, lower limb
  - upper limb — *see* Defect, reduction, upper limb
    - intercalary, humeral, radioulnar — *see* Agenesis, arm, with hand present
- **MERRF syndrome** (myoclonic epilepsy associated with ragged-red fiber) E88.42
- **Merzbacher-Pelizaeus disease** E75.27
- **Mesaortitis** — *see* Aortitis
- **Mesarteritis** — *see* Arteritis
- **Mesencephalitis** — *see* Encephalitis
- **Mesenchymoma** — *see also* Neoplasm, connective tissue, uncertain behavior
  - benign — *see* Neoplasm, connective tissue, benign
  - malignant — *see* Neoplasm, connective tissue, malignant
- **Mesenteritis**
  - retractile K65.4
  - sclerosing K65.4
- **Mesentery, mesenteric** — *see* condition
- **Mesiodens, mesiodentes** KØØ.1
- **Mesio-occlusion** M26.213
- **Mesocolon** — *see* condition
- **Mesonephroma** (malignant) — *see* Neoplasm, malignant, by site
  - benign — *see* Neoplasm, benign, by site
- **Mesophlebitis** — *see* Phlebitis
- **Mesostromal dysgenesia** Q13.89
- **Mesothelioma** (malignant) C45.9
  - benign
    - mesentery D19.1
    - mesocolon D19.1
    - omentum D19.1
    - peritoneum D19.1
    - pleura D19.Ø
    - specified site NEC D19.7
    - unspecified site D19.9
  - biphasic C45.9
    - benign
      - mesentery D19.1
      - mesocolon D19.1
      - omentum D19.1
      - peritoneum D19.1
      - pleura D19.Ø
      - specified site NEC D19.7
      - unspecified site D19.9
  - cystic D48.4
  - epithelioid C45.9
    - benign
      - mesentery D19.1
      - mesocolon D19.1
      - omentum D19.1
      - peritoneum D19.1
      - pleura D19.Ø
      - specified site NEC D19.7
      - unspecified site D19.9
  - fibrous C45.9
    - benign
      - mesentery D19.1
      - mesocolon D19.1
      - omentum D19.1
      - peritoneum D19.1
      - pleura D19.Ø
      - specified site NEC D19.7
      - unspecified site D19.9
  - site classification
    - liver C45.7
    - lung C45.7
    - mediastinum C45.7
    - mesentery C45.1
    - mesocolon C45.1
    - omentum C45.1
    - pericardium C45.2
    - peritoneum C45.1
    - pleura C45.Ø
      - parietal C45.Ø
    - retroperitoneum C45.7
    - specified site NEC C45.7
    - unspecified C45.9
- **Metabolic syndrome** E88.81Ø
- **Metagonimiasis** B66.8
- **Metagonimus infestation** (intestine) B66.8
- **Metal**
  - pigmentation L81.8
  - polisher's disease J62.8
- **Metamorphopsia** H53.15
- **Metaplasia**
  - apocrine (breast) — *see* Dysplasia, mammary, specified type NEC
  - cervix (squamous) — *see* Dysplasia, cervix
  - endometrium (squamous) (uterus) N85.8
  - esophagus K22.7- ☑
  - gastric intestinal K31.AØ
    - with dysplasia K31.A29
      - high grade K31.A22
      - low grade K31.A21
    - indefinite for dysplasia K31.AØ
    - without dysplasia K31.A19

Migraine — *continued*
- ophthalmoplegic — *continued*
  - not intractable G43.BØ (*following* G43.7)
    - without refractory migraine G43.BØ (*following* G43.7)
- persistent aura (with, without) cerebral infarction — *see* Migraine, with aura, persistent
- preceded or accompanied by transient focal neurological phenomena — *see* Migraine, with aura
- pre-menstrual — *see* Migraine, menstrual
- pure menstrual — *see* Migraine, menstrual
- retinal — *see* Migraine, with aura
- specified NEC G43.8Ø9
  - intractable G43.819
    - with status migrainosus G43.811
    - without status migrainosus G43.819
  - not intractable G43.8Ø9
    - with status migrainosus G43.8Ø1
    - without status migrainosus G43.8Ø9
- sporadic — *see* Migraine, hemiplegic
- transformed — *see* Migraine, without aura, chronic
- triggered seizures — *see* Migraine, with aura
- without aura G43.ØØ9
  - with refractory migraine G43.Ø19
    - with status migrainosus G43.Ø11
    - without status migrainosus G43.Ø19
  - chronic G43.7Ø9
    - with refractory migraine G43.719
      - with status migrainosus G43.711
      - without status migrainosus G43.719
    - intractable
      - with status migrainosus G43.711
      - without status migrainosus G43.719
    - not intractable
      - with status migrainosus G43.7Ø1
      - without status migrainosus G43.7Ø9
    - without refractory migraine G43.7Ø9
      - with status migrainosus G43.7Ø1
      - without status migrainosus G43.7Ø9
  - intractable
    - with status migrainosus G43.Ø11
    - without status migrainosus G43.Ø19
  - not intractable
    - with status migrainosus G43.ØØ1
    - without status migrainosus G43.ØØ9
  - without mention of refractory migraine G43.ØØ9
    - with status migrainosus G43.ØØ1
    - without status migrainosus G43.ØØ9
- without refractory migraine G43.9Ø9
  - with status migrainosus G43.9Ø1
  - without status migrainosus G43.9Ø9

Migrant, social Z59.ØØ
Migration, anxiety concerning Z6Ø.3
Migratory, migrating — *see also* condition
- person Z59.ØØ
- testis Q55.29

Mikity-Wilson disease or syndrome P27.Ø
Mikulicz' disease or syndrome K11.8
Miliaria L74.3
- alba L74.1
- apocrine L75.2
- crystallina L74.1
- profunda L74.2
- rubra L74.Ø
- tropicalis L74.2

Miliary — *see* condition
Milium L72.Ø
- colloid L57.8

Milk
- crust L21.Ø
- excessive secretion O92.6
- poisoning — *see* Poisoning, food, noxious
- retention O92.79
- sickness — *see* Poisoning, food, noxious
- spots I31.Ø

Milk-alkali disease or syndrome E83.52
Milk-leg (deep vessels) (nonpuerperal) — *see* Embolism, vein, lower extremity
- complicating pregnancy O22.3- ☑
- puerperal, postpartum, childbirth O87.1

Milkman's disease or syndrome M83.8
Milky urine — *see* Chyluria
Millard-Gubler (-Foville) **paralysis or syndrome** G46.3
Millar's asthma J38.5
Miller Fisher syndrome G61.Ø
Mills' disease — *see* Hemiplegia
Millstone maker's pneumoconiosis J62.8
Milroy's disease (chronic hereditary edema) Q82.Ø
Minamata disease T56.1 ☑
Miners' asthma or lung J6Ø
Minkowski-Chauffard syndrome — *see* Spherocytosis
Minor — *see* condition
Minor's disease (hematomyelia) G95.19
Minot's disease (hemorrhagic disease), newborn P53
Minot-von Willebrand-Jurgens disease or syndrome (angiohemophilia) — *see* Disease, von Willebrand
Minus (and plus) **hand** (intrinsic) — *see* Deformity, limb, specified type NEC, forearm
Miosis (pupil) H57.Ø3
Mirizzi's syndrome (hepatic duct stenosis) K83.1
Mirror writing F81.Ø
MIS-A M35.81
Misadventure (of) (prophylactic) (therapeutic) — *see also* Complications T88.9 ☑
- administration of insulin (by accident) — *see* subcategory T38.3 ☑
- infusion — *see* Complications, infusion
- local applications (of fomentations, plasters, etc.) T88.9 ☑
  - burn or scald — *see* Burn
  - specified NEC T88.8 ☑
- medical care (early) (late) T88.9 ☑
  - adverse effect of drugs or chemicals — *see* Table of Drugs and Chemicals
  - burn or scald — *see* Burn
  - specified NEC T88.8 ☑
- specified NEC T88.8 ☑
- surgical procedure (early) (late) — *see* Complications, surgical procedure
- transfusion — *see* Complications, transfusion
- vaccination or other immunological procedure — *see* Complications, vaccination

MIS-C M35.81
Miscarriage OØ3.9
Misdirection, aqueous H4Ø.83- ☑
Misperception, sleep state F51.Ø2
Misplaced, misplacement
- ear Q17.4
- kidney (acquired) N28.89
  - congenital Q63.2
- organ or site, congenital NEC — *see* Malposition, congenital

Missed
- abortion OØ2.1
- delivery O36.4 ☑

Missing — *see also* Absence
- string of intrauterine contraceptive device T83.32- ☑

Misuse of drugs F19.99
Mitchell's disease (erythromelalgia) I73.81
Mite(s) (infestation) B88.9
- diarrhea B88.Ø
- grain (itch) B88.Ø
- hair follicle (itch) B88.Ø
- in sputum B88.Ø

Mitral — *see* condition
Mittelschmerz N94.Ø
Mixed — *see* condition
MMN (multifocal motor neuropathy) G61.82
MNGIE (Mitochondrial Neurogastrointestinal Encephalopathy) **syndrome** E88.49
Mobile, mobility
- cecum Q43.3
- excessive — *see* Hypermobility
- gallbladder, congenital Q44.1
- kidney N28.89
- organ or site, congenital NEC — *see* Malposition, congenital

Mobitz heart block (atrioventricular) I44.1
Moebius, Möbius
- disease (ophthalmoplegic migraine) — *see* Migraine, ophthalmoplegic
- syndrome Q87.Ø
  - congenital oculofacial paralysis (with other anomalies) Q87.Ø
  - ophthalmoplegic migraine — *see* Migraine, ophthalmoplegic

Moeller's glossitis K14.Ø
MOGAD (myelin oligodendrocyte glycoprotein antibody disease) G37.81
Mohr's syndrome (Types I and II) Q87.Ø
Mola destruens D39.2
Molar pregnancy OØ2.Ø
Molarization of premolars KØØ.2
Molding, head (during birth) — *omit code*
Mole (pigmented) — *see also* Nevus
- blood OØ2.Ø

Mole — *continued*
- Breus' OØ2.Ø
- cancerous — *see* Melanoma
- carneous OØ2.Ø
- destructive D39.2
- fleshy OØ2.Ø
- hydatid, hydatidiform (benign) (complicating pregnancy) (delivered) (undelivered) OØ1.9
  - classical OØ1.Ø
  - complete OØ1.Ø
  - incomplete OØ1.1
  - invasive D39.2
  - malignant D39.2
  - partial OØ1.1
- intrauterine OØ2.Ø
- invasive (hydatidiform) D39.2
- malignant
  - meaning
    - malignant hydatidiform mole D39.2
    - melanoma — *see* Melanoma
- nonhydatidiform OØ2.Ø
- nonpigmented — *see* Nevus
- pregnancy NEC OØ2.Ø
- skin — *see* Nevus
- tubal OØØ.1Ø- ☑
  - with intrauterine pregnancy OØØ.11- ☑
- vesicular — *see* Mole, hydatidiform

Molimen, molimina (menstrual) N94.3
Molluscum contagiosum (epitheliale) BØ8.1
Monckeberg's arteriosclerosis, disease, or sclerosis — *see* Arteriosclerosis, extremities
Mondini's malformation (cochlea) Q16.5
Mondor's disease I8Ø.8
Monge's disease T7Ø.29 ☑
Monilethrix (congenital) Q84.1
Moniliasis — *see also* Candidiasis B37.9
- neonatal P37.5

Monitoring (encounter for)
- therapeutic drug level Z51.81

Monkey malaria B53.1
Monkeypox BØ4
Monoarthritis M13.1Ø
- ankle M13.17- ☑
- elbow M13.12- ☑
- foot joint M13.17- ☑
- hand joint M13.14- ☑
- hip M13.15- ☑
- knee M13.16- ☑
- shoulder M13.11- ☑
- wrist M13.13- ☑

Monoblastic — *see* condition
Monochromat (ism), monochromatopsia (acquired) (congenital) H53.51
Monocytic — *see* condition
Monocytopenia D72.818
Monocytosis (symptomatic) D72.821
Monomania — *see* Psychosis
Mononeuritis G58.9
- cranial nerve — *see* Disorder, nerve, cranial
- femoral nerve G57.2- ☑
- lateral
  - cutaneous nerve of thigh G57.1- ☑
  - popliteal nerve G57.3- ☑
- lower limb G57.9- ☑
  - specified nerve NEC G57.8- ☑
- medial popliteal nerve G57.4- ☑
- median nerve G56.1- ☑
- multiplex G58.7
- plantar nerve G57.6- ☑
- posterior tibial nerve G57.5- ☑
- radial nerve G56.3- ☑
- sciatic nerve G57.Ø- ☑
- specified NEC G58.8
- tibial nerve G57.4- ☑
- ulnar nerve G56.2- ☑
- upper limb G56.9- ☑
  - specified nerve NEC G56.8- ☑
- vestibular — *see* subcategory H93.3 ☑

Mononeuropathy G58.9
- carpal tunnel syndrome — *see* Syndrome, carpal tunnel
- diabetic NEC — *see* EØ8-E13 with .41
- femoral nerve — *see* Lesion, nerve, femoral
- ilioinguinal nerve G57.8- ☑
- in diseases classified elsewhere — *see* category G59
- intercostal G58.Ø
- lower limb G57.9- ☑
  - causalgia — *see* Causalgia, lower limb

☑ **Additional Character Required — Refer to the Tabular List for Character Selection**

Mononeuropathy — *continued*
- lower limb — *continued*
  - femoral nerve — *see* Lesion, nerve, femoral
  - meralgia paresthetica G57.1- ☑
  - plantar nerve — *see* Lesion, nerve, plantar
  - popliteal nerve — *see* Lesion, nerve, popliteal
  - sciatic nerve — *see* Lesion, nerve, sciatic
  - specified NEC G57.8- ☑
  - tarsal tunnel syndrome — *see* Syndrome, tarsal tunnel
- median nerve — *see* Lesion, nerve, median
- multiplex G58.7
- obturator nerve G57.8- ☑
- popliteal nerve — *see* Lesion, nerve, popliteal
- radial nerve — *see* Lesion, nerve, radial
- saphenous nerve G57.8- ☑
- specified NEC G58.8
- tarsal tunnel syndrome — *see* Syndrome, tarsal tunnel
- tuberculous A17.83
- ulnar nerve — *see* Lesion, nerve, ulnar
- upper limb G56.9- ☑
  - carpal tunnel syndrome — *see* Syndrome, carpal tunnel
  - causalgia — *see* Causalgia
  - median nerve — *see* Lesion, nerve, median
  - radial nerve — *see* Lesion, nerve, radial
  - specified site NEC G56.8- ☑
  - ulnar nerve — *see* Lesion, nerve, ulnar

Mononucleosis, infectious B27.9Ø
- with
  - complication NEC B27.99
  - meningitis B27.92
  - polyneuropathy B27.91
- cytomegaloviral B27.1Ø
  - with
    - complication NEC B27.19
    - meningitis B27.12
    - polyneuropathy B27.11
- Epstein-Barr (virus) B27.ØØ
  - with
    - complication NEC B27.Ø9
    - meningitis B27.Ø2
    - polyneuropathy B27.Ø1
- gammaherpesviral B27.ØØ
  - with
    - complication NEC B27.Ø9
    - meningitis B27.Ø2
    - polyneuropathy B27.Ø1
- specified NEC B27.8Ø
  - with
    - complication NEC B27.89
    - meningitis B27.82
    - polyneuropathy B27.81

Monoparesis — *see* Monoplegia

Monoplegia G83.3- ☑
- congenital (cerebral) G8Ø.8
  - spastic G8Ø.1
- embolic (current episode) I63.4- ☑
- following
  - cerebrovascular disease
    - cerebral infarction
      - lower limb I69.34- ☑
      - upper limb I69.33- ☑
    - intracerebral hemorrhage
      - lower limb I69.14- ☑
      - upper limb I69.13- ☑
    - lower limb I69.94- ☑
    - nontraumatic intracranial hemorrhage NEC
      - lower limb I69.24- ☑
      - upper limb I69.23- ☑
    - specified disease NEC
      - lower limb I69.84- ☑
      - upper limb I69.83- ☑
    - stroke NOS
      - lower limb I69.34- ☑
      - upper limb I69.33- ☑
    - subarachnoid hemorrhage
      - lower limb I69.Ø4- ☑
      - upper limb I69.Ø3- ☑
    - upper limb I69.93- ☑
- hysterical (transient) F44.4
- lower limb G83.1- ☑
- psychogenic (conversion reaction) F44.4
- thrombotic (current episode) I63.3- ☑
- transient R29.818
- upper limb G83.2- ☑

Monorchism, monorchidism Q55.Ø

Monosomy — *see also* Deletion, chromosome Q93.9
- specified NEC Q93.89
- whole chromosome
  - meiotic nondisjunction Q93.Ø
  - mitotic nondisjunction Q93.1
  - mosaicism Q93.1
- X Q96.9

Monster, monstrosity (single) Q89.7
- acephalic QØØ.Ø
- twin Q89.4

Monteggia's fracture (-dislocation) S52.27- ☑

Mooren's ulcer (cornea) — *see* Ulcer, cornea, Mooren's

Moore's syndrome — *see* Epilepsy, specified NEC

Mooser-Neill reaction A75.2

Mooser's bodies A75.2

Morbidity not stated or unknown R69

Morbilli — *see* Measles

Morbus — *see also* Disease
- angelicus, anglorum E55.Ø
- Beigel B36.2
- caducus — *see* Epilepsy
- celiacus K9Ø.Ø
- comitialis — *see* Epilepsy
- cordis — *see also* Disease, heart I51.9
  - valvulorum — *see* Endocarditis
- coxae senilis M16.9
  - tuberculous A18.Ø2
- hemorrhagicus neonatorum P53
- maculosus neonatorum P54.5

Morel (-Stewart)(-Morgagni) **syndrome** M85.2

Morel-Kraepelin disease — *see* Schizophrenia

Morel-Moore syndrome M85.2

Morgagni's
- cyst, organ, hydatid, or appendage
  - female Q5Ø.5
  - male (epididymal) Q55.4
    - testicular Q55.29
- syndrome M85.2

Morgagni-Stewart-Morel syndrome M85.2

Morgagni-Stokes-Adams syndrome I45.9

Morgagni-Turner (-Albright) **syndrome** Q96.9

Moria FØ7.Ø

Moron (I.Q. 5Ø-69) F7Ø

Morphea L94.Ø

Morphinism (without remission) F11.2Ø
- with remission F11.21

Morphinomania (without remission) F11.2Ø
- with remission F11.21

Morquio (-Ullrich)(-Brailsford) **disease or syndrome** — *see* Mucopolysaccharidosis

Mortification (dry) (moist) — *see* Gangrene

Morton's metatarsalgia (neuralgia) (neuroma) (syndrome) G57.6- ☑

Morvan's disease or syndrome G6Ø.8

Mosaicism, mosaic (autosomal) (chromosomal)
- 45,X/46,XX Q96.3
- 45,X/other cell lines NEC with abnormal sex chromosome Q96.4
- sex chromosome
  - female Q97.8
  - lines with various numbers of X chromosomes Q97.2
  - male Q98.7
- XY Q96.3

Moschowitz' disease M31.19

Mother yaw A66.Ø

Motion sickness (from travel, any vehicle) (from roundabouts or swings) T75.3 ☑

Mottled, mottling, teeth (enamel) (endemic) (nonendemic) KØØ.3

Mounier-Kuhn syndrome Q32.4
- with bronchiectasis J47.9
  - exacerbation (acute) J47.1
  - lower respiratory infection J47.Ø
- acquired J98.Ø9
  - with bronchiectasis J47.9
    - with
      - exacerbation (acute) J47.1
      - lower respiratory infection J47.Ø

Mountain
- sickness T7Ø.29 ☑
  - with polycythemia , acquired (acute) D75.1
- tick fever A93.2

Mouse, joint — *see* Loose, body, joint
- knee M23.4- ☑

Mouth — *see* condition

Movable
- coccyx — *see* subcategory M53.2 ☑

Movable — *continued*
- kidney N28.89
  - congenital Q63.8
- spleen D73.89

Movements, dystonic R25.8

Moyamoya disease I67.5

MRSA (Methicillin resistant Staphylococcus aureus)
- infection A49.Ø2
  - as the cause of diseases classified elsewhere B95.62
- sepsis A41.Ø2

MSD (multiple sulfatase deficiency) E75.26

MSSA (Methicillin susceptible Staphylococcus aureus)
- infection A49.Ø1
  - as the cause of diseases classified elsewhere B95.61
- sepsis A41.Ø1

Mucha-Habermann disease L41.Ø

Mucinosis (cutaneous) (focal) (papular) (skin) L98.5
- oral K13.79

Mucocele
- appendix K38.8
- buccal cavity K13.79
- gallbladder K82.1
- lacrimal sac, chronic HØ4.43- ☑
- nasal sinus J34.1
- nose J34.1
- salivary gland (any) K11.6
- sinus (accessory) (nasal) J34.1
- turbinate (bone) (middle) (nasal) J34.1
- uterus N85.8

Mucolipidosis
- I E77.1
- II, III E77.Ø
- IV E75.11

Mucopolysaccharidosis E76.3
- beta-gluduronidase deficiency E76.29
- cardiopathy E76.3 *[I52]*
- Hunter's syndrome E76.1
- Hurler's syndrome E76.Ø1
- Hurler-Scheie syndrome E76.Ø2
- Maroteaux-Lamy syndrome E76.29
- Morquio syndrome E76.219
  - A E76.21Ø
  - B E76.211
  - classic E76.21Ø
- Sanfilippo syndrome E76.22
- Scheie's syndrome E76.Ø3
- specified NEC E76.29
- type
  - I
    - Hurler's syndrome E76.Ø1
    - Hurler-Scheie syndrome E76.Ø2
    - Scheie's syndrome E76.Ø3
  - II E76.1
  - III E76.22
  - IV E76.219
  - IVA E76.21Ø
  - IVB E76.211
  - VI E76.29
  - VII E76.29

Mucormycosis B46.5
- cutaneous B46.3
- disseminated B46.4
- gastrointestinal B46.2
- generalized B46.4
- pulmonary B46.Ø
- rhinocerebral B46.1
- skin B46.3
- subcutaneous B46.3

Mucositis (ulcerative) K12.3Ø
- due to drugs NEC K12.32
- gastrointestinal K92.81
- mouth (oral) (oropharyngeal) K12.3Ø
  - due to antineoplastic therapy K12.31
  - due to drugs NEC K12.32
  - due to radiation K12.33
  - specified NEC K12.39
  - viral K12.39
- nasal J34.81
- oral cavity — *see* Mucositis, mouth
- oral soft tissues — *see* Mucositis, mouth
- vagina and vulva N76.81

Mucositis necroticans agranulocytica — *see* Agranulocytosis

Mucous — *see also* condition
- patches (syphilitic) A51.39
  - congenital A5Ø.Ø7

Mucoviscidosis E84.9
- with meconium obstruction E84.11

Mucus
- asphyxia or suffocation — *see* Asphyxia, mucus
- in stool R19.5
- plug — *see* Asphyxia, mucus

Muguet B37.Ø
Mulberry molars (congenital syphilis) A5Ø.52
Mullerian mixed tumor
- specified site — *see* Neoplasm, malignant, by site
- unspecified site C54.9

Multicystic kidney (development) Q61.4
Multiparity (grand) Z64.1
- affecting management of pregnancy, labor and delivery (supervision only) OØ9.4- ☑
- requiring contraceptive management — *see* Contraception

Multipartita placenta O43.19- ☑
Multiple, multiplex — *see also* condition
- digits (congenital) Q69.9
- endocrine neoplasia — *see* Neoplasia, endocrine, multiple (MEN)
- personality F44.81

Multisystem inflammatory syndrome (in adult) (in children) M35.81
Mumps B26.9
- arthritis B26.85
- complication NEC B26.89
- encephalitis B26.2
- hepatitis B26.81
- meningitis (aseptic) B26.1
- meningoencephalitis B26.2
- myocarditis B26.82
- oophoritis B26.89
- orchitis B26.Ø
- pancreatitis B26.3
- polyneuropathy B26.84

Mumu — *see also* Infestation, filarial B74.9 *[N51]*
Munchhausen's syndrome — *see* Disorder, factitious
Munchmeyer's syndrome — *see* Myositis, ossificans, progressiva
Mural — *see* condition
Murmur (cardiac) (heart) (organic) RØ1.1
- abdominal R19.15
- aortic (valve) — *see* Endocarditis, aortic
- benign RØ1.Ø
- diastolic — *see* Endocarditis
- Flint I35.1
- functional RØ1.Ø
- Graham Steell I37.1
- innocent RØ1.Ø
- mitral (valve) — *see* Insufficiency, mitral
- nonorganic RØ1.Ø
- presystolic, mitral — *see* Insufficiency, mitral
- pulmonic (valve) I37.8
- systolic RØ1.1
- tricuspid (valve) IØ7.9
- valvular — *see* Endocarditis

Murri's disease (intermittent hemoglobinuria) D59.6
Muscle, muscular — *see also* condition
- carnitine (palmityltransferase) deficiency E71.314

Musculoneuralgia — *see* Neuralgia
Mushrooming hip — *see* Derangement, joint, specified NEC, hip
Mushroom-workers' (pickers') **disease or lung** J67.5
Mutation(s)
- factor V Leiden D68.51
- prothrombin gene D68.52
- surfactant, of lung J84.83

Mutism — *see also* Aphasia
- deaf (acquired) (congenital) NEC H91.3
- elective (adjustment reaction) (childhood) F94.Ø
- hysterical F44.4
- selective (childhood) F94.Ø

MVD (microvillus inclusion disease) Q43.8
MVID (microvillus inclusion disease) Q43.8
Myalgia M79.1Ø
- auxiliary muscles, head and neck M79.12
- epidemic (cervical) B33.Ø
- mastication muscle M79.11
- site specified NEC M79.18
- traumatic NEC T14.8 ☑

Myasthenia G7Ø.9
- congenital G7Ø.2
- cordis — *see* Failure, heart
- developmental G7Ø.2
- gravis G7Ø.ØØ
  - with exacerbation (acute) G7Ø.Ø1
  - in crisis G7Ø.Ø1

Myasthenia — *continued*
- gravis — *continued*
  - neonatal, transient P94.Ø
  - pseudoparalytica G7Ø.ØØ
    - with exacerbation (acute) G7Ø.Ø1
    - in crisis G7Ø.Ø1
- stomach, psychogenic F45.8
- syndrome
  - in
    - diabetes mellitus — *see* EØ8-E13 with .44
    - neoplastic disease — *see also* Neoplasm D49.9 *[G73.3]*
    - pernicious anemia D51.Ø *[G73.3]*
    - thyrotoxicosis EØ5.9Ø *[G73.3]*
      - with thyroid storm EØ5.91 *[G73.3]*

Myasthenic M62.81
Mycelium infection B49
Mycetismus — *see* Poisoning, food, noxious, mushroom
Mycetoma B47.9
- actinomycotic B47.1
- bone (mycotic) B47.9 *[M9Ø.8Ø]*
- eumycotic B47.Ø
- foot B47.9
  - actinomycotic B47.1
  - mycotic B47.Ø
- madurae NEC B47.9
  - mycotic B47.Ø
- maduromycotic B47.Ø
- mycotic B47.Ø
- nocardial B47.1

Mycobacteriosis — *see* Mycobacterium
Mycobacterium, mycobacterial (infection) A31.9
- anonymous A31.9
- atypical A31.9
  - cutaneous A31.1
  - pulmonary A31.Ø
    - tuberculous — *see* Tuberculosis, pulmonary
  - specified site NEC A31.8
- avium (intracellulare complex) A31.Ø
- balnei A31.1
- Battey A31.Ø
- chelonei A31.8
- cutaneous A31.1
- extrapulmonary systemic A31.8
- fortuitum A31.8
- intracellulare (Battey bacillus) A31.Ø
- kakaferifu A31.8
- kansasii (yellow bacillus) A31.Ø
- kasongo A31.8
- leprae — *see also* Leprosy A3Ø.9
- luciflavum A31.1
- marinum (M. balnei) A31.1
- nonspecific — *see* Mycobacterium, atypical
- pulmonary (atypical) A31.Ø
  - tuberculous — *see* Tuberculosis, pulmonary
- scrofulaceum A31.8
- simiae A31.8
- systemic, extrapulmonary A31.8
- szulgai A31.8
- terrae A31.8
- triviale A31.8
- tuberculosis (human, bovine) — *see* Tuberculosis
- ulcerans A31.1
- xenopi A31.8

Mycoplasma (M.) **pneumoniae, as cause of disease classified elsewhere** B96.Ø
Mycosis, mycotic B49
- cutaneous NEC B36.9
- ear B36.9
  - in
    - aspergillosis B44.89
    - candidiasis B37.84
    - moniliasis B37.84
- fungoides (extranodal) (solid organ) C84.Ø- ☑
- mouth B37.Ø
- nails B35.1
- opportunistic B48.8
- skin NEC B36.9
- specified NEC B48.8
- stomatitis B37.Ø
- vagina, vaginitis (candidal) (acute) B37.31
  - chronic (recurrent) B37.32

Mydriasis (pupil) H57.Ø4
Myelatelia QØ6.1
Myelinolysis, pontine, central G37.2

Myelitis (acute) (ascending) (childhood) (chronic) (descending) (diffuse) (disseminated) (idiopathic) (pressure) (progressive) (spinal cord) (subacute) — *see also* Encephalitis GØ4.91
- flaccid GØ4.82
- herpes simplex BØØ.82
- herpes zoster BØ2.24
- in diseases classified elsewhere GØ5.4
- necrotizing, subacute G37.4
- optic neuritis in G36.Ø
- postchickenpox BØ1.12
- postherpetic BØ2.24
- postimmunization GØ4.Ø2
- postinfectious NEC GØ4.89
- postvaccinal GØ4.Ø2
- specified NEC GØ4.89
- syphilitic (transverse) A52.14
- toxic G92.9
- transverse (in demyelinating diseases of central nervous system) G37.3
- tuberculous A17.82
- varicella BØ1.12

Myeloblastic — *see* condition
Myeloblastoma
- granular cell — *see also* Neoplasm, connective tissue
  - malignant — *see* Neoplasm, connective tissue, malignant
  - tongue D1Ø.1

Myelocele — *see* Spina bifida
Myelocystocele — *see* Spina bifida
Myelocytic — *see* condition
Myelodysplasia D46.9
- specified NEC D46.Z (*following* D46.4)
- spinal cord (congenital) QØ6.1

Myelodysplastic syndrome — *see also* Syndrome, myelodysplastic D46.9
- with
  - 5q deletion D46.C (*following* D46.2)
  - isolated del (5q) chromosomal abnormality D46.C (*following* D46.2)
- specified NEC D46.Z (*following* D46.4)

Myeloencephalitis — *see* Encephalitis
Myelofibrosis D75.81
- with myeloid metaplasia D47.4
- acute C94.4- ☑
- idiopathic (chronic) D47.4
- primary D47.1
- secondary D75.81
  - in myeloproliferative disease D47.4

Myelogenous — *see* condition
Myeloid — *see* condition
Myelokathexis D7Ø.9
Myeloleukodystrophy E75.29
Myelolipoma — *see* Lipoma
Myeloma (multiple) C9Ø.Ø- ☑
- monostotic C9Ø.3 ☑
  - plasma cell C9Ø.Ø- ☑
- plasma cell C9Ø.Ø- ☑
- solitary — *see also* Plasmacytoma, solitary C9Ø.3- ☑

Myelomalacia G95.89
Myelomatosis C9Ø.Ø- ☑
Myelomeningitis — *see* Meningoencephalitis
Myelomeningocele (spinal cord) — *see* Spina bifida
Myelo-osteo-musculodysplasia hereditaria Q79.8
Myelopathic
- anemia D64.89
- muscle atrophy — *see* Atrophy, muscle, spinal
- pain syndrome G89.Ø

Myelopathy (spinal cord) G95.9
- drug-induced G95.89
- in (due to)
  - degeneration or displacement, intervertebral disc NEC — *see* Disorder, disc, with, myelopathy
  - disease classified elsewhere G99.2
  - infection — *see* Encephalitis
  - intervertebral disc disorder — *see also* Disorder, disc, with, myelopathy
  - mercury — *see* subcategory T56.1 ☑
  - neoplastic disease — *see also* Neoplasm D49.9 *[G99.2]*
  - pernicious anemia D51.Ø *[G99.2]*
  - spondylosis — *see* Spondylosis, with myelopathy NEC
- necrotic (subacute) (vascular) G95.19
- radiation-induced G95.89
- spondylogenic NEC — *see* Spondylosis, with myelopathy NEC

N

- **Naegeli's**
  - disease Q82.8
  - leukemia, monocytic C93.1- ☑
- **Naegleriasis** (with meningoencephalitis) B6Ø.2
- **Naffziger's syndrome** G54.Ø
- **Naga sore** — *see* Ulcer, skin
- **Nägele's pelvis** M95.5
  - with disproportion (fetopelvic) O33.Ø
    - causing obstructed labor O65.Ø
- **Nail** — *see also* condition
  - biting F98.8
  - patella syndrome Q87.2
- **Nanism, nanosomia** — *see* Dwarfism
- **Nanophyetiasis** B66.8
- **Nanukayami** A27.89
- **Napkin rash** L22
- **Narcolepsy** G47.419
  - with cataplexy G47.411
  - in conditions classified elsewhere G47.429
    - with cataplexy G47.421
- **Narcosis** RØ6.89
- **Narcotism** — *see* Dependence
- **NARP** (Neuropathy, Ataxia and Retinitis pigmentosa) syndrome E88.49
- **Narrow**
  - anterior chamber angle H4Ø.Ø3- ☑
  - gingival width (of periodontal soft tissue) KØ5.5
  - pelvis — *see* Contraction, pelvis
- **Narrowing** — *see also* Stenosis
  - artery I77.1
    - auditory, internal I65.8
    - basilar — *see* Occlusion, artery, basilar
    - carotid — *see* Occlusion, artery, carotid
    - cerebellar — *see* Occlusion, artery, cerebellar
    - cerebral — *see* Occlusion artery, cerebral
    - choroidal — *see* Occlusion, artery, precerebral, specified NEC
    - communicating posterior — *see* Occlusion, artery, precerebral, specified NEC
    - coronary — *see also* Disease, heart, ischemic, atherosclerotic
      - congenital Q24.5
        - syphilitic A5Ø.54 *[I52]*
      - due to syphilis NEC A52.Ø6
    - hypophyseal — *see* Occlusion, artery, precerebral, specified NEC
    - pontine — *see* Occlusion, artery, precerebral, specified NEC
    - precerebral — *see* Occlusion, artery, precerebral
    - vertebral — *see* Occlusion, artery, vertebral
  - auditory canal (external) — *see* Stenosis, external ear canal
  - eustachian tube — *see* Obstruction, eustachian tube
  - eyelid — *see* Disorder, eyelid function
  - larynx J38.6
  - mesenteric artery — *see also* Ischemia, intestine, acute K55.Ø59
  - palate M26.89
  - palpebral fissure — *see* Disorder, eyelid function
  - ureter N13.5
    - with infection N13.6
  - urethra — *see* Stricture, urethra
- **Narrowness, abnormal, eyelid** Q1Ø.3
- **Nasal** — *see* condition
- **Nasolachrymal, nasolacrimal** — *see* condition
- **Nasopharyngeal** — *see also* condition
  - pituitary gland Q89.2
  - torticollis M43.6
- **Nasopharyngitis** (acute) (infective) (streptococcal) (subacute) JØØ
  - chronic (suppurative) (ulcerative) J31.1
- **Nasopharynx, nasopharyngeal** — *see* condition
- **Natal tooth, teeth** KØØ.6
- **Nausea** (without vomiting) R11.Ø
  - with vomiting R11.2
  - gravidarum — *see* Hyperemesis, gravidarum
  - marina T75.3 ☑
  - navalis T75.3 ☑
- **Navel** — *see* condition
- **Neapolitan fever** — *see* Brucellosis
- **Near drowning** T75.1 ☑
- **Nearsightedness** — *see* Myopia
- **Near-syncope** R55
- **Nebula, cornea** — *see* Opacity, cornea
- **Necator americanus infestation** B76.1
- **Necatoriasis** B76.1
- **Neck** — *see* condition
- **Necrobiosis** R68.89
  - lipoidica NEC L92.1
    - with diabetes — *see* EØ8-E13 with .62Ø
- **Necrolysis, toxic epidermal** L51.2
  - due to drug
    - correct substance properly administered — *see* Table of Drugs and Chemicals, by drug, adverse effect
    - overdose or wrong substance given or taken — *see* Table of Drugs and Chemicals, by drug, poisoning
- **Necrophilia** F65.89
- **Necrosis, necrotic** (ischemic) — *see also* Gangrene
  - adrenal (capsule) (gland) E27.49
  - amputation stump (surgical) (late) T87.5Ø
    - arm T87.5- ☑
    - leg T87.5- ☑
  - antrum J32.Ø
  - aorta (hyaline) — *see also* Aneurysm, aorta
    - cystic medial — *see* Dissection, aorta
  - artery I77.5
  - bladder (aseptic) (sphincter) N32.89
  - bone — *see also* Osteonecrosis M87.9
    - aseptic or avascular — *see* Osteonecrosis
      - idiopathic M87.ØØ
    - ethmoid J32.2
    - jaw M27.2
    - tuberculous — *see* Tuberculosis, bone
  - brain I67.89
  - breast (aseptic) (fat) (segmental) N64.1
  - bronchus J98.Ø9
  - central nervous system NEC I67.89
  - cerebellar I67.89
  - cerebral I67.89
  - colon — *see also* Infarct, intestine K55.Ø49
  - cornea H18.89- ☑
  - cortical (acute) (renal) N17.1
  - cystic medial (aorta) — *see* Dissection, aorta
  - dental pulp KØ4.1
  - esophagus K22.89
  - ethmoid (bone) J32.2
  - eyelid — *see* Disorder, eyelid, degenerative
  - fat, fatty (generalized) — *see also* Disorder, soft tissue, specified type NEC)
    - abdominal wall K65.4
    - breast (aseptic) (segmental) N64.1
    - localized — *see* Degeneration, by site, fatty
    - mesentery K65.4
    - omentum K65.4
    - pancreas K86.89
    - peritoneum K65.4
    - skin (subcutaneous), newborn P83.Ø
    - subcutaneous, due to birth injury P15.6
  - gallbladder — *see* Cholecystitis, acute
  - heart — *see* Infarct, myocardium
  - hip, aseptic or avascular — *see* Osteonecrosis, by type, femur
  - intestine (acute) (hemorrhagic) (massive) — *see also* Infarct, intestine K55.Ø69
  - jaw M27.2
  - kidney (bilateral) N28.Ø
    - acute N17.9
    - cortical (acute) (bilateral) N17.1
      - with ectopic or molar pregnancy OØ8.4
    - medullary (bilateral) (in acute renal failure) (papillary) N17.2
    - papillary (bilateral) (in acute renal failure) N17.2
    - tubular N17.Ø
      - with ectopic or molar pregnancy OØ8.4
      - complicating
        - abortion — *see* Abortion, by type, complicated by, tubular necrosis
        - ectopic or molar pregnancy OØ8.4
        - pregnancy — *see* Pregnancy, complicated by, diseases of, specified type or system NEC
      - following ectopic or molar pregnancy OØ8.4
      - traumatic T79.5 ☑
  - larynx J38.7
  - liver (with hepatic failure) (cell) — *see* Failure, hepatic
    - hemorrhagic, central K76.2
  - lung J85.Ø
  - lymphatic gland — *see* Lymphadenitis, acute
  - mammary gland (fat) (segmental) N64.1
  - mastoid (chronic) — *see* Mastoiditis, chronic

Necrosis, necrotic — *continued*

  - medullary (acute) (renal) N17.2
  - mesentery — *see also* Infarct, intestine K55.Ø69
    - fat K65.4
  - mitral valve — *see* Insufficiency, mitral
  - myocardium, myocardial — *see* Infarct, myocardium
  - nose J34.Ø
  - omentum (with mesenteric infarction) — *see also* Infarct, intestine K55.Ø69
    - fat K65.4
  - orbit, orbital — *see* Osteomyelitis, orbit
  - ossicles, ear — *see* Abnormal, ear ossicles
  - ovary N7Ø.92
  - pancreas (aseptic) (duct) (fat) K86.89
    - acute (infective) — *see* Pancreatitis, acute
    - infective — *see* Pancreatitis, acute
  - papillary (acute) (renal) N17.2
  - perineum N9Ø.89
  - peritoneum (with mesenteric infarction) — *see also* Infarct, intestine K55.Ø69
    - fat K65.4
  - pharynx JØ2.9
    - in granulocytopenia — *see* Neutropenia
    - Vincent's A69.1
  - phosphorus — *see* subcategory T54.2 ☑
  - pituitary (gland) E23.Ø
    - postpartum O99.285
    - Sheehan O99.285
  - pressure — *see* Ulcer, pressure, by site
  - pulmonary J85.Ø
  - pulp (dental) KØ4.1
  - radiation — *see* Necrosis, by site
  - radium — *see* Necrosis, by site
  - renal — *see* Necrosis, kidney
  - sclera H15.89
  - scrotum N5Ø.89
  - skin or subcutaneous tissue NEC I96
  - spine, spinal (column) — *see also* Osteonecrosis, by type, vertebra
    - cord G95.19
  - spleen D73.5
  - stomach K31.89
  - stomatitis (ulcerative) A69.Ø
  - subcutaneous fat, newborn P83.88
  - subendocardial (acute) I21.4
    - chronic I25.89
  - suprarenal (capsule) (gland) E27.49
  - testis N5Ø.89
  - thymus (gland) E32.8
  - tonsil J35.8
  - trachea J39.8
  - tuberculous NEC — *see* Tuberculosis
  - tubular (acute) (anoxic) (renal) (toxic) N17.Ø
    - postprocedural N99.Ø
  - vagina N89.8
  - vertebra — *see also* Osteonecrosis, by type, vertebra
    - tuberculous A18.Ø1
  - vulva N9Ø.89
  - X-ray — *see* Necrosis, by site
- **Necrospermia** — *see* Infertility, male
- **Need** (for)
  - care provider because (of)
    - assistance with personal care Z74.1
    - continuous supervision required Z74.3
    - impaired mobility Z74.Ø9
    - no other household member able to render care Z74.2
    - specified reason NEC Z74.8
  - immunization — *see* Vaccination
  - vaccination — *see* Vaccination
- **Neglect**
  - adult
    - confirmed T74.Ø1 ☑
    - history of Z91.412
    - suspected T76.Ø1 ☑
  - child (childhood)
    - confirmed T74.Ø2 ☑
    - history of Z62.812
    - suspected T76.Ø2 ☑
  - emotional, in childhood Z62.898
  - hemispatial R41.4
  - left-sided R41.4
  - sensory R41.4
  - visuospatial R41.4
- **Neisserian infection NEC** — *see* Gonococcus
- **Nelaton's syndrome** G6Ø.8
- **Nelson's syndrome** E24.1
- **Nematodiasis** (intestinal) B82.Ø

- **Nematodiasis** — *continued*
  - Ancylostoma B76.Ø
- **Neonatal** — *see also* Newborn
  - acne L7Ø.4
  - bradycardia P29.12
  - screening, abnormal findings on — *see* Abnormal, neonatal screening
  - tachycardia P29.11
  - tooth, teeth KØØ.6
- **Neonatorum** — *see* condition
- **Neoplasia**
  - endocrine, multiple (MEN) E31.2Ø
    - type I E31.21
    - type IIA E31.22
    - type IIB E31.23
  - intraepithelial (histologically confirmed)
    - anal (AIN) (histologically confirmed) K62.82
      - grade I K62.82
      - grade II K62.82
      - severe DØ1.3
    - cervical glandular (histologically confirmed) DØ6.9
    - cervix (uteri) (CIN) (histologically confirmed) N87.9
      - glandular DØ6.9
      - grade I N87.Ø
      - grade II N87.1
      - grade III (severe dysplasia) — *see also* Carcinoma, cervix uteri, in situ DØ6.9
    - prostate (histologically confirmed) (PIN) N42.31
      - grade I N42.31
      - grade II N42.31
      - grade III (severe dysplasia) DØ7.5
    - vagina (histologically confirmed) (VAIN) N89.3
      - grade I N89.Ø
      - grade II N89.1
      - grade III (severe dysplasia) DØ7.2
    - vulva (histologically confirmed) (VIN) N9Ø.3
      - grade I N9Ø.Ø
      - grade II N9Ø.1
      - grade III (severe dysplasia) DØ7.1
- **Neoplasm, neoplastic** — *see also* Table of Neoplasms
  - lipomatous, benign — *see* Lipoma
  - malignant mast cell C96.2Ø
    - specified type NEC C96.29
  - mast cell, of uncertain behavior NEC D47.Ø9
  - myelodysplastic/myeloproliferative, unclassifiable C94.6
- **Neovascularization**
  - ciliary body — *see* Disorder, iris, vascular
  - cornea H16.4Ø- ☑
    - deep H16.44- ☑
    - ghost vessels — *see* Ghost, vessels
    - localized H16.43- ☑
    - pannus — *see* Pannus
  - iris — *see* Disorder, iris, vascular
  - retina H35.Ø5- ☑
- **Nephralgia** N23
- **Nephritis, nephritic** (albuminuric) (azotemic) (congenital) (disseminated) (epithelial) (familial) (focal) (granulomatous) (hemorrhagic) (infantile) (nonsuppurative, excretory) (uremic) NØ5.9
  - with
    - C3
      - glomerulonephritis NØ5.A
      - glomerulopathy NØ5.A
        - with dense deposit disease NØ5.6
    - dense deposit disease NØ5.6
    - diffuse
      - crescentic glomerulonephritis NØ5.7
      - endocapillary proliferative glomerulonephritis NØ5.4
      - membranous glomerulonephritis NØ5.2
      - mesangial proliferative glomerulonephritis NØ5.3
      - mesangiocapillary glomerulonephritis NØ5.5
    - edema — *see* Nephrosis
    - focal and segmental glomerular lesions NØ5.1
    - foot process disease NØ4.9
    - glomerular lesion
      - diffuse sclerosing NØ5.8
      - hypocomplementemic — *see* Nephritis, membranoproliferative
      - IgA — *see* Nephropathy, IgA
      - lobular, lobulonodular — *see* Nephritis, membranoproliferative
      - nodular — *see* Nephritis, membranoproliferative
    - lesion of
      - glomerulonephritis, proliferative NØ5.8
      - renal necrosis NØ5.9
    - minor glomerular abnormality NØ5.Ø

- **Nephritis, nephritic** — *continued*
  - with — *continued*
    - specified morphological changes NEC NØ5.8
  - acute NØØ.9
    - with
      - C3
        - glomerulonephritis NØØ.A
        - glomerulopathy NØØ.A
          - with dense deposit disease NØØ.6
      - dense deposit disease NØØ.6
      - diffuse
        - crescentic glomerulonephritis NØØ.7
        - endocapillary proliferative glomerulonephritis NØØ.4
        - membranous glomerulonephritis NØØ.2
        - mesangial proliferative glomerulonephritis NØØ.3
        - mesangiocapillary glomerulonephritis NØØ.5
      - focal and segmental glomerular lesions NØØ.1
      - minor glomerular abnormality NØØ.Ø
      - specified morphological changes NEC NØØ.8
  - amyloid E85.4 *[NØ8]*
  - antiglomerular basement membrane (anti-GBM) antibody NEC
    - in Goodpasture's syndrome M31.Ø
  - antitubular basement membrane (tubulo-interstitial) NEC N12
    - toxic — *see* Nephropathy, toxic
  - arteriolar — *see* Hypertension, kidney
  - arteriosclerotic — *see* Hypertension, kidney
  - ascending — *see* Nephritis, tubulo-interstitial
  - atrophic NØ3.9
  - Balkan (endemic) N15.Ø
  - calculous, calculus — *see* Calculus, kidney
  - cardiac — *see* Hypertension, kidney
  - cardiovascular — *see* Hypertension, kidney
  - chronic NØ3.9
    - with
      - C3
        - glomerulonephritis NØ3.A
        - glomerulopathy NØ3.A
          - with dense deposit disease NØ3.6
      - dense deposit disease NØ3.6
      - diffuse
        - crescentic glomerulonephritis NØ3.7
        - endocapillary proliferative glomerulonephritis NØ3.4
        - membranous glomerulonephritis NØ3.2
        - mesangial proliferative glomerulonephritis NØ3.3
        - mesangiocapillary glomerulonephritis NØ3.5
      - focal and segmental glomerular lesions NØ3.1
      - minor glomerular abnormality NØ3.Ø
      - specified morphological changes NEC NØ3.8
    - arteriosclerotic — *see* Hypertension, kidney
  - cirrhotic N26.9
  - complicating pregnancy O26.83- ☑
  - croupous NØØ.9
  - degenerative — *see* Nephrosis
  - diffuse sclerosing NØ5.8
  - due to
    - diabetes mellitus — *see* EØ8-E13 with .21
    - subacute bacterial endocarditis I33.Ø
    - systemic lupus erythematosus (chronic) M32.14
    - typhoid fever AØ1.Ø9
  - gonococcal (acute) (chronic) A54.21
  - hypocomplementemic — *see* Nephritis, membranoproliferative
  - IgA — *see* Nephropathy, IgA
  - immune complex (circulating) NEC NØ5.8
  - infective — *see* Nephritis, tubulo-interstitial
  - interstitial — *see* Nephritis, tubulo-interstitial
  - lead N14.3
  - membranoproliferative (diffuse) (type 1 or 3) — *see also* NØØ-NØ7 with fourth character .5 NØ5.5
    - type 2 — *see also* NØØ-NØ7 with fourth character .6 NØ5.6
  - minimal change NØ5.Ø
  - necrotic, necrotizing NEC — *see also* NØØ-NØ7 with fourth character .8 NØ5.8
  - nephrotic — *see* Nephrosis
  - nodular — *see* Nephritis, membranoproliferative
  - polycystic Q61.3
    - adult type Q61.2
    - autosomal
      - dominant Q61.2
      - recessive NEC Q61.19
    - childhood type NEC Q61.19

- **Nephritis, nephritic** — *continued*
  - polycystic — *continued*
    - infantile type NEC Q61.19
  - poststreptococcal NØ5.9
    - acute NØØ.9
    - chronic NØ3.9
    - rapidly progressive NØ1.9
  - proliferative NEC — *see also* NØØ-NØ7 with fourth character .8 NØ5.8
  - purulent — *see* Nephritis, tubulo-interstitial
  - rapidly progressive NØ1.9
    - with
      - C3
        - glomerulonephritis NØ1.A
        - glomerulopathy NØ1.A
          - with dense deposit disease NØ1.6
      - dense deposit disease NØ1.6
      - diffuse
        - crescentic glomerulonephritis NØ1.7
        - endocapillary proliferative glomerulonephritis NØ1.4
        - membranous glomerulonephritis NØ1.2
        - mesangial proliferative glomerulonephritis NØ1.3
        - mesangiocapillary glomerulonephritis NØ1.5
      - focal and segmental glomerular lesions NØ1.1
      - minor glomerular abnormality NØ1.Ø
      - specified morphological changes NEC NØ1.8
  - salt losing or wasting NEC N28.89
  - saturnine N14.3
  - sclerosing, diffuse NØ5.8
  - septic — *see* Nephritis, tubulo-interstitial
  - specified pathology NEC — *see also* NØØ-NØ7 with fourth character .8 NØ5.8
  - subacute NØ1.9
  - suppurative — *see* Nephritis, tubulo-interstitial
  - syphilitic (late) A52.75
    - congenital A5Ø.59 *[NØ8]*
    - early (secondary) A51.44
  - toxic — *see* Nephropathy, toxic
  - tubal, tubular — *see* Nephritis, tubulo-interstitial
  - tuberculous A18.11
  - tubulo-interstitial (in) N12
    - acute (infectious) N1Ø
    - chronic (infectious) N11.9
      - nonobstructive N11.8
        - reflux-associated N11.Ø
      - obstructive N11.1
      - specified NEC N11.8
    - due to
      - brucellosis A23.9 *[N16]*
      - cryoglobulinemia D89.1 *[N16]*
      - glycogen storage disease E74.ØØ *[N16]*
    - Sjogren's syndrome M35.Ø4
  - vascular — *see* Hypertension, kidney
  - war NØØ.9
- **Nephroblastoma** (epithelial) (mesenchymal) C64- ☑
- **Nephrocalcinosis** E83.59 *[N29]*
- **Nephrocystitis, pustular** — *see* Nephritis, tubulo-interstitial
- **Nephrolithiasis** (congenital) (pelvis) (recurrent) — *see also* Calculus, kidney
- **Nephroma** C64- ☑
  - mesoblastic D41.Ø- ☑
- **Nephronephritis** — *see* Nephrosis
- **Nephronophthisis** Q61.5
- **Nephropathia epidemica** A98.5
- **Nephropathy** — *see also* Nephritis N28.9
  - with
    - edema — *see* Nephrosis
    - glomerular lesion — *see* Glomerulonephritis
  - amyloid, hereditary E85.Ø
  - analgesic N14.Ø
    - with medullary necrosis, acute N17.2
  - Balkan (endemic) N15.Ø
  - chemical — *see* Nephropathy, toxic
  - contrast medium, radiography N14.11
  - contrast-induced N14.11
  - diabetic — *see* EØ8-E13 with .21
  - drug-induced N14.2
    - contrast-induced N14.11
    - specified NEC N14.19
  - focal and segmental hyalinosis or sclerosis NØ2.1
  - heavy metal-induced N14.3
  - hereditary NEC NØ7.9
    - with
      - C3
        - glomerulonephritis NØ7.A

- **Neuritis** — *continued*
  - retrobulbar — *see also* Neuritis, optic, retrobulbar — *continued*
    - in (due to)
      - late syphilis A52.15
        - meningococcal infection A39.82
    - meningococcal A39.82
    - syphilitic A52.15
  - sciatic (nerve) — *see also* Sciatica
    - due to displacement of intervertebral disc — *see* Disorder, disc, with, radiculopathy
  - serum — *see also* Reaction, serum T8Ø.69 ☑
  - shoulder-girdle G54.5
  - specified nerve NEC G58.8
  - spinal (nerve) root — *see* Radiculopathy
  - syphilitic A52.15
  - thenar (median) G56.1- ☑
  - thoracic M54.14
  - toxic NEC G62.2
  - trochlear (nerve) — *see* Strabismus, paralytic, fourth nerve
  - vagus (nerve) G52.2
- **Neuroastrocytoma** — *see* Neoplasm, uncertain behavior, by site
- **Neuroavitaminosis** E56.9 *[G99.8]*
- **Neuroblastoma**
  - olfactory C3Ø.Ø
  - specified site — *see* Neoplasm, malignant, by site
  - unspecified site C74.9Ø
- **Neurochorioretinitis** — *see* Chorioretinitis
- **Neurocirculatory asthenia** F45.8
- **Neurocysticercosis** B69.Ø
- **Neurocytoma** — *see* Neoplasm, benign, by site
- **Neurodermatitis** (circumscribed) (circumscripta) (local) L28.Ø
  - atopic L2Ø.81
  - diffuse (Brocq) L2Ø.81
  - disseminated L2Ø.81
- **Neuroencephalomyelopathy, optic** G36.Ø
- **Neuroepithelioma** — *see also* Neoplasm, malignant, by site
  - olfactory C3Ø.Ø
- **Neurofibroma** — *see also* Neoplasm, nerve, benign
  - melanotic — *see* Neoplasm, nerve, benign
  - multiple — *see* Neurofibromatosis
  - plexiform — *see* Neoplasm, nerve, benign
- **Neurofibromatosis** (multiple) (nonmalignant) Q85.ØØ
  - acoustic Q85.Ø2
  - malignant — *see* Neoplasm, nerve, malignant
  - specified NEC Q85.Ø9
  - type 1 (von Recklinghausen) Q85.Ø1
  - type 2 Q85.Ø2
- **Neurofibrosarcoma** — *see* Neoplasm, nerve, malignant
- **Neurogenic** — *see also* condition
  - bladder — *see also* Dysfunction, bladder, neuromuscular N31.9
    - cauda equina syndrome G83.4
  - bowel NEC K59.2
  - heart F45.8
- **Neuroglioma** — *see* Neoplasm, uncertain behavior, by site
- **Neurolabyrinthitis** (of Dix and Hallpike) — *see* Neuronitis, vestibular
- **Neurolathyrism** — *see* Poisoning, food, noxious, plant
- **Neuroleprosy** A3Ø.9
- **Neuroma** — *see also* Neoplasm, nerve, benign
  - acoustic (nerve) D33.3
  - amputation (stump) (traumatic) (surgical complication) (late) T87.3- ☑
    - arm T87.3- ☑
    - leg T87.3- ☑
  - digital (toe) G57.6- ☑
  - interdigital G58.8
    - lower limb (toe) G57.8- ☑
    - upper limb G56.8- ☑
  - intermetatarsal G57.8- ☑
  - Morton's G57.6- ☑
  - nonneoplastic
    - arm G56.9- ☑
    - leg G57.9- ☑
    - lower extremity G57.9- ☑
    - upper extremity G56.9- ☑
  - optic (nerve) D33.3
  - plantar G57.6- ☑
  - plexiform — *see* Neoplasm, nerve, benign
  - surgical (nonneoplastic)
    - arm G56.9- ☑
- **Neuroma** — *continued*
  - surgical — *continued*
    - leg G57.9- ☑
    - lower extremity G57.9- ☑
    - upper extremity G56.9- ☑
- **Neuromyalgia** — *see* Neuralgia
- **Neuromyasthenia** (epidemic) (postinfectious) G93.39
- **Neuromyelitis** G36.9
  - ascending G61.Ø
  - optica G36.Ø
- **Neuromyopathy** G7Ø.9
  - paraneoplastic — *see also*, Neoplasm, by site, if known D49.9 *[G13.Ø]*
- **Neuromyotonia** (Isaacs) G71.19
- **Neuronevus** — *see* Nevus
- **Neuronitis** G58.9
  - ascending (acute) G57.2- ☑
  - vestibular H81.2- ☑
- **Neuroparalytic** — *see* condition
- **Neuropathy, neuropathic** G62.9
  - acute motor G62.81
  - alcoholic G62.1
    - with psychosis — *see* Psychosis, alcoholic
  - arm G56.9- ☑
  - autonomic, peripheral — *see* Neuropathy, peripheral, autonomic
  - axillary G56.9- ☑
  - bladder N31.9
    - atonic (motor) (sensory) N31.2
    - autonomous N31.2
    - flaccid N31.2
    - nonreflex N31.2
    - reflex N31.1
    - uninhibited N31.Ø
  - brachial plexus G54.Ø
  - cervical plexus G54.2
  - chronic
    - progressive segmentally demyelinating G62.89
    - relapsing demyelinating G62.89
  - Dejerine-Sottas G6Ø.Ø
  - diabetic — *see* EØ8-E13 with .4Ø
    - mononeuropathy — *see* EØ8-E13 with .41
    - polyneuropathy — *see* EØ8-E13 with .42
  - entrapment G58.9
    - iliohypogastric nerve G57.8- ☑
    - ilioinguinal nerve G57.8- ☑
    - lateral cutaneous nerve of thigh G57.1- ☑
    - median nerve G56.Ø- ☑
    - obturator nerve G57.8- ☑
    - peroneal nerve G57.3- ☑
    - posterior tibial nerve G57.5- ☑
    - saphenous nerve G57.8- ☑
    - ulnar nerve G56.2- ☑
  - facial nerve G51.9
  - hereditary G6Ø.9
    - motor and sensory (types I-IV) G6Ø.Ø
    - sensory G6Ø.8
    - specified NEC G6Ø.8
  - hypertrophic G6Ø.Ø
    - Charcot-Marie-Tooth G6Ø.Ø
    - Dejerine-Sottas G6Ø.Ø
    - interstitial progressive G6Ø.Ø
    - of infancy G6Ø.Ø
    - Refsum G6Ø.1
  - idiopathic G6Ø.9
    - progressive G6Ø.3
    - specified NEC G6Ø.8
  - in association with hereditary ataxia G6Ø.2
  - intercostal G58.Ø
  - ischemic — *see* Disorder, nerve
  - Jamaica (ginger) G62.2
  - leg NEC G57.9- ☑
  - lower extremity G57.9- ☑
  - lumbar plexus G54.1
  - median nerve G56.1- ☑
  - motor and sensory — *see also* Polyneuropathy
    - hereditary (types I-IV) G6Ø.Ø
  - multifocal motor (MMN) G61.82
  - multiple (acute) (chronic) — *see* Polyneuropathy
  - optic (nerve) — *see also* Neuritis, optic
    - ischemic H47.Ø1- ☑
  - paraneoplastic (sensorial) (Denny Brown) — *see also*, Neoplasm, by site, if known D49.9 *[G13.Ø]*
  - peripheral (nerve) — *see also* Polyneuropathy G62.9
    - autonomic G9Ø.9
      - idiopathic G9Ø.Ø9
- **Neuropathy, neuropathic** — *continued*
  - peripheral — *see also* Polyneuropathy — *continued*
    - autonomic — *continued*
      - in (due to)
        - amyloidosis E85.4 *[G99.Ø]*
        - diabetes mellitus — *see* EØ8-E13 with .43
        - endocrine disease NEC E34.9 *[G99.Ø]*
        - gout M1Ø.ØØ *[G99.Ø]*
        - hyperthyroidism EØ5.9Ø *[G99.Ø]*
          - with thyroid storm EØ5.91 *[G99.Ø]*
        - metabolic disease NEC E88.9 *[G99.Ø]*
    - idiopathic G6Ø.9
      - progressive G6Ø.3
    - in (due to)
      - antitetanus serum G62.Ø
      - arsenic G62.2
      - drugs NEC G62.Ø
      - lead G62.2
      - organophosphate compounds G62.2
      - toxic agent NEC G62.2
  - plantar nerves G57.6- ☑
  - progressive
    - hypertrophic interstitial G6Ø.Ø
    - inflammatory G62.81
  - radicular NEC — *see* Radiculopathy
  - sacral plexus G54.1
  - sciatic G57.Ø- ☑
  - serum G61.1
  - toxic NEC G62.2
  - trigeminal sensory G5Ø.8
  - ulnar nerve G56.2- ☑
  - uremic N18.9 *[G63]*
  - vitamin B12 E53.8 *[G63]*
    - with anemia (pernicious) D51.Ø *[G63]*
      - due to dietary deficiency D51.3 *[G63]*
- **Neurophthisis** — *see also* Disorder, nerve
  - peripheral, diabetic — *see* EØ8-E13 with .42
- **Neuroretinitis** — *see* Chorioretinitis
- **Neuroretinopathy, hereditary optic** H47.22
- **Neurosarcoma** — *see* Neoplasm, nerve, malignant
- **Neurosclerosis** — *see* Disorder, nerve
- **Neurosis, neurotic** F48.9
  - anankastic F42.8
  - anxiety (state) F41.1
    - panic type F41.Ø
  - asthenic F48.8
  - bladder F45.8
  - cardiac (reflex) F45.8
  - cardiovascular F45.8
  - character F6Ø.9
  - colon F45.8
  - compensation F68.1Ø
  - compulsive, compulsion F42.8
  - conversion F44.9
  - craft F48.8
  - cutaneous F45.8
  - depersonalization F48.1
  - depressive (reaction) (type) F34.1
  - environmental F48.8
  - excoriation L98.1
  - fatigue F48.8
  - functional — *see* Disorder, somatoform
  - gastric F45.8
  - gastrointestinal F45.8
  - heart F45.8
  - hypochondriacal F45.21
  - hysterical F44.9
  - incoordination F45.8
    - larynx F45.8
    - vocal cord F45.8
  - intestine F45.8
  - larynx (sensory) F45.8
    - hysterical F44.4
  - mixed NEC F48.8
  - musculoskeletal F45.8
  - obsessional F42.8
  - obsessive-compulsive F42.8
  - occupational F48.8
  - ocular NEC F45.8
  - organ — *see* Disorder, somatoform
  - pharynx F45.8
  - phobic F4Ø.9
  - posttraumatic (situational) F43.1Ø
    - acute F43.11
    - chronic F43.12
  - psychasthenic (type) F48.8
  - railroad F48.8
  - rectum F45.8

Neurosis, neurotic — *continued*
- respiratory F45.8
- rumination F45.8
- sexual F65.9
- situational F48.8
- social F4Ø.1Ø
  - generalized F4Ø.11
- specified type NEC F48.8
- state F48.9
  - with depersonalization episode F48.1
- stomach F45.8
- traumatic F43.1Ø
  - acute F43.11
  - chronic F43.12
- vasomotor F45.8
- visceral F45.8
- war F48.8

Neurospongioblastosis diffusa Q85.1

Neurosyphilis (arrested) (early) (gumma) (late) (latent) (recurrent) (relapse) A52.3
- with ataxia (cerebellar) (locomotor) (spastic) (spinal) A52.19
- aneurysm (cerebral) A52.Ø5
- arachnoid (adhesive) A52.13
- arteritis (any artery) (cerebral) A52.Ø4
- asymptomatic A52.2
- congenital A5Ø.4Ø
- dura (mater) A52.13
- general paresis A52.17
- hemorrhagic A52.Ø5
- juvenile (asymptomatic) (meningeal) A5Ø.4Ø
- leptomeninges (aseptic) A52.13
- meningeal, meninges (adhesive) A52.13
- meningitis A52.13
- meningovascular (diffuse) A52.13
- optic atrophy A52.15
- parenchymatous (degenerative) A52.19
- paresis, paretic A52.17
  - juvenile A5Ø.45
- remission in (sustained) A52.3
- serological (without symptoms) A52.2
- specified nature or site NEC A52.19
- tabes, tabetic (dorsalis) A52.11
  - juvenile A5Ø.45
- taboparesis A52.17
  - juvenile A5Ø.45
- thrombosis (cerebral) A52.Ø5
- vascular (cerebral) NEC A52.Ø5

Neurothekeoma — *see* Neoplasm, nerve, benign

Neurotic — *see* Neurosis

Neurotoxemia — *see* Toxemia

Neutroclusion M26.211

Neutropenia, neutropenic (chronic) (genetic) (idiopathic) (immune) (infantile) (malignant) (pernicious) (splenic) D7Ø.9
- congenital (primary) D7Ø.Ø
- cyclic D7Ø.4
- cytoreductive cancer chemotherapy sequela D7Ø.1
- drug-induced D7Ø.2
  - due to cytoreductive cancer chemotherapy D7Ø.1
- due to infection D7Ø.3
- fever D7Ø.9
- neonatal, transitory (isoimmune) (maternal transfer) P61.5
- periodic D7Ø.4
- secondary (cyclic) (periodic) (splenic) D7Ø.4
  - drug-induced D7Ø.2
    - due to cytoreductive cancer chemotherapy D7Ø.1
- specified NEC D7Ø.8
- toxic D7Ø.8

Neutrophilia, hereditary giant D72.Ø

Nevocarcinoma — *see* Melanoma

Nevus D22.9
- achromic — *see* Neoplasm, skin, benign
- amelanotic — *see* Neoplasm, skin, benign
- angiomatous D18.ØØ
  - intra-abdominal D18.Ø3
  - intracranial D18.Ø2
  - skin D18.Ø1
  - specified site NEC D18.Ø9
- araneus I78.1
- balloon cell — *see* Neoplasm, skin, benign
- bathing trunk D48.5
- blue — *see* Neoplasm, skin, benign
  - cellular — *see* Neoplasm, skin, benign
  - giant — *see* Neoplasm, skin, benign
  - Jadassohn's — *see* Neoplasm, skin, benign
  - malignant — *see* Melanoma

Nevus — *continued*
- capillary D18.ØØ
  - intra-abdominal D18.Ø3
  - intracranial D18.Ø2
  - skin D18.Ø1
  - specified site NEC D18.Ø9
- cavernous D18.ØØ
  - intra-abdominal D18.Ø3
  - intracranial D18.Ø2
  - skin D18.Ø1
  - specified site NEC D18.Ø9
- cellular — *see* Neoplasm, skin, benign
  - blue — *see* Neoplasm, skin, benign
- choroid D31.3- ☑
- comedonicus Q82.5
- conjunctiva D31.Ø- ☑
- dermal — *see* Neoplasm, skin, benign
  - with epidermal nevus — *see* Neoplasm, skin, benign
- dysplastic — *see* Neoplasm, skin, benign
- eye D31.9- ☑
- flammeus Q82.5
- hemangiomatous D18.ØØ
  - intra-abdominal D18.Ø3
  - intracranial D18.Ø2
  - skin D18.Ø1
  - specified site NEC D18.Ø9
- iris D31.4- ☑
- lacrimal gland D31.5- ☑
- lymphatic D18.1
- magnocellular
  - specified site — *see* Neoplasm, benign, by site
  - unspecified site D31.4Ø
- malignant — *see* Melanoma
- meaning hemangioma D18.ØØ
  - intra-abdominal D18.Ø3
  - intracranial D18.Ø2
  - skin D18.Ø1
  - specified site NEC D18.Ø9
- mouth (mucosa) D1Ø.3Ø
  - specified site NEC D1Ø.39
  - white sponge Q38.6
- multiplex Q85.1
- non-neoplastic I78.1
- oral mucosa D1Ø.3Ø
  - specified site NEC D1Ø.39
  - white sponge Q38.6
- orbit D31.6- ☑
- pigmented
  - giant — *see also* Neoplasm, skin, uncertain behavior D48.5
    - malignant melanoma in — *see* Melanoma
- portwine Q82.5
- retina D31.2- ☑
- retrobulbar D31.6- ☑
- sanguineous Q82.5
- senile I78.1
- skin D22.9
  - abdominal wall D22.5
  - ala nasi D22.39
  - ankle D22.7- ☑
  - anus, anal D22.5
  - arm D22.6- ☑
  - auditory canal (external) D22.2- ☑
  - auricle (ear) D22.2- ☑
  - auricular canal (external) D22.2- ☑
  - axilla, axillary fold D22.5
  - back D22.5
  - breast D22.5
  - brow D22.39
  - buttock D22.5
  - canthus (eye) D22.1- ☑
  - cheek (external) D22.39
  - chest wall D22.5
  - chin D22.39
  - ear (external) D22.2- ☑
  - external meatus (ear) D22.2- ☑
  - eyebrow D22.39
  - eyelid (lower) (upper) D22.1- ☑
  - face D22.3Ø
    - specified NEC D22.39
  - female genital organ (external) NEC D28.Ø
  - finger D22.6- ☑
  - flank D22.5
  - foot D22.7- ☑
  - forearm D22.6- ☑
  - forehead D22.39
  - foreskin D29.Ø

Nevus — *continued*
- skin — *continued*
  - genital organ (external) NEC
    - female D28.Ø
    - male D29.9
  - gluteal region D22.5
  - groin D22.5
  - hand D22.6- ☑
  - heel D22.7- ☑
  - helix D22.2- ☑
  - hip D22.7- ☑
  - interscapular region D22.5
  - jaw D22.39
  - knee D22.7- ☑
  - labium (majus) (minus) D28.Ø
  - leg D22.7- ☑
  - lip (lower) (upper) D22.Ø
  - lower limb D22.7- ☑
  - male genital organ (external) D29.9
  - nail D22.9
    - finger D22.6- ☑
    - toe D22.7- ☑
  - nasolabial groove D22.39
  - nates D22.5
  - neck D22.4
  - nose (external) D22.39
  - palpebra D22.1- ☑
  - penis D29.Ø
  - perianal skin D22.5
  - perineum D22.5
  - pinna D22.2- ☑
  - popliteal fossa or space D22.7- ☑
  - prepuce D29.Ø
  - pudendum D28.Ø
  - scalp D22.4
  - scrotum D29.4
  - shoulder D22.6- ☑
  - submammary fold D22.5
  - temple D22.39
  - thigh D22.7- ☑
  - toe D22.7- ☑
  - trunk NEC D22.5
  - umbilicus D22.5
  - upper limb D22.6- ☑
  - vulva D28.Ø
- specified site NEC — *see* Neoplasm, by site, benign
- spider I78.1
- stellar I78.1
- strawberry Q82.5
- Sutton's benign D22.9
- unius lateris Q82.5
- Unna's Q82.5
- vascular Q82.5
- verrucous Q82.5

Newborn (infant) (liveborn) (singleton) Z38.2
- abstinence syndrome P96.1
- acne L7Ø.4
- affected by
  - abnormalities of membranes PØ2.9
    - specified NEC PØ2.8
  - abruptio placenta PØ2.1
  - amino-acid metabolic disorder, transitory P74.8
  - amniocentesis (while in utero) PØØ.6
  - amnionitis PØ2.78
  - apparent life threatening event (ALTE) R68.13
  - bleeding (into)
    - cerebral cortex P52.22
    - germinal matrix P52.Ø
    - ventricles P52.1
  - breech delivery PØ3.Ø
  - cardiac arrest P29.81
  - cardiomyopathy I42.8
    - congenital I42.4
  - cerebral ischemia P91.Ø
  - Cesarean delivery PØ3.4
  - chemotherapy agents PØ4.11
  - chorioamnionitis PØ2.78
  - cocaine (crack) PØ4.41
  - complications of labor and delivery PØ3.9
    - specified NEC PØ3.89
  - compression of umbilical cord NEC PØ2.5
  - contracted pelvis PØ3.1
  - cyanosis P28.2
  - delivery PØ3.9
    - Cesarean PØ3.4
    - forceps PØ3.2
    - vacuum extractor PØ3.3
  - drugs of addiction PØ4.4Ø

Obesity — *continued*
- due to
  - drug E66.1
  - excess calories E66.Ø9
    - morbid E66.Ø1
    - severe E66.Ø1
- endocrine E66.8
- endogenous E66.8
- exogenous E66.Ø9
- familial E66.8
- glandular E66.8
- hypothyroid — *see* Hypothyroidism
- hypoventilation syndrome (OHS) E66.2
- morbid E66.Ø1
  - with
    - alveolar hypoventilation E66.2
    - obesity hypoventilation syndrome (OHS) E66.2
  - due to excess calories E66.Ø1
- nutritional E66.Ø9
- pituitary E23.6
- severe E66.Ø1
- specified type NEC E66.8

Oblique — *see* condition

Obliteration
- appendix (lumen) K38.8
- artery I77.1
- bile duct (noncalculous) K83.1
- common duct (noncalculous) K83.1
- cystic duct — *see* Obstruction, gallbladder
- disease, arteriolar I77.1
- endometrium N85.8
- eye, anterior chamber — *see* Disorder, globe, hypotony
- fallopian tube N97.1
- lymphatic vessel I89.Ø
  - due to mastectomy I97.2
- organ or site, congenital NEC — *see* Atresia, by site
- ureter N13.5
  - with infection N13.6
- urethra — *see* Stricture, urethra
- vein I87.8
- vestibule (oral) KØ8.89

Observation (following) (for) (without need for further medical care) ZØ4.9
- accident NEC ZØ4.3
  - at work ZØ4.2
  - transport ZØ4.1
- adverse effect of drug ZØ3.6
- alleged rape or sexual assault (victim), ruled out
  - adult ZØ4.41
  - child ZØ4.42
- criminal assault ZØ4.89
- development state
  - adolescent ZØØ.3
  - period of rapid growth in childhood ZØØ.2
  - puberty ZØØ.3
- disease, specified NEC ZØ3.89
- following work accident ZØ4.2
- forced sexual exploitation ZØ4.81
- forced labor exploitation ZØ4.82
- growth and development state — *see* Observation, development state
- injuries (accidental) NEC — *see also* Observation, accident
- newborn (for)
  - suspected condition, related to exposure from the mother or birth process — *see* Newborn, affected by, maternal
    - ruled out ZØ5.9
      - cardiac ZØ5.Ø
      - connective tissue ZØ5.73
      - gastrointestinal ZØ5.5
      - genetic ZØ5.41
      - genitourinary ZØ5.6
      - immunologic ZØ5.43
      - infectious ZØ5.1
      - metabolic ZØ5.42
      - musculoskeletal ZØ5.72
      - neurological ZØ5.2
      - respiratory ZØ5.3
      - skin and subcutaneous tissue ZØ5.71
      - specified condition NEC ZØ5.89
- postpartum
  - immediately after delivery Z39.Ø
  - routine follow-up Z39.2
- pregnancy (normal) (without complication) Z34.9- ☑
  - high risk OØ9.9- ☑
- suicide attempt, alleged NEC ZØ3.89
  - self-poisoning ZØ3.6

Observation — *continued*
- suspected, ruled out — *see also* Suspected condition, ruled out
  - abuse, physical
    - adult ZØ4.71
    - child ZØ4.72
  - accident at work ZØ4.2
  - adult battering victim ZØ4.71
  - child battering victim ZØ4.72
  - condition NEC ZØ3.89
    - newborn — *see also* Observation, newborn (for), suspected condition, ruled out ZØ5.9
  - drug poisoning or adverse effect ZØ3.6
  - exposure (to)
    - anthrax ZØ3.81Ø
    - biological agent NEC ZØ3.818
  - foreign body
    - aspirated (inhaled) ZØ3.822
    - ingested ZØ3.821
    - inserted (injected), in (eye) (orifice) (skin) ZØ3.823
  - inflicted injury NEC ZØ4.89
  - suicide attempt, alleged ZØ3.89
    - self-poisoning ZØ3.6
  - toxic effects from ingested substance (drug) (poison) ZØ3.6
- toxic effects from ingested substance (drug) (poison) ZØ3.6

Obsession, obsessional state F42.8
- mixed thoughts and acts F42.2

Obsessive-compulsive neurosis or reaction F42.8

Obstetric embolism, septic — *see* Embolism, obstetric, septic

Obstetrical trauma (complicating delivery) O71.9
- with or following ectopic or molar pregnancy OØ8.6
- specified type NEC O71.89

Obstipation — *see* Constipation

Obstruction, obstructed, obstructive
- airway J98.8
  - with
    - allergic alveolitis J67.9
    - asthma J45.9Ø9
      - with
        - exacerbation (acute) J45.9Ø1
        - status asthmaticus J45.9Ø2
    - bronchiectasis J47.9
      - with
        - exacerbation (acute) J47.1
        - lower respiratory infection J47.Ø
    - bronchitis (chronic) J44.89
    - emphysema J43.9
  - chronic J44.9
    - with
      - allergic alveolitis — *see* Pneumonitis, hypersensitivity
      - bronchiectasis J47.9
        - with
          - exacerbation (acute) J47.1
          - lower respiratory infection J47.Ø
  - due to
    - foreign body — *see* Foreign body, by site, causing asphyxia
    - inhalation of fumes or vapors J68.9
    - laryngospasm J38.5
- ampulla of Vater K83.1
- aortic (heart) (valve) — *see* Stenosis, aortic
- aortoiliac I74.Ø9
- aqueduct of Sylvius G91.1
  - congenital QØ3.Ø
    - with spina bifida — *see* Spina bifida, by site, with hydrocephalus
- Arnold-Chiari — *see* Arnold-Chiari disease
- artery — *see also* Atherosclerosis, artery I7Ø.9 ☑
  - basilar (complete) (partial) — *see* Occlusion, artery, basilar
  - carotid (complete) (partial) — *see* Occlusion, artery, carotid
  - cerebellar — *see* Occlusion, artery, cerebellar
  - cerebral (anterior) (middle) (posterior) — *see* Occlusion, artery, cerebral
  - precerebral — *see* Occlusion, artery, precerebral
  - renal N28.Ø
  - retinal NEC — *see* Occlusion, artery, retina
  - stent — *see* Restenosis, stent
  - vertebral (complete) (partial) — *see* Occlusion, artery, vertebral
- band (intestinal) — *see also* Obstruction, intestine, specified NEC K56.699

Obstruction, obstructed, obstructive — *continued*
- bile duct or passage (common) (hepatic) (noncalculous) K83.1
  - with calculus K8Ø.51
  - congenital (causing jaundice) Q44.3
- biliary (duct) (tract) K83.1
  - gallbladder K82.Ø
- bladder-neck (acquired) N32.Ø
  - congenital Q64.31
  - due to hyperplasia (hypertrophy) of prostate — *see* Hyperplasia, prostate
- bowel — *see* Obstruction, intestine
- bronchus J98.Ø9
- canal, ear — *see* Stenosis, external ear canal
- cardia K22.2
- caval veins (inferior) (superior) I87.1
- cecum — *see* Obstruction, intestine
- circulatory I99.8
- colon — *see* Obstruction, intestine
- common duct (noncalculous) K83.1
- coronary (artery) — *see* Occlusion, coronary
- cystic duct — *see also* Obstruction, gallbladder
  - with calculus K8Ø.21
- device, implant or graft — *see also* Complications, by site and type, mechanical T85.698 ☑
  - arterial graft NEC — *see* Complication, cardiovascular device, mechanical, vascular
  - catheter NEC T85.628 ☑
    - cystostomy T83.Ø9Ø ☑
    - dialysis (renal) T82.49 ☑
      - intraperitoneal T85.691 ☑
    - Hopkins T83.Ø98 ☑
    - ileostomy T83.Ø98 ☑
    - infusion NEC T82.594 ☑
      - spinal (epidural) (subdural) T85.69Ø ☑
    - nephrostomy T83.Ø92 ☑
    - urethral indwelling T83.Ø91 ☑
    - urinary T83.Ø98 ☑
    - urostomy T83.Ø98 ☑
  - due to infection T85.79 ☑
  - gastrointestinal — *see* Complications, prosthetic device, mechanical, gastrointestinal device
  - genital NEC T83.498 ☑
    - intrauterine contraceptive device T83.39 ☑
    - penile prosthesis (cylinder) (implanted) (pump) (resevoir) T83.49Ø ☑
    - testicular prosthesis T83.491 ☑
  - heart NEC — *see* Complication, cardiovascular device, mechanical
  - joint prosthesis — *see* Complications, joint prosthesis, mechanical, specified NEC, by site
  - orthopedic NEC — *see* Complication, orthopedic, device, mechanical
  - specified NEC T85.628 ☑
  - urinary NEC — *see also* Complication, genitourinary, device, urinary, mechanical
    - graft T83.29 ☑
  - vascular NEC — *see* Complication, cardiovascular device, mechanical
  - ventricular intracranial shunt T85.Ø9 ☑
- due to foreign body accidentally left in operative wound T81.529 ☑
- duodenum K31.5
- ejaculatory duct N5Ø.89
- esophagus K22.2
- eustachian tube (complete) (partial) H68.1Ø- ☑
  - cartilagenous (extrinsic) H68.13- ☑
  - intrinsic H68.12- ☑
  - osseous H68.11- ☑
- fallopian tube (bilateral) N97.1
- fecal K56.41
  - with hernia — *see* Hernia, by site, with obstruction
- foramen of Monro (congenital) QØ3.8
  - with spina bifida — *see* Spina bifida, by site, with hydrocephalus
- foreign body — *see* Foreign body
- gallbladder K82.Ø
  - with calculus, stones K8Ø.21
  - congenital Q44.1
- gastric outlet K31.1
- gastrointestinal — *see* Obstruction, intestine
- hepatic K76.89
  - duct (noncalculous) K83.1
- ileum — *see* Obstruction, intestine
- iliofemoral (artery) I74.5
- intestine K56.6Ø9

Obstruction, obstructed, obstructive — *continued*
- intestine — *continued*
  - with
    - adhesions (intestinal) (peritoneal) K56.50
      - complete K56.52
      - incomplete K56.51
      - partial K56.51
  - adynamic K56.0
  - by gallstone K56.3
  - complete K56.601
  - congenital (small) Q41.9
    - large Q42.9
      - specified part NEC Q42.8
  - incomplete K56.600
  - neurogenic K56.0
    - Hirschsprung's disease or megacolon Q43.1
  - newborn P76.9
    - due to
      - fecaliths P76.8
      - inspissated milk P76.2
      - meconium (plug) P76.0
        - in mucoviscidosis E84.11
    - specified NEC P76.8
  - partial K56.600
  - postoperative K91.30
    - complete K91.32
    - incomplete K91.31
    - partial K91.31
  - reflex K56.0
  - specified NEC K56.699
    - complete K56.691
    - incomplete K56.690
    - partial K56.690
  - volvulus K56.2
- intracardiac ball valve prosthesis T82.09 ☑
- jejunum — *see* Obstruction, intestine
- joint prosthesis — *see* Complications, joint prosthesis, mechanical, specified NEC, by site
- kidney (calices) — *see also* Hydronephrosis N28.89
- labor — *see* Delivery
- lacrimal (passages) (duct)
  - by
    - dacryolith — *see* Dacryolith
    - stenosis — *see* Stenosis, lacrimal
  - congenital Q10.5
  - neonatal H04.53- ☑
- lacrimonasal duct — *see* Obstruction, lacrimal
- lacteal, with steatorrhea K90.2
- laryngitis — *see* Laryngitis
- larynx NEC J38.6
  - congenital Q31.8
- lung J98.4
  - disease, chronic J44.9
- lymphatic I89.0
- meconium (plug)
  - newborn P76.0
    - due to fecaliths P76.0
    - in mucoviscidosis E84.11
- mitral — *see* Stenosis, mitral
- nasal J34.89
- nasolacrimal duct — *see also* Obstruction, lacrimal
  - congenital Q10.5
- nasopharynx J39.2
- nose J34.89
- organ or site, congenital NEC — *see* Atresia, by site
- pancreatic duct K86.89
- parotid duct or gland K11.8
- pelviureteral junction N13.5
  - with hydronephrosis N13.0
  - congenital Q62.39
- pharynx J39.2
- portal (circulation) (vein) I81
- prostate — *see also* Hyperplasia, prostate
  - valve (urinary) N32.0
- pulmonary valve (heart) I37.0
- pyelonephritis (chronic) N11.1
- pylorus
  - adult K31.1
  - congenital or infantile Q40.0
- rectosigmoid — *see* Obstruction, intestine
- rectum K62.4
- renal — *see also* Hydronephrosis N28.89
  - outflow N13.8
  - pelvis, congenital Q62.39
- respiratory J98.8
  - chronic J44.9
- retinal (vessels) H34.9
- salivary duct (any) K11.8

Obstruction, obstructed, obstructive — *continued*
- salivary duct — *continued*
  - with calculus K11.5
- sigmoid — *see* Obstruction, intestine
- sinus (accessory) (nasal) J34.89
- Stensen's duct K11.8
- stomach NEC K31.89
  - acute K31.0
  - congenital Q40.2
  - due to pylorospasm K31.3
- submandibular duct K11.8
- submaxillary gland K11.8
  - with calculus K11.5
- thoracic duct I89.0
- thrombotic — *see* Thrombosis
- trachea J39.8
- tracheostomy airway J95.03
- tricuspid (valve) — *see* Stenosis, tricuspid
- upper respiratory, congenital Q34.8
- ureter (functional) (pelvic junction) NEC N13.5
  - with
    - hydronephrosis N13.1
      - with infection N13.6
      - congenital Q62.39
    - pyelonephritis (chronic) N11.1
  - congenital Q62.39
  - due to calculus — *see* Calculus, ureter
- urethra NEC N36.8
  - congenital Q64.39
- urinary (moderate) N13.9
  - due to hyperplasia (hypertrophy) of prostate — *see* Hyperplasia, prostate
  - organ or tract (lower) N13.9
  - prostatic valve N32.0
  - specified NEC N13.8
- uropathy N13.9
- uterus N85.8
- vagina N89.5
- valvular — *see* Endocarditis
- vein, venous I87.1
  - caval (inferior) (superior) I87.1
  - thrombotic — *see* Thrombosis
- vena cava (inferior) (superior) I87.1
- vesical NEC N32.0
- vesicourethral orifice N32.0
  - congenital Q64.31
- vessel NEC I99.8
  - stent — *see* Restenosis, stent

Obturator — *see* condition

Occlusal wear, teeth K03.0

Occlusio pupillae — *see* Membrane, pupillary

Occlusion, occluded
- anus K62.4
  - congenital Q42.3
    - with fistula Q42.2
- aortoiliac (chronic) I74.09
- aqueduct of Sylvius G91.1
  - congenital Q03.0
    - with spina bifida — *see* Spina bifida, by site, with hydrocephalus
- artery — *see also* Atherosclerosis, artery I70.9 ☑
  - auditory, internal I65.8
  - basilar I65.1
    - with
      - infarction I63.22
        - due to
          - embolism I63.12
          - thrombosis I63.02
  - brain or cerebral I66.9
    - with infarction (due to) I63.5- ☑
      - embolism I63.4- ☑
      - thrombosis I63.3- ☑
  - carotid I65.2- ☑
    - with
      - infarction I63.23- ☑
        - due to
          - embolism I63.13- ☑
          - thrombosis I63.03- ☑
  - cerebellar (anterior inferior) (posterior inferior) (superior) I66.3
    - with infarction I63.54- ☑
      - due to
        - embolism I63.44- ☑
        - thrombosis I63.34- ☑
  - cerebral I66.9
    - with infarction I63.50
      - due to
        - embolism I63.40

Occlusion, occluded — *continued*
- artery — *see also* Atherosclerosis, artery — *continued*
  - cerebral — *continued*
    - with infarction — *continued*
      - due to — *continued*
        - embolism — *continued*
          - specified NEC I63.49
        - thrombosis I63.30
          - specified NEC I63.39
    - anterior I66.1- ☑
      - with infarction I63.52- ☑
        - due to
          - embolism I63.42- ☑
          - thrombosis I63.32- ☑
    - middle I66.0- ☑
      - with infarction I63.51- ☑
        - due to
          - embolism I63.41- ☑
          - thrombosis I63.31- ☑
    - posterior I66.2- ☑
      - with infarction I63.53- ☑
        - due to
          - embolism I63.43- ☑
          - thrombosis I63.33- ☑
    - specified NEC I66.8
      - with infarction I63.59
        - due to
          - embolism I63.4- ☑
          - thrombosis I63.3- ☑
  - choroidal (anterior) — *see* Occlusion, artery, precerebral, specified NEC
  - communicating posterior — *see* Occlusion, artery, precerebral, specified NEC
  - complete
    - coronary I25.82
    - extremities I70.92
  - coronary (acute) (thrombotic) (without myocardial infarction) I24.0
    - with myocardial infarction — *see* Infarction, myocardium
    - chronic total I25.82
    - complete I25.82
    - healed or old I25.2
    - total (chronic) I25.82
  - hypophyseal — *see* Occlusion, artery, precerebral, specified NEC
  - iliac I74.5
  - lower extremities due to stenosis or stricture I77.1
  - mesenteric (embolic) (thrombotic) — *see also* Infarct, intestine K55.069
  - perforating — *see* Occlusion, artery, cerebral, specified NEC
  - peripheral I77.9
    - thrombotic or embolic I74.4
  - pontine — *see* Occlusion, artery, precerebral, specified NEC
  - precerebral I65.9
    - with infarction I63.20
      - specified NEC I63.29
      - due to
        - embolism I63.10
          - specified NEC I63.19
        - thrombosis I63.00
          - specified NEC I63.09
    - basilar — *see* Occlusion, artery, basilar
    - carotid — *see* Occlusion, artery, carotid
    - puerperal O88.23
    - specified NEC I65.8
      - with infarction I63.29
        - due to
          - embolism I63.19
          - thrombosis I63.09
    - vertebral — *see* Occlusion, artery, vertebral
  - renal N28.0
  - retinal
    - branch H34.23- ☑
    - central H34.1- ☑
    - partial H34.21- ☑
    - transient H34.0- ☑
  - spinal — *see* Occlusion, artery, precerebral, vertebral
  - total (chronic)
    - coronary I25.82
    - extremities I70.92
  - vertebral I65.0- ☑
    - with
      - infarction I63.21- ☑

Occlusion, occluded — *continued*
- artery — *see also* Atherosclerosis, artery — *continued*
  - vertebral — *continued*
    - with — *continued*
      - infarction — *continued*
        - due to
          - embolism I63.11- ☑
          - thrombosis I63.Ø1- ☑
- basilar artery — *see* Occlusion, artery, basilar
- bile duct (common) (hepatic) (noncalculous) K83.1
- bowel — *see* Obstruction, intestine
- carotid (artery) (common) (internal) — *see* Occlusion, artery, carotid
- centric (of teeth) M26.59
  - maximum intercuspation discrepancy M26.55
- cerebellar (artery) — *see* Occlusion, artery, cerebellar
- cerebral (artery) — *see* Occlusion, artery, cerebral
- cerebrovascular — *see also* Occlusion, artery, cerebral
  - with infarction I63.5- ☑
- cervical canal — *see* Stricture, cervix
- cervix (uteri) — *see* Stricture, cervix
- choanal Q3Ø.Ø
- choroidal (artery) — *see* Occlusion, artery, precerebral, specified NEC
- colon — *see* Obstruction, intestine
- communicating posterior artery — *see* Occlusion, artery, precerebral, specified NEC
- coronary (artery) (vein) (thrombotic) — *see also* Infarct, myocardium
  - chronic total I25.82
  - healed or old I25.2
  - not resulting in infarction I24.Ø
  - total (chronic) I25.82
- cystic duct — *see* Obstruction, gallbladder
- embolic — *see* Embolism
- fallopian tube N97.1
  - congenital Q5Ø.6
- gallbladder — *see also* Obstruction, gallbladder
  - congenital (causing jaundice) Q44.1
- gingiva, traumatic KØ6.2
- hymen N89.6
  - congenital Q52.3
- hypophyseal (artery) — *see* Occlusion, artery, precerebral, specified NEC
- iliac artery I74.5
- intestine — *see* Obstruction, intestine
- lacrimal passages — *see* Obstruction, lacrimal
- lung J98.4
- lymph or lymphatic channel I89.Ø
- mammary duct N64.89
- mesenteric artery (embolic) (thrombotic) — *see also* Infarct, intestine K55.Ø69
- nose J34.89
  - congenital Q3Ø.Ø
- organ or site, congenital NEC — *see* Atresia, by site
- oviduct N97.1
  - congenital Q5Ø.6
- peripheral arteries
  - due to stricture or stenosis I77.1
  - upper extremity I74.2
- pontine (artery) — *see* Occlusion, artery, precerebral, specified NEC
- posterior lingual, of mandibular teeth M26.29
- precerebral artery — *see* Occlusion, artery, precerebral
- punctum lacrimale — *see* Obstruction, lacrimal
- pupil — *see* Membrane, pupillary
- pylorus, adult — *see also* Stricture, pylorus K31.1
- renal artery N28.Ø
- retina, retinal
  - artery — *see* Occlusion, artery, retinal
  - vein (central) H34.81- ☑
    - engorgement H34.82- ☑
    - tributary H34.83- ☑
  - vessels H34.9
- spinal artery — *see* Occlusion, artery, precerebral, vertebral
- teeth (mandibular) (posterior lingual) M26.29
- thoracic duct I89.Ø
- thrombotic — *see* Thrombosis, artery
- traumatic
  - edentulous (alveolar) ridge KØ6.2
  - gingiva KØ6.2
  - periodontal KØ5.5
- tubal N97.1
- ureter (complete) (partial) N13.5
  - congenital Q62.1Ø
- ureteropelvic junction N13.5
  - congenital Q62.11
- ureterovesical orifice N13.5
  - congenital Q62.12
- urethra — *see* Stricture, urethra
- uterus N85.8
- vagina N89.5
- vascular NEC I99.8
- vein — *see* Thrombosis
  - retinal — *see* Occlusion, retinal, vein
- vena cava (inferior) (superior) — *see* Embolism, vena cava
- ventricle (brain) NEC G91.1
- vertebral (artery) — *see* Occlusion, artery, vertebral
- vessel (blood) I99.8
- vulva N9Ø.5

Occult
- blood in feces (stools) R19.5

Occupational
- problems NEC Z56.89

Ochlophobia — *see* Agoraphobia

Ochronosis (endogenous) E7Ø.29

Ocular muscle — *see* condition

Oculogyric crisis or disturbance H51.8
- psychogenic F45.8

Oculomotor syndrome H51.9

Oculopathy
- syphilitic NEC A52.71
  - congenital
    - early A5Ø.Ø1
    - late A5Ø.3Ø
  - early (secondary) A51.43
  - late A52.71

Oddi's sphincter spasm K83.4

Odontalgia KØ8.89

Odontoameloblastoma — *see* Cyst, calcifying odontogenic

Odontoclasia KØ3.89

Odontodysplasia, regional KØØ.4

Odontogenesis imperfecta KØØ.5

Odontoma (ameloblastic) (complex) (compound) (fibroameloblastic) — *see* Cyst, calcifying odontogenic

Odontomyelitis (closed) (open) KØ4.Ø1
- irreversible KØ4.Ø2
- reversible KØ4.Ø1

Odontorrhagia KØ8.89

Odontosarcoma, ameloblastic C41.1
- upper jaw (bone) C41.Ø

Oestriasis — *see* Myiasis

Oguchi's disease H53.63

Ohara's disease — *see* Tularemia

OHS (obesity hypoventilation syndrome) E66.2

Oidiomycosis — *see* Candidiasis

Oidium albicans infection — *see* Candidiasis

Old age (without mention of debility) R54
- dementia FØ3 ☑

Old (previous) **myocardial infarction** I25.2

Olfactory — *see* condition

Oligemia — *see* Anemia

Oligoastrocytoma
- specified site — *see* Neoplasm, malignant, by site
- unspecified site C71.9

Oligocythemia D64.9

Oligodendroblastoma
- specified site — *see* Neoplasm, malignant
- unspecified site C71.9

Oligodendroglioma
- anaplastic type
  - specified site — *see* Neoplasm, malignant, by site
  - unspecified site C71.9
- specified site — *see* Neoplasm, malignant, by site
- unspecified site C71.9

Oligodontia — *see* Anodontia

Oligoencephalon QØ2

Oligohidrosis L74.4

Oligohydramnios O41.Ø- ☑

Oligohydrosis L74.4

Oligomenorrhea N91.5
- primary N91.3
- secondary N91.4

Oligophrenia — *see also* Disability, intellectual
- phenylpyruvic E7Ø.Ø

Oligospermia N46.11
- due to
  - drug therapy N46.121
  - efferent duct obstruction N46.123
  - infection N46.122
  - radiation N46.124
  - specified cause NEC N46.129
  - systemic disease N46.125

Oligotrichia — *see* Alopecia

Oliguria R34
- with, complicating or following ectopic or molar pregnancy OØ8.4
- postprocedural N99.Ø
- puerperal O9Ø.49

Ollier's disease Q78.4

Omenotocele — *see* Hernia, abdomen, specified site NEC

Omentitis — *see* Peritonitis

Omentum, omental — *see* condition

Omphalitis (congenital) (newborn) P38.9
- with mild hemorrhage P38.1
- without hemorrhage P38.9
- not of newborn LØ8.82
- tetanus A33

Omphalocele Q79.2

Omphalomesenteric duct, persistent Q43.Ø

Omphalorrhagia, newborn P51.9

Omsk hemorrhagic fever A98.1

Onanism (excessive) F98.8

Onchocerciasis, onchocercosis B73.1
- with
  - eye disease B73.ØØ
    - endophthalmitis B73.Ø1
    - eyelid B73.Ø9
    - glaucoma B73.Ø2
    - specified NEC B73.Ø9
  - eyelid B73.Ø9
  - eye NEC B73.ØØ

Oncocytoma — *see* Neoplasm, benign, by site

Oncovirus, as cause of disease classified elsewhere B97.32

Ondine's curse — *see* Apnea, sleep

Oneirophrenia F23

Onychauxis L6Ø.2
- congenital Q84.5

Onychia — *see also* Cellulitis, digit
- with lymphangitis — *see* Lymphangitis, acute, digit
- candidal B37.2
- dermatophytic B35.1

Onychitis — *see also* Cellulitis, digit
- with lymphangitis — *see* Lymphangitis, acute, digit

Onychocryptosis L6Ø.Ø

Onychodystrophy L6Ø.3
- congenital Q84.6

Onychogryphosis, onychogryposis L6Ø.2

Onycholysis L6Ø.1

Onychomadesis L6Ø.8

Onychomalacia L6Ø.3

Onychomycosis (finger) (toe) B35.1

Onycho-osteodysplasia Q87.2

Onychophagia F98.8

Onychophosis L6Ø.8

Onychoptosis L6Ø.8

Onychorrhexis L6Ø.3
- congenital Q84.6

Onychoschizia L6Ø.3

Onyxis (finger) (toe) L6Ø.Ø

Onyxitis — *see also* Cellulitis, digit
- with lymphangitis — *see* Lymphangitis, acute, digit

Oophoritis (cystic) (infectional) (interstitial) N7Ø.92
- with salpingitis N7Ø.93
- acute N7Ø.Ø2
  - with salpingitis N7Ø.Ø3
- chronic N7Ø.12
  - with salpingitis N7Ø.13
- complicating abortion — *see* Abortion, by type, complicated by, oophoritis

Oophorocele N83.4- ☑

Opacity, opacities
- cornea H17.- ☑
  - central H17.1- ☑
  - congenital Q13.3
  - degenerative — *see* Degeneration, cornea
  - hereditary — *see* Dystrophy, cornea
  - inflammatory — *see* Keratitis
  - minor H17.81- ☑
  - peripheral H17.82- ☑
  - sequelae of trachoma (healed) B94.Ø
  - specified NEC H17.89
- enamel (teeth) (fluoride) (nonfluoride) KØØ.3

Opacity, opacities — *continued*
- lens — *see* Cataract
- snowball — *see* Deposit, crystalline
- vitreous (humor) NEC H43.39- ☑
  - congenital Q14.0
  - membranes and strands H43.31- ☑

Opalescent dentin (hereditary) K00.5

Open, opening
- abnormal, organ or site, congenital — *see* Imperfect, closure
- angle with
  - borderline
    - findings
      - high risk H40.02- ☑
      - low risk H40.01- ☑
    - intraocular pressure H40.00- ☑
  - cupping of discs H40.01- ☑
  - glaucoma (primary) — *see* Glaucoma, open angle
- bite
  - anterior M26.220
  - posterior M26.221
- false — *see* Imperfect, closure
- margin on tooth restoration K08.51
- restoration margins of tooth K08.51
- wound — *see* Wound, open

Operational fatigue F48.8

Operative — *see* condition

Operculitis — *see* Periodontitis

Operculum — *see* Break, retina

Ophiasis L63.2

Ophthalmia — *see also* Conjunctivitis H10.9
- actinic rays — *see* Photokeratitis
- allergic (acute) — *see* Conjunctivitis, acute, atopic
- blennorrhagic (gonococcal) (neonatorum) A54.31
- diphtheritic A36.86
- Egyptian A71.1
- electrica — *see* Photokeratitis
- gonococcal (neonatorum) A54.31
- metastatic — *see* Endophthalmitis, purulent
- migraine — *see* Migraine, ophthalmoplegic
- neonatorum, newborn P39.1
  - gonococcal A54.31
- nodosa H16.24- ☑
- purulent — *see* Conjunctivitis, acute, mucopurulent
- spring — *see* Conjunctivitis, acute, atopic
- sympathetic — *see* Uveitis, sympathetic

Ophthalmitis — *see* Ophthalmia

Ophthalmocele (congenital) Q15.8

Ophthalmoneuromyelitis G36.0

Ophthalmoplegia — *see also* Strabismus, paralytic
- anterior internuclear — *see* Ophthalmoplegia, internuclear
- ataxia-areflexia G61.0
- diabetic — *see* E08-E13 with .39
- exophthalmic E05.00
  - with thyroid storm E05.01
- external H49.88- ☑
  - progressive H49.4- ☑
    - with pigmentary retinopathy — *see* Kearns-Sayre syndrome
  - total H49.3- ☑
- internal (complete) (total) H52.51- ☑
- internuclear H51.2- ☑
- migraine — *see* Migraine, ophthalmoplegic
- Parinaud's H49.88- ☑
- progressive external — *see* Ophthalmoplegia, external, progressive
- supranuclear, progressive G23.1
- total (external) — *see* Ophthalmoplegia, external, total

Opioid(s)
- abuse — *see* Abuse, drug, opioids
- dependence — *see* Dependence, drug, opioids
- induced, without use disorder
  - anxiety disorder F11.988
  - delirium F11.921
  - depressive disorder F11.94
  - sexual dysfunction F11.981
  - sleep disorder F11.982

Opisthognathism M26.09

Opisthorchiasis (felineus) (viverrini) B66.0

Opitz' disease D73.2

Opiumism — *see* Dependence, drug, opioid

Oppenheim's disease G70.2

Oppenheim-Urbach disease (necrobiosis lipoidica diabeticorum) — *see* E08-E13 with .620

Optic nerve — *see* condition

Orbit — *see* condition

Orchioblastoma C62.9- ☑

Orchitis (gangrenous) (nonspecific) (septic) (suppurative) N45.2
- blennorrhagic (gonococcal) (acute) (chronic) A54.23
- chlamydial A56.19
- filarial — *see also* Infestation, filarial B74.9 *[N51]*
- gonococcal (acute) (chronic) A54.23
- mumps B26.0
- syphilitic A52.76
- tuberculous A18.15

Orf (virus disease) B08.02

Organic — *see also* condition
- brain syndrome F09
- heart — *see* Disease, heart
- mental disorder F09
- psychosis F09

Orgasm
- anejaculatory N53.13

Oriental
- bilharziasis B65.2
- schistosomiasis B65.2

Orifice — *see* condition

Origin of both great vessels from right ventricle Q20.1

Ormond's disease (with ureteral obstruction) N13.5
- with infection N13.6

Ornithine metabolism disorder E72.4

Ornithinemia (Type I) (Type II) E72.4

Ornithosis A70

Orotaciduria, oroticaciduria (congenital) (hereditary) (pyrimidine deficiency) E79.89
- anemia D53.0

Orthodontics
- adjustment Z46.4
- fitting Z46.4

Orthopnea R06.01

Orthopoxvirus B08.09

Os, uterus — *see* condition

Osgood-Schlatter disease or osteochondrosis M92.52- ☑

Osler (-Weber)-**Rendu disease** I78.0

Osler's nodes I33.0

Osmidrosis L75.0

Osseous — *see* condition

Ossification
- artery — *see* Arteriosclerosis
- auricle (ear) — *see* Disorder, pinna, specified type NEC
- bronchial J98.09
- cardiac — *see* Degeneration, myocardial
- cartilage (senile) — *see* Disorder, cartilage, specified type NEC
- coronary (artery) — *see* Disease, heart, ischemic, atherosclerotic
- diaphragm J98.6
- ear, middle — *see* Otosclerosis
- falx cerebri G96.198
- fontanel, premature Q75.009
- heart — *see also* Degeneration, myocardial
  - valve — *see* Endocarditis
- larynx J38.7
- ligament — *see* Disorder, tendon, specified type NEC
  - posterior longitudinal — *see* Spondylopathy, specified NEC
- meninges (cerebral) (spinal) G96.198
- multiple, eccentric centers — *see* Disorder, bone, development or growth
- muscle — *see also* Calcification, muscle
  - due to burns — *see* Myositis, ossificans, in, burns
  - paralytic — *see* Myositis, ossificans, in, quadriplegia
  - progressive — *see* Myositis, ossificans, progressiva
  - specified NEC M61.50
    - ankle M61.57- ☑
    - foot M61.57- ☑
    - forearm M61.53- ☑
    - hand M61.54- ☑
    - lower leg M61.56- ☑
    - multiple sites M61.59
    - pelvic region M61.55- ☑
    - shoulder region M61.51- ☑
    - specified site NEC M61.58
    - thigh M61.55- ☑
    - upper arm M61.52- ☑
  - traumatic — *see* Myositis, ossificans, traumatica
- myocardium, myocardial — *see* Degeneration, myocardial
- penis N48.89
- periarticular — *see* Disorder, joint, specified type NEC

Ossification — *continued*
- pinna — *see* Disorder, pinna, specified type NEC
- rider's bone — *see* Ossification, muscle, specified NEC
- sclera H15.89
- subperiosteal, post-traumatic M89.8X- ☑
- tendon — *see* Disorder, tendon, specified type NEC
- trachea J39.8
- tympanic membrane — *see* Disorder, tympanic membrane, specified NEC
- vitreous (humor) — *see* Deposit, crystalline

Osteitis — *see also* Osteomyelitis
- alveolar M27.3
- condensans M85.30
  - ankle M85.37- ☑
  - foot M85.37- ☑
  - forearm M85.33- ☑
  - hand M85.34- ☑
  - lower leg M85.36- ☑
  - multiple site M85.39
  - neck M85.38
  - rib M85.38
  - shoulder M85.31- ☑
  - skull M85.38
  - specified site NEC M85.38
  - thigh M85.35- ☑
  - toe M85.37- ☑
  - upper arm M85.32- ☑
  - vertebra M85.38
- deformans — *see also* Paget's disease, bone M88.9
  - in (due to)
    - malignant neoplasm of bone — *see also* Neoplasm, malignant, by site C41.9 *[M90.60]*
    - neoplastic disease — *see also* Neoplasm, by type and site D49.9 *[M90.60]*
      - carpus D49.2 *[M90.64-]* ☑
      - clavicle D49.2 *[M90.61-]* ☑
      - femur D49.2 *[M90.65-]* ☑
      - fibula D49.2 *[M90.66-]* ☑
      - finger D49.2 *[M90.64-]* ☑
      - humerus D49.2 *[M90.62-]* ☑
      - ilium D49.2 *[M90.68]*
      - ischium D49.2 *[M90.68]*
      - metacarpus D49.2 *[M90.64-]* ☑
      - metatarsus D49.2 *[M90.67-]* ☑
      - multiple sites D49.89 *[M90.69]*
      - neck D49.2 *[M90.68]*
      - pubic ramus D49.2 *[M90.68]*
      - radius D49.2 *[M90.63-]* ☑
      - rib D49.2 *[M90.68]*
      - scapula D49.2 *[M90.61-]* ☑
      - skull D49.2 *[M90.68]*
      - tarsus D49.2 *[M90.67-]* ☑
      - tibia D49.2 *[M90.66-]* ☑
      - toe D49.2 *[M90.67-]* ☑
      - ulna D49.2 *[M90.63-]* ☑
      - vertebra D49.2 *[M90.68]*
  - skull M88.0
  - specified NEC — *see* Paget's disease, bone, by site
  - vertebra M88.1
- due to yaws A66.6
- fibrosa NEC — *see* Cyst, bone, by site
  - circumscripta — *see* Dysplasia, fibrous, bone NEC
  - cystica (generalisata) E21.0
  - disseminata Q78.1
  - osteoplastica E21.0
- fragilitans Q78.0
- Garr's (sclerosing) — *see* Osteomyelitis, specified type NEC
- jaw (acute) (chronic) (lower) (suppurative) (upper) M27.2
- parathyroid E21.0
- petrous bone (acute) (chronic) — *see* Petrositis
- sclerotic, nonsuppurative — *see* Osteomyelitis, specified type NEC
- tuberculosa A18.09
  - cystica D86.89
  - multiplex cystoides D86.89

Osteoarthritis M19.90
- ankle M19.07- ☑
  - post-traumatic M19.17- ☑
  - primary M19.07- ☑
  - secondary M19.27- ☑
- elbow M19.02- ☑
  - post-traumatic M19.12- ☑
  - primary M19.02- ☑
  - secondary M19.22- ☑

- **Osteoarthritis** — *continued*
  - foot joint M19.Ø7- ☑
    - post-traumatic M19.17- ☑
    - primary M19.Ø7- ☑
    - secondary M19.27- ☑
  - generalized (multiple joints) M15.9
    - erosive M15.4
    - primary M15.Ø
    - specified NEC M15.8
  - hand joint M19.Ø4- ☑
    - first carpometacarpal joint M18.9
      - post-traumatic — *see* Osteoarthritis, post-traumatic NEC, hand joint, first carpometacarpal joint
      - primary — *see* Osteoarthritis, primary, hand joint, first carpometacarpal joint
      - secondary — *see* Osteoarthritis, secondary, hand joint, first carpometacarpal joint
    - post-traumatic M19.14- ☑
    - primary M19.Ø4- ☑
    - secondary M19.24- ☑
  - hip M16.9
    - bilateral M16.Ø
      - due to hip dysplasia M16.2
      - post-traumatic M16.4
      - secondary M16.6
    - due to hip dysplasia (unilateral) M16.3- ☑
      - bilateral M16.2
    - post-traumatic — *see* Osteoarthritis, post-traumatic, hip
    - primary M16.1- ☑
    - secondary — *see* Osteoarthritis, secondary, hip
    - unilateral M16.1- ☑
      - due to hip dysplasia M16.3- ☑
      - post-traumatic M16.5- ☑
      - primary M16.1- ☑
      - secondary NEC M16.7
  - interphalangeal
    - distal (Heberden) M15.1
    - proximal (Bouchard) M15.2
  - knee M17.9
    - bilateral M17.Ø
      - post-traumatic M17.2
      - secondary M17.4
    - post-traumatic — *see* Osteoarthritis, post-traumatic, knee
    - primary M17.1- ☑
      - bilateral M17.Ø
    - secondary — *see* Osteoarthritis, secondary, knee
    - unilateral M17.1- ☑
      - post-traumatic M17.3- ☑
      - primary M17.1- ☑
      - secondary NEC M17.5
  - post-traumatic NEC M19.92
    - ankle M19.17- ☑
    - elbow M19.12- ☑
    - foot joint M19.17- ☑
    - hand joint M19.14- ☑
      - first carpometacarpal joint M18.3- ☑
        - bilateral M18.2
    - hip M16.5- ☑
      - bilateral M16.4
    - knee M17.3- ☑
      - bilateral M17.2
    - shoulder M19.11- ☑
    - specified site NEC M19.19
    - wrist M19.13- ☑
  - primary M19.91
    - ankle M19.Ø7- ☑
    - elbow M19.Ø2- ☑
    - foot joint M19.Ø7- ☑
    - hand joint M19.Ø4- ☑
      - first carpometacarpal joint M18.1- ☑
        - bilateral M18.Ø
    - hip M16.1- ☑
      - bilateral M16.Ø
    - knee M17.1- ☑
      - bilateral M17.Ø
    - multiple sites M15.9
    - shoulder M19.Ø1- ☑
    - specified site NEC M19.Ø9
    - spine — *see* Spondylosis
    - wrist M19.Ø3- ☑
  - secondary M19.93
    - ankle M19.27- ☑
    - elbow M19.22- ☑
    - foot joint M19.27- ☑

- **Osteoarthritis** — *continued*
  - secondary — *continued*
    - hand joint M19.24- ☑
      - first carpometacarpal joint M18.5- ☑
        - bilateral M18.4
    - hip M16.7-
      - bilateral M16.6
    - knee M17.5-
      - bilateral M17.4
    - multiple M15.3
    - shoulder M19.21- ☑
    - specified site NEC M19.29
    - spine — *see* Spondylosis
    - wrist M19.23- ☑
  - shoulder M19.Ø1- ☑
    - post-traumatic M19.11- ☑
    - primary M19.Ø1- ☑
    - secondary M19.21- ☑
  - specified site NEC M19.Ø9
  - spine — *see* Spondylosis
  - wrist M19.Ø3- ☑
    - first carpometacarpal joint — *see* Osteoarthritis, hand joint, first carpometacarpal joint
    - post-traumatic M19.13- ☑
    - primary M19.Ø3- ☑
    - secondary M19.23 ☑
- **Osteoarthropathy** (hypertrophic) M19.9Ø
  - ankle — *see* Osteoarthritis, primary, ankle
  - elbow — *see* Osteoarthritis, primary, elbow
  - foot joint — *see* Osteoarthritis, primary, foot
  - hand joint — *see* Osteoarthritis, primary, hand joint
  - knee joint — *see* Osteoarthritis, primary, knee
  - multiple site — *see* Osteoarthritis, primary, multiple joint
  - pulmonary — *see also* Osteoarthropathy, specified type NEC
    - hypertrophic — *see* Osteoarthropathy, hypertrophic, specified type NEC
  - secondary — *see* Osteoarthropathy, specified type NEC
  - secondary hypertrophic — *see* Osteoarthropathy, specified type NEC
  - shoulder — *see* Osteoarthritis, primary, shoulder
  - specified joint NEC — *see* Osteoarthritis, primary, specified joint NEC
  - specified type NEC M89.4Ø
    - carpus M89.44- ☑
    - clavicle M89.41- ☑
    - femur M89.45- ☑
    - fibula M89.46- ☑
    - finger M89.44- ☑
    - humerus M89.42- ☑
    - ilium M89.48
    - ischium M89.48
    - metacarpus M89.44- ☑
    - metatarsus M89.47- ☑
    - multiple sites M89.49
    - neck M89.48
    - pubic ramus M89.48
    - radius M89.43- ☑
    - rib M89.48
    - scapula M89.41- ☑
    - skull M89.48
    - tarsus M89.47- ☑
    - tibia M89.46- ☑
    - toe M89.47- ☑
    - ulna M89.43- ☑
    - vertebra M89.48
  - spine — *see* Spondylosis
  - wrist — *see* Osteoarthritis, primary, wrist
- **Osteoarthrosis** (degenerative) (hypertrophic) (joint) — *see also* Osteoarthritis
  - deformans alkaptonurica E7Ø.29 *[M36.8]*
  - erosive M15.4
  - generalized M15.9
    - primary M15.Ø
  - polyarticular M15.9
  - spine — *see* Spondylosis
- **Osteoblastoma** — *see* Neoplasm, bone, benign
  - aggressive — *see* Neoplasm, bone, uncertain behavior
- **Osteochondritis** — *see also* Osteochondropathy, by site
  - Brailsford's — *see* Osteochondrosis, juvenile, radius
  - dissecans M93.2Ø
    - ankle M93.27- ☑
    - elbow M93.22- ☑
    - foot M93.27- ☑
    - hand M93.24- ☑
    - hip M93.25- ☑

- **Osteochondritis** — *continued*
  - dissecans — *continued*
    - knee M93.26- ☑
    - multiple sites M93.29
    - shoulder joint M93.21- ☑
    - specified site NEC M93.28
    - wrist M93.23- ☑
  - juvenile M92.9
    - patellar — *see* Osteochondrosis, juvenile, patella
  - syphilitic (congenital) (early) A5Ø.Ø2 *[M9Ø.8Ø]*
    - ankle A5Ø.Ø2 *[M9Ø.87-]* ☑
    - elbow A5Ø.Ø2 *[M9Ø.82-]* ☑
    - foot A5Ø.Ø2 *[M9Ø.87-]* ☑
    - forearm A5Ø.Ø2 *[M9Ø.83-]* ☑
    - hand A5Ø.Ø2 *[M9Ø.84-]* ☑
    - hip A5Ø.Ø2 *[M9Ø.85-]* ☑
    - knee A5Ø.Ø2 *[M9Ø.86-]* ☑
    - multiple sites A5Ø.Ø2 *[M9Ø.89]*
    - shoulder joint A5Ø.Ø2 *[M9Ø.81-]* ☑
    - specified site NEC A5Ø.Ø2 *[M9Ø.88]*
- **Osteochondroarthrosis deformans endemica** — *see* Disease, Kaschin-Beck
- **Osteochondrodysplasia** Q78.9
  - with defects of growth of tubular bones and spine Q77.9
    - specified NEC Q77.8
  - specified NEC Q78.8
- **Osteochondrodystrophy** E78.9
- **Osteochondrolysis** — *see* Osteochondritis, dissecans
- **Osteochondroma** — *see* Neoplasm, bone, benign
- **Osteochondromatosis** D16.9
  - syndrome Q78.4
- **Osteochondromyxosarcoma** — *see* Neoplasm, bone, malignant
- **Osteochondropathy** M93.9Ø
  - ankle M93.97- ☑
  - elbow M93.92- ☑
  - foot M93.97- ☑
  - hand M93.94- ☑
  - hip M93.95- ☑
  - Kienbock's disease of adults M93.1
  - knee M93.96- ☑
  - multiple joints M93.99
  - osteochondritis dissecans — *see* Osteochondritis, dissecans
  - osteochondrosis — *see* Osteochondrosis
  - shoulder region M93.91- ☑
  - slipped upper femoral epiphysis — *see* Slipped, epiphysis, upper femoral
  - specified joint NEC M93.98
  - specified type NEC M93.8Ø
    - ankle M93.87- ☑
    - elbow M93.82- ☑
    - foot M93.87- ☑
    - hand M93.84- ☑
    - hip M93.85- ☑
    - knee M93.86- ☑
    - multiple joints M93.89
    - shoulder region M93.81- ☑
    - specified joint NEC M93.88
    - wrist M93.83- ☑
  - syphilitic, congenital
    - early A5Ø.Ø2 *[M9Ø.8Ø]*
    - late A5Ø.56 *[M9Ø.8Ø]*
  - wrist M93.93- ☑
- **Osteochondrosarcoma** — *see* Neoplasm, bone, malignant
- **Osteochondrosis** — *see also* Osteochondropathy, by site
  - acetabulum (juvenile) M91.Ø
  - adult — *see* Osteochondropathy, specified type NEC, by site
  - astragalus (juvenile) — *see* Osteochondrosis, juvenile, tarsus
  - Blount M92.51- ☑
  - Buchanan's M91.Ø
  - Burns' — *see* Osteochondrosis, juvenile, ulna
  - calcaneus (juvenile) — *see* Osteochondrosis, juvenile, tarsus
  - capitular epiphysis (femur) (juvenile) — *see* Legg-Calve-Perthes disease
  - carpal (juvenile) (lunate) (scaphoid) — *see* Osteochondrosis, juvenile, hand, carpal lunate
    - adult M93.1
  - coxae juvenilis — *see* Legg-Calve-Perthes disease
  - deformans juvenilis, coxae — *see* Legg-Calve-Perthes disease

Osteochondrosis — *continued*
- Diaz's — *see* Osteochondrosis, juvenile, tarsus
- dissecans (knee) (shoulder) — *see* Osteochondritis, dissecans
- femoral capital epiphysis (juvenile) — *see* Legg-Calve-Perthes disease
- femur (head), juvenile — *see* Legg-Calve-Perthes disease
- fibula (juvenile) — *see* Osteochondrosis, juvenile, fibula
- foot NEC (juvenile) M92.8
- Freiberg's — *see* Osteochondrosis, juvenile, metatarsus
- Haas' (juvenile) — *see* Osteochondrosis, juvenile, humerus
- Haglund's — *see* Osteochondrosis, juvenile, tarsus
- hip (juvenile) — *see* Legg-Calve-Perthes disease
- humerus (capitulum) (head) (juvenile) — *see* Osteochondrosis, juvenile, humerus
- ilium, iliac crest (juvenile) M91.Ø
- ischiopubic synchondrosis M91.Ø
- Iselin's — *see* Osteochondrosis, juvenile, metatarsus
- juvenile, juvenilis M92.9
  - after congenital dislocation of hip reduction — *see* Osteochondrosis, juvenile, hip, specified NEC
  - arm — *see* Osteochondrosis, juvenile, upper limb NEC
  - capitular epiphysis (femur) — *see* Legg-Calve-Perthes disease
  - clavicle, sternal epiphysis — *see* Osteochondrosis, juvenile, upper limb NEC
  - coxae — *see* Legg-Calve-Perthes disease
  - deformans M92.9
  - fibula M92.5Ø- ☑
  - foot NEC M92.8
  - hand M92.2Ø- ☑
    - carpal lunate M92.21- ☑
    - metacarpal head M92.22- ☑
    - specified site NEC M92.29- ☑
  - head of femur — *see* Legg-Calve-Perthes disease
  - hip and pelvis M91.9- ☑
    - coxa plana — *see* Coxa, plana
    - femoral head — *see* Legg-Calve-Perthes disease
    - pelvis M91.Ø
    - pseudocoxalgia — *see* Pseudocoxalgia
    - specified NEC M91.8- ☑
  - humerus M92.Ø- ☑
  - limb
    - lower NEC M92.8
    - upper NEC — *see* Osteochondrosis, juvenile, upper limb NEC
  - medial cuneiform bone — *see* Osteochondrosis, juvenile, tarsus
  - metatarsus M92.7- ☑
  - patella M92.4- ☑
  - radius M92.1- ☑
  - specified
    - site NEC M92.8
    - type NEC M92.8
      - tibia and fibula M92.59- ☑
  - spine M42.ØØ
    - cervical region M42.Ø2
    - cervicothoracic region M42.Ø3
    - lumbar region M42.Ø6
    - lumbosacral region M42.Ø7
    - multiple sites M42.Ø9
    - occipito-atlanto-axial region M42.Ø1
    - sacrococcygeal region M42.Ø8
    - thoracic region M42.Ø4
    - thoracolumbar region M42.Ø5
  - tarsus M92.6- ☑
  - tibia M92.5Ø- ☑
    - proximal M92.51- ☑
    - tubercle M92.52- ☑
  - ulna M92.1- ☑
  - upper limb NEC M92.3- ☑
  - vertebra (body) (epiphyseal plates) (Calve's) (Scheuermann's) — *see* Osteochondrosis, juvenile, spine
- Kienbock's — *see* Osteochondrosis, juvenile, hand, carpal lunate
  - adult M93.1
- Kohler's
  - patellar — *see* Osteochondrosis, juvenile, patella
  - tarsal navicular — *see* Osteochondrosis, juvenile, tarsus
- Legg-Perthes (-Calve) (-Waldenstrom) — *see* Legg-Calve-Perthes disease

Osteochondrosis — *continued*
- limb
  - lower NEC (juvenile) M92.8
    - tibia and fibula M92.59- ☑
  - upper NEC (juvenile) — *see* Osteochondrosis, juvenile, upper limb NEC
- lunate bone (carpal) (juvenile) — *see also* Osteochondrosis, juvenile, hand, carpal lunate
  - adult M93.1
- Mauclaire's — *see* Osteochondrosis, juvenile, hand, metacarpal
- metacarpal (head) (juvenile) — *see* Osteochondrosis, juvenile, hand, metacarpal
- metatarsus (fifth) (head) (juvenile) (second) — *see* Osteochondrosis, juvenile, metatarsus
- navicular (juvenile) — *see* Osteochondrosis, juvenile, tarsus
- os
  - calcis (juvenile) — *see* Osteochondrosis, juvenile, tarsus
  - tibiale externum (juvenile) — *see* Osteochondrosis, juvenile, tarsus
- Osgood-Schlatter M92.52- ☑
- Panner's — *see* Osteochondrosis, juvenile, humerus
- patellar center (juvenile) (primary) (secondary) — *see* Osteochondrosis, juvenile, patella
- pelvis (juvenile) M91.Ø
- Pierson's M91.Ø
- radius (head) (juvenile) — *see* Osteochondrosis, juvenile, radius
- Scheuermann's — *see* Osteochondrosis, juvenile, spine
- Sever's — *see* Osteochondrosis, juvenile, tarsus
- Sinding-Larsen — *see* Osteochondrosis, juvenile, patella
- spine M42.9
  - adult M42.1Ø
    - cervical region M42.12
    - cervicothoracic region M42.13
    - lumbar region M42.16
    - lumbosacral region M42.17
    - multiple sites M42.19
    - occipito-atlanto-axial region M42.11
    - sacrococcygeal region M42.18
    - thoracic region M42.14
    - thoracolumbar region M42.15
  - juvenile — *see* Osteochondrosis, juvenile, spine
- symphysis pubis (juvenile) M91.Ø
- syphilitic (congenital) A5Ø.Ø2
- talus (juvenile) — *see* Osteochondrosis, juvenile, tarsus
- tarsus (navicular) (juvenile) — *see* Osteochondrosis, juvenile, tarsus
- tibia (proximal) (tubercle) (juvenile) — *see* Osteochondrosis, juvenile, tibia
- tuberculous — *see* Tuberculosis, bone
- ulna (lower) (juvenile) — *see* Osteochondrosis, juvenile, ulna
- van Neck's M91.Ø
- vertebral — *see* Osteochondrosis, spine

Osteoclastoma D48.Ø
- malignant — *see* Neoplasm, bone, malignant

Osteodynia — *see* Disorder, bone, specified type NEC

Osteodystrophy Q78.9
- azotemic N25.Ø
- congenital Q78.9
- parathyroid, secondary E21.1
- renal N25.Ø

Osteofibroma — *see* Neoplasm, bone, benign

Osteofibrosarcoma — *see* Neoplasm, bone, malignant

Osteogenesis imperfecta Q78.Ø

Osteogenic — *see* condition

Osteolysis M89.5Ø
- carpus M89.54- ☑
- clavicle M89.51- ☑
- femur M89.55- ☑
- fibula M89.56- ☑
- finger M89.54- ☑
- humerus M89.52- ☑
- ilium M89.58
- ischium M89.58
- joint prosthesis (periprosthetic) — *see* Complications, joint prosthesis, mechanical, periprosthetic, osteolysis, by site
- metacarpus M89.54- ☑
- metatarsus M89.57- ☑
- multiple sites M89.59
- neck M89.58

Osteolysis — *continued*
- periprosthetic — *see* Complications, joint prosthesis, mechanical, periprosthetic, osteolysis, by site
- pubic ramus M89.58
- radius M89.53- ☑
- rib M89.58
- scapula M89.51- ☑
- skull M89.58
- tarsus M89.57- ☑
- tibia M89.56- ☑
- toe M89.57- ☑
- ulna M89.53- ☑
- vertebra M89.58

Osteoma — *see also* Neoplasm, bone, benign
- osteoid — *see also* Neoplasm, bone, benign
  - giant — *see* Neoplasm, bone, benign

Osteomalacia M83.9
- adult M83.9
  - drug-induced NEC M83.5
  - due to
    - malabsorption (postsurgical) M83.2
    - malnutrition M83.3
  - specified NEC M83.8
- aluminium-induced M83.4
- infantile — *see* Rickets
- juvenile — *see* Rickets
- oncogenic E83.89
- pelvis M83.8
- puerperal M83.Ø
- senile M83.1
- vitamin-D-resistant in adults E83.31 *[M9Ø.8-]* ☑
  - carpus E83.31 *[M9Ø.84-]* ☑
  - clavicle E83.31 *[M9Ø.81-]* ☑
  - femur E83.31 *[M9Ø.85-]* ☑
  - fibula E83.31 *[M9Ø.86-]* ☑
  - finger E83.31 *[M9Ø.84-]* ☑
  - humerus E83.31 *[M9Ø.82-]* ☑
  - ilium E83.31 *[M9Ø.88]*
  - ischium E83.31 *[M9Ø.88]*
  - metacarpus E83.31 *[M9Ø.84-]* ☑
  - metatarsus E83.31 *[M9Ø.87-]* ☑
  - multiple sites E83.31 *[M9Ø.89]*
  - neck E83.31 *[M9Ø.88]*
  - pubic ramus E83.31 *[M9Ø.88]*
  - radius E83.31 *[M9Ø.83-]* ☑
  - rib E83.31 *[M9Ø.88]*
  - scapula E83.31 *[M9Ø.819]*
  - skull E83.31 *[M9Ø.88]*
  - tarsus E83.31 *[M9Ø.879]*
  - tibia E83.31 *[M9Ø.869]*
  - toe E83.31 *[M9Ø.879]*
  - ulna E83.31 *[M9Ø.839]*
  - vertebra E83.31 *[M9Ø.88]*

Osteomyelitis (general) (infective) (localized) (neonatal) (purulent) (septic) (staphylococcal) (streptococcal) (suppurative) (with periostitis) M86.9
- acute M86.1Ø
  - carpus M86.14- ☑
  - clavicle M86.11- ☑
  - femur M86.15- ☑
  - fibula M86.16- ☑
  - finger M86.14- ☑
  - hematogenous M86.ØØ
    - carpus M86.Ø4- ☑
    - clavicle M86.Ø1- ☑
    - femur M86.Ø5- ☑
    - fibula M86.Ø6- ☑
    - finger M86.Ø4- ☑
    - humerus M86.Ø2- ☑
    - ilium M86.Ø8
    - ischium M86.Ø8
    - mandible M27.2
    - metacarpus M86.Ø4- ☑
    - metatarsus M86.Ø7- ☑
    - multiple sites M86.Ø9
    - neck M86.Ø8
    - orbit HØ5.Ø2- ☑
    - petrous bone — *see* Petrositis
    - radius M86.Ø3- ☑
    - rib M86.Ø8
    - scapula M86.Ø1- ☑
    - skull M86.Ø8
    - tarsus M86.Ø7- ☑
    - tibia M86.Ø6- ☑
    - toe M86.Ø7- ☑
    - ulna M86.Ø3- ☑

- **Osteomyelitis** — *continued*
  - acute — *continued*
    - hematogenous — *continued*
      - vertebra — *see* Osteomyelitis, vertebra
    - humerus M86.12- ☑
    - ilium M86.18
    - ischium M86.18
    - mandible M27.2
    - metacarpus M86.14- ☑
    - metatarsus M86.17- ☑
    - multiple sites M86.19
    - neck M86.18
    - orbit HØ5.Ø2- ☑
    - petrous bone — *see* Petrositis
    - radius M86.13- ☑
    - rib M86.18
    - scapula M86.11- ☑
    - skull M86.18
    - tarsus M86.17- ☑
    - tibia M86.16- ☑
    - toe M86.17- ☑
    - ulna M86.13- ☑
    - vertebra — *see* Osteomyelitis, vertebra
  - chronic (or old) M86.6Ø
    - with draining sinus M86.4Ø
      - carpus M86.44- ☑
      - clavicle M86.41- ☑
      - femur M86.45- ☑
      - fibula M86.46- ☑
      - finger M86.44- ☑
      - humerus M86.42- ☑
      - ilium M86.48
      - ischium M86.48
      - mandible M27.2
      - metacarpus M86.44- ☑
      - metatarsus M86.47- ☑
      - multiple sites M86.49
      - neck M86.48
      - orbit HØ5.Ø2- ☑
      - petrous bone — *see* Petrositis
      - pubic ramus M86.48
      - radius M86.43- ☑
      - rib M86.48
      - scapula M86.41- ☑
      - skull M86.48
      - tarsus M86.47- ☑
      - tibia M86.46- ☑
      - toe M86.47- ☑
      - ulna M86.43- ☑
      - vertebra — *see* Osteomyelitis, vertebra
    - carpus M86.64- ☑
    - clavicle M86.61- ☑
    - femur M86.65- ☑
    - fibula M86.66- ☑
    - finger M86.64- ☑
    - hematogenous NEC M86.5Ø
      - carpus M86.54- ☑
      - clavicle M86.51- ☑
      - femur M86.55- ☑
      - fibula M86.56- ☑
      - finger M86.54- ☑
      - humerus M86.52- ☑
      - ilium M86.58
      - ischium M86.58
      - mandible M27.2
      - metacarpus M86.54- ☑
      - metatarsus M86.57- ☑
      - multifocal M86.3Ø
        - carpus M86.34- ☑
        - clavicle M86.31- ☑
        - femur M86.35- ☑
        - fibula M86.36- ☑
        - finger M86.34- ☑
        - humerus M86.32- ☑
        - ilium M86.38
        - ischium M86.38
        - metacarpus M86.34- ☑
        - metatarsus M86.37- ☑
        - multiple sites M86.39
        - neck M86.38
        - pubic ramus M86.38
        - radius M86.33- ☑
        - rib M86.38
        - scapula M86.31- ☑
        - skull M86.38
        - tarsus M86.37- ☑
        - tibia M86.36- ☑

- **Osteomyelitis** — *continued*
  - chronic — *continued*
    - hematogenous — *continued*
      - multifocal — *continued*
        - toe M86.37- ☑
        - ulna M86.33- ☑
        - vertebra — *see* Osteomyelitis, vertebra
      - multiple sites M86.59
      - neck M86.58
      - orbit HØ5.Ø2- ☑
      - petrous bone — *see* Petrositis
      - pubic ramus M86.58
      - radius M86.53- ☑
      - rib M86.58
      - scapula M86.51- ☑
      - skull M86.58
      - tarsus M86.57- ☑
      - tibia M86.56- ☑
      - toe M86.57- ☑
      - ulna M86.53- ☑
      - vertebra — *see* Osteomyelitis, vertebra
    - humerus M86.62- ☑
    - ilium M86.659
    - ischium M86.659
    - mandible M27.2
    - metacarpus M86.64- ☑
    - metatarsus M86.67- ☑
    - multifocal — *see* Osteomyelitis, chronic, hematogenous, multifocal
    - multiple sites M86.69
    - neck M86.68
    - orbit HØ5.Ø2- ☑
    - petrous bone — *see* Petrositis
    - radius M86.63- ☑
    - rib M86.68
    - scapula M86.61- ☑
    - skull M86.68
    - tarsus M86.67- ☑
    - tibia M86.66- ☑
    - toe M86.67- ☑
    - ulna M86.63- ☑
    - vertebra — *see* Osteomyelitis, vertebra
  - echinococcal B67.2
  - Garr's — *see* Osteomyelitis, specified type NEC
  - in diabetes mellitus — *see* EØ8-E13 with .69
  - jaw (acute) (chronic) (lower) (neonatal) (suppurative) (upper) M27.2
  - nonsuppurating — *see* Osteomyelitis, specified type NEC
  - orbit HØ5.Ø2- ☑
  - petrous bone — *see* Petrositis
  - Salmonella (arizonae) (cholerae-suis) (enteritidis) (typhimurium) AØ2.24
  - sclerosing, nonsuppurative — *see* Osteomyelitis, specified type NEC
  - specified type NEC — *see also* subcategory M86.8X- ☑
    - mandible M27.2
    - orbit HØ5.Ø2- ☑
    - petrous bone — *see* Petrositis
    - vertebra — *see* Osteomyelitis, vertebra
  - subacute M86.2Ø
    - carpus M86.24- ☑
    - clavicle M86.21- ☑
    - femur M86.25- ☑
    - fibula M86.26- ☑
    - finger M86.24- ☑
    - humerus M86.22- ☑
    - mandible M27.2
    - metacarpus M86.24- ☑
    - metatarsus M86.27- ☑
    - multiple sites M86.29
    - neck M86.28
    - orbit HØ5.Ø2- ☑
    - petrous bone — *see* Petrositis
    - radius M86.23- ☑
    - rib M86.28
    - scapula M86.21- ☑
    - skull M86.28
    - tarsus M86.27- ☑
    - tibia M86.26- ☑
    - toe M86.27- ☑
    - ulna M86.23- ☑
    - vertebra — *see* Osteomyelitis, vertebra
  - syphilitic A52.77
    - congenital (early) A5Ø.Ø2 *[M9Ø.8Ø]*
  - tuberculous — *see* Tuberculosis, bone
  - typhoid AØ1.Ø5

- **Osteomyelitis** — *continued*
  - vertebra M46.2Ø
    - cervical region M46.22
    - cervicothoracic region M46.23
    - lumbar region M46.26
    - lumbosacral region M46.27
    - occipito-atlanto-axial region M46.21
    - sacrococcygeal region M46.28
    - thoracic region M46.24
    - thoracolumbar region M46.25
- **Osteomyelofibrosis** D47.4
- **Osteomyelosclerosis** D75.89
- **Osteonecrosis** M87.9
  - due to
    - drugs — *see* Osteonecrosis, secondary, due to, drugs
    - trauma — *see* Osteonecrosis, secondary, due to, trauma
  - idiopathic aseptic M87.ØØ
    - ankle M87.Ø7- ☑
    - carpus M87.Ø3- ☑
    - clavicle M87.Ø1- ☑
    - femur M87.Ø5- ☑
    - fibula M87.Ø6- ☑
    - finger M87.Ø4- ☑
    - humerus M87.Ø2- ☑
    - ilium M87.Ø5Ø
    - ischium M87.Ø5Ø
    - metacarpus M87.Ø4- ☑
    - metatarsus M87.Ø7- ☑
    - multiple sites M87.Ø9
    - neck M87.Ø8
    - pelvis M87.Ø5Ø
    - pubic ramus M87.Ø5Ø
    - radius M87.Ø3- ☑
    - rib M87.Ø8
    - scapula M87.Ø1- ☑
    - skull M87.Ø8
    - tarsus M87.Ø7- ☑
    - tibia M87.Ø6- ☑
    - toe M87.Ø7- ☑
    - ulna M87.Ø3- ☑
    - vertebra M87.Ø8
  - secondary NEC M87.3Ø
    - carpus M87.33- ☑
    - clavicle M87.31- ☑
    - due to
      - drugs M87.1Ø
        - carpus M87.13- ☑
        - clavicle M87.11- ☑
        - femur M87.15- ☑
        - fibula M87.16- ☑
        - finger M87.14- ☑
        - humerus M87.12- ☑
        - ilium M87.15Ø
        - ischium M87.15Ø
        - jaw M87.18Ø
        - metacarpus M87.14- ☑
        - metatarsus M87.17- ☑
        - multiple sites M87.19
        - neck M87.18 ☑
        - pubic ramus M87.15Ø
        - radius M87.13- ☑
        - rib M87.18 ☑
        - scapula M87.11- ☑
        - skull M87.18 ☑
        - tarsus M87.17- ☑
        - tibia M87.16- ☑
        - toe M87.17- ☑
        - ulna M87.13- ☑
        - vertebra M87.18 ☑
      - hemoglobinopathy NEC D58.2 *[M9Ø.5Ø]*
        - carpus D58.2 *[M9Ø.54-]* ☑
        - clavicle D58.2 *[M9Ø.51-]* ☑
        - femur D58.2 *[M9Ø.55-]* ☑
        - fibula D58.2 *[M9Ø.56-]* ☑
        - finger D58.2 *[M9Ø.54-]* ☑
        - humerus D58.2 *[M9Ø.52-]* ☑
        - ilium D58.2 *[M9Ø.58]*
        - ischium D58.2 *[M9Ø.58]*
        - metacarpus D58.2 *[M9Ø.54-]* ☑
        - metatarsus D58.2 *[M9Ø.57-]* ☑
        - multiple sites D58.2 *[M9Ø.58]*
        - neck D58.2 *[M9Ø.58]*
        - pubic ramus D58.2 *[M9Ø.58]*
        - radius D58.2 *[M9Ø.53-]* ☑
        - rib D58.2 *[M9Ø.58]*

- **Osteonecrosis** — *continued*
  - secondary — *continued*
    - due to — *continued*
      - hemoglobinopathy — *continued*
        - scapula D58.2 *[M90.51-]* ☑
        - skull D58.2 *[M90.58]*
        - tarsus D58.2 *[M90.57-]* ☑
        - tibia D58.2 *[M90.56-]* ☑
        - toe D58.2 *[M90.57-]* ☑
        - ulna D58.2 *[M90.53-]* ☑
        - vertebra D58.2 *[M90.58]*
      - trauma (previous) M87.20
        - carpus M87.23- ☑
        - clavicle M87.21- ☑
        - femur M87.25- ☑
        - fibula M87.26- ☑
        - finger M87.24- ☑
        - humerus M87.22- ☑
        - ilium M87.250
        - ischium M87.250
        - metacarpus M87.24- ☑
        - metatarsus M87.27- ☑
        - multiple sites M87.29
        - neck M87.28
        - pubic ramus M87.250
        - radius M87.23- ☑
        - rib M87.28
        - scapula M87.21- ☑
        - skull M87.28
        - tarsus M87.27- ☑
        - tibia M87.26- ☑
        - toe M87.27- ☑
        - ulna M87.23- ☑
        - vertebra M87.28
    - femur M87.35- ☑
    - fibula M87.36- ☑
    - finger M87.34- ☑
    - humerus M87.32- ☑
    - ilium M87.350
    - in
      - caisson disease T70.3 ☑ *[M90.50]*
        - carpus T70.3 ☑ *[M90.54-]* ☑
        - clavicle T70.3 ☑ *[M90.51-]* ☑
        - femur T70.3 ☑ *[M90.55-]* ☑
        - fibula T70.3 ☑ *[M90.56-]* ☑
        - finger T70.3 ☑ *[M90.54-]* ☑
        - humerus T70.3 ☑ *[M90.52-]* ☑
        - ilium T70.3 ☑ *[M90.58]*
        - ischium T70.3 ☑ *[M90.58]*
        - metacarpus T70.3 ☑ *[M90.54-]* ☑
        - metatarsus T70.3 ☑ *[M90.57-]* ☑
        - multiple sites T70.3 ☑ *[M90.59]*
        - neck T70.3 ☑ *[M90.58]*
        - pubic ramus T70.3 ☑ *[M90.58]*
        - radius T70.3 ☑ *[M90.53-]* ☑
        - rib T70.3 ☑ *[M90.58]*
        - scapula T70.3 ☑ *[M90.51-]* ☑
        - skull T70.3 ☑ *[M90.58]*
        - tarsus T70.3 ☑ *[M90.57-]* ☑
        - tibia T70.3 ☑ *[M90.56-]* ☑
        - toe T70.3 ☑ *[M90.57-]* ☑
        - ulna T70.3 ☑ *[M90.53-]* ☑
        - vertebra T70.3 ☑ *[M90.58]*
    - ischium M87.350
    - metacarpus M87.34- ☑
    - metatarsus M87.37- ☑
    - multiple site M87.39
    - neck M87.38
    - pubic ramus M87.350
    - radius M87.33- ☑
    - rib M87.38
    - scapula M87.319
    - skull M87.38
    - tarsus M87.379
    - tibia M87.366
    - toe M87.379
    - ulna M87.33- ☑
    - vertebra M87.38
  - specified type NEC M87.80
    - carpus M87.83- ☑
    - clavicle M87.81- ☑
    - femur M87.85- ☑
    - fibula M87.86- ☑
    - finger M87.84- ☑
    - humerus M87.82- ☑
    - ilium M87.850
    - ischium M87.850
    - metacarpus M87.84- ☑
    - metatarsus M87.87- ☑
    - multiple sites M87.89
    - neck M87.88
    - pubic ramus M87.850
    - radius M87.83- ☑
    - rib M87.88
    - scapula M87.81- ☑
    - skull M87.88
    - tarsus M87.87- ☑
    - tibia M87.86- ☑
    - toe M87.87- ☑
    - ulna M87.83- ☑
    - vertebra M87.88
- **Osteo-onycho-arthro-dysplasia** Q87.2
- **Osteo-onychodysplasia, hereditary** Q87.2
- **Osteopathia condensans disseminata** Q78.8
- **Osteopathy** — *see also* Osteomyelitis, Osteonecrosis, Osteoporosis
  - after poliomyelitis M89.60
    - carpus M89.64- ☑
    - clavicle M89.61- ☑
    - femur M89.65- ☑
    - fibula M89.66- ☑
    - finger M89.64- ☑
    - humerus M89.62- ☑
    - ilium M89.68
    - ischium M89.68
    - metacarpus M89.64- ☑
    - metatarsus M89.67- ☑
    - multiple sites M89.69
    - neck M89.68
    - pubic ramus M89.68
    - radius M89.63- ☑
    - rib M89.68
    - scapula M89.61- ☑
    - skull M89.68
    - tarsus M89.67- ☑
    - tibia M89.66- ☑
    - toe M89.67- ☑
    - ulna M89.63- ☑
    - vertebra M89.68
  - in (due to)
    - renal osteodystrophy N25.0
    - specified diseases classified elsewhere — *see* subcategory M90.8 ☑
- **Osteopenia** M85.8- ☑
  - borderline M85.8- ☑
- **Osteoperiostitis** — *see* Osteomyelitis, specified type NEC
- **Osteopetrosis** (familial) Q78.2
- **Osteophyte** M25.70
  - ankle M25.77- ☑
  - elbow M25.72- ☑
  - foot joint M25.77- ☑
  - hand joint M25.74- ☑
  - hip M25.75- ☑
  - knee M25.76- ☑
  - shoulder M25.71- ☑
  - spine M25.78
  - vertebrae M25.78
  - wrist M25.73- ☑
- **Osteopoikilosis** Q78.8
- **Osteoporosis** (female) (male) M81.0
  - with current pathological fracture M80.00 ☑
  - age-related M81.0
    - with current pathologic fracture M80.00 ☑
      - carpus M80.04- ☑
      - clavicle M80.01- ☑
      - femur M80.05- ☑
      - fibula M80.06- ☑
      - finger M80.04- ☑
      - hip M80.05- ☑
      - humerus M80.02- ☑
      - ilium M80.0A ☑
      - ischium M80.0A ☑
      - metacarpus M80.04- ☑
      - metatarsus M80.07- ☑
      - pelvis M80.0B- ☑
      - pubis ramus M80.0A ☑
      - radius M80.03- ☑
      - rib(s) M80.0A ☑
      - scapula M80.01- ☑
      - site specified NEC M80.0A ☑
      - specified site NEC M80.0A ☑
      - tarsus M80.07- ☑
      - tibia M80.06- ☑
      - toe M80.07- ☑
      - ulna M80.03- ☑
      - vertebra M80.08 ☑
  - disuse M81.8
    - with current pathological fracture M80.80 ☑
      - carpus M80.84- ☑
      - clavicle M80.81- ☑
      - femur M80.85- ☑
      - fibula M80.86- ☑
      - finger M80.84- ☑
      - hip M80.85- ☑
      - humerus M80.82- ☑
      - ilium M80.8A ☑
      - ischium M80.8A ☑
      - metacarpus M80.84- ☑
      - metatarsus M80.87- ☑
      - pelvis M80.8B- ☑
      - pubis ramus M80.8A ☑
      - radius M80.83- ☑
      - scapula M80.81- ☑
      - site specified NEC M80.8A ☑
      - tarsus M80.87- ☑
      - tibia M80.86- ☑
      - toe M80.87- ☑
      - ulna M80.83- ☑
      - vertebra M80.88 ☑
  - drug-induced — *see* Osteoporosis, specified type NEC
  - idiopathic — *see* Osteoporosis, specified type NEC
  - involutional — *see* Osteoporosis, age-related
  - Lequesne M81.6
  - localized M81.6
  - postmenopausal M81.0
    - with pathological fracture M80.00 ☑
      - carpus M80.04- ☑
      - clavicle M80.01- ☑
      - femur M80.05- ☑
      - fibula M80.06- ☑
      - finger M80.04- ☑
      - hip M80.05- ☑
      - humerus M80.02- ☑
      - ilium M80.0A ☑
      - ischium M80.0A ☑
      - metacarpus M80.04- ☑
      - metatarsus M80.07- ☑
      - pelvis M80.0B- ☑
      - pubis ramus M80.0A ☑
      - radius M80.03- ☑
      - scapula M80.01- ☑
      - site specified NEC M80.0A ☑
      - tarsus M80.07- ☑
      - tibia M80.06- ☑
      - toe M80.07- ☑
      - ulna M80.03- ☑
      - vertebra M80.08 ☑
  - postoophorectomy — *see* Osteoporosis, specified type NEC
  - postsurgical malabsorption — *see* Osteoporosis, specified type NEC
  - post-traumatic — *see* Osteoporosis, specified type NEC
  - senile — *see* Osteoporosis, age-related
  - specified type NEC M81.8
    - with pathological fracture M80.80 ☑
      - carpus M80.84- ☑
      - clavicle M80.81- ☑
      - femur M80.85- ☑
      - fibula M80.86- ☑
      - finger M80.84- ☑
      - hip M80.85- ☑
      - humerus M80.82- ☑
      - ilium M80.8A ☑
      - ischium M80.8A ☑
      - metacarpus M80.84- ☑
      - metatarsus M80.87- ☑
      - pelvis M80.8B- ☑
      - pubis ramus M80.8A ☑
      - radius M80.83- ☑
      - scapula M80.81- ☑
      - site specified NEC M80.8A ☑
      - tarsus M80.87- ☑

- **Overdistension** — *see* Distension
- **Overdose, overdosage** (drug) — *see* Table of Drugs and Chemicals, by drug, poisoning
- **Overeating** R63.2
  - nonorganic origin F5Ø.89
  - psychogenic F5Ø.89
- **Overexertion** (effects) (exhaustion) T73.3 ☑
- **Overexposure** (effects) T73.9 ☑
  - exhaustion T73.2 ☑
- **Overfeeding** — *see* Overeating
  - newborn P92.4
- **Overfill, endodontic** M27.52
- **Overgrowth**
  - bacterial
    - small intestinal K63.8219
      - fungal K63.822
      - hydrogen-subtype K63.8211
      - hydrogen sulfide-subtype K63.8212
  - bone — *see* Hypertrophy, bone
  - intestinal methanogen K63.829
- **Overhanging of dental restorative material** (unrepairable) KØ8.52
- **Overheated** (places) (effects) — *see* Heat
- **Overjet** (excessive horizontal) M26.23
- **Overlaid, overlying** (suffocation) — *see* Asphyxia, traumatic, due to mechanical threat
- **Overlap, excessive horizontal** (teeth) M26.23
- **Overlapping toe** (acquired) — *see also* Deformity, toe, specified NEC
  - congenital (fifth toe) Q66.89
- **Overload**
  - circulatory, due to transfusion (blood) (blood components) (TACO) E87.71
  - fluid E87.7Ø
    - due to transfusion (blood) (blood components) E87.71
    - specified NEC E87.79
  - iron, due to repeated red blood cell transfusions E83.111
  - potassium (K) E87.5
  - sodium (Na) E87.Ø
- **Overnutrition** — *see* Hyperalimentation
- **Overproduction** — *see also* Hypersecretion
  - ACTH E27.Ø
  - catecholamine E27.5
  - growth hormone E22.Ø
- **Overprotection, child by parent** Z62.1
- **Overriding**
  - aorta Q25.49
  - finger (acquired) — *see* Deformity, finger
    - congenital Q68.1
  - toe (acquired) — *see also* Deformity, toe, specified NEC
    - congenital Q66.89
- **Overstrained** R53.83
  - heart — *see* Hypertrophy, cardiac
- **Overuse, muscle NEC** M7Ø.8- ☑
- **Overweight** E66.3
- **Overworked** R53.83
- **Oviduct** — *see* condition
- **Ovotestis** Q56.Ø
- **Ovulation** (cycle)
  - failure or lack of N97.Ø
  - pain N94.Ø
- **Ovum** — *see* condition
- **Owren's disease or syndrome** (parahemophilia) D68.2
- **Ox heart** — *see* Hypertrophy, cardiac
- **Oxalosis** E72.53
- **Oxaluria** E72.53
- **Oxycephaly, oxycephalic** Q75.ØØ9
  - syphilitic, congenital A5Ø.Ø2
- **Oxyuriasis** B8Ø
- **Oxyuris vermicularis** (infestation) B8Ø
- **Ozena** J31.Ø

P

- **Pachyderma, pachydermia** L85.9
  - larynx (verrucosa) J38.7
- **Pachydermatocele** (congenital) Q82.8
- **Pachydermoperiostosis** — *see also* Osteoarthropathy, hypertrophic, specified type NEC
  - clubbed nail M89.4Ø *[L62]*
- **Pachygyria** QØ4.3
- **Pachymeningitis** (adhesive) (basal) (brain) (cervical) (chronic) (circumscribed) (external) (fibrous) (hemorrhagic) (hypertrophic) (internal) (purulent) (spinal) (suppurative) — *see* Meningitis
- **Pachyonychia** (congenital) Q84.5
- **Pacinian tumor** — *see* Neoplasm, skin, benign
- **Pad, knuckle or Garrod's** M72.1
- **Paget's disease**
  - with infiltrating duct carcinoma — *see* Neoplasm, breast, malignant
  - bone M88.9
    - carpus M88.84- ☑
    - clavicle M88.81- ☑
    - femur M88.85- ☑
    - fibula M88.86- ☑
    - finger M88.84- ☑
    - humerus M88.82- ☑
    - ilium M88.88
    - in neoplastic disease — *see* Osteitis, deformans, in neoplastic disease
    - ischium M88.88
    - metacarpus M88.84- ☑
    - metatarsus M88.87- ☑
    - multiple sites M88.89
    - neck M88.88
    - pubic ramus M88.88
    - radius M88.83- ☑
    - rib M88.88
    - scapula M88.81- ☑
    - skull M88.Ø
    - specified NEC M88.88
    - tarsus M88.87- ☑
    - tibia M88.86- ☑
    - toe M88.87- ☑
    - ulna M88.83- ☑
    - vertebra M88.1
  - breast (female) C5Ø.Ø1- ☑
    - male C5Ø.Ø2- ☑
  - extramammary — *see also* Neoplasm, skin, malignant
    - anus C21.Ø
      - margin C44.59Ø
      - skin C44.59Ø
  - intraductal carcinoma — *see* Neoplasm, breast, malignant
  - malignant — *see* Neoplasm, skin, malignant
    - breast (female) C5Ø.Ø1- ☑
      - male C5Ø.Ø2- ☑
    - unspecified site (female) C5Ø.Ø1- ☑
      - male C5Ø.Ø2- ☑
  - mammary — *see* Paget's disease, breast
  - nipple — *see* Paget's disease, breast
  - osteitis deformans — *see* Paget's disease, bone
- **Paget-Schroetter syndrome** I82.89Ø
- **Pain**(s) — *see also* Painful R52
  - abdominal R1Ø.9
    - colic R1Ø.83
    - generalized R1Ø.84
      - with acute abdomen R1Ø.Ø
    - lower R1Ø.3Ø
      - left quadrant R1Ø.32
      - pelvic or perineal R1Ø.2
      - periumbilical R1Ø.33
      - right quadrant R1Ø.31
    - rebound — *see* Tenderness, abdominal, rebound
    - severe with abdominal rigidity R1Ø.Ø
    - tenderness — *see* Tenderness, abdominal
    - upper R1Ø.1Ø
      - epigastric R1Ø.13
      - left quadrant R1Ø.12
      - right quadrant R1Ø.11
  - acute R52
    - due to trauma G89.11
    - neoplasm related G89.3
    - postprocedural NEC G89.18
    - post-thoracotomy G89.12
    - specified by site — *code to* Pain, by site
  - adnexa (uteri) R1Ø.2
  - anginoid — *see* Pain, precordial
  - anus K62.89
  - arm — *see* Pain, limb, upper
  - axillary (axilla) M79.62- ☑
  - back (postural) M54.9
  - bladder R39.89
    - associated with micturition — *see* Micturition, painful
    - chronic R39.82
  - bone — *see* Disorder, bone, specified type NEC
  - breast N64.4
  - broad ligament R1Ø.2
  - cancer associated (acute) (chronic) G89.3
  - cecum — *see* Pain, abdominal

Pain(s) — *continued*

  - cervicobrachial M53.1
  - chest (central) RØ7.9
    - anterior wall RØ7.89
    - atypical RØ7.89
    - ischemic I2Ø.9
    - musculoskeletal RØ7.89
    - non-cardiac RØ7.89
    - on breathing RØ7.1
    - pleurodynia RØ7.81
    - precordial RØ7.2
    - wall (anterior) RØ7.89
  - chronic G89.29
    - associated with significant psychosocial dysfunction G89.4
    - due to trauma G89.21
    - neoplasm related G89.3
    - postoperative NEC G89.28
    - postprocedural NEC G89.28
    - post-thoracotomy G89.22
    - specified NEC G89.29
  - coccyx M53.3
  - colon — *see* Pain, abdominal
  - coronary — *see* Angina
  - costochondral RØ7.1
  - diaphragm RØ7.1
  - due to cancer G89.3
  - due to device, implant or graft — *see also* Complications, by site and type, specified NEC T85.848 ☑
    - arterial graft NEC T82.848 ☑
    - breast (implant) T85.848 ☑
    - catheter NEC T85.848 ☑
      - dialysis (renal) T82.848 ☑
        - intraperitoneal T85.848 ☑
      - infusion NEC T82.848 ☑
        - spinal (epidural) (subdural) T85.84Ø ☑
      - urinary (indwelling) T83.84 ☑
    - electronic (electrode) (pulse generator) (stimulator)
      - bone T85.84Ø ☑
      - cardiac T82.847 ☑
      - nervous system (brain) (peripheral nerve) (spinal) T85.84 ☑
      - urinary T83.84 ☑
    - fixation, internal (orthopedic) NEC T84.84 ☑
    - gastrointestinal (bile duct) (esophagus) T85.848 ☑
    - genital NEC T83.84 ☑
    - heart NEC T82.847 ☑
    - infusion NEC T85.848 ☑
    - joint prosthesis T84.84 ☑
    - ocular (corneal graft) (orbital implant) NEC T85.848 ☑
    - orthopedic NEC T84.84 ☑
    - specified NEC T85.848 ☑
    - urinary NEC T83.84 ☑
    - vascular NEC T82.848 ☑
    - ventricular intracranial shunt T85.84Ø ☑
  - due to malignancy (primary) (secondary) G89.3
  - ear — *see* subcategory H92.Ø ☑
  - epigastric, epigastrium R1Ø.13
  - eye — *see* Pain, ocular
  - face, facial R51.9
    - atypical G5Ø.1
  - female genital organs NEC N94.89
  - finger — *see* Pain, limb, upper
  - flank — *see* Pain, abdominal
  - foot — *see* Pain, limb, lower
  - gallbladder K82.9
  - gas (intestinal) R14.1
  - gastric — *see* Pain, abdominal
  - generalized NOS R52
  - genital organ
    - female N94.89
    - male N5Ø.89
  - groin — *see* Pain, abdominal, lower
  - hand — *see* Pain, limb, upper
  - head — *see* Headache
  - heart — *see* Pain, precordial
  - infra-orbital — *see* Neuralgia, trigeminal
  - intercostal RØ7.82
  - intermenstrual N94.Ø
  - jaw R68.84
  - joint M25.5Ø
    - ankle M25.57- ☑
    - elbow M25.52- ☑
    - finger M25.54- ☑
    - foot M25.57- ☑
    - hand M25.54- ☑

Index

Overdistension — Pain

- **Pain(s)** — *continued*
  - joint — *continued*
    - hip M25.55- ☑
    - knee M25.56- ☑
    - shoulder M25.51- ☑
    - specified site NEC M25.59
    - toe M25.57- ☑
    - wrist M25.53- ☑
  - kidney N23
  - laryngeal RØ7.Ø
  - leg — *see* Pain, limb, lower
  - limb M79.6Ø9
    - lower M79.6Ø- ☑
      - foot M79.67- ☑
      - lower leg M79.66- ☑
      - thigh M79.65- ☑
      - toe M79.67- ☑
    - upper M79.6Ø- ☑
      - axilla M79.62- ☑
      - finger M79.64- ☑
      - forearm M79.63- ☑
      - hand M79.64- ☑
      - upper arm M79.62- ☑
  - loin M54.5Ø
  - low back M54.5Ø
    - specified NEC M54.59
    - vertebral end plate M54.51
    - vertebrogenic M54.51
  - lumbar region M54.5Ø
    - vertebral end plate M54.51
    - vertebrogenic M54.51
  - mandibular R68.84
  - mastoid — *see* subcategory H92.Ø ☑
  - maxilla R68.84
  - menstrual — *see also* Dysmenorrhea N94.6
  - metacarpophalangeal (joint) — *see* Pain, joint, hand
  - metatarsophalangeal (joint) — *see* Pain, joint, foot
  - mouth K13.79
  - muscle — *see* Myalgia
  - musculoskeletal — *see also* Pain, by site M79.18
  - myofascial M79.18
  - nasal J34.89
  - nasopharynx J39.2
  - neck NEC M54.2
  - nerve NEC — *see* Neuralgia
  - neuromuscular — *see* Neuralgia
  - nose J34.89
  - ocular H57.1- ☑
  - ophthalmic — *see* Pain, ocular
  - orbital region — *see* Pain, ocular
  - ovary N94.89
  - over heart — *see* Pain, precordial
  - ovulation N94.Ø
  - pelvic (female) R1Ø.2
  - penis N48.89
  - pericardial — *see* Pain, precordial
  - perineal, perineum R1Ø.2
  - pharynx J39.2
  - pleura, pleural, pleuritic RØ7.81
  - postoperative NOS G89.18
  - postprocedural NOS G89.18
  - post-thoracotomy G89.12
  - precordial (region) RØ7.2
  - premenstrual N94.3
  - psychogenic (persistent) (any site) F45.41
  - radicular (spinal) — *see* Radiculopathy
  - rectum K62.89
  - respiration RØ7.1
  - retrosternal RØ7.2
  - rheumatoid, muscular — *see* Myalgia
  - rib RØ7.81
  - root (spinal) — *see* Radiculopathy
  - round ligament (stretch) R1Ø.2
  - sacroiliac M53.3
  - sciatic — *see* Sciatica
  - scrotum N5Ø.82
  - seminal vesicle N5Ø.89
  - shoulder M25.51- ☑
  - spermatic cord N5Ø.89
  - spinal root — *see* Radiculopathy
  - spine M54.9
    - cervical M54.2
    - low back M54.5Ø
      - with sciatica M54.4- ☑
    - thoracic M54.6
  - stomach — *see* Pain, abdominal
  - substernal RØ7.2
  - temporomandibular (joint) M26.62- ☑
  - testis N5Ø.81- ☑
  - thoracic spine M54.6
    - with radicular and visceral pain M54.14
  - throat RØ7.Ø
  - tibia — *see* Pain, limb, lower
  - toe — *see* Pain, limb, lower
  - tongue K14.6
  - tooth KØ8.89
  - trigeminal — *see* Neuralgia, trigeminal
  - tumor associated G89.3
  - ureter N23
  - urinary (organ) (system) N23
  - uterus NEC N94.89
  - vagina R1Ø.2
  - vertebral end plate — *see* Pain, vertebrogenic
  - vertebrogenic M54.89
    - low back M54.51
    - lumbar M54.51
    - syndrome M54.89
  - vesical R39.89
    - associated with micturition — *see* Micturition, painful
  - vulva R1Ø.2
- **Painful** — *see also* Pain
  - coitus
    - female N94.1Ø
    - male N53.12
    - psychogenic F52.6
  - ejaculation (semen) N53.12
    - psychogenic F52.6
  - erection — *see* Priapism
  - feet syndrome E53.8
  - joint replacement (hip) (knee) T84.84 ☑
  - menstruation — *see* Dysmenorrhea
    - psychogenic F45.8
  - micturition — *see* Micturition, painful
  - respiration RØ7.1
  - scar NEC L9Ø.5
  - wire sutures T81.89 ☑
- **Painter's colic** — *see* subcategory T56.Ø ☑
- **Palate** — *see* condition
- **Palatoplegia** K13.79
- **Palatoschisis** — *see* Cleft, palate
- **Palilalia** R48.8
- **Palliative care** Z51.5
- **Pallor** R23.1
  - optic disc, temporal — *see* Atrophy, optic
- **Palmar** — *see also* condition
  - fascia — *see* condition
- **Palpable**
  - cecum K63.89
  - kidney N28.89
  - ovary N83.8
  - prostate N42.9
  - spleen — *see* Splenomegaly
- **Palpitations** (heart) RØØ.2
  - psychogenic F45.8
- **Palsy** — *see also* Paralysis G83.9
  - atrophic diffuse (progressive) G12.22
  - Bell's — *see also* Palsy, facial
    - newborn P11.3
  - brachial plexus NEC G54.Ø
    - newborn (birth injury) P14.3
  - brain — *see* Palsy, cerebral
  - bulbar (progressive) (chronic) G12.22
    - of childhood (Fazio-Londe) G12.1
    - pseudo NEC G12.29
    - supranuclear (progressive) G23.1
  - cerebral (congenital) G8Ø.9
    - ataxic G8Ø.4
    - athetoid G8Ø.3
    - choreathetoid G8Ø.3
    - diplegic G8Ø.8
      - spastic G8Ø.1
    - dyskinetic G8Ø.3
      - athetoid G8Ø.3
      - choreathetoid G8Ø.3
      - distonic G8Ø.3
    - dystonic G8Ø.3
    - hemiplegic G8Ø.8
      - spastic G8Ø.2
    - mixed G8Ø.8
    - monoplegic G8Ø.8
      - spastic G8Ø.1
    - paraplegic G8Ø.8
      - spastic G8Ø.1
    - quadriplegic G8Ø.8
      - spastic G8Ø.Ø
    - spastic G8Ø.1
      - diplegic G8Ø.1
      - hemiplegic G8Ø.2
      - monoplegic G8Ø.1
      - quadriplegic G8Ø.Ø
      - specified NEC G8Ø.1
      - tetrapelgic G8Ø.Ø
    - specified NEC G8Ø.8
    - syphilitic A52.12
      - congenital A5Ø.49
    - tetraplegic G8Ø.8
      - spastic G8Ø.Ø
  - cranial nerve — *see also* Disorder, nerve, cranial
    - multiple G52.7
      - in
        - infectious disease B99 ☑ *[G53]*
        - neoplastic disease — *see also* Neoplasm D49.9 *[G53]*
        - parasitic disease B89 *[G53]*
        - sarcoidosis D86.82
  - creeping G12.22
  - diver's T7Ø.3 ☑
  - Erb's P14.Ø
  - facial G51.Ø
    - newborn (birth injury) P11.3
  - glossopharyngeal G52.1
  - Klumpke (-Dejerine) P14.1
  - lead — *see* subcategory T56.Ø ☑
  - median nerve (tardy) G56.1- ☑
  - nerve G58.9
    - specified NEC G58.8
  - peroneal nerve (acute) (tardy) G57.3- ☑
  - progressive supranuclear G23.1
  - pseudobulbar NEC G12.29
  - radial nerve (acute) G56.3- ☑
  - seventh nerve — *see also* Palsy, facial
    - newborn P11.3
  - shaking — *see* Parkinsonism
  - spastic (cerebral) (spinal) G8Ø.1
  - ulnar nerve (tardy) G56.2- ☑
  - wasting G12.29
- **Paludism** — *see* Malaria
- **Panangiitis** M3Ø.Ø
- **Panaris, panaritium** — *see also* Cellulitis, digit
  - with lymphangitis — *see* Lymphangitis, acute, digit
- **Panarteritis nodosa** M3Ø.Ø
  - brain or cerebral I67.7
- **Pancake heart** R93.1
  - with cor pulmonale (chronic) I27.81
- **Pancarditis** (acute) (chronic) I51.89
  - rheumatic IØ9.89
    - active or acute IØ1.8
- **Pancoast's syndrome or tumor** C34.1- ☑
- **Pancolitis** — *see also* Colitis
  - ulcerative (chronic) K51.ØØ
    - with
      - abscess K51.Ø14
      - complication K51.Ø19
      - fistula K51.Ø13
      - obstruction K51.Ø12
      - rectal bleeding K51.Ø11
      - specified complication NEC K51.Ø18
- **Pancreas, pancreatic** — *see* condition
- **Pancreatitis** (annular) (apoplectic) (calcareous) (edematous) (hemorrhagic) (malignant) (subacute) (suppurative) K85.9Ø
  - with necrosis (uninfected) K85.91
    - infected K85.92
  - acute (without necrosis or infection) K85.9Ø
    - with necrosis (uninfected) K85.91
      - infected K85.92
    - alcohol induced (without necrosis or infection) K85.2Ø
      - with necrosis (uninfected) K85.21
        - infected K85.22
    - biliary (without necrosis or infection) K85.1Ø
      - with necrosis (uninfected) K85.11
        - infected K85.12
    - drug induced (without necrosis or infection) K85.3Ø
      - with necrosis (uninfected) K85.31
        - infected K85.32
    - gallstone (without necrosis or infection) K85.1Ø
      - with necrosis (uninfected) K85.11
        - infected K85.12

Pancreatitis — *continued*
- acute — *continued*
  - idiopathic (without necrosis or infection) K85.ØØ
    - with necrosis (uninfected) K85.Ø1
      - infected K85.Ø2
  - specified NEC (without necrosis or infection) K85.8Ø
    - with necrosis (uninfected) K85.81
      - infected K85.82
- chronic (infectious) K86.1
  - alcohol-induced K86.Ø
  - recurrent K86.1
  - relapsing K86.1
- cystic (chronic) K86.1
- cytomegaloviral B25.2
- fibrous (chronic) K86.1
- gallstone (without necrosis or infection) K85.1Ø
  - with necrosis (uninfected) K85.11
    - infected K85.12
- gangrenous — *see* Pancreatitis, acute
- interstitial (chronic) K86.1
  - acute — *see also* Pancreatitis, acute K85.8Ø
- mumps B26.3
- recurrent
  - acute — *see* Pancreatitis, acute by type
  - chronic K86.1
- relapsing, chronic K86.1
- syphilitic A52.74

Pancreatoblastoma — *see* Neoplasm, pancreas, malignant
Pancreolithiasis K86.89
Pancytolysis D75.89
Pancytopenia (acquired) D61.818
- with
  - malformations D61.Ø9
  - myelodysplastic syndrome — *see* Syndrome, myelodysplastic
- antineoplastic chemotherapy induced D61.81Ø
- congenital D61.Ø9
- drug-induced NEC D61.811

PANDAS (pediatric autoimmune neuropsychiatric disorders associated with streptococcal infections syndrome) D89.89
Panencephalitis, subacute, sclerosing A81.1
Panhematopenia D61.9
- congenital D61.Ø9
- constitutional D61.Ø9
- splenic, primary D73.1

Panhemocytopenia D61.9
- congenital D61.Ø9
- constitutional D61.Ø9

Panhypogonadism E29.1
Panhypopituitarism E23.Ø
- prepubertal E23.Ø

Panic (attack) (state) F41.Ø
- reaction to exceptional stress (transient) F43.Ø

Panmyelopathy, familial, constitutional D61.Ø9
Panmyelophthisis D61.82
- congenital D61.Ø9

Panmyelosis (acute) (with myelofibrosis) C94.4- ☑
Panner's disease — *see* Osteochondrosis, juvenile, humerus
Panneuritis endemica E51.11
Panniculitis (nodular) (nonsuppurative) M79.3
- back M54.ØØ
  - cervical region M54.Ø2
  - cervicothoracic region M54.Ø3
  - lumbar region M54.Ø6
  - lumbosacral region M54.Ø7
  - multiple sites M54.Ø9
  - occipito-atlanto-axial region M54.Ø1
  - sacrococcygeal region M54.Ø8
  - thoracic region M54.Ø4
  - thoracolumbar region M54.Ø5
- lupus L93.2
- mesenteric K65.4
- neck M54.Ø2
  - cervicothoracic region M54.Ø3
  - occipito-atlanto-axial region M54.Ø1
- relapsing M35.6

Panniculus adiposus (abdominal) E65
Pannus (allergic) (cornea) (degenerativus) (keratic) H16.42- ☑
- abdominal (symptomatic) E65
- trachomatosus, trachomatous (active) A71.1

Panophthalmitis H44.Ø1- ☑
Pansinusitis (chronic) (hyperplastic) (nonpurulent) (purulent) J32.4
- acute JØ1.4Ø

Pansinusitis — *continued*
- acute — *continued*
  - recurrent JØ1.41
- tuberculous A15.8

Pansynostosis Q75.Ø52
Panuveitis (sympathetic) H44.11- ☑
Panvalvular disease IØ8.9
- specified NEC IØ8.8

PAPA (pyogenic arthritis, pyoderma gangrenosum, and acne syndrome) MØ4.8
Papanicolaou smear, cervix Z12.4
- as part of routine gynecological examination ZØ1.419
  - with abnormal findings ZØ1.411
- for suspected neoplasm Z12.4
- nonspecific abnormal finding R87.619
- routine ZØ1.419
  - with abnormal findings ZØ1.411

Papilledema (choked disc) H47.1Ø
- associated with
  - decreased ocular pressure H47.12
  - increased intracranial pressure H47.11
  - retinal disorder H47.13
- Foster-Kennedy syndrome H47.14- ☑

Papillitis H46.ØØ
- anus K62.89
- chronic lingual K14.4
- necrotizing, kidney N17.2
- optic H46.Ø- ☑
- rectum K62.89
- renal, necrotizing N17.2
- tongue K14.Ø

Papilloma — *see also* Neoplasm, benign, by site
- acuminatum (female) (male) (anogenital) A63.Ø
- basal cell L82.1
  - inflamed L82.Ø
- benign pinta (primary) A67.Ø
- bladder (urinary) (transitional cell) D41.4
- choroid plexus (lateral ventricle) (third ventricle) D33.Ø
  - anaplastic C71.5
  - fourth ventricle D33.1
  - malignant C71.5
- renal pelvis (transitional cell) D41.1- ☑
  - benign D3Ø.1- ☑
- Schneiderian
  - specified site — *see* Neoplasm, benign, by site
  - unspecified site D14.Ø
- serous surface
  - borderline malignancy
    - specified site — *see* Neoplasm, uncertain behavior, by site
    - unspecified site D39.1Ø
  - specified site — *see* Neoplasm, benign, by site
  - unspecified site D27.9
- transitional (cell)
  - bladder (urinary) D41.4
  - inverted type — *see* Neoplasm, uncertain behavior, by site
  - renal pelvis D41.1- ☑
  - ureter D41.2- ☑
- ureter (transitional cell) D41.2- ☑
  - benign D3Ø.2- ☑
- urothelial — *see* Neoplasm, uncertain behavior, by site
- villous — *see* Neoplasm, uncertain behavior, by site
  - adenocarcinoma in — *see* Neoplasm, malignant, by site
    - in situ — *see* Neoplasm, in situ
- yaws, plantar or palmar A66.1

Papillomata, multiple, of yaws A66.1
Papillomatosis — *see also* Neoplasm, benign, by site
- confluent and reticulated L83
- cystic, breast — *see* Mastopathy, cystic
- ductal, breast — *see* Mastopathy, cystic
- intraductal (diffuse) — *see* Neoplasm, benign, by site
- subareolar duct D24- ☑

Papillomavirus, as cause of disease classified elsewhere B97.7
Papillon-Léage and Psaume syndrome Q87.Ø
Papule(s) R23.8
- carate (primary) A67.Ø
- fibrous, of nose D22.39
- Gottron's L94.4
- pinta (primary) A67.Ø

Papulosis
- lymphomatoid C86.6
- malignant I77.89

Papyraceous fetus O31.Ø- ☑
Para-albuminemia E88.Ø9
Paracephalus Q89.7
Parachute mitral valve Q23.2
Paracoccidioidomycosis B41.9
- disseminated B41.7
- generalized B41.7
- mucocutaneous-lymphangitic B41.8
- pulmonary B41.Ø
- specified NEC B41.8
- visceral B41.8

Paradentosis KØ5.4
Paraffinoma T88.8 ☑
Paraganglioma D44.7
- adrenal D35.Ø- ☑
  - malignant C74.1- ☑
- aortic body D44.7
  - malignant C75.5
- carotid body D44.6
  - malignant C75.4
- chromaffin — *see also* Neoplasm, benign, by site
  - malignant — *see* Neoplasm, malignant, by site
- extra-adrenal D44.7
  - malignant C75.5
    - specified site — *see* Neoplasm, malignant, by site
    - unspecified site C75.5
  - specified site — *see* Neoplasm, uncertain behavior, by site
  - unspecified site D44.7
- gangliocytic D13.2
  - specified site — *see* Neoplasm, benign, by site
  - unspecified site D13.2
- glomus jugulare D44.7
  - malignant C75.5
- jugular D44.7
- malignant C75.5
  - specified site — *see* Neoplasm, malignant, by site
  - unspecified site C75.5
- nonchromaffin D44.7
  - malignant C75.5
    - specified site — *see* Neoplasm, malignant, by site
    - unspecified site C75.5
  - specified site — *see* Neoplasm, uncertain behavior, by site
  - unspecified site D44.7
- parasympathetic D44.7
  - specified site — *see* Neoplasm, uncertain behavior, by site
  - unspecified site D44.7
- specified site — *see* Neoplasm, uncertain behavior, by site
- sympathetic D44.7
  - specified site — *see* Neoplasm, uncertain behavior, by site
  - unspecified site D44.7
- unspecified site D44.7

Parageusia R43.2
- psychogenic F45.8

Paragonimiasis B66.4
Paragranuloma, Hodgkin — *see* Lymphoma, Hodgkin, specified NEC
Parahemophilia — *see also* Defect, coagulation D68.2
Parakeratosis R23.4
- variegata L41.Ø

Paralysis, paralytic (complete) (incomplete) G83.9
- with
  - syphilis A52.17
- abducens, abducent (nerve) — *see* Strabismus, paralytic, sixth nerve
- abductor, lower extremity G57.9- ☑
- accessory nerve G52.8
- accommodation — *see also* Paresis, of accommodation
  - hysterical F44.89
- acoustic nerve (except Deafness) H93.3 ☑
- agitans — *see also* Parkinsonism G2Ø.C
  - arteriosclerotic G21.4
- alternating (oculomotor) G83.89
- amyotrophic G12.21
- ankle G57.9- ☑
- anus (sphincter) K62.89
- arm — *see* Monoplegia, upper limb
- ascending (spinal), acute G61.Ø
- association G12.29
- asthenic bulbar G7Ø.ØØ
  - with exacerbation (acute) G7Ø.Ø1
  - in crisis G7Ø.Ø1
- ataxic (hereditary) G11.9
  - general (syphilitic) A52.17

- **Parkinson's disease, syndrome or tremor** — *see* Parkinsonism
- **Parodontitis** — *see* Periodontitis
- **Parodontosis** KØ5.4
- **Paronychia** — *see also* Cellulitis, digit
  - with lymphangitis — *see* Lymphangitis, acute, digit
  - candidal (chronic) B37.2
  - tuberculous (primary) A18.4
- **Parorexia** (psychogenic) F5Ø.89
- **Parosmia** R43.1
  - psychogenic F45.8
- **Parotid gland** — *see* condition
- **Parotitis, parotiditis** (allergic) (nonspecific toxic) (purulent) (septic) (suppurative) — *see also* Sialoadenitis
  - epidemic — *see* Mumps
  - infectious — *see* Mumps
  - postoperative K91.89
  - surgical K91.89
- **Parrot fever** A7Ø
- **Parrot's disease** (early congenital syphilitic pseudoparalysis) A5Ø.Ø2
- **Parry-Romberg syndrome** G51.8
- **Parry's disease or syndrome** EØ5.ØØ
  - with thyroid storm EØ5.Ø1
- **Pars planitis** — *see* Cyclitis
- **Parsonage** (-Aldren)-**Turner syndrome** G54.5
- **Parson's disease** (exophthalmic goiter) EØ5.ØØ
  - with thyroid storm EØ5.Ø1
- **Particolored infant** Q82.8
- **Parturition** — *see* Delivery
- **Parulis** KØ4.7
  - with sinus KØ4.6
- **Parvovirus, as cause of disease classified elsewhere** B97.6
- **Pasini and Pierini's atrophoderma** L9Ø.3
- **Passage**
  - false, urethra N36.5
  - meconium (newborn) during delivery PØ3.82
  - of sounds or bougies — *see* Attention to, artificial, opening
- **Passive** — *see* condition
  - smoking Z77.22
- **Past due on rent or mortgage** Z59.81- ☑
- **Pasteurella septica** A28.Ø
- **Pasteurellosis** — *see* Infection, Pasteurella
- **PAT** (paroxysmal atrial tachycardia) I47.19
- **Patau's syndrome** — *see* Trisomy, 13
- **Patches**
  - mucous (syphilitic) A51.39
    - congenital A5Ø.Ø7
  - smokers' (mouth) K13.24
- **Patellar** — *see* condition
- **Patent** — *see also* Imperfect, closure
  - canal of Nuck Q52.4
  - cervix N88.3
  - ductus arteriosus or Botallo's Q25.Ø
  - foramen
    - botalli Q21.12
    - ovale Q21.12
  - interauricular septum Q21.19
  - interventricular septum Q21.Ø
  - omphalomesenteric duct Q43.Ø
  - os (uteri) — *see* Patent, cervix
  - ostium secundum (type II) Q21.11
  - urachus Q64.4
  - vitelline duct Q43.Ø
- **Paterson** (-Brown) (-Kelly) **syndrome or web** D5Ø.1
- **Pathologic, pathological** — *see also* condition
  - asphyxia RØ9.Ø1
  - fire-setting F63.1
  - gambling F63.Ø
  - ovum OØ2.Ø
  - resorption, tooth KØ3.3
  - stealing F63.2
- **Pathology** (of) — *see* Disease
  - periradicular, associated with previous endodontic treatment NEC M27.59
- **Pattern, sleep-wake, irregular** G47.23
- **Patulous** — *see also* Imperfect, closure (congenital)
  - alimentary tract Q45.8
    - lower Q43.8
    - upper Q4Ø.8
  - eustachian tube H69.Ø- ☑
- **Pause, sinoatrial** I49.5
- **Paxton's disease** B36.2
- **Pearl(s)**
  - enamel KØØ.2
- **Pearl(s)** — *continued*
  - Epstein's KØ9.8
- **Pearl-worker's disease** — *see* Osteomyelitis, specified type NEC
- **Pectenosis** K62.4
- **Pectoral** — *see* condition
- **Pectus**
  - carinatum (congenital) Q67.7
    - acquired M95.4
    - rachitic sequelae (late effect) E64.3
  - excavatum (congenital) Q67.6
    - acquired M95.4
    - rachitic sequelae (late effect) E64.3
  - recurvatum (congenital) Q67.6
- **Pedatrophia** E41
- **Pederosis** F65.4
- **Pediatric inflammatory multisystem syndrome** M35.81
- **Pediculosis** (infestation) B85.2
  - capitis (head-louse) (any site) B85.Ø
  - corporis (body-louse) (any site) B85.1
  - eyelid B85.Ø
  - mixed (classifiable to more than one of the titles B85.Ø-B85.3) B85.4
  - pubis (pubic louse) (any site) B85.3
  - vestimenti B85.1
  - vulvae B85.3
- **Pediculus** (infestation) — *see* Pediculosis
- **Pedophilia** F65.4
- **Peg-shaped teeth** KØØ.2
- **Pelade** — *see* Alopecia, areata
- **Pelger-Huet anomaly or syndrome** D72.Ø
- **Peliosis** (rheumatica) D69.Ø
  - hepatis K76.4
    - with toxic liver disease K71.8
- **Pelizaeus-Merzbacher disease** E75.27
- **Pellagra** (alcoholic) E52
  - with
    - polyneuropathy E52 *[G63]*
- **Pellagra-cerebellar-ataxia-renal aminoaciduria syndrome** E72.Ø2
- **Pellegrini** (-Stieda) **disease or syndrome** — *see* Bursitis, tibial collateral
- **Pellizzi's syndrome** E34.8
- **Pel's crisis** A52.11
- **Pelvic** — *see also* condition
  - examination (periodic) (routine) ZØ1.419
    - with abnormal findings ZØ1.411
  - kidney, congenital Q63.2
- **Pelviolithiasis** — *see* Calculus, kidney
- **Pelviperitonitis** — *see also* Peritonitis, pelvic
  - gonococcal A54.24
  - puerperal O85
- **Pelvis** — *see* condition or type
- **Pemphigoid** L12.9
  - benign, mucous membrane L12.1
  - bullous L12.Ø
  - cicatricial L12.1
  - juvenile L12.2
  - ocular L12.1
  - specified NEC L12.8
- **Pemphigus** L1Ø.9
  - benign familial (chronic) Q82.8
  - Brazilian L1Ø.3
  - circinatus L13.Ø
  - conjunctiva L12.1
  - drug-induced L1Ø.5
  - erythematosus L1Ø.4
  - foliaceous L1Ø.2
  - gangrenous — *see* Gangrene
  - neonatorum LØ1.Ø3
  - ocular L12.1
  - paraneoplastic L1Ø.81
  - specified NEC L1Ø.89
  - syphilitic (congenital) A5Ø.Ø6
  - vegetans L1Ø.1
  - vulgaris L1Ø.Ø
  - wildfire L1Ø.3
- **Pendred's syndrome** EØ7.1
- **Pendulous**
  - abdomen, in pregnancy — *see* Pregnancy, complicated by, abnormal, pelvic organs or tissues NEC
  - breast N64.89
- **Penetrating wound** — *see also* Puncture
  - with internal injury — *see* Injury, by site
  - eyeball — *see* Puncture, eyeball
  - orbit (with or without foreign body) — *see* Puncture, orbit
- **Penetrating wound** — *continued*
  - uterus by instrument with or following ectopic or molar pregnancy OØ8.6
- **Penicillosis** B48.4
- **Penis** — *see* condition
- **Penitis** N48.29
- **Pentalogy of Fallot** Q21.8
- **Pentasomy X syndrome** Q97.1
- **Pentosuria** (essential) E74.89
- **Percreta placenta** - O43.23 ☑
- **Peregrinating patient** — *see* Disorder, factitious
- **Perforation, perforated** (nontraumatic) (of)
  - accidental during procedure (blood vessel) (nerve) (organ) — *see* Complication, accidental puncture or laceration
  - antrum — *see* Sinusitis, maxillary
  - appendix K35.32
    - with localized peritonitis K35.32
  - atrial septum, multiple Q21.19
  - attic, ear — *see* Perforation, tympanum, attic
  - bile duct (common) (hepatic) K83.2
    - cystic K82.2
  - bladder (urinary)
    - with or following ectopic or molar pregnancy OØ8.6
    - obstetrical trauma O71.5
    - traumatic S37.29 ☑
      - at delivery O71.5
  - bowel K63.1
    - with or following ectopic or molar pregnancy OØ8.6
    - newborn P78.Ø
    - obstetrical trauma O71.5
    - traumatic — *see* Laceration, intestine
  - broad ligament N83.8
    - with or following ectopic or molar pregnancy OØ8.6
    - obstetrical trauma O71.6
  - by
    - device, implant or graft — *see also* Complications, by site and type, mechanical T85.628 ☑
      - arterial graft NEC — *see* Complication, cardiovascular device, mechanical, vascular
      - breast (implant) T85.49 ☑
      - catheter NEC T85.698 ☑
        - cystostomy T83.Ø9Ø ☑
        - dialysis (renal) T82.49 ☑
          - intraperitoneal T85.691 ☑
        - infusion NEC T82.594 ☑
          - spinal (epidural) (subdural) T85.69Ø ☑
        - urinary — *see also* Complications, catheter, urinary T83.Ø98 ☑
      - electronic (electrode) (pulse generator) (stimulator)
        - bone T84.39Ø ☑
        - cardiac T82.199 ☑
          - electrode T82.19Ø ☑
          - pulse generator T82.191 ☑
          - specified type NEC T82.198 ☑
        - nervous system — *see* Complication, prosthetic device, mechanical, electronic nervous system stimulator
        - urinary — *see* Complication, genitourinary, device, urinary, mechanical
      - fixation, internal (orthopedic) NEC — *see* Complication, fixation device, mechanical
      - gastrointestinal — *see* Complications, prosthetic device, mechanical, gastrointestinal device
      - genital NEC T83.498 ☑
        - intrauterine contraceptive device T83.39 ☑
        - penile prosthesis T83.49Ø ☑
      - heart NEC — *see* Complication, cardiovascular device, mechanical
      - joint prosthesis — *see* Complications, joint prosthesis, mechanical, specified NEC, by site
      - ocular NEC — *see* Complications, prosthetic device, mechanical, ocular device
      - orthopedic NEC — *see* Complication, orthopedic, device, mechanical
      - specified NEC T85.628 ☑
      - urinary NEC — *see also* Complication, genitourinary, device, urinary, mechanical
        - graft T83.29 ☑
      - vascular NEC — *see* Complication, cardiovascular device, mechanical
      - ventricular intracranial shunt T85.Ø9 ☑
    - foreign body left accidentally in operative wound T81.539 ☑

- **Perforation, perforated** — *continued*
  - by — *continued*
    - instrument (any) during a procedure, accidental — *see* Puncture, accidental complicating surgery
  - cecum K35.32
    - with localized peritonitis K35.32
  - cervix (uteri) N88.8
    - with or following ectopic or molar pregnancy OØ8.6
    - obstetrical trauma O71.3
  - colon K63.1
    - newborn P78.Ø
    - obstetrical trauma O71.5
    - traumatic — *see* Laceration, intestine, large
  - common duct (bile) K83.2
  - cornea (due to ulceration) — *see* Ulcer, cornea, perforated
  - cystic duct K82.2
  - diverticulum (intestine) K57.8Ø
    - with bleeding K57.81
    - large intestine K57.2Ø
      - with
        - bleeding K57.21
        - small intestine K57.4Ø
          - with bleeding K57.41
    - small intestine K57.ØØ
      - with
        - bleeding K57.Ø1
        - large intestine K57.4Ø
          - with bleeding K57.41
  - ear drum — *see* Perforation, tympanum
  - esophagus K22.3
  - ethmoidal sinus — *see* Sinusitis, ethmoidal
  - frontal sinus — *see* Sinusitis, frontal
  - gallbladder K82.2
  - heart valve — *see* Endocarditis
  - ileum K63.1
    - newborn P78.Ø
    - obstetrical trauma O71.5
    - traumatic — *see* Laceration, intestine, small
  - instrumental, surgical (accidental) (blood vessel) (nerve) (organ) — *see* Puncture, accidental complicating surgery
  - intestine NEC K63.1
    - with ectopic or molar pregnancy OØ8.6
    - newborn P78.Ø
    - obstetrical trauma O71.5
    - traumatic — *see* Laceration, intestine
    - ulcerative NEC K63.1
      - newborn P78.Ø
  - jejunum, jejunal K63.1
    - obstetrical trauma O71.5
    - traumatic — *see* Laceration, intestine, small
    - ulcer — *see* Ulcer, gastrojejunal, with perforation
  - joint prosthesis — *see* Complications, joint prosthesis, mechanical, specified NEC, by site
  - mastoid (antrum) (cell) — *see* Disorder, mastoid, specified NEC
  - maxillary sinus — *see* Sinusitis, maxillary
  - membrana tympani — *see* Perforation, tympanum
  - nasal
    - septum J34.89
      - congenital Q3Ø.3
      - syphilitic A52.73
    - sinus J34.89
      - congenital Q3Ø.8
      - due to sinusitis — *see* Sinusitis
  - palate — *see also* Cleft, palate Q35.9
    - syphilitic A52.79
  - palatine vault — *see also* Cleft, palate, hard Q35.1
    - syphilitic A52.79
      - congenital A5Ø.59
  - pars flaccida (ear drum) — *see* Perforation, tympanum, attic
  - pelvic
    - floor S31.Ø3Ø ☑
      - with
        - ectopic or molar pregnancy OØ8.6
        - penetration into retroperitoneal space S31.Ø31 ☑
        - retained foreign body S31.Ø4Ø ☑
          - with penetration into retroperitoneal space S31.Ø41 ☑
      - following ectopic or molar pregnancy OØ8.6
      - obstetrical trauma O7Ø.1
    - organ S37.99 ☑
      - adrenal gland S37.818 ☑
      - bladder — *see* Perforation, bladder
      - fallopian tube S37.599 ☑

- **Perforation, perforated** — *continued*
  - pelvic — *continued*
    - organ — *continued*
      - fallopian tube — *continued*
        - bilateral S37.592 ☑
        - unilateral S37.591 ☑
      - kidney S37.Ø9- ☑
      - obstetrical trauma O71.5
      - ovary S37.499 ☑
        - bilateral S37.492 ☑
        - unilateral S37.491 ☑
      - prostate S37.828 ☑
      - specified organ NEC S37.898 ☑
      - ureter — *see* Perforation, ureter
      - urethra — *see* Perforation, urethra
      - uterus — *see* Perforation, uterus
  - perineum — *see* Laceration, perineum
  - pharynx J39.2
  - rectum K63.1
    - newborn P78.Ø
    - obstetrical trauma O71.5
    - traumatic S36.63 ☑
  - root canal space due to endodontic treatment M27.51
  - sigmoid K63.1
    - newborn P78.Ø
    - obstetrical trauma O71.5
    - traumatic S36.533 ☑
  - sinus (accessory) (chronic) (nasal) J34.89
  - sphenoidal sinus — *see* Sinusitis, sphenoidal
  - surgical (accidental) (by instrument) (blood vessel) (nerve) (organ) — *see* Puncture, accidental complicating surgery
  - traumatic
    - external — *see* Puncture
    - eye — *see* Puncture, eyeball
    - internal organ — *see* Injury, by site
  - tympanum, tympanic (membrane) (persistent post-traumatic) (postinflammatory) H72.9- ☑
    - attic H72.1- ☑
      - multiple — *see* Perforation, tympanum, multiple
      - total — *see* Perforation, tympanum, total
    - central H72.Ø- ☑
      - multiple — *see* Perforation, tympanum, multiple
      - total — *see* Perforation, tympanum, total
    - marginal NEC — *see* subcategory H72.2 ☑
    - multiple H72.81- ☑
    - pars flaccida — *see* Perforation, tympanum, attic
    - total H72.82- ☑
    - traumatic, current episode SØ9.2- ☑
  - typhoid, gastrointestinal — *see* Typhoid
  - ulcer — *see* Ulcer, by site, with perforation
  - ureter N28.89
    - traumatic S37.19 ☑
  - urethra N36.8
    - with ectopic or molar pregnancy OØ8.6
    - following ectopic or molar pregnancy OØ8.6
    - obstetrical trauma O71.5
    - traumatic S37.39 ☑
      - at delivery O71.5
  - uterus
    - with ectopic or molar pregnancy OØ8.6
    - by intrauterine contraceptive device T83.39 ☑
    - following ectopic or molar pregnancy OØ8.6
    - obstetrical trauma O71.1
    - traumatic S37.69 ☑
      - obstetric O71.1
  - uvula K13.79
    - syphilitic A52.79
  - vagina O71.4
    - obstetrical trauma O71.4
    - other trauma — *see* Puncture, vagina
- **Periadenitis mucosa necrotica recurrens** K12.Ø
- **Periappendicitis** (acute) — *see* Appendicitis
- **Periarteritis nodosa** (disseminated) (infectious) (necrotizing) M3Ø.Ø
- **Periarthritis** (joint) — *see also* Enthesopathy
  - Duplay's M75.Ø- ☑
  - gonococcal A54.42
  - humeroscapularis — *see* Capsulitis, adhesive
  - scapulohumeral — *see* Capsulitis, adhesive
  - shoulder — *see* Capsulitis, adhesive
  - wrist M77.2- ☑
- **Periarthrosis** (angioneural) — *see* Enthesopathy
- **Pericapsulitis, adhesive** (shoulder) — *see* Capsulitis, adhesive
- **Pericarditis** (with decompensation) (with effusion) I31.9

- **Pericarditis** — *continued*
  - with rheumatic fever (conditions in IØØ)
    - active — *see* Pericarditis, rheumatic
    - inactive or quiescent IØ9.2
  - acute (hemorrhagic) (nonrheumatic) (Sicca) I3Ø.9
    - with chorea (acute) (rheumatic) (Sydenham's) IØ2.Ø
    - benign I3Ø.8
    - nonspecific I3Ø.Ø
    - rheumatic IØ1.Ø
      - with chorea (acute) (Sydenham's) IØ2.Ø
  - adhesive or adherent (chronic) (external) (internal) I31.Ø
    - acute — *see* Pericarditis, acute
    - rheumatic IØ9.2
  - bacterial (acute) (subacute) (with serous or seropurulent effusion) I3Ø.1
  - calcareous I31.1
  - cholesterol (chronic) I31.8
    - acute I3Ø.9
  - chronic (nonrheumatic) I31.9
    - rheumatic IØ9.2
  - constrictive (chronic) I31.1
  - coxsackie B33.23
  - fibrinocaseous (tuberculous) A18.84
  - fibrinopurulent I3Ø.1
  - fibrinous I3Ø.8
  - fibrous I31.Ø
  - gonococcal A54.83
  - idiopathic I3Ø.Ø
  - in systemic lupus erythematosus M32.12
  - infective I3Ø.1
  - meningococcal A39.53
  - neoplastic (chronic) I31.8
    - acute I3Ø.9
  - obliterans, obliterating I31.Ø
  - plastic I31.Ø
  - pneumococcal I3Ø.1
  - postinfarction I24.1
  - purulent I3Ø.1
  - rheumatic (active) (acute) (with effusion) (with pneumonia) IØ1.Ø
    - with chorea (acute) (rheumatic) (Sydenham's) IØ2.Ø
    - chronic or inactive (with chorea) IØ9.2
  - rheumatoid — *see* Rheumatoid, carditis
  - septic I3Ø.1
  - serofibrinous I3Ø.8
  - staphylococcal I3Ø.1
  - streptococcal I3Ø.1
  - suppurative I3Ø.1
  - syphilitic A52.Ø6
  - tuberculous A18.84
  - uremic N18.9 *[I32]*
  - viral I3Ø.1
- **Pericardium, pericardial** — *see* condition
- **Pericellulitis** — *see* Cellulitis
- **Pericementitis** (chronic) (suppurative) — *see also* Periodontitis
  - acute KØ5.2Ø
    - generalized — *see* Periodontitis, aggressive, generalized
    - localized — *see* Periodontitis, aggressive, localized
- **Perichondritis**
  - auricle — *see* Perichondritis, ear
  - bronchus J98.Ø9
  - ear (external) H61.ØØ- ☑
    - acute H61.Ø1- ☑
    - chronic H61.Ø2- ☑
  - external auditory canal — *see* Perichondritis, ear
  - larynx J38.7
    - syphilitic A52.73
    - typhoid AØ1.Ø9
  - nose J34.89
  - pinna — *see* Perichondritis, ear
  - trachea J39.8
- **Periclasia** KØ5.4
- **Pericoronitis** — *see* Periodontitis
- **Pericystitis** N3Ø.9Ø
  - with hematuria N3Ø.91
- **Peridiverticulitis** (intestine) K57.92
  - cecum — *see* Diverticulitis, intestine, large
  - colon — *see* Diverticulitis, intestine, large
  - duodenum — *see* Diverticulitis, intestine, small
  - intestine — *see* Diverticulitis, intestine
  - jejunum — *see* Diverticulitis, intestine, small
  - rectosigmoid — *see* Diverticulitis, intestine, large
  - rectum — *see* Diverticulitis, intestine, large
  - sigmoid — *see* Diverticulitis, intestine, large
- **Periendocarditis** — *see* Endocarditis
- **Periepididymitis** N45.1

Perifolliculitis LØ1.Ø2
abscedens, caput, scalp L66.3
capitis, abscedens (et suffodiens) L66.3
superficial pustular LØ1.Ø2
Perihepatitis K65.8
Perilabyrinthitis (acute) — *see* subcategory H83.Ø ☑
Perimeningitis — *see* Meningitis
Perimetritis — *see* Endometritis
Perimetrosalpingitis — *see* Salpingo-oophoritis
Perineocele N81.81
Perinephric, perinephritic — *see* condition
Perinephritis — *see also* Infection, kidney
purulent — *see* Abscess, kidney
Perineum, perineal — *see* condition
Perineuritis NEC — *see* Neuralgia
Periodic — *see* condition
Periodontitis (chronic) (complex) (compound) (local) (simplex) KØ5.3Ø
acute KØ5.2Ø
generalized KØ5.229
moderate KØ5.222
severe KØ5.223
slight KØ5.221
localized KØ5.219
moderate KØ5.212
severe KØ5.213
slight KØ5.211
aggressive KØ5.2Ø
generalized KØ5.229
moderate KØ5.222
severe KØ5.223
slight KØ5.221
localized KØ5.219
moderate KØ5.212
severe KØ5.213
slight KØ5.211
apical KØ4.5
acute (pulpal origin) KØ4.4
generalized KØ5.329
moderate KØ5.322
severe KØ5.323
slight KØ5.321
localized KØ5.319
moderate KØ5.312
severe KØ5.313
slight KØ5.311
Periodontoclasia KØ5.4
Periodontosis (juvenile) KØ5.4
Periods — *see also* Menstruation
heavy N92.Ø
irregular N92.6
shortened intervals (irregular) N92.1
Perionychia — *see also* Cellulitis, digit
with lymphangitis — *see* Lymphangitis, acute, digit
Perioophoritis — *see* Salpingo-oophoritis
Periorchitis N45.2
Periosteum, periosteal — *see* condition
Periostitis (albuminosa) (circumscribed) (diffuse) (infective) (monomelic) — *see also* Osteomyelitis
alveolar M27.3
alveolodental M27.3
dental M27.3
gonorrheal A54.43
jaw (lower) (upper) M27.2
orbit HØ5.Ø3- ☑
syphilitic A52.77
congenital (early) A5Ø.Ø2 *[M9Ø.8Ø]*
secondary A51.46
tuberculous — *see* Tuberculosis, bone
yaws (hypertrophic) (early) (late) A66.6 *[M9Ø.8Ø]*
Periostosis (hyperplastic) — *see also* Disorder, bone, specified type NEC
with osteomyelitis — *see* Osteomyelitis, specified type NEC
Peripartum
cardiomyopathy O9Ø.3
Periphlebitis — *see* Phlebitis
Periproctitis K62.89
Periprostatitis — *see* Prostatitis
Perirectal — *see* condition
Perirenal — *see* condition
Perisalpingitis — *see* Salpingo-oophoritis
Perisplenitis (infectional) D73.89
Peristalsis, visible or reversed R19.2
Peritendinitis — *see* Enthesopathy
Peritoneum, peritoneal — *see* condition
Peritonitis (adhesive) (bacterial) (fibrinous) (hemorrhagic) (idiopathic) (localized) (perforative) (primary) (with adhesions) (with effusion) K65.9
with or following
abscess K65.1
appendicitis
with perforation or rupture K35.32
generalized — *see also* Appendicitis K35.2Ø9
localized — *see also* Appendicitis K35.3Ø
diverticular disease (intestine) K57.8Ø
with bleeding K57.81
ectopic or molar pregnancy OØ8.Ø
large intestine K57.2Ø
with
bleeding K57.21
small intestine K57.4Ø
with bleeding K57.41
small intestine K57.ØØ
with
bleeding K57.Ø1
large intestine K57.4Ø
with bleeding K57.41
acute (generalized) K65.Ø
aseptic T81.61 ☑
bile, biliary K65.3
chemical T81.61 ☑
chlamydial A74.81
chronic proliferative K65.8
complicating abortion — *see* Abortion, by type, complicated by, pelvic peritonitis
congenital P78.1
diaphragmatic K65.Ø
diffuse K65.Ø
diphtheritic A36.89
disseminated K65.Ø
due to
bile K65.3
foreign
body or object accidentally left during a procedure (instrument) (sponge) (swab) T81.599 ☑
substance accidentally left during a procedure (chemical) (powder) (talc) T81.61 ☑
talc T81.61 ☑
urine K65.8
eosinophilic K65.8
acute K65.Ø
fibrocaseous (tuberculous) A18.31
fibropurulent K65.Ø
following ectopic or molar pregnancy OØ8.Ø
general (ized) K65.Ø
gonococcal A54.85
meconium (newborn) P78.Ø
neonatal P78.1
meconium P78.Ø
pancreatic K65.Ø
paroxysmal, familial E85.Ø
benign E85.Ø
pelvic
female N73.5
acute N73.3
chronic N73.4
with adhesions N73.6
male K65.Ø
periodic, familial E85.Ø
proliferative, chronic K65.8
puerperal, postpartum, childbirth O85
purulent K65.Ø
septic K65.Ø
specified NEC K65.8
spontaneous bacterial K65.2
subdiaphragmatic K65.Ø
subphrenic K65.Ø
suppurative K65.Ø
syphilitic A52.74
congenital (early) A5Ø.Ø8 *[K67]*
talc T81.61 ☑
tuberculous A18.31
urine K65.8
Peritonsillar — *see* condition
Peritonsillitis J36
Perityphlitis — *see also* Cecitis K37
Periureteritis N28.89
Periurethral — *see* condition
Periurethritis (gangrenous) — *see* Urethritis
Periuterine — *see* condition
Perivaginitis — *see* Vaginitis
Perivasculitis, retinal H35.Ø6- ☑
Perivasitis (chronic) N49.1
Perivesiculitis (seminal) — *see* Vesiculitis
Perlèche NEC K13.Ø
due to
candidiasis B37.83
moniliasis B37.83
riboflavin deficiency E53.Ø
vitamin B2 (riboflavin) deficiency E53.Ø
Pernicious — *see* condition
Pernio, perniosis T69.1 ☑
Perpetrator (of abuse) — *see* Index to External Causes of Injury, Perpetrator
Persecution
delusion F22
social Z6Ø.5
Perseveration (tonic) R48.8
Persistence, persistent (congenital)
anal membrane Q42.3
with fistula Q42.2
arteria stapedia Q16.3
atrioventricular canal Q21.2Ø
branchial cleft NOS Q18.2
cyst Q18.Ø
fistula Q18.Ø
sinus Q18.Ø
bulbus cordis in left ventricle Q21.8
canal of Cloquet Q14.Ø
capsule (opaque) Q12.8
cilioretinal artery or vein Q14.8
cloaca Q43.7
communication — *see* Fistula, congenital
convolutions
aortic arch Q25.46
fallopian tube Q5Ø.6
oviduct Q5Ø.6
uterine tube Q5Ø.6
double aortic arch Q25.45
ductus arteriosus (Botalli) Q25.Ø
fetal
circulation P29.38
form of cervix (uteri) Q51.828
hemoglobin, hereditary (HPFH) D56.4
foramen
Botalli Q21.12
ovale Q21.12
Gartner's duct Q52.4
hemoglobin, fetal (hereditary) (HPFH) D56.4
hyaloid
artery (generally incomplete) Q14.Ø
system Q14.8
hymen, in pregnancy or childbirth — *see* Pregnancy, complicated by, abnormal, vulva
lanugo Q84.2
left
posterior cardinal vein Q26.8
root with right arch of aorta Q25.49
superior vena cava Q26.1
Meckel's diverticulum Q43.Ø
malignant — *see* Table of Neoplasms, small intestine, malignant
mucosal disease (middle ear) — *see* Otitis, media, suppurative, chronic, tubotympanic
nail(s), anomalous Q84.6
omphalomesenteric duct Q43.Ø
organ or site not listed — *see* Anomaly, by site
ostium
atrioventriculare commune Q21.23
primum Q21.2Ø
secundum Q21.11
ovarian rests in fallopian tube Q5Ø.6
pancreatic tissue in intestinal tract Q43.8
primary (deciduous)
teeth KØØ.6
vitreous hyperplasia Q14.Ø
pupillary membrane Q13.89
rhesus (Rh) titer — *see* Complication(s), transfusion, incompatibility reaction, Rh (factor)
right aortic arch Q25.47
sinus
urogenitalis
female Q52.8
male Q55.8
venosus with imperfect incorporation in right auricle Q26.8
thymus (gland) (hyperplasia) E32.Ø
thyroglossal duct Q89.2
thyrolingual duct Q89.2
truncus arteriosus or communis Q2Ø.Ø

- **Persistence, persistent** — *continued*
  - tunica vasculosa lentis Q12.2
  - umbilical sinus Q64.4
  - urachus Q64.4
  - vitelline duct Q43.Ø
- **Person** (with)
  - admitted for clinical research, as a control subject (normal comparison) (participant) ZØØ.6
  - awaiting admission to adequate facility elsewhere Z75.1
  - concern (normal) about sick person in family Z63.6
  - consulting on behalf of another Z71.Ø
  - feigning illness Z76.5
  - living (in)
    - alone Z6Ø.2
    - boarding school Z59.3
    - residential institution Z59.3
    - without
      - adequate housing Z59.1Ø
        - air conditioning Z59.11
        - environmental temperature Z59.11
        - heating Z59.11
        - space Z59.19
      - housing (permanent) (temporary) Z59.ØØ
      - person able to render necessary care Z74.2
      - shelter Z59.Ø2
  - on waiting list Z75.1
  - sick or handicapped in family Z63.6
- **Personality** (disorder) F6Ø.9
  - accentuation of traits (type A pattern) Z73.1
  - affective F34.Ø
  - aggressive F6Ø.3
  - amoral F6Ø.2
  - anacastic, anankastic F6Ø.5
  - antisocial F6Ø.2
  - anxious F6Ø.6
  - asocial F6Ø.2
  - asthenic F6Ø.7
  - avoidant F6Ø.6
  - borderline F6Ø.3
  - change due to organic condition (enduring) FØ7.Ø
  - compulsive F6Ø.5
  - cycloid F34.Ø
  - cyclothymic F34.Ø
  - dependent F6Ø.7
  - depressive F34.1
  - dissocial F6Ø.2
  - dual F44.81
  - eccentric F6Ø.89
  - emotionally unstable F6Ø.3
  - expansive paranoid F6Ø.Ø
  - explosive F6Ø.3
  - fanatic F6Ø.Ø
  - haltlose type F6Ø.89
  - histrionic F6Ø.4
  - hyperthymic F34.Ø
  - hypothymic F34.1
  - hysterical F6Ø.4
  - immature F6Ø.89
  - inadequate F6Ø.7
  - labile (emotional) F6Ø.3
  - mixed (nonspecific) F6Ø.89
  - morally defective F6Ø.2
  - multiple F44.81
  - narcissistic F6Ø.81
  - obsessional F6Ø.5
  - obsessive (-compulsive) F6Ø.5
  - organic FØ7.Ø
  - overconscientious F6Ø.5
  - paranoid F6Ø.Ø
  - passive (-dependent) F6Ø.7
  - passive-aggressive F6Ø.89
  - pathologic F6Ø.9
  - pattern defect or disturbance F6Ø.9
  - pseudopsychopathic (organic) FØ7.Ø
  - pseudoretarded (organic) FØ7.Ø
  - psychoinfantile F6Ø.4
  - psychoneurotic NEC F6Ø.89
  - psychopathic F6Ø.2
  - querulant F6Ø.Ø
  - sadistic F6Ø.89
  - schizoid F6Ø.1
  - self-defeating F6Ø.89
  - sensitive paranoid F6Ø.Ø
  - sociopathic (amoral) (antisocial) (asocial) (dissocial) F6Ø.2
  - specified NEC F6Ø.89
  - type A Z73.1
  - unstable (emotional) F6Ø.3
- **Perthes' disease** — *see* Legg-Calve-Perthes disease
- **Pertussis** — *see also* Whooping cough A37.9Ø
- **Perversion, perverted**
  - appetite F5Ø.89
    - psychogenic F5Ø.89
  - function
    - pituitary gland E23.2
      - posterior lobe E22.2
  - sense of smell and taste R43.8
    - psychogenic F45.8
  - sexual — *see* Deviation, sexual
- **Pervious, congenital** — *see also* Imperfect, closure
  - ductus arteriosus Q25.Ø
- **Pes** (congenital) — *see also* Talipes
  - acquired — *see also* Deformity, limb, foot, specified NEC
    - planus — *see* Deformity, limb, flat foot
  - adductus Q66.89
  - cavus Q66.7- ☑
  - deformity NEC, acquired — *see* Deformity, limb, foot, specified NEC
  - planus (acquired) (any degree) — *see also* Deformity, limb, flat foot
    - rachitic sequelae (late effect) E64.3
  - valgus Q66.6
- **Pest, pestis** — *see* Plague
- **Petechia, petechiae** R23.3
  - newborn P54.5
- **Petechial typhus** A75.9
- **Peter's anomaly** Q13.4
- **Petit mal seizure** — *see* Epilepsy, childhood, absence
- **Petit's hernia** — *see* Hernia, abdomen, specified site NEC
- **Petrellidosis** B48.2
- **Petrositis** H7Ø.2Ø- ☑
  - acute H7Ø.21- ☑
  - chronic H7Ø.22- ☑
- **Peutz-Jeghers disease or syndrome** Q85.89
- **Peyronie's disease** N48.6
- **PFAPA** (periodic fever, aphthous stomatitis, pharyngitis, and adenopathy syndrome) MØ4.8
- **Pfeiffer's disease** — *see* Mononucleosis, infectious
- **Phagedena** (dry) (moist) (sloughing) — *see also* Gangrene
  - geometric L88
  - penis N48.29
  - tropical — *see* Ulcer, skin
  - vulva N76.6
- **Phagedenic** — *see* condition
- **Phakoma** H35.89
- **Phakomatosis** — *see also* specific eponymous syndromes Q85.9
  - Bourneville's Q85.1
  - specified NEC Q85.89
- **Phantom limb syndrome** (without pain) G54.7
  - with pain G54.6
- **Pharyngeal pouch syndrome** D82.1
- **Pharyngitis** (acute) (catarrhal) (gangrenous) (infective) (malignant) (membranous) (phlegmonous) (pseudomembranous) (simple) (subacute) (suppurative) (ulcerative) (viral) JØ2.9
  - with influenza, flu, or grippe — *see* Influenza, with, pharyngitis
  - aphthous BØ8.5
  - atrophic J31.2
  - chlamydial A56.4
  - chronic (atrophic) (granular) (hypertrophic) J31.2
  - coxsackievirus BØ8.5
  - diphtheritic A36.Ø
  - enteroviral vesicular BØ8.5
  - follicular (chronic) J31.2
  - fusospirochetal A69.1
  - gonococcal A54.5
  - granular (chronic) J31.2
  - herpesviral BØØ.2
  - hypertrophic J31.2
  - infectional, chronic J31.2
  - influenzal — *see* Influenza, with, respiratory manifestations NEC
  - lymphonodular, acute (enteroviral) BØ8.8
  - pneumococcal JØ2.8
  - purulent JØ2.9
  - putrid JØ2.9
  - septic JØ2.Ø
  - sicca J31.2
  - specified organism NEC JØ2.8
  - staphylococcal JØ2.8
  - streptococcal JØ2.Ø
  - syphilitic, congenital (early) A5Ø.Ø3
- **Pharyngitis** — *continued*
  - tuberculous A15.8
  - vesicular, enteroviral BØ8.5
  - viral NEC JØ2.8
- **Pharyngoconjunctivitis, viral** B3Ø.2
- **Pharyngolaryngitis** (acute) JØ6.Ø
  - chronic J37.Ø
- **Pharyngoplegia** J39.2
- **Pharyngotonsillitis, herpesviral** BØØ.2
- **Pharyngotracheitis, chronic** J42
- **Pharynx, pharyngeal** — *see* condition
- **Phelan-McDermid syndrome** Q93.52
- **Phencyclidine-induced**
  - anxiety disorder F16.98Ø
  - bipolar and related disorder F16.94
  - depressive disorder F16.94
  - psychotic disorder F16.959
- **Phenomenon**
  - Arthus' — *see* Arthus' phenomenon
  - jaw-winking QØ7.8
  - lupus erythematosus (LE) cell M32.9
  - Raynaud's (secondary) I73.ØØ
    - with gangrene I73.Ø1
  - vasomotor R55
  - vasospastic I73.9
  - vasovagal R55
  - Wenckebach's I44.1
- **Phenylketonuria** E7Ø.1
  - classical E7Ø.Ø
  - maternal E7Ø.1
- **Pheochromoblastoma**
  - specified site — *see* Neoplasm, malignant, by site
  - unspecified site C74.1Ø
- **Pheochromocytoma**
  - malignant
    - specified site — *see* Neoplasm, malignant, by site
    - unspecified site C74.1Ø
  - specified site — *see* Neoplasm, benign, by site
  - unspecified site D35.ØØ
- **Pheohyphomycosis** — *see* Chromomycosis
- **Pheomycosis** — *see* Chromomycosis
- **Phimosis** (congenital) (due to infection) N47.1
  - chancroidal A57
- **Phlebectasia** — *see also* Varix
  - congenital Q27.4
- **Phlebitis** (infective) (pyemic) (septic) (suppurative) I8Ø.9
  - antepartum — *see* Thrombophlebitis, antepartum
  - blue — *see* Phlebitis, leg, deep
  - breast, superficial I8Ø.8
  - calf muscular vein (NOS) I8Ø.25- ☑
  - cavernous (venous) sinus — *see* Phlebitis, intracranial (venous) sinus
  - cerebral (venous) sinus — *see* Phlebitis, intracranial (venous) sinus
  - chest wall, superficial I8Ø.8
  - cranial (venous) sinus — *see* Phlebitis, intracranial (venous) sinus
  - deep (vessels) — *see* Phlebitis, leg, deep
  - due to implanted device — *see* Complications, by site and type, specified NEC
  - during or resulting from a procedure T81.72 ☑
  - femoral vein (superficial) I8Ø.1- ☑
  - femoropopliteal vein I8Ø.Ø- ☑
  - gastrocnemial vein I8Ø.25- ☑
  - gestational — *see* Phlebopathy, gestational
  - hepatic veins I8Ø.8
  - iliac vein (common) (external) (internal) I8Ø.21- ☑
  - iliofemoral — *see* Phlebitis, femoral vein
  - intracranial (venous) sinus (any) GØ8
    - nonpyogenic I67.6
  - intraspinal venous sinuses and veins GØ8
    - nonpyogenic G95.19
  - lateral (venous) sinus — *see* Phlebitis, intracranial (venous) sinus
  - leg I8Ø.3
    - antepartum — *see* Thrombophlebitis, antepartum
    - deep (vessels) NEC I8Ø.2Ø- ☑
      - iliac I8Ø.21- ☑
      - popliteal vein I8Ø.22- ☑
      - specified vessel NEC I8Ø.29- ☑
      - tibial vein (anterior) (posterior) I8Ø.23- ☑
    - femoral vein (superficial) I8Ø.1- ☑
    - superficial (vessels) I8Ø.Ø- ☑
  - longitudinal sinus — *see* Phlebitis, intracranial (venous) sinus
  - lower limb — *see* Phlebitis, leg
  - migrans, migrating (superficial) I82.1

- **Phlebitis** — *continued*
  - pelvic
    - with ectopic or molar pregnancy O08.Ø
    - following ectopic or molar pregnancy O08.Ø
    - puerperal, postpartum O87.1
  - peroneal vein I8Ø.24- ☑
  - popliteal vein — *see* Phlebitis, leg, deep, popliteal
  - portal (vein) K75.1
  - postoperative T81.72 ☑
  - pregnancy — *see* Thrombophlebitis, antepartum
  - puerperal, postpartum, childbirth O87.Ø
    - deep O87.1
    - pelvic O87.1
    - superficial O87.Ø
  - retina — *see* Vasculitis, retina
  - saphenous (accessory) (great) (long) (small) — *see* Phlebitis, leg, superficial
  - sinus (meninges) — *see* Phlebitis, intracranial (venous) sinus
  - soleal vein I8Ø.25- ☑
  - specified site NEC I8Ø.8
  - syphilitic A52.Ø9
  - tibial vein — *see* Phlebitis, leg, deep, tibial
  - ulcerative I8Ø.9
    - leg — *see* Phlebitis, leg
  - umbilicus I8Ø.8
  - uterus (septic) — *see* Endometritis
  - varicose (leg) (lower limb) — *see* Varix, leg, with, inflammation
- **Phlebofibrosis** I87.8
- **Phleboliths** I87.8
- **Phlebopathy,**
  - gestational O22.9- ☑
  - puerperal O87.9
- **Phlebosclerosis** I87.8
- **Phlebothrombosis** — *see also* Thrombosis
  - antepartum — *see* Thrombophlebitis, antepartum
  - pregnancy — *see* Thrombophlebitis, antepartum
  - puerperal — *see* Thrombophlebitis, puerperal
- **Phlebotomus fever** A93.1
- **Phlegmasia**
  - alba dolens O87.1
    - nonpuerperal — *see* Phlebitis, femoral vein
  - cerulea dolens — *see* Phlebitis, leg, deep
- **Phlegmon** — *see* Abscess
- **Phlegmonous** — *see* condition
- **Phlyctenulosis** (allergic) (keratoconjunctivitis) (nontuberculous) — *see also* Keratoconjunctivitis
  - cornea — *see* Keratoconjunctivitis
  - tuberculous A18.52
- **Phobia, phobic** F4Ø.9
  - animal F4Ø.218
    - spiders F4Ø.21Ø
  - examination F4Ø.298
  - reaction F4Ø.9
  - simple F4Ø.298
  - social F4Ø.1Ø
    - generalized F4Ø.11
  - specific (isolated) F4Ø.298
    - animal F4Ø.218
      - spiders F4Ø.21Ø
    - blood F4Ø.23Ø
    - injection F4Ø.231
    - injury F4Ø.233
    - men F4Ø.29Ø
    - natural environment F4Ø.228
      - thunderstorms F4Ø.22Ø
    - situational F4Ø.248
      - bridges F4Ø.242
      - closed in spaces F4Ø.24Ø
      - flying F4Ø.243
      - heights F4Ø.241
    - specified focus NEC F4Ø.298
    - transfusion F4Ø.231
    - women F4Ø.291
  - specified NEC F4Ø.8
    - medical care NEC F4Ø.232
  - state F4Ø.9
- **Phocas' disease** — *see* Mastopathy, cystic
- **Phocomelia** Q73.1
  - lower limb — *see* Agenesis, leg, with foot present
  - upper limb — *see* Agenesis, arm, with hand present
- **Phoria** H5Ø.5Ø
- **Phosphate-losing tubular disorder** N25.Ø
- **Phosphatemia** E83.39
- **Phosphaturia** E83.39
- **Photodermatitis** (sun) L56.8
- **Photodermatitis** — *continued*
  - chronic L57.8
  - due to drug L56.8
  - light other than sun L59.8
- **Photokeratitis** H16.13- ☑
- **Photophobia** H53.14- ☑
- **Photophthalmia** — *see* Photokeratitis
- **Photopsia** H53.19
- **Photoretinitis** — *see* Retinopathy, solar
- **Photosensitivity, photosensitization** (sun) skin L56.8
  - light other than sun L59.8
- **Phrenitis** — *see* Encephalitis
- **Phrynoderma** (vitamin A deficiency) E5Ø.8
- **Phthiriasis** (pubis) B85.3
  - with any infestation classifiable to B85.Ø-B85.2 B85.4
- **Phthirus infestation** — *see* Phthiriasis
- **Phthisis** — *see also* Tuberculosis
  - bulbi (infectional) — *see* Disorder, globe, degenerated condition, atrophy
  - eyeball (due to infection) — *see* Disorder, globe, degenerated condition, atrophy
- **PHTS** Q85.81
- **Phycomycosis** — *see* Zygomycosis
- **Physalopteriasis** B81.8
- **Physical restraint status** Z78.1
- **Phytobezoar** T18.9 ☑
  - intestine T18.3 ☑
  - stomach T18.2 ☑
- **Pian** — *see* Yaws
- **Pianoma** A66.1
- **Pica** F5Ø.89
  - in adults F5Ø.89
  - infant or child F98.3
- **Picking, nose** F98.8
- **Pick-Niemann disease** — *see* Niemann-Pick disease or syndrome
- **Pick's**
  - cerebral atrophy — *see also* Dementia, in, diseases specified elsewhere G31.Ø1 *[FØ2.8Ø]*
    - with behavioral disturbance — *see also* Dementia, in, diseases specified elsewhere G31.Ø1 *[FØ2.81-]* ☑
  - disease or syndrome (brain) — *see also* Dementia, in, diseases specified elsewhere G31.Ø1 *[FØ2.8Ø]*
    - with behavioral disturbance — *see also* Dementia, in, diseases specified elsewhere G31.Ø1 *[FØ2.81-]* ☑
    - brain — *see also* Dementia, in, diseases specified elsewhere G31.Ø1 *[FØ2.8Ø]*
      - with behavioral disturbance — *see also* Dementia, in, diseases specified elsewhere G31.Ø1 *[FØ2.81-]* ☑
    - pericardium (pericardial pseudocirrhosis of liver) I31.1
  - syndrome
    - brain — *see also* Dementia, in, diseases specified elsewhere G31.Ø1 *[FØ2.8Ø]*
      - with behavioral disturbance — *see also* Dementia, in, diseases specified elsewhere G31.Ø1 *[FØ2.81-]* ☑
    - of heart (pericardial pseudocirrhosis of liver) I31.1
- **Pickwickian syndrome** E66.2
- **Piebaldism** E7Ø.39
- **Piedra** (beard) (scalp) B36.8
  - black B36.3
  - white B36.2
- **Pierre Robin deformity or syndrome** Q87.Ø
- **Pierson's disease or osteochondrosis** M91.Ø
- **Pig-bel** AØ5.2
- **Pigeon**
  - breast or chest (acquired) M95.4
    - congenital Q67.7
    - rachitic sequelae (late effect) E64.3
  - breeder's disease or lung J67.2
  - fancier's disease or lung J67.2
  - toe — *see* Deformity, toe, specified NEC
- **Pigmentation** (abnormal) (anomaly) L81.9
  - conjunctiva H11.13- ☑
  - cornea (anterior) H18.Ø1- ☑
    - posterior H18.Ø5- ☑
    - stromal H18.Ø6- ☑
  - diminished melanin formation NEC L81.6
  - iron L81.8
  - lids, congenital Q82.8
  - limbus corneae — *see* Pigmentation, cornea
  - metals L81.8
  - optic papilla, congenital Q14.2
- **Pigmentation** — *continued*
  - retina, congenital (grouped) (nevoid) Q14.1
  - scrotum, congenital Q82.8
  - tattoo L81.8
- **Piles** — *see also* Hemorrhoids K64.9
- **Pili**
  - annulati or torti (congenital) Q84.1
  - incarnati L73.1
- **Pill roller hand** (intrinsic) — *see* Parkinsonism
- **Pilomatrixoma** — *see* Neoplasm, skin, benign
  - malignant — *see* Neoplasm, skin, malignant
- **Pilonidal** — *see* condition
- **Pimple** R23.8
- **PIMS** M35.81
- **PIN** — *see* Neoplasia, intraepithelial, prostate
- **Pinched nerve** — *see* Neuropathy, entrapment
- **Pindborg tumor** — *see* Cyst, calcifying odontogenic
- **Pineal body or gland** — *see* condition
- **Pinealoblastoma** C75.3
- **Pinealoma** D44.5
  - malignant C75.3
- **Pineoblastoma** C75.3
- **Pineocytoma** D44.5
- **Pinguecula** H11.15- ☑
- **Pingueculitis** H1Ø.81- ☑
- **Pinhole meatus** — *see also* Stricture, urethra N35.919
- **Pink**
  - disease — *see* subcategory T56.1 ☑
  - eye — *see* Conjunctivitis, acute, mucopurulent
- **Pinkus' disease** (lichen nitidus) L44.1
- **Pinpoint**
  - meatus — *see* Stricture, urethra
  - os (uteri) — *see* Stricture, cervix
- **Pins and needles** R2Ø.2
- **Pinta** A67.9
  - cardiovascular lesions A67.2
  - chancre (primary) A67.Ø
  - erythematous plaques A67.1
  - hyperchromic lesions A67.1
  - hyperkeratosis A67.1
  - lesions A67.9
    - cardiovascular A67.2
    - hyperchromic A67.1
    - intermediate A67.1
    - late A67.2
    - mixed A67.3
    - primary A67.Ø
    - skin (achromic) (cicatricial) (dyschromic) A67.2
      - hyperchromic A67.1
      - mixed (achromic and hyperchromic) A67.3
  - papule (primary) A67.Ø
  - skin lesions (achromic) (cicatricial) (dyschromic) A67.2
    - hyperchromic A67.1
    - mixed (achromic and hyperchromic) A67.3
  - vitiligo A67.2
- **Pintids** A67.1
- **Pinworm** (disease) (infection) (infestation) B8Ø
- **Piroplasmosis** — *see also* Babesiosis B6Ø.ØØ
  - specified NEC B6Ø.Ø9
- **Pistol wound** — *see* Gunshot wound
- **Pitchers' elbow** — *see* Derangement, joint, specified type NEC, elbow
- **Pithecoid pelvis** Q74.2
  - with disproportion (fetopelvic) O33.Ø
    - causing obstructed labor O65.Ø
- **Pithiatism** F48.8
- **Pitted** — *see* Pitting
- **Pitting** — *see also* Edema R6Ø.9
  - lip R6Ø.Ø
  - nail L6Ø.8
  - teeth KØØ.4
- **Pituitary gland** — *see* condition
- **Pituitary-snuff-taker's disease** J67.8
- **Pityriasis** (capitis) L21.Ø
  - alba L3Ø.5
  - circinata (et maculata) L42
  - furfuracea L21.Ø
  - Hebra's L26
  - lichenoides L41.Ø
    - chronica L41.1
    - et varioliformis (acuta) L41.Ø
  - maculata (et circinata) L3Ø.5
  - nigra B36.1
  - pilaris, Hebra's L44.Ø
  - rosea L42
  - rotunda L44.8
  - rubra (Hebra) pilaris L44.Ø

Pityriasis — *continued*
- simplex L3Ø.5
- specified type NEC L3Ø.5
- streptogenes L3Ø.5
- versicolor (scrotal) B36.Ø

Placenta, placental — *see* Pregnancy, complicated by (care of) (management affected by), specified condition
Placentitis O41.14- ☑
Plagiocephaly Q67.3
- non-deformational
  - anterior Q75.Ø21
  - posterior Q75.Ø4- ☑

Plague A2Ø.9
- abortive A2Ø.8
- ambulatory A2Ø.8
- asymptomatic A2Ø.8
- bubonic A2Ø.Ø
- cellulocutaneous A2Ø.1
- cutaneobubonic A2Ø.1
- lymphatic gland A2Ø.Ø
- meningitis A2Ø.3
- pharyngeal A2Ø.8
- pneumonic (primary) (secondary) A2Ø.2
- pulmonary, pulmonic A2Ø.2
- septicemic A2Ø.7
- tonsillar A2Ø.8
  - septicemic A2Ø.7

Planning, family
- contraception Z3Ø.9
- procreation Z31.69

Plaque(s)
- artery, arterial — *see* Arteriosclerosis
- calcareous — *see* Calcification
- coronary, lipid rich I25.83
- epicardial I31.8
- erythematous, of pinta A67.1
- Hollenhorst's — *see* Occlusion, artery, retina
- lipid rich, coronary I25.83
- pleural (without asbestos) J92.9
  - with asbestos J92.Ø
- tongue K13.29

Plasmacytoma C9Ø.3- ☑
- extramedullary C9Ø.2- ☑
- medullary C9Ø.Ø- ☑
- solitary C9Ø.3- ☑

Plasmacytopenia D72.818
Plasmacytosis D72.822
Plaster ulcer — *see* Ulcer, pressure, by site
Plateau iris syndrome (post-iridectomy) (postprocedural) (without glaucoma) H21.82
- with glaucoma H4Ø.22- ☑

Platybasia Q75.8
Platyonychia (congenital) Q84.6
- acquired L6Ø.8

Platypelloid pelvis M95.5
- with disproportion (fetopelvic) O33.Ø
  - causing obstructed labor O65.Ø
- congenital Q74.2

Platyspondylisis Q76.49
Plaut (-Vincent) **disease** — *see also* Vincent's A69.1
Plethora R23.2
- newborn P61.1

Pleura, pleural — *see* condition
Pleuralgia RØ7.81
Pleurisy (acute) (adhesive) (chronic) (costal) (diaphragmatic) (double) (dry) (fibrinous) (fibrous) (interlobar) (latent) (plastic) (primary) (residual) (sicca) (sterile) (subacute) (unresolved) RØ9.1
- with
  - adherent pleura J86.Ø
  - effusion J9Ø
    - chylous, chyliform J94.Ø
    - tuberculous (non primary) A15.6
      - primary (progressive) A15.7
  - tuberculosis — *see* Pleurisy, tuberculous (non primary)
- encysted — *see* Pleurisy, with effusion
- exudative — *see* Pleurisy, with effusion
- fibrinopurulent, fibropurulent — *see* Pyothorax
- hemorrhagic — *see* Hemothorax
- pneumococcal J9Ø
- purulent — *see* Pyothorax
- septic — *see* Pyothorax
- serofibrinous — *see* Pleurisy, with effusion
- seropurulent — *see* Pyothorax
- serous — *see* Pleurisy, with effusion

Pleurisy — *continued*
- staphylococcal J86.9
- streptococcal J9Ø
- suppurative — *see* Pyothorax
- traumatic (post) (current) — *see* Injury, intrathoracic, pleura
- tuberculous (with effusion) (non primary) A15.6
  - primary (progressive) A15.7

Pleuritis sicca — *see* Pleurisy
Pleurobronchopneumonia — *see* Pneumonia, broncho-
Pleurodynia RØ7.81
- epidemic B33.Ø
- viral B33.Ø

Pleuropericarditis — *see also* Pericarditis
- acute I3Ø.9

Pleuropneumonia (acute) (bilateral) (double) (septic) — *see also* Pneumonia J18.8
- chronic — *see* Fibrosis, lung

Pleuro-pneumonia-like-organism (PPLO), as cause of disease classified elsewhere B96.Ø
Pleurorrhea — *see* Pleurisy, with effusion
Plexitis, brachial G54.Ø
Plica
- polonica B85.Ø
- syndrome, knee M67.5- ☑
- tonsil J35.8

Plicated tongue K14.5
Plug
- bronchus NEC J98.Ø9
- meconium (newborn) NEC syndrome P76.Ø
- mucus — *see* Asphyxia, mucus

Plumbism — *see* subcategory T56.Ø ☑
Plummer's disease EØ5.2Ø
- with thyroid storm EØ5.21

Plummer-Vinson syndrome D5Ø.1
Pluricarential syndrome of infancy E4Ø
Plus (and minus) **hand** (intrinsic) — *see* Deformity, limb, specified type NEC, forearm
PMEI (polymorphic epilepsy in infancy) G4Ø.83- ☑
Pneumathemia — *see* Air, embolism
Pneumatic hammer (drill) syndrome T75.21 ☑
Pneumatocele (lung) J98.4
- intracranial G93.89
- tension J98.8

Pneumatosis
- cystoides intestinalis K63.89
- intestinalis K63.89
- peritonei K66.8

Pneumaturia R39.89
Pneumoblastoma — *see* Neoplasm, lung, malignant
Pneumocephalus G93.89
Pneumococcemia A4Ø.3
Pneumococcus, pneumococcal — *see* condition
Pneumoconiosis (due to) (inhalation of) J64
- with tuberculosis (any type in A15) J65
- aluminum J63.Ø
- asbestos J61
- bagasse, bagassosis J67.1
- bauxite J63.1
- beryllium J63.2
- coal miners' (simple) J6Ø
- coalworkers' (simple) J6Ø
- collier's J6Ø
- cotton dust J66.Ø
- diatomite (diatomaceous earth) J62.8
- dust
  - inorganic NEC J63.6
  - lime J62.8
  - marble J62.8
  - organic NEC J66.8
- fumes or vapors (from silo) J68.9
- graphite J63.3
- grinder's J62.8
- kaolin J62.8
- mica J62.8
- millstone maker's J62.8
- mineral fibers NEC J61
- miner's J6Ø
- moldy hay J67.Ø
- potter's J62.8
- rheumatoid — *see* Rheumatoid, lung
- sandblaster's J62.8
- silica, silicate NEC J62.8
  - with carbon J6Ø
- stonemason's J62.8
- talc (dust) J62.Ø

Pneumocystis carinii pneumonia B59
Pneumocystis jiroveci (pneumonia) B59
Pneumocystosis (with pneumonia) B59
Pneumohemopericardium I31.2
Pneumohemothorax J94.2
- traumatic S27.2 ☑

Pneumohydropericardium — *see* Pericarditis
Pneumohydrothorax — *see* Hydrothorax
Pneumomediastinum J98.2
- congenital or perinatal P25.2

Pneumomycosis B49 *[J99]*
Pneumonia (acute) (double) (migratory) (purulent) (septic) (unresolved) J18.9
- with
  - influenza — *see* Influenza, with, pneumonia
  - lung abscess J85.1
    - due to specified organism — *see* Pneumonia, in (due to)
- 2Ø19 (novel) coronavirus J12.82
- adenoviral J12.Ø
- adynamic J18.2
- alba A5Ø.Ø4
- allergic — *see also* Pneumonitis, hypersensitivity J82.89
- alveolar — *see* Pneumonia, lobar
- anaerobes J15.8
- anthrax A22.1
- apex, apical — *see* Pneumonia, lobar
- Ascaris B77.81
- aspiration J69.Ø
  - due to
    - aspiration of microorganisms
      - bacterial J15.9
      - viral J12.9
    - food (regurgitated) J69.Ø
    - gastric secretions J69.Ø
    - milk (regurgitated) J69.Ø
    - oils, essences J69.1
    - solids, liquids NEC J69.8
    - vomitus J69.Ø
  - newborn P24.81
    - amniotic fluid (clear) P24.11
    - blood P24.21
    - food (regurgitated) P24.31
    - liquor (amnii) P24.11
    - meconium P24.Ø1
    - milk P24.31
    - mucus P24.11
    - specified NEC P24.81
    - stomach contents P24.31
  - postprocedural J95.4
- atypical NEC J18.9
- bacillus J15.9
  - specified NEC J15.8
- bacterial J15.9
  - specified NEC J15.8
- Bacteroides (fragilis) (oralis) (melaninogenicus) J15.8
- basal, basic, basilar — *see* Pneumonia, by type
- bronchiolitis obliterans organized (BOOP) J84.89
- broncho-, bronchial (confluent) (croupous) (diffuse) (disseminated) (hemorrhagic) (involving lobes) (lobar) (terminal) J18.Ø
  - allergic — *see also* Pneumonitis, hypersensitivity J82.89
  - aspiration — *see* Pneumonia, aspiration
  - bacterial J15.9
    - specified NEC J15.8
  - chronic — *see* Fibrosis, lung
  - diplococcal J13
  - Eaton's agent J15.7
  - Escherichia coli (E. coli) J15.5
  - Friedlander's bacillus J15.Ø
  - Hemophilus influenzae J14
  - hypostatic J18.2
  - inhalation — *see also* Pneumonia, aspiration
    - due to fumes or vapors (chemical) J68.Ø
    - of oils or essences J69.1
  - Klebsiella (pneumoniae) J15.Ø
  - lipid, lipoid J69.1
    - endogenous J84.89
  - Mycoplasma (pneumoniae) J15.7
  - pleuro-pneumonia-like-organisms (PPLO) J15.7
  - pneumococcal J13
  - Proteus J15.69
  - Pseudomonas J15.1
  - Serratia marcescens J15.69
  - specified organism NEC J16.8
  - staphylococcal — *see* Pneumonia, staphylococcal
  - streptococcal NEC J15.4
    - group B J15.3
    - pneumoniae J13

Pneumonia — *continued*
  broncho-, bronchial — *continued*
    viral, virus — *see* Pneumonia, viral
  Butyrivibrio (fibriosolvens) J15.8
  Candida B37.1
  caseous — *see* Tuberculosis, pulmonary
  catarrhal — *see* Pneumonia, broncho
  chlamydial J16.Ø
    congenital P23.1
  cholesterol J84.89
  cirrhotic (chronic) — *see* Fibrosis, lung
  Clostridium (haemolyticum) (novyi) J15.8
  confluent — *see* Pneumonia, broncho
  congenital (infective) P23.9
    due to
      bacterium NEC P23.6
      Chlamydia P23.1
      Escherichia coli P23.4
      Haemophilus influenzae P23.6
      infective organism NEC P23.8
      Klebsiella pneumoniae P23.6
      Mycoplasma P23.6
      Pseudomonas P23.5
      Staphylococcus P23.2
      Streptococcus (except group B) P23.6
        group B P23.3
      viral agent P23.Ø
    specified NEC P23.8
  coronavirus (novel) (disease) 2Ø19 J12.82
  COVID-19 J12.82
  croupous — *see* Pneumonia, lobar
  cryptogenic organizing J84.116
  cytomegalic inclusion B25.Ø
  cytomegaloviral B25.Ø
  deglutition — *see* Pneumonia, aspiration
  desquamative interstitial J84.117
  diffuse — *see* Pneumonia, broncho
  diplococcal, diplococcus (broncho-) (lobar) J13
  disseminated (focal) — *see* Pneumonia, broncho
  Eaton's agent J15.7
  embolic, embolism — *see* Embolism, pulmonary
  Enterobacter J15.69
  eosinophilic J82.81
    acute J82.82
    chronic J82.81
  Escherichia coli (E. coli) J15.5
  Eubacterium J15.8
  fibrinous — *see* Pneumonia, lobar
  fibroid, fibrous (chronic) — *see* Fibrosis, lung
  Friedlander's bacillus J15.Ø
  Fusobacterium (nucleatum) J15.8
  gangrenous J85.Ø
  giant cell (measles) BØ5.2
  gonococcal A54.84
  gram-negative bacteria NEC J15.69
    anaerobic J15.8
  Hemophilus influenzae (broncho) (lobar) J14
  human metapneumovirus J12.3
  hypostatic (broncho) (lobar) J18.2
  in (due to)
    Acinetobacter baumannii J15.61
    actinomycosis A42.Ø
    adenovirus J12.Ø
    anthrax A22.1
    ascariasis B77.81
    aspergillosis B44.9
    Bacillus anthracis A22.1
    Bacterium anitratum J15.69
    candidiasis B37.1
    chickenpox BØ1.2
    Chlamydia J16.Ø
      neonatal P23.1
    coccidioidomycosis B38.2
      acute B38.Ø
      chronic B38.1
    cytomegalovirus disease B25.Ø
    Diplococcus (pneumoniae) J13
    Eaton's agent J15.7
    Enterobacter J15.69
    Escherichia coli (E. coli) J15.5
    Friedlander's bacillus J15.Ø
    fumes and vapors (chemical) (inhalation) J68.Ø
    gonorrhea A54.84
    Hemophilus influenzae (H. influenzae) J14
    Herellea J15.69
    histoplasmosis B39.2
      acute B39.Ø
      chronic B39.1

Pneumonia — *continued*
  in — *continued*
    human metapneumovirus J12.3
    Klebsiella (pneumoniae) J15.Ø
    measles BØ5.2
    Mycoplasma (pneumoniae) J15.7
    nocardiosis, nocardiasis A43.Ø
    ornithosis A7Ø
    parainfluenza virus J12.2
    pleuro-pneumonia-like-organism (PPLO) J15.7
    pneumococcus J13
    pneumocystosis (Pneumocystis carinii) (Pneumocystis jiroveci) B59
    Proteus J15.69
    Pseudomonas NEC J15.1
      pseudomallei A24.1
    psittacosis A7Ø
    Q fever A78
    respiratory syncytial virus (RSV) J12.1
    rheumatic fever IØØ *[J17]*
    rubella BØ6.81
    Salmonella (infection) AØ2.22
      typhi AØ1.Ø3
    schistosomiasis B65.9 *[J17]*
    Serratia marcescens J15.69
    specified
      bacterium NEC J15.8
      organism NEC J16.8
    spirochetal NEC A69.8
    Staphylococcus J15.2Ø
      aureus (methicillin susceptible) (MSSA) J15.211
        methicillin resistant (MRSA) J15.212
      specified NEC J15.29
    Streptococcus J15.4
      group B J15.3
      pneumoniae J13
      specified NEC J15.4
    toxoplasmosis B58.3
    tularemia A21.2
    typhoid (fever) AØ1.Ø3
    varicella BØ1.2
    virus — *see* Pneumonia, viral
    whooping cough A37.91
      due to
        Bordetella parapertussis A37.11
        Bordetella pertussis A37.Ø1
        specified NEC A37.81
    Yersinia pestis A2Ø.2
  inhalation of food or vomit — *see* Pneumonia, aspiration
  interstitial J84.9
    chronic J84.111
    desquamative J84.117
    due to
      collagen vascular disease J84.178
      known underlying cause J84.178
    idiopathic NOS J84.111
    in disease classified elsewhere J84.178
    lymphocytic (due to collagen vascular disease) (in diseases classified elsewhere) J84.178
    lymphoid J84.2
    non-specific J84.89
      due to
        collagen vascular disease J84.178
        known underlying cause J84.178
      idiopathic J84.113
      in diseases classified elsewhere J84.178
    plasma cell B59
    pseudomonas J15.1
    usual J84.112
      due to collagen vascular disease J84.178
      idiopathic J84.112
      in diseases classified elsewhere J84.178
  Klebsiella (pneumoniae) J15.Ø
  lipid, lipoid (exogenous) J69.1
    endogenous J84.89
  lobar (disseminated) (double) (interstitial) J18.1
    bacterial J15.9
      specified NEC J15.8
    chronic — *see* Fibrosis, lung
    Escherichia coli (E. coli) J15.5
    Friedlander's bacillus J15.Ø
    Hemophilus influenzae J14
    hypostatic J18.2
    Klebsiella (pneumoniae) J15.Ø
    pneumococcal J13
    Proteus J15.69
    Pseudomonas J15.1
    specified organism NEC J16.8

Pneumonia — *continued*
  lobar — *continued*
    staphylococcal — *see* Pneumonia, staphylococcal
    streptococcal NEC J15.4
    Streptococcus pneumoniae J13
    viral, virus — *see* Pneumonia, viral
  lobular — *see* Pneumonia, broncho
  Loffler's J82.89
  lymphoid interstitial J84.2
  massive — *see* Pneumonia, lobar
  meconium P24.Ø1
  MRSA (methicillin resistant Staphylococcus aureus) J15.212
  MSSA (methicillin susceptible Staphylococcus aureus) J15.211
  multilobar — *see* Pneumonia, by type
  Mycoplasma (pneumoniae) J15.7
  necrotic J85.Ø
  neonatal P23.9
    aspiration — *see* Aspiration, by substance, with pneumonia
  nitrogen dioxide J68.Ø
  organizing J84.89
    due to
      collagen vascular disease J84.178
      known underlying cause J84.178
    in diseases classified elsewhere J84.178
  orthostatic J18.2
  parainfluenza virus J12.2
  parenchymatous — *see* Fibrosis, lung
  passive J18.2
  patchy — *see* Pneumonia, broncho
  Peptococcus J15.8
  Peptostreptococcus J15.8
  plasma cell (of infants) B59
  pleurolobar — *see* Pneumonia, lobar
  pleuro-pneumonia-like organism (PPLO) J15.7
  pneumococcal (broncho) (lobar) J13
  Pneumocystis (carinii) (jiroveci) B59
  postinfectional NEC B99 ☑ *[J17]*
  postmeasles BØ5.2
  Proteus J15.69
  Pseudomonas J15.1
  psittacosis A7Ø
  radiation J7Ø.Ø
  respiratory syncytial virus (RSV) J12.1
  resulting from a procedure J95.89
  rheumatic IØØ *[J17]*
  Salmonella (arizonae) (cholerae-suis) (enteritidis) (typhimurium) AØ2.22
    typhi AØ1.Ø3
    typhoid fever AØ1.Ø3
  SARS-associated coronavirus J12.81
  SARS-CoV-2 J12.82
  segmented, segmental — *see* Pneumonia, broncho-
  Serratia marcescens J15.69
  specified NEC J18.8
    bacterium NEC J15.8
    organism NEC J16.8
    virus NEC J12.89
  spirochetal NEC A69.8
  staphylococcal (broncho) (lobar) J15.2Ø
    aureus (methicillin susceptible) (MSSA) J15.211
      methicillin resistant (MRSA) J15.212
    specified NEC J15.29
  static, stasis J18.2
  streptococcal NEC (broncho) (lobar) J15.4
    group
      A J15.4
      B J15.3
      specified NEC J15.4
  Streptococcus pneumoniae J13
  syphilitic, congenital (early) A5Ø.Ø4
  traumatic (complication) (early) (secondary) T79.8 ☑
  tuberculous (any) — *see* Tuberculosis, pulmonary
  tularemic A21.2
  varicella BØ1.2
  Veillonella J15.8
  ventilator associated J95.851
  viral, virus (broncho) (interstitial) (lobar) J12.9
    adenoviral J12.Ø
    congenital P23.Ø
    human metapneumovirus J12.3
    parainfluenza J12.2
    respiratory syncytial (RSV) J12.1
    SARS-associated coronavirus J12.81
    specified NEC J12.89
  white (congenital) A5Ø.Ø4

Polyp, polypus — *continued*
  colon — *continued*
    inflammatory — *continued*
      with — *continued*
        complication K51.419
          specified NEC K51.418
        fistula K51.413
        intestinal obstruction K51.412
        rectal bleeding K51.411
    sigmoid K63.5
    transverse K63.5
  corpus uteri N84.Ø
  dental KØ4.Ø1
    irreversible KØ4.Ø2
    reversible KØ4.Ø1
  duodenum K31.7
  ear (middle) H74.4- ☑
  endometrium N84.Ø
  esophageal K22.81
  esophagogastric junction K22.82
  ethmoidal (sinus) J33.8
  fallopian tube N84.8
  female genital tract N84.9
    specified NEC N84.8
  frontal (sinus) J33.8
  gallbladder K82.4
  gingiva, gum KØ6.8
  labia, labium (majus) (minus) N84.3
  larynx (mucous) J38.1
    adenomatous D14.1
  malignant — *see* Neoplasm, malignant, by site
  maxillary (sinus) J33.8
  middle ear — *see* Polyp, ear (middle)
  myometrium N84.Ø
  nares
    anterior J33.9
    posterior J33.Ø
  nasal (mucous) J33.9
    cavity J33.Ø
    septum J33.Ø
  nasopharyngeal J33.Ø
  nose (mucous) J33.9
  oviduct N84.8
  pharynx J39.2
  placenta O9Ø.89
  prostate — *see* Enlargement, enlarged, prostate
  pudenda, pudendum N84.3
  pulpal (dental) KØ4.Ø1
    irreversible KØ4.Ø2
    reversible KØ4.Ø1
  rectum (nonadenomatous) K62.1
    adenomatous — *see* Polyp, adenomatous
  septum (nasal) J33.Ø
  sinus (accessory) (ethmoidal) (frontal) (maxillary) (sphenoidal) J33.8
  sphenoidal (sinus) J33.8
  stomach K31.7
    adenomatous D13.1
  tube, fallopian N84.8
  turbinate, mucous membrane J33.8
  umbilical, newborn P83.6
  ureter N28.89
  urethra N36.2
  uterus (body) (corpus) (mucous) N84.Ø
    cervix N84.1
    in pregnancy or childbirth — *see* Pregnancy, complicated by, tumor, uterus
  vagina N84.2
  vocal cord (mucous) J38.1
  vulva N84.3
Polyphagia R63.2
Polyploidy Q92.7
Polypoid — *see* condition
Polyposis — *see also* Polyp
  adenomatous D13.91
  coli (adenomatous) D12.6
    adenocarcinoma in C18.9
    adenocarcinoma in situ in — *see* Neoplasm, in situ, by site
    carcinoma in C18.9
  colon (adenomatous) D12.6
  familial D12.6
    adenocarcinoma in situ in — *see* Neoplasm, in situ, by site
    adenomatous D13.91
  intestinal D12.6
    adenomatous D13.91
  malignant lymphomatous C83.1- ☑

Polyposis — *continued*
  multiple, adenomatous — *see also* Neoplasm, benign D36.9
Polyradiculitis — *see* Polyneuropathy
Polyradiculoneuropathy (acute) (postinfective) (segmentally demyelinating) G61.Ø
Polyserositis
  due to pericarditis I31.1
  pericardial I31.1
  periodic, familial E85.Ø
  tuberculous A19.9
    acute A19.1
    chronic A19.8
Polysplenia syndrome Q89.Ø9
Polysyndactyly — *see also* Syndactylism, syndactyly Q7Ø.4
Polytrichia L68.3
Polyunguia Q84.6
Polyuria R35.89
  nocturnal R35.81
  psychogenic F45.8
  specified NEC R35.89
Pompe's disease (glycogen storage) E74.Ø2
Pompholyx L3Ø.1
Poncet's disease (tuberculous rheumatism) A18.Ø9
Pond fracture — *see* Fracture, skull
Ponos B55.Ø
Pons, pontine — *see* condition
Poor
  aesthetic of existing restoration of tooth KØ8.56
  contractions, labor O62.2
  gingival margin to tooth restoration KØ8.51
  personal hygiene R46.Ø
  prenatal care, affecting management of pregnancy — *see* Pregnancy, complicated by, insufficient, prenatal care
  sucking reflex (newborn) R29.2
  urinary stream R39.12
  vision NEC H54.7
Poradenitis, nostras inguinalis or venerea A55
Porencephaly (congenital) (developmental) (true) QØ4.6
  acquired G93.Ø
  nondevelopmental G93.Ø
  traumatic (post) FØ7.89
Porocephaliasis B88.8
Porokeratosis Q82.8
Poroma, eccrine — *see* Neoplasm, skin, benign
Porphyria (South African) E8Ø.2Ø
  acquired E8Ø.2Ø
  acute intermittent (hepatic) (Swedish) E8Ø.21
  cutanea tarda (hereditary) (symptomatic) E8Ø.1
  due to drugs E8Ø.2Ø
    correct substance properly administered — *see* Table of Drugs and Chemicals, by drug, adverse effect
    overdose or wrong substance given or taken — *see* Table of Drugs and Chemicals, by drug, poisoning
  erythropoietic (congenital) (hereditary) E8Ø.Ø
  hepatocutaneous type E8Ø.1
  secondary E8Ø.2Ø
  toxic NEC E8Ø.2Ø
  variegata E8Ø.2Ø
Porphyrinuria — *see* Porphyria
Porphyruria — *see* Porphyria
Port wine nevus, mark, or stain Q82.5
Portal — *see* condition
Posadas-Wernicke disease B38.9
Positive
  culture (nonspecific)
    blood R78.81
    bronchial washings R84.5
    cerebrospinal fluid R83.5
    cervix uteri R87.5
    nasal secretions R84.5
    nipple discharge R89.5
    nose R84.5
      staphylococcus (Methicillin susceptible) Z22.321
        Methicillin resistant Z22.322
    peritoneal fluid R85.5
    pleural fluid R84.5
    prostatic secretions R86.5
    saliva R85.5
    seminal fluid R86.5
    sputum R84.5
    synovial fluid R89.5
    throat scrapings R84.5
    urine R82.79

Positive — *continued*
  culture — *continued*
    vagina R87.5
    vulva R87.5
    wound secretions R89.5
  PPD (skin test) R76.11
  serology for syphilis A53.Ø
    false R76.8
    with signs or symptoms — *code as* Syphilis, by site and stage
  skin test, tuberculin (without active tuberculosis) R76.11
  test, human immunodeficiency virus (HIV) R75
  VDRL A53.Ø
    with signs or symptoms — *code by* site and stage under Syphilis A53.9
  Wassermann reaction A53.Ø
Post COVID-19 condition, unspecified UØ9.9
Postcardiotomy syndrome I97.Ø
Postcaval ureter Q62.62
Postcholecystectomy syndrome K91.5
Postclimacteric bleeding N95.Ø
Postcommissurotomy syndrome I97.Ø
Postconcussional syndrome FØ7.81
Postcontusional syndrome FØ7.81
Postcricoid region — *see* condition
Post-dates (4Ø-42 weeks) (pregnancy) (mother) O48.Ø
  more than 42 weeks gestation O48.1
Postencephalitic syndrome FØ7.89
Posterior — *see* condition
Posterolateral sclerosis (spinal cord) — *see* Degeneration, combined
Postexanthematous — *see* condition
Postfebrile — *see* condition
Postgastrectomy dumping syndrome K91.1
Posthemiplegic chorea — *see* Monoplegia
Posthemorrhagic anemia (chronic) D5Ø.Ø
  acute D62
  newborn P61.3
Postherpetic neuralgia (zoster) BØ2.29
  trigeminal BØ2.22
Posthitis N47.7
Postimmunization complication or reaction — *see* Complications, vaccination
Postinfectious — *see* condition
Postlaminectomy syndrome NEC M96.1
Postleukotomy syndrome FØ7.Ø
Postmastectomy lymphedema (syndrome) I97.2
Postmaturity, postmature (over 42 weeks)
  maternal (over 42 weeks gestation) O48.1
  newborn PØ8.22
Postmeasles complication NEC — *see also* condition BØ5.89
Postmenopausal
  endometrium (atrophic) N95.8
    suppurative — *see also* Endometritis N71.9
  osteoporosis — *see* Osteoporosis, postmenopausal
Postnasal drip RØ9.82
  due to
    allergic rhinitis — *see* Rhinitis, allergic
    common cold JØØ
    gastroesophageal reflux — *see* Reflux, gastroesophageal
    nasopharyngitis — *see* Nasopharyngitis
    other known condition — *code to* condition
    sinusitis — *see* Sinusitis
Postnatal — *see* condition
Postoperative (postprocedural) — *see also* Complication, postoperative
  pneumothorax, therapeutic Z98.3
  state NEC Z98.89Ø
  visit — *see* Aftercare
  wound check — *see* Aftercare
Postpancreatectomy hyperglycemia E89.1
Postpartum — *see* Puerperal
Postphlebitic syndrome — *see* Syndrome, postthrombotic
Postpolio (myelitic) **syndrome** G14
Postpoliomyelitic — *see also* condition
  osteopathy — *see* Osteopathy, after poliomyelitis
Postprocedural — *see also* Postoperative
  hypoinsulinemia E89.1
Postschizophrenic depression F32.89
Postsurgery status — *see also* Status (post)
  pneumothorax, therapeutic Z98.3
Post-term (4Ø-42 weeks) (pregnancy) (mother) O48.Ø
  infant PØ8.21
  more than 42 weeks gestation (mother) O48.1

- **Post-traumatic brain syndrome, nonpsychotic** FØ7.81
- **Post-typhoid abscess** AØ1.Ø9
- **Postures, hysterical** F44.2
- **Postvaccinal reaction or complication** — *see* Complications, vaccination
- **Postvalvulotomy syndrome** I97.Ø
- **Potain's**
  - disease (pulmonary edema) — *see* Edema, lung
  - syndrome (gastrectasis with dyspepsia) K31.Ø
- **POTS** (postural orthostatic tachycardia syndrome) G9Ø.A
- **Potter's**
  - asthma J62.8
  - facies Q6Ø.6
  - lung J62.8
  - syndrome (with renal agenesis) Q6Ø.6
- **Pott's**
  - curvature (spinal) A18.Ø1
  - disease or paraplegia A18.Ø1
  - spinal curvature A18.Ø1
  - tumor, puffy — *see* Osteomyelitis, specified type NEC
- **Pouch**
  - bronchus Q32.4
  - Douglas' — *see* condition
  - esophagus, esophageal, congenital Q39.6
    - acquired K22.5
  - gastric K31.4
  - Hartmann's K82.8
  - pharynx, pharyngeal (congenital) Q38.7
- **Pouchitis** K91.85Ø
- **Poultrymen's itch** B88.Ø
- **Poverty NEC** Z59.6
  - extreme Z59.5
- **Poxvirus NEC** BØ8.8
- **Prader-Willi syndrome** Q87.11
- **Prader-Willi-like syndrome** Q87.19
- **Preauricular appendage or tag** Q17.Ø
- **Prebetalipoproteinemia** (acquired) (essential) (familial) (hereditary) (primary) (secondary) E78.1
  - with chylomicronemia E78.3
- **Precipitate labor or delivery** O62.3
- **Preclimacteric bleeding** (menorrhagia) N92.4
- **Precocious**
  - adrenarche E3Ø.1
  - menarche E3Ø.1
  - menstruation E3Ø.1
  - pubarche E3Ø.1
  - puberty E3Ø.1
    - central E22.8
  - sexual development NEC E3Ø.1
  - thelarche E3Ø.8
- **Precocity, sexual** (constitutional) (cryptogenic) (female) (idiopathic) (male) E3Ø.1
  - with adrenal hyperplasia E25.9
    - congenital E25.Ø
- **Precordial pain** RØ7.2
- **Predeciduous teeth** KØØ.2
- **Prediabetes, prediabetic** R73.Ø3
  - complicating
    - pregnancy — *see* Pregnancy, complicated by, diseases of, specified type or system NEC
    - puerperium O99.893
- **Predislocation status of hip at birth** Q65.6
- **Pre-eclampsia** O14.9- ☑
  - with pre-existing hypertension — *see* Hypertension, complicating pregnancy, pre-existing, with, pre-eclampsia
  - complicating
    - childbirth O14.94
    - puerperium O14.95
  - mild O14.Ø- ☑
    - complicating
      - childbirth O14.Ø4
      - puerperium O14.Ø5
  - moderate O14.Ø- ☑
    - complicating
      - childbirth O14.Ø4
      - puerperium O14.Ø5
  - severe O14.1- ☑
    - with hemolysis, elevated liver enzymes and low platelet count (HELLP) O14.2- ☑
      - complicating
        - childbirth O14.24
        - puerperium O14.25
    - complicating
      - childbirth O14.14
      - puerperium O14.15
- **Pre-eruptive color change, teeth, tooth** KØØ.8
- **Pre-excitation atrioventricular conduction** I45.6
- **Preglaucoma** H4Ø.ØØ- ☑
- **Pregnancy** (single) (uterine) — *see also* Delivery and Puerperal Z33.1

> *Note: The Tabular must be reviewed for assignment of appropriate seventh character for multiple gestation codes in Chapter 15*

> *Note: The Tabular must be reviewed for assignment of the appropriate character indicating the trimester of the pregnancy*

  - abdominal (ectopic) OØØ.ØØ
    - with intrauterine pregnancy OØØ.Ø1
    - with viable fetus O36.7- ☑
  - ampullar OØØ.1Ø- ☑
    - with intrauterine pregnancy OØØ.11- ☑
  - biochemical OØ2.81
  - broad ligament OØØ.8Ø
    - with intrauterine pregnancy OØØ.81
  - cervical OØØ.8
    - with intrauterine pregnancy OØØ.81
  - chemical OØ2.81
  - complicated by (care of) (management affected by)
    - abnormal, abnormality
      - cervix O34.4- ☑
        - causing obstructed labor O65.5
      - cord (umbilical) O69.9 ☑
      - fetal heart rate or rhythm O36.83- ☑
      - findings on antenatal screening of mother O28.9
        - biochemical O28.1
        - chromosomal O28.5
        - cytological O28.2
        - genetic O28.5
        - hematological O28.Ø
        - radiological O28.4
        - specified NEC O28.8
        - ultrasonic O28.3
      - glucose (tolerance) NEC O99.81Ø
      - pelvic organs O34.9- ☑
        - specified NEC O34.8- ☑
          - causing obstructed labor O65.5
      - pelvis (bony) (major) NEC O33.Ø
      - perineum O34.7- ☑
      - position
        - placenta O44.Ø- ☑
          - with hemorrhage O44.1- ☑
        - uterus O34.59- ☑
      - uterus O34.59- ☑
        - causing obstructed labor O65.5
        - congenital O34.Ø- ☑
      - vagina O34.6- ☑
        - causing obstructed labor O65.5
      - vulva O34.7- ☑
        - causing obstructed labor O65.5
    - abruptio placentae — *see* Abruptio placentae
    - abscess or cellulitis
      - bladder O23.1- ☑
      - breast O91.11- ☑
      - genital organ or tract O23.9- ☑
    - abuse
      - physical O9A.31 ☑ (*following* O99)
      - psychological O9A.51 ☑ (*following* O99)
      - sexual O9A.41 ☑ (*following* O99)
    - adverse effect anesthesia O29.9- ☑
      - aspiration pneumonitis O29.Ø1- ☑
      - cardiac arrest O29.11- ☑
      - cardiac complication NEC O29.19- ☑
      - cardiac failure O29.12- ☑
      - central nervous system complication NEC O29.29- ☑
      - cerebral anoxia O29.21- ☑
      - failed or difficult intubation O29.6- ☑
      - inhalation of stomach contents or secretions NOS O29.Ø1- ☑
      - local, toxic reaction O29.3X ☑
      - Mendelson's syndrome O29.Ø1- ☑
      - pressure collapse of lung O29.Ø2- ☑
      - pulmonary complications NEC O29.Ø9- ☑
      - specified NEC O29.8X- ☑
      - spinal and epidural type NEC O29.5X ☑
        - induced headache O29.4- ☑
    - albuminuria — *see also* Proteinuria, gestational O12.1- ☑
    - alcohol use O99.31- ☑
    - amnionitis O41.12- ☑
    - anaphylactoid syndrome of pregnancy O88.Ø1- ☑

Pregnancy — *continued*

  - complicated by — *continued*
    - anemia (conditions in D5Ø-D64) (pre-existing) O99.Ø1- ☑
      - complicating the puerperium O99.Ø3
    - antepartum hemorrhage O46.9- ☑
      - with coagulation defect — *see* Hemorrhage, antepartum, with coagulation defect
      - specified NEC O46.8X- ☑
    - appendicitis O99.61- ☑
    - atrophy (yellow) (acute) liver (subacute) O26.61- ☑
    - bariatric surgery status O99.84- ☑
    - bicornis or bicornuate uterus O34.Ø- ☑
    - biliary tract problems O26.61- ☑
    - breech presentation O32.1 ☑
    - cardiovascular diseases (conditions in IØØ-IØ9, I2Ø-I52, I7Ø-I99) O99.41- ☑
    - cerebrovascular disorders (conditions in I6Ø-I69) O99.41- ☑
    - cervical shortening O26.87- ☑
    - cervicitis O23.51- ☑
    - cesarean scar defect (isthmocele) O34.22
    - chloasma (gravidarum) O26.89- ☑
    - cholecystitis O99.61- ☑
    - cholestasis (intrahepatic) O26.64- ☑
    - chorioamnionitis O41.12- ☑
    - circulatory system disorder (conditions in IØØ-IØ9, I2Ø-I99, O99.41-)
    - compound presentation O32.6 ☑
    - conjoined twins O3Ø.Ø2- ☑
    - connective system disorders (conditions in MØØ-M99) O99.891
    - contracted pelvis (general) O33.1
      - inlet O33.2
      - outlet O33.3 ☑
    - convulsions (eclamptic) (uremic) — *see also* Eclampsia O15.9
    - cracked nipple O92.11- ☑
    - cystitis O23.1- ☑
    - cystocele O34.8- ☑
    - death of fetus (near term) O36.4 ☑
      - early pregnancy OØ2.1
      - of one fetus or more in multiple gestation O31.2- ☑
    - deciduitis O41.14- ☑
    - decreased fetal movement O36.81- ☑
    - dental problems O99.61- ☑
    - diabetes (mellitus) O24.91- ☑
      - gestational (pregnancy induced) — *see* Diabetes, gestational
      - pre-existing O24.31- ☑
        - specified NEC O24.81- ☑
        - type 1 O24.Ø1- ☑
        - type 2 O24.11- ☑
    - digestive system disorders (conditions in KØØ-K93) O99.61- ☑
    - diseases of — *see* Pregnancy, complicated by, specified body system disease
      - biliary tract O26.61- ☑
      - blood NEC (conditions in D65-D77) O99.11- ☑
      - liver O26.61- ☑
      - specified NEC O99.891
    - disorders of — *see* Pregnancy, complicated by, specified body system disorder
      - amniotic fluid and membranes O41.9- ☑
        - specified NEC O41.8X- ☑
      - biliary tract O26.61- ☑
      - ear and mastoid process (conditions in H6Ø-H95) O99.891
      - eye and adnexa (conditions in HØØ-H59) O99.891
      - liver O26.61- ☑
      - skin (conditions in LØØ-L99) O99.71- ☑
      - specified NEC O99.891
    - displacement, uterus NEC O34.59- ☑
      - causing obstructed labor O65.5
    - disproportion (due to) O33.9
      - fetal (ascites) (hydrops) (meningomyelocele) (sacral teratoma) (tumor) deformities NEC O33.7 ☑
      - generally contracted pelvis O33.1
      - hydrocephalic fetus O33.6 ☑
      - inlet contraction of pelvis O33.2
      - mixed maternal and fetal origin O33.4 ☑
      - specified NEC O33.8
    - double uterus O34.Ø- ☑
      - causing obstructed labor O65.5
    - drug use (conditions in F11-F19) O99.32- ☑

- **Pregnancy** — *continued*
  - complicated by — *continued*
    - eclampsia, eclamptic (coma) (convulsions) (delirium) (nephritis) (uremia) — *see also* Eclampsia O15.- ☑
    - ectopic pregnancy — *see* Pregnancy, ectopic
    - edema O12.Ø- ☑
      - with
        - gestational hypertension, mild — *see also* Pre-eclampsia O14.Ø- ☑
        - proteinuria O12.2- ☑
    - effusion, amniotic fluid — *see* Pregnancy, complicated by, premature rupture of membranes
    - elderly
      - multigravida OØ9.52- ☑
      - primigravida OØ9.51- ☑
    - embolism — *see also* Embolism, obstetric, pregnancy O88.- ☑
    - endocrine diseases NEC O99.28- ☑
    - endometritis O86.12
    - excessive weight gain O26.Ø- ☑
    - exhaustion O26.81- ☑
      - during labor and delivery O75.81
    - face presentation O32.3 ☑
    - failed induction of labor O61.9
      - instrumental O61.1
      - mechanical O61.1
      - medical O61.Ø
      - specified NEC O61.8
      - surgical O61.1
    - failed or difficult intubation for anesthesia O29.6- ☑
    - false labor (pains) O47.9
      - at or after 37 completed weeks of pregnancy O47.1
      - before 37 completed weeks of pregnancy O47.Ø- ☑
    - fatigue O26.81- ☑
      - during labor and delivery O75.81
    - fatty metamorphosis of liver O26.61- ☑
    - female genital mutilation O34.8- ☑ *[N9Ø.81-]* ☑
    - fetal (maternal care for)
      - abnormality or damage O35.9 ☑
        - acid-base balance O68
        - specified type NEC O35.8 ☑
      - acidemia O68
      - acidosis O68
      - agenesis of corpus callosum O35.Ø1 ☑
      - alkalosis O68
      - anemia and thrombocytopenia O36.82- ☑
      - anencephaly O35.Ø2 ☑
      - bradycardia O36.83- ☑
      - cardiac anomalies O35.B ☑
      - central nervous system malformation or damage O35.ØØ ☑
        - specified type NEC O35.Ø9 ☑
      - choroid plexus cysts O35.Ø3 ☑
      - chromosomal abnormality (conditions in Q9Ø-Q99) O35.1Ø ☑
        - sex chromosome O35.15 ☑
        - specified NEC O35.19 ☑
        - Trisomy 13 O35.11 ☑
        - Trisomy 18 O35.12 ☑
        - Trisomy 21 O35.13 ☑
        - Turner Syndrome O35.14 ☑
      - conjoined twins O3Ø.Ø2- ☑
      - damage from
        - amniocentesis O35.7 ☑
        - biopsy procedures O35.7 ☑
        - drug addiction O35.5 ☑
        - hematological investigation O35.7 ☑
        - intrauterine contraceptive device O35.7 ☑
        - maternal
          - alcohol addiction O35.4 ☑
          - cytomegalovirus infection O35.3 ☑
          - disease NEC O35.8 ☑
          - drug addiction O35.5 ☑
          - listeriosis O35.8 ☑
          - rubella O35.3 ☑
          - toxoplasmosis O35.8 ☑
          - viral infection O35.3 ☑
        - medical procedure NEC O35.7 ☑
        - radiation O35.6 ☑
      - death (near term) O36.4 ☑
        - early pregnancy OØ2.1
      - decreased movement O36.81- ☑
      - depressed heart rate tones O36.83- ☑
      - disproportion due to deformity (fetal) O33.7 ☑

- **Pregnancy** — *continued*
  - complicated by — *continued*
    - fetal — *continued*
      - encephalocele O35.Ø4 ☑
      - excessive growth (large for dates) O36.6- ☑
      - facial anomalies O35.A ☑
      - gastrointestinal anomalies O35.D ☑
      - genitourinary anomalies O35.E ☑
      - growth retardation O36.59- ☑
        - light for dates O36.59- ☑
        - small for dates O36.59- ☑
      - heart rate irregularity (abnormal variability) (bradycardia) (decelerations) (tachycardia) O36.83- ☑
      - hereditary disease O35.2 ☑
      - holoprosencephaly O35.Ø5 ☑
      - hydrocephalus O35.Ø6 ☑
      - hydrocephaly O35.Ø6 ☑
      - intrauterine death O36.4 ☑
      - microcephaly O35.Ø7 ☑
      - musculoskeletal anomalies
        - lower extremities O35.H ☑
        - trunk O35.F ☑
        - upper extremities O35.G ☑
      - non-reassuring heart rate or rhythm O36.83- ☑
      - poor growth O36.59- ☑
        - light for dates O36.59- ☑
        - small for dates O36.59- ☑
      - problem O36.9- ☑
        - specified NEC O36.89- ☑
      - pulmonary anomalies O35.C ☑
      - reduction (elective) O31.3- ☑
      - selective termination O31.3- ☑
      - spina bifida O35.Ø8 ☑
      - thrombocytopenia O36.82- ☑
    - fibroid (tumor) (uterus) O34.1- ☑
    - fissure of nipple O92.11- ☑
    - gallstones O99.61- ☑
    - gastric banding status O99.84- ☑
    - gastric bypass status O99.84- ☑
    - genital herpes (asymptomatic) (history of) (inactive) O98.3- ☑
    - genital tract infection O23.9- ☑
    - glomerular diseases (conditions in NØØ-NØ7) O26.83- ☑
      - with hypertension, pre-existing — *see* Hypertension, complicating, pregnancy, pre-existing, with, renal disease
    - gonorrhea O98.21- ☑
    - grand multiparity OØ9.4 ☑
    - habitual aborter — *see* Pregnancy, complicated by, recurrent pregnancy loss
    - HELLP syndrome (hemolysis, elevated liver enzymes and low platelet count) O14.2- ☑
    - hemorrhage
      - antepartum — *see* Hemorrhage, antepartum
      - before 2Ø completed weeks gestation O2Ø.9
        - specified NEC O2Ø.8
      - due to premature separation, placenta — *see also* Abruptio placentae O45.9- ☑
      - early O2Ø.9
        - specified NEC O2Ø.8
      - threatened abortion O2Ø.Ø
    - hemorrhoids O22.4- ☑
    - hepatitis (viral) O98.41- ☑
    - herniation of uterus O34.59- ☑
    - high
      - head at term O32.4 ☑
      - risk — *see* Supervision (of) (for), high-risk
    - history of in utero procedure during previous pregnancy OØ9.82- ☑
    - HIV O98.71- ☑
    - human immunodeficiency virus (HIV) disease O98.71- ☑
    - hydatidiform mole — *see also* Mole, hydatidiform OØ1.9
    - hydramnios O4Ø.- ☑
    - hydrocephalic fetus (disproportion) O33.6 ☑
    - hydrops
      - amnii O4Ø.- ☑
      - fetalis O36.2- ☑
        - associated with isoimmunization — *see also* Pregnancy, complicated by, isoimmunization O36.11- ☑
    - hydrorrhea O42.9Ø

- **Pregnancy** — *continued*
  - complicated by — *continued*
    - hyperemesis (gravidarum) (mild) — *see also* Hyperemesis, gravidarum O21.Ø
    - hypertension — *see* Hypertension, complicating pregnancy
    - hypertensive
      - heart and renal disease, pre-existing — *see* Hypertension, complicating, pregnancy, pre-existing, with, heart disease, with renal disease
      - heart disease, pre-existing — *see* Hypertension, complicating, pregnancy, pre-existing, with, heart disease
      - renal disease, pre-existing — *see* Hypertension, complicating, pregnancy, pre-existing, with, renal disease
    - hypotension O26.5- ☑
    - immune disorders NEC (conditions in D8Ø-D89) O99.11- ☑
    - incarceration, uterus O34.51- ☑
    - incompetent cervix O34.3- ☑
    - inconclusive fetal viability O36.8Ø ☑
    - infection(s) O98.91- ☑
      - amniotic fluid or sac O41.1Ø- ☑
      - bladder O23.1- ☑
      - carrier state NEC O99.83Ø
        - streptococcus B O99.82Ø
      - genital organ or tract O23.9- ☑
        - specified NEC O23.59- ☑
      - genitourinary tract O23.9- ☑
      - gonorrhea O98.21- ☑
      - hepatitis (viral) O98.41- ☑
      - HIV O98.71- ☑
      - human immunodeficiency virus (HIV) O98.71- ☑
      - intrauterine O41.12 ☑
      - kidney O23.Ø- ☑
      - nipple O91.Ø1- ☑
      - parasitic disease O98.91- ☑
        - specified NEC O98.81- ☑
      - protozoal disease O98.61- ☑
      - sexually transmitted NEC O98.31- ☑
      - specified type NEC O98.81- ☑
      - syphilis O98.11- ☑
      - tuberculosis O98.Ø1- ☑
      - urethra O23.2- ☑
      - urinary (tract) O23.4- ☑
        - specified NEC O23.3- ☑
      - viral disease O98.51- ☑
    - inflammation
      - intrauterine O41.12 ☑
    - injury or poisoning (conditions in SØØ-T88) O9A.21- ☑ (*following* O99)
      - due to abuse
        - physical O9A.31- ☑ (*following* O99)
        - psychological O9A.51- ☑ (*following* O99)
        - sexual O9A.41- ☑ (*following* O99)
    - insufficient
      - prenatal care OØ9.3- ☑
      - weight gain O26.1- ☑
    - insulin resistance O26.89 ☑
    - intrauterine fetal death (near term) O36.4 ☑
      - early pregnancy OØ2.1
      - multiple gestation (one fetus or more) O31.2- ☑
    - isoimmunization O36.11- ☑
      - anti-A sensitization O36.11- ☑
      - anti-B sensitization O36.19- ☑
      - Rh O36.Ø9- ☑
        - anti-D antibody O36.Ø1- ☑
      - specified NEC O36.19- ☑
    - laceration of uterus NEC O71.81
    - malformation
      - central nervous system O35.ØØ ☑
        - specified type NEC O35.Ø9 ☑
      - placenta, placental (vessel) O43.1Ø- ☑
        - specified NEC O43.19- ☑
      - uterus (congenital) O34.Ø- ☑
    - malnutrition (conditions in E4Ø-E46) O25.1- ☑
    - maternal hypotension syndrome O26.5- ☑
    - mental disorders (conditions in FØ1-FØ9, F2Ø-F52 and F54-F99) O99.34- ☑
      - alcohol use O99.31- ☑
      - drug use O99.32- ☑
      - smoking O99.33- ☑
    - mentum presentation O32.3 ☑
    - metabolic disorders O99.28- ☑

Pregnancy — *continued*
weeks of gestation — *continued*
36 weeks Z3A.36 (*following* Z36)
37 weeks Z3A.37 (*following* Z36)
38 weeks Z3A.38 (*following* Z36)
39 weeks Z3A.39 (*following* Z36)
40 weeks Z3A.40 (*following* Z36)
41 weeks Z3A.41 (*following* Z36)
42 weeks Z3A.42 (*following* Z36)
greater than 42 weeks Z3A.49 (*following* Z36)
less than 8 weeks Z3A.01 (*following* Z36)
not specified Z3A.00 (*following* Z36)
Preiser's disease — *see* Osteonecrosis, secondary, due to, trauma, metacarpus
Pre-kwashiorkor — *see* Malnutrition, severe
Preleukemia (syndrome) D46.9
Preluxation, hip, congenital Q65.6
Premature — *see also* condition
adrenarche E27.0
aging E34.8
beats I49.40
atrial I49.1
auricular I49.1
supraventricular I49.1
birth NEC — *see* Preterm, newborn
closure, foramen ovale Q21.8
contraction
atrial I49.1
atrioventricular I49.2
auricular I49.1
auriculoventricular I49.49
heart (extrasystole) I49.49
junctional I49.2
ventricular I49.3
delivery — *see also* Pregnancy, complicated by, preterm labor O60.10 ☑
ejaculation F52.4
infant NEC — *see* Preterm, newborn
light-for-dates — *see* Light for dates
labor — *see* Pregnancy, complicated by, preterm labor
lungs P28.0
menopause E28.319
asymptomatic E28.319
symptomatic E28.310
newborn
extreme (less than 28 completed weeks) — *see* Immaturity, extreme
less than 37 completed weeks — *see* Preterm, newborn
puberty E30.1
rupture membranes or amnion — *see* Pregnancy, complicated by, premature rupture of membranes
senility E34.8
thelarche E30.8
ventricular systole I49.3
Prematurity NEC (less than 37 completed weeks) — *see* Preterm, newborn
extreme (less than 28 completed weeks) — *see* Immaturity, extreme
Premenstrual
dysphoric disorder (PMDD) F32.81
tension (syndrome) N94.3
Premolarization, cuspids K00.2
Prenatal
care, normal pregnancy — *see* Pregnancy, normal
screening of mother — *see also* Encounter, antenatal screening Z36.9
teeth K00.6
Preparatory care for subsequent treatment NEC
for dialysis Z49.01
peritoneal Z49.02
Prepartum — *see* condition
Preponderance, left or right ventricular I51.7
Prepuce — *see* condition
PRES (posterior reversible encephalopathy syndrome) I67.83
Presbycardia R54
Presbycusis, presbyacusia H91.1- ☑
Presbyesophagus K22.89
Presbyophrenia F03 ☑
Presbyopia H52.4
Prescription of contraceptives (initial) Z30.019
barrier Z30.018
diaphragm Z30.018
emergency (postcoital) Z30.012
implantable subdermal Z30.017
injectable Z30.013

Prescription of contraceptives — *continued*
intrauterine contraceptive device Z30.014
pills Z30.011
postcoital (emergency) Z30.012
repeat Z30.40
barrier Z30.49
diaphragm Z30.49
implantable subdermal Z30.46
injectable Z30.42
pills Z30.41
specified type NEC Z30.49
transdermal patch hormonal Z30.45
vaginal ring hormonal Z30.44
specified type NEC Z30.018
transdermal patch hormonal Z30.016
vaginal ring hormonal Z30.015
Presence (of)
ankle-joint implant (functional) (prosthesis) Z96.66- ☑
aortocoronary (bypass) graft Z95.1
arterial-venous shunt (dialysis) Z99.2
artificial
eye (globe) Z97.0
heart (fully implantable) (mechanical) Z95.812
valve Z95.2
larynx Z96.3
lens (intraocular) Z96.1
limb (complete) (partial) Z97.1- ☑
arm Z97.1- ☑
bilateral Z97.15
leg Z97.1- ☑
bilateral Z97.16
audiological implant (functional) Z96.29
bladder implant (functional) Z96.0
bone
conduction hearing device Z96.29
implant (functional) NEC Z96.7
joint (prosthesis) — *see* Presence, joint implant
cardiac
defibrillator (functional) (with synchronous cardiac pacemaker) Z95.810
implant or graft Z95.9
specified type NEC Z95.818
pacemaker Z95.0
resynchronization therapy
defibrillator Z95.810
pacemaker Z95.0
cardioverter-defibrillator (ICD) Z95.810
cerebrospinal fluid drainage device Z98.2
cochlear implant (functional) Z96.21
contact lens (es) Z97.3
coronary artery graft or prosthesis Z95.5
CRT-D (cardiac resynchronization therapy defibrillator) Z95.810
CRT-P (cardiac resynchronization therapy pacemaker) Z95.0
CSF shunt Z98.2
dental prosthesis device Z97.2
dentures Z97.2
device (external) NEC Z97.8
cardiac NEC Z95.818
heart assist Z95.811
implanted (functional) Z96.9
specified NEC Z96.89
prosthetic Z97.8
ear implant Z96.20
cochlear implant Z96.21
myringotomy tube Z96.22
specified type NEC Z96.29
elbow-joint implant (functional) (prosthesis) Z96.62- ☑
endocrine implant (functional) NEC Z96.49
eustachian tube stent or device (functional) Z96.29
external hearing-aid or device Z97.4
finger-joint implant (functional) (prosthetic) Z96.69- ☑
functional implant Z96.9
specified NEC Z96.89
graft
cardiac NEC Z95.818
vascular NEC Z95.828
hearing-aid or device (external) Z97.4
implant (bone) (cochlear) (functional) Z96.21
heart assist device Z95.811
heart valve implant (functional) Z95.2
prosthetic Z95.2
specified type NEC Z95.4
xenogenic Z95.3
hip-joint implant (functional) (prosthesis) Z96.64- ☑
ICD (cardioverter-defibrillator) Z95.810

Presence — *continued*
implanted device (artificial) (functional) (prosthetic) Z96.9
automatic cardiac defibrillator (with synchronous cardiac pacemaker) Z95.810
cardiac pacemaker Z95.0
cochlear Z96.21
dental Z96.5
heart Z95.812
heart valve Z95.2
prosthetic Z95.2
specified NEC Z95.4
xenogenic Z95.3
insulin pump Z96.41
intraocular lens Z96.1
joint Z96.60
ankle Z96.66- ☑
elbow Z96.62- ☑
finger Z96.69- ☑
hip Z96.64- ☑
knee Z96.65- ☑
shoulder Z96.61- ☑
specified NEC Z96.698
wrist Z96.63- ☑
larynx Z96.3
myringotomy tube Z96.22
otological Z96.20
cochlear Z96.21
eustachian stent Z96.29
myringotomy Z96.22
specified NEC Z96.29
stapes Z96.29
skin Z96.81
skull plate Z96.7
specified NEC Z96.89
urogenital Z96.0
insulin pump (functional) Z96.41
intestinal bypass or anastomosis Z98.0
intraocular lens (functional) Z96.1
intrauterine contraceptive device (IUD) Z97.5
intravascular implant (functional) (prosthetic) NEC Z95.9
coronary artery Z95.5
defibrillator (with synchronous cardiac pacemaker) Z95.810
peripheral vessel (with angioplasty) Z95.820
joint implant (prosthetic) (any) Z96.60
ankle — *see* Presence, ankle joint implant
elbow — *see* Presence, elbow joint implant
finger — *see* Presence, finger joint implant
hip — *see* Presence, hip joint implant
knee — *see* Presence, knee joint implant
shoulder — *see* Presence, shoulder joint implant
specified joint NEC Z96.698
wrist — *see* Presence, wrist joint implant
knee-joint implant (functional) (prosthesis) Z96.65- ☑
laryngeal implant (functional) Z96.3
mandibular implant (dental) Z96.5
myringotomy tube(s) Z96.22
neurostimulator (brain) (gastric) (peripheral nerve) (sacral nerve) (spinal cord) (vagus nerve) Z96.82
orthopedic-joint implant (prosthetic) (any) — *see* Presence, joint implant
otological implant (functional) Z96.29
shoulder-joint implant (functional) (prosthesis) Z96.61- ☑
skull-plate implant Z96.7
spectacles Z97.3
stapes implant (functional) Z96.29
systemic lupus erythematosus [SLE] inhibitor D68.62
tendon implant (functional) (graft) Z96.7
tooth root(s) implant Z96.5
ureteral stent Z96.0
urethral stent Z96.0
urogenital implant (functional) Z96.0
vascular implant or device Z95.9
access port device Z95.828
specified type NEC Z95.828
wrist-joint implant (functional) (prosthesis) Z96.63- ☑
Presenile — *see also* condition
dementia F03 ☑
premature aging E34.8
Presentation, fetal — *see* Delivery, complicated by, malposition
Prespondylolisthesis (congenital) Q76.2
Pressure
area, skin — *see* Ulcer, pressure, by site
brachial plexus G54.0

Pressure — *continued*
- brain G93.5
  - injury at birth NEC P11.1
- cerebral — *see* Pressure, brain
- chest R07.89
- cone, tentorial G93.5
- hyposystolic — *see also* Hypotension
  - incidental reading, without diagnosis of hypotension R03.1
- increased
  - intracranial benign G93.2
    - injury at birth P11.0
  - intraocular H40.05- ☑
- injury — *see* Ulcer, pressure, by site
- lumbosacral plexus G54.1
- mediastinum J98.59
- necrosis (chronic) — *see* Ulcer, pressure, by site
- parental, inappropriate (excessive) Z62.6
- sore (chronic) — *see* Ulcer, pressure, by site
- spinal cord G95.20
- ulcer (chronic) — *see* Ulcer, pressure, by site
- venous, increased I87.8

Pre-syncope R55

Preterm
- delivery — *see also* Pregnancy, complicated by, preterm labor O60.10 ☑
- labor — *see* Pregnancy, complicated by, preterm labor
- newborn (infant) P07.30
  - gestational age
    - 28 completed weeks (28 weeks, 0 days through 28 weeks, 6 days) P07.31
    - 29 completed weeks (29 weeks, 0 days through 29 weeks, 6 days) P07.32
    - 30 completed weeks (30 weeks, 0 days through 30 weeks, 6 days) P07.33
    - 31 completed weeks (31 weeks, 0 days through 31 weeks, 6 days) P07.34
    - 32 completed weeks (32 weeks, 0 days through 32 weeks, 6 days) P07.35
    - 33 completed weeks (33 weeks, 0 days through 33 weeks, 6 days) P07.36
    - 34 completed weeks (34 weeks, 0 days through 34 weeks, 6 days) P07.37
    - 35 completed weeks (35 weeks, 0 days through 35 weeks, 6 days) P07.38
    - 36 completed weeks (36 weeks, 0 days through 36 weeks, 6 days) P07.39

Previa
- placenta (total) (without hemorrhage) O44.0- ☑
  - with hemorrhage O44.1- ☑
  - complete O44.0- ☑
    - with hemorrhage O44.1- ☑
  - low — *see also* Delivery, complicated, by, placenta, low O44.4- ☑
    - with hemorrhage O44.5- ☑
  - marginal O44.2- ☑
    - with hemorrhage O44.3- ☑
  - partial O44.2- ☑
    - with hemorrhage O44.3- ☑
- vasa O69.4 ☑

Priapism N48.30
- due to
  - disease classified elsewhere N48.32
  - drug N48.33
  - specified cause NEC N48.39
  - trauma N48.31

Prickling sensation (skin) R20.2

Prickly heat L74.0

Primary — *see* condition

Primigravida
- elderly, affecting management of pregnancy, labor and delivery (supervision only) — *see* Pregnancy, complicated by, elderly, primigravida
- older, affecting management of pregnancy, labor and delivery (supervision only) — *see* Pregnancy, complicated by, elderly, primigravida
- very young, affecting management of pregnancy, labor and delivery (supervision only) — *see* Pregnancy, complicated by, young mother, primigravida

Primipara
- elderly, affecting management of pregnancy, labor and delivery (supervision only) — *see* Pregnancy, complicated by, elderly, primigravida
- older, affecting management of pregnancy, labor and delivery (supervision only) — *see* Pregnancy, complicated by, elderly, primigravida

Primipara — *continued*
- very young, affecting management of pregnancy, labor and delivery (supervision only) — *see* Pregnancy, complicated by, young mother, primigravida

Primus varus Q66.21- ☑

PRIND (Prolonged reversible ischemic neurologic deficit) I63.9

Pringle's disease (tuberous sclerosis) Q85.1

Prinzmetal angina I20.1

Prizefighter ear — *see* Cauliflower ear

Problem (with) (related to)
- academic Z55.8
- acculturation Z60.3
- adjustment (to)
  - change of job Z56.1
  - life-cycle transition Z60.0
  - pension Z60.0
  - retirement Z60.0
- adopted child Z62.821
- alcoholism in family Z63.72
- atypical parenting situation Z62.9
- bankruptcy Z59.89
- behavioral (adult) F69
  - drug seeking Z76.5
- birth of sibling affecting child Z62.898
- care (of)
  - provider dependency Z74.9
    - specified NEC Z74.8
  - sick or handicapped person in family or household Z63.6
- child
  - abuse (affecting the child) — *see* Maltreatment, child
  - custody or support proceedings Z65.3
  - in
    - care of non-parental family member Z62.23
    - custody of
      - grandparent Z62.23
      - non-parental relative Z62.23
      - non-relative guardian Z62.24
    - foster care Z62.21
    - kinship care Z62.23
    - welfare
      - custody Z62.21
      - guardianship Z62.21
  - leaving living situation without permission Z62.892
  - living in
    - group home Z62.22
    - orphanage Z62.22
- child-rearing Z62.9
  - specified NEC Z62.898
- communication (developmental) F80.9
- completing medical forms Z55.6
- conflict or discord (with)
  - boss Z56.4
  - classmates Z55.4
  - counselor Z64.4
  - employer Z56.4
  - family Z63.9
    - specified NEC Z63.8
  - probation officer Z64.4
  - social worker Z64.4
  - teachers Z55.4
  - workmates Z56.4
- conviction in legal proceedings Z65.0
  - with imprisonment Z65.1
- counselor Z64.4
- creditors Z59.89
- digestive K92.9
- drug addict in family Z63.72
- ear — *see* Disorder, ear
- economic Z59.9
  - affecting care Z59.9
  - specified NEC Z59.89
  - strain Z59.86
- education Z55.9
  - specified NEC Z55.8
- employment Z56.9
  - change of job Z56.1
  - discord Z56.4
  - environment Z56.5
  - sexual harassment Z56.81
  - specified NEC Z56.89
  - stressful schedule Z56.3
  - stress NEC Z56.6
  - threat of job loss Z56.2
  - unemployment Z56.0
- enuresis, child F98.0

Problem — *continued*
- eye H57.9
- failed examinations (school) Z55.2
- falling Z91.81
- family — *see also* Disruption, family Z63.9
  - specified NEC Z63.8
- feeding (elderly) (infant) NOS R63.39
  - newborn P92.9
    - breast P92.5
    - overfeeding P92.4
    - slow P92.2
    - specified NEC P92.8
    - underfeeding P92.3
  - nonorganic F50.89
- finance Z59.9
  - specified NEC Z59.89
- foreclosure on loan Z59.89
- foster child Z62.822
- frightening experience(s) in childhood Z62.898
- genital NEC
  - female N94.9
  - male N50.9
- health care Z75.9
  - specified NEC Z75.8
- health literacy Z55.6
- hearing — *see* Deafness
- homelessness Z59.00
- housing Z59.9
  - inadequate Z59.10
  - isolated Z59.89
  - specified NEC Z59.89
- identity (of childhood) F93.8
- illegitimate pregnancy (unwanted) Z64.0
- illiteracy Z55.0
- impaired mobility Z74.09
- imprisonment or incarceration Z65.1
- inadequate teaching affecting education Z55.8
- inappropriate (excessive) parental pressure Z62.6
- influencing health status NEC Z78.9
- in-law Z63.1
- institutionalization, affecting child Z62.22
- intrafamilial communication Z63.8
- jealousy, child F93.8
- landlord Z59.2
- language (developmental) F80.9
- learning (developmental) F81.9
- legal Z65.3
  - conviction without imprisonment Z65.0
  - imprisonment Z65.1
  - release from prison Z65.2
- life-management Z73.9
  - specified NEC Z73.89
- life-style Z72.9
  - gambling Z72.6
  - high-risk sexual behavior (heterosexual) Z72.51
    - bisexual Z72.53
    - homosexual Z72.52
  - inappropriate eating habits NEC Z72.4
  - self-damaging behavior NEC Z72.89
  - specified NEC Z72.89
  - tobacco use Z72.0
- literacy Z55.9
  - low level Z55.0
  - specified NEC Z55.8
- living alone Z60.2
- lodgers Z59.2
- loss of love relationship in childhood Z62.898
- marital Z63.0
  - involving
    - divorce Z63.5
    - estrangement Z63.5
    - gender identity F66
- mastication K08.89
- medical
  - care, within family Z63.6
  - facilities Z75.9
    - specified NEC Z75.8
- mental F48.9
- money Z59.86
- multiparity Z64.1
- negative life events in childhood Z62.9
  - altered pattern of family relationships Z62.898
  - frightening experience Z62.898
  - loss of
    - love relationship Z62.898
    - self-esteem Z62.898
  - physical abuse (alleged) — *see* Maltreatment, child
  - removal from home Z62.29
  - specified event NEC Z62.898

- **Pseudopuberty, precocious** — *continued*
  - male isosexual E25.8
- **Pseudorickets** (renal) N25.Ø
- **Pseudorubella** BØ8.2Ø
- **Pseudosclerema, newborn** P83.88
- **Pseudosclerosis** (brain)
  - Jakob's — *see* Creutzfeldt-Jakob disease or syndrome
  - of Westphal (Strumpell) E83.Ø1
  - spastic — *see* Creutzfeldt-Jakob disease or syndrome
- **Pseudotetanus** — *see* Convulsions
- **Pseudotetany** R29.Ø
  - hysterical F44.5
- **Pseudotruncus arteriosus** Q25.49
- **Pseudotuberculosis** A28.2
  - enterocolitis AØ4.8
  - pasteurella (infection) A28.Ø
- **Pseudotumor** G93.2
  - cerebri G93.2
  - orbital HØ5.11 ☑
- **Pseudoxanthoma elasticum** Q82.8
- **Psilosis** (sprue) (tropical) K9Ø.1
  - nontropical K9Ø.Ø
- **Psittacosis** A7Ø
- **Psoitis** M6Ø.88
- **Psoriasis** L4Ø.9
  - arthropathic L4Ø.5Ø
    - arthritis mutilans L4Ø.52
    - distal interphalangeal L4Ø.51
    - juvenile L4Ø.54
    - other specified L4Ø.59
    - spondylitis L4Ø.53
  - buccal K13.29
  - flexural L4Ø.8
  - guttate L4Ø.4
  - mouth K13.29
  - nummular L4Ø.Ø
  - plaque L4Ø.Ø
  - psychogenic F54
  - pustular (generalized) L4Ø.1
    - palmaris et plantaris L4Ø.3
  - specified NEC L4Ø.8
  - vulgaris L4Ø.Ø
- **Psychasthenia** F48.8
- **Psychiatric disorder or problem** F99
- **Psychogenic** — *see also* condition
  - factors associated with physical conditions F54
- **Psychological and behavioral factors affecting medical condition** F59
- **Psychoneurosis, psychoneurotic** — *see also* Neurosis
  - anxiety (state) F41.1
  - depersonalization F48.1
  - hypochondriacal F45.21
  - hysteria F44.9
  - neurasthenic F48.8
  - personality NEC F6Ø.89
- **Psychopathy, psychopathic**
  - affectionless F94.2
  - autistic F84.5
  - constitution, post-traumatic FØ7.81
  - personality — *see* Disorder, personality
  - sexual — *see* Deviation, sexual
  - state F6Ø.2
- **Psychosexual identity disorder of childhood** F64.2
- **Psychosis, psychotic** F29
  - acute (transient) F23
    - hysterical F44.9
  - affective — *see* Disorder, mood
  - alcoholic F1Ø.959
    - with
      - abuse F1Ø.159
      - anxiety disorder F1Ø.98Ø
        - with
          - abuse F1Ø.18Ø
          - dependence F1Ø.28Ø
      - delirium tremens F1Ø.231
      - delusions F1Ø.95Ø
        - with
          - abuse F1Ø.15Ø
          - dependence F1Ø.25Ø
      - dementia F1Ø.97
        - with dependence F1Ø.27
      - dependence F1Ø.259
      - hallucinosis F1Ø.951
        - with
          - abuse F1Ø.151
          - dependence F1Ø.251
      - mood disorder F1Ø.94

- **Psychosis, psychotic** — *continued*
  - alcoholic — *continued*
    - with — *continued*
      - mood disorder — *continued*
        - with
          - abuse F1Ø.14
          - dependence F1Ø.24
      - paranoia F1Ø.95Ø
        - with
          - abuse F1Ø.15Ø
          - dependence F1Ø.25Ø
      - persisting amnesia F1Ø.96
        - with dependence F1Ø.26
    - amnestic confabulatory F1Ø.96
      - with dependence F1Ø.26
    - delirium tremens F1Ø.231
    - Korsakoff's, Korsakov's, Korsakow's F1Ø.26
    - paranoid type F1Ø.95Ø
      - with
        - abuse F1Ø.15Ø
        - dependence F1Ø.25Ø
  - anergastic — *see* Psychosis, organic
  - arteriosclerotic (simple type) (uncomplicated) — *see also* Dementia, vascular FØ1.5Ø
    - with behavioral disturbance — *see* Dementia, vascular
  - childhood F84.Ø
    - atypical F84.8
  - climacteric — *see* Psychosis, involutional
  - confusional F29
    - acute or subacute FØ5
    - reactive F23
  - cycloid F23
  - depressive — *see* Disorder, depressive
  - disintegrative (childhood) F84.3
  - drug-induced — *see* F11-F19 with .X59
    - paranoid and hallucinatory states — *see* F11-F19 with .X5Ø or .X51
  - due to or associated with
    - addiction, drug — *see* F11-F19 with .X59
    - dependence
      - alcohol F1Ø.259
      - drug — *see* F11-F19 with .X59
    - epilepsy FØ6.8
    - Huntington's chorea FØ6.8
    - ischemia, cerebrovascular (generalized) FØ6.8
    - multiple sclerosis FØ6.8
    - physical disease FØ6.8
    - presenile dementia FØ3 ☑
    - senile dementia FØ3 ☑
    - vascular disease (arteriosclerotic) (cerebral) — *see also* Dementia, vascular FØ1.5Ø
      - with behavioral disturbance — *see* Dementia, vascular
  - epileptic FØ6.8
  - episode F23
    - due to or associated with physical condition FØ6.8
  - exhaustive F43.Ø
  - hallucinatory, chronic F28
  - hypomanic F3Ø.8
  - hysterical (acute) F44.9
  - induced F24
  - infantile F84.Ø
    - atypical F84.8
  - infective (acute) (subacute) FØ5
  - involutional F28
    - depressive — *see* Disorder, depressive
    - melancholic — *see* Disorder, depressive
    - paranoid (state) F22
  - Korsakoff's, Korsakov's, Korsakow's (nonalcoholic) FØ4
    - alcoholic F1Ø.96
      - in dependence F1Ø.26
    - induced by other psychoactive substance — *see* categories F11-F19 with .X5X
  - mania, manic (single episode) F3Ø.2
    - recurrent type F31.89
  - manic-depressive — *see* Disorder, bipolar
  - menopausal — *see* Psychosis, involutional
  - mixed schizophrenic and affective F25.8
  - multi-infarct (cerebrovascular) — *see also* Dementia, vascular FØ1.5Ø
    - with behavioral disturbance — *see* Dementia, vascular
  - nonorganic F29
    - specified NEC F28
  - organic FØ9

- **Psychosis, psychotic** — *continued*
  - organic — *continued*
    - due to or associated with
      - arteriosclerosis (cerebral) — *see* Psychosis, arteriosclerotic
      - cerebrovascular disease, arteriosclerotic — *see* Psychosis, arteriosclerotic
      - childbirth — *see* Psychosis, puerperal
      - Creutzfeldt-Jakob disease or syndrome — *see* Creutzfeldt-Jakob disease or syndrome
      - dependence, alcohol F1Ø.259
      - disease
        - alcoholic liver F1Ø.259
        - brain, arteriosclerotic — *see* Psychosis, arteriosclerotic
        - cerebrovascular — *see also* Dementia, vascular FØ1.5Ø
          - with behavioral disturbance — *see* Dementia, vascular
        - Creutzfeldt-Jakob — *see* Creutzfeldt-Jakob disease or syndrome
        - endocrine or metabolic FØ6.8
          - acute or subacute FØ5
        - liver, alcoholic F1Ø.259
      - epilepsy transient (acute) FØ5
      - infection
        - brain (intracranial) FØ6.8
          - acute or subacute FØ5
      - intoxication
        - alcoholic (acute) F1Ø.259
        - drug F11-F19 with .x59
      - ischemia, cerebrovascular (generalized) — *see* Psychosis, arteriosclerotic
      - puerperium — *see* Psychosis, puerperal
      - trauma, brain (birth) (from electric current) (surgical) FØ6.8
        - acute or subacute FØ5
    - infective FØ6.8
      - acute or subacute FØ5
    - post-traumatic FØ6.8
      - acute or subacute FØ5
  - paranoiac F22
  - paranoid (climacteric) (involutional) (menopausal) F22
    - psychogenic (acute) F23
    - schizophrenic F2Ø.Ø
    - senile FØ3 ☑
  - postpartum (NOS) F53.1
  - presbyophrenic (type) FØ3 ☑
  - presenile FØ3 ☑
  - psychogenic (paranoid) F23
    - depressive F32.3
  - puerperal (NOS) F53.1
    - specified type — *see* Psychosis, by type
  - reactive (brief) (transient) (emotional stress) (psychological trauma) F23
    - depressive F32.3
      - recurrent F33.3
    - excitative type F3Ø.8
  - schizoaffective F25.9
    - depressive type F25.1
    - manic type F25.Ø
  - schizophrenia, schizophrenic — *see* Schizophrenia
  - schizophrenia-like, in epilepsy FØ6.2
  - schizophreniform F2Ø.81
    - affective type F25.9
    - brief F23
    - confusional type F23
    - mixed type F25.Ø
  - senile NEC FØ3 ☑
    - depressed or paranoid type FØ3 ☑
    - simple deterioration FØ3 ☑
    - specified type — *code to* condition
  - shared F24
  - situational (reactive) F23
  - symbiotic (childhood) F84.3
  - symptomatic FØ9
- **Psychosomatic** — *see* Disorder, psychosomatic
- **Psychosyndrome, organic** FØ7.9
- **Psychotic episode due to or associated with physical condition** FØ6.8
- **Pterygium** (eye) H11.ØØ- ☑
  - amyloid H11.Ø1- ☑
  - central H11.Ø2- ☑
  - colli Q18.3
  - double H11.Ø3- ☑
  - peripheral
    - progressive H11.Ø5- ☑
    - stationary H11.Ø4- ☑

- **Puncture** — *continued*
  - finger(s) — *continued*
    - index — *continued*
      - left — *continued*
        - with
          - damage to nail S61.331 ☑
            - with
              - foreign body S61.341 ☑
          - foreign body S61.241 ☑
      - right S61.23Ø ☑
        - with
          - damage to nail S61.33Ø ☑
            - with
              - foreign body S61.34Ø ☑
          - foreign body S61.24Ø ☑
    - little S61.238 ☑
      - with
        - damage to nail S61.338 ☑
          - with
            - foreign body S61.348 ☑
        - foreign body S61.248 ☑
      - left S61.237 ☑
        - with
          - damage to nail S61.337 ☑
            - with
              - foreign body S61.347 ☑
          - foreign body S61.247 ☑
      - right S61.236 ☑
        - with
          - damage to nail S61.336 ☑
            - with
              - foreign body S61.346 ☑
          - foreign body S61.246 ☑
    - middle S61.238 ☑
      - with
        - damage to nail S61.338 ☑
          - with
            - foreign body S61.348 ☑
        - foreign body S61.248 ☑
      - left S61.233 ☑
        - with
          - damage to nail S61.333 ☑
            - with
              - foreign body S61.343 ☑
          - foreign body S61.243 ☑
      - right S61.232 ☑
        - with
          - damage to nail S61.332 ☑
            - with
              - foreign body S61.342 ☑
          - foreign body S61.242 ☑
    - ring S61.238 ☑
      - with
        - damage to nail S61.338 ☑
          - with
            - foreign body S61.348 ☑
        - foreign body S61.248 ☑
      - left S61.235 ☑
        - with
          - damage to nail S61.335 ☑
            - with
              - foreign body S61.345 ☑
          - foreign body S61.245 ☑
      - right S61.234 ☑
        - with
          - damage to nail S61.334 ☑
            - with
              - foreign body S61.344 ☑
          - foreign body S61.244 ☑
  - flank S31.139 ☑
    - with foreign body S31.149 ☑
  - foot (except toe(s) alone) S91.339 ☑
    - with foreign body S91.349 ☑
    - left S91.332 ☑
      - with foreign body S91.342 ☑
    - right S91.331 ☑
      - with foreign body S91.341 ☑
    - toe — *see* Puncture, toe
  - forearm S51.839 ☑
    - with
      - foreign body S51.849 ☑
    - elbow only — *see* Puncture, elbow
    - left S51.832 ☑
      - with
        - foreign body S51.842 ☑
    - right S51.831 ☑

- **Puncture** — *continued*
  - forearm — *continued*
    - right — *continued*
      - with
        - foreign body S51.841 ☑
  - forehead — *see* Puncture, head, specified site NEC
  - genital organs, external
    - female S31.532 ☑
      - with foreign body S31.542 ☑
      - vagina — *see* Puncture, vagina
      - vulva — *see* Puncture, vulva
    - male S31.531 ☑
      - with foreign body S31.541 ☑
      - penis — *see* Puncture, penis
      - scrotum — *see* Puncture, scrotum
      - testis — *see* Puncture, testis
  - groin — *see* Puncture, abdomen, wall
  - gum — *see* Puncture, oral cavity
  - hand S61.439 ☑
    - with
      - foreign body S61.449 ☑
    - finger — *see* Puncture, finger
    - left S61.432 ☑
      - with
        - foreign body S61.442 ☑
    - right S61.431 ☑
      - with
        - foreign body S61.441 ☑
    - thumb — *see* Puncture, thumb
  - head SØ1.93 ☑
    - with foreign body SØ1.94 ☑
    - cheek — *see* Puncture, cheek
    - ear — *see* Puncture, ear
    - eyelid — *see* Puncture, eyelid
    - lip — *see* Puncture, oral cavity
    - nose — *see* Puncture, nose
    - oral cavity — *see* Puncture, oral cavity
    - scalp SØ1.Ø3 ☑
      - with foreign body SØ1.Ø4 ☑
    - specified site NEC SØ1.83 ☑
      - with foreign body SØ1.84 ☑
    - temporomandibular area — *see* Puncture, cheek
  - heart S26.99 ☑
    - with hemopericardium S26.Ø9 ☑
    - without hemopericardium S26.19 ☑
  - heel — *see* Puncture, foot
  - hip S71.Ø39 ☑
    - with foreign body S71.Ø49 ☑
    - left S71.Ø32 ☑
      - with foreign body S71.Ø42 ☑
    - right S71.Ø31 ☑
      - with foreign body S71.Ø41 ☑
  - hymen — *see* Puncture, vagina
  - hypochondrium — *see* Puncture, abdomen, wall
  - hypogastric region — *see* Puncture, abdomen, wall
  - inguinal region — *see* Puncture, abdomen, wall
  - instep — *see* Puncture, foot
  - internal organs — *see* Injury, by site
  - interscapular region — *see* Puncture, thorax, back
  - intestine
    - large
      - colon S36.599 ☑
        - ascending S36.59Ø ☑
        - descending S36.592 ☑
        - sigmoid S36.593 ☑
        - specified site NEC S36.598 ☑
        - transverse S36.591 ☑
      - rectum S36.69 ☑
    - small S36.499 ☑
      - duodenum S36.49Ø ☑
      - specified site NEC S36.498 ☑
  - intra-abdominal organ S36.99 ☑
    - gallbladder S36.128 ☑
    - intestine — *see* Puncture, intestine
    - liver S36.118 ☑
    - pancreas — *see* Puncture, pancreas
    - peritoneum S36.81 ☑
    - specified site NEC S36.898 ☑
    - spleen S36.Ø9 ☑
    - stomach S36.39 ☑
  - jaw — *see* Puncture, head, specified site NEC
  - knee S81.Ø39 ☑
    - with foreign body S81.Ø49 ☑
    - left S81.Ø32 ☑
      - with foreign body S81.Ø42 ☑
    - right S81.Ø31 ☑

- **Puncture** — *continued*
  - knee — *continued*
    - right — *continued*
      - with foreign body S81.Ø41 ☑
  - labium (majus) (minus) — *see* Puncture, vulva
  - lacrimal duct — *see* Puncture, eyelid
  - larynx S11.Ø13 ☑
    - with foreign body S11.Ø14 ☑
  - leg (lower) S81.839 ☑
    - with foreign body S81.849 ☑
    - foot — *see* Puncture, foot
    - knee — *see* Puncture, knee
    - left S81.832 ☑
      - with foreign body S81.842 ☑
    - right S81.831 ☑
      - with foreign body S81.841 ☑
    - upper — *see* Puncture, thigh
  - lip SØ1.531 ☑
    - with foreign body SØ1.541 ☑
  - loin — *see* Puncture, abdomen, wall
  - lower back — *see* Puncture, back, lower
  - lumbar region — *see* Puncture, back, lower
  - malar region — *see* Puncture, head, specified site NEC
  - mammary — *see* Puncture, breast
  - mastoid region — *see* Puncture, head, specified site NEC
  - mouth — *see* Puncture, oral cavity
  - nail
    - finger — *see* Puncture, finger, with damage to nail
    - toe — *see* Puncture, toe, with damage to nail
  - nasal (septum) (sinus) — *see* Puncture, nose
  - nasopharynx — *see* Puncture, head, specified site NEC
  - neck S11.93 ☑
    - with foreign body S11.94 ☑
    - involving
      - cervical esophagus — *see* Puncture, cervical esophagus
      - larynx — *see* Puncture, larynx
      - pharynx — *see* Puncture, pharynx
      - thyroid gland — *see* Puncture, thyroid gland
      - trachea — *see* Puncture, trachea
    - specified site NEC S11.83 ☑
      - with foreign body S11.84 ☑
  - nose (septum) (sinus) SØ1.23 ☑
    - with foreign body SØ1.24 ☑
  - ocular — *see* Puncture, eyeball
  - oral cavity SØ1.532 ☑
    - with foreign body SØ1.542 ☑
  - orbit SØ5.4- ☑
  - palate — *see* Puncture, oral cavity
  - palm — *see* Puncture, hand
  - pancreas S36.299 ☑
    - body S36.291 ☑
    - head S36.29Ø ☑
    - tail S36.292 ☑
  - pelvis — *see* Puncture, back, lower
  - penis S31.23 ☑
    - with foreign body S31.24 ☑
  - perineum
    - female S31.43 ☑
      - with foreign body S31.44 ☑
    - male S31.139 ☑
      - with foreign body S31.149 ☑
  - periocular area (with or without lacrimal passages) — *see* Puncture, eyelid
  - phalanges
    - finger — *see* Puncture, finger
    - toe — *see* Puncture, toe
  - pharynx S11.23 ☑
    - with foreign body S11.24 ☑
  - pinna — *see* Puncture, ear
  - popliteal space — *see* Puncture, knee
  - prepuce — *see* Puncture, penis
  - pubic region S31.139 ☑
    - with foreign body S31.149 ☑
  - pudendum — *see* Puncture, genital organs, external
  - rectovaginal septum — *see* Puncture, vagina
  - sacral region — *see* Puncture, back, lower
  - sacroiliac region — *see* Puncture, back, lower
  - salivary gland — *see* Puncture, oral cavity
  - scalp SØ1.Ø3 ☑
    - with foreign body SØ1.Ø4 ☑
  - scapular region — *see* Puncture, shoulder
  - scrotum S31.33 ☑
    - with foreign body S31.34 ☑
  - shin — *see* Puncture, leg

- **Pyelonephritis** — *continued*
  - in — *continued*
    - Sjogren's disease M35.Ø4
    - toxoplasmosis B58.83
    - transplant rejection T86.91 *[N16]*
    - Wilson's disease E83.Ø1 *[N16]*
  - nonobstructive N12
    - with reflux (vesicoureteral) N11.Ø
    - chronic N11.8
  - syphilitic A52.75
- **Pyelonephrosis** (obstructive) N11.1
  - chronic N11.9
- **Pyelophlebitis** I8Ø.8
- **Pyeloureteritis cystica** N28.85
- **Pyemia, pyemic** (fever) (infection) (purulent) — *see also* Sepsis
  - joint — *see* Arthritis, pyogenic or pyemic
  - liver K75.1
  - pneumococcal A4Ø.3
  - portal K75.1
  - postvaccinal T88.Ø ☑
  - puerperal, postpartum, childbirth O85
  - specified organism NEC A41.89
  - tuberculous — *see* Tuberculosis, miliary
- **Pygopagus** Q89.4
- **Pyknoepilepsy** (idiopathic) — *see* Pyknolepsy
- **Pyknolepsy** G4Ø.AØ9 (*following* G4Ø.3)
  - intractable G4Ø.A19 (*following* G4Ø.3)
    - with status epilepticus G4Ø.A11 (*following* G4Ø.3)
    - without status epilepticus G4Ø.A19 (*following* G4Ø.3)
  - not intractable G4Ø.AØ9 (*following* G4Ø.3)
    - with status epilepticus G4Ø.AØ1 (*following* G4Ø.3)
    - without status epilepticus G4Ø.AØ9 (*following* G4Ø.3)
- **Pylephlebitis** K75.1
- **Pyle's syndrome** Q78.5
- **Pylethrombophlebitis** K75.1
- **Pylethrombosis** K75.1
- **Pyloritis** K29.9Ø
  - with bleeding K29.91
- **Pylorospasm** (reflex) **NEC** K31.3
  - congenital or infantile Q4Ø.Ø
  - neurotic F45.8
  - newborn Q4Ø.Ø
  - psychogenic F45.8
- **Pylorus, pyloric** — *see* condition
- **Pyoarthrosis** — *see* Arthritis, pyogenic or pyemic
- **Pyocele**
  - mastoid — *see* Mastoiditis, acute
  - sinus (accessory) — *see* Sinusitis
  - turbinate (bone) J32.9
  - urethra — *see also* Urethritis N34.Ø
- **Pyocolpos** — *see* Vaginitis
- **Pyocystitis** N3Ø.8Ø
  - with hematuria N3Ø.81
- **Pyoderma, pyodermia** LØ8.Ø
  - gangrenosum L88
  - newborn P39.4
  - phagedenic L88
  - vegetans LØ8.81
- **Pyodermatitis** LØ8.Ø
  - vegetans LØ8.81
- **Pyogenic** — *see* condition
- **Pyohydronephrosis** N13.6
- **Pyometra, pyometrium, pyometritis** — *see* Endometritis
- **Pyomyositis** (tropical) — *see* Myositis, infective
- **Pyonephritis** N12
- **Pyonephrosis** N13.6
  - tuberculous A18.11
- **Pyo-oophoritis** — *see* Salpingo-oophoritis
- **Pyo-ovarium** — *see* Salpingo-oophoritis
- **Pyopericarditis, pyopericardium** I3Ø.1
- **Pyophlebitis** — *see* Phlebitis
- **Pyopneumopericardium** I3Ø.1
- **Pyopneumothorax** (infective) J86.9
  - with fistula J86.Ø
  - tuberculous NEC A15.6
- **Pyosalpinx, pyosalpingitis** — *see also* Salpingo-oophoritis
- **Pyothorax** J86.9
  - with fistula J86.Ø
  - tuberculous NEC A15.6
- **Pyoureter** N28.89
  - tuberculous A18.11
- **Pyramidopallidonigral syndrome** G2Ø.C
- **Pyrexia** (of unknown origin) R5Ø.9
  - atmospheric T67.Ø1 ☑
- **Pyrexia** — *continued*
  - during labor NEC O75.2
  - heat T67.Ø1 ☑
  - newborn P81.9
    - environmentally-induced P81.Ø
  - persistent R5Ø.9
  - puerperal O86.4
- **Pyroglobulinemia NEC** E88.Ø9
- **Pyromania** F63.1
- **Pyrosis** R12
- **Pyuria** (bacterial) (sterile) R82.81

Q

- **Q fever** A78
  - with pneumonia A78
- **Quadricuspid aortic valve** Q23.8
- **Quadrilateral fever** A78
- **Quadriparesis** — *see* Quadriplegia
  - meaning muscle weakness M62.81
- **Quadriplegia** G82.5Ø
  - complete
    - C1-C4 level G82.51
    - C5-C7 level G82.53
  - congenital (cerebral) (spinal) G8Ø.8
    - spastic G8Ø.Ø
  - embolic (current episode) I63.4- ☑
  - functional R53.2
  - incomplete
    - C1-C4 level G82.52
    - C5-C7 level G82.54
  - thrombotic (current episode) I63.3- ☑
  - traumatic — *code to* injury with seventh character S
    - current episode — *see* Injury, spinal (cord), cervical
- **Quadruplet, pregnancy** — *see* Pregnancy, quadruplet
- **Quarrelsomeness** F6Ø.3
- **Queensland fever** A77.3
- **Quervain's disease** M65.4
  - thyroid EØ6.1
- **Queyrat's erythroplasia** DØ7.4
  - penis DØ7.4
  - specified site — *see* Neoplasm, skin, in situ
  - unspecified site DØ7.4
- **Quincke's disease or edema** T78.3 ☑
  - hereditary D84.1
- **Quinsy** (gangrenous) J36
- **Quintan fever** A79.Ø
- **Quintuplet, pregnancy** — *see* Pregnancy, quintuplet

R

- **Rabbit fever** — *see* Tularemia
- **Rabies** A82.9
  - contact Z2Ø.3
  - exposure to Z2Ø.3
  - inoculation reaction — *see* Complications, vaccination
  - sylvatic A82.Ø
  - urban A82.1
- **Rachischisis** — *see* Spina bifida
- **Rachitic** — *see also* condition
  - deformities of spine (late effect) (sequelae) E64.3
  - pelvis (late effect) (sequelae) E64.3
    - with disproportion (fetopelvic) O33.Ø
      - causing obstructed labor O65.Ø
- **Rachitis, rachitism** (acute) (tarda) — *see also* Rickets
  - renalis N25.Ø
  - sequelae E64.3
- **Radial nerve** — *see* condition
- **Radiation**
  - burn — *see* Burn
  - effects NOS T66 ☑
  - sickness NOS T66 ☑
  - therapy, encounter for Z51.Ø
- **Radiculitis** (pressure) (vertebrogenic) — *see* Radiculopathy
- **Radiculomyelitis** — *see also* Encephalitis
  - toxic, due to
    - Clostridium tetani A35
    - Corynebacterium diphtheriae A36.82
- **Radiculopathy** M54.1Ø
  - cervical region M54.12
  - cervicothoracic region M54.13
  - due to
    - disc disorder
      - C3 M5Ø.11
      - C4 M5Ø.11
      - C5 M5Ø.121
- **Radiculopathy** — *continued*
  - due to — *continued*
    - disc disorder — *continued*
      - C6 M5Ø.122
      - C7 M5Ø.123
    - displacement of intervertebral disc — *see* Disorder, disc, with, radiculopathy
  - leg M54.1- ☑
  - lumbar region M54.16
  - lumbosacral region M54.17
  - occipito-atlanto-axial region M54.11
  - postherpetic BØ2.29
  - sacrococcygeal region M54.18
  - syphilitic A52.11
  - thoracic region (with visceral pain) M54.14
  - thoracolumbar region M54.15
- **Radiodermal burns** (acute, chronic, or occupational) — *see* Burn
- **Radiodermatitis** L58.9
  - acute L58.Ø
  - chronic L58.1
- **Radiotherapy session** Z51.Ø
- **RAEB** (refractory anemia with excess blasts) D46.2- ☑
- **Rage, meaning rabies** — *see* Rabies
- **Ragpicker's disease** A22.1
- **Ragsorter's disease** A22.1
- **Raillietiniasis** B71.8
- **Railroad neurosis** F48.8
- **Railway spine** F48.8
- **Raised** — *see also* Elevated
  - antibody titer R76.Ø
- **Rake teeth, tooth** M26.39
- **Rales** RØ9.89
- **Ramifying renal pelvis** Q63.8
- **Ramsay-Hunt disease or syndrome** — *see also* Hunt's, disease BØ2.21
  - meaning dyssynergia cerebellaris myoclonica G11.19
- **Ranula** K11.6
  - congenital Q38.4
- **Rape**
  - adult
    - confirmed T74.21 ☑
    - suspected T76.21 ☑
  - alleged, observation or examination, ruled out
    - adult ZØ4.41
    - child ZØ4.42
  - child
    - confirmed T74.22 ☑
    - suspected T76.22 ☑
- **Rapid**
  - feeble pulse, due to shock, following injury T79.4 ☑
  - heart (beat) RØØ.Ø
    - psychogenic F45.8
  - second stage (delivery) O62.3
  - time-zone change syndrome G47.25
- **Rarefaction, bone** — *see* Disorder, bone, density and structure, specified NEC
- **Rash** (toxic) R21
  - canker A38.9
  - diaper L22
  - drug (internal use) L27.Ø
    - contact — *see also* Dermatitis, due to, drugs, external L25.1
  - following immunization T88.1 ☑
  - food — *see* Dermatitis, due to, food
  - heat L74.Ø
  - napkin (psoriasiform) L22
  - nettle — *see* Urticaria
  - pustular LØ8.Ø
  - rose R21
    - epidemic BØ6.9
  - scarlet A38.9
  - serum — *see also* Reaction, serum T8Ø.69 ☑
  - wandering tongue K14.1
- **Rasmussen aneurysm** — *see* Tuberculosis, pulmonary
- **Rasmussen encephalitis** GØ4.81
- **Rat-bite fever** A25.9
  - due to Streptobacillus moniliformis A25.1
  - spirochetal (morsus muris) A25.Ø
- **Rathke's pouch tumor** D44.3
- **Raymond** (-Cestan) **syndrome** I65.8
- **Raynaud's disease, phenomenon or syndrome** (secondary) I73.ØØ
  - with gangrene (symmetric) I73.Ø1
- **RDS** (newborn) (type I) P22.Ø
  - type II P22.1
- **Reaction** — *see also* Disorder

- **Reaction** — *continued*
  - withdrawing, child or adolescent F93.8
  - adaptation — *see* Disorder, adjustment
  - adjustment (anxiety) (conduct disorder) (depressiveness) (distress) — *see* Disorder, adjustment
    - with
      - mutism, elective (child) (adolescent) F94.Ø
  - adverse
    - food (any) (ingested) NEC T78.1 ☑
      - anaphylactic — *see* Shock, anaphylactic, due to food
  - affective — *see* Disorder, mood
  - allergic — *see* Allergy
  - anaphylactic — *see* Shock, anaphylactic
  - anaphylactoid — *see* Shock, anaphylactic
  - anesthesia — *see* Anesthesia, complication
  - antitoxin (prophylactic) (therapeutic) — *see* Complications, vaccination
  - anxiety F41.1
  - Arthus — *see* Arthus' phenomenon
  - asthenic F48.8
  - combat and operational stress F43.Ø
  - compulsive F42.8
  - conversion F44.9
  - crisis, acute F43.Ø
  - deoxyribonuclease (DNA) (DNase) hypersensitivity D69.2
  - depressive (single episode) F32.9
    - affective (single episode) F31.4
      - recurrent episode F33.9
    - neurotic F34.1
    - psychoneurotic F34.1
    - psychotic F32.3
    - recurrent — *see* Disorder, depressive, recurrent
  - dissociative F44.9
  - drug NEC T88.7 ☑
    - addictive — *see* Dependence, drug
      - transmitted via placenta or breast milk — *see* Absorption, drug, addictive, through placenta
    - allergic — *see* Allergy, drug
    - lichenoid L43.2
    - newborn P93.8
      - gray baby syndrome P93.Ø
    - overdose or poisoning (by accident) — *see* Table of Drugs and Chemicals, by drug, poisoning
    - photoallergic L56.1
    - phototoxic L56.Ø
    - withdrawal — *see* Dependence, by drug, with, withdrawal
      - infant of dependent mother P96.1
      - newborn P96.1
    - wrong substance given or taken (by accident) — *see* Table of Drugs and Chemicals, by drug, poisoning
  - fear F4Ø.9
    - child (abnormal) F93.8
  - febrile nonhemolytic transfusion (FNHTR) R5Ø.84
  - fluid loss, cerebrospinal G97.1
  - foreign
    - body NEC — *see* Granuloma, foreign body
      - in operative wound (inadvertently left) — *see* Foreign body, accidentally left during a procedure
    - substance accidentally left during a procedure (chemical) (powder) (talc) T81.6Ø ☑
      - aseptic peritonitis T81.61 ☑
      - body or object (instrument) (sponge) (swab) — *see* Foreign body, accidentally left during a procedure
      - specified reaction NEC T81.69 ☑
  - grief — *see* Disorder, adjustment
  - Herxheimer's R68.89
  - hyperkinetic — *see* Hyperkinesia
  - hypochondriacal F45.2Ø
  - hypoglycemic, due to insulin E16.Ø
    - with coma (diabetic) — *see* Diabetes, coma
      - nondiabetic E15
    - therapeutic misadventure — *see* subcategory T38.3 ☑
  - hypomanic F3Ø.8
  - hysterical F44.9
  - immunization — *see* Complications, vaccination
  - incompatibility
    - ABO blood group (infusion) (transfusion) — *see* Complication(s), transfusion, incompatibility reaction, ABO
      - delayed serologic T8Ø.39 ☑
- **Reaction** — *continued*
  - incompatibility — *continued*
    - minor blood group (Duffy) (E) (K) (Kell) (Kidd) (Lewis) (M) (N) (P) (S) T8Ø.89 ☑
    - Rh (factor) (infusion) (transfusion) — *see* Complication(s), transfusion, incompatibility reaction, Rh (factor)
  - inflammatory — *see* Infection
  - infusion — *see* Complications, infusion
  - inoculation (immune serum) — *see* Complications, vaccination
  - insulin T38.3- ☑
  - involutional psychotic — *see* Disorder, depressive
  - leukemoid D72.823
    - basophilic D72.823
    - lymphocytic D72.823
    - monocytic D72.823
    - myelocytic D72.823
    - neutrophilic D72.823
  - LSD (acute)
    - due to drug abuse — *see* Abuse, drug, hallucinogen
    - due to drug dependence — *see* Dependence, drug, hallucinogen
  - lumbar puncture G97.1
  - manic-depressive — *see* Disorder, bipolar
  - neurasthenic F48.8
  - neurogenic — *see* Neurosis
  - neurotic F48.9
  - neurotic-depressive F34.1
  - nitritoid — *see* Crisis, nitritoid
  - nonspecific
    - to
      - cell mediated immunity measurement of gamma interferon antigen response without active tuberculosis R76.12
      - QuantiFERON-TB test (QFT) without active tuberculosis R76.12
      - tuberculin test — *see also* Reaction, tuberculin skin test R76.11
  - obsessive-compulsive F42.8
  - organic, acute or subacute — *see* Delirium
  - paranoid (acute) F23
    - chronic F22
    - senile FØ3 ☑
  - passive dependency F6Ø.7
  - phobic F4Ø.9
  - post-traumatic stress, uncomplicated Z73.3
  - psychogenic F99
  - psychoneurotic — *see also* Neurosis
    - compulsive F42.8
    - depersonalization F48.1
    - depressive F34.1
    - hypochondriacal F45.2Ø
    - neurasthenic F48.8
    - obsessive F42.8
  - psychophysiologic — *see* Disorder, somatoform
  - psychosomatic — *see* Disorder, somatoform
  - psychotic — *see* Psychosis
  - scarlet fever toxin — *see* Complications, vaccination
  - schizophrenic F23
    - acute (brief) (undifferentiated) F23
    - latent F21
    - undifferentiated (acute) (brief) F23
  - serological for syphilis — *see* Serology for syphilis
  - serum T8Ø.69 ☑
    - anaphylactic (immediate) — *see also* Shock, anaphylactic T8Ø.59 ☑
    - specified reaction NEC
      - due to
        - administration of blood and blood products T8Ø.61 ☑
        - immunization T8Ø.62 ☑
        - serum specified NEC T8Ø.69 ☑
        - vaccination T8Ø.62 ☑
  - situational — *see* Disorder, adjustment
  - somatization — *see* Disorder, somatoform
  - spinal puncture G97.1
    - dural G97.1
  - stress (severe) F43.9
    - acute (agitation) ("daze") (disorientation) (disturbance of consciousness) (flight reaction) (fugue) F43.Ø
    - specified NEC F43.89
  - surgical procedure — *see* Complications, surgical procedure
  - tetanus antitoxin — *see* Complications, vaccination
  - toxic, to local anesthesia T88.59 ☑
    - in labor and delivery O74.4
- **Reaction** — *continued*
  - toxic, to local anesthesia — *continued*
    - in pregnancy O29.3X- ☑
    - postpartum, puerperal O89.3
  - toxin-antitoxin — *see* Complications, vaccination
  - transfusion (blood) (bone marrow) (lymphocytes) (allergic) — *see* Complications, transfusion
  - tuberculin skin test, abnormal R76.11
  - vaccination (any) — *see* Complications, vaccination
- **Reactive airway disease** — *see* Asthma
- **Reactive depression** — *see* Reaction, depressive
- **Rearrangement**
  - chromosomal
    - balanced (in) Q95.9
      - abnormal individual (autosomal) Q95.2
        - non-sex (autosomal) chromosomes Q95.2
        - sex/non-sex chromosomes Q95.3
      - specified NEC Q95.8
- **Recalcitrant patient** — *see* Noncompliance
- **Recanalization, thrombus** — *see* Thrombosis
- **Recession, receding**
  - chamber angle (eye) H21.55- ☑
  - chin M26.Ø9
  - gingival (postinfective) (postoperative)
    - generalized KØ6.Ø2Ø
      - minimal KØ6.Ø21
      - moderate KØ6.Ø22
      - severe KØ6.Ø23
    - localized KØ6.Ø1Ø
      - minimal KØ6.Ø11
      - moderate KØ6.Ø12
      - severe KØ6.Ø13
- **Recklinghausen disease** Q85.Ø1
  - bones E21.Ø
- **Reclus' disease** (cystic) — *see* Mastopathy, cystic
- **Recrudescence**
  - deficit
    - cerebral infarction — *see* Sequelae, infarction, cerebral
    - stroke — *see* Sequelae, infarction, cerebral
  - sequelae
    - cerebral infarction — *see* Sequelae, infarction, cerebral
    - stroke — *see* Sequelae, infarction, cerebral
- **Recrudescent typhus** (fever) A75.1
- **Recruitment, auditory** H93.21- ☑
- **Rectalgia** K62.89
- **Rectitis** K62.89
- **Rectocele**
  - female (without uterine prolapse) N81.6
    - with uterine prolapse N81.4
      - complete N81.3
      - incomplete N81.2
  - in pregnancy — *see* Pregnancy, complicated by, abnormal, pelvic organs or tissues NEC
  - male K62.3
- **Rectosigmoid junction** — *see* condition
- **Rectosigmoiditis** K63.89
  - ulcerative (chronic) K51.3Ø
    - with
      - complication K51.319
        - abscess K51.314
        - fistula K51.313
        - obstruction K51.312
        - rectal bleeding K51.311
        - specified NEC K51.318
- **Rectourethral** — *see* condition
- **Rectovaginal** — *see* condition
- **Rectovesical** — *see* condition
- **Rectum, rectal** — *see* condition
- **Recurrent** — *see* condition
  - pregnancy loss — *see* Loss (of), pregnancy, recurrent
- **Red bugs** B88.Ø
- **Red tide** — *see also* Table of Drugs and Chemicals T65.82- ☑
- **Red-cedar lung or pneumonitis** J67.8
- **Reduced**
  - mobility Z74.Ø9
  - ventilatory or vital capacity R94.2
- **Redundant, redundancy**
  - anus (congenital) Q43.8
  - clitoris N9Ø.89
  - colon (congenital) Q43.8
  - foreskin (congenital) N47.8
  - intestine (congenital) Q43.8
  - labia N9Ø.69
  - organ or site, congenital NEC — *see* Accessory

Residual — *continued*
- urine R39.198

Resistance, resistant (to)
- activated protein C D68.51
- insulin E88.819
  - complicating pregnancy O26.89- ☑
  - specified type NEC E88.818
- organism(s)
  - to
    - drug Z16.3Ø
      - aminoglycosides Z16.29
      - amoxicillin Z16.11
      - ampicillin Z16.11
      - antibiotic(s) Z16.2Ø
        - multiple Z16.24
        - specified NEC Z16.29
      - antifungal Z16.32
      - antimicrobial (single) Z16.3Ø
        - multiple Z16.35
        - specified NEC Z16.39
      - antimycobacterial (single) Z16.341
        - multiple Z16.342
      - antiparasitic Z16.31
      - antiviral Z16.33
      - beta lactam antibiotics Z16.1Ø
        - specified NEC Z16.19
      - carbapenem Z16.13
      - cephalosporins Z16.19
      - extended beta lactamase (ESBL) Z16.12
      - fluoroquinolones Z16.23
      - macrolides Z16.29
      - methicillin — *see* MRSA
      - multiple drugs (MDRO)
        - antibiotics Z16.24
        - antimicrobial Z16.35
        - antimycobacterials Z16.342
      - penicillins Z16.11
      - quinine (and related compounds) Z16.31
      - quinolones Z16.23
      - sulfonamides Z16.29
      - tetracyclines Z16.29
      - tuberculostatics (single) Z16.341
        - multiple Z16.342
      - vancomycin Z16.21
        - related antibiotics Z16.22
- thyroid hormone E07.89

Resorption
- dental (roots) KØ3.3
  - alveoli M26.79
- teeth (external) (internal) (pathological) (roots) KØ3.3

Respiration
- Cheyne-Stokes RØ6.3
- decreased due to shock, following injury T79.4 ☑
- disorder of, psychogenic F45.8
- insufficient, or poor RØ6.89
  - newborn P28.5
- painful RØ7.1
- sighing, psychogenic F45.8

Respiratory — *see also* condition
- distress syndrome (newborn) (type I) P22.Ø
  - type II P22.1
- syncytial virus, as cause of disease classified elsewhere — *see also* Virus, respiratory syncytial (RSV) B97.4

Respite care Z75.5

Response (drug)
- photoallergic L56.1
- phototoxic L56.Ø

Restenosis
- stent
  - vascular
    - end stent
      - adjacent to stent — *see* Arteriosclerosis
      - within the stent
        - coronary T82.855 ☑
        - peripheral T82.856 ☑
    - in stent
      - coronary vessel T82.855 ☑
      - peripheral vessel T82.856 ☑

Restless legs (syndrome) G25.81

Restlessness R45.1

Restoration (of)
- dental
  - aesthetically inadequate or displeasing KØ8.56
  - defective KØ8.5Ø
    - specified NEC KØ8.59
  - failure of marginal integrity KØ8.51
  - failure of periodontal anatomical intergrity KØ8.54

Restoration — *continued*
- organ continuity from previous sterilization (tuboplasty) (vasoplasty) Z31.Ø
  - aftercare Z31.42
- tooth (existing)
  - contours biologically incompatible with oral health KØ8.54
  - open margins KØ8.51
  - overhanging KØ8.52
  - poor aesthetic KØ8.56
  - poor gingival margins KØ8.51
- unsatisfactory, of tooth KØ8.5Ø
  - specified NEC KØ8.59

Restorative material (dental)
- allergy to KØ8.55
- fractured KØ8.539
  - with loss of material KØ8.531
  - without loss of material KØ8.53Ø
- unrepairable overhanging of KØ8.52

Restriction of housing space Z59.19

Rests, ovarian, in fallopian tube Q5Ø.6

Restzustand (schizophrenic) F2Ø.5

Retained — *see also* Retention
- cholelithiasis following cholecystectomy K91.86
- foreign body fragments (type of) Z18.9
  - acrylics Z18.2
  - animal quill(s) or spines Z18.31
  - cement Z18.83
  - concrete Z18.83
  - crystalline Z18.83
  - depleted isotope Z18.Ø9
  - depleted uranium Z18.Ø1
  - diethylhexyl phthalates Z18.2
  - glass Z18.81
  - isocyanate Z18.2
  - magnetic metal Z18.11
  - metal Z18.1Ø
  - nonmagnectic metal Z18.12
  - nontherapeutic radioactive Z18.Ø9
  - organic NEC Z18.39
  - plastic Z18.2
  - quill(s) (animal) Z18.31
  - radioactive (nontherapeutic) NEC Z18.Ø9
  - specified NEC Z18.89
  - spine(s) (animal) Z18.31
  - stone Z18.83
  - tooth (teeth) Z18.32
  - wood Z18.33
- fragments (type of) Z18.9
  - acrylics Z18.2
  - animal quill(s) or spines Z18.31
  - cement Z18.83
  - concrete Z18.83
  - crystalline Z18.83
  - depleted isotope Z18.Ø9
  - depleted uranium Z18.Ø1
  - diethylhexyl phthalates Z18.2
  - glass Z18.81
  - isocyanate Z18.2
  - magnetic metal Z18.11
  - metal Z18.1Ø
  - nonmagnectic metal Z18.12
  - nontherapeutic radioactive Z18.Ø9
  - organic NEC Z18.39
  - plastic Z18.2
  - quill(s) (animal) Z18.31
  - radioactive (nontherapeutic) NEC Z18.Ø9
  - specified NEC Z18.89
  - spine(s) (animal) Z18.31
  - stone Z18.83
  - tooth (teeth) Z18.32
  - wood Z18.33
- gallstones, following cholecystectomy K91.86

Retardation
- development, developmental, specific — *see* Disorder, developmental
- endochondral bone growth — *see* Disorder, bone, development or growth
- growth R62.5Ø
  - due to malnutrition E45
- mental — *see* Disability, intellectual
- motor function, specific F82
- physical (child) R62.52
  - due to malnutrition E45
- reading (specific) F81.Ø
- spelling (specific) (without reading disorder) F81.81

Retching — *see* Vomiting

Retention — *see also* Retained

Retention — *continued*
- bladder — *see* Retention, urine
- carbon dioxide E87.29
- cholelithiasis following cholecystectomy K91.86
- cyst — *see* Cyst
- dead
  - fetus (at or near term) (mother) O36.4 ☑
    - early fetal death OØ2.1
  - ovum OØ2.Ø
- decidua (fragments) (following delivery) (with hemorrhage) O72.2
  - without hemorrhage O73.1
- deciduous tooth KØØ.6
- dental root KØ8.3
- fecal — *see* Constipation
- fetus
  - dead O36.4 ☑
    - early OØ2.1
- fluid R6Ø.9
- foreign body — *see also* Foreign body, retained
  - current trauma — *code as* Foreign body, by site or type
- gallstones, following cholecystectomy K91.86
- gastric K31.89
- intrauterine contraceptive device, in pregnancy — *see* Pregnancy, complicated by, retention, intrauterine device
- membranes (complicating delivery) (with hemorrhage) O72.2
  - with abortion — *see* Abortion, by type
  - without hemorrhage O73.1
- meniscus — *see* Derangement, meniscus
- menses N94.89
- milk (puerperal, postpartum) O92.79
- nitrogen, extrarenal R39.2
- ovary syndrome N99.83
- placenta (total) (with hemorrhage) O72.Ø
  - without hemorrhage O73.Ø
  - portions or fragments (with hemorrhage) O72.2
    - without hemorrhage O73.1
- products of conception
  - early pregnancy (dead fetus) OØ2.1
  - following
    - delivery (with hemorrhage) O72.2
      - without hemorrhage O73.1
- secundines (following delivery) (with hemorrhage) O72.Ø
  - without hemorrhage O73.Ø
  - complicating puerperium (delayed hemorrhage) O72.2
  - partial O72.2
    - without hemorrhage O73.1
- smegma, clitoris N9Ø.89
- urine R33.9
  - due to hyperplasia (hypertrophy) of prostate — *see* Hyperplasia, prostate
  - drug-induced R33.Ø
  - organic R33.8
    - drug-induced R33.Ø
  - psychogenic F45.8
  - specified NEC R33.8
- water (in tissues) — *see* Edema

Reticulation, dust — *see* Pneumoconiosis

Reticulocytosis R7Ø.1

Reticuloendotheliosis
- acute infantile C96.Ø
- leukemic C91.4- ☑
- nonlipid C96.Ø

Reticulohistiocytoma (giant-cell) D76.3

Reticuloid, actinic L57.1

Reticulosis (skin)
- acute of infancy C96.Ø
- hemophagocytic, familial D76.1
- histiocytic medullary C96.A (*following* C96.6)
- lipomelanotic I89.8
- malignant (midline) C86.Ø
- polymorphic C83.8- ☑
- Sezary — *see* Sezary disease

Retina, retinal — *see also* condition
- dark area D49.81

Retinitis — *see also* Inflammation, chorioretinal
- albuminurica N18.9 *[H32]*
- diabetic — *see* Diabetes, retinitis
- disciformis — *see* Degeneration, macula
- focal — *see* Inflammation, chorioretinal, focal
- gravidarum — *see* Pregnancy, complicated by, specified pregnancy-related condition NEC

- **Retinitis** — *continued*
  - juxtapapillaris — *see* Inflammation, chorioretinal, focal, juxtapapillary
  - luetic — *see* Retinitis, syphilitic
  - pigmentosa H35.52
  - proliferans — *see* Disorder, globe, degenerative, specified type NEC
  - proliferating — *see* Disorder, globe, degenerative, specified type NEC
  - renal N18.9 *[H32]*
  - syphilitic (early) (secondary) A51.43
    - central, recurrent A52.71
    - congenital (early) A50.01 *[H32]*
    - late A52.71
  - tuberculous A18.53
- **Retinoblastoma** C69.2- ☑
  - differentiated C69.2- ☑
  - undifferentiated C69.2- ☑
- **Retinochoroiditis** — *see also* Inflammation, chorioretinal
  - disseminated — *see* Inflammation, chorioretinal, disseminated
    - syphilitic A52.71
  - focal — *see* Inflammation, chorioretinal
  - juxtapapillaris — *see* Inflammation, chorioretinal, focal, juxtapapillary
- **Retinopathy** (background) H35.ØØ
  - arteriosclerotic I7Ø.8 *[H35.Ø-]* ☑
  - atherosclerotic I7Ø.8 *[H35.Ø-]* ☑
  - central serous — *see* Chorioretinopathy, central serous
  - Coats H35.Ø2- ☑
  - diabetic — *see* Diabetes, retinopathy
  - exudative H35.Ø2- ☑
  - hypertensive H35.Ø3- ☑
  - in (due to)
    - diabetes — *see* Diabetes, retinopathy
    - sickle-cell disorders
      - nonproliferative D57.- ☑ *[H36.81-]* ☑
      - proliferative D57.- ☑ *[H36.82-]* ☑
  - of prematurity H35.1Ø- ☑
    - stage Ø H35.11- ☑
    - stage 1 H35.12- ☑
    - stage 2 H35.13- ☑
    - stage 3 H35.14- ☑
    - stage 4 H35.15- ☑
    - stage 5 H35.16- ☑
  - pigmentary, congenital — *see* Dystrophy, retina
  - proliferative NEC H35.2- ☑
    - diabetic — *see* Diabetes, retinopathy, proliferative
    - sickle-cell D57.- ☑ *[H36.82-]* ☑
    - thaslassemia H35.2 ☑
  - solar H31.Ø2- ☑
- **Retinoschisis** H33.1Ø- ☑
  - congenital Q14.1
  - specified type NEC H33.19- ☑
- **Retortamoniasis** AØ7.8
- **Retractile testis** Q55.22
- **Retraction**
  - cervix — *see* Retroversion, uterus
  - drum (membrane) — *see* Disorder, tympanic membrane, specified NEC
  - finger — *see* Deformity, finger
  - lid HØ2.539
    - left HØ2.536
      - lower HØ2.535
      - upper HØ2.534
    - right HØ2.533
      - lower HØ2.532
      - upper HØ2.531
  - lung J98.4
  - mediastinum J98.59
  - nipple N64.53
    - associated with
      - lactation O92.Ø3
      - pregnancy O92.Ø1- ☑
      - puerperium O92.Ø2
    - congenital Q83.8
  - palmar fascia M72.Ø
  - pleura — *see* Pleurisy
  - ring, uterus (Bandl's) (pathological) O62.4
  - sternum (congenital) Q76.7
    - acquired M95.4
  - uterus — *see* Retroversion, uterus
  - valve (heart) — *see* Endocarditis
- **Retrobulbar** — *see* condition
- **Retrocecal** — *see* condition
- **Retrocession** — *see* Retroversion
- **Retrodisplacement** — *see* Retroversion
- **Retroflection, retroflexion** — *see* Retroversion
- **Retrognathia, retrognathism** (mandibular) (maxillary) M26.19
- **Retrograde menstruation** N92.5
- **Retroperineal** — *see* condition
- **Retroperitoneal** — *see* condition
- **Retroperitonitis** K68.9
- **Retropharyngeal** — *see* condition
- **Retroplacental** — *see* condition
- **Retroposition** — *see* Retroversion
- **Retroprosthetic membrane** T85.398 ☑
- **Retrosternal thyroid** (congenital) Q89.2
- **Retroversion, retroverted**
  - cervix — *see* Retroversion, uterus
  - female NEC — *see* Retroversion, uterus
  - iris H21.89
  - testis (congenital) Q55.29
  - uterus (acquired) (acute) (any degree) (asymptomatic) (cervix) (postinfectional) (postpartal, old) N85.4
    - congenital Q51.818
    - in pregnancy O34.53- ☑
- **Retrovirus, as cause of disease classified elsewhere** B97.3Ø
  - human
    - immunodeficiency, type 2 (HIV 2) B97.35
    - T-cell lymphotropic
      - type I (HTLV-I) B97.33
      - type II (HTLV-II) B97.34
  - lentivirus B97.31
  - oncovirus B97.32
  - specified NEC B97.39
- **Retrusion, premaxilla** (developmental) M26.Ø9
- **Rett's disease or syndrome** F84.2
- **Reverse peristalsis** R19.2
- **Reye's syndrome** G93.7
- **Rh** (factor)
  - hemolytic disease (newborn) P55.Ø
  - incompatibility, immunization or sensitization
    - affecting management of pregnancy NEC O36.Ø9- ☑
      - anti-D antibody O36.Ø1- ☑
    - newborn P55.Ø
    - transfusion reaction — *see* Complication(s), transfusion, incompatibility reaction, Rh (factor)
  - negative mother affecting newborn P55.Ø
  - titer elevated — *see* Complication(s), transfusion, incompatibility reaction, Rh (factor)
  - transfusion reaction — *see* Complication(s), transfusion, incompatibility reaction, Rh (factor)
- **Rhabdomyolysis** (idiopathic) NEC M62.82
  - traumatic T79.6 ☑
- **Rhabdomyoma** — *see also* Neoplasm, connective tissue, benign
  - adult — *see* Neoplasm, connective tissue, benign
  - fetal — *see* Neoplasm, connective tissue, benign
  - glycogenic — *see* Neoplasm, connective tissue, benign
- **Rhabdomyosarcoma** (any type) — *see* Neoplasm, connective tissue, malignant
- **Rhabdosarcoma** — *see* Rhabdomyosarcoma
- **Rhesus** (factor) **incompatibility** — *see* Rh, incompatibility
- **Rheumatic** (acute) (subacute)
  - adherent pericardium IØ9.2
  - chronic IØ9.89
  - coronary arteritis IØ1.8
  - degeneration, myocardium IØ9.Ø
  - fever (acute) — *see* Fever, rheumatic
  - heart — *see* Disease, heart, rheumatic
  - myocardial degeneration — *see* Degeneration, myocardium
  - myocarditis (chronic) (inactive) (with chorea) IØ9.Ø
    - active or acute IØ1.2
    - with chorea (acute) (rheumatic) (Sydenham's) IØ2.Ø
  - pancarditis, acute IØ1.8
    - with chorea (acute (rheumatic) Sydenham's) IØ2.Ø
  - pericarditis (active) (acute) (with effusion) (with pneumonia) IØ1.Ø
    - with chorea (acute) (rheumatic) (Sydenham's) IØ2.Ø
    - chronic or inactive IØ9.2
  - pneumonia IØØ *[J17]*
  - torticollis M43.6
  - typhoid fever AØ1.Ø9
- **Rheumatism** (articular) (neuralgic) (nonarticular) M79.Ø
  - gout — *see* Arthritis, rheumatoid
  - intercostal, meaning Tietze's disease M94.Ø
  - palindromic (any site) M12.3Ø
    - ankle M12.37- ☑
    - elbow M12.32- ☑
    - foot joint M12.37- ☑
    - hand joint M12.34- ☑
    - hip M12.35- ☑
    - knee M12.36- ☑
    - multiple site M12.39
    - shoulder M12.31- ☑
    - specified joint NEC M12.38
    - vertebrae M12.38
    - wrist M12.33- ☑
  - sciatic M54.4- ☑
- **Rheumatoid** — *see also* condition
  - arthritis — *see also* Arthritis, rheumatoid
    - with involvement of organs NEC MØ5.6Ø
      - ankle MØ5.67- ☑
      - elbow MØ5.62- ☑
      - foot joint MØ5.67- ☑
      - hand joint MØ5.64- ☑
      - hip MØ5.65- ☑
      - knee MØ5.66- ☑
      - multiple site MØ5.69
      - shoulder MØ5.61- ☑
      - vertebra — *see* Spondylitis, ankylosing
      - wrist MØ5.63- ☑
    - seronegative — *see* Arthritis, rheumatoid, seronegative
    - seropositive — *see* Arthritis, rheumatoid, seropositive
  - carditis MØ5.3Ø
    - ankle MØ5.37- ☑
    - elbow MØ5.32- ☑
    - foot joint MØ5.37- ☑
    - hand joint MØ5.34- ☑
    - hip MØ5.35- ☑
    - knee MØ5.36- ☑
    - multiple site MØ5.39
    - shoulder MØ5.31- ☑
    - vertebra — *see* Spondylitis, ankylosing
    - wrist MØ5.33- ☑
  - endocarditis — *see* Rheumatoid, carditis
  - lung (disease) MØ5.1Ø
    - ankle MØ5.17- ☑
    - elbow MØ5.12- ☑
    - foot joint MØ5.17- ☑
    - hand joint MØ5.14- ☑
    - hip MØ5.15- ☑
    - knee MØ5.16- ☑
    - multiple site MØ5.19
    - shoulder MØ5.11- ☑
    - vertebra — *see* Spondylitis, ankylosing
    - wrist MØ5.13- ☑
  - myocarditis — *see* Rheumatoid, carditis
  - myopathy MØ5.4Ø
    - ankle MØ5.47- ☑
    - elbow MØ5.42- ☑
    - foot joint MØ5.47- ☑
    - hand joint MØ5.44- ☑
    - hip MØ5.45- ☑
    - knee MØ5.46- ☑
    - multiple site MØ5.49
    - shoulder MØ5.41- ☑
    - vertebra — *see* Spondylitis, ankylosing
    - wrist MØ5.43- ☑
  - pericarditis — *see* Rheumatoid, carditis
  - polyarthritis — *see* Arthritis, rheumatoid
  - polyneuropathy MØ5.5Ø
    - ankle MØ5.57- ☑
    - elbow MØ5.52- ☑
    - foot joint MØ5.57- ☑
    - hand joint MØ5.54- ☑
    - hip MØ5.55- ☑
    - knee MØ5.56- ☑
    - multiple site MØ5.59
    - shoulder MØ5.51- ☑
    - vertebra — *see* Spondylitis, ankylosing
    - wrist MØ5.53- ☑
  - vasculitis MØ5.2Ø
    - ankle MØ5.27- ☑
    - elbow MØ5.22- ☑
    - foot joint MØ5.27- ☑
    - hand joint MØ5.24- ☑
    - hip MØ5.25- ☑
    - knee MØ5.26- ☑
    - multiple site MØ5.29
    - shoulder MØ5.21- ☑

- **Rheumatoid** — *continued*
  - vasculitis — *continued*
    - vertebra — *see* Spondylitis, ankylosing
    - wrist MØ5.23- ☑
- **Rhinitis** (atrophic) (catarrhal) (chronic) (croupous) (fibrinous) (granulomatous) (hyperplastic) (hypertrophic) (membranous) (obstructive) (purulent) (suppurative) (ulcerative) J31.Ø
  - with
    - sore throat — *see* Nasopharyngitis
  - acute JØØ
  - allergic J3Ø.9
    - with asthma J45.9Ø9
      - with
        - exacerbation (acute) J45.9Ø1
        - status asthmaticus J45.9Ø2
    - due to
      - food J3Ø.5
      - pollen J3Ø.1
    - nonseasonal J3Ø.89
    - perennial J3Ø.89
    - seasonal NEC J3Ø.2
    - specified NEC J3Ø.89
  - infective JØØ
  - pneumococcal JØØ
  - syphilitic A52.73
    - congenital A5Ø.Ø5 *[J99]*
  - tuberculous A15.8
  - vasomotor J3Ø.Ø
- **Rhinoantritis** (chronic) — *see* Sinusitis, maxillary
- **Rhinodacryolith** — *see* Dacryolith
- **Rhinolith** (nasal sinus) J34.89
- **Rhinomegaly** J34.89
- **Rhinopharyngitis** (acute) (subacute) — *see also* Nasopharyngitis
  - chronic J31.1
  - destructive ulcerating A66.5
  - mutilans A66.5
- **Rhinophyma** L71.1
- **Rhinorrhea** J34.89
  - cerebrospinal (fluid) G96.Ø1
    - postoperative G96.Ø8
    - specified NEC G96.Ø8
    - spontaneous G96.Ø1
    - traumatic G96.Ø8
  - paroxysmal — *see* Rhinitis, allergic
  - spasmodic — *see* Rhinitis, allergic
- **Rhinosalpingitis** — *see* Salpingitis, eustachian
- **Rhinoscleroma** A48.8
- **Rhinosinusitis** — *see* Sinusitis
- **Rhinosporidiosis** B48.1
- **Rhinovirus infection NEC** B34.8
- **Rhizomelic chondrodysplasia punctata** E71.54Ø
- **Rhythm**
  - atrioventricular nodal I49.8
  - disorder I49.9
    - coronary sinus I49.8
    - ectopic I49.8
    - nodal I49.8
  - escape I49.9
  - heart, abnormal I49.9
  - idioventricular I44.2
  - nodal I49.8
  - sleep, inversion G47.2- ☑
    - nonorganic origin — *see* Disorder, sleep, circadian rhythm, psychogenic
- **Rhytidosis facialis** L98.8
- **Rib** — *see also* condition
  - cervical Q76.5
- **Riboflavin deficiency** E53.Ø
- **Rice bodies** — *see also* Loose, body, joint
  - knee M23.4- ☑
- **Richter syndrome** — *see* Leukemia, chronic lymphocytic, B-cell type
- **Richter's hernia** — *see* Hernia, abdomen, with obstruction
- **Ricinism** — *see* Poisoning, food, noxious, plant
- **Rickets** (active) (acute) (adolescent) (chest wall) (congenital) (current) (infantile) (intestinal) E55.Ø
  - adult — *see* Osteomalacia
  - celiac K9Ø.Ø
  - hypophosphatemic with nephrotic-glycosuric dwarfism E72.Ø9
  - inactive E64.3
  - kidney N25.Ø
  - renal N25.Ø
  - sequelae, any E64.3
  - vitamin-D-resistant E83.31 *[M9Ø.8Ø]*
- **Rickettsia 364D/R. philipii** (Pacific Coast tick fever) A77.8
- **Rickettsial disease** A79.9
  - specified type NEC A79.89
- **Rickettsialpox** (Rickettsia akari) A79.1
- **Rickettsiosis** A79.9
  - due to
    - Ehrlichia sennetsu A79.81
    - Neorickettsia sennetsu A79.81
    - Rickettsia akari (rickettsialpox) A79.1
  - specified type NEC A79.89
  - tick-borne A77.9
  - vesicular A79.1
- **Rider's bone** — *see* Ossification, muscle, specified NEC
- **Ridge, alveolus** — *see also* condition
  - flabby KØ6.8
- **Ridged ear, congenital** Q17.3
- **Riedel's**
  - lobe, liver Q44.79
  - struma, thyroiditis or disease EØ6.5
- **Rieger's anomaly or syndrome** Q13.81
- **Riehl's melanosis** L81.4
- **Rietti-Greppi-Micheli anemia** D56.9
- **Rieux's hernia** — *see* Hernia, abdomen, specified site NEC
- **Riga** (-Fede) **disease** K14.Ø
- **Riggs' disease** — *see* Periodontitis
- **Right aortic arch** Q25.47
- **Right middle lobe syndrome** J98.11
- **Rigid, rigidity** — *see also* condition
  - abdominal R19.3Ø
    - with severe abdominal pain R1Ø.Ø
    - epigastric R19.36
    - generalized R19.37
    - left lower quadrant R19.34
    - left upper quadrant R19.32
    - periumbilic R19.35
    - right lower quadrant R19.33
    - right upper quadrant R19.31
  - articular, multiple, congenital Q68.8
  - cervix (uteri) in pregnancy — *see* Pregnancy, complicated by, abnormal, cervix
  - hymen (acquired) (congenital) N89.6
  - nuchal R29.1
  - pelvic floor in pregnancy — *see* Pregnancy, complicated by, abnormal, pelvic organs or tissues NEC
  - perineum or vulva in pregnancy — *see* Pregnancy, complicated by, abnormal, vulva
  - spine — *see* Dorsopathy, specified NEC
  - vagina in pregnancy — *see* Pregnancy, complicated by, abnormal, vagina
- **Rigors** R68.89
  - with fever R5Ø.9
- **Riley-Day syndrome** G9Ø.1
- **RIND** (reversible ischemic neurologic deficit) I63.9
- **Ring(s)**
  - aorta (vascular) Q25.45
  - Bandl's O62.4
  - contraction, complicating delivery O62.4
  - esophageal, lower (muscular) K22.2
  - Fleischer's (cornea) H18.Ø4- ☑
  - hymenal, tight (acquired) (congenital) N89.6
  - Kayser-Fleischer (cornea) H18.Ø4- ☑
  - retraction, uterus, pathological O62.4
  - Schatzki's (esophagus) (lower) K22.2
    - congenital Q39.3
  - Soemmerring's — *see* Cataract, secondary
  - vascular (congenital) Q25.8
    - aorta Q25.45
- **Ringed hair** (congenital) Q84.1
- **Ringworm** B35.9
  - beard B35.Ø
  - black dot B35.Ø
  - body B35.4
  - Burmese B35.5
  - corporeal B35.4
  - foot B35.3
  - groin B35.6
  - hand B35.2
  - honeycomb B35.Ø
  - nails B35.1
  - perianal (area) B35.6
  - scalp B35.Ø
  - specified NEC B35.8
  - Tokelau B35.5
- **Rise, venous pressure** I87.8
- **Rising, PSA following treatment for malignant neoplasm of prostate** R97.21
- **Risk**
  - for
    - dental caries Z91.849
      - high Z91.843
      - low Z91.841
      - moderate Z91.842
    - homelessness, imminent Z59.811
    - suffocation (smothering) under another while sleeping Z72.823
  - suicidal
    - meaning personal history of attempted suicide Z91.51
    - meaning suicidal ideation — *see* Ideation, suicidal
- **Ritter's disease** LØØ
- **Rivalry, sibling** Z62.891
- **Rivalta's disease** A42.2
- **River blindness** B73.Ø1
- **Robert's pelvis** Q74.2
  - with disproportion (fetopelvic) O33.Ø
    - causing obstructed labor O65.Ø
- **Robin** (-Pierre) **syndrome** Q87.Ø
- **Robinow-Silvermann-Smith syndrome** Q87.19
- **Robinson's** (hidrotic) **ectodermal dysplasia or syndrome** Q82.4
- **Robles' disease** B73.Ø1
- **Rocky Mountain** (spotted) **fever** A77.Ø
- **Roetheln** — *see* Rubella
- **Roger's disease** Q21.Ø
- **Rokitansky-Aschoff sinuses** (gallbladder) K82.8
- **Rolando's fracture** (displaced) S62.22- ☑
  - nondisplaced S62.22- ☑
- **Romano-Ward** (prolonged QT interval) **syndrome** I45.81
- **Romberg's disease or syndrome** G51.8
- **Roof, mouth** — *see* condition
- **Rosacea** L71.9
  - acne L71.9
  - keratitis L71.8
  - specified NEC L71.8
- **Rosary, rachitic** E55.Ø
- **Rose**
  - cold J3Ø.1
  - fever J3Ø.1
  - rash R21
    - epidemic BØ6.9
- **Rosenbach's erysipeloid** A26.Ø
- **Rosenthal's disease or syndrome** D68.1
- **Roseola** BØ9
  - infantum BØ8.2Ø
    - due to human herpesvirus 6 BØ8.21
    - due to human herpesvirus 7 BØ8.22
- **Ross River disease or fever** B33.1
- **Rossbach's disease** K31.89
  - psychogenic F45.8
- **Rostan's asthma** (cardiac) — *see* Failure, ventricular, left
- **Rotation**
  - anomalous, incomplete or insufficient, intestine Q43.3
  - cecum (congenital) Q43.3
  - colon (congenital) Q43.3
  - spine, incomplete or insufficient — *see* Dorsopathy, deforming, specified NEC
  - tooth, teeth, fully erupted M26.35
  - vertebra, incomplete or insufficient — *see* Dorsopathy, deforming, specified NEC
- **Rotes Querol disease or syndrome** — *see* Hyperostosis, ankylosing
- **Roth** (-Bernhardt) **disease or syndrome** — *see* Meralgia paraesthetica
- **Rothmund** (-Thomson) **syndrome** Q82.8
- **Rotor's disease or syndrome** E8Ø.6
- **Round**
  - back (with wedging of vertebrae) — *see* Kyphosis
    - sequelae (late effect) of rickets E64.3
  - worms (large) (infestation) NEC B82.Ø
    - Ascariasis — *see also* Ascariasis B77.9
- **Roussy-Levy syndrome** G6Ø.Ø
- **Rubella** (German measles) BØ6.9
  - complication NEC BØ6.Ø9
    - neurological BØ6.ØØ
  - congenital P35.Ø
  - contact Z2Ø.4
  - exposure to Z2Ø.4
  - maternal
    - care for (suspected) damage to fetus O35.3 ☑
    - manifest rubella in infant P35.Ø
    - suspected damage to fetus affecting management of pregnancy O35.3 ☑
  - specified complications NEC BØ6.89

- **Rubeola** (meaning measles) — *see* Measles
  - meaning rubella — *see* Rubella
- **Rubeosis, iris** — *see* Disorder, iris, vascular
- **Rubinstein-Taybi syndrome** Q87.2
- **Rudimentary** (congenital) — *see also* Agenesis
  - arm — *see* Defect, reduction, upper limb
  - bone Q79.9
  - cervix uteri Q51.828
  - eye Q11.2
  - lobule of ear Q17.3
  - patella Q74.1
  - respiratory organs in thoracopagus Q89.4
  - tracheal bronchus Q32.4
  - uterus Q51.818
    - in male Q56.1
  - vagina Q52.0
- **Ruled out condition** — *see* Observation, suspected
- **Rumination** R11.10
  - with nausea R11.2
  - disorder of infancy F98.21
  - neurotic F42.8
  - newborn P92.1
  - obsessional F42.8
  - psychogenic F42.8
- **Runaway** [from current living environment] Z62.892
- **Runeberg's disease** D51.0
- **Running out of money** Z59.86
- **Runny nose** R09.89
- **Rupia** (syphilitic) A51.39
  - congenital A50.06
  - tertiary A52.79
- **Rupture, ruptured**
  - abscess (spontaneous) — *code by* site under Abscess
  - aneurysm — *see* Aneurysm
  - anus (sphincter) — *see* Laceration, anus
  - aorta, aortic I71.8
    - abdominal I71.30
      - infrarenal I71.33
      - juxtarenal I71.32
      - pararenal I71.31
    - arch I71.12
    - ascending I71.11
    - descending I71.8
      - abdominal I71.30
      - thoracic I71.13
    - syphilitic A52.01
    - thoracoabdominal I71.50
      - paravisceral I71.52
      - supraceliac I71.51
    - thorax, thoracic I71.10
    - transverse I71.12
    - traumatic — *see* Injury, aorta, laceration, major
    - valve or cusp — *see also* Endocarditis, aortic I35.8
  - appendix (with peritonitis) — *see also* Appendicitis K35.32
    - with localized peritonitis — *see also* Appendicitis K35.32
  - arteriovenous fistula, brain — *see* Fistula, arteriovenous, brain, ruptured
  - artery I77.2
    - brain — *see* Hemorrhage, intracranial, intracerebral
    - coronary — *see* Infarct, myocardium
    - heart — *see* Infarct, myocardium
    - pulmonary I28.8
    - traumatic (complication) — *see* Injury, blood vessel
  - bile duct (common) (hepatic) K83.2
    - cystic K82.2
  - bladder (sphincter) (nontraumatic) (spontaneous) N32.89
    - following ectopic or molar pregnancy O08.6
    - obstetrical trauma O71.5
    - traumatic S37.29 ☑
  - blood vessel — *see also* Hemorrhage
    - brain — *see* Hemorrhage, intracranial, intracerebral
    - heart — *see* Infarct, myocardium
    - traumatic (complication) — *see* Injury, blood vessel, laceration; major, by site
  - bone — *see* Fracture
  - bowel (nontraumatic) K63.1
  - brain
    - aneurysm (congenital) — *see also* Hemorrhage, intracranial, subarachnoid
      - syphilitic A52.05
    - hemorrhagic — *see* Hemorrhage, intracranial, intracerebral
  - capillaries I78.8
  - cardiac (auricle) (ventricle) (wall) I23.3
    - with hemopericardium I23.0

Rupture, ruptured — *continued*

  - cardiac — *continued*
    - infectional I40.9
    - traumatic — *see* Injury, heart
  - cartilage (articular) (current) — *see also* Sprain
    - knee S83.3- ☑
    - semilunar — *see* Tear, meniscus
  - cecum (with peritonitis) K65.0
    - with peritoneal abscess K35.33
    - traumatic S36.598 ☑
  - celiac artery, traumatic — *see* Injury, blood vessel, celiac artery, laceration, major
  - cerebral aneurysm (congenital) (see Hemorrhage, intracranial, subarachnoid)
  - cervix (uteri)
    - with ectopic or molar pregnancy O08.6
    - following ectopic or molar pregnancy O08.6
    - obstetrical trauma O71.3
    - traumatic S37.69 ☑
  - chordae tendineae NEC I51.1
    - concurrent with acute myocardial infarction — *see* Infarct, myocardium
    - following acute myocardial infarction (current complication) I23.4
  - choroid (direct) (indirect) (traumatic) H31.32- ☑
  - circle of Willis I60.6
  - colon (nontraumatic) K63.1
    - traumatic — *see* Injury, intestine, large
  - cornea (traumatic) — *see* Injury, eye, laceration
  - coronary (artery) (thrombotic) — *see* Infarct, myocardium
  - corpus luteum (infected) (ovary) N83.1- ☑
  - cyst — *see* Cyst
  - cystic duct K82.2
  - Descemet's membrane — *see* Change, corneal membrane, Descemet's, rupture
    - traumatic — *see* Injury, eye, laceration
  - diaphragm, traumatic — *see* Injury, intrathoracic, diaphragm
  - disc — *see* Rupture, intervertebral disc
  - diverticulum (intestine) K57.80
    - with bleeding K57.81
    - bladder N32.3
    - large intestine K57.20
      - with
        - bleeding K57.21
        - small intestine K57.40
          - with bleeding K57.41
    - small intestine K57.00
      - with
        - bleeding K57.01
        - large intestine K57.40
          - with bleeding K57.41
  - duodenal stump K31.89
  - ear drum (nontraumatic) — *see also* Perforation, tympanum
    - traumatic S09.2- ☑
      - due to blast injury — *see* Injury, blast, ear
  - esophagus K22.3
  - eye (without prolapse or loss of intraocular tissue) — *see* Injury, eye, laceration
  - fallopian tube NEC (nonobstetric) (nontraumatic) N83.8
    - due to pregnancy O00.10- ☑
      - with intrauterine pregnancy O00.11- ☑
  - fontanel P13.1
  - gallbladder K82.2
    - traumatic S36.128 ☑
  - gastric — *see also* Rupture, stomach
    - vessel K92.2
  - globe (eye) (traumatic) — *see* Injury, eye, laceration
  - graafian follicle (hematoma) N83.0- ☑
  - heart — *see* Rupture, cardiac
  - hymen (nontraumatic) (nonintentional) N89.8
  - internal organ, traumatic — *see* Injury, by site
  - intervertebral disc — *see* Displacement, intervertebral disc
    - traumatic — *see* Rupture, traumatic, intervertebral disc
  - intestine NEC (nontraumatic) K63.1
    - traumatic — *see* Injury, intestine
  - iris — *see also* Abnormality, pupillary
    - traumatic — *see* Injury, eye, laceration
  - joint capsule, traumatic — *see* Sprain
  - kidney (traumatic) S37.06- ☑
    - birth injury P15.8
    - nontraumatic N28.89

Rupture, ruptured — *continued*

  - lacrimal duct (traumatic) — *see* Injury, eye, specified site NEC
  - lens (cataract) (traumatic) — *see* Cataract, traumatic
  - ligament, traumatic — *see* Rupture, traumatic, ligament, by site
  - liver S36.116 ☑
    - birth injury P15.0
  - lymphatic vessel I89.8
  - marginal sinus (placental) (with hemorrhage) — *see* Hemorrhage, antepartum, specified cause NEC
  - membrana tympani (nontraumatic) — *see* Perforation, tympanum
  - membranes (spontaneous)
    - artificial
      - delayed delivery following O75.5
    - delayed delivery following — *see* Pregnancy, complicated by, premature rupture of membranes
  - meningeal artery I60.8
  - meniscus (knee) — *see also* Tear, meniscus
    - old — *see* Derangement, meniscus
    - site other than knee — *code as* Sprain
  - mesenteric artery, traumatic — *see* Injury, mesenteric, artery, laceration, major
  - mesentery (nontraumatic) K66.8
    - traumatic — *see* Injury, intra-abdominal, specified, site NEC
  - mitral (valve) I34.89
  - muscle (traumatic) — *see also* Strain
    - diastasis — *see* Diastasis, muscle
    - nontraumatic M62.10
      - ankle M62.17- ☑
      - foot M62.17- ☑
      - forearm M62.13- ☑
      - hand M62.14- ☑
      - lower leg M62.16- ☑
      - pelvic region M62.15- ☑
      - shoulder region M62.11- ☑
      - specified site NEC M62.18
      - thigh M62.15- ☑
      - upper arm M62.12- ☑
    - traumatic — *see* Strain, by site
  - musculotendinous junction NEC, nontraumatic — *see* Rupture, tendon, spontaneous
  - mycotic aneurysm causing cerebral hemorrhage — *see* Hemorrhage, intracranial, subarachnoid
  - myocardium, myocardial — *see* Rupture, cardiac
    - traumatic — *see* Injury, heart
  - nontraumatic, meaning hernia — *see* Hernia
  - obstructed — *see* Hernia, by site, obstructed
  - operation wound — *see* Disruption, wound, operation
  - ovary, ovarian N83.8
    - corpus luteum cyst N83.1- ☑
    - follicle (graafian) N83.0- ☑
  - oviduct (nonobstetric) (nontraumatic) N83.8
    - due to pregnancy O00.10- ☑
      - with intrauterine pregnancy O00.11- ☑
  - pancreas (nontraumatic) K86.89
    - traumatic S36.299 ☑
  - papillary muscle NEC I51.2
    - following acute myocardial infarction (current complication) I23.5
  - pelvic
    - floor, complicating delivery O70.1
    - organ NEC, obstetrical trauma O71.5
  - perineum (nonobstetric) (nontraumatic) N90.89
    - complicating delivery — *see* Delivery, complicated, by, laceration, anus (sphincter)
  - postoperative wound — *see* Disruption, wound, operation
  - prostate (traumatic) S37.828 ☑
  - pulmonary
    - artery I28.8
    - valve (heart) I37.8
    - vein I28.8
    - vessel I28.8
  - pus tube — *see* Salpingitis
  - pyosalpinx — *see* Salpingitis
  - rectum (nontraumatic) K63.1
    - traumatic S36.69 ☑
  - retina, retinal (traumatic) (without detachment) — *see also* Break, retina
    - with detachment — *see* Detachment, retina, with retinal, break
  - rotator cuff (nontraumatic) M75.10- ☑
    - complete M75.12- ☑
    - incomplete M75.11- ☑

S

- **Sclerosis, sclerotic** — *continued*
  - insular G35
  - kidney — *see* Sclerosis, renal
  - larynx J38.7
  - lateral (amyotrophic) (descending) (spinal) G12.21
    - primary G12.23
  - lens, senile nuclear — *see* Cataract, senile, nuclear
  - liver K74.1
    - with fibrosis K74.2
      - alcoholic K70.2
    - alcoholic K70.2
    - cardiac K76.1
  - lung — *see* Fibrosis, lung
  - mastoid — *see* Mastoiditis, chronic
  - mesial temporal G93.81
  - mitral I05.8
  - Monckeberg's (medial) — *see* Arteriosclerosis, extremities
  - multiple (brain stem) (cerebral) (generalized) (spinal cord) G35
  - myocardium, myocardial — *see* Disease, heart, ischemic, atherosclerotic
  - nuclear (senile), eye — *see* Cataract, senile, nuclear
  - ovary N83.8
  - pancreas K86.89
  - penis N48.6
  - peripheral arteries — *see* Arteriosclerosis, extremities
  - plaques G35
  - pluriglandular E31.8
  - polyglandular E31.8
  - posterolateral (spinal cord) — *see* Degeneration, combined
  - presenile (Alzheimer's) — *see* Disease, Alzheimer's, early onset
  - primary, lateral G12.23
  - progressive, systemic M34.0
  - pulmonary — *see* Fibrosis, lung
    - artery I27.0
    - valve (heart) — *see* Endocarditis, pulmonary
  - renal N26.9
    - with
      - cystine storage disease E72.09
      - hypertensive heart disease (conditions in I11) — *see* Hypertension, cardiorenal
    - arteriolar (hyaline) (hyperplastic) — *see* Hypertension, kidney
  - retina (senile) (vascular) H35.00
  - senile (vascular) — *see* Arteriosclerosis
  - spinal (cord) (progressive) G95.89
    - ascending G61.0
    - combined — *see also* Degeneration, combined
      - multiple G35
      - syphilitic A52.11
    - disseminated G35
    - dorsolateral — *see* Degeneration, combined
    - hereditary (Friedreich's) (mixed form) G11.11
    - lateral (amyotrophic) G12.21
      - progressive G12.23
    - multiple G35
    - posterior (syphilitic) A52.11
  - stomach K31.89
  - subendocardial, congenital I42.4
  - systemic M34.9
    - with
      - lung involvement M34.81
      - myopathy M34.82
      - polyneuropathy M34.83
    - drug-induced M34.2
    - due to chemicals NEC M34.2
    - progressive M34.0
    - specified NEC M34.89
  - temporal (mesial) G93.81
  - tricuspid (heart) (valve) I07.8
  - tuberous (brain) Q85.1
  - tympanic membrane — *see* Disorder, tympanic membrane, specified NEC
  - valve, valvular (heart) — *see* Endocarditis
  - vascular — *see* Arteriosclerosis
  - vein I87.8
- **Scoliosis** (acquired) (postural) M41.9
  - adolescent (idiopathic) — *see* Scoliosis, idiopathic, adolescent
  - congenital Q67.5
    - due to bony malformation Q76.3
    - failure of segmentation (hemivertebra) Q76.3
    - hemivertebra fusion Q76.3
    - postural Q67.5
  - degenerative M41.5- ☑
- **Scoliosis** — *continued*
  - idiopathic M41.20
    - adolescent M41.129
      - cervical region M41.122
      - cervicothoracic region M41.123
      - lumbar region M41.126
      - lumbosacral region M41.127
      - thoracic region M41.124
      - thoracolumbar region M41.125
    - cervical region M41.22
    - cervicothoracic region M41.23
    - infantile M41.00
      - cervical region M41.02
      - cervicothoracic region M41.03
      - lumbar region M41.06
      - lumbosacral region M41.07
      - sacrococcygeal region M41.08
      - thoracic region M41.04
      - thoracolumbar region M41.05
    - juvenile M41.119
      - cervical region M41.112
      - cervicothoracic region M41.113
      - lumbar region M41.116
      - lumbosacral region M41.117
      - thoracic region M41.114
      - thoracolumbar region M41.115
    - lumbar region M41.26
    - lumbosacral region M41.27
    - thoracic region M41.24
    - thoracolumbar region M41.25
  - infantile — *see* Scoliosis, idiopathic, infantile
  - neuromuscular M41.40
    - cervical region M41.42
    - cervicothoracic region M41.43
    - lumbar region M41.46
    - lumbosacral region M41.47
    - occipito-atlanto-axial region M41.41
    - thoracic region M41.44
    - thoracolumbar region M41.45
  - paralytic — *see* Scoliosis, neuromuscular
  - postprocedural M96.89
  - postradiation therapy M96.5
  - rachitic (late effect or sequelae) E64.3 *[M49.80]*
    - cervical region E64.3 *[M49.82]*
    - cervicothoracic region E64.3 *[M49.83]*
    - lumbar region E64.3 *[M49.86]*
    - lumbosacral region E64.3 *[M49.87]*
    - multiple sites E64.3 *[M49.89]*
    - occipito-atlanto-axial region E64.3 *[M49.81]*
    - sacrococcygeal region E64.3 *[M49.88]*
    - thoracic region E64.3 *[M49.84]*
    - thoracolumbar region E64.3 *[M49.85]*
  - sciatic M54.4- ☑
  - secondary (to) NEC M41.50
    - cerebral palsy, Friedreich's ataxia, poliomyelitis, neuromuscular disorders — *see* Scoliosis, neuromuscular
    - cervical region M41.52
    - cervicothoracic region M41.53
    - lumbar region M41.56
    - lumbosacral region M41.57
    - thoracic region M41.54
    - thoracolumbar region M41.55
  - specified form NEC M41.80
    - cervical region M41.82
    - cervicothoracic region M41.83
    - lumbar region M41.86
    - lumbosacral region M41.87
    - thoracic region M41.84
    - thoracolumbar region M41.85
  - thoracogenic M41.30
    - thoracic region M41.34
    - thoracolumbar region M41.35
  - tuberculous A18.01
- **Scoliotic pelvis**
  - with disproportion (fetopelvic) O33.0
    - causing obstructed labor O65.0
- **Scorbutus, scorbutic** — *see also* Scurvy
  - anemia D53.2
- **Score, NIHSS** (National Institutes of Health Stroke Scale) R29.7- ☑
- **Scotoma** (arcuate) (Bjerrum) (central) (ring) — *see also* Defect, visual field, localized, scotoma
  - scintillating H53.12- ☑
- **Scratch** — *see* Abrasion
- **Scratchy throat** R09.89
- **Screening** (for) Z13.9
  - alcoholism Z13.39
- **Screening** — *continued*
  - anemia Z13.0
  - anomaly, congenital Z13.89
  - antenatal, of mother — *see also* Encounter, antenatal screening Z36.9
  - arterial hypertension Z13.6
  - arthropod-borne viral disease NEC Z11.59
  - autism Z13.41
  - bacteriuria, asymptomatic Z13.89
  - behavioral disorder Z13.30
    - specified NEC Z13.39
  - brain injury, traumatic Z13.850
  - bronchitis, chronic Z13.83
  - brucellosis Z11.2
  - cardiovascular disorder Z13.6
  - cataract Z13.5
  - chlamydial diseases Z11.8
  - cholera Z11.0
  - chromosomal abnormalities (nonprocreative) NEC Z13.79
  - colonoscopy Z12.11
  - congenital
    - dislocation of hip Z13.89
    - eye disorder Z13.5
    - malformation or deformation Z13.89
  - contamination NEC Z13.88
  - coronavirus (disease) (novel) 2019 Z11.52
  - COVID-19 Z11.52
  - cystic fibrosis Z13.228
  - dengue fever Z11.59
  - dental disorder Z13.84
  - depression (adult) (adolescent) (child) Z13.31
    - maternal Z13.32
    - perinatal Z13.32
  - developmental
    - delays Z13.40
      - global (milestones) Z13.42
      - specified NEC Z13.49
    - handicap Z13.42
      - in early childhood Z13.42
  - diabetes mellitus Z13.1
  - diphtheria Z11.2
  - disability, intellectual Z13.39
  - disease or disorder Z13.9
    - bacterial NEC Z11.2
      - intestinal infectious Z11.0
      - respiratory tuberculosis Z11.1
    - behavioral Z13.30
      - specified NEC Z13.39
    - blood or blood-forming organ Z13.0
    - cardiovascular Z13.6
    - Chagas' Z11.6
    - chlamydial Z11.8
    - coronavirus (novel) 2019 Z11.52
    - COVID-19 Z11.52
    - dental Z13.89
    - developmental delays Z13.40
      - global (milestones) Z13.42
      - specified NEC Z13.49
    - digestive tract NEC Z13.818
      - lower GI Z13.811
      - upper GI Z13.810
    - ear Z13.5
    - endocrine Z13.29
    - eye Z13.5
    - genitourinary Z13.89
    - heart Z13.6
    - human immunodeficiency virus (HIV) infection Z11.4
    - immunity Z13.0
    - infection
      - intestinal Z11.0
        - specified NEC Z11.6
    - infectious Z11.9
    - mental health and behavioral Z13.30
      - specified NEC Z13.39
    - metabolic Z13.228
    - neurological Z13.89
    - nutritional Z13.21
      - metabolic Z13.228
        - lipoid disorders Z13.220
    - protozoal Z11.6
      - intestinal Z11.0
    - respiratory Z13.83
    - rheumatic Z13.828
    - rickettsial Z11.8
    - sexually-transmitted NEC Z11.3
      - human immunodeficiency virus (HIV) Z11.4
    - sickle-cell (trait) Z13.0
    - skin Z13.89

Septic — *continued*
- nail — *see also* Cellulitis, digit
  - with lymphangitis — *see* Lymphangitis, acute, digit
- sore — *see also* Abscess
  - throat J02.Ø
    - streptococcal J02.Ø
- spleen (acute) D73.89
- teeth, tooth (pulpal origin) KØ4.4
- throat — *see* Pharyngitis
- thrombus — *see* Thrombosis
- toe — *see* Cellulitis, digit
  - with lymphangitis — *see* Lymphangitis, acute, digit
- tonsils, chronic J35.Ø1
  - with adenoiditis J35.Ø3
- uterus — *see* Endometritis

Septicemia A41.9
- meaning sepsis — *see* Sepsis

Septum, septate (congenital) — *see also* Anomaly, by site
- anal Q42.3
  - with fistula Q42.2
- aqueduct of Sylvius QØ3.Ø
  - with spina bifida — *see* Spina bifida, by site, with hydrocephalus
- uterus Q51.28
  - complete Q51.21
  - partial Q51.22
  - specified NEC Q51.28
- vagina Q52.1Ø
  - in pregnancy — *see* Pregnancy, complicated by, abnormal vagina
    - causing obstructed labor O65.5
  - longitudinal Q52.129
    - microperforate
      - left side Q52.124
      - right side Q52.123
    - nonobstruction Q52.12Ø
    - obstructing Q52.129
      - left side Q52.122
      - right side Q52.121
  - transverse Q52.11

Sequelae (of) — *see also* condition
- abscess, intracranial or intraspinal (conditions in GØ6) GØ9
- amputation — *code to* injury with seventh character S
- burn and corrosion — *code to* injury with seventh character S
- calcium deficiency E64.8
- cerebrovascular disease — *see* Sequelae, disease, cerebrovascular
- childbirth O94
- contusion — *code to* injury with seventh character S
- corrosion — *see* Sequelae, burn and corrosion
- COVID-19 (post acute) UØ9.9
- crushing injury — *code to* injury with seventh character S
- disease
  - cerebrovascular I69.9Ø
    - alteration of sensation I69.998
    - aphasia I69.92Ø
    - apraxia I69.99Ø
    - ataxia I69.993
    - cognitive deficits I69.91 ☑
    - disturbance of vision I69.998
    - dysarthria I69.922
    - dysphagia I69.991
    - dysphasia I69.921
    - facial droop I69.992
    - facial weakness I69.992
    - fluency disorder I69.923
    - hemiplegia I69.95- ☑
    - hemorrhage
      - intracerebral — *see* Sequelae, hemorrhage, intracerebral
      - intracranial, nontraumatic NEC — *see* Sequelae, hemorrhage, intracranial, nontraumatic
      - subarachnoid — *see* Sequelae, hemorrhage, subarachnoid
    - language deficit I69.928
    - monoplegia
      - lower limb I69.94- ☑
      - upper limb I69.93- ☑
    - paralytic syndrome I69.96- ☑
    - specified effect NEC I69.998
    - specified type NEC I69.8Ø
      - alteration of sensation I69.898

Sequelae — *continued*
- disease — *continued*
  - cerebrovascular — *continued*
    - specified type — *continued*
      - aphasia I69.82Ø
      - apraxia I69.89Ø
      - ataxia I69.893
      - cognitive deficits I69.81 ☑
      - disturbance of vision I69.898
      - dysarthria I69.822
      - dysphagia I69.891
      - dysphasia I69.821
      - facial droop I69.892
      - facial weakness I69.892
      - fluency disorder I69.823
      - hemiplegia I69.85- ☑
      - language deficit I69.828
      - monoplegia
        - lower limb I69.84- ☑
        - upper limb I69.83- ☑
      - paralytic syndrome I69.86- ☑
      - specified effect NEC I69.898
    - speech deficit I69.928
      - speech deficit I69.828
    - stroke NOS — *see* Sequelae, stroke NOS
- dislocation — *code to* injury with seventh character S
- encephalitis or encephalomyelitis (conditions in GØ4) GØ9
  - in infectious disease NEC B94.8
  - viral B94.1
- external cause — *code to* injury with seventh character S
- foreign body entering natural orifice — *code to* injury with seventh character S
- fracture — *code to* injury with seventh character S
- frostbite — *code to* injury with seventh character S
- Hansen's disease B92
- hemorrhage
  - intracerebral I69.1Ø
    - alteration of sensation I69.198
    - aphasia I69.12Ø
    - apraxia I69.19Ø
    - ataxia I69.193
    - cognitive deficits I69.11 ☑
    - disturbance of vision I69.198
    - dysarthria I69.122
    - dysphagia I69.191
    - dysphasia I69.121
    - facial droop I69.192
    - facial weakness I69.192
    - fluency disorder I69.123
    - hemiplegia I69.15- ☑
    - language deficit NEC I69.128
    - monoplegia
      - lower limb I69.14- ☑
      - upper limb I69.13- ☑
    - paralytic syndrome I69.16- ☑
    - specified effect NEC I69.198
    - speech deficit NEC I69.128
  - intracranial, nontraumatic NEC I69.2Ø
    - alteration of sensation I69.298
    - aphasia I69.22Ø
    - apraxia I69.29Ø
    - ataxia I69.293
    - cognitive deficits I69.21 ☑
    - disturbance of vision I69.298
    - dysarthria I69.222
    - dysphagia I69.291
    - dysphasia I69.221
    - facial droop I69.292
    - facial weakness I69.292
    - fluency disorder I69.223
    - hemiplegia I69.25- ☑
    - language deficit NEC I69.228
    - monoplegia
      - lower limb I69.24- ☑
      - upper limb I69.23- ☑
    - paralytic syndrome I69.26- ☑
    - specified effect NEC I69.298
    - speech deficit NEC I69.228
  - subarachnoid I69.ØØ
    - alteration of sensation I69.Ø98
    - aphasia I69.Ø2Ø
    - apraxia I69.Ø9Ø
    - ataxia I69.Ø93
    - cognitive deficits — *see* subcategory I69.Ø1- ☑
    - disturbance of vision I69.Ø98
    - dysarthria I69.Ø22

Sequelae — *continued*
- hemorrhage — *continued*
  - subarachnoid — *continued*
    - dysphagia I69.Ø91
    - dysphasia I69.Ø21
    - facial droop I69.Ø92
    - facial weakness I69.Ø92
    - fluency disorder I69.Ø23
    - hemiplegia I69.Ø5- ☑
    - language deficit NEC I69.Ø28
    - monoplegia
      - lower limb I69.Ø4- ☑
      - upper limb I69.Ø3- ☑
    - paralytic syndrome I69.Ø6- ☑
    - specified effect NEC I69.Ø98
    - speech deficit NEC I69.Ø28
- hepatitis, viral B94.2
- hyperalimentation E68
- infarction
  - cerebral I69.3Ø
    - alteration of sensation I69.398
    - aphasia I69.32Ø
    - apraxia I69.39Ø
    - ataxia I69.393
    - cognitive deficits I69.31 ☑
    - disturbance of vision I69.398
    - dysarthria I69.322
    - dysphagia I69.391
    - dysphasia I69.321
    - facial droop I69.392
    - facial weakness I69.392
    - fluency disorder I69.323
    - hemiplegia I69.35- ☑
    - language deficit NEC I69.328
    - monoplegia
      - lower limb I69.34- ☑
      - upper limb I69.33- ☑
    - paralytic syndrome I69.36- ☑
    - specified effect NEC I69.398
    - speech deficit NEC I69.328
- infection, pyogenic, intracranial or intraspinal GØ9
- infectious disease B94.9
  - specified NEC B94.8
- injury — *code to* injury with seventh character S
- leprosy B92
- meningitis
  - bacterial (conditions in GØØ) GØ9
  - other or unspecified cause (conditions in GØ3) GØ9
- muscle (and tendon) injury — *code to* injury with seventh character S
- myelitis — *see* Sequelae, encephalitis
- niacin deficiency E64.8
- nutritional deficiency E64.9
  - specified NEC E64.8
- obstetrical condition O94
- parasitic disease B94.9
- phlebitis or thrombophlebitis of intracranial or intraspinal venous sinuses and veins (conditions in GØ8) GØ9
- poisoning — *code to* poisoning with seventh character S
  - nonmedicinal substance — *see* Sequelae, toxic effect, nonmedicinal substance
- poliomyelitis (acute) B91
- pregnancy O94
- protein-energy malnutrition E64.Ø
- puerperium O94
- rickets E64.3
- SARS-CoV-2 (post acute) UØ9.9
- selenium deficiency E64.8
- sprain and strain — *code to* injury with seventh character S
- stroke NOS I69.3Ø
  - alteration in sensation I69.398
  - aphasia I69.32Ø
  - apraxia I69.39Ø
  - ataxia I69.393
  - cognitive deficits I69.31 ☑
  - disturbance of vision I69.398
  - dysarthria I69.322
  - dysphagia I69.391
  - dysphasia I69.321
  - facial droop I69.392
  - facial weakness I69.392
  - hemiplegia I69.35- ☑
  - language deficit NEC I69.328
  - monoplegia
    - lower limb I69.34- ☑

Shock — *continued*
- therapeutic misadventure NEC T81.1Ø ☑
- thyroxin
  - overdose or wrong substance given or taken — *see* Table of Drugs and Chemicals, by drug, poisoning
- toxic, syndrome A48.3
- transfusion — *see* Complications, transfusion
- traumatic (immediate) (delayed) T79.4 ☑

Shoemaker's chest M95.4

Short, shortening, shortness
- arm (acquired) — *see also* Deformity, limb, unequal length
  - congenital Q71.81- ☑
  - forearm — *see* Deformity, limb, unequal length
- bowel syndrome K91.2
- breath RØ6.Ø2
- cervical (complicating pregnancy) O26.87- ☑
  - non-gravid uterus N88.3
- common bile duct, congenital Q44.5
- cord (umbilical), complicating delivery O69.3 ☑
- cystic duct, congenital Q44.5
- esophagus (congenital) Q39.8
- femur (acquired) — *see* Deformity, limb, unequal length, femur
  - congenital — *see* Defect, reduction, lower limb, longitudinal, femur
- frenum, frenulum, linguae (congenital) Q38.1
- hip (acquired) — *see also* Deformity, limb, unequal length
  - congenital Q65.89
- leg (acquired) — *see also* Deformity, limb, unequal length
  - congenital Q72.81- ☑
  - lower leg — *see also* Deformity, limb, unequal length
- limbed stature, with immunodeficiency D82.2
- lower limb (acquired) — *see also* Deformity, limb, unequal length
  - congenital Q72.81- ☑
- organ or site, congenital NEC — *see* Distortion
- palate, congenital Q38.5
- radius (acquired) — *see also* Deformity, limb, unequal length
  - congenital — *see* Defect, reduction, upper limb, longitudinal, radius
- rib syndrome Q77.2
- stature (child) (hereditary) (idiopathic) NEC R62.52
  - constitutional E34.31
  - due to
    - endocrine disorder E34.3Ø
      - specified type NEC, due to endocrine dosorder E34.39
    - genetic causes E34.329
      - ACAN gene variant E34.328
      - acid-labile subunit gene (IGFALS) defect E34.321
      - aggrecan deficiency E34.328
      - genetic syndrome with resistance to insulin-like growth factor-1 E34.322
      - growth hormone gene 1 (GH1) defect with growth hormone neutralizing antibodies E34.321
      - growth hormone insensitivity syndrome (GHIS) E34.321
      - insulin-like growth factor 1 gene (IGF1) defect E34.321
      - insulin-like growth factor-1 receptor (IGF-1R) defect E34.322
      - insulin-like growth factor-1 (IGF-1) resistance E34.322
      - NPR-2 gene variant E34.328
      - post-insulin-like growth factor-1 receptor signaling defect E34.322
      - primary insulin-like growth factor-1 (IGF-1) deficiency E34.321
      - severe primary insulin-like growth factor-1 deficiency (SPIGFD) E34.321
      - signal transducer and activator of transcription 5B gene (STAT5b) defect E34.321
      - specified genetic cause NEC E34.328
  - Laron-type E34.321
- tendon — *see also* Contraction, tendon
  - with contracture of joint — *see* Contraction, joint
  - Achilles (acquired) M67.Ø- ☑
    - congenital Q66.89
  - congenital Q79.8

Short, shortening, shortness — *continued*
- thigh (acquired) — *see also* Deformity, limb, unequal length, femur
  - congenital — *see* Defect, reduction, lower limb, longitudinal, femur
- tibialis anterior (tendon) — *see* Contraction, tendon
- umbilical cord
  - complicating delivery O69.3 ☑
- upper limb, congenital — *see* Defect, reduction, upper limb, specified type NEC
- urethra N36.8
- uvula, congenital Q38.5
- vagina (congenital) Q52.4

Shortsightedness — *see* Myopia

Shoshin (acute fulminating beriberi) E51.11

Shoulder — *see* condition

Shovel-shaped incisors KØØ.2

Shower, thromboembolic — *see* Embolism

Shunt
- arterial-venous (dialysis) Z99.2
- arteriovenous, pulmonary (acquired) I28.Ø
  - congenital Q25.72
- cerebral ventricle (communicating) in situ Z98.2
- surgical, prosthetic, with complications — *see* Complications, cardiovascular, device or implant

Shutdown, renal N28.9

Shy-Drager syndrome G9Ø.3

Sialadenitis, sialadenosis (any gland) (chronic) (periodic) (suppurative) — *see* Sialoadenitis

Sialectasia K11.8

Sialidosis E77.1

Sialitis, silitis (any gland) (chronic) (suppurative) — *see* Sialoadenitis

Sialoadenitis (any gland) (periodic) (suppurative) K11.2Ø
- acute K11.21
  - recurrent K11.22
- chronic K11.23

Sialoadenopathy K11.9

Sialoangitis — *see* Sialoadenitis

Sialodochitis (fibrinosa) — *see* Sialoadenitis

Sialodocholithiasis K11.5

Sialolithiasis K11.5

Sialometaplasia, necrotizing K11.8

Sialorrhea — *see also* Ptyalism
- periodic — *see* Sialoadenitis

Sialosis K11.7

Siamese twin Q89.4

Sibling rivalry Z62.891

Sicard's syndrome G52.7

Sicca syndrome — *see* Syndrome, Sjogren

Sick R69
- or handicapped person in family Z63.79
  - needing care at home Z63.6
- sinus (syndrome) I49.5

Sick-euthyroid syndrome EØ7.81

Sickle-cell
- anemia — *see* Disease, sickle-cell
- beta plus — *see* Disease, sickle-cell, thalassemia, beta plus
- beta zero — *see* Disease, sickle-cell, thalassemia, beta zero
- trait D57.3

Sicklemia — *see also* Disease, sickle-cell
- trait D57.3

Sickness
- air (travel) T75.3 ☑
- airplane T75.3 ☑
- alpine T7Ø.29 ☑
- altitude T7Ø.2Ø ☑
- Andes T7Ø.29 ☑
- aviator's T7Ø.29 ☑
- balloon T7Ø.29 ☑
- car T75.3 ☑
- compressed air T7Ø.3 ☑
- decompression T7Ø.3 ☑
- green D5Ø.8
- milk — *see* Poisoning, food, noxious
- motion T75.3 ☑
- mountain T7Ø.29 ☑
  - acute D75.1
- protein — *see also* Reaction, serum T8Ø.69 ☑
- radiation T66 ☑
- roundabout (motion) T75.3 ☑
- sea T75.3 ☑
- serum NEC — *see also* Reaction, serum T8Ø.69 ☑
- sleeping (African) B56.9
  - by Trypanosoma B56.9

Sickness — *continued*
- sleeping — *continued*
  - by Trypanosoma — *continued*
    - brucei
      - gambiense B56.Ø
      - rhodesiense B56.1
    - East African B56.1
    - Gambian B56.Ø
    - Rhodesian B56.1
    - West African B56.Ø
- swing (motion) T75.3 ☑
- train (railway) (travel) T75.3 ☑
- travel (any vehicle) T75.3 ☑

Sideropenia — *see* Anemia, iron deficiency

Siderosilicosis J62.8

Siderosis (lung) J63.4
- brain G93.89
- eye (globe) — *see* Disorder, globe, degenerative, siderosis

Siemens' syndrome (ectodermal dysplasia) Q82.8

Sighing RØ6.89
- psychogenic F45.8

Sigmoid — *see also* condition
- flexure — *see* condition
- kidney Q63.1

Sigmoiditis — *see also* Enteritis K52.9
- infectious AØ9
- noninfectious K52.9

Silfverskold's syndrome Q78.9

Silicosiderosis J62.8

Silicosis, silicotic (simple) (complicated) J62.8
- with tuberculosis J65

Silicotuberculosis J65

Silo-fillers' disease J68.8
- bronchitis J68.Ø
- pneumonitis J68.Ø
- pulmonary edema J68.1

Silver's syndrome Q87.19

Simian malaria B53.1

Simmonds' cachexia or disease E23.Ø

Simons' disease or syndrome (progressive lipodystrophy) E88.1

Simple, simplex — *see* condition

Simulation, conscious (of illness) Z76.5

Simultanagnosia (asimultagnosia) R48.3

Sin Nombre virus disease (Hantavirus) (cardio)-pulmonary syndrome) B33.4

Sinding-Larsen disease or osteochondrosis — *see* Osteochondrosis, juvenile, patella

Singapore hemorrhagic fever A91

Singer's node or nodule J38.2

Single
- atrium Q21.2Ø
- coronary artery Q24.5
- umbilical artery Q27.Ø
- ventricle Q2Ø.4

Singultus RØ6.6
- epidemicus B33.Ø

Sinus — *see also* Fistula
- abdominal K63.89
- arrest I45.5
- arrhythmia I49.8
- bradycardia RØØ.1
- branchial cleft (internal) (external) Q18.Ø
- coccygeal — *see* Sinus, pilonidal
- dental KØ4.6
- dermal (congenital) QØ6.8
  - with abscess QØ6.8
  - coccygeal, pilonidal — *see* Sinus, coccygeal
- infected, skin NEC LØ8.89
- marginal, ruptured or bleeding — *see* Hemorrhage, antepartum, specified cause NEC
- medial, face and neck Q18.8
- pause I45.5
- pericranii QØ1.9
- pilonidal (infected) (rectum) LØ5.92
  - with abscess LØ5.Ø2
- preauricular Q18.1
- rectovaginal N82.3
- Rokitansky-Aschoff (gallbladder) K82.8
- sacrococcygeal (dermoid) (infected) — *see* Sinus, pilonidal
- tachycardia RØØ.Ø
  - paroxysmal I47.19
- tarsi syndrome M25.57- ☑
- testis N5Ø.89
- tract (postinfective) — *see* Fistula
- urachus Q64.4

- **Sinusitis** (accessory) (chronic) (hyperplastic) (nasal) (nonpurulent) (purulent) J32.9
  - acute JØ1.9Ø
    - ethmoidal JØ1.2Ø
      - recurrent JØ1.21
    - frontal JØ1.1Ø
      - recurrent JØ1.11
    - involving more than one sinus, other than pansinusitis JØ1.8Ø
      - recurrent JØ1.81
    - maxillary JØ1.ØØ
      - recurrent JØ1.Ø1
    - pansinusitis JØ1.4Ø
      - recurrent JØ1.41
    - recurrent JØ1.91
    - specified NEC JØ1.8Ø
      - recurrent JØ1.81
    - sphenoidal JØ1.3Ø
      - recurrent JØ1.31
  - allergic — *see* Rhinitis, allergic
  - due to high altitude T7Ø.1 ☑
  - ethmoidal J32.2
    - acute JØ1.2Ø
      - recurrent JØ1.21
  - frontal J32.1
    - acute JØ1.1Ø
      - recurrent JØ1.11
  - influenzal — *see* Influenza, with, respiratory manifestations NEC
  - involving more than one sinus but not pansinusitis J32.8
    - acute JØ1.8Ø
      - recurrent JØ1.81
  - maxillary J32.Ø
    - acute JØ1.ØØ
      - recurrent JØ1.Ø1
  - sphenoidal J32.3
    - acute JØ1.3Ø
      - recurrent JØ1.31
  - tuberculous, any sinus A15.8
- **Sinusitis-bronchiectasis-situs inversus** (syndrome) (triad) Q89.3
- **Sipple's syndrome** E31.22
- **Sirenomelia** (syndrome) Q87.2
- **Siriasis** T67.Ø1 ☑
- **Sirkari's disease** B55.Ø
- **Siti** A65
- **Situation, psychiatric** F99
- **Situational**
  - disturbance (transient) — *see* Disorder, adjustment
    - acute F43.Ø
  - maladjustment — *see* Disorder, adjustment
  - reaction — *see* Disorder, adjustment
    - acute F43.Ø
- **Situs inversus or transversus** (abdominalis) (thoracis) Q89.3
- **Sixth disease** BØ8.2Ø
  - due to human herpesvirus 6 BØ8.21
  - due to human herpesvirus 7 BØ8.22
- **Sjogren-Larsson syndrome** Q87.19
- **Sjogren's syndrome or disease** — *see* Syndrome, Sjogren
- **Skeletal** — *see* condition
- **Skene's gland** — *see* condition
- **Skenitis** — *see* Urethritis
- **Skerljevo** A65
- **Skevas-Zerfus disease** — *see* Toxicity, venom, marine animal, sea anemone
- **Skin** — *see also* condition
  - clammy R23.1
  - donor — *see* Donor, skin
  - dry L85.3
  - hidebound M35.9
- **Slate-dressers' or slate-miners' lung** J62.8
- **Sleep**
  - apnea — *see* Apnea, sleep
  - deprivation Z72.82Ø
  - disorder or disturbance G47.9
    - child F51.9
    - nonorganic origin F51.9
    - specified NEC G47.8
  - disturbance G47.9
    - nonorganic origin F51.9
  - drunkenness F51.9
  - rhythm inversion G47.2- ☑
  - terrors F51.4
  - walking F51.3
    - hysterical F44.89
- **Sleep hygiene**
  - abuse Z72.821
  - inadequate Z72.821
  - poor Z72.821
- **Sleeping sickness** — *see* Sickness, sleeping
- **Sleeplessness** — *see* Insomnia
  - menopausal N95.1
- **Sleep-wake schedule disorder** G47.2Ø
- **Slim disease** (in HIV infection) B2Ø
- **Slipped, slipping**
  - epiphysis (traumatic) — *see also* Osteochondropathy, specified type NEC
    - capital femoral (traumatic) [SCFE]
      - acute (on chronic) S79.Ø1- ☑
      - nontraumatic M93.ØØ- ☑
    - current traumatic — *code as* Fracture, by site
    - upper femoral (nontraumatic) [SUFE] M93.ØØ- ☑
      - acute M93.Ø1- ☑
        - on chronic M93.Ø3- ☑
      - chronic M93.Ø2- ☑
  - intervertebral disc — *see* Displacement, intervertebral disc
  - ligature, umbilical P51.8
  - patella — *see* Disorder, patella, derangement NEC
  - rib M89.8X8
  - sacroiliac joint — *see* subcategory M53.2 ☑
  - tendon — *see* Disorder, tendon
  - ulnar nerve, nontraumatic — *see* Lesion, nerve, ulnar
  - vertebra NEC — *see* Spondylolisthesis
- **Slocumb's syndrome** E27.Ø
- **Sloughing** (multiple) (phagedena) (skin) — *see also* Gangrene
  - abscess — *see* Abscess
  - appendix K38.8
  - fascia — *see* Disorder, soft tissue, specified type NEC
  - scrotum N5Ø.89
  - tendon — *see* Disorder, tendon
  - transplanted organ — *see* Rejection, transplant
  - ulcer — *see* Ulcer, skin
- **Slow**
  - feeding, newborn P92.2
  - flow syndrome, coronary I2Ø.89
  - heart (beat) RØØ.1
- **Slowing, urinary stream** R39.198
- **Sluder's neuralgia** (syndrome) G44.89
- **Slurred, slurring speech** R47.81
- **Small** (ness)
  - for gestational age — *see* Small for dates
  - introitus, vagina N89.6
  - kidney (unknown cause) N27.9
    - bilateral N27.1
    - unilateral N27.Ø
  - ovary (congenital) Q5Ø.39
  - pelvis
    - with disproportion (fetopelvic) O33.1
      - causing obstructed labor O65.1
  - uterus N85.8
  - white kidney NØ3.9
- **Small-and-light-for-dates** — *see* Small for dates
- **Small-for-dates** (infant) PØ5.1Ø
  - with weight of
    - 499 grams or less PØ5.11
    - 5ØØ-749 grams PØ5.12
    - 75Ø-999 grams PØ5.13
    - 1ØØØ-1249 grams PØ5.14
    - 125Ø-1499 grams PØ5.15
    - 15ØØ-1749 grams PØ5.16
    - 175Ø-1999 grams PØ5.17
    - 2ØØØ-2499 grams PØ5.18
    - 25ØØ grams and over PØ5.19
  - specified NEC PØ5.19
- **Smallpox** BØ3
- **Smearing, fecal** R15.1
- **SMEI** (severe myoclonic epilepsy in infancy) G4Ø.83- ☑
- **Smith-Lemli-Opitz syndrome** E78.72
- **Smith's fracture** S52.54- ☑
- **Smoker** — *see* Dependence, drug, nicotine
- **Smoker's**
  - bronchitis J41.Ø
  - cough J41.Ø
  - palate K13.24
  - throat J31.2
  - tongue K13.24
- **Smoking**
  - passive Z77.22
- **Smothering spells** RØ6.81
- **Snaggle teeth, tooth** M26.39
- **Snapping**
  - finger — *see* Trigger finger
  - hip — *see* Derangement, joint, specified type NEC, hip
    - involving the iliotiblial band M76.3- ☑
  - knee — *see* Derangement, knee
    - involving the iliotiblial band M76.3- ☑
- **Sneddon-Wilkinson disease or syndrome** (sub-corneal pustular dermatosis) L13.1
- **Sneezing** (intractable) RØ6.7
- **Sniffing**
  - cocaine
    - abuse — *see* Abuse, drug, cocaine
    - dependence — *see* Dependence, drug, cocaine
  - gasoline
    - abuse — *see* Abuse, drug, inhalant
    - dependence — *see* Dependence, drug, inhalant
  - glue (airplane)
    - abuse — *see* Abuse, drug, inhalant
    - drug dependence — *see* Dependence, drug, inhalant
- **Sniffles**
  - newborn P28.89
- **Snoring** RØ6.83
- **Snow blindness** — *see* Photokeratitis
- **Snuffles** (non-syphilitic) RØ6.5
  - newborn P28.89
  - syphilitic (infant) A5Ø.Ø5 *[J99]*
- **Social**
  - exclusion Z6Ø.4
    - due to discrimination or persecution (perceived) Z6Ø.5
  - migrant Z59.ØØ
    - acculturation difficulty Z6Ø.3
  - rejection Z6Ø.4
    - due to discrimination or persecution Z6Ø.5
  - role conflict NEC Z73.5
  - skills inadequacy NEC Z73.4
  - transplantation Z6Ø.3
- **Sodoku** A25.Ø
- **Soemmerring's ring** — *see* Cataract, secondary
- **Soft** — *see also* condition
  - nails L6Ø.3
- **Softening**
  - bone — *see* Osteomalacia
  - brain (necrotic) (progressive) G93.89
    - congenital QØ4.8
    - embolic I63.4- ☑
    - hemorrhagic — *see* Hemorrhage, intracranial, intracerebral
    - occlusive I63.5- ☑
    - thrombotic I63.3- ☑
  - cartilage M94.2- ☑
    - patella M22.4- ☑
  - cerebellar — *see* Softening, brain
  - cerebral — *see* Softening, brain
  - cerebrospinal — *see* Softening, brain
  - myocardial, heart — *see* Degeneration, myocardial
  - spinal cord G95.89
  - stomach K31.89
- **Soldier's**
  - heart F45.8
  - patches I31.Ø
- **Solitary**
  - cyst, kidney N28.1
  - kidney, congenital Q6Ø.Ø
- **Solvent abuse** — *see* Abuse, drug, inhalant
  - dependence — *see* Dependence, drug, inhalant
- **Somatization reaction, somatic reaction** — *see* Disorder, somatoform
- **Somnambulism** F51.3
  - hysterical F44.89
- **Somnolence** R4Ø.Ø
  - nonorganic origin F51.11
- **Sonne dysentery** AØ3.3
- **Soor** B37.Ø
- **Sore**
  - bed — *see* Ulcer, pressure, by site
  - chiclero B55.1
  - Delhi B55.1
  - desert — *see* Ulcer, skin
  - eye H57.1- ☑
  - Lahore B55.1
  - mouth K13.79
    - canker K12.Ø
  - muscle M79.1Ø
  - Naga — *see* Ulcer, skin
  - of skin — *see* Ulcer, skin

- **Sore** — *continued*
  - oriental B55.1
  - pressure — *see* Ulcer, pressure, by site
  - skin L98.9
  - soft A57
  - throat (acute) — *see also* Pharyngitis
    - with influenza, flu, or grippe — *see* Influenza, with, respiratory manifestations NEC
    - chronic J31.2
    - coxsackie (virus) BØ8.5
    - diphtheritic A36.Ø
    - herpesviral BØØ.2
    - influenzal — *see* Influenza, with, respiratory manifestations NEC
    - septic JØ2.Ø
    - streptococcal (ulcerative) JØ2.Ø
    - viral NEC JØ2.8
      - coxsackie BØ8.5
  - tropical — *see* Ulcer, skin
  - veldt — *see* Ulcer, skin
- **Soto's syndrome** (cerebral gigantism) Q87.3
- **South African cardiomyopathy syndrome** I42.8
- **Southeast Asian hemorrhagic fever** A91
- **Spacing**
  - abnormal, tooth, teeth, fully erupted M26.3Ø
  - excessive, tooth, fully erupted M26.32
- **Spade-like hand** (congenital) Q68.1
- **Spading nail** L6Ø.8
  - congenital Q84.6
- **Spanish collar** N47.1
- **Sparganosis** B7Ø.1
- **Spasm**(s), **spastic, spasticity** — *see also* condition R25.2
  - accommodation — *see* Spasm, of accommodation
  - ampulla of Vater K83.4
  - anus, ani (sphincter) (reflex) K59.4
    - psychogenic F45.8
  - artery I73.9
    - cerebral G45.9
  - Bell's G51.3- ☑
  - bladder (sphincter, external or internal) N32.89
    - psychogenic F45.8
  - bronchus, bronchiole J98.Ø1
  - cardia K22.Ø
  - cardiac I2Ø.1
  - carpopedal — *see* Tetany
  - cerebral (arteries) (vascular) G45.9
  - cervix, complicating delivery O62.4
  - ciliary body (of accommodation) — *see* Spasm, of accommodation
  - colon — *see also* Irritable, bowel K58.9
    - with diarrhea K58.Ø
    - psychogenic F45.8
  - common duct K83.8
  - compulsive — *see* Tic
  - conjugate H51.8
  - coronary (artery) I2Ø.1
  - diaphragm (reflex) RØ6.6
    - epidemic B33.Ø
    - psychogenic F45.8
  - duodenum K59.89
  - epidemic diaphragmatic (transient) B33.Ø
  - esophagus (diffuse) K22.4
    - psychogenic F45.8
  - facial G51.3- ☑
  - fallopian tube N83.8
  - gastrointestinal (tract) K31.89
    - psychogenic F45.8
  - glottis J38.5
    - hysterical F44.4
    - psychogenic F45.8
      - conversion reaction F44.4
    - reflex through recurrent laryngeal nerve J38.5
  - habit — *see* Tic
  - heart I2Ø.1
  - hemifacial (clonic) G51.3- ☑
  - hourglass — *see* Contraction, hourglass
  - hysterical F44.4
  - infantile — *see* Epilepsy, spasms
  - inferior oblique, eye H51.8
  - intestinal — *see also* Syndrome, irritable bowel K58.9
    - psychogenic F45.8
  - larynx, laryngeal J38.5
    - hysterical F44.4
    - psychogenic F45.8
      - conversion reaction F44.4
  - levator palpebrae superioris — *see* Disorder, eyelid function
  - muscle NEC M62.838

- **Spasm(s), spastic, spasticity** — *continued*
  - muscle — *continued*
    - back M62.83Ø
  - nerve, trigeminal G51.Ø
  - nervous F45.8
  - nodding F98.4
  - occupational F48.8
  - oculogyric H51.8
    - psychogenic F45.8
  - of accommodation H52.53- ☑
  - ophthalmic artery — *see* Occlusion, artery, retina
  - perineal, female N94.89
  - peroneo-extensor — *see also* Deformity, limb, flat foot
  - pharynx (reflex) J39.2
    - hysterical F45.8
    - psychogenic F45.8
  - psychogenic F45.8
  - pylorus NEC K31.3
    - adult hypertrophic K31.89
    - congenital or infantile Q4Ø.Ø
    - psychogenic F45.8
  - rectum (sphincter) K59.4
    - psychogenic F45.8
  - retinal (artery) — *see* Occlusion, artery, retina
  - sigmoid — *see also* Syndrome, irritable bowel K58.9
    - psychogenic F45.8
  - sphincter of Oddi K83.4
  - stomach K31.89
    - neurotic F45.8
  - throat J39.2
    - hysterical F45.8
    - psychogenic F45.8
  - tic F95.9
    - chronic F95.1
    - transient of childhood F95.Ø
  - tongue K14.8
  - torsion (progressive) G24.1
  - trigeminal nerve — *see* Neuralgia, trigeminal
  - ureter N13.5
  - urethra (sphincter) N35.919
  - uterus N85.8
    - complicating labor O62.4
  - vagina N94.2
    - psychogenic F52.5
  - vascular I73.9
  - vasomotor I73.9
  - vein NEC I87.8
  - viscera — *see* Pain, abdominal
- **Spasmodic** — *see* condition
- **Spasmophilia** — *see* Tetany
- **Spasmus nutans** F98.4
- **Spastic, spasticity** — *see also* Spasm
  - child (cerebral) (congenital) (paralysis) G8Ø.1
- **Speaker's throat** R49.8
- **Specific, specified** — *see* condition
- **Speech**
  - defect, disorder, disturbance, impediment — *see* Disorder, speech R47.9
    - psychogenic, in childhood and adolescence F98.8
    - slurring R47.81
    - specified NEC R47.89
- **Spells, transient oxygen desaturation of newborn** — *see also* Apnea, newborn P28.4Ø
  - during sleep — *see also* Apnea, newborn, sleep, primary P28.3Ø
- **Spencer's disease** AØ8.19
- **Spens' syndrome** (syncope with heart block) I45.9
- **Sperm counts** (fertility testing) Z31.41
  - postvasectomy Z3Ø.8
    - reversal Z31.42
- **Spermatic cord** — *see* condition
- **Spermatocele** N43.4Ø
  - congenital Q55.4
  - multiple N43.42
  - single N43.41
- **Spermatocystitis** N49.Ø
- **Spermatocytoma** C62.9- ☑
  - specified site — *see* Neoplasm, malignant, by site
- **Spermatorrhea** N5Ø.89
- **Sphacelus** — *see* Gangrene
- **Sphenoidal** — *see* condition
- **Sphenoiditis** (chronic) — *see* Sinusitis, sphenoidal
- **Sphenopalatine ganglion neuralgia** G9Ø.Ø9
- **Sphericity, increased, lens** (congenital) Q12.4
- **Spherocytosis** (congenital) (familial) (hereditary) D58.Ø
  - hemoglobin disease D58.Ø
  - sickle-cell (disease) D57.8- ☑
- **Spherophakia** Q12.4

- **Sphincter** — *see* condition
- **Sphincteritis, sphincter of Oddi** — *see* Cholangitis
- **Sphingolipidosis** E75.3
  - specified NEC E75.29
- **Sphingomyelinosis** E75.3
- **Spicule tooth** KØØ.2
- **Spider**
  - bite — *see* Toxicity, venom, spider
    - nonvenomous — *see* Bite, by site, superficial, insect
  - fingers — *see* Syndrome, Marfan
  - nevus I78.1
  - toes — *see* Syndrome, Marfan
  - vascular I78.1
- **Spiegler-Fendt**
  - benign lymphocytoma L98.8
  - sarcoid LØ8.89
- **Spielmeyer-Vogt disease** E75.4
- **Spina bifida** (aperta) QØ5.9
  - with hydrocephalus NEC QØ5.4
  - cervical QØ5.5
    - with hydrocephalus QØ5.Ø
  - dorsal QØ5.6
    - with hydrocephalus QØ5.1
  - lumbar QØ5.7
    - with hydrocephalus QØ5.2
  - lumbosacral QØ5.7
    - with hydrocephalus QØ5.2
  - occulta Q76.Ø
  - sacral QØ5.8
    - with hydrocephalus QØ5.3
  - thoracic QØ5.6
    - with hydrocephalus QØ5.1
  - thoracolumbar QØ5.6
    - with hydrocephalus QØ5.1
- **Spindle, Krukenberg's** — *see* Pigmentation, cornea, posterior
- **Spine, spinal** — *see* condition
- **Spiradenoma** (eccrine) — *see* Neoplasm, skin, benign
- **Spirillosis** A25.Ø
- **Spirillum**
  - minus A25.Ø
  - obermeieri infection A68.Ø
- **Spirochetal** — *see* condition
- **Spirochetosis** A69.9
  - arthritic, arthritica A69.9
  - bronchopulmonary A69.8
  - icterohemorrhagic A27.Ø
  - lung A69.8
- **Spirometrosis** B7Ø.1
- **Spitting blood** — *see* Hemoptysis
- **Splanchnoptosis** K63.4
- **Spleen, splenic** — *see* condition
- **Splenectasis** — *see* Splenomegaly
- **Splenitis** (interstitial) (malignant) (nonspecific) D73.89
  - malarial — *see also* Malaria B54 *[D77]*
  - tuberculous A18.85
- **Splenocele** D73.89
- **Splenomegaly, splenomegalia** (Bengal) (cryptogenic) (idiopathic) (tropical) R16.1
  - with hepatomegaly R16.2
  - cirrhotic D73.2
  - congenital Q89.Ø9
  - congestive, chronic D73.2
  - Egyptian B65.1
  - Gaucher's E75.22
  - malarial — *see also* Malaria B54 *[D77]*
  - neutropenic D73.81
  - Niemann-Pick — *see* Niemann-Pick disease or syndrome
  - siderotic D73.2
  - syphilitic A52.79
    - congenital (early) A5Ø.Ø8 *[D77]*
- **Splenopathy** D73.9
- **Splenoptosis** D73.89
- **Splenosis** D73.89
- **Splinter** — *see* Foreign body, superficial, by site
- **Split, splitting**
  - foot Q72.7- ☑
  - hand Q71.6 ☑
  - heart sounds RØ1.2
  - lip, congenital — *see* Cleft, lip
  - nails L6Ø.3
  - urinary stream R39.13
- **Spondylarthrosis** — *see* Spondylosis
- **Spondylitis** (chronic) — *see also* Spondylopathy, inflammatory
  - ankylopoietica — *see* Spondylitis, ankylosing

Spondylitis — *continued*
- ankylosing (chronic) M45.9
  - with lung involvement M45.9 *[J99]*
  - cervical region M45.2
  - cervicothoracic region M45.3
  - juvenile M08.1
  - lumbar region M45.6
  - lumbosacral region M45.7
  - multiple sites M45.0
  - occipito-atlanto-axial region M45.1
  - sacrococcygeal region M45.8
  - thoracic region M45.4
  - thoracolumbar region M45.5
- atrophic (ligamentous) — *see* Spondylitis, ankylosing
- deformans (chronic) — *see* Spondylosis
- gonococcal A54.41
- gouty — *see also* Gout, by type, vertebrae M10.08
- in (due to)
  - brucellosis A23.9 *[M49.80]*
    - cervical region A23.9 *[M49.82]*
    - cervicothoracic region A23.9 *[M49.83]*
    - lumbar region A23.9 *[M49.86]*
    - lumbosacral region A23.9 *[M49.87]*
    - multiple sites A23.9 *[M49.89]*
    - occipito-atlanto-axial region A23.9 *[M49.81]*
    - sacrococcygeal region A23.9 *[M49.88]*
    - thoracic region A23.9 *[M49.84]*
    - thoracolumbar region A23.9 *[M49.85]*
  - enterobacteria — *see also* subcategory M49.8 A04.9
  - tuberculosis A18.01
- infectious NEC — *see* Spondylopathy, infective
- juvenile ankylosing (chronic) M08.1
- Kummell's — *see* Spondylopathy, traumatic
- Marie-Strumpell — *see* Spondylitis, ankylosing
- muscularis — *see* Spondylopathy, specified NEC
- psoriatic L40.53
- rheumatoid — *see* Spondylitis, ankylosing
- rhizomelica — *see* Spondylitis, ankylosing
- sacroiliac NEC M46.1
- senescent, senile — *see* Spondylosis
- traumatic (chronic) or post-traumatic — *see* Spondylopathy, traumatic
- tuberculous A18.01
- typhosa A01.05

Spondyloarthritis
- axial — *see also* Spondylitis, ankylosing
  - non-radiographic M45.A0
    - cervical M45.A2
    - cervicothoracic M45.A3
    - lumbar M45.A6
    - lumbosacral M45.A7
    - multiple sites M45.AB
    - occipito-atlanto-axial region M45.A1
    - sacral and sacrococcygeal M45.A8
    - thoracic M45.A4
    - thoracolumbar M45.A5

Spondylolisthesis (acquired) (degenerative) M43.10
- with disproportion (fetopelvic) O33.0
  - causing obstructed labor O65.0
- cervical region M43.12
- cervicothoracic region M43.13
- congenital Q76.2
- lumbar region M43.16
- lumbosacral region M43.17
- multiple sites M43.19
- occipito-atlanto-axial region M43.11
- sacrococcygeal region M43.18
- thoracic region M43.14
- thoracolumbar region M43.15
- traumatic (old) M43.10
  - acute
    - fifth cervical (displaced) S12.430 ☑
      - nondisplaced S12.431 ☑
      - specified type NEC (displaced) S12.450 ☑
        - nondisplaced S12.451 ☑
      - type III S12.44 ☑
    - fourth cervical (displaced) S12.330 ☑
      - nondisplaced S12.331 ☑
      - specified type NEC (displaced) S12.350 ☑
        - nondisplaced S12.351 ☑
      - type III S12.34 ☑
    - second cervical (displaced) S12.130 ☑
      - nondisplaced S12.131 ☑
      - specified type NEC (displaced) S12.150 ☑
        - nondisplaced S12.151 ☑
      - type III S12.14 ☑
    - seventh cervical (displaced) S12.630 ☑

Spondylolisthesis — *continued*
- traumatic — *continued*
  - acute — *continued*
    - seventh cervical — *continued*
      - nondisplaced S12.631 ☑
      - specified type NEC (displaced) S12.650 ☑
        - nondisplaced S12.651 ☑
      - type III S12.64 ☑
    - sixth cervical (displaced) S12.530 ☑
      - nondisplaced S12.531 ☑
      - specified type NEC (displaced) S12.550 ☑
        - nondisplaced S12.551 ☑
      - type III S12.54 ☑
    - third cervical (displaced) S12.230 ☑
      - nondisplaced S12.231 ☑
      - specified type NEC (displaced) S12.250 ☑
        - nondisplaced S12.251 ☑
      - type III S12.24 ☑

Spondylolysis (acquired) M43.00
- cervical region M43.02
- cervicothoracic region M43.03
- congenital Q76.2
- lumbar region M43.06
- lumbosacral region M43.07
  - with disproportion (fetopelvic) O33.0
    - causing obstructed labor O65.8
- multiple sites M43.09
- occipito-atlanto-axial region M43.01
- sacrococcygeal region M43.08
- thoracic region M43.04
- thoracolumbar region M43.05

Spondylopathy M48.9
- infective NEC M46.50
  - cervical region M46.52
  - cervicothoracic region M46.53
  - lumbar region M46.56
  - lumbosacral region M46.57
  - multiple sites M46.59
  - occipito-atlanto-axial region M46.51
  - sacrococcygeal region M46.58
  - thoracic region M46.54
  - thoracolumbar region M46.55
- inflammatory M46.90
  - cervical region M46.92
  - cervicothoracic region M46.93
  - lumbar region M46.96
  - lumbosacral region M46.97
  - multiple sites M46.99
  - occipito-atlanto-axial region M46.91
  - sacrococcygeal region M46.98
  - specified type NEC M46.80
    - cervical region M46.82
    - cervicothoracic region M46.83
    - lumbar region M46.86
    - lumbosacral region M46.87
    - multiple sites M46.89
    - occipito-atlanto-axial region M46.81
    - sacrococcygeal region M46.88
    - thoracic region M46.84
    - thoracolumbar region M46.85
  - thoracic region M46.94
  - thoracolumbar region M46.95
- neuropathic, in
  - syringomyelia and syringobulbia G95.0
  - tabes dorsalis A52.11
- specified NEC — *see* subcategory M48.8 ☑
- traumatic M48.30
  - cervical region M48.32
  - cervicothoracic region M48.33
  - lumbar region M48.36
  - lumbosacral region M48.37
  - occipito-atlanto-axial region M48.31
  - sacrococcygeal region M48.38
  - thoracic region M48.34
  - thoracolumbar region M48.35

Spondylosis M47.9
- with
  - disproportion (fetopelvic) O33.0
    - causing obstructed labor O65.0
  - myelopathy NEC M47.10
    - cervical region M47.12
    - cervicothoracic region M47.13
    - lumbar region M47.16
    - occipito-atlanto-axial region M47.11
    - thoracic region M47.14
    - thoracolumbar region M47.15
  - radiculopathy M47.20
    - cervical region M47.22

Spondylosis — *continued*
- with — *continued*
  - radiculopathy — *continued*
    - cervicothoracic region M47.23
    - lumbar region M47.26
    - lumbosacral region M47.27
    - occipito-atlanto-axial region M47.21
    - sacrococcygeal region M47.28
    - thoracic region M47.24
    - thoracolumbar region M47.25
- specified NEC M47.899
  - cervical region M47.892
  - cervicothoracic region M47.893
  - facet joint M47.819
  - lumbar region M47.896
  - lumbosacral region M47.897
  - occipito-atlanto-axial region M47.891
  - sacrococcygeal region M47.898
  - thoracic region M47.894
  - thoracolumbar region M47.895
- traumatic — *see* Spondylopathy, traumatic
- without myelopathy or radiculopathy M47.819
  - cervical region M47.812
  - cervicothoracic region M47.813
  - lumbar region M47.816
  - lumbosacral region M47.817
  - occipito-atlanto-axial region M47.811
  - sacrococcygeal region M47.818
  - thoracic region M47.814
  - thoracolumbar region M47.815

Sponge
- inadvertently left in operation wound — *see* Foreign body, accidentally left during a procedure
- kidney (medullary) Q61.5

Sponge-diver's disease — *see* Toxicity, venom, marine animal, sea anemone

Spongioblastoma (any type) — *see* Neoplasm, malignant, by site
- specified site — *see* Neoplasm, malignant, by site
- unspecified site C71.9

Spongioneuroblastoma — *see* Neoplasm, malignant, by site

Spontaneous — *see also* condition
- fracture (cause unknown) — *see* Fracture, pathological

Spoon nail L60.3
- congenital Q84.6

Sporadic — *see* condition

Sporothrix schenckii infection — *see* Sporotrichosis

Sporotrichosis B42.9
- arthritis B42.82
- disseminated B42.7
- generalized B42.7
- lymphocutaneous (fixed) (progressive) B42.1
- pulmonary B42.0
- specified NEC B42.89

Spots, spotting (in) (of)
- Bitot's — *see also* Pigmentation, conjunctiva
  - in the young child E50.1
  - vitamin A deficiency E50.1
- cafe, au lait L81.3
- Cayenne pepper I78.1
- cotton wool, retina — *see* Occlusion, artery, retina
- de Morgan's (senile angiomas) I78.1
- Fuchs' black (myopic) — *see also* Myopia, degenerative H44.2- ☑
- intermenstrual (regular) N92.0
  - irregular N92.1
- Koplik's B05.9
- liver L81.4
- pregnancy O26.85- ☑
- purpuric R23.3
- ruby I78.1

Spotted fever — *see* Fever, spotted A77.9

Sprain (joint) (ligament)
- acromioclavicular joint or ligament S43.5- ☑
- ankle S93.40- ☑
  - calcaneofibular ligament S93.41- ☑
  - deltoid ligament S93.42- ☑
  - internal collateral ligament — *see* Sprain, ankle, specified ligament NEC
  - specified ligament NEC S93.49- ☑
  - talofibular ligament — *see* Sprain, ankle, specified ligament NEC
  - tibiofibular ligament S93.43- ☑
- anterior longitudinal, cervical S13.4 ☑
- atlas, atlanto-axial, atlanto-occipital S13.4 ☑
- breast bone — *see* Sprain, sternum
- calcaneofibular — *see* Sprain, ankle

Stahli's line (cornea) (pigment) — *see* Pigmentation, cornea, anterior

Stain, staining
- meconium (newborn) P96.83
- port wine Q82.5
- tooth, teeth (hard tissues) (extrinsic) K03.6
  - due to
    - accretions K03.6
    - deposits (betel) (black) (green) (materia alba) (orange) (soft) (tobacco) K03.6
    - metals (copper) (silver) K03.7
    - nicotine K03.6
    - pulpal bleeding K03.7
    - tobacco K03.6
  - intrinsic K00.8

Stammering — *see also* Disorder, fluency F80.81

Standstill
- auricular I45.5
- cardiac — *see* Arrest, cardiac
- sinoatrial I45.5
- ventricular — *see* Arrest, cardiac

Stannosis J63.5

Stanton's disease — *see* Melioidosis

Staphylitis (acute) (catarrhal) (chronic) (gangrenous) (membranous) (suppurative) (ulcerative) K12.2

Staphylococcal scalded skin syndrome L00

Staphylococcemia A41.2

Staphylococcus, staphylococcal — *see also* condition
- as cause of disease classified elsewhere B95.8
  - aureus (methicillin susceptible) (MSSA) B95.61
    - methicillin resistant (MRSA) B95.62
- specified NEC, as cause of disease classified elsewhere B95.7

Staphyloma (sclera)
- cornea H18.72- ☑
- equatorial H15.81- ☑
- localized (anterior) H15.82- ☑
- posticum H15.83- ☑
- ring H15.85- ☑

Stargardt's disease — *see* Dystrophy, retina

Starvation (inanition) (due to lack of food) T73.0 ☑
- edema — *see* Malnutrition, severe

Stasis
- bile (noncalculous) K83.1
- bronchus J98.09
  - with infection — *see* Bronchitis
- cardiac — *see* Failure, heart, congestive
- cecum K59.89
- colon K59.89
- dermatitis I87.2
  - with
    - varicose ulcer — *see* Varix, leg, with ulcer, with inflammation
    - varicose veins — *see* Varix, leg, with, inflammation
  - due to postthrombotic syndrome — *see* Syndrome, postthrombotic
- duodenal K31.5
- eczema — *see* Varix, leg, with, inflammation
- edema — *see* Hypertension, venous (chronic), idiopathic
- foot T69.0- ☑
- ileocecal coil K59.89
- ileum K59.89
- intestinal K59.89
- jejunum K59.89
- kidney N19
- liver (cirrhotic) K76.1
- lymphatic I89.8
- pneumonia J18.2
- pulmonary — *see* Edema, lung
- rectal K59.89
- renal N19
  - tubular N17.0
- ulcer — *see* Varix, leg, with, ulcer
  - without varicose veins — *see also* Ulcer, by site I87.2
- urine — *see* Retention, urine
- venous I87.8

State (of)
- affective and paranoid, mixed, organic psychotic F06.8
- agitated R45.1
  - acute reaction to stress F43.0
- anxiety (neurotic) F41.1
- apprehension F41.1
- burn-out Z73.0
- climacteric, female Z78.0
  - symptomatic N95.1
- compulsive F42.8

State — *continued*
- compulsive — *continued*
  - mixed with obsessional thoughts F42.2
- confusional (psychogenic) F44.89
  - acute — *see also* Delirium
    - with
      - arteriosclerotic dementia — *see also* Dementia, vascular F01.50
        - with behavioral disturbance — *see* Dementia, vascular
      - senility or dementia F05
    - alcoholic F10.231
  - epileptic F05
  - reactive (from emotional stress, psychological trauma) F44.89
  - subacute — *see* Delirium
- convulsive — *see* Convulsions
- crisis F43.0
- depressive F32.A
  - neurotic F34.1
- dissociative F44.9
- emotional shock (stress) R45.7
- hypercoagulation — *see* Hypercoagulable
- locked-in G83.5
- menopausal Z78.0
  - symptomatic N95.1
- neurotic F48.9
  - with depersonalization F48.1
- obsessional F42.8
- oneiroid (schizophrenia-like) F23
- organic
  - hallucinatory (nonalcoholic) F06.0
  - paranoid (-hallucinatory) F06.2
- panic F41.0
- paranoid F22
  - climacteric F22
  - involutional F22
  - menopausal F22
  - organic F06.2
  - senile F03 ☑
  - simple F22
- persistent vegetative R40.3
- phobic F40.9
- postleukotomy F07.0
- pregnant
  - gestational carrier Z33.3
  - incidental Z33.1
- psychogenic, twilight F44.89
- psychopathic (constitutional) F60.2
- psychotic, organic — *see also* Psychosis, organic
  - mixed paranoid and affective F06.8
  - senile or presenile F03 ☑
  - transient NEC F06.8
    - with
      - depression F06.31
      - hallucinations F06.0
- residual schizophrenic F20.5
- restlessness R45.1
- stress (emotional) R45.7
- tension (mental) F48.9
  - specified NEC F48.8
- transient organic psychotic NEC F06.8
  - depressive type F06.31
  - hallucinatory type F06.0
- twilight
  - epileptic F05
  - psychogenic F44.89
- vegetative, persistent R40.3
- vital exhaustion Z73.0
- withdrawal, — *see* Withdrawal, state

Status (post) — *see also* Presence (of)
- absence, epileptic — *see* Epilepsy, by type, with status epilepticus
- administration of tPA (rtPA) in a different facility within the last 24 hours prior to admission to current facility Z92.82
- adrenalectomy (unilateral) (bilateral) E89.6
- anastomosis Z98.0
- anginosus I20.9
- angioplasty (peripheral) Z98.62
  - with implant Z95.820
  - coronary artery Z98.61
    - with implant Z95.5
- aortocoronary bypass Z95.1
- arthrodesis Z98.1
- artificial opening (of) Z93.9
  - gastrointestinal tract Z93.4
  - specified NEC Z93.8

Status — *continued*
- artificial opening — *continued*
  - urinary tract Z93.6
  - vagina Z93.8
- asthmaticus — *see* Asthma, by type, with status asthmaticus
- awaiting organ transplant Z76.82
- bariatric surgery Z98.84
- bed confinement Z74.01
- bleb, filtering (vitreous), after glaucoma surgery Z98.83
- breast implant Z98.82
  - removal Z98.86
- cataract extraction Z98.4- ☑
- cholecystectomy Z90.49
- clitorectomy N90.811
  - with excision of labia minora N90.812
- colectomy (complete) (partial) Z90.49
- colonization — *see* Carrier (suspected) of
- colostomy Z93.3
- convulsivus idiopathicus — *see* Epilepsy, by type, with status epilepticus
- coronary artery angioplasty — *see* Status, angioplasty, coronary artery
- coronary artery bypass graft Z95.1
- cystectomy (urinary bladder) Z90.6
- cystostomy Z93.50
  - appendico-vesicostomy Z93.52
  - cutaneous Z93.51
  - specified NEC Z93.59
- delinquent immunization Z28.39
  - COVID-19 Z28.31- ☑
- dental Z98.818
  - crown Z98.811
  - fillings Z98.811
  - restoration Z98.811
  - sealant Z98.810
  - specified NEC Z98.818
- deployment (current) (military) Z56.82
- dialysis (hemodialysis) (peritoneal) Z99.2
- do not resuscitate (DNR) Z66
- donor — *see* Donor
- embedded fragments — *see* Retained, foreign body fragments (type of)
- embedded splinter — *see* Retained, foreign body fragments (type of)
- enterostomy Z93.4
- epileptic, epilepticus — *see also* Epilepsy, by type, with status epilepticus G40.901
- estrogen receptor
  - negative Z17.1
  - positive Z17.0
- female genital cutting — *see* Female genital mutilation status
- female genital mutilation — *see* Female genital mutilation status
- filtering (vitreous) bleb after glaucoma surgery Z98.83
- gastrectomy (complete) (partial) Z90.3
- gastric banding Z98.84
- gastric bypass for obesity Z98.84
- gastrostomy Z93.1
- human immunodeficiency virus (HIV) infection, asymptomatic Z21
- hysterectomy (complete) (total) Z90.710
  - partial (with remaining cervial stump) Z90.711
- ileostomy Z93.2
- implant
  - breast Z98.82
- infibulation N90.813
- intestinal bypass Z98.0
- jejunostomy Z93.4
- lapsed immunization schedule Z28.39
- laryngectomy Z90.02
- lymphaticus E32.8
- malignancy
  - castrate resistant prostate Z19.2
  - hormone resistant Z19.2
  - hormone sensitive Z19.1
- marmoratus G80.3
- mastectomy (unilateral) (bilateral) Z90.1- ☑
- military deployment status (current) Z56.82
  - in theater or in support of military war, peacekeeping and humanitarian operations Z56.82
- nephrectomy (unilateral) (bilateral) Z90.5
- nephrostomy Z93.6
- obesity surgery Z98.84
- oophorectomy
  - bilateral Z90.722
  - unilateral Z90.721

Status — *continued*
- organ replacement
  - by artificial or mechanical device or prosthesis of
    - artery Z95.828
    - bladder Z96.Ø
    - blood vessel Z95.828
    - breast Z97.8
    - eye globe Z97.Ø
    - heart Z95.812
      - valve Z95.2
    - intestine Z97.8
    - joint Z96.6Ø
      - hip — *see* Presence, hip joint implant
      - knee — *see* Presence, knee joint implant
      - specified site NEC Z96.698
    - kidney Z97.8
    - larynx Z96.3
    - lens Z96.1
    - limbs — *see* Presence, artificial, limb
    - liver Z97.8
    - lung Z97.8
    - pancreas Z97.8
  - by organ transplant (heterologous) (homologous) — *see* Transplant
- pacemaker
  - brain Z96.89
  - cardiac Z95.Ø
  - specified NEC Z96.89
- pancreatectomy Z9Ø.41Ø
  - complete Z9Ø.41Ø
  - partial Z9Ø.411
  - total Z9Ø.41Ø
- physical restraint Z78.1
- pneumonectomy (complete) (partial) Z9Ø.2
- pneumothorax, therapeutic Z98.3
- postcommotio cerebri FØ7.81
- postoperative (postprocedural) NEC Z98.89Ø
  - breast implant Z98.82
  - dental Z98.818
    - crown Z98.811
    - fillings Z98.811
    - restoration Z98.811
    - sealant Z98.81Ø
    - specified NEC Z98.818
  - pneumothorax, therapeutic Z98.3
  - uterine scar Z98.891
- postpartum (routine follow-up) Z39.2
  - care immediately after delivery Z39.Ø
- postsurgical (postprocedural) NEC Z98.89Ø
  - pneumothorax, therapeutic Z98.3
- pregnancy, incidental Z33.1
- prosthesis coronary angioplasty Z95.5
- pseudophakia Z96.1
- renal dialysis (hemodialysis) (peritoneal) Z99.2
- retained foreign body — *see* Retained, foreign body fragments (type of)
- reversed jejunal transposition (for bypass) Z98.Ø
- salpingo-oophorectomy
  - bilateral Z9Ø.722
  - unilateral Z9Ø.721
- sex reassignment surgery status Z87.89Ø
- shunt
  - arteriovenous (for dialysis) Z99.2
  - cerebrospinal fluid Z98.2
  - ventricular (communicating) (for drainage) Z98.2
- splenectomy Z9Ø.81
- thymicolymphaticus E32.8
- thymicus E32.8
- thymolymphaticus E32.8
- thyroidectomy (hypothyroidism) E89.Ø
- tooth (teeth) extraction — *see also* Absence, teeth, acquired KØ8.4Ø9
- tPA (rtPA) administration in a different facility within the last 24 hours prior to admission to current facility Z92.82
- tracheostomy Z93.Ø
- transplant — *see* Transplant
  - organ removed Z98.85
- tubal ligation Z98.51
- underimmunization Z28.39
  - COVID-19 Z28.31- ☑
    - partially vaccinated (for) Z28.311
    - unvaccinated (for) Z28.31Ø
- ureterostomy Z93.6
- urethrostomy Z93.6
- vagina, artificial Z93.8
- vasectomy Z98.52
- wheelchair confinement Z99.3

Stealing
- child problem F91.8
  - in company with others Z72.81Ø
- pathological (compulsive) F63.2

Steam burn — *see* Burn

Steatocystoma multiplex L72.2

Steatohepatitis (nonalcoholic) (NASH) K75.81

Steatoma L72.3
- eyelid (cystic) — *see* Dermatosis, eyelid
  - infected — *see* Hordeolum

Steatorrhea (chronic) K9Ø.9
- with lacteal obstruction K9Ø.2
- idiopathic (adult) (infantile) K9Ø.9
- pancreatic K9Ø.3
- primary K9Ø.Ø
- tropical K9Ø.1

Steatosis E88.89
- heart — *see* Degeneration, myocardial
- kidney N28.89
- liver NEC K76.Ø

Steele-Richardson-Olszewski disease or syndrome G23.1

Steinbrocker's syndrome G9Ø.8

Steinert's disease G71.11

Stein-Leventhal syndrome E28.2

Stein's syndrome E28.2

STEMI — *see also* Infarct, myocardium, ST elevation I21.3

Stenocardia I2Ø.89

Stenocephaly Q75.8

Stenosis, stenotic (cicatricial) — *see also* Stricture
- ampulla of Vater K83.1
- anus, anal (canal) (sphincter) K62.4
  - and rectum K62.4
  - congenital Q42.3
    - with fistula Q42.2
- aorta (ascending) (supraventricular) (congenital) Q25.1
  - arteriosclerotic I7Ø.Ø
  - calcified I7Ø.Ø
  - supravalvular Q25.3
- aortic (valve) I35.Ø
  - with insufficiency I35.2
  - congenital Q23.Ø
  - rheumatic IØ6.Ø
    - with
      - incompetency, insufficiency or regurgitation IØ6.2
        - with mitral (valve) disease IØ8.Ø
          - with tricuspid (valve) disease IØ8.3
      - mitral (valve) disease IØ8.Ø
        - with tricuspid (valve) disease IØ8.3
      - tricuspid (valve) disease IØ8.2
        - with mitral (valve) disease IØ8.3
  - specified cause NEC I35.Ø
  - syphilitic A52.Ø3
- aqueduct of Sylvius (congenital) QØ3.Ø
  - with spina bifida — *see* Spina bifida, by site, with hydrocephalus
  - acquired G91.1
- artery NEC — *see also* Arteriosclerosis I77.1
  - celiac I77.4
  - cerebral — *see* Occlusion, artery, cerebral
  - extremities — *see* Arteriosclerosis, extremities
  - precerebral — *see* Occlusion, artery, precerebral
  - pulmonary (congenital) Q25.6
    - acquired I28.8
  - renal I7Ø.1
  - stent
    - coronary T82.855 ☑
    - peripheral T82.856 ☑
- bile duct (common) (hepatic) K83.1
  - congenital Q44.3
- bladder-neck (acquired) N32.Ø
  - congenital Q64.31
- brain G93.89
- bronchus J98.Ø9
  - congenital Q32.3
  - syphilitic A52.72
- cardia (stomach) K22.2
  - congenital Q39.3
- cardiovascular — *see* Disease, cardiovascular
- caudal M48.Ø8
- cervix, cervical (canal) N88.2
  - congenital Q51.828
  - in pregnancy or childbirth — *see* Pregnancy, complicated by, abnormal cervix
- colon — *see also* Obstruction, intestine
  - congenital Q42.9
    - specified NEC Q42.8

Stenosis, stenotic — *continued*
- colostomy K94.Ø3
- common (bile) duct K83.1
  - congenital Q44.3
- coronary (artery) — *see* Disease, heart, ischemic, atherosclerotic
- cystic duct — *see* Obstruction, gallbladder
- due to presence of device, implant or graft — *see also* Complications, by site and type, specified NEC T85.858 ☑
  - arterial graft NEC T82.858 ☑
  - breast (implant) T85.858 ☑
  - catheter T85.858 ☑
    - dialysis (renal) T82.858 ☑
      - intraperitoneal T85.858 ☑
    - infusion NEC T82.858 ☑
      - spinal (epidural) (subdural) T85.85Ø ☑
    - urinary (indwelling) T83.85 ☑
  - fixation, internal (orthopedic) NEC T84.85 ☑
  - gastrointestinal (bile duct) (esophagus) T85.858 ☑
  - genital NEC T83.85 ☑
  - heart NEC T82.857 ☑
  - joint prosthesis T84.85 ☑
  - ocular (corneal graft) (orbital implant) NEC T85.858 ☑
  - orthopedic NEC T84.85 ☑
  - specified NEC T85.858 ☑
  - urinary NEC T83.85 ☑
  - vascular NEC T82.858 ☑
  - ventricular intracranial shunt T85.85Ø ☑
- duodenum K31.5
  - congenital Q41.Ø
- ejaculatory duct NEC N5Ø.89
  - stent
    - vascular
      - end stent
        - adjacent to stent — *see* Arteriosclerosis
        - within the stent
          - coronary T82.855 ☑
          - peripheral T82.856 ☑
      - in stent
        - coronary vessel T82.855 ☑
        - peripheral vessel T82.856 ☑
- endocervical os — *see* Stenosis, cervix
- enterostomy K94.13
- esophagus K22.2
  - congenital Q39.3
  - syphilitic A52.79
    - congenital A5Ø.59 *[K23]*
- eustachian tube — *see* Obstruction, eustachian tube
- external ear canal (acquired) H61.3Ø- ☑
  - congenital Q16.1
  - due to
    - inflammation H61.32- ☑
    - trauma H61.31- ☑
  - postprocedural H95.81- ☑
  - specified cause NEC H61.39- ☑
- gallbladder — *see* Obstruction, gallbladder
- glottis J38.6
- heart valve — *see also* Endocarditis I38
  - aortic — *see* Stenosis, aortic
  - congenital Q24.8
  - mitral — *see* Stenosis, mitral
  - pulmonary — *see* Stenosis, pulmonary valve
  - tricuspid — *see* Stenosis, tricuspid
- hepatic duct K83.1
- hymen N89.6
- hypertrophic subaortic (idiopathic) I42.1
- ileum — *see also* Obstruction, intestine, specified NEC K56.699
  - congenital Q41.2
- infundibulum cardia Q24.3
- intervertebral foramina — *see also* Lesion, biomechanical, specified NEC
  - connective tissue M99.79
    - abdomen M99.79
    - cervical region M99.71
    - cervicothoracic M99.71
    - head region M99.7Ø
    - lumbar region M99.73
    - lumbosacral M99.73
    - occipitocervical M99.7Ø
    - sacral region M99.74
    - sacrococcygeal M99.74
    - sacroiliac M99.74
    - specified NEC M99.79
    - thoracic region M99.72

Stenosis, stenotic — *continued*
  intervertebral foramina — *see also* Lesion, biomechanical, specified — *continued*
    connective tissue — *continued*
      thoracolumbar M99.72
    disc M99.79
      abdomen M99.79
      cervical region M99.71
      cervicothoracic M99.71
      head region M99.7Ø
      lower extremity M99.76
      lumbar region M99.73
      lumbosacral M99.73
      occipitocervical M99.7Ø
      pelvic M99.75
      rib cage M99.78
      sacral region M99.74
      sacrococcygeal M99.74
      sacroiliac M99.74
      specified NEC M99.79
      thoracic region M99.72
      thoracolumbar M99.72
      upper extremity M99.77
    osseous M99.69
      abdomen M99.69
      cervical region M99.61
      cervicothoracic M99.61
      head region M99.6Ø
      lower extremity M99.66
      lumbar region M99.63
      lumbosacral M99.63
      occipitocervical M99.6Ø
      pelvic M99.65
      rib cage M99.68
      sacral region M99.64
      sacrococcygeal M99.64
      sacroiliac M99.64
      specified NEC M99.69
      thoracic region M99.62
      thoracolumbar M99.62
      upper extremity M99.67
    subluxation — *see* Stenosis, intervertebral foramina, osseous
  intestine — *see also* Obstruction, intestine
    congenital (small) Q41.9
      large Q42.9
        specified NEC Q42.8
      specified NEC Q41.8
  jejunum — *see also* Obstruction, intestine, specified NEC K56.699
    congenital Q41.1
  lacrimal (passage)
    canaliculi HØ4.54- ☑
    congenital Q1Ø.5
    duct HØ4.55- ☑
    punctum HØ4.56- ☑
    sac HØ4.57- ☑
  lacrimonasal duct — *see* Stenosis, lacrimal, duct
    congenital Q1Ø.5
  larynx J38.6
    congenital NEC Q31.8
      subglottic Q31.1
    syphilitic A52.73
      congenital A5Ø.59 *[J99]*
  mitral (chronic) (inactive) (valve) IØ5.Ø
    with
      aortic valve disease IØ8.Ø
      incompetency, insufficiency or regurgitation IØ5.2
    active or acute IØ1.1
      with rheumatic or Sydenham's chorea IØ2.Ø
    congenital Q23.2
    specified cause, except rheumatic I34.2
    syphilitic A52.Ø3
  myocardium, myocardial — *see also* Degeneration, myocardial
    hypertrophic subaortic (idiopathic) I42.1
  nares (anterior) (posterior) J34.89
    congenital Q3Ø.Ø
  nasal duct — *see also* Stenosis, lacrimal, duct
    congenital Q1Ø.5
  nasolacrimal duct — *see also* Stenosis, lacrimal, duct
    congenital Q1Ø.5
  neural canal — *see also* Lesion, biomechanical, specified NEC
    connective tissue M99.49
      abdomen M99.49
      cervical region M99.41

Stenosis, stenotic — *continued*
  neural canal — *see also* Lesion, biomechanical, specified — *continued*
    connective tissue — *continued*
      cervicothoracic M99.41
      head region M99.4Ø
      lower extremity M99.46
      lumbar region M99.43
      lumbosacral M99.43
      occipitocervical M99.4Ø
      pelvic M99.45
      rib cage M99.48
      sacral region M99.44
      sacrococcygeal M99.44
      sacroiliac M99.44
      specified NEC M99.49
      thoracic region M99.42
      thoracolumbar M99.42
      upper extremity M99.47
    intervertebral disc M99.59
      abdomen M99.59
      cervical region M99.51
      cervicothoracic M99.51
      head region M99.5Ø
      lower extremity M99.56
      lumbar region M99.53
      lumbosacral M99.53
      occipitocervical M99.5Ø
      pelvic M99.55
      rib cage M99.58
      sacral region M99.54
      sacrococcygeal M99.54
      sacroiliac M99.54
      specified NEC M99.59
      thoracic region M99.52
      thoracolumbar M99.52
      upper extremity M99.57
    osseous M99.39
      abdomen M99.39
      cervical region M99.31
      cervicothoracic M99.31
      head region M99.3Ø
      lower extremity M99.36
      lumbar region M99.33
      lumbosacral M99.33
      occipitocervical M99.3Ø
      pelvic M99.35
      rib cage M99.38
      sacral region M99.34
      sacrococcygeal M99.34
      sacroiliac M99.34
      specified NEC M99.39
      thoracic region M99.32
      thoracolumbar M99.32
      upper extremity M99.37
    subluxation M99.29
      cervical region M99.21
      cervicothoracic M99.21
      head region M99.2Ø
      lower extremity M99.26
      lumbar region M99.23
      lumbosacral M99.23
      occipitocervical M99.2Ø
      pelvic M99.25
      rib cage M99.28
      sacral region M99.24
      sacrococcygeal M99.24
      sacroiliac M99.24
      specified NEC M99.29
      thoracic region M99.22
      thoracolumbar M99.22
      upper extremity M99.27
  organ or site, congenital NEC — *see* Atresia, by site
  papilla of Vater K83.1
  pulmonary (artery) (congenital) Q25.6
    with ventricular septal defect, transposition of aorta, and hypertrophy of right ventricle Q21.3
    acquired I28.8
    in tetralogy of Fallot Q21.3
    infundibular Q24.3
    subvalvular Q24.3
    supravalvular Q25.6
    valve I37.Ø
      with insufficiency I37.2
      congenital Q22.1
      rheumatic IØ9.89
        with aortic, mitral or tricuspid (valve) disease IØ8.8
    vein, acquired I28.8

Stenosis, stenotic — *continued*
  pulmonary — *continued*
    vessel NEC I28.8
  pulmonic (congenital) Q22.1
    infundibular Q24.3
    subvalvular Q24.3
  pylorus (hypertrophic) (acquired) K31.1
    adult K31.1
    congenital Q4Ø.Ø
    infantile Q4Ø.Ø
  rectum (sphincter) — *see* Stricture, rectum
  renal artery I7Ø.1
    congenital Q27.1
  salivary duct (any) K11.8
  sphincter of Oddi K83.1
  spinal M48.ØØ
    cervical region M48.Ø2
    cervicothoracic region M48.Ø3
    lumbar region (NOS) (without neurogenic claudication) M48.Ø61
      with neurogenic claudication M48.Ø62
    lumbosacral region M48.Ø7
    occipito-atlanto-axial region M48.Ø1
    sacrococcygeal region M48.Ø8
    thoracic region M48.Ø4
    thoracolumbar region M48.Ø5
  stomach, hourglass K31.2
  subaortic (congenital) Q24.4
    hypertrophic (idiopathic) I42.1
  subglottic J38.6
    congenital Q31.1
    postprocedural J95.5
  trachea J39.8
    congenital Q32.1
    syphilitic A52.73
    tuberculous NEC A15.5
  tracheostomy J95.Ø3
  tricuspid (valve) IØ7.Ø
    with
      aortic (valve) disease IØ8.2
      incompetency, insufficiency or regurgitation IØ7.2
        with aortic (valve) disease IØ8.2
          with mitral (valve) disease IØ8.3
      mitral (valve) disease IØ8.1
        with aortic (valve) disease IØ8.3
    congenital Q22.4
    nonrheumatic I36.Ø
      with insufficiency I36.2
  tubal N97.1
  ureter — *see* Atresia, ureter
  ureteropelvic junction, congenital Q62.11
  ureterovesical orifice, congenital Q62.12
  urethra (valve) *see also* Stricture, urethra
    congenital Q64.32
  urinary meatus, congenital Q64.33
  vagina N89.5
    congenital Q52.4
    in pregnancy — *see* Pregnancy, complicated by, abnormal vagina
      causing obstructed labor O65.5
  valve (cardiac) (heart) — *see also* Endocarditis I38
    congenital Q24.8
      aortic Q23.Ø
      mitral Q23.2
      pulmonary Q22.1
      tricuspid Q22.4
  vena cava (inferior) (superior) I87.1
    congenital Q26.Ø
  vesicourethral orifice Q64.31
  vulva N9Ø.5
Stent jail T82.897 ☑
Stercolith (impaction) K56.41
  appendix K38.1
Stercoraceous, stercoral ulcer K63.3
  anus or rectum K62.6
Stereotypies NEC F98.4
Sterility — *see* Infertility
Sterilization — *see* Encounter (for), sterilization
Sternalgia — *see* Angina
Sternopagus Q89.4
Sternum bifidum Q76.7
Steroid
  effects (adverse) (adrenocortical) (iatrogenic)
    cushingoid E24.2
      correct substance properly administered — *see* Table of Drugs and Chemicals, by drug, adverse effect

Steroid — *continued*
- effects — *continued*
  - cushingoid — *continued*
    - overdose or wrong substance given or taken — *see* Table of Drugs and Chemicals, by drug, poisoning
  - diabetes — *see* subcategory E09 ☑
    - correct substance properly administered — *see* Table of Drugs and Chemicals, by drug, adverse effect
    - overdose or wrong substance given or taken — *see* Table of Drugs and Chemicals, by drug, poisoning
  - fever R50.2
  - insufficiency E27.3
    - correct substance properly administered — *see* Table of Drugs and Chemicals, by drug, adverse effect
    - overdose or wrong substance given or taken — *see* Table of Drugs and Chemicals, by drug, poisoning
- responder H40.04- ☑

Stevens-Johnson disease or syndrome L51.1
- toxic epidermal necrolysis overlap L51.3

Stewart-Morel syndrome M85.2

Sticker's disease B08.3

Sticky eye — *see* Conjunctivitis, acute, mucopurulent

Stieda's disease — *see* Bursitis, tibial collateral

Stiff neck — *see* Torticollis

Stiff-man syndrome G25.82

Stiffness, joint NEC M25.60
- ankle M25.67- ☑
- ankylosis — *see* Ankylosis, joint
- contracture — *see* Contraction, joint
- elbow M25.62- ☑
- foot M25.67- ☑
- hand M25.64- ☑
- hip M25.65- ☑
- knee M25.66- ☑
- shoulder M25.61- ☑
- specified site NEC M25.69
- wrist M25.63- ☑

Stigmata congenital syphilis A50.59

Stillbirth P95

Still-Felty syndrome — *see* Felty's syndrome

Still's disease or syndrome (juvenile) M08.20
- adult-onset M06.1
- ankle M08.27- ☑
- elbow M08.22- ☑
- foot joint M08.27- ☑
- hand joint M08.24- ☑
- hip M08.25- ☑
- knee M08.26- ☑
- multiple site M08.29
- shoulder M08.21- ☑
- specified site NEC M08.2A
- vertebra M08.28
- wrist M08.23- ☑

Stimulation, ovary E28.1

Sting (venomous) (with allergic or anaphylactic shock) — *see* Table of Drugs and Chemicals, by animal or substance, poisoning

Stippled epiphyses Q78.8

Stitch
- abscess T81.41 ☑
- burst (in operation wound) — *see* Disruption, wound, operation

Stokes' disease E05.00
- with thyroid storm E05.01

Stokes-Adams disease or syndrome I45.9

Stokvis (-Talma) **disease** D74.8

Stoma malfunction
- colostomy K94.03
- enterostomy K94.13
- gastrostomy K94.23
- ileostomy K94.13
- tracheostomy J95.03

Stomach — *see* condition

Stomatitis (denture) (ulcerative) K12.1
- angular K13.0
  - due to dietary or vitamin deficiency E53.0
- aphthous K12.0
- bovine B08.61
- candidal B37.0
- catarrhal K12.1
- diphtheritic A36.89

Stomatitis — *continued*
- due to
  - dietary deficiency E53.0
  - thrush B37.0
  - vitamin deficiency
    - B group NEC E53.9
    - B2 (riboflavin) E53.0
- epidemic B08.8
- epizootic B08.8
- follicular K12.1
- gangrenous A69.0
- Geotrichum B48.3
- herpesviral, herpetic B00.2
- herpetiformis K12.0
- malignant K12.1
- membranous acute K12.1
- monilial B37.0
- mycotic B37.0
- necrotizing ulcerative A69.0
- parasitic B37.0
- septic K12.1
- spirochetal A69.1
- suppurative (acute) K12.2
- ulceromembranous A69.1
- vesicular K12.1
  - with exanthem (enteroviral) B08.4
  - virus disease A93.8
- Vincent's A69.1

Stomatocytosis D58.8

Stomatomycosis B37.0

Stomatorrhagia K13.79

Stone(s) — *see also* Calculus
- bladder (diverticulum) N21.0
- cystine E72.09
- heart syndrome I50.1
- kidney N20.0
- prostate N42.0
- pulpal (dental) K04.2
- renal N20.0
- salivary gland or duct (any) K11.5
- urethra (impacted) N21.1
- urinary (duct) (impacted) (passage) N20.9
  - bladder (diverticulum) N21.0
  - lower tract N21.9
  - specified NEC N21.8
- xanthine E79.82 *[N22]*

Stonecutter's lung J62.8

Stonemason's asthma, disease, lung or pneumoconiosis J62.8

Stoppage
- heart — *see* Arrest, cardiac
- urine — *see* Retention, urine

Storm, thyroid — *see* Thyrotoxicosis

Strabismus (congenital) (nonparalytic) H50.9
- concomitant H50.40
  - convergent — *see* Strabismus, convergent concomitant
  - divergent — *see* Strabismus, divergent concomitant
- convergent concomitant H50.00
  - accommodative component H50.43
  - alternating H50.05
    - with
      - A pattern H50.06
      - specified noncomitances NEC H50.08
      - V pattern H50.07
  - monocular H50.01- ☑
    - with
      - A pattern H50.02- ☑
      - specified noncomitances NEC H50.04- ☑
      - V pattern H50.03- ☑
    - intermittent H50.31- ☑
      - alternating H50.32
- cyclotropia H50.41 ☑
- divergent concomitant H50.10
  - alternating H50.15
    - with
      - A pattern H50.16
      - specified noncomitances NEC H50.18
      - V pattern H50.17
  - monocular H50.11- ☑
    - with
      - A pattern H50.12- ☑
      - specified noncomitances NEC H50.14- ☑
      - V pattern H50.13- ☑
    - intermittent H50.33 ☑
      - alternating H50.34
- Duane's syndrome H50.81- ☑
- due to adhesions, scars H50.69

Strabismus — *continued*
- heterophoria H50.50
  - alternating H50.55
  - cyclophoria H50.54
  - esophoria H50.51
  - exophoria H50.52
  - vertical H50.53
- heterotropia H50.40
  - intermittent H50.30
- hypertropia H50.2- ☑
- hypotropia — *see* Hypertropia
- latent H50.50
- mechanical H50.60
  - Brown's sheath syndrome H50.61- ☑
  - specified type NEC H50.69
- monofixation syndrome H50.42
- paralytic H49.9
  - abducens nerve H49.2- ☑
  - fourth nerve H49.1- ☑
  - Kearns-Sayre syndrome H49.81- ☑
  - ophthalmoplegia (external)
    - progressive H49.4- ☑
      - with pigmentary retinopathy H49.81- ☑
    - total H49.3- ☑
  - sixth nerve H49.2- ☑
  - specified type NEC H49.88- ☑
  - third nerve H49.0- ☑
  - trochlear nerve H49.1- ☑
- specified type NEC H50.89
- vertical H50.2- ☑

Strain
- back S39.012 ☑
- cervical S16.1 ☑
- eye NEC — *see* Disturbance, vision, subjective
- heart — *see* Disease, heart
- low back S39.012 ☑
- mental NOS Z73.3
  - work-related Z56.6
- muscle (tendon) — *see* Injury, muscle, by site, strain
- neck S16.1 ☑
- physical NOS Z73.3
  - work-related Z56.6
- postural — *see also* Disorder, soft tissue, due to use
- psychological NEC Z73.3
- tendon — *see* Injury, muscle, by site, strain

Straining, on urination R39.16

Strand, vitreous — *see* Opacity, vitreous, membranes and strands

Strangulation, strangulated — *see also* Asphyxia, traumatic
- appendix K38.8
- bladder-neck N32.0
- bowel or colon K56.2
- food or foreign body — *see* Foreign body, by site
- hemorrhoids — *see* Hemorrhoids, with complication
- hernia — *see also* Hernia, by site, with obstruction
  - with gangrene — *see* Hernia, by site, with gangrene
- intestine (large) (small) K56.2
  - with hernia — *see also* Hernia, by site, with obstruction
    - with gangrene — *see* Hernia, by site, with gangrene
- mesentery K56.2
- mucus — *see* Asphyxia, mucus
- omentum K56.2
- organ or site, congenital NEC — *see* Atresia, by site
- ovary — *see* Torsion, ovary
- penis N48.89
  - foreign body T19.4 ☑
- rupture — *see* Hernia, by site, with obstruction
- stomach due to hernia — *see also* Hernia, by site, with obstruction
  - with gangrene — *see* Hernia, by site, with gangrene
- vesicourethral orifice N32.0

Strangury R30.0

Straw itch B88.0

Strawberry
- gallbladder K82.4
- mark Q82.5
- tongue (red) (white) K14.3

Streak(s)
- macula, angioid H35.33
- ovarian Q50.32

Strephosymbolia F81.0
- secondary to organic lesion R48.8

Streptobacillary fever A25.1

Streptobacillosis A25.1

- **Stricture** — *continued*
  - urethra — *see also* Stricture, urethra, male — *continued*
    - male — *continued*
      - meatal N35.911
      - membranous urethra N35.913
      - overlapping sites N35.916
    - postcatheterization — *see* Stricture, urethra, postprocedural
    - postinfective NEC
      - female N35.12
      - male N35.119
        - anterior urethra N35.114
        - bulbous urethra N35.112
        - meatal N35.111
        - membranous urethra N35.113
        - overlapping sites N35.116
    - postobstetric N35.Ø21
    - postoperative — *see* Stricture, urethra, postprocedural
    - postprocedural
      - female N99.12
      - male N99.114
        - anterior bulbous urethra N99.113
        - bulbous urethra N99.111
        - fossa navicularis N99.115
        - meatal N99.11Ø
        - membranous urethra N99.112
        - overlapping sites N99.116
    - post-traumatic
      - female N35.Ø28
        - due to childbirth N35.Ø21
      - male N35.Ø14
        - anterior urethra N35.Ø13
        - bulbous urethra N35.Ø11
        - meatal N35.Ø1Ø
        - membranous urethra N35.Ø12
        - overlapping sites N35.Ø16
    - sequela (late effect) of
      - childbirth N35.Ø21
      - injury — *see* Stricture, urethra, post-traumatic
    - specified cause NEC
      - female N35.82
      - male N35.819
        - anterior urethra N35.814
        - bulbous urethra N35.812
        - meatal N35.811
        - membranous urethra N35.813
        - overlapping sites N35.816
    - syphilitic A52.76
    - traumatic — *see* Stricture, urethra, post-traumatic
    - valvular (posterior), congenital Q64.2
  - urinary meatus — *see* Stricture, urethra
  - uterus, uterine (synechiae) N85.6
    - os (external) (internal) — *see* Stricture, cervix
  - vagina (outlet) — *see* Stenosis, vagina
  - valve (cardiac) (heart) — *see also* Endocarditis
    - congenital
      - aortic Q23.Ø
      - mitral Q23.2
      - pulmonary Q22.1
      - tricuspid Q22.4
  - vas deferens N5Ø.89
    - congenital Q55.4
  - vein I87.1
  - vena cava (inferior) (superior) NEC I87.1
    - congenital Q26.Ø
  - vesicourethral orifice N32.Ø
    - congenital Q64.31
  - vulva (acquired) N9Ø.5
- **Stridor** RØ6.1
  - congenital (larynx) P28.89
- **Stridulous** — *see* condition
- **Stroke** (apoplectic) (brain) (ischemic) (paralytic) I63.9
  - cerebral, perinatal P91.82- ☑
  - cerebrovascular (ischemic) I63.9
    - chronic (old) (remote) (imaging) (without sequelae) Z86.73
      - with residual defects — *see* Sequelae, disease, cerebrovascular
    - embolic I63.- ☑
    - thrombolic I63.- ☑
  - cryptogenic — *see also* infarction, cerebral I63.9
  - epileptic — *see* Epilepsy
  - heat T67.Ø1 ☑
    - exertional T67.Ø2 ☑
    - specified NEC T67.Ø9 ☑
  - in evolution I63.9
- **Stroke** — *continued*
  - intraoperative
    - during cardiac surgery I97.81Ø
    - during other surgery I97.811
  - ischemic, perinatal arterial P91.82- ☑
  - lightning — *see* Lightning
  - meaning
    - cerebral hemorrhage — *code to* Hemorrhage, intracranial
    - cerebral infarction — *code to* Infarction, cerebral
  - neonatal P91.82- ☑
  - postprocedural
    - following cardiac surgery I97.82Ø
    - following other surgery I97.821
  - sun T67.Ø1 ☑
    - specified NEC T67.Ø9 ☑
  - unspecified (NOS) I63.9
- **Stromatosis, endometrial** D39.Ø
- **Strongyloidiasis, strongyloidosis** B78.9
  - cutaneous B78.1
  - disseminated B78.7
  - intestinal B78.Ø
- **Strophulus pruriginosus** L28.2
- **Struck by lightning** — *see* Lightning
- **Struma** — *see also* Goiter
  - Hashimoto EØ6.3
  - lymphomatosa EØ6.3
  - nodosa (simplex) EØ4.9
    - endemic EØ1.2
      - multinodular EØ1.1
    - multinodular EØ4.2
      - iodine-deficiency related EØ1.1
    - toxic or with hyperthyroidism EØ5.2Ø
      - with thyroid storm EØ5.21
      - multinodular EØ5.2Ø
        - with thyroid storm EØ5.21
      - uninodular EØ5.1Ø
        - with thyroid storm EØ5.11
    - toxicosa EØ5.2Ø
      - with thyroid storm EØ5.21
      - multinodular EØ5.2Ø
        - with thyroid storm EØ5.21
      - uninodular EØ5.1Ø
        - with thyroid storm EØ5.11
    - uninodular EØ4.1
  - ovarii D27.- ☑
  - Riedel's EØ6.5
- **Strumipriva cachexia** EØ3.4
- **Strumpell-Marie spine** — *see* Spondylitis, ankylosing
- **Strumpell-Westphal pseudosclerosis** E83.Ø1
- **Stuart deficiency disease** (factor X) D68.2
- **Stuart-Prower factor deficiency** (factor X) D68.2
- **Student's elbow** — *see* Bursitis, elbow, olecranon
- **Stump** — *see* Amputation
- **Stunting, nutritional** E45
- **Stupor** (catatonic) R4Ø.1
  - depressive (single episode) F32.89
    - recurrent episode F33.8
  - dissociative F44.2
  - manic F3Ø.2
  - manic-depressive F31.89
  - psychogenic (anergic) F44.2
  - reaction to exceptional stress (transient) F43.Ø
- **Sturge** (-Weber) (-Dimitri) (-Kalischer) **disease or syndrome** Q85.89
- **Stuttering** F8Ø.81
  - adult onset F98.5
  - childhood onset F8Ø.81
  - following cerebrovascular disease — *see* Disorder, fluency. following cerebrovascular disease
  - in conditions classified elsewhere R47.82
- **Sty, stye** (external) (internal) (meibomian) (zeisian) — *see* Hordeolum
- **Subacidity, gastric** K31.89
  - psychogenic F45.8
- **Subacute** — *see* condition
- **Subarachnoid** — *see* condition
- **Subcortical** — *see* condition
- **Subcostal syndrome, nerve compression** — *see* Mononeuropathy, upper limb, specified site NEC
- **Subcutaneous, subcuticular** — *see* condition
- **Subdural** — *see* condition
- **Subendocardium** — *see* condition
- **Subependymoma**
  - specified site — *see* Neoplasm, uncertain behavior, by site
  - unspecified site D43.2
- **Suberosis** J67.3
- **Subglossitis** — *see* Glossitis
- **Subhemophilia** D66
- **Subinvolution**
  - breast (postlactational) (postpuerperal) N64.89
  - puerperal O9Ø.89
  - uterus (chronic) (nonpuerperal) N85.3
    - puerperal O9Ø.89
- **Sublingual** — *see* condition
- **Sublinguitis** — *see* Sialoadenitis
- **Subluxatable hip** Q65.6
- **Subluxation** — *see also* Dislocation
  - acromioclavicular S43.11- ☑
  - ankle S93.Ø- ☑
  - atlantoaxial, recurrent M43.4
    - with myelopathy M43.3
  - carpometacarpal (joint) NEC S63.Ø5- ☑
    - thumb S63.Ø4- ☑
  - complex, vertebral — *see* Complex, subluxation
  - congenital — *see also* Malposition, congenital
    - hip — *see* Dislocation, hip, congenital, partial
    - joint (excluding hip)
      - lower limb Q68.8
      - shoulder Q68.8
      - upper limb Q68.8
  - elbow (traumatic) S53.1Ø- ☑
    - anterior S53.11- ☑
    - lateral S53.14- ☑
    - medial S53.13- ☑
    - posterior S53.12- ☑
    - specified type NEC S53.19- ☑
  - finger S63.2Ø- ☑
    - index S63.2Ø- ☑
    - interphalangeal S63.22- ☑
      - distal S63.24- ☑
        - index S63.24- ☑
        - little S63.24- ☑
        - middle S63.24- ☑
        - ring S63.24- ☑
      - index S63.22- ☑
      - little S63.22- ☑
      - middle S63.22- ☑
      - proximal S63.23- ☑
        - index S63.23- ☑
        - little S63.23- ☑
        - middle S63.23- ☑
        - ring S63.23- ☑
      - ring S63.22- ☑
    - little S63.2Ø- ☑
    - metacarpophalangeal S63.21- ☑
      - index S63.21- ☑
      - little S63.21- ☑
      - middle S63.21- ☑
      - ring S63.21- ☑
    - middle S63.2Ø- ☑
    - ring S63.2Ø- ☑
  - foot S93.3Ø- ☑
    - specified site NEC S93.33- ☑
    - tarsal joint S93.31- ☑
    - tarsometatarsal joint S93.32- ☑
    - toe — *see* Subluxation, toe
  - hip S73.ØØ- ☑
    - anterior S73.Ø3- ☑
      - obturator S73.Ø2- ☑
    - central S73.Ø4- ☑
    - posterior S73.Ø1- ☑
  - interphalangeal (joint)
    - finger S63.22- ☑
      - distal joint S63.24- ☑
        - index S63.24- ☑
        - little S63.24- ☑
        - middle S63.24- ☑
        - ring S63.24- ☑
      - index S63.22- ☑
      - little S63.22- ☑
      - middle S63.22- ☑
      - proximal joint S63.23- ☑
        - index S63.23- ☑
        - little S63.23- ☑
        - middle S63.23- ☑
        - ring S63.23- ☑
      - ring S63.22- ☑
    - thumb S63.12- ☑
    - toe S93.13- ☑
      - great S93.13- ☑
      - lesser S93.13- ☑

- **Synchondrosis** — *continued*
  - ischiopubic M91.0
- **Synchysis** (scintillans) (senile) (vitreous body) H43.89
- **Syncope** (near) (pre-) R55
  - anginosa I20.89
  - bradycardia R00.1
  - cardiac R55
  - carotid sinus G90.01
  - due to spinal (lumbar) puncture G97.1
  - heart R55
  - heat T67.1 ☑
  - laryngeal R05.4
  - psychogenic F48.8
  - tussive R05.8
  - vasoconstriction R55
  - vasodepressor R55
  - vasomotor R55
  - vasovagal R55
- **Syndactylism, syndactyly** Q70.9
  - complex (with synostosis)
    - fingers Q70.0- ☑
    - toes Q70.2- ☑
  - simple (without synostosis)
    - fingers Q70.1- ☑
    - toes Q70.3- ☑
- **Syndrome** — *see also* Disease
  - 22q13.3 deletion Q93.52
  - 48,XXXX Q97.1
  - 49,XXXXX Q97.1
  - 4H G11.5
  - 5q minus NOS D46.C (*following* D46.2)
  - abdominal
    - acute R10.0
    - muscle deficiency Q79.4
  - abnormal innervation H02.519
    - left H02.516
      - lower H02.515
      - upper H02.514
    - right H02.513
      - lower H02.512
      - upper H02.511
  - abstinence, neonatal P96.1
  - acid pulmonary aspiration, obstetric O74.0
  - acquired immunodeficiency — *see* Human, immunodeficiency virus (HIV) disease
  - activated phosphoinositide 3-kinase delta syndrome [APDS] D81.82
  - acute abdominal R10.0
  - acute respiratory distress (adult) (child) J80
    - idiopathic J84.114
  - Adair-Dighton Q78.0
  - Adams-Stokes (-Morgagni) I45.9
  - adiposogenital E23.6
  - adrenal
    - hemorrhage (meningococcal) A39.1
    - meningococcic A39.1
  - adrenocortical — *see* Cushing's, syndrome
  - adrenogenital E25.9
    - congenital, associated with enzyme deficiency E25.0
  - afferent loop NEC K91.89
  - Aicardi-Goutières E79.81
  - Alagille (-Watson) Q44.71
  - alcohol withdrawal (without convulsions) — *see* Dependence, alcohol, with, withdrawal
  - Alder's D72.0
  - Aldrich (-Wiskott) D82.0
  - alien hand R41.4
  - Alport Q87.81
  - alveolar hypoventilation E66.2
  - alveolocapillary block J84.10
  - amnesic, amnestic (confabulatory) (due to) — *see* Disorder, amnesic
  - amyostatic (Wilson's disease) E83.01
  - androgen insensitivity E34.50
    - complete E34.51
    - partial E34.52
  - androgen resistance — *see also* Syndrome, androgen insensitivity E34.50
  - Angelman Q93.51
  - anginal — *see* Angina
  - ankyloglossia superior Q38.1
  - anterior
    - chest wall R07.89
    - cord G83.82
    - spinal artery G95.19
      - compression M47.019
        - cervical region M47.012
        - cervicothoracic region M47.013

- **Syndrome** — *continued*
  - anterior — *continued*
    - spinal artery — *continued*
      - compression — *continued*
        - lumbar region M47.016
        - occipito-atlanto-axial region M47.011
        - thoracic region M47.014
        - thoracolumbar region M47.015
    - tibial M76.81- ☑
  - antibody deficiency D80.9
    - agammaglobulinemic D80.1
      - hereditary D80.0
    - congenital D80.0
    - hypogammaglobulinemic D80.1
      - hereditary D80.0
  - anticardiolipin (-antibody) D68.61
  - antidepressant discontinuation T43.205 ☑
  - antiphospholipid (-antibody) D68.61
  - aortic
    - arch M31.4
    - bifurcation I74.09
  - aortomesenteric duodenum occlusion K31.5
  - apical ballooning (transient left ventricular) I51.81
  - arcuate ligament I77.4
  - argentaffin, argintaffinoma E34.0
  - Arnold-Chiari — *see* Arnold-Chiari disease
  - Arrillaga-Ayerza I27.0
  - arterial tortuosity Q87.82
  - arteriovenous steal T82.898- ☑
  - Asherman's N85.6
  - aspiration, of newborn — *see* Aspiration, by substance, with pneumonia
    - meconium P24.01
  - ataxia-telangiectasia G11.3
  - auriculotemporal G50.8
  - autoerythrocyte sensitization (Gardner-Diamond) D69.2
  - autoimmune lymphoproliferative [ALPS] D89.82
  - autoimmune polyglandular E31.0
  - autoinflammatory M04.9
    - specified type NEC M04.8
  - autosomal — *see* Abnormal, autosomes
  - Avellis' G46.8
  - Ayerza (-Arrillaga) I27.0
  - Babinski-Nageotte G83.89
  - Bakwin-Krida Q78.5
  - Bardet-Biedl Q87.83
  - bare lymphocyte D81.6
  - Barre-Guillain G61.0
  - Barre-Lieou M53.0
  - Barrett's — *see* Barrett's, esophagus
  - Barsony-Polgar K22.4
  - Barsony-Teschendorf K22.4
  - Barth E78.71
  - Bartter's E26.81
  - basal cell nevus Q87.89
  - Basedow's E05.00
    - with thyroid storm E05.01
  - basilar artery G45.0
  - Batten-Steinert G71.11
  - battered
    - baby or child — *see* Maltreatment, child, physical abuse
    - spouse — *see* Maltreatment, adult, physical abuse
  - Beals Q87.40
  - Beau's I51.5
  - Beck's I65.8
  - Benedikt's G46.3
  - Bequez Cesar (-Steinbrinck-Chediak-Higashi) E70.330
  - Bernhardt-Roth — *see* Meralgia paresthetica
  - Bernheim's — *see* Failure, heart, right
  - big spleen D73.1
  - bilateral polycystic ovarian E28.2
  - Bing-Horton's — *see* Horton's headache
  - Birt-Hogg-Dube syndrome Q87.89
  - Bjorck (-Thorsen) E34.0
  - black
    - lung J60
    - widow spider bite — *see* Toxicity, venom, spider, black widow
  - Blackfan-Diamond D61.01
  - Blau M04.8
  - blind loop K90.2
    - congenital Q43.8
    - postsurgical K91.2
  - blue sclera Q78.0
  - blue toe I75.02- ☑
  - Boder-Sedgewick G11.3
  - Boerhaave's K22.3

- **Syndrome** — *continued*
  - Borjeson Forssman Lehmann Q89.8
  - Bouillaud's I01.9
  - Bourneville (-Pringle) Q85.1
  - Bouveret (-Hoffman) I47.9
  - brachial plexus G54.0
  - bradycardia-tachycardia I49.5
  - brain (nonpsychotic) F09
    - with psychosis, psychotic reaction F09
    - acute or subacute — *see* Delirium
    - congenital — *see* Disability, intellectual
    - organic F09
      - post-traumatic (nonpsychotic) F07.81
        - psychotic F09
    - personality change F07.0
    - postcontusional F07.81
    - post-traumatic, nonpsychotic F07.81
    - psycho-organic F09
    - psychotic F06.8
  - brain stem stroke G46.3
  - Brandt's (acrodermatitis enteropathica) E83.2
  - broad ligament laceration N83.8
  - Brock's J98.11
  - bronchiolitis obliterans — *see also* Bronchiolitis, obliterative J44.81
  - bronze baby P83.88
  - Brown-Sequard G83.81
  - Brugada I49.8
  - bubbly lung P27.0
  - Buchem's M85.2
  - Budd-Chiari I82.0
  - bulbar (progressive) G12.22
  - Burger-Grutz E78.3
  - Burke's K86.89
  - Burnett's (milk-alkali) E83.52
  - burning feet E53.9
  - Bywaters' T79.5 ☑
  - Call-Fleming I67.841
  - carbohydrate-deficient glycoprotein (CDGS) E77.8
  - carcinogenic thrombophlebitis I82.1
  - carcinoid E34.0
  - cardiac asthma I50.1
  - cardiacos negros I27.0
  - cardiofaciocutaneous Q87.89
  - cardiopulmonary-obesity E66.2
  - cardiorenal — *see* Hypertension, cardiorenal
  - cardiorespiratory distress (idiopathic), newborn P22.0
  - cardiovascular renal — *see* Hypertension, cardiorenal
  - carotid
    - artery (hemispheric) (internal) G45.1
    - body G90.01
    - sinus G90.01
  - carpal tunnel G56.0- ☑
  - Cassidy (-Scholte) E34.0
  - cat cry Q93.4
  - cat eye Q92.8
  - cauda equina G83.4
  - causalgia — *see* Causalgia
  - celiac K90.0
    - artery compression I77.4
    - axis I77.4
  - central pain G89.0
  - cerebellar
    - hereditary G11.9
    - stroke G46.4
  - cerebellomedullary malformation — *see* Spina bifida
  - cerebral
    - artery
      - anterior G46.1
      - middle G46.0
      - posterior G46.2
    - gigantism E22.0
  - cervical (root) M53.1
    - disc — *see* Disorder, disc, cervical, with neuritis
    - fusion Q76.1
    - posterior, sympathicus M53.0
    - rib Q76.5
    - sympathetic paralysis G90.2
  - cervicobrachial (diffuse) M53.1
  - cervicocranial M53.0
  - cervicodorsal outlet G54.2
  - cervicothoracic outlet G54.0
  - Cestan (-Raymond) I65.8
  - Charcot's (angina cruris) (intermittent claudication) I73.9
  - Charcot-Weiss-Baker G90.09
  - CHARGE Q89.8
  - Chediak-Higashi (-Steinbrinck) E70.330

Syndrome — *continued*
- chest wall RØ7.1
- Chiari's (hepatic vein thrombosis) I82.Ø
- Chilaiditi's Q43.3
- child maltreatment — *see* Maltreatment, child
- chondrocostal junction M94.Ø
- chondroectodermal dysplasia Q77.6
- chromosome 4 short arm deletion Q93.3
- chromosome 5 short arm deletion Q93.4
- chronic
  - infantile neurological, cutaneous and articular (CINCA) MØ4.2
  - pain G89.4
    - personality F68.8
- Churg-Strauss M3Ø.1
- Clarke-Hadfield K86.89
- Clerambault's automatism G93.89
- Clouston's (hidrotic ectodermal dysplasia) Q82.4
- clumsiness, clumsy child F82
- cluster headache G44.ØØ9
  - intractable G44.ØØ1
  - not intractable G44.ØØ9
- Coffin-Lowry Q89.8
- cold injury (newborn) P8Ø.Ø
- combined immunity deficiency D81.9
- compartment (deep) (posterior) (traumatic) T79.AØ ☑ (*following* T79.7)
  - abdomen T79.A3 ☑ (*following* T79.7)
  - lower extremity (hip, buttock, thigh, leg, foot, toes) T79.A2 ☑ (*following* T79.7)
  - nontraumatic
    - abdomen M79.A3 (*following* M79.7)
    - lower extremity (hip, buttock, thigh, leg, foot, toes) M79.A2- ☑ (*following* M79.7)
    - specified site NEC M79.A9 (*following* M79.7)
    - upper extremity (shoulder, arm, forearm, wrist, hand, fingers) M79.A1- ☑ (*following* M79.7)
  - postprocedural — *see* Syndrome, compartment, nontraumatic
  - specified site NEC T79.A9 ☑ (*following* T79.7)
  - upper extremity (shoulder, arm, forearm, wrist, hand, fingers) T79.A1 ☑ (*following* T79.7)
- complex regional pain — *see* Syndrome, pain, complex regional
- compression T79.5 ☑
  - anterior spinal — *see* Syndrome, anterior, spinal artery, compression
  - cauda equina G83.4
  - celiac artery I77.4
  - vertebral artery M47.Ø29
    - cervical region M47.Ø22
    - occipito-atlanto-axial region M47.Ø21
- concussion FØ7.81
- congenital
  - affecting multiple systems NEC Q87.89
  - central alveolar hypoventilation G47.35
  - facial diplegia Q87.Ø
  - muscular hypertrophy-cerebral Q87.89
  - oculo-auriculovertebral Q87.Ø
  - oculofacial diplegia (Moebius) Q87.Ø
  - rubella (manifest) P35.Ø
- congestion-fibrosis (pelvic), female N94.89
- congestive dysmenorrhea N94.6
- connective tissue M35.9
  - overlap NEC M35.1
- Conn's E26.Ø1
- conus medullaris G95.81
- cord
  - anterior G83.82
  - posterior G83.83
- coronary
  - acute NEC I24.9
  - insufficiency or intermediate I2Ø.Ø
  - slow flow I2Ø.89
- Costen's (complex) M26.69
- costochondral junction M94.Ø
- costoclavicular G54.Ø
- costovertebral E22.Ø
- Cowden
  - PTEN related Q85.81
  - specified NEC Q85.82
- craniovertebral M53.Ø
- Creutzfeldt-Jakob — *see* Creutzfeldt-Jakob disease or syndrome
- crib death R99
- cricopharyngeal — *see* Dysphagia
- cri-du-chat Q93.4
- croup JØ5.Ø
- CRPS I — *see* Syndrome, pain, complex regional I
- crush T79.5 ☑
- cryopyrin-associated perodic MØ4.2
- cryptophthalmos Q87.Ø
- cubital tunnel — *see* Lesion, nerve, ulnar
- Curschmann (-Batten) (-Steinert) G71.11
- Cushing's E24.9
  - alcohol-induced E24.4
  - due to
    - alcohol
    - drugs E24.2
    - ectopic ACTH E24.3
    - overproduction of pituitary ACTH E24.Ø
  - drug-induced E24.2
  - overdose or wrong substance given or taken — *see* Table of Drugs and Chemicals, by drug, poisoning
  - pituitary-dependent E24.Ø
  - specified type NEC E24.8
- cystic duct stump K91.5
- cytokine release D89.839
  - grade 1 D89.831
  - grade 2 D89.832
  - grade 3 D89.833
  - grade 4 D89.834
  - grade 5 D89.835
- Dana-Putnam D51.Ø
- Danbolt (-Cross) (acrodermatitis enteropathica) E83.2
- Dandy-Walker QØ3.1
  - with spina bifida QØ7.Ø1
- Danlos' — *see also* Syndrome, Ehlers-Danlos Q79.6Ø
- De Quervain E34.51
- de Toni-Fanconi (-Debre) E72.Ø9
  - with cystinosis E72.Ø4
- de Vivo syndrome E74.81Ø
- defibrination — *see also* Fibrinolysis
  - with
    - antepartum hemorrhage — *see* Hemorrhage, antepartum, with coagulation defect
    - intrapartum hemorrhage — *see* Hemorrhage, complicating, delivery
  - newborn P6Ø
  - postpartum O72.3
- Degos' I77.89
- Dejerine-Roussy G89.Ø
- delayed sleep phase G47.21
- demyelinating G37.9
- dependence — *see* F1Ø-F19 with fourth character .2
- depersonalization (-derealization) F48.1
- di George's D82.1
- diabetes mellitus in newborn infant P7Ø.2
- diabetes mellitus-hypertension-nephrosis — *see* Diabetes, nephrosis
- diabetes-nephrosis — *see* Diabetes, nephrosis
- diabetic amyotrophy — *see* Diabetes, amyotrophy
- dialysis associated steal T82.898- ☑
- Diamond-Blackfan D61.Ø1
- Diamond-Gardener D69.2
- DIC (diffuse or disseminated intravascular coagulopathy) D65
- Dighton's Q78.Ø
- disequilibrium E87.8
- Dohle body-panmyelopathic D72.Ø
- dorsolateral medullary G46.4
- double athetosis G8Ø.3
- Down — *see also* Down syndrome Q9Ø.9
- Dravet (intractable) G4Ø.834
  - with status epilepticus G4Ø.833
  - without status epilepticus G4Ø.834
- Dresbach's (elliptocytosis) D58.1
- DRESS (drug rash with eosinophilia and systemic symptoms) D72.12
- Dressler's (postmyocardial infarction) I24.1
  - postcardiotomy I97.Ø
- drug rash with eosinophilia and systemic symptoms (DRESS) D72.12
- drug withdrawal, infant of dependent mother P96.1
- dry eye HØ4.12- ☑
  - due to abnormality
    - chromosomal Q99.9
      - sex
        - female phenotype Q97.9
        - male phenotype Q98.9
      - specified NEC Q99.8
- dumping (postgastrectomy) K91.1
  - nonsurgical K31.89

Syndrome — *continued*
- Dupre's (meningism) R29.1
- dysmetabolic X E88.81Ø
- dyspraxia, developmental F82
- Eagle-Barrett Q79.4
- Eaton-Lambert — *see* Syndrome, Lambert-Eaton
- Ebstein's Q22.5
- ectopic ACTH E24.3
- eczema-thrombocytopenia D82.Ø
- Eddowes' Q78.Ø
- effort (psychogenic) F45.8
- Ehlers-Danlos Q79.6Ø
  - classical (cEDS) (classical EDS) Q79.61
  - hypermobile (hEDS) (hypermobile EDS) Q79.62
  - specified NEC Q79.69
  - vascular (vascular EDS) (vEDS) Q79.63
- Eisenmenger's I27.83
- Ekman's Q78.Ø
- electric feet E53.8
- Ellis-van Creveld Q77.6
- empty nest Z6Ø.Ø
- endocrine-hypertensive E27.Ø
- entrapment — *see* Neuropathy, entrapment
- eosinophilia-myalgia M35.89
- epileptic — *see also* Epilepsy, by type
  - absence G4Ø.AØ9 (*following* G4Ø.3)
    - intractable G4Ø.A19 (*following* G4Ø.3)
      - with status epilepticus G4Ø.A11 (*following* G4Ø.3)
      - without status epilepticus G4Ø.A19 (*following* G4Ø.3)
    - not intractable G4Ø.AØ9 (*following* G4Ø.3)
      - with status epilepticus G4Ø.AØ1 (*following* G4Ø.3)
      - without status epilepticus G4Ø.AØ9 (*following* G4Ø.3)
- Erdheim-Chester (ECD) E88.89
- Erdheim's E22.Ø
- erythrocyte fragmentation D59.4
- Evans D69.41
- exhaustion F48.8
- extrapyramidal G25.9
  - specified NEC G25.89
- eye retraction — *see* Strabismus
- eyelid-malar-mandible Q87.Ø
- Faber's D5Ø.9
- facet M47.89- ☑
- facet joint — *see also* Spondylosis M47.819
- facial pain, paroxysmal G5Ø.Ø
- Fallot's Q21.3
- familial cold autoinflammatory MØ4.2
- familial eczema-thrombocytopenia (Wiskott-Aldrich) D82.Ø
- Fanconi (-de Toni) (-Debre) E72.Ø9
  - with cystinosis E72.Ø4
- Fanconi's (anemia) (congenital pancytopenia) D61.Ø9
- fatigue
  - chronic G93.32
  - postviral G93.31
  - psychogenic F48.8
- faulty bowel habit K59.39
- Feil-Klippel (brevicollis) Q76.1
- Felty's — *see* Felty's syndrome
- fertile eunuch E23.Ø
- fetal
  - alcohol (dysmorphic) Q86.Ø
  - hydantoin Q86.1
- Fiedler's I4Ø.1
- first arch Q87.Ø
- fish odor E72.89
- Fisher's G61.Ø
- Fitzhugh-Curtis
  - due to
    - Chlamydia trachomatis A74.81
    - Neisseria gonorrhorea (gonococcal peritonitis) A54.85
- Fitz's — *see also* Pancreatitis, acute K85.8Ø
- Flajani (-Basedow) EØ5.ØØ
  - with thyroid storm EØ5.Ø1
- flatback — *see* Flatback syndrome
- floppy
  - baby P94.2
  - iris (intraoeprative) (IFIS) H21.81
  - mitral valve I34.1
- flush E34.Ø
- Foix-Alajouanine G95.19
- Fong's Q87.2
- food protein-induced enterocolitis (FPIES) K52.21

Syndrome — *continued*
- foramen magnum G93.5
- Foster-Kennedy H47.14- ☑
- Foville's (peduncular) G46.3
- fragile X Q99.2
- Franceschetti Q75.4
- Frey's
  - auriculotemporal G5Ø.8
  - hyperhidrosis L74.52
- Friderichsen-Waterhouse A39.1
- Froin's G95.89
- frontal lobe FØ7.Ø
- Fukuhara E88.49
- functional
  - bowel K59.9
  - prepubertal castrate E29.1
- Gaisbock's D75.1
- ganglion (basal ganglia brain) G25.9
  - geniculi G51.1
- Gardner-Diamond D69.2
- gastroesophageal
  - junction K22.Ø
  - laceration-hemorrhage K22.6
- gastrojejunal loop obstruction K91.89
- Gee-Herter-Heubner K9Ø.Ø
- Gelineau's G47.419
  - with cataplexy G47.411
- genito-anorectal A55
- Gerstmann-Straussler-Scheinker (GSS) A81.82
- Gianotti-Crosti L44.4
- giant platelet (Bernard-Soulier) D69.1
- Gilles de la Tourette's F95.2
- Glass Q87.89
- Gleich's D72.118
- goiter-deafness EØ7.1
- Goldberg Q89.8
- Goldberg-Maxwell E34.51
- Good's D83.8
- Gopalan' (burning feet) E53.8
- Gorlin's Q87.89
- Gougerot-Blum L81.7
- Gouley's I31.1
- Gower's R55
- gray or grey (newborn) P93.Ø
  - platelet D69.1
- Gubler-Millard G46.3
- Guillain-Barre (-Strohl) G61.Ø
- gustatory sweating G5Ø.8
- Hadfield-Clarke K86.89
- hair tourniquet — *see* Constriction, external, by site
- Hamman's J98.19
- hand-foot L27.1
- hand-shoulder G9Ø.8
- hantavirus (cardio)-pulmonary (HPS) (HCPS) B33.4
- happy puppet Q93.51
- Harada's H3Ø.81- ☑
- Hayem-Faber D5Ø.9
- headache NEC G44.89
  - complicated NEC G44.59
- Heberden's I2Ø.89
- Hedinger's E34.Ø
- Hegglin's D72.Ø
- HELLP (hemolysis, elevated liver enzymes and low platelet count) O14.2- ☑
  - complicating
    - childbirth O14.24
    - puerperium O14.25
- hemolytic-uremic D59.3Ø
  - atypical D59.39
    - genetic D59.32
    - hereditary D59.32
    - infection-associated D59.31
    - secondary D59.39
    - specified NEC D59.39
  - due to genetic disorder D59.32
  - familial D59.32
  - hereditary D59.32
  - infection-associated D59.31
  - secondary D59.39
  - Shiga toxin-producing E. coli [STEC] related D59.31
  - specified NEC D59.39
  - typical D59.31
- hemophagocytic, infection-associated D76.2
- Henoch-Schonlein D69.Ø
- hepatic flexure K59.89
- hepatopulmonary K76.81
- hepatorenal K76.7
  - following delivery O9Ø.41
  - postoperative or postprocedural K91.83

Syndrome — *continued*
- hepatorenal — *continued*
  - postpartum, puerperal O9Ø.41
- hepatourologic K76.7
- hereditary alpha tryptasemia D89.44
- Herter (-Gee) (nontropical sprue) K9Ø.Ø
- Heubner-Herter K9Ø.Ø
- Heyd's K76.7
- Hilger's G9Ø.Ø9
- histamine-like (fish poisoning) — *see* Poisoning, fish
- histiocytic D76.3
- histiocytosis NEC D76.3
- HIV infection, acute B2Ø
- Hoffmann-Werdnig G12.Ø
- Hollander-Simons E88.1
- Hoppe-Goldflam G7Ø.ØØ
  - with exacerbation (acute) G7Ø.Ø1
  - in crisis G7Ø.Ø1
- Horner's G9Ø.2
- hungry bone E83.81
- hunterian glossitis D51.Ø
- Hunt's (herpetic geniculate ganglionitis) (neuralgia) BØ2.21
  - dyssynergia cerebellaris myoclonica G11.19
- Hutchinson's triad A5Ø.53
- hyperabduction G54.Ø
- hyperammonemia-hyperornithinemia-homocitrullinemia E72.4
- hypereosinophilic (HES) D72.119
  - idiopathic (IHES) D72.11Ø
  - lymphocytic variant (LHES) D72.111
  - myeloid D72.118
  - specified NEC D72.118
- hyperimmunoglobulin D MØ4.1
- hyperimmunoglobulin E (IgE) D82.4
- hyperkalemic E87.5
- hyperkinetic — *see* Hyperkinesia
- hypermobility M35.7
- hypernatremia E87.Ø
- hyperosmolarity — *see also* Diabetes, by type, with hyperosmolarity E87.Ø
- hyperperfusion G97.82
- hypersplenic D73.1
- hypertransfusion, newborn P61.1
- hyperventilation F45.8
- hyperviscosity (of serum)
  - polycythemic D75.1
  - sclerothymic D58.8
- hypoglycemic (familial) (neonatal) E16.2
- hypokalemic E87.6
- hyponatremic E87.1
- hypopituitarism E23.Ø
- hypoplastic left-heart Q23.4
- hypopotassemia E87.6
- hyposmolality E87.1
- hypotension, maternal O26.5- ☑
- hypothenar hammer I73.89
- hypoventilation, obesity (OHS) E66.2
- ICF (intravascular coagulation-fibrinolysis) D65
- idiopathic
  - cardiorespiratory distress, newborn P22.Ø
  - nephrotic (infantile) NØ4.9
- iliotibial band M76.3- ☑
- immobility, immobilization (paraplegic) M62.3
- immune effector cell-associated neurotoxicity (ICANS) G92.ØØ
  - grade
    - 1 G92.Ø1
    - 2 G92.Ø2
    - 3 G92.Ø3
    - 4 G92.Ø4
    - 5 G92.Ø5
    - unspecified G92.ØØ
- immune reconstitution D89.3
- immune reconstitution inflammatory [IRIS] D89.3
- immunity deficiency, combined D81.9
- immunodeficiency
  - acquired — *see* Human, immunodeficiency virus (HIV) disease
  - combined D81.9
- impending coronary I2Ø.Ø
- impingement, shoulder M75.4- ☑
- inappropriate secretion of antidiuretic hormone E22.2
- infant
  - gestational diabetes P7Ø.Ø
  - of diabetic mother P7Ø.1
- infantilism (pituitary) E23.Ø
- inferior vena cava I87.1

Syndrome — *continued*
- inspissated bile (newborn) P59.1
- institutional (childhood) F94.2
- insufficient sleep F51.12
- insulin resistance
  - type A E88.811
  - type B E88.818
- intermediate coronary (artery) I2Ø.Ø
- interspinous ligament — *see* Spondylopathy, specified NEC
- intestinal
  - carcinoid E34.Ø
  - knot K56.2
- intravascular coagulation-fibrinolysis (ICF) D65
- iodine-deficiency, congenital EØØ.9
  - type
    - mixed EØØ.2
    - myxedematous EØØ.1
    - neurological EØØ.Ø
- IRDS (idiopathic respiratory distress, newborn) P22.Ø
- irritable
  - bowel K58.9
    - with
      - constipation K58.1
      - diarrhea K58.Ø
    - mixed K58.2
    - psychogenic F45.8
    - specified NEC K58.8
  - heart (psychogenic) F45.8
  - weakness F48.8
- ischemic
  - bowel (transient) K55.9
    - chronic K55.1
    - due to mesenteric artery insufficiency K55.1
  - steal T82.898 ☑
- IVC (intravascular coagulopathy) D65
- Ivemark's Q89.Ø1
- Jaccoud's — *see* Arthropathy, postrheumatic, chronic
- Jackson's G83.89
- Jakob-Creutzfeldt — *see* Creutzfeldt-Jakob disease or syndrome
- jaw-winking QØ7.8
- Jervell-Lange-Nielsen I45.81
- jet lag G47.25
- Job's D71
- Joseph-Diamond-Blackfan D61.Ø1
- jugular foramen G52.7
- Kabuki Q89.8
- Kanner's (autism) F84.Ø
- Kartagener's Q89.3
- Kelly's D5Ø.1
- Kimmelstiel-Wilson — *see* Diabetes, specified type, with Kimmelstiel-Wilson disease
- Klein (e)-Levine G47.13
- Klippel-Feil (brevicollis) Q76.1
- Kohler-Pellegrini-Steida — *see* Bursitis, tibial collateral
- Konig's K59.89
- Korsakoff (-Wernicke) (nonalcoholic) FØ4
  - alcoholic F1Ø.26
- Kostmann's D7Ø.Ø
- Krabbe's congenital muscle hypoplasia Q79.8
- labyrinthine — *see* subcategory H83.2 ☑
- lacunar NEC G46.7
- Lambert-Eaton G7Ø.8Ø
  - in
    - neoplastic disease G73.1
    - specified disease NEC G7Ø.81
- Landau-Kleffner — *see* Epilepsy, specified NEC
- Larsen's Q74.8
- lateral
  - cutaneous nerve of thigh G57.1- ☑
  - medullary G46.4
- Launois' E22.Ø
- Laurence-Moon Q87.84
- lazy
  - leukocyte D7Ø.8
  - posture M62.3
- Lemiere I8Ø.8
- Lennox-Gastaut G4Ø.812
  - intractable G4Ø.814
    - with status epilepticus G4Ø.813
    - without status epilepticus G4Ø.814
  - not intractable G4Ø.812
    - with status epilepticus G4Ø.811
    - without status epilepticus G4Ø.812
- lenticular, progressive E83.Ø1
- Leopold-Levi's EØ5.9Ø
- Lev's I44.2

☑ **Additional Character Required — Refer to the Tabular List for Character Selection**

Syndrome — *continued*
- pluridefiency E4Ø
- pluriglandular (compensatory) E31.8
  - autoimmune E31.Ø
- pneumatic hammer T75.21 ☑
- polyangiitis overlap M3Ø.8
- polycarential of infancy E4Ø
- polyglandular E31.8
  - autoimmune E31.Ø
- polysplenia Q89.Ø9
- pontine NEC G93.89
- popliteal
  - artery entrapment I77.89
  - web Q87.89
- post chemoembolization — *code to* associated conditions
- post endometrial ablation N99.85
- postbacterial fatigue G93.39
- postcardiac injury
  - postcardiotomy I97.Ø
  - postmyocardial infarction I24.1
- postcardiotomy I97.Ø
- postcholecystectomy K91.5
- postcommissurotomy I97.Ø
- postconcussional FØ7.81
- postcontusional FØ7.81
- post-COVID (-19) UØ9.9
- postencephalitic FØ7.89
- posterior
  - cervical sympathetic M53.Ø
  - cord G83.83
  - fossa compression G93.5
  - reversible encephalopathy (PRES) I67.83
- postgastrectomy (dumping) K91.1
- postgastric surgery K91.1
- postinfarction I24.1
- postinfectious fatigue G93.39
- postlaminectomy NEC M96.1
- postleukotomy FØ7.Ø
- postmastectomy lymphedema I97.2
- postmyocardial infarction I24.1
- postoperative NEC T81.9 ☑
  - blind loop K9Ø.2
- postpartum panhypopituitary (Sheehan) E23.Ø
- postpolio (myelitic) G14
- postthrombotic I87.ØØ9
  - with
    - inflammation I87.Ø2- ☑
      - with ulcer I87.Ø3- ☑
    - specified complication NEC I87.Ø9- ☑
    - ulcer I87.Ø1- ☑
      - with inflammation I87.Ø3- ☑
  - asymptomatic I87.ØØ- ☑
- postural
  - orthostatic tachycardia [POTS] G9Ø.A
  - tachycardia G9Ø.A
- postvagotomy K91.1
- postvalvulotomy I97.Ø
- postviral NEC G93.31
  - fatigue G93.31
- Potain's K31.Ø
- potassium intoxication E87.5
- Prader-Willi Q87.11
- Prader-Willi-like Q87.19
- precerebral artery (multiple) (bilateral) G45.2
- preinfarction I2Ø.Ø
- preleukemic D46.9
- premature senility E34.8
- premenstrual dysphoric F32.81
- premenstrual tension N94.3
- Prinzmetal-Massumi RØ7.1
- prune belly Q79.4
- pseudo -Turner's Q87.19
- pseudocarpal tunnel (sublimis) — *see* Syndrome, carpal tunnel
- pseudoparalytica G7Ø.ØØ
  - with exacerbation (acute) G7Ø.Ø1
  - in crisis G7Ø.Ø1
- psycho-organic (nonpsychotic severity) FØ7.9
  - acute or subacute FØ5
  - depressive type FØ6.31
  - hallucinatory type FØ6.Ø
  - nonpsychotic severity FØ7.Ø
  - specified NEC FØ7.89
- PTEN (hamartoma) tumor Q85.81
- pulmonary
  - arteriosclerosis I27.Ø
  - dysmaturity (Wilson-Mikity) P27.Ø

Syndrome — *continued*
- pulmonary — *continued*
  - hypoperfusion (idiopathic) P22.Ø
  - renal (hemorrhagic) (Goodpasture's) M31.Ø
- pure
  - motor lacunar G46.5
  - sensory lacunar G46.6
- Putnam-Dana D51.Ø
- pyogenic arthritis, pyoderma gangrenosum, and acne [PAPA] MØ4.8
- pyramidopallidonigral G2Ø.C
- pyriformis — *see* Lesion, nerve, sciatic
- QT interval prolongation I45.81
- radicular NEC — *see* Radiculopathy
  - upper limbs, newborn (birth injury) P14.3
- rapid time-zone change G47.25
- Rasmussen GØ4.81
- Raymond (-Cestan) I65.8
- Raynaud's I73.ØØ
  - with gangrene I73.Ø1
- RDS (respiratory distress syndrome, newborn) P22.Ø
- reactive airways dysfunction J68.3
- Refsum's G6Ø.1
- Reifenstein E34.52
- renal glomerulohyalinosis-diabetic — *see* Diabetes, nephrosis
- Rendu-Osler-Weber I78.Ø
- residual ovary N99.83
- resistant ovary E28.39
- respiratory
  - distress
    - acute J8Ø
      - adult J8Ø
      - child J8Ø
      - idiopathic J84.114
    - newborn (idiopathic) (type I) P22.Ø
      - type II P22.1
- restless legs G25.81
- restrictive allograft J4A.Ø
- retinoblastoma (familial) C69.2 ☑
- retroperitoneal fibrosis K68.2
- retroviral seroconversion (acute) Z21
- Reye's G93.7
- Richter — *see* Leukemia, chronic lymphocytic, B-cell type
- Ridley's I5Ø.1
- right
  - heart, hypoplastic Q22.6
  - ventricular obstruction — *see* Failure, heart, right
- Romano-Ward (prolonged QT interval) I45.81
- rotator cuff, shoulder — *see also* Tear, rotator cuff M75.1Ø- ☑
- Rotes Querol — *see* Hyperostosis, ankylosing
- Roth — *see* Meralgia paresthetica
- rubella (congenital) P35.Ø
- Ruvalcaba-Myhre-Smith E71.44Ø
- Rytand-Lipsitch I44.2
- salt
  - depletion E87.1
    - due to heat NEC T67.8 ☑
      - causing heat exhaustion or prostration T67.4 ☑
  - low E87.1
- salt-losing N28.89
- SATB2-associated Q87.89
- Scaglietti-Dagnini E22.Ø
- scalenus anticus (anterior) G54.Ø
- scapulocostal — *see* Mononeuropathy, upper limb, specified site NEC
- scapuloperoneal G71.Ø9
- schizophrenic, of childhood NEC F2Ø.9
- Schnitzler D47.2
- Scholte's E34.Ø
- Schroeder's E27.Ø
- Schuller-Christian C96.5
- Schwachman (-Diamond) D61.Ø2
- Schwartz (-Jampel) G71.13
- Schwartz-Bartter E22.2
- scimitar Q26.8
- sclerocystic ovary E28.2
- Seitelberger's G31.89
- septicemic adrenal hemorrhage A39.1
- seroconversion, retroviral (acute) Z21
- serous meningitis G93.2
- severe acute respiratory (SARS) J12.81
  - coronavirus 2 (*see also* COVID-19) UØ7.1
    - pneumonia J12.82
- shaken infant T74.4 ☑

Syndrome — *continued*
- shock (traumatic) T79.4 ☑
  - kidney N17.Ø
    - following crush injury T79.5 ☑
  - toxic A48.3
- shock-lung J8Ø
- Shone's — *code to* specific anomalies
- short
  - bowel K9Ø.829
    - with
      - colon in continuity K9Ø.821
      - iliocolonic anastomosis K9Ø.821
    - without colon in continuity K9Ø.822
  - gut — *see* Syndrome, short, bowel
  - rib Q77.2
- shoulder-hand — *see* Algoneurodystrophy
- Shwachman (-Diamond) D61.Ø2
- sicca — *see* Syndrome, Sjogren
- sick
  - cell E87.1
  - sinus I49.5
- sick-euthyroid EØ7.81
- sideropenic D5Ø.1
- Siemens' ectodermal dysplasia Q82.4
- Silfverskold's Q78.9
- Simons' E88.1
- sinus tarsi M25.57- ☑
- sinusitis-bronchiectasis-situs inversus Q89.3
- Sipple's E31.22
- sirenomelia Q87.2
- Sjogren M35.ØØ
  - with
    - central nervous system involvement M35.Ø7
    - dental involvement M35.ØC
    - gastrointestinal involvement M35.Ø8
    - glomerular disease M35.ØA
    - inflammatory arthritis M35.Ø5
    - keratoconjunctivitis M35.Ø1
    - lung involvement M35.Ø2
    - myopathy M35.Ø3
    - peripheral nervous system involvement M35.Ø6
    - renal tubular acidosis M35.Ø4
    - specified organ involvement, NEC M35.Ø9
    - tubulo-interstitial nephropathy M35.Ø4
    - vasculitis M35.ØB
- Slocumb's E27.Ø
- slow flow, coronary I2Ø.89
- Sluder's G44.89
- Smith-Magenis Q93.88
- Sneddon-Wilkinson L13.1
- Snyder-Robinson Q87.89
- Sotos' Q87.3
- South African cardiomyopathy I42.8
- spasmodic
  - upward movement, eyes H51.8
  - winking F95.8
- Spen's I45.9
- splenic
  - agenesis Q89.Ø1
  - flexure K59.89
  - neutropenia D73.81
- Spurway's Q78.Ø
- staphylococcal scalded skin LØØ
- steal
  - arteriovenous T82.898- ☑
  - ischemic T82.898- ☑
  - subclavian G45.8
- Stein-Leventhal E28.2
- Stein's E28.2
- Stevens-Johnson syndrome L51.1
  - toxic epidermal necrolysis overlap L51.3
- Stewart-Morel M85.2
- Stickler Q89.8
- stiff baby Q89.8
- stiff man G25.82
- Still-Felty — *see* Felty's syndrome
- Stokes (-Adams) I45.9
- stone heart I5Ø.1
- straight back, congenital Q76.49
- Sturge-Weber (-Dimitri) Q85.89
- subclavian steal G45.8
- subcoracoid-pectoralis minor G54.Ø
- subcostal nerve compression I77.89
- subphrenic interposition Q43.3
- superior
  - cerebellar artery I63.89
  - mesenteric artery K55.1
  - semi-circular canal dehiscence H83.8X- ☑

Syndrome — *continued*
superior — *continued*
vena cava I87.1
supine hypotensive (maternal) — *see* Syndrome, hypotension, maternal
suprarenal cortical E27.Ø
supraspinatus — *see also* Tear, rotator cuff M75.1Ø- ☑
Susac G93.49
swallowed blood P78.2
sweat retention L74.Ø
Swyer Q99.1
Symond's G93.2
sympathetic
cervical paralysis G9Ø.2
pelvic, female N94.89
systemic inflammatory response (SIRS), of non-infectious origin (without organ dysfunction) R65.1Ø
with acute organ dysfunction R65.11
tachycardia-bradycardia I49.5
takotsubo I51.81
TAR (thrombocytopenia with absent radius) Q87.2
tarsal tunnel G57.5- ☑
teething KØØ.7
tegmental G93.89
telangiectasic-pigmentation-cataract Q82.8
temporal pyramidal apex — *see* Otitis, media, suppurative, acute
temporomandibular joint-pain-dysfunction M26.62- ☑
Terry's — *see also* Myopia, degenerative H44.2- ☑
testicular feminization — *see also* Syndrome, androgen insensitivity E34.51
thalamic pain (hyperesthetic) G89.Ø
thoracic outlet (compression) G54.Ø
Thorson-Bjorck E34.Ø
thrombocytopenia with absent radius (TAR) Q87.2
thrombosis with thrombocytopenia D75.84
thyroid-adrenocortical insufficiency E31.Ø
tibial
anterior M76.81- ☑
posterior M76.82- ☑
Tietze's M94.Ø
time-zone (rapid) G47.25
Toni-Fanconi E72.Ø9
with cystinosis E72.Ø4
Touraine's Q79.8
tourniquet — *see* Constriction, external, by site
toxic shock A48.3
transient left ventricular apical ballooning I51.81
traumatic vasospastic T75.22 ☑
Treacher Collins Q75.4
triple X, female Q97.Ø
trisomy Q92.9
13 Q91.7
meiotic nondisjunction Q91.4
mitotic nondisjunction Q91.5
mosaicism Q91.5
translocation Q91.6
18 Q91.3
meiotic nondisjunction Q91.Ø
mitotic nondisjunction Q91.1
mosaicism Q91.1
translocation Q91.2
2Ø (q)(p) Q92.8
21 Q9Ø.9
meiotic nondisjunction Q9Ø.Ø
mitotic nondisjunction Q9Ø.1
mosaicism Q9Ø.1
translocation Q9Ø.2
22 Q92.8
tropical wet feet T69.Ø- ☑
Trousseau's I82.1
tumor lysis (following antineoplastic chemotherapy) (spontaneous) NEC E88.3
tumor necrosis factor receptor associated periodic (TRAPS) MØ4.1
Twiddler's (due to)
automatic implantable defibrillator T82.198 ☑
cardiac pacemaker T82.198 ☑
Unverricht (-Lundborg) — *see* Epilepsy, generalized, idiopathic
upward gaze H51.8
uremia, chronic — *see also* Disease, kidney, chronic N18.9
urethral N34.3
urethro-oculo-articular — *see* Reiter's disease
urohepatic K76.7
vago-hypoglossal G52.7
van Buchem's M85.2

Syndrome — *continued*
van der Hoeve's Q78.Ø
vascular NEC in cerebrovascular disease G46.8
vasoconstriction, reversible cerebrovascular I67.841
vasomotor I73.9
vasospastic (traumatic) T75.22 ☑
vasovagal R55
VATER Q87.2
velo-cardio-facial Q93.81
vena cava (inferior) (superior) (obstruction) I87.1
vertebral
artery G45.Ø
compression — *see* Syndrome, anterior, spinal artery, compression
steal G45.Ø
vertebro-basilar artery G45.Ø
vertebrogenic (pain) — *see also* Pain, vertebrogenic M54.89
vertiginous — *see* Disorder, vestibular function
Vinson-Plummer D5Ø.1
virus B34.9
visceral larva migrans B83.Ø
visual disorientation H53.8
vitamin B6 deficiency E53.1
vitreal corneal H59.Ø1- ☑
vitreous (touch) H59.Ø1- ☑
Vogt-Koyanagi H2Ø.82- ☑
Volkmann's T79.6 ☑
von Hippel-Lindau Q85.83
von Schroetter's I82.89Ø
von Willebrand (-Jurgen) — *see* Disease, von Willebrand
acquired — *see also* Disease, von Willebrand D68.Ø4
Waldenstrom-Kjellberg D5Ø.1
Wallenberg's G46.3
wasting (syndrome) due to underlying condition E88.A
water retention E87.79
Waterhouse (-Friderichsen) A39.1
Weber-Gubler G46.3
Weber-Leyden G46.3
Weber's G46.3
Wegener's M31.3Ø
with
kidney involvement M31.31
lung involvement M31.3Ø
with kidney involvement M31.31
Weingarten's (tropical eosinophilia) J82.89
Weiss-Baker G9Ø.Ø9
Werdnig-Hoffman G12.Ø
Wermer's E31.21
Werner's E34.8
Wernicke-Korsakoff (nonalcoholic) FØ4
alcoholic F1Ø.26
Westphal-Strumpell E83.Ø1
West's — *see* Epilepsy, spasms
wet
feet (maceration) (tropical) T69.Ø- ☑
lung, newborn P22.1
whiplash S13.4 ☑
whistling face Q87.Ø
Wilkie's K55.1
Wilkinson-Sneddon L13.1
Willebrand (-Jurgens) — *see* Disease, von Willebrand
Williams Q93.82
Wilson's (hepatolenticular degeneration) E83.Ø1
Wiskott-Aldrich D82.Ø
withdrawal — *see* Withdrawal, state
drug
infant of dependent mother P96.1
therapeutic use, newborn P96.2
Woakes' (ethmoiditis) J33.1
Wright's (hyperabduction) G54.Ø
X I2Ø.9
XXXX Q97.1
XXXXX Q97.1
XXXXY Q98.1
XXY Q98.Ø
Yao MØ4.8
yellow nail L6Ø.5
Zahorsky's BØ8.5
Zellweger syndrome E71.51Ø
Zellweger-like syndrome E71.541

Synechia (anterior) (iris) (posterior) (pupil) — *see also* Adhesions, iris
intra-uterine (traumatic) N85.6

Synesthesia R2Ø.8

Syngamiasis, syngamosis B83.3

Synodontia KØØ.2

Synorchidism, synorchism Q55.1

Synostosis (congenital) Q78.8
astragalo-scaphoid Q74.2
radioulnar Q74.Ø

Synovial sarcoma — *see* Neoplasm, connective tissue, malignant

Synovioma (malignant) — *see also* Neoplasm, connective tissue, malignant
benign — *see* Neoplasm, connective tissue, benign

Synoviosarcoma — *see* Neoplasm, connective tissue, malignant

Synovitis — *see also* Tenosynovitis M65.9
crepitant
hand M7Ø.Ø- ☑
wrist M7Ø.Ø3- ☑
gonococcal A54.49
gouty — *see* Gout
in (due to)
crystals M65.8- ☑
gonorrhea A54.49
syphilis (late) A52.78
use, overuse, pressure — *see* Disorder, soft tissue, due to use
infective NEC — *see* Tenosynovitis, infective NEC
specified NEC — *see* Tenosynovitis, specified type NEC
syphilitic A52.78
congenital (early) A5Ø.Ø2
toxic — *see* Synovitis, transient
transient M67.3- ☑
ankle M67.37- ☑
elbow M67.32- ☑
foot joint M67.37- ☑
hand joint M67.34- ☑
hip M67.35- ☑
knee M67.36- ☑
multiple site M67.39
pelvic region M67.35- ☑
shoulder M67.31- ☑
specified joint NEC M67.38
wrist M67.33- ☑
traumatic, current — *see* Sprain
tuberculous — *see* Tuberculosis, synovitis
villonodular (pigmented) M12.2- ☑
ankle M12.27- ☑
elbow M12.22- ☑
foot joint M12.27- ☑
hand joint M12.24- ☑
hip M12.25- ☑
knee M12.26- ☑
multiple site M12.29
pelvic region M12.25- ☑
shoulder M12.21- ☑
specified joint NEC M12.28
vertebrae M12.28
wrist M12.23- ☑

Syphilid A51.39
congenital A5Ø.Ø6
newborn A5Ø.Ø6
tubercular (late) A52.79

Syphilis, syphilitic (acquired) A53.9
abdomen (late) A52.79
acoustic nerve A52.15
adenopathy (secondary) A51.49
adrenal (gland) (with cortical hypofunction) A52.79
age under 2 years NOS — *see also* Syphilis, congenital, early
acquired A51.9
alopecia (secondary) A51.32
anemia (late) A52.79 *[D63.8]*
aneurysm (aorta) (ruptured) A52.Ø1
central nervous system A52.Ø5
congenital A5Ø.54 *[I79.Ø]*
anus (late) A52.74
primary A51.1
secondary A51.39
aorta (arch) (abdominal) (thoracic) A52.Ø2
aneurysm A52.Ø1
aortic (insufficiency) (regurgitation) (stenosis) A52.Ø3
aneurysm A52.Ø1
arachnoid (adhesive) (cerebral) (spinal) A52.13
asymptomatic — *see* Syphilis, latent
ataxia (locomotor) A52.11
atrophoderma maculatum A51.39
auricular fibrillation A52.Ø6
bladder (late) A52.76
bone A52.77
secondary A51.46

Syphilis, syphilitic — *continued*
- brain A52.17
- breast (late) A52.79
- bronchus (late) A52.72
- bubo (primary) A51.0
- bulbar palsy A52.19
- bursa (late) A52.78
- cardiac decompensation A52.06
- cardiovascular A52.00
- central nervous system (late) (recurrent) (relapse) (tertiary) A52.3
  - with
    - ataxia A52.11
    - general paralysis A52.17
      - juvenile A50.45
    - paresis (general) A52.17
      - juvenile A50.45
    - tabes (dorsalis) A52.11
      - juvenile A50.45
    - taboparesis A52.17
      - juvenile A50.45
  - aneurysm A52.05
  - congenital A50.40
  - juvenile A50.40
  - remission in (sustained) A52.3
  - serology doubtful, negative, or positive A52.3
  - specified nature or site NEC A52.19
  - vascular A52.05
- cerebral A52.17
  - meningovascular A52.13
  - nerves (multiple palsies) A52.15
  - sclerosis A52.17
  - thrombosis A52.05
- cerebrospinal (tabetic type) A52.12
- cerebrovascular A52.05
- cervix (late) A52.76
- chancre (multiple) A51.0
  - extragenital A51.2
  - Rollet's A51.0
- Charcot's joint A52.16
- chorioretinitis A51.43
  - congenital A50.01
  - late A52.71
  - prenatal A50.01
- choroiditis — *see* Syphilitic chorioretinitis
- choroidoretinitis — *see* Syphilitic chorioretinitis
- ciliary body (secondary) A51.43
  - late A52.71
- colon (late) A52.74
- combined spinal sclerosis A52.11
- condyloma (latum) A51.31
- congenital A50.9
  - with
    - paresis (general) A50.45
    - tabes (dorsalis) A50.45
    - taboparesis A50.45
  - chorioretinitis, choroiditis A50.01 *[H32]*
  - early, or less than 2 years after birth NEC A50.2
    - with manifestations — *see* Syphilis, congenital, early, symptomatic
    - latent (without manifestations) A50.1
      - negative spinal fluid test A50.1
      - serology positive A50.1
    - symptomatic A50.09
      - cutaneous A50.06
      - mucocutaneous A50.07
      - oculopathy A50.01
      - osteochondropathy A50.02
      - pharyngitis A50.03
      - pneumonia A50.04
      - rhinitis A50.05
      - visceral A50.08
  - interstitial keratitis A50.31
  - juvenile neurosyphilis A50.45
  - late, or 2 years or more after birth NEC A50.7
    - chorioretinitis, choroiditis A50.32
    - interstitial keratitis A50.31
    - juvenile neurosyphilis A50.45
    - latent (without manifestations) A50.6
      - negative spinal fluid test A50.6
      - serology positive A50.6
    - symptomatic or with manifestations NEC A50.59
      - arthropathy A50.55
      - cardiovascular A50.54
      - Clutton's joints A50.51
      - Hutchinson's teeth A50.52
      - Hutchinson's triad A50.53
      - osteochondropathy A50.56
      - saddle nose A50.57

Syphilis, syphilitic — *continued*
- conjugal A53.9
  - tabes A52.11
- conjunctiva (late) A52.71
- contact Z20.2
- cord bladder A52.19
- cornea, late A52.71
- coronary (artery) (sclerosis) A52.06
- coryza, congenital A50.05
- cranial nerve A52.15
  - multiple palsies A52.15
- cutaneous — *see* Syphilis, skin
- dacryocystitis (late) A52.71
- degeneration, spinal cord A52.12
- dementia paralytica A52.17
  - juvenilis A50.45
- destruction of bone A52.77
- dilatation, aorta A52.01
- due to blood transfusion A53.9
- dura mater A52.13
- ear A52.79
  - inner A52.79
    - nerve (eighth) A52.15
    - neurorecurrence A52.15
- early A51.9
  - cardiovascular A52.00
  - central nervous system A52.3
  - latent (without manifestations) (less than 2 years after infection) A51.5
    - negative spinal fluid test A51.5
    - serological relapse after treatment A51.5
    - serology positive A51.5
  - relapse (treated, untreated) A51.9
  - skin A51.39
  - symptomatic A51.9
    - extragenital chancre A51.2
    - primary, except extragenital chancre A51.0
    - secondary — *see also* Syphilis, secondary A51.39
      - relapse (treated, untreated) A51.49
  - ulcer A51.39
- eighth nerve (neuritis) A52.15
- endemic A65
- endocarditis A52.03
  - aortic A52.03
  - pulmonary A52.03
- epididymis (late) A52.76
- epiglottis (late) A52.73
- epiphysitis (congenital) (early) A50.02
- episcleritis (late) A52.71
- esophagus A52.79
- eustachian tube A52.73
- exposure to Z20.2
- eye A52.71
- eyelid (late) (with gumma) A52.71
- fallopian tube (late) A52.76
- fracture A52.77
- gallbladder (late) A52.74
- gastric (polyposis) (late) A52.74
- general A53.9
  - paralysis A52.17
    - juvenile A50.45
- genital (primary) A51.0
- glaucoma A52.71
- gumma NEC A52.79
  - cardiovascular system A52.00
  - central nervous system A52.3
  - congenital A50.59
- heart (block) (decompensation) (disease) (failure) A52.06 *[I52]*
  - valve NEC A52.03
- hemianesthesia A52.19
- hemianopsia A52.71
- hemiparesis A52.17
- hemiplegia A52.17
- hepatic artery A52.09
- hepatis A52.74
- hepatomegaly, congenital A50.08
- hereditaria tarda — *see* Syphilis, congenital, late
- hereditary — *see* Syphilis, congenital
- Hutchinson's teeth A50.52
- hyalitis A52.71
- inactive — *see* Syphilis, latent
- infantum — *see* Syphilis, congenital
- inherited — *see* Syphilis, congenital
- internal ear A52.79
- intestine (late) A52.74
- iris, iritis (secondary) A51.43
  - late A52.71

Syphilis, syphilitic — *continued*
- joint (late) A52.77
- keratitis (congenital) (interstitial) (late) A50.31
- kidney (late) A52.75
- lacrimal passages (late) A52.71
- larynx (late) A52.73
- late A52.9
  - cardiovascular A52.00
  - central nervous system A52.3
  - kidney A52.75
  - latent or 2 years or more after infection (without manifestations) A52.8
    - negative spinal fluid test A52.8
    - serology positive A52.8
  - paresis A52.17
  - specified site NEC A52.79
  - symptomatic or with manifestations A52.79
  - tabes A52.11
- latent A53.0
  - with signs or symptoms — *code by* site and stage under Syphilis
  - central nervous system A52.2
  - date of infection unspecified A53.0
  - early, or less than 2 years after infection A51.5
  - follow-up of latent syphilis A53.0
    - date of infection unspecified A53.0
    - late, or 2 years or more after infection A52.8
  - late, or 2 years or more after infection A52.8
  - positive serology (only finding) A53.0
    - date of infection unspecified A53.0
    - early, or less than 2 years after infection A51.5
    - late, or 2 years or more after infection A52.8
- lens (late) A52.71
- leukoderma A51.39
  - late A52.79
- lienitis A52.79
- lip A51.39
  - chancre (primary) A51.2
  - late A52.79
- Lissauer's paralysis A52.17
- liver A52.74
- locomotor ataxia A52.11
- lung A52.72
- lymph gland (early) (secondary) A51.49
  - late A52.79
- lymphadenitis (secondary) A51.49
- macular atrophy of skin A51.39
  - striated A52.79
- mediastinum (late) A52.73
- meninges (adhesive) (brain) (spinal cord) A52.13
- meningitis A52.13
  - acute (secondary) A51.41
  - congenital A50.41
- meningoencephalitis A52.14
- meningovascular A52.13
  - congenital A50.41
- mesarteritis A52.09
  - brain A52.04
- middle ear A52.77
- mitral stenosis A52.03
- monoplegia A52.17
- mouth (secondary) A51.39
  - late A52.79
- mucocutaneous (secondary) A51.39
  - late A52.79
- mucous
  - membrane (secondary) A51.39
    - late A52.79
  - patches A51.39
    - congenital A50.07
- mulberry molars A50.52
- muscle A52.78
- myocardium A52.06
- nasal sinus (late) A52.73
- neonatorum — *see* Syphilis, congenital
- nephrotic syndrome (secondary) A51.44
- nerve palsy (any cranial nerve) A52.15
  - multiple A52.15
- nervous system, central A52.3
- neuritis A52.15
  - acoustic A52.15
- neurorecidive of retina A52.19
- neuroretinitis A52.19
- newborn — *see* Syphilis, congenital
- nodular superficial (late) A52.79
- nonvenereal A65
- nose (late) A52.73
  - saddle back deformity A50.57
- occlusive arterial disease A52.09

- **Tabacism, tabacosis, tabagism** — *see also* Poisoning, tobacco
  - meaning dependence (without remission) F17.200
    - with
      - disorder F17.299
        - in remission F17.211
        - specified disorder NEC F17.298
        - withdrawal F17.203
- **Tabardillo** A75.9
  - flea-borne A75.2
  - louse-borne A75.0
- **Tabes, tabetic** A52.10
  - with
    - central nervous system syphilis A52.10
    - Charcot's joint A52.16
    - cord bladder A52.19
    - crisis, viscera (any) A52.19
    - paralysis, general A52.17
    - paresis (general) A52.17
    - perforating ulcer (foot) A52.19
  - arthropathy (Charcot) A52.16
  - bladder A52.19
  - bone A52.11
  - cerebrospinal A52.12
  - congenital A50.45
  - conjugal A52.10
  - dorsalis A52.11
    - juvenile A50.49
  - juvenile A50.49
  - latent A52.19
  - mesenterica A18.39
  - paralysis, insane, general A52.17
  - spasmodic A52.17
  - syphilis (cerebrospinal) A52.12
- **Taboparalysis** A52.17
- **Taboparesis** (remission) A52.17
  - juvenile A50.45
- **TAC** (trigeminal autonomic cephalgia) **NEC** G44.099
  - intractable G44.091
  - not intractable G44.099
- **Tache noir** S60.22- ☑
- **Tachyalimentation** K91.2
- **Tachyarrhythmia, tachyrhythmia** — *see* Tachycardia
- **Tachycardia** R00.0
  - atrial (paroxysmal) I47.19
  - auricular I47.19
  - AV nodal re-entry (re-entrant) I47.19
  - junctional (paroxysmal) I47.19
  - newborn P29.11
  - nodal (paroxysmal) I47.19
  - non-paroxysmal AV nodal I45.89
  - paroxysmal (sustained) (nonsustained) I47.9
    - with sinus bradycardia I49.5
    - atrial (PAT) I47.19
    - atrioventricular (AV) (re-entrant) I47.19
      - psychogenic F54
    - junctional I47.19
      - ectopic I47.19
    - nodal I47.19
    - psychogenic (atrial) (supraventricular) (ventricular) F54
    - supraventricular (sustained) I47.10
      - psychogenic F54
    - ventricular I47.20
      - psychogenic F54
      - specified type NEC I47.29
  - psychogenic F45.8
  - sick sinus I49.5
  - sinoauricular NOS R00.0
    - paroxysmal I47.19
  - sinus [sinusal] NOS R00.0
    - inappropriate, so stated (IST) I47.11
    - paroxysmal I47.19
  - supraventricular I47.10
  - ventricular (paroxysmal) (sustained) I47.20
    - psychogenic F54
    - specified NEC I47.29
- **Tachygastria** K31.89
- **Tachypnea** R06.82
  - hysterical F45.8
  - newborn (idiopathic) (transitory) P22.1
  - psychogenic F45.8
  - transitory, of newborn P22.1
- **TACO** (transfusion associated circulatory overload) E87.71
- **TAD** (transfusion-associated dyspnea) J95.87
- **Taenia** (infection) (infestation) B68.9
  - diminuta B71.0
  - echinococcal infestation B67.90
  - mediocanellata B68.1
  - nana B71.0
  - saginata B68.1
  - solium (intestinal form) B68.0
    - larval form — *see* Cysticercosis
- **Taeniasis** (intestine) — *see* Taenia
- **Tag** (hypertrophied skin) (infected) L91.8
  - adenoid J35.8
  - anus K64.4
  - hemorrhoidal K64.4
  - hymen N89.8
  - perineal N90.89
  - preauricular Q17.0
  - sentinel K64.4
  - skin L91.8
    - accessory (congenital) Q82.8
    - anus K64.4
    - congenital Q82.8
    - preauricular Q17.0
  - tonsil J35.8
  - urethra, urethral N36.8
  - vulva N90.89
- **Tahyna fever** B33.8
- **Takahara's disease** E80.3
- **Takayasu's disease or syndrome** M31.4
- **Talaromycosis** B48.4
- **Talcosis** (pulmonary) J62.0
- **Talipes** (congenital) Q66.89
  - acquired, planus — *see* Deformity, limb, flat foot
  - asymmetric Q66.89
  - calcaneovalgus Q66.4- ☑
  - calcaneovarus Q66.1- ☑
  - calcaneus Q66.89
  - cavus Q66.7- ☑
  - equinovalgus Q66.6
  - equinovarus Q66.0- ☑
  - equinus Q66.89
  - percavus Q66.7- ☑
  - planovalgus Q66.6
  - planus (acquired) (any degree) — *see also* Deformity, limb, flat foot
    - congenital Q66.5- ☑
    - due to rickets (sequelae) E64.3
  - valgus Q66.6
  - varus Q66.3- ☑
- **Tall stature, constitutional** E34.4
- **Talma's disease** M62.89
- **Talon noir** S90.3- ☑
  - hand S60.22- ☑
  - heel S90.3- ☑
  - toe S90.1- ☑
- **Tamponade, heart** I31.4
- **Tanapox** (virus disease) B08.71
- **Tangier disease** E78.6
- **Tantrum, child problem** F91.8
- **Tapeworm** (infection) (infestation) — *see* Infestation, tapeworm
- **Tapia's syndrome** G52.7
- **TAR** (thrombocytopenia with absent radius) **syndrome** Q87.2
- **Tarral-Besnier disease** L44.0
- **Tarsal tunnel syndrome** — *see* Syndrome, tarsal tunnel
- **Tarsalgia** — *see* Pain, limb, lower
- **Tarsitis** (eyelid) H01.8
  - syphilitic A52.71
  - tuberculous A18.4
- **Tartar** (teeth) (dental calculus) K03.6
- **Tattoo** (mark) L81.8
- **Tauri's disease** E74.09
- **Taurodontism** K00.2
- **Taussig-Bing syndrome** Q20.1
- **Taybi's syndrome** Q87.2
- **Tay-Sachs amaurotic familial idiocy or disease** E75.02
- **TBI** (traumatic brain injury) S06.9 ☑
- **Teacher's node or nodule** J38.2
- **Tear, torn** (traumatic) — *see also* Laceration
  - with abortion — *see* Abortion
  - annular fibrosis M51.35
  - anus, anal (sphincter) S31.831 ☑
    - complicating delivery
      - with third degree perineal laceration — *see also* Delivery, complicated, by, laceration, perineum, third degree O70.20
        - with mucosa O70.3
- **Tear, torn** — *continued*
  - anus, anal — *continued*
    - complicating delivery — *continued*
      - without third degree perineal laceration O70.4
    - nontraumatic (healed) (old) K62.81
  - articular cartilage, old — *see* Derangement, joint, articular cartilage, by site
  - bladder
    - with ectopic or molar pregnancy O08.6
    - following ectopic or molar pregnancy O08.6
    - obstetrical O71.5
    - traumatic — *see* Injury, bladder
  - bowel
    - with ectopic or molar pregnancy O08.6
    - following ectopic or molar pregnancy O08.6
    - obstetrical trauma O71.5
  - broad ligament
    - with ectopic or molar pregnancy O08.6
    - following ectopic or molar pregnancy O08.6
    - obstetrical trauma O71.6
  - bucket handle (knee) (meniscus) — *see* Tear, meniscus
  - capsule, joint — *see* Sprain
  - cartilage — *see also* Sprain
    - articular, old — *see* Derangement, joint, articular cartilage, by site
  - cervix
    - with ectopic or molar pregnancy O08.6
    - following ectopic or molar pregnancy O08.6
    - obstetrical trauma (current) O71.3
    - old N88.1
    - traumatic — *see* Injury, uterus
  - dural G97.41
    - nontraumatic G96.11
  - internal organ — *see* Injury, by site
  - knee cartilage
    - articular (current) S83.3- ☑
    - old — *see* Derangement, knee, meniscus, due to old tear
  - ligament — *see* Sprain
  - meniscus (knee) (current injury) S83.209 ☑
    - bucket-handle S83.20- ☑
    - lateral
      - bucket-handle S83.25- ☑
      - complex S83.27- ☑
      - peripheral S83.26- ☑
      - specified type NEC S83.28- ☑
    - medial
      - bucket-handle S83.21- ☑
      - complex S83.23- ☑
      - peripheral S83.22- ☑
      - specified type NEC S83.24- ☑
    - old — *see* Derangement, knee, meniscus, due to old tear
    - site other than knee — *code as* Sprain
    - specified type NEC S83.20- ☑
  - muscle — *see* Strain
  - pelvic
    - floor, complicating delivery O70.1
    - organ NEC, obstetrical trauma O71.5
      - with ectopic or molar pregnancy O08.6
      - following ectopic or molar pregnancy O08.6
  - perineal, secondary O90.1
  - periurethral tissue, obstetrical trauma O71.82
    - with ectopic or molar pregnancy O08.6
    - following ectopic or molar pregnancy O08.6
  - rectovaginal septum — *see* Laceration, vagina
  - retina, retinal (without detachment) (horseshoe) — *see also* Break, retina, horseshoe
    - with detachment — *see* Detachment, retina, with retinal, break
  - rotator cuff (nontraumatic) M75.10- ☑
    - complete M75.12- ☑
    - incomplete M75.11- ☑
    - traumatic S46.01- ☑
      - capsule S43.42- ☑
  - semilunar cartilage, knee — *see* Tear, meniscus
  - supraspinatus (complete) (incomplete) (nontraumatic) — *see also* Tear, rotator cuff M75.10- ☑
  - tendon — *see* Strain
  - tentorial, at birth P10.4
  - umbilical cord
    - complicating delivery O69.89 ☑
  - urethra
    - with ectopic or molar pregnancy O08.6
    - following ectopic or molar pregnancy O08.6
    - obstetrical trauma O71.5
  - uterus — *see* Injury, uterus

Tear, torn — *continued*
- vagina — *see* Laceration, vagina
- vessel, from catheter — *see* Puncture, accidental complicating surgery
- vulva, complicating delivery O70.0

Tear-stone — *see* Dacryolith

Teeth — *see also* condition
- grinding
  - psychogenic F45.8
  - sleep related G47.63

Teething (syndrome) K00.7

Telangiectasia, telangiectasis (verrucous) I78.1
- ataxic (cerebellar) (Louis-Bar) G11.3
- familial I78.0
- hemorrhagic, hereditary (congenital) (senile) I78.0
- hereditary, hemorrhagic (congenital) (senile) I78.0
- juxtafoveal H35.07- ☑
- macular H35.07- ☑
- macularis eruptiva perstans D47.01
- parafoveal H35.07- ☑
- retinal (idiopathic) (juxtafoveal) (macular) (parafoveal) H35.07- ☑
- spider I78.1

Telephone scatologia F65.89

Telescoped bowel or intestine K56.1
- congenital Q43.8

Temperature
- body, high (of unknown origin) R50.9
- cold, trauma from T69.9 ☑
  - newborn P80.0
  - specified effect NEC T69.8 ☑

Temple — *see* condition

Temporal — *see* condition

Temporomandibular joint pain-dysfunction syndrome M26.62- ☑

Temporosphenoidal — *see* condition

Tendency
- bleeding — *see* Defect, coagulation
- suicide
  - meaning personal history of attempted suicide Z91.51
  - meaning suicidal ideation — *see* Ideation, suicidal
- to fall R29.6

Tenderness, abdominal R10.819
- epigastric R10.816
- generalized R10.817
- left lower quadrant R10.814
- left upper quadrant R10.812
- periumbilic R10.815
- rebound R10.829
  - epigastric R10.826
  - generalized R10.827
  - left lower quadrant R10.824
  - left upper quadrant R10.822
  - periumbilic R10.825
  - right lower quadrant R10.823
  - right upper quadrant R10.821
- right lower quadrant R10.813
- right upper quadrant R10.811

Tendinitis, tendonitis — *see also* Enthesopathy
- Achilles M76.6- ☑
- adhesive — *see* Tenosynovitis, specified type NEC
  - shoulder — *see* Capsulitis, adhesive
- bicipital M75.2- ☑
- calcific M65.2- ☑
  - ankle M65.27- ☑
  - foot M65.27- ☑
  - forearm M65.23- ☑
  - hand M65.24- ☑
  - lower leg M65.26- ☑
  - multiple sites M65.29
  - pelvic region M65.25- ☑
  - shoulder M75.3- ☑
  - specified site NEC M65.28
  - thigh M65.25- ☑
  - upper arm M65.22- ☑
- due to use, overuse, pressure — *see also* Disorder, soft tissue, due to use
  - specified NEC — *see* Disorder, soft tissue, due to use, specified NEC
- gluteal M76.0- ☑
- patellar M76.5- ☑
- peroneal M76.7- ☑
- psoas M76.1- ☑
- tibial (posterior) M76.82- ☑
  - anterior M76.81- ☑
- trochanteric — *see* Bursitis, hip, trochanteric

Tendon — *see* condition

Tendosynovitis — *see* Tenosynovitis

Tenesmus (rectal) R19.8
- vesical R30.1

Tennis elbow — *see* Epicondylitis, lateral

Tenonitis — *see also* Tenosynovitis
- eye (capsule) H05.04- ☑

Tenontosynovitis — *see* Tenosynovitis

Tenontothecitis — *see* Tenosynovitis

Tenophyte — *see* Disorder, synovium, specified type NEC

Tenosynovitis — *see also* Synovitis M65.9
- adhesive — *see* Tenosynovitis, specified type NEC
  - shoulder — *see* Capsulitis, adhesive
- bicipital (calcifying) — *see* Tendinitis, bicipital
- gonococcal A54.49
- in (due to)
  - crystals M65.8- ☑
  - gonorrhea A54.49
  - syphilis (late) A52.78
  - use, overuse, pressure — *see also* Disorder, soft tissue, due to use
    - specified NEC — *see* Disorder, soft tissue, due to use, specified NEC
- infective NEC M65.1- ☑
  - ankle M65.17- ☑
  - foot M65.17- ☑
  - forearm M65.13- ☑
  - hand M65.14- ☑
  - lower leg M65.16- ☑
  - multiple sites M65.19
  - pelvic region M65.15- ☑
  - shoulder region M65.11- ☑
  - specified site NEC M65.18
  - thigh M65.15- ☑
  - upper arm M65.12- ☑
- radial styloid M65.4
- shoulder region M65.81- ☑
  - adhesive — *see* Capsulitis, adhesive
- specified type NEC M65.88
  - ankle M65.87- ☑
  - foot M65.87- ☑
  - forearm M65.83- ☑
  - hand M65.84- ☑
  - lower leg M65.86- ☑
  - multiple sites M65.89
  - pelvic region M65.85- ☑
  - shoulder region M65.81- ☑
  - specified site NEC M65.88
  - thigh M65.85- ☑
  - upper arm M65.82- ☑
- tuberculous — *see* Tuberculosis, tenosynovitis

Tenovaginitis — *see* Tenosynovitis

Tension
- arterial, high — *see also* Hypertension
  - without diagnosis of hypertension R03.0
- headache G44.209
  - intractable G44.201
  - not intractable G44.209
- nervous R45.0
- pneumothorax J93.0
- premenstrual N94.3
- state (mental) F48.9

Tentorium — *see* condition

Teratencephalus Q89.8

Teratism Q89.7

Teratoblastoma (malignant) — *see* Neoplasm, malignant, by site

Teratocarcinoma — *see also* Neoplasm, malignant, by site
- liver C22.7

Teratoma (solid) — *see also* Neoplasm, uncertain behavior, by site
- with embryonal carcinoma, mixed — *see* Neoplasm, malignant, by site
- with malignant transformation — *see* Neoplasm, malignant, by site
- adult (cystic) — *see* Neoplasm, benign, by site
- benign — *see* Neoplasm, benign, by site
- combined with choriocarcinoma — *see* Neoplasm, malignant, by site
- cystic (adult) — *see* Neoplasm, benign, by site
- differentiated — *see* Neoplasm, benign, by site
- embryonal — *see also* Neoplasm, malignant, by site
  - liver C22.7
- immature — *see* Neoplasm, malignant, by site
  - liver C22.7

Teratoma — *continued*
- liver — *continued*
  - adult, benign, cystic, differentiated type or mature D13.4
- malignant — *see also* Neoplasm, malignant, by site
  - anaplastic — *see* Neoplasm, malignant, by site
  - intermediate — *see* Neoplasm, malignant, by site
    - specified site — *see* Neoplasm, malignant, by site
    - unspecified site C62.90
  - undifferentiated — *see* Neoplasm, malignant, by site
- mature — *see* Neoplasm, uncertain behavior, by site
  - malignant — *see* Neoplasm, by site, malignant, by site
- ovary D27.- ☑
  - embryonal, immature or malignant C56- ☑
- solid — *see* Neoplasm, uncertain behavior, by site
- testis C62.9- ☑
  - adult, benign, cystic, differentiated type or mature D29.2- ☑
  - scrotal C62.1- ☑
  - undescended C62.0- ☑

Termination
- anomalous — *see also* Malposition, congenital
  - right pulmonary vein Q26.3
- pregnancy, elective Z33.2

Ternidens diminutus infestation B81.8

Ternidensiasis B81.8

Terror(s) night (child) F51.4

Terrorism, victim of Z65.4

Terry's syndrome — *see also* Myopia, degenerative H44.2- ☑

Tertiary — *see* condition

Test, tests, testing (for)
- adequacy (for dialysis)
  - hemodialysis Z49.31
  - peritoneal Z49.32
- blood pressure Z01.30
  - abnormal reading — *see* Blood, pressure
- blood typing Z01.83
  - Rh typing Z01.83
- blood-alcohol Z02.83
  - positive — *see* Findings, abnormal, in blood
- blood-drug Z02.83
  - positive — *see* Findings, abnormal, in blood
- cardiac pulse generator (battery) Z45.010
- fertility Z31.41
- genetic
  - disease carrier status for procreative management
    - female Z31.430
    - male Z31.440
  - male partner of patient with recurrent pregnancy loss Z31.441
  - procreative management NEC
    - female Z31.438
    - male Z31.448
- hearing Z01.10
  - with abnormal findings NEC Z01.118
  - infant or child (over 28 days old) Z00.129
    - with abnormal findings Z00.121
- HIV (human immunodeficiency virus)
  - nonconclusive (in infants) R75
  - positive Z21
  - seropositive Z21
- immunity status Z01.84
- intelligence NEC Z01.89
- laboratory (as part of a general medical examination) Z00.00
  - with abnormal finding Z00.01
  - for medicolegal reason NEC Z04.89
- male partner of patient with recurrent pregnancy loss Z31.441
- Mantoux (for tuberculosis) Z11.1
  - abnormal result R76.11
- pregnancy, positive first pregnancy — *see* Pregnancy, normal, first
- procreative Z31.49
  - fertility Z31.41
- skin, diagnostic
  - allergy Z01.82
    - special screening examination — *see* Screening, by name of disease
  - Mantoux Z11.1
  - tuberculin Z11.1
- specified NEC Z01.89
- tuberculin Z11.1
  - abnormal result R76.11

- **Test, tests, testing** — *continued*
  - vision Z01.00
    - with abnormal findings Z01.01
    - following failed vision screening Z01.020
      - with abnormal findings Z01.021
    - infant or child (over 28 days old) Z00.129
      - with abnormal findings Z00.121
  - Wassermann Z11.3
    - positive — *see* Serology for syphilis, positive
- **Testicle, testicular, testis** — *see also* condition
  - feminization syndrome — *see also* Syndrome, androgen insensitivity E34.51
  - migrans Q55.29
- **Tetanus, tetanic** (cephalic) (convulsions) A35
  - with
    - abortion A34
    - ectopic or molar pregnancy O08.0
  - following ectopic or molar pregnancy O08.0
  - inoculation reaction (due to serum) — *see* Complications, vaccination
  - neonatorum A33
  - obstetrical A34
  - puerperal, postpartum, childbirth A34
- **Tetany** (due to) R29.0
  - alkalosis E87.3
  - associated with rickets E55.0
  - convulsions R29.0
    - hysterical F44.5
  - functional (hysterical) F44.5
  - hyperkinetic R29.0
    - hysterical F44.5
  - hyperpnea R06.4
    - hysterical F44.5
    - psychogenic F45.8
  - hyperventilation — *see also* Hyperventilation R06.4
    - hysterical F44.5
  - neonatal (without calcium or magnesium deficiency) P71.3
  - parathyroid (gland) E20.9
  - parathyroprival E89.2
  - post- (para)thyroidectomy E89.2
  - postoperative E89.2
  - pseudotetany R29.0
  - psychogenic (conversion reaction) F44.5
- **Tetralogy of Fallot** Q21.3
- **Tetraplegia** (chronic) — *see also* Quadriplegia G82.50
- **Thailand hemorrhagic fever** A91
- **Thalassanemia** — *see* Thalassemia
- **Thalassemia** (anemia) (disease) D56.9
  - with other hemoglobinopathy D56.8
  - alpha (major) (severe) (triple gene defect) D56.0
    - minor D56.3
    - silent carrier D56.3
    - trait D56.3
  - beta (severe) D56.1
    - homozygous D56.1
    - major D56.1
    - minor D56.3
    - trait D56.3
  - delta-beta (homozygous) D56.2
    - minor D56.3
    - trait D56.3
  - dominant D56.8
  - hemoglobin
    - C D56.8
    - E-beta D56.5
  - intermedia D56.1
  - major D56.1
  - minor D56.3
  - mixed D56.8
  - sickle-cell — *see* Disease, sickle-cell, thalassemia
  - specified type NEC D56.8
  - trait D56.3
  - variants D56.8
- **Thanatophoric dwarfism or short stature** Q77.1
- **Thaysen-Gee disease** (nontropical sprue) K90.0
- **Thaysen's disease** K90.0
- **Thecoma** D27- ☑
  - luteinized D27- ☑
  - malignant C56- ☑
- **Thelarche, premature** E30.8
- **Thelaziasis** B83.8
- **Thelitis** N61.0
  - puerperal, postpartum or gestational — *see* Infection, nipple
- **Therapeutic** — *see* condition
- **Therapy**
  - drug, long-term (current) (prophylactic)
    - agents affecting estrogen receptors and estrogen levels NEC Z79.818
    - anastrozole (Arimidex) Z79.811
    - antibiotics Z79.2
      - short-term use — *omit code*
    - anticoagulants Z79.01
    - anti-inflammatory Z79.1
    - antiplatelet Z79.02
    - antithrombotics Z79.02
    - aromatase inhibitors Z79.811
    - aspirin Z79.82
    - birth control pill or patch Z79.3
    - bisphosphonates Z79.83
    - contraceptive, oral Z79.3
    - drug, specified NEC Z79.899
    - estrogen receptor downregulators Z79.818
    - Evista Z79.810
    - exemestane (Aromasin) Z79.811
    - Fareston Z79.810
    - fulvestrant (Faslodex) Z79.818
    - gonadotropin-releasing hormone (GnRH) agonist Z79.818
    - goserelin acetate (Zoladex) Z79.818
    - hormone replacement Z79.890
    - insulin Z79.4
    - letrozole (Femara) Z79.811
    - leuprolide acetate (leuprorelin) (Lupron) Z79.818
    - megestrol acetate (Megace) Z79.818
    - methadone
      - for pain management Z79.891
      - maintenance therapy F11.20
    - Nolvadex Z79.810
    - opiate analgesic Z79.891
    - oral antidiabetic Z79.84
    - oral contraceptive Z79.3
    - oral hypoglycemic Z79.84
    - raloxifene (Evista) Z79.810
    - selective estrogen receptor modulators (SERMs) Z79.810
    - short term — *omit code*
    - steroids
      - inhaled Z79.51
      - systemic Z79.52
    - tamoxifen (Nolvadex) Z79.810
    - toremifene (Fareston) Z79.810
- **Thermic** — *see* condition
- **Thermography** (abnormal) — *see also* Abnormal, diagnostic imaging R93.89
  - breast R92.8
- **Thermoplegia** T67.01 ☑
- **Thesaurismosis, glycogen** — *see* Disease, glycogen storage
- **Thiamin deficiency** E51.9
  - specified NEC E51.8
- **Thiaminic deficiency with beriberi** E51.11
- **Thibierge-Weissenbach syndrome** — *see* Sclerosis, systemic
- **Thickening**
  - bone — *see* Hypertrophy, bone
  - breast N64.59
  - endometrium R93.89
  - epidermal L85.9
    - specified NEC L85.8
  - hymen N89.6
  - larynx J38.7
  - nail L60.2
    - congenital Q84.5
  - periosteal — *see* Hypertrophy, bone
  - pleura J92.9
    - with asbestos J92.0
  - skin R23.4
  - subepiglottic J38.7
  - tongue K14.8
  - valve, heart — *see* Endocarditis
- **Thigh** — *see* condition
- **Thinning vertebra** — *see* Spondylopathy, specified NEC
- **Thirst, excessive** R63.1
  - due to deprivation of water T73.1 ☑
- **Thomsen disease** G71.12
- **Thoracic** — *see also* condition
  - kidney Q63.2
  - outlet syndrome G54.0
- **Thoracogastroschisis** (congenital) Q79.8
- **Thoracopagus** Q89.4
- **Thorax** — *see* condition
- **Thorn's syndrome** N28.89
- **Thorson-Bjorck syndrome** E34.0
- **Threadworm** (infection) (infestation) B80
- **Threatened**
  - abortion O20.0
    - with subsequent abortion O03.9
  - abuse (harm) — *see* Maltreatment
  - job loss, anxiety concerning Z56.2
  - labor (without delivery) O47.9
    - at or after 37 completed weeks of gestation O47.1
    - before 37 completed weeks of gestation O47.0- ☑
  - loss of job, anxiety concerning Z56.2
  - miscarriage O20.0
  - unemployment, anxiety concerning Z56.2
- **Three-day fever** A93.1
- **Threshers' lung** J67.0
- **Thrix annulata** (congenital) Q84.1
- **Throat** — *see* condition
- **Thrombasthenia** (Glanzmann) (hemorrhagic) (hereditary) D69.1
- **Thromboangiitis** I73.1
  - obliterans (general) I73.1
    - cerebral I67.89
    - vessels
      - brain I67.89
      - spinal cord I67.89
- **Thromboarteritis** — *see* Arteritis
- **Thromboasthenia** (Glanzmann) (hemorrhagic) (hereditary) D69.1
- **Thrombocytasthenia** (Glanzmann) D69.1
- **Thrombocythemia** (hemorrhagic) *see also* Thrombocytosis D75.839
  - essential D47.3
  - idiopathic D47.3
  - primary D47.3
- **Thrombocytopathy** (dystrophic) (granulopenic) D69.1
- **Thrombocytopenia, thrombocytopenic** D69.6
  - with absent radius (TAR) Q87.2
  - congenital D69.42
  - dilutional D69.59
  - due to
    - (massive) blood transfusion D69.59
    - drugs D69.59
    - extracorporeal circulation of blood D69.59
    - platelet alloimmunization D69.59
  - essential D69.3
  - heparin induced (HIT) D75.829
    - delayed-onset D75.828
    - immune-mediated D75.822
    - non-immune D75.821
    - persisting D75.828
    - syndrome
      - autoimmune D75.828
      - specified NEC D75.828
      - spontaneous (without heparin exposure) D75.84
    - type 1 D75.821
    - type 2 D75.822
  - heparin-associated D75.821
  - hereditary D69.42
  - idiopathic D69.3
  - neonatal, transitory P61.0
    - due to
      - exchange transfusion P61.0
      - idiopathic maternal thrombocytopenia P61.0
      - isoimmunization P61.0
  - primary NEC D69.49
    - idiopathic D69.3
  - puerperal, postpartum O72.3
  - secondary D69.59
  - transient neonatal P61.0
  - vaccine-induced thrombotic D75.84
- **Thrombocytosis** D75.839
  - essential D47.3
  - idiopathic D47.3
  - primary D47.3
  - reactive D75.838
  - secondary D75.838
  - specified NEC D75.838
- **Thromboembolism** — *see* Embolism
- **Thrombopathy** (Bernard-Soulier) D69.1
  - constitutional — *see* Disease, von Willebrand
  - Willebrand-Jurgens — *see* Disease, von Willebrand
- **Thrombopenia** — *see* Thrombocytopenia
- **Thrombophilia** D68.59
  - primary NEC D68.59
  - secondary NEC D68.69
  - specified NEC D68.69
- **Thrombophlebitis** I80.9
  - antepartum O22.2- ☑

Thrombosis, thrombotic — *continued*
- tricuspid I07.8
- tumor — *see* Neoplasm, unspecified behavior, by site
- tunica vaginalis N50.1
- umbilical cord (vessels), complicating delivery O69.5 ☑
- vas deferens N50.1
- vein (acute) I82.90
  - antecubital I82.61- ☑
    - chronic I82.71- ☑
  - axillary I82.A1- ☑ (*following* I82.7)
    - chronic I82.A2- ☑ (*following* I82.7)
  - basilic I82.61- ☑
    - chronic I82.71- ☑
  - brachial I82.62- ☑
    - chronic I82.72- ☑
  - brachiocephalic (innominate) I82.290
    - chronic I82.291
  - calf muscular I82.46- ☑
    - chronic I82.56- ☑
  - cephalic I82.61- ☑
    - chronic I82.71- ☑
  - cerebral, nonpyogenic I67.6
  - chronic I82.91
  - deep (DVT) I82.40- ☑
    - calf I82.4Z- ☑
      - chronic I82.5Z- ☑
    - lower leg I82.4Z- ☑
      - chronic I82.5Z- ☑
    - thigh I82.4Y- ☑
      - chronic I82.5Y- ☑
    - upper leg I82.4Y- ☑
      - chronic I82.5Y- ☑
  - femoral I82.41- ☑
    - chronic I82.51- ☑
  - iliac (iliofemoral) I82.42- ☑
    - chronic I82.52- ☑
  - innominate I82.290
    - chronic I82.291
  - internal jugular I82.C1- ☑ (*following* I82.7)
    - chronic I82.C2- ☑ (*following* I82.7)
  - lower extremity
    - deep I82.40- ☑
      - chronic I82.50- ☑
      - specified NEC I82.49- ☑
        - chronic NEC I82.59- ☑
    - distal
      - deep I82.4Z- ☑
    - proximal
      - deep I82.4Y- ☑
        - chronic I82.5Y- ☑
    - superficial I82.81- ☑
  - perianal K64.5
  - peroneal I82.45- ☑
    - chronic I82.55- ☑
  - popliteal I82.43- ☑
    - chronic I82.53- ☑
  - radial I82.62- ☑
    - chronic I82.72- ☑
  - renal I82.3
  - saphenous (greater) (lesser) I82.81- ☑
  - specified NEC I82.890
    - chronic NEC I82.891
  - subclavian I82.B1- ☑ (*following* I82.7)
    - chronic I82.B2- ☑ (*following* I82.7)
  - thoracic NEC I82.290
    - chronic I82.291
  - tibial I82.44- ☑
    - chronic I82.54- ☑
  - ulnar I82.62- ☑
    - chronic I82.72- ☑
  - upper extremity I82.60- ☑
    - chronic I82.70- ☑
    - deep I82.62- ☑
      - chronic I82.72- ☑
    - superficial I82.61- ☑
      - chronic I82.71- ☑
- vena cava
  - inferior I82.220
    - chronic I82.221
  - superior I82.210
    - chronic I82.211
- venous, perianal K64.5
- ventricle — *see also* Infarct, myocardium
  - following acute myocardial infarction (current complication) I23.6
  - not resulting in infarction I24.0

Thrombosis, thrombotic — *continued*
- ventricle — *see also* Infarct, myocardium — *continued*
  - old I51.3

Thrombus — *see* Thrombosis

Thrush — *see also* Candidiasis
- newborn P37.5
- oral B37.0
- vaginal (acute) B37.31
  - chronic (recurrent) B37.32

Thumb — *see also* condition
- sucking (child problem) F98.8

Thymitis E32.8

Thymoma — *see also* Neoplasm, thymus, by type
- malignant C37
- metaplastic C37
- microscopic D15.0
- sclerosing C37
- type A C37
- type AB C37
- type B1 C37
- type B2 C37
- type B3 C37

Thymus, thymic (gland) — *see* condition

Thyrocele — *see* Goiter

Thyroglossal — *see also* condition
- cyst Q89.2
- duct, persistent Q89.2

Thyroid (gland) (body) — *see also* condition
- hormone resistance E07.89
- lingual Q89.2
- nodule (cystic) (nontoxic) (single) E04.1

Thyroiditis E06.9
- acute (nonsuppurative) (pyogenic) (suppurative) E06.0
- autoimmune E06.3
- chronic (nonspecific) (sclerosing) E06.5
  - with thyrotoxicosis, transient E06.2
  - fibrous E06.5
  - lymphadenoid E06.3
  - lymphocytic E06.3
  - lymphoid E06.3
- de Quervain's E06.1
- drug-induced E06.4
- fibrous (chronic) E06.5
- giant-cell (follicular) E06.1
- granulomatous (de Quervain) (subacute) E06.1
- Hashimoto's (struma lymphomatosa) E06.3
- iatrogenic E06.4
- ligneous E06.5
- lymphocytic (chronic) E06.3
- lymphoid E06.3
- lymphomatous E06.3
- nonsuppurative E06.1
- postpartum, puerperal O90.5
- pseudotuberculous E06.1
- pyogenic E06.0
- radiation E06.4
- Riedel's E06.5
- subacute (granulomatous) E06.1
- suppurative E06.0
- tuberculous A18.81
- viral E06.1
- woody E06.5

Thyrolingual duct, persistent Q89.2

Thyromegaly E01.0

Thyrotoxic
- crisis — *see* Thyrotoxicosis
- heart disease or failure — *see also* Thyrotoxicosis E05.90 *[I43]*
  - with thyroid storm E05.91 *[I43]*
- storm — *see* Thyrotoxicosis

Thyrotoxicosis (recurrent) E05.90
- with
  - goiter (diffuse) E05.00
    - with thyroid storm E05.01
    - adenomatous uninodular E05.10
      - with thyroid storm E05.11
    - multinodular E05.20
      - with thyroid storm E05.21
    - nodular E05.20
      - with thyroid storm E05.21
    - uninodular E05.10
      - with thyroid storm E05.11
  - infiltrative
    - dermopathy E05.00
      - with thyroid storm E05.01
    - ophthalmopathy E05.00
      - with thyroid storm E05.01

Thyrotoxicosis — *continued*
- with — *continued*
  - single thyroid nodule E05.10
    - with thyroid storm E05.11
  - thyroid storm E05.91
- due to
  - ectopic thyroid nodule or tissue E05.30
    - with thyroid storm E05.31
  - ingestion of (excessive) thyroid material E05.40
    - with thyroid storm E05.41
  - overproduction of thyroid-stimulating hormone E05.80
    - with thyroid storm E05.81
  - specified cause NEC E05.80
    - with thyroid storm E05.81
- factitia E05.40
  - with thyroid storm E05.41
- heart — *see also* Failure, heart, high-output E05.90 *[I43]*
  - with thyroid storm — *see also* Failure, heart, high-output E05.91 *[I43]*
  - failure — *see also* Failure, heart, high-output E05.90 *[I43]*
- neonatal (transient) P72.1
- transient with chronic thyroiditis E06.2

Tibia vara M92.51- ☑

Tic (disorder) F95.9
- breathing F95.8
- child problem F95.0
- compulsive F95.1
- de la Tourette F95.2
- degenerative (generalized) (localized) G25.69
  - facial G25.69
- disorder
  - chronic
    - motor F95.1
    - vocal F95.1
  - combined vocal and multiple motor F95.2
  - transient F95.0
- douloureux G50.0
  - atypical G50.1
  - postherpetic, postzoster B02.22
- drug-induced G25.61
- eyelid F95.8
- habit F95.9
  - chronic F95.1
  - transient of childhood F95.0
- lid, transient of childhood F95.0
- motor-verbal F95.2
- occupational F48.8
- orbicularis F95.8
  - transient of childhood F95.0
- organic origin G25.69
- postchoreic G25.69
- provisional F95.0
- psychogenic, compulsive F95.1
- salaam R25.8
- spasm (motor or vocal) F95.9
  - chronic F95.1
  - transient of childhood F95.0
- specified NEC F95.8

Tick-borne — *see* condition

Tietze's disease or syndrome M94.0

Tight, tightness
- anus K62.89
- chest R07.89
- fascia (lata) M62.89
- foreskin (congenital) N47.1
- hymen, hymenal ring N89.6
- introitus (acquired) (congenital) N89.6
- rectal sphincter K62.89
- tendon — *see* Short, tendon
- urethral sphincter N35.919

Tilting vertebra — *see* Dorsopathy, deforming, specified NEC

Timidity, child F93.8

Tinea (intersecta) (tarsi) B35.9
- amiantacea L44.8
- asbestina B35.0
- barbae B35.0
- beard B35.0
- black dot B35.0
- blanca B36.2
- capitis B35.0
- corporis B35.4
- cruris B35.6
- flava B36.0
- foot B35.3
- furfuracea B36.0

Tracheobronchomegaly — *continued*
- with bronchiectasis — *continued*
  - with
    - exacerbation (acute) J47.1
    - lower respiratory infection J47.Ø
- acquired J98.Ø9
  - with bronchiectasis J47.9
    - with
      - exacerbation (acute) J47.1
      - lower respiratory infection J47.Ø

Tracheobronchopneumonitis — *see* Pneumonia, broncho-

Tracheocele (external) (internal) J39.8
- congenital Q32.1

Tracheomalacia J39.8
- congenital Q32.Ø

Tracheopharyngitis (acute) JØ6.9
- chronic J42
- due to external agent — *see* Inflammation, respiratory, upper, due to

Tracheostenosis J39.8

Tracheostomy
- complication — *see* Complication, tracheostomy
- status Z93.Ø
  - attention to Z43.Ø
  - malfunctioning J95.Ø3

Trachoma, trachomatous A71.9
- active (stage) A71.1
- contraction of conjunctiva A71.1
- dubium A71.Ø
- healed or sequelae B94.Ø
- initial (stage) A71.Ø
- pannus A71.1
- Türck's J37.Ø

Traction, vitreomacular H43.82- ☑

Train sickness T75.3 ☑

Trait(s)
- Hb-S D57.3
- hemoglobin
  - abnormal NEC D58.2
    - with thalassemia D56.3
  - C — *see* Disease, hemoglobin C
  - S (Hb-S) D57.3
- Lepore D56.3
- personality, accentuated Z73.1
- sickle-cell D57.3
  - with elliptocytosis or spherocytosis D57.3
- type A personality Z73.1

Tramp Z59.ØØ

Trance R41.89
- hysterical F44.89

Transaminasemia R74.Ø1

Transection
- abdomen (partial) S38.3 ☑
- aorta (incomplete) — *see also* Injury, aorta
  - complete — *see* Injury, aorta, laceration, major
- carotid artery (incomplete) — *see also* Injury, blood vessel, carotid, laceration
  - complete — *see* Injury, blood vessel, carotid, laceration, major
- celiac artery (incomplete) S35.211 ☑
  - branch (incomplete) S35.291 ☑
    - complete S35.292 ☑
  - complete S35.212 ☑
- innominate
  - artery (incomplete) — *see also* Injury, blood vessel, thoracic, innominate, artery, laceration
    - complete — *see* Injury, blood vessel, thoracic, innominate, artery, laceration, major
  - vein (incomplete) — *see also* Injury, blood vessel, thoracic, innominate, vein, laceration
    - complete — *see* Injury, blood vessel, thoracic, innominate, vein, laceration, major
- jugular vein (external) (incomplete) — *see also* Injury, blood vessel, jugular vein, laceration
  - complete — *see* Injury, blood vessel, jugular vein, laceration, major
  - internal (incomplete) — *see also* Injury, blood vessel, jugular vein, internal, laceration
    - complete — *see* Injury, blood vessel, jugular vein, internal, laceration, major
- mesenteric artery (incomplete) — *see also* Injury, mesenteric, artery, laceration
  - complete — *see* Injury, mesenteric artery, laceration, major
- pulmonary vessel (incomplete) — *see also* Injury, blood vessel, thoracic, pulmonary, laceration

Transection — *continued*
- pulmonary vessel — *see also* Injury, blood vessel, thoracic, pulmonary, laceration — *continued*
  - complete — *see* Injury, blood vessel, thoracic, pulmonary, laceration, major
- subclavian — *see* Transection, innominate
- vena cava (incomplete) — *see also* Injury, vena cava
  - complete — *see* Injury, vena cava, laceration, major
- vertebral artery (incomplete) — *see also* Injury, blood vessel, vertebral, laceration
  - complete — *see* Injury, blood vessel, vertebral, laceration, major

Transfusion
- associated (red blood cell) hemochromatosis E83.111
- blood
  - ABO incompatible — *see* Complication(s), transfusion, incompatibility reaction, ABO
  - minor blood group (Duffy) (E) (K) (Kell) (Kidd) (Lewis) (M) (N) (P) (S) T8Ø.89 ☑
  - reaction or complication — *see* Complications, transfusion
- fetomaternal (mother) — *see* Pregnancy, complicated by, placenta, transfusion syndrome
- maternofetal (mother) — *see* Pregnancy, complicated by, placenta, transfusion syndrome
- placental (syndrome) (mother) — *see* Pregnancy, complicated by, placenta, transfusion syndrome
- reaction (adverse) — *see* Complications, transfusion
- related acute lung injury (TRALI) J95.84
- twin-to-twin — *see* Pregnancy, complicated by, placenta, transfusion syndrome, fetus to fetus

Transgender F64.Ø

Transient (meaning homeless) — *see also* condition Z59.ØØ

Translocation
- balanced autosomal Q95.9
  - in normal individual Q95.Ø
- chromosomes NEC Q99.8
  - balanced and insertion in normal individual Q95.Ø
- Down syndrome Q9Ø.2
- trisomy
  - 13 Q91.6
  - 18 Q91.2
  - 21 Q9Ø.2

Translucency, iris — *see* Degeneration, iris

Transmission of chemical substances through the placenta — *see* Absorption, chemical, through placenta

Transparency, lung, unilateral J43.Ø

Transplant (ed) (status) Z94.9
- awaiting organ Z76.82
- bone Z94.6
  - marrow Z94.81
- candidate Z76.82
- complication — *see* Complication, transplant
- cornea Z94.7
- heart Z94.1
  - and lung(s) Z94.3
  - valve Z95.2
    - prosthetic Z95.2
    - specified NEC Z95.4
    - xenogenic Z95.3
- intestine Z94.82
- kidney Z94.Ø
- liver Z94.4
- lung(s) Z94.2
  - and heart Z94.3
- organ (failure) (infection) (rejection) Z94.9
  - removal status Z98.85
- pancreas Z94.83
- skin Z94.5
- social Z6Ø.3
- specified organ or tissue NEC Z94.89
- stem cells Z94.84
- tissue Z94.9

Transplants, ovarian, endometrial N8Ø.1Ø- ☑

Transposed — *see* Transposition

Transposition (congenital) — *see also* Malposition, congenital
- abdominal viscera Q89.3
- aorta (dextra) Q2Ø.3
- appendix Q43.8
- colon Q43.8
- corrected Q2Ø.5
- great vessels (complete) (partial) Q2Ø.3
- heart Q24.Ø
  - with complete transposition of viscera Q89.3
- intestine (large) (small) Q43.8

Transposition — *continued*
- reversed jejunal (for bypass) (status) Z98.Ø
- scrotum Q55.23
- stomach Q4Ø.2
  - with general transposition of viscera Q89.3
- tooth, teeth, fully erupted M26.3Ø
- vessels, great (complete) (partial) Q2Ø.3
- viscera (abdominal) (thoracic) Q89.3

Transsexualism F64.Ø

Transverse — *see also* condition
- arrest (deep), in labor O64.Ø ☑
- lie (mother) O32.2 ☑
  - causing obstructed labor O64.8 ☑

Transvestism, transvestitism (dual-role) F64.1
- fetishistic F65.1

Trapped placenta (with hemorrhage) O72.Ø
- without hemorrhage O73.Ø

TRAPS (tumor necrosis factor receptor associated periodic syndrome) MØ4.1

Trauma, traumatism — *see also* Injury
- acoustic — *see* subcategory H83.3 ☑
- birth — *see* Birth, injury
- complicating ectopic or molar pregnancy OØ8.6
- during delivery O71.9
- following ectopic or molar pregnancy OØ8.6
- non-accidental — *see* Abuse, physical
- obstetric O71.9
  - specified NEC O71.89
- occusal
  - primary KØ8.81
  - secondary KØ8.82

Traumatic — *see also* condition
- brain injury SØ6.9 ☑

Treacher Collins syndrome Q75.4

Treitz's hernia — *see* Hernia, abdomen, specified site NEC

Trematode infestation — *see* Infestation, fluke

Trematodiasis — *see* Infestation, fluke

Trembling paralysis — *see* Parkinsonism

Tremor(s) R25.1
- drug induced G25.1
- essential (benign) G25.Ø
- familial G25.Ø
- hereditary G25.Ø
- hysterical F44.4
- intention G25.2
- medication induced postural G25.1
- mercurial — *see* subcategory T56.1 ☑
- Parkinson's — *see* Parkinsonism
- psychogenic (conversion reaction) F44.4
- senilis R54
- specified type NEC G25.2

Trench
- fever A79.Ø
- foot — *see* Immersion, foot
- mouth A69.1

Treponema pallidum infection — *see* Syphilis

Treponematosis
- due to
  - T. pallidum — *see* Syphilis
  - T. pertenue — *see* Yaws

Triad
- Hutchinson's (congenital syphilis) A5Ø.53
- Kartagener's Q89.3
- Saint's — *see* Hernia, diaphragm

Trichiasis (eyelid) HØ2.Ø59
- with entropion — *see* Entropion
- left HØ2.Ø56
  - lower HØ2.Ø55
  - upper HØ2.Ø54
- right HØ2.Ø53
  - lower HØ2.Ø52
  - upper HØ2.Ø51

Trichinella spiralis (infection) (infestation) B75

Trichinellosis, trichiniasis, trichinelliasis, trichinosis B75
- with muscle disorder B75 *[M63.8Ø]*
  - ankle B75 *[M63.87-]* ☑
  - foot B75 *[M63.87-]* ☑
  - forearm B75 *[M63.83-]* ☑
  - hand B75 *[M63.84-]* ☑
  - lower leg B75 *[M63.86-]* ☑
  - multiple sites B75 *[M63.89]*
  - pelvic region B75 *[M63.85-]* ☑
  - shoulder region B75 *[M63.81-]* ☑
  - specified site NEC B75 *[M63.88]*
  - thigh B75 *[M63.85-]* ☑

- **Trichinellosis, trichiniasis, trichinelliasis, trichinosis** — *continued*
  - with muscle disorder — *continued*
    - upper arm B75 *[M63.82-]* ☑
- **Trichobezoar** T18.9 ☑
  - intestine T18.3 ☑
  - stomach T18.2 ☑
- **Trichocephaliasis, trichocephalosis** B79
- **Trichocephalus infestation** B79
- **Trichoclasis** L67.8
- **Trichoepithelioma** — *see also* Neoplasm, skin, benign
  - malignant — *see* Neoplasm, skin, malignant
- **Trichofolliculoma** — *see* Neoplasm, skin, benign
- **Tricholemmoma** — *see* Neoplasm, skin, benign
- **Trichomoniasis** A59.9
  - bladder A59.Ø3
  - cervix A59.Ø9
  - intestinal AØ7.8
  - prostate A59.Ø2
  - seminal vesicles A59.Ø9
  - specified site NEC A59.8
  - urethra A59.Ø3
  - urogenitalis A59.ØØ
  - vagina A59.Ø1
  - vulva A59.Ø1
- **Trichomycosis**
  - axillaris A48.8
  - nodosa, nodularis B36.8
- **Trichonodosis** L67.8
- **Trichophytid, trichophyton infection** — *see* Dermatophytosis
- **Trichophytobezoar** T18.9 ☑
  - intestine T18.3 ☑
  - stomach T18.2 ☑
- **Trichophytosis** — *see* Dermatophytosis
- **Trichoptilosis** L67.8
- **Trichorrhexis** (nodosa) (invaginata) L67.Ø
- **Trichosis axillaris** A48.8
- **Trichosporosis nodosa** B36.2
- **Trichostasis spinulosa** (congenital) Q84.1
- **Trichostrongyliasis, trichostrongylosis** (small intestine) B81.2
- **Trichostrongylus infection** B81.2
- **Trichotillomania** F63.3
- **Trichromat, trichromatopsia, anomalous** (congenital) H53.55
- **Trichuriasis** B79
- **Trichuris trichiura** (infection) (infestation) (any site) B79
- **Tricuspid** (valve) — *see* condition
- **Trifid** — *see also* Accessory
  - kidney (pelvis) Q63.8
  - tongue Q38.3
- **Trigeminal neuralgia** — *see* Neuralgia, trigeminal
- **Trigeminy** RØØ.8
- **Trigger finger** (acquired) M65.3Ø
  - congenital Q74.Ø
  - index finger M65.32- ☑
  - little finger M65.35- ☑
  - middle finger M65.33- ☑
  - ring finger M65.34- ☑
  - thumb M65.31- ☑
- **Trigonitis** (bladder) (chronic) (pseudomembranous) N3Ø.3Ø
  - with hematuria N3Ø.31
- **Trigonocephaly** Q75.Ø3
- **Trilocular heart** — *see* Cor triloculare
- **Trimethylaminuria** E72.52
- **Tripartite placenta** O43.19- ☑
- **Triphalangeal thumb** Q74.Ø
- **Triple** — *see also* Accessory
  - kidneys Q63.Ø
  - uteri Q51.818
  - X, female Q97.Ø
- **Triple I** O41.12- ☑
- **Triplegia** G83.89
  - congenital G8Ø.8
- **Triplet** (newborn) — *see also* Newborn, triplet
  - complicating pregnancy — *see* Pregnancy, triplet
- **Triplication** — *see* Accessory
- **Triploidy** Q92.7
- **Trismus** R25.2
  - neonatorum A33
  - newborn A33
- **Trisomy** (syndrome) Q92.9
  - 13 (partial) Q91.7
    - meiotic nondisjunction Q91.4
    - mitotic nondisjunction Q91.5
- **Trisomy** — *continued*
  - 13 — *continued*
    - mosaicism Q91.5
    - translocation Q91.6
  - 18 (partial) Q91.3
    - meiotic nondisjunction Q91.Ø
    - mitotic nondisjunction Q91.1
    - mosaicism Q91.1
    - translocation Q91.2
  - 2Ø Q92.8
  - 21 (partial) Q9Ø.9
    - meiotic nondisjunction Q9Ø.Ø
    - mitotic nondisjunction Q9Ø.1
    - mosaicism Q9Ø.1
    - translocation Q9Ø.2
  - 22 Q92.8
  - autosomes Q92.9
  - chromosome specified NEC Q92.8
    - partial Q92.2
      - due to unbalanced translocation Q92.5
    - specified NEC Q92.8
    - whole (nonsex chromosome)
      - meiotic nondisjunction Q92.Ø
      - mitotic nondisjunction Q92.1
      - mosaicism Q92.1
  - due to
    - dicentrics — *see* Extra, marker chromosomes
    - extra rings — *see* Extra, marker chromosomes
    - isochromosomes — *see* Extra, marker chromosomes
  - specified NEC Q92.8
  - whole chromosome Q92.9
    - meiotic nondisjunction Q92.Ø
    - mitotic nondisjunction Q92.1
    - mosaicism Q92.1
    - partial Q92.9
    - specified NEC Q92.8
- **Tritanomaly, tritanopia** H53.55
- **Trombiculosis, trombiculiasis, trombidiosis** B88.Ø
- **Trophedema** (congenital) (hereditary) Q82.Ø
- **Trophoblastic disease** — *see also* Mole, hydatidiform OØ1.9
- **Tropholymphedema** Q82.Ø
- **Trophoneurosis NEC** G96.89
  - disseminated M34.9
- **Tropical** — *see* condition
- **Trouble** — *see also* Disease
  - heart — *see* Disease, heart
  - kidney — *see* Disease, renal
  - nervous R45.Ø
  - sinus — *see* Sinusitis
- **Trousseau's syndrome** (thrombophlebitis migrans) I82.1
- **Truancy, childhood**
  - from school Z72.81Ø
- **Truncus**
  - arteriosus (persistent) Q2Ø.Ø
  - communis Q2Ø.Ø
- **Trunk** — *see* condition
- **Trypanosomiasis**
  - African B56.9
    - by Trypanosoma brucei
      - gambiense B56.Ø
      - rhodesiense B56.1
  - American — *see* Chagas' disease
  - Brazilian — *see* Chagas' disease
  - by Trypanosoma
    - brucei gambiense B56.Ø
    - brucei rhodesiense B56.1
    - cruzi — *see* Chagas' disease
  - gambiensis, Gambian B56.Ø
  - rhodesiensis, Rhodesian B56.1
  - South American — *see* Chagas' disease
  - where
    - African trypanosomiasis is prevalent B56.9
    - Chagas' disease is prevalent B57.2
- **Tryptasemia, hereditary alpha** D89.44
- **T-shaped incisors** KØØ.2
- **Tsutsugamushi** (disease) (fever) A75.3
- **Tube, tubal, tubular** — *see* condition
- **Tubercle** — *see also* Tuberculosis
  - brain, solitary A17.81
  - Darwin's Q17.8
  - Ghon, primary infection A15.7
- **Tuberculid, tuberculide** (indurating, subcutaneous) (lichenoid) (miliary) (papulonecrotic) (primary) (skin) A18.4
- **Tuberculoma** — *see also* Tuberculosis
  - brain A17.81
  - meninges (cerebral) (spinal) A17.1
- **Tuberculoma** — *continued*
  - spinal cord A17.81
- **Tuberculosis, tubercular, tuberculous** (calcification) (calcified) (caseous) (chromogenic acid-fast bacilli) (degeneration) (fibrocaseous) (fistula) (interstitial) (isolated circumscribed lesions) (necrosis) (parenchymatous) (ulcerative) A15.9
  - with pneumoconiosis (any condition in J6Ø-J64) J65
  - abdomen (lymph gland) A18.39
  - abscess (respiratory) A15.9
    - bone A18.Ø3
      - hip A18.Ø2
      - knee A18.Ø2
      - sacrum A18.Ø1
      - specified site NEC A18.Ø3
      - spinal A18.Ø1
      - vertebra A18.Ø1
    - brain A17.81
    - breast A18.89
    - Cowper's gland A18.15
    - dura (mater) (cerebral) (spinal) A17.81
    - epidural (cerebral) (spinal) A17.81
    - female pelvis A18.17
    - frontal sinus A15.8
    - genital organs NEC A18.1Ø
    - genitourinary A18.1Ø
    - gland (lymphatic) — *see* Tuberculosis, lymph gland
    - hip A18.Ø2
    - intestine A18.32
    - ischiorectal A18.32
    - joint NEC A18.Ø2
      - hip A18.Ø2
      - knee A18.Ø2
      - specified NEC A18.Ø2
      - vertebral A18.Ø1
    - kidney A18.11
    - knee A18.Ø2
    - latent Z22.7
    - lumbar (spine) A18.Ø1
    - lung — *see* Tuberculosis, pulmonary
    - meninges (cerebral) (spinal) A17.Ø
    - muscle A18.Ø9
    - perianal (fistula) A18.32
    - perinephritic A18.11
    - perirectal A18.32
    - rectum A18.32
    - retropharyngeal A15.8
    - sacrum A18.Ø1
    - scrofulous A18.2
    - scrotum A18.15
    - skin (primary) A18.4
    - spinal cord A17.81
    - spine or vertebra (column) A18.Ø1
    - subdiaphragmatic A18.31
    - testis A18.15
    - urinary A18.13
    - uterus A18.17
  - accessory sinus — *see* Tuberculosis, sinus
  - Addison's disease A18.7
  - adenitis — *see* Tuberculosis, lymph gland
  - adenoids A15.8
  - adenopathy — *see* Tuberculosis, lymph gland
  - adherent pericardium A18.84
  - adnexa (uteri) A18.17
  - adrenal (capsule) (gland) A18.7
  - alimentary canal A18.32
  - anemia A18.89
  - ankle (joint) (bone) A18.Ø2
  - anus A18.32
  - apex, apical — *see* Tuberculosis, pulmonary
  - appendicitis, appendix A18.32
  - arachnoid A17.Ø
  - artery, arteritis A18.89
    - cerebral A18.89
  - arthritis (chronic) (synovial) A18.Ø2
    - spine or vertebra (column) A18.Ø1
  - articular — *see* Tuberculosis, joint
  - ascites A18.31
  - asthma — *see* Tuberculosis, pulmonary
  - axilla, axillary (gland) A18.2
  - bladder A18.12
  - bone A18.Ø3
    - hip A18.Ø2
    - knee A18.Ø2
    - limb NEC A18.Ø3
    - sacrum A18.Ø1
    - spine or vertebral column A18.Ø1
  - bowel (miliary) A18.32

Tumor — *continued*
- cells — *see also* Neoplasm, unspecified behavior, by site
  - benign — *see* Neoplasm, benign, by site
  - malignant — *see* Neoplasm, malignant, by site
  - uncertain whether benign or malignant — *see* Neoplasm, uncertain behavior, by site
- cervix, in pregnancy or childbirth — *see* Pregnancy, complicated by, tumor, cervix
- chondromatous giant cell — *see* Neoplasm, bone, benign
- chromaffin — *see also* Neoplasm, benign, by site
  - malignant — *see* Neoplasm, malignant, by site
- Cock's peculiar L72.3
- Codman's — *see* Neoplasm, bone, benign
- dentigerous, mixed — *see* Cyst, calcifying odontogenic
- dermoid — *see* Neoplasm, benign, by site
  - with malignant transformation C56- ☑
- desmoid (extra-abdominal) — *see also* Neoplasm, connective tissue, uncertain behavior
  - abdominal — *see* Neoplasm, connective tissue, uncertain behavior
- embolus — *see* Neoplasm, secondary, by site
- embryonal (mixed) — *see also* Neoplasm, uncertain behavior, by site
  - liver C22.7
- endodermal sinus
  - specified site — *see* Neoplasm, malignant, by site
  - unspecified site
    - female C56.- ☑
    - male C62.90
- epithelial
  - benign — *see* Neoplasm, benign, by site
  - malignant — *see* Neoplasm, malignant, by site
- Ewing's — *see* Neoplasm, bone, malignant, by site
- fatty — *see* Lipoma
- fibroid — *see* Leiomyoma
- G cell
  - malignant
    - pancreas C25.4
    - specified site NEC — *see* Neoplasm, malignant, by site
    - unspecified site C25.4
  - specified site — *see* Neoplasm, uncertain behavior, by site
  - unspecified site D37.8
- germ cell — *see also* Neoplasm, malignant, by site
  - mixed — *see* Neoplasm, malignant, by site
- ghost cell, odontogenic — *see* Cyst, calcifying odontogenic
- giant cell — *see also* Neoplasm, uncertain behavior, by site
  - bone D48.0
    - malignant — *see* Neoplasm, bone, malignant
  - chondromatous — *see* Neoplasm, bone, benign
  - malignant — *see* Neoplasm, malignant, by site
  - soft parts — *see* Neoplasm, connective tissue, uncertain behavior
    - malignant — *see* Neoplasm, connective tissue, malignant
- glomus D18.00
  - intra-abdominal D18.03
  - intracranial D18.02
  - jugulare D44.7
    - malignant C75.5
  - skin D18.01
  - specified site NEC D18.09
- gonadal stromal — *see* Neoplasm, uncertain behavior, by site
- granular cell — *see also* Neoplasm, connective tissue, benign
  - malignant — *see* Neoplasm, connective tissue, malignant
- granulosa cell D39.1- ☑
  - juvenile D39.1- ☑
  - malignant C56- ☑
- granulosa cell-theca cell D39.1- ☑
  - malignant C56- ☑
- Grawitz's C64- ☑
- hemorrhoidal — *see* Hemorrhoids
- hilar cell D27- ☑
- hilus cell D27- ☑
- Hurthle cell (benign) D34
  - malignant C73
- hydatid — *see* Echinococcus
- hypernephroid — *see also* Neoplasm, uncertain behavior, by site
- interstitial cell — *see also* Neoplasm, uncertain behavior, by site
  - benign — *see* Neoplasm, benign, by site
  - malignant — *see* Neoplasm, malignant, by site
- intravascular bronchial alveolar D38.1
- islet cell — *see* Neoplasm, benign, by site
  - malignant — *see* Neoplasm, malignant, by site
    - pancreas C25.4
    - specified site NEC — *see* Neoplasm, malignant, by site
    - unspecified site C25.4
  - pancreas D13.7
  - specified site NEC — *see* Neoplasm, benign, by site
  - unspecified site D13.7
- juxtaglomerular D41.0- ☑
- Klatskin's C22.1
- Krukenberg's C79.6- ☑
- Leydig cell — *see* Neoplasm, uncertain behavior, by site
  - benign — *see* Neoplasm, benign, by site
    - specified site — *see* Neoplasm, benign, by site
    - unspecified site
      - female D27.9
      - male D29.20
  - malignant — *see* Neoplasm, malignant, by site
    - specified site — *see* Neoplasm, malignant, by site
    - unspecified site
      - female C56.9
      - male C62.90
  - specified site — *see* Neoplasm, uncertain behavior, by site
  - unspecified site
    - female D39.10
    - male D40.10
- lipid cell, ovary D27- ☑
- lipoid cell, ovary D27- ☑
- malignant — *see also* Neoplasm, malignant, by site C80.1
  - fusiform cell (type) C80.1
  - giant cell (type) C80.1
  - localized, plasma cell — *see* Plasmacytoma, solitary
  - mixed NEC C80.1
  - small cell (type) C80.1
  - spindle cell (type) C80.1
  - unclassified C80.1
- mast cell D47.09
- melanotic, neuroectodermal — *see* Neoplasm, benign, by site
- Merkel cell — *see* Carcinoma, Merkel cell
- mesenchymal
  - malignant — *see* Neoplasm, connective tissue, malignant
  - mixed — *see* Neoplasm, connective tissue, uncertain behavior
- mesodermal, mixed — *see also* Neoplasm, malignant, by site
  - liver C22.4
- mesonephric — *see also* Neoplasm, uncertain behavior, by site
  - malignant — *see* Neoplasm, malignant, by site
- metastatic
  - from specified site — *see* Neoplasm, malignant, by site
  - of specified site — *see* Neoplasm, malignant, by site
  - to specified site — *see* Neoplasm, secondary, by site
- mixed NEC — *see also* Neoplasm, benign, by site
  - malignant — *see* Neoplasm, malignant, by site
- mucinous of low malignant potential
  - specified site — *see* Neoplasm, malignant, by site
  - unspecified site C56.9
- mucocarcinoid
  - specified site — *see* Neoplasm, malignant, by site
  - unspecified site C18.1
- mucoepidermoid — *see* Neoplasm, uncertain behavior, by site
- Mullerian, mixed
  - specified site — *see* Neoplasm, malignant, by site
  - unspecified site C54.9
- myoepithelial — *see* Neoplasm, benign, by site
- neuroectodermal (peripheral) — *see* Neoplasm, malignant, by site
  - primitive
    - specified site — *see* Neoplasm, malignant, by site
    - unspecified site C71.9
- neuroendocrine D3A.8 (*following* D36)
  - malignant poorly differentiated C7A.1 (*following* C75)
  - secondary NEC C7B.8 (*following* C75)
  - specified NEC C7A.8 (*following* C75)
- neurogenic olfactory C30.0
- nonencapsulated sclerosing C73
- odontogenic (adenomatoid) (benign) (calcifying epithelial) (keratocystic) (squamous) — *see* Cyst, calcifying odontogenic
  - malignant C41.1
    - upper jaw (bone) C41.0
- ovarian stromal D39.1- ☑
- ovary, in pregnancy — *see* Pregnancy, complicated by
- pacinian — *see* Neoplasm, skin, benign
- Pancoast's — *see* Pancoast's syndrome
- papillary — *see also* Papilloma
  - cystic D37.9
  - mucinous of low malignant potential C56- ☑
    - specified site — *see* Neoplasm, malignant, by site
    - unspecified site C56.9
  - serous of low malignant potential
    - specified site — *see* Neoplasm, malignant, by site
    - unspecified site C56.9
- pelvic, in pregnancy or childbirth — *see* Pregnancy, complicated by
- phantom F45.8
- phyllodes D48.6- ☑
  - benign D24- ☑
  - malignant — *see* Neoplasm, breast, malignant
- Pindborg — *see* Cyst, calcifying odontogenic
- placental site trophoblastic D39.2
- plasma cell (malignant) (localized) — *see* Plasmacytoma, solitary
- polyvesicular vitelline
  - specified site — *see* Neoplasm, malignant, by site
  - unspecified site
    - female C56.9
    - male C62.90
- Pott's puffy — *see* Osteomyelitis, specified NEC
- Rathke's pouch D44.3
- retinal anlage — *see* Neoplasm, benign, by site
- salivary gland type, mixed — *see* Neoplasm, salivary gland, benign
  - malignant — *see* Neoplasm, salivary gland, malignant
- Sampson's N80.10- ☑
- Schmincke's — *see* Neoplasm, nasopharynx, malignant
- sclerosing stromal D27- ☑
- sebaceous — *see* Cyst, sebaceous
- secondary — *see* Neoplasm, secondary, by site
  - carcinoid C7B.00 (*following* C75)
    - bone C7B.03 (*following* C75)
    - distant lymph nodes C7B.01 (*following* C75)
    - liver C7B.02 (*following* C75)
    - peritoneum C7B.04 (*following* C75)
    - specified NEC C7B.09 (*following* C75)
  - neuroendocrine NEC C7B.8 (*following* C75)
- serous of low malignant potential
  - specified site — *see* Neoplasm, malignant, by site
  - unspecified site C56.9
- Sertoli cell — *see* Neoplasm, benign, by site
  - with lipid storage
    - specified site — *see* Neoplasm, benign, by site
    - unspecified site
      - female D27.9
      - male D29.20
  - specified site — *see* Neoplasm, benign, by site
  - unspecified site
    - female D27.9
    - male D29.20
- Sertoli-Leydig cell — *see* Neoplasm, benign, by site
  - specified site — *see* Neoplasm, benign, by site
  - unspecified site
    - female D27.9
    - male D29.20
- sex cord (-stromal) — *see* Neoplasm, uncertain behavior, by site
  - with annular tubules D39.1- ☑
- skin appendage — *see* Neoplasm, skin, benign
- smooth muscle — *see* Neoplasm, connective tissue, uncertain behavior
- soft tissue
  - benign — *see* Neoplasm, connective tissue, benign

Tumor — *continued*
- soft tissue — *continued*
  - malignant — *see* Neoplasm, connective tissue, malignant
- sternomastoid (congenital) Q68.Ø
- stromal
  - endometrial D39.Ø
  - gastric D48.19
    - benign D21.4
    - malignant C16.9
    - uncertain behavior D48.19
  - gastrointestinal C49.A- ☑
    - benign D21.4
    - esophagus C49.A1
    - malignant C49.AØ
      - colon C49.A4
      - duodenum C49.A3
      - esophagus C49.A1
      - ileum C49.A3
      - jejunum C49.A3
      - large intestine C49.A4
      - Meckel diverticulum C49.A3
      - omentum C49.A9
      - peritoneum C49.A9
      - rectum C49.A5
      - small intestine C49.A3
      - specified site NEC C49.A9
      - stomach C49.A2
    - rectum C49.A5
    - small intestine C49.A3
    - specified site NEC C49.A9
    - stomach C49.A2
    - uncertain behavior D48.19
  - intestine
    - benign D21.4
    - malignant
      - large C49.A4
      - small C49.A3
    - uncertain behavior D48.19
  - ovarian D39.1- ☑
  - stomach C49.A2
    - benign D21.4
    - malignant C49.A2
    - uncertain behavior D48.19
- sweat gland — *see also* Neoplasm, skin, uncertain behavior
  - benign — *see* Neoplasm, skin, benign
  - malignant — *see* Neoplasm, skin, malignant
- syphilitic, brain A52.17
- testicular D4Ø.1Ø
- testicular stromal D4Ø.1- ☑
- theca cell D27.- ☑
- theca cell-granulosa cell D39.1- ☑
- Triton, malignant — *see* Neoplasm, nerve, malignant
- trophoblastic, placental site D39.2
- turban D23.4
- uterus (body), in pregnancy or childbirth — *see* Pregnancy, complicated by, tumor, uterus
- vagina, in pregnancy or childbirth — *see* Pregnancy, complicated by
- varicose — *see* Varix
- von Recklinghausen's — *see* Neurofibromatosis
- vulva or perineum, in pregnancy or childbirth — *see* Pregnancy, complicated by
  - causing obstructed labor O65.5
- Warthin's — *see* Neoplasm, salivary gland, benign
- Wilms' C64- ☑
- yolk sac — *see* Neoplasm, malignant, by site
  - specified site — *see* Neoplasm, malignant, by site
  - unspecified site
    - female C56.9
    - male C62.9Ø

Tumor lysis syndrome (following antineoplastic chemotherapy) (spontaneous) NEC E88.3

Tumorlet — *see* Neoplasm, uncertain behavior, by site

Tungiasis B88.1

Tunica vasculosa lentis Q12.2

Turban tumor D23.4

Türck's trachoma J37.Ø

Turner-Kieser syndrome Q87.2

Turner-like syndrome Q87.19

Turner's
- hypoplasia (tooth) KØØ.4
- syndrome Q96.9
  - specified NEC Q96.8
- tooth KØØ.4

Turner-Ullrich syndrome Q96.9

Tussis convulsiva — *see* Whooping cough

Twiddler's syndrome (due to)
- automatic implantable defibrillatorT82.198
- cardiac pacemaker T82.198 ☑

Twilight state
- epileptic FØ5
- psychogenic F44.89

Twin (newborn) — *see also* Newborn, twin
- conjoined Q89.4
- pregnancy — *see* Pregnancy, twin

Twinning, teeth KØØ.2

Twist, twisted
- bowel, colon or intestine K56.2
- hair (congenital) Q84.1
- mesentery K56.2
- omentum K56.2
- organ or site, congenital NEC — *see* Anomaly, by site
- ovarian pedicle — *see* Torsion, ovary

Twitching R25.3

Tylosis (acquired) L84
- buccalis K13.29
- linguae K13.29
- palmaris et plantaris (congenital) (inherited) Q82.8
  - acquired L85.1

Tympanism R14.Ø

Tympanites (abdominal) (intestinal) R14.Ø

Tympanitis — *see* Myringitis

Tympanosclerosis H74.Ø ☑

Tympanum — *see* condition

Tympany
- abdomen R14.Ø
- chest RØ9.89

Type A behavior pattern Z73.1

Typhlitis — *see* Cecitis

Typhoenteritis — *see* Typhoid

Typhoid (abortive) (ambulant) (any site) (clinical) (fever) (hemorrhagic) (infection) (intermittent) (malignant) (rheumatic) (Widal negative) AØ1.ØØ
- with pneumonia AØ1.Ø3
- abdominal AØ1.Ø9
- arthritis AØ1.Ø4
- carrier (suspected) of Z22.Ø
- cholecystitis (current) AØ1.Ø9
- endocarditis AØ1.Ø2
- heart involvement AØ1.Ø2
- inoculation reaction — *see* Complications, vaccination
- meningitis AØ1.Ø1
- mesenteric lymph nodes AØ1.Ø9
- myocarditis AØ1.Ø2
- osteomyelitis AØ1.Ø5
- perichondritis, larynx AØ1.Ø9
- pneumonia AØ1.Ø3
- specified NEC AØ1.Ø9
- spine AØ1.Ø5
- ulcer (perforating) AØ1.Ø9

Typhomalaria (fever) — *see* Malaria

Typhomania AØ1.ØØ

Typhoperitonitis AØ1.Ø9

Typhus (fever) A75.9
- abdominal, abdominalis — *see* Typhoid
- African tick A77.1
- amarillic A95.9
- brain A75.9 *[G94]*
- cerebral A75.9 *[G94]*
- classical A75.Ø
- due to Rickettsia
  - prowazekii A75.Ø
    - recrudescent A75.1
  - tsutsugamushi A75.3
  - typhi A75.2
- endemic (flea-borne) A75.2
- epidemic (louse-borne) A75.Ø
- exanthematicus SAI A75.Ø
  - brillii SAI A75.1
  - mexicanus SAI A75.2
  - typhus murinus A75.2
- exanthematic NEC A75.Ø
- flea-borne A75.2
- India tick A77.1
- Kenya (tick) A77.1
- louse-borne A75.Ø
- Mexican A75.2
- mite-borne A75.3
- murine A75.2
- North Asian tick-borne A77.2
- Orientia Tsutsugamushi (scrub typhus) A75.3
- petechial A75.9
- Queensland tick A77.3
- rat A75.2

Typhus — *continued*
- recrudescent A75.1
- recurrens — *see* Fever, relapsing
- Sao Paulo A77.Ø
- scrub (China) (India) (Malaysia) (New Guinea) A75.3
- shop (of Malaysia) A75.2
- Siberian tick A77.2
- tick-borne A77.9
- tropical (mite-borne) A75.3

Tyrosinemia E7Ø.21
- newborn, transitory P74.5

Tyrosinosis E7Ø.21

Tyrosinuria E7Ø.29

U

Uhl's anomaly or disease Q24.8

Ulcer, ulcerated, ulcerating, ulceration, ulcerative
- alveolar process M27.3
- amebic (intestine) AØ6.1
  - skin AØ6.7
- anastomotic — *see* Ulcer, gastrojejunal
- anorectal K62.6
- antral — *see* Ulcer, stomach
- anus (sphincter) (solitary) K62.6
- aorta — *see* Aneurysm
- aphthous (oral) (recurrent) K12.Ø
  - genital organ(s)
    - female N76.6
    - male N5Ø.89
- artery I77.2
- atrophic — *see* Ulcer, skin
  - decubitus — *see* Ulcer, pressure, by site
- back L98.429
  - with
    - bone involvement without evidence of necrosis L98.426
    - bone necrosis L98.424
    - exposed fat layer L98.422
    - muscle involvement without evidence of necrosis L98.425
    - muscle necrosis L98.423
    - skin breakdown only L98.421
    - specified severity NEC L98.428
- Barrett's (esophagus) K22.1Ø
  - with bleeding K22.11
- bile duct (common) (hepatic) K83.8
- bladder (solitary) (sphincter) NEC N32.89
  - bilharzial B65.9 *[N33]*
  - in schistosomiasis (bilharzial) B65.9 *[N33]*
  - submucosal — *see* Cystitis, interstitial
  - tuberculous A18.12
- bleeding K27.4
- bone — *see* Osteomyelitis, specified type NEC
- bowel — *see* Ulcer, intestine
- breast N61.1
- bronchus J98.Ø9
- buccal (cavity) (traumatic) K12.1
- Buruli A31.1
- buttock L98.419
  - with
    - bone involvement without evidence of necrosis L98.416
    - bone necrosis L98.414
    - exposed fat layer L98.412
    - muscle involvement without evidence of necrosis L98.415
    - muscle necrosis L98.413
    - skin breakdown only L98.411
    - specified severity NEC L98.418
- cameron *see* Ulcer, stomach
- cancerous — *see* Neoplasm, malignant, by site
- cardia K22.1Ø
  - with bleeding K22.11
- cardioesophageal (peptic) K22.1Ø
  - with bleeding K22.11
- cecum — *see* Ulcer, intestine
- cervix (uteri) (decubitus) (trophic) N86
  - with cervicitis N72
- chancroidal A57
- chiclero B55.1
- chronic (cause unknown) — *see* Ulcer, skin
- Cochin-China B55.1
- colon — *see* Ulcer, intestine
- conjunctiva H1Ø.89
- cornea H16.ØØ- ☑
  - with hypopyon H16.Ø3- ☑
  - central H16.Ø1- ☑

Ulcer, ulcerated, ulcerating, ulceration, ulcerative — *continued*
- lower limb — *continued*
  - heel — *continued*
    - left — *continued*
      - with — *continued*
        - bone necrosis L97.424
        - exposed fat layer L97.422
        - muscle involvement without evidence of necrosis L97.425
        - muscle necrosis L97.423
        - skin breakdown only L97.421
        - specified severity NEC L97.428
    - right L97.419
      - with
        - bone involvement without evidence of necrosis L97.416
        - bone necrosis L97.414
        - exposed fat layer L97.412
        - muscle involvement without evidence of necrosis L97.415
        - muscle necrosis L97.413
        - skin breakdown only L97.411
        - specified severity NEC L97.418
  - left L97.929
    - with
      - bone involvement without evidence of necrosis L97.926
      - bone necrosis L97.924
      - exposed fat layer L97.922
      - muscle involvement without evidence of necrosis L97.925
      - muscle necrosis L97.923
      - skin breakdown only L97.921
      - specified severity NEC L97.928
  - leprous A3Ø.1
  - lower leg NOS L97.9Ø9
    - with
      - bone involvement without evidence of necrosis L97.9Ø6
      - bone necrosis L97.9Ø4
      - exposed fat layer L97.9Ø2
      - muscle involvement without evidence of necrosis L97.9Ø5
      - muscle necrosis L97.9Ø3
      - skin breakdown only L97.9Ø1
      - specified severity NEC L97.9Ø8
    - left L97.929
      - with
        - bone involvement without evidence of necrosis L97.926
        - bone necrosis L97.924
        - exposed fat layer L97.922
        - muscle involvement without evidence of necrosis L97.925
        - muscle necrosis L97.923
        - skin breakdown only L97.921
        - specified severity NEC L97.928
    - right L97.919
      - with
        - bone involvement without evidence of necrosis L97.916
        - bone necrosis L97.914
        - exposed fat layer L97.912
        - muscle involvement without evidence of necrosis L97.915
        - muscle necrosis L97.913
        - skin breakdown only L97.911
        - specified severity NEC L97.918
    - specified site NEC L97.8Ø9
      - with
        - bone involvement without evidence of necrosis L97.8Ø6
        - bone necrosis L97.8Ø4
        - exposed fat layer L97.8Ø2
        - muscle involvement without evidence of necrosis L97.8Ø5
        - muscle necrosis L97.8Ø3
        - skin breakdown only L97.8Ø1
        - specified severity NEC L97.8Ø8
      - left L97.829
        - with
          - bone involvement without evidence of necrosis L97.826
          - bone necrosis L97.824
          - exposed fat layer L97.822
          - muscle involvement without evidence of necrosis L97.825
          - muscle necrosis L97.823

Ulcer, ulcerated, ulcerating, ulceration, ulcerative — *continued*
- lower limb — *continued*
  - lower leg — *continued*
    - specified site — *continued*
      - left — *continued*
        - with — *continued*
          - skin breakdown only L97.821
          - specified severity NEC L97.828
      - right L97.819
        - with
          - bone involvement without evidence of necrosis L97.816
          - bone necrosis L97.814
          - exposed fat layer L97.812
          - muscle involvement without evidence of necrosis L97.815
          - muscle necrosis L97.813
          - skin breakdown only L97.811
          - specified severity NEC L97.818
  - midfoot L97.4Ø9
    - with
      - bone involvement without evidence of necrosis L97.4Ø6
      - bone necrosis L97.4Ø4
      - exposed fat layer L97.4Ø2
      - muscle involvement without evidence of necrosis L97.4Ø5
      - muscle necrosis L97.4Ø3
      - skin breakdown only L97.4Ø1
      - specified severity NEC L97.4Ø8
    - left L97.429
      - with
        - bone involvement without evidence of necrosis L97.426
        - bone necrosis L97.424
        - exposed fat layer L97.422
        - muscle involvement without evidence of necrosis L97.425
        - muscle necrosis L97.423
        - skin breakdown only L97.421
        - specified severity NEC L97.428
    - right L97.419
      - with
        - bone involvement without evidence of necrosis L97.416
        - bone necrosis L97.414
        - exposed fat layer L97.412
        - muscle involvement without evidence of necrosis L97.415
        - muscle necrosis L97.413
        - skin breakdown only L97.411
        - specified severity NEC L97.418
  - right L97.919
    - with
      - bone involvement without evidence of necrosis L97.916
      - bone necrosis L97.914
      - exposed fat layer L97.912
      - muscle involvement without evidence of necrosis L97.915
      - muscle necrosis L97.913
      - skin breakdown only L97.911
      - specified severity NEC L97.918
  - syphilitic A52.19
  - thigh L97.1Ø9
    - with
      - bone involvement without evidence of necrosis L97.1Ø6
      - bone necrosis L97.1Ø4
      - exposed fat layer L97.1Ø2
      - muscle involvement without evidence of necrosis L97.1Ø5
      - muscle necrosis L97.1Ø3
      - skin breakdown only L97.1Ø1
      - specified severity NEC L97.1Ø8
    - left L97.129
      - with
        - bone involvement without evidence of necrosis L97.126
        - bone necrosis L97.124
        - exposed fat layer L97.122
        - muscle involvement without evidence of necrosis L97.125
        - muscle necrosis L97.123
        - skin breakdown only L97.121
        - specified severity NEC L97.128
    - right L97.119

Ulcer, ulcerated, ulcerating, ulceration, ulcerative — *continued*
- lower limb — *continued*
  - thigh — *continued*
    - right — *continued*
      - with
        - bone involvement without evidence of necrosis L97.116
        - bone necrosis L97.114
        - exposed fat layer L97.112
        - muscle involvement without evidence of necrosis L97.115
        - muscle necrosis L97.113
        - skin breakdown only L97.111
        - specified severity NEC L97.118
  - toe L97.5Ø9
    - with
      - bone involvement without evidence of necrosis L97.5Ø6
      - bone necrosis L97.5Ø4
      - exposed fat layer L97.5Ø2
      - muscle involvement without evidence of necrosis L97.5Ø5
      - muscle necrosis L97.5Ø3
      - skin breakdown only L97.5Ø1
      - specified severity NEC L97.5Ø8
    - left L97.529
      - with
        - bone involvement without evidence of necrosis L97.526
        - bone necrosis L97.524
        - exposed fat layer L97.522
        - muscle involvement without evidence of necrosis L97.525
        - muscle necrosis L97.523
        - skin breakdown only L97.521
        - specified severity NEC L97.528
    - right L97.519
      - with
        - bone involvement without evidence of necrosis L97.516
        - bone necrosis L97.514
        - exposed fat layer L97.512
        - muscle involvement without evidence of necrosis L97.515
        - muscle necrosis L97.513
        - skin breakdown only L97.511
        - specified severity NEC L97.518
  - varicose — *see* Varix, leg, with, ulcer
- luetic — *see* Ulcer, syphilitic
- lung J98.4
  - tuberculous — *see* Tuberculosis, pulmonary
- malignant — *see* Neoplasm, malignant, by site
- marginal NEC — *see* Ulcer, gastrojejunal
- meatus (urinarius) N34.2
- Meckel's diverticulum Q43.Ø
  - malignant — *see* Table of Neoplasms, small intestine, malignant
- Meleney's (chronic undermining) — *see* Ulcer, skin
- Mooren's (cornea) — *see* Ulcer, cornea, Mooren's
- mycobacterial (skin) A31.1
- nasopharynx J39.2
- neck, uterus N86
- neurogenic NEC — *see* Ulcer, skin
- nose, nasal (passage) (infective) (septum) J34.Ø
  - skin — *see* Ulcer, skin
  - spirochetal A69.8
  - varicose (bleeding) I86.8
- oral mucosa (traumatic) K12.1
- palate (soft) K12.1
- penis (chronic) N48.5
- peptic (site unspecified) K27.9
  - with
    - hemorrhage K27.4
      - and perforation K27.6
    - perforation K27.5
  - acute K27.3
    - with
      - hemorrhage K27.Ø
        - and perforation K27.2
      - perforation K27.1
  - chronic K27.7
    - with
      - hemorrhage K27.4
        - and perforation K27.6
      - perforation K27.5
  - esophagus K22.1Ø
    - with bleeding K22.11

- **Ulcer, ulcerated, ulcerating, ulceration, ulcerative** — *continued*
  - peptic — *continued*
    - newborn P78.82
  - perforating K27.5
    - skin — *see* Ulcer, skin
  - peritonsillar J35.8
  - phagedenic (tropical) — *see* Ulcer, skin
  - pharynx J39.2
  - phlebitis — *see* Phlebitis
  - plaster — *see* Ulcer, pressure, by site
  - popliteal space — *see* Ulcer, lower limb
  - postpyloric — *see* Ulcer, duodenum
  - prepuce N47.7
  - prepyloric — *see* Ulcer, stomach
  - pressure (pressure area) L89.9- ☑
    - ankle L89.5- ☑
    - back L89.1- ☑
    - buttock L89.3- ☑
    - coccyx L89.15- ☑
    - contiguous site of back, buttock, hip L89.4- ☑
    - elbow L89.Ø- ☑
    - face L89.81- ☑
    - head L89.81- ☑
    - heel L89.6- ☑
    - hip L89.2- ☑
    - sacral region (tailbone) L89.15- ☑
    - specified site NEC L89.89- ☑
    - stage 1 (healing) (pre-ulcer skin changes limited to persistent focal edema)
      - ankle L89.5- ☑
      - back L89.1- ☑
      - buttock L89.3- ☑
      - coccyx L89.15- ☑
      - contiguous site of back, buttock, hip L89.4- ☑
      - elbow L89.Ø- ☑
      - face L89.81- ☑
      - head L89.81- ☑
      - heel L89.6- ☑
      - hip L89.2- ☑
      - sacral region (tailbone) L89.15- ☑
      - specified site NEC L89.89- ☑
    - stage 2 (healing) (abrasion, blister, partial thickness skin loss involving epidermis and/or dermis)
      - ankle L89.5- ☑
      - back L89.1- ☑
      - buttock L89.3- ☑
      - coccyx L89.15- ☑
      - contiguous site of back, buttock, hip L89.4- ☑
      - elbow L89.Ø- ☑
      - face L89.81- ☑
      - head L89.81- ☑
      - heel L89.6- ☑
      - hip L89.2- ☑
      - sacral region (tailbone) L89.15- ☑
      - specified site NEC L89.89- ☑
    - stage 3 (healing) (full thickness skin loss involving damage or necrosis of subcutaneous tissue)
      - ankle L89.5- ☑
      - back L89.1- ☑
      - buttock L89.3- ☑
      - coccyx L89.15- ☑
      - contiguous site of back, buttock, hip L89.4- ☑
      - elbow L89.Ø- ☑
      - face L89.81- ☑
      - head L89.81- ☑
      - heel L89.6- ☑
      - hip L89.2- ☑
      - sacral region (tailbone) L89.15- ☑
      - specified site NEC L89.89- ☑
    - stage 4 (healing) (necrosis of soft tissues through to underlying muscle, tendon, or bone)
      - ankle L89.5- ☑
      - back L89.1- ☑
      - buttock L89.3- ☑
      - coccyx L89.15- ☑
      - contiguous site of back, buttock, hip L89.4- ☑
      - elbow L89.Ø- ☑
      - face L89.81- ☑
      - head L89.81- ☑
      - heel L89.6- ☑
      - hip L89.2- ☑
      - sacral region (tailbone) L89.15- ☑
      - specified site NEC L89.89- ☑
    - unspecified stage
      - ankle L89.5- ☑

- **Ulcer, ulcerated, ulcerating, ulceration, ulcerative** — *continued*
  - pressure — *continued*
    - unspecified stage — *continued*
      - back L89.1- ☑
      - buttock L89.3- ☑
      - coccyx L89.15- ☑
      - contiguous site of back, buttock, hip L89.4- ☑
      - elbow L89.Ø- ☑
      - face L89.81- ☑
      - head L89.81- ☑
      - heel L89.6- ☑
      - hip L89.2- ☑
      - sacral region (tailbone) L89.15- ☑
      - specified site NEC L89.89- ☑
    - unstageable
      - ankle L89.5- ☑
      - back L89.1- ☑
      - buttock L89.3- ☑
      - coccyx L89.15- ☑
      - contiguous site of back, buttock, hip L89.4- ☑
      - elbow L89.Ø- ☑
      - face L89.81- ☑
      - head L89.81- ☑
      - heel L89.6- ☑
      - hip L89.2- ☑
      - sacral region (tailbone) L89.15- ☑
      - specified site NEC L89.89- ☑
  - primary of intestine K63.3
    - with perforation K63.1
  - prostate N41.9
  - pyloric — *see* Ulcer, stomach
  - rectosigmoid K63.3
    - with perforation K63.1
  - rectum (sphincter) (solitary) K62.6
    - stercoraceous, stercoral K62.6
  - retina — *see* Inflammation, chorioretinal
  - rodent — *see also* Neoplasm, skin, malignant
  - sclera — *see* Scleritis
  - scrofulous (tuberculous) A18.2
  - scrotum N5Ø.89
    - tuberculous A18.15
    - varicose I86.1
  - seminal vesicle N5Ø.89
  - sigmoid — *see* Ulcer, intestine
  - skin (atrophic) (chronic) (neurogenic) (non-healing) (perforating) (pyogenic) (trophic) (tropical) L98.499
    - with gangrene — *see* Gangrene
    - amebic AØ6.7
    - back — *see* Ulcer, back
    - buttock — *see* Ulcer, buttock
    - decubitus — *see* Ulcer, pressure
    - lower limb — *see* Ulcer, lower limb
    - mycobacterial A31.1
    - specified site NEC L98.499
      - with
        - bone involvement without evidence of necrosis L98.496
        - bone necrosis L98.494
        - exposed fat layer L98.492
        - muscle involvement without evidence of necrosis L98.495
        - muscle necrosis L98.493
        - skin breakdown only L98.491
        - specified severity NEC L98.498
    - tuberculous (primary) A18.4
    - varicose — *see* Ulcer, varicose
  - sloughing — *see* Ulcer, skin
  - solitary, anus or rectum (sphincter) K62.6
  - sore throat JØ2.9
    - streptococcal JØ2.Ø
  - spermatic cord N5Ø.89
  - spine (tuberculous) A18.Ø1
  - stasis (venous) — *see* Varix, leg, with, ulcer
    - without varicose veins — *see also* Ulcer, by site I87.2
  - stercoraceous, stercoral K63.3
    - with perforation K63.1
    - anus or rectum K62.6
  - stoma, stomal — *see* Ulcer, gastrojejunal
  - stomach (eroded) (peptic) (round) K25.9
    - with
      - hemorrhage K25.4
        - and perforation K25.6
      - perforation K25.5
    - acute K25.3

- **Ulcer, ulcerated, ulcerating, ulceration, ulcerative** — *continued*
  - stomach — *continued*
    - acute — *continued*
      - with
        - hemorrhage K25.Ø
          - and perforation K25.2
        - perforation K25.1
    - chronic K25.7
      - with
        - hemorrhage K25.4
          - and perforation K25.6
        - perforation K25.5
  - stomal — *see* Ulcer, gastrojejunal
  - stomatitis K12.1
  - stress — *see* Ulcer, peptic
  - strumous (tuberculous) A18.2
  - submucosal, bladder — *see* Cystitis, interstitial
  - syphilitic (any site) (early) (secondary) A51.39
    - late A52.79
    - perforating A52.79
      - foot A52.11
  - testis N5Ø.89
  - thigh — *see* Ulcer, lower limb
  - throat J39.2
    - diphtheritic A36.Ø
  - toe — *see* Ulcer, lower limb
  - tongue (traumatic) K14.Ø
  - tonsil J35.8
    - diphtheritic A36.Ø
  - trachea J39.8
  - trophic — *see* Ulcer, skin
  - tropical — *see* Ulcer, skin
  - tuberculous — *see* Tuberculosis, ulcer
  - tunica vaginalis N5Ø.89
  - turbinate J34.89
  - typhoid (perforating) — *see* Typhoid
  - unspecified site — *see* Ulcer, skin
  - urethra (meatus) — *see* Urethritis
  - uterus N85.8
    - cervix N86
      - with cervicitis N72
    - neck N86
      - with cervicitis N72
  - vagina N76.5
    - in Behcet's disease M35.2 *[N77.Ø]*
    - pessary N89.8
  - valve, heart I33.Ø
  - varicose (lower limb, any part) — *see also* Varix, leg, with, ulcer
    - broad ligament I86.2
    - esophagus — *see* Varix, esophagus
    - inflamed or infected — *see* Varix, leg, with ulcer, with inflammation
    - nasal septum I86.8
    - perineum I86.3
    - scrotum I86.1
    - specified site NEC I86.8
    - sublingual I86.Ø
    - vulva I86.3
  - vas deferens N5Ø.89
  - vulva (acute) (infectional) N76.6
    - in (due to)
      - Behcet's disease M35.2 *[N77.Ø]*
      - herpesviral (herpes simplex) infection A6Ø.Ø4
      - tuberculosis A18.18
  - vulvobuccal, recurring N76.6
  - X-ray L58.1
  - yaws A66.4
- **Ulcerosa scarlatina** A38.8
- **Ulcus** — *see also* Ulcer
  - cutis tuberculosum A18.4
  - duodeni — *see* Ulcer, duodenum
  - durum (syphilitic) A51.Ø
    - extragenital A51.2
  - gastrojejunale — *see* Ulcer, gastrojejunal
  - hypostaticum — *see* Ulcer, varicose
  - molle (cutis) (skin) A57
  - serpens corneae — *see* Ulcer, cornea, central
  - ventriculi — *see* Ulcer, stomach
- **Ulegyria** QØ4.8
- **Ulerythema**
  - ophryogenes, congenital Q84.2
  - sycosiforme L73.8
- **Ullrich** (-Bonnevie) (-Turner) **syndrome** — *see also* Turner's syndrome Q87.19
- **Ullrich-Feichtiger syndrome** Q87.Ø
- **Ulnar** — *see* condition

Ulorrhagia, ulorrhea KØ6.8

Umbilicus, umbilical — *see* condition

Unable to
- make ends meet Z59.86
- obtain
  - adequate
    - childcare due to limited financial resources, specified NEC Z59.87
    - clothing due to limited financial resources, specified NEC Z59.87
    - utilities due to limited financial resources, specified NEC Z59.87
  - basic
    - needs due to limited financial resources, specified NEC Z59.87
    - services in physical environment Z58.81
  - internet service, due to unavailability in geographic area Z58.81
  - telephone service, due to unavailability in geographic area Z58.81
  - utilities, due to inadequate physical environment Z58.81

Unacceptable
- contours of tooth KØ8.54
- morphology of tooth KØ8.54

Unaffordable transportation Z59.82

Unavailability (of)
- bed at medical facility Z75.1
- health service-related agencies Z75.4
- medical facilities (at) Z75.3
  - due to
    - investigation by social service agency Z75.2
    - lack of services at home Z75.Ø
    - remoteness from facility Z75.3
    - waiting list Z75.1
  - home Z75.Ø
  - outpatient clinic Z75.3
- schooling Z55.1
- social service agencies Z75.4

Uncinaria americana infestation B76.1

Uncinariasis B76.9

Uncongenial work Z56.5

Unconscious (ness) — *see* Coma

Under observation — *see* Observation

Underachievement in school Z55.3

Underdevelopment — *see also* Undeveloped
- nose Q3Ø.1
- sexual E3Ø.Ø

Underdosing — *see also* Table of Drugs and Chemicals, categories T36-T5Ø, with final character 6 Z91.14 ☑
- intentional NEC Z91.128
  - due to financial hardship of patient Z91.12Ø
- unintentional NEC Z91.138
  - due to patient's age related debility Z91.13Ø

Underfeeding, newborn P92.3

Underfill, endodontic M27.53

Underimmunization status Z28.39
- COVID-19 Z28.31- ☑
  - partially vaccinated (for) Z28.311
  - unvaccinated (for) Z28.31Ø

Undernourishment — *see* Malnutrition

Undernutrition — *see* Malnutrition

Underweight R63.6
- for gestational age — *see* Light for dates

Underwood's disease P83.Ø

Undescended — *see also* Malposition, congenital
- cecum Q43.3
- colon Q43.3
- testicle — *see* Cryptorchid

Undeveloped, undevelopment — *see also* Hypoplasia
- brain (congenital) QØ2
- cerebral (congenital) QØ2
- heart Q24.8
- lung Q33.6
- testis E29.1
- uterus E3Ø.Ø

Undiagnosed (disease) R69

Undulant fever — *see* Brucellosis

Unemployment, anxiety concerning Z56.Ø
- threatened Z56.2

Unequal length (acquired) (limb) — *see also* Deformity, limb, unequal length
- leg — *see also* Deformity, limb, unequal length
  - congenital Q72.9- ☑

Unextracted dental root KØ8.3

Unguis incarnatus L6Ø.Ø

Unhappiness R45.2

Unicornate uterus Q51.4

Unicornate uterus — *continued*
- in pregnancy or childbirth O34.ØØ

Unilateral — *see also* condition
- development, breast N64.89
- organ or site, congenital NEC — *see* Agenesis, by site

Unilocular heart Q2Ø.8

Unimmunized — *see also* Underimmunization status
- for COVID-19 Z28.31Ø

Union, abnormal — *see also* Fusion
- larynx and trachea Q34.8

Universal mesentery Q43.3

Unreliable transportation Z59.82

Unrepairable overhanging of dental restorative materials KØ8.52

Unroofed coronary sinus Q21.13

Unsafe transportation Z59.82

Unsatisfactory
- restoration of tooth KØ8.5Ø
  - specified NEC KØ8.59
- sample of cytologic smear
  - anus R85.615
  - cervix R87.615
  - vagina R87.625
- surroundings Z59.19
  - work Z56.5

Unsoundness of mind — *see* Psychosis

Unstable
- back NEC — *see* Instability, joint, spine
- hip (congenital) Q65.6
  - acquired — *see* Derangement, joint, specified type NEC, hip
- joint — *see* Instability, joint
  - secondary to removal of joint prosthesis M96.89
- lie (mother) O32.Ø ☑
- lumbosacral joint (congenital) — *see* subcategory M53.2
- sacroiliac — *see* subcategory M53.2 ☑
- spine NEC — *see* Instability, joint, spine

Unsteadiness on feet R26.81

Untruthfulness, child problem F91.8

Unvaccinated — *see also* Underimmunization status
- for COVID-19 Z28.31Ø

Unverricht (-Lundborg) **disease or epilepsy** — *see* Epilepsy, generalized, idiopathic

Unwanted
- multiple moves in the last 12 months Z59.81- ☑
- pregnancy Z64.Ø

Upbringing, institutional Z62.22
- away from parents NEC Z62.29
- in care of non-parental family member Z62.21
- in foster care Z62.21
- in orphanage or group home Z62.22
- in welfare custody Z62.21

Upper respiratory — *see* condition

Upset
- gastric K3Ø
- gastrointestinal K3Ø
  - psychogenic F45.8
- intestinal (large) (small) K59.9
  - psychogenic F45.8
- menstruation N93.9
- mental F48.9
- stomach K3Ø
  - psychogenic F45.8

Urachus — *see also* condition
- patent or persistent Q64.4

Urbach-Oppenheim disease (necrobiosis lipoidica diabeticorum) — *see* EØ8-E13 with .62Ø

Urbach's lipoid proteinosis E78.89

Urbach-Wiethe disease E78.89

Urban yellow fever A95.1

Urea
- blood, high — *see* Uremia
- cycle metabolism disorder — *see* Disorder, urea cycle metabolism

Uremia, uremic N19
- with
  - ectopic or molar pregnancy OØ8.4
  - polyneuropathy N18.9 *[G63]*
- chronic NOS — *see also* Disease, kidney, chronic N18.9
  - due to hypertension — *see* Hypertensive, kidney
- complicating
  - ectopic or molar pregnancy OØ8.4
- congenital P96.Ø
- extrarenal R39.2
- following ectopic or molar pregnancy OØ8.4
- newborn P96.Ø

Uremia, uremic — *continued*
- prerenal R39.2

Ureter, ureteral — *see* condition

Ureteralgia N23

Ureterectasis — *see* Hydroureter

Ureteritis N28.89
- cystica N28.86
- due to calculus N2Ø.1
  - with calculus, kidney N2Ø.2
    - with hydronephrosis N13.2
- gonococcal (acute) (chronic) A54.21
- nonspecific N28.89

Ureterocele N28.89
- congenital (orthotopic) Q62.31
  - ectopic Q62.32

Ureterolith, ureterolithiasis — *see* Calculus, ureter

Ureterostomy
- attention to Z43.6
- status Z93.6

Urethra, urethral — *see* condition

Urethralgia R39.89

Urethritis (anterior) (posterior) N34.2
- calculous N21.1
- candidal B37.41
- chlamydial A56.Ø1
- diplococcal (gonococcal) A54.Ø1
  - with abscess (accessory gland) (periurethral) A54.1
- gonococcal A54.Ø1
  - with abscess (accessory gland) (periurethral) A54.1
- nongonococcal N34.1
  - Reiter's — *see* Reiter's disease
- nonspecific N34.1
- nonvenereal N34.1
- postmenopausal N34.2
- puerperal O86.22
- Reiter's — *see* Reiter's disease
- specified NEC N34.2
- trichomonal or due to Trichomonas (vaginalis) A59.Ø3

Urethrocele N81.Ø
- with
  - cystocele — *see* Cystocele
  - prolapse of uterus — *see* Prolapse, uterus

Urethrolithiasis (with colic or infection) N21.1

Urethrorectal — *see* condition

Urethrorrhagia N36.8

Urethrorrhea R36.9

Urethrostomy
- attention to Z43.6
- status Z93.6

Urethrotrigonitis — *see* Trigonitis

Urethrovaginal — *see* condition

Urgency
- fecal R15.2
- hypertensive — *see* Hypertension
- urinary R39.15

Urhidrosis, uridrosis L74.8

Uric acid in blood (increased) E79.Ø

Uricacidemia (asymptomatic) E79.Ø

Uricemia (asymptomatic) E79.Ø

Uricosuria R82.998

Urinary — *see* condition

Urination
- frequent R35.Ø
- painful R3Ø.9

Urine
- blood in — *see* Hematuria
- discharge, excessive R35.89
- enuresis, nonorganic origin F98.Ø
- extravasation R39.Ø
- frequency R35.Ø
- incontinence R32
  - nonorganic origin F98.Ø
- intermittent stream R39.198
- pus in N39.Ø
- retention or stasis R33.9
  - organic R33.8
    - drug-induced R33.Ø
  - psychogenic F45.8
- secretion
  - deficient R34
  - excessive R35.89
  - frequency R35.Ø
- stream
  - intermittent R39.198
  - slowing R39.198
  - splitting R39.13
  - weak R39.12

Urinemia — *see* Uremia

☑ **Additional Character Required — Refer to the Tabular List for Character Selection**

- **Urinoma, urethra** N36.8
- **Uroarthritis, infectious** (Reiter's) — *see* Reiter's disease
- **Urodialysis** R34
- **Urolithiasis** — *see* Calculus, urinary
- **Uronephrosis** — *see* Hydronephrosis
- **Uropathy** N39.9
  - obstructive N13.9
    - specified NEC N13.8
  - reflux N13.9
    - specified NEC N13.8
  - vesicoureteral reflux-associated — *see* Reflux, vesicoureteral
- **Urosepsis** — *code to* condition
- **Urticaria** L50.9
  - with angioneurotic edema T78.3 ☑
    - hereditary D84.1
  - allergic L50.0
  - cholinergic L50.5
  - chronic L50.8
  - cold, familial L50.2
  - contact L50.6
  - dermatographic L50.3
  - due to
    - cold or heat L50.2
    - drugs L50.0
    - food L50.0
    - inhalants L50.0
    - plants L50.6
    - serum — *see also* Reaction, serum T80.69 ☑
  - factitial L50.3
  - familial cold M04.2
  - giant T78.3 ☑
    - hereditary D84.1
  - gigantea T78.3 ☑
  - idiopathic L50.1
  - larynx T78.3 ☑
    - hereditary D84.1
  - neonatorum P83.88
  - nonallergic L50.1
  - papulosa (Hebra) L28.2
  - pigmentosa D47.01
    - congenital Q82.2
    - of neonatal onset Q82.2
    - of newborn onset Q82.2
  - recurrent periodic L50.8
  - serum — *see also* Reaction, serum T80.69 ☑
  - solar L56.3
  - specified type NEC L50.8
  - thermal (cold) (heat) L50.2
  - vibratory L50.4
  - xanthelasmoidea — *see* Urticaria pigmentosa
- **Use** (of)
  - alcohol F10.90
    - with
      - intoxication F10.929
      - sleep disorder F10.982
      - withdrawal F10.939
        - with
          - perceptual disturbance F10.932
        - delirium F10.931
        - uncomplicated F10.930
    - harmful — *see* Abuse, alcohol
    - in remission F10.91
  - amphetamines — *see* Use, stimulant NEC
  - caffeine — *see* Use, stimulant NEC
  - cannabis F12.90
    - with
      - anxiety disorder F12.980
      - intoxication F12.929
        - with
          - delirium F12.921
          - perceptual disturbance F12.922
        - uncomplicated F12.920
      - other specified disorder F12.988
      - psychosis F12.959
        - delusions F12.950
        - hallucinations F12.951
      - unspecified disorder F12.99
      - withdrawal F12.93
    - in remission F12.91
  - cocaine F14.90
    - with
      - anxiety disorder F14.980
      - intoxication F14.929
        - with
          - delirium F14.921
          - perceptual disturbance F14.922
        - uncomplicated F14.920

Use — *continued*

- cocaine — *continued*
  - with — *continued*
    - other specified disorder F14.988
    - psychosis F14.959
      - delusions F14.950
      - hallucinations F14.951
    - sexual dysfunction F14.981
    - sleep disorder F14.982
    - unspecified disorder F14.99
    - withdrawal F14.93
  - harmful — *see* Abuse, drug, cocaine
  - in remission F14.91
- drug(s) NEC F19.90
  - with sleep disorder F19.982
  - harmful — *see* Abuse, drug, by type
- hallucinogen NEC F16.90
  - with
    - anxiety disorder F16.980
    - intoxication F16.929
      - with
        - delirium F16.921
      - uncomplicated F16.920
    - mood disorder F16.94
    - other specified disorder F16.988
    - perception disorder (flashbacks) F16.983
    - psychosis F16.959
      - delusions F16.950
      - hallucinations F16.951
    - unspecified disorder F16.99
  - harmful — *see* Abuse, drug, hallucinogen NEC
  - in remission F16.91
- inhalants F18.90
  - with
    - anxiety disorder F18.980
    - intoxication F18.929
      - with delirium F18.921
      - uncomplicated F18.920
    - mood disorder F18.94
    - other specified disorder F18.988
    - persisting dementia F18.97
    - psychosis F18.959
      - delusions F18.950
      - hallucinations F18.951
    - unspecified disorder F18.99
  - harmful — *see* Abuse, drug, inhalant
  - in remission F18.91
- methadone — *see* Use, opioid
- nonprescribed drugs F19.90
  - harmful — *see* Abuse, non-psychoactive substance
- opioid F11.90
  - with
    - disorder F11.99
      - mood F11.94
      - sleep F11.982
      - specified type NEC F11.988
    - intoxication F11.929
      - with
        - delirium F11.921
        - perceptual disturbance F11.922
      - uncomplicated F11.920
    - opioid-associated amnestic syndrome F11.988
    - withdrawal F11.93
  - harmful — *see* Abuse, drug, opioid
  - in remission F11.91
- patent medicines F19.90
  - harmful — *see* Abuse, non-psychoactive substance
- psychoactive drug NEC F19.90
  - with
    - anxiety disorder F19.980
    - intoxication F19.929
      - with
        - delirium F19.921
        - perceptual disturbance F19.922
      - uncomplicated F19.920
    - mood disorder F19.94
    - other specified disorder F19.988
    - persisting
      - amnestic disorder F19.96
      - dementia F19.97
    - psychosis F19.959
      - delusions F19.950
      - hallucinations F19.951
    - sexual dysfunction F19.981
    - sleep disorder F19.982
    - unspecified disorder F19.99
    - withdrawal F19.939

Use — *continued*

- psychoactive drug — *continued*
  - with — *continued*
    - withdrawal — *continued*
      - with
        - delirium F19.931
        - perceptual disturbance F19.932
      - uncomplicated F19.930
  - harmful — *see* Abuse, drug NEC, psychoactive NEC
  - in remission F19.91
- sedative, hypnotic, or anxiolytic F13.90
  - with
    - anxiety disorder F13.980
    - intoxication F13.929
      - with
        - delirium F13.921
      - uncomplicated F13.920
    - other specified disorder F13.988
    - persisting
      - amnestic disorder F13.96
      - dementia F13.97
    - psychosis F13.959
      - delusions F13.950
      - hallucinations F13.951
    - sexual dysfunction F13.981
    - sleep disorder F13.982
    - unspecified disorder F13.99
  - harmful — *see* Abuse, drug, sedative, hypnotic, or anxiolytic
  - in remission F13.91
- stimulant NEC F15.90
  - with
    - anxiety disorder F15.980
    - intoxication F15.929
      - with
        - delirium F15.921
        - perceptual disturbance F15.922
      - uncomplicated F15.920
    - mood disorder F15.94
    - other specified disorder F15.988
    - psychosis F15.959
      - delusions F15.950
      - hallucinations F15.951
    - sexual dysfunction F15.981
    - sleep disorder F15.982
    - unspecified disorder F15.99
    - withdrawal F15.93
  - harmful — *see* Abuse, drug, stimulant NEC
  - in remission F15.91
- tobacco Z72.0
  - with dependence — *see* Dependence, drug, nicotine
- volatile solvents — *see also* Use, inhalant F18.90
  - harmful — *see* Abuse, drug, inhalant

- **Usher-Senear disease or syndrome** L10.4
- **Uta** B55.1
- **Uteromegaly** N85.2
- **Uterovaginal** — *see* condition
- **Uterovesical** — *see* condition
- **Uveal** — *see* condition
- **Uveitis** (anterior) — *see also* Iridocyclitis
  - acute — *see* Iridocyclitis, acute
  - chronic — *see* Iridocyclitis, chronic
  - due to toxoplasmosis (acquired) B58.09
    - congenital P37.1
  - granulomatous — *see* Iridocyclitis, chronic
  - heterochromic — *see* Cyclitis, Fuchs' heterochromic
  - lens-induced — *see* Iridocyclitis, lens-induced
  - posterior — *see* Chorioretinitis
  - sympathetic H44.13- ☑
  - syphilitic (secondary) A51.43
    - congenital (early) A50.01
    - late A52.71
  - tuberculous A18.54
- **Uveoencephalitis** — *see* Inflammation, chorioretinal
- **Uveokeratitis** — *see* Iridocyclitis
- **Uveoparotitis** D86.89
- **Uvula** — *see* condition
- **Uvulitis** (acute) (catarrhal) (chronic) (membranous) (suppurative) (ulcerative) K12.2

V

- **Vaccination** (prophylactic)
  - complication or reaction — *see* Complications, vaccination
  - delayed Z28.9
  - encounter for Z23
  - not done — *see* Immunization, not done

- **Vaccination** — *continued*
  - partial — *see also* Underimmunization status
    - for COVID-19 Z28.311
- **Vaccinia** (generalized) (localized) T88.1 ☑
  - congenital P35.8
  - without vaccination BØ8.Ø11
- **Vacuum, in sinus** (accessory) (nasal) J34.89
- **Vagabond, vagabondage** Z59.ØØ
- **Vagabond's disease** B85.1
- **Vagina, vaginal** — *see* condition
- **Vaginalitis** (tunica) (testis) N49.1
- **Vaginismus** (reflex) N94.2
  - functional F52.5
  - nonorganic F52.5
  - psychogenic F52.5
  - secondary N94.2
- **Vaginitis** (acute) (circumscribed) (diffuse) (emphysematous) (nonvenereal) (ulcerative) N76.Ø
  - with ectopic or molar pregnancy OØ8.Ø
  - amebic AØ6.82
  - atrophic, postmenopausal N95.2
  - bacterial N76.Ø
  - blennorrhagic (gonococcal) A54.Ø2
  - candidal (acute) B37.31
    - chronic (recurrent) B37.32
  - chlamydial A56.Ø2
  - chronic N76.1
  - due to Trichomonas (vaginalis) A59.Ø1
  - following ectopic or molar pregnancy OØ8.Ø
  - gonococcal A54.Ø2
    - with abscess (accessory gland) (periurethral) A54.1
  - granuloma A58
  - in (due to)
    - candidiasis (acute) B37.31
      - chronic (recurrent) B37.32
    - herpesviral (herpes simplex) infection A6Ø.Ø4
    - pinworm infection B8Ø *[N77.1]*
  - monilial (acute) B37.31
    - chronic (recurrent) B37.32
  - mycotic (candidal) (acute) B37.31
    - chronic (recurrent) B37.32
  - postmenopausal atrophic N95.2
  - puerperal (postpartum) O86.13
  - senile (atrophic) N95.2
  - subacute or chronic N76.1
  - syphilitic (early) A51.Ø
    - late A52.76
  - trichomonal A59.Ø1
  - tuberculous A18.18
- **Vaginosis** — *see* Vaginitis
- **Vagotonia** G52.2
- **Vagrancy** Z59.ØØ
- **VAIN** — *see* Neoplasia, intraepithelial, vagina
- **Vallecula** — *see* condition
- **Valley fever** B38.Ø
- **Valsuani's disease** — *see* Anemia, obstetric
- **Valve, valvular** (formation) — *see also* condition
  - cerebral ventricle (communicating) in situ Z98.2
  - cervix, internal os Q51.828
  - congenital NEC — *see* Atresia, by site
  - ureter (pelvic junction) (vesical orifice) Q62.39
  - urethra (congenital) (posterior) Q64.2
- **Valvulitis** (chronic) — *see* Endocarditis
- **Valvulopathy** — *see* Endocarditis
- **Van Bogaert's leukoencephalopathy** (sclerosing) (subacute) A81.1
- **Van Bogaert-Scherer-Epstein disease or syndrome** E75.5
- **Van Buchem's syndrome** M85.2
- **Van Creveld-von Gierke disease** E74.Ø1
- **Van der Hoeve** (-de Kleyn) **syndrome** Q78.Ø
- **Van der Woude's syndrome** Q38.Ø
- **Van Neck's disease or osteochondrosis** M91.Ø
- **Vanishing lung** J44.89
- **Vapor asphyxia or suffocation** T59.9 ☑
  - specified agent — *see* Table of Drugs and Chemicals
- **Variance, lethal ball, prosthetic heart valve** T82.Ø9 ☑
- **Variants, thalassemic** D56.8
- **Variations in hair color** L67.1
- **Varicella** BØ1.9
  - with
    - complications NEC BØ1.89
    - encephalitis BØ1.11
    - encephalomyelitis BØ1.11
    - meningitis BØ1.Ø
    - myelitis BØ1.12
    - pneumonia BØ1.2
  - congenital P35.8
- **Varices** — *see* Varix
- **Varicocele** (scrotum) (thrombosed) I86.1
  - ovary I86.2
  - perineum I86.3
  - spermatic cord (ulcerated) I86.1
- **Varicose**
  - aneurysm (ruptured) I77.Ø
  - dermatitis — *see* Varix, leg, with, inflammation
  - eczema — *see* Varix, leg, with, inflammation
  - phlebitis — *see* Varix, with, inflammation
  - tumor — *see* Varix
  - ulcer (lower limb, any part) — *see also* Varix, leg, with, ulcer
    - anus — *see also* Hemorrhoids K64.8
    - esophagus — *see* Varix, esophagus
    - inflamed or infected — *see* Varix, leg, with ulcer, with inflammation
    - nasal septum I86.8
    - perineum I86.3
    - scrotum I86.1
    - specified site NEC I86.8
  - vein — *see* Varix
  - vessel — *see* Varix, leg
- **Varicosis, varicosities, varicosity** — *see* Varix
- **Variola** (major) (minor) BØ3
- **Varioloid** BØ3
- **Varix** (lower limb) I83.9Ø
  - with
    - bleeding I83.899
    - edema I83.899
    - inflammation I83.1Ø
      - with ulcer (venous) I83.2Ø9
    - pain I83.819
    - rupture I83.899
    - specified complication NEC I83.899
    - stasis dermatitis I83.1Ø
      - with ulcer (venous) I83.2Ø9
    - swelling I83.899
    - ulcer I83.ØØ9
      - with inflammation I83.2Ø9
  - aneurysmal I77.Ø
  - asymptomatic I83.9- ☑
  - bladder I86.2
  - broad ligament I86.2
  - complicating
    - childbirth (lower extremity) O87.4
      - anus or rectum O87.2
      - genital (vagina, vulva or perineum) O87.8
    - pregnancy (lower extremity) O22.Ø- ☑
      - anus or rectum O22.4- ☑
      - genital (vagina, vulva or perineum) O22.1- ☑
    - puerperium (lower extremity) O87.4
      - anus or rectum O87.2
      - genital (vagina, vulva, perineum) O87.8
  - congenital (any site) Q27.8
  - esophagus (idiopathic) (primary) (ulcerated) I85.ØØ
    - bleeding I85.Ø1
    - congenital Q27.8
    - in (due to)
      - alcoholic liver disease I85.1Ø
        - bleeding I85.11
      - cirrhosis of liver I85.1Ø
        - bleeding I85.11
      - portal hypertension I85.1Ø
        - bleeding I85.11
      - schistosomiasis I85.1Ø
        - bleeding I85.11
      - toxic liver disease I85.1Ø
        - bleeding I85.11
    - secondary I85.1Ø
      - bleeding I85.11
  - gastric I86.4
  - inflamed or infected I83.1Ø
    - ulcerated I83.2Ø9
  - labia (majora) I86.3
  - leg (asymptomatic) I83.9- ☑
    - with
      - edema I83.899
      - inflammation I83.1Ø
        - with ulcer — *see* Varix, leg, with, ulcer, with inflammation by site
      - pain I83.819
      - specified complication NEC I83.899
      - swelling I83.899
      - ulcer I83.Ø- ☑
        - with inflammation I83.2- ☑
        - ankle I83.ØØ3
          - with inflammation I83.2Ø3

- **Varix** — *continued*
  - leg — *continued*
    - with — *continued*
      - ulcer — *continued*
        - calf I83.ØØ2
          - with inflammation I83.2Ø2
        - foot NEC I83.ØØ5
          - with inflammation I83.2Ø5
        - heel I83.ØØ4
          - with inflammation I83.2Ø4
        - lower leg NEC I83.ØØ8
          - with inflammation I83.2Ø8
        - midfoot I83.ØØ4
          - with inflammation I83.2Ø4
        - thigh I83.ØØ1
          - with inflammation I83.2Ø1
    - bilateral (asymptomatic) I83.93
      - with
        - edema I83.893
        - pain I83.813
        - specified complication NEC I83.893
        - swelling I83.893
        - ulcer I83.Ø- ☑
          - with inflammation I83.2Ø9
    - left (asymptomatic) I83.92
      - with
        - edema I83.892
        - inflammation I83.12
          - with ulcer — *see* Varix, leg, with, ulcer, with inflammation by site
        - pain I83.812
        - specified complication NEC I83.892
        - swelling I83.892
        - ulcer I83.Ø29
          - with inflammation I83.229
          - ankle I83.Ø23
            - with inflammation I83.223
          - calf I83.Ø22
            - with inflammation I83.222
          - foot NEC I83.Ø25
            - with inflammation I83.225
          - heel I83.Ø24
            - with inflammation I83.224
          - lower leg NEC I83.Ø28
            - with inflammation I83.228
          - midfoot I83.Ø24
            - with inflammation I83.224
          - thigh I83.Ø21
            - with inflammation I83.221
    - right (asymptomatic) I83.91
      - with
        - edema I83.891
        - inflammation I83.11
          - with ulcer — *see* Varix, leg, with, ulcer, with inflammation by site
        - pain I83.811
        - specified complication NEC I83.891
        - swelling I83.891
        - ulcer I83.Ø19
          - with inflammation I83.219
          - ankle I83.Ø13
            - with inflammation I83.213
          - calf I83.Ø12
            - with inflammation I83.212
          - foot NEC I83.Ø15
            - with inflammation I83.215
          - heel I83.Ø14
            - with inflammation I83.214
          - lower leg NEC I83.Ø18
            - with inflammation I83.218
          - midfoot I83.Ø14
            - with inflammation I83.214
          - thigh I83.Ø11
            - with inflammation I83.211
  - nasal septum I86.8
  - orbit I86.8
    - congenital Q27.8
  - ovary I86.2
  - papillary I78.1
  - pelvis I86.2
  - perineum I86.3
  - pharynx I86.8
  - placenta O43.89- ☑
  - renal papilla I86.8
  - retina H35.Ø9
  - scrotum (ulcerated) I86.1
  - sigmoid colon I86.8
  - specified site NEC I86.8
  - spinal (cord) (vessels) I86.8

Varix — *continued*
- spleen, splenic (vein) (with phlebolith) I86.8
- stomach I86.4
- sublingual I86.Ø
- ulcerated I83.ØØ9
  - inflamed or infected I83.2Ø9
- uterine ligament I86.2
- vagina I86.8
- vocal cord I86.8
- vulva I86.3

Vas deferens — *see* condition
Vas deferentitis N49.1
Vasa previa O69.4 ☑
- hemorrhage from, affecting newborn P5Ø.Ø

Vascular — *see also* condition
- loop on optic papilla Q14.2
- spasm I73.9
- spider I78.1

Vascularization, cornea — *see* Neovascularization, cornea
Vasculitis I77.6
- allergic D69.Ø
- ANCA (antineutrophilic cytoplasmic antibody) associated I77.82
- ANCA (antineutrophilic cytoplasmic antibody) positive I77.82
- antineutrophilic cytoplasmic antibody [ANCA] I77.82
- cryoglobulinemic D89.1
- disseminated I77.6
- hypocomplementemic M31.8
- kidney I77.89
- leukocytoclastic M31.Ø
- livedoid L95.Ø
- nodular L95.8
- retina H35.Ø6- ☑
- rheumatic — *see* Fever, rheumatic
- rheumatoid — *see* Rheumatoid, vasculitis
- skin (limited to) L95.9
  - specified NEC L95.8
- systemic M31.8

Vasculopathy, necrotizing M31.9
- cardiac allograft T86.29Ø
- specified NEC M31.8

Vasitis (nodosa) N49.1
- tuberculous A18.15

Vasodilation I73.9
Vasomotor — *see* condition
Vasoplasty, after previous sterilization Z31.Ø
- aftercare Z31.42

Vasospasm (vasoconstriction) — *see also* Angiospasm I73.9
- cerebral (cerebrovascular) (artery) I67.848
  - reversible I67.841
- coronary I2Ø.1
- nerve
  - arm — *see* Mononeuropathy, upper limb
  - brachial plexus G54.Ø
  - cervical plexus G54.2
  - leg — *see* Mononeuropathy, lower limb
- peripheral NOS I73.9
- retina (artery) — *see* Occlusion, artery, retina

Vasospastic — *see* condition
Vasovagal attack (paroxysmal) R55
- psychogenic F45.8

VATER syndrome Q87.2
Vater's ampulla — *see* condition
Vegetation, vegetative
- adenoid (nasal fossa) J35.8
- endocarditis (acute) (any valve) (subacute) I33.Ø
- heart (mycotic) (valve) I33.Ø

Veil
- Jackson's Q43.3

Vein, venous — *see* condition
Veldt sore — *see* Ulcer, skin
Velpeau's hernia — *see* Hernia, femoral
Venereal
- bubo A55
- disease A64
- granuloma inguinale A58
- lymphogranuloma (Durand-Nicolas-Favre) A55

Venofibrosis I87.8
Venom, venomous — *see* Table of Drugs and Chemicals, by animal or substance, poisoning
Venous — *see* condition
Ventilator lung, newborn P27.8
Ventral — *see* condition
Ventricle, ventricular — *see also* condition
- escape I49.3

Ventricle, ventricular — *continued*
- inversion Q2Ø.5

Ventriculitis (cerebral) — *see also* Encephalitis GØ4.9Ø
Ventriculostomy status Z98.2
Vernet's syndrome G52.7
Verneuil's disease (syphilitic bursitis) A52.78
Verruca (due to HPV) (filiformis) (simplex) (viral) (vulgaris) BØ7.9
- acuminata A63.Ø
- necrogenica (primary) (tuberculosa) A18.4
- plana BØ7.8
- plantaris BØ7.Ø
- seborrheica L82.1
  - inflamed L82.Ø
- senile (seborrheic) L82.1
  - inflamed L82.Ø
- tuberculosa (primary) A18.4
- venereal A63.Ø

Verrucosities — *see* Verruca
Verruga peruana, peruviana A44.1
Version
- cervix — *see* Malposition, uterus
- uterus (postinfectional) (postpartal, old) — *see* Malposition, uterus

Vertebra, vertebral — *see* condition
Vertical talus (congenital) Q66.8Ø
- left foot Q66.82
- right foot Q66.81

Vertigo R42
- auditory — *see* Vertigo, aural
- aural H81.31- ☑
- benign paroxysmal (positional) H81.1- ☑
- central (origin) H81.4
- cerebral H81.4
- Dix and Hallpike (epidemic) — *see* Neuronitis, vestibular
- due to infrasound T75.23 ☑
- epidemic A88.1
  - Dix and Hallpike — *see* Neuronitis, vestibular
  - Pedersen's — *see* Neuronitis, vestibular
  - vestibular neuronitis — *see* Neuronitis, vestibular
- hysterical F44.89
- infrasound T75.23 ☑
- labyrinthine — *see* subcategory H81.Ø ☑
- laryngeal RØ5.4
- malignant positional H81.4
- Meniere's — *see* subcategory H81.Ø ☑
- menopausal N95.1
- otogenic — *see* Vertigo, aural
- paroxysmal positional, benign — *see* Vertigo, benign paroxysmal
- Pedersen's (epidemic) — *see* Neuronitis, vestibular
- peripheral NEC H81.39- ☑
- positional
  - benign paroxysmal — *see* Vertigo, benign paroxysmal
  - malignant H81.4

Very-low-density-lipoprotein-type (VLDL) **hyperlipoproteinemia** E78.1
Vesania — *see* Psychosis
Vesical — *see* condition
Vesicle
- cutaneous R23.8
- seminal — *see* condition
- skin R23.8

Vesicocolic — *see* condition
Vesicoperineal — *see* condition
Vesicorectal — *see* condition
Vesicourethrorectal — *see* condition
Vesicovaginal — *see* condition
Vesicular — *see* condition
Vesiculitis (seminal) N49.Ø
- amebic AØ6.82
- gonorrheal (acute) (chronic) A54.23
- trichomonal A59.Ø9
- tuberculous A18.15

Vestibulitis (ear) — *see also* subcategory H83.Ø ☑
- nose (external) J34.89
- vulvar N94.81Ø

Vestibulopathy , acute peripheral (recurrent) — *see* Neuronitis, vestibular
Vestige, vestigial — *see also* Persistence
- branchial Q18.Ø
- structures in vitreous Q14.Ø

Vibration
- adverse effects T75.2Ø ☑
  - pneumatic hammer syndrome T75.21 ☑

Vibration — *continued*
- adverse effects — *continued*
  - specified effect NEC T75.29 ☑
  - vasospastic syndrome T75.22 ☑
  - vertigo from infrasound T75.23 ☑
- exposure (occupational) Z57.7
- vertigo T75.23 ☑

Vibriosis A28.9
Victim (of)
- crime Z65.4
- disaster Z65.5
- terrorism Z65.4
- torture Z65.4
- war Z65.5

Vidal's disease L28.Ø
Villaret's syndrome G52.7
Villous — *see* condition
VIN — *see* Neoplasia, intraepithelial, vulva
Vincent's infection (angina) (gingivitis) A69.1
- stomatitis NEC A69.1

Vinson-Plummer syndrome D5Ø.1
Violence, physical R45.6
Viosterol deficiency — *see* Deficiency, calciferol
Vipoma — *see* Neoplasm, malignant, by site
Viremia B34.9
Virilism (adrenal) E25.9
- congenital E25.Ø

Virilization (female) (suprarenal) E25.9
- congenital E25.Ø
- isosexual E28.2

Virulent bubo A57
Virus, viral — *see also* condition
- as cause of disease classified elsewhere B97.89
  - respiratory syncytial virus (RSV) — *see* Virus, respiratory syncytial (RSV)
- cytomegalovirus B25.9
- human immunodeficiency (HIV) — *see* Human, immunodeficiency virus (HIV) disease
- infection — *see* Infection, virus
- respiratory syncytial (RSV)
  - as cause of disease classified elsewhere B97.4
  - bronchiolitis J21.Ø
  - bronchitis J2Ø.5
  - bronchopneumonia J12.1
  - otitis media H65.- ☑ *[B97.4]*
  - pneumonia J12.1
  - upper respiratory infection JØ6.9 *[B97.4]*
- specified NEC B34.8
- swine influenza (viruses that normally cause infections in pigs) — *see also* Influenza, due to, identified novel influenza A virus JØ9.X2
- West Nile (fever) A92.3Ø
  - with
    - complications NEC A92.39
    - cranial nerve disorders A92.32
    - encephalitis A92.31
    - encephalomyelitis A92.31
    - neurologic manifestation NEC A92.32
    - optic neuritis A92.32
    - polyradiculitis A92.32

Viscera, visceral — *see* condition
Visceroptosis K63.4
Visible peristalsis R19.2
Vision, visual
- binocular, suppression H53.34
- blurred, blurring H53.8
  - hysterical F44.6
- defect, defective NEC H54.7
- disorientation (syndrome) H53.8
- disturbance H53.9
  - hysterical F44.6
- double H53.2
- examination ZØ1.ØØ
  - with abnormal findings ZØ1.Ø1
  - following failed vision screening ZØ1.Ø2Ø
    - with abnormal findings ZØ1.Ø21
- field, limitation (defect) — *see* Defect, visual field
- hallucinations R44.1
- halos H53.19
- loss — *see* Loss, vision
  - sudden — *see* Disturbance, vision, subjective, loss, sudden
- low (both eyes) — *see* Low, vision
- perception, simultaneous without fusion H53.33

Vitality, lack or want of R53.83
- newborn P96.89

Vitamin deficiency — *see* Deficiency, vitamin

Vitelline duct, persistent Q43.Ø
Vitiligo L8Ø
- eyelid HØ2.739
  - left HØ2.736
    - lower HØ2.735
    - upper HØ2.734
  - right HØ2.733
    - lower HØ2.732
    - upper HØ2.731
- pinta A67.2
- vulva N9Ø.89

Vitreal corneal syndrome H59.Ø1- ☑
Vitreoretinopathy, proliferative — *see also* Retinopathy, proliferative
- with retinal detachment — *see* Detachment, retina, traction

Vitreous — *see also* condition
- touch syndrome — *see* Complication, postprocedural, following cataract surgery

Vocal cord — *see* condition
Vogt-Koyanagi syndrome H2Ø.82- ☑
Vogt's disease or syndrome G8Ø.3
Vogt-Spielmeyer amaurotic idiocy or disease E75.4
Voice
- change R49.9
  - specified NEC R49.8
- loss — *see* Aphonia

Volhynian fever A79.Ø
Volkmann's ischemic contracture or paralysis (complicating trauma) T79.6 ☑
Volvulus (bowel) (colon) (intestine) K56.2
- with perforation K56.2
- congenital Q43.8
- duodenum K31.5
- fallopian tube — *see* Torsion, fallopian tube
- oviduct — *see* Torsion, fallopian tube
- stomach (due to absence of gastrocolic ligament) K31.89

Vomiting R11.1Ø
- with nausea R11.2
- asphyxia — *see* Foreign body, by site, causing asphyxia, gastric contents
- bilious (cause unknown) R11.14
  - following gastro-intestinal surgery K91.Ø
  - in newborn P92.Ø1
- blood — *see* Hematemesis
- causing asphyxia, choking, or suffocation — *see* Foreign body, by site
- cyclical, in migraine G43.AØ (*following* G43.7)
  - with refractory migraine G43.A1 (*following* G43.7)
  - intractable G43.A1 (*following* G43.7)
  - not intractable G43.AØ (*following* G43.7)
  - psychogenic F5Ø.89
  - without refractory migraine G43.AØ (*following* G43.7)
- cyclical syndrome NOS (unrelated to migraine) R11.15
- fecal mater R11.13
- following gastrointestinal surgery K91.Ø
  - psychogenic F5Ø.89
- functional K31.89
- hysterical F5Ø.89
- nervous F5Ø.89
- neurotic F5Ø.89
- newborn NEC P92.Ø9
  - bilious P92.Ø1
- periodic R11.1Ø
  - psychogenic F5Ø.89
- persistent R11.15
- projectile R11.12
- psychogenic F5Ø.89
- uremic — *see* Uremia
- without nausea R11.11

Vomito negro — *see* Fever, yellow
Von Bezold's abscess — *see* Mastoiditis, acute
Von Economo-Cruchet disease A85.8
Von Eulenburg's disease G71.19
Von Gierke's disease E74.Ø1
Von Hippel (-Lindau) **disease or syndrome** Q85.83
Von Jaksch's anemia or disease D64.89
Von Recklinghausen
- disease (neurofibromatosis) Q85.Ø1
  - bones E21.Ø

Von Schroetter's syndrome I82.89Ø
Von Willebrand (-Jurgens) (-Minot) **disease or syndrome** — *see* Disease, von Willebrand
Von Zumbusch's disease L4Ø.1
Voyeurism F65.3
Vrolik's disease Q78.Ø
Vulva — *see* condition
Vulvismus N94.2
Vulvitis (acute) (allergic) (atrophic) (hypertrophic) (intertriginous) (senile) N76.2
- with ectopic or molar pregnancy OØ8.Ø
- adhesive, congenital Q52.79
- blennorrhagic (gonococcal) A54.Ø2
- candidal (acute) B37.31
  - chronic (recurrent) B37.32
- chlamydial A56.Ø2
- due to Haemophilus ducreyi A57
- following ectopic or molar pregnancy OØ8.Ø
- gonococcal A54.Ø2
  - with abscess (accessory gland) (periurethral) A54.1
- herpesviral A6Ø.Ø4
- leukoplakic N9Ø.4
- monilial (acute) B37.31
  - chronic (recurrent) B37.32
- puerperal (postpartum) O86.19
- subacute or chronic N76.3
- syphilitic (early) A51.Ø
  - late A52.76
- trichomonal A59.Ø1
- tuberculous A18.18

Vulvodynia N94.819
- specified NEC N94.818

Vulvorectal — *see* condition
Vulvovaginitis (acute) — *see* Vaginitis

W

Waiting list, person on Z75.1
- for organ transplant Z76.82
- undergoing social agency investigation Z75.2

Waldenstrom
- hypergammaglobulinemia D89.Ø
- syndrome or macroglobulinemia C88.Ø

Waldenstrom-Kjellberg syndrome D5Ø.1
Walking
- difficulty R26.2
  - psychogenic F44.4
- sleep F51.3
  - hysterical F44.89

Wall, abdominal — *see* condition
Wallenberg's disease or syndrome G46.3
Wallgren's disease I87.8
Wandering
- gallbladder, congenital Q44.1
- in diseases classified elsewhere Z91.83
- kidney, congenital Q63.8
- organ or site, congenital NEC — *see* Malposition, congenital, by site
- pacemaker (heart) I49.8
- spleen D73.89

War neurosis F48.8
Wart (due to HPV) (filiform) (infectious) (viral) BØ7.9
- anogenital region (venereal) A63.Ø
- common BØ7.8
- external genital organs (venereal) A63.Ø
- flat BØ7.8
- Hassal-Henle's (of cornea) H18.49
- Peruvian A44.1
- plantar BØ7.Ø
- prosector (tuberculous) A18.4
- seborrheic L82.1
  - inflamed L82.Ø
- senile (seborrheic) L82.1
  - inflamed L82.Ø
- tuberculous A18.4
- venereal A63.Ø

Warthin's tumor — *see* Neoplasm, salivary gland, benign
Wassilieff's disease A27.Ø
Wasting
- disease (syndrome) E88.A
  - due to
    - malnutrition E43
      - with marasmus E41
    - underlying condition E88.A
- extreme (due to malnutrition) E43
  - with marasmus E41
- muscle NEC — *see* Atrophy, muscle

Water
- clefts (senile cataract) — *see* Cataract, senile, incipient
- deprivation of T73.1 ☑
- intoxication E87.79
- itch B76.9
- lack of T73.1 ☑
  - safe drinking Z58.6

Water — *continued*
- loading E87.7Ø
- on
  - brain — *see* Hydrocephalus
  - chest J94.8
- poisoning E87.79

Waterbrash R12
Waterhouse (-Friderichsen) **syndrome or disease** (meningococcal) A39.1
Water-losing nephritis N25.89
Watermelon stomach K31.819
- with hemorrhage K31.811
- without hemorrhage K31.819

Watsoniasis B66.8
Wax in ear — *see* Impaction, cerumen
Weak, weakening, weakness (generalized) R53.1
- arches (acquired) — *see also* Deformity, limb, flat foot
- bladder (sphincter) R32
- facial R29.81Ø
  - following
    - cerebrovascular disease I69.992
      - cerebral infarction I69.392
      - intracerebral hemorrhage I69.192
      - nontraumatic intracranial hemorrhage NEC I69.292
      - specified disease NEC I69.892
      - stroke I69.392
      - subarachnoid hemorrhage I69.Ø92
- foot (double) — *see also* Weak, arches
- heart, cardiac — *see* Failure, heart
- mind F7Ø
- muscle M62.81
- myocardium — *see* Failure, heart
- newborn P96.89
- pelvic fundus N81.89
- pubocervical tissue N81.82
- rectovaginal tissue N81.83
- senile R54
- urinary stream R39.12
- valvular — *see* Endocarditis

Wear, worn (with normal or routine use)
- articular bearing surface of internal joint prosthesis — *see* Complications, joint prosthesis, mechanical, wear of articular bearing surfaces, by site
- device, implant or graft — *see* Complications, by site, mechanical complication
- tooth, teeth (approximal) (hard tissues) (interproximal) (occlusal) KØ3.Ø

Weather, weathered
- effects of
  - cold T69.9 ☑
    - specified effect NEC T69.8 ☑
  - hot — *see* Heat
- skin L57.8

Weaver's syndrome Q87.3
Web, webbed (congenital)
- duodenal Q43.8
- esophagus Q39.4
- fingers Q7Ø.1- ☑
- larynx (glottic) (subglottic) Q31.Ø
- neck (pterygium colli) Q18.3
- Paterson-Kelly D5Ø.1
- popliteal syndrome Q87.89
- toes Q7Ø.3- ☑

Weber-Christian disease M35.6
Weber-Cockayne syndrome (epidermolysis bullosa) Q81.8
Weber-Gubler syndrome G46.3
Weber-Leyden syndrome G46.3
Weber-Osler syndrome I78.Ø
Weber's paralysis or syndrome G46.3
Wedge-shaped or wedging vertebra — *see* Collapse, vertebra NEC
Wegener's granulomatosis or syndrome M31.3Ø
- with
  - kidney involvement M31.31
  - lung involvement M31.3Ø
    - with kidney involvement M31.31

Wegner's disease A5Ø.Ø2
Weight
- 1ØØØ-2499 grams at birth (low) — *see* Low, birthweight
- 999 grams or less at birth (extremely low) — *see* Low, birthweight, extreme
- and length below 1Øth percentile for gestational age PØ5.1- ☑
- below but length above 1Øth percentile for gestational age PØ5.Ø- ☑

- **Wound, open** — *continued*
  - buttock S31.809 ☑
    - bite — *see* Bite, buttock
    - laceration — *see* Laceration, buttock
    - left S31.829 ☑
    - puncture — *see* Puncture, buttock
    - right S31.819 ☑
  - calf — *see* Wound, open, leg
  - canaliculus lacrimalis — *see* Wound, open, eyelid
  - canthus, eye — *see* Wound, open, eyelid
  - cervical esophagus S11.20 ☑
    - bite S11.25 ☑
    - laceration — *see* Laceration, esophagus, traumatic, cervical
    - puncture — *see* Puncture, cervical esophagus
  - cheek (external) S01.40- ☑
    - bite — *see* Bite, cheek
    - internal — *see* Wound, open, oral cavity
    - laceration — *see* Laceration, cheek
    - puncture — *see* Puncture, cheek
  - chest wall — *see* Wound, open, thorax
  - chin — *see* Wound, open, head, specified site NEC
  - choroid — *see* Wound, open, ocular
  - ciliary body (eye) — *see* Wound, open, ocular
  - clitoris S31.40 ☑
    - with amputation — *see* Amputation, traumatic, clitoris
    - bite S31.45 ☑
    - laceration — *see* Laceration, vulva
    - puncture — *see* Puncture, vulva
  - conjunctiva — *see* Wound, open, ocular
  - cornea — *see* Wound, open, ocular
  - costal region — *see* Wound, open, thorax
  - Descemet's membrane — *see* Wound, open, ocular
  - digit(s)
    - foot — *see* Wound, open, toe
    - hand — *see* Wound, open, finger
  - ear (canal) (external) S01.30- ☑
    - with amputation — *see* Amputation, traumatic, ear
    - bite — *see* Bite, ear
    - drum S09.2- ☑
    - laceration — *see* Laceration, ear
    - puncture — *see* Puncture, ear
  - elbow S51.00- ☑
    - bite — *see* Bite, elbow
    - laceration — *see* Laceration, elbow
    - puncture — *see* Puncture, elbow
  - epididymis — *see* Wound, open, testis
  - epigastric region S31.102 ☑
    - with penetration into peritoneal cavity S31.602 ☑
    - bite — *see* Bite, abdomen, wall, epigastric region
    - laceration — *see* Laceration, abdomen, wall, epigastric region
    - puncture — *see* Puncture, abdomen, wall, epigastric region
  - epiglottis — *see* Wound, open, neck, specified site NEC
  - esophagus (thoracic) S27.819 ☑
    - cervical — *see* Wound, open, cervical esophagus
    - laceration S27.813 ☑
    - specified type NEC S27.818 ☑
  - eye — *see* Wound, open, ocular
  - eyeball — *see* Wound, open, ocular
  - eyebrow — *see* Wound, open, eyelid
  - eyelid S01.10- ☑
    - bite — *see* Bite, eyelid
    - laceration — *see* Laceration, eyelid
    - puncture — *see* Puncture, eyelid
  - face NEC — *see* Wound, open, head, specified site NEC
  - finger(s) S61.209 ☑
    - with
      - amputation — *see* Amputation, traumatic, finger
      - damage to nail S61.309 ☑
    - bite — *see* Bite, finger
    - index S61.208 ☑
      - with
        - damage to nail S61.308 ☑
      - left S61.201 ☑
        - with
          - damage to nail S61.301 ☑
      - right S61.200 ☑
        - with
          - damage to nail S61.300 ☑
    - laceration — *see* Laceration, finger
    - little S61.208 ☑
      - with
        - damage to nail S61.308 ☑

- **Wound, open** — *continued*
  - finger(s) — *continued*
    - little — *continued*
      - left S61.207 ☑
        - with damage to nail S61.307 ☑
      - right S61.206 ☑
        - with damage to nail S61.306 ☑
    - middle S61.208 ☑
      - with
        - damage to nail S61.308 ☑
      - left S61.203 ☑
        - with damage to nail S61.303 ☑
      - right S61.202 ☑
        - with damage to nail S61.302 ☑
    - puncture — *see* Puncture, finger
    - ring S61.208 ☑
      - with
        - damage to nail S61.308 ☑
      - left S61.205 ☑
        - with damage to nail S61.305 ☑
      - right S61.204 ☑
        - with damage to nail S61.304 ☑
  - flank — *see* Wound, open, abdomen, wall
  - foot (except toe(s) alone) S91.30- ☑
    - with amputation — *see* Amputation, traumatic, foot
    - bite — *see* Bite, foot
    - laceration — *see* Laceration, foot
    - puncture — *see* Puncture, foot
    - toe — *see* Wound, open, toe
  - forearm S51.80- ☑
    - with
      - amputation — *see* Amputation, traumatic, forearm
    - bite — *see* Bite, forearm
    - elbow only — *see* Wound, open, elbow
    - laceration — *see* Laceration, forearm
    - puncture — *see* Puncture, forearm
  - forehead — *see* Wound, open, head, specified site NEC
  - genital organs, external
    - with amputation — *see* Amputation, traumatic, genital organs
    - bite — *see* Bite, genital organ
    - female S31.502 ☑
      - vagina S31.40 ☑
      - vulva S31.40 ☑
    - laceration — *see* Laceration, genital organ
    - male S31.501 ☑
      - penis S31.20 ☑
      - scrotum S31.30 ☑
      - testes S31.30 ☑
    - puncture — *see* Puncture, genital organ
  - globe (eye) — *see* Wound, open, ocular
  - groin — *see* Wound, open, abdomen, wall
  - gum — *see* Wound, open, oral cavity
  - hand S61.40- ☑
    - with
      - amputation — *see* Amputation, traumatic, hand
    - bite — *see* Bite, hand
    - finger(s) — *see* Wound, open, finger
    - laceration — *see* Laceration, hand
    - puncture — *see* Puncture, hand
    - thumb — *see* Wound, open, thumb
  - head S01.90 ☑
    - bite — *see* Bite, head
    - cheek — *see* Wound, open, cheek
    - ear — *see* Wound, open, ear
    - eyelid — *see* Wound, open, eyelid
    - laceration — *see* Laceration, head
    - lip — *see* Wound, open, lip
    - nose S01.20 ☑
    - oral cavity — *see* Wound, open, oral cavity
    - puncture — *see* Puncture, head
    - scalp — *see* Wound, open, scalp
    - specified site NEC S01.80 ☑
    - temporomandibular area — *see* Wound, open, cheek
  - heel — *see* Wound, open, foot
  - hip S71.00- ☑
    - with amputation — *see* Amputation, traumatic, hip
    - bite — *see* Bite, hip
    - laceration — *see* Laceration, hip
    - puncture — *see* Puncture, hip
  - hymen S31.40 ☑
    - bite — *see* Bite, vulva
    - laceration — *see* Laceration, vagina
    - puncture — *see* Puncture, vagina

- **Wound, open** — *continued*
  - hypochondrium S31.109 ☑
    - bite — *see* Bite, hypochondrium
    - laceration — *see* Laceration, hypochondrium
    - puncture — *see* Puncture, hypochondrium
  - hypogastric region S31.109 ☑
    - bite — *see* Bite, hypogastric region
    - laceration — *see* Laceration, hypogastric region
    - puncture — *see* Puncture, hypogastric region
  - iliac (region) — *see* Wound, open, inguinal region
  - inguinal region S31.109 ☑
    - bite — *see* Bite, abdomen, wall, lower quadrant
    - laceration — *see* Laceration, inguinal region
    - puncture — *see* Puncture, inguinal region
  - instep — *see* Wound, open, foot
  - interscapular region — *see* Wound, open, thorax, back
  - intraocular — *see* Wound, open, ocular
  - iris — *see* Wound, open, ocular
  - jaw — *see* Wound, open, head, specified site NEC
  - knee S81.00- ☑
    - bite — *see* Bite, knee
    - laceration — *see* Laceration, knee
    - puncture — *see* Puncture, knee
  - labium (majus) (minus) — *see* Wound, open, vulva
  - laceration — *see* Laceration, by site
  - lacrimal duct — *see* Wound, open, eyelid
  - larynx S11.019 ☑
    - bite — *see* Bite, larynx
    - laceration — *see* Laceration, larynx
    - puncture — *see* Puncture, larynx
  - left
    - lower quadrant S31.104 ☑
      - with penetration into peritoneal cavity S31.604 ☑
      - bite — *see* Bite, abdomen, wall, left, lower quadrant
      - laceration — *see* Laceration, abdomen, wall, left, lower quadrant
      - puncture — *see* Puncture, abdomen, wall, left, lower quadrant
    - upper quadrant S31.101 ☑
      - with penetration into peritoneal cavity S31.601 ☑
      - bite — *see* Bite, abdomen, wall, left, upper quadrant
      - laceration — *see* Laceration, abdomen, wall, left, upper quadrant
      - puncture — *see* Puncture, abdomen, wall, left, upper quadrant
  - leg (lower) S81.80- ☑
    - with amputation — *see* Amputation, traumatic, leg
    - ankle — *see* Wound, open, ankle
    - bite — *see* Bite, leg
    - foot — *see* Wound, open, foot
    - knee — *see* Wound, open, knee
    - laceration — *see* Laceration, leg
    - puncture — *see* Puncture, leg
    - toe — *see* Wound, open, toe
    - upper — *see* Wound, open, thigh
  - lip S01.501 ☑
    - bite — *see* Bite, lip
    - laceration — *see* Laceration, lip
    - puncture — *see* Puncture, lip
  - loin S31.109 ☑
    - bite — *see* Bite, abdomen, wall
    - laceration — *see* Laceration, loin
    - puncture — *see* Puncture, loin
  - lower back — *see* Wound, open, back, lower
  - lumbar region — *see* Wound, open, back, lower
  - malar region — *see* Wound, open, head, specified site NEC
  - mammary — *see* Wound, open, breast
  - mastoid region — *see* Wound, open, head, specified site NEC
  - mouth — *see* Wound, open, oral cavity
  - nail
    - finger — *see* Wound, open, finger, with damage to nail
    - toe — *see* Wound, open, toe, with damage to nail
  - nape (neck) — *see* Wound, open, neck
  - nasal (septum) (sinus) — *see* Wound, open, nose
  - nasopharynx — *see* Wound, open, head, specified site NEC
  - neck S11.90 ☑
    - bite — *see* Bite, neck

X

Y

Z

Note: The list below gives the code number for neoplasms by anatomical site. For each site there are six possible code numbers according to whether the neoplasm in question is malignant, benign, in situ, of uncertain behavior, or of unspecified nature. The description of the neoplasm will often indicate which of the six columns is appropriate; e.g., malignant melanoma of skin, benign fibroadenoma of breast, carcinoma in situ of cervix uteri. Where such descriptors are not present, the remainder of the Index should be consulted where guidance is given to the appropriate column for each morphological (histological) variety listed; e.g., Mesonephroma – see Neoplasm, malignant; Embryoma — see also Neoplasm, uncertain behavior; Disease, Bowen's – see Neoplasm, skin, in situ. However, the guidance in the Index can be overridden if one of the descriptors mentioned above is present; e.g., malignant adenoma of colon is coded to C18.9 and not to D12.6 as the adjective "malignant" overrides the Index entry "Adenoma — *see also* Neoplasm, benign, by site." Codes listed with a dash -, following the code have a required additional character for laterality. The tabular list must be reviewed for the complete code.

	Malignant Primary	Malignant Secondary	Ca in situ	Benign	Uncertain Behavior	Unspecified Behavior
Neoplasm, neoplastic	C8Ø.1	C79.9	DØ9.9	D36.9	D48.9	D49.9
abdomen, abdominal	C76.2	C79.8-☑	DØ9.8	D36.7	D48.7	D49.89
cavity	C76.2	C79.8-☑	DØ9.8	D36.7	D48.7	D49.89
organ	C76.2	C79.8-☑	DØ9.8	D36.7	D48.7	D49.89
viscera	C76.2	C79.8-☑	DØ9.8	D36.7	D48.7	D49.89
wall — *see also* Neoplasm, abdomen, wall, skin	C44.5Ø9	C79.2	DØ4.5	D23.5	D48.5	D49.2
connective tissue	C49.4	C79.8-☑	—	D21.4	D48.1☑	D49.2
skin	C44.5Ø9	—	—	—	—	—
basal cell carcinoma	C44.519	—	—	—	—	—
specified type NEC	C44.599	—	—	—	—	—
squamous cell carcinoma	C44.529	—	—	—	—	—
abdominopelvic	C76.8	C79.8-☑	—	D36.7	D48.7	D49.89
accessory sinus — *see* Neoplasm, sinus						
acoustic nerve	C72.4-☑	C79.49	—	D33.3	D43.3	D49.7
adenoid (pharynx) (tissue)	C11.1	C79.89	DØØ.Ø8	D1Ø.6	D37.Ø5	D49.Ø
adipose tissue — *see also* Neoplasm, connective tissue	C49.4	C79.89	—	D21.9	D48.1☑	D49.2
adnexa (uterine)	C57.4	C79.89	DØ7.39	D28.7	D39.8	D49.59
adrenal	C74.9-☑	C79.7-☑	DØ9.3	D35.Ø-☑	D44.1-☑	D49.7
capsule	C74.9-☑	C79.7-☑	DØ9.3	D35.Ø-☑	D44.1-☑	D49.7
cortex	C74.Ø-☑	C79.7-☑	DØ9.3	D35.Ø-☑	D44.1-☑	D49.7
gland	C74.9-☑	C79.7-☑	DØ9.3	D35.Ø-☑	D44.1-☑	D49.7
medulla	C74.1-☑	C79.7-☑	DØ9.3	D35.Ø-☑	D44.1-☑	D49.7
ala nasi (external) — *see also* Neoplasm, skin, nose	C44.3Ø1	C79.2	DØ4.39	D23.39	D48.5	D49.2
alimentary canal or tract NEC	C26.9	C78.8Ø	DØ1.9	D13.99	D37.9	D49.Ø
alveolar	CØ3.9	C79.89	DØØ.Ø3	D1Ø.39	D37.Ø9	D49.Ø
mucosa	CØ3.9	C79.89	DØØ.Ø3	D1Ø.39	D37.Ø9	D49.Ø
lower	CØ3.1	C79.89	DØØ.Ø3	D1Ø.39	D37.Ø9	D49.Ø
upper	CØ3.Ø	C79.89	DØØ.Ø3	D1Ø.39	D37.Ø9	D49.Ø
ridge or process	C41.1	C79.51	—	D16.5	D48.Ø	D49.2
carcinoma	CØ3.9	C79.8-☑	—	—	—	—
lower	CØ3.1	C79.8-☑	—	—	—	—
upper	CØ3.Ø	C79.8-☑	—	—	—	—
lower	C41.1	C79.51	—	D16.5	D48.Ø	D49.2
mucosa	CØ3.9	C79.89	DØØ.Ø3	D1Ø.39	D37.Ø9	D49.Ø
lower	CØ3.1	C79.89	DØØ.Ø3	D1Ø.39	D37.Ø9	D49.Ø
upper	CØ3.Ø	C79.89	DØØ.Ø3	D1Ø.39	D37.Ø9	D49.Ø
upper	C41.Ø	C79.51	—	D16.4	D48.Ø	D49.2
sulcus	CØ6.1	C79.89	DØØ.Ø2	D1Ø.39	D37.Ø9	D49.Ø
alveolus	CØ3.9	C79.89	DØØ.Ø3	D1Ø.39	D37.Ø9	D49.Ø
lower	CØ3.1	C79.89	DØØ.Ø3	D1Ø.39	D37.Ø9	D49.Ø
upper	CØ3.Ø	C79.89	DØØ.Ø3	D1Ø.39	D37.Ø9	D49.Ø
ampulla of Vater	C24.1	C78.89	DØ1.5	D13.5	D37.6	D49.Ø
ankle NEC	C76.5-☑	C79.89	DØ4.7-☑	D36.7	D48.7	D49.89
anorectum, anorectal (junction)	C21.8	C78.5	DØ1.3	D12.9	D37.8	D49.Ø
antecubital fossa or space	C76.4-☑	C79.89	DØ4.6-☑	D36.7	D48.7	D49.89
Neoplasm, neoplastic — *continued*						
antrum (Highmore) (maxillary)	C31.Ø	C78.39	DØ2.3	D14.Ø	D38.5	D49.1
pyloric	C16.3	C78.89	DØØ.2	D13.1	D37.1	D49.Ø
tympanicum	C3Ø.1	C78.39	DØ2.3	D14.Ø	D38.5	D49.1
anus, anal	C21.Ø	C78.5	DØ1.3	D12.9	D37.8	D49.Ø
canal	C21.1	C78.5	DØ1.3	D12.9	D37.8	D49.Ø
cloacogenic zone	C21.2	C78.5	DØ1.3	D12.9	D37.8	D49.Ø
margin — *see also* Neoplasm, anus, skin	C44.5ØØ	C79.2	DØ4.5	D23.5	D48.5	D49.2
overlapping lesion with rectosigmoid junction or rectum	C21.8	—	—	—	—	—
skin	C44.5ØØ	C79.2	DØ4.5	D23.5	D48.5	D49.2
basal cell carcinoma	C44.51Ø	—	—	—	—	—
specified type NEC	C44.59Ø	—	—	—	—	—
squamous cell carcinoma	C44.52Ø	—	—	—	—	—
sphincter	C21.1	C78.5	DØ1.3	D12.9	D37.8	D49.Ø
aorta (thoracic)	C49.3	C79.89	—	D21.3	D48.1☑	D49.2
abdominal	C49.4	C79.89	—	D21.4	D48.1☑	D49.2
aortic body	C75.5	C79.89	—	D35.6	D44.7	D49.7
aponeurosis	C49.9	C79.89	—	D21.9	D48.1☑	D49.2
palmar	C49.1-☑	C79.89	—	D21.1-☑	D48.1☑	D49.2
plantar	C49.2-☑	C79.89	—	D21.2-☑	D48.1☑	D49.2
appendix	C18.1	C78.5	DØ1.Ø	D12.1	D37.3	D49.Ø
arachnoid	C7Ø.9	C79.49	—	D32.9	D42.9	D49.7
cerebral	C7Ø.Ø	C79.32	—	D32.Ø	D42.Ø	D49.7
spinal	C7Ø.1	C79.49	—	D32.1	D42.1	D49.7
areola	C5Ø.Ø-☑	C79.81	DØ5-☑	D24-☑	D48.6-☑	D49.3
arm NEC	C76.4-☑	C79.89	DØ4.6-☑	D36.7	D48.7	D49.89
artery — *see* Neoplasm, connective tissue						
aryepiglottic fold	C13.1	C79.89	DØØ.Ø8	D1Ø.7	D37.Ø5	D49.Ø
hypopharyngeal aspect	C13.1	C79.89	DØØ.Ø8	D1Ø.7	D37.Ø5	D49.Ø
laryngeal aspect	C32.1	C78.39	DØ2.Ø	D14.1	D38.Ø	D49.1
marginal zone	C13.1	C79.89	DØØ.Ø8	D1Ø.7	D37.Ø5	D49.Ø
arytenoid (cartilage)	C32.3	C78.39	DØ2.Ø	D14.1	D38.Ø	D49.1
fold — *see* Neoplasm, aryepiglottic						
associated with transplanted organ	C8Ø.2	—	—	—	—	—
atlas	C41.2	C79.51	—	D16.6	D48.Ø	D49.2
atrium, cardiac	C38.Ø	C79.89	—	D15.1	D48.7	D49.89
auditory						
canal (external) (skin)	C44.2Ø-☑	C79.2	DØ4.2-☑	D23.2-☑	D48.5	D49.2
internal	C3Ø.1	C78.39	DØ2.3	D14.Ø	D38.5	D49.1
nerve	C72.4-☑	C79.49	—	D33.3	D43.3	D49.7
tube	C3Ø.1	C78.39	DØ2.3	D14.Ø	D38.5	D49.1
opening	C11.2	C79.89	DØØ.Ø8	D1Ø.6	D37.Ø5	D49.Ø
auricle, ear — *see also* Neoplasm, skin, ear	C44.2Ø-☑	C79.2	DØ4.2-☑	D23.2-☑	D48.5	D49.2
auricular canal (external) — *see also* Neoplasm, skin, ear	C44.2Ø-☑	C79.2	DØ4.2-☑	D23.2-☑	D48.5	D49.2
internal	C3Ø.1	C78.39	DØ2.3	D14.Ø	D38.5	D49.2
autonomic nerve or nervous system NEC (see Neoplasm, nerve, peripheral)						
axilla, axillary	C76.1	C79.89	DØ9.8	D36.7	D48.7	D49.89
fold — *see also* Neoplasm, skin, trunk	C44.5Ø9	C79.2	DØ4.5	D23.5	D48.5	D49.2
back NEC	C76.8	C79.89	DØ4.5	D36.7	D48.7	D49.89
Bartholin's gland	C51.Ø	C79.82	DØ7.1	D28.Ø	D39.8	D49.59
basal ganglia	C71.Ø	C79.31	—	D33.Ø	D43.Ø	D49.6
basis pedunculi	C71.7	C79.31	—	D33.1	D43.1	D49.6
bile or biliary (tract)	C24.9	C78.89	DØ1.5	D13.5	D37.6	D49.Ø

	Malignant Primary	Malignant Secondary	Ca in situ	Benign	Uncertain Behavior	Unspecified Behavior
Neoplasm, neoplastic *— continued*						
bile or biliary — *continued*						
canaliculi (biliferi) (intrahepatic)	C22.1	C78.7	DØ1.5	D13.4	D37.6	D49.Ø
canals, interlobular	C22.1	C78.89	DØ1.5	D13.4	D37.6	D49.Ø
duct or passage (common) (cystic) (extrahepatic)	C24.Ø	C78.89	DØ1.5	D13.5	D37.6	D49.Ø
interlobular	C22.1	C78.89	DØ1.5	D13.4	D37.6	D49.Ø
intrahepatic	C22.1	C78.7	DØ1.5	D13.4	D37.6	D49.Ø
and extrahepatic	C24.8	C78.89	DØ1.5	D13.5	D37.6	D49.Ø
bladder (urinary)	C67.9	C79.11	DØ9.Ø	D3Ø.3	D41.4	D49.4
dome	C67.1	C79.11	DØ9.Ø	D3Ø.3	D41.4	D49.4
neck	C67.5	C79.11	DØ9.Ø	D3Ø.3	D41.4	D49.4
orifice	C67.9	C79.11	DØ9.Ø	D3Ø.3	D41.4	D49.4
ureteric	C67.6	C79.11	DØ9.Ø	D3Ø.3	D41.4	D49.4
urethral	C67.5	C79.11	DØ9.Ø	D3Ø.3	D41.4	D49.4
overlapping lesion	C67.8	—	—	—	—	—
sphincter	C67.8	C79.11	DØ9.Ø	D3Ø.3	D41.4	D49.4
trigone	C67.Ø	C79.11	DØ9.Ø	D3Ø.3	D41.4	D49.4
urachus	C67.7	C79.11	DØ9.Ø	D3Ø.3	D41.4	D49.4
wall	C67.9	C79.11	DØ9.Ø	D3Ø.3	D41.4	D49.4
anterior	C67.3	C79.11	DØ9.Ø	D3Ø.3	D41.4	D49.4
lateral	C67.2	C79.11	DØ9.Ø	D3Ø.3	D41.4	D49.4
posterior	C67.4	C79.11	DØ9.Ø	D3Ø.3	D41.4	D49.4
blood vessel — *see* Neoplasm, connective tissue						
bone (periosteum)	C41.9	C79.51	—	D16.9-	D48.Ø	D49.2
acetabulum						
ankle	C4Ø.3-☑	C79.51	—	D16.3-☑	—	—
arm NEC	C4Ø.Ø-☑	C79.51	—	D16.Ø-☑	—	—
astragalus	C4Ø.3-☑	C79.51	—	D16.3-☑	—	—
atlas	C41.2	C79.51	—	D16.6	D48.Ø	D49.2
axis	C41.2	C79.51	—	D16.6	D48.Ø	D49.2
back NEC	C41.2	C79.51	—	D16.6	D48.Ø	D49.2
calcaneus	C4Ø.3-☑	C79.51	—	D16.3-☑	—	—
calvarium	C41.Ø	C79.51	—	D16.4	D48.Ø	D49.2
carpus (any)	C4Ø.1-☑	C79.51	—	D16.1-☑	—	—
cartilage NEC	C41.9	C79.51	—	D16.9	D48.Ø	D49.2
clavicle	C41.3	C79.51	—	D16.7	D48.Ø	D49.2
clivus	C41.Ø	C79.51	—	D16.4	D48.Ø	D49.2
coccygeal vertebra	C41.4	C79.51	—	D16.8	D48.Ø	D49.2
coccyx	C41.4	C79.51	—	D16.8	D48.Ø	D49.2
costal cartilage	C41.3	C79.51	—	D16.7	D48.Ø	D49.2
costovertebral joint	C41.3	C79.51	—	D16.7	D48.Ø	D49.2
cranial	C41.Ø	C79.51	—	D16.4	D48.Ø	D49.2
cuboid	C4Ø.3-☑	C79.51	—	D16.3-☑	—	—
cuneiform	C41.9	C79.51	—	D16.9	D48.Ø	D49.2
elbow	C4Ø.Ø-☑	C79.51	—	D16.Ø-☑	—	—
ethmoid (labyrinth)	C41.Ø	C79.51	—	D16.4	D48.Ø	D49.2
face	C41.Ø	C79.51	—	D16.4	D48.Ø	D49.2
femur (any part)	C4Ø.2-☑	C79.51	—	D16.2-☑	—	—
fibula (any part)	C4Ø.2-☑	C79.51	—	D16.2-☑	—	—
finger (any)	C4Ø.1-☑	C79.51	—	D16.1-☑	—	—
foot	C4Ø.3-☑	C79.51	—	D16.3-☑	—	—
forearm	C4Ø.Ø-☑	C79.51	—	D16.Ø-☑	—	—
frontal	C41.Ø	C79.51	—	D16.4	D48.Ø	D49.2
hand	C4Ø.1-☑	C79.51	—	D16.1-☑	—	—
heel	C4Ø.3-☑	C79.51	—	D16.3-☑	—	—
hip	C41.4	C79.51	—	D16.8	D48.Ø	D49.2
humerus (any part)	C4Ø.Ø-☑	C79.51	—	D16.Ø-☑	—	—
hyoid	C41.Ø	C79.51	—	D16.4	D48.Ø	D49.2
ilium	C41.4	C79.51	—	D16.8	D48.Ø	D49.2
innominate	C41.4	C79.51	—	D16.8	D48.Ø	D49.2
intervertebral cartilage or disc	C41.2	C79.51	—	D16.6	D48.Ø	D49.2
ischium	C41.4	C79.51	—	D16.8	D48.Ø	D49.2
jaw (lower)	C41.1	C79.51	—	D16.5	D48.Ø	D49.2
knee	C4Ø.2-☑	C79.51	—	D16.2-☑	—	—
leg NEC	C4Ø.2-☑	C79.51	—	D16.2-☑	—	—
limb NEC	C4Ø.9-☑	C79.51	—	D16.9	—	—
Neoplasm, neoplastic *— continued*						
bone — *continued*						
limb — *continued*						
lower (long bones)	C4Ø.2-☑	C79.51	—	D16.2-☑	—	—
short bones	C4Ø.3-☑	C79.51	—	D16.3-☑	—	—
upper (long bones)	C4Ø.Ø-☑	C79.51	—	D16.Ø-☑	—	—
short bones	C4Ø.1-☑	C79.51	—	D16.1-☑	—	—
malar	C41.Ø	C79.51	—	D16.4	D48.Ø	D49.2
mandible	C41.1	C79.51	—	D16.5	D48.Ø	D49.2
marrow NEC (any bone)	C96.9	C79.52	—	—	D47.9	D49.89
mastoid	C41.Ø	C79.51	—	D16.4	D48.Ø	D49.2
maxilla, maxillary (superior)	C41.Ø	C79.51	—	D16.4	D48.Ø	D49.2
inferior	C41.1	C79.51	—	D16.5	D48.Ø	D49.2
metacarpus (any)	C4Ø.1-☑	C79.51	—	D16.1-☑	—	—
metatarsus (any)	C4Ø.3-☑	C79.51	—	D16.3-☑	—	—
navicular						
ankle	C4Ø.3-☑	C79.51	—	—	—	—
hand	C4Ø.1-☑	C79.51	—	—	—	—
nose, nasal	C41.Ø	C79.51	—	D16.4	D48.Ø	D49.2
occipital	C41.Ø	C79.51	—	D16.4	D48.Ø	D49.2
orbit	C41.Ø	C79.51	—	D16.4	D48.Ø	D49.2
overlapping sites	C4Ø.8-☑	—	—	—	—	—
parietal	C41.Ø	C79.51	—	D16.4	D48.Ø	D49.2
patella	C4Ø.2-☑	C79.51	—	—	—	—
pelvic	C41.4	C79.51	—	D16.8	D48.Ø	D49.2
phalanges						
foot	C4Ø.3-☑	C79.51	—	—	—	—
hand	C4Ø.1-☑	C79.51	—	—	—	—
pubic	C41.4	C79.51	—	D16.8	D48.Ø	D49.2
radius (any part)	C4Ø.Ø-☑	C79.51	—	D16.Ø-☑	—	—
rib	C41.3	C79.51	—	D16.7	D48.Ø	D49.2
sacral vertebra	C41.4	C79.51	—	D16.8	D48.Ø	D49.2
sacrum	C41.4	C79.51	—	D16.8	D48.Ø	D49.2
scaphoid						
of ankle	C4Ø.3-☑	C79.51	—	—	—	—
of hand	C4Ø.1-☑	C79.51	—	—	—	—
scapula (any part)	C4Ø.Ø-☑	C79.51	—	D16.Ø-☑	—	—
sella turcica	C41.Ø	C79.51	—	D16.4	D48.Ø	D49.2
shoulder	C4Ø.Ø-☑	C79.51	—	D16.Ø-☑	—	—
skull	C41.Ø	C79.51	—	D16.4	D48.Ø	D49.2
sphenoid	C41.Ø	C79.51	—	D16.4	D48.Ø	D49.2
spine, spinal (column)	C41.2	C79.51	—	D16.6	D48.Ø	D49.2
coccyx	C41.4	C79.51	—	D16.8	D48.Ø	D49.2
sacrum	C41.4	C79.51	—	D16.8	D48.Ø	D49.2
sternum	C41.3	C79.51	—	D16.7	D48.Ø	D49.2
tarsus (any)	C4Ø.3-☑	C79.51	—	—	—	—
temporal	C41.Ø	C79.51	—	D16.4	D48.Ø	D49.2
thumb	C4Ø.1-☑	C79.51	—	—	—	—
tibia (any part)	C4Ø.2-☑	C79.51	—	—	—	—
toe (any)	C4Ø.3-☑	C79.51	—	—	—	—
trapezium	C4Ø.1-☑	C79.51	—	—	—	—
trapezoid	C4Ø.1-☑	C79.51	—	—	—	—
turbinate	C41.Ø	C79.51	—	D16.4	D48.Ø	D49.2
ulna (any part)	C4Ø.Ø-☑	C79.51	—	D16.Ø-☑	—	—
unciform	C4Ø.1-☑	C79.51	—	—	—	—
vertebra (column)	C41.2	C79.51	—	D16.6	D48.Ø	D49.2
coccyx	C41.4	C79.51	—	D16.8	D48.Ø	D49.2
sacrum	C41.4	C79.51	—	D16.8	D48.Ø	D49.2
vomer	C41.Ø	C79.51	—	D16.4	D48.Ø	D49.2
wrist	C4Ø.1-☑	C79.51	—	—	—	—
xiphoid process	C41.3	C79.51	—	D16.7	D48.Ø	D49.2
zygomatic	C41.Ø	C79.51	—	D16.4	D48.Ø	D49.2
book-leaf (mouth) — *ventral surface of tongue and floor of mouth*	CØ6.89	C79.89	DØØ.ØØ	D1Ø.39	D37.Ø9	D49.Ø
bowel — *see* Neoplasm, intestine						
brachial plexus	C47.1-☑	C79.89	—	D36.12	D48.2	D49.2
brain NEC	C71.9	C79.31	—	D33.2	D43.2	D49.6

☑ **Additional Character Required — Refer to the Tabular List for Character Selection**

	Malignant Primary	Malignant Secondary	Ca in situ	Benign	Uncertain Behavior	Unspecified Behavior
Neoplasm, neoplastic — *continued*						
brain — *continued*						
basal ganglia	C71.0	C79.31	—	D33.0	D43.0	D49.6
cerebellopontine angle	C71.6	C79.31	—	D33.1	D43.1	D49.6
cerebellum NOS	C71.6	C79.31	—	D33.1	D43.1	D49.6
cerebrum	C71.0	C79.31	—	D33.0	D43.0	D49.6
choroid plexus	C71.7	C79.31	—	D33.1	D43.1	D49.6
corpus callosum	C71.8	C79.31	—	D33.2	D43.2	D49.6
corpus striatum	C71.0	C79.31	—	D33.0	D43.0	D49.6
cortex (cerebral)	C71.0	C79.31	—	D33.0	D43.0	D49.6
frontal lobe	C71.1	C79.31	—	D33.0	D43.0	D49.6
globus pallidus	C71.0	C79.31	—	D33.0	D43.0	D49.6
hippocampus	C71.2	C79.31	—	D33.0	D43.0	D49.6
hypothalamus	C71.0	C79.31	—	D33.0	D43.0	D49.6
internal capsule	C71.0	C79.31	—	D33.0	D43.0	D49.6
medulla oblongata	C71.7	C79.31	—	D33.1	D43.1	D49.6
meninges	C70.0	C79.32	—	D32.0	D42.0	D49.7
midbrain	C71.7	C79.31	—	D33.1	D43.1	D49.6
occipital lobe	C71.4	C79.31	—	D33.0	D43.0	D49.6
overlapping lesion	C71.8	C79.31	—	—	—	—
parietal lobe	C71.3	C79.31	—	D33.0	D43.0	D49.6
peduncle	C71.7	C79.31	—	D33.1	D43.1	D49.6
pons	C71.7	C79.31	—	D33.1	D43.1	D49.6
stem	C71.7	C79.31	—	D33.1	D43.1	D49.6
tapetum	C71.8	C79.31	—	D33.2	D43.2	D49.6
temporal lobe	C71.2	C79.31	—	D33.0	D43.0	D49.6
thalamus	C71.0	C79.31	—	D33.0	D43.0	D49.6
uncus	C71.2	C79.31	—	D33.0	D43.0	D49.6
ventricle (floor)	C71.5	C79.31	—	D33.0	D43.0	D49.6
fourth	C71.7	C79.31	—	D33.1	D43.1	D49.6
branchial (cleft) (cyst) (vestiges)	C10.4	C79.89	D00.08	D10.5	D37.05	D49.0
breast (connective tissue) (glandular tissue) (soft parts)	C50.9-☑	C79.81	D05.-☑	D24.-☑	D48.6-☑	D49.3
areola	C50.0-☑	C79.81	D05.-☑	D24.-☑	D48.6-☑	D49.3
axillary tail	C50.6-☑	C79.81	D05.-☑	D24.-☑	D48.6-☑	D49.3
central portion	C50.1-☑	C79.81	D05.-☑	D24.-☑	D48.6-☑	D49.3
inner	C50.8-☑	C79.81	D05.-☑	D24.-☑	D48.6-☑	D49.3
lower	C50.8-☑	C79.81	D05.-☑	D24.-☑	D48.6-☑	D49.3
lower-inner quadrant	C50.3-☑	C79.81	D05.-☑	D24.-☑	D48.6-☑	D49.3
lower-outer quadrant	C50.5-☑	C79.81	D05.-☑	D24.-☑	D48.6-☑	D49.3
mastectomy site (skin) — *see also* Neoplasm, breast, skin	C44.501	C79.2	—	—	—	—
specified as breast tissue	C50.8-☑	C79.81	—	—	—	—
midline	C50.8-☑	C79.81	D05.-☑	D24.-☑	D48.6-☑	D49.3
nipple	C50.0-☑	C79.81	D05.-☑	D24.-☑	D48.6-☑	D49.3
outer	C50.8-☑	C79.81	D05.-☑	D24.-☑	D48.6-☑	D49.3
overlapping lesion	C50.8-☑	—	—	—	—	—
skin	C44.501	C79.2	D04.5	D23.5	D48.5	D49.2
basal cell carcinoma	C44.511	—	—	—	—	—
specified type NEC	C44.591	—	—	—	—	—
squamous cell carcinoma	C44.521	—	—	—	—	—
tail (axillary)	C50.6-☑	C79.81	D05.-☑	D24.-☑	D48.6-☑	D49.3
upper	C50.8-☑	C79.81	D05.-☑	D24.-☑	D48.6-☑	D49.3
upper-inner quadrant	C50.2-☑	C79.81	D05.-☑	D24.-☑	D48.6-☑	D49.3
upper-outer quadrant	C50.4-☑	C79.81	D05.-☑	D24.-☑	D48.6-☑	D49.3
broad ligament	C57.1-☑	C79.82	D07.39	D28.2	D39.8	D49.59
bronchiogenic, bronchogenic (lung)	C34.9-☑	C78.0-☑	D02.2-☑	D14.3-☑	D38.1	D49.1
bronchiole	C34.9-☑	C78.0-☑	D02.2-☑	D14.3-☑	D38.1	D49.1
bronchus	C34.9-☑	C78.0-☑	D02.2-☑	D14.3-☑	D38.1	D49.1
carina	C34.0-☑	C78.0-☑	D02.2-☑	D14.3-☑	D38.1	D49.1
lower lobe of lung	C34.3-☑	C78.0-☑	D02.2-☑	D14.3-☑	D38.1	D49.1

	Malignant Primary	Malignant Secondary	Ca in situ	Benign	Uncertain Behavior	Unspecified Behavior
Neoplasm, neoplastic — *continued*						
bronchus — *continued*						
main	C34.0-☑	C78.0-☑	D02.2-☑	D14.3-☑	D38.1	D49.1
middle lobe of lung	C34.2	C78.0-☑	D02.21	D14.31	D38.1	D49.1
overlapping lesion	C34.8-☑	—	—	—	—	—
upper lobe of lung	C34.1-☑	C78.0-☑	D02.2-☑	D14.3-☑	D38.1	D49.1
brow	C44.309	C79.2	D04.39	D23.39	D48.5	D49.2
basal cell carcinoma	C44.319	—	—	—	—	—
specified type NEC	C44.399	—	—	—	—	—
squamous cell carcinoma	C44.329	—	—	—	—	—
buccal (cavity)	C06.9	C79.89	D00.00	D10.39	D37.09	D49.0
commissure	C06.0	C79.89	D00.02	D10.39	D37.09	D49.0
groove (lower) (upper)	C06.1	C79.89	D00.02	D10.39	D37.09	D49.0
mucosa	C06.0	C79.89	D00.02	D10.39	D37.09	D49.0
sulcus (lower) (upper)	C06.1	C79.89	D00.02	D10.39	D37.09	D49.0
bulbourethral gland	C68.0	C79.19	D09.19	D30.4	D41.3	D49.59
bursa — *see* Neoplasm, connective tissue						
buttock NEC	C76.3	C79.89	D04.5	D36.7	D48.7	D49.89
calf	C76.5-☑	C79.89	D04.7-☑	D36.7	D48.7	D49.89
calvarium	C41.0	C79.51	—	D16.4	D48.0	D49.2
calyx, renal	C65.-☑	C79.0-☑	D09.19	D30.1-☑	D41.1-☑	D49.51-☑
canal						
anal	C21.1	C78.5	D01.3	D12.9	D37.8	D49.0
auditory (external) — *see also* Neoplasm, skin, ear	C44.20-☑	C79.2	D04.2-☑	D23.2-☑	D48.5	D49.2
auricular (external) — *see also* Neoplasm, skin, ear	C44.20-☑	C79.2	D04.2-☑	D23.2-☑	D48.5	D49.2
canaliculi, biliary (biliferi) (intrahepatic)	C22.1	C78.7	D01.5	D13.4	D37.6	D49.0
canthus (eye) (inner) (outer)	C44.10-☑	C79.2	D04.1-☑	D23.1-☑	D48.5	D49.2
basal cell carcinoma	C44.11-☑	—	—	—	—	—
sebaceous cell	C44.13-☑	—	—	—	—	—
specified type NEC	C44.19-☑	—	—	—	—	—
squamous cell carcinoma	C44.12-☑	—	—	—	—	—
capillary — *see* Neoplasm, connective tissue						
caput coli	C18.0	C78.5	D01.0	D12.0	D37.4	D49.0
carcinoid — *see* Tumor, carcinoid						
cardia (gastric)	C16.0	C78.89	D00.2	D13.1	D37.1	D49.0
cardiac orifice (stomach)	C16.0	C78.89	D00.2	D13.1	D37.1	D49.0
cardio-esophageal junction	C16.0	C78.89	D00.2	D13.1	D37.1	D49.0
cardio-esophagus	C16.0	C78.89	D00.2	D13.1	D37.1	D49.0
carina (bronchus)	C34.0-☑	C78.0-☑	D02.2-☑	D14.3-☑	D38.1	D49.1
carotid (artery)	C49.0	C79.89	—	D21.0	D48.1☑	D49.2
body	C75.4	C79.89	—	D35.5	D44.6	D49.7
carpus (any bone)	C40.1-☑	C79.51	—	D16.1-☑	—	—
cartilage (articular) (joint) NEC — *see also* Neoplasm, bone	C41.9	C79.51	—	D16.9	D48.0	D49.2
arytenoid	C32.3	C78.39	D02.0	D14.1	D38.0	D49.1
auricular	C49.0	C79.89	—	D21.0	D48.1☑	D49.2
bronchi	C34.0-☑	C78.39	—	D14.3-☑	D38.1	D49.1
costal	C41.3	C79.51	—	D16.7	D48.0	D49.2
cricoid	C32.3	C78.39	D02.0	D14.1	D38.0	D49.1
cuneiform	C32.3	C78.39	D02.0	D14.1	D38.0	D49.1
ear (external)	C49.0	C79.89	—	D21.0	D48.1☑	D49.2
ensiform	C41.3	C79.51	—	D16.7	D48.0	D49.2
epiglottis	C32.1	C78.39	D02.0	D14.1	D38.0	D49.1

	Malignant Primary	Malignant Secondary	Ca in situ	Benign	Uncertain Behavior	Unspecified Behavior
Neoplasm, neoplastic — *continued*						
cartilage — *see also* Neoplasm, bone — *continued*						
epiglottis — *continued*						
anterior surface	C1Ø.1	C79.89	DØØ.Ø8	D1Ø.5	D37.Ø5	D49.Ø
eyelid	C49.Ø	C79.89	—	D21.Ø	D48.1☑	D49.2
intervertebral	C41.2	C79.51	—	D16.6	D48.Ø	D49.2
larynx, laryngeal	C32.3	C78.39	DØ2.Ø	D14.1	D38.Ø	D49.1
nose, nasal	C3Ø.Ø	C78.39	DØ2.3	D14.Ø	D38.5	D49.1
pinna	C49.Ø	C79.89	—	D21.Ø	D48.1☑	D49.2
rib	C41.3	C79.51	—	D16.7	D48.Ø	D49.2
semilunar (knee)	C4Ø.2-☑	C79.51	—	D16.2-☑	D48.Ø	D49.2
thyroid	C32.3	C78.39	DØ2.Ø	D14.1	D38.Ø	D49.1
trachea	C33	C78.39	DØ2.1	D14.2	D38.1	D49.1
cauda equina	C72.1	C79.49	—	D33.4	D43.4	D49.7
cavity						
buccal	CØ6.9	C79.89	DØØ.ØØ	D1Ø.3Ø	D37.Ø9	D49.Ø
nasal	C3Ø.Ø	C78.39	DØ2.3	D14.Ø	D38.5	D49.1
oral	CØ6.9	C79.89	DØØ.ØØ	D1Ø.3Ø	D37.Ø9	D49.Ø
peritoneal	C48.2	C78.6	—	D2Ø.1	D48.4	D49.Ø
tympanic	C3Ø.1	C78.39	DØ2.3	D14.Ø	D38.5	D49.1
cecum	C18.Ø	C78.5	DØ1.Ø	D12.Ø	D37.4	D49.Ø
central nervous system	C72.9	C79.4Ø	—	—	—	—
cerebellopontine (angle)	C71.6	C79.31	—	D33.1	D43.1	D49.6
cerebellum, cerebellar	C71.6	C79.31	—	D33.1	D43.1	D49.6
cerebrum, cerebra (cortex) (hemisphere) (white matter)	C71.Ø	C79.31	—	D33.Ø	D43.Ø	D49.6
meninges	C7Ø.Ø	C79.32	—	D32.Ø	D42.Ø	D49.7
peduncle	C71.7	C79.31	—	D33.1	D43.1	D49.6
ventricle	C71.5	C79.31	—	D33.Ø	D43.Ø	D49.6
fourth	C71.7	C79.31	—	D33.1	D43.1	D49.6
cervical region	C76.Ø	C79.89	DØ9.8	D36.7	D48.7	D49.89
cervix (cervical) (uteri) (uterus)	C53.9	C79.82	DØ6.9	D26.Ø	D39.Ø	D49.59
canal	C53.Ø	C79.82	DØ6.Ø	D26.Ø	D39.Ø	D49.59
endocervix (canal) (gland)	C53.Ø	C79.82	DØ6.Ø	D26.Ø	D39.Ø	D49.59
exocervix	C53.1	C79.82	DØ6.1	D26.Ø	D39.Ø	D49.59
external os	C53.1	C79.82	DØ6.1	D26.Ø	D39.Ø	D49.59
internal os	C53.Ø	C79.82	DØ6.Ø	D26.Ø	D39.Ø	D49.59
nabothian gland	C53.Ø	C79.82	DØ6.Ø	D26.Ø	D39.Ø	D49.59
overlapping lesion	C53.8	—	—	—	—	—
squamocolumnar junction	C53.8	C79.82	DØ6.7	D26.Ø	D39.Ø	D49.59
stump	C53.8	C79.82	DØ6.7	D26.Ø	D39.Ø	D49.59
cheek	C76.Ø	C79.89	DØ9.8	D36.7	D48.7	D49.89
external	C44.3Ø9	C79.2	DØ4.39	D23.39	D48.5	D49.2
basal cell carcinoma	C44.319	—	—	—	—	—
specified type NEC	C44.399	—	—	—	—	—
squamous cell carcinoma	C44.329	—	—	—	—	—
inner aspect	CØ6.Ø	C79.89	DØØ.Ø2	D1Ø.39	D37.Ø9	D49.Ø
internal	CØ6.Ø	C79.89	DØØ.Ø2	D1Ø.39	D37.Ø9	D49.Ø
mucosa	CØ6.Ø	C79.89	DØØ.Ø2	D1Ø.39	D37.Ø9	D49.Ø
chest (wall) NEC	C76.1	C79.89	DØ9.8	D36.7	D48.7	D49.89
chiasma opticum	C72.3-☑	C79.49	—	D33.3	D43.3	D49.7
chin	C44.3Ø9	C79.2	DØ4.39	D23.39	D48.5	D49.2
basal cell carcinoma	C44.319	—	—	—	—	—
specified type NEC	C44.399	—	—	—	—	—
squamous cell carcinoma	C44.329	—	—	—	—	—
choana	C11.3	C79.89	DØØ.Ø8	D1Ø.6	D37.Ø5	D49.Ø
cholangiole	C22.1	C78.89	DØ1.5	D13.4	D37.6	D49.Ø
choledochal duct	C24.Ø	C78.89	DØ1.5	D13.5	D37.6	D49.Ø
choroid	C69.3-☑	C79.49	DØ9.2-☑	D31.3-☑	D48.7	D49.81
plexus	C71.5	C79.31	—	D33.Ø	D43.Ø	D49.6
ciliary body	C69.4-☑	C79.49	DØ9.2-☑	D31.4-☑	D48.7	D49.89
clavicle	C41.3	C79.51	—	D16.7	D48.Ø	D49.2

	Malignant Primary	Malignant Secondary	Ca in situ	Benign	Uncertain Behavior	Unspecified Behavior
Neoplasm, neoplastic — *continued*						
clitoris	C51.2	C79.82	DØ7.1	D28.Ø	D39.8	D49.59
clivus	C41.Ø	C79.51	—	D16.4	D48.Ø	D49.2
cloacogenic zone	C21.2	C78.5	DØ1.3	D12.9	D37.8	D49.Ø
coccygeal						
body or glomus	C49.5	C79.89	—	D21.5	D48.1☑	D49.2
vertebra	C41.4	C79.51	—	D16.8	D48.Ø	D49.2
coccyx	C41.4	C79.51	—	D16.8	D48.Ø	D49.2
colon — *see also* Neoplasm, intestine, large	C18.9	C78.5	—	—	—	—
with rectum	C19	C78.5	DØ1.1	D12.7	D37.5	D49.Ø
columnella — *see also* Neoplasm, skin, face	C44.39Ø	C79.2	DØ4.39	D23.39	D48.5	D49.2
column, spinal — *see* Neoplasm, spine						
commissure						
labial, lip	CØØ.6	C79.89	DØØ.Ø1	D1Ø.39	D37.Ø1	D49.Ø
laryngeal	C32.Ø	C78.39	DØ2.Ø	D14.1	D38.Ø	D49.1
common (bile) duct	C24.Ø	C78.89	DØ1.5	D13.5	D37.6	D49.Ø
concha — *see also* Neoplasm, skin, ear	C44.2Ø-☑	C79.2	DØ4.2-☑	D23.2-☑	D48.5	D49.2
nose	C3Ø.Ø	C78.39	DØ2.3	D14.Ø	D38.5	D49.1
conjunctiva	C69.Ø-☑	C79.49	DØ9.2-☑	D31.Ø-☑	D48.7	D49.89
connective tissue NEC	C49.9	C79.89	—	D21.9	D48.1☑	D49.2

Note: For neoplasms of connective tissue (blood vessel, bursa, fascia, ligament, muscle, peripheral nerves, sympathetic and parasympathetic nerves and ganglia, synovia, tendon, etc.) or of morphological types that indicate connective tissue, code according to the list under "Neoplasm, connective tissue". For sites that do not appear in this list, code to neoplasm of that site; e.g., fibrosarcoma, pancreas (C25.9)

Note: Morphological types that indicate connective tissue appear in their proper place in the alphabetic index with the instruction "see Neoplasm, connective tissue ...."

	Malignant Primary	Malignant Secondary	Ca in situ	Benign	Uncertain Behavior	Unspecified Behavior
abdomen	C49.4	C79.89	—	D21.4	D48.1☑	D49.2
abdominal wall	C49.4	C79.89	—	D21.4	D48.1☑	D49.2
ankle	C49.2-☑	C79.89	—	D21.2-☑	D48.1☑	D49.2
antecubital fossa or space	C49.1-☑	C79.89	—	D21.1-☑	D48.1☑	D49.2
arm	C49.1-☑	C79.89	—	D21.1-☑	D48.1☑	D49.2
auricle (ear)	C49.Ø	C79.89	—	D21.Ø	D48.1☑	D49.2
axilla	C49.3	C79.89	—	D21.3	D48.1☑	D49.2
back	C49.6	C79.89	—	D21.6	D48.1☑	D49.2
breast — *see* Neoplasm, breast						
buttock	C49.5	C79.89	—	D21.5	D48.1☑	D49.2
calf	C49.2-☑	C79.89	—	D21.2-☑	D48.1☑	D49.2
cervical region	C49.Ø	C79.89	—	D21.Ø	D48.1☑	D49.2
cheek	C49.Ø	C79.89	—	D21.Ø	D48.1☑	D49.2
chest (wall)	C49.3	C79.89	—	D21.3	D48.1☑	D49.2
chin	C49.Ø	C79.89	—	D21.Ø	D48.1☑	D49.2
diaphragm	C49.3	C79.89	—	D21.3	D48.1☑	D49.2
ear (external)	C49.Ø	C79.89	—	D21.Ø	D48.1☑	D49.2
elbow	C49.1-☑	C79.89	—	D21.1-☑	D48.1☑	D49.2
extrarectal	C49.5	C79.89	—	D21.5	D48.1☑	D49.2
extremity	C49.9	C79.89	—	D21.9	D48.1☑	D49.2
lower	C49.2-☑	C79.89	—	D21.2-☑	D48.1☑	D49.2
upper	C49.1-☑	C79.89	—	D21.1-☑	D48.1☑	D49.2
eyelid	C49.Ø	C79.89	—	D21.Ø	D48.1☑	D49.2
face	C49.Ø	C79.89	—	D21.Ø	D48.1☑	D49.2
finger	C49.1-☑	C79.89	—	D21.1-☑	D48.1☑	D49.2
flank	C49.6	C79.89	—	D21.6	D48.1☑	D49.2
foot	C49.2-☑	C79.89	—	D21.2-☑	D48.1☑	D49.2
forearm	C49.1-☑	C79.89	—	D21.1-☑	D48.1☑	D49.2
forehead	C49.Ø	C79.89	—	D21.Ø	D48.1☑	D49.2
gastric	C49.4	C79.89	—	D21.4	D48.1☑	D49.2
gastrointestinal	C49.4	C79.89	—	D21.4	D48.1☑	D49.2
gluteal region	C49.5	C79.89	—	D21.5	D48.1☑	D49.2
great vessels NEC	C49.3	C79.89	—	D21.3	D48.1☑	D49.2
groin	C49.5	C79.89	—	D21.5	D48.1☑	D49.2

	Malignant Primary	Malignant Secondary	Ca in situ	Benign	Uncertain Behavior	Unspecified Behavior
Neoplasm, neoplastic — *continued*						
connective tissue — *continued*						
hand	C49.1-☑	C79.89	—	D21.1-☑	D48.1☑	D49.2
head	C49.0	C79.89	—	D21.0	D48.1☑	D49.2
heel	C49.2-☑	C79.89	—	D21.2-☑	D48.1☑	D49.2
hip	C49.2-☑	C79.89	—	D21.2-☑	D48.1☑	D49.2
hypochondrium	C49.4	C79.89	—	D21.4	D48.1☑	D49.2
iliopsoas muscle	C49.5	C79.89	—	D21.5	D48.1☑	D49.2
infraclavicular region	C49.3	C79.89	—	D21.3	D48.1☑	D49.2
inguinal (canal) (region)	C49.5	C79.89	—	D21.5	D48.1☑	D49.2
intestinal	C49.4	C79.89	—	D21.4	D48.1☑	D49.2
intrathoracic	C49.3	C79.89	—	D21.3	D48.1☑	D49.2
ischiorectal fossa	C49.5	C79.89	—	D21.5	D48.1☑	D49.2
jaw	C03.9	C79.89	D00.03	D10.39	D48.1☑	D49.0
knee	C49.2-☑	C79.89	—	D21.2-☑	D48.1☑	D49.2
leg	C49.2-☑	C79.89	—	D21.2-☑	D48.1☑	D49.2
limb NEC	C49.9	C79.89	—	D21.9	D48.1☑	D49.2
lower	C49.2-☑	C79.89	—	D21.2-☑	D48.1☑	D49.2
upper	C49.1-☑	C79.89	—	D21.1-☑	D48.1☑	D49.2
nates	C49.5	C79.89	—	D21.5	D48.1☑	D49.2
neck	C49.0	C79.89	—	D21.0	D48.1☑	D49.2
orbit	C69.6-☑	C79.49	D09.2-☑	D31.6-☑	D48.1☑	D49.89
overlapping lesion	C49.8	—	—	—	—	—
pararectal	C49.5	C79.89	—	D21.5	D48.1☑	D49.2
para-urethral	C49.5	C79.89	—	D21.5	D48.1☑	D49.2
paravaginal	C49.5	C79.89	—	D21.5	D48.1☑	D49.2
pelvis (floor)	C49.5	C79.89	—	D21.5	D48.1☑	D49.2
pelvo-abdominal	C49.8	C79.89	—	D21.6	D48.1☑	D49.2
perineum	C49.5	C79.89	—	D21.5	D48.1☑	D49.2
perirectal (tissue)	C49.5	C79.89	—	D21.5	D48.1☑	D49.2
periurethral (tissue)	C49.5	C79.89	—	D21.5	D48.1☑	D49.2
popliteal fossa or space	C49.2-☑	C79.89	—	D21.2-☑	D48.1☑	D49.2
presacral	C49.5	C79.89	—	D21.5	D48.1☑	D49.2
psoas muscle	C49.4	C79.89	—	D21.4	D48.1☑	D49.2
pterygoid fossa	C49.0	C79.89	—	D21.0	D48.1☑	D49.2
rectovaginal septum or wall	C49.5	C79.89	—	D21.5	D48.1☑	D49.2
rectovesical	C49.5	C79.89	—	D21.5	D48.1☑	D49.2
retroperitoneum	C48.0	C78.6	—	D20.0	D48.3	D49.0
sacrococcygeal region	C49.5	C79.89	—	D21.5	D48.1☑	D49.2
scalp	C49.0	C79.89	—	D21.0	D48.1☑	D49.2
scapular region	C49.3	C79.89	—	D21.3	D48.1☑	D49.2
shoulder	C49.1-☑	C79.89	—	D21.1-☑	D48.1☑	D49.2
skin (dermis) NEC — *see also* Neoplasm, skin, by site	C44.90	C79.2	D04.9	D23.9	D48.5	D49.2
stomach	C49.4	C79.89	—	D21.4	D48.1☑	D49.2
submental	C49.0	C79.89	—	D21.0	D48.1☑	D49.2
supraclavicular region	C49.0	C79.89	—	D21.0	D48.1☑	D49.2
temple	C49.0	C79.89	—	D21.0	D48.1☑	D49.2
temporal region	C49.0	C79.89	—	D21.0	D48.1☑	D49.2
thigh	C49.2-☑	C79.89	—	D21.2-☑	D48.1☑	D49.2
thoracic (duct) (wall)	C49.3	C79.89	—	D21.3	D48.1☑	D49.2
thorax	C49.3	C79.89	—	D21.3	D48.1☑	D49.2
thumb	C49.1-☑	C79.89	—	D21.1-☑	D48.1☑	D49.2
toe	C49.2-☑	C79.89	—	D21.2-☑	D48.1☑	D49.2
trunk	C49.6	C79.89	—	D21.6	D48.1☑	D49.2
umbilicus	C49.4	C79.89	—	D21.4	D48.1☑	D49.2
vesicorectal	C49.5	C79.89	—	D21.5	D48.1☑	D49.2
wrist	C49.1-☑	C79.89	—	D21.1-☑	D48.1☑	D49.2
conus medullaris	C72.0	C79.49	—	D33.4	D43.4	D49.7
cord (true) (vocal)	C32.0	C78.39	D02.0	D14.1	D38.0	D49.1
false	C32.1	C78.39	D02.0	D14.1	D38.0	D49.1
spermatic	C63.1-☑	C79.82	D07.69	D29.8	D40.8	D49.59
spinal (cervical) (lumbar) (thoracic)	C72.0	C79.49	—	D33.4	D43.4	D49.7

	Malignant Primary	Malignant Secondary	Ca in situ	Benign	Uncertain Behavior	Unspecified Behavior
Neoplasm, neoplastic — *continued*						
cornea (limbus)	C69.1-☑	C79.49	D09.2-☑	D31.1-☑	D48.7	D49.89
corpus						
albicans	C56.-☑	C79.6-☑	D07.39	D27.-☑	D39.1-☑	D49.59
callosum, brain	C71.0	C79.31	—	D33.2	D43.2	D49.6
cavernosum	C60.2	C79.82	D07.4	D29.0	D40.8	D49.59
gastric	C16.2	C78.89	D00.2	D13.1	D37.1	D49.0
overlapping sites	C54.8	—	—	—	—	—
penis	C60.2	C79.82	D07.4	D29.0	D40.8	D49.59
striatum, cerebrum	C71.0	C79.31	—	D33.0	D43.0	D49.6
uteri	C54.9	C79.82	D07.0	D26.1	D39.0	D49.59
isthmus	C54.0	C79.82	D07.0	D26.1	D39.0	D49.59
cortex						
adrenal	C74.0-☑	C79.7-☑	D09.3	D35.0-☑	D44.1-☑	D49.7
cerebral	C71.0	C79.31	—	D33.0	D43.0	D49.6
costal cartilage	C41.3	C79.51	—	D16.7	D48.0	D49.2
costovertebral joint	C41.3	C79.51	—	D16.7	D48.0	D49.2
Cowper's gland	C68.0	C79.19	D09.19	D30.4	D41.3	D49.59
cranial (fossa, any)	C71.9	C79.31	—	D33.2	D43.2	D49.6
meninges	C70.0	C79.32	—	D32.0	D42.0	D49.7
nerve	C72.50	C79.49	—	D33.3	D43.3	D49.7
specified NEC	C72.59	C79.49	—	D33.3	D43.3	D49.7
craniobuccal pouch	C75.2	C79.89	D09.3	D35.2	D44.3	D49.7
craniopharyngeal (duct) (pouch)	C75.2	C79.89	D09.3	D35.3	D44.4	D49.7
cricoid	C13.0	C79.89	D00.08	D10.7	D37.05	D49.0
cartilage	C32.3	C78.39	D02.0	D14.1	D38.0	D49.1
cricopharynx	C13.0	C79.89	D00.08	D10.7	D37.05	D49.0
crypt of Morgagni	C21.8	C78.5	D01.3	D12.9	D37.8	D49.0
crystalline lens	C69.4-☑	C79.49	D09.2-☑	D31.4-☑	D48.7	D49.89
cul-de-sac (Douglas')	C48.1	C78.6	—	D20.1	D48.4	D49.0
cuneiform cartilage	C32.3	C78.39	D02.0	D14.1	D38.0	D49.1
cutaneous — *see* Neoplasm, skin						
cutis — *see* Neoplasm, skin						
cystic (bile) duct (common)	C24.0	C78.89	D01.5	D13.5	D37.6	D49.0
dermis — *see* Neoplasm, skin						
diaphragm	C49.3	C79.89	—	D21.3	D48.1☑	D49.2
digestive organs, system, tube, or tract NEC	C26.9	C78.89	D01.9	D13.99	D37.9	D49.0
disc, intervertebral	C41.2	C79.51	—	D16.6	D48.0	D49.2
disease, generalized	C80.0	—	—	—	—	—
disseminated	C80.0	—	—	—	—	—
Douglas' cul-de-sac or pouch	C48.1	C78.6	—	D20.1	D48.4	D49.0
duodenojejunal junction	C17.8	C78.4	D01.49	D13.39	D37.2	D49.0
duodenum	C17.0	C78.4	D01.49	D13.2	D37.2	D49.0
dura (cranial) (mater)	C70.9	C79.49	—	D32.9	D42.9	D49.7
cerebral	C70.0	C79.32	—	D32.0	D42.0	D49.7
spinal	C70.1	C79.49	—	D32.1	D42.1	D49.7
ear (external) — *see also* Neoplasm, skin, ear	C44.20-☑	C79.2	D04.2-☑	D23.2-☑	D48.5	D49.2
auricle or auris — *see also* Neoplasm, skin, ear	C44.20-☑	C79.2	D04.2-☑	D23.2-☑	D48.5	D49.2
canal, external — *see also* Neoplasm, skin, ear	C44.20-☑	C79.2	D04.2-☑	D23.2-☑	D48.5	D49.2
cartilage	C49.0	C79.89	—	D21.0	D48.1☑	D49.2
external meatus — *see also* Neoplasm, skin, ear	C44.20-☑	C79.2	D04.2-☑	D23.2-☑	D48.5	D49.2
inner	C30.1	C78.39	D02.3	D14.0	D38.5	D49.1
lobule — *see also* Neoplasm, skin, ear	C44.20-☑	C79.2	D04.2-☑	D23.2-☑	D48.5	D49.2

	Malignant Primary	Malignant Secondary	Ca in situ	Benign	Uncertain Behavior	Unspecified Behavior
Neoplasm, neoplastic — *continued*						
ear — *see also* Neoplasm, skin, ear — *continued*						
middle	C30.1	C78.39	D02.3	D14.0	D38.5	D49.1
overlapping lesion with accessory sinuses	C31.8	—	—	—	—	—
skin	C44.20-☑	C79.2	D04.2-☑	D23.2-☑	D48.5	D49.2
basal cell carcinoma	C44.21-☑	—	—	—	—	—
specified type NEC	C44.29-☑	—	—	—	—	—
squamous cell carcinoma	C44.22-☑	—	—	—	—	—
earlobe	C44.20-☑	C79.2	D04.2-☑	D23.2-☑	D48.5	D49.2
basal cell carcinoma	C44.21-☑	—	—	—	—	—
specified type NEC	C44.29-☑	—	—	—	—	—
squamous cell carcinoma	C44.22-☑	—	—	—	—	—
ejaculatory duct	C63.7	C79.82	D07.69	D29.8	D40.8	D49.59
elbow NEC	C76.4-☑	C79.89	D04.6-☑	D36.7	D48.7	D49.89
endocardium	C38.0	C79.89	—	D15.1	D48.7	D49.89
endocervix (canal) (gland)	C53.0	C79.82	D06.0	D26.0	D39.0	D49.59
endocrine gland NEC	C75.9	C79.89	D09.3	D35.9	D44.9	D49.7
pluriglandular	C75.8	C79.89	D09.3	D35.7	D44.9	D49.7
endometrium (gland) (stroma)	C54.1	C79.82	D07.0	D26.1	D39.0	D49.59
ensiform cartilage	C41.3	C79.51	—	D16.7	D48.0	D49.2
enteric — *see* Neoplasm, intestine						
ependyma (brain)	C71.5	C79.31	—	D33.0	D43.0	D49.6
fourth ventricle	C71.7	C79.31	—	D33.1	D43.1	D49.6
epicardium	C38.0	C79.89	—	D15.1	D48.7	D49.89
epididymis	C63.0-☑	C79.82	D07.69	D29.3-☑	D40.8	D49.59
epidural	C72.9	C79.49	—	D33.9	D43.9	D49.7
epiglottis	C32.1	C78.39	D02.0	D14.1	D38.0	D49.1
anterior aspect or surface	C10.1	C79.89	D00.08	D10.5	D37.05	D49.0
cartilage	C32.3	C78.39	D02.0	D14.1	D38.0	D49.1
free border (margin)	C10.1	C79.89	D00.08	D10.5	D37.05	D49.0
junctional region	C10.8	C79.89	D00.08	D10.5	D37.05	D49.0
posterior (laryngeal) surface	C32.1	C78.39	D02.0	D14.1	D38.0	D49.1
suprahyoid portion	C32.1	C78.39	D02.0	D14.1	D38.0	D49.1
esophagogastric junction	C16.0	C78.89	D00.2	D13.1	D37.1	D49.0
esophagus	C15.9	C78.89	D00.1	D13.0	D37.8	D49.0
abdominal	C15.5	C78.89	D00.1	D13.0	D37.8	D49.0
cervical	C15.3	C78.89	D00.1	D13.0	D37.8	D49.0
distal (third)	C15.5	C78.89	D00.1	D13.0	D37.8	D49.0
lower (third)	C15.5	C78.89	D00.1	D13.0	D37.8	D49.0
middle (third)	C15.4	C78.89	D00.1	D13.0	D37.8	D49.0
overlapping lesion	C15.8	—	—	—	—	—
proximal (third)	C15.3	C78.89	D00.1	D13.0	D37.8	D49.0
thoracic	C15.4	C78.89	D00.1	D13.0	D37.8	D49.0
upper (third)	C15.3	C78.89	D00.1	D13.0	D37.8	D49.0
ethmoid (sinus)	C31.1	C78.39	D02.3	D14.0	D38.5	D49.1
bone or labyrinth	C41.0	C79.51	—	D16.4	D48.0	D49.2
eustachian tube	C30.1	C78.39	D02.3	D14.0	D38.5	D49.1
exocervix	C53.1	C79.82	D06.1	D26.0	D39.0	D49.59
external						
meatus (ear) — *see also* Neoplasm, skin, ear	C44.20-☑	C79.2	D04.2-☑	D23.2-☑	D48.5	D49.2
os, cervix uteri	C53.1	C79.82	D06.1	D26.0	D39.0	D49.59
extradural	C72.9	C79.49	—	D33.9	D43.9	D49.7
extrahepatic (bile) duct	C24.0	C78.89	D01.5	D13.5	D37.6	D49.0
overlapping lesion with gallbladder	C24.8	—	—	—	—	—

	Malignant Primary	Malignant Secondary	Ca in situ	Benign	Uncertain Behavior	Unspecified Behavior
Neoplasm, neoplastic — *continued*						
extraocular muscle	C69.6-☑	C79.49	D09.2-☑	D31.6-☑	D48.7	D49.89
extrarectal	C76.3	C79.89	D09.8	D36.7	D48.7	D49.89
extremity	C76.8	C79.89	D04.8	D36.7	D48.7	D49.89
lower	C76.5-☑	C79.89	D04.7-☑	D36.7	D48.7	D49.89
upper	C76.4-☑	C79.89	D04.6-☑	D36.7	D48.7	D49.89
eyeball	C69.9-☑	C79.49	D09.2-☑	D31.9-☑	D48.7	D49.89
eyebrow	C44.309	C79.2	D04.39	D23.39	D48.5	D49.2
basal cell carcinoma	C44.319	—	—	—	—	—
specified type NEC	C44.399	—	—	—	—	—
squamous cell carcinoma	C44.329	—	—	—	—	—
eyelid (lower) (skin) (upper)	C44.10-☑	—	—	—	—	—
basal cell carcinoma	C44.11-☑	—	—	—	—	—
cartilage	C49.0	C79.89	—	D21.0	D48.1☑	D49.2
sebaceous cell	C44.13-☑	—	—	—	—	—
specified type NEC	C44.19-☑	—	—	—	—	—
squamous cell carcinoma	C44.12-☑	—	—	—	—	—
eye NEC	C69.9-☑	C79.49	D09.2-☑	D31.9-☑	D48.7	D49.89
overlapping sites	C69.8-☑	—	—	—	—	—
face NEC	C76.0	C79.89	D04.39	D36.7	D48.7	D49.89
fallopian tube (accessory)	C57.0-☑	C79.82	D07.39	D28.2	D39.8	D49.59
falx (cerebella) (cerebri)	C70.0	C79.32	—	D32.0	D42.0	D49.7
fascia — *see also* Neoplasm, connective tissue						
palmar	C49.1-☑	C79.89	—	D21.1-☑	D48.1☑	D49.2
plantar	C49.2-☑	C79.89	—	D21.2-☑	D48.1☑	D49.2
fatty tissue — *see* Neoplasm, connective tissue						
fauces, faucial NEC	C10.9	C79.89	D00.08	D10.5	D37.05	D49.0
pillars	C09.1	C79.89	D00.08	D10.5	D37.05	D49.0
tonsil	C09.9	C79.89	D00.08	D10.4	D37.05	D49.0
femur (any part)	C40.2-☑	—	—	D16.2-☑	—	—
fetal membrane	C58	C79.82	D07.0	D26.7	D39.2	D49.59
fibrous tissue — *see* Neoplasm, connective tissue						
fibula (any part)	C40.2-☑	C79.51	—	D16.2-☑	—	—
filum terminale	C72.0	C79.49	—	D33.4	D43.4	D49.7
finger NEC	C76.4-☑	C79.89	D04.6-☑	D36.7	D48.7	D49.89
flank NEC	C76.8	C79.89	D04.5	D36.7	D48.7	D49.89
follicle, nabothian	C53.0	C79.82	D06.0	D26.0	D39.0	D49.59
foot NEC	C76.5-☑	C79.89	D04.7-☑	D36.7	D48.7	D49.89
forearm NEC	C76.4-☑	C79.89	D04.6-☑	D36.7	D48.7	D49.89
forehead (skin)	C44.309	C79.2	D04.39	D23.39	D48.5	D49.2
basal cell carcinoma	C44.319	—	—	—	—	—
specified type NEC	C44.399	—	—	—	—	—
squamous cell carcinoma	C44.329	—	—	—	—	—
foreskin	C60.0	C79.82	D07.4	D29.0	D40.8	D49.59
fornix						
pharyngeal	C11.3	C79.89	D00.08	D10.6	D37.05	D49.0
vagina	C52	C79.82	D07.2	D28.1	D39.8	D49.59
fossa (of)						
anterior (cranial)	C71.9	C79.31	—	D33.2	D43.2	D49.6
cranial	C71.9	C79.31	—	D33.2	D43.2	D49.6
ischiorectal	C76.3	C79.89	D09.8	D36.7	D48.7	D49.89
middle (cranial)	C71.9	C79.31	—	D33.2	D43.2	D49.6
piriform	C12	C79.89	D00.08	D10.7	D37.05	D49.0
pituitary	C75.1	C79.89	D09.3	D35.2	D44.3	D49.7
posterior (cranial)	C71.9	C79.31	—	D33.2	D43.2	D49.6
pterygoid	C49.0	C79.89	—	D21.0	D48.1☑	D49.2
pyriform	C12	C79.89	D00.08	D10.7	D37.05	D49.0
Rosenmuller	C11.2	C79.89	D00.08	D10.6	D37.05	D49.0
tonsillar	C09.0	C79.89	D00.08	D10.5	D37.05	D49.0
fourchette	C51.9	C79.82	D07.1	D28.0	D39.8	D49.59

☑ **Additional Character Required — Refer to the Tabular List for Character Selection**

	Malignant Primary	Malignant Secondary	Ca in situ	Benign	Uncertain Behavior	Unspecified Behavior
Neoplasm, neoplastic — *continued*						
frenulum						
labii — *see* Neoplasm, lip, internal						
linguae	C02.2	C79.89	D00.07	D10.1	D37.02	D49.0
frontal						
bone	C41.0	C79.51	—	D16.4	D48.0	D49.2
lobe, brain	C71.1	C79.31	—	D33.0	D43.0	D49.6
pole	C71.1	C79.31	—	D33.0	D43.0	D49.6
sinus	C31.2	C78.39	D02.3	D14.0	D38.5	D49.1
fundus						
stomach	C16.1	C78.89	D00.2	D13.1	D37.1	D49.0
uterus	C54.3	C79.82	D07.0	D26.1	D39.0	D49.59
gallbladder	C23	C78.89	D01.5	D13.5	D37.6	D49.0
overlapping lesion with extrahepatic bile ducts	C24.8	—	—	—	—	—
gall duct (extrahepatic)	C24.0	C78.89	D01.5	D13.5	D37.6	D49.0
intrahepatic	C22.1	C78.7	D01.5	D13.4	D37.6	D49.0
ganglia — *see also* Neoplasm, nerve, peripheral	C47.9	C79.89	—	D36.10	D48.2	D49.2
basal	C71.0	C79.31	—	D33.0	D43.0	D49.6
cranial nerve	C72.50	C79.49	—	D33.3	D43.3	D49.7
Gartner's duct	C52	C79.82	D07.2	D28.1	D39.8	D49.59
gastric — *see* Neoplasm, stomach						
gastrocolic	C26.9	C78.89	D01.9	D13.99	D37.9	D49.0
gastroesophageal junction	C16.0	C78.89	D00.2	D13.1	D37.1	D49.0
gastrointestinal (tract) NEC	C26.9	C78.89	D01.9	D13.99	D37.9	D49.0
generalized	C80.0	—	—	—	—	—
genital organ or tract						
female NEC	C57.9	C79.82	D07.30	D28.9	D39.9	D49.59
overlapping lesion	C57.8	—	—	—	—	—
specified site NEC	C57.7	C79.82	D07.39	D28.7	D39.8	D49.59
male NEC	C63.9	C79.82	D07.60	D29.9	D40.9	D49.59
overlapping lesion	C63.8	—	—	—	—	—
specified site NEC	C63.7	C79.82	D07.69	D29.8	D40.8	D49.59
genitourinary tract						
female	C57.9	C79.82	D07.30	D28.9	D39.9	D49.59
male	C63.9	C79.82	D07.60	D29.9	D40.9	D49.59
gingiva (alveolar) (marginal)	C03.9	C79.89	D00.03	D10.39	D37.09	D49.0
lower	C03.1	C79.89	D00.03	D10.39	D37.09	D49.0
mandibular	C03.1	C79.89	D00.03	D10.39	D37.09	D49.0
maxillary	C03.0	C79.89	D00.03	D10.39	D37.09	D49.0
upper	C03.0	C79.89	D00.03	D10.39	D37.09	D49.0
gland, glandular (lymphatic) (system) — *see also* Neoplasm, lymph gland						
endocrine NEC	C75.9	C79.89	D09.3	D35.9	D44.9	D49.7
salivary — *see* Neoplasm, salivary gland						
glans penis	C60.1	C79.82	D07.4	D29.0	D40.8	D49.59
globus pallidus	C71.0	C79.31	—	D33.0	D43.0	D49.6
glomus						
coccygeal	C49.5	C79.89	—	D21.5	D48.1☑	D49.2
jugularis	C75.5	C79.89	—	D35.6	D44.7	D49.7
glosso-epiglottic fold(s)	C10.1	C79.89	D00.08	D10.5	D37.05	D49.0
glossopalatine fold	C09.1	C79.89	D00.08	D10.5	D37.05	D49.0
glossopharyngeal sulcus	C09.0	C79.89	D00.08	D10.5	D37.05	D49.0
glottis	C32.0	C78.39	D02.0	D14.1	D38.0	D49.1
gluteal region	C76.3	C79.89	D04.5	D36.7	D48.7	D49.89
great vessels NEC	C49.3	C79.89	—	D21.3	D48.1☑	D49.2
groin NEC	C76.3	C79.89	D04.5	D36.7	D48.7	D49.89
gum	C03.9	C79.89	D00.03	D10.39	D37.09	D49.0
lower	C03.1	C79.89	D00.03	D10.39	D37.09	D49.0
upper	C03.0	C79.89	D00.03	D10.39	D37.09	D49.0

	Malignant Primary	Malignant Secondary	Ca in situ	Benign	Uncertain Behavior	Unspecified Behavior
Neoplasm, neoplastic — *continued*						
hand NEC	C76.4-☑	C79.89	D04.6-☑	D36.7	D48.7	D49.89
head NEC	C76.0	C79.89	D04.4	D36.7	D48.7	D49.89
heart	C38.0	C79.89	—	D15.1	D48.7	D49.89
heel NEC	C76.5-☑	C79.89	D04.7-☑	D36.7	D48.7	D49.89
helix — *see also* Neoplasm, skin, ear	C44.20-☑	C79.2	D04.2-☑	D23.2-☑	D48.5	D49.2
hematopoietic, hemopoietic tissue NEC	C96.9	—	—	—	—	—
specified NEC	C96.Z	—	—	—	—	—
hemisphere, cerebral	C71.0	C79.31	—	D33.0	D43.0	D49.6
hemorrhoidal zone	C21.1	C78.5	D01.3	D12.9	D37.8	D49.0
hepatic — *see also* Index to disease, by histology	C22.9	C78.7	D01.5	D13.4	D37.6	D49.0
duct (bile)	C24.0	C78.89	D01.5	D13.5	D37.6	D49.0
flexure (colon)	C18.3	C78.5	D01.0	D12.3	D37.4	D49.0
primary	C22.8	C78.7	D01.5	D13.4	D37.6	D49.0
hepatobiliary	C24.9	C78.89	D01.5	D13.5	D37.6	D49.0
hepatoblastoma	C22.2	C78.7	D01.5	D13.4	D37.6	D49.0
hepatoma	C22.0	C78.7	D01.5	D13.4	D37.6	D49.0
hilus of lung	C34.0-☑	C78.0-☑	D02.2-☑	D14.3-☑	D38.1	D49.1
hippocampus, brain	C71.2	C79.31	—	D33.0	D43.0	D49.6
hip NEC	C76.5-☑	C79.89	D04.7-☑	D36.7	D48.7	D49.89
humerus (any part)	C40.0-☑	C79.51	—	D16.0-☑	—	—
hymen	C52	C79.82	D07.2	D28.1	D39.8	D49.59
hypopharynx, hypopharyngeal NEC	C13.9	C79.89	D00.08	D10.7	D37.05	D49.0
overlapping lesion	C13.8	—	—	—	—	—
postcricoid region	C13.0	C79.89	D00.08	D10.7	D37.05	D49.0
posterior wall	C13.2	C79.89	D00.08	D10.7	D37.05	D49.0
pyriform fossa (sinus)	C12	C79.89	D00.08	D10.7	D37.05	D49.0
hypophysis	C75.1	C79.89	D09.3	D35.2	D44.3	D49.7
hypothalamus	C71.0	C79.31	—	D33.0	D43.0	D49.6
ileocecum, ileocecal (coil) (junction) (valve)	C18.0	C78.5	D01.0	D12.0	D37.4	D49.0
ileum	C17.2	C78.4	D01.49	D13.39	D37.2	D49.0
ilium	C41.4	C79.51	—	D16.8	D48.0	D49.2
immunoproliferative NEC	C88.9	—	—	—	—	—
infraclavicular (region)	C76.1	C79.89	D04.5	D36.7	D48.7	D49.89
inguinal (region)	C76.3	C79.89	D04.5	D36.7	D48.7	D49.89
insula	C71.0	C79.31	—	D33.0	D43.0	D49.6
insular tissue (pancreas)	C25.4	C78.89	D01.7	D13.7	D37.8	D49.0
brain	C71.0	C79.31	—	D33.0	D43.0	D49.6
interarytenoid fold	C13.1	C78.39	D00.08	D10.7	D37.05	D49.0
hypopharyngeal aspect	C13.1	C79.89	D00.08	D10.7	D37.05	D49.0
laryngeal aspect	C32.1	C78.39	D02.0	D14.1	D38.0	D49.1
marginal zone	C13.1	C79.89	D00.08	D10.7	D37.05	D49.0
interdental papillae	C03.9	C79.89	D00.03	D10.39	D37.09	D49.0
lower	C03.1	C79.89	D00.03	D10.39	D37.09	D49.0
upper	C03.0	C79.89	D00.03	D10.39	D37.09	D49.0
internal						
capsule	C71.0	C79.31	—	D33.0	D43.0	D49.6
os (cervix)	C53.0	C79.82	D06.0	D26.0	D39.0	D49.59
intervertebral cartilage or disc	C41.2	C79.51	—	D16.6	D48.0	D49.2
intestine, intestinal	C26.0	C78.80	D01.40	D13.99	D37.8	D49.0
large	C18.9	C78.5	D01.0	D12.6	D37.4	D49.0
appendix	C18.1	C78.5	D01.0	D12.1	D37.3	D49.0
caput coli	C18.0	C78.5	D01.0	D12.0	D37.4	D49.0
cecum	C18.0	C78.5	D01.0	D12.0	D37.4	D49.0
colon	C18.9	C78.5	D01.0	D12.6	D37.4	D49.0
and rectum	C19	C78.5	D01.1	D12.7	D37.5	D49.0
ascending	C18.2	C78.5	D01.0	D12.2	D37.4	D49.0

	Malignant Primary	Malignant Secondary	Ca in situ	Benign	Uncertain Behavior	Unspecified Behavior
Neoplasm, neoplastic — *continued*						
intestine, intestinal — *continued*						
large — *continued*						
colon — *continued*						
caput	C18.0	C78.5	D01.0	D12.0	D37.4	D49.0
descending	C18.6	C78.5	D01.0	D12.4	D37.4	D49.0
distal	C18.6	C78.5	D01.0	D12.4	D37.4	D49.0
left	C18.6	C78.5	D01.0	D12.4	D37.4	D49.0
overlapping lesion	C18.8	—	—	—	—	—
pelvic	C18.7	C78.5	D01.0	D12.5	D37.4	D49.0
right	C18.2	C78.5	D01.0	D12.2	D37.4	D49.0
sigmoid (flexure)	C18.7	C78.5	D01.0	D12.5	D37.4	D49.0
transverse	C18.4	C78.5	D01.0	D12.3	D37.4	D49.0
hepatic flexure	C18.3	C78.5	D01.0	D12.3	D37.4	D49.0
ileocecum, ileocecal (coil) (valve)	C18.0	C78.5	D01.0	D12.0	D37.4	D49.0
overlapping lesion	C18.8	—	—	—	—	—
sigmoid flexure (lower) (upper)	C18.7	C78.5	D01.0	D12.5	D37.4	D49.0
splenic flexure	C18.5	C78.5	D01.0	D12.3	D37.4	D49.0
small	C17.9	C78.4	D01.40	D13.30	D37.2	D49.0
duodenum	C17.0	C78.4	D01.49	D13.2	D37.2	D49.0
ileum	C17.2	C78.4	D01.49	D13.39	D37.2	D49.0
jejunum	C17.1	C78.4	D01.49	D13.39	D37.2	D49.0
overlapping lesion	C17.8	—	—	—	—	—
tract NEC	C26.0	C78.89	D01.40	D13.99	D37.8	D49.0
intra-abdominal	C76.2	C79.89	D09.8	D36.7	D48.7	D49.89
intracranial NEC	C71.9	C79.31	—	D33.2	D43.2	D49.6
intrahepatic (bile) duct	C22.1	C78.7	D01.5	D13.4	D37.6	D49.0
intraocular	C69.9-☑	C79.49	D09.2-☑	D31.9-☑	D48.7	D49.89
intraorbital	C69.6-☑	C79.49	D09.2-☑	D31.6-☑	D48.7	D49.89
intrasellar	C75.1	C79.89	D09.3	D35.2	D44.3	D49.7
intrathoracic (cavity) (organs)	C76.1	C79.89	D09.8	D15.9	D48.7	D49.89
specified NEC	C76.1	C79.89	D09.8	D15.7	—	—
iris	C69.4-☑	C79.49	D09.2-☑	D31.4-☑	D48.7	D49.89
ischiorectal (fossa)	C76.3	C79.89	D09.8	D36.7	D48.7	D49.89
ischium	C41.4	C79.51	—	D16.8	D48.0	D49.2
island of Reil	C71.0	C79.31	—	D33.0	D43.0	D49.6
islands or islets of Langerhans	C25.4	C78.89	D01.7	D13.7	D37.8	D49.0
isthmus uteri	C54.0	C79.82	D07.0	D26.1	D39.0	D49.59
jaw	C76.0	C79.89	D09.8	D36.7	D48.7	D49.89
bone	C41.1	C79.51	—	D16.5	D48.0	D49.2
lower	C41.1	C79.51	—	D16.5	—	—
upper	C41.0	C79.51	—	D16.4	—	—
carcinoma (any type) (lower) (upper)	C76.0	C79.89	—	—	—	—
skin — *see also* Neoplasm, skin, face	C44.309	C79.2	D04.39	D23.39	D48.5	D49.2
soft tissues	C03.9	C79.89	D00.03	D10.39	D37.09	D49.0
lower	C03.1	C79.89	D00.03	D10.39	D37.09	D49.0
upper	C03.0	C79.89	D00.03	D10.39	D37.09	D49.0
jejunum	C17.1	C78.4	D01.49	D13.39	D37.2	D49.0
joint NEC — *see also* Neoplasm, bone	C41.9	C79.51	—	D16.9	D48.0	D49.2
acromioclavicular	C40.0-☑	C79.51	—	D16.0-☑	—	—
bursa or synovial membrane — *see* Neoplasm, connective tissue						
costovertebral	C41.3	C79.51	—	D16.7	D48.0	D49.2
sternocostal	C41.3	C79.51	—	D16.7	D48.0	D49.2
temporomandibular	C41.1	C79.51	—	D16.5	D48.0	D49.2
junction						
anorectal	C21.8	C78.5	D01.3	D12.9	D37.8	D49.0
cardioesophageal	C16.0	C78.89	D00.2	D13.1	D37.1	D49.0
esophagogastric	C16.0	C78.89	D00.2	D13.1	D37.1	D49.0
gastroesophageal	C16.0	C78.89	D00.2	D13.1	D37.1	D49.0

	Malignant Primary	Malignant Secondary	Ca in situ	Benign	Uncertain Behavior	Unspecified Behavior
Neoplasm, neoplastic — *continued*						
junction — *continued*						
hard and soft palate	C05.9	C79.89	D00.00	D10.39	D37.09	D49.0
ileocecal	C18.0	C78.5	D01.0	D12.0	D37.4	D49.0
pelvirectal	C19	C78.5	D01.1	D12.7	D37.5	D49.0
pelviureteric	C65.-☑	C79.0-☑	D09.19	D30.1-☑	D41.1-☑	D49.59
rectosigmoid	C19	C78.5	D01.1	D12.7	D37.5	D49.0
squamocolumnar, of cervix	C53.8	C79.82	D06.7	D26.0	D39.0	D49.59
Kaposi's sarcoma — *see* Kaposi's, sarcoma						
kidney (parenchymal)	C64.-☑	C79.0-☑	D09.19	D30.0-☑	D41.0-☑	D49.51-☑
calyx	C65.-☑	C79.0-☑	D09.19	D30.1-☑	D41.1-☑	D49.51-☑
hilus	C65.-☑	C79.0-☑	D09.19	D30.1-☑	D41.1-☑	D49.51-☑
pelvis	C65.-☑	C79.0-☑	D09.19	D30.1-☑	D41.1-☑	D49.51-☑
knee NEC	C76.5-☑	C79.89	D04.7-☑	D36.7	D48.7	D49.89
labia (skin)	C51.9	C79.82	D07.1	D28.0	D39.8	D49.59
majora	C51.0	C79.82	D07.1	D28.0	D39.8	D49.59
minora	C51.1	C79.82	D07.1	D28.0	D39.8	D49.59
labial — *see also* Neoplasm, lip	C00.9	C79.89	D00.01	D10.0	D37.01	D49.0
sulcus (lower) (upper)	C06.1	C79.89	D00.02	D10.39	D37.09	D49.0
labium (skin)	C51.9	C79.82	D07.1	D28.0	D39.8	D49.59
majus	C51.0	C79.82	D07.1	D28.0	D39.8	D49.59
minus	C51.1	C79.82	D07.1	D28.0	D39.8	D49.59
lacrimal						
canaliculi	C69.5-☑	C79.49	D09.2-☑	D31.5-☑	D48.7	D49.89
duct (nasal)	C69.5-☑	C79.49	D09.2-☑	D31.5-☑	D48.7	D49.89
gland	C69.5-☑	C79.49	D09.2-☑	D31.5-☑	D48.7	D49.89
punctum	C69.5-☑	C79.49	D09.2-☑	D31.5-☑	D48.7	D49.89
sac	C69.5-☑	C79.49	D09.2-☑	D31.5-☑	D48.7	D49.89
Langerhans, islands or islets	C25.4	C78.89	D01.7	D13.7	D37.8	D49.0
laryngopharynx	C13.9	C79.89	D00.08	D10.7	D37.05	D49.0
larynx, laryngeal NEC	C32.9	C78.39	D02.0	D14.1	D38.0	D49.1
aryepiglottic fold	C32.1	C78.39	D02.0	D14.1	D38.0	D49.1
cartilage (arytenoid) (cricoid) (cuneiform) (thyroid)	C32.3	C78.39	D02.0	D14.1	D38.0	D49.1
commissure (anterior) (posterior)	C32.0	C78.39	D02.0	D14.1	D38.0	D49.1
extrinsic NEC	C32.1	C78.39	D02.0	D14.1	D38.0	D49.1
meaning hypopharynx	C13.9	C79.89	D00.08	D10.7	D37.05	D49.0
interarytenoid fold	C32.1	C78.39	D02.0	D14.1	D38.0	D49.1
intrinsic	C32.0	C78.39	D02.0	D14.1	D38.0	D49.1
overlapping lesion	C32.8	—	—	—	—	—
ventricular band	C32.1	C78.39	D02.0	D14.1	D38.0	D49.1
leg NEC	C76.5-☑	C79.89	D04.7-☑	D36.7	D48.7	D49.89
lens, crystalline	C69.4-☑	C79.49	D09.2-☑	D31.4-☑	D48.7	D49.89
lid (lower) (upper)	C44.10-☑	C79.2	D04.1-☑	D23.1-☑	D48.5	D49.2
basal cell carcinoma	C44.11-☑	—	—	—	—	—
sebaceous cell	C44.13-☑	—	—	—	—	—
specified type NEC	C44.19-☑	—	—	—	—	—
squamous cell carcinoma	C44.12-☑	—	—	—	—	—
ligament — *see also* Neoplasm, connective tissue						
broad	C57.1-☑	C79.82	D07.39	D28.2	D39.8	D49.59
Mackenrodt's	C57.7	C79.82	D07.39	D28.7	D39.8	D49.59
non-uterine — *see* Neoplasm, connective tissue						
round	C57.2-☑	C79.82	—	D28.2	D39.8	D49.59
sacro-uterine	C57.3	C79.82	—	D28.2	D39.8	D49.59
uterine	C57.3	C79.82	—	D28.2	D39.8	D49.59
utero-ovarian	C57.7	C79.82	D07.39	D28.2	D39.8	D49.59
uterosacral	C57.3	C79.82	—	D28.2	D39.8	D49.59
limb	C76.8	C79.89	D04.8	D36.7	D48.7	D49.89

	Malignant Primary	Malignant Secondary	Ca in situ	Benign	Uncertain Behavior	Unspecified Behavior
Neoplasm, neoplastic — *continued*						
limb — *continued*						
lower	C76.5-☑	C79.89	DØ4.7-☑	D36.7	D48.7	D49.89
upper	C76.4-☑	C79.89	DØ4.6-☑	D36.7	D48.7	D49.89
limbus of cornea	C69.1-☑	C79.49	DØ9.2-☑	D31.1-☑	D48.7	D49.89
lingual NEC — *see also* Neoplasm, tongue	CØ2.9	C79.89	DØØ.Ø7	D1Ø.1	D37.Ø2	D49.Ø
lingula, lung	C34.1-☑	C78.Ø-☑	DØ2.2-☑	D14.3-☑	D38.1	D49.1
lip	CØØ.9	C79.89	DØØ.Ø1	D1Ø.Ø	D37.Ø1	D49.Ø
buccal aspect — *see* Neoplasm, lip, internal						
commissure	CØØ.6	C79.89	DØØ.Ø1	D1Ø.Ø	D37.Ø1	D49.Ø
external	CØØ.2	C79.89	DØØ.Ø1	D1Ø.Ø	D37.Ø1	D49.Ø
lower	CØØ.1	C79.89	DØØ.Ø1	D1Ø.Ø	D37.Ø1	D49.Ø
upper	CØØ.Ø	C79.89	DØØ.Ø1	D1Ø.Ø	D37.Ø1	D49.Ø
frenulum — *see* Neoplasm, lip, internal						
inner aspect — *see* Neoplasm, lip, internal						
internal	CØØ.5	C79.89	DØØ.Ø1	D1Ø.Ø	D37.Ø1	D49.Ø
lower	CØØ.4	C79.89	DØØ.Ø1	D1Ø.Ø	D37.Ø1	D49.Ø
upper	CØØ.3	C79.89	DØØ.Ø1	D1Ø.Ø	D37.Ø1	D49.Ø
lipstick area	CØØ.2	C79.89	DØØ.Ø1	D1Ø.Ø	D37.Ø1	D49.Ø
lower	CØØ.1	C79.89	DØØ.Ø1	D1Ø.Ø	D37.Ø1	D49.Ø
upper	CØØ.Ø	C79.89	DØØ.Ø1	D1Ø.Ø	D37.Ø1	D49.Ø
lower	CØØ.1	C79.89	DØØ.Ø1	D1Ø.Ø	D37.Ø1	D49.Ø
internal	CØØ.4	C79.89	DØØ.Ø1	D1Ø.Ø	D37.Ø1	D49.Ø
mucosa — *see* Neoplasm, lip, internal						
oral aspect — *see* Neoplasm, lip, internal						
overlapping lesion	CØØ.8	—	—	—	—	—
with oral cavity or pharynx	C14.8	—	—	—	—	—
skin (commissure) (lower) (upper)	C44.ØØ	C79.2	DØ4.Ø	D23.Ø	D48.5	D49.2
basal cell carcinoma	C44.Ø1	—	—	—	—	—
specified type NEC	C44.Ø9	—	—	—	—	—
squamous cell carcinoma	C44.Ø2	—	—	—	—	—
upper	CØØ.Ø	C79.89	DØØ.Ø1	D1Ø.Ø	D37.Ø1	D49.Ø
internal	CØØ.3	C79.89	DØØ.Ø1	D1Ø.Ø	D37.Ø1	D49.Ø
vermilion border	CØØ.2	C79.89	DØØ.Ø1	D1Ø.Ø	D37.Ø1	D49.Ø
lower	CØØ.1	C79.89	DØØ.Ø1	D1Ø.Ø	D37.Ø1	D49.Ø
upper	CØØ.Ø	C79.89	DØØ.Ø1	D1Ø.Ø	D37.Ø1	D49.Ø
lipomatous — *see* Lipoma, by site						
liver — *see also* Index to disease, by histology	C22.9	C78.7	DØ1.5	D13.4	D37.6	D49.Ø
primary	C22.8	C78.7	DØ1.5	D13.4	D37.6	D49.Ø
lumbosacral plexus	C47.5	C79.89	—	D36.16	D48.2	D49.2
lung	C34.9-☑	C78.Ø-☑	DØ2.2-☑	D14.3-☑	D38.1	D49.1
azygos lobe	C34.1-☑	C78.Ø-☑	DØ2.2-☑	D14.3-☑	D38.1	D49.1
carina	C34.Ø-☑	C78.Ø-☑	DØ2.2-☑	D14.3-☑	D38.1	D49.1
hilus	C34.Ø-☑	C78.Ø-☑	DØ2.2-☑	D14.3-☑	D38.1	D49.1
linqula	C34.1-☑	C78.Ø-☑	DØ2.2-☑	D14.3-☑	D38.1	D49.1
lobe NEC	C34.9-☑	C78.Ø-☑	DØ2.2-☑	D14.3-☑	D38.1	D49.1
lower lobe	C34.3-☑	C78.Ø-☑	DØ2.2-☑	D14.3-☑	D38.1	D49.1
main bronchus	C34.Ø-☑	C78.Ø-☑	DØ2.2-☑	D14.3-☑	D38.1	D49.1
mesothelioma — *see* Mesothelioma						
middle lobe	C34.2	C78.Ø-☑	DØ2.21	D14.31	D38.1	D49.1
overlapping lesion	C34.8-☑	—	—	—	—	—
upper lobe	C34.1-☑	C78.Ø-☑	DØ2.2-☑	D14.3-☑	D38.1	D49.1
lymph, lymphatic channel NEC	C49.9	C79.89	—	D21.9	D48.1☑	D49.2

	Malignant Primary	Malignant Secondary	Ca in situ	Benign	Uncertain Behavior	Unspecified Behavior
Neoplasm, neoplastic — *continued*						
lymph, lymphatic channel — *continued*						
gland (secondary)	—	C77.9	—	D36.Ø	D48.7	D49.89
abdominal	—	C77.2	—	D36.Ø	D48.7	D49.89
aortic	—	C77.2	—	D36.Ø	D48.7	D49.89
arm	—	C77.3	—	D36.Ø	D48.7	D49.89
auricular (anterior) (posterior)	—	C77.Ø	—	D36.Ø	D48.7	D49.89
axilla, axillary	—	C77.3	—	D36.Ø	D48.7	D49.89
brachial	—	C77.3	—	D36.Ø	D48.7	D49.89
bronchial	—	C77.1	—	D36.Ø	D48.7	D49.89
bronchopulmonary	—	C77.1	—	D36.Ø	D48.7	D49.89
celiac	—	C77.2	—	D36.Ø	D48.7	D49.89
cervical	—	C77.Ø	—	D36.Ø	D48.7	D49.89
cervicofacial	—	C77.Ø	—	D36.Ø	D48.7	D49.89
Cloquet	—	C77.4	—	D36.Ø	D48.7	D49.89
colic	—	C77.2	—	D36.Ø	D48.7	D49.89
common duct	—	C77.2	—	D36.Ø	D48.7	D49.89
cubital	—	C77.3	—	D36.Ø	D48.7	D49.89
diaphragmatic	—	C77.1	—	D36.Ø	D48.7	D49.89
epigastric, inferior	—	C77.1	—	D36.Ø	D48.7	D49.89
epitrochlear	—	C77.3	—	D36.Ø	D48.7	D49.89
esophageal	—	C77.1	—	D36.Ø	D48.7	D49.89
face	—	C77.Ø	—	D36.Ø	D48.7	D49.89
femoral	—	C77.4	—	D36.Ø	D48.7	D49.89
gastric	—	C77.2	—	D36.Ø	D48.7	D49.89
groin	—	C77.4	—	D36.Ø	D48.7	D49.89
head	—	C77.Ø	—	D36.Ø	D48.7	D49.89
hepatic	—	C77.2	—	D36.Ø	D48.7	D49.89
hilar (pulmonary)	—	C77.1	—	D36.Ø	D48.7	D49.89
splenic	—	C77.2	—	D36.Ø	D48.7	D49.89
hypogastric	—	C77.5	—	D36.Ø	D48.7	D49.89
ileocolic	—	C77.2	—	D36.Ø	D48.7	D49.89
iliac	—	C77.5	—	D36.Ø	D48.7	D49.89
infraclavicular	—	C77.3	—	D36.Ø	D48.7	D49.89
inguina, inguinal	—	C77.4	—	D36.Ø	D48.7	D49.89
innominate	—	C77.1	—	D36.Ø	D48.7	D49.89
intercostal	—	C77.1	—	D36.Ø	D48.7	D49.89
intestinal	—	C77.2	—	D36.Ø	D48.7	D49.89
intrabdominal	—	C77.2	—	D36.Ø	D48.7	D49.89
intrapelvic	—	C77.5	—	D36.Ø	D48.7	D49.89
intrathoracic	—	C77.1	—	D36.Ø	D48.7	D49.89
jugular	—	C77.Ø	—	D36.Ø	D48.7	D49.89
leg	—	C77.4	—	D36.Ø	D48.7	D49.89
limb						
lower	—	C77.4	—	D36.Ø	D48.7	D49.89
upper	—	C77.3	—	D36.Ø	D48.7	D49.89
lower limb	—	C77.4	—	D36.Ø	D48.7	D49.89
lumbar	—	C77.2	—	D36.Ø	D48.7	D49.89
mandibular	—	C77.Ø	—	D36.Ø	D48.7	D49.89
mediastinal	—	C77.1	—	D36.Ø	D48.7	D49.89
mesenteric (inferior) (superior)	—	C77.2	—	D36.Ø	D48.7	D49.89
midcolic	—	C77.2	—	D36.Ø	D48.7	D49.89
multiple sites in categories C77.0 - C77.5	—	C77.8	—	D36.Ø	D48.7	D49.89
neck	—	C77.Ø	—	D36.Ø	D48.7	D49.89
obturator	—	C77.5	—	D36.Ø	D48.7	D49.89
occipital	—	C77.Ø	—	D36.Ø	D48.7	D49.89
pancreatic	—	C77.2	—	D36.Ø	D48.7	D49.89
para-aortic	—	C77.2	—	D36.Ø	D48.7	D49.89
paracervical	—	C77.5	—	D36.Ø	D48.7	D49.89
parametrial	—	C77.5	—	D36.Ø	D48.7	D49.89
parasternal	—	C77.1	—	D36.Ø	D48.7	D49.89
parotid	—	C77.Ø	—	D36.Ø	D48.7	D49.89
pectoral	—	C77.3	—	D36.Ø	D48.7	D49.89
pelvic	—	C77.5	—	D36.Ø	D48.7	D49.89
peri-aortic	—	C77.2	—	D36.Ø	D48.7	D49.89
peripancreatic	—	C77.2	—	D36.Ø	D48.7	D49.89
popliteal	—	C77.4	—	D36.Ø	D48.7	D49.89
porta hepatis	—	C77.2	—	D36.Ø	D48.7	D49.89
portal	—	C77.2	—	D36.Ø	D48.7	D49.89
preauricular	—	C77.Ø	—	D36.Ø	D48.7	D49.89
prelaryngeal	—	C77.Ø	—	D36.Ø	D48.7	D49.89

	Malignant Primary	Malignant Secondary	Ca in situ	Benign	Uncertain Behavior	Unspecified Behavior
Neoplasm, neoplastic — *continued*						
lymph, lymphatic channel — *continued*						
gland — *continued*						
presymphysial	—	C77.5	—	D36.Ø	D48.7	D49.89
pretracheal	—	C77.Ø	—	D36.Ø	D48.7	D49.89
primary (any site) NEC	C96.9	—	—	—	—	—
pulmonary (hiler)	—	C77.1	—	D36.Ø	D48.7	D49.89
pyloric	—	C77.2	—	D36.Ø	D48.7	D49.89
retroperitoneal	—	C77.2	—	D36.Ø	D48.7	D49.89
retropharyngeal	—	C77.Ø	—	D36.Ø	D48.7	D49.89
Rosenmuller's	—	C77.4	—	D36.Ø	D48.7	D49.89
sacral	—	C77.5	—	D36.Ø	D48.7	D49.89
scalene	—	C77.Ø	—	D36.Ø	D48.7	D49.89
site NEC	—	C77.9	—	D36.Ø	D48.7	D49.89
splenic (hilar)	—	C77.2	—	D36.Ø	D48.7	D49.89
subclavicular	—	C77.3	—	D36.Ø	D48.7	D49.89
subinguinal	—	C77.4	—	D36.Ø	D48.7	D49.89
sublingual	—	C77.Ø	—	D36.Ø	D48.7	D49.89
submandibular	—	C77.Ø	—	D36.Ø	D48.7	D49.89
submaxillary	—	C77.Ø	—	D36.Ø	D48.7	D49.89
submental	—	C77.Ø	—	D36.Ø	D48.7	D49.89
subscapular	—	C77.3	—	D36.Ø	D48.7	D49.89
supraclavicular	—	C77.Ø	—	D36.Ø	D48.7	D49.89
thoracic	—	C77.1	—	D36.Ø	D48.7	D49.89
tibial	—	C77.4	—	D36.Ø	D48.7	D49.89
tracheal	—	C77.1	—	D36.Ø	D48.7	D49.89
tracheobronchial	—	C77.1	—	D36.Ø	D48.7	D49.89
upper limb	—	C77.3	—	D36.Ø	D48.7	D49.89
Virchow's	—	C77.Ø	—	D36.Ø	D48.7	D49.89
node — *see also* Neoplasm, lymph gland						
primary NEC	C96.9	—	—	—	—	—
vessel — *see also* Neoplasm, connective tissue	C49.9	C79.89	—	D21.9	D48.1☑	D49.2
Mackenrodt's ligament	C57.7	C79.82	DØ7.39	D28.7	D39.8	D49.59
malar	C41.Ø	C79.51	—	D16.4	D48.Ø	D49.2
region — *see* Neoplasm, cheek						
mammary gland — *see* Neoplasm, breast						
mandible	C41.1	C79.51	—	D16.5	D48.Ø	D49.2
alveolar						
mucosa (carcinoma)	CØ3.1	C79.89	DØØ.Ø3	D1Ø.39	D37.Ø9	D49.Ø
ridge or process	C41.1	C79.51	—	D16.5	D48.Ø	D49.2
marrow (bone) NEC	C96.9	C79.52	—	—	D47.9	D49.89
mastectomy site (skin) — *see also* Neoplasm, breast, skin	C44.5Ø1	C79.2	—	—	—	—
specified as breast tissue	C5Ø.8-☑	C79.81	—	—	—	—
mastoid (air cells) (antrum) (cavity)	C3Ø.1	C78.39	DØ2.3	D14.Ø	D38.5	D49.1
bone or process	C41.Ø	C79.51	—	D16.4	D48.Ø	D49.2
maxilla, maxillary (superior)	C41.Ø	C79.51	—	D16.4	D48.Ø	D49.2
alveolar						
mucosa	CØ3.Ø	C79.89	DØØ.Ø3	D1Ø.39	D37.Ø9	D49.Ø
ridge or process (carcinoma)	C41.Ø	C79.51	—	D16.4	D48.Ø	D49.2
antrum	C31.Ø	C78.39	DØ2.3	D14.Ø	D38.5	D49.1
carcinoma	CØ3.Ø	C79.51	—	—	—	—
inferior — *see* Neoplasm, mandible						
sinus	C31.Ø	C78.39	DØ2.3	D14.Ø	D38.5	D49.1
meatus external (ear) — *see also* Neoplasm, skin, ear	C44.2Ø-☑	C79.2	DØ4.2-☑	D23.2-☑	D48.5	D49.2

	Malignant Primary	Malignant Secondary	Ca in situ	Benign	Uncertain Behavior	Unspecified Behavior
Neoplasm, neoplastic — *continued*						
Meckel diverticulum, malignant	C17.3	C78.4	DØ1.49	D13.39	D37.2	D49.Ø
mediastinum, mediastinal	C38.3	C78.1	—	D15.2	D38.3	D49.89
anterior	C38.1	C78.1	—	D15.2	D38.3	D49.89
posterior	C38.2	C78.1	—	D15.2	D38.3	D49.89
medulla						
adrenal	C74.1-☑	C79.7-☑	DØ9.3	D35.Ø-☑	D44.1-☑	D49.7
oblongata	C71.7	C79.31	—	D33.1	D43.1	D49.6
meibomian gland	C44.1Ø-☑	C79.2	DØ4.1-☑	D23.1-☑	D48.5	D49.2
basal cell carcinoma	C44.11-☑	—	—	—	—	—
sebaceous cell	C44.13-☑	—	—	—	—	—
specified type NEC	C44.19-☑	—	—	—	—	—
squamous cell carcinoma	C44.12-☑	—	—	—	—	—
melanoma — *see* Melanoma						
meninges	C7Ø.9	C79.49	—	D32.9	D42.9	D49.7
brain	C7Ø.Ø	C79.32	—	D32.Ø	D42.Ø	D49.7
cerebral	C7Ø.Ø	C79.32	—	D32.Ø	D42.Ø	D49.7
crainial	C7Ø.Ø	C79.32	—	D32.Ø	D42.Ø	D49.7
intracranial	C7Ø.Ø	C79.32	—	D32.Ø	D42.Ø	D49.7
spinal (cord)	C7Ø.1	C79.49	—	D32.1	D42.1	D49.7
meniscus, knee joint (lateral) (medial)	C4Ø.2-☑	C79.51	—	D16.2-☑	D48.Ø	D49.2
Merkel cell — *see* Carcinoma, Merkel cell						
mesentery, mesenteric	C48.1	C78.6	—	D2Ø.1	D48.4	D49.Ø
mesoappendix	C48.1	C78.6	—	D2Ø.1	D48.4	D49.Ø
mesocolon	C48.1	C78.6	—	D2Ø.1	D48.4	D49.Ø
mesopharynx — *see* Neoplasm, oropharynx						
mesosalpinx	C57.1-☑	C79.82	DØ7.39	D28.2	D39.8	D49.59
mesothelial tissue — *see* Mesothelioma						
mesothelioma — *see* Mesothelioma						
mesovarium	C57.1-☑	C79.82	DØ7.39	D28.2	D39.8	D49.59
metacarpus (any bone)	C4Ø.1-☑	C79.51	—	D16.1-☑	—	—
metastatic NEC — *see also* Neoplasm, by site, secondary	—	C79.9	—	—	—	—
metatarsus (any bone)	C4Ø.3-☑	C79.51	—	D16.3-☑	—	—
midbrain	C71.7	C79.31	—	D33.1	D43.1	D49.6
milk duct — *see* Neoplasm, breast						
mons						
pubis	C51.9	C79.82	DØ7.1	D28.Ø	D39.8	D49.59
veneris	C51.9	C79.82	DØ7.1	D28.Ø	D39.8	D49.59
motor tract	C72.9	C79.49	—	D33.9	D43.9	D49.7
brain	C71.9	C79.31	—	D33.2	D43.2	D49.6
cauda equina	C72.1	C79.49	—	D33.4	D43.4	D49.7
spinal	C72.Ø	C79.49	—	D33.4	D43.4	D49.7
mouth	CØ6.9	C79.89	DØØ.ØØ	D1Ø.3Ø	D37.Ø9	D49.Ø
book-leaf	CØ6.89	C79.89	—	—	—	—
floor	CØ4.9	C79.89	DØØ.Ø6	D1Ø.2	D37.Ø9	D49.Ø
anterior portion	CØ4.Ø	C79.89	DØØ.Ø6	D1Ø.2	D37.Ø9	D49.Ø
lateral portion	CØ4.1	C79.89	DØØ.Ø6	D1Ø.2	D37.Ø9	D49.Ø
overlapping lesion	CØ4.8	—	—	—	—	—
overlapping NEC	CØ6.8Ø	—	—	—	—	—
roof	CØ5.9	C79.89	DØØ.ØØ	D1Ø.39	D37.Ø9	D49.Ø
specified part NEC	CØ6.89	C79.89	DØØ.ØØ	D1Ø.39	D37.Ø9	D49.Ø
vestibule	CØ6.1	C79.89	DØØ.ØØ	D1Ø.39	D37.Ø9	D49.Ø
mucosa						
alveolar (ridge or process)	CØ3.9	C79.89	DØØ.Ø3	D1Ø.39	D37.Ø9	D49.Ø
lower	CØ3.1	C79.89	DØØ.Ø3	D1Ø.39	D37.Ø9	D49.Ø
upper	CØ3.Ø	C79.89	DØØ.Ø3	D1Ø.39	D37.Ø9	D49.Ø

☑ **Additional Character Required — Refer to the Tabular List for Character Selection**

	Malignant Primary	Malignant Secondary	Ca in situ	Benign	Uncertain Behavior	Unspecified Behavior
Neoplasm, neoplastic — *continued*						
mucosa — *continued*						
buccal	CØ6.Ø	C79.89	DØØ.Ø2	D1Ø.39	D37.Ø9	D49.Ø
cheek	CØ6.Ø	C79.89	DØØ.Ø2	D1Ø.39	D37.Ø9	D49.Ø
lip — *see* Neoplasm, lip, internal						
nasal	C3Ø.Ø	C78.39	DØ2.3	D14.Ø	D38.5	D49.1
oral	CØ6.Ø	C79.89	DØØ.Ø2	D1Ø.39	D37.Ø9	D49.Ø
Mullerian duct						
female	C57.7	C79.82	DØ7.39	D28.7	D39.8	D49.59
male	C63.7	C79.82	DØ7.69	D29.8	D4Ø.8	D49.59
muscle — *see also* Neoplasm, connective tissue						
extraocular	C69.6-☑	C79.49	DØ9.2-☑	D31.6-☑	D48.7	D49.89
myocardium	C38.Ø	C79.89	—	D15.1	D48.7	D49.89
myometrium	C54.2	C79.82	DØ7.Ø	D26.1	D39.Ø	D49.59
myopericardium	C38.Ø	C79.89	—	D15.1	D48.7	D49.89
nabothian gland (follicle)	C53.Ø	C79.82	DØ6.Ø	D26.Ø	D39.Ø	D49.59
nail — *see also* Neoplasm, skin, limb	C44.9Ø	C79.2	DØ4.9	D23.9	D48.5	D49.2
finger — *see also* Neoplasm, skin, limb, upper	C44.6Ø-☑	C79.2	DØ4.6-☑	D23.6-☑	D48.5	D49.2
toe — *see also* Neoplasm, skin, limb, lower	C44.7Ø-☑	C79.2	DØ4.7-☑	D23.7-☑	D48.5	D49.2
nares, naris (anterior) (posterior)	C3Ø.Ø	C78.39	DØ2.3	D14.Ø	D38.5	D49.1
nasal — *see* Neoplasm, nose						
nasolabial groove — *see also* Neoplasm, skin, face	C44.3Ø9	C79.2	DØ4.39	D23.39	D48.5	D49.2
nasolacrimal duct	C69.5-☑	C79.49	DØ9.2-☑	D31.5-☑	D48.7	D49.89
nasopharynx, nasopharyngeal	C11.9	C79.89	DØØ.Ø8	D1Ø.6	D37.Ø5	D49.Ø
floor	C11.3	C79.89	DØØ.Ø8	D1Ø.6	D37.Ø5	D49.Ø
overlapping lesion	C11.8	—	—	—	—	—
roof	C11.Ø	C79.89	DØØ.Ø8	D1Ø.6	D37.Ø5	D49.Ø
wall	C11.9	C79.89	DØØ.Ø8	D1Ø.6	D37.Ø5	D49.Ø
anterior	C11.3	C79.89	DØØ.Ø8	D1Ø.6	D37.Ø5	D49.Ø
lateral	C11.2	C79.89	DØØ.Ø8	D1Ø.6	D37.Ø5	D49.Ø
posterior	C11.1	C79.89	DØØ.Ø8	D1Ø.6	D37.Ø5	D49.Ø
superior	C11.Ø	C79.89	DØØ.Ø8	D1Ø.6	D37.Ø5	D49.Ø
nates — *see also* Neoplasm, skin, trunk	C44.5Ø9	C79.2	DØ4.5	D23.5	D48.5	D49.2
neck NEC	C76.Ø	C79.89	DØ9.8	D36.7	D48.7	D49.89
skin	C44.4Ø	—	—	—	—	—
basal cell carcinoma	C44.41	—	—	—	—	—
specified type NEC	C44.49	—	—	—	—	—
squamous cell carcinoma	C44.42	—	—	—	—	—
nerve (ganglion)	C47.9	C79.89	—	D36.1Ø	D48.2	D49.2
abducens	C72.59	C79.49	—	D33.3	D43.3	D49.7
accessory (spinal)	C72.59	C79.49	—	D33.3	D43.3	D49.7
acoustic	C72.4-☑	C79.49	—	D33.3	D43.3	D49.7
auditory	C72.4-☑	C79.49	—	D33.3	D43.3	D49.7
autonomic NEC — *see also* Neoplasm, nerve, peripheral	C47.9	C79.89	—	D36.1Ø	D48.2	D49.2
brachial	C47.1-☑	C79.89	—	D36.12	D48.2	D49.2
cranial	C72.5Ø	C79.49	—	D33.3	D43.3	D49.7
specified NEC	C72.59	C79.49	—	D33.3	D43.3	D49.7
facial	C72.59	C79.49	—	D33.3	D43.3	D49.7
femoral	C47.2-☑	C79.89	—	D36.13	D48.2	D49.2
ganglion NEC — *see also* Neoplasm, nerve, peripheral	C47.9	C79.89	—	D36.1Ø	D48.2	D49.2
glossopharyngeal	C72.59	C79.49	—	D33.3	D43.3	D49.7
hypoglossal	C72.59	C79.49	—	D33.3	D43.3	D49.7
intercostal	C47.3	C79.89	—	D36.14	D48.2	D49.2
lumbar	C47.6	C79.89	—	D36.17	D48.2	D49.2
Neoplasm, neoplastic — *continued*						
nerve — *continued*						
median	C47.1-☑	C79.89	—	D36.12	D48.2	D49.2
obturator	C47.2-☑	C79.89	—	D36.13	D48.2	D49.2
oculomotor	C72.59	C79.49	—	D33.3	D43.3	D49.7
olfactory	C47.2-☑	C79.49	—	D33.3	D43.3	D49.7
optic	C72.3-☑	C79.49	—	D33.3	D43.3	D49.7
parasympathetic NEC	C47.9	C79.89	—	D36.1Ø	D48.2	D49.2
peripheral NEC	C47.9	C79.89	—	D36.1Ø	D48.2	D49.2
abdomen	C47.4	C79.89	—	D36.15	D48.2	D49.2
abdominal wall	C47.4	C79.89	—	D36.15	D48.2	D49.2
ankle	C47.2-☑	C79.89	—	D36.13	D48.2	D49.2
antecubital fossa or space	C47.1-☑	C79.89	—	D36.12	D48.2	D49.2
arm	C47.1-☑	C79.89	—	D36.12	D48.2	D49.2
auricle (ear)	C47.Ø	C79.89	—	D36.11	D48.2	D49.2
axilla	C47.3	C79.89	—	D36.12	D48.2	D49.2
back	C47.6	C79.89	—	D36.17	D48.2	D49.2
buttock	C47.5	C79.89	—	D36.16	D48.2	D49.2
calf	C47.2-☑	C79.89	—	D36.13	D48.2	D49.2
cervical region	C47.Ø	C79.89	—	D36.11	D48.2	D49.2
cheek	C47.Ø	C79.89	—	D36.11	D48.2	D49.2
chest (wall)	C47.3	C79.89	—	D36.14	D48.2	D49.2
chin	C47.Ø	C79.89	—	D36.11	D48.2	D49.2
ear (external)	C47.Ø	C79.89	—	D36.11	D48.2	D49.2
elbow	C47.1-☑	C79.89	—	D36.12	D48.2	D49.2
extrarectal	C47.5	C79.89	—	D36.16	D48.2	D49.2
extremity	C47.9	C79.89	—	D36.1Ø	D48.2	D49.2
lower	C47.2-☑	C79.89	—	D36.13	D48.2	D49.2
upper	C47.1-☑	C79.89	—	D36.12	D48.2	D49.2
eyelid	C47.Ø	C79.89	—	D36.11	D48.2	D49.2
face	C47.Ø	C79.89	—	D36.11	D48.2	D49.2
finger	C47.1-☑	C79.89	—	D36.12	D48.2	D49.2
flank	C47.6	C79.89	—	D36.17	D48.2	D49.2
foot	C47.2-☑	C79.89	—	D36.13	D48.2	D49.2
forearm	C47.1-☑	C79.89	—	D36.12	D48.2	D49.2
forehead	C47.Ø	C79.89	—	D36.11	D48.2	D49.2
gluteal region	C47.5	C79.89	—	D36.16	D48.2	D49.2
groin	C47.5	C79.89	—	D36.16	D48.2	D49.2
hand	C47.1-☑	C79.89	—	D36.12	D48.2	D49.2
head	C47.Ø	C79.89	—	D36.11	D48.2	D49.2
heel	C47.2-☑	C79.89	—	D36.13	D48.2	D49.2
hip	C47.2-☑	C79.89	—	D36.13	D48.2	D49.2
infraclavicular region	C47.3	C79.89	—	D36.14	D48.2	D49.2
inguinal (canal) (region)	C47.5	C79.89	—	D36.16	D48.2	D49.2
intrathoracic	C47.3	C79.89	—	D36.14	D48.2	D49.2
ischiorectal fossa	C47.5	C79.89	—	D36.16	D48.2	D49.2
knee	C47.2-☑	C79.89	—	D36.13	D48.2	D49.2
leg	C47.2-☑	C79.89	—	D36.13	D48.2	D49.2
limb NEC	C47.9	C79.89	—	D36.1Ø	D48.2	D49.2
lower	C47.2-☑	C79.89	—	D36.13	D48.2	D49.2
upper	C47.1-☑	C79.89	—	D36.12	D48.2	D49.2
nates	C47.5	C79.89	—	D36.16	D48.2	D49.2
neck	C47.Ø	C79.89	—	D36.11	D48.2	D49.2
orbit	C69.6-☑	C79.49	—	D31.6-☑	D48.7	D49.2
pararectal	C47.5	C79.89	—	D36.16	D48.2	D49.2
paraurethral	C47.5	C79.89	—	D36.16	D48.2	D49.2
paravaginal	C47.5	C79.89	—	D36.16	D48.2	D49.2
pelvis (floor)	C47.5	C79.89	—	D36.16	D48.2	D49.2
pelvoabdominal	C47.8	C79.89	—	D36.17	D48.2	D49.2
perineum	C47.5	C79.89	—	D36.16	D48.2	D49.2
perirectal (tissue)	C47.5	C79.89	—	D36.16	D48.2	D49.2
periurethral (tissue)	C47.5	C79.89	—	D36.16	D48.2	D49.2
popliteal fossa or space	C47.2-☑	C79.89	—	D36.13	D48.2	D49.2
presacral	C47.5	C79.89	—	D36.16	D48.2	D49.2
pterygoid fossa	C47.Ø	C79.89	—	D36.11	D48.2	D49.2
rectovaginal septum or wall	C47.5	C79.89	—	D36.16	D48.2	D49.2
rectovesical	C47.5	C79.89	—	D36.16	D48.2	D49.2
sacrococcygeal region	C47.5	C79.89	—	D36.16	D48.2	D49.2

	Malignant Primary	Malignant Secondary	Ca in situ	Benign	Uncertain Behavior	Unspecified Behavior
Neoplasm, neoplastic — *continued*						
nerve — *continued*						
peripheral — *continued*						
scalp	C47.Ø	C79.89	—	D36.11	D48.2	D49.2
scapular region	C47.3	C79.89	—	D36.14	D48.2	D49.2
shoulder	C47.1-☑	C79.89	—	D36.12	D48.2	D49.2
submental	C47.Ø	C79.89	—	D36.11	D48.2	D49.2
supraclavicular region	C47.Ø	C79.89	—	D36.11	D48.2	D49.2
temple	C47.Ø	C79.89	—	D36.11	D48.2	D49.2
temporal region	C47.Ø	C79.89	—	D36.11	D48.2	D49.2
thigh	C47.2-☑	C79.89	—	D36.13	D48.2	D49.2
thoracic (duct) (wall)	C47.3	C79.89	—	D36.14	D48.2	D49.2
thorax	C47.3	C79.89	—	D36.14	D48.2	D49.2
thumb	C47.1-☑	C79.89	—	D36.12	D48.2	D49.2
toe	C47.2-☑	C79.89	—	D36.13	D48.2	D49.2
trunk	C47.6	C79.89	—	D36.17	D48.2	D49.2
umbilicus	C47.4	C79.89	—	D36.15	D48.2	D49.2
vesicorectal	C47.5	C79.89	—	D36.16	D48.2	D49.2
wrist	C47.1-☑	C79.89	—	D36.12	D48.2	D49.2
radial	C47.1-☑	C79.89	—	D36.12	D48.2	D49.2
sacral	C47.5	C79.89	—	D36.16	D48.2	D49.2
sciatic	C47.2-☑	C79.89	—	D36.13	D48.2	D49.2
spinal NEC	C47.9	C79.89	—	D36.1Ø	D48.2	D49.2
accessory	C72.59	C79.49	—	D33.3	D43.3	D49.7
sympathetic NEC — *see also* Neoplasm, nerve, peripheral	C47.9	C79.89	—	D36.1Ø	D48.2	D49.2
trigeminal	C72.59	C79.49	—	D33.3	D43.3	D49.7
trochlear	C72.59	C79.49	—	D33.3	D43.3	D49.7
ulnar	C47.1-☑	C79.89	—	D36.12	D48.2	D49.2
vagus	C72.59	C79.49	—	D33.3	D43.3	D49.7
nervous system (central)	C72.9	C79.4Ø	—	D33.9	D43.9	D49.7
autonomic — *see* Neoplasm, nerve, peripheral						
parasympathetic — *see* Neoplasm, nerve, peripheral						
specified site NEC	—	C79.49	—	D33.7	D43.8	—
sympathetic — *see* Neoplasm, nerve, peripheral						
nevus — *see* Nevus						
nipple	C5Ø.Ø-☑	C79.81	DØ5.-☑	D24.-☑	—	—
nose, nasal	C76.Ø	C79.89	DØ9.8	D36.7	D48.7	D49.89
ala (external) (nasi) — *see also* Neoplasm, nose, skin	C44.3Ø1	C79.2	DØ4.39	D23.39	D48.5	D49.2
bone	C41.Ø	C79.51	—	D16.4	D48.Ø	D49.2
cartilage	C3Ø.Ø	C78.39	DØ2.3	D14.Ø	D38.5	D49.1
cavity	C3Ø.Ø	C78.39	DØ2.3	D14.Ø	D38.5	D49.1
choana	C11.3	C79.89	DØØ.Ø8	D1Ø.6	D37.Ø5	D49.Ø
external (skin) — *see also* Neoplasm, nose, skin	C44.3Ø1	C79.2	DØ4.39	D23.39	D48.5	D49.2
fossa	C3Ø.Ø	C78.39	DØ2.3	D14.Ø	D38.5	D49.1
internal	C3Ø.Ø	C78.39	DØ2.3	D14.Ø	D38.5	D49.1
mucosa	C3Ø.Ø	C78.39	DØ2.3	D14.Ø	D38.5	D49.1
septum	C3Ø.Ø	C78.39	DØ2.3	D14.Ø	D38.5	D49.1
posterior margin	C11.3	C79.89	DØØ.Ø8	D1Ø.6	D37.Ø5	D49.Ø
sinus — *see* Neoplasm, sinus						
skin	C44.3Ø1	C79.2	DØ4.39	D23.39	D48.5	D49.2
basal cell carcinoma	C44.311	—	—	—	—	—
specified type NEC	C44.391	—	—	—	—	—
squamous cell carcinoma	C44.321	—	—	—	—	—
turbinate (mucosa)	C3Ø.Ø	C78.39	DØ2.3	D14.Ø	D38.5	D49.1
bone	C41.Ø	C79.51	—	D16.4	D48.Ø	D49.2

	Malignant Primary	Malignant Secondary	Ca in situ	Benign	Uncertain Behavior	Unspecified Behavior
Neoplasm, neoplastic — *continued*						
nose, nasal — *continued*						
vestibule	C3Ø.Ø	C78.39	DØ2.3	D14.Ø	D38.5	D49.1
nostril	C3Ø.Ø	C78.39	DØ2.3	D14.Ø	D38.5	D49.1
nucleus pulposus	C41.2	C79.51	—	D16.6	D48.Ø	D49.2
occipital						
bone	C41.Ø	C79.51	—	D16.4	D48.Ø	D49.2
lobe or pole, brain	C71.4	C79.31	—	D33.Ø	D43.Ø	D49.6
odontogenic — *see* Neoplasm, jaw bone						
olfactory nerve or bulb	C72.2-☑	C79.49	—	D33.3	D43.3	D49.7
olive (brain)	C71.7	C79.31	—	D33.1	D43.1	D49.6
omentum	C48.1	C78.6	—	D2Ø.1	D48.4	D49.Ø
operculum (brain)	C71.Ø	C79.31	—	D33.Ø	D43.Ø	D49.6
optic nerve, chiasm, or tract	C72.3-☑	C79.49	—	D33.3	D43.3	D49.7
oral (cavity)	CØ6.9	C79.89	DØØ.ØØ	D1Ø.3Ø	D37.Ø9	D49.Ø
ill-defined	C14.8	C79.89	DØØ.ØØ	D1Ø.3Ø	D37.Ø9	D49.Ø
mucosa	CØ6.Ø	C79.89	DØØ.Ø2	D1Ø.39	D37.Ø9	D49.Ø
orbit	C69.6-☑	C79.49	DØ9.2-☑	D31.6-☑	D48.7	D49.89
autonomic nerve	C69.6-☑	C79.49	—	D31.6-☑	D48.7	D49.2
bone	C41.Ø	C79.51	—	D16.4	D48.Ø	D49.2
eye	C69.6-☑	C79.49	DØ9.2-☑	D31.6-☑	D48.7	D49.89
peripheral nerves	C69.6-☑	C79.49	—	D31.6-☑	D48.7	D49.2
soft parts	C69.6-☑	C79.49	DØ9.2-☑	D31.6-☑	D48.7	D49.89
organ of Zuckerkandl	C75.5	C79.89	—	D35.6	D44.7	D49.7
oropharynx	C1Ø.9	C79.89	DØØ.Ø8	D1Ø.5	D37.Ø5	D49.Ø
branchial cleft (vestige)	C1Ø.4	C79.89	DØØ.Ø8	D1Ø.5	D37.Ø5	D49.Ø
junctional region	C1Ø.8	C79.89	DØØ.Ø8	D1Ø.5	D37.Ø5	D49.Ø
lateral wall	C1Ø.2	C79.89	DØØ.Ø8	D1Ø.5	D37.Ø5	D49.Ø
overlapping lesion	C1Ø.8	—	—	—	—	—
pillars or fauces	CØ9.1	C79.89	DØØ.Ø8	D1Ø.5	D37.Ø5	D49.Ø
posterior wall	C1Ø.3	C79.89	DØØ.Ø8	D1Ø.5	D37.Ø5	D49.Ø
vallecula	C1Ø.Ø	C79.89	DØØ.Ø8	D1Ø.5	D37.Ø5	D49.Ø
os						
external	C53.1	C79.82	DØ6.1	D26.Ø	D39.Ø	D49.59
internal	C53.Ø	C79.82	DØ6.Ø	D26.Ø	D39.Ø	D49.59
ovary	C56.-☑	C79.6-☑	DØ7.39	D27.-☑	D39.1-☑	D49.59
oviduct	C57.Ø-☑	C79.82	DØ7.39	D28.2	D39.8	D49.59
palate	CØ5.9	C79.89	DØØ.ØØ	D1Ø.39	D37.Ø9	D49.Ø
hard	CØ5.Ø	C79.89	DØØ.Ø5	D1Ø.39	D37.Ø9	D49.Ø
junction of hard and soft palate	CØ5.9	C79.89	DØØ.ØØ	D1Ø.39	D37.Ø9	D49.Ø
overlapping lesions	CØ5.8	—	—	—	—	—
soft	CØ5.1	C79.89	DØØ.Ø4	D1Ø.39	D37.Ø9	D49.Ø
nasopharyngeal surface	C11.3	C79.89	DØØ.Ø8	D1Ø.6	D37.Ø5	D49.Ø
posterior surface	C11.3	C79.89	DØØ.Ø8	D1Ø.6	D37.Ø5	D49.Ø
superior surface	C11.3	C79.89	DØØ.Ø8	D1Ø.6	D37.Ø5	D49.Ø
palatoglossal arch	CØ9.1	C79.89	DØØ.ØØ	D1Ø.5	D37.Ø9	D49.Ø
palatopharyngeal arch	CØ9.1	C79.89	DØØ.ØØ	D1Ø.5	D37.Ø9	D49.Ø
pallium	C71.Ø	C79.31	—	D33.Ø	D43.Ø	D49.6
palpebra	C44.1Ø-☑	C79.2	DØ4.1-☑	D23.1-☑	D48.5	D49.2
basal cell carcinoma	C44.11-☑	—	—	—	—	—
sebaceous cell	C44.13-☑	—	—	—	—	—
specified type NEC	C44.19-☑	—	—	—	—	—
squamous cell carcinoma	C44.12-☑	—	—	—	—	—
pancreas	C25.9	C78.89	DØ1.7	D13.6	D37.8	D49.Ø
body	C25.1	C78.89	DØ1.7	D13.6	D37.8	D49.Ø
duct (of Santorini) (of Wirsung)	C25.3	C78.89	DØ1.7	D13.6	D37.8	D49.Ø
ectopic tissue	C25.7	C78.89	—	D13.6	D37.8	D49.Ø
head	C25.Ø	C78.89	DØ1.7	D13.6	D37.8	D49.Ø
islet cells	C25.4	C78.89	DØ1.7	D13.7	D37.8	D49.Ø
neck	C25.7	C78.89	DØ1.7	D13.6	D37.8	D49.Ø

	Malignant Primary	Malignant Secondary	Ca in situ	Benign	Uncertain Behavior	Unspecified Behavior
Neoplasm, neoplastic — *continued*						
pancreas — *continued*						
overlapping lesion	C25.8	—	—	—	—	—
tail	C25.2	C78.89	DØ1.7	D13.6	D37.8	D49.Ø
para-aortic body	C75.5	C79.89	—	D35.6	D44.7	D49.7
paraganglion NEC	C75.5	C79.89	—	D35.6	D44.7	D49.7
parametrium	C57.3	C79.82	—	D28.2	D39.8	D49.59
paranephric	C48.Ø	C78.6	—	D2Ø.Ø	D48.3	D49.Ø
pararectal	C76.3	C79.89	—	D36.7	D48.7	D49.89
parasagittal (region)	C76.Ø	C79.89	DØ9.8	D36.7	D48.7	D49.89
parasellar	C72.9	C79.49	—	D33.9	D43.8	D49.7
parathyroid (gland)	C75.Ø	C79.89	DØ9.3	D35.1	D44.2	D49.7
paraurethral	C76.3	C79.89	—	D36.7	D48.7	D49.89
gland	C68.1	C79.19	DØ9.19	D3Ø.8	D41.8	D49.59
paravaginal	C76.3	C79.89	—	D36.7	D48.7	D49.89
parenchyma, kidney	C64.-☑	C79.Ø-☑	DØ9.19	D3Ø.Ø-☑	D41.Ø-☑	D49.51-☑
parietal						
bone	C41.Ø	C79.51	—	D16.4	D48.Ø	D49.2
lobe, brain	C71.3	C79.31	—	D33.Ø	D43.Ø	D49.6
paroophoron	C57.1-☑	C79.82	DØ7.39	D28.2	D39.8	D49.59
parotid (duct) (gland)	CØ7	C79.89	DØØ.ØØ	D11.Ø	D37.Ø3Ø	D49.Ø
parovarium	C57.1-☑	C79.82	DØ7.39	D28.2	D39.8	D49.59
patella	C4Ø.2Ø	C79.51	—	—	—	—
peduncle, cerebral	C71.7	C79.31	—	D33.1	D43.1	D49.6
pelvirectal junction	C19	C78.5	DØ1.1	D12.7	D37.5	D49.Ø
pelvis, pelvic	C76.3	C79.89	DØ9.8	D36.7	D48.7	D49.89
bone	C41.4	C79.51	—	D16.8	D48.Ø	D49.2
floor	C76.3	C79.89	DØ9.8	D36.7	D48.7	D49.89
renal	C65.-☑	C79.Ø-☑	DØ9.19	D3Ø.1-☑	D41.1-☑	D49.51-☑
viscera	C76.3	C79.89	DØ9.8	D36.7	D48.7	D49.89
wall	C76.3	C79.89	DØ9.8	D36.7	D48.7	D49.89
pelvo-abdominal	C76.8	C79.89	DØ9.8	D36.7	D48.7	D49.89
penis	C6Ø.9	C79.82	DØ7.4	D29.Ø	D4Ø.8	D49.59
body	C6Ø.2	C79.82	DØ7.4	D29.Ø	D4Ø.8	D49.59
corpus (cavernosum)	C6Ø.2	C79.82	DØ7.4	D29.Ø	D4Ø.8	D49.59
glans	C6Ø.1	C79.82	DØ7.4	D29.Ø	D4Ø.8	D49.59
overlapping sites	C6Ø.8	—	—	—	—	—
skin NEC	C6Ø.9	C79.82	DØ7.4	D29.Ø	D4Ø.8	D49.59
periadrenal (tissue)	C48.Ø	C78.6	—	D2Ø.Ø	D48.3	D49.Ø
perianal (skin) — *see also* Neoplasm, anus, skin	C44.5ØØ	C79.2	DØ4.5	D23.5	D48.5	D49.2
pericardium	C38.Ø	C79.89	—	D15.1	D48.7	D49.89
perinephric	C48.Ø	C78.6	—	D2Ø.Ø	D48.3	D49.Ø
perineum	C76.3	C79.89	DØ9.8	D36.7	D48.7	D49.89
periodontal tissue NEC	CØ3.9	C79.89	DØØ.Ø3	D1Ø.39	D37.Ø9	D49.Ø
periosteum — *see* Neoplasm, bone						
peripancreatic	C48.Ø	C78.6	—	D2Ø.Ø	D48.3	D49.Ø
peripheral nerve NEC	C47.9	C79.89	—	D36.1Ø	D48.2	D49.2
perirectal (tissue)	C76.3	C79.89	—	D36.7	D48.7	D49.89
perirenal (tissue)	C48.Ø	C78.6	—	D2Ø.Ø	D48.3	D49.Ø
peritoneum, peritoneal (cavity)	C48.2	C78.6	—	D2Ø.1	D48.4	D49.Ø
benign mesothelial tissue — *see* Mesothelioma, benign						
overlapping lesion	C48.8	—	—	—	—	—
with digestive organs	C26.9	—	—	—	—	—
parietal	C48.1	C78.6	—	D2Ø.1	D48.4	D49.Ø
pelvic	C48.1	C78.6	—	D2Ø.1	D48.4	D49.Ø
specified part NEC	C48.1	C78.6	—	D2Ø.1	D48.4	D49.Ø
peritonsillar (tissue)	C76.Ø	C79.89	DØ9.8	D36.7	D48.7	D49.89
periurethral tissue	C76.3	C79.89	—	D36.7	D48.7	D49.89
phalanges						
foot	C4Ø.3-☑	C79.51	—	D16.3-☑	—	—
Neoplasm, neoplastic — *continued*						
phalanges — *continued*						
hand	C4Ø.1-☑	C79.51	—	D16.1-☑	—	—
pharynx, pharyngeal	C14.Ø	C79.89	DØØ.Ø8	D1Ø.9	D37.Ø5	D49.Ø
bursa	C11.1	C79.89	DØØ.Ø8	D1Ø.6	D37.Ø5	D49.Ø
fornix	C11.3	C79.89	DØØ.Ø8	D1Ø.6	D37.Ø5	D49.Ø
recess	C11.2	C79.89	DØØ.Ø8	D1Ø.6	D37.Ø5	D49.Ø
region	C14.Ø	C79.89	DØØ.Ø8	D1Ø.9	D37.Ø5	D49.Ø
tonsil	C11.1	C79.89	DØØ.Ø8	D1Ø.6	D37.Ø5	D49.Ø
wall (lateral) (posterior)	C14.Ø	C79.89	DØØ.Ø8	D1Ø.9	D37.Ø5	D49.Ø
pia mater	C7Ø.9	C79.4Ø	—	D32.9	D42.9	D49.7
cerebral	C7Ø.Ø	C79.32	—	D32.Ø	D42.Ø	D49.7
cranial	C7Ø.Ø	C79.32	—	D32.Ø	D42.Ø	D49.7
spinal	C7Ø.1	C79.49	—	D32.1	D42.1	D49.7
pillars of fauces	CØ9.1	C79.89	DØØ.Ø8	D1Ø.5	D37.Ø5	D49.Ø
pineal (body) (gland)	C75.3	C79.89	DØ9.3	D35.4	D44.5	D49.7
pinna (ear) NEC — *see also* Neoplasm, skin, ear	C44.2Ø-☑	C79.2	DØ4.2-☑	D23.2-☑	D48.5	D49.2
piriform fossa or sinus	C12	C79.89	DØØ.Ø8	D1Ø.7	D37.Ø5	D49.Ø
pituitary (body) (fossa) (gland) (lobe)	C75.1	C79.89	DØ9.3	D35.2	D44.3	D49.7
placenta	C58	C79.82	DØ7.Ø	D26.7	D39.2	D49.59
pleura, pleural (cavity)	C38.4	C78.2	—	D19.Ø	D38.2	D49.1
overlapping lesion with heart or mediastinum	C38.8	—	—	—	—	—
parietal	C38.4	C78.2	—	D19.Ø	D38.2	D49.1
visceral	C38.4	C78.2	—	D19.Ø	D38.2	D49.1
plexus						
brachial	C47.1-☑	C79.89	—	D36.12	D48.2	D49.2
cervical	C47.Ø	C79.89	—	D36.11	D48.2	D49.2
choroid	C71.5	C79.31	—	D33.Ø	D43.Ø	D49.6
lumbosacral	C47.5	C79.89	—	D36.16	D48.2	D49.2
sacral	C47.5	C79.89	—	D36.16	D48.2	D49.2
pluriendocrine	C75.8	C79.89	DØ9.3	D35.7	D44.9	D49.7
pole						
frontal	C71.1	C79.31	—	D33.Ø	D43.Ø	D49.6
occipital	C71.4	C79.31	—	D33.Ø	D43.Ø	D49.6
pons (varolii)	C71.7	C79.31	—	D33.1	D43.1	D49.6
popliteal fossa or space	C76.5-☑	C79.89	DØ4.7-☑	D36.7	D48.7	D49.89
postcricoid (region)	C13.Ø	C79.89	DØØ.Ø8	D1Ø.7	D37.Ø5	D49.Ø
posterior fossa (cranial)	C71.9	C79.31	—	D33.2	D43.2	D49.6
postnasal space	C11.9	C79.89	DØØ.Ø8	D1Ø.6	D37.Ø5	D49.Ø
prepuce	C6Ø.Ø	C79.82	DØ7.4	D29.Ø	D4Ø.8	D49.59
prepylorus	C16.4	C78.89	DØØ.2	D13.1	D37.1	D49.Ø
presacral (region)	C76.3	C79.89	—	D36.7	D48.7	D49.89
prostate (gland)	C61	C79.82	DØ7.5	D29.1	D4Ø.Ø	D49.59
utricle	C68.Ø	C79.19	DØ9.19	D3Ø.4	D41.3	D49.59
pterygoid fossa	C49.Ø	C79.89	—	D21.Ø	D48.1☑	D49.2
pubic bone	C41.4	C79.51	—	D16.8	D48.Ø	D49.2
pudenda, pudendum (female)	C51.9	C79.82	DØ7.1	D28.Ø	D39.8	D49.59
pulmonary — *see also* Neoplasm, lung	C34.9-☑	C78.Ø-☑	DØ2.2-☑	D14.3-☑	D38.1	D49.1
putamen	C71.Ø	C79.31	—	D33.Ø	D43.Ø	D49.6
pyloric						
antrum	C16.3	C78.89	DØØ.2	D13.1	D37.1	D49.Ø
canal	C16.4	C78.89	DØØ.2	D13.1	D37.1	D49.Ø
pylorus	C16.4	C78.89	DØØ.2	D13.1	D37.1	D49.Ø
pyramid (brain)	C71.7	C79.31	—	D33.1	D43.1	D49.6
pyriform fossa or sinus	C12	C79.89	DØØ.Ø8	D1Ø.7	D37.Ø5	D49.Ø
radius (any part)	C4Ø.Ø-☑	C79.51	—	D16.Ø-☑	—	—
Rathke's pouch	C75.1	C79.89	DØ9.3	D35.2	D44.3	D49.7
rectosigmoid (junction)	C19	C78.5	DØ1.1	D12.7	D37.5	D49.Ø
overlapping lesion with anus or rectum	C21.8	—	—	—	—	—
rectouterine pouch	C48.1	C78.6	—	D2Ø.1	D48.4	D49.Ø

	Malignant Primary	Malignant Secondary	Ca in situ	Benign	Uncertain Behavior	Unspecified Behavior
Neoplasm, neoplastic *— continued*						
rectovaginal septum or wall	C76.3	C79.89	DØ9.8	D36.7	D48.7	D49.89
rectovesical septum	C76.3	C79.89	DØ9.8	D36.7	D48.7	D49.89
rectum (ampulla)	C2Ø	C78.5	DØ1.2	D12.8	D37.5	D49.Ø
and colon	C19	C78.5	DØ1.1	D12.7	D37.5	D49.Ø
overlapping lesion with anus or rectosigmoid junction	C21.8	—	—	—	—	—
renal	C64.-☑	C79.Ø-☑	DØ9.19	D3Ø.Ø-☑	D41.Ø-☑	D49.51-☑
calyx	C65.-☑	C79.Ø-☑	DØ9.19	D3Ø.1-☑	D41.1-☑	D49.51-☑
hilus	C65.-☑	C79.Ø-☑	DØ9.19	D3Ø.1-☑	D41.1-☑	D49.51-☑
parenchyma	C64.-☑	C79.Ø-☑	DØ9.19	D3Ø.Ø-☑	D41.Ø-☑	D49.51-☑
pelvis	C65.-☑	C79.Ø-☑	DØ9.19	D3Ø.1-☑	D41.1-☑	D49.51-☑
respiratory						
organs or system NEC	C39.9	C78.3Ø	DØ2.4	D14.4	D38.6	D49.1
tract NEC	C39.9	C78.3Ø	DØ2.4	D14.4	D38.5	D49.1
upper	C39.Ø	C78.3Ø	DØ2.4	D14.4	D38.5	D49.1
retina	C69.2-☑	C79.49	DØ9.2-☑	D31.2-☑	D48.7	D49.81
retrobulbar	C69.6-☑	C79.49	—	D31.6-☑	D48.7	D49.89
retrocecal	C48.Ø	C78.6	—	D2Ø.Ø	D48.3	D49.Ø
retromolar (area) (triangle) (trigone)	CØ6.2	C79.89	DØØ.ØØ	D1Ø.39	D37.Ø9	D49.Ø
retro-orbital	C76.Ø	C79.89	DØ9.8	D36.7	D48.7	D49.89
retroperitoneal (space) (tissue)	C48.Ø	C78.6	—	D2Ø.Ø	D48.3	D49.Ø
retroperitoneum	C48.Ø	C78.6	—	D2Ø.Ø	D48.3	D49.Ø
retropharyngeal	C14.Ø	C79.89	DØØ.Ø8	D1Ø.9	D37.Ø5	D49.Ø
retrovesical (septum)	C76.3	C79.89	DØ9.8	D36.7	D48.7	D49.89
rhinencephalon	C71.Ø	C79.31	—	D33.Ø	D43.Ø	D49.6
rib	C41.3	C79.51	—	D16.7	D48.Ø	D49.2
Rosenmuller's fossa	C11.2	C79.89	DØØ.Ø8	D1Ø.6	D37.Ø5	D49.Ø
round ligament	C57.2-☑	C79.82	—	D28.2	D39.8	D49.59
sacrococcyx, sacrococcygeal	C41.4	C79.51	—	D16.8	D48.Ø	D49.2
region	C76.3	C79.89	DØ9.8	D36.7	D48.7	D49.89
sacrouterine ligament	C57.3	C79.82	—	D28.2	D39.8	D49.59
sacrum, sacral (vertebra)	C41.4	C79.51	—	D16.8	D48.Ø	D49.2
salivary gland or duct (major)	CØ8.9	C79.89	DØØ.ØØ	D11.9	D37.Ø39	D49.Ø
minor NEC	CØ6.9	C79.89	DØØ.ØØ	D1Ø.39	D37.Ø4	D49.Ø
overlapping lesion	CØ8.9	—	—	—	—	—
parotid	CØ7	C79.89	DØØ.ØØ	D11.Ø	D37.Ø3Ø	D49.Ø
pluriglandular	CØ8.9	C79.89	DØØ.ØØ	D11.9	D37.Ø39	D49.Ø
sublingual	CØ8.1	C79.89	DØØ.ØØ	D11.7	D37.Ø31	D49.Ø
submandibular	CØ8.Ø	C79.89	DØØ.ØØ	D11.7	D37.Ø32	D49.Ø
submaxillary	CØ8.Ø	C79.89	DØØ.ØØ	D11.7	D37.Ø32	D49.Ø
salpinx (uterine)	C57.Ø-☑	C79.82	DØ7.39	D28.2	D39.8	D49.59
Santorini's duct	C25.3	C78.89	DØ1.7	D13.6	D37.8	D49.Ø
scalp	C44.4Ø	C79.2	DØ4.4	D23.4	D48.5	D49.2
basal cell carcinoma	C44.41	—	—	—	—	—
specified type NEC	C44.49	—	—	—	—	—
squamous cell carcinoma	C44.42	—	—	—	—	—
scapula (any part)	C4Ø.Ø-☑	C79.51	—	D16.Ø-☑	—	—
scapular region	C76.1	C79.89	DØ9.8	D36.7	D48.7	D49.89
scar NEC *— see also* Neoplasm, skin, by site	C44.9Ø	C79.2	DØ4.9	D23.9	D48.5	D49.2
sciatic nerve	C47.2-☑	C79.89	—	D36.13	D48.2	D49.2
sclera	C69.4-☑	C79.49	DØ9.2-☑	D31.4-☑	D48.7	D49.89
scrotum (skin)	C63.2	C79.82	DØ7.61	D29.4	D4Ø.8	D49.59
sebaceous gland *— see* Neoplasm, skin						
sella turcica	C75.1	C79.89	DØ9.3	D35.2	D44.3	D49.7
bone	C41.Ø	C79.51	—	D16.4	D48.Ø	D49.2
semilunar cartilage (knee)	C4Ø.2-☑	C79.51	—	D16.2-☑	D48.Ø	D49.2
seminal vesicle	C63.7	C79.82	DØ7.69	D29.8	D4Ø.8	D49.59
septum						
nasal	C3Ø.Ø	C78.39	DØ2.3	D14.Ø	D38.5	D49.1
Neoplasm, neoplastic *— continued*						
septum *— continued*						
nasal *— continued*						
posterior margin	C11.3	C79.89	DØØ.Ø8	D1Ø.6	D37.Ø5	D49.Ø
rectovaginal	C76.3	C79.89	DØ9.8	D36.7	D48.7	D49.89
rectovesical	C76.3	C79.89	DØ9.8	D36.7	D48.7	D49.89
urethrovaginal	C57.9	C79.82	DØ7.3Ø	D28.9	D39.9	D49.59
vesicovaginal	C57.9	C79.82	DØ7.3Ø	D28.9	D39.9	D49.59
shoulder NEC	C76.4-☑	C79.89	DØ4.6-☑	D36.7	D48.7	D49.89
sigmoid flexure (lower) (upper)	C18.7	C78.5	DØ1.Ø	D12.5	D37.4	D49.Ø
sinus (accessory)	C31.9	C78.39	DØ2.3	D14.Ø	D38.5	D49.1
bone (any)	C41.Ø	C79.51	—	D16.4	D48.Ø	D49.2
ethmoidal	C31.1	C78.39	DØ2.3	D14.Ø	D38.5	D49.1
frontal	C31.2	C78.39	DØ2.3	D14.Ø	D38.5	D49.1
maxillary	C31.Ø	C78.39	DØ2.3	D14.Ø	D38.5	D49.1
nasal, paranasal NEC	C31.9	C78.39	DØ2.3	D14.Ø	D38.5	D49.1
overlapping lesion	C31.8	—	—	—	—	—
pyriform	C12	C79.89	DØØ.Ø8	D1Ø.7	D37.Ø5	D49.Ø
sphenoid	C31.3	C78.39	DØ2.3	D14.Ø	D38.5	D49.1
skeleton, skeletal NEC	C41.9	C79.51	—	D16.9	D48.Ø	D49.2
Skene's gland	C68.1	C79.19	DØ9.19	D3Ø.8	D41.8	D49.59
skin NOS	C44.9Ø	C79.2	DØ4.9	D23.9	D48.5	D49.2
abdominal wall	C44.5Ø9	C79.2	DØ4.5	D23.5	D48.5	D49.2
basal cell carcinoma	C44.519	—	—	—	—	—
specified type NEC	C44.599	—	—	—	—	—
squamous cell carcinoma	C44.529	—	—	—	—	—
ala nasi *— see also* Neoplasm, nose, skin	C44.3Ø1	C79.2	DØ4.39	D23.39	D48.5	D49.2
ankle *— see also* Neoplasm, skin, limb, lower	C44.7Ø-☑	C79.2	DØ4.7-☑	D23.7-☑	D48.5	D49.2
antecubital space *— see also* Neoplasm, skin, limb, upper	C44.6Ø-☑	C79.2	DØ4.6-☑	D23.6-☑	D48.5	D49.2
anus	C44.5ØØ	C79.2	DØ4.5	D23.5	D48.5	D49.2
basal cell carcinoma	C44.51Ø	—	—	—	—	—
specified type NEC	C44.59Ø	—	—	—	—	—
squamous cell carcinoma	C44.52Ø	—	—	—	—	—
arm *— see also* Neoplasm, skin, limb, upper	C44.6Ø-☑	C79.2	DØ4.6-☑	D23.6-☑	D48.5	D49.2
auditory canal (external) *— see also* Neoplasm, skin, ear	C44.2Ø-☑	C79.2	DØ4.2-☑	D23.2-☑	D48.5	D49.2
auricle (ear) *— see also* Neoplasm, skin, ear	C44.2Ø-☑	C79.2	DØ4.2-☑	D23.2-☑	D48.5	D49.2
auricular canal (external) *— see also* Neoplasm, skin, ear	C44.2Ø-☑	C79.2	DØ4.2-☑	D23.2-☑	D48.5	D49.2
axilla, axillary fold *— see also* Neoplasm, skin, trunk	C44.5Ø9	C79.2	DØ4.5	D23.5	D48.5	D49.2
back *— see also* Neoplasm, skin, trunk	C44.5Ø9	C79.2	DØ4.5	D23.5	D48.5	D49.2
basal cell carcinoma	C44.91	—	—	—	—	—
breast	C44.5Ø1	C79.2	DØ4.5	D23.5	D48.5	D49.2
basal cell carcinoma	C44.511	—	—	—	—	—
specified type NEC	C44.591	—	—	—	—	—
squamous cell carcinoma	C44.521	—	—	—	—	—

	Malignant Primary	Malignant Secondary	Ca in situ	Benign	Uncertain Behavior	Unspecified Behavior
Neoplasm, neoplastic — *continued*						
skin — *continued*						
brow — *see also* Neoplasm, skin, face	C44.3Ø9	C79.2	DØ4.39	D23.39	D48.5	D49.2
buttock — *see also* Neoplasm, skin, trunk	C44.5Ø9	C79.2	DØ4.5	D23.5	D48.5	D49.2
calf — *see also* Neoplasm, skin, limb, lower	C44.7Ø-☑	C79.2	DØ4.7-☑	D23.7-☑	D48.5	D49.2
canthus (eye) (inner) (outer)	C44.1Ø-☑	C79.2	DØ4.1-☑	D23.1-☑	D48.5	D49.2
basal cell carcinoma	C44.11-☑	—	—	—	—	—
sebaceous cell	C44.13-☑	—	—	—	—	—
specified type NEC	C44.19-☑	—	—	—	—	—
squamous cell carcinoma	C44.12-☑	—	—	—	—	—
cervical region — *see also* Neoplasm, skin, neck	C44.4Ø	C79.2	DØ4.4	D23.4	D48.5	D49.2
cheek (external) — *see also* Neoplasm, skin, face	C44.3Ø9	C79.2	DØ4.39	D23.39	D48.5	D49.2
chest (wall) — *see also* Neoplasm, skin, trunk	C44.5Ø9	C79.2	DØ4.5	D23.5	D48.5	D49.2
chin — *see also* Neoplasm, skin, face	C44.3Ø9	C79.2	DØ4.39	D23.39	D48.5	D49.2
clavicular area — *see also* Neoplasm, skin, trunk	C44.5Ø9	C79.2	DØ4.5	D23.5	D48.5	D49.2
clitoris	C51.2	C79.82	DØ7.1	D28.Ø	D39.8	D49.59
columnella — *see also* Neoplasm, skin, face	C44.3Ø9	C79.2	DØ4.39	D23.39	D48.5	D49.2
concha — *see also* Neoplasm, skin, ear	C44.2Ø-☑	C79.2	DØ4.2-☑	D23.2-☑	D48.5	D49.2
ear (external)	C44.2Ø-☑	C79.2	DØ4.2-☑	D23.2-☑	D48.5	D49.2
basal cell carcinoma	C44.21-☑	—	—	—	—	—
specified type NEC	C44.29-☑	—	—	—	—	—
squamous cell carcinoma	C44.22-☑	—	—	—	—	—
elbow — *see also* Neoplasm, skin, limb, upper	C44.6Ø-☑	C79.2	DØ4.6-☑	D23.6-☑	D48.5	D49.2
eyebrow — *see also* Neoplasm, skin, face	C44.3Ø9	C79.2	DØ4.39	D23.39	D48.5	D49.2
eyelid	C44.1Ø-☑	C79.2	DØ4.1-☑	D23.1-☑	D48.5	D49.2
basal cell carcinoma	C44.11-☑	—	—	—	—	—
sebaceous cell	C44.13-☑	—	—	—	—	—
specified type NEC	C44.19-☑	—	—	—	—	—
squamous cell carcinoma	C44.12-☑	—	—	—	—	—
face NOS	C44.3ØØ	C79.2	DØ4.3Ø	D23.3Ø	D48.5	D49.2
basal cell carcinoma	C44.31Ø	—	—	—	—	—
specified type NEC	C44.39Ø	—	—	—	—	—
squamous cell carcinoma	C44.32Ø	—	—	—	—	—
female genital organs (external)	C51.9	C79.82	DØ7.1	D28.Ø	D39.8	D49.59
clitoris	C51.2	C79.82	DØ7.1	D28.Ø	D39.8	D49.59
labium NEC	C51.9	C79.82	DØ7.1	D28.Ø	D39.8	D49.59
majus	C51.Ø	C79.82	DØ7.1	D28.Ø	D39.8	D49.59
minus	C51.1	C79.82	DØ7.1	D28.Ø	D39.8	D49.59
pudendum	C51.9	C79.82	DØ7.1	D28.Ø	D39.8	D49.59
vulva	C51.9	C79.82	DØ7.1	D28.Ø	D39.8	D49.59
finger — *see also* Neoplasm, skin, limb, upper	C44.6Ø-☑	C79.2	DØ4.6-☑	D23.6-☑	D48.5	D49.2
Neoplasm, neoplastic — *continued*						
skin — *continued*						
flank — *see also* Neoplasm, skin, trunk	C44.5Ø9	C79.2	DØ4.5	D23.5	D48.5	D49.2
foot — *see also* Neoplasm, skin, limb, lower	C44.7Ø-☑	C79.2	DØ4.7-☑	D23.7-☑	D48.5	D49.2
forearm — *see also* Neoplasm, skin, limb, upper	C44.6Ø-☑	C79.2	DØ4.6-☑	D23.6-☑	D48.5	D49.2
forehead — *see also* Neoplasm, skin, face	C44.3Ø9	C79.2	DØ4.39	D23.39	D48.5	D49.2
glabella — *see also* Neoplasm, skin, face	C44.3Ø9	C79.2	DØ4.39	D23.39	D48.5	D49.2
gluteal region — *see also* Neoplasm, skin, trunk	C44.5Ø9	C79.2	DØ4.5	D23.5	D48.5	D49.2
groin — *see also* Neoplasm, skin, trunk	C44.5Ø9	C79.2	DØ4.5	D23.5	D48.5	D49.2
hand — *see also* Neoplasm, skin, limb, upper	C44.6Ø-☑	C79.2	DØ4.6-☑	D23.6-☑	D48.5	D49.2
head NEC — *see also* Neoplasm, skin, scalp	C44.4Ø	C79.2	DØ4.4	D23.4	D48.5	D49.2
heel — *see also* Neoplasm, skin, limb, lower	C44.7Ø-☑	C79.2	DØ4.7-☑	D23.7-☑	D48.5	D49.2
helix — *see also* Neoplasm, skin, ear	C44.2Ø-☑	C79.2	DØ4.2-☑	D23.2-☑	D48.5	D49.2
hip — *see also* Neoplasm, skin, limb, lower	C44.7Ø-☑	C79.2	DØ4.7-☑	D23.7-☑	D48.5	D49.2
infraclavicular region — *see also* Neoplasm, skin, trunk	C44.5Ø9	C79.2	DØ4.5	D23.5	D48.5	D49.2
inguinal region — *see also* Neoplasm, skin, trunk	C44.5Ø9	C79.2	DØ4.5	D23.5	D48.5	D49.2
jaw — *see also* Neoplasm, skin, face	C44.3Ø9	C79.2	DØ4.39	D23.39	D48.5	D49.2
Kaposi's sarcoma — *see* Kaposi's, sarcoma, skin						
knee — *see also* Neoplasm, skin, limb, lower	C44.7Ø-☑	C79.2	DØ4.7-☑	D23.7-☑	D48.5	D49.2
labia						
majora	C51.Ø	C79.82	DØ7.1	D28.Ø	D39.8	D49.59
minora	C51.1	C79.82	DØ7.1	D28.Ø	D39.8	D49.59
leg — *see also* Neoplasm, skin, limb, lower	C44.7Ø-☑	C79.2	DØ4.7-☑	D23.7-☑	D48.5	D49.2
lid (lower) (upper)	C44.1Ø-☑	C79.2	DØ4.1-☑	D23.1-☑	D48.5	D49.2
basal cell carcinoma	C44.11-☑	—	—	—	—	—
sebaceous cell	C44.13-☑	—	—	—	—	—
specified type NEC	C44.19-☑	—	—	—	—	—
squamous cell carcinoma	C44.12-☑	—	—	—	—	—
limb NEC	C44.9Ø	C79.2	DØ4.9	D23.9	D48.5	D49.2
basal cell carcinoma	C44.91	—	—	—	—	—
lower	C44.7Ø-☑	C79.2	DØ4.7-☑	D23.7-☑	D48.5	D49.2
basal cell carcinoma	C44.71-☑	—	—	—	—	—
specified type NEC	C44.79-☑	—	—	—	—	—
squamous cell carcinoma	C44.72-☑	—	—	—	—	—
upper	C44.6Ø-☑	C79.2	DØ4.6-☑	D23.6-☑	D48.5	D49.2
basal cell carcinoma	C44.61-☑	—	—	—	—	—

	Malignant Primary	Malignant Secondary	Ca in situ	Benign	Uncertain Behavior	Unspecified Behavior
Neoplasm, neoplastic — *continued*						
skin — *continued*						
limb — *continued*						
upper — *continued*						
specified type NEC	C44.69-☑	—	—	—	—	—
squamous cell carcinoma	C44.62-☑	—	—	—	—	—
lip (lower) (upper)	C44.00	C79.2	D04.0	D23.0	D48.5	D49.2
basal cell carcinoma	C44.01	—	—	—	—	—
specified type NEC	C44.09	—	—	—	—	—
squamous cell carcinoma	C44.02	—	—	—	—	—
male genital organs	C63.9	C79.82	D07.60	D29.9	D40.8	D49.59
penis	C60.9	C79.82	D07.4	D29.0	D40.8	D49.59
prepuce	C60.0	C79.82	D07.4	D29.0	D40.8	D49.59
scrotum	C63.2	C79.82	D07.61	D29.4	D40.8	D49.59
mastectomy site (skin) — *see also* Neoplasm, skin, breast	C44.501	C79.2	—	—	—	—
specified as breast tissue	C50.8-☑	C79.81	—	—	—	—
meatus, acoustic (external) — *see also* Neoplasm, skin, ear	C44.20-☑	C79.2	D04.2-☑	D23.2-☑	D48.5	D49.2
melanotic — *see* Melanoma						
Merkel cell — *see* Carcinoma, Merkel cell						
nates — *see also* Neoplasm, skin, trunk	C44.509	C79.2	D04.5	D23.5	D48.5	D49.2
neck	C44.40	C79.2	D04.4	D23.4	D48.5	D49.2
basal cell carcinoma	C44.41	—	—	—	—	—
specified type NEC	C44.49	—	—	—	—	—
squamous cell carcinoma	C44.42	—	—	—	—	—
nevus — *see* Nevus, skin						
nose (external) — *see also* Neoplasm, nose, skin	C44.301	C79.2	D04.39	D23.39	D48.5	D49.2
overlapping lesion	C44.80	—	—	—	—	—
basal cell carcinoma	C44.81	—	—	—	—	—
specified type NEC	C44.89	—	—	—	—	—
squamous cell carcinoma	C44.82	—	—	—	—	—
palm — *see also* Neoplasm, skin, limb, upper	C44.60-☑	C79.2	D04.6-☑	D23.6-☑	D48.5	D49.2
palpebra	C44.10-☑	C79.2	D04.1-☑	D23.1-☑	D48.5	D49.2
basal cell carcinoma	C44.11-☑	—	—	—	—	—
sebaceous cell	C44.13-☑	—	—	—	—	—
specified type NEC	C44.19-☑	—	—	—	—	—
squamous cell carcinoma	C44.12-☑	—	—	—	—	—
penis NEC	C60.9	C79.82	D07.4	D29.0	D40.8	D49.59
perianal — *see also* Neoplasm, skin, anus	C44.500	C79.2	D04.5	D23.5	D48.5	D49.2
perineum — *see also* Neoplasm, skin, anus	C44.500	C79.2	D04.5	D23.5	D48.5	D49.2
pinna — *see also* Neoplasm, skin, ear	C44.20-☑	C79.2	D04.2-☑	D23.2-☑	D48.5	D49.2
plantar — *see also* Neoplasm, skin, limb, lower	C44.70-☑	C79.2	D04.7-☑	D23.7-☑	D48.5	D49.2
Neoplasm, neoplastic — *continued*						
skin — *continued*						
popliteal fossa or space — *see also* Neoplasm, skin, limb, lower	C44.70-☑	C79.2	D04.7-☑	D23.7-☑	D48.5	D49.2
prepuce	C60.0	C79.82	D07.4	D29.0	D40.8	D49.59
pubes — *see also* Neoplasm, skin, trunk	C44.509	C79.2	D04.5	D23.5	D48.5	D49.2
sacrococcygeal region — *see also* Neoplasm, skin, trunk	C44.509	C79.2	D04.5	D23.5	D48.5	D49.2
scalp	C44.40	C79.2	D04.4	D23.4	D48.5	D49.2
basal cell carcinoma	C44.41	—	—	—	—	—
specified type NEC	C44.49	—	—	—	—	—
squamous cell carcinoma	C44.42	—	—	—	—	—
scapular region — *see also* Neoplasm, skin, trunk	C44.509	C79.2	D04.5	D23.5	D48.5	D49.2
scrotum	C63.2	C79.82	D07.61	D29.4	D40.8	D49.59
shoulder — *see also* Neoplasm, skin, limb, upper	C44.60-☑	C79.2	D04.6-☑	D23.6-☑	D48.5	D49.2
sole (foot) — *see also* Neoplasm, skin, limb, lower	C44.70-☑	C79.2	D04.7-☑	D23.7-☑	D48.5	D49.2
specified sites NEC	C44.80	C79.2	D04.8	D23.9	D48.5	D49.2
basal cell carcinoma	C44.81	—	—	—	—	—
specified type NEC	C44.89	—	—	—	—	—
squamous cell carcinoma	C44.82	—	—	—	—	—
specified type NEC	C44.99	—	—	—	—	—
squamous cell carcinoma	C44.92	—	—	—	—	—
submammary fold — *see also* Neoplasm, skin, trunk	C44.509	C79.2	D04.5	D23.5	D48.5	D49.2
supraclavicular region — *see also* Neoplasm, skin, neck	C44.40	C79.2	D04.4	D23.4	D48.5	D49.2
temple — *see also* Neoplasm, skin, face	C44.309	C79.2	D04.39	D23.39	D48.5	D49.2
thigh — *see also* Neoplasm, skin, limb, lower	C44.70-☑	C79.2	D04.7-☑	D23.7-☑	D48.5	D49.2
thoracic wall — *see also* Neoplasm, skin, trunk	C44.509	C79.2	D04.5	D23.5	D48.5	D49.2
thumb — *see also* Neoplasm, skin, limb, upper	C44.60-☑	C79.2	D04.6-☑	D23.6-☑	D48.5	D49.2
toe — *see also* Neoplasm, skin, limb, lower	C44.70-☑	C79.2	D04.7-☑	D23.7-☑	D48.5	D49.2
tragus — *see also* Neoplasm, skin, ear	C44.20-☑	C79.2	D04.2-☑	D23.2-☑	D48.5	D49.2
trunk	C44.509	C79.2	D04.5	D23.5	D48.5	D49.2
basal cell carcinoma	C44.519	—	—	—	—	—
specified type NEC	C44.599	—	—	—	—	—
squamous cell carcinoma	C44.529	—	—	—	—	—
umbilicus — *see also* Neoplasm, skin, trunk	C44.509	C79.2	D04.5	D23.5	D48.5	D49.2
vulva	C51.9	C79.82	D07.1	D28.0	D39.8	D49.59
overlapping lesion	C51.8	—	—	—	—	—

	Malignant Primary	Malignant Secondary	Ca in situ	Benign	Uncertain Behavior	Unspecified Behavior
Neoplasm, neoplastic — *continued*						
skin — *continued*						
wrist — *see also* Neoplasm, skin, limb, upper	C44.60-☑	C79.2	D04.6-☑	D23.6-☑	D48.5	D49.2
skull	C41.0	C79.51	—	D16.4	D48.0	D49.2
soft parts or tissues — *see* Neoplasm, connective tissue						
specified site NEC	C76.8	C79.89	D09.8	D36.7	D48.7	D49.89
spermatic cord	C63.1-☑	C79.82	D07.69	D29.8	D40.8	D49.59
sphenoid	C31.3	C78.39	D02.3	D14.0	D38.5	D49.1
bone	C41.0	C79.51	—	D16.4	D48.0	D49.2
sinus	C31.3	C78.39	D02.3	D14.0	D38.5	D49.1
sphincter						
anal	C21.1	C78.5	D01.3	D12.9	D37.8	D49.0
of Oddi	C24.0	C78.89	D01.5	D13.5	D37.6	D49.0
spine, spinal (column)	C41.2	C79.51	—	D16.6	D48.0	D49.2
bulb	C71.7	C79.31	—	D33.1	D43.1	D49.6
coccyx	C41.4	C79.51	—	D16.8	D48.0	D49.2
cord (cervical) (lumbar) (sacral) (thoracic)	C72.0	C79.49	—	D33.4	D43.4	D49.7
dura mater	C70.1	C79.49	—	D32.1	D42.1	D49.7
lumbosacral	C41.2	C79.51	—	D16.6	D48.0	D49.2
marrow NEC	C96.9	C79.52	—	—	D47.9	D49.89
membrane	C70.1	C79.49	—	D32.1	D42.1	D49.7
meninges	C70.1	C79.49	—	D32.1	D42.1	D49.7
nerve (root)	C47.9	C79.89	—	D36.10	D48.2	D49.2
pia mater	C70.1	C79.49	—	D32.1	D42.1	D49.7
root	C47.9	C79.89	—	D36.10	D48.2	D49.2
sacrum	C41.4	C79.51	—	D16.8	D48.0	D49.2
spleen, splenic NEC	C26.1	C78.89	D01.7	D13.99	D37.8	D49.0
flexure (colon)	C18.5	C78.5	D01.0	D12.3	D37.4	D49.0
stem, brain	C71.7	C79.31	—	D33.1	D43.1	D49.6
Stensen's duct	C07	C79.89	D00.00	D11.0	D37.030	D49.0
sternum	C41.3	C79.51	—	D16.7	D48.0	D49.2
stomach	C16.9	C78.89	D00.2	D13.1	D37.1	D49.0
antrum (pyloric)	C16.3	C78.89	D00.2	D13.1	D37.1	D49.0
body	C16.2	C78.89	D00.2	D13.1	D37.1	D49.0
cardia	C16.0	C78.89	D00.2	D13.1	D37.1	D49.0
cardiac orifice	C16.0	C78.89	D00.2	D13.1	D37.1	D49.0
corpus	C16.2	C78.89	D00.2	D13.1	D37.1	D49.0
fundus	C16.1	C78.89	D00.2	D13.1	D37.1	D49.0
greater curvature NEC	C16.6	C78.89	D00.2	D13.1	D37.1	D49.0
lesser curvature NEC	C16.5	C78.89	D00.2	D13.1	D37.1	D49.0
overlapping lesion	C16.8	—	—	—	—	—
prepylorus	C16.4	C78.89	D00.2	D13.1	D37.1	D49.0
pylorus	C16.4	C78.89	D00.2	D13.1	D37.1	D49.0
wall NEC	C16.9	C78.89	D00.2	D13.1	D37.1	D49.0
anterior NEC	C16.8	C78.89	D00.2	D13.1	D37.1	D49.0
posterior NEC	C16.8	C78.89	D00.2	D13.1	D37.1	D49.0
stroma, endometrial	C54.1	C79.82	D07.0	D26.1	D39.0	D49.59
stump, cervical	C53.8	C79.82	D06.7	D26.0	D39.0	D49.59
subcutaneous (nodule) (tissue) NEC — *see* Neoplasm, connective tissue						
subdural	C70.9	C79.32	—	D32.9	D42.9	D49.7
subglottis, subglottic	C32.2	C78.39	D02.0	D14.1	D38.0	D49.1
sublingual	C04.9	C79.89	D00.06	D10.2	D37.09	D49.0
gland or duct	C08.1	C79.89	D00.00	D11.7	D37.031	D49.0
submandibular gland	C08.0	C79.89	D00.00	D11.7	D37.032	D49.0
submaxillary gland or duct	C08.0	C79.89	D00.00	D11.7	D37.032	D49.0
submental	C76.0	C79.89	D09.8	D36.7	D48.7	D49.89
subpleural	C34.9-☑	C78.0-☑	D02.2-☑	D14.3-☑	D38.1	D49.1
substernal	C38.1	C78.1	—	D15.2	D38.3	D49.89
sudoriferous, sudoriparous gland, site unspecified	C44.90	C79.2	D04.9	D23.9	D48.5	D49.2
specified site — *see* Neoplasm, skin						

	Malignant Primary	Malignant Secondary	Ca in situ	Benign	Uncertain Behavior	Unspecified Behavior
Neoplasm, neoplastic — *continued*						
supraclavicular region	C76.0	C79.89	D09.8	D36.7	D48.7	D49.89
supraglottis	C32.1	C78.39	D02.0	D14.1	D38.0	D49.1
suprarenal	C74.9-☑	C79.7-☑	D09.3	D35.0-☑	D44.1-☑	D49.7
capsule	C74.9-☑	C79.7-☑	D09.3	D35.0-☑	D44.1-☑	D49.7
cortex	C74.0-☑	C79.7-☑	D09.3	D35.0-☑	D44.1-☑	D49.7
gland	C74.9-☑	C79.7-☑	D09.3	D35.0-☑	D44.1-☑	D49.7
medulla	C74.1-☑	C79.7-☑	D09.3	D35.0-☑	D44.1-☑	D49.7
suprasellar (region)	C71.9	C79.31	—	D33.2	D43.2	D49.6
supratentorial (brain) NEC	C71.0	C79.31	—	D33.0	D43.0	D49.6
sweat gland (apocrine) (eccrine), site unspecified	C44.90	C79.2	D04.9	D23.9	D48.5	D49.2
specified site — *see* Neoplasm, skin						
sympathetic nerve or nervous system NEC	C47.9	C79.89	—	D36.10	D48.2	D49.2
symphysis pubis	C41.4	C79.51	—	D16.8	D48.0	D49.2
synovial membrane — *see* Neoplasm, connective tissue						
tapetum, brain	C71.8	C79.31	—	D33.2	D43.2	D49.6
tarsus (any bone)	C40.3-☑	C79.51	—	D16.3-☑	—	—
temple (skin) — *see also* Neoplasm, skin, face	C44.309	C79.2	D04.39	D23.39	D48.5	D49.2
temporal						
bone	C41.0	C79.51	—	D16.4	D48.0	D49.2
lobe or pole	C71.2	C79.31	—	D33.0	D43.0	D49.6
region	C76.0	C79.89	D09.8	D36.7	D48.7	D49.89
skin — *see also* Neoplasm, skin, face	C44.309	C79.2	D04.39	D23.39	D48.5	D49.2
tendon (sheath) — *see* Neoplasm, connective tissue						
tentorium (cerebelli)	C70.0	C79.32	—	D32.0	D42.0	D49.7
testis, testes	C62.9-☑	C79.82	D07.69	D29.2-☑	D40.1-☑	D49.59
descended	C62.1-☑	C79.82	D07.69	D29.2-☑	D40.1-☑	D49.59
ectopic	C62.0-☑	C79.82	D07.69	D29.2-☑	D40.1-☑	D49.59
retained	C62.0-☑	C79.82	D07.69	D29.2-☑	D40.1-☑	D49.59
scrotal	C62.1-☑	C79.82	D07.69	D29.2-☑	D40.1-☑	D49.59
undescended	C62.0-☑	C79.82	D07.69	D29.2-☑	D40.1-☑	D49.59
unspecified whether descended or undescended	C62.9-☑	C79.82	D07.69	D29.2-☑	D40.1-☑	D49.59
thalamus	C71.0	C79.31	—	D33.0	D43.0	D49.6
thigh NEC	C76.5-☑	C79.89	D04.7-☑	D36.7	D48.7	D49.89
thorax, thoracic (cavity) (organs NEC)	C76.1	C79.89	D09.8	D36.7	D48.7	D49.89
duct	C49.3	C79.89	—	D21.3	D48.1☑	D49.2
wall NEC	C76.1	C79.89	D09.8	D36.7	D48.7	D49.89
throat	C14.0	C79.89	D00.08	D10.9	D37.05	D49.0
thumb NEC	C76.4-☑	C79.89	D04.6-☑	D36.7	D48.7	D49.89
thymus (gland)	C37	C79.89	D09.3	D15.0	D38.4	D49.89
thyroglossal duct	C73	C79.89	D09.3	D34	D44.0	D49.7
thyroid (gland)	C73	C79.89	D09.3	D34	D44.0	D49.7
cartilage	C32.3	C78.39	D02.0	D14.1	D38.0	D49.1
tibia (any part)	C40.2-☑	C79.51	—	D16.2-☑	—	—
toe NEC	C76.5-☑	C79.89	D04.7-☑	D36.7	D48.7	D49.89
tongue	C02.9	C79.89	D00.07	D10.1	D37.02	D49.0
anterior (two-thirds) NEC	C02.3	C79.89	D00.07	D10.1	D37.02	D49.0
dorsal surface	C02.0	C79.89	D00.07	D10.1	D37.02	D49.0
ventral surface	C02.2	C79.89	D00.07	D10.1	D37.02	D49.0
base (dorsal surface)	C01	C79.89	D00.07	D10.1	D37.02	D49.0
border (lateral)	C02.1	C79.89	D00.07	D10.1	D37.02	D49.0
dorsal surface NEC	C02.0	C79.89	D00.07	D10.1	D37.02	D49.0
fixed part NEC	C01	C79.89	D00.07	D10.1	D37.02	D49.0
foreamen cecum	C02.0	C79.89	D00.07	D10.1	D37.02	D49.0
frenulum linguae	C02.2	C79.89	D00.07	D10.1	D37.02	D49.0
junctional zone	C02.8	C79.89	D00.07	D10.1	D37.02	D49.0

	Malignant Primary	Malignant Secondary	Ca in situ	Benign	Uncertain Behavior	Unspecified Behavior
Neoplasm, neoplastic — *continued*						
tongue — *continued*						
margin (lateral)	C02.1	C79.89	D00.07	D10.1	D37.02	D49.0
midline NEC	C02.0	C79.89	D00.07	D10.1	D37.02	D49.0
mobile part NEC	C02.3	C79.89	D00.07	D10.1	D37.02	D49.0
overlapping lesion	C02.8	—	—	—	—	—
posterior (third)	C01	C79.89	D00.07	D10.1	D37.02	D49.0
root	C01	C79.89	D00.07	D10.1	D37.02	D49.0
surface (dorsal)	C02.0	C79.89	D00.07	D10.1	D37.02	D49.0
base	C01	C79.89	D00.07	D10.1	D37.02	D49.0
ventral	C02.2	C79.89	D00.07	D10.1	D37.02	D49.0
tip	C02.1	C79.89	D00.07	D10.1	D37.02	D49.0
tonsil	C02.4	C79.89	D00.07	D10.1	D37.02	D49.0
tonsil	C09.9	C79.89	D00.08	D10.4	D37.05	D49.0
fauces, faucial	C09.9	C79.89	D00.08	D10.4	D37.05	D49.0
lingual	C02.4	C79.89	D00.07	D10.1	D37.02	D49.0
overlapping sites	C09.8	—	—	—	—	—
palatine	C09.9	C79.89	D00.08	D10.4	D37.05	D49.0
pharyngeal	C11.1	C79.89	D00.08	D10.6	D37.05	D49.0
pillar (anterior) (posterior)	C09.1	C79.89	D00.08	D10.5	D37.05	D49.0
tonsillar fossa	C09.0	C79.89	D00.08	D10.5	D37.05	D49.0
tooth socket NEC	C03.9	C79.89	D00.03	D10.39	D37.09	D49.0
trachea (cartilage) (mucosa)	C33	C78.39	D02.1	D14.2	D38.1	D49.1
overlapping lesion with bronchus or lung	C34.8-☑	—	—	—	—	—
tracheobronchial	C34.8-☑	C78.39	D02.1	D14.2	D38.1	D49.1
overlapping lesion with lung	C34.8-☑	—	—	—	—	—
tragus — *see also* Neoplasm, skin, ear	C44.20-☑	C79.2	D04.2-☑	D23.2-☑	D48.5	D49.2
trunk NEC	C76.8	C79.89	D04.5	D36.7	D48.7	D49.89
tubo-ovarian	C57.8	C79.82	D07.39	D28.7	D39.8	D49.59
tunica vaginalis	C63.7	C79.82	D07.69	D29.8	D40.8	D49.59
turbinate (bone)	C41.0	C79.51	—	D16.4	D48.0	D49.2
nasal	C30.0	C78.39	D02.3	D14.0	D38.5	D49.1
tympanic cavity	C30.1	C78.39	D02.3	D14.0	D38.5	D49.1
ulna (any part)	C40.0-☑	C79.51	—	D16.0-☑	—	—
umbilicus, umbilical — *see also* Neoplasm, skin, trunk	C44.509	C79.2	D04.5	D23.5	D48.5	D49.2
uncus, brain	C71.2	C79.31	—	D33.0	D43.0	D49.6
unknown site or unspecified	C80.1	C79.9	D09.9	D36.9	D48.9	D49.9
urachus	C67.7	C79.11	D09.0	D30.3	D41.4	D49.4
ureter-bladder (junction)	C67.6	C79.11	D09.0	D30.3	D41.4	D49.4
ureter, ureteral	C66.-☑	C79.19	D09.19	D30.2-☑	D41.2-☑	D49.59
orifice (bladder)	C67.6	C79.11	D09.0	D30.3	D41.4	D49.4
urethra, urethral (gland)	C68.0	C79.19	D09.19	D30.4	D41.3	D49.59
orifice, internal	C67.5	C79.11	D09.0	D30.3	D41.4	D49.4
urethrovaginal (septum)	C57.9	C79.82	D07.30	D28.9	D39.8	D49.59
urinary organ or system	C68.9	C79.10	D09.10	D30.9	D41.9	D49.59
bladder — *see* Neoplasm, bladder						
overlapping lesion	C68.8	—	—	—	—	—
specified sites NEC	C68.8	C79.19	D09.19	D30.8	D41.8	D49.59
utero-ovarian	C57.8	C79.82	D07.39	D28.7	D39.8	D49.59
ligament	C57.1-☑	C79.82	D07.39	D28.2	D39.8	D49.59
uterosacral ligament	C57.3	C79.82	—	D28.2	D39.8	D49.59
uterus, uteri, uterine	C55	C79.82	D07.0	D26.9	D39.0	D49.59
adnexa NEC	C57.4	C79.82	D07.39	D28.7	D39.8	D49.59
body	C54.9	C79.82	D07.0	D26.1	D39.0	D49.59
cervix	C53.9	C79.82	D06.9	D26.0	D39.0	D49.59
cornu	C54.9	C79.82	D07.0	D26.1	D39.0	D49.59
corpus	C54.9	C79.82	D07.0	D26.1	D39.0	D49.59
endocervix (canal) (gland)	C53.0	C79.82	D06.0	D26.0	D39.0	D49.59
endometrium	C54.1	C79.82	D07.0	D26.1	D39.0	D49.59
Neoplasm, neoplastic — *continued*						
uterus, uteri, uterine — *continued*						
exocervix	C53.1	C79.82	D06.1	D26.0	D39.0	D49.59
external os	C53.1	C79.82	D06.1	D26.0	D39.0	D49.59
fundus	C54.3	C79.82	D07.0	D26.1	D39.0	D49.59
internal os	C53.0	C79.82	D06.0	D26.0	D39.0	D49.59
isthmus	C54.0	C79.82	D07.0	D26.1	D39.0	D49.59
ligament	C57.3	C79.82	—	D28.2	D39.8	D49.59
broad	C57.1-☑	C79.82	D07.39	D28.2	D39.8	D49.59
round	C57.2-☑	C79.82	—	D28.2	D39.8	D49.59
lower segment	C54.0	C79.82	D07.0	D26.1	D39.0	D49.59
myometrium	C54.2	C79.82	D07.0	D26.1	D39.0	D49.59
overlapping sites	C54.8	—	—	—	—	—
squamocolumnar junction	C53.8	C79.82	D06.7	D26.0	D39.0	D49.59
tube	C57.0-☑	C79.82	D07.39	D28.2	D39.8	D49.59
utricle, prostatic	C68.0	C79.19	D09.19	D30.4	D41.3	D49.59
uveal tract	C69.4-☑	C79.49	D09.2-☑	D31.4-☑	D48.7	D49.89
uvula	C05.2	C79.89	D00.04	D10.39	D37.09	D49.0
vagina, vaginal (fornix) (vault) (wall)	C52	C79.82	D07.2	D28.1	D39.8	D49.59
vaginovesical	C57.9	C79.82	D07.30	D28.9	D39.9	D49.59
septum	C57.9	C79.82	D07.30	D28.9	D39.9	D49.59
vallecula (epiglottis)	C10.0	C79.89	D00.08	D10.5	D37.05	D49.0
vascular — *see* Neoplasm, connective tissue						
vas deferens	C63.1-☑	C79.82	D07.69	D29.8	D40.8	D49.59
Vater's ampulla	C24.1	C78.89	D01.5	D13.5	D37.6	D49.0
vein, venous — *see* Neoplasm, connective tissue						
vena cava (abdominal) (inferior)	C49.4	C79.89	—	D21.4	D48.1☑	D49.2
superior	C49.3	C79.89	—	D21.3	D48.1☑	D49.2
ventricle (cerebral) (floor) (lateral) (third)	C71.5	C79.31	—	D33.0	D43.0	D49.6
cardiac (left) (right)	C38.0	C79.89	—	D15.1	D48.7	D49.89
fourth	C71.7	C79.31	—	D33.1	D43.1	D49.6
ventricular band of larynx	C32.1	C78.39	D02.0	D14.1	D38.0	D49.1
ventriculus — *see* Neoplasm, stomach						
vermillion border — *see* Neoplasm, lip						
vermis, cerebellum	C71.6	C79.31	—	D33.1	D43.1	D49.6
vertebra (column)	C41.2	C79.51	—	D16.6	D48.0	D49.2
coccyx	C41.4	C79.51	—	D16.8	D48.0	D49.2
marrow NEC	C96.9	C79.52	—	—	D47.9	D49.89
sacrum	C41.4	C79.51	—	D16.8	D48.0	D49.2
vesical — *see* Neoplasm, bladder						
vesicle, seminal	C63.7	C79.82	D07.69	D29.8	D40.8	D49.59
vesicocervical tissue	C57.9	C79.82	D07.30	D28.9	D39.9	D49.59
vesicorectal	C76.3	C79.82	D09.8	D36.7	D48.7	D49.89
vesicovaginal	C57.9	C79.82	D07.30	D28.9	D39.9	D49.59
septum	C57.9	C79.82	D07.30	D28.9	D39.8	D49.59
vessel (blood) — *see* Neoplasm, connective tissue						
vestibular gland, greater	C51.0	C79.82	D07.1	D28.0	D39.8	D49.59
vestibule						
mouth	C06.1	C79.89	D00.00	D10.39	D37.09	D49.0
nose	C30.0	C78.39	D02.3	D14.0	D38.5	D49.1
Virchow's gland	C77.0	C77.0	—	D36.0	D48.7	D49.89
viscera NEC	C76.8	C79.89	D09.8	D36.7	D48.7	D49.89
vocal cords (true)	C32.0	C78.39	D02.0	D14.1	D38.0	D49.1
false	C32.1	C78.39	D02.0	D14.1	D38.0	D49.1
vomer	C41.0	C79.51	—	D16.4	D48.0	D49.2
vulva	C51.9	C79.82	D07.1	D28.0	D39.8	D49.59
vulvovaginal gland	C51.0	C79.82	D07.1	D28.0	D39.8	D49.59
Waldeyer's ring	C14.2	C79.89	D00.08	D10.9	D37.05	D49.0

☑ **Additional Character Required — Refer to the Tabular List for Character Selection**

	Malignant Primary	Malignant Secondary	Ca in situ	Benign	Uncertain Behavior	Unspecified Behavior
Neoplasm, neoplastic — *continued*						
Wharton's duct	C08.0	C79.89	D00.00	D11.7	D37.032	D49.0
white matter (central) (cerebral)	C71.0	C79.31	—	D33.0	D43.0	D49.6
windpipe	C33	C78.39	D02.1	D14.2	D38.1	D49.1
Wirsung's duct	C25.3	C78.89	D01.7	D13.6	D37.8	D49.0
wolffian (body) (duct)						
female	C57.7	C79.82	D07.39	D28.7	D39.8	D49.59
male	C63.7	C79.82	D07.69	D29.8	D40.8	D49.59
womb — *see* Neoplasm, uterus						
wrist NEC	C76.4-☑	C79.89	D04.6-☑	D36.7	D48.7	D49.89
xiphoid process	C41.3	C79.51	—	D16.7	D48.0	D49.2
Zuckerkandl organ	C75.5	C79.89	—	D35.6	D44.7	D49.7

Substance	Poisoning, Accidental (unintentional)	Poisoning, Intentional Self-harm	Poisoning, Assault	Poisoning, Undetermined	Adverse Effect	Under-dosing
14-hydroxydihydro-morphinone	T40.2X1	T40.2X2	T40.2X3	T40.2X4	T40.2X5	T40.2X6
1-Propanol	T51.3X1	T51.3X2	T51.3X3	T51.3X4	—	—
2,3,7,8-Tetrachlorodibenzo-p-dioxin	T53.7X1	T53.7X2	T53.7X3	T53.7X4	—	—
2,4,5-T (trichloro-phenoxyacetic acid)	T60.1X1	T60.1X2	T60.1X3	T60.1X4	—	—
2,4,5-Trichlorophen-oxyacetic acid	T60.3X1	T60.3X2	T60.3X3	T60.3X4	—	—
2,4-D (dichlorophen-oxyacetic acid)	T60.3X1	T60.3X2	T60.3X3	T60.3X4	—	—
2,4-Toluene diisocyanate	T65.0X1	T65.0X2	T65.0X3	T65.0X4	—	—
2-Deoxy-5-fluorouridine	T45.1X1	T45.1X2	T45.1X3	T45.1X4	T45.1X5	T45.1X6
2-Ethoxyethanol	T52.3X1	T52.3X2	T52.3X3	T52.3X4	—	—
2-Methoxyethanol	T52.3X1	T52.3X2	T52.3X3	T52.3X4	—	—
2-Propanol	T51.2X1	T51.2X2	T51.2X3	T51.2X4	—	—
3,4-methylenedioxymeth-amphetamine	T43.641	T43.642	T43.643	T43.644	—	—
4-Aminobutyric acid	T43.8X1	T43.8X2	T43.8X3	T43.8X4	T43.8X5	T43.8X6
4-Aminophenol derivatives	T39.1X1	T39.1X2	T39.1X3	T39.1X4	T39.1X5	T39.1X6
5-Deoxy-5-fluorouridine	T45.1X1	T45.1X2	T45.1X3	T45.1X4	T45.1X5	T45.1X6
5-Methoxypsoralen (5-MOP)	T50.991	T50.992	T50.993	T50.994	T50.995	T50.996
8-Aminoquinoline drugs	T37.2X1	T37.2X2	T37.2X3	T37.2X4	T37.2X5	T37.2X6
8-Methoxypsoralen (8-MOP)	T50.991	T50.992	T50.993	T50.994	T50.995	T50.996
9-hydoxyrisperidone*	T43.591	T43.592	T43.593	T43.594	T43.595	T43.596
ABOB	T37.5X1	T37.5X2	T37.5X3	T37.5X4	T37.5X5	T37.5X6
Abrine	T62.2X1	T62.2X2	T62.2X3	T62.2X4	—	—
Abrus (seed)	T62.2X1	T62.2X2	T62.2X3	T62.2X4	—	—
Absinthe	T51.0X1	T51.0X2	T51.0X3	T51.0X4	—	—
beverage	T51.0X1	T51.0X2	T51.0X3	T51.0X4	—	—
Acaricide	T60.8X1	T60.8X2	T60.8X3	T60.8X4	—	—
Acebutolol	T44.7X1	T44.7X2	T44.7X3	T44.7X4	T44.7X5	T44.7X6
Acecarbromal	T42.6X1	T42.6X2	T42.6X3	T42.6X4	T42.6X5	T42.6X6
Aceclidine	T44.1X1	T44.1X2	T44.1X3	T44.1X4	T44.1X5	T44.1X6
Acedapsone	T37.0X1	T37.0X2	T37.0X3	T37.0X4	T37.0X5	T37.0X6
Acefylline piperazine	T48.6X1	T48.6X2	T48.6X3	T48.6X4	T48.6X5	T48.6X6
Acemorphan	T40.2X1	T40.2X2	T40.2X3	T40.2X4	T40.2X5	T40.2X6
Acenocoumarin	T45.511	T45.512	T45.513	T45.514	T45.515	T45.516
Acenocoumarol	T45.511	T45.512	T45.513	T45.514	T45.515	T45.516
Aceon*	T46.4X1	T46.4X2	T46.4X3	T46.4X4	T46.4X5	T46.4X6
Acepifylline	T48.6X1	T48.6X2	T48.6X3	T48.6X4	T48.6X5	T48.6X6
Acepromazine	T43.3X1	T43.3X2	T43.3X3	T43.3X4	T43.3X5	T43.3X6
Acesulfamethoxypyridazine	T37.0X1	T37.0X2	T37.0X3	T37.0X4	T37.0X5	T37.0X6
Acetal	T52.8X1	T52.8X2	T52.8X3	T52.8X4	—	—
Acetaldehyde (vapor)	T52.8X1	T52.8X2	T52.8X3	T52.8X4	—	—
liquid	T65.891	T65.892	T65.893	T65.894	—	—
Acetaminophen	T39.1X1	T39.1X2	T39.1X3	T39.1X4	T39.1X5	T39.1X6
Acetaminosalol	T39.1X1	T39.1X2	T39.1X3	T39.1X4	T39.1X5	T39.1X6
Acetanilide	T39.1X1	T39.1X2	T39.1X3	T39.1X4	T39.1X5	T39.1X6
Acetarsol	T37.3X1	T37.3X2	T37.3X3	T37.3X4	T37.3X5	T37.3X6
Acetazolamide	T50.2X1	T50.2X2	T50.2X3	T50.2X4	T50.2X5	T50.2X6
Acetiamine	T45.2X1	T45.2X2	T45.2X3	T45.2X4	T45.2X5	T45.2X6
Acetic						
acid	T54.2X1	T54.2X2	T54.2X3	T54.2X4	—	—
with sodium acetate (ointment)	T49.3X1	T49.3X2	T49.3X3	T49.3X4	T49.3X5	T49.3X6
ester (solvent)(vapor)	T52.8X1	T52.8X2	T52.8X3	T52.8X4	—	—
irrigating solution	T50.3X1	T50.3X2	T50.3X3	T50.3X4	T50.3X5	T50.3X6
medicinal (lotion)	T49.2X1	T49.2X2	T49.2X3	T49.2X4	T49.2X5	T49.2X6
anhydride	T65.891	T65.892	T65.893	T65.894	—	—
ether (vapor)	T52.8X1	T52.8X2	T52.8X3	T52.8X4	—	—
Acetohexamide	T38.3X1	T38.3X2	T38.3X3	T38.3X4	T38.3X5	T38.3X6
Acetohydroxamic acid	T50.991	T50.992	T50.993	T50.994	T50.995	T50.996
Acetomenaphthone	T45.7X1	T45.7X2	T45.7X3	T45.7X4	T45.7X5	T45.7X6
Acetomorphine	T40.1X1	T40.1X2	T40.1X3	T40.1X4	—	—
Acetone (oils)	T52.4X1	T52.4X2	T52.4X3	T52.4X4	—	—
chlorinated	T52.4X1	T52.4X2	T52.4X3	T52.4X4	—	—
vapor	T52.4X1	T52.4X2	T52.4X3	T52.4X4	—	—
Acetonitrile	T52.8X1	T52.8X2	T52.8X3	T52.8X4	—	—
Acetophenazine	T43.3X1	T43.3X2	T43.3X3	T43.3X4	T43.3X5	T43.3X6
Acetophenetedin	T39.1X1	T39.1X2	T39.1X3	T39.1X4	T39.1X5	T39.1X6
Acetophenone	T52.4X1	T52.4X2	T52.4X3	T52.4X4	—	—
Acetorphine	T40.2X1	T40.2X2	T40.2X3	T40.2X4	—	—
Acetosulfone (sodium)	T37.1X1	T37.1X2	T37.1X3	T37.1X4	T37.1X5	T37.1X6
Acetrizoate (sodium)	T50.8X1	T50.8X2	T50.8X3	T50.8X4	T50.8X5	T50.8X6
Acetrizoic acid	T50.8X1	T50.8X2	T50.8X3	T50.8X4	T50.8X5	T50.8X6
Acetyl						
bromide	T53.6X1	T53.6X2	T53.6X3	T53.6X4	—	—
chloride	T53.6X1	T53.6X2	T53.6X3	T53.6X4	—	—
Acetylcarbromal	T42.6X1	T42.6X2	T42.6X3	T42.6X4	T42.6X5	T42.6X6
Acetylcholine						
Acetylcholine — *continued*						
chloride	T44.1X1	T44.1X2	T44.1X3	T44.1X4	T44.1X5	T44.1X6
derivative	T44.1X1	T44.1X2	T44.1X3	T44.1X4	T44.1X5	T44.1X6
Acetylcysteine	T48.4X1	T48.4X2	T48.4X3	T48.4X4	T48.4X5	T48.4X6
Acetyldigitoxin	T46.0X1	T46.0X2	T46.0X3	T46.0X4	T46.0X5	T46.0X6
Acetyldigoxin	T46.0X1	T46.0X2	T46.0X3	T46.0X4	T46.0X5	T46.0X6
Acetyldihydrocodeine	T40.2X1	T40.2X2	T40.2X3	T40.2X4	—	—
Acetyldihydrocodeinone	T40.2X1	T40.2X2	T40.2X3	T40.2X4	—	—
Acetylene (gas)	T59.891	T59.892	T59.893	T59.894	—	—
dichloride	T53.6X1	T53.6X2	T53.6X3	T53.6X4	—	—
incomplete combustion of	T58.11	T58.12	T58.13	T58.14	—	—
industrial	T59.891	T59.892	T59.893	T59.894	—	—
tetrachloride	T53.6X1	T53.6X2	T53.6X3	T53.6X4	—	—
vapor	T53.6X1	T53.6X2	T53.6X3	T53.6X4	—	—
Acetylpheneturide	T42.6X1	T42.6X2	T42.6X3	T42.6X4	T42.6X5	T42.6X6
Acetylphenylhydrazine	T39.8X1	T39.8X2	T39.8X3	T39.8X4	T39.8X5	T39.8X6
Acetylsalicylic acid (salts)	T39.011	T39.012	T39.013	T39.014	T39.015	T39.016
enteric coated	T39.011	T39.012	T39.013	T39.014	T39.015	T39.016
Acetylsulfamethoxypyridazine	T37.0X1	T37.0X2	T37.0X3	T37.0X4	T37.0X5	T37.0X6
Achromycin	T36.4X1	T36.4X2	T36.4X3	T36.4X4	T36.4X5	T36.4X6
ophthalmic preparation	T49.5X1	T49.5X2	T49.5X3	T49.5X4	T49.5X5	T49.5X6
topical NEC	T49.0X1	T49.0X2	T49.0X3	T49.0X4	T49.0X5	T49.0X6
Aciclovir	T37.5X1	T37.5X2	T37.5X3	T37.5X4	T37.5X5	T37.5X6
Acidifying agent NEC	T50.901	T50.902	T50.903	T50.904	T50.905	T50.906
Acid (corrosive) **NEC**	T54.2X1	T54.2X2	T54.2X3	T54.2X4	—	—
AcipHex*	T47.1X1	T47.1X2	T47.1X3	T47.1X4	T47.1X5	T47.1X6
Acipimox	T46.6X1	T46.6X2	T46.6X3	T46.6X4	T46.6X5	T46.6X6
Acitretin	T50.991	T50.992	T50.993	T50.994	T50.995	T50.996
Aclarubicin	T45.1X1	T45.1X2	T45.1X3	T45.1X4	T45.1X5	T45.1X6
Aclatonium napadisilate	T48.1X1	T48.1X2	T48.1X3	T48.1X4	T48.1X5	T48.1X6
Aconite (wild)	T46.991	T46.992	T46.993	T46.994	T46.995	T46.996
Aconitine	T46.991	T46.992	T46.993	T46.994	T46.995	T46.996
Aconitum ferox	T46.991	T46.992	T46.993	T46.994	T46.995	T46.996
Acridine	T65.6X1	T65.6X2	T65.6X3	T65.6X4	—	—
vapor	T59.891	T59.892	T59.893	T59.894	—	—
Acriflavine	T37.91	T37.92	T37.93	T37.94	T37.95	T37.96
Acriflavinium chloride	T49.0X1	T49.0X2	T49.0X3	T49.0X4	T49.0X5	T49.0X6
Acrinol	T49.0X1	T49.0X2	T49.0X3	T49.0X4	T49.0X5	T49.0X6
Acrisorcin	T49.0X1	T49.0X2	T49.0X3	T49.0X4	T49.0X5	T49.0X6
Acrivastine	T45.0X1	T45.0X2	T45.0X3	T45.0X4	T45.0X5	T45.0X6
Acrolein (gas)	T59.891	T59.892	T59.893	T59.894	—	—
liquid	T54.1X1	T54.1X2	T54.1X3	T54.1X4	—	—
Acrylamide	T65.891	T65.892	T65.893	T65.894	—	—
Acrylic resin	T49.3X1	T49.3X2	T49.3X3	T49.3X4	T49.3X5	T49.3X6
Acrylonitrile	T65.891	T65.892	T65.893	T65.894	—	—
Actaea spicata	T62.2X1	T62.2X2	T62.2X3	T62.2X4	—	—
berry	T62.1X1	T62.1X2	T62.1X3	T62.1X4	—	—
Acterol	T37.3X1	T37.3X2	T37.3X3	T37.3X4	T37.3X5	T37.3X6
ACTH	T38.811	T38.812	T38.813	T38.814	T38.815	T38.816
Actinomycin C	T45.1X1	T45.1X2	T45.1X3	T45.1X4	T45.1X5	T45.1X6
Actinomycin D	T45.1X1	T45.1X2	T45.1X3	T45.1X4	T45.1X5	T45.1X6
Activated charcoal — *see also* Charcoal, medicinal	T47.6X1	T47.6X2	T47.6X3	T47.6X4	T47.6X5	T47.6X6
Activella*	T38.5X1	T38.5X2	T38.5X3	T38.5X4	T38.5X5	T38.5X6
Acyclovir	T37.5X1	T37.5X2	T37.5X3	T37.5X4	T37.5X5	T37.5X6
Adderall*	T43.621	T43.622	T43.623	T43.624	T43.625	T43.626
Adenine	T45.2X1	T45.2X2	T45.2X3	T45.2X4	T45.2X5	T45.2X6
arabinoside	T37.5X1	T37.5X2	T37.5X3	T37.5X4	T37.5X5	T37.5X6
Adenosine (phosphate)	T46.2X1	T46.2X2	T46.2X3	T46.2X4	T46.2X5	T46.2X6
ADH	T38.891	T38.892	T38.893	T38.894	T38.895	T38.896
Adhesive NEC	T65.891	T65.892	T65.893	T65.894	—	—
Adicillin	T36.0X1	T36.0X2	T36.0X3	T36.0X4	T36.0X5	T36.0X6
Adiphenine	T44.3X1	T44.3X2	T44.3X3	T44.3X4	T44.3X5	T44.3X6
Adipiodone	T50.8X1	T50.8X2	T50.8X3	T50.8X4	T50.8X5	T50.8X6
Adjunct, pharmaceutical	T50.901	T50.902	T50.903	T50.904	T50.905	T50.906
Adrenal (extract, cortex or medulla) (glucocorticoids) (hormones) (mineralocorticoids)	T38.0X1	T38.0X2	T38.0X3	T38.0X4	T38.0X5	T38.0X6
ENT agent	T49.6X1	T49.6X2	T49.6X3	T49.6X4	T49.6X5	T49.6X6
ophthalmic preparation	T49.5X1	T49.5X2	T49.5X3	T49.5X4	T49.5X5	T49.5X6
topical NEC	T49.0X1	T49.0X2	T49.0X3	T49.0X4	T49.0X5	T49.0X6
Adrenalin — *see* Adrenaline						
Adrenaline	T44.5X1	T44.5X2	T44.5X3	T44.5X4	T44.5X5	T44.5X6
Adrenergic NEC	T44.901	T44.902	T44.903	T44.904	T44.905	T44.906
blocking agent NEC	T44.8X1	T44.8X2	T44.8X3	T44.8X4	T44.8X5	T44.8X6
beta, heart	T44.7X1	T44.7X2	T44.7X3	T44.7X4	T44.7X5	T44.7X6
specified NEC	T44.991	T44.992	T44.993	T44.994	T44.995	T44.996
Adrenochrome						
derivative	T46.991	T46.992	T46.993	T46.994	T46.995	T46.996
(mono) semicarbazone	T46.991	T46.992	T46.993	T46.994	T46.995	T46.996
Adrenocorticotrophic hormone	T38.811	T38.812	T38.813	T38.814	T38.815	T38.816

Substance	Poisoning, Accidental (unintentional)	Poisoning, Intentional Self-harm	Poisoning, Assault	Poisoning, Undetermined	Adverse Effect	Under-dosing
Adrenocorticotrophin	T38.811	T38.812	T38.813	T38.814	T38.815	T38.816
Adriamycin	T45.1X1	T45.1X2	T45.1X3	T45.1X4	T45.1X5	T45.1X6
Adrucil*	T45.1X1	T45.1X2	T45.1X3	T45.1X4	T45.1X5	T45.1X6
Aerosol spray NEC	T65.91	T65.92	T65.93	T65.94	—	—
Aerosporin	T36.8X1	T36.8X2	T36.8X3	T36.8X4	T36.8X5	T36.8X6
ENT agent	T49.6X1	T49.6X2	T49.6X3	T49.6X4	T49.6X5	T49.6X6
ophthalmic preparation	T49.5X1	T49.5X2	T49.5X3	T49.5X4	T49.5X5	T49.5X6
topical NEC	T49.ØX1	T49.ØX2	T49.ØX3	T49.ØX4	T49.ØX5	T49.ØX6
Aethusa cynapium	T62.2X1	T62.2X2	T62.2X3	T62.2X4	—	—
Afghanistan black	T4Ø.711	T4Ø.712	T4Ø.713	T4Ø.714	T4Ø.715	T4Ø.716
Aflatoxin	T64.Ø1	T64.Ø2	T64.Ø3	T64.Ø4	—	—
Afloqualone	T42.8X1	T42.8X2	T42.8X3	T42.8X4	T42.8X5	T42.8X6
African boxwood	T62.2X1	T62.2X2	T62.2X3	T62.2X4	—	—
Agar	T47.4X1	T47.4X2	T47.4X3	T47.4X4	T47.4X5	T47.4X6
Agonist						
predominantly						
alpha-adrenoreceptor	T44.4X1	T44.4X2	T44.4X3	T44.4X4	T44.4X5	T44.4X6
beta-adrenoreceptor	T44.5X1	T44.5X2	T44.5X3	T44.5X4	T44.5X5	T44.5X6
Agricultural agent NEC	T65.91	T65.92	T65.93	T65.94	—	—
Agrypnal	T42.3X1	T42.3X2	T42.3X3	T42.3X4	T42.3X5	T42.3X6
AHLG	T5Ø.Z11	T5Ø.Z12	T5Ø.Z13	T5Ø.Z14	T5Ø.Z15	T5Ø.Z16
Air contaminant(s), **source/type NOS**	T65.91	T65.92	T65.93	T65.94	—	—
Ajmaline	T46.2X1	T46.2X2	T46.2X3	T46.2X4	T46.2X5	T46.2X6
Akee	T62.1X1	T62.1X2	T62.1X3	T62.1X4	—	—
Akne-Mycin*	T49.ØX1	T49.ØX2	T49.ØX3	T49.ØX4	T49.ØX5	T49.ØX6
Akrinol	T49.ØX1	T49.ØX2	T49.ØX3	T49.ØX4	T49.ØX5	T49.ØX6
Akritoin	T37.8X1	T37.8X2	T37.8X3	T37.8X4	T37.8X5	T37.8X6
Alacepril	T46.4X1	T46.4X2	T46.4X3	T46.4X4	T46.4X5	T46.4X6
Alantolactone	T37.4X1	T37.4X2	T37.4X3	T37.4X4	T37.4X5	T37.4X6
Albamycin	T36.8X1	T36.8X2	T36.8X3	T36.8X4	T36.8X5	T36.8X6
Albendazole	T37.4X1	T37.4X2	T37.4X3	T37.4X4	T37.4X5	T37.4X6
Albigutide*	T38.3X1	T38.3X2	T38.3X3	T38.3X4	T38.3X5	T38.3X6
Albumin						
bovine	T45.8X1	T45.8X2	T45.8X3	T45.8X4	T45.8X5	T45.8X6
human serum	T45.8X1	T45.8X2	T45.8X3	T45.8X4	T45.8X5	T45.8X6
salt-poor	T45.8X1	T45.8X2	T45.8X3	T45.8X4	T45.8X5	T45.8X6
normal human serum	T45.8X1	T45.8X2	T45.8X3	T45.8X4	T45.8X5	T45.8X6
Albuterol	T48.6X1	T48.6X2	T48.6X3	T48.6X4	T48.6X5	T48.6X6
Albutoin	T42.ØX1	T42.ØX2	T42.ØX3	T42.ØX4	T42.ØX5	T42.ØX6
Alclometasone	T49.ØX1	T49.ØX2	T49.ØX3	T49.ØX4	T49.ØX5	T49.ØX6
Alcohol	T51.91	T51.92	T51.93	T51.94	—	—
absolute	T51.ØX1	T51.ØX2	T51.ØX3	T51.ØX4	—	—
beverage	T51.ØX1	T51.ØX2	T51.ØX3	T51.ØX4	—	—
allyl	T51.8X1	T51.8X2	T51.8X3	T51.8X4	—	—
amyl	T51.3X1	T51.3X2	T51.3X3	T51.3X4	—	—
antifreeze	T51.1X1	T51.1X2	T51.1X3	T51.1X4	—	—
beverage	T51.ØX1	T51.ØX2	T51.ØX3	T51.ØX4	—	—
butyl	T51.3X1	T51.3X2	T51.3X3	T51.3X4	—	—
dehydrated	T51.ØX1	T51.ØX2	T51.ØX3	T51.ØX4	—	—
beverage	T51.ØX1	T51.ØX2	T51.ØX3	T51.ØX4	—	—
denatured	T51.ØX1	T51.ØX2	T51.ØX3	T51.ØX4	—	—
deterrent NEC	T5Ø.6X1	T5Ø.6X2	T5Ø.6X3	T5Ø.6X4	T5Ø.6X5	T5Ø.6X6
diagnostic (gastric function)	T5Ø.8X1	T5Ø.8X2	T5Ø.8X3	T5Ø.8X4	T5Ø.8X5	T5Ø.8X6
ethyl	T51.ØX1	T51.ØX2	T51.ØX3	T51.ØX4	—	—
beverage	T51.ØX1	T51.ØX2	T51.ØX3	T51.ØX4	—	—
grain	T51.ØX1	T51.ØX2	T51.ØX3	T51.ØX4	—	—
beverage	T51.ØX1	T51.ØX2	T51.ØX3	T51.ØX4	—	—
industrial	T51.ØX1	T51.ØX2	T51.ØX3	T51.ØX4	—	—
isopropyl	T51.2X1	T51.2X2	T51.2X3	T51.2X4	—	—
methyl	T51.1X1	T51.1X2	T51.1X3	T51.1X4	—	—
preparation for consumption	T51.ØX1	T51.ØX2	T51.ØX3	T51.ØX4	—	—
propyl	T51.3X1	T51.3X2	T51.3X3	T51.3X4	—	—
secondary	T51.2X1	T51.2X2	T51.2X3	T51.2X4	—	—
radiator	T51.1X1	T51.1X2	T51.1X3	T51.1X4	—	—
rubbing	T51.2X1	T51.2X2	T51.2X3	T51.2X4	—	—
specified type NEC	T51.8X1	T51.8X2	T51.8X3	T51.8X4	—	—
surgical	T51.ØX1	T51.ØX2	T51.ØX3	T51.ØX4	—	—
vapor (from any type of Alcohol)	T59.891	T59.892	T59.893	T59.894	—	—
wood	T51.1X1	T51.1X2	T51.1X3	T51.1X4	—	—
Alcuronium (chloride)	T48.1X1	T48.1X2	T48.1X3	T48.1X4	T48.1X5	T48.1X6
Aldactone	T5Ø.ØX1	T5Ø.ØX2	T5Ø.ØX3	T5Ø.ØX4	T5Ø.ØX5	T5Ø.ØX6
Aldesulfone sodium	T37.1X1	T37.1X2	T37.1X3	T37.1X4	T37.1X5	T37.1X6
Aldicarb	T6Ø.ØX1	T6Ø.ØX2	T6Ø.ØX3	T6Ø.ØX4	—	—
Aldomet	T46.5X1	T46.5X2	T46.5X3	T46.5X4	T46.5X5	T46.5X6
Aldosterone	T5Ø.ØX1	T5Ø.ØX2	T5Ø.ØX3	T5Ø.ØX4	T5Ø.ØX5	T5Ø.ØX6
Aldrin (dust)	T6Ø.1X1	T6Ø.1X2	T6Ø.1X3	T6Ø.1X4	—	—
Aleve — *see* Naproxen						
Alexitol sodium	T47.1X1	T47.1X2	T47.1X3	T47.1X4	T47.1X5	T47.1X6
Alfacalcidol	T45.2X1	T45.2X2	T45.2X3	T45.2X4	T45.2X5	T45.2X6

Substance	Poisoning, Accidental (unintentional)	Poisoning, Intentional Self-harm	Poisoning, Assault	Poisoning, Undetermined	Adverse Effect	Under-dosing
Alfadolone	T41.1X1	T41.1X2	T41.1X3	T41.1X4	T41.1X5	T41.1X6
Alfaxalone	T41.1X1	T41.1X2	T41.1X3	T41.1X4	T41.1X5	T41.1X6
Alfentanil	T4Ø.411	T4Ø.412	T4Ø.413	T4Ø.414	T4Ø.415	T4Ø.416
Alfuzosin (hydrochloride)	T44.8X1	T44.8X2	T44.8X3	T44.8X4	T44.8X5	T44.8X6
Algae (harmful) (toxin)	T65.821	T65.822	T65.823	T65.824	—	—
Algeldrate	T47.1X1	T47.1X2	T47.1X3	T47.1X4	T47.1X5	T47.1X6
Algin	T47.8X1	T47.8X2	T47.8X3	T47.8X4	T47.8X5	T47.8X6
Alglucerase	T45.3X1	T45.3X2	T45.3X3	T45.3X4	T45.3X5	T45.3X6
Alidase	T45.3X1	T45.3X2	T45.3X3	T45.3X4	T45.3X5	T45.3X6
Alimemazine	T43.3X1	T43.3X2	T43.3X3	T43.3X4	T43.3X5	T43.3X6
Aliphatic thiocyanates	T65.ØX1	T65.ØX2	T65.ØX3	T65.ØX4	—	—
Alitretinoin*	T49.ØX1	T49.ØX2	T49.ØX3	T49.ØX4	T49.ØX5	T49.ØX6
Alizapride	T45.ØX1	T45.ØX2	T45.ØX3	T45.ØX4	T45.ØX5	T45.ØX6
Alkali (caustic)	T54.3X1	T54.3X2	T54.3X3	T54.3X4	—	—
Alkaline antiseptic solution (aromatic)	T49.6X1	T49.6X2	T49.6X3	T49.6X4	T49.6X5	T49.6X6
Alkalinizing agents (medicinal)	T5Ø.9Ø1	T5Ø.9Ø2	T5Ø.9Ø3	T5Ø.9Ø4	T5Ø.9Ø5	T5Ø.9Ø6
Alkalizing agent NEC	T5Ø.9Ø1	T5Ø.9Ø2	T5Ø.9Ø3	T5Ø.9Ø4	T5Ø.9Ø5	T5Ø.9Ø6
Alka-seltzer	T39.Ø11	T39.Ø12	T39.Ø13	T39.Ø14	T39.Ø15	T39.Ø16
Alkavervir	T46.5X1	T46.5X2	T46.5X3	T46.5X4	T46.5X5	T46.5X6
Alkeran*	T45.1X1	T45.1X2	T45.1X3	T45.1X4	T45.1X5	T45.1X6
Alkonium (bromide)	T49.ØX1	T49.ØX2	T49.ØX3	T49.ØX4	T49.ØX5	T49.ØX6
Alkylating drug NEC	T45.1X1	T45.1X2	T45.1X3	T45.1X4	T45.1X5	T45.1X6
antimyeloproliferative	T45.1X1	T45.1X2	T45.1X3	T45.1X4	T45.1X5	T45.1X6
lymphatic	T45.1X1	T45.1X2	T45.1X3	T45.1X4	T45.1X5	T45.1X6
Alkylisocyanate	T65.ØX1	T65.ØX2	T65.ØX3	T65.ØX4	—	—
Allantoin	T49.4X1	T49.4X2	T49.4X3	T49.4X4	T49.4X5	T49.4X6
Allegron	T43.Ø11	T43.Ø12	T43.Ø13	T43.Ø14	T43.Ø15	T43.Ø16
Allethrin	T49.ØX1	T49.ØX2	T49.ØX3	T49.ØX4	T49.ØX5	T49.ØX6
Allobarbital	T42.3X1	T42.3X2	T42.3X3	T42.3X4	T42.3X5	T42.3X6
Allopurinol	T5Ø.4X1	T5Ø.4X2	T5Ø.4X3	T5Ø.4X4	T5Ø.4X5	T5Ø.4X6
Allyl						
alcohol	T51.8X1	T51.8X2	T51.8X3	T51.8X4	—	—
disulfide	T46.6X1	T46.6X2	T46.6X3	T46.6X4	T46.6X5	T46.6X6
Allylestrenol	T38.5X1	T38.5X2	T38.5X3	T38.5X4	T38.5X5	T38.5X6
Allylisopropylacetylurea	T42.6X1	T42.6X2	T42.6X3	T42.6X4	T42.6X5	T42.6X6
Allylisopropylmalonylurea	T42.3X1	T42.3X2	T42.3X3	T42.3X4	T42.3X5	T42.3X6
Allylthiourea	T49.3X1	T49.3X2	T49.3X3	T49.3X4	T49.3X5	T49.3X6
Allyltribromide	T42.6X1	T42.6X2	T42.6X3	T42.6X4	T42.6X5	T42.6X6
Allypropymal	T42.3X1	T42.3X2	T42.3X3	T42.3X4	T42.3X5	T42.3X6
Almagate	T47.1X1	T47.1X2	T47.1X3	T47.1X4	T47.1X5	T47.1X6
Almasilate	T47.1X1	T47.1X2	T47.1X3	T47.1X4	T47.1X5	T47.1X6
Almitrine	T5Ø.7X1	T5Ø.7X2	T5Ø.7X3	T5Ø.7X4	T5Ø.7X5	T5Ø.7X6
Aloes	T47.2X1	T47.2X2	T47.2X3	T47.2X4	T47.2X5	T47.2X6
Aloglutamol	T47.1X1	T47.1X2	T47.1X3	T47.1X4	T47.1X5	T47.1X6
Aloin	T47.2X1	T47.2X2	T47.2X3	T47.2X4	T47.2X5	T47.2X6
Aloxidone	T42.2X1	T42.2X2	T42.2X3	T42.2X4	T42.2X5	T42.2X6
Alpha						
acetyldigoxin	T46.ØX1	T46.ØX2	T46.ØX3	T46.ØX4	T46.ØX5	T46.ØX6
adrenergic blocking drug	T44.6X1	T44.6X2	T44.6X3	T44.6X4	T44.6X5	T44.6X6
amylase	T45.3X1	T45.3X2	T45.3X3	T45.3X4	T45.3X5	T45.3X6
tocoferol (acetate)	T45.2X1	T45.2X2	T45.2X3	T45.2X4	T45.2X5	T45.2X6
tocopherol	T45.2X1	T45.2X2	T45.2X3	T45.2X4	T45.2X5	T45.2X6
Alphadolone	T41.1X1	T41.1X2	T41.1X3	T41.1X4	T41.1X5	T41.1X6
Alphaprodine	T4Ø.491	T4Ø.492	T4Ø.493	T4Ø.494	T4Ø.495	T4Ø.496
Alphaxalone	T41.1X1	T41.1X2	T41.1X3	T41.1X4	T41.1X5	T41.1X6
Alprazolam	T42.4X1	T42.4X2	T42.4X3	T42.4X4	T42.4X5	T42.4X6
Alprenolol	T44.7X1	T44.7X2	T44.7X3	T44.7X4	T44.7X5	T44.7X6
Alprostadil	T46.7X1	T46.7X2	T46.7X3	T46.7X4	T46.7X5	T46.7X6
Alsactide	T38.811	T38.812	T38.813	T38.814	T38.815	T38.816
Alseroxylon	T46.5X1	T46.5X2	T46.5X3	T46.5X4	T46.5X5	T46.5X6
Alteplase	T45.611	T45.612	T45.613	T45.614	T45.615	T45.616
Altizide	T5Ø.2X1	T5Ø.2X2	T5Ø.2X3	T5Ø.2X4	T5Ø.2X5	T5Ø.2X6
Altoprev*	T46.6X1	T46.6X2	T46.6X3	T46.6X4	T46.6X5	T46.6X6
Altretamine	T45.1X1	T45.1X2	T45.1X3	T45.1X4	T45.1X5	T45.1X6
Alum (medicinal)	T49.4X1	T49.4X2	T49.4X3	T49.4X4	T49.4X5	T49.4X6
nonmedicinal (ammonium) (potassium)	T56.891	T56.892	T56.893	T56.894	—	—
Aluminium, aluminum						
acetate	T49.2X1	T49.2X2	T49.2X3	T49.2X4	T49.2X5	T49.2X6
solution	T49.ØX1	T49.ØX2	T49.ØX3	T49.ØX4	T49.ØX5	T49.ØX6
aspirin	T39.Ø11	T39.Ø12	T39.Ø13	T39.Ø14	T39.Ø15	T39.Ø16
bis (acetylsalicylate)	T39.Ø11	T39.Ø12	T39.Ø13	T39.Ø14	T39.Ø15	T39.Ø16
carbonate (gel, basic)	T47.1X1	T47.1X2	T47.1X3	T47.1X4	T47.1X5	T47.1X6
chlorhydroxide-complex	T47.1X1	T47.1X2	T47.1X3	T47.1X4	T47.1X5	T47.1X6
chloride	T49.2X1	T49.2X2	T49.2X3	T49.2X4	T49.2X5	T49.2X6
clofibrate	T46.6X1	T46.6X2	T46.6X3	T46.6X4	T46.6X5	T46.6X6
diacetate	T49.2X1	T49.2X2	T49.2X3	T49.2X4	T49.2X5	T49.2X6
glycinate	T47.1X1	T47.1X2	T47.1X3	T47.1X4	T47.1X5	T47.1X6
hydroxide (gel)	T47.1X1	T47.1X2	T47.1X3	T47.1X4	T47.1X5	T47.1X6
hydroxide-magnesium carb. gel	T47.1X1	T47.1X2	T47.1X3	T47.1X4	T47.1X5	T47.1X6

Substance	Poisoning, Accidental (unintentional)	Poisoning, Intentional Self-harm	Poisoning, Assault	Poisoning, Undetermined	Adverse Effect	Under-dosing
Aluminium, aluminum — *continued*						
magnesium silicate	T47.1X1	T47.1X2	T47.1X3	T47.1X4	T47.1X5	T47.1X6
nicotinate	T46.7X1	T46.7X2	T46.7X3	T46.7X4	T46.7X5	T46.7X6
ointment (surgical) (topical)	T49.3X1	T49.3X2	T49.3X3	T49.3X4	T49.3X5	T49.3X6
phosphate	T47.1X1	T47.1X2	T47.1X3	T47.1X4	T47.1X5	T47.1X6
salicylate	T39.Ø91	T39.Ø92	T39.Ø93	T39.Ø94	T39.Ø95	T39.Ø96
silicate	T47.1X1	T47.1X2	T47.1X3	T47.1X4	T47.1X5	T47.1X6
sodium silicate	T47.1X1	T47.1X2	T47.1X3	T47.1X4	T47.1X5	T47.1X6
subacetate	T49.2X1	T49.2X2	T49.2X3	T49.2X4	T49.2X5	T49.2X6
sulfate	T49.ØX1	T49.ØX2	T49.ØX3	T49.ØX4	T49.ØX5	T49.ØX6
tannate	T47.6X1	T47.6X2	T47.6X3	T47.6X4	T47.6X5	T47.6X6
topical NEC	T49.3X1	T49.3X2	T49.3X3	T49.3X4	T49.3X5	T49.3X6
Alurate	T42.3X1	T42.3X2	T42.3X3	T42.3X4	T42.3X5	T42.3X6
Alverine	T44.3X1	T44.3X2	T44.3X3	T44.3X4	T44.3X5	T44.3X6
Alvodine	T4Ø.2X1	T4Ø.2X2	T4Ø.2X3	T4Ø.2X4	T4Ø.2X5	T4Ø.2X6
Amanita phalloides	T62.ØX1	T62.ØX2	T62.ØX3	T62.ØX4	—	—
Amanitine	T62.ØX1	T62.ØX2	T62.ØX3	T62.ØX4	—	—
Amantadine	T42.8X1	T42.8X2	T42.8X3	T42.8X4	T42.8X5	T42.8X6
Ambazone	T49.6X1	T49.6X2	T49.6X3	T49.6X4	T49.6X5	T49.6X6
Ambenonium (chloride)	T44.ØX1	T44.ØX2	T44.ØX3	T44.ØX4	T44.ØX5	T44.ØX6
Ambien*	T42.6X1	T42.6X2	T42.6X3	T42.6X4	T42.6X5	T42.6X6
Ambroxol	T48.4X1	T48.4X2	T48.4X3	T48.4X4	T48.4X5	T48.4X6
Ambuphylline	T48.6X1	T48.6X2	T48.6X3	T48.6X4	T48.6X5	T48.6X6
Ambutonium bromide	T44.3X1	T44.3X2	T44.3X3	T44.3X4	T44.3X5	T44.3X6
Amcinonide	T49.ØX1	T49.ØX2	T49.ØX3	T49.ØX4	T49.ØX5	T49.ØX6
Amdinocilline	T36.ØX1	T36.ØX2	T36.ØX3	T36.ØX4	T36.ØX5	T36.ØX6
Americaine*	T41.3X1	T41.3X2	T41.3X3	T41.3X4	T41.3X5	T41.3X6
Ametazole	T5Ø.8X1	T5Ø.8X2	T5Ø.8X3	T5Ø.8X4	T5Ø.8X5	T5Ø.8X6
Amethocaine	T41.3X1	T41.3X2	T41.3X3	T41.3X4	T41.3X5	T41.3X6
regional	T41.3X1	T41.3X2	T41.3X3	T41.3X4	T41.3X5	T41.3X6
spinal	T41.3X1	T41.3X2	T41.3X3	T41.3X4	T41.3X5	T41.3X6
Amethopterin	T45.1X1	T45.1X2	T45.1X3	T45.1X4	T45.1X5	T45.1X6
Amezinium metilsulfate	T44.991	T44.992	T44.993	T44.994	T44.995	T44.996
Amfebutamone	T43.291	T43.292	T43.293	T43.294	T43.295	T43.296
Amfepramone	T5Ø.5X1	T5Ø.5X2	T5Ø.5X3	T5Ø.5X4	T5Ø.5X5	T5Ø.5X6
Amfetamine	T43.621	T43.622	T43.623	T43.624	T43.625	T43.626
Amfetaminil	T43.621	T43.622	T43.623	T43.624	T43.625	T43.626
Amfomycin	T36.8X1	T36.8X2	T36.8X3	T36.8X4	T36.8X5	T36.8X6
Amidefrine mesilate	T48.5X1	T48.5X2	T48.5X3	T48.5X4	T48.5X5	T48.5X6
Amidone	T4Ø.3X1	T4Ø.3X2	T4Ø.3X3	T4Ø.3X4	T4Ø.3X5	T4Ø.3X6
Amidopyrine	T39.2X1	T39.2X2	T39.2X3	T39.2X4	T39.2X5	T39.2X6
Amidotrizoate	T5Ø.8X1	T5Ø.8X2	T5Ø.8X3	T5Ø.8X4	T5Ø.8X5	T5Ø.8X6
Amiflamine	T43.1X1	T43.1X2	T43.1X3	T43.1X4	T43.1X5	T43.1X6
Amikacin	T36.5X1	T36.5X2	T36.5X3	T36.5X4	T36.5X5	T36.5X6
Amikhelline	T46.3X1	T46.3X2	T46.3X3	T46.3X4	T46.3X5	T46.3X6
Amiloride	T5Ø.2X1	T5Ø.2X2	T5Ø.2X3	T5Ø.2X4	T5Ø.2X5	T5Ø.2X6
Aminacrine	T49.ØX1	T49.ØX2	T49.ØX3	T49.ØX4	T49.ØX5	T49.ØX6
Amineptine	T43.Ø11	T43.Ø12	T43.Ø13	T43.Ø14	T43.Ø15	T43.Ø16
Aminitrozole	T37.3X1	T37.3X2	T37.3X3	T37.3X4	T37.3X5	T37.3X6
Aminoacetic acid (derivatives)	T5Ø.3X1	T5Ø.3X2	T5Ø.3X3	T5Ø.3X4	T5Ø.3X5	T5Ø.3X6
Amino acids	T5Ø.3X1	T5Ø.3X2	T5Ø.3X3	T5Ø.3X4	T5Ø.3X5	T5Ø.3X6
Aminoacridine	T49.ØX1	T49.ØX2	T49.ØX3	T49.ØX4	T49.ØX5	T49.ØX6
Aminobenzoic acid (-p)	T49.3X1	T49.3X2	T49.3X3	T49.3X4	T49.3X5	T49.3X6
Aminocaproic acid	T45.621	T45.622	T45.623	T45.624	T45.625	T45.626
Aminoethylisothiourium	T45.8X1	T45.8X2	T45.8X3	T45.8X4	T45.8X5	T45.8X6
Aminofenazone	T39.2X1	T39.2X2	T39.2X3	T39.2X4	T39.2X5	T39.2X6
Aminoglutethimide	T45.1X1	T45.1X2	T45.1X3	T45.1X4	T45.1X5	T45.1X6
Aminoglycosides*	T36.5X1	T36.5X2	T36.5X3	T36.5X4	T36.5X5	T36.5X6
Aminohippuric acid	T5Ø.8X1	T5Ø.8X2	T5Ø.8X3	T5Ø.8X4	T5Ø.8X5	T5Ø.8X6
Aminomethylbenzoic acid	T45.691	T45.692	T45.693	T45.694	T45.695	T45.696
Aminometradine	T5Ø.2X1	T5Ø.2X2	T5Ø.2X3	T5Ø.2X4	T5Ø.2X5	T5Ø.2X6
Aminopentamide	T44.3X1	T44.3X2	T44.3X3	T44.3X4	T44.3X5	T44.3X6
Aminophenazone	T39.2X1	T39.2X2	T39.2X3	T39.2X4	T39.2X5	T39.2X6
Aminophenol	T54.ØX1	T54.ØX2	T54.ØX3	T54.ØX4	—	—
Aminophenylpyridone	T43.591	T43.592	T43.593	T43.594	T43.595	T43.596
Aminophylline	T48.6X1	T48.6X2	T48.6X3	T48.6X4	T48.6X5	T48.6X6
Aminopterin sodium	T45.1X1	T45.1X2	T45.1X3	T45.1X4	T45.1X5	T45.1X6
Aminopyrine	T39.2X1	T39.2X2	T39.2X3	T39.2X4	T39.2X5	T39.2X6
Aminorex	T5Ø.5X1	T5Ø.5X2	T5Ø.5X3	T5Ø.5X4	T5Ø.5X5	T5Ø.5X6
Aminosalicylic acid	T37.1X1	T37.1X2	T37.1X3	T37.1X4	T37.1X5	T37.1X6
Aminosalylum	T37.1X1	T37.1X2	T37.1X3	T37.1X4	T37.1X5	T37.1X6
Amiodarone	T46.2X1	T46.2X2	T46.2X3	T46.2X4	T46.2X5	T46.2X6
Amiphenazole	T5Ø.7X1	T5Ø.7X2	T5Ø.7X3	T5Ø.7X4	T5Ø.7X5	T5Ø.7X6
Amiquinsin	T46.5X1	T46.5X2	T46.5X3	T46.5X4	T46.5X5	T46.5X6
Amisometradine	T5Ø.2X1	T5Ø.2X2	T5Ø.2X3	T5Ø.2X4	T5Ø.2X5	T5Ø.2X6
Amisulpride	T43.591	T43.592	T43.593	T43.594	T43.595	T43.596
Amitriptyline	T43.Ø11	T43.Ø12	T43.Ø13	T43.Ø14	T43.Ø15	T43.Ø16
Amitriptylinoxide	T43.Ø11	T43.Ø12	T43.Ø13	T43.Ø14	T43.Ø15	T43.Ø16
Amlexanox	T48.6X1	T48.6X2	T48.6X3	T48.6X4	T48.6X5	T48.6X6

Substance	Poisoning, Accidental (unintentional)	Poisoning, Intentional Self-harm	Poisoning, Assault	Poisoning, Undetermined	Adverse Effect	Under-dosing
Ammonia (fumes) (gas) (vapor)	T59.891	T59.892	T59.893	T59.894	—	—
aromatic spirit	T48.991	T48.992	T48.993	T48.994	T48.995	T48.996
liquid (household)	T54.3X1	T54.3X2	T54.3X3	T54.3X4	—	—
Ammoniated mercury	T49.ØX1	T49.ØX2	T49.ØX3	T49.ØX4	T49.ØX5	T49.ØX6
Ammonium						
acid tartrate	T49.5X1	T49.5X2	T49.5X3	T49.5X4	T49.5X5	T49.5X6
bromide	T42.6X1	T42.6X2	T42.6X3	T42.6X4	T42.6X5	T42.6X6
carbonate	T54.3X1	T54.3X2	T54.3X3	T54.3X4	—	—
chloride	T5Ø.991	T5Ø.992	T5Ø.993	T5Ø.994	T5Ø.995	T5Ø.996
expectorant	T48.4X1	T48.4X2	T48.4X3	T48.4X4	T48.4X5	T48.4X6
compounds (household) NEC	T54.3X1	T54.3X2	T54.3X3	T54.3X4	—	—
fumes (any usage)	T59.891	T59.892	T59.893	T59.894	—	—
industrial	T54.3X1	T54.3X2	T54.3X3	T54.3X4	—	—
ichthyosulronate	T49.4X1	T49.4X2	T49.4X3	T49.4X4	T49.4X5	T49.4X6
mandelate	T37.91	T37.92	T37.93	T37.94	T37.95	T37.96
sulfamate	T6Ø.3X1	T6Ø.3X2	T6Ø.3X3	T6Ø.3X4	—	—
sulfonate resin	T47.8X1	T47.8X2	T47.8X3	T47.8X4	T47.8X5	T47.8X6
Amobarbital (sodium)	T42.3X1	T42.3X2	T42.3X3	T42.3X4	T42.3X5	T42.3X6
Amodiaquine	T37.2X1	T37.2X2	T37.2X3	T37.2X4	T37.2X5	T37.2X6
Amopyroquin (e)	T37.2X1	T37.2X2	T37.2X3	T37.2X4	T37.2X5	T37.2X6
Amoxapine	T43.Ø11	T43.Ø12	T43.Ø13	T43.Ø14	T43.Ø15	T43.Ø16
Amoxicillin	T36.ØX1	T36.ØX2	T36.ØX3	T36.ØX4	T36.ØX5	T36.ØX6
Amperozide	T43.591	T43.592	T43.593	T43.594	T43.595	T43.596
Amphenidone	T43.591	T43.592	T43.593	T43.594	T43.595	T43.596
Amphetamine NEC	T43.621	T43.622	T43.623	T43.624	T43.625	T43.626
Amphogel*	T47.1X1	T47.1X2	T47.1X3	T47.1X4	T47.1X5	T47.1X6
Amphomycin	T36.8X1	T36.8X2	T36.8X3	T36.8X4	T36.8X5	T36.8X6
Amphotalide	T37.4X1	T37.4X2	T37.4X3	T37.4X4	T37.4X5	T37.4X6
Amphotericin B	T36.7X1	T36.7X2	T36.7X3	T36.7X4	T36.7X5	T36.7X6
topical	T49.ØX1	T49.ØX2	T49.ØX3	T49.ØX4	T49.ØX5	T49.ØX6
Ampicillin	T36.ØX1	T36.ØX2	T36.ØX3	T36.ØX4	T36.ØX5	T36.ØX6
Amprotropine	T44.3X1	T44.3X2	T44.3X3	T44.3X4	T44.3X5	T44.3X6
Amsacrine	T45.1X1	T45.1X2	T45.1X3	T45.1X4	T45.1X5	T45.1X6
Amygdaline	T62.2X1	T62.2X2	T62.2X3	T62.2X4	—	—
Amyl						
acetate	T52.8X1	T52.8X2	T52.8X3	T52.8X4	—	—
vapor	T59.891	T59.892	T59.893	T59.894	—	—
alcohol	T51.3X1	T51.3X2	T51.3X3	T51.3X4	—	—
chloride	T53.6X1	T53.6X2	T53.6X3	T53.6X4	—	—
formate	T52.8X1	T52.8X2	T52.8X3	T52.8X4	—	—
nitrite	T46.3X1	T46.3X2	T46.3X3	T46.3X4	T46.3X5	T46.3X6
propionate	T65.891	T65.892	T65.893	T65.894	—	—
Amylase	T47.5X1	T47.5X2	T47.5X3	T47.5X4	T47.5X5	T47.5X6
Amyleine, regional	T41.3X1	T41.3X2	T41.3X3	T41.3X4	T41.3X5	T41.3X6
Amylene						
dichloride	T53.6X1	T53.6X2	T53.6X3	T53.6X4	—	—
hydrate	T51.3X1	T51.3X2	T51.3X3	T51.3X4	—	—
Amylmetacresol	T49.6X1	T49.6X2	T49.6X3	T49.6X4	T49.6X5	T49.6X6
Amylobarbitone	T42.3X1	T42.3X2	T42.3X3	T42.3X4	T42.3X5	T42.3X6
Amylocaine, regional	T41.3X1	T41.3X2	T41.3X3	T41.3X4	T41.3X5	T41.3X6
infiltration (subcutaneous)	T41.3X1	T41.3X2	T41.3X3	T41.3X4	T41.3X5	T41.3X6
nerve block (peripheral) (plexus)	T41.3X1	T41.3X2	T41.3X3	T41.3X4	T41.3X5	T41.3X6
spinal	T41.3X1	T41.3X2	T41.3X3	T41.3X4	T41.3X5	T41.3X6
topical (surface)	T41.3X1	T41.3X2	T41.3X3	T41.3X4	T41.3X5	T41.3X6
Amylopectin	T47.6X1	T47.6X2	T47.6X3	T47.6X4	T47.6X5	T47.6X6
Amytal (sodium)	T42.3X1	T42.3X2	T42.3X3	T42.3X4	T42.3X5	T42.3X6
Anabolic steroid	T38.7X1	T38.7X2	T38.7X3	T38.7X4	T38.7X5	T38.7X6
Anacaine*	T41.3X1	T41.3X2	T41.3X3	T41.3X4	T41.3X5	T41.3X6
Analeptic NEC	T5Ø.7X1	T5Ø.7X2	T5Ø.7X3	T5Ø.7X4	T5Ø.7X5	T5Ø.7X6
Analgesic	T39.91	T39.92	T39.93	T39.94	T39.95	T39.96
anti-inflammatory NEC	T39.91	T39.92	T39.93	T39.94	T39.95	T39.96
propionic acid derivative	T39.311	T39.312	T39.313	T39.314	T39.315	T39.316
antirheumatic NEC	T39.4X1	T39.4X2	T39.4X3	T39.4X4	T39.4X5	T39.4X6
aromatic NEC	T39.1X1	T39.1X2	T39.1X3	T39.1X4	T39.1X5	T39.1X6
narcotic NEC	T4Ø.6Ø1	T4Ø.6Ø2	T4Ø.6Ø3	T4Ø.6Ø4	T4Ø.6Ø5	T4Ø.6Ø6
combination	T4Ø.6Ø1	T4Ø.6Ø2	T4Ø.6Ø3	T4Ø.6Ø4	T4Ø.6Ø5	T4Ø.6Ø6
obstetric	T4Ø.6Ø1	T4Ø.6Ø2	T4Ø.6Ø3	T4Ø.6Ø4	T4Ø.6Ø5	T4Ø.6Ø6
non-narcotic NEC	T39.91	T39.92	T39.93	T39.94	T39.95	T39.96
combination	T39.91	T39.92	T39.93	T39.94	T39.95	T39.96
pyrazole	T39.2X1	T39.2X2	T39.2X3	T39.2X4	T39.2X5	T39.2X6
specified NEC	T39.8X1	T39.8X2	T39.8X3	T39.8X4	T39.8X5	T39.8X6
Analgin	T39.2X1	T39.2X2	T39.2X3	T39.2X4	T39.2X5	T39.2X6
Anamirta cocculus	T62.1X1	T62.1X2	T62.1X3	T62.1X4	—	—
Ancillin	T36.ØX1	T36.ØX2	T36.ØX3	T36.ØX4	T36.ØX5	T36.ØX6
Ancrod	T45.691	T45.692	T45.693	T45.694	T45.695	T45.696
Androgen	T38.7X1	T38.7X2	T38.7X3	T38.7X4	T38.7X5	T38.7X6
Androgen-estrogen mixture	T38.7X1	T38.7X2	T38.7X3	T38.7X4	T38.7X5	T38.7X6
Androstalone	T38.7X1	T38.7X2	T38.7X3	T38.7X4	T38.7X5	T38.7X6
Androstanolone	T38.7X1	T38.7X2	T38.7X3	T38.7X4	T38.7X5	T38.7X6

Substance	Poisoning, Accidental (unintentional)	Poisoning, Intentional Self-harm	Poisoning, Assault	Poisoning, Undetermined	Adverse Effect	Under-dosing
Androsterone	T38.7X1	T38.7X2	T38.7X3	T38.7X4	T38.7X5	T38.7X6
Anemone pulsatilla	T62.2X1	T62.2X2	T62.2X3	T62.2X4	—	—
Anesthesia						
caudal	T41.3X1	T41.3X2	T41.3X3	T41.3X4	T41.3X5	T41.3X6
endotracheal	T41.ØX1	T41.ØX2	T41.ØX3	T41.ØX4	T41.ØX5	T41.ØX6
epidural	T41.3X1	T41.3X2	T41.3X3	T41.3X4	T41.3X5	T41.3X6
inhalation	T41.ØX1	T41.ØX2	T41.ØX3	T41.ØX4	T41.ØX5	T41.ØX6
local	T41.3X1	T41.3X2	T41.3X3	T41.3X4	T41.3X5	T41.3X6
mucosal	T41.3X1	T41.3X2	T41.3X3	T41.3X4	T41.3X5	T41.3X6
muscle relaxation	T48.1X1	T48.1X2	T48.1X3	T48.1X4	T48.1X5	T48.1X6
nerve blocking	T41.3X1	T41.3X2	T41.3X3	T41.3X4	T41.3X5	T41.3X6
plexus blocking	T41.3X1	T41.3X2	T41.3X3	T41.3X4	T41.3X5	T41.3X6
potentiated	T41.2Ø1	T41.2Ø2	T41.2Ø3	T41.2Ø4	T41.2Ø5	T41.2Ø6
rectal	T41.2Ø1	T41.2Ø2	T41.2Ø3	T41.2Ø4	T41.2Ø5	T41.2Ø6
general	T41.2Ø1	T41.2Ø2	T41.2Ø3	T41.2Ø4	T41.2Ø5	T41.2Ø6
local	T41.3X1	T41.3X2	T41.3X3	T41.3X4	T41.3X5	T41.3X6
regional	T41.3X1	T41.3X2	T41.3X3	T41.3X4	T41.3X5	T41.3X6
surface	T41.3X1	T41.3X2	T41.3X3	T41.3X4	T41.3X5	T41.3X6
Anesthetic NEC — *see also* Anesthesia	T41.41	T41.42	T41.43	T41.44	T41.45	T41.46
with muscle relaxant	T41.2Ø1	T41.2Ø2	T41.2Ø3	T41.2Ø4	T41.2Ø5	T41.2Ø6
general	T41.2Ø1	T41.2Ø2	T41.2Ø3	T41.2Ø4	T41.2Ø5	T41.2Ø6
local	T41.3X1	T41.3X2	T41.3X3	T41.3X4	T41.3X5	T41.3X6
gaseous NEC	T41.ØX1	T41.ØX2	T41.ØX3	T41.ØX4	T41.ØX5	T41.ØX6
general NEC	T41.2Ø1	T41.2Ø2	T41.2Ø3	T41.2Ø4	T41.2Ø5	T41.2Ø6
halogenated hydrocarbon derivatives NEC	T41.ØX1	T41.ØX2	T41.ØX3	T41.ØX4	T41.ØX5	T41.ØX6
infiltration NEC	T41.3X1	T41.3X2	T41.3X3	T41.3X4	T41.3X5	T41.3X6
intravenous NEC	T41.1X1	T41.1X2	T41.1X3	T41.1X4	T41.1X5	T41.1X6
local NEC	T41.3X1	T41.3X2	T41.3X3	T41.3X4	T41.3X5	T41.3X6
rectal	T41.2Ø1	T41.2Ø2	T41.2Ø3	T41.2Ø4	T41.2Ø5	T41.2Ø6
general	T41.2Ø1	T41.2Ø2	T41.2Ø3	T41.2Ø4	T41.2Ø5	T41.2Ø6
local	T41.3X1	T41.3X2	T41.3X3	T41.3X4	T41.3X5	T41.3X6
regional NEC	T41.3X1	T41.3X2	T41.3X3	T41.3X4	T41.3X5	T41.3X6
spinal NEC	T41.3X1	T41.3X2	T41.3X3	T41.3X4	T41.3X5	T41.3X6
thiobarbiturate	T41.1X1	T41.1X2	T41.1X3	T41.1X4	T41.1X5	T41.1X6
topical	T41.3X1	T41.3X2	T41.3X3	T41.3X4	T41.3X5	T41.3X6
Aneurine	T45.2X1	T45.2X2	T45.2X3	T45.2X4	T45.2X5	T45.2X6
Angeliq*	T38.5X1	T38.5X2	T38.5X3	T38.5X4	T38.5X5	T38.5X6
Angio-Conray	T5Ø.8X1	T5Ø.8X2	T5Ø.8X3	T5Ø.8X4	T5Ø.8X5	T5Ø.8X6
Angiotensin	T44.5X1	T44.5X2	T44.5X3	T44.5X4	T44.5X5	T44.5X6
Angiotensinamide	T44.991	T44.992	T44.993	T44.994	T44.995	T44.996
Anhydrohydroxy-progesterone	T38.5X1	T38.5X2	T38.5X3	T38.5X4	T38.5X5	T38.5X6
Anhydron	T5Ø.2X1	T5Ø.2X2	T5Ø.2X3	T5Ø.2X4	T5Ø.2X5	T5Ø.2X6
Anileridine	T4Ø.491	T4Ø.492	T4Ø.493	T4Ø.494	T4Ø.495	T4Ø.496
Aniline (dye) (liquid)	T65.3X1	T65.3X2	T65.3X3	T65.3X4	—	—
analgesic	T39.1X1	T39.1X2	T39.1X3	T39.1X4	T39.1X5	T39.1X6
derivatives, therapeutic NEC	T39.1X1	T39.1X2	T39.1X3	T39.1X4	T39.1X5	T39.1X6
vapor	T65.3X1	T65.3X2	T65.3X3	T65.3X4	—	—
Aniscoropine	T44.3X1	T44.3X2	T44.3X3	T44.3X4	T44.3X5	T44.3X6
Anise oil	T47.5X1	T47.5X2	T47.5X3	T47.5X4	T47.5X5	T47.5X6
Anisidine	T65.3X1	T65.3X2	T65.3X3	T65.3X4	—	—
Anisindione	T45.511	T45.512	T45.513	T45.514	T45.515	T45.516
Anisotropine methyl-bromide	T44.3X1	T44.3X2	T44.3X3	T44.3X4	T44.3X5	T44.3X6
Anistreplase	T45.611	T45.612	T45.613	T45.614	T45.615	T45.616
Anorexiant (central)	T5Ø.5X1	T5Ø.5X2	T5Ø.5X3	T5Ø.5X4	T5Ø.5X5	T5Ø.5X6
Anorexic agents	T5Ø.5X1	T5Ø.5X2	T5Ø.5X3	T5Ø.5X4	T5Ø.5X5	T5Ø.5X6
Ansaid*	T39.311	T39.312	T39.313	T39.314	T39.315	T39.316
Ansamycin	T36.6X1	T36.6X2	T36.6X3	T36.6X4	T36.6X5	T36.6X6
Ant (bite) (sting)	T63.421	T63.422	T63.423	T63.424	—	—
Antabuse	T5Ø.6X1	T5Ø.6X2	T5Ø.6X3	T5Ø.6X4	T5Ø.6X5	T5Ø.6X6
Antacid NEC	T47.1X1	T47.1X2	T47.1X3	T47.1X4	T47.1X5	T47.1X6
Antagonist						
Aldosterone	T5Ø.ØX1	T5Ø.ØX2	T5Ø.ØX3	T5Ø.ØX4	T5Ø.ØX5	T5Ø.ØX6
alpha-adrenoreceptor	T44.6X1	T44.6X2	T44.6X3	T44.6X4	T44.6X5	T44.6X6
anticoagulant	T45.7X1	T45.7X2	T45.7X3	T45.7X4	T45.7X5	T45.7X6
beta-adrenoreceptor	T44.7X1	T44.7X2	T44.7X3	T44.7X4	T44.7X5	T44.7X6
extrapyramidal NEC	T44.3X1	T44.3X2	T44.3X3	T44.3X4	T44.3X5	T44.3X6
folic acid	T45.1X1	T45.1X2	T45.1X3	T45.1X4	T45.1X5	T45.1X6
H2 receptor	T47.ØX1	T47.ØX2	T47.ØX3	T47.ØX4	T47.ØX5	T47.ØX6
heavy metal	T45.8X1	T45.8X2	T45.8X3	T45.8X4	T45.8X5	T45.8X6
narcotic analgesic	T5Ø.7X1	T5Ø.7X2	T5Ø.7X3	T5Ø.7X4	T5Ø.7X5	T5Ø.7X6
opiate	T5Ø.7X1	T5Ø.7X2	T5Ø.7X3	T5Ø.7X4	T5Ø.7X5	T5Ø.7X6
pyrimidine	T45.1X1	T45.1X2	T45.1X3	T45.1X4	T45.1X5	T45.1X6
serotonin	T46.5X1	T46.5X2	T46.5X3	T46.5X4	T46.5X5	T46.5X6
Antazolin (e)	T45.ØX1	T45.ØX2	T45.ØX3	T45.ØX4	T45.ØX5	T45.ØX6
Anterior pituitary hormone NEC	T38.811	T38.812	T38.813	T38.814	T38.815	T38.816
Anthelmintic NEC	T37.4X1	T37.4X2	T37.4X3	T37.4X4	T37.4X5	T37.4X6
Anthiolimine	T37.4X1	T37.4X2	T37.4X3	T37.4X4	T37.4X5	T37.4X6
Anthralin	T49.4X1	T49.4X2	T49.4X3	T49.4X4	T49.4X5	T49.4X6

Substance	Poisoning, Accidental (unintentional)	Poisoning, Intentional Self-harm	Poisoning, Assault	Poisoning, Undetermined	Adverse Effect	Under-dosing
Anthramycin	T45.1X1	T45.1X2	T45.1X3	T45.1X4	T45.1X5	T45.1X6
Antiadrenergic NEC	T44.8X1	T44.8X2	T44.8X3	T44.8X4	T44.8X5	T44.8X6
Antiallergic NEC	T45.ØX1	T45.ØX2	T45.ØX3	T45.ØX4	T45.ØX5	T45.ØX6
Antiandrogen NEC	T38.6X1	T38.6X2	T38.6X3	T38.6X4	T38.6X5	T38.6X6
Anti-anemic (drug) (preparation)	T45.8X1	T45.8X2	T45.8X3	T45.8X4	T45.8X5	T45.8X6
Antianxiety drug NEC	T43.5Ø1	T43.5Ø2	T43.5Ø3	T43.5Ø4	T43.5Ø5	T43.5Ø6
Antiaris toxicaria	T65.891	T65.892	T65.893	T65.894	—	—
Antiarteriosclerotic drug	T46.6X1	T46.6X2	T46.6X3	T46.6X4	T46.6X5	T46.6X6
Antiasthmatic drug NEC	T48.6X1	T48.6X2	T48.6X3	T48.6X4	T48.6X5	T48.6X6
Antibiotic Otic Suspension (Solution)*	T49.6X1	T49.6X2	T49.6X3	T49.6X4	T49.6X5	T49.6X6
Antibiotic NEC	T36.91	T36.92	T36.93	T36.94	T36.95	T36.96
aminoglycoside	T36.5X1	T36.5X2	T36.5X3	T36.5X4	T36.5X5	T36.5X6
anticancer	T45.1X1	T45.1X2	T45.1X3	T45.1X4	T45.1X5	T45.1X6
antifungal	T36.7X1	T36.7X2	T36.7X3	T36.7X4	T36.7X5	T36.7X6
antimycobacterial	T36.5X1	T36.5X2	T36.5X3	T36.5X4	T36.5X5	T36.5X6
antineoplastic	T45.1X1	T45.1X2	T45.1X3	T45.1X4	T45.1X5	T45.1X6
b-lactam NEC	T36.1X1	T36.1X2	T36.1X3	T36.1X4	T36.1X5	T36.1X6
cephalosporin (group)	T36.1X1	T36.1X2	T36.1X3	T36.1X4	T36.1X5	T36.1X6
chloramphenicol (group)	T36.2X1	T36.2X2	T36.2X3	T36.2X4	T36.2X5	T36.2X6
ENT	T49.6X1	T49.6X2	T49.6X3	T49.6X4	T49.6X5	T49.6X6
eye	T49.5X1	T49.5X2	T49.5X3	T49.5X4	T49.5X5	T49.5X6
fungicidal (local)	T49.ØX1	T49.ØX2	T49.ØX3	T49.ØX4	T49.ØX5	T49.ØX6
intestinal	T36.8X1	T36.8X2	T36.8X3	T36.8X4	T36.8X5	T36.8X6
local	T49.ØX1	T49.ØX2	T49.ØX3	T49.ØX4	T49.ØX5	T49.ØX6
macrolides	T36.3X1	T36.3X2	T36.3X3	T36.3X4	T36.3X5	T36.3X6
polypeptide	T36.8X1	T36.8X2	T36.8X3	T36.8X4	T36.8X5	T36.8X6
specified NEC	T36.8X1	T36.8X2	T36.8X3	T36.8X4	T36.8X5	T36.8X6
tetracycline (group)	T36.4X1	T36.4X2	T36.4X3	T36.4X4	T36.4X5	T36.4X6
throat	T49.6X1	T49.6X2	T49.6X3	T49.6X4	T49.6X5	T49.6X6
Anticancer agents NEC	T45.1X1	T45.1X2	T45.1X3	T45.1X4	T45.1X5	T45.1X6
Anticholesterolemic drug NEC	T46.6X1	T46.6X2	T46.6X3	T46.6X4	T46.6X5	T46.6X6
Anticholinergic NEC	T44.3X1	T44.3X2	T44.3X3	T44.3X4	T44.3X5	T44.3X6
Anticholinesterase	T44.ØX1	T44.ØX2	T44.ØX3	T44.ØX4	T44.ØX5	T44.ØX6
organophosphorus	T44.ØX1	T44.ØX2	T44.ØX3	T44.ØX4	T44.ØX5	T44.ØX6
insecticide	T6Ø.ØX1	T6Ø.ØX2	T6Ø.ØX3	T6Ø.ØX4	—	—
nerve gas	T59.891	T59.892	T59.893	T59.894	—	—
reversible	T44.ØX1	T44.ØX2	T44.ØX3	T44.ØX4	T44.ØX5	T44.ØX6
ophthalmological	T49.5X1	T49.5X2	T49.5X3	T49.5X4	T49.5X5	T49.5X6
Anticoagulant NEC	T45.511	T45.512	T45.513	T45.514	T45.515	T45.516
Antagonist	T45.7X1	T45.7X2	T45.7X3	T45.7X4	T45.7X5	T45.7X6
Anti-common-cold drug NEC	T48.5X1	T48.5X2	T48.5X3	T48.5X4	T48.5X5	T48.5X6
Anticonvulsant	T42.71	T42.72	T42.73	T42.74	T42.75	T42.76
barbiturate	T42.3X1	T42.3X2	T42.3X3	T42.3X4	T42.3X5	T42.3X6
combination (with barbiturate)	T42.3X1	T42.3X2	T42.3X3	T42.3X4	T42.3X5	T42.3X6
hydantoin	T42.ØX1	T42.ØX2	T42.ØX3	T42.ØX4	T42.ØX5	T42.ØX6
hypnotic NEC	T42.6X1	T42.6X2	T42.6X3	T42.6X4	T42.6X5	T42.6X6
oxazolidinedione	T42.2X1	T42.2X2	T42.2X3	T42.2X4	T42.2X5	T42.2X6
pyrimidinedione	T42.6X1	T42.6X2	T42.6X3	T42.6X4	T42.6X5	T42.6X6
specified NEC	T42.6X1	T42.6X2	T42.6X3	T42.6X4	T42.6X5	T42.6X6
succinimide	T42.2X1	T42.2X2	T42.2X3	T42.2X4	T42.2X5	T42.2X6
Antidepressant	T43.2Ø1	T43.2Ø2	T43.2Ø3	T43.2Ø4	T43.2Ø5	T43.2Ø6
monoamine oxidase inhibitor	T43.1X1	T43.1X2	T43.1X3	T43.1X4	T43.1X5	T43.1X6
selective serotonin norepinephrine reuptake inhibitor	T43.211	T43.212	T43.213	T43.214	T43.215	T43.216
selective serotonin reuptake inhibitor	T43.221	T43.222	T43.223	T43.224	T43.225	T43.226
specified NEC	T43.291	T43.292	T43.293	T43.294	T43.295	T43.296
tetracyclic	T43.Ø21	T43.Ø22	T43.Ø23	T43.Ø24	T43.Ø25	T43.Ø26
triazolopyridine	T43.211	T43.212	T43.213	T43.214	T43.215	T43.216
tricyclic	T43.Ø11	T43.Ø12	T43.Ø13	T43.Ø14	T43.Ø15	T43.Ø16
Antidiabetic NEC	T38.3X1	T38.3X2	T38.3X3	T38.3X4	T38.3X5	T38.3X6
biguanide	T38.3X1	T38.3X2	T38.3X3	T38.3X4	T38.3X5	T38.3X6
and sulfonyl combined	T38.3X1	T38.3X2	T38.3X3	T38.3X4	T38.3X5	T38.3X6
combined	T38.3X1	T38.3X2	T38.3X3	T38.3X4	T38.3X5	T38.3X6
sulfonylurea	T38.3X1	T38.3X2	T38.3X3	T38.3X4	T38.3X5	T38.3X6
Antidiarrheal drug NEC	T47.6X1	T47.6X2	T47.6X3	T47.6X4	T47.6X5	T47.6X6
absorbent	T47.6X1	T47.6X2	T47.6X3	T47.6X4	T47.6X5	T47.6X6
Anti-D immunoglobulin (human)	T5Ø.Z11	T5Ø.Z12	T5Ø.Z13	T5Ø.Z14	T5Ø.Z15	T5Ø.Z16
Antidiphtheria serum	T5Ø.Z11	T5Ø.Z12	T5Ø.Z13	T5Ø.Z14	T5Ø.Z15	T5Ø.Z16
Antidiuretic hormone	T38.891	T38.892	T38.893	T38.894	T38.895	T38.896
Antidote NEC	T5Ø.6X1	T5Ø.6X2	T5Ø.6X3	T5Ø.6X4	T5Ø.6X5	T5Ø.6X6
heavy metal	T45.8X1	T45.8X2	T45.8X3	T45.8X4	T45.8X5	T45.8X6
Antidysrhythmic NEC	T46.2X1	T46.2X2	T46.2X3	T46.2X4	T46.2X5	T46.2X6
Antiemetic drug	T45.ØX1	T45.ØX2	T45.ØX3	T45.ØX4	T45.ØX5	T45.ØX6
Antiepilepsy agent	T42.71	T42.72	T42.73	T42.74	T42.75	T42.76

Substance	Poisoning, Accidental (unintentional)	Poisoning, Intentional Self-harm	Poisoning, Assault	Poisoning, Undetermined	Adverse Effect	Under-dosing
Antiepilepsy agent — *continued*						
combination	T42.5X1	T42.5X2	T42.5X3	T42.5X4	T42.5X5	T42.5X6
mixed	T42.5X1	T42.5X2	T42.5X3	T42.5X4	T42.5X5	T42.5X6
specified, NEC	T42.6X1	T42.6X2	T42.6X3	T42.6X4	T42.6X5	T42.6X6
Antiestrogen NEC	T38.6X1	T38.6X2	T38.6X3	T38.6X4	T38.6X5	T38.6X6
Antifertility pill	T38.4X1	T38.4X2	T38.4X3	T38.4X4	T38.4X5	T38.4X6
Antifibrinolytic drug	T45.621	T45.622	T45.623	T45.624	T45.625	T45.626
Antifilarial drug	T37.4X1	T37.4X2	T37.4X3	T37.4X4	T37.4X5	T37.4X6
Antiflatulent	T47.5X1	T47.5X2	T47.5X3	T47.5X4	T47.5X5	T47.5X6
Antifreeze	T65.91	T65.92	T65.93	T65.94	—	—
alcohol	T51.1X1	T51.1X2	T51.1X3	T51.1X4	—	—
ethylene glycol	T51.8X1	T51.8X2	T51.8X3	T51.8X4	—	—
Antifungal						
antibiotic (systemic)	T36.7X1	T36.7X2	T36.7X3	T36.7X4	T36.7X5	T36.7X6
anti-infective NEC	T37.91	T37.92	T37.93	T37.94	T37.95	T37.96
disinfectant, local	T49.ØX1	T49.ØX2	T49.ØX3	T49.ØX4	T49.ØX5	T49.ØX6
nonmedicinal (spray)	T6Ø.3X1	T6Ø.3X2	T6Ø.3X3	T6Ø.3X4	—	—
topical	T49.ØX1	T49.ØX2	T49.ØX3	T49.ØX4	T49.ØX5	T49.ØX6
Anti-gastric-secretion drug NEC	T47.1X1	T47.1X2	T47.1X3	T47.1X4	T47.1X5	T47.1X6
Antigonadotrophin NEC	T38.6X1	T38.6X2	T38.6X3	T38.6X4	T38.6X5	T38.6X6
Antihallucinogen	T43.5Ø1	T43.5Ø2	T43.5Ø3	T43.5Ø4	T43.5Ø5	T43.5Ø6
Antihelmintics	T37.4X1	T37.4X2	T37.4X3	T37.4X4	T37.4X5	T37.4X6
Antihemophilic						
factor	T45.8X1	T45.8X2	T45.8X3	T45.8X4	T45.8X5	T45.8X6
fraction	T45.8X1	T45.8X2	T45.8X3	T45.8X4	T45.8X5	T45.8X6
globulin concentrate	T45.7X1	T45.7X2	T45.7X3	T45.7X4	T45.7X5	T45.7X6
human plasma	T45.8X1	T45.8X2	T45.8X3	T45.8X4	T45.8X5	T45.8X6
plasma, dried	T45.7X1	T45.7X2	T45.7X3	T45.7X4	T45.7X5	T45.7X6
Antihemorrhoidal preparation	T49.2X1	T49.2X2	T49.2X3	T49.2X4	T49.2X5	T49.2X6
Antiheparin drug	T45.7X1	T45.7X2	T45.7X3	T45.7X4	T45.7X5	T45.7X6
Antihistamine	T45.ØX1	T45.ØX2	T45.ØX3	T45.ØX4	T45.ØX5	T45.ØX6
Antihookworm drug	T37.4X1	T37.4X2	T37.4X3	T37.4X4	T37.4X5	T37.4X6
Anti-human lymphocytic globulin	T5Ø.Z11	T5Ø.Z12	T5Ø.Z13	T5Ø.Z14	T5Ø.Z15	T5Ø.Z16
Antihyperlipidemic drug	T46.6X1	T46.6X2	T46.6X3	T46.6X4	T46.6X5	T46.6X6
Antihypertensive drug NEC	T46.5X1	T46.5X2	T46.5X3	T46.5X4	T46.5X5	T46.5X6
Anti-infective NEC	T37.91	T37.92	T37.93	T37.94	T37.95	T37.96
anthelmintic	T37.4X1	T37.4X2	T37.4X3	T37.4X4	T37.4X5	T37.4X6
antibiotics	T36.91	T36.92	T36.93	T36.94	T36.95	T36.96
specified NEC	T36.8X1	T36.8X2	T36.8X3	T36.8X4	T36.8X5	T36.8X6
antimalarial	T37.2X1	T37.2X2	T37.2X3	T37.2X4	T37.2X5	T37.2X6
antimycobacterial NEC	T37.1X1	T37.1X2	T37.1X3	T37.1X4	T37.1X5	T37.1X6
antibiotics	T36.5X1	T36.5X2	T36.5X3	T36.5X4	T36.5X5	T36.5X6
antiprotozoal NEC	T37.3X1	T37.3X2	T37.3X3	T37.3X4	T37.3X5	T37.3X6
blood	T37.2X1	T37.2X2	T37.2X3	T37.2X4	T37.2X5	T37.2X6
antiviral	T37.5X1	T37.5X2	T37.5X3	T37.5X4	T37.5X5	T37.5X6
arsenical	T37.8X1	T37.8X2	T37.8X3	T37.8X4	T37.8X5	T37.8X6
bismuth, local	T49.ØX1	T49.ØX2	T49.ØX3	T49.ØX4	T49.ØX5	T49.ØX6
ENT	T49.6X1	T49.6X2	T49.6X3	T49.6X4	T49.6X5	T49.6X6
eye NEC	T49.5X1	T49.5X2	T49.5X3	T49.5X4	T49.5X5	T49.5X6
heavy metals NEC	T37.8X1	T37.8X2	T37.8X3	T37.8X4	T37.8X5	T37.8X6
local NEC	T49.ØX1	T49.ØX2	T49.ØX3	T49.ØX4	T49.ØX5	T49.ØX6
specified NEC	T49.ØX1	T49.ØX2	T49.ØX3	T49.ØX4	T49.ØX5	T49.ØX6
mixed	T37.91	T37.92	T37.93	T37.94	T37.95	T37.96
ophthalmic preparation	T49.5X1	T49.5X2	T49.5X3	T49.5X4	T49.5X5	T49.5X6
topical NEC	T49.ØX1	T49.ØX2	T49.ØX3	T49.ØX4	T49.ØX5	T49.ØX6
Anti-inflammatory drug NEC	T39.391	T39.392	T39.393	T39.394	T39.395	T39.396
local	T49.ØX1	T49.ØX2	T49.ØX3	T49.ØX4	T49.ØX5	T49.ØX6
nonsteroidal NEC	T39.391	T39.392	T39.393	T39.394	T39.395	T39.396
propionic acid derivative	T39.311	T39.312	T39.313	T39.314	T39.315	T39.316
specified NEC	T39.391	T39.392	T39.393	T39.394	T39.395	T39.396
Antikaluretic	T5Ø.3X1	T5Ø.3X2	T5Ø.3X3	T5Ø.3X4	T5Ø.3X5	T5Ø.3X6
Antiknock (tetraethyl lead)	T56.ØX1	T56.ØX2	T56.ØX3	T56.ØX4	—	—
Antilipemic drug NEC	T46.6X1	T46.6X2	T46.6X3	T46.6X4	T46.6X5	T46.6X6
Antilysin*	T45.621	T45.622	T45.623	T45.624	T45.625	T45.626
Antimalarial	T37.2X1	T37.2X2	T37.2X3	T37.2X4	T37.2X5	T37.2X6
prophylactic NEC	T37.2X1	T37.2X2	T37.2X3	T37.2X4	T37.2X5	T37.2X6
pyrimidine derivative	T37.2X1	T37.2X2	T37.2X3	T37.2X4	T37.2X5	T37.2X6
Antimetabolite	T45.1X1	T45.1X2	T45.1X3	T45.1X4	T45.1X5	T45.1X6
Antimitotic agent	T45.1X1	T45.1X2	T45.1X3	T45.1X4	T45.1X5	T45.1X6
Antimony (compounds) (vapor) **NEC**	T56.891	T56.892	T56.893	T56.894	—	—
anti-infectives	T37.8X1	T37.8X2	T37.8X3	T37.8X4	T37.8X5	T37.8X6
dimercaptosuccinate	T37.3X1	T37.3X2	T37.3X3	T37.3X4	T37.3X5	T37.3X6
hydride	T56.891	T56.892	T56.893	T56.894	—	—
pesticide (vapor)	T6Ø.8X1	T6Ø.8X2	T6Ø.8X3	T6Ø.8X4	—	—
potassium (sodium) tartrate	T37.8X1	T37.8X2	T37.8X3	T37.8X4	T37.8X5	T37.8X6
Antimony (compounds) (vapor) **NEC** — *continued*						
sodium dimercaptosuccinate	T37.3X1	T37.3X2	T37.3X3	T37.3X4	T37.3X5	T37.3X6
tartrated	T37.8X1	T37.8X2	T37.8X3	T37.8X4	T37.8X5	T37.8X6
Antimuscarinic NEC	T44.3X1	T44.3X2	T44.3X3	T44.3X4	T44.3X5	T44.3X6
Antimycobacterial drug NEC	T37.1X1	T37.1X2	T37.1X3	T37.1X4	T37.1X5	T37.1X6
antibiotics	T36.5X1	T36.5X2	T36.5X3	T36.5X4	T36.5X5	T36.5X6
combination	T37.1X1	T37.1X2	T37.1X3	T37.1X4	T37.1X5	T37.1X6
Antinausea drug	T45.ØX1	T45.ØX2	T45.ØX3	T45.ØX4	T45.ØX5	T45.ØX6
Antinematode drug	T37.4X1	T37.4X2	T37.4X3	T37.4X4	T37.4X5	T37.4X6
Antineoplastic NEC	T45.1X1	T45.1X2	T45.1X3	T45.1X4	T45.1X5	T45.1X6
alkaloidal	T45.1X1	T45.1X2	T45.1X3	T45.1X4	T45.1X5	T45.1X6
antibiotics	T45.1X1	T45.1X2	T45.1X3	T45.1X4	T45.1X5	T45.1X6
combination	T45.1X1	T45.1X2	T45.1X3	T45.1X4	T45.1X5	T45.1X6
estrogen	T38.5X1	T38.5X2	T38.5X3	T38.5X4	T38.5X5	T38.5X6
steroid	T38.7X1	T38.7X2	T38.7X3	T38.7X4	T38.7X5	T38.7X6
Antiparasitic drug (systemic)	T37.91	T37.92	T37.93	T37.94	T37.95	T37.96
local	T49.ØX1	T49.ØX2	T49.ØX3	T49.ØX4	T49.ØX5	T49.ØX6
specified NEC	T37.8X1	T37.8X2	T37.8X3	T37.8X4	T37.8X5	T37.8X6
Antiparkinsonism drug NEC	T42.8X1	T42.8X2	T42.8X3	T42.8X4	T42.8X5	T42.8X6
Antiperspirant NEC	T49.2X1	T49.2X2	T49.2X3	T49.2X4	T49.2X5	T49.2X6
Antiphlogistic NEC	T39.4X1	T39.4X2	T39.4X3	T39.4X4	T39.4X5	T39.4X6
Antiplatyhelmintic drug	T37.4X1	T37.4X2	T37.4X3	T37.4X4	T37.4X5	T37.4X6
Antiprotozoal drug NEC	T37.3X1	T37.3X2	T37.3X3	T37.3X4	T37.3X5	T37.3X6
blood	T37.2X1	T37.2X2	T37.2X3	T37.2X4	T37.2X5	T37.2X6
local	T49.ØX1	T49.ØX2	T49.ØX3	T49.ØX4	T49.ØX5	T49.ØX6
Antipruritic drug NEC	T49.1X1	T49.1X2	T49.1X3	T49.1X4	T49.1X5	T49.1X6
Antipsychotic drug	T43.5Ø1	T43.5Ø2	T43.5Ø3	T43.5Ø4	T43.5Ø5	T43.5Ø6
specified NEC	T43.591	T43.592	T43.593	T43.594	T43.595	T43.596
Antipyretic	T39.91	T39.92	T39.93	T39.94	T39.95	T39.96
specified NEC	T39.8X1	T39.8X2	T39.8X3	T39.8X4	T39.8X5	T39.8X6
Antipyrine	T39.2X1	T39.2X2	T39.2X3	T39.2X4	T39.2X5	T39.2X6
Antirabies hyperimmune serum	T5Ø.Z11	T5Ø.Z12	T5Ø.Z13	T5Ø.Z14	T5Ø.Z15	T5Ø.Z16
Antirheumatic NEC	T39.4X1	T39.4X2	T39.4X3	T39.4X4	T39.4X5	T39.4X6
Antirigidity drug NEC	T42.8X1	T42.8X2	T42.8X3	T42.8X4	T42.8X5	T42.8X6
Antischistosomal drug	T37.4X1	T37.4X2	T37.4X3	T37.4X4	T37.4X5	T37.4X6
Antiscorpion sera	T5Ø.Z11	T5Ø.Z12	T5Ø.Z13	T5Ø.Z14	T5Ø.Z15	T5Ø.Z16
Antiseborrheics	T49.4X1	T49.4X2	T49.4X3	T49.4X4	T49.4X5	T49.4X6
Antiseptics (external) (medicinal)	T49.ØX1	T49.ØX2	T49.ØX3	T49.ØX4	T49.ØX5	T49.ØX6
Antistine	T45.ØX1	T45.ØX2	T45.ØX3	T45.ØX4	T45.ØX5	T45.ØX6
Antitapeworm drug	T37.4X1	T37.4X2	T37.4X3	T37.4X4	T37.4X5	T37.4X6
Antitetanus immunoglobulin	T5Ø.Z11	T5Ø.Z12	T5Ø.Z13	T5Ø.Z14	T5Ø.Z15	T5Ø.Z16
Antithrombin III*	T45.511	T45.512	T45.513	T45.514	T45.515	T45.516
Antithrombotic	T45.521	T45.522	T45.523	T45.524	T45.525	T45.526
Antithyroid drug NEC	T38.2X1	T38.2X2	T38.2X3	T38.2X4	T38.2X5	T38.2X6
Antitoxin	T5Ø.Z11	T5Ø.Z12	T5Ø.Z13	T5Ø.Z14	T5Ø.Z15	T5Ø.Z16
diphtheria	T5Ø.Z11	T5Ø.Z12	T5Ø.Z13	T5Ø.Z14	T5Ø.Z15	T5Ø.Z16
gas gangrene	T5Ø.Z11	T5Ø.Z12	T5Ø.Z13	T5Ø.Z14	T5Ø.Z15	T5Ø.Z16
tetanus	T5Ø.Z11	T5Ø.Z12	T5Ø.Z13	T5Ø.Z14	T5Ø.Z15	T5Ø.Z16
Antitrichomonal drug	T37.3X1	T37.3X2	T37.3X3	T37.3X4	T37.3X5	T37.3X6
Antituberculars	T37.1X1	T37.1X2	T37.1X3	T37.1X4	T37.1X5	T37.1X6
antibiotics	T36.5X1	T36.5X2	T36.5X3	T36.5X4	T36.5X5	T36.5X6
Antitussive NEC	T48.3X1	T48.3X2	T48.3X3	T48.3X4	T48.3X5	T48.3X6
codeine mixture	T4Ø.2X1	T4Ø.2X2	T4Ø.2X3	T4Ø.2X4	T4Ø.2X5	T4Ø.2X6
opiate	T4Ø.2X1	T4Ø.2X2	T4Ø.2X3	T4Ø.2X4	T4Ø.2X5	T4Ø.2X6
Antivaricose drug	T46.8X1	T46.8X2	T46.8X3	T46.8X4	T46.8X5	T46.8X6
Antivenin, antivenom (sera)	T5Ø.Z11	T5Ø.Z12	T5Ø.Z13	T5Ø.Z14	T5Ø.Z15	T5Ø.Z16
crotaline	T5Ø.Z11	T5Ø.Z12	T5Ø.Z13	T5Ø.Z14	T5Ø.Z15	T5Ø.Z16
spider bite	T5Ø.Z11	T5Ø.Z12	T5Ø.Z13	T5Ø.Z14	T5Ø.Z15	T5Ø.Z16
Antivert*	T45.ØX1	T45.ØX2	T45.ØX3	T45.ØX4	T45.ØX5	T45.ØX6
Antivertigo drug	T45.ØX1	T45.ØX2	T45.ØX3	T45.ØX4	T45.ØX5	T45.ØX6
Antiviral drug NEC	T37.5X1	T37.5X2	T37.5X3	T37.5X4	T37.5X5	T37.5X6
eye	T49.5X1	T49.5X2	T49.5X3	T49.5X4	T49.5X5	T49.5X6
Antiwhipworm drug	T37.4X1	T37.4X2	T37.4X3	T37.4X4	T37.4X5	T37.4X6
Ant poison — *see* Insecticide						
Antrol — *see also* by specific chemical substance	T6Ø.91	T6Ø.92	T6Ø.93	T6Ø.94	—	—
fungicide	T6Ø.91	T6Ø.92	T6Ø.93	T6Ø.94	—	—
ANTU (alpha naphthylthiourea)	T6Ø.4X1	T6Ø.4X2	T6Ø.4X3	T6Ø.4X4	—	—
Apalcillin	T36.ØX1	T36.ØX2	T36.ØX3	T36.ØX4	T36.ØX5	T36.ØX6
APC	T48.5X1	T48.5X2	T48.5X3	T48.5X4	T48.5X5	T48.5X6
Aplonidine	T44.4X1	T44.4X2	T44.4X3	T44.4X4	T44.4X5	T44.4X6
Apomorphine	T47.7X1	T47.7X2	T47.7X3	T47.7X4	T47.7X5	T47.7X6

Substance	Poisoning, Accidental (unintentional)	Poisoning, Intentional Self-harm	Poisoning, Assault	Poisoning, Undetermined	Adverse Effect	Under-dosing
Appetite depressants, central	T5Ø.5X1	T5Ø.5X2	T5Ø.5X3	T5Ø.5X4	T5Ø.5X5	T5Ø.5X6
Apraclonidine (hydrochloride)	T44.4X1	T44.4X2	T44.4X3	T44.4X4	T44.4X5	T44.4X6
Apresoline	T46.5X1	T46.5X2	T46.5X3	T46.5X4	T46.5X5	T46.5X6
Apri*	T38.4X1	T38.4X2	T38.4X3	T38.4X4	T38.4X5	T38.4X6
Aprindine	T46.2X1	T46.2X2	T46.2X3	T46.2X4	T46.2X5	T46.2X6
Aprobarbital	T42.3X1	T42.3X2	T42.3X3	T42.3X4	T42.3X5	T42.3X6
Apronalide	T42.6X1	T42.6X2	T42.6X3	T42.6X4	T42.6X5	T42.6X6
Aprotinin	T45.621	T45.622	T45.623	T45.624	T45.625	T45.626
Aptocaine	T41.3X1	T41.3X2	T41.3X3	T41.3X4	T41.3X5	T41.3X6
Aqua fortis	T54.2X1	T54.2X2	T54.2X3	T54.2X4	—	—
Ara-A	T37.5X1	T37.5X2	T37.5X3	T37.5X4	T37.5X5	T37.5X6
Ara-C	T45.1X1	T45.1X2	T45.1X3	T45.1X4	T45.1X5	T45.1X6
Arachis oil	T49.3X1	T49.3X2	T49.3X3	T49.3X4	T49.3X5	T49.3X6
cathartic	T47.4X1	T47.4X2	T47.4X3	T47.4X4	T47.4X5	T47.4X6
Aralen	T37.2X1	T37.2X2	T37.2X3	T37.2X4	T37.2X5	T37.2X6
Arecoline	T44.1X1	T44.1X2	T44.1X3	T44.1X4	T44.1X5	T44.1X6
Arginine	T5Ø.991	T5Ø.992	T5Ø.993	T5Ø.994	T5Ø.995	T5Ø.996
glutamate	T5Ø.991	T5Ø.992	T5Ø.993	T5Ø.994	T5Ø.995	T5Ø.996
Argyrol	T49.ØX1	T49.ØX2	T49.ØX3	T49.ØX4	T49.ØX5	T49.ØX6
ENT agent	T49.6X1	T49.6X2	T49.6X3	T49.6X4	T49.6X5	T49.6X6
ophthalmic preparation	T49.5X1	T49.5X2	T49.5X3	T49.5X4	T49.5X5	T49.5X6
Aristocort	T38.ØX1	T38.ØX2	T38.ØX3	T38.ØX4	T38.ØX5	T38.ØX6
ENT agent	T49.6X1	T49.6X2	T49.6X3	T49.6X4	T49.6X5	T49.6X6
ophthalmic preparation	T49.5X1	T49.5X2	T49.5X3	T49.5X4	T49.5X5	T49.5X6
topical NEC	T49.ØX1	T49.ØX2	T49.ØX3	T49.ØX4	T49.ØX5	T49.ØX6
Armour*	T38.1X1	T38.1X2	T38.1X3	T38.1X4	T38.1X5	T38.1X6
Aromatics, corrosive	T54.1X1	T54.1X2	T54.1X3	T54.1X4	—	—
disinfectants	T54.1X1	T54.1X2	T54.1X3	T54.1X4	—	—
Arsenate of lead	T57.ØX1	T57.ØX2	T57.ØX3	T57.ØX4	—	—
herbicide	T57.ØX1	T57.ØX2	T57.ØX3	T57.ØX4	—	—
Arsenic, arsenicals (compounds) (dust) (vapor) **NEC**	T57.ØX1	T57.ØX2	T57.ØX3	T57.ØX4	—	—
anti-infectives	T37.8X1	T37.8X2	T37.8X3	T37.8X4	T37.8X5	T37.8X6
pesticide (dust) (fumes)	T57.ØX1	T57.ØX2	T57.ØX3	T57.ØX4	—	—
Arsine (gas)	T57.ØX1	T57.ØX2	T57.ØX3	T57.ØX4	—	—
Arsobal*	T37.3X1	T37.3X2	T37.3X3	T37.3X4	T37.3X5	T37.3X6
Arsphenamine (silver)	T37.8X1	T37.8X2	T37.8X3	T37.8X4	T37.8X5	T37.8X6
Arsthinol	T37.3X1	T37.3X2	T37.3X3	T37.3X4	T37.3X5	T37.3X6
Artane	T44.3X1	T44.3X2	T44.3X3	T44.3X4	T44.3X5	T44.3X6
Arthropod (venomous) **NEC**	T63.481	T63.482	T63.483	T63.484	—	—
Articaine	T41.3X1	T41.3X2	T41.3X3	T41.3X4	T41.3X5	T41.3X6
Asbestos	T57.8X1	T57.8X2	T57.8X3	T57.8X4	—	—
Ascaridole	T37.4X1	T37.4X2	T37.4X3	T37.4X4	T37.4X5	T37.4X6
Ascorbic acid	T45.2X1	T45.2X2	T45.2X3	T45.2X4	T45.2X5	T45.2X6
Asiaticoside	T49.ØX1	T49.ØX2	T49.ØX3	T49.ØX4	T49.ØX5	T49.ØX6
Asparaginase	T45.1X1	T45.1X2	T45.1X3	T45.1X4	T45.1X5	T45.1X6
Aspidium (oleoresin)	T37.4X1	T37.4X2	T37.4X3	T37.4X4	T37.4X5	T37.4X6
Aspirin (aluminum) (soluble)	T39.Ø11	T39.Ø12	T39.Ø13	T39.Ø14	T39.Ø15	T39.Ø16
Aspoxicillin	T36.ØX1	T36.ØX2	T36.ØX3	T36.ØX4	T36.ØX5	T36.ØX6
Astemizole	T45.ØX1	T45.ØX2	T45.ØX3	T45.ØX4	T45.ØX5	T45.ØX6
Astringent (local)	T49.2X1	T49.2X2	T49.2X3	T49.2X4	T49.2X5	T49.2X6
specified NEC	T49.2X1	T49.2X2	T49.2X3	T49.2X4	T49.2X5	T49.2X6
Astromicin	T36.5X1	T36.5X2	T36.5X3	T36.5X4	T36.5X5	T36.5X6
Ataractic drug NEC	T43.5Ø1	T43.5Ø2	T43.5Ø3	T43.5Ø4	T43.5Ø5	T43.5Ø6
Atenolol	T44.7X1	T44.7X2	T44.7X3	T44.7X4	T44.7X5	T44.7X6
Atonia drug, intestinal	T47.4X1	T47.4X2	T47.4X3	T47.4X4	T47.4X5	T47.4X6
Atophan	T5Ø.4X1	T5Ø.4X2	T5Ø.4X3	T5Ø.4X4	T5Ø.4X5	T5Ø.4X6
Atracurium besilate	T48.1X1	T48.1X2	T48.1X3	T48.1X4	T48.1X5	T48.1X6
Atropine	T44.3X1	T44.3X2	T44.3X3	T44.3X4	T44.3X5	T44.3X6
derivative	T44.3X1	T44.3X2	T44.3X3	T44.3X4	T44.3X5	T44.3X6
methonitrate	T44.3X1	T44.3X2	T44.3X3	T44.3X4	T44.3X5	T44.3X6
Atrovent*	T48.6X1	T48.6X2	T48.6X3	T48.6X4	T48.6X5	T48.6X6
Attapulgite	T47.6X1	T47.6X2	T47.6X3	T47.6X4	T47.6X5	T47.6X6
Augmentin (ES-600) (XR)*	T36.ØX1	T36.ØX2	T36.ØX3	T36.ØX4	T36.ØX5	T36.ØX6
Auramine	T65.891	T65.892	T65.893	T65.894	—	—
dye	T65.6X1	T65.6X2	T65.6X3	T65.6X4	—	—
fungicide	T6Ø.3X1	T6Ø.3X2	T6Ø.3X3	T6Ø.3X4	—	—
Auranofin	T39.4X1	T39.4X2	T39.4X3	T39.4X4	T39.4X5	T39.4X6
Aurantiin	T46.991	T46.992	T46.993	T46.994	T46.995	T46.996
Aureomycin	T36.4X1	T36.4X2	T36.4X3	T36.4X4	T36.4X5	T36.4X6
ophthalmic preparation	T49.5X1	T49.5X2	T49.5X3	T49.5X4	T49.5X5	T49.5X6
topical NEC	T49.ØX1	T49.ØX2	T49.ØX3	T49.ØX4	T49.ØX5	T49.ØX6
Aurothioglucose	T39.4X1	T39.4X2	T39.4X3	T39.4X4	T39.4X5	T39.4X6
Aurothioglycanide	T39.4X1	T39.4X2	T39.4X3	T39.4X4	T39.4X5	T39.4X6
Aurothiomalate sodium	T39.4X1	T39.4X2	T39.4X3	T39.4X4	T39.4X5	T39.4X6
Aurotioprol	T39.4X1	T39.4X2	T39.4X3	T39.4X4	T39.4X5	T39.4X6
Automobile fuel	T52.ØX1	T52.ØX2	T52.ØX3	T52.ØX4	—	—
Autonomic nervous system agent NEC	T44.9Ø1	T44.9Ø2	T44.9Ø3	T44.9Ø4	T44.9Ø5	T44.9Ø6
Avelox*	T36.8X1	T36.8X2	T36.8X3	T36.8X4	T36.8X5	T36.8X6

Substance	Poisoning, Accidental (unintentional)	Poisoning, Intentional Self-harm	Poisoning, Assault	Poisoning, Undetermined	Adverse Effect	Under-dosing
Avlosulfon	T37.1X1	T37.1X2	T37.1X3	T37.1X4	T37.1X5	T37.1X6
Avomine	T42.6X1	T42.6X2	T42.6X3	T42.6X4	T42.6X5	T42.6X6
Axerophthol	T45.2X1	T45.2X2	T45.2X3	T45.2X4	T45.2X5	T45.2X6
Azacitidine	T45.1X1	T45.1X2	T45.1X3	T45.1X4	T45.1X5	T45.1X6
Azacyclonol	T43.591	T43.592	T43.593	T43.594	T43.595	T43.596
Azadirachta	T6Ø.2X1	T6Ø.2X2	T6Ø.2X3	T6Ø.2X4	—	—
Azanidazole	T37.3X1	T37.3X2	T37.3X3	T37.3X4	T37.3X5	T37.3X6
Azapetine	T46.7X1	T46.7X2	T46.7X3	T46.7X4	T46.7X5	T46.7X6
Azapropazone	T39.2X1	T39.2X2	T39.2X3	T39.2X4	T39.2X5	T39.2X6
Azaribine	T45.1X1	T45.1X2	T45.1X3	T45.1X4	T45.1X5	T45.1X6
Azaserine	T45.1X1	T45.1X2	T45.1X3	T45.1X4	T45.1X5	T45.1X6
Azatadine	T45.ØX1	T45.ØX2	T45.ØX3	T45.ØX4	T45.ØX5	T45.ØX6
Azatepa	T45.1X1	T45.1X2	T45.1X3	T45.1X4	T45.1X5	T45.1X6
Azathioprine	T45.1X1	T45.1X2	T45.1X3	T45.1X4	T45.1X5	T45.1X6
Azelaic acid	T49.ØX1	T49.ØX2	T49.ØX3	T49.ØX4	T49.ØX5	T49.ØX6
Azelastine	T45.ØX1	T45.ØX2	T45.ØX3	T45.ØX4	T45.ØX5	T45.ØX6
Azidocillin	T36.ØX1	T36.ØX2	T36.ØX3	T36.ØX4	T36.ØX5	T36.ØX6
Azidothymidine	T37.5X1	T37.5X2	T37.5X3	T37.5X4	T37.5X5	T37.5X6
Azinphos (ethyl) (methyl)	T6Ø.ØX1	T6Ø.ØX2	T6Ø.ØX3	T6Ø.ØX4	—	—
Aziridine (chelating)	T54.1X1	T54.1X2	T54.1X3	T54.1X4	—	—
Azithromycin	T36.3X1	T36.3X2	T36.3X3	T36.3X4	T36.3X5	T36.3X6
Azlocillin	T36.ØX1	T36.ØX2	T36.ØX3	T36.ØX4	T36.ØX5	T36.ØX6
Azobenzene smoke	T65.3X1	T65.3X2	T65.3X3	T65.3X4	—	—
acaricide	T6Ø.8X1	T6Ø.8X2	T6Ø.8X3	T6Ø.8X4	—	—
Azo-Standard*	T49.ØX1	T49.ØX2	T49.ØX3	T49.ØX4	T49.ØX5	T49.ØX6
Azosulfamide	T37.ØX1	T37.ØX2	T37.ØX3	T37.ØX4	T37.ØX5	T37.ØX6
AZT	T37.5X1	T37.5X2	T37.5X3	T37.5X4	T37.5X5	T37.5X6
Aztreonam	T36.1X1	T36.1X2	T36.1X3	T36.1X4	T36.1X5	T36.1X6
Azulfidine	T37.ØX1	T37.ØX2	T37.ØX3	T37.ØX4	T37.ØX5	T37.ØX6
Azuresin	T5Ø.8X1	T5Ø.8X2	T5Ø.8X3	T5Ø.8X4	T5Ø.8X5	T5Ø.8X6
b-acetyldigoxin	T46.ØX1	T46.ØX2	T46.ØX3	T46.ØX4	T46.ØX5	T46.ØX6
P-Acetamidophenol	T39.1X1	T39.1X2	T39.1X3	T39.1X4	T39.1X5	T39.1X6
Bacampicillin	T36.ØX1	T36.ØX2	T36.ØX3	T36.ØX4	T36.ØX5	T36.ØX6
Bacillus						
lactobacillus	T47.8X1	T47.8X2	T47.8X3	T47.8X4	T47.8X5	T47.8X6
subtilis	T47.6X1	T47.6X2	T47.6X3	T47.6X4	T47.6X5	T47.6X6
Bacimycin	T49.ØX1	T49.ØX2	T49.ØX3	T49.ØX4	T49.ØX5	T49.ØX6
ophthalmic preparation	T49.5X1	T49.5X2	T49.5X3	T49.5X4	T49.5X5	T49.5X6
Bacitracin zinc	T49.ØX1	T49.ØX2	T49.ØX3	T49.ØX4	T49.ØX5	T49.ØX6
with neomycin	T49.ØX1	T49.ØX2	T49.ØX3	T49.ØX4	T49.ØX5	T49.ØX6
ENT agent	T49.6X1	T49.6X2	T49.6X3	T49.6X4	T49.6X5	T49.6X6
ophthalmic preparation	T49.5X1	T49.5X2	T49.5X3	T49.5X4	T49.5X5	T49.5X6
topical NEC	T49.ØX1	T49.ØX2	T49.ØX3	T49.ØX4	T49.ØX5	T49.ØX6
Baclofen	T42.8X1	T42.8X2	T42.8X3	T42.8X4	T42.8X5	T42.8X6
Bactrim*	T36.8X1	T36.8X2	T36.8X3	T36.8X4	T36.8X5	T36.8X6
Baking soda	T5Ø.991	T5Ø.992	T5Ø.993	T5Ø.994	T5Ø.995	T5Ø.996
BAL	T45.8X1	T45.8X2	T45.8X3	T45.8X4	T45.8X5	T45.8X6
Bambuterol	T48.6X1	T48.6X2	T48.6X3	T48.6X4	T48.6X5	T48.6X6
Bamethan (sulfate)	T46.7X1	T46.7X2	T46.7X3	T46.7X4	T46.7X5	T46.7X6
Bamifylline	T48.6X1	T48.6X2	T48.6X3	T48.6X4	T48.6X5	T48.6X6
Bamipine	T45.ØX1	T45.ØX2	T45.ØX3	T45.ØX4	T45.ØX5	T45.ØX6
Baneberry — *see* Actaea spicata						
Banewort — *see* Belladonna						
Barbenyl	T42.3X1	T42.3X2	T42.3X3	T42.3X4	T42.3X5	T42.3X6
Barbexaclone	T42.6X1	T42.6X2	T42.6X3	T42.6X4	T42.6X5	T42.6X6
Barbital	T42.3X1	T42.3X2	T42.3X3	T42.3X4	T42.3X5	T42.3X6
sodium	T42.3X1	T42.3X2	T42.3X3	T42.3X4	T42.3X5	T42.3X6
Barbitone	T42.3X1	T42.3X2	T42.3X3	T42.3X4	T42.3X5	T42.3X6
Barbiturate NEC	T42.3X1	T42.3X2	T42.3X3	T42.3X4	T42.3X5	T42.3X6
with tranquilizer	T42.3X1	T42.3X2	T42.3X3	T42.3X4	T42.3X5	T42.3X6
anesthetic (intravenous)	T41.1X1	T41.1X2	T41.1X3	T41.1X4	T41.1X5	T41.1X6
Barium (carbonate) (chloride) (sulfite)	T57.8X1	T57.8X2	T57.8X3	T57.8X4	—	—
diagnostic agent	T5Ø.8X1	T5Ø.8X2	T5Ø.8X3	T5Ø.8X4	T5Ø.8X5	T5Ø.8X6
pesticide	T6Ø.4X1	T6Ø.4X2	T6Ø.4X3	T6Ø.4X4	—	—
rodenticide	T6Ø.4X1	T6Ø.4X2	T6Ø.4X3	T6Ø.4X4	—	—
sulfate (medicinal)	T5Ø.8X1	T5Ø.8X2	T5Ø.8X3	T5Ø.8X4	T5Ø.8X5	T5Ø.8X6
Barrier cream	T49.3X1	T49.3X2	T49.3X3	T49.3X4	T49.3X5	T49.3X6
Basic fuchsin	T49.ØX1	T49.ØX2	T49.ØX3	T49.ØX4	T49.ØX5	T49.ØX6
Basiliximab*	T45.1X1	T45.1X2	T45.1X3	T45.1X4	T45.1X5	T45.1X6
Battery acid or fluid	T54.2X1	T54.2X2	T54.2X3	T54.2X4	—	—
Bay rum	T51.8X1	T51.8X2	T51.8X3	T51.8X4	—	—
b-benzalbutyramide	T46.6X1	T46.6X2	T46.6X3	T46.6X4	T46.6X5	T46.6X6
BCG (vaccine)	T5Ø.A91	T5Ø.A92	T5Ø.A93	T5Ø.A94	T5Ø.A95	T5Ø.A96
BCNU	T45.1X1	T45.1X2	T45.1X3	T45.1X4	T45.1X5	T45.1X6
Bearsfoot	T62.2X1	T62.2X2	T62.2X3	T62.2X4	—	—
Beclamide	T42.6X1	T42.6X2	T42.6X3	T42.6X4	T42.6X5	T42.6X6
Beclomethasone	T44.5X1	T44.5X2	T44.5X3	T44.5X4	T44.5X5	T44.5X6
Bee (sting) (venom)	T63.441	T63.442	T63.443	T63.444	—	—
Befunolol	T49.5X1	T49.5X2	T49.5X3	T49.5X4	T49.5X5	T49.5X6
Bekanamycin	T36.5X1	T36.5X2	T36.5X3	T36.5X4	T36.5X5	T36.5X6
Belladonna — *see also* Nightshade						

Substance	Poisoning, Accidental (unintentional)	Poisoning, Intentional Self-harm	Poisoning, Assault	Poisoning, Undetermined	Adverse Effect	Under-dosing
Belladonna — *see also* Nightshade — *continued*						
alkaloids	T44.3X1	T44.3X2	T44.3X3	T44.3X4	T44.3X5	T44.3X6
extract	T44.3X1	T44.3X2	T44.3X3	T44.3X4	T44.3X5	T44.3X6
herb	T44.3X1	T44.3X2	T44.3X3	T44.3X4	T44.3X5	T44.3X6
Belviq*	T5Ø.5X1	T5Ø.5X2	T5Ø.5X3	T5Ø.5X4	T5Ø.5X5	T5Ø.5X6
Bemegride	T5Ø.7X1	T5Ø.7X2	T5Ø.7X3	T5Ø.7X4	T5Ø.7X5	T5Ø.7X6
Benactyzine	T44.3X1	T44.3X2	T44.3X3	T44.3X4	T44.3X5	T44.3X6
Benadryl	T45.ØX1	T45.ØX2	T45.ØX3	T45.ØX4	T45.ØX5	T45.ØX6
Benaprizine	T44.3X1	T44.3X2	T44.3X3	T44.3X4	T44.3X5	T44.3X6
Benazepril	T46.4X1	T46.4X2	T46.4X3	T46.4X4	T46.4X5	T46.4X6
Bencyclane	T46.7X1	T46.7X2	T46.7X3	T46.7X4	T46.7X5	T46.7X6
Bendazol	T46.3X1	T46.3X2	T46.3X3	T46.3X4	T46.3X5	T46.3X6
Bendrofluazide	T5Ø.2X1	T5Ø.2X2	T5Ø.2X3	T5Ø.2X4	T5Ø.2X5	T5Ø.2X6
Bendroflumethiazide	T5Ø.2X1	T5Ø.2X2	T5Ø.2X3	T5Ø.2X4	T5Ø.2X5	T5Ø.2X6
Benemid	T5Ø.4X1	T5Ø.4X2	T5Ø.4X3	T5Ø.4X4	T5Ø.4X5	T5Ø.4X6
Benethamine penicillin	T36.ØX1	T36.ØX2	T36.ØX3	T36.ØX4	T36.ØX5	T36.ØX6
Benexate	T47.1X1	T47.1X2	T47.1X3	T47.1X4	T47.1X5	T47.1X6
Benfluorex	T46.6X1	T46.6X2	T46.6X3	T46.6X4	T46.6X5	T46.6X6
Benfotiamine	T45.2X1	T45.2X2	T45.2X3	T45.2X4	T45.2X5	T45.2X6
Benisone	T49.ØX1	T49.ØX2	T49.ØX3	T49.ØX4	T49.ØX5	T49.ØX6
Benomyl	T6Ø.ØX1	T6Ø.ØX2	T6Ø.ØX3	T6Ø.ØX4	—	—
Benoquin	T49.8X1	T49.8X2	T49.8X3	T49.8X4	T49.8X5	T49.8X6
Benoxinate	T41.3X1	T41.3X2	T41.3X3	T41.3X4	T41.3X5	T41.3X6
Benperidol	T43.4X1	T43.4X2	T43.4X3	T43.4X4	T43.4X5	T43.4X6
Benproperine	T48.3X1	T48.3X2	T48.3X3	T48.3X4	T48.3X5	T48.3X6
Benserazide	T42.8X1	T42.8X2	T42.8X3	T42.8X4	T42.8X5	T42.8X6
Bentazepam	T42.4X1	T42.4X2	T42.4X3	T42.4X4	T42.4X5	T42.4X6
Bentiromide	T5Ø.8X1	T5Ø.8X2	T5Ø.8X3	T5Ø.8X4	T5Ø.8X5	T5Ø.8X6
Bentonite	T49.3X1	T49.3X2	T49.3X3	T49.3X4	T49.3X5	T49.3X6
Benzalbutyramide	T46.6X1	T46.6X2	T46.6X3	T46.6X4	T46.6X5	T46.6X6
Benzalkonium (chloride)	T49.ØX1	T49.ØX2	T49.ØX3	T49.ØX4	T49.ØX5	T49.ØX6
ophthalmic preparation	T49.5X1	T49.5X2	T49.5X3	T49.5X4	T49.5X5	T49.5X6
Benzamidosalicylate (calcium)	T37.1X1	T37.1X2	T37.1X3	T37.1X4	T37.1X5	T37.1X6
Benzamine	T41.3X1	T41.3X2	T41.3X3	T41.3X4	T41.3X5	T41.3X6
lactate	T49.1X1	T49.1X2	T49.1X3	T49.1X4	T49.1X5	T49.1X6
Benzamphetamine	T5Ø.5X1	T5Ø.5X2	T5Ø.5X3	T5Ø.5X4	T5Ø.5X5	T5Ø.5X6
Benzapril hydrochloride	T46.5X1	T46.5X2	T46.5X3	T46.5X4	T46.5X5	T46.5X6
Benzathine benzylpenicillin	T36.ØX1	T36.ØX2	T36.ØX3	T36.ØX4	T36.ØX5	T36.ØX6
Benzathine penicillin	T36.ØX1	T36.ØX2	T36.ØX3	T36.ØX4	T36.ØX5	T36.ØX6
Benzatropine	T42.8X1	T42.8X2	T42.8X3	T42.8X4	T42.8X5	T42.8X6
Benzbromarone	T5Ø.4X1	T5Ø.4X2	T5Ø.4X3	T5Ø.4X4	T5Ø.4X5	T5Ø.4X6
Benzcarbimine	T45.1X1	T45.1X2	T45.1X3	T45.1X4	T45.1X5	T45.1X6
Benzedrex	T44.991	T44.992	T44.993	T44.994	T44.995	T44.996
Benzedrine (amphetamine)	T43.621	T43.622	T43.623	T43.624	T43.625	T43.626
Benzenamine	T65.3X1	T65.3X2	T65.3X3	T65.3X4	—	—
Benzene	T52.1X1	T52.1X2	T52.1X3	T52.1X4	—	—
homologues (acetyl) (dimethyl) (methyl) (solvent)	T52.2X1	T52.2X2	T52.2X3	T52.2X4	—	—
Benzethonium (chloride)	T49.ØX1	T49.ØX2	T49.ØX3	T49.ØX4	T49.ØX5	T49.ØX6
Benzfetamine	T5Ø.5X1	T5Ø.5X2	T5Ø.5X3	T5Ø.5X4	T5Ø.5X5	T5Ø.5X6
Benzhexol	T44.3X1	T44.3X2	T44.3X3	T44.3X4	T44.3X5	T44.3X6
Benzhydramine (chloride)	T45.ØX1	T45.ØX2	T45.ØX3	T45.ØX4	T45.ØX5	T45.ØX6
Benzidine	T65.891	T65.892	T65.893	T65.894	—	—
Benzilonium bromide	T44.3X1	T44.3X2	T44.3X3	T44.3X4	T44.3X5	T44.3X6
Benzimidazole	T6Ø.3X1	T6Ø.3X2	T6Ø.3X3	T6Ø.3X4	—	—
Benzin (e) — *see* Ligroin						
Benziodarone	T46.3X1	T46.3X2	T46.3X3	T46.3X4	T46.3X5	T46.3X6
Benznidazole	T37.3X1	T37.3X2	T37.3X3	T37.3X4	T37.3X5	T37.3X6
Benzocaine	T41.3X1	T41.3X2	T41.3X3	T41.3X4	T41.3X5	T41.3X6
Benzocol*	T41.3X1	T41.3X2	T41.3X3	T41.3X4	T41.3X5	T41.3X6
Benzodiapin	T42.4X1	T42.4X2	T42.4X3	T42.4X4	T42.4X5	T42.4X6
Benzodiazepine NEC	T42.4X1	T42.4X2	T42.4X3	T42.4X4	T42.4X5	T42.4X6
Benzoic acid	T49.ØX1	T49.ØX2	T49.ØX3	T49.ØX4	T49.ØX5	T49.ØX6
with salicylic acid	T49.ØX1	T49.ØX2	T49.ØX3	T49.ØX4	T49.ØX5	T49.ØX6
Benzoin (tincture)	T48.5X1	T48.5X2	T48.5X3	T48.5X4	T48.5X5	T48.5X6
Benzol (benzene)	T52.1X1	T52.1X2	T52.1X3	T52.1X4	—	—
vapor	T52.ØX1	T52.ØX2	T52.ØX3	T52.ØX4	—	—
Benzomorphan	T4Ø.2X1	T4Ø.2X2	T4Ø.2X3	T4Ø.2X4	T4Ø.2X5	T4Ø.2X6
Benzonatate	T48.3X1	T48.3X2	T48.3X3	T48.3X4	T48.3X5	T48.3X6
Benzophenones	T49.3X1	T49.3X2	T49.3X3	T49.3X4	T49.3X5	T49.3X6
Benzopyrone	T46.991	T46.992	T46.993	T46.994	T46.995	T46.996
Benzothiadiazides	T5Ø.2X1	T5Ø.2X2	T5Ø.2X3	T5Ø.2X4	T5Ø.2X5	T5Ø.2X6
Benzoxonium chloride	T49.ØX1	T49.ØX2	T49.ØX3	T49.ØX4	T49.ØX5	T49.ØX6
Benzoylpas calcium	T37.1X1	T37.1X2	T37.1X3	T37.1X4	T37.1X5	T37.1X6
Benzoyl peroxide	T49.ØX1	T49.ØX2	T49.ØX3	T49.ØX4	T49.ØX5	T49.ØX6
Benzperidin	T43.591	T43.592	T43.593	T43.594	T43.595	T43.596
Benzperidol	T43.591	T43.592	T43.593	T43.594	T43.595	T43.596
Benzphetamine	T5Ø.5X1	T5Ø.5X2	T5Ø.5X3	T5Ø.5X4	T5Ø.5X5	T5Ø.5X6
Benzpyrinium bromide	T44.1X1	T44.1X2	T44.1X3	T44.1X4	T44.1X5	T44.1X6
Benzquinamide	T45.ØX1	T45.ØX2	T45.ØX3	T45.ØX4	T45.ØX5	T45.ØX6

Substance	Poisoning, Accidental (unintentional)	Poisoning, Intentional Self-harm	Poisoning, Assault	Poisoning, Undetermined	Adverse Effect	Under-dosing
Benzthiazide	T5Ø.2X1	T5Ø.2X2	T5Ø.2X3	T5Ø.2X4	T5Ø.2X5	T5Ø.2X6
Benztropine						
anticholinergic	T44.3X1	T44.3X2	T44.3X3	T44.3X4	T44.3X5	T44.3X6
antiparkinson	T42.8X1	T42.8X2	T42.8X3	T42.8X4	T42.8X5	T42.8X6
Benzydamine	T49.ØX1	T49.ØX2	T49.ØX3	T49.ØX4	T49.ØX5	T49.ØX6
Benzyl						
acetate	T52.8X1	T52.8X2	T52.8X3	T52.8X4	—	—
alcohol	T49.ØX1	T49.ØX2	T49.ØX3	T49.ØX4	T49.ØX5	T49.ØX6
benzoate	T49.ØX1	T49.ØX2	T49.ØX3	T49.ØX4	T49.ØX5	T49.ØX6
Benzoic acid	T49.ØX1	T49.ØX2	T49.ØX3	T49.ØX4	T49.ØX5	T49.ØX6
hydroquinone*	T49.4X1	T49.4X2	T49.4X3	T49.4X4	T49.4X5	T49.4X6
morphine	T4Ø.2X1	T4Ø.2X2	T4Ø.2X3	T4Ø.2X4	—	—
nicotinate	T46.6X1	T46.6X2	T46.6X3	T46.6X4	T46.6X5	T46.6X6
penicillin	T36.ØX1	T36.ØX2	T36.ØX3	T36.ØX4	T36.ØX5	T36.ØX6
Benzylhydrochlorthiazide	T5Ø.2X1	T5Ø.2X2	T5Ø.2X3	T5Ø.2X4	T5Ø.2X5	T5Ø.2X6
Benzylpenicillin	T36.ØX1	T36.ØX2	T36.ØX3	T36.ØX4	T36.ØX5	T36.ØX6
Benzylthiouracil	T38.2X1	T38.2X2	T38.2X3	T38.2X4	T38.2X5	T38.2X6
Bephenium hydroxynaphthoate	T37.4X1	T37.4X2	T37.4X3	T37.4X4	T37.4X5	T37.4X6
Bepridil	T46.1X1	T46.1X2	T46.1X3	T46.1X4	T46.1X5	T46.1X6
Bergamot oil	T65.891	T65.892	T65.893	T65.894	—	—
Bergapten	T5Ø.991	T5Ø.992	T5Ø.993	T5Ø.994	T5Ø.995	T5Ø.996
Berries, poisonous	T62.1X1	T62.1X2	T62.1X3	T62.1X4	—	—
Beryllium (compounds)	T56.7X1	T56.7X2	T56.7X3	T56.7X4	—	—
beta adrenergic blocking agent, heart	T44.7X1	T44.7X2	T44.7X3	T44.7X4	T44.7X5	T44.7X6
Betacarotene	T45.2X1	T45.2X2	T45.2X3	T45.2X4	T45.2X5	T45.2X6
Beta-Chlor	T42.6X1	T42.6X2	T42.6X3	T42.6X4	T42.6X5	T42.6X6
Betahistine	T46.7X1	T46.7X2	T46.7X3	T46.7X4	T46.7X5	T46.7X6
Betaine	T47.5X1	T47.5X2	T47.5X3	T47.5X4	T47.5X5	T47.5X6
Betamethasone	T49.ØX1	T49.ØX2	T49.ØX3	T49.ØX4	T49.ØX5	T49.ØX6
topical	T49.ØX1	T49.ØX2	T49.ØX3	T49.ØX4	T49.ØX5	T49.ØX6
Betamicin	T36.8X1	T36.8X2	T36.8X3	T36.8X4	T36.8X5	T36.8X6
Betanidine	T46.5X1	T46.5X2	T46.5X3	T46.5X4	T46.5X5	T46.5X6
Betaxolol	T44.7X1	T44.7X2	T44.7X3	T44.7X4	T44.7X5	T44.7X6
Betazole	T5Ø.8X1	T5Ø.8X2	T5Ø.8X3	T5Ø.8X4	T5Ø.8X5	T5Ø.8X6
Bethanechol	T44.1X1	T44.1X2	T44.1X3	T44.1X4	T44.1X5	T44.1X6
chloride	T44.1X1	T44.1X2	T44.1X3	T44.1X4	T44.1X5	T44.1X6
Bethanidine	T46.5X1	T46.5X2	T46.5X3	T46.5X4	T46.5X5	T46.5X6
Betoxycaine	T41.3X1	T41.3X2	T41.3X3	T41.3X4	T41.3X5	T41.3X6
Betula oil	T49.3X1	T49.3X2	T49.3X3	T49.3X4	T49.3X5	T49.3X6
Bevantolol	T44.7X1	T44.7X2	T44.7X3	T44.7X4	T44.7X5	T44.7X6
Bevonium metilsulfate	T44.3X1	T44.3X2	T44.3X3	T44.3X4	T44.3X5	T44.3X6
Bezafibrate	T46.6X1	T46.6X2	T46.6X3	T46.6X4	T46.6X5	T46.6X6
Bezitramide	T4Ø.491	T4Ø.492	T4Ø.493	T4Ø.494	T4Ø.495	T4Ø.496
BHA	T5Ø.991	T5Ø.992	T5Ø.993	T5Ø.994	T5Ø.995	T5Ø.996
Bhang	T4Ø.711	T4Ø.712	T4Ø.713	T4Ø.714	T4Ø.715	T4Ø.716
BHC (medicinal)	T49.ØX1	T49.ØX2	T49.ØX3	T49.ØX4	T49.ØX5	T49.ØX6
nonmedicinal (vapor)	T53.6X1	T53.6X2	T53.6X3	T53.6X4	—	—
Bialamicol	T37.3X1	T37.3X2	T37.3X3	T37.3X4	T37.3X5	T37.3X6
Bibenzonium bromide	T48.3X1	T48.3X2	T48.3X3	T48.3X4	T48.3X5	T48.3X6
Bibrocathol	T49.5X1	T49.5X2	T49.5X3	T49.5X4	T49.5X5	T49.5X6
Bichloride of mercury — *see* Mercury, chloride						
Bichromates (calcium) (potassium)(sodium) (crystals)	T57.8X1	T57.8X2	T57.8X3	T57.8X4	—	—
fumes	T56.2X1	T56.2X2	T56.2X3	T56.2X4	—	—
Biclotymol	T49.6X1	T49.6X2	T49.6X3	T49.6X4	T49.6X5	T49.6X6
BiCNU*	T45.1X1	T45.1X2	T45.1X3	T45.1X4	T45.1X5	T45.1X6
Bicucculine	T5Ø.7X1	T5Ø.7X2	T5Ø.7X3	T5Ø.7X4	T5Ø.7X5	T5Ø.7X6
Bifemelane	T43.291	T43.292	T43.293	T43.294	T43.295	T43.296
Biguanide derivatives, oral	T38.3X1	T38.3X2	T38.3X3	T38.3X4	T38.3X5	T38.3X6
Bile salts	T47.5X1	T47.5X2	T47.5X3	T47.5X4	T47.5X5	T47.5X6
Biligrafin	T5Ø.8X1	T5Ø.8X2	T5Ø.8X3	T5Ø.8X4	T5Ø.8X5	T5Ø.8X6
Bilopaque	T5Ø.8X1	T5Ø.8X2	T5Ø.8X3	T5Ø.8X4	T5Ø.8X5	T5Ø.8X6
Binifibrate	T46.6X1	T46.6X2	T46.6X3	T46.6X4	T46.6X5	T46.6X6
Binitrobenzol	T65.3X1	T65.3X2	T65.3X3	T65.3X4	—	—
Bioflavonoid(s)	T46.991	T46.992	T46.993	T46.994	T46.995	T46.996
Biological substance NEC	T5Ø.9Ø1	T5Ø.9Ø2	T5Ø.9Ø3	T5Ø.9Ø4	T5Ø.9Ø5	T5Ø.9Ø6
Biotin	T45.2X1	T45.2X2	T45.2X3	T45.2X4	T45.2X5	T45.2X6
Biperiden	T44.3X1	T44.3X2	T44.3X3	T44.3X4	T44.3X5	T44.3X6
Bisacodyl	T47.2X1	T47.2X2	T47.2X3	T47.2X4	T47.2X5	T47.2X6
Bisbentiamine	T45.2X1	T45.2X2	T45.2X3	T45.2X4	T45.2X5	T45.2X6
Bisbutiamine	T45.2X1	T45.2X2	T45.2X3	T45.2X4	T45.2X5	T45.2X6
Bisdequalinium (salts) (diacetate)	T49.6X1	T49.6X2	T49.6X3	T49.6X4	T49.6X5	T49.6X6
Bishydroxycoumarin	T45.511	T45.512	T45.513	T45.514	T45.515	T45.516
Bismarsen	T37.8X1	T37.8X2	T37.8X3	T37.8X4	T37.8X5	T37.8X6
Bismuth salts	T47.6X1	T47.6X2	T47.6X3	T47.6X4	T47.6X5	T47.6X6
aluminate	T47.1X1	T47.1X2	T47.1X3	T47.1X4	T47.1X5	T47.1X6
anti-infectives	T37.8X1	T37.8X2	T37.8X3	T37.8X4	T37.8X5	T37.8X6

Substance	Poisoning, Accidental (unintentional)	Poisoning, Intentional Self-harm	Poisoning, Assault	Poisoning, Undetermined	Adverse Effect	Under-dosing
Bismuth salts — *continued*						
formic iodide	T49.ØX1	T49.ØX2	T49.ØX3	T49.ØX4	T49.ØX5	T49.ØX6
glycolylarsenate	T49.ØX1	T49.ØX2	T49.ØX3	T49.ØX4	T49.ØX5	T49.ØX6
nonmedicinal (compounds) NEC	T65.91	T65.92	T65.93	T65.94	—	—
subcarbonate	T47.6X1	T47.6X2	T47.6X3	T47.6X4	T47.6X5	T47.6X6
subsalicylate	T37.8X1	T37.8X2	T37.8X3	T37.8X4	T37.8X5	T37.8X6
sulfarsphenamine	T37.8X1	T37.8X2	T37.8X3	T37.8X4	T37.8X5	T37.8X6
Bisoprolol	T44.7X1	T44.7X2	T44.7X3	T44.7X4	T44.7X5	T44.7X6
Bisoxatin	T47.2X1	T47.2X2	T47.2X3	T47.2X4	T47.2X5	T47.2X6
Bisulepin (hydrochloride)	T45.ØX1	T45.ØX2	T45.ØX3	T45.ØX4	T45.ØX5	T45.ØX6
Bithionol	T37.8X1	T37.8X2	T37.8X3	T37.8X4	T37.8X5	T37.8X6
anthelminthic	T37.4X1	T37.4X2	T37.4X3	T37.4X4	T37.4X5	T37.4X6
Bitolterol	T48.6X1	T48.6X2	T48.6X3	T48.6X4	T48.6X5	T48.6X6
Bitoscanate	T37.4X1	T37.4X2	T37.4X3	T37.4X4	T37.4X5	T37.4X6
Bitter almond oil	T62.8X1	T62.8X2	T62.8X3	T62.8X4	—	—
Bittersweet	T62.2X1	T62.2X2	T62.2X3	T62.2X4	—	—
Bivalirudin*	T45.511	T45.512	T45.513	T45.514	T45.515	T45.516
Black						
flag	T6Ø.91	T6Ø.92	T6Ø.93	T6Ø.94	—	—
henbane	T62.2X1	T62.2X2	T62.2X3	T62.2X4	—	—
leaf (40)	T6Ø.91	T6Ø.92	T6Ø.93	T6Ø.94	—	—
widow spider (bite)	T63.311	T63.312	T63.313	T63.314	—	—
antivenin	T5Ø.Z11	T5Ø.Z12	T5Ø.Z13	T5Ø.Z14	T5Ø.Z15	T5Ø.Z16
Blast furnace gas (carbon monoxide from)	T58.8X1	T58.8X2	T58.8X3	T58.8X4	—	—
Bleach	T54.91	T54.92	T54.93	T54.94	—	—
Bleaching agent (medicinal)	T49.4X1	T49.4X2	T49.4X3	T49.4X4	T49.4X5	T49.4X6
Bleomycin	T45.1X1	T45.1X2	T45.1X3	T45.1X4	T45.1X5	T45.1X6
Blockain	T41.3X1	T41.3X2	T41.3X3	T41.3X4	T41.3X5	T41.3X6
infiltration (subcutaneous)	T41.3X1	T41.3X2	T41.3X3	T41.3X4	T41.3X5	T41.3X6
nerve block (peripheral) (plexus)	T41.3X1	T41.3X2	T41.3X3	T41.3X4	T41.3X5	T41.3X6
topical (surface)	T41.3X1	T41.3X2	T41.3X3	T41.3X4	T41.3X5	T41.3X6
Blockers, calcium channel	T46.1X1	T46.1X2	T46.1X3	T46.1X4	T46.1X5	T46.1X6
Blood (derivatives) (natural) (plasma) (whole)	T45.8X1	T45.8X2	T45.8X3	T45.8X4	T45.8X5	T45.8X6
dried	T45.8X1	T45.8X2	T45.8X3	T45.8X4	T45.8X5	T45.8X6
drug affecting NEC	T45.91	T45.92	T45.93	T45.94	T45.95	T45.96
expander NEC	T45.8X1	T45.8X2	T45.8X3	T45.8X4	T45.8X5	T45.8X6
fraction NEC	T45.8X1	T45.8X2	T45.8X3	T45.8X4	T45.8X5	T45.8X6
substitute (macromolecular)	T45.8X1	T45.8X2	T45.8X3	T45.8X4	T45.8X5	T45.8X6
Blue velvet	T4Ø.2X1	T4Ø.2X2	T4Ø.2X3	T4Ø.2X4	—	—
Bone meal	T62.8X1	T62.8X2	T62.8X3	T62.8X4	—	—
Bonine	T45.ØX1	T45.ØX2	T45.ØX3	T45.ØX4	T45.ØX5	T45.ØX6
Bontril*	T5Ø.5X1	T5Ø.5X2	T5Ø.5X3	T5Ø.5X4	T5Ø.5X5	T5Ø.5X6
Bopindolol	T44.7X1	T44.7X2	T44.7X3	T44.7X4	T44.7X5	T44.7X6
Boracic acid	T49.ØX1	T49.ØX2	T49.ØX3	T49.ØX4	T49.ØX5	T49.ØX6
ENT agent	T49.6X1	T49.6X2	T49.6X3	T49.6X4	T49.6X5	T49.6X6
ophthalmic preparation	T49.5X1	T49.5X2	T49.5X3	T49.5X4	T49.5X5	T49.5X6
Borane complex	T57.8X1	T57.8X2	T57.8X3	T57.8X4	—	—
Borate(s)	T57.8X1	T57.8X2	T57.8X3	T57.8X4	—	—
buffer	T5Ø.991	T5Ø.992	T5Ø.993	T5Ø.994	T5Ø.995	T5Ø.996
cleanser	T54.91	T54.92	T54.93	T54.94	—	—
sodium	T57.8X1	T57.8X2	T57.8X3	T57.8X4	—	—
Borax (cleanser)	T54.91	T54.92	T54.93	T54.94	—	—
Bordeaux mixture	T6Ø.3X1	T6Ø.3X2	T6Ø.3X3	T6Ø.3X4	—	—
Boric acid	T49.ØX1	T49.ØX2	T49.ØX3	T49.ØX4	T49.ØX5	T49.ØX6
ENT agent	T49.6X1	T49.6X2	T49.6X3	T49.6X4	T49.6X5	T49.6X6
ophthalmic preparation	T49.5X1	T49.5X2	T49.5X3	T49.5X4	T49.5X5	T49.5X6
Bornaprine	T44.3X1	T44.3X2	T44.3X3	T44.3X4	T44.3X5	T44.3X6
Boron	T57.8X1	T57.8X2	T57.8X3	T57.8X4	—	—
hydride NEC	T57.8X1	T57.8X2	T57.8X3	T57.8X4	—	—
fumes or gas	T57.8X1	T57.8X2	T57.8X3	T57.8X4	—	—
trifluoride	T59.891	T59.892	T59.893	T59.894	—	—
Botox	T48.291	T48.292	T48.293	T48.294	T48.295	T48.296
Botulinus anti-toxin (type A, B)	T5Ø.Z11	T5Ø.Z12	T5Ø.Z13	T5Ø.Z14	T5Ø.Z15	T5Ø.Z16
Brake fluid vapor	T59.891	T59.892	T59.893	T59.894	—	—
Brallobarbital	T42.3X1	T42.3X2	T42.3X3	T42.3X4	T42.3X5	T42.3X6
Bran (wheat)	T47.4X1	T47.4X2	T47.4X3	T47.4X4	T47.4X5	T47.4X6
Brass (fumes)	T56.891	T56.892	T56.893	T56.894	—	—
Brasso	T52.ØX1	T52.ØX2	T52.ØX3	T52.ØX4	—	—
Bretylium tosilate	T46.2X1	T46.2X2	T46.2X3	T46.2X4	T46.2X5	T46.2X6
Brevital (sodium)	T41.1X1	T41.1X2	T41.1X3	T41.1X4	T41.1X5	T41.1X6
Brinase	T45.3X1	T45.3X2	T45.3X3	T45.3X4	T45.3X5	T45.3X6
British antilewisite	T45.8X1	T45.8X2	T45.8X3	T45.8X4	T45.8X5	T45.8X6
Brodalumab*	T5Ø.991	T5Ø.992	T5Ø.993	T5Ø.994	T5Ø.995	T5Ø.996
Brodifacoum	T6Ø.4X1	T6Ø.4X2	T6Ø.4X3	T6Ø.4X4	—	—
Bromal (hydrate)	T42.6X1	T42.6X2	T42.6X3	T42.6X4	T42.6X5	T42.6X6
Bromazepam	T42.4X1	T42.4X2	T42.4X3	T42.4X4	T42.4X5	T42.4X6

Substance	Poisoning, Accidental (unintentional)	Poisoning, Intentional Self-harm	Poisoning, Assault	Poisoning, Undetermined	Adverse Effect	Under-dosing
Bromazine	T45.ØX1	T45.ØX2	T45.ØX3	T45.ØX4	T45.ØX5	T45.ØX6
Brombenzylcyanide	T59.3X1	T59.3X2	T59.3X3	T59.3X4	—	—
Bromelains	T45.3X1	T45.3X2	T45.3X3	T45.3X4	T45.3X5	T45.3X6
Bromethalin	T6Ø.4X1	T6Ø.4X2	T6Ø.4X3	T6Ø.4X4	—	—
Bromhexine	T48.4X1	T48.4X2	T48.4X3	T48.4X4	T48.4X5	T48.4X6
Bromide salts	T42.6X1	T42.6X2	T42.6X3	T42.6X4	T42.6X5	T42.6X6
Bromindione	T45.511	T45.512	T45.513	T45.514	T45.515	T45.516
Bromine						
compounds (medicinal)	T42.6X1	T42.6X2	T42.6X3	T42.6X4	T42.6X5	T42.6X6
sedative	T42.6X1	T42.6X2	T42.6X3	T42.6X4	T42.6X5	T42.6X6
vapor	T59.891	T59.892	T59.893	T59.894	—	—
Bromisoval	T42.6X1	T42.6X2	T42.6X3	T42.6X4	T42.6X5	T42.6X6
Bromisovalum	T42.6X1	T42.6X2	T42.6X3	T42.6X4	T42.6X5	T42.6X6
Bromobenzylcyanide	T59.3X1	T59.3X2	T59.3X3	T59.3X4	—	—
Bromochlorosalicylani-lide	T49.ØX1	T49.ØX2	T49.ØX3	T49.ØX4	T49.ØX5	T49.ØX6
Bromocriptine	T42.8X1	T42.8X2	T42.8X3	T42.8X4	T42.8X5	T42.8X6
Bromodiphenhydramine	T45.ØX1	T45.ØX2	T45.ØX3	T45.ØX4	T45.ØX5	T45.ØX6
Bromoform	T42.6X1	T42.6X2	T42.6X3	T42.6X4	T42.6X5	T42.6X6
Bromophenol blue reagent	T5Ø.991	T5Ø.992	T5Ø.993	T5Ø.994	T5Ø.995	T5Ø.996
Bromopride	T47.8X1	T47.8X2	T47.8X3	T47.8X4	T47.8X5	T47.8X6
Bromosalicylchloranitide	T49.ØX1	T49.ØX2	T49.ØX3	T49.ØX4	T49.ØX5	T49.ØX6
Bromosalicylhydroxamic acid	T37.1X1	T37.1X2	T37.1X3	T37.1X4	T37.1X5	T37.1X6
Bromo-seltzer	T39.1X1	T39.1X2	T39.1X3	T39.1X4	T39.1X5	T39.1X6
Bromoxynil	T6Ø.3X1	T6Ø.3X2	T6Ø.3X3	T6Ø.3X4	—	—
Bromperidol	T43.4X1	T43.4X2	T43.4X3	T43.4X4	T43.4X5	T43.4X6
Brompheniramine	T45.ØX1	T45.ØX2	T45.ØX3	T45.ØX4	T45.ØX5	T45.ØX6
Bromsulfophthalein	T5Ø.8X1	T5Ø.8X2	T5Ø.8X3	T5Ø.8X4	T5Ø.8X5	T5Ø.8X6
Bromural	T42.6X1	T42.6X2	T42.6X3	T42.6X4	T42.6X5	T42.6X6
Bromvaletone	T42.6X1	T42.6X2	T42.6X3	T42.6X4	T42.6X5	T42.6X6
Bronchodilator NEC	T48.6X1	T48.6X2	T48.6X3	T48.6X4	T48.6X5	T48.6X6
Brotizolam	T42.4X1	T42.4X2	T42.4X3	T42.4X4	T42.4X5	T42.4X6
Brovincamine	T46.7X1	T46.7X2	T46.7X3	T46.7X4	T46.7X5	T46.7X6
Brown recluse spider (bite) (venom)	T63.331	T63.332	T63.333	T63.334	—	—
Brown spider (bite) (venom)	T63.391	T63.392	T63.393	T63.394	—	—
Broxaterol	T48.6X1	T48.6X2	T48.6X3	T48.6X4	T48.6X5	T48.6X6
Broxuridine	T45.1X1	T45.1X2	T45.1X3	T45.1X4	T45.1X5	T45.1X6
Broxyquinoline	T37.8X1	T37.8X2	T37.8X3	T37.8X4	T37.8X5	T37.8X6
Bruceine	T48.291	T48.292	T48.293	T48.294	T48.295	T48.296
Brucia	T62.2X1	T62.2X2	T62.2X3	T62.2X4	—	—
Brucine	T65.1X1	T65.1X2	T65.1X3	T65.1X4	—	—
Brunswick green — *see* Copper						
Bruten — *see* Ibuprofen						
Bryonia	T47.2X1	T47.2X2	T47.2X3	T47.2X4	T47.2X5	T47.2X6
Buclizine	T45.ØX1	T45.ØX2	T45.ØX3	T45.ØX4	T45.ØX5	T45.ØX6
Buclosamide	T49.ØX1	T49.ØX2	T49.ØX3	T49.ØX4	T49.ØX5	T49.ØX6
Budesonide	T44.5X1	T44.5X2	T44.5X3	T44.5X4	T44.5X5	T44.5X6
Budralazine	T46.5X1	T46.5X2	T46.5X3	T46.5X4	T46.5X5	T46.5X6
Bufferin	T39.Ø11	T39.Ø12	T39.Ø13	T39.Ø14	T39.Ø15	T39.Ø16
Buflomedil	T46.7X1	T46.7X2	T46.7X3	T46.7X4	T46.7X5	T46.7X6
Buformin	T38.3X1	T38.3X2	T38.3X3	T38.3X4	T38.3X5	T38.3X6
Bufotenine	T4Ø.991	T4Ø.992	T4Ø.993	T4Ø.994	—	—
Bufrolin	T48.6X1	T48.6X2	T48.6X3	T48.6X4	T48.6X5	T48.6X6
Bufylline	T48.6X1	T48.6X2	T48.6X3	T48.6X4	T48.6X5	T48.6X6
Bulgaricum IB*	T47.6X1	T47.6X2	T47.6X3	T47.6X4	T47.6X5	T47.6X6
Bulk filler	T5Ø.5X1	T5Ø.5X2	T5Ø.5X3	T5Ø.5X4	T5Ø.5X5	T5Ø.5X6
cathartic	T47.4X1	T47.4X2	T47.4X3	T47.4X4	T47.4X5	T47.4X6
Bumetanide	T5Ø.1X1	T5Ø.1X2	T5Ø.1X3	T5Ø.1X4	T5Ø.1X5	T5Ø.1X6
Bunaftine	T46.2X1	T46.2X2	T46.2X3	T46.2X4	T46.2X5	T46.2X6
Bunamiodyl	T5Ø.8X1	T5Ø.8X2	T5Ø.8X3	T5Ø.8X4	T5Ø.8X5	T5Ø.8X6
Bunazosin	T44.6X1	T44.6X2	T44.6X3	T44.6X4	T44.6X5	T44.6X6
Bunitrolol	T44.7X1	T44.7X2	T44.7X3	T44.7X4	T44.7X5	T44.7X6
Buphenine	T46.7X1	T46.7X2	T46.7X3	T46.7X4	T46.7X5	T46.7X6
Bupivacaine	T41.3X1	T41.3X2	T41.3X3	T41.3X4	T41.3X5	T41.3X6
infiltration (subcutaneous)	T41.3X1	T41.3X2	T41.3X3	T41.3X4	T41.3X5	T41.3X6
nerve block (peripheral) (plexus)	T41.3X1	T41.3X2	T41.3X3	T41.3X4	T41.3X5	T41.3X6
spinal	T41.3X1	T41.3X2	T41.3X3	T41.3X4	T41.3X5	T41.3X6
Bupranolol	T44.7X1	T44.7X2	T44.7X3	T44.7X4	T44.7X5	T44.7X6
Buprenorphine	T4Ø.491	T4Ø.492	T4Ø.493	T4Ø.494	T4Ø.495	T4Ø.496
Bupropion	T43.291	T43.292	T43.293	T43.294	T43.295	T43.296
Burimamide	T47.1X1	T47.1X2	T47.1X3	T47.1X4	T47.1X5	T47.1X6
Buserelin	T38.891	T38.892	T38.893	T38.894	T38.895	T38.896
Buspirone	T43.591	T43.592	T43.593	T43.594	T43.595	T43.596
Busulfan, busulphan	T45.1X1	T45.1X2	T45.1X3	T45.1X4	T45.1X5	T45.1X6
Busulfex*	T45.1X1	T45.1X2	T45.1X3	T45.1X4	T45.1X5	T45.1X6
Butabarbital (sodium)	T42.3X1	T42.3X2	T42.3X3	T42.3X4	T42.3X5	T42.3X6
Butabarbitone	T42.3X1	T42.3X2	T42.3X3	T42.3X4	T42.3X5	T42.3X6
Butabarpal	T42.3X1	T42.3X2	T42.3X3	T42.3X4	T42.3X5	T42.3X6
Butacaine	T41.3X1	T41.3X2	T41.3X3	T41.3X4	T41.3X5	T41.3X6

Substance	Poisoning, Accidental (unintentional)	Poisoning, Intentional Self-harm	Poisoning, Assault	Poisoning, Undetermined	Adverse Effect	Under-dosing
Butalamine	T46.7X1	T46.7X2	T46.7X3	T46.7X4	T46.7X5	T46.7X6
Butalbital	T42.3X1	T42.3X2	T42.3X3	T42.3X4	T42.3X5	T42.3X6
Butallylonal	T42.3X1	T42.3X2	T42.3X3	T42.3X4	T42.3X5	T42.3X6
Butamben	T41.3X1	T41.3X2	T41.3X3	T41.3X4	T41.3X5	T41.3X6
Butamirate	T48.3X1	T48.3X2	T48.3X3	T48.3X4	T48.3X5	T48.3X6
Butane (distributed in mobile container)	T59.891	T59.892	T59.893	T59.894	—	—
distributed through pipes	T59.891	T59.892	T59.893	T59.894	—	—
incomplete combustion	T58.11	T58.12	T58.13	T58.14	—	—
Butanilicaine	T41.3X1	T41.3X2	T41.3X3	T41.3X4	T41.3X5	T41.3X6
Butanol	T51.3X1	T51.3X2	T51.3X3	T51.3X4	—	—
Butanone, 2-butanone	T52.4X1	T52.4X2	T52.4X3	T52.4X4	—	—
Butantrone	T49.4X1	T49.4X2	T49.4X3	T49.4X4	T49.4X5	T49.4X6
Butaperazine	T43.3X1	T43.3X2	T43.3X3	T43.3X4	T43.3X5	T43.3X6
Butazolidin	T39.2X1	T39.2X2	T39.2X3	T39.2X4	T39.2X5	T39.2X6
Butetamate	T48.6X1	T48.6X2	T48.6X3	T48.6X4	T48.6X5	T48.6X6
Butethal	T42.3X1	T42.3X2	T42.3X3	T42.3X4	T42.3X5	T42.3X6
Butethamate	T44.3X1	T44.3X2	T44.3X3	T44.3X4	T44.3X5	T44.3X6
Buthalitone (sodium)	T41.1X1	T41.1X2	T41.1X3	T41.1X4	T41.1X5	T41.1X6
Butisol (sodium)	T42.3X1	T42.3X2	T42.3X3	T42.3X4	T42.3X5	T42.3X6
Butizide	T5Ø.2X1	T5Ø.2X2	T5Ø.2X3	T5Ø.2X4	T5Ø.2X5	T5Ø.2X6
Butobarbital	T42.3X1	T42.3X2	T42.3X3	T42.3X4	T42.3X5	T42.3X6
sodium	T42.3X1	T42.3X2	T42.3X3	T42.3X4	T42.3X5	T42.3X6
Butobarbitone	T42.3X1	T42.3X2	T42.3X3	T42.3X4	T42.3X5	T42.3X6
Butoconazole (nitrate)	T49.ØX1	T49.ØX2	T49.ØX3	T49.ØX4	T49.ØX5	T49.ØX6
Butorphanol	T4Ø.491	T4Ø.492	T4Ø.493	T4Ø.494	T4Ø.495	T4Ø.496
Butriptyline	T43.Ø11	T43.Ø12	T43.Ø13	T43.Ø14	T43.Ø15	T43.Ø16
Butropium bromide	T44.3X1	T44.3X2	T44.3X3	T44.3X4	T44.3X5	T44.3X6
Buttercups	T62.2X1	T62.2X2	T62.2X3	T62.2X4	—	—
Butter of antimony — *see* Antimony						
Butyl						
acetate (secondary)	T52.8X1	T52.8X2	T52.8X3	T52.8X4	—	—
alcohol	T51.3X1	T51.3X2	T51.3X3	T51.3X4	—	—
aminobenzoate	T41.3X1	T41.3X2	T41.3X3	T41.3X4	T41.3X5	T41.3X6
butyrate	T52.8X1	T52.8X2	T52.8X3	T52.8X4	—	—
carbinol	T51.3X1	T51.3X2	T51.3X3	T51.3X4	—	—
carbitol	T52.3X1	T52.3X2	T52.3X3	T52.3X4	—	—
cellosolve	T52.3X1	T52.3X2	T52.3X3	T52.3X4	—	—
chloral (hydrate)	T42.6X1	T42.6X2	T42.6X3	T42.6X4	T42.6X5	T42.6X6
formate	T52.8X1	T52.8X2	T52.8X3	T52.8X4	—	—
lactate	T52.8X1	T52.8X2	T52.8X3	T52.8X4	—	—
propionate	T52.8X1	T52.8X2	T52.8X3	T52.8X4	—	—
scopolamine bromide	T44.3X1	T44.3X2	T44.3X3	T44.3X4	T44.3X5	T44.3X6
thiobarbital sodium	T41.1X1	T41.1X2	T41.1X3	T41.1X4	T41.1X5	T41.1X6
Butylated hydroxyanisole	T5Ø.991	T5Ø.992	T5Ø.993	T5Ø.994	T5Ø.995	T5Ø.996
Butylchloral hydrate	T42.6X1	T42.6X2	T42.6X3	T42.6X4	T42.6X5	T42.6X6
Butyltoluene	T52.2X1	T52.2X2	T52.2X3	T52.2X4	—	—
Butyn	T41.3X1	T41.3X2	T41.3X3	T41.3X4	T41.3X5	T41.3X6
Butyrophenone (-based tranquilizers)	T43.4X1	T43.4X2	T43.4X3	T43.4X4	T43.4X5	T43.4X6
Cabazitaxel*	T45.1X1	T45.1X2	T45.1X3	T45.1X4	T45.1X5	T45.1X6
Cabergoline	T42.8X1	T42.8X2	T42.8X3	T42.8X4	T42.8X5	T42.8X6
Cacodyl, cacodylic acid	T57.ØX1	T57.ØX2	T57.ØX3	T57.ØX4	—	—
Cactinomycin	T45.1X1	T45.1X2	T45.1X3	T45.1X4	T45.1X5	T45.1X6
Cade oil	T49.4X1	T49.4X2	T49.4X3	T49.4X4	T49.4X5	T49.4X6
Cadexomer iodine	T49.ØX1	T49.ØX2	T49.ØX3	T49.ØX4	T49.ØX5	T49.ØX6
Cadmium (chloride) (fumes) (oxide)	T56.3X1	T56.3X2	T56.3X3	T56.3X4	—	—
sulfide (medicinal) NEC	T49.4X1	T49.4X2	T49.4X3	T49.4X4	T49.4X5	T49.4X6
Cadralazine	T46.5X1	T46.5X2	T46.5X3	T46.5X4	T46.5X5	T46.5X6
Caffeine	T43.611	T43.612	T43.613	T43.614	T43.615	T43.616
Calabar bean	T62.2X1	T62.2X2	T62.2X3	T62.2X4	—	—
Caladium seguinum	T62.2X1	T62.2X2	T62.2X3	T62.2X4	—	—
Calamine (lotion)	T49.3X1	T49.3X2	T49.3X3	T49.3X4	T49.3X5	T49.3X6
Calcifediol	T45.2X1	T45.2X2	T45.2X3	T45.2X4	T45.2X5	T45.2X6
Calciferol	T45.2X1	T45.2X2	T45.2X3	T45.2X4	T45.2X5	T45.2X6
Calcijex*	T45.2X1	T45.2X2	T45.2X3	T45.2X4	T45.2X5	T45.2X6
Calcitonin	T5Ø.991	T5Ø.992	T5Ø.993	T5Ø.994	T5Ø.995	T5Ø.996
Calcitriol	T45.2X1	T45.2X2	T45.2X3	T45.2X4	T45.2X5	T45.2X6
Calcium	T5Ø.3X1	T5Ø.3X2	T5Ø.3X3	T5Ø.3X4	T5Ø.3X5	T5Ø.3X6
actylsalicylate	T39.Ø11	T39.Ø12	T39.Ø13	T39.Ø14	T39.Ø15	T39.Ø16
benzamidosalicylate	T37.1X1	T37.1X2	T37.1X3	T37.1X4	T37.1X5	T37.1X6
bromide	T42.6X1	T42.6X2	T42.6X3	T42.6X4	T42.6X5	T42.6X6
bromolactobionate	T42.6X1	T42.6X2	T42.6X3	T42.6X4	T42.6X5	T42.6X6
carbaspirin	T39.Ø11	T39.Ø12	T39.Ø13	T39.Ø14	T39.Ø15	T39.Ø16
carbimide	T5Ø.6X1	T5Ø.6X2	T5Ø.6X3	T5Ø.6X4	T5Ø.6X5	T5Ø.6X6
carbonate	T47.1X1	T47.1X2	T47.1X3	T47.1X4	T47.1X5	T47.1X6
chloride	T5Ø.991	T5Ø.992	T5Ø.993	T5Ø.994	T5Ø.995	T5Ø.996
anhydrous	T5Ø.991	T5Ø.992	T5Ø.993	T5Ø.994	T5Ø.995	T5Ø.996
cyanide	T57.8X1	T57.8X2	T57.8X3	T57.8X4	—	—
dioctyl sulfosuccinate	T47.4X1	T47.4X2	T47.4X3	T47.4X4	T47.4X5	T47.4X6
disodium edathamil	T45.8X1	T45.8X2	T45.8X3	T45.8X4	T45.8X5	T45.8X6
Calcium — *continued*						
disodium edetate	T45.8X1	T45.8X2	T45.8X3	T45.8X4	T45.8X5	T45.8X6
dobesilate	T46.991	T46.992	T46.993	T46.994	T46.995	T46.996
EDTA	T45.8X1	T45.8X2	T45.8X3	T45.8X4	T45.8X5	T45.8X6
ferrous citrate	T45.4X1	T45.4X2	T45.4X3	T45.4X4	T45.4X5	T45.4X6
folinate	T45.8X1	T45.8X2	T45.8X3	T45.8X4	T45.8X5	T45.8X6
glubionate	T5Ø.3X1	T5Ø.3X2	T5Ø.3X3	T5Ø.3X4	T5Ø.3X5	T5Ø.3X6
gluconate	T5Ø.3X1	T5Ø.3X2	T5Ø.3X3	T5Ø.3X4	T5Ø.3X5	T5Ø.3X6
gluconogalactogluconate	T5Ø.3X1	T5Ø.3X2	T5Ø.3X3	T5Ø.3X4	T5Ø.3X5	T5Ø.3X6
hydrate, hydroxide	T54.3X1	T54.3X2	T54.3X3	T54.3X4	—	—
hypochlorite	T54.3X1	T54.3X2	T54.3X3	T54.3X4	—	—
iodide	T48.4X1	T48.4X2	T48.4X3	T48.4X4	T48.4X5	T48.4X6
ipodate	T5Ø.8X1	T5Ø.8X2	T5Ø.8X3	T5Ø.8X4	T5Ø.8X5	T5Ø.8X6
lactate	T5Ø.3X1	T5Ø.3X2	T5Ø.3X3	T5Ø.3X4	T5Ø.3X5	T5Ø.3X6
leucovorin	T45.8X1	T45.8X2	T45.8X3	T45.8X4	T45.8X5	T45.8X6
mandelate	T37.91	T37.92	T37.93	T37.94	T37.95	T37.96
oxide	T54.3X1	T54.3X2	T54.3X3	T54.3X4	—	—
pantothenate	T45.2X1	T45.2X2	T45.2X3	T45.2X4	T45.2X5	T45.2X6
phosphate	T5Ø.3X1	T5Ø.3X2	T5Ø.3X3	T5Ø.3X4	T5Ø.3X5	T5Ø.3X6
salicylate	T39.Ø91	T39.Ø92	T39.Ø93	T39.Ø94	T39.Ø95	T39.Ø96
salts	T5Ø.3X1	T5Ø.3X2	T5Ø.3X3	T5Ø.3X4	T5Ø.3X5	T5Ø.3X6
Calculus-dissolving drug	T5Ø.991	T5Ø.992	T5Ø.993	T5Ø.994	T5Ø.995	T5Ø.996
Calomel	T49.ØX1	T49.ØX2	T49.ØX3	T49.ØX4	T49.ØX5	T49.ØX6
Caloric agent	T5Ø.3X1	T5Ø.3X2	T5Ø.3X3	T5Ø.3X4	T5Ø.3X5	T5Ø.3X6
Calusterone	T38.7X1	T38.7X2	T38.7X3	T38.7X4	T38.7X5	T38.7X6
Camazepam	T42.4X1	T42.4X2	T42.4X3	T42.4X4	T42.4X5	T42.4X6
Camomile	T49.ØX1	T49.ØX2	T49.ØX3	T49.ØX4	T49.ØX5	T49.ØX6
Camoquin	T37.2X1	T37.2X2	T37.2X3	T37.2X4	T37.2X5	T37.2X6
Camphor						
insecticide	T6Ø.2X1	T6Ø.2X2	T6Ø.2X3	T6Ø.2X4	—	—
medicinal	T49.8X1	T49.8X2	T49.8X3	T49.8X4	T49.8X5	T49.8X6
Camylofin	T44.3X1	T44.3X2	T44.3X3	T44.3X4	T44.3X5	T44.3X6
Cancer chemotherapy drug regimen	T45.1X1	T45.1X2	T45.1X3	T45.1X4	T45.1X5	T45.1X6
Candeptin	T49.ØX1	T49.ØX2	T49.ØX3	T49.ØX4	T49.ØX5	T49.ØX6
Candicidin	T49.ØX1	T49.ØX2	T49.ØX3	T49.ØX4	T49.ØX5	T49.ØX6
Cankaid*	T49.6X1	T49.6X2	T49.6X3	T49.6X4	T49.6X5	T49.6X6
Cannabinoids, synthetic	T4Ø.721	T4Ø.722	T4Ø.723	T4Ø.724	T4Ø.725	T4Ø.726
Cannabinol	T4Ø.711	T4Ø.712	T4Ø.713	T4Ø.714	T4Ø.715	T4Ø.716
Cannabis (derivatives)	T4Ø.711	T4Ø.712	T4Ø.713	T4Ø.714	T4Ø.715	T4Ø.716
Canned heat	T51.1X1	T51.1X2	T51.1X3	T51.1X4	—	—
Canrenoic acid	T5Ø.ØX1	T5Ø.ØX2	T5Ø.ØX3	T5Ø.ØX4	T5Ø.ØX5	T5Ø.ØX6
Canrenone	T5Ø.ØX1	T5Ø.ØX2	T5Ø.ØX3	T5Ø.ØX4	T5Ø.ØX5	T5Ø.ØX6
Cantharides, cantharidin, cantharis	T49.8X1	T49.8X2	T49.8X3	T49.8X4	T49.8X5	T49.8X6
Canthaxanthin	T5Ø.991	T5Ø.992	T5Ø.993	T5Ø.994	T5Ø.995	T5Ø.996
Capillary-active drug NEC	T46.9Ø1	T46.9Ø2	T46.9Ø3	T46.9Ø4	T46.9Ø5	T46.9Ø6
Capreomycin	T36.8X1	T36.8X2	T36.8X3	T36.8X4	T36.8X5	T36.8X6
Capresla*	T45.1X1	T45.1X2	T45.1X3	T45.1X4	T45.1X5	T45.1X6
Capsicum	T49.4X1	T49.4X2	T49.4X3	T49.4X4	T49.4X5	T49.4X6
Captafol	T6Ø.3X1	T6Ø.3X2	T6Ø.3X3	T6Ø.3X4	—	—
Captan	T6Ø.3X1	T6Ø.3X2	T6Ø.3X3	T6Ø.3X4	—	—
Captodiame, captodiamine	T43.591	T43.592	T43.593	T43.594	T43.595	T43.596
Captopril	T46.4X1	T46.4X2	T46.4X3	T46.4X4	T46.4X5	T46.4X6
Caramiphen	T44.3X1	T44.3X2	T44.3X3	T44.3X4	T44.3X5	T44.3X6
Carazolol	T44.7X1	T44.7X2	T44.7X3	T44.7X4	T44.7X5	T44.7X6
Carbachol	T44.1X1	T44.1X2	T44.1X3	T44.1X4	T44.1X5	T44.1X6
Carbacrylamine (resin)	T5Ø.3X1	T5Ø.3X2	T5Ø.3X3	T5Ø.3X4	T5Ø.3X5	T5Ø.3X6
Carbamate (insecticide)	T6Ø.ØX1	T6Ø.ØX2	T6Ø.ØX3	T6Ø.ØX4	—	—
Carbamate (sedative)	T42.6X1	T42.6X2	T42.6X3	T42.6X4	T42.6X5	T42.6X6
herbicide	T6Ø.ØX1	T6Ø.ØX2	T6Ø.ØX3	T6Ø.ØX4	—	—
insecticide	T6Ø.ØX1	T6Ø.ØX2	T6Ø.ØX3	T6Ø.ØX4	—	—
Carbamazepine	T42.1X1	T42.1X2	T42.1X3	T42.1X4	T42.1X5	T42.1X6
Carbamide	T47.3X1	T47.3X2	T47.3X3	T47.3X4	T47.3X5	T47.3X6
peroxide	T49.ØX1	T49.ØX2	T49.ØX3	T49.ØX4	T49.ØX5	T49.ØX6
topical	T49.8X1	T49.8X2	T49.8X3	T49.8X4	T49.8X5	T49.8X6
Carbamylcholine chloride	T44.1X1	T44.1X2	T44.1X3	T44.1X4	T44.1X5	T44.1X6
Carbaril	T6Ø.ØX1	T6Ø.ØX2	T6Ø.ØX3	T6Ø.ØX4	—	—
Carbarsone	T37.3X1	T37.3X2	T37.3X3	T37.3X4	T37.3X5	T37.3X6
Carbaryl	T6Ø.ØX1	T6Ø.ØX2	T6Ø.ØX3	T6Ø.ØX4	—	—
Carbaspirin	T39.Ø11	T39.Ø12	T39.Ø13	T39.Ø14	T39.Ø15	T39.Ø16
Carbastat*	T49.5X1	T49.5X2	T49.5X3	T49.5X4	T49.5X5	T49.5X6
Carbazochrome (salicylate) (sodium sulfonate)	T49.4X1	T49.4X2	T49.4X3	T49.4X4	T49.4X5	T49.4X6
Carbenicillin	T36.ØX1	T36.ØX2	T36.ØX3	T36.ØX4	T36.ØX5	T36.ØX6
Carbenoxolone	T47.1X1	T47.1X2	T47.1X3	T47.1X4	T47.1X5	T47.1X6
Carbetapentane	T48.3X1	T48.3X2	T48.3X3	T48.3X4	T48.3X5	T48.3X6
Carbethyl salicylate	T39.Ø91	T39.Ø92	T39.Ø93	T39.Ø94	T39.Ø95	T39.Ø96
Carbidopa (with levodopa)	T42.8X1	T42.8X2	T42.8X3	T42.8X4	T42.8X5	T42.8X6
Carbimazole	T38.2X1	T38.2X2	T38.2X3	T38.2X4	T38.2X5	T38.2X6
Carbinol	T51.1X1	T51.1X2	T51.1X3	T51.1X4	—	—
Carbinoxamine	T45.ØX1	T45.ØX2	T45.ØX3	T45.ØX4	T45.ØX5	T45.ØX6

Substance	Poisoning, Accidental (unintentional)	Poisoning, Intentional Self-harm	Poisoning, Assault	Poisoning, Undetermined	Adverse Effect	Under-dosing
Carbiphene	T39.8X1	T39.8X2	T39.8X3	T39.8X4	T39.8X5	T39.8X6
Carbitol	T52.3X1	T52.3X2	T52.3X3	T52.3X4	—	—
Carbocaine	T41.3X1	T41.3X2	T41.3X3	T41.3X4	T41.3X5	T41.3X6
infiltration (subcutaneous)	T41.3X1	T41.3X2	T41.3X3	T41.3X4	T41.3X5	T41.3X6
nerve block (peripheral) (plexus)	T41.3X1	T41.3X2	T41.3X3	T41.3X4	T41.3X5	T41.3X6
topical (surface)	T41.3X1	T41.3X2	T41.3X3	T41.3X4	T41.3X5	T41.3X6
Carbocisteine	T48.4X1	T48.4X2	T48.4X3	T48.4X4	T48.4X5	T48.4X6
Carbocromen	T46.3X1	T46.3X2	T46.3X3	T46.3X4	T46.3X5	T46.3X6
Carbol fuchsin	T49.ØX1	T49.ØX2	T49.ØX3	T49.ØX4	T49.ØX5	T49.ØX6
Carbolic acid — *see also* Phenol	T54.ØX1	T54.ØX2	T54.ØX3	T54.ØX4	—	—
Carbolonium (bromide)	T48.1X1	T48.1X2	T48.1X3	T48.1X4	T48.1X5	T48.1X6
Carbo medicinalis	T47.6X1	T47.6X2	T47.6X3	T47.6X4	T47.6X5	T47.6X6
Carbomycin	T36.8X1	T36.8X2	T36.8X3	T36.8X4	T36.8X5	T36.8X6
Carbon						
bisulfide (liquid)	T65.4X1	T65.4X2	T65.4X3	T65.4X4	—	—
vapor	T65.4X1	T65.4X2	T65.4X3	T65.4X4	—	—
dioxide (gas)	T59.7X1	T59.7X2	T59.7X3	T59.7X4	—	—
medicinal	T41.5X1	T41.5X2	T41.5X3	T41.5X4	T41.5X5	T41.5X6
nonmedicinal	T59.7X1	T59.7X2	T59.7X3	T59.7X4	—	—
snow	T49.4X1	T49.4X2	T49.4X3	T49.4X4	T49.4X5	T49.4X6
disulfide (liquid)	T65.4X1	T65.4X2	T65.4X3	T65.4X4	—	—
vapor	T65.4X1	T65.4X2	T65.4X3	T65.4X4	—	—
monoxide (from incomplete combustion)	T58.91	T58.92	T58.93	T58.94	—	—
blast furnace gas	T58.8X1	T58.8X2	T58.8X3	T58.8X4	—	—
butane (distributed in mobile container)	T58.11	T58.12	T58.13	T58.14	—	—
distributed through pipes	T58.11	T58.12	T58.13	T58.14	—	—
charcoal fumes	T58.2X1	T58.2X2	T58.2X3	T58.2X4	—	—
coal	T58.2X1	T58.2X2	T58.2X3	T58.2X4	—	—
coke (in domestic stoves, fireplaces)	T58.2X1	T58.2X2	T58.2X3	T58.2X4	—	—
exhaust gas (motor) not in transit	T58.Ø1	T58.Ø2	T58.Ø3	T58.Ø4	—	—
combustion engine, any not in watercraft	T58.Ø1	T58.Ø2	T58.Ø3	T58.Ø4	—	—
farm tractor, not in transit	T58.Ø1	T58.Ø2	T58.Ø3	T58.Ø4	—	—
gas engine	T58.Ø1	T58.Ø2	T58.Ø3	T58.Ø4	—	—
motor pump	T58.Ø1	T58.Ø2	T58.Ø3	T58.Ø4	—	—
motor vehicle, not in transit	T58.Ø1	T58.Ø2	T58.Ø3	T58.Ø4	—	—
fuel (in domestic use)	T58.2X1	T58.2X2	T58.2X3	T58.2X4	—	—
gas (piped)	T58.11	T58.12	T58.13	T58.14	—	—
in mobile container	T58.11	T58.12	T58.13	T58.14	—	—
piped (natural)	T58.11	T58.12	T58.13	T58.14	—	—
utility	T58.11	T58.12	T58.13	T58.14	—	—
in mobile container	T58.11	T58.12	T58.13	T58.14	—	—
gas (piped)	T58.11	T58.12	T58.13	T58.14	—	—
illuminating gas	T58.11	T58.12	T58.13	T58.14	—	—
industrial fuels or gases, any	T58.8X1	T58.8X2	T58.8X3	T58.8X4	—	—
kerosene (in domestic stoves, fireplaces)	T58.2X1	T58.2X2	T58.2X3	T58.2X4	—	—
kiln gas or vapor	T58.8X1	T58.8X2	T58.8X3	T58.8X4	—	—
motor exhaust gas, not in transit	T58.Ø1	T58.Ø2	T58.Ø3	T58.Ø4	—	—
piped gas (manufactured) (natural)	T58.11	T58.12	T58.13	T58.14	—	—
producer gas	T58.8X1	T58.8X2	T58.8X3	T58.8X4	—	—
propane (distributed in mobile container)	T58.11	T58.12	T58.13	T58.14	—	—
distributed through pipes	T58.11	T58.12	T58.13	T58.14	—	—
solid (in domestic stoves, fireplaces)	T58.2X1	T58.2X2	T58.2X3	T58.2X4	—	—
specified source NEC	T58.8X1	T58.8X2	T58.8X3	T58.8X4	—	—
stove gas	T58.11	T58.12	T58.13	T58.14	—	—
piped	T58.11	T58.12	T58.13	T58.14	—	—
utility gas	T58.11	T58.12	T58.13	T58.14	—	—
piped	T58.11	T58.12	T58.13	T58.14	—	—
water gas	T58.11	T58.12	T58.13	T58.14	—	—
wood (in domestic stoves, fireplaces)	T58.2X1	T58.2X2	T58.2X3	T58.2X4	—	—
tetrachloride (vapor) NEC	T53.ØX1	T53.ØX2	T53.ØX3	T53.ØX4	—	—
liquid (cleansing agent) NEC	T53.ØX1	T53.ØX2	T53.ØX3	T53.ØX4	—	—
solvent	T53.ØX1	T53.ØX2	T53.ØX3	T53.ØX4	—	—
Carbonic acid gas	T59.7X1	T59.7X2	T59.7X3	T59.7X4	—	—
anhydrase inhibitor NEC	T5Ø.2X1	T5Ø.2X2	T5Ø.2X3	T5Ø.2X4	T5Ø.2X5	T5Ø.2X6

Substance	Poisoning, Accidental (unintentional)	Poisoning, Intentional Self-harm	Poisoning, Assault	Poisoning, Undetermined	Adverse Effect	Under-dosing
Carbophenothion	T6Ø.ØX1	T6Ø.ØX2	T6Ø.ØX3	T6Ø.ØX4	—	—
Carboplatin	T45.1X1	T45.1X2	T45.1X3	T45.1X4	T45.1X5	T45.1X6
Carboprost	T48.ØX1	T48.ØX2	T48.ØX3	T48.ØX4	T48.ØX5	T48.ØX6
Carboquone	T45.1X1	T45.1X2	T45.1X3	T45.1X4	T45.1X5	T45.1X6
Carbowax	T49.3X1	T49.3X2	T49.3X3	T49.3X4	T49.3X5	T49.3X6
Carboxymethylcellulose	T47.4X1	T47.4X2	T47.4X3	T47.4X4	T47.4X5	T47.4X6
Carbrital	T42.3X1	T42.3X2	T42.3X3	T42.3X4	T42.3X5	T42.3X6
Carbromal	T42.6X1	T42.6X2	T42.6X3	T42.6X4	T42.6X5	T42.6X6
Carbutamide	T38.3X1	T38.3X2	T38.3X3	T38.3X4	T38.3X5	T38.3X6
Carbuterol	T48.6X1	T48.6X2	T48.6X3	T48.6X4	T48.6X5	T48.6X6
Cardiac						
depressants	T46.2X1	T46.2X2	T46.2X3	T46.2X4	T46.2X5	T46.2X6
rhythm regulator	T46.2X1	T46.2X2	T46.2X3	T46.2X4	T46.2X5	T46.2X6
specified NEC	T46.2X1	T46.2X2	T46.2X3	T46.2X4	T46.2X5	T46.2X6
Cardiografin	T5Ø.8X1	T5Ø.8X2	T5Ø.8X3	T5Ø.8X4	T5Ø.8X5	T5Ø.8X6
Cardiogreen	T5Ø.8X1	T5Ø.8X2	T5Ø.8X3	T5Ø.8X4	T5Ø.8X5	T5Ø.8X6
Cardiotonic (glycoside) **NEC**	T46.ØX1	T46.ØX2	T46.ØX3	T46.ØX4	T46.ØX5	T46.ØX6
Cardiovascular drug NEC	T46.9Ø1	T46.9Ø2	T46.9Ø3	T46.9Ø4	T46.9Ø5	T46.9Ø6
Cardizem*	T46.1X1	T46.1X2	T46.1X3	T46.1X4	T46.1X5	T46.1X6
Cardrase	T5Ø.2X1	T5Ø.2X2	T5Ø.2X3	T5Ø.2X4	T5Ø.2X5	T5Ø.2X6
Carfecillin	T36.ØX1	T36.ØX2	T36.ØX3	T36.ØX4	T36.ØX5	T36.ØX6
Carfenazine	T43.3X1	T43.3X2	T43.3X3	T43.3X4	T43.3X5	T43.3X6
Carfusin	T49.ØX1	T49.ØX2	T49.ØX3	T49.ØX4	T49.ØX5	T49.ØX6
Carindacillin	T36.ØX1	T36.ØX2	T36.ØX3	T36.ØX4	T36.ØX5	T36.ØX6
Carisoprodol	T42.8X1	T42.8X2	T42.8X3	T42.8X4	T42.8X5	T42.8X6
Carmellose	T47.4X1	T47.4X2	T47.4X3	T47.4X4	T47.4X5	T47.4X6
Carminative	T47.5X1	T47.5X2	T47.5X3	T47.5X4	T47.5X5	T47.5X6
Carmofur	T45.1X1	T45.1X2	T45.1X3	T45.1X4	T45.1X5	T45.1X6
Carmustine	T45.1X1	T45.1X2	T45.1X3	T45.1X4	T45.1X5	T45.1X6
Carotene	T45.2X1	T45.2X2	T45.2X3	T45.2X4	T45.2X5	T45.2X6
Carphenazine	T43.3X1	T43.3X2	T43.3X3	T43.3X4	T43.3X5	T43.3X6
Carpipramine	T42.4X1	T42.4X2	T42.4X3	T42.4X4	T42.4X5	T42.4X6
Carprofen	T39.311	T39.312	T39.313	T39.314	T39.315	T39.316
Carpronium chloride	T44.3X1	T44.3X2	T44.3X3	T44.3X4	T44.3X5	T44.3X6
Carrageenan	T47.8X1	T47.8X2	T47.8X3	T47.8X4	T47.8X5	T47.8X6
Carteolol	T44.7X1	T44.7X2	T44.7X3	T44.7X4	T44.7X5	T44.7X6
Carter's Little Pills	T47.2X1	T47.2X2	T47.2X3	T47.2X4	T47.2X5	T47.2X6
Cartia*	T46.1X1	T46.1X2	T46.1X3	T46.1X4	T46.1X5	T46.1X6
Cascara (sagrada)	T47.2X1	T47.2X2	T47.2X3	T47.2X4	T47.2X5	T47.2X6
Cassava	T62.2X1	T62.2X2	T62.2X3	T62.2X4	—	—
Castellani's paint	T49.ØX1	T49.ØX2	T49.ØX3	T49.ØX4	T49.ØX5	T49.ØX6
Castor						
bean	T62.2X1	T62.2X2	T62.2X3	T62.2X4	—	—
oil	T47.2X1	T47.2X2	T47.2X3	T47.2X4	T47.2X5	T47.2X6
Catalase	T45.3X1	T45.3X2	T45.3X3	T45.3X4	T45.3X5	T45.3X6
Caterpillar (sting)	T63.431	T63.432	T63.433	T63.434	—	—
Catha (edulis) (tea)	T43.691	T43.692	T43.693	T43.694	—	—
Cathartic NEC	T47.4X1	T47.4X2	T47.4X3	T47.4X4	T47.4X5	T47.4X6
anthacene derivative	T47.2X1	T47.2X2	T47.2X3	T47.2X4	T47.2X5	T47.2X6
bulk	T47.4X1	T47.4X2	T47.4X3	T47.4X4	T47.4X5	T47.4X6
contact	T47.2X1	T47.2X2	T47.2X3	T47.2X4	T47.2X5	T47.2X6
emollient NEC	T47.4X1	T47.4X2	T47.4X3	T47.4X4	T47.4X5	T47.4X6
irritant NEC	T47.2X1	T47.2X2	T47.2X3	T47.2X4	T47.2X5	T47.2X6
mucilage	T47.4X1	T47.4X2	T47.4X3	T47.4X4	T47.4X5	T47.4X6
saline	T47.3X1	T47.3X2	T47.3X3	T47.3X4	T47.3X5	T47.3X6
vegetable	T47.2X1	T47.2X2	T47.2X3	T47.2X4	T47.2X5	T47.2X6
Cathine	T5Ø.5X1	T5Ø.5X2	T5Ø.5X3	T5Ø.5X4	T5Ø.5X5	T5Ø.5X6
Cathomycin	T36.8X1	T36.8X2	T36.8X3	T36.8X4	T36.8X5	T36.8X6
Cation exchange resin	T5Ø.3X1	T5Ø.3X2	T5Ø.3X3	T5Ø.3X4	T5Ø.3X5	T5Ø.3X6
Caustic(s) **NEC**	T54.91	T54.92	T54.93	T54.94	—	—
alkali	T54.3X1	T54.3X2	T54.3X3	T54.3X4	—	—
hydroxide	T54.3X1	T54.3X2	T54.3X3	T54.3X4	—	—
potash	T54.3X1	T54.3X2	T54.3X3	T54.3X4	—	—
soda	T54.3X1	T54.3X2	T54.3X3	T54.3X4	—	—
specified NEC	T54.91	T54.92	T54.93	T54.94	—	—
Ceepryn	T49.ØX1	T49.ØX2	T49.ØX3	T49.ØX4	T49.ØX5	T49.ØX6
ENT agent	T49.6X1	T49.6X2	T49.6X3	T49.6X4	T49.6X5	T49.6X6
lozenges	T49.6X1	T49.6X2	T49.6X3	T49.6X4	T49.6X5	T49.6X6
Cefacetrile	T36.1X1	T36.1X2	T36.1X3	T36.1X4	T36.1X5	T36.1X6
Cefaclor	T36.1X1	T36.1X2	T36.1X3	T36.1X4	T36.1X5	T36.1X6
Cefadroxil	T36.1X1	T36.1X2	T36.1X3	T36.1X4	T36.1X5	T36.1X6
Cefalexin	T36.1X1	T36.1X2	T36.1X3	T36.1X4	T36.1X5	T36.1X6
Cefaloglycin	T36.1X1	T36.1X2	T36.1X3	T36.1X4	T36.1X5	T36.1X6
Cefaloridine	T36.1X1	T36.1X2	T36.1X3	T36.1X4	T36.1X5	T36.1X6
Cefalosporins	T36.1X1	T36.1X2	T36.1X3	T36.1X4	T36.1X5	T36.1X6
Cefalotin	T36.1X1	T36.1X2	T36.1X3	T36.1X4	T36.1X5	T36.1X6
Cefamandole	T36.1X1	T36.1X2	T36.1X3	T36.1X4	T36.1X5	T36.1X6
Cefamycin antibiotic	T36.1X1	T36.1X2	T36.1X3	T36.1X4	T36.1X5	T36.1X6
Cefapirin	T36.1X1	T36.1X2	T36.1X3	T36.1X4	T36.1X5	T36.1X6
Cefatrizine	T36.1X1	T36.1X2	T36.1X3	T36.1X4	T36.1X5	T36.1X6
Cefazedone	T36.1X1	T36.1X2	T36.1X3	T36.1X4	T36.1X5	T36.1X6
Cefazolin	T36.1X1	T36.1X2	T36.1X3	T36.1X4	T36.1X5	T36.1X6
Cefbuperazone	T36.1X1	T36.1X2	T36.1X3	T36.1X4	T36.1X5	T36.1X6

*Optum Value-Add

Substance	Poisoning, Accidental (unintentional)	Poisoning, Intentional Self-harm	Poisoning, Assault	Poisoning, Undetermined	Adverse Effect	Under-dosing
Cefetamet	T36.1X1	T36.1X2	T36.1X3	T36.1X4	T36.1X5	T36.1X6
Cefixime	T36.1X1	T36.1X2	T36.1X3	T36.1X4	T36.1X5	T36.1X6
Cefmenoxime	T36.1X1	T36.1X2	T36.1X3	T36.1X4	T36.1X5	T36.1X6
Cefmetazole	T36.1X1	T36.1X2	T36.1X3	T36.1X4	T36.1X5	T36.1X6
Cefminox	T36.1X1	T36.1X2	T36.1X3	T36.1X4	T36.1X5	T36.1X6
Cefonicid	T36.1X1	T36.1X2	T36.1X3	T36.1X4	T36.1X5	T36.1X6
Cefoperazone	T36.1X1	T36.1X2	T36.1X3	T36.1X4	T36.1X5	T36.1X6
Ceforanide	T36.1X1	T36.1X2	T36.1X3	T36.1X4	T36.1X5	T36.1X6
Cefotaxime	T36.1X1	T36.1X2	T36.1X3	T36.1X4	T36.1X5	T36.1X6
Cefotetan	T36.1X1	T36.1X2	T36.1X3	T36.1X4	T36.1X5	T36.1X6
Cefotiam	T36.1X1	T36.1X2	T36.1X3	T36.1X4	T36.1X5	T36.1X6
Cefoxitin	T36.1X1	T36.1X2	T36.1X3	T36.1X4	T36.1X5	T36.1X6
Cefpimizole	T36.1X1	T36.1X2	T36.1X3	T36.1X4	T36.1X5	T36.1X6
Cefpiramide	T36.1X1	T36.1X2	T36.1X3	T36.1X4	T36.1X5	T36.1X6
Cefradine	T36.1X1	T36.1X2	T36.1X3	T36.1X4	T36.1X5	T36.1X6
Cefroxadine	T36.1X1	T36.1X2	T36.1X3	T36.1X4	T36.1X5	T36.1X6
Cefsulodin	T36.1X1	T36.1X2	T36.1X3	T36.1X4	T36.1X5	T36.1X6
Ceftazidime	T36.1X1	T36.1X2	T36.1X3	T36.1X4	T36.1X5	T36.1X6
Cefteram	T36.1X1	T36.1X2	T36.1X3	T36.1X4	T36.1X5	T36.1X6
Ceftezole	T36.1X1	T36.1X2	T36.1X3	T36.1X4	T36.1X5	T36.1X6
Ceftin*	T36.1X1	T36.1X2	T36.1X3	T36.1X4	T36.1X5	T36.1X6
Ceftizoxime	T36.1X1	T36.1X2	T36.1X3	T36.1X4	T36.1X5	T36.1X6
Ceftriaxone	T36.1X1	T36.1X2	T36.1X3	T36.1X4	T36.1X5	T36.1X6
Cefuroxime	T36.1X1	T36.1X2	T36.1X3	T36.1X4	T36.1X5	T36.1X6
Cefuzonam	T36.1X1	T36.1X2	T36.1X3	T36.1X4	T36.1X5	T36.1X6
Celestone	T38.0X1	T38.0X2	T38.0X3	T38.0X4	T38.0X5	T38.0X6
topical	T49.0X1	T49.0X2	T49.0X3	T49.0X4	T49.0X5	T49.0X6
Celexa*	T43.221	T43.222	T43.223	T43.224	T43.225	T43.226
Celiprolol	T44.7X1	T44.7X2	T44.7X3	T44.7X4	T44.7X5	T44.7X6
Cellosolve	T52.91	T52.92	T52.93	T52.94	—	—
Cell stimulants and proliferants	T49.8X1	T49.8X2	T49.8X3	T49.8X4	T49.8X5	T49.8X6
Cellulose						
cathartic	T47.4X1	T47.4X2	T47.4X3	T47.4X4	T47.4X5	T47.4X6
hydroxyethyl	T47.4X1	T47.4X2	T47.4X3	T47.4X4	T47.4X5	T47.4X6
nitrates (topical)	T49.3X1	T49.3X2	T49.3X3	T49.3X4	T49.3X5	T49.3X6
oxidized	T49.4X1	T49.4X2	T49.4X3	T49.4X4	T49.4X5	T49.4X6
Centipede (bite)	T63.411	T63.412	T63.413	T63.414	—	—
Central nervous system						
depressants	T42.71	T42.72	T42.73	T42.74	T42.75	T42.76
anesthetic (general) NEC	T41.201	T41.202	T41.203	T41.204	T41.205	T41.206
gases NEC	T41.0X1	T41.0X2	T41.0X3	T41.0X4	T41.0X5	T41.0X6
intravenous	T41.1X1	T41.1X2	T41.1X3	T41.1X4	T41.1X5	T41.1X6
barbiturates	T42.3X1	T42.3X2	T42.3X3	T42.3X4	T42.3X5	T42.3X6
benzodiazepines	T42.4X1	T42.4X2	T42.4X3	T42.4X4	T42.4X5	T42.4X6
bromides	T42.6X1	T42.6X2	T42.6X3	T42.6X4	T42.6X5	T42.6X6
cannabis sativa	T40.711	T40.712	T40.713	T40.714	T40.715	T40.716
chloral hydrate	T42.6X1	T42.6X2	T42.6X3	T42.6X4	T42.6X5	T42.6X6
ethanol	T51.0X1	T51.0X2	T51.0X3	T51.0X4	—	—
hallucinogenics	T40.901	T40.902	T40.903	T40.904	T40.905	T40.906
hypnotics	T42.71	T42.72	T42.73	T42.74	T42.75	T42.76
specified NEC	T42.6X1	T42.6X2	T42.6X3	T42.6X4	T42.6X5	T42.6X6
muscle relaxants	T42.8X1	T42.8X2	T42.8X3	T42.8X4	T42.8X5	T42.8X6
paraldehyde	T42.6X1	T42.6X2	T42.6X3	T42.6X4	T42.6X5	T42.6X6
sedatives; sedative-hypnotics	T42.71	T42.72	T42.73	T42.74	T42.75	T42.76
mixed NEC	T42.6X1	T42.6X2	T42.6X3	T42.6X4	T42.6X5	T42.6X6
specified NEC	T42.6X1	T42.6X2	T42.6X3	T42.6X4	T42.6X5	T42.6X6
muscle-tone depressants	T42.8X1	T42.8X2	T42.8X3	T42.8X4	T42.8X5	T42.8X6
stimulants	T43.601	T43.602	T43.603	T43.604	T43.605	T43.606
amphetamines	T43.621	T43.622	T43.623	T43.624	T43.625	T43.626
analeptics	T50.7X1	T50.7X2	T50.7X3	T50.7X4	T50.7X5	T50.7X6
antidepressants	T43.201	T43.202	T43.203	T43.204	T43.205	T43.206
opiate antagonists	T50.7X1	T50.7X2	T50.7X3	T50.7X4	T50.7X5	T50.7X6
specified NEC	T43.691	T43.692	T43.693	T43.694	T43.695	T43.696
Cepacol*	T41.3X1	T41.3X2	T41.3X3	T41.3X4	T41.3X5	T41.3X6
Cephalexin	T36.1X1	T36.1X2	T36.1X3	T36.1X4	T36.1X5	T36.1X6
Cephaloglycin	T36.1X1	T36.1X2	T36.1X3	T36.1X4	T36.1X5	T36.1X6
Cephaloridine	T36.1X1	T36.1X2	T36.1X3	T36.1X4	T36.1X5	T36.1X6
Cephalosporins	T36.1X1	T36.1X2	T36.1X3	T36.1X4	T36.1X5	T36.1X6
N (adicillin)	T36.0X1	T36.0X2	T36.0X3	T36.0X4	T36.0X5	T36.0X6
Cephalothin	T36.1X1	T36.1X2	T36.1X3	T36.1X4	T36.1X5	T36.1X6
Cephalotin	T36.1X1	T36.1X2	T36.1X3	T36.1X4	T36.1X5	T36.1X6
Cephradine	T36.1X1	T36.1X2	T36.1X3	T36.1X4	T36.1X5	T36.1X6
Cerbera (odallam)	T62.2X1	T62.2X2	T62.2X3	T62.2X4	—	—
Cerberin	T46.0X1	T46.0X2	T46.0X3	T46.0X4	T46.0X5	T46.0X6
Cerebral stimulants	T43.601	T43.602	T43.603	T43.604	T43.605	T43.606
psychotherapeutic	T43.601	T43.602	T43.603	T43.604	T43.605	T43.606
specified NEC	T43.691	T43.692	T43.693	T43.694	T43.695	T43.696
Cerium oxalate	T45.0X1	T45.0X2	T45.0X3	T45.0X4	T45.0X5	T45.0X6
Cerous oxalate	T45.0X1	T45.0X2	T45.0X3	T45.0X4	T45.0X5	T45.0X6
Ceruletide	T50.8X1	T50.8X2	T50.8X3	T50.8X4	T50.8X5	T50.8X6
Cetacort*	T49.0X1	T49.0X2	T49.0X3	T49.0X4	T49.0X5	T49.0X6
Cetalkonium (chloride)	T49.0X1	T49.0X2	T49.0X3	T49.0X4	T49.0X5	T49.0X6
Cethexonium chloride	T49.0X1	T49.0X2	T49.0X3	T49.0X4	T49.0X5	T49.0X6
Cetiedil	T46.7X1	T46.7X2	T46.7X3	T46.7X4	T46.7X5	T46.7X6
Cetirizine	T45.0X1	T45.0X2	T45.0X3	T45.0X4	T45.0X5	T45.0X6
Cetomacrogol	T50.991	T50.992	T50.993	T50.994	T50.995	T50.996
Cetotiamine	T45.2X1	T45.2X2	T45.2X3	T45.2X4	T45.2X5	T45.2X6
Cetoxime	T45.0X1	T45.0X2	T45.0X3	T45.0X4	T45.0X5	T45.0X6
Cetraxate	T47.1X1	T47.1X2	T47.1X3	T47.1X4	T47.1X5	T47.1X6
Cetrimide	T49.0X1	T49.0X2	T49.0X3	T49.0X4	T49.0X5	T49.0X6
Cetrimonium (bromide)	T49.0X1	T49.0X2	T49.0X3	T49.0X4	T49.0X5	T49.0X6
Cetylpyridinium chloride	T49.0X1	T49.0X2	T49.0X3	T49.0X4	T49.0X5	T49.0X6
ENT agent	T49.6X1	T49.6X2	T49.6X3	T49.6X4	T49.6X5	T49.6X6
lozenges	T49.6X1	T49.6X2	T49.6X3	T49.6X4	T49.6X5	T49.6X6
Cevadilla — *see* Sabadilla						
Cevitamic acid	T45.2X1	T45.2X2	T45.2X3	T45.2X4	T45.2X5	T45.2X6
Chalk, precipitated	T47.1X1	T47.1X2	T47.1X3	T47.1X4	T47.1X5	T47.1X6
Chamomile	T49.0X1	T49.0X2	T49.0X3	T49.0X4	T49.0X5	T49.0X6
Ch'an su	T46.0X1	T46.0X2	T46.0X3	T46.0X4	T46.0X5	T46.0X6
Charcoal	T47.6X1	T47.6X2	T47.6X3	T47.6X4	T47.6X5	T47.6X6
activated — *see also* Charcoal, medicinal	T47.6X1	T47.6X2	T47.6X3	T47.6X4	T47.6X5	T47.6X6
fumes (Carbon monoxide)	T58.2X1	T58.2X2	T58.2X3	T58.2X4	—	—
industrial	T58.8X1	T58.8X2	T58.8X3	T58.8X4	—	—
medicinal (activated)	T47.6X1	T47.6X2	T47.6X3	T47.6X4	T47.6X5	T47.6X6
antidiarrheal	T47.6X1	T47.6X2	T47.6X3	T47.6X4	T47.6X5	T47.6X6
poison control	T47.8X1	T47.8X2	T47.8X3	T47.8X4	T47.8X5	T47.8X6
specified use other than for diarrhea	T47.8X1	T47.8X2	T47.8X3	T47.8X4	T47.8X5	T47.8X6
topical	T49.8X1	T49.8X2	T49.8X3	T49.8X4	T49.8X5	T49.8X6
Chaulmosulfone	T37.1X1	T37.1X2	T37.1X3	T37.1X4	T37.1X5	T37.1X6
Chelating agent NEC	T50.6X1	T50.6X2	T50.6X3	T50.6X4	T50.6X5	T50.6X6
Chelidonium majus	T62.2X1	T62.2X2	T62.2X3	T62.2X4	—	—
Chemical substance NEC	T65.91	T65.92	T65.93	T65.94	—	—
Chenodeoxycholic acid	T47.5X1	T47.5X2	T47.5X3	T47.5X4	T47.5X5	T47.5X6
Chenodiol	T47.5X1	T47.5X2	T47.5X3	T47.5X4	T47.5X5	T47.5X6
Chenopodium	T37.4X1	T37.4X2	T37.4X3	T37.4X4	T37.4X5	T37.4X6
Cherry laurel	T62.2X1	T62.2X2	T62.2X3	T62.2X4	—	—
Chiggertox*	T41.3X1	T41.3X2	T41.3X3	T41.3X4	T41.3X5	T41.3X6
Chinidin (e)	T46.2X1	T46.2X2	T46.2X3	T46.2X4	T46.2X5	T46.2X6
Chiniofon	T37.8X1	T37.8X2	T37.8X3	T37.8X4	T37.8X5	T37.8X6
Chlophedianol	T48.3X1	T48.3X2	T48.3X3	T48.3X4	T48.3X5	T48.3X6
Chloral	T42.6X1	T42.6X2	T42.6X3	T42.6X4	T42.6X5	T42.6X6
derivative	T42.6X1	T42.6X2	T42.6X3	T42.6X4	T42.6X5	T42.6X6
hydrate	T42.6X1	T42.6X2	T42.6X3	T42.6X4	T42.6X5	T42.6X6
Chloralamide	T42.6X1	T42.6X2	T42.6X3	T42.6X4	T42.6X5	T42.6X6
Chloralodol	T42.6X1	T42.6X2	T42.6X3	T42.6X4	T42.6X5	T42.6X6
Chloralose	T60.4X1	T60.4X2	T60.4X3	T60.4X4	—	—
Chlorambucil	T45.1X1	T45.1X2	T45.1X3	T45.1X4	T45.1X5	T45.1X6
Chloramine	T57.8X1	T57.8X2	T57.8X3	T57.8X4	—	—
T	T49.0X1	T49.0X2	T49.0X3	T49.0X4	T49.0X5	T49.0X6
topical	T49.0X1	T49.0X2	T49.0X3	T49.0X4	T49.0X5	T49.0X6
Chloramphenicol	T36.2X1	T36.2X2	T36.2X3	T36.2X4	T36.2X5	T36.2X6
ENT agent	T49.6X1	T49.6X2	T49.6X3	T49.6X4	T49.6X5	T49.6X6
ophthalmic preparation	T49.5X1	T49.5X2	T49.5X3	T49.5X4	T49.5X5	T49.5X6
topical NEC	T49.0X1	T49.0X2	T49.0X3	T49.0X4	T49.0X5	T49.0X6
Chlorate (potassium) (sodium) **NEC**	T60.3X1	T60.3X2	T60.3X3	T60.3X4	—	—
herbicide	T60.3X1	T60.3X2	T60.3X3	T60.3X4	—	—
Chlorazanil	T50.2X1	T50.2X2	T50.2X3	T50.2X4	T50.2X5	T50.2X6
Chlorbenzene, chlorbenzol	T53.7X1	T53.7X2	T53.7X3	T53.7X4	—	—
Chlorbenzoxamine	T44.3X1	T44.3X2	T44.3X3	T44.3X4	T44.3X5	T44.3X6
Chlorbutol	T42.6X1	T42.6X2	T42.6X3	T42.6X4	T42.6X5	T42.6X6
Chlorcyclizine	T45.0X1	T45.0X2	T45.0X3	T45.0X4	T45.0X5	T45.0X6
Chlordan (e) (dust)	T60.1X1	T60.1X2	T60.1X3	T60.1X4	—	—
Chlordantoin	T49.0X1	T49.0X2	T49.0X3	T49.0X4	T49.0X5	T49.0X6
Chlordiazepoxide	T42.4X1	T42.4X2	T42.4X3	T42.4X4	T42.4X5	T42.4X6
Chlordiethyl benzamide	T49.3X1	T49.3X2	T49.3X3	T49.3X4	T49.3X5	T49.3X6
Chloresium	T49.8X1	T49.8X2	T49.8X3	T49.8X4	T49.8X5	T49.8X6
Chlorethiazol	T42.6X1	T42.6X2	T42.6X3	T42.6X4	T42.6X5	T42.6X6
Chlorethyl — *see* Ethyl, chloride						
Chloretone	T42.6X1	T42.6X2	T42.6X3	T42.6X4	T42.6X5	T42.6X6
Chlorex	T53.6X1	T53.6X2	T53.6X3	T53.6X4	—	—
insecticide	T60.1X1	T60.1X2	T60.1X3	T60.1X4	—	—
Chlorfenvinphos	T60.0X1	T60.0X2	T60.0X3	T60.0X4	—	—
Chlorhexadol	T42.6X1	T42.6X2	T42.6X3	T42.6X4	T42.6X5	T42.6X6
Chlorhexamide	T45.1X1	T45.1X2	T45.1X3	T45.1X4	T45.1X5	T45.1X6
Chlorhexidine	T49.0X1	T49.0X2	T49.0X3	T49.0X4	T49.0X5	T49.0X6
Chlorhexidine Gluconate Oral Rinse*	T49.6X1	T49.6X2	T49.6X3	T49.6X4	T49.6X5	T49.6X6
Chlorhydroxyquinolin	T49.0X1	T49.0X2	T49.0X3	T49.0X4	T49.0X5	T49.0X6
Chloride of lime (bleach)	T54.3X1	T54.3X2	T54.3X3	T54.3X4	—	—
Chlorimipramine	T43.011	T43.012	T43.013	T43.014	T43.015	T43.016

Substance	Poisoning, Accidental (unintentional)	Poisoning, Intentional Self-harm	Poisoning, Assault	Poisoning, Undetermined	Adverse Effect	Under-dosing
Chlorinated						
camphene	T53.6X1	T53.6X2	T53.6X3	T53.6X4	—	—
diphenyl	T53.7X1	T53.7X2	T53.7X3	T53.7X4	—	—
hydrocarbons NEC	T53.91	T53.92	T53.93	T53.94	—	—
solvents	T53.91	T53.92	T53.93	T53.94	—	—
lime (bleach)	T54.3X1	T54.3X2	T54.3X3	T54.3X4	—	—
and boric acid solution	T49.ØX1	T49.ØX2	T49.ØX3	T49.ØX4	T49.ØX5	T49.ØX6
naphthalene (insecticide)	T6Ø.1X1	T6Ø.1X2	T6Ø.1X3	T6Ø.1X4	—	—
industrial (non-pesticide)	T53.7X1	T53.7X2	T53.7X3	T53.7X4	—	—
pesticide NEC	T6Ø.8X1	T6Ø.8X2	T6Ø.8X3	T6Ø.8X4	—	—
soda — *see also* sodium hypochlorite						
solution	T49.ØX1	T49.ØX2	T49.ØX3	T49.ØX4	T49.ØX5	T49.ØX6
Chlorine (fumes) (gas)	T59.4X1	T59.4X2	T59.4X3	T59.4X4	—	—
bleach	T54.3X1	T54.3X2	T54.3X3	T54.3X4	—	—
compound gas NEC	T59.4X1	T59.4X2	T59.4X3	T59.4X4	—	—
disinfectant	T59.4X1	T59.4X2	T59.4X3	T59.4X4	—	—
releasing agents NEC	T59.4X1	T59.4X2	T59.4X3	T59.4X4	—	—
Chlorisondamine chloride	T46.991	T46.992	T46.993	T46.994	T46.995	T46.996
Chlormadinone	T38.5X1	T38.5X2	T38.5X3	T38.5X4	T38.5X5	T38.5X6
Chlormephos	T6Ø.ØX1	T6Ø.ØX2	T6Ø.ØX3	T6Ø.ØX4	—	—
Chlormerodrin	T5Ø.2X1	T5Ø.2X2	T5Ø.2X3	T5Ø.2X4	T5Ø.2X5	T5Ø.2X6
Chlormethiazole	T42.6X1	T42.6X2	T42.6X3	T42.6X4	T42.6X5	T42.6X6
Chlormethine	T45.1X1	T45.1X2	T45.1X3	T45.1X4	T45.1X5	T45.1X6
Chlormethylenecycline	T36.4X1	T36.4X2	T36.4X3	T36.4X4	T36.4X5	T36.4X6
Chlormezanone	T42.6X1	T42.6X2	T42.6X3	T42.6X4	T42.6X5	T42.6X6
Chloroacetic acid	T6Ø.3X1	T6Ø.3X2	T6Ø.3X3	T6Ø.3X4	—	—
Chloroacetone	T59.3X1	T59.3X2	T59.3X3	T59.3X4	—	—
Chloroacetophenone	T59.3X1	T59.3X2	T59.3X3	T59.3X4	—	—
Chloroaniline	T53.7X1	T53.7X2	T53.7X3	T53.7X4	—	—
Chlorobenzene, chlorobenzol	T53.7X1	T53.7X2	T53.7X3	T53.7X4	—	—
Chlorobromomethane (fire extinguisher)	T53.6X1	T53.6X2	T53.6X3	T53.6X4	—	—
Chlorobutanol	T49.ØX1	T49.ØX2	T49.ØX3	T49.ØX4	T49.ØX5	T49.ØX6
Chlorocresol	T49.ØX1	T49.ØX2	T49.ØX3	T49.ØX4	T49.ØX5	T49.ØX6
Chlorodehydromethyltestosterone	T38.7X1	T38.7X2	T38.7X3	T38.7X4	T38.7X5	T38.7X6
Chlorodeoxyadenosine*	T45.1X1	T45.1X2	T45.1X3	T45.1X4	T45.1X5	T45.1X6
Chlorodinitrobenzene	T53.7X1	T53.7X2	T53.7X3	T53.7X4	—	—
dust or vapor	T53.7X1	T53.7X2	T53.7X3	T53.7X4	—	—
Chlorodiphenyl	T53.7X1	T53.7X2	T53.7X3	T53.7X4	—	—
Chloroethane — *see* Ethyl, chloride						
Chloroethylene	T53.6X1	T53.6X2	T53.6X3	T53.6X4	—	—
Chlorofluorocarbons	T53.5X1	T53.5X2	T53.5X3	T53.5X4	—	—
Chloroform (fumes) (vapor)	T53.1X1	T53.1X2	T53.1X3	T53.1X4	—	—
anesthetic	T41.ØX1	T41.ØX2	T41.ØX3	T41.ØX4	T41.ØX5	T41.ØX6
solvent	T53.1X1	T53.1X2	T53.1X3	T53.1X4	—	—
water, concentrated	T41.ØX1	T41.ØX2	T41.ØX3	T41.ØX4	T41.ØX5	T41.ØX6
Chloroguanide	T37.2X1	T37.2X2	T37.2X3	T37.2X4	T37.2X5	T37.2X6
Chloromycetin	T36.2X1	T36.2X2	T36.2X3	T36.2X4	T36.2X5	T36.2X6
ENT agent	T49.6X1	T49.6X2	T49.6X3	T49.6X4	T49.6X5	T49.6X6
ophthalmic preparation	T49.5X1	T49.5X2	T49.5X3	T49.5X4	T49.5X5	T49.5X6
otic solution	T49.6X1	T49.6X2	T49.6X3	T49.6X4	T49.6X5	T49.6X6
topical NEC	T49.ØX1	T49.ØX2	T49.ØX3	T49.ØX4	T49.ØX5	T49.ØX6
Chloronitrobenzene	T53.7X1	T53.7X2	T53.7X3	T53.7X4	—	—
dust or vapor	T53.7X1	T53.7X2	T53.7X3	T53.7X4	—	—
Chlorophacinone	T6Ø.4X1	T6Ø.4X2	T6Ø.4X3	T6Ø.4X4	—	—
Chlorophenol	T53.7X1	T53.7X2	T53.7X3	T53.7X4	—	—
Chlorophenothane	T6Ø.1X1	T6Ø.1X2	T6Ø.1X3	T6Ø.1X4	—	—
Chlorophyll	T5Ø.991	T5Ø.992	T5Ø.993	T5Ø.994	T5Ø.995	T5Ø.996
Chloropicrin (fumes)	T53.6X1	T53.6X2	T53.6X3	T53.6X4	—	—
fumigant	T6Ø.8X1	T6Ø.8X2	T6Ø.8X3	T6Ø.8X4	—	—
fungicide	T6Ø.3X1	T6Ø.3X2	T6Ø.3X3	T6Ø.3X4	—	—
pesticide	T6Ø.8X1	T6Ø.8X2	T6Ø.8X3	T6Ø.8X4	—	—
Chloroprocaine	T41.3X1	T41.3X2	T41.3X3	T41.3X4	T41.3X5	T41.3X6
infiltration (subcutaneous)	T41.3X1	T41.3X2	T41.3X3	T41.3X4	T41.3X5	T41.3X6
nerve block (peripheral) (plexus)	T41.3X1	T41.3X2	T41.3X3	T41.3X4	T41.3X5	T41.3X6
spinal	T41.3X1	T41.3X2	T41.3X3	T41.3X4	T41.3X5	T41.3X6
Chloroptic	T49.5X1	T49.5X2	T49.5X3	T49.5X4	T49.5X5	T49.5X6
Chloropurine	T45.1X1	T45.1X2	T45.1X3	T45.1X4	T45.1X5	T45.1X6
Chloropyramine	T45.ØX1	T45.ØX2	T45.ØX3	T45.ØX4	T45.ØX5	T45.ØX6
Chloropyrifos	T6Ø.ØX1	T6Ø.ØX2	T6Ø.ØX3	T6Ø.ØX4	—	—
Chloropyrilene	T45.ØX1	T45.ØX2	T45.ØX3	T45.ØX4	T45.ØX5	T45.ØX6
Chloroquine	T37.2X1	T37.2X2	T37.2X3	T37.2X4	T37.2X5	T37.2X6
Chlorostat*	T49.ØX1	T49.ØX2	T49.ØX3	T49.ØX4	T49.ØX5	T49.ØX6
Chlorothalonil	T6Ø.3X1	T6Ø.3X2	T6Ø.3X3	T6Ø.3X4	—	—
Chlorothen	T45.ØX1	T45.ØX2	T45.ØX3	T45.ØX4	T45.ØX5	T45.ØX6
Chlorothiazide	T5Ø.2X1	T5Ø.2X2	T5Ø.2X3	T5Ø.2X4	T5Ø.2X5	T5Ø.2X6
Chlorothymol	T49.4X1	T49.4X2	T49.4X3	T49.4X4	T49.4X5	T49.4X6
Chlorotrianisene	T38.5X1	T38.5X2	T38.5X3	T38.5X4	T38.5X5	T38.5X6
Chlorovinyldichloroarsine, not in war	T57.ØX1	T57.ØX2	T57.ØX3	T57.ØX4	—	—
Chloroxine	T49.4X1	T49.4X2	T49.4X3	T49.4X4	T49.4X5	T49.4X6
Chloroxylenol	T49.ØX1	T49.ØX2	T49.ØX3	T49.ØX4	T49.ØX5	T49.ØX6
Chlorphenamine	T45.ØX1	T45.ØX2	T45.ØX3	T45.ØX4	T45.ØX5	T45.ØX6
Chlorphenesin	T42.8X1	T42.8X2	T42.8X3	T42.8X4	T42.8X5	T42.8X6
topical (antifungal)	T49.ØX1	T49.ØX2	T49.ØX3	T49.ØX4	T49.ØX5	T49.ØX6
Chlorpheniramine	T45.ØX1	T45.ØX2	T45.ØX3	T45.ØX4	T45.ØX5	T45.ØX6
Chlorphenoxamine	T45.ØX1	T45.ØX2	T45.ØX3	T45.ØX4	T45.ØX5	T45.ØX6
Chlorphentermine	T5Ø.5X1	T5Ø.5X2	T5Ø.5X3	T5Ø.5X4	T5Ø.5X5	T5Ø.5X6
Chlorprocaine — *see* Chloroprocaine						
Chlorproguanil	T37.2X1	T37.2X2	T37.2X3	T37.2X4	T37.2X5	T37.2X6
Chlorpromazine	T43.3X1	T43.3X2	T43.3X3	T43.3X4	T43.3X5	T43.3X6
Chlorpropamide	T38.3X1	T38.3X2	T38.3X3	T38.3X4	T38.3X5	T38.3X6
Chlorprothixene	T43.4X1	T43.4X2	T43.4X3	T43.4X4	T43.4X5	T43.4X6
Chlorquinaldol	T49.ØX1	T49.ØX2	T49.ØX3	T49.ØX4	T49.ØX5	T49.ØX6
Chlorquinol	T49.ØX1	T49.ØX2	T49.ØX3	T49.ØX4	T49.ØX5	T49.ØX6
Chlortalidone	T5Ø.2X1	T5Ø.2X2	T5Ø.2X3	T5Ø.2X4	T5Ø.2X5	T5Ø.2X6
Chlortetracycline	T36.4X1	T36.4X2	T36.4X3	T36.4X4	T36.4X5	T36.4X6
Chlorthalidone	T5Ø.2X1	T5Ø.2X2	T5Ø.2X3	T5Ø.2X4	T5Ø.2X5	T5Ø.2X6
Chlorthion	T6Ø.ØX1	T6Ø.ØX2	T6Ø.ØX3	T6Ø.ØX4	—	—
Chlorthiophos	T6Ø.ØX1	T6Ø.ØX2	T6Ø.ØX3	T6Ø.ØX4	—	—
Chlortrianisene	T38.5X1	T38.5X2	T38.5X3	T38.5X4	T38.5X5	T38.5X6
Chlor-Trimeton	T45.ØX1	T45.ØX2	T45.ØX3	T45.ØX4	T45.ØX5	T45.ØX6
Chlorzoxazone	T42.8X1	T42.8X2	T42.8X3	T42.8X4	T42.8X5	T42.8X6
Choke damp	T59.7X1	T59.7X2	T59.7X3	T59.7X4	—	—
Cholagogues	T47.5X1	T47.5X2	T47.5X3	T47.5X4	T47.5X5	T47.5X6
Cholebrine	T5Ø.8X1	T5Ø.8X2	T5Ø.8X3	T5Ø.8X4	T5Ø.8X5	T5Ø.8X6
Cholecalciferol	T45.2X1	T45.2X2	T45.2X3	T45.2X4	T45.2X5	T45.2X6
Cholecystokinin	T5Ø.8X1	T5Ø.8X2	T5Ø.8X3	T5Ø.8X4	T5Ø.8X5	T5Ø.8X6
Cholera vaccine	T5Ø.A91	T5Ø.A92	T5Ø.A93	T5Ø.A94	T5Ø.A95	T5Ø.A96
Choleretic	T47.5X1	T47.5X2	T47.5X3	T47.5X4	T47.5X5	T47.5X6
Cholesterol-lowering agents	T46.6X1	T46.6X2	T46.6X3	T46.6X4	T46.6X5	T46.6X6
Cholestyramine (resin)	T46.6X1	T46.6X2	T46.6X3	T46.6X4	T46.6X5	T46.6X6
Cholic acid	T47.5X1	T47.5X2	T47.5X3	T47.5X4	T47.5X5	T47.5X6
Choline	T48.6X1	T48.6X2	T48.6X3	T48.6X4	T48.6X5	T48.6X6
chloride	T5Ø.991	T5Ø.992	T5Ø.993	T5Ø.994	T5Ø.995	T5Ø.996
dihydrogen citrate	T5Ø.991	T5Ø.992	T5Ø.993	T5Ø.994	T5Ø.995	T5Ø.996
salicylate	T39.Ø91	T39.Ø92	T39.Ø93	T39.Ø94	T39.Ø95	T39.Ø96
theophyllinate	T48.6X1	T48.6X2	T48.6X3	T48.6X4	T48.6X5	T48.6X6
Cholinergic (drug) **NEC**	T44.1X1	T44.1X2	T44.1X3	T44.1X4	T44.1X5	T44.1X6
muscle tone enhancer	T44.1X1	T44.1X2	T44.1X3	T44.1X4	T44.1X5	T44.1X6
organophosphorus	T44.ØX1	T44.ØX2	T44.ØX3	T44.ØX4	T44.ØX5	T44.ØX6
insecticide	T6Ø.ØX1	T6Ø.ØX2	T6Ø.ØX3	T6Ø.ØX4	—	—
nerve gas	T59.891	T59.892	T59.893	T59.894	—	—
trimethyl ammonium propanediol	T44.1X1	T44.1X2	T44.1X3	T44.1X4	T44.1X5	T44.1X6
Cholinesterase reactivator	T5Ø.6X1	T5Ø.6X2	T5Ø.6X3	T5Ø.6X4	T5Ø.6X5	T5Ø.6X6
Cholografin	T5Ø.8X1	T5Ø.8X2	T5Ø.8X3	T5Ø.8X4	T5Ø.8X5	T5Ø.8X6
Chorionic gonadotropin	T38.891	T38.892	T38.893	T38.894	T38.895	T38.896
Chromate	T56.2X1	T56.2X2	T56.2X3	T56.2X4	—	—
dust or mist	T56.2X1	T56.2X2	T56.2X3	T56.2X4	—	—
lead — *see also* lead	T56.ØX1	T56.ØX2	T56.ØX3	T56.ØX4	—	—
paint	T56.ØX1	T56.ØX2	T56.ØX3	T56.ØX4	—	—
Chromelin*	T49.3X1	T49.3X2	T49.3X3	T49.3X4	T49.3X5	T49.3X6
Chromic						
acid	T56.2X1	T56.2X2	T56.2X3	T56.2X4	—	—
dust or mist	T56.2X1	T56.2X2	T56.2X3	T56.2X4	—	—
phosphate 32P	T45.1X1	T45.1X2	T45.1X3	T45.1X4	T45.1X5	T45.1X6
Chromium	T56.2X1	T56.2X2	T56.2X3	T56.2X4	—	—
compounds — *see* Chromate						
sesquioxide	T5Ø.8X1	T5Ø.8X2	T5Ø.8X3	T5Ø.8X4	T5Ø.8X5	T5Ø.8X6
Chromomycin A3	T45.1X1	T45.1X2	T45.1X3	T45.1X4	T45.1X5	T45.1X6
Chromonar	T46.3X1	T46.3X2	T46.3X3	T46.3X4	T46.3X5	T46.3X6
Chromyl chloride	T56.2X1	T56.2X2	T56.2X3	T56.2X4	—	—
Chrysarobin	T49.4X1	T49.4X2	T49.4X3	T49.4X4	T49.4X5	T49.4X6
Chrysazin	T47.2X1	T47.2X2	T47.2X3	T47.2X4	T47.2X5	T47.2X6
Chymar	T45.3X1	T45.3X2	T45.3X3	T45.3X4	T45.3X5	T45.3X6
ophthalmic preparation	T49.5X1	T49.5X2	T49.5X3	T49.5X4	T49.5X5	T49.5X6
Chymopapain	T45.3X1	T45.3X2	T45.3X3	T45.3X4	T45.3X5	T45.3X6
Chymotrypsin	T45.3X1	T45.3X2	T45.3X3	T45.3X4	T45.3X5	T45.3X6
ophthalmic preparation	T49.5X1	T49.5X2	T49.5X3	T49.5X4	T49.5X5	T49.5X6
Cialis*	T46.7X1	T46.7X2	T46.7X3	T46.7X4	T46.7X5	T46.7X6
Cianidanol	T5Ø.991	T5Ø.992	T5Ø.993	T5Ø.994	T5Ø.995	T5Ø.996
Cianopramine	T43.Ø11	T43.Ø12	T43.Ø13	T43.Ø14	T43.Ø15	T43.Ø16
Cibenzoline	T46.2X1	T46.2X2	T46.2X3	T46.2X4	T46.2X5	T46.2X6
Ciclacillin	T36.ØX1	T36.ØX2	T36.ØX3	T36.ØX4	T36.ØX5	T36.ØX6
Ciclobarbital — *see* Hexobarbital						
Ciclonicate	T46.7X1	T46.7X2	T46.7X3	T46.7X4	T46.7X5	T46.7X6

Substance	Poisoning, Accidental (unintentional)	Poisoning, Intentional Self-harm	Poisoning, Assault	Poisoning, Undetermined	Adverse Effect	Under-dosing
Ciclopirox (olamine)	T49.ØX1	T49.ØX2	T49.ØX3	T49.ØX4	T49.ØX5	T49.ØX6
Ciclosporin	T45.1X1	T45.1X2	T45.1X3	T45.1X4	T45.1X5	T45.1X6
Cicuta maculata or virosa	T62.2X1	T62.2X2	T62.2X3	T62.2X4	—	—
Cicutoxin	T62.2X1	T62.2X2	T62.2X3	T62.2X4	—	—
Cigarette lighter fluid	T52.ØX1	T52.ØX2	T52.ØX3	T52.ØX4	—	—
Cigarettes (tobacco)	T65.221	T65.222	T65.223	T65.224	—	—
Ciguatoxin	T61.Ø1	T61.Ø2	T61.Ø3	T61.Ø4	—	—
Cilazapril	T46.4X1	T46.4X2	T46.4X3	T46.4X4	T46.4X5	T46.4X6
Cimetidine	T47.ØX1	T47.ØX2	T47.ØX3	T47.ØX4	T47.ØX5	T47.ØX6
Cimetropium bromide	T44.3X1	T44.3X2	T44.3X3	T44.3X4	T44.3X5	T44.3X6
Cinchocaine	T41.3X1	T41.3X2	T41.3X3	T41.3X4	T41.3X5	T41.3X6
topical (surface)	T41.3X1	T41.3X2	T41.3X3	T41.3X4	T41.3X5	T41.3X6
Cinchona	T37.2X1	T37.2X2	T37.2X3	T37.2X4	T37.2X5	T37.2X6
Cinchonine alkaloids	T37.2X1	T37.2X2	T37.2X3	T37.2X4	T37.2X5	T37.2X6
Cinchophen	T5Ø.4X1	T5Ø.4X2	T5Ø.4X3	T5Ø.4X4	T5Ø.4X5	T5Ø.4X6
Cinepazide	T46.7X1	T46.7X2	T46.7X3	T46.7X4	T46.7X5	T46.7X6
Cinnamedrine	T48.5X1	T48.5X2	T48.5X3	T48.5X4	T48.5X5	T48.5X6
Cinnarizine	T45.ØX1	T45.ØX2	T45.ØX3	T45.ØX4	T45.ØX5	T45.ØX6
Cinoxacin	T37.8X1	T37.8X2	T37.8X3	T37.8X4	T37.8X5	T37.8X6
Ciprofibrate	T46.6X1	T46.6X2	T46.6X3	T46.6X4	T46.6X5	T46.6X6
Ciprofloxacin	T36.8X1	T36.8X2	T36.8X3	T36.8X4	T36.8X5	T36.8X6
Cisapride	T47.8X1	T47.8X2	T47.8X3	T47.8X4	T47.8X5	T47.8X6
Cisplatin	T45.1X1	T45.1X2	T45.1X3	T45.1X4	T45.1X5	T45.1X6
Citalopram	T43.221	T43.222	T43.223	T43.224	T43.225	T43.226
Citanest	T41.3X1	T41.3X2	T41.3X3	T41.3X4	T41.3X5	T41.3X6
infiltration (subcutaneous)	T41.3X1	T41.3X2	T41.3X3	T41.3X4	T41.3X5	T41.3X6
nerve block (peripheral) (plexus)	T41.3X1	T41.3X2	T41.3X3	T41.3X4	T41.3X5	T41.3X6
Citracel*	T5Ø.3X1	T5Ø.3X2	T5Ø.3X3	T5Ø.3X4	T5Ø.3X5	T5Ø.3X6
Citric acid	T47.5X1	T47.5X2	T47.5X3	T47.5X4	T47.5X5	T47.5X6
Citrovorum (factor)	T45.8X1	T45.8X2	T45.8X3	T45.8X4	T45.8X5	T45.8X6
Claviceps purpurea	T62.2X1	T62.2X2	T62.2X3	T62.2X4	—	—
Clavulanic acid	T36.1X1	T36.1X2	T36.1X3	T36.1X4	T36.1X5	T36.1X6
Cleaner, cleansing agent, type not specified	T65.891	T65.892	T65.893	T65.894	—	—
of paint or varnish	T52.91	T52.92	T52.93	T52.94	—	—
specified type NEC	T65.891	T65.892	T65.893	T65.894	—	—
Clebopride	T47.8X1	T47.8X2	T47.8X3	T47.8X4	T47.8X5	T47.8X6
Clefamide	T37.3X1	T37.3X2	T37.3X3	T37.3X4	T37.3X5	T37.3X6
Clemastine	T45.ØX1	T45.ØX2	T45.ØX3	T45.ØX4	T45.ØX5	T45.ØX6
Clematis vitalba	T62.2X1	T62.2X2	T62.2X3	T62.2X4	—	—
Clemizole	T45.ØX1	T45.ØX2	T45.ØX3	T45.ØX4	T45.ØX5	T45.ØX6
penicillin	T36.ØX1	T36.ØX2	T36.ØX3	T36.ØX4	T36.ØX5	T36.ØX6
Clenbuterol	T48.6X1	T48.6X2	T48.6X3	T48.6X4	T48.6X5	T48.6X6
Clidinium bromide	T44.3X1	T44.3X2	T44.3X3	T44.3X4	T44.3X5	T44.3X6
Clinda-Derm*	T49.ØX1	T49.ØX2	T49.ØX3	T49.ØX4	T49.ØX5	T49.ØX6
Clindamycin	T36.8X1	T36.8X2	T36.8X3	T36.8X4	T36.8X5	T36.8X6
Clinofibrate	T46.6X1	T46.6X2	T46.6X3	T46.6X4	T46.6X5	T46.6X6
Clioquinol	T37.8X1	T37.8X2	T37.8X3	T37.8X4	T37.8X5	T37.8X6
Cliradon	T4Ø.2X1	T4Ø.2X2	T4Ø.2X3	T4Ø.2X4	—	—
Clobazam	T42.4X1	T42.4X2	T42.4X3	T42.4X4	T42.4X5	T42.4X6
Clobenzorex	T5Ø.5X1	T5Ø.5X2	T5Ø.5X3	T5Ø.5X4	T5Ø.5X5	T5Ø.5X6
Clobetasol	T49.ØX1	T49.ØX2	T49.ØX3	T49.ØX4	T49.ØX5	T49.ØX6
Clobetasone	T49.ØX1	T49.ØX2	T49.ØX3	T49.ØX4	T49.ØX5	T49.ØX6
Clobutinol	T48.3X1	T48.3X2	T48.3X3	T48.3X4	T48.3X5	T48.3X6
Clocortolone	T38.ØX1	T38.ØX2	T38.ØX3	T38.ØX4	T38.ØX5	T38.ØX6
Clodantoin	T49.ØX1	T49.ØX2	T49.ØX3	T49.ØX4	T49.ØX5	T49.ØX6
Clodronic acid	T5Ø.991	T5Ø.992	T5Ø.993	T5Ø.994	T5Ø.995	T5Ø.996
Clofazimine	T37.1X1	T37.1X2	T37.1X3	T37.1X4	T37.1X5	T37.1X6
Clofedanol	T48.3X1	T48.3X2	T48.3X3	T48.3X4	T48.3X5	T48.3X6
Clofenamide	T5Ø.2X1	T5Ø.2X2	T5Ø.2X3	T5Ø.2X4	T5Ø.2X5	T5Ø.2X6
Clofenotane	T49.ØX1	T49.ØX2	T49.ØX3	T49.ØX4	T49.ØX5	T49.ØX6
Clofezone	T39.2X1	T39.2X2	T39.2X3	T39.2X4	T39.2X5	T39.2X6
Clofibrate	T46.6X1	T46.6X2	T46.6X3	T46.6X4	T46.6X5	T46.6X6
Clofibride	T46.6X1	T46.6X2	T46.6X3	T46.6X4	T46.6X5	T46.6X6
Cloforex	T5Ø.5X1	T5Ø.5X2	T5Ø.5X3	T5Ø.5X4	T5Ø.5X5	T5Ø.5X6
Clomethiazole	T42.6X1	T42.6X2	T42.6X3	T42.6X4	T42.6X5	T42.6X6
Clometocillin	T36.ØX1	T36.ØX2	T36.ØX3	T36.ØX4	T36.ØX5	T36.ØX6
Clomifene	T38.5X1	T38.5X2	T38.5X3	T38.5X4	T38.5X5	T38.5X6
Clomiphene	T38.5X1	T38.5X2	T38.5X3	T38.5X4	T38.5X5	T38.5X6
Clomipramine	T43.Ø11	T43.Ø12	T43.Ø13	T43.Ø14	T43.Ø15	T43.Ø16
Clomocycline	T36.4X1	T36.4X2	T36.4X3	T36.4X4	T36.4X5	T36.4X6
Clonazepam	T42.4X1	T42.4X2	T42.4X3	T42.4X4	T42.4X5	T42.4X6
Clonidine	T46.5X1	T46.5X2	T46.5X3	T46.5X4	T46.5X5	T46.5X6
Clonixin	T39.8X1	T39.8X2	T39.8X3	T39.8X4	T39.8X5	T39.8X6
Clopamide	T5Ø.2X1	T5Ø.2X2	T5Ø.2X3	T5Ø.2X4	T5Ø.2X5	T5Ø.2X6
Clopenthixol	T43.4X1	T43.4X2	T43.4X3	T43.4X4	T43.4X5	T43.4X6
Cloperastine	T48.3X1	T48.3X2	T48.3X3	T48.3X4	T48.3X5	T48.3X6
Clophedianol	T48.3X1	T48.3X2	T48.3X3	T48.3X4	T48.3X5	T48.3X6
Cloponone	T36.2X1	T36.2X2	T36.2X3	T36.2X4	T36.2X5	T36.2X6
Cloprednol	T38.ØX1	T38.ØX2	T38.ØX3	T38.ØX4	T38.ØX5	T38.ØX6
Cloral betaine	T42.6X1	T42.6X2	T42.6X3	T42.6X4	T42.6X5	T42.6X6
Cloramfenicol	T36.2X1	T36.2X2	T36.2X3	T36.2X4	T36.2X5	T36.2X6
Clorazepate (dipotassium)	T42.4X1	T42.4X2	T42.4X3	T42.4X4	T42.4X5	T42.4X6
Clorexolone	T5Ø.2X1	T5Ø.2X2	T5Ø.2X3	T5Ø.2X4	T5Ø.2X5	T5Ø.2X6
Clorfenamine	T45.ØX1	T45.ØX2	T45.ØX3	T45.ØX4	T45.ØX5	T45.ØX6
Clorgiline	T43.1X1	T43.1X2	T43.1X3	T43.1X4	T43.1X5	T43.1X6
Clorotepine	T44.3X1	T44.3X2	T44.3X3	T44.3X4	T44.3X5	T44.3X6
Clorox (bleach)	T54.91	T54.92	T54.93	T54.94	—	—
Clorprenaline	T48.6X1	T48.6X2	T48.6X3	T48.6X4	T48.6X5	T48.6X6
Clortermine	T5Ø.5X1	T5Ø.5X2	T5Ø.5X3	T5Ø.5X4	T5Ø.5X5	T5Ø.5X6
Clotiapine	T43.591	T43.592	T43.593	T43.594	T43.595	T43.596
Clotiazepam	T42.4X1	T42.4X2	T42.4X3	T42.4X4	T42.4X5	T42.4X6
Clotibric acid	T46.6X1	T46.6X2	T46.6X3	T46.6X4	T46.6X5	T46.6X6
Clotrimazole	T49.ØX1	T49.ØX2	T49.ØX3	T49.ØX4	T49.ØX5	T49.ØX6
Cloxacillin	T36.ØX1	T36.ØX2	T36.ØX3	T36.ØX4	T36.ØX5	T36.ØX6
Cloxazolam	T42.4X1	T42.4X2	T42.4X3	T42.4X4	T42.4X5	T42.4X6
Cloxiquine	T49.ØX1	T49.ØX2	T49.ØX3	T49.ØX4	T49.ØX5	T49.ØX6
Clozapine	T42.4X1	T42.4X2	T42.4X3	T42.4X4	T42.4X5	T42.4X6
Coagulant NEC	T45.7X1	T45.7X2	T45.7X3	T45.7X4	T45.7X5	T45.7X6
Coal (carbon monoxide from) — *see also* Carbon, monoxide, coal	T58.2X1	T58.2X2	T58.2X3	T58.2X4	—	—
oil — *see* Kerosene						
tar	T49.1X1	T49.1X2	T49.1X3	T49.1X4	T49.1X5	T49.1X6
fumes	T59.891	T59.892	T59.893	T59.894	—	—
medicinal (ointment)	T49.4X1	T49.4X2	T49.4X3	T49.4X4	T49.4X5	T49.4X6
analgesics NEC	T39.2X1	T39.2X2	T39.2X3	T39.2X4	T39.2X5	T39.2X6
naphtha (solvent)	T52.ØX1	T52.ØX2	T52.ØX3	T52.ØX4	—	—
Coartem*	T37.2X1	T37.2X2	T37.2X3	T37.2X4	T37.2X5	T37.2X6
Cobalamine	T45.2X1	T45.2X2	T45.2X3	T45.2X4	T45.2X5	T45.2X6
Cobalt (nonmedicinal) (fumes) (industrial)	T56.891	T56.892	T56.893	T56.894	—	—
medicinal (trace) (chloride)	T45.8X1	T45.8X2	T45.8X3	T45.8X4	T45.8X5	T45.8X6
Cobra (venom)	T63.Ø41	T63.Ø42	T63.Ø43	T63.Ø44	—	—
Coca (leaf)	T4Ø.5X1	T4Ø.5X2	T4Ø.5X3	T4Ø.5X4	T4Ø.5X5	T4Ø.5X6
Cocaine	T4Ø.5X1	T4Ø.5X2	T4Ø.5X3	T4Ø.5X4	T4Ø.5X5	T4Ø.5X6
topical anesthetic	T41.3X1	T41.3X2	T41.3X3	T41.3X4	T41.3X5	T41.3X6
Cocarboxylase	T45.3X1	T45.3X2	T45.3X3	T45.3X4	T45.3X5	T45.3X6
Coccidioidin	T5Ø.8X1	T5Ø.8X2	T5Ø.8X3	T5Ø.8X4	T5Ø.8X5	T5Ø.8X6
Cocculus indicus	T62.1X1	T62.1X2	T62.1X3	T62.1X4	—	—
Cochineal	T65.6X1	T65.6X2	T65.6X3	T65.6X4	—	—
medicinal products	T5Ø.991	T5Ø.992	T5Ø.993	T5Ø.994	T5Ø.995	T5Ø.996
Codeine	T4Ø.2X1	T4Ø.2X2	T4Ø.2X3	T4Ø.2X4	T4Ø.2X5	T4Ø.2X6
Cod-liver oil	T45.2X1	T45.2X2	T45.2X3	T45.2X4	T45.2X5	T45.2X6
Coenzyme A	T5Ø.991	T5Ø.992	T5Ø.993	T5Ø.994	T5Ø.995	T5Ø.996
Coffee	T62.8X1	T62.8X2	T62.8X3	T62.8X4	—	—
Cogalactoisomerase	T5Ø.991	T5Ø.992	T5Ø.993	T5Ø.994	T5Ø.995	T5Ø.996
Cogentin	T44.3X1	T44.3X2	T44.3X3	T44.3X4	T44.3X5	T44.3X6
Coke fumes or gas (carbon monoxide)	T58.2X1	T58.2X2	T58.2X3	T58.2X4	—	—
industrial use	T58.8X1	T58.8X2	T58.8X3	T58.8X4	—	—
Colace	T47.4X1	T47.4X2	T47.4X3	T47.4X4	T47.4X5	T47.4X6
Colaspase	T45.1X1	T45.1X2	T45.1X3	T45.1X4	T45.1X5	T45.1X6
Colazal*	T47.8X1	T47.8X2	T47.8X3	T47.8X4	T47.8X5	T47.8X6
Colchicine	T5Ø.4X1	T5Ø.4X2	T5Ø.4X3	T5Ø.4X4	T5Ø.4X5	T5Ø.4X6
Colchicum	T62.2X1	T62.2X2	T62.2X3	T62.2X4	—	—
Cold cream	T49.3X1	T49.3X2	T49.3X3	T49.3X4	T49.3X5	T49.3X6
Colecalciferol	T45.2X1	T45.2X2	T45.2X3	T45.2X4	T45.2X5	T45.2X6
Colestipol	T46.6X1	T46.6X2	T46.6X3	T46.6X4	T46.6X5	T46.6X6
Colestyramine	T46.6X1	T46.6X2	T46.6X3	T46.6X4	T46.6X5	T46.6X6
Colimycin	T36.8X1	T36.8X2	T36.8X3	T36.8X4	T36.8X5	T36.8X6
Colistimethate	T36.8X1	T36.8X2	T36.8X3	T36.8X4	T36.8X5	T36.8X6
Colistin	T36.8X1	T36.8X2	T36.8X3	T36.8X4	T36.8X5	T36.8X6
sulfate (eye preparation)	T49.5X1	T49.5X2	T49.5X3	T49.5X4	T49.5X5	T49.5X6
Collagen	T5Ø.991	T5Ø.992	T5Ø.993	T5Ø.994	T5Ø.995	T5Ø.996
Collagenase	T49.4X1	T49.4X2	T49.4X3	T49.4X4	T49.4X5	T49.4X6
Collodion	T49.3X1	T49.3X2	T49.3X3	T49.3X4	T49.3X5	T49.3X6
Colocynth	T47.2X1	T47.2X2	T47.2X3	T47.2X4	T47.2X5	T47.2X6
Colophony adhesive	T49.3X1	T49.3X2	T49.3X3	T49.3X4	T49.3X5	T49.3X6
Colorant — *see also* Dye	T5Ø.991	T5Ø.992	T5Ø.993	T5Ø.994	T5Ø.995	T5Ø.996
Coloring matter — *see* Dye(s)						
Combustion gas (after combustion) — *see* Carbon, monoxide						
prior to combustion	T59.891	T59.892	T59.893	T59.894	—	—
Cometriq*	T45.1X1	T45.1X2	T45.1X3	T45.1X4	T45.1X5	T45.1X6
Compazine	T43.3X1	T43.3X2	T43.3X3	T43.3X4	T43.3X5	T43.3X6
Compound						
1080 (sodium fluoroacetate)	T6Ø.4X1	T6Ø.4X2	T6Ø.4X3	T6Ø.4X4	—	—
269 (endrin)	T6Ø.1X1	T6Ø.1X2	T6Ø.1X3	T6Ø.1X4	—	—
3422 (parathion)	T6Ø.ØX1	T6Ø.ØX2	T6Ø.ØX3	T6Ø.ØX4	—	—
3911 (phorate)	T6Ø.ØX1	T6Ø.ØX2	T6Ø.ØX3	T6Ø.ØX4	—	—
3956 (toxaphene)	T6Ø.1X1	T6Ø.1X2	T6Ø.1X3	T6Ø.1X4	—	—
4049 (malathion)	T6Ø.ØX1	T6Ø.ØX2	T6Ø.ØX3	T6Ø.ØX4	—	—

Substance	Poisoning, Accidental (unintentional)	Poisoning, Intentional Self-harm	Poisoning, Assault	Poisoning, Undetermined	Adverse Effect	Under-dosing
Compound — *continued*						
4069 (malathion)	T6Ø.ØX1	T6Ø.ØX2	T6Ø.ØX3	T6Ø.ØX4	—	—
4124 (dicapthon)	T6Ø.ØX1	T6Ø.ØX2	T6Ø.ØX3	T6Ø.ØX4	—	—
42 (warfarin)	T6Ø.4X1	T6Ø.4X2	T6Ø.4X3	T6Ø.4X4	—	—
497 (dieldrin)	T6Ø.1X1	T6Ø.1X2	T6Ø.1X3	T6Ø.1X4	—	—
E (cortisone)	T38.ØX1	T38.ØX2	T38.ØX3	T38.ØX4	T38.ØX5	T38.ØX6
F (hydrocortisone)	T38.ØX1	T38.ØX2	T38.ØX3	T38.ØX4	T38.ØX5	T38.ØX6
Comvax*	T5Ø.A21	T5Ø.A22	T5Ø.A23	T5Ø.A24	T5Ø.A25	T5Ø.A26
Congener, anabolic	T38.7X1	T38.7X2	T38.7X3	T38.7X4	T38.7X5	T38.7X6
Congo red	T5Ø.8X1	T5Ø.8X2	T5Ø.8X3	T5Ø.8X4	T5Ø.8X5	T5Ø.8X6
Coniine, conine	T62.2X1	T62.2X2	T62.2X3	T62.2X4	—	—
Conium (maculatum)	T62.2X1	T62.2X2	T62.2X3	T62.2X4	—	—
Conjugated estrogenic substances	T38.5X1	T38.5X2	T38.5X3	T38.5X4	T38.5X5	T38.5X6
Contac	T48.5X1	T48.5X2	T48.5X3	T48.5X4	T48.5X5	T48.5X6
Contact lens solution	T49.5X1	T49.5X2	T49.5X3	T49.5X4	T49.5X5	T49.5X6
Contraceptive (oral)	T38.4X1	T38.4X2	T38.4X3	T38.4X4	T38.4X5	T38.4X6
vaginal	T49.8X1	T49.8X2	T49.8X3	T49.8X4	T49.8X5	T49.8X6
Contrast medium, radiography	T5Ø.8X1	T5Ø.8X2	T5Ø.8X3	T5Ø.8X4	T5Ø.8X5	T5Ø.8X6
Convallaria glycosides	T46.ØX1	T46.ØX2	T46.ØX3	T46.ØX4	T46.ØX5	T46.ØX6
Convallaria majalis	T62.2X1	T62.2X2	T62.2X3	T62.2X4	—	—
berry	T62.1X1	T62.1X2	T62.1X3	T62.1X4	—	—
Copperhead snake (bite) (venom)	T63.Ø61	T63.Ø62	T63.Ø63	T63.Ø64	—	—
Copper (dust) (fumes) (nonmedicinal) **NEC**	T56.4X1	T56.4X2	T56.4X3	T56.4X4	—	—
arsenate, arsenite	T57.ØX1	T57.ØX2	T57.ØX3	T57.ØX4	—	—
insecticide	T6Ø.2X1	T6Ø.2X2	T6Ø.2X3	T6Ø.2X4	—	—
emetic	T47.7X1	T47.7X2	T47.7X3	T47.7X4	T47.7X5	T47.7X6
fungicide	T6Ø.3X1	T6Ø.3X2	T6Ø.3X3	T6Ø.3X4	—	—
gluconate	T49.ØX1	T49.ØX2	T49.ØX3	T49.ØX4	T49.ØX5	T49.ØX6
insecticide	T6Ø.2X1	T6Ø.2X2	T6Ø.2X3	T6Ø.2X4	—	—
medicinal (trace)	T45.8X1	T45.8X2	T45.8X3	T45.8X4	T45.8X5	T45.8X6
oleate	T49.ØX1	T49.ØX2	T49.ØX3	T49.ØX4	T49.ØX5	T49.ØX6
sulfate	T56.4X1	T56.4X2	T56.4X3	T56.4X4	—	—
cupric	T56.4X1	T56.4X2	T56.4X3	T56.4X4	—	—
fungicide	T6Ø.3X1	T6Ø.3X2	T6Ø.3X3	T6Ø.3X4	—	—
medicinal						
ear	T49.6X1	T49.6X2	T49.6X3	T49.6X4	T49.6X5	T49.6X6
emetic	T47.7X1	T47.7X2	T47.7X3	T47.7X4	T47.7X5	T47.7X6
eye	T49.5X1	T49.5X2	T49.5X3	T49.5X4	T49.5X5	T49.5X6
cuprous	T56.4X1	T56.4X2	T56.4X3	T56.4X4	—	—
fungicide	T6Ø.3X1	T6Ø.3X2	T6Ø.3X3	T6Ø.3X4	—	—
medicinal						
ear	T49.6X1	T49.6X2	T49.6X3	T49.6X4	T49.6X5	T49.6X6
emetic	T47.7X1	T47.7X2	T47.7X3	T47.7X4	T47.7X5	T47.7X6
eye	T49.5X1	T49.5X2	T49.5X3	T49.5X4	T49.5X5	T49.5X6
Coral (sting)	T63.691	T63.692	T63.693	T63.694	—	—
snake (bite) (venom)	T63.Ø21	T63.Ø22	T63.Ø23	T63.Ø24	—	—
Corbadrine	T49.6X1	T49.6X2	T49.6X3	T49.6X4	T49.6X5	T49.6X6
Cordite	T65.891	T65.892	T65.893	T65.894	—	—
vapor	T59.891	T59.892	T59.893	T59.894	—	—
Cordran	T49.ØX1	T49.ØX2	T49.ØX3	T49.ØX4	T49.ØX5	T49.ØX6
Cormax*	T49.ØX1	T49.ØX2	T49.ØX3	T49.ØX4	T49.ØX5	T49.ØX6
Corn cures	T49.4X1	T49.4X2	T49.4X3	T49.4X4	T49.4X5	T49.4X6
Cornhusker's lotion	T49.3X1	T49.3X2	T49.3X3	T49.3X4	T49.3X5	T49.3X6
Corn starch	T49.3X1	T49.3X2	T49.3X3	T49.3X4	T49.3X5	T49.3X6
Coronary vasodilator NEC	T46.3X1	T46.3X2	T46.3X3	T46.3X4	T46.3X5	T46.3X6
Corrosive NEC	T54.91	T54.92	T54.93	T54.94	—	—
acid NEC	T54.2X1	T54.2X2	T54.2X3	T54.2X4	—	—
aromatics	T54.1X1	T54.1X2	T54.1X3	T54.1X4	—	—
disinfectant	T54.1X1	T54.1X2	T54.1X3	T54.1X4	—	—
fumes NEC	T54.91	T54.92	T54.93	T54.94	—	—
specified NEC	T54.91	T54.92	T54.93	T54.94	—	—
sublimate	T56.1X1	T56.1X2	T56.1X3	T56.1X4	—	—
Cortate	T38.ØX1	T38.ØX2	T38.ØX3	T38.ØX4	T38.ØX5	T38.ØX6
Cort-Dome	T38.ØX1	T38.ØX2	T38.ØX3	T38.ØX4	T38.ØX5	T38.ØX6
ENT agent	T49.6X1	T49.6X2	T49.6X3	T49.6X4	T49.6X5	T49.6X6
ophthalmic preparation	T49.5X1	T49.5X2	T49.5X3	T49.5X4	T49.5X5	T49.5X6
topical NEC	T49.ØX1	T49.ØX2	T49.ØX3	T49.ØX4	T49.ØX5	T49.ØX6
Cortef	T38.ØX1	T38.ØX2	T38.ØX3	T38.ØX4	T38.ØX5	T38.ØX6
ENT agent	T49.6X1	T49.6X2	T49.6X3	T49.6X4	T49.6X5	T49.6X6
ophthalmic preparation	T49.5X1	T49.5X2	T49.5X3	T49.5X4	T49.5X5	T49.5X6
topical NEC	T49.ØX1	T49.ØX2	T49.ØX3	T49.ØX4	T49.ØX5	T49.ØX6
Corticosteroid	T38.ØX1	T38.ØX2	T38.ØX3	T38.ØX4	T38.ØX5	T38.ØX6
ENT agent	T49.6X1	T49.6X2	T49.6X3	T49.6X4	T49.6X5	T49.6X6
mineral	T5Ø.ØX1	T5Ø.ØX2	T5Ø.ØX3	T5Ø.ØX4	T5Ø.ØX5	T5Ø.ØX6
ophthalmic	T49.5X1	T49.5X2	T49.5X3	T49.5X4	T49.5X5	T49.5X6
topical NEC	T49.ØX1	T49.ØX2	T49.ØX3	T49.ØX4	T49.ØX5	T49.ØX6
Corticotropin	T38.811	T38.812	T38.813	T38.814	T38.815	T38.816
Cortisol	T49.ØX1	T49.ØX2	T49.ØX3	T49.ØX4	T49.ØX5	T49.ØX6
ENT agent	T49.6X1	T49.6X2	T49.6X3	T49.6X4	T49.6X5	T49.6X6

Substance	Poisoning, Accidental (unintentional)	Poisoning, Intentional Self-harm	Poisoning, Assault	Poisoning, Undetermined	Adverse Effect	Under-dosing
Cortisol — *continued*						
ophthalmic preparation	T49.5X1	T49.5X2	T49.5X3	T49.5X4	T49.5X5	T49.5X6
topical NEC	T49.ØX1	T49.ØX2	T49.ØX3	T49.ØX4	T49.ØX5	T49.ØX6
Cortisone (acetate)	T38.ØX1	T38.ØX2	T38.ØX3	T38.ØX4	T38.ØX5	T38.ØX6
ENT agent	T49.6X1	T49.6X2	T49.6X3	T49.6X4	T49.6X5	T49.6X6
ophthalmic preparation	T49.5X1	T49.5X2	T49.5X3	T49.5X4	T49.5X5	T49.5X6
topical NEC	T49.ØX1	T49.ØX2	T49.ØX3	T49.ØX4	T49.ØX5	T49.ØX6
Cortisporin*	T49.ØX1	T49.ØX2	T49.ØX3	T49.ØX4	T49.ØX5	T49.ØX6
Cortivazol	T38.ØX1	T38.ØX2	T38.ØX3	T38.ØX4	T38.ØX5	T38.ØX6
Cortogen	T38.ØX1	T38.ØX2	T38.ØX3	T38.ØX4	T38.ØX5	T38.ØX6
ENT agent	T49.6X1	T49.6X2	T49.6X3	T49.6X4	T49.6X5	T49.6X6
ophthalmic preparation	T49.5X1	T49.5X2	T49.5X3	T49.5X4	T49.5X5	T49.5X6
Cortone	T38.ØX1	T38.ØX2	T38.ØX3	T38.ØX4	T38.ØX5	T38.ØX6
ENT agent	T49.6X1	T49.6X2	T49.6X3	T49.6X4	T49.6X5	T49.6X6
ophthalmic preparation	T49.5X1	T49.5X2	T49.5X3	T49.5X4	T49.5X5	T49.5X6
Cortril	T38.ØX1	T38.ØX2	T38.ØX3	T38.ØX4	T38.ØX5	T38.ØX6
ENT agent	T49.6X1	T49.6X2	T49.6X3	T49.6X4	T49.6X5	T49.6X6
ophthalmic preparation	T49.5X1	T49.5X2	T49.5X3	T49.5X4	T49.5X5	T49.5X6
topical NEC	T49.ØX1	T49.ØX2	T49.ØX3	T49.ØX4	T49.ØX5	T49.ØX6
Corynebacterium parvum	T45.1X1	T45.1X2	T45.1X3	T45.1X4	T45.1X5	T45.1X6
Cosmetic preparation	T49.8X1	T49.8X2	T49.8X3	T49.8X4	T49.8X5	T49.8X6
Cosmetics	T49.8X1	T49.8X2	T49.8X3	T49.8X4	T49.8X5	T49.8X6
Cosyntropin	T38.811	T38.812	T38.813	T38.814	T38.815	T38.816
Cotarnine	T45.7X1	T45.7X2	T45.7X3	T45.7X4	T45.7X5	T45.7X6
Co-trimoxazole	T36.8X1	T36.8X2	T36.8X3	T36.8X4	T36.8X5	T36.8X6
Cottonseed oil	T49.3X1	T49.3X2	T49.3X3	T49.3X4	T49.3X5	T49.3X6
Cough mixture (syrup)	T48.4X1	T48.4X2	T48.4X3	T48.4X4	T48.4X5	T48.4X6
containing opiates	T4Ø.2X1	T4Ø.2X2	T4Ø.2X3	T4Ø.2X4	T4Ø.2X5	T4Ø.2X6
expectorants	T48.4X1	T48.4X2	T48.4X3	T48.4X4	T48.4X5	T48.4X6
Coumadin	T45.511	T45.512	T45.513	T45.514	T45.515	T45.516
rodenticide	T6Ø.4X1	T6Ø.4X2	T6Ø.4X3	T6Ø.4X4	—	—
Coumaphos	T6Ø.ØX1	T6Ø.ØX2	T6Ø.ØX3	T6Ø.ØX4	—	—
Coumarin	T45.511	T45.512	T45.513	T45.514	T45.515	T45.516
Coumetarol	T45.511	T45.512	T45.513	T45.514	T45.515	T45.516
Cowbane	T62.2X1	T62.2X2	T62.2X3	T62.2X4	—	—
Cozaar*	T46.5X1	T46.5X2	T46.5X3	T46.5X4	T46.5X5	T46.5X6
Cozyme	T45.2X1	T45.2X2	T45.2X3	T45.2X4	T45.2X5	T45.2X6
Crack	T4Ø.5X1	T4Ø.5X2	T4Ø.5X3	T4Ø.5X4	—	—
Crataegus extract	T46.ØX1	T46.ØX2	T46.ØX3	T46.ØX4	T46.ØX5	T46.ØX6
Creolin	T54.1X1	T54.1X2	T54.1X3	T54.1X4	—	—
disinfectant	T54.1X1	T54.1X2	T54.1X3	T54.1X4	—	—
Creosol (compound)	T49.ØX1	T49.ØX2	T49.ØX3	T49.ØX4	T49.ØX5	T49.ØX6
Creosote (coal tar) (beechwood)	T49.ØX1	T49.ØX2	T49.ØX3	T49.ØX4	T49.ØX5	T49.ØX6
medicinal (expectorant)	T48.4X1	T48.4X2	T48.4X3	T48.4X4	T48.4X5	T48.4X6
syrup	T48.4X1	T48.4X2	T48.4X3	T48.4X4	T48.4X5	T48.4X6
Cresol(s)	T49.ØX1	T49.ØX2	T49.ØX3	T49.ØX4	T49.ØX5	T49.ØX6
and soap solution	T49.ØX1	T49.ØX2	T49.ØX3	T49.ØX4	T49.ØX5	T49.ØX6
Crestor*	T46.6X1	T46.6X2	T46.6X3	T46.6X4	T46.6X5	T46.6X6
Cresyl acetate	T49.ØX1	T49.ØX2	T49.ØX3	T49.ØX4	T49.ØX5	T49.ØX6
Cresylic acid	T49.ØX1	T49.ØX2	T49.ØX3	T49.ØX4	T49.ØX5	T49.ØX6
Crimidine	T6Ø.4X1	T6Ø.4X2	T6Ø.4X3	T6Ø.4X4	—	—
Croconazole	T37.8X1	T37.8X2	T37.8X3	T37.8X4	T37.8X5	T37.8X6
Cromoglicic acid	T48.6X1	T48.6X2	T48.6X3	T48.6X4	T48.6X5	T48.6X6
Cromolyn	T48.6X1	T48.6X2	T48.6X3	T48.6X4	T48.6X5	T48.6X6
Cromonar	T46.3X1	T46.3X2	T46.3X3	T46.3X4	T46.3X5	T46.3X6
Cropropamide	T39.8X1	T39.8X2	T39.8X3	T39.8X4	T39.8X5	T39.8X6
with crotethamide	T5Ø.7X1	T5Ø.7X2	T5Ø.7X3	T5Ø.7X4	T5Ø.7X5	T5Ø.7X6
Crotamiton	T49.ØX1	T49.ØX2	T49.ØX3	T49.ØX4	T49.ØX5	T49.ØX6
Crotethamide	T39.8X1	T39.8X2	T39.8X3	T39.8X4	T39.8X5	T39.8X6
with cropropamide	T5Ø.7X1	T5Ø.7X2	T5Ø.7X3	T5Ø.7X4	T5Ø.7X5	T5Ø.7X6
Croton (oil)	T47.2X1	T47.2X2	T47.2X3	T47.2X4	T47.2X5	T47.2X6
chloral	T42.6X1	T42.6X2	T42.6X3	T42.6X4	T42.6X5	T42.6X6
Crude oil	T52.ØX1	T52.ØX2	T52.ØX3	T52.ØX4	—	—
Cryogenine	T39.8X1	T39.8X2	T39.8X3	T39.8X4	T39.8X5	T39.8X6
Cryolite (vapor)	T6Ø.1X1	T6Ø.1X2	T6Ø.1X3	T6Ø.1X4	—	—
insecticide	T6Ø.1X1	T6Ø.1X2	T6Ø.1X3	T6Ø.1X4	—	—
Cryptenamine (tannates)	T46.5X1	T46.5X2	T46.5X3	T46.5X4	T46.5X5	T46.5X6
Crystal violet	T49.ØX1	T49.ØX2	T49.ØX3	T49.ØX4	T49.ØX5	T49.ØX6
Cuckoopint	T62.2X1	T62.2X2	T62.2X3	T62.2X4	—	—
Cumetharol	T45.511	T45.512	T45.513	T45.514	T45.515	T45.516
Cupric						
acetate	T6Ø.3X1	T6Ø.3X2	T6Ø.3X3	T6Ø.3X4	—	—
acetoarsenite	T57.ØX1	T57.ØX2	T57.ØX3	T57.ØX4	—	—
arsenate	T57.ØX1	T57.ØX2	T57.ØX3	T57.ØX4	—	—
gluconate	T49.ØX1	T49.ØX2	T49.ØX3	T49.ØX4	T49.ØX5	T49.ØX6
oleate	T49.ØX1	T49.ØX2	T49.ØX3	T49.ØX4	T49.ØX5	T49.ØX6
sulfate	T56.4X1	T56.4X2	T56.4X3	T56.4X4	—	—
Cuprimine*	T5Ø.6X1	T5Ø.6X2	T5Ø.6X3	T5Ø.6X4	T5Ø.6X5	T5Ø.6X6
Cuprous sulfate — *see also* Copper, sulfate	T56.4X1	T56.4X2	T56.4X3	T56.4X4	—	—
Curare, curarine	T48.1X1	T48.1X2	T48.1X3	T48.1X4	T48.1X5	T48.1X6
Cyamemazine	T43.3X1	T43.3X2	T43.3X3	T43.3X4	T43.3X5	T43.3X6

Substance	Poisoning, Accidental (unintentional)	Poisoning, Intentional Self-harm	Poisoning, Assault	Poisoning, Undetermined	Adverse Effect	Under-dosing
Cyamopsis tetragonoloba	T46.6X1	T46.6X2	T46.6X3	T46.6X4	T46.6X5	T46.6X6
Cyanacetyl hydrazide	T37.1X1	T37.1X2	T37.1X3	T37.1X4	T37.1X5	T37.1X6
Cyanic acid (gas)	T59.891	T59.892	T59.893	T59.894	—	—
Cyanide(s) (compounds) (potassium) (sodium) **NEC**	T65.ØX1	T65.ØX2	T65.ØX3	T65.ØX4	—	—
dust or gas (inhalation) NEC	T57.3X1	T57.3X2	T57.3X3	T57.3X4	—	—
fumigant	T65.ØX1	T65.ØX2	T65.ØX3	T65.ØX4	—	—
hydrogen	T57.3X1	T57.3X2	T57.3X3	T57.3X4	—	—
mercuric — *see* Mercury						
pesticide (dust) (fumes)	T65.ØX1	T65.ØX2	T65.ØX3	T65.ØX4	—	—
Cyanoacrylate adhesive	T49.3X1	T49.3X2	T49.3X3	T49.3X4	T49.3X5	T49.3X6
Cyanocobalamin	T45.8X1	T45.8X2	T45.8X3	T45.8X4	T45.8X5	T45.8X6
Cyanogen (chloride) (gas) **NEC**	T59.891	T59.892	T59.893	T59.894	—	—
Cyclacillin	T36.ØX1	T36.ØX2	T36.ØX3	T36.ØX4	T36.ØX5	T36.ØX6
Cyclaine	T41.3X1	T41.3X2	T41.3X3	T41.3X4	T41.3X5	T41.3X6
Cyclamate	T50.991	T50.992	T50.993	T50.994	T50.995	T50.996
Cyclamen europaeum	T62.2X1	T62.2X2	T62.2X3	T62.2X4	—	—
Cyclandelate	T46.7X1	T46.7X2	T46.7X3	T46.7X4	T46.7X5	T46.7X6
Cyclazocine	T50.7X1	T50.7X2	T50.7X3	T50.7X4	T50.7X5	T50.7X6
Cyclizine	T45.ØX1	T45.ØX2	T45.ØX3	T45.ØX4	T45.ØX5	T45.ØX6
Cyclobarbital	T42.3X1	T42.3X2	T42.3X3	T42.3X4	T42.3X5	T42.3X6
Cyclobarbitone	T42.3X1	T42.3X2	T42.3X3	T42.3X4	T42.3X5	T42.3X6
Cyclobenzaprine	T48.1X1	T48.1X2	T48.1X3	T48.1X4	T48.1X5	T48.1X6
Cyclodrine	T44.3X1	T44.3X2	T44.3X3	T44.3X4	T44.3X5	T44.3X6
Cycloguanil embonate	T37.2X1	T37.2X2	T37.2X3	T37.2X4	T37.2X5	T37.2X6
Cyclohexane	T52.8X1	T52.8X2	T52.8X3	T52.8X4	—	—
Cyclohexanol	T51.8X1	T51.8X2	T51.8X3	T51.8X4	—	—
Cyclohexanone	T52.4X1	T52.4X2	T52.4X3	T52.4X4	—	—
Cycloheximide	T60.3X1	T60.3X2	T60.3X3	T60.3X4	—	—
Cyclohexyl acetate	T52.8X1	T52.8X2	T52.8X3	T52.8X4	—	—
Cycloleucin	T45.1X1	T45.1X2	T45.1X3	T45.1X4	T45.1X5	T45.1X6
Cyclomethycaine	T41.3X1	T41.3X2	T41.3X3	T41.3X4	T41.3X5	T41.3X6
Cyclopentamine	T44.4X1	T44.4X2	T44.4X3	T44.4X4	T44.4X5	T44.4X6
Cyclopenthiazide	T50.2X1	T50.2X2	T50.2X3	T50.2X4	T50.2X5	T50.2X6
Cyclopentolate	T44.3X1	T44.3X2	T44.3X3	T44.3X4	T44.3X5	T44.3X6
Cyclophosphamide	T45.1X1	T45.1X2	T45.1X3	T45.1X4	T45.1X5	T45.1X6
Cycloplegic drug	T49.5X1	T49.5X2	T49.5X3	T49.5X4	T49.5X5	T49.5X6
Cyclopropane	T41.291	T41.292	T41.293	T41.294	T41.295	T41.296
Cyclopyrabital	T39.8X1	T39.8X2	T39.8X3	T39.8X4	T39.8X5	T39.8X6
Cycloserine	T37.1X1	T37.1X2	T37.1X3	T37.1X4	T37.1X5	T37.1X6
Cyclosporin	T45.1X1	T45.1X2	T45.1X3	T45.1X4	T45.1X5	T45.1X6
Cyclothiazide	T50.2X1	T50.2X2	T50.2X3	T50.2X4	T50.2X5	T50.2X6
Cycrimine	T44.3X1	T44.3X2	T44.3X3	T44.3X4	T44.3X5	T44.3X6
Cyhalothrin	T60.1X1	T60.1X2	T60.1X3	T60.1X4	—	—
Cymarin	T46.ØX1	T46.ØX2	T46.ØX3	T46.ØX4	T46.ØX5	T46.ØX6
Cymbalta*	T43.221	T43.222	T43.223	T43.224	T43.225	T43.226
Cypermethrin	T60.1X1	T60.1X2	T60.1X3	T60.1X4	—	—
Cyphenothrin	T60.2X1	T60.2X2	T60.2X3	T60.2X4	—	—
Cyproheptadine	T45.ØX1	T45.ØX2	T45.ØX3	T45.ØX4	T45.ØX5	T45.ØX6
Cyproterone	T38.6X1	T38.6X2	T38.6X3	T38.6X4	T38.6X5	T38.6X6
Cystaran*	T49.5X1	T49.5X2	T49.5X3	T49.5X4	T49.5X5	T49.5X6
Cysteamine	T50.6X1	T50.6X2	T50.6X3	T50.6X4	T50.6X5	T50.6X6
Cytarabine	T45.1X1	T45.1X2	T45.1X3	T45.1X4	T45.1X5	T45.1X6
Cytisus						
laburnum	T62.2X1	T62.2X2	T62.2X3	T62.2X4	—	—
scoparius	T62.2X1	T62.2X2	T62.2X3	T62.2X4	—	—
Cytochrome C	T47.5X1	T47.5X2	T47.5X3	T47.5X4	T47.5X5	T47.5X6
Cytomel	T38.1X1	T38.1X2	T38.1X3	T38.1X4	T38.1X5	T38.1X6
Cytosine arabinoside	T45.1X1	T45.1X2	T45.1X3	T45.1X4	T45.1X5	T45.1X6
Cytoxan	T45.1X1	T45.1X2	T45.1X3	T45.1X4	T45.1X5	T45.1X6
Cytozyme	T45.7X1	T45.7X2	T45.7X3	T45.7X4	T45.7X5	T45.7X6
S-Carboxymethylcysteine	T48.4X1	T48.4X2	T48.4X3	T48.4X4	T48.4X5	T48.4X6
Dabigatran*	T45.511	T45.512	T45.513	T45.514	T45.515	T45.516
Dacarbazine	T45.1X1	T45.1X2	T45.1X3	T45.1X4	T45.1X5	T45.1X6
Dactinomycin	T45.1X1	T45.1X2	T45.1X3	T45.1X4	T45.1X5	T45.1X6
DADPS	T37.1X1	T37.1X2	T37.1X3	T37.1X4	T37.1X5	T37.1X6
Dakin's solution	T49.ØX1	T49.ØX2	T49.ØX3	T49.ØX4	T49.ØX5	T49.ØX6
Dalapon (sodium)	T60.3X1	T60.3X2	T60.3X3	T60.3X4	—	—
Dalmane	T42.4X1	T42.4X2	T42.4X3	T42.4X4	T42.4X5	T42.4X6
Danazol	T38.6X1	T38.6X2	T38.6X3	T38.6X4	T38.6X5	T38.6X6
Danilone	T45.511	T45.512	T45.513	T45.514	T45.515	T45.516
Danthron	T47.2X1	T47.2X2	T47.2X3	T47.2X4	T47.2X5	T47.2X6
Dantrolene	T42.8X1	T42.8X2	T42.8X3	T42.8X4	T42.8X5	T42.8X6
Dantron	T47.2X1	T47.2X2	T47.2X3	T47.2X4	T47.2X5	T47.2X6
Daphne (gnidium) (mezereum)	T62.2X1	T62.2X2	T62.2X3	T62.2X4	—	—
berry	T62.1X1	T62.1X2	T62.1X3	T62.1X4	—	—
Dapsone	T37.1X1	T37.1X2	T37.1X3	T37.1X4	T37.1X5	T37.1X6
Daraprim	T37.2X1	T37.2X2	T37.2X3	T37.2X4	T37.2X5	T37.2X6
Darnel	T62.2X1	T62.2X2	T62.2X3	T62.2X4	—	—

Substance	Poisoning, Accidental (unintentional)	Poisoning, Intentional Self-harm	Poisoning, Assault	Poisoning, Undetermined	Adverse Effect	Under-dosing
Darvon	T39.8X1	T39.8X2	T39.8X3	T39.8X4	T39.8X5	T39.8X6
Daunomycin	T45.1X1	T45.1X2	T45.1X3	T45.1X4	T45.1X5	T45.1X6
Daunorubicin	T45.1X1	T45.1X2	T45.1X3	T45.1X4	T45.1X5	T45.1X6
DBI	T38.3X1	T38.3X2	T38.3X3	T38.3X4	T38.3X5	T38.3X6
D-Con	T60.91	T60.92	T60.93	T60.94	—	—
insecticide	T60.2X1	T60.2X2	T60.2X3	T60.2X4	—	—
rodenticide	T60.4X1	T60.4X2	T60.4X3	T60.4X4	—	—
DDAVP	T38.891	T38.892	T38.893	T38.894	T38.895	T38.896
DDE (bis(chlorophenyl)-dichloroethylene)	T60.2X1	T60.2X2	T60.2X3	T60.2X4	—	—
DDS	T37.1X1	T37.1X2	T37.1X3	T37.1X4	T37.1X5	T37.1X6
DDT (dust)	T60.1X1	T60.1X2	T60.1X3	T60.1X4	—	—
Deadly nightshade — *see also* Belladonna	T62.2X1	T62.2X2	T62.2X3	T62.2X4	—	—
berry	T62.1X1	T62.1X2	T62.1X3	T62.1X4	—	—
Deamino-D-arginine vasopressin	T38.891	T38.892	T38.893	T38.894	T38.895	T38.896
Deanol (aceglumate)	T50.991	T50.992	T50.993	T50.994	T50.995	T50.996
Debrisoquine	T46.5X1	T46.5X2	T46.5X3	T46.5X4	T46.5X5	T46.5X6
Decaborane	T57.8X1	T57.8X2	T57.8X3	T57.8X4	—	—
fumes	T59.891	T59.892	T59.893	T59.894	—	—
Decadron	T38.ØX1	T38.ØX2	T38.ØX3	T38.ØX4	T38.ØX5	T38.ØX6
ENT agent	T49.6X1	T49.6X2	T49.6X3	T49.6X4	T49.6X5	T49.6X6
ophthalmic preparation	T49.5X1	T49.5X2	T49.5X3	T49.5X4	T49.5X5	T49.5X6
topical NEC	T49.ØX1	T49.ØX2	T49.ØX3	T49.ØX4	T49.ØX5	T49.ØX6
Decahydronaphthalene	T52.8X1	T52.8X2	T52.8X3	T52.8X4	—	—
Decalin	T52.8X1	T52.8X2	T52.8X3	T52.8X4	—	—
Decamethonium (bromide)	T48.1X1	T48.1X2	T48.1X3	T48.1X4	T48.1X5	T48.1X6
Decholin	T47.5X1	T47.5X2	T47.5X3	T47.5X4	T47.5X5	T47.5X6
Declomycin	T36.4X1	T36.4X2	T36.4X3	T36.4X4	T36.4X5	T36.4X6
Decongestant, nasal (mucosa)	T48.5X1	T48.5X2	T48.5X3	T48.5X4	T48.5X5	T48.5X6
combination	T48.5X1	T48.5X2	T48.5X3	T48.5X4	T48.5X5	T48.5X6
Deet	T60.8X1	T60.8X2	T60.8X3	T60.8X4	—	—
Deferoxamine	T45.8X1	T45.8X2	T45.8X3	T45.8X4	T45.8X5	T45.8X6
Deflazacort	T38.ØX1	T38.ØX2	T38.ØX3	T38.ØX4	T38.ØX5	T38.ØX6
Deglycyrrhizinized extract of licorice	T48.4X1	T48.4X2	T48.4X3	T48.4X4	T48.4X5	T48.4X6
Dehydrocholic acid	T47.5X1	T47.5X2	T47.5X3	T47.5X4	T47.5X5	T47.5X6
Dehydroemetine	T37.3X1	T37.3X2	T37.3X3	T37.3X4	T37.3X5	T37.3X6
Dekalin	T52.8X1	T52.8X2	T52.8X3	T52.8X4	—	—
Delafloxacin*	T36.8X1	T36.8X2	T36.8X3	T36.8X4	T36.8X5	T36.8X6
Delalutin	T38.5X1	T38.5X2	T38.5X3	T38.5X4	T38.5X5	T38.5X6
Delorazepam	T42.4X1	T42.4X2	T42.4X3	T42.4X4	T42.4X5	T42.4X6
Delphinium	T62.2X1	T62.2X2	T62.2X3	T62.2X4	—	—
Deltacortisone*	T38.ØX1	T38.ØX2	T38.ØX3	T38.ØX4	T38.ØX5	T38.ØX6
Deltamethrin	T60.1X1	T60.1X2	T60.1X3	T60.1X4	—	—
Deltasone	T38.ØX1	T38.ØX2	T38.ØX3	T38.ØX4	T38.ØX5	T38.ØX6
Deltra	T38.ØX1	T38.ØX2	T38.ØX3	T38.ØX4	T38.ØX5	T38.ØX6
Delvinal	T42.3X1	T42.3X2	T42.3X3	T42.3X4	T42.3X5	T42.3X6
Demecarium (bromide)	T49.5X1	T49.5X2	T49.5X3	T49.5X4	T49.5X5	T49.5X6
Demeclocycline	T36.4X1	T36.4X2	T36.4X3	T36.4X4	T36.4X5	T36.4X6
Demecolcine	T45.1X1	T45.1X2	T45.1X3	T45.1X4	T45.1X5	T45.1X6
Demegestone	T38.5X1	T38.5X2	T38.5X3	T38.5X4	T38.5X5	T38.5X6
Demelanizing agents	T49.8X1	T49.8X2	T49.8X3	T49.8X4	T49.8X5	T49.8X6
Demephion -O and -S	T60.ØX1	T60.ØX2	T60.ØX3	T60.ØX4	—	—
Demerol	T40.2X1	T40.2X2	T40.2X3	T40.2X4	T40.2X5	T40.2X6
Demethylchlortetracycline	T36.4X1	T36.4X2	T36.4X3	T36.4X4	T36.4X5	T36.4X6
Demethyltetracycline	T36.4X1	T36.4X2	T36.4X3	T36.4X4	T36.4X5	T36.4X6
Demeton -O and -S	T60.ØX1	T60.ØX2	T60.ØX3	T60.ØX4	—	—
Demulcent (external)	T49.3X1	T49.3X2	T49.3X3	T49.3X4	T49.3X5	T49.3X6
specified NEC	T49.3X1	T49.3X2	T49.3X3	T49.3X4	T49.3X5	T49.3X6
Demulen	T38.4X1	T38.4X2	T38.4X3	T38.4X4	T38.4X5	T38.4X6
Denatured alcohol	T51.ØX1	T51.ØX2	T51.ØX3	T51.ØX4	—	—
Dendrid	T49.5X1	T49.5X2	T49.5X3	T49.5X4	T49.5X5	T49.5X6
Dental drug, topical application NEC	T49.7X1	T49.7X2	T49.7X3	T49.7X4	T49.7X5	T49.7X6
Dentifrice	T49.7X1	T49.7X2	T49.7X3	T49.7X4	T49.7X5	T49.7X6
Deodorant spray (feminine hygiene)	T49.8X1	T49.8X2	T49.8X3	T49.8X4	T49.8X5	T49.8X6
Deoxycortone	T50.ØX1	T50.ØX2	T50.ØX3	T50.ØX4	T50.ØX5	T50.ØX6
Deoxyribonuclease (pancreatic)	T45.3X1	T45.3X2	T45.3X3	T45.3X4	T45.3X5	T45.3X6
Depilatory	T49.4X1	T49.4X2	T49.4X3	T49.4X4	T49.4X5	T49.4X6
Deprenalin	T42.8X1	T42.8X2	T42.8X3	T42.8X4	T42.8X5	T42.8X6
Deprenyl	T42.8X1	T42.8X2	T42.8X3	T42.8X4	T42.8X5	T42.8X6
Depressant						
appetite (central)	T50.5X1	T50.5X2	T50.5X3	T50.5X4	T50.5X5	T50.5X6
cardiac	T46.2X1	T46.2X2	T46.2X3	T46.2X4	T46.2X5	T46.2X6
central nervous system (anesthetic) — *see also* Central nervous system, depressants	T42.71	T42.72	T42.73	T42.74	T42.75	T42.76

Substance	Poisoning, Accidental (unintentional)	Poisoning, Intentional Self-harm	Poisoning, Assault	Poisoning, Undetermined	Adverse Effect	Under-dosing
Depressant — *continued*						
central nervous system — *see also* Central nervous system, depressants — *continued*						
general anesthetic	T41.2Ø1	T41.2Ø2	T41.2Ø3	T41.2Ø4	T41.2Ø5	T41.2Ø6
muscle tone	T42.8X1	T42.8X2	T42.8X3	T42.8X4	T42.8X5	T42.8X6
muscle tone, central	T42.8X1	T42.8X2	T42.8X3	T42.8X4	T42.8X5	T42.8X6
psychotherapeutic	T43.5Ø1	T43.5Ø2	T43.5Ø3	T43.5Ø4	T43.5Ø5	T43.5Ø6
Depressant, appetite	T5Ø.5X1	T5Ø.5X2	T5Ø.5X3	T5Ø.5X4	T5Ø.5X5	T5Ø.5X6
Deptropine	T45.ØX1	T45.ØX2	T45.ØX3	T45.ØX4	T45.ØX5	T45.ØX6
Dequalinium (chloride)	T49.ØX1	T49.ØX2	T49.ØX3	T49.ØX4	T49.ØX5	T49.ØX6
Derris root	T6Ø.2X1	T6Ø.2X2	T6Ø.2X3	T6Ø.2X4	—	—
Deserpidine	T46.5X1	T46.5X2	T46.5X3	T46.5X4	T46.5X5	T46.5X6
Desferrioxamine	T45.8X1	T45.8X2	T45.8X3	T45.8X4	T45.8X5	T45.8X6
Desipramine	T43.Ø11	T43.Ø12	T43.Ø13	T43.Ø14	T43.Ø15	T43.Ø16
Deslanoside	T46.ØX1	T46.ØX2	T46.ØX3	T46.ØX4	T46.ØX5	T46.ØX6
Desloughing agent	T49.4X1	T49.4X2	T49.4X3	T49.4X4	T49.4X5	T49.4X6
Desmethylimipramine	T43.Ø11	T43.Ø12	T43.Ø13	T43.Ø14	T43.Ø15	T43.Ø16
Desmopressin	T38.891	T38.892	T38.893	T38.894	T38.895	T38.896
Desocodeine	T4Ø.2X1	T4Ø.2X2	T4Ø.2X3	T4Ø.2X4	T4Ø.2X5	T4Ø.2X6
Desogestrel	T38.5X1	T38.5X2	T38.5X3	T38.5X4	T38.5X5	T38.5X6
Desomorphine	T4Ø.2X1	T4Ø.2X2	T4Ø.2X3	T4Ø.2X4	—	—
Desonide	T49.ØX1	T49.ØX2	T49.ØX3	T49.ØX4	T49.ØX5	T49.ØX6
Desoximetasone	T49.ØX1	T49.ØX2	T49.ØX3	T49.ØX4	T49.ØX5	T49.ØX6
Desoxycorticosteroid	T5Ø.ØX1	T5Ø.ØX2	T5Ø.ØX3	T5Ø.ØX4	T5Ø.ØX5	T5Ø.ØX6
Desoxycortone	T5Ø.ØX1	T5Ø.ØX2	T5Ø.ØX3	T5Ø.ØX4	T5Ø.ØX5	T5Ø.ØX6
Desoxyephedrine	T43.651	T43.652	T43.653	T43.654	T43.655	T43.656
Detaxtran	T46.6X1	T46.6X2	T46.6X3	T46.6X4	T46.6X5	T46.6X6
Detergent	T49.2X1	T49.2X2	T49.2X3	T49.2X4	T49.2X5	T49.2X6
external medication	T49.2X1	T49.2X2	T49.2X3	T49.2X4	T49.2X5	T49.2X6
local	T49.2X1	T49.2X2	T49.2X3	T49.2X4	T49.2X5	T49.2X6
medicinal	T49.2X1	T49.2X2	T49.2X3	T49.2X4	T49.2X5	T49.2X6
nonmedicinal	T55.1X1	T55.1X2	T55.1X3	T55.1X4	—	—
specified NEC	T55.1X1	T55.1X2	T55.1X3	T55.1X4	—	—
Deterrent, alcohol	T5Ø.6X1	T5Ø.6X2	T5Ø.6X3	T5Ø.6X4	T5Ø.6X5	T5Ø.6X6
Detoxifying agent	T5Ø.6X1	T5Ø.6X2	T5Ø.6X3	T5Ø.6X4	T5Ø.6X5	T5Ø.6X6
Detrothyronine	T38.1X1	T38.1X2	T38.1X3	T38.1X4	T38.1X5	T38.1X6
Dettol (external medication)	T49.ØX1	T49.ØX2	T49.ØX3	T49.ØX4	T49.ØX5	T49.ØX6
Dexamethasone	T38.ØX1	T38.ØX2	T38.ØX3	T38.ØX4	T38.ØX5	T38.ØX6
ENT agent	T49.6X1	T49.6X2	T49.6X3	T49.6X4	T49.6X5	T49.6X6
ophthalmic preparation	T49.5X1	T49.5X2	T49.5X3	T49.5X4	T49.5X5	T49.5X6
topical NEC	T49.ØX1	T49.ØX2	T49.ØX3	T49.ØX4	T49.ØX5	T49.ØX6
Dexamfetamine	T43.621	T43.622	T43.623	T43.624	T43.625	T43.626
Dexamphetamine	T43.621	T43.622	T43.623	T43.624	T43.625	T43.626
Dexbrompheniramine	T45.ØX1	T45.ØX2	T45.ØX3	T45.ØX4	T45.ØX5	T45.ØX6
Dexchlorpheniramine	T45.ØX1	T45.ØX2	T45.ØX3	T45.ØX4	T45.ØX5	T45.ØX6
Dexedrine	T43.621	T43.622	T43.623	T43.624	T43.625	T43.626
Dexetimide	T44.3X1	T44.3X2	T44.3X3	T44.3X4	T44.3X5	T44.3X6
Dexfenfluramine	T5Ø.5X1	T5Ø.5X2	T5Ø.5X3	T5Ø.5X4	T5Ø.5X5	T5Ø.5X6
Dexpanthenol	T45.2X1	T45.2X2	T45.2X3	T45.2X4	T45.2X5	T45.2X6
Dextran (40) (70) (150)	T45.8X1	T45.8X2	T45.8X3	T45.8X4	T45.8X5	T45.8X6
Dextriferron	T45.4X1	T45.4X2	T45.4X3	T45.4X4	T45.4X5	T45.4X6
Dextroamphetamine	T43.621	T43.622	T43.623	T43.624	T43.625	T43.626
Dextro calcium pantothenate	T45.2X1	T45.2X2	T45.2X3	T45.2X4	T45.2X5	T45.2X6
Dextromethorphan	T48.3X1	T48.3X2	T48.3X3	T48.3X4	T48.3X5	T48.3X6
Dextromoramide	T4Ø.491	T4Ø.492	T4Ø.493	T4Ø.494	—	—
topical	T49.8X1	T49.8X2	T49.8X3	T49.8X4	T49.8X5	T49.8X6
Dextro pantothenyl alcohol	T45.2X1	T45.2X2	T45.2X3	T45.2X4	T45.2X5	T45.2X6
Dextropropoxyphene	T4Ø.491	T4Ø.492	T4Ø.493	T4Ø.494	T4Ø.495	T4Ø.496
Dextrorphan	T4Ø.2X1	T4Ø.2X2	T4Ø.2X3	T4Ø.2X4	T4Ø.2X5	T4Ø.2X6
Dextrose	T5Ø.3X1	T5Ø.3X2	T5Ø.3X3	T5Ø.3X4	T5Ø.3X5	T5Ø.3X6
concentrated solution, intravenous	T46.8X1	T46.8X2	T46.8X3	T46.8X4	T46.8X5	T46.8X6
Dextrothyroxin	T38.1X1	T38.1X2	T38.1X3	T38.1X4	T38.1X5	T38.1X6
Dextrothyroxine sodium	T38.1X1	T38.1X2	T38.1X3	T38.1X4	T38.1X5	T38.1X6
DFP	T44.ØX1	T44.ØX2	T44.ØX3	T44.ØX4	T44.ØX5	T44.ØX6
DHE	T37.3X1	T37.3X2	T37.3X3	T37.3X4	T37.3X5	T37.3X6
45	T46.5X1	T46.5X2	T46.5X3	T46.5X4	T46.5X5	T46.5X6
DiaBeta*	T38.3X1	T38.3X2	T38.3X3	T38.3X4	T38.3X5	T38.3X6
Diabinese	T38.3X1	T38.3X2	T38.3X3	T38.3X4	T38.3X5	T38.3X6
Diacetone alcohol	T52.4X1	T52.4X2	T52.4X3	T52.4X4	—	—
Diacetyl monoxime	T5Ø.991	T5Ø.992	T5Ø.993	T5Ø.994	—	—
Diacetylmorphine	T4Ø.1X1	T4Ø.1X2	T4Ø.1X3	T4Ø.1X4	—	—
Diachylon plaster	T49.4X1	T49.4X2	T49.4X3	T49.4X4	T49.4X5	T49.4X6
Diaethylstilboestrolum	T38.5X1	T38.5X2	T38.5X3	T38.5X4	T38.5X5	T38.5X6
Diagnostic agent NEC	T5Ø.8X1	T5Ø.8X2	T5Ø.8X3	T5Ø.8X4	T5Ø.8X5	T5Ø.8X6
Dial (soap)	T49.2X1	T49.2X2	T49.2X3	T49.2X4	T49.2X5	T49.2X6
sedative	T42.3X1	T42.3X2	T42.3X3	T42.3X4	T42.3X5	T42.3X6
Dialkyl carbonate	T52.91	T52.92	T52.93	T52.94	—	—
Diallylbarbituric acid	T42.3X1	T42.3X2	T42.3X3	T42.3X4	T42.3X5	T42.3X6
Diallymal	T42.3X1	T42.3X2	T42.3X3	T42.3X4	T42.3X5	T42.3X6

Substance	Poisoning, Accidental (unintentional)	Poisoning, Intentional Self-harm	Poisoning, Assault	Poisoning, Undetermined	Adverse Effect	Under-dosing
Dialysis solution (intraperitoneal)	T5Ø.3X1	T5Ø.3X2	T5Ø.3X3	T5Ø.3X4	T5Ø.3X5	T5Ø.3X6
Diaminodiphenylsulfone	T37.1X1	T37.1X2	T37.1X3	T37.1X4	T37.1X5	T37.1X6
Diamorphine	T4Ø.1X1	T4Ø.1X2	T4Ø.1X3	T4Ø.1X4	—	—
Diamox	T5Ø.2X1	T5Ø.2X2	T5Ø.2X3	T5Ø.2X4	T5Ø.2X5	T5Ø.2X6
Diamthazole	T49.ØX1	T49.ØX2	T49.ØX3	T49.ØX4	T49.ØX5	T49.ØX6
Dianthone	T47.2X1	T47.2X2	T47.2X3	T47.2X4	T47.2X5	T47.2X6
Diaphenylsulfone	T37.ØX1	T37.ØX2	T37.ØX3	T37.ØX4	T37.ØX5	T37.ØX6
Diasone (sodium)	T37.1X1	T37.1X2	T37.1X3	T37.1X4	T37.1X5	T37.1X6
Diastase	T47.5X1	T47.5X2	T47.5X3	T47.5X4	T47.5X5	T47.5X6
Diastat*	T42.4X1	T42.4X2	T42.4X3	T42.4X4	T42.4X5	T42.4X6
Diatrizoate	T5Ø.8X1	T5Ø.8X2	T5Ø.8X3	T5Ø.8X4	T5Ø.8X5	T5Ø.8X6
Diazepam	T42.4X1	T42.4X2	T42.4X3	T42.4X4	T42.4X5	T42.4X6
Diazinon	T6Ø.ØX1	T6Ø.ØX2	T6Ø.ØX3	T6Ø.ØX4	—	—
Diazomethane (gas)	T59.891	T59.892	T59.893	T59.894	—	—
Diazoxide	T46.5X1	T46.5X2	T46.5X3	T46.5X4	T46.5X5	T46.5X6
Dibekacin	T36.5X1	T36.5X2	T36.5X3	T36.5X4	T36.5X5	T36.5X6
Dibenamine	T44.6X1	T44.6X2	T44.6X3	T44.6X4	T44.6X5	T44.6X6
Dibenzepin	T43.Ø11	T43.Ø12	T43.Ø13	T43.Ø14	T43.Ø15	T43.Ø16
Dibenzheptropine	T45.ØX1	T45.ØX2	T45.ØX3	T45.ØX4	T45.ØX5	T45.ØX6
Dibenzyline	T44.6X1	T44.6X2	T44.6X3	T44.6X4	T44.6X5	T44.6X6
Diborane (gas)	T59.891	T59.892	T59.893	T59.894	—	—
Dibromochloropropane	T6Ø.8X1	T6Ø.8X2	T6Ø.8X3	T6Ø.8X4	—	—
Dibromodulcitol	T45.1X1	T45.1X2	T45.1X3	T45.1X4	T45.1X5	T45.1X6
Dibromoethane	T53.6X1	T53.6X2	T53.6X3	T53.6X4	—	—
Dibromomannitol	T45.1X1	T45.1X2	T45.1X3	T45.1X4	T45.1X5	T45.1X6
Dibromopropamidine isethionate	T49.ØX1	T49.ØX2	T49.ØX3	T49.ØX4	T49.ØX5	T49.ØX6
Dibrompropamidine	T49.ØX1	T49.ØX2	T49.ØX3	T49.ØX4	T49.ØX5	T49.ØX6
Dibucaine	T41.3X1	T41.3X2	T41.3X3	T41.3X4	T41.3X5	T41.3X6
topical (surface)	T41.3X1	T41.3X2	T41.3X3	T41.3X4	T41.3X5	T41.3X6
Dibunate sodium	T48.3X1	T48.3X2	T48.3X3	T48.3X4	T48.3X5	T48.3X6
Dibutoline sulfate	T44.3X1	T44.3X2	T44.3X3	T44.3X4	T44.3X5	T44.3X6
Dicamba	T6Ø.3X1	T6Ø.3X2	T6Ø.3X3	T6Ø.3X4	—	—
Dicapthon	T6Ø.ØX1	T6Ø.ØX2	T6Ø.ØX3	T6Ø.ØX4	—	—
Dichlobenil	T6Ø.3X1	T6Ø.3X2	T6Ø.3X3	T6Ø.3X4	—	—
Dichlone	T6Ø.3X1	T6Ø.3X2	T6Ø.3X3	T6Ø.3X4	—	—
Dichloralphenozone	T42.6X1	T42.6X2	T42.6X3	T42.6X4	T42.6X5	T42.6X6
Dichlorbenzidine	T65.3X1	T65.3X2	T65.3X3	T65.3X4	—	—
Dichlorhydrin	T52.8X1	T52.8X2	T52.8X3	T52.8X4	—	—
Dichlorhydroxyquinoline	T37.8X1	T37.8X2	T37.8X3	T37.8X4	T37.8X5	T37.8X6
Dichlorobenzene	T53.7X1	T53.7X2	T53.7X3	T53.7X4	—	—
Dichlorobenzyl alcohol	T49.6X1	T49.6X2	T49.6X3	T49.6X4	T49.6X5	T49.6X6
Dichlorodifluoromethane	T53.5X1	T53.5X2	T53.5X3	T53.5X4	—	—
Dichloroethane	T52.8X1	T52.8X2	T52.8X3	T52.8X4	—	—
Dichloroethylene	T53.6X1	T53.6X2	T53.6X3	T53.6X4	—	—
Dichloroethyl sulfide, not in war	T59.891	T59.892	T59.893	T59.894	—	—
Dichloroformoxine, not in war	T59.891	T59.892	T59.893	T59.894	—	—
Dichlorohydrin, alpha-dichlorohydrin	T52.8X1	T52.8X2	T52.8X3	T52.8X4	—	—
Dichloromethane (solvent)	T53.4X1	T53.4X2	T53.4X3	T53.4X4	—	—
vapor	T53.4X1	T53.4X2	T53.4X3	T53.4X4	—	—
Dichloronaphthoquinone	T6Ø.3X1	T6Ø.3X2	T6Ø.3X3	T6Ø.3X4	—	—
Dichlorophen	T37.4X1	T37.4X2	T37.4X3	T37.4X4	T37.4X5	T37.4X6
Dichloropropene	T6Ø.3X1	T6Ø.3X2	T6Ø.3X3	T6Ø.3X4	—	—
Dichloropropionic acid	T6Ø.3X1	T6Ø.3X2	T6Ø.3X3	T6Ø.3X4	—	—
Dichlorphenamide	T5Ø.2X1	T5Ø.2X2	T5Ø.2X3	T5Ø.2X4	T5Ø.2X5	T5Ø.2X6
Dichlorvos	T6Ø.ØX1	T6Ø.ØX2	T6Ø.ØX3	T6Ø.ØX4	—	—
Dichysterol*	T45.2X1	T45.2X2	T45.2X3	T45.2X4	T45.2X5	T45.2X6
Diclofenac	T39.391	T39.392	T39.393	T39.394	T39.395	T39.396
Diclofenamide	T5Ø.2X1	T5Ø.2X2	T5Ø.2X3	T5Ø.2X4	T5Ø.2X5	T5Ø.2X6
Diclofensine	T43.291	T43.292	T43.293	T43.294	T43.295	T43.296
Diclonixine	T39.8X1	T39.8X2	T39.8X3	T39.8X4	T39.8X5	T39.8X6
Dicloxacillin	T36.ØX1	T36.ØX2	T36.ØX3	T36.ØX4	T36.ØX5	T36.ØX6
Dicophane	T49.ØX1	T49.ØX2	T49.ØX3	T49.ØX4	T49.ØX5	T49.ØX6
Dicoumarol, dicoumarin, dicumarol	T45.511	T45.512	T45.513	T45.514	T45.515	T45.516
Dicrotophos	T6Ø.ØX1	T6Ø.ØX2	T6Ø.ØX3	T6Ø.ØX4	—	—
Dicyanogen (gas)	T65.ØX1	T65.ØX2	T65.ØX3	T65.ØX4	—	—
Dicyclomine	T44.3X1	T44.3X2	T44.3X3	T44.3X4	T44.3X5	T44.3X6
Dicycloverine	T44.3X1	T44.3X2	T44.3X3	T44.3X4	T44.3X5	T44.3X6
Didanosine*	T37.5X1	T37.5X2	T37.5X3	T37.5X4	T37.5X5	T37.5X6
Dideoxycytidine	T37.5X1	T37.5X2	T37.5X3	T37.5X4	T37.5X5	T37.5X6
Dideoxyinosine	T37.5X1	T37.5X2	T37.5X3	T37.5X4	T37.5X5	T37.5X6
Dieldrin (vapor)	T6Ø.1X1	T6Ø.1X2	T6Ø.1X3	T6Ø.1X4	—	—
Diemal	T42.3X1	T42.3X2	T42.3X3	T42.3X4	T42.3X5	T42.3X6
Dienestrol	T38.5X1	T38.5X2	T38.5X3	T38.5X4	T38.5X5	T38.5X6
Dienoestrol	T38.5X1	T38.5X2	T38.5X3	T38.5X4	T38.5X5	T38.5X6
Dietetic drug NEC	T5Ø.9Ø1	T5Ø.9Ø2	T5Ø.9Ø3	T5Ø.9Ø4	T5Ø.9Ø5	T5Ø.9Ø6
Diethazine	T42.8X1	T42.8X2	T42.8X3	T42.8X4	T42.8X5	T42.8X6

Substance	Poisoning, Accidental (unintentional)	Poisoning, Intentional Self-harm	Poisoning, Assault	Poisoning, Undetermined	Adverse Effect	Under-dosing
Diethyl						
barbituric acid	T42.3X1	T42.3X2	T42.3X3	T42.3X4	T42.3X5	T42.3X6
carbamazine	T37.4X1	T37.4X2	T37.4X3	T37.4X4	T37.4X5	T37.4X6
carbinol	T51.3X1	T51.3X2	T51.3X3	T51.3X4	—	—
carbonate	T52.8X1	T52.8X2	T52.8X3	T52.8X4	—	—
ether (vapor) — *see also* ether	T41.0X1	T41.0X2	T41.0X3	T41.0X4	T41.0X5	T41.0X6
oxide	T52.8X1	T52.8X2	T52.8X3	T52.8X4	—	—
propion	T50.5X1	T50.5X2	T50.5X3	T50.5X4	T50.5X5	T50.5X6
stilbestrol	T38.5X1	T38.5X2	T38.5X3	T38.5X4	T38.5X5	T38.5X6
toluamide (nonmedicinal)	T60.8X1	T60.8X2	T60.8X3	T60.8X4	—	—
medicinal	T49.3X1	T49.3X2	T49.3X3	T49.3X4	T49.3X5	T49.3X6
Diethylcarbamazine	T37.4X1	T37.4X2	T37.4X3	T37.4X4	T37.4X5	T37.4X6
Diethylene						
dioxide	T52.8X1	T52.8X2	T52.8X3	T52.8X4	—	—
glycol (monoacetate) (monobutyl ether) (monoethyl ether)	T52.3X1	T52.3X2	T52.3X3	T52.3X4	—	—
Diethylhexylphthalate	T65.891	T65.892	T65.893	T65.894	—	—
Diethylpropion	T50.5X1	T50.5X2	T50.5X3	T50.5X4	T50.5X5	T50.5X6
Diethylstilbestrol	T38.5X1	T38.5X2	T38.5X3	T38.5X4	T38.5X5	T38.5X6
Diethylstilboestrol	T38.5X1	T38.5X2	T38.5X3	T38.5X4	T38.5X5	T38.5X6
Diethylsulfone-diethylmethane	T42.6X1	T42.6X2	T42.6X3	T42.6X4	T42.6X5	T42.6X6
Diethyltoluamide	T49.0X1	T49.0X2	T49.0X3	T49.0X4	T49.0X5	T49.0X6
Diethyltryptamine (DET)	T40.991	T40.992	T40.993	T40.994	—	—
Difebarbamate	T42.3X1	T42.3X2	T42.3X3	T42.3X4	T42.3X5	T42.3X6
Difencloxazine	T40.2X1	T40.2X2	T40.2X3	T40.2X4	T40.2X5	T40.2X6
Difenidol	T45.0X1	T45.0X2	T45.0X3	T45.0X4	T45.0X5	T45.0X6
Difenoxin	T47.6X1	T47.6X2	T47.6X3	T47.6X4	T47.6X5	T47.6X6
Difetarsone	T37.3X1	T37.3X2	T37.3X3	T37.3X4	T37.3X5	T37.3X6
Diffusin	T45.3X1	T45.3X2	T45.3X3	T45.3X4	T45.3X5	T45.3X6
Diflorasone	T49.0X1	T49.0X2	T49.0X3	T49.0X4	T49.0X5	T49.0X6
Diflos	T44.0X1	T44.0X2	T44.0X3	T44.0X4	T44.0X5	T44.0X6
Diflubenzuron	T60.1X1	T60.1X2	T60.1X3	T60.1X4	—	—
Diflucan*	T37.8X1	T37.8X2	T37.8X3	T37.8X4	T37.8X5	T37.8X6
Diflucortolone	T49.0X1	T49.0X2	T49.0X3	T49.0X4	T49.0X5	T49.0X6
Diflunisal	T39.091	T39.092	T39.093	T39.094	T39.095	T39.096
Difluoromethyldopa	T42.8X1	T42.8X2	T42.8X3	T42.8X4	T42.8X5	T42.8X6
Difluorophate	T44.0X1	T44.0X2	T44.0X3	T44.0X4	T44.0X5	T44.0X6
Digestant NEC	T47.5X1	T47.5X2	T47.5X3	T47.5X4	T47.5X5	T47.5X6
Digitalin (e)	T46.0X1	T46.0X2	T46.0X3	T46.0X4	T46.0X5	T46.0X6
Digitalis (leaf)(glycoside)	T46.0X1	T46.0X2	T46.0X3	T46.0X4	T46.0X5	T46.0X6
lanata	T46.0X1	T46.0X2	T46.0X3	T46.0X4	T46.0X5	T46.0X6
purpurea	T46.0X1	T46.0X2	T46.0X3	T46.0X4	T46.0X5	T46.0X6
Digitoxin	T46.0X1	T46.0X2	T46.0X3	T46.0X4	T46.0X5	T46.0X6
Digitoxose	T46.0X1	T46.0X2	T46.0X3	T46.0X4	T46.0X5	T46.0X6
Digoxin	T46.0X1	T46.0X2	T46.0X3	T46.0X4	T46.0X5	T46.0X6
Digoxine	T46.0X1	T46.0X2	T46.0X3	T46.0X4	T46.0X5	T46.0X6
Dihydralazine	T46.5X1	T46.5X2	T46.5X3	T46.5X4	T46.5X5	T46.5X6
Dihydrazine	T46.5X1	T46.5X2	T46.5X3	T46.5X4	T46.5X5	T46.5X6
Dihydrocodeine	T40.2X1	T40.2X2	T40.2X3	T40.2X4	T40.2X5	T40.2X6
Dihydrocodeinone	T40.2X1	T40.2X2	T40.2X3	T40.2X4	T40.2X5	T40.2X6
Dihydroergocornine	T46.7X1	T46.7X2	T46.7X3	T46.7X4	T46.7X5	T46.7X6
Dihydroergocristine (mesilate)	T46.7X1	T46.7X2	T46.7X3	T46.7X4	T46.7X5	T46.7X6
Dihydroergokryptine	T46.7X1	T46.7X2	T46.7X3	T46.7X4	T46.7X5	T46.7X6
Dihydroergotamine	T46.5X1	T46.5X2	T46.5X3	T46.5X4	T46.5X5	T46.5X6
Dihydroergotoxine	T46.7X1	T46.7X2	T46.7X3	T46.7X4	T46.7X5	T46.7X6
mesilate	T46.7X1	T46.7X2	T46.7X3	T46.7X4	T46.7X5	T46.7X6
Dihydrohydroxycodeinone	T40.2X1	T40.2X2	T40.2X3	T40.2X4	T40.2X5	T40.2X6
Dihydrohydroxymorphinone	T40.2X1	T40.2X2	T40.2X3	T40.2X4	T40.2X5	T40.2X6
Dihydroisocodeine	T40.2X1	T40.2X2	T40.2X3	T40.2X4	T40.2X5	T40.2X6
Dihydromorphine	T40.2X1	T40.2X2	T40.2X3	T40.2X4	—	—
Dihydromorphinone	T40.2X1	T40.2X2	T40.2X3	T40.2X4	T40.2X5	T40.2X6
Dihydrostreptomycin	T36.5X1	T36.5X2	T36.5X3	T36.5X4	T36.5X5	T36.5X6
Dihydrotachysterol	T45.2X1	T45.2X2	T45.2X3	T45.2X4	T45.2X5	T45.2X6
Dihydroxyacetone*	T49.3X1	T49.3X2	T49.3X3	T49.3X4	T49.3X5	T49.3X6
Dihydroxyaluminum aminoacetate	T47.1X1	T47.1X2	T47.1X3	T47.1X4	T47.1X5	T47.1X6
Dihydroxyaluminum sodium carbonate	T47.1X1	T47.1X2	T47.1X3	T47.1X4	T47.1X5	T47.1X6
Dihydroxyanthraquinone	T47.2X1	T47.2X2	T47.2X3	T47.2X4	T47.2X5	T47.2X6
Dihydroxycodeinone	T40.2X1	T40.2X2	T40.2X3	T40.2X4	T40.2X5	T40.2X6
Dihydroxypropyl theophylline	T50.2X1	T50.2X2	T50.2X3	T50.2X4	T50.2X5	T50.2X6
Diiodohydroxyquin	T37.8X1	T37.8X2	T37.8X3	T37.8X4	T37.8X5	T37.8X6
topical	T49.0X1	T49.0X2	T49.0X3	T49.0X4	T49.0X5	T49.0X6
Diiodohydroxyquinoline	T37.8X1	T37.8X2	T37.8X3	T37.8X4	T37.8X5	T37.8X6
Diiodotyrosine	T38.2X1	T38.2X2	T38.2X3	T38.2X4	T38.2X5	T38.2X6
Diisopromine	T44.3X1	T44.3X2	T44.3X3	T44.3X4	T44.3X5	T44.3X6
Diisopropylamine	T46.3X1	T46.3X2	T46.3X3	T46.3X4	T46.3X5	T46.3X6

Substance	Poisoning, Accidental (unintentional)	Poisoning, Intentional Self-harm	Poisoning, Assault	Poisoning, Undetermined	Adverse Effect	Under-dosing
Diisopropylfluorophosphonate	T44.0X1	T44.0X2	T44.0X3	T44.0X4	T44.0X5	T44.0X6
Dilantin	T42.0X1	T42.0X2	T42.0X3	T42.0X4	T42.0X5	T42.0X6
Dilatrate*	T46.3X1	T46.3X2	T46.3X3	T46.3X4	T46.3X5	T46.3X6
Dilaudid	T40.2X1	T40.2X2	T40.2X3	T40.2X4	T40.2X5	T40.2X6
Dilazep	T46.3X1	T46.3X2	T46.3X3	T46.3X4	T46.3X5	T46.3X6
Dill	T47.5X1	T47.5X2	T47.5X3	T47.5X4	T47.5X5	T47.5X6
Diloxanide	T37.3X1	T37.3X2	T37.3X3	T37.3X4	T37.3X5	T37.3X6
Diltiazem	T46.1X1	T46.1X2	T46.1X3	T46.1X4	T46.1X5	T46.1X6
Dimazole	T49.0X1	T49.0X2	T49.0X3	T49.0X4	T49.0X5	T49.0X6
Dimefline	T50.7X1	T50.7X2	T50.7X3	T50.7X4	T50.7X5	T50.7X6
Dimefox	T60.0X1	T60.0X2	T60.0X3	T60.0X4	—	—
Dimemorfan	T48.3X1	T48.3X2	T48.3X3	T48.3X4	T48.3X5	T48.3X6
Dimenhydrinate	T45.0X1	T45.0X2	T45.0X3	T45.0X4	T45.0X5	T45.0X6
Dimercaprol (British anti-lewisite)	T45.8X1	T45.8X2	T45.8X3	T45.8X4	T45.8X5	T45.8X6
Dimercaptopropanol	T45.8X1	T45.8X2	T45.8X3	T45.8X4	T45.8X5	T45.8X6
Dimestrol	T38.5X1	T38.5X2	T38.5X3	T38.5X4	T38.5X5	T38.5X6
Dimetane	T45.0X1	T45.0X2	T45.0X3	T45.0X4	T45.0X5	T45.0X6
Dimethicone	T47.1X1	T47.1X2	T47.1X3	T47.1X4	T47.1X5	T47.1X6
Dimethindene	T45.0X1	T45.0X2	T45.0X3	T45.0X4	T45.0X5	T45.0X6
Dimethisoquin	T49.1X1	T49.1X2	T49.1X3	T49.1X4	T49.1X5	T49.1X6
Dimethisterone	T38.5X1	T38.5X2	T38.5X3	T38.5X4	T38.5X5	T38.5X6
Dimethoate	T60.0X1	T60.0X2	T60.0X3	T60.0X4	—	—
Dimethocaine	T41.3X1	T41.3X2	T41.3X3	T41.3X4	T41.3X5	T41.3X6
Dimethoxanate	T48.3X1	T48.3X2	T48.3X3	T48.3X4	T48.3X5	T48.3X6
Dimethyl						
arsine, arsinic acid	T57.0X1	T57.0X2	T57.0X3	T57.0X4	—	—
carbinol	T51.2X1	T51.2X2	T51.2X3	T51.2X4	—	—
carbonate	T52.8X1	T52.8X2	T52.8X3	T52.8X4	—	—
diguanide	T38.3X1	T38.3X2	T38.3X3	T38.3X4	T38.3X5	T38.3X6
ketone	T52.4X1	T52.4X2	T52.4X3	T52.4X4	—	—
vapor	T52.4X1	T52.4X2	T52.4X3	T52.4X4	—	—
meperidine	T40.2X1	T40.2X2	T40.2X3	T40.2X4	T40.2X5	T40.2X6
parathion	T60.0X1	T60.0X2	T60.0X3	T60.0X4	—	—
phthlate	T49.3X1	T49.3X2	T49.3X3	T49.3X4	T49.3X5	T49.3X6
polysiloxane	T47.8X1	T47.8X2	T47.8X3	T47.8X4	T47.8X5	T47.8X6
sulfate (fumes)	T59.891	T59.892	T59.893	T59.894	—	—
liquid	T65.891	T65.892	T65.893	T65.894	—	—
sulfoxide (nonmedicinal)	T52.8X1	T52.8X2	T52.8X3	T52.8X4	—	—
medicinal	T49.4X1	T49.4X2	T49.4X3	T49.4X4	T49.4X5	T49.4X6
tryptamine	T40.991	T40.992	T40.993	T40.994	—	—
tubocurarine	T48.1X1	T48.1X2	T48.1X3	T48.1X4	T48.1X5	T48.1X6
Dimethylamine sulfate	T49.4X1	T49.4X2	T49.4X3	T49.4X4	T49.4X5	T49.4X6
Dimethylcysteine*	T50.6X1	T50.6X2	T50.6X3	T50.6X4	T50.6X5	T50.6X6
Dimethylformamide	T52.8X1	T52.8X2	T52.8X3	T52.8X4	—	—
Dimethyltubocurarinium chloride	T48.1X1	T48.1X2	T48.1X3	T48.1X4	T48.1X5	T48.1X6
Dimeticone	T47.1X1	T47.1X2	T47.1X3	T47.1X4	T47.1X5	T47.1X6
Dimetilan	T60.0X1	T60.0X2	T60.0X3	T60.0X4	—	—
Dimetindene	T45.0X1	T45.0X2	T45.0X3	T45.0X4	T45.0X5	T45.0X6
Dimetotiazine	T43.3X1	T43.3X2	T43.3X3	T43.3X4	T43.3X5	T43.3X6
Dimorpholamine	T50.7X1	T50.7X2	T50.7X3	T50.7X4	T50.7X5	T50.7X6
Dimoxyline	T46.3X1	T46.3X2	T46.3X3	T46.3X4	T46.3X5	T46.3X6
Dinitrobenzene	T65.3X1	T65.3X2	T65.3X3	T65.3X4	—	—
vapor	T59.891	T59.892	T59.893	T59.894	—	—
Dinitrobenzol	T65.3X1	T65.3X2	T65.3X3	T65.3X4	—	—
vapor	T59.891	T59.892	T59.893	T59.894	—	—
Dinitrobutylphenol	T65.3X1	T65.3X2	T65.3X3	T65.3X4	—	—
Dinitro (-ortho-)cresol (pesticide) (spray)	T65.3X1	T65.3X2	T65.3X3	T65.3X4	—	—
Dinitrocyclohexylphenol	T65.3X1	T65.3X2	T65.3X3	T65.3X4	—	—
Dinitrophenol	T65.3X1	T65.3X2	T65.3X3	T65.3X4	—	—
Dinoprost	T48.0X1	T48.0X2	T48.0X3	T48.0X4	T48.0X5	T48.0X6
Dinoprostone	T48.0X1	T48.0X2	T48.0X3	T48.0X4	T48.0X5	T48.0X6
Dinoseb	T60.3X1	T60.3X2	T60.3X3	T60.3X4	—	—
Dioctyl sulfosuccinate (calcium) (sodium)	T47.4X1	T47.4X2	T47.4X3	T47.4X4	T47.4X5	T47.4X6
Diodone	T50.8X1	T50.8X2	T50.8X3	T50.8X4	T50.8X5	T50.8X6
Diodoquin	T37.8X1	T37.8X2	T37.8X3	T37.8X4	T37.8X5	T37.8X6
Dionin	T40.2X1	T40.2X2	T40.2X3	T40.2X4	T40.2X5	T40.2X6
Diosmin	T46.991	T46.992	T46.993	T46.994	T46.995	T46.996
Diovan*	T46.5X1	T46.5X2	T46.5X3	T46.5X4	T46.5X5	T46.5X6
Dioxane	T52.8X1	T52.8X2	T52.8X3	T52.8X4	—	—
Dioxathion	T60.0X1	T60.0X2	T60.0X3	T60.0X4	—	—
Dioxin	T53.7X1	T53.7X2	T53.7X3	T53.7X4	—	—
Dioxopromethazine	T43.3X1	T43.3X2	T43.3X3	T43.3X4	T43.3X5	T43.3X6
Dioxyline	T46.3X1	T46.3X2	T46.3X3	T46.3X4	T46.3X5	T46.3X6
Dipentene	T52.8X1	T52.8X2	T52.8X3	T52.8X4	—	—
Diperodon	T41.3X1	T41.3X2	T41.3X3	T41.3X4	T41.3X5	T41.3X6
Diphacinone	T60.4X1	T60.4X2	T60.4X3	T60.4X4	—	—
Diphemanil	T44.3X1	T44.3X2	T44.3X3	T44.3X4	T44.3X5	T44.3X6
metilsulfate	T44.3X1	T44.3X2	T44.3X3	T44.3X4	T44.3X5	T44.3X6

Substance	Poisoning, Accidental (unintentional)	Poisoning, Intentional Self-harm	Poisoning, Assault	Poisoning, Undetermined	Adverse Effect	Under-dosing
Diphenadione	T45.511	T45.512	T45.513	T45.514	T45.515	T45.516
rodenticide	T6Ø.4X1	T6Ø.4X2	T6Ø.4X3	T6Ø.4X4	—	—
Diphenhydramine	T45.ØX1	T45.ØX2	T45.ØX3	T45.ØX4	T45.ØX5	T45.ØX6
Diphenidol	T45.ØX1	T45.ØX2	T45.ØX3	T45.ØX4	T45.ØX5	T45.ØX6
Diphenoxylate	T47.6X1	T47.6X2	T47.6X3	T47.6X4	T47.6X5	T47.6X6
Diphenylamine	T65.3X1	T65.3X2	T65.3X3	T65.3X4	—	—
Diphenylbutazone	T39.2X1	T39.2X2	T39.2X3	T39.2X4	T39.2X5	T39.2X6
Diphenylchloroarsine, not in war	T57.ØX1	T57.ØX2	T57.ØX3	T57.ØX4	—	—
Diphenylhydantoin	T42.ØX1	T42.ØX2	T42.ØX3	T42.ØX4	T42.ØX5	T42.ØX6
Diphenylmethane dye	T52.1X1	T52.1X2	T52.1X3	T52.1X4	—	—
Diphenylpyraline	T45.ØX1	T45.ØX2	T45.ØX3	T45.ØX4	T45.ØX5	T45.ØX6
Diphtheria						
antitoxin	T5Ø.Z11	T5Ø.Z12	T5Ø.Z13	T5Ø.Z14	T5Ø.Z15	T5Ø.Z16
toxoid	T5Ø.A91	T5Ø.A92	T5Ø.A93	T5Ø.A94	T5Ø.A95	T5Ø.A96
with tetanus toxoid	T5Ø.A21	T5Ø.A22	T5Ø.A23	T5Ø.A24	T5Ø.A25	T5Ø.A26
with pertussis component	T5Ø.A11	T5Ø.A12	T5Ø.A13	T5Ø.A14	T5Ø.A15	T5Ø.A16
vaccine	T5Ø.A91	T5Ø.A92	T5Ø.A93	T5Ø.A94	T5Ø.A95	T5Ø.A96
combination						
without pertussis	T5Ø.A21	T5Ø.A22	T5Ø.A23	T5Ø.A24	T5Ø.A25	T5Ø.A26
including pertussis	T5Ø.A11	T5Ø.A12	T5Ø.A13	T5Ø.A14	T5Ø.A15	T5Ø.A16
Diphylline	T5Ø.2X1	T5Ø.2X2	T5Ø.2X3	T5Ø.2X4	T5Ø.2X5	T5Ø.2X6
Dipipanone	T4Ø.491	T4Ø.492	T4Ø.493	T4Ø.494	—	—
Dipivefrine	T49.5X1	T49.5X2	T49.5X3	T49.5X4	T49.5X5	T49.5X6
Diplovax	T5Ø.B91	T5Ø.B92	T5Ø.B93	T5Ø.B94	T5Ø.B95	T5Ø.B96
Diprophylline	T5Ø.2X1	T5Ø.2X2	T5Ø.2X3	T5Ø.2X4	T5Ø.2X5	T5Ø.2X6
Dipropyline	T48.291	T48.292	T48.293	T48.294	T48.295	T48.296
Dipyridamole	T46.3X1	T46.3X2	T46.3X3	T46.3X4	T46.3X5	T46.3X6
Dipyrone	T39.2X1	T39.2X2	T39.2X3	T39.2X4	T39.2X5	T39.2X6
Diquat (dibromide)	T6Ø.3X1	T6Ø.3X2	T6Ø.3X3	T6Ø.3X4	—	—
Disinfectant	T65.891	T65.892	T65.893	T65.894	—	—
alkaline	T54.3X1	T54.3X2	T54.3X3	T54.3X4	—	—
aromatic	T54.1X1	T54.1X2	T54.1X3	T54.1X4	—	—
intestinal	T37.8X1	T37.8X2	T37.8X3	T37.8X4	T37.8X5	T37.8X6
Disipal	T42.8X1	T42.8X2	T42.8X3	T42.8X4	T42.8X5	T42.8X6
Disodium edetate	T5Ø.6X1	T5Ø.6X2	T5Ø.6X3	T5Ø.6X4	T5Ø.6X5	T5Ø.6X6
Disoprofol	T41.291	T41.292	T41.293	T41.294	T41.295	T41.296
Disopyramide*	T46.2X1	T46.2X2	T46.2X3	T46.2X4	T46.2X5	T46.2X6
Distigmine (bromide)	T44.ØX1	T44.ØX2	T44.ØX3	T44.ØX4	T44.ØX5	T44.ØX6
Disulfamide	T5Ø.2X1	T5Ø.2X2	T5Ø.2X3	T5Ø.2X4	T5Ø.2X5	T5Ø.2X6
Disulfanilamide	T37.ØX1	T37.ØX2	T37.ØX3	T37.ØX4	T37.ØX5	T37.ØX6
Disulfiram	T5Ø.6X1	T5Ø.6X2	T5Ø.6X3	T5Ø.6X4	T5Ø.6X5	T5Ø.6X6
Disulfoton	T6Ø.ØX1	T6Ø.ØX2	T6Ø.ØX3	T6Ø.ØX4	—	—
Dithiazanine iodide	T37.4X1	T37.4X2	T37.4X3	T37.4X4	T37.4X5	T37.4X6
Dithiocarbamate	T6Ø.ØX1	T6Ø.ØX2	T6Ø.ØX3	T6Ø.ØX4	—	—
Dithranol	T49.4X1	T49.4X2	T49.4X3	T49.4X4	T49.4X5	T49.4X6
Diucardin	T5Ø.2X1	T5Ø.2X2	T5Ø.2X3	T5Ø.2X4	T5Ø.2X5	T5Ø.2X6
Diupres	T5Ø.2X1	T5Ø.2X2	T5Ø.2X3	T5Ø.2X4	T5Ø.2X5	T5Ø.2X6
Diuretic NEC	T5Ø.2X1	T5Ø.2X2	T5Ø.2X3	T5Ø.2X4	T5Ø.2X5	T5Ø.2X6
benzothiadiazine	T5Ø.2X1	T5Ø.2X2	T5Ø.2X3	T5Ø.2X4	T5Ø.2X5	T5Ø.2X6
carbonic acid anhydrase inhibitors	T5Ø.2X1	T5Ø.2X2	T5Ø.2X3	T5Ø.2X4	T5Ø.2X5	T5Ø.2X6
furfuryl NEC	T5Ø.2X1	T5Ø.2X2	T5Ø.2X3	T5Ø.2X4	T5Ø.2X5	T5Ø.2X6
loop (high-ceiling)	T5Ø.1X1	T5Ø.1X2	T5Ø.1X3	T5Ø.1X4	T5Ø.1X5	T5Ø.1X6
mercurial NEC	T5Ø.2X1	T5Ø.2X2	T5Ø.2X3	T5Ø.2X4	T5Ø.2X5	T5Ø.2X6
osmotic	T5Ø.2X1	T5Ø.2X2	T5Ø.2X3	T5Ø.2X4	T5Ø.2X5	T5Ø.2X6
purine NEC	T5Ø.2X1	T5Ø.2X2	T5Ø.2X3	T5Ø.2X4	T5Ø.2X5	T5Ø.2X6
saluretic NEC	T5Ø.2X1	T5Ø.2X2	T5Ø.2X3	T5Ø.2X4	T5Ø.2X5	T5Ø.2X6
sulfonamide	T5Ø.2X1	T5Ø.2X2	T5Ø.2X3	T5Ø.2X4	T5Ø.2X5	T5Ø.2X6
thiazide NEC	T5Ø.2X1	T5Ø.2X2	T5Ø.2X3	T5Ø.2X4	T5Ø.2X5	T5Ø.2X6
xanthine	T5Ø.2X1	T5Ø.2X2	T5Ø.2X3	T5Ø.2X4	T5Ø.2X5	T5Ø.2X6
Diurgin	T5Ø.2X1	T5Ø.2X2	T5Ø.2X3	T5Ø.2X4	T5Ø.2X5	T5Ø.2X6
Diuril	T5Ø.2X1	T5Ø.2X2	T5Ø.2X3	T5Ø.2X4	T5Ø.2X5	T5Ø.2X6
Diuron	T6Ø.3X1	T6Ø.3X2	T6Ø.3X3	T6Ø.3X4	—	—
Divalproex	T42.6X1	T42.6X2	T42.6X3	T42.6X4	T42.6X5	T42.6X6
Divinyl ether	T41.ØX1	T41.ØX2	T41.ØX3	T41.ØX4	T41.ØX5	T41.ØX6
Dixanthogen	T49.ØX1	T49.ØX2	T49.ØX3	T49.ØX4	T49.ØX5	T49.ØX6
Dixyrazine	T43.3X1	T43.3X2	T43.3X3	T43.3X4	T43.3X5	T43.3X6
D-lysergic acid diethylamide	T4Ø.8X1	T4Ø.8X2	T4Ø.8X3	T4Ø.8X4	—	—
DMCT	T36.4X1	T36.4X2	T36.4X3	T36.4X4	T36.4X5	T36.4X6
DMSO — *see* Dimethyl, sulfoxide						
DNBP	T6Ø.3X1	T6Ø.3X2	T6Ø.3X3	T6Ø.3X4	—	—
DNOC	T65.3X1	T65.3X2	T65.3X3	T65.3X4	—	—
Dobutamine	T44.5X1	T44.5X2	T44.5X3	T44.5X4	T44.5X5	T44.5X6
DOCA	T38.ØX1	T38.ØX2	T38.ØX3	T38.ØX4	T38.ØX5	T38.ØX6
Docusate sodium	T47.4X1	T47.4X2	T47.4X3	T47.4X4	T47.4X5	T47.4X6
Dodicin	T49.ØX1	T49.ØX2	T49.ØX3	T49.ØX4	T49.ØX5	T49.ØX6
Dofamium chloride	T49.ØX1	T49.ØX2	T49.ØX3	T49.ØX4	T49.ØX5	T49.ØX6
Dolophine	T4Ø.3X1	T4Ø.3X2	T4Ø.3X3	T4Ø.3X4	T4Ø.3X5	T4Ø.3X6
Doloxene	T39.8X1	T39.8X2	T39.8X3	T39.8X4	T39.8X5	T39.8X6

Substance	Poisoning, Accidental (unintentional)	Poisoning, Intentional Self-harm	Poisoning, Assault	Poisoning, Undetermined	Adverse Effect	Under-dosing
Domestic gas (after combustion) — *see* Gas, utility						
prior to combustion	T59.891	T59.892	T59.893	T59.894	—	—
Domiodol	T48.4X1	T48.4X2	T48.4X3	T48.4X4	T48.4X5	T48.4X6
Domiphen (bromide)	T49.ØX1	T49.ØX2	T49.ØX3	T49.ØX4	T49.ØX5	T49.ØX6
Domperidone	T45.ØX1	T45.ØX2	T45.ØX3	T45.ØX4	T45.ØX5	T45.ØX6
Donepezil*	T44.ØX1	T44.ØX2	T44.ØX3	T44.ØX4	T44.ØX5	T44.ØX6
Dopa	T42.8X1	T42.8X2	T42.8X3	T42.8X4	T42.8X5	T42.8X6
Dopamine	T44.991	T44.992	T44.993	T44.994	T44.995	T44.996
Doriden	T42.6X1	T42.6X2	T42.6X3	T42.6X4	T42.6X5	T42.6X6
Dormiral	T42.3X1	T42.3X2	T42.3X3	T42.3X4	T42.3X5	T42.3X6
Dormison	T42.6X1	T42.6X2	T42.6X3	T42.6X4	T42.6X5	T42.6X6
Dornase	T48.4X1	T48.4X2	T48.4X3	T48.4X4	T48.4X5	T48.4X6
Dorsacaine	T41.3X1	T41.3X2	T41.3X3	T41.3X4	T41.3X5	T41.3X6
Dosulepin	T43.Ø11	T43.Ø12	T43.Ø13	T43.Ø14	T43.Ø15	T43.Ø16
Dothiepin	T43.Ø11	T43.Ø12	T43.Ø13	T43.Ø14	T43.Ø15	T43.Ø16
Doxantrazole	T48.6X1	T48.6X2	T48.6X3	T48.6X4	T48.6X5	T48.6X6
Doxapram	T5Ø.7X1	T5Ø.7X2	T5Ø.7X3	T5Ø.7X4	T5Ø.7X5	T5Ø.7X6
Doxazosin	T44.6X1	T44.6X2	T44.6X3	T44.6X4	T44.6X5	T44.6X6
Doxepin	T43.Ø11	T43.Ø12	T43.Ø13	T43.Ø14	T43.Ø15	T43.Ø16
Doxifluridine	T45.1X1	T45.1X2	T45.1X3	T45.1X4	T45.1X5	T45.1X6
Doxil*	T45.1X1	T45.1X2	T45.1X3	T45.1X4	T45.1X5	T45.1X6
Doxorubicin	T45.1X1	T45.1X2	T45.1X3	T45.1X4	T45.1X5	T45.1X6
Doxycycline	T36.4X1	T36.4X2	T36.4X3	T36.4X4	T36.4X5	T36.4X6
Doxylamine	T45.ØX1	T45.ØX2	T45.ØX3	T45.ØX4	T45.ØX5	T45.ØX6
Dramamine	T45.ØX1	T45.ØX2	T45.ØX3	T45.ØX4	T45.ØX5	T45.ØX6
Drano (drain cleaner)	T54.3X1	T54.3X2	T54.3X3	T54.3X4	—	—
Dressing, live pulp	T49.7X1	T49.7X2	T49.7X3	T49.7X4	T49.7X5	T49.7X6
Drocode	T4Ø.2X1	T4Ø.2X2	T4Ø.2X3	T4Ø.2X4	T4Ø.2X5	T4Ø.2X6
Dromoran	T4Ø.2X1	T4Ø.2X2	T4Ø.2X3	T4Ø.2X4	T4Ø.2X5	T4Ø.2X6
Dromostanolone	T38.7X1	T38.7X2	T38.7X3	T38.7X4	T38.7X5	T38.7X6
Dronabinol	T4Ø.711	T4Ø.712	T4Ø.713	T4Ø.714	T4Ø.715	T4Ø.716
Droperidol	T43.591	T43.592	T43.593	T43.594	T43.595	T43.596
Dropropizine	T48.3X1	T48.3X2	T48.3X3	T48.3X4	T48.3X5	T48.3X6
Drostanolone	T38.7X1	T38.7X2	T38.7X3	T38.7X4	T38.7X5	T38.7X6
Drotaverine	T44.3X1	T44.3X2	T44.3X3	T44.3X4	T44.3X5	T44.3X6
Drotrecogin alfa	T45.511	T45.512	T45.513	T45.514	T45.515	T45.516
Drug NEC	T5Ø.9Ø1	T5Ø.9Ø2	T5Ø.9Ø3	T5Ø.9Ø4	T5Ø.9Ø5	T5Ø.9Ø6
specified NEC	T5Ø.991	T5Ø.992	T5Ø.993	T5Ø.994	T5Ø.995	T5Ø.996
DTIC	T45.1X1	T45.1X2	T45.1X3	T45.1X4	T45.1X5	T45.1X6
Duboisine	T44.3X1	T44.3X2	T44.3X3	T44.3X4	T44.3X5	T44.3X6
Dulcolax	T47.2X1	T47.2X2	T47.2X3	T47.2X4	T47.2X5	T47.2X6
Duponol (C) (EP)	T49.2X1	T49.2X2	T49.2X3	T49.2X4	T49.2X5	T49.2X6
Durabolin	T38.7X1	T38.7X2	T38.7X3	T38.7X4	T38.7X5	T38.7X6
Durezol*	T49.5X1	T49.5X2	T49.5X3	T49.5X4	T49.5X5	T49.5X6
Dyclone	T41.3X1	T41.3X2	T41.3X3	T41.3X4	T41.3X5	T41.3X6
Dyclonine	T41.3X1	T41.3X2	T41.3X3	T41.3X4	T41.3X5	T41.3X6
Dydrogesterone	T38.5X1	T38.5X2	T38.5X3	T38.5X4	T38.5X5	T38.5X6
Dye NEC	T65.6X1	T65.6X2	T65.6X3	T65.6X4	—	—
antiseptic	T49.ØX1	T49.ØX2	T49.ØX3	T49.ØX4	T49.ØX5	T49.ØX6
diagnostic agents	T5Ø.8X1	T5Ø.8X2	T5Ø.8X3	T5Ø.8X4	T5Ø.8X5	T5Ø.8X6
pharmaceutical NEC	T5Ø.9Ø1	T5Ø.9Ø2	T5Ø.9Ø3	T5Ø.9Ø4	T5Ø.9Ø5	T5Ø.9Ø6
Dyflos	T44.ØX1	T44.ØX2	T44.ØX3	T44.ØX4	T44.ØX5	T44.ØX6
Dymelor	T38.3X1	T38.3X2	T38.3X3	T38.3X4	T38.3X5	T38.3X6
Dynamite	T65.3X1	T65.3X2	T65.3X3	T65.3X4	—	—
fumes	T59.891	T59.892	T59.893	T59.894	—	—
Dyphylline	T44.3X1	T44.3X2	T44.3X3	T44.3X4	T44.3X5	T44.3X6
b-eucaine	T49.1X1	T49.1X2	T49.1X3	T49.1X4	T49.1X5	T49.1X6
Ear drug NEC	T49.6X1	T49.6X2	T49.6X3	T49.6X4	T49.6X5	T49.6X6
Ear preparations	T49.6X1	T49.6X2	T49.6X3	T49.6X4	T49.6X5	T49.6X6
Echothiophate, echothiopate, ecothiopate	T49.5X1	T49.5X2	T49.5X3	T49.5X4	T49.5X5	T49.5X6
Econazole	T49.ØX1	T49.ØX2	T49.ØX3	T49.ØX4	T49.ØX5	T49.ØX6
Ecothiopate iodide	T49.5X1	T49.5X2	T49.5X3	T49.5X4	T49.5X5	T49.5X6
Ecstasy	T43.641	T43.642	T43.643	T43.644	—	—
Ectylurea	T42.6X1	T42.6X2	T42.6X3	T42.6X4	T42.6X5	T42.6X6
Edathamil disodium	T45.8X1	T45.8X2	T45.8X3	T45.8X4	T45.8X5	T45.8X6
Edecrin	T5Ø.1X1	T5Ø.1X2	T5Ø.1X3	T5Ø.1X4	T5Ø.1X5	T5Ø.1X6
Edetate, disodium (calcium)	T45.8X1	T45.8X2	T45.8X3	T45.8X4	T45.8X5	T45.8X6
Edoxudine	T49.5X1	T49.5X2	T49.5X3	T49.5X4	T49.5X5	T49.5X6
Edrophonium	T44.ØX1	T44.ØX2	T44.ØX3	T44.ØX4	T44.ØX5	T44.ØX6
chloride	T44.ØX1	T44.ØX2	T44.ØX3	T44.ØX4	T44.ØX5	T44.ØX6
EDTA	T5Ø.6X1	T5Ø.6X2	T5Ø.6X3	T5Ø.6X4	T5Ø.6X5	T5Ø.6X6
Effexor*	T43.221	T43.222	T43.223	T43.224	T43.225	T43.226
Eflornithine	T37.2X1	T37.2X2	T37.2X3	T37.2X4	T37.2X5	T37.2X6
Efloxate	T46.3X1	T46.3X2	T46.3X3	T46.3X4	T46.3X5	T46.3X6
Elase	T49.8X1	T49.8X2	T49.8X3	T49.8X4	T49.8X5	T49.8X6
Elastase	T47.5X1	T47.5X2	T47.5X3	T47.5X4	T47.5X5	T47.5X6
Elaterium	T47.2X1	T47.2X2	T47.2X3	T47.2X4	T47.2X5	T47.2X6
Elcatonin	T5Ø.991	T5Ø.992	T5Ø.993	T5Ø.994	T5Ø.995	T5Ø.996
Elder	T62.2X1	T62.2X2	T62.2X3	T62.2X4	—	—
berry, (unripe)	T62.1X1	T62.1X2	T62.1X3	T62.1X4	—	—

*Optum Value-Add

Substance	Poisoning, Accidental (unintentional)	Poisoning, Intentional Self-harm	Poisoning, Assault	Poisoning, Undetermined	Adverse Effect	Under-dosing
Electrolyte balance drug	T5Ø.3X1	T5Ø.3X2	T5Ø.3X3	T5Ø.3X4	T5Ø.3X5	T5Ø.3X6
Electrolytes NEC	T5Ø.3X1	T5Ø.3X2	T5Ø.3X3	T5Ø.3X4	T5Ø.3X5	T5Ø.3X6
Electrolytic agent NEC	T5Ø.3X1	T5Ø.3X2	T5Ø.3X3	T5Ø.3X4	T5Ø.3X5	T5Ø.3X6
Elemental diet	T5Ø.9Ø1	T5Ø.9Ø2	T5Ø.9Ø3	T5Ø.9Ø4	T5Ø.9Ø5	T5Ø.9Ø6
Elliptinium acetate	T45.1X1	T45.1X2	T45.1X3	T45.1X4	T45.1X5	T45.1X6
Elocon*	T49.ØX1	T49.ØX2	T49.ØX3	T49.ØX4	T49.ØX5	T49.ØX6
Embramine	T45.ØX1	T45.ØX2	T45.ØX3	T45.ØX4	T45.ØX5	T45.ØX6
Emepronium (salts)	T44.3X1	T44.3X2	T44.3X3	T44.3X4	T44.3X5	T44.3X6
bromide	T44.3X1	T44.3X2	T44.3X3	T44.3X4	T44.3X5	T44.3X6
Emetic NEC	T47.7X1	T47.7X2	T47.7X3	T47.7X4	T47.7X5	T47.7X6
Emetine	T37.3X1	T37.3X2	T37.3X3	T37.3X4	T37.3X5	T37.3X6
Emollient NEC	T49.3X1	T49.3X2	T49.3X3	T49.3X4	T49.3X5	T49.3X6
Emorfazone	T39.8X1	T39.8X2	T39.8X3	T39.8X4	T39.8X5	T39.8X6
Emylcamate	T43.591	T43.592	T43.593	T43.594	T43.595	T43.596
Enalapril	T46.4X1	T46.4X2	T46.4X3	T46.4X4	T46.4X5	T46.4X6
Enalaprilat	T46.4X1	T46.4X2	T46.4X3	T46.4X4	T46.4X5	T46.4X6
Enbrel*	T39.4X1	T39.4X2	T39.4X3	T39.4X4	T39.4X5	T39.4X6
Encainide	T46.2X1	T46.2X2	T46.2X3	T46.2X4	T46.2X5	T46.2X6
Endocaine	T41.3X1	T41.3X2	T41.3X3	T41.3X4	T41.3X5	T41.3X6
Endosulfan	T6Ø.2X1	T6Ø.2X2	T6Ø.2X3	T6Ø.2X4	—	—
Endothall	T6Ø.3X1	T6Ø.3X2	T6Ø.3X3	T6Ø.3X4	—	—
Endralazine	T46.5X1	T46.5X2	T46.5X3	T46.5X4	T46.5X5	T46.5X6
Endrin	T6Ø.1X1	T6Ø.1X2	T6Ø.1X3	T6Ø.1X4	—	—
Enflurane	T41.ØX1	T41.ØX2	T41.ØX3	T41.ØX4	T41.ØX5	T41.ØX6
Enfuvirtide*	T37.5X1	T37.5X2	T37.5X3	T37.5X4	T37.5X5	T37.5X6
Enhexymal	T42.3X1	T42.3X2	T42.3X3	T42.3X4	T42.3X5	T42.3X6
Enocitabine	T45.1X1	T45.1X2	T45.1X3	T45.1X4	T45.1X5	T45.1X6
Enovid	T38.4X1	T38.4X2	T38.4X3	T38.4X4	T38.4X5	T38.4X6
Enoxacin	T36.8X1	T36.8X2	T36.8X3	T36.8X4	T36.8X5	T36.8X6
Enoxaparin (sodium)	T45.511	T45.512	T45.513	T45.514	T45.515	T45.516
Enpiprazole	T43.591	T43.592	T43.593	T43.594	T43.595	T43.596
Enprofylline	T48.6X1	T48.6X2	T48.6X3	T48.6X4	T48.6X5	T48.6X6
Enprostil	T47.1X1	T47.1X2	T47.1X3	T47.1X4	T47.1X5	T47.1X6
Enterogastrone	T38.891	T38.892	T38.893	T38.894	T38.895	T38.896
ENT preparations (anti-infectives)	T49.6X1	T49.6X2	T49.6X3	T49.6X4	T49.6X5	T49.6X6
Enviomycin	T36.8X1	T36.8X2	T36.8X3	T36.8X4	T36.8X5	T36.8X6
Enzodase	T45.3X1	T45.3X2	T45.3X3	T45.3X4	T45.3X5	T45.3X6
Enzyme NEC	T45.3X1	T45.3X2	T45.3X3	T45.3X4	T45.3X5	T45.3X6
depolymerizing	T49.8X1	T49.8X2	T49.8X3	T49.8X4	T49.8X5	T49.8X6
fibrolytic	T45.3X1	T45.3X2	T45.3X3	T45.3X4	T45.3X5	T45.3X6
gastric	T47.5X1	T47.5X2	T47.5X3	T47.5X4	T47.5X5	T47.5X6
intestinal	T47.5X1	T47.5X2	T47.5X3	T47.5X4	T47.5X5	T47.5X6
local action	T49.4X1	T49.4X2	T49.4X3	T49.4X4	T49.4X5	T49.4X6
proteolytic	T49.4X1	T49.4X2	T49.4X3	T49.4X4	T49.4X5	T49.4X6
thrombolytic	T45.3X1	T45.3X2	T45.3X3	T45.3X4	T45.3X5	T45.3X6
EPAB	T41.3X1	T41.3X2	T41.3X3	T41.3X4	T41.3X5	T41.3X6
Epanutin	T42.ØX1	T42.ØX2	T42.ØX3	T42.ØX4	T42.ØX5	T42.ØX6
Ephedra	T44.991	T44.992	T44.993	T44.994	T44.995	T44.996
Ephedrine	T44.991	T44.992	T44.993	T44.994	T44.995	T44.996
Epichlorhydrin, epichlorohydrin	T52.8X1	T52.8X2	T52.8X3	T52.8X4	—	—
Epicillin	T36.ØX1	T36.ØX2	T36.ØX3	T36.ØX4	T36.ØX5	T36.ØX6
Epiestriol	T38.5X1	T38.5X2	T38.5X3	T38.5X4	T38.5X5	T38.5X6
Epilim — *see* Sodium, valproate						
Epimestrol	T38.5X1	T38.5X2	T38.5X3	T38.5X4	T38.5X5	T38.5X6
Epinephrine	T44.5X1	T44.5X2	T44.5X3	T44.5X4	T44.5X5	T44.5X6
EpiPen*	T44.5X1	T44.5X2	T44.5X3	T44.5X4	T44.5X5	T44.5X6
Epirubicin	T45.1X1	T45.1X2	T45.1X3	T45.1X4	T45.1X5	T45.1X6
Epitiostanol	T38.7X1	T38.7X2	T38.7X3	T38.7X4	T38.7X5	T38.7X6
Epitizide	T5Ø.2X1	T5Ø.2X2	T5Ø.2X3	T5Ø.2X4	T5Ø.2X5	T5Ø.2X6
EPN	T6Ø.ØX1	T6Ø.ØX2	T6Ø.ØX3	T6Ø.ØX4	—	—
EPO	T45.8X1	T45.8X2	T45.8X3	T45.8X4	T45.8X5	T45.8X6
Epoetin alpha	T45.8X1	T45.8X2	T45.8X3	T45.8X4	T45.8X5	T45.8X6
Epomediol	T5Ø.991	T5Ø.992	T5Ø.993	T5Ø.994	T5Ø.995	T5Ø.996
Epoprostenol	T45.521	T45.522	T45.523	T45.524	T45.525	T45.526
Epoxy resin	T65.891	T65.892	T65.893	T65.894	—	—
Eprazinone	T48.4X1	T48.4X2	T48.4X3	T48.4X4	T48.4X5	T48.4X6
Epsilon aminocaproic acid	T45.621	T45.622	T45.623	T45.624	T45.625	T45.626
Epsom salt	T47.3X1	T47.3X2	T47.3X3	T47.3X4	T47.3X5	T47.3X6
Eptazocine	T4Ø.491	T4Ø.492	T4Ø.493	T4Ø.494	T4Ø.495	T4Ø.496
Equanil	T43.591	T43.592	T43.593	T43.594	T43.595	T43.596
Equisetum	T62.2X1	T62.2X2	T62.2X3	T62.2X4	—	—
diuretic	T5Ø.2X1	T5Ø.2X2	T5Ø.2X3	T5Ø.2X4	T5Ø.2X5	T5Ø.2X6
Ergobasine	T48.ØX1	T48.ØX2	T48.ØX3	T48.ØX4	T48.ØX5	T48.ØX6
Ergocalciferol	T45.2X1	T45.2X2	T45.2X3	T45.2X4	T45.2X5	T45.2X6
Ergoloid mesylates	T46.7X1	T46.7X2	T46.7X3	T46.7X4	T46.7X5	T46.7X6
Ergometrine	T48.ØX1	T48.ØX2	T48.ØX3	T48.ØX4	T48.ØX5	T48.ØX6
Ergonovine	T48.ØX1	T48.ØX2	T48.ØX3	T48.ØX4	T48.ØX5	T48.ØX6
Ergotamine	T46.5X1	T46.5X2	T46.5X3	T46.5X4	T46.5X5	T46.5X6
Ergotocine	T48.ØX1	T48.ØX2	T48.ØX3	T48.ØX4	T48.ØX5	T48.ØX6
Ergotrate	T48.ØX1	T48.ØX2	T48.ØX3	T48.ØX4	T48.ØX5	T48.ØX6
Ergot NEC	T64.81	T64.82	T64.83	T64.84	—	—
Ergot — *continued*						
derivative	T48.ØX1	T48.ØX2	T48.ØX3	T48.ØX4	T48.ØX5	T48.ØX6
medicinal (alkaloids)	T48.ØX1	T48.ØX2	T48.ØX3	T48.ØX4	T48.ØX5	T48.ØX6
prepared	T48.ØX1	T48.ØX2	T48.ØX3	T48.ØX4	T48.ØX5	T48.ØX6
Eritrityl tetranitrate	T46.3X1	T46.3X2	T46.3X3	T46.3X4	T46.3X5	T46.3X6
Erythrityl tetranitrate	T46.3X1	T46.3X2	T46.3X3	T46.3X4	T46.3X5	T46.3X6
Erythrol tetranitrate	T46.3X1	T46.3X2	T46.3X3	T46.3X4	T46.3X5	T46.3X6
Erythromycin (salts)	T36.3X1	T36.3X2	T36.3X3	T36.3X4	T36.3X5	T36.3X6
ophthalmic preparation	T49.5X1	T49.5X2	T49.5X3	T49.5X4	T49.5X5	T49.5X6
topical NEC	T49.ØX1	T49.ØX2	T49.ØX3	T49.ØX4	T49.ØX5	T49.ØX6
Erythropoietin	T45.8X1	T45.8X2	T45.8X3	T45.8X4	T45.8X5	T45.8X6
human	T45.8X1	T45.8X2	T45.8X3	T45.8X4	T45.8X5	T45.8X6
Esbriet*	T48.991	T48.992	T48.993	T48.994	T48.995	T48.996
Escin	T46.991	T46.992	T46.993	T46.994	T46.995	T46.996
Escitalopram*	T43.221	T43.222	T43.223	T43.224	T43.225	T43.226
Esculin	T45.2X1	T45.2X2	T45.2X3	T45.2X4	T45.2X5	T45.2X6
Esculoside	T45.2X1	T45.2X2	T45.2X3	T45.2X4	T45.2X5	T45.2X6
ESDT (ether-soluble tar distillate)	T49.1X1	T49.1X2	T49.1X3	T49.1X4	T49.1X5	T49.1X6
Eserine	T49.5X1	T49.5X2	T49.5X3	T49.5X4	T49.5X5	T49.5X6
Esflurbiprofen	T39.311	T39.312	T39.313	T39.314	T39.315	T39.316
Eskabarb	T42.3X1	T42.3X2	T42.3X3	T42.3X4	T42.3X5	T42.3X6
Eskalith	T43.8X1	T43.8X2	T43.8X3	T43.8X4	T43.8X5	T43.8X6
Esmolol	T44.7X1	T44.7X2	T44.7X3	T44.7X4	T44.7X5	T44.7X6
Estanozolol	T38.7X1	T38.7X2	T38.7X3	T38.7X4	T38.7X5	T38.7X6
Estazolam	T42.4X1	T42.4X2	T42.4X3	T42.4X4	T42.4X5	T42.4X6
Estradiol	T38.5X1	T38.5X2	T38.5X3	T38.5X4	T38.5X5	T38.5X6
with testosterone	T38.7X1	T38.7X2	T38.7X3	T38.7X4	T38.7X5	T38.7X6
benzoate	T38.5X1	T38.5X2	T38.5X3	T38.5X4	T38.5X5	T38.5X6
Estramustine	T45.1X1	T45.1X2	T45.1X3	T45.1X4	T45.1X5	T45.1X6
Estriol	T38.5X1	T38.5X2	T38.5X3	T38.5X4	T38.5X5	T38.5X6
Estrogen	T38.5X1	T38.5X2	T38.5X3	T38.5X4	T38.5X5	T38.5X6
with progesterone	T38.5X1	T38.5X2	T38.5X3	T38.5X4	T38.5X5	T38.5X6
conjugated	T38.5X1	T38.5X2	T38.5X3	T38.5X4	T38.5X5	T38.5X6
Estrone	T38.5X1	T38.5X2	T38.5X3	T38.5X4	T38.5X5	T38.5X6
Estropipate	T38.5X1	T38.5X2	T38.5X3	T38.5X4	T38.5X5	T38.5X6
Etacrynate sodium	T5Ø.1X1	T5Ø.1X2	T5Ø.1X3	T5Ø.1X4	T5Ø.1X5	T5Ø.1X6
Etacrynic acid	T5Ø.1X1	T5Ø.1X2	T5Ø.1X3	T5Ø.1X4	T5Ø.1X5	T5Ø.1X6
Etafedrine	T48.6X1	T48.6X2	T48.6X3	T48.6X4	T48.6X5	T48.6X6
Etafenone	T46.3X1	T46.3X2	T46.3X3	T46.3X4	T46.3X5	T46.3X6
Etambutol	T37.1X1	T37.1X2	T37.1X3	T37.1X4	T37.1X5	T37.1X6
Etamiphyllin	T48.6X1	T48.6X2	T48.6X3	T48.6X4	T48.6X5	T48.6X6
Etamivan	T5Ø.7X1	T5Ø.7X2	T5Ø.7X3	T5Ø.7X4	T5Ø.7X5	T5Ø.7X6
Etamsylate	T45.7X1	T45.7X2	T45.7X3	T45.7X4	T45.7X5	T45.7X6
Etebenecid	T5Ø.4X1	T5Ø.4X2	T5Ø.4X3	T5Ø.4X4	T5Ø.4X5	T5Ø.4X6
Ethacridine	T49.ØX1	T49.ØX2	T49.ØX3	T49.ØX4	T49.ØX5	T49.ØX6
Ethacrynate*	T5Ø.1X1	T5Ø.1X2	T5Ø.1X3	T5Ø.1X4	T5Ø.1X5	T5Ø.1X6
Ethacrynic acid	T5Ø.1X1	T5Ø.1X2	T5Ø.1X3	T5Ø.1X4	T5Ø.1X5	T5Ø.1X6
Ethadione	T42.2X1	T42.2X2	T42.2X3	T42.2X4	T42.2X5	T42.2X6
Ethambutol	T37.1X1	T37.1X2	T37.1X3	T37.1X4	T37.1X5	T37.1X6
Ethamide	T5Ø.2X1	T5Ø.2X2	T5Ø.2X3	T5Ø.2X4	T5Ø.2X5	T5Ø.2X6
Ethamivan	T5Ø.7X1	T5Ø.7X2	T5Ø.7X3	T5Ø.7X4	T5Ø.7X5	T5Ø.7X6
Ethamsylate	T45.7X1	T45.7X2	T45.7X3	T45.7X4	T45.7X5	T45.7X6
Ethanol	T51.ØX1	T51.ØX2	T51.ØX3	T51.ØX4	—	—
beverage	T51.ØX1	T51.ØX2	T51.ØX3	T51.ØX4	—	—
Ethanolamine oleate	T46.8X1	T46.8X2	T46.8X3	T46.8X4	T46.8X5	T46.8X6
Ethaverine	T44.3X1	T44.3X2	T44.3X3	T44.3X4	T44.3X5	T44.3X6
Ethchlorvynol	T42.6X1	T42.6X2	T42.6X3	T42.6X4	T42.6X5	T42.6X6
Ethebenecid	T5Ø.4X1	T5Ø.4X2	T5Ø.4X3	T5Ø.4X4	T5Ø.4X5	T5Ø.4X6
Ether (vapor)	T41.ØX1	T41.ØX2	T41.ØX3	T41.ØX4	T41.ØX5	T41.ØX6
anesthetic	T41.ØX1	T41.ØX2	T41.ØX3	T41.ØX4	T41.ØX5	T41.ØX6
divinyl	T41.ØX1	T41.ØX2	T41.ØX3	T41.ØX4	T41.ØX5	T41.ØX6
ethyl (medicinal)	T41.ØX1	T41.ØX2	T41.ØX3	T41.ØX4	T41.ØX5	T41.ØX6
nonmedicinal	T52.8X1	T52.8X2	T52.8X3	T52.8X4	—	—
petroleum — *see* Ligroin						
solvent	T52.8X1	T52.8X2	T52.8X3	T52.8X4	—	—
Ethiazide	T5Ø.2X1	T5Ø.2X2	T5Ø.2X3	T5Ø.2X4	T5Ø.2X5	T5Ø.2X6
Ethidium chloride (vapor)	T59.891	T59.892	T59.893	T59.894	—	—
Ethinamate	T42.6X1	T42.6X2	T42.6X3	T42.6X4	T42.6X5	T42.6X6
Ethinylestradiol, ethinyloestradiol	T38.5X1	T38.5X2	T38.5X3	T38.5X4	T38.5X5	T38.5X6
with						
levonorgestrel	T38.4X1	T38.4X2	T38.4X3	T38.4X4	T38.4X5	T38.4X6
norethisterone	T38.4X1	T38.4X2	T38.4X3	T38.4X4	T38.4X5	T38.4X6
Ethiodized oil (131 I)	T5Ø.8X1	T5Ø.8X2	T5Ø.8X3	T5Ø.8X4	T5Ø.8X5	T5Ø.8X6
Ethiofos*	T5Ø.991	T5Ø.992	T5Ø.993	T5Ø.994	T5Ø.995	T5Ø.996
Ethion	T6Ø.ØX1	T6Ø.ØX2	T6Ø.ØX3	T6Ø.ØX4	—	—
Ethionamide	T37.1X1	T37.1X2	T37.1X3	T37.1X4	T37.1X5	T37.1X6
Ethioniamide	T37.1X1	T37.1X2	T37.1X3	T37.1X4	T37.1X5	T37.1X6
Ethisterone	T38.5X1	T38.5X2	T38.5X3	T38.5X4	T38.5X5	T38.5X6
Ethobral	T42.3X1	T42.3X2	T42.3X3	T42.3X4	T42.3X5	T42.3X6
Ethocaine (infiltration) (topical)	T41.3X1	T41.3X2	T41.3X3	T41.3X4	T41.3X5	T41.3X6

Substance	Poisoning, Accidental (unintentional)	Poisoning, Intentional Self-harm	Poisoning, Assault	Poisoning, Undetermined	Adverse Effect	Under-dosing
Ethocaine — *continued*						
nerve block (peripheral) (plexus)	T41.3X1	T41.3X2	T41.3X3	T41.3X4	T41.3X5	T41.3X6
spinal	T41.3X1	T41.3X2	T41.3X3	T41.3X4	T41.3X5	T41.3X6
Ethoheptazine	T4Ø.491	T4Ø.492	T4Ø.493	T4Ø.494	T4Ø.495	T4Ø.496
Ethopropazine	T44.3X1	T44.3X2	T44.3X3	T44.3X4	T44.3X5	T44.3X6
Ethosuximide	T42.2X1	T42.2X2	T42.2X3	T42.2X4	T42.2X5	T42.2X6
Ethotoin	T42.ØX1	T42.ØX2	T42.ØX3	T42.ØX4	T42.ØX5	T42.ØX6
Ethoxazene	T37.91	T37.92	T37.93	T37.94	T37.95	T37.96
Ethoxazorutoside	T46.991	T46.992	T46.993	T46.994	T46.995	T46.996
Ethoxzolamide	T5Ø.2X1	T5Ø.2X2	T5Ø.2X3	T5Ø.2X4	T5Ø.2X5	T5Ø.2X6
Ethyl						
acetate	T52.8X1	T52.8X2	T52.8X3	T52.8X4	—	—
alcohol	T51.ØX1	T51.ØX2	T51.ØX3	T51.ØX4	—	—
beverage	T51.ØX1	T51.ØX2	T51.ØX3	T51.ØX4	—	—
aldehyde (vapor)	T59.891	T59.892	T59.893	T59.894	—	—
liquid	T52.8X1	T52.8X2	T52.8X3	T52.8X4	—	—
aminobenzoate	T41.3X1	T41.3X2	T41.3X3	T41.3X4	T41.3X5	T41.3X6
aminophenothiazine	T43.3X1	T43.3X2	T43.3X3	T43.3X4	T43.3X5	T43.3X6
benzoate	T52.8X1	T52.8X2	T52.8X3	T52.8X4	—	—
biscoumacetate	T45.511	T45.512	T45.513	T45.514	T45.515	T45.516
bromide (anesthetic)	T41.ØX1	T41.ØX2	T41.ØX3	T41.ØX4	T41.ØX5	T41.ØX6
carbamate	T45.1X1	T45.1X2	T45.1X3	T45.1X4	T45.1X5	T45.1X6
carbinol	T51.3X1	T51.3X2	T51.3X3	T51.3X4	—	—
carbonate	T52.8X1	T52.8X2	T52.8X3	T52.8X4	—	—
chaulmoograte	T37.1X1	T37.1X2	T37.1X3	T37.1X4	T37.1X5	T37.1X6
chloride (anesthetic)	T41.ØX1	T41.ØX2	T41.ØX3	T41.ØX4	T41.ØX5	T41.ØX6
anesthetic (local)	T41.3X1	T41.3X2	T41.3X3	T41.3X4	T41.3X5	T41.3X6
inhaled	T41.ØX1	T41.ØX2	T41.ØX3	T41.ØX4	T41.ØX5	T41.ØX6
local	T49.4X1	T49.4X2	T49.4X3	T49.4X4	T49.4X5	T49.4X6
solvent	T53.6X1	T53.6X2	T53.6X3	T53.6X4	—	—
dibunate	T48.3X1	T48.3X2	T48.3X3	T48.3X4	T48.3X5	T48.3X6
dichloroarsine (vapor)	T57.ØX1	T57.ØX2	T57.ØX3	T57.ØX4	—	—
estranol	T38.7X1	T38.7X2	T38.7X3	T38.7X4	T38.7X5	T38.7X6
ether — *see also* ether	T52.8X1	T52.8X2	T52.8X3	T52.8X4	—	—
formate NEC (solvent)	T52.ØX1	T52.ØX2	T52.ØX3	T52.ØX4	—	—
fumarate	T49.4X1	T49.4X2	T49.4X3	T49.4X4	T49.4X5	T49.4X6
hydroxyisobutyrate NEC (solvent)	T52.8X1	T52.8X2	T52.8X3	T52.8X4	—	—
iodoacetate	T59.3X1	T59.3X2	T59.3X3	T59.3X4	—	—
lactate NEC (solvent)	T52.8X1	T52.8X2	T52.8X3	T52.8X4	—	—
loflazepate	T42.4X1	T42.4X2	T42.4X3	T42.4X4	T42.4X5	T42.4X6
mercuric chloride	T56.1X1	T56.1X2	T56.1X3	T56.1X4	—	—
methylcarbinol	T51.8X1	T51.8X2	T51.8X3	T51.8X4	—	—
morphine	T4Ø.2X1	T4Ø.2X2	T4Ø.2X3	T4Ø.2X4	T4Ø.2X5	T4Ø.2X6
noradrenaline	T48.6X1	T48.6X2	T48.6X3	T48.6X4	T48.6X5	T48.6X6
oxybutyrate NEC (solvent)	T52.8X1	T52.8X2	T52.8X3	T52.8X4	—	—
Ethylene (gas)	T59.891	T59.892	T59.893	T59.894	—	—
anesthetic (general)	T41.ØX1	T41.ØX2	T41.ØX3	T41.ØX4	T41.ØX5	T41.ØX6
chlorohydrin	T52.8X1	T52.8X2	T52.8X3	T52.8X4	—	—
vapor	T53.6X1	T53.6X2	T53.6X3	T53.6X4	—	—
dichloride	T52.8X1	T52.8X2	T52.8X3	T52.8X4	—	—
vapor	T53.6X1	T53.6X2	T53.6X3	T53.6X4	—	—
dinitrate	T52.3X1	T52.3X2	T52.3X3	T52.3X4	—	—
glycol(s)	T52.8X1	T52.8X2	T52.8X3	T52.8X4	—	—
dinitrate	T52.3X1	T52.3X2	T52.3X3	T52.3X4	—	—
monobutyl ether	T52.3X1	T52.3X2	T52.3X3	T52.3X4	—	—
imine	T54.1X1	T54.1X2	T54.1X3	T54.1X4	—	—
oxide (fumigant) (nonmedicinal)	T59.891	T59.892	T59.893	T59.894	—	—
medicinal	T49.ØX1	T49.ØX2	T49.ØX3	T49.ØX4	T49.ØX5	T49.ØX6
Ethylenediaminetetra-acetic acid	T5Ø.6X1	T5Ø.6X2	T5Ø.6X3	T5Ø.6X4	T5Ø.6X5	T5Ø.6X6
Ethylenediamine theophylline	T48.6X1	T48.6X2	T48.6X3	T48.6X4	T48.6X5	T48.6X6
Ethylenedinitrilotetra-acetate	T5Ø.6X1	T5Ø.6X2	T5Ø.6X3	T5Ø.6X4	T5Ø.6X5	T5Ø.6X6
Ethylestrenol	T38.7X1	T38.7X2	T38.7X3	T38.7X4	T38.7X5	T38.7X6
Ethylhydroxycellulose	T47.4X1	T47.4X2	T47.4X3	T47.4X4	T47.4X5	T47.4X6
Ethylidene						
chloride NEC	T53.6X1	T53.6X2	T53.6X3	T53.6X4	—	—
diacetate	T6Ø.3X1	T6Ø.3X2	T6Ø.3X3	T6Ø.3X4	—	—
dicoumarin	T45.511	T45.512	T45.513	T45.514	T45.515	T45.516
dicoumarol	T45.511	T45.512	T45.513	T45.514	T45.515	T45.516
diethyl ether	T52.ØX1	T52.ØX2	T52.ØX3	T52.ØX4	—	—
Ethylmorphine	T4Ø.2X1	T4Ø.2X2	T4Ø.2X3	T4Ø.2X4	T4Ø.2X5	T4Ø.2X6
Ethylnorepinephrine	T48.6X1	T48.6X2	T48.6X3	T48.6X4	T48.6X5	T48.6X6
Ethylparachlorophen-oxyisobutyrate	T46.6X1	T46.6X2	T46.6X3	T46.6X4	T46.6X5	T46.6X6
Ethynodiol	T38.4X1	T38.4X2	T38.4X3	T38.4X4	T38.4X5	T38.4X6
with mestranol diacetate	T38.4X1	T38.4X2	T38.4X3	T38.4X4	T38.4X5	T38.4X6
Ethyol*	T5Ø.991	T5Ø.992	T5Ø.993	T5Ø.994	T5Ø.995	T5Ø.996
Etidocaine	T41.3X1	T41.3X2	T41.3X3	T41.3X4	T41.3X5	T41.3X6
infiltration (subcutaneous)	T41.3X1	T41.3X2	T41.3X3	T41.3X4	T41.3X5	T41.3X6

Substance	Poisoning, Accidental (unintentional)	Poisoning, Intentional Self-harm	Poisoning, Assault	Poisoning, Undetermined	Adverse Effect	Under-dosing
Etidocaine — *continued*						
nerve (peripheral) (plexus)	T41.3X1	T41.3X2	T41.3X3	T41.3X4	T41.3X5	T41.3X6
Etidronate	T5Ø.991	T5Ø.992	T5Ø.993	T5Ø.994	T5Ø.995	T5Ø.996
Etidronic acid (disodium salt)	T5Ø.991	T5Ø.992	T5Ø.993	T5Ø.994	T5Ø.995	T5Ø.996
Etifoxine	T42.6X1	T42.6X2	T42.6X3	T42.6X4	T42.6X5	T42.6X6
Etilefrine	T44.4X1	T44.4X2	T44.4X3	T44.4X4	T44.4X5	T44.4X6
Etilfen	T42.3X1	T42.3X2	T42.3X3	T42.3X4	T42.3X5	T42.3X6
Etinodiol	T38.4X1	T38.4X2	T38.4X3	T38.4X4	T38.4X5	T38.4X6
Etiroxate	T46.6X1	T46.6X2	T46.6X3	T46.6X4	T46.6X5	T46.6X6
Etizolam	T42.4X1	T42.4X2	T42.4X3	T42.4X4	T42.4X5	T42.4X6
Etodolac	T39.391	T39.392	T39.393	T39.394	T39.395	T39.396
Etofamide	T37.3X1	T37.3X2	T37.3X3	T37.3X4	T37.3X5	T37.3X6
Etofibrate	T46.6X1	T46.6X2	T46.6X3	T46.6X4	T46.6X5	T46.6X6
Etofylline	T46.7X1	T46.7X2	T46.7X3	T46.7X4	T46.7X5	T46.7X6
clofibrate	T46.6X1	T46.6X2	T46.6X3	T46.6X4	T46.6X5	T46.6X6
Etoglucid	T45.1X1	T45.1X2	T45.1X3	T45.1X4	T45.1X5	T45.1X6
Etomidate	T41.1X1	T41.1X2	T41.1X3	T41.1X4	T41.1X5	T41.1X6
Etomide	T39.8X1	T39.8X2	T39.8X3	T39.8X4	T39.8X5	T39.8X6
Etomidoline	T44.3X1	T44.3X2	T44.3X3	T44.3X4	T44.3X5	T44.3X6
Etoposide	T45.1X1	T45.1X2	T45.1X3	T45.1X4	T45.1X5	T45.1X6
Etorphine	T4Ø.2X1	T4Ø.2X2	T4Ø.2X3	T4Ø.2X4	T4Ø.2X5	T4Ø.2X6
Etoval	T42.3X1	T42.3X2	T42.3X3	T42.3X4	T42.3X5	T42.3X6
Etozolin	T5Ø.1X1	T5Ø.1X2	T5Ø.1X3	T5Ø.1X4	T5Ø.1X5	T5Ø.1X6
Etravirine*	T37.5X1	T37.5X2	T37.5X3	T37.5X4	T37.5X5	T37.5X6
Etretinate	T5Ø.991	T5Ø.992	T5Ø.993	T5Ø.994	T5Ø.995	T5Ø.996
Etryptamine	T43.691	T43.692	T43.693	T43.694	T43.695	T43.696
Etybenzatropine	T44.3X1	T44.3X2	T44.3X3	T44.3X4	T44.3X5	T44.3X6
Etynodiol	T38.4X1	T38.4X2	T38.4X3	T38.4X4	T38.4X5	T38.4X6
Eucaine	T41.3X1	T41.3X2	T41.3X3	T41.3X4	T41.3X5	T41.3X6
Eucalyptus oil	T49.7X1	T49.7X2	T49.7X3	T49.7X4	T49.7X5	T49.7X6
Eucatropine	T49.5X1	T49.5X2	T49.5X3	T49.5X4	T49.5X5	T49.5X6
Eucodal	T4Ø.2X1	T4Ø.2X2	T4Ø.2X3	T4Ø.2X4	T4Ø.2X5	T4Ø.2X6
Euneryl	T42.3X1	T42.3X2	T42.3X3	T42.3X4	T42.3X5	T42.3X6
Euphthalmine	T44.3X1	T44.3X2	T44.3X3	T44.3X4	T44.3X5	T44.3X6
Eurax	T49.ØX1	T49.ØX2	T49.ØX3	T49.ØX4	T49.ØX5	T49.ØX6
Euresol	T49.4X1	T49.4X2	T49.4X3	T49.4X4	T49.4X5	T49.4X6
Euthroid	T38.1X1	T38.1X2	T38.1X3	T38.1X4	T38.1X5	T38.1X6
Evans blue	T5Ø.8X1	T5Ø.8X2	T5Ø.8X3	T5Ø.8X4	T5Ø.8X5	T5Ø.8X6
Evipal	T42.3X1	T42.3X2	T42.3X3	T42.3X4	T42.3X5	T42.3X6
sodium	T41.1X1	T41.1X2	T41.1X3	T41.1X4	T41.1X5	T41.1X6
Evipan	T42.3X1	T42.3X2	T42.3X3	T42.3X4	T42.3X5	T42.3X6
sodium	T41.1X1	T41.1X2	T41.1X3	T41.1X4	T41.1X5	T41.1X6
Exalamide	T49.ØX1	T49.ØX2	T49.ØX3	T49.ØX4	T49.ØX5	T49.ØX6
Exalgin	T39.1X1	T39.1X2	T39.1X3	T39.1X4	T39.1X5	T39.1X6
Excipients, pharmaceutical	T5Ø.901	T5Ø.902	T5Ø.903	T5Ø.904	T5Ø.905	T5Ø.906
Exhaust gas (engine) (motor vehicle)	T58.Ø1	T58.Ø2	T58.Ø3	T58.Ø4	—	—
Ex-Lax (phenolphthalein)	T47.2X1	T47.2X2	T47.2X3	T47.2X4	T47.2X5	T47.2X6
Expectorant NEC	T48.4X1	T48.4X2	T48.4X3	T48.4X4	T48.4X5	T48.4X6
Extended insulin zinc suspension	T38.3X1	T38.3X2	T38.3X3	T38.3X4	T38.3X5	T38.3X6
External medications (skin) (mucous membrane)	T49.91	T49.92	T49.93	T49.94	T49.95	T49.96
dental agent	T49.7X1	T49.7X2	T49.7X3	T49.7X4	T49.7X5	T49.7X6
ENT agent	T49.6X1	T49.6X2	T49.6X3	T49.6X4	T49.6X5	T49.6X6
ophthalmic preparation	T49.5X1	T49.5X2	T49.5X3	T49.5X4	T49.5X5	T49.5X6
specified NEC	T49.8X1	T49.8X2	T49.8X3	T49.8X4	T49.8X5	T49.8X6
Extina*	T49.ØX1	T49.ØX2	T49.ØX3	T49.ØX4	T49.ØX5	T49.ØX6
Extrapyramidal antagonist NEC	T44.3X1	T44.3X2	T44.3X3	T44.3X4	T44.3X5	T44.3X6
Eye agents (anti-infective)	T49.5X1	T49.5X2	T49.5X3	T49.5X4	T49.5X5	T49.5X6
Eye drug NEC	T49.5X1	T49.5X2	T49.5X3	T49.5X4	T49.5X5	T49.5X6
FAC (fluorouracil + doxorubicin + cyclophosphamide)	T45.1X1	T45.1X2	T45.1X3	T45.1X4	T45.1X5	T45.1X6
Factor						
I (fibrinogen)	T45.8X1	T45.8X2	T45.8X3	T45.8X4	T45.8X5	T45.8X6
III (thromboplastin)	T45.8X1	T45.8X2	T45.8X3	T45.8X4	T45.8X5	T45.8X6
IX complex	T45.7X1	T45.7X2	T45.7X3	T45.7X4	T45.7X5	T45.7X6
human	T45.8X1	T45.8X2	T45.8X3	T45.8X4	T45.8X5	T45.8X6
VIII (antihemophilic Factor) (concentrate)	T45.8X1	T45.8X2	T45.8X3	T45.8X4	T45.8X5	T45.8X6
Famotidine	T47.ØX1	T47.ØX2	T47.ØX3	T47.ØX4	T47.ØX5	T47.ØX6
Fat suspension, intravenous	T5Ø.991	T5Ø.992	T5Ø.993	T5Ø.994	T5Ø.995	T5Ø.996
Fazadinium bromide	T48.1X1	T48.1X2	T48.1X3	T48.1X4	T48.1X5	T48.1X6
Febarbamate	T42.3X1	T42.3X2	T42.3X3	T42.3X4	T42.3X5	T42.3X6
Fecal softener	T47.4X1	T47.4X2	T47.4X3	T47.4X4	T47.4X5	T47.4X6
Fedrilate	T48.3X1	T48.3X2	T48.3X3	T48.3X4	T48.3X5	T48.3X6
Felodipine	T46.1X1	T46.1X2	T46.1X3	T46.1X4	T46.1X5	T46.1X6
Felypressin	T38.891	T38.892	T38.893	T38.894	T38.895	T38.896
Femizol*	T49.ØX1	T49.ØX2	T49.ØX3	T49.ØX4	T49.ØX5	T49.ØX6

Substance	Poisoning, Accidental (unintentional)	Poisoning, Intentional Self-harm	Poisoning, Assault	Poisoning, Undetermined	Adverse Effect	Under-dosing
Femoxetine	T43.221	T43.222	T43.223	T43.224	T43.225	T43.226
Fenalcomine	T46.3X1	T46.3X2	T46.3X3	T46.3X4	T46.3X5	T46.3X6
Fenamisal	T37.1X1	T37.1X2	T37.1X3	T37.1X4	T37.1X5	T37.1X6
Fenazone	T39.2X1	T39.2X2	T39.2X3	T39.2X4	T39.2X5	T39.2X6
Fenbendazole	T37.4X1	T37.4X2	T37.4X3	T37.4X4	T37.4X5	T37.4X6
Fenbutrazate	T5Ø.5X1	T5Ø.5X2	T5Ø.5X3	T5Ø.5X4	T5Ø.5X5	T5Ø.5X6
Fencamfamine	T43.691	T43.692	T43.693	T43.694	T43.695	T43.696
Fendiline	T46.1X1	T46.1X2	T46.1X3	T46.1X4	T46.1X5	T46.1X6
Fenetylline	T43.691	T43.692	T43.693	T43.694	T43.695	T43.696
Fenflumizole	T39.391	T39.392	T39.393	T39.394	T39.395	T39.396
Fenfluramine	T5Ø.5X1	T5Ø.5X2	T5Ø.5X3	T5Ø.5X4	T5Ø.5X5	T5Ø.5X6
Fenobarbital	T42.3X1	T42.3X2	T42.3X3	T42.3X4	T42.3X5	T42.3X6
Fenofibrate	T46.6X1	T46.6X2	T46.6X3	T46.6X4	T46.6X5	T46.6X6
Fenoprofen	T39.311	T39.312	T39.313	T39.314	T39.315	T39.316
Fenoterol	T48.6X1	T48.6X2	T48.6X3	T48.6X4	T48.6X5	T48.6X6
Fenoverine	T44.3X1	T44.3X2	T44.3X3	T44.3X4	T44.3X5	T44.3X6
Fenoxazoline	T48.5X1	T48.5X2	T48.5X3	T48.5X4	T48.5X5	T48.5X6
Fenproporex	T5Ø.5X1	T5Ø.5X2	T5Ø.5X3	T5Ø.5X4	T5Ø.5X5	T5Ø.5X6
Fenquizone	T5Ø.2X1	T5Ø.2X2	T5Ø.2X3	T5Ø.2X4	T5Ø.2X5	T5Ø.2X6
Fentanyl (analogs)	T4Ø.411	T4Ø.412	T4Ø.413	T4Ø.414	T4Ø.415	T4Ø.416
Fentazin	T43.3X1	T43.3X2	T43.3X3	T43.3X4	T43.3X5	T43.3X6
Fenthion	T6Ø.ØX1	T6Ø.ØX2	T6Ø.ØX3	T6Ø.ØX4	—	—
Fenticlor	T49.ØX1	T49.ØX2	T49.ØX3	T49.ØX4	T49.ØX5	T49.ØX6
Fenylbutazone	T39.2X1	T39.2X2	T39.2X3	T39.2X4	T39.2X5	T39.2X6
Feprazone	T39.2X1	T39.2X2	T39.2X3	T39.2X4	T39.2X5	T39.2X6
Fer de lance (bite) (venom)	T63.Ø61	T63.Ø62	T63.Ø63	T63.Ø64	—	—
Ferrex*	T45.4X1	T45.4X2	T45.4X3	T45.4X4	T45.4X5	T45.4X6
Ferric — *see also* Iron						
chloride	T45.4X1	T45.4X2	T45.4X3	T45.4X4	T45.4X5	T45.4X6
citrate	T45.4X1	T45.4X2	T45.4X3	T45.4X4	T45.4X5	T45.4X6
hydroxide						
colloidal	T45.4X1	T45.4X2	T45.4X3	T45.4X4	T45.4X5	T45.4X6
polymaltose	T45.4X1	T45.4X2	T45.4X3	T45.4X4	T45.4X5	T45.4X6
pyrophosphate	T45.4X1	T45.4X2	T45.4X3	T45.4X4	T45.4X5	T45.4X6
Ferritin	T45.4X1	T45.4X2	T45.4X3	T45.4X4	T45.4X5	T45.4X6
Ferrocholinate	T45.4X1	T45.4X2	T45.4X3	T45.4X4	T45.4X5	T45.4X6
Ferrodextrane	T45.4X1	T45.4X2	T45.4X3	T45.4X4	T45.4X5	T45.4X6
Ferropolimaler	T45.4X1	T45.4X2	T45.4X3	T45.4X4	T45.4X5	T45.4X6
Ferrous — *see also* Iron						
phosphate	T45.4X1	T45.4X2	T45.4X3	T45.4X4	T45.4X5	T45.4X6
salt	T45.4X1	T45.4X2	T45.4X3	T45.4X4	T45.4X5	T45.4X6
with folic acid	T45.4X1	T45.4X2	T45.4X3	T45.4X4	T45.4X5	T45.4X6
Ferrous fumerate, gluconate, lactate, salt NEC, sulfate (medicinal)	T45.4X1	T45.4X2	T45.4X3	T45.4X4	T45.4X5	T45.4X6
Ferrovanadium (fumes)	T59.891	T59.892	T59.893	T59.894	—	—
Ferrum — *see* Iron						
Fertilizers NEC	T65.891	T65.892	T65.893	T65.894	—	—
with herbicide mixture	T6Ø.3X1	T6Ø.3X2	T6Ø.3X3	T6Ø.3X4	—	—
Fetoxilate	T47.6X1	T47.6X2	T47.6X3	T47.6X4	T47.6X5	T47.6X6
Fiber, dietary	T47.4X1	T47.4X2	T47.4X3	T47.4X4	T47.4X5	T47.4X6
Fiberglass	T65.831	T65.832	T65.833	T65.834	—	—
Fibrinogen (human)	T45.8X1	T45.8X2	T45.8X3	T45.8X4	T45.8X5	T45.8X6
Fibrinolysin (human)	T45.691	T45.692	T45.693	T45.694	T45.695	T45.696
Fibrinolysis						
affecting drug	T45.6Ø1	T45.6Ø2	T45.6Ø3	T45.6Ø4	T45.6Ø5	T45.6Ø6
inhibitor NEC	T45.621	T45.622	T45.623	T45.624	T45.625	T45.626
Fibrinolytic drug	T45.611	T45.612	T45.613	T45.614	T45.615	T45.616
Filix mas	T37.4X1	T37.4X2	T37.4X3	T37.4X4	T37.4X5	T37.4X6
Filtering cream	T49.3X1	T49.3X2	T49.3X3	T49.3X4	T49.3X5	T49.3X6
Finacea*	T49.ØX1	T49.ØX2	T49.ØX3	T49.ØX4	T49.ØX5	T49.ØX6
Fiorinal	T39.Ø11	T39.Ø12	T39.Ø13	T39.Ø14	T39.Ø15	T39.Ø16
Firedamp	T59.891	T59.892	T59.893	T59.894	—	—
Fish, noxious, nonbacterial	T61.91	T61.92	T61.93	T61.94	—	—
ciguatera	T61.Ø1	T61.Ø2	T61.Ø3	T61.Ø4	—	—
scombroid	T61.11	T61.12	T61.13	T61.14	—	—
shell	T61.781	T61.782	T61.783	T61.784	—	—
specified NEC	T61.771	T61.772	T61.773	T61.774	—	—
Flagyl	T37.3X1	T37.3X2	T37.3X3	T37.3X4	T37.3X5	T37.3X6
Flavine adenine dinucleotide	T45.2X1	T45.2X2	T45.2X3	T45.2X4	T45.2X5	T45.2X6
Flavodic acid	T46.991	T46.992	T46.993	T46.994	T46.995	T46.996
Flavoxate	T44.3X1	T44.3X2	T44.3X3	T44.3X4	T44.3X5	T44.3X6
Flaxedil	T48.1X1	T48.1X2	T48.1X3	T48.1X4	T48.1X5	T48.1X6
Flaxseed (medicinal)	T49.3X1	T49.3X2	T49.3X3	T49.3X4	T49.3X5	T49.3X6
Flecainide	T46.2X1	T46.2X2	T46.2X3	T46.2X4	T46.2X5	T46.2X6
Fleroxacin	T36.8X1	T36.8X2	T36.8X3	T36.8X4	T36.8X5	T36.8X6
Floctafenine	T39.8X1	T39.8X2	T39.8X3	T39.8X4	T39.8X5	T39.8X6
Flomax	T44.6X1	T44.6X2	T44.6X3	T44.6X4	T44.6X5	T44.6X6
Flomoxef	T36.1X1	T36.1X2	T36.1X3	T36.1X4	T36.1X5	T36.1X6
Flonase*	T49.6X1	T49.6X2	T49.6X3	T49.6X4	T49.6X5	T49.6X6
Flopropione	T44.3X1	T44.3X2	T44.3X3	T44.3X4	T44.3X5	T44.3X6

Substance	Poisoning, Accidental (unintentional)	Poisoning, Intentional Self-harm	Poisoning, Assault	Poisoning, Undetermined	Adverse Effect	Under-dosing
FLORAjen*	T47.6X1	T47.6X2	T47.6X3	T47.6X4	T47.6X5	T47.6X6
Florantyrone	T47.5X1	T47.5X2	T47.5X3	T47.5X4	T47.5X5	T47.5X6
Floraquin	T37.8X1	T37.8X2	T37.8X3	T37.8X4	T37.8X5	T37.8X6
Florinef	T38.ØX1	T38.ØX2	T38.ØX3	T38.ØX4	T38.ØX5	T38.ØX6
ENT agent	T49.6X1	T49.6X2	T49.6X3	T49.6X4	T49.6X5	T49.6X6
ophthalmic preparation	T49.5X1	T49.5X2	T49.5X3	T49.5X4	T49.5X5	T49.5X6
topical NEC	T49.ØX1	T49.ØX2	T49.ØX3	T49.ØX4	T49.ØX5	T49.ØX6
Flovent*	T49.1X1	T49.1X2	T49.1X3	T49.1X4	T49.1X5	T49.1X6
Flowers of sulfur	T49.4X1	T49.4X2	T49.4X3	T49.4X4	T49.4X5	T49.4X6
Floxuridine	T45.1X1	T45.1X2	T45.1X3	T45.1X4	T45.1X5	T45.1X6
Fluanisone	T43.4X1	T43.4X2	T43.4X3	T43.4X4	T43.4X5	T43.4X6
Flubendazole	T37.4X1	T37.4X2	T37.4X3	T37.4X4	T37.4X5	T37.4X6
Fluclorolone acetonide	T49.ØX1	T49.ØX2	T49.ØX3	T49.ØX4	T49.ØX5	T49.ØX6
Flucloxacillin	T36.ØX1	T36.ØX2	T36.ØX3	T36.ØX4	T36.ØX5	T36.ØX6
Fluconazole	T37.8X1	T37.8X2	T37.8X3	T37.8X4	T37.8X5	T37.8X6
Flucytosine	T37.8X1	T37.8X2	T37.8X3	T37.8X4	T37.8X5	T37.8X6
Fludeoxyglucose (18F)	T5Ø.8X1	T5Ø.8X2	T5Ø.8X3	T5Ø.8X4	T5Ø.8X5	T5Ø.8X6
Fludiazepam	T42.4X1	T42.4X2	T42.4X3	T42.4X4	T42.4X5	T42.4X6
Fludrocortisone	T5Ø.ØX1	T5Ø.ØX2	T5Ø.ØX3	T5Ø.ØX4	T5Ø.ØX5	T5Ø.ØX6
ENT agent	T49.6X1	T49.6X2	T49.6X3	T49.6X4	T49.6X5	T49.6X6
ophthalmic preparation	T49.5X1	T49.5X2	T49.5X3	T49.5X4	T49.5X5	T49.5X6
topical NEC	T49.ØX1	T49.ØX2	T49.ØX3	T49.ØX4	T49.ØX5	T49.ØX6
Fludroxycortide	T49.ØX1	T49.ØX2	T49.ØX3	T49.ØX4	T49.ØX5	T49.ØX6
Flufenamic acid	T39.391	T39.392	T39.393	T39.394	T39.395	T39.396
Fluindione	T45.511	T45.512	T45.513	T45.514	T45.515	T45.516
Flumequine	T37.8X1	T37.8X2	T37.8X3	T37.8X4	T37.8X5	T37.8X6
Flumethasone	T49.ØX1	T49.ØX2	T49.ØX3	T49.ØX4	T49.ØX5	T49.ØX6
Flumethiazide	T5Ø.2X1	T5Ø.2X2	T5Ø.2X3	T5Ø.2X4	T5Ø.2X5	T5Ø.2X6
Flumidin	T37.5X1	T37.5X2	T37.5X3	T37.5X4	T37.5X5	T37.5X6
Flunarizine	T46.7X1	T46.7X2	T46.7X3	T46.7X4	T46.7X5	T46.7X6
Flunidazole	T37.8X1	T37.8X2	T37.8X3	T37.8X4	T37.8X5	T37.8X6
Flunisolide	T48.6X1	T48.6X2	T48.6X3	T48.6X4	T48.6X5	T48.6X6
Flunitrazepam	T42.4X1	T42.4X2	T42.4X3	T42.4X4	T42.4X5	T42.4X6
Fluocinolone (acetonide)	T49.ØX1	T49.ØX2	T49.ØX3	T49.ØX4	T49.ØX5	T49.ØX6
Fluocinonide	T49.ØX1	T49.ØX2	T49.ØX3	T49.ØX4	T49.ØX5	T49.ØX6
Fluocortin (butyl)	T49.ØX1	T49.ØX2	T49.ØX3	T49.ØX4	T49.ØX5	T49.ØX6
Fluocortolone	T49.ØX1	T49.ØX2	T49.ØX3	T49.ØX4	T49.ØX5	T49.ØX6
Fluohydrocortisone	T38.ØX1	T38.ØX2	T38.ØX3	T38.ØX4	T38.ØX5	T38.ØX6
ENT agent	T49.6X1	T49.6X2	T49.6X3	T49.6X4	T49.6X5	T49.6X6
ophthalmic preparation	T49.5X1	T49.5X2	T49.5X3	T49.5X4	T49.5X5	T49.5X6
topical NEC	T49.ØX1	T49.ØX2	T49.ØX3	T49.ØX4	T49.ØX5	T49.ØX6
Fluonid	T49.ØX1	T49.ØX2	T49.ØX3	T49.ØX4	T49.ØX5	T49.ØX6
Fluopromazine	T43.3X1	T43.3X2	T43.3X3	T43.3X4	T43.3X5	T43.3X6
Fluoracetate	T6Ø.8X1	T6Ø.8X2	T6Ø.8X3	T6Ø.8X4	—	—
Fluorescein	T5Ø.8X1	T5Ø.8X2	T5Ø.8X3	T5Ø.8X4	T5Ø.8X5	T5Ø.8X6
Fluorhydrocortisone	T5Ø.ØX1	T5Ø.ØX2	T5Ø.ØX3	T5Ø.ØX4	T5Ø.ØX5	T5Ø.ØX6
Fluoride (nonmedicinal) (pesticide) (sodium) **NEC**	T6Ø.8X1	T6Ø.8X2	T6Ø.8X3	T6Ø.8X4	—	—
hydrogen — *see* Hydrofluoric acid						
medicinal NEC	T5Ø.991	T5Ø.992	T5Ø.993	T5Ø.994	T5Ø.995	T5Ø.996
dental use	T49.7X1	T49.7X2	T49.7X3	T49.7X4	T49.7X5	T49.7X6
not pesticide NEC	T54.91	T54.92	T54.93	T54.94	—	—
stannous	T49.7X1	T49.7X2	T49.7X3	T49.7X4	T49.7X5	T49.7X6
Fluorigard*	T47.7X1	T47.7X2	T47.7X3	T47.7X4	T47.7X5	T47.7X6
Fluorinated corticosteroids	T38.ØX1	T38.ØX2	T38.ØX3	T38.ØX4	T38.ØX5	T38.ØX6
Fluorine (gas)	T59.5X1	T59.5X2	T59.5X3	T59.5X4	—	—
salt — *see* Fluoride(s)						
Fluoristan	T49.7X1	T49.7X2	T49.7X3	T49.7X4	T49.7X5	T49.7X6
Fluormetholone	T49.ØX1	T49.ØX2	T49.ØX3	T49.ØX4	T49.ØX5	T49.ØX6
Fluoroacetate	T6Ø.8X1	T6Ø.8X2	T6Ø.8X3	T6Ø.8X4	—	—
Fluorocarbon monomer	T53.6X1	T53.6X2	T53.6X3	T53.6X4	—	—
Fluorocytosine	T37.8X1	T37.8X2	T37.8X3	T37.8X4	T37.8X5	T37.8X6
Fluorodeoxyuridine	T45.1X1	T45.1X2	T45.1X3	T45.1X4	T45.1X5	T45.1X6
Fluorometholone	T49.ØX1	T49.ØX2	T49.ØX3	T49.ØX4	T49.ØX5	T49.ØX6
ophthalmic preparation	T49.5X1	T49.5X2	T49.5X3	T49.5X4	T49.5X5	T49.5X6
Fluorophosphate insecticide	T6Ø.ØX1	T6Ø.ØX2	T6Ø.ØX3	T6Ø.ØX4	—	—
Fluorosol	T46.3X1	T46.3X2	T46.3X3	T46.3X4	T46.3X5	T46.3X6
Fluorouracil	T45.1X1	T45.1X2	T45.1X3	T45.1X4	T45.1X5	T45.1X6
Fluorphenylalanine	T49.5X1	T49.5X2	T49.5X3	T49.5X4	T49.5X5	T49.5X6
Fluothane	T41.ØX1	T41.ØX2	T41.ØX3	T41.ØX4	T41.ØX5	T41.ØX6
Fluoxetine	T43.221	T43.222	T43.223	T43.224	T43.225	T43.226
Fluoxymesterone	T38.7X1	T38.7X2	T38.7X3	T38.7X4	T38.7X5	T38.7X6
Flupenthixol	T43.4X1	T43.4X2	T43.4X3	T43.4X4	T43.4X5	T43.4X6
Flupentixol	T43.4X1	T43.4X2	T43.4X3	T43.4X4	T43.4X5	T43.4X6
Fluphenazine	T43.3X1	T43.3X2	T43.3X3	T43.3X4	T43.3X5	T43.3X6
Fluprednidene	T49.ØX1	T49.ØX2	T49.ØX3	T49.ØX4	T49.ØX5	T49.ØX6
Fluprednisolone	T38.ØX1	T38.ØX2	T38.ØX3	T38.ØX4	T38.ØX5	T38.ØX6
Fluradoline	T39.8X1	T39.8X2	T39.8X3	T39.8X4	T39.8X5	T39.8X6
Flurandrenolide	T49.ØX1	T49.ØX2	T49.ØX3	T49.ØX4	T49.ØX5	T49.ØX6
Flurandrenolone	T49.ØX1	T49.ØX2	T49.ØX3	T49.ØX4	T49.ØX5	T49.ØX6

Substance	Poisoning, Accidental (unintentional)	Poisoning, Intentional Self-harm	Poisoning, Assault	Poisoning, Undetermined	Adverse Effect	Under-dosing
Flurazepam	T42.4X1	T42.4X2	T42.4X3	T42.4X4	T42.4X5	T42.4X6
Flurbiprofen	T39.311	T39.312	T39.313	T39.314	T39.315	T39.316
Flurobate	T49.ØX1	T49.ØX2	T49.ØX3	T49.ØX4	T49.ØX5	T49.ØX6
Fluroxene	T41.ØX1	T41.ØX2	T41.ØX3	T41.ØX4	T41.ØX5	T41.ØX6
Fluspirilene	T43.591	T43.592	T43.593	T43.594	T43.595	T43.596
Flutamide	T38.6X1	T38.6X2	T38.6X3	T38.6X4	T38.6X5	T38.6X6
Flutazolam	T38.ØX1	T38.ØX2	T38.ØX3	T38.ØX4	T38.ØX5	T38.ØX6
Fluticasone propionate	T38.ØX1	T38.ØX2	T38.ØX3	T38.ØX4	T38.ØX5	T38.ØX6
Flutoprazepam	T42.4X1	T42.4X2	T42.4X3	T42.4X4	T42.4X5	T42.4X6
Flutropium bromide	T48.6X1	T48.6X2	T48.6X3	T48.6X4	T48.6X5	T48.6X6
Fluvoxamine	T43.221	T43.222	T43.223	T43.224	T43.225	T43.226
Folacin	T45.8X1	T45.8X2	T45.8X3	T45.8X4	T45.8X5	T45.8X6
Folic acid	T45.8X1	T45.8X2	T45.8X3	T45.8X4	T45.8X5	T45.8X6
with ferrous salt	T45.2X1	T45.2X2	T45.2X3	T45.2X4	T45.2X5	T45.2X6
antagonist	T45.1X1	T45.1X2	T45.1X3	T45.1X4	T45.1X5	T45.1X6
Folinic acid	T45.8X1	T45.8X2	T45.8X3	T45.8X4	T45.8X5	T45.8X6
Folium stramoniae	T48.6X1	T48.6X2	T48.6X3	T48.6X4	T48.6X5	T48.6X6
Follicle-stimulating hormone, human	T38.811	T38.812	T38.813	T38.814	T38.815	T38.816
Folpet	T6Ø.3X1	T6Ø.3X2	T6Ø.3X3	T6Ø.3X4	—	—
Fomepizole*	T5Ø.6X1	T5Ø.6X2	T5Ø.6X3	T5Ø.6X4	T5Ø.6X5	T5Ø.6X6
Fominoben	T48.3X1	T48.3X2	T48.3X3	T48.3X4	T48.3X5	T48.3X6
Food, foodstuffs, noxious, nonbacterial, NEC	T62.91	T62.92	T62.93	T62.94	—	—
berries	T62.1X1	T62.1X2	T62.1X3	T62.1X4	—	—
fish — *see also* Fish	T61.91	T61.92	T61.93	T61.94	—	—
mushrooms	T62.ØX1	T62.ØX2	T62.ØX3	T62.ØX4	—	—
plants	T62.2X1	T62.2X2	T62.2X3	T62.2X4	—	—
seafood	T61.91	T61.92	T61.93	T61.94	—	—
specified NEC	T61.8X1	T61.8X2	T61.8X3	T61.8X4	—	—
seeds	T62.2X1	T62.2X2	T62.2X3	T62.2X4	—	—
shellfish	T61.781	T61.782	T61.783	T61.784	—	—
specified NEC	T62.8X1	T62.8X2	T62.8X3	T62.8X4	—	—
Fool's parsley	T62.2X1	T62.2X2	T62.2X3	T62.2X4	—	—
Formaldehyde (solution), gas or vapor	T59.2X1	T59.2X2	T59.2X3	T59.2X4	—	—
fungicide	T6Ø.3X1	T6Ø.3X2	T6Ø.3X3	T6Ø.3X4	—	—
Formalin	T59.2X1	T59.2X2	T59.2X3	T59.2X4	—	—
fungicide	T6Ø.3X1	T6Ø.3X2	T6Ø.3X3	T6Ø.3X4	—	—
vapor	T59.2X1	T59.2X2	T59.2X3	T59.2X4	—	—
Formic acid	T54.2X1	T54.2X2	T54.2X3	T54.2X4	—	—
vapor	T59.891	T59.892	T59.893	T59.894	—	—
Formoterol*	T48.6X1	T48.6X2	T48.6X3	T48.6X4	T48.6X5	T48.6X6
Fortaz*	T36.1X1	T36.1X2	T36.1X3	T36.1X4	T36.1X5	T36.1X6
Foscarnet sodium	T37.5X1	T37.5X2	T37.5X3	T37.5X4	T37.5X5	T37.5X6
Fosfestrol	T38.5X1	T38.5X2	T38.5X3	T38.5X4	T38.5X5	T38.5X6
Fosfomycin	T36.8X1	T36.8X2	T36.8X3	T36.8X4	T36.8X5	T36.8X6
Fosfonet sodium	T37.5X1	T37.5X2	T37.5X3	T37.5X4	T37.5X5	T37.5X6
Fosinopril	T46.4X1	T46.4X2	T46.4X3	T46.4X4	T46.4X5	T46.4X6
sodium	T46.4X1	T46.4X2	T46.4X3	T46.4X4	T46.4X5	T46.4X6
Fowler's solution	T57.ØX1	T57.ØX2	T57.ØX3	T57.ØX4	—	—
Foxglove	T62.2X1	T62.2X2	T62.2X3	T62.2X4	—	—
Framycetin	T36.5X1	T36.5X2	T36.5X3	T36.5X4	T36.5X5	T36.5X6
Frangula	T47.2X1	T47.2X2	T47.2X3	T47.2X4	T47.2X5	T47.2X6
extract	T47.2X1	T47.2X2	T47.2X3	T47.2X4	T47.2X5	T47.2X6
Frei antigen	T5Ø.8X1	T5Ø.8X2	T5Ø.8X3	T5Ø.8X4	T5Ø.8X5	T5Ø.8X6
Freon	T53.5X1	T53.5X2	T53.5X3	T53.5X4	—	—
Fructose	T5Ø.3X1	T5Ø.3X2	T5Ø.3X3	T5Ø.3X4	T5Ø.3X5	T5Ø.3X6
Frusemide	T5Ø.1X1	T5Ø.1X2	T5Ø.1X3	T5Ø.1X4	T5Ø.1X5	T5Ø.1X6
FSH	T38.811	T38.812	T38.813	T38.814	T38.815	T38.816
Ftorafur	T45.1X1	T45.1X2	T45.1X3	T45.1X4	T45.1X5	T45.1X6
Fuel						
automobile	T52.ØX1	T52.ØX2	T52.ØX3	T52.ØX4	—	—
exhaust gas, not in transit	T58.Ø1	T58.Ø2	T58.Ø3	T58.Ø4	—	—
vapor NEC	T52.ØX1	T52.ØX2	T52.ØX3	T52.ØX4	—	—
gas (domestic use) — *see also* Carbon, monoxide, fuel, utility	T59.891	T59.892	T59.893	T59.894	—	—
utility	T59.891	T59.892	T59.893	T59.894	—	—
incomplete combustion of — *see* Carbon, monoxide, fuel, utility						
in mobile container	T59.891	T59.892	T59.893	T59.894	—	—
piped (natural)	T59.891	T59.892	T59.893	T59.894	—	—
industrial, incomplete combustion	T58.8X1	T58.8X2	T58.8X3	T58.8X4	—	—
Fugillin	T36.8X1	T36.8X2	T36.8X3	T36.8X4	T36.8X5	T36.8X6
Fulminate of mercury	T56.1X1	T56.1X2	T56.1X3	T56.1X4	—	—
Fulvicin	T36.7X1	T36.7X2	T36.7X3	T36.7X4	T36.7X5	T36.7X6
Fumadil	T36.8X1	T36.8X2	T36.8X3	T36.8X4	T36.8X5	T36.8X6
Fumagillin	T36.8X1	T36.8X2	T36.8X3	T36.8X4	T36.8X5	T36.8X6
Fumaric acid	T49.4X1	T49.4X2	T49.4X3	T49.4X4	T49.4X5	T49.4X6

Substance	Poisoning, Accidental (unintentional)	Poisoning, Intentional Self-harm	Poisoning, Assault	Poisoning, Undetermined	Adverse Effect	Under-dosing
Fumes (from)	T59.91	T59.92	T59.93	T59.94	—	—
carbon monoxide — *see* Carbon, monoxide						
charcoal (domestic use) — *see* Charcoal, fumes						
chloroform — *see* Chloroform						
coke (in domestic stoves, fireplaces) — *see* Coke fumes						
corrosive NEC	T54.91	T54.92	T54.93	T54.94	—	—
ether — *see* ether						
freons	T53.5X1	T53.5X2	T53.5X3	T53.5X4	—	—
hydrocarbons	T59.891	T59.892	T59.893	T59.894	—	—
petroleum (liquefied)	T59.891	T59.892	T59.893	T59.894	—	—
distributed through pipes (pure or mixed with air)	T59.891	T59.892	T59.893	T59.894	—	—
lead — *see* lead						
metal — *see* Metals, or the specified metal						
nitrogen dioxide	T59.ØX1	T59.ØX2	T59.ØX3	T59.ØX4	—	—
pesticides — *see* Pesticide						
petroleum (liquefied)	T59.891	T59.892	T59.893	T59.894	—	—
distributed through pipes (pure or mixed with air)	T59.891	T59.892	T59.893	T59.894	—	—
polyester	T59.891	T59.892	T59.893	T59.894	—	—
specified source NEC — *see also* substance specified	T59.891	T59.892	T59.893	T59.894	—	—
sulfur dioxide	T59.1X1	T59.1X2	T59.1X3	T59.1X4	—	—
Fumigant NEC	T6Ø.91	T6Ø.92	T6Ø.93	T6Ø.94	—	—
Fungicide NEC (nonmedicinal)	T6Ø.3X1	T6Ø.3X2	T6Ø.3X3	T6Ø.3X4	—	—
Fungi, noxious, used as food	T62.ØX1	T62.ØX2	T62.ØX3	T62.ØX4	—	—
Fungizone	T36.7X1	T36.7X2	T36.7X3	T36.7X4	T36.7X5	T36.7X6
topical	T49.ØX1	T49.ØX2	T49.ØX3	T49.ØX4	T49.ØX5	T49.ØX6
Fungoid*	T49.ØX1	T49.ØX2	T49.ØX3	T49.ØX4	T49.ØX5	T49.ØX6
Furacin	T49.ØX1	T49.ØX2	T49.ØX3	T49.ØX4	T49.ØX5	T49.ØX6
Furadantin	T37.91	T37.92	T37.93	T37.94	T37.95	T37.96
Furazolidone	T37.8X1	T37.8X2	T37.8X3	T37.8X4	T37.8X5	T37.8X6
Furazolium chloride	T49.ØX1	T49.ØX2	T49.ØX3	T49.ØX4	T49.ØX5	T49.ØX6
Furfural	T52.8X1	T52.8X2	T52.8X3	T52.8X4	—	—
Furnace (coal burning) (domestic), gas from	T58.2X1	T58.2X2	T58.2X3	T58.2X4	—	—
industrial	T58.8X1	T58.8X2	T58.8X3	T58.8X4	—	—
Furniture polish	T65.891	T65.892	T65.893	T65.894	—	—
Furosemide	T5Ø.1X1	T5Ø.1X2	T5Ø.1X3	T5Ø.1X4	T5Ø.1X5	T5Ø.1X6
Furoxone	T37.91	T37.92	T37.93	T37.94	T37.95	T37.96
Fursultiamine	T45.2X1	T45.2X2	T45.2X3	T45.2X4	T45.2X5	T45.2X6
Fusafungine	T36.8X1	T36.8X2	T36.8X3	T36.8X4	T36.8X5	T36.8X6
Fusel oil (any) (amyl) (butyl) (propyl), vapor	T51.3X1	T51.3X2	T51.3X3	T51.3X4	—	—
Fusidate (ethanolamine) (sodium)	T36.8X1	T36.8X2	T36.8X3	T36.8X4	T36.8X5	T36.8X6
Fusidic acid	T36.8X1	T36.8X2	T36.8X3	T36.8X4	T36.8X5	T36.8X6
Fytic acid, nonasodium	T5Ø.6X1	T5Ø.6X2	T5Ø.6X3	T5Ø.6X4	T5Ø.6X5	T5Ø.6X6
b-Galactosidase	T47.5X1	T47.5X2	T47.5X3	T47.5X4	T47.5X5	T47.5X6
GABA	T43.8X1	T43.8X2	T43.8X3	T43.8X4	T43.8X5	T43.8X6
Gabapentin*	T42.6X1	T42.6X2	T42.6X3	T42.6X4	T42.6X5	T42.6X6
Gabitril*	T42.6X1	T42.6X2	T42.6X3	T42.6X4	T42.6X5	T42.6X6
Gadolinium	T56.821	T56.822	T56.823	T56.824	—	—
Gadopentetic acid	T5Ø.8X1	T5Ø.8X2	T5Ø.8X3	T5Ø.8X4	T5Ø.8X5	T5Ø.8X6
Galactose	T5Ø.3X1	T5Ø.3X2	T5Ø.3X3	T5Ø.3X4	T5Ø.3X5	T5Ø.3X6
Galantamine	T44.ØX1	T44.ØX2	T44.ØX3	T44.ØX4	T44.ØX5	T44.ØX6
Gallamine (triethiodide)	T48.1X1	T48.1X2	T48.1X3	T48.1X4	T48.1X5	T48.1X6
Gallium citrate	T5Ø.991	T5Ø.992	T5Ø.993	T5Ø.994	T5Ø.995	T5Ø.996
Gallopamil	T46.1X1	T46.1X2	T46.1X3	T46.1X4	T46.1X5	T46.1X6
Gamboge	T47.2X1	T47.2X2	T47.2X3	T47.2X4	T47.2X5	T47.2X6
Gamimune	T5Ø.Z11	T5Ø.Z12	T5Ø.Z13	T5Ø.Z14	T5Ø.Z15	T5Ø.Z16
Gamma-aminobutyric acid	T43.8X1	T43.8X2	T43.8X3	T43.8X4	T43.8X5	T43.8X6
Gamma-benzene hexachloride (medicinal)	T49.ØX1	T49.ØX2	T49.ØX3	T49.ØX4	T49.ØX5	T49.ØX6
nonmedicinal, vapor	T53.6X1	T53.6X2	T53.6X3	T53.6X4	—	—
Gamma-BHC (medicinal) — *see also* Gamma-benzene hexachloride	T49.ØX1	T49.ØX2	T49.ØX3	T49.ØX4	T49.ØX5	T49.ØX6
Gamma globulin	T5Ø.Z11	T5Ø.Z12	T5Ø.Z13	T5Ø.Z14	T5Ø.Z15	T5Ø.Z16
Gamulin	T5Ø.Z11	T5Ø.Z12	T5Ø.Z13	T5Ø.Z14	T5Ø.Z15	T5Ø.Z16
Ganciclovir (sodium)	T37.5X1	T37.5X2	T37.5X3	T37.5X4	T37.5X5	T37.5X6
Ganglionic blocking drug NEC	T44.2X1	T44.2X2	T44.2X3	T44.2X4	T44.2X5	T44.2X6
specified NEC	T44.2X1	T44.2X2	T44.2X3	T44.2X4	T44.2X5	T44.2X6

Substance	Poisoning, Accidental (unintentional)	Poisoning, Intentional Self-harm	Poisoning, Assault	Poisoning, Undetermined	Adverse Effect	Under-dosing
Ganja	T4Ø.711	T4Ø.712	T4Ø.713	T4Ø.714	T4Ø.715	T4Ø.716
Garamycin	T36.5X1	T36.5X2	T36.5X3	T36.5X4	T36.5X5	T36.5X6
ophthalmic preparation	T49.5X1	T49.5X2	T49.5X3	T49.5X4	T49.5X5	T49.5X6
topical NEC	T49.ØX1	T49.ØX2	T49.ØX3	T49.ØX4	T49.ØX5	T49.ØX6
Gardenal	T42.3X1	T42.3X2	T42.3X3	T42.3X4	T42.3X5	T42.3X6
Gardepanyl	T42.3X1	T42.3X2	T42.3X3	T42.3X4	T42.3X5	T42.3X6
Gaseous substance — *see* Gas						
Gasoline	T52.ØX1	T52.ØX2	T52.ØX3	T52.ØX4	—	—
vapor	T52.ØX1	T52.ØX2	T52.ØX3	T52.ØX4	—	—
Gastric enzymes	T47.5X1	T47.5X2	T47.5X3	T47.5X4	T47.5X5	T47.5X6
Gastrografin	T5Ø.8X1	T5Ø.8X2	T5Ø.8X3	T5Ø.8X4	T5Ø.8X5	T5Ø.8X6
Gastrointestinal drug	T47.91	T47.92	T47.93	T47.94	T47.95	T47.96
biological	T47.8X1	T47.8X2	T47.8X3	T47.8X4	T47.8X5	T47.8X6
specified NEC	T47.8X1	T47.8X2	T47.8X3	T47.8X4	T47.8X5	T47.8X6
Gas NEC	T59.91	T59.92	T59.93	T59.94	—	—
acetylene	T59.891	T59.892	T59.893	T59.894	—	—
incomplete combustion of	T58.11	T58.12	T58.13	T58.14	—	—
air contaminants, source or type not specified	T59.91	T59.92	T59.93	T59.94	—	—
anesthetic	T41.ØX1	T41.ØX2	T41.ØX3	T41.ØX4	T41.ØX5	T41.ØX6
blast furnace	T58.8X1	T58.8X2	T58.8X3	T58.8X4	—	—
butane — *see* butane						
carbon monoxide — *see* Carbon, monoxide						
chlorine	T59.4X1	T59.4X2	T59.4X3	T59.4X4	—	—
coal	T58.2X1	T58.2X2	T58.2X3	T58.2X4	—	—
cyanide	T57.3X1	T57.3X2	T57.3X3	T57.3X4	—	—
dicyanogen	T65.ØX1	T65.ØX2	T65.ØX3	T65.ØX4	—	—
domestic — *see* Domestic gas						
exhaust	T58.Ø1	T58.Ø2	T58.Ø3	T58.Ø4	—	—
from utility (for cooking, heating, or lighting) (after combustion) — *see* Carbon, monoxide, fuel, utility						
prior to combustion	T59.891	T59.892	T59.893	T59.894	—	—
from wood- or coal-burning stove or fireplace	T58.2X1	T58.2X2	T58.2X3	T58.2X4	—	—
fuel (domestic use) (after combustion) — *see also* Carbon, monoxide, fuel						
industrial use	T58.8X1	T58.8X2	T58.8X3	T58.8X4	—	—
prior to combustion	T59.891	T59.892	T59.893	T59.894	—	—
utility	T59.891	T59.892	T59.893	T59.894	—	—
incomplete combustion of — *see* Carbon, monoxide, fuel, utility						
in mobile container	T59.891	T59.892	T59.893	T59.894	—	—
piped (natural)	T59.891	T59.892	T59.893	T59.894	—	—
garage	T58.Ø1	T58.Ø2	T58.Ø3	T58.Ø4	—	—
hydrocarbon NEC	T59.891	T59.892	T59.893	T59.894	—	—
incomplete combustion of — *see* Carbon, monoxide, fuel, utility						
liquefied — *see* butane						
piped	T59.891	T59.892	T59.893	T59.894	—	—
hydrocyanic acid	T65.ØX1	T65.ØX2	T65.ØX3	T65.ØX4	—	—
illuminating (after combustion)	T58.11	T58.12	T58.13	T58.14	—	—
prior to combustion	T59.891	T59.892	T59.893	T59.894	—	—
incomplete combustion, any — *see* Carbon, monoxide						
kiln	T58.8X1	T58.8X2	T58.8X3	T58.8X4	—	—
lacrimogenic	T59.3X1	T59.3X2	T59.3X3	T59.3X4	—	—
liquefied petroleum — *see* butane						
marsh	T59.891	T59.892	T59.893	T59.894	—	—
motor exhaust, not in transit	T58.Ø1	T58.Ø2	T58.Ø3	T58.Ø4	—	—
mustard, not in war	T59.891	T59.892	T59.893	T59.894	—	—
natural	T59.891	T59.892	T59.893	T59.894	—	—
nerve, not in war	T59.91	T59.92	T59.93	T59.94	—	—
oil	T52.ØX1	T52.ØX2	T52.ØX3	T52.ØX4	—	—
petroleum (liquefied) (distributed in mobile containers)	T59.891	T59.892	T59.893	T59.894	—	—
piped (pure or mixed with air)	T59.891	T59.892	T59.893	T59.894	—	—
piped (manufactured) (natural) NEC	T59.891	T59.892	T59.893	T59.894	—	—
producer	T58.8X1	T58.8X2	T58.8X3	T58.8X4	—	—
propane — *see* propane						
Gas — *continued*						
refrigerant (chlorofluoro-carbon)	T53.5X1	T53.5X2	T53.5X3	T53.5X4	—	—
not chlorofluoro-carbon	T59.891	T59.892	T59.893	T59.894	—	—
sewer	T59.91	T59.92	T59.93	T59.94	—	—
specified source NEC	T59.91	T59.92	T59.93	T59.94	—	—
stove (after combustion)	T58.11	T58.12	T58.13	T58.14	—	—
prior to combustion	T59.891	T59.892	T59.893	T59.894	—	—
tear	T59.3X1	T59.3X2	T59.3X3	T59.3X4	—	—
therapeutic	T41.5X1	T41.5X2	T41.5X3	T41.5X4	T41.5X5	T41.5X6
utility (for cooking, heating, or lighting) (piped) NEC	T59.891	T59.892	T59.893	T59.894	—	—
incomplete combustion of — *see* Carbon, monoxide, fuel, utility						
in mobile container	T59.891	T59.892	T59.893	T59.894	—	—
piped (natural)	T59.891	T59.892	T59.893	T59.894	—	—
water	T58.11	T58.12	T58.13	T58.14	—	—
incomplete combustion of — *see* Carbon, monoxide, fuel, utility						
Gaultheria procumbens	T62.2X1	T62.2X2	T62.2X3	T62.2X4	—	—
Gaviscon*	T47.1X1	T47.1X2	T47.1X3	T47.1X4	T47.1X5	T47.1X6
Gefarnate	T44.3X1	T44.3X2	T44.3X3	T44.3X4	T44.3X5	T44.3X6
Gelatin (intravenous)	T45.8X1	T45.8X2	T45.8X3	T45.8X4	T45.8X5	T45.8X6
absorbable (sponge)	T45.7X1	T45.7X2	T45.7X3	T45.7X4	T45.7X5	T45.7X6
Gelfilm	T49.8X1	T49.8X2	T49.8X3	T49.8X4	T49.8X5	T49.8X6
Gelfoam	T45.7X1	T45.7X2	T45.7X3	T45.7X4	T45.7X5	T45.7X6
Gelsemine	T5Ø.991	T5Ø.992	T5Ø.993	T5Ø.994	T5Ø.995	T5Ø.996
Gelsemium (sempervirens)	T62.2X1	T62.2X2	T62.2X3	T62.2X4	—	—
Gemeprost	T48.ØX1	T48.ØX2	T48.ØX3	T48.ØX4	T48.ØX5	T48.ØX6
Gemfibrozil	T46.6X1	T46.6X2	T46.6X3	T46.6X4	T46.6X5	T46.6X6
Gemonil	T42.3X1	T42.3X2	T42.3X3	T42.3X4	T42.3X5	T42.3X6
Gentamicin	T36.5X1	T36.5X2	T36.5X3	T36.5X4	T36.5X5	T36.5X6
ophthalmic preparation	T49.5X1	T49.5X2	T49.5X3	T49.5X4	T49.5X5	T49.5X6
topical NEC	T49.ØX1	T49.ØX2	T49.ØX3	T49.ØX4	T49.ØX5	T49.ØX6
Gentasol*	T49.5X1	T49.5X2	T49.5X3	T49.5X4	T49.5X5	T49.5X6
Gentian	T47.5X1	T47.5X2	T47.5X3	T47.5X4	T47.5X5	T47.5X6
violet	T49.ØX1	T49.ØX2	T49.ØX3	T49.ØX4	T49.ØX5	T49.ØX6
Gepefrine	T44.4X1	T44.4X2	T44.4X3	T44.4X4	T44.4X5	T44.4X6
Gestonorone caproate	T38.5X1	T38.5X2	T38.5X3	T38.5X4	T38.5X5	T38.5X6
Gexane	T49.ØX1	T49.ØX2	T49.ØX3	T49.ØX4	T49.ØX5	T49.ØX6
Gila monster (venom)	T63.111	T63.112	T63.113	T63.114	—	—
Ginger	T47.5X1	T47.5X2	T47.5X3	T47.5X4	T47.5X5	T47.5X6
Jamaica — *see* Jamaica, ginger						
Gitalin	T46.ØX1	T46.ØX2	T46.ØX3	T46.ØX4	T46.ØX5	T46.ØX6
amorphous	T46.ØX1	T46.ØX2	T46.ØX3	T46.ØX4	T46.ØX5	T46.ØX6
Gitaloxin	T46.ØX1	T46.ØX2	T46.ØX3	T46.ØX4	T46.ØX5	T46.ØX6
Gitoxin	T46.ØX1	T46.ØX2	T46.ØX3	T46.ØX4	T46.ØX5	T46.ØX6
Glafenine	T39.8X1	T39.8X2	T39.8X3	T39.8X4	T39.8X5	T39.8X6
Glandular extract (medicinal) **NEC**	T5Ø.Z91	T5Ø.Z92	T5Ø.Z93	T5Ø.Z94	T5Ø.Z95	T5Ø.Z96
Glaucarubin	T37.3X1	T37.3X2	T37.3X3	T37.3X4	T37.3X5	T37.3X6
Glibenclamide	T38.3X1	T38.3X2	T38.3X3	T38.3X4	T38.3X5	T38.3X6
Glibornuride	T38.3X1	T38.3X2	T38.3X3	T38.3X4	T38.3X5	T38.3X6
Gliclazide	T38.3X1	T38.3X2	T38.3X3	T38.3X4	T38.3X5	T38.3X6
Glimidine	T38.3X1	T38.3X2	T38.3X3	T38.3X4	T38.3X5	T38.3X6
Glipizide	T38.3X1	T38.3X2	T38.3X3	T38.3X4	T38.3X5	T38.3X6
Gliquidone	T38.3X1	T38.3X2	T38.3X3	T38.3X4	T38.3X5	T38.3X6
Glisolamide	T38.3X1	T38.3X2	T38.3X3	T38.3X4	T38.3X5	T38.3X6
Glisoxepide	T38.3X1	T38.3X2	T38.3X3	T38.3X4	T38.3X5	T38.3X6
Globin zinc insulin	T38.3X1	T38.3X2	T38.3X3	T38.3X4	T38.3X5	T38.3X6
Globulin						
antilymphocytic	T5Ø.Z11	T5Ø.Z12	T5Ø.Z13	T5Ø.Z14	T5Ø.Z15	T5Ø.Z16
antirhesus	T5Ø.Z11	T5Ø.Z12	T5Ø.Z13	T5Ø.Z14	T5Ø.Z15	T5Ø.Z16
antivenin	T5Ø.Z11	T5Ø.Z12	T5Ø.Z13	T5Ø.Z14	T5Ø.Z15	T5Ø.Z16
antiviral	T5Ø.Z11	T5Ø.Z12	T5Ø.Z13	T5Ø.Z14	T5Ø.Z15	T5Ø.Z16
Glucagon	T38.3X1	T38.3X2	T38.3X3	T38.3X4	T38.3X5	T38.3X6
Glucocorticoids	T38.ØX1	T38.ØX2	T38.ØX3	T38.ØX4	T38.ØX5	T38.ØX6
Glucocorticosteroid	T38.ØX1	T38.ØX2	T38.ØX3	T38.ØX4	T38.ØX5	T38.ØX6
Gluconic acid	T5Ø.991	T5Ø.992	T5Ø.993	T5Ø.994	T5Ø.995	T5Ø.996
Glucosamine sulfate	T39.4X1	T39.4X2	T39.4X3	T39.4X4	T39.4X5	T39.4X6
Glucose	T5Ø.3X1	T5Ø.3X2	T5Ø.3X3	T5Ø.3X4	T5Ø.3X5	T5Ø.3X6
with sodium chloride	T5Ø.3X1	T5Ø.3X2	T5Ø.3X3	T5Ø.3X4	T5Ø.3X5	T5Ø.3X6
Glucosulfone sodium	T37.1X1	T37.1X2	T37.1X3	T37.1X4	T37.1X5	T37.1X6
Glucotrol*	T38.3X1	T38.3X2	T38.3X3	T38.3X4	T38.3X5	T38.3X6
Glucurolactone	T47.8X1	T47.8X2	T47.8X3	T47.8X4	T47.8X5	T47.8X6
Glue NEC	T52.8X1	T52.8X2	T52.8X3	T52.8X4	—	—
Glutamic acid	T47.5X1	T47.5X2	T47.5X3	T47.5X4	T47.5X5	T47.5X6
Glutaral (medicinal)	T49.ØX1	T49.ØX2	T49.ØX3	T49.ØX4	T49.ØX5	T49.ØX6
nonmedicinal	T65.891	T65.892	T65.893	T65.894	—	—
Glutaraldehyde (nonmedicinal)	T65.891	T65.892	T65.893	T65.894	—	—

Substance	Poisoning, Accidental (unintentional)	Poisoning, Intentional Self-harm	Poisoning, Assault	Poisoning, Undetermined	Adverse Effect	Under-dosing
Glutaraldehyde — *continued*						
medicinal	T49.ØX1	T49.ØX2	T49.ØX3	T49.ØX4	T49.ØX5	T49.ØX6
Glutathione	T5Ø.6X1	T5Ø.6X2	T5Ø.6X3	T5Ø.6X4	T5Ø.6X5	T5Ø.6X6
Glutethimide	T42.6X1	T42.6X2	T42.6X3	T42.6X4	T42.6X5	T42.6X6
Glyburide	T38.3X1	T38.3X2	T38.3X3	T38.3X4	T38.3X5	T38.3X6
Glycerin	T47.4X1	T47.4X2	T47.4X3	T47.4X4	T47.4X5	T47.4X6
Glycerol	T47.4X1	T47.4X2	T47.4X3	T47.4X4	T47.4X5	T47.4X6
borax	T49.6X1	T49.6X2	T49.6X3	T49.6X4	T49.6X5	T49.6X6
intravenous	T5Ø.3X1	T5Ø.3X2	T5Ø.3X3	T5Ø.3X4	T5Ø.3X5	T5Ø.3X6
iodinated	T48.4X1	T48.4X2	T48.4X3	T48.4X4	T48.4X5	T48.4X6
Glycerophosphate	T5Ø.991	T5Ø.992	T5Ø.993	T5Ø.994	T5Ø.995	T5Ø.996
Glyceryl						
gualacolate	T48.4X1	T48.4X2	T48.4X3	T48.4X4	T48.4X5	T48.4X6
nitrate	T46.3X1	T46.3X2	T46.3X3	T46.3X4	T46.3X5	T46.3X6
triacetate (topical)	T49.ØX1	T49.ØX2	T49.ØX3	T49.ØX4	T49.ØX5	T49.ØX6
trinitrate	T46.3X1	T46.3X2	T46.3X3	T46.3X4	T46.3X5	T46.3X6
Glycine	T5Ø.3X1	T5Ø.3X2	T5Ø.3X3	T5Ø.3X4	T5Ø.3X5	T5Ø.3X6
Glyclopyramide	T38.3X1	T38.3X2	T38.3X3	T38.3X4	T38.3X5	T38.3X6
Glycobiarsol	T37.3X1	T37.3X2	T37.3X3	T37.3X4	T37.3X5	T37.3X6
Glycols (ether)	T52.3X1	T52.3X2	T52.3X3	T52.3X4	—	—
Glyconiazide	T37.1X1	T37.1X2	T37.1X3	T37.1X4	T37.1X5	T37.1X6
Glycopyrrolate	T44.3X1	T44.3X2	T44.3X3	T44.3X4	T44.3X5	T44.3X6
Glycopyrronium	T44.3X1	T44.3X2	T44.3X3	T44.3X4	T44.3X5	T44.3X6
bromide	T44.3X1	T44.3X2	T44.3X3	T44.3X4	T44.3X5	T44.3X6
Glycoside, cardiac (stimulant)	T46.ØX1	T46.ØX2	T46.ØX3	T46.ØX4	T46.ØX5	T46.ØX6
Glycyclamide	T38.3X1	T38.3X2	T38.3X3	T38.3X4	T38.3X5	T38.3X6
Glycyrrhiza extract	T48.4X1	T48.4X2	T48.4X3	T48.4X4	T48.4X5	T48.4X6
Glycyrrhizic acid	T48.4X1	T48.4X2	T48.4X3	T48.4X4	T48.4X5	T48.4X6
Glycyrrhizinate potassium	T48.4X1	T48.4X2	T48.4X3	T48.4X4	T48.4X5	T48.4X6
Glymidine sodium	T38.3X1	T38.3X2	T38.3X3	T38.3X4	T38.3X5	T38.3X6
Glyphosate	T6Ø.3X1	T6Ø.3X2	T6Ø.3X3	T6Ø.3X4	—	—
Glyphylline	T48.6X1	T48.6X2	T48.6X3	T48.6X4	T48.6X5	T48.6X6
Gold						
colloidal (I98Au)	T45.1X1	T45.1X2	T45.1X3	T45.1X4	T45.1X5	T45.1X6
salts	T39.4X1	T39.4X2	T39.4X3	T39.4X4	T39.4X5	T39.4X6
Golden sulfide of antimony	T56.891	T56.892	T56.893	T56.894	—	—
Goldylocks	T62.2X1	T62.2X2	T62.2X3	T62.2X4	—	—
Gonadal tissue extract	T38.9Ø1	T38.9Ø2	T38.9Ø3	T38.9Ø4	T38.9Ø5	T38.9Ø6
female	T38.5X1	T38.5X2	T38.5X3	T38.5X4	T38.5X5	T38.5X6
male	T38.7X1	T38.7X2	T38.7X3	T38.7X4	T38.7X5	T38.7X6
Gonadorelin	T38.891	T38.892	T38.893	T38.894	T38.895	T38.896
Gonadotropin	T38.891	T38.892	T38.893	T38.894	T38.895	T38.896
chorionic	T38.891	T38.892	T38.893	T38.894	T38.895	T38.896
pituitary	T38.811	T38.812	T38.813	T38.814	T38.815	T38.816
Goserelin	T45.1X1	T45.1X2	T45.1X3	T45.1X4	T45.1X5	T45.1X6
Grain alcohol	T51.ØX1	T51.ØX2	T51.ØX3	T51.ØX4	—	—
Gralise*	T42.6X1	T42.6X2	T42.6X3	T42.6X4	T42.6X5	T42.6X6
Gramicidin	T49.ØX1	T49.ØX2	T49.ØX3	T49.ØX4	T49.ØX5	T49.ØX6
Granisetron	T45.ØX1	T45.ØX2	T45.ØX3	T45.ØX4	T45.ØX5	T45.ØX6
Gratiola officinalis	T62.2X1	T62.2X2	T62.2X3	T62.2X4	—	—
Grease	T65.891	T65.892	T65.893	T65.894	—	—
Green hellebore	T62.2X1	T62.2X2	T62.2X3	T62.2X4	—	—
Green soap	T49.2X1	T49.2X2	T49.2X3	T49.2X4	T49.2X5	T49.2X6
Grifulvin	T36.7X1	T36.7X2	T36.7X3	T36.7X4	T36.7X5	T36.7X6
Griseofulvin	T36.7X1	T36.7X2	T36.7X3	T36.7X4	T36.7X5	T36.7X6
Growth hormone	T38.811	T38.812	T38.813	T38.814	T38.815	T38.816
Guaiacol derivatives	T48.4X1	T48.4X2	T48.4X3	T48.4X4	T48.4X5	T48.4X6
Guaiac reagent	T5Ø.991	T5Ø.992	T5Ø.993	T5Ø.994	T5Ø.995	T5Ø.996
Guaifenesin	T48.4X1	T48.4X2	T48.4X3	T48.4X4	T48.4X5	T48.4X6
Guaimesal	T48.4X1	T48.4X2	T48.4X3	T48.4X4	T48.4X5	T48.4X6
Guaiphenesin	T48.4X1	T48.4X2	T48.4X3	T48.4X4	T48.4X5	T48.4X6
Guaituss*	T48.4X1	T48.4X2	T48.4X3	T48.4X4	T48.4X5	T48.4X6
Guamecycline	T36.4X1	T36.4X2	T36.4X3	T36.4X4	T36.4X5	T36.4X6
Guanabenz	T46.5X1	T46.5X2	T46.5X3	T46.5X4	T46.5X5	T46.5X6
Guanacline	T46.5X1	T46.5X2	T46.5X3	T46.5X4	T46.5X5	T46.5X6
Guanadrel	T46.5X1	T46.5X2	T46.5X3	T46.5X4	T46.5X5	T46.5X6
Guanatol	T37.2X1	T37.2X2	T37.2X3	T37.2X4	T37.2X5	T37.2X6
Guanethidine	T46.5X1	T46.5X2	T46.5X3	T46.5X4	T46.5X5	T46.5X6
Guanfacine	T46.5X1	T46.5X2	T46.5X3	T46.5X4	T46.5X5	T46.5X6
Guano	T65.891	T65.892	T65.893	T65.894	—	—
Guanochlor	T46.5X1	T46.5X2	T46.5X3	T46.5X4	T46.5X5	T46.5X6
Guanoclor	T46.5X1	T46.5X2	T46.5X3	T46.5X4	T46.5X5	T46.5X6
Guanoctine	T46.5X1	T46.5X2	T46.5X3	T46.5X4	T46.5X5	T46.5X6
Guanoxabenz	T46.5X1	T46.5X2	T46.5X3	T46.5X4	T46.5X5	T46.5X6
Guanoxan	T46.5X1	T46.5X2	T46.5X3	T46.5X4	T46.5X5	T46.5X6
Guar gum (medicinal)	T46.6X1	T46.6X2	T46.6X3	T46.6X4	T46.6X5	T46.6X6
Hachimycin	T36.7X1	T36.7X2	T36.7X3	T36.7X4	T36.7X5	T36.7X6
Hair						
dye	T49.4X1	T49.4X2	T49.4X3	T49.4X4	T49.4X5	T49.4X6
preparation NEC	T49.4X1	T49.4X2	T49.4X3	T49.4X4	T49.4X5	T49.4X6
Halazepam	T42.4X1	T42.4X2	T42.4X3	T42.4X4	T42.4X5	T42.4X6

Substance	Poisoning, Accidental (unintentional)	Poisoning, Intentional Self-harm	Poisoning, Assault	Poisoning, Undetermined	Adverse Effect	Under-dosing
Halcinolone	T49.ØX1	T49.ØX2	T49.ØX3	T49.ØX4	T49.ØX5	T49.ØX6
Halcinonide	T49.ØX1	T49.ØX2	T49.ØX3	T49.ØX4	T49.ØX5	T49.ØX6
Halethazole	T49.ØX1	T49.ØX2	T49.ØX3	T49.ØX4	T49.ØX5	T49.ØX6
Hallucinogen NOS	T4Ø.9Ø1	T4Ø.9Ø2	T4Ø.9Ø3	T4Ø.9Ø4	T4Ø.9Ø5	T4Ø.9Ø6
specified NEC	T4Ø.991	T4Ø.992	T4Ø.993	T4Ø.994	T4Ø.995	T4Ø.996
Halofantrine	T37.2X1	T37.2X2	T37.2X3	T37.2X4	T37.2X5	T37.2X6
Halofenate	T46.6X1	T46.6X2	T46.6X3	T46.6X4	T46.6X5	T46.6X6
Halometasone	T49.ØX1	T49.ØX2	T49.ØX3	T49.ØX4	T49.ØX5	T49.ØX6
Haloperidol	T43.4X1	T43.4X2	T43.4X3	T43.4X4	T43.4X5	T43.4X6
Haloprogin	T49.ØX1	T49.ØX2	T49.ØX3	T49.ØX4	T49.ØX5	T49.ØX6
Halotex	T49.ØX1	T49.ØX2	T49.ØX3	T49.ØX4	T49.ØX5	T49.ØX6
Halothane	T41.ØX1	T41.ØX2	T41.ØX3	T41.ØX4	T41.ØX5	T41.ØX6
Haloxazolam	T42.4X1	T42.4X2	T42.4X3	T42.4X4	T42.4X5	T42.4X6
Halquinols	T49.ØX1	T49.ØX2	T49.ØX3	T49.ØX4	T49.ØX5	T49.ØX6
Hamamelis	T49.2X1	T49.2X2	T49.2X3	T49.2X4	T49.2X5	T49.2X6
Haptendextran	T45.8X1	T45.8X2	T45.8X3	T45.8X4	T45.8X5	T45.8X6
Harmonyl	T46.5X1	T46.5X2	T46.5X3	T46.5X4	T46.5X5	T46.5X6
Hartmann's solution	T5Ø.3X1	T5Ø.3X2	T5Ø.3X3	T5Ø.3X4	T5Ø.3X5	T5Ø.3X6
Hashish	T4Ø.711	T4Ø.712	T4Ø.713	T4Ø.714	T4Ø.715	T4Ø.716
Havrix*	T5Ø.B91	T5Ø.B92	T5Ø.B93	T5Ø.B94	T5Ø.B95	T5Ø.B96
Hawaiian Woodrose seeds	T4Ø.991	T4Ø.992	T4Ø.993	T4Ø.994	—	—
HCB	T6Ø.3X1	T6Ø.3X2	T6Ø.3X3	T6Ø.3X4	—	—
HCH	T53.6X1	T53.6X2	T53.6X3	T53.6X4	—	—
medicinal	T49.ØX1	T49.ØX2	T49.ØX3	T49.ØX4	T49.ØX5	T49.ØX6
HCN	T57.3X1	T57.3X2	T57.3X3	T57.3X4	—	—
Headache cures, drugs, powders NEC	T5Ø.9Ø1	T5Ø.9Ø2	T5Ø.9Ø3	T5Ø.9Ø4	T5Ø.9Ø5	T5Ø.9Ø6
Heavenly Blue (morning glory)	T4Ø.991	T4Ø.992	T4Ø.993	T4Ø.994	—	—
Heavy metal antidote	T45.8X1	T45.8X2	T45.8X3	T45.8X4	T45.8X5	T45.8X6
Hedaquinium	T49.ØX1	T49.ØX2	T49.ØX3	T49.ØX4	T49.ØX5	T49.ØX6
Hedge hyssop	T62.2X1	T62.2X2	T62.2X3	T62.2X4	—	—
Heet	T49.8X1	T49.8X2	T49.8X3	T49.8X4	T49.8X5	T49.8X6
Helenin	T37.4X1	T37.4X2	T37.4X3	T37.4X4	T37.4X5	T37.4X6
Helium (nonmedicinal) **NEC**	T59.891	T59.892	T59.893	T59.894	—	—
medicinal	T48.991	T48.992	T48.993	T48.994	T48.995	T48.996
Hellebore (black) (green) (white)	T62.2X1	T62.2X2	T62.2X3	T62.2X4	—	—
Hematin	T45.8X1	T45.8X2	T45.8X3	T45.8X4	T45.8X5	T45.8X6
Hematinic preparation	T45.8X1	T45.8X2	T45.8X3	T45.8X4	T45.8X5	T45.8X6
Hematological agent	T45.91	T45.92	T45.93	T45.94	T45.95	T45.96
specified NEC	T45.8X1	T45.8X2	T45.8X3	T45.8X4	T45.8X5	T45.8X6
Hemlock	T62.2X1	T62.2X2	T62.2X3	T62.2X4	—	—
Hemostatic	T45.621	T45.622	T45.623	T45.624	T45.625	T45.626
drug, systemic	T45.621	T45.622	T45.623	T45.624	T45.625	T45.626
Hemostyptic	T49.4X1	T49.4X2	T49.4X3	T49.4X4	T49.4X5	T49.4X6
Henbane	T62.2X1	T62.2X2	T62.2X3	T62.2X4	—	—
Heparin (sodium)	T45.511	T45.512	T45.513	T45.514	T45.515	T45.516
action reverser	T45.7X1	T45.7X2	T45.7X3	T45.7X4	T45.7X5	T45.7X6
Heparin-fraction	T45.511	T45.512	T45.513	T45.514	T45.515	T45.516
Heparinoid (systemic)	T45.511	T45.512	T45.513	T45.514	T45.515	T45.516
Hepatic secretion stimulant	T47.8X1	T47.8X2	T47.8X3	T47.8X4	T47.8X5	T47.8X6
Hepatitis A vaccine*	T5Ø.B91	T5Ø.B92	T5Ø.B93	T5Ø.B94	T5Ø.B95	T5Ø.B96
Hepatitis B						
immune globulin	T5Ø.Z11	T5Ø.Z12	T5Ø.Z13	T5Ø.Z14	T5Ø.Z15	T5Ø.Z16
vaccine	T5Ø.B91	T5Ø.B92	T5Ø.B93	T5Ø.B94	T5Ø.B95	T5Ø.B96
Hepronicate	T46.7X1	T46.7X2	T46.7X3	T46.7X4	T46.7X5	T46.7X6
Heptabarb	T42.3X1	T42.3X2	T42.3X3	T42.3X4	T42.3X5	T42.3X6
Heptabarbital	T42.3X1	T42.3X2	T42.3X3	T42.3X4	T42.3X5	T42.3X6
Heptabarbitone	T42.3X1	T42.3X2	T42.3X3	T42.3X4	T42.3X5	T42.3X6
Heptachlor	T6Ø.1X1	T6Ø.1X2	T6Ø.1X3	T6Ø.1X4	—	—
Heptalgin	T4Ø.2X1	T4Ø.2X2	T4Ø.2X3	T4Ø.2X4	T4Ø.2X5	T4Ø.2X6
Heptaminol	T46.3X1	T46.3X2	T46.3X3	T46.3X4	T46.3X5	T46.3X6
Herbicide NEC	T6Ø.3X1	T6Ø.3X2	T6Ø.3X3	T6Ø.3X4	—	—
Heroin	T4Ø.1X1	T4Ø.1X2	T4Ø.1X3	T4Ø.1X4	—	—
Herplex	T49.5X1	T49.5X2	T49.5X3	T49.5X4	T49.5X5	T49.5X6
HES	T45.8X1	T45.8X2	T45.8X3	T45.8X4	T45.8X5	T45.8X6
Hesperidin	T46.991	T46.992	T46.993	T46.994	T46.995	T46.996
Hetacillin	T36.ØX1	T36.ØX2	T36.ØX3	T36.ØX4	T36.ØX5	T36.ØX6
Hetastarch	T45.8X1	T45.8X2	T45.8X3	T45.8X4	T45.8X5	T45.8X6
HETP	T6Ø.ØX1	T6Ø.ØX2	T6Ø.ØX3	T6Ø.ØX4	—	—
Hexachlorobenzene (vapor)	T6Ø.3X1	T6Ø.3X2	T6Ø.3X3	T6Ø.3X4	—	—
Hexachlorocyclohexane	T53.6X1	T53.6X2	T53.6X3	T53.6X4	—	—
Hexachlorophene	T49.ØX1	T49.ØX2	T49.ØX3	T49.ØX4	T49.ØX5	T49.ØX6
Hexadiline	T46.3X1	T46.3X2	T46.3X3	T46.3X4	T46.3X5	T46.3X6
Hexadimethrine (bromide)	T45.7X1	T45.7X2	T45.7X3	T45.7X4	T45.7X5	T45.7X6
Hexadylamine	T46.3X1	T46.3X2	T46.3X3	T46.3X4	T46.3X5	T46.3X6
Hexaethyl tetraphosphate	T6Ø.ØX1	T6Ø.ØX2	T6Ø.ØX3	T6Ø.ØX4	—	—
Hexafluorenium bromide	T48.1X1	T48.1X2	T48.1X3	T48.1X4	T48.1X5	T48.1X6
Hexafluronium (bromide)	T48.1X1	T48.1X2	T48.1X3	T48.1X4	T48.1X5	T48.1X6
Hexa-germ	T49.2X1	T49.2X2	T49.2X3	T49.2X4	T49.2X5	T49.2X6

Substance	Poisoning, Accidental (unintentional)	Poisoning, Intentional Self-harm	Poisoning, Assault	Poisoning, Undetermined	Adverse Effect	Under-dosing
Hexahydrobenzol	T52.8X1	T52.8X2	T52.8X3	T52.8X4	—	—
Hexahydrocresol(s)	T51.8X1	T51.8X2	T51.8X3	T51.8X4	—	—
arsenide	T57.ØX1	T57.ØX2	T57.ØX3	T57.ØX4	—	—
arseniurated	T57.ØX1	T57.ØX2	T57.ØX3	T57.ØX4	—	—
cyanide	T57.3X1	T57.3X2	T57.3X3	T57.3X4	—	—
gas	T59.891	T59.892	T59.893	T59.894	—	—
Fluoride (liquid)	T57.8X1	T57.8X2	T57.8X3	T57.8X4	—	—
vapor	T59.891	T59.892	T59.893	T59.894	—	—
phophorated	T6Ø.ØX1	T6Ø.ØX2	T6Ø.ØX3	T6Ø.ØX4	—	—
sulfate	T57.8X1	T57.8X2	T57.8X3	T57.8X4	—	—
sulfide (gas)	T59.6X1	T59.6X2	T59.6X3	T59.6X4	—	—
arseniurated	T57.ØX1	T57.ØX2	T57.ØX3	T57.ØX4	—	—
sulfurated	T57.8X1	T57.8X2	T57.8X3	T57.8X4	—	—
Hexahydrophenol	T51.8X1	T51.8X2	T51.8X3	T51.8X4	—	—
Hexalen	T51.8X1	T51.8X2	T51.8X3	T51.8X4	—	—
Hexamethonium bromide	T44.2X1	T44.2X2	T44.2X3	T44.2X4	T44.2X5	T44.2X6
Hexamethylene	T52.8X1	T52.8X2	T52.8X3	T52.8X4	—	—
Hexamethylmelamine	T45.1X1	T45.1X2	T45.1X3	T45.1X4	T45.1X5	T45.1X6
Hexamidine	T49.ØX1	T49.ØX2	T49.ØX3	T49.ØX4	T49.ØX5	T49.ØX6
Hexamine (mandelate)	T37.8X1	T37.8X2	T37.8X3	T37.8X4	T37.8X5	T37.8X6
Hexanone, 2-hexanone	T52.4X1	T52.4X2	T52.4X3	T52.4X4	—	—
Hexanuorenium	T48.1X1	T48.1X2	T48.1X3	T48.1X4	T48.1X5	T48.1X6
Hexapropymate	T42.6X1	T42.6X2	T42.6X3	T42.6X4	T42.6X5	T42.6X6
Hexasonium iodide	T44.3X1	T44.3X2	T44.3X3	T44.3X4	T44.3X5	T44.3X6
Hexcarbacholine bromide	T48.1X1	T48.1X2	T48.1X3	T48.1X4	T48.1X5	T48.1X6
Hexemal	T42.3X1	T42.3X2	T42.3X3	T42.3X4	T42.3X5	T42.3X6
Hexestrol	T38.5X1	T38.5X2	T38.5X3	T38.5X4	T38.5X5	T38.5X6
Hexethal (sodium)	T42.3X1	T42.3X2	T42.3X3	T42.3X4	T42.3X5	T42.3X6
Hexetidine	T37.8X1	T37.8X2	T37.8X3	T37.8X4	T37.8X5	T37.8X6
Hexobarbital	T42.3X1	T42.3X2	T42.3X3	T42.3X4	T42.3X5	T42.3X6
rectal	T41.291	T41.292	T41.293	T41.294	T41.295	T41.296
sodium	T41.1X1	T41.1X2	T41.1X3	T41.1X4	T41.1X5	T41.1X6
Hexobendine	T46.3X1	T46.3X2	T46.3X3	T46.3X4	T46.3X5	T46.3X6
Hexocyclium	T44.3X1	T44.3X2	T44.3X3	T44.3X4	T44.3X5	T44.3X6
metilsulfate	T44.3X1	T44.3X2	T44.3X3	T44.3X4	T44.3X5	T44.3X6
Hexoestrol	T38.5X1	T38.5X2	T38.5X3	T38.5X4	T38.5X5	T38.5X6
Hexone	T52.4X1	T52.4X2	T52.4X3	T52.4X4	—	—
Hexoprenaline	T48.6X1	T48.6X2	T48.6X3	T48.6X4	T48.6X5	T48.6X6
Hexylcaine	T41.3X1	T41.3X2	T41.3X3	T41.3X4	T41.3X5	T41.3X6
Hexylresorcinol	T52.2X1	T52.2X2	T52.2X3	T52.2X4	—	—
HGH (human growth hormone)	T38.811	T38.812	T38.813	T38.814	T38.815	T38.816
Hibistat*	T49.ØX1	T49.ØX2	T49.ØX3	T49.ØX4	T49.ØX5	T49.ØX6
Hinkle's pills	T47.2X1	T47.2X2	T47.2X3	T47.2X4	T47.2X5	T47.2X6
Histalog	T5Ø.8X1	T5Ø.8X2	T5Ø.8X3	T5Ø.8X4	T5Ø.8X5	T5Ø.8X6
Histamine (phosphate)	T5Ø.8X1	T5Ø.8X2	T5Ø.8X3	T5Ø.8X4	T5Ø.8X5	T5Ø.8X6
Histolyn*	T5Ø.8X1	T5Ø.8X2	T5Ø.8X3	T5Ø.8X4	T5Ø.8X5	T5Ø.8X6
Histoplasmin	T5Ø.8X1	T5Ø.8X2	T5Ø.8X3	T5Ø.8X4	T5Ø.8X5	T5Ø.8X6
Holly berries	T62.2X1	T62.2X2	T62.2X3	T62.2X4	—	—
Homatropine	T44.3X1	T44.3X2	T44.3X3	T44.3X4	T44.3X5	T44.3X6
methylbromide	T44.3X1	T44.3X2	T44.3X3	T44.3X4	T44.3X5	T44.3X6
Homochlorcyclizine	T45.ØX1	T45.ØX2	T45.ØX3	T45.ØX4	T45.ØX5	T45.ØX6
Homosalate	T49.3X1	T49.3X2	T49.3X3	T49.3X4	T49.3X5	T49.3X6
Homo-tet	T5Ø.Z11	T5Ø.Z12	T5Ø.Z13	T5Ø.Z14	T5Ø.Z15	T5Ø.Z16
Hormone	T38.8Ø1	T38.8Ø2	T38.8Ø3	T38.8Ø4	T38.8Ø5	T38.8Ø6
adrenal cortical steroids	T38.ØX1	T38.ØX2	T38.ØX3	T38.ØX4	T38.ØX5	T38.ØX6
androgenic	T38.7X1	T38.7X2	T38.7X3	T38.7X4	T38.7X5	T38.7X6
anterior pituitary NEC	T38.811	T38.812	T38.813	T38.814	T38.815	T38.816
antidiabetic agents	T38.3X1	T38.3X2	T38.3X3	T38.3X4	T38.3X5	T38.3X6
antidiuretic	T38.891	T38.892	T38.893	T38.894	T38.895	T38.896
cancer therapy	T45.1X1	T45.1X2	T45.1X3	T45.1X4	T45.1X5	T45.1X6
follicle stimulating	T38.811	T38.812	T38.813	T38.814	T38.815	T38.816
gonadotropic	T38.891	T38.892	T38.893	T38.894	T38.895	T38.896
pituitary	T38.811	T38.812	T38.813	T38.814	T38.815	T38.816
growth	T38.811	T38.812	T38.813	T38.814	T38.815	T38.816
luteinizing	T38.811	T38.812	T38.813	T38.814	T38.815	T38.816
ovarian	T38.5X1	T38.5X2	T38.5X3	T38.5X4	T38.5X5	T38.5X6
oxytocic	T48.ØX1	T48.ØX2	T48.ØX3	T48.ØX4	T48.ØX5	T48.ØX6
parathyroid (derivatives)	T5Ø.991	T5Ø.992	T5Ø.993	T5Ø.994	T5Ø.995	T5Ø.996
pituitary (posterior) NEC	T38.891	T38.892	T38.893	T38.894	T38.895	T38.896
anterior	T38.811	T38.812	T38.813	T38.814	T38.815	T38.816
specified, NEC	T38.891	T38.892	T38.893	T38.894	T38.895	T38.896
thyroid	T38.1X1	T38.1X2	T38.1X3	T38.1X4	T38.1X5	T38.1X6
Hornet (sting)	T63.451	T63.452	T63.453	T63.454	—	—
Horse anti-human lymphocytic serum	T5Ø.Z11	T5Ø.Z12	T5Ø.Z13	T5Ø.Z14	T5Ø.Z15	T5Ø.Z16
Horticulture agent NEC	T65.91	T65.92	T65.93	T65.94	—	—
with pesticide	T6Ø.91	T6Ø.92	T6Ø.93	T6Ø.94	—	—
Human						
albumin	T45.8X1	T45.8X2	T45.8X3	T45.8X4	T45.8X5	T45.8X6
growth hormone (HGH)	T38.811	T38.812	T38.813	T38.814	T38.815	T38.816
immune serum	T5Ø.Z11	T5Ø.Z12	T5Ø.Z13	T5Ø.Z14	T5Ø.Z15	T5Ø.Z16
Hyaluronidase	T45.3X1	T45.3X2	T45.3X3	T45.3X4	T45.3X5	T45.3X6

Substance	Poisoning, Accidental (unintentional)	Poisoning, Intentional Self-harm	Poisoning, Assault	Poisoning, Undetermined	Adverse Effect	Under-dosing
Hyazyme	T45.3X1	T45.3X2	T45.3X3	T45.3X4	T45.3X5	T45.3X6
Hycodan	T4Ø.2X1	T4Ø.2X2	T4Ø.2X3	T4Ø.2X4	T4Ø.2X5	T4Ø.2X6
Hydantoin derivative NEC	T42.ØX1	T42.ØX2	T42.ØX3	T42.ØX4	T42.ØX5	T42.ØX6
Hydeltra	T38.ØX1	T38.ØX2	T38.ØX3	T38.ØX4	T38.ØX5	T38.ØX6
Hydergine	T44.6X1	T44.6X2	T44.6X3	T44.6X4	T44.6X5	T44.6X6
Hydrabamine penicillin	T36.ØX1	T36.ØX2	T36.ØX3	T36.ØX4	T36.ØX5	T36.ØX6
Hydralazine	T46.5X1	T46.5X2	T46.5X3	T46.5X4	T46.5X5	T46.5X6
Hydrargaphen	T49.ØX1	T49.ØX2	T49.ØX3	T49.ØX4	T49.ØX5	T49.ØX6
Hydrargyri aminochloridum	T49.ØX1	T49.ØX2	T49.ØX3	T49.ØX4	T49.ØX5	T49.ØX6
Hydrastine	T48.291	T48.292	T48.293	T48.294	T48.295	T48.296
Hydrazine	T54.1X1	T54.1X2	T54.1X3	T54.1X4	—	—
monoamine oxidase inhibitors	T43.1X1	T43.1X2	T43.1X3	T43.1X4	T43.1X5	T43.1X6
Hydrazoic acid, azides	T54.2X1	T54.2X2	T54.2X3	T54.2X4	—	—
Hydriodic acid	T48.4X1	T48.4X2	T48.4X3	T48.4X4	T48.4X5	T48.4X6
Hydrisalic*	T49.4X1	T49.4X2	T49.4X3	T49.4X4	T49.4X5	T49.4X6
Hydrocarbon gas	T59.891	T59.892	T59.893	T59.894	—	—
incomplete combustion of — *see* Carbon, monoxide, fuel, utility						
liquefied (mobile container)	T59.891	T59.892	T59.893	T59.894	—	—
piped (natural)	T59.891	T59.892	T59.893	T59.894	—	—
Hydrochloric acid (liquid)	T54.2X1	T54.2X2	T54.2X3	T54.2X4	—	—
medicinal (digestant)	T47.5X1	T47.5X2	T47.5X3	T47.5X4	T47.5X5	T47.5X6
vapor	T59.891	T59.892	T59.893	T59.894	—	—
Hydrochlorothiazide	T5Ø.2X1	T5Ø.2X2	T5Ø.2X3	T5Ø.2X4	T5Ø.2X5	T5Ø.2X6
Hydrocodone	T4Ø.2X1	T4Ø.2X2	T4Ø.2X3	T4Ø.2X4	T4Ø.2X5	T4Ø.2X6
Hydrocortisone (derivatives)	T38.ØX1	T38.ØX2	T38.ØX3	T38.ØX4	T38.ØX5	T38.ØX6
aceponate	T49.ØX1	T49.ØX2	T49.ØX3	T49.ØX4	T49.ØX5	T49.ØX6
ENT agent	T49.6X1	T49.6X2	T49.6X3	T49.6X4	T49.6X5	T49.6X6
ophthalmic preparation	T49.5X1	T49.5X2	T49.5X3	T49.5X4	T49.5X5	T49.5X6
topical NEC	T49.ØX1	T49.ØX2	T49.ØX3	T49.ØX4	T49.ØX5	T49.ØX6
Hydrocortone	T38.ØX1	T38.ØX2	T38.ØX3	T38.ØX4	T38.ØX5	T38.ØX6
ENT agent	T49.6X1	T49.6X2	T49.6X3	T49.6X4	T49.6X5	T49.6X6
ophthalmic preparation	T49.5X1	T49.5X2	T49.5X3	T49.5X4	T49.5X5	T49.5X6
topical NEC	T49.ØX1	T49.ØX2	T49.ØX3	T49.ØX4	T49.ØX5	T49.ØX6
Hydrocyanic acid (liquid)	T57.3X1	T57.3X2	T57.3X3	T57.3X4	—	—
gas	T65.ØX1	T65.ØX2	T65.ØX3	T65.ØX4	—	—
Hydroflumethiazide	T5Ø.2X1	T5Ø.2X2	T5Ø.2X3	T5Ø.2X4	T5Ø.2X5	T5Ø.2X6
Hydrofluoric acid (liquid)	T54.2X1	T54.2X2	T54.2X3	T54.2X4	—	—
vapor	T59.891	T59.892	T59.893	T59.894	—	—
Hydrogen	T59.891	T59.892	T59.893	T59.894	—	—
arsenide	T57.ØX1	T57.ØX2	T57.ØX3	T57.ØX4	—	—
arseniureted	T57.ØX1	T57.ØX2	T57.ØX3	T57.ØX4	—	—
chloride	T57.8X1	T57.8X2	T57.8X3	T57.8X4	—	—
cyanide (salts)	T57.3X1	T57.3X2	T57.3X3	T57.3X4	—	—
gas	T57.3X1	T57.3X2	T57.3X3	T57.3X4	—	—
Fluoride	T59.5X1	T59.5X2	T59.5X3	T59.5X4	—	—
vapor	T59.5X1	T59.5X2	T59.5X3	T59.5X4	—	—
peroxide	T49.ØX1	T49.ØX2	T49.ØX3	T49.ØX4	T49.ØX5	T49.ØX6
phosphureted	T57.1X1	T57.1X2	T57.1X3	T57.1X4	—	—
sulfide	T59.6X1	T59.6X2	T59.6X3	T59.6X4	—	—
arseniureted	T57.ØX1	T57.ØX2	T57.ØX3	T57.ØX4	—	—
sulfureted	T59.6X1	T59.6X2	T59.6X3	T59.6X4	—	—
Hydromethylpyridine	T46.7X1	T46.7X2	T46.7X3	T46.7X4	T46.7X5	T46.7X6
Hydromorphinol	T4Ø.2X1	T4Ø.2X2	T4Ø.2X3	T4Ø.2X4	—	—
Hydromorphinone	T4Ø.2X1	T4Ø.2X2	T4Ø.2X3	T4Ø.2X4	T4Ø.2X5	T4Ø.2X6
Hydromorphone	T4Ø.2X1	T4Ø.2X2	T4Ø.2X3	T4Ø.2X4	T4Ø.2X5	T4Ø.2X6
Hydromox	T5Ø.2X1	T5Ø.2X2	T5Ø.2X3	T5Ø.2X4	T5Ø.2X5	T5Ø.2X6
Hydrophilic lotion	T49.3X1	T49.3X2	T49.3X3	T49.3X4	T49.3X5	T49.3X6
Hydroquinidine	T46.2X1	T46.2X2	T46.2X3	T46.2X4	T46.2X5	T46.2X6
Hydroquinone	T52.2X1	T52.2X2	T52.2X3	T52.2X4	—	—
vapor	T59.891	T59.892	T59.893	T59.894	—	—
Hydro-ride*	T5Ø.2X1	T5Ø.2X2	T5Ø.2X3	T5Ø.2X4	T5Ø.2X5	T5Ø.2X6
Hydrosulfuric acid (gas)	T59.6X1	T59.6X2	T59.6X3	T59.6X4	—	—
Hydrotalcite	T47.1X1	T47.1X2	T47.1X3	T47.1X4	T47.1X5	T47.1X6
Hydrous wool fat	T49.3X1	T49.3X2	T49.3X3	T49.3X4	T49.3X5	T49.3X6
Hydroxide, caustic	T54.3X1	T54.3X2	T54.3X3	T54.3X4	—	—
Hydroxocobalamin	T45.8X1	T45.8X2	T45.8X3	T45.8X4	T45.8X5	T45.8X6
Hydroxyamphetamine	T49.5X1	T49.5X2	T49.5X3	T49.5X4	T49.5X5	T49.5X6
Hydroxycarbamide	T45.1X1	T45.1X2	T45.1X3	T45.1X4	T45.1X5	T45.1X6
Hydroxychloroquine	T37.8X1	T37.8X2	T37.8X3	T37.8X4	T37.8X5	T37.8X6
Hydroxydaunorubicin*	T45.1X1	T45.1X2	T45.1X3	T45.1X4	T45.1X5	T45.1X6
Hydroxydihydrocodeinone	T4Ø.2X1	T4Ø.2X2	T4Ø.2X3	T4Ø.2X4	T4Ø.2X5	T4Ø.2X6
Hydroxyestrone	T38.5X1	T38.5X2	T38.5X3	T38.5X4	T38.5X5	T38.5X6
Hydroxyethyl starch	T45.8X1	T45.8X2	T45.8X3	T45.8X4	T45.8X5	T45.8X6
Hydroxymethylpentanone	T52.4X1	T52.4X2	T52.4X3	T52.4X4	—	—
Hydroxyphenamate	T43.591	T43.592	T43.593	T43.594	T43.595	T43.596
Hydroxyphenylbutazone	T39.2X1	T39.2X2	T39.2X3	T39.2X4	T39.2X5	T39.2X6
Hydroxyprogesterone	T38.5X1	T38.5X2	T38.5X3	T38.5X4	T38.5X5	T38.5X6

Substance	Poisoning, Accidental (unintentional)	Poisoning, Intentional Self-harm	Poisoning, Assault	Poisoning, Undetermined	Adverse Effect	Under-dosing
Hydroxyprogesterone — *continued*						
caproate	T38.5X1	T38.5X2	T38.5X3	T38.5X4	T38.5X5	T38.5X6
Hydroxyquinoline (derivatives) **NEC**	T37.8X1	T37.8X2	T37.8X3	T37.8X4	T37.8X5	T37.8X6
Hydroxystilbamidine	T37.3X1	T37.3X2	T37.3X3	T37.3X4	T37.3X5	T37.3X6
Hydroxytoluene (nonmedicinal)	T54.ØX1	T54.ØX2	T54.ØX3	T54.ØX4	—	—
medicinal	T49.ØX1	T49.ØX2	T49.ØX3	T49.ØX4	T49.ØX5	T49.ØX6
Hydroxyurea	T45.1X1	T45.1X2	T45.1X3	T45.1X4	T45.1X5	T45.1X6
Hydroxyzine	T43.591	T43.592	T43.593	T43.594	T43.595	T43.596
Hyoscine	T44.3X1	T44.3X2	T44.3X3	T44.3X4	T44.3X5	T44.3X6
Hyoscyamine	T44.3X1	T44.3X2	T44.3X3	T44.3X4	T44.3X5	T44.3X6
Hyoscyamus	T44.3X1	T44.3X2	T44.3X3	T44.3X4	T44.3X5	T44.3X6
dry extract	T44.3X1	T44.3X2	T44.3X3	T44.3X4	T44.3X5	T44.3X6
Hypaque	T5Ø.8X1	T5Ø.8X2	T5Ø.8X3	T5Ø.8X4	T5Ø.8X5	T5Ø.8X6
HyperRAB*	T5Ø.Z11	T5Ø.Z12	T5Ø.Z13	T5Ø.Z14	T5Ø.Z15	T5Ø.Z16
Hypertussis	T5Ø.Z11	T5Ø.Z12	T5Ø.Z13	T5Ø.Z14	T5Ø.Z15	T5Ø.Z16
Hypnotic	T42.71	T42.72	T42.73	T42.74	T42.75	T42.76
anticonvulsant	T42.71	T42.72	T42.73	T42.74	T42.75	T42.76
specified NEC	T42.6X1	T42.6X2	T42.6X3	T42.6X4	T42.6X5	T42.6X6
Hypochlorite	T49.ØX1	T49.ØX2	T49.ØX3	T49.ØX4	T49.ØX5	T49.ØX6
Hypophysis, posterior	T38.891	T38.892	T38.893	T38.894	T38.895	T38.896
Hypotensive NEC	T46.5X1	T46.5X2	T46.5X3	T46.5X4	T46.5X5	T46.5X6
Hypromellose	T49.5X1	T49.5X2	T49.5X3	T49.5X4	T49.5X5	T49.5X6
Ibacitabine	T37.5X1	T37.5X2	T37.5X3	T37.5X4	T37.5X5	T37.5X6
Ibopamine	T44.991	T44.992	T44.993	T44.994	T44.995	T44.996
Ibufenac	T39.311	T39.312	T39.313	T39.314	T39.315	T39.316
Ibuprofen	T39.311	T39.312	T39.313	T39.314	T39.315	T39.316
Ibuproxam	T39.311	T39.312	T39.313	T39.314	T39.315	T39.316
Ibuterol	T48.6X1	T48.6X2	T48.6X3	T48.6X4	T48.6X5	T48.6X6
Ichthammol	T49.ØX1	T49.ØX2	T49.ØX3	T49.ØX4	T49.ØX5	T49.ØX6
Ichthyol	T49.4X1	T49.4X2	T49.4X3	T49.4X4	T49.4X5	T49.4X6
Idarubicin	T45.1X1	T45.1X2	T45.1X3	T45.1X4	T45.1X5	T45.1X6
Idrocilamide	T42.8X1	T42.8X2	T42.8X3	T42.8X4	T42.8X5	T42.8X6
Ifenprodil	T46.7X1	T46.7X2	T46.7X3	T46.7X4	T46.7X5	T46.7X6
Ifosfamide	T45.1X1	T45.1X2	T45.1X3	T45.1X4	T45.1X5	T45.1X6
Iletin	T38.3X1	T38.3X2	T38.3X3	T38.3X4	T38.3X5	T38.3X6
Ilex	T62.2X1	T62.2X2	T62.2X3	T62.2X4	—	—
Illuminating gas (after combustion)	T58.11	T58.12	T58.13	T58.14	—	—
prior to combustion	T59.891	T59.892	T59.893	T59.894	—	—
Ilopan	T45.2X1	T45.2X2	T45.2X3	T45.2X4	T45.2X5	T45.2X6
Iloprost	T46.7X1	T46.7X2	T46.7X3	T46.7X4	T46.7X5	T46.7X6
Ilotycin	T36.3X1	T36.3X2	T36.3X3	T36.3X4	T36.3X5	T36.3X6
ophthalmic preparation	T49.5X1	T49.5X2	T49.5X3	T49.5X4	T49.5X5	T49.5X6
topical NEC	T49.ØX1	T49.ØX2	T49.ØX3	T49.ØX4	T49.ØX5	T49.ØX6
Imdur*	T46.3X1	T46.3X2	T46.3X3	T46.3X4	T46.3X5	T46.3X6
Imidazole-4-carboxamide	T45.1X1	T45.1X2	T45.1X3	T45.1X4	T45.1X5	T45.1X6
Iminostilbene	T42.1X1	T42.1X2	T42.1X3	T42.1X4	T42.1X5	T42.1X6
Imipenem	T36.ØX1	T36.ØX2	T36.ØX3	T36.ØX4	T36.ØX5	T36.ØX6
Imipramine	T43.Ø11	T43.Ø12	T43.Ø13	T43.Ø14	T43.Ø15	T43.Ø16
Immu-G	T5Ø.Z11	T5Ø.Z12	T5Ø.Z13	T5Ø.Z14	T5Ø.Z15	T5Ø.Z16
Immuglobin	T5Ø.Z11	T5Ø.Z12	T5Ø.Z13	T5Ø.Z14	T5Ø.Z15	T5Ø.Z16
Immune						
globulin	T5Ø.Z11	T5Ø.Z12	T5Ø.Z13	T5Ø.Z14	T5Ø.Z15	T5Ø.Z16
serum globulin	T5Ø.Z11	T5Ø.Z12	T5Ø.Z13	T5Ø.Z14	T5Ø.Z15	T5Ø.Z16
Immunoglobin human (intravenous) (normal)	T5Ø.Z11	T5Ø.Z12	T5Ø.Z13	T5Ø.Z14	T5Ø.Z15	T5Ø.Z16
unmodified	T5Ø.Z11	T5Ø.Z12	T5Ø.Z13	T5Ø.Z14	T5Ø.Z15	T5Ø.Z16
Immunosuppressive drug	T45.1X1	T45.1X2	T45.1X3	T45.1X4	T45.1X5	T45.1X6
Immu-tetanus	T5Ø.Z11	T5Ø.Z12	T5Ø.Z13	T5Ø.Z14	T5Ø.Z15	T5Ø.Z16
Indalpine	T43.221	T43.222	T43.223	T43.224	T43.225	T43.226
Indanazoline	T48.5X1	T48.5X2	T48.5X3	T48.5X4	T48.5X5	T48.5X6
Indandione (derivatives)	T45.511	T45.512	T45.513	T45.514	T45.515	T45.516
Indapamide	T46.5X1	T46.5X2	T46.5X3	T46.5X4	T46.5X5	T46.5X6
Indendione (derivatives)	T45.511	T45.512	T45.513	T45.514	T45.515	T45.516
Indenolol	T44.7X1	T44.7X2	T44.7X3	T44.7X4	T44.7X5	T44.7X6
Inderal	T44.7X1	T44.7X2	T44.7X3	T44.7X4	T44.7X5	T44.7X6
Indian						
hemp	T4Ø.711	T4Ø.712	T4Ø.713	T4Ø.714	T4Ø.715	T4Ø.716
tobacco	T62.2X1	T62.2X2	T62.2X3	T62.2X4	—	—
Indigo carmine	T5Ø.8X1	T5Ø.8X2	T5Ø.8X3	T5Ø.8X4	T5Ø.8X5	T5Ø.8X6
Indobufen	T45.521	T45.522	T45.523	T45.524	T45.525	T45.526
Indocin	T39.2X1	T39.2X2	T39.2X3	T39.2X4	T39.2X5	T39.2X6
Indocyanine green	T5Ø.8X1	T5Ø.8X2	T5Ø.8X3	T5Ø.8X4	T5Ø.8X5	T5Ø.8X6
Indometacin	T39.391	T39.392	T39.393	T39.394	T39.395	T39.396
Indomethacin	T39.391	T39.392	T39.393	T39.394	T39.395	T39.396
farnesil	T39.4X1	T39.4X2	T39.4X3	T39.4X4	T39.4X5	T39.4X6
Indoramin	T44.6X1	T44.6X2	T44.6X3	T44.6X4	T44.6X5	T44.6X6
Industrial						
alcohol	T51.ØX1	T51.ØX2	T51.ØX3	T51.ØX4	—	—
fumes	T59.891	T59.892	T59.893	T59.894	—	—

Substance	Poisoning, Accidental (unintentional)	Poisoning, Intentional Self-harm	Poisoning, Assault	Poisoning, Undetermined	Adverse Effect	Under-dosing
Industrial — *continued*						
solvents (fumes) (vapors)	T52.91	T52.92	T52.93	T52.94	—	—
Inflectra*	T39.4X1	T39.4X2	T39.4X3	T39.4X4	T39.4X5	T39.4X6
Influenza vaccine	T5Ø.B91	T5Ø.B92	T5Ø.B93	T5Ø.B94	T5Ø.B95	T5Ø.B96
Ingested substance NEC	T65.91	T65.92	T65.93	T65.94	—	—
INH	T37.1X1	T37.1X2	T37.1X3	T37.1X4	T37.1X5	T37.1X6
Inhalation, gas (noxious) — *see* Gas						
Inhibitor						
angiotensin-converting enzyme	T46.4X1	T46.4X2	T46.4X3	T46.4X4	T46.4X5	T46.4X6
carbonic anhydrase	T5Ø.2X1	T5Ø.2X2	T5Ø.2X3	T5Ø.2X4	T5Ø.2X5	T5Ø.2X6
fibrinolysis	T45.621	T45.622	T45.623	T45.624	T45.625	T45.626
monoamine oxidase NEC	T43.1X1	T43.1X2	T43.1X3	T43.1X4	T43.1X5	T43.1X6
hydrazine	T43.1X1	T43.1X2	T43.1X3	T43.1X4	T43.1X5	T43.1X6
postsynaptic	T43.8X1	T43.8X2	T43.8X3	T43.8X4	T43.8X5	T43.8X6
prothrombin synthesis	T45.511	T45.512	T45.513	T45.514	T45.515	T45.516
Ink	T65.891	T65.892	T65.893	T65.894	—	—
Innopran*	T44.7X1	T44.7X2	T44.7X3	T44.7X4	T44.7X5	T44.7X6
Inorganic substance NEC	T57.91	T57.92	T57.93	T57.94	—	—
Inosine pranobex	T37.5X1	T37.5X2	T37.5X3	T37.5X4	T37.5X5	T37.5X6
Inositol	T5Ø.991	T5Ø.992	T5Ø.993	T5Ø.994	T5Ø.995	T5Ø.996
nicotinate	T46.7X1	T46.7X2	T46.7X3	T46.7X4	T46.7X5	T46.7X6
Inproquone	T45.1X1	T45.1X2	T45.1X3	T45.1X4	T45.1X5	T45.1X6
Insecticide NEC	T6Ø.91	T6Ø.92	T6Ø.93	T6Ø.94	—	—
carbamate	T6Ø.ØX1	T6Ø.ØX2	T6Ø.ØX3	T6Ø.ØX4	—	—
chlorinated	T6Ø.1X1	T6Ø.1X2	T6Ø.1X3	T6Ø.1X4	—	—
mixed	T6Ø.91	T6Ø.92	T6Ø.93	T6Ø.94	—	—
organochlorine	T6Ø.1X1	T6Ø.1X2	T6Ø.1X3	T6Ø.1X4	—	—
organophosphorus	T6Ø.ØX1	T6Ø.ØX2	T6Ø.ØX3	T6Ø.ØX4	—	—
Insect (sting), venomous	T63.481	T63.482	T63.483	T63.484	—	—
ant	T63.421	T63.422	T63.423	T63.424	—	—
bee	T63.441	T63.442	T63.443	T63.444	—	—
caterpillar	T63.431	T63.432	T63.433	T63.434	—	—
hornet	T63.451	T63.452	T63.453	T63.454	—	—
wasp	T63.461	T63.462	T63.463	T63.464	—	—
Insular tissue extract	T38.3X1	T38.3X2	T38.3X3	T38.3X4	T38.3X5	T38.3X6
Insulin (amorphous) (globin) (isophane) (Lente) (NPH) (Semilente) (Ultralente)	T38.3X1	T38.3X2	T38.3X3	T38.3X4	T38.3X5	T38.3X6
defalan	T38.3X1	T38.3X2	T38.3X3	T38.3X4	T38.3X5	T38.3X6
human	T38.3X1	T38.3X2	T38.3X3	T38.3X4	T38.3X5	T38.3X6
injection, soluble	T38.3X1	T38.3X2	T38.3X3	T38.3X4	T38.3X5	T38.3X6
biphasic	T38.3X1	T38.3X2	T38.3X3	T38.3X4	T38.3X5	T38.3X6
intermediate acting	T38.3X1	T38.3X2	T38.3X3	T38.3X4	T38.3X5	T38.3X6
protamine zinc	T38.3X1	T38.3X2	T38.3X3	T38.3X4	T38.3X5	T38.3X6
slow acting	T38.3X1	T38.3X2	T38.3X3	T38.3X4	T38.3X5	T38.3X6
zinc						
protamine injection	T38.3X1	T38.3X2	T38.3X3	T38.3X4	T38.3X5	T38.3X6
suspension (amorphous) (crystalline)	T38.3X1	T38.3X2	T38.3X3	T38.3X4	T38.3X5	T38.3X6
Interferon (alpha) (beta) (gamma)	T37.5X1	T37.5X2	T37.5X3	T37.5X4	T37.5X5	T37.5X6
Intestinal motility control drug	T47.6X1	T47.6X2	T47.6X3	T47.6X4	T47.6X5	T47.6X6
biological	T47.8X1	T47.8X2	T47.8X3	T47.8X4	T47.8X5	T47.8X6
Intranarcon	T41.1X1	T41.1X2	T41.1X3	T41.1X4	T41.1X5	T41.1X6
Intravenous						
amino acids	T5Ø.991	T5Ø.992	T5Ø.993	T5Ø.994	T5Ø.995	T5Ø.996
fat suspension	T5Ø.991	T5Ø.992	T5Ø.993	T5Ø.994	T5Ø.995	T5Ø.996
Inulin	T5Ø.8X1	T5Ø.8X2	T5Ø.8X3	T5Ø.8X4	T5Ø.8X5	T5Ø.8X6
Invanz*	T36.1X1	T36.1X2	T36.1X3	T36.1X4	T36.1X5	T36.1X6
Invert sugar	T5Ø.3X1	T5Ø.3X2	T5Ø.3X3	T5Ø.3X4	T5Ø.3X5	T5Ø.3X6
Inza — *see* Naproxen						
Iobenzamic acid	T5Ø.8X1	T5Ø.8X2	T5Ø.8X3	T5Ø.8X4	T5Ø.8X5	T5Ø.8X6
Iocarmic acid	T5Ø.8X1	T5Ø.8X2	T5Ø.8X3	T5Ø.8X4	T5Ø.8X5	T5Ø.8X6
Iocetamic acid	T5Ø.8X1	T5Ø.8X2	T5Ø.8X3	T5Ø.8X4	T5Ø.8X5	T5Ø.8X6
Iodamide	T5Ø.8X1	T5Ø.8X2	T5Ø.8X3	T5Ø.8X4	T5Ø.8X5	T5Ø.8X6
Iodide NEC — *see also* Iodine	T49.ØX1	T49.ØX2	T49.ØX3	T49.ØX4	T49.ØX5	T49.ØX6
mercury (ointment)	T49.ØX1	T49.ØX2	T49.ØX3	T49.ØX4	T49.ØX5	T49.ØX6
methylate	T49.ØX1	T49.ØX2	T49.ØX3	T49.ØX4	T49.ØX5	T49.ØX6
potassium (expectorant) NEC	T48.4X1	T48.4X2	T48.4X3	T48.4X4	T48.4X5	T48.4X6
Iodinated						
contrast medium	T5Ø.8X1	T5Ø.8X2	T5Ø.8X3	T5Ø.8X4	T5Ø.8X5	T5Ø.8X6
glycerol	T48.4X1	T48.4X2	T48.4X3	T48.4X4	T48.4X5	T48.4X6
human serum albumin (131I)	T5Ø.8X1	T5Ø.8X2	T5Ø.8X3	T5Ø.8X4	T5Ø.8X5	T5Ø.8X6
Iodine (antiseptic, external) (tincture) **NEC**	T49.ØX1	T49.ØX2	T49.ØX3	T49.ØX4	T49.ØX5	T49.ØX6

Substance	Poisoning, Accidental (unintentional)	Poisoning, Intentional Self-harm	Poisoning, Assault	Poisoning, Undetermined	Adverse Effect	Under-dosing
Iodine (antiseptic, external) (tincture) **NEC** — *continued*						
125 — *see also* Radiation sickness, and exposure to radioactive isotopes	T5Ø.8X1	T5Ø.8X2	T5Ø.8X3	T5Ø.8X4	T5Ø.8X5	T5Ø.8X6
therapeutic	T5Ø.991	T5Ø.992	T5Ø.993	T5Ø.994	T5Ø.995	T5Ø.996
131 — *see also* Radiation sickness, and exposure to radioactive isotopes	T5Ø.8X1	T5Ø.8X2	T5Ø.8X3	T5Ø.8X4	T5Ø.8X5	T5Ø.8X6
therapeutic	T38.2X1	T38.2X2	T38.2X3	T38.2X4	T38.2X5	T38.2X6
diagnostic	T5Ø.8X1	T5Ø.8X2	T5Ø.8X3	T5Ø.8X4	T5Ø.8X5	T5Ø.8X6
for thyroid conditions (antithyroid)	T38.2X1	T38.2X2	T38.2X3	T38.2X4	T38.2X5	T38.2X6
solution	T49.ØX1	T49.ØX2	T49.ØX3	T49.ØX4	T49.ØX5	T49.ØX6
vapor	T59.891	T59.892	T59.893	T59.894	—	—
Iodipamide	T5Ø.8X1	T5Ø.8X2	T5Ø.8X3	T5Ø.8X4	T5Ø.8X5	T5Ø.8X6
Iodized (poppy seed) oil	T5Ø.8X1	T5Ø.8X2	T5Ø.8X3	T5Ø.8X4	T5Ø.8X5	T5Ø.8X6
Iodobismitol	T37.8X1	T37.8X2	T37.8X3	T37.8X4	T37.8X5	T37.8X6
Iodochlorhydroxyquin	T37.8X1	T37.8X2	T37.8X3	T37.8X4	T37.8X5	T37.8X6
topical	T49.ØX1	T49.ØX2	T49.ØX3	T49.ØX4	T49.ØX5	T49.ØX6
Iodochlorhydroxyquinoline	T37.8X1	T37.8X2	T37.8X3	T37.8X4	T37.8X5	T37.8X6
Iodocholesterol (131I)	T5Ø.8X1	T5Ø.8X2	T5Ø.8X3	T5Ø.8X4	T5Ø.8X5	T5Ø.8X6
Iodoform	T49.ØX1	T49.ØX2	T49.ØX3	T49.ØX4	T49.ØX5	T49.ØX6
Iodohippuric acid	T5Ø.8X1	T5Ø.8X2	T5Ø.8X3	T5Ø.8X4	T5Ø.8X5	T5Ø.8X6
Iodopanoic acid	T5Ø.8X1	T5Ø.8X2	T5Ø.8X3	T5Ø.8X4	T5Ø.8X5	T5Ø.8X6
Iodophthalein (sodium)	T5Ø.8X1	T5Ø.8X2	T5Ø.8X3	T5Ø.8X4	T5Ø.8X5	T5Ø.8X6
Iodopyracet	T5Ø.8X1	T5Ø.8X2	T5Ø.8X3	T5Ø.8X4	T5Ø.8X5	T5Ø.8X6
Iodoquinol	T37.8X1	T37.8X2	T37.8X3	T37.8X4	T37.8X5	T37.8X6
Iodoxamic acid	T5Ø.8X1	T5Ø.8X2	T5Ø.8X3	T5Ø.8X4	T5Ø.8X5	T5Ø.8X6
Iofendylate	T5Ø.8X1	T5Ø.8X2	T5Ø.8X3	T5Ø.8X4	T5Ø.8X5	T5Ø.8X6
Ioglycamic acid	T5Ø.8X1	T5Ø.8X2	T5Ø.8X3	T5Ø.8X4	T5Ø.8X5	T5Ø.8X6
Iohexol	T5Ø.8X1	T5Ø.8X2	T5Ø.8X3	T5Ø.8X4	T5Ø.8X5	T5Ø.8X6
Ion exchange resin						
anion	T47.8X1	T47.8X2	T47.8X3	T47.8X4	T47.8X5	T47.8X6
cation	T5Ø.3X1	T5Ø.3X2	T5Ø.3X3	T5Ø.3X4	T5Ø.3X5	T5Ø.3X6
cholestyramine	T46.6X1	T46.6X2	T46.6X3	T46.6X4	T46.6X5	T46.6X6
intestinal	T47.8X1	T47.8X2	T47.8X3	T47.8X4	T47.8X5	T47.8X6
Iopamidol	T5Ø.8X1	T5Ø.8X2	T5Ø.8X3	T5Ø.8X4	T5Ø.8X5	T5Ø.8X6
Iopanoic acid	T5Ø.8X1	T5Ø.8X2	T5Ø.8X3	T5Ø.8X4	T5Ø.8X5	T5Ø.8X6
Iophenoic acid	T5Ø.8X1	T5Ø.8X2	T5Ø.8X3	T5Ø.8X4	T5Ø.8X5	T5Ø.8X6
Iopodate, sodium	T5Ø.8X1	T5Ø.8X2	T5Ø.8X3	T5Ø.8X4	T5Ø.8X5	T5Ø.8X6
Iopodic acid	T5Ø.8X1	T5Ø.8X2	T5Ø.8X3	T5Ø.8X4	T5Ø.8X5	T5Ø.8X6
Iopromide	T5Ø.8X1	T5Ø.8X2	T5Ø.8X3	T5Ø.8X4	T5Ø.8X5	T5Ø.8X6
Iopydol	T5Ø.8X1	T5Ø.8X2	T5Ø.8X3	T5Ø.8X4	T5Ø.8X5	T5Ø.8X6
Iotalamic acid	T5Ø.8X1	T5Ø.8X2	T5Ø.8X3	T5Ø.8X4	T5Ø.8X5	T5Ø.8X6
Iothalamate	T5Ø.8X1	T5Ø.8X2	T5Ø.8X3	T5Ø.8X4	T5Ø.8X5	T5Ø.8X6
Iothiouracil	T38.2X1	T38.2X2	T38.2X3	T38.2X4	T38.2X5	T38.2X6
Iotrol	T5Ø.8X1	T5Ø.8X2	T5Ø.8X3	T5Ø.8X4	T5Ø.8X5	T5Ø.8X6
Iotrolan	T5Ø.8X1	T5Ø.8X2	T5Ø.8X3	T5Ø.8X4	T5Ø.8X5	T5Ø.8X6
Iotroxate	T5Ø.8X1	T5Ø.8X2	T5Ø.8X3	T5Ø.8X4	T5Ø.8X5	T5Ø.8X6
Iotroxic acid	T5Ø.8X1	T5Ø.8X2	T5Ø.8X3	T5Ø.8X4	T5Ø.8X5	T5Ø.8X6
Ioversol	T5Ø.8X1	T5Ø.8X2	T5Ø.8X3	T5Ø.8X4	T5Ø.8X5	T5Ø.8X6
Ioxaglate	T5Ø.8X1	T5Ø.8X2	T5Ø.8X3	T5Ø.8X4	T5Ø.8X5	T5Ø.8X6
Ioxaglic acid	T5Ø.8X1	T5Ø.8X2	T5Ø.8X3	T5Ø.8X4	T5Ø.8X5	T5Ø.8X6
Ioxitalamic acid	T5Ø.8X1	T5Ø.8X2	T5Ø.8X3	T5Ø.8X4	T5Ø.8X5	T5Ø.8X6
Ipecac	T47.7X1	T47.7X2	T47.7X3	T47.7X4	T47.7X5	T47.7X6
Ipecacuanha	T48.4X1	T48.4X2	T48.4X3	T48.4X4	T48.4X5	T48.4X6
Ipodate, calcium	T5Ø.8X1	T5Ø.8X2	T5Ø.8X3	T5Ø.8X4	T5Ø.8X5	T5Ø.8X6
IPOL*	T5Ø.B91	T5Ø.B92	T5Ø.B93	T5Ø.B94	T5Ø.B95	T5Ø.B96
Ipral	T42.3X1	T42.3X2	T42.3X3	T42.3X4	T42.3X5	T42.3X6
Ipratropium (bromide)	T48.6X1	T48.6X2	T48.6X3	T48.6X4	T48.6X5	T48.6X6
Ipriflavone	T46.3X1	T46.3X2	T46.3X3	T46.3X4	T46.3X5	T46.3X6
Iprindole	T43.Ø11	T43.Ø12	T43.Ø13	T43.Ø14	T43.Ø15	T43.Ø16
Iproclozide	T43.1X1	T43.1X2	T43.1X3	T43.1X4	T43.1X5	T43.1X6
Iprofenin	T5Ø.8X1	T5Ø.8X2	T5Ø.8X3	T5Ø.8X4	T5Ø.8X5	T5Ø.8X6
Iproheptine	T49.2X1	T49.2X2	T49.2X3	T49.2X4	T49.2X5	T49.2X6
Iproniazid	T43.1X1	T43.1X2	T43.1X3	T43.1X4	T43.1X5	T43.1X6
Iproplatin	T45.1X1	T45.1X2	T45.1X3	T45.1X4	T45.1X5	T45.1X6
Iproveratril	T46.1X1	T46.1X2	T46.1X3	T46.1X4	T46.1X5	T46.1X6
Irinotecan*	T45.1X1	T45.1X2	T45.1X3	T45.1X4	T45.1X5	T45.1X6
Iron (compounds) (medicinal) **NEC**	T45.4X1	T45.4X2	T45.4X3	T45.4X4	T45.4X5	T45.4X6
ammonium	T45.4X1	T45.4X2	T45.4X3	T45.4X4	T45.4X5	T45.4X6
dextran injection	T45.4X1	T45.4X2	T45.4X3	T45.4X4	T45.4X5	T45.4X6
nonmedicinal	T56.891	T56.892	T56.893	T56.894	—	—
salts	T45.4X1	T45.4X2	T45.4X3	T45.4X4	T45.4X5	T45.4X6
sorbitex	T45.4X1	T45.4X2	T45.4X3	T45.4X4	T45.4X5	T45.4X6
sorbitol citric acid complex	T45.4X1	T45.4X2	T45.4X3	T45.4X4	T45.4X5	T45.4X6
Irrigating fluid (vaginal)	T49.8X1	T49.8X2	T49.8X3	T49.8X4	T49.8X5	T49.8X6
eye	T49.5X1	T49.5X2	T49.5X3	T49.5X4	T49.5X5	T49.5X6
Isepamicin	T36.5X1	T36.5X2	T36.5X3	T36.5X4	T36.5X5	T36.5X6
Isoaminile (citrate)	T48.3X1	T48.3X2	T48.3X3	T48.3X4	T48.3X5	T48.3X6
Isoamyl nitrite	T46.3X1	T46.3X2	T46.3X3	T46.3X4	T46.3X5	T46.3X6

Substance	Poisoning, Accidental (unintentional)	Poisoning, Intentional Self-harm	Poisoning, Assault	Poisoning, Undetermined	Adverse Effect	Under-dosing
Isobenzan	T6Ø.1X1	T6Ø.1X2	T6Ø.1X3	T6Ø.1X4	—	—
Isobutyl acetate	T52.8X1	T52.8X2	T52.8X3	T52.8X4	—	—
Isocarboxazid	T43.1X1	T43.1X2	T43.1X3	T43.1X4	T43.1X5	T43.1X6
Isoconazole	T49.ØX1	T49.ØX2	T49.ØX3	T49.ØX4	T49.ØX5	T49.ØX6
Isocyanate	T65.ØX1	T65.ØX2	T65.ØX3	T65.ØX4	—	—
Isoephedrine	T44.991	T44.992	T44.993	T44.994	T44.995	T44.996
Isoetarine	T48.6X1	T48.6X2	T48.6X3	T48.6X4	T48.6X5	T48.6X6
Isoethadione	T42.2X1	T42.2X2	T42.2X3	T42.2X4	T42.2X5	T42.2X6
Isoetharine	T44.5X1	T44.5X2	T44.5X3	T44.5X4	T44.5X5	T44.5X6
Isoflurane	T41.ØX1	T41.ØX2	T41.ØX3	T41.ØX4	T41.ØX5	T41.ØX6
Isoflurophate	T44.ØX1	T44.ØX2	T44.ØX3	T44.ØX4	T44.ØX5	T44.ØX6
Isomaltose, ferric complex	T45.4X1	T45.4X2	T45.4X3	T45.4X4	T45.4X5	T45.4X6
Isometheptene	T44.3X1	T44.3X2	T44.3X3	T44.3X4	T44.3X5	T44.3X6
Isoniazid	T37.1X1	T37.1X2	T37.1X3	T37.1X4	T37.1X5	T37.1X6
with						
rifampicin	T36.6X1	T36.6X2	T36.6X3	T36.6X4	T36.6X5	T36.6X6
thioacetazone	T37.1X1	T37.1X2	T37.1X3	T37.1X4	T37.1X5	T37.1X6
Isonicotinic acid hydrazide	T37.1X1	T37.1X2	T37.1X3	T37.1X4	T37.1X5	T37.1X6
Isonipecaine	T4Ø.491	T4Ø.492	T4Ø.493	T4Ø.494	T4Ø.495	T4Ø.496
Isopentaquine	T37.2X1	T37.2X2	T37.2X3	T37.2X4	T37.2X5	T37.2X6
Isophane insulin	T38.3X1	T38.3X2	T38.3X3	T38.3X4	T38.3X5	T38.3X6
Isophorone	T65.891	T65.892	T65.893	T65.894	—	—
Isophosphamide	T45.1X1	T45.1X2	T45.1X3	T45.1X4	T45.1X5	T45.1X6
Isopregnenone	T38.5X1	T38.5X2	T38.5X3	T38.5X4	T38.5X5	T38.5X6
Isoprenaline	T48.6X1	T48.6X2	T48.6X3	T48.6X4	T48.6X5	T48.6X6
Isopromethazine	T43.3X1	T43.3X2	T43.3X3	T43.3X4	T43.3X5	T43.3X6
Isopropamide	T44.3X1	T44.3X2	T44.3X3	T44.3X4	T44.3X5	T44.3X6
iodide	T44.3X1	T44.3X2	T44.3X3	T44.3X4	T44.3X5	T44.3X6
Isopropanol	T51.2X1	T51.2X2	T51.2X3	T51.2X4	—	—
Isopropyl						
acetate	T52.8X1	T52.8X2	T52.8X3	T52.8X4	—	—
alcohol	T51.2X1	T51.2X2	T51.2X3	T51.2X4	—	—
medicinal	T49.4X1	T49.4X2	T49.4X3	T49.4X4	T49.4X5	T49.4X6
ether	T52.8X1	T52.8X2	T52.8X3	T52.8X4	—	—
Isopropylaminophenazone	T39.2X1	T39.2X2	T39.2X3	T39.2X4	T39.2X5	T39.2X6
Isoproterenol	T48.6X1	T48.6X2	T48.6X3	T48.6X4	T48.6X5	T48.6X6
Isosorbide dinitrate	T46.3X1	T46.3X2	T46.3X3	T46.3X4	T46.3X5	T46.3X6
Isothipendyl	T45.ØX1	T45.ØX2	T45.ØX3	T45.ØX4	T45.ØX5	T45.ØX6
Isotretinoin	T5Ø.991	T5Ø.992	T5Ø.993	T5Ø.994	T5Ø.995	T5Ø.996
Isoxazolyl penicillin	T36.ØX1	T36.ØX2	T36.ØX3	T36.ØX4	T36.ØX5	T36.ØX6
Isoxicam	T39.391	T39.392	T39.393	T39.394	T39.395	T39.396
Isoxsuprine	T46.7X1	T46.7X2	T46.7X3	T46.7X4	T46.7X5	T46.7X6
Ispagula	T47.4X1	T47.4X2	T47.4X3	T47.4X4	T47.4X5	T47.4X6
husk	T47.4X1	T47.4X2	T47.4X3	T47.4X4	T47.4X5	T47.4X6
Isradipine	T46.1X1	T46.1X2	T46.1X3	T46.1X4	T46.1X5	T46.1X6
I-thyroxine sodium	T38.1X1	T38.1X2	T38.1X3	T38.1X4	T38.1X5	T38.1X6
Itraconazole	T37.8X1	T37.8X2	T37.8X3	T37.8X4	T37.8X5	T37.8X6
Itramin tosilate	T46.3X1	T46.3X2	T46.3X3	T46.3X4	T46.3X5	T46.3X6
Ivarest*	T41.3X1	T41.3X2	T41.3X3	T41.3X4	T41.3X5	T41.3X6
Ivermectin	T37.4X1	T37.4X2	T37.4X3	T37.4X4	T37.4X5	T37.4X6
Izoniazid	T37.1X1	T37.1X2	T37.1X3	T37.1X4	T37.1X5	T37.1X6
with thioacetazone	T37.1X1	T37.1X2	T37.1X3	T37.1X4	T37.1X5	T37.1X6
Jalap	T47.2X1	T47.2X2	T47.2X3	T47.2X4	T47.2X5	T47.2X6
Jamaica						
dogwood (bark)	T39.8X1	T39.8X2	T39.8X3	T39.8X4	T39.8X5	T39.8X6
ginger	T65.891	T65.892	T65.893	T65.894	—	—
root	T62.2X1	T62.2X2	T62.2X3	T62.2X4	—	—
Jantoven*	T45.511	T45.512	T45.513	T45.514	T45.515	T45.516
Jatropha	T62.2X1	T62.2X2	T62.2X3	T62.2X4	—	—
curcas	T62.2X1	T62.2X2	T62.2X3	T62.2X4	—	—
Jectofer	T45.4X1	T45.4X2	T45.4X3	T45.4X4	T45.4X5	T45.4X6
Jellyfish (sting)	T63.621	T63.622	T63.623	T63.624	—	—
Jequirity (bean)	T62.2X1	T62.2X2	T62.2X3	T62.2X4	—	—
Jimson weed (stramonium)	T62.2X1	T62.2X2	T62.2X3	T62.2X4	—	—
seeds	T62.2X1	T62.2X2	T62.2X3	T62.2X4	—	—
Josamycin	T36.3X1	T36.3X2	T36.3X3	T36.3X4	T36.3X5	T36.3X6
Juniper tar	T49.1X1	T49.1X2	T49.1X3	T49.1X4	T49.1X5	T49.1X6
Kaletra*	T37.5X1	T37.5X2	T37.5X3	T37.5X4	T37.5X5	T37.5X6
Kallidinogenase	T46.7X1	T46.7X2	T46.7X3	T46.7X4	T46.7X5	T46.7X6
Kallikrein	T46.7X1	T46.7X2	T46.7X3	T46.7X4	T46.7X5	T46.7X6
Kanamycin	T36.5X1	T36.5X2	T36.5X3	T36.5X4	T36.5X5	T36.5X6
Kantrex	T36.5X1	T36.5X2	T36.5X3	T36.5X4	T36.5X5	T36.5X6
Kaolin	T47.6X1	T47.6X2	T47.6X3	T47.6X4	T47.6X5	T47.6X6
light	T47.6X1	T47.6X2	T47.6X3	T47.6X4	T47.6X5	T47.6X6
Karaya (gum)	T47.4X1	T47.4X2	T47.4X3	T47.4X4	T47.4X5	T47.4X6
Kebuzone	T39.2X1	T39.2X2	T39.2X3	T39.2X4	T39.2X5	T39.2X6
Keflex*	T36.1X1	T36.1X2	T36.1X3	T36.1X4	T36.1X5	T36.1X6
Kelevan	T6Ø.1X1	T6Ø.1X2	T6Ø.1X3	T6Ø.1X4	—	—
Kemithal	T41.1X1	T41.1X2	T41.1X3	T41.1X4	T41.1X5	T41.1X6
Kenacort	T38.ØX1	T38.ØX2	T38.ØX3	T38.ØX4	T38.ØX5	T38.ØX6
Keratolytic drug NEC	T49.4X1	T49.4X2	T49.4X3	T49.4X4	T49.4X5	T49.4X6
anthracene	T49.4X1	T49.4X2	T49.4X3	T49.4X4	T49.4X5	T49.4X6
Keratoplastic NEC	T49.4X1	T49.4X2	T49.4X3	T49.4X4	T49.4X5	T49.4X6

Substance	Poisoning, Accidental (unintentional)	Poisoning, Intentional Self-harm	Poisoning, Assault	Poisoning, Undetermined	Adverse Effect	Under-dosing
Kerosene, kerosine (fuel) (solvent) **NEC**	T52.0X1	T52.0X2	T52.0X3	T52.0X4	—	—
- insecticide	T52.0X1	T52.0X2	T52.0X3	T52.0X4	—	—
- vapor	T52.0X1	T52.0X2	T52.0X3	T52.0X4	—	—
Ketamine	T41.291	T41.292	T41.293	T41.294	T41.295	T41.296
Ketazolam	T42.4X1	T42.4X2	T42.4X3	T42.4X4	T42.4X5	T42.4X6
Ketazon	T39.2X1	T39.2X2	T39.2X3	T39.2X4	T39.2X5	T39.2X6
Ketobemidone	T40.491	T40.492	T40.493	T40.494	—	—
Ketoconazole	T49.0X1	T49.0X2	T49.0X3	T49.0X4	T49.0X5	T49.0X6
Ketols	T52.4X1	T52.4X2	T52.4X3	T52.4X4	—	—
Ketone oils	T52.4X1	T52.4X2	T52.4X3	T52.4X4	—	—
Ketoprofen	T39.311	T39.312	T39.313	T39.314	T39.315	T39.316
Ketorolac	T39.8X1	T39.8X2	T39.8X3	T39.8X4	T39.8X5	T39.8X6
Ketotifen	T45.0X1	T45.0X2	T45.0X3	T45.0X4	T45.0X5	T45.0X6
Keytruda*	T45.1X1	T45.1X2	T45.1X3	T45.1X4	T45.1X5	T45.1X6
Khat	T43.691	T43.692	T43.693	T43.694	—	—
Khellin	T46.3X1	T46.3X2	T46.3X3	T46.3X4	T46.3X5	T46.3X6
Khelloside	T46.3X1	T46.3X2	T46.3X3	T46.3X4	T46.3X5	T46.3X6
Kiln gas or vapor (carbon monoxide)	T58.8X1	T58.8X2	T58.8X3	T58.8X4	—	—
Kineret*	T39.4X1	T39.4X2	T39.4X3	T39.4X4	T39.4X5	T39.4X6
Kitasamycin	T36.3X1	T36.3X2	T36.3X3	T36.3X4	T36.3X5	T36.3X6
Komgiblyze*	T38.3X1	T38.3X2	T38.3X3	T38.3X4	T38.3X5	T38.3X6
Konsyl	T47.4X1	T47.4X2	T47.4X3	T47.4X4	T47.4X5	T47.4X6
Kosam seed	T62.2X1	T62.2X2	T62.2X3	T62.2X4	—	—
Krait (venom)	T63.091	T63.092	T63.093	T63.094	—	—
Kwell (insecticide)	T60.1X1	T60.1X2	T60.1X3	T60.1X4	—	—
- anti-infective (topical)	T49.0X1	T49.0X2	T49.0X3	T49.0X4	T49.0X5	T49.0X6
Labetalol	T44.8X1	T44.8X2	T44.8X3	T44.8X4	T44.8X5	T44.8X6
Laburnum (seeds)	T62.2X1	T62.2X2	T62.2X3	T62.2X4	—	—
- leaves	T62.2X1	T62.2X2	T62.2X3	T62.2X4	—	—
Lachesine	T49.5X1	T49.5X2	T49.5X3	T49.5X4	T49.5X5	T49.5X6
Lacidipine	T46.5X1	T46.5X2	T46.5X3	T46.5X4	T46.5X5	T46.5X6
Lacquer	T65.6X1	T65.6X2	T65.6X3	T65.6X4	—	—
Lacrimogenic gas	T59.3X1	T59.3X2	T59.3X3	T59.3X4	—	—
Lactated potassic saline	T50.3X1	T50.3X2	T50.3X3	T50.3X4	T50.3X5	T50.3X6
Lactic acid	T49.8X1	T49.8X2	T49.8X3	T49.8X4	T49.8X5	T49.8X6
Lactobacillus						
- acidophilus	T47.6X1	T47.6X2	T47.6X3	T47.6X4	T47.6X5	T47.6X6
- - compound	T47.6X1	T47.6X2	T47.6X3	T47.6X4	T47.6X5	T47.6X6
- bifidus, lyophilized	T47.6X1	T47.6X2	T47.6X3	T47.6X4	T47.6X5	T47.6X6
- bulgaricus	T47.6X1	T47.6X2	T47.6X3	T47.6X4	T47.6X5	T47.6X6
- sporogenes	T47.6X1	T47.6X2	T47.6X3	T47.6X4	T47.6X5	T47.6X6
Lactoflavin	T45.2X1	T45.2X2	T45.2X3	T45.2X4	T45.2X5	T45.2X6
Lactose (as excipient)	T50.901	T50.902	T50.903	T50.904	T50.905	T50.906
Lactuca (virosa) (extract)	T42.6X1	T42.6X2	T42.6X3	T42.6X4	T42.6X5	T42.6X6
Lactucarium	T42.6X1	T42.6X2	T42.6X3	T42.6X4	T42.6X5	T42.6X6
Lactulose	T47.3X1	T47.3X2	T47.3X3	T47.3X4	T47.3X5	T47.3X6
Laevo — *see* Levo-						
Lanatosides	T46.0X1	T46.0X2	T46.0X3	T46.0X4	T46.0X5	T46.0X6
Lanolin	T49.3X1	T49.3X2	T49.3X3	T49.3X4	T49.3X5	T49.3X6
Lanoxin*	T46.0X1	T46.0X2	T46.0X3	T46.0X4	T46.0X5	T46.0X6
Largactil	T43.3X1	T43.3X2	T43.3X3	T43.3X4	T43.3X5	T43.3X6
Larkspur	T62.2X1	T62.2X2	T62.2X3	T62.2X4	—	—
Laroxyl	T43.011	T43.012	T43.013	T43.014	T43.015	T43.016
Lasix	T50.1X1	T50.1X2	T50.1X3	T50.1X4	T50.1X5	T50.1X6
Lassar's paste	T49.4X1	T49.4X2	T49.4X3	T49.4X4	T49.4X5	T49.4X6
Latamoxef	T36.1X1	T36.1X2	T36.1X3	T36.1X4	T36.1X5	T36.1X6
Latex	T65.811	T65.812	T65.813	T65.814	—	—
Lathyrus (seed)	T62.2X1	T62.2X2	T62.2X3	T62.2X4	—	—
Laudanum	T40.0X1	T40.0X2	T40.0X3	T40.0X4	T40.0X5	T40.0X6
Laudexium	T48.1X1	T48.1X2	T48.1X3	T48.1X4	T48.1X5	T48.1X6
Laughing gas	T41.0X1	T41.0X2	T41.0X3	T41.0X4	T41.0X5	T41.0X6
Laurel, black or cherry	T62.2X1	T62.2X2	T62.2X3	T62.2X4	—	—
Laurolinium	T49.0X1	T49.0X2	T49.0X3	T49.0X4	T49.0X5	T49.0X6
Lauryl sulfoacetate	T49.2X1	T49.2X2	T49.2X3	T49.2X4	T49.2X5	T49.2X6
Laxative NEC	T47.4X1	T47.4X2	T47.4X3	T47.4X4	T47.4X5	T47.4X6
- osmotic	T47.3X1	T47.3X2	T47.3X3	T47.3X4	T47.3X5	T47.3X6
- saline	T47.3X1	T47.3X2	T47.3X3	T47.3X4	T47.3X5	T47.3X6
- stimulant	T47.2X1	T47.2X2	T47.2X3	T47.2X4	T47.2X5	T47.2X6
L-dopa	T42.8X1	T42.8X2	T42.8X3	T42.8X4	T42.8X5	T42.8X6
Lead (dust) (fumes) (vapor) **NEC**	T56.0X1	T56.0X2	T56.0X3	T56.0X4	—	—
- acetate	T49.2X1	T49.2X2	T49.2X3	T49.2X4	T49.2X5	T49.2X6
- alkyl (fuel additive)	T56.0X1	T56.0X2	T56.0X3	T56.0X4	—	—
- anti-infectives	T37.8X1	T37.8X2	T37.8X3	T37.8X4	T37.8X5	T37.8X6
- antiknock compound (tetraethyl)	T56.0X1	T56.0X2	T56.0X3	T56.0X4	—	—
- arsenate, arsenite (dust)(herbicide) (insecticide) (vapor)	T57.0X1	T57.0X2	T57.0X3	T57.0X4	—	—
- carbonate	T56.0X1	T56.0X2	T56.0X3	T56.0X4	—	—
- - paint	T56.0X1	T56.0X2	T56.0X3	T56.0X4	—	—
Lead (dust) (fumes) (vapor) **NEC** *— continued*						
- chromate	T56.0X1	T56.0X2	T56.0X3	T56.0X4	—	—
- - paint	T56.0X1	T56.0X2	T56.0X3	T56.0X4	—	—
- dioxide	T56.0X1	T56.0X2	T56.0X3	T56.0X4	—	—
- inorganic	T56.0X1	T56.0X2	T56.0X3	T56.0X4	—	—
- iodide	T56.0X1	T56.0X2	T56.0X3	T56.0X4	—	—
- - pigment (paint)	T56.0X1	T56.0X2	T56.0X3	T56.0X4	—	—
- monoxide (dust)	T56.0X1	T56.0X2	T56.0X3	T56.0X4	—	—
- - paint	T56.0X1	T56.0X2	T56.0X3	T56.0X4	—	—
- organic	T56.0X1	T56.0X2	T56.0X3	T56.0X4	—	—
- oxide	T56.0X1	T56.0X2	T56.0X3	T56.0X4	—	—
- - paint	T56.0X1	T56.0X2	T56.0X3	T56.0X4	—	—
- paint	T56.0X1	T56.0X2	T56.0X3	T56.0X4	—	—
- salts	T56.0X1	T56.0X2	T56.0X3	T56.0X4	—	—
- specified compound NEC	T56.0X1	T56.0X2	T56.0X3	T56.0X4	—	—
- tetra-ethyl	T56.0X1	T56.0X2	T56.0X3	T56.0X4	—	—
Lebanese red	T40.711	T40.712	T40.713	T40.714	T40.715	T40.716
Lefetamine	T39.8X1	T39.8X2	T39.8X3	T39.8X4	T39.8X5	T39.8X6
Lenperone	T43.4X1	T43.4X2	T43.4X3	T43.4X4	T43.4X5	T43.4X6
Lente lietin (insulin)	T38.3X1	T38.3X2	T38.3X3	T38.3X4	T38.3X5	T38.3X6
Leptazol	T50.7X1	T50.7X2	T50.7X3	T50.7X4	T50.7X5	T50.7X6
Leptophos	T60.0X1	T60.0X2	T60.0X3	T60.0X4	—	—
Leritine	T40.2X1	T40.2X2	T40.2X3	T40.2X4	T40.2X5	T40.2X6
Lescol*	T46.6X1	T46.6X2	T46.6X3	T46.6X4	T46.6X5	T46.6X6
Letosteine	T48.4X1	T48.4X2	T48.4X3	T48.4X4	T48.4X5	T48.4X6
Letter	T38.1X1	T38.1X2	T38.1X3	T38.1X4	T38.1X5	T38.1X6
Lettuce opium	T42.6X1	T42.6X2	T42.6X3	T42.6X4	T42.6X5	T42.6X6
Leucinocaine	T41.3X1	T41.3X2	T41.3X3	T41.3X4	T41.3X5	T41.3X6
Leucocianidol	T46.991	T46.992	T46.993	T46.994	T46.995	T46.996
Leucovorin (factor)	T45.8X1	T45.8X2	T45.8X3	T45.8X4	T45.8X5	T45.8X6
Leukeran	T45.1X1	T45.1X2	T45.1X3	T45.1X4	T45.1X5	T45.1X6
Leuprolide	T38.891	T38.892	T38.893	T38.894	T38.895	T38.896
Levalbuterol	T48.6X1	T48.6X2	T48.6X3	T48.6X4	T48.6X5	T48.6X6
Levallorphan	T50.7X1	T50.7X2	T50.7X3	T50.7X4	T50.7X5	T50.7X6
Levamisole	T37.4X1	T37.4X2	T37.4X3	T37.4X4	T37.4X5	T37.4X6
Levanil	T42.6X1	T42.6X2	T42.6X3	T42.6X4	T42.6X5	T42.6X6
Levarterenol	T44.4X1	T44.4X2	T44.4X3	T44.4X4	T44.4X5	T44.4X6
Levdropropizine	T48.3X1	T48.3X2	T48.3X3	T48.3X4	T48.3X5	T48.3X6
Levobunolol	T49.5X1	T49.5X2	T49.5X3	T49.5X4	T49.5X5	T49.5X6
Levocabastine (hydrochloride)	T45.0X1	T45.0X2	T45.0X3	T45.0X4	T45.0X5	T45.0X6
Levocarnitine	T50.991	T50.992	T50.993	T50.994	T50.995	T50.996
Levodopa	T42.8X1	T42.8X2	T42.8X3	T42.8X4	T42.8X5	T42.8X6
- with carbidopa	T42.8X1	T42.8X2	T42.8X3	T42.8X4	T42.8X5	T42.8X6
Levo-dromoran	T40.2X1	T40.2X2	T40.2X3	T40.2X4	T40.2X5	T40.2X6
Levoglutamide	T50.991	T50.992	T50.993	T50.994	T50.995	T50.996
Levoid	T38.1X1	T38.1X2	T38.1X3	T38.1X4	T38.1X5	T38.1X6
Levo-isomethadone	T40.3X1	T40.3X2	T40.3X3	T40.3X4	T40.3X5	T40.3X6
Levomepromazine	T43.3X1	T43.3X2	T43.3X3	T43.3X4	T43.3X5	T43.3X6
Levonordefrin	T49.6X1	T49.6X2	T49.6X3	T49.6X4	T49.6X5	T49.6X6
Levonorgestrel	T38.4X1	T38.4X2	T38.4X3	T38.4X4	T38.4X5	T38.4X6
- with ethinylestradiol	T38.5X1	T38.5X2	T38.5X3	T38.5X4	T38.5X5	T38.5X6
Levopromazine	T43.3X1	T43.3X2	T43.3X3	T43.3X4	T43.3X5	T43.3X6
Levoprome	T42.6X1	T42.6X2	T42.6X3	T42.6X4	T42.6X5	T42.6X6
Levopropoxyphene	T40.491	T40.492	T40.493	T40.494	T40.495	T40.496
Levopropylhexedrine	T50.5X1	T50.5X2	T50.5X3	T50.5X4	T50.5X5	T50.5X6
Levoproxyphylline	T48.6X1	T48.6X2	T48.6X3	T48.6X4	T48.6X5	T48.6X6
Levorphanol	T40.491	T40.492	T40.493	T40.494	T40.495	T40.496
Levothroid*	T38.1X1	T38.1X2	T38.1X3	T38.1X4	T38.1X5	T38.1X6
Levothyroxine	T38.1X1	T38.1X2	T38.1X3	T38.1X4	T38.1X5	T38.1X6
- sodium	T38.1X1	T38.1X2	T38.1X3	T38.1X4	T38.1X5	T38.1X6
Levsin	T44.3X1	T44.3X2	T44.3X3	T44.3X4	T44.3X5	T44.3X6
Levulose	T50.3X1	T50.3X2	T50.3X3	T50.3X4	T50.3X5	T50.3X6
Lewisite (gas), not in war	T57.0X1	T57.0X2	T57.0X3	T57.0X4	—	—
Lexapro*	T43.221	T43.222	T43.223	T43.224	T43.225	T43.226
Librium	T42.4X1	T42.4X2	T42.4X3	T42.4X4	T42.4X5	T42.4X6
Lidex	T49.0X1	T49.0X2	T49.0X3	T49.0X4	T49.0X5	T49.0X6
Lidocaine	T41.3X1	T41.3X2	T41.3X3	T41.3X4	T41.3X5	T41.3X6
- regional	T41.3X1	T41.3X2	T41.3X3	T41.3X4	T41.3X5	T41.3X6
- spinal	T41.3X1	T41.3X2	T41.3X3	T41.3X4	T41.3X5	T41.3X6
Lidofenin	T50.8X1	T50.8X2	T50.8X3	T50.8X4	T50.8X5	T50.8X6
Lidoflazine	T46.1X1	T46.1X2	T46.1X3	T46.1X4	T46.1X5	T46.1X6
Lighter fluid	T52.0X1	T52.0X2	T52.0X3	T52.0X4	—	—
Lignin hemicellulose	T47.6X1	T47.6X2	T47.6X3	T47.6X4	T47.6X5	T47.6X6
Lignocaine	T41.3X1	T41.3X2	T41.3X3	T41.3X4	T41.3X5	T41.3X6
- regional	T41.3X1	T41.3X2	T41.3X3	T41.3X4	T41.3X5	T41.3X6
- spinal	T41.3X1	T41.3X2	T41.3X3	T41.3X4	T41.3X5	T41.3X6
Ligroin (e) (solvent)	T52.0X1	T52.0X2	T52.0X3	T52.0X4	—	—
- vapor	T59.891	T59.892	T59.893	T59.894	—	—
Ligustrum vulgare	T62.2X1	T62.2X2	T62.2X3	T62.2X4	—	—
Lily of the valley	T62.2X1	T62.2X2	T62.2X3	T62.2X4	—	—
Lime (chloride)	T54.3X1	T54.3X2	T54.3X3	T54.3X4	—	—

Substance	Poisoning, Accidental (unintentional)	Poisoning, Intentional Self-harm	Poisoning, Assault	Poisoning, Undetermined	Adverse Effect	Under-dosing
Limonene	T52.8X1	T52.8X2	T52.8X3	T52.8X4	—	—
Lincomycin	T36.8X1	T36.8X2	T36.8X3	T36.8X4	T36.8X5	T36.8X6
Lindane (insecticide) (nonmedicinal) (vapor)	T53.6X1	T53.6X2	T53.6X3	T53.6X4	—	—
medicinal	T49.ØX1	T49.ØX2	T49.ØX3	T49.ØX4	T49.ØX5	T49.ØX6
Liniments NEC	T49.91	T49.92	T49.93	T49.94	T49.95	T49.96
Linoleic acid	T46.6X1	T46.6X2	T46.6X3	T46.6X4	T46.6X5	T46.6X6
Linolenic acid	T46.6X1	T46.6X2	T46.6X3	T46.6X4	T46.6X5	T46.6X6
Linseed	T47.4X1	T47.4X2	T47.4X3	T47.4X4	T47.4X5	T47.4X6
Liothyronine	T38.1X1	T38.1X2	T38.1X3	T38.1X4	T38.1X5	T38.1X6
Liotrix	T38.1X1	T38.1X2	T38.1X3	T38.1X4	T38.1X5	T38.1X6
Lipancreatin	T47.5X1	T47.5X2	T47.5X3	T47.5X4	T47.5X5	T47.5X6
Lipitor*	T46.6X1	T46.6X2	T46.6X3	T46.6X4	T46.6X5	T46.6X6
Lipo-alprostadil	T46.7X1	T46.7X2	T46.7X3	T46.7X4	T46.7X5	T46.7X6
Lipo-Lutin	T38.5X1	T38.5X2	T38.5X3	T38.5X4	T38.5X5	T38.5X6
Lipotropic drug NEC	T5Ø.9Ø1	T5Ø.9Ø2	T5Ø.9Ø3	T5Ø.9Ø4	T5Ø.9Ø5	T5Ø.9Ø6
Liquefied petroleum gases	T59.891	T59.892	T59.893	T59.894	—	—
piped (pure or mixed with air)	T59.891	T59.892	T59.893	T59.894	—	—
Liquid						
paraffin	T47.4X1	T47.4X2	T47.4X3	T47.4X4	T47.4X5	T47.4X6
petrolatum	T47.4X1	T47.4X2	T47.4X3	T47.4X4	T47.4X5	T47.4X6
topical	T49.3X1	T49.3X2	T49.3X3	T49.3X4	T49.3X5	T49.3X6
specified NEC	T65.891	T65.892	T65.893	T65.894	—	—
substance	T65.91	T65.92	T65.93	T65.94	—	—
Liquor creosolis compositus	T65.891	T65.892	T65.893	T65.894	—	—
Liquorice	T48.4X1	T48.4X2	T48.4X3	T48.4X4	T48.4X5	T48.4X6
extract	T47.8X1	T47.8X2	T47.8X3	T47.8X4	T47.8X5	T47.8X6
Liraglutide*	T38.3X1	T38.3X2	T38.3X3	T38.3X4	T38.3X5	T38.3X6
Lisinopril	T46.4X1	T46.4X2	T46.4X3	T46.4X4	T46.4X5	T46.4X6
Lisuride	T42.8X1	T42.8X2	T42.8X3	T42.8X4	T42.8X5	T42.8X6
Lithane	T43.8X1	T43.8X2	T43.8X3	T43.8X4	T43.8X5	T43.8X6
Lithium	T56.891	T56.892	T56.893	T56.894	—	—
gluconate	T43.591	T43.592	T43.593	T43.594	T43.595	T43.596
salts (carbonate)	T43.591	T43.592	T43.593	T43.594	T43.595	T43.596
Lithonate	T43.8X1	T43.8X2	T43.8X3	T43.8X4	T43.8X5	T43.8X6
Liver						
extract	T45.8X1	T45.8X2	T45.8X3	T45.8X4	T45.8X5	T45.8X6
for parenteral use	T45.8X1	T45.8X2	T45.8X3	T45.8X4	T45.8X5	T45.8X6
fraction 1	T45.8X1	T45.8X2	T45.8X3	T45.8X4	T45.8X5	T45.8X6
hydrolysate	T45.8X1	T45.8X2	T45.8X3	T45.8X4	T45.8X5	T45.8X6
Lizard (bite) (venom)	T63.121	T63.122	T63.123	T63.124	—	—
LMD	T45.8X1	T45.8X2	T45.8X3	T45.8X4	T45.8X5	T45.8X6
Lobelia	T62.2X1	T62.2X2	T62.2X3	T62.2X4	—	—
Lobeline	T5Ø.7X1	T5Ø.7X2	T5Ø.7X3	T5Ø.7X4	T5Ø.7X5	T5Ø.7X6
Local action drug NEC	T49.8X1	T49.8X2	T49.8X3	T49.8X4	T49.8X5	T49.8X6
Locorten	T49.ØX1	T49.ØX2	T49.ØX3	T49.ØX4	T49.ØX5	T49.ØX6
Lofepramine	T43.Ø11	T43.Ø12	T43.Ø13	T43.Ø14	T43.Ø15	T43.Ø16
Lolium temulentum	T62.2X1	T62.2X2	T62.2X3	T62.2X4	—	—
Lomotil	T47.6X1	T47.6X2	T47.6X3	T47.6X4	T47.6X5	T47.6X6
Lomustine	T45.1X1	T45.1X2	T45.1X3	T45.1X4	T45.1X5	T45.1X6
Lonidamine	T45.1X1	T45.1X2	T45.1X3	T45.1X4	T45.1X5	T45.1X6
LoOvral*	T38.4X1	T38.4X2	T38.4X3	T38.4X4	T38.4X5	T38.4X6
Loperamide	T47.6X1	T47.6X2	T47.6X3	T47.6X4	T47.6X5	T47.6X6
Loprazolam	T42.4X1	T42.4X2	T42.4X3	T42.4X4	T42.4X5	T42.4X6
Lorajmine	T46.2X1	T46.2X2	T46.2X3	T46.2X4	T46.2X5	T46.2X6
Loratidine	T45.ØX1	T45.ØX2	T45.ØX3	T45.ØX4	T45.ØX5	T45.ØX6
Lorazepam	T42.4X1	T42.4X2	T42.4X3	T42.4X4	T42.4X5	T42.4X6
Lorcainide	T46.2X1	T46.2X2	T46.2X3	T46.2X4	T46.2X5	T46.2X6
Lormetazepam	T42.4X1	T42.4X2	T42.4X3	T42.4X4	T42.4X5	T42.4X6
Lotions NEC	T49.91	T49.92	T49.93	T49.94	T49.95	T49.96
Lotrimin*	T49.ØX1	T49.ØX2	T49.ØX3	T49.ØX4	T49.ØX5	T49.ØX6
Lotusate	T42.3X1	T42.3X2	T42.3X3	T42.3X4	T42.3X5	T42.3X6
Lovastatin	T46.6X1	T46.6X2	T46.6X3	T46.6X4	T46.6X5	T46.6X6
Lowila	T49.2X1	T49.2X2	T49.2X3	T49.2X4	T49.2X5	T49.2X6
Loxapine	T43.591	T43.592	T43.593	T43.594	T43.595	T43.596
Lozenges (throat)	T49.6X1	T49.6X2	T49.6X3	T49.6X4	T49.6X5	T49.6X6
LSD	T4Ø.8X1	T4Ø.8X2	T4Ø.8X3	T4Ø.8X4	—	—
L-Tryptophan — *see* amino acid						
Lubricant, eye	T49.5X1	T49.5X2	T49.5X3	T49.5X4	T49.5X5	T49.5X6
Lubricating oil NEC	T52.ØX1	T52.ØX2	T52.ØX3	T52.ØX4	—	—
Lucanthone	T37.4X1	T37.4X2	T37.4X3	T37.4X4	T37.4X5	T37.4X6
Luminal	T42.3X1	T42.3X2	T42.3X3	T42.3X4	T42.3X5	T42.3X6
Lung irritant (gas) **NEC**	T59.91	T59.92	T59.93	T59.94	—	—
Luteinizing hormone	T38.811	T38.812	T38.813	T38.814	T38.815	T38.816
Lutocylol	T38.5X1	T38.5X2	T38.5X3	T38.5X4	T38.5X5	T38.5X6
Lutromone	T38.5X1	T38.5X2	T38.5X3	T38.5X4	T38.5X5	T38.5X6
Lututrin	T48.291	T48.292	T48.293	T48.294	T48.295	T48.296
Luveris*	T38.891	T38.892	T38.893	T38.894	T38.895	T38.896
Lye (concentrated)	T54.3X1	T54.3X2	T54.3X3	T54.3X4	—	—
Lygranum (skin test)	T5Ø.8X1	T5Ø.8X2	T5Ø.8X3	T5Ø.8X4	T5Ø.8X5	T5Ø.8X6
Lymecycline	T36.4X1	T36.4X2	T36.4X3	T36.4X4	T36.4X5	T36.4X6
Lymphogranuloma venereum antigen	T5Ø.8X1	T5Ø.8X2	T5Ø.8X3	T5Ø.8X4	T5Ø.8X5	T5Ø.8X6
Lynestrenol	T38.4X1	T38.4X2	T38.4X3	T38.4X4	T38.4X5	T38.4X6
Lyovac Sodium Edecrin	T5Ø.1X1	T5Ø.1X2	T5Ø.1X3	T5Ø.1X4	T5Ø.1X5	T5Ø.1X6
Lypressin	T38.891	T38.892	T38.893	T38.894	T38.895	T38.896
Lysergic acid diethylamide	T4Ø.8X1	T4Ø.8X2	T4Ø.8X3	T4Ø.8X4	—	—
Lysergide	T4Ø.8X1	T4Ø.8X2	T4Ø.8X3	T4Ø.8X4	—	—
Lysine vasopressin	T38.891	T38.892	T38.893	T38.894	T38.895	T38.896
Lysol	T54.1X1	T54.1X2	T54.1X3	T54.1X4	—	—
Lysozyme	T49.ØX1	T49.ØX2	T49.ØX3	T49.ØX4	T49.ØX5	T49.ØX6
Lytta (vitatta)	T49.8X1	T49.8X2	T49.8X3	T49.8X4	T49.8X5	T49.8X6
Mace	T59.3X1	T59.3X2	T59.3X3	T59.3X4	—	—
Macrogol	T5Ø.991	T5Ø.992	T5Ø.993	T5Ø.994	T5Ø.995	T5Ø.996
Macrolide						
anabolic drug	T38.7X1	T38.7X2	T38.7X3	T38.7X4	T38.7X5	T38.7X6
antibiotic	T36.3X1	T36.3X2	T36.3X3	T36.3X4	T36.3X5	T36.3X6
Mafenide	T49.ØX1	T49.ØX2	T49.ØX3	T49.ØX4	T49.ØX5	T49.ØX6
Magaldrate	T47.1X1	T47.1X2	T47.1X3	T47.1X4	T47.1X5	T47.1X6
Magic mushroom	T4Ø.991	T4Ø.992	T4Ø.993	T4Ø.994	—	—
Magnamycin	T36.8X1	T36.8X2	T36.8X3	T36.8X4	T36.8X5	T36.8X6
Magnesia magma	T47.1X1	T47.1X2	T47.1X3	T47.1X4	T47.1X5	T47.1X6
Magnesium NEC	T56.891	T56.892	T56.893	T56.894	—	—
carbonate	T47.1X1	T47.1X2	T47.1X3	T47.1X4	T47.1X5	T47.1X6
citrate	T47.4X1	T47.4X2	T47.4X3	T47.4X4	T47.4X5	T47.4X6
hydroxide	T47.1X1	T47.1X2	T47.1X3	T47.1X4	T47.1X5	T47.1X6
oxide	T47.1X1	T47.1X2	T47.1X3	T47.1X4	T47.1X5	T47.1X6
peroxide	T49.ØX1	T49.ØX2	T49.ØX3	T49.ØX4	T49.ØX5	T49.ØX6
salicylate	T39.Ø91	T39.Ø92	T39.Ø93	T39.Ø94	T39.Ø95	T39.Ø96
silicofluoride	T5Ø.3X1	T5Ø.3X2	T5Ø.3X3	T5Ø.3X4	T5Ø.3X5	T5Ø.3X6
sulfate	T47.4X1	T47.4X2	T47.4X3	T47.4X4	T47.4X5	T47.4X6
thiosulfate	T45.ØX1	T45.ØX2	T45.ØX3	T45.ØX4	T45.ØX5	T45.ØX6
trisilicate	T47.1X1	T47.1X2	T47.1X3	T47.1X4	T47.1X5	T47.1X6
Malathion (medicinal)	T49.ØX1	T49.ØX2	T49.ØX3	T49.ØX4	T49.ØX5	T49.ØX6
insecticide	T6Ø.ØX1	T6Ø.ØX2	T6Ø.ØX3	T6Ø.ØX4	—	—
Male fern extract	T37.4X1	T37.4X2	T37.4X3	T37.4X4	T37.4X5	T37.4X6
M-AMSA	T45.1X1	T45.1X2	T45.1X3	T45.1X4	T45.1X5	T45.1X6
Mandelic acid	T37.8X1	T37.8X2	T37.8X3	T37.8X4	T37.8X5	T37.8X6
Manganese (dioxide) (salts)	T57.2X1	T57.2X2	T57.2X3	T57.2X4	—	—
medicinal	T5Ø.991	T5Ø.992	T5Ø.993	T5Ø.994	T5Ø.995	T5Ø.996
Mannitol	T47.3X1	T47.3X2	T47.3X3	T47.3X4	T47.3X5	T47.3X6
hexanitrate	T46.3X1	T46.3X2	T46.3X3	T46.3X4	T46.3X5	T46.3X6
Mannomustine	T45.1X1	T45.1X2	T45.1X3	T45.1X4	T45.1X5	T45.1X6
MAO inhibitors	T43.1X1	T43.1X2	T43.1X3	T43.1X4	T43.1X5	T43.1X6
Mapharsen	T37.8X1	T37.8X2	T37.8X3	T37.8X4	T37.8X5	T37.8X6
Maphenide	T49.ØX1	T49.ØX2	T49.ØX3	T49.ØX4	T49.ØX5	T49.ØX6
Maprotiline	T43.Ø21	T43.Ø22	T43.Ø23	T43.Ø24	T43.Ø25	T43.Ø26
Marcaine	T41.3X1	T41.3X2	T41.3X3	T41.3X4	T41.3X5	T41.3X6
infiltration (subcutaneous)	T41.3X1	T41.3X2	T41.3X3	T41.3X4	T41.3X5	T41.3X6
nerve block (peripheral) (plexus)	T41.3X1	T41.3X2	T41.3X3	T41.3X4	T41.3X5	T41.3X6
Marezine	T45.ØX1	T45.ØX2	T45.ØX3	T45.ØX4	T45.ØX5	T45.ØX6
Marihuana	T4Ø.711	T4Ø.712	T4Ø.713	T4Ø.714	T4Ø.715	T4Ø.716
Marijuana	T4Ø.711	T4Ø.712	T4Ø.713	T4Ø.714	T4Ø.715	T4Ø.716
Marine (sting)	T63.691	T63.692	T63.693	T63.694	—	—
animals (sting)	T63.691	T63.692	T63.693	T63.694	—	—
plants (sting)	T63.711	T63.712	T63.713	T63.714	—	—
Marplan	T43.1X1	T43.1X2	T43.1X3	T43.1X4	T43.1X5	T43.1X6
Marsh gas	T59.891	T59.892	T59.893	T59.894	—	—
Marsilid	T43.1X1	T43.1X2	T43.1X3	T43.1X4	T43.1X5	T43.1X6
Massengill*	T49.ØX1	T49.ØX2	T49.ØX3	T49.ØX4	T49.ØX5	T49.ØX6
Matulane	T45.1X1	T45.1X2	T45.1X3	T45.1X4	T45.1X5	T45.1X6
Mazindol	T5Ø.5X1	T5Ø.5X2	T5Ø.5X3	T5Ø.5X4	T5Ø.5X5	T5Ø.5X6
MCPA	T6Ø.3X1	T6Ø.3X2	T6Ø.3X3	T6Ø.3X4	—	—
MDMA	T43.641	T43.642	T43.643	T43.644	—	—
Meadow saffron	T62.2X1	T62.2X2	T62.2X3	T62.2X4	—	—
Measles virus vaccine (attenuated)	T5Ø.B91	T5Ø.B92	T5Ø.B93	T5Ø.B94	T5Ø.B95	T5Ø.B96
Meat, noxious	T62.8X1	T62.8X2	T62.8X3	T62.8X4	—	—
Meballymal	T42.3X1	T42.3X2	T42.3X3	T42.3X4	T42.3X5	T42.3X6
Mebanazine	T43.1X1	T43.1X2	T43.1X3	T43.1X4	T43.1X5	T43.1X6
Mebaral	T42.3X1	T42.3X2	T42.3X3	T42.3X4	T42.3X5	T42.3X6
Mebendazole	T37.4X1	T37.4X2	T37.4X3	T37.4X4	T37.4X5	T37.4X6
Mebeverine	T44.3X1	T44.3X2	T44.3X3	T44.3X4	T44.3X5	T44.3X6
Mebhydrolin	T45.ØX1	T45.ØX2	T45.ØX3	T45.ØX4	T45.ØX5	T45.ØX6
Mebumal	T42.3X1	T42.3X2	T42.3X3	T42.3X4	T42.3X5	T42.3X6
Mebutamate	T43.591	T43.592	T43.593	T43.594	T43.595	T43.596
Mecamylamine	T44.2X1	T44.2X2	T44.2X3	T44.2X4	T44.2X5	T44.2X6
Mechlorethamine	T45.1X1	T45.1X2	T45.1X3	T45.1X4	T45.1X5	T45.1X6
Mecillinam	T36.ØX1	T36.ØX2	T36.ØX3	T36.ØX4	T36.ØX5	T36.ØX6
Meclizine (hydrochloride)	T45.ØX1	T45.ØX2	T45.ØX3	T45.ØX4	T45.ØX5	T45.ØX6
Meclocycline	T36.4X1	T36.4X2	T36.4X3	T36.4X4	T36.4X5	T36.4X6
Meclofenamate	T39.391	T39.392	T39.393	T39.394	T39.395	T39.396
Meclofenamic acid	T39.391	T39.392	T39.393	T39.394	T39.395	T39.396

Substance	Poisoning, Accidental (unintentional)	Poisoning, Intentional Self-harm	Poisoning, Assault	Poisoning, Undetermined	Adverse Effect	Under-dosing
Meclofenoxate	T43.691	T43.692	T43.693	T43.694	T43.695	T43.696
Meclozine	T45.0X1	T45.0X2	T45.0X3	T45.0X4	T45.0X5	T45.0X6
Mecobalamin	T45.8X1	T45.8X2	T45.8X3	T45.8X4	T45.8X5	T45.8X6
Mecoprop	T60.3X1	T60.3X2	T60.3X3	T60.3X4	—	—
Mecrilate	T49.3X1	T49.3X2	T49.3X3	T49.3X4	T49.3X5	T49.3X6
Mecysteine	T48.4X1	T48.4X2	T48.4X3	T48.4X4	T48.4X5	T48.4X6
Medazepam	T42.4X1	T42.4X2	T42.4X3	T42.4X4	T42.4X5	T42.4X6
Medicament NEC	T50.901	T50.902	T50.903	T50.904	T50.905	T50.906
Medinal	T42.3X1	T42.3X2	T42.3X3	T42.3X4	T42.3X5	T42.3X6
Medomin	T42.3X1	T42.3X2	T42.3X3	T42.3X4	T42.3X5	T42.3X6
Medrogestone	T38.5X1	T38.5X2	T38.5X3	T38.5X4	T38.5X5	T38.5X6
Medrol*	T38.0X1	T38.0X2	T38.0X3	T38.0X4	T38.0X5	T38.0X6
Medroxalol	T44.8X1	T44.8X2	T44.8X3	T44.8X4	T44.8X5	T44.8X6
Medroxyprogesterone acetate (depot)	T38.5X1	T38.5X2	T38.5X3	T38.5X4	T38.5X5	T38.5X6
Medrysone	T49.0X1	T49.0X2	T49.0X3	T49.0X4	T49.0X5	T49.0X6
Mefenamic acid	T39.391	T39.392	T39.393	T39.394	T39.395	T39.396
Mefenorex	T50.5X1	T50.5X2	T50.5X3	T50.5X4	T50.5X5	T50.5X6
Mefloquine	T37.2X1	T37.2X2	T37.2X3	T37.2X4	T37.2X5	T37.2X6
Mefoxin*	T36.1X1	T36.1X2	T36.1X3	T36.1X4	T36.1X5	T36.1X6
Mefruside	T50.2X1	T50.2X2	T50.2X3	T50.2X4	T50.2X5	T50.2X6
Megahallucinogen	T40.901	T40.902	T40.903	T40.904	T40.905	T40.906
Megestrol	T38.5X1	T38.5X2	T38.5X3	T38.5X4	T38.5X5	T38.5X6
Meglumine						
antimoniate	T37.8X1	T37.8X2	T37.8X3	T37.8X4	T37.8X5	T37.8X6
diatrizoate	T50.8X1	T50.8X2	T50.8X3	T50.8X4	T50.8X5	T50.8X6
iodipamide	T50.8X1	T50.8X2	T50.8X3	T50.8X4	T50.8X5	T50.8X6
iotroxate	T50.8X1	T50.8X2	T50.8X3	T50.8X4	T50.8X5	T50.8X6
MEK (methyl ethyl ketone)	T52.4X1	T52.4X2	T52.4X3	T52.4X4	—	—
Meladinin	T49.3X1	T49.3X2	T49.3X3	T49.3X4	T49.3X5	T49.3X6
Meladrazine	T44.3X1	T44.3X2	T44.3X3	T44.3X4	T44.3X5	T44.3X6
Melaleuca alternifolia oil	T49.0X1	T49.0X2	T49.0X3	T49.0X4	T49.0X5	T49.0X6
Melanizing agents	T49.3X1	T49.3X2	T49.3X3	T49.3X4	T49.3X5	T49.3X6
Melanocyte-stimulating hormone	T38.891	T38.892	T38.893	T38.894	T38.895	T38.896
Melarsonyl potassium	T37.3X1	T37.3X2	T37.3X3	T37.3X4	T37.3X5	T37.3X6
Melarsoprol	T37.3X1	T37.3X2	T37.3X3	T37.3X4	T37.3X5	T37.3X6
Melia azedarach	T62.2X1	T62.2X2	T62.2X3	T62.2X4	—	—
Melitracen	T43.011	T43.012	T43.013	T43.014	T43.015	T43.016
Mellaril	T43.3X1	T43.3X2	T43.3X3	T43.3X4	T43.3X5	T43.3X6
Meloxicam*	T39.391	T39.392	T39.393	T39.394	T39.395	T39.396
Meloxine	T49.3X1	T49.3X2	T49.3X3	T49.3X4	T49.3X5	T49.3X6
Melperone	T43.4X1	T43.4X2	T43.4X3	T43.4X4	T43.4X5	T43.4X6
Melphalan	T45.1X1	T45.1X2	T45.1X3	T45.1X4	T45.1X5	T45.1X6
Memantine	T43.8X1	T43.8X2	T43.8X3	T43.8X4	T43.8X5	T43.8X6
Menadiol	T45.7X1	T45.7X2	T45.7X3	T45.7X4	T45.7X5	T45.7X6
sodium sulfate	T45.7X1	T45.7X2	T45.7X3	T45.7X4	T45.7X5	T45.7X6
Menadione	T45.7X1	T45.7X2	T45.7X3	T45.7X4	T45.7X5	T45.7X6
sodium bisulfite	T45.7X1	T45.7X2	T45.7X3	T45.7X4	T45.7X5	T45.7X6
Menaphthone	T45.7X1	T45.7X2	T45.7X3	T45.7X4	T45.7X5	T45.7X6
Menaquinone	T45.7X1	T45.7X2	T45.7X3	T45.7X4	T45.7X5	T45.7X6
Menatetrenone	T45.7X1	T45.7X2	T45.7X3	T45.7X4	T45.7X5	T45.7X6
Meningococcal vaccine	T50.A91	T50.A92	T50.A93	T50.A94	T50.A95	T50.A96
Menningovax (-AC) (-C)	T50.A91	T50.A92	T50.A93	T50.A94	T50.A95	T50.A96
Menotropins	T38.811	T38.812	T38.813	T38.814	T38.815	T38.816
Menthol	T48.5X1	T48.5X2	T48.5X3	T48.5X4	T48.5X5	T48.5X6
Mepacrine	T37.2X1	T37.2X2	T37.2X3	T37.2X4	T37.2X5	T37.2X6
Meparfynol	T42.6X1	T42.6X2	T42.6X3	T42.6X4	T42.6X5	T42.6X6
Mepartricin	T36.7X1	T36.7X2	T36.7X3	T36.7X4	T36.7X5	T36.7X6
Mepazine	T43.3X1	T43.3X2	T43.3X3	T43.3X4	T43.3X5	T43.3X6
Mepenzolate	T44.3X1	T44.3X2	T44.3X3	T44.3X4	T44.3X5	T44.3X6
bromide	T44.3X1	T44.3X2	T44.3X3	T44.3X4	T44.3X5	T44.3X6
Meperidine	T40.491	T40.492	T40.493	T40.494	T40.495	T40.496
Mephebarbital	T42.3X1	T42.3X2	T42.3X3	T42.3X4	T42.3X5	T42.3X6
Mephenamin (e)	T42.8X1	T42.8X2	T42.8X3	T42.8X4	T42.8X5	T42.8X6
Mephenesin	T42.8X1	T42.8X2	T42.8X3	T42.8X4	T42.8X5	T42.8X6
Mephenhydramine	T45.0X1	T45.0X2	T45.0X3	T45.0X4	T45.0X5	T45.0X6
Mephenoxalone	T42.8X1	T42.8X2	T42.8X3	T42.8X4	T42.8X5	T42.8X6
Mephentermine	T44.991	T44.992	T44.993	T44.994	T44.995	T44.996
Mephenytoin	T42.0X1	T42.0X2	T42.0X3	T42.0X4	T42.0X5	T42.0X6
with phenobarbital	T42.3X1	T42.3X2	T42.3X3	T42.3X4	T42.3X5	T42.3X6
Mephobarbital	T42.3X1	T42.3X2	T42.3X3	T42.3X4	T42.3X5	T42.3X6
Mephosfolan	T60.0X1	T60.0X2	T60.0X3	T60.0X4	—	—
Mepindolol	T44.7X1	T44.7X2	T44.7X3	T44.7X4	T44.7X5	T44.7X6
Mepiperphenidol	T44.3X1	T44.3X2	T44.3X3	T44.3X4	T44.3X5	T44.3X6
Mepitiostane	T38.7X1	T38.7X2	T38.7X3	T38.7X4	T38.7X5	T38.7X6
Mepivacaine	T41.3X1	T41.3X2	T41.3X3	T41.3X4	T41.3X5	T41.3X6
epidural	T41.3X1	T41.3X2	T41.3X3	T41.3X4	T41.3X5	T41.3X6
Meprednisone	T38.0X1	T38.0X2	T38.0X3	T38.0X4	T38.0X5	T38.0X6
Meprobam	T43.591	T43.592	T43.593	T43.594	T43.595	T43.596
Meprobamate	T43.591	T43.592	T43.593	T43.594	T43.595	T43.596
Meproscillarin	T46.0X1	T46.0X2	T46.0X3	T46.0X4	T46.0X5	T46.0X6
Meprylcaine	T41.3X1	T41.3X2	T41.3X3	T41.3X4	T41.3X5	T41.3X6
Meptazinol	T39.8X1	T39.8X2	T39.8X3	T39.8X4	T39.8X5	T39.8X6
Mepyramine	T45.0X1	T45.0X2	T45.0X3	T45.0X4	T45.0X5	T45.0X6
Mequinol*	T49.8X1	T49.8X2	T49.8X3	T49.8X4	T49.8X5	T49.8X6
Mequitazine	T43.3X1	T43.3X2	T43.3X3	T43.3X4	T43.3X5	T43.3X6
Meralluride	T50.2X1	T50.2X2	T50.2X3	T50.2X4	T50.2X5	T50.2X6
Merbaphen	T50.2X1	T50.2X2	T50.2X3	T50.2X4	T50.2X5	T50.2X6
Merbromin	T49.0X1	T49.0X2	T49.0X3	T49.0X4	T49.0X5	T49.0X6
Mercaptobenzothiazole salts	T49.0X1	T49.0X2	T49.0X3	T49.0X4	T49.0X5	T49.0X6
Mercaptomerin	T50.2X1	T50.2X2	T50.2X3	T50.2X4	T50.2X5	T50.2X6
Mercaptopurine	T45.1X1	T45.1X2	T45.1X3	T45.1X4	T45.1X5	T45.1X6
Mercumatilin	T50.2X1	T50.2X2	T50.2X3	T50.2X4	T50.2X5	T50.2X6
Mercuramide	T50.2X1	T50.2X2	T50.2X3	T50.2X4	T50.2X5	T50.2X6
Mercurochrome	T49.0X1	T49.0X2	T49.0X3	T49.0X4	T49.0X5	T49.0X6
Mercurophylline	T50.2X1	T50.2X2	T50.2X3	T50.2X4	T50.2X5	T50.2X6
Mercury, mercurial, mercuric, mercurous (compounds) (cyanide) (fumes) (nonmedicinal) (vapor) **NEC**	T56.1X1	T56.1X2	T56.1X3	T56.1X4	—	—
ammoniated	T49.0X1	T49.0X2	T49.0X3	T49.0X4	T49.0X5	T49.0X6
anti-infective						
local	T49.0X1	T49.0X2	T49.0X3	T49.0X4	T49.0X5	T49.0X6
systemic	T37.8X1	T37.8X2	T37.8X3	T37.8X4	T37.8X5	T37.8X6
topical	T49.0X1	T49.0X2	T49.0X3	T49.0X4	T49.0X5	T49.0X6
chloride (ammoniated)	T49.0X1	T49.0X2	T49.0X3	T49.0X4	T49.0X5	T49.0X6
fungicide	T56.1X1	T56.1X2	T56.1X3	T56.1X4	—	—
diuretic NEC	T50.2X1	T50.2X2	T50.2X3	T50.2X4	T50.2X5	T50.2X6
fungicide	T56.1X1	T56.1X2	T56.1X3	T56.1X4	—	—
organic (fungicide)	T56.1X1	T56.1X2	T56.1X3	T56.1X4	—	—
oxide, yellow	T49.0X1	T49.0X2	T49.0X3	T49.0X4	T49.0X5	T49.0X6
Mersalyl	T50.2X1	T50.2X2	T50.2X3	T50.2X4	T50.2X5	T50.2X6
Merthiolate	T49.0X1	T49.0X2	T49.0X3	T49.0X4	T49.0X5	T49.0X6
ophthalmic preparation	T49.5X1	T49.5X2	T49.5X3	T49.5X4	T49.5X5	T49.5X6
Meruvax	T50.B91	T50.B92	T50.B93	T50.B94	T50.B95	T50.B96
Mesalazine	T47.8X1	T47.8X2	T47.8X3	T47.8X4	T47.8X5	T47.8X6
Mescal buttons	T40.991	T40.992	T40.993	T40.994	—	—
Mescaline	T40.991	T40.992	T40.993	T40.994	—	—
Mesna	T48.4X1	T48.4X2	T48.4X3	T48.4X4	T48.4X5	T48.4X6
Mesoglycan	T46.6X1	T46.6X2	T46.6X3	T46.6X4	T46.6X5	T46.6X6
Mesoridazine	T43.3X1	T43.3X2	T43.3X3	T43.3X4	T43.3X5	T43.3X6
Mestanolone	T38.7X1	T38.7X2	T38.7X3	T38.7X4	T38.7X5	T38.7X6
Mesterolone	T38.7X1	T38.7X2	T38.7X3	T38.7X4	T38.7X5	T38.7X6
Mestranol	T38.5X1	T38.5X2	T38.5X3	T38.5X4	T38.5X5	T38.5X6
Mesulergine	T42.8X1	T42.8X2	T42.8X3	T42.8X4	T42.8X5	T42.8X6
Mesulfen	T49.0X1	T49.0X2	T49.0X3	T49.0X4	T49.0X5	T49.0X6
Mesuximide	T42.2X1	T42.2X2	T42.2X3	T42.2X4	T42.2X5	T42.2X6
Metabutethamine	T41.3X1	T41.3X2	T41.3X3	T41.3X4	T41.3X5	T41.3X6
Metactesylacetate	T49.0X1	T49.0X2	T49.0X3	T49.0X4	T49.0X5	T49.0X6
Metacycline	T36.4X1	T36.4X2	T36.4X3	T36.4X4	T36.4X5	T36.4X6
Metaldehyde (snail killer) **NEC**	T60.8X1	T60.8X2	T60.8X3	T60.8X4	—	—
Metals (heavy) (nonmedicinal)	T56.91	T56.92	T56.93	T56.94	—	—
dust, fumes, or vapor NEC	T56.91	T56.92	T56.93	T56.94	—	—
gadolinium	T56.821	T56.822	T56.823	T56.824	—	—
light NEC	T56.91	T56.92	T56.93	T56.94	—	—
dust, fumes, or vapor NEC	T56.91	T56.92	T56.93	T56.94	—	—
specified NEC	T56.891	T56.892	T56.893	T56.894	—	—
thallium	T56.811	T56.812	T56.813	T56.814	—	—
Metamfetamine	T43.651	T43.652	T43.653	T43.654	T43.655	T43.656
Metamizole sodium	T39.2X1	T39.2X2	T39.2X3	T39.2X4	T39.2X5	T39.2X6
Metampicillin	T36.0X1	T36.0X2	T36.0X3	T36.0X4	T36.0X5	T36.0X6
Metamucil	T47.4X1	T47.4X2	T47.4X3	T47.4X4	T47.4X5	T47.4X6
Metandienone	T38.7X1	T38.7X2	T38.7X3	T38.7X4	T38.7X5	T38.7X6
Metandrostenolone	T38.7X1	T38.7X2	T38.7X3	T38.7X4	T38.7X5	T38.7X6
Metaphen	T49.0X1	T49.0X2	T49.0X3	T49.0X4	T49.0X5	T49.0X6
Metaphos	T60.0X1	T60.0X2	T60.0X3	T60.0X4	—	—
Metapramine	T43.011	T43.012	T43.013	T43.014	T43.015	T43.016
Metaproterenol	T48.291	T48.292	T48.293	T48.294	T48.295	T48.296
Metaraminol	T44.4X1	T44.4X2	T44.4X3	T44.4X4	T44.4X5	T44.4X6
Metaxalone	T42.8X1	T42.8X2	T42.8X3	T42.8X4	T42.8X5	T42.8X6
Meted*	T49.4X1	T49.4X2	T49.4X3	T49.4X4	T49.4X5	T49.4X6
Metenolone	T38.7X1	T38.7X2	T38.7X3	T38.7X4	T38.7X5	T38.7X6
Metergoline	T42.8X1	T42.8X2	T42.8X3	T42.8X4	T42.8X5	T42.8X6
Metescufylline	T46.991	T46.992	T46.993	T46.994	T46.995	T46.996
Metetoin	T42.0X1	T42.0X2	T42.0X3	T42.0X4	T42.0X5	T42.0X6
Metformin	T38.3X1	T38.3X2	T38.3X3	T38.3X4	T38.3X5	T38.3X6
Methacholine	T44.1X1	T44.1X2	T44.1X3	T44.1X4	T44.1X5	T44.1X6
Methacycline	T36.4X1	T36.4X2	T36.4X3	T36.4X4	T36.4X5	T36.4X6
Methadone	T40.3X1	T40.3X2	T40.3X3	T40.3X4	T40.3X5	T40.3X6
Methadose*	T40.3X1	T40.3X2	T40.3X3	T40.3X4	T40.3X5	T40.3X6

*Optum Value-Add

Substance	Poisoning, Accidental (unintentional)	Poisoning, Intentional Self-harm	Poisoning, Assault	Poisoning, Undetermined	Adverse Effect	Under-dosing
Methallenestril	T38.5X1	T38.5X2	T38.5X3	T38.5X4	T38.5X5	T38.5X6
Methallenoestril	T38.5X1	T38.5X2	T38.5X3	T38.5X4	T38.5X5	T38.5X6
Methamphetamine	T43.651	T43.652	T43.653	T43.654	T43.655	T43.656
Methampyrone	T39.2X1	T39.2X2	T39.2X3	T39.2X4	T39.2X5	T39.2X6
Methandienone	T38.7X1	T38.7X2	T38.7X3	T38.7X4	T38.7X5	T38.7X6
Methandriol	T38.7X1	T38.7X2	T38.7X3	T38.7X4	T38.7X5	T38.7X6
Methandrostenolone	T38.7X1	T38.7X2	T38.7X3	T38.7X4	T38.7X5	T38.7X6
Methane	T59.891	T59.892	T59.893	T59.894	—	—
Methanethiol	T59.891	T59.892	T59.893	T59.894	—	—
Methaniazide	T37.1X1	T37.1X2	T37.1X3	T37.1X4	T37.1X5	T37.1X6
Methanol (vapor)	T51.1X1	T51.1X2	T51.1X3	T51.1X4	—	—
Methantheline	T44.3X1	T44.3X2	T44.3X3	T44.3X4	T44.3X5	T44.3X6
Methanthelinium bromide	T44.3X1	T44.3X2	T44.3X3	T44.3X4	T44.3X5	T44.3X6
Methaphenilene	T45.ØX1	T45.ØX2	T45.ØX3	T45.ØX4	T45.ØX5	T45.ØX6
Methapyrilene	T45.ØX1	T45.ØX2	T45.ØX3	T45.ØX4	T45.ØX5	T45.ØX6
Methaqualone (compound)	T42.6X1	T42.6X2	T42.6X3	T42.6X4	T42.6X5	T42.6X6
Metharbital	T42.3X1	T42.3X2	T42.3X3	T42.3X4	T42.3X5	T42.3X6
Methazolamide	T5Ø.2X1	T5Ø.2X2	T5Ø.2X3	T5Ø.2X4	T5Ø.2X5	T5Ø.2X6
Methdilazine	T43.3X1	T43.3X2	T43.3X3	T43.3X4	T43.3X5	T43.3X6
Methedrine	T43.651	T43.652	T43.653	T43.654	T43.655	T43.656
Methenamine (mandelate)	T37.8X1	T37.8X2	T37.8X3	T37.8X4	T37.8X5	T37.8X6
Methenolone	T38.7X1	T38.7X2	T38.7X3	T38.7X4	T38.7X5	T38.7X6
Methergine	T48.ØX1	T48.ØX2	T48.ØX3	T48.ØX4	T48.ØX5	T48.ØX6
Methetoin	T42.ØX1	T42.ØX2	T42.ØX3	T42.ØX4	T42.ØX5	T42.ØX6
Methiacil	T38.2X1	T38.2X2	T38.2X3	T38.2X4	T38.2X5	T38.2X6
Methicillin	T36.ØX1	T36.ØX2	T36.ØX3	T36.ØX4	T36.ØX5	T36.ØX6
Methimazole	T38.2X1	T38.2X2	T38.2X3	T38.2X4	T38.2X5	T38.2X6
Methiodal sodium	T5Ø.8X1	T5Ø.8X2	T5Ø.8X3	T5Ø.8X4	T5Ø.8X5	T5Ø.8X6
Methionine	T5Ø.991	T5Ø.992	T5Ø.993	T5Ø.994	T5Ø.995	T5Ø.996
Methisazone	T37.5X1	T37.5X2	T37.5X3	T37.5X4	T37.5X5	T37.5X6
Methisoprinol	T37.5X1	T37.5X2	T37.5X3	T37.5X4	T37.5X5	T37.5X6
Methitural	T42.3X1	T42.3X2	T42.3X3	T42.3X4	T42.3X5	T42.3X6
Methixene	T44.3X1	T44.3X2	T44.3X3	T44.3X4	T44.3X5	T44.3X6
Methobarbital, methobarbitone	T42.3X1	T42.3X2	T42.3X3	T42.3X4	T42.3X5	T42.3X6
Methocarbamol	T42.8X1	T42.8X2	T42.8X3	T42.8X4	T42.8X5	T42.8X6
skeletal muscle relaxant	T48.1X1	T48.1X2	T48.1X3	T48.1X4	T48.1X5	T48.1X6
Methohexital	T41.1X1	T41.1X2	T41.1X3	T41.1X4	T41.1X5	T41.1X6
Methohexitone	T41.1X1	T41.1X2	T41.1X3	T41.1X4	T41.1X5	T41.1X6
Methoin	T42.ØX1	T42.ØX2	T42.ØX3	T42.ØX4	T42.ØX5	T42.ØX6
Metholpholine	T39.8X1	T39.8X2	T39.8X3	T39.8X4	T39.8X5	T39.8X6
Methopromazine	T43.3X1	T43.3X2	T43.3X3	T43.3X4	T43.3X5	T43.3X6
Methorate	T48.3X1	T48.3X2	T48.3X3	T48.3X4	T48.3X5	T48.3X6
Methoserpidine	T46.5X1	T46.5X2	T46.5X3	T46.5X4	T46.5X5	T46.5X6
Methotrexate	T45.1X1	T45.1X2	T45.1X3	T45.1X4	T45.1X5	T45.1X6
Methotrimeprazine	T43.3X1	T43.3X2	T43.3X3	T43.3X4	T43.3X5	T43.3X6
Methoxa-Dome	T49.3X1	T49.3X2	T49.3X3	T49.3X4	T49.3X5	T49.3X6
Methoxamine	T44.4X1	T44.4X2	T44.4X3	T44.4X4	T44.4X5	T44.4X6
Methoxsalen	T5Ø.991	T5Ø.992	T5Ø.993	T5Ø.994	T5Ø.995	T5Ø.996
Methoxyaniline	T65.3X1	T65.3X2	T65.3X3	T65.3X4	—	—
Methoxybenzyl penicillin	T36.ØX1	T36.ØX2	T36.ØX3	T36.ØX4	T36.ØX5	T36.ØX6
Methoxychlor	T53.7X1	T53.7X2	T53.7X3	T53.7X4	—	—
Methoxy-DDT	T53.7X1	T53.7X2	T53.7X3	T53.7X4	—	—
Methoxyflurane	T41.ØX1	T41.ØX2	T41.ØX3	T41.ØX4	T41.ØX5	T41.ØX6
Methoxyphenamine	T48.6X1	T48.6X2	T48.6X3	T48.6X4	T48.6X5	T48.6X6
Methoxypromazine	T43.3X1	T43.3X2	T43.3X3	T43.3X4	T43.3X5	T43.3X6
Methscopolamine bromide	T44.3X1	T44.3X2	T44.3X3	T44.3X4	T44.3X5	T44.3X6
Methsuximide	T42.2X1	T42.2X2	T42.2X3	T42.2X4	T42.2X5	T42.2X6
Methyclothiazide	T5Ø.2X1	T5Ø.2X2	T5Ø.2X3	T5Ø.2X4	T5Ø.2X5	T5Ø.2X6
Methyl						
acetate	T52.4X1	T52.4X2	T52.4X3	T52.4X4	—	—
acetone	T52.4X1	T52.4X2	T52.4X3	T52.4X4	—	—
acrylate	T65.891	T65.892	T65.893	T65.894	—	—
alcohol	T51.1X1	T51.1X2	T51.1X3	T51.1X4	—	—
aminophenol	T65.3X1	T65.3X2	T65.3X3	T65.3X4	—	—
amphetamine	T43.651	T43.652	T43.653	T43.654	T43.655	T43.656
androstanolone	T38.7X1	T38.7X2	T38.7X3	T38.7X4	T38.7X5	T38.7X6
atropine	T44.3X1	T44.3X2	T44.3X3	T44.3X4	T44.3X5	T44.3X6
benzene	T52.2X1	T52.2X2	T52.2X3	T52.2X4	—	—
benzoate	T52.8X1	T52.8X2	T52.8X3	T52.8X4	—	—
benzol	T52.2X1	T52.2X2	T52.2X3	T52.2X4	—	—
bromide (gas)	T59.891	T59.892	T59.893	T59.894	—	—
fumigant	T6Ø.8X1	T6Ø.8X2	T6Ø.8X3	T6Ø.8X4	—	—
butanol	T51.3X1	T51.3X2	T51.3X3	T51.3X4	—	—
carbinol	T51.1X1	T51.1X2	T51.1X3	T51.1X4	—	—
carbonate	T52.8X1	T52.8X2	T52.8X3	T52.8X4	—	—
CCNU	T45.1X1	T45.1X2	T45.1X3	T45.1X4	T45.1X5	T45.1X6
cellosolve	T52.91	T52.92	T52.93	T52.94	—	—
cellulose	T47.4X1	T47.4X2	T47.4X3	T47.4X4	T47.4X5	T47.4X6
chloride (gas)	T59.891	T59.892	T59.893	T59.894	—	—
chloroformate	T59.3X1	T59.3X2	T59.3X3	T59.3X4	—	—
cyclohexane	T52.8X1	T52.8X2	T52.8X3	T52.8X4	—	—
Methyl — *continued*						
cyclohexanol	T51.8X1	T51.8X2	T51.8X3	T51.8X4	—	—
cyclohexanone	T52.8X1	T52.8X2	T52.8X3	T52.8X4	—	—
cyclohexyl acetate	T52.8X1	T52.8X2	T52.8X3	T52.8X4	—	—
demeton	T6Ø.ØX1	T6Ø.ØX2	T6Ø.ØX3	T6Ø.ØX4	—	—
dihydromorphinone	T4Ø.2X1	T4Ø.2X2	T4Ø.2X3	T4Ø.2X4	T4Ø.2X5	T4Ø.2X6
ergometrine	T48.ØX1	T48.ØX2	T48.ØX3	T48.ØX4	T48.ØX5	T48.ØX6
ergonovine	T48.ØX1	T48.ØX2	T48.ØX3	T48.ØX4	T48.ØX5	T48.ØX6
ethyl ketone	T52.4X1	T52.4X2	T52.4X3	T52.4X4	—	—
glucamine antimonate	T37.8X1	T37.8X2	T37.8X3	T37.8X4	T37.8X5	T37.8X6
hydrazine	T65.891	T65.892	T65.893	T65.894	—	—
iodide	T65.891	T65.892	T65.893	T65.894	—	—
isobutyl ketone	T52.4X1	T52.4X2	T52.4X3	T52.4X4	—	—
isothiocyanate	T6Ø.3X1	T6Ø.3X2	T6Ø.3X3	T6Ø.3X4	—	—
mercaptan	T59.891	T59.892	T59.893	T59.894	—	—
morphine NEC	T4Ø.2X1	T4Ø.2X2	T4Ø.2X3	T4Ø.2X4	T4Ø.2X5	T4Ø.2X6
nicotinate	T49.4X1	T49.4X2	T49.4X3	T49.4X4	T49.4X5	T49.4X6
paraben	T49.ØX1	T49.ØX2	T49.ØX3	T49.ØX4	T49.ØX5	T49.ØX6
parafynol	T42.6X1	T42.6X2	T42.6X3	T42.6X4	T42.6X5	T42.6X6
parathion	T6Ø.ØX1	T6Ø.ØX2	T6Ø.ØX3	T6Ø.ØX4	—	—
peridol	T43.4X1	T43.4X2	T43.4X3	T43.4X4	T43.4X5	T43.4X6
phenidate	T43.631	T43.632	T43.633	T43.634	T43.635	T43.636
prednisolone	T38.ØX1	T38.ØX2	T38.ØX3	T38.ØX4	T38.ØX5	T38.ØX6
ENT agent	T49.6X1	T49.6X2	T49.6X3	T49.6X4	T49.6X5	T49.6X6
ophthalmic preparation	T49.5X1	T49.5X2	T49.5X3	T49.5X4	T49.5X5	T49.5X6
topical NEC	T49.ØX1	T49.ØX2	T49.ØX3	T49.ØX4	T49.ØX5	T49.ØX6
propylcarbinol	T51.3X1	T51.3X2	T51.3X3	T51.3X4	—	—
rosaniline NEC	T49.ØX1	T49.ØX2	T49.ØX3	T49.ØX4	T49.ØX5	T49.ØX6
salicylate	T49.2X1	T49.2X2	T49.2X3	T49.2X4	T49.2X5	T49.2X6
sulfate (fumes)	T59.891	T59.892	T59.893	T59.894	—	—
liquid	T52.8X1	T52.8X2	T52.8X3	T52.8X4	—	—
sulfonal	T42.6X1	T42.6X2	T42.6X3	T42.6X4	T42.6X5	T42.6X6
testosterone	T38.7X1	T38.7X2	T38.7X3	T38.7X4	T38.7X5	T38.7X6
thiouracil	T38.2X1	T38.2X2	T38.2X3	T38.2X4	T38.2X5	T38.2X6
Methylacetoxyprogesterone*	T38.5X1	T38.5X2	T38.5X3	T38.5X4	T38.5X5	T38.5X6
Methylamphetamine	T43.651	T43.652	T43.653	T43.654	T43.655	T43.656
Methylated spirit	T51.1X1	T51.1X2	T51.1X3	T51.1X4	—	—
Methylatropine nitrate	T44.3X1	T44.3X2	T44.3X3	T44.3X4	T44.3X5	T44.3X6
Methylbenactyzium bromide	T44.3X1	T44.3X2	T44.3X3	T44.3X4	T44.3X5	T44.3X6
Methylbenzethonium chloride	T49.ØX1	T49.ØX2	T49.ØX3	T49.ØX4	T49.ØX5	T49.ØX6
Methylcellulose	T47.4X1	T47.4X2	T47.4X3	T47.4X4	T47.4X5	T47.4X6
laxative	T47.4X1	T47.4X2	T47.4X3	T47.4X4	T47.4X5	T47.4X6
Methylchlorophenoxyacetic acid	T6Ø.3X1	T6Ø.3X2	T6Ø.3X3	T6Ø.3X4	—	—
Methyldopa	T46.5X1	T46.5X2	T46.5X3	T46.5X4	T46.5X5	T46.5X6
Methyldopate	T46.5X1	T46.5X2	T46.5X3	T46.5X4	T46.5X5	T46.5X6
Methylene						
blue	T5Ø.6X1	T5Ø.6X2	T5Ø.6X3	T5Ø.6X4	T5Ø.6X5	T5Ø.6X6
chloride or dichloride (solvent) NEC	T53.4X1	T53.4X2	T53.4X3	T53.4X4	—	—
Methylenedioxyamphetamine	T43.621	T43.622	T43.623	T43.624	T43.625	T43.626
Methylenedioxymeth-amphetamine	T43.641	T43.642	T43.643	T43.644	—	—
Methylergometrine	T48.ØX1	T48.ØX2	T48.ØX3	T48.ØX4	T48.ØX5	T48.ØX6
Methylergonovine	T48.ØX1	T48.ØX2	T48.ØX3	T48.ØX4	T48.ØX5	T48.ØX6
Methylestrenolone	T38.5X1	T38.5X2	T38.5X3	T38.5X4	T38.5X5	T38.5X6
Methylethyl cellulose	T5Ø.991	T5Ø.992	T5Ø.993	T5Ø.994	T5Ø.995	T5Ø.996
Methylhexabital	T42.3X1	T42.3X2	T42.3X3	T42.3X4	T42.3X5	T42.3X6
Methylmorphine	T4Ø.2X1	T4Ø.2X2	T4Ø.2X3	T4Ø.2X4	T4Ø.2X5	T4Ø.2X6
Methylparaben (ophthalmic)	T49.5X1	T49.5X2	T49.5X3	T49.5X4	T49.5X5	T49.5X6
Methylparafynol	T42.6X1	T42.6X2	T42.6X3	T42.6X4	T42.6X5	T42.6X6
Methylpentynol, methylpenthynol	T42.6X1	T42.6X2	T42.6X3	T42.6X4	T42.6X5	T42.6X6
Methylphenidate	T43.631	T43.632	T43.633	T43.634	T43.635	T43.636
Methylphenobarbital	T42.3X1	T42.3X2	T42.3X3	T42.3X4	T42.3X5	T42.3X6
Methylpolysiloxane	T47.1X1	T47.1X2	T47.1X3	T47.1X4	T47.1X5	T47.1X6
Methylprednisolone — *see* Methyl, prednisolone						
Methylrosaniline	T49.ØX1	T49.ØX2	T49.ØX3	T49.ØX4	T49.ØX5	T49.ØX6
Methylrosanilinium chloride	T49.ØX1	T49.ØX2	T49.ØX3	T49.ØX4	T49.ØX5	T49.ØX6
Methyltestosterone	T38.7X1	T38.7X2	T38.7X3	T38.7X4	T38.7X5	T38.7X6
Methylthionine chloride	T5Ø.6X1	T5Ø.6X2	T5Ø.6X3	T5Ø.6X4	T5Ø.6X5	T5Ø.6X6
Methylthioninium chloride	T5Ø.6X1	T5Ø.6X2	T5Ø.6X3	T5Ø.6X4	T5Ø.6X5	T5Ø.6X6
Methylthiouracil	T38.2X1	T38.2X2	T38.2X3	T38.2X4	T38.2X5	T38.2X6
Methyprylon	T42.6X1	T42.6X2	T42.6X3	T42.6X4	T42.6X5	T42.6X6
Methysergide	T46.5X1	T46.5X2	T46.5X3	T46.5X4	T46.5X5	T46.5X6
Metiamide	T47.1X1	T47.1X2	T47.1X3	T47.1X4	T47.1X5	T47.1X6
Meticillin	T36.ØX1	T36.ØX2	T36.ØX3	T36.ØX4	T36.ØX5	T36.ØX6

Substance	Poisoning, Accidental (unintentional)	Poisoning, Intentional Self-harm	Poisoning, Assault	Poisoning, Undetermined	Adverse Effect	Under-dosing
Meticrane	T5Ø.2X1	T5Ø.2X2	T5Ø.2X3	T5Ø.2X4	T5Ø.2X5	T5Ø.2X6
Metildigoxin	T46.ØX1	T46.ØX2	T46.ØX3	T46.ØX4	T46.ØX5	T46.ØX6
Metipranolol	T49.5X1	T49.5X2	T49.5X3	T49.5X4	T49.5X5	T49.5X6
Metirosine	T46.5X1	T46.5X2	T46.5X3	T46.5X4	T46.5X5	T46.5X6
Metisazone	T37.5X1	T37.5X2	T37.5X3	T37.5X4	T37.5X5	T37.5X6
Metixene	T44.3X1	T44.3X2	T44.3X3	T44.3X4	T44.3X5	T44.3X6
Metizoline	T48.5X1	T48.5X2	T48.5X3	T48.5X4	T48.5X5	T48.5X6
Metoclopramide	T45.ØX1	T45.ØX2	T45.ØX3	T45.ØX4	T45.ØX5	T45.ØX6
Metofenazate	T43.3X1	T43.3X2	T43.3X3	T43.3X4	T43.3X5	T43.3X6
Metofoline	T39.8X1	T39.8X2	T39.8X3	T39.8X4	T39.8X5	T39.8X6
Metolazone	T5Ø.2X1	T5Ø.2X2	T5Ø.2X3	T5Ø.2X4	T5Ø.2X5	T5Ø.2X6
Metopon	T4Ø.2X1	T4Ø.2X2	T4Ø.2X3	T4Ø.2X4	T4Ø.2X5	T4Ø.2X6
Metoprine	T45.1X1	T45.1X2	T45.1X3	T45.1X4	T45.1X5	T45.1X6
Metoprolol	T44.7X1	T44.7X2	T44.7X3	T44.7X4	T44.7X5	T44.7X6
Metrifonate	T6Ø.ØX1	T6Ø.ØX2	T6Ø.ØX3	T6Ø.ØX4	—	—
Metrizamide	T5Ø.8X1	T5Ø.8X2	T5Ø.8X3	T5Ø.8X4	T5Ø.8X5	T5Ø.8X6
Metrizoic acid	T5Ø.8X1	T5Ø.8X2	T5Ø.8X3	T5Ø.8X4	T5Ø.8X5	T5Ø.8X6
Metronidazole	T37.8X1	T37.8X2	T37.8X3	T37.8X4	T37.8X5	T37.8X6
Metycaine	T41.3X1	T41.3X2	T41.3X3	T41.3X4	T41.3X5	T41.3X6
infiltration (subcutaneous)	T41.3X1	T41.3X2	T41.3X3	T41.3X4	T41.3X5	T41.3X6
nerve block (peripheral) (plexus)	T41.3X1	T41.3X2	T41.3X3	T41.3X4	T41.3X5	T41.3X6
topical (surface)	T41.3X1	T41.3X2	T41.3X3	T41.3X4	T41.3X5	T41.3X6
Metyrapone	T5Ø.8X1	T5Ø.8X2	T5Ø.8X3	T5Ø.8X4	T5Ø.8X5	T5Ø.8X6
Mevacor*	T46.6X1	T46.6X2	T46.6X3	T46.6X4	T46.6X5	T46.6X6
Mevinphos	T6Ø.ØX1	T6Ø.ØX2	T6Ø.ØX3	T6Ø.ØX4	—	—
Mexazolam	T42.4X1	T42.4X2	T42.4X3	T42.4X4	T42.4X5	T42.4X6
Mexenone	T49.3X1	T49.3X2	T49.3X3	T49.3X4	T49.3X5	T49.3X6
Mexiletine	T46.2X1	T46.2X2	T46.2X3	T46.2X4	T46.2X5	T46.2X6
Mezereon	T62.2X1	T62.2X2	T62.2X3	T62.2X4	—	—
berries	T62.1X1	T62.1X2	T62.1X3	T62.1X4	—	—
Mezlocillin	T36.ØX1	T36.ØX2	T36.ØX3	T36.ØX4	T36.ØX5	T36.ØX6
Mianserin	T43.Ø21	T43.Ø22	T43.Ø23	T43.Ø24	T43.Ø25	T43.Ø26
Micatin	T49.ØX1	T49.ØX2	T49.ØX3	T49.ØX4	T49.ØX5	T49.ØX6
Miconazole	T49.ØX1	T49.ØX2	T49.ØX3	T49.ØX4	T49.ØX5	T49.ØX6
Micronomicin	T36.5X1	T36.5X2	T36.5X3	T36.5X4	T36.5X5	T36.5X6
Microzide*	T5Ø.2X1	T5Ø.2X2	T5Ø.2X3	T5Ø.2X4	T5Ø.2X5	T5Ø.2X6
Midazolam	T42.4X1	T42.4X2	T42.4X3	T42.4X4	T42.4X5	T42.4X6
Midecamycin	T36.3X1	T36.3X2	T36.3X3	T36.3X4	T36.3X5	T36.3X6
Mifepristone	T38.6X1	T38.6X2	T38.6X3	T38.6X4	T38.6X5	T38.6X6
Milk of magnesia	T47.1X1	T47.1X2	T47.1X3	T47.1X4	T47.1X5	T47.1X6
Millipede (tropical) (venomous)	T63.411	T63.412	T63.413	T63.414	—	—
Miltown	T43.591	T43.592	T43.593	T43.594	T43.595	T43.596
Milverine	T44.3X1	T44.3X2	T44.3X3	T44.3X4	T44.3X5	T44.3X6
Minaprine	T43.291	T43.292	T43.293	T43.294	T43.295	T43.296
Minaxolone	T41.291	T41.292	T41.293	T41.294	T41.295	T41.296
Mineral						
acids	T54.2X1	T54.2X2	T54.2X3	T54.2X4	—	—
oil (laxative)(medicinal)	T47.4X1	T47.4X2	T47.4X3	T47.4X4	T47.4X5	T47.4X6
emulsion	T47.2X1	T47.2X2	T47.2X3	T47.2X4	T47.2X5	T47.2X6
nonmedicinal	T52.ØX1	T52.ØX2	T52.ØX3	T52.ØX4	—	—
topical	T49.3X1	T49.3X2	T49.3X3	T49.3X4	T49.3X5	T49.3X6
salt NEC	T5Ø.3X1	T5Ø.3X2	T5Ø.3X3	T5Ø.3X4	T5Ø.3X5	T5Ø.3X6
spirits	T52.ØX1	T52.ØX2	T52.ØX3	T52.ØX4	—	—
Mineralocorticosteroid	T5Ø.ØX1	T5Ø.ØX2	T5Ø.ØX3	T5Ø.ØX4	T5Ø.ØX5	T5Ø.ØX6
Minocycline	T36.4X1	T36.4X2	T36.4X3	T36.4X4	T36.4X5	T36.4X6
Minoxidil	T46.7X1	T46.7X2	T46.7X3	T46.7X4	T46.7X5	T46.7X6
Miokamycin	T36.3X1	T36.3X2	T36.3X3	T36.3X4	T36.3X5	T36.3X6
Miotic drug	T49.5X1	T49.5X2	T49.5X3	T49.5X4	T49.5X5	T49.5X6
Mipafox	T6Ø.ØX1	T6Ø.ØX2	T6Ø.ØX3	T6Ø.ØX4	—	—
Mipomerson*	T46.6X1	T46.6X2	T46.6X3	T46.6X4	T46.6X5	T46.6X6
Mirex	T6Ø.1X1	T6Ø.1X2	T6Ø.1X3	T6Ø.1X4	—	—
Mirtazapine	T43.Ø21	T43.Ø22	T43.Ø23	T43.Ø24	T43.Ø25	T43.Ø26
Misonidazole	T37.3X1	T37.3X2	T37.3X3	T37.3X4	T37.3X5	T37.3X6
Misoprostol	T47.1X1	T47.1X2	T47.1X3	T47.1X4	T47.1X5	T47.1X6
Mithramycin	T45.1X1	T45.1X2	T45.1X3	T45.1X4	T45.1X5	T45.1X6
Mitobronitol	T45.1X1	T45.1X2	T45.1X3	T45.1X4	T45.1X5	T45.1X6
Mitoguazone	T45.1X1	T45.1X2	T45.1X3	T45.1X4	T45.1X5	T45.1X6
Mitolactol	T45.1X1	T45.1X2	T45.1X3	T45.1X4	T45.1X5	T45.1X6
Mitomycin	T45.1X1	T45.1X2	T45.1X3	T45.1X4	T45.1X5	T45.1X6
Mitopodozide	T45.1X1	T45.1X2	T45.1X3	T45.1X4	T45.1X5	T45.1X6
Mitotane	T45.1X1	T45.1X2	T45.1X3	T45.1X4	T45.1X5	T45.1X6
Mitoxantrone	T45.1X1	T45.1X2	T45.1X3	T45.1X4	T45.1X5	T45.1X6
Mivacurium chloride	T48.1X1	T48.1X2	T48.1X3	T48.1X4	T48.1X5	T48.1X6
Miyari bacteria	T47.6X1	T47.6X2	T47.6X3	T47.6X4	T47.6X5	T47.6X6
Moclobemide	T43.1X1	T43.1X2	T43.1X3	T43.1X4	T43.1X5	T43.1X6
Moderil	T46.5X1	T46.5X2	T46.5X3	T46.5X4	T46.5X5	T46.5X6
Mofebutazone	T39.2X1	T39.2X2	T39.2X3	T39.2X4	T39.2X5	T39.2X6
Mogadon — *see* Nitrazepam						
Molindone	T43.591	T43.592	T43.593	T43.594	T43.595	T43.596
Molsidomine	T46.3X1	T46.3X2	T46.3X3	T46.3X4	T46.3X5	T46.3X6
Mometasone	T49.ØX1	T49.ØX2	T49.ØX3	T49.ØX4	T49.ØX5	T49.ØX6

Substance	Poisoning, Accidental (unintentional)	Poisoning, Intentional Self-harm	Poisoning, Assault	Poisoning, Undetermined	Adverse Effect	Under-dosing
Monistat	T49.ØX1	T49.ØX2	T49.ØX3	T49.ØX4	T49.ØX5	T49.ØX6
Monkshood	T62.2X1	T62.2X2	T62.2X3	T62.2X4	—	—
Monoamine oxidase inhibitor NEC	T43.1X1	T43.1X2	T43.1X3	T43.1X4	T43.1X5	T43.1X6
hydrazine	T43.1X1	T43.1X2	T43.1X3	T43.1X4	T43.1X5	T43.1X6
Monobenzone	T49.4X1	T49.4X2	T49.4X3	T49.4X4	T49.4X5	T49.4X6
Monochloroacetic acid	T6Ø.3X1	T6Ø.3X2	T6Ø.3X3	T6Ø.3X4	—	—
Monochlorobenzene	T53.7X1	T53.7X2	T53.7X3	T53.7X4	—	—
Monoethanolamine	T46.8X1	T46.8X2	T46.8X3	T46.8X4	T46.8X5	T46.8X6
oleate	T46.8X1	T46.8X2	T46.8X3	T46.8X4	T46.8X5	T46.8X6
Monooctanoin	T5Ø.991	T5Ø.992	T5Ø.993	T5Ø.994	T5Ø.995	T5Ø.996
Monophenylbutazone	T39.2X1	T39.2X2	T39.2X3	T39.2X4	T39.2X5	T39.2X6
Monopril*	T46.4X1	T46.4X2	T46.4X3	T46.4X4	T46.4X5	T46.4X6
Monosodium glutamate	T65.891	T65.892	T65.893	T65.894	—	—
Monosulfiram	T49.ØX1	T49.ØX2	T49.ØX3	T49.ØX4	T49.ØX5	T49.ØX6
Monoxide, carbon — *see* Carbon, monoxide						
Monoxidine hydrochloride	T46.1X1	T46.1X2	T46.1X3	T46.1X4	T46.1X5	T46.1X6
Monuron	T6Ø.3X1	T6Ø.3X2	T6Ø.3X3	T6Ø.3X4	—	—
Moperone	T43.4X1	T43.4X2	T43.4X3	T43.4X4	T43.4X5	T43.4X6
Mopidamol	T45.1X1	T45.1X2	T45.1X3	T45.1X4	T45.1X5	T45.1X6
MOPP (mechloreth-amine + vincristine + prednisone + procarba-zine)	T45.1X1	T45.1X2	T45.1X3	T45.1X4	T45.1X5	T45.1X6
Morfin	T4Ø.2X1	T4Ø.2X2	T4Ø.2X3	T4Ø.2X4	T4Ø.2X5	T4Ø.2X6
Morinamide	T37.1X1	T37.1X2	T37.1X3	T37.1X4	T37.1X5	T37.1X6
Morning glory seeds	T4Ø.991	T4Ø.992	T4Ø.993	T4Ø.994	—	—
Moroxydine	T37.5X1	T37.5X2	T37.5X3	T37.5X4	T37.5X5	T37.5X6
Morphazinamide	T37.1X1	T37.1X2	T37.1X3	T37.1X4	T37.1X5	T37.1X6
Morphine	T4Ø.2X1	T4Ø.2X2	T4Ø.2X3	T4Ø.2X4	T4Ø.2X5	T4Ø.2X6
antagonist	T5Ø.7X1	T5Ø.7X2	T5Ø.7X3	T5Ø.7X4	T5Ø.7X5	T5Ø.7X6
Morpholinylethylmorphine	T4Ø.2X1	T4Ø.2X2	T4Ø.2X3	T4Ø.2X4	—	—
Morsuximide	T42.2X1	T42.2X2	T42.2X3	T42.2X4	T42.2X5	T42.2X6
Mosapramine	T43.591	T43.592	T43.593	T43.594	T43.595	T43.596
Moth balls — *see also* Pesticide	T6Ø.2X1	T6Ø.2X2	T6Ø.2X3	T6Ø.2X4	—	—
naphthalene	T6Ø.2X1	T6Ø.2X2	T6Ø.2X3	T6Ø.2X4	—	—
paradichlorobenzene	T6Ø.1X1	T6Ø.1X2	T6Ø.1X3	T6Ø.1X4	—	—
Motor exhaust gas	T58.Ø1	T58.Ø2	T58.Ø3	T58.Ø4	—	—
Motrin*	T39.311	T39.312	T39.313	T39.314	T39.315	T39.316
Mouthwash (antiseptic) (zinc chloride)	T49.6X1	T49.6X2	T49.6X3	T49.6X4	T49.6X5	T49.6X6
Moxastine	T45.ØX1	T45.ØX2	T45.ØX3	T45.ØX4	T45.ØX5	T45.ØX6
Moxaverine	T44.3X1	T44.3X2	T44.3X3	T44.3X4	T44.3X5	T44.3X6
Moxisylyte	T46.7X1	T46.7X2	T46.7X3	T46.7X4	T46.7X5	T46.7X6
Mucilage, plant	T47.4X1	T47.4X2	T47.4X3	T47.4X4	T47.4X5	T47.4X6
Mucolytic drug	T48.4X1	T48.4X2	T48.4X3	T48.4X4	T48.4X5	T48.4X6
Mucomyst	T48.4X1	T48.4X2	T48.4X3	T48.4X4	T48.4X5	T48.4X6
Mucous membrane agents (external)	T49.91	T49.92	T49.93	T49.94	T49.95	T49.96
specified NEC	T49.8X1	T49.8X2	T49.8X3	T49.8X4	T49.8X5	T49.8X6
Multaq*	T46.2X1	T46.2X2	T46.2X3	T46.2X4	T46.2X5	T46.2X6
Multiple unspecified drugs, medicaments and biological substances	T5Ø.911	T5Ø.912	T5Ø.913	T5Ø.914	T5Ø.915	T5Ø.916
Mumps						
immune globulin (human)	T5Ø.Z11	T5Ø.Z12	T5Ø.Z13	T5Ø.Z14	T5Ø.Z15	T5Ø.Z16
skin test antigen	T5Ø.8X1	T5Ø.8X2	T5Ø.8X3	T5Ø.8X4	T5Ø.8X5	T5Ø.8X6
vaccine	T5Ø.B91	T5Ø.B92	T5Ø.B93	T5Ø.B94	T5Ø.B95	T5Ø.B96
Mumpsvax	T5Ø.B91	T5Ø.B92	T5Ø.B93	T5Ø.B94	T5Ø.B95	T5Ø.B96
Mupirocin	T49.ØX1	T49.ØX2	T49.ØX3	T49.ØX4	T49.ØX5	T49.ØX6
Muriatic acid — *see* Hydrochloric acid						
Muromonab-CD3	T45.1X1	T45.1X2	T45.1X3	T45.1X4	T45.1X5	T45.1X6
Muscle-action drug NEC	T48.2Ø1	T48.2Ø2	T48.2Ø3	T48.2Ø4	T48.2Ø5	T48.2Ø6
Muscle affecting agents NEC	T48.2Ø1	T48.2Ø2	T48.2Ø3	T48.2Ø4	T48.2Ø5	T48.2Ø6
oxytocic	T48.ØX1	T48.ØX2	T48.ØX3	T48.ØX4	T48.ØX5	T48.ØX6
relaxants	T48.2Ø1	T48.2Ø2	T48.2Ø3	T48.2Ø4	T48.2Ø5	T48.2Ø6
central nervous system	T42.8X1	T42.8X2	T42.8X3	T42.8X4	T42.8X5	T42.8X6
skeletal	T48.1X1	T48.1X2	T48.1X3	T48.1X4	T48.1X5	T48.1X6
smooth	T44.3X1	T44.3X2	T44.3X3	T44.3X4	T44.3X5	T44.3X6
Muscle relaxant — *see* Relaxant, muscle						
Muscle-tone depressant, central NEC	T42.8X1	T42.8X2	T42.8X3	T42.8X4	T42.8X5	T42.8X6
specified NEC	T42.8X1	T42.8X2	T42.8X3	T42.8X4	T42.8X5	T42.8X6
Mushroom, noxious	T62.ØX1	T62.ØX2	T62.ØX3	T62.ØX4	—	—
Mussel, noxious	T61.781	T61.782	T61.783	T61.784	—	—
Mustard (emetic)	T47.7X1	T47.7X2	T47.7X3	T47.7X4	T47.7X5	T47.7X6
black	T47.7X1	T47.7X2	T47.7X3	T47.7X4	T47.7X5	T47.7X6
gas, not in war	T59.91	T59.92	T59.93	T59.94	—	—
nitrogen	T45.1X1	T45.1X2	T45.1X3	T45.1X4	T45.1X5	T45.1X6

*Optum Value-Add

Table of Drugs and Chemicals

Substance	Poisoning, Accidental (unintentional)	Poisoning, Intentional Self-harm	Poisoning, Assault	Poisoning, Undetermined	Adverse Effect	Under-dosing
Mustine	T45.1X1	T45.1X2	T45.1X3	T45.1X4	T45.1X5	T45.1X6
M-vac	T45.1X1	T45.1X2	T45.1X3	T45.1X4	T45.1X5	T45.1X6
Mycifradin	T36.5X1	T36.5X2	T36.5X3	T36.5X4	T36.5X5	T36.5X6
topical	T49.ØX1	T49.ØX2	T49.ØX3	T49.ØX4	T49.ØX5	T49.ØX6
Mycitracin	T36.8X1	T36.8X2	T36.8X3	T36.8X4	T36.8X5	T36.8X6
ophthalmic preparation	T49.5X1	T49.5X2	T49.5X3	T49.5X4	T49.5X5	T49.5X6
Mycostatin	T36.7X1	T36.7X2	T36.7X3	T36.7X4	T36.7X5	T36.7X6
topical	T49.ØX1	T49.ØX2	T49.ØX3	T49.ØX4	T49.ØX5	T49.ØX6
Mycotoxins	T64.81	T64.82	T64.83	T64.84	—	—
aflatoxin	T64.Ø1	T64.Ø2	T64.Ø3	T64.Ø4	—	—
specified NEC	T64.81	T64.82	T64.83	T64.84	—	—
Mydriacyl	T44.3X1	T44.3X2	T44.3X3	T44.3X4	T44.3X5	T44.3X6
Mydriatic drug	T49.5X1	T49.5X2	T49.5X3	T49.5X4	T49.5X5	T49.5X6
Myelobromal	T45.1X1	T45.1X2	T45.1X3	T45.1X4	T45.1X5	T45.1X6
Myleran	T45.1X1	T45.1X2	T45.1X3	T45.1X4	T45.1X5	T45.1X6
Myochrysin (e)	T39.2X1	T39.2X2	T39.2X3	T39.2X4	T39.2X5	T39.2X6
Myoneural blocking agents	T48.1X1	T48.1X2	T48.1X3	T48.1X4	T48.1X5	T48.1X6
Myrac*	T36.4X1	T36.4X2	T36.4X3	T36.4X4	T36.4X5	T36.4X6
Myralact	T49.ØX1	T49.ØX2	T49.ØX3	T49.ØX4	T49.ØX5	T49.ØX6
Myristica fragrans	T62.2X1	T62.2X2	T62.2X3	T62.2X4	—	—
Myristicin	T65.891	T65.892	T65.893	T65.894	—	—
Mysoline	T42.3X1	T42.3X2	T42.3X3	T42.3X4	T42.3X5	T42.3X6
Nabilone	T4Ø.711	T4Ø.712	T4Ø.713	T4Ø.714	T4Ø.715	T4Ø.716
Nabumetone	T39.391	T39.392	T39.393	T39.394	T39.395	T39.396
Nadolol	T44.7X1	T44.7X2	T44.7X3	T44.7X4	T44.7X5	T44.7X6
Nafcillin	T36.ØX1	T36.ØX2	T36.ØX3	T36.ØX4	T36.ØX5	T36.ØX6
Nafoxidine	T38.6X1	T38.6X2	T38.6X3	T38.6X4	T38.6X5	T38.6X6
Naftazone	T46.991	T46.992	T46.993	T46.994	T46.995	T46.996
Naftidrofuryl (oxalate)	T46.7X1	T46.7X2	T46.7X3	T46.7X4	T46.7X5	T46.7X6
Naftifine	T49.ØX1	T49.ØX2	T49.ØX3	T49.ØX4	T49.ØX5	T49.ØX6
Nail polish remover	T52.91	T52.92	T52.93	T52.94	—	—
Nalbuphine	T4Ø.491	T4Ø.492	T4Ø.493	T4Ø.494	T4Ø.495	T4Ø.496
Naled	T6Ø.ØX1	T6Ø.ØX2	T6Ø.ØX3	T6Ø.ØX4	—	—
Nalidixic acid	T37.8X1	T37.8X2	T37.8X3	T37.8X4	T37.8X5	T37.8X6
Nalorphine	T5Ø.7X1	T5Ø.7X2	T5Ø.7X3	T5Ø.7X4	T5Ø.7X5	T5Ø.7X6
Naloxone	T5Ø.7X1	T5Ø.7X2	T5Ø.7X3	T5Ø.7X4	T5Ø.7X5	T5Ø.7X6
Naltrexone	T5Ø.7X1	T5Ø.7X2	T5Ø.7X3	T5Ø.7X4	T5Ø.7X5	T5Ø.7X6
Namenda	T43.8X1	T43.8X2	T43.8X3	T43.8X4	T43.8X5	T43.8X6
Nandrolone	T38.7X1	T38.7X2	T38.7X3	T38.7X4	T38.7X5	T38.7X6
Naphazoline	T48.5X1	T48.5X2	T48.5X3	T48.5X4	T48.5X5	T48.5X6
Naphtha (painters') (petroleum)	T52.ØX1	T52.ØX2	T52.ØX3	T52.ØX4	—	—
solvent	T52.ØX1	T52.ØX2	T52.ØX3	T52.ØX4	—	—
vapor	T52.ØX1	T52.ØX2	T52.ØX3	T52.ØX4	—	—
Naphthalene (non-chlorinated)	T6Ø.2X1	T6Ø.2X2	T6Ø.2X3	T6Ø.2X4	—	—
chlorinated	T6Ø.1X1	T6Ø.1X2	T6Ø.1X3	T6Ø.1X4	—	—
vapor	T6Ø.1X1	T6Ø.1X2	T6Ø.1X3	T6Ø.1X4	—	—
insecticide or moth repellent	T6Ø.2X1	T6Ø.2X2	T6Ø.2X3	T6Ø.2X4	—	—
chlorinated	T6Ø.1X1	T6Ø.1X2	T6Ø.1X3	T6Ø.1X4	—	—
vapor	T6Ø.2X1	T6Ø.2X2	T6Ø.2X3	T6Ø.2X4	—	—
chlorinated	T6Ø.1X1	T6Ø.1X2	T6Ø.1X3	T6Ø.1X4	—	—
Naphthol	T65.891	T65.892	T65.893	T65.894	—	—
Naphthylamine	T65.891	T65.892	T65.893	T65.894	—	—
Naphthylthiourea (ANTU)	T6Ø.4X1	T6Ø.4X2	T6Ø.4X3	T6Ø.4X4	—	—
Naprosyn — *see* Naproxen						
Naproxen	T39.311	T39.312	T39.313	T39.314	T39.315	T39.316
Narcotic (drug)	T4Ø.6Ø1	T4Ø.6Ø2	T4Ø.6Ø3	T4Ø.6Ø4	T4Ø.6Ø5	T4Ø.6Ø6
analgesic NEC	T4Ø.6Ø1	T4Ø.6Ø2	T4Ø.6Ø3	T4Ø.6Ø4	T4Ø.6Ø5	T4Ø.6Ø6
antagonist	T5Ø.7X1	T5Ø.7X2	T5Ø.7X3	T5Ø.7X4	T5Ø.7X5	T5Ø.7X6
specified NEC	T4Ø.691	T4Ø.692	T4Ø.693	T4Ø.694	T4Ø.695	T4Ø.696
synthetic	T4Ø.491	T4Ø.492	T4Ø.493	T4Ø.494	T4Ø.495	T4Ø.496
Narcotine	T48.3X1	T48.3X2	T48.3X3	T48.3X4	T48.3X5	T48.3X6
Nardil	T43.1X1	T43.1X2	T43.1X3	T43.1X4	T43.1X5	T43.1X6
Nasacort*	T49.5X1	T49.5X2	T49.5X3	T49.5X4	T49.5X5	T49.5X6
Nasal drug NEC	T49.6X1	T49.6X2	T49.6X3	T49.6X4	T49.6X5	T49.6X6
Natamycin	T49.ØX1	T49.ØX2	T49.ØX3	T49.ØX4	T49.ØX5	T49.ØX6
Natrium cyanide — *see* Cyanide(s)						
Natural						
blood (product)	T45.8X1	T45.8X2	T45.8X3	T45.8X4	T45.8X5	T45.8X6
gas (piped)	T59.891	T59.892	T59.893	T59.894	—	—
incomplete combustion	T58.11	T58.12	T58.13	T58.14	—	—
Nealbarbital	T42.3X1	T42.3X2	T42.3X3	T42.3X4	T42.3X5	T42.3X6
Nectadon	T48.3X1	T48.3X2	T48.3X3	T48.3X4	T48.3X5	T48.3X6
Nedocromil	T48.6X1	T48.6X2	T48.6X3	T48.6X4	T48.6X5	T48.6X6
Nefopam	T39.8X1	T39.8X2	T39.8X3	T39.8X4	T39.8X5	T39.8X6
Nematocyst (sting)	T63.691	T63.692	T63.693	T63.694	—	—
Nembutal	T42.3X1	T42.3X2	T42.3X3	T42.3X4	T42.3X5	T42.3X6
Nemonapride	T43.591	T43.592	T43.593	T43.594	T43.595	T43.596
Neoarsphenamine	T37.8X1	T37.8X2	T37.8X3	T37.8X4	T37.8X5	T37.8X6

Substance	Poisoning, Accidental (unintentional)	Poisoning, Intentional Self-harm	Poisoning, Assault	Poisoning, Undetermined	Adverse Effect	Under-dosing
Neocinchophen	T5Ø.4X1	T5Ø.4X2	T5Ø.4X3	T5Ø.4X4	T5Ø.4X5	T5Ø.4X6
Neomycin (derivatives)	T36.5X1	T36.5X2	T36.5X3	T36.5X4	T36.5X5	T36.5X6
with						
bacitracin	T49.ØX1	T49.ØX2	T49.ØX3	T49.ØX4	T49.ØX5	T49.ØX6
neostigmine	T44.ØX1	T44.ØX2	T44.ØX3	T44.ØX4	T44.ØX5	T44.ØX6
ENT agent	T49.6X1	T49.6X2	T49.6X3	T49.6X4	T49.6X5	T49.6X6
ophthalmic preparation	T49.5X1	T49.5X2	T49.5X3	T49.5X4	T49.5X5	T49.5X6
topical NEC	T49.ØX1	T49.ØX2	T49.ØX3	T49.ØX4	T49.ØX5	T49.ØX6
Neonal	T42.3X1	T42.3X2	T42.3X3	T42.3X4	T42.3X5	T42.3X6
Neopham*	T5Ø.3X1	T5Ø.3X2	T5Ø.3X3	T5Ø.3X4	T5Ø.3X5	T5Ø.3X6
Neoprontosil	T37.ØX1	T37.ØX2	T37.ØX3	T37.ØX4	T37.ØX5	T37.ØX6
Neosalvarsan	T37.8X1	T37.8X2	T37.8X3	T37.8X4	T37.8X5	T37.8X6
Neosilversalvarsan	T37.8X1	T37.8X2	T37.8X3	T37.8X4	T37.8X5	T37.8X6
Neosporin	T36.8X1	T36.8X2	T36.8X3	T36.8X4	T36.8X5	T36.8X6
ENT agent	T49.6X1	T49.6X2	T49.6X3	T49.6X4	T49.6X5	T49.6X6
opthalmic preparation	T49.5X1	T49.5X2	T49.5X3	T49.5X4	T49.5X5	T49.5X6
topical NEC	T49.ØX1	T49.ØX2	T49.ØX3	T49.ØX4	T49.ØX5	T49.ØX6
Neostigmine bromide	T44.ØX1	T44.ØX2	T44.ØX3	T44.ØX4	T44.ØX5	T44.ØX6
Neraval	T42.3X1	T42.3X2	T42.3X3	T42.3X4	T42.3X5	T42.3X6
Neravan	T42.3X1	T42.3X2	T42.3X3	T42.3X4	T42.3X5	T42.3X6
Nerium oleander	T62.2X1	T62.2X2	T62.2X3	T62.2X4	—	—
Nerlynx*	T45.1X1	T45.1X2	T45.1X3	T45.1X4	T45.1X5	T45.1X6
Nerve gas, not in war	T59.91	T59.92	T59.93	T59.94	—	—
Nesacaine	T41.3X1	T41.3X2	T41.3X3	T41.3X4	T41.3X5	T41.3X6
infiltration (subcutaneous)	T41.3X1	T41.3X2	T41.3X3	T41.3X4	T41.3X5	T41.3X6
nerve block (peripheral) (plexus)	T41.3X1	T41.3X2	T41.3X3	T41.3X4	T41.3X5	T41.3X6
Netilmicin	T36.5X1	T36.5X2	T36.5X3	T36.5X4	T36.5X5	T36.5X6
Neurobarb	T42.3X1	T42.3X2	T42.3X3	T42.3X4	T42.3X5	T42.3X6
Neuroleptic drug NEC	T43.5Ø1	T43.5Ø2	T43.5Ø3	T43.5Ø4	T43.5Ø5	T43.5Ø6
Neuromuscular blocking drug	T48.1X1	T48.1X2	T48.1X3	T48.1X4	T48.1X5	T48.1X6
Neutral insulin injection	T38.3X1	T38.3X2	T38.3X3	T38.3X4	T38.3X5	T38.3X6
Neutral spirits	T51.ØX1	T51.ØX2	T51.ØX3	T51.ØX4	—	—
beverage	T51.ØX1	T51.ØX2	T51.ØX3	T51.ØX4	—	—
Niacin	T46.7X1	T46.7X2	T46.7X3	T46.7X4	T46.7X5	T46.7X6
Niacinamide	T45.2X1	T45.2X2	T45.2X3	T45.2X4	T45.2X5	T45.2X6
Nialamide	T43.1X1	T43.1X2	T43.1X3	T43.1X4	T43.1X5	T43.1X6
Niaprazine	T42.6X1	T42.6X2	T42.6X3	T42.6X4	T42.6X5	T42.6X6
Nicametate	T46.7X1	T46.7X2	T46.7X3	T46.7X4	T46.7X5	T46.7X6
Nicardipine	T46.1X1	T46.1X2	T46.1X3	T46.1X4	T46.1X5	T46.1X6
Nicergoline	T46.7X1	T46.7X2	T46.7X3	T46.7X4	T46.7X5	T46.7X6
Nickel (carbonyl) (tetra-carbonyl) (fumes) (vapor)	T56.891	T56.892	T56.893	T56.894	—	—
Nickelocene	T56.891	T56.892	T56.893	T56.894	—	—
Niclosamide	T37.4X1	T37.4X2	T37.4X3	T37.4X4	T37.4X5	T37.4X6
Nicofuranose	T46.7X1	T46.7X2	T46.7X3	T46.7X4	T46.7X5	T46.7X6
Nicomorphine	T4Ø.2X1	T4Ø.2X2	T4Ø.2X3	T4Ø.2X4	—	—
Nicorandil	T46.3X1	T46.3X2	T46.3X3	T46.3X4	T46.3X5	T46.3X6
Nicotiana (plant)	T62.2X1	T62.2X2	T62.2X3	T62.2X4	—	—
Nicotinamide	T45.2X1	T45.2X2	T45.2X3	T45.2X4	T45.2X5	T45.2X6
Nicotine (insecticide) (spray) (sulfate) **NEC**	T6Ø.2X1	T6Ø.2X2	T6Ø.2X3	T6Ø.2X4	—	—
from tobacco	T65.291	T65.292	T65.293	T65.294	—	—
cigarettes	T65.221	T65.222	T65.223	T65.224	—	—
not insecticide	T65.291	T65.292	T65.293	T65.294	—	—
Nicotinic acid	T46.7X1	T46.7X2	T46.7X3	T46.7X4	T46.7X5	T46.7X6
Nicotinyl alcohol	T46.7X1	T46.7X2	T46.7X3	T46.7X4	T46.7X5	T46.7X6
Nicoumalone	T45.511	T45.512	T45.513	T45.514	T45.515	T45.516
Nifedipine	T46.1X1	T46.1X2	T46.1X3	T46.1X4	T46.1X5	T46.1X6
Nifenazone	T39.2X1	T39.2X2	T39.2X3	T39.2X4	T39.2X5	T39.2X6
Nifuraldezone	T37.91	T37.92	T37.93	T37.94	T37.95	T37.96
Nifuratel	T37.8X1	T37.8X2	T37.8X3	T37.8X4	T37.8X5	T37.8X6
Nifurtimox	T37.3X1	T37.3X2	T37.3X3	T37.3X4	T37.3X5	T37.3X6
Nifurtoinol	T37.8X1	T37.8X2	T37.8X3	T37.8X4	T37.8X5	T37.8X6
Nightshade, deadly (solanum) — *see also* Belladonna	T62.2X1	T62.2X2	T62.2X3	T62.2X4	—	—
berry	T62.1X1	T62.1X2	T62.1X3	T62.1X4	—	—
Nikethamide	T5Ø.7X1	T5Ø.7X2	T5Ø.7X3	T5Ø.7X4	T5Ø.7X5	T5Ø.7X6
Nilstat	T36.7X1	T36.7X2	T36.7X3	T36.7X4	T36.7X5	T36.7X6
topical	T49.ØX1	T49.ØX2	T49.ØX3	T49.ØX4	T49.ØX5	T49.ØX6
Nilutamide	T38.6X1	T38.6X2	T38.6X3	T38.6X4	T38.6X5	T38.6X6
Nimesulide	T39.391	T39.392	T39.393	T39.394	T39.395	T39.396
Nimetazepam	T42.4X1	T42.4X2	T42.4X3	T42.4X4	T42.4X5	T42.4X6
Nimodipine	T46.1X1	T46.1X2	T46.1X3	T46.1X4	T46.1X5	T46.1X6
Nimorazole	T37.3X1	T37.3X2	T37.3X3	T37.3X4	T37.3X5	T37.3X6
Nimustine	T45.1X1	T45.1X2	T45.1X3	T45.1X4	T45.1X5	T45.1X6
Nipent*	T45.1X1	T45.1X2	T45.1X3	T45.1X4	T45.1X5	T45.1X6
Niridazole	T37.4X1	T37.4X2	T37.4X3	T37.4X4	T37.4X5	T37.4X6
Nisentil	T4Ø.2X1	T4Ø.2X2	T4Ø.2X3	T4Ø.2X4	T4Ø.2X5	T4Ø.2X6
Nisoldipine	T46.1X1	T46.1X2	T46.1X3	T46.1X4	T46.1X5	T46.1X6
Nitramine	T65.3X1	T65.3X2	T65.3X3	T65.3X4	—	—
Nitrate, organic	T46.3X1	T46.3X2	T46.3X3	T46.3X4	T46.3X5	T46.3X6

Mustine — Nitrate, organic

Substance	Poisoning, Accidental (unintentional)	Poisoning, Intentional Self-harm	Poisoning, Assault	Poisoning, Undetermined	Adverse Effect	Under-dosing
Nitrazepam	T42.4X1	T42.4X2	T42.4X3	T42.4X4	T42.4X5	T42.4X6
Nitrefazole	T5Ø.6X1	T5Ø.6X2	T5Ø.6X3	T5Ø.6X4	T5Ø.6X5	T5Ø.6X6
Nitrendipine	T46.1X1	T46.1X2	T46.1X3	T46.1X4	T46.1X5	T46.1X6
Nitric						
acid (liquid)	T54.2X1	T54.2X2	T54.2X3	T54.2X4	—	—
vapor	T59.891	T59.892	T59.893	T59.894	—	—
oxide (gas)	T59.ØX1	T59.ØX2	T59.ØX3	T59.ØX4	—	—
Nitrimidazine	T37.3X1	T37.3X2	T37.3X3	T37.3X4	T37.3X5	T37.3X6
Nitrite, amyl (medicinal) (vapor)	T46.3X1	T46.3X2	T46.3X3	T46.3X4	T46.3X5	T46.3X6
Nitroaniline	T65.3X1	T65.3X2	T65.3X3	T65.3X4	—	—
vapor	T59.891	T59.892	T59.893	T59.894	—	—
Nitrobenzene, nitrobenzol	T65.3X1	T65.3X2	T65.3X3	T65.3X4	—	—
vapor	T65.3X1	T65.3X2	T65.3X3	T65.3X4	—	—
Nitrocellulose	T65.891	T65.892	T65.893	T65.894	—	—
lacquer	T65.891	T65.892	T65.893	T65.894	—	—
Nitrodiphenyl	T65.3X1	T65.3X2	T65.3X3	T65.3X4	—	—
Nitrofural	T49.ØX1	T49.ØX2	T49.ØX3	T49.ØX4	T49.ØX5	T49.ØX6
Nitrofurantoin	T37.8X1	T37.8X2	T37.8X3	T37.8X4	T37.8X5	T37.8X6
Nitrofurazone	T49.ØX1	T49.ØX2	T49.ØX3	T49.ØX4	T49.ØX5	T49.ØX6
Nitrogen	T59.ØX1	T59.ØX2	T59.ØX3	T59.ØX4	—	—
mustard	T45.1X1	T45.1X2	T45.1X3	T45.1X4	T45.1X5	T45.1X6
Nitroglycerin, nitroglycerol (medicinal)	T46.3X1	T46.3X2	T46.3X3	T46.3X4	T46.3X5	T46.3X6
nonmedicinal	T65.5X1	T65.5X2	T65.5X3	T65.5X4	—	—
fumes	T65.5X1	T65.5X2	T65.5X3	T65.5X4	—	—
Nitroglycol	T52.3X1	T52.3X2	T52.3X3	T52.3X4	—	—
Nitrohydrochloric acid	T54.2X1	T54.2X2	T54.2X3	T54.2X4	—	—
Nitromersol	T49.ØX1	T49.ØX2	T49.ØX3	T49.ØX4	T49.ØX5	T49.ØX6
Nitronaphthalene	T65.891	T65.892	T65.893	T65.894	—	—
Nitrophenol	T54.ØX1	T54.ØX2	T54.ØX3	T54.ØX4	—	—
Nitropropane	T52.8X1	T52.8X2	T52.8X3	T52.8X4	—	—
Nitroprusside	T46.5X1	T46.5X2	T46.5X3	T46.5X4	T46.5X5	T46.5X6
Nitrosodimethylamine	T65.3X1	T65.3X2	T65.3X3	T65.3X4	—	—
Nitrothiazol	T37.4X1	T37.4X2	T37.4X3	T37.4X4	T37.4X5	T37.4X6
Nitrotoluene, nitrotoluol	T65.3X1	T65.3X2	T65.3X3	T65.3X4	—	—
vapor	T65.3X1	T65.3X2	T65.3X3	T65.3X4	—	—
Nitrous						
acid (liquid)	T54.2X1	T54.2X2	T54.2X3	T54.2X4	—	—
fumes	T59.891	T59.892	T59.893	T59.894	—	—
ether spirit	T46.3X1	T46.3X2	T46.3X3	T46.3X4	T46.3X5	T46.3X6
oxide	T41.ØX1	T41.ØX2	T41.ØX3	T41.ØX4	T41.ØX5	T41.ØX6
Nitroxoline	T37.8X1	T37.8X2	T37.8X3	T37.8X4	T37.8X5	T37.8X6
Nitrozone	T49.ØX1	T49.ØX2	T49.ØX3	T49.ØX4	T49.ØX5	T49.ØX6
Nizatidine	T47.ØX1	T47.ØX2	T47.ØX3	T47.ØX4	T47.ØX5	T47.ØX6
Nizofenone	T43.8X1	T43.8X2	T43.8X3	T43.8X4	T43.8X5	T43.8X6
Noctec	T42.6X1	T42.6X2	T42.6X3	T42.6X4	T42.6X5	T42.6X6
No Doz*	T43.611	T43.612	T43.613	T43.614	T43.615	T43.616
Noludar	T42.6X1	T42.6X2	T42.6X3	T42.6X4	T42.6X5	T42.6X6
Nomegestrol	T38.5X1	T38.5X2	T38.5X3	T38.5X4	T38.5X5	T38.5X6
Nomifensine	T43.291	T43.292	T43.293	T43.294	T43.295	T43.296
Nonoxinol	T49.8X1	T49.8X2	T49.8X3	T49.8X4	T49.8X5	T49.8X6
Nonylphenoxy (polyethoxyethanol)	T49.8X1	T49.8X2	T49.8X3	T49.8X4	T49.8X5	T49.8X6
Noptil	T42.3X1	T42.3X2	T42.3X3	T42.3X4	T42.3X5	T42.3X6
Noradrenaline	T44.4X1	T44.4X2	T44.4X3	T44.4X4	T44.4X5	T44.4X6
Noramidopyrine	T39.2X1	T39.2X2	T39.2X3	T39.2X4	T39.2X5	T39.2X6
methanesulfonate sodium	T39.2X1	T39.2X2	T39.2X3	T39.2X4	T39.2X5	T39.2X6
Norbormide	T6Ø.4X1	T6Ø.4X2	T6Ø.4X3	T6Ø.4X4	—	—
Nordazepam	T42.4X1	T42.4X2	T42.4X3	T42.4X4	T42.4X5	T42.4X6
Norepinephrine	T44.4X1	T44.4X2	T44.4X3	T44.4X4	T44.4X5	T44.4X6
Norethandrolone	T38.7X1	T38.7X2	T38.7X3	T38.7X4	T38.7X5	T38.7X6
Norethindrone	T38.4X1	T38.4X2	T38.4X3	T38.4X4	T38.4X5	T38.4X6
Norethisterone (acetate) (enantate)	T38.4X1	T38.4X2	T38.4X3	T38.4X4	T38.4X5	T38.4X6
with ethinylestradiol	T38.5X1	T38.5X2	T38.5X3	T38.5X4	T38.5X5	T38.5X6
Noretynodrel	T38.5X1	T38.5X2	T38.5X3	T38.5X4	T38.5X5	T38.5X6
Norfenefrine	T44.4X1	T44.4X2	T44.4X3	T44.4X4	T44.4X5	T44.4X6
Norfloxacin	T36.8X1	T36.8X2	T36.8X3	T36.8X4	T36.8X5	T36.8X6
Norgestrel	T38.4X1	T38.4X2	T38.4X3	T38.4X4	T38.4X5	T38.4X6
Norgestrienone	T38.4X1	T38.4X2	T38.4X3	T38.4X4	T38.4X5	T38.4X6
Norlestrin	T38.4X1	T38.4X2	T38.4X3	T38.4X4	T38.4X5	T38.4X6
Norlutin	T38.4X1	T38.4X2	T38.4X3	T38.4X4	T38.4X5	T38.4X6
Normal serum albumin (human), salt-poor	T45.8X1	T45.8X2	T45.8X3	T45.8X4	T45.8X5	T45.8X6
Normethandrone	T38.5X1	T38.5X2	T38.5X3	T38.5X4	T38.5X5	T38.5X6
Normison — *see* Benzodiazepines						
Normorphine	T4Ø.2X1	T4Ø.2X2	T4Ø.2X3	T4Ø.2X4	—	—
Norpseudoephedrine	T5Ø.5X1	T5Ø.5X2	T5Ø.5X3	T5Ø.5X4	T5Ø.5X5	T5Ø.5X6
Nortestosterone (furanpropionate)	T38.7X1	T38.7X2	T38.7X3	T38.7X4	T38.7X5	T38.7X6
Nortriptyline	T43.Ø11	T43.Ø12	T43.Ø13	T43.Ø14	T43.Ø15	T43.Ø16
Norvasc*	T46.1X1	T46.1X2	T46.1X3	T46.1X4	T46.1X5	T46.1X6
Noscapine	T48.3X1	T48.3X2	T48.3X3	T48.3X4	T48.3X5	T48.3X6
Nose preparations	T49.6X1	T49.6X2	T49.6X3	T49.6X4	T49.6X5	T49.6X6
Novobiocin	T36.5X1	T36.5X2	T36.5X3	T36.5X4	T36.5X5	T36.5X6
Novocain (infiltration) (topical)	T41.3X1	T41.3X2	T41.3X3	T41.3X4	T41.3X5	T41.3X6
nerve block (peripheral) (plexus)	T41.3X1	T41.3X2	T41.3X3	T41.3X4	T41.3X5	T41.3X6
spinal	T41.3X1	T41.3X2	T41.3X3	T41.3X4	T41.3X5	T41.3X6
Noxious foodstuff	T62.91	T62.92	T62.93	T62.94	—	—
specified NEC	T62.8X1	T62.8X2	T62.8X3	T62.8X4	—	—
Noxiptiline	T43.Ø11	T43.Ø12	T43.Ø13	T43.Ø14	T43.Ø15	T43.Ø16
Noxytiolin	T49.ØX1	T49.ØX2	T49.ØX3	T49.ØX4	T49.ØX5	T49.ØX6
NPH Iletin (insulin)	T38.3X1	T38.3X2	T38.3X3	T38.3X4	T38.3X5	T38.3X6
Numorphan	T4Ø.2X1	T4Ø.2X2	T4Ø.2X3	T4Ø.2X4	T4Ø.2X5	T4Ø.2X6
Nunol	T42.3X1	T42.3X2	T42.3X3	T42.3X4	T42.3X5	T42.3X6
Nupercaine (spinal anesthetic)	T41.3X1	T41.3X2	T41.3X3	T41.3X4	T41.3X5	T41.3X6
topical (surface)	T41.3X1	T41.3X2	T41.3X3	T41.3X4	T41.3X5	T41.3X6
Nutmeg oil (liniment)	T49.3X1	T49.3X2	T49.3X3	T49.3X4	T49.3X5	T49.3X6
Nutrilipid*	T5Ø.991	T5Ø.992	T5Ø.993	T5Ø.994	T5Ø.995	T5Ø.996
Nutritional supplement	T5Ø.9Ø1	T5Ø.9Ø2	T5Ø.9Ø3	T5Ø.9Ø4	T5Ø.9Ø5	T5Ø.9Ø6
Nux vomica	T65.1X1	T65.1X2	T65.1X3	T65.1X4	—	—
Nydrazid	T37.1X1	T37.1X2	T37.1X3	T37.1X4	T37.1X5	T37.1X6
Nylidrin	T46.7X1	T46.7X2	T46.7X3	T46.7X4	T46.7X5	T46.7X6
Nystatin	T36.7X1	T36.7X2	T36.7X3	T36.7X4	T36.7X5	T36.7X6
topical	T49.ØX1	T49.ØX2	T49.ØX3	T49.ØX4	T49.ØX5	T49.ØX6
Nytol	T45.ØX1	T45.ØX2	T45.ØX3	T45.ØX4	T45.ØX5	T45.ØX6
Obidoxime chloride	T5Ø.6X1	T5Ø.6X2	T5Ø.6X3	T5Ø.6X4	T5Ø.6X5	T5Ø.6X6
Octafonium (chloride)	T49.3X1	T49.3X2	T49.3X3	T49.3X4	T49.3X5	T49.3X6
Octamethyl pyrophosphoramide	T6Ø.ØX1	T6Ø.ØX2	T6Ø.ØX3	T6Ø.ØX4	—	—
Octanoin	T5Ø.991	T5Ø.992	T5Ø.993	T5Ø.994	T5Ø.995	T5Ø.996
Octatropine methylbromide	T44.3X1	T44.3X2	T44.3X3	T44.3X4	T44.3X5	T44.3X6
Octotiamine	T45.2X1	T45.2X2	T45.2X3	T45.2X4	T45.2X5	T45.2X6
Octoxinol (9)	T49.8X1	T49.8X2	T49.8X3	T49.8X4	T49.8X5	T49.8X6
Octreotide	T38.991	T38.992	T38.993	T38.994	T38.995	T38.996
Octyl nitrite	T46.3X1	T46.3X2	T46.3X3	T46.3X4	T46.3X5	T46.3X6
Oestradiol	T38.5X1	T38.5X2	T38.5X3	T38.5X4	T38.5X5	T38.5X6
Oestriol	T38.5X1	T38.5X2	T38.5X3	T38.5X4	T38.5X5	T38.5X6
Oestrogen	T38.5X1	T38.5X2	T38.5X3	T38.5X4	T38.5X5	T38.5X6
Oestrone	T38.5X1	T38.5X2	T38.5X3	T38.5X4	T38.5X5	T38.5X6
Ofloxacin	T36.8X1	T36.8X2	T36.8X3	T36.8X4	T36.8X5	T36.8X6
Oil (of)	T65.891	T65.892	T65.893	T65.894	—	—
bitter almond	T62.8X1	T62.8X2	T62.8X3	T62.8X4	—	—
cloves	T49.7X1	T49.7X2	T49.7X3	T49.7X4	T49.7X5	T49.7X6
colors	T65.6X1	T65.6X2	T65.6X3	T65.6X4	—	—
fumes	T59.891	T59.892	T59.893	T59.894	—	—
lubricating	T52.ØX1	T52.ØX2	T52.ØX3	T52.ØX4	—	—
Niobe	T52.8X1	T52.8X2	T52.8X3	T52.8X4	—	—
vitriol (liquid)	T54.2X1	T54.2X2	T54.2X3	T54.2X4	—	—
fumes	T54.2X1	T54.2X2	T54.2X3	T54.2X4	—	—
wintergreen (bitter) NEC	T49.3X1	T49.3X2	T49.3X3	T49.3X4	T49.3X5	T49.3X6
Oily preparation (for skin)	T49.3X1	T49.3X2	T49.3X3	T49.3X4	T49.3X5	T49.3X6
Ointment NEC	T49.3X1	T49.3X2	T49.3X3	T49.3X4	T49.3X5	T49.3X6
Olanzapine	T43.591	T43.592	T43.593	T43.594	T43.595	T43.596
Oleander	T62.2X1	T62.2X2	T62.2X3	T62.2X4	—	—
Oleandomycin	T36.3X1	T36.3X2	T36.3X3	T36.3X4	T36.3X5	T36.3X6
Oleandrin	T46.ØX1	T46.ØX2	T46.ØX3	T46.ØX4	T46.ØX5	T46.ØX6
Oleic acid	T46.6X1	T46.6X2	T46.6X3	T46.6X4	T46.6X5	T46.6X6
Oleovitamin A	T45.2X1	T45.2X2	T45.2X3	T45.2X4	T45.2X5	T45.2X6
Oleum ricini	T47.2X1	T47.2X2	T47.2X3	T47.2X4	T47.2X5	T47.2X6
Olive oil (medicinal) **NEC**	T47.4X1	T47.4X2	T47.4X3	T47.4X4	T47.4X5	T47.4X6
Olivomycin	T45.1X1	T45.1X2	T45.1X3	T45.1X4	T45.1X5	T45.1X6
Olodaterol*	T48.6X1	T48.6X2	T48.6X3	T48.6X4	T48.6X5	T48.6X6
Olsalazine	T47.8X1	T47.8X2	T47.8X3	T47.8X4	T47.8X5	T47.8X6
Omeprazole	T47.1X1	T47.1X2	T47.1X3	T47.1X4	T47.1X5	T47.1X6
OMPA	T6Ø.ØX1	T6Ø.ØX2	T6Ø.ØX3	T6Ø.ØX4	—	—
Oncovin	T45.1X1	T45.1X2	T45.1X3	T45.1X4	T45.1X5	T45.1X6
Ondansetron	T45.ØX1	T45.ØX2	T45.ØX3	T45.ØX4	T45.ØX5	T45.ØX6
Ophthaine	T41.3X1	T41.3X2	T41.3X3	T41.3X4	T41.3X5	T41.3X6
Ophthetic	T41.3X1	T41.3X2	T41.3X3	T41.3X4	T41.3X5	T41.3X6
Opiate NEC	T4Ø.6Ø1	T4Ø.6Ø2	T4Ø.6Ø3	T4Ø.6Ø4	T4Ø.6Ø5	T4Ø.6Ø6
antagonists	T5Ø.7X1	T5Ø.7X2	T5Ø.7X3	T5Ø.7X4	T5Ø.7X5	T5Ø.7X6
Opioid NEC	T4Ø.2X1	T4Ø.2X2	T4Ø.2X3	T4Ø.2X4	T4Ø.2X5	T4Ø.2X6
Opipramol	T43.Ø11	T43.Ø12	T43.Ø13	T43.Ø14	T43.Ø15	T43.Ø16
Opium alkaloids (total)	T4Ø.ØX1	T4Ø.ØX2	T4Ø.ØX3	T4Ø.ØX4	T4Ø.ØX5	T4Ø.ØX6
standardized powdered	T4Ø.ØX1	T4Ø.ØX2	T4Ø.ØX3	T4Ø.ØX4	T4Ø.ØX5	T4Ø.ØX6
tincture (camphorated)	T4Ø.ØX1	T4Ø.ØX2	T4Ø.ØX3	T4Ø.ØX4	T4Ø.ØX5	T4Ø.ØX6
Optivar*	T49.5X1	T49.5X2	T49.5X3	T49.5X4	T49.5X5	T49.5X6
Oracon	T38.4X1	T38.4X2	T38.4X3	T38.4X4	T38.4X5	T38.4X6
Oragrafin	T5Ø.8X1	T5Ø.8X2	T5Ø.8X3	T5Ø.8X4	T5Ø.8X5	T5Ø.8X6

Substance	Poisoning, Accidental (unintentional)	Poisoning, Intentional Self-harm	Poisoning, Assault	Poisoning, Undetermined	Adverse Effect	Under-dosing
Oral contraceptives	T38.4X1	T38.4X2	T38.4X3	T38.4X4	T38.4X5	T38.4X6
Oral rehydration salts	T5Ø.3X1	T5Ø.3X2	T5Ø.3X3	T5Ø.3X4	T5Ø.3X5	T5Ø.3X6
Orazamide	T5Ø.991	T5Ø.992	T5Ø.993	T5Ø.994	T5Ø.995	T5Ø.996
Orciprenaline	T48.291	T48.292	T48.293	T48.294	T48.295	T48.296
Organidin	T48.4X1	T48.4X2	T48.4X3	T48.4X4	T48.4X5	T48.4X6
Organonitrate NEC	T46.3X1	T46.3X2	T46.3X3	T46.3X4	T46.3X5	T46.3X6
Organophosphates	T6Ø.ØX1	T6Ø.ØX2	T6Ø.ØX3	T6Ø.ØX4	—	—
Orimune	T5Ø.B91	T5Ø.B92	T5Ø.B93	T5Ø.B94	T5Ø.B95	T5Ø.B96
Orinase	T38.3X1	T38.3X2	T38.3X3	T38.3X4	T38.3X5	T38.3X6
Ormeloxifene	T38.6X1	T38.6X2	T38.6X3	T38.6X4	T38.6X5	T38.6X6
Ornidazole	T37.3X1	T37.3X2	T37.3X3	T37.3X4	T37.3X5	T37.3X6
Ornithine aspartate	T5Ø.991	T5Ø.992	T5Ø.993	T5Ø.994	T5Ø.995	T5Ø.996
Ornoprostil	T47.1X1	T47.1X2	T47.1X3	T47.1X4	T47.1X5	T47.1X6
Orphenadrine (hydrochloride)	T42.8X1	T42.8X2	T42.8X3	T42.8X4	T42.8X5	T42.8X6
Ortal (sodium)	T42.3X1	T42.3X2	T42.3X3	T42.3X4	T42.3X5	T42.3X6
Orthoboric acid	T49.ØX1	T49.ØX2	T49.ØX3	T49.ØX4	T49.ØX5	T49.ØX6
ENT agent	T49.6X1	T49.6X2	T49.6X3	T49.6X4	T49.6X5	T49.6X6
ophthalmic preparation	T49.5X1	T49.5X2	T49.5X3	T49.5X4	T49.5X5	T49.5X6
Orthocaine	T41.3X1	T41.3X2	T41.3X3	T41.3X4	T41.3X5	T41.3X6
Orthodichlorobenzene	T53.7X1	T53.7X2	T53.7X3	T53.7X4	—	—
Ortho-Novum	T38.4X1	T38.4X2	T38.4X3	T38.4X4	T38.4X5	T38.4X6
Orthotolidine (reagent)	T54.2X1	T54.2X2	T54.2X3	T54.2X4	—	—
Osmic acid (liquid)	T54.2X1	T54.2X2	T54.2X3	T54.2X4	—	—
fumes	T54.2X1	T54.2X2	T54.2X3	T54.2X4	—	—
Osmotic diuretics	T5Ø.2X1	T5Ø.2X2	T5Ø.2X3	T5Ø.2X4	T5Ø.2X5	T5Ø.2X6
Otilonium bromide	T44.3X1	T44.3X2	T44.3X3	T44.3X4	T44.3X5	T44.3X6
Otorhinolaryngological drug NEC	T49.6X1	T49.6X2	T49.6X3	T49.6X4	T49.6X5	T49.6X6
Ouabain (e)	T46.ØX1	T46.ØX2	T46.ØX3	T46.ØX4	T46.ØX5	T46.ØX6
Ovarian						
hormone	T38.5X1	T38.5X2	T38.5X3	T38.5X4	T38.5X5	T38.5X6
stimulant	T38.5X1	T38.5X2	T38.5X3	T38.5X4	T38.5X5	T38.5X6
Ovide*	T49.ØX1	T49.ØX2	T49.ØX3	T49.ØX4	T49.ØX5	T49.ØX6
Ovral	T38.4X1	T38.4X2	T38.4X3	T38.4X4	T38.4X5	T38.4X6
Ovulen	T38.4X1	T38.4X2	T38.4X3	T38.4X4	T38.4X5	T38.4X6
Oxacillin	T36.ØX1	T36.ØX2	T36.ØX3	T36.ØX4	T36.ØX5	T36.ØX6
Oxalic acid	T54.2X1	T54.2X2	T54.2X3	T54.2X4	—	—
ammonium salt	T5Ø.991	T5Ø.992	T5Ø.993	T5Ø.994	T5Ø.995	T5Ø.996
Oxamniquine	T37.4X1	T37.4X2	T37.4X3	T37.4X4	T37.4X5	T37.4X6
Oxanamide	T43.591	T43.592	T43.593	T43.594	T43.595	T43.596
Oxandrolone	T38.7X1	T38.7X2	T38.7X3	T38.7X4	T38.7X5	T38.7X6
Oxantel	T37.4X1	T37.4X2	T37.4X3	T37.4X4	T37.4X5	T37.4X6
Oxapium iodide	T44.3X1	T44.3X2	T44.3X3	T44.3X4	T44.3X5	T44.3X6
Oxaprotiline	T43.Ø21	T43.Ø22	T43.Ø23	T43.Ø24	T43.Ø25	T43.Ø26
Oxaprozin	T39.311	T39.312	T39.313	T39.314	T39.315	T39.316
Oxatomide	T45.ØX1	T45.ØX2	T45.ØX3	T45.ØX4	T45.ØX5	T45.ØX6
Oxazepam	T42.4X1	T42.4X2	T42.4X3	T42.4X4	T42.4X5	T42.4X6
Oxazimedrine	T5Ø.5X1	T5Ø.5X2	T5Ø.5X3	T5Ø.5X4	T5Ø.5X5	T5Ø.5X6
Oxazolam	T42.4X1	T42.4X2	T42.4X3	T42.4X4	T42.4X5	T42.4X6
Oxazolidine derivatives	T42.2X1	T42.2X2	T42.2X3	T42.2X4	T42.2X5	T42.2X6
Oxazolidinedione (derivative)	T42.2X1	T42.2X2	T42.2X3	T42.2X4	T42.2X5	T42.2X6
Ox bile extract	T47.5X1	T47.5X2	T47.5X3	T47.5X4	T47.5X5	T47.5X6
Oxcarbazepine	T42.1X1	T42.1X2	T42.1X3	T42.1X4	T42.1X5	T42.1X6
Oxedrine	T44.4X1	T44.4X2	T44.4X3	T44.4X4	T44.4X5	T44.4X6
Oxeladin (citrate)	T48.3X1	T48.3X2	T48.3X3	T48.3X4	T48.3X5	T48.3X6
Oxendolone	T38.5X1	T38.5X2	T38.5X3	T38.5X4	T38.5X5	T38.5X6
Oxetacaine	T41.3X1	T41.3X2	T41.3X3	T41.3X4	T41.3X5	T41.3X6
Oxethazine	T41.3X1	T41.3X2	T41.3X3	T41.3X4	T41.3X5	T41.3X6
Oxetorone	T39.8X1	T39.8X2	T39.8X3	T39.8X4	T39.8X5	T39.8X6
Oxiconazole	T49.ØX1	T49.ØX2	T49.ØX3	T49.ØX4	T49.ØX5	T49.ØX6
Oxidizing agent NEC	T54.91	T54.92	T54.93	T54.94	—	—
Oxipurinol	T5Ø.4X1	T5Ø.4X2	T5Ø.4X3	T5Ø.4X4	T5Ø.4X5	T5Ø.4X6
Oxitriptan	T43.291	T43.292	T43.293	T43.294	T43.295	T43.296
Oxitropium bromide	T48.6X1	T48.6X2	T48.6X3	T48.6X4	T48.6X5	T48.6X6
Oxodipine	T46.1X1	T46.1X2	T46.1X3	T46.1X4	T46.1X5	T46.1X6
Oxolamine	T48.3X1	T48.3X2	T48.3X3	T48.3X4	T48.3X5	T48.3X6
Oxolinic acid	T37.8X1	T37.8X2	T37.8X3	T37.8X4	T37.8X5	T37.8X6
Oxomemazine	T43.3X1	T43.3X2	T43.3X3	T43.3X4	T43.3X5	T43.3X6
Oxophenarsine	T37.3X1	T37.3X2	T37.3X3	T37.3X4	T37.3X5	T37.3X6
Oxprenolol	T44.7X1	T44.7X2	T44.7X3	T44.7X4	T44.7X5	T44.7X6
Oxsoralen	T49.3X1	T49.3X2	T49.3X3	T49.3X4	T49.3X5	T49.3X6
Oxtriphylline	T48.6X1	T48.6X2	T48.6X3	T48.6X4	T48.6X5	T48.6X6
Oxybate sodium	T41.291	T41.292	T41.293	T41.294	T41.295	T41.296
Oxybuprocaine	T41.3X1	T41.3X2	T41.3X3	T41.3X4	T41.3X5	T41.3X6
Oxybutynin	T44.3X1	T44.3X2	T44.3X3	T44.3X4	T44.3X5	T44.3X6
Oxychlorosene	T49.ØX1	T49.ØX2	T49.ØX3	T49.ØX4	T49.ØX5	T49.ØX6
Oxycodone	T4Ø.2X1	T4Ø.2X2	T4Ø.2X3	T4Ø.2X4	T4Ø.2X5	T4Ø.2X6
OxyContin*	T4Ø.2X1	T4Ø.2X2	T4Ø.2X3	T4Ø.2X4	T4Ø.2X5	T4Ø.2X6
Oxyfedrine	T46.3X1	T46.3X2	T46.3X3	T46.3X4	T46.3X5	T46.3X6
Oxygen	T41.5X1	T41.5X2	T41.5X3	T41.5X4	T41.5X5	T41.5X6
Oxylone	T49.ØX1	T49.ØX2	T49.ØX3	T49.ØX4	T49.ØX5	T49.ØX6
Oxylone — *continued*						
ophthalmic preparation	T49.5X1	T49.5X2	T49.5X3	T49.5X4	T49.5X5	T49.5X6
Oxymesterone	T38.7X1	T38.7X2	T38.7X3	T38.7X4	T38.7X5	T38.7X6
Oxymetazoline	T48.5X1	T48.5X2	T48.5X3	T48.5X4	T48.5X5	T48.5X6
Oxymetholone	T38.7X1	T38.7X2	T38.7X3	T38.7X4	T38.7X5	T38.7X6
Oxymorphone	T4Ø.2X1	T4Ø.2X2	T4Ø.2X3	T4Ø.2X4	T4Ø.2X5	T4Ø.2X6
Oxypertine	T43.591	T43.592	T43.593	T43.594	T43.595	T43.596
Oxyphenbutazone	T39.2X1	T39.2X2	T39.2X3	T39.2X4	T39.2X5	T39.2X6
Oxyphencyclimine	T44.3X1	T44.3X2	T44.3X3	T44.3X4	T44.3X5	T44.3X6
Oxyphenisatine	T47.2X1	T47.2X2	T47.2X3	T47.2X4	T47.2X5	T47.2X6
Oxyphenonium bromide	T44.3X1	T44.3X2	T44.3X3	T44.3X4	T44.3X5	T44.3X6
Oxypolygelatin	T45.8X1	T45.8X2	T45.8X3	T45.8X4	T45.8X5	T45.8X6
Oxyquinoline (derivatives)	T37.8X1	T37.8X2	T37.8X3	T37.8X4	T37.8X5	T37.8X6
Oxytetracycline	T36.4X1	T36.4X2	T36.4X3	T36.4X4	T36.4X5	T36.4X6
Oxytocic drug NEC	T48.ØX1	T48.ØX2	T48.ØX3	T48.ØX4	T48.ØX5	T48.ØX6
Oxytocin (synthetic)	T48.ØX1	T48.ØX2	T48.ØX3	T48.ØX4	T48.ØX5	T48.ØX6
Oxytrol*	T44.3X1	T44.3X2	T44.3X3	T44.3X4	T44.3X5	T44.3X6
Ozone	T59.891	T59.892	T59.893	T59.894	—	—
PABA	T49.3X1	T49.3X2	T49.3X3	T49.3X4	T49.3X5	T49.3X6
Packed red cells	T45.8X1	T45.8X2	T45.8X3	T45.8X4	T45.8X5	T45.8X6
Padimate	T49.3X1	T49.3X2	T49.3X3	T49.3X4	T49.3X5	T49.3X6
Paint NEC	T65.6X1	T65.6X2	T65.6X3	T65.6X4	—	—
cleaner	T52.91	T52.92	T52.93	T52.94	—	—
fumes NEC	T59.891	T59.892	T59.893	T59.894	—	—
lead (fumes)	T56.ØX1	T56.ØX2	T56.ØX3	T56.ØX4	—	—
solvent NEC	T52.8X1	T52.8X2	T52.8X3	T52.8X4	—	—
stripper	T52.8X1	T52.8X2	T52.8X3	T52.8X4	—	—
Palfium	T4Ø.2X1	T4Ø.2X2	T4Ø.2X3	T4Ø.2X4	—	—
Palm kernel oil	T5Ø.991	T5Ø.992	T5Ø.993	T5Ø.994	T5Ø.995	T5Ø.996
Paludrine	T37.2X1	T37.2X2	T37.2X3	T37.2X4	T37.2X5	T37.2X6
PAM (pralidoxime)	T5Ø.6X1	T5Ø.6X2	T5Ø.6X3	T5Ø.6X4	T5Ø.6X5	T5Ø.6X6
Pamaquine (naphthoute)	T37.2X1	T37.2X2	T37.2X3	T37.2X4	T37.2X5	T37.2X6
Panadol	T39.1X1	T39.1X2	T39.1X3	T39.1X4	T39.1X5	T39.1X6
Pancreatic						
digestive secretion stimulant	T47.8X1	T47.8X2	T47.8X3	T47.8X4	T47.8X5	T47.8X6
dornase	T45.3X1	T45.3X2	T45.3X3	T45.3X4	T45.3X5	T45.3X6
Pancreatin	T47.5X1	T47.5X2	T47.5X3	T47.5X4	T47.5X5	T47.5X6
Pancrelipase	T47.5X1	T47.5X2	T47.5X3	T47.5X4	T47.5X5	T47.5X6
Pancuronium (bromide)	T48.1X1	T48.1X2	T48.1X3	T48.1X4	T48.1X5	T48.1X6
Pangamic acid	T45.2X1	T45.2X2	T45.2X3	T45.2X4	T45.2X5	T45.2X6
Panthenol	T45.2X1	T45.2X2	T45.2X3	T45.2X4	T45.2X5	T45.2X6
topical	T49.8X1	T49.8X2	T49.8X3	T49.8X4	T49.8X5	T49.8X6
Pantopon	T4Ø.ØX1	T4Ø.ØX2	T4Ø.ØX3	T4Ø.ØX4	T4Ø.ØX5	T4Ø.ØX6
Pantoprazole*	T47.1X1	T47.1X2	T47.1X3	T47.1X4	T47.1X5	T47.1X6
Pantothenic acid	T45.2X1	T45.2X2	T45.2X3	T45.2X4	T45.2X5	T45.2X6
Panwarfin	T45.511	T45.512	T45.513	T45.514	T45.515	T45.516
Papain	T47.5X1	T47.5X2	T47.5X3	T47.5X4	T47.5X5	T47.5X6
digestant	T47.5X1	T47.5X2	T47.5X3	T47.5X4	T47.5X5	T47.5X6
Papaveretum	T4Ø.ØX1	T4Ø.ØX2	T4Ø.ØX3	T4Ø.ØX4	T4Ø.ØX5	T4Ø.ØX6
Papaverine	T44.3X1	T44.3X2	T44.3X3	T44.3X4	T44.3X5	T44.3X6
Para-acetamidophenol	T39.1X1	T39.1X2	T39.1X3	T39.1X4	T39.1X5	T39.1X6
Para-aminobenzoic acid	T49.3X1	T49.3X2	T49.3X3	T49.3X4	T49.3X5	T49.3X6
Para-aminophenol derivatives	T39.1X1	T39.1X2	T39.1X3	T39.1X4	T39.1X5	T39.1X6
Para-aminosalicylic acid	T37.1X1	T37.1X2	T37.1X3	T37.1X4	T37.1X5	T37.1X6
Paracetaldehyde	T42.6X1	T42.6X2	T42.6X3	T42.6X4	T42.6X5	T42.6X6
Paracetamol	T39.1X1	T39.1X2	T39.1X3	T39.1X4	T39.1X5	T39.1X6
Parachlorophenol (camphorated)	T49.ØX1	T49.ØX2	T49.ØX3	T49.ØX4	T49.ØX5	T49.ØX6
Paracodin	T4Ø.2X1	T4Ø.2X2	T4Ø.2X3	T4Ø.2X4	T4Ø.2X5	T4Ø.2X6
Paradione	T42.2X1	T42.2X2	T42.2X3	T42.2X4	T42.2X5	T42.2X6
Paraffin(s) (wax)	T52.ØX1	T52.ØX2	T52.ØX3	T52.ØX4	—	—
liquid (medicinal)	T47.4X1	T47.4X2	T47.4X3	T47.4X4	T47.4X5	T47.4X6
nonmedicinal	T52.ØX1	T52.ØX2	T52.ØX3	T52.ØX4	—	—
Paraformaldehyde	T6Ø.3X1	T6Ø.3X2	T6Ø.3X3	T6Ø.3X4	—	—
Paraldehyde	T42.6X1	T42.6X2	T42.6X3	T42.6X4	T42.6X5	T42.6X6
Paramethadione	T42.2X1	T42.2X2	T42.2X3	T42.2X4	T42.2X5	T42.2X6
Paramethasone	T38.ØX1	T38.ØX2	T38.ØX3	T38.ØX4	T38.ØX5	T38.ØX6
acetate	T49.ØX1	T49.ØX2	T49.ØX3	T49.ØX4	T49.ØX5	T49.ØX6
Paraoxon	T6Ø.ØX1	T6Ø.ØX2	T6Ø.ØX3	T6Ø.ØX4	—	—
Paraquat	T6Ø.3X1	T6Ø.3X2	T6Ø.3X3	T6Ø.3X4	—	—
Parasympatholytic NEC	T44.3X1	T44.3X2	T44.3X3	T44.3X4	T44.3X5	T44.3X6
Parasympathomimetic drug NEC	T44.1X1	T44.1X2	T44.1X3	T44.1X4	T44.1X5	T44.1X6
Parathion	T6Ø.ØX1	T6Ø.ØX2	T6Ø.ØX3	T6Ø.ØX4	—	—
Parathormone	T5Ø.991	T5Ø.992	T5Ø.993	T5Ø.994	T5Ø.995	T5Ø.996
Parathyroid extract	T5Ø.991	T5Ø.992	T5Ø.993	T5Ø.994	T5Ø.995	T5Ø.996
Paratyphoid vaccine	T5Ø.A91	T5Ø.A92	T5Ø.A93	T5Ø.A94	T5Ø.A95	T5Ø.A96
Paredrine	T44.4X1	T44.4X2	T44.4X3	T44.4X4	T44.4X5	T44.4X6
Paregoric	T4Ø.ØX1	T4Ø.ØX2	T4Ø.ØX3	T4Ø.ØX4	T4Ø.ØX5	T4Ø.ØX6
Pargyline	T46.5X1	T46.5X2	T46.5X3	T46.5X4	T46.5X5	T46.5X6
Paris green	T57.ØX1	T57.ØX2	T57.ØX3	T57.ØX4	—	—

Substance	Poisoning, Accidental (unintentional)	Poisoning, Intentional Self-harm	Poisoning, Assault	Poisoning, Undetermined	Adverse Effect	Under-dosing
Paris green — *continued*						
insecticide	T57.ØX1	T57.ØX2	T57.ØX3	T57.ØX4	—	—
Parnate	T43.1X1	T43.1X2	T43.1X3	T43.1X4	T43.1X5	T43.1X6
Paromomycin	T36.5X1	T36.5X2	T36.5X3	T36.5X4	T36.5X5	T36.5X6
Paroxypropione	T45.1X1	T45.1X2	T45.1X3	T45.1X4	T45.1X5	T45.1X6
Parsabiv*	T5Ø.991	T5Ø.992	T5Ø.993	T5Ø.994	T5Ø.995	T5Ø.996
Parzone	T4Ø.2X1	T4Ø.2X2	T4Ø.2X3	T4Ø.2X4	T4Ø.2X5	T4Ø.2X6
PAS	T37.1X1	T37.1X2	T37.1X3	T37.1X4	T37.1X5	T37.1X6
Pasiniazid	T37.1X1	T37.1X2	T37.1X3	T37.1X4	T37.1X5	T37.1X6
PBB (polybrominated biphenyls)	T65.891	T65.892	T65.893	T65.894	—	—
PCB	T65.891	T65.892	T65.893	T65.894	—	—
PCP						
meaning pentachlorophenol	T6Ø.1X1	T6Ø.1X2	T6Ø.1X3	T6Ø.1X4	—	—
fungicide	T6Ø.3X1	T6Ø.3X2	T6Ø.3X3	T6Ø.3X4	—	—
herbicide	T6Ø.3X1	T6Ø.3X2	T6Ø.3X3	T6Ø.3X4	—	—
insecticide	T6Ø.1X1	T6Ø.1X2	T6Ø.1X3	T6Ø.1X4	—	—
meaning phencyclidine	T4Ø.991	T4Ø.992	T4Ø.993	T4Ø.994	—	—
Peach kernel oil (emulsion)	T47.4X1	T47.4X2	T47.4X3	T47.4X4	T47.4X5	T47.4X6
Peanut oil (emulsion) **NEC**	T47.4X1	T47.4X2	T47.4X3	T47.4X4	T47.4X5	T47.4X6
topical	T49.3X1	T49.3X2	T49.3X3	T49.3X4	T49.3X5	T49.3X6
Pearly Gates (morning glory seeds)	T4Ø.991	T4Ø.992	T4Ø.993	T4Ø.994	—	—
Pecazine	T43.3X1	T43.3X2	T43.3X3	T43.3X4	T43.3X5	T43.3X6
Pectin	T47.6X1	T47.6X2	T47.6X3	T47.6X4	T47.6X5	T47.6X6
Pediaflor*	T49.7X1	T49.7X2	T49.7X3	T49.7X4	T49.7X5	T49.7X6
Pefloxacin	T37.8X1	T37.8X2	T37.8X3	T37.8X4	T37.8X5	T37.8X6
Pegademase, bovine	T5Ø.Z91	T5Ø.Z92	T5Ø.Z93	T5Ø.Z94	T5Ø.Z95	T5Ø.Z96
Pelletierine tannate	T37.4X1	T37.4X2	T37.4X3	T37.4X4	T37.4X5	T37.4X6
Pemirolast (potassium)	T48.6X1	T48.6X2	T48.6X3	T48.6X4	T48.6X5	T48.6X6
Pemoline	T5Ø.7X1	T5Ø.7X2	T5Ø.7X3	T5Ø.7X4	T5Ø.7X5	T5Ø.7X6
Pempidine	T44.2X1	T44.2X2	T44.2X3	T44.2X4	T44.2X5	T44.2X6
Penamecillin	T36.ØX1	T36.ØX2	T36.ØX3	T36.ØX4	T36.ØX5	T36.ØX6
Penbutolol	T44.7X1	T44.7X2	T44.7X3	T44.7X4	T44.7X5	T44.7X6
Penethamate	T36.ØX1	T36.ØX2	T36.ØX3	T36.ØX4	T36.ØX5	T36.ØX6
Penfluridol	T43.591	T43.592	T43.593	T43.594	T43.595	T43.596
Penflutizide	T5Ø.2X1	T5Ø.2X2	T5Ø.2X3	T5Ø.2X4	T5Ø.2X5	T5Ø.2X6
Pengitoxin	T46.ØX1	T46.ØX2	T46.ØX3	T46.ØX4	T46.ØX5	T46.ØX6
Penicillamine	T5Ø.6X1	T5Ø.6X2	T5Ø.6X3	T5Ø.6X4	T5Ø.6X5	T5Ø.6X6
Penicillin (any)	T36.ØX1	T36.ØX2	T36.ØX3	T36.ØX4	T36.ØX5	T36.ØX6
Penicillinase	T45.3X1	T45.3X2	T45.3X3	T45.3X4	T45.3X5	T45.3X6
Penicilloyl polylysine	T5Ø.8X1	T5Ø.8X2	T5Ø.8X3	T5Ø.8X4	T5Ø.8X5	T5Ø.8X6
Penimepicycline	T36.4X1	T36.4X2	T36.4X3	T36.4X4	T36.4X5	T36.4X6
Pentacel*	T5Ø.A11	T5Ø.A12	T5Ø.A13	T5Ø.A14	T5Ø.A15	T5Ø.A16
Pentachloroethane	T53.6X1	T53.6X2	T53.6X3	T53.6X4	—	—
Pentachloronaphthalene	T53.7X1	T53.7X2	T53.7X3	T53.7X4	—	—
Pentachlorophenol (pesticide)	T6Ø.1X1	T6Ø.1X2	T6Ø.1X3	T6Ø.1X4	—	—
fungicide	T6Ø.3X1	T6Ø.3X2	T6Ø.3X3	T6Ø.3X4	—	—
herbicide	T6Ø.3X1	T6Ø.3X2	T6Ø.3X3	T6Ø.3X4	—	—
insecticide	T6Ø.1X1	T6Ø.1X2	T6Ø.1X3	T6Ø.1X4	—	—
Pentaerythritol	T46.3X1	T46.3X2	T46.3X3	T46.3X4	T46.3X5	T46.3X6
chloral	T42.6X1	T42.6X2	T42.6X3	T42.6X4	T42.6X5	T42.6X6
tetranitrate NEC	T46.3X1	T46.3X2	T46.3X3	T46.3X4	T46.3X5	T46.3X6
Pentaerythrityl tetranitrate	T46.3X1	T46.3X2	T46.3X3	T46.3X4	T46.3X5	T46.3X6
Pentagastrin	T5Ø.8X1	T5Ø.8X2	T5Ø.8X3	T5Ø.8X4	T5Ø.8X5	T5Ø.8X6
Pentalin	T53.6X1	T53.6X2	T53.6X3	T53.6X4	—	—
Pentamethonium bromide	T44.2X1	T44.2X2	T44.2X3	T44.2X4	T44.2X5	T44.2X6
Pentamidine	T37.3X1	T37.3X2	T37.3X3	T37.3X4	T37.3X5	T37.3X6
Pentanol	T51.3X1	T51.3X2	T51.3X3	T51.3X4	—	—
Pentapyrrolinium (bitartrate)	T44.2X1	T44.2X2	T44.2X3	T44.2X4	T44.2X5	T44.2X6
Pentaquine	T37.2X1	T37.2X2	T37.2X3	T37.2X4	T37.2X5	T37.2X6
Pentazocine	T4Ø.491	T4Ø.492	T4Ø.493	T4Ø.494	T4Ø.495	T4Ø.496
Pentetrazole	T5Ø.7X1	T5Ø.7X2	T5Ø.7X3	T5Ø.7X4	T5Ø.7X5	T5Ø.7X6
Penthienate bromide	T44.3X1	T44.3X2	T44.3X3	T44.3X4	T44.3X5	T44.3X6
Pentifylline	T46.7X1	T46.7X2	T46.7X3	T46.7X4	T46.7X5	T46.7X6
Pentobarbital	T42.3X1	T42.3X2	T42.3X3	T42.3X4	T42.3X5	T42.3X6
sodium	T42.3X1	T42.3X2	T42.3X3	T42.3X4	T42.3X5	T42.3X6
Pentobarbitone	T42.3X1	T42.3X2	T42.3X3	T42.3X4	T42.3X5	T42.3X6
Pentolonium tartrate	T44.2X1	T44.2X2	T44.2X3	T44.2X4	T44.2X5	T44.2X6
Pentosan polysulfate (sodium)	T39.8X1	T39.8X2	T39.8X3	T39.8X4	T39.8X5	T39.8X6
Pentostatin	T45.1X1	T45.1X2	T45.1X3	T45.1X4	T45.1X5	T45.1X6
Pentothal	T41.1X1	T41.1X2	T41.1X3	T41.1X4	T41.1X5	T41.1X6
Pentoxifylline	T46.7X1	T46.7X2	T46.7X3	T46.7X4	T46.7X5	T46.7X6
Pentoxyverine	T48.3X1	T48.3X2	T48.3X3	T48.3X4	T48.3X5	T48.3X6
Pentrinat	T46.3X1	T46.3X2	T46.3X3	T46.3X4	T46.3X5	T46.3X6
Pentylenetetrazole	T5Ø.7X1	T5Ø.7X2	T5Ø.7X3	T5Ø.7X4	T5Ø.7X5	T5Ø.7X6
Pentylsalicylamide	T37.1X1	T37.1X2	T37.1X3	T37.1X4	T37.1X5	T37.1X6
Pentymal	T42.3X1	T42.3X2	T42.3X3	T42.3X4	T42.3X5	T42.3X6

Substance	Poisoning, Accidental (unintentional)	Poisoning, Intentional Self-harm	Poisoning, Assault	Poisoning, Undetermined	Adverse Effect	Under-dosing
Pepcid*	T47.ØX1	T47.ØX2	T47.ØX3	T47.ØX4	T47.ØX5	T47.ØX6
Peplomycin	T45.1X1	T45.1X2	T45.1X3	T45.1X4	T45.1X5	T45.1X6
Peppermint (oil)	T47.5X1	T47.5X2	T47.5X3	T47.5X4	T47.5X5	T47.5X6
Pepsin	T47.5X1	T47.5X2	T47.5X3	T47.5X4	T47.5X5	T47.5X6
digestant	T47.5X1	T47.5X2	T47.5X3	T47.5X4	T47.5X5	T47.5X6
Pepstatin	T47.1X1	T47.1X2	T47.1X3	T47.1X4	T47.1X5	T47.1X6
Peptavlon	T5Ø.8X1	T5Ø.8X2	T5Ø.8X3	T5Ø.8X4	T5Ø.8X5	T5Ø.8X6
Perazine	T43.3X1	T43.3X2	T43.3X3	T43.3X4	T43.3X5	T43.3X6
Percaine (spinal)	T41.3X1	T41.3X2	T41.3X3	T41.3X4	T41.3X5	T41.3X6
topical (surface)	T41.3X1	T41.3X2	T41.3X3	T41.3X4	T41.3X5	T41.3X6
Perchloroethylene	T53.3X1	T53.3X2	T53.3X3	T53.3X4	—	—
medicinal	T37.4X1	T37.4X2	T37.4X3	T37.4X4	T37.4X5	T37.4X6
vapor	T53.3X1	T53.3X2	T53.3X3	T53.3X4	—	—
Percodan	T4Ø.2X1	T4Ø.2X2	T4Ø.2X3	T4Ø.2X4	T4Ø.2X5	T4Ø.2X6
Percogesic — *see also* acetaminophen	T45.ØX1	T45.ØX2	T45.ØX3	T45.ØX4	T45.ØX5	T45.ØX6
Percorten	T38.ØX1	T38.ØX2	T38.ØX3	T38.ØX4	T38.ØX5	T38.ØX6
Pergolide	T42.8X1	T42.8X2	T42.8X3	T42.8X4	T42.8X5	T42.8X6
Pergonal	T38.811	T38.812	T38.813	T38.814	T38.815	T38.816
Perhexilene	T46.3X1	T46.3X2	T46.3X3	T46.3X4	T46.3X5	T46.3X6
Perhexiline (maleate)	T46.3X1	T46.3X2	T46.3X3	T46.3X4	T46.3X5	T46.3X6
Periactin	T45.ØX1	T45.ØX2	T45.ØX3	T45.ØX4	T45.ØX5	T45.ØX6
Periciazine	T43.3X1	T43.3X2	T43.3X3	T43.3X4	T43.3X5	T43.3X6
Periclor	T42.6X1	T42.6X2	T42.6X3	T42.6X4	T42.6X5	T42.6X6
Perindopril	T46.4X1	T46.4X2	T46.4X3	T46.4X4	T46.4X5	T46.4X6
Perisoxal	T39.8X1	T39.8X2	T39.8X3	T39.8X4	T39.8X5	T39.8X6
Peritoneal dialysis solution	T5Ø.3X1	T5Ø.3X2	T5Ø.3X3	T5Ø.3X4	T5Ø.3X5	T5Ø.3X6
Peritrate	T46.3X1	T46.3X2	T46.3X3	T46.3X4	T46.3X5	T46.3X6
Perlapine	T42.4X1	T42.4X2	T42.4X3	T42.4X4	T42.4X5	T42.4X6
Permanganate	T65.891	T65.892	T65.893	T65.894	—	—
Permapen*	T36.ØX1	T36.ØX2	T36.ØX3	T36.ØX4	T36.ØX5	T36.ØX6
Permethrin	T6Ø.1X1	T6Ø.1X2	T6Ø.1X3	T6Ø.1X4	—	—
Pernocton	T42.3X1	T42.3X2	T42.3X3	T42.3X4	T42.3X5	T42.3X6
Pernoston	T42.3X1	T42.3X2	T42.3X3	T42.3X4	T42.3X5	T42.3X6
Peronine	T4Ø.2X1	T4Ø.2X2	T4Ø.2X3	T4Ø.2X4	—	—
Perphenazine	T43.3X1	T43.3X2	T43.3X3	T43.3X4	T43.3X5	T43.3X6
Pertofrane	T43.Ø11	T43.Ø12	T43.Ø13	T43.Ø14	T43.Ø15	T43.Ø16
Pertussis						
immune serum (human)	T5Ø.Z11	T5Ø.Z12	T5Ø.Z13	T5Ø.Z14	T5Ø.Z15	T5Ø.Z16
vaccine (with diphtheria toxoid) (with tetanus toxoid)	T5Ø.A11	T5Ø.A12	T5Ø.A13	T5Ø.A14	T5Ø.A15	T5Ø.A16
Peruvian balsam	T49.ØX1	T49.ØX2	T49.ØX3	T49.ØX4	T49.ØX5	T49.ØX6
Peruvoside	T46.ØX1	T46.ØX2	T46.ØX3	T46.ØX4	T46.ØX5	T46.ØX6
Pesticide (dust) (fumes) (vapor) **NEC**	T6Ø.91	T6Ø.92	T6Ø.93	T6Ø.94	—	—
arsenic	T57.ØX1	T57.ØX2	T57.ØX3	T57.ØX4	—	—
chlorinated	T6Ø.1X1	T6Ø.1X2	T6Ø.1X3	T6Ø.1X4	—	—
cyanide	T65.ØX1	T65.ØX2	T65.ØX3	T65.ØX4	—	—
kerosene	T52.ØX1	T52.ØX2	T52.ØX3	T52.ØX4	—	—
mixture (of compounds)	T6Ø.91	T6Ø.92	T6Ø.93	T6Ø.94	—	—
naphthalene	T6Ø.2X1	T6Ø.2X2	T6Ø.2X3	T6Ø.2X4	—	—
organochlorine (compounds)	T6Ø.1X1	T6Ø.1X2	T6Ø.1X3	T6Ø.1X4	—	—
petroleum (distillate) (products) NEC	T6Ø.8X1	T6Ø.8X2	T6Ø.8X3	T6Ø.8X4	—	—
specified ingredient NEC	T6Ø.8X1	T6Ø.8X2	T6Ø.8X3	T6Ø.8X4	—	—
strychnine	T65.1X1	T65.1X2	T65.1X3	T65.1X4	—	—
thallium	T6Ø.4X1	T6Ø.4X2	T6Ø.4X3	T6Ø.4X4	—	—
Pethidine	T4Ø.491	T4Ø.492	T4Ø.493	T4Ø.494	T4Ø.495	T4Ø.496
Petrichloral	T42.6X1	T42.6X2	T42.6X3	T42.6X4	T42.6X5	T42.6X6
Petrol	T52.ØX1	T52.ØX2	T52.ØX3	T52.ØX4	—	—
vapor	T52.ØX1	T52.ØX2	T52.ØX3	T52.ØX4	—	—
Petrolatum	T49.3X1	T49.3X2	T49.3X3	T49.3X4	T49.3X5	T49.3X6
hydrophilic	T49.3X1	T49.3X2	T49.3X3	T49.3X4	T49.3X5	T49.3X6
liquid	T47.4X1	T47.4X2	T47.4X3	T47.4X4	T47.4X5	T47.4X6
topical	T49.3X1	T49.3X2	T49.3X3	T49.3X4	T49.3X5	T49.3X6
nonmedicinal	T52.ØX1	T52.ØX2	T52.ØX3	T52.ØX4	—	—
red veterinary	T49.3X1	T49.3X2	T49.3X3	T49.3X4	T49.3X5	T49.3X6
white	T49.3X1	T49.3X2	T49.3X3	T49.3X4	T49.3X5	T49.3X6
Petroleum (products) **NEC**	T52.ØX1	T52.ØX2	T52.ØX3	T52.ØX4	—	—
benzine(s) — *see* Ligroin						
ether — *see* Ligroin						
jelly — *see* Petrolatum						
naphtha — *see* Ligroin						
pesticide	T6Ø.8X1	T6Ø.8X2	T6Ø.8X3	T6Ø.8X4	—	—
solids	T52.ØX1	T52.ØX2	T52.ØX3	T52.ØX4	—	—
solvents	T52.ØX1	T52.ØX2	T52.ØX3	T52.ØX4	—	—
vapor	T52.ØX1	T52.ØX2	T52.ØX3	T52.ØX4	—	—
Peyote	T4Ø.991	T4Ø.992	T4Ø.993	T4Ø.994	—	—
Phanodorm, phanodorn	T42.3X1	T42.3X2	T42.3X3	T42.3X4	T42.3X5	T42.3X6
Phanquinone	T37.3X1	T37.3X2	T37.3X3	T37.3X4	T37.3X5	T37.3X6
Phanquone	T37.3X1	T37.3X2	T37.3X3	T37.3X4	T37.3X5	T37.3X6

Substance	Poisoning, Accidental (unintentional)	Poisoning, Intentional Self-harm	Poisoning, Assault	Poisoning, Undetermined	Adverse Effect	Under-dosing
Pharmaceutical						
adjunct NEC	T5Ø.9Ø1	T5Ø.9Ø2	T5Ø.9Ø3	T5Ø.9Ø4	T5Ø.9Ø5	T5Ø.9Ø6
excipient NEC	T5Ø.9Ø1	T5Ø.9Ø2	T5Ø.9Ø3	T5Ø.9Ø4	T5Ø.9Ø5	T5Ø.9Ø6
sweetener	T5Ø.9Ø1	T5Ø.9Ø2	T5Ø.9Ø3	T5Ø.9Ø4	T5Ø.9Ø5	T5Ø.9Ø6
viscous agent	T5Ø.9Ø1	T5Ø.9Ø2	T5Ø.9Ø3	T5Ø.9Ø4	T5Ø.9Ø5	T5Ø.9Ø6
Phazyme*	T47.1X1	T47.1X2	T47.1X3	T47.1X4	T47.1X5	T47.1X6
Phemitone	T42.3X1	T42.3X2	T42.3X3	T42.3X4	T42.3X5	T42.3X6
Phenacaine	T41.3X1	T41.3X2	T41.3X3	T41.3X4	T41.3X5	T41.3X6
Phenacemide	T42.6X1	T42.6X2	T42.6X3	T42.6X4	T42.6X5	T42.6X6
Phenacetin	T39.1X1	T39.1X2	T39.1X3	T39.1X4	T39.1X5	T39.1X6
Phenadoxone	T4Ø.2X1	T4Ø.2X2	T4Ø.2X3	T4Ø.2X4	—	—
Phenaglycodol	T43.591	T43.592	T43.593	T43.594	T43.595	T43.596
Phenantoin	T42.ØX1	T42.ØX2	T42.ØX3	T42.ØX4	T42.ØX5	T42.ØX6
Phenaphthazine reagent	T5Ø.991	T5Ø.992	T5Ø.993	T5Ø.994	T5Ø.995	T5Ø.996
Phenazocine	T4Ø.491	T4Ø.492	T4Ø.493	T4Ø.494	T4Ø.495	T4Ø.496
Phenazone	T39.2X1	T39.2X2	T39.2X3	T39.2X4	T39.2X5	T39.2X6
Phenazopyridine	T39.8X1	T39.8X2	T39.8X3	T39.8X4	T39.8X5	T39.8X6
Phenbenicillin	T36.ØX1	T36.ØX2	T36.ØX3	T36.ØX4	T36.ØX5	T36.ØX6
Phenbutrazate	T5Ø.5X1	T5Ø.5X2	T5Ø.5X3	T5Ø.5X4	T5Ø.5X5	T5Ø.5X6
Phencyclidine	T4Ø.991	T4Ø.992	T4Ø.993	T4Ø.994	T4Ø.995	T4Ø.996
Phendimetrazine	T5Ø.5X1	T5Ø.5X2	T5Ø.5X3	T5Ø.5X4	T5Ø.5X5	T5Ø.5X6
Phenelzine	T43.1X1	T43.1X2	T43.1X3	T43.1X4	T43.1X5	T43.1X6
Phenemal	T42.3X1	T42.3X2	T42.3X3	T42.3X4	T42.3X5	T42.3X6
Phenergan	T42.6X1	T42.6X2	T42.6X3	T42.6X4	T42.6X5	T42.6X6
Pheneticillin	T36.ØX1	T36.ØX2	T36.ØX3	T36.ØX4	T36.ØX5	T36.ØX6
Pheneturide	T42.6X1	T42.6X2	T42.6X3	T42.6X4	T42.6X5	T42.6X6
Phenformin	T38.3X1	T38.3X2	T38.3X3	T38.3X4	T38.3X5	T38.3X6
Phenglutarimide	T44.3X1	T44.3X2	T44.3X3	T44.3X4	T44.3X5	T44.3X6
Phenicarbazide	T39.8X1	T39.8X2	T39.8X3	T39.8X4	T39.8X5	T39.8X6
Phenindamine	T45.ØX1	T45.ØX2	T45.ØX3	T45.ØX4	T45.ØX5	T45.ØX6
Phenindione	T45.511	T45.512	T45.513	T45.514	T45.515	T45.516
Pheniprazine	T43.1X1	T43.1X2	T43.1X3	T43.1X4	T43.1X5	T43.1X6
Pheniramine	T45.ØX1	T45.ØX2	T45.ØX3	T45.ØX4	T45.ØX5	T45.ØX6
Phenisatin	T47.2X1	T47.2X2	T47.2X3	T47.2X4	T47.2X5	T47.2X6
Phenmetrazine	T5Ø.5X1	T5Ø.5X2	T5Ø.5X3	T5Ø.5X4	T5Ø.5X5	T5Ø.5X6
Phenobal	T42.3X1	T42.3X2	T42.3X3	T42.3X4	T42.3X5	T42.3X6
Phenobarbital	T42.3X1	T42.3X2	T42.3X3	T42.3X4	T42.3X5	T42.3X6
with						
mephenytoin	T42.3X1	T42.3X2	T42.3X3	T42.3X4	T42.3X5	T42.3X6
phenytoin	T42.3X1	T42.3X2	T42.3X3	T42.3X4	T42.3X5	T42.3X6
sodium	T42.3X1	T42.3X2	T42.3X3	T42.3X4	T42.3X5	T42.3X6
Phenobarbitone	T42.3X1	T42.3X2	T42.3X3	T42.3X4	T42.3X5	T42.3X6
Phenobutiodil	T5Ø.8X1	T5Ø.8X2	T5Ø.8X3	T5Ø.8X4	T5Ø.8X5	T5Ø.8X6
Phenoctide	T49.ØX1	T49.ØX2	T49.ØX3	T49.ØX4	T49.ØX5	T49.ØX6
Phenol	T49.ØX1	T49.ØX2	T49.ØX3	T49.ØX4	T49.ØX5	T49.ØX6
disinfectant	T54.ØX1	T54.ØX2	T54.ØX3	T54.ØX4	—	—
in oil injection	T46.8X1	T46.8X2	T46.8X3	T46.8X4	T46.8X5	T46.8X6
medicinal	T49.1X1	T49.1X2	T49.1X3	T49.1X4	T49.1X5	T49.1X6
nonmedicinal NEC	T54.ØX1	T54.ØX2	T54.ØX3	T54.ØX4	—	—
pesticide	T6Ø.8X1	T6Ø.8X2	T6Ø.8X3	T6Ø.8X4	—	—
red	T5Ø.8X1	T5Ø.8X2	T5Ø.8X3	T5Ø.8X4	T5Ø.8X5	T5Ø.8X6
Phenolic preparation	T49.1X1	T49.1X2	T49.1X3	T49.1X4	T49.1X5	T49.1X6
Phenolphthalein	T47.2X1	T47.2X2	T47.2X3	T47.2X4	T47.2X5	T47.2X6
Phenolsulfonphthalein	T5Ø.8X1	T5Ø.8X2	T5Ø.8X3	T5Ø.8X4	T5Ø.8X5	T5Ø.8X6
Phenomorphan	T4Ø.2X1	T4Ø.2X2	T4Ø.2X3	T4Ø.2X4	—	—
Phenonyl	T42.3X1	T42.3X2	T42.3X3	T42.3X4	T42.3X5	T42.3X6
Phenoperidine	T4Ø.491	T4Ø.492	T4Ø.493	T4Ø.494	—	—
Phenopyrazone	T46.991	T46.992	T46.993	T46.994	T46.995	T46.996
Phenoquin	T5Ø.4X1	T5Ø.4X2	T5Ø.4X3	T5Ø.4X4	T5Ø.4X5	T5Ø.4X6
Phenothiazine (psychotropic) **NEC**	T43.3X1	T43.3X2	T43.3X3	T43.3X4	T43.3X5	T43.3X6
insecticide	T6Ø.2X1	T6Ø.2X2	T6Ø.2X3	T6Ø.2X4	—	—
Phenothrin	T49.ØX1	T49.ØX2	T49.ØX3	T49.ØX4	T49.ØX5	T49.ØX6
Phenoxybenzamine	T46.7X1	T46.7X2	T46.7X3	T46.7X4	T46.7X5	T46.7X6
Phenoxyethanol	T49.ØX1	T49.ØX2	T49.ØX3	T49.ØX4	T49.ØX5	T49.ØX6
Phenoxymethyl penicillin	T36.ØX1	T36.ØX2	T36.ØX3	T36.ØX4	T36.ØX5	T36.ØX6
Phenprobamate	T42.8X1	T42.8X2	T42.8X3	T42.8X4	T42.8X5	T42.8X6
Phenprocoumon	T45.511	T45.512	T45.513	T45.514	T45.515	T45.516
Phensuximide	T42.2X1	T42.2X2	T42.2X3	T42.2X4	T42.2X5	T42.2X6
Phentermine	T5Ø.5X1	T5Ø.5X2	T5Ø.5X3	T5Ø.5X4	T5Ø.5X5	T5Ø.5X6
Phenthicillin	T36.ØX1	T36.ØX2	T36.ØX3	T36.ØX4	T36.ØX5	T36.ØX6
Phentolamine	T46.7X1	T46.7X2	T46.7X3	T46.7X4	T46.7X5	T46.7X6
Phenyl						
butazone	T39.2X1	T39.2X2	T39.2X3	T39.2X4	T39.2X5	T39.2X6
enediamine	T65.3X1	T65.3X2	T65.3X3	T65.3X4	—	—
hydrazine	T65.3X1	T65.3X2	T65.3X3	T65.3X4	—	—
antineoplastic	T45.1X1	T45.1X2	T45.1X3	T45.1X4	T45.1X5	T45.1X6
mercuric compounds — *see* Mercury						
salicylate	T49.3X1	T49.3X2	T49.3X3	T49.3X4	T49.3X5	T49.3X6
Phenylalanine mustard	T45.1X1	T45.1X2	T45.1X3	T45.1X4	T45.1X5	T45.1X6
Phenylbutazone	T39.2X1	T39.2X2	T39.2X3	T39.2X4	T39.2X5	T39.2X6
Phenylenediamine	T65.3X1	T65.3X2	T65.3X3	T65.3X4	—	—

Substance	Poisoning, Accidental (unintentional)	Poisoning, Intentional Self-harm	Poisoning, Assault	Poisoning, Undetermined	Adverse Effect	Under-dosing
Phenylephrine	T44.4X1	T44.4X2	T44.4X3	T44.4X4	T44.4X5	T44.4X6
Phenylethylbiguanide	T38.3X1	T38.3X2	T38.3X3	T38.3X4	T38.3X5	T38.3X6
Phenylmercuric						
acetate	T49.ØX1	T49.ØX2	T49.ØX3	T49.ØX4	T49.ØX5	T49.ØX6
borate	T49.ØX1	T49.ØX2	T49.ØX3	T49.ØX4	T49.ØX5	T49.ØX6
nitrate	T49.ØX1	T49.ØX2	T49.ØX3	T49.ØX4	T49.ØX5	T49.ØX6
Phenylmethylbarbitone	T42.3X1	T42.3X2	T42.3X3	T42.3X4	T42.3X5	T42.3X6
Phenylpropanol	T47.5X1	T47.5X2	T47.5X3	T47.5X4	T47.5X5	T47.5X6
Phenylpropanolamine	T44.991	T44.992	T44.993	T44.994	T44.995	T44.996
Phenylsulfthion	T6Ø.ØX1	T6Ø.ØX2	T6Ø.ØX3	T6Ø.ØX4	—	—
Phenyltoloxamine	T45.ØX1	T45.ØX2	T45.ØX3	T45.ØX4	T45.ØX5	T45.ØX6
Phenyramidol, phenyramidon	T39.8X1	T39.8X2	T39.8X3	T39.8X4	T39.8X5	T39.8X6
Phenytek*	T42.ØX1	T42.ØX2	T42.ØX3	T42.ØX4	T42.ØX5	T42.ØX6
Phenytoin	T42.ØX1	T42.ØX2	T42.ØX3	T42.ØX4	T42.ØX5	T42.ØX6
with Phenobarbital	T42.3X1	T42.3X2	T42.3X3	T42.3X4	T42.3X5	T42.3X6
pHisoHex	T49.2X1	T49.2X2	T49.2X3	T49.2X4	T49.2X5	T49.2X6
Pholcodine	T48.3X1	T48.3X2	T48.3X3	T48.3X4	T48.3X5	T48.3X6
Pholedrine	T46.991	T46.992	T46.993	T46.994	T46.995	T46.996
Phorate	T6Ø.ØX1	T6Ø.ØX2	T6Ø.ØX3	T6Ø.ØX4	—	—
Phosdrin	T6Ø.ØX1	T6Ø.ØX2	T6Ø.ØX3	T6Ø.ØX4	—	—
Phosfolan	T6Ø.ØX1	T6Ø.ØX2	T6Ø.ØX3	T6Ø.ØX4	—	—
Phosgene (gas)	T59.891	T59.892	T59.893	T59.894	—	—
Phosphamidon	T6Ø.ØX1	T6Ø.ØX2	T6Ø.ØX3	T6Ø.ØX4	—	—
Phosphate	T65.891	T65.892	T65.893	T65.894	—	—
laxative	T47.4X1	T47.4X2	T47.4X3	T47.4X4	T47.4X5	T47.4X6
organic	T6Ø.ØX1	T6Ø.ØX2	T6Ø.ØX3	T6Ø.ØX4	—	—
solvent	T52.91	T52.92	T52.93	T52.94	—	—
tricresyl	T65.891	T65.892	T65.893	T65.894	—	—
Phosphine	T57.1X1	T57.1X2	T57.1X3	T57.1X4	—	—
fumigant	T57.1X1	T57.1X2	T57.1X3	T57.1X4	—	—
Phospholine	T49.5X1	T49.5X2	T49.5X3	T49.5X4	T49.5X5	T49.5X6
Phosphoric acid	T54.2X1	T54.2X2	T54.2X3	T54.2X4	—	—
Phosphorus (compound) **NEC**	T57.1X1	T57.1X2	T57.1X3	T57.1X4	—	—
pesticide	T6Ø.ØX1	T6Ø.ØX2	T6Ø.ØX3	T6Ø.ØX4	—	—
Photrexa*	T49.5X1	T49.5X2	T49.5X3	T49.5X4	T49.5X5	T49.5X6
Phthalates	T65.891	T65.892	T65.893	T65.894	—	—
Phthalic anhydride	T65.891	T65.892	T65.893	T65.894	—	—
Phthalimidoglutarimide	T42.6X1	T42.6X2	T42.6X3	T42.6X4	T42.6X5	T42.6X6
Phthalylsulfathiazole	T37.ØX1	T37.ØX2	T37.ØX3	T37.ØX4	T37.ØX5	T37.ØX6
Phylloquinone	T45.7X1	T45.7X2	T45.7X3	T45.7X4	T45.7X5	T45.7X6
Physeptone	T4Ø.3X1	T4Ø.3X2	T4Ø.3X3	T4Ø.3X4	T4Ø.3X5	T4Ø.3X6
Physostigma venenosum	T62.2X1	T62.2X2	T62.2X3	T62.2X4	—	—
Physostigmine	T49.5X1	T49.5X2	T49.5X3	T49.5X4	T49.5X5	T49.5X6
Phytolacca decandra	T62.2X1	T62.2X2	T62.2X3	T62.2X4	—	—
berries	T62.1X1	T62.1X2	T62.1X3	T62.1X4	—	—
Phytomenadione	T45.7X1	T45.7X2	T45.7X3	T45.7X4	T45.7X5	T45.7X6
Phytonadione	T45.7X1	T45.7X2	T45.7X3	T45.7X4	T45.7X5	T45.7X6
Picoperine	T48.3X1	T48.3X2	T48.3X3	T48.3X4	T48.3X5	T48.3X6
Picosulfate (sodium)	T47.2X1	T47.2X2	T47.2X3	T47.2X4	T47.2X5	T47.2X6
Picric (acid)	T54.2X1	T54.2X2	T54.2X3	T54.2X4	—	—
Picrotoxin	T5Ø.7X1	T5Ø.7X2	T5Ø.7X3	T5Ø.7X4	T5Ø.7X5	T5Ø.7X6
Piketoprofen	T49.ØX1	T49.ØX2	T49.ØX3	T49.ØX4	T49.ØX5	T49.ØX6
Pilocarpine	T44.1X1	T44.1X2	T44.1X3	T44.1X4	T44.1X5	T44.1X6
Pilocarpus (jaborandi) extract	T44.1X1	T44.1X2	T44.1X3	T44.1X4	T44.1X5	T44.1X6
Pilsicainide (hydrochloride)	T46.2X1	T46.2X2	T46.2X3	T46.2X4	T46.2X5	T46.2X6
Pimaricin	T36.7X1	T36.7X2	T36.7X3	T36.7X4	T36.7X5	T36.7X6
Pimeclone	T5Ø.7X1	T5Ø.7X2	T5Ø.7X3	T5Ø.7X4	T5Ø.7X5	T5Ø.7X6
Pimelic ketone	T52.8X1	T52.8X2	T52.8X3	T52.8X4	—	—
Pimethixene	T45.ØX1	T45.ØX2	T45.ØX3	T45.ØX4	T45.ØX5	T45.ØX6
Piminodine	T4Ø.2X1	T4Ø.2X2	T4Ø.2X3	T4Ø.2X4	T4Ø.2X5	T4Ø.2X6
Pimozide	T43.591	T43.592	T43.593	T43.594	T43.595	T43.596
Pinacidil	T46.5X1	T46.5X2	T46.5X3	T46.5X4	T46.5X5	T46.5X6
Pinaverium bromide	T44.3X1	T44.3X2	T44.3X3	T44.3X4	T44.3X5	T44.3X6
Pinazepam	T42.4X1	T42.4X2	T42.4X3	T42.4X4	T42.4X5	T42.4X6
Pindolol	T44.7X1	T44.7X2	T44.7X3	T44.7X4	T44.7X5	T44.7X6
Pindone	T6Ø.4X1	T6Ø.4X2	T6Ø.4X3	T6Ø.4X4	—	—
Pine oil (disinfectant)	T65.891	T65.892	T65.893	T65.894	—	—
Pinkroot	T37.4X1	T37.4X2	T37.4X3	T37.4X4	T37.4X5	T37.4X6
Pipadone	T4Ø.2X1	T4Ø.2X2	T4Ø.2X3	T4Ø.2X4	—	—
Pipamazine	T45.ØX1	T45.ØX2	T45.ØX3	T45.ØX4	T45.ØX5	T45.ØX6
Pipamperone	T43.4X1	T43.4X2	T43.4X3	T43.4X4	T43.4X5	T43.4X6
Pipazetate	T48.3X1	T48.3X2	T48.3X3	T48.3X4	T48.3X5	T48.3X6
Pipemidic acid	T37.8X1	T37.8X2	T37.8X3	T37.8X4	T37.8X5	T37.8X6
Pipenzolate bromide	T44.3X1	T44.3X2	T44.3X3	T44.3X4	T44.3X5	T44.3X6
Piperacetazine	T43.3X1	T43.3X2	T43.3X3	T43.3X4	T43.3X5	T43.3X6
Piperacillin	T36.ØX1	T36.ØX2	T36.ØX3	T36.ØX4	T36.ØX5	T36.ØX6
Piperazine	T37.4X1	T37.4X2	T37.4X3	T37.4X4	T37.4X5	T37.4X6
estrone sulfate	T38.5X1	T38.5X2	T38.5X3	T38.5X4	T38.5X5	T38.5X6
Piper cubeba	T62.2X1	T62.2X2	T62.2X3	T62.2X4	—	—
Piperidione	T48.3X1	T48.3X2	T48.3X3	T48.3X4	T48.3X5	T48.3X6

Substance	Poisoning, Accidental (unintentional)	Poisoning, Intentional Self-harm	Poisoning, Assault	Poisoning, Undetermined	Adverse Effect	Under-dosing
Piperidolate	T44.3X1	T44.3X2	T44.3X3	T44.3X4	T44.3X5	T44.3X6
Piperocaine	T41.3X1	T41.3X2	T41.3X3	T41.3X4	T41.3X5	T41.3X6
infiltration (subcutaneous)	T41.3X1	T41.3X2	T41.3X3	T41.3X4	T41.3X5	T41.3X6
nerve block (peripheral) (plexus)	T41.3X1	T41.3X2	T41.3X3	T41.3X4	T41.3X5	T41.3X6
topical (surface)	T41.3X1	T41.3X2	T41.3X3	T41.3X4	T41.3X5	T41.3X6
Piperonyl butoxide	T6Ø.8X1	T6Ø.8X2	T6Ø.8X3	T6Ø.8X4	—	—
Pipethanate	T44.3X1	T44.3X2	T44.3X3	T44.3X4	T44.3X5	T44.3X6
Pipobroman	T45.1X1	T45.1X2	T45.1X3	T45.1X4	T45.1X5	T45.1X6
Pipotiazine	T43.3X1	T43.3X2	T43.3X3	T43.3X4	T43.3X5	T43.3X6
Pipoxizine	T45.ØX1	T45.ØX2	T45.ØX3	T45.ØX4	T45.ØX5	T45.ØX6
Pipradrol	T43.691	T43.692	T43.693	T43.694	T43.695	T43.696
Piprinhydrinate	T45.ØX1	T45.ØX2	T45.ØX3	T45.ØX4	T45.ØX5	T45.ØX6
Pirarubicin	T45.1X1	T45.1X2	T45.1X3	T45.1X4	T45.1X5	T45.1X6
Pirazinamide	T37.1X1	T37.1X2	T37.1X3	T37.1X4	T37.1X5	T37.1X6
Pirbuterol	T48.6X1	T48.6X2	T48.6X3	T48.6X4	T48.6X5	T48.6X6
Pirenzepine	T47.1X1	T47.1X2	T47.1X3	T47.1X4	T47.1X5	T47.1X6
Piretanide	T5Ø.1X1	T5Ø.1X2	T5Ø.1X3	T5Ø.1X4	T5Ø.1X5	T5Ø.1X6
Pirfenidone*	T48.991	T48.992	T48.993	T48.994	T48.995	T48.996
Piribedil	T42.8X1	T42.8X2	T42.8X3	T42.8X4	T42.8X5	T42.8X6
Piridoxilate	T46.3X1	T46.3X2	T46.3X3	T46.3X4	T46.3X5	T46.3X6
Piritramide	T4Ø.491	T4Ø.492	T4Ø.493	T4Ø.494	—	—
Piromidic acid	T37.8X1	T37.8X2	T37.8X3	T37.8X4	T37.8X5	T37.8X6
Piroxicam	T39.391	T39.392	T39.393	T39.394	T39.395	T39.396
beta-cyclodextrin complex	T39.8X1	T39.8X2	T39.8X3	T39.8X4	T39.8X5	T39.8X6
Pirozadil	T46.6X1	T46.6X2	T46.6X3	T46.6X4	T46.6X5	T46.6X6
Piscidia (bark) (erythrina)	T39.8X1	T39.8X2	T39.8X3	T39.8X4	T39.8X5	T39.8X6
Pitch	T65.891	T65.892	T65.893	T65.894	—	—
Pitkin's solution	T41.3X1	T41.3X2	T41.3X3	T41.3X4	T41.3X5	T41.3X6
Pitocin	T48.ØX1	T48.ØX2	T48.ØX3	T48.ØX4	T48.ØX5	T48.ØX6
Pitressin (tannate)	T38.891	T38.892	T38.893	T38.894	T38.895	T38.896
Pituitary extracts (posterior)	T38.891	T38.892	T38.893	T38.894	T38.895	T38.896
anterior	T38.811	T38.812	T38.813	T38.814	T38.815	T38.816
Pituitrin	T38.891	T38.892	T38.893	T38.894	T38.895	T38.896
Pivampicillin	T36.ØX1	T36.ØX2	T36.ØX3	T36.ØX4	T36.ØX5	T36.ØX6
Pivmecillinam	T36.ØX1	T36.ØX2	T36.ØX3	T36.ØX4	T36.ØX5	T36.ØX6
Placental hormone	T38.891	T38.892	T38.893	T38.894	T38.895	T38.896
Placidyl	T42.6X1	T42.6X2	T42.6X3	T42.6X4	T42.6X5	T42.6X6
Plague vaccine	T5Ø.A91	T5Ø.A92	T5Ø.A93	T5Ø.A94	T5Ø.A95	T5Ø.A96
Plant						
food or fertilizer NEC	T65.891	T65.892	T65.893	T65.894	—	—
containing herbicide	T6Ø.3X1	T6Ø.3X2	T6Ø.3X3	T6Ø.3X4	—	—
noxious, used as food	T62.2X1	T62.2X2	T62.2X3	T62.2X4	—	—
berries	T62.1X1	T62.1X2	T62.1X3	T62.1X4	—	—
seeds	T62.2X1	T62.2X2	T62.2X3	T62.2X4	—	—
specified type NEC	T62.2X1	T62.2X2	T62.2X3	T62.2X4	—	—
Plasma	T45.8X1	T45.8X2	T45.8X3	T45.8X4	T45.8X5	T45.8X6
expander NEC	T45.8X1	T45.8X2	T45.8X3	T45.8X4	T45.8X5	T45.8X6
protein fraction (human)	T45.8X1	T45.8X2	T45.8X3	T45.8X4	T45.8X5	T45.8X6
Plasmanate	T45.8X1	T45.8X2	T45.8X3	T45.8X4	T45.8X5	T45.8X6
Plasminogen (tissue) activator	T45.611	T45.612	T45.613	T45.614	T45.615	T45.616
Plaster dressing	T49.3X1	T49.3X2	T49.3X3	T49.3X4	T49.3X5	T49.3X6
Plastic dressing	T49.3X1	T49.3X2	T49.3X3	T49.3X4	T49.3X5	T49.3X6
Plavix*	T45.521	T45.522	T45.523	T45.524	T45.525	T45.526
Plegicil	T43.3X1	T43.3X2	T43.3X3	T43.3X4	T43.3X5	T43.3X6
Plicamycin	T45.1X1	T45.1X2	T45.1X3	T45.1X4	T45.1X5	T45.1X6
Podophyllotoxin	T49.8X1	T49.8X2	T49.8X3	T49.8X4	T49.8X5	T49.8X6
Podophyllum (resin)	T49.4X1	T49.4X2	T49.4X3	T49.4X4	T49.4X5	T49.4X6
Poisonous berries	T62.1X1	T62.1X2	T62.1X3	T62.1X4	—	—
Poison NEC	T65.91	T65.92	T65.93	T65.94	—	—
Pokeweed (any part)	T62.2X1	T62.2X2	T62.2X3	T62.2X4	—	—
Poldine metilsulfate	T44.3X1	T44.3X2	T44.3X3	T44.3X4	T44.3X5	T44.3X6
Polidexide (sulfate)	T46.6X1	T46.6X2	T46.6X3	T46.6X4	T46.6X5	T46.6X6
Polidocanol	T46.8X1	T46.8X2	T46.8X3	T46.8X4	T46.8X5	T46.8X6
Poliomyelitis vaccine	T5Ø.B91	T5Ø.B92	T5Ø.B93	T5Ø.B94	T5Ø.B95	T5Ø.B96
Polish (car) (floor) (furniture) (metal) (porcelain) (silver)	T65.891	T65.892	T65.893	T65.894	—	—
abrasive	T65.891	T65.892	T65.893	T65.894	—	—
porcelain	T65.891	T65.892	T65.893	T65.894	—	—
Poloxalkol	T47.4X1	T47.4X2	T47.4X3	T47.4X4	T47.4X5	T47.4X6
Poloxamer	T47.4X1	T47.4X2	T47.4X3	T47.4X4	T47.4X5	T47.4X6
Polyaminostyrene resins	T5Ø.3X1	T5Ø.3X2	T5Ø.3X3	T5Ø.3X4	T5Ø.3X5	T5Ø.3X6
Polycarbophil	T47.4X1	T47.4X2	T47.4X3	T47.4X4	T47.4X5	T47.4X6
Polychlorinated biphenyl	T65.891	T65.892	T65.893	T65.894	—	—
Polycycline	T36.4X1	T36.4X2	T36.4X3	T36.4X4	T36.4X5	T36.4X6
Polyester fumes	T59.891	T59.892	T59.893	T59.894	—	—
Polyester resin hardener	T52.91	T52.92	T52.93	T52.94	—	—
fumes	T59.891	T59.892	T59.893	T59.894	—	—
Polyestradiol phosphate	T38.5X1	T38.5X2	T38.5X3	T38.5X4	T38.5X5	T38.5X6
Polyethanolamine alkyl sulfate	T49.2X1	T49.2X2	T49.2X3	T49.2X4	T49.2X5	T49.2X6
Polyethylene adhesive	T49.3X1	T49.3X2	T49.3X3	T49.3X4	T49.3X5	T49.3X6
Polyferose	T45.4X1	T45.4X2	T45.4X3	T45.4X4	T45.4X5	T45.4X6
Polygeline	T45.8X1	T45.8X2	T45.8X3	T45.8X4	T45.8X5	T45.8X6
Polymyxin	T36.8X1	T36.8X2	T36.8X3	T36.8X4	T36.8X5	T36.8X6
B	T36.8X1	T36.8X2	T36.8X3	T36.8X4	T36.8X5	T36.8X6
ENT agent	T49.6X1	T49.6X2	T49.6X3	T49.6X4	T49.6X5	T49.6X6
ophthalmic preparation	T49.5X1	T49.5X2	T49.5X3	T49.5X4	T49.5X5	T49.5X6
topical NEC	T49.ØX1	T49.ØX2	T49.ØX3	T49.ØX4	T49.ØX5	T49.ØX6
E sulfate (eye preparation)	T49.5X1	T49.5X2	T49.5X3	T49.5X4	T49.5X5	T49.5X6
Polynoxylin	T49.ØX1	T49.ØX2	T49.ØX3	T49.ØX4	T49.ØX5	T49.ØX6
Polyoestradiol phosphate	T38.5X1	T38.5X2	T38.5X3	T38.5X4	T38.5X5	T38.5X6
Polyoxymethyleneurea	T49.ØX1	T49.ØX2	T49.ØX3	T49.ØX4	T49.ØX5	T49.ØX6
Poly-Pred*	T49.5X1	T49.5X2	T49.5X3	T49.5X4	T49.5X5	T49.5X6
Polysilane	T47.8X1	T47.8X2	T47.8X3	T47.8X4	T47.8X5	T47.8X6
Polytetrafluoroethylene (inhaled)	T59.891	T59.892	T59.893	T59.894	—	—
Polythiazide	T5Ø.2X1	T5Ø.2X2	T5Ø.2X3	T5Ø.2X4	T5Ø.2X5	T5Ø.2X6
Polyvidone	T45.8X1	T45.8X2	T45.8X3	T45.8X4	T45.8X5	T45.8X6
Polyvinylpyrrolidone	T45.8X1	T45.8X2	T45.8X3	T45.8X4	T45.8X5	T45.8X6
Pontocaine (hydrochloride) (infiltration) (topical)	T41.3X1	T41.3X2	T41.3X3	T41.3X4	T41.3X5	T41.3X6
nerve block (peripheral) (plexus)	T41.3X1	T41.3X2	T41.3X3	T41.3X4	T41.3X5	T41.3X6
spinal	T41.3X1	T41.3X2	T41.3X3	T41.3X4	T41.3X5	T41.3X6
Porfiromycin	T45.1X1	T45.1X2	T45.1X3	T45.1X4	T45.1X5	T45.1X6
Portactant alfa*	T48.991	T48.992	T48.993	T48.994	T48.995	T48.996
Posterior pituitary hormone NEC	T38.891	T38.892	T38.893	T38.894	T38.895	T38.896
Pot	T4Ø.711	T4Ø.712	T4Ø.713	T4Ø.714	T4Ø.715	T4Ø.716
Potash (caustic)	T54.3X1	T54.3X2	T54.3X3	T54.3X4	—	—
Potassic saline injection (lactated)	T5Ø.3X1	T5Ø.3X2	T5Ø.3X3	T5Ø.3X4	T5Ø.3X5	T5Ø.3X6
Potassium (salts) **NEC**	T5Ø.3X1	T5Ø.3X2	T5Ø.3X3	T5Ø.3X4	T5Ø.3X5	T5Ø.3X6
aminobenzoate	T45.8X1	T45.8X2	T45.8X3	T45.8X4	T45.8X5	T45.8X6
aminosalicylate	T37.1X1	T37.1X2	T37.1X3	T37.1X4	T37.1X5	T37.1X6
antimony ' tartrate'	T37.8X1	T37.8X2	T37.8X3	T37.8X4	T37.8X5	T37.8X6
arsenite (solution)	T57.ØX1	T57.ØX2	T57.ØX3	T57.ØX4	—	—
bichromate	T56.2X1	T56.2X2	T56.2X3	T56.2X4	—	—
bisulfate	T47.3X1	T47.3X2	T47.3X3	T47.3X4	T47.3X5	T47.3X6
bromide	T42.6X1	T42.6X2	T42.6X3	T42.6X4	T42.6X5	T42.6X6
canrenoate	T5Ø.ØX1	T5Ø.ØX2	T5Ø.ØX3	T5Ø.ØX4	T5Ø.ØX5	T5Ø.ØX6
carbonate	T54.3X1	T54.3X2	T54.3X3	T54.3X4	—	—
chlorate NEC	T65.891	T65.892	T65.893	T65.894	—	—
chloride	T5Ø.3X1	T5Ø.3X2	T5Ø.3X3	T5Ø.3X4	T5Ø.3X5	T5Ø.3X6
citrate	T5Ø.991	T5Ø.992	T5Ø.993	T5Ø.994	T5Ø.995	T5Ø.996
cyanide	T65.ØX1	T65.ØX2	T65.ØX3	T65.ØX4	—	—
ferric hexacyanoferrate (medicinal)	T5Ø.6X1	T5Ø.6X2	T5Ø.6X3	T5Ø.6X4	T5Ø.6X5	T5Ø.6X6
nonmedicinal	T65.891	T65.892	T65.893	T65.894	—	—
Fluoride	T57.8X1	T57.8X2	T57.8X3	T57.8X4	—	—
glucaldrate	T47.1X1	T47.1X2	T47.1X3	T47.1X4	T47.1X5	T47.1X6
hydroxide	T54.3X1	T54.3X2	T54.3X3	T54.3X4	—	—
iodate	T49.ØX1	T49.ØX2	T49.ØX3	T49.ØX4	T49.ØX5	T49.ØX6
iodide	T48.4X1	T48.4X2	T48.4X3	T48.4X4	T48.4X5	T48.4X6
nitrate	T57.8X1	T57.8X2	T57.8X3	T57.8X4	—	—
oxalate	T65.891	T65.892	T65.893	T65.894	—	—
perchlorate (nonmedicinal) NEC	T65.891	T65.892	T65.893	T65.894	—	—
antithyroid	T38.2X1	T38.2X2	T38.2X3	T38.2X4	T38.2X5	T38.2X6
medicinal	T38.2X1	T38.2X2	T38.2X3	T38.2X4	T38.2X5	T38.2X6
Permanganate (nonmedicinal)	T65.891	T65.892	T65.893	T65.894	—	—
medicinal	T49.ØX1	T49.ØX2	T49.ØX3	T49.ØX4	T49.ØX5	T49.ØX6
sulfate	T47.2X1	T47.2X2	T47.2X3	T47.2X4	T47.2X5	T47.2X6
Potassium-removing resin	T5Ø.3X1	T5Ø.3X2	T5Ø.3X3	T5Ø.3X4	T5Ø.3X5	T5Ø.3X6
Potassium-retaining drug	T5Ø.3X1	T5Ø.3X2	T5Ø.3X3	T5Ø.3X4	T5Ø.3X5	T5Ø.3X6
Povidone	T45.8X1	T45.8X2	T45.8X3	T45.8X4	T45.8X5	T45.8X6
iodine	T49.ØX1	T49.ØX2	T49.ØX3	T49.ØX4	T49.ØX5	T49.ØX6
Practolol	T44.7X1	T44.7X2	T44.7X3	T44.7X4	T44.7X5	T44.7X6
Prajmalium bitartrate	T46.2X1	T46.2X2	T46.2X3	T46.2X4	T46.2X5	T46.2X6
Pralidoxime (iodide)	T5Ø.6X1	T5Ø.6X2	T5Ø.6X3	T5Ø.6X4	T5Ø.6X5	T5Ø.6X6
chloride	T5Ø.6X1	T5Ø.6X2	T5Ø.6X3	T5Ø.6X4	T5Ø.6X5	T5Ø.6X6
Pramiverine	T44.3X1	T44.3X2	T44.3X3	T44.3X4	T44.3X5	T44.3X6
Pramlintide*	T38.3X1	T38.3X2	T38.3X3	T38.3X4	T38.3X5	T38.3X6
Pramocaine	T49.1X1	T49.1X2	T49.1X3	T49.1X4	T49.1X5	T49.1X6
Pramoxine	T49.1X1	T49.1X2	T49.1X3	T49.1X4	T49.1X5	T49.1X6
Prasterone	T38.7X1	T38.7X2	T38.7X3	T38.7X4	T38.7X5	T38.7X6
Pravachol*	T46.6X1	T46.6X2	T46.6X3	T46.6X4	T46.6X5	T46.6X6
Pravastatin	T46.6X1	T46.6X2	T46.6X3	T46.6X4	T46.6X5	T46.6X6
Prazepam	T42.4X1	T42.4X2	T42.4X3	T42.4X4	T42.4X5	T42.4X6
Praziquantel	T37.4X1	T37.4X2	T37.4X3	T37.4X4	T37.4X5	T37.4X6

Substance	Poisoning, Accidental (unintentional)	Poisoning, Intentional Self-harm	Poisoning, Assault	Poisoning, Undetermined	Adverse Effect	Under-dosing
Prazitone	T43.291	T43.292	T43.293	T43.294	T43.295	T43.296
Prazosin	T44.6X1	T44.6X2	T44.6X3	T44.6X4	T44.6X5	T44.6X6
Prednicarbate	T49.ØX1	T49.ØX2	T49.ØX3	T49.ØX4	T49.ØX5	T49.ØX6
Prednimustine	T45.1X1	T45.1X2	T45.1X3	T45.1X4	T45.1X5	T45.1X6
Prednisolone	T38.ØX1	T38.ØX2	T38.ØX3	T38.ØX4	T38.ØX5	T38.ØX6
ENT agent	T49.6X1	T49.6X2	T49.6X3	T49.6X4	T49.6X5	T49.6X6
ophthalmic preparation	T49.5X1	T49.5X2	T49.5X3	T49.5X4	T49.5X5	T49.5X6
steaglate	T49.ØX1	T49.ØX2	T49.ØX3	T49.ØX4	T49.ØX5	T49.ØX6
topical NEC	T49.ØX1	T49.ØX2	T49.ØX3	T49.ØX4	T49.ØX5	T49.ØX6
Prednisone	T38.ØX1	T38.ØX2	T38.ØX3	T38.ØX4	T38.ØX5	T38.ØX6
Prednylidene	T38.ØX1	T38.ØX2	T38.ØX3	T38.ØX4	T38.ØX5	T38.ØX6
Pregnandiol	T38.5X1	T38.5X2	T38.5X3	T38.5X4	T38.5X5	T38.5X6
Pregneninolone	T38.5X1	T38.5X2	T38.5X3	T38.5X4	T38.5X5	T38.5X6
Preludin	T43.691	T43.692	T43.693	T43.694	T43.695	T43.696
Premarin	T38.5X1	T38.5X2	T38.5X3	T38.5X4	T38.5X5	T38.5X6
Premedication anesthetic	T41.2Ø1	T41.2Ø2	T41.2Ø3	T41.2Ø4	T41.2Ø5	T41.2Ø6
Prenalterol	T44.5X1	T44.5X2	T44.5X3	T44.5X4	T44.5X5	T44.5X6
Prenoxdiazine	T48.3X1	T48.3X2	T48.3X3	T48.3X4	T48.3X5	T48.3X6
Prenylamine	T46.3X1	T46.3X2	T46.3X3	T46.3X4	T46.3X5	T46.3X6
Preparation H	T49.8X1	T49.8X2	T49.8X3	T49.8X4	T49.8X5	T49.8X6
Preparation, local	T49.4X1	T49.4X2	T49.4X3	T49.4X4	T49.4X5	T49.4X6
Preservative (nonmedicinal)	T65.891	T65.892	T65.893	T65.894	—	—
medicinal	T5Ø.9Ø1	T5Ø.9Ø2	T5Ø.9Ø3	T5Ø.9Ø4	T5Ø.9Ø5	T5Ø.9Ø6
wood	T6Ø.91	T6Ø.92	T6Ø.93	T6Ø.94	—	—
Prethcamide	T5Ø.7X1	T5Ø.7X2	T5Ø.7X3	T5Ø.7X4	T5Ø.7X5	T5Ø.7X6
Prevacid*	T47.1X1	T47.1X2	T47.1X3	T47.1X4	T47.1X5	T47.1X6
Pride of China	T62.2X1	T62.2X2	T62.2X3	T62.2X4	—	—
Pridinol	T44.3X1	T44.3X2	T44.3X3	T44.3X4	T44.3X5	T44.3X6
Prifinium bromide	T44.3X1	T44.3X2	T44.3X3	T44.3X4	T44.3X5	T44.3X6
Prilocaine	T41.3X1	T41.3X2	T41.3X3	T41.3X4	T41.3X5	T41.3X6
infiltration (subcutaneous)	T41.3X1	T41.3X2	T41.3X3	T41.3X4	T41.3X5	T41.3X6
nerve block (peripheral) (plexus)	T41.3X1	T41.3X2	T41.3X3	T41.3X4	T41.3X5	T41.3X6
regional	T41.3X1	T41.3X2	T41.3X3	T41.3X4	T41.3X5	T41.3X6
Prilosec*	T47.1X1	T47.1X2	T47.1X3	T47.1X4	T47.1X5	T47.1X6
Primaquine	T37.2X1	T37.2X2	T37.2X3	T37.2X4	T37.2X5	T37.2X6
Primidone	T42.6X1	T42.6X2	T42.6X3	T42.6X4	T42.6X5	T42.6X6
Primula (veris)	T62.2X1	T62.2X2	T62.2X3	T62.2X4	—	—
Prinadol	T4Ø.2X1	T4Ø.2X2	T4Ø.2X3	T4Ø.2X4	T4Ø.2X5	T4Ø.2X6
Priscol, Priscoline	T44.6X1	T44.6X2	T44.6X3	T44.6X4	T44.6X5	T44.6X6
Pristinamycin	T36.3X1	T36.3X2	T36.3X3	T36.3X4	T36.3X5	T36.3X6
Pristiq*	T43.211	T43.212	T43.213	T43.214	T43.215	T43.216
Privet	T62.2X1	T62.2X2	T62.2X3	T62.2X4	—	—
berries	T62.1X1	T62.1X2	T62.1X3	T62.1X4	—	—
Privine	T44.4X1	T44.4X2	T44.4X3	T44.4X4	T44.4X5	T44.4X6
Pro-Banthine	T44.3X1	T44.3X2	T44.3X3	T44.3X4	T44.3X5	T44.3X6
Probarbital	T42.3X1	T42.3X2	T42.3X3	T42.3X4	T42.3X5	T42.3X6
Probenecid	T5Ø.4X1	T5Ø.4X2	T5Ø.4X3	T5Ø.4X4	T5Ø.4X5	T5Ø.4X6
Probucol	T46.6X1	T46.6X2	T46.6X3	T46.6X4	T46.6X5	T46.6X6
Procainamide	T46.2X1	T46.2X2	T46.2X3	T46.2X4	T46.2X5	T46.2X6
Procaine	T41.3X1	T41.3X2	T41.3X3	T41.3X4	T41.3X5	T41.3X6
benzylpenicillin	T36.ØX1	T36.ØX2	T36.ØX3	T36.ØX4	T36.ØX5	T36.ØX6
nerve block (periphreal) (plexus)	T41.3X1	T41.3X2	T41.3X3	T41.3X4	T41.3X5	T41.3X6
penicillin G	T36.ØX1	T36.ØX2	T36.ØX3	T36.ØX4	T36.ØX5	T36.ØX6
regional	T41.3X1	T41.3X2	T41.3X3	T41.3X4	T41.3X5	T41.3X6
spinal	T41.3X1	T41.3X2	T41.3X3	T41.3X4	T41.3X5	T41.3X6
Procalmidol	T43.591	T43.592	T43.593	T43.594	T43.595	T43.596
Procarbazine	T45.1X1	T45.1X2	T45.1X3	T45.1X4	T45.1X5	T45.1X6
Procaterol	T44.5X1	T44.5X2	T44.5X3	T44.5X4	T44.5X5	T44.5X6
Prochlorperazine	T43.3X1	T43.3X2	T43.3X3	T43.3X4	T43.3X5	T43.3X6
Procyclidine	T44.3X1	T44.3X2	T44.3X3	T44.3X4	T44.3X5	T44.3X6
Producer gas	T58.8X1	T58.8X2	T58.8X3	T58.8X4	—	—
Profadol	T4Ø.491	T4Ø.492	T4Ø.493	T4Ø.494	T4Ø.495	T4Ø.496
Profenamine	T44.3X1	T44.3X2	T44.3X3	T44.3X4	T44.3X5	T44.3X6
Profenil	T44.3X1	T44.3X2	T44.3X3	T44.3X4	T44.3X5	T44.3X6
Proflavine	T49.ØX1	T49.ØX2	T49.ØX3	T49.ØX4	T49.ØX5	T49.ØX6
Progabide	T42.6X1	T42.6X2	T42.6X3	T42.6X4	T42.6X5	T42.6X6
Progesterone	T38.5X1	T38.5X2	T38.5X3	T38.5X4	T38.5X5	T38.5X6
Progestin	T38.5X1	T38.5X2	T38.5X3	T38.5X4	T38.5X5	T38.5X6
oral contraceptive	T38.4X1	T38.4X2	T38.4X3	T38.4X4	T38.4X5	T38.4X6
Progestogen NEC	T38.5X1	T38.5X2	T38.5X3	T38.5X4	T38.5X5	T38.5X6
Progestone	T38.5X1	T38.5X2	T38.5X3	T38.5X4	T38.5X5	T38.5X6
Proglumide	T47.1X1	T47.1X2	T47.1X3	T47.1X4	T47.1X5	T47.1X6
Prograf*	T45.1X1	T45.1X2	T45.1X3	T45.1X4	T45.1X5	T45.1X6
Proguanil	T37.2X1	T37.2X2	T37.2X3	T37.2X4	T37.2X5	T37.2X6
Prolactin	T38.811	T38.812	T38.813	T38.814	T38.815	T38.816
Prolintane	T43.691	T43.692	T43.693	T43.694	T43.695	T43.696
Proloid	T38.1X1	T38.1X2	T38.1X3	T38.1X4	T38.1X5	T38.1X6
Proluton	T38.5X1	T38.5X2	T38.5X3	T38.5X4	T38.5X5	T38.5X6
Promacetin	T37.1X1	T37.1X2	T37.1X3	T37.1X4	T37.1X5	T37.1X6
Promazine	T43.3X1	T43.3X2	T43.3X3	T43.3X4	T43.3X5	T43.3X6

Substance	Poisoning, Accidental (unintentional)	Poisoning, Intentional Self-harm	Poisoning, Assault	Poisoning, Undetermined	Adverse Effect	Under-dosing
Promedol	T4Ø.2X1	T4Ø.2X2	T4Ø.2X3	T4Ø.2X4	—	—
Promegestone	T38.5X1	T38.5X2	T38.5X3	T38.5X4	T38.5X5	T38.5X6
Promethazine (teoclate)	T43.3X1	T43.3X2	T43.3X3	T43.3X4	T43.3X5	T43.3X6
Promin	T37.1X1	T37.1X2	T37.1X3	T37.1X4	T37.1X5	T37.1X6
Pronase	T45.3X1	T45.3X2	T45.3X3	T45.3X4	T45.3X5	T45.3X6
Pronestyl (hydrochloride)	T46.2X1	T46.2X2	T46.2X3	T46.2X4	T46.2X5	T46.2X6
Pronetalol	T44.7X1	T44.7X2	T44.7X3	T44.7X4	T44.7X5	T44.7X6
Prontosil	T37.ØX1	T37.ØX2	T37.ØX3	T37.ØX4	T37.ØX5	T37.ØX6
Propachlor	T6Ø.3X1	T6Ø.3X2	T6Ø.3X3	T6Ø.3X4	—	—
Propafenone	T46.2X1	T46.2X2	T46.2X3	T46.2X4	T46.2X5	T46.2X6
Propallylonal	T42.3X1	T42.3X2	T42.3X3	T42.3X4	T42.3X5	T42.3X6
Propamidine	T49.ØX1	T49.ØX2	T49.ØX3	T49.ØX4	T49.ØX5	T49.ØX6
Propane (distributed in mobile container)	T59.891	T59.892	T59.893	T59.894	—	—
distributed through pipes	T59.891	T59.892	T59.893	T59.894	—	—
incomplete combustion	T58.11	T58.12	T58.13	T58.14	—	—
Propanidid	T41.291	T41.292	T41.293	T41.294	T41.295	T41.296
Propanil	T6Ø.3X1	T6Ø.3X2	T6Ø.3X3	T6Ø.3X4	—	—
Propantheline	T44.3X1	T44.3X2	T44.3X3	T44.3X4	T44.3X5	T44.3X6
bromide	T44.3X1	T44.3X2	T44.3X3	T44.3X4	T44.3X5	T44.3X6
Proparacaine	T41.3X1	T41.3X2	T41.3X3	T41.3X4	T41.3X5	T41.3X6
Propatylnitrate	T46.3X1	T46.3X2	T46.3X3	T46.3X4	T46.3X5	T46.3X6
Propicillin	T36.ØX1	T36.ØX2	T36.ØX3	T36.ØX4	T36.ØX5	T36.ØX6
Propine*	T49.5X1	T49.5X2	T49.5X3	T49.5X4	T49.5X5	T49.5X6
Propiolactone	T49.ØX1	T49.ØX2	T49.ØX3	T49.ØX4	T49.ØX5	T49.ØX6
Propiomazine	T45.ØX1	T45.ØX2	T45.ØX3	T45.ØX4	T45.ØX5	T45.ØX6
Propionaldehyde (medicinal)	T42.6X1	T42.6X2	T42.6X3	T42.6X4	T42.6X5	T42.6X6
Propionate (calcium) (sodium)	T49.ØX1	T49.ØX2	T49.ØX3	T49.ØX4	T49.ØX5	T49.ØX6
Propion gel	T49.ØX1	T49.ØX2	T49.ØX3	T49.ØX4	T49.ØX5	T49.ØX6
Propitocaine	T41.3X1	T41.3X2	T41.3X3	T41.3X4	T41.3X5	T41.3X6
infiltration (subcutaneous)	T41.3X1	T41.3X2	T41.3X3	T41.3X4	T41.3X5	T41.3X6
nerve block (peripheral) (plexus)	T41.3X1	T41.3X2	T41.3X3	T41.3X4	T41.3X5	T41.3X6
Propofol	T41.291	T41.292	T41.293	T41.294	T41.295	T41.296
Propoxur	T6Ø.ØX1	T6Ø.ØX2	T6Ø.ØX3	T6Ø.ØX4	—	—
Propoxycaine	T41.3X1	T41.3X2	T41.3X3	T41.3X4	T41.3X5	T41.3X6
infiltration (subcutaneous)	T41.3X1	T41.3X2	T41.3X3	T41.3X4	T41.3X5	T41.3X6
nerve block (peripheral) (plexus)	T41.3X1	T41.3X2	T41.3X3	T41.3X4	T41.3X5	T41.3X6
topical (surface)	T41.3X1	T41.3X2	T41.3X3	T41.3X4	T41.3X5	T41.3X6
Propoxyphene	T4Ø.491	T4Ø.492	T4Ø.493	T4Ø.494	T4Ø.495	T4Ø.496
Propranolol	T44.7X1	T44.7X2	T44.7X3	T44.7X4	T44.7X5	T44.7X6
Propyl						
alcohol	T51.3X1	T51.3X2	T51.3X3	T51.3X4	—	—
carbinol	T51.3X1	T51.3X2	T51.3X3	T51.3X4	—	—
hexadrine	T44.4X1	T44.4X2	T44.4X3	T44.4X4	T44.4X5	T44.4X6
iodone	T5Ø.8X1	T5Ø.8X2	T5Ø.8X3	T5Ø.8X4	T5Ø.8X5	T5Ø.8X6
thiouracil	T38.2X1	T38.2X2	T38.2X3	T38.2X4	T38.2X5	T38.2X6
Propylaminophenothiazine	T43.3X1	T43.3X2	T43.3X3	T43.3X4	T43.3X5	T43.3X6
Propylene	T59.891	T59.892	T59.893	T59.894	—	—
Propylhexedrine	T48.5X1	T48.5X2	T48.5X3	T48.5X4	T48.5X5	T48.5X6
Propyliodone	T5Ø.8X1	T5Ø.8X2	T5Ø.8X3	T5Ø.8X4	T5Ø.8X5	T5Ø.8X6
Propylparaben (ophthalmic)	T49.5X1	T49.5X2	T49.5X3	T49.5X4	T49.5X5	T49.5X6
Propylthiouracil	T38.2X1	T38.2X2	T38.2X3	T38.2X4	T38.2X5	T38.2X6
Propyphenazone	T39.2X1	T39.2X2	T39.2X3	T39.2X4	T39.2X5	T39.2X6
Proquazone	T39.391	T39.392	T39.393	T39.394	T39.395	T39.396
Proscar*	T38.6X1	T38.6X2	T38.6X3	T38.6X4	T38.6X5	T38.6X6
Proscillaridin	T46.ØX1	T46.ØX2	T46.ØX3	T46.ØX4	T46.ØX5	T46.ØX6
Prostacyclin	T45.521	T45.522	T45.523	T45.524	T45.525	T45.526
Prostaglandin (I2)	T45.521	T45.522	T45.523	T45.524	T45.525	T45.526
E1	T46.7X1	T46.7X2	T46.7X3	T46.7X4	T46.7X5	T46.7X6
E2	T48.ØX1	T48.ØX2	T48.ØX3	T48.ØX4	T48.ØX5	T48.ØX6
F2 alpha	T48.ØX1	T48.ØX2	T48.ØX3	T48.ØX4	T48.ØX5	T48.ØX6
Prostigmin	T44.ØX1	T44.ØX2	T44.ØX3	T44.ØX4	T44.ØX5	T44.ØX6
Prosultiamine	T45.2X1	T45.2X2	T45.2X3	T45.2X4	T45.2X5	T45.2X6
Protamine sulfate	T45.7X1	T45.7X2	T45.7X3	T45.7X4	T45.7X5	T45.7X6
zinc insulin	T38.3X1	T38.3X2	T38.3X3	T38.3X4	T38.3X5	T38.3X6
Protease	T47.5X1	T47.5X2	T47.5X3	T47.5X4	T47.5X5	T47.5X6
Protectant, skin NEC	T49.3X1	T49.3X2	T49.3X3	T49.3X4	T49.3X5	T49.3X6
Protein hydrolysate	T5Ø.991	T5Ø.992	T5Ø.993	T5Ø.994	T5Ø.995	T5Ø.996
Prothiaden — *see* Dothiepin hydrochloride						
Prothionamide	T37.1X1	T37.1X2	T37.1X3	T37.1X4	T37.1X5	T37.1X6
Prothipendyl	T43.591	T43.592	T43.593	T43.594	T43.595	T43.596
Prothoate	T6Ø.ØX1	T6Ø.ØX2	T6Ø.ØX3	T6Ø.ØX4	—	—
Prothrombin						
activator	T45.7X1	T45.7X2	T45.7X3	T45.7X4	T45.7X5	T45.7X6
synthesis inhibitor	T45.511	T45.512	T45.513	T45.514	T45.515	T45.516
Protionamide	T37.1X1	T37.1X2	T37.1X3	T37.1X4	T37.1X5	T37.1X6
Protirelin	T38.891	T38.892	T38.893	T38.894	T38.895	T38.896

Substance	Poisoning, Accidental (unintentional)	Poisoning, Intentional Self-harm	Poisoning, Assault	Poisoning, Undetermined	Adverse Effect	Under-dosing
Protokylol	T48.6X1	T48.6X2	T48.6X3	T48.6X4	T48.6X5	T48.6X6
Protopam	T50.6X1	T50.6X2	T50.6X3	T50.6X4	T50.6X5	T50.6X6
Protoveratrine(s) (A) (B)	T46.5X1	T46.5X2	T46.5X3	T46.5X4	T46.5X5	T46.5X6
Protriptyline	T43.011	T43.012	T43.013	T43.014	T43.015	T43.016
Proventil*	T48.6X1	T48.6X2	T48.6X3	T48.6X4	T48.6X5	T48.6X6
Provera	T38.5X1	T38.5X2	T38.5X3	T38.5X4	T38.5X5	T38.5X6
Provitamin A	T45.2X1	T45.2X2	T45.2X3	T45.2X4	T45.2X5	T45.2X6
Proxibarbal	T42.3X1	T42.3X2	T42.3X3	T42.3X4	T42.3X5	T42.3X6
Proxymetacaine	T41.3X1	T41.3X2	T41.3X3	T41.3X4	T41.3X5	T41.3X6
Proxyphylline	T48.6X1	T48.6X2	T48.6X3	T48.6X4	T48.6X5	T48.6X6
Prozac — *see* Fluoxetine hydrochloride						
Prunus						
laurocerasus	T62.2X1	T62.2X2	T62.2X3	T62.2X4	—	—
virginiana	T62.2X1	T62.2X2	T62.2X3	T62.2X4	—	—
Prussian blue						
commercial	T65.891	T65.892	T65.893	T65.894	—	—
therapeutic	T50.6X1	T50.6X2	T50.6X3	T50.6X4	T50.6X5	T50.6X6
Prussic acid	T65.0X1	T65.0X2	T65.0X3	T65.0X4	—	—
vapor	T57.3X1	T57.3X2	T57.3X3	T57.3X4	—	—
Pseudoephedrine	T44.991	T44.992	T44.993	T44.994	T44.995	T44.996
Psilocin	T40.991	T40.992	T40.993	T40.994	—	—
Psilocybin	T40.991	T40.992	T40.993	T40.994	—	—
Psilocybine	T40.991	T40.992	T40.993	T40.994	—	—
Psoralene (nonmedicinal)	T65.891	T65.892	T65.893	T65.894	—	—
Psoralens (medicinal)	T50.991	T50.992	T50.993	T50.994	T50.995	T50.996
PSP (phenolsulfonphthalein)	T50.8X1	T50.8X2	T50.8X3	T50.8X4	T50.8X5	T50.8X6
Psychodysleptic drug NOS	T40.901	T40.902	T40.903	T40.904	T40.905	T40.906
specified NEC	T40.991	T40.992	T40.993	T40.994	T40.995	T40.996
Psychostimulant	T43.601	T43.602	T43.603	T43.604	T43.605	T43.606
amphetamine	T43.621	T43.622	T43.623	T43.624	T43.625	T43.626
caffeine	T43.611	T43.612	T43.613	T43.614	T43.615	T43.616
methylphenidate	T43.631	T43.632	T43.633	T43.634	T43.635	T43.636
specified NEC	T43.691	T43.692	T43.693	T43.694	T43.695	T43.696
Psychotherapeutic drug NEC	T43.91	T43.92	T43.93	T43.94	T43.95	T43.96
antidepressants — *see also* Antidepressant	T43.201	T43.202	T43.203	T43.204	T43.205	T43.206
specified NEC	T43.8X1	T43.8X2	T43.8X3	T43.8X4	T43.8X5	T43.8X6
tranquilizers NEC	T43.501	T43.502	T43.503	T43.504	T43.505	T43.506
Psychotomimetic agents	T40.901	T40.902	T40.903	T40.904	T40.905	T40.906
Psychotropic drug NEC	T43.91	T43.92	T43.93	T43.94	T43.95	T43.96
specified NEC	T43.8X1	T43.8X2	T43.8X3	T43.8X4	T43.8X5	T43.8X6
Psyllium hydrophilic mucilloid	T47.4X1	T47.4X2	T47.4X3	T47.4X4	T47.4X5	T47.4X6
Pteroylglutamic acid	T45.8X1	T45.8X2	T45.8X3	T45.8X4	T45.8X5	T45.8X6
Pteroyltriglutamate	T45.1X1	T45.1X2	T45.1X3	T45.1X4	T45.1X5	T45.1X6
PTFE — *see* Polytetrafluoroethylene						
Pulmicort*	T44.5X1	T44.5X2	T44.5X3	T44.5X4	T44.5X5	T44.5X6
Pulp						
devitalizing paste	T49.7X1	T49.7X2	T49.7X3	T49.7X4	T49.7X5	T49.7X6
dressing	T49.7X1	T49.7X2	T49.7X3	T49.7X4	T49.7X5	T49.7X6
Pulsatilla	T62.2X1	T62.2X2	T62.2X3	T62.2X4	—	—
Pumpkin seed extract	T37.4X1	T37.4X2	T37.4X3	T37.4X4	T37.4X5	T37.4X6
Purex (bleach)	T54.91	T54.92	T54.93	T54.94	—	—
Purgative NEC — *see also* Cathartic	T47.4X1	T47.4X2	T47.4X3	T47.4X4	T47.4X5	T47.4X6
Purine analogue (antineoplastic)	T45.1X1	T45.1X2	T45.1X3	T45.1X4	T45.1X5	T45.1X6
Purine diuretics	T50.2X1	T50.2X2	T50.2X3	T50.2X4	T50.2X5	T50.2X6
Purinethol	T45.1X1	T45.1X2	T45.1X3	T45.1X4	T45.1X5	T45.1X6
PVP	T45.8X1	T45.8X2	T45.8X3	T45.8X4	T45.8X5	T45.8X6
Pyrabital	T39.8X1	T39.8X2	T39.8X3	T39.8X4	T39.8X5	T39.8X6
Pyramidon	T39.2X1	T39.2X2	T39.2X3	T39.2X4	T39.2X5	T39.2X6
Pyrantel	T37.4X1	T37.4X2	T37.4X3	T37.4X4	T37.4X5	T37.4X6
Pyrathiazine	T45.0X1	T45.0X2	T45.0X3	T45.0X4	T45.0X5	T45.0X6
Pyrazinamide	T37.1X1	T37.1X2	T37.1X3	T37.1X4	T37.1X5	T37.1X6
Pyrazinoic acid (amide)	T37.1X1	T37.1X2	T37.1X3	T37.1X4	T37.1X5	T37.1X6
Pyrazole (derivatives)	T39.2X1	T39.2X2	T39.2X3	T39.2X4	T39.2X5	T39.2X6
Pyrazolone analgesic NEC	T39.2X1	T39.2X2	T39.2X3	T39.2X4	T39.2X5	T39.2X6
Pyrethrin, pyrethrum (nonmedicinal)	T60.2X1	T60.2X2	T60.2X3	T60.2X4	—	—
Pyrethrum extract	T49.0X1	T49.0X2	T49.0X3	T49.0X4	T49.0X5	T49.0X6
Pyribenzamine	T45.0X1	T45.0X2	T45.0X3	T45.0X4	T45.0X5	T45.0X6
Pyridine	T52.8X1	T52.8X2	T52.8X3	T52.8X4	—	—
aldoxime methiodide	T50.6X1	T50.6X2	T50.6X3	T50.6X4	T50.6X5	T50.6X6
aldoxime methyl chloride	T50.6X1	T50.6X2	T50.6X3	T50.6X4	T50.6X5	T50.6X6
vapor	T59.891	T59.892	T59.893	T59.894	—	—
Pyridium	T39.8X1	T39.8X2	T39.8X3	T39.8X4	T39.8X5	T39.8X6
Pyridostigmine bromide	T44.0X1	T44.0X2	T44.0X3	T44.0X4	T44.0X5	T44.0X6
Pyridoxal phosphate	T45.2X1	T45.2X2	T45.2X3	T45.2X4	T45.2X5	T45.2X6
Pyridoxine	T45.2X1	T45.2X2	T45.2X3	T45.2X4	T45.2X5	T45.2X6
Pyrilamine	T45.0X1	T45.0X2	T45.0X3	T45.0X4	T45.0X5	T45.0X6
Pyrimethamine	T37.2X1	T37.2X2	T37.2X3	T37.2X4	T37.2X5	T37.2X6
with sulfadoxine	T37.2X1	T37.2X2	T37.2X3	T37.2X4	T37.2X5	T37.2X6
Pyrimidine antagonist	T45.1X1	T45.1X2	T45.1X3	T45.1X4	T45.1X5	T45.1X6
Pyriminil	T60.4X1	T60.4X2	T60.4X3	T60.4X4	—	—
Pyrithione zinc	T49.4X1	T49.4X2	T49.4X3	T49.4X4	T49.4X5	T49.4X6
Pyrithyldione	T42.6X1	T42.6X2	T42.6X3	T42.6X4	T42.6X5	T42.6X6
Pyrogallic acid	T49.0X1	T49.0X2	T49.0X3	T49.0X4	T49.0X5	T49.0X6
Pyrogallol	T49.0X1	T49.0X2	T49.0X3	T49.0X4	T49.0X5	T49.0X6
Pyroxylin	T49.3X1	T49.3X2	T49.3X3	T49.3X4	T49.3X5	T49.3X6
Pyrrobutamine	T45.0X1	T45.0X2	T45.0X3	T45.0X4	T45.0X5	T45.0X6
Pyrrolizidine alkaloids	T62.8X1	T62.8X2	T62.8X3	T62.8X4	—	—
Pyrvinium chloride	T37.4X1	T37.4X2	T37.4X3	T37.4X4	T37.4X5	T37.4X6
PZI	T38.3X1	T38.3X2	T38.3X3	T38.3X4	T38.3X5	T38.3X6
Qbrelis*	T46.4X1	T46.4X2	T46.4X3	T46.4X4	T46.4X5	T46.4X6
Quaalude	T42.6X1	T42.6X2	T42.6X3	T42.6X4	T42.6X5	T42.6X6
Quarternary ammonium						
anti-infective	T49.0X1	T49.0X2	T49.0X3	T49.0X4	T49.0X5	T49.0X6
ganglion blocking	T44.2X1	T44.2X2	T44.2X3	T44.2X4	T44.2X5	T44.2X6
parasympatholytic	T44.3X1	T44.3X2	T44.3X3	T44.3X4	T44.3X5	T44.3X6
Quazepam	T42.4X1	T42.4X2	T42.4X3	T42.4X4	T42.4X5	T42.4X6
Quicklime	T54.3X1	T54.3X2	T54.3X3	T54.3X4	—	—
Quilbron-T*	T48.6X1	T48.6X2	T48.6X3	T48.6X4	T48.6X5	T48.6X6
Quillaja extract	T48.4X1	T48.4X2	T48.4X3	T48.4X4	T48.4X5	T48.4X6
Quinacrine	T37.2X1	T37.2X2	T37.2X3	T37.2X4	T37.2X5	T37.2X6
Quinaglute	T46.2X1	T46.2X2	T46.2X3	T46.2X4	T46.2X5	T46.2X6
Quinalbarbital	T42.3X1	T42.3X2	T42.3X3	T42.3X4	T42.3X5	T42.3X6
Quinalbarbitone sodium	T42.3X1	T42.3X2	T42.3X3	T42.3X4	T42.3X5	T42.3X6
Quinalphos	T60.0X1	T60.0X2	T60.0X3	T60.0X4	—	—
Quinapril	T46.4X1	T46.4X2	T46.4X3	T46.4X4	T46.4X5	T46.4X6
Quinestradiol	T38.5X1	T38.5X2	T38.5X3	T38.5X4	T38.5X5	T38.5X6
Quinestradol	T38.5X1	T38.5X2	T38.5X3	T38.5X4	T38.5X5	T38.5X6
Quinestrol	T38.5X1	T38.5X2	T38.5X3	T38.5X4	T38.5X5	T38.5X6
Quinethazone	T50.2X1	T50.2X2	T50.2X3	T50.2X4	T50.2X5	T50.2X6
Quingestanol	T38.4X1	T38.4X2	T38.4X3	T38.4X4	T38.4X5	T38.4X6
Quinidine	T46.2X1	T46.2X2	T46.2X3	T46.2X4	T46.2X5	T46.2X6
Quinine	T37.2X1	T37.2X2	T37.2X3	T37.2X4	T37.2X5	T37.2X6
Quiniobine	T37.8X1	T37.8X2	T37.8X3	T37.8X4	T37.8X5	T37.8X6
Quinisocaine	T49.1X1	T49.1X2	T49.1X3	T49.1X4	T49.1X5	T49.1X6
Quinocide	T37.2X1	T37.2X2	T37.2X3	T37.2X4	T37.2X5	T37.2X6
Quinoline (derivatives) **NEC**	T37.8X1	T37.8X2	T37.8X3	T37.8X4	T37.8X5	T37.8X6
Quinupramine	T43.011	T43.012	T43.013	T43.014	T43.015	T43.016
Quixin*	T49.5X1	T49.5X2	T49.5X3	T49.5X4	T49.5X5	T49.5X6
Quotane	T41.3X1	T41.3X2	T41.3X3	T41.3X4	T41.3X5	T41.3X6
Rabies						
immune globulin (human)	T50.Z11	T50.Z12	T50.Z13	T50.Z14	T50.Z15	T50.Z16
vaccine	T50.B91	T50.B92	T50.B93	T50.B94	T50.B95	T50.B96
Racemoramide	T40.2X1	T40.2X2	T40.2X3	T40.2X4	—	—
Racemorphan	T40.2X1	T40.2X2	T40.2X3	T40.2X4	T40.2X5	T40.2X6
Racepinefrin	T44.5X1	T44.5X2	T44.5X3	T44.5X4	T44.5X5	T44.5X6
Raclopride	T43.591	T43.592	T43.593	T43.594	T43.595	T43.596
Radiator alcohol	T51.1X1	T51.1X2	T51.1X3	T51.1X4	—	—
Radioactive drug NEC	T50.8X1	T50.8X2	T50.8X3	T50.8X4	T50.8X5	T50.8X6
Radio-opaque (drugs) (materials)	T50.8X1	T50.8X2	T50.8X3	T50.8X4	T50.8X5	T50.8X6
Ramifenazone	T39.2X1	T39.2X2	T39.2X3	T39.2X4	T39.2X5	T39.2X6
Ramipril	T46.4X1	T46.4X2	T46.4X3	T46.4X4	T46.4X5	T46.4X6
Ranitidine	T47.0X1	T47.0X2	T47.0X3	T47.0X4	T47.0X5	T47.0X6
Ranunculus	T62.2X1	T62.2X2	T62.2X3	T62.2X4	—	—
Rat poison NEC	T60.4X1	T60.4X2	T60.4X3	T60.4X4	—	—
Rattlesnake (venom)	T63.011	T63.012	T63.013	T63.014	—	—
Raubasine	T46.7X1	T46.7X2	T46.7X3	T46.7X4	T46.7X5	T46.7X6
Raudixin	T46.5X1	T46.5X2	T46.5X3	T46.5X4	T46.5X5	T46.5X6
Rautensin	T46.5X1	T46.5X2	T46.5X3	T46.5X4	T46.5X5	T46.5X6
Rautina	T46.5X1	T46.5X2	T46.5X3	T46.5X4	T46.5X5	T46.5X6
Rautotal	T46.5X1	T46.5X2	T46.5X3	T46.5X4	T46.5X5	T46.5X6
Rauwiloid	T46.5X1	T46.5X2	T46.5X3	T46.5X4	T46.5X5	T46.5X6
Rauwoldin	T46.5X1	T46.5X2	T46.5X3	T46.5X4	T46.5X5	T46.5X6
Rauwolfia (alkaloids)	T46.5X1	T46.5X2	T46.5X3	T46.5X4	T46.5X5	T46.5X6
Razadyne*	T44.0X1	T44.0X2	T44.0X3	T44.0X4	T44.0X5	T44.0X6
Razoxane	T45.1X1	T45.1X2	T45.1X3	T45.1X4	T45.1X5	T45.1X6
Realgar	T57.0X1	T57.0X2	T57.0X3	T57.0X4	—	—
Recombinant (R) — *see* specific protein						
Red blood cells, packed	T45.8X1	T45.8X2	T45.8X3	T45.8X4	T45.8X5	T45.8X6
Red squill (scilliroside)	T60.4X1	T60.4X2	T60.4X3	T60.4X4	—	—
Reducing agent, industrial NEC	T65.891	T65.892	T65.893	T65.894	—	—
Refrigerant gas (chlorofluorocarbon)	T53.5X1	T53.5X2	T53.5X3	T53.5X4	—	—
not chlorofluorocarbon	T59.891	T59.892	T59.893	T59.894	—	—
Regroton	T50.2X1	T50.2X2	T50.2X3	T50.2X4	T50.2X5	T50.2X6

Substance	Poisoning, Accidental (unintentional)	Poisoning, Intentional Self-harm	Poisoning, Assault	Poisoning, Undetermined	Adverse Effect	Under-dosing
Rehydration salts (oral)	T50.3X1	T50.3X2	T50.3X3	T50.3X4	T50.3X5	T50.3X6
Rela	T42.8X1	T42.8X2	T42.8X3	T42.8X4	T42.8X5	T42.8X6
Relaxant, muscle						
anesthetic	T48.1X1	T48.1X2	T48.1X3	T48.1X4	T48.1X5	T48.1X6
central nervous system	T42.8X1	T42.8X2	T42.8X3	T42.8X4	T42.8X5	T42.8X6
skeletal NEC	T48.1X1	T48.1X2	T48.1X3	T48.1X4	T48.1X5	T48.1X6
smooth NEC	T44.3X1	T44.3X2	T44.3X3	T44.3X4	T44.3X5	T44.3X6
Remoxipride	T43.591	T43.592	T43.593	T43.594	T43.595	T43.596
Renese	T50.2X1	T50.2X2	T50.2X3	T50.2X4	T50.2X5	T50.2X6
Renografin	T50.8X1	T50.8X2	T50.8X3	T50.8X4	T50.8X5	T50.8X6
Replacement solution	T50.3X1	T50.3X2	T50.3X3	T50.3X4	T50.3X5	T50.3X6
Reproterol	T48.6X1	T48.6X2	T48.6X3	T48.6X4	T48.6X5	T48.6X6
Rescinnamine	T46.5X1	T46.5X2	T46.5X3	T46.5X4	T46.5X5	T46.5X6
Reserpin (e)	T46.5X1	T46.5X2	T46.5X3	T46.5X4	T46.5X5	T46.5X6
Resorcin, resorcinol (nonmedicinal)	T65.891	T65.892	T65.893	T65.894	—	—
medicinal	T49.4X1	T49.4X2	T49.4X3	T49.4X4	T49.4X5	T49.4X6
Respaire	T48.4X1	T48.4X2	T48.4X3	T48.4X4	T48.4X5	T48.4X6
Respiratory drug NEC	T48.901	T48.902	T48.903	T48.904	T48.905	T48.906
antiasthmatic NEC	T48.6X1	T48.6X2	T48.6X3	T48.6X4	T48.6X5	T48.6X6
anti-common-cold NEC	T48.5X1	T48.5X2	T48.5X3	T48.5X4	T48.5X5	T48.5X6
expectorant NEC	T48.4X1	T48.4X2	T48.4X3	T48.4X4	T48.4X5	T48.4X6
stimulant	T48.901	T48.902	T48.903	T48.904	T48.905	T48.906
Restoril*	T42.4X1	T42.4X2	T42.4X3	T42.4X4	T42.4X5	T42.4X6
Retinoic acid	T49.0X1	T49.0X2	T49.0X3	T49.0X4	T49.0X5	T49.0X6
Retinol	T45.2X1	T45.2X2	T45.2X3	T45.2X4	T45.2X5	T45.2X6
Rh (D) **immune globulin** (human)	T50.Z11	T50.Z12	T50.Z13	T50.Z14	T50.Z15	T50.Z16
Rhodine	T39.011	T39.012	T39.013	T39.014	T39.015	T39.016
RhoGAM	T50.Z11	T50.Z12	T50.Z13	T50.Z14	T50.Z15	T50.Z16
Rhubarb						
dry extract	T47.2X1	T47.2X2	T47.2X3	T47.2X4	T47.2X5	T47.2X6
tincture, compound	T47.2X1	T47.2X2	T47.2X3	T47.2X4	T47.2X5	T47.2X6
Ribavirin	T37.5X1	T37.5X2	T37.5X3	T37.5X4	T37.5X5	T37.5X6
Riboflavin	T45.2X1	T45.2X2	T45.2X3	T45.2X4	T45.2X5	T45.2X6
Ribostamycin	T36.5X1	T36.5X2	T36.5X3	T36.5X4	T36.5X5	T36.5X6
Ricin	T62.2X1	T62.2X2	T62.2X3	T62.2X4	—	—
Ricinus communis	T62.2X1	T62.2X2	T62.2X3	T62.2X4	—	—
Rickettsial vaccine NEC	T50.A91	T50.A92	T50.A93	T50.A94	T50.A95	T50.A96
Rifabutin	T36.6X1	T36.6X2	T36.6X3	T36.6X4	T36.6X5	T36.6X6
Rifamide	T36.6X1	T36.6X2	T36.6X3	T36.6X4	T36.6X5	T36.6X6
Rifampicin	T36.6X1	T36.6X2	T36.6X3	T36.6X4	T36.6X5	T36.6X6
with isoniazid	T37.1X1	T37.1X2	T37.1X3	T37.1X4	T37.1X5	T37.1X6
Rifampin	T36.6X1	T36.6X2	T36.6X3	T36.6X4	T36.6X5	T36.6X6
Rifamycin	T36.6X1	T36.6X2	T36.6X3	T36.6X4	T36.6X5	T36.6X6
Rifaximin	T36.6X1	T36.6X2	T36.6X3	T36.6X4	T36.6X5	T36.6X6
Rimantadine	T37.5X1	T37.5X2	T37.5X3	T37.5X4	T37.5X5	T37.5X6
Rimazolium metilsulfate	T39.8X1	T39.8X2	T39.8X3	T39.8X4	T39.8X5	T39.8X6
Rimifon	T37.1X1	T37.1X2	T37.1X3	T37.1X4	T37.1X5	T37.1X6
Rimiterol	T48.6X1	T48.6X2	T48.6X3	T48.6X4	T48.6X5	T48.6X6
Ringer (lactate) **solution**	T50.3X1	T50.3X2	T50.3X3	T50.3X4	T50.3X5	T50.3X6
Risperdal*	T43.591	T43.592	T43.593	T43.594	T43.595	T43.596
Ristocetin	T36.8X1	T36.8X2	T36.8X3	T36.8X4	T36.8X5	T36.8X6
Ritalin	T43.631	T43.632	T43.633	T43.634	T43.635	T43.636
Ritodrine	T44.5X1	T44.5X2	T44.5X3	T44.5X4	T44.5X5	T44.5X6
Roach killer — *see* Insecticide						
Robaxin*	T48.1X1	T48.1X2	T48.1X3	T48.1X4	T48.1X5	T48.1X6
Robitussin*	T48.3X1	T48.3X2	T48.3X3	T48.3X4	T48.3X5	T48.3X6
Rociverine	T44.3X1	T44.3X2	T44.3X3	T44.3X4	T44.3X5	T44.3X6
Rocky Mountain spotted fever vaccine	T50.A91	T50.A92	T50.A93	T50.A94	T50.A95	T50.A96
Rodenticide NEC	T60.4X1	T60.4X2	T60.4X3	T60.4X4	—	—
Rohypnol	T42.4X1	T42.4X2	T42.4X3	T42.4X4	T42.4X5	T42.4X6
Rokitamycin	T36.3X1	T36.3X2	T36.3X3	T36.3X4	T36.3X5	T36.3X6
Rolaids	T47.1X1	T47.1X2	T47.1X3	T47.1X4	T47.1X5	T47.1X6
Rolitetracycline	T36.4X1	T36.4X2	T36.4X3	T36.4X4	T36.4X5	T36.4X6
Romilar	T48.3X1	T48.3X2	T48.3X3	T48.3X4	T48.3X5	T48.3X6
Ronifibrate	T46.6X1	T46.6X2	T46.6X3	T46.6X4	T46.6X5	T46.6X6
Rosaprostol	T47.1X1	T47.1X2	T47.1X3	T47.1X4	T47.1X5	T47.1X6
Rose bengal sodium (131I)	T50.8X1	T50.8X2	T50.8X3	T50.8X4	T50.8X5	T50.8X6
Rose water ointment	T49.3X1	T49.3X2	T49.3X3	T49.3X4	T49.3X5	T49.3X6
Rosoxacin	T37.8X1	T37.8X2	T37.8X3	T37.8X4	T37.8X5	T37.8X6
Rotenone	T60.2X1	T60.2X2	T60.2X3	T60.2X4	—	—
Rotoxamine	T45.0X1	T45.0X2	T45.0X3	T45.0X4	T45.0X5	T45.0X6
Rough-on-rats	T60.4X1	T60.4X2	T60.4X3	T60.4X4	—	—
Roxatidine	T47.0X1	T47.0X2	T47.0X3	T47.0X4	T47.0X5	T47.0X6
Roxithromycin	T36.3X1	T36.3X2	T36.3X3	T36.3X4	T36.3X5	T36.3X6
Rt-PA	T45.611	T45.612	T45.613	T45.614	T45.615	T45.616
Rubbing alcohol	T51.2X1	T51.2X2	T51.2X3	T51.2X4	—	—
Rubefacient	T49.4X1	T49.4X2	T49.4X3	T49.4X4	T49.4X5	T49.4X6
Rubella vaccine	T50.B91	T50.B92	T50.B93	T50.B94	T50.B95	T50.B96
Rubeola vaccine	T50.B91	T50.B92	T50.B93	T50.B94	T50.B95	T50.B96
Rubidium chloride Rb82	T50.8X1	T50.8X2	T50.8X3	T50.8X4	T50.8X5	T50.8X6
Rubidomycin	T45.1X1	T45.1X2	T45.1X3	T45.1X4	T45.1X5	T45.1X6
Rue	T62.2X1	T62.2X2	T62.2X3	T62.2X4	—	—
Rufocromomycin	T45.1X1	T45.1X2	T45.1X3	T45.1X4	T45.1X5	T45.1X6
Russel's viper venin	T45.7X1	T45.7X2	T45.7X3	T45.7X4	T45.7X5	T45.7X6
Ruta (graveolens)	T62.2X1	T62.2X2	T62.2X3	T62.2X4	—	—
Rutinum	T46.991	T46.992	T46.993	T46.994	T46.995	T46.996
Rutoside	T46.991	T46.992	T46.993	T46.994	T46.995	T46.996
b-sitosterol(s)	T46.6X1	T46.6X2	T46.6X3	T46.6X4	T46.6X5	T46.6X6
Sabadilla (plant)	T62.2X1	T62.2X2	T62.2X3	T62.2X4	—	—
pesticide	T60.2X1	T60.2X2	T60.2X3	T60.2X4	—	—
Sabril*	T42.6X1	T42.6X2	T42.6X3	T42.6X4	T42.6X5	T42.6X6
Saccharated iron oxide	T45.8X1	T45.8X2	T45.8X3	T45.8X4	T45.8X5	T45.8X6
Saccharin	T50.901	T50.902	T50.903	T50.904	T50.905	T50.906
Saccharomyces boulardii	T47.6X1	T47.6X2	T47.6X3	T47.6X4	T47.6X5	T47.6X6
Safflower oil	T46.6X1	T46.6X2	T46.6X3	T46.6X4	T46.6X5	T46.6X6
Safrazine	T43.1X1	T43.1X2	T43.1X3	T43.1X4	T43.1X5	T43.1X6
Salazosulfapyridine	T37.0X1	T37.0X2	T37.0X3	T37.0X4	T37.0X5	T37.0X6
Salbutamol	T48.6X1	T48.6X2	T48.6X3	T48.6X4	T48.6X5	T48.6X6
Salicylamide	T39.091	T39.092	T39.093	T39.094	T39.095	T39.096
Salicylate NEC	T39.091	T39.092	T39.093	T39.094	T39.095	T39.096
methyl	T49.3X1	T49.3X2	T49.3X3	T49.3X4	T49.3X5	T49.3X6
theobromine calcium	T50.2X1	T50.2X2	T50.2X3	T50.2X4	T50.2X5	T50.2X6
Salicylazosulfapyridine	T37.0X1	T37.0X2	T37.0X3	T37.0X4	T37.0X5	T37.0X6
Salicylhydroxamic acid	T49.0X1	T49.0X2	T49.0X3	T49.0X4	T49.0X5	T49.0X6
Salicylic acid	T49.4X1	T49.4X2	T49.4X3	T49.4X4	T49.4X5	T49.4X6
with benzoic acid	T49.4X1	T49.4X2	T49.4X3	T49.4X4	T49.4X5	T49.4X6
congeners	T39.091	T39.092	T39.093	T39.094	T39.095	T39.096
derivative	T39.091	T39.092	T39.093	T39.094	T39.095	T39.096
salts	T39.091	T39.092	T39.093	T39.094	T39.095	T39.096
Salinazid	T37.1X1	T37.1X2	T37.1X3	T37.1X4	T37.1X5	T37.1X6
Salmeterol	T48.6X1	T48.6X2	T48.6X3	T48.6X4	T48.6X5	T48.6X6
Salol	T49.3X1	T49.3X2	T49.3X3	T49.3X4	T49.3X5	T49.3X6
Salsalate	T39.091	T39.092	T39.093	T39.094	T39.095	T39.096
Salt-replacing drug	T50.901	T50.902	T50.903	T50.904	T50.905	T50.906
Salt-retaining mineralocorticoid	T50.0X1	T50.0X2	T50.0X3	T50.0X4	T50.0X5	T50.0X6
Salt substitute	T50.901	T50.902	T50.903	T50.904	T50.905	T50.906
Saluretic NEC	T50.2X1	T50.2X2	T50.2X3	T50.2X4	T50.2X5	T50.2X6
Saluron	T50.2X1	T50.2X2	T50.2X3	T50.2X4	T50.2X5	T50.2X6
Salvarsan 606 (neosilver) (silver)	T37.8X1	T37.8X2	T37.8X3	T37.8X4	T37.8X5	T37.8X6
Sambucus canadensis	T62.2X1	T62.2X2	T62.2X3	T62.2X4	—	—
berry	T62.1X1	T62.1X2	T62.1X3	T62.1X4	—	—
Sandril	T46.5X1	T46.5X2	T46.5X3	T46.5X4	T46.5X5	T46.5X6
Sanguinaria canadensis	T62.2X1	T62.2X2	T62.2X3	T62.2X4	—	—
Saniflush (cleaner)	T54.2X1	T54.2X2	T54.2X3	T54.2X4	—	—
Santonin	T37.4X1	T37.4X2	T37.4X3	T37.4X4	T37.4X5	T37.4X6
Santyl	T49.8X1	T49.8X2	T49.8X3	T49.8X4	T49.8X5	T49.8X6
Saralasin	T46.5X1	T46.5X2	T46.5X3	T46.5X4	T46.5X5	T46.5X6
Sarcolysin	T45.1X1	T45.1X2	T45.1X3	T45.1X4	T45.1X5	T45.1X6
Sarilumab*	T39.4X1	T39.4X2	T39.4X3	T39.4X4	T39.4X5	T39.4X6
Sarkomycin	T45.1X1	T45.1X2	T45.1X3	T45.1X4	T45.1X5	T45.1X6
Saroten	T43.011	T43.012	T43.013	T43.014	T43.015	T43.016
Saturnine — *see* Lead						
Savin (oil)	T49.4X1	T49.4X2	T49.4X3	T49.4X4	T49.4X5	T49.4X6
Scammony	T47.2X1	T47.2X2	T47.2X3	T47.2X4	T47.2X5	T47.2X6
Scarlet red	T49.8X1	T49.8X2	T49.8X3	T49.8X4	T49.8X5	T49.8X6
Scheele's green	T57.0X1	T57.0X2	T57.0X3	T57.0X4	—	—
insecticide	T57.0X1	T57.0X2	T57.0X3	T57.0X4	—	—
Schizontozide (blood) (tissue)	T37.2X1	T37.2X2	T37.2X3	T37.2X4	T37.2X5	T37.2X6
Schradan	T60.0X1	T60.0X2	T60.0X3	T60.0X4	—	—
Schweinfurth green	T57.0X1	T57.0X2	T57.0X3	T57.0X4	—	—
insecticide	T57.0X1	T57.0X2	T57.0X3	T57.0X4	—	—
Scilla, rat poison	T60.4X1	T60.4X2	T60.4X3	T60.4X4	—	—
Scillaren	T60.4X1	T60.4X2	T60.4X3	T60.4X4	—	—
Sclerosing agent	T46.8X1	T46.8X2	T46.8X3	T46.8X4	T46.8X5	T46.8X6
Scombrotoxin	T61.11	T61.12	T61.13	T61.14	—	—
Scopolamine	T44.3X1	T44.3X2	T44.3X3	T44.3X4	T44.3X5	T44.3X6
Scopolia extract	T44.3X1	T44.3X2	T44.3X3	T44.3X4	T44.3X5	T44.3X6
Scouring powder	T65.891	T65.892	T65.893	T65.894	—	—
Sea						
anemone (sting)	T63.631	T63.632	T63.633	T63.634	—	—
cucumber (sting)	T63.691	T63.692	T63.693	T63.694	—	—
snake (bite) (venom)	T63.091	T63.092	T63.093	T63.094	—	—
urchin spine (puncture)	T63.691	T63.692	T63.693	T63.694	—	—
Seafood	T61.91	T61.92	T61.93	T61.94	—	—
specified NEC	T61.8X1	T61.8X2	T61.8X3	T61.8X4	—	—
Secbutabarbital	T42.3X1	T42.3X2	T42.3X3	T42.3X4	T42.3X5	T42.3X6
Secbutabarbitone	T42.3X1	T42.3X2	T42.3X3	T42.3X4	T42.3X5	T42.3X6
Secnidazole	T37.3X1	T37.3X2	T37.3X3	T37.3X4	T37.3X5	T37.3X6
Secobarbital	T42.3X1	T42.3X2	T42.3X3	T42.3X4	T42.3X5	T42.3X6
Seconal	T42.3X1	T42.3X2	T42.3X3	T42.3X4	T42.3X5	T42.3X6

Substance	Poisoning, Accidental (unintentional)	Poisoning, Intentional Self-harm	Poisoning, Assault	Poisoning, Undetermined	Adverse Effect	Under-dosing
Secretin	T5Ø.8X1	T5Ø.8X2	T5Ø.8X3	T5Ø.8X4	T5Ø.8X5	T5Ø.8X6
Sectral*	T44.7X1	T44.7X2	T44.7X3	T44.7X4	T44.7X5	T44.7X6
Sedative NEC	T42.71	T42.72	T42.73	T42.74	T42.75	T42.76
mixed NEC	T42.6X1	T42.6X2	T42.6X3	T42.6X4	T42.6X5	T42.6X6
Sedormid	T42.6X1	T42.6X2	T42.6X3	T42.6X4	T42.6X5	T42.6X6
Seed disinfectant or dressing	T6Ø.8X1	T6Ø.8X2	T6Ø.8X3	T6Ø.8X4	—	—
Seeds (poisonous)	T62.2X1	T62.2X2	T62.2X3	T62.2X4	—	—
Selegiline	T42.8X1	T42.8X2	T42.8X3	T42.8X4	T42.8X5	T42.8X6
Selenium NEC	T56.891	T56.892	T56.893	T56.894	—	—
disulfide or sulfide	T49.4X1	T49.4X2	T49.4X3	T49.4X4	T49.4X5	T49.4X6
fumes	T59.891	T59.892	T59.893	T59.894	—	—
sulfide	T49.4X1	T49.4X2	T49.4X3	T49.4X4	T49.4X5	T49.4X6
Selenomethionine (75Se)	T5Ø.8X1	T5Ø.8X2	T5Ø.8X3	T5Ø.8X4	T5Ø.8X5	T5Ø.8X6
Selsun	T49.4X1	T49.4X2	T49.4X3	T49.4X4	T49.4X5	T49.4X6
Semustine	T45.1X1	T45.1X2	T45.1X3	T45.1X4	T45.1X5	T45.1X6
Senega syrup	T48.4X1	T48.4X2	T48.4X3	T48.4X4	T48.4X5	T48.4X6
Senna	T47.2X1	T47.2X2	T47.2X3	T47.2X4	T47.2X5	T47.2X6
Sennoside A+B	T47.2X1	T47.2X2	T47.2X3	T47.2X4	T47.2X5	T47.2X6
Septisol	T49.2X1	T49.2X2	T49.2X3	T49.2X4	T49.2X5	T49.2X6
Seractide	T38.811	T38.812	T38.813	T38.814	T38.815	T38.816
Serax	T42.4X1	T42.4X2	T42.4X3	T42.4X4	T42.4X5	T42.4X6
Serenesil	T42.6X1	T42.6X2	T42.6X3	T42.6X4	T42.6X5	T42.6X6
Serenium (hydrochloride)	T37.91	T37.92	T37.93	T37.94	T37.95	T37.96
Serepax — *see* Oxazepam						
Serevent*	T48.6X1	T48.6X2	T48.6X3	T48.6X4	T48.6X5	T48.6X6
Sermorelin	T38.891	T38.892	T38.893	T38.894	T38.895	T38.896
Sernyl	T41.1X1	T41.1X2	T41.1X3	T41.1X4	T41.1X5	T41.1X6
Serotonin	T5Ø.991	T5Ø.992	T5Ø.993	T5Ø.994	T5Ø.995	T5Ø.996
Serpasil	T46.5X1	T46.5X2	T46.5X3	T46.5X4	T46.5X5	T46.5X6
Serrapeptase	T45.3X1	T45.3X2	T45.3X3	T45.3X4	T45.3X5	T45.3X6
Sertraline*	T43.221	T43.222	T43.223	T43.224	T43.225	T43.226
Serum						
antibotulinus	T5Ø.Z11	T5Ø.Z12	T5Ø.Z13	T5Ø.Z14	T5Ø.Z15	T5Ø.Z16
anticytotoxic	T5Ø.Z11	T5Ø.Z12	T5Ø.Z13	T5Ø.Z14	T5Ø.Z15	T5Ø.Z16
antidiphtheria	T5Ø.Z11	T5Ø.Z12	T5Ø.Z13	T5Ø.Z14	T5Ø.Z15	T5Ø.Z16
antimeningococcus	T5Ø.Z11	T5Ø.Z12	T5Ø.Z13	T5Ø.Z14	T5Ø.Z15	T5Ø.Z16
anti-Rh	T5Ø.Z11	T5Ø.Z12	T5Ø.Z13	T5Ø.Z14	T5Ø.Z15	T5Ø.Z16
anti-snake-bite	T5Ø.Z11	T5Ø.Z12	T5Ø.Z13	T5Ø.Z14	T5Ø.Z15	T5Ø.Z16
antitetanic	T5Ø.Z11	T5Ø.Z12	T5Ø.Z13	T5Ø.Z14	T5Ø.Z15	T5Ø.Z16
antitoxic	T5Ø.Z11	T5Ø.Z12	T5Ø.Z13	T5Ø.Z14	T5Ø.Z15	T5Ø.Z16
complement (inhibitor)	T45.8X1	T45.8X2	T45.8X3	T45.8X4	T45.8X5	T45.8X6
convalescent	T5Ø.Z11	T5Ø.Z12	T5Ø.Z13	T5Ø.Z14	T5Ø.Z15	T5Ø.Z16
hemolytic complement	T45.8X1	T45.8X2	T45.8X3	T45.8X4	T45.8X5	T45.8X6
immune (human)	T5Ø.Z11	T5Ø.Z12	T5Ø.Z13	T5Ø.Z14	T5Ø.Z15	T5Ø.Z16
protective NEC	T5Ø.Z11	T5Ø.Z12	T5Ø.Z13	T5Ø.Z14	T5Ø.Z15	T5Ø.Z16
Setastine	T45.ØX1	T45.ØX2	T45.ØX3	T45.ØX4	T45.ØX5	T45.ØX6
Setoperone	T43.591	T43.592	T43.593	T43.594	T43.595	T43.596
Sewer gas	T59.91	T59.92	T59.93	T59.94	—	—
Shampoo	T55.ØX1	T55.ØX2	T55.ØX3	T55.ØX4	—	—
Shellfish, noxious, nonbacterial	T61.781	T61.782	T61.783	T61.784	—	—
Sildenafil	T46.7X1	T46.7X2	T46.7X3	T46.7X4	T46.7X5	T46.7X6
Silibinin	T5Ø.991	T5Ø.992	T5Ø.993	T5Ø.994	T5Ø.995	T5Ø.996
Silicone NEC	T65.891	T65.892	T65.893	T65.894	—	—
medicinal	T49.3X1	T49.3X2	T49.3X3	T49.3X4	T49.3X5	T49.3X6
Silvadene	T49.ØX1	T49.ØX2	T49.ØX3	T49.ØX4	T49.ØX5	T49.ØX6
Silver	T49.ØX1	T49.ØX2	T49.ØX3	T49.ØX4	T49.ØX5	T49.ØX6
anti-infectives	T49.ØX1	T49.ØX2	T49.ØX3	T49.ØX4	T49.ØX5	T49.ØX6
arsphenamine	T37.8X1	T37.8X2	T37.8X3	T37.8X4	T37.8X5	T37.8X6
colloidal	T49.ØX1	T49.ØX2	T49.ØX3	T49.ØX4	T49.ØX5	T49.ØX6
nitrate	T49.ØX1	T49.ØX2	T49.ØX3	T49.ØX4	T49.ØX5	T49.ØX6
ophthalmic preparation	T49.5X1	T49.5X2	T49.5X3	T49.5X4	T49.5X5	T49.5X6
toughened (keratolytic)	T49.4X1	T49.4X2	T49.4X3	T49.4X4	T49.4X5	T49.4X6
nonmedicinal (dust)	T56.891	T56.892	T56.893	T56.894	—	—
protein	T49.5X1	T49.5X2	T49.5X3	T49.5X4	T49.5X5	T49.5X6
salvarsan	T37.8X1	T37.8X2	T37.8X3	T37.8X4	T37.8X5	T37.8X6
sulfadiazine	T49.4X1	T49.4X2	T49.4X3	T49.4X4	T49.4X5	T49.4X6
Silymarin	T5Ø.991	T5Ø.992	T5Ø.993	T5Ø.994	T5Ø.995	T5Ø.996
Simaldrate	T47.1X1	T47.1X2	T47.1X3	T47.1X4	T47.1X5	T47.1X6
Simazine	T6Ø.3X1	T6Ø.3X2	T6Ø.3X3	T6Ø.3X4	—	—
Simethicone	T47.1X1	T47.1X2	T47.1X3	T47.1X4	T47.1X5	T47.1X6
Simfibrate	T46.6X1	T46.6X2	T46.6X3	T46.6X4	T46.6X5	T46.6X6
Simvastatin	T46.6X1	T46.6X2	T46.6X3	T46.6X4	T46.6X5	T46.6X6
Sincalide	T5Ø.8X1	T5Ø.8X2	T5Ø.8X3	T5Ø.8X4	T5Ø.8X5	T5Ø.8X6
Sinequan	T43.Ø11	T43.Ø12	T43.Ø13	T43.Ø14	T43.Ø15	T43.Ø16
Singoserp	T46.5X1	T46.5X2	T46.5X3	T46.5X4	T46.5X5	T46.5X6
Singulair*	T48.6X1	T48.6X2	T48.6X3	T48.6X4	T48.6X5	T48.6X6
Sintrom	T45.511	T45.512	T45.513	T45.514	T45.515	T45.516
Sisomicin	T36.5X1	T36.5X2	T36.5X3	T36.5X4	T36.5X5	T36.5X6
Sitosterols	T46.6X1	T46.6X2	T46.6X3	T46.6X4	T46.6X5	T46.6X6
Skeletal muscle relaxants	T48.1X1	T48.1X2	T48.1X3	T48.1X4	T48.1X5	T48.1X6

Substance	Poisoning, Accidental (unintentional)	Poisoning, Intentional Self-harm	Poisoning, Assault	Poisoning, Undetermined	Adverse Effect	Under-dosing
Skin						
agents (external)	T49.91	T49.92	T49.93	T49.94	T49.95	T49.96
specified NEC	T49.8X1	T49.8X2	T49.8X3	T49.8X4	T49.8X5	T49.8X6
test antigen	T5Ø.8X1	T5Ø.8X2	T5Ø.8X3	T5Ø.8X4	T5Ø.8X5	T5Ø.8X6
Sleep-eze	T45.ØX1	T45.ØX2	T45.ØX3	T45.ØX4	T45.ØX5	T45.ØX6
Sleeping draught, pill	T42.71	T42.72	T42.73	T42.74	T42.75	T42.76
Smallpox vaccine	T5Ø.B11	T5Ø.B12	T5Ø.B13	T5Ø.B14	T5Ø.B15	T5Ø.B16
Smelter fumes NEC	T56.91	T56.92	T56.93	T56.94	—	—
Smog	T59.1X1	T59.1X2	T59.1X3	T59.1X4	—	—
Smoke NEC	T59.811	T59.812	T59.813	T59.814	—	—
Smooth muscle relaxant	T44.3X1	T44.3X2	T44.3X3	T44.3X4	T44.3X5	T44.3X6
Snail killer NEC	T6Ø.8X1	T6Ø.8X2	T6Ø.8X3	T6Ø.8X4	—	—
Snake venom or bite	T63.ØØ1	T63.ØØ2	T63.ØØ3	T63.ØØ4	—	—
hemocoagulase	T45.7X1	T45.7X2	T45.7X3	T45.7X4	T45.7X5	T45.7X6
Snuff	T65.211	T65.212	T65.213	T65.214	—	—
Soap (powder) (product)	T55.ØX1	T55.ØX2	T55.ØX3	T55.ØX4	—	—
enema	T47.4X1	T47.4X2	T47.4X3	T47.4X4	T47.4X5	T47.4X6
medicinal, soft	T49.2X1	T49.2X2	T49.2X3	T49.2X4	T49.2X5	T49.2X6
superfatted	T49.2X1	T49.2X2	T49.2X3	T49.2X4	T49.2X5	T49.2X6
Sobrerol	T48.4X1	T48.4X2	T48.4X3	T48.4X4	T48.4X5	T48.4X6
Soda (caustic)	T54.3X1	T54.3X2	T54.3X3	T54.3X4	—	—
bicarb	T47.1X1	T47.1X2	T47.1X3	T47.1X4	T47.1X5	T47.1X6
chlorinated — *see* Sodium, hypochlorite						
Sodium						
acetosulfone	T37.1X1	T37.1X2	T37.1X3	T37.1X4	T37.1X5	T37.1X6
acetrizoate	T5Ø.8X1	T5Ø.8X2	T5Ø.8X3	T5Ø.8X4	T5Ø.8X5	T5Ø.8X6
acid phosphate	T5Ø.3X1	T5Ø.3X2	T5Ø.3X3	T5Ø.3X4	T5Ø.3X5	T5Ø.3X6
alginate	T47.8X1	T47.8X2	T47.8X3	T47.8X4	T47.8X5	T47.8X6
amidotrizoate	T5Ø.8X1	T5Ø.8X2	T5Ø.8X3	T5Ø.8X4	T5Ø.8X5	T5Ø.8X6
aminohippurate*	T5Ø.8X1	T5Ø.8X2	T5Ø.8X3	T5Ø.8X4	T5Ø.8X5	T5Ø.8X6
aminopterin	T45.1X1	T45.1X2	T45.1X3	T45.1X4	T45.1X5	T45.1X6
amylosulfate	T47.8X1	T47.8X2	T47.8X3	T47.8X4	T47.8X5	T47.8X6
amytal	T42.3X1	T42.3X2	T42.3X3	T42.3X4	T42.3X5	T42.3X6
antimony gluconate	T37.3X1	T37.3X2	T37.3X3	T37.3X4	T37.3X5	T37.3X6
arsenate	T57.ØX1	T57.ØX2	T57.ØX3	T57.ØX4	—	—
aurothiomalate	T39.4X1	T39.4X2	T39.4X3	T39.4X4	T39.4X5	T39.4X6
aurothiosulfate	T39.4X1	T39.4X2	T39.4X3	T39.4X4	T39.4X5	T39.4X6
barbiturate	T42.3X1	T42.3X2	T42.3X3	T42.3X4	T42.3X5	T42.3X6
basic phosphate	T47.4X1	T47.4X2	T47.4X3	T47.4X4	T47.4X5	T47.4X6
bicarbonate	T47.1X1	T47.1X2	T47.1X3	T47.1X4	T47.1X5	T47.1X6
bichromate	T57.8X1	T57.8X2	T57.8X3	T57.8X4	—	—
biphosphate	T5Ø.3X1	T5Ø.3X2	T5Ø.3X3	T5Ø.3X4	T5Ø.3X5	T5Ø.3X6
bisulfate	T65.891	T65.892	T65.893	T65.894	—	—
borate						
cleanser	T57.8X1	T57.8X2	T57.8X3	T57.8X4	—	—
eye	T49.5X1	T49.5X2	T49.5X3	T49.5X4	T49.5X5	T49.5X6
therapeutic	T49.8X1	T49.8X2	T49.8X3	T49.8X4	T49.8X5	T49.8X6
bromide	T42.6X1	T42.6X2	T42.6X3	T42.6X4	T42.6X5	T42.6X6
cacodylate (nonmedicinal) NEC	T5Ø.8X1	T5Ø.8X2	T5Ø.8X3	T5Ø.8X4	T5Ø.8X5	T5Ø.8X6
anti-infective	T37.8X1	T37.8X2	T37.8X3	T37.8X4	T37.8X5	T37.8X6
herbicide	T6Ø.3X1	T6Ø.3X2	T6Ø.3X3	T6Ø.3X4	—	—
calcium edetate	T45.8X1	T45.8X2	T45.8X3	T45.8X4	T45.8X5	T45.8X6
carbonate NEC	T54.3X1	T54.3X2	T54.3X3	T54.3X4	—	—
chlorate NEC	T65.891	T65.892	T65.893	T65.894	—	—
herbicide	T54.91	T54.92	T54.93	T54.94	—	—
chloride	T5Ø.3X1	T5Ø.3X2	T5Ø.3X3	T5Ø.3X4	T5Ø.3X5	T5Ø.3X6
with glucose	T5Ø.3X1	T5Ø.3X2	T5Ø.3X3	T5Ø.3X4	T5Ø.3X5	T5Ø.3X6
chromate	T65.891	T65.892	T65.893	T65.894	—	—
citrate	T5Ø.991	T5Ø.992	T5Ø.993	T5Ø.994	T5Ø.995	T5Ø.996
cromoglicate	T48.6X1	T48.6X2	T48.6X3	T48.6X4	T48.6X5	T48.6X6
cyanide	T65.ØX1	T65.ØX2	T65.ØX3	T65.ØX4	—	—
cyclamate	T5Ø.3X1	T5Ø.3X2	T5Ø.3X3	T5Ø.3X4	T5Ø.3X5	T5Ø.3X6
dehydrocholate	T45.8X1	T45.8X2	T45.8X3	T45.8X4	T45.8X5	T45.8X6
diatrizoate	T5Ø.8X1	T5Ø.8X2	T5Ø.8X3	T5Ø.8X4	T5Ø.8X5	T5Ø.8X6
dibunate	T48.4X1	T48.4X2	T48.4X3	T48.4X4	T48.4X5	T48.4X6
dioctyl sulfosuccinate	T47.4X1	T47.4X2	T47.4X3	T47.4X4	T47.4X5	T47.4X6
dipantoyl ferrate	T45.8X1	T45.8X2	T45.8X3	T45.8X4	T45.8X5	T45.8X6
edetate	T45.8X1	T45.8X2	T45.8X3	T45.8X4	T45.8X5	T45.8X6
ethacrynate	T5Ø.1X1	T5Ø.1X2	T5Ø.1X3	T5Ø.1X4	T5Ø.1X5	T5Ø.1X6
etidronate*	T5Ø.991	T5Ø.992	T5Ø.993	T5Ø.994	T5Ø.995	T5Ø.996
feredetate	T45.8X1	T45.8X2	T45.8X3	T45.8X4	T45.8X5	T45.8X6
Fluoride — *see* Fluoride						
fluoroacetate (dust) (pesticide)	T6Ø.4X1	T6Ø.4X2	T6Ø.4X3	T6Ø.4X4	—	—
free salt	T5Ø.3X1	T5Ø.3X2	T5Ø.3X3	T5Ø.3X4	T5Ø.3X5	T5Ø.3X6
fusidate	T36.8X1	T36.8X2	T36.8X3	T36.8X4	T36.8X5	T36.8X6
glucaldrate	T47.1X1	T47.1X2	T47.1X3	T47.1X4	T47.1X5	T47.1X6
glucosulfone	T37.1X1	T37.1X2	T37.1X3	T37.1X4	T37.1X5	T37.1X6
glutamate	T45.8X1	T45.8X2	T45.8X3	T45.8X4	T45.8X5	T45.8X6
hydrogen carbonate	T5Ø.3X1	T5Ø.3X2	T5Ø.3X3	T5Ø.3X4	T5Ø.3X5	T5Ø.3X6
hydroxide	T54.3X1	T54.3X2	T54.3X3	T54.3X4	—	—

*Optum Value-Add

Substance	Poisoning, Accidental (unintentional)	Poisoning, Intentional Self-harm	Poisoning, Assault	Poisoning, Undetermined	Adverse Effect	Under-dosing
Sodium — *continued*						
hypochlorite (bleach) NEC	T54.3X1	T54.3X2	T54.3X3	T54.3X4	—	—
disinfectant	T54.3X1	T54.3X2	T54.3X3	T54.3X4	—	—
medicinal (anti-infective) (external)	T49.ØX1	T49.ØX2	T49.ØX3	T49.ØX4	T49.ØX5	T49.ØX6
vapor	T54.3X1	T54.3X2	T54.3X3	T54.3X4	—	—
hyposulfite	T49.ØX1	T49.ØX2	T49.ØX3	T49.ØX4	T49.ØX5	T49.ØX6
indigotin disulfonate	T5Ø.8X1	T5Ø.8X2	T5Ø.8X3	T5Ø.8X4	T5Ø.8X5	T5Ø.8X6
iodide	T5Ø.991	T5Ø.992	T5Ø.993	T5Ø.994	T5Ø.995	T5Ø.996
I-131	T5Ø.8X1	T5Ø.8X2	T5Ø.8X3	T5Ø.8X4	T5Ø.8X5	T5Ø.8X6
therapeutic	T38.2X1	T38.2X2	T38.2X3	T38.2X4	T38.2X5	T38.2X6
iodohippurate (131I)	T5Ø.8X1	T5Ø.8X2	T5Ø.8X3	T5Ø.8X4	T5Ø.8X5	T5Ø.8X6
iopodate	T5Ø.8X1	T5Ø.8X2	T5Ø.8X3	T5Ø.8X4	T5Ø.8X5	T5Ø.8X6
iothalamate	T5Ø.8X1	T5Ø.8X2	T5Ø.8X3	T5Ø.8X4	T5Ø.8X5	T5Ø.8X6
iron edetate	T45.4X1	T45.4X2	T45.4X3	T45.4X4	T45.4X5	T45.4X6
lactate (compound solution)	T45.8X1	T45.8X2	T45.8X3	T45.8X4	T45.8X5	T45.8X6
lauryl (sulfate)	T49.2X1	T49.2X2	T49.2X3	T49.2X4	T49.2X5	T49.2X6
L-triiodothyronine	T38.1X1	T38.1X2	T38.1X3	T38.1X4	T38.1X5	T38.1X6
magnesium citrate	T5Ø.991	T5Ø.992	T5Ø.993	T5Ø.994	T5Ø.995	T5Ø.996
mersalate	T5Ø.2X1	T5Ø.2X2	T5Ø.2X3	T5Ø.2X4	T5Ø.2X5	T5Ø.2X6
metasilicate	T65.891	T65.892	T65.893	T65.894	—	—
metrizoate	T5Ø.8X1	T5Ø.8X2	T5Ø.8X3	T5Ø.8X4	T5Ø.8X5	T5Ø.8X6
monofluoroacetate (pesticide)	T6Ø.1X1	T6Ø.1X2	T6Ø.1X3	T6Ø.1X4	—	—
morrhuate	T46.8X1	T46.8X2	T46.8X3	T46.8X4	T46.8X5	T46.8X6
nafcillin	T36.ØX1	T36.ØX2	T36.ØX3	T36.ØX4	T36.ØX5	T36.ØX6
nitrate (oxidizing agent)	T65.891	T65.892	T65.893	T65.894	—	—
nitrite	T5Ø.6X1	T5Ø.6X2	T5Ø.6X3	T5Ø.6X4	T5Ø.6X5	T5Ø.6X6
nitroferricyanide	T46.5X1	T46.5X2	T46.5X3	T46.5X4	T46.5X5	T46.5X6
nitroprusside	T46.5X1	T46.5X2	T46.5X3	T46.5X4	T46.5X5	T46.5X6
oxalate	T65.891	T65.892	T65.893	T65.894	—	—
oxide/peroxide	T65.891	T65.892	T65.893	T65.894	—	—
oxybate	T41.291	T41.292	T41.293	T41.294	T41.295	T41.296
para-aminohippurate	T5Ø.8X1	T5Ø.8X2	T5Ø.8X3	T5Ø.8X4	T5Ø.8X5	T5Ø.8X6
perborate (nonmedicinal) NEC	T65.891	T65.892	T65.893	T65.894	—	—
medicinal	T49.ØX1	T49.ØX2	T49.ØX3	T49.ØX4	T49.ØX5	T49.ØX6
soap	T55.ØX1	T55.ØX2	T55.ØX3	T55.ØX4	—	—
percarbonate — *see* Sodium, perborate						
pertechnetate Tc99m	T5Ø.8X1	T5Ø.8X2	T5Ø.8X3	T5Ø.8X4	T5Ø.8X5	T5Ø.8X6
phosphate						
cellulose	T45.8X1	T45.8X2	T45.8X3	T45.8X4	T45.8X5	T45.8X6
dibasic	T47.2X1	T47.2X2	T47.2X3	T47.2X4	T47.2X5	T47.2X6
monobasic	T47.2X1	T47.2X2	T47.2X3	T47.2X4	T47.2X5	T47.2X6
phytate	T5Ø.6X1	T5Ø.6X2	T5Ø.6X3	T5Ø.6X4	T5Ø.6X5	T5Ø.6X6
picosulfate	T47.2X1	T47.2X2	T47.2X3	T47.2X4	T47.2X5	T47.2X6
polyhydroxyaluminium monocarbonate	T47.1X1	T47.1X2	T47.1X3	T47.1X4	T47.1X5	T47.1X6
polystyrene sulfonate	T5Ø.3X1	T5Ø.3X2	T5Ø.3X3	T5Ø.3X4	T5Ø.3X5	T5Ø.3X6
propionate	T49.ØX1	T49.ØX2	T49.ØX3	T49.ØX4	T49.ØX5	T49.ØX6
propyl hydroxybenzoate	T5Ø.991	T5Ø.992	T5Ø.993	T5Ø.994	T5Ø.995	T5Ø.996
psylliate	T46.8X1	T46.8X2	T46.8X3	T46.8X4	T46.8X5	T46.8X6
removing resins	T5Ø.3X1	T5Ø.3X2	T5Ø.3X3	T5Ø.3X4	T5Ø.3X5	T5Ø.3X6
salicylate	T39.Ø91	T39.Ø92	T39.Ø93	T39.Ø94	T39.Ø95	T39.Ø96
salt NEC	T5Ø.3X1	T5Ø.3X2	T5Ø.3X3	T5Ø.3X4	T5Ø.3X5	T5Ø.3X6
selenate	T6Ø.2X1	T6Ø.2X2	T6Ø.2X3	T6Ø.2X4	—	—
stibogluconate	T37.3X1	T37.3X2	T37.3X3	T37.3X4	T37.3X5	T37.3X6
sulfate	T47.4X1	T47.4X2	T47.4X3	T47.4X4	T47.4X5	T47.4X6
sulfoxone	T37.1X1	T37.1X2	T37.1X3	T37.1X4	T37.1X5	T37.1X6
tetradecyl sulfate	T46.8X1	T46.8X2	T46.8X3	T46.8X4	T46.8X5	T46.8X6
thiopental	T41.1X1	T41.1X2	T41.1X3	T41.1X4	T41.1X5	T41.1X6
thiosalicylate	T39.Ø91	T39.Ø92	T39.Ø93	T39.Ø94	T39.Ø95	T39.Ø96
thiosulfate	T5Ø.6X1	T5Ø.6X2	T5Ø.6X3	T5Ø.6X4	T5Ø.6X5	T5Ø.6X6
tolbutamide	T38.3X1	T38.3X2	T38.3X3	T38.3X4	T38.3X5	T38.3X6
(L)-triiodothyronine	T38.1X1	T38.1X2	T38.1X3	T38.1X4	T38.1X5	T38.1X6
tyropanoate	T5Ø.8X1	T5Ø.8X2	T5Ø.8X3	T5Ø.8X4	T5Ø.8X5	T5Ø.8X6
valproate	T42.6X1	T42.6X2	T42.6X3	T42.6X4	T42.6X5	T42.6X6
versenate	T5Ø.6X1	T5Ø.6X2	T5Ø.6X3	T5Ø.6X4	T5Ø.6X5	T5Ø.6X6
Sodium-free salt	T5Ø.9Ø1	T5Ø.9Ø2	T5Ø.9Ø3	T5Ø.9Ø4	T5Ø.9Ø5	T5Ø.9Ø6
Sodium-removing resin	T5Ø.3X1	T5Ø.3X2	T5Ø.3X3	T5Ø.3X4	T5Ø.3X5	T5Ø.3X6
Soft soap	T55.ØX1	T55.ØX2	T55.ØX3	T55.ØX4	—	—
Solanine	T62.2X1	T62.2X2	T62.2X3	T62.2X4	—	—
berries	T62.1X1	T62.1X2	T62.1X3	T62.1X4	—	—
Solanum dulcamara	T62.2X1	T62.2X2	T62.2X3	T62.2X4	—	—
berries	T62.1X1	T62.1X2	T62.1X3	T62.1X4	—	—
Solapsone	T37.1X1	T37.1X2	T37.1X3	T37.1X4	T37.1X5	T37.1X6
Solaquin*	T49.8X1	T49.8X2	T49.8X3	T49.8X4	T49.8X5	T49.8X6
Solar lotion	T49.3X1	T49.3X2	T49.3X3	T49.3X4	T49.3X5	T49.3X6
Solasulfone	T37.1X1	T37.1X2	T37.1X3	T37.1X4	T37.1X5	T37.1X6
Soldering fluid	T65.891	T65.892	T65.893	T65.894	—	—
Solid substance	T65.91	T65.92	T65.93	T65.94	—	—

Substance	Poisoning, Accidental (unintentional)	Poisoning, Intentional Self-harm	Poisoning, Assault	Poisoning, Undetermined	Adverse Effect	Under-dosing
Solid substance — *continued*						
specified NEC	T65.891	T65.892	T65.893	T65.894	—	—
Solvent, industrial NEC	T52.91	T52.92	T52.93	T52.94	—	—
naphtha	T52.ØX1	T52.ØX2	T52.ØX3	T52.ØX4	—	—
petroleum	T52.ØX1	T52.ØX2	T52.ØX3	T52.ØX4	—	—
specified NEC	T52.8X1	T52.8X2	T52.8X3	T52.8X4	—	—
Soma	T42.8X1	T42.8X2	T42.8X3	T42.8X4	T42.8X5	T42.8X6
Somatorelin	T38.891	T38.892	T38.893	T38.894	T38.895	T38.896
Somatostatin	T38.991	T38.992	T38.993	T38.994	T38.995	T38.996
Somatotropin	T38.811	T38.812	T38.813	T38.814	T38.815	T38.816
Somatrem	T38.811	T38.812	T38.813	T38.814	T38.815	T38.816
Somatropin	T38.811	T38.812	T38.813	T38.814	T38.815	T38.816
Sominex	T45.ØX1	T45.ØX2	T45.ØX3	T45.ØX4	T45.ØX5	T45.ØX6
Somnos	T42.6X1	T42.6X2	T42.6X3	T42.6X4	T42.6X5	T42.6X6
Somonal	T42.3X1	T42.3X2	T42.3X3	T42.3X4	T42.3X5	T42.3X6
Soneryl	T42.3X1	T42.3X2	T42.3X3	T42.3X4	T42.3X5	T42.3X6
Soothing syrup	T5Ø.9Ø1	T5Ø.9Ø2	T5Ø.9Ø3	T5Ø.9Ø4	T5Ø.9Ø5	T5Ø.9Ø6
Sopor	T42.6X1	T42.6X2	T42.6X3	T42.6X4	T42.6X5	T42.6X6
Soporific	T42.71	T42.72	T42.73	T42.74	T42.75	T42.76
Soporific drug	T42.71	T42.72	T42.73	T42.74	T42.75	T42.76
specified type NEC	T42.6X1	T42.6X2	T42.6X3	T42.6X4	T42.6X5	T42.6X6
Sorbide nitrate	T46.3X1	T46.3X2	T46.3X3	T46.3X4	T46.3X5	T46.3X6
Sorbitol	T47.4X1	T47.4X2	T47.4X3	T47.4X4	T47.4X5	T47.4X6
Sotalol	T44.7X1	T44.7X2	T44.7X3	T44.7X4	T44.7X5	T44.7X6
Sotradecol	T46.8X1	T46.8X2	T46.8X3	T46.8X4	T46.8X5	T46.8X6
Soysterol	T46.6X1	T46.6X2	T46.6X3	T46.6X4	T46.6X5	T46.6X6
Spacoline	T44.3X1	T44.3X2	T44.3X3	T44.3X4	T44.3X5	T44.3X6
Spanish fly	T49.8X1	T49.8X2	T49.8X3	T49.8X4	T49.8X5	T49.8X6
Sparine	T43.3X1	T43.3X2	T43.3X3	T43.3X4	T43.3X5	T43.3X6
Sparteine	T48.ØX1	T48.ØX2	T48.ØX3	T48.ØX4	T48.ØX5	T48.ØX6
Spasmolytic						
anticholinergics	T44.3X1	T44.3X2	T44.3X3	T44.3X4	T44.3X5	T44.3X6
autonomic	T44.3X1	T44.3X2	T44.3X3	T44.3X4	T44.3X5	T44.3X6
bronchial NEC	T48.6X1	T48.6X2	T48.6X3	T48.6X4	T48.6X5	T48.6X6
quaternary ammonium	T44.3X1	T44.3X2	T44.3X3	T44.3X4	T44.3X5	T44.3X6
skeletal muscle NEC	T48.1X1	T48.1X2	T48.1X3	T48.1X4	T48.1X5	T48.1X6
Spectinomycin	T36.5X1	T36.5X2	T36.5X3	T36.5X4	T36.5X5	T36.5X6
Spectracef*	T36.1X1	T36.1X2	T36.1X3	T36.1X4	T36.1X5	T36.1X6
Speed	T43.651	T43.652	T43.653	T43.654	T43.655	T43.656
Spermicide	T49.8X1	T49.8X2	T49.8X3	T49.8X4	T49.8X5	T49.8X6
Spider (bite) (venom)	T63.391	T63.392	T63.393	T63.394	—	—
antivenin	T5Ø.Z11	T5Ø.Z12	T5Ø.Z13	T5Ø.Z14	T5Ø.Z15	T5Ø.Z16
Spigelia (root)	T37.4X1	T37.4X2	T37.4X3	T37.4X4	T37.4X5	T37.4X6
Spindle inactivator	T5Ø.4X1	T5Ø.4X2	T5Ø.4X3	T5Ø.4X4	T5Ø.4X5	T5Ø.4X6
Spiperone	T43.4X1	T43.4X2	T43.4X3	T43.4X4	T43.4X5	T43.4X6
Spiramycin	T36.3X1	T36.3X2	T36.3X3	T36.3X4	T36.3X5	T36.3X6
Spirapril	T46.4X1	T46.4X2	T46.4X3	T46.4X4	T46.4X5	T46.4X6
Spirilene	T43.591	T43.592	T43.593	T43.594	T43.595	T43.596
Spirit(s) (neutral) **NEC**	T51.ØX1	T51.ØX2	T51.ØX3	T51.ØX4	—	—
beverage	T51.ØX1	T51.ØX2	T51.ØX3	T51.ØX4	—	—
industrial	T51.ØX1	T51.ØX2	T51.ØX3	T51.ØX4	—	—
mineral	T52.ØX1	T52.ØX2	T52.ØX3	T52.ØX4	—	—
of salt — *see* Hydrochloric acid						
surgical	T51.ØX1	T51.ØX2	T51.ØX3	T51.ØX4	—	—
Spiriva*	T44.3X1	T44.3X2	T44.3X3	T44.3X4	T44.3X5	T44.3X6
Spironolactone	T5Ø.ØX1	T5Ø.ØX2	T5Ø.ØX3	T5Ø.ØX4	T5Ø.ØX5	T5Ø.ØX6
Spiroperidol	T43.4X1	T43.4X2	T43.4X3	T43.4X4	T43.4X5	T43.4X6
Sponge, absorbable (gelatin)	T45.7X1	T45.7X2	T45.7X3	T45.7X4	T45.7X5	T45.7X6
Sporostacin	T49.ØX1	T49.ØX2	T49.ØX3	T49.ØX4	T49.ØX5	T49.ØX6
Spray (aerosol)	T65.91	T65.92	T65.93	T65.94	—	—
cosmetic	T65.891	T65.892	T65.893	T65.894	—	—
medicinal NEC	T5Ø.9Ø1	T5Ø.9Ø2	T5Ø.9Ø3	T5Ø.9Ø4	T5Ø.9Ø5	T5Ø.9Ø6
pesticides — *see* Pesticide						
specified content — *see* specific substance						
Spurge flax	T62.2X1	T62.2X2	T62.2X3	T62.2X4	—	—
Spurges	T62.2X1	T62.2X2	T62.2X3	T62.2X4	—	—
Sputum viscosity-lowering drug	T48.4X1	T48.4X2	T48.4X3	T48.4X4	T48.4X5	T48.4X6
Squill	T46.ØX1	T46.ØX2	T46.ØX3	T46.ØX4	T46.ØX5	T46.ØX6
rat poison	T6Ø.4X1	T6Ø.4X2	T6Ø.4X3	T6Ø.4X4	—	—
Squirting cucumber (cathartic)	T47.2X1	T47.2X2	T47.2X3	T47.2X4	T47.2X5	T47.2X6
Stains	T65.6X1	T65.6X2	T65.6X3	T65.6X4	—	—
Stannous fluoride	T49.7X1	T49.7X2	T49.7X3	T49.7X4	T49.7X5	T49.7X6
Stanolone	T38.7X1	T38.7X2	T38.7X3	T38.7X4	T38.7X5	T38.7X6
Stanozolol	T38.7X1	T38.7X2	T38.7X3	T38.7X4	T38.7X5	T38.7X6
Staphisagria or stavesacre (pediculicide)	T49.ØX1	T49.ØX2	T49.ØX3	T49.ØX4	T49.ØX5	T49.ØX6
Starch	T5Ø.9Ø1	T5Ø.9Ø2	T5Ø.9Ø3	T5Ø.9Ø4	T5Ø.9Ø5	T5Ø.9Ø6
Stavzor*	T42.6X1	T42.6X2	T42.6X3	T42.6X4	T42.6X5	T42.6X6
Stelazine	T43.3X1	T43.3X2	T43.3X3	T43.3X4	T43.3X5	T43.3X6

Substance	Poisoning, Accidental (unintentional)	Poisoning, Intentional Self-harm	Poisoning, Assault	Poisoning, Undetermined	Adverse Effect	Under-dosing
Stemetil	T43.3X1	T43.3X2	T43.3X3	T43.3X4	T43.3X5	T43.3X6
Stepronin	T48.4X1	T48.4X2	T48.4X3	T48.4X4	T48.4X5	T48.4X6
Sterculia	T47.4X1	T47.4X2	T47.4X3	T47.4X4	T47.4X5	T47.4X6
Sternutator gas	T59.891	T59.892	T59.893	T59.894	—	—
Steroid	T38.ØX1	T38.ØX2	T38.ØX3	T38.ØX4	T38.ØX5	T38.ØX6
anabolic	T38.7X1	T38.7X2	T38.7X3	T38.7X4	T38.7X5	T38.7X6
androgenic	T38.7X1	T38.7X2	T38.7X3	T38.7X4	T38.7X5	T38.7X6
antineoplastic, hormone	T38.7X1	T38.7X2	T38.7X3	T38.7X4	T38.7X5	T38.7X6
estrogen	T38.5X1	T38.5X2	T38.5X3	T38.5X4	T38.5X5	T38.5X6
ENT agent	T49.6X1	T49.6X2	T49.6X3	T49.6X4	T49.6X5	T49.6X6
ophthalmic preparation	T49.5X1	T49.5X2	T49.5X3	T49.5X4	T49.5X5	T49.5X6
topical NEC	T49.ØX1	T49.ØX2	T49.ØX3	T49.ØX4	T49.ØX5	T49.ØX6
Stibine	T56.891	T56.892	T56.893	T56.894	—	—
Stibogluconate	T37.3X1	T37.3X2	T37.3X3	T37.3X4	T37.3X5	T37.3X6
Stibophen	T37.4X1	T37.4X2	T37.4X3	T37.4X4	T37.4X5	T37.4X6
Stilbamidine (isetionate)	T37.3X1	T37.3X2	T37.3X3	T37.3X4	T37.3X5	T37.3X6
Stilbestrol	T38.5X1	T38.5X2	T38.5X3	T38.5X4	T38.5X5	T38.5X6
Stilboestrol	T38.5X1	T38.5X2	T38.5X3	T38.5X4	T38.5X5	T38.5X6
Stimulant						
central nervous system — *see also* Psychostimulant	T43.6Ø1	T43.6Ø2	T43.6Ø3	T43.6Ø4	T43.6Ø5	T43.6Ø6
analeptics	T5Ø.7X1	T5Ø.7X2	T5Ø.7X3	T5Ø.7X4	T5Ø.7X5	T5Ø.7X6
opiate antagonist	T5Ø.7X1	T5Ø.7X2	T5Ø.7X3	T5Ø.7X4	T5Ø.7X5	T5Ø.7X6
psychotherapeutic NEC — *see also* Psychotherapeutic drug	T43.6Ø1	T43.6Ø2	T43.6Ø3	T43.6Ø4	T43.6Ø5	T43.6Ø6
specified NEC	T43.691	T43.692	T43.693	T43.694	T43.695	T43.696
respiratory	T48.9Ø1	T48.9Ø2	T48.9Ø3	T48.9Ø4	T48.9Ø5	T48.9Ø6
Stone-dissolving drug	T5Ø.9Ø1	T5Ø.9Ø2	T5Ø.9Ø3	T5Ø.9Ø4	T5Ø.9Ø5	T5Ø.9Ø6
Storage battery (cells) (acid)	T54.2X1	T54.2X2	T54.2X3	T54.2X4	—	—
Stovaine	T41.3X1	T41.3X2	T41.3X3	T41.3X4	T41.3X5	T41.3X6
infiltration (subcutaneous)	T41.3X1	T41.3X2	T41.3X3	T41.3X4	T41.3X5	T41.3X6
nerve block (peripheral) (plexus)	T41.3X1	T41.3X2	T41.3X3	T41.3X4	T41.3X5	T41.3X6
spinal	T41.3X1	T41.3X2	T41.3X3	T41.3X4	T41.3X5	T41.3X6
topical (surface)	T41.3X1	T41.3X2	T41.3X3	T41.3X4	T41.3X5	T41.3X6
Stovarsal	T37.8X1	T37.8X2	T37.8X3	T37.8X4	T37.8X5	T37.8X6
Stove gas — *see* Gas, stove						
Stoxil	T49.5X1	T49.5X2	T49.5X3	T49.5X4	T49.5X5	T49.5X6
Stramonium	T48.6X1	T48.6X2	T48.6X3	T48.6X4	T48.6X5	T48.6X6
natural state	T62.2X1	T62.2X2	T62.2X3	T62.2X4	—	—
Streptodornase	T45.3X1	T45.3X2	T45.3X3	T45.3X4	T45.3X5	T45.3X6
Streptoduocin	T36.5X1	T36.5X2	T36.5X3	T36.5X4	T36.5X5	T36.5X6
Streptokinase	T45.611	T45.612	T45.613	T45.614	T45.615	T45.616
Streptomycin (derivative)	T36.5X1	T36.5X2	T36.5X3	T36.5X4	T36.5X5	T36.5X6
Streptonivicin	T36.5X1	T36.5X2	T36.5X3	T36.5X4	T36.5X5	T36.5X6
Streptovarycin	T36.5X1	T36.5X2	T36.5X3	T36.5X4	T36.5X5	T36.5X6
Streptozocin	T45.1X1	T45.1X2	T45.1X3	T45.1X4	T45.1X5	T45.1X6
Streptozotocin	T45.1X1	T45.1X2	T45.1X3	T45.1X4	T45.1X5	T45.1X6
Stripper (paint) (solvent)	T52.8X1	T52.8X2	T52.8X3	T52.8X4	—	—
Strobane	T6Ø.1X1	T6Ø.1X2	T6Ø.1X3	T6Ø.1X4	—	—
Strofantina	T46.ØX1	T46.ØX2	T46.ØX3	T46.ØX4	T46.ØX5	T46.ØX6
Stromectol*	T37.4X1	T37.4X2	T37.4X3	T37.4X4	T37.4X5	T37.4X6
Strophanthin (g) (k)	T46.ØX1	T46.ØX2	T46.ØX3	T46.ØX4	T46.ØX5	T46.ØX6
Strophanthus	T46.ØX1	T46.ØX2	T46.ØX3	T46.ØX4	T46.ØX5	T46.ØX6
Strophantin	T46.ØX1	T46.ØX2	T46.ØX3	T46.ØX4	T46.ØX5	T46.ØX6
Strophantin-g	T46.ØX1	T46.ØX2	T46.ØX3	T46.ØX4	T46.ØX5	T46.ØX6
Strychnine (nonmedicinal) (pesticide) (salts)	T65.1X1	T65.1X2	T65.1X3	T65.1X4	—	—
medicinal	T48.291	T48.292	T48.293	T48.294	T48.295	T48.296
Strychnos (ignatii) — *see* Strychnine						
Styramate	T42.8X1	T42.8X2	T42.8X3	T42.8X4	T42.8X5	T42.8X6
Styrene	T65.891	T65.892	T65.893	T65.894	—	—
Succinimide, antiepileptic or anticonvulsant	T42.2X1	T42.2X2	T42.2X3	T42.2X4	T42.2X5	T42.2X6
mercuric — *see* Mercury						
Succinylcholine	T48.1X1	T48.1X2	T48.1X3	T48.1X4	T48.1X5	T48.1X6
Succinylsulfathiazole	T37.ØX1	T37.ØX2	T37.ØX3	T37.ØX4	T37.ØX5	T37.ØX6
Sucralfate	T47.1X1	T47.1X2	T47.1X3	T47.1X4	T47.1X5	T47.1X6
Sucrose	T5Ø.3X1	T5Ø.3X2	T5Ø.3X3	T5Ø.3X4	T5Ø.3X5	T5Ø.3X6
Sufentanil	T4Ø.411	T4Ø.412	T4Ø.413	T4Ø.414	T4Ø.415	T4Ø.416
Sulbactam	T36.ØX1	T36.ØX2	T36.ØX3	T36.ØX4	T36.ØX5	T36.ØX6
Sulbenicillin	T36.ØX1	T36.ØX2	T36.ØX3	T36.ØX4	T36.ØX5	T36.ØX6
Sulbentine	T49.ØX1	T49.ØX2	T49.ØX3	T49.ØX4	T49.ØX5	T49.ØX6
Sulconazole*	T49.ØX1	T49.ØX2	T49.ØX3	T49.ØX4	T49.ØX5	T49.ØX6
Sulfacetamide	T49.ØX1	T49.ØX2	T49.ØX3	T49.ØX4	T49.ØX5	T49.ØX6
ophthalmic preparation	T49.5X1	T49.5X2	T49.5X3	T49.5X4	T49.5X5	T49.5X6
Sulfachlorpyridazine	T37.ØX1	T37.ØX2	T37.ØX3	T37.ØX4	T37.ØX5	T37.ØX6
Sulfacitine	T37.ØX1	T37.ØX2	T37.ØX3	T37.ØX4	T37.ØX5	T37.ØX6
Sulfadiasulfone sodium	T37.ØX1	T37.ØX2	T37.ØX3	T37.ØX4	T37.ØX5	T37.ØX6
Sulfadiazine	T37.ØX1	T37.ØX2	T37.ØX3	T37.ØX4	T37.ØX5	T37.ØX6

Substance	Poisoning, Accidental (unintentional)	Poisoning, Intentional Self-harm	Poisoning, Assault	Poisoning, Undetermined	Adverse Effect	Under-dosing
Sulfadiazine — *continued*						
silver (topical)	T49.ØX1	T49.ØX2	T49.ØX3	T49.ØX4	T49.ØX5	T49.ØX6
Sulfadimethoxine	T37.ØX1	T37.ØX2	T37.ØX3	T37.ØX4	T37.ØX5	T37.ØX6
Sulfadimidine	T37.ØX1	T37.ØX2	T37.ØX3	T37.ØX4	T37.ØX5	T37.ØX6
Sulfadoxine	T37.ØX1	T37.ØX2	T37.ØX3	T37.ØX4	T37.ØX5	T37.ØX6
with pyrimethamine	T37.2X1	T37.2X2	T37.2X3	T37.2X4	T37.2X5	T37.2X6
Sulfaethidole	T37.ØX1	T37.ØX2	T37.ØX3	T37.ØX4	T37.ØX5	T37.ØX6
Sulfafurazole	T37.ØX1	T37.ØX2	T37.ØX3	T37.ØX4	T37.ØX5	T37.ØX6
Sulfaguanidine	T37.ØX1	T37.ØX2	T37.ØX3	T37.ØX4	T37.ØX5	T37.ØX6
Sulfalene	T37.ØX1	T37.ØX2	T37.ØX3	T37.ØX4	T37.ØX5	T37.ØX6
Sulfaloxate	T37.ØX1	T37.ØX2	T37.ØX3	T37.ØX4	T37.ØX5	T37.ØX6
Sulfaloxic acid	T37.ØX1	T37.ØX2	T37.ØX3	T37.ØX4	T37.ØX5	T37.ØX6
Sulfamazone	T39.2X1	T39.2X2	T39.2X3	T39.2X4	T39.2X5	T39.2X6
Sulfamerazine	T37.ØX1	T37.ØX2	T37.ØX3	T37.ØX4	T37.ØX5	T37.ØX6
Sulfameter	T37.ØX1	T37.ØX2	T37.ØX3	T37.ØX4	T37.ØX5	T37.ØX6
Sulfamethazine	T37.ØX1	T37.ØX2	T37.ØX3	T37.ØX4	T37.ØX5	T37.ØX6
Sulfamethizole	T37.ØX1	T37.ØX2	T37.ØX3	T37.ØX4	T37.ØX5	T37.ØX6
Sulfamethoxazole	T37.ØX1	T37.ØX2	T37.ØX3	T37.ØX4	T37.ØX5	T37.ØX6
with trimethoprim	T36.8X1	T36.8X2	T36.8X3	T36.8X4	T36.8X5	T36.8X6
Sulfamethoxydiazine	T37.ØX1	T37.ØX2	T37.ØX3	T37.ØX4	T37.ØX5	T37.ØX6
Sulfamethoxypyridazine	T37.ØX1	T37.ØX2	T37.ØX3	T37.ØX4	T37.ØX5	T37.ØX6
Sulfamethylthiazole	T37.ØX1	T37.ØX2	T37.ØX3	T37.ØX4	T37.ØX5	T37.ØX6
Sulfametoxydiazine	T37.ØX1	T37.ØX2	T37.ØX3	T37.ØX4	T37.ØX5	T37.ØX6
Sulfamidopyrine	T39.2X1	T39.2X2	T39.2X3	T39.2X4	T39.2X5	T39.2X6
Sulfamonomethoxine	T37.ØX1	T37.ØX2	T37.ØX3	T37.ØX4	T37.ØX5	T37.ØX6
Sulfamoxole	T37.ØX1	T37.ØX2	T37.ØX3	T37.ØX4	T37.ØX5	T37.ØX6
Sulfamylon	T49.ØX1	T49.ØX2	T49.ØX3	T49.ØX4	T49.ØX5	T49.ØX6
Sulfan blue (diagnostic dye)	T5Ø.8X1	T5Ø.8X2	T5Ø.8X3	T5Ø.8X4	T5Ø.8X5	T5Ø.8X6
Sulfanilamide	T37.ØX1	T37.ØX2	T37.ØX3	T37.ØX4	T37.ØX5	T37.ØX6
Sulfanilylguanidine	T37.ØX1	T37.ØX2	T37.ØX3	T37.ØX4	T37.ØX5	T37.ØX6
Sulfaperin	T37.ØX1	T37.ØX2	T37.ØX3	T37.ØX4	T37.ØX5	T37.ØX6
Sulfaphenazole	T37.ØX1	T37.ØX2	T37.ØX3	T37.ØX4	T37.ØX5	T37.ØX6
Sulfaphenylthiazole	T37.ØX1	T37.ØX2	T37.ØX3	T37.ØX4	T37.ØX5	T37.ØX6
Sulfaproxyline	T37.ØX1	T37.ØX2	T37.ØX3	T37.ØX4	T37.ØX5	T37.ØX6
Sulfapyridine	T37.ØX1	T37.ØX2	T37.ØX3	T37.ØX4	T37.ØX5	T37.ØX6
Sulfapyrimidine	T37.ØX1	T37.ØX2	T37.ØX3	T37.ØX4	T37.ØX5	T37.ØX6
Sulfarsphenamine	T37.8X1	T37.8X2	T37.8X3	T37.8X4	T37.8X5	T37.8X6
Sulfasalazine	T37.ØX1	T37.ØX2	T37.ØX3	T37.ØX4	T37.ØX5	T37.ØX6
Sulfasuxidine	T37.ØX1	T37.ØX2	T37.ØX3	T37.ØX4	T37.ØX5	T37.ØX6
Sulfasymazine	T37.ØX1	T37.ØX2	T37.ØX3	T37.ØX4	T37.ØX5	T37.ØX6
Sulfated amylopectin	T47.8X1	T47.8X2	T47.8X3	T47.8X4	T47.8X5	T47.8X6
Sulfathiazole	T37.ØX1	T37.ØX2	T37.ØX3	T37.ØX4	T37.ØX5	T37.ØX6
Sulfatostearate	T49.2X1	T49.2X2	T49.2X3	T49.2X4	T49.2X5	T49.2X6
Sulfatrim*	T36.8X1	T36.8X2	T36.8X3	T36.8X4	T36.8X5	T36.8X6
Sulfinpyrazone	T5Ø.4X1	T5Ø.4X2	T5Ø.4X3	T5Ø.4X4	T5Ø.4X5	T5Ø.4X6
Sulfiram	T49.ØX1	T49.ØX2	T49.ØX3	T49.ØX4	T49.ØX5	T49.ØX6
Sulfisomidine	T37.ØX1	T37.ØX2	T37.ØX3	T37.ØX4	T37.ØX5	T37.ØX6
Sulfisoxazole	T37.ØX1	T37.ØX2	T37.ØX3	T37.ØX4	T37.ØX5	T37.ØX6
ophthalmic preparation	T49.5X1	T49.5X2	T49.5X3	T49.5X4	T49.5X5	T49.5X6
Sulfobromophthalein (sodium)	T5Ø.8X1	T5Ø.8X2	T5Ø.8X3	T5Ø.8X4	T5Ø.8X5	T5Ø.8X6
Sulfobromphthalein	T5Ø.8X1	T5Ø.8X2	T5Ø.8X3	T5Ø.8X4	T5Ø.8X5	T5Ø.8X6
Sulfogaiacol	T48.4X1	T48.4X2	T48.4X3	T48.4X4	T48.4X5	T48.4X6
Sulfomyxin	T36.8X1	T36.8X2	T36.8X3	T36.8X4	T36.8X5	T36.8X6
Sulfonal	T42.6X1	T42.6X2	T42.6X3	T42.6X4	T42.6X5	T42.6X6
Sulfonamide NEC	T37.ØX1	T37.ØX2	T37.ØX3	T37.ØX4	T37.ØX5	T37.ØX6
eye	T49.5X1	T49.5X2	T49.5X3	T49.5X4	T49.5X5	T49.5X6
Sulfonazide	T37.1X1	T37.1X2	T37.1X3	T37.1X4	T37.1X5	T37.1X6
Sulfones	T37.1X1	T37.1X2	T37.1X3	T37.1X4	T37.1X5	T37.1X6
Sulfonethylmethane	T42.6X1	T42.6X2	T42.6X3	T42.6X4	T42.6X5	T42.6X6
Sulfonmethane	T42.6X1	T42.6X2	T42.6X3	T42.6X4	T42.6X5	T42.6X6
Sulfonphthal, sulfonphthol	T5Ø.8X1	T5Ø.8X2	T5Ø.8X3	T5Ø.8X4	T5Ø.8X5	T5Ø.8X6
Sulfonylurea derivatives, oral	T38.3X1	T38.3X2	T38.3X3	T38.3X4	T38.3X5	T38.3X6
Sulforidazine	T43.3X1	T43.3X2	T43.3X3	T43.3X4	T43.3X5	T43.3X6
Sulfoxone	T37.1X1	T37.1X2	T37.1X3	T37.1X4	T37.1X5	T37.1X6
Sulfuric acid	T54.2X1	T54.2X2	T54.2X3	T54.2X4	—	—
Sulfur, sulfurated, sulfuric, sulfurous, sulfuryl (compounds NEC) (medicinal)	T49.4X1	T49.4X2	T49.4X3	T49.4X4	T49.4X5	T49.4X6
acid	T54.2X1	T54.2X2	T54.2X3	T54.2X4	—	—
dioxide (gas)	T59.1X1	T59.1X2	T59.1X3	T59.1X4	—	—
ether — *see* Ether(s)						
hydrogen	T59.6X1	T59.6X2	T59.6X3	T59.6X4	—	—
medicinal (keratolytic) (ointment) NEC	T49.4X1	T49.4X2	T49.4X3	T49.4X4	T49.4X5	T49.4X6
ointment	T49.ØX1	T49.ØX2	T49.ØX3	T49.ØX4	T49.ØX5	T49.ØX6
pesticide (vapor)	T6Ø.91	T6Ø.92	T6Ø.93	T6Ø.94	—	—
vapor NEC	T59.891	T59.892	T59.893	T59.894	—	—
Sulglicotide	T47.1X1	T47.1X2	T47.1X3	T47.1X4	T47.1X5	T47.1X6
Sulindac	T39.391	T39.392	T39.393	T39.394	T39.395	T39.396

Substance	Poisoning, Accidental (unintentional)	Poisoning, Intentional Self-harm	Poisoning, Assault	Poisoning, Undetermined	Adverse Effect	Under-dosing
Sulisatin	T47.2X1	T47.2X2	T47.2X3	T47.2X4	T47.2X5	T47.2X6
Sulisobenzone	T49.3X1	T49.3X2	T49.3X3	T49.3X4	T49.3X5	T49.3X6
Sulkowitch's reagent	T5Ø.8X1	T5Ø.8X2	T5Ø.8X3	T5Ø.8X4	T5Ø.8X5	T5Ø.8X6
Sulmetozine	T44.3X1	T44.3X2	T44.3X3	T44.3X4	T44.3X5	T44.3X6
Suloctidil	T46.7X1	T46.7X2	T46.7X3	T46.7X4	T46.7X5	T46.7X6
Sulph- — *see also* Sulf-						
Sulphadiazine	T37.ØX1	T37.ØX2	T37.ØX3	T37.ØX4	T37.ØX5	T37.ØX6
Sulphadimethoxine	T37.ØX1	T37.ØX2	T37.ØX3	T37.ØX4	T37.ØX5	T37.ØX6
Sulphadimidine	T37.ØX1	T37.ØX2	T37.ØX3	T37.ØX4	T37.ØX5	T37.ØX6
Sulphadione	T37.1X1	T37.1X2	T37.1X3	T37.1X4	T37.1X5	T37.1X6
Sulphafurazole	T37.ØX1	T37.ØX2	T37.ØX3	T37.ØX4	T37.ØX5	T37.ØX6
Sulphamethizole	T37.ØX1	T37.ØX2	T37.ØX3	T37.ØX4	T37.ØX5	T37.ØX6
Sulphamethoxazole	T37.ØX1	T37.ØX2	T37.ØX3	T37.ØX4	T37.ØX5	T37.ØX6
Sulphan blue	T5Ø.8X1	T5Ø.8X2	T5Ø.8X3	T5Ø.8X4	T5Ø.8X5	T5Ø.8X6
Sulphaphenazole	T37.ØX1	T37.ØX2	T37.ØX3	T37.ØX4	T37.ØX5	T37.ØX6
Sulphapyridine	T37.ØX1	T37.ØX2	T37.ØX3	T37.ØX4	T37.ØX5	T37.ØX6
Sulphasalazine	T37.ØX1	T37.ØX2	T37.ØX3	T37.ØX4	T37.ØX5	T37.ØX6
Sulphinpyrazone	T5Ø.4X1	T5Ø.4X2	T5Ø.4X3	T5Ø.4X4	T5Ø.4X5	T5Ø.4X6
Sulpiride	T43.591	T43.592	T43.593	T43.594	T43.595	T43.596
Sulprostone	T48.ØX1	T48.ØX2	T48.ØX3	T48.ØX4	T48.ØX5	T48.ØX6
Sulpyrine	T39.2X1	T39.2X2	T39.2X3	T39.2X4	T39.2X5	T39.2X6
Sultamicillin	T36.ØX1	T36.ØX2	T36.ØX3	T36.ØX4	T36.ØX5	T36.ØX6
Sulthiame	T42.6X1	T42.6X2	T42.6X3	T42.6X4	T42.6X5	T42.6X6
Sultiame	T42.6X1	T42.6X2	T42.6X3	T42.6X4	T42.6X5	T42.6X6
Sultopride	T43.591	T43.592	T43.593	T43.594	T43.595	T43.596
Sumatriptan	T39.8X1	T39.8X2	T39.8X3	T39.8X4	T39.8X5	T39.8X6
Sumavel*	T39.8X1	T39.8X2	T39.8X3	T39.8X4	T39.8X5	T39.8X6
Sunflower seed oil	T46.6X1	T46.6X2	T46.6X3	T46.6X4	T46.6X5	T46.6X6
Superinone	T48.4X1	T48.4X2	T48.4X3	T48.4X4	T48.4X5	T48.4X6
Suprofen	T39.311	T39.312	T39.313	T39.314	T39.315	T39.316
Suramin (sodium)	T37.4X1	T37.4X2	T37.4X3	T37.4X4	T37.4X5	T37.4X6
Surfacaine	T41.3X1	T41.3X2	T41.3X3	T41.3X4	T41.3X5	T41.3X6
Surital	T41.1X1	T41.1X2	T41.1X3	T41.1X4	T41.1X5	T41.1X6
Sutilains	T45.3X1	T45.3X2	T45.3X3	T45.3X4	T45.3X5	T45.3X6
Suxamethonium (chloride)	T48.1X1	T48.1X2	T48.1X3	T48.1X4	T48.1X5	T48.1X6
Suxethonium (chloride)	T48.1X1	T48.1X2	T48.1X3	T48.1X4	T48.1X5	T48.1X6
Suxibuzone	T39.2X1	T39.2X2	T39.2X3	T39.2X4	T39.2X5	T39.2X6
Sweetener	T5Ø.9Ø1	T5Ø.9Ø2	T5Ø.9Ø3	T5Ø.9Ø4	T5Ø.9Ø5	T5Ø.9Ø6
Sweet niter spirit	T46.3X1	T46.3X2	T46.3X3	T46.3X4	T46.3X5	T46.3X6
Sweet oil (birch)	T49.3X1	T49.3X2	T49.3X3	T49.3X4	T49.3X5	T49.3X6
Sylvant*	T45.1X1	T45.1X2	T45.1X3	T45.1X4	T45.1X5	T45.1X6
Sym-dichloroethyl ether	T53.6X1	T53.6X2	T53.6X3	T53.6X4	—	—
Sympatholytic NEC	T44.8X1	T44.8X2	T44.8X3	T44.8X4	T44.8X5	T44.8X6
haloalkylamine	T44.8X1	T44.8X2	T44.8X3	T44.8X4	T44.8X5	T44.8X6
Sympathomimetic NEC	T44.9Ø1	T44.9Ø2	T44.9Ø3	T44.9Ø4	T44.9Ø5	T44.9Ø6
anti-common-cold	T48.5X1	T48.5X2	T48.5X3	T48.5X4	T48.5X5	T48.5X6
bronchodilator	T48.6X1	T48.6X2	T48.6X3	T48.6X4	T48.6X5	T48.6X6
specified NEC	T44.991	T44.992	T44.993	T44.994	T44.995	T44.996
Synagis	T5Ø.B91	T5Ø.B92	T5Ø.B93	T5Ø.B94	T5Ø.B95	T5Ø.B96
Synalar	T49.ØX1	T49.ØX2	T49.ØX3	T49.ØX4	T49.ØX5	T49.ØX6
Synthetic cannabinoids	T4Ø.721	T4Ø.722	T4Ø.723	T4Ø.724	T4Ø.725	T4Ø.726
Synthroid	T38.1X1	T38.1X2	T38.1X3	T38.1X4	T38.1X5	T38.1X6
Syntocinon	T48.ØX1	T48.ØX2	T48.ØX3	T48.ØX4	T48.ØX5	T48.ØX6
Syrosingopine	T46.5X1	T46.5X2	T46.5X3	T46.5X4	T46.5X5	T46.5X6
Systemic drug	T45.91	T45.92	T45.93	T45.94	T45.95	T45.96
specified NEC	T45.8X1	T45.8X2	T45.8X3	T45.8X4	T45.8X5	T45.8X6
Tablets — *see also* specified substance	T5Ø.9Ø1	T5Ø.9Ø2	T5Ø.9Ø3	T5Ø.9Ø4	T5Ø.9Ø5	T5Ø.9Ø6
Tace	T38.5X1	T38.5X2	T38.5X3	T38.5X4	T38.5X5	T38.5X6
Tacrine	T44.ØX1	T44.ØX2	T44.ØX3	T44.ØX4	T44.ØX5	T44.ØX6
Tadalafil	T46.7X1	T46.7X2	T46.7X3	T46.7X4	T46.7X5	T46.7X6
Talampicillin	T36.ØX1	T36.ØX2	T36.ØX3	T36.ØX4	T36.ØX5	T36.ØX6
Talbutal	T42.3X1	T42.3X2	T42.3X3	T42.3X4	T42.3X5	T42.3X6
Talc powder	T49.3X1	T49.3X2	T49.3X3	T49.3X4	T49.3X5	T49.3X6
Talcum	T49.3X1	T49.3X2	T49.3X3	T49.3X4	T49.3X5	T49.3X6
Taleranol	T38.6X1	T38.6X2	T38.6X3	T38.6X4	T38.6X5	T38.6X6
Taltz*	T39.391	T39.392	T39.393	T39.394	T39.395	T39.396
Tamoxifen	T38.6X1	T38.6X2	T38.6X3	T38.6X4	T38.6X5	T38.6X6
Tamsulosin	T44.6X1	T44.6X2	T44.6X3	T44.6X4	T44.6X5	T44.6X6
Tandearil, tanderil	T39.2X1	T39.2X2	T39.2X3	T39.2X4	T39.2X5	T39.2X6
Tannic acid	T49.2X1	T49.2X2	T49.2X3	T49.2X4	T49.2X5	T49.2X6
medicinal (astringent)	T49.2X1	T49.2X2	T49.2X3	T49.2X4	T49.2X5	T49.2X6
Tannin — *see* Tannic acid						
Tansy	T62.2X1	T62.2X2	T62.2X3	T62.2X4	—	—
TAO	T36.3X1	T36.3X2	T36.3X3	T36.3X4	T36.3X5	T36.3X6
Tapazole	T38.2X1	T38.2X2	T38.2X3	T38.2X4	T38.2X5	T38.2X6
Taractan	T43.591	T43.592	T43.593	T43.594	T43.595	T43.596
Tarantula (venomous)	T63.321	T63.322	T63.323	T63.324	—	—
Tartar emetic	T37.8X1	T37.8X2	T37.8X3	T37.8X4	T37.8X5	T37.8X6
Tartaric acid	T65.891	T65.892	T65.893	T65.894	—	—
Tartrated antimony (anti-infective)	T37.8X1	T37.8X2	T37.8X3	T37.8X4	T37.8X5	T37.8X6
Tartrate, laxative	T47.4X1	T47.4X2	T47.4X3	T47.4X4	T47.4X5	T47.4X6

Substance	Poisoning, Accidental (unintentional)	Poisoning, Intentional Self-harm	Poisoning, Assault	Poisoning, Undetermined	Adverse Effect	Under-dosing
Tar NEC	T52.ØX1	T52.ØX2	T52.ØX3	T52.ØX4	—	—
camphor	T6Ø.1X1	T6Ø.1X2	T6Ø.1X3	T6Ø.1X4	—	—
distillate	T49.1X1	T49.1X2	T49.1X3	T49.1X4	T49.1X5	T49.1X6
fumes	T59.891	T59.892	T59.893	T59.894	—	—
medicinal	T49.1X1	T49.1X2	T49.1X3	T49.1X4	T49.1X5	T49.1X6
ointment	T49.1X1	T49.1X2	T49.1X3	T49.1X4	T49.1X5	T49.1X6
Tauromustine	T45.1X1	T45.1X2	T45.1X3	T45.1X4	T45.1X5	T45.1X6
TCA — *see* Trichloroacetic acid						
TCDD	T53.7X1	T53.7X2	T53.7X3	T53.7X4	—	—
TDI (vapor)	T65.ØX1	T65.ØX2	T65.ØX3	T65.ØX4	—	—
Tear						
gas	T59.3X1	T59.3X2	T59.3X3	T59.3X4	—	—
solution	T49.5X1	T49.5X2	T49.5X3	T49.5X4	T49.5X5	T49.5X6
Tecentriq*	T45.1X1	T45.1X2	T45.1X3	T45.1X4	T45.1X5	T45.1X6
Teclothiazide	T5Ø.2X1	T5Ø.2X2	T5Ø.2X3	T5Ø.2X4	T5Ø.2X5	T5Ø.2X6
Teclozan	T37.3X1	T37.3X2	T37.3X3	T37.3X4	T37.3X5	T37.3X6
Tegafur	T45.1X1	T45.1X2	T45.1X3	T45.1X4	T45.1X5	T45.1X6
Tegretol	T42.1X1	T42.1X2	T42.1X3	T42.1X4	T42.1X5	T42.1X6
Teicoplanin	T36.8X1	T36.8X2	T36.8X3	T36.8X4	T36.8X5	T36.8X6
Telepaque	T5Ø.8X1	T5Ø.8X2	T5Ø.8X3	T5Ø.8X4	T5Ø.8X5	T5Ø.8X6
Tellurium	T56.891	T56.892	T56.893	T56.894	—	—
fumes	T56.891	T56.892	T56.893	T56.894	—	—
TEM	T45.1X1	T45.1X2	T45.1X3	T45.1X4	T45.1X5	T45.1X6
Temazepam	T42.4X1	T42.4X2	T42.4X3	T42.4X4	T42.4X5	T42.4X6
Temocillin	T36.ØX1	T36.ØX2	T36.ØX3	T36.ØX4	T36.ØX5	T36.ØX6
Tenamfetamine	T43.621	T43.622	T43.623	T43.624	T43.625	T43.626
Tenecteplase*	T45.611	T45.612	T45.613	T45.614	T45.615	T45.616
Teniposide	T45.1X1	T45.1X2	T45.1X3	T45.1X4	T45.1X5	T45.1X6
Tenitramine	T46.3X1	T46.3X2	T46.3X3	T46.3X4	T46.3X5	T46.3X6
Tenoglicin	T48.4X1	T48.4X2	T48.4X3	T48.4X4	T48.4X5	T48.4X6
Tenonitrozole	T37.3X1	T37.3X2	T37.3X3	T37.3X4	T37.3X5	T37.3X6
Tenoxicam	T39.391	T39.392	T39.393	T39.394	T39.395	T39.396
TEPA	T45.1X1	T45.1X2	T45.1X3	T45.1X4	T45.1X5	T45.1X6
TEPP	T6Ø.ØX1	T6Ø.ØX2	T6Ø.ØX3	T6Ø.ØX4	—	—
Teprotide	T46.5X1	T46.5X2	T46.5X3	T46.5X4	T46.5X5	T46.5X6
Terazosin	T44.6X1	T44.6X2	T44.6X3	T44.6X4	T44.6X5	T44.6X6
Terbufos	T6Ø.ØX1	T6Ø.ØX2	T6Ø.ØX3	T6Ø.ØX4	—	—
Terbutaline	T48.6X1	T48.6X2	T48.6X3	T48.6X4	T48.6X5	T48.6X6
Terconazole	T49.ØX1	T49.ØX2	T49.ØX3	T49.ØX4	T49.ØX5	T49.ØX6
Terfenadine	T45.ØX1	T45.ØX2	T45.ØX3	T45.ØX4	T45.ØX5	T45.ØX6
Teriparatide (acetate)	T5Ø.991	T5Ø.992	T5Ø.993	T5Ø.994	T5Ø.995	T5Ø.996
Terizidone	T37.1X1	T37.1X2	T37.1X3	T37.1X4	T37.1X5	T37.1X6
Terlipressin	T38.891	T38.892	T38.893	T38.894	T38.895	T38.896
Terodiline	T46.3X1	T46.3X2	T46.3X3	T46.3X4	T46.3X5	T46.3X6
Teroxalene	T37.4X1	T37.4X2	T37.4X3	T37.4X4	T37.4X5	T37.4X6
Terpin (cis) **hydrate**	T48.4X1	T48.4X2	T48.4X3	T48.4X4	T48.4X5	T48.4X6
Terramycin	T36.4X1	T36.4X2	T36.4X3	T36.4X4	T36.4X5	T36.4X6
Tertatolol	T44.7X1	T44.7X2	T44.7X3	T44.7X4	T44.7X5	T44.7X6
Tessalon	T48.3X1	T48.3X2	T48.3X3	T48.3X4	T48.3X5	T48.3X6
Testolactone	T38.7X1	T38.7X2	T38.7X3	T38.7X4	T38.7X5	T38.7X6
Testosterone	T38.7X1	T38.7X2	T38.7X3	T38.7X4	T38.7X5	T38.7X6
Tetanus toxoid or vaccine	T5Ø.A91	T5Ø.A92	T5Ø.A93	T5Ø.A94	T5Ø.A95	T5Ø.A96
antitoxin	T5Ø.Z11	T5Ø.Z12	T5Ø.Z13	T5Ø.Z14	T5Ø.Z15	T5Ø.Z16
immune globulin (human)	T5Ø.Z11	T5Ø.Z12	T5Ø.Z13	T5Ø.Z14	T5Ø.Z15	T5Ø.Z16
toxoid	T5Ø.A91	T5Ø.A92	T5Ø.A93	T5Ø.A94	T5Ø.A95	T5Ø.A96
with diphtheria toxoid	T5Ø.A21	T5Ø.A22	T5Ø.A23	T5Ø.A24	T5Ø.A25	T5Ø.A26
with pertussis	T5Ø.A11	T5Ø.A12	T5Ø.A13	T5Ø.A14	T5Ø.A15	T5Ø.A16
Tetrabenazine	T43.591	T43.592	T43.593	T43.594	T43.595	T43.596
Tetracaine	T41.3X1	T41.3X2	T41.3X3	T41.3X4	T41.3X5	T41.3X6
nerve block (peripheral) (plexus)	T41.3X1	T41.3X2	T41.3X3	T41.3X4	T41.3X5	T41.3X6
regional	T41.3X1	T41.3X2	T41.3X3	T41.3X4	T41.3X5	T41.3X6
spinal	T41.3X1	T41.3X2	T41.3X3	T41.3X4	T41.3X5	T41.3X6
Tetrachlorethylene — *see* Tetrachloroethylene						
Tetrachlormethiazide	T5Ø.2X1	T5Ø.2X2	T5Ø.2X3	T5Ø.2X4	T5Ø.2X5	T5Ø.2X6
Tetrachloroethane	T53.6X1	T53.6X2	T53.6X3	T53.6X4	—	—
vapor	T53.6X1	T53.6X2	T53.6X3	T53.6X4	—	—
paint or varnish	T53.6X1	T53.6X2	T53.6X3	T53.6X4	—	—
Tetrachloroethylene (liquid)	T53.3X1	T53.3X2	T53.3X3	T53.3X4	—	—
medicinal	T37.4X1	T37.4X2	T37.4X3	T37.4X4	T37.4X5	T37.4X6
vapor	T53.3X1	T53.3X2	T53.3X3	T53.3X4	—	—
Tetrachloromethane — *see* Carbon tetrachloride						
Tetracosactide	T38.811	T38.812	T38.813	T38.814	T38.815	T38.816
Tetracosactrin	T38.811	T38.812	T38.813	T38.814	T38.815	T38.816
Tetracycline	T36.4X1	T36.4X2	T36.4X3	T36.4X4	T36.4X5	T36.4X6
ophthalmic preparation	T49.5X1	T49.5X2	T49.5X3	T49.5X4	T49.5X5	T49.5X6
topical NEC	T49.ØX1	T49.ØX2	T49.ØX3	T49.ØX4	T49.ØX5	T49.ØX6
Tetradifon	T6Ø.8X1	T6Ø.8X2	T6Ø.8X3	T6Ø.8X4	—	—
Tetradotoxin	T61.771	T61.772	T61.773	T61.774	—	—

Substance	Poisoning, Accidental (unintentional)	Poisoning, Intentional Self-harm	Poisoning, Assault	Poisoning, Undetermined	Adverse Effect	Under-dosing
Tetraethyl						
lead	T56.0X1	T56.0X2	T56.0X3	T56.0X4	—	—
pyrophosphate	T60.0X1	T60.0X2	T60.0X3	T60.0X4	—	—
Tetraethylammonium chloride	T44.2X1	T44.2X2	T44.2X3	T44.2X4	T44.2X5	T44.2X6
Tetraethylthiuram disulfide	T50.6X1	T50.6X2	T50.6X3	T50.6X4	T50.6X5	T50.6X6
Tetrahydroaminoacridine	T44.0X1	T44.0X2	T44.0X3	T44.0X4	T44.0X5	T44.0X6
Tetrahydrocannabinol	T40.711	T40.712	T40.713	T40.714	T40.715	T40.716
Tetrahydrofuran	T52.8X1	T52.8X2	T52.8X3	T52.8X4	—	—
Tetrahydrolipstatin*	T47.8X1	T47.8X2	T47.8X3	T47.8X4	T47.8X5	T47.8X6
Tetrahydronaphthalene	T52.8X1	T52.8X2	T52.8X3	T52.8X4	—	—
Tetrahydrozoline	T49.5X1	T49.5X2	T49.5X3	T49.5X4	T49.5X5	T49.5X6
Tetralin	T52.8X1	T52.8X2	T52.8X3	T52.8X4	—	—
Tetramethrin	T60.2X1	T60.2X2	T60.2X3	T60.2X4	—	—
Tetramethylthiuram (disulfide) NEC	T60.3X1	T60.3X2	T60.3X3	T60.3X4	—	—
medicinal	T49.0X1	T49.0X2	T49.0X3	T49.0X4	T49.0X5	T49.0X6
Tetramisole	T37.4X1	T37.4X2	T37.4X3	T37.4X4	T37.4X5	T37.4X6
Tetranicotinoyl fructose	T46.7X1	T46.7X2	T46.7X3	T46.7X4	T46.7X5	T46.7X6
Tetrazepam	T42.4X1	T42.4X2	T42.4X3	T42.4X4	T42.4X5	T42.4X6
Tetronal	T42.6X1	T42.6X2	T42.6X3	T42.6X4	T42.6X5	T42.6X6
Tetryl	T65.3X1	T65.3X2	T65.3X3	T65.3X4	—	—
Tetrylammonium chloride	T44.2X1	T44.2X2	T44.2X3	T44.2X4	T44.2X5	T44.2X6
Tetryzoline	T49.5X1	T49.5X2	T49.5X3	T49.5X4	T49.5X5	T49.5X6
Thalidomide	T45.1X1	T45.1X2	T45.1X3	T45.1X4	T45.1X5	T45.1X6
Thallium (compounds) (dust) NEC	T56.811	T56.812	T56.813	T56.814	—	—
pesticide	T60.4X1	T60.4X2	T60.4X3	T60.4X4	—	—
THC	T40.711	T40.712	T40.713	T40.714	T40.715	T40.716
Thebacon	T48.3X1	T48.3X2	T48.3X3	T48.3X4	T48.3X5	T48.3X6
Thebaine	T40.2X1	T40.2X2	T40.2X3	T40.2X4	T40.2X5	T40.2X6
Thenoic acid	T49.6X1	T49.6X2	T49.6X3	T49.6X4	T49.6X5	T49.6X6
Thenyldiamine	T45.0X1	T45.0X2	T45.0X3	T45.0X4	T45.0X5	T45.0X6
Theobromine (calcium salicylate)	T48.6X1	T48.6X2	T48.6X3	T48.6X4	T48.6X5	T48.6X6
sodium salicylate	T48.6X1	T48.6X2	T48.6X3	T48.6X4	T48.6X5	T48.6X6
Theolair*	T48.6X1	T48.6X2	T48.6X3	T48.6X4	T48.6X5	T48.6X6
Theophyllamine	T48.6X1	T48.6X2	T48.6X3	T48.6X4	T48.6X5	T48.6X6
Theophylline	T48.6X1	T48.6X2	T48.6X3	T48.6X4	T48.6X5	T48.6X6
aminobenzoic acid	T48.6X1	T48.6X2	T48.6X3	T48.6X4	T48.6X5	T48.6X6
ethylenediamine	T48.6X1	T48.6X2	T48.6X3	T48.6X4	T48.6X5	T48.6X6
piperazine p-amino-benzoate	T48.6X1	T48.6X2	T48.6X3	T48.6X4	T48.6X5	T48.6X6
Therevac*	T47.4X1	T47.4X2	T47.4X3	T47.4X4	T47.4X5	T47.4X6
Thiabendazole	T37.4X1	T37.4X2	T37.4X3	T37.4X4	T37.4X5	T37.4X6
Thialbarbital	T41.1X1	T41.1X2	T41.1X3	T41.1X4	T41.1X5	T41.1X6
Thiamazole	T38.2X1	T38.2X2	T38.2X3	T38.2X4	T38.2X5	T38.2X6
Thiambutosine	T37.1X1	T37.1X2	T37.1X3	T37.1X4	T37.1X5	T37.1X6
Thiamine	T45.2X1	T45.2X2	T45.2X3	T45.2X4	T45.2X5	T45.2X6
Thiamphenicol	T36.2X1	T36.2X2	T36.2X3	T36.2X4	T36.2X5	T36.2X6
Thiamylal	T41.1X1	T41.1X2	T41.1X3	T41.1X4	T41.1X5	T41.1X6
sodium	T41.1X1	T41.1X2	T41.1X3	T41.1X4	T41.1X5	T41.1X6
Thiazesim	T43.291	T43.292	T43.293	T43.294	T43.295	T43.296
Thiazides (diuretics)	T50.2X1	T50.2X2	T50.2X3	T50.2X4	T50.2X5	T50.2X6
Thiazinamium metilsulfate	T43.3X1	T43.3X2	T43.3X3	T43.3X4	T43.3X5	T43.3X6
Thiethylperazine	T43.3X1	T43.3X2	T43.3X3	T43.3X4	T43.3X5	T43.3X6
Thimerosal	T49.0X1	T49.0X2	T49.0X3	T49.0X4	T49.0X5	T49.0X6
ophthalmic preparation	T49.5X1	T49.5X2	T49.5X3	T49.5X4	T49.5X5	T49.5X6
Thioacetazone	T37.1X1	T37.1X2	T37.1X3	T37.1X4	T37.1X5	T37.1X6
with isoniazid	T37.1X1	T37.1X2	T37.1X3	T37.1X4	T37.1X5	T37.1X6
Thiobarbital sodium	T41.1X1	T41.1X2	T41.1X3	T41.1X4	T41.1X5	T41.1X6
Thiobarbiturate anesthetic	T41.1X1	T41.1X2	T41.1X3	T41.1X4	T41.1X5	T41.1X6
Thiobismol	T37.8X1	T37.8X2	T37.8X3	T37.8X4	T37.8X5	T37.8X6
Thiobutabarbital sodium	T41.1X1	T41.1X2	T41.1X3	T41.1X4	T41.1X5	T41.1X6
Thiocarbamate (insecticide)	T60.0X1	T60.0X2	T60.0X3	T60.0X4	—	—
Thiocarbamide	T38.2X1	T38.2X2	T38.2X3	T38.2X4	T38.2X5	T38.2X6
Thiocarbarsone	T37.8X1	T37.8X2	T37.8X3	T37.8X4	T37.8X5	T37.8X6
Thiocarlide	T37.1X1	T37.1X2	T37.1X3	T37.1X4	T37.1X5	T37.1X6
Thioctamide	T50.991	T50.992	T50.993	T50.994	T50.995	T50.996
Thioctic acid	T50.991	T50.992	T50.993	T50.994	T50.995	T50.996
Thiofos	T60.0X1	T60.0X2	T60.0X3	T60.0X4	—	—
Thioglycolate	T49.4X1	T49.4X2	T49.4X3	T49.4X4	T49.4X5	T49.4X6
Thioglycolic acid	T65.891	T65.892	T65.893	T65.894	—	—
Thioguanine	T45.1X1	T45.1X2	T45.1X3	T45.1X4	T45.1X5	T45.1X6
Thiomercaptomerin	T50.2X1	T50.2X2	T50.2X3	T50.2X4	T50.2X5	T50.2X6
Thiomerin	T50.2X1	T50.2X2	T50.2X3	T50.2X4	T50.2X5	T50.2X6
Thiomersal	T49.0X1	T49.0X2	T49.0X3	T49.0X4	T49.0X5	T49.0X6
Thionazin	T60.0X1	T60.0X2	T60.0X3	T60.0X4	—	—
Thiopental (sodium)	T41.1X1	T41.1X2	T41.1X3	T41.1X4	T41.1X5	T41.1X6
Thiopentone (sodium)	T41.1X1	T41.1X2	T41.1X3	T41.1X4	T41.1X5	T41.1X6
Thiopropazate	T43.3X1	T43.3X2	T43.3X3	T43.3X4	T43.3X5	T43.3X6
Thioproperazine	T43.3X1	T43.3X2	T43.3X3	T43.3X4	T43.3X5	T43.3X6
Thioridazine	T43.3X1	T43.3X2	T43.3X3	T43.3X4	T43.3X5	T43.3X6
Thiosinamine	T49.3X1	T49.3X2	T49.3X3	T49.3X4	T49.3X5	T49.3X6
Thiotepa	T45.1X1	T45.1X2	T45.1X3	T45.1X4	T45.1X5	T45.1X6
Thiothixene	T43.4X1	T43.4X2	T43.4X3	T43.4X4	T43.4X5	T43.4X6
Thiouracil (benzyl) (methyl) (propyl)	T38.2X1	T38.2X2	T38.2X3	T38.2X4	T38.2X5	T38.2X6
Thiourea	T38.2X1	T38.2X2	T38.2X3	T38.2X4	T38.2X5	T38.2X6
Thiphenamil	T44.3X1	T44.3X2	T44.3X3	T44.3X4	T44.3X5	T44.3X6
Thiram	T60.3X1	T60.3X2	T60.3X3	T60.3X4	—	—
medicinal	T49.2X1	T49.2X2	T49.2X3	T49.2X4	T49.2X5	T49.2X6
Thonzylamine (systemic)	T45.0X1	T45.0X2	T45.0X3	T45.0X4	T45.0X5	T45.0X6
mucosal decongestant	T48.5X1	T48.5X2	T48.5X3	T48.5X4	T48.5X5	T48.5X6
Thorazine	T43.3X1	T43.3X2	T43.3X3	T43.3X4	T43.3X5	T43.3X6
Thorium dioxide suspension	T50.8X1	T50.8X2	T50.8X3	T50.8X4	T50.8X5	T50.8X6
Thornapple	T62.2X1	T62.2X2	T62.2X3	T62.2X4	—	—
Throat drug NEC	T49.6X1	T49.6X2	T49.6X3	T49.6X4	T49.6X5	T49.6X6
Thrombate 111*	T45.511	T45.512	T45.513	T45.514	T45.515	T45.516
Thrombin	T45.7X1	T45.7X2	T45.7X3	T45.7X4	T45.7X5	T45.7X6
Thrombolysin	T45.611	T45.612	T45.613	T45.614	T45.615	T45.616
Thromboplastin	T45.7X1	T45.7X2	T45.7X3	T45.7X4	T45.7X5	T45.7X6
Thurfyl nicotinate	T46.7X1	T46.7X2	T46.7X3	T46.7X4	T46.7X5	T46.7X6
Thymol	T49.0X1	T49.0X2	T49.0X3	T49.0X4	T49.0X5	T49.0X6
Thymopentin	T37.5X1	T37.5X2	T37.5X3	T37.5X4	T37.5X5	T37.5X6
Thymoxamine	T46.7X1	T46.7X2	T46.7X3	T46.7X4	T46.7X5	T46.7X6
Thymus extract	T38.891	T38.892	T38.893	T38.894	T38.895	T38.896
Thyreotrophic hormone	T38.811	T38.812	T38.813	T38.814	T38.815	T38.816
Thyroglobulin	T38.1X1	T38.1X2	T38.1X3	T38.1X4	T38.1X5	T38.1X6
Thyroid (hormone)	T38.1X1	T38.1X2	T38.1X3	T38.1X4	T38.1X5	T38.1X6
Thyrolar	T38.1X1	T38.1X2	T38.1X3	T38.1X4	T38.1X5	T38.1X6
Thyrotrophin	T38.811	T38.812	T38.813	T38.814	T38.815	T38.816
Thyrotropic hormone	T38.811	T38.812	T38.813	T38.814	T38.815	T38.816
Thyroxine	T38.1X1	T38.1X2	T38.1X3	T38.1X4	T38.1X5	T38.1X6
Tiabendazole	T37.4X1	T37.4X2	T37.4X3	T37.4X4	T37.4X5	T37.4X6
Tiamizide	T50.2X1	T50.2X2	T50.2X3	T50.2X4	T50.2X5	T50.2X6
Tianeptine	T43.291	T43.292	T43.293	T43.294	T43.295	T43.296
Tiapamil	T46.1X1	T46.1X2	T46.1X3	T46.1X4	T46.1X5	T46.1X6
Tiapride	T43.591	T43.592	T43.593	T43.594	T43.595	T43.596
Tiaprofenic acid	T39.311	T39.312	T39.313	T39.314	T39.315	T39.316
Tiaramide	T39.8X1	T39.8X2	T39.8X3	T39.8X4	T39.8X5	T39.8X6
Ticagrelor*	T45.521	T45.522	T45.523	T45.524	T45.525	T45.526
Ticarcillin	T36.0X1	T36.0X2	T36.0X3	T36.0X4	T36.0X5	T36.0X6
Ticlatone	T49.0X1	T49.0X2	T49.0X3	T49.0X4	T49.0X5	T49.0X6
Ticlopidine	T45.521	T45.522	T45.523	T45.524	T45.525	T45.526
Ticrynafen	T50.1X1	T50.1X2	T50.1X3	T50.1X4	T50.1X5	T50.1X6
Tidiacic	T50.991	T50.992	T50.993	T50.994	T50.995	T50.996
Tiemonium	T44.3X1	T44.3X2	T44.3X3	T44.3X4	T44.3X5	T44.3X6
iodide	T44.3X1	T44.3X2	T44.3X3	T44.3X4	T44.3X5	T44.3X6
Tienilic acid	T50.1X1	T50.1X2	T50.1X3	T50.1X4	T50.1X5	T50.1X6
Tifenamil	T44.3X1	T44.3X2	T44.3X3	T44.3X4	T44.3X5	T44.3X6
Tigan	T45.0X1	T45.0X2	T45.0X3	T45.0X4	T45.0X5	T45.0X6
Tigloidine	T44.3X1	T44.3X2	T44.3X3	T44.3X4	T44.3X5	T44.3X6
Tilactase	T47.5X1	T47.5X2	T47.5X3	T47.5X4	T47.5X5	T47.5X6
Tiletamine	T41.291	T41.292	T41.293	T41.294	T41.295	T41.296
Tilidine	T40.491	T40.492	T40.493	T40.494	—	—
Timepidium bromide	T44.3X1	T44.3X2	T44.3X3	T44.3X4	T44.3X5	T44.3X6
Timiperone	T43.4X1	T43.4X2	T43.4X3	T43.4X4	T43.4X5	T43.4X6
Timolol	T44.7X1	T44.7X2	T44.7X3	T44.7X4	T44.7X5	T44.7X6
Tincture, iodine — *see* Iodine						
Tindal	T43.3X1	T43.3X2	T43.3X3	T43.3X4	T43.3X5	T43.3X6
Tinidazole	T37.3X1	T37.3X2	T37.3X3	T37.3X4	T37.3X5	T37.3X6
Tin (chloride) (dust) (oxide) **NEC**	T56.6X1	T56.6X2	T56.6X3	T56.6X4	—	—
anti-infectives	T37.8X1	T37.8X2	T37.8X3	T37.8X4	T37.8X5	T37.8X6
Tinoridine	T39.8X1	T39.8X2	T39.8X3	T39.8X4	T39.8X5	T39.8X6
Tiocarlide	T37.1X1	T37.1X2	T37.1X3	T37.1X4	T37.1X5	T37.1X6
Tioclomarol	T45.511	T45.512	T45.513	T45.514	T45.515	T45.516
Tioconazole	T49.0X1	T49.0X2	T49.0X3	T49.0X4	T49.0X5	T49.0X6
Tioguanine	T45.1X1	T45.1X2	T45.1X3	T45.1X4	T45.1X5	T45.1X6
Tiopronin	T50.991	T50.992	T50.993	T50.994	T50.995	T50.996
Tiotixene	T43.4X1	T43.4X2	T43.4X3	T43.4X4	T43.4X5	T43.4X6
Tioxolone	T49.4X1	T49.4X2	T49.4X3	T49.4X4	T49.4X5	T49.4X6
Tipepidine	T48.3X1	T48.3X2	T48.3X3	T48.3X4	T48.3X5	T48.3X6
Tiquizium bromide	T44.3X1	T44.3X2	T44.3X3	T44.3X4	T44.3X5	T44.3X6
Tiratricol	T38.1X1	T38.1X2	T38.1X3	T38.1X4	T38.1X5	T38.1X6
Tisopurine	T50.4X1	T50.4X2	T50.4X3	T50.4X4	T50.4X5	T50.4X6
Titanium (compounds) (vapor)	T56.891	T56.892	T56.893	T56.894	—	—
dioxide	T49.3X1	T49.3X2	T49.3X3	T49.3X4	T49.3X5	T49.3X6
ointment	T49.3X1	T49.3X2	T49.3X3	T49.3X4	T49.3X5	T49.3X6

Substance	Poisoning, Accidental (unintentional)	Poisoning, Intentional Self-harm	Poisoning, Assault	Poisoning, Undetermined	Adverse Effect	Under-dosing
Titanium — *continued*						
oxide	T49.3X1	T49.3X2	T49.3X3	T49.3X4	T49.3X5	T49.3X6
tetrachloride	T56.891	T56.892	T56.893	T56.894	—	—
Titanocene	T56.891	T56.892	T56.893	T56.894	—	—
Titroid	T38.1X1	T38.1X2	T38.1X3	T38.1X4	T38.1X5	T38.1X6
Tizanidine	T42.8X1	T42.8X2	T42.8X3	T42.8X4	T42.8X5	T42.8X6
TMTD	T60.3X1	T60.3X2	T60.3X3	T60.3X4	—	—
TNT (fumes)	T65.3X1	T65.3X2	T65.3X3	T65.3X4	—	—
Toadstool	T62.0X1	T62.0X2	T62.0X3	T62.0X4	—	—
Tobacco NEC	T65.291	T65.292	T65.293	T65.294	—	—
cigarettes	T65.221	T65.222	T65.223	T65.224	—	—
Indian	T62.2X1	T62.2X2	T62.2X3	T62.2X4	—	—
smoke, second-hand	T65.221	T65.222	T65.223	T65.224	—	—
Tobraflex*	T49.5X1	T49.5X2	T49.5X3	T49.5X4	T49.5X5	T49.5X6
Tobramycin	T36.5X1	T36.5X2	T36.5X3	T36.5X4	T36.5X5	T36.5X6
Tocainide	T46.2X1	T46.2X2	T46.2X3	T46.2X4	T46.2X5	T46.2X6
Tocoferol	T45.2X1	T45.2X2	T45.2X3	T45.2X4	T45.2X5	T45.2X6
Tocopherol	T45.2X1	T45.2X2	T45.2X3	T45.2X4	T45.2X5	T45.2X6
acetate	T45.2X1	T45.2X2	T45.2X3	T45.2X4	T45.2X5	T45.2X6
Tocosamine	T48.0X1	T48.0X2	T48.0X3	T48.0X4	T48.0X5	T48.0X6
Todralazine	T46.5X1	T46.5X2	T46.5X3	T46.5X4	T46.5X5	T46.5X6
Tofisopam	T42.4X1	T42.4X2	T42.4X3	T42.4X4	T42.4X5	T42.4X6
Tofranil	T43.011	T43.012	T43.013	T43.014	T43.015	T43.016
Toilet deodorizer	T65.891	T65.892	T65.893	T65.894	—	—
Tolamolol	T44.7X1	T44.7X2	T44.7X3	T44.7X4	T44.7X5	T44.7X6
Tolazamide	T38.3X1	T38.3X2	T38.3X3	T38.3X4	T38.3X5	T38.3X6
Tolazoline	T46.7X1	T46.7X2	T46.7X3	T46.7X4	T46.7X5	T46.7X6
Tolbutamide (sodium)	T38.3X1	T38.3X2	T38.3X3	T38.3X4	T38.3X5	T38.3X6
Tolciclate	T49.0X1	T49.0X2	T49.0X3	T49.0X4	T49.0X5	T49.0X6
Tolmetin	T39.391	T39.392	T39.393	T39.394	T39.395	T39.396
Tolnaftate	T49.0X1	T49.0X2	T49.0X3	T49.0X4	T49.0X5	T49.0X6
Tolonidine	T46.5X1	T46.5X2	T46.5X3	T46.5X4	T46.5X5	T46.5X6
Toloxatone	T42.6X1	T42.6X2	T42.6X3	T42.6X4	T42.6X5	T42.6X6
Tolperisone	T44.3X1	T44.3X2	T44.3X3	T44.3X4	T44.3X5	T44.3X6
Tolserol	T42.8X1	T42.8X2	T42.8X3	T42.8X4	T42.8X5	T42.8X6
Toluene (liquid)	T52.2X1	T52.2X2	T52.2X3	T52.2X4	—	—
diisocyanate	T65.0X1	T65.0X2	T65.0X3	T65.0X4	—	—
Toluidine	T65.891	T65.892	T65.893	T65.894	—	—
vapor	T59.891	T59.892	T59.893	T59.894	—	—
Toluol (liquid)	T52.2X1	T52.2X2	T52.2X3	T52.2X4	—	—
vapor	T52.2X1	T52.2X2	T52.2X3	T52.2X4	—	—
Toluylenediamine	T65.3X1	T65.3X2	T65.3X3	T65.3X4	—	—
Tolylene-2,4-diisocyanate	T65.0X1	T65.0X2	T65.0X3	T65.0X4	—	—
Tonic NEC	T50.901	T50.902	T50.903	T50.904	T50.905	T50.906
Topical action drug NEC	T49.91	T49.92	T49.93	T49.94	T49.95	T49.96
ear, nose or throat	T49.6X1	T49.6X2	T49.6X3	T49.6X4	T49.6X5	T49.6X6
eye	T49.5X1	T49.5X2	T49.5X3	T49.5X4	T49.5X5	T49.5X6
skin	T49.91	T49.92	T49.93	T49.94	T49.95	T49.96
specified NEC	T49.8X1	T49.8X2	T49.8X3	T49.8X4	T49.8X5	T49.8X6
Toprol*	T44.7X1	T44.7X2	T44.7X3	T44.7X4	T44.7X5	T44.7X6
Toquizine	T44.3X1	T44.3X2	T44.3X3	T44.3X4	T44.3X5	T44.3X6
Toremifene	T38.6X1	T38.6X2	T38.6X3	T38.6X4	T38.6X5	T38.6X6
Tosylchloramide sodium	T49.8X1	T49.8X2	T49.8X3	T49.8X4	T49.8X5	T49.8X6
Toxaphene (dust) (spray)	T60.1X1	T60.1X2	T60.1X3	T60.1X4	—	—
Toxin, diphtheria (Schick Test)	T50.8X1	T50.8X2	T50.8X3	T50.8X4	T50.8X5	T50.8X6
Toxoid						
combined	T50.A21	T50.A22	T50.A23	T50.A24	T50.A25	T50.A26
diphtheria	T50.A91	T50.A92	T50.A93	T50.A94	T50.A95	T50.A96
tetanus	T50.A91	T50.A92	T50.A93	T50.A94	T50.A95	T50.A96
Trace element NEC	T45.8X1	T45.8X2	T45.8X3	T45.8X4	T45.8X5	T45.8X6
Tractor fuel NEC	T52.0X1	T52.0X2	T52.0X3	T52.0X4	—	—
Tragacanth	T50.991	T50.992	T50.993	T50.994	T50.995	T50.996
Tramadol	T40.421	T40.422	T40.423	T40.424	T40.425	T40.426
Tramazoline	T48.5X1	T48.5X2	T48.5X3	T48.5X4	T48.5X5	T48.5X6
Tranexamic acid	T45.621	T45.622	T45.623	T45.624	T45.625	T45.626
Tranilast	T45.0X1	T45.0X2	T45.0X3	T45.0X4	T45.0X5	T45.0X6
Tranquilizer NEC	T43.501	T43.502	T43.503	T43.504	T43.505	T43.506
with hypnotic or sedative	T42.6X1	T42.6X2	T42.6X3	T42.6X4	T42.6X5	T42.6X6
benzodiazepine NEC	T42.4X1	T42.4X2	T42.4X3	T42.4X4	T42.4X5	T42.4X6
butyrophenone NEC	T43.4X1	T43.4X2	T43.4X3	T43.4X4	T43.4X5	T43.4X6
carbamate	T43.591	T43.592	T43.593	T43.594	T43.595	T43.596
dimethylamine	T43.3X1	T43.3X2	T43.3X3	T43.3X4	T43.3X5	T43.3X6
ethylamine	T43.3X1	T43.3X2	T43.3X3	T43.3X4	T43.3X5	T43.3X6
hydroxyzine	T43.591	T43.592	T43.593	T43.594	T43.595	T43.596
major NEC	T43.501	T43.502	T43.503	T43.504	T43.505	T43.506
penothiazine NEC	T43.3X1	T43.3X2	T43.3X3	T43.3X4	T43.3X5	T43.3X6
phenothiazine-based	T43.3X1	T43.3X2	T43.3X3	T43.3X4	T43.3X5	T43.3X6
piperazine NEC	T43.3X1	T43.3X2	T43.3X3	T43.3X4	T43.3X5	T43.3X6
piperidine	T43.3X1	T43.3X2	T43.3X3	T43.3X4	T43.3X5	T43.3X6
propylamine	T43.3X1	T43.3X2	T43.3X3	T43.3X4	T43.3X5	T43.3X6
specified NEC	T43.591	T43.592	T43.593	T43.594	T43.595	T43.596
thioxanthene NEC	T43.591	T43.592	T43.593	T43.594	T43.595	T43.596

Substance	Poisoning, Accidental (unintentional)	Poisoning, Intentional Self-harm	Poisoning, Assault	Poisoning, Undetermined	Adverse Effect	Under-dosing
Tranxene	T42.4X1	T42.4X2	T42.4X3	T42.4X4	T42.4X5	T42.4X6
Tranylcypromine	T43.1X1	T43.1X2	T43.1X3	T43.1X4	T43.1X5	T43.1X6
Trapidil	T46.3X1	T46.3X2	T46.3X3	T46.3X4	T46.3X5	T46.3X6
Trasentine	T44.3X1	T44.3X2	T44.3X3	T44.3X4	T44.3X5	T44.3X6
Travert	T50.3X1	T50.3X2	T50.3X3	T50.3X4	T50.3X5	T50.3X6
Trazodone	T43.211	T43.212	T43.213	T43.214	T43.215	T43.216
Treanda*	T45.1X1	T45.1X2	T45.1X3	T45.1X4	T45.1X5	T45.1X6
Trecator	T37.1X1	T37.1X2	T37.1X3	T37.1X4	T37.1X5	T37.1X6
Treosulfan	T45.1X1	T45.1X2	T45.1X3	T45.1X4	T45.1X5	T45.1X6
Tretamine	T45.1X1	T45.1X2	T45.1X3	T45.1X4	T45.1X5	T45.1X6
Tretinoin	T49.0X1	T49.0X2	T49.0X3	T49.0X4	T49.0X5	T49.0X6
Tretoquinol	T48.6X1	T48.6X2	T48.6X3	T48.6X4	T48.6X5	T48.6X6
Triacetin	T49.0X1	T49.0X2	T49.0X3	T49.0X4	T49.0X5	T49.0X6
Triacetoxyanthracene	T49.4X1	T49.4X2	T49.4X3	T49.4X4	T49.4X5	T49.4X6
Triacetyloleandomycin	T36.3X1	T36.3X2	T36.3X3	T36.3X4	T36.3X5	T36.3X6
Triamcinolone	T38.0X1	T38.0X2	T38.0X3	T38.0X4	T38.0X5	T38.0X6
ENT agent	T49.6X1	T49.6X2	T49.6X3	T49.6X4	T49.6X5	T49.6X6
hexacetonide	T49.0X1	T49.0X2	T49.0X3	T49.0X4	T49.0X5	T49.0X6
ophthalmic preparation	T49.5X1	T49.5X2	T49.5X3	T49.5X4	T49.5X5	T49.5X6
topical NEC	T49.0X1	T49.0X2	T49.0X3	T49.0X4	T49.0X5	T49.0X6
Triampyzine	T44.3X1	T44.3X2	T44.3X3	T44.3X4	T44.3X5	T44.3X6
Triamterene	T50.2X1	T50.2X2	T50.2X3	T50.2X4	T50.2X5	T50.2X6
Triazine (herbicide)	T60.3X1	T60.3X2	T60.3X3	T60.3X4	—	—
Triaziquone	T45.1X1	T45.1X2	T45.1X3	T45.1X4	T45.1X5	T45.1X6
Triazolam	T42.4X1	T42.4X2	T42.4X3	T42.4X4	T42.4X5	T42.4X6
Triazole (herbicide)	T60.3X1	T60.3X2	T60.3X3	T60.3X4	—	—
Tribavirin*	T37.5X1	T37.5X2	T37.5X3	T37.5X4	T37.5X5	T37.5X6
Tribenoside	T46.991	T46.992	T46.993	T46.994	T46.995	T46.996
Tribromacetaldehyde	T42.6X1	T42.6X2	T42.6X3	T42.6X4	T42.6X5	T42.6X6
Tribromoethanol, rectal	T41.291	T41.292	T41.293	T41.294	T41.295	T41.296
Tribromomethane	T42.6X1	T42.6X2	T42.6X3	T42.6X4	T42.6X5	T42.6X6
Trichlorethane	T53.2X1	T53.2X2	T53.2X3	T53.2X4	—	—
Trichlorethylene	T53.2X1	T53.2X2	T53.2X3	T53.2X4	—	—
Trichlorfon	T60.0X1	T60.0X2	T60.0X3	T60.0X4	—	—
Trichlormethiazide	T50.2X1	T50.2X2	T50.2X3	T50.2X4	T50.2X5	T50.2X6
Trichlormethine	T45.1X1	T45.1X2	T45.1X3	T45.1X4	T45.1X5	T45.1X6
Trichloroacetic acid, Trichloracetic acid	T54.2X1	T54.2X2	T54.2X3	T54.2X4	—	—
medicinal	T49.4X1	T49.4X2	T49.4X3	T49.4X4	T49.4X5	T49.4X6
Trichloroethane	T53.2X1	T53.2X2	T53.2X3	T53.2X4	—	—
Trichloroethanol	T42.6X1	T42.6X2	T42.6X3	T42.6X4	T42.6X5	T42.6X6
Trichloroethylene (liquid) (vapor)	T53.2X1	T53.2X2	T53.2X3	T53.2X4	—	—
anesthetic (gas)	T41.0X1	T41.0X2	T41.0X3	T41.0X4	T41.0X5	T41.0X6
vapor NEC	T53.2X1	T53.2X2	T53.2X3	T53.2X4	—	—
Trichloroethyl phosphate	T42.6X1	T42.6X2	T42.6X3	T42.6X4	T42.6X5	T42.6X6
Trichlorofluoromethane NEC	T53.5X1	T53.5X2	T53.5X3	T53.5X4	—	—
Trichloronate	T60.0X1	T60.0X2	T60.0X3	T60.0X4	—	—
Trichloropropane	T53.6X1	T53.6X2	T53.6X3	T53.6X4	—	—
Trichlorotriethylamine	T45.1X1	T45.1X2	T45.1X3	T45.1X4	T45.1X5	T45.1X6
Trichomonacides NEC	T37.3X1	T37.3X2	T37.3X3	T37.3X4	T37.3X5	T37.3X6
Trichomycin	T36.7X1	T36.7X2	T36.7X3	T36.7X4	T36.7X5	T36.7X6
Triclobisonium chloride	T49.0X1	T49.0X2	T49.0X3	T49.0X4	T49.0X5	T49.0X6
Triclocarban	T49.0X1	T49.0X2	T49.0X3	T49.0X4	T49.0X5	T49.0X6
Triclofos	T42.6X1	T42.6X2	T42.6X3	T42.6X4	T42.6X5	T42.6X6
Triclosan	T49.0X1	T49.0X2	T49.0X3	T49.0X4	T49.0X5	T49.0X6
Tricosal*	T39.091	T39.092	T39.093	T39.094	T39.095	T39.096
Tricresyl phosphate	T65.891	T65.892	T65.893	T65.894	—	—
solvent	T52.91	T52.92	T52.93	T52.94	—	—
Tricyclamol chloride	T44.3X1	T44.3X2	T44.3X3	T44.3X4	T44.3X5	T44.3X6
Tridesilon	T49.0X1	T49.0X2	T49.0X3	T49.0X4	T49.0X5	T49.0X6
Tridihexethyl iodide	T44.3X1	T44.3X2	T44.3X3	T44.3X4	T44.3X5	T44.3X6
Tridione	T42.2X1	T42.2X2	T42.2X3	T42.2X4	T42.2X5	T42.2X6
Trientine	T45.8X1	T45.8X2	T45.8X3	T45.8X4	T45.8X5	T45.8X6
Triethanolamine NEC	T54.3X1	T54.3X2	T54.3X3	T54.3X4	—	—
detergent	T54.3X1	T54.3X2	T54.3X3	T54.3X4	—	—
trinitrate (biphosphate)	T46.3X1	T46.3X2	T46.3X3	T46.3X4	T46.3X5	T46.3X6
Triethanomelamine	T45.1X1	T45.1X2	T45.1X3	T45.1X4	T45.1X5	T45.1X6
Triethylenemelamine	T45.1X1	T45.1X2	T45.1X3	T45.1X4	T45.1X5	T45.1X6
Triethylenephosphoramide	T45.1X1	T45.1X2	T45.1X3	T45.1X4	T45.1X5	T45.1X6
Triethylenethiophosphoramide	T45.1X1	T45.1X2	T45.1X3	T45.1X4	T45.1X5	T45.1X6
Trifluoperazine	T43.3X1	T43.3X2	T43.3X3	T43.3X4	T43.3X5	T43.3X6
Trifluoroethyl vinyl ether	T41.0X1	T41.0X2	T41.0X3	T41.0X4	T41.0X5	T41.0X6
Trifluperidol	T43.4X1	T43.4X2	T43.4X3	T43.4X4	T43.4X5	T43.4X6
Triflupromazine	T43.3X1	T43.3X2	T43.3X3	T43.3X4	T43.3X5	T43.3X6
Trifluridine	T37.5X1	T37.5X2	T37.5X3	T37.5X4	T37.5X5	T37.5X6
Triflusal	T45.521	T45.522	T45.523	T45.524	T45.525	T45.526
Trihexyphenidyl	T44.3X1	T44.3X2	T44.3X3	T44.3X4	T44.3X5	T44.3X6
Triiodothyronine	T38.1X1	T38.1X2	T38.1X3	T38.1X4	T38.1X5	T38.1X6
Trilene	T41.0X1	T41.0X2	T41.0X3	T41.0X4	T41.0X5	T41.0X6
Trilostane	T38.991	T38.992	T38.993	T38.994	T38.995	T38.996

Substance	Poisoning, Accidental (unintentional)	Poisoning, Intentional Self-harm	Poisoning, Assault	Poisoning, Undetermined	Adverse Effect	Under-dosing
Trimebutine	T44.3X1	T44.3X2	T44.3X3	T44.3X4	T44.3X5	T44.3X6
Trimecaine	T41.3X1	T41.3X2	T41.3X3	T41.3X4	T41.3X5	T41.3X6
Trimeprazine (tartrate)	T44.3X1	T44.3X2	T44.3X3	T44.3X4	T44.3X5	T44.3X6
Trimetaphan camsilate	T44.2X1	T44.2X2	T44.2X3	T44.2X4	T44.2X5	T44.2X6
Trimetazidine	T46.7X1	T46.7X2	T46.7X3	T46.7X4	T46.7X5	T46.7X6
Trimethadione	T42.2X1	T42.2X2	T42.2X3	T42.2X4	T42.2X5	T42.2X6
Trimethaphan	T44.2X1	T44.2X2	T44.2X3	T44.2X4	T44.2X5	T44.2X6
Trimethidinium	T44.2X1	T44.2X2	T44.2X3	T44.2X4	T44.2X5	T44.2X6
Trimethobenzamide	T45.ØX1	T45.ØX2	T45.ØX3	T45.ØX4	T45.ØX5	T45.ØX6
Trimethoprim	T37.8X1	T37.8X2	T37.8X3	T37.8X4	T37.8X5	T37.8X6
with sulfamethoxazole	T36.8X1	T36.8X2	T36.8X3	T36.8X4	T36.8X5	T36.8X6
Trimethylcarbinol	T51.3X1	T51.3X2	T51.3X3	T51.3X4	—	—
Trimethylpsoralen	T49.3X1	T49.3X2	T49.3X3	T49.3X4	T49.3X5	T49.3X6
Trimeton	T45.ØX1	T45.ØX2	T45.ØX3	T45.ØX4	T45.ØX5	T45.ØX6
Trimetrexate	T45.1X1	T45.1X2	T45.1X3	T45.1X4	T45.1X5	T45.1X6
Trimipramine	T43.Ø11	T43.Ø12	T43.Ø13	T43.Ø14	T43.Ø15	T43.Ø16
Trimox*	T36.ØX1	T36.ØX2	T36.ØX3	T36.ØX4	T36.ØX5	T36.ØX6
Trimustine	T45.1X1	T45.1X2	T45.1X3	T45.1X4	T45.1X5	T45.1X6
Trinitrine	T46.3X1	T46.3X2	T46.3X3	T46.3X4	T46.3X5	T46.3X6
Trinitrobenzol	T65.3X1	T65.3X2	T65.3X3	T65.3X4	—	—
Trinitrophenol	T65.3X1	T65.3X2	T65.3X3	T65.3X4	—	—
Trinitrotoluene (fumes)	T65.3X1	T65.3X2	T65.3X3	T65.3X4	—	—
Trional	T42.6X1	T42.6X2	T42.6X3	T42.6X4	T42.6X5	T42.6X6
Triorthocresyl phosphate	T65.891	T65.892	T65.893	T65.894	—	—
Trioxide of arsenic	T57.ØX1	T57.ØX2	T57.ØX3	T57.ØX4	—	—
Trioxysalen	T49.4X1	T49.4X2	T49.4X3	T49.4X4	T49.4X5	T49.4X6
Tripamide	T5Ø.2X1	T5Ø.2X2	T5Ø.2X3	T5Ø.2X4	T5Ø.2X5	T5Ø.2X6
Triparanol	T46.6X1	T46.6X2	T46.6X3	T46.6X4	T46.6X5	T46.6X6
Tripelennamine	T45.ØX1	T45.ØX2	T45.ØX3	T45.ØX4	T45.ØX5	T45.ØX6
Triperiden	T44.3X1	T44.3X2	T44.3X3	T44.3X4	T44.3X5	T44.3X6
Triperidol	T43.4X1	T43.4X2	T43.4X3	T43.4X4	T43.4X5	T43.4X6
Triphenylphosphate	T65.891	T65.892	T65.893	T65.894	—	—
Triple						
bromides	T42.6X1	T42.6X2	T42.6X3	T42.6X4	T42.6X5	T42.6X6
carbonate	T47.1X1	T47.1X2	T47.1X3	T47.1X4	T47.1X5	T47.1X6
vaccine						
DPT	T5Ø.A11	T5Ø.A12	T5Ø.A13	T5Ø.A14	T5Ø.A15	T5Ø.A16
including pertussis	T5Ø.A11	T5Ø.A12	T5Ø.A13	T5Ø.A14	T5Ø.A15	T5Ø.A16
MMR	T5Ø.B91	T5Ø.B92	T5Ø.B93	T5Ø.B94	T5Ø.B95	T5Ø.B96
Triprolidine	T45.ØX1	T45.ØX2	T45.ØX3	T45.ØX4	T45.ØX5	T45.ØX6
Trisodium hydrogen edetate	T5Ø.6X1	T5Ø.6X2	T5Ø.6X3	T5Ø.6X4	T5Ø.6X5	T5Ø.6X6
Trisoralen	T49.3X1	T49.3X2	T49.3X3	T49.3X4	T49.3X5	T49.3X6
Trisulfapyrimidines	T37.ØX1	T37.ØX2	T37.ØX3	T37.ØX4	T37.ØX5	T37.ØX6
Trithiozine	T44.3X1	T44.3X2	T44.3X3	T44.3X4	T44.3X5	T44.3X6
Tritiozine	T44.3X1	T44.3X2	T44.3X3	T44.3X4	T44.3X5	T44.3X6
Tritoqualine	T45.ØX1	T45.ØX2	T45.ØX3	T45.ØX4	T45.ØX5	T45.ØX6
Trizivir*	T37.5X1	T37.5X2	T37.5X3	T37.5X4	T37.5X5	T37.5X6
Trofosfamide	T45.1X1	T45.1X2	T45.1X3	T45.1X4	T45.1X5	T45.1X6
Troleandomycin	T36.3X1	T36.3X2	T36.3X3	T36.3X4	T36.3X5	T36.3X6
Trolnitrate (phosphate)	T46.3X1	T46.3X2	T46.3X3	T46.3X4	T46.3X5	T46.3X6
Tromantadine	T37.5X1	T37.5X2	T37.5X3	T37.5X4	T37.5X5	T37.5X6
Trometamol	T5Ø.2X1	T5Ø.2X2	T5Ø.2X3	T5Ø.2X4	T5Ø.2X5	T5Ø.2X6
Tromethamine	T5Ø.2X1	T5Ø.2X2	T5Ø.2X3	T5Ø.2X4	T5Ø.2X5	T5Ø.2X6
Tronothane	T41.3X1	T41.3X2	T41.3X3	T41.3X4	T41.3X5	T41.3X6
Tropacine	T44.3X1	T44.3X2	T44.3X3	T44.3X4	T44.3X5	T44.3X6
Tropatepine	T44.3X1	T44.3X2	T44.3X3	T44.3X4	T44.3X5	T44.3X6
Tropicamide	T44.3X1	T44.3X2	T44.3X3	T44.3X4	T44.3X5	T44.3X6
Trospium chloride	T44.3X1	T44.3X2	T44.3X3	T44.3X4	T44.3X5	T44.3X6
Troxerutin	T46.991	T46.992	T46.993	T46.994	T46.995	T46.996
Troxidone	T42.2X1	T42.2X2	T42.2X3	T42.2X4	T42.2X5	T42.2X6
Tryparsamide	T37.3X1	T37.3X2	T37.3X3	T37.3X4	T37.3X5	T37.3X6
Trypsin	T45.3X1	T45.3X2	T45.3X3	T45.3X4	T45.3X5	T45.3X6
Tryptizol	T43.Ø11	T43.Ø12	T43.Ø13	T43.Ø14	T43.Ø15	T43.Ø16
TSH	T38.811	T38.812	T38.813	T38.814	T38.815	T38.816
Tuaminoheptane	T48.5X1	T48.5X2	T48.5X3	T48.5X4	T48.5X5	T48.5X6
Tuberculin, purified protein derivative (PPD)	T5Ø.8X1	T5Ø.8X2	T5Ø.8X3	T5Ø.8X4	T5Ø.8X5	T5Ø.8X6
Tubocurare	T48.1X1	T48.1X2	T48.1X3	T48.1X4	T48.1X5	T48.1X6
Tubocurarine (chloride)	T48.1X1	T48.1X2	T48.1X3	T48.1X4	T48.1X5	T48.1X6
Tulobuterol	T48.6X1	T48.6X2	T48.6X3	T48.6X4	T48.6X5	T48.6X6
Turpentine (spirits of)	T52.8X1	T52.8X2	T52.8X3	T52.8X4	—	—
vapor	T52.8X1	T52.8X2	T52.8X3	T52.8X4	—	—
Twinrix*	T5Ø.B91	T5Ø.B92	T5Ø.B93	T5Ø.B94	T5Ø.B95	T5Ø.B96
Tybamate	T43.591	T43.592	T43.593	T43.594	T43.595	T43.596
Tygacil*	T36.4X1	T36.4X2	T36.4X3	T36.4X4	T36.4X5	T36.4X6
Tyloxapol	T48.4X1	T48.4X2	T48.4X3	T48.4X4	T48.4X5	T48.4X6
Tymazoline	T48.5X1	T48.5X2	T48.5X3	T48.5X4	T48.5X5	T48.5X6
Tymlos*	T5Ø.991	T5Ø.992	T5Ø.993	T5Ø.994	T5Ø.995	T5Ø.996
Typhoid-paratyphoid vaccine	T5Ø.A91	T5Ø.A92	T5Ø.A93	T5Ø.A94	T5Ø.A95	T5Ø.A96
Typhus vaccine	T5Ø.A91	T5Ø.A92	T5Ø.A93	T5Ø.A94	T5Ø.A95	T5Ø.A96
Tyropanoate	T5Ø.8X1	T5Ø.8X2	T5Ø.8X3	T5Ø.8X4	T5Ø.8X5	T5Ø.8X6

Substance	Poisoning, Accidental (unintentional)	Poisoning, Intentional Self-harm	Poisoning, Assault	Poisoning, Undetermined	Adverse Effect	Under-dosing
Tyrothricin	T49.6X1	T49.6X2	T49.6X3	T49.6X4	T49.6X5	T49.6X6
ENT agent	T49.6X1	T49.6X2	T49.6X3	T49.6X4	T49.6X5	T49.6X6
ophthalmic preparation	T49.5X1	T49.5X2	T49.5X3	T49.5X4	T49.5X5	T49.5X6
Ufenamate	T39.391	T39.392	T39.393	T39.394	T39.395	T39.396
Ultraviolet light protectant	T49.3X1	T49.3X2	T49.3X3	T49.3X4	T49.3X5	T49.3X6
Unasyn*	T36.ØX1	T36.ØX2	T36.ØX3	T36.ØX4	T36.ØX5	T36.ØX6
Undecenoic acid	T49.ØX1	T49.ØX2	T49.ØX3	T49.ØX4	T49.ØX5	T49.ØX6
Undecoylium	T49.ØX1	T49.ØX2	T49.ØX3	T49.ØX4	T49.ØX5	T49.ØX6
Undecylenic acid (derivatives)	T49.ØX1	T49.ØX2	T49.ØX3	T49.ØX4	T49.ØX5	T49.ØX6
Unna's boot	T49.3X1	T49.3X2	T49.3X3	T49.3X4	T49.3X5	T49.3X6
Unsaturated fatty acid	T46.6X1	T46.6X2	T46.6X3	T46.6X4	T46.6X5	T46.6X6
Uracil mustard	T45.1X1	T45.1X2	T45.1X3	T45.1X4	T45.1X5	T45.1X6
Uramustine	T45.1X1	T45.1X2	T45.1X3	T45.1X4	T45.1X5	T45.1X6
Urapidil	T46.5X1	T46.5X2	T46.5X3	T46.5X4	T46.5X5	T46.5X6
Urari	T48.1X1	T48.1X2	T48.1X3	T48.1X4	T48.1X5	T48.1X6
Urate oxidase	T5Ø.4X1	T5Ø.4X2	T5Ø.4X3	T5Ø.4X4	T5Ø.4X5	T5Ø.4X6
Urea	T47.3X1	T47.3X2	T47.3X3	T47.3X4	T47.3X5	T47.3X6
peroxide	T49.ØX1	T49.ØX2	T49.ØX3	T49.ØX4	T49.ØX5	T49.ØX6
stibamine	T37.4X1	T37.4X2	T37.4X3	T37.4X4	T37.4X5	T37.4X6
topical	T49.8X1	T49.8X2	T49.8X3	T49.8X4	T49.8X5	T49.8X6
Ureaphil*	T48.ØX1	T48.ØX2	T48.ØX3	T48.ØX4	T48.ØX5	T48.ØX6
Urethane	T45.1X1	T45.1X2	T45.1X3	T45.1X4	T45.1X5	T45.1X6
Urginea (maritima) (scilla) — *see* Squill						
Uric acid metabolism drug NEC	T5Ø.4X1	T5Ø.4X2	T5Ø.4X3	T5Ø.4X4	T5Ø.4X5	T5Ø.4X6
Uricosuric agent	T5Ø.4X1	T5Ø.4X2	T5Ø.4X3	T5Ø.4X4	T5Ø.4X5	T5Ø.4X6
Urinary anti-infective	T37.8X1	T37.8X2	T37.8X3	T37.8X4	T37.8X5	T37.8X6
Urofollitropin	T38.811	T38.812	T38.813	T38.814	T38.815	T38.816
Urokinase	T45.611	T45.612	T45.613	T45.614	T45.615	T45.616
Urokon	T5Ø.8X1	T5Ø.8X2	T5Ø.8X3	T5Ø.8X4	T5Ø.8X5	T5Ø.8X6
Ursodeoxycholic acid	T5Ø.991	T5Ø.992	T5Ø.993	T5Ø.994	T5Ø.995	T5Ø.996
Ursodiol	T5Ø.991	T5Ø.992	T5Ø.993	T5Ø.994	T5Ø.995	T5Ø.996
Urtica	T62.2X1	T62.2X2	T62.2X3	T62.2X4	—	—
Utility gas — *see* Gas, utility						
Vaccine NEC	T5Ø.Z91	T5Ø.Z92	T5Ø.Z93	T5Ø.Z94	T5Ø.Z95	T5Ø.Z96
antineoplastic	T5Ø.Z91	T5Ø.Z92	T5Ø.Z93	T5Ø.Z94	T5Ø.Z95	T5Ø.Z96
bacterial NEC	T5Ø.A91	T5Ø.A92	T5Ø.A93	T5Ø.A94	T5Ø.A95	T5Ø.A96
with						
other bacterial component	T5Ø.A21	T5Ø.A22	T5Ø.A23	T5Ø.A24	T5Ø.A25	T5Ø.A26
pertussis component	T5Ø.A11	T5Ø.A12	T5Ø.A13	T5Ø.A14	T5Ø.A15	T5Ø.A16
viral-rickettsial component	T5Ø.A21	T5Ø.A22	T5Ø.A23	T5Ø.A24	T5Ø.A25	T5Ø.A26
mixed NEC	T5Ø.A21	T5Ø.A22	T5Ø.A23	T5Ø.A24	T5Ø.A25	T5Ø.A26
BCG	T5Ø.A91	T5Ø.A92	T5Ø.A93	T5Ø.A94	T5Ø.A95	T5Ø.A96
cholera	T5Ø.A91	T5Ø.A92	T5Ø.A93	T5Ø.A94	T5Ø.A95	T5Ø.A96
diphtheria	T5Ø.A91	T5Ø.A92	T5Ø.A93	T5Ø.A94	T5Ø.A95	T5Ø.A96
with tetanus	T5Ø.A21	T5Ø.A22	T5Ø.A23	T5Ø.A24	T5Ø.A25	T5Ø.A26
and pertussis	T5Ø.A11	T5Ø.A12	T5Ø.A13	T5Ø.A14	T5Ø.A15	T5Ø.A16
influenza	T5Ø.B91	T5Ø.B92	T5Ø.B93	T5Ø.B94	T5Ø.B95	T5Ø.B96
measles	T5Ø.B91	T5Ø.B92	T5Ø.B93	T5Ø.B94	T5Ø.B95	T5Ø.B96
with mumps and rubella	T5Ø.B91	T5Ø.B92	T5Ø.B93	T5Ø.B94	T5Ø.B95	T5Ø.B96
meningococcal	T5Ø.A91	T5Ø.A92	T5Ø.A93	T5Ø.A94	T5Ø.A95	T5Ø.A96
mumps	T5Ø.B91	T5Ø.B92	T5Ø.B93	T5Ø.B94	T5Ø.B95	T5Ø.B96
paratyphoid	T5Ø.A91	T5Ø.A92	T5Ø.A93	T5Ø.A94	T5Ø.A95	T5Ø.A96
pertussis	T5Ø.A11	T5Ø.A12	T5Ø.A13	T5Ø.A14	T5Ø.A15	T5Ø.A16
with diphtheria	T5Ø.A11	T5Ø.A12	T5Ø.A13	T5Ø.A14	T5Ø.A15	T5Ø.A16
and tetanus	T5Ø.A11	T5Ø.A12	T5Ø.A13	T5Ø.A14	T5Ø.A15	T5Ø.A16
with other component	T5Ø.A11	T5Ø.A12	T5Ø.A13	T5Ø.A14	T5Ø.A15	T5Ø.A16
plague	T5Ø.A91	T5Ø.A92	T5Ø.A93	T5Ø.A94	T5Ø.A95	T5Ø.A96
poliomyelitis	T5Ø.B91	T5Ø.B92	T5Ø.B93	T5Ø.B94	T5Ø.B95	T5Ø.B96
poliovirus	T5Ø.B91	T5Ø.B92	T5Ø.B93	T5Ø.B94	T5Ø.B95	T5Ø.B96
rabies	T5Ø.B91	T5Ø.B92	T5Ø.B93	T5Ø.B94	T5Ø.B95	T5Ø.B96
respiratory syncytial virus	T5Ø.B91	T5Ø.B92	T5Ø.B93	T5Ø.B94	T5Ø.B95	T5Ø.B96
rickettsial NEC	T5Ø.A91	T5Ø.A92	T5Ø.A93	T5Ø.A94	T5Ø.A95	T5Ø.A96
with						
bacterial component	T5Ø.A21	T5Ø.A22	T5Ø.A23	T5Ø.A24	T5Ø.A25	T5Ø.A26
Rocky Mountain spotted fever	T5Ø.A91	T5Ø.A92	T5Ø.A93	T5Ø.A94	T5Ø.A95	T5Ø.A96
rubella	T5Ø.B91	T5Ø.B92	T5Ø.B93	T5Ø.B94	T5Ø.B95	T5Ø.B96
sabin oral	T5Ø.B91	T5Ø.B92	T5Ø.B93	T5Ø.B94	T5Ø.B95	T5Ø.B96
smallpox	T5Ø.B11	T5Ø.B12	T5Ø.B13	T5Ø.B14	T5Ø.B15	T5Ø.B16
TAB	T5Ø.A91	T5Ø.A92	T5Ø.A93	T5Ø.A94	T5Ø.A95	T5Ø.A96
tetanus	T5Ø.A91	T5Ø.A92	T5Ø.A93	T5Ø.A94	T5Ø.A95	T5Ø.A96
typhoid	T5Ø.A91	T5Ø.A92	T5Ø.A93	T5Ø.A94	T5Ø.A95	T5Ø.A96
typhus	T5Ø.A91	T5Ø.A92	T5Ø.A93	T5Ø.A94	T5Ø.A95	T5Ø.A96
viral NEC	T5Ø.B91	T5Ø.B92	T5Ø.B93	T5Ø.B94	T5Ø.B95	T5Ø.B96
yellow fever	T5Ø.B91	T5Ø.B92	T5Ø.B93	T5Ø.B94	T5Ø.B95	T5Ø.B96
Vaccinia immune globulin	T5Ø.Z11	T5Ø.Z12	T5Ø.Z13	T5Ø.Z14	T5Ø.Z15	T5Ø.Z16
Vaginal contraceptives	T49.8X1	T49.8X2	T49.8X3	T49.8X4	T49.8X5	T49.8X6

*Optum Value-Add

Substance	Poisoning, Accidental (unintentional)	Poisoning, Intentional Self-harm	Poisoning, Assault	Poisoning, Undetermined	Adverse Effect	Under-dosing
Valacyclovir*	T37.5X1	T37.5X2	T37.5X3	T37.5X4	T37.5X5	T37.5X6
Valerian						
root	T42.6X1	T42.6X2	T42.6X3	T42.6X4	T42.6X5	T42.6X6
tincture	T42.6X1	T42.6X2	T42.6X3	T42.6X4	T42.6X5	T42.6X6
Valethamate bromide	T44.3X1	T44.3X2	T44.3X3	T44.3X4	T44.3X5	T44.3X6
Valisone	T49.ØX1	T49.ØX2	T49.ØX3	T49.ØX4	T49.ØX5	T49.ØX6
Valium	T42.4X1	T42.4X2	T42.4X3	T42.4X4	T42.4X5	T42.4X6
Valmid	T42.6X1	T42.6X2	T42.6X3	T42.6X4	T42.6X5	T42.6X6
Valnoctamide	T42.6X1	T42.6X2	T42.6X3	T42.6X4	T42.6X5	T42.6X6
Valproate (sodium)	T42.6X1	T42.6X2	T42.6X3	T42.6X4	T42.6X5	T42.6X6
Valproic acid	T42.6X1	T42.6X2	T42.6X3	T42.6X4	T42.6X5	T42.6X6
Valpromide	T42.6X1	T42.6X2	T42.6X3	T42.6X4	T42.6X5	T42.6X6
Vanadium	T56.891	T56.892	T56.893	T56.894	—	—
Vancomycin	T36.8X1	T36.8X2	T36.8X3	T36.8X4	T36.8X5	T36.8X6
Vandazole*	T49.ØX1	T49.ØX2	T49.ØX3	T49.ØX4	T49.ØX5	T49.ØX6
Vapor — *see also* Gas	T59.91	T59.92	T59.93	T59.94	—	—
kiln (carbon monoxide)	T58.8X1	T58.8X2	T58.8X3	T58.8X4	—	—
lead — *see* lead						
specified source NEC	T59.891	T59.892	T59.893	T59.894	—	—
Vardenafil	T46.7X1	T46.7X2	T46.7X3	T46.7X4	T46.7X5	T46.7X6
Varicose reduction drug	T46.8X1	T46.8X2	T46.8X3	T46.8X4	T46.8X5	T46.8X6
Varnish	T65.4X1	T65.4X2	T65.4X3	T65.4X4	—	—
cleaner	T52.91	T52.92	T52.93	T52.94	—	—
Vaseline	T49.3X1	T49.3X2	T49.3X3	T49.3X4	T49.3X5	T49.3X6
Vasodilan	T46.7X1	T46.7X2	T46.7X3	T46.7X4	T46.7X5	T46.7X6
Vasodilator						
coronary NEC	T46.3X1	T46.3X2	T46.3X3	T46.3X4	T46.3X5	T46.3X6
peripheral NEC	T46.7X1	T46.7X2	T46.7X3	T46.7X4	T46.7X5	T46.7X6
Vasopressin	T38.891	T38.892	T38.893	T38.894	T38.895	T38.896
Vasopressor drugs	T38.891	T38.892	T38.893	T38.894	T38.895	T38.896
Vecuronium bromide	T48.1X1	T48.1X2	T48.1X3	T48.1X4	T48.1X5	T48.1X6
Vegetable extract, astringent	T49.2X1	T49.2X2	T49.2X3	T49.2X4	T49.2X5	T49.2X6
Venlafaxine	T43.211	T43.212	T43.213	T43.214	T43.215	T43.216
Venom, venomous (bite) (sting)	T63.91	T63.92	T63.93	T63.94	—	—
amphibian NEC	T63.831	T63.832	T63.833	T63.834	—	—
animal NEC	T63.891	T63.892	T63.893	T63.894	—	—
ant	T63.421	T63.422	T63.423	T63.424	—	—
arthropod NEC	T63.481	T63.482	T63.483	T63.484	—	—
bee	T63.441	T63.442	T63.443	T63.444	—	—
centipede	T63.411	T63.412	T63.413	T63.414	—	—
fish	T63.591	T63.592	T63.593	T63.594	—	—
frog	T63.811	T63.812	T63.813	T63.814	—	—
hornet	T63.451	T63.452	T63.453	T63.454	—	—
insect NEC	T63.481	T63.482	T63.483	T63.484	—	—
lizard	T63.121	T63.122	T63.123	T63.124	—	—
marine						
animals	T63.691	T63.692	T63.693	T63.694	—	—
bluebottle	T63.611	T63.612	T63.613	T63.614	—	—
jellyfish NEC	T63.621	T63.622	T63.623	T63.624	—	—
Portuguese Man-o-war	T63.611	T63.612	T63.613	T63.614	—	—
sea anemone	T63.631	T63.632	T63.633	T63.634	—	—
specified NEC	T63.691	T63.692	T63.693	T63.694	—	—
fish	T63.591	T63.592	T63.593	T63.594	—	—
plants	T63.711	T63.712	T63.713	T63.714	—	—
sting ray	T63.511	T63.512	T63.513	T63.514	—	—
millipede (tropical)	T63.411	T63.412	T63.413	T63.414	—	—
plant NEC	T63.791	T63.792	T63.793	T63.794	—	—
marine	T63.711	T63.712	T63.713	T63.714	—	—
reptile	T63.191	T63.192	T63.193	T63.194	—	—
gila monster	T63.111	T63.112	T63.113	T63.114	—	—
lizard NEC	T63.121	T63.122	T63.123	T63.124	—	—
scorpion	T63.2X1	T63.2X2	T63.2X3	T63.2X4	—	—
snake	T63.ØØ1	T63.ØØ2	T63.ØØ3	T63.ØØ4	—	—
African NEC	T63.Ø81	T63.Ø82	T63.Ø83	T63.Ø84	—	—
American (North) (South) NEC	T63.Ø61	T63.Ø62	T63.Ø63	T63.Ø64	—	—
Asian	T63.Ø81	T63.Ø82	T63.Ø83	T63.Ø84	—	—
Australian	T63.Ø71	T63.Ø72	T63.Ø73	T63.Ø74	—	—
cobra	T63.Ø41	T63.Ø42	T63.Ø43	T63.Ø44	—	—
coral snake	T63.Ø21	T63.Ø22	T63.Ø23	T63.Ø24	—	—
rattlesnake	T63.Ø11	T63.Ø12	T63.Ø13	T63.Ø14	—	—
specified NEC	T63.Ø91	T63.Ø92	T63.Ø93	T63.Ø94	—	—
taipan	T63.Ø31	T63.Ø32	T63.Ø33	T63.Ø34	—	—
specified NEC	T63.891	T63.892	T63.893	T63.894	—	—
spider	T63.3Ø1	T63.3Ø2	T63.3Ø3	T63.3Ø4	—	—
black widow	T63.311	T63.312	T63.313	T63.314	—	—
brown recluse	T63.331	T63.332	T63.333	T63.334	—	—
specified NEC	T63.391	T63.392	T63.393	T63.394	—	—
tarantula	T63.321	T63.322	T63.323	T63.324	—	—
sting ray	T63.511	T63.512	T63.513	T63.514	—	—
toad	T63.821	T63.822	T63.823	T63.824	—	—

Substance	Poisoning, Accidental (unintentional)	Poisoning, Intentional Self-harm	Poisoning, Assault	Poisoning, Undetermined	Adverse Effect	Under-dosing
Venom, venomous — *continued*						
wasp	T63.461	T63.462	T63.463	T63.464	—	—
Venous sclerosing drug NEC	T46.8X1	T46.8X2	T46.8X3	T46.8X4	T46.8X5	T46.8X6
Ventavis*	T46.7X1	T46.7X2	T46.7X3	T46.7X4	T46.7X5	T46.7X6
Ventolin — *see* Albuterol						
Veramon	T42.3X1	T42.3X2	T42.3X3	T42.3X4	T42.3X5	T42.3X6
Verapamil	T46.1X1	T46.1X2	T46.1X3	T46.1X4	T46.1X5	T46.1X6
Veratrine	T46.5X1	T46.5X2	T46.5X3	T46.5X4	T46.5X5	T46.5X6
Veratrum						
album	T62.2X1	T62.2X2	T62.2X3	T62.2X4	—	—
alkaloids	T46.5X1	T46.5X2	T46.5X3	T46.5X4	T46.5X5	T46.5X6
viride	T62.2X1	T62.2X2	T62.2X3	T62.2X4	—	—
Verdigris	T6Ø.3X1	T6Ø.3X2	T6Ø.3X3	T6Ø.3X4	—	—
Veronal	T42.3X1	T42.3X2	T42.3X3	T42.3X4	T42.3X5	T42.3X6
Veroxil	T37.4X1	T37.4X2	T37.4X3	T37.4X4	T37.4X5	T37.4X6
Versenate	T5Ø.6X1	T5Ø.6X2	T5Ø.6X3	T5Ø.6X4	T5Ø.6X5	T5Ø.6X6
Versidyne	T39.8X1	T39.8X2	T39.8X3	T39.8X4	T39.8X5	T39.8X6
Vetrabutine	T48.ØX1	T48.ØX2	T48.ØX3	T48.ØX4	T48.ØX5	T48.ØX6
Vexol*	T49.5X1	T49.5X2	T49.5X3	T49.5X4	T49.5X5	T49.5X6
Vibramycin*	T36.4X1	T36.4X2	T36.4X3	T36.4X4	T36.4X5	T36.4X6
Victrelis*	T37.5X1	T37.5X2	T37.5X3	T37.5X4	T37.5X5	T37.5X6
Vidarabine	T37.5X1	T37.5X2	T37.5X3	T37.5X4	T37.5X5	T37.5X6
Vienna						
green	T57.ØX1	T57.ØX2	T57.ØX3	T57.ØX4	—	—
insecticide	T6Ø.2X1	T6Ø.2X2	T6Ø.2X3	T6Ø.2X4	—	—
red	T57.ØX1	T57.ØX2	T57.ØX3	T57.ØX4	—	—
pharmaceutical dye	T5Ø.991	T5Ø.992	T5Ø.993	T5Ø.994	T5Ø.995	T5Ø.996
Vigabatrin	T42.6X1	T42.6X2	T42.6X3	T42.6X4	T42.6X5	T42.6X6
Viloxazine	T43.291	T43.292	T43.293	T43.294	T43.295	T43.296
Viminol	T39.8X1	T39.8X2	T39.8X3	T39.8X4	T39.8X5	T39.8X6
Vinbarbital, vinbarbitone	T42.3X1	T42.3X2	T42.3X3	T42.3X4	T42.3X5	T42.3X6
Vinblastine	T45.1X1	T45.1X2	T45.1X3	T45.1X4	T45.1X5	T45.1X6
Vinburnine	T46.7X1	T46.7X2	T46.7X3	T46.7X4	T46.7X5	T46.7X6
Vincamine	T45.1X1	T45.1X2	T45.1X3	T45.1X4	T45.1X5	T45.1X6
Vincristine	T45.1X1	T45.1X2	T45.1X3	T45.1X4	T45.1X5	T45.1X6
Vindesine	T45.1X1	T45.1X2	T45.1X3	T45.1X4	T45.1X5	T45.1X6
Vinesthene, vinethene	T41.ØX1	T41.ØX2	T41.ØX3	T41.ØX4	T41.ØX5	T41.ØX6
Vinorelbine tartrate	T45.1X1	T45.1X2	T45.1X3	T45.1X4	T45.1X5	T45.1X6
Vinpocetine	T46.7X1	T46.7X2	T46.7X3	T46.7X4	T46.7X5	T46.7X6
Vinyl						
acetate	T65.891	T65.892	T65.893	T65.894	—	—
bital	T42.3X1	T42.3X2	T42.3X3	T42.3X4	T42.3X5	T42.3X6
bromide	T65.891	T65.892	T65.893	T65.894	—	—
chloride	T59.891	T59.892	T59.893	T59.894	—	—
ether	T41.ØX1	T41.ØX2	T41.ØX3	T41.ØX4	T41.ØX5	T41.ØX6
Vinylbital	T42.3X1	T42.3X2	T42.3X3	T42.3X4	T42.3X5	T42.3X6
Vinylidene chloride	T65.891	T65.892	T65.893	T65.894	—	—
Vioform	T37.8X1	T37.8X2	T37.8X3	T37.8X4	T37.8X5	T37.8X6
topical	T49.ØX1	T49.ØX2	T49.ØX3	T49.ØX4	T49.ØX5	T49.ØX6
Viokase*	T47.5X1	T47.5X2	T47.5X3	T47.5X4	T47.5X5	T47.5X6
Viomycin	T36.8X1	T36.8X2	T36.8X3	T36.8X4	T36.8X5	T36.8X6
Viosterol	T45.2X1	T45.2X2	T45.2X3	T45.2X4	T45.2X5	T45.2X6
Viper (venom)	T63.Ø91	T63.Ø92	T63.Ø93	T63.Ø94	—	—
Viprynium	T37.4X1	T37.4X2	T37.4X3	T37.4X4	T37.4X5	T37.4X6
Viquidil	T46.7X1	T46.7X2	T46.7X3	T46.7X4	T46.7X5	T46.7X6
Viral vaccine NEC	T5Ø.B91	T5Ø.B92	T5Ø.B93	T5Ø.B94	T5Ø.B95	T5Ø.B96
Virginiamycin	T36.8X1	T36.8X2	T36.8X3	T36.8X4	T36.8X5	T36.8X6
Virugon	T37.5X1	T37.5X2	T37.5X3	T37.5X4	T37.5X5	T37.5X6
Viscous agent	T5Ø.9Ø1	T5Ø.9Ø2	T5Ø.9Ø3	T5Ø.9Ø4	T5Ø.9Ø5	T5Ø.9Ø6
Visine	T49.5X1	T49.5X2	T49.5X3	T49.5X4	T49.5X5	T49.5X6
Visnadine	T46.3X1	T46.3X2	T46.3X3	T46.3X4	T46.3X5	T46.3X6
Vitamin NEC	T45.2X1	T45.2X2	T45.2X3	T45.2X4	T45.2X5	T45.2X6
A	T45.2X1	T45.2X2	T45.2X3	T45.2X4	T45.2X5	T45.2X6
B1	T45.2X1	T45.2X2	T45.2X3	T45.2X4	T45.2X5	T45.2X6
B2	T45.2X1	T45.2X2	T45.2X3	T45.2X4	T45.2X5	T45.2X6
B6	T45.2X1	T45.2X2	T45.2X3	T45.2X4	T45.2X5	T45.2X6
B12	T45.2X1	T45.2X2	T45.2X3	T45.2X4	T45.2X5	T45.2X6
B15	T45.2X1	T45.2X2	T45.2X3	T45.2X4	T45.2X5	T45.2X6
B NEC	T45.2X1	T45.2X2	T45.2X3	T45.2X4	T45.2X5	T45.2X6
nicotinic acid	T46.7X1	T46.7X2	T46.7X3	T46.7X4	T46.7X5	T46.7X6
C	T45.2X1	T45.2X2	T45.2X3	T45.2X4	T45.2X5	T45.2X6
D	T45.2X1	T45.2X2	T45.2X3	T45.2X4	T45.2X5	T45.2X6
D2	T45.2X1	T45.2X2	T45.2X3	T45.2X4	T45.2X5	T45.2X6
D3	T45.2X1	T45.2X2	T45.2X3	T45.2X4	T45.2X5	T45.2X6
E	T45.2X1	T45.2X2	T45.2X3	T45.2X4	T45.2X5	T45.2X6
E acetate	T45.2X1	T45.2X2	T45.2X3	T45.2X4	T45.2X5	T45.2X6
hematopoietic	T45.8X1	T45.8X2	T45.8X3	T45.8X4	T45.8X5	T45.8X6
K1	T45.7X1	T45.7X2	T45.7X3	T45.7X4	T45.7X5	T45.7X6
K2	T45.7X1	T45.7X2	T45.7X3	T45.7X4	T45.7X5	T45.7X6
K NEC	T45.7X1	T45.7X2	T45.7X3	T45.7X4	T45.7X5	T45.7X6
PP	T45.2X1	T45.2X2	T45.2X3	T45.2X4	T45.2X5	T45.2X6
ulceroprotectant	T47.1X1	T47.1X2	T47.1X3	T47.1X4	T47.1X5	T47.1X6

Substance	Poisoning, Accidental (unintentional)	Poisoning, Intentional Self-harm	Poisoning, Assault	Poisoning, Undetermined	Adverse Effect	Under-dosing
Vleminckx's solution	T49.4X1	T49.4X2	T49.4X3	T49.4X4	T49.4X5	T49.4X6
Voltaren — *see* Diclofenac sodium						
Voraxaze*	T5Ø.6X1	T5Ø.6X2	T5Ø.6X3	T5Ø.6X4	T5Ø.6X5	T5Ø.6X6
Warfarin	T45.511	T45.512	T45.513	T45.514	T45.515	T45.516
rodenticide	T6Ø.4X1-	T6Ø.4X2-	T6Ø.4X3-	T6Ø.4X4-	—	—
sodium	T45.511	T45.512	T45.513	T45.514	T45.515	T45.516
Wasp (sting)	T63.461	T63.462	T63.463	T63.464	—	—
Water						
balance drug	T5Ø.3X1	T5Ø.3X2	T5Ø.3X3	T5Ø.3X4	T5Ø.3X5	T5Ø.3X6
distilled	T5Ø.3X1	T5Ø.3X2	T5Ø.3X3	T5Ø.3X4	T5Ø.3X5	T5Ø.3X6
gas — *see* Gas, water						
incomplete combustion of — *see* Carbon, monoxide, fuel, utility						
hemlock	T62.2X1	T62.2X2	T62.2X3	T62.2X4	—	—
moccasin (venom)	T63.Ø61	T63.Ø62	T63.Ø63	T63.Ø64	—	—
purified	T5Ø.3X1	T5Ø.3X2	T5Ø.3X3	T5Ø.3X4	T5Ø.3X5	T5Ø.3X6
Wax (paraffin) (petroleum)	T52.ØX1	T52.ØX2	T52.ØX3	T52.ØX4	—	—
automobile	T65.891	T65.892	T65.893	T65.894	—	—
floor	T52.ØX1	T52.ØX2	T52.ØX3	T52.ØX4	—	—
Weed killers NEC	T6Ø.3X1	T6Ø.3X2	T6Ø.3X3	T6Ø.3X4	—	—
Wellbutrin*	T43.291	T43.292	T43.293	T43.294	T43.295	T43.296
Welldorm	T42.6X1	T42.6X2	T42.6X3	T42.6X4	T42.6X5	T42.6X6
Westcort*	T49.ØX1	T49.ØX2	T49.ØX3	T49.ØX4	T49.ØX5	T49.ØX6
White						
arsenic	T57.ØX1	T57.ØX2	T57.ØX3	T57.ØX4	—	—
hellebore	T62.2X1	T62.2X2	T62.2X3	T62.2X4	—	—
lotion (keratolytic)	T49.4X1	T49.4X2	T49.4X3	T49.4X4	T49.4X5	T49.4X6
spirit	T52.ØX1	T52.ØX2	T52.ØX3	T52.ØX4	—	—
Whitewash	T65.891	T65.892	T65.893	T65.894	—	—
Whole blood (human)	T45.8X1	T45.8X2	T45.8X3	T45.8X4	T45.8X5	T45.8X6
Wild						
black cherry	T62.2X1	T62.2X2	T62.2X3	T62.2X4	—	—
poisonous plants NEC	T62.2X1	T62.2X2	T62.2X3	T62.2X4	—	—
Window cleaning fluid	T65.891	T65.892	T65.893	T65.894	—	—
Wintergreen (oil)	T49.3X1	T49.3X2	T49.3X3	T49.3X4	T49.3X5	T49.3X6
Wisterine	T62.2X1	T62.2X2	T62.2X3	T62.2X4	—	—
Witch hazel	T49.2X1	T49.2X2	T49.2X3	T49.2X4	T49.2X5	T49.2X6
Wood alcohol or spirit	T51.1X1	T51.1X2	T51.1X3	T51.1X4	—	—
Wool fat (hydrous)	T49.3X1	T49.3X2	T49.3X3	T49.3X4	T49.3X5	T49.3X6
Woorali	T48.1X1	T48.1X2	T48.1X3	T48.1X4	T48.1X5	T48.1X6
Wormseed, American	T37.4X1	T37.4X2	T37.4X3	T37.4X4	T37.4X5	T37.4X6
Xamoterol	T44.5X1	T44.5X2	T44.5X3	T44.5X4	T44.5X5	T44.5X6
Xanax*	T42.4X1	T42.4X2	T42.4X3	T42.4X4	T42.4X5	T42.4X6
Xanthine diuretics	T5Ø.2X1	T5Ø.2X2	T5Ø.2X3	T5Ø.2X4	T5Ø.2X5	T5Ø.2X6
Xanthinol nicotinate	T46.7X1	T46.7X2	T46.7X3	T46.7X4	T46.7X5	T46.7X6
Xanthotoxin	T49.3X1	T49.3X2	T49.3X3	T49.3X4	T49.3X5	T49.3X6
Xantinol nicotinate	T46.7X1	T46.7X2	T46.7X3	T46.7X4	T46.7X5	T46.7X6
Xantocillin	T36.ØX1	T36.ØX2	T36.ØX3	T36.ØX4	T36.ØX5	T36.ØX6
Xenon (127Xe) (133Xe)	T5Ø.8X1	T5Ø.8X2	T5Ø.8X3	T5Ø.8X4	T5Ø.8X5	T5Ø.8X6
Xenysalate	T49.4X1	T49.4X2	T49.4X3	T49.4X4	T49.4X5	T49.4X6
Xibornol	T37.8X1	T37.8X2	T37.8X3	T37.8X4	T37.8X5	T37.8X6
Xigris	T45.511	T45.512	T45.513	T45.514	T45.515	T45.516
Xipamide	T5Ø.2X1	T5Ø.2X2	T5Ø.2X3	T5Ø.2X4	T5Ø.2X5	T5Ø.2X6
Xylene (vapor)	T52.2X1	T52.2X2	T52.2X3	T52.2X4	—	—
Xylocaine (infiltration) (topical)	T41.3X1	T41.3X2	T41.3X3	T41.3X4	T41.3X5	T41.3X6
nerve block (peripheral) (plexus)	T41.3X1	T41.3X2	T41.3X3	T41.3X4	T41.3X5	T41.3X6
spinal	T41.3X1	T41.3X2	T41.3X3	T41.3X4	T41.3X5	T41.3X6
Xylol (vapor)	T52.2X1	T52.2X2	T52.2X3	T52.2X4	—	—
Xylometazoline	T48.5X1	T48.5X2	T48.5X3	T48.5X4	T48.5X5	T48.5X6
Xylose*	T5Ø.8X1	T5Ø.8X2	T5Ø.8X3	T5Ø.8X4	T5Ø.8X5	T5Ø.8X6
Yaz*	T38.4X1	T38.4X2	T38.4X3	T38.4X4	T38.4X5	T38.4X6
Yeast	T45.2X1	T45.2X2	T45.2X3	T45.2X4	T45.2X5	T45.2X6
dried	T45.2X1	T45.2X2	T45.2X3	T45.2X4	T45.2X5	T45.2X6
Yellow						
fever vaccine	T5Ø.B91	T5Ø.B92	T5Ø.B93	T5Ø.B94	T5Ø.B95	T5Ø.B96
jasmine	T62.2X1	T62.2X2	T62.2X3	T62.2X4	—	—
phenolphthalein	T47.2X1	T47.2X2	T47.2X3	T47.2X4	T47.2X5	T47.2X6
Yervoy*	T45.1X1	T45.1X2	T45.1X3	T45.1X4	T45.1X5	T45.1X6
Yew	T62.2X1	T62.2X2	T62.2X3	T62.2X4	—	—
Yohimbic acid	T4Ø.991	T4Ø.992	T4Ø.993	T4Ø.994	T4Ø.995	T4Ø.996
Zactane	T39.8X1	T39.8X2	T39.8X3	T39.8X4	T39.8X5	T39.8X6
Zalcitabine	T37.5X1	T37.5X2	T37.5X3	T37.5X4	T37.5X5	T37.5X6
Zanaflex*	T48.1X1	T48.1X2	T48.1X3	T48.1X4	T48.1X5	T48.1X6
Zaroxolyn	T5Ø.2X1	T5Ø.2X2	T5Ø.2X3	T5Ø.2X4	T5Ø.2X5	T5Ø.2X6
Zephiran (topical)	T49.ØX1	T49.ØX2	T49.ØX3	T49.ØX4	T49.ØX5	T49.ØX6
ophthalmic preparation	T49.5X1	T49.5X2	T49.5X3	T49.5X4	T49.5X5	T49.5X6
Zeranol	T38.7X1	T38.7X2	T38.7X3	T38.7X4	T38.7X5	T38.7X6
Zerone	T51.1X1	T51.1X2	T51.1X3	T51.1X4	—	—
Zidovudine	T37.5X1	T37.5X2	T37.5X3	T37.5X4	T37.5X5	T37.5X6
Zilactin*	T41.3X1	T41.3X2	T41.3X3	T41.3X4	T41.3X5	T41.3X6
Zimeldine	T43.221	T43.222	T43.223	T43.224	T43.225	T43.226
Zinc (compounds) (fumes) (vapor) **NEC**	T56.5X1	T56.5X2	T56.5X3	T56.5X4	—	—
anti-infectives	T49.ØX1	T49.ØX2	T49.ØX3	T49.ØX4	T49.ØX5	T49.ØX6
antivaricose	T46.8X1	T46.8X2	T46.8X3	T46.8X4	T46.8X5	T46.8X6
bacitracin	T49.ØX1	T49.ØX2	T49.ØX3	T49.ØX4	T49.ØX5	T49.ØX6
chloride (mouthwash)	T49.6X1	T49.6X2	T49.6X3	T49.6X4	T49.6X5	T49.6X6
chromate	T56.5X1	T56.5X2	T56.5X3	T56.5X4	—	—
gelatin	T49.3X1	T49.3X2	T49.3X3	T49.3X4	T49.3X5	T49.3X6
oxide	T49.3X1	T49.3X2	T49.3X3	T49.3X4	T49.3X5	T49.3X6
plaster	T49.3X1	T49.3X2	T49.3X3	T49.3X4	T49.3X5	T49.3X6
peroxide	T49.ØX1	T49.ØX2	T49.ØX3	T49.ØX4	T49.ØX5	T49.ØX6
pesticides	T56.5X1	T56.5X2	T56.5X3	T56.5X4	—	—
phosphide	T6Ø.4X1	T6Ø.4X2	T6Ø.4X3	T6Ø.4X4	—	—
pyrithionate	T49.4X1	T49.4X2	T49.4X3	T49.4X4	T49.4X5	T49.4X6
stearate	T49.3X1	T49.3X2	T49.3X3	T49.3X4	T49.3X5	T49.3X6
sulfate	T49.5X1	T49.5X2	T49.5X3	T49.5X4	T49.5X5	T49.5X6
ENT agent	T49.6X1	T49.6X2	T49.6X3	T49.6X4	T49.6X5	T49.6X6
ophthalmic solution	T49.5X1	T49.5X2	T49.5X3	T49.5X4	T49.5X5	T49.5X6
topical NEC	T49.ØX1	T49.ØX2	T49.ØX3	T49.ØX4	T49.ØX5	T49.ØX6
undecylenate	T49.ØX1	T49.ØX2	T49.ØX3	T49.ØX4	T49.ØX5	T49.ØX6
Zineb	T6Ø.ØX1	T6Ø.ØX2	T6Ø.ØX3	T6Ø.ØX4	—	—
Zinostatin	T45.1X1	T45.1X2	T45.1X3	T45.1X4	T45.1X5	T45.1X6
Zipeprol	T48.3X1	T48.3X2	T48.3X3	T48.3X4	T48.3X5	T48.3X6
Zocor*	T46.6X1	T46.6X2	T46.6X3	T46.6X4	T46.6X5	T46.6X6
Zofenopril	T46.4X1	T46.4X2	T46.4X3	T46.4X4	T46.4X5	T46.4X6
Zoloft*	T43.221	T43.222	T43.223	T43.224	T43.225	T43.226
Zolpidem	T42.6X1	T42.6X2	T42.6X3	T42.6X4	T42.6X5	T42.6X6
Zomepirac	T39.391	T39.392	T39.393	T39.394	T39.395	T39.396
Zopiclone	T42.6X1	T42.6X2	T42.6X3	T42.6X4	T42.6X5	T42.6X6
Zorubicin	T45.1X1	T45.1X2	T45.1X3	T45.1X4	T45.1X5	T45.1X6
Zotepine	T43.591	T43.592	T43.593	T43.594	T43.595	T43.596
Zovant	T45.511	T45.512	T45.513	T45.514	T45.515	T45.516
Zoxazolamine	T42.8X1	T42.8X2	T42.8X3	T42.8X4	T42.8X5	T42.8X6
Zuclopenthixol	T43.4X1	T43.4X2	T43.4X3	T43.4X4	T43.4X5	T43.4X6
Zyflo*	T48.6X1	T48.6X2	T48.6X3	T48.6X4	T48.6X5	T48.6X6
Zygadenus (venenosus)	T62.2X1	T62.2X2	T62.2X3	T62.2X4	—	—
Zyprexa	T43.591	T43.592	T43.593	T43.594	T43.595	T43.596
Zyzal*	T45.ØX1	T45.ØX2	T45.ØX3	T45.ØX4	T45.ØX5	T45.ØX6

A

- **Abandonment** (causing exposure to weather conditions) (with intent to injure or kill) NEC X58 ☑
- **Abuse** (adult) (child) (mental) (physical) (sexual) X58 ☑
- **Accident** (to) X58 ☑
  - aircraft (in transit) (powered) — *see also* Accident, transport, aircraft
    - due to, caused by cataclysm — *see* Forces of nature, by type
  - animal-drawn vehicle — *see* Accident, transport, animal-drawn vehicle occupant
  - animal-rider — *see* Accident, transport, animal-rider
  - automobile — *see* Accident, transport, car occupant
  - bare foot water skier V94.4 ☑
  - boat, boating — *see also* Accident, watercraft
    - striking swimmer
      - powered V94.11 ☑
      - unpowered V94.12 ☑
  - bus — *see* Accident, transport, bus occupant
  - cable car, not on rails V98.0 ☑
    - on rails — *see* Accident, transport, streetcar occupant
  - car — *see* Accident, transport, car occupant
  - caused by, due to
    - animal NEC W64 ☑
    - chain hoist W24.0 ☑
    - cold (excessive) — *see* Exposure, cold
    - corrosive liquid, substance — *see* Table of Drugs and Chemicals
    - cutting or piercing instrument — *see* Contact, with, by type of instrument
    - drive belt W24.0 ☑
    - electric
      - current — *see* Exposure, electric current
      - motor — *see also* Contact, with, by type of machine W31.3 ☑
        - current (of) W86.8 ☑
    - environmental factor NEC X58 ☑
    - explosive material — *see* Explosion
    - fire, flames — *see* Exposure, fire
    - firearm missile — *see* Discharge, firearm by type
    - heat (excessive) — *see* Heat
    - hot — *see* Contact, with, hot
    - ignition — *see* Ignition
    - lifting device W24.0 ☑
    - lightning — *see* subcategory T75.0 ☑
      - causing fire — *see* Exposure, fire
    - machine, machinery — *see* Contact, with, by type of machine
    - natural factor NEC X58 ☑
    - pulley (block) W24.0 ☑
    - radiation — *see* Radiation
    - steam X13.1 ☑
      - inhalation X13.0 ☑
      - pipe X16 ☑
    - thunderbolt — *see* subcategory T75.0 ☑
      - causing fire — *see* Exposure, fire
    - transmission device W24.1 ☑
  - coach — *see* Accident, transport, bus occupant
  - coal car — *see* Accident, transport, industrial vehicle occupant
  - diving — *see also* Fall, into, water
    - with
      - drowning or submersion — *see* Drowning
  - forklift — *see* Accident, transport, industrial vehicle occupant
  - heavy transport vehicle NOS — *see* Accident, transport, truck occupant
  - ice yacht V98.2 ☑
  - in
    - medical, surgical procedure
      - as, or due to misadventure — *see* Misadventure
      - causing an abnormal reaction or later complication without mention of misadventure — *see also* Complication of or following, by type of procedure Y84.9
  - land yacht V98.1 ☑
  - late effect of — *see* W00-X58 with 7th character S
  - logging car — *see* Accident, transport, industrial vehicle occupant
  - machine, machinery — *see also* Contact, with, by type of machine
    - on board watercraft V93.69 ☑
      - explosion — *see* Explosion, in, watercraft

- **Accident** — *continued*
  - machine, machinery — *see also* Contact, with, by type of machine — *continued*
    - on board watercraft — *continued*
      - fire — *see* Burn, on board watercraft
      - powered craft V93.63 ☑
        - ferry boat V93.61 ☑
        - fishing boat V93.62 ☑
        - jetskis V93.63 ☑
        - liner V93.61 ☑
        - merchant ship V93.60 ☑
        - passenger ship V93.61 ☑
        - sailboat V93.64 ☑
  - mine tram — *see* Accident, transport, industrial vehicle occupant
  - mobility scooter (motorized) — *see* Accident, transport, pedestrian, conveyance, specified type NEC
  - motor scooter — *see* Accident, transport, motorcycle
  - motor vehicle NOS (traffic) — *see also* Accident, transport V89.2 ☑
    - nontraffic V89.0 ☑
    - three-wheeled NOS — *see* Accident, transport, three-wheeled motor vehicle occupant
  - motorcycle NOS — *see* Accident, transport, motorcycle
  - nonmotor vehicle NOS (nontraffic) — *see also* Accident, transport V89.1 ☑
    - traffic NOS V89.3 ☑
  - nontraffic (victim's mode of transport NOS) V88.9 ☑
    - collision (between) V88.7 ☑
      - bus and truck V88.5 ☑
      - car and:
        - bus V88.3 ☑
        - pickup V88.2 ☑
        - three-wheeled motor vehicle V88.0 ☑
        - train V88.6 ☑
        - truck V88.4 ☑
        - two-wheeled motor vehicle V88.0 ☑
        - van V88.2 ☑
      - specified vehicle NEC and:
        - three-wheeled motor vehicle V88.1 ☑
        - two-wheeled motor vehicle V88.1 ☑
    - known mode of transport — *see* Accident, transport, by type of vehicle
    - noncollision V88.8 ☑
  - on board watercraft V93.89 ☑
    - powered craft V93.83 ☑
      - ferry boat V93.81 ☑
      - fishing boat V93.82 ☑
      - jetskis V93.83 ☑
      - liner V93.81 ☑
      - merchant ship V93.80 ☑
      - passenger ship V93.81 ☑
    - unpowered craft V93.88 ☑
      - canoe V93.85 ☑
      - inflatable V93.86 ☑
        - in tow
          - recreational V94.31 ☑
          - specified NEC V94.32 ☑
      - kayak V93.85 ☑
      - sailboat V93.84 ☑
      - surf-board V93.88 ☑
      - water skis V93.87 ☑
      - windsurfer V93.88 ☑
  - parachutist V97.29 ☑
    - entangled in object V97.21 ☑
    - injured on landing V97.22 ☑
  - pedal cycle — *see* Accident, transport, pedal cyclist
  - pedestrian (on foot)
    - with
      - another pedestrian W51 ☑
        - on pedestrian conveyance NEC V00.09 ☑
        - with fall W03 ☑
          - due to ice or snow W00.0 ☑
      - rider of
        - hoverboard V00.038 ☑
        - Segway V00.038 ☑
        - standing
          - electric scooter V00.031 ☑
          - micro-mobility pedestrian conveyance NEC V00.038 ☑
      - roller skater (in-line) V00.01 ☑
      - skate boarder V00.02 ☑
      - transport vehicle — *see* Accident, transport
    - on pedestrian conveyance — *see* Accident, transport, pedestrian, conveyance

- **Accident** — *continued*
  - pick-up truck or van — *see* Accident, transport, pickup truck occupant
  - quarry truck — *see* Accident, transport, industrial vehicle occupant
  - railway vehicle (any) (in motion) — *see* Accident, transport, railway vehicle occupant
    - due to cataclysm — *see* Forces of nature, by type
  - scooter (non-motorized) — *see* Accident, transport, pedestrian, conveyance, scooter
  - sequelae of — *see* categories W00-X58 with 7th character S
  - skateboard — *see* Accident, transport, pedestrian, conveyance, skateboard
  - ski(ing) — *see* Accident, transport, pedestrian, conveyance
    - lift V98.3 ☑
  - specified cause NEC X58 ☑
  - streetcar — *see* Accident, transport, streetcar occupant
  - traffic (victim's mode of transport NOS) V87.9 ☑
    - collision (between) V87.7 ☑
      - bus and truck V87.5 ☑
      - car and:
        - bus V87.3 ☑
        - pickup V87.2 ☑
        - three-wheeled motor vehicle V87.0 ☑
        - train V87.6 ☑
        - truck V87.4 ☑
        - two-wheeled motor vehicle V87.0 ☑
        - van V87.2 ☑
      - specified vehicle NEC V86.39 ☑
        - and
          - three-wheeled motor vehicle V87.1 ☑
          - two-wheeled motor vehicle V87.1 ☑
        - driver V86.09 ☑
        - passenger V86.19 ☑
        - person on outside V86.29 ☑
        - while boarding or alighting V86.49 ☑
    - known mode of transport — *see* Accident, transport, by type of vehicle
    - noncollision V87.8 ☑
  - transport (involving injury to) V99 ☑
    - 18 wheeler — *see* Accident, transport, truck occupant
    - agricultural vehicle occupant (nontraffic) V84.9 ☑
      - driver V84.5 ☑
      - hanger-on V84.7 ☑
      - passenger V84.6 ☑
      - traffic V84.3 ☑
        - driver V84.0 ☑
        - hanger-on V84.2 ☑
        - passenger V84.1 ☑
      - while boarding or alighting V84.4 ☑
    - aircraft NEC V97.89 ☑
      - military NEC V97.818 ☑
        - civilian injured by V97.811 ☑
        - with civilian aircraft V97.810 ☑
      - occupant injured (in)
        - nonpowered craft accident V96.9 ☑
          - balloon V96.00 ☑
            - collision V96.03 ☑
            - crash V96.01 ☑
            - explosion V96.05 ☑
            - fire V96.04 ☑
            - forced landing V96.02 ☑
            - specified type NEC V96.09 ☑
          - glider V96.20 ☑
            - collision V96.23 ☑
            - crash V96.21 ☑
            - explosion V96.25 ☑
            - fire V96.24 ☑
            - forced landing V96.22 ☑
            - specified type NEC V96.29 ☑
          - hang glider V96.10 ☑
            - collision V96.13 ☑
            - crash V96.11 ☑
            - explosion V96.15 ☑
            - fire V96.14 ☑
            - forced landing V96.12 ☑
            - specified type NEC V96.19 ☑
          - specified craft NEC V96.8 ☑
        - powered craft accident V95.9 ☑
          - fixed wing NEC
            - commercial V95.30 ☑
              - collision V95.33 ☑
              - crash V95.31 ☑

- **Accident** — *continued*
  - transport — *continued*
    - bus occupant — *continued*
      - hanger-on — *continued*
        - collision — *continued*
          - three wheeled motor vehicle (traffic) V72.7 ☑
            - nontraffic V72.2 ☑
          - truck (traffic) V74.7 ☑
            - nontraffic V74.2 ☑
          - two wheeled motor vehicle (traffic) V72.7 ☑
            - nontraffic V72.2 ☑
          - van (traffic) V73.7 ☑
            - nontraffic V73.2 ☑
        - noncollision accident (traffic) V78.7 ☑
          - nontraffic V78.2 ☑
      - noncollision accident (traffic) V78.9 ☑
        - nontraffic V78.3 ☑
        - while boarding or alighting V78.4 ☑
      - nontraffic V79.3 ☑
      - passenger
        - collision (with)
          - animal (traffic) V70.6 ☑
            - being ridden (traffic) V76.6 ☑
              - nontraffic V76.1 ☑
            - nontraffic V70.1 ☑
          - animal-drawn vehicle (traffic) V76.6 ☑
            - nontraffic V76.1 ☑
          - bus (traffic) V74.6 ☑
            - nontraffic V74.1 ☑
          - car (traffic) V73.6 ☑
            - nontraffic V73.1 ☑
          - motor vehicle NOS (traffic) V79.50 ☑
            - nontraffic V79.10 ☑
            - specified type NEC (traffic) V79.59 ☑
              - nontraffic V79.19 ☑
          - pedal cycle (traffic) V71.6 ☑
            - nontraffic V71.1 ☑
          - pickup truck (traffic) V73.6 ☑
            - nontraffic V73.1 ☑
          - railway vehicle (traffic) V75.6 ☑
            - nontraffic V75.1 ☑
          - specified vehicle NEC (traffic) V76.6 ☑
            - nontraffic V76.1 ☑
          - stationary object (traffic) V77.6 ☑
            - nontraffic V77.1 ☑
          - streetcar (traffic) V76.6 ☑
            - nontraffic V76.1 ☑
          - three wheeled motor vehicle (traffic) V72.6 ☑
            - nontraffic V72.1 ☑
          - truck (traffic) V74.6 ☑
            - nontraffic V74.1 ☑
          - two wheeled motor vehicle (traffic) V72.6 ☑
            - nontraffic V72.1 ☑
          - van (traffic) V73.6 ☑
            - nontraffic V73.1 ☑
        - noncollision accident (traffic) V78.6 ☑
          - nontraffic V78.1 ☑
      - specified type NEC V79.88 ☑
        - military vehicle V79.81 ☑
    - cable car, not on rails V98.0 ☑
      - on rails — *see* Accident, transport, streetcar occupant
    - car occupant V49.9 ☑
      - ambulance occupant — *see* Accident, transport, ambulance occupant
      - collision (with)
        - animal (traffic) V40.9 ☑
          - being ridden (traffic) V46.9 ☑
            - nontraffic V46.3 ☑
            - while boarding or alighting V46.4 ☑
          - nontraffic V40.3 ☑
          - while boarding or alighting V40.4 ☑
        - animal-drawn vehicle (traffic) V46.9 ☑
          - nontraffic V46.3 ☑
          - while boarding or alighting V46.4 ☑
        - bus (traffic) V44.9 ☑
          - nontraffic V44.3 ☑
          - while boarding or alighting V44.4 ☑
        - car (traffic) V43.92 ☑
          - nontraffic V43.32 ☑
          - while boarding or alighting V43.42 ☑
        - motor vehicle NOS (traffic) V49.60 ☑

- **Accident** — *continued*
  - transport — *continued*
    - car occupant — *continued*
      - collision — *continued*
        - motor vehicle — *continued*
          - nontraffic V49.20 ☑
          - specified type NEC (traffic) V49.69 ☑
            - nontraffic V49.29 ☑
        - pedal cycle (traffic) V41.9 ☑
          - nontraffic V41.3 ☑
          - while boarding or alighting V41.4 ☑
        - pickup truck (traffic) V43.93 ☑
          - nontraffic V43.33 ☑
          - while boarding or alighting V43.43 ☑
        - railway vehicle (traffic) V45.9 ☑
          - nontraffic V45.3 ☑
          - while boarding or alighting V45.4 ☑
        - specified vehicle NEC (traffic) V46.9 ☑
          - nontraffic V46.3 ☑
          - while boarding or alighting V46.4 ☑
        - sport utility vehicle (traffic) V43.91 ☑
          - nontraffic V43.31 ☑
          - while boarding or alighting V43.41 ☑
        - stationary object (traffic) V47.9 ☑
          - nontraffic V47.3 ☑
          - while boarding or alighting V47.4 ☑
        - streetcar (traffic) V46.9 ☑
          - nontraffic V46.3 ☑
          - while boarding or alighting V46.4 ☑
        - three wheeled motor vehicle (traffic) V42.9 ☑
          - nontraffic V42.3 ☑
          - while boarding or alighting V42.4 ☑
        - truck (traffic) V44.9 ☑
          - nontraffic V44.3 ☑
          - while boarding or alighting V44.4 ☑
        - two wheeled motor vehicle (traffic) V42.9 ☑
          - nontraffic V42.3 ☑
          - while boarding or alighting V42.4 ☑
        - van (traffic) V43.94 ☑
          - nontraffic V43.34 ☑
          - while boarding or alighting V43.44 ☑
      - driver
        - collision (with)
          - animal (traffic) V40.5 ☑
            - being ridden (traffic) V46.5 ☑
              - nontraffic V46.0 ☑
            - nontraffic V40.0 ☑
          - animal-drawn vehicle (traffic) V46.5 ☑
            - nontraffic V46.0 ☑
          - bus (traffic) V44.5 ☑
            - nontraffic V44.0 ☑
          - car (traffic) V43.52 ☑
            - nontraffic V43.02 ☑
          - motor vehicle NOS (traffic) V49.40 ☑
            - nontraffic V49.00 ☑
            - specified type NEC (traffic) V49.49 ☑
              - nontraffic V49.09 ☑
          - pedal cycle (traffic) V41.5 ☑
            - nontraffic V41.0 ☑
          - pickup truck (traffic) V43.53 ☑
            - nontraffic V43.03 ☑
          - railway vehicle (traffic) V45.5 ☑
            - nontraffic V45.0 ☑
          - specified vehicle NEC (traffic) V46.5 ☑
            - nontraffic V46.0 ☑
          - sport utility vehicle (traffic) V43.51 ☑
            - nontraffic V43.01 ☑
          - stationary object (traffic) V47.5 ☑
            - nontraffic V47.0 ☑
          - streetcar (traffic) V46.5 ☑
            - nontraffic V46.0 ☑
          - three wheeled motor vehicle (traffic) V42.5 ☑
            - nontraffic V42.0 ☑
          - truck (traffic) V44.5 ☑
            - nontraffic V44.0 ☑
          - two wheeled motor vehicle (traffic) V42.5 ☑
            - nontraffic V42.0 ☑
          - van (traffic) V43.54 ☑
            - nontraffic V43.04 ☑
        - noncollision accident (traffic) V48.5 ☑
          - nontraffic V48.0 ☑
      - hanger-on
        - collision (with)
          - animal (traffic) V40.7 ☑

- **Accident** — *continued*
  - transport — *continued*
    - car occupant — *continued*
      - hanger-on — *continued*
        - collision — *continued*
          - animal — *continued*
            - being ridden (traffic) V46.7 ☑
              - nontraffic V46.2 ☑
            - nontraffic V40.2 ☑
          - animal-drawn vehicle (traffic) V46.7 ☑
            - nontraffic V46.2 ☑
          - bus (traffic) V44.7 ☑
            - nontraffic V44.2 ☑
          - car (traffic) V43.72 ☑
            - nontraffic V43.22 ☑
          - pedal cycle (traffic) V41.7 ☑
            - nontraffic V41.2 ☑
          - pickup truck (traffic) V43.73 ☑
            - nontraffic V43.23 ☑
          - railway vehicle (traffic) V45.7 ☑
            - nontraffic V45.2 ☑
          - specified vehicle NEC (traffic) V46.7 ☑
            - nontraffic V46.2 ☑
          - sport utility vehicle (traffic) V43.71 ☑
            - nontraffic V43.21 ☑
          - stationary object (traffic) V47.7 ☑
            - nontraffic V47.2 ☑
          - streetcar (traffic) V46.7 ☑
            - nontraffic V46.2 ☑
          - three wheeled motor vehicle (traffic) V42.7 ☑
            - nontraffic V42.2 ☑
          - truck (traffic) V44.7 ☑
            - nontraffic V44.2 ☑
          - two wheeled motor vehicle (traffic) V42.7 ☑
            - nontraffic V42.2 ☑
          - van (traffic) V43.74 ☑
            - nontraffic V43.24 ☑
        - noncollision accident (traffic) V48.7 ☑
          - nontraffic V48.2 ☑
      - noncollision accident (traffic) V48.9 ☑
        - nontraffic V48.3 ☑
        - while boarding or alighting V48.4 ☑
      - nontraffic V49.3 ☑
      - passenger
        - collision (with)
          - animal (traffic) V40.6 ☑
            - being ridden (traffic) V46.6 ☑
              - nontraffic V46.1 ☑
            - nontraffic V40.1 ☑
          - animal-drawn vehicle (traffic) V46.6 ☑
            - nontraffic V46.1 ☑
          - bus (traffic) V44.6 ☑
            - nontraffic V44.1 ☑
          - car (traffic) V43.62 ☑
            - nontraffic V43.12 ☑
          - motor vehicle NOS (traffic) V49.50 ☑
            - nontraffic V49.10 ☑
            - specified type NEC (traffic) V49.59 ☑
              - nontraffic V49.19 ☑
          - pedal cycle (traffic) V41.6 ☑
            - nontraffic V41.1 ☑
          - pickup truck (traffic) V43.63 ☑
            - nontraffic V43.13 ☑
          - railway vehicle (traffic) V45.6 ☑
            - nontraffic V45.1 ☑
          - specified vehicle NEC (traffic) V46.6 ☑
            - nontraffic V46.1 ☑
          - sport utility vehicle (traffic) V43.61 ☑
            - nontraffic V43.11 ☑
          - stationary object (traffic) V47.6 ☑
            - nontraffic V47.1 ☑
          - streetcar (traffic) V46.6 ☑
            - nontraffic V46.1 ☑
          - three wheeled motor vehicle (traffic) V42.6 ☑
            - nontraffic V42.1 ☑
          - truck (traffic) V44.6 ☑
            - nontraffic V44.1 ☑
          - two wheeled motor vehicle (traffic) V42.6 ☑
            - nontraffic V42.1 ☑
          - van (traffic) V43.64 ☑
            - nontraffic V43.14 ☑
        - noncollision accident (traffic) V48.6 ☑

- **Accident** — *continued*
  - transport — *continued*
    - pedestrian — *continued*
      - conveyance — *continued*
        - flat-bottomed — *continued*
          - collision — *continued*
            - vehicle — *continued*
              - motor — *continued*
                - traffic V09.20 ☑
          - fall V00.381 ☑
          - nontraffic V09.1 ☑
            - involving motor vehicle NEC V09.00 ☑
          - snow
            - board — *see* Accident, transport, pedestrian, conveyance, snow board
            - ski — *see* Accident, transport, pedestrian, conveyance, skis (snow)
          - traffic V09.3 ☑
            - involving motor vehicle NEC V09.20 ☑
        - gliding type NEC V00.288 ☑
          - collision (with) V09.9 ☑
            - animal being ridden or animal drawn vehicle V06.99 ☑
              - nontraffic V06.09 ☑
              - traffic V06.19 ☑
            - bus or heavy transport V04.99 ☑
              - nontraffic V04.09 ☑
              - traffic V04.19 ☑
            - car V03.99 ☑
              - nontraffic V03.09 ☑
              - traffic V03.19 ☑
            - pedal cycle V01.99 ☑
              - nontraffic V01.09 ☑
              - traffic V01.19 ☑
            - pick-up truck or van V03.99 ☑
              - nontraffic V03.09 ☑
              - traffic V03.19 ☑
            - railway (train) (vehicle) V05.99 ☑
              - nontraffic V05.09 ☑
              - traffic V05.19 ☑
            - stationary object V00.282 ☑
            - streetcar V06.99 ☑
              - nontraffic V06.09 ☑
              - traffic V02.19 ☑
            - two- or three-wheeled motor vehicle V02.99 ☑
              - nontraffic V02.09 ☑
              - traffic V02.19 ☑
            - vehicle V09.9 ☑
              - animal-drawn V06.99 ☑
                - nontraffic V06.09 ☑
                - traffic V06.19 ☑
              - motor
                - nontraffic V09.00 ☑
                - traffic V09.20 ☑
          - fall V00.281 ☑
          - heelies — *see* Accident, transport, pedestrian, conveyance, heelies
          - ice skate — *see* Accident, transport, pedestrian, conveyance, ice skate
          - nontraffic V09.1 ☑
            - involving motor vehicle NEC V09.00 ☑
          - sled — *see* Accident, transport, pedestrian, conveyance, sled
          - traffic V09.3 ☑
            - involving motor vehicle NEC V09.20 ☑
            - wheelies — *see* Accident, transport, pedestrian, conveyance, heelies
        - heelies V00.158 ☑
          - colliding with stationary object V00.152 ☑
          - fall V00.151 ☑
        - hoverboard
          - collision with
            - animal being ridden or animal drawn vehicle V06.938 ☑
              - nontraffic V06.038 ☑
              - traffic V06.138 ☑
            - bus or heavy transport V04.938 ☑
              - nontraffic V04.038 ☑
              - traffic V04.138 ☑
            - car V03.938 ☑
              - nontraffic V03.038 ☑
              - traffic V03.138 ☑
            - pedal cycle V01.938 ☑

- **Accident** — *continued*
  - transport — *continued*
    - pedestrian — *continued*
      - conveyance — *continued*
        - hoverboard — *continued*
          - collision with — *continued*
            - pedal cycle — *continued*
              - nontraffic V01.038 ☑
              - traffic V01.138 ☑
            - pick-up or van V03.938 ☑
              - nontraffic V03.038 ☑
              - traffic V03.138 ☑
            - railway (train) (vehicle) V05.938 ☑
              - nontraffic V05.038 ☑
              - traffic V05.138 ☑
            - streetcar V06.938 ☑
              - nontraffic V06.038 ☑
              - traffic V06.138 ☑
            - three-wheeled motor vehicle V02.938 ☑
              - nontraffic V02.038 ☑
              - traffic V02.138 ☑
            - two-wheeled motor vehicle V02.938 ☑
              - nontraffic V02.038 ☑
              - traffic V02.138 ☑
            - vehicle, nonmotor, specified NEC V06.938 ☑
              - nontraffic V06.038 ☑
              - traffic V06.138 ☑
          - fall V00.848 ☑
        - ice skates V00.218 ☑
          - collision (with) V09.9 ☑
            - animal being ridden or animal drawn vehicle V06.99 ☑
              - nontraffic V06.09 ☑
              - traffic V06.19 ☑
            - bus or heavy transport V04.99 ☑
              - nontraffic V04.09 ☑
              - traffic V04.19 ☑
            - car V03.99 ☑
              - nontraffic V03.09 ☑
              - traffic V03.19 ☑
            - pedal cycle V01.99 ☑
              - nontraffic V01.09 ☑
              - traffic V01.19 ☑
            - pick-up truck or van V03.99 ☑
              - nontraffic V03.09 ☑
              - traffic V03.19 ☑
            - railway (train) (vehicle) V05.99 ☑
              - nontraffic V05.09 ☑
              - traffic V05.19 ☑
            - stationary object V00.212 ☑
            - streetcar V06.99 ☑
              - nontraffic V06.09 ☑
              - traffic V06.19 ☑
            - two- or three-wheeled motor vehicle V02.99 ☑
              - nontraffic V02.09 ☑
              - traffic V02.19 ☑
            - vehicle V09.9 ☑
              - animal-drawn V06.99 ☑
                - nontraffic V06.09 ☑
                - traffic V06.19 ☑
              - motor
                - nontraffic V09.00 ☑
                - traffic V09.20 ☑
          - fall V00.211 ☑
          - nontraffic V09.1 ☑
            - involving motor vehicle NEC V09.00 ☑
          - traffic V09.3 ☑
            - involving motor vehicle NEC V09.20 ☑
        - motorized mobility scooter V00.838 ☑
          - collision with stationary object V00.832 ☑
          - fall from V00.831 ☑
        - nontraffic V09.1 ☑
          - involving motor vehicle V09.00 ☑
            - military V09.01 ☑
            - specified type NEC V09.09 ☑
        - roller skates (non in-line) V00.128 ☑
          - collision (with) V09.9 ☑
            - animal being ridden or animal drawn vehicle V06.91 ☑
              - nontraffic V06.01 ☑
              - traffic V06.11 ☑

- **Accident** — *continued*
  - transport — *continued*
    - pedestrian — *continued*
      - conveyance — *continued*
        - roller skates — *continued*
          - collision — *continued*
            - bus or heavy transport V04.91 ☑
              - nontraffic V04.01 ☑
              - traffic V04.11 ☑
            - car V03.91 ☑
              - nontraffic V03.01 ☑
              - traffic V03.11 ☑
            - pedal cycle V01.91 ☑
              - nontraffic V01.01 ☑
              - traffic V01.11 ☑
            - pick-up truck or van V03.91 ☑
              - nontraffic V03.01 ☑
              - traffic V03.11 ☑
            - railway (train) (vehicle) V05.91 ☑
              - nontraffic V05.01 ☑
              - traffic V05.11 ☑
            - stationary object V00.122 ☑
            - streetcar V06.91 ☑
              - nontraffic V06.01 ☑
              - traffic V06.11 ☑
            - two- or three-wheeled motor vehicle V02.91 ☑
              - nontraffic V02.01 ☑
              - traffic V02.11 ☑
            - vehicle V09.9 ☑
              - animal-drawn V06.91 ☑
                - nontraffic V06.01 ☑
                - traffic V06.11 ☑
              - motor
                - nontraffic V09.00 ☑
                - traffic V09.20 ☑
          - fall V00.121 ☑
          - in-line V00.118 ☑
            - collision — *see* also Accident, transport, pedestrian, conveyance occupant, roller skates, collision
              - with stationary object V00.112 ☑
            - fall V00.111 ☑
            - nontraffic V09.1 ☑
              - involving motor vehicle NEC V09.00 ☑
            - traffic V09.3 ☑
              - involving motor vehicle NEC V09.20 ☑
        - rolling shoes V00.158 ☑
          - colliding with stationary object V00.152 ☑
          - fall V00.151 ☑
        - rolling type NEC V00.188 ☑
          - collision (with) V09.9 ☑
            - animal being ridden or animal drawn vehicle V06.99 ☑
              - nontraffic V06.09 ☑
              - traffic V06.19 ☑
            - bus or heavy transport V04.99 ☑
              - nontraffic V04.09 ☑
              - traffic V04.19 ☑
            - car V03.99 ☑
              - nontraffic V03.09 ☑
              - traffic V03.19 ☑
            - pedal cycle V01.99 ☑
              - nontraffic V01.09 ☑
              - traffic V01.19 ☑
            - pick-up truck or van V03.99 ☑
              - nontraffic V03.09 ☑
              - traffic V03.19 ☑
            - railway (train) (vehicle) V05.99 ☑
              - nontraffic V05.09 ☑
              - traffic V05.19 ☑
            - stationary object V00.182 ☑
            - streetcar V06.99 ☑
              - nontraffic V06.09 ☑
              - traffic V06.19 ☑
            - two- or three-wheeled motor vehicle V02.99 ☑
              - nontraffic V02.09 ☑
              - traffic V02.19 ☑
            - vehicle V09.9 ☑
              - animal-drawn V06.99 ☑
                - nontraffic V06.09 ☑
                - traffic V06.19 ☑
              - motor
                - nontraffic V09.00 ☑

- **Accident** — *continued*
  - transport — *continued*
    - person — *continued*
      - collision — *continued*
        - car — *continued*
          - heavy transport vehicle — *continued*
            - nontraffic V88.4 ☑
          - nontraffic V88.5 ☑
          - pick-up truck or van (traffic) V87.2 ☑
            - nontraffic V88.2 ☑
          - train or railway vehicle (traffic) V87.6 ☑
            - nontraffic V88.6 ☑
          - two-or three-wheeled motor vehicle (traffic) V87.Ø ☑
            - nontraffic V88.Ø ☑
        - motor vehicle (traffic) NEC V87.7 ☑
          - nontraffic V88.7 ☑
        - two-or three-wheeled vehicle (with) (traffic) motor vehicle NEC V87.1 ☑
          - nontraffic V88.1 ☑
      - nonmotor vehicle (collision) (noncollision) (traffic) V87.9 ☑
        - nontraffic V88.9 ☑
    - pickup truck occupant V59.9 ☑
      - collision (with)
        - animal (traffic) V5Ø.9 ☑
          - being ridden (traffic) V56.9 ☑
            - nontraffic V56.3 ☑
            - while boarding or alighting V56.4 ☑
          - nontraffic V5Ø.3 ☑
          - while boarding or alighting V5Ø.4 ☑
        - animal-drawn vehicle (traffic) V56.9 ☑
          - nontraffic V56.3 ☑
          - while boarding or alighting V56.4 ☑
        - bus (traffic) V54.9 ☑
          - nontraffic V54.3 ☑
          - while boarding or alighting V54.4 ☑
        - car (traffic) V53.9 ☑
          - nontraffic V53.3 ☑
          - while boarding or alighting V53.4 ☑
        - motor vehicle NOS (traffic) V59.6Ø ☑
          - nontraffic V59.2Ø ☑
          - specified type NEC (traffic) V59.69 ☑
            - nontraffic V59.29 ☑
        - pedal cycle (traffic) V51.9 ☑
          - nontraffic V51.3 ☑
          - while boarding or alighting V51.4 ☑
        - pickup truck (traffic) V53.9 ☑
          - nontraffic V53.3 ☑
          - while boarding or alighting V53.4 ☑
        - railway vehicle (traffic) V55.9 ☑
          - nontraffic V55.3 ☑
          - while boarding or alighting V55.4 ☑
        - specified vehicle NEC (traffic) V56.9 ☑
          - nontraffic V56.3 ☑
          - while boarding or alighting V56.4 ☑
        - stationary object (traffic) V57.9 ☑
          - nontraffic V57.3 ☑
          - while boarding or alighting V57.4 ☑
        - streetcar (traffic) V56.9 ☑
          - nontraffic V56.3 ☑
          - while boarding or alighting V56.4 ☑
        - three wheeled motor vehicle (traffic) V52.9 ☑
          - nontraffic V52.3 ☑
          - while boarding or alighting V52.4 ☑
        - truck (traffic) V54.9 ☑
          - nontraffic V54.3 ☑
          - while boarding or alighting V54.4 ☑
        - two wheeled motor vehicle (traffic) V52.9 ☑
          - nontraffic V52.3 ☑
          - while boarding or alighting V52.4 ☑
        - van (traffic) V53.9 ☑
          - nontraffic V53.3 ☑
          - while boarding or alighting V53.4 ☑
      - driver
        - collision (with)
          - animal (traffic) V5Ø.5 ☑
            - being ridden (traffic) V56.5 ☑
              - nontraffic V56.Ø ☑
            - nontraffic V5Ø.Ø ☑
          - animal-drawn vehicle (traffic) V56.5 ☑
            - nontraffic V56.Ø ☑
          - bus (traffic) V54.5 ☑
            - nontraffic V54.Ø ☑
          - car (traffic) V53.5 ☑
            - nontraffic V53.Ø ☑

- **Accident** — *continued*
  - transport — *continued*
    - pickup truck occupant — *continued*
      - driver — *continued*
        - collision — *continued*
          - motor vehicle NOS (traffic) V59.4Ø ☑
            - nontraffic V59.ØØ ☑
            - specified type NEC (traffic) V59.49 ☑
              - nontraffic V59.Ø9 ☑
          - pedal cycle (traffic) V51.5 ☑
            - nontraffic V51.Ø ☑
          - pickup truck (traffic) V53.5 ☑
            - nontraffic V53.Ø ☑
          - railway vehicle (traffic) V55.5 ☑
            - nontraffic V55.Ø ☑
          - specified vehicle NEC (traffic) V56.5 ☑
            - nontraffic V56.Ø ☑
          - stationary object (traffic) V57.5 ☑
            - nontraffic V57.Ø ☑
          - streetcar (traffic) V56.5 ☑
            - nontraffic V56.Ø ☑
          - three wheeled motor vehicle (traffic) V52.5 ☑
            - nontraffic V52.Ø ☑
          - truck (traffic) V54.5 ☑
            - nontraffic V54.Ø ☑
          - two wheeled motor vehicle (traffic) V52.5 ☑
            - nontraffic V52.Ø ☑
          - van (traffic) V53.5 ☑
            - nontraffic V53.Ø ☑
        - noncollision accident (traffic) V58.5 ☑
          - nontraffic V58.Ø ☑
      - hanger-on
        - collision (with)
          - animal (traffic) V5Ø.7 ☑
            - being ridden (traffic) V56.7 ☑
              - nontraffic V56.2 ☑
            - nontraffic V5Ø.2 ☑
          - animal-drawn vehicle (traffic) V56.7 ☑
            - nontraffic V56.2 ☑
          - bus (traffic) V54.7 ☑
            - nontraffic V54.2 ☑
          - car (traffic) V53.7 ☑
            - nontraffic V53.2 ☑
          - pedal cycle (traffic) V51.7 ☑
            - nontraffic V51.2 ☑
          - pickup truck (traffic) V53.7 ☑
            - nontraffic V53.2 ☑
          - railway vehicle (traffic) V55.7 ☑
            - nontraffic V55.2 ☑
          - specified vehicle NEC (traffic) V56.7 ☑
            - nontraffic V56.2 ☑
          - stationary object (traffic) V57.7 ☑
            - nontraffic V57.2 ☑
          - streetcar (traffic) V56.7 ☑
            - nontraffic V56.2 ☑
          - three wheeled motor vehicle (traffic) V52.7 ☑
            - nontraffic V52.2 ☑
          - truck (traffic) V54.7 ☑
            - nontraffic V54.2 ☑
          - two wheeled motor vehicle (traffic) V52.7 ☑
            - nontraffic V52.2 ☑
          - van (traffic) V53.7 ☑
            - nontraffic V53.2 ☑
        - noncollision accident (traffic) V58.7 ☑
          - nontraffic V58.2 ☑
      - noncollision accident (traffic) V58.9 ☑
        - nontraffic V58.3 ☑
        - while boarding or alighting V58.4 ☑
      - nontraffic V59.3 ☑
      - passenger
        - collision (with)
          - animal (traffic) V5Ø.6 ☑
            - being ridden (traffic) V56.6 ☑
              - nontraffic V56.1 ☑
            - nontraffic V5Ø.1 ☑
          - animal-drawn vehicle (traffic) V56.6 ☑
            - nontraffic V56.1 ☑
          - bus (traffic) V54.6 ☑
            - nontraffic V54.1 ☑
          - car (traffic) V53.6 ☑
            - nontraffic V53.1 ☑
          - motor vehicle NOS (traffic) V59.5Ø ☑

- **Accident** — *continued*
  - transport — *continued*
    - pickup truck occupant — *continued*
      - passenger — *continued*
        - collision — *continued*
          - motor vehicle — *continued*
            - nontraffic V59.1Ø ☑
            - specified type NEC (traffic) V59.59 ☑
              - nontraffic V59.19 ☑
          - pedal cycle (traffic) V51.6 ☑
            - nontraffic V51.1 ☑
          - pickup truck (traffic) V53.6 ☑
            - nontraffic V53.1 ☑
          - railway vehicle (traffic) V55.6 ☑
            - nontraffic V55.1 ☑
          - specified vehicle NEC (traffic) V56.6 ☑
            - nontraffic V56.1 ☑
          - stationary object (traffic) V57.6 ☑
            - nontraffic V57.1 ☑
          - streetcar (traffic) V56.6 ☑
            - nontraffic V56.1 ☑
          - three wheeled motor vehicle (traffic) V52.6 ☑
            - nontraffic V52.1 ☑
          - truck (traffic) V54.6 ☑
            - nontraffic V54.1 ☑
          - two wheeled motor vehicle (traffic) V52.6 ☑
            - nontraffic V52.1 ☑
          - van (traffic) V53.6 ☑
            - nontraffic V53.1 ☑
        - noncollision accident (traffic) V58.6 ☑
          - nontraffic V58.1 ☑
      - specified type NEC V59.88 ☑
        - military vehicle V59.81 ☑
    - quarry truck — *see* Accident, transport, industrial vehicle occupant
    - race car — *see* Accident, transport, motor vehicle NEC occupant
    - railway vehicle occupant V81.9 ☑
      - collision (with) V81.3 ☑
        - motor vehicle (non-military) (traffic) V81.1 ☑
          - military V81.83 ☑
          - nontraffic V81.Ø ☑
        - rolling stock V81.2 ☑
        - specified object NEC V81.3 ☑
      - during derailment V81.7 ☑
        - with antecedent collision — *see* Accident, transport, railway vehicle occupant, collision
      - explosion V81.81 ☑
      - fall (in railway vehicle) V81.5 ☑
        - during derailment V81.7 ☑
          - with antecedent collision — *see* Accident, transport, railway vehicle occupant, collision
        - from railway vehicle V81.6 ☑
          - during derailment V81.7 ☑
            - with antecedent collision — *see* Accident, transport, railway vehicle occupant, collision
        - while boarding or alighting V81.4 ☑
      - fire V81.81 ☑
      - object falling onto train V81.82 ☑
      - specified type NEC V81.89 ☑
      - while boarding or alighting V81.4 ☑
    - Segway VØØ.848 ☑
    - ski lift V98.3 ☑
    - snowmobile occupant (nontraffic) V86.92 ☑
      - driver V86.52 ☑
      - hanger-on V86.72 ☑
      - passenger V86.62 ☑
      - traffic V86.32 ☑
        - driver V86.Ø2 ☑
        - hanger-on V86.22 ☑
        - passenger V86.12 ☑
      - while boarding or alighting V86.42 ☑
    - specified NEC V98.8 ☑
    - sport utility vehicle occupant — *see also* Accident, transport, pickup truck occupant
    - streetcar occupant V82.9 ☑
      - collision (with) V82.3 ☑
        - motor vehicle (traffic) V82.1 ☑
          - nontraffic V82.Ø ☑
        - rolling stock V82.2 ☑
      - during derailment V82.7 ☑

☑ **Additional Character Required — Refer to the Tabular List for Character Selection**

Activity — *continued*
- elliptical machine Y93.A1 (*following* Y93.7)
- exercise(s)
  - machines ((primarily) for)
    - cardiorespiratory conditioning Y93.A1 (*following* Y93.7)
    - muscle strengthening Y93.B1 (*following* Y93.7)
  - muscle strengthening (non-machine) NEC Y93.B9 (*following* Y93.7)
- external motion NEC Y93.I9 (*following* Y93.7)
  - rollercoaster Y93.I1 (*following* Y93.7)
- fainting game Y93.85
- field hockey Y93.65
- figure skating (pairs) (singles) Y93.21
- flag football Y93.62
- floor mopping and cleaning Y93.E5 (*following* Y93.7)
- food preparation and clean up Y93.G1 (*following* Y93.7)
- football (American) NOS Y93.61
  - flag Y93.62
  - tackle Y93.61
  - touch Y93.62
- four square Y93.6A
- free weights Y93.B3 (*following* Y93.7)
- frisbee (ultimate) Y93.74
- furniture
  - building Y93.D3 (*following* Y93.7)
  - finishing Y93.D3 (*following* Y93.7)
  - repair Y93.D3 (*following* Y93.7)
- game playing (electronic)
  - using interactive device Y93.C2 (*following* Y93.7)
  - using keyboard or other stationary device Y93.C1 (*following* Y93.7)
- gardening Y93.H2 (*following* Y93.7)
- golf Y93.53
- grass drills Y93.A6 (*following* Y93.7)
- grilling and smoking food Y93.G2 (*following* Y93.7)
- grooming and shearing an animal Y93.K3 (*following* Y93.7)
- guerilla drills Y93.A6 (*following* Y93.7)
- gymnastics (rhythmic) Y93.43
- hand held interactive electronic device Y93.C2 (*following* Y93.7)
- handball Y93.73
- handcrafts NEC Y93.D9 (*following* Y93.7)
- hang gliding Y93.35
- hiking (on level or elevated terrain) Y93.Ø1
- hockey (ice) Y93.22
  - field Y93.65
- horseback riding Y93.52
- household (interior) maintenance NEC Y93.E9 (*following* Y93.7)
- ice NEC Y93.29
  - dancing Y93.21
  - hockey Y93.22
  - skating Y93.21
- inline roller skating Y93.51
- ironing Y93.E4 (*following* Y93.7)
- judo Y93.75
- jumping jacks Y93.A2 (*following* Y93.7)
- jumping rope Y93.56
- jumping (off) NEC Y93.39
  - BASE (Building, Antenna, Span, Earth) Y93.33
  - bungee Y93.34
  - jacks Y93.A2 (*following* Y93.7)
  - rope Y93.56
- karate Y93.75
- kayaking (in calm and turbulent water) Y93.16
- keyboarding (computer) Y93.C1 (*following* Y93.7)
- kickball Y93.6A
- knitting Y93.D1 (*following* Y93.7)
- lacrosse Y93.65
- land maintenance NEC Y93.H9 (*following* Y93.7)
- landscaping Y93.H2 (*following* Y93.7)
- laundry Y93.E2 (*following* Y93.7)
- machines (exercise)
  - primarily for cardiorespiratory conditioning Y93.A1 (*following* Y93.7)
  - primarily for muscle strengthening Y93.B1 (*following* Y93.7)
- maintenance
  - exterior building NEC Y93.H9 (*following* Y93.7)
  - household (interior) NEC Y93.E9 (*following* Y93.7)
  - land Y93.H9 (*following* Y93.7)
  - property Y93.H9 (*following* Y93.7)
- marching (on level or elevated terrain) Y93.Ø1
- martial arts Y93.75
- microwave oven Y93.G3 (*following* Y93.7)
- milking an animal Y93.K2 (*following* Y93.7)
- mopping (floor) Y93.E5 (*following* Y93.7)

Activity — *continued*
- mountain climbing Y93.31
- muscle strengthening
  - exercises (non-machine) NEC Y93.B9 (*following* Y93.7)
  - machines Y93.B1 (*following* Y93.7)
- musical keyboard (electronic) playing Y93.J1 (*following* Y93.7)
- nordic skiing Y93.24
- obstacle course Y93.A5 (*following* Y93.7)
- oven (microwave) Y93.G3 (*following* Y93.7)
- packing up and unpacking in moving to a new residence Y93.E6 (*following* Y93.7)
- parasailing Y93.19
- pass out game Y93.85
- percussion instrument playing NEC Y93.J2 (*following* Y93.7)
- personal
  - bathing and showering Y93.E1 (*following* Y93.7)
  - hygiene NEC Y93.E8 (*following* Y93.7)
  - showering Y93.E1 (*following* Y93.7)
- physical games generally associated with school recess, summer camp and children Y93.6A
- physical training NEC Y93.A9 (*following* Y93.7)
- piano playing Y93.J1 (*following* Y93.7)
- pilates Y93.B4 (*following* Y93.7)
- platform diving Y93.12
- playing musical instrument
  - brass instrument Y93.J4 (*following* Y93.7)
  - drum Y93.J2 (*following* Y93.7)
  - musical keyboard (electronic) Y93.J1 (*following* Y93.7)
  - percussion instrument NEC Y93.J2 (*following* Y93.7)
  - piano Y93.J1 (*following* Y93.7)
  - string instrument Y93.J3 (*following* Y93.7)
  - winds instrument Y93.J4 (*following* Y93.7)
- property maintenance
  - exterior NEC Y93.H9 (*following* Y93.7)
  - interior NEC Y93.E9 (*following* Y93.7)
- pruning (garden and lawn) Y93.H2 (*following* Y93.7)
- pull-ups Y93.B2 (*following* Y93.7)
- push-ups Y93.B2 (*following* Y93.7)
- racquetball Y93.73
- rafting (in calm and turbulent water) Y93.16
- raking (leaves) Y93.H1 (*following* Y93.7)
- rappelling Y93.32
- refereeing a sports activity Y93.81
- residential relocation Y93.E6 (*following* Y93.7)
- rhythmic gymnastics Y93.43
- rhythmic movement NEC Y93.49
- riding
  - horseback Y93.52
  - rollercoaster Y93.I1 (*following* Y93.7)
- rock climbing Y93.31
- roller skating (inline) Y93.51
- rollercoaster riding Y93.I1 (*following* Y93.7)
- rough housing and horseplay Y93.83
- rowing (in calm and turbulent water) Y93.16
- rugby Y93.63
- running Y93.Ø2
- SCUBA diving Y93.15
- sewing Y93.D2 (*following* Y93.7)
- shoveling Y93.H1 (*following* Y93.7)
  - dirt Y93.H1 (*following* Y93.7)
  - snow Y93.H1 (*following* Y93.7)
- showering (personal) Y93.E1 (*following* Y93.7)
- sit-ups Y93.B2 (*following* Y93.7)
- skateboarding Y93.51
- skating (ice) Y93.21
  - roller Y93.51
- skiing (alpine) (downhill) Y93.23
  - cross country Y93.24
  - nordic Y93.24
  - water Y93.17
- sledding (snow) Y93.23
- sleeping (sleep) Y93.84
- smoking and grilling food Y93.G2 (*following* Y93.7)
- snorkeling Y93.15
- snow NEC Y93.29
  - boarding Y93.23
  - shoveling Y93.H1 (*following* Y93.7)
  - sledding Y93.23
  - tubing Y93.23
- soccer Y93.66
- softball Y93.64
- specified NEC Y93.89
- spectator at an event Y93.82
- sports NEC Y93.79
  - sports played as a team or group NEC Y93.69

Activity — *continued*
- sports — *continued*
  - sports played individually NEC Y93.59
- springboard diving Y93.12
- squash Y93.73
- stationary bike Y93.A1 (*following* Y93.7)
- step (stepping) exercise (class) Y93.A3 (*following* Y93.7)
- stepper machine Y93.A1 (*following* Y93.7)
- stove Y93.G3 (*following* Y93.7)
- string instrument playing Y93.J3 (*following* Y93.7)
- surfing Y93.18
  - wind Y93.18
- swimming Y93.11
- tackle football Y93.61
- tap dancing Y93.41
- tennis Y93.73
- tobogganing Y93.23
- touch football Y93.62
- track and field events (non-running) Y93.57
  - running Y93.Ø2
- trampoline Y93.44
- treadmill Y93.A1 (*following* Y93.7)
- trimming shrubs Y93.H2 (*following* Y93.7)
- tubing (in calm and turbulent water) Y93.16
  - snow Y93.23
- ultimate frisbee Y93.74
- underwater diving Y93.15
- unpacking in moving to a new residence Y93.E6 (*following* Y93.7)
- use of stove, oven and microwave oven Y93.G3 (*following* Y93.7)
- vacuuming Y93.E3 (*following* Y93.7)
- volleyball (beach) (court) Y93.68
- wake boarding Y93.17
- walking (on level or elevated terrain) Y93.Ø1
  - an animal Y93.K1 (*following* Y93.7)
- walking an animal Y93.K1 (*following* Y93.7)
- wall climbing Y93.31
- warm up and cool down exercises Y93.A2 (*following* Y93.7)
- water NEC Y93.19
  - aerobics Y93.14
  - craft NEC Y93.19
  - exercise Y93.14
  - polo Y93.13
  - skiing Y93.17
  - sliding Y93.18
  - survival training and testing Y93.19
- weeding (garden and lawn) Y93.H2 (*following* Y93.7)
- wind instrument playing Y93.J4 (*following* Y93.7)
- windsurfing Y93.18
- wrestling Y93.72
- yoga Y93.42

Adverse effect of drugs — *see* Table of Drugs and Chemicals

Aerosinusitis — *see* Air, pressure

After-effect, late — *see* Sequelae

Air
- blast in war operations — *see* War operations, air blast
- pressure
  - change, rapid
    - during
      - ascent W94.29 ☑
        - while (in) (surfacing from)
          - aircraft W94.23 ☑
          - deep water diving W94.21 ☑
          - underground W94.22 ☑
      - descent W94.39 ☑
        - in
          - aircraft W94.31 ☑
          - water W94.32 ☑
  - high, prolonged W94.Ø ☑
  - low, prolonged W94.12 ☑
    - due to residence or long visit at high altitude W94.11 ☑

Alpine sickness W94.11 ☑

Altitude sickness W94.11 ☑

Anaphylactic shock, anaphylaxis — *see* Table of Drugs and Chemicals

Andes disease W94.11 ☑

Arachnidism, arachnoidism X58 ☑

Arson (with intent to injure or kill) X97 ☑

Asphyxia, asphyxiation
- by
  - food (bone) (seed) — *see* categories T17 and T18 ☑
  - gas — *see also* Table of Drugs and Chemicals
    - legal
      - execution — *see* Legal, intervention, gas

- **Asphyxia, asphyxiation** — *continued*
  - by — *continued*
    - gas — *see also* Table of Drugs and Chemicals — *continued*
      - legal — *continued*
        - intervention — *see* Legal, intervention, gas
  - from
    - fire — *see also* Exposure, fire
      - in war operations — *see* War operations, fire
    - ignition — *see* Ignition
    - vomitus T17.81 ☑
  - in war operations — *see* War operations, restriction of airway
- **Aspiration**
  - food (any type) (into respiratory tract) (with asphyxia, obstruction respiratory tract, suffocation) — *see* categories T17 and T18 ☑
  - foreign body — *see* Foreign body, aspiration
  - vomitus (with asphyxia, obstruction respiratory tract, suffocation) T17.81 ☑
- **Assassination** (attempt) — *see* Assault
- **Assault** (homicidal) (by) (in) Y09
  - arson X97 ☑
  - bite (of human being) Y04.1 ☑
  - bodily force Y04.8 ☑
    - bite Y04.1 ☑
    - bumping into Y04.2 ☑
    - sexual — *see* subcategories T74.Ø, T76.Ø ☑
    - unarmed fight Y04.Ø ☑
  - bomb X96.9 ☑
    - antipersonnel X96.Ø ☑
    - fertilizer X96.3 ☑
    - gasoline X96.1 ☑
    - letter X96.2 ☑
    - petrol X96.1 ☑
    - pipe X96.3 ☑
    - specified NEC X96.8 ☑
  - brawl (hand) (fists) (foot) (unarmed) Y04.Ø ☑
  - burning, burns (by fire) NEC X97 ☑
    - acid Y08.89 ☑
    - caustic, corrosive substance Y08.89 ☑
    - chemical from swallowing caustic, corrosive substance — *see* Table of Drugs and Chemicals
    - cigarette(s) X97 ☑
    - hot object X98.9 ☑
      - fluid NEC X98.2 ☑
      - household appliance X98.3 ☑
      - specified NEC X98.8 ☑
      - steam X98.Ø ☑
      - tap water X98.1 ☑
      - vapors X98.Ø ☑
    - scalding — *see* Assault, burning
    - steam X98.Ø ☑
    - vitriol Y08.89 ☑
  - caustic, corrosive substance (gas) Y08.89 ☑
  - crashing of
    - aircraft Y08.81 ☑
    - motor vehicle Y03.8 ☑
      - pushed in front of Y02.Ø ☑
      - run over Y03.Ø ☑
      - specified NEC Y03.8 ☑
  - cutting or piercing instrument X99.9 ☑
    - dagger X99.2 ☑
    - glass X99.Ø ☑
    - knife X99.1 ☑
    - specified NEC X99.8 ☑
    - sword X99.2 ☑
  - dagger X99.2 ☑
  - drowning (in) X92.9 ☑
    - bathtub X92.Ø ☑
    - natural water X92.3 ☑
    - specified NEC X92.8 ☑
    - swimming pool X92.1 ☑
      - following fall X92.2 ☑
  - dynamite X96.8 ☑
  - explosive(s) (material) X96.9 ☑
  - fight (hand) (fists) (foot) (unarmed) Y04.Ø ☑
    - with weapon — *see* Assault, by type of weapon
  - fire X97 ☑
  - firearm X95.9 ☑
    - airgun X95.Ø1 ☑
    - handgun X93 ☑
    - hunting rifle X94.1 ☑
    - larger X94.9 ☑
      - specified NEC X94.8 ☑
    - machine gun X94.2 ☑
- **Assault** — *continued*
  - firearm — *continued*
    - shotgun X94.Ø ☑
    - specified NEC X95.8 ☑
  - from high place Y01 ☑
  - gunshot (wound) NEC — *see* Assault, firearm, by type
  - incendiary device X97 ☑
  - injury Y09
    - to child due to criminal abortion attempt NEC Y08.89 ☑
  - knife X99.1 ☑
  - late effect of — *see* categories X92-Y08 with 7th character S
  - placing before moving object NEC Y02.8 ☑
    - motor vehicle Y02.Ø ☑
  - poisoning — *see* categories T36-T65 with 7th character S
  - puncture, any part of body — *see* Assault, cutting or piercing instrument
  - pushing
    - before moving object NEC Y02.8 ☑
      - motor vehicle Y02.Ø ☑
      - subway train Y02.1 ☑
      - train Y02.1 ☑
    - from high place Y01 ☑
  - rape T74.2- ☑
  - scalding — *see* Assault, burning
  - sequelae of — *see* categories X92-Y08 with 7th character S
  - sexual (by bodily force) T74.2- ☑
  - shooting — *see* Assault, firearm
  - specified means NEC Y08.89 ☑
  - stab, any part of body — *see* Assault, cutting or piercing instrument
  - steam X98.Ø ☑
  - striking against
    - other person Y04.2 ☑
    - sports equipment Y08.09 ☑
      - baseball bat Y08.02 ☑
      - hockey stick Y08.01 ☑
  - struck by
    - sports equipment Y08.09 ☑
      - baseball bat Y08.02 ☑
      - hockey stick Y08.01 ☑
  - submersion — *see* Assault, drowning
  - violence Y09
  - weapon Y09
    - blunt Y00 ☑
    - cutting or piercing — *see* Assault, cutting or piercing instrument
    - firearm — *see* Assault, firearm
  - wound Y09
    - cutting — *see* Assault, cutting or piercing instrument
    - gunshot — *see* Assault, firearm
    - knife X99.1 ☑
    - piercing — *see* Assault, cutting or piercing instrument
    - puncture — *see* Assault, cutting or piercing instrument
    - stab — *see* Assault, cutting or piercing instrument
- **Attack by mammals NEC** W55.89 ☑
- **Avalanche** — *see* Landslide
- **Aviator's disease** — *see* Air, pressure

B

- **Barotitis, barodontalgia, barosinusitis, barotrauma** (otitic) (sinus) — *see* Air, pressure
- **Battered** (baby) (child) (person) (syndrome) X58 ☑
- **Bayonet wound** W26.1 ☑
  - in
    - legal intervention — *see* Legal, intervention, sharp object, bayonet
    - war operations — *see* War operations, combat
  - stated as undetermined whether accidental or intentional Y28.8 ☑
  - suicide (attempt) X78.2 ☑
- **Bean in nose** — *see* categories T17 and T18 ☑
- **Bed set on fire NEC** — *see* Exposure, fire, uncontrolled, building, bed
- **Beheading** (by guillotine)
  - homicide X99.9 ☑
  - legal execution — *see* Legal, intervention
- **Bending, injury in** (prolonged) (static) X50.1 ☑
- **Bends** — *see* Air, pressure, change
- **Bite, bitten by**
  - alligator W58.01 ☑
  - arthropod (nonvenomous) NEC W57 ☑
  - bull W55.21 ☑
  - cat W55.01 ☑
  - cow W55.21 ☑
  - crocodile W58.11 ☑
  - dog W54.Ø ☑
  - goat W55.31 ☑
  - hoof stock NEC W55.31 ☑
  - horse W55.11 ☑
  - human being (accidentally) W50.3 ☑
    - with intent to injure or kill Y04.1 ☑
    - as, or caused by, a crowd or human stampede (with fall) W52 ☑
    - assault Y04.1 ☑
    - homicide (attempt) Y04.1 ☑
    - in
      - fight Y04.1 ☑
  - insect (nonvenomous) W57 ☑
  - lizard (nonvenomous) W59.01 ☑
  - mammal NEC W55.81 ☑
    - marine W56.31 ☑
  - marine animal (nonvenomous) W56.81 ☑
  - millipede W57 ☑
  - moray eel W56.51 ☑
  - mouse W53.01 ☑
  - person(s) (accidentally) W50.3 ☑
    - with intent to injure or kill Y04.1 ☑
    - as, or caused by, a crowd or human stampede (with fall) W52 ☑
    - assault Y04.1 ☑
    - homicide (attempt) Y04.1 ☑
    - in
      - fight Y04.1 ☑
  - pig W55.41 ☑
  - raccoon W55.51 ☑
  - rat W53.11 ☑
  - reptile W59.81 ☑
    - lizard W59.01 ☑
    - snake W59.11 ☑
    - turtle W59.21 ☑
      - terrestrial W59.81 ☑
  - rodent W53.81 ☑
    - mouse W53.01 ☑
    - rat W53.11 ☑
    - specified NEC W53.81 ☑
    - squirrel W53.21 ☑
  - shark W56.41 ☑
  - sheep W55.31 ☑
  - snake (nonvenomous) W59.11 ☑
  - spider (nonvenomous) W57 ☑
  - squirrel W53.21 ☑
- **Blast** (air) in war operations — *see* War operations, blast
- **Blizzard** X37.2 ☑
- **Blood alcohol level** Y90.9
  - less than 2Ømg/1ØØml Y90.Ø
  - presence in blood, level not specified Y90.9
  - 2Ø-39mg/1ØØml Y90.1
  - 4Ø-59mg/1ØØml Y90.2
  - 6Ø-79mg/1ØØml Y90.3
  - 8Ø-99mg/1ØØml Y90.4
  - 1ØØ-119mg/1ØØml Y90.5
  - 12Ø-199mg/1ØØml Y90.6
  - 2ØØ-239mg/1ØØml Y90.7
- **Blow** X58 ☑
  - by law-enforcing agent, police (on duty) — *see* Legal, intervention, manhandling
    - blunt object — *see* Legal, intervention, blunt object
- **Blowing up** — *see* Explosion
- **Brawl** (hand) (fists) (foot) Y04.Ø ☑
- **Breakage** (accidental) (part of)
  - ladder (causing fall) W11 ☑
  - scaffolding (causing fall) W12 ☑
- **Broken**
  - glass, contact with — *see* Contact, with, glass
  - power line (causing electric shock) W85 ☑
- **Bumping against, into** (accidentally)
  - object NEC W22.8 ☑
    - caused by crowd or human stampede (with fall) W52 ☑
    - sports equipment W21.9 ☑
    - with fall — *see* Fall, due to, bumping against, object
  - person(s) W51 ☑
    - with fall W03 ☑
      - due to ice or snow W00.Ø ☑

Bumping against, into — *continued*
- person(s) — *continued*
  - assault Y04.2 ☑
  - caused by, a crowd or human stampede (with fall) W52 ☑
  - homicide (attempt) Y04.2 ☑
- sports equipment W21.9 ☑

Burn, burned, burning (accidental) (by) (from) (on)
- acid NEC — *see* Table of Drugs and Chemicals
- bed linen — *see* Exposure, fire, uncontrolled, in building, bed
- blowtorch X08.8 ☑
  - with ignition of clothing NEC X06.2 ☑
    - nightwear X05 ☑
- bonfire, campfire (controlled) — *see also* Exposure, fire, controlled, not in building)
  - uncontrolled — *see* Exposure, fire, uncontrolled, not in building
- candle X08.8 ☑
  - with ignition of clothing NEC X06.2 ☑
    - nightwear X05 ☑
- caustic liquid, substance (external) (internal) NEC — *see* Table of Drugs and Chemicals
- chemical (external) (internal) — *see also* Table of Drugs and Chemicals
  - in war operations — *see* War operations. fire
- cigar(s) or cigarette(s) X08.8 ☑
  - with ignition of clothing NEC X06.2 ☑
    - nightwear X05 ☑
- clothes, clothing NEC (from controlled fire) X06.2 ☑
  - with conflagration — *see* Exposure, fire, uncontrolled, building
    - not in building or structure — *see* Exposure, fire, uncontrolled, not in building
- cooker (hot) X15.8 ☑
  - stated as undetermined whether accidental or intentional Y27.3 ☑
  - suicide (attempt) X77.3 ☑
- electric blanket X16 ☑
- engine (hot) X17 ☑
- fire, flames — *see* Exposure, fire
- flare, Very pistol — *see* Discharge, firearm NEC
- heat
  - from appliance (electrical) (household) X15.8 ☑
    - cooker X15.8 ☑
    - hotplate X15.2 ☑
    - kettle X15.8 ☑
    - light bulb X15.8 ☑
    - saucepan X15.3 ☑
    - skillet X15.3 ☑
    - stated as undetermined whether accidental or intentional Y27.3 ☑
    - stove X15.0 ☑
    - suicide (attempt) X77.3 ☑
    - toaster X15.1 ☑
  - in local application or packing during medical or surgical procedure Y63.5
- heating
  - appliance, radiator or pipe X16 ☑
- homicide (attempt) — *see* Assault, burning
- hot
  - air X14.1 ☑
  - cooker X15.8 ☑
  - drink X10.0 ☑
  - engine X17 ☑
  - fat X10.2 ☑
  - fluid NEC X12 ☑
  - food X10.1 ☑
  - gases X14.1 ☑
  - heating appliance X16 ☑
  - household appliance NEC X15.8 ☑
  - kettle X15.8 ☑
  - liquid NEC X12 ☑
  - machinery X17 ☑
  - metal (molten) (liquid) NEC X18 ☑
  - object (not producing fire or flames) NEC X19 ☑
  - oil (cooking) X10.2 ☑
  - pipe(s) X16 ☑
  - radiator X16 ☑
  - saucepan (glass) (metal) X15.3 ☑
  - stove (kitchen) X15.0 ☑
  - substance NEC X19 ☑
    - caustic or corrosive NEC — *see* Table of Drugs and Chemicals
  - toaster X15.1 ☑
  - tool X17 ☑

Burn, burned, burning — *continued*
- hot — *continued*
  - vapor X13.1 ☑
  - water (tap) — *see* Contact, with, hot, tap water
- hotplate X15.2 ☑
  - suicide (attempt) X77.3 ☑
- ignition — *see* Ignition
- in war operations — *see* War operations, fire
- inflicted by other person X97 ☑
  - by hot objects, hot vapor, and steam — *see* Assault, burning, hot object
- internal, from swallowed caustic, corrosive liquid, substance — *see* Table of Drugs and Chemicals
- iron (hot) X15.8 ☑
  - stated as undetermined whether accidental or intentional Y27.3 ☑
  - suicide (attempt) X77.3 ☑
- kettle (hot) X15.8 ☑
  - stated as undetermined whether accidental or intentional Y27.3 ☑
  - suicide (attempt) X77.3 ☑
- lamp (flame) X08.8 ☑
  - with ignition of clothing NEC X06.2 ☑
    - nightwear X05 ☑
- lighter (cigar) (cigarette) X08.8 ☑
  - with ignition of clothing NEC X06.2 ☑
    - nightwear X05 ☑
- lightning — *see* subcategory T75.0 ☑
  - causing fire — *see* Exposure, fire
- liquid (boiling) (hot) NEC X12 ☑
  - stated as undetermined whether accidental or intentional Y27.2 ☑
  - suicide (attempt) X77.2 ☑
- local application of externally applied substance in medical or surgical care Y63.5
- machinery (hot) X17 ☑
- matches X08.8 ☑
  - with ignition of clothing NEC X06.2 ☑
    - nightwear X05 ☑
- mattress — *see* Exposure, fire, uncontrolled, building, bed
- medicament, externally applied Y63.5
- metal (hot) (liquid) (molten) NEC X18 ☑
- nightwear (nightclothes, nightdress, gown, pajamas, robe) X05 ☑
- object (hot) NEC X19 ☑
- on board watercraft
  - due to
    - accident to watercraft V91.09 ☑
      - powered craft V91.03 ☑
        - ferry boat V91.01 ☑
        - fishing boat V91.02 ☑
        - jetskis V91.03 ☑
        - liner V91.01 ☑
        - merchant ship V91.00 ☑
        - passenger ship V91.01 ☑
      - unpowered craft V91.08 ☑
        - canoe V91.05 ☑
        - inflatable V91.06 ☑
        - kayak V91.05 ☑
        - sailboat V91.04 ☑
        - surf-board V91.08 ☑
        - water skis V91.07 ☑
        - windsurfer V91.08 ☑
    - fire on board V93.09 ☑
      - ferry boat V93.01 ☑
      - fishing boat V93.02 ☑
      - jetskis V93.03 ☑
      - liner V93.01 ☑
      - merchant ship V93.00 ☑
      - passenger ship V93.01 ☑
      - powered craft NEC V93.03 ☑
      - sailboat V93.04 ☑
    - specified heat source NEC on board V93.19 ☑
      - ferry boat V93.11 ☑
      - fishing boat V93.12 ☑
      - jetskis V93.13 ☑
      - liner V93.11 ☑
      - merchant ship V93.10 ☑
      - passenger ship V93.11 ☑
      - powered craft NEC V93.13 ☑
      - sailboat V93.14 ☑
- pipe (hot) X16 ☑
  - smoking X08.8 ☑
    - with ignition of clothing NEC X06.2 ☑
      - nightwear X05 ☑

Burn, burned, burning — *continued*
- powder — *see* Powder burn
- radiator (hot) X16 ☑
- saucepan (hot) (glass) (metal) X15.3 ☑
  - stated as undetermined whether accidental or intentional Y27.3 ☑
  - suicide (attempt) X77.3 ☑
- self-inflicted X76 ☑
  - stated as undetermined whether accidental or intentional Y26 ☑
- stated as undetermined whether accidental or intentional Y27.0 ☑
- steam X13.1 ☑
  - pipe X16 ☑
    - stated as undetermined whether accidental or intentional Y27.8 ☑
  - stated as undetermined whether accidental or intentional Y27.0 ☑
  - suicide (attempt) X77.0 ☑
- stove (hot) (kitchen) X15.0 ☑
  - stated as undetermined whether accidental or intentional Y27.3 ☑
  - suicide (attempt) X77.3 ☑
- substance (hot) NEC X19 ☑
  - boiling X12 ☑
    - stated as undetermined whether accidental or intentional Y27.2 ☑
    - suicide (attempt) X77.2 ☑
  - molten (metal) X18 ☑
- suicide (attempt) NEC X76 ☑
  - hot
    - household appliance X77.3 ☑
    - object X77.9 ☑
- therapeutic misadventure
  - heat in local application or packing during medical or surgical procedure Y63.5
  - overdose of radiation Y63.2
- toaster (hot) X15.1 ☑
  - stated as undetermined whether accidental or intentional Y27.3 ☑
  - suicide (attempt) X77.3 ☑
- tool (hot) X17 ☑
- torch, welding X08.8 ☑
  - with ignition of clothing NEC X06.2 ☑
    - nightwear X05 ☑
- trash fire (controlled) — *see* Exposure, fire, controlled, not in building
  - uncontrolled — *see* Exposure, fire, uncontrolled, not in building
- vapor (hot) X13.1 ☑
  - stated as undetermined whether accidental or intentional Y27.0 ☑
  - suicide (attempt) X77.0 ☑
- Very pistol — *see* Discharge, firearm NEC

Butted by animal W55.82 ☑
- bull W55.22 ☑
- cow W55.22 ☑
- goat W55.32 ☑
- horse W55.12 ☑
- pig W55.42 ☑
- sheep W55.32 ☑

C

Caisson disease — *see* Air, pressure, change

Campfire (exposure to) (controlled) — *see also* Exposure, fire, controlled, not in building
- uncontrolled — *see* Exposure, fire, uncontrolled, not in building

Capital punishment (any means) — *see* Legal, intervention

Car sickness T75.3 ☑

Casualty (not due to war) NEC X58 ☑
- war — *see* War operations

Cat
- bite W55.01 ☑
- scratch W55.03 ☑

Cataclysm, cataclysmic (any injury) NEC — *see* Forces of nature

Catching fire — *see* Exposure, fire

Caught
- between
  - folding object W23.0 ☑
  - objects (moving) W23.0 ☑

- **Caught** — *continued*
  - between — *continued*
    - objects — *continued*
      - and
        - machinery — *see* Contact, with, by type of machine
        - stationary W23.2 ☑
      - stationary W23.1 ☑
        - and moving W23.2 ☑
    - sliding door and door frame W23.Ø ☑
  - by, in
    - machinery (moving parts of) — *see* Contact, with, by type of machine
    - washing-machine wringer W23.Ø ☑
  - under packing crate (due to losing grip) W23.1 ☑
- **Cave-in caused by cataclysmic earth surface movement or eruption** — *see* Landslide
- **Change**(s) in air pressure — *see* Air, pressure, change
- **Choked, choking** (on) (any object except food or vomitus)
  - food (bone) (seed) — *see* categories T17 and T18 ☑
  - vomitus T17.81- ☑
- **Civil insurrection** — *see* War operations
- **Cloudburst** (any injury) X37.8 ☑
- **Cold, exposure to** (accidental) (excessive) (extreme) (natural) (place) NEC — *see* Exposure, cold
- **Collapse**
  - building W2Ø.1 ☑
    - burning (uncontrolled fire) XØØ.2 ☑
  - dam or man-made structure (causing earth movement) X36.Ø ☑
  - machinery — *see* Contact, with, by type of machine
  - structure W2Ø.1 ☑
    - burning (uncontrolled fire) XØØ.2 ☑
- **Collision** (accidental) NEC — *see also* Accident, transport V89.9 ☑
  - pedestrian W51 ☑
    - with fall WØ3 ☑
      - due to ice or snow WØØ.Ø ☑
      - involving pedestrian conveyance — *see* Accident, transport, pedestrian, conveyance
    - and
      - crowd or human stampede (with fall) W52 ☑
      - object W22.8 ☑
        - with fall — *see* Fall, due to, bumping against, object
  - person(s) — *see* Collision, pedestrian
  - transport vehicle NEC V89.9 ☑
    - and
      - avalanche, fallen or not moving — *see* Accident, transport
        - falling or moving — *see* Landslide
      - landslide, fallen or not moving — *see* Accident, transport
        - falling or moving — *see* Landslide
    - due to cataclysm — *see* Forces of nature, by type
    - intentional, purposeful suicide (attempt) — *see* Suicide, collision
- **Combustion, spontaneous** — *see* Ignition
- **Complication** (delayed) **of or following** (medical or surgical procedure) Y84.9
  - with misadventure — *see* Misadventure
  - amputation of limb(s) Y83.5
  - anastomosis (arteriovenous) (blood vessel) (gastrojejunal) (tendon) (natural or artificial material) Y83.2
  - aspiration (of fluid) Y84.4
    - tissue Y84.8
  - biopsy Y84.8
  - blood
    - sampling Y84.7
    - transfusion
      - procedure Y84.8
  - bypass Y83.2
  - catheterization (urinary) Y84.6
    - cardiac Y84.Ø
  - colostomy Y83.3
  - cystostomy Y83.3
  - dialysis (kidney) Y84.1
  - drug — *see* Table of Drugs and Chemicals
  - due to misadventure — *see* Misadventure
  - duodenostomy Y83.3
  - electroshock therapy Y84.3
  - external stoma, creation of Y83.3
  - formation of external stoma Y83.3
  - gastrostomy Y83.3
  - graft Y83.2
  - hypothermia (medically-induced) Y84.8
- **Complication** (delayed) **of or following** — *continued*
  - implant, implantation (of)
    - artificial
      - internal device (cardiac pacemaker) (electrodes in brain) (heart valve prosthesis) (orthopedic) Y83.1
      - material or tissue (for anastomosis or bypass) Y83.2
        - with creation of external stoma Y83.3
    - natural tissues (for anastomosis or bypass) Y83.2
      - with creation of external stoma Y83.3
  - infusion
    - procedure Y84.8
  - injection — *see* Table of Drugs and Chemicals
    - procedure Y84.8
  - insertion of gastric or duodenal sound Y84.5
  - insulin-shock therapy Y84.3
  - paracentesis (abdominal) (thoracic) (aspirative) Y84.4
  - procedures other than surgical operation — *see* Complication of or following, by type of procedure
  - radiological procedure or therapy Y84.2
  - removal of organ (partial) (total) NEC Y83.6
  - sampling
    - blood Y84.7
    - fluid NEC Y84.4
    - tissue Y84.8
  - shock therapy Y84.3
  - surgical operation NEC — *see also* Complication of or following, by type of operation Y83.9
    - reconstructive NEC Y83.4
      - with
        - anastomosis, bypass or graft Y83.2
        - formation of external stoma Y83.3
    - specified NEC Y83.8
  - transfusion — *see also* Table of Drugs and Chemicals
    - procedure Y84.8
  - transplant, transplantation (heart) (kidney) (liver) (whole organ, any) Y83.Ø
    - partial organ Y83.4
  - ureterostomy Y83.3
  - vaccination — *see also* Table of Drugs and Chemicals
    - procedure Y84.8
- **Compression**
  - divers' squeeze — *see* Air, pressure, change
  - trachea by
    - food (lodged in esophagus) — *see* categories T17 and T18 ☑
    - vomitus (lodged in esophagus) T17.81- ☑
- **Conflagration** — *see* Exposure, fire, uncontrolled
- **Constriction** (external)
  - hair W49.Ø1 ☑
  - jewelry W49.Ø4 ☑
  - ring W49.Ø4 ☑
  - rubber band W49.Ø3 ☑
  - specified item NEC W49.Ø9 ☑
  - string W49.Ø2 ☑
  - thread W49.Ø2 ☑
- **Contact** (accidental)
  - with
    - abrasive wheel (metalworking) W31.1 ☑
    - alligator W58.Ø9 ☑
      - bite W58.Ø1 ☑
      - crushing W58.Ø3 ☑
      - strike W58.Ø2 ☑
    - amphibian W62.9 ☑
      - frog W62.Ø ☑
      - toad W62.1 ☑
    - animal (nonvenomous) NEC W64 ☑
      - marine W56.89 ☑
        - bite W56.81 ☑
        - dolphin — *see* Contact, with, dolphin
        - fish NEC — *see* Contact, with, fish
        - mammal — *see* Contact, with, mammal, marine
        - orca — *see* Contact, with, orca
        - sea lion — *see* Contact, with, sea lion
        - shark — *see* Contact, with, shark
        - strike W56.82 ☑
    - animate mechanical force NEC W64 ☑
    - arrow W21.89 ☑
      - not thrown, projected or falling W45.8 ☑
    - arthropods (nonvenomous) W57 ☑
    - axe W27.Ø ☑
    - band-saw (industrial) W31.2 ☑
    - bayonet — *see* Bayonet wound
    - bee(s) X58 ☑
- **Contact** — *continued*
  - with — *continued*
    - bench-saw (industrial) W31.2 ☑
    - bird W61.99 ☑
      - bite W61.91 ☑
      - chicken — *see* Contact, with, chicken
      - duck — *see* Contact, with, duck
      - goose — *see* Contact, with, goose
      - macaw — *see* Contact, with, macaw
      - parrot — *see* Contact, with, parrot
      - psittacine — *see* Contact, with, psittacine
      - strike W61.92 ☑
      - turkey — *see* Contact, with, turkey
    - blender W29.Ø ☑
    - boiling water X12 ☑
      - stated as undetermined whether accidental or intentional Y27.2 ☑
      - suicide (attempt) X77.2 ☑
    - bore, earth-drilling or mining (land) (seabed) W31.Ø ☑
    - buffalo — *see* Contact, with, hoof stock NEC
    - bull W55.29 ☑
      - bite W55.21 ☑
      - gored W55.22 ☑
      - strike W55.22 ☑
    - bumper cars W31.81 ☑
    - camel — *see* Contact, with, hoof stock NEC
    - can
      - lid W26.8 ☑
      - opener W27.4 ☑
        - powered W29.Ø ☑
    - cat W55.Ø9 ☑
      - bite W55.Ø1 ☑
      - scratch W55.Ø3 ☑
    - caterpillar (venomous) X58 ☑
    - centipede (venomous) X58 ☑
    - chain
      - hoist W24.Ø ☑
        - agricultural operations W3Ø.89 ☑
      - saw W29.3 ☑
    - chicken W61.39 ☑
      - peck W61.33 ☑
      - strike W61.32 ☑
    - chisel W27.Ø ☑
    - circular saw W31.2 ☑
    - cobra X58 ☑
    - combine (harvester) W3Ø.Ø ☑
    - conveyer belt W24.1 ☑
    - cooker (hot) X15.8 ☑
      - stated as undetermined whether accidental or intentional Y27.3 ☑
      - suicide (attempt) X77.3 ☑
    - coral X58 ☑
    - cotton gin W31.82 ☑
    - cow W55.29 ☑
      - bite W55.21 ☑
      - strike W55.22 ☑
    - crane W24.Ø ☑
      - agricultural operations W3Ø.89 ☑
    - crocodile W58.19 ☑
      - bite W58.11 ☑
      - crushing W58.13 ☑
      - strike W58.12 ☑
    - dagger W26.1 ☑
      - stated as undetermined whether accidental or intentional Y28.2 ☑
      - suicide (attempt) X78.2 ☑
    - dairy equipment W31.82 ☑
    - dart W21.89 ☑
      - not thrown, projected or falling W45.8 ☑
    - deer — *see* Contact, with, hoof stock NEC
    - derrick W24.Ø ☑
      - agricultural operations W3Ø.89 ☑
        - hay W3Ø.2 ☑
    - dog W54.8 ☑
      - bite W54.Ø ☑
      - strike W54.1 ☑
    - dolphin W56.Ø9 ☑
      - bite W56.Ø1 ☑
      - strike W56.Ø2 ☑
    - donkey — *see* Contact, with, hoof stock NEC
    - drill (powered) W29.8 ☑
      - earth (land) (seabed) W31.Ø ☑
      - nonpowered W27.8 ☑
    - drive belt W24.Ø ☑
      - agricultural operations W3Ø.89 ☑

- **Contact** — *continued*
  - with — *continued*
    - mammal — *continued*
      - cat — *see* Contact, with, cat
      - cow — *see* Contact, with, cow
      - goat — *see* Contact, with, goat
      - hoof stock — *see* Contact, with, hoof stock
      - horse — *see* Contact, with, horse
      - marine W56.39 ☑
        - dolphin — *see* Contact, with, dolphin
        - orca — *see* Contact, with, orca
        - sea lion — *see* Contact, with, sea lion
        - specified NEC W56.39 ☑
          - bite W56.31 ☑
          - strike W56.32 ☑
      - pig — *see* Contact, with, pig
      - raccoon — *see* Contact, with, raccoon
      - rodent — *see* Contact, with, rodent
      - sheep — *see* Contact, with, sheep
      - specified NEC W55.89 ☑
        - bite W55.81 ☑
        - strike W55.82 ☑
    - marine
      - animal W56.89 ☑
        - bite W56.81 ☑
        - dolphin — *see* Contact, with, dolphin
        - fish NEC — *see* Contact, with, fish
        - mammal — *see* Contact, with, mammal, marine
        - orca — *see* Contact, with, orca
        - sea lion — *see* Contact, with, sea lion
        - shark — *see* Contact, with, shark
        - strike W56.82 ☑
    - meat
      - grinder (domestic) W29.Ø ☑
        - industrial W31.82 ☑
        - nonpowered W27.4 ☑
      - slicer (domestic) W29.Ø ☑
        - industrial W31.82 ☑
    - merry go round W31.81 ☑
    - metal, hot (liquid) (molten) NEC X18 ☑
    - millipede W57 ☑
    - nail W45.Ø ☑
      - gun W29.4 ☑
    - needle (sewing) W27.3 ☑
      - hypodermic W46.Ø ☑
        - contaminated W46.1 ☑
    - object (blunt) NEC
      - hot NEC X19 ☑
      - legal intervention — *see* Legal, intervention, blunt object
      - sharp NEC W45.8 ☑
        - inflicted by other person NEC W45.8 ☑
          - stated as
            - intentional homicide (attempt) — *see* Assault, cutting or piercing instrument
        - legal intervention — *see* Legal, intervention, sharp object
        - self-inflicted X78.9 ☑
    - orca W56.29 ☑
      - bite W56.21 ☑
      - strike W56.22 ☑
    - overhead plane W31.2 ☑
    - paper (as sharp object) W26.2 ☑
    - paper-cutter W27.5 ☑
    - parrot W61.Ø9 ☑
      - bite W61.Ø1 ☑
      - strike W61.Ø2 ☑
    - pig W55.49 ☑
      - bite W55.41 ☑
      - strike W55.42 ☑
    - pipe, hot X16 ☑
    - pitchfork W27.1 ☑
    - plane (metal) (wood) W27.Ø ☑
      - overhead W31.2 ☑
    - plant thorns, spines, sharp leaves or other mechanisms W6Ø ☑
    - powered
      - garden cultivator W29.3 ☑
      - household appliance, implement, or machine W29.8 ☑
      - saw (industrial) W31.2 ☑
        - hand W29.8 ☑
    - printing machine W31.89 ☑
    - psittacine bird W61.29 ☑
- **Contact** — *continued*
  - with — *continued*
    - psittacine bird — *continued*
      - bite W61.21 ☑
      - macaw — *see* Contact, with, macaw
      - parrot — *see* Contact, with, parrot
      - strike W61.22 ☑
    - pulley (block) (transmission) W24.Ø ☑
      - agricultural operations W3Ø.89 ☑
    - raccoon W55.59 ☑
      - bite W55.51 ☑
      - strike W55.52 ☑
    - radial-saw (industrial) W31.2 ☑
    - radiator (hot) X16 ☑
    - rake W27.1 ☑
    - rattlesnake X58 ☑
    - reaper W3Ø.Ø ☑
    - reptile W59.89 ☑
      - lizard — *see* Contact, with, lizard
      - snake — *see* Contact, with, snake
      - specified NEC W59.89 ☑
        - bite W59.81 ☑
        - crushing W59.83 ☑
        - strike W59.82 ☑
      - turtle — *see* Contact, with, turtle
    - rivet gun (powered) W29.4 ☑
    - road scraper — *see* Accident, transport, construction vehicle
    - rodent (feces) (urine) W53.89 ☑
      - bite W53.81 ☑
      - mouse W53.Ø9 ☑
        - bite W53.Ø1 ☑
      - rat W53.19 ☑
        - bite W53.11 ☑
      - specified NEC W53.89 ☑
        - bite W53.81 ☑
      - squirrel W53.29 ☑
        - bite W53.21 ☑
    - roller coaster W31.81 ☑
    - rope NEC W24.Ø ☑
      - agricultural operations W3Ø.89 ☑
    - saliva — *see* Contact, with, by type of animal
    - sander W29.8 ☑
      - industrial W31.2 ☑
    - saucepan (hot) (glass) (metal) X15.3 ☑
    - saw W27.Ø ☑
      - band (industrial) W31.2 ☑
      - bench (industrial) W31.2 ☑
      - chain W29.3 ☑
      - hand W27.Ø ☑
    - sawing machine, metal W31.1 ☑
    - scissors W27.2 ☑
    - scorpion X58 ☑
    - screwdriver W27.Ø ☑
      - powered W29.8 ☑
    - sea
      - anemone, cucumber or urchin (spine) X58 ☑
      - lion W56.19 ☑
        - bite W56.11 ☑
        - strike W56.12 ☑
    - serpent — *see* Contact, with, snake, by type
    - sewing-machine (electric) (powered) W29.2 ☑
      - not powered W27.8 ☑
    - shaft (hoist) (lift) (transmission) NEC W24.Ø ☑
      - agricultural W3Ø.89 ☑
    - shark W56.49 ☑
      - bite W56.41 ☑
      - strike W56.42 ☑
    - sharp object(s) W26.9 ☑
      - specified NEC W26.8 ☑
    - shears (hand) W27.2 ☑
      - powered (industrial) W31.1 ☑
        - domestic W29.2 ☑
    - sheep W55.39 ☑
      - bite W55.31 ☑
      - strike W55.32 ☑
    - shovel W27.8 ☑
      - steam — *see* Accident, transport, construction vehicle
    - snake (nonvenomous) W59.19 ☑
      - bite W59.11 ☑
      - crushing W59.13 ☑
      - strike W59.12 ☑
    - spade W27.1 ☑
    - spider (venomous) X58 ☑
    - spin-drier W29.2 ☑
- **Contact** — *continued*
  - with — *continued*
    - spinning machine W31.89 ☑
    - splinter W45.8 ☑
    - sports equipment W21.9 ☑
    - staple gun (powered) W29.8 ☑
    - steam X13.1 ☑
      - engine W31.3 ☑
      - inhalation X13.Ø ☑
      - pipe X16 ☑
      - shovel W31.89 ☑
    - stove (hot) (kitchen) X15.Ø ☑
    - substance, hot NEC X19 ☑
      - molten (metal) X18 ☑
    - sword W26.1 ☑
      - assault X99.2 ☑
      - stated as undetermined whether accidental or intentional Y28.2 ☑
      - suicide (attempt) X78.2 ☑
    - tarantula X58 ☑
    - thresher W3Ø.Ø ☑
    - tin can lid W26.8 ☑
    - toad W62.1 ☑
    - toaster (hot) X15.1 ☑
    - tool W27.8 ☑
      - hand (not powered) W27.8 ☑
        - auger W27.Ø ☑
        - axe W27.Ø ☑
        - can opener W27.4 ☑
        - chisel W27.Ø ☑
        - fork W27.4 ☑
        - garden W27.1 ☑
        - handsaw W27.Ø ☑
        - hoe W27.1 ☑
        - ice-pick W27.4 ☑
        - kitchen utensil W27.4 ☑
        - manual
          - lawn mower W27.1 ☑
          - sewing machine W27.8 ☑
        - meat grinder W27.4 ☑
        - needle (sewing) W27.3 ☑
          - hypodermic W46.Ø ☑
            - contaminated W46.1 ☑
        - paper cutter W27.5 ☑
        - pitchfork W27.1 ☑
        - rake W27.1 ☑
        - scissors W27.2 ☑
        - screwdriver W27.Ø ☑
        - specified NEC W27.8 ☑
        - workbench W27.Ø ☑
      - hot X17 ☑
      - powered W29.8 ☑
        - blender W29.Ø ☑
          - commercial W31.82 ☑
        - can opener W29.Ø ☑
          - commercial W31.82 ☑
        - chainsaw W29.3 ☑
        - clothes dryer W29.2 ☑
          - commercial W31.82 ☑
        - dishwasher W29.2 ☑
          - commercial W31.82 ☑
        - edger W29.3 ☑
        - electric fan W29.2 ☑
          - commercial W31.82 ☑
        - electric knife W29.1 ☑
        - food processor W29.Ø ☑
          - commercial W31.82 ☑
        - garbage disposal W29.Ø ☑
          - commercial W31.82 ☑
        - garden tool W29.3 ☑
        - hedge trimmer W29.3 ☑
        - ice maker W29.Ø ☑
          - commercial W31.82 ☑
        - kitchen appliance W29.Ø ☑
          - commercial W31.82 ☑
        - lawn mower W28 ☑
        - meat grinder W29.Ø ☑
          - commercial W31.82 ☑
        - mixer W29.Ø ☑
          - commercial W31.82 ☑
        - rototiller W29.3 ☑
        - sewing machine W29.2 ☑
          - commercial W31.82 ☑
        - washing machine W29.2 ☑
          - commercial W31.82 ☑

- **Contact** — *continued*
  - with — *continued*
    - transmission device (belt, cable, chain, gear, pinion, shaft) W24.1 ☑
      - agricultural operations W30.89 ☑
    - turbine (gas) (water-driven) W31.3 ☑
    - turkey W61.49 ☑
      - peck W61.43 ☑
      - strike W61.42 ☑
    - turtle (nonvenomous) W59.29 ☑
      - bite W59.21 ☑
      - strike W59.22 ☑
      - terrestrial W59.89 ☑
        - bite W59.81 ☑
        - crushing W59.83 ☑
        - strike W59.82 ☑
    - under-cutter W31.0 ☑
    - urine — *see* Contact, with, by type of animal
    - vehicle
      - agricultural use (transport) — *see* Accident, transport, agricultural vehicle
        - not on public highway W30.81 ☑
      - industrial use (transport) — *see* Accident, transport, industrial vehicle
        - not on public highway W31.83 ☑
      - off-road use (transport) — *see* Accident, transport, all-terrain or off-road vehicle
        - not on public highway W31.83 ☑
      - special construction use (transport) — *see* Accident, transport, construction vehicle
        - not on public highway W31.83 ☑
    - venomous
      - animal X58 ☑
      - arthropods X58 ☑
      - lizard X58 ☑
      - marine animal NEC X58 ☑
      - marine plant NEC X58 ☑
      - millipedes (tropical) X58 ☑
      - plant(s) X58 ☑
      - snake X58 ☑
      - spider X58 ☑
    - viper X58 ☑
    - washing-machine (powered) W29.2 ☑
    - wasp X58 ☑
    - weaving-machine W31.89 ☑
    - winch W24.0 ☑
      - agricultural operations W30.89 ☑
    - wire NEC W24.0 ☑
      - agricultural operations W30.89 ☑
    - wood slivers W45.8 ☑
    - yellow jacket X58 ☑
    - zebra — *see* Contact, with, hoof stock NEC
  - pressure X50.9 ☑
  - stress X50.9 ☑
- **Coup de soleil** X32 ☑
- **Crash**
  - aircraft (in transit) (powered) V95.9 ☑
    - balloon V96.01 ☑
    - fixed wing NEC (private) V95.21 ☑
      - commercial V95.31 ☑
    - glider V96.21 ☑
      - hang V96.11 ☑
      - powered V95.11 ☑
    - helicopter V95.01 ☑
    - in war operations — *see* War operations, destruction of aircraft
    - microlight V95.11 ☑
    - nonpowered V96.9 ☑
      - specified NEC V96.8 ☑
    - powered NEC V95.8 ☑
    - stated as
      - homicide (attempt) Y08.81 ☑
      - suicide (attempt) X83.0 ☑
    - ultralight V95.11 ☑
  - spacecraft V95.41 ☑
  - transport vehicle NEC — *see also* Accident, transport V89.9 ☑
    - homicide (attempt) Y03.8 ☑
    - motor NEC (traffic) V89.2 ☑
      - homicide (attempt) Y03.8 ☑
      - suicide (attempt) — *see* Suicide, collision
- **Cruelty** (mental) (physical) (sexual) X58 ☑
- **Crushed** (accidentally) X58 ☑
  - between objects (moving) (stationary and moving) W23.0 ☑
    - stationary W23.1 ☑
- **Crushed** — *continued*
  - by
    - alligator W58.03 ☑
    - avalanche NEC — *see* Landslide
    - cave-in W20.0 ☑
      - caused by cataclysmic earth surface movement — *see* Landslide
    - crocodile W58.13 ☑
    - crowd or human stampede W52 ☑
    - falling
      - aircraft V97.39 ☑
        - in war operations — *see* War operations, destruction of aircraft
      - earth, material W20.0 ☑
        - caused by cataclysmic earth surface movement — *see* Landslide
      - object NEC W20.8 ☑
    - landslide NEC — *see* Landslide
    - lizard (nonvenomous) W59.09 ☑
    - machinery — *see* Contact, with, by type of machine
    - reptile NEC W59.89 ☑
    - snake (nonvenomous) W59.13 ☑
  - in
    - machinery — *see* Contact, with, by type of machine
- **Cut, cutting** (any part of body) (accidental) — *see also* Contact, with, by object or machine
  - during medical or surgical treatment as misadventure — *see* Index to Diseases and Injuries, Complications
  - homicide (attempt) — *see* Assault, cutting or piercing instrument
  - inflicted by other person — *see* Assault, cutting or piercing instrument
  - legal
    - execution — *see* Legal, intervention
    - intervention — *see* Legal, intervention, sharp object
  - machine NEC — *see also* Contact, with, by type of machine W31.9 ☑
  - self-inflicted — *see* Suicide, cutting or piercing instrument
  - suicide (attempt) — *see* Suicide, cutting or piercing instrument
- **Cyclone** (any injury) X37.1 ☑

D

- **Decapitation** (accidental circumstances) NEC X58 ☑
  - homicide X99.9 ☑
  - legal execution — *see* Legal, intervention
- **Dehydration from lack of water** X58 ☑
- **Deprivation** X58 ☑
- **Derailment** (accidental)
  - railway (rolling stock) (train) (vehicle) (without antecedent collision) V81.7 ☑
    - with antecedent collision — *see* Accident, transport, railway vehicle occupant
  - streetcar (without antecedent collision) V82.7 ☑
    - with antecedent collision — *see* Accident, transport, streetcar occupant
- **Descent**
  - parachute (voluntary) (without accident to aircraft) V97.29 ☑
    - due to accident to aircraft — *see* Accident, transport, aircraft
- **Desertion** X58 ☑
- **Destitution** X58 ☑
- **Disability, late effect or sequela of injury** — *see* Sequelae
- **Discharge** (accidental)
  - airgun W34.010 ☑
    - assault X95.01 ☑
    - homicide (attempt) X95.01 ☑
    - stated as undetermined whether accidental or intentional Y24.0 ☑
    - suicide (attempt) X74.01 ☑
  - BB gun — *see* Discharge, airgun
  - firearm (accidental) W34.00 ☑
    - assault X95.9 ☑
    - handgun (pistol) (revolver) W32.0 ☑
      - assault X93 ☑
      - homicide (attempt) X93 ☑
      - legal intervention — *see* Legal, intervention, firearm, handgun
      - stated as undetermined whether accidental or intentional Y22 ☑
      - suicide (attempt) X72 ☑
- **Discharge** — *continued*
  - firearm — *continued*
    - homicide (attempt) X95.9 ☑
    - hunting rifle W33.02 ☑
      - assault X94.1 ☑
      - homicide (attempt) X94.1 ☑
      - legal intervention
        - injuring
          - bystander Y35.032 ☑
          - law enforcement personnel Y35.031 ☑
          - suspect Y35.033 ☑
          - unspecified person Y35.039 ☑
      - stated as undetermined whether accidental or intentional Y23.1 ☑
      - suicide (attempt) X73.1 ☑
    - larger W33.00 ☑
      - assault X94.9 ☑
      - homicide (attempt) X94.9 ☑
      - hunting rifle — *see* Discharge, firearm, hunting rifle
      - legal intervention — *see* Legal, intervention, firearm by type of firearm
      - machine gun — *see* Discharge, firearm, machine gun
      - shotgun — *see* Discharge, firearm, shotgun
      - specified NEC W33.09 ☑
        - assault X94.8 ☑
        - homicide (attempt) X94.8 ☑
        - legal intervention
          - injuring
            - bystander Y35.092 ☑
            - law enforcement personnel Y35.091 ☑
            - suspect Y35.093 ☑
            - unspecified person Y35.099 ☑
        - stated as undetermined whether accidental or intentional Y23.8 ☑
        - suicide (attempt) X73.8 ☑
      - stated as undetermined whether accidental or intentional Y23.9 ☑
      - suicide (attempt) X73.9 ☑
    - legal intervention
      - injuring
        - bystander Y35.002 ☑
        - law enforcement personnel Y35.001 ☑
        - suspect Y35.03 ☑
        - unspecified person Y35.009 ☑
      - using rubber bullet
        - injuring
          - bystander Y35.042 ☑
          - law enforcement personnel Y35.041 ☑
          - suspect Y35.043 ☑
          - unspecified person Y35.049 ☑
    - machine gun W33.03 ☑
      - assault X94.2 ☑
      - homicide (attempt) X94.2 ☑
      - legal intervention — *see* Legal, intervention, firearm, machine gun
      - stated as undetermined whether accidental or intentional Y23.3 ☑
      - suicide (attempt) X73.2 ☑
    - pellet gun — *see* Discharge, airgun
    - shotgun W33.01 ☑
      - assault X94.0 ☑
      - homicide (attempt) X94.0 ☑
      - legal intervention — *see* Legal, intervention, firearm, specified NEC
      - stated as undetermined whether accidental or intentional Y23.0 ☑
      - suicide (attempt) X73.0 ☑
    - specified NEC W34.09 ☑
      - assault X95.8 ☑
      - homicide (attempt) X95.8 ☑
      - legal intervention — *see* Legal, intervention, firearm, specified NEC
      - stated as undetermined whether accidental or intentional Y24.8 ☑
      - suicide (attempt) X74.8 ☑
    - stated as undetermined whether accidental or intentional Y24.9 ☑
    - suicide (attempt) X74.9 ☑
    - Very pistol W34.09 ☑
      - assault X95.8 ☑
      - homicide (attempt) X95.8 ☑
      - stated as undetermined whether accidental or intentional Y24.8 ☑

Discharge — *continued*
- firearm — *continued*
  - Very pistol — *continued*
    - suicide (attempt) X74.8 ☑
- firework(s) W39 ☑
  - stated as undetermined whether accidental or intentional Y25 ☑
- gas-operated gun NEC W34.Ø18 ☑
  - airgun — *see* Discharge, airgun
  - assault X95.Ø9 ☑
  - homicide (attempt) X95.Ø9 ☑
  - paintball gun — *see* Discharge, paintball gun
  - stated as undetermined whether accidental or intentional Y24.8 ☑
  - suicide (attempt) X74.Ø9 ☑
- gun NEC — *see also* Discharge, firearm NEC
  - air — *see* Discharge, airgun
  - BB — *see* Discharge, airgun
  - for single hand use — *see* Discharge, firearm, handgun
  - hand — *see* Discharge, firearm, handgun
  - machine — *see* Discharge, firearm, machine gun
  - other specified — *see* Discharge, firearm NEC
  - paintball — *see* Discharge, paintball gun
  - pellet — *see* Discharge, airgun
- handgun — *see* Discharge, firearm, handgun
- machine gun — *see* Discharge, firearm, machine gun
- paintball gun W34.Ø11 ☑
  - assault X95.Ø2 ☑
  - homicide (attempt) X95.Ø2 ☑
  - stated as undetermined whether accidental or intentional Y24.8 ☑
  - suicide (attempt) X74.Ø2 ☑
- pistol — *see* Discharge, firearm, handgun
  - flare — *see* Discharge, firearm, Very pistol
  - pellet — *see* Discharge, airgun
  - Very — *see* Discharge, firearm, Very pistol
- revolver — *see* Discharge, firearm, handgun
- rifle (hunting) — *see* Discharge, firearm, hunting rifle
- shotgun — *see* Discharge, firearm, shotgun
- spring-operated gun NEC W34.Ø18 ☑
  - assault X95.Ø9 ☑
  - homicide (attempt) X95.Ø9 ☑
  - stated as undetermined whether accidental or intentional Y24.8 ☑
  - suicide (attempt) X74.Ø9 ☑

Disease
- Andes W94.11 ☑
- aviator's — *see* Air, pressure
- range W94.11 ☑

Diver's disease, palsy, paralysis, squeeze — *see* Air, pressure

Diving (into water) — *see* Accident, diving

Dog bite W54.Ø ☑

Dragged by transport vehicle NEC — *see also* Accident, transport VØ9.9 ☑

Drinking poison (accidental) — *see* Table of Drugs and Chemicals

Dropped (accidentally) **while being carried or supported by other person** WØ4 ☑

Drowning (accidental) W74 ☑
- assault X92.9 ☑
- due to
  - accident (to)
    - machinery — *see* Contact, with, by type of machine
    - watercraft V9Ø.89 ☑
      - burning V9Ø.29 ☑
        - powered V9Ø.23 ☑
          - fishing boat V9Ø.22 ☑
          - jetskis V9Ø.23 ☑
          - merchant ship V9Ø.2Ø ☑
          - passenger ship V9Ø.21 ☑
        - unpowered V9Ø.28 ☑
          - canoe V9Ø.25 ☑
          - inflatable V9Ø.26 ☑
          - kayak V9Ø.25 ☑
          - sailboat V9Ø.24 ☑
          - water skis V9Ø.27 ☑
      - crushed V9Ø.39 ☑
        - powered V9Ø.33 ☑
          - fishing boat V9Ø.32 ☑
          - jetskis V9Ø.33 ☑
          - merchant ship V9Ø.3Ø ☑
          - passenger ship V9Ø.31 ☑
        - unpowered V9Ø.38 ☑

Drowning — *continued*
- due to — *continued*
  - accident — *continued*
    - watercraft — *continued*
      - crushed — *continued*
        - unpowered — *continued*
          - canoe V9Ø.35 ☑
          - inflatable V9Ø.36 ☑
          - kayak V9Ø.35 ☑
          - sailboat V9Ø.34 ☑
          - water skis V9Ø.37 ☑
      - overturning V9Ø.Ø9 ☑
        - powered V9Ø.Ø3 ☑
          - fishing boat V9Ø.Ø2 ☑
          - jetskis V9Ø.Ø3 ☑
          - merchant ship V9Ø.ØØ ☑
          - passenger ship V9Ø.Ø1 ☑
        - unpowered V9Ø.Ø8 ☑
          - canoe V9Ø.Ø5 ☑
          - inflatable V9Ø.Ø6 ☑
          - kayak V9Ø.Ø5 ☑
          - sailboat V9Ø.Ø4 ☑
      - sinking V9Ø.19 ☑
        - powered V9Ø.13 ☑
          - fishing boat V9Ø.12 ☑
          - jetskis V9Ø.13 ☑
          - merchant ship V9Ø.1Ø ☑
          - passenger ship V9Ø.11 ☑
        - unpowered V9Ø.18 ☑
          - canoe V9Ø.15 ☑
          - inflatable V9Ø.16 ☑
          - kayak V9Ø.15 ☑
          - sailboat V9Ø.14 ☑
      - specified type NEC V9Ø.89 ☑
        - powered V9Ø.83 ☑
          - fishing boat V9Ø.82 ☑
          - jetskis V9Ø.83 ☑
          - merchant ship V9Ø.8Ø ☑
          - passenger ship V9Ø.81 ☑
        - unpowered V9Ø.88 ☑
          - canoe V9Ø.85 ☑
          - inflatable V9Ø.86 ☑
          - kayak V9Ø.85 ☑
          - sailboat V9Ø.84 ☑
          - water skis V9Ø.87 ☑
  - avalanche — *see* Landslide
  - cataclysmic
    - earth surface movement NEC — *see* Forces of nature, earth movement
    - storm — *see* Forces of nature, cataclysmic storm
  - cloudburst X37.8 ☑
  - cyclone X37.1 ☑
  - fall overboard (from) V92.Ø9 ☑
    - powered craft V92.Ø3 ☑
      - ferry boat V92.Ø1 ☑
      - fishing boat V92.Ø2 ☑
      - jetskis V92.Ø3 ☑
      - liner V92.Ø1 ☑
      - merchant ship V92.ØØ ☑
      - passenger ship V92.Ø1 ☑
    - resulting from
      - accident to watercraft — *see* Drowning, due to, accident to, watercraft
      - being washed overboard (from) V92.29 ☑
        - powered craft V92.23 ☑
          - ferry boat V92.21 ☑
          - fishing boat V92.22 ☑
          - jetskis V92.23 ☑
          - liner V92.21 ☑
          - merchant ship V92.2Ø ☑
          - passenger ship V92.21 ☑
        - unpowered craft V92.28 ☑
          - canoe V92.25 ☑
          - inflatable V92.26 ☑
          - kayak V92.25 ☑
          - sailboat V92.24 ☑
          - surf-board V92.28 ☑
          - water skis V92.27 ☑
          - windsurfer V92.28 ☑
      - motion of watercraft V92.19 ☑
        - powered craft V92.13 ☑
          - ferry boat V92.11 ☑
          - fishing boat V92.12 ☑
          - jetskis V92.13 ☑
          - liner V92.11 ☑
          - merchant ship V92.1Ø ☑

Drowning — *continued*
- due to — *continued*
  - fall overboard — *continued*
    - resulting from — *continued*
      - motion of watercraft — *continued*
        - powered craft — *continued*
          - passenger ship V92.11 ☑
        - unpowered craft
          - canoe V92.15 ☑
          - inflatable V92.16 ☑
          - kayak V92.15 ☑
          - sailboat V92.14 ☑
    - unpowered craft V92.Ø8 ☑
      - canoe V92.Ø5 ☑
      - inflatable V92.Ø6 ☑
      - kayak V92.Ø5 ☑
      - sailboat V92.Ø4 ☑
      - surf-board V92.Ø8 ☑
      - water skis V92.Ø7 ☑
      - windsurfer V92.Ø8 ☑
  - hurricane X37.Ø ☑
  - jumping into water from watercraft (involved in accident) — *see also* Drowning, due to, accident to, watercraft
    - without accident to or on watercraft W16.711 ☑
  - tidal wave NEC — *see* Forces of nature, tidal wave
  - torrential rain X37.8 ☑
- following
  - fall
    - into
      - bathtub W16.211 ☑
      - bucket W16.221 ☑
      - fountain — *see* Drowning, following, fall, into, water, specified NEC
      - quarry — *see* Drowning, following, fall, into, water, specified NEC
      - reservoir — *see* Drowning, following, fall, into, water, specified NEC
      - swimming-pool W16.Ø11 ☑
        - stated as undetermined whether accidental or intentional Y21.3 ☑
        - striking
          - bottom W16.Ø21 ☑
          - wall W16.Ø31 ☑
        - suicide (attempt) X71.2 ☑
      - water NOS W16.41 ☑
        - natural (lake) (open sea) (river) (stream) (pond) W16.111 ☑
          - striking
            - bottom W16.121 ☑
            - side W16.131 ☑
        - specified NEC W16.311 ☑
          - striking
            - bottom W16.321 ☑
            - wall W16.331 ☑
    - overboard NEC — *see* Drowning, due to, fall overboard
  - jump or dive
    - from boat W16.711 ☑
      - striking bottom W16.721 ☑
    - into
      - fountain — *see* Drowning, following, jump or dive, into, water, specified NEC
      - quarry — *see* Drowning, following, jump or dive, into, water, specified NEC
      - reservoir — *see* Drowning, following, jump or dive, into, water, specified NEC
      - swimming-pool W16.511 ☑
        - striking
          - bottom W16.521 ☑
          - wall W16.531 ☑
        - suicide (attempt) X71.2 ☑
      - water NOS W16.91 ☑
        - natural (lake) (open sea) (river) (stream) (pond) W16.611 ☑
        - specified NEC W16.811 ☑
          - bottom W16.821 ☑
          - striking
            - bottom W16.821 ☑
            - wall W16.831 ☑
        - striking
          - bottom W16.821 ☑
          - wall W16.831 ☑
        - striking bottom W16.621 ☑
- homicide (attempt) X92.9 ☑
- in
  - bathtub (accidental) W65 ☑

- **Drowning** — *continued*
  - in — *continued*
    - bathtub — *continued*
      - assault X92.0 ☑
      - following fall W16.211 ☑
        - stated as undetermined whether accidental or intentional Y21.1 ☑
      - stated as undetermined whether accidental or intentional Y21.0 ☑
      - suicide (attempt) X71.0 ☑
    - lake — *see* Drowning, in, natural water
    - natural water (lake) (open sea) (river) (stream) (pond) W69 ☑
      - assault X92.3 ☑
      - following
        - dive or jump W16.611 ☑
          - striking bottom W16.621 ☑
        - fall W16.111 ☑
          - striking
            - bottom W16.121 ☑
            - side W16.131 ☑
      - stated as undetermined whether accidental or intentional Y21.4 ☑
      - suicide (attempt) X71.3 ☑
    - quarry — *see* Drowning, in, specified place NEC
    - quenching tank — *see* Drowning, in, specified place NEC
    - reservoir — *see* Drowning, in, specified place NEC
    - river — *see* Drowning, in, natural water
    - sea — *see* Drowning, in, natural water
    - specified place NEC W73 ☑
      - assault X92.8 ☑
      - following
        - dive or jump W16.811 ☑
          - striking
            - bottom W16.821 ☑
            - wall W16.831 ☑
        - fall W16.311 ☑
          - striking
            - bottom W16.321 ☑
            - wall W16.331 ☑
      - stated as undetermined whether accidental or intentional Y21.8 ☑
      - suicide (attempt) X71.8 ☑
    - stream — *see* Drowning, in, natural water
    - swimming-pool W67 ☑
      - assault X92.1 ☑
        - following fall X92.2 ☑
      - following
        - dive or jump W16.511 ☑
          - striking
            - bottom W16.521 ☑
            - wall W16.531 ☑
        - fall W16.011 ☑
          - striking
            - bottom W16.021 ☑
            - wall W16.031 ☑
      - stated as undetermined whether accidental or intentional Y21.2 ☑
        - following fall Y21.3 ☑
      - suicide (attempt) X71.1 ☑
        - following fall X71.2 ☑
    - war operations — *see* War operations, restriction of airway
  - resulting from accident to watercraft — *see* Drowning, due to, accident, watercraft
  - self-inflicted X71.9 ☑
  - stated as undetermined whether accidental or intentional Y21.9 ☑
  - suicide (attempt) X71.9 ☑

E

- **Earth falling** (on) W20.0 ☑
  - caused by cataclysmic earth surface movement or eruption — *see* Landslide
- **Earth** (surface) **movement NEC** — *see* Forces of nature, earth movement
- **Earthquake** (any injury) X34 ☑
- **Effect**(s) (adverse) **of**
  - air pressure (any) — *see* Air, pressure
  - cold, excessive (exposure to) — *see* Exposure, cold
  - heat (excessive) — *see* Heat
  - hot place (weather) — *see* Heat
  - insolation X30 ☑
  - late — *see* Sequelae
- **Effect**(s) (adverse) **of** — *continued*
  - motion — *see* Motion
  - nuclear explosion or weapon in war operations — *see* War operations, nuclear weapon
  - radiation — *see* Radiation
  - travel — *see* Travel
- **Electric shock** (accidental) (by) (in) — *see* Exposure, electric current
- **Electrocution** (accidental) — *see* Exposure, electric current
- **Endotracheal tube wrongly placed during anesthetic procedure**
- **Entanglement**
  - in
    - bed linen, causing suffocation T71 ☑
    - wheel of pedal cycle V19.88 ☑
- **Entry of foreign body or material** — *see* Foreign body
- **Environmental pollution related condition** — *see* category Z57 ☑
- **Execution, legal** (any method) — *see* Legal, intervention
- **Exhaustion**
  - cold — *see* Exposure, cold
  - due to excessive exertion — *see also* Overexertion X50.9 ☑
  - heat — *see* Heat
- **Explosion** (accidental) (of) (with secondary fire) W40.9 ☑
  - acetylene W40.1 ☑
  - aerosol can W36.1 ☑
  - air tank (compressed) (in machinery) W36.2 ☑
  - aircraft (in transit) (powered) NEC V95.9 ☑
    - balloon V96.05 ☑
    - fixed wing NEC (private) V95.25 ☑
      - commercial V95.35 ☑
    - glider V96.25 ☑
      - hang V96.15 ☑
      - powered V95.15 ☑
    - helicopter V95.05 ☑
    - in war operations — *see* War operations, destruction of aircraft
    - microlight V95.15 ☑
    - nonpowered V96.9 ☑
      - specified NEC V96.8 ☑
    - powered NEC V95.8 ☑
    - stated as
      - homicide (attempt) Y03.8 ☑
      - suicide (attempt) X83.0 ☑
    - ultralight V95.15 ☑
  - anesthetic gas in operating room W40.1 ☑
  - antipersonnel bomb W40.8 ☑
    - assault X96.0 ☑
    - homicide (attempt) X96.0 ☑
    - suicide (attempt) X75 ☑
  - assault X96.9 ☑
  - bicycle tire W37.0 ☑
  - blasting (cap) (materials) W40.0 ☑
  - boiler (machinery), not on transport vehicle W35 ☑
    - on watercraft — *see* Explosion, in, watercraft
  - butane W40.1 ☑
  - caused by other person X96.9 ☑
  - coal gas W40.1 ☑
  - detonator W40.0 ☑
  - dump (munitions) W40.8 ☑
  - dynamite W40.0 ☑
    - in
      - assault X96.8 ☑
      - homicide (attempt) X96.8 ☑
      - legal intervention
        - injuring
          - bystander Y35.112 ☑
          - law enforcement personnel Y35.111 ☑
          - suspect Y35.113 ☑
          - unspecified person Y35.119 ☑
      - suicide (attempt) X75 ☑
  - explosive (material) W40.9 ☑
    - gas W40.1 ☑
    - in blasting operation W40.0 ☑
    - specified NEC W40.8 ☑
      - in
        - assault X96.8 ☑
        - homicide (attempt) X96.8 ☑
        - legal intervention
          - injuring
            - bystander Y35.192 ☑
            - law enforcement personnel Y35.191 ☑
            - suspect Y35.193 ☑
- **Explosion** — *continued*
  - explosive — *continued*
    - specified — *continued*
      - in — *continued*
        - legal intervention — *continued*
          - injuring — *continued*
            - unspecified person Y35.199 ☑
        - suicide (attempt) X75 ☑
  - factory (munitions) W40.8 ☑
  - fertilizer bomb W40.8 ☑
    - assault X96.3 ☑
    - homicide (attempt) X96.3 ☑
    - suicide (attempt) X75 ☑
  - firearm (parts) NEC W34.19 ☑
    - airgun W34.110 ☑
    - BB gun W34.110 ☑
    - gas, air or spring-operated gun NEC W34.118 ☑
    - hangun W32.1 ☑
    - hunting rifle W33.12 ☑
    - larger firearm W33.10 ☑
      - specified NEC W33.19 ☑
    - machine gun W33.13 ☑
    - paintball gun W34.111 ☑
    - pellet gun W34.110 ☑
    - shotgun W33.11 ☑
    - Very pistol [flare] W34.19 ☑
  - fire-damp W40.1 ☑
  - fireworks W39 ☑
  - gas (coal) (explosive) W40.1 ☑
    - cylinder W36.9 ☑
      - aerosol can W36.1 ☑
      - air tank W36.2 ☑
      - pressurized W36.3 ☑
      - specified NEC W36.8 ☑
  - gasoline (fumes) (tank) not in moving motor vehicle W40.1 ☑
    - bomb W40.8 ☑
      - assault X96.1 ☑
      - homicide (attempt) X96.1 ☑
      - suicide (attempt) X75 ☑
    - in motor vehicle — *see* Accident, transport, by type of vehicle
  - grain store W40.8 ☑
  - grenade W40.8 ☑
    - in
      - assault X96.8 ☑
      - homicide (attempt) X96.8 ☑
      - legal intervention
        - injuring
          - bystander Y35.192 ☑
          - law enforcement personnel Y35.191 ☑
          - suspect Y35.193 ☑
          - unspecified person Y35.199 ☑
      - suicide (attempt) X75 ☑
  - handgun (parts) — *see* Explosion, firearm, hangun (parts)
  - homicide (attempt) X96.9 ☑
    - antipersonnel bomb — *see* Explosion, antipersonnel bomb
    - fertilizer bomb — *see* Explosion, fertilizer bomb
    - gasoline bomb — *see* Explosion, gasoline bomb
    - letter bomb — *see* Explosion, letter bomb
    - pipe bomb — *see* Explosion, pipe bomb
    - specified NEC X96.8 ☑
  - hose, pressurized W37.8 ☑
  - hot water heater, tank (in machinery) W35 ☑
    - on watercraft — *see* Explosion, in, watercraft
  - in, on
    - dump W40.8 ☑
    - factory W40.8 ☑
    - mine (of explosive gases) NEC W40.1 ☑
    - watercraft V93.59 ☑
      - powered craft V93.53 ☑
        - ferry boat V93.51 ☑
        - fishing boat V93.52 ☑
        - jetskis V93.53 ☑
        - liner V93.51 ☑
        - merchant ship V93.50 ☑
        - passenger ship V93.51 ☑
        - sailboat V93.54 ☑
  - letter bomb W40.8 ☑
    - assault X96.2 ☑
    - homicide (attempt) X96.2 ☑
    - suicide (attempt) X75 ☑
  - machinery — *see also* Contact, with, by type of machine

External Causes Index

Drowning — Explosion

Exposure — *continued*
- gravitational forces (abnormal) W49.9 ☑
- heat (natural) NEC — *see* Heat
- high-pressure jet (hydraulic) (pneumatic) W49.9 ☑
- hydraulic jet W49.9 ☑
- inanimate mechanical force W49.9 ☑
- jet, high-pressure (hydraulic) (pneumatic) W49.9 ☑
- lightning — *see* subcategory T75.Ø ☑
  - causing fire — *see* Exposure, fire
- mechanical forces NEC W49.9 ☑
  - animate NEC W64 ☑
  - inanimate NEC W49.9 ☑
- noise W42.9 ☑
  - supersonic W42.Ø ☑
- noxious substance — *see* Table of Drugs and Chemicals
- pneumatic jet W49.9 ☑
- prolonged in deep-freeze unit or refrigerator W93.2 ☑
- radiation — *see* Radiation
- smoke — *see also* Exposure, fire
  - tobacco, second hand Z77.22
- specified factors NEC X58 ☑
- sunlight X32 ☑
  - man-made (sun lamp) W89.8 ☑
    - tanning bed W89.1 ☑
- supersonic waves W42.Ø ☑
- transmission line(s), electric W85 ☑
- vibration W49.9 ☑
- waves
  - infrasound W49.9 ☑
  - sound W42.9 ☑
  - supersonic W42.Ø ☑
- weather NEC — *see* Forces of nature

External cause status Y99.9
- child assisting in compensated work for family Y99.8
- civilian activity done for financial or other compensation Y99.Ø
- civilian activity done for income or pay Y99.Ø
- family member assisting in compensated work for other family member Y99.8
- hobby not done for income Y99.8
- leisure activity Y99.8
- military activity Y99.1
- off-duty activity of military personnel Y99.8
- recreation or sport not for income or while a student Y99.8
- specified NEC Y99.8
- student activity Y99.8
- volunteer activity Y99.2

F

Factors, supplemental
- alcohol
  - blood level
    - less than 2Ømg/1ØØml Y9Ø.Ø
    - presence in blood, level not specified Y9Ø.9
    - 2Ø-39mg/1ØØml Y9Ø.1
    - 4Ø-59mg/1ØØml Y9Ø.2
    - 6Ø-79mg/1ØØml Y9Ø.3
    - 8Ø-99mg/1ØØml Y9Ø.4
    - 1ØØ-119mg/1ØØml Y9Ø.5
    - 12Ø-199mg/1ØØml Y9Ø.6
    - 2ØØ-239mg/1ØØml Y9Ø.7
    - 24Ømg/1ØØml or more Y9Ø.8
  - presence in blood, but level not specified Y9Ø.9
- environmental-pollution-related condition- see Z57 ☑
- nosocomial condition Y95
- work-related condition Y99.Ø

Failure
- in suture or ligature during surgical procedure Y65.2
- mechanical, of instrument or apparatus (any) (during any medical or surgical procedure) Y65.8
- sterile precautions (during medical and surgical care) — *see* Misadventure, failure, sterile precautions, by type of procedure
- to
  - introduce tube or instrument Y65.4
    - endotracheal tube during anesthesia Y65.3
  - make curve (transport vehicle) NEC — *see* Accident, transport
  - remove tube or instrument Y65.4

Fall, falling (accidental) W19 ☑
- building W2Ø.1 ☑
  - burning (uncontrolled fire) XØØ.3 ☑
- down
  - embankment W17.81 ☑
  - escalator W1Ø.Ø ☑
  - hill W17.81 ☑
  - ladder W11 ☑
  - ramp W1Ø.2 ☑
  - stairs, steps W1Ø.9 ☑
- due to
  - bumping against
    - object W18.ØØ ☑
      - sharp glass W18.Ø2 ☑
      - specified NEC W18.Ø9 ☑
      - sports equipment W18.Ø1 ☑
    - person WØ3 ☑
      - due to ice or snow WØØ.Ø ☑
      - on pedestrian conveyance — *see* Accident, transport, pedestrian, conveyance
  - collision with another person WØ3 ☑
    - due to ice or snow WØØ.Ø ☑
    - involving pedestrian conveyance — *see* Accident, transport, pedestrian, conveyance
  - grocery cart tipping over W17.82 ☑
  - ice or snow WØØ.9 ☑
    - from one level to another WØØ.2 ☑
      - on stairs or steps WØØ.1 ☑
    - involving pedestrian conveyance — *see* Accident, transport, pedestrian, conveyance
    - on same level WØØ.Ø ☑
  - slipping (on moving sidewalk) WØ1.Ø ☑
    - with subsequent striking against object WØ1.1Ø ☑
      - furniture WØ1.19Ø ☑
      - sharp object WØ1.119 ☑
        - glass WØ1.11Ø ☑
        - power tool or machine WØ1.111 ☑
        - specified NEC WØ1.118 ☑
      - specified NEC WØ1.198 ☑
  - striking against
    - object W18.ØØ ☑
      - sharp glass W18.Ø2 ☑
      - specified NEC W18.Ø9 ☑
      - sports equipment W18.Ø1 ☑
    - person WØ3 ☑
      - due to ice or snow WØØ.Ø ☑
      - on pedestrian conveyance — *see* Accident, transport, pedestrian, conveyance
- earth (with asphyxia or suffocation (by pressure)) — *see* Earth, falling
- from, off, out of
  - aircraft NEC (with accident to aircraft NEC) V97.Ø ☑
    - while boarding or alighting V97.1 ☑
  - balcony W13.Ø ☑
  - bed WØ6 ☑
  - boat, ship, watercraft NEC (with drowning or submersion) — *see* Drowning, due to, fall overboard
    - with hitting bottom or object V94.Ø ☑
  - bridge W13.1 ☑
  - building W13.9 ☑
    - burning (uncontrolled fire) XØØ.3 ☑
  - cavity W17.2 ☑
  - chair WØ7 ☑
  - cherry picker W17.89 ☑
  - cliff W15 ☑
  - dock W17.4 ☑
  - embankment W17.81 ☑
  - escalator W1Ø.Ø ☑
  - flagpole W13.8 ☑
  - furniture NEC WØ8 ☑
  - grocery cart W17.82 ☑
  - haystack W17.89 ☑
  - high place NEC W17.89 ☑
    - stated as undetermined whether accidental or intentional Y3Ø ☑
  - hole W17.2 ☑
  - incline W1Ø.2 ☑
  - ladder W11 ☑
  - lifting device W17.89 ☑
  - machine, machinery — *see also* Contact, with, by type of machine
    - not in operation W17.89 ☑
  - manhole W17.1 ☑
  - mobile elevated work platform [MEWP] W17.89 ☑
  - motorized mobility scooter WØ5.2 ☑
  - one level to another NEC W17.89 ☑
    - intentional, purposeful, suicide (attempt) X8Ø ☑
    - stated as undetermined whether accidental or intentional Y3Ø ☑
  - pit W17.2 ☑
  - playground equipment WØ9.8 ☑
    - jungle gym WØ9.2 ☑
    - slide WØ9.Ø ☑
    - swing WØ9.1 ☑
  - quarry W17.89 ☑
  - railing W13.9 ☑
  - ramp W1Ø.2 ☑
  - roof W13.2 ☑
  - scaffolding W12 ☑
  - scooter (nonmotorized) WØ5.1 ☑
    - motorized mobility WØ5.2 ☑
  - sky lift W17.89 ☑
  - stairs, steps W1Ø.9 ☑
    - curb W1Ø.1 ☑
    - due to ice or snow WØØ.1 ☑
    - escalator W1Ø.Ø ☑
    - incline W1Ø.2 ☑
    - ramp W1Ø.2 ☑
    - sidewalk curb W1Ø.1 ☑
    - specified NEC W1Ø.8 ☑
    - standing
      - electric scooter VØØ.841 ☑
      - micro-mobility pedestrian conveyance VØØ.848 ☑
  - stepladder W11 ☑
  - stool WØ8 ☑
  - storm drain W17.1 ☑
  - streetcar NEC V82.6 ☑
    - while boarding or alighting V82.4 ☑
    - with antecedent collision — *see* Accident, transport, streetcar occupant
  - structure NEC W13.8 ☑
    - burning (uncontrolled fire) XØØ.3 ☑
  - table WØ8 ☑
  - toilet W18.11 ☑
    - with subsequent striking against object W18.12 ☑
  - train NEC V81.6 ☑
    - during derailment (without antecedent collision) V81.7 ☑
      - with antecedent collision — *see* Accident, transport, railway vehicle occupant
    - while boarding or alighting V81.4 ☑
  - transport vehicle after collision — *see* Accident, transport, by type of vehicle, collision
  - tree W14 ☑
  - vehicle (in motion) NEC — *see also* Accident, transport V89.9 ☑
    - motor NEC — *see also* Accident, transport, occupant, by type of vehicle V87.8 ☑
    - stationary W17.89 ☑
      - while boarding or alighting — *see* Accident, transport, by type of vehicle, while boarding or alighting
  - viaduct W13.8 ☑
  - wall W13.8 ☑
  - watercraft — *see also* Drowning, due to, fall overboard
    - with hitting bottom or object V94.Ø ☑
  - well W17.Ø ☑
  - wheelchair, non-moving WØ5.Ø ☑
    - powered — *see* Accident, transport, pedestrian, conveyance occupant, specified type NEC
  - window W13.4 ☑
- in, on
  - aircraft NEC V97.Ø ☑
    - while boarding or alighting V97.1 ☑
    - with accident to aircraft V97.Ø ☑
  - bathtub (empty) W18.2 ☑
    - filled W16.212 ☑
      - causing drowning W16.211 ☑
  - escalator W1Ø.Ø ☑
  - incline W1Ø.2 ☑
  - ladder W11 ☑
  - machine, machinery — *see* Contact, with, by type of machine
  - object, edged, pointed or sharp (with cut) — *see* Fall, by type
  - playground equipment WØ9.8 ☑
    - jungle gym WØ9.2 ☑

- **Fall, falling** — *continued*
  - in, on — *continued*
    - playground equipment — *continued*
      - slide W09.0 ☑
      - swing W09.1 ☑
    - ramp W10.2 ☑
    - scaffolding W12 ☑
    - shower W18.2 ☑
      - causing drowning W16.211 ☑
    - staircase, stairs, steps W10.9 ☑
      - curb W10.1 ☑
      - due to ice or snow W00.1 ☑
      - escalator W10.0 ☑
      - incline W10.2 ☑
      - specified NEC W10.8 ☑
    - streetcar (without antecedent collision) V82.5 ☑
      - with antecedent collision — *see* Accident, transport, streetcar occupant
      - while boarding or alighting V82.4 ☑
    - train (without antecedent collision) V81.5 ☑
      - with antecedent collision — *see* Accident, transport, railway vehicle occupant
      - during derailment (without antecedent collision) V81.7 ☑
        - with antecedent collision — *see* Accident, transport, railway vehicle occupant
      - while boarding or alighting V81.4 ☑
    - transport vehicle after collision — *see* Accident, transport, by type of vehicle, collision
    - watercraft V93.39 ☑
      - due to
        - accident to craft V91.29 ☑
          - powered craft V91.23 ☑
            - ferry boat V91.21 ☑
            - fishing boat V91.22 ☑
            - jetskis V91.23 ☑
            - liner V91.21 ☑
            - merchant ship V91.20 ☑
            - passenger ship V91.21 ☑
          - unpowered craft
            - canoe V91.25 ☑
            - inflatable V91.26 ☑
            - kayak V91.25 ☑
            - sailboat V91.24 ☑
      - powered craft V93.33 ☑
        - ferry boat V93.31 ☑
        - fishing boat V93.32 ☑
        - jetskis V93.33 ☑
        - liner V93.31 ☑
        - merchant ship V93.30 ☑
        - passenger ship V93.31 ☑
      - unpowered craft V93.38 ☑
        - canoe V93.35 ☑
        - inflatable V93.36 ☑
        - kayak V93.35 ☑
        - sailboat V93.34 ☑
        - surf-board V93.38 ☑
        - windsurfer V93.38 ☑
  - into
    - cavity W17.2 ☑
    - dock W17.4 ☑
    - fire — *see* Exposure, fire, by type
    - haystack W17.89 ☑
    - hole W17.2 ☑
    - lake — *see* Fall, into, water
    - manhole W17.1 ☑
    - moving part of machinery — *see* Contact, with, by type of machine
    - ocean — *see* Fall, into, water
    - opening in surface NEC W17.89 ☑
    - pit W17.2 ☑
    - pond — *see* Fall, into, water
    - quarry W17.89 ☑
    - river — *see* Fall, into, water
    - shaft W17.89 ☑
    - storm drain W17.1 ☑
    - stream — *see* Fall, into, water
    - swimming pool — *see also* Fall, into, water, in, swimming pool
      - empty W17.3 ☑
    - tank W17.89 ☑
    - water W16.42 ☑
      - causing drowning W16.41 ☑
      - from watercraft — *see* Drowning, due to, fall overboard
      - hitting diving board W21.4 ☑

- **Fall, falling** — *continued*
  - into — *continued*
    - water — *continued*
      - in
        - bathtub W16.212 ☑
          - causing drowning W16.211 ☑
        - bucket W16.222 ☑
          - causing drowning W16.221 ☑
        - natural body of water W16.112 ☑
          - causing drowning W16.111 ☑
          - striking
            - bottom W16.122 ☑
              - causing drowning W16.121 ☑
            - side W16.132 ☑
              - causing drowning W16.131 ☑
        - specified water NEC W16.312 ☑
          - causing drowning W16.311 ☑
          - striking
            - bottom W16.322 ☑
              - causing drowning W16.321 ☑
            - wall W16.332 ☑
              - causing drowning W16.331 ☑
        - swimming pool W16.012 ☑
          - causing drowning W16.011 ☑
          - striking
            - bottom W16.022 ☑
              - causing drowning W16.031 ☑
            - wall W16.032 ☑
              - causing drowning W16.021 ☑
        - utility bucket W16.222 ☑
          - causing drowning W16.221 ☑
    - well W17.0 ☑
  - involving
    - bed W06 ☑
    - chair W07 ☑
    - furniture NEC W08 ☑
    - glass — *see* Fall, by type
    - playground equipment W09.8 ☑
      - jungle gym W09.2 ☑
      - slide W09.0 ☑
      - swing W09.1 ☑
    - roller blades — *see* Accident, transport, pedestrian, conveyance
    - skateboard(s) — *see* Accident, transport, pedestrian, conveyance
    - skates (ice) (in line) (roller) — *see* Accident, transport, pedestrian, conveyance
    - skis — *see* Accident, transport, pedestrian, conveyance
    - table W08 ☑
    - wheelchair, non-moving W05.0 ☑
      - powered — *see* Accident, transport, pedestrian, conveyance, specified type NEC
  - object — *see* Struck by, object, falling
  - off
    - toilet W18.11 ☑
      - with subsequent striking against object W18.12 ☑
  - on same level W18.30 ☑
    - due to
      - specified NEC W18.39 ☑
      - stepping on an object W18.31 ☑
  - out of
    - bed W06 ☑
    - building NEC W13.8 ☑
    - chair W07 ☑
    - furniture NEC W08 ☑
    - wheelchair, non-moving W05.0 ☑
      - powered — *see* Accident, transport, pedestrian, conveyance, specified type NEC
    - window W13.4 ☑
  - over
    - animal W01.0 ☑
    - cliff W15 ☑
    - embankment W17.81 ☑
    - small object W01.0 ☑
  - rock W20.8 ☑
  - same level W18.30 ☑
    - from
      - being crushed, pushed, or stepped on by a crowd or human stampede W52 ☑
      - collision, pushing, shoving, by or with other person W03 ☑
      - slipping, stumbling, tripping W01.0 ☑
    - involving ice or snow W00.0 ☑

- **Fall, falling** — *continued*
  - same level — *continued*
    - involving ice or snow — *continued*
      - involving skates (ice) (roller), skateboard, skis — *see* Accident, transport, pedestrian, conveyance
  - snowslide (avalanche) — *see* Landslide
  - stone W20.8 ☑
  - structure W20.1 ☑
    - burning (uncontrolled fire) X00.3 ☑
  - through
    - bridge W13.1 ☑
    - floor W13.3 ☑
    - roof W13.2 ☑
    - wall W13.8 ☑
    - window W13.4 ☑
  - timber W20.8 ☑
  - tree (caused by lightning) W20.8 ☑
  - while being carried or supported by other person(s) W04 ☑
- **Fallen on by**
  - animal (not being ridden) NEC W55.89 ☑
- **Felo-de-se** — *see* Suicide
- **Fight** (hand) (fists) (foot) — *see* Assault, fight
- **Fire** (accidental) — *see* Exposure, fire
- **Firearm discharge** — *see* Discharge, firearm
- **Fireball effects from nuclear explosion in war operations** — *see* War operations, nuclear weapons
- **Fireworks** (explosion) W39 ☑
- **Flash burns from explosion** — *see* Explosion
- **Flood** (any injury) (caused by) X38 ☑
  - collapse of man-made structure causing earth movement X36.0 ☑
  - tidal wave — *see* Forces of nature, tidal wave
- **Food** (any type) **in**
  - air passages (with asphyxia, obstruction, or suffocation) — *see* categories T17 and T18 ☑
  - alimentary tract causing asphyxia (due to compression of trachea) — *see* categories T17 and T18 ☑
- **Forces of nature** X39.8 ☑
  - avalanche X36.1 ☑
    - causing transport accident — *see* Accident, transport, by type of vehicle
  - blizzard X37.2 ☑
  - cataclysmic storm X37.9 ☑
    - with flood X38 ☑
    - blizzard X37.2 ☑
    - cloudburst X37.8 ☑
    - cyclone X37.1 ☑
    - dust storm X37.3 ☑
    - hurricane X37.0 ☑
    - specified storm NEC X37.8 ☑
    - storm surge X37.0 ☑
    - tornado X37.1 ☑
    - twister X37.1 ☑
    - typhoon X37.0 ☑
  - cloudburst X37.8 ☑
  - cold (natural) X31 ☑
  - cyclone X37.1 ☑
  - dam collapse causing earth movement X36.0 ☑
  - dust storm X37.3 ☑
  - earth movement X36.1 ☑
    - caused by dam or structure collapse X36.0 ☑
    - earthquake X34 ☑
  - earthquake X34 ☑
  - flood (caused by) X38 ☑
    - dam collapse X36.0 ☑
    - tidal wave — *see* Forces of nature, tidal wave
  - heat (natural) X30 ☑
  - hurricane X37.0 ☑
  - landslide X36.1 ☑
    - causing transport accident — *see* Accident, transport, by type of vehicle
  - lightning — *see* subcategory T75.0 ☑
    - causing fire — *see* Exposure, fire
  - mudslide X36.1 ☑
    - causing transport accident — *see* Accident, transport, by type of vehicle
  - radiation (natural) X39.08 ☑
    - radon X39.01 ☑
  - radon X39.01 ☑
  - specified force NEC X39.8 ☑
  - storm surge X37.0 ☑
  - structure collapse causing earth movement X36.0 ☑
  - sunlight X32 ☑
  - tidal wave X37.41 ☑

- **Incident, adverse** — *continued*
  - device — *continued*
    - obstetrical — *continued*
      - miscellaneous Y76.8
      - monitoring Y76.Ø
      - prosthetic Y76.2
      - rehabilitative Y76.1
      - surgical Y76.3
      - therapeutic Y76.1
    - ophthalmic Y77.8
      - accessory Y77.2
      - contact lens (rigid gas permeable) (soft (hydrophilic)) Y77.11
      - diagnostic Y77.Ø
      - miscellaneous Y77.8
      - monitoring Y77.Ø
      - prosthetic Y77.2
      - rehabilitative Y77.19
      - surgical Y77.3
      - therapeutic Y77.19
    - orthopedic Y79.8
      - accessory Y79.2
      - diagnostic Y79.Ø
      - miscellaneous Y79.8
      - monitoring Y79.Ø
      - prosthetic Y79.2
      - rehabilitative Y79.1
      - surgical Y79.3
      - therapeutic Y79.1
    - otorhinolaryngological Y72.8
      - accessory Y72.2
      - diagnostic Y72.Ø
      - miscellaneous Y72.8
      - monitoring Y72.Ø
      - prosthetic Y72.2
      - rehabilitative Y72.1
      - surgical Y72.3
      - therapeutic Y72.1
    - personal use Y74.8
      - accessory Y74.2
      - diagnostic Y74.Ø
      - miscellaneous Y74.8
      - monitoring Y74.Ø
      - prosthetic Y74.2
      - rehabilitative Y74.1
      - surgical Y74.3
      - therapeutic Y74.1
    - physical medicine Y8Ø.8
      - accessory Y8Ø.2
      - diagnostic Y8Ø.Ø
      - miscellaneous Y8Ø.8
      - monitoring Y8Ø.Ø
      - prosthetic Y8Ø.2
      - rehabilitative Y8Ø.1
      - surgical Y8Ø.3
      - therapeutic Y8Ø.1
    - plastic surgical Y81.8
      - accessory Y81.2
      - diagnostic Y81.Ø
      - miscellaneous Y81.8
      - monitoring Y81.Ø
      - prosthetic Y81.2
      - rehabilitative Y81.1
      - surgical Y81.3
      - therapeutic Y81.1
    - radiological Y78.8
      - accessory Y78.2
      - diagnostic Y78.Ø
      - miscellaneous Y78.8
      - monitoring Y78.Ø
      - prosthetic Y78.2
      - rehabilitative Y78.1
      - surgical Y78.3
      - therapeutic Y78.1
    - urology Y73.8
      - accessory Y73.2
      - diagnostic Y73.Ø
      - miscellaneous Y73.8
      - monitoring Y73.Ø
      - prosthetic Y73.2
      - rehabilitative Y73.1
      - surgical Y73.3
      - therapeutic Y73.1
- **Incineration** (accidental) — *see* Exposure, fire
- **Infanticide** — *see* Assault
- **Infrasound waves** (causing injury) W49.9 ☑
- **Ingestion**
  - foreign body (causing injury) (with obstruction) — *see* Foreign body, alimentary canal
  - poisonous
    - plant(s) X58 ☑
    - substance NEC — *see* Table of Drugs and Chemicals
- **Inhalation**
  - excessively cold substance, man-made — *see* Exposure, cold, man-made
  - food (any type) (into respiratory tract) (with asphyxia, obstruction respiratory tract, suffocation) — *see* categories T17 and T18 ☑
  - foreign body — *see* Foreign body, aspiration
  - gastric contents (with asphyxia, obstruction respiratory passage, suffocation) T17.81- ☑
  - hot air or gases X14.Ø ☑
  - liquid air, hydrogen, nitrogen W93.12 ☑
    - suicide (attempt) X83.2 ☑
  - steam X13.Ø ☑
    - assault X98.Ø ☑
    - stated as undetermined whether accidental or intentional Y27.Ø ☑
    - suicide (attempt) X77.Ø ☑
  - toxic gas — *see* Table of Drugs and Chemicals
  - vomitus (with asphyxia, obstruction respiratory passage, suffocation) T17.81- ☑
- **Injury, injured** (accidental(ly)) NOS X58 ☑
  - by, caused by, from
    - assault — *see* Assault
    - law-enforcing agent, police, in course of legal intervention — *see* Legal intervention
    - suicide (attempt) X83.8 ☑
  - due to, in
    - civil insurrection — *see* War operations
    - fight — *see also* Assault, fight YØ4.Ø ☑
    - war operations — *see* War operations
  - homicide — *see also* Assault YØ9
  - inflicted (by)
    - in course of arrest (attempted), suppression of disturbance, maintenance of order, by law-enforcing agents — *see* Legal intervention
    - other person
      - stated as
        - accidental X58 ☑
        - intentional, homicide (attempt) — *see* Assault
        - undetermined whether accidental or intentional Y33 ☑
  - purposely (inflicted) by other person(s) — *see* Assault
  - self-inflicted X83.8 ☑
    - stated as accidental X58 ☑
  - specified cause NEC X58 ☑
  - undetermined whether accidental or intentional Y33 ☑
- **Insolation, effects** X3Ø ☑
- **Insufficient nourishment** X58 ☑
- **Interruption of respiration** (by)
  - food (lodged in esophagus) — *see* categories T17 and T18 ☑
  - vomitus (lodged in esophagus) T17.81- ☑
- **Intervention, legal** — *see* Legal intervention
- **Intoxication**
  - drug — *see* Table of Drugs and Chemicals
  - poison — *see* Table of Drugs and Chemicals

J

- **Jammed** (accidentally)
  - between objects (moving) (stationary and moving) W23.Ø ☑
    - stationary W23.1 ☑
- **Jumped, jumping**
  - before moving object NEC X81.8 ☑
    - motor vehicle X81.Ø ☑
    - subway train X81.1 ☑
    - train X81.1 ☑
    - undetermined whether accidental or intentional Y31 ☑
  - from
    - boat (into water) voluntarily, without accident (to or on boat) W16.712 ☑
      - striking bottom W16.722 ☑
        - causing drowning W16.721 ☑
      - with
        - accident to or on boat — *see* Accident, watercraft
        - drowning or submersion W16.711 ☑
          - suicide (attempt) X71.3 ☑
    - building — *see also* Jumped, from, high place W13.9 ☑
      - burning (uncontrolled fire) XØØ.5 ☑
    - high place NEC W17.89 ☑
      - suicide (attempt) X8Ø ☑
      - undetermined whether accidental or intentional Y3Ø ☑
    - structure — *see also* Jumped, from, high place W13.9 ☑
      - burning (uncontrolled fire) XØØ.5 ☑
  - into water W16.92 ☑
    - causing drowning W16.91 ☑
    - from, off watercraft — *see* Jumped, from, boat
    - in
      - natural body W16.612 ☑
        - causing drowning W16.611 ☑
        - striking bottom W16.622 ☑
          - causing drowning W16.621 ☑
      - specified place NEC W16.812 ☑
        - causing drowning W16.811 ☑
        - striking
          - bottom W16.822 ☑
            - causing drowning W16.821 ☑
          - wall W16.832 ☑
            - causing drowning W16.831 ☑
      - swimming pool W16.512 ☑
        - causing drowning W16.511 ☑
        - striking
          - bottom W16.522 ☑
            - causing drowning W16.521 ☑
          - wall W16.532 ☑
            - causing drowning W16.531 ☑
    - suicide (attempt) X71.3 ☑

K

- **Kicked by**
  - animal NEC W55.82 ☑
  - person(s) (accidentally) W5Ø.1 ☑
    - with intent to injure or kill YØ4.Ø ☑
    - as, or caused by, a crowd or human stampede (with fall) W52 ☑
    - assault YØ4.Ø ☑
    - homicide (attempt) YØ4.Ø ☑
    - in
      - fight YØ4.Ø ☑
      - legal intervention
        - injuring
          - bystander Y35.812 ☑
          - law enforcement personnel Y35.811 ☑
          - suspect Y35.813 ☑
          - unspecified person Y35.819 ☑
- **Kicking**
  - against
    - object W22.8 ☑
      - sports equipment W21.9 ☑
      - stationary W22.Ø9 ☑
        - sports equipment W21.89 ☑
    - person — *see* Striking against, person
    - sports equipment W21.9 ☑
  - carpet stretcher with knee X5Ø.3 ☑
- **Killed, killing** (accidentally) NOS — *see also* Injury X58 ☑
  - in
    - action — *see* War operations
    - brawl, fight (hand) (fists) (foot) YØ4.Ø ☑
      - by weapon — *see also* Assault
        - cutting, piercing — *see* Assault, cutting or piercing instrument
        - firearm — *see* Discharge, firearm, by type, homicide
  - self
    - stated as
      - accident NOS X58 ☑
      - suicide — *see* Suicide
      - undetermined whether accidental or intentional Y33 ☑
- **Kneeling** (prolonged (static) X5Ø.1 ☑
- **Knocked down** (accidentally) (by) NOS X58 ☑
  - animal (not being ridden) NEC — *see also* Struck by, by type of animal
  - crowd or human stampede W52 ☑
  - person W51 ☑
    - in brawl, fight YØ4.Ø ☑

Knocked down — *continued*
- transport vehicle NEC — *see also* Accident, transport V09.9 ☑

L

Laceration NEC — *see* Injury

Lack of
- care (helpless person) (infant) (newborn) X58 ☑
- food except as result of abandonment or neglect X58 ☑
  - due to abandonment or neglect X58 ☑
- water except as result of transport accident X58 ☑
  - due to transport accident — *see* Accident, transport, by type
  - helpless person, infant, newborn X58 ☑

Landslide (falling on transport vehicle) X36.1 ☑
- caused by collapse of man-made structure X36.0 ☑

Late effect — *see* Sequelae

Legal
- execution (any method) — *see* Legal, intervention
- intervention (by)
  - baton — *see* Legal, intervention, blunt object, baton
  - bayonet — *see* Legal, intervention, sharp object, bayonet
  - blow — *see* Legal, intervention, manhandling
  - blunt object
    - baton
      - injuring
        - bystander Y35.312 ☑
        - law enforcement personnel Y35.311 ☑
        - suspect Y35.313 ☑
        - unspecified person Y35.319 ☑
    - injuring
      - bystander Y35.302 ☑
      - law enforcement personnel Y35.301 ☑
      - suspect Y35.303 ☑
      - unspecified person Y35.309 ☑
    - specified NEC
      - injuring
        - bystander Y35.392 ☑
        - law enforcement personnel Y35.391 ☑
        - suspect Y35.393 ☑
        - unspecified person Y35.399 ☑
    - stave
      - injuring
        - bystander Y35.392 ☑
        - law enforcement personnel Y35.391 ☑
        - suspect Y35.393 ☑
        - unspecified person Y35.399 ☑
  - bomb — *see* Legal, intervention, explosive
  - conducted energy device
    - injuring
      - bystander Y35.832 ☑
      - law enforcement personnel Y35.831 ☑
      - suspect Y35.833 ☑
      - unspecified person Y35.839 ☑
  - cutting or piercing instrument — *see* Legal, intervention, sharp object
  - dynamite — *see* Legal, intervention, explosive, dynamite
  - electroshock device (taser)
    - injuring
      - bystander Y35.832 ☑
      - law enforcement personnel Y35.831 ☑
      - suspect Y35.833 ☑
      - unspecified person Y35.839 ☑
  - explosive(s)
    - dynamite
      - injuring
        - bystander Y35.112 ☑
        - law enforcement personnel Y35.111 ☑
        - suspect Y35.113 ☑
        - unspecified person Y35.119 ☑
    - grenade
      - injuring
        - bystander Y35.192 ☑
        - law enforcement personnel Y35.191 ☑
        - suspect Y35.193 ☑
        - unspecified person Y35.199 ☑
    - injuring
      - bystander Y35.102 ☑
      - law enforcement personnel Y35.101 ☑
      - suspect Y35.103 ☑
      - unspecified person Y35.109 ☑

Legal — *continued*
- intervention — *continued*
  - explosive(s) — *continued*
    - mortar bomb
      - injuring
        - bystander Y35.192 ☑
        - law enforcement personnel Y35.191 ☑
        - suspect Y35.193 ☑
        - unspecified person Y35.199 ☑
    - shell
      - injuring
        - bystander Y35.122 ☑
        - law enforcement personnel Y35.121 ☑
        - suspect Y35.123 ☑
        - unspecified person Y35.129 ☑
    - specified NEC
      - injuring
        - bystander Y35.192 ☑
        - law enforcement personnel Y35.191 ☑
        - suspect Y35.193 ☑
        - unspecified person Y35.199 ☑
  - firearm(s) (discharge)
    - handgun
      - injuring
        - bystander Y35.022 ☑
        - law enforcement personnel Y35.021 ☑
        - suspect Y35.023 ☑
        - unspecified person Y35.029 ☑
    - injuring
      - bystander Y35.002 ☑
      - law enforcement personnel Y35.001 ☑
      - suspect Y35.003 ☑
      - unspecified person Y35.009 ☑
    - machine gun
      - injuring
        - bystander Y35.012 ☑
        - law enforcement personnel Y35.011 ☑
        - suspect Y35.013 ☑
        - unspecified person Y35.019 ☑
    - rifle pellet
      - injuring
        - bystander Y35.032 ☑
        - law enforcement personnel Y35.031 ☑
        - suspect Y35.033 ☑
        - unspecified person Y35.039 ☑
    - rubber bullet
      - injuring
        - bystander Y35.042 ☑
        - law enforcement personnel Y35.041 ☑
        - suspect Y35.043 ☑
        - unspecified person Y35.049 ☑
    - shotgun — *see* Legal, intervention, firearm, specified NEC
    - specified NEC
      - injuring
        - bystander Y35.092 ☑
        - law enforcement personnel Y35.091 ☑
        - suspect Y35.093 ☑
        - unspecified person Y35.099 ☑
  - gas (asphyxiation) (poisoning)
    - injuring
      - bystander Y35.202 ☑
      - law enforcement personnel Y35.201 ☑
      - suspect Y35.203 ☑
      - unspecified person Y35.209 ☑
    - specified NEC
      - injuring
        - bystander Y35.292 ☑
        - law enforcement personnel Y35.291 ☑
        - suspect Y35.293 ☑
        - unspecified person Y35.299 ☑
    - tear gas
      - injuring
        - bystander Y35.212 ☑
        - law enforcement personnel Y35.211 ☑
        - suspect Y35.213 ☑
        - unspecified person Y35.219 ☑
  - grenade — *see* Legal, intervention, explosive, grenade
  - injuring
    - bystander Y35.92 ☑
    - law enforcement personnel Y35.91 ☑
    - suspect Y35.93 ☑
    - unspecified person Y35.99 ☑
  - late effect (of) — *see* with 7th character S Y35 ☑

Legal — *continued*
- intervention — *continued*
  - manhandling
    - injuring
      - bystander Y35.812 ☑
      - law enforcement personnel Y35.811 ☑
      - suspect Y35.813 ☑
      - unspecified person Y35.819 ☑
  - sequelae (of) — *see* with 7th character S Y35 ☑
  - sharp objects
    - bayonet
      - injuring
        - bystander Y35.412 ☑
        - law enforcement personnel Y35.411 ☑
        - suspect Y35.413 ☑
        - unspecified person Y35.419 ☑
    - injuring
      - bystander Y35.402 ☑
      - law enforcement personnel Y35.401 ☑
      - suspect Y35.403 ☑
      - unspecified person Y35.409 ☑
    - specified NEC
      - injuring
        - bystander Y35.492 ☑
        - law enforcement personnel Y35.491 ☑
        - suspect Y35.493 ☑
        - unspecified person Y35.499 ☑
  - specified means NEC
    - injuring
      - bystander Y35.892 ☑
      - law enforcement personnel Y35.891 ☑
      - suspect Y35.893 ☑
      - unspecified person Y35.899 ☑
  - stabbing — *see* Legal, intervention, sharp object
  - stave — *see* Legal, intervention, blunt object, stave
  - stun gun
    - injuring
      - bystander Y35.832 ☑
      - law enforcement personnel Y35.831 ☑
      - suspect Y35.833 ☑
      - unspecified person Y35.839 ☑
  - taser
    - injuring
      - bystander Y35.832 ☑
      - law enforcement personnel Y35.831 ☑
      - suspect Y35.833 ☑
      - unspecified person Y35.839 ☑
  - tear gas — *see* Legal, intervention, gas, tear gas
  - truncheon — *see* Legal, intervention, blunt object, stave

Lifting — *see also* Overexertion
- heavy objects X50.0 ☑
- weights X50.0 ☑

Lightning (shock) (stroke) (struck by) — *see* subcategory T75.0 ☑
- causing fire — *see* Exposure, fire

Loss of control (transport vehicle) NEC — *see* Accident, transport

Lost at sea NOS — *see* Drowning, due to, fall overboard

Low
- pressure (effects) — *see* Air, pressure, low
- temperature (effects) — *see* Exposure, cold

Lying before train, vehicle or other moving object X81.8 ☑
- subway train X81.1 ☑
- train X81.1 ☑
- undetermined whether accidental or intentional Y31 ☑

Lynching — *see* Assault

M

Malfunction (mechanism or component) (of)
- firearm W34.10 ☑
  - airgun W34.110 ☑
  - BB gun W34.110 ☑
  - gas, air or spring-operated gun NEC W34.118 ☑
  - handgun W32.1 ☑
  - hunting rifle W33.12 ☑
  - larger firearm W33.10 ☑
    - specified NEC W33.19 ☑
  - machine gun W33.13 ☑
  - paintball gun W34.111 ☑
  - pellet gun W34.110 ☑
  - shotgun W33.11 ☑
  - specified NEC W34.19 ☑
  - Very pistol [flare] W34.19 ☑

N

O

P

External Causes Index

Misadventure — Place of occurrence

Place of occurrence — *continued*
- football field Y92.321
- forest Y92.821
- freeway Y92.411
- gallery Y92.250
- garage (commercial) Y92.59
  - boarding house Y92.044
  - military base Y92.135
  - mobile home Y92.025
  - nursing home Y92.124
  - orphanage Y92.114
  - private house Y92.015
  - reform school Y92.155
- gas station Y92.524
- gasworks Y92.69
- golf course Y92.39
- gravel pit Y92.64
- grocery Y92.512
- gymnasium Y92.39
- handball court Y92.318
- harbor Y92.89
- harness racing course Y92.39
- healthcare provider office Y92.531
- highway Y92.410
  - interstate Y92.411
- hill Y92.828
- hockey rink Y92.330
- home — *see* Place of occurrence, residence
- hospice — *see* Place of occurrence, residence, institutional, nursing home
- hospital Y92.239
  - cafeteria Y92.233
  - corridor Y92.232
  - operating room Y92.234
  - patient
    - bathroom Y92.231
    - room Y92.230
  - specified NEC Y92.238
- hotel Y92.59
- house — *see also* Place of occurrence, residence
  - abandoned Y92.89
  - under construction Y92.61
- industrial and construction area (yard) Y92.69
  - building under construction Y92.61
  - dock Y92.62
  - dry dock Y92.62
  - factory Y92.63
  - gasworks Y92.69
  - mine Y92.64
  - oil rig Y92.65
  - pit Y92.64
  - power station Y92.69
  - shipyard Y92.62
  - specified NEC Y92.69
  - tunnel under construction Y92.69
  - workshop Y92.69
- interstate Y92.411
- kindergarten Y92.211
- lacrosse field Y92.328
- lake Y92.838
  - wilderness Y92.828
- library Y92.241
- mall Y92.59
- market Y92.512
- marsh Y92.828
- military
  - base — *see* Place of occurrence, residence, institutional, military base
  - training ground Y92.84
- mine Y92.64
- mosque Y92.22
- motel Y92.59
- motorway (interstate) Y92.411
- mountain Y92.828
- movie-house Y92.26
- museum Y92.251
- music-hall Y92.252
- not applicable Y92.9
- nuclear power station Y92.69
- nursing home — *see* Place of occurrence, residence, institutional, nursing home
- office building Y92.59
- offshore installation Y92.65
- oil rig Y92.65
- old people's home — *see* Place of occurrence, residence, institutional, specified NEC
- opera-house Y92.253

Place of occurrence — *continued*
- orphanage — *see* Place of occurrence, residence, institutional, orphanage
- outpatient surgery center Y92.530
- park (public) Y92.830
  - amusement Y92.831
- parking garage Y92.89
  - lot Y92.481
- pavement Y92.480
- physician office Y92.531
- polo field Y92.328
- pond Y92.828
- post office Y92.242
- power station Y92.69
- prairie Y92.828
- prison — *see* Place of occurrence, residence, institutional, prison
- public
  - administration building Y92.248
    - city hall Y92.243
    - courthouse Y92.240
    - library Y92.241
    - post office Y92.242
    - specified NEC Y92.248
  - building NEC Y92.29
  - hall Y92.29
  - place NOS Y92.89
- race course Y92.39
- radio station Y92.59
- railway line (bridge) Y92.85
- ranch (outbuildings) — *see* Place of occurrence, farm
- recreation area Y92.838
  - amusement park Y92.831
  - beach Y92.832
  - campsite Y92.833
  - park (public) Y92.830
  - seashore Y92.832
  - specified NEC Y92.838
- reform school - — *see* Place of occurrence, residence, institutional, reform school
- religious institution Y92.22
- residence (non-institutional) (private) Y92.009
  - apartment Y92.039
    - bathroom Y92.031
    - bedroom Y92.032
    - kitchen Y92.030
    - specified NEC Y92.038
  - bathroom Y92.002
  - bedroom Y92.003
  - boarding house Y92.049
    - bathroom Y92.041
    - bedroom Y92.042
    - driveway Y92.043
    - garage Y92.044
    - garden Y92.046
    - kitchen Y92.040
    - specified NEC Y92.048
    - swimming pool Y92.045
    - yard Y92.046
  - dining room Y92.001
  - garden Y92.007
  - home Y92.009
  - house, single family Y92.019
    - bathroom Y92.012
    - bedroom Y92.013
    - dining room Y92.011
    - driveway Y92.014
    - garage Y92.015
    - garden Y92.017
    - kitchen Y92.010
    - specified NEC Y92.018
    - swimming pool Y92.016
    - yard Y92.017
  - institutional Y92.10
    - children's home — *see* Place of occurrence, residence, institutional, orphanage
    - hospice — *see* Place of occurrence, residence, institutional, nursing home
    - military base Y92.139
      - barracks Y92.133
      - garage Y92.135
      - garden Y92.137
      - kitchen Y92.130
      - mess hall Y92.131
      - specified NEC Y92.138
      - swimming pool Y92.136
      - yard Y92.137
    - nursing home Y92.129
      - bathroom Y92.121

Place of occurrence — *continued*
- residence — *continued*
  - institutional — *continued*
    - nursing home — *continued*
      - bedroom Y92.122
      - driveway Y92.123
      - garage Y92.124
      - garden Y92.126
      - kitchen Y92.120
      - specified NEC Y92.128
      - swimming pool Y92.125
      - yard Y92.126
    - orphanage Y92.119
      - bathroom Y92.111
      - bedroom Y92.112
      - driveway Y92.113
      - garage Y92.114
      - garden Y92.116
      - kitchen Y92.110
      - specified NEC Y92.118
      - swimming pool Y92.115
      - yard Y92.116
    - prison Y92.149
      - bathroom Y92.142
      - cell Y92.143
      - courtyard Y92.147
      - dining room Y92.141
      - kitchen Y92.140
      - specified NEC Y92.148
      - swimming pool Y92.146
    - reform school Y92.159
      - bathroom Y92.152
      - bedroom Y92.153
      - dining room Y92.151
      - driveway Y92.154
      - garage Y92.155
      - garden Y92.157
      - kitchen Y92.150
      - specified NEC Y92.158
      - swimming pool Y92.156
      - yard Y92.157
    - school dormitory Y92.169
      - bathroom Y92.162
      - bedroom Y92.163
      - dining room Y92.161
      - kitchen Y92.160
      - specified NEC Y92.168
    - specified NEC Y92.199
      - bathroom Y92.192
      - bedroom Y92.193
      - dining room Y92.191
      - driveway Y92.194
      - garage Y92.195
      - garden Y92.197
      - kitchen Y92.190
      - specified NEC Y92.198
      - swimming pool Y92.196
      - yard Y92.197
  - kitchen Y92.000
  - mobile home Y92.029
    - bathroom Y92.022
    - bedroom Y92.023
    - dining room Y92.021
    - driveway Y92.024
    - garage Y92.025
    - garden Y92.027
    - kitchen Y92.020
    - specified NEC Y92.028
    - swimming pool Y92.026
    - yard Y92.027
  - specified place in residence NEC Y92.008
  - specified residence type NEC Y92.099
    - bathroom Y92.091
    - bedroom Y92.092
    - driveway Y92.093
    - garage Y92.094
    - garden Y92.096
    - kitchen Y92.090
    - specified NEC Y92.098
    - swimming pool Y92.095
    - yard Y92.096
- restaurant Y92.511
- riding school Y92.39
- river Y92.828
- road Y92.410
- rodeo ring Y92.39
- rugby field Y92.328
- same day surgery center Y92.530
- sand pit Y92.64

Place of occurrence — *continued*
- school (private) (public) (state) Y92.219
  - college Y92.214
  - daycare center Y92.210
  - elementary school Y92.211
  - high school Y92.213
  - kindergarten Y92.211
  - middle school Y92.212
  - specified NEC Y92.218
  - trace school Y92.215
  - university Y92.214
  - vocational school Y92.215
- sea (shore) Y92.832
- senior citizen center Y92.29
- service area
  - airport Y92.520
  - bus station Y92.521
  - gas station Y92.524
  - highway rest stop Y92.523
  - railway station Y92.522
- shipyard Y92.62
- shop (commercial) Y92.513
- sidewalk Y92.480
- silo Y92.79
- skating rink (roller) Y92.331
  - ice Y92.330
- slaughter house Y92.86
- soccer field Y92.322
- specified place NEC Y92.89
- sports area Y92.39
  - athletic
    - court Y92.318
      - basketball Y92.310
      - specified NEC Y92.318
      - squash Y92.311
      - tennis Y92.312
    - field Y92.328
      - baseball Y92.320
      - cricket ground Y92.328
      - football Y92.321
      - hockey Y92.328
      - soccer Y92.322
      - specified NEC Y92.328
  - golf course Y92.39
  - gymnasium Y92.39
  - riding school Y92.39
  - skating rink (roller) Y92.331
    - ice Y92.330
  - stadium Y92.39
  - swimming pool Y92.34
- squash court Y92.311
- stadium Y92.39
- steeplechasing course Y92.39
- store Y92.512
- stream Y92.828
- street and highway Y92.410
  - bike path Y92.482
  - freeway Y92.411
  - highway ramp Y92.415
  - interstate highway Y92.411
  - local residential or business street Y92.414
  - motorway Y92.411
  - parking lot Y92.481
  - parkway Y92.412
  - sidewalk Y92.480
  - specified NEC Y92.488
  - state road Y92.413
- subway car Y92.816
- supermarket Y92.512
- swamp Y92.828
- swimming pool (public) Y92.34
  - private (at) Y92.095
    - boarding house Y92.045
    - military base Y92.136
    - mobile home Y92.026
    - nursing home Y92.125
    - orphanage Y92.115
    - prison Y92.146
    - reform school Y92.156
    - single family residence Y92.016
- synagogue Y92.22
- tavern Y92.59
- television station Y92.59
- tennis court Y92.312
- theater Y92.254
- trade area Y92.59
  - bank Y92.510
  - cafe Y92.511
  - casino Y92.59

Place of occurrence — *continued*
- trade area — *continued*
  - garage Y92.59
  - hotel Y92.59
  - market Y92.512
  - office building Y92.59
  - radio station Y92.59
  - restaurant Y92.511
  - shop Y92.513
  - shopping mall Y92.59
  - store Y92.512
  - supermarket Y92.512
  - television station Y92.59
  - warehouse Y92.59
- trailer park, residential — *see* Place of occurrence, residence, mobile home
- trailer site NOS Y92.89
- train Y92.815
  - station Y92.522
- truck Y92.812
- tunnel under construction Y92.69
- university Y92.214
- urgent (health) care center Y92.532
- vehicle (transport) Y92.818
  - airplane Y92.813
  - boat Y92.814
  - bus Y92.811
  - car Y92.810
  - specified NEC Y92.818
  - subway car Y92.816
  - train Y92.815
  - truck Y92.812
- warehouse Y92.59
- water reservoir Y92.89
- wilderness area Y92.828
  - desert Y92.820
  - forest Y92.821
  - marsh Y92.828
  - mountain Y92.828
  - prairie Y92.828
  - specified NEC Y92.828
  - swamp Y92.828
- workshop Y92.69
- yard, private Y92.096
  - boarding house Y92.046
  - mobile home Y92.027
  - single family house Y92.017
- youth center Y92.29
- zoo (zoological garden) Y92.834

Plumbism — *see* Table of Drugs and Chemicals, lead

Poisoning (accidental) (by) — *see also* Table of Drugs and Chemicals
- by plant, thorns, spines, sharp leaves or other mechanisms NEC X58 ☑
- carbon monoxide
  - generated by
    - motor vehicle — *see* Accident, transport
    - watercraft (in transit) (not in transit) V93.89 ☑
      - ferry boat V93.81 ☑
      - fishing boat V93.82 ☑
      - jet skis V93.83 ☑
      - liner V93.81 ☑
      - merchant ship V93.80 ☑
      - passenger ship V93.81 ☑
      - powered craft NEC V93.83 ☑
- caused by injection of poisons into skin by plant thorns, spines, sharp leaves X58 ☑
  - marine or sea plants (venomous) X58 ☑
- execution — *see* Legal, intervention, gas
  - intervention
    - by gas — *see* Legal, intervention, gas
    - other specified means — *see* Legal, intervention, specified means NEC
- exhaust gas
  - generated by
    - motor vehicle — *see* Accident, transport
    - watercraft (in transit) (not in transit) V93.89 ☑
      - ferry boat V93.81 ☑
      - fishing boat V93.82 ☑
      - jet skis V93.83 ☑
      - liner V93.81 ☑
      - merchant ship V93.80 ☑
      - passenger ship V93.81 ☑
      - powered craft NEC V93.83 ☑
- fumes or smoke due to
  - explosion — *see also* Explosion W40.9 ☑
  - fire — *see* Exposure, fire
  - ignition — *see* Ignition

Poisoning — *continued*
- gas
  - in legal intervention — *see* Legal, intervention, gas
  - legal execution — *see* Legal, intervention, gas
- in war operations — *see* War operations
- legal

Powder burn (by) (from)
- airgun W34.110 ☑
- BB gun W34.110 ☑
- firearn NEC W34.19 ☑
- gas, air or spring-operated gun NEC W34.118 ☑
- handgun W32.1 ☑
- hunting rifle W33.12 ☑
- larger firearm W33.10 ☑
  - specified NEC W33.19 ☑
- machine gun W33.13 ☑
- paintball gun W34.111 ☑
- pellet gun W34.110 ☑
- shotgun W33.11 ☑
- Very pistol [flare] W34.19 ☑

Premature cessation (of) **surgical and medical care** Y66

Privation (food) (water) X58 ☑

Procedure (operation)
- correct, on wrong side or body part (wrong side) (wrong site) Y65.53
- intended for another patient done on wrong patient Y65.52
- performed on patient not scheduled for surgery Y65.52
- performed on wrong patient Y65.52
- wrong, performed on correct patient Y65.51

Prolonged
- sitting in transport vehicle — *see* Sitting
- stay in
  - high altitude as cause of anoxia, barodontalgia, barotitis or hypoxia W94.11 ☑
  - weightless environment X52 ☑

Pulling, excessive — *see also* Overexertion X50.9- ☑

Puncture, puncturing — *see also* Contact, with, by type of object or machine
- by
  - plant thorns, spines, sharp leaves or other mechanisms NEC W60 ☑
- during medical or surgical treatment as misadventure — *see* Index to Diseases and Injuries, Complication(s)

Pushed, pushing (accidental) (injury in)
- by other person(s) (accidental) W51 ☑
  - as, or caused by, a crowd or human stampede (with fall) W52 ☑
  - before moving object NEC Y02.8 ☑
    - motor vehicle Y02.0 ☑
    - subway train Y02.1 ☑
    - train Y02.1 ☑
  - from
    - high place NEC
      - in accidental circumstances W17.89 ☑
      - stated as
        - intentional, homicide (attempt) Y01 ☑
        - undetermined whether accidental or intentional Y30 ☑
    - transport vehicle NEC — *see also* Accident, transport V89.9 ☑
      - stated as
        - intentional, homicide (attempt) Y08.89 ☑
  - with fall W03 ☑
    - due to ice or snow W00.0 ☑
- overexertion X50.9 ☑

R

Radiation (exposure to)
- arc lamps W89.0 ☑
- atomic power plant (malfunction) NEC W88.1 ☑
- complication of or abnormal reaction to medical radiotherapy Y84.2
- electromagnetic, ionizing W88.0 ☑
- gamma rays W88.1 ☑
- in
  - war operations (from or following nuclear explosion) — *see* War operations
- inadvertent exposure of patient (receiving test or therapy) Y63.3
- infrared (heaters and lamps) W90.1 ☑
  - excessive heat from W92 ☑
- ionized, ionizing (particles, artificially accelerated)
  - radioisotopes W88.1 ☑

- **Radiation** — *continued*
  - ionized, ionizing — *continued*
    - specified NEC W88.8 ☑
    - x-rays W88.Ø ☑
  - isotopes, radioactive — *see* Radiation, radioactive isotopes
  - laser(s) W9Ø.2 ☑
    - in war operations — *see* War operations
    - misadventure in medical care Y63.2
  - light sources (man-made visible and ultraviolet) W89.9 ☑
    - natural X32 ☑
    - specified NEC W89.8 ☑
    - tanning bed W89.1 ☑
    - welding light W89.Ø ☑
  - man-made visible light W89.9 ☑
    - specified NEC W89.8 ☑
    - tanning bed W89.1 ☑
    - welding light W89.Ø ☑
  - microwave W9Ø.8 ☑
  - misadventure in medical or surgical procedure Y63.2
  - natural NEC X39.Ø8 ☑
    - radon X39.Ø1 ☑
  - overdose (in medical or surgical procedure) Y63.2
  - radar W9Ø.Ø ☑
  - radioactive isotopes (any) W88.1 ☑
    - atomic power plant malfunction W88.1 ☑
    - misadventure in medical or surgical treatment Y63.2
  - radiofrequency W9Ø.Ø ☑
  - radium NEC W88.1 ☑
  - sun X32 ☑
  - ultraviolet (light) (man-made) W89.9 ☑
    - natural X32 ☑
    - specified NEC W89.8 ☑
    - tanning bed W89.1 ☑
    - welding light W89.Ø ☑
  - welding arc, torch, or light W89.Ø ☑
    - excessive heat from W92 ☑
  - x-rays (hard) (soft) W88.Ø ☑
- **Range disease** W94.11 ☑
- **Rape** (attempted) T74.2- ☑
- **Rat bite** W53.11 ☑
- **Reaching** (prolonged) (static) X5Ø.1 ☑
- **Reaction, abnormal to medical procedure** — *see also* Complication of or following, by type of procedure Y84.9
  - biologicals — *see* Table of Drugs and Chemicals
  - drugs — *see* Table of Drugs and Chemicals
  - vaccine — *see* Table of Drugs and Chemicals
  - with misadventure — *see* Misadventure
- **Recoil**
  - airgun W34.11Ø ☑
  - BB gun W34.11Ø ☑
  - firearn NEC W34.19 ☑
  - gas, air or spring-operated gun NEC W34.118 ☑
  - handgun W32.1 ☑
  - hunting rifle W33.12 ☑
  - larger firearm W33.1Ø ☑
    - specified NEC W33.19 ☑
  - machine gun W33.13 ☑
  - paintball gun W34.111 ☑
  - pellet W34.11Ø ☑
  - shotgun W33.11 ☑
  - Very pistol [flare] W34.19 ☑
- **Reduction in**
  - atmospheric pressure — *see* Air, pressure, change
- **Rock falling on or hitting** (accidentally) (person) W2Ø.8 ☑
  - in cave-in W2Ø.Ø ☑
- **Run over** (accidentally) (by)
  - animal (not being ridden) NEC W55.89 ☑
  - machinery — *see* Contact, with, by specified type of machine
  - transport vehicle NEC — *see also* Accident, transport VØ9.9 ☑
    - intentional homicide (attempt) YØ3.Ø ☑
    - motor NEC VØ9.2Ø ☑
      - intentional homicide (attempt) YØ3.Ø ☑
- **Running**
  - before moving object X81.8 ☑
    - motor vehicle X81.Ø ☑
- **Running off, away**
  - animal (being ridden) — *see also* Accident, transport V8Ø.918 ☑
    - not being ridden W55.89 ☑
- **Running off, away** — *continued*
  - animal-drawn vehicle NEC — *see also* Accident, transport V8Ø.928 ☑
  - highway, road(way), street
    - transport vehicle NEC — *see also* Accident, transport V89.9 ☑
- **Rupture pressurized devices** — *see* Explosion, by type of device

S

- **Saturnism** — *see* Table of Drugs and Chemicals, lead
- **Scald, scalding** (accidental) (by) (from) (in) X19 ☑
  - air (hot) X14.1 ☑
  - gases (hot) X14.1 ☑
  - homicide (attempt) — *see* Assault, burning, hot object
  - inflicted by other person
    - stated as intentional, homicide (attempt) — *see* Assault, burning, hot object
  - liquid (boiling) (hot) NEC X12 ☑
    - stated as undetermined whether accidental or intentional Y27.2 ☑
    - suicide (attempt) X77.2 ☑
  - local application of externally applied substance in medical or surgical care Y63.5
  - metal (molten) (liquid) (hot) NEC X18 ☑
  - self-inflicted X77.9 ☑
  - stated as undetermined whether accidental or intentional Y27.8 ☑
  - steam X13.1 ☑
    - assault X98.Ø ☑
    - stated as undetermined whether accidental or intentional Y27.Ø ☑
    - suicide (attempt) X77.Ø ☑
  - suicide (attempt) X77.9 ☑
  - vapor (hot) X13.1 ☑
    - assault X98.Ø ☑
    - stated as undetermined whether accidental or intentional Y27.Ø ☑
    - suicide (attempt) X77.Ø ☑
- **Scratched by**
  - cat W55.Ø3 ☑
  - person(s) (accidentally) W5Ø.4 ☑
    - with intent to injure or kill YØ4.Ø ☑
    - as, or caused by, a crowd or human stampede (with fall) W52 ☑
    - assault YØ4.Ø ☑
    - homicide (attempt) YØ4.Ø ☑
    - in
      - fight YØ4.Ø ☑
      - legal intervention
        - injuring
          - bystander Y35.892 ☑
          - law enforcement personnel Y35.891 ☑
          - suspect Y35.893 ☑
          - unspecified person Y35.899 ☑
- **Seasickness** T75.3 ☑
- **Self-harm NEC** — *see also* External cause by type, undetermined whether accidental or intentional
  - intentional — *see* Suicide
  - poisoning NEC — *see* Table of Drugs and Chemicals, poisoning, accidental
- **Self-inflicted** (injury) **NEC** — *see also* External cause by type, undetermined whether accidental or intentional
  - intentional — *see* Suicide
  - poisoning NEC — *see* Table of Drugs and Chemicals, poisoning, accidental
- **Sequelae** (of)
  - accident NEC — *see* WØØ-X58 with 7th character S
  - assault (homicidal) (any means) — *see* X92-YØ8 with 7th character S
  - homicide, attempt (any means) — *see* X92-YØ8 with 7th character S
  - injury undetermined whether accidentally or purposely inflicted — *see* Y21-Y33 with 7th character S
  - intentional self-harm (classifiable to X71-X83) — *see* X71-X83 with 7th character S
  - legal intervention — *see* with 7th character S Y35 ☑
  - motor vehicle accident — *see* VØØ-V99 with 7th character S
  - suicide, attempt (any means) — *see* X71-X83 with 7th character S
  - transport accident — *see* VØØ-V99 with 7th character S
  - war operations — *see* War operations
- **Shock**
  - electric — *see* Exposure, electric current
  - from electric appliance (any) (faulty) W86.8 ☑
    - domestic W86.Ø ☑
    - suicide (attempt) X83.1 ☑
- **Shooting, shot** (accidental(ly)) — *see also* Discharge, firearm, by type
  - herself or himself — *see* Discharge, firearm by type, self-inflicted
  - homicide (attempt) — *see* Discharge, firearm by type, homicide
  - in war operations — *see* War operations
  - inflicted by other person — *see* Discharge, firearm by type, homicide
    - accidental — *see* Discharge, firearm, by type of firearm
  - legal
    - execution — *see* Legal, intervention, firearm
    - intervention — *see* Legal, intervention, firearm
  - self-inflicted — *see* Discharge, firearm by type, suicide
    - accidental — *see* Discharge, firearm, by type of firearm
  - suicide (attempt) — *see* Discharge, firearm by type, suicide
- **Shoving** (accidentally) **by other person** — *see* Pushed, by other person
- **Sickness**
  - alpine W94.11 ☑
  - motion — *see* Motion
  - mountain W94.11 ☑
- **Sinking** (accidental)
  - watercraft (causing drowning, submersion) — *see also* Drowning, due to, accident to, watercraft, sinking
    - causing injury except drowning or submersion — *see* Accident, watercraft, causing, injury NEC
- **Siriasis** X32 ☑
- **Sitting** (prolonged) (static) X5Ø.1 ☑
- **Slashed wrists** — *see* Cut, self-inflicted
- **Slipping** (accidental) (on same level) (with fall) WØ1.Ø ☑
  - on
    - ice WØØ.Ø ☑
      - with skates — *see* Accident, transport, pedestrian, conveyance
    - mud WØ1.Ø ☑
    - oil WØ1.Ø ☑
    - snow WØØ.Ø ☑
      - with skis — *see* Accident, transport, pedestrian, conveyance
    - surface (slippery) (wet) NEC WØ1.Ø ☑
  - without fall W18.4Ø ☑
    - due to
      - specified NEC W18.49 ☑
      - stepping from one level to another W18.43 ☑
      - stepping into hole or opening W18.42 ☑
      - stepping on object W18.41 ☑
- **Sliver, wood, contact with** W45.8 ☑
- **Smoldering** (due to fire) — *see* Exposure, fire
- **Sodomy** (attempted) **by force** T74.2 ☑
- **Sound waves** (causing injury) W42.9 ☑
  - supersonic W42.Ø ☑
- **Splinter, contact with** W45.8 ☑
- **Stab, stabbing** — *see* Cut
- **Standing** (prolonged) (static) X5Ø.1 ☑
- **Starvation** X58 ☑
- **Status of external cause** Y99.9
  - child assisting in compensated work for family Y99.8
  - civilian activity done for financial or other compensation Y99.Ø
  - civilian activity done for income or pay Y99.Ø
  - family member assisting in compensated work for other family member Y99.8
  - hobby not done for income Y99.8
  - leisure activity Y99.8
  - military activity Y99.1
  - off-duty activity of military personnel Y99.8
  - recreation or sport not for income or while a student Y99.8
  - specified NEC Y99.8
  - student activity Y99.8
  - volunteer activity Y99.2
- **Stepped on**
  - by
    - animal (not being ridden) NEC W55.89 ☑
    - crowd or human stampede W52 ☑
    - person W5Ø.Ø ☑
- **Stepping on**
  - object W22.8 ☑

- **Stepping on** — *continued*
  - object — *continued*
    - sports equipment W21.9 ☑
    - stationary W22.Ø9 ☑
      - sports equipment W21.89 ☑
    - with fall W18.31 ☑
  - person W51 ☑
    - by crowd or human stampede W52 ☑
  - sports equipment W21.9 ☑
- **Sting**
  - arthropod, nonvenomous W57 ☑
  - insect, nonvenomous W57 ☑
- **Storm** (cataclysmic) — *see* Forces of nature, cataclysmic storm
- **Straining, excessive** — *see also* Overexertion X5Ø.9 ☑
- **Strangling** — *see* Strangulation
- **Strangulation** (accidental) T71 ☑
- **Strenuous movements** — *see also* Overexertion X5Ø.9 ☑
- **Striking against**
  - airbag (automobile) W22.1Ø ☑
    - driver side W22.11 ☑
    - front passenger side W22.12 ☑
    - specified NEC W22.19 ☑
  - bottom when
    - diving or jumping into water (in) W16.822 ☑
      - causing drowning W16.821 ☑
      - from boat W16.722 ☑
        - causing drowning W16.721 ☑
      - natural body W16.622 ☑
        - causing drowning W16.821 ☑
      - swimming pool W16.522 ☑
        - causing drowning W16.521 ☑
    - falling into water (in) W16.322 ☑
      - causing drowning W16.321 ☑
      - fountain — *see* Striking against, bottom when, falling into water, specified NEC
      - natural body W16.122 ☑
        - causing drowning W16.121 ☑
      - reservoir — *see* Striking against, bottom when, falling into water, specified NEC
      - specified NEC W16.322 ☑
        - causing drowning W16.321 ☑
      - swimming pool W16.Ø22 ☑
        - causing drowning W16.Ø21 ☑
  - diving board (swimming-pool) W21.4 ☑
  - object W22.8 ☑
    - caused by crowd or human stampede (with fall) W52 ☑
    - furniture W22.Ø3 ☑
    - lamppost W22.Ø2 ☑
    - sports equipment W21.9 ☑
    - stationary W22.Ø9 ☑
      - sports equipment W21.89 ☑
    - wall W22.Ø1 ☑
    - with
      - drowning or submersion — *see* Drowning
      - fall — *see* Fall, due to, bumping against, object
  - person(s) W51 ☑
    - as, or caused by, a crowd or human stampede (with fall) W52 ☑
    - assault YØ4.2 ☑
    - homicide (attempt) YØ4.2 ☑
    - with fall WØ3 ☑
      - due to ice or snow WØØ.Ø ☑
  - sports equipment W21.9 ☑
  - wall (when) W22.Ø1 ☑
    - diving or jumping into water (in) W16.832 ☑
      - causing drowning W16.831 ☑
      - swimming pool W16.532 ☑
        - causing drowning W16.531 ☑
    - falling into water (in) W16.332 ☑
      - causing drowning W16.331 ☑
      - fountain — *see* Striking against, wall when, falling into water, specified NEC
      - natural body W16.132 ☑
        - causing drowning W16.131 ☑
      - reservoir — *see* Striking against, wall when, falling into water, specified NEC
      - specified NEC W16.332 ☑
        - causing drowning W16.331 ☑
      - swimming pool W16.Ø32 ☑
        - causing drowning W16.Ø31 ☑
    - swimming pool (when) W22.Ø42 ☑
      - causing drowning W22.Ø41 ☑
      - diving or jumping into water W16.532 ☑
- **Striking against** — *continued*
  - wall — *continued*
    - swimming pool — *continued*
      - diving or jumping into water — *continued*
        - causing drowning W16.531 ☑
      - falling into water W16.Ø32 ☑
        - causing drowning W16.Ø31 ☑
- **Struck** (accidentally) **by**
  - airbag (automobile) W22.1Ø ☑
    - driver side W22.11 ☑
    - front passenger side W22.12 ☑
    - specified NEC W22.19 ☑
  - alligator W58.Ø2 ☑
  - animal (not being ridden) NEC W55.89 ☑
  - avalanche — *see* Landslide
  - ball (hit) (thrown) W21.ØØ ☑
    - assault YØ8.Ø9 ☑
    - baseball W21.Ø3 ☑
    - basketball W21.Ø5 ☑
    - football W21.Ø1 ☑
    - golf ball W21.Ø4 ☑
    - soccer W21.Ø2 ☑
    - softball W21.Ø7 ☑
    - specified NEC W21.Ø9 ☑
    - volleyball W21.Ø6 ☑
  - bat or racquet
    - baseball bat W21.11 ☑
      - assault YØ8.Ø2 ☑
    - golf club W21.13 ☑
      - assault YØ8.Ø9 ☑
    - specified NEC W21.19 ☑
      - assault YØ8.Ø9 ☑
    - tennis racquet W21.12 ☑
      - assault YØ8.Ø9 ☑
  - bullet — *see also* Discharge, firearm by type
    - in war operations — *see* War operations
  - crocodile W58.12 ☑
  - dog W54.1 ☑
  - flare, Very pistol — *see* Discharge, firearm NEC
  - hailstones X39.8 ☑
  - hockey (ice)
    - field
      - puck W21.221 ☑
      - stick W21.211 ☑
    - puck W21.22Ø ☑
    - stick W21.21Ø ☑
      - assault YØ8.Ø1 ☑
  - landslide — *see* Landslide
  - law-enforcement agent (on duty) — *see* Legal, intervention, manhandling
    - with blunt object — *see* Legal, intervention, blunt object
  - lightning T75.Ø ☑
    - causing fire — *see* Exposure, fire
  - machine — *see* Contact, with, by type of machine
  - mammal NEC W55.89 ☑
    - marine W56.32 ☑
  - marine animal W56.82 ☑
  - missile
    - firearm — *see* Discharge, firearm by type
    - in war operations — *see* War operations, missile
  - object W22.8 ☑
    - blunt W22.8 ☑
      - assault YØØ ☑
      - suicide (attempt) X79 ☑
      - undetermined whether accidental or intentional Y29 ☑
    - falling W2Ø.8 ☑
      - from, in, on
        - building W2Ø.1 ☑
          - burning (uncontrolled fire) XØØ.4 ☑
        - cataclysmic
          - earth surface movement NEC — *see* Landslide
          - storm — *see* Forces of nature, cataclysmic storm
        - cave-in W2Ø.Ø ☑
        - earthquake X34 ☑
        - machine (in operation) — *see* Contact, with, by type of machine
        - structure W2Ø.1 ☑
          - burning XØØ.4 ☑
        - transport vehicle (in motion) — *see* Accident, transport, by type of vehicle
        - watercraft V93.49 ☑
- **Struck** (accidentally) **by** — *continued*
  - object — *continued*
    - falling — *continued*
      - from, in, on — *continued*
        - watercraft — *continued*
          - due to
            - accident to craft V91.39 ☑
              - powered craft V91.33 ☑
                - ferry boat V91.31 ☑
                - fishing boat V91.32 ☑
                - jetskis V91.33 ☑
                - liner V91.31 ☑
                - merchant ship V91.3Ø ☑
                - passenger ship V91.31 ☑
              - unpowered craft V91.38 ☑
                - canoe V91.35 ☑
                - inflatable V91.36 ☑
                - kayak V91.35 ☑
                - sailboat V91.34 ☑
                - surf-board V91.38 ☑
                - windsurfer V91.38 ☑
          - powered craft V93.43 ☑
            - ferry boat V93.41 ☑
            - fishing boat V93.42 ☑
            - jetskis V93.43 ☑
            - liner V93.41 ☑
            - merchant ship V93.4Ø ☑
            - passenger ship V93.41 ☑
          - unpowered craft V93.48 ☑
            - sailboat V93.44 ☑
            - surf-board V93.48 ☑
            - windsurfer V93.48 ☑
    - moving NEC W2Ø.8 ☑
    - projected W2Ø.8 ☑
      - assault YØØ ☑
      - in sports W21.9 ☑
        - assault YØ8.Ø9 ☑
        - ball W21.ØØ ☑
          - baseball W21.Ø3 ☑
          - basketball W21.Ø5 ☑
          - football W21.Ø1 ☑
          - golf ball W21.Ø4 ☑
          - soccer W21.Ø2 ☑
          - softball W21.Ø7 ☑
          - specified NEC W21.Ø9 ☑
          - volleyball W21.Ø6 ☑
        - bat or racquet
          - baseball bat W21.11 ☑
            - assault YØ8.Ø2 ☑
          - golf club W21.13 ☑
            - assault YØ8.Ø9 ☑
          - specified NEC W21.19 ☑
            - assault YØ8.Ø9 ☑
          - tennis racquet W21.12 ☑
            - assault YØ8.Ø9 ☑
        - hockey (ice)
          - field
            - puck W21.221 ☑
            - stick W21.211 ☑
          - puck W21.22Ø ☑
          - stick W21.21Ø ☑
            - assault YØ8.Ø1 ☑
        - specified NEC W21.89 ☑
    - set in motion by explosion — *see* Explosion
    - thrown W2Ø.8 ☑
      - assault YØØ ☑
      - in sports W21.9 ☑
        - assault YØ8.Ø9 ☑
        - ball W21.ØØ ☑
          - baseball W21.Ø3 ☑
          - basketball W21.Ø5 ☑
          - football W21.Ø1 ☑
          - golf ball W21.Ø4 ☑
          - soccer W21.Ø2 ☑
          - soft ball W21.Ø7 ☑
          - specified NEC W21.Ø9 ☑
          - volleyball W21.Ø6 ☑
        - bat or racquet
          - baseball bat W21.11 ☑
            - assault YØ8.Ø2 ☑
          - golf club W21.13 ☑
            - assault YØ8.Ø9 ☑
          - specified NEC W21.19 ☑
            - assault YØ8.Ø9 ☑
          - tennis racquet W21.12 ☑
            - assault YØ8.Ø9 ☑

T

U

V

W

ICD-10-CM Tabular List of Diseases and Injuries

Chapter 1. Certain Infectious and Parasitic Diseases (AØØ–B99), UØ7.1, UØ9.9

Chapter-specific Guidelines with Coding Examples

The chapter-specific guidelines from the ICD-10-CM Official Guidelines for Coding and Reporting have been provided below. Along with these guidelines are coding examples, contained in the shaded boxes, that have been developed to help illustrate the coding and/or sequencing guidance found in these guidelines.

a. Human immunodeficiency virus (HIV) infections

1) Code only confirmed cases

Code only confirmed cases of HIV infection/illness. This is an exception to the hospital inpatient guideline Section II, H.

In this context, "confirmation" does not require documentation of positive serology or culture for HIV; the provider's diagnostic statement that the patient is HIV positive or has an HIV-related illness is sufficient.

> Patient admitted with anemia with possible HIV infection
>
> **D64.9 Anemia, unspecified**
>
> *Explanation:* Only the anemia is coded in this scenario because it has not been confirmed that an HIV infection is present. This is an exception to the guideline Section II, H for hospital inpatient coding.

2) Selection and sequencing of HIV codes

(a) Patient admitted for HIV-related condition

If a patient is admitted for an HIV-related condition, the principal diagnosis should be B2Ø, Human immunodeficiency virus [HIV] disease followed by additional diagnosis codes for all reported HIV-related conditions.

An exception to this guideline is if the reason for admission is hemolytic-uremic syndrome associated with HIV disease. Assign code D59.31, Infection-associated hemolytic-uremic syndrome, followed by code B2Ø, Human immunodeficiency virus [HIV] disease.

(b) Patient with HIV disease admitted for unrelated condition

If a patient with HIV disease is admitted for an unrelated condition (such as a traumatic injury), the code for the unrelated condition (e.g., the nature of injury code) should be the principal diagnosis. Other diagnoses would be B2Ø followed by additional diagnosis codes for all reported HIV-related conditions.

> Unstable angina, native coronary artery atherosclerosis, HIV
>
> **I25.11Ø Atherosclerotic heart disease of native coronary artery with unstable angina pectoris**
>
> **B2Ø Human immunodeficiency virus [HIV] disease**
>
> *Explanation:* The arteriosclerotic coronary artery disease and the unstable angina are not related to HIV, so those conditions are reported first using a combination code, and HIV is reported secondarily.

(c) Whether the patient is newly diagnosed

Whether the patient is newly diagnosed or has had previous admissions/encounters for HIV conditions is irrelevant to the sequencing decision.

(d) Asymptomatic human immunodeficiency virus

Z21, Asymptomatic human immunodeficiency virus [HIV] infection status, is to be applied when the patient without any documentation of symptoms is listed as being "HIV positive," "known HIV," "HIV test positive," or similar terminology. Do not use this code if the term "AIDS" or "HIV disease" is used or if the patient is treated for any HIV-related illness or is described as having any condition(s) resulting from his/her HIV positive status; use B2Ø in these cases.

(e) Patients with inconclusive HIV serology

Patients with inconclusive HIV serology, but no definitive diagnosis or manifestations of the illness, may be assigned code R75, Inconclusive laboratory evidence of human immunodeficiency virus [HIV].

(f) Previously diagnosed HIV-related illness

Patients with any known prior diagnosis of an HIV-related illness should be coded to B2Ø. Once a patient has developed an HIV-related illness, the patient should always be assigned code B2Ø on every subsequent admission/encounter. Patients previously diagnosed with any HIV illness (B2Ø) should never be assigned to R75 or Z21, Asymptomatic human immunodeficiency virus [HIV] infection status.

(g) HIV infection in pregnancy, childbirth and the puerperium

During pregnancy, childbirth or the puerperium, a patient admitted (or presenting for a health care encounter) because of an HIV-related illness should receive a principal diagnosis code of O98.7-, Human immunodeficiency [HIV] disease complicating pregnancy, childbirth and the puerperium, followed by B2Ø and the code(s) for the HIV-related illness(es). Codes from Chapter 15 always take sequencing priority.

Patients with asymptomatic HIV infection status admitted (or presenting for a health care encounter) during pregnancy, childbirth, or the puerperium should receive codes of O98.7- and Z21.

(h) Encounters for testing for HIV

If a patient is being seen to determine his/her HIV status, use code Z11.4, Encounter for screening for human immunodeficiency virus [HIV]. Use additional codes for any associated high-risk behavior, if applicable.

If a patient with signs or symptoms is being seen for HIV testing, code the signs and symptoms. An additional counseling code Z71.7, Human immunodeficiency virus [HIV] counseling, may be used if counseling is provided during the encounter for the test.

When a patient returns to be informed of his/her HIV test results and the test result is negative, use code Z71.7, Human immunodeficiency virus [HIV] counseling.

If the results are positive, see previous guidelines and assign codes as appropriate.

(i) HIV managed by antiretroviral medication

If a patient with documented HIV disease, HIV-related illness or AIDS is currently managed on antiretroviral medications, assign code B2Ø, Human immunodeficiency virus [HIV] disease. Code Z79.899, Other long term (current) drug therapy, may be assigned as an additional code to identify the long-term (current) use of antiretroviral medications.

(j) Encounter for HIV Prophylaxis Measure

When a patient is seen for administration of pre-exposure prophylaxis medication for HIV, assign code Z29.81, Encounter for HIV pre-exposure prophylaxis. Pre-exposure prophylaxis (PrEP) is intended to prevent infection in people who are at risk for getting HIV through sex or injection drug use. Any risk factors for HIV should also be coded.

b. Infectious agents as the cause of diseases classified to other chapters

Certain infections are classified in chapters other than Chapter 1 and no organism is identified as part of the infection code. In these instances, it is necessary to use an additional code from Chapter 1 to identify the organism. A code from category B95, Streptococcus, Staphylococcus, and Enterococcus as the cause of diseases classified to other chapters, B96, Other bacterial agents as the cause of diseases classified to other chapters, or B97, Viral agents as the cause of diseases classified to other chapters, is to be used as an additional code to identify the organism. An instructional note will be found at the infection code advising that an additional organism code is required.

c. Infections resistant to antibiotics

Many bacterial infections are resistant to current antibiotics. It is necessary to identify all infections documented as antibiotic resistant. Assign a code from category Z16, Resistance to antimicrobial drugs, following the infection code only if the infection code does not identify drug resistance.

d. Sepsis, severe sepsis, and septic shock infections resistant to antibiotics

1) Coding of sepsis and severe sepsis

(a) Sepsis

For a diagnosis of sepsis, assign the appropriate code for the underlying systemic infection. If the type of infection or causal organism is not further specified, assign code A41.9, Sepsis, unspecified organism.

A code from subcategory R65.2, Severe sepsis, should not be assigned unless severe sepsis or an associated acute organ dysfunction is documented.

(i) Negative or inconclusive blood cultures and sepsis

Negative or inconclusive blood cultures do not preclude a diagnosis of sepsis in patients with clinical evidence of the condition; however, the provider should be queried.

(ii) Urosepsis

The term urosepsis is a nonspecific term. It is not to be considered synonymous with sepsis. It has no default code in the Alphabetic Index. Should a provider use this term, he/she must be queried for clarification.

(iii) Sepsis with organ dysfunction

If a patient has sepsis and associated acute organ dysfunction or multiple organ dysfunction (MOD), follow the instructions for coding severe sepsis.

(iv) Acute organ dysfunction that is not clearly associated with the sepsis

If a patient has sepsis and an acute organ dysfunction, but the medical record documentation indicates that the acute organ dysfunction is related to a medical condition other than the sepsis, do not assign a code from subcategory R65.2, Severe sepsis. An acute organ dysfunction must be associated with the sepsis in order to assign the severe sepsis code. If the documentation is not clear as to whether an acute organ dysfunction is related to the sepsis or another medical condition, query the provider.

Sepsis and acute respiratory failure due to COPD exacerbation

A41.9	**Sepsis, unspecified organism**
J44.1	**Chronic obstructive pulmonary disease with (acute) exacerbation**
J96.ØØ	**Acute respiratory failure, unspecified whether with hypoxia or hypercapnia**

Explanation: Although acute organ dysfunction is present in the form of acute respiratory failure, severe sepsis (R65.2) is not coded in this example, as the acute respiratory failure is attributed to the COPD exacerbation rather than the sepsis. Sequencing of these codes would be determined by the circumstances of the admission.

(b) Severe sepsis

The coding of severe sepsis requires a minimum of 2 codes: first a code for the underlying systemic infection, followed by a code from subcategory R65.2, Severe sepsis. If the causal organism is not documented, assign code A41.9, Sepsis, unspecified organism, for the infection. Additional code(s) for the associated acute organ dysfunction are also required.

Due to the complex nature of severe sepsis, some cases may require querying the provider prior to assignment of the codes.

2) Septic shock

Septic shock generally refers to circulatory failure associated with severe sepsis, and therefore, it represents a type of acute organ dysfunction.

For cases of septic shock, the code for the systemic infection should be sequenced first, followed by code R65.21, Severe sepsis with septic shock or code T81.12, Postprocedural septic shock. Any additional codes for the other acute organ dysfunctions should also be assigned. As noted in the sequencing instructions in the Tabular List, the code for septic shock cannot be assigned as a principal diagnosis.

Sepsis with septic shock

A41.9	**Sepsis, unspecified organism**
R65.21	**Severe sepsis with septic shock**

Explanation: Documentation of septic shock automatically implies severe sepsis as it is a form of acute organ dysfunction. Septic shock is not coded as the principal diagnosis; it is always preceded by the code for the systemic infection.

3) Sequencing of severe sepsis

If severe sepsis is present on admission, and meets the definition of principal diagnosis, the underlying systemic infection should be assigned as principal diagnosis followed by the appropriate code from subcategory R65.2 as required by the sequencing rules in the Tabular List. A code from subcategory R65.2 can never be assigned as a principal diagnosis.

When severe sepsis develops during an encounter (it was not present on admission), the underlying systemic infection and the appropriate code from subcategory R65.2 should be assigned as secondary diagnoses.

Severe sepsis may be present on admission, but the diagnosis may not be confirmed until sometime after admission. If the documentation is not clear whether severe sepsis was present on admission, the provider should be queried.

For infection-associated hemolytic-uremic syndrome with severe sepsis, see guideline I.C.1.d.9.

4) Sepsis or severe sepsis with a localized infection

If the reason for admission is sepsis or severe sepsis and a localized infection, such as pneumonia or cellulitis, a code(s) for the underlying systemic infection should be assigned first and the code for the localized infection should be assigned as a secondary diagnosis. If the patient has severe sepsis, a code from subcategory R65.2 should also be assigned as a secondary diagnosis. If the patient is admitted with a localized infection, such as pneumonia, and sepsis/severe sepsis doesn't develop until after admission, the localized infection should be assigned first, followed by the appropriate sepsis/severe sepsis codes.

For hemolytic-uremic syndrome associated with sepsis, see guideline I.C.1.d.9.

Patient presents with acute renal failure due to severe sepsis from *Pseudomonas* pneumonia

A41.52	**Sepsis due to Pseudomonas**
J15.1	**Pneumonia due to Pseudomonas**
R65.2Ø	**Severe sepsis without septic shock**
N17.9	**Acute kidney failure, unspecified**

Explanation: If all conditions are present on admission, the systemic infection (sepsis) is sequenced first followed by the codes for the localized infection (pneumonia), severe sepsis and any organ dysfunction. If only the pneumonia was present on admission with the sepsis and resulting renal failure developing later in the admission, then the pneumonia would be sequenced first.

5) Sepsis due to a postprocedural infection

(a) Documentation of causal relationship

As with all postprocedural complications, code assignment is based on the provider's documentation of the relationship between the infection and the procedure.

(b) Sepsis due to a postprocedural infection

For **sepsis** following a **postprocedural wound (surgical site) infection,** a code from T81.41 to T81.43, Infection following a procedure, or a code from O86.ØØ to O86.Ø3, Infection of obstetric surgical wound, that identifies the site of the infection should be **sequenced** first, if known. Assign an additional code for sepsis following a procedure (T81.44) or sepsis following an obstetrical procedure (O86.Ø4). Use an additional code to identify the infectious agent. If the patient has severe sepsis, the appropriate code from subcategory R65.2 should also be assigned with the additional code(s) for any acute organ dysfunction.

For infections following infusion, transfusion, therapeutic injection, or immunization, a code from subcategory T8Ø.2, Infections following infusion, transfusion, and therapeutic injection, or code T88.Ø-, Infection following immunization, should be coded first, followed by the code for the specific infection. If the patient has severe sepsis, the appropriate code from subcategory R65.2 should also be assigned, with the additional codes(s) for any acute organ dysfunction.

(c) Postprocedural infection and postprocedural septic shock

If a postprocedural infection has resulted in postprocedural septic shock, assign the codes indicated above for sepsis due to a postprocedural infection, followed by code T81.12-, Postprocedural septic shock. Do not assign code R65.21, Severe sepsis with septic shock. Additional code(s) should be assigned for any acute organ dysfunction.

Septic shock following abdominal procedure with intramuscular abscess

T81.42XA	**Infection following a procedure, deep incisional surgical site, initial encounter**
T81.44XA	**Sepsis following a procedure, initial encounter**
A41.9	**Sepsis, unspecified organism**
T81.12XA	**Postprocedural septic shock, initial encounter**

Explanation: The first code reported identifies the site of the postprocedural infection with intramuscular abscess coded to "deep incisional surgical site." If sepsis occurred as a result of the postprocedural infection, code T81.44- should be coded as a secondary diagnosis, followed by a code for the specific type of sepsis. Postprocedural septic shock is captured by code T81.12- and not with code R65.21. If any other acute organ dysfunction was documented as associated with the postprocedural sepsis, additional codes could be assigned to represent those conditions.

6) Sepsis and severe sepsis associated with a noninfectious process (condition)

In some cases, a noninfectious process (condition) such as trauma, may lead to an infection which can result in sepsis or severe sepsis. If sepsis or severe sepsis is documented as associated with a noninfectious condition, such as a burn or serious injury, and this condition meets the definition for principal diagnosis, the code for the noninfectious condition should be sequenced first, followed by the code for the resulting infection. If severe sepsis is present, a code from subcategory R65.2 should also be assigned with any associated organ dysfunction(s) codes. It is not necessary to assign a code from subcategory R65.1, Systemic inflammatory response syndrome (SIRS) of non-infectious origin, for these cases.

If the infection meets the definition of principal diagnosis, it should be sequenced before the non-infectious condition. When both the associated non-infectious condition and the infection meet the definition of principal diagnosis, either may be assigned as principal diagnosis.

Only one code from category R65, Symptoms and signs specifically associated with systemic inflammation and infection, should be assigned. Therefore, when a non-infectious condition leads to an infection resulting in severe sepsis, assign the appropriate code from subcategory R65.2, Severe sepsis. Do not additionally assign a code from subcategory R65.1, Systemic inflammatory response syndrome (SIRS) of non-infectious origin.

See Section I.C.18. SIRS due to non-infectious process.

Patient admitted with multiple third-degree burns of right upper arm develops severe MSSA sepsis with septic shock, three days into admission

T22.391A	**Burn of third degree of multiple sites of right shoulder and upper arm limb, except wrist and hand, initial encounter**
A41.Ø1	**Sepsis due to Methicillin susceptible Staphylococcus aureus**
R65.21	**Severe sepsis with septic shock**

Explanation: Severe sepsis is coded rather than SIRS from R65 because it is documented as a severe systemic infectious response with septic shock to a noninfectious condition. The code for the systemic infection is not used as the principal diagnosis because it was not present on admission. The patient was admitted for the burn injury.

7) Sepsis and septic shock complicating abortion, pregnancy, childbirth, and the puerperium

See Section I.C.15. Sepsis and septic shock complicating abortion, pregnancy, childbirth and the puerperium

8) Newborn sepsis

See Section I.C.16. f. Bacterial sepsis of Newborn

9) Hemolytic-uremic syndrome associated with sepsis

If the reason for admission is hemolytic-uremic syndrome that is associated with sepsis, assign code D59.31, Infection-associated hemolytic-uremic syndrome, as the principal diagnosis. Codes for the underlying systemic infection and any other conditions (such as severe sepsis) should be assigned as secondary diagnoses.

e. Methicillin resistant Staphylococcus aureus (MRSA) conditions

1) Selection and sequencing of MRSA codes

(a) Combination codes for MRSA infection

When a patient is diagnosed with an infection that is due to methicillin resistant *Staphylococcus aureus* (MRSA), and that infection has a combination code that includes the causal organism (e.g., sepsis, pneumonia) assign the appropriate combination code for the condition (e.g., code A41.Ø2, Sepsis due to Methicillin resistant Staphylococcus aureus or code J15.212, Pneumonia due to Methicillin resistant Staphylococcus aureus). Do not assign code B95.62, Methicillin resistant Staphylococcus aureus infection as the cause of diseases classified elsewhere, as an additional code, because the combination code includes the type of infection and the MRSA organism. Do not assign a code from subcategory Z16.11, Resistance to penicillins, as an additional diagnosis.

See Section C.1. for instructions on coding and sequencing of sepsis and severe sepsis.

(b) Other codes for MRSA infection

When there is documentation of a current infection (e.g., wound infection, stitch abscess, urinary tract infection) due to MRSA, and that infection does not have a combination code that includes the causal organism, assign the appropriate code to identify the condition along with code B95.62, Methicillin resistant Staphylococcus aureus infection as the cause of diseases classified elsewhere for the MRSA infection. Do not assign a code from subcategory Z16.11, Resistance to penicillins.

(c) Methicillin susceptible Staphylococcus aureus (MSSA) and MRSA colonization

The condition or state of being colonized or carrying MSSA or MRSA is called colonization or carriage, while an individual person is described as being colonized or being a carrier.

Colonization means that MSSA or MSRA is present on or in the body without necessarily causing illness. A positive MRSA colonization test might be documented by the provider as "MRSA screen positive" or "MRSA nasal swab positive".

Assign code Z22.322, Carrier or suspected carrier of Methicillin resistant Staphylococcus aureus, for patients documented as having MRSA colonization. Assign code Z22.321, Carrier or suspected carrier of Methicillin susceptible Staphylococcus aureus, for patients documented as having MSSA colonization. Colonization is not necessarily indicative of a disease process or as the cause of a specific condition the patient may have unless documented as such by the provider.

(d) MRSA colonization and infection

If a patient is documented as having both MRSA colonization and infection during a hospital admission, code Z22.322, Carrier or suspected carrier of Methicillin resistant Staphylococcus aureus, and a code for the MRSA infection may both be assigned.

f. Zika virus infections

1) Code only confirmed cases

Code only a confirmed diagnosis of Zika virus (A92.5, Zika virus disease) as documented by the provider. This is an exception to the hospital inpatient guideline Section II, H. In this context, "confirmation" does not require documentation of the type of test performed; the provider's diagnostic statement that the condition is confirmed is sufficient. This code should be assigned regardless of the stated mode of transmission.

If the provider documents "suspected", "possible" or "probable" Zika, do not assign code A92.5. Assign a code(s) explaining the reason for encounter (such as fever, rash, or joint pain) or Z2Ø.821, Contact with and (suspected) exposure to Zika virus.

g. Coronavirus infections

1) COVID-19 infection (infection due to SARS-CoV-2)

(a) Code only confirmed cases

Code only a confirmed diagnosis of the 2019 novel coronavirus disease (COVID-19) as documented by the provider, or documentation of a positive COVID-19 test result. For a confirmed diagnosis, assign code UØ7.1, COVID-19. This is an exception to the hospital inpatient guideline Section II, H. In this context, "confirmation" does not require documentation of a positive test result for COVID-19; the provider's documentation that the individual has COVID-19 is sufficient.

If the provider documents "suspected," "possible," "probable," or "inconclusive" COVID-19, do not assign code UØ7.1. Instead, code the signs and symptoms reported. See guideline I.C.1.g.1.g.

An elderly patient who is a former smoker is admitted with a productive cough, fatigue, and chest discomfort. CXR and PFTs indicate acute bronchitis. Treatment includes cough suppressants and anti-inflammatory medication, along with isolation precautions. The provider documents acute bronchitis likely due to COVID-19. Laboratory tests were inconclusive.

J2Ø.9	**Acute bronchitis, unspecified**
Z87.891	**History of tobacco dependence**

Explanation: Because the COVID-19 diagnosis was documented as likely by the provider, code UØ7.1 cannot be assigned. Instead a code explaining the reason for the encounter is used, in this case the acute bronchitis. Code J2Ø.9 Acute bronchitis, unspecified, is used because the causative organism, specifically that which causes COVID-19, is not confirmed. Without further documentation of COVID-19 or another causative organism being present, code J2Ø.8 Acute bronchitis due to other specified organisms, does not apply.

(b) Sequencing of codes

When COVID-19 meets the definition of principal diagnosis, code UØ7.1, COVID-19, should be sequenced first, followed by the appropriate codes for associated manifestations, except when another guideline requires that certain codes be sequenced first, such as obstetrics, sepsis, or transplant complications.

The patient presents with acute hypoxic respiratory failure due to sepsis from COVID-19 related pneumonia.

A41.89	**Other specified sepsis**
UØ7.1	**COVID-19**
J12.82	**Pneumonia due to coronavirus disease 2019**
J96.Ø1	**Acute respiratory failure with hypoxia**
R65.2Ø	**Severe sepsis without septic shock**

Explanation: If all conditions are present on admission, the systemic infection (sepsis) is sequenced first, followed by the code(s) for the localized infection (COVID-19 and pneumonia). The acute respiratory failure (acute organ dysfunction) is clearly documented as being associated with the sepsis, and therefore a severe sepsis code from subcategory R65.2- can also be assigned. If the sepsis had developed later in the admission, with or without any associated respiratory failure, the COVID-19 code would be sequenced first.

For a COVID-19 infection that progresses to sepsis, see Section I.C.1.d. Sepsis, Severe Sepsis, and Septic Shock

See Section I.C.15.s. for COVID-19 infection in pregnancy, childbirth, and the puerperium

See Section I.C.16.h. for COVID-19 infection in newborn

For a COVID-19 infection in a lung transplant patient, see Section I.C.19.g.3.a. Transplant complications other than kidney.

(c) Acute respiratory manifestations of COVID-19

When the reason for the encounter/admission is a respiratory manifestation of COVID-19, assign code U07.1, COVID-19, as the principal/first-listed diagnosis and assign code(s) for the respiratory manifestation(s) as additional diagnoses.

The following conditions are examples of common respiratory manifestations of COVID-19.

(i) Pneumonia

For a patient with pneumonia confirmed as due to COVID-19, assign codes U07.1, COVID-19, and J12.82, Pneumonia due to coronavirus disease 2019.

(ii) Acute bronchitis

For a patient with acute bronchitis confirmed as due to COVID-19, assign codes U07.1, and J20.8, Acute bronchitis due to other specified organisms.

Bronchitis not otherwise specified (NOS) due to COVID-19 should be coded using code U07.1 and J40, Bronchitis, not specified as acute or chronic.

(iii) Lower respiratory infection

If the COVID-19 is documented as being associated with a lower respiratory infection, not otherwise specified (NOS), or an acute respiratory infection, NOS, codes U07.1 and J22, Unspecified acute lower respiratory infection, should be assigned.

If the COVID-19 is documented as being associated with a respiratory infection, NOS, codes U07.1 and J98.8, Other specified respiratory disorders, should be assigned.

(iv) Acute respiratory distress syndrome

For acute respiratory distress syndrome (ARDS) due to COVID-19, assign codes U07.1, and J80, Acute respiratory distress syndrome.

(v) Acute respiratory failure

For acute respiratory failure due to COVID-19, assign code U07.1, and code J96.0-, Acute respiratory failure.

(d) Non-respiratory manifestations of COVID-19

When the reason for the encounter/admission is a non-respiratory manifestation (e.g., viral enteritis) of COVID-19, assign code U07.1, COVID-19, as the principal/first-listed diagnosis and assign code(s) for the manifestation(s) as additional diagnoses.

(e) Exposure to COVID-19

For asymptomatic individuals with actual or suspected exposure to COVID-19, assign code Z20.822, Contact with and (suspected) exposure to COVID-19.

For symptomatic individuals with actual or suspected exposure to COVID-19 and the infection has been ruled out, or test results are inconclusive or unknown, assign code Z20.822, Contact with and (suspected) exposure to COVID-19. See guideline I.C.21.c.1, Contact/Exposure, for additional guidance regarding the use of category Z20 codes.

If COVID-19 is confirmed, see guideline I.C.1.g.1.a.

(f) Screening for COVID-19

For screening for COVID-19, including preoperative testing, assign code Z11.52, Encounter for screening for COVID-19.

(g) Signs and symptoms without definitive diagnosis of COVID-19

For patients presenting with any signs/symptoms associated with COVID-19 (such as fever, etc.) but a definitive diagnosis has not been established, assign the appropriate code(s) for each of the presenting signs and symptoms such as:

- R05.1, Acute cough, or R05.9, Cough, unspecified
- R06.02 Shortness of breath
- R50.9 Fever, unspecified

If a patient with signs/symptoms associated with COVID-19 also has an actual or suspected contact with or exposure to COVID-19, assign Z20.822, Contact with and (suspected) exposure to COVID19, as an additional code.

(h) Asymptomatic individuals who test positive for COVID-19

For asymptomatic individuals who test positive for COVID-19, see guideline I.C.1.g.1.a. Although the individual is asymptomatic, the individual has tested positive and is considered to have the COVID-19 infection.

(i) Personal history of COVID-19

For patients with a history of COVID-19, assign code Z86.16, Personal history of COVID-19.

(j) Follow-up visits after COVID-19 infection has resolved

For individuals who previously had COVID-19, without residual symptom(s) or condition(s), and are being seen for follow-up evaluation, and COVID-19 test results are negative, assign codes Z09, Encounter for follow-up examination after completed treatment for conditions other than malignant neoplasm, and Z86.16, Personal history of COVID-19.

For follow-up visits for individuals with symptom(s) or condition(s) related to a previous COVID-19 infection, see guideline I.C.1.g.1.m.

See Section I.C.21.c.8, Factors influencing health states and contact with health services, Follow-up

(k) Encounter for antibody testing

For an encounter for antibody testing that is not being performed to confirm a current COVID-19 infection, nor is a follow-up test after resolution of COVID-19, assign Z01.84, Encounter for antibody response examination.

Follow the applicable guidelines above if the individual is being tested to confirm a current COVID-19 infection.

For follow-up testing after a COVID-19 infection, see guideline I.C.1.g.1.j.

(l) Multisystem inflammatory syndrome

For individuals with multisystem inflammatory syndrome (MIS) and COVID-19, assign code U07.1, COVID-19, as the principal/first-listed diagnosis and assign code M35.81, Multisystem inflammatory syndrome, as an additional diagnosis.

If an individual with a history of COVID-19 develops MIS, assign codes M35.81, Multisystem inflammatory syndrome, and U09.9, Post COVID-19 condition, unspecified.

If an individual with a known or suspected exposure to COVID-19, and no current COVID-19 infection or history of COVID-19, develops MIS, assign codes M35.81, Multisystem inflammatory syndrome, and Z20.822, Contact with and (suspected) exposure to COVID-19.

Additional codes should be assigned for any associated complications of MIS.

(m) Post COVID-19 condition

For sequela of COVID-19, or associated symptoms or conditions that develop following a previous COVID-19 infection, assign a code(s) for the specific symptom(s) or condition(s) related to the previous COVID-19 infection, if known, and code U09.9, Post COVID-19 condition, unspecified.

Code U09.9 should not be assigned for manifestations of an active (current) COVID-19 infection.

If a patient has a condition(s) associated with a previous COVID-19 infection and develops a new active (current) COVID-19 infection, code U09.9 may be assigned in conjunction with code U07.1, COVID-19, to identify that the patient also has a condition(s) associated with a previous COVID-19 infection. Code(s) for the specific condition(s) associated with the previous COVID-19 infection and code(s) for manifestation(s) of the new active (current) COVID-19 infection should also be assigned.

(n) Underimmunization for COVID-19 Status

Code Z28.310, Unvaccinated for COVID-19, may be assigned when the patient has not received a COVID-19 vaccine of any type. Code Z28.311, Partially vaccinated for COVID-19, may be assigned when the patient has been partially vaccinated for COVID-19 as per the recommendations of the Centers for Disease Control and Prevention (CDC) in place at the time of the encounter. For information, visit the CDC's website https://www.cdc.gov/coronavirus/2019-ncov/vaccines/.

See Section I.B.14. for underimmunization documentation by clinicians other than patient's provider.

Chapter 1. Certain Infectious and Parasitic Diseases (A00-B99)

INCLUDES diseases generally recognized as communicable or transmissible

Use additional code to identify resistance to antimicrobial drugs (Z16.-)

EXCLUDES 1 *certain localized infections - see body system-related chapters*

EXCLUDES 2 *carrier or suspected carrier of infectious disease (Z22.-)*
infectious and parasitic diseases complicating pregnancy, childbirth and the puerperium (O98.-)
infectious and parasitic diseases specific to the perinatal period (P35-P39)
influenza and other acute respiratory infections (J00-J22)

This chapter contains the following blocks:

A00-A09 Intestinal infectious diseases
A15-A19 Tuberculosis
A20-A28 Certain zoonotic bacterial diseases
A30-A49 Other bacterial diseases
A50-A64 Infections with a predominantly sexual mode of transmission
A65-A69 Other spirochetal diseases
A70-A74 Other diseases caused by chlamydiae
A75-A79 Rickettsioses
A80-A89 Viral and prion infections of the central nervous system
A90-A99 Arthropod-borne viral fevers and viral hemorrhagic fevers
B00-B09 Viral infections characterized by skin and mucous membrane lesions
B10 Other human herpesviruses
B15-B19 Viral hepatitis
B20 Human immunodeficiency virus [HIV] disease
B25-B34 Other viral diseases
B35-B49 Mycoses
B50-B64 Protozoal diseases
B65-B83 Helminthiases
B85-B89 Pediculosis, acariasis and other infestations
B90-B94 Sequelae of infectious and parasitic diseases
B95-B97 Bacterial and viral infectious agents
B99 Other infectious diseases

Intestinal infectious diseases (A00-A09)

✓4th **A00 Cholera**

DEF: Acute infection of the bowel due to *Vibrio cholerae* that presents with profuse diarrhea, cramps, and vomiting, resulting in severe dehydration, electrolyte imbalance, and death. It is spread through ingestion of food or water contaminated with feces of infected persons.

A00.0 Cholera due to Vibrio cholerae 01, biovar cholerae CC
Classical cholera

A00.1 Cholera due to Vibrio cholerae 01, biovar eltor CC
Cholera eltor

A00.9 Cholera, unspecified CC

✓4th **A01 Typhoid and paratyphoid fevers**

DEF: Typhoid fever: Acute generalized illness caused by *Salmonella typhi*. Clinical features include fever, headache, abdominal pain, cough, toxemia, leukopenia, abnormal pulse, rose spots on the skin, bacteremia, hyperplasia of intestinal lymph nodes, mesenteric lymphadenopathy, and Peyer's patches in the intestines.

DEF: Paratyphoid fever: Prolonged febrile illness, caused by *Salmonella* serotypes other than *S. typhi*, especially *S. enterica* serotypes paratyphi A, B, and C.

✓5th **A01.0 Typhoid fever**
Infection due to Salmonella typhi

A01.00 Typhoid fever, unspecified CC
A01.01 Typhoid meningitis CC
A01.02 Typhoid fever with heart involvement CC
Typhoid endocarditis
Typhoid myocarditis
A01.03 Typhoid pneumonia CC HCC
A01.04 Typhoid arthritis CC HCC
A01.05 Typhoid osteomyelitis CC HCC
A01.09 Typhoid fever with other complications CC

A01.1 Paratyphoid fever A CC
A01.2 Paratyphoid fever B CC
A01.3 Paratyphoid fever C CC
A01.4 Paratyphoid fever, unspecified CC
Infection due to Salmonella paratyphi NOS

✓4th **A02 Other salmonella infections**

INCLUDES infection or foodborne intoxication due to any Salmonella species other than S. typhi and S. paratyphi

A02.0 Salmonella enteritis CC
Salmonellosis
TIP: Dehydration (E86.0) is a complication of salmonella enteritis and may be reported separately.

A02.1 Salmonella sepsis HIV MCC HCC

✓5th **A02.2 Localized salmonella infections**

A02.20 Localized salmonella infection, unspecified HIV
A02.21 Salmonella meningitis HIV MCC
A02.22 Salmonella pneumonia HIV MCC HCC
A02.23 Salmonella arthritis HIV CC HCC
A02.24 Salmonella osteomyelitis HIV CC HCC
A02.25 Salmonella pyelonephritis HIV CC
Salmonella tubulo-interstitial nephropathy
A02.29 Salmonella with other localized infection HIV CC

A02.8 Other specified salmonella infections HIV CC
A02.9 Salmonella infection, unspecified HIV CC

✓4th **A03 Shigellosis**

DEF: Infection caused by the genus *Shigella*, of the family *Enterobacteriaceae* that is known to cause an acute dysenteric infection of the bowel with fever, drowsiness, anorexia, nausea, vomiting, bloody diarrhea, abdominal cramps, and distention.

A03.0 Shigellosis due to Shigella dysenteriae CC
Group A shigellosis [Shiga-Kruse dysentery]

A03.1 Shigellosis due to Shigella flexneri
Group B shigellosis

A03.2 Shigellosis due to Shigella boydii
Group C shigellosis

A03.3 Shigellosis due to Shigella sonnei
Group D shigellosis

A03.8 Other shigellosis

A03.9 Shigellosis, unspecified
Bacillary dysentery NOS

✓4th **A04 Other bacterial intestinal infections**

EXCLUDES 1 *bacterial foodborne intoxications, NEC (A05.-)*
tuberculous enteritis (A18.32)

DEF: *Escherichia coli*: Gram-negative, anaerobic bacteria of the family *Enterobacteriaceae* found in the large intestine of warm-blooded animals, generally as a nonpathologic entity aiding in digestion. They become pathogenic when an opportunity to grow somewhere outside this relationship presents itself, such as ingestion of fecal-contaminated food or water.

A04.0 Enteropathogenic Escherichia coli infection CC
A04.1 Enterotoxigenic Escherichia coli infection CC
A04.2 Enteroinvasive Escherichia coli infection CC
A04.3 Enterohemorrhagic Escherichia coli infection CC
DEF: *E. coli* infection penetrating the intestinal mucosa, producing microscopic ulceration and bleeding.

A04.4 Other intestinal Escherichia coli infections CC
Escherichia coli enteritis NOS

A04.5 Campylobacter enteritis CC
TIP: For Guillain-Barre syndrome occurring as a sequela of *Campylobacter enteritis*, assign code G61.0 as the first-listed diagnosis followed by B94.8 for the sequelae.

A04.6 Enteritis due to Yersinia enterocolitica CC
EXCLUDES 1 *extraintestinal yersiniosis (A28.2)*

✓5th **A04.7 Enterocolitis due to Clostridium difficile**
Foodborne intoxication by Clostridium difficile
Pseudomembraneous colitis
AHA: 2017,4Q,4

A04.71 Enterocolitis due to Clostridium difficile, recurrent CC
AHA: 2020,1Q,18

A04.72 Enterocolitis due to Clostridium difficile, not specified as recurrent CC

A04.8 Other specified bacterial intestinal infections CC

A04.9 Bacterial intestinal infection, unspecified CC
Bacterial enteritis NOS

✓4th **A05 Other bacterial foodborne intoxications, not elsewhere classified**

EXCLUDES 1 *Clostridium difficile foodborne intoxication and infection (A04.7-)*
Escherichia coli infection (A04.0-A04.4)
listeriosis (A32.-)
salmonella foodborne intoxication and infection (A02.-)
toxic effect of noxious foodstuffs (T61-T62)

A05.0 Foodborne staphylococcal intoxication CC
TIP: Assign code A04.8 to report a staphylococcal infection when it is caused by the ingestion of contaminated food but not caused by *S. aureus* toxins.

AØ5.1 Botulism food poisoning CC
Botulism NOS
Classical foodborne intoxication due to Clostridium botulinum
EXCLUDES 1 *infant botulism (A48.51)*
wound botulism (A48.52)
DEF: Muscle-paralyzing neurotoxic disease caused by ingesting pre-formed toxin from the bacterium *Clostridium botulinum*. It causes vomiting and diarrhea, vision problems, slurred speech, difficulty swallowing, paralysis, and death.

AØ5.2 Foodborne Clostridium perfringens [Clostridium welchii] intoxication CC
Enteritis necroticans
Pig-bel

AØ5.3 Foodborne Vibrio parahaemolyticus intoxication CC

AØ5.4 Foodborne Bacillus cereus intoxication CC

AØ5.5 Foodborne Vibrio vulnificus intoxication CC

AØ5.8 Other specified bacterial foodborne intoxications CC

AØ5.9 Bacterial foodborne intoxication, unspecified

✓4th **AØ6 Amebiasis**
INCLUDES infection due to Entamoeba histolytica
EXCLUDES 1 *other protozoal intestinal diseases (AØ7.-)*
EXCLUDES 2 *acanthamebiasis (B6Ø.1-)*
Naegleriasis (B6Ø.2)
DEF: Infection with a single cell protozoan known as the amoeba. Transmission occurs through ingestion of feces, contaminated food or water, use of human feces as fertilizer, or person-to-person contact.

AØ6.Ø Acute amebic dysentery CC
Acute amebiasis
Intestinal amebiasis NOS

AØ6.1 Chronic intestinal amebiasis CC

AØ6.2 Amebic nondysenteric colitis CC

AØ6.3 Ameboma of intestine CC
Ameboma NOS

AØ6.4 Amebic liver abscess MCC
Hepatic amebiasis

AØ6.5 Amebic lung abscess MCC HCC
Amebic abscess of lung (and liver)

AØ6.6 Amebic brain abscess MCC
Amebic abscess of brain (and liver) (and lung)

AØ6.7 Cutaneous amebiasis

✓5th **AØ6.8 Amebic infection of other sites**

AØ6.81 Amebic cystitis CC

AØ6.82 Other amebic genitourinary infections CC
Amebic balanitis
Amebic vesiculitis
Amebic vulvovaginitis

AØ6.89 Other amebic infections CC
Amebic appendicitis
Amebic splenic abscess

AØ6.9 Amebiasis, unspecified

✓4th **AØ7 Other protozoal intestinal diseases**
DEF: Protozoa: Group comprised of the simplest, single celled organisms, ranging in size from micro to macroscopic. They can live alone or in colonies, and do not show any differentiation in tissues. Most are motile and can live free in nature, but some are parasitic, causing disease in the variety of hosts they inhabit.

AØ7.Ø Balantidiasis
Balantidial dysentery

AØ7.1 Giardiasis [lambliasis] CC
DEF: Infection caused by the flagellate protozoan *Giardia lamblia* causing gastrointestinal problems such as vomiting, chronic diarrhea, and weight loss. The most common parasite in the U.S., this is usually transmitted by ingesting contaminated water while in the cyst state, after which it latches onto the wall of the small intestine.

AØ7.2 Cryptosporidiosis CC HCC
DEF: Microscopic parasite found in water and one of the most common causes of waterborne gastrointestinal infectious disease in the United States. It is usually transmitted by ingesting contaminated drinking water or recreational water and causes profuse watery diarrhea, flatulence, abdominal pain, and cramping.

AØ7.3 Isosporiasis HIV CC
Infection due to Isospora belli and Isospora hominis
Intestinal coccidiosis
Isosporosis

AØ7.4 Cyclosporiasis CC

AØ7.8 Other specified protozoal intestinal diseases CC
Intestinal microsporidiosis
Intestinal trichomoniasis
Sarcocystosis
Sarcosporidiosis

AØ7.9 Protozoal intestinal disease, unspecified CC
Flagellate diarrhea
Protozoal colitis
Protozoal diarrhea
Protozoal dysentery

✓4th **AØ8 Viral and other specified intestinal infections**
EXCLUDES 1 *influenza with involvement of gastrointestinal tract (JØ9.X3, J1Ø.2, J11.2)*

AØ8.Ø Rotaviral enteritis CC

✓5th **AØ8.1 Acute gastroenteropathy due to Norwalk agent and other small round viruses**

AØ8.11 Acute gastroenteropathy due to Norwalk agent CC
Acute gastroenteropathy due to Norovirus
Acute gastroenteropathy due to Norwalk-like agent

AØ8.19 Acute gastroenteropathy due to other small round viruses CC
Acute gastroenteropathy due to small round virus [SRV] NOS

AØ8.2 Adenoviral enteritis CC

✓5th **AØ8.3 Other viral enteritis**

AØ8.31 Calicivirus enteritis CC

AØ8.32 Astrovirus enteritis CC

AØ8.39 Other viral enteritis CC
Coxsackie virus enteritis
Echovirus enteritis
Enterovirus enteritis NEC
Torovirus enteritis

AØ8.4 Viral intestinal infection, unspecified
Viral enteritis NOS
Viral gastroenteritis NOS
Viral gastroenteropathy NOS
AHA: 2016,3Q,12

AØ8.8 Other specified intestinal infections

AØ9 Infectious gastroenteritis and colitis, unspecified CC
Infectious colitis NOS
Infectious enteritis NOS
Infectious gastroenteritis NOS
EXCLUDES 1 *colitis NOS (K52.9)*
diarrhea NOS (R19.7)
enteritis NOS (K52.9)
gastroenteritis NOS (K52.9)
noninfective gastroenteritis and colitis, unspecified (K52.9)
DEF: Colitis: Inflammation of mucous membranes of the colon.
DEF: Enteritis: Inflammation of mucous membranes of the small intestine.
DEF: Gastroenteritis: Inflammation of mucous membranes of the stomach and intestines.

Tuberculosis (A15-A19)

INCLUDES infections due to Mycobacterium tuberculosis and Mycobacterium bovis

EXCLUDES 1 *congenital tuberculosis (P37.Ø)*
nonspecific reaction to test for tuberculosis without active tuberculosis (R76.1-)
pneumoconiosis associated with tuberculosis, any type in A15 (J65)
positive PPD (R76.11)
positive tuberculin skin test without active tuberculosis (R76.11)
sequelae of tuberculosis (B9Ø.-)
silicotuberculosis (J65)

DEF: Bacterial infection that typically spreads by inhalation of an airborne agent that usually attacks the lungs, but may also affect other organs.

✓4th A15 Respiratory tuberculosis

A15.Ø Tuberculosis of lung HIV CC
Tuberculous bronchiectasis
Tuberculous fibrosis of lung
Tuberculous pneumonia
Tuberculous pneumothorax

Tuberculosis of Lung

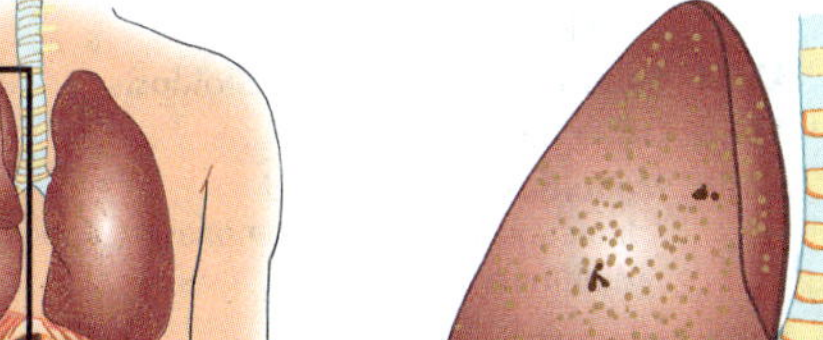

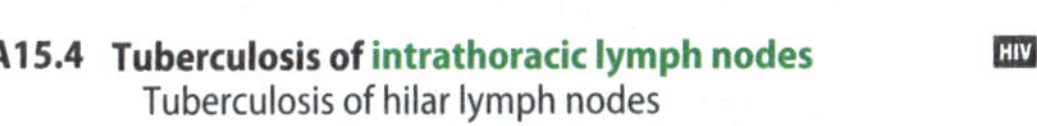

A15.4 Tuberculosis of intrathoracic lymph nodes HIV CC
Tuberculosis of hilar lymph nodes
Tuberculosis of mediastinal lymph nodes
Tuberculosis of tracheobronchial lymph nodes
EXCLUDES 1 *tuberculosis specified as primary (A15.7)*

A15.5 Tuberculosis of larynx, trachea and bronchus HIV CC
Tuberculosis of bronchus
Tuberculosis of glottis
Tuberculosis of larynx
Tuberculosis of trachea

A15.6 Tuberculous pleurisy HIV CC
Tuberculosis of pleura Tuberculous empyema
EXCLUDES 1 *primary respiratory tuberculosis (A15.7)*

A15.7 Primary respiratory tuberculosis HIV CC

A15.8 Other respiratory tuberculosis HIV CC
Mediastinal tuberculosis
Nasopharyngeal tuberculosis
Tuberculosis of nose
Tuberculosis of sinus [any nasal]

A15.9 Respiratory tuberculosis unspecified HIV CC

✓4th A17 Tuberculosis of nervous system

A17.Ø Tuberculous meningitis HIV MCC
Tuberculosis of meninges (cerebral)(spinal)
Tuberculous leptomeningitis
EXCLUDES 1 *tuberculous meningoencephalitis (A17.82)*

A17.1 Meningeal tuberculoma HIV MCC
Tuberculoma of meninges (cerebral) (spinal)
EXCLUDES 2 *tuberculoma of brain and spinal cord (A17.81)*

✓5th A17.8 Other tuberculosis of nervous system

A17.81 Tuberculoma of brain and spinal cord HIV MCC
Tuberculous abscess of brain and spinal cord

A17.82 Tuberculous meningoencephalitis HIV MCC
Tuberculous myelitis

A17.83 Tuberculous neuritis HIV MCC
Tuberculous mononeuropathy

A17.89 Other tuberculosis of nervous system HIV MCC
Tuberculous polyneuropathy

A17.9 Tuberculosis of nervous system, unspecified HIV CC

✓4th A18 Tuberculosis of other organs

✓5th A18.Ø Tuberculosis of bones and joints

A18.Ø1 Tuberculosis of spine HIV CC
Pott's disease or curvature of spine
Tuberculous arthritis
Tuberculous osteomyelitis of spine
Tuberculous spondylitis

A18.Ø2 Tuberculous arthritis of other joints HIV CC
Tuberculosis of hip (joint)
Tuberculosis of knee (joint)

A18.Ø3 Tuberculosis of other bones HIV CC
Tuberculous mastoiditis
Tuberculous osteomyelitis

A18.Ø9 Other musculoskeletal tuberculosis HIV CC
Tuberculous myositis
Tuberculous synovitis
Tuberculous tenosynovitis

✓5th A18.1 Tuberculosis of genitourinary system

A18.1Ø Tuberculosis of genitourinary system, unspecified HIV CC

A18.11 Tuberculosis of kidney and ureter HIV CC

A18.12 Tuberculosis of bladder HIV CC

A18.13 Tuberculosis of other urinary organs HIV CC
Tuberculous urethritis

A18.14 Tuberculosis of prostate HIV CC A ♂

A18.15 Tuberculosis of other male genital organs HIV CC ♂

A18.16 Tuberculosis of cervix HIV CC ♀

A18.17 Tuberculous female pelvic inflammatory disease HIV CC ♀
Tuberculous endometritis
Tuberculous oophoritis and salpingitis

A18.18 Tuberculosis of other female genital organs HIV CC ♀
Tuberculous ulceration of vulva

A18.2 Tuberculous peripheral lymphadenopathy HIV CC
Tuberculous adenitis
EXCLUDES 2 *tuberculosis of bronchial and mediastinal lymph nodes (A15.4)*
tuberculosis of mesenteric and retroperitoneal lymph nodes (A18.39)
tuberculous tracheobronchial adenopathy (A15.4)

✓5th A18.3 Tuberculosis of intestines, peritoneum and mesenteric glands

A18.31 Tuberculous peritonitis HIV MCC
Tuberculous ascites
DEF: Tuberculous inflammation of the membrane lining the abdomen.

A18.32 Tuberculous enteritis HIV CC
Tuberculosis of anus and rectum
Tuberculosis of intestine (large) (small)

A18.39 Retroperitoneal tuberculosis HIV CC
Tuberculosis of mesenteric glands
Tuberculosis of retroperitoneal (lymph glands)

A18.4 Tuberculosis of skin and subcutaneous tissue HIV CC
Erythema induratum, tuberculous
Lupus excedens
Lupus vulgaris NOS
Lupus vulgaris of eyelid
Scrofuloderma
Tuberculosis of external ear
EXCLUDES 2 *lupus erythematosus (L93.-)*
systemic lupus erythematosus (M32.-)

✓5th A18.5 Tuberculosis of eye
EXCLUDES 2 *lupus vulgaris of eyelid (A18.4)*

A18.5Ø Tuberculosis of eye, unspecified HIV CC

A18.51 Tuberculous episcleritis HIV CC

A18.52 Tuberculous keratitis HIV CC
Tuberculous interstitial keratitis
Tuberculous keratoconjunctivitis (interstitial) (phlyctenular)

A18.53 Tuberculous chorioretinitis HIV CC

A18.54 Tuberculous iridocyclitis HIV CC

A18.59 Other tuberculosis of eye HIV CC
Tuberculous conjunctivitis

A18.6 Tuberculosis of (inner) (middle) ear HIV CC
Tuberculous otitis media
EXCLUDES 2 *tuberculosis of external ear (A18.4)*
tuberculous mastoiditis (A18.03)

A18.7 Tuberculosis of adrenal glands HIV CC
Tuberculous Addison's disease

✓5th **A18.8 Tuberculosis of other specified organs**

A18.81 Tuberculosis of thyroid gland HIV CC

A18.82 Tuberculosis of other endocrine glands HIV CC
Tuberculosis of pituitary gland
Tuberculosis of thymus gland

A18.83 Tuberculosis of digestive tract organs, not elsewhere classified HIV CC
EXCLUDES 1 *tuberculosis of intestine (A18.32)*

A18.84 Tuberculosis of heart HIV CC
Tuberculous cardiomyopathy
Tuberculous endocarditis
Tuberculous myocarditis
Tuberculous pericarditis

A18.85 Tuberculosis of spleen HIV CC

A18.89 Tuberculosis of other sites HIV CC
Tuberculosis of muscle
Tuberculous cerebral arteritis

✓4th **A19 Miliary tuberculosis**
INCLUDES disseminated tuberculosis
generalized tuberculosis
tuberculous polyserositis

A19.0 Acute miliary tuberculosis of a single specified site HIV MCC

A19.1 Acute miliary tuberculosis of multiple sites HIV MCC

A19.2 Acute miliary tuberculosis, unspecified HIV MCC

A19.8 Other miliary tuberculosis HIV MCC

A19.9 Miliary tuberculosis, unspecified HIV MCC

Certain zoonotic bacterial diseases (A20-A28)

✓4th **A20 Plague**
INCLUDES infection due to Yersinia pestis

A20.0 Bubonic plague MCC

A20.1 Cellulocutaneous plague MCC

A20.2 Pneumonic plague MCC HCC

A20.3 Plague meningitis MCC

A20.7 Septicemic plague MCC HCC

A20.8 Other forms of plague MCC
Abortive plague
Asymptomatic plague
Pestis minor

A20.9 Plague, unspecified MCC

✓4th **A21 Tularemia**
INCLUDES deer-fly fever
infection due to Francisella tularensis
rabbit fever

DEF: Febrile disease transmitted to humans by the bites of deer flies, fleas, and ticks, by inhaling aerosolized *F. tularensis*, or by ingesting contaminated food or water. Patients quickly develop fever, chills, weakness, headache, backache, and malaise.

A21.0 Ulceroglandular tularemia CC

A21.1 Oculoglandular tularemia CC
Ophthalmic tularemia

A21.2 Pulmonary tularemia CC HCC

A21.3 Gastrointestinal tularemia CC
Abdominal tularemia

A21.7 Generalized tularemia CC

A21.8 Other forms of tularemia CC

A21.9 Tularemia, unspecified CC

✓4th **A22 Anthrax**
INCLUDES infection due to Bacillus anthracis

A22.0 Cutaneous anthrax CC
Malignant carbuncle
Malignant pustule

A22.1 Pulmonary anthrax MCC HCC
Inhalation anthrax
Ragpicker's disease
Woolsorter's disease

A22.2 Gastrointestinal anthrax CC

A22.7 Anthrax sepsis MCC HCC

A22.8 Other forms of anthrax CC
Anthrax meningitis

A22.9 Anthrax, unspecified CC

✓4th **A23 Brucellosis**
INCLUDES Malta fever
Mediterranean fever
undulant fever

A23.0 Brucellosis due to Brucella melitensis

A23.1 Brucellosis due to Brucella abortus

A23.2 Brucellosis due to Brucella suis

A23.3 Brucellosis due to Brucella canis

A23.8 Other brucellosis CC

A23.9 Brucellosis, unspecified CC

✓4th **A24 Glanders and melioidosis**

A24.0 Glanders CC
Infection due to Pseudomonas mallei
Malleus

A24.1 Acute and fulminating melioidosis CC
Melioidosis pneumonia
Melioidosis sepsis

A24.2 Subacute and chronic melioidosis CC

A24.3 Other melioidosis CC

A24.9 Melioidosis, unspecified CC
Infection due to Pseudomonas pseudomallei NOS
Whitmore's disease

✓4th **A25 Rat-bite fevers**

A25.0 Spirillosis CC
Sodoku

A25.1 Streptobacillosis CC
Epidemic arthritic erythema
Haverhill fever
Streptobacillary rat-bite fever

A25.9 Rat-bite fever, unspecified CC

✓4th **A26 Erysipeloid**
DEF: Acute cutaneous infection typically caused by trauma to the skin. Presenting as cellulitis, it may become systemic, affecting other organs. It is a gram-positive bacillus and mainly acquired by those who routinely handle meat.

A26.0 Cutaneous erysipeloid
Erythema migrans

A26.7 Erysipelothrix sepsis MCC HCC

A26.8 Other forms of erysipeloid

A26.9 Erysipeloid, unspecified

✓4th **A27 Leptospirosis**

A27.0 Leptospirosis icterohemorrhagica CC
Leptospiral or spirochetal jaundice (hemorrhagic)
Weil's disease

✓5th **A27.8 Other forms of leptospirosis**

A27.81 Aseptic meningitis in leptospirosis MCC

A27.89 Other forms of leptospirosis CC

A27.9 Leptospirosis, unspecified CC

✓4th **A28 Other zoonotic bacterial diseases, not elsewhere classified**

A28.0 Pasteurellosis CC

A28.1 Cat-scratch disease CC
Cat-scratch fever

A28.2 Extraintestinal yersiniosis CC
EXCLUDES 1 *enteritis due to Yersinia enterocolitica (A04.6)*
plague (A20.-)

A28.8 Other specified zoonotic bacterial diseases, not elsewhere classified CC

A28.9 Zoonotic bacterial disease, unspecified CC

Other bacterial diseases (A30-A49)

AHA: 2016,3Q,8-14

✓4th **A30 Leprosy [Hansen's disease]**
INCLUDES infection due to Mycobacterium leprae
EXCLUDES 1 *sequelae of leprosy (B92)*

A30.0 Indeterminate leprosy CC
I leprosy

A30.1 Tuberculoid leprosy CC
TT leprosy

A30.2 Borderline tuberculoid leprosy CC
BT leprosy

A30.3 Borderline leprosy CC
BB leprosy

A30.4 Borderline lepromatous leprosy CC
BL leprosy

A30.5 Lepromatous leprosy CC
LL leprosy

A30.8 Other forms of leprosy CC

A30.9 Leprosy, unspecified CC

✓4th **A31 Infection due to other mycobacteria**
EXCLUDES 2 *leprosy (A30.-)*
tuberculosis (A15-A19)

A31.0 Pulmonary mycobacterial infection CC HCC
Infection due to Mycobacterium avium
Infection due to Mycobacterium intracellulare [Battey bacillus]
Infection due to Mycobacterium kansasii

A31.1 Cutaneous mycobacterial infection CC
Buruli ulcer
Infection due to Mycobacterium marinum
Infection due to Mycobacterium ulcerans

A31.2 Disseminated mycobacterium avium-intracellulare complex (DMAC) HIV CC HCC
MAC sepsis

A31.8 Other mycobacterial infections HIV CC

A31.9 Mycobacterial infection, unspecified HIV CC
Atypical mycobacterial infection NOS
Mycobacteriosis NOS

✓4th **A32 Listeriosis**
INCLUDES listerial foodborne infection
EXCLUDES 1 *neonatal (disseminated) listeriosis (P37.2)*

A32.0 Cutaneous listeriosis CC

✓5th A32.1 Listerial meningitis and meningoencephalitis

A32.11 Listerial meningitis CC

A32.12 Listerial meningoencephalitis CC

A32.7 Listerial sepsis MCC HCC

✓5th A32.8 Other forms of listeriosis

A32.81 Oculoglandular listeriosis CC

A32.82 Listerial endocarditis CC

A32.89 Other forms of listeriosis CC
Listerial cerebral arteritis

A32.9 Listeriosis, unspecified CC

A33 Tetanus neonatorum MCC N

A34 Obstetrical tetanus CC M ♀

A35 Other tetanus MCC
Tetanus NOS
EXCLUDES 1 *obstetrical tetanus (A34)*
tetanus neonatorum (A33)

DEF: Tetanus: Acute, often fatal, infectious disease caused by the anaerobic, spore-forming bacillus *Clostridium tetani.* The bacillus enters the body through a contaminated wound, burns, surgical wounds, or cutaneous ulcers. Symptoms include lockjaw, spasms, seizures, and paralysis.

✓4th **A36 Diphtheria**

A36.0 Pharyngeal diphtheria CC
Diphtheritic membranous angina
Tonsillar diphtheria

A36.1 Nasopharyngeal diphtheria CC

A36.2 Laryngeal diphtheria CC
Diphtheritic laryngotracheitis

A36.3 Cutaneous diphtheria CC
EXCLUDES 2 *erythrasma (L08.1)*

✓5th A36.8 Other diphtheria

A36.81 Diphtheritic cardiomyopathy CC HCC
Diphtheritic myocarditis

A36.82 Diphtheritic radiculomyelitis CC

A36.83 Diphtheritic polyneuritis CC

A36.84 Diphtheritic tubulo-interstitial nephropathy CC

A36.85 Diphtheritic cystitis CC

A36.86 Diphtheritic conjunctivitis CC

A36.89 Other diphtheritic complications CC
Diphtheritic peritonitis

A36.9 Diphtheria, unspecified CC

✓4th **A37 Whooping cough**
DEF: Acute, highly contagious respiratory tract infection caused by *Bordetella pertussis* and *B. bronchiseptica.* Whooping cough is known by its characteristic paroxysmal cough.

✓5th A37.0 Whooping cough due to Bordetella pertussis

A37.00 Whooping cough due to Bordetella pertussis without pneumonia CC
Paroxysmal cough due to Bordetella pertussis without pneumonia

A37.01 Whooping cough due to Bordetella pertussis with pneumonia MCC
Paroxysmal cough due to Bordetella pertussis with pneumonia

✓5th A37.1 Whooping cough due to Bordetella parapertussis

A37.10 Whooping cough due to Bordetella parapertussis without pneumonia CC

A37.11 Whooping cough due to Bordetella parapertussis with pneumonia MCC

✓5th A37.8 Whooping cough due to other Bordetella species

A37.80 Whooping cough due to other Bordetella species without pneumonia CC

A37.81 Whooping cough due to other Bordetella species with pneumonia MCC

✓5th A37.9 Whooping cough, unspecified species

A37.90 Whooping cough, unspecified species without pneumonia CC

A37.91 Whooping cough, unspecified species with pneumonia MCC

✓4th **A38 Scarlet fever**
INCLUDES scarlatina
EXCLUDES 2 *streptococcal sore throat (J02.0)*
DEF: Acute contagious disease caused by Group A bacteria, the same bacterium that causes strep throat. Individuals with strep throat can develop scarlet fever particularly if the infection is not treated with antibiotics. It is characterized by a red blush to the skin of the chest and abdomen and swelling of the nose, throat, and mouth.

A38.0 Scarlet fever with otitis media CC

A38.1 Scarlet fever with myocarditis CC

A38.8 Scarlet fever with other complications CC

A38.9 Scarlet fever, uncomplicated CC
Scarlet fever, NOS

✓4th **A39 Meningococcal infection**
DEF: Condition caused by *Neisseria meningitidis*, a bacteria that may invade the spinal cord, brain, heart, joints, optic nerve, or bloodstream.

A39.0 Meningococcal meningitis MCC

A39.1 Waterhouse-Friderichsen syndrome MCC HCC
Meningococcal hemorrhagic adrenalitis
Meningococcic adrenal syndrome

A39.2 Acute meningococcemia MCC HCC

A39.3 Chronic meningococcemia MCC HCC

A39.4 Meningococcemia, unspecified MCC HCC

✓5th A39.5 Meningococcal heart disease

A39.50 Meningococcal carditis, unspecified MCC

A39.51 Meningococcal endocarditis MCC

A39.52 Meningococcal myocarditis MCC

A39.53 Meningococcal pericarditis MCC

✓5th A39.8 Other meningococcal infections

A39.81 Meningococcal encephalitis MCC

A39.82 Meningococcal retrobulbar neuritis CC

A39.83 Meningococcal arthritis CC HCC

A39.84 Postmeningococcal arthritis CC HCC

A39.89 Other meningococcal infections CC
Meningococcal conjunctivitis

A39.9 Meningococcal infection, unspecified CC
Meningococcal disease NOS

Chapter 1. Certain Infectious and Parasitic Diseases

A30.2–A39.9

A4Ø Streptococcal sepsis (4th)

▶Code first, if applicable, postprocedural sepsis (T81.44-)◀
~~postprocedural streptococcal sepsis (T81.4-)~~
▶sepsis due to central venous catheter (T8Ø.211-)◀
streptococcal sepsis during labor (O75.3)
streptococcal sepsis following abortion or ectopic or molar pregnancy ▶(OØ3.37, OØ3.87, OØ4.87, OØ7.37, OØ8.82)◀
streptococcal sepsis following immunization ▶(T88.Ø-)◀
streptococcal sepsis following infusion, transfusion or therapeutic injection ▶(T8Ø.22-, T8Ø.29-)◀

EXCLUDES 1 *neonatal (P36.Ø-P36.1)*
puerperal sepsis (O85)
sepsis due to Streptococcus, group D (A41.81)

AHA: 2020,2Q,8,28; 2019,4Q,65; 2018,4Q,89; 2018,1Q,16; 2016,1Q,32

A4Ø.Ø Sepsis due to streptococcus, group A MCC HCC
A4Ø.1 Sepsis due to streptococcus, group B MCC HCC
AHA: 2019,1Q,14
A4Ø.3 Sepsis due to Streptococcus pneumoniae MCC HCC
Pneumococcal sepsis
A4Ø.8 Other streptococcal sepsis MCC HCC
A4Ø.9 Streptococcal sepsis, unspecified HIV MCC HCC

A41 Other sepsis (4th)

▶Code first, if applicable, postprocedural sepsis (T81.44-)◀
~~postprocedural sepsis (T81.4-)~~
▶sepsis due to central venous catheter (T8Ø.211-)◀
sepsis during labor (O75.3)
sepsis following abortion, ectopic or molar pregnancy ▶(OØ3.37, OØ3.87, OØ4.87, OØ7.37, OØ8.82)◀
sepsis following immunization ▶(T88.Ø-)◀
sepsis following infusion, transfusion or therapeutic injection ▶(T8Ø.22-, T8Ø.29-)◀

EXCLUDES 1 *bacteremia NOS (R78.81)*
neonatal (P36.-)
puerperal sepsis (O85)
streptococcal sepsis (A4Ø.-)

EXCLUDES 2 *sepsis (due to) (in) actinomycotic (A42.7)*
sepsis (due to) (in) anthrax (A22.7)
sepsis (due to) (in) candidal (B37.7)
sepsis (due to) (in) Erysipelothrix (A26.7)
sepsis (due to) (in) extraintestinal yersiniosis (A28.2)
sepsis (due to) (in) gonococcal (A54.86)
sepsis (due to) (in) herpesviral (BØØ.7)
sepsis (due to) (in) listerial (A32.7)
sepsis (due to) (in) melioidosis (A24.1)
sepsis (due to) (in) meningococcal (A39.2-A39.4)
sepsis (due to) (in) plague (A2Ø.7)
sepsis (due to) (in) tularemia (A21.7)
toxic shock syndrome (A48.3)

AHA: 2020,2Q,8,28; 2019,4Q,65; 2019,3Q,17; 2018,4Q,18; 2018,1Q,16; 2016,1Q,32; 2014,2Q,13

A41.Ø Sepsis due to Staphylococcus aureus (5th)
A41.Ø1 Sepsis due to Methicillin susceptible Staphylococcus aureus HIV MCC HCC
MSSA sepsis
Staphylococcus aureus sepsis NOS
AHA: 2020,2Q,17
A41.Ø2 Sepsis due to Methicillin resistant Staphylococcus aureus HIV MCC HCC
A41.1 Sepsis due to other specified staphylococcus HIV MCC HCC
Coagulase negative staphylococcus sepsis
A41.2 Sepsis due to unspecified staphylococcus HIV MCC HCC
A41.3 Sepsis due to Hemophilus influenzae HIV MCC HCC
A41.4 Sepsis due to anaerobes HIV MCC HCC
EXCLUDES 1 *gas gangrene (A48.Ø)*

A41.5 Sepsis due to other Gram-negative organisms (5th)
A41.5Ø Gram-negative sepsis, unspecified HIV MCC HCC
Gram-negative sepsis NOS
AHA: 2020,2Q,28
A41.51 Sepsis due to Escherichia coli [E. coli] HIV MCC HCC
AHA: 2020,2Q,17
A41.52 Sepsis due to Pseudomonas HIV MCC HCC
▶Pseudomonas aeruginosa◀
A41.53 Sepsis due to Serratia HIV MCC HCC
● **A41.54 Sepsis due to Acinetobacter baumannii** MCC
A41.59 Other Gram-negative sepsis HIV MCC HCC

A41.8 Other specified sepsis (5th)
A41.81 Sepsis due to Enterococcus HIV MCC HCC
TIP: *E. faecium,* is a species of *Enterococcus* that is highly resistant to multiple antibiotics. Assign a code from category Z16 when resistance to antimicrobial drugs is documented.
A41.89 Other specified sepsis HIV MCC HCC
AHA: 2020,2Q,8; 2017,1Q,51; 2016,3Q,8-14
TIP: Viral sepsis is coded here; assign an additional code to identify the specific viral agent or illness.
A41.9 Sepsis, unspecified organism HIV MCC HCC
Septicemia NOS
AHA: 2022,2Q,5; 2022,1Q,35; 2020,2Q,28

A42 Actinomycosis (4th)
EXCLUDES 1 *actinomycetoma (B47.1)*
A42.Ø Pulmonary actinomycosis HIV CC HCC
A42.1 Abdominal actinomycosis HIV CC
A42.2 Cervicofacial actinomycosis HIV CC
A42.7 Actinomycotic sepsis HIV MCC HCC
A42.8 Other forms of actinomycosis (5th)
A42.81 Actinomycotic meningitis HIV CC
A42.82 Actinomycotic encephalitis HIV CC
A42.89 Other forms of actinomycosis HIV CC
A42.9 Actinomycosis, unspecified HIV CC

A43 Nocardiosis (4th)
DEF: Rare bacterial infection occurring most often in those with weakened immune systems. Can be acquired in soil, decaying plants, or standing water. It typically begins in the lungs and has a tendency to spread to other body systems.
A43.Ø Pulmonary nocardiosis HIV CC HCC
A43.1 Cutaneous nocardiosis HIV CC
A43.8 Other forms of nocardiosis HIV CC
A43.9 Nocardiosis, unspecified HIV CC

A44 Bartonellosis (4th)
A44.Ø Systemic bartonellosis CC
Oroya fever
A44.1 Cutaneous and mucocutaneous bartonellosis CC
Verruga peruana
A44.8 Other forms of bartonellosis CC
A44.9 Bartonellosis, unspecified CC

A46 Erysipelas
EXCLUDES 1 *postpartum or puerperal erysipelas (O86.89)*
DEF: Skin infection affecting the upper dermis and superficial dermal lymphatics. Lesion edges are well-demarcated with distinct raised borders. It is often caused by group A *Streptococci.*

A48 Other bacterial diseases, not elsewhere classified (4th)
EXCLUDES 1 *actinomycetoma (B47.1)*
A48.Ø Gas gangrene MCC HCC
Clostridial cellulitis
Clostridial myonecrosis
AHA: 2017,4Q,102
A48.1 Legionnaires' disease HIV MCC HCC
DEF: Severe and often fatal infection by *Legionella pneumophila.* Symptoms include high fever, gastrointestinal pain, headache, myalgia, dry cough, and pneumonia and it is usually transmitted through airborne water droplets via air conditioning systems or hot tubs.
A48.2 Nonpneumonic Legionnaires' disease [Pontiac fever]
A48.3 Toxic shock syndrome MCC HCC
Use additional code to identify the organism (B95, B96)
EXCLUDES 1 *endotoxic shock NOS (R57.8)*
sepsis NOS (A41.9)
AHA: 2022,1Q,35
DEF: Bacteria producing an endotoxin, such as *Staphylococci,* flood the body with the toxins producing a high fever, vomiting and diarrhea, decreasing blood pressure, a skin rash, and shock.
Synonym(s): *TSS.*
A48.4 Brazilian purpuric fever
Systemic Hemophilus aegyptius infection
A48.5 Other specified botulism (5th)
Non-foodborne intoxication due to toxins of Clostridium botulinum [C. botulinum]
EXCLUDES 1 *food poisoning due to toxins of Clostridium botulinum (AØ5.1)*
A48.51 Infant botulism CC P

A48.52 **Wound botulism** CC
Non-foodborne botulism NOS
Use additional code for associated wound

A48.8 **Other specified bacterial diseases**

A49 Bacterial infection of unspecified site

EXCLUDES 1 *bacterial agents as the cause of diseases classified elsewhere (B95-B96)*
chlamydial infection NOS (A74.9)
meningococcal infection NOS (A39.9)
rickettsial infection NOS (A79.9)
spirochetal infection NOS (A69.9)

A49.Ø **Staphylococcal infection, unspecified site**

A49.Ø1 **Methicillin susceptible Staphylococcus aureus infection, unspecified site**
Methicillin susceptible Staphylococcus aureus (MSSA) infection
Staphylococcus aureus infection NOS

A49.Ø2 **Methicillin resistant Staphylococcus aureus infection, unspecified site**
Methicillin resistant Staphylococcus aureus (MRSA) infection

A49.1 **Streptococcal infection, unspecified site**

A49.2 **Hemophilus influenzae infection, unspecified site**

A49.3 **Mycoplasma infection, unspecified site**

A49.8 **Other bacterial infections of unspecified site**

A49.9 **Bacterial infection, unspecified**
EXCLUDES 1 *bacteremia NOS (R78.81)*

Infections with a predominantly sexual mode of transmission (AØ5–A64)

EXCLUDES 1 ~~*human immunodeficiency virus [HIV] disease (B2Ø)*~~
nonspecific and nongonococcal urethritis (N34.1)
Reiter's disease (MØ2.3-)

EXCLUDES 2 ▶*human immunodeficiency virus [HIV] disease (B2Ø)*◀

AHA: 2021,2Q,6

A5Ø Congenital syphilis

A5Ø.Ø **Early congenital syphilis, symptomatic**
Any congenital syphilitic condition specified as early or manifest less than two years after birth.

A5Ø.Ø1 **Early congenital syphilitic oculopathy** CC

A5Ø.Ø2 **Early congenital syphilitic osteochondropathy** CC

A5Ø.Ø3 **Early congenital syphilitic pharyngitis** CC
Early congenital syphilitic laryngitis

A5Ø.Ø4 **Early congenital syphilitic pneumonia** CC

A5Ø.Ø5 **Early congenital syphilitic rhinitis** CC

A5Ø.Ø6 **Early cutaneous congenital syphilis** CC

A5Ø.Ø7 **Early mucocutaneous congenital syphilis** CC

A5Ø.Ø8 **Early visceral congenital syphilis** CC

A5Ø.Ø9 **Other early congenital syphilis, symptomatic** CC

A5Ø.1 **Early congenital syphilis, latent**
Congenital syphilis without clinical manifestations, with positive serological reaction and negative spinal fluid test, less than two years after birth.

A5Ø.2 **Early congenital syphilis, unspecified** CC
Congenital syphilis NOS less than two years after birth.

A5Ø.3 **Late congenital syphilitic oculopathy**
EXCLUDES 1 *Hutchinson's triad (A5Ø.53)*

A5Ø.3Ø **Late congenital syphilitic oculopathy, unspecified** CC

A5Ø.31 **Late congenital syphilitic interstitial keratitis** CC

A5Ø.32 **Late congenital syphilitic chorioretinitis** CC

A5Ø.39 **Other late congenital syphilitic oculopathy** CC

A5Ø.4 **Late congenital neurosyphilis [juvenile neurosyphilis]**
Use additional code to identify any associated mental disorder
EXCLUDES 1 *Hutchinson's triad (A5Ø.53)*

A5Ø.4Ø **Late congenital neurosyphilis, unspecified** CC
Juvenile neurosyphilis NOS

A5Ø.41 **Late congenital syphilitic meningitis** MCC

A5Ø.42 **Late congenital syphilitic encephalitis** MCC

A5Ø.43 **Late congenital syphilitic polyneuropathy** CC

A5Ø.44 **Late congenital syphilitic optic nerve atrophy** CC

A5Ø.45 **Juvenile general paresis** CC
Dementia paralytica juvenilis
Juvenile tabetoparetic neurosyphilis

A5Ø.49 **Other late congenital neurosyphilis** CC
Juvenile tabes dorsalis

A5Ø.5 **Other late congenital syphilis, symptomatic**
Any congenital syphilitic condition specified as late or manifest two years or more after birth.

A5Ø.51 **Clutton's joints** CC

A5Ø.52 **Hutchinson's teeth** CC

A5Ø.53 **Hutchinson's triad** CC

A5Ø.54 **Late congenital cardiovascular syphilis** CC

A5Ø.55 **Late congenital syphilitic arthropathy** CC HCC

A5Ø.56 **Late congenital syphilitic osteochondropathy** CC

A5Ø.57 **Syphilitic saddle nose** CC

A5Ø.59 **Other late congenital syphilis, symptomatic** CC

A5Ø.6 **Late congenital syphilis, latent**
Congenital syphilis without clinical manifestations, with positive serological reaction and negative spinal fluid test, two years or more after birth.

A5Ø.7 **Late congenital syphilis, unspecified**
Congenital syphilis NOS two years or more after birth.

A5Ø.9 **Congenital syphilis, unspecified**

A51 Early syphilis

DEF: Syphilis: Sexually transmitted disease caused by the *Treponema pallidum* spirochete. Syphilis usually exhibits cutaneous manifestations and may exist for years without symptoms.

A51.Ø **Primary genital syphilis**
Syphilitic chancre NOS

A51.1 **Primary anal syphilis**

A51.2 **Primary syphilis of other sites**

A51.3 **Secondary syphilis of skin and mucous membranes**
DEF: Transitory or chronic cutaneous eruptions that present within two to 10 weeks following an initial syphilis infection that may include nontender lymphadenopathy along with alopecia and condylomata lata.

A51.31 **Condyloma latum** CC

A51.32 **Syphilitic alopecia** CC

A51.39 **Other secondary syphilis of skin** CC
Syphilitic leukoderma
Syphilitic mucous patch
EXCLUDES 1 *late syphilitic leukoderma (A52.79)*

A51.4 **Other secondary syphilis**

A51.41 **Secondary syphilitic meningitis** MCC

A51.42 **Secondary syphilitic female pelvic disease** CC ♀

A51.43 **Secondary syphilitic oculopathy** CC
Secondary syphilitic chorioretinitis
Secondary syphilitic iridocyclitis, iritis
Secondary syphilitic uveitis

A51.44 **Secondary syphilitic nephritis** CC

A51.45 **Secondary syphilitic hepatitis** CC

A51.46 **Secondary syphilitic osteopathy** CC

A51.49 **Other secondary syphilitic conditions** CC
Secondary syphilitic lymphadenopathy
Secondary syphilitic myositis

A51.5 **Early syphilis, latent**
Syphilis (acquired) without clinical manifestations, with positive serological reaction and negative spinal fluid test, less than two years after infection.

A51.9 **Early syphilis, unspecified**

A52 Late syphilis

A52.Ø **Cardiovascular and cerebrovascular syphilis**

A52.ØØ **Cardiovascular syphilis, unspecified** CC

A52.Ø1 **Syphilitic aneurysm of aorta** CC

A52.Ø2 **Syphilitic aortitis** CC

A52.Ø3 **Syphilitic endocarditis** CC
Syphilitic aortic valve incompetence or stenosis
Syphilitic mitral valve stenosis
Syphilitic pulmonary valve regurgitation

A52.Ø4 **Syphilitic cerebral arteritis** CC

A52.Ø5 **Other cerebrovascular syphilis** CC
Syphilitic cerebral aneurysm (ruptured) (non-ruptured)
Syphilitic cerebral thrombosis

A52.Ø6 Other syphilitic heart involvement CC
Syphilitic coronary artery disease
Syphilitic myocarditis
Syphilitic pericarditis

A52.Ø9 Other cardiovascular syphilis CC

√5th **A52.1 Symptomatic neurosyphilis**

A52.1Ø Symptomatic neurosyphilis, unspecified CC

A52.11 Tabes dorsalis CC
Locomotor ataxia (progressive)
Tabetic neurosyphilis

A52.12 Other cerebrospinal syphilis CC

A52.13 Late syphilitic meningitis MCC

A52.14 Late syphilitic encephalitis MCC

A52.15 Late syphilitic neuropathy CC
Late syphilitic acoustic neuritis
Late syphilitic optic (nerve) atrophy
Late syphilitic polyneuropathy
Late syphilitic retrobulbar neuritis

A52.16 Charcôt's arthropathy (tabetic) CC
DEF: Progressive neurologic arthropathy in which chronic degeneration of joints in the weight-bearing areas with peripheral hypertrophy occurs as a complication of a neuropathy disorder. Supporting structures relax from a loss of sensation resulting in chronic joint instability.

A52.17 General paresis CC
Dementia paralytica

A52.19 Other symptomatic neurosyphilis CC
Syphilitic parkinsonism

A52.2 Asymptomatic neurosyphilis CC

A52.3 Neurosyphilis, unspecified CC
Gumma (syphilitic)
Syphilis (late)
Syphiloma
AHA: 2021,2Q,6

√5th **A52.7 Other symptomatic late syphilis**

A52.71 Late syphilitic oculopathy CC
Late syphilitic chorioretinitis
Late syphilitic episcleritis

A52.72 Syphilis of lung and bronchus CC

A52.73 Symptomatic late syphilis of other respiratory organs CC

A52.74 Syphilis of liver and other viscera CC
Late syphilitic peritonitis

A52.75 Syphilis of kidney and ureter CC
Syphilitic glomerular disease

A52.76 Other genitourinary symptomatic late syphilis CC
Late syphilitic female pelvic inflammatory disease

A52.77 Syphilis of bone and joint CC

A52.78 Syphilis of other musculoskeletal tissue CC
Late syphilitic bursitis
Syphilis [stage unspecified] of bursa
Syphilis [stage unspecified] of muscle
Syphilis [stage unspecified] of synovium
Syphilis [stage unspecified] of tendon

A52.79 Other symptomatic late syphilis CC
Late syphilitic leukoderma
Syphilis of adrenal gland
Syphilis of pituitary gland
Syphilis of thyroid gland
Syphilitic splenomegaly
EXCLUDES 1 *syphilitic leukoderma (secondary) (A51.39)*

A52.8 Late syphilis, latent
Syphilis (acquired) without clinical manifestations, with positive serological reaction and negative spinal fluid test, two years or more after infection

A52.9 Late syphilis, unspecified

√4th **A53 Other and unspecified syphilis**

A53.Ø Latent syphilis, unspecified as early or late
Latent syphilis NOS
Positive serological reaction for syphilis

A53.9 Syphilis, unspecified
Infection due to Treponema pallidum NOS
Syphilis (acquired) NOS
EXCLUDES 1 *syphilis NOS under two years of age (A5Ø.2)*

√4th **A54 Gonococcal infection**
DEF: Sexually transmitted bacterial infection caused by *Neisseria gonorrhoeae*. Women are often asymptomatic, while men tend to develop urinary symptoms quickly.

√5th **A54.Ø Gonococcal infection of lower genitourinary tract without periurethral or accessory gland abscess**
EXCLUDES 1 *gonococcal infection with genitourinary gland abscess (A54.1)*
gonococcal infection with periurethral abscess (A54.1)

A54.ØØ Gonococcal infection of lower genitourinary tract, unspecified CC

A54.Ø1 Gonococcal cystitis and urethritis, unspecified CC

A54.Ø2 Gonococcal vulvovaginitis, unspecified CC ♀

A54.Ø3 Gonococcal cervicitis, unspecified CC ♀

A54.Ø9 Other gonococcal infection of lower genitourinary tract CC

A54.1 Gonococcal infection of lower genitourinary tract with periurethral and accessory gland abscess CC
Gonococcal Bartholin's gland abscess

√5th **A54.2 Gonococcal pelviperitonitis and other gonococcal genitourinary infection**

A54.21 Gonococcal infection of kidney and ureter CC

A54.22 Gonococcal prostatitis CC ♂

A54.23 Gonococcal infection of other male genital organs CC ♂
Gonococcal epididymitis
Gonococcal orchitis

A54.24 Gonococcal female pelvic inflammatory disease CC ♀
Gonococcal pelviperitonitis
EXCLUDES 1 *gonococcal peritonitis (A54.85)*

A54.29 Other gonococcal genitourinary infections CC

√5th **A54.3 Gonococcal infection of eye**

A54.3Ø Gonococcal infection of eye, unspecified CC

A54.31 Gonococcal conjunctivitis CC
Ophthalmia neonatorum due to gonococcus

A54.32 Gonococcal iridocyclitis CC

A54.33 Gonococcal keratitis CC

A54.39 Other gonococcal eye infection CC
Gonococcal endophthalmia

√5th **A54.4 Gonococcal infection of musculoskeletal system**

A54.4Ø Gonococcal infection of musculoskeletal system, unspecified CC HCC

A54.41 Gonococcal spondylopathy CC HCC

A54.42 Gonococcal arthritis CC HCC
EXCLUDES 2 *gonococcal infection of spine (A54.41)*

A54.43 Gonococcal osteomyelitis CC HCC
EXCLUDES 2 *gonococcal infection of spine (A54.41)*

A54.49 Gonococcal infection of other musculoskeletal tissue CC HCC
Gonococcal bursitis
Gonococcal myositis
Gonococcal synovitis
Gonococcal tenosynovitis

A54.5 Gonococcal pharyngitis

A54.6 Gonococcal infection of anus and rectum

√5th **A54.8 Other gonococcal infections**

A54.81 Gonococcal meningitis MCC

A54.82 Gonococcal brain abscess CC

A54.83 Gonococcal heart infection CC
Gonococcal endocarditis
Gonococcal myocarditis
Gonococcal pericarditis

A54.84 Gonococcal pneumonia CC HCC

A54.85 Gonococcal peritonitis CC HCC
EXCLUDES 1 *gonococcal pelviperitonitis (A54.24)*

A54.86 Gonococcal sepsis MCC HCC

A54.89 Other gonococcal infections CC
Gonococcal keratoderma
Gonococcal lymphadenitis

A54.9 Gonococcal infection, unspecified CC

A55 Chlamydial lymphogranuloma (venereum)
Climatic or tropical bubo
Durand-Nicolas-Favre disease
Esthiomene
Lymphogranuloma inguinale

A56 Other sexually transmitted chlamydial diseases
INCLUDES sexually transmitted diseases due to Chlamydia trachomatis
EXCLUDES 1 *neonatal chlamydial conjunctivitis (P39.1)*
neonatal chlamydial pneumonia (P23.1)
EXCLUDES 2 *chlamydial lymphogranuloma (A55)*
conditions classified to A74.-
DEF: *Chlamydia trachomatis*: Bacterium that causes a common venereal disease. Symptoms of chlamydia are usually mild or absent, however, serious complications may cause irreversible damage, including cystitis, pelvic inflammatory disease, and infertility in women and discharge from the penis, prostatitis, and infertility in men. Genital chlamydial infection can cause arthritis, skin lesions, and inflammation of the eye and urethra.
Synonym(s): *Reiter's syndrome.*

A56.0 Chlamydial infection of lower genitourinary tract
A56.00 Chlamydial infection of lower genitourinary tract, unspecified
A56.01 Chlamydial cystitis and urethritis
A56.02 Chlamydial vulvovaginitis ♀
A56.09 Other chlamydial infection of lower genitourinary tract
Chlamydial cervicitis
A56.1 Chlamydial infection of pelviperitoneum and other genitourinary organs
A56.11 Chlamydial female pelvic inflammatory disease ♀
A56.19 Other chlamydial genitourinary infection
Chlamydial epididymitis
Chlamydial orchitis
A56.2 Chlamydial infection of genitourinary tract, unspecified
A56.3 Chlamydial infection of anus and rectum
A56.4 Chlamydial infection of pharynx
A56.8 Sexually transmitted chlamydial infection of other sites

A57 Chancroid
Ulcus molle
DEF: Localized infection by *Haemophilus ducreyi*, causing genital ulcers and infecting the inguinal lymph nodes.

A58 Granuloma inguinale
Donovanosis

A59 Trichomoniasis
EXCLUDES 2 *intestinal trichomoniasis (A07.8)*
DEF: Infection with the parasitic, flagellated protozoa of the genus *Trichomonas*. This protozoon is found in the intestinal and genitourinary tracts of humans and in the mouth around tartar, cavities, and areas of periodontal disease.
A59.0 Urogenital trichomoniasis
A59.00 Urogenital trichomoniasis, unspecified
Fluor (vaginalis) due to Trichomonas
Leukorrhea (vaginalis) due to Trichomonas
A59.01 Trichomonal vulvovaginitis ♀
A59.02 Trichomonal prostatitis ♂
A59.03 Trichomonal cystitis and urethritis
A59.09 Other urogenital trichomoniasis
Trichomonas cervicitis
A59.8 Trichomoniasis of other sites
A59.9 Trichomoniasis, unspecified

A60 Anogenital herpesviral [herpes simplex] infections
A60.0 Herpesviral infection of genitalia and urogenital tract
A60.00 Herpesviral infection of urogenital system, unspecified HIV
A60.01 Herpesviral infection of penis HIV ♂
A60.02 Herpesviral infection of other male genital organs ♂
A60.03 Herpesviral cervicitis ♀
A60.04 Herpesviral vulvovaginitis HIV ♀
Herpesviral [herpes simplex] ulceration
Herpesviral [herpes simplex] vaginitis
Herpesviral [herpes simplex] vulvitis
A60.09 Herpesviral infection of other urogenital tract HIV
AHA: 2020,1Q,20
A60.1 Herpesviral infection of perianal skin and rectum HIV
A60.9 Anogenital herpesviral infection, unspecified HIV

A63 Other predominantly sexually transmitted diseases, not elsewhere classified
EXCLUDES 2 *molluscum contagiosum (B08.1)*
papilloma of cervix (D26.0)
A63.0 Anogenital (venereal) warts
Anogenital warts due to (human) papillomavirus [HPV]
Condyloma acuminatum
A63.8 Other specified predominantly sexually transmitted diseases

A64 Unspecified sexually transmitted disease

Other spirochetal diseases (A65-A69)

EXCLUDES 2 *leptospirosis (A27.-)*
syphilis (A50-A53)

A65 Nonvenereal syphilis
Bejel
Endemic syphilis
Njovera

A66 Yaws
INCLUDES bouba
frambesia (tropica)
pian
A66.0 Initial lesions of yaws
Chancre of yaws
Frambesia, initial or primary
Initial frambesial ulcer
Mother yaw
A66.1 Multiple papillomata and wet crab yaws
Frambesioma
Pianoma
Plantar or palmar papilloma of yaws
A66.2 Other early skin lesions of yaws
Cutaneous yaws, less than five years after infection
Early yaws (cutaneous) (macular) (maculopapular) (micropapular) (papular)
Frambeside of early yaws
A66.3 Hyperkeratosis of yaws
Ghoul hand
Hyperkeratosis, palmar or plantar (early) (late) due to yaws
Worm-eaten soles
A66.4 Gummata and ulcers of yaws
Gummatous frambeside
Nodular late yaws (ulcerated)
A66.5 Gangosa
Rhinopharyngitis mutilans
A66.6 Bone and joint lesions of yaws HCC
Yaws ganglion
Yaws goundou
Yaws gumma, bone
Yaws gummatous osteitis or periostitis
Yaws hydrarthrosis
Yaws osteitis
Yaws periostitis (hypertrophic)
A66.7 Other manifestations of yaws
Juxta-articular nodules of yaws
Mucosal yaws
A66.8 Latent yaws
Yaws without clinical manifestations, with positive serology
A66.9 Yaws, unspecified

A67 Pinta [carate]
A67.0 Primary lesions of pinta
Chancre (primary) of pinta
Papule (primary) of pinta
A67.1 Intermediate lesions of pinta
Erythematous plaques of pinta
Hyperchromic lesions of pinta
Hyperkeratosis of pinta
Pintids
A67.2 Late lesions of pinta
Achromic skin lesions of pinta
Cicatricial skin lesions of pinta
Dyschromic skin lesions of pinta
A67.3 Mixed lesions of pinta
Achromic with hyperchromic skin lesions of pinta [carate]
A67.9 Pinta, unspecified

Chapter 1. Certain Infectious and Parasitic Diseases

A55–A67.9

A68 Relapsing fevers
INCLUDES recurrent fever
EXCLUDES 2 *Lyme disease (A69.2-)*

A68.0 Louse-borne relapsing fever CC
Relapsing fever due to Borrelia recurrentis

A68.1 Tick-borne relapsing fever CC
Relapsing fever due to any Borrelia species other than Borrelia recurrentis

A68.9 Relapsing fever, unspecified CC

A69 Other spirochetal infections

A69.0 Necrotizing ulcerative stomatitis
Cancrum oris
Fusospirochetal gangrene
Noma
Stomatitis gangrenosa

A69.1 Other Vincent's infections CC
Fusospirochetal pharyngitis
Necrotizing ulcerative (acute) gingivitis
Necrotizing ulcerative (acute) gingivostomatitis
Spirochetal stomatitis
Trench mouth
Vincent's angina
Vincent's gingivitis

A69.2 Lyme disease
Erythema chronicum migrans due to Borrelia burgdorferi
DEF: Recurrent multisystem disorder through tick bites that begins with lesions of erythema chronicum migrans and is followed by arthritis of the large joints, myalgia, malaise, and neurological and cardiac manifestations.

A69.20 Lyme disease, unspecified CC
AHA: 2021,4Q,5

A69.21 Meningitis due to Lyme disease CC

A69.22 Other neurologic disorders in Lyme disease CC
Cranial neuritis
Meningoencephalitis
Polyneuropathy

A69.23 Arthritis due to Lyme disease CC HCC

A69.29 Other conditions associated with Lyme disease CC
Myopericarditis due to Lyme disease
AHA: 2016,3Q,12

A69.8 Other specified spirochetal infections

A69.9 Spirochetal infection, unspecified

Other diseases caused by chlamydiae (A70-A74)

EXCLUDES 1 *sexually transmitted chlamydial diseases (A55-A56)*

A70 Chlamydia psittaci infections CC
Ornithosis
Parrot fever
Psittacosis

A71 Trachoma
EXCLUDES 1 *sequelae of trachoma (B94.0)*

A71.0 Initial stage of trachoma
Trachoma dubium

A71.1 Active stage of trachoma
Granular conjunctivitis (trachomatous)
Trachomatous follicular conjunctivitis
Trachomatous pannus

A71.9 Trachoma, unspecified

A74 Other diseases caused by chlamydiae
EXCLUDES 1 *neonatal chlamydial conjunctivitis (P39.1)*
neonatal chlamydial pneumonia (P23.1)
Reiter's disease (M02.3-)
sexually transmitted chlamydial diseases (A55-A56)
EXCLUDES 2 *chlamydial pneumonia (J16.0)*

A74.0 Chlamydial conjunctivitis
Paratrachoma

A74.8 Other chlamydial diseases

A74.81 Chlamydial peritonitis

A74.89 Other chlamydial diseases

A74.9 Chlamydial infection, unspecified
Chlamydiosis NOS

Rickettsioses (A75-A79)

DEF: Rickettsia: Condition caused by bacteria that live in lice/ticks transmitted to humans through bites.

A75 Typhus fever
EXCLUDES 1 *rickettsiosis due to Ehrlichia sennetsu (A79.81)*

A75.0 Epidemic louse-borne typhus fever due to Rickettsia prowazekii CC
Classical typhus (fever)
Epidemic (louse-borne) typhus

A75.1 Recrudescent typhus [Brill's disease] CC
Brill-Zinsser disease

A75.2 Typhus fever due to Rickettsia typhi CC
Murine (flea-borne) typhus

A75.3 Typhus fever due to Rickettsia tsutsugamushi CC
Scrub (mite-borne) typhus
Tsutsugamushi fever
Typhus fever due to Orientia Tsutsugamushi (scrub typhus)

A75.9 Typhus fever, unspecified CC
Typhus (fever) NOS

A77 Spotted fever [tick-borne rickettsioses]

A77.0 Spotted fever due to Rickettsia rickettsii CC
Rocky Mountain spotted fever
Sao Paulo fever

A77.1 Spotted fever due to Rickettsia conorii CC
African tick typhus
Boutonneuse fever
India tick typhus
Kenya tick typhus
Marseilles fever
Mediterranean tick fever

A77.2 Spotted fever due to Rickettsia siberica CC
North Asian tick fever
Siberian tick typhus

A77.3 Spotted fever due to Rickettsia australis CC
Queensland tick typhus

A77.4 Ehrlichiosis
EXCLUDES 1 *anaplasmosis [A. phagocytophilum] (A79.82)*
rickettsiosis due to Ehrlichia sennetsu (A79.81)
AHA: 2021,4Q,5

A77.40 Ehrlichiosis, unspecified CC

A77.41 Ehrlichiosis chafeensis [E. chafeensis] CC

A77.49 Other ehrlichiosis CC
Ehrlichiosis due to E. ewingii
Ehrlichiosis due to E. muris euclairensis

A77.8 Other spotted fevers CC
Rickettsia 364D/R. philipii (Pacific Coast tick fever)
Spotted fever due to Rickettsia africae (African tick bite fever)
Spotted fever due to Rickettsia parkeri

A77.9 Spotted fever, unspecified CC
Tick-borne typhus NOS

A78 Q fever CC
Infection due to Coxiella burnetii
Nine Mile fever
Quadrilateral fever

A79 Other rickettsioses

A79.0 Trench fever CC
Quintan fever
Wolhynian fever

A79.1 Rickettsialpox due to Rickettsia akari CC
Kew Garden fever
Vesicular rickettsiosis

A79.8 Other specified rickettsioses

A79.81 Rickettsiosis due to Ehrlichia sennetsu CC
Rickettsiosis due to Neorickettsia sennetsu

A79.82 Anaplasmosis [A. phagocytophilum] CC
Transfusion transmitted A. phagocytophilum
AHA: 2021,4Q,4-5

A79.89 Other specified rickettsioses CC

A79.9 Rickettsiosis, unspecified CC
Rickettsial infection NOS

Viral and prion infections of the central nervous system (A80-A89)

EXCLUDES 1 *postpolio syndrome (G14)*
sequelae of poliomyelitis (B91)
sequelae of viral encephalitis (B94.1)

A80 Acute poliomyelitis

EXCLUDES 1 *acute flaccid myelitis (G04.82)*

A80.0 Acute paralytic poliomyelitis, vaccine-associated MCC
A80.1 Acute paralytic poliomyelitis, wild virus, imported MCC
A80.2 Acute paralytic poliomyelitis, wild virus, indigenous MCC
A80.3 Acute paralytic poliomyelitis, other and unspecified
A80.30 Acute paralytic poliomyelitis, unspecified MCC
A80.39 Other acute paralytic poliomyelitis MCC
A80.4 Acute nonparalytic poliomyelitis
A80.9 Acute poliomyelitis, unspecified

A81 Atypical virus infections of central nervous system

INCLUDES diseases of the central nervous system caused by prions

Use additional code, if applicable, to identify:
dementia with anxiety (F02.84, F02.A4, F02.B4, F02.C4)
dementia with behavioral disturbance (F02.81-, F02.A1-, F02.B1-, F02.C1-)
dementia with mood disturbance (F02.83, F02.A3, F02.B3, F02.C3)
dementia with psychotic disturbance (F02.82, F02.A2, F02.B2, F02.C2)
dementia without behavioral disturbance (F02.80, F02.A0, F02.B0, F02.C0)
mild neurocognitive disorder due to known physiological condition (F06.7-)

A81.0 Creutzfeldt-Jakob disease

DEF: Communicable, rare spongiform encephalopathy occurring later in life with progressive destruction of the pyramidal and extrapyramidal systems eventually leading to death. Progressive dementia, wasting of muscles, tremor, and other symptoms are present.

A81.00 Creutzfeldt-Jakob disease, unspecified CC HCC
Jakob-Creutzfeldt disease, unspecified
A81.01 Variant Creutzfeldt-Jakob disease CC HCC
vCJD
A81.09 Other Creutzfeldt-Jakob disease CC HCC
CJD
Familial Creutzfeldt-Jakob disease
Iatrogenic Creutzfeldt-Jakob disease
Sporadic Creutzfeldt-Jakob disease
Subacute spongiform encephalopathy (with dementia)

A81.1 Subacute sclerosing panencephalitis CC HCC
Dawson's inclusion body encephalitis
Van Bogaert's sclerosing leukoencephalopathy
A81.2 Progressive multifocal leukoencephalopathy HIV CC HCC
Multifocal leukoencephalopathy NOS
A81.8 Other atypical virus infections of central nervous system
A81.81 Kuru CC HCC
A81.82 Gerstmann-Straussler-Scheinker syndrome HIV CC HCC
GSS syndrome
A81.83 Fatal familial insomnia HIV CC HCC
FFI
A81.89 Other atypical virus infections of central nervous system HIV CC HCC
A81.9 Atypical virus infection of central nervous system, unspecified HIV CC HCC
Prion diseases of the central nervous system NOS

A82 Rabies

A82.0 Sylvatic rabies CC
A82.1 Urban rabies CC
A82.9 Rabies, unspecified CC

A83 Mosquito-borne viral encephalitis

INCLUDES mosquito-borne viral meningoencephalitis

EXCLUDES 2 *Venezuelan equine encephalitis (A92.2)*
West Nile fever (A92.3-)
West Nile virus (A92.3-)

A83.0 Japanese encephalitis MCC
A83.1 Western equine encephalitis MCC
A83.2 Eastern equine encephalitis MCC
A83.3 St Louis encephalitis MCC
A83.4 Australian encephalitis MCC
Kunjin virus disease
A83.5 California encephalitis MCC
California meningoencephalitis
La Crosse encephalitis
A83.6 Rocio virus disease MCC
A83.8 Other mosquito-borne viral encephalitis MCC
A83.9 Mosquito-borne viral encephalitis, unspecified MCC

A84 Tick-borne viral encephalitis

INCLUDES tick-borne viral meningoencephalitis

A84.0 Far Eastern tick-borne encephalitis [Russian spring-summer encephalitis] MCC
A84.1 Central European tick-borne encephalitis MCC
A84.8 Other tick-borne viral encephalitis
AHA: 2020,4Q,4-5
A84.81 Powassan virus disease MCC
A84.89 Other tick-borne viral encephalitis MCC
Louping ill
Code first, if applicable, transfusion related infection (T80.22-)
A84.9 Tick-borne viral encephalitis, unspecified MCC

A85 Other viral encephalitis, not elsewhere classified

INCLUDES specified viral encephalomyelitis NEC
specified viral meningoencephalitis NEC

EXCLUDES 1 *encephalitis due to cytomegalovirus (B25.8)*
encephalitis due to herpesvirus NEC (B10.0-)
encephalitis due to herpesvirus [herpes simplex] (B00.4)
encephalitis due to measles virus (B05.0)
encephalitis due to mumps virus (B26.2)
encephalitis due to poliomyelitis virus (A80.-)
encephalitis due to zoster (B02.0)
lymphocytic choriomeningitis (A87.2)
myalgic encephalomyelitis (G93.32)

A85.0 Enteroviral encephalitis HIV CC
Enteroviral encephalomyelitis
A85.1 Adenoviral encephalitis HIV CC
Adenoviral meningoencephalitis
A85.2 Arthropod-borne viral encephalitis, unspecified MCC
EXCLUDES 1 *West nile virus with encephalitis (A92.31)*
A85.8 Other specified viral encephalitis HIV CC
Encephalitis lethargica
Von Economo-Cruchet disease

A86 Unspecified viral encephalitis HIV CC
Viral encephalomyelitis NOS
Viral meningoencephalitis NOS

A87 Viral meningitis

EXCLUDES 1 *meningitis due to herpesvirus [herpes simplex] (B00.3)*
meningitis due to measles virus (B05.1)
meningitis due to mumps virus (B26.1)
meningitis due to poliomyelitis virus (A80.-)
meningitis due to zoster (B02.1)

DEF: Meningitis: Inflammation of the meningeal layers of the brain and spine.

A87.0 Enteroviral meningitis CC
Coxsackievirus meningitis
Echovirus meningitis
A87.1 Adenoviral meningitis CC
A87.2 Lymphocytic choriomeningitis CC
Lymphocytic meningoencephalitis
A87.8 Other viral meningitis CC
A87.9 Viral meningitis, unspecified CC

A88 Other viral infections of central nervous system, not elsewhere classified

EXCLUDES 1 *viral encephalitis NOS (A86)*
viral meningitis NOS (A87.9)

A88.0 Enteroviral exanthematous fever [Boston exanthem] CC
A88.1 Epidemic vertigo
A88.8 Other specified viral infections of central nervous system HIV CC

A89 Unspecified viral infection of central nervous system HIV CC

Arthropod-borne viral fevers and viral hemorrhagic fevers (A90-A99)

A90 Dengue fever [classical dengue] CC
EXCLUDES 1 *dengue hemorrhagic fever (A91)*
AHA: 2016,3Q,13

A91 Dengue hemorrhagic fever CC

✓4th **A92 Other mosquito-borne viral fevers**
EXCLUDES 1 *Ross River disease (B33.1)*

A92.0 Chikungunya virus disease CC
Chikungunya (hemorrhagic) fever

A92.1 O'nyong-nyong fever CC

A92.2 Venezuelan equine fever CC
Venezuelan equine encephalitis
Venezuelan equine encephalomyelitis virus disease

✓5th **A92.3 West Nile virus infection**
West Nile fever
AHA: 2016,3Q,12

A92.30 West Nile virus infection, unspecified MCC
West Nile fever NOS
West Nile fever without complications
West Nile virus NOS

A92.31 West Nile virus infection with encephalitis MCC
West Nile encephalitis
West Nile encephalomyelitis

A92.32 West Nile virus infection with other neurologic manifestation MCC
Use additional code to specify the neurologic manifestation

A92.39 West Nile virus infection with other complications MCC
Use additional code to specify the other conditions

A92.4 Rift Valley fever CC

A92.5 Zika virus disease CC
Zika virus fever
Zika virus infection
Zika NOS
EXCLUDES 1 *congenital Zika virus disease (P35.4)*
AHA: 2016,4Q,4-7
DEF: Virus transmitted via a bite from an infected Aedes species mosquito. Common symptoms of the virus include fever, rash, joint pain, and conjunctivitis; they are usually mild in nature and may last from several days to a week. Most people who have the Zika virus do not require medical attention; however, in pregnant women, the Zika virus can cause a serious birth defect called microcephaly, as well as other severe fetal brain defects.
TIP: Code only confirmed diagnoses of Zika virus; documentation by the physician that the disease is confirmed is sufficient.

A92.8 Other specified mosquito-borne viral fevers CC

A92.9 Mosquito-borne viral fever, unspecified CC

✓4th **A93 Other arthropod-borne viral fevers, not elsewhere classified**

A93.0 Oropouche virus disease CC
Oropouche fever

A93.1 Sandfly fever CC
Pappataci fever
Phlebotomus fever

A93.2 Colorado tick fever CC

A93.8 Other specified arthropod-borne viral fevers CC
Piry virus disease
Vesicular stomatitis virus disease [Indiana fever]

A94 Unspecified arthropod-borne viral fever CC
Arboviral fever NOS
Arbovirus infection NOS

✓4th **A95 Yellow fever**

A95.0 Sylvatic yellow fever CC
Jungle yellow fever

A95.1 Urban yellow fever CC

A95.9 Yellow fever, unspecified CC

✓4th **A96 Arenaviral hemorrhagic fever**

A96.0 Junin hemorrhagic fever CC
Argentinian hemorrhagic fever

A96.1 Machupo hemorrhagic fever CC
Bolivian hemorrhagic fever

A96.2 Lassa fever

A96.8 Other arenaviral hemorrhagic fevers CC

A96.9 Arenaviral hemorrhagic fever, unspecified CC

✓4th **A98 Other viral hemorrhagic fevers, not elsewhere classified**
EXCLUDES 1 *chikungunya hemorrhagic fever (A92.0)*
dengue hemorrhagic fever (A91)

A98.0 Crimean-Congo hemorrhagic fever CC
Central Asian hemorrhagic fever

A98.1 Omsk hemorrhagic fever CC

A98.2 Kyasanur Forest disease CC

A98.3 Marburg virus disease

A98.4 Ebola virus disease

A98.5 Hemorrhagic fever with renal syndrome CC
Epidemic hemorrhagic fever
Korean hemorrhagic fever
Russian hemorrhagic fever
Hantaan virus disease
Hantavirus disease with renal manifestations
Nephropathia epidemica
Songo fever
EXCLUDES 1 *hantavirus (cardio)-pulmonary syndrome (B33.4)*

A98.8 Other specified viral hemorrhagic fevers CC

A99 Unspecified viral hemorrhagic fever CC

Viral infections characterized by skin and mucous membrane lesions (B00-B09)

✓4th **B00 Herpesviral [herpes simplex] infections**
EXCLUDES 1 *congenital herpesviral infections (P35.2)*
EXCLUDES 2 *anogenital herpesviral infection (A60.-)*
gammaherpesviral mononucleosis (B27.0-)
herpangina (B08.5)

B00.0 Eczema herpeticum HIV
Kaposi's varicelliform eruption

B00.1 Herpesviral vesicular dermatitis HIV
Herpes simplex facialis
Herpes simplex labialis
Herpes simplex otitis externa
Vesicular dermatitis of ear
Vesicular dermatitis of lip

B00.2 Herpesviral gingivostomatitis and pharyngotonsillitis HIV CC
Herpesviral pharyngitis

B00.3 Herpesviral meningitis HIV MCC

B00.4 Herpesviral encephalitis HIV MCC
Herpesviral meningoencephalitis
Simian B disease
EXCLUDES 1 *herpesviral encephalitis due to herpesvirus 6 and 7 (B10.01, B10.09)*
non-simplex herpesviral encephalitis (B10.0-)

✓5th **B00.5 Herpesviral ocular disease**

B00.50 Herpesviral ocular disease, unspecified HIV CC

B00.51 Herpesviral iridocyclitis HIV CC
Herpesviral iritis
Herpesviral uveitis, anterior

B00.52 Herpesviral keratitis HIV CC
Herpesviral keratoconjunctivitis

B00.53 Herpesviral conjunctivitis HIV CC

B00.59 Other herpesviral disease of eye HIV CC
Herpesviral dermatitis of eyelid

B00.7 Disseminated herpesviral disease HIV MCC HCC
Herpesviral sepsis

✓5th **B00.8 Other forms of herpesviral infections**

B00.81 Herpesviral hepatitis HIV CC

B00.82 Herpes simplex myelitis MCC HCC

B00.89 Other herpesviral infection HIV CC
Herpesviral whitlow

B00.9 Herpesviral infection, unspecified HIV
Herpes simplex infection NOS

✓4th **B01 Varicella [chickenpox]**

B01.0 Varicella meningitis CC

✓5th **B01.1 Varicella encephalitis, myelitis and encephalomyelitis**
Postchickenpox encephalitis, myelitis and encephalomyelitis

B01.11 Varicella encephalitis and encephalomyelitis MCC
Postchickenpox encephalitis and encephalomyelitis

B01.12 Varicella myelitis MCC HCC
Postchickenpox myelitis

B01.2 Varicella pneumonia MCC

✓5th **B01.8 Varicella with other complications**

B01.81 Varicella keratitis CC

B01.89 Other varicella complications CC

B01.9 Varicella without complication CC
Varicella NOS

✓4th **B02 Zoster [herpes zoster]**

INCLUDES shingles
zona

B02.0 Zoster encephalitis HIV CC
Zoster meningoencephalitis

B02.1 Zoster meningitis HIV MCC
AHA: 2019,1Q,18

✓5th **B02.2 Zoster with other nervous system involvement**

B02.21 Postherpetic geniculate ganglionitis HIV CC

B02.22 Postherpetic trigeminal neuralgia HIV CC

B02.23 Postherpetic polyneuropathy HIV CC

B02.24 Postherpetic myelitis MCC HCC
Herpes zoster myelitis

B02.29 Other postherpetic nervous system involvement HIV CC
Postherpetic radiculopathy

✓5th **B02.3 Zoster ocular disease**

B02.30 Zoster ocular disease, unspecified HIV CC

B02.31 Zoster conjunctivitis HIV CC

B02.32 Zoster iridocyclitis HIV CC

B02.33 Zoster keratitis HIV CC
Herpes zoster keratoconjunctivitis

B02.34 Zoster scleritis HIV CC

B02.39 Other herpes zoster eye disease HIV CC
Zoster blepharitis

B02.7 Disseminated zoster HIV CC

B02.8 Zoster with other complications HIV CC
Herpes zoster otitis externa

B02.9 Zoster without complications HIV
Zoster NOS

B03 Smallpox CC

NOTE In 1980 the 33rd World Health Assembly declared that smallpox had been eradicated.

The classification is maintained for surveillance purposes.

B04 Monkeypox CC
AHA: 2022,3Q,3-4

✓4th **B05 Measles**

INCLUDES morbilli

EXCLUDES 1 *subacute sclerosing panencephalitis (A81.1)*

B05.0 Measles complicated by encephalitis MCC
Postmeasles encephalitis

B05.1 Measles complicated by meningitis CC
Postmeasles meningitis

B05.2 Measles complicated by pneumonia MCC
Postmeasles pneumonia

B05.3 Measles complicated by otitis media
Postmeasles otitis media

B05.4 Measles with intestinal complications CC

✓5th **B05.8 Measles with other complications**

B05.81 Measles keratitis and keratoconjunctivitis CC

B05.89 Other measles complications CC

B05.9 Measles without complication
Measles NOS

✓4th **B06 Rubella [German measles]**

EXCLUDES 1 *congenital rubella (P35.0)*

DEF: Highly contagious virus in which the symptoms are mild and short-lived in most people. Rubella during pregnancy, however, can result in abortion, stillbirth, or congenital defects.

✓5th **B06.0 Rubella with neurological complications**

B06.00 Rubella with neurological complication, unspecified CC

B06.01 Rubella encephalitis MCC
Rubella meningoencephalitis

B06.02 Rubella meningitis CC

B06.09 Other neurological complications of rubella CC

✓5th **B06.8 Rubella with other complications**

B06.81 Rubella pneumonia CC

B06.82 Rubella arthritis CC HCC

B06.89 Other rubella complications CC

B06.9 Rubella without complication
Rubella NOS

✓4th **B07 Viral warts**

INCLUDES verruca simplex
verruca vulgaris
viral warts due to human papillomavirus

EXCLUDES 2 *anogenital (venereal) warts (A63.0)*
papilloma of bladder (D41.4)
papilloma of cervix (D26.0)
papilloma larynx (D14.1)

B07.0 Plantar wart
Verruca plantaris

B07.8 Other viral warts
Common wart
Flat wart
Verruca plana

B07.9 Viral wart, unspecified

✓4th **B08 Other viral infections characterized by skin and mucous membrane lesions, not elsewhere classified**

EXCLUDES 1 *vesicular stomatitis virus disease (A93.8)*

✓5th **B08.0 Other orthopoxvirus infections**

EXCLUDES 2 *monkeypox (B04)*

✓6th **B08.01 Cowpox and vaccinia not from vaccine**

B08.010 Cowpox
DEF: Disease contracted by milking infected cows. The vesicles usually appear on the fingers, hands, and adjacent areas and usually disappear without scarring. Other symptoms include local edema, lymphangitis, and regional lymphadenitis with or without fever.

B08.011 Vaccinia not from vaccine
EXCLUDES 1 *vaccinia (from vaccination) (generalized) (T88.1)*

B08.02 Orf virus disease
Contagious pustular dermatitis
Ecthyma contagiosum

B08.03 Pseudocowpox [milker's node]

B08.04 Paravaccinia, unspecified

B08.09 Other orthopoxvirus infections
Orthopoxvirus infection NOS

B08.1 Molluscum contagiosum
DEF: Benign poxvirus infection causing small bumps on the skin or conjunctiva, transmitted by close contact.

✓5th **B08.2 Exanthema subitum [sixth disease]**
Roseola infantum

B08.20 Exanthema subitum [sixth disease], unspecified P
Roseola infantum, unspecified

B08.21 Exanthema subitum [sixth disease] due to human herpesvirus 6 P
Roseola infantum due to human herpesvirus 6

B08.22 Exanthema subitum [sixth disease] due to human herpesvirus 7 P
Roseola infantum due to human herpesvirus 7

B08.3 Erythema infectiosum [fifth disease] CC
DEF: Infection with human parvovirus B19, mainly occurring in children. Symptoms include a low-grade fever, malaise, or a "cold" a few days before the appearance of a mild rash illness that presents as a "slapped-cheek" rash on the face and a lacy red rash on the trunk and limbs.

B08.4 Enteroviral vesicular stomatitis with exanthem
Hand, foot and mouth disease

B08.5 Enteroviral vesicular pharyngitis
Herpangina
DEF: Acute infectious Coxsackie virus infection causing throat lesions, fever, and vomiting that generally affects children in the summer.

✓5th **B08.6 Parapoxvirus infections**

B08.60 Parapoxvirus infection, unspecified

B08.61 Bovine stomatitis

B08.62 Sealpox

B08.69 Other parapoxvirus infections

✓5th **B08.7 Yatapoxvirus infections**
- **B08.70 Yatapoxvirus infection, unspecified**
- **B08.71 Tanapox virus disease** CC
- **B08.72 Yaba pox virus disease**
  Yaba monkey tumor disease
- **B08.79 Other yatapoxvirus infections**

B08.8 Other specified viral infections characterized by skin and mucous membrane lesions
Enteroviral lymphonodular pharyngitis
Foot-and-mouth disease
Poxvirus NEC

B09 Unspecified viral infection characterized by skin and mucous membrane lesions
Viral enanthema NOS
Viral exanthema NOS

Other human herpesviruses (B10)

✓4th **B10 Other human herpesviruses**
EXCLUDES 2 *cytomegalovirus (B25.9)*
Epstein-Barr virus (B27.0-)
herpes NOS (B00.9)
herpes simplex (B00.-)
herpes zoster (B02.-)
human herpesvirus NOS (B00.-)
human herpesvirus 1 and 2 (B00.-)
human herpesvirus 3 (B01.-, B02.-)
human herpesvirus 4 (B27.0-)
human herpesvirus 5 (B25.-)
varicella (B01.-)
zoster (B02.-)

✓5th **B10.0 Other human herpesvirus encephalitis**
EXCLUDES 2 *herpes encephalitis NOS (B00.4)*
herpes simplex encephalitis (B00.4)
human herpesvirus encephalitis (B00.4)
simian B herpes virus encephalitis (B00.4)
- **B10.01 Human herpesvirus 6 encephalitis** HIV MCC
- **B10.09 Other human herpesvirus encephalitis** HIV MCC
  Human herpesvirus 7 encephalitis

✓5th **B10.8 Other human herpesvirus infection**
- **B10.81 Human herpesvirus 6 infection**
- **B10.82 Human herpesvirus 7 infection**
- **B10.89 Other human herpesvirus infection**
  Human herpesvirus 8 infection
  Kaposi's sarcoma-associated herpesvirus infection

Viral hepatitis (B15-B19)

EXCLUDES 1 *sequelae of viral hepatitis (B94.2)*
EXCLUDES 2 *cytomegaloviral hepatitis (B25.1)*
herpesviral [herpes simplex] hepatitis (B00.81)

DEF: Hepatitis A: HAV infection that is self-limiting with flulike symptoms. Transmission is fecal-oral.
DEF: Hepatitis B: HBV infection that can be chronic and systemic. Transmission is bodily fluids.
DEF: Hepatitis C: HCV infection that can be chronic and systemic. Transmission is blood transfusion and unidentified agents.
DEF: Hepatitis D (delta): HDV that occurs only in the presence of hepatitis B virus. Transmission is contaminated blood in contact with mucous membranes.
DEF: Hepatitis E: HEV is an epidemic form. Transmission is fecal-oral, most often from contaminated water.

✓4th **B15 Acute hepatitis A**
- **B15.0 Hepatitis A with hepatic coma** MCC
- **B15.9 Hepatitis A without hepatic coma** CC
  Hepatitis A (acute)(viral) NOS

✓4th **B16 Acute hepatitis B**
AHA: 2016,3Q,13
- **B16.0 Acute hepatitis B with delta-agent with hepatic coma** MCC
- **B16.1 Acute hepatitis B with delta-agent without hepatic coma** CC
- **B16.2 Acute hepatitis B without delta-agent with hepatic coma** MCC
- **B16.9 Acute hepatitis B without delta-agent and without hepatic coma** CC
  Hepatitis B (acute) (viral) NOS

✓4th **B17 Other acute viral hepatitis**
- **B17.0 Acute delta-(super) infection of hepatitis B carrier** CC

✓5th **B17.1 Acute hepatitis C**
- **B17.10 Acute hepatitis C without hepatic coma** CC
  Acute hepatitis C NOS
- **B17.11 Acute hepatitis C with hepatic coma** MCC

B17.2 Acute hepatitis E CC
B17.8 Other specified acute viral hepatitis CC
Hepatitis non-A non-B (acute) (viral) NEC
B17.9 Acute viral hepatitis, unspecified CC
Acute hepatitis NOS
Acute infectious hepatitis NOS

✓4th **B18 Chronic viral hepatitis**
INCLUDES carrier of viral hepatitis
AHA: 2017,1Q,41
- **B18.0 Chronic viral hepatitis B with delta-agent** CC HCC
- **B18.1 Chronic viral hepatitis B without delta-agent** CC HCC
  Carrier of viral hepatitis B
  Chronic (viral) hepatitis B
- **B18.2 Chronic viral hepatitis C** HCC
  Carrier of viral hepatitis C
  AHA: 2018,1Q,4
- **B18.8 Other chronic viral hepatitis** CC HCC
  Carrier of other viral hepatitis
- **B18.9 Chronic viral hepatitis, unspecified** CC HCC
  Carrier of unspecified viral hepatitis

✓4th **B19 Unspecified viral hepatitis**
- **B19.0 Unspecified viral hepatitis with hepatic coma** MCC

✓5th **B19.1 Unspecified viral hepatitis B**
- **B19.10 Unspecified viral hepatitis B without hepatic coma** CC
  Unspecified viral hepatitis B NOS
- **B19.11 Unspecified viral hepatitis B with hepatic coma** MCC

✓5th **B19.2 Unspecified viral hepatitis C**
- **B19.20 Unspecified viral hepatitis C without hepatic coma**
  Viral hepatitis C NOS
- **B19.21 Unspecified viral hepatitis C with hepatic coma** MCC

B19.9 Unspecified viral hepatitis without hepatic coma CC
Viral hepatitis NOS

Human immunodeficiency virus [HIV] disease (B20)

B20 Human immunodeficiency virus [HIV] disease CC HCC
INCLUDES acquired immune deficiency syndrome [AIDS]
AIDS-related complex [ARC]
HIV infection, symptomatic
Code first human immunodeficiency virus [HIV] disease complicating pregnancy, childbirth and the puerperium, if applicable (O98.7-)
Use additional code(s) to identify all manifestations of HIV infection
EXCLUDES 1 *asymptomatic human immunodeficiency virus [HIV] infection status (Z21)*
exposure to HIV virus (Z20.6)
inconclusive serologic evidence of HIV (R75)
AHA: 2022,1Q,36; 2021,2Q,6; 2021,1Q,52; 2020,4Q,97; 2020,2Q,12; 2019,1Q,8-11

Other viral diseases (B25-B34)

✓4th **B25 Cytomegaloviral disease**
EXCLUDES 1 *congenital cytomegalovirus infection (P35.1)*
cytomegaloviral mononucleosis (B27.1-)
- **B25.0 Cytomegaloviral pneumonitis** MCC HCC
- **B25.1 Cytomegaloviral hepatitis** CC HCC
- **B25.2 Cytomegaloviral pancreatitis** MCC HCC
- **B25.8 Other cytomegaloviral diseases** HIV CC HCC
  Cytomegaloviral encephalitis
- **B25.9 Cytomegaloviral disease, unspecified** HIV CC HCC

✓4th **B26 Mumps**
INCLUDES epidemic parotitis
infectious parotitis
- **B26.0 Mumps orchitis** CC ♂
- **B26.1 Mumps meningitis** MCC
- **B26.2 Mumps encephalitis** MCC
- **B26.3 Mumps pancreatitis** CC

B26.8 Mumps with other complications

- **B26.81 Mumps hepatitis** CC
- **B26.82 Mumps myocarditis** CC
- **B26.83 Mumps nephritis** CC
- **B26.84 Mumps polyneuropathy** CC
- **B26.85 Mumps arthritis** CC HCC
- **B26.89 Other mumps complications** CC

B26.9 Mumps without complication
Mumps NOS
Mumps parotitis NOS

B27 Infectious mononucleosis

INCLUDES glandular fever
monocytic angina
Pfeiffer's disease

B27.Ø Gammaherpesviral mononucleosis
Mononucleosis due to Epstein-Barr virus

- **B27.ØØ Gammaherpesviral mononucleosis without complication**
- **B27.Ø1 Gammaherpesviral mononucleosis with polyneuropathy**
- **B27.Ø2 Gammaherpesviral mononucleosis with meningitis**
- **B27.Ø9 Gammaherpesviral mononucleosis with other complications**
  Hepatomegaly in gammaherpesviral mononucleosis

B27.1 Cytomegaloviral mononucleosis

- **B27.1Ø Cytomegaloviral mononucleosis without complications**
- **B27.11 Cytomegaloviral mononucleosis with polyneuropathy**
- **B27.12 Cytomegaloviral mononucleosis with meningitis**
- **B27.19 Cytomegaloviral mononucleosis with other complication**
  Hepatomegaly in cytomegaloviral mononucleosis

B27.8 Other infectious mononucleosis

- **B27.8Ø Other infectious mononucleosis without complication**
- **B27.81 Other infectious mononucleosis with polyneuropathy**
- **B27.82 Other infectious mononucleosis with meningitis**
- **B27.89 Other infectious mononucleosis with other complication**
  Hepatomegaly in other infectious mononucleosis

B27.9 Infectious mononucleosis, unspecified

- **B27.9Ø Infectious mononucleosis, unspecified without complication**
- **B27.91 Infectious mononucleosis, unspecified with polyneuropathy**
- **B27.92 Infectious mononucleosis, unspecified with meningitis**
- **B27.99 Infectious mononucleosis, unspecified with other complication**
  Hepatomegaly in unspecified infectious mononucleosis

B3Ø Viral conjunctivitis

EXCLUDES 1 *herpesviral [herpes simplex] ocular disease (BØØ.5)*
ocular zoster (BØ2.3)

Viral Conjunctivitis

B3Ø.Ø Keratoconjunctivitis due to adenovirus
Epidemic keratoconjunctivitis
Shipyard eye

B3Ø.1 Conjunctivitis due to adenovirus
Acute adenoviral follicular conjunctivitis
Swimming-pool conjunctivitis

B3Ø.2 Viral pharyngoconjunctivitis

B3Ø.3 Acute epidemic hemorrhagic conjunctivitis (enteroviral)
Conjunctivitis due to coxsackievirus 24
Conjunctivitis due to enterovirus 7Ø
Hemorrhagic conjunctivitis (acute)(epidemic)

B3Ø.8 Other viral conjunctivitis
Newcastle conjunctivitis

B3Ø.9 Viral conjunctivitis, unspecified

B33 Other viral diseases, not elsewhere classified

B33.Ø Epidemic myalgia
Bornholm disease

B33.1 Ross River disease CC
Epidemic polyarthritis and exanthema
Ross River fever

B33.2 Viral carditis
Coxsackie (virus) carditis

- **B33.2Ø Viral carditis, unspecified** CC
- **B33.21 Viral endocarditis** CC
- **B33.22 Viral myocarditis** CC
- **B33.23 Viral pericarditis** CC
- **B33.24 Viral cardiomyopathy** HCC

B33.3 Retrovirus infections, not elsewhere classified
Retrovirus infection NOS

B33.4 Hantavirus (cardio)-pulmonary syndrome [HPS] [HCPS] CC
Hantavirus disease with pulmonary manifestations
Sin nombre virus disease
Use additional code to identify any associated acute kidney failure (N17.9)
EXCLUDES 1 *hantavirus disease with renal manifestations (A98.5)*
hemorrhagic fever with renal manifestations (A98.5)

B33.8 Other specified viral diseases
EXCLUDES 1 *anogenital human papillomavirus infection (A63.Ø)*
viral warts due to human papillomavirus infection (BØ7)

B34 Viral infection of unspecified site

EXCLUDES 1 *anogenital human papillomavirus infection (A63.Ø)*
cytomegaloviral disease NOS (B25.9)
herpesvirus [herpes simplex] infection NOS (BØØ.9)
retrovirus infection NOS (B33.3)
viral agents as the cause of diseases classified elsewhere (B97.-)
viral warts due to human papillomavirus infection (BØ7)

B34.Ø Adenovirus infection, unspecified

B34.1 Enterovirus infection, unspecified
Coxsackievirus infection NOS
Echovirus infection NOS

B34.2 Coronavirus infection, unspecified
EXCLUDES 1 *COVID-19 (UØ7.1)*
pneumonia due to SARS-associated coronavirus (J12.81)
AHA: 2020,1Q,34-36

B34.3 Parvovirus infection, unspecified CC

B34.4 Papovavirus infection, unspecified

B34.8 Other viral infections of unspecified site

B34.9 Viral infection, unspecified
Viremia NOS
AHA: 2016,3Q,10

Mycoses (B35-B49)

EXCLUDES 2 *hypersensitivity pneumonitis due to organic dust (J67.-)*
mycosis fungoides (C84.Ø-)

B35 Dermatophytosis

INCLUDES favus
infections due to species of Epidermophyton, Micro-sporum and Trichophyton
tinea, any type except those in B36.-

DEF: Contagious superficial fungal infection of the skin that invades and grows in dead keratin.

B35.Ø Tinea barbae and tinea capitis
Beard ringworm
Kerion
Scalp ringworm
Sycosis, mycotic

B35.1 Tinea unguium
Dermatophytic onychia
Dermatophytosis of nail
Onychomycosis
Ringworm of nails

B35.2 Tinea manuum
Dermatophytosis of hand
Hand ringworm

B35.3 Tinea pedis
Athlete's foot
Dermatophytosis of foot
Foot ringworm

B35.4 Tinea corporis
Ringworm of the body

B35.5 Tinea imbricata
Tokelau

B35.6 Tinea cruris
Dhobi itch
Groin ringworm
Jock itch

B35.8 Other dermatophytoses
Disseminated dermatophytosis
Granulomatous dermatophytosis

B35.9 Dermatophytosis, unspecified
Ringworm NOS

✓4th B36 Other superficial mycoses

B36.0 Pityriasis versicolor
Tinea flava
Tinea versicolor

B36.1 Tinea nigra
Keratomycosis nigricans palmaris
Microsporosis nigra
Pityriasis nigra

B36.2 White piedra
Tinea blanca

B36.3 Black piedra

B36.8 Other specified superficial mycoses

B36.9 Superficial mycosis, unspecified

✓4th B37 Candidiasis

INCLUDES candidosis
moniliasis

EXCLUDES 1 *neonatal candidiasis (P37.5)*

DEF: *Candida:* Genus of yeast-like fungi that are commonly found in the mouth, skin, intestinal tract, and vagina. It may cause a white, cheesy discharge.

B37.0 Candidal stomatitis HIV CC
Oral thrush

B37.1 Pulmonary candidiasis HIV MCC HCC
Candidal bronchitis
Candidal pneumonia

B37.2 Candidiasis of skin and nail HIV
Candidal onychia
Candidal paronychia

EXCLUDES 2 *diaper dermatitis (L22)*

✓5th B37.3 Candidiasis of vulva and vagina
Candidal vulvovaginitis
Monilial vulvovaginitis
Vaginal thrush

AHA: 2022,4Q,4-5

B37.31 Acute candidiasis of vulva and vagina ♀
Candidiasis of vulva and vagina NOS

B37.32 Chronic candidiasis of vulva and vagina ♀
Recurrent candidiasis of vulva and vagina

✓5th B37.4 Candidiasis of other urogenital sites

B37.41 Candidal cystitis and urethritis CC H6

B37.42 Candidal balanitis ♂

B37.49 Other urogenital candidiasis CC H6
Candidal pyelonephritis

B37.5 Candidal meningitis HIV MCC

B37.6 Candidal endocarditis HIV MCC

B37.7 Candidal sepsis MCC HCC
Disseminated candidiasis
Systemic candidiasis

AHA: 2014,4Q,46

TIP: This code is assigned when sepsis is documented as due to any *Candida* type. If the nonspecific term "non-*Candida albicans*" is documented, code B48.8 Other specified mycoses, is assigned.

✓5th B37.8 Candidiasis of other sites

B37.81 Candidal esophagitis HIV CC HCC

B37.82 Candidal enteritis HIV CC
Candidal proctitis

B37.83 Candidal cheilitis HIV CC

B37.84 Candidal otitis externa HIV CC

B37.89 Other sites of candidiasis HIV CC
Candidal osteomyelitis

B37.9 Candidiasis, unspecified HIV
Thrush NOS

✓4th B38 Coccidioidomycosis

B38.0 Acute pulmonary coccidioidomycosis HIV CC HCC

B38.1 Chronic pulmonary coccidioidomycosis HIV CC HCC

B38.2 Pulmonary coccidioidomycosis, unspecified HIV CC HCC

B38.3 Cutaneous coccidioidomycosis HIV CC

B38.4 Coccidioidomycosis meningitis HIV MCC

DEF: *Coccidioides immitis* infection of the lining of the brain and/or spinal cord.

B38.7 Disseminated coccidioidomycosis HIV CC
Generalized coccidioidomycosis

✓5th B38.8 Other forms of coccidioidomycosis

B38.81 Prostatic coccidioidomycosis HIV CC ♂

B38.89 Other forms of coccidioidomycosis HIV CC

B38.9 Coccidioidomycosis, unspecified HIV CC

✓4th B39 Histoplasmosis

Code first associated AIDS (B20)

Use additional code for any associated manifestations, such as:
endocarditis (I39)
meningitis (G02)
pericarditis (I32)
retinitis (H32)

DEF: Type of lung infection caused by breathing in fungal spores often found in the droppings of bats and birds or soil contaminated by their droppings.

Histoplasmosis

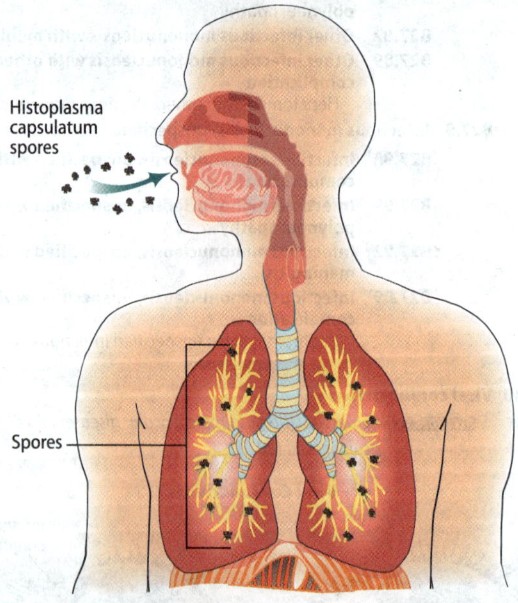

B39.0 Acute pulmonary histoplasmosis capsulati HIV MCC HCC

B39.1 Chronic pulmonary histoplasmosis capsulati HIV MCC HCC

B39.2 Pulmonary histoplasmosis capsulati, unspecified HIV MCC HCC

B39.3 Disseminated histoplasmosis capsulati HIV CC
Generalized histoplasmosis capsulati

B39.4 Histoplasmosis capsulati, unspecified HIV
American histoplasmosis

B39.5 Histoplasmosis duboisii HIV
African histoplasmosis

B39.9 Histoplasmosis, unspecified HIV

B40 Blastomycosis ✓4th

EXCLUDES 1 *Brazilian blastomycosis (B41.-)*
keloidal blastomycosis (B48.0)

- **B40.0 Acute pulmonary blastomycosis** CC HCC
- **B40.1 Chronic pulmonary blastomycosis** CC HCC
- **B40.2 Pulmonary blastomycosis, unspecified** CC HCC
- **B40.3 Cutaneous blastomycosis** CC
- **B40.7 Disseminated blastomycosis** CC
  Generalized blastomycosis
- ✓5th **B40.8 Other forms of blastomycosis**
  - **B40.81 Blastomycotic meningoencephalitis** CC
    Meningomyelitis due to blastomycosis
  - **B40.89 Other forms of blastomycosis** CC
- **B40.9 Blastomycosis, unspecified** CC

B41 Paracoccidioidomycosis ✓4th

INCLUDES Brazilian blastomycosis
Lutz' disease

- **B41.0 Pulmonary paracoccidioidomycosis** CC HCC
- **B41.7 Disseminated paracoccidioidomycosis** CC
  Generalized paracoccidioidomycosis
- **B41.8 Other forms of paracoccidioidomycosis** CC
- **B41.9 Paracoccidioidomycosis, unspecified** CC

B42 Sporotrichosis ✓4th

- **B42.0 Pulmonary sporotrichosis**
- **B42.1 Lymphocutaneous sporotrichosis**
- **B42.7 Disseminated sporotrichosis**
  Generalized sporotrichosis
- ✓5th **B42.8 Other forms of sporotrichosis**
  - **B42.81 Cerebral sporotrichosis**
    Meningitis due to sporotrichosis
  - **B42.82 Sporotrichosis arthritis** HCC
  - **B42.89 Other forms of sporotrichosis**
- **B42.9 Sporotrichosis, unspecified**

B43 Chromomycosis and pheomycotic abscess ✓4th

- **B43.0 Cutaneous chromomycosis**
  Dermatitis verrucosa
- **B43.1 Pheomycotic brain abscess**
  Cerebral chromomycosis
- **B43.2 Subcutaneous pheomycotic abscess and cyst**
- **B43.8 Other forms of chromomycosis**
- **B43.9 Chromomycosis, unspecified**

B44 Aspergillosis ✓4th

INCLUDES aspergilloma

- **B44.0 Invasive pulmonary aspergillosis** MCC HCC
- **B44.1 Other pulmonary aspergillosis** CC HCC
- **B44.2 Tonsillar aspergillosis** CC HCC
- **B44.7 Disseminated aspergillosis** CC HCC
  Generalized aspergillosis
- ✓5th **B44.8 Other forms of aspergillosis**
  - **B44.81 Allergic bronchopulmonary aspergillosis** CC HCC
  - **B44.89 Other forms of aspergillosis** CC HCC
- **B44.9 Aspergillosis, unspecified** CC HCC

B45 Cryptococcosis ✓4th

- **B45.0 Pulmonary cryptococcosis** HIV CC HCC
- **B45.1 Cerebral cryptococcosis** MCC HCC
  Cryptococcal meningitis
  Cryptococcosis meningocerebralis
- **B45.2 Cutaneous cryptococcosis** HIV CC HCC
- **B45.3 Osseous cryptococcosis** HIV CC HCC
- **B45.7 Disseminated cryptococcosis** HIV CC HCC
  Generalized cryptococcosis
- **B45.8 Other forms of cryptococcosis** HIV CC HCC
- **B45.9 Cryptococcosis, unspecified** HIV CC HCC

B46 Zygomycosis ✓4th

- **B46.0 Pulmonary mucormycosis** MCC HCC
- **B46.1 Rhinocerebral mucormycosis** MCC HCC
- **B46.2 Gastrointestinal mucormycosis** MCC HCC
- **B46.3 Cutaneous mucormycosis** MCC HCC
  Subcutaneous mucormycosis
- **B46.4 Disseminated mucormycosis** MCC HCC
  Generalized mucormycosis
- **B46.5 Mucormycosis, unspecified** MCC HCC
- **B46.8 Other zygomycoses** MCC HCC
  Entomophthoromycosis
- **B46.9 Zygomycosis, unspecified** MCC HCC
  Phycomycosis NOS

B47 Mycetoma ✓4th

- **B47.0 Eumycetoma** CC
  Madura foot, mycotic
  Maduromycosis
- **B47.1 Actinomycetoma** HIV CC
- **B47.9 Mycetoma, unspecified** HIV CC
  Madura foot NOS

B48 Other mycoses, not elsewhere classified ✓4th

- **B48.0 Lobomycosis**
  Keloidal blastomycosis
  Lobo's disease
- **B48.1 Rhinosporidiosis**
- **B48.2 Allescheriasis** CC
  Infection due to Pseudallescheria boydii
  EXCLUDES 1 *eumycetoma (B47.0)*
- **B48.3 Geotrichosis** CC
  Geotrichum stomatitis
- **B48.4 Penicillosis** CC HCC
  Talaromycosis
- **B48.8 Other specified mycoses** HIV CC HCC
  Adiaspiromycosis
  Infection of tissue and organs by Alternaria
  Infection of tissue and organs by Drechslera
  Infection of tissue and organs by Fusarium
  Infection of tissue and organs by saprophytic fungi NEC
  AHA: 2014,4Q,46; 2014,2Q,13
  TIP: This code is assigned when the nonspecific term "non-*Candida albicans*" sepsis is documented. If sepsis is documented as due to any *Candida* type, code B37.7 Candidal sepsis, is assigned.

B49 Unspecified mycosis CC
Fungemia NOS

Protozoal diseases (B50-B64)

EXCLUDES 1 *amebiasis (A06.-)*
other protozoal intestinal diseases (A07.-)

B50 Plasmodium falciparum malaria ✓4th

INCLUDES mixed infections of Plasmodium falciparum with any other Plasmodium species

- **B50.0 Plasmodium falciparum malaria with cerebral complications** CC
  Cerebral malaria NOS
- **B50.8 Other severe and complicated Plasmodium falciparum malaria** CC
  Severe or complicated Plasmodium falciparum malaria NOS
- **B50.9 Plasmodium falciparum malaria, unspecified** MCC

B51 Plasmodium vivax malaria ✓4th

INCLUDES mixed infections of Plasmodium vivax with other Plasmodium species, except Plasmodium falciparum

EXCLUDES 1 *Plasmodium vivax with Plasmodium falciparum (B50.-)*

- **B51.0 Plasmodium vivax malaria with rupture of spleen** CC
- **B51.8 Plasmodium vivax malaria with other complications** CC
- **B51.9 Plasmodium vivax malaria without complication** CC
  Plasmodium vivax malaria NOS

B52 Plasmodium malariae malaria ✓4th

INCLUDES mixed infections of Plasmodium malariae with other Plasmodium species, except Plasmodium falciparum and Plasmodium vivax

EXCLUDES 1 *Plasmodium falciparum (B50.-)*
Plasmodium vivax (B51.-)

- **B52.0 Plasmodium malariae malaria with nephropathy** CC
- **B52.8 Plasmodium malariae malaria with other complications** CC
- **B52.9 Plasmodium malariae malaria without complication** CC
  Plasmodium malariae malaria NOS

Chapter 1. Certain Infectious and Parasitic Diseases

B40–B52.9

✓4th **B53 Other specified malaria**

B53.Ø Plasmodium ovale malaria CC

EXCLUDES 1 *Plasmodium ovale with Plasmodium falciparum (B5Ø.-)*
Plasmodium ovale with Plasmodium malariae (B52.-)
Plasmodium ovale with Plasmodium vivax (B51.-)

B53.1 Malaria due to simian plasmodia CC

EXCLUDES 1 *malaria due to simian plasmodia with Plasmodium falciparum (B5Ø.-)*
malaria due to simian plasmodia with Plasmodium malariae (B52.-)
malaria due to simian plasmodia with Plasmodium ovale (B53.Ø)
malaria due to simian plasmodia with Plasmodium vivax (B51.-)

B53.8 Other malaria, not elsewhere classified CC

B54 Unspecified malaria CC

✓4th **B55 Leishmaniasis**

B55.Ø Visceral leishmaniasis CC
Kala-azar
Post-kala-azar dermal leishmaniasis

B55.1 Cutaneous leishmaniasis CC

B55.2 Mucocutaneous leishmaniasis CC

B55.9 Leishmaniasis, unspecified CC

✓4th **B56 African trypanosomiasis**

B56.Ø Gambiense trypanosomiasis CC
Infection due to Trypanosoma brucei gambiense
West African sleeping sickness

B56.1 Rhodesiense trypanosomiasis CC
East African sleeping sickness
Infection due to Trypanosoma brucei rhodesiense

B56.9 African trypanosomiasis, unspecified CC
Sleeping sickness NOS

✓4th **B57 Chagas' disease**

INCLUDES American trypanosomiasis
infection due to Trypanosoma cruzi

B57.Ø Acute Chagas' disease with heart involvement CC
Acute Chagas' disease with myocarditis

B57.1 Acute Chagas' disease without heart involvement CC
Acute Chagas' disease NOS

B57.2 Chagas' disease (chronic) with heart involvement CC
American trypanosomiasis NOS
Chagas' disease (chronic) NOS
Chagas' disease (chronic) with myocarditis
Trypanosomiasis NOS

✓5th **B57.3 Chagas' disease (chronic) with digestive system involvement**

B57.3Ø Chagas' disease with digestive system involvement, unspecified CC

B57.31 Megaesophagus in Chagas' disease CC

B57.32 Megacolon in Chagas' disease CC

B57.39 Other digestive system involvement in Chagas' disease CC

✓5th **B57.4 Chagas' disease (chronic) with nervous system involvement**

B57.4Ø Chagas' disease with nervous system involvement, unspecified CC

B57.41 Meningitis in Chagas' disease CC

B57.42 Meningoencephalitis in Chagas' disease CC

B57.49 Other nervous system involvement in Chagas' disease CC

B57.5 Chagas' disease (chronic) with other organ involvement CC

✓4th **B58 Toxoplasmosis**

INCLUDES infection due to Toxoplasma gondii

EXCLUDES 1 *congenital toxoplasmosis (P37.1)*

✓5th **B58.Ø Toxoplasma oculopathy**

B58.ØØ Toxoplasma oculopathy, unspecified HIV CC

B58.Ø1 Toxoplasma chorioretinitis HIV CC

B58.Ø9 Other toxoplasma oculopathy HIV CC
Toxoplasma uveitis

B58.1 Toxoplasma hepatitis HIV CC

B58.2 Toxoplasma meningoencephalitis HIV MCC HCC

B58.3 Pulmonary toxoplasmosis HIV MCC HCC

✓5th **B58.8 Toxoplasmosis with other organ involvement**

B58.81 Toxoplasma myocarditis HIV MCC

B58.82 Toxoplasma myositis HIV CC

B58.83 Toxoplasma tubulo-interstitial nephropathy HIV CC
Toxoplasma pyelonephritis

B58.89 Toxoplasmosis with other organ involvement HIV CC

B58.9 Toxoplasmosis, unspecified HIV CC

B59 Pneumocystosis HIV MCC HCC
Pneumonia due to Pneumocystis carinii
Pneumonia due to Pneumocystis jiroveci

✓4th **B6Ø Other protozoal diseases, not elsewhere classified**

EXCLUDES 1 *cryptosporidiosis (AØ7.2)*
intestinal microsporidiosis (AØ7.8)
isosporiasis (AØ7.3)

✓5th **B6Ø.Ø Babesiosis**

AHA: 2020,4Q,5-6

B6Ø.ØØ Babesiosis, unspecified CC
Babesiosis due to unspecified Babesia species
Piroplasmosis, unspecified

B6Ø.Ø1 Babesiosis due to Babesia microti CC
Infection due to B. microti

B6Ø.Ø2 Babesiosis due to Babesia duncani CC
Infection due to B. duncani and B. duncani-type species

B6Ø.Ø3 Babesiosis due to Babesia divergens CC
Babesiosis due to Babesia MO-1
Infection due to B. divergens and B. divergens-like strains

B6Ø.Ø9 Other babesiosis CC
Babesiosis due to Babesia KO-1
Babesiosis due to Babesia venatorum
Infection due to other Babesia species
Infection due to other protozoa of the order Piroplasmida
Other piroplasmosis

✓5th **B6Ø.1 Acanthamebiasis**

B6Ø.1Ø Acanthamebiasis, unspecified CC

B6Ø.11 Meningoencephalitis due to Acanthamoeba (culbertsoni)

B6Ø.12 Conjunctivitis due to Acanthamoeba

B6Ø.13 Keratoconjunctivitis due to Acanthamoeba

B6Ø.19 Other acanthamebic disease CC

B6Ø.2 Naegleriasis CC
Primary amebic meningoencephalitis

B6Ø.8 Other specified protozoal diseases HIV
Microsporidiosis

B64 Unspecified protozoal disease

Helminthiases (B65-B83)

✓4th **B65 Schistosomiasis [bilharziasis]**

INCLUDES snail fever

B65.Ø Schistosomiasis due to Schistosoma haematobium [urinary schistosomiasis] CC

B65.1 Schistosomiasis due to Schistosoma mansoni [intestinal schistosomiasis] CC

B65.2 Schistosomiasis due to Schistosoma japonicum CC
Asiatic schistosomiasis

B65.3 Cercarial dermatitis CC
Swimmer's itch

B65.8 Other schistosomiasis CC
Infection due to Schistosoma intercalatum
Infection due to Schistosoma mattheei
Infection due to Schistosoma mekongi

B65.9 Schistosomiasis, unspecified CC

✓4th **B66 Other fluke infections**

B66.Ø Opisthorchiasis CC
Infection due to cat liver fluke
Infection due to Opisthorchis (felineus)(viverrini)

B66.1 Clonorchiasis CC
Chinese liver fluke disease
Infection due to Clonorchis sinensis
Oriental liver fluke disease

B66.2 Dicroceliasis CC
Infection due to Dicrocoelium dendriticum
Lancet fluke infection

B66.3 Fascioliasis CC
Infection due to Fasciola gigantica
Infection due to Fasciola hepatica
Infection due to Fasciola indica
Sheep liver fluke disease

B66.4 Paragonimiasis CC HCC
Infection due to Paragonimus species
Lung fluke disease
Pulmonary distomiasis

B66.5 Fasciolopsiasis CC
Infection due to Fasciolopsis buski
Intestinal distomiasis

B66.8 Other specified fluke infections CC
Echinostomiasis
Heterophyiasis
Metagonimiasis
Nanophyetiasis
Watsoniasis

B66.9 Fluke infection, unspecified

✓4th B67 Echinococcosis
INCLUDES hydatidosis

B67.0 Echinococcus granulosus infection of liver CC
B67.1 Echinococcus granulosus infection of lung CC HCC
B67.2 Echinococcus granulosus infection of bone CC
✓5th B67.3 Echinococcus granulosus infection, other and multiple sites
B67.31 Echinococcus granulosus infection, thyroid gland CC
B67.32 Echinococcus granulosus infection, multiple sites CC
B67.39 Echinococcus granulosus infection, other sites CC
B67.4 Echinococcus granulosus infection, unspecified CC
Dog tapeworm (infection)
B67.5 Echinococcus multilocularis infection of liver CC
✓5th B67.6 Echinococcus multilocularis infection, other and multiple sites
B67.61 Echinococcus multilocularis infection, multiple sites CC
B67.69 Echinococcus multilocularis infection, other sites CC
B67.7 Echinococcus multilocularis infection, unspecified CC
B67.8 Echinococcosis, unspecified, of liver CC
✓5th B67.9 Echinococcosis, other and unspecified
B67.90 Echinococcosis, unspecified CC
Echinococcosis NOS
B67.99 Other echinococcosis CC

✓4th B68 Taeniasis
EXCLUDES 1 *cysticercosis (B69.-)*

B68.0 Taenia solium taeniasis CC
Pork tapeworm (infection)
B68.1 Taenia saginata taeniasis CC
Beef tapeworm (infection)
Infection due to adult tapeworm Taenia saginata
B68.9 Taeniasis, unspecified CC

✓4th B69 Cysticercosis
INCLUDES cysticerciasis infection due to larval form of Taenia solium

DEF: Condition that is developed when larvae or eggs of the tapeworm *Taenia solium* are ingested, most commonly in fecally contaminated water or undercooked pork.

B69.0 Cysticercosis of central nervous system CC
B69.1 Cysticercosis of eye CC
✓5th B69.8 Cysticercosis of other sites
B69.81 Myositis in cysticercosis CC
B69.89 Cysticercosis of other sites CC
B69.9 Cysticercosis, unspecified CC

✓4th B70 Diphyllobothriasis and sparganosis

B70.0 Diphyllobothriasis CC
Diphyllobothrium (adult) (latum) (pacificum) infection
Fish tapeworm (infection)
EXCLUDES 2 *larval diphyllobothriasis (B70.1)*

B70.1 Sparganosis CC
Infection due to Sparganum (mansoni) (proliferum)
Infection due to Spirometra larva
Larval diphyllobothriasis
Spirometrosis

✓4th B71 Other cestode infections

B71.0 Hymenolepiasis CC
Dwarf tapeworm infection
Rat tapeworm (infection)
B71.1 Dipylidiasis CC
B71.8 Other specified cestode infections CC
Coenurosis
B71.9 Cestode infection, unspecified
Tapeworm (infection) NOS

B72 Dracunculiasis CC
INCLUDES guinea worm infection
infection due to Dracunculus medinensis

✓4th B73 Onchocerciasis
INCLUDES onchocerca volvulus infection
onchocercosis
river blindness

✓5th B73.0 Onchocerciasis with eye disease
B73.00 Onchocerciasis with eye involvement, unspecified CC
B73.01 Onchocerciasis with endophthalmitis CC
B73.02 Onchocerciasis with glaucoma CC
B73.09 Onchocerciasis with other eye involvement CC
Infestation of eyelid due to onchocerciasis
B73.1 Onchocerciasis without eye disease CC

✓4th B74 Filariasis
EXCLUDES 2 *onchocerciasis (B73)*
tropical (pulmonary) eosinophilia NOS (J82.89)

B74.0 Filariasis due to Wuchereria bancrofti CC
Bancroftian elephantiasis
Bancroftian filariasis
B74.1 Filariasis due to Brugia malayi CC
B74.2 Filariasis due to Brugia timori CC
B74.3 Loiasis CC
Calabar swelling
Eyeworm disease of Africa
Loa loa infection
B74.4 Mansonelliasis CC
Infection due to Mansonella ozzardi
Infection due to Mansonella perstans
Infection due to Mansonella streptocerca
B74.8 Other filariases CC
Dirofilariasis
B74.9 Filariasis, unspecified CC

B75 Trichinellosis CC
INCLUDES infection due to Trichinella species
trichiniasis

DEF: Infection by *Trichinella spiralis,* the smallest of the parasitic nematodes, that is transmitted by eating undercooked pork or bear meat.
Synonym(s): *Trichinosis.*

✓4th B76 Hookworm diseases
INCLUDES uncinariasis

B76.0 Ancylostomiasis CC
Infection due to Ancylostoma species
B76.1 Necatoriasis CC
Infection due to Necator americanus
B76.8 Other hookworm diseases CC
B76.9 Hookworm disease, unspecified CC
Cutaneous larva migrans NOS

✓4th B77 Ascariasis
INCLUDES ascaridiasis
roundworm infection

B77.0 Ascariasis with intestinal complications CC
✓5th B77.8 Ascariasis with other complications
B77.81 Ascariasis pneumonia MCC
B77.89 Ascariasis with other complications CC
B77.9 Ascariasis, unspecified CC

B78 Strongyloidiasis

EXCLUDES 1 *trichostrongyliasis (B81.2)*

B78.0 Intestinal strongyloidiasis HIV CC

B78.1 Cutaneous strongyloidiasis

B78.7 Disseminated strongyloidiasis HIV CC

B78.9 Strongyloidiasis, unspecified HIV CC

B79 Trichuriasis CC

INCLUDES trichocephaliasis
whipworm (disease)(infection)

B80 Enterobiasis CC

INCLUDES oxyuriasis
pinworm infection
threadworm infection

B81 Other intestinal helminthiases, not elsewhere classified

EXCLUDES 1 *angiostrongyliasis due to:*
angiostrongylus cantonensis (B83.2)
parastrongylus cantonensis (B83.2)

B81.0 Anisakiasis CC

Infection due to Anisakis larva

B81.1 Intestinal capillariasis CC

Capillariasis NOS
Infection due to Capillaria philippinensis

EXCLUDES 2 *hepatic capillariasis (B83.8)*

B81.2 Trichostrongyliasis CC

B81.3 Intestinal angiostrongyliasis CC

Angiostrongyliasis due to:
Angiostrongylus costaricensis
Parastrongylus costaricensis

B81.4 Mixed intestinal helminthiases CC

Infection due to intestinal helminths classified to more than one of the categories B65.0-B81.3 and B81.8
Mixed helminthiasis NOS

B81.8 Other specified intestinal helminthiases CC

Infection due to Oesophagostomum species [esophagostomiasis]
Infection due to Ternidens diminutus [ternidensiasis]

B82 Unspecified intestinal parasitism

B82.0 Intestinal helminthiasis, unspecified CC

B82.9 Intestinal parasitism, unspecified

B83 Other helminthiases

EXCLUDES 1 *capillariasis NOS (B81.1)*

EXCLUDES 2 *intestinal capillariasis (B81.1)*

B83.0 Visceral larva migrans

Toxocariasis

B83.1 Gnathostomiasis

Wandering swelling

B83.2 Angiostrongyliasis due to Parastrongylus cantonensis

Eosinophilic meningoencephalitis due to Parastrongylus cantonensis

EXCLUDES 2 *intestinal angiostrongyliasis (B81.3)*

B83.3 Syngamiasis

Syngamosis

B83.4 Internal hirudiniasis

EXCLUDES 2 *external hirudiniasis (B88.3)*

B83.8 Other specified helminthiases

Acanthocephaliasis
Gongylonemiasis
Hepatic capillariasis
Metastrongyliasis
Thelaziasis

B83.9 Helminthiasis, unspecified

Worms NOS

EXCLUDES 1 *intestinal helminthiasis NOS (B82.0)*

Pediculosis, acariasis and other infestations (B85-B89)

B85 Pediculosis and phthiriasis

B85.0 Pediculosis due to Pediculus humanus capitis

Head-louse infestation

B85.1 Pediculosis due to Pediculus humanus corporis

Body-louse infestation

B85.2 Pediculosis, unspecified

B85.3 Phthiriasis

Infestation by crab-louse
Infestation by Phthirus pubis

B85.4 Mixed pediculosis and phthiriasis

Infestation classifiable to more than one of the categories B85.0-B85.3

B86 Scabies

Sarcoptic itch

DEF: Mite infestation that is caused by *Sarcoptes scabiei.* Scabies causes intense itching and sometimes secondary infection.

B87 Myiasis

INCLUDES infestation by larva of flies

B87.0 Cutaneous myiasis

Creeping myiasis

B87.1 Wound myiasis

Traumatic myiasis

B87.2 Ocular myiasis

B87.3 Nasopharyngeal myiasis

Laryngeal myiasis

B87.4 Aural myiasis

B87.8 Myiasis of other sites

B87.81 Genitourinary myiasis

B87.82 Intestinal myiasis

B87.89 Myiasis of other sites

B87.9 Myiasis, unspecified

B88 Other infestations

B88.0 Other acariasis

Acarine dermatitis
Dermatitis due to Demodex species
Dermatitis due to Dermanyssus gallinae
Dermatitis due to Liponyssoides sanguineus
Trombiculosis

EXCLUDES 2 *scabies (B86)*

B88.1 Tungiasis [sandflea infestation]

B88.2 Other arthropod infestations

Scarabiasis

B88.3 External hirudiniasis

Leech infestation NOS

EXCLUDES 2 *internal hirudiniasis (B83.4)*

B88.8 Other specified infestations

Ichthyoparasitism due to Vandellia cirrhosa
Linguatulosis
Porocephaliasis

B88.9 Infestation, unspecified

Infestation (skin) NOS
Infestation by mites NOS
Skin parasites NOS

B89 Unspecified parasitic disease

Sequelae of infectious and parasitic diseases (B90-B94)

NOTE Categories B90-B94 are to be used to indicate conditions in categories A00-B89 as the cause of sequelae, which are themselves classified elsewhere. The "sequelae" include conditions specified as such; they also include residuals of diseases classifiable to the above categories if there is evidence that the disease itself is no longer present. Codes from these categories are not to be used for chronic infections. Code chronic current infections to active infectious disease as appropriate.

Code first condition resulting from (sequela) the infectious or parasitic disease

B90 Sequelae of tuberculosis

B90.0 Sequelae of central nervous system tuberculosis

B90.1 Sequelae of genitourinary tuberculosis

B90.2 Sequelae of tuberculosis of bones and joints

B90.8 Sequelae of tuberculosis of other organs

EXCLUDES 2 *sequelae of respiratory tuberculosis (B90.9)*

B90.9 Sequelae of respiratory and unspecified tuberculosis

Sequelae of tuberculosis NOS

B91 Sequelae of poliomyelitis

EXCLUDES 1 *postpolio syndrome (G14)*

B92 Sequelae of leprosy

B94 Sequelae of other and unspecified infectious and parasitic diseases

B94.0 Sequelae of trachoma

B94.1 Sequelae of viral encephalitis

B94.2 Sequelae of viral hepatitis

B94.8 Sequelae of other specified infectious and parasitic diseases

AHA: 2021,1Q,25-30,31-49; 2020,3Q,10-14; 2017,4Q,109

N Newborn: 0 P Pediatric: 0-17 M Maternity: 9-64 A Adult: 15-124 UNS Unspecified Site MCC Major Complication/Comorbidity CC Complication/Comorbidity

B94.9 Sequelae of unspecified infectious and parasitic disease UPD
EXCLUDES 2 *post COVID-19 condition (UØ9.9)*

Bacterial and viral infectious agents (B95-B97)

NOTE These categories are provided for use as supplementary or additional codes to identify the infectious agent(s) in diseases classified elsewhere.

AHA: 2020,2Q,18; 2018,4Q,34; 2018,1Q,16

B95 Streptococcus, Staphylococcus, and Enterococcus as the cause of diseases classified elsewhere

B95.Ø Streptococcus, group A, as the cause of diseases classified elsewhere UPD

B95.1 Streptococcus, group B, as the cause of diseases classified elsewhere UPD
AHA: 2020,1Q,10; 2019,2Q,8-10

B95.2 Enterococcus as the cause of diseases classified elsewhere UPD

B95.3 Streptococcus pneumoniae as the cause of diseases classified elsewhere UPD

B95.4 Other streptococcus as the cause of diseases classified elsewhere UPD

B95.5 Unspecified streptococcus as the cause of diseases classified elsewhere UPD

B95.6 Staphylococcus aureus as the cause of diseases classified elsewhere

B95.61 Methicillin susceptible Staphylococcus aureus infection as the cause of diseases classified elsewhere UPD
Methicillin susceptible Staphylococcus aureus (MSSA) infection as the cause of diseases classified elsewhere
Staphylococcus aureus infection NOS as the cause of diseases classified elsewhere

B95.62 Methicillin resistant Staphylococcus aureus infection as the cause of diseases classified elsewhere UPD
Methicillin resistant staphylococcus aureus (MRSA) infection as the cause of diseases classified elsewhere
AHA: 2016,1Q,12

B95.7 Other staphylococcus as the cause of diseases classified elsewhere UPD

B95.8 Unspecified staphylococcus as the cause of diseases classified elsewhere UPD

B96 Other bacterial agents as the cause of diseases classified elsewhere

B96.Ø Mycoplasma pneumoniae [M. pneumoniae] as the cause of diseases classified elsewhere UPD
Pleuro-pneumonia-like-organism [PPLO]

B96.1 Klebsiella pneumoniae [K. pneumoniae] as the cause of diseases classified elsewhere UPD

B96.2 Escherichia coli [E. coli] as the cause of diseases classified elsewhere
AHA: 2022,1Q,31

B96.2Ø Unspecified Escherichia coli [E. coli] as the cause of diseases classified elsewhere UPD
Escherichia coli [E. coli] NOS

B96.21 Shiga toxin-producing Escherichia coli [E. coli] [STEC] O157 as the cause of diseases classified elsewhere UPD
E. coli O157:H- (nonmotile) with confirmation of Shiga toxin
E. coli O157 with confirmation of Shiga toxin when H antigen is unknown, or is not H7
O157:H7 Escherichia coli [E.coli] with or without confirmation of Shiga toxin-production
Shiga toxin-producing Escherichia coli [E.coli] O157:H7 with or without confirmation of Shiga toxin-production
STEC O157:H7 with or without confirmation of Shiga toxin-production

B96.22 Other specified Shiga toxin-producing Escherichia coli [E. coli] [STEC] as the cause of diseases classified elsewhere UPD
Non-O157 Shiga toxin-producing Escherichia coli [E.coli]
Non-O157 Shiga toxin-producing Escherichia coli [E.coli] with known O group

B96.23 Unspecified Shiga toxin-producing Escherichia coli [E. coli] [STEC] as the cause of diseases classified elsewhere UPD
Shiga toxin-producing Escherichia coli [E. coli] with unspecified O group
STEC NOS

B96.29 Other Escherichia coli [E. coli] as the cause of diseases classified elsewhere UPD
Non-Shiga toxin-producing E. coli

B96.3 Hemophilus influenzae [H. influenzae] as the cause of diseases classified elsewhere UPD

B96.4 Proteus (mirabilis) (morganii) as the cause of diseases classified elsewhere UPD

B96.5 Pseudomonas (aeruginosa) (mallei) (pseudomallei) as the cause of diseases classified elsewhere UPD
AHA: 2015,1Q,18

B96.6 Bacteroides fragilis [B. fragilis] as the cause of diseases classified elsewhere UPD

B96.7 Clostridium perfringens [C. perfringens] as the cause of diseases classified elsewhere UPD

B96.8 Other specified bacterial agents as the cause of diseases classified elsewhere

B96.81 Helicobacter pylori [H. pylori] as the cause of diseases classified elsewhere UPD

B96.82 Vibrio vulnificus as the cause of diseases classified elsewhere UPD

● **B96.83 Acinetobacter baumannii as the cause of diseases classified elsewhere**

B96.89 Other specified bacterial agents as the cause of diseases classified elsewhere UPD

B97 Viral agents as the cause of diseases classified elsewhere
AHA: 2016,3Q,8-10,14

B97.Ø Adenovirus as the cause of diseases classified elsewhere UPD

B97.1 Enterovirus as the cause of diseases classified elsewhere

B97.1Ø Unspecified enterovirus as the cause of diseases classified elsewhere UPD

B97.11 Coxsackievirus as the cause of diseases classified elsewhere UPD

B97.12 Echovirus as the cause of diseases classified elsewhere UPD

B97.19 Other enterovirus as the cause of diseases classified elsewhere UPD

B97.2 Coronavirus as the cause of diseases classified elsewhere
TIP: Do not report a code from this subcategory for COVID-19; refer to U07.1.

B97.21 SARS-associated coronavirus as the cause of diseases classified elsewhere CC UPD
EXCLUDES 1 *pneumonia due to SARS-associated coronavirus (J12.81)*

B97.29 Other coronavirus as the cause of diseases classified elsewhere UPD
AHA: 2020,2Q,5; 2020,1Q,34-36

B97.3 Retrovirus as the cause of diseases classified elsewhere
EXCLUDES 1 *human immunodeficiency virus [HIV] disease (B2Ø)*

B97.3Ø Unspecified retrovirus as the cause of diseases classified elsewhere UPD

B97.31 Lentivirus as the cause of diseases classified elsewhere UPD

B97.32 Oncovirus as the cause of diseases classified elsewhere UPD

B97.33 Human T-cell lymphotrophic virus, type I [HTLV-I] as the cause of diseases classified elsewhere CC UPD

B97.34 Human T-cell lymphotrophic virus, type II [HTLV-II] as the cause of diseases classified elsewhere CC UPD

B97.35 Human immunodeficiency virus, type 2 [HIV 2] as the cause of diseases classified elsewhere CC UPD HCC

B97.39 Other retrovirus as the cause of diseases classified elsewhere UPD

B97.4 Respiratory syncytial virus as the cause of diseases classified elsewhere UPD
RSV as the cause of diseases classified elsewhere
Code first related disorders, such as:
otitis media (H65.-)
upper respiratory infection (JØ6.9)
EXCLUDES 1 *acute bronchiolitis due to respiratory syncytial virus (RSV) (J21.Ø)*
acute bronchitis due to respiratory syncytial virus (RSV) (J2Ø.5)
respiratory syncytial virus (RSV) pneumonia (J12.1)

B97.5 Reovirus as the cause of diseases classified elsewhere UPD

B97.6 Parvovirus as the cause of diseases classified elsewhere UPD

B97.7 Papillomavirus as the cause of diseases classified elsewhere UPD

√5th **B97.8 Other viral agents as the cause of diseases classified elsewhere**

B97.81 Human metapneumovirus as the cause of diseases classified elsewhere UPD

B97.89 Other viral agents as the cause of diseases classified elsewhere UPD

Other infectious diseases (B99)

√4th **B99 Other and unspecified infectious diseases**

B99.8 Other infectious disease HIV

B99.9 Unspecified infectious disease

Chapter 2. Neoplasms (CØØ–D49)

Chapter-specific Guidelines with Coding Examples

The chapter-specific guidelines from the ICD-10-CM Official Guidelines for Coding and Reporting have been provided below. Along with these guidelines are coding examples, contained in the shaded boxes, that have been developed to help illustrate the coding and/or sequencing guidance found in these guidelines.

General guidelines

Chapter 2 of the ICD-10-CM contains the codes for most benign and all malignant neoplasms. Certain benign neoplasms, such as prostatic adenomas, may be found in the specific body system chapters. To properly code a neoplasm, it is necessary to determine from the record if the neoplasm is benign, in-situ, malignant, or of uncertain histologic behavior. If malignant, any secondary (metastatic) sites should also be determined.

Primary malignant neoplasms overlapping site boundaries

A primary malignant neoplasm that overlaps two or more contiguous (next to each other) sites should be classified to the subcategory/code .8 ('overlapping lesion'), unless the combination is specifically indexed elsewhere. For multiple neoplasms of the same site that are not contiguous such as tumors in different quadrants of the same breast, codes for each site should be assigned.

A 73-year-old white female with a large rapidly growing malignant tumor in the left breast extending from the upper outer quadrant into the axillary tail

C5Ø.812	**Malignant neoplasm of overlapping sites of left female breast**

Explanation: Because this is a single large tumor that overlaps two contiguous sites, a single code for overlapping sites is assigned.

A 52-year old white female with two distinct lesions of the right breast, one (Ø.5 cm) in the upper outer quadrant and a second (1.5 cm) in the lower outer quadrant; path report indicates both lesions are malignant

C5Ø.411	**Malignant neoplasm of upper-outer quadrant of right female breast**
C5Ø.511	**Malignant neoplasm of lower-outer quadrant of right female breast**

Explanation: This patient has two distinct malignant lesions of right breast in adjacent quadrants. Because the lesions are not contiguous, two codes are reported.

Malignant neoplasm of ectopic tissue

Malignant neoplasms of ectopic tissue are to be coded to the site of origin mentioned, e.g., ectopic pancreatic malignant neoplasms involving the stomach are coded to malignant neoplasm of pancreas, unspecified (C25.9).

The neoplasm table in the Alphabetic Index should be referenced first. However, if the histological term is documented, that term should be referenced first, rather than going immediately to the Neoplasm Table, in order to determine which column in the Neoplasm Table is appropriate. For example, if the documentation indicates "adenoma," refer to the term in the Alphabetic Index to review the entries under this term and the instructional note to "see also neoplasm, by site, benign." The table provides the proper code based on the type of neoplasm and the site. It is important to select the proper column in the table that corresponds to the type of neoplasm. The Tabular List should then be referenced to verify that the correct code has been selected from the table and that a more specific site code does not exist.

See Section I.C.21. Factors influencing health status and contact with health services, Status, for information regarding Z15.Ø, codes for genetic susceptibility to cancer.

a. Admission/Encounter for treatment of primary site

If the malignancy is chiefly responsible for occasioning the patient admission/encounter and treatment is directed at the primary site, designate the primary malignancy as the principal/first-listed diagnosis.

The only exception to this guideline is if the administration of chemotherapy, immunotherapy or external beam radiation therapy is chiefly responsible for occasioning the admission/encounter. In that case, assign the appropriate Z51.-- code as the first-listed or principal diagnosis, and the underlying diagnosis or problem for which the service is being performed as a secondary diagnosis.

b. Admission/Encounter for treatment of secondary site

When a patient is admitted because of a primary neoplasm with metastasis and treatment is directed toward the secondary site only, the secondary neoplasm is designated as the principal diagnosis even though the primary malignancy is still present.

Patient with primary prostate cancer with metastasis to lungs admitted for wedge resection of mass in right lung

C78.Ø1	**Secondary malignant neoplasm of right lung**
C61	**Malignant neoplasm of prostate**

Explanation: Since the admission is for treatment of the lung metastasis, the secondary lung metastasis is sequenced before the primary prostate cancer.

c. Coding and sequencing of complications

Coding and sequencing of complications associated with the malignancies or with the therapy thereof are subject to the following guidelines:

1) Anemia associated with malignancy

When admission/encounter is for management of an anemia associated with the malignancy, and the treatment is only for anemia, the appropriate code for the malignancy is sequenced as the principal or first-listed diagnosis followed by the appropriate code for the anemia (such as code D63.Ø, Anemia in neoplastic disease).

Patient is admitted for treatment of anemia in advanced colon cancer

C18.9	**Malignant neoplasm of colon, unspecified**
D63.Ø	**Anemia in neoplastic disease**

Explanation: Even though the admission was solely to treat the anemia, this guideline indicates that the code for the malignancy is sequenced first.

2) Anemia associated with chemotherapy, immunotherapy and radiation therapy

When the admission/encounter is for management of an anemia associated with an adverse effect of the administration of chemotherapy or immunotherapy and the only treatment is for the anemia, the anemia code is sequenced first followed by the appropriate codes for the neoplasm and the adverse effect (T45.1X5, Adverse effect of antineoplastic and immunosuppressive drugs).

A 56-year-old Hispanic male with grade II follicular lymphoma involving multiple lymph node sites referred for blood transfusion to treat anemia due to chemotherapy

D64.81	**Anemia due to antineoplastic chemotherapy**
C82.18	**Follicular lymphoma grade II, lymph nodes of multiple sites**
T45.1X5A	**Adverse effect of antineoplastic and immunosuppressive drugs, initial encounter**

Explanation: The code for the anemia is sequenced first followed by the code for the malignant neoplasm and lastly the code for the adverse effect.

When the admission/encounter is for management of an anemia associated with an adverse effect of radiotherapy, the anemia code should be sequenced first, followed by the appropriate neoplasm code and code Y84.2, Radiological procedure and radiotherapy as the cause of abnormal reaction of the patient, or of later complication, without mention of misadventure at the time of the procedure.

A 55-year-old male with a large malignant rectal tumor has been receiving external radiation therapy to shrink the tumor prior to planned surgery. He is admitted today for a blood transfusion to treat anemia related to radiation therapy.

D64.89	**Other specified anemias**
C2Ø	**Malignant neoplasm of rectum**
Y84.2	**Radiological procedure and radiotherapy as the cause of abnormal reaction of the patient, or of later complication, without mention of misadventure at the time of the procedure**

Explanation: The code for the anemia is sequenced first, followed by the code for the malignancy, and lastly the code for the abnormal reaction due to radiotherapy.

3) Management of dehydration due to the malignancy

When the admission/encounter is for management of dehydration due to the malignancy and only the dehydration is being treated (intravenous rehydration), the dehydration is sequenced first, followed by the code(s) for the malignancy.

4) Treatment of a complication resulting from a surgical procedure

When the admission/encounter is for treatment of a complication resulting from a surgical procedure, designate the complication as the principal or first-listed diagnosis if treatment is directed at resolving the complication.

d. Primary malignancy previously excised

When a primary malignancy has been previously excised or eradicated from its site and there is no further treatment directed to that site and there is no evidence of any existing primary malignancy at that site, a code from category Z85, Personal history of malignant neoplasm, should be used to indicate the former site of the malignancy. Any mention of extension, invasion, or metastasis to another site is coded as a secondary malignant neoplasm to that site. The secondary site may be the principal or first-listed diagnosis with the Z85 code used as a secondary code.

See section I.C.2.t. Secondary malignant neoplasm of lymphoid tissue.

History of breast cancer, left radical mastectomy 18 months ago with no current treatment; bronchoscopy with lung biopsy shows metastatic disease in the right lung

C78.Ø1	**Secondary malignant neoplasm of right lung**
Z85.3	**Personal history of malignant neoplasm of breast**

Explanation: The patient has undergone a diagnostic procedure that revealed metastatic breast cancer in the right lung. The code for the secondary (metastatic) site is sequenced first followed by a personal history code to identify the former site of the primary malignancy.

e. Admissions/encounters involving chemotherapy, immunotherapy and radiation therapy

1) Episode of care involves surgical removal of neoplasm

When an episode of care involves the surgical removal of a neoplasm, primary or secondary site, followed by adjunct chemotherapy or radiation treatment during the same episode of care, the code for the neoplasm should be assigned as principal or first-listed diagnosis.

2) Patient admission/encounter chiefly for administration of chemotherapy, immunotherapy and radiation therapy

If a patient admission/encounter is **chiefly** for the administration of chemotherapy, immunotherapy or external beam radiation therapy assign code Z51.Ø, Encounter for antineoplastic radiation therapy, or Z51.11, Encounter for antineoplastic chemotherapy, or Z51.12, Encounter for antineoplastic immunotherapy as the first-listed or principal diagnosis. If a patient receives more than one of these therapies during the same admission, more than one of these codes may be assigned, in any sequence.

The malignancy for which the therapy is being administered should be assigned as a secondary diagnosis.

If a patient admission/encounter is for the insertion or implantation of radioactive elements (e.g., brachytherapy) the appropriate code for the malignancy is sequenced as the principal or first-listed diagnosis. Code Z51.Ø should not be assigned.

3) Patient admitted for radiation therapy, chemotherapy or immunotherapy and develops complications

When a patient is admitted for the purpose of external beam radiotherapy, immunotherapy or chemotherapy and develops complications such as uncontrolled nausea and vomiting or dehydration, the principal or first-listed diagnosis is Z51.Ø, Encounter for antineoplastic radiation therapy, or Z51.11, Encounter for antineoplastic chemotherapy, or Z51.12, Encounter for antineoplastic immunotherapy followed by any codes for the complications.

When a patient is admitted for the purpose of insertion or implantation of radioactive elements (e.g., brachytherapy) and develops complications such as uncontrolled nausea and vomiting or dehydration, the principal or first-listed diagnosis is the appropriate code for the malignancy followed by any codes for the complications.

A patient with prostate cancer was admitted for brachytherapy seed implantation and consequently developed urinary retention.

C61	**Malignant neoplasm of prostate**
R33.9	**Retention of urine, unspecified**

Explanation: A code for the malignancy should be listed as the principal diagnosis when insertion of a radioactive element is the reason for admission, even when a complication related to that radioactive element occurs. Codes describing the complications should be listed as secondary codes.

f. Admission/encounter to determine extent of malignancy

When the reason for admission/encounter is to determine the extent of the malignancy, or for a procedure such as paracentesis or thoracentesis, the primary malignancy or appropriate metastatic site is designated as the principal or first-listed diagnosis, even though chemotherapy or radiotherapy is administered.

Patient with left lung cancer with malignant pleural effusion admitted for paracentesis and initiation/administration of chemotherapy

C34.92	**Malignant neoplasm of unspecified part of left bronchus or lung**
J91.Ø	**Malignant pleural effusion**
Z51.11	**Encounter for antineoplastic chemotherapy**

Explanation: The lung cancer is sequenced before the chemotherapy in this instance because the paracentesis for the malignant effusion is also being performed. An instructional note under the malignant effusion instructs that the lung cancer be sequenced first.

g. Symptoms, signs, and abnormal findings listed in Chapter 18 associated with neoplasms

Symptoms, signs, and ill-defined conditions listed in Chapter 18 characteristic of, or associated with, an existing primary or secondary site malignancy cannot be used to replace the malignancy as principal or first-listed diagnosis, regardless of the number of admissions or encounters for treatment and care of the neoplasm.

See Section I.C.21. Factors influencing health status and contact with health services, Encounter for prophylactic organ removal.

h. Admission/encounter for pain control/management

See Section I.C.6. for information on coding admission/encounter for pain control/management.

i. Malignancy in two or more noncontiguous sites

A patient may have more than one malignant tumor in the same organ. These tumors may represent different primaries or metastatic disease, depending on the site. Should the documentation be unclear, the provider should be queried as to the status of each tumor so that the correct codes can be assigned.

j. Disseminated malignant neoplasm, unspecified

Code C8Ø.Ø, Disseminated malignant neoplasm, unspecified, is for use only in those cases where the patient has advanced metastatic disease and no known primary or secondary sites are specified. It should not be used in place of assigning codes for the primary site and all known secondary sites.

Patient who has had no medical care for many years is seen today and diagnosed with carcinomatosis

C8Ø.Ø	**Disseminated malignant neoplasm, unspecified**

Explanation: Carcinomatosis NOS is an "includes" note under this code. Should seldom be used but is available for use in cases such as this.

k. Malignant neoplasm without specification of site

Code C8Ø.1, Malignant (primary) neoplasm, unspecified, equates to Cancer, unspecified. This code should only be used when no determination can be made as to the primary site of a malignancy. This code should rarely be used in the inpatient setting.

l. Sequencing of neoplasm codes

1) Encounter for treatment of primary malignancy

If the reason for the encounter is for treatment of a primary malignancy, assign the malignancy as the principal/first-listed diagnosis. The primary site is to be sequenced first, followed by any metastatic sites.

2) Encounter for treatment of secondary malignancy

When an encounter is for a primary malignancy with metastasis and treatment is directed toward the metastatic (secondary) site(s) only, the metastatic site(s) is designated as the principal/first-listed diagnosis. The primary malignancy is coded as an additional code.

Patient has primary colon cancer with metastasis to rib and is evaluated for possible excision of portion of rib bone

C79.51 Secondary malignant neoplasm of bone

C18.9 Malignant neoplasm of colon, unspecified

Explanation: The treatment for this encounter is focused on the metastasis to the rib bone rather than the primary colon cancer, thus indicating that the bone metastasis is sequenced as the first-listed code.

3) Malignant neoplasm in a pregnant patient

When a pregnant patient has a malignant neoplasm, a code from subcategory O9A.1-, Malignant neoplasm complicating pregnancy, childbirth, and the puerperium, should be sequenced first, followed by the appropriate code from Chapter 2 to indicate the type of neoplasm.

A 30-year-old pregnant female in second trimester evaluated for thyroid malignancy

O9A.112 Malignant neoplasm complicating pregnancy, second trimester

C73 Malignant neoplasm of thyroid gland

Explanation: Codes from chapter 15 describing complications of pregnancy are sequenced as first-listed codes, further specified by codes from other chapters such as neoplastic, unless the pregnancy is documented as incidental to the condition. See also guideline 1.C.15.a.1.

4) Encounter for complication associated with a neoplasm

When an encounter is for management of a complication associated with a neoplasm, such as dehydration, and the treatment is only for the complication, the complication is coded first, followed by the appropriate code(s) for the neoplasm.

The exception to this guideline is anemia. When the admission/encounter is for management of an anemia associated with the malignancy, and the treatment is only for anemia, the appropriate code for the malignancy is sequenced as the principal or first-listed diagnosis followed by code D63.Ø, Anemia in neoplastic disease.

Patient with pancreatic cancer is seen for initiation of TPN for cancer-related moderate protein-calorie malnutrition

E44.Ø Moderate protein-calorie malnutrition

C25.9 Malignant neoplasm of pancreas, unspecified

Explanation: The encounter is to initiate treatment for malnutrition, a common complication of many types of neoplasms, and is sequenced first.

5) Complication from surgical procedure for treatment of a neoplasm

When an encounter is for treatment of a complication resulting from a surgical procedure performed for the treatment of the neoplasm, designate the complication as the principal/first-listed diagnosis. See the guideline regarding the coding of a current malignancy versus personal history to determine if the code for the neoplasm should also be assigned.

6) Pathologic fracture due to a neoplasm

When an encounter is for a pathological fracture due to a neoplasm, and the focus of treatment is the fracture, a code from subcategory M84.5, Pathological fracture in neoplastic disease, should be sequenced first, followed by the code for the neoplasm.

If the focus of treatment is the neoplasm with an associated pathological fracture, the neoplasm code should be sequenced first, followed by a code from M84.5 for the pathological fracture.

m. Current malignancy versus personal history of malignancy

When a primary malignancy has been excised but further treatment, such as an additional surgery for the malignancy, radiation therapy or chemotherapy is directed to that site, the primary malignancy code should be used until treatment is completed.

Female patient with ongoing chemotherapy after right mastectomy for breast cancer

C5Ø.911 Malignant neoplasm of unspecified site of right female breast

Z9Ø.11 Acquired absence of right breast and nipple

Explanation: Even though the breast has been removed, the breast cancer is still being treated with chemotherapy and therefore is still coded as a current condition rather than personal history.

When a primary malignancy has been previously excised or eradicated from its site, there is no further treatment (of the malignancy) directed to that site, and there is no evidence of any existing primary malignancy at that site, a code from category Z85, Personal history of malignant neoplasm, should be used to indicate the former site of the malignancy.

Codes from subcategories Z85.Ø – Z85.85 should only be assigned for the former site of a primary malignancy, not the site of a secondary malignancy. Code Z85.89 may be assigned for the former site(s) of either a primary or secondary malignancy.

See Section I.C.21. Factors influencing health status and contact with health services, History (of)

n. Leukemia, multiple myeloma, and malignant plasma cell neoplasms in remission versus personal history

The categories for leukemia, and category C9Ø, Multiple myeloma and malignant plasma cell neoplasms, have codes indicating whether or not the leukemia has achieved remission. There are also codes Z85.6, Personal history of leukemia, and Z85.79, Personal history of other malignant neoplasms of lymphoid, hematopoietic and related tissues. If the documentation is unclear as to whether the leukemia has achieved remission, the provider should be queried.

See Section I.C.21. Factors influencing health status and contact with health services, History (of)

o. Aftercare following surgery for neoplasm

See Section I.C.21. Factors influencing health status and contact with health services, Aftercare

p. Follow-up care for completed treatment of a malignancy

See Section I.C.21. Factors influencing health status and contact with health services, Follow-up

q. Prophylactic organ removal for prevention of malignancy

See Section I.C. 21, Factors influencing health status and contact with health services, Prophylactic organ removal

r. Malignant neoplasm associated with transplanted organ

A malignant neoplasm of a transplanted organ should be coded as a transplant complication. Assign first the appropriate code from category T86.-, Complications of transplanted organs and tissue, followed by code C8Ø.2, Malignant neoplasm associated with transplanted organ. Use an additional code for the specific malignancy.

s. Breast implant associated anaplastic large cell lymphoma

Breast implant associated anaplastic large cell lymphoma (BIA-ALCL) is a type of lymphoma that can develop around breast implants. Assign code C84.7A, Anaplastic large cell lymphoma, ALK-negative, breast, for BIA-ALCL. Do not assign a complication code from chapter 19.

t. Secondary malignant neoplasm of lymphoid tissue

When a malignant neoplasm of lymphoid tissue metastasizes beyond the lymph nodes, a code from categories C81–C85 with a final character "9" should be assigned identifying "extranodal and solid organ sites" rather than a code for the secondary neoplasm of the affected solid organ. For example, for metastasis of **diffuse large** B-cell lymphoma to the lung, brain and left adrenal gland, assign code C83.39, Diffuse large B-cell lymphoma, extranodal and solid organ sites.

Chapter 2. Neoplasms (C00-D49)

NOTE

Functional activity
All neoplasms are classified in this chapter, whether they are functionally active or not. An additional code from Chapter 4 may be used, to identify functional activity associated with any neoplasm.

Morphology [Histology]
Chapter 2 classifies neoplasms primarily by site (topography), with broad groupings for behavior, malignant, in situ, benign, etc. The Table of Neoplasms should be used to identify the correct topography code. In a few cases, such as for malignant melanoma and certain neuroendocrine tumors, the morphology (histologic type) is included in the category and codes.

Primary malignant neoplasms overlapping site boundaries
A primary malignant neoplasm that overlaps two or more contiguous (next to each other) sites should be classified to the subcategory/code .8 ("overlapping lesion"), unless the combination is specifically indexed elsewhere. For multiple neoplasms of the same site that are not contiguous, such as tumors in different quadrants of the same breast, codes for each site should be assigned.

Malignant neoplasm of ectopic tissue
Malignant neoplasms of ectopic tissue are to be coded to the site mentioned, e.g., ectopic pancreatic malignant neoplasms are coded to pancreas, unspecified (C25.9).

AHA: 2023,2Q,6; 2017,4Q,103; 2017,1Q,4,5-6,8

This chapter contains the following blocks:

- C00-C14 Malignant neoplasms of lip, oral cavity and pharynx
- C15-C26 Malignant neoplasms of digestive organs
- C30-C39 Malignant neoplasms of respiratory and intrathoracic organs
- C40-C41 Malignant neoplasms of bone and articular cartilage
- C43-C44 Melanoma and other malignant neoplasms of skin
- C45-C49 Malignant neoplasms of mesothelial and soft tissue
- C50 Malignant neoplasms of breast
- C51-C58 Malignant neoplasms of female genital organs
- C60-C63 Malignant neoplasms of male genital organs
- C64-C68 Malignant neoplasms of urinary tract
- C69-C72 Malignant neoplasms of eye, brain and other parts of central nervous system
- C73-C75 Malignant neoplasms of thyroid and other endocrine glands
- C7A Malignant neuroendocrine tumors
- C7B Secondary neuroendocrine tumors
- C76-C80 Malignant neoplasms of ill-defined, other secondary and unspecified sites
- C81-C96 Malignant neoplasms of lymphoid, hematopoietic and related tissue
- D00-D09 In situ neoplasms
- D10-D36 Benign neoplasms, except benign neuroendocrine tumors
- D3A Benign neuroendocrine tumors
- D37-D48 Neoplasms of uncertain behavior, polycythemia vera and myelodysplastic syndromes
- D49 Neoplasms of unspecified behavior

MALIGNANT NEOPLASMS (C00-C96)

Malignant neoplasms, stated or presumed to be primary (of specified sites), and certain specified histologies, except neuroendocrine, and of lymphoid, hematopoietic and related tissue (C00-C75)

AHA: 2022,1Q,16

Malignant neoplasms of lip, oral cavity and pharynx (C00-C14)

4th C00 Malignant neoplasm of lip
Use additional code to identify:
alcohol abuse and dependence (F10.-)
history of tobacco dependence (Z87.891)
tobacco dependence (F17.-)
tobacco use (Z72.0)

EXCLUDES 1 *malignant melanoma of lip (C43.0)*
Merkel cell carcinoma of lip (C4A.0)
other and unspecified malignant neoplasm of skin of lip (C44.0-)

C00.0 Malignant neoplasm of external upper lip
Malignant neoplasm of lipstick area of upper lip
Malignant neoplasm of upper lip NOS
Malignant neoplasm of vermilion border of upper lip

C00.1 Malignant neoplasm of external lower lip
Malignant neoplasm of lower lip NOS
Malignant neoplasm of lipstick area of lower lip
Malignant neoplasm of vermilion border of lower lip

C00.2 Malignant neoplasm of external lip, unspecified
Malignant neoplasm of vermilion border of lip NOS

C00.3 Malignant neoplasm of upper lip, inner aspect
Malignant neoplasm of buccal aspect of upper lip
Malignant neoplasm of frenulum of upper lip
Malignant neoplasm of mucosa of upper lip
Malignant neoplasm of oral aspect of upper lip

C00.4 Malignant neoplasm of lower lip, inner aspect
Malignant neoplasm of buccal aspect of lower lip
Malignant neoplasm of frenulum of lower lip
Malignant neoplasm of mucosa of lower lip
Malignant neoplasm of oral aspect of lower lip

C00.5 Malignant neoplasm of lip, unspecified, inner aspect
Malignant neoplasm of buccal aspect of lip, unspecified
Malignant neoplasm of frenulum of lip, unspecified
Malignant neoplasm of mucosa of lip, unspecified
Malignant neoplasm of oral aspect of lip, unspecified

C00.6 Malignant neoplasm of commissure of lip, unspecified

C00.8 Malignant neoplasm of overlapping sites of lip

C00.9 Malignant neoplasm of lip, unspecified

C01 Malignant neoplasm of base of tongue HCC
Malignant neoplasm of dorsal surface of base of tongue
Malignant neoplasm of fixed part of tongue NOS
Malignant neoplasm of posterior third of tongue
Use additional code to identify:
alcohol abuse and dependence (F10.-)
history of tobacco dependence (Z87.891)
tobacco dependence (F17.-)
tobacco use (Z72.0)

Malignant Neoplasm of Tongue

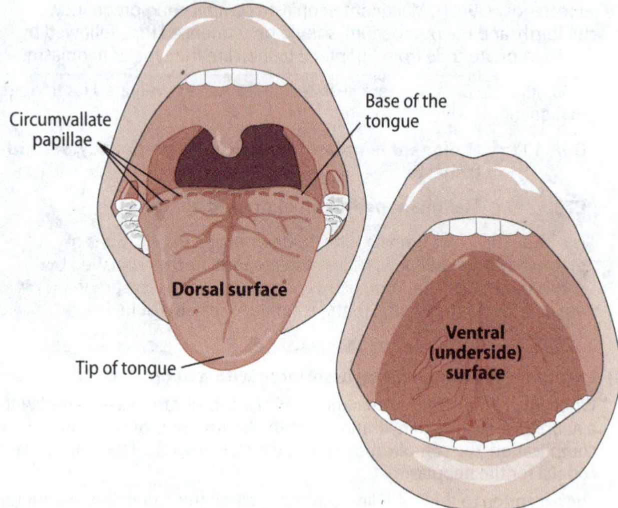

4th C02 Malignant neoplasm of other and unspecified parts of tongue
Use additional code to identify:
alcohol abuse and dependence (F10.-)
history of tobacco dependence (Z87.891)
tobacco dependence (F17.-)
tobacco use (Z72.0)

C02.0 Malignant neoplasm of dorsal surface of tongue HCC
Malignant neoplasm of anterior two-thirds of tongue, dorsal surface
EXCLUDES 2 *malignant neoplasm of dorsal surface of base of tongue (C01)*

C02.1 Malignant neoplasm of border of tongue HCC
Malignant neoplasm of tip of tongue

C02.2 Malignant neoplasm of ventral surface of tongue HCC
Malignant neoplasm of anterior two-thirds of tongue, ventral surface
Malignant neoplasm of frenulum linguae

C02.3 Malignant neoplasm of anterior two-thirds of tongue, part unspecified HCC
Malignant neoplasm of middle third of tongue NOS
Malignant neoplasm of mobile part of tongue NOS

C02.4 Malignant neoplasm of lingual tonsil HCC
EXCLUDES 2 *malignant neoplasm of tonsil NOS (C09.9)*

C02.8 Malignant neoplasm of overlapping sites of tongue HCC
Malignant neoplasm of two or more contiguous sites of tongue

C02.9 Malignant neoplasm of tongue, unspecified HCC

C03 Malignant neoplasm of gum

INCLUDES malignant neoplasm of alveolar (ridge) mucosa
malignant neoplasm of gingiva

Use additional code to identify:
alcohol abuse and dependence (F10.-)
history of tobacco dependence (Z87.891)
tobacco dependence (F17.-)
tobacco use (Z72.0)

EXCLUDES 2 *malignant odontogenic neoplasms (C41.0-C41.1)*

C03.0 Malignant neoplasm of upper gum HCC
C03.1 Malignant neoplasm of lower gum HCC
C03.9 Malignant neoplasm of gum, unspecified HCC

C04 Malignant neoplasm of floor of mouth

Use additional code to identify:
alcohol abuse and dependence (F10.-)
history of tobacco dependence (Z87.891)
tobacco dependence (F17.-)
tobacco use (Z72.0)

C04.0 Malignant neoplasm of anterior floor of mouth HCC
Malignant neoplasm of anterior to the premolar-canine junction
C04.1 Malignant neoplasm of lateral floor of mouth HCC
C04.8 Malignant neoplasm of overlapping sites of floor of mouth HCC
C04.9 Malignant neoplasm of floor of mouth, unspecified HCC

C05 Malignant neoplasm of palate

Use additional code to identify:
alcohol abuse and dependence (F10.-)
history of tobacco dependence (Z87.891)
tobacco dependence (F17.-)
tobacco use (Z72.0)

EXCLUDES 1 *Kaposi's sarcoma of palate (C46.2)*

C05.0 Malignant neoplasm of hard palate HCC
C05.1 Malignant neoplasm of soft palate HCC
EXCLUDES 2 *malignant neoplasm of nasopharyngeal surface of soft palate (C11.3)*
C05.2 Malignant neoplasm of uvula HCC
C05.8 Malignant neoplasm of overlapping sites of palate HCC
C05.9 Malignant neoplasm of palate, unspecified HCC
Malignant neoplasm of roof of mouth

C06 Malignant neoplasm of other and unspecified parts of mouth

Use additional code to identify:
alcohol abuse and dependence (F10.-)
history of tobacco dependence (Z87.891)
tobacco dependence (F17.-)
tobacco use (Z72.0)

C06.0 Malignant neoplasm of cheek mucosa HCC
Malignant neoplasm of buccal mucosa NOS
Malignant neoplasm of internal cheek
C06.1 Malignant neoplasm of vestibule of mouth HCC
Malignant neoplasm of buccal sulcus (upper) (lower)
Malignant neoplasm of labial sulcus (upper) (lower)
C06.2 Malignant neoplasm of retromolar area HCC
C06.8 Malignant neoplasm of overlapping sites of other and unspecified parts of mouth
C06.80 Malignant neoplasm of overlapping sites of unspecified parts of mouth HCC
C06.89 Malignant neoplasm of overlapping sites of other parts of mouth HCC
"book leaf" neoplasm [ventral surface of tongue and floor of mouth]
C06.9 Malignant neoplasm of mouth, unspecified HCC
Malignant neoplasm of minor salivary gland, unspecified site
Malignant neoplasm of oral cavity NOS

C07 Malignant neoplasm of parotid gland HCC

Use additional code to identify:
alcohol abuse and dependence (F10.-)
exposure to environmental tobacco smoke (Z77.22)
exposure to tobacco smoke in the perinatal period (P96.81)
history of tobacco dependence (Z87.891)
occupational exposure to environmental tobacco smoke (Z57.31)
tobacco dependence (F17.-)
tobacco use (Z72.0)

C08 Malignant neoplasm of other and unspecified major salivary glands

INCLUDES malignant neoplasm of salivary ducts

Use additional code to identify:
alcohol abuse and dependence (F10.-)
exposure to environmental tobacco smoke (Z77.22)
exposure to tobacco smoke in the perinatal period (P96.81)
history of tobacco dependence (Z87.891)
occupational exposure to environmental tobacco smoke (Z57.31)
tobacco dependence (F17.-)
tobacco use (Z72.0)

EXCLUDES 1 *malignant neoplasms of specified minor salivary glands which are classified according to their anatomical location*
EXCLUDES 2 *malignant neoplasms of minor salivary glands NOS (C06.9)*
malignant neoplasm of parotid gland (C07)

C08.0 Malignant neoplasm of submandibular gland HCC
Malignant neoplasm of submaxillary gland
C08.1 Malignant neoplasm of sublingual gland HCC
C08.9 Malignant neoplasm of major salivary gland, unspecified HCC
Malignant neoplasm of salivary gland (major) NOS

C09 Malignant neoplasm of tonsil

Use additional code to identify:
alcohol abuse and dependence (F10.-)
exposure to environmental tobacco smoke (Z77.22)
exposure to tobacco smoke in the perinatal period (P96.81)
history of tobacco dependence (Z87.891)
occupational exposure to environmental tobacco smoke (Z57.31)
tobacco dependence (F17.-)
tobacco use (Z72.0)

EXCLUDES 2 *malignant neoplasm of lingual tonsil (C02.4)*
malignant neoplasm of pharyngeal tonsil (C11.1)

C09.0 Malignant neoplasm of tonsillar fossa HCC
C09.1 Malignant neoplasm of tonsillar pillar (anterior) (posterior) HCC
C09.8 Malignant neoplasm of overlapping sites of tonsil HCC
C09.9 Malignant neoplasm of tonsil, unspecified HCC
Malignant neoplasm of faucial tonsils
Malignant neoplasm of palatine tonsils
Malignant neoplasm of tonsil NOS

C10 Malignant neoplasm of oropharynx

Use additional code to identify:
alcohol abuse and dependence (F10.-)
exposure to environmental tobacco smoke (Z77.22)
exposure to tobacco smoke in the perinatal period (P96.81)
history of tobacco dependence (Z87.891)
occupational exposure to environmental tobacco smoke (Z57.31)
tobacco dependence (F17.-)
tobacco use (Z72.0)

EXCLUDES 2 *malignant neoplasm of tonsil (C09.-)*

DEF: Oropharynx: Middle portion of pharynx (throat); communicates with the oral cavity, nasopharynx and laryngopharynx.

C10.0 Malignant neoplasm of vallecula HCC
C10.1 Malignant neoplasm of anterior surface of epiglottis HCC
Malignant neoplasm of epiglottis, free border [margin]
Malignant neoplasm of glossoepiglottic fold(s)
EXCLUDES 2 *malignant neoplasm of epiglottis (suprahyoid portion) NOS (C32.1)*
C10.2 Malignant neoplasm of lateral wall of oropharynx HCC
C10.3 Malignant neoplasm of posterior wall of oropharynx HCC
C10.4 Malignant neoplasm of branchial cleft HCC
Malignant neoplasm of branchial cyst [site of neoplasm]
C10.8 Malignant neoplasm of overlapping sites of oropharynx HCC
Malignant neoplasm of junctional region of oropharynx
C10.9 Malignant neoplasm of oropharynx, unspecified HCC

Chapter 2. Neoplasms

C03–C10.9

C11 Malignant neoplasm of nasopharynx

Use additional code to identify:
exposure to environmental tobacco smoke (Z77.22)
exposure to tobacco smoke in the perinatal period (P96.81)
history of tobacco dependence (Z87.891)
occupational exposure to environmental tobacco smoke (Z57.31)
tobacco dependence (F17.-)
tobacco use (Z72.Ø)

DEF: Nasopharynx: Upper portion of pharynx (throat); communicates with the nasal cavities, oropharynx and tympanic cavities.

C11.Ø Malignant neoplasm of superior wall of nasopharynx HCC
Malignant neoplasm of roof of nasopharynx

C11.1 Malignant neoplasm of posterior wall of nasopharynx HCC
Malignant neoplasm of adenoid
Malignant neoplasm of pharyngeal tonsil

C11.2 Malignant neoplasm of lateral wall of nasopharynx HCC
Malignant neoplasm of fossa of Rosenmuller
Malignant neoplasm of opening of auditory tube
Malignant neoplasm of pharyngeal recess

C11.3 Malignant neoplasm of anterior wall of nasopharynx HCC
Malignant neoplasm of floor of nasopharynx
Malignant neoplasm of nasopharyngeal (anterior) (posterior) surface of soft palate
Malignant neoplasm of posterior margin of nasal choana
Malignant neoplasm of posterior margin of nasal septum

C11.8 Malignant neoplasm of overlapping sites of nasopharynx HCC

C11.9 Malignant neoplasm of nasopharynx, unspecified HCC
Malignant neoplasm of nasopharyngeal wall NOS

C12 Malignant neoplasm of pyriform sinus HCC
Malignant neoplasm of pyriform fossa
Use additional code to identify:
exposure to environmental tobacco smoke (Z77.22)
exposure to tobacco smoke in the perinatal period (P96.81)
history of tobacco dependence (Z87.891)
occupational exposure to environmental tobacco smoke (Z57.31)
tobacco dependence (F17.-)
tobacco use (Z72.Ø)

C13 Malignant neoplasm of hypopharynx

Use additional code to identify:
exposure to environmental tobacco smoke (Z77.22)
exposure to tobacco smoke in the perinatal period (P96.81)
history of tobacco dependence (Z87.891)
occupational exposure to environmental tobacco smoke (Z57.31)
tobacco dependence (F17.-)
tobacco use (Z72.Ø)

EXCLUDES 2 *malignant neoplasm of pyriform sinus (C12)*

DEF: Hypopharynx: Lower portion of pharynx (throat); communicates with the oropharynx and the esophagus. ***Synonym(s):*** *laryngopharynx.*

C13.Ø Malignant neoplasm of postcricoid region HCC

C13.1 Malignant neoplasm of aryepiglottic fold, hypopharyngeal aspect HCC
Malignant neoplasm of aryepiglottic fold, marginal zone
Malignant neoplasm of aryepiglottic fold NOS
Malignant neoplasm of interarytenoid fold, marginal zone
Malignant neoplasm of interarytenoid fold NOS
EXCLUDES 2 *malignant neoplasm of aryepiglottic fold or interarytenoid fold, laryngeal aspect (C32.1)*

C13.2 Malignant neoplasm of posterior wall of hypopharynx HCC

C13.8 Malignant neoplasm of overlapping sites of hypopharynx HCC

C13.9 Malignant neoplasm of hypopharynx, unspecified HCC
Malignant neoplasm of hypopharyngeal wall NOS

C14 Malignant neoplasm of other and ill-defined sites in the lip, oral cavity and pharynx

Use additional code to identify:
alcohol abuse and dependence (F1Ø.-)
exposure to environmental tobacco smoke (Z77.22)
exposure to tobacco smoke in the perinatal period (P96.81)
history of tobacco dependence (Z87.891)
occupational exposure to environmental tobacco smoke (Z57.31)
tobacco dependence (F17.-)
tobacco use (Z72.Ø)

EXCLUDES 1 *malignant neoplasm of oral cavity NOS (CØ6.9)*

C14.Ø Malignant neoplasm of pharynx, unspecified HCC

C14.2 Malignant neoplasm of Waldeyer's ring HCC
DEF: Waldeyer's ring: Ring of lymphoid tissue that is made up of the two palatine tonsils, the pharyngeal tonsil (adenoid), and the lingual tonsil. It functions as the defense against infection and assists with the development of the immune system.

C14.8 Malignant neoplasm of overlapping sites of lip, oral cavity and pharynx HCC
Primary malignant neoplasm of two or more contiguous sites of lip, oral cavity and pharynx
EXCLUDES 1 *"book leaf" neoplasm [ventral surface of tongue and floor of mouth] (CØ6.89)*

Malignant neoplasms of digestive organs (C15-C26)

EXCLUDES 1 *Kaposi's sarcoma of gastrointestinal sites (C46.4)*
EXCLUDES 2 *gastrointestinal stromal tumors (C49.A-)*

C15 Malignant neoplasm of esophagus

Use additional code to identify:
alcohol abuse and dependence (F1Ø.-)

AHA: 2022,3Q,10

C15.3 Malignant neoplasm of upper third of esophagus CC HCC

C15.4 Malignant neoplasm of middle third of esophagus CC HCC

C15.5 Malignant neoplasm of lower third of esophagus CC HCC
EXCLUDES 1 *malignant neoplasm of cardio-esophageal junction (C16.Ø)*

C15.8 Malignant neoplasm of overlapping sites of esophagus CC HCC

C15.9 Malignant neoplasm of esophagus, unspecified CC HCC

C16 Malignant neoplasm of stomach

Use additional code to identify:
alcohol abuse and dependence (F1Ø.-)
EXCLUDES 2 *malignant carcinoid tumor of the stomach (C7A.Ø92)*

C16.Ø Malignant neoplasm of cardia CC HCC
Malignant neoplasm of cardiac orifice
Malignant neoplasm of cardio-esophageal junction
Malignant neoplasm of esophagus and stomach
Malignant neoplasm of gastro-esophageal junction

C16.1 Malignant neoplasm of fundus of stomach CC HCC

C16.2 Malignant neoplasm of body of stomach CC HCC

C16.3 Malignant neoplasm of pyloric antrum CC HCC
Malignant neoplasm of gastric antrum

C16.4 Malignant neoplasm of pylorus CC HCC
Malignant neoplasm of prepylorus
Malignant neoplasm of pyloric canal

C16.5 Malignant neoplasm of lesser curvature of stomach, unspecified CC HCC
Malignant neoplasm of lesser curvature of stomach, not classifiable to C16.1-C16.4

C16.6 Malignant neoplasm of greater curvature of stomach, unspecified CC HCC
Malignant neoplasm of greater curvature of stomach, not classifiable to C16.Ø-C16.4

C16.8 Malignant neoplasm of overlapping sites of stomach CC HCC

C16.9 Malignant neoplasm of stomach, unspecified CC HCC
Gastric cancer NOS

C17 Malignant neoplasm of small intestine

EXCLUDES 1 *malignant carcinoid tumors of the small intestine (C7A.Ø1)*

AHA: 2016,1Q,19

C17.Ø Malignant neoplasm of duodenum CC HCC

C17.1 Malignant neoplasm of jejunum CC HCC

C17.2 Malignant neoplasm of ileum CC HCC
EXCLUDES 1 *malignant neoplasm of ileocecal valve (C18.Ø)*

C17.3 Meckel's diverticulum, malignant CC HCC
EXCLUDES 1 *Meckel's diverticulum, congenital (Q43.Ø)*
DEF: Congenital, abnormal remnant of embryonic digestive system development that leaves a sacculation or outpouching from the wall of the small intestine near the terminal part of the ileum made of acid-secreting tissue as in the stomach.

C17.8 Malignant neoplasm of overlapping sites of small intestine CC HCC

C17.9 Malignant neoplasm of small intestine, unspecified CC HCC

C18 Malignant neoplasm of colon

EXCLUDES 1 *malignant carcinoid tumors of the colon (C7A.Ø2-)*

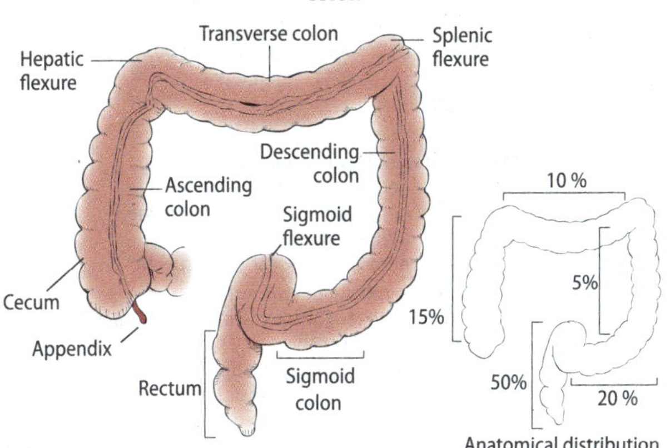

Anatomical distribution of large bowel cancers

C18.Ø Malignant neoplasm of cecum CC HCC
Malignant neoplasm of ileocecal valve

C18.1 Malignant neoplasm of appendix CC HCC

C18.2 Malignant neoplasm of ascending colon CC HCC

C18.3 Malignant neoplasm of hepatic flexure CC HCC

C18.4 Malignant neoplasm of transverse colon CC HCC

C18.5 Malignant neoplasm of splenic flexure CC HCC

C18.6 Malignant neoplasm of descending colon CC HCC

C18.7 Malignant neoplasm of sigmoid colon CC HCC
Malignant neoplasm of sigmoid (flexure)
EXCLUDES 1 *malignant neoplasm of rectosigmoid junction (C19)*

C18.8 Malignant neoplasm of overlapping sites of colon CC HCC

C18.9 Malignant neoplasm of colon, unspecified CC HCC
Malignant neoplasm of large intestine NOS

C19 Malignant neoplasm of rectosigmoid junction CC HCC
Malignant neoplasm of colon with rectum
Malignant neoplasm of rectosigmoid (colon)
EXCLUDES 1 *malignant carcinoid tumors of the colon (C7A.Ø2-)*

C2Ø Malignant neoplasm of rectum CC HCC
Malignant neoplasm of rectal ampulla
EXCLUDES 1 *malignant carcinoid tumor of the rectum (C7A.Ø26)*

C21 Malignant neoplasm of anus and anal canal

EXCLUDES 2 *malignant carcinoid tumors of the colon (C7A.Ø2-)*
malignant melanoma of anal margin (C43.51)
malignant melanoma of anal skin (C43.51)
malignant melanoma of perianal skin (C43.51)
other and unspecified malignant neoplasm of anal margin (C44.5ØØ, C44.51Ø, C44.52Ø, C44.59Ø)
other and unspecified malignant neoplasm of anal skin (C44.5ØØ, C44.51Ø, C44.52Ø, C44.59Ø)
other and unspecified malignant neoplasm of perianal skin (C44.5ØØ, C44.51Ø, C44.52Ø, C44.59Ø)

C21.Ø Malignant neoplasm of anus, unspecified CC HCC

C21.1 Malignant neoplasm of anal canal CC HCC
Malignant neoplasm of anal sphincter

C21.2 Malignant neoplasm of cloacogenic zone CC HCC

C21.8 Malignant neoplasm of overlapping sites of rectum, anus and anal canal CC HCC
Malignant neoplasm of anorectal junction
Malignant neoplasm of anorectum
Primary malignant neoplasm of two or more contiguous sites of rectum, anus and anal canal

C22 Malignant neoplasm of liver and intrahepatic bile ducts

EXCLUDES 1 *malignant neoplasm of biliary tract NOS (C24.9)*
secondary malignant neoplasm of liver and intrahepatic bile duct (C78.7)

Use additional code to identify:
alcohol abuse and dependence (F1Ø.-)
hepatitis B (B16.-, B18.Ø-B18.1)
hepatitis C (B17.1-, B18.2)

C22.Ø Liver cell carcinoma CC HCC
Hepatocellular carcinoma
Hepatoma
AHA: 2016,1Q,18

C22.1 Intrahepatic bile duct carcinoma CC HCC
Cholangiocarcinoma
EXCLUDES 1 *malignant neoplasm of hepatic duct (C24.Ø)*
AHA: 2023,1Q,24

C22.2 Hepatoblastoma CC HCC

C22.3 Angiosarcoma of liver CC HCC
Kupffer cell sarcoma

C22.4 Other sarcomas of liver CC HCC

C22.7 Other specified carcinomas of liver CC HCC

C22.8 Malignant neoplasm of liver, primary, unspecified as to type CC HCC

C22.9 Malignant neoplasm of liver, not specified as primary or secondary CC HCC

C23 Malignant neoplasm of gallbladder CC HCC

C24 Malignant neoplasm of other and unspecified parts of biliary tract

EXCLUDES 1 *malignant neoplasm of intrahepatic bile duct (C22.1)*

C24.Ø Malignant neoplasm of extrahepatic bile duct CC HCC
Malignant neoplasm of biliary duct or passage NOS
Malignant neoplasm of common bile duct
Malignant neoplasm of cystic duct
Malignant neoplasm of hepatic duct

C24.1 Malignant neoplasm of ampulla of Vater CC HCC
DEF: Malignant neoplasm in the area of dilation at the juncture of the common bile and pancreatic ducts near the opening into the lumen of the duodenum.

C24.8 Malignant neoplasm of overlapping sites of biliary tract CC HCC
Malignant neoplasm involving both intrahepatic and extrahepatic bile ducts
Primary malignant neoplasm of two or more contiguous sites of biliary tract

C24.9 Malignant neoplasm of biliary tract, unspecified CC HCC

C25 Malignant neoplasm of pancreas

Code also if applicable exocrine pancreatic insufficiency (K86.81)
Use additional code to identify:
alcohol abuse and dependence (F1Ø.-)

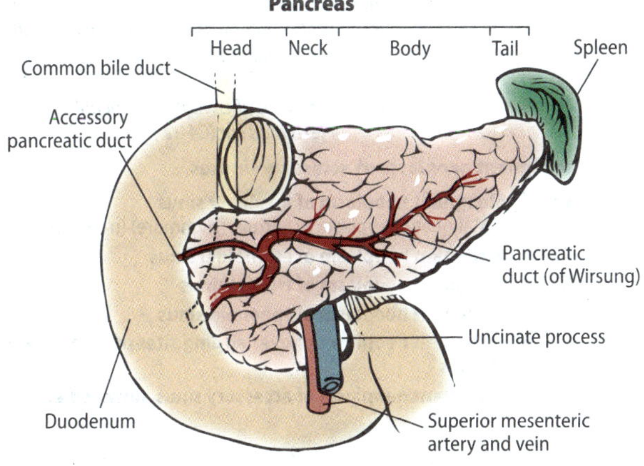

C25.Ø Malignant neoplasm of head of pancreas CC HCC

C25.1 Malignant neoplasm of body of pancreas CC HCC

C25.2 Malignant neoplasm of tail of pancreas CC HCC

C25.3 Malignant neoplasm of pancreatic duct CC HCC

C25.4 Malignant neoplasm of endocrine pancreas CC HCC
Malignant neoplasm of islets of Langerhans
Use additional code to identify any functional activity

C25.7 Malignant neoplasm of other parts of pancreas CC HCC
Malignant neoplasm of neck of pancreas

C25.8 Malignant neoplasm of overlapping sites of pancreas CC HCC

C25.9 Malignant neoplasm of pancreas, unspecified CC HCC

C26 Malignant neoplasm of other and ill-defined digestive organs
EXCLUDES 1 *malignant neoplasm of peritoneum and retroperitoneum (C48.-)*

C26.0 Malignant neoplasm of intestinal tract, part unspecified HCC
Malignant neoplasm of intestine NOS

C26.1 Malignant neoplasm of spleen HCC
EXCLUDES 1 *Hodgkin lymphoma (C81.-)*
non-Hodgkin lymphoma (C82-C85)

C26.9 Malignant neoplasm of ill-defined sites within the digestive system HCC
Malignant neoplasm of alimentary canal or tract NOS
Malignant neoplasm of gastrointestinal tract NOS
EXCLUDES 1 *malignant neoplasm of abdominal NOS (C76.2)*
malignant neoplasm of intra-abdominal NOS (C76.2)

Malignant neoplasms of respiratory and intrathoracic organs (C30-C39)

INCLUDES malignant neoplasm of middle ear
EXCLUDES 1 *mesothelioma (C45.-)*

C30 Malignant neoplasm of nasal cavity and middle ear

C30.0 Malignant neoplasm of nasal cavity HCC
Malignant neoplasm of cartilage of nose
Malignant neoplasm of nasal concha
Malignant neoplasm of internal nose
Malignant neoplasm of septum of nose
Malignant neoplasm of vestibule of nose
EXCLUDES 1 *malignant neoplasm of nasal bone (C41.0)*
malignant neoplasm of nose NOS (C76.0)
malignant neoplasm of olfactory bulb (C72.2-)
malignant neoplasm of posterior margin of nasal septum and choana (C11.3)
malignant melanoma of skin of nose (C43.31)
malignant neoplasm of turbinates (C41.0)
other and unspecified malignant neoplasm of skin of nose (C44.301, C44.311, C44.321, C44.391)

C30.1 Malignant neoplasm of middle ear HCC
Malignant neoplasm of antrum tympanicum
Malignant neoplasm of auditory tube
Malignant neoplasm of eustachian tube
Malignant neoplasm of inner ear
Malignant neoplasm of mastoid air cells
Malignant neoplasm of tympanic cavity
EXCLUDES 1 *malignant neoplasm of auricular canal (external) (C43.2-,C44.2-)*
malignant neoplasm of bone of ear (meatus) (C41.0)
malignant neoplasm of cartilage of ear (C49.0)
malignant melanoma of skin of (external) ear (C43.2-)
other and unspecified malignant neoplasm of skin of (external) ear (C44.2-)

C31 Malignant neoplasm of accessory sinuses

C31.0 Malignant neoplasm of maxillary sinus HCC
Malignant neoplasm of antrum (Highmore) (maxillary)

C31.1 Malignant neoplasm of ethmoidal sinus HCC

C31.2 Malignant neoplasm of frontal sinus HCC

C31.3 Malignant neoplasm of sphenoid sinus HCC

C31.8 Malignant neoplasm of overlapping sites of accessory sinuses HCC

C31.9 Malignant neoplasm of accessory sinus, unspecified HCC

C32 Malignant neoplasm of larynx
Use additional code to identify:
alcohol abuse and dependence (F10.-)
exposure to environmental tobacco smoke (Z77.22)
exposure to tobacco smoke in the perinatal period (P96.81)
history of tobacco dependence (Z87.891)
occupational exposure to environmental tobacco smoke (Z57.31)
tobacco dependence (F17.-)
tobacco use (Z72.0)

C32.0 Malignant neoplasm of glottis HCC
Malignant neoplasm of intrinsic larynx
Malignant neoplasm of laryngeal commissure (anterior)(posterior)
Malignant neoplasm of vocal cord (true) NOS

C32.1 Malignant neoplasm of supraglottis HCC
Malignant neoplasm of aryepiglottic fold or interarytenoid fold, laryngeal aspect
Malignant neoplasm of epiglottis (suprahyoid portion) NOS
Malignant neoplasm of extrinsic larynx
Malignant neoplasm of false vocal cord
Malignant neoplasm of posterior (laryngeal) surface of epiglottis
Malignant neoplasm of ventricular bands
EXCLUDES 2 *malignant neoplasm of anterior surface of epiglottis (C10.1)*
malignant neoplasm of aryepiglottic fold or interarytenoid fold, hypopharyngeal aspect (C13.1)
malignant neoplasm of aryepiglottic fold or interarytenoid fold, marginal zone (C13.1)
malignant neoplasm of aryepiglottic fold or interarytenoid fold NOS (C13.1)

C32.2 Malignant neoplasm of subglottis HCC

C32.3 Malignant neoplasm of laryngeal cartilage HCC

C32.8 Malignant neoplasm of overlapping sites of larynx HCC

C32.9 Malignant neoplasm of larynx, unspecified HCC

C33 Malignant neoplasm of trachea CC HCC
Use additional code to identify:
exposure to environmental tobacco smoke (Z77.22)
exposure to tobacco smoke in the perinatal period (P96.81)
history of tobacco dependence (Z87.891)
occupational exposure to environmental tobacco smoke (Z57.31)
tobacco dependence (F17.-)
tobacco use (Z72.0)

C34 Malignant neoplasm of bronchus and lung
Use additional code to identify:
exposure to environmental tobacco smoke (Z77.22)
exposure to tobacco smoke in the perinatal period (P96.81)
history of tobacco dependence (Z87.891)
occupational exposure to environmental tobacco smoke (Z57.31)
tobacco dependence (F17.-)
tobacco use (Z72.0)
EXCLUDES 1 *Kaposi's sarcoma of lung (C46.5-)*
malignant carcinoid tumor of the bronchus and lung (C7A.090)

AHA: 2023,1Q,20-21; 2022,4Q,22; 2019,1Q,16

TIP: When documented, assign code I31.31 for associated malignant pericardial effusion. The neoplasm code should be sequenced first.

C34.0 Malignant neoplasm of main bronchus
Malignant neoplasm of carina
Malignant neoplasm of hilus (of lung)

C34.00 Malignant neoplasm of unspecified main bronchus CC HCC

C34.01 Malignant neoplasm of right main bronchus CC HCC

C34.02 Malignant neoplasm of left main bronchus CC HCC

C34.1 Malignant neoplasm of upper lobe, bronchus or lung

C34.10 Malignant neoplasm of upper lobe, unspecified bronchus or lung CC HCC

C34.11 Malignant neoplasm of upper lobe, right bronchus or lung CC HCC

C34.12 Malignant neoplasm of upper lobe, left bronchus or lung CC HCC

C34.2 Malignant neoplasm of middle lobe, bronchus or lung CC HCC

C34.3 Malignant neoplasm of lower lobe, bronchus or lung

C34.30 Malignant neoplasm of lower lobe, unspecified bronchus or lung CC HCC

C34.31 **Malignant neoplasm of lower lobe, right bronchus or lung** CC HCC

C34.32 **Malignant neoplasm of lower lobe, left bronchus or lung** CC HCC

✓5th C34.8 **Malignant neoplasm of overlapping sites of bronchus and lung**

C34.80 **Malignant neoplasm of overlapping sites of unspecified bronchus and lung** CC HCC

C34.81 **Malignant neoplasm of overlapping sites of right bronchus and lung** CC HCC

C34.82 **Malignant neoplasm of overlapping sites of left bronchus and lung** CC HCC

✓5th C34.9 **Malignant neoplasm of unspecified part of bronchus or lung**

C34.90 **Malignant neoplasm of unspecified part of unspecified bronchus or lung** CC HCC
Lung cancer NOS

C34.91 **Malignant neoplasm of unspecified part of right bronchus or lung** CC HCC

C34.92 **Malignant neoplasm of unspecified part of left bronchus or lung** CC HCC

C37 **Malignant neoplasm of thymus** CC HCC
EXCLUDES 1 *malignant carcinoid tumor of the thymus (C7A.Ø91)*

✓4th C38 **Malignant neoplasm of heart, mediastinum and pleura**
EXCLUDES 1 *mesothelioma (C45.-)*

C38.Ø **Malignant neoplasm of heart** CC HCC
Malignant neoplasm of pericardium
EXCLUDES 1 *malignant neoplasm of great vessels (C49.3)*

C38.1 **Malignant neoplasm of anterior mediastinum** CC HCC

C38.2 **Malignant neoplasm of posterior mediastinum** CC HCC

C38.3 **Malignant neoplasm of mediastinum, part unspecified** CC HCC

C38.4 **Malignant neoplasm of pleura** CC HCC

C38.8 **Malignant neoplasm of overlapping sites of heart, mediastinum and pleura** CC HCC

✓4th C39 **Malignant neoplasm of other and ill-defined sites in the respiratory system and intrathoracic organs**
Use additional code to identify:
exposure to environmental tobacco smoke (Z77.22)
exposure to tobacco smoke in the perinatal period (P96.81)
history of tobacco dependence (Z87.891)
occupational exposure to environmental tobacco smoke (Z57.31)
tobacco dependence (F17.-)
tobacco use (Z72.Ø)
EXCLUDES 1 *intrathoracic malignant neoplasm NOS (C76.1)*
thoracic malignant neoplasm NOS (C76.1)

C39.Ø **Malignant neoplasm of upper respiratory tract, part unspecified** HCC

C39.9 **Malignant neoplasm of lower respiratory tract, part unspecified** HCC
Malignant neoplasm of respiratory tract NOS

Malignant neoplasms of bone and articular cartilage (C4Ø-C41)

INCLUDES malignant neoplasm of cartilage (articular) (joint)
malignant neoplasm of periosteum
EXCLUDES 1 *malignant neoplasm of bone marrow NOS (C96.9)*
malignant neoplasm of synovia (C49.-)

✓4th C4Ø **Malignant neoplasm of bone and articular cartilage of limbs**
Use additional code to identify major osseous defect, if applicable (M89.7-)

✓5th C4Ø.Ø **Malignant neoplasm of scapula and long bones of upper limb**

C4Ø.ØØ **Malignant neoplasm of scapula and long bones of unspecified upper limb** CC HCC

C4Ø.Ø1 **Malignant neoplasm of scapula and long bones of right upper limb** CC HCC

C4Ø.Ø2 **Malignant neoplasm of scapula and long bones of left upper limb** CC HCC

✓5th C4Ø.1 **Malignant neoplasm of short bones of upper limb**

C4Ø.1Ø **Malignant neoplasm of short bones of unspecified upper limb** CC HCC

C4Ø.11 **Malignant neoplasm of short bones of right upper limb** CC HCC

C4Ø.12 **Malignant neoplasm of short bones of left upper limb** CC HCC

✓5th C4Ø.2 **Malignant neoplasm of long bones of lower limb**

C4Ø.2Ø **Malignant neoplasm of long bones of unspecified lower limb** CC HCC

C4Ø.21 **Malignant neoplasm of long bones of right lower limb** CC HCC

C4Ø.22 **Malignant neoplasm of long bones of left lower limb** CC HCC

✓5th C4Ø.3 **Malignant neoplasm of short bones of lower limb**

C4Ø.3Ø **Malignant neoplasm of short bones of unspecified lower limb** CC HCC

C4Ø.31 **Malignant neoplasm of short bones of right lower limb** CC HCC

C4Ø.32 **Malignant neoplasm of short bones of left lower limb** CC HCC

✓5th C4Ø.8 **Malignant neoplasm of overlapping sites of bone and articular cartilage of limb**

C4Ø.8Ø **Malignant neoplasm of overlapping sites of bone and articular cartilage of unspecified limb** CC HCC

C4Ø.81 **Malignant neoplasm of overlapping sites of bone and articular cartilage of right limb** CC HCC

C4Ø.82 **Malignant neoplasm of overlapping sites of bone and articular cartilage of left limb** CC HCC

✓5th C4Ø.9 **Malignant neoplasm of unspecified bones and articular cartilage of limb**

C4Ø.9Ø **Malignant neoplasm of unspecified bones and articular cartilage of unspecified limb** CC HCC

C4Ø.91 **Malignant neoplasm of unspecified bones and articular cartilage of right limb** CC HCC

C4Ø.92 **Malignant neoplasm of unspecified bones and articular cartilage of left limb** CC HCC

✓4th C41 **Malignant neoplasm of bone and articular cartilage of other and unspecified sites**
EXCLUDES 1 *malignant neoplasm of bones of limbs (C4Ø.-)*
malignant neoplasm of cartilage of ear (C49.Ø)
malignant neoplasm of cartilage of eyelid (C49.Ø)
malignant neoplasm of cartilage of larynx (C32.3)
malignant neoplasm of cartilage of limbs (C4Ø.-)
malignant neoplasm of cartilage of nose (C3Ø.Ø)

C41.Ø **Malignant neoplasm of bones of skull and face** CC HCC
Malignant neoplasm of maxilla (superior)
Malignant neoplasm of orbital bone
EXCLUDES 2 *carcinoma, any type except intraosseous or odontogenic of:*
maxillary sinus (C31.Ø)
upper jaw (CØ3.Ø)
malignant neoplasm of jaw bone (lower) (C41.1)

C41.1 **Malignant neoplasm of mandible** CC HCC
Malignant neoplasm of inferior maxilla
Malignant neoplasm of lower jaw bone
EXCLUDES 2 *carcinoma, any type except intraosseous or odontogenic of:*
jaw NOS (CØ3.9)
lower (CØ3.1)
malignant neoplasm of upper jaw bone (C41.Ø)

C41.2 **Malignant neoplasm of vertebral column** CC HCC
EXCLUDES 1 *malignant neoplasm of sacrum and coccyx (C41.4)*

C41.3 **Malignant neoplasm of ribs, sternum and clavicle** CC HCC

C41.4 **Malignant neoplasm of pelvic bones, sacrum and coccyx** CC HCC

C41.9 **Malignant neoplasm of bone and articular cartilage, unspecified** CC HCC

Melanoma and other malignant neoplasms of skin (C43-C44)

✓4th C43 **Malignant melanoma of skin**
EXCLUDES 1 *melanoma in situ (DØ3.-)*
EXCLUDES 2 *malignant melanoma of skin of genital organs (C51-C52, C6Ø.-, C63.-)*
Merkel cell carcinoma (C4A.-)
sites other than skin - code to malignant neoplasm of the site

C43.Ø **Malignant melanoma of lip** HCC
EXCLUDES 1 *malignant neoplasm of vermilion border of lip (CØØ.Ø-CØØ.2)*

✓5th C43.1 **Malignant melanoma of eyelid, including canthus**
AHA: 2018,4Q,4

C43.1Ø **Malignant melanoma of unspecified eyelid, including canthus** HCC

✓6th C43.11 **Malignant melanoma of right eyelid, including canthus**

C43.111 **Malignant melanoma of right upper eyelid, including canthus** HCC

C43.112 **Malignant melanoma of right lower eyelid, including canthus** HCC

✓6th C43.12 **Malignant melanoma of left eyelid, including canthus**

C43.121 **Malignant melanoma of left upper eyelid, including canthus** HCC

C43.122 **Malignant melanoma of left lower eyelid, including canthus** HCC

✓5th C43.2 **Malignant melanoma of ear and external auricular canal**

C43.2Ø **Malignant melanoma of unspecified ear and external auricular canal** HCC

C43.21 **Malignant melanoma of right ear and external auricular canal** HCC

C43.22 **Malignant melanoma of left ear and external auricular canal** HCC

✓5th C43.3 **Malignant melanoma of other and unspecified parts of face**

C43.3Ø **Malignant melanoma of unspecified part of face** HCC

C43.31 **Malignant melanoma of nose** HCC

C43.39 **Malignant melanoma of other parts of face** HCC

C43.4 **Malignant melanoma of scalp and neck** HCC

✓5th C43.5 **Malignant melanoma of trunk**

EXCLUDES 2 *malignant neoplasm of anus NOS (C21.Ø)*
malignant neoplasm of scrotum (C63.2)

C43.51 **Malignant melanoma of anal skin** HCC
Malignant melanoma of anal margin
Malignant melanoma of perianal skin

C43.52 **Malignant melanoma of skin of breast** HCC

C43.59 **Malignant melanoma of other part of trunk** HCC

✓5th C43.6 **Malignant melanoma of upper limb, including shoulder**

C43.6Ø **Malignant melanoma of unspecified upper limb, including shoulder** HCC

C43.61 **Malignant melanoma of right upper limb, including shoulder** HCC

C43.62 **Malignant melanoma of left upper limb, including shoulder** HCC

✓5th C43.7 **Malignant melanoma of lower limb, including hip**

C43.7Ø **Malignant melanoma of unspecified lower limb, including hip** HCC

C43.71 **Malignant melanoma of right lower limb, including hip** HCC

C43.72 **Malignant melanoma of left lower limb, including hip** HCC

C43.8 **Malignant melanoma of overlapping sites of skin** HCC

C43.9 **Malignant melanoma of skin, unspecified** HCC
Malignant melanoma of unspecified site of skin
Melanoma (malignant) NOS

✓4th **C4A Merkel cell carcinoma**

DEF: Malignant cutaneous cancer predominantly found in elderly patients with sun exposure that usually presents as a flesh-colored or bluish-red lump typically seen on the neck, head, and face.

C4A.Ø **Merkel cell carcinoma of lip** HCC

EXCLUDES 1 *malignant neoplasm of vermilion border of lip (CØØ.Ø-CØØ.2)*

✓5th C4A.1 **Merkel cell carcinoma of eyelid, including canthus**

AHA: 2018,4Q,4

C4A.1Ø **Merkel cell carcinoma of unspecified eyelid, including canthus** HCC

✓6th C4A.11 **Merkel cell carcinoma of right eyelid, including canthus**

C4A.111 **Merkel cell carcinoma of right upper eyelid, including canthus** HCC

C4A.112 **Merkel cell carcinoma of right lower eyelid, including canthus** HCC

✓6th C4A.12 **Merkel cell carcinoma of left eyelid, including canthus**

C4A.121 **Merkel cell carcinoma of left upper eyelid, including canthus** HCC

C4A.122 **Merkel cell carcinoma of left lower eyelid, including canthus** HCC

✓5th C4A.2 **Merkel cell carcinoma of ear and external auricular canal**

C4A.2Ø **Merkel cell carcinoma of unspecified ear and external auricular canal** HCC

C4A.21 **Merkel cell carcinoma of right ear and external auricular canal** HCC

C4A.22 **Merkel cell carcinoma of left ear and external auricular canal** HCC

✓5th C4A.3 **Merkel cell carcinoma of other and unspecified parts of face**

C4A.3Ø **Merkel cell carcinoma of unspecified part of face** HCC

C4A.31 **Merkel cell carcinoma of nose** HCC

C4A.39 **Merkel cell carcinoma of other parts of face** HCC

C4A.4 **Merkel cell carcinoma of scalp and neck** HCC

✓5th C4A.5 **Merkel cell carcinoma of trunk**

EXCLUDES 2 *malignant neoplasm of anus NOS (C21.Ø)*
malignant neoplasm of scrotum (C63.2)

C4A.51 **Merkel cell carcinoma of anal skin** HCC
Merkel cell carcinoma of anal margin
Merkel cell carcinoma of perianal skin

C4A.52 **Merkel cell carcinoma of skin of breast** HCC

C4A.59 **Merkel cell carcinoma of other part of trunk** HCC

✓5th C4A.6 **Merkel cell carcinoma of upper limb, including shoulder**

C4A.6Ø **Merkel cell carcinoma of unspecified upper limb, including shoulder** HCC

C4A.61 **Merkel cell carcinoma of right upper limb, including shoulder** HCC

C4A.62 **Merkel cell carcinoma of left upper limb, including shoulder** HCC

✓5th C4A.7 **Merkel cell carcinoma of lower limb, including hip**

C4A.7Ø **Merkel cell carcinoma of unspecified lower limb, including hip** HCC

C4A.71 **Merkel cell carcinoma of right lower limb, including hip** HCC

C4A.72 **Merkel cell carcinoma of left lower limb, including hip** HCC

C4A.8 **Merkel cell carcinoma of overlapping sites** HCC

C4A.9 **Merkel cell carcinoma, unspecified** HCC
Merkel cell carcinoma of unspecified site
Merkel cell carcinoma NOS

✓4th **C44 Other and unspecified malignant neoplasm of skin**

INCLUDES malignant neoplasm of sebaceous glands
malignant neoplasm of sweat glands

EXCLUDES 1 *Kaposi's sarcoma of skin (C46.Ø)*
malignant melanoma of skin (C43.-)
malignant neoplasm of skin of genital organs (C51-C52, C6Ø.-, C63.2)
Merkel cell carcinoma (C4A.-)

DEF: Basal cell carcinoma: Abnormal growth of skin cells that arises from the deepest layer of the epidermis and may present as an open sore, red patches, pink growth, or scar. Typically caused by sun exposure, it is one of the most common forms of skin cancer.

DEF: Squamous cell carcinoma: Uncontrolled growth of abnormal skin cells that arises from the outer layers of the skin (epidermis) and may present as an open sore. It is characterized by a firm, red nodule, elevated growth with a central depression, or a flat sore with a scaly crust.

✓5th C44.Ø **Other and unspecified malignant neoplasm of skin of lip**

EXCLUDES 1 *malignant neoplasm of lip (CØØ.-)*

C44.ØØ **Unspecified malignant neoplasm of skin of lip**

C44.Ø1 **Basal cell carcinoma of skin of lip**

C44.Ø2 **Squamous cell carcinoma of skin of lip**

C44.Ø9 **Other specified malignant neoplasm of skin of lip**

✓5th C44.1 **Other and unspecified malignant neoplasm of skin of eyelid, including canthus**

EXCLUDES 1 *connective tissue of eyelid (C49.Ø)*

AHA: 2018,4Q,4

✓6th C44.1Ø **Unspecified malignant neoplasm of skin of eyelid, including canthus**

C44.1Ø1 **Unspecified malignant neoplasm of skin of unspecified eyelid, including canthus**

✓7th C44.1Ø2 **Unspecified malignant neoplasm of skin of right eyelid, including canthus**

C44.1Ø21 **Unspecified malignant neoplasm of skin of right upper eyelid, including canthus**

C44.1Ø22 **Unspecified malignant neoplasm of skin of right lower eyelid, including canthus**

✓7th C44.1Ø9 **Unspecified malignant neoplasm of skin of left eyelid, including canthus**

C44.1Ø91 **Unspecified malignant neoplasm of skin of left upper eyelid, including canthus**

C44.1Ø92 **Unspecified malignant neoplasm of skin of left lower eyelid, including canthus**

C44.11 Basal cell carcinoma of skin of eyelid, including canthus
C44.111 Basal cell carcinoma of skin of unspecified eyelid, including canthus
C44.112 Basal cell carcinoma of skin of right eyelid, including canthus
C44.1121 Basal cell carcinoma of skin of right upper eyelid, including canthus
C44.1122 Basal cell carcinoma of skin of right lower eyelid, including canthus
C44.119 Basal cell carcinoma of skin of left eyelid, including canthus
C44.1191 Basal cell carcinoma of skin of left upper eyelid, including canthus
C44.1192 Basal cell carcinoma of skin of left lower eyelid, including canthus
C44.12 Squamous cell carcinoma of skin of eyelid, including canthus
C44.121 Squamous cell carcinoma of skin of unspecified eyelid, including canthus
C44.122 Squamous cell carcinoma of skin of right eyelid, including canthus
C44.1221 Squamous cell carcinoma of skin of right upper eyelid, including canthus
C44.1222 Squamous cell carcinoma of skin of right lower eyelid, including canthus
C44.129 Squamous cell carcinoma of skin of left eyelid, including canthus
C44.1291 Squamous cell carcinoma of skin of left upper eyelid, including canthus
C44.1292 Squamous cell carcinoma of skin of left lower eyelid, including canthus
C44.13 Sebaceous cell carcinoma of skin of eyelid, including canthus
C44.131 Sebaceous cell carcinoma of skin of unspecified eyelid, including canthus
C44.132 Sebaceous cell carcinoma of skin of right eyelid, including canthus
C44.1321 Sebaceous cell carcinoma of skin of right upper eyelid, including canthus
C44.1322 Sebaceous cell carcinoma of skin of right lower eyelid, including canthus
C44.139 Sebaceous cell carcinoma of skin of left eyelid, including canthus
C44.1391 Sebaceous cell carcinoma of skin of left upper eyelid, including canthus
C44.1392 Sebaceous cell carcinoma of skin of left lower eyelid, including canthus
C44.19 Other specified malignant neoplasm of skin of eyelid, including canthus
C44.191 Other specified malignant neoplasm of skin of unspecified eyelid, including canthus
C44.192 Other specified malignant neoplasm of skin of right eyelid, including canthus
C44.1921 Other specified malignant neoplasm of skin of right upper eyelid, including canthus
C44.1922 Other specified malignant neoplasm of skin of right lower eyelid, including canthus
C44.199 Other specified malignant neoplasm of skin of left eyelid, including canthus
C44.1991 Other specified malignant neoplasm of skin of left upper eyelid, including canthus
C44.1992 Other specified malignant neoplasm of skin of left lower eyelid, including canthus

C44.2 Other and unspecified malignant neoplasm of skin of ear and external auricular canal
EXCLUDES 1 *connective tissue of ear (C49.Ø)*
C44.2Ø Unspecified malignant neoplasm of skin of ear and external auricular canal
C44.2Ø1 Unspecified malignant neoplasm of skin of unspecified ear and external auricular canal
C44.2Ø2 Unspecified malignant neoplasm of skin of right ear and external auricular canal
C44.2Ø9 Unspecified malignant neoplasm of skin of left ear and external auricular canal
C44.21 Basal cell carcinoma of skin of ear and external auricular canal
C44.211 Basal cell carcinoma of skin of unspecified ear and external auricular canal
C44.212 Basal cell carcinoma of skin of right ear and external auricular canal
C44.219 Basal cell carcinoma of skin of left ear and external auricular canal
C44.22 Squamous cell carcinoma of skin of ear and external auricular canal
C44.221 Squamous cell carcinoma of skin of unspecified ear and external auricular canal
C44.222 Squamous cell carcinoma of skin of right ear and external auricular canal
C44.229 Squamous cell carcinoma of skin of left ear and external auricular canal
C44.29 Other specified malignant neoplasm of skin of ear and external auricular canal
C44.291 Other specified malignant neoplasm of skin of unspecified ear and external auricular canal
C44.292 Other specified malignant neoplasm of skin of right ear and external auricular canal
C44.299 Other specified malignant neoplasm of skin of left ear and external auricular canal
C44.3 Other and unspecified malignant neoplasm of skin of other and unspecified parts of face
C44.3Ø Unspecified malignant neoplasm of skin of other and unspecified parts of face
C44.3ØØ Unspecified malignant neoplasm of skin of unspecified part of face
C44.3Ø1 Unspecified malignant neoplasm of skin of nose
C44.3Ø9 Unspecified malignant neoplasm of skin of other parts of face
C44.31 Basal cell carcinoma of skin of other and unspecified parts of face
C44.31Ø Basal cell carcinoma of skin of unspecified parts of face
C44.311 Basal cell carcinoma of skin of nose
C44.319 Basal cell carcinoma of skin of other parts of face
C44.32 Squamous cell carcinoma of skin of other and unspecified parts of face
C44.32Ø Squamous cell carcinoma of skin of unspecified parts of face
C44.321 Squamous cell carcinoma of skin of nose
C44.329 Squamous cell carcinoma of skin of other parts of face
C44.39 Other specified malignant neoplasm of skin of other and unspecified parts of face
C44.39Ø Other specified malignant neoplasm of skin of unspecified parts of face
C44.391 Other specified malignant neoplasm of skin of nose
C44.399 Other specified malignant neoplasm of skin of other parts of face
C44.4 Other and unspecified malignant neoplasm of skin of scalp and neck
C44.4Ø Unspecified malignant neoplasm of skin of scalp and neck
C44.41 Basal cell carcinoma of skin of scalp and neck
C44.42 Squamous cell carcinoma of skin of scalp and neck
C44.49 Other specified malignant neoplasm of skin of scalp and neck

C44.5 Other and unspecified malignant neoplasm of skin of trunk
EXCLUDES 1 *anus NOS (C21.0)*
scrotum (C63.2)

C44.50 Unspecified malignant neoplasm of skin of trunk
C44.500 Unspecified malignant neoplasm of anal skin
Unspecified malignant neoplasm of anal margin
Unspecified malignant neoplasm of perianal skin
C44.501 Unspecified malignant neoplasm of skin of breast
C44.509 Unspecified malignant neoplasm of skin of other part of trunk

C44.51 Basal cell carcinoma of skin of trunk
C44.510 Basal cell carcinoma of anal skin
Basal cell carcinoma of anal margin
Basal cell carcinoma of perianal skin
C44.511 Basal cell carcinoma of skin of breast
C44.519 Basal cell carcinoma of skin of other part of trunk

C44.52 Squamous cell carcinoma of skin of trunk
C44.520 Squamous cell carcinoma of anal skin
Squamous cell carcinoma of anal margin
Squamous cell carcinoma of perianal skin
C44.521 Squamous cell carcinoma of skin of breast
C44.529 Squamous cell carcinoma of skin of other part of trunk

C44.59 Other specified malignant neoplasm of skin of trunk
C44.590 Other specified malignant neoplasm of anal skin
Other specified malignant neoplasm of anal margin
Other specified malignant neoplasm of perianal skin
C44.591 Other specified malignant neoplasm of skin of breast
C44.599 Other specified malignant neoplasm of skin of other part of trunk

C44.6 Other and unspecified malignant neoplasm of skin of upper limb, including shoulder

C44.60 Unspecified malignant neoplasm of skin of upper limb, including shoulder
C44.601 Unspecified malignant neoplasm of skin of unspecified upper limb, including shoulder
C44.602 Unspecified malignant neoplasm of skin of right upper limb, including shoulder
C44.609 Unspecified malignant neoplasm of skin of left upper limb, including shoulder

C44.61 Basal cell carcinoma of skin of upper limb, including shoulder
C44.611 Basal cell carcinoma of skin of unspecified upper limb, including shoulder
C44.612 Basal cell carcinoma of skin of right upper limb, including shoulder
C44.619 Basal cell carcinoma of skin of left upper limb, including shoulder

C44.62 Squamous cell carcinoma of skin of upper limb, including shoulder
C44.621 Squamous cell carcinoma of skin of unspecified upper limb, including shoulder
C44.622 Squamous cell carcinoma of skin of right upper limb, including shoulder
C44.629 Squamous cell carcinoma of skin of left upper limb, including shoulder

C44.69 Other specified malignant neoplasm of skin of upper limb, including shoulder
C44.691 Other specified malignant neoplasm of skin of unspecified upper limb, including shoulder
C44.692 Other specified malignant neoplasm of skin of right upper limb, including shoulder
C44.699 Other specified malignant neoplasm of skin of left upper limb, including shoulder

C44.7 Other and unspecified malignant neoplasm of skin of lower limb, including hip

C44.70 Unspecified malignant neoplasm of skin of lower limb, including hip
C44.701 Unspecified malignant neoplasm of skin of unspecified lower limb, including hip
C44.702 Unspecified malignant neoplasm of skin of right lower limb, including hip
C44.709 Unspecified malignant neoplasm of skin of left lower limb, including hip

C44.71 Basal cell carcinoma of skin of lower limb, including hip
C44.711 Basal cell carcinoma of skin of unspecified lower limb, including hip
C44.712 Basal cell carcinoma of skin of right lower limb, including hip
C44.719 Basal cell carcinoma of skin of left lower limb, including hip

C44.72 Squamous cell carcinoma of skin of lower limb, including hip
C44.721 Squamous cell carcinoma of skin of unspecified lower limb, including hip
C44.722 Squamous cell carcinoma of skin of right lower limb, including hip
C44.729 Squamous cell carcinoma of skin of left lower limb, including hip

C44.79 Other specified malignant neoplasm of skin of lower limb, including hip
C44.791 Other specified malignant neoplasm of skin of unspecified lower limb, including hip
C44.792 Other specified malignant neoplasm of skin of right lower limb, including hip
C44.799 Other specified malignant neoplasm of skin of left lower limb, including hip

C44.8 Other and unspecified malignant neoplasm of overlapping sites of skin
C44.80 Unspecified malignant neoplasm of overlapping sites of skin
C44.81 Basal cell carcinoma of overlapping sites of skin
C44.82 Squamous cell carcinoma of overlapping sites of skin
C44.89 Other specified malignant neoplasm of overlapping sites of skin

C44.9 Other and unspecified malignant neoplasm of skin, unspecified
C44.90 Unspecified malignant neoplasm of skin, unspecified
Malignant neoplasm of unspecified site of skin
C44.91 Basal cell carcinoma of skin, unspecified
C44.92 Squamous cell carcinoma of skin, unspecified
C44.99 Other specified malignant neoplasm of skin, unspecified

Malignant neoplasms of mesothelial and soft tissue (C45-C49)

C45 Mesothelioma
DEF: Rare type of cancer that forms in the thin layer of protective tissue that covers the majority of internal organs (mesothelium).

C45.0 Mesothelioma of pleura CC HCC
EXCLUDES 1 *other malignant neoplasm of pleura (C38.4)*
AHA: 2017,2Q,11
TIP: For pleural mesothelioma that has metastasized to the chest wall, assign this code for the primary site along with C79.89 for metastatic cancer in the chest wall.

C45.1 Mesothelioma of peritoneum CC HCC
Mesothelioma of cul-de-sac
Mesothelioma of mesentery
Mesothelioma of mesocolon
Mesothelioma of omentum
Mesothelioma of peritoneum (parietal) (pelvic)
EXCLUDES 1 *other malignant neoplasm of soft tissue of peritoneum (C48.-)*

C45.2 Mesothelioma of pericardium CC HCC
EXCLUDES 1 *other malignant neoplasm of pericardium (C38.0)*

C45.7 Mesothelioma of other sites HCC
C45.9 Mesothelioma, unspecified HCC

C46 Kaposi's sarcoma

Code first any human immunodeficiency virus [HIV] disease (B2Ø)

DEF: Malignant neoplasm that causes patches of abnormal tissue to grow under the skin, in the lining of the mouth, nose, and throat, in lymph nodes, or in other visceral organs. Kaposi's sarcoma is caused by human herpesvirus8 (HHV8).

C46.Ø Kaposi's sarcoma of skin HIV CC HCC

C46.1 Kaposi's sarcoma of soft tissue HIV CC HCC

Kaposi's sarcoma of blood vessel
Kaposi's sarcoma of connective tissue
Kaposi's sarcoma of fascia
Kaposi's sarcoma of ligament
Kaposi's sarcoma of lymphatic(s) NEC
Kaposi's sarcoma of muscle

EXCLUDES 2 *Kaposi's sarcoma of lymph glands and nodes (C46.3)*

C46.2 Kaposi's sarcoma of palate HIV CC HCC

C46.3 Kaposi's sarcoma of lymph nodes HIV CC HCC

C46.4 Kaposi's sarcoma of gastrointestinal sites HIV CC HCC

C46.5 Kaposi's sarcoma of lung

AHA: 2019,1Q,16

TIP: When documented, assign code I31.31 for associated malignant pericardial effusion. The neoplasm code should be sequenced first.

C46.5Ø Kaposi's sarcoma of unspecified lung HIV CC HCC

C46.51 Kaposi's sarcoma of right lung HIV CC HCC

C46.52 Kaposi's sarcoma of left lung HIV CC HCC

C46.7 Kaposi's sarcoma of other sites HIV CC HCC

C46.9 Kaposi's sarcoma, unspecified HIV CC HCC

Kaposi's sarcoma of unspecified site

C47 Malignant neoplasm of peripheral nerves and autonomic nervous system

INCLUDES malignant neoplasm of sympathetic and parasympathetic nerves and ganglia

EXCLUDES 1 *Kaposi's sarcoma of soft tissue (C46.1)*

C47.Ø Malignant neoplasm of peripheral nerves of head, face and neck CC HCC

EXCLUDES 1 *malignant neoplasm of peripheral nerves of orbit (C69.6-)*

C47.1 Malignant neoplasm of peripheral nerves of upper limb, including shoulder

C47.1Ø Malignant neoplasm of peripheral nerves of unspecified upper limb, including shoulder CC HCC

C47.11 Malignant neoplasm of peripheral nerves of right upper limb, including shoulder CC HCC

C47.12 Malignant neoplasm of peripheral nerves of left upper limb, including shoulder CC HCC

C47.2 Malignant neoplasm of peripheral nerves of lower limb, including hip

C47.2Ø Malignant neoplasm of peripheral nerves of unspecified lower limb, including hip CC HCC

C47.21 Malignant neoplasm of peripheral nerves of right lower limb, including hip CC HCC

C47.22 Malignant neoplasm of peripheral nerves of left lower limb, including hip CC HCC

C47.3 Malignant neoplasm of peripheral nerves of thorax CC HCC

C47.4 Malignant neoplasm of peripheral nerves of abdomen CC HCC

C47.5 Malignant neoplasm of peripheral nerves of pelvis CC HCC

C47.6 Malignant neoplasm of peripheral nerves of trunk, unspecified CC HCC

Malignant neoplasm of peripheral nerves of unspecified part of trunk

C47.8 Malignant neoplasm of overlapping sites of peripheral nerves and autonomic nervous system CC HCC

C47.9 Malignant neoplasm of peripheral nerves and autonomic nervous system, unspecified CC HCC

Malignant neoplasm of unspecified site of peripheral nerves and autonomic nervous system

C48 Malignant neoplasm of retroperitoneum and peritoneum

EXCLUDES 1 *Kaposi's sarcoma of connective tissue (C46.1)*
mesothelioma (C45.-)

C48.Ø Malignant neoplasm of retroperitoneum CC HCC

C48.1 Malignant neoplasm of specified parts of peritoneum CC HCC

Malignant neoplasm of cul-de-sac
Malignant neoplasm of mesentery
Malignant neoplasm of mesocolon
Malignant neoplasm of omentum
Malignant neoplasm of parietal peritoneum
Malignant neoplasm of pelvic peritoneum

C48.2 Malignant neoplasm of peritoneum, unspecified CC HCC

C48.8 Malignant neoplasm of overlapping sites of retroperitoneum and peritoneum CC HCC

C49 Malignant neoplasm of other connective and soft tissue

INCLUDES malignant neoplasm of blood vessel
malignant neoplasm of bursa
malignant neoplasm of cartilage
malignant neoplasm of fascia
malignant neoplasm of fat
malignant neoplasm of ligament, except uterine
malignant neoplasm of lymphatic vessel
malignant neoplasm of muscle
malignant neoplasm of synovia
malignant neoplasm of tendon (sheath)

EXCLUDES 1 *malignant neoplasm of cartilage (of):*
articular (C4Ø-C41)
larynx (C32.3)
nose (C3Ø.Ø)
malignant neoplasm of connective tissue of breast (C5Ø.-)

EXCLUDES 2 *Kaposi's sarcoma of soft tissue (C46.1)*
malignant neoplasm of heart (C38.Ø)
malignant neoplasm of peripheral nerves and autonomic nervous system (C47.-)
malignant neoplasm of peritoneum (C48.2)
malignant neoplasm of retroperitoneum (C48.Ø)
malignant neoplasm of uterine ligament (C57.3)
mesothelioma (C45.-)

C49.Ø Malignant neoplasm of connective and soft tissue of head, face and neck CC HCC

Malignant neoplasm of connective tissue of ear
Malignant neoplasm of connective tissue of eyelid

EXCLUDES 1 *connective tissue of orbit (C69.6-)*

C49.1 Malignant neoplasm of connective and soft tissue of upper limb, including shoulder

C49.1Ø Malignant neoplasm of connective and soft tissue of unspecified upper limb, including shoulder CC HCC

C49.11 Malignant neoplasm of connective and soft tissue of right upper limb, including shoulder CC HCC

C49.12 Malignant neoplasm of connective and soft tissue of left upper limb, including shoulder CC HCC

C49.2 Malignant neoplasm of connective and soft tissue of lower limb, including hip

C49.2Ø Malignant neoplasm of connective and soft tissue of unspecified lower limb, including hip CC HCC

C49.21 Malignant neoplasm of connective and soft tissue of right lower limb, including hip CC HCC

C49.22 Malignant neoplasm of connective and soft tissue of left lower limb, including hip CC HCC

C49.3 Malignant neoplasm of connective and soft tissue of thorax CC HCC

Malignant neoplasm of axilla
Malignant neoplasm of diaphragm
Malignant neoplasm of great vessels

EXCLUDES 1 *malignant neoplasm of breast (C5Ø.-)*
malignant neoplasm of heart (C38.Ø)
malignant neoplasm of mediastinum (C38.1-C38.3)
malignant neoplasm of thymus (C37)

AHA: 2015,3Q,19

C49.4 Malignant neoplasm of connective and soft tissue of abdomen CC HCC

Malignant neoplasm of abdominal wall
Malignant neoplasm of hypochondrium

C49.5 Malignant neoplasm of connective and soft tissue of pelvis CC HCC

Malignant neoplasm of buttock
Malignant neoplasm of groin
Malignant neoplasm of perineum

C49.6 Malignant neoplasm of connective and soft tissue of trunk, unspecified CC HCC

Malignant neoplasm of back NOS

C49.8 **Malignant neoplasm of overlapping sites of connective and soft tissue** CC HCC
Primary malignant neoplasm of two or more contiguous sites of connective and soft tissue

C49.9 **Malignant neoplasm of connective and soft tissue, unspecified** CC HCC

✓5th C49.A **Gastrointestinal stromal tumor**
AHA: 2016,4Q,8
DEF: Uncommon malignant tumor found in the GI tract that originates from interstitial cells of the autonomic nervous system. Most occur in the stomach or small intestine but can originate anywhere in the GI tract.

C49.AØ **Gastrointestinal stromal tumor, unspecified site** CC HCC
C49.A1 **Gastrointestinal stromal tumor of esophagus** CC HCC
C49.A2 **Gastrointestinal stromal tumor of stomach** CC HCC
C49.A3 **Gastrointestinal stromal tumor of small intestine** CC HCC
C49.A4 **Gastrointestinal stromal tumor of large intestine** CC HCC
C49.A5 **Gastrointestinal stromal tumor of rectum** CC HCC
C49.A9 **Gastrointestinal stromal tumor of other sites** CC HCC

Malignant neoplasms of breast (C5Ø)

✓4th **C5Ø Malignant neoplasm of breast**
INCLUDES connective tissue of breast
Paget's disease of breast
Paget's disease of nipple
Use additional code to identify estrogen receptor status (Z17.Ø, Z17.1)
EXCLUDES 1 *skin of breast (C44.5Ø1, C44.511, C44.521, C44.591)*
AHA: 2017,4Q,19

Female Breast

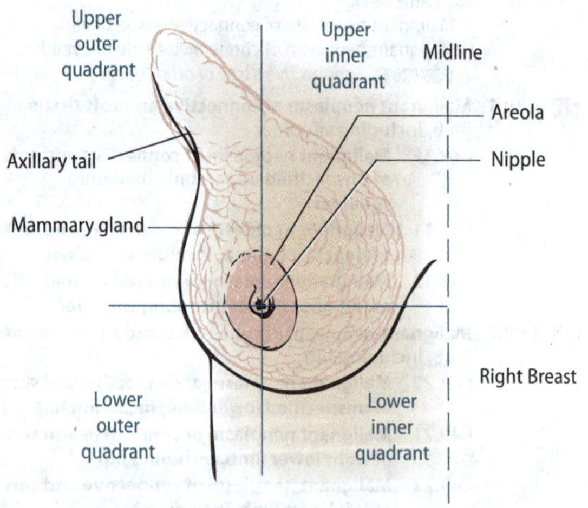

Upper outer quadrant
Upper inner quadrant
Midline
Areola
Axillary tail
Nipple
Mammary gland
Right Breast
Lower outer quadrant
Lower inner quadrant

✓5th C5Ø.Ø **Malignant neoplasm of nipple and areola**
✓6th C5Ø.Ø1 **Malignant neoplasm of nipple and areola, female**
C5Ø.Ø11 **Malignant neoplasm of nipple and areola, right female breast** HCC ♀
C5Ø.Ø12 **Malignant neoplasm of nipple and areola, left female breast** HCC ♀
C5Ø.Ø19 **Malignant neoplasm of nipple and areola, unspecified female breast** HCC ♀
✓6th C5Ø.Ø2 **Malignant neoplasm of nipple and areola, male**
C5Ø.Ø21 **Malignant neoplasm of nipple and areola, right male breast** HCC ♂
C5Ø.Ø22 **Malignant neoplasm of nipple and areola, left male breast** HCC ♂
C5Ø.Ø29 **Malignant neoplasm of nipple and areola, unspecified male breast** HCC ♂

✓5th C5Ø.1 **Malignant neoplasm of central portion of breast**
✓6th C5Ø.11 **Malignant neoplasm of central portion of breast, female**
C5Ø.111 **Malignant neoplasm of central portion of right female breast** HCC ♀
C5Ø.112 **Malignant neoplasm of central portion of left female breast** HCC ♀
C5Ø.119 **Malignant neoplasm of central portion of unspecified female breast** HCC ♀
✓6th C5Ø.12 **Malignant neoplasm of central portion of breast, male**
C5Ø.121 **Malignant neoplasm of central portion of right male breast** HCC ♂
C5Ø.122 **Malignant neoplasm of central portion of left male breast** HCC ♂
C5Ø.129 **Malignant neoplasm of central portion of unspecified male breast** HCC ♂

✓5th C5Ø.2 **Malignant neoplasm of upper-inner quadrant of breast**
✓6th C5Ø.21 **Malignant neoplasm of upper-inner quadrant of breast, female**
C5Ø.211 **Malignant neoplasm of upper-inner quadrant of right female breast** HCC ♀
C5Ø.212 **Malignant neoplasm of upper-inner quadrant of left female breast** HCC ♀
C5Ø.219 **Malignant neoplasm of upper-inner quadrant of unspecified female breast** HCC ♀
✓6th C5Ø.22 **Malignant neoplasm of upper-inner quadrant of breast, male**
C5Ø.221 **Malignant neoplasm of upper-inner quadrant of right male breast** HCC ♂
C5Ø.222 **Malignant neoplasm of upper-inner quadrant of left male breast** HCC ♂
C5Ø.229 **Malignant neoplasm of upper-inner quadrant of unspecified male breast** HCC ♂

✓5th C5Ø.3 **Malignant neoplasm of lower-inner quadrant of breast**
✓6th C5Ø.31 **Malignant neoplasm of lower-inner quadrant of breast, female**
C5Ø.311 **Malignant neoplasm of lower-inner quadrant of right female breast** HCC ♀
C5Ø.312 **Malignant neoplasm of lower-inner quadrant of left female breast** HCC ♀
C5Ø.319 **Malignant neoplasm of lower-inner quadrant of unspecified female breast** HCC ♀
✓6th C5Ø.32 **Malignant neoplasm of lower-inner quadrant of breast, male**
C5Ø.321 **Malignant neoplasm of lower-inner quadrant of right male breast** HCC ♂
C5Ø.322 **Malignant neoplasm of lower-inner quadrant of left male breast** HCC ♂
C5Ø.329 **Malignant neoplasm of lower-inner quadrant of unspecified male breast** HCC ♂

✓5th C5Ø.4 **Malignant neoplasm of upper-outer quadrant of breast**
✓6th C5Ø.41 **Malignant neoplasm of upper-outer quadrant of breast, female**
C5Ø.411 **Malignant neoplasm of upper-outer quadrant of right female breast** HCC ♀
C5Ø.412 **Malignant neoplasm of upper-outer quadrant of left female breast** HCC ♀
C5Ø.419 **Malignant neoplasm of upper-outer quadrant of unspecified female breast** HCC ♀
✓6th C5Ø.42 **Malignant neoplasm of upper-outer quadrant of breast, male**
C5Ø.421 **Malignant neoplasm of upper-outer quadrant of right male breast** HCC ♂
C5Ø.422 **Malignant neoplasm of upper-outer quadrant of left male breast** HCC ♂
C5Ø.429 **Malignant neoplasm of upper-outer quadrant of unspecified male breast** HCC ♂

✓5th C5Ø.5 **Malignant neoplasm of lower-outer quadrant of breast**
✓6th C5Ø.51 **Malignant neoplasm of lower-outer quadrant of breast, female**
C5Ø.511 **Malignant neoplasm of lower-outer quadrant of right female breast** HCC ♀
C5Ø.512 **Malignant neoplasm of lower-outer quadrant of left female breast** HCC ♀
C5Ø.519 **Malignant neoplasm of lower-outer quadrant of unspecified female breast** HCC ♀
✓6th C5Ø.52 **Malignant neoplasm of lower-outer quadrant of breast, male**
C5Ø.521 **Malignant neoplasm of lower-outer quadrant of right male breast** HCC ♂

C50.522 Malignant neoplasm of lower-outer quadrant of left male breast HCC ♂
C50.529 Malignant neoplasm of lower-outer quadrant of unspecified male breast HCC ♂

C50.6 Malignant neoplasm of axillary tail of breast
C50.61 Malignant neoplasm of axillary tail of breast, female
C50.611 Malignant neoplasm of axillary tail of right female breast HCC ♀
C50.612 Malignant neoplasm of axillary tail of left female breast HCC ♀
C50.619 Malignant neoplasm of axillary tail of unspecified female breast HCC ♀
C50.62 Malignant neoplasm of axillary tail of breast, male
C50.621 Malignant neoplasm of axillary tail of right male breast HCC ♂
C50.622 Malignant neoplasm of axillary tail of left male breast HCC ♂
C50.629 Malignant neoplasm of axillary tail of unspecified male breast HCC ♂

C50.8 Malignant neoplasm of overlapping sites of breast
C50.81 Malignant neoplasm of overlapping sites of breast, female
C50.811 Malignant neoplasm of overlapping sites of right female breast HCC ♀
C50.812 Malignant neoplasm of overlapping sites of left female breast HCC ♀
C50.819 Malignant neoplasm of overlapping sites of unspecified female breast HCC ♀
C50.82 Malignant neoplasm of overlapping sites of breast, male
C50.821 Malignant neoplasm of overlapping sites of right male breast HCC ♂
C50.822 Malignant neoplasm of overlapping sites of left male breast HCC ♂
C50.829 Malignant neoplasm of overlapping sites of unspecified male breast HCC ♂

C50.9 Malignant neoplasm of breast of unspecified site
C50.91 Malignant neoplasm of breast of unspecified site, female
AHA: 2022,3Q,10,14
C50.911 Malignant neoplasm of unspecified site of right female breast HCC ♀
C50.912 Malignant neoplasm of unspecified site of left female breast HCC ♀
C50.919 Malignant neoplasm of unspecified site of unspecified female breast HCC ♀
C50.92 Malignant neoplasm of breast of unspecified site, male
C50.921 Malignant neoplasm of unspecified site of right male breast HCC ♂
C50.922 Malignant neoplasm of unspecified site of left male breast HCC ♂
C50.929 Malignant neoplasm of unspecified site of unspecified male breast HCC ♂

Malignant neoplasms of female genital organs (C51-C58)

INCLUDES malignant neoplasm of skin of female genital organs

C51 Malignant neoplasm of vulva
EXCLUDES 1 *carcinoma in situ of vulva (D07.1)*
C51.0 Malignant neoplasm of labium majus HCC ♀
Malignant neoplasm of Bartholin's [greater vestibular] gland
C51.1 Malignant neoplasm of labium minus HCC ♀
C51.2 Malignant neoplasm of clitoris HCC ♀
C51.8 Malignant neoplasm of overlapping sites of vulva HCC ♀
C51.9 Malignant neoplasm of vulva, unspecified HCC ♀
Malignant neoplasm of external female genitalia NOS
Malignant neoplasm of pudendum

C52 Malignant neoplasm of vagina HCC ♀
EXCLUDES 1 *carcinoma in situ of vagina (D07.2)*

C53 Malignant neoplasm of cervix uteri
EXCLUDES 1 *carcinoma in situ of cervix uteri (D06.-)*
AHA: 2017,4Q,103
C53.0 Malignant neoplasm of endocervix HCC ♀
C53.1 Malignant neoplasm of exocervix HCC ♀
C53.8 Malignant neoplasm of overlapping sites of cervix uteri HCC ♀
C53.9 Malignant neoplasm of cervix uteri, unspecified HCC ♀

C54 Malignant neoplasm of corpus uteri
C54.0 Malignant neoplasm of isthmus uteri HCC ♀
Malignant neoplasm of lower uterine segment
C54.1 Malignant neoplasm of endometrium HCC ♀
C54.2 Malignant neoplasm of myometrium HCC ♀
C54.3 Malignant neoplasm of fundus uteri HCC ♀
C54.8 Malignant neoplasm of overlapping sites of corpus uteri HCC ♀
C54.9 Malignant neoplasm of corpus uteri, unspecified HCC ♀

C55 Malignant neoplasm of uterus, part unspecified HCC ♀

C56 Malignant neoplasm of ovary
Use additional code to identify any functional activity
C56.1 Malignant neoplasm of right ovary CC HCC ♀
C56.2 Malignant neoplasm of left ovary CC HCC ♀
C56.3 Malignant neoplasm of bilateral ovaries CC HCC ♀
C56.9 Malignant neoplasm of unspecified ovary CC HCC ♀

C57 Malignant neoplasm of other and unspecified female genital organs
C57.0 Malignant neoplasm of fallopian tube
Malignant neoplasm of oviduct
Malignant neoplasm of uterine tube
C57.00 Malignant neoplasm of unspecified fallopian tube HCC ♀
C57.01 Malignant neoplasm of right fallopian tube HCC ♀
C57.02 Malignant neoplasm of left fallopian tube HCC ♀
C57.1 Malignant neoplasm of broad ligament
C57.10 Malignant neoplasm of unspecified broad ligament HCC ♀
C57.11 Malignant neoplasm of right broad ligament HCC ♀
C57.12 Malignant neoplasm of left broad ligament HCC ♀
C57.2 Malignant neoplasm of round ligament
C57.20 Malignant neoplasm of unspecified round ligament HCC ♀
C57.21 Malignant neoplasm of right round ligament HCC ♀
C57.22 Malignant neoplasm of left round ligament HCC ♀
C57.3 Malignant neoplasm of parametrium HCC ♀
Malignant neoplasm of uterine ligament NOS
C57.4 Malignant neoplasm of uterine adnexa, unspecified HCC ♀
C57.7 Malignant neoplasm of other specified female genital organs HCC ♀
Malignant neoplasm of wolffian body or duct
C57.8 Malignant neoplasm of overlapping sites of female genital organs HCC ♀
Primary malignant neoplasm of two or more contiguous sites of the female genital organs whose point of origin cannot be determined
Primary tubo-ovarian malignant neoplasm whose point of origin cannot be determined
Primary utero-ovarian malignant neoplasm whose point of origin cannot be determined
C57.9 Malignant neoplasm of female genital organ, unspecified HCC ♀
Malignant neoplasm of female genitourinary tract NOS

C58 Malignant neoplasm of placenta HCC M ♀
INCLUDES choriocarcinoma NOS
chorionepithelioma NOS
EXCLUDES 1 *chorioadenoma (destruens) (D39.2)*
hydatidiform mole NOS (O01.9)
invasive hydatidiform mole (D39.2)
male choriocarcinoma NOS (C62.9-)
malignant hydatidiform mole (D39.2)

Malignant neoplasms of male genital organs (C60-C63)

INCLUDES malignant neoplasm of skin of male genital organs

C60 Malignant neoplasm of penis
C60.0 Malignant neoplasm of prepuce HCC ♂
Malignant neoplasm of foreskin
C60.1 Malignant neoplasm of glans penis HCC ♂

C60.2 Malignant neoplasm of body of penis HCC ♂
Malignant neoplasm of corpus cavernosum

C60.8 Malignant neoplasm of overlapping sites of penis HCC ♂

C60.9 Malignant neoplasm of penis, unspecified HCC ♂
Malignant neoplasm of skin of penis NOS

C61 Malignant neoplasm of prostate HCC ♂
Use additional code, if applicable, to identify:
hormone sensitivity status (Z19.1-Z19.2)
rising PSA following treatment for malignant neoplasm of prostate (R97.21)
EXCLUDES 1 *malignant neoplasm of seminal vesicle (C63.7)*
AHA: 2017,1Q,17

C62 Malignant neoplasm of testis
Use additional code to identify any functional activity

C62.0 Malignant neoplasm of undescended testis
Malignant neoplasm of ectopic testis
Malignant neoplasm of retained testis

C62.00 Malignant neoplasm of unspecified undescended testis HCC ♂

C62.01 Malignant neoplasm of undescended right testis HCC ♂

C62.02 Malignant neoplasm of undescended left testis HCC ♂

C62.1 Malignant neoplasm of descended testis
Malignant neoplasm of scrotal testis

C62.10 Malignant neoplasm of unspecified descended testis HCC ♂

C62.11 Malignant neoplasm of descended right testis HCC ♂

C62.12 Malignant neoplasm of descended left testis HCC ♂

C62.9 Malignant neoplasm of testis, unspecified whether descended or undescended

C62.90 Malignant neoplasm of unspecified testis, unspecified whether descended or undescended HCC ♂
Malignant neoplasm of testis NOS

C62.91 Malignant neoplasm of right testis, unspecified whether descended or undescended HCC ♂

C62.92 Malignant neoplasm of left testis, unspecified whether descended or undescended HCC ♂

C63 Malignant neoplasm of other and unspecified male genital organs

C63.0 Malignant neoplasm of epididymis

C63.00 Malignant neoplasm of unspecified epididymis HCC ♂

C63.01 Malignant neoplasm of right epididymis HCC ♂

C63.02 Malignant neoplasm of left epididymis HCC ♂

C63.1 Malignant neoplasm of spermatic cord

C63.10 Malignant neoplasm of unspecified spermatic cord HCC ♂

C63.11 Malignant neoplasm of right spermatic cord HCC ♂

C63.12 Malignant neoplasm of left spermatic cord HCC ♂

C63.2 Malignant neoplasm of scrotum HCC ♂
Malignant neoplasm of skin of scrotum

C63.7 Malignant neoplasm of other specified male genital organs HCC ♂
Malignant neoplasm of seminal vesicle
Malignant neoplasm of tunica vaginalis

C63.8 Malignant neoplasm of overlapping sites of male genital organs HCC ♂
Primary malignant neoplasm of two or more contiguous sites of male genital organs whose point of origin cannot be determined

C63.9 Malignant neoplasm of male genital organ, unspecified HCC ♂
Malignant neoplasm of male genitourinary tract NOS

Malignant neoplasms of urinary tract (C64-C68)

C64 Malignant neoplasm of kidney, except renal pelvis
EXCLUDES 1 *malignant carcinoid tumor of the kidney (C7A.093)*
malignant neoplasm of renal calyces (C65.-)
malignant neoplasm of renal pelvis (C65.-)

C64.1 Malignant neoplasm of right kidney, except renal pelvis CC HCC

C64.2 Malignant neoplasm of left kidney, except renal pelvis CC HCC

C64.9 Malignant neoplasm of unspecified kidney, except renal pelvis CC HCC

C65 Malignant neoplasm of renal pelvis
INCLUDES malignant neoplasm of pelviureteric junction
malignant neoplasm of renal calyces

C65.1 Malignant neoplasm of right renal pelvis CC HCC

C65.2 Malignant neoplasm of left renal pelvis CC HCC

C65.9 Malignant neoplasm of unspecified renal pelvis CC HCC

C66 Malignant neoplasm of ureter
EXCLUDES 1 *malignant neoplasm of ureteric orifice of bladder (C67.6)*

C66.1 Malignant neoplasm of right ureter CC HCC

C66.2 Malignant neoplasm of left ureter CC HCC

C66.9 Malignant neoplasm of unspecified ureter CC HCC

C67 Malignant neoplasm of bladder

C67.0 Malignant neoplasm of trigone of bladder HCC

C67.1 Malignant neoplasm of dome of bladder HCC

C67.2 Malignant neoplasm of lateral wall of bladder HCC

C67.3 Malignant neoplasm of anterior wall of bladder HCC

C67.4 Malignant neoplasm of posterior wall of bladder HCC

C67.5 Malignant neoplasm of bladder neck HCC
Malignant neoplasm of internal urethral orifice

C67.6 Malignant neoplasm of ureteric orifice HCC

C67.7 Malignant neoplasm of urachus HCC

C67.8 Malignant neoplasm of overlapping sites of bladder HCC

C67.9 Malignant neoplasm of bladder, unspecified HCC
AHA: 2016,1Q,19

C68 Malignant neoplasm of other and unspecified urinary organs
EXCLUDES 1 *malignant neoplasm of female genitourinary tract NOS (C57.9)*
malignant neoplasm of male genitourinary tract NOS (C63.9)

C68.0 Malignant neoplasm of urethra CC HCC
EXCLUDES 1 *malignant neoplasm of urethral orifice of bladder (C67.5)*

C68.1 Malignant neoplasm of paraurethral glands CC HCC

C68.8 Malignant neoplasm of overlapping sites of urinary organs CC HCC
Primary malignant neoplasm of two or more contiguous sites of urinary organs whose point of origin cannot be determined

C68.9 Malignant neoplasm of urinary organ, unspecified CC HCC
Malignant neoplasm of urinary system NOS

Malignant neoplasms of eye, brain and other parts of central nervous system (C69-C72)

C69 Malignant neoplasm of eye and adnexa
EXCLUDES 1 *malignant neoplasm of connective tissue of eyelid (C49.0)*
malignant neoplasm of eyelid (skin) (C43.1-, C44.1-)
malignant neoplasm of optic nerve (C72.3-)

C69.0 Malignant neoplasm of conjunctiva

C69.00 Malignant neoplasm of unspecified conjunctiva HCC

C69.01 Malignant neoplasm of right conjunctiva HCC

C69.02 Malignant neoplasm of left conjunctiva HCC

C69.1 Malignant neoplasm of cornea

C69.10 Malignant neoplasm of unspecified cornea HCC

C69.11 Malignant neoplasm of right cornea HCC

C69.12 Malignant neoplasm of left cornea HCC

C69.2 Malignant neoplasm of retina
EXCLUDES 1 *dark area on retina (D49.81)*
neoplasm of unspecified behavior of retina and choroid (D49.81)
retinal freckle (D49.81)

C69.20 Malignant neoplasm of unspecified retina HCC

C69.21 Malignant neoplasm of right retina HCC

C69.22 Malignant neoplasm of left retina HCC

C69.3 Malignant neoplasm of choroid

C69.30 Malignant neoplasm of unspecified choroid HCC

C69.31 Malignant neoplasm of right choroid HCC

C69.32 Malignant neoplasm of left choroid HCC

✓5th **C69.4 Malignant neoplasm of ciliary body**

C69.40 Malignant neoplasm of unspecified ciliary body HCC

C69.41 Malignant neoplasm of right ciliary body HCC

C69.42 Malignant neoplasm of left ciliary body HCC

✓5th **C69.5 Malignant neoplasm of lacrimal gland and duct**

Malignant neoplasm of lacrimal sac
Malignant neoplasm of nasolacrimal duct

C69.50 Malignant neoplasm of unspecified lacrimal gland and duct HCC

C69.51 Malignant neoplasm of right lacrimal gland and duct HCC

C69.52 Malignant neoplasm of left lacrimal gland and duct HCC

✓5th **C69.6 Malignant neoplasm of orbit**

Malignant neoplasm of connective tissue of orbit
Malignant neoplasm of extraocular muscle
Malignant neoplasm of peripheral nerves of orbit
Malignant neoplasm of retrobulbar tissue
Malignant neoplasm of retro-ocular tissue

EXCLUDES 1 *malignant neoplasm of orbital bone (C41.0)*

C69.60 Malignant neoplasm of unspecified orbit HCC

C69.61 Malignant neoplasm of right orbit HCC

C69.62 Malignant neoplasm of left orbit HCC

✓5th **C69.8 Malignant neoplasm of overlapping sites of eye and adnexa**

C69.80 Malignant neoplasm of overlapping sites of unspecified eye and adnexa HCC

C69.81 Malignant neoplasm of overlapping sites of right eye and adnexa HCC

C69.82 Malignant neoplasm of overlapping sites of left eye and adnexa HCC

✓5th **C69.9 Malignant neoplasm of unspecified site of eye**

Malignant neoplasm of eyeball

C69.90 Malignant neoplasm of unspecified site of unspecified eye HCC

C69.91 Malignant neoplasm of unspecified site of right eye HCC

C69.92 Malignant neoplasm of unspecified site of left eye HCC

✓4th **C70 Malignant neoplasm of meninges**

C70.0 Malignant neoplasm of cerebral meninges CC HCC

C70.1 Malignant neoplasm of spinal meninges CC HCC

C70.9 Malignant neoplasm of meninges, unspecified CC HCC

✓4th **C71 Malignant neoplasm of brain**

EXCLUDES 1 *malignant neoplasm of cranial nerves (C72.2-C72.5)*
retrobulbar malignant neoplasm (C69.6-)

Lobes of the Brain

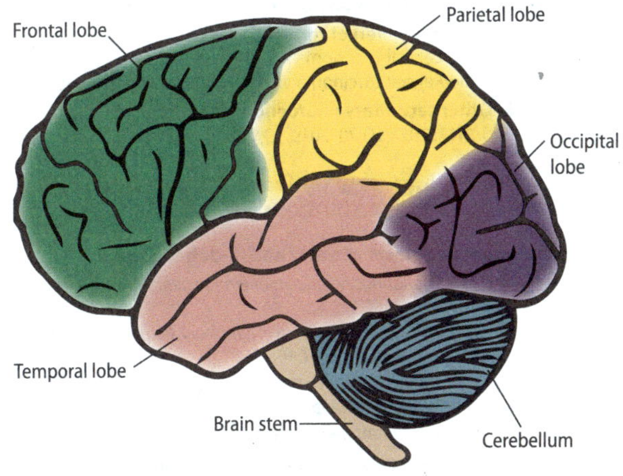

C71.0 Malignant neoplasm of cerebrum, except lobes and ventricles CC HCC

Malignant neoplasm of supratentorial NOS

C71.1 Malignant neoplasm of frontal lobe CC HCC

C71.2 Malignant neoplasm of temporal lobe CC HCC

C71.3 Malignant neoplasm of parietal lobe CC HCC

C71.4 Malignant neoplasm of occipital lobe CC HCC

C71.5 Malignant neoplasm of cerebral ventricle CC HCC

EXCLUDES 1 *malignant neoplasm of fourth cerebral ventricle (C71.7)*

C71.6 Malignant neoplasm of cerebellum CC HCC

C71.7 Malignant neoplasm of brain stem CC HCC

Malignant neoplasm of fourth cerebral ventricle
Infratentorial malignant neoplasm NOS

C71.8 Malignant neoplasm of overlapping sites of brain CC HCC

C71.9 Malignant neoplasm of brain, unspecified CC HCC

AHA: 2014,3Q,3

✓4th **C72 Malignant neoplasm of spinal cord, cranial nerves and other parts of central nervous system**

EXCLUDES 1 *malignant neoplasm of meninges (C70.-)*
malignant neoplasm of peripheral nerves and autonomic nervous system (C47.-)

C72.0 Malignant neoplasm of spinal cord CC HCC

C72.1 Malignant neoplasm of cauda equina CC HCC

✓5th **C72.2 Malignant neoplasm of olfactory nerve**

Malignant neoplasm of olfactory bulb

C72.20 Malignant neoplasm of unspecified olfactory nerve CC HCC

C72.21 Malignant neoplasm of right olfactory nerve CC HCC

C72.22 Malignant neoplasm of left olfactory nerve CC HCC

✓5th **C72.3 Malignant neoplasm of optic nerve**

C72.30 Malignant neoplasm of unspecified optic nerve CC HCC

C72.31 Malignant neoplasm of right optic nerve CC HCC

C72.32 Malignant neoplasm of left optic nerve CC HCC

✓5th **C72.4 Malignant neoplasm of acoustic nerve**

C72.40 Malignant neoplasm of unspecified acoustic nerve CC HCC

C72.41 Malignant neoplasm of right acoustic nerve CC HCC

C72.42 Malignant neoplasm of left acoustic nerve CC HCC

✓5th **C72.5 Malignant neoplasm of other and unspecified cranial nerves**

C72.50 Malignant neoplasm of unspecified cranial nerve CC HCC

Malignant neoplasm of cranial nerve NOS

C72.59 Malignant neoplasm of other cranial nerves CC HCC

C72.9 Malignant neoplasm of central nervous system, unspecified CC HCC

Malignant neoplasm of unspecified site of central nervous system
Malignant neoplasm of nervous system NOS

Malignant neoplasms of thyroid and other endocrine glands (C73-C75)

C73 Malignant neoplasm of thyroid gland HCC

Use additional code to identify any functional activity

✓4th **C74 Malignant neoplasm of adrenal gland**

TIP: If an adrenal gland tumor is described as functioning (producing too much of a hormone), additional codes should be assigned to report the functional activity.

✓5th **C74.0 Malignant neoplasm of cortex of adrenal gland**

C74.00 Malignant neoplasm of cortex of unspecified adrenal gland CC HCC

C74.01 Malignant neoplasm of cortex of right adrenal gland CC HCC

C74.02 Malignant neoplasm of cortex of left adrenal gland CC HCC

✓5th **C74.1 Malignant neoplasm of medulla of adrenal gland**

C74.10 Malignant neoplasm of medulla of unspecified adrenal gland CC HCC

C74.11 Malignant neoplasm of medulla of right adrenal gland CC HCC

C74.12 Malignant neoplasm of medulla of left adrenal gland CC HCC

✓5th **C74.9 Malignant neoplasm of unspecified part of adrenal gland**

C74.90 Malignant neoplasm of unspecified part of unspecified adrenal gland CC HCC

C74.91 Malignant neoplasm of unspecified part of right adrenal gland CC HCC

C74.92 **Malignant neoplasm of unspecified part of left adrenal gland** CC HCC

C75 Malignant neoplasm of other endocrine glands and related structures

EXCLUDES 1 *malignant carcinoid tumors (C7A.0-)*
malignant neoplasm of adrenal gland (C74.-)
malignant neoplasm of endocrine pancreas (C25.4)
malignant neoplasm of islets of Langerhans (C25.4)
malignant neoplasm of ovary (C56.-)
malignant neoplasm of testis (C62.-)
malignant neoplasm of thymus (C37)
malignant neoplasm of thyroid gland (C73)
malignant neuroendocrine tumors (C7A.-)

C75.0 Malignant neoplasm of parathyroid gland CC HCC

C75.1 Malignant neoplasm of pituitary gland CC HCC

C75.2 Malignant neoplasm of craniopharyngeal duct CC HCC

C75.3 Malignant neoplasm of pineal gland CC HCC

C75.4 Malignant neoplasm of carotid body CC HCC

C75.5 Malignant neoplasm of aortic body and other paraganglia CC HCC

C75.8 Malignant neoplasm with pluriglandular involvement, unspecified CC HCC

C75.9 Malignant neoplasm of endocrine gland, unspecified CC HCC

Malignant neuroendocrine tumors (C7A)

C7A Malignant neuroendocrine tumors

Code also any associated multiple endocrine neoplasia [MEN] syndromes (E31.2-)

Use additional code to identify any associated endocrine syndrome, such as:
carcinoid syndrome (E34.0)

EXCLUDES 2 *malignant pancreatic islet cell tumors (C25.4)*
Merkel cell carcinoma (C4A.-)

AHA: 2019,3Q,7

DEF: Tumors comprised of cells that are capable of producing hormonal syndromes in which the normal hormonal balance required to support body system function is adversely affected.

C7A.0 Malignant carcinoid tumors

AHA: 2019,3Q,7

DEF: Specific type of slow-growing neuroendocrine tumors. Carcinoid tumors occur most commonly in the hormone producing cells of the gastrointestinal tracts and can also occur in the pancreas, testes, ovaries, or lungs.

C7A.00 Malignant carcinoid tumor of unspecified site CC HCC

C7A.01 Malignant carcinoid tumors of the small intestine

C7A.010 Malignant carcinoid tumor of the duodenum CC HCC

C7A.011 Malignant carcinoid tumor of the jejunum CC HCC

C7A.012 Malignant carcinoid tumor of the ileum CC HCC

C7A.019 Malignant carcinoid tumor of the small intestine, unspecified portion CC HCC

C7A.02 Malignant carcinoid tumors of the appendix, large intestine, and rectum

C7A.020 Malignant carcinoid tumor of the appendix CC HCC

C7A.021 Malignant carcinoid tumor of the cecum CC HCC

C7A.022 Malignant carcinoid tumor of the ascending colon CC HCC

C7A.023 Malignant carcinoid tumor of the transverse colon CC HCC

C7A.024 Malignant carcinoid tumor of the descending colon CC HCC

C7A.025 Malignant carcinoid tumor of the sigmoid colon CC HCC

C7A.026 Malignant carcinoid tumor of the rectum CC HCC

C7A.029 Malignant carcinoid tumor of the large intestine, unspecified portion CC HCC
Malignant carcinoid tumor of the colon NOS

C7A.09 Malignant carcinoid tumors of other sites

C7A.090 Malignant carcinoid tumor of the bronchus and lung CC HCC

AHA: 2019,1Q,16

TIP: When documented, assign code I31.31 for associated malignant pericardial effusion. The neoplasm code should be sequenced first.

C7A.091 Malignant carcinoid tumor of the thymus CC HCC

C7A.092 Malignant carcinoid tumor of the stomach CC HCC

C7A.093 Malignant carcinoid tumor of the kidney CC HCC

C7A.094 Malignant carcinoid tumor of the foregut, unspecified CC HCC

C7A.095 Malignant carcinoid tumor of the midgut, unspecified CC HCC

C7A.096 Malignant carcinoid tumor of the hindgut, unspecified CC HCC

C7A.098 Malignant carcinoid tumors of other sites CC HCC

C7A.1 Malignant poorly differentiated neuroendocrine tumors CC HCC
Malignant poorly differentiated neuroendocrine tumor NOS
Malignant poorly differentiated neuroendocrine carcinoma, any site
High grade neuroendocrine carcinoma, any site

AHA: 2023,1Q,20-21

C7A.8 Other malignant neuroendocrine tumors CC HCC

AHA: 2019,3Q,7

Secondary neuroendocrine tumors (C7B)

C7B Secondary neuroendocrine tumors

Use additional code to identify any functional activity

C7B.0 Secondary carcinoid tumors

AHA: 2019,3Q,7

DEF: Specific type of slow-growing neuroendocrine tumors. Carcinoid tumors occur most commonly in the hormone producing cells of the gastrointestinal tracts and can also occur in the pancreas, testes, ovaries, or lungs.

C7B.00 Secondary carcinoid tumors, unspecified site HCC

C7B.01 Secondary carcinoid tumors of distant lymph nodes CC HCC

C7B.02 Secondary carcinoid tumors of liver CC HCC

C7B.03 Secondary carcinoid tumors of bone CC HCC

C7B.04 Secondary carcinoid tumors of peritoneum CC HCC
Mesentary metastasis of carcinoid tumor

C7B.09 Secondary carcinoid tumors of other sites CC HCC

C7B.1 Secondary Merkel cell carcinoma HCC
Merkel cell carcinoma nodal presentation
Merkel cell carcinoma visceral metastatic presentation

C7B.8 Other secondary neuroendocrine tumors CC HCC

AHA: 2023,1Q,20; 2019,3Q,7

Malignant neoplasms of ill-defined, other secondary and unspecified sites (C76-C80)

C76 Malignant neoplasm of other and ill-defined sites

EXCLUDES 1 *malignant neoplasm of female genitourinary tract NOS (C57.9)*
malignant neoplasm of lymphoid, hematopoietic and related tissue (C81-C96)
malignant neoplasm of male genitourinary tract NOS (C63.9)
malignant neoplasm of skin (C44.-)
malignant neoplasm of unspecified site NOS (C80.1)

C76.0 Malignant neoplasm of head, face and neck HCC
Malignant neoplasm of cheek NOS
Malignant neoplasm of nose NOS

C76.1 Malignant neoplasm of thorax HCC
Intrathoracic malignant neoplasm NOS
Malignant neoplasm of axilla NOS
Thoracic malignant neoplasm NOS

C76.2 Malignant neoplasm of abdomen HCC

C76.3 **Malignant neoplasm of pelvis** HCC
Malignant neoplasm of groin NOS
Malignant neoplasm of sites overlapping systems within the pelvis
Rectovaginal (septum) malignant neoplasm
Rectovesical (septum) malignant neoplasm

✓5th C76.4 **Malignant neoplasm of upper limb**
C76.40 **Malignant neoplasm of unspecified upper limb** HCC
C76.41 **Malignant neoplasm of right upper limb** HCC
C76.42 **Malignant neoplasm of left upper limb** HCC

✓5th C76.5 **Malignant neoplasm of lower limb**
C76.50 **Malignant neoplasm of unspecified lower limb** HCC
C76.51 **Malignant neoplasm of right lower limb** HCC
C76.52 **Malignant neoplasm of left lower limb** HCC

C76.8 **Malignant neoplasm of other specified ill-defined sites** HCC
Malignant neoplasm of overlapping ill-defined sites

✓4th **C77 Secondary and unspecified malignant neoplasm of lymph nodes**
EXCLUDES 1 *malignant neoplasm of lymph nodes, specified as primary (C81-C86, C88, C96.-)*
mesentary metastasis of carcinoid tumor (C7B.Ø4)
secondary carcinoid tumors of distant lymph nodes (C7B.Ø1)

C77.Ø **Secondary and unspecified malignant neoplasm of lymph nodes of head, face and neck** CC HCC
Secondary and unspecified malignant neoplasm of supraclavicular lymph nodes
AHA: 2022,3Q,14

C77.1 **Secondary and unspecified malignant neoplasm of intrathoracic lymph nodes** CC HCC
C77.2 **Secondary and unspecified malignant neoplasm of intra-abdominal lymph nodes** CC HCC
C77.3 **Secondary and unspecified malignant neoplasm of axilla and upper limb lymph nodes** CC HCC
Secondary and unspecified malignant neoplasm of pectoral lymph nodes
C77.4 **Secondary and unspecified malignant neoplasm of inguinal and lower limb lymph nodes** CC HCC
C77.5 **Secondary and unspecified malignant neoplasm of intrapelvic lymph nodes** CC HCC
C77.8 **Secondary and unspecified malignant neoplasm of lymph nodes of multiple regions** CC HCC
C77.9 **Secondary and unspecified malignant neoplasm of lymph node, unspecified** CC HCC

✓4th **C78 Secondary malignant neoplasm of respiratory and digestive organs**
EXCLUDES 1 *secondary carcinoid tumors of liver (C7B.Ø2)*
secondary carcinoid tumors of peritoneum (C7B.Ø4)
EXCLUDES 2 *lymph node metastases (C77.Ø)*
AHA: 2023,1Q,22

✓5th C78.Ø **Secondary malignant neoplasm of lung**
AHA: 2022,3Q,9; 2019,1Q,16
C78.ØØ **Secondary malignant neoplasm of unspecified lung** CC HCC
C78.Ø1 **Secondary malignant neoplasm of right lung** CC HCC
C78.Ø2 **Secondary malignant neoplasm of left lung** CC HCC
C78.1 **Secondary malignant neoplasm of mediastinum** CC HCC
C78.2 **Secondary malignant neoplasm of pleura** CC HCC

✓5th C78.3 **Secondary malignant neoplasm of other and unspecified respiratory organs**
C78.3Ø **Secondary malignant neoplasm of unspecified respiratory organ** CC HCC
C78.39 **Secondary malignant neoplasm of other respiratory organs** CC HCC
C78.4 **Secondary malignant neoplasm of small intestine** CC HCC
C78.5 **Secondary malignant neoplasm of large intestine and rectum** CC HCC
C78.6 **Secondary malignant neoplasm of retroperitoneum and peritoneum** CC HCC
AHA: 2017,2Q,12
C78.7 **Secondary malignant neoplasm of liver and intrahepatic bile duct** CC HCC
AHA: 2022,3Q,14

✓5th C78.8 **Secondary malignant neoplasm of other and unspecified digestive organs**
C78.8Ø **Secondary malignant neoplasm of unspecified digestive organ** CC HCC
C78.89 **Secondary malignant neoplasm of other digestive organs** CC HCC
Code also exocrine pancreatic insufficiency (K86.81)

✓4th **C79 Secondary malignant neoplasm of other and unspecified sites**
EXCLUDES 1 *secondary carcinoid tumors (C7B.-)*
secondary neuroendocrine tumors (C7B.-)
AHA: 2023,1Q,22

✓5th C79.Ø **Secondary malignant neoplasm of kidney and renal pelvis**
C79.ØØ **Secondary malignant neoplasm of unspecified kidney and renal pelvis** CC HCC
C79.Ø1 **Secondary malignant neoplasm of right kidney and renal pelvis** CC HCC
C79.Ø2 **Secondary malignant neoplasm of left kidney and renal pelvis** CC HCC

✓5th C79.1 **Secondary malignant neoplasm of bladder and other and unspecified urinary organs**
C79.1Ø **Secondary malignant neoplasm of unspecified urinary organs** CC HCC
C79.11 **Secondary malignant neoplasm of bladder** CC HCC
EXCLUDES 2 *lymph node metastases (C77.Ø)*
C79.19 **Secondary malignant neoplasm of other urinary organs** CC HCC
C79.2 **Secondary malignant neoplasm of skin** CC HCC
EXCLUDES 1 *secondary Merkel cell carcinoma (C7B.1)*

✓5th C79.3 **Secondary malignant neoplasm of brain and cerebral meninges**
C79.31 **Secondary malignant neoplasm of brain** CC HCC
AHA: 2022,3Q,9-10
C79.32 **Secondary malignant neoplasm of cerebral meninges** CC HCC
AHA: 2020,1Q,13

✓5th C79.4 **Secondary malignant neoplasm of other and unspecified parts of nervous system**
C79.4Ø **Secondary malignant neoplasm of unspecified part of nervous system** CC HCC
C79.49 **Secondary malignant neoplasm of other parts of nervous system** CC HCC

✓5th C79.5 **Secondary malignant neoplasm of bone and bone marrow**
EXCLUDES 1 *secondary carcinoid tumors of bone (C7B.Ø3)*
C79.51 **Secondary malignant neoplasm of bone** CC HCC
AHA: 2022,3Q,14
TIP: Do not assign in addition to a code from subcategory C90.0 when multiple myeloma is described as metastatic to the bone; bone involvement is integral to multiple myeloma.
C79.52 **Secondary malignant neoplasm of bone marrow** CC HCC

✓5th C79.6 **Secondary malignant neoplasm of ovary**
C79.6Ø **Secondary malignant neoplasm of unspecified ovary** CC HCC ♀
C79.61 **Secondary malignant neoplasm of right ovary** CC HCC ♀
C79.62 **Secondary malignant neoplasm of left ovary** CC HCC ♀
C79.63 **Secondary malignant neoplasm of bilateral ovaries** CC HCC ♀

✓5th C79.7 **Secondary malignant neoplasm of adrenal gland**
C79.7Ø **Secondary malignant neoplasm of unspecified adrenal gland** CC HCC
C79.71 **Secondary malignant neoplasm of right adrenal gland** CC HCC
C79.72 **Secondary malignant neoplasm of left adrenal gland** CC HCC

✓5th C79.8 **Secondary malignant neoplasm of other specified sites**
C79.81 **Secondary malignant neoplasm of breast** CC HCC
C79.82 **Secondary malignant neoplasm of genital organs** CC HCC
C79.89 **Secondary malignant neoplasm of other specified sites** CC HCC
AHA: 2017,2Q,11

C79.9 Secondary malignant neoplasm of unspecified site CC HCC
Metastatic cancer NOS
Metastatic disease NOS
EXCLUDES 1 *carcinomatosis NOS (C80.0)*
generalized cancer NOS (C80.0)
malignant (primary) neoplasm of unspecified site (C80.1)
AHA: 2023,2Q,5

4th C80 Malignant neoplasm without specification of site
EXCLUDES 1 *malignant carcinoid tumor of unspecified site (C7A.00)*
malignant neoplasm of specified multiple sites - code to each site

C80.0 Disseminated malignant neoplasm, unspecified CC HCC
Carcinomatosis NOS
Generalized cancer, unspecified site (primary) (secondary)
Generalized malignancy, unspecified site (primary) (secondary)

C80.1 Malignant (primary) neoplasm, unspecified HCC
Cancer NOS
Cancer unspecified site (primary)
Carcinoma unspecified site (primary)
Malignancy unspecified site (primary)
EXCLUDES 1 *secondary malignant neoplasm of unspecified site (C79.9)*

C80.2 Malignant neoplasm associated with transplanted organ CC UPD HCC
Code first complication of transplanted organ (T86.-)
Use additional code to identify the specific malignancy

Malignant neoplasms of lymphoid, hematopoietic and related tissue (C81-C96)

EXCLUDES 2 *Kaposi's sarcoma of lymph nodes (C46.3)*
secondary and unspecified neoplasm of lymph nodes (C77.-)
secondary neoplasm of bone marrow (C79.52)
secondary neoplasm of spleen (C78.89)

4th C81 Hodgkin lymphoma
EXCLUDES 1 *personal history of Hodgkin lymphoma (Z85.71)*
AHA: 2023,1Q,22
DEF: Malignant disorder of lymphoid cells characterized by the presence of progressively swollen lymph nodes and spleen that may also involve the liver. A diagnosis of Hodgkin's lymphoma can be confirmed by the presence of Reed-Sternberg cells. ***Synonym(s):*** *Hodgkin disease.*

5th C81.0 Nodular lymphocyte predominant Hodgkin lymphoma
C81.00 Nodular lymphocyte predominant Hodgkin lymphoma, unspecified site CC HCC
C81.01 Nodular lymphocyte predominant Hodgkin lymphoma, lymph nodes of head, face, and neck CC HCC
C81.02 Nodular lymphocyte predominant Hodgkin lymphoma, intrathoracic lymph nodes CC HCC
C81.03 Nodular lymphocyte predominant Hodgkin lymphoma, intra-abdominal lymph nodes CC HCC
C81.04 Nodular lymphocyte predominant Hodgkin lymphoma, lymph nodes of axilla and upper limb CC HCC
C81.05 Nodular lymphocyte predominant Hodgkin lymphoma, lymph nodes of inguinal region and lower limb CC HCC
C81.06 Nodular lymphocyte predominant Hodgkin lymphoma, intrapelvic lymph nodes CC HCC
C81.07 Nodular lymphocyte predominant Hodgkin lymphoma, spleen CC HCC
C81.08 Nodular lymphocyte predominant Hodgkin lymphoma, lymph nodes of multiple sites CC HCC
C81.09 Nodular lymphocyte predominant Hodgkin lymphoma, extranodal and solid organ sites CC HCC

5th C81.1 Nodular sclerosis Hodgkin lymphoma
Nodular sclerosis classical Hodgkin lymphoma
C81.10 Nodular sclerosis Hodgkin lymphoma, unspecified site CC HCC
C81.11 Nodular sclerosis Hodgkin lymphoma, lymph nodes of head, face, and neck CC HCC
C81.12 Nodular sclerosis Hodgkin lymphoma, intrathoracic lymph nodes CC HCC
C81.13 Nodular sclerosis Hodgkin lymphoma, intra-abdominal lymph nodes CC HCC
C81.14 Nodular sclerosis Hodgkin lymphoma, lymph nodes of axilla and upper limb CC HCC
C81.15 Nodular sclerosis Hodgkin lymphoma, lymph nodes of inguinal region and lower limb CC HCC
C81.16 Nodular sclerosis Hodgkin lymphoma, intrapelvic lymph nodes CC HCC
C81.17 Nodular sclerosis Hodgkin lymphoma, spleen CC HCC
C81.18 Nodular sclerosis Hodgkin lymphoma, lymph nodes of multiple sites CC HCC
C81.19 Nodular sclerosis Hodgkin lymphoma, extranodal and solid organ sites CC HCC

5th C81.2 Mixed cellularity Hodgkin lymphoma
Mixed cellularity classical Hodgkin lymphoma
C81.20 Mixed cellularity Hodgkin lymphoma, unspecified site CC HCC
C81.21 Mixed cellularity Hodgkin lymphoma, lymph nodes of head, face, and neck CC HCC
C81.22 Mixed cellularity Hodgkin lymphoma, intrathoracic lymph nodes CC HCC
C81.23 Mixed cellularity Hodgkin lymphoma, intra-abdominal lymph nodes CC HCC
C81.24 Mixed cellularity Hodgkin lymphoma, lymph nodes of axilla and upper limb CC HCC
C81.25 Mixed cellularity Hodgkin lymphoma, lymph nodes of inguinal region and lower limb CC HCC
C81.26 Mixed cellularity Hodgkin lymphoma, intrapelvic lymph nodes CC HCC
C81.27 Mixed cellularity Hodgkin lymphoma, spleen CC HCC
C81.28 Mixed cellularity Hodgkin lymphoma, lymph nodes of multiple sites CC HCC
C81.29 Mixed cellularity Hodgkin lymphoma, extranodal and solid organ sites CC HCC

5th C81.3 Lymphocyte depleted Hodgkin lymphoma
Lymphocyte depleted classical Hodgkin lymphoma
C81.30 Lymphocyte depleted Hodgkin lymphoma, unspecified site CC HCC
C81.31 Lymphocyte depleted Hodgkin lymphoma, lymph nodes of head, face, and neck CC HCC
C81.32 Lymphocyte depleted Hodgkin lymphoma, intrathoracic lymph nodes CC HCC
C81.33 Lymphocyte depleted Hodgkin lymphoma, intra-abdominal lymph nodes CC HCC
C81.34 Lymphocyte depleted Hodgkin lymphoma, lymph nodes of axilla and upper limb CC HCC
C81.35 Lymphocyte depleted Hodgkin lymphoma, lymph nodes of inguinal region and lower limb CC HCC
C81.36 Lymphocyte depleted Hodgkin lymphoma, intrapelvic lymph nodes CC HCC
C81.37 Lymphocyte depleted Hodgkin lymphoma, spleen CC HCC
C81.38 Lymphocyte depleted Hodgkin lymphoma, lymph nodes of multiple sites CC HCC
C81.39 Lymphocyte depleted Hodgkin lymphoma, extranodal and solid organ sites CC HCC

5th C81.4 Lymphocyte-rich Hodgkin lymphoma
Lymphocyte-rich classical Hodgkin lymphoma
EXCLUDES 1 *nodular lymphocyte predominant Hodgkin lymphoma (C81.0-)*
C81.40 Lymphocyte-rich Hodgkin lymphoma, unspecified site CC HCC
C81.41 Lymphocyte-rich Hodgkin lymphoma, lymph nodes of head, face, and neck CC HCC
C81.42 Lymphocyte-rich Hodgkin lymphoma, intrathoracic lymph nodes CC HCC
C81.43 Lymphocyte-rich Hodgkin lymphoma, intra-abdominal lymph nodes CC HCC
C81.44 Lymphocyte-rich Hodgkin lymphoma, lymph nodes of axilla and upper limb CC HCC
C81.45 Lymphocyte-rich Hodgkin lymphoma, lymph nodes of inguinal region and lower limb CC HCC
C81.46 Lymphocyte-rich Hodgkin lymphoma, intrapelvic lymph nodes CC HCC
C81.47 Lymphocyte-rich Hodgkin lymphoma, spleen CC HCC
C81.48 Lymphocyte-rich Hodgkin lymphoma, lymph nodes of multiple sites CC HCC
C81.49 Lymphocyte-rich Hodgkin lymphoma, extranodal and solid organ sites CC HCC

C81.7 Other Hodgkin lymphoma
Classical Hodgkin lymphoma NOS
Other classical Hodgkin lymphoma
C81.70 Other Hodgkin lymphoma, unspecified site CC HCC
C81.71 Other Hodgkin lymphoma, lymph nodes of head, face, and neck CC HCC
C81.72 Other Hodgkin lymphoma, intrathoracic lymph nodes CC HCC
C81.73 Other Hodgkin lymphoma, intra-abdominal lymph nodes CC HCC
C81.74 Other Hodgkin lymphoma, lymph nodes of axilla and upper limb CC HCC
C81.75 Other Hodgkin lymphoma, lymph nodes of inguinal region and lower limb CC HCC
C81.76 Other Hodgkin lymphoma, intrapelvic lymph nodes CC HCC
C81.77 Other Hodgkin lymphoma, spleen CC HCC
C81.78 Other Hodgkin lymphoma, lymph nodes of multiple sites CC HCC
C81.79 Other Hodgkin lymphoma, extranodal and solid organ sites CC HCC

C81.9 Hodgkin lymphoma, unspecified
C81.90 Hodgkin lymphoma, unspecified, unspecified site CC HCC
C81.91 Hodgkin lymphoma, unspecified, lymph nodes of head, face, and neck CC HCC
C81.92 Hodgkin lymphoma, unspecified, intrathoracic lymph nodes CC HCC
C81.93 Hodgkin lymphoma, unspecified, intra-abdominal lymph nodes CC HCC
C81.94 Hodgkin lymphoma, unspecified, lymph nodes of axilla and upper limb CC HCC
C81.95 Hodgkin lymphoma, unspecified, lymph nodes of inguinal region and lower limb CC HCC
C81.96 Hodgkin lymphoma, unspecified, intrapelvic lymph nodes CC HCC
C81.97 Hodgkin lymphoma, unspecified, spleen CC HCC
C81.98 Hodgkin lymphoma, unspecified, lymph nodes of multiple sites CC HCC
C81.99 Hodgkin lymphoma, unspecified, extranodal and solid organ sites CC HCC

C82 Follicular lymphoma
INCLUDES follicular lymphoma with or without diffuse areas
EXCLUDES 1 *mature T/NK-cell lymphomas (C84.-)*
personal history of non-Hodgkin lymphoma (Z85.72)
AHA: 2023,1Q,22
DEF: Most common subgroup of non-Hodgkin lymphomas (NHL), accounting for 20 to 30 percent of all NHLs. NHL is a B-cell lymphoma that is slow growing and characterized by the circular pattern of malignant cell growth with the cells clustered into identifiable nodules or follicles.

C82.0 Follicular lymphoma grade I
C82.00 Follicular lymphoma grade I, unspecified site CC HCC
C82.01 Follicular lymphoma grade I, lymph nodes of head, face, and neck CC HCC
C82.02 Follicular lymphoma grade I, intrathoracic lymph nodes CC HCC
C82.03 Follicular lymphoma grade I, intra-abdominal lymph nodes CC HCC
C82.04 Follicular lymphoma grade I, lymph nodes of axilla and upper limb CC HCC
C82.05 Follicular lymphoma grade I, lymph nodes of inguinal region and lower limb CC HCC
C82.06 Follicular lymphoma grade I, intrapelvic lymph nodes CC HCC
C82.07 Follicular lymphoma grade I, spleen CC HCC
C82.08 Follicular lymphoma grade I, lymph nodes of multiple sites CC HCC
C82.09 Follicular lymphoma grade I, extranodal and solid organ sites CC HCC

C82.1 Follicular lymphoma grade II
C82.10 Follicular lymphoma grade II, unspecified site CC HCC
C82.11 Follicular lymphoma grade II, lymph nodes of head, face, and neck CC HCC
C82.12 Follicular lymphoma grade II, intrathoracic lymph nodes CC HCC
C82.13 Follicular lymphoma grade II, intra-abdominal lymph nodes CC HCC
C82.14 Follicular lymphoma grade II, lymph nodes of axilla and upper limb CC HCC
C82.15 Follicular lymphoma grade II, lymph nodes of inguinal region and lower limb CC HCC
C82.16 Follicular lymphoma grade II, intrapelvic lymph nodes CC HCC
C82.17 Follicular lymphoma grade II, spleen CC HCC
C82.18 Follicular lymphoma grade II, lymph nodes of multiple sites CC HCC
C82.19 Follicular lymphoma grade II, extranodal and solid organ sites CC HCC

C82.2 Follicular lymphoma grade III, unspecified
C82.20 Follicular lymphoma grade III, unspecified, unspecified site CC HCC
C82.21 Follicular lymphoma grade III, unspecified, lymph nodes of head, face, and neck CC HCC
C82.22 Follicular lymphoma grade III, unspecified, intrathoracic lymph nodes CC HCC
C82.23 Follicular lymphoma grade III, unspecified, intra-abdominal lymph nodes CC HCC
C82.24 Follicular lymphoma grade III, unspecified, lymph nodes of axilla and upper limb CC HCC
C82.25 Follicular lymphoma grade III, unspecified, lymph nodes of inguinal region and lower limb CC HCC
C82.26 Follicular lymphoma grade III, unspecified, intrapelvic lymph nodes CC HCC
C82.27 Follicular lymphoma grade III, unspecified, spleen CC HCC
C82.28 Follicular lymphoma grade III, unspecified, lymph nodes of multiple sites CC HCC
C82.29 Follicular lymphoma grade III, unspecified, extranodal and solid organ sites CC HCC

C82.3 Follicular lymphoma grade IIIa
C82.30 Follicular lymphoma grade IIIa, unspecified site CC HCC
C82.31 Follicular lymphoma grade IIIa, lymph nodes of head, face, and neck CC HCC
C82.32 Follicular lymphoma grade IIIa, intrathoracic lymph nodes CC HCC
C82.33 Follicular lymphoma grade IIIa, intra-abdominal lymph nodes CC HCC
C82.34 Follicular lymphoma grade IIIa, lymph nodes of axilla and upper limb CC HCC
C82.35 Follicular lymphoma grade IIIa, lymph nodes of inguinal region and lower limb CC HCC
C82.36 Follicular lymphoma grade IIIa, intrapelvic lymph nodes CC HCC
C82.37 Follicular lymphoma grade IIIa, spleen CC HCC
C82.38 Follicular lymphoma grade IIIa, lymph nodes of multiple sites CC HCC
C82.39 Follicular lymphoma grade IIIa, extranodal and solid organ sites CC HCC

C82.4 Follicular lymphoma grade IIIb
C82.40 Follicular lymphoma grade IIIb, unspecified site CC HCC
C82.41 Follicular lymphoma grade IIIb, lymph nodes of head, face, and neck CC HCC
C82.42 Follicular lymphoma grade IIIb, intrathoracic lymph nodes CC HCC
C82.43 Follicular lymphoma grade IIIb, intra-abdominal lymph nodes CC HCC
C82.44 Follicular lymphoma grade IIIb, lymph nodes of axilla and upper limb CC HCC
C82.45 Follicular lymphoma grade IIIb, lymph nodes of inguinal region and lower limb CC HCC
C82.46 Follicular lymphoma grade IIIb, intrapelvic lymph nodes CC HCC
C82.47 Follicular lymphoma grade IIIb, spleen CC HCC
C82.48 Follicular lymphoma grade IIIb, lymph nodes of multiple sites CC HCC
C82.49 Follicular lymphoma grade IIIb, extranodal and solid organ sites CC HCC

C82.5 Diffuse follicle center lymphoma
C82.50 Diffuse follicle center lymphoma, unspecified site HIV CC HCC
C82.51 Diffuse follicle center lymphoma, lymph nodes of head, face, and neck HIV CC HCC

C82.52 Diffuse follicle center lymphoma, intrathoracic lymph nodes HIV CC HCC
C82.53 Diffuse follicle center lymphoma, intra-abdominal lymph nodes HIV CC HCC
C82.54 Diffuse follicle center lymphoma, lymph nodes of axilla and upper limb HIV CC HCC
C82.55 Diffuse follicle center lymphoma, lymph nodes of inguinal region and lower limb HIV CC HCC
C82.56 Diffuse follicle center lymphoma, intrapelvic lymph nodes HIV CC HCC
C82.57 Diffuse follicle center lymphoma, spleen HIV CC HCC
C82.58 Diffuse follicle center lymphoma, lymph nodes of multiple sites HIV CC HCC
C82.59 Diffuse follicle center lymphoma, extranodal and solid organ sites HIV CC HCC

✓5th C82.6 Cutaneous follicle center lymphoma

C82.60 Cutaneous follicle center lymphoma, unspecified site CC HCC
C82.61 Cutaneous follicle center lymphoma, lymph nodes of head, face, and neck CC HCC
C82.62 Cutaneous follicle center lymphoma, intrathoracic lymph nodes CC HCC
C82.63 Cutaneous follicle center lymphoma, intra-abdominal lymph nodes CC HCC
C82.64 Cutaneous follicle center lymphoma, lymph nodes of axilla and upper limb CC HCC
C82.65 Cutaneous follicle center lymphoma, lymph nodes of inguinal region and lower limb CC HCC
C82.66 Cutaneous follicle center lymphoma, intrapelvic lymph nodes CC HCC
C82.67 Cutaneous follicle center lymphoma, spleen CC HCC
C82.68 Cutaneous follicle center lymphoma, lymph nodes of multiple sites CC HCC
C82.69 Cutaneous follicle center lymphoma, extranodal and solid organ sites CC HCC

✓5th C82.8 Other types of follicular lymphoma

C82.80 Other types of follicular lymphoma, unspecified site CC HCC
C82.81 Other types of follicular lymphoma, lymph nodes of head, face, and neck CC HCC
C82.82 Other types of follicular lymphoma, intrathoracic lymph nodes CC HCC
C82.83 Other types of follicular lymphoma, intra-abdominal lymph nodes CC HCC
C82.84 Other types of follicular lymphoma, lymph nodes of axilla and upper limb CC HCC
C82.85 Other types of follicular lymphoma, lymph nodes of inguinal region and lower limb CC HCC
C82.86 Other types of follicular lymphoma, intrapelvic lymph nodes CC HCC
C82.87 Other types of follicular lymphoma, spleen CC HCC
C82.88 Other types of follicular lymphoma, lymph nodes of multiple sites CC HCC
C82.89 Other types of follicular lymphoma, extranodal and solid organ sites CC HCC

✓5th C82.9 Follicular lymphoma, unspecified

C82.90 Follicular lymphoma, unspecified, unspecified site CC HCC
C82.91 Follicular lymphoma, unspecified, lymph nodes of head, face, and neck CC HCC
C82.92 Follicular lymphoma, unspecified, intrathoracic lymph nodes CC HCC
C82.93 Follicular lymphoma, unspecified, intra-abdominal lymph nodes CC HCC
C82.94 Follicular lymphoma, unspecified, lymph nodes of axilla and upper limb CC HCC
C82.95 Follicular lymphoma, unspecified, lymph nodes of inguinal region and lower limb CC HCC
C82.96 Follicular lymphoma, unspecified, intrapelvic lymph nodes CC HCC
C82.97 Follicular lymphoma, unspecified, spleen CC HCC
C82.98 Follicular lymphoma, unspecified, lymph nodes of multiple sites CC HCC
C82.99 Follicular lymphoma, unspecified, extranodal and solid organ sites CC HCC

✓4th C83 Non-follicular lymphoma

EXCLUDES 1 *personal history of non-Hodgkin lymphoma (Z85.72)*

AHA: 2023,1Q,22

✓5th C83.0 Small cell B-cell lymphoma

Lymphoplasmacytic lymphoma
Nodal marginal zone lymphoma
Non-leukemic variant of B-CLL
Splenic marginal zone lymphoma

EXCLUDES 1 *chronic lymphocytic leukemia (C91.1)*
mature T/NK-cell lymphomas (C84.-)
Waldenstrom macroglobulinemia (C88.0)

AHA: 2023,1Q,18

DEF: Nonfollicular lymphoma that is rare, slow growing, and usually found in the older population.

C83.00 Small cell B-cell lymphoma, unspecified site HIV CC HCC
C83.01 Small cell B-cell lymphoma, lymph nodes of head, face, and neck HIV CC HCC
C83.02 Small cell B-cell lymphoma, intrathoracic lymph nodes HIV CC HCC
C83.03 Small cell B-cell lymphoma, intra-abdominal lymph nodes HIV CC HCC
C83.04 Small cell B-cell lymphoma, lymph nodes of axilla and upper limb HIV CC HCC
C83.05 Small cell B-cell lymphoma, lymph nodes of inguinal region and lower limb HIV CC HCC
C83.06 Small cell B-cell lymphoma, intrapelvic lymph nodes HIV CC HCC
C83.07 Small cell B-cell lymphoma, spleen HIV CC HCC
C83.08 Small cell B-cell lymphoma, lymph nodes of multiple sites HIV CC HCC
C83.09 Small cell B-cell lymphoma, extranodal and solid organ sites HIV CC HCC

✓5th C83.1 Mantle cell lymphoma

Centrocytic lymphoma
Malignant lymphomatous polyposis

DEF: Rare form of B-cell non-Hodgkin lymphoma named for the location of the tumor cell production, the mantle zone of the lymph nodes.

C83.10 Mantle cell lymphoma, unspecified site HIV CC HCC
C83.11 Mantle cell lymphoma, lymph nodes of head, face, and neck HIV CC HCC
C83.12 Mantle cell lymphoma, intrathoracic lymph nodes HIV CC HCC
C83.13 Mantle cell lymphoma, intra-abdominal lymph nodes HIV CC HCC
C83.14 Mantle cell lymphoma, lymph nodes of axilla and upper limb HIV CC HCC
C83.15 Mantle cell lymphoma, lymph nodes of inguinal region and lower limb HIV CC HCC
C83.16 Mantle cell lymphoma, intrapelvic lymph nodes HIV CC HCC
C83.17 Mantle cell lymphoma, spleen HIV CC HCC
C83.18 Mantle cell lymphoma, lymph nodes of multiple sites HIV CC HCC
C83.19 Mantle cell lymphoma, extranodal and solid organ sites HIV CC HCC

✓5th C83.3 Diffuse large B-cell lymphoma

Anaplastic diffuse large B-cell lymphoma
CD30-positive diffuse large B-cell lymphoma
Centroblastic diffuse large B-cell lymphoma
Diffuse large B-cell lymphoma, subtype not specified
Immunoblastic diffuse large B-cell lymphoma
Plasmablastic diffuse large B-cell lymphoma
T-cell rich diffuse large B-cell lymphoma

EXCLUDES 1 *mediastinal (thymic) large B-cell lymphoma (C85.2-)*
mature T/NK-cell lymphomas (C84.-)

DEF: Nonfollicular lymphoma that is one of the more common types of lymphoma. This cancer is fast growing and affects any age but is found mostly in the older population.

C83.30 Diffuse large B-cell lymphoma, unspecified site HIV CC HCC
C83.31 Diffuse large B-cell lymphoma, lymph nodes of head, face, and neck HIV CC HCC
C83.32 Diffuse large B-cell lymphoma, intrathoracic lymph nodes HIV CC HCC
C83.33 Diffuse large B-cell lymphoma, intra-abdominal lymph nodes HIV CC HCC

C83.34 Diffuse large B-cell lymphoma, lymph nodes of axilla and upper limb HIV CC HCC

C83.35 Diffuse large B-cell lymphoma, lymph nodes of inguinal region and lower limb HIV CC HCC

C83.36 Diffuse large B-cell lymphoma, intrapelvic lymph nodes HIV CC HCC

C83.37 Diffuse large B-cell lymphoma, spleen HIV CC HCC

C83.38 Diffuse large B-cell lymphoma, lymph nodes of multiple sites HIV CC HCC
AHA: 2023,1Q,22

C83.39 Diffuse large B-cell lymphoma, extranodal and solid organ sites HIV CC HCC
AHA: 2023,1Q,22

✓5th C83.5 Lymphoblastic (diffuse) lymphoma

B-precursor lymphoma
Lymphoblastic B-cell lymphoma
Lymphoblastic lymphoma NOS
Lymphoblastic T-cell lymphoma
T-precursor lymphoma

DEF: Type of non-Hodgkin lymphoma considered lymphoma or leukemia—the determination is made based on the amount of bone marrow involvement. The cells are small to medium immature T-cells that often originate in the thymus where many of the T-cells are made.

C83.50 Lymphoblastic (diffuse) lymphoma, unspecified site CC HCC

C83.51 Lymphoblastic (diffuse) lymphoma, lymph nodes of head, face, and neck CC HCC

C83.52 Lymphoblastic (diffuse) lymphoma, intrathoracic lymph nodes CC HCC

C83.53 Lymphoblastic (diffuse) lymphoma, intra-abdominal lymph nodes CC HCC

C83.54 Lymphoblastic (diffuse) lymphoma, lymph nodes of axilla and upper limb CC HCC

C83.55 Lymphoblastic (diffuse) lymphoma, lymph nodes of inguinal region and lower limb CC HCC

C83.56 Lymphoblastic (diffuse) lymphoma, intrapelvic lymph nodes CC HCC

C83.57 Lymphoblastic (diffuse) lymphoma, spleen CC HCC

C83.58 Lymphoblastic (diffuse) lymphoma, lymph nodes of multiple sites CC HCC

C83.59 Lymphoblastic (diffuse) lymphoma, extranodal and solid organ sites CC HCC

✓5th C83.7 Burkitt lymphoma

Atypical Burkitt lymphoma
Burkitt-like lymphoma

EXCLUDES 1 *mature B-cell leukemia Burkitt type (C91.A-)*

DEF: Malignancy of the lymphatic system, most often seen as a large bone-deteriorating lesion within the jaw or as an abdominal mass. It is a form of non-Hodgkin's lymphoma and is recognized as the fastest growing human tumor.

C83.70 Burkitt lymphoma, unspecified site HIV CC HCC

C83.71 Burkitt lymphoma, lymph nodes of head, face, and neck HIV CC HCC

C83.72 Burkitt lymphoma, intrathoracic lymph nodes HIV CC HCC

C83.73 Burkitt lymphoma, intra-abdominal lymph nodes HIV CC HCC

C83.74 Burkitt lymphoma, lymph nodes of axilla and upper limb HIV CC HCC

C83.75 Burkitt lymphoma, lymph nodes of inguinal region and lower limb HIV CC HCC

C83.76 Burkitt lymphoma, intrapelvic lymph nodes HIV CC HCC

C83.77 Burkitt lymphoma, spleen HIV CC HCC

C83.78 Burkitt lymphoma, lymph nodes of multiple sites HIV CC HCC

C83.79 Burkitt lymphoma, extranodal and solid organ sites HIV CC HCC

✓5th C83.8 Other non-follicular lymphoma

Intravascular large B-cell lymphoma
Lymphoid granulomatosis
Primary effusion B-cell lymphoma

EXCLUDES 1 *mediastinal (thymic) large B-cell lymphoma (C85.2-)*
T-cell rich B-cell lymphoma (C83.3-)

C83.80 Other non-follicular lymphoma, unspecified site HIV CC HCC

C83.81 Other non-follicular lymphoma, lymph nodes of head, face, and neck HIV CC HCC

C83.82 Other non-follicular lymphoma, intrathoracic lymph nodes HIV CC HCC

C83.83 Other non-follicular lymphoma, intra-abdominal lymph nodes HIV CC HCC

C83.84 Other non-follicular lymphoma, lymph nodes of axilla and upper limb HIV CC HCC

C83.85 Other non-follicular lymphoma, lymph nodes of inguinal region and lower limb HIV CC HCC

C83.86 Other non-follicular lymphoma, intrapelvic lymph nodes HIV CC HCC

C83.87 Other non-follicular lymphoma, spleen HIV CC HCC

C83.88 Other non-follicular lymphoma, lymph nodes of multiple sites HIV CC HCC

C83.89 Other non-follicular lymphoma, extranodal and solid organ sites HIV CC HCC

✓5th C83.9 Non-follicular (diffuse) lymphoma, unspecified

C83.90 Non-follicular (diffuse) lymphoma, unspecified, unspecified site HIV CC HCC

C83.91 Non-follicular (diffuse) lymphoma, unspecified, lymph nodes of head, face, and neck HIV CC HCC

C83.92 Non-follicular (diffuse) lymphoma, unspecified, intrathoracic lymph nodes HIV CC HCC

C83.93 Non-follicular (diffuse) lymphoma, unspecified, intra-abdominal lymph nodes HIV CC HCC

C83.94 Non-follicular (diffuse) lymphoma, unspecified, lymph nodes of axilla and upper limb HIV CC HCC

C83.95 Non-follicular (diffuse) lymphoma, unspecified, lymph nodes of inguinal region and lower limb HIV CC HCC

C83.96 Non-follicular (diffuse) lymphoma, unspecified, intrapelvic lymph nodes HIV CC HCC

C83.97 Non-follicular (diffuse) lymphoma, unspecified, spleen HIV CC HCC

C83.98 Non-follicular (diffuse) lymphoma, unspecified, lymph nodes of multiple sites HIV CC HCC

C83.99 Non-follicular (diffuse) lymphoma, unspecified, extranodal and solid organ sites HIV CC HCC

✓4th C84 Mature T/NK-cell lymphomas

EXCLUDES 1 *personal history of non-Hodgkin lymphoma (Z85.72)*

AHA: 2023,1Q,22

✓5th C84.0 Mycosis fungoides

EXCLUDES 1 *peripheral T-cell lymphoma, not elsewhere classified (C84.4-)*

DEF: Most common form of cutaneous T-cell lymphoma. A type of non-Hodgkin lymphoma in which white blood cells become cancerous and affect the skin and sometimes internal organs.
Synonym(s): *Alibert-Bazin syndrome.*

C84.00 Mycosis fungoides, unspecified site CC HCC

C84.01 Mycosis fungoides, lymph nodes of head, face, and neck CC HCC

C84.02 Mycosis fungoides, intrathoracic lymph nodes CC HCC

C84.03 Mycosis fungoides, intra-abdominal lymph nodes CC HCC

C84.04 Mycosis fungoides, lymph nodes of axilla and upper limb CC HCC

C84.05 Mycosis fungoides, lymph nodes of inguinal region and lower limb CC HCC

C84.06 Mycosis fungoides, intrapelvic lymph nodes CC HCC

C84.07 Mycosis fungoides, spleen CC HCC

C84.08 Mycosis fungoides, lymph nodes of multiple sites CC HCC

C84.09 Mycosis fungoides, extranodal and solid organ sites CC HCC

✓5th C84.1 Sezary disease

DEF: Extension of mycosis fungoides that affects the blood and all of the skin, appearing as sunburn, rather than patches. It spreads to the lymph nodes and is often linked to a weakened immune system.

C84.10 Sezary disease, unspecified site CC HCC

C84.11 Sezary disease, lymph nodes of head, face, and neck CC HCC

C84.12 Sezary disease, intrathoracic lymph nodes CC HCC

C84.13 Sezary disease, intra-abdominal lymph nodes CC HCC

C84.14 **Sezary disease, lymph nodes of axilla and upper limb** CC HCC

C84.15 **Sezary disease, lymph nodes of inguinal region and lower limb** CC HCC

C84.16 **Sezary disease, intrapelvic lymph nodes** CC HCC

C84.17 **Sezary disease, spleen** CC HCC

C84.18 **Sezary disease, lymph nodes of multiple sites** CC HCC

C84.19 **Sezary disease, extranodal and solid organ sites** CC HCC

✓5th **C84.4 Peripheral T-cell lymphoma, not elsewhere classified**

Lennert's lymphoma
Lymphoepithelioid lymphoma
Mature T-cell lymphoma, not elsewhere classified

C84.4Ø **Peripheral T-cell lymphoma, not elsewhere classified, unspecified site** HIV CC HCC

C84.41 **Peripheral T-cell lymphoma, not elsewhere classified, lymph nodes of head, face, and neck** HIV CC HCC

C84.42 **Peripheral T-cell lymphoma, not elsewhere classified, intrathoracic lymph nodes** HIV CC HCC

C84.43 **Peripheral T-cell lymphoma, not elsewhere classified, intra-abdominal lymph nodes** HIV CC HCC

C84.44 **Peripheral T-cell lymphoma, not elsewhere classified, lymph nodes of axilla and upper limb** HIV CC HCC

C84.45 **Peripheral T-cell lymphoma, not elsewhere classified, lymph nodes of inguinal region and lower limb** HIV CC HCC

C84.46 **Peripheral T-cell lymphoma, not elsewhere classified, intrapelvic lymph nodes** HIV CC HCC

C84.47 **Peripheral T-cell lymphoma, not elsewhere classified, spleen** HIV CC HCC

C84.48 **Peripheral T-cell lymphoma, not elsewhere classified, lymph nodes of multiple sites** HIV CC HCC

C84.49 **Peripheral T-cell lymphoma, not elsewhere classified, extranodal and solid organ sites** HIV CC HCC

✓5th **C84.6 Anaplastic large cell lymphoma, ALK-positive**

Anaplastic large cell lymphoma, CD3Ø-positive

C84.6Ø **Anaplastic large cell lymphoma, ALK-positive, unspecified site** HIV CC HCC

C84.61 **Anaplastic large cell lymphoma, ALK-positive, lymph nodes of head, face, and neck** HIV CC HCC

C84.62 **Anaplastic large cell lymphoma, ALK-positive, intrathoracic lymph nodes** HIV CC HCC

C84.63 **Anaplastic large cell lymphoma, ALK-positive, intra-abdominal lymph nodes** HIV CC HCC

C84.64 **Anaplastic large cell lymphoma, ALK-positive, lymph nodes of axilla and upper limb** HIV CC HCC

C84.65 **Anaplastic large cell lymphoma, ALK-positive, lymph nodes of inguinal region and lower limb** HIV CC HCC

C84.66 **Anaplastic large cell lymphoma, ALK-positive, intrapelvic lymph nodes** HIV CC HCC

C84.67 **Anaplastic large cell lymphoma, ALK-positive, spleen** HIV CC HCC

C84.68 **Anaplastic large cell lymphoma, ALK-positive, lymph nodes of multiple sites** HIV CC HCC

C84.69 **Anaplastic large cell lymphoma, ALK-positive, extranodal and solid organ sites** HIV CC HCC

✓5th **C84.7 Anaplastic large cell lymphoma, ALK-negative**

EXCLUDES 1 *primary cutaneous CD3Ø-positive T-cell proliferations (C86.6-)*

C84.7Ø **Anaplastic large cell lymphoma, ALK-negative, unspecified site** HIV CC HCC

C84.71 **Anaplastic large cell lymphoma, ALK-negative, lymph nodes of head, face, and neck** HIV CC HCC

C84.72 **Anaplastic large cell lymphoma, ALK-negative, intrathoracic lymph nodes** HIV CC HCC

C84.73 **Anaplastic large cell lymphoma, ALK-negative, intra-abdominal lymph nodes** HIV CC HCC

C84.74 **Anaplastic large cell lymphoma, ALK-negative, lymph nodes of axilla and upper limb** HIV CC HCC

C84.75 **Anaplastic large cell lymphoma, ALK-negative, lymph nodes of inguinal region and lower limb** HIV CC HCC

C84.76 **Anaplastic large cell lymphoma, ALK-negative, intrapelvic lymph nodes** HIV CC HCC

C84.77 **Anaplastic large cell lymphoma, ALK-negative, spleen** HIV CC HCC

C84.78 **Anaplastic large cell lymphoma, ALK-negative, lymph nodes of multiple sites** HIV CC HCC

C84.79 **Anaplastic large cell lymphoma, ALK-negative, extranodal and solid organ sites** HIV CC HCC

C84.7A **Anaplastic large cell lymphoma, ALK-negative, breast** HIV CC HCC

Breast implant associated anaplastic large cell lymphoma (BIA-ALCL)

Use additional code to identify:
breast implant status (Z98.82)
personal history of breast implant removal (Z98.86)

AHA: 2021,4Q,6

✓5th **C84.A Cutaneous T-cell lymphoma, unspecified**

AHA: 2021,2Q,6

C84.AØ **Cutaneous T-cell lymphoma, unspecified, unspecified site** HIV CC HCC

C84.A1 **Cutaneous T-cell lymphoma, unspecified lymph nodes of head, face, and neck** HIV CC HCC

C84.A2 **Cutaneous T-cell lymphoma, unspecified, intrathoracic lymph nodes** HIV CC HCC

C84.A3 **Cutaneous T-cell lymphoma, unspecified, intra-abdominal lymph nodes** HIV CC HCC

C84.A4 **Cutaneous T-cell lymphoma, unspecified, lymph nodes of axilla and upper limb** HIV CC HCC

C84.A5 **Cutaneous T-cell lymphoma, unspecified, lymph nodes of inguinal region and lower limb** HIV CC HCC

C84.A6 **Cutaneous T-cell lymphoma, unspecified, intrapelvic lymph nodes** HIV CC HCC

C84.A7 **Cutaneous T-cell lymphoma, unspecified, spleen** HIV CC HCC

C84.A8 **Cutaneous T-cell lymphoma, unspecified, lymph nodes of multiple sites** HIV CC HCC

C84.A9 **Cutaneous T-cell lymphoma, unspecified, extranodal and solid organ sites** HIV CC HCC

✓5th **C84.Z Other mature T/NK-cell lymphomas**

NOTE If T-cell lineage or involvement is mentioned in conjunction with a specific lymphoma, code to the more specific description.

EXCLUDES 1 *angioimmunoblastic T-cell lymphoma (C86.5)*
blastic NK-cell lymphoma (C86.4)
enteropathy-type T-cell lymphoma (C86.2)
extranodal NK-cell lymphoma, nasal type (C86.Ø)
hepatosplenic T-cell lymphoma (C86.1)
primary cutaneous CD3Ø-positive T-cell proliferations (C86.6)
subcutaneous panniculitis-like T-cell lymphoma (C86.3)
T-cell leukemia (C91.1-)

C84.ZØ **Other mature T/NK-cell lymphomas, unspecified site** HIV CC HCC

C84.Z1 **Other mature T/NK-cell lymphomas, lymph nodes of head, face, and neck** HIV CC HCC

C84.Z2 **Other mature T/NK-cell lymphomas, intrathoracic lymph nodes** HIV CC HCC

C84.Z3 **Other mature T/NK-cell lymphomas, intra-abdominal lymph nodes** HIV CC HCC

C84.Z4 **Other mature T/NK-cell lymphomas, lymph nodes of axilla and upper limb** HIV CC HCC

C84.Z5 **Other mature T/NK-cell lymphomas, lymph nodes of inguinal region and lower limb** HIV CC HCC

C84.Z6 **Other mature T/NK-cell lymphomas, intrapelvic lymph nodes** HIV CC HCC

C84.Z7 **Other mature T/NK-cell lymphomas, spleen** HIV CC HCC

C84.Z8 **Other mature T/NK-cell lymphomas, lymph nodes of multiple sites** HIV CC HCC

C84.Z9 **Other mature T/NK-cell lymphomas, extranodal and solid organ sites** HIV CC HCC

✓5th **C84.9 Mature T/NK-cell lymphomas, unspecified**

NK/T cell lymphoma NOS

EXCLUDES 1 *mature T-cell lymphoma, not elsewhere classified (C84.4-)*

C84.9Ø **Mature T/NK-cell lymphomas, unspecified, unspecified site** HIV CC HCC

C84.91 Mature T/NK-cell lymphomas, unspecified, lymph nodes of head, face, and neck HIV CC HCC
C84.92 Mature T/NK-cell lymphomas, unspecified, intrathoracic lymph nodes HIV CC HCC
C84.93 Mature T/NK-cell lymphomas, unspecified, intra-abdominal lymph nodes HIV CC HCC
C84.94 Mature T/NK-cell lymphomas, unspecified, lymph nodes of axilla and upper limb HIV CC HCC
C84.95 Mature T/NK-cell lymphomas, unspecified, lymph nodes of inguinal region and lower limb HIV CC HCC
C84.96 Mature T/NK-cell lymphomas, unspecified, intrapelvic lymph nodes HIV CC HCC
C84.97 Mature T/NK-cell lymphomas, unspecified, spleen HIV CC HCC
C84.98 Mature T/NK-cell lymphomas, unspecified, lymph nodes of multiple sites HIV CC HCC
C84.99 Mature T/NK-cell lymphomas, unspecified, extranodal and solid organ sites HIV CC HCC

✓4th C85 Other specified and unspecified types of non-Hodgkin lymphoma

EXCLUDES 1 *other specified types of T/NK-cell lymphoma (C86.-)*
personal history of non-Hodgkin lymphoma (Z85.72)

AHA: 2023,1Q,22

✓5th C85.1 Unspecified B-cell lymphoma

NOTE If B-cell lineage or involvement is mentioned in conjunction with a specific lymphoma, code to the more specific description.

C85.10 Unspecified B-cell lymphoma, unspecified site HIV CC HCC
C85.11 Unspecified B-cell lymphoma, lymph nodes of head, face, and neck HIV CC HCC
C85.12 Unspecified B-cell lymphoma, intrathoracic lymph nodes HIV CC HCC
C85.13 Unspecified B-cell lymphoma, intra-abdominal lymph nodes HIV CC HCC
C85.14 Unspecified B-cell lymphoma, lymph nodes of axilla and upper limb HIV CC HCC
C85.15 Unspecified B-cell lymphoma, lymph nodes of inguinal region and lower limb HIV CC HCC
C85.16 Unspecified B-cell lymphoma, intrapelvic lymph nodes HIV CC HCC
C85.17 Unspecified B-cell lymphoma, spleen HIV CC HCC
C85.18 Unspecified B-cell lymphoma, lymph nodes of multiple sites HIV CC HCC
C85.19 Unspecified B-cell lymphoma, extranodal and solid organ sites HIV CC HCC

✓5th C85.2 Mediastinal (thymic) large B-cell lymphoma

C85.20 Mediastinal (thymic) large B-cell lymphoma, unspecified site HIV CC HCC
C85.21 Mediastinal (thymic) large B-cell lymphoma, lymph nodes of head, face, and neck HIV CC HCC
C85.22 Mediastinal (thymic) large B-cell lymphoma, intrathoracic lymph nodes HIV CC HCC
C85.23 Mediastinal (thymic) large B-cell lymphoma, intra-abdominal lymph nodes HIV CC HCC
C85.24 Mediastinal (thymic) large B-cell lymphoma, lymph nodes of axilla and upper limb HIV CC HCC
C85.25 Mediastinal (thymic) large B-cell lymphoma, lymph nodes of inguinal region and lower limb HIV CC HCC
C85.26 Mediastinal (thymic) large B-cell lymphoma, intrapelvic lymph nodes HIV CC HCC
C85.27 Mediastinal (thymic) large B-cell lymphoma, spleen HIV CC HCC
C85.28 Mediastinal (thymic) large B-cell lymphoma, lymph nodes of multiple sites HIV CC HCC
C85.29 Mediastinal (thymic) large B-cell lymphoma, extranodal and solid organ sites HIV CC HCC

✓5th C85.8 Other specified types of non-Hodgkin lymphoma

C85.80 Other specified types of non-Hodgkin lymphoma, unspecified site HIV CC HCC
C85.81 Other specified types of non-Hodgkin lymphoma, lymph nodes of head, face, and neck HIV CC HCC
C85.82 Other specified types of non-Hodgkin lymphoma, intrathoracic lymph nodes HIV CC HCC
C85.83 Other specified types of non-Hodgkin lymphoma, intra-abdominal lymph nodes HIV CC HCC
C85.84 Other specified types of non-Hodgkin lymphoma, lymph nodes of axilla and upper limb HIV CC HCC
C85.85 Other specified types of non-Hodgkin lymphoma, lymph nodes of inguinal region and lower limb HIV CC HCC
C85.86 Other specified types of non-Hodgkin lymphoma, intrapelvic lymph nodes HIV CC HCC
C85.87 Other specified types of non-Hodgkin lymphoma, spleen HIV CC HCC
C85.88 Other specified types of non-Hodgkin lymphoma, lymph nodes of multiple sites HIV CC HCC
C85.89 Other specified types of non-Hodgkin lymphoma, extranodal and solid organ sites HIV CC HCC

✓5th C85.9 Non-Hodgkin lymphoma, unspecified

Lymphoma NOS
Malignant lymphoma NOS
Non-Hodgkin lymphoma NOS

C85.90 Non-Hodgkin lymphoma, unspecified, unspecified site HIV CC HCC
C85.91 Non-Hodgkin lymphoma, unspecified, lymph nodes of head, face, and neck HIV CC HCC
C85.92 Non-Hodgkin lymphoma, unspecified, intrathoracic lymph nodes HIV CC HCC
C85.93 Non-Hodgkin lymphoma, unspecified, intra-abdominal lymph nodes HIV CC HCC
C85.94 Non-Hodgkin lymphoma, unspecified, lymph nodes of axilla and upper limb HIV CC HCC
C85.95 Non-Hodgkin lymphoma, unspecified, lymph nodes of inguinal region and lower limb HIV CC HCC
C85.96 Non-Hodgkin lymphoma, unspecified, intrapelvic lymph nodes HIV CC HCC
C85.97 Non-Hodgkin lymphoma, unspecified, spleen HIV CC HCC
C85.98 Non-Hodgkin lymphoma, unspecified, lymph nodes of multiple sites HIV CC HCC
C85.99 Non-Hodgkin lymphoma, unspecified, extranodal and solid organ sites HIV CC HCC

✓4th C86 Other specified types of T/NK-cell lymphoma

EXCLUDES 1 *anaplastic large cell lymphoma, ALK negative (C84.7-)*
anaplastic large cell lymphoma, ALK positive (C84.6-)
mature T/NK-cell lymphomas (C84.-)
other specified types of non-Hodgkin lymphoma (C85.8-)

C86.0 Extranodal NK/T-cell lymphoma, nasal type HIV CC HCC
C86.1 Hepatosplenic T-cell lymphoma HIV CC HCC
Alpha-beta and gamma delta types
C86.2 Enteropathy-type (intestinal) T-cell lymphoma HIV CC HCC
Enteropathy associated T-cell lymphoma
C86.3 Subcutaneous panniculitis-like T-cell lymphoma HIV CC HCC
C86.4 Blastic NK-cell lymphoma HIV CC HCC
Blastic plasmacytoid dendritic cell neoplasm (BPDCN)
C86.5 Angioimmunoblastic T-cell lymphoma HIV CC HCC
Angioimmunoblastic lymphadenopathy with dysproteinemia (AILD)
C86.6 Primary cutaneous CD30-positive T-cell proliferations HIV CC HCC
Lymphomatoid papulosis
Primary cutaneous anaplastic large cell lymphoma
Primary cutaneous CD30-positive large T-cell lymphoma

✓4th C88 Malignant immunoproliferative diseases and certain other B-cell lymphomas

EXCLUDES 1 *B-cell lymphoma, unspecified (C85.1-)*
personal history of other malignant neoplasms of lymphoid, hematopoietic and related tissues (Z85.79)

C88.0 Waldenstrom macroglobulinemia HCC
Lymphoplasmacytic lymphoma with IgM-production
Macroglobulinemia (idiopathic) (primary)
EXCLUDES 1 *small cell B-cell lymphoma (C83.0)*
C88.2 Heavy chain disease CC HCC
Franklin disease
Gamma heavy chain disease
Mu heavy chain disease
C88.3 Immunoproliferative small intestinal disease CC HCC
Alpha heavy chain disease
Mediterranean lymphoma

C88.4 Extranodal marginal zone B-cell lymphoma of mucosa-associated lymphoid tissue [MALT-lymphoma] HIV CC HCC

Lymphoma of skin-associated lymphoid tissue [SALT-lymphoma]

Lymphoma of bronchial-associated lymphoid tissue [BALT-lymphoma]

EXCLUDES 1 *high malignant (diffuse large B-cell) lymphoma (C83.3-)*

C88.8 Other malignant immunoproliferative diseases CC HCC

C88.9 Malignant immunoproliferative disease, unspecified CC HCC

Immunoproliferative disease NOS

✓4th **C90 Multiple myeloma and malignant plasma cell neoplasms**

EXCLUDES 1 *personal history of other malignant neoplasms of lymphoid, hematopoietic and related tissues (Z85.79)*

AHA: 2019,2Q,30

✓5th **C90.0 Multiple myeloma**

Kahler's disease

Medullary plasmacytoma

Myelomatosis

Plasma cell myeloma

EXCLUDES 1 *solitary myeloma (C90.3-)*
solitary plasmactyoma (C90.3-)

AHA: 2021,3Q,5

TIP: Smoldering multiple myeloma (SMM) is a plasma cell disorder that has not yet progressed to active multiple myeloma. Code D47.Z2 should be used when only SMM is documented.

TIP: Do not assign an additional code for bone metastasis (C79.51) when multiple myeloma is described as metastatic to the bone; bone involvement is integral to this disease process.

C90.00 Multiple myeloma not having achieved remission CC HCC

Multiple myeloma with failed remission

Multiple myeloma NOS

C90.01 Multiple myeloma in remission CC HCC

C90.02 Multiple myeloma in relapse CC HCC

✓5th **C90.1 Plasma cell leukemia**

Plasmacytic leukemia

AHA: 2019,2Q,30

C90.10 Plasma cell leukemia not having achieved remission CC HCC

Plasma cell leukemia with failed remission

Plasma cell leukemia NOS

C90.11 Plasma cell leukemia in remission CC HCC

C90.12 Plasma cell leukemia in relapse CC HCC

✓5th **C90.2 Extramedullary plasmacytoma**

C90.20 Extramedullary plasmacytoma not having achieved remission CC HCC

Extramedullary plasmacytoma with failed remission

Extramedullary plasmacytoma NOS

C90.21 Extramedullary plasmacytoma in remission CC HCC

C90.22 Extramedullary plasmacytoma in relapse CC HCC

✓5th **C90.3 Solitary plasmacytoma**

Localized malignant plasma cell tumor NOS

Plasmacytoma NOS

Solitary myeloma

C90.30 Solitary plasmacytoma not having achieved remission CC HCC

Solitary plasmacytoma with failed remission

Solitary plasmacytoma NOS

C90.31 Solitary plasmacytoma in remission CC HCC

C90.32 Solitary plasmacytoma in relapse CC HCC

✓4th **C91 Lymphoid leukemia**

EXCLUDES 1 *personal history of leukemia (Z85.6)*

AHA: 2020,1Q,13

DEF: Malignant proliferation of immature lymphocytes (white blood cells that make up lymphoid tissue), called lymphoblasts, that originate in the bone marrow. Can be acute (ALL) or chronic (CLL).

✓5th **C91.0 Acute lymphoblastic leukemia [ALL]**

NOTE Codes in subcategory C91.0- should only be used for T-cell and B-cell precursor leukemia

C91.00 Acute lymphoblastic leukemia not having achieved remission CC HCC

Acute lymphoblastic leukemia with failed remission

Acute lymphoblastic leukemia NOS

C91.01 Acute lymphoblastic leukemia, in remission CC HCC

C91.02 Acute lymphoblastic leukemia, in relapse CC HCC

✓5th **C91.1 Chronic lymphocytic leukemia of B-cell type**

Lymphoplasmacytic leukemia

Richter syndrome

EXCLUDES 1 *lymphoplasmacytic lymphoma (C83.0-)*

AHA: 2023,1Q,18

C91.10 Chronic lymphocytic leukemia of B-cell type not having achieved remission CC HCC

Chronic lymphocytic leukemia of B-cell type with failed remission

Chronic lymphocytic leukemia of B-cell type NOS

C91.11 Chronic lymphocytic leukemia of B-cell type in remission CC HCC

C91.12 Chronic lymphocytic leukemia of B-cell type in relapse CC HCC

✓5th **C91.3 Prolymphocytic leukemia of B-cell type**

C91.30 Prolymphocytic leukemia of B-cell type not having achieved remission CC HCC

Prolymphocytic leukemia of B-cell type with failed remission

Prolymphocytic leukemia of B-cell type NOS

C91.31 Prolymphocytic leukemia of B-cell type, in remission CC HCC

C91.32 Prolymphocytic leukemia of B-cell type, in relapse CC HCC

✓5th **C91.4 Hairy cell leukemia**

Leukemic reticuloendotheliosis

DEF: Rare type of leukemia that is slow growing and often also considered a type of lymphoma. The small B-cell lymphocytes appear with "hairy" projections under a microscope and are found mostly in the bone marrow, spleen, and blood.

C91.40 Hairy cell leukemia not having achieved remission CC HCC

Hairy cell leukemia with failed remission

Hairy cell leukemia NOS

C91.41 Hairy cell leukemia, in remission CC HCC

C91.42 Hairy cell leukemia, in relapse CC HCC

✓5th **C91.5 Adult T-cell lymphoma/leukemia (HTLV-1-associated)**

Acute variant of adult T-cell lymphoma/leukemia (HTLV-1-associated)

Chronic variant of adult T-cell lymphoma/leukemia (HTLV-1-associated)

Lymphomatoid variant of adult T-cell lymphoma/leukemia (HTLV-1-associated)

Smouldering variant of adult T-cell lymphoma/leukemia (HTLV-1-associated)

C91.50 Adult T-cell lymphoma/leukemia (HTLV-1-associated) not having achieved remission CC HCC A

Adult T-cell lymphoma/leukemia (HTLV-1-associated) with failed remission

Adult T-cell lymphoma/leukemia (HTLV-1-associated) NOS

C91.51 Adult T-cell lymphoma/leukemia (HTLV-1-associated), in remission CC HCC A

C91.52 Adult T-cell lymphoma/leukemia (HTLV-1-associated), in relapse CC HCC A

✓5th **C91.6 Prolymphocytic leukemia of T-cell type**

C91.60 Prolymphocytic leukemia of T-cell type not having achieved remission CC HCC

Prolymphocytic leukemia of T-cell type with failed remission

Prolymphocytic leukemia of T-cell type NOS

C91.61 Prolymphocytic leukemia of T-cell type, in remission CC HCC

C91.62 Prolymphocytic leukemia of T-cell type, in relapse CC HCC

✓5th **C91.A Mature B-cell leukemia Burkitt-type**

EXCLUDES 1 *Burkitt lymphoma (C83.7-)*

C91.A0 Mature B-cell leukemia Burkitt-type not having achieved remission CC HCC

Mature B-cell leukemia Burkitt-type with failed remission

Mature B-cell leukemia Burkitt-type NOS

C91.A1 Mature B-cell leukemia Burkitt-type, in remission CC HCC

C91.A2 **Mature B-cell leukemia Burkitt-type, in relapse** CC HCC

✓5th C91.Z **Other lymphoid leukemia**

T-cell large granular lymphocytic leukemia (associated with rheumatoid arthritis)

C91.Z0 **Other lymphoid leukemia not having achieved remission** CC HCC

Other lymphoid leukemia with failed remission
Other lymphoid leukemia NOS

C91.Z1 **Other lymphoid leukemia, in remission** CC HCC

C91.Z2 **Other lymphoid leukemia, in relapse** CC HCC

✓5th C91.9 **Lymphoid leukemia, unspecified**

C91.90 **Lymphoid leukemia, unspecified not having achieved remission** CC HCC

Lymphoid leukemia with failed remission
Lymphoid leukemia NOS

C91.91 **Lymphoid leukemia, unspecified, in remission** CC HCC

C91.92 **Lymphoid leukemia, unspecified, in relapse** CC HCC

✓4th C92 **Myeloid leukemia**

INCLUDES granulocytic leukemia
myelogenous leukemia

▶Code also, if applicable, pancytopenia (acquired) (D61.818)◀

EXCLUDES 1 *personal history of leukemia (Z85.6)*

AHA: 2020,1Q,13; 2019,1Q,16

DEF: Cancer that develops in immature myelocytes called myeloblasts. These are the cells that become white blood cells (except lymphocytes), red blood cells, or platelet-making cells. Can be acute (AML) or chronic (CML).

TIP: Pancytopenia, although common in some types of myeloid leukemias, is not always inherent. When it is documented, code D61.818 can be assigned in addition to a code from this category.

✓5th C92.0 **Acute myeloblastic leukemia**

Acute myeloblastic leukemia, minimal differentiation
Acute myeloblastic leukemia (with maturation)
Acute myeloblastic leukemia 1/ETO
Acute myeloblastic leukemia M0
Acute myeloblastic leukemia M1
Acute myeloblastic leukemia M2
Acute myeloblastic leukemia with t(8;21)
Acute myeloblastic leukemia (without a FAB classification) NOS
Refractory anemia with excess blasts in transformation [RAEBT]

EXCLUDES 1 *acute exacerbation of chronic myeloid leukemia (C92.10)*
refractory anemia with excess of blasts not in transformation (D46.2-)

AHA: 2018,4Q,87

C92.00 **Acute myeloblastic leukemia, not having achieved remission** CC HCC

Acute myeloblastic leukemia with failed remission
Acute myeloblastic leukemia NOS

C92.01 **Acute myeloblastic leukemia, in remission** CC HCC

AHA: 2021,3Q,4

C92.02 **Acute myeloblastic leukemia, in relapse** CC HCC

AHA: 2023,1Q,23

✓5th C92.1 **Chronic myeloid leukemia, BCR/ABL-positive**

Chronic myelogenous leukemia, Philadelphia chromosome (Ph1) positive
Chronic myelogenous leukemia, t(9;22) (q34;q11)
Chronic myelogenous leukemia with crisis of blast cells

EXCLUDES 1 *atypical chronic myeloid leukemia BCR/ABL-negative (C92.2-)*
chronic myelomonocytic leukemia (C93.1-)
chronic myeloproliferative disease (D47.1)

C92.10 **Chronic myeloid leukemia, BCR/ABL-positive, not having achieved remission** CC HCC

Chronic myeloid leukemia, BCR/ABL-positive with failed remission
Chronic myeloid leukemia, BCR/ABL-positive NOS

C92.11 **Chronic myeloid leukemia, BCR/ABL-positive, in remission** CC HCC

C92.12 **Chronic myeloid leukemia, BCR/ABL-positive, in relapse** CC HCC

✓5th C92.2 **Atypical chronic myeloid leukemia, BCR/ABL-negative**

C92.20 **Atypical chronic myeloid leukemia, BCR/ABL-negative, not having achieved remission** CC HCC

Atypical chronic myeloid leukemia, BCR/ABL-negative with failed remission
Atypical chronic myeloid leukemia, BCR/ABL-negative NOS

C92.21 **Atypical chronic myeloid leukemia, BCR/ABL-negative, in remission** CC HCC

C92.22 **Atypical chronic myeloid leukemia, BCR/ABL-negative, in relapse** CC HCC

✓5th C92.3 **Myeloid sarcoma**

A malignant tumor of immature myeloid cells
Chloroma
Granulocytic sarcoma

C92.30 **Myeloid sarcoma, not having achieved remission** CC HCC

Myeloid sarcoma with failed remission
Myeloid sarcoma NOS

C92.31 **Myeloid sarcoma, in remission** CC HCC

C92.32 **Myeloid sarcoma, in relapse** CC HCC

✓5th C92.4 **Acute promyelocytic leukemia**

AML M3
AML Me with t(15;17) and variants

C92.40 **Acute promyelocytic leukemia, not having achieved remission** CC HCC

Acute promyelocytic leukemia with failed remission
Acute promyelocytic leukemia NOS

C92.41 **Acute promyelocytic leukemia, in remission** CC HCC

C92.42 **Acute promyelocytic leukemia, in relapse** CC HCC

✓5th C92.5 **Acute myelomonocytic leukemia**

AML M4
AML M4 Eo with inv(16) or t(16;16)

C92.50 **Acute myelomonocytic leukemia, not having achieved remission** CC HCC

Acute myelomonocytic leukemia with failed remission
Acute myelomonocytic leukemia NOS

C92.51 **Acute myelomonocytic leukemia, in remission** CC HCC

C92.52 **Acute myelomonocytic leukemia, in relapse** CC HCC

✓5th C92.6 **Acute myeloid leukemia with 11q23-abnormality**

Acute myeloid leukemia with variation of MLL-gene

C92.60 **Acute myeloid leukemia with 11q23-abnormality not having achieved remission** CC HCC

Acute myeloid leukemia with 11q23-abnormality with failed remission
Acute myeloid leukemia with 11q23-abnormality NOS

C92.61 **Acute myeloid leukemia with 11q23-abnormality in remission** CC HCC

C92.62 **Acute myeloid leukemia with 11q23-abnormality in relapse** CC HCC

✓5th C92.A **Acute myeloid leukemia with multilineage dysplasia**

Acute myeloid leukemia with dysplasia of remaining hematopoesis and/or myelodysplastic disease in its history

C92.A0 **Acute myeloid leukemia with multilineage dysplasia, not having achieved remission** CC HCC

Acute myeloid leukemia with multilineage dysplasia with failed remission
Acute myeloid leukemia with multilineage dysplasia NOS

C92.A1 **Acute myeloid leukemia with multilineage dysplasia, in remission** CC HCC

C92.A2 **Acute myeloid leukemia with multilineage dysplasia, in relapse** CC HCC

✓5th C92.Z **Other myeloid leukemia**

C92.Z0 **Other myeloid leukemia not having achieved remission** CC HCC

Myeloid leukemia NEC with failed remission
Myeloid leukemia NEC

C92.Z1 **Other myeloid leukemia, in remission** CC HCC

C92.Z2 **Other myeloid leukemia, in relapse** CC HCC

✓5th **C92.9 Myeloid leukemia, unspecified**

C92.90 Myeloid leukemia, unspecified, not having achieved remission CC HCC
Myeloid leukemia, unspecified with failed remission
Myeloid leukemia, unspecified NOS

C92.91 Myeloid leukemia, unspecified in remission CC HCC

C92.92 Myeloid leukemia, unspecified in relapse CC HCC

✓4th **C93 Monocytic leukemia**

INCLUDES monocytoid leukemia
EXCLUDES 1 *personal history of leukemia (Z85.6)*

AHA: 2020,1Q,13

✓5th **C93.0 Acute monoblastic/monocytic leukemia**
AML M5
AML M5a
AML M5b

C93.00 Acute monoblastic/monocytic leukemia, not having achieved remission CC HCC
Acute monoblastic/monocytic leukemia with failed remission
Acute monoblastic/monocytic leukemia NOS

C93.01 Acute monoblastic/monocytic leukemia, in remission CC HCC

C93.02 Acute monoblastic/monocytic leukemia, in relapse CC HCC

✓5th **C93.1 Chronic myelomonocytic leukemia**
Chronic monocytic leukemia
CMML-1
CMML-2
CMML with eosinophilia
Code also, if applicable, eosinophilia (D72.18)

C93.10 Chronic myelomonocytic leukemia not having achieved remission CC HCC
Chronic myelomonocytic leukemia with failed remission
Chronic myelomonocytic leukemia NOS

C93.11 Chronic myelomonocytic leukemia, in remission CC HCC

C93.12 Chronic myelomonocytic leukemia, in relapse CC HCC

✓5th **C93.3 Juvenile myelomonocytic leukemia**

C93.30 Juvenile myelomonocytic leukemia, not having achieved remission CC HCC P
Juvenile myelomonocytic leukemia with failed remission
Juvenile myelomonocytic leukemia NOS

C93.31 Juvenile myelomonocytic leukemia, in remission CC HCC P

C93.32 Juvenile myelomonocytic leukemia, in relapse CC HCC P

✓5th **C93.Z Other monocytic leukemia**

C93.Z0 Other monocytic leukemia, not having achieved remission CC HCC
Other monocytic leukemia NOS

C93.Z1 Other monocytic leukemia, in remission CC HCC

C93.Z2 Other monocytic leukemia, in relapse CC HCC

✓5th **C93.9 Monocytic leukemia, unspecified**

C93.90 Monocytic leukemia, unspecified, not having achieved remission CC HCC
Monocytic leukemia, unspecified with failed remission
Monocytic leukemia, unspecified NOS

C93.91 Monocytic leukemia, unspecified in remission CC HCC

C93.92 Monocytic leukemia, unspecified in relapse CC HCC

✓4th **C94 Other leukemias of specified cell type**

EXCLUDES 1 *leukemic reticuloendotheliosis (C91.4-)*
myelodysplastic syndromes (D46.-)
personal history of leukemia (Z85.6)
plasma cell leukemia (C90.1-)

AHA: 2020,1Q,13

✓5th **C94.0 Acute erythroid leukemia**
Acute myeloid leukemia M6(a)(b)
Erythroleukemia
DEF: Erythroleukemia: Malignant blood dyscrasia (a myeloproliferative disorder).

C94.00 Acute erythroid leukemia, not having achieved remission CC HCC
Acute erythroid leukemia with failed remission
Acute erythroid leukemia NOS

C94.01 Acute erythroid leukemia, in remission CC HCC

C94.02 Acute erythroid leukemia, in relapse CC HCC

✓5th **C94.2 Acute megakaryoblastic leukemia**
Acute megakaryocytic leukemia
Acute myeloid leukemia M7

C94.20 Acute megakaryoblastic leukemia not having achieved remission CC HCC
Acute megakaryoblastic leukemia with failed remission
Acute megakaryoblastic leukemia NOS

C94.21 Acute megakaryoblastic leukemia, in remission CC HCC

C94.22 Acute megakaryoblastic leukemia, in relapse CC HCC

✓5th **C94.3 Mast cell leukemia**

AHA: 2017,4Q,5

C94.30 Mast cell leukemia not having achieved remission CC HCC
Mast cell leukemia with failed remission
Mast cell leukemia NOS

C94.31 Mast cell leukemia, in remission CC HCC

C94.32 Mast cell leukemia, in relapse CC HCC

✓5th **C94.4 Acute panmyelosis with myelofibrosis**
Acute myelofibrosis

EXCLUDES 1 *myelofibrosis NOS (D75.81)*
secondary myelofibrosis NOS (D75.81)

C94.40 Acute panmyelosis with myelofibrosis not having achieved remission CC HCC
Acute myelofibrosis NOS
Acute panmyelosis with myelofibrosis with failed remission
Acute panmyelosis NOS

C94.41 Acute panmyelosis with myelofibrosis, in remission CC HCC

C94.42 Acute panmyelosis with myelofibrosis, in relapse CC HCC

C94.6 Myelodysplastic disease, not elsewhere classified CC HCC
Myelodysplastic/myeloproliferative neoplasm, unclassifiable
Myeloproliferative disease, not elsewhere classified

✓5th **C94.8 Other specified leukemias**
Aggressive NK-cell leukemia
Acute basophilic leukemia
►Code also, if applicable, eosinophilia (D72.18)◄

C94.80 Other specified leukemias not having achieved remission CC HCC
Other specified leukemia with failed remission
Other specified leukemias NOS

C94.81 Other specified leukemias, in remission CC HCC

C94.82 Other specified leukemias, in relapse CC HCC

C95 Leukemia of unspecified cell type
EXCLUDES 1 *personal history of leukemia (Z85.6)*
AHA: 2020,1Q,13

C95.0 Acute leukemia of unspecified cell type
Acute bilineal leukemia
Acute mixed lineage leukemia
Biphenotypic acute leukemia
Stem cell leukemia of unclear lineage
EXCLUDES 1 *acute exacerbation of unspecified chronic leukemia (C95.10)*

C95.00 Acute leukemia of unspecified cell type not having achieved remission CC HCC
Acute leukemia of unspecified cell type with failed remission
Acute leukemia NOS

C95.01 Acute leukemia of unspecified cell type, in remission CC HCC

C95.02 Acute leukemia of unspecified cell type, in relapse CC HCC

C95.1 Chronic leukemia of unspecified cell type

C95.10 Chronic leukemia of unspecified cell type not having achieved remission CC HCC
Chronic leukemia of unspecified cell type with failed remission
Chronic leukemia NOS

C95.11 Chronic leukemia of unspecified cell type, in remission CC HCC

C95.12 Chronic leukemia of unspecified cell type, in relapse CC HCC

C95.9 Leukemia, unspecified

C95.90 Leukemia, unspecified not having achieved remission CC HCC
Leukemia, unspecified with failed remission
Leukemia NOS

C95.91 Leukemia, unspecified, in remission CC HCC

C95.92 Leukemia, unspecified, in relapse CC HCC

C96 Other and unspecified malignant neoplasms of lymphoid, hematopoietic and related tissue
EXCLUDES 1 *personal history of other malignant neoplasms of lymphoid, hematopoietic and related tissues (Z85.79)*

C96.0 Multifocal and multisystemic (disseminated) Langerhans-cell histiocytosis CC HCC
Histiocytosis X, multisystemic
Letterer-Siwe disease
EXCLUDES 1 *adult pulmonary Langerhans cell histiocytosis (J84.82)*
multifocal and unisystemic Langerhans-cell histiocytosis (C96.5)
unifocal Langerhans-cell histiocytosis (C96.6)

C96.2 Malignant mast cell neoplasm
EXCLUDES 1 *indolent mastocytosis (D47.02)*
mast cell leukemia (C94.30)
mastocytosis (congenital) (cutaneous) (Q82.2)
AHA: 2017,4Q,5
DEF: Mast cell: Type of white blood cell found in the loose connective tissue of blood vessels and bronchioles responsible for acute hypersensitivity reactions, including anaphylactic shock. The IgE receptors on these cells bind with allergens causing cell degranulation and diffuse, widespread histamine release that results in airway constriction and vasodilation with decreased systemic blood pressure.

C96.20 Malignant mast cell neoplasm, unspecified CC HCC

C96.21 Aggressive systemic mastocytosis CC HCC

C96.22 Mast cell sarcoma CC HCC

C96.29 Other malignant mast cell neoplasm CC HCC

C96.4 Sarcoma of dendritic cells (accessory cells) CC HCC
Follicular dendritic cell sarcoma
Interdigitating dendritic cell sarcoma
Langerhans cell sarcoma

C96.5 Multifocal and unisystemic Langerhans-cell histiocytosis CC HCC
Hand-Schuller-Christian disease
Histiocytosis X, multifocal
EXCLUDES 1 *multifocal and multisystemic (disseminated) Langerhans-cell histiocytosis (C96.0)*
unifocal Langerhans-cell histiocytosis (C96.6)

C96.6 Unifocal Langerhans-cell histiocytosis CC HCC
Eosinophilic granuloma
Histiocytosis X, unifocal
Histiocytosis X NOS
Langerhans-cell histiocytosis NOS
EXCLUDES 1 *multifocal and multisysemic (disseminated) Langerhans-cell histiocytosis (C96.0)*
multifocal and unisystemic Langerhans-cell histiocytosis (C96.5)

C96.A Histiocytic sarcoma CC HCC
Malignant histiocytosis

C96.Z Other specified malignant neoplasms of lymphoid, hematopoietic and related tissue CC HCC

C96.9 Malignant neoplasm of lymphoid, hematopoietic and related tissue, unspecified CC HCC

In situ neoplasms (D00-D09)

INCLUDES Bowen's disease
erythroplasia
grade III intraepithelial neoplasia
Queyrat's erythroplasia

D00 Carcinoma in situ of oral cavity, esophagus and stomach
EXCLUDES 1 *melanoma in situ (D03.-)*

D00.0 Carcinoma in situ of lip, oral cavity and pharynx
Use additional code to identify:
exposure to environmental tobacco smoke (Z77.22)
exposure to tobacco smoke in the perinatal period (P96.81)
history of tobacco dependence (Z87.891)
occupational exposure to environmental tobacco smoke (Z57.31)
tobacco dependence (F17.-)
tobacco use (Z72.0)
EXCLUDES 1 *carcinoma in situ of aryepiglottic fold or interarytenoid fold, laryngeal aspect (D02.0)*
carcinoma in situ of epiglottis NOS (D02.0)
carcinoma in situ of epiglottis suprahyoid portion (D02.0)
carcinoma in situ of skin of lip (D03.0, D04.0)

D00.00 Carcinoma in situ of oral cavity, unspecified site

D00.01 Carcinoma in situ of labial mucosa and vermilion border

D00.02 Carcinoma in situ of buccal mucosa

D00.03 Carcinoma in situ of gingiva and edentulous alveolar ridge

D00.04 Carcinoma in situ of soft palate

D00.05 Carcinoma in situ of hard palate

D00.06 Carcinoma in situ of floor of mouth

D00.07 Carcinoma in situ of tongue

D00.08 Carcinoma in situ of pharynx
Carcinoma in situ of aryepiglottic fold NOS
Carcinoma in situ of hypopharyngeal aspect of aryepiglottic fold
Carcinoma in situ of marginal zone of aryepiglottic fold

D00.1 Carcinoma in situ of esophagus

D00.2 Carcinoma in situ of stomach

D01 Carcinoma in situ of other and unspecified digestive organs
EXCLUDES 1 *melanoma in situ (D03.-)*

D01.0 Carcinoma in situ of colon
EXCLUDES 1 *carcinoma in situ of rectosigmoid junction (D01.1)*

D01.1 Carcinoma in situ of rectosigmoid junction

D01.2 Carcinoma in situ of rectum

D01.3 Carcinoma in situ of anus and anal canal
Anal intraepithelial neoplasia III [AIN III]
Severe dysplasia of anus
EXCLUDES 1 *anal intraepithelial neoplasia I and II [AIN I and AIN II] (K62.82)*
carcinoma in situ of anal margin (D04.5)
carcinoma in situ of anal skin (D04.5)
carcinoma in situ of perianal skin (D04.5)

D01.4 Carcinoma in situ of other and unspecified parts of intestine
EXCLUDES 1 *carcinoma in situ of ampulla of Vater (D01.5)*

D01.40 Carcinoma in situ of unspecified part of intestine

D01.49 Carcinoma in situ of other parts of intestine

D01.5 Carcinoma in situ of liver, gallbladder and bile ducts
Carcinoma in situ of ampulla of Vater

DØ1.7 Carcinoma in situ of other specified digestive organs
Carcinoma in situ of pancreas

DØ1.9 Carcinoma in situ of digestive organ, unspecified

DØ2 Carcinoma in situ of middle ear and respiratory system
Use additional code to identify:
exposure to environmental tobacco smoke (Z77.22)
exposure to tobacco smoke in the perinatal period (P96.81)
history of tobacco dependence (Z87.891)
occupational exposure to environmental tobacco smoke (Z57.31)
tobacco dependence (F17.-)
tobacco use (Z72.Ø)
EXCLUDES 1 *melanoma in situ (DØ3.-)*

DØ2.Ø Carcinoma in situ of larynx
Carcinoma in situ of aryepiglottic fold or interarytenoid fold, laryngeal aspect
Carcinoma in situ of epiglottis (suprahyoid portion)
EXCLUDES 1 *carcinoma in situ of aryepiglottic fold or interarytenoid fold NOS (DØØ.Ø8)*
carcinoma in situ of hypopharyngeal aspect (DØØ.Ø8)
carcinoma in situ of marginal zone (DØØ.Ø8)

DØ2.1 Carcinoma in situ of trachea

DØ2.2 Carcinoma in situ of bronchus and lung
DØ2.2Ø Carcinoma in situ of unspecified bronchus and lung
DØ2.21 Carcinoma in situ of right bronchus and lung
DØ2.22 Carcinoma in situ of left bronchus and lung

DØ2.3 Carcinoma in situ of other parts of respiratory system
Carcinoma in situ of accessory sinuses
Carcinoma in situ of middle ear
Carcinoma in situ of nasal cavities
EXCLUDES 1 *carcinoma in situ of ear (external) (skin) (DØ4.2-)*
carcinoma in situ of nose NOS (DØ9.8)
carcinoma in situ of skin of nose (DØ4.3)

DØ2.4 Carcinoma in situ of respiratory system, unspecified

DØ3 Melanoma in situ
DØ3.Ø Melanoma in situ of lip HCC

DØ3.1 Melanoma in situ of eyelid, including canthus
AHA: 2018,4Q,4
DØ3.1Ø Melanoma in situ of unspecified eyelid, including canthus HCC
DØ3.11 Melanoma in situ of right eyelid, including canthus
DØ3.111 Melanoma in situ of right upper eyelid, including canthus HCC
DØ3.112 Melanoma in situ of right lower eyelid, including canthus HCC
DØ3.12 Melanoma in situ of left eyelid, including canthus
DØ3.121 Melanoma in situ of left upper eyelid, including canthus HCC
DØ3.122 Melanoma in situ of left lower eyelid, including canthus HCC

DØ3.2 Melanoma in situ of ear and external auricular canal
DØ3.2Ø Melanoma in situ of unspecified ear and external auricular canal HCC
DØ3.21 Melanoma in situ of right ear and external auricular canal HCC
DØ3.22 Melanoma in situ of left ear and external auricular canal HCC

DØ3.3 Melanoma in situ of other and unspecified parts of face
DØ3.3Ø Melanoma in situ of unspecified part of face HCC
DØ3.39 Melanoma in situ of other parts of face HCC

DØ3.4 Melanoma in situ of scalp and neck HCC

DØ3.5 Melanoma in situ of trunk
DØ3.51 Melanoma in situ of anal skin HCC
Melanoma in situ of anal margin
Melanoma in situ of perianal skin
DØ3.52 Melanoma in situ of breast (skin) (soft tissue) HCC
DØ3.59 Melanoma in situ of other part of trunk HCC

DØ3.6 Melanoma in situ of upper limb, including shoulder
DØ3.6Ø Melanoma in situ of unspecified upper limb, including shoulder HCC
DØ3.61 Melanoma in situ of right upper limb, including shoulder HCC
DØ3.62 Melanoma in situ of left upper limb, including shoulder HCC

DØ3.7 Melanoma in situ of lower limb, including hip
DØ3.7Ø Melanoma in situ of unspecified lower limb, including hip HCC
DØ3.71 Melanoma in situ of right lower limb, including hip HCC
DØ3.72 Melanoma in situ of left lower limb, including hip HCC

DØ3.8 Melanoma in situ of other sites HCC
Melanoma in situ of scrotum
EXCLUDES 1 *carcinoma in situ of scrotum (DØ7.61)*

DØ3.9 Melanoma in situ, unspecified HCC

DØ4 Carcinoma in situ of skin
EXCLUDES 1 *erythroplasia of Queyrat (penis) NOS (DØ7.4)*
melanoma in situ (DØ3.-)

DØ4.Ø Carcinoma in situ of skin of lip
EXCLUDES 2 *carcinoma in situ of vermilion border of lip (DØØ.Ø1)*

DØ4.1 Carcinoma in situ of skin of eyelid, including canthus
AHA: 2018,4Q,4
DØ4.1Ø Carcinoma in situ of skin of unspecified eyelid, including canthus
DØ4.11 Carcinoma in situ of skin of right eyelid, including canthus
DØ4.111 Carcinoma in situ of skin of right upper eyelid, including canthus
DØ4.112 Carcinoma in situ of skin of right lower eyelid, including canthus
DØ4.12 Carcinoma in situ of skin of left eyelid, including canthus
DØ4.121 Carcinoma in situ of skin of left upper eyelid, including canthus
DØ4.122 Carcinoma in situ of skin of left lower eyelid, including canthus

DØ4.2 Carcinoma in situ of skin of ear and external auricular canal
DØ4.2Ø Carcinoma in situ of skin of unspecified ear and external auricular canal
DØ4.21 Carcinoma in situ of skin of right ear and external auricular canal
DØ4.22 Carcinoma in situ of skin of left ear and external auricular canal

DØ4.3 Carcinoma in situ of skin of other and unspecified parts of face
DØ4.3Ø Carcinoma in situ of skin of unspecified part of face
DØ4.39 Carcinoma in situ of skin of other parts of face

DØ4.4 Carcinoma in situ of skin of scalp and neck

DØ4.5 Carcinoma in situ of skin of trunk
Carcinoma in situ of anal margin
Carcinoma in situ of anal skin
Carcinoma in situ of perianal skin
Carcinoma in situ of skin of breast
EXCLUDES 1 *carcinoma in situ of anus NOS (DØ1.3)*
carcinoma in situ of scrotum (DØ7.61)
carcinoma in situ of skin of genital organs (DØ7.-)

DØ4.6 Carcinoma in situ of skin of upper limb, including shoulder
DØ4.6Ø Carcinoma in situ of skin of unspecified upper limb, including shoulder
DØ4.61 Carcinoma in situ of skin of right upper limb, including shoulder
DØ4.62 Carcinoma in situ of skin of left upper limb, including shoulder

DØ4.7 Carcinoma in situ of skin of lower limb, including hip
DØ4.7Ø Carcinoma in situ of skin of unspecified lower limb, including hip
DØ4.71 Carcinoma in situ of skin of right lower limb, including hip
DØ4.72 Carcinoma in situ of skin of left lower limb, including hip

DØ4.8 Carcinoma in situ of skin of other sites

DØ4.9 Carcinoma in situ of skin, unspecified

DØ5 Carcinoma in situ of breast
EXCLUDES 1 *carcinoma in situ of skin of breast (DØ4.5)*
melanoma in situ of breast (skin) (DØ3.5)
Paget's disease of breast or nipple (C5Ø.-)

DØ5.Ø Lobular carcinoma in situ of breast
DØ5.ØØ Lobular carcinoma in situ of unspecified breast
DØ5.Ø1 Lobular carcinoma in situ of right breast
DØ5.Ø2 Lobular carcinoma in situ of left breast

D05.1 Intraductal carcinoma in situ of breast
D05.10 Intraductal carcinoma in situ of unspecified breast
D05.11 Intraductal carcinoma in situ of right breast
D05.12 Intraductal carcinoma in situ of left breast
D05.8 Other specified type of carcinoma in situ of breast
D05.80 Other specified type of carcinoma in situ of unspecified breast
D05.81 Other specified type of carcinoma in situ of right breast
D05.82 Other specified type of carcinoma in situ of left breast
D05.9 Unspecified type of carcinoma in situ of breast
D05.90 Unspecified type of carcinoma in situ of unspecified breast
D05.91 Unspecified type of carcinoma in situ of right breast
D05.92 Unspecified type of carcinoma in situ of left breast

D06 Carcinoma in situ of cervix uteri
INCLUDES cervical adenocarcinoma in situ
cervical intraepithelial glandular neoplasia
cervical intraepithelial neoplasia III [CIN III]
severe dysplasia of cervix uteri
EXCLUDES 1 *cervical intraepithelial neoplasia II [CIN II] (N87.1)*
cytologic evidence of malignancy of cervix without histologic confirmation (R87.614)
high grade squamous intraepithelial lesion (HGSIL) of cervix (R87.613)
melanoma in situ of cervix (D03.5)
moderate cervical dysplasia (N87.1)
D06.0 Carcinoma in situ of endocervix ♀
D06.1 Carcinoma in situ of exocervix ♀
D06.7 Carcinoma in situ of other parts of cervix ♀
D06.9 Carcinoma in situ of cervix, unspecified ♀

D07 Carcinoma in situ of other and unspecified genital organs
EXCLUDES 1 *melanoma in situ of trunk (D03.5)*
D07.0 Carcinoma in situ of endometrium ♀
D07.1 Carcinoma in situ of vulva ♀
Severe dysplasia of vulva
Vulvar intraepithelial neoplasia III [VIN III]
EXCLUDES 1 *moderate dysplasia of vulva (N90.1)*
vulvar intraepithelial neoplasia II [VIN II] (N90.1)
D07.2 Carcinoma in situ of vagina ♀
Severe dysplasia of vagina
Vaginal intraepithelial neoplasia III [VAIN III]
EXCLUDES 1 *moderate dysplasia of vagina (N89.1)*
vaginal intraepithelial neoplasia II [VIN II] (N89.1)
D07.3 Carcinoma in situ of other and unspecified female genital organs
D07.30 Carcinoma in situ of unspecified female genital organs ♀
D07.39 Carcinoma in situ of other female genital organs ♀
D07.4 Carcinoma in situ of penis ♂
Erythroplasia of Queyrat NOS
D07.5 Carcinoma in situ of prostate ♂
Prostatic intraepithelial neoplasia III (PIN III)
Severe dysplasia of prostate
EXCLUDES 1 *dysplasia (mild) (moderate) of prostate (N42.3-)*
prostatic intraepithelial neoplasia II [PIN II] (N42.3-)
D07.6 Carcinoma in situ of other and unspecified male genital organs
D07.60 Carcinoma in situ of unspecified male genital organs ♂
D07.61 Carcinoma in situ of scrotum ♂
D07.69 Carcinoma in situ of other male genital organs ♂

D09 Carcinoma in situ of other and unspecified sites
EXCLUDES 1 *melanoma in situ (D03.-)*
D09.0 Carcinoma in situ of bladder
D09.1 Carcinoma in situ of other and unspecified urinary organs
D09.10 Carcinoma in situ of unspecified urinary organ
D09.19 Carcinoma in situ of other urinary organs
D09.2 Carcinoma in situ of eye
EXCLUDES 1 *carcinoma in situ of skin of eyelid (D04.1-)*
D09.20 Carcinoma in situ of unspecified eye
D09.21 Carcinoma in situ of right eye
D09.22 Carcinoma in situ of left eye
D09.3 Carcinoma in situ of thyroid and other endocrine glands
EXCLUDES 1 *carcinoma in situ of endocrine pancreas (D01.7)*
carcinoma in situ of ovary (D07.39)
carcinoma in situ of testis (D07.69)
D09.8 Carcinoma in situ of other specified sites
D09.9 Carcinoma in situ, unspecified

Benign neoplasms, except benign neuroendocrine tumors (D10-D36)

D10 Benign neoplasm of mouth and pharynx
D10.0 Benign neoplasm of lip
Benign neoplasm of lip (frenulum) (inner aspect) (mucosa) (vermilion border)
EXCLUDES 1 *benign neoplasm of skin of lip (D22.0, D23.0)*
D10.1 Benign neoplasm of tongue
Benign neoplasm of lingual tonsil
D10.2 Benign neoplasm of floor of mouth
D10.3 Benign neoplasm of other and unspecified parts of mouth
D10.30 Benign neoplasm of unspecified part of mouth
D10.39 Benign neoplasm of other parts of mouth
Benign neoplasm of minor salivary gland NOS
EXCLUDES 1 *benign odontogenic neoplasms (D16.4-D16.5)*
benign neoplasm of mucosa of lip (D10.0)
benign neoplasm of nasopharyngeal surface of soft palate (D10.6)
D10.4 Benign neoplasm of tonsil
Benign neoplasm of tonsil (faucial) (palatine)
EXCLUDES 1 *benign neoplasm of lingual tonsil (D10.1)*
benign neoplasm of pharyngeal tonsil (D10.6)
benign neoplasm of tonsillar fossa (D10.5)
benign neoplasm of tonsillar pillars (D10.5)
D10.5 Benign neoplasm of other parts of oropharynx
Benign neoplasm of epiglottis, anterior aspect
Benign neoplasm of tonsillar fossa
Benign neoplasm of tonsillar pillars
Benign neoplasm of vallecula
EXCLUDES 1 *benign neoplasm of epiglottis NOS (D14.1)*
benign neoplasm of epiglottis, suprahyoid portion (D14.1)
DEF: Oropharynx: Middle portion of pharynx (throat); communicates with the oral cavity, nasopharynx and laryngopharynx.
D10.6 Benign neoplasm of nasopharynx
Benign neoplasm of pharyngeal tonsil
Benign neoplasm of posterior margin of septum and choanae
DEF: Nasopharynx: Upper portion of pharynx (throat); communicates with the nasal cavities, oropharynx and tympanic cavities.
D10.7 Benign neoplasm of hypopharynx
DEF: Hypopharynx: Lower portion of pharynx (throat); communicates with the oropharynx and the esophagus.
Synonym(s): *laryngopharynx.*
D10.9 Benign neoplasm of pharynx, unspecified

D11 Benign neoplasm of major salivary glands
EXCLUDES 1 *benign neoplasms of specified minor salivary glands which are classified according to their anatomical location*
benign neoplasms of minor salivary glands NOS (D10.39)
D11.0 Benign neoplasm of parotid gland
D11.7 Benign neoplasm of other major salivary glands
Benign neoplasm of sublingual salivary gland
Benign neoplasm of submandibular salivary gland
D11.9 Benign neoplasm of major salivary gland, unspecified

D12 Benign neoplasm of colon, rectum, anus and anal canal
EXCLUDES 1 ~~*benign carcinoid tumors of the large intestine, and rectum (D3A.02-)*~~
~~*polyp of colon NOS (K63.5)*~~
EXCLUDES 2 ▶*benign carcinoid tumors of the large intestine, and rectum (D3A.02-)*◀
▶*polyp of colon NOS (K63.5)*◀
AHA: 2018,2Q,14; 2017,1Q,15; 2015,2Q,14
TIP: Code K63.5 Polyp of colon, is assigned when documentation states hyperplastic colon polyps, regardless of the site in the colon. Slow-growing, hyperplastic polyps are not precancerous and are classified differently from benign or adenomatous polyps.
D12.0 Benign neoplasm of cecum
Benign neoplasm of ileocecal valve

D12.1 Benign neoplasm of appendix
EXCLUDES 1 *benign carcinoid tumor of the appendix (D3A.020)*

D12.2 Benign neoplasm of ascending colon

D12.3 Benign neoplasm of transverse colon
Benign neoplasm of hepatic flexure
Benign neoplasm of splenic flexure
AHA: 2017,1Q,16

D12.4 Benign neoplasm of descending colon

D12.5 Benign neoplasm of sigmoid colon

D12.6 Benign neoplasm of colon, unspecified
Adenomatosis of colon
Benign neoplasm of large intestine NOS
Polyposis (hereditary) of colon
EXCLUDES 1 *inflammatory polyp of colon (K51.4-)*

D12.7 Benign neoplasm of rectosigmoid junction

D12.8 Benign neoplasm of rectum
EXCLUDES 1 *benign carcinoid tumor of the rectum (D3A.026)*
AHA: 2018,1Q,6

D12.9 Benign neoplasm of anus and anal canal
Benign neoplasm of anus NOS
EXCLUDES 1 *benign neoplasm of anal margin (D22.5, D23.5)*
benign neoplasm of anal skin (D22.5, D23.5)
benign neoplasm of perianal skin (D22.5, D23.5)

✓4th **D13 Benign neoplasm of other and ill-defined parts of digestive system**
EXCLUDES 1 *benign stromal tumors of digestive system (D21.4)*

D13.0 Benign neoplasm of esophagus

D13.1 Benign neoplasm of stomach
EXCLUDES 1 *benign carcinoid tumor of the stomach (D3A.092)*

D13.2 Benign neoplasm of duodenum
EXCLUDES 1 *benign carcinoid tumor of the duodenum (D3A.010)*

✓5th **D13.3 Benign neoplasm of other and unspecified parts of small intestine**
EXCLUDES 1 *benign carcinoid tumors of the small intestine (D3A.01-)*
benign neoplasm of ileocecal valve (D12.0)

D13.30 Benign neoplasm of unspecified part of small intestine

D13.39 Benign neoplasm of other parts of small intestine

D13.4 Benign neoplasm of liver
Benign neoplasm of intrahepatic bile ducts

D13.5 Benign neoplasm of extrahepatic bile ducts

D13.6 Benign neoplasm of pancreas
EXCLUDES 1 *benign neoplasm of endocrine pancreas (D13.7)*

D13.7 Benign neoplasm of endocrine pancreas
Benign neoplasm of islets of Langerhans
Islet cell tumor
Use additional code to identify any functional activity

▲ ✓5th **D13.9 Benign neoplasm of ill-defined sites within the digestive system**
~~Benign neoplasm of digestive system NOS~~
~~Benign neoplasm of intestine NOS~~
~~Benign neoplasm of spleen~~

● **D13.91 Familial adenomatous polyposis**
Code also associated conditions, such as:
benign neoplasm of colon (D12.6)
malignant neoplasm of colon (C18.-)

● **D13.99 Benign neoplasm of ill-defined sites within the digestive system**
Benign neoplasm of digestive system NOS
Benign neoplasm of intestine NOS
Benign neoplasm of spleen

✓4th **D14 Benign neoplasm of middle ear and respiratory system**

D14.0 Benign neoplasm of middle ear, nasal cavity and accessory sinuses
Benign neoplasm of cartilage of nose
EXCLUDES 1 *benign neoplasm of auricular canal (external) (D22.2-, D23.2-)*
benign neoplasm of bone of ear (D16.4)
benign neoplasm of bone of nose (D16.4)
benign neoplasm of cartilage of ear (D21.0)
benign neoplasm of ear (external)(skin) (D22.2-, D23.2-)
benign neoplasm of nose NOS (D36.7)
benign neoplasm of skin of nose (D22.39, D23.39)
benign neoplasm of olfactory bulb (D33.3)
benign neoplasm of posterior margin of septum and choanae (D10.6)
polyp of accessory sinus (J33.8)
polyp of ear (middle) (H74.4)
polyp of nasal (cavity) (J33.-)

D14.1 Benign neoplasm of larynx
Adenomatous polyp of larynx
Benign neoplasm of epiglottis (suprahyoid portion)
EXCLUDES 1 *benign neoplasm of epiglottis, anterior aspect (D10.5)*
polyp (nonadenomatous) of vocal cord or larynx (J38.1)

D14.2 Benign neoplasm of trachea

✓5th **D14.3 Benign neoplasm of bronchus and lung**
EXCLUDES 1 *benign carcinoid tumor of the bronchus and lung (D3A.090)*

D14.30 Benign neoplasm of unspecified bronchus and lung

D14.31 Benign neoplasm of right bronchus and lung

D14.32 Benign neoplasm of left bronchus and lung

D14.4 Benign neoplasm of respiratory system, unspecified

✓4th **D15 Benign neoplasm of other and unspecified intrathoracic organs**
EXCLUDES 1 *benign neoplasm of mesothelial tissue (D19.-)*

D15.0 Benign neoplasm of thymus
EXCLUDES 1 *benign carcinoid tumor of the thymus (D3A.091)*

D15.1 Benign neoplasm of heart
EXCLUDES 1 *benign neoplasm of great vessels (D21.3)*

D15.2 Benign neoplasm of mediastinum

D15.7 Benign neoplasm of other specified intrathoracic organs

D15.9 Benign neoplasm of intrathoracic organ, unspecified

✓4th **D16 Benign neoplasm of bone and articular cartilage**
EXCLUDES 1 *benign neoplasm of connective tissue of ear (D21.0)*
benign neoplasm of connective tissue of eyelid (D21.0)
benign neoplasm of connective tissue of larynx (D14.1)
benign neoplasm of connective tissue of nose (D14.0)
benign neoplasm of synovia (D21.-)

✓5th **D16.0 Benign neoplasm of scapula and long bones of upper limb**

D16.00 Benign neoplasm of scapula and long bones of unspecified upper limb

D16.01 Benign neoplasm of scapula and long bones of right upper limb

D16.02 Benign neoplasm of scapula and long bones of left upper limb

✓5th **D16.1 Benign neoplasm of short bones of upper limb**

D16.10 Benign neoplasm of short bones of unspecified upper limb

D16.11 Benign neoplasm of short bones of right upper limb

D16.12 Benign neoplasm of short bones of left upper limb

✓5th **D16.2 Benign neoplasm of long bones of lower limb**

D16.20 Benign neoplasm of long bones of unspecified lower limb

D16.21 Benign neoplasm of long bones of right lower limb

D16.22 Benign neoplasm of long bones of left lower limb

✓5th **D16.3 Benign neoplasm of short bones of lower limb**

D16.30 Benign neoplasm of short bones of unspecified lower limb

D16.31 Benign neoplasm of short bones of right lower limb

D16.32 Benign neoplasm of short bones of left lower limb

D16.4 Benign neoplasm of bones of skull and face
Benign neoplasm of maxilla (superior)
Benign neoplasm of orbital bone
Keratocyst of maxilla
Keratocystic odontogenic tumor of maxilla
EXCLUDES 2 *benign neoplasm of lower jaw bone (D16.5)*

D16.5 Benign neoplasm of lower jaw bone
Keratocyst of mandible
Keratocystic odontogenic tumor of mandible

D16.6 Benign neoplasm of vertebral column
EXCLUDES 1 *benign neoplasm of sacrum and coccyx (D16.8)*

D16.7 Benign neoplasm of ribs, sternum and clavicle

D16.8 Benign neoplasm of pelvic bones, sacrum and coccyx

D16.9 Benign neoplasm of bone and articular cartilage, unspecified

D17 Benign lipomatous neoplasm

D17.0 Benign lipomatous neoplasm of skin and subcutaneous tissue of head, face and neck

D17.1 Benign lipomatous neoplasm of skin and subcutaneous tissue of trunk

D17.2 Benign lipomatous neoplasm of skin and subcutaneous tissue of limb

D17.20 Benign lipomatous neoplasm of skin and subcutaneous tissue of unspecified limb

D17.21 Benign lipomatous neoplasm of skin and subcutaneous tissue of right arm

D17.22 Benign lipomatous neoplasm of skin and subcutaneous tissue of left arm

D17.23 Benign lipomatous neoplasm of skin and subcutaneous tissue of right leg

D17.24 Benign lipomatous neoplasm of skin and subcutaneous tissue of left leg

D17.3 Benign lipomatous neoplasm of skin and subcutaneous tissue of other and unspecified sites

D17.30 Benign lipomatous neoplasm of skin and subcutaneous tissue of unspecified sites

D17.39 Benign lipomatous neoplasm of skin and subcutaneous tissue of other sites

D17.4 Benign lipomatous neoplasm of intrathoracic organs

D17.5 Benign lipomatous neoplasm of intra-abdominal organs
EXCLUDES 1 *benign lipomatous neoplasm of peritoneum and retroperitoneum (D17.79)*

D17.6 Benign lipomatous neoplasm of spermatic cord ♂

D17.7 Benign lipomatous neoplasm of other sites

D17.71 Benign lipomatous neoplasm of kidney

D17.72 Benign lipomatous neoplasm of other genitourinary organ

D17.79 Benign lipomatous neoplasm of other sites
Benign lipomatous neoplasm of peritoneum
Benign lipomatous neoplasm of retroperitoneum

D17.9 Benign lipomatous neoplasm, unspecified
Lipoma NOS

D18 Hemangioma and lymphangioma, any site
EXCLUDES 1 *benign neoplasm of glomus jugulare (D35.6)*
blue or pigmented nevus (D22.-)
nevus NOS (D22.-)
vascular nevus (Q82.5)

D18.0 Hemangioma
Angioma NOS
Cavernous nevus
DEF: Common benign tumor usually occurring in infancy that is composed of newly formed blood vessels due to malformation of the angioblastic tissue.

D18.00 Hemangioma unspecified site

D18.01 Hemangioma of skin and subcutaneous tissue

D18.02 Hemangioma of intracranial structures HCC

D18.03 Hemangioma of intra-abdominal structures

D18.09 Hemangioma of other sites

D18.1 Lymphangioma, any site
AHA: 2018,3Q,31; 2018,2Q,13

D19 Benign neoplasm of mesothelial tissue

D19.0 Benign neoplasm of mesothelial tissue of pleura

D19.1 Benign neoplasm of mesothelial tissue of peritoneum

D19.7 Benign neoplasm of mesothelial tissue of other sites

D19.9 Benign neoplasm of mesothelial tissue, unspecified
Benign mesothelioma NOS

D20 Benign neoplasm of soft tissue of retroperitoneum and peritoneum
EXCLUDES 1 *benign lipomatous neoplasm of peritoneum and retroperitoneum (D17.79)*
benign neoplasm of mesothelial tissue (D19.-)

D20.0 Benign neoplasm of soft tissue of retroperitoneum

D20.1 Benign neoplasm of soft tissue of peritoneum

D21 Other benign neoplasms of connective and other soft tissue
INCLUDES benign neoplasm of blood vessel
benign neoplasm of bursa
benign neoplasm of cartilage
benign neoplasm of fascia
benign neoplasm of fat
benign neoplasm of ligament, except uterine
benign neoplasm of lymphatic channel
benign neoplasm of muscle
benign neoplasm of synovia
benign neoplasm of tendon (sheath)
benign stromal tumors
EXCLUDES 1 *benign neoplasm of articular cartilage (D16.-)*
benign neoplasm of cartilage of larynx (D14.1)
benign neoplasm of cartilage of nose (D14.0)
benign neoplasm of connective tissue of breast (D24.-)
benign neoplasm of peripheral nerves and autonomic nervous system (D36.1-)
benign neoplasm of peritoneum (D20.1)
benign neoplasm of retroperitoneum (D20.0)
benign neoplasm of uterine ligament, any (D28.2)
benign neoplasm of vascular tissue (D18.-)
hemangioma (D18.0-)
lipomatous neoplasm (D17.-)
lymphangioma (D18.1)
uterine leiomyoma (D25.-)

D21.0 Benign neoplasm of connective and other soft tissue of head, face and neck
Benign neoplasm of connective tissue of ear
Benign neoplasm of connective tissue of eyelid
EXCLUDES 1 *benign neoplasm of connective tissue of orbit (D31.6-)*

D21.1 Benign neoplasm of connective and other soft tissue of upper limb, including shoulder

D21.10 Benign neoplasm of connective and other soft tissue of unspecified upper limb, including shoulder

D21.11 Benign neoplasm of connective and other soft tissue of right upper limb, including shoulder

D21.12 Benign neoplasm of connective and other soft tissue of left upper limb, including shoulder

D21.2 Benign neoplasm of connective and other soft tissue of lower limb, including hip

D21.20 Benign neoplasm of connective and other soft tissue of unspecified lower limb, including hip

D21.21 Benign neoplasm of connective and other soft tissue of right lower limb, including hip

D21.22 Benign neoplasm of connective and other soft tissue of left lower limb, including hip

D21.3 Benign neoplasm of connective and other soft tissue of thorax
Benign neoplasm of axilla
Benign neoplasm of diaphragm
Benign neoplasm of great vessels
EXCLUDES 1 *benign neoplasm of heart (D15.1)*
benign neoplasm of mediastinum (D15.2)
benign neoplasm of thymus (D15.0)

D21.4 Benign neoplasm of connective and other soft tissue of abdomen
Benign stromal tumors of abdomen

D21.5 Benign neoplasm of connective and other soft tissue of pelvis
EXCLUDES 1 *benign neoplasm of any uterine ligament (D28.2)*
uterine leiomyoma (D25.-)

D21.6 Benign neoplasm of connective and other soft tissue of trunk, unspecified
Benign neoplasm of connective and other soft tissue of back NOS

D21.9 Benign neoplasm of connective and other soft tissue, unspecified

D22 Melanocytic nevi

INCLUDES atypical nevus
blue hairy pigmented nevus
nevus NOS

D22.0 Melanocytic nevi of lip

D22.1 Melanocytic nevi of eyelid, including canthus

AHA: 2018,4Q,4

D22.10 Melanocytic nevi of unspecified eyelid, including canthus

D22.11 Melanocytic nevi of right eyelid, including canthus

D22.111 Melanocytic nevi of right upper eyelid, including canthus

D22.112 Melanocytic nevi of right lower eyelid, including canthus

D22.12 Melanocytic nevi of left eyelid, including canthus

D22.121 Melanocytic nevi of left upper eyelid, including canthus

D22.122 Melanocytic nevi of left lower eyelid, including canthus

D22.2 Melanocytic nevi of ear and external auricular canal

D22.20 Melanocytic nevi of unspecified ear and external auricular canal

D22.21 Melanocytic nevi of right ear and external auricular canal

D22.22 Melanocytic nevi of left ear and external auricular canal

D22.3 Melanocytic nevi of other and unspecified parts of face

D22.30 Melanocytic nevi of unspecified part of face

D22.39 Melanocytic nevi of other parts of face

D22.4 Melanocytic nevi of scalp and neck

D22.5 Melanocytic nevi of trunk

Melanocytic nevi of anal margin
Melanocytic nevi of anal skin
Melanocytic nevi of perianal skin
Melanocytic nevi of skin of breast

D22.6 Melanocytic nevi of upper limb, including shoulder

D22.60 Melanocytic nevi of unspecified upper limb, including shoulder

D22.61 Melanocytic nevi of right upper limb, including shoulder

D22.62 Melanocytic nevi of left upper limb, including shoulder

D22.7 Melanocytic nevi of lower limb, including hip

D22.70 Melanocytic nevi of unspecified lower limb, including hip

D22.71 Melanocytic nevi of right lower limb, including hip

D22.72 Melanocytic nevi of left lower limb, including hip

D22.9 Melanocytic nevi, unspecified

D23 Other benign neoplasms of skin

INCLUDES benign neoplasm of hair follicles
benign neoplasm of sebaceous glands
benign neoplasm of sweat glands

EXCLUDES 1 *benign lipomatous neoplasms of skin (D17.0-D17.3)*

EXCLUDES 2 *melanocytic nevi (D22.-)*

D23.0 Other benign neoplasm of skin of lip

EXCLUDES 1 *benign neoplasm of vermilion border of lip (D10.0)*

D23.1 Other benign neoplasm of skin of eyelid, including canthus

AHA: 2018,4Q,4

D23.10 Other benign neoplasm of skin of unspecified eyelid, including canthus

D23.11 Other benign neoplasm of skin of right eyelid, including canthus

D23.111 Other benign neoplasm of skin of right upper eyelid, including canthus

D23.112 Other benign neoplasm of skin of right lower eyelid, including canthus

D23.12 Other benign neoplasm of skin of left eyelid, including canthus

D23.121 Other benign neoplasm of skin of left upper eyelid, including canthus

D23.122 Other benign neoplasm of skin of left lower eyelid, including canthus

D23.2 Other benign neoplasm of skin of ear and external auricular canal

D23.20 Other benign neoplasm of skin of unspecified ear and external auricular canal

D23.21 Other benign neoplasm of skin of right ear and external auricular canal

D23.22 Other benign neoplasm of skin of left ear and external auricular canal

D23.3 Other benign neoplasm of skin of other and unspecified parts of face

D23.30 Other benign neoplasm of skin of unspecified part of face

D23.39 Other benign neoplasm of skin of other parts of face

D23.4 Other benign neoplasm of skin of scalp and neck

D23.5 Other benign neoplasm of skin of trunk

Other benign neoplasm of anal margin
Other benign neoplasm of anal skin
Other benign neoplasm of perianal skin
Other benign neoplasm of skin of breast

EXCLUDES 1 *benign neoplasm of anus NOS (D12.9)*

D23.6 Other benign neoplasm of skin of upper limb, including shoulder

D23.60 Other benign neoplasm of skin of unspecified upper limb, including shoulder

D23.61 Other benign neoplasm of skin of right upper limb, including shoulder

D23.62 Other benign neoplasm of skin of left upper limb, including shoulder

D23.7 Other benign neoplasm of skin of lower limb, including hip

D23.70 Other benign neoplasm of skin of unspecified lower limb, including hip

D23.71 Other benign neoplasm of skin of right lower limb, including hip

D23.72 Other benign neoplasm of skin of left lower limb, including hip

D23.9 Other benign neoplasm of skin, unspecified

D24 Benign neoplasm of breast

INCLUDES benign neoplasm of connective tissue of breast
benign neoplasm of soft parts of breast
fibroadenoma of breast

EXCLUDES 2 *adenofibrosis of breast (N60.2)*
benign cyst of breast (N60.-)
benign mammary dysplasia (N60.-)
benign neoplasm of skin of breast (D22.5, D23.5)
fibrocystic disease of breast (N60.-)

D24.1 Benign neoplasm of right breast

D24.2 Benign neoplasm of left breast

D24.9 Benign neoplasm of unspecified breast

D25 Leiomyoma of uterus

INCLUDES uterine fibroid
uterine fibromyoma
uterine myoma

Uterine Leiomyomas (Fibroids)

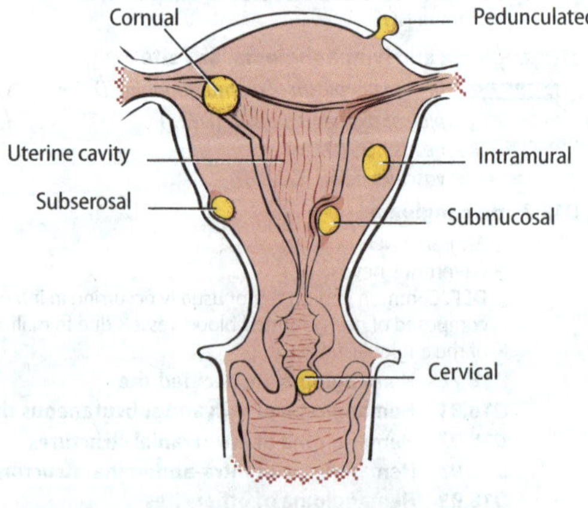

D25.0 Submucous leiomyoma of uterus ♀

D25.1 Intramural leiomyoma of uterus ♀

Interstitial leiomyoma of uterus

D25.2 Subserosal leiomyoma of uterus ♀

Subperitoneal leiomyoma of uterus

D25.9 Leiomyoma of uterus, unspecified ♀

D26 Other benign neoplasms of uterus

D26.0 Other benign neoplasm of cervix uteri ♀

D26.1 Other benign neoplasm of corpus uteri ♀

D26.7 Other benign neoplasm of other parts of uterus ♀

D26.9 Other benign neoplasm of uterus, unspecified ♀

D27 Benign neoplasm of ovary

Use additional code to identify any functional activity

EXCLUDES 2 *corpus albicans cyst (N83.2-)*
corpus luteum cyst (N83.1-)
endometrial cyst (N80.1-)
follicular (atretic) cyst (N83.0-)
graafian follicle cyst (N83.0-)
ovarian cyst NEC (N83.2-)
ovarian retention cyst (N83.2-)

D27.0 Benign neoplasm of right ovary ♀

D27.1 Benign neoplasm of left ovary ♀

D27.9 Benign neoplasm of unspecified ovary ♀

D28 Benign neoplasm of other and unspecified female genital organs

INCLUDES adenomatous polyp
benign neoplasm of skin of female genital organs
benign teratoma

EXCLUDES 1 *epoophoron cyst (Q50.5)*
fimbrial cyst (Q50.4)
Gartner's duct cyst (Q52.4)
parovarian cyst (Q50.5)

D28.0 Benign neoplasm of vulva ♀

D28.1 Benign neoplasm of vagina ♀

D28.2 Benign neoplasm of uterine tubes and ligaments ♀
Benign neoplasm of fallopian tube
Benign neoplasm of uterine ligament (broad) (round)

D28.7 Benign neoplasm of other specified female genital organs ♀

D28.9 Benign neoplasm of female genital organ, unspecified ♀

D29 Benign neoplasm of male genital organs

INCLUDES benign neoplasm of skin of male genital organs

D29.0 Benign neoplasm of penis ♂

D29.1 Benign neoplasm of prostate ♂
EXCLUDES 1 *enlarged prostate (N40.-)*

D29.2 Benign neoplasm of testis

Use additional code to identify any functional activity

D29.20 Benign neoplasm of unspecified testis ♂

D29.21 Benign neoplasm of right testis ♂

D29.22 Benign neoplasm of left testis ♂

D29.3 Benign neoplasm of epididymis

D29.30 Benign neoplasm of unspecified epididymis ♂

D29.31 Benign neoplasm of right epididymis ♂

D29.32 Benign neoplasm of left epididymis ♂

D29.4 Benign neoplasm of scrotum ♂
Benign neoplasm of skin of scrotum

D29.8 Benign neoplasm of other specified male genital organs ♂
Benign neoplasm of seminal vesicle
Benign neoplasm of spermatic cord
Benign neoplasm of tunica vaginalis

D29.9 Benign neoplasm of male genital organ, unspecified ♂

D30 Benign neoplasm of urinary organs

D30.0 Benign neoplasm of kidney

EXCLUDES 1 *benign carcinoid tumor of the kidney (D3A.093)*
benign neoplasm of renal calyces (D30.1-)
benign neoplasm of renal pelvis (D30.1-)

D30.00 Benign neoplasm of unspecified kidney

D30.01 Benign neoplasm of right kidney

D30.02 Benign neoplasm of left kidney

D30.1 Benign neoplasm of renal pelvis

D30.10 Benign neoplasm of unspecified renal pelvis

D30.11 Benign neoplasm of right renal pelvis

D30.12 Benign neoplasm of left renal pelvis

D30.2 Benign neoplasm of ureter

EXCLUDES 1 *benign neoplasm of ureteric orifice of bladder (D30.3)*

D30.20 Benign neoplasm of unspecified ureter

D30.21 Benign neoplasm of right ureter

D30.22 Benign neoplasm of left ureter

D30.3 Benign neoplasm of bladder
Benign neoplasm of ureteric orifice of bladder
Benign neoplasm of urethral orifice of bladder

D30.4 Benign neoplasm of urethra
EXCLUDES 1 *benign neoplasm of urethral orifice of bladder (D30.3)*

D30.8 Benign neoplasm of other specified urinary organs
Benign neoplasm of paraurethral glands

D30.9 Benign neoplasm of urinary organ, unspecified
Benign neoplasm of urinary system NOS

D31 Benign neoplasm of eye and adnexa

EXCLUDES 1 *benign neoplasm of connective tissue of eyelid (D21.0)*
benign neoplasm of optic nerve (D33.3)
benign neoplasm of skin of eyelid (D22.1-, D23.1-)

D31.0 Benign neoplasm of conjunctiva

D31.00 Benign neoplasm of unspecified conjunctiva

D31.01 Benign neoplasm of right conjunctiva

D31.02 Benign neoplasm of left conjunctiva

D31.1 Benign neoplasm of cornea

D31.10 Benign neoplasm of unspecified cornea

D31.11 Benign neoplasm of right cornea

D31.12 Benign neoplasm of left cornea

D31.2 Benign neoplasm of retina

EXCLUDES 1 *dark area on retina (D49.81)*
hemangioma of retina (D49.81)
neoplasm of unspecified behavior of retina and choroid (D49.81)
retinal freckle (D49.81)

D31.20 Benign neoplasm of unspecified retina

D31.21 Benign neoplasm of right retina

D31.22 Benign neoplasm of left retina

D31.3 Benign neoplasm of choroid

D31.30 Benign neoplasm of unspecified choroid

D31.31 Benign neoplasm of right choroid

D31.32 Benign neoplasm of left choroid

D31.4 Benign neoplasm of ciliary body

D31.40 Benign neoplasm of unspecified ciliary body

D31.41 Benign neoplasm of right ciliary body

D31.42 Benign neoplasm of left ciliary body

D31.5 Benign neoplasm of lacrimal gland and duct
Benign neoplasm of lacrimal sac
Benign neoplasm of nasolacrimal duct

D31.50 Benign neoplasm of unspecified lacrimal gland and duct

D31.51 Benign neoplasm of right lacrimal gland and duct

D31.52 Benign neoplasm of left lacrimal gland and duct

D31.6 Benign neoplasm of unspecified site of orbit
Benign neoplasm of connective tissue of orbit
Benign neoplasm of extraocular muscle
Benign neoplasm of peripheral nerves of orbit
Benign neoplasm of retrobulbar tissue
Benign neoplasm of retro-ocular tissue
EXCLUDES 1 *benign neoplasm of orbital bone (D16.4)*

D31.60 Benign neoplasm of unspecified site of unspecified orbit

D31.61 Benign neoplasm of unspecified site of right orbit

D31.62 Benign neoplasm of unspecified site of left orbit

D31.9 Benign neoplasm of unspecified part of eye
Benign neoplasm of eyeball

D31.90 Benign neoplasm of unspecified part of unspecified eye

D31.91 Benign neoplasm of unspecified part of right eye

D31.92 Benign neoplasm of unspecified part of left eye

D32 Benign neoplasm of meninges

D32.0 Benign neoplasm of cerebral meninges HCC

D32.1 Benign neoplasm of spinal meninges HCC

D32.9 Benign neoplasm of meninges, unspecified HCC
Meningioma NOS

D33 Benign neoplasm of brain and other parts of central nervous system

EXCLUDES 1 *angioma (D18.Ø-)*
benign neoplasm of meninges (D32.-)
benign neoplasm of peripheral nerves and autonomic nervous system (D36.1-)
hemangioma (D18.Ø-)
neurofibromatosis (Q85.Ø-)
retro-ocular benign neoplasm (D31.6-)

D33.Ø Benign neoplasm of brain, supratentorial HCC
Benign neoplasm of cerebral ventricle
Benign neoplasm of cerebrum
Benign neoplasm of frontal lobe
Benign neoplasm of occipital lobe
Benign neoplasm of parietal lobe
Benign neoplasm of temporal lobe
EXCLUDES 1 *benign neoplasm of fourth ventricle (D33.1)*

D33.1 Benign neoplasm of brain, infratentorial HCC
Benign neoplasm of brain stem
Benign neoplasm of cerebellum
Benign neoplasm of fourth ventricle

D33.2 Benign neoplasm of brain, unspecified HCC

D33.3 Benign neoplasm of cranial nerves HCC
Benign neoplasm of olfactory bulb

D33.4 Benign neoplasm of spinal cord HCC

D33.7 Benign neoplasm of other specified parts of central nervous system HCC

D33.9 Benign neoplasm of central nervous system, unspecified HCC
Benign neoplasm of nervous system (central) NOS

D34 Benign neoplasm of thyroid gland
Use additional code to identify any functional activity

D35 Benign neoplasm of other and unspecified endocrine glands
Use additional code to identify any functional activity
EXCLUDES 1 *benign neoplasm of endocrine pancreas (D13.7)*
benign neoplasm of ovary (D27.-)
benign neoplasm of testis (D29.2.-)
benign neoplasm of thymus (D15.Ø)

D35.Ø Benign neoplasm of adrenal gland
D35.ØØ Benign neoplasm of unspecified adrenal gland
D35.Ø1 Benign neoplasm of right adrenal gland
D35.Ø2 Benign neoplasm of left adrenal gland

D35.1 Benign neoplasm of parathyroid gland

D35.2 Benign neoplasm of pituitary gland HCC
AHA: 2014,3Q,22

D35.3 Benign neoplasm of craniopharyngeal duct HCC

D35.4 Benign neoplasm of pineal gland HCC

D35.5 Benign neoplasm of carotid body

D35.6 Benign neoplasm of aortic body and other paraganglia
Benign tumor of glomus jugulare

D35.7 Benign neoplasm of other specified endocrine glands

D35.9 Benign neoplasm of endocrine gland, unspecified
Benign neoplasm of unspecified endocrine gland

D36 Benign neoplasm of other and unspecified sites

D36.Ø Benign neoplasm of lymph nodes
EXCLUDES 1 *lymphangioma (D18.1)*

D36.1 Benign neoplasm of peripheral nerves and autonomic nervous system
EXCLUDES 1 *benign neoplasm of peripheral nerves of orbit (D31.6-)*
neurofibromatosis (Q85.Ø-)

D36.1Ø Benign neoplasm of peripheral nerves and autonomic nervous system, unspecified
D36.11 Benign neoplasm of peripheral nerves and autonomic nervous system of face, head, and neck
D36.12 Benign neoplasm of peripheral nerves and autonomic nervous system, upper limb, including shoulder
D36.13 Benign neoplasm of peripheral nerves and autonomic nervous system of lower limb, including hip
D36.14 Benign neoplasm of peripheral nerves and autonomic nervous system of thorax
D36.15 Benign neoplasm of peripheral nerves and autonomic nervous system of abdomen
D36.16 Benign neoplasm of peripheral nerves and autonomic nervous system of pelvis
D36.17 Benign neoplasm of peripheral nerves and autonomic nervous system of trunk, unspecified

D36.7 Benign neoplasm of other specified sites
Benign neoplasm of back NOS
Benign neoplasm of nose NOS

D36.9 Benign neoplasm, unspecified site

Benign neuroendocrine tumors (D3A)

D3A Benign neuroendocrine tumors
Code also any associated multiple endocrine neoplasia [MEN] syndromes (E31.2-)
Use additional code to identify any associated endocrine syndrome, such as:
carcinoid syndrome (E34.Ø)
EXCLUDES 2 *benign pancreatic islet cell tumors (D13.7)*

D3A.Ø Benign carcinoid tumors
DEF: Specific type of slow-growing neuroendocrine tumors. Carcinoid tumors occur most commonly in the hormone producing cells of the gastrointestinal tracts and can also occur in the pancreas, testes, ovaries, or lungs.

D3A.ØØ Benign carcinoid tumor of unspecified site
Carcinoid tumor NOS

D3A.Ø1 Benign carcinoid tumors of the small intestine
D3A.Ø1Ø Benign carcinoid tumor of the duodenum
D3A.Ø11 Benign carcinoid tumor of the jejunum
D3A.Ø12 Benign carcinoid tumor of the ileum
D3A.Ø19 Benign carcinoid tumor of the small intestine, unspecified portion

D3A.Ø2 Benign carcinoid tumors of the appendix, large intestine, and rectum
D3A.Ø2Ø Benign carcinoid tumor of the appendix
D3A.Ø21 Benign carcinoid tumor of the cecum
D3A.Ø22 Benign carcinoid tumor of the ascending colon
D3A.Ø23 Benign carcinoid tumor of the transverse colon
D3A.Ø24 Benign carcinoid tumor of the descending colon
D3A.Ø25 Benign carcinoid tumor of the sigmoid colon
D3A.Ø26 Benign carcinoid tumor of the rectum
D3A.Ø29 Benign carcinoid tumor of the large intestine, unspecified portion
Benign carcinoid tumor of the colon NOS

D3A.Ø9 Benign carcinoid tumors of other sites
D3A.Ø9Ø Benign carcinoid tumor of the bronchus and lung
D3A.Ø91 Benign carcinoid tumor of the thymus
D3A.Ø92 Benign carcinoid tumor of the stomach
D3A.Ø93 Benign carcinoid tumor of the kidney
D3A.Ø94 Benign carcinoid tumor of the foregut, unspecified
D3A.Ø95 Benign carcinoid tumor of the midgut, unspecified
D3A.Ø96 Benign carcinoid tumor of the hindgut, unspecified
D3A.Ø98 Benign carcinoid tumors of other sites

D3A.8 Other benign neuroendocrine tumors
Neuroendocrine tumor NOS

Neoplasms of uncertain behavior, polycythemia vera and myelodysplastic syndromes (D37-D48)

NOTE Categories D37-D44, and D48 classify by site neoplasms of uncertain behavior, i.e., histologic confirmation whether the neoplasm is malignant or benign cannot be made.

EXCLUDES 1 *neoplasms of unspecified behavior (D49.-)*

D37 Neoplasm of uncertain behavior of oral cavity and digestive organs

EXCLUDES 1 *stromal tumors of uncertain behavior of digestive system ▶(D48.1-)◀*

D37.0 Neoplasm of uncertain behavior of lip, oral cavity and pharynx

EXCLUDES 1 *neoplasm of uncertain behavior of aryepiglottic fold or interarytenoid fold, laryngeal aspect (D38.0)*
neoplasm of uncertain behavior of epiglottis NOS (D38.0)
neoplasm of uncertain behavior of skin of lip (D48.5)
neoplasm of uncertain behavior of suprahyoid portion of epiglottis (D38.0)

D37.01 Neoplasm of uncertain behavior of lip
Neoplasm of uncertain behavior of vermilion border of lip

D37.02 Neoplasm of uncertain behavior of tongue

D37.03 Neoplasm of uncertain behavior of the major salivary glands

D37.030 Neoplasm of uncertain behavior of the parotid salivary glands

D37.031 Neoplasm of uncertain behavior of the sublingual salivary glands

D37.032 Neoplasm of uncertain behavior of the submandibular salivary glands

D37.039 Neoplasm of uncertain behavior of the major salivary glands, unspecified

D37.04 Neoplasm of uncertain behavior of the minor salivary glands
Neoplasm of uncertain behavior of submucosal salivary glands of cheek
Neoplasm of uncertain behavior of submucosal salivary glands of hard palate
Neoplasm of uncertain behavior of submucosal salivary glands of lip
Neoplasm of uncertain behavior of submucosal salivary glands of soft palate

D37.05 Neoplasm of uncertain behavior of pharynx
Neoplasm of uncertain behavior of aryepiglottic fold of pharynx NOS
Neoplasm of uncertain behavior of hypopharyngeal aspect of aryepiglottic fold of pharynx
Neoplasm of uncertain behavior of marginal zone of aryepiglottic fold of pharynx

D37.09 Neoplasm of uncertain behavior of other specified sites of the oral cavity

D37.1 Neoplasm of uncertain behavior of stomach

D37.2 Neoplasm of uncertain behavior of small intestine

D37.3 Neoplasm of uncertain behavior of appendix

D37.4 Neoplasm of uncertain behavior of colon

D37.5 Neoplasm of uncertain behavior of rectum
Neoplasm of uncertain behavior of rectosigmoid junction

D37.6 Neoplasm of uncertain behavior of liver, gallbladder and bile ducts
Neoplasm of uncertain behavior of ampulla of Vater

D37.8 Neoplasm of uncertain behavior of other specified digestive organs
Neoplasm of uncertain behavior of anal canal
Neoplasm of uncertain behavior of anal sphincter
Neoplasm of uncertain behavior of anus NOS
Neoplasm of uncertain behavior of esophagus
Neoplasm of uncertain behavior of intestine NOS
Neoplasm of uncertain behavior of pancreas

EXCLUDES 1 *neoplasm of uncertain behavior of anal margin (D48.5)*
neoplasm of uncertain behavior of anal skin (D48.5)
neoplasm of uncertain behavior of perianal skin (D48.5)

D37.9 Neoplasm of uncertain behavior of digestive organ, unspecified

D38 Neoplasm of uncertain behavior of middle ear and respiratory and intrathoracic organs

EXCLUDES 1 *neoplasm of uncertain behavior of heart (D48.7)*

D38.0 Neoplasm of uncertain behavior of larynx
Neoplasm of uncertain behavior of aryepiglottic fold or interarytenoid fold, laryngeal aspect
Neoplasm of uncertain behavior of epiglottis (suprahyoid portion)

EXCLUDES 1 *neoplasm of uncertain behavior of aryepiglottic fold or interarytenoid fold NOS (D37.05)*
neoplasm of uncertain behavior of hypopharyngeal aspect of aryepiglottic fold (D37.05)
neoplasm of uncertain behavior of marginal zone of aryepiglottic fold (D37.05)

D38.1 Neoplasm of uncertain behavior of trachea, bronchus and lung

D38.2 Neoplasm of uncertain behavior of pleura

D38.3 Neoplasm of uncertain behavior of mediastinum

D38.4 Neoplasm of uncertain behavior of thymus

D38.5 Neoplasm of uncertain behavior of other respiratory organs
Neoplasm of uncertain behavior of accessory sinuses
Neoplasm of uncertain behavior of cartilage of nose
Neoplasm of uncertain behavior of middle ear
Neoplasm of uncertain behavior of nasal cavities

EXCLUDES 1 *neoplasm of uncertain behavior of ear (external) (skin) (D48.5)*
neoplasm of uncertain behavior of nose NOS (D48.7)
neoplasm of uncertain behavior of skin of nose (D48.5)

D38.6 Neoplasm of uncertain behavior of respiratory organ, unspecified

D39 Neoplasm of uncertain behavior of female genital organs

D39.0 Neoplasm of uncertain behavior of uterus ♀

D39.1 Neoplasm of uncertain behavior of ovary
Use additional code to identify any functional activity

D39.10 Neoplasm of uncertain behavior of unspecified ovary ♀

D39.11 Neoplasm of uncertain behavior of right ovary ♀

D39.12 Neoplasm of uncertain behavior of left ovary ♀

D39.2 Neoplasm of uncertain behavior of placenta M ♀
Chorioadenoma destruens
Invasive hydatidiform mole
Malignant hydatidiform mole

EXCLUDES 1 *hydatidiform mole NOS (O01.9)*

D39.8 Neoplasm of uncertain behavior of other specified female genital organs ♀
Neoplasm of uncertain behavior of skin of female genital organs

D39.9 Neoplasm of uncertain behavior of female genital organ, unspecified ♀

D40 Neoplasm of uncertain behavior of male genital organs

D40.0 Neoplasm of uncertain behavior of prostate ♂

D40.1 Neoplasm of uncertain behavior of testis

D40.10 Neoplasm of uncertain behavior of unspecified testis ♂

D40.11 Neoplasm of uncertain behavior of right testis ♂

D40.12 Neoplasm of uncertain behavior of left testis ♂

D40.8 Neoplasm of uncertain behavior of other specified male genital organs ♂
Neoplasm of uncertain behavior of skin of male genital organs

D40.9 Neoplasm of uncertain behavior of male genital organ, unspecified ♂

D41 Neoplasm of uncertain behavior of urinary organs

D41.0 Neoplasm of uncertain behavior of kidney

EXCLUDES 1 *neoplasm of uncertain behavior of renal pelvis (D41.1-)*

D41.00 Neoplasm of uncertain behavior of unspecified kidney

D41.01 Neoplasm of uncertain behavior of right kidney

D41.02 Neoplasm of uncertain behavior of left kidney

D41.1 Neoplasm of uncertain behavior of renal pelvis

D41.10 Neoplasm of uncertain behavior of unspecified renal pelvis

D41.11 Neoplasm of uncertain behavior of right renal pelvis

D41.12 Neoplasm of uncertain behavior of left renal pelvis

D41.2 Neoplasm of uncertain behavior of ureter

D41.20 Neoplasm of uncertain behavior of unspecified ureter

D41.21 Neoplasm of uncertain behavior of right ureter
D41.22 Neoplasm of uncertain behavior of left ureter
D41.3 Neoplasm of uncertain behavior of urethra
D41.4 Neoplasm of uncertain behavior of bladder
D41.8 Neoplasm of uncertain behavior of other specified urinary organs
D41.9 Neoplasm of uncertain behavior of unspecified urinary organ

D42 Neoplasm of uncertain behavior of meninges
D42.Ø Neoplasm of uncertain behavior of cerebral meninges HCC
D42.1 Neoplasm of uncertain behavior of spinal meninges HCC
D42.9 Neoplasm of uncertain behavior of meninges, unspecified HCC

D43 Neoplasm of uncertain behavior of brain and central nervous system
EXCLUDES 1 *neoplasm of uncertain behavior of peripheral nerves and autonomic nervous system (D48.2)*
D43.Ø Neoplasm of uncertain behavior of brain, supratentorial HCC
Neoplasm of uncertain behavior of cerebral ventricle
Neoplasm of uncertain behavior of cerebrum
Neoplasm of uncertain behavior of frontal lobe
Neoplasm of uncertain behavior of occipital lobe
Neoplasm of uncertain behavior of parietal lobe
Neoplasm of uncertain behavior of temporal lobe
EXCLUDES 1 *neoplasm of uncertain behavior of fourth ventricle (D43.1)*
D43.1 Neoplasm of uncertain behavior of brain, infratentorial HCC
Neoplasm of uncertain behavior of brain stem
Neoplasm of uncertain behavior of cerebellum
Neoplasm of uncertain behavior of fourth ventricle
AHA: 2023,2Q,16
D43.2 Neoplasm of uncertain behavior of brain, unspecified HCC
D43.3 Neoplasm of uncertain behavior of cranial nerves HCC
D43.4 Neoplasm of uncertain behavior of spinal cord HCC
D43.8 Neoplasm of uncertain behavior of other specified parts of central nervous system HCC
D43.9 Neoplasm of uncertain behavior of central nervous system, unspecified HCC
Neoplasm of uncertain behavior of nervous system (central) NOS

D44 Neoplasm of uncertain behavior of endocrine glands
EXCLUDES 1 *multiple endocrine adenomatosis (E31.2-)*
multiple endocrine neoplasia (E31.2-)
neoplasm of uncertain behavior of endocrine pancreas (D37.8)
neoplasm of uncertain behavior of ovary (D39.1-)
neoplasm of uncertain behavior of testis (DØ.1-)
neoplasm of uncertain behavior of thymus (D38.4)
D44.Ø Neoplasm of uncertain behavior of thyroid gland
D44.1 Neoplasm of uncertain behavior of adrenal gland
Use additional code to identify any functional activity
D44.1Ø Neoplasm of uncertain behavior of unspecified adrenal gland
D44.11 Neoplasm of uncertain behavior of right adrenal gland
D44.12 Neoplasm of uncertain behavior of left adrenal gland
D44.2 Neoplasm of uncertain behavior of parathyroid gland
D44.3 Neoplasm of uncertain behavior of pituitary gland HCC
Use additional code to identify any functional activity
D44.4 Neoplasm of uncertain behavior of craniopharyngeal duct HCC
D44.5 Neoplasm of uncertain behavior of pineal gland HCC
D44.6 Neoplasm of uncertain behavior of carotid body HCC
D44.7 Neoplasm of uncertain behavior of aortic body and other paraganglia HCC
AHA: 2021,2Q,7; 2016,4Q,26
D44.9 Neoplasm of uncertain behavior of unspecified endocrine gland

D45 Polycythemia vera HCC
EXCLUDES 1 *familial polycythemia (D75.Ø)*
secondary polycythemia (D75.1)
DEF: Abnormal proliferation of all bone marrow elements, increased red cell mass, and total blood volume. The etiology is unknown, but it is frequently associated with splenomegaly, leukocytosis, and thrombocythemia.

D46 Myelodysplastic syndromes
Use additional code for adverse effect, if applicable, to identify drug (T36-T5Ø with fifth or sixth character 5)
EXCLUDES 2 *drug-induced aplastic anemia (D61.1)*
D46.Ø Refractory anemia without ring sideroblasts, so stated HCC
Refractory anemia without sideroblasts, without excess of blasts
D46.1 Refractory anemia with ring sideroblasts HCC
RARS
D46.2 Refractory anemia with excess of blasts [RAEB]
D46.2Ø Refractory anemia with excess of blasts, unspecified HCC
RAEB NOS
D46.21 Refractory anemia with excess of blasts 1 HCC
RAEB 1
D46.22 Refractory anemia with excess of blasts 2 CC HCC
RAEB 2
D46.A Refractory cytopenia with multilineage dysplasia HCC
D46.B Refractory cytopenia with multilineage dysplasia and ring sideroblasts HCC
RCMD RS
D46.C Myelodysplastic syndrome with isolated del(5q) chromosomal abnormality CC HCC
Myelodysplastic syndrome with 5q deletion
5q minus syndrome NOS
D46.4 Refractory anemia, unspecified HCC
D46.Z Other myelodysplastic syndromes HCC
EXCLUDES 1 *chronic myelomonocytic leukemia (C93.1-)*
D46.9 Myelodysplastic syndrome, unspecified HCC
Myelodysplasia NOS

D47 Other neoplasms of uncertain behavior of lymphoid, hematopoietic and related tissue
D47.Ø Mast cell neoplasms of uncertain behavior
EXCLUDES 1 *congenital cutaneous mastocytosis (Q82.2)*
histiocytic neoplasms of uncertain behavior (D47.Z9)
malignant mast cell neoplasm (C96.2-)
AHA: 2017,4Q,5
D47.Ø1 Cutaneous mastocytosis CC
Diffuse cutaneous mastocytosis
Maculopapular cutaneous mastocytosis
Solitary mastocytoma
Telangiectasia macularis eruptiva perstans
Urticaria pigmentosa
EXCLUDES 1 *congenital (diffuse) (maculopapular) cutaneous mastocytosis (Q82.2)*
congenital urticaria pigmentosa (Q82.2)
extracutaneous mastocytoma (D47.Ø9)
D47.Ø2 Systemic mastocytosis CC
Indolent systemic mastocytosis
Isolated bone marrow mastocytosis
Smoldering systemic mastocytosis
Systemic mastocytosis, with an associated hematological non-mast cell lineage disease (SM-AHNMD)
Code also, if applicable, any associated hematological non-mast cell lineage disease, such as:
acute myeloid leukemia (C92.6-, C92.A-)
chronic myelomonocytic leukemia (C93.1-)
essential thrombocytosis (D47.3)
hypereosinophilic syndrome (D72.1)
myelodysplastic syndrome (D46.9)
myeloproliferative syndrome (D47.1)
non-Hodgkin lymphoma (C82-C85)
plasma cell myeloma (C9Ø.Ø-)
polycythemia vera (D45)
EXCLUDES 1 *aggressive systemic mastocytosis (C96.21)*
mast cell leukemia (C94.3-)
D47.Ø9 Other mast cell neoplasms of uncertain behavior CC
Extracutaneous mastocytoma
Mast cell tumor NOS
Mastocytoma NOS
Mastocytosis NOS

D47.1 Chronic myeloproliferative disease CC HCC
Chronic neutrophilic leukemia
Myeloproliferative disease, unspecified
EXCLUDES 1 *atypical chronic myeloid leukemia BCR/ABL-negative (C92.2-)*
chronic myeloid leukemia BCR/ABL-positive (C92.1-)
myelofibrosis NOS (D75.81)
myelophthisic anemia (D61.82)
myelophthisis (D61.82)
secondary myelofibrosis NOS (D75.81)

D47.2 Monoclonal gammopathy
Monoclonal gammopathy of undetermined significance [MGUS]
AHA: 2021,3Q,5
TIP: Smoldering multiple myeloma (SMM) is coded here.

D47.3 Essential (hemorrhagic) thrombocythemia HCC
Essential thrombocytosis
Idiopathic hemorrhagic thrombocythemia
Primary thrombocytosis
EXCLUDES 2 *reactive thrombocytosis (D75.838)*
secondary thrombocytosis (D75.838)
thrombocythemia NOS (D75.839)
thrombocytosis NOS (D75.839)
DEF: Chronic myeloproliferative neoplasm involving production of excess blood platelets that may result in abnormal clotting or hemorrhaging.

D47.4 Osteomyelofibrosis HCC
Chronic idiopathic myelofibrosis
Myelofibrosis (idiopathic) (with myeloid metaplasia)
Myelosclerosis (megakaryocytic) with myeloid metaplasia
Secondary myelofibrosis in myeloproliferative disease
EXCLUDES 1 *acute myelofibrosis (C94.4-)*

✓5th **D47.Z Other specified neoplasms of uncertain behavior of lymphoid, hematopoietic and related tissue**
AHA: 2016,4Q,8

D47.Z1 Post-transplant lymphoproliferative disorder (PTLD) CC UPD HCC
Code first complications of transplanted organs and tissue (T86.-)
DEF: Excessive proliferation of B-cell lymphocytes following Epstein-Barr virus infection in organ transplant patients. It may progress to non-Hodgkin lymphoma.

D47.Z2 Castleman disease CC HCC
Code also, if applicable, human herpesvirus 8 infection (B10.89)
EXCLUDES 2 *Kaposi's sarcoma (C46.-)*
DEF: Rare disease of the lymph nodes and lymphoid tissues that closely mimics lymphoma.

D47.Z9 Other specified neoplasms of uncertain behavior of lymphoid, hematopoietic and related tissue CC HCC
Histiocytic tumors of uncertain behavior

D47.9 Neoplasm of uncertain behavior of lymphoid, hematopoietic and related tissue, unspecified CC HCC
Lymphoproliferative disease NOS

✓4th **D48 Neoplasm of uncertain behavior of other and unspecified sites**
EXCLUDES 1 *neurofibromatosis (nonmalignant) (Q85.0-)*

D48.0 Neoplasm of uncertain behavior of bone and articular cartilage
EXCLUDES 1 *neoplasm of uncertain behavior of cartilage of ear ▶(D48.1-)◀*
neoplasm of uncertain behavior of cartilage of larynx (D38.0)
neoplasm of uncertain behavior of cartilage of nose (D38.5)
neoplasm of uncertain behavior of connective tissue of eyelid ▶(D48.1-)◀
neoplasm of uncertain behavior of synovia ▶(D48.1-)◀

▲ ✓5th **D48.1 Neoplasm of uncertain behavior of connective and other soft tissue**
Neoplasm of uncertain behavior of connective tissue of ear
Neoplasm of uncertain behavior of connective tissue of eyelid
Stromal tumors of uncertain behavior of digestive system
EXCLUDES 1 *neoplasm of uncertain behavior of articular cartilage (D48.0)*
neoplasm of uncertain behavior of cartilage of larynx (D38.0)
neoplasm of uncertain behavior of cartilage of nose (D38.5)
neoplasm of uncertain behavior of connective tissue of breast (D48.6-)

● ✓6th **D48.11 Desmoid tumor**
● **D48.110 Desmoid tumor of head and neck**
● **D48.111 Desmoid tumor of chest wall**
● **D48.112 Desmoid tumor, intrathoracic**
● **D48.113 Desmoid tumor of abdominal wall**
● **D48.114 Desmoid tumor, intraabdominal**
Desmoid tumor of pelvic cavity
Desmoid tumor, peritoneal, retroperitoneal
● **D48.115 Desmoid tumor of upper extremity and shoulder girdle**
● **D48.116 Desmoid tumor of lower extremity and pelvic girdle**
Desmoid tumor of buttock
● **D48.117 Desmoid tumor of back**
● **D48.118 Desmoid tumor of other site**
● **D48.119 Desmoid tumor of unspecified site**
● **D48.19 Other specified neoplasm of uncertain behavior of connective and other soft tissue**

D48.2 Neoplasm of uncertain behavior of peripheral nerves and autonomic nervous system
EXCLUDES 1 *neoplasm of uncertain behavior of peripheral nerves of orbit (D48.7)*

D48.3 Neoplasm of uncertain behavior of retroperitoneum

D48.4 Neoplasm of uncertain behavior of peritoneum

D48.5 Neoplasm of uncertain behavior of skin
Neoplasm of uncertain behavior of anal margin
Neoplasm of uncertain behavior of anal skin
Neoplasm of uncertain behavior of perianal skin
Neoplasm of uncertain behavior of skin of breast
EXCLUDES 1 *neoplasm of uncertain behavior of anus NOS (D37.8)*
neoplasm of uncertain behavior of skin of genital organs (D39.8, D40.8)
neoplasm of uncertain behavior of vermilion border of lip (D37.0)

✓5th **D48.6 Neoplasm of uncertain behavior of breast**
Cystosarcoma phyllodes
Neoplasm of uncertain behavior of connective tissue of breast
EXCLUDES 1 *neoplasm of uncertain behavior of skin of breast (D48.5)*

D48.60 Neoplasm of uncertain behavior of unspecified breast
D48.61 Neoplasm of uncertain behavior of right breast
D48.62 Neoplasm of uncertain behavior of left breast

D48.7 Neoplasm of uncertain behavior of other specified sites
Neoplasm of uncertain behavior of eye
Neoplasm of uncertain behavior of heart
Neoplasm of uncertain behavior of peripheral nerves of orbit
EXCLUDES 1 *neoplasm of uncertain behavior of connective tissue ▶(D48.1-)◀*
neoplasm of uncertain behavior of skin of eyelid (D48.5)

D48.9 Neoplasm of uncertain behavior, unspecified

Neoplasms of unspecified behavior (D49)

D49 Neoplasms of unspecified behavior

NOTE Category D49 classifies by site neoplasms of unspecified morphology and behavior. The term "mass", unless otherwise stated, is not to be regarded as a neoplastic growth.

INCLUDES "growth" NOS
neoplasm NOS
new growth NOS
tumor NOS

EXCLUDES 1 *neoplasms of uncertain behavior (D37-D44, D48)*

D49.Ø Neoplasm of unspecified behavior of digestive system

EXCLUDES 1 *neoplasm of unspecified behavior of margin of anus (D49.2)*
neoplasm of unspecified behavior of perianal skin (D49.2)
neoplasm of unspecified behavior of skin of anus (D49.2)

D49.1 Neoplasm of unspecified behavior of respiratory system

D49.2 Neoplasm of unspecified behavior of bone, soft tissue, and skin

EXCLUDES 1 *neoplasm of unspecified behavior of anal canal (D49.Ø)*
neoplasm of unspecified behavior of anus NOS (D49.Ø)
neoplasm of unspecified behavior of bone marrow (D49.89)
neoplasm of unspecified behavior of cartilage of larynx (D49.1)
neoplasm of unspecified behavior of cartilage of nose (D49.1)
neoplasm of unspecified behavior of connective tissue of breast (D49.3)
neoplasm of unspecified behavior of skin of genital organs (D49.59)
neoplasm of unspecified behavior of vermilion border of lip (D49.Ø)

D49.3 Neoplasm of unspecified behavior of breast

EXCLUDES 1 *neoplasm of unspecified behavior of skin of breast (D49.2)*

D49.4 Neoplasm of unspecified behavior of bladder

D49.5 Neoplasm of unspecified behavior of other genitourinary organs

AHA: 2016,4Q,9

D49.51 Neoplasm of unspecified behavior of kidney

D49.511 Neoplasm of unspecified behavior of right kidney

D49.512 Neoplasm of unspecified behavior of left kidney

D49.519 Neoplasm of unspecified behavior of unspecified kidney

D49.59 Neoplasm of unspecified behavior of other genitourinary organ

D49.6 Neoplasm of unspecified behavior of brain HCC

EXCLUDES 1 *neoplasm of unspecified behavior of cerebral meninges (D49.7)*
neoplasm of unspecified behavior of cranial nerves (D49.7)

D49.7 Neoplasm of unspecified behavior of endocrine glands and other parts of nervous system

EXCLUDES 1 *neoplasm of unspecified behavior of peripheral, sympathetic, and parasympathetic nerves and ganglia (D49.2)*

D49.8 Neoplasm of unspecified behavior of other specified sites

EXCLUDES 1 *neoplasm of unspecified behavior of eyelid (skin) (D49.2)*
neoplasm of unspecified behavior of eyelid cartilage (D49.2)
neoplasm of unspecified behavior of great vessels (D49.2)
neoplasm of unspecified behavior of optic nerve (D49.7)

D49.81 Neoplasm of unspecified behavior of retina and choroid

Dark area on retina
Retinal freckle

D49.89 Neoplasm of unspecified behavior of other specified sites

D49.9 Neoplasm of unspecified behavior of unspecified site

Chapter 3. Diseases of the Blood and Blood-forming Organs and Certain Disorders Involving the Immune Mechanism (D5Ø–D89)

Chapter-specific Guidelines with Coding Examples

Reserved for future guideline expansion

Chapter 3. Diseases of the Blood and Blood-forming Organs and Certain Disorders Involving the Immune Mechanism (D5Ø-D89)

EXCLUDES 2 *autoimmune disease (systemic) NOS (M35.9)*
certain conditions originating in the perinatal period (PØØ-P96)
complications of pregnancy, childbirth and the puerperium (OØØ-O9A)
congenital malformations, deformations and chromosomal abnormalities (QØØ-Q99)
endocrine, nutritional and metabolic diseases (EØØ-E88)
human immunodeficiency virus [HIV] disease (B2Ø)
injury, poisoning and certain other consequences of external causes (SØØ-T88)
neoplasms (CØØ-D49)
symptoms, signs and abnormal clinical and laboratory findings, not elsewhere classified (RØØ-R94)

This chapter contains the following blocks:

D5Ø-D53 Nutritional anemias
D55-D59 Hemolytic anemias
D6Ø-D64 Aplastic and other anemias and other bone marrow failure syndromes
D65-D69 Coagulation defects, purpura and other hemorrhagic conditions
D7Ø-D77 Other disorders of blood and blood-forming organs
D78 Intraoperative and postprocedural complications of the spleen
D8Ø-D89 Certain disorders involving the immune mechanism

Nutritional anemias (D5Ø-D53)

DEF: Nutritional anemia: The result of inadequate intake or absorption of a vitamin or mineral that impacts the production of red blood cells or causes them to develop abnormally affecting the size and shape.

TIP: Documentation must identify a link between anemia and the nutritional deficiency; low levels of a particular nutrient may occur concurrently with anemia but not cause the anemia.

✓4th **D5Ø Iron deficiency anemia**

INCLUDES asiderotic anemia
hypochromic anemia

D5Ø.Ø Iron deficiency anemia secondary to blood loss (chronic)
Posthemorrhagic anemia (chronic)
EXCLUDES 1 *acute posthemorrhagic anemia (D62)*
congenital anemia from fetal blood loss (P61.3)
AHA: 2019,3Q,17

D5Ø.1 Sideropenic dysphagia
Kelly-Paterson syndrome
Plummer-Vinson syndrome

D5Ø.8 Other iron deficiency anemias
Iron deficiency anemia due to inadequate dietary iron intake

D5Ø.9 Iron deficiency anemia, unspecified

✓4th **D51 Vitamin B12 deficiency anemia**

EXCLUDES 1 *vitamin B12 deficiency (E53.8)*

D51.Ø Vitamin B12 deficiency anemia due to intrinsic factor deficiency
Addison anemia
Biermer anemia
Congenital intrinsic factor deficiency
Pernicious (congenital) anemia
DEF: Chronic progressive anemia due to vitamin B12 malabsorption, caused by lack of secretion of intrinsic factor, which is produced by the gastric mucosa of the stomach.

D51.1 Vitamin B12 deficiency anemia due to selective vitamin B12 malabsorption with proteinuria
Imerslund (Gräsbeck) syndrome
Megaloblastic hereditary anemia

D51.2 Transcobalamin II deficiency

D51.3 Other dietary vitamin B12 deficiency anemia
Vegan anemia

D51.8 Other vitamin B12 deficiency anemias

D51.9 Vitamin B12 deficiency anemia, unspecified

✓4th **D52 Folate deficiency anemia**

EXCLUDES 1 *folate deficiency without anemia (E53.8)*

DEF: Deficiency in a B complex vitamin needed for the production of healthy red blood cells. Lack of folate, or folic acid, and other absorption conditions can cause anemia resulting in large, misshapen red blood cells called megaloblasts.

D52.Ø Dietary folate deficiency anemia
Nutritional megaloblastic anemia
DEF: Result of a poor diet with inadequate intake of folate, which is needed to produce healthy red blood cells.

D52.1 Drug-induced folate deficiency anemia
Use additional code for adverse effect, if applicable, to identify drug (T36-T5Ø with fifth or sixth character 5)

D52.8 Other folate deficiency anemias

D52.9 Folate deficiency anemia, unspecified
Folic acid deficiency anemia NOS

✓4th **D53 Other nutritional anemias**

INCLUDES megaloblastic anemia unresponsive to vitamin B12 or folate therapy

D53.Ø Protein deficiency anemia
Amino-acid deficiency anemia
Orotaciduric anemia
EXCLUDES 1 *Lesch-Nyhan syndrome (E79.1)*

D53.1 Other megaloblastic anemias, not elsewhere classified
Megaloblastic anemia NOS
EXCLUDES 1 *Di Guglielmo's disease (C94.Ø)*

D53.2 Scorbutic anemia
EXCLUDES 1 *scurvy (E54)*

D53.8 Other specified nutritional anemias
Anemia associated with deficiency of copper
Anemia associated with deficiency of molybdenum
Anemia associated with deficiency of zinc
EXCLUDES 1 *nutritional deficiencies without anemia, such as:*
copper deficiency NOS (E61.Ø)
molybdenum deficiency NOS (E61.5)
zinc deficiency NOS (E6Ø)

D53.9 Nutritional anemia, unspecified
Simple chronic anemia
EXCLUDES 1 *anemia NOS (D64.9)*
AHA: 2018,4Q,88

Hemolytic anemias (D55-D59)

✓4th **D55 Anemia due to enzyme disorders**

EXCLUDES 1 *drug-induced enzyme deficiency anemia (D59.2)*

D55.Ø Anemia due to glucose-6-phosphate dehydrogenase [G6PD] deficiency HCC
Favism
G6PD deficiency anemia
EXCLUDES 1 *glucose-6-phosphate dehydrogenase (G6PD) deficiency without anemia (D75.A)*

D55.1 Anemia due to other disorders of glutathione metabolism HCC
Anemia (due to) enzyme deficiencies, except G6PD, related to the hexose monophosphate [HMP] shunt pathway
Anemia (due to) hemolytic nonspherocytic (hereditary), type I

✓5th **D55.2 Anemia due to disorders of glycolytic enzymes**
EXCLUDES 1 *disorders of glycolysis not associated with anemia (E74.81-)*
AHA: 2021,4Q,6-7

D55.21 Anemia due to pyruvate kinase deficiency HCC
PK deficiency anemia
Pyruvate kinase deficiency anemia

D55.29 Anemia due to other disorders of glycolytic enzymes HCC
Hexokinase deficiency anemia
Triose-phosphate isomerase deficiency anemia

D55.3 Anemia due to disorders of nucleotide metabolism HCC

D55.8 Other anemias due to enzyme disorders HCC

D55.9 Anemia due to enzyme disorder, unspecified HCC

D56 Thalassemia

EXCLUDES 1 *sickle-cell thalassemia (D57.4-)*

DEF: Group of inherited disorders of hemoglobin metabolism causing mild to severe anemia. It is usually found in people of Mediterranean, African, Chinese, or Asian descent.

Thalassemia

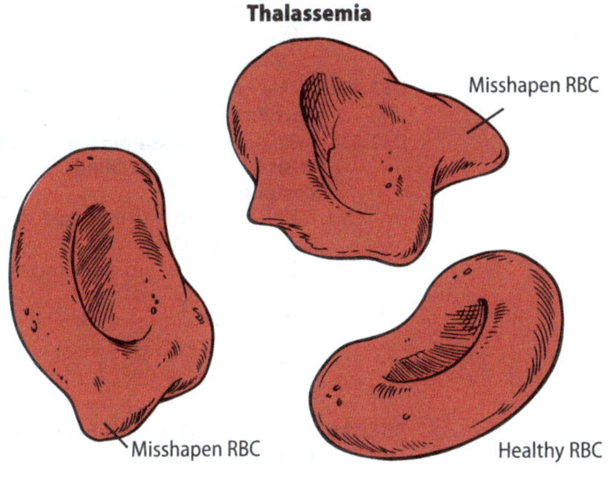

D56.Ø Alpha thalassemia HCC

Alpha thalassemia major
Hemoglobin H Constant Spring
Hemoglobin H disease
Hydrops fetalis due to alpha thalassemia
Severe alpha thalassemia
Triple gene defect alpha thalassemia

Use additional code, if applicable, for hydrops fetalis due to alpha thalassemia (P56.99)

EXCLUDES 1 *alpha thalassemia trait or minor (D56.3)*
asymptomatic alpha thalassemia (D56.3)
hydrops fetalis due to isoimmunization (P56.Ø)
hydrops fetalis not due to immune hemolysis (P83.2)

DEF: HBA1 and HBA2 genetic variant of chromosome 16 prevalent among those of African and Southeast Asian descent. Alpha thalassemia is associated with a wide spectrum of anemic presentation and includes hemoglobin H disease subtypes.

D56.1 Beta thalassemia HCC

Beta thalassemia major
Cooley's anemia
Homozygous beta thalassemia
Severe beta thalassemia
Thalassemia intermedia
Thalassemia major

EXCLUDES 1 *beta thalassemia minor (D56.3)*
beta thalassemia trait (D56.3)
delta-beta thalassemia (D56.2)
hemoglobin E-beta thalassemia (D56.5)
sickle-cell beta thalassemia (D57.4-)

D56.2 Delta-beta thalassemia HCC

Homozygous delta-beta thalassemia

EXCLUDES 1 *delta-beta thalassemia minor (D56.3)*
delta-beta thalassemia trait (D56.3)

D56.3 Thalassemia minor

Alpha thalassemia minor
Alpha thalassemia silent carrier
Alpha thalassemia trait
Beta thalassemia minor
Beta thalassemia trait
Delta-beta thalassemia minor
Delta-beta thalassemia trait
Thalassemia trait NOS

EXCLUDES 1 *alpha thalassemia (D56.Ø)*
beta thalassemia (D56.1)
delta-beta thalassemia (D56.2)
hemoglobin E-beta thalassemia (D56.5)
sickle-cell trait (D57.3)

DEF: Solitary abnormal gene that identifies a carrier of the disease, yet with an absence of symptoms or a clinically mild anemic presentation.

D56.4 Hereditary persistence of fetal hemoglobin [HPFH] HCC

D56.5 Hemoglobin E-beta thalassemia HCC

EXCLUDES 1 *beta thalassemia (D56.1)*
beta thalassemia minor (D56.3)
beta thalassemia trait (D56.3)
delta-beta thalassemia (D56.2)
delta-beta thalassemia trait (D56.3)
hemoglobin E disease (D58.2)
other hemoglobinopathies (D58.2)
sickle-cell beta thalassemia (D57.4-)

D56.8 Other thalassemias HCC

Dominant thalassemia
Hemoglobin C thalassemia
Mixed thalassemia
Thalassemia with other hemoglobinopathy

EXCLUDES 1 *hemoglobin C disease (D58.2)*
hemoglobin E disease (D58.2)
other hemoglobinopathies (D58.2)
sickle-cell anemia (D57.-)
sickle-cell thalassemia ▶(D57.4-)◀

D56.9 Thalassemia, unspecified

Mediterranean anemia (with other hemoglobinopathy)

D57 Sickle-cell disorders

Use additional code for any associated fever (R50.81)

EXCLUDES 1 *other hemoglobinopathies (D58.-)*

AHA: 2022,2Q,28

DEF: Severe, chronic inherited diseases caused by a genetic variation in hemoglobin protein of the red blood cell. The gene mutation causes the red blood cell to become hard, sticky, and crescent or sickle shaped, making it harder for red blood cells to travel through the bloodstream, disrupting blood flow and decreasing oxygen transport to tissues.

Sickle cell

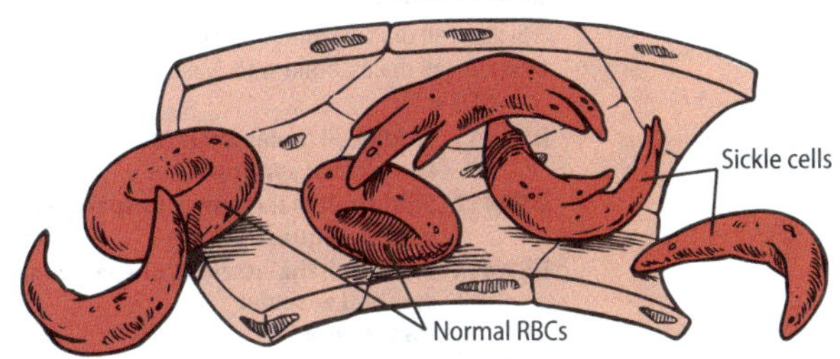

D57.Ø Hb-SS disease with crisis

Sickle-cell disease with crisis
▶Hb-SS disease with (vaso-occlusive) pain◀

AHA: 2020,4Q,6-7

D57.ØØ Hb-SS disease with crisis, unspecified MCC HCC

Hb-SS disease with (painful) crisis NOS
▶Hb-SS disease with (vaso-occlusive) pain NOS◀

D57.Ø1 Hb-SS disease with acute chest syndrome MCC HCC

D57.Ø2 Hb-SS disease with splenic sequestration MCC HCC

D57.Ø3 Hb-SS disease with cerebral vascular involvement MCC HCC

Code also, if applicable, cerebral infarction (I63.-)

● **D57.Ø4 Hb-SS disease with dactylitis** MCC

D57.Ø9 Hb-SS disease with crisis with other specified complication MCC HCC

Use additional code to identify complications, such as:
cholelithiasis (K8Ø.-)
priapism (N48.32)

D57.1 Sickle-cell disease without crisis HCC

Hb-SS disease without crisis
Sickle-cell anemia NOS
Sickle-cell disease NOS
Sickle-cell disorder NOS

D57.2 Sickle-cell/Hb-C disease

Hb-SC disease
Hb-S/Hb-C disease

AHA: 2020,4Q,6-7

D57.2Ø Sickle-cell/Hb-C disease without crisis HCC

D57.21 Sickle-cell/Hb-C disease with crisis

D57.211 Sickle-cell/Hb-C disease with acute chest syndrome MCC HCC

D57.212 Sickle-cell/Hb-C disease with splenic sequestration MCC HCC

D57.213 Sickle-cell/Hb-C disease with cerebral vascular involvement MCC HCC
Code also, if applicable, cerebral infarction (I63.-)

● **D57.214 Sickle-cell/Hb-C disease with dactylitis** MCC

D57.218 Sickle-cell/Hb-C disease with crisis with other specified complication MCC HCC
Use additional code to identify complications, such as:
cholelithiasis (K80.-)
priapism (N48.32)

D57.219 Sickle-cell/Hb-C disease with crisis, unspecified MCC HCC
Sickle-cell/Hb-C disease with crisis NOS
▶Sickle-cell/Hb-C disease with (vaso-occlusive) pain NOS◀

D57.3 Sickle-cell trait HCC
Hb-S trait
Heterozygous hemoglobin S
DEF: Heterozygous genetic makeup characterized by one gene for normal hemoglobin and one for sickle-cell hemoglobin. The clinical disease is rarely present.

√5th **D57.4 Sickle-cell thalassemia**
Sickle-cell beta thalassemia
Thalassemia Hb-S disease
AHA: 2020,4Q,6-7

D57.40 Sickle-cell thalassemia without crisis HCC
Microdrepanocytosis
Sickle-cell thalassemia NOS

√6th **D57.41 Sickle-cell thalassemia, unspecified, with crisis**
Sickle-cell thalassemia with (painful) crisis NOS
▶Sickle-cell thalassemia with (vaso-occlusive) pain NOS◀

D57.411 Sickle-cell thalassemia, unspecified, with acute chest syndrome MCC HCC

D57.412 Sickle-cell thalassemia, unspecified, with splenic sequestration MCC HCC

D57.413 Sickle-cell thalassemia, unspecified, with cerebral vascular involvement MCC HCC
Code also, if applicable cerebral infarction (I63.-)

● **D57.414 Sickle-cell thalassemia, unspecified, with dactylitis** MCC

D57.418 Sickle-cell thalassemia, unspecified, with crisis with other specified complication MCC HCC
Use additional code to identify complications, such as:
cholelithiasis (K80.-)
priapism (N48.32)

D57.419 Sickle-cell thalassemia, unspecified, with crisis MCC HCC
Sickle-cell thalassemia with (painful) crisis NOS
▶Sickle-cell thalassemia with (vaso-occlusive) pain NOS◀

D57.42 Sickle-cell thalassemia beta zero without crisis HCC
HbS-beta zero without crisis
Sickle-cell beta zero without crisis

√6th **D57.43 Sickle-cell thalassemia beta zero with crisis**
HbS-beta zero with crisis
Sickle-cell beta zero with crisis

D57.431 Sickle-cell thalassemia beta zero with acute chest syndrome MCC HCC
HbS-beta zero with acute chest syndrome
Sickle-cell beta zero with acute chest syndrome

D57.432 Sickle-cell thalassemia beta zero with splenic sequestration MCC HCC
HbS-beta zero with splenic sequestration
Sickle-cell beta zero with splenic sequestration

D57.433 Sickle-cell thalassemia beta zero with cerebral vascular involvement MCC HCC
HbS-beta zero with cerebral vascular involvement
Sickle-cell beta zero with cerebral vascular involvement
Code also, if applicable cerebral infarction (I63.-)

● **D57.434 Sickle-cell thalassemia beta zero with dactylitis** MCC

D57.438 Sickle-cell thalassemia beta zero with crisis with other specified complication MCC HCC
HbS-beta zero with other specified complication
Sickle-cell beta zero with other specified complication
Use additional code to identify complications, such as:
cholelithiasis (K80.-)
priapism (N48.32)

D57.439 Sickle-cell thalassemia beta zero with crisis, unspecified MCC HCC
HbS-beta zero with other specified complication
Sickle-cell beta zero with crisis unspecified
Sickle-cell thalassemia beta zero with (painful) crisis NOS
▶Sickle-cell thalassemia beta zero with (vaso-occlusive) pain NOS◀

D57.44 Sickle-cell thalassemia beta plus without crisis HCC
HbS-beta plus without crisis
Sickle-cell beta plus without crisis

√6th **D57.45 Sickle-cell thalassemia beta plus with crisis**
HbS-beta plus with crisis
Sickle-cell beta plus with crisis

D57.451 Sickle-cell thalassemia beta plus with acute chest syndrome MCC HCC
HbS-beta plus with acute chest syndrome
Sickle-cell beta plus with acute chest syndrome

D57.452 Sickle-cell thalassemia beta plus with splenic sequestration MCC HCC
HbS-beta plus with splenic sequestration
Sickle-cell beta plus with splenic sequestration

D57.453 Sickle-cell thalassemia beta plus with cerebral vascular involvement MCC HCC
HbS-beta plus with cerebral vascular involvement
Sickle-cell beta plus with cerebral vascular involvement
Code also, if applicable cerebral infarction (I63.-)

● **D57.454 Sickle-cell thalassemia beta plus with dactylitis** MCC

D57.458 Sickle-cell thalassemia beta plus with crisis with other specified complication MCC HCC
HbS-beta plus with crisis with other specified complication
Sickle-cell beta plus with crisis with other specified complication
Use additional code to identify complications, such as:
cholelithiasis (K80.-)
priapism (N48.32)

D57.459 Sickle-cell thalassemia beta plus with crisis, unspecified MCC HCC
HbS-beta plus with crisis with unspecified complication
Sickle-cell beta plus with crisis with unspecified complication
Sickle-cell thalassemia beta plus with (painful) crisis NOS
▶Sickle-cell thalassemia beta plus with (vaso-occlusive) pain NOS◀

D57.8 Other sickle-cell disorders
Hb-SD disease
Hb-SE disease
AHA: 2020,4Q,6-7

D57.80 Other sickle-cell disorders without crisis HCC

D57.81 Other sickle-cell disorders with crisis

D57.811 Other sickle-cell disorders with acute chest syndrome MCC HCC

D57.812 Other sickle-cell disorders with splenic sequestration MCC HCC

D57.813 Other sickle-cell disorders with cerebral vascular involvement MCC HCC
Code also, if applicable: cerebral infarction (I63.-)

● **D57.814 Other sickle-cell disorders with dactylitis** MCC

D57.818 Other sickle-cell disorders with crisis with other specified complication MCC HCC
Use additional code to identify complications, such as:
cholelithiasis (K80.-)
priapism (N48.32)

D57.819 Other sickle-cell disorders with crisis, unspecified MCC HCC
Other sickle-cell disorders with crisis NOS
▶Other sickle-cell disorders with (vaso-occlusive) pain NOS◀

D58 Other hereditary hemolytic anemias
EXCLUDES 1 *hemolytic anemia of the newborn (P55.-)*

D58.0 Hereditary spherocytosis HCC
Acholuric (familial) jaundice
Congenital (spherocytic) hemolytic icterus
Minkowski-Chauffard syndrome
DEF: Inherited condition caused by mutations to genes responsible for the production of proteins that form the membranes of red blood cells. The shape and flexibility of the red blood cell membrane is altered, diminishing the cell's ability to traverse the spleen, therefore becoming trapped and destroyed before the red blood cell has reached maturity.

D58.1 Hereditary elliptocytosis HCC
Elliptocytosis (congenital)
Ovalocytosis (congenital) (hereditary)

D58.2 Other hemoglobinopathies HCC
Abnormal hemoglobin NOS
Congenital Heinz body anemia
Hb-C disease
Hb-D disease
Hb-E disease
Hemoglobinopathy NOS
Unstable hemoglobin hemolytic disease
EXCLUDES 1 *familial polycythemia (D75.0)*
Hb-M disease (D74.0)
hemoglobin E-beta thalassemia (D56.5)
hereditary persistence of fetal hemoglobin [HPFH] (D56.4)
high-altitude polycythemia (D75.1)
methemoglobinemia (D74.-)
other hemoglobinopathies with thalassemia (D56.8)

D58.8 Other specified hereditary hemolytic anemias CC HCC
Stomatocytosis

D58.9 Hereditary hemolytic anemia, unspecified CC HCC

D59 Acquired hemolytic anemia
DEF: Non-hereditary anemia characterized by premature destruction of red blood cells caused by infectious organisms, poisons, and physical agents.

D59.0 Drug-induced autoimmune hemolytic anemia CC HCC
Use additional code for adverse effect, if applicable, to identify drug (T36-T50 with fifth or sixth character 5)

D59.1 Other autoimmune hemolytic anemias
EXCLUDES 2 *Evans syndrome (D69.41)*
hemolytic disease of newborn (P55.-)
paroxysmal cold hemoglobinuria (D59.6)
AHA: 2020,4Q,7-8

D59.10 Autoimmune hemolytic anemia, unspecified CC HCC

D59.11 Warm autoimmune hemolytic anemia CC HCC
Warm type (primary) (secondary) (symptomatic) autoimmune hemolytic anemia
Warm type autoimmune hemolytic disease

D59.12 Cold autoimmune hemolytic anemia CC HCC
Chronic cold hemagglutinin disease
Cold agglutinin disease
Cold agglutinin hemoglobinuria
Cold type (primary) (secondary) (symptomatic) autoimmune hemolytic anemia
Cold type autoimmune hemolytic disease

D59.13 Mixed type autoimmune hemolytic anemia CC HCC
Mixed type autoimmune hemolytic disease
Mixed type, cold and warm, (primary) (secondary) (symptomatic) autoimmune hemolytic anemia

D59.19 Other autoimmune hemolytic anemia CC HCC

D59.2 Drug-induced nonautoimmune hemolytic anemia CC HCC
Drug-induced enzyme deficiency anemia
Use additional code for adverse effect, if applicable, to identify drug (T36-T50 with fifth or sixth character 5)

D59.3 Hemolytic-uremic syndrome
Code also, if applicable, any associated:
acute kidney failure (N17.-)
chronic kidney disease (N18.-)
AHA: 2022,4Q,5-6
DEF: Condition typically precipitated by infection causing low platelets and destruction of red blood cells resulting in hemolytic anemia. This cell damage and blockage of renal capillaries lead to kidney failure. Mainly affects children.

D59.30 Hemolytic-uremic syndrome, unspecified MCC HCC
Hemolytic-uremic syndrome NOS

D59.31 Infection-associated hemolytic-uremic syndrome MCC HCC
Shiga toxin-producing E. coli [STEC] related hemolytic uremic syndrome
Typical hemolytic uremic syndrome
Use additional code to identify associated infection, such as:
E. coli infection (B96.2-)
human immunodeficiency virus [HIV] disease (B20)
pneumococcal meningitis (G00.1)
pneumococcal pneumonia (J13)
sepsis due to Streptococcus pneumoniae (A40.3)
Shigella dysenteriae (A03.9)
streptococcus pneumoniae as the cause of diseases classified elsewhere (B95.3)

D59.32 Hereditary hemolytic-uremic syndrome MCC HCC
Atypical hemolytic uremic syndrome with an identified genetic cause
Code also, if applicable:
defects in the complement system (D84.1)
methylmalonic acidemia (E71.120)

D59.39 Other hemolytic-uremic syndrome MCC HCC
Atypical (nongenetic) hemolytic uremic syndrome
Secondary hemolytic-uremic syndrome
Code first, if applicable, any associated:
COVID-19 (U07.1)
complications of heart transplant (T86.2-)
complications of kidney transplant (T86.1-)
complications of liver transplant (T86.4-)
Code also, if applicable, any associated condition, such as:
hypertensive emergency (I16.1)
malignant neoplasm (C00-C96)
systemic lupus erythematosus (M32.-)
Use additional code, if applicable, for adverse effect to identify drug (T36-T50 with fifth or sixth character 5)
AHA: 2022,4Q,6

D59.4 Other nonautoimmune hemolytic anemias CC HCC
Mechanical hemolytic anemia
Microangiopathic hemolytic anemia
Toxic hemolytic anemia

D59.5 Paroxysmal nocturnal hemoglobinuria [Marchiafava-Micheli] HCC
EXCLUDES 1 *hemoglobinuria NOS (R82.3)*

Chapter 3. Diseases of the Blood and Blood-forming Organs
D57.8–D59.5

D59.6 Hemoglobinuria due to hemolysis from other external causes HCC
Hemoglobinuria from exertion
March hemoglobinuria
Paroxysmal cold hemoglobinuria
Use additional code (Chapter 20) to identify external cause
EXCLUDES 1 *hemoglobinuria NOS (R82.3)*

D59.8 Other acquired hemolytic anemias HCC

D59.9 Acquired hemolytic anemia, unspecified CC HCC
Idiopathic hemolytic anemia, chronic

Aplastic and other anemias and other bone marrow failure syndromes (D60-D64)

✓4th D60 Acquired pure red cell aplasia [erythroblastopenia]
INCLUDES red cell aplasia (acquired) (adult) (with thymoma)
EXCLUDES 1 *congenital red cell aplasia (D61.01)*
DEF: Bone marrow failure characterized by underproduction of red blood cells while white blood cell and platelet production remains normal.

D60.0 Chronic acquired pure red cell aplasia MCC HCC

D60.1 Transient acquired pure red cell aplasia MCC HCC

D60.8 Other acquired pure red cell aplasias MCC HCC

D60.9 Acquired pure red cell aplasia, unspecified MCC HCC

✓4th D61 Other aplastic anemias and other bone marrow failure syndromes
EXCLUDES 2 *neutropenia (D70.-)*
AHA: 2020,3Q,22; 2014,4Q,22
DEF: Aplastic anemia: Bone marrow failure characterized by underproduction of red bloods cells, white blood cells and platelets.

✓5th D61.0 Constitutional aplastic anemia

D61.01 Constitutional (pure) red blood cell aplasia CC HCC
Blackfan-Diamond syndrome
Congenital (pure) red cell aplasia
Familial hypoplastic anemia
Primary (pure) red cell aplasia
Red cell (pure) aplasia of infants
EXCLUDES 1 *acquired red cell aplasia (D60.9)*

● **D61.02 Shwachman-Diamond syndrome** CC
Code also, if applicable, associated conditions such as:
acute myeloblastic leukemia (C92.0-)
exocrine pancreatic insufficiency (K86.81)
myelodysplastic syndrome (D46.-)
Use additional code, if applicable, for genetic susceptibility to other malignant neoplasm (Z15.09)

D61.09 Other constitutional aplastic anemia CC HCC
Fanconi's anemia
Pancytopenia with malformations

D61.1 Drug-induced aplastic anemia MCC HCC
Use additional code for adverse effect, if applicable, to identify drug (T36-T50 with fifth or sixth character 5)

D61.2 Aplastic anemia due to other external agents MCC HCC
Code first, if applicable, toxic effects of substances chiefly nonmedicinal as to source (T51-T65)

D61.3 Idiopathic aplastic anemia MCC HCC

✓5th D61.8 Other specified aplastic anemias and other bone marrow failure syndromes

✓6th D61.81 Pancytopenia
EXCLUDES 1 *pancytopenia (due to) (with) aplastic anemia (D61.9)*
pancytopenia (due to) (with) bone marrow infiltration (D61.82)
pancytopenia (due to) (with) congenital (pure) red cell aplasia (D61.01)
pancytopenia (due to) (with) hairy cell leukemia (C91.4-)
pancytopenia (due to) (with) human immunodeficiency virus disease (B20)
pancytopenia (due to) (with) leukoerythroblastic anemia (D61.82)
pancytopenia (due to) (with) myeloproliferative disease (D47.1)
EXCLUDES 2 *pancytopenia (due to) (with) myelodysplastic syndromes (D46.-)*
DEF: Shortage of all three blood cells: white, red, and platelets.

D61.810 Antineoplastic chemotherapy induced pancytopenia MCC HCC
EXCLUDES 2 *aplastic anemia due to antineoplastic chemotherapy (D61.1)*
AHA: 2020,3Q,22

D61.811 Other drug-induced pancytopenia MCC HCC
EXCLUDES 2 *aplastic anemia due to drugs (D61.1)*

D61.818 Other pancytopenia CC HCC
AHA: 2023,1Q,23; 2020,3Q,24; 2019,1Q,16
TIP: Assign this code in addition to myeloid leukemia codes (C92.-) when pancytopenia is documented. Although common in some types of myeloid leukemia, pancytopenia is not always inherent.

D61.82 Myelophthisis CC HCC
Leukoerythroblastic anemia
Myelophthisic anemia
Panmyelophthisis
Code also the underlying disorder, such as:
malignant neoplasm of breast (C50.-)
tuberculosis (A15.-)
EXCLUDES 1 *idiopathic myelofibrosis (D47.1)*
myelofibrosis NOS (D75.81)
myelofibrosis with myeloid metaplasia (D47.4)
primary myelofibrosis (D47.1)
secondary myelofibrosis (D75.81)
DEF: Condition that occurs when normal hematopoietic tissue in the bone marrow is replaced with abnormal tissue, such as fibrous tissue or tumors. Most commonly seen during the advanced stages of cancer.

D61.89 Other specified aplastic anemias and other bone marrow failure syndromes MCC HCC

D61.9 Aplastic anemia, unspecified CC HCC
Hypoplastic anemia NOS
Medullary hypoplasia

D62 Acute posthemorrhagic anemia CC
EXCLUDES 1 *anemia due to chronic blood loss (D50.0)*
blood loss anemia NOS (D50.0)
congenital anemia from fetal blood loss (P61.3)
AHA: 2023,1Q,15,16; 2019,3Q,11,17

✓4th D63 Anemia in chronic diseases classified elsewhere

D63.0 Anemia in neoplastic disease
Code first neoplasm (C00-D49)
EXCLUDES 1 *aplastic anemia due to antineoplastic chemotherapy (D61.1)*
EXCLUDES 2 *anemia due to antineoplastic chemotherapy (D64.81)*

D63.1 Anemia in chronic kidney disease
Erythropoietin resistant anemia (EPO resistant anemia)
Code first underlying chronic kidney disease (CKD) (N18.-)

D63.8 Anemia in other chronic diseases classified elsewhere
Code first underlying disease, such as:
diphyllobothriasis (B7Ø.Ø)
hookworm disease (B76.Ø-B76.9)
hypothyroidism (EØØ.Ø-EØ3.9)
malaria (B5Ø.Ø-B54)
symptomatic late syphilis (A52.79)
tuberculosis (A18.89)

D64 Other anemias
EXCLUDES 1 *refractory anemia (D46.-)*
refractory anemia with excess blasts in transformation [RAEB T] (C92.Ø-)

DEF: Sideroblastic anemia: Hereditary or secondary disorder in which the red blood cells cannot effectively use iron, a nutrient needed to make hemoglobin. Although the iron can enter the red blood cell it is not assimilated into the hemoglobin molecule and builds up ringed sideroblasts around the cell nucleus.

D64.Ø Hereditary sideroblastic anemia HCC
Sex-linked hypochromic sideroblastic anemia

D64.1 Secondary sideroblastic anemia due to disease HCC
Code first underlying disease

D64.2 Secondary sideroblastic anemia due to drugs and toxins HCC
Code first poisoning due to drug or toxin, if applicable ▶(T36-T65 with fifth or sixth character 1-4)◀
Use additional code for adverse effect, if applicable, to identify drug (T36-T5Ø with fifth or sixth character 5)

D64.3 Other sideroblastic anemias HCC
Sideroblastic anemia NOS
Pyridoxine-responsive sideroblastic anemia NEC

D64.4 Congenital dyserythropoietic anemia
Dyshematopoietic anemia (congenital)
EXCLUDES 1 *Blackfan-Diamond syndrome (D61.Ø1)*
Di Guglielmo's disease (C94.Ø)

D64.8 Other specified anemias

D64.81 Anemia due to antineoplastic chemotherapy
Antineoplastic chemotherapy induced anemia
EXCLUDES 2 *anemia in neoplastic disease (D63.Ø)*
aplastic anemia due to antineoplastic chemotherapy (D61.1)
AHA: 2023,2Q,17; 2021,3Q,4; 2014,4Q,22

D64.89 Other specified anemias
Infantile pseudoleukemia

D64.9 Anemia, unspecified
AHA: 2020,3Q,24; 2018,4Q,88; 2017,1Q,7

Coagulation defects, purpura and other hemorrhagic conditions (D65-D69)

D65 Disseminated intravascular coagulation [defibrination syndrome] MCC HCC
Afibrinogenemia, acquired
Consumption coagulopathy
▶COVID-19 associated diffuse or disseminated intravascular coagulopathy◀
Diffuse or disseminated intravascular coagulation [DIC]
Fibrinolytic hemorrhage, acquired
Fibrinolytic purpura
Purpura fulminans
▶Code also, if applicable, associated condition◀
EXCLUDES 1 *disseminated intravascular coagulation (complicating):*
abortion or ectopic or molar pregnancy (OØØ-OØ7, OØ8.1)
in newborn (P6Ø)
pregnancy, childbirth and the puerperium (O45.Ø, O46.Ø, O67.Ø, O72.3)
AHA: 2021,1Q,39

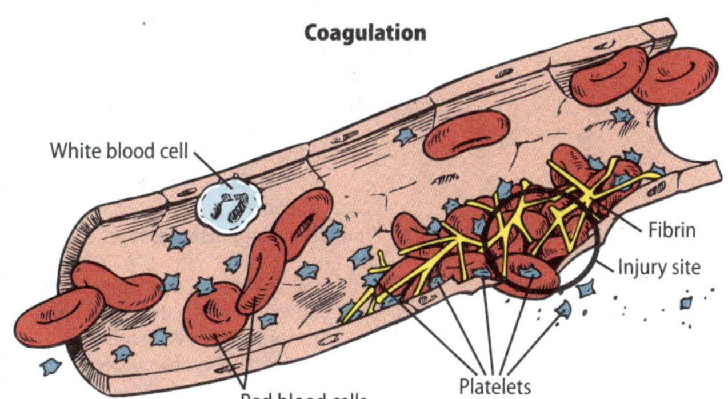

D66 Hereditary factor VIII deficiency MCC HCC
Classical hemophilia
Deficiency factor VIII (with functional defect)
Hemophilia A
Hemophilia NOS
EXCLUDES 1 *factor VIII deficiency with vascular defect (D68.Ø-)*
AHA: 2022,4Q,9
DEF: Hereditary, sex-linked lack of antihemophilic globulin (AHG) (factor VIII) that causes abnormal coagulation characterized by increased bleeding; large bruises of skin; bleeding in the mouth, nose, and gastrointestinal tract; and hemorrhages into joints, resulting in swelling and impaired function.
TIP: Factor VIII deficiency may also be documented in patients with VWD. Only a code for the VWD should be reported; do not report code D66.

D67 Hereditary factor IX deficiency MCC HCC
Christmas disease
Factor IX deficiency (with functional defect)
Hemophilia B
Plasma thromboplastin component [PTC] deficiency

D68 Other coagulation defects
EXCLUDES 1 *abnormal coagulation profile NOS (R79.1)*
EXCLUDES 2 *coagulation defects complicating abortion or ectopic or molar pregnancy (OØØ-OØ7, OØ8.1)*
coagulation defects complicating pregnancy, childbirth and the puerperium (O45.Ø, O46.Ø, O67.Ø, O72.3)
AHA: 2016,1Q,14

D68.Ø Von Willebrand disease
EXCLUDES 1 *capillary fragility (hereditary) (D69.8)*
factor VIII deficiency NOS (D66)
factor VIII deficiency with functional defect (D66)
AHA: 2022,4Q,7-9
DEF: Congenital, abnormal blood coagulation caused by deficient blood factor VII. Symptoms include excess or prolonged bleeding.
TIP: Factor VIII deficiency may also be documented in patients with VWD. Only a code for the VWD should be reported; do not report code D66.

D68.ØØ Von Willebrand disease, unspecified CC HCC

D68.01 Von Willebrand disease, type 1 CC HCC
Partial quantitative deficiency of von Willebrand factor
Type 1C von Willebrand disease
AHA: 2022,4Q,9

✓6th **D68.02 Von Willebrand disease, type 2**
Qualitative defects of von Willebrand factor

D68.020 Von Willebrand disease, type 2A CC HCC
Qualitative defects of von Willebrand factor with decreased platelet adhesion and selective deficiency of high-molecular-weight multimers

D68.021 Von Willebrand disease, type 2B CC HCC
Qualitative defects of von Willebrand factor with high-molecular-weight von Willebrand factor loss
Qualitative defects of von Willebrand factor with hyper-adhesive forms
Qualitative defects of von Willebrand factor with increased affinity for platelet glycoprotein Ib

D68.022 Von Willebrand disease, type 2M CC HCC
Qualitative defects of von Willebrand factor with defective platelet adhesion with a normal size distribution of von Willebrand factor multimers

D68.023 Von Willebrand disease, type 2N CC HCC
Qualitative defects of von Willebrand factor with defective von Willebrand factor to factor VIII binding
Qualitative defects of von Willebrand factor with markedly decreased affinity for factor VIII

D68.029 Von Willebrand disease, type 2, unspecified CC HCC
Qualitative defect in von Willebrand factor function, with no further subtyping

D68.03 Von Willebrand disease, type 3 CC HCC
(Near) complete absence of von Willebrand factor
Total quantitative deficiency of von Willebrand factor

D68.04 Acquired von Willebrand disease CC HCC
Acquired von Willebrand syndrome

D68.09 Other von Willebrand disease CC HCC
Platelet-type von Willebrand disease
Pseudo-von Willebrand disease
Code also, if applicable, qualitative platelet defects (D69.1)

D68.1 Hereditary factor XI deficiency CC HCC
Hemophilia C
Plasma thromboplastin antecedent [PTA] deficiency
Rosenthal's disease

D68.2 Hereditary deficiency of other clotting factors CC HCC
AC globulin deficiency
Congenital afibrinogenemia
Deficiency of factor I [fibrinogen]
Deficiency of factor II [prothrombin]
Deficiency of factor V [labile]
Deficiency of factor VII [stable]
Deficiency of factor X [Stuart-Prower]
Deficiency of factor XII [Hageman]
Deficiency of factor XIII [fibrin stabilizing]
Dysfibrinogenemia (congenital)
Hypoproconvertinemia
Owren's disease
Proaccelerin deficiency

✓5th **D68.3 Hemorrhagic disorder due to circulating anticoagulants**

✓6th **D68.31 Hemorrhagic disorder due to intrinsic circulating anticoagulants, antibodies, or inhibitors**

D68.311 Acquired hemophilia CC HCC
Autoimmune hemophilia
Autoimmune inhibitors to clotting factors
Secondary hemophilia

D68.312 Antiphospholipid antibody with hemorrhagic disorder CC HCC
Lupus anticoagulant (LAC) with hemorrhagic disorder
Systemic lupus erythematosus [SLE] inhibitor with hemorrhagic disorder
EXCLUDES 1 *antiphospholipid antibody, finding without diagnosis (R76.0)*
antiphospholipid antibody syndrome (D68.61)
antiphospholipid antibody with hypercoagulable state (D68.61)
lupus anticoagulant (LAC) finding without diagnosis (R76.0)
lupus anticoagulant (LAC) with hypercoagulable state (D68.62)
systemic lupus erythematosus [SLE] inhibitor finding without diagnosis (R76.0)
systemic lupus erythematosus [SLE] inhibitor with hypercoagulable state (D68.62)

D68.318 Other hemorrhagic disorder due to intrinsic circulating anticoagulants, antibodies, or inhibitors CC HCC
Antithromboplastinemia
Antithromboplastinogenemia
Hemorrhagic disorder due to intrinsic increase in antithrombin
Hemorrhagic disorder due to intrinsic increase in anti-VIIIa
Hemorrhagic disorder due to intrinsic increase in anti-IXa
Hemorrhagic disorder due to intrinsic increase in anti-XIa

D68.32 Hemorrhagic disorder due to extrinsic circulating anticoagulants CC HCC
Drug-induced hemorrhagic disorder
Hemorrhagic disorder due to increase in anti-IIa
Hemorrhagic disorder due to increase in anti-Xa
Hyperheparinemia
Use additional code for adverse effect, if applicable, to identify drug (T45.515, T45.525)
AHA: 2021,1Q,4; 2016,1Q,14-15
TIP: Do not assign to identify routine therapeutic anticoagulation effects; assign only for documented adverse effects.

D68.4 Acquired coagulation factor deficiency CC HCC
Deficiency of coagulation factor due to liver disease
Deficiency of coagulation factor due to vitamin K deficiency
EXCLUDES 1 *vitamin K deficiency of newborn (P53)*

✓5th **D68.5 Primary thrombophilia**
Primary hypercoagulable states
EXCLUDES 1 *antiphospholipid syndrome (D68.61)*
lupus anticoagulant (D68.62)
secondary activated protein C resistance (D68.69)
secondary antiphospholipid antibody syndrome (D68.69)
secondary lupus anticoagulant with hypercoagulable state (D68.69)
secondary systemic lupus erythematosus [SLE] inhibitor with hypercoagulable state (D68.69)
systemic lupus erythematosus [SLE] inhibitor finding without diagnosis (R76.0)
systemic lupus erythematosus [SLE] inhibitor with hemorrhagic disorder (D68.312)
thrombotic thrombocytopenic purpura (M31.19)
DEF: Thrombophilia: Increased tendency of the blood to clot, which can lead to thrombus or embolus formation.

D68.51 Activated protein C resistance CC HCC
Factor V Leiden mutation

D68.52 Prothrombin gene mutation CC HCC

D68.59 **Other primary thrombophilia** CC HCC
Antithrombin III deficiency
Hypercoagulable state NOS
Primary hypercoagulable state NEC
Primary thrombophilia NEC
Protein C deficiency
Protein S deficiency
Thrombophilia NOS
AHA: 2021,2Q,8

√5th D68.6 **Other thrombophilia**
Other hypercoagulable states
EXCLUDES 1 *diffuse or disseminated intravascular coagulation [DIC] (D65)*
heparin induced thrombocytopenia (HIT) (D75.82-)
hyperhomocysteinemia (E72.11)

D68.61 **Antiphospholipid syndrome** CC HCC
Anticardiolipin syndrome
Antiphospholipid antibody syndrome
EXCLUDES 1 *anti-phospholipid antibody, finding without diagnosis (R76.Ø)*
anti-phospholipid antibody with hemorrhagic disorder (D68.312)
lupus anticoagulant syndrome (D68.62)

D68.62 **Lupus anticoagulant syndrome** CC HCC
Lupus anticoagulant
Presence of systemic lupus erythematosus [SLE] inhibitor
EXCLUDES 1 *anticardiolipin syndrome (D68.61)*
antiphospholipid syndrome (D68.61)
lupus anticoagulant (LAC) finding without diagnosis (R76.Ø)
lupus anticoagulant (LAC) with hemorrhagic disorder (D68.312)

D68.69 **Other thrombophilia** CC HCC
▶COVID-19 associated hypercoagulability◀
Hypercoagulable states NEC
Secondary hypercoagulable state NOS
▶Code also, if applicable, associated condition◀
AHA: 2021,2Q,8

D68.8 **Other specified coagulation defects** CC HCC
▶COVID-19 associated coagulopathy◀
▶Code also, if applicable, associated condition◀
EXCLUDES 1 *hemorrhagic disease of newborn (P53)*
AHA: 2021,1Q,39

D68.9 **Coagulation defect, unspecified** CC HCC

√4th D69 **Purpura and other hemorrhagic conditions**
EXCLUDES 1 *benign hypergammaglobulinemic purpura (D89.Ø)*
cryoglobulinemic purpura (D89.1)
essential (hemorrhagic) thrombocythemia (D47.3)
hemorrhagic thrombocythemia (D47.3)
purpura fulminans (D65)
thrombotic thrombocytopenic purpura (M31.19)
Waldenstrom hypergammaglobulinemic purpura (D89.Ø)

D69.Ø **Allergic purpura** CC HCC
Allergic vasculitis
Nonthrombocytopenic hemorrhagic purpura
Nonthrombocytopenic idiopathic purpura
Purpura anaphylactoid
Purpura Henoch(-Schonlein)
Purpura rheumatica
Vascular purpura
EXCLUDES 1 *thrombocytopenic hemorrhagic purpura (D69.3)*
AHA: 2020,3Q,26
DEF: Any hemorrhagic condition, thrombocytic or nonthrombocytopenic in origin, caused by a presumed allergic reaction.

D69.1 **Qualitative platelet defects** HCC
Bernard-Soulier [giant platelet] syndrome
Glanzmann's disease
Grey platelet syndrome
Thromboasthenia (hemorrhagic) (hereditary)
Thrombocytopathy
EXCLUDES 1 *hemolytic-uremic syndrome (D59.3-)*
EXCLUDES 2 *von Willebrand disease (D68.Ø-)*

D69.2 **Other nonthrombocytopenic purpura** HCC
Purpura NOS
Purpura simplex
Senile purpura

D69.3 **Immune thrombocytopenic purpura** CC HCC
Hemorrhagic (thrombocytopenic) purpura
Idiopathic thrombocytopenic purpura
Tidal platelet dysgenesis
DEF: Tidal platelet dysgenesis: Fluctuation of platelet counts from normal to very low within periods of 20 to 40 days and may involve autoimmune platelet destruction.

√5th D69.4 **Other primary thrombocytopenia**
EXCLUDES 1 *transient neonatal thrombocytopenia (P61.Ø)*
Wiskott-Aldrich syndrome (D82.Ø)

D69.41 **Evans syndrome** CC HCC

D69.42 **Congenital and hereditary thrombocytopenia purpura** CC HCC
Congenital thrombocytopenia
Hereditary thrombocytopenia
Code first congenital or hereditary disorder, such as: thrombocytopenia with absent radius (TAR syndrome) (Q87.2)

D69.49 **Other primary thrombocytopenia** HCC
Megakaryocytic hypoplasia
Primary thrombocytopenia NOS

√5th D69.5 **Secondary thrombocytopenia**
EXCLUDES 1 *heparin induced thrombocytopenia (HIT) (D75.82-)*
transient thrombocytopenia of newborn (P61.Ø)

D69.51 **Posttransfusion purpura**
Posttransfusion purpura from whole blood (fresh) or blood products
PTP

D69.59 **Other secondary thrombocytopenia**
AHA: 2014,4Q,22

D69.6 **Thrombocytopenia, unspecified** HCC
AHA: 2020,3Q,24

D69.8 **Other specified hemorrhagic conditions** HCC
Capillary fragility (hereditary)
Vascular pseudohemophilia

D69.9 **Hemorrhagic condition, unspecified** HCC

Other disorders of blood and blood-forming organs (D7Ø-D77)

√4th D7Ø **Neutropenia**
INCLUDES agranulocytosis
decreased absolute neurophile count (ANC)
Use additional code for any associated:
fever (R5Ø.81)
~~mucositis (J34.81, K12.3-, K92.81, N76.81)~~
▶Code also, if applicable, mucositis (J34.81, K12.3-, K92.81, N76.81)◀
EXCLUDES 1 *neutropenic splenomegaly (D73.81)*
transient neonatal neutropenia (P61.5)
DEF: Abnormally low number of neutrophils. Neutrophils are phagocytic, meaning they surround and consume harmful pathogens, primarily bacteria. When neutrophil counts decrease the risk of infection increases.

D7Ø.Ø **Congenital agranulocytosis** HCC
Congenital neutropenia
Infantile genetic agranulocytosis
Kostmann's disease

D7Ø.1 **Agranulocytosis secondary to cancer chemotherapy** HCC
Code also underlying neoplasm
Use additional code for adverse effect, if applicable, to identify drug (T45.1X5)
AHA: 2020,3Q,22; 2014,4Q,22

D7Ø.2 **Other drug-induced agranulocytosis** HCC
Use additional code for adverse effect, if applicable, to identify drug (T36-T5Ø with fifth or sixth character 5)

D7Ø.3 **Neutropenia due to infection** HCC

D7Ø.4 **Cyclic neutropenia** HCC
Cyclic hematopoiesis
Periodic neutropenia

D7Ø.8 **Other neutropenia** HCC

D7Ø.9 **Neutropenia, unspecified** HCC
AHA: 2020,3Q,24

D71 **Functional disorders of polymorphonuclear neutrophils** HCC
Cell membrane receptor complex [CR3] defect
Chronic (childhood) granulomatous disease
Congenital dysphagocytosis
Progressive septic granulomatosis

√4th D72 Other disorders of white blood cells

EXCLUDES 1 *basophilia (D72.824)*
immunity disorders (D8Ø-D89)
neutropenia (D7Ø)
preleukemia (syndrome) (D46.9)

D72.Ø Genetic anomalies of leukocytes HCC
Alder (granulation) (granulocyte) anomaly
Alder syndrome
Hereditary leukocytic hypersegmentation
Hereditary leukocytic hyposegmentation
Hereditary leukomelanopathy
May-Hegglin (granulation) (granulocyte) anomaly
May-Hegglin syndrome
Pelger-Huet (granulation) (granulocyte) anomaly
Pelger-Huet syndrome
EXCLUDES 1 *Chediak (-Steinbrinck)-Higashi syndrome (E7Ø.33Ø)*

√5th D72.1 Eosinophilia
EXCLUDES 2 *Loffler's syndrome (J82.89)*
pulmonary eosinophilia (J82.-)
AHA: 2020,4Q,8-10
DEF: Abnormally large accumulation or formation of eosinophils (nucleated, granular leukocytes) in the blood, characteristic of allergic states and infection.

D72.1Ø Eosinophilia, unspecified

√6th D72.11 Hypereosinophilic syndrome [HES]

D72.11Ø Idiopathic hypereosinophilic syndrome [IHES]

D72.111 Lymphocytic Variant Hypereosinophilic Syndrome [LHES]
Lymphocyte variant hypereosinophilia
Code also, if applicable, any associated lymphocytic neoplastic disorder

D72.118 Other hypereosinophilic syndrome
Episodic angioedema with eosinophilia
Gleich's syndrome

D72.119 Hypereosinophilic syndrome [HES], unspecified

D72.12 Drug rash with eosinophilia and systemic symptoms syndrome
DRESS syndrome
Use additional code for adverse effect, if applicable, to identify drug (T36-T5Ø with fifth or sixth character 5)

D72.18 Eosinophilia in diseases classified elsewhere
Code first underlying disease, such as:
chronic myelomonocytic leukemia (C93.1-)

D72.19 Other eosinophilia
Familial eosinophilia
Hereditary eosinophilia

√5th D72.8 Other specified disorders of white blood cells
EXCLUDES 1 *leukemia (C91-C95)*

√6th D72.81 Decreased white blood cell count
EXCLUDES 1 *neutropenia (D7Ø.-)*

D72.81Ø Lymphocytopenia
Decreased lymphocytes

D72.818 Other decreased white blood cell count
Basophilic leukopenia
Eosinophilic leukopenia
Monocytopenia
Other decreased leukocytes
Plasmacytopenia

D72.819 Decreased white blood cell count, unspecified
Decreased leukocytes, unspecified
Leukocytopenia, unspecified
Leukopenia
EXCLUDES 1 *malignant leukopenia (D7Ø.9)*

√6th D72.82 Elevated white blood cell count
EXCLUDES 1 *eosinophilia (D72.1)*

D72.82Ø Lymphocytosis (symptomatic)
Elevated lymphocytes

D72.821 Monocytosis (symptomatic)
EXCLUDES 1 *infectious mononucleosis (B27.-)*

D72.822 Plasmacytosis

D72.823 Leukemoid reaction
Basophilic leukemoid reaction
Leukemoid reaction NOS
Lymphocytic leukemoid reaction
Monocytic leukemoid reaction
Myelocytic leukemoid reaction
Neutrophilic leukemoid reaction

D72.824 Basophilia
DEF: Increase in the basophils of the blood, a type of white blood cell, often seen in conjunction with neoplastic disorders.

D72.825 Bandemia
Bandemia without diagnosis of specific infection
EXCLUDES 1 *confirmed infection - code to infection*
leukemia (C91.-, C92.-, C93.-, C94.-, C95.-)
DEF: Increase in early neutrophil cells, called band cells, that may indicate infection.

D72.828 Other elevated white blood cell count

D72.829 Elevated white blood cell count, unspecified
Elevated leukocytes, unspecified
Leukocytosis, unspecified

D72.89 Other specified disorders of white blood cells
Abnormality of white blood cells NEC

D72.9 Disorder of white blood cells, unspecified
Abnormal leukocyte differential NOS

√4th D73 Diseases of spleen

D73.Ø Hyposplenism
Atrophy of spleen
EXCLUDES 1 *asplenia (congenital) (Q89.Ø1)*
postsurgical absence of spleen (Z9Ø.81)

D73.1 Hypersplenism
EXCLUDES 1 *neutropenic splenomegaly (D73.81)*
primary splenic neutropenia (D73.81)
splenitis, splenomegaly in late syphilis (A52.79)
splenitis, splenomegaly in tuberculosis (A18.85)
splenomegaly NOS (R16.1)
splenomegaly congenital (Q89.Ø)

D73.2 Chronic congestive splenomegaly

D73.3 Abscess of spleen

D73.4 Cyst of spleen

D73.5 Infarction of spleen
Splenic rupture, nontraumatic
Torsion of spleen
EXCLUDES 1 *rupture of spleen due to Plasmodium vivax malaria (B51.Ø)*
traumatic rupture of spleen (S36.Ø3-)

√5th D73.8 Other diseases of spleen

D73.81 Neutropenic splenomegaly
Werner-Schultz disease

D73.89 Other diseases of spleen
Fibrosis of spleen NOS
Perisplenitis
Splenitis NOS

D73.9 Disease of spleen, unspecified

√4th D74 Methemoglobinemia

D74.Ø Congenital methemoglobinemia CC
Congenital NADH-methemoglobin reductase deficiency
Hemoglobin-M [Hb-M] disease
Methemoglobinemia, hereditary

D74.8 Other methemoglobinemias CC
Acquired methemoglobinemia (with sulfhemoglobinemia)
Toxic methemoglobinemia

D74.9 Methemoglobinemia, unspecified CC

D75 Other and unspecified diseases of blood and blood-forming organs

EXCLUDES 2 *acute lymphadenitis (LØ4.-)*
chronic lymphadenitis (I88.1)
enlarged lymph nodes (R59.-)
hypergammaglobulinemia NOS (D89.2)
lymphadenitis NOS (I88.9)
mesenteric lymphadenitis (acute) (chronic) (I88.Ø)

D75.Ø Familial erythrocytosis
Benign polycythemia
Familial polycythemia
EXCLUDES 1 *hereditary ovalocytosis (D58.1)*

D75.1 Secondary polycythemia
Acquired polycythemia
Emotional polycythemia
Erythrocytosis NOS
Hypoxemic polycythemia
Nephrogenous polycythemia
Polycythemia due to erythropoietin
Polycythemia due to fall in plasma volume
Polycythemia due to high altitude
Polycythemia due to stress
Polycythemia NOS
Relative polycythemia
EXCLUDES 1 *polycythemia neonatorum (P61.1)*
polycythemia vera (D45)
DEF: Elevated number of red blood cells in circulating blood as a result of reduced oxygen supply to the tissues.

D75.8 Other specified diseases of blood and blood-forming organs

D75.81 ***Myelofibrosis*** CC HCC
Myelofibrosis NOS
Secondary myelofibrosis NOS
Code first the underlying disorder, such as:
malignant neoplasm of breast (C5Ø.-)
Use additional code, if applicable, for associated therapy-related myelodysplastic syndrome (D46.-)
Use additional code for adverse effect, if applicable, to identify drug (T45.1X5)
EXCLUDES 1 *acute myelofibrosis (C94.4-)*
idiopathic myelofibrosis (D47.1)
leukoerythroblastic anemia (D61.82)
myelofibrosis with myeloid metaplasia (D47.4)
myelophthisic anemia (D61.82)
myelophthisis (D61.82)
primary myelofibrosis (D47.1)

D75.82 Heparin induced thrombocytopenia (HIT)
Use additional code, if applicable, for adverse effect of heparin (T45.515-)
AHA: 2022,4Q,9-10
DEF: Immune-mediated reaction to heparin therapy causing an abrupt fall in platelet count and serious complications such as pulmonary embolism, stroke, AMI, or DVT.

D75.821 Non-immune heparin-induced thrombocytopenia HCC
Non-immune HIT
Type 1 heparin-induced thrombocytopenia

D75.822 Immune-mediated heparin-induced thrombocytopenia HCC
Immune-mediated HIT
Type 2 heparin-induced thrombocytopenia

D75.828 Other heparin-induced thrombocytopenia syndrome HCC
Autoimmune heparin-induced thrombocytopenia syndrome
Delayed-onset heparin-induced thrombocytopenia
Persisting heparin-induced thrombocytopenia

D75.829 Heparin-induced thrombocytopenia, unspecified HCC

D75.83 Thrombocytosis
EXCLUDES 2 *essential thrombocythemia (D47.3)*
AHA: 2021,4Q,7-8

D75.838 Other thrombocytosis
Reactive thrombocytosis
Secondary thrombocytosis
Code also underlying condition, if known and applicable

D75.839 Thrombocytosis, unspecified
Thrombocythemia NOS
Thrombocytosis NOS

D75.84 Other platelet-activating anti-PF4 disorders HCC
Spontaneous heparin-induced thrombocytopenia syndrome (without heparin exposure)
Thrombosis with thrombocytopenia syndrome
Vaccine-induced thrombotic thrombocytopenia
Use additional code, if applicable, for adverse effect of other viral vaccine (T5Ø.B95-)
AHA: 2022,4Q,9-10

D75.89 Other specified diseases of blood and blood-forming organs

D75.9 Disease of blood and blood-forming organs, unspecified

D75.A Glucose-6-phosphate dehydrogenase (G6PD) deficiency without anemia
EXCLUDES 1 *glucose-6-phosphate dehydrogenase (G6PD) deficiency with anemia (D55.Ø)*
AHA: 2019,4Q,4-5

D76 Other specified diseases with participation of lymphoreticular and reticulohistiocytic tissue
EXCLUDES 1 *(Abt-) Letterer-Siwe disease (C96.Ø)*
eosinophilic granuloma (C96.6)
Hand-Schuller-Christian disease (C96.5)
histiocytic medullary reticulosis (C96.9)
histiocytic sarcoma (C96.A)
histiocytosis X, multifocal (C96.5)
histiocytosis X, unifocal (C96.6)
Langerhans-cell histiocytosis, multifocal (C96.5)
Langerhans-cell histiocytosis NOS (C96.6)
Langerhans-cell histiocytosis, unifocal (C96.6)
leukemic reticuloendotheliosis (C91.4-)
lipomelanotic reticulosis (I89.8)
malignant histiocytosis (C96.A)
malignant reticulosis (C86.Ø)
nonlipid reticuloendotheliosis (C96.Ø)

D76.1 Hemophagocytic lymphohistiocytosis CC HCC
Familial hemophagocytic reticulosis
Histiocytoses of mononuclear phagocytes

D76.2 Hemophagocytic syndrome, infection-associated CC HCC
Use additional code to identify infectious agent or disease

D76.3 Other histiocytosis syndromes CC HCC
Reticulohistiocytoma (giant-cell)
Sinus histiocytosis with massive lymphadenopathy
Xanthogranuloma

D77 ***Other disorders of blood and blood-forming organs in diseases classified elsewhere***
Code first underlying disease, such as:
amyloidosis (E85.-)
congenital early syphilis ▶(A5Ø.Ø-)◀
echinococcosis (B67.Ø-B67.9)
malaria (B5Ø.Ø-B54)
schistosomiasis [bilharziasis] (B65.Ø-B65.9)
vitamin C deficiency (E54)
EXCLUDES 1 *rupture of spleen due to Plasmodium vivax malaria (B51.Ø)*
splenitis, splenomegaly in late syphilis (A52.79)
splenitis, splenomegaly in tuberculosis (A18.85)

Intraoperative and postprocedural complications of the spleen (D78)

D78 Intraoperative and postprocedural complications of the spleen
AHA: 2016,4Q,9-10

D78.Ø Intraoperative hemorrhage and hematoma of the spleen complicating a procedure
EXCLUDES 1 *intraoperative hemorrhage and hematoma of the spleen due to accidental puncture or laceration during a procedure (D78.1-)*

D78.Ø1 Intraoperative hemorrhage and hematoma of the spleen complicating a procedure on the spleen CC

D78.02 Intraoperative hemorrhage and hematoma of the spleen complicating other procedure CC

✓5th D78.1 Accidental puncture and laceration of the spleen during a procedure

D78.11 Accidental puncture and laceration of the spleen during a procedure on the spleen CC

D78.12 Accidental puncture and laceration of the spleen during other procedure CC

AHA: 2022,1Q,22

✓5th D78.2 Postprocedural hemorrhage of the spleen following a procedure

D78.21 Postprocedural hemorrhage of the spleen following a procedure on the spleen CC

D78.22 Postprocedural hemorrhage of the spleen following other procedure CC

✓5th D78.3 Postprocedural hematoma and seroma of the spleen following a procedure

D78.31 Postprocedural hematoma of the spleen following a procedure on the spleen CC

D78.32 Postprocedural hematoma of the spleen following other procedure CC

D78.33 Postprocedural seroma of the spleen following a procedure on the spleen CC

D78.34 Postprocedural seroma of the spleen following other procedure CC

✓5th D78.8 Other intraoperative and postprocedural complications of the spleen

Use additional code, if applicable, to further specify disorder

D78.81 Other intraoperative complications of the spleen CC

D78.89 Other postprocedural complications of the spleen CC

Certain disorders involving the immune mechanism (D80-D89)

INCLUDES defects in the complement system
immunodeficiency disorders, except human immunodeficiency virus [HIV] disease
sarcoidosis

EXCLUDES 1 *autoimmune disease (systemic) NOS (M35.9)*
functional disorders of polymorphonuclear neutrophils (D71)
human immunodeficiency virus [HIV] disease (B20)

✓4th **D80 Immunodeficiency with predominantly antibody defects**

D80.0 Hereditary hypogammaglobulinemia CC HCC
Autosomal recessive agammaglobulinemia (Swiss type)
X-linked agammaglobulinemia [Bruton] (with growth hormone deficiency)

D80.1 Nonfamilial hypogammaglobulinemia CC HCC
Agammaglobulinemia with immunoglobulin-bearing B-lymphocytes
Common variable agammaglobulinemia [CVAgamma]
Hypogammaglobulinemia NOS

D80.2 Selective deficiency of immunoglobulin A [IgA] CC HCC

D80.3 Selective deficiency of immunoglobulin G [IgG] subclasses CC HCC

D80.4 Selective deficiency of immunoglobulin M [IgM] CC HCC

D80.5 Immunodeficiency with increased immunoglobulin M [IgM] CC HCC

D80.6 Antibody deficiency with near-normal immunoglobulins or with hyperimmunoglobulinemia CC HCC

D80.7 Transient hypogammaglobulinemia of infancy CC HCC

D80.8 Other immunodeficiencies with predominantly antibody defects CC HCC
Kappa light chain deficiency

D80.9 Immunodeficiency with predominantly antibody defects, unspecified CC HCC

✓4th **D81 Combined immunodeficiencies**

EXCLUDES 1 *autosomal recessive agammaglobulinemia (Swiss type) (D80.0)*

D81.0 Severe combined immunodeficiency [SCID] with reticular dysgenesis CC HCC

D81.1 Severe combined immunodeficiency [SCID] with low T- and B-cell numbers CC HCC

D81.2 Severe combined immunodeficiency [SCID] with low or normal B-cell numbers CC HCC

✓5th D81.3 Adenosine deaminase [ADA] deficiency

AHA: 2019,4Q,5-6

D81.30 Adenosine deaminase deficiency, unspecified CC HCC
ADA deficiency NOS

D81.31 Severe combined immunodeficiency due to adenosine deaminase deficiency CC HCC
ADA deficiency with SCID
Adenosine deaminase [ADA] deficiency with severe combined immunodeficiency

D81.32 Adenosine deaminase 2 deficiency CC HCC
ADA2 deficiency
Adenosine deaminase deficiency type 2
Code also, if applicable, any associated manifestations, such as:
polyarteritis nodosa (M30.0)
stroke (I63.-)

D81.39 Other adenosine deaminase deficiency CC HCC
Adenosine deaminase [ADA] deficiency type 1, NOS
Adenosine deaminase [ADA] deficiency type 1, without SCID
Adenosine deaminase [ADA] deficiency type 1, without severe combined immunodeficiency
Partial ADA deficiency (type 1)
Partial adenosine deaminase deficiency (type 1)

D81.4 Nezelof's syndrome CC HCC

D81.5 Purine nucleoside phosphorylase [PNP] deficiency CC HCC

D81.6 Major histocompatibility complex class I deficiency CC HCC
Bare lymphocyte syndrome

D81.7 Major histocompatibility complex class II deficiency CC HCC

✓5th D81.8 Other combined immunodeficiencies

✓6th D81.81 Biotin-dependent carboxylase deficiency
Multiple carboxylase deficiency

EXCLUDES 1 *biotin-dependent carboxylase deficiency due to dietary deficiency of biotin (E53.8)*

D81.810 Biotinidase deficiency

D81.818 Other biotin-dependent carboxylase deficiency
Holocarboxylase synthetase deficiency
Other multiple carboxylase deficiency

D81.819 Biotin-dependent carboxylase deficiency, unspecified
Multiple carboxylase deficiency, unspecified

D81.82 Activated Phosphoinositide 3-kinase Delta Syndrome [APDS] CC HCC
p110d-activating mutation causing senescent T cells, lymphadenopathy, and immunodeficiency [PASLI] disease
Code also, if applicable, any associated manifestations, such as:
bronchiectasis (J47.-)
herpes virus infections (B00.-)
other acute respiratory tract infections (J00-J06; J20-J22)
other infections (A00-B99)
pneumonia (J12-J18)
AHA: 2022,4Q,11

D81.89 Other combined immunodeficiencies CC HCC

D81.9 Combined immunodeficiency, unspecified CC HCC
Severe combined immunodeficiency disorder [SCID] NOS

✓4th **D82 Immunodeficiency associated with other major defects**

EXCLUDES 1 *ataxia telangiectasia [Louis-Bar] (G11.3)*

D82.0 Wiskott-Aldrich syndrome CC HCC
Immunodeficiency with thrombocytopenia and eczema

D82.1 Di George's syndrome CC HCC
Pharyngeal pouch syndrome
Thymic alymphoplasia
Thymic aplasia or hypoplasia with immunodeficiency
AHA: 2019,3Q,14

D82.2 Immunodeficiency with short-limbed stature HCC

D82.3 Immunodeficiency following hereditary defective response to Epstein-Barr virus HCC
X-linked lymphoproliferative disease

D82.4 Hyperimmunoglobulin E [IgE] syndrome HCC

D82.8 Immunodeficiency associated with other specified major defects HCC

D82.9 Immunodeficiency associated with major defect, unspecified HCC

✓4th **D83 Common variable immunodeficiency**

D83.0 Common variable immunodeficiency with predominant abnormalities of B-cell numbers and function CC HCC

D83.1 Common variable immunodeficiency with predominant immunoregulatory T-cell disorders CC HCC

D83.2 Common variable immunodeficiency with autoantibodies to B- or T-cells CC HCC

D83.8 Other common variable immunodeficiencies CC HCC

D83.9 Common variable immunodeficiency, unspecified CC HCC

✓4th **D84 Other immunodeficiencies**

D84.0 Lymphocyte function antigen-1 [LFA-1] defect HCC

D84.1 Defects in the complement system HCC
C1 esterase inhibitor [C1-INH] deficiency

✓5th D84.8 Other specified immunodeficiencies
AHA: 2020,4Q,10-12

D84.81 Immunodeficiency due to conditions classified elsewhere CC HCC
Code first underlying condition, such as:
chromosomal abnormalities (Q90-Q99)
diabetes mellitus (E08-E13)
malignant neoplasms (C00-C96)
EXCLUDES 1 *certain disorders involving the immune mechanism (D80-D83, D84.0, D84.1, D84.9)*
human immunodeficiency virus [HIV] disease (B20)
AHA: 2021,1Q,52

✓6th D84.82 Immunodeficiency due to drugs and external causes

D84.821 Immunodeficiency due to drugs CC HCC
Immunodeficiency due to (current or past) medication
Use additional code for adverse effect if applicable, to identify adverse effect of drug (T36-T50 with fifth or six character 5)
Use additional code, if applicable, for associated long term (current) drug therapy drug or medication such as:
long term (current) drug therapy systemic steroids (Z79.52)
other long term (current) drug therapy (Z79.899)

D84.822 Immunodeficiency due to external causes CC HCC
Code also, if applicable, radiological procedure and radiotherapy (Y84.2)
Use additional code for external cause such as:
exposure to ionizing radiation (W88)

D84.89 Other immunodeficiencies CC HCC

D84.9 Immunodeficiency, unspecified CC HCC
Immunocompromised NOS
Immunodeficient NOS
Immunosuppressed NOS
AHA: 2020,4Q,10

✓4th **D86 Sarcoidosis**
DEF: Clustering of immune cells resulting in granuloma formation. Often affects the lungs and lymphatic system but can occur in other body sites.

D86.0 Sarcoidosis of lung HCC

D86.1 Sarcoidosis of lymph nodes

D86.2 Sarcoidosis of lung with sarcoidosis of lymph nodes HCC

D86.3 Sarcoidosis of skin

✓5th D86.8 Sarcoidosis of other sites

D86.81 Sarcoid meningitis

D86.82 Multiple cranial nerve palsies in sarcoidosis HCC

D86.83 Sarcoid iridocyclitis

D86.84 Sarcoid pyelonephritis
Tubulo-interstitial nephropathy in sarcoidosis

D86.85 Sarcoid myocarditis

D86.86 Sarcoid arthropathy
Polyarthritis in sarcoidosis

D86.87 Sarcoid myositis

D86.89 Sarcoidosis of other sites
Hepatic granuloma
Uveoparotid fever [Heerfordt]

D86.9 Sarcoidosis, unspecified

✓4th **D89 Other disorders involving the immune mechanism, not elsewhere classified**
EXCLUDES 1 *hyperglobulinemia NOS (R77.1)*
monoclonal gammopathy (of undetermined significance) (D47.2)
EXCLUDES 2 *transplant failure and rejection (T86.-)*

D89.0 Polyclonal hypergammaglobulinemia
Benign hypergammaglobulinemic purpura
Polyclonal gammopathy NOS

D89.1 Cryoglobulinemia HCC
Cryoglobulinemic purpura
Cryoglobulinemic vasculitis
Essential cryoglobulinemia
Idiopathic cryoglobulinemia
Mixed cryoglobulinemia
Primary cryoglobulinemia
Secondary cryoglobulinemia

D89.2 Hypergammaglobulinemia, unspecified

D89.3 Immune reconstitution syndrome HCC
Immune reconstitution inflammatory syndrome [IRIS]
Use additional code for adverse effect, if applicable, to identify drug (T36-T50 with fifth or sixth character 5)

✓5th D89.4 Mast cell activation syndrome and related disorders
EXCLUDES 1 *aggressive systemic mastocytosis (C96.21)*
congenital cutaneous mastocytosis (Q82.2)
(non-congenital) cutaneous mastocytosis (D47.01)
(indolent) systemic mastocytosis (D47.02)
malignant mast cell neoplasm (C96.2-)
malignant mastocytoma (C96.29)
mast cell leukemia (C94.3-)
mast cell sarcoma (C96.22)
mastocytoma NOS (D47.09)
other mast cell neoplasms of uncertain behavior (D47.09)
systemic mastocytosis associated with a clonal hematologic non-mast cell lineage disease (SM-AHNMD) (D47.02)
AHA: 2016,4Q,11

D89.40 Mast cell activation, unspecified HCC
Mast cell activation disorder, unspecified
Mast cell activation syndrome, NOS

D89.41 Monoclonal mast cell activation syndrome HCC

D89.42 Idiopathic mast cell activation syndrome HCC

D89.43 Secondary mast cell activation HCC
Secondary mast cell activation syndrome
Code also underlying etiology, if known

D89.44 Hereditary alpha tryptasemia HCC
Use additional code, if applicable, for:
allergy status, other than to drugs and biological substances (Z91.0-)
personal history of anaphylaxis (Z87.892)
AHA: 2021,4Q,8

D89.49 Other mast cell activation disorder HCC
Other mast cell activation syndrome

✓5th D89.8 Other specified disorders involving the immune mechanism, not elsewhere classified

✓6th D89.81 Graft-versus-host disease
Code first underlying cause, such as:
complications of blood transfusion (T80.89)
complications of transplanted organs and tissue (T86.-)
Use additional code to identify associated manifestations, such as:
desquamative dermatitis (L30.8)
diarrhea (R19.7)
elevated bilirubin (R17)
hair loss (L65.9)

D89.810 Acute graft-versus-host disease CC UPD HCC

D89.811 Chronic graft-versus-host disease CC UPD HCC

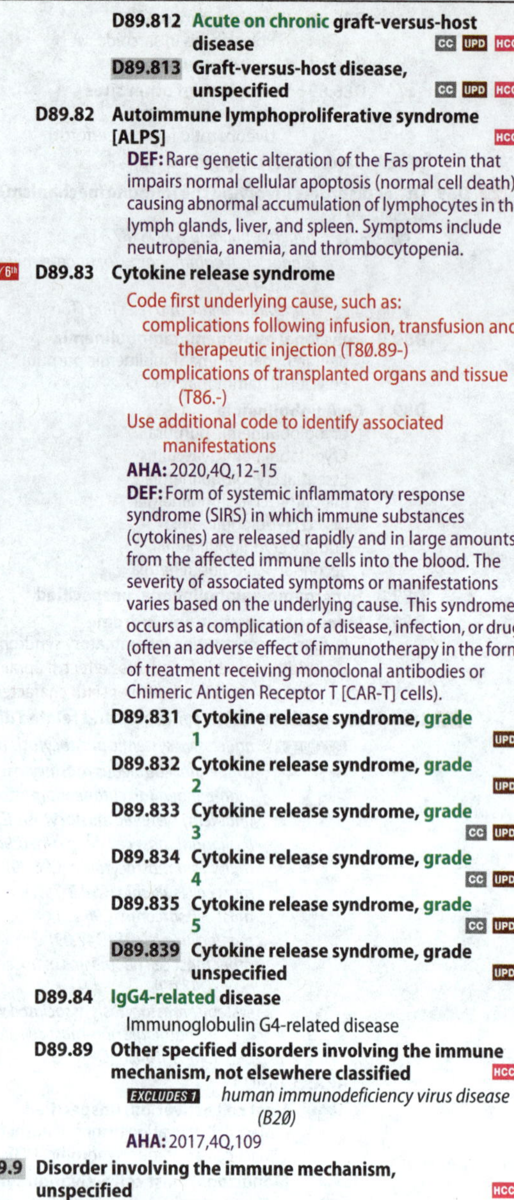

D89.812 Acute on chronic graft-versus-host disease CC UPD HCC

D89.813 Graft-versus-host disease, unspecified CC UPD HCC

D89.82 Autoimmune lymphoproliferative syndrome [ALPS] HCC

DEF: Rare genetic alteration of the Fas protein that impairs normal cellular apoptosis (normal cell death), causing abnormal accumulation of lymphocytes in the lymph glands, liver, and spleen. Symptoms include neutropenia, anemia, and thrombocytopenia.

✓6th **D89.83 Cytokine release syndrome**

Code first underlying cause, such as:
- complications following infusion, transfusion and therapeutic injection (T8Ø.89-)
- complications of transplanted organs and tissue (T86.-)

Use additional code to identify associated manifestations

AHA: 2020,4Q,12-15

DEF: Form of systemic inflammatory response syndrome (SIRS) in which immune substances (cytokines) are released rapidly and in large amounts from the affected immune cells into the blood. The severity of associated symptoms or manifestations varies based on the underlying cause. This syndrome occurs as a complication of a disease, infection, or drug (often an adverse effect of immunotherapy in the form of treatment receiving monoclonal antibodies or Chimeric Antigen Receptor T [CAR-T] cells).

D89.831 Cytokine release syndrome, grade 1 UPD

D89.832 Cytokine release syndrome, grade 2 UPD

D89.833 Cytokine release syndrome, grade 3 CC UPD

D89.834 Cytokine release syndrome, grade 4 CC UPD

D89.835 Cytokine release syndrome, grade 5 CC UPD

D89.839 Cytokine release syndrome, grade unspecified UPD

● **D89.84 IgG4-related disease**

Immunoglobulin G4-related disease

D89.89 Other specified disorders involving the immune mechanism, not elsewhere classified HCC

EXCLUDES 1 *human immunodeficiency virus disease (B2Ø)*

AHA: 2017,4Q,109

D89.9 Disorder involving the immune mechanism, unspecified HCC

Immune disease NOS

AHA: 2015,3Q,22

Chapter 4. Endocrine, Nutritional, and Metabolic Diseases (EØØ–E89)

Chapter-specific Guidelines with Coding Examples

The chapter-specific guidelines from the ICD-10-CM Official Guidelines for Coding and Reporting have been provided below. Along with these guidelines are coding examples, contained in the shaded boxes, that have been developed to help illustrate the coding and/or sequencing guidance found in these guidelines.

a. Diabetes mellitus

The diabetes mellitus codes are combination codes that include the type of diabetes mellitus, the body system affected, and the complications affecting that body system. As many codes within a particular category as are necessary to describe all of the complications of the disease may be used. They should be sequenced based on the reason for a particular encounter. Assign as many codes from categories EØ8–E13 as needed to identify all of the associated conditions that the patient has.

Patient is seen for poorly controlled diabetes, type 2, with diabetic polyneuropathy and diabetic retinopathy with macular edema

E11.65 **Type 2 diabetes mellitus with hyperglycemia**

E11.311 **Type 2 diabetes mellitus with unspecified diabetic retinopathy with macular edema**

E11.42 **Type 2 diabetes mellitus with diabetic polyneuropathy**

Explanation: Use as many codes to describe the diabetic complications as needed. Many are combination codes that describe more than one condition. Code first the reason for the encounter. "Poorly controlled" is described as "with hyperglycemia." Diabetes documented as "uncontrolled" is not assumed to be hyperglycemic but can be classified to either hyperglycemia or hypoglycemia. If documentation is not clear, the provider must be queried so that the appropriate code can be reported.

1) Type of diabetes

The age of a patient is not the sole determining factor, though most type 1 diabetics develop the condition before reaching puberty. For this reason, type 1 diabetes mellitus is also referred to as juvenile diabetes.

A 45-year-old patient is diagnosed with type 1 diabetes

E1Ø.9 **Type 1 diabetes mellitus without complications**

Explanation: Although most type 1 diabetics are diagnosed in childhood or adolescence, it can also begin in adults.

2) Type of diabetes mellitus not documented

If the type of diabetes mellitus is not documented in the medical record the default is E11.-, Type 2 diabetes mellitus.

H & P lists diabetes and hypertension on patient problem list

E11.9 **Type 2 diabetes mellitus without complications**

I1Ø **Essential (primary) hypertension**

Explanation: Since the type of diabetes was not documented and no complications were noted, the default code is E11.9.

3) Diabetes mellitus and the use of insulin, oral hypoglycemics, and injectable non-insulin drugs

If the documentation in a medical record does not indicate the type of diabetes but does indicate that the patient uses insulin, code E11-, Type 2 diabetes mellitus, should be assigned. Additional code(s) should be assigned from category Z79 to identify the long-term (current) use of insulin, oral hypoglycemic drugs, or injectable non-insulin antidiabetic, as follows:

If the patient is treated with both oral hypoglycemic drugs and insulin, both code Z79.4, Long term (current) use of insulin, and code Z79.84, Long term (current) use of oral hypoglycemic drugs, should be assigned.

If the patient is treated with both insulin and an injectable non-insulin antidiabetic drug, assign codes Z79.4, Long term (current) use of insulin, and Z79.85, Long-term (current) use of injectable non-insulin antidiabetic drugs.

If the patient is treated with both oral hypoglycemic drugs and an injectable non-insulin antidiabetic drug, assign codes Z79.84, Long term (current) use of oral hypoglycemic drugs, and Z79.85, Long-term (current) use of injectable non-insulin antidiabetic drugs.

Code Z79.4 should not be assigned if insulin is given temporarily to bring a type 2 patient's blood sugar under control during an encounter.

Type 2 diabetic patient on daily metformin and Victoza is admitted in ketoacidosis, insulin given to stabilize blood sugars and discontinued at discharge

E11.1Ø **Type 2 diabetes mellitus with ketoacidosis without coma**

Z79.84 **Long term (current) use of oral hypoglycemic drugs**

Z79.85 **Long term (current) use of injectable non-insulin anti-diabetic drugs**

Explanation: Documentation indicates the patient is on an oral antidiabetic medication (metformin) and an injectable noninsulin antidiabetic medication (Victoza). Although insulin was given to the patient during the encounter, it was discontinued at discharge, indicating that the patient does not regularly use insulin. A Z code representing long-term use of the oral drug and long-term use of the injectable medication can be applied. Applying code Z79.4 to represent long-term use of insulin would be inappropriate.

4) Diabetes mellitus in pregnancy and gestational diabetes

See Section I.C.15. Diabetes mellitus in pregnancy.

See Section I.C.15. Gestational (pregnancy induced) diabetes

5) Complications due to insulin pump malfunction

(a) Underdose of insulin due to insulin pump failure

An underdose of insulin due to an insulin pump failure should be assigned to a code from subcategory T85.6, Mechanical complication of other specified internal and external prosthetic devices, implants and grafts, that specifies the type of pump malfunction, as the principal or first-listed code, followed by code T38.3X6-, Underdosing of insulin and oral hypoglycemic [antidiabetic] drugs. Additional codes for the type of diabetes mellitus and any associated complications due to the underdosing should also be assigned.

A 24-year-old type 1 diabetic male treated in ED for hyperglycemia; insulin pump found to be malfunctioning and underdosing

T85.614A **Breakdown (mechanical) of insulin pump, initial encounter**

T38.3X6A **Underdosing of insulin and oral hypoglycemic [antidiabetic] drugs, initial encounter**

E1Ø.65 **Type 1 diabetes mellitus with hyperglycemia**

Explanation: The complication code for the mechanical breakdown of the pump is sequenced first, followed by the underdosing code and type of diabetes with complication. Code all other diabetic complication codes necessary to describe the patient's condition.

(b) Overdose of insulin due to insulin pump failure

The principal or first-listed code for an encounter due to an insulin pump malfunction resulting in an overdose of insulin, should also be T85.6-, Mechanical complication of other specified internal and external prosthetic devices, implants and grafts, followed by code T38.3X1-, Poisoning by insulin and oral hypoglycemic [antidiabetic] drugs, accidental (unintentional).

A 24-year-old type 1 diabetic male found down with diabetic coma, brought into ED and treated for hypoglycemia; insulin pump found to be malfunctioning and overdosing

T85.614A **Breakdown (mechanical) of insulin pump, initial encounter**

T38.3X1A **Poisoning by insulin and oral hypoglycemic [antidiabetic] drugs, accidental (unintentional), initial encounter**

E1Ø.641 **Type 1 diabetes mellitus with hypoglycemia with coma**

Explanation: The complication code for the mechanical breakdown of the pump is sequenced first, followed by the poisoning code and type of diabetes with complication. All the characters in the combination code must be used to form a valid code and to fully describe the type of diabetes, the hypoglycemia, and the coma.

6) **Secondary diabetes mellitus**

Codes under categories EØ8, Diabetes mellitus due to underlying condition, EØ9, Drug or chemical induced diabetes mellitus, and E13, Other specified diabetes mellitus, identify complications/manifestations associated with secondary diabetes mellitus. Secondary diabetes is always caused by another condition or event (e.g., cystic fibrosis, malignant neoplasm of pancreas, pancreatectomy, adverse effect of drug, or poisoning).

(a) **Secondary diabetes mellitus and the use of insulin or oral hypoglycemic drugs**

For patients with secondary diabetes mellitus who routinely use insulin, oral hypoglycemic drugs, or injectable non-insulin drugs, additional code(s) from category Z79 should be assigned to identify the long-term (current) use of insulin, oral hypoglycemic drugs, or non-injectable non-insulin drugs as follows:

If the patient is treated with both oral hypoglycemic drugs and insulin, both code Z79.4, Long term (current) use of insulin, and code Z79.84, Long term (current) use of oral hypoglycemic drugs, should be assigned.

If the patient is treated with both insulin and an injectable non-insulin antidiabetic drug, assign codes Z79.4, Long-term (current) use of insulin, and Z79.85, Long-term (current) use of injectable non-insulin antidiabetic drugs.

If the patient is treated with both oral hypoglycemic drugs and an injectable non-insulin antidiabetic drug, assign codes Z79.84, Long-term (current) use of oral hypoglycemic drugs, and Z79.85, Long-term (current) use of injectable non-insulin antidiabetic drugs.

Code Z79.4 should not be assigned if insulin is given temporarily to bring a secondary diabetic patient's blood sugar under control during an encounter

The patient, maintained on metformin and insulin, was admitted for treatment of diabetic gangrene. The patient developed diabetes secondary to Nelson's syndrome.

E24.1	**Nelson's syndrome**
EØ8.52	**Diabetes mellitus due to underlying condition with diabetic peripheral angiopathy with gangrene**
Z79.4	**Long term (current) use of insulin**
Z79.84	**Long term (current) use of oral hypoglycemic drugs**

Explanation: When diabetes is caused by an underlying condition, the underlying condition should always be sequenced before any codes representing the diabetes. Patients with secondary diabetes may be maintained on both insulin and an oral hypoglycemic. When maintained on both, report a code for the long term use of insulin and a code for the long term use of oral hypoglycemic.

(b) **Assigning and sequencing secondary diabetes codes and its causes**

The sequencing of the secondary diabetes codes in relationship to codes for the cause of the diabetes is based on the Tabular List instructions for categories EØ8, EØ9 and E13.

(i) **Secondary diabetes mellitus due to pancreatectomy**

For postpancreatectomy diabetes mellitus (lack of insulin due to the surgical removal of all or part of the pancreas), assign code E89.1, Postprocedural hypoinsulinemia. Assign a code from category E13 and a code from subcategory Z9Ø.41, Acquired absence of pancreas, as additional codes.

Patient with newly diagnosed diabetes after surgical removal of part of pancreas is discharged with referral for consult to initiate insulin.

E89.1	**Postprocedural hypoinsulinemia**
E13.9	**Other specified diabetes mellitus without complications**
Z9Ø.411	**Acquired partial absence of pancreas**

Explanation: Sequence the postprocedural complication of the hypoinsulinemia due to the partial removal of the pancreas as the first-listed code, followed by codes for other specified diabetes (NEC) without complications and partial acquired absence of the pancreas. Code Z79.4 Long term (current) use of insulin, is not added because the insulin has not yet been started.

(ii) **Secondary diabetes due to drugs**

Secondary diabetes may be caused by an adverse effect of correctly administered medications, poisoning or sequela of poisoning.

See section I.C.19.e. for coding of adverse effects and poisoning, and section I.C.20 for external cause code reporting.

Initial encounter for corticosteroid-induced diabetes mellitus

EØ9.9	**Drug or chemical induced diabetes mellitus without complications**
T38.ØX5A	**Adverse effect of glucocorticoids and synthetic analogues, initial encounter**

Explanation: If the diabetes is caused by an adverse effect of a drug, the diabetic condition is coded first. If it occurs from a poisoning or overdose, the poisoning code causing the diabetes is sequenced first.

Chapter 4. Endocrine, Nutritional and Metabolic Diseases (E00-E89)

NOTE All neoplasms, whether functionally active or not, are classified in Chapter 2. Appropriate codes in this chapter (i.e. E05.8, E07.0, E16-E31, E34.-) may be used as additional codes to indicate either functional activity by neoplasms and ectopic endocrine tissue or hyperfunction and hypofunction of endocrine glands associated with neoplasms and other conditions classified elsewhere.

EXCLUDES 1 *transitory endocrine and metabolic disorders specific to newborn (P70-P74)*

AHA: 2018,2Q,6

This chapter contains the following blocks:

E00-E07 Disorders of thyroid gland
E08-E13 Diabetes mellitus
E15-E16 Other disorders of glucose regulation and pancreatic internal secretion
E20-E35 Disorders of other endocrine glands
E36 Intraoperative complications of endocrine system
E40-E46 Malnutrition
E50-E64 Other nutritional deficiencies
E65-E68 Overweight, obesity and other hyperalimentation
E70-E88 Metabolic disorders
E89 Postprocedural endocrine and metabolic complications and disorders, not elsewhere classified

Disorders of thyroid gland (E00-E07)

✓4th **E00 Congenital iodine-deficiency syndrome**
Use additional code (F70-F79) to identify associated intellectual disabilities
EXCLUDES 1 *subclinical iodine-deficiency hypothyroidism (E02)*

E00.0 Congenital iodine-deficiency syndrome, neurological type
Endemic cretinism, neurological type

E00.1 Congenital iodine-deficiency syndrome, myxedematous type
Endemic hypothyroid cretinism
Endemic cretinism, myxedematous type

E00.2 Congenital iodine-deficiency syndrome, mixed type
Endemic cretinism, mixed type

E00.9 Congenital iodine-deficiency syndrome, unspecified
Congenital iodine-deficiency hypothyroidism NOS
Endemic cretinism NOS

✓4th **E01 Iodine-deficiency related thyroid disorders and allied conditions**
EXCLUDES 1 *congenital iodine-deficiency syndrome (E00.-)*
subclinical iodine-deficiency hypothyroidism (E02)

E01.0 Iodine-deficiency related diffuse (endemic) goiter

E01.1 Iodine-deficiency related multinodular (endemic) goiter
Iodine-deficiency related nodular goiter

E01.2 Iodine-deficiency related (endemic) goiter, unspecified
Endemic goiter NOS

E01.8 Other iodine-deficiency related thyroid disorders and allied conditions
Acquired iodine-deficiency hypothyroidism NOS

E02 Subclinical iodine-deficiency hypothyroidism
AHA: 2021,1Q,8

✓4th **E03 Other hypothyroidism**
EXCLUDES 1 *iodine-deficiency related hypothyroidism (E00-E02)*
postprocedural hypothyroidism (E89.0)
DEF: Hypothyroidism: Underproduction of thyroid hormone.

E03.0 Congenital hypothyroidism with diffuse goiter
Congenital parenchymatous goiter (nontoxic)
Congenital goiter (nontoxic) NOS
EXCLUDES 1 *transitory congenital goiter with normal function (P72.0)*

E03.1 Congenital hypothyroidism without goiter
Aplasia of thyroid (with myxedema)
Congenital atrophy of thyroid
Congenital hypothyroidism NOS

E03.2 Hypothyroidism due to medicaments and other exogenous substances
Code first poisoning due to drug or toxin, if applicable ▶(T36-T65 with fifth or sixth character 1-4)◀
Use additional code for adverse effect, if applicable, to identify drug (T36-T50 with fifth or sixth character 5)

E03.3 Postinfectious hypothyroidism

E03.4 Atrophy of thyroid (acquired)
EXCLUDES 1 *congenital atrophy of thyroid (E03.1)*

E03.5 Myxedema coma MCC HCC

E03.8 Other specified hypothyroidism
AHA: 2021,1Q,8

E03.9 Hypothyroidism, unspecified
Myxedema NOS

✓4th **E04 Other nontoxic goiter**
EXCLUDES 1 *congenital goiter (NOS) (diffuse) (parenchymatous) (E03.0)*
iodine-deficiency related goiter (E00-E02)

E04.0 Nontoxic diffuse goiter
Diffuse (colloid) nontoxic goiter
Simple nontoxic goiter

E04.1 Nontoxic single thyroid nodule
Colloid nodule (cystic) (thyroid)
Nontoxic uninodular goiter
Thyroid (cystic) nodule NOS
DEF: Enlarged thyroid, commonly due to decreased thyroid production, with a single nodule. No clinical hypothyroidism.

E04.2 Nontoxic multinodular goiter
Cystic goiter NOS
Multinodular (cystic) goiter NOS
DEF: Enlarged thyroid, commonly due to decreased thyroid production with multiple nodules. No clinical hypothyroidism.

E04.8 Other specified nontoxic goiter

E04.9 Nontoxic goiter, unspecified
Goiter NOS
Nodular goiter (nontoxic) NOS

✓4th **E05 Thyrotoxicosis [hyperthyroidism]**
EXCLUDES 1 *chronic thyroiditis with transient thyrotoxicosis (E06.2)*
neonatal thyrotoxicosis (P72.1)
DEF: Excessive quantities of hormones from the thyroid gland caused by overproduction or loss of storage ability.

✓5th **E05.0 Thyrotoxicosis with diffuse goiter**
Exophthalmic or toxic goiter NOS
Graves' disease
Toxic diffuse goiter
DEF: Diffuse thyroid enlargement accompanied by hyperthyroidism, bulging eyes, and dermopathy.

E05.00 Thyrotoxicosis with diffuse goiter without thyrotoxic crisis or storm

E05.01 Thyrotoxicosis with diffuse goiter with thyrotoxic crisis or storm MCC

Goiter

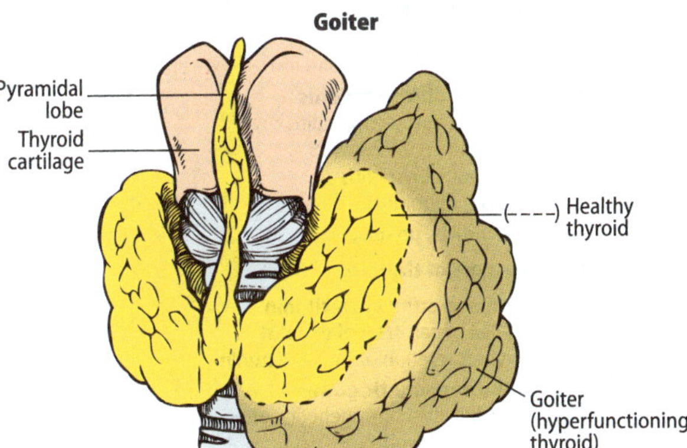

✓5th **E05.1 Thyrotoxicosis with toxic single thyroid nodule**
Thyrotoxicosis with toxic uninodular goiter
DEF: Symptomatic hyperthyroidism with a single nodule on the enlarged thyroid gland. Onset of symptoms can be abrupt and include extreme nervousness, insomnia, weight loss, tremors, and psychosis or coma.

E05.10 Thyrotoxicosis with toxic single thyroid nodule without thyrotoxic crisis or storm

E05.11 Thyrotoxicosis with toxic single thyroid nodule with thyrotoxic crisis or storm MCC

✓5th **E05.2 Thyrotoxicosis with toxic multinodular goiter**
Toxic nodular goiter NOS

E05.20 Thyrotoxicosis with toxic multinodular goiter without thyrotoxic crisis or storm

E05.21 Thyrotoxicosis with toxic multinodular goiter with thyrotoxic crisis or storm MCC

✓5th **E05.3 Thyrotoxicosis from ectopic thyroid tissue**

E05.30 Thyrotoxicosis from ectopic thyroid tissue without thyrotoxic crisis or storm

E05.31 Thyrotoxicosis from ectopic thyroid tissue with thyrotoxic crisis or storm MCC

E05.4 Thyrotoxicosis factitia

E05.40 Thyrotoxicosis factitia without thyrotoxic crisis or storm

E05.41 Thyrotoxicosis factitia with thyrotoxic crisis or storm MCC

E05.8 Other thyrotoxicosis

Overproduction of thyroid-stimulating hormone

E05.80 Other thyrotoxicosis without thyrotoxic crisis or storm

E05.81 Other thyrotoxicosis with thyrotoxic crisis or storm MCC

E05.9 Thyrotoxicosis, unspecified

Hyperthyroidism NOS

E05.90 Thyrotoxicosis, unspecified without thyrotoxic crisis or storm

E05.91 Thyrotoxicosis, unspecified with thyrotoxic crisis or storm MCC

E06 Thyroiditis

EXCLUDES 1 *postpartum thyroiditis (O90.5)*

DEF: Inflammation of the thyroid gland.

E06.0 Acute thyroiditis CC

Abscess of thyroid
Pyogenic thyroiditis
Suppurative thyroiditis
Use additional code (B95-B97) to identify infectious agent

E06.1 Subacute thyroiditis

de Quervain thyroiditis
Giant-cell thyroiditis
Granulomatous thyroiditis
Nonsuppurative thyroiditis
Viral thyroiditis

EXCLUDES 1 *autoimmune thyroiditis (E06.3)*

E06.2 Chronic thyroiditis with transient thyrotoxicosis

EXCLUDES 1 *autoimmune thyroiditis (E06.3)*

E06.3 Autoimmune thyroiditis

Hashimoto's thyroiditis
Hashitoxicosis (transient)
Lymphadenoid goiter
Lymphocytic thyroiditis
Struma lymphomatosa

E06.4 Drug-induced thyroiditis

Use additional code for adverse effect, if applicable, to identify drug (T36-T50 with fifth or sixth character 5)

E06.5 Other chronic thyroiditis

Chronic fibrous thyroiditis
Chronic thyroiditis NOS
Ligneous thyroiditis
Riedel thyroiditis

E06.9 Thyroiditis, unspecified

E07 Other disorders of thyroid

E07.0 Hypersecretion of calcitonin

C-cell hyperplasia of thyroid
Hypersecretion of thyrocalcitonin

E07.1 Dyshormogenetic goiter

Familial dyshormogenetic goiter
Pendred's syndrome

EXCLUDES 1 *transitory congenital goiter with normal function (P72.0)*

E07.8 Other specified disorders of thyroid

E07.81 Sick-euthyroid syndrome

Euthyroid sick-syndrome

DEF: Thyroid dysfunction caused by abnormal levels of thyroid hormones T3 and/or T4. This syndrome is often associated with starvation or critical illness.

E07.89 Other specified disorders of thyroid

Abnormality of thyroid-binding globulin
Hemorrhage of thyroid
Infarction of thyroid

E07.9 Disorder of thyroid, unspecified

Diabetes mellitus (E08-E13)

AHA: 2020,1Q,12; 2018,2Q,6; 2017,4Q,100-101; 2016,2Q,36; 2016,1Q,11-13; 2013,4Q,114; 2013,3Q,20

E08 Diabetes mellitus due to underlying condition

Code first the underlying condition, such as:
congenital rubella (P35.0)
Cushing's syndrome (E24.-)
cystic fibrosis (E84.-)
malignant neoplasm (C00-C96)
malnutrition (E40-E46)
pancreatitis and other diseases of the pancreas (K85-K86.-)

Use additional code to identify control using:
insulin (Z79.4)
oral antidiabetic drugs (Z79.84)
oral hypoglycemic drugs (Z79.84)

EXCLUDES 1 *drug or chemical induced diabetes mellitus (E09.-)*
gestational diabetes (O24.4-)
neonatal diabetes mellitus (P70.2)
postpancreatectomy diabetes mellitus (E13.-)
postprocedural diabetes mellitus (E13.-)
secondary diabetes mellitus NEC (E13.-)
type 1 diabetes mellitus (E10.-)
type 2 diabetes mellitus (E11.-)

E08.0 Diabetes mellitus due to underlying condition with hyperosmolarity

DEF: Diabetic hyperosmolarity: Extremely high levels of glucose in the blood without ketones.

E08.00 Diabetes mellitus due to underlying condition with hyperosmolarity without nonketotic hyperglycemic-hyperosmolar coma (NKHHC) MCC H9 HCC

E08.01 Diabetes mellitus due to underlying condition with hyperosmolarity with coma MCC H9 HCC

E08.1 Diabetes mellitus due to underlying condition with ketoacidosis

DEF: Diabetic ketoacidosis: Potentially life-threatening complication due to a shortage of insulin in which the body switches to burning fatty acids and producing acidic ketone bodies.

E08.10 Diabetes mellitus due to underlying condition with ketoacidosis without coma MCC H9 HCC

E08.11 Diabetes mellitus due to underlying condition with ketoacidosis with coma MCC H9 HCC

E08.2 Diabetes mellitus due to underlying condition with kidney complications

AHA: 2019,3Q,3; 2018,4Q,88

E08.21 Diabetes mellitus due to underlying condition with diabetic nephropathy HCC

Diabetes mellitus due to underlying condition with intercapillary glomerulosclerosis
Diabetes mellitus due to underlying condition with intracapillary glomerulonephrosis
Diabetes mellitus due to underlying condition with Kimmelstiel-Wilson disease

E08.22 Diabetes mellitus due to underlying condition with diabetic chronic kidney disease HCC

Use additional code to identify stage of chronic kidney disease (N18.1-N18.6)

E08.29 Diabetes mellitus due to underlying condition with other diabetic kidney complication HCC

Renal tubular degeneration in diabetes mellitus due to underlying condition

E08.3 Diabetes mellitus due to underlying condition with ophthalmic complications

AHA: 2016,4Q,11-13

One of the following 7th characters is to be assigned to codes in subcategories E08.32, E08.33, E08.34, E08.35, and E08.37 to designate laterality of the disease:
1 right eye
2 left eye
3 bilateral
9 unspecified eye

E08.31 Diabetes mellitus due to underlying condition with unspecified diabetic retinopathy

DEF: Diabetic retinopathy: Diabetic complication from damage to the retinal vessels resulting in vision problems that can progress to blindness.

E08.311 Diabetes mellitus due to underlying condition with unspecified diabetic retinopathy with macular edema HCC

E08.319 Diabetes mellitus due to underlying condition with unspecified diabetic retinopathy without macular edema HCC

E08.32 Diabetes mellitus due to underlying condition with mild nonproliferative diabetic retinopathy

Diabetes mellitus due to underlying condition with nonproliferative diabetic retinopathy NOS

E08.321 Diabetes mellitus due to underlying condition with mild nonproliferative diabetic retinopathy with macular edema HCC

E08.329 Diabetes mellitus due to underlying condition with mild nonproliferative diabetic retinopathy without macular edema HCC

E08.33 Diabetes mellitus due to underlying condition with moderate nonproliferative diabetic retinopathy

E08.331 Diabetes mellitus due to underlying condition with moderate nonproliferative diabetic retinopathy with macular edema HCC

E08.339 Diabetes mellitus due to underlying condition with moderate nonproliferative diabetic retinopathy without macular edema HCC

E08.34 Diabetes mellitus due to underlying condition with severe nonproliferative diabetic retinopathy

E08.341 Diabetes mellitus due to underlying condition with severe nonproliferative diabetic retinopathy with macular edema HCC

E08.349 Diabetes mellitus due to underlying condition with severe nonproliferative diabetic retinopathy without macular edema HCC

E08.35 Diabetes mellitus due to underlying condition with proliferative diabetic retinopathy

E08.351 Diabetes mellitus due to underlying condition with proliferative diabetic retinopathy with macular edema HCC

E08.352 Diabetes mellitus due to underlying condition with proliferative diabetic retinopathy with traction retinal detachment involving the macula HCC

E08.353 Diabetes mellitus due to underlying condition with proliferative diabetic retinopathy with traction retinal detachment not involving the macula HCC

E08.354 Diabetes mellitus due to underlying condition with proliferative diabetic retinopathy with combined traction retinal detachment and rhegmatogenous retinal detachment HCC

E08.355 Diabetes mellitus due to underlying condition with stable proliferative diabetic retinopathy HCC

E08.359 Diabetes mellitus due to underlying condition with proliferative diabetic retinopathy without macular edema HCC

E08.36 Diabetes mellitus due to underlying condition with diabetic cataract HCC

AHA: 2019,2Q,30-31; 2016,4Q,142

E08.37 Diabetes mellitus due to underlying condition with diabetic macular edema, resolved following treatment HCC

E08.39 Diabetes mellitus due to underlying condition with other diabetic ophthalmic complication HCC

Use additional code to identify manifestation, such as:
diabetic glaucoma (H40-H42)

E08.4 Diabetes mellitus due to underlying condition with neurological complications

E08.40 Diabetes mellitus due to underlying condition with diabetic neuropathy, unspecified HCC

E08.41 Diabetes mellitus due to underlying condition with diabetic mononeuropathy HCC

E08.42 Diabetes mellitus due to underlying condition with diabetic polyneuropathy HCC

Diabetes mellitus due to underlying condition with diabetic neuralgia

E08.43 Diabetes mellitus due to underlying condition with diabetic autonomic (poly)neuropathy HCC

Diabetes mellitus due to underlying condition with diabetic gastroparesis

AHA: 2013,4Q,114

E08.44 Diabetes mellitus due to underlying condition with diabetic amyotrophy HCC

E08.49 Diabetes mellitus due to underlying condition with other diabetic neurological complication HCC

E08.5 Diabetes mellitus due to underlying condition with circulatory complications

E08.51 Diabetes mellitus due to underlying condition with diabetic peripheral angiopathy without gangrene HCC

AHA: 2018,3Q,3-4; 2018,2Q,7

E08.52 Diabetes mellitus due to underlying condition with diabetic peripheral angiopathy with gangrene CC HCC

Diabetes mellitus due to underlying condition with diabetic gangrene

AHA: 2020,2Q,18; 2018,3Q,3; 2018,2Q,7; 2017,4Q,102

E08.59 Diabetes mellitus due to underlying condition with other circulatory complications HCC

E08.6 Diabetes mellitus due to underlying condition with other specified complications

E08.61 Diabetes mellitus due to underlying condition with diabetic arthropathy

E08.610 Diabetes mellitus due to underlying condition with diabetic neuropathic arthropathy HCC

Diabetes mellitus due to underlying condition with Charcôt's joints

DEF: Charcot's joint: Progressive neurologic arthropathy in which chronic degeneration of joints in the weight-bearing areas with peripheral hypertrophy occurs as a complication of a neuropathy disorder. Supporting structures relax from a loss of sensation resulting in chronic joint instability.

E08.618 Diabetes mellitus due to underlying condition with other diabetic arthropathy HCC

AHA: 2018,2Q,6

E08.62 Diabetes mellitus due to underlying condition with skin complications

E08.620 Diabetes mellitus due to underlying condition with diabetic dermatitis HCC

Diabetes mellitus due to underlying condition with diabetic necrobiosis lipoidica

E08.621 Diabetes mellitus due to underlying condition with foot ulcer HCC

Use additional code to identify site of ulcer (L97.4-, L97.5-)

AHA: 2020,2Q,19

EØ8.622 *Diabetes mellitus due to underlying condition with other skin ulcer* HCC
Use additional code to identify site of ulcer (L97.1-L97.9, L98.41-L98.49)
AHA: 2021,1Q,7; 2017,4Q,17

EØ8.628 *Diabetes mellitus due to underlying condition with other skin complications* HCC

6th **EØ8.63** **Diabetes mellitus due to underlying condition with oral complications**

EØ8.630 *Diabetes mellitus due to underlying condition with periodontal disease* HCC

EØ8.638 *Diabetes mellitus due to underlying condition with other oral complications* HCC

6th **EØ8.64** **Diabetes mellitus due to underlying condition with hypoglycemia**
AHA: 2017,1Q,42

EØ8.641 *Diabetes mellitus due to underlying condition with hypoglycemia with coma* MCC HCC

EØ8.649 *Diabetes mellitus due to underlying condition with hypoglycemia without coma* HCC
AHA: 2016,3Q,42; 2015,3Q,21

EØ8.65 *Diabetes mellitus due to underlying condition with hyperglycemia* HCC
AHA: 2017,1Q,42; 2013,3Q,20

EØ8.69 *Diabetes mellitus due to underlying condition with other specified complication* HCC
Use additional code to identify complication
AHA: 2016,4Q,141; 2016,1Q,13

EØ8.8 *Diabetes mellitus due to underlying condition with unspecified complications* HCC

EØ8.9 *Diabetes mellitus due to underlying condition without complications* HCC
AHA: 2020,2Q,18

4th **EØ9** **Drug or chemical induced diabetes mellitus**

Code first poisoning due to drug or toxin, if applicable ►(T36-T65 with fifth or sixth character 1-4)◄
Use additional code for adverse effect, if applicable, to identify drug (T36-T5Ø with fifth or sixth character 5)
Use additional code to identify control using:
insulin (Z79.4)
oral antidiabetic drugs (Z79.84)
oral hypoglycemic drugs (Z79.84)

EXCLUDES 1 *diabetes mellitus due to underlying condition (EØ8.-)*
gestational diabetes (O24.4-)
neonatal diabetes mellitus (P7Ø.2)
postpancreatectomy diabetes mellitus (E13.-)
postprocedural diabetes mellitus (E13.-)
secondary diabetes mellitus NEC (E13.-)
type 1 diabetes mellitus (E1Ø.-)
type 2 diabetes mellitus (E11.-)

5th **EØ9.Ø** **Drug or chemical induced diabetes mellitus with hyperosmolarity**
DEF: Diabetic hyperosmolarity: Extremely high levels of glucose in the blood without ketones.

EØ9.ØØ **Drug or chemical induced diabetes mellitus with hyperosmolarity without nonketotic hyperglycemic-hyperosmolar coma (NKHHC)** MCC H9 HCC

EØ9.Ø1 **Drug or chemical induced diabetes mellitus with hyperosmolarity with coma** MCC H9 HCC

5th **EØ9.1** **Drug or chemical induced diabetes mellitus with ketoacidosis**
DEF: Diabetic ketoacidosis: Potentially life-threatening complication due to a shortage of insulin in which the body switches to burning fatty acids and producing acidic ketone bodies.

EØ9.1Ø **Drug or chemical induced diabetes mellitus with ketoacidosis without coma** MCC H9 HCC

EØ9.11 **Drug or chemical induced diabetes mellitus with ketoacidosis with coma** MCC H9 HCC

5th **EØ9.2** **Drug or chemical induced diabetes mellitus with kidney complications**
AHA: 2019,3Q,3; 2018,4Q,88

EØ9.21 **Drug or chemical induced diabetes mellitus with diabetic nephropathy** HCC
Drug or chemical induced diabetes mellitus with intercapillary glomerulosclerosis
Drug or chemical induced diabetes mellitus with intracapillary glomerulonephrosis
Drug or chemical induced diabetes mellitus with Kimmelstiel-Wilson disease

EØ9.22 **Drug or chemical induced diabetes mellitus with diabetic chronic kidney disease** HCC
Use additional code to identify stage of chronic kidney disease (N18.1-N18.6)

EØ9.29 **Drug or chemical induced diabetes mellitus with other diabetic kidney complication** HCC
Drug or chemical induced diabetes mellitus with renal tubular degeneration

5th **EØ9.3** **Drug or chemical induced diabetes mellitus with ophthalmic complications**
AHA: 2016,4Q,11-13

One of the following 7th characters is to be assigned to codes in subcategories EØ9.32, EØ9.33, EØ9.34, EØ9.35, and EØ9.37 to designate laterality of the disease:
1 right eye
2 left eye
3 bilateral
9 unspecified eye

6th **EØ9.31** **Drug or chemical induced diabetes mellitus with unspecified diabetic retinopathy**
DEF: Diabetic retinopathy: Diabetic complication from damage to the retinal vessels resulting in vision problems that can progress to blindness.

EØ9.311 **Drug or chemical induced diabetes mellitus with unspecified diabetic retinopathy with macular edema** HCC

EØ9.319 **Drug or chemical induced diabetes mellitus with unspecified diabetic retinopathy without macular edema** HCC

6th **EØ9.32** **Drug or chemical induced diabetes mellitus with mild nonproliferative diabetic retinopathy**
Drug or chemical induced diabetes mellitus with nonproliferative diabetic retinopathy NOS

7th **EØ9.321** **Drug or chemical induced diabetes mellitus with mild nonproliferative diabetic retinopathy with macular edema** HCC

7th **EØ9.329** **Drug or chemical induced diabetes mellitus with mild nonproliferative diabetic retinopathy without macular edema** HCC

6th **EØ9.33** **Drug or chemical induced diabetes mellitus with moderate nonproliferative diabetic retinopathy**

7th **EØ9.331** **Drug or chemical induced diabetes mellitus with moderate nonproliferative diabetic retinopathy with macular edema** HCC

7th **EØ9.339** **Drug or chemical induced diabetes mellitus with moderate nonproliferative diabetic retinopathy without macular edema** HCC

6th **EØ9.34** **Drug or chemical induced diabetes mellitus with severe nonproliferative diabetic retinopathy**

7th **EØ9.341** **Drug or chemical induced diabetes mellitus with severe nonproliferative diabetic retinopathy with macular edema** HCC

7th **EØ9.349** **Drug or chemical induced diabetes mellitus with severe nonproliferative diabetic retinopathy without macular edema** HCC

6th **EØ9.35** **Drug or chemical induced diabetes mellitus with proliferative diabetic retinopathy**

7th **EØ9.351** **Drug or chemical induced diabetes mellitus with proliferative diabetic retinopathy with macular edema** HCC

7th **EØ9.352** **Drug or chemical induced diabetes mellitus with proliferative diabetic retinopathy with traction retinal detachment involving the macula** HCC

√7th E09.353 **Drug or chemical induced diabetes mellitus with proliferative diabetic retinopathy with traction retinal detachment not involving the macula** HCC

√7th E09.354 **Drug or chemical induced diabetes mellitus with proliferative diabetic retinopathy with combined traction retinal detachment and rhegmatogenous retinal detachment** HCC

√7th E09.355 **Drug or chemical induced diabetes mellitus with stable proliferative diabetic retinopathy** HCC

√7th E09.359 **Drug or chemical induced diabetes mellitus with proliferative diabetic retinopathy without macular edema** HCC

E09.36 **Drug or chemical induced diabetes mellitus with diabetic cataract** HCC
AHA: 2019,2Q,30-31; 2016,4Q,142

√x7th E09.37 **Drug or chemical induced diabetes mellitus with diabetic macular edema, resolved following treatment** HCC

E09.39 **Drug or chemical induced diabetes mellitus with other diabetic ophthalmic complication** HCC
Use additional code to identify manifestation, such as:
diabetic glaucoma (H40-H42)

√5th E09.4 **Drug or chemical induced diabetes mellitus with neurological complications**

E09.40 **Drug or chemical induced diabetes mellitus with neurological complications with diabetic neuropathy, unspecified** HCC

E09.41 **Drug or chemical induced diabetes mellitus with neurological complications with diabetic mononeuropathy** HCC

E09.42 **Drug or chemical induced diabetes mellitus with neurological complications with diabetic polyneuropathy** HCC
Drug or chemical induced diabetes mellitus with diabetic neuralgia

E09.43 **Drug or chemical induced diabetes mellitus with neurological complications with diabetic autonomic (poly)neuropathy** HCC
Drug or chemical induced diabetes mellitus with diabetic gastroparesis
AHA: 2013,4Q,114

E09.44 **Drug or chemical induced diabetes mellitus with neurological complications with diabetic amyotrophy** HCC

E09.49 **Drug or chemical induced diabetes mellitus with neurological complications with other diabetic neurological complication** HCC

√5th E09.5 **Drug or chemical induced diabetes mellitus with circulatory complications**

E09.51 **Drug or chemical induced diabetes mellitus with diabetic peripheral angiopathy without gangrene** HCC
AHA: 2018,3Q,3-4; 2018,2Q,7

E09.52 **Drug or chemical induced diabetes mellitus with diabetic peripheral angiopathy with gangrene** CC HCC
Drug or chemical induced diabetes mellitus with diabetic gangrene
AHA: 2020,2Q,18; 2018,3Q,3; 2018,2Q,7; 2017,4Q,102

E09.59 **Drug or chemical induced diabetes mellitus with other circulatory complications** HCC

√5th E09.6 **Drug or chemical induced diabetes mellitus with other specified complications**

√6th E09.61 **Drug or chemical induced diabetes mellitus with diabetic arthropathy**

E09.610 **Drug or chemical induced diabetes mellitus with diabetic neuropathic arthropathy** HCC
Drug or chemical induced diabetes mellitus with Charcôt's joints
DEF: Charcot's joint: Progressive neurologic arthropathy in which chronic degeneration of joints in the weight-bearing areas with peripheral hypertrophy occurs as a complication of a neuropathy disorder. Supporting structures relax from a loss of sensation resulting in chronic joint instability.

E09.618 **Drug or chemical induced diabetes mellitus with other diabetic arthropathy** HCC
AHA: 2018,2Q,6

√6th E09.62 **Drug or chemical induced diabetes mellitus with skin complications**

E09.620 **Drug or chemical induced diabetes mellitus with diabetic dermatitis** HCC
Drug or chemical induced diabetes mellitus with diabetic necrobiosis lipoidica

E09.621 **Drug or chemical induced diabetes mellitus with foot ulcer** HCC
Use additional code to identify site of ulcer (L97.4-, L97.5-)
AHA: 2020,2Q,19

E09.622 **Drug or chemical induced diabetes mellitus with other skin ulcer** HCC
Use additional code to identify site of ulcer (L97.1-L97.9, L98.41-L98.49)
AHA: 2021,1Q,7; 2017,4Q,17

E09.628 **Drug or chemical induced diabetes mellitus with other skin complications** HCC

√6th E09.63 **Drug or chemical induced diabetes mellitus with oral complications**

E09.630 **Drug or chemical induced diabetes mellitus with periodontal disease** HCC

E09.638 **Drug or chemical induced diabetes mellitus with other oral complications** HCC

√6th E09.64 **Drug or chemical induced diabetes mellitus with hypoglycemia**
AHA: 2017,1Q,42

E09.641 **Drug or chemical induced diabetes mellitus with hypoglycemia with coma** MCC HCC

E09.649 **Drug or chemical induced diabetes mellitus with hypoglycemia without coma** HCC
AHA: 2016,3Q,42; 2015,3Q,21

E09.65 **Drug or chemical induced diabetes mellitus with hyperglycemia** HCC
AHA: 2017,1Q,42; 2013,3Q,20

E09.69 **Drug or chemical induced diabetes mellitus with other specified complication** HCC
Use additional code to identify complication
AHA: 2016,4Q,141; 2016,1Q,13

E09.8 **Drug or chemical induced diabetes mellitus with unspecified complications** HCC

E09.9 **Drug or chemical induced diabetes mellitus without complications** HCC
AHA: 2020,2Q,18

E10 Type 1 diabetes mellitus

INCLUDES brittle diabetes (mellitus)
diabetes (mellitus) due to autoimmune process
diabetes (mellitus) due to immune mediated pancreatic islet beta-cell destruction
idiopathic diabetes (mellitus)
juvenile onset diabetes (mellitus)
ketosis-prone diabetes (mellitus)

EXCLUDES 1 *diabetes mellitus due to underlying condition (E08.-)*
drug or chemical induced diabetes mellitus (E09.-)
gestational diabetes (O24.4-)
hyperglycemia NOS (R73.9)
neonatal diabetes mellitus (P70.2)
postpancreatectomy diabetes mellitus (E13.-)
postprocedural diabetes mellitus (E13.-)
secondary diabetes mellitus NEC (E13.-)
type 2 diabetes mellitus (E11.-)

AHA: 2023,2Q,10; 2020,3Q,30

E10.1 Type 1 diabetes mellitus with ketoacidosis

AHA: 2013,3Q,20

DEF: Diabetic ketoacidosis: Potentially life-threatening complication due to a shortage of insulin in which the body switches to burning fatty acids and producing acidic ketone bodies.

E10.10 Type 1 diabetes mellitus with ketoacidosis without coma MCC H9 HCC

E10.11 Type 1 diabetes mellitus with ketoacidosis with coma MCC H9 HCC

E10.2 Type 1 diabetes mellitus with kidney complications

AHA: 2019,3Q,3; 2018,4Q,88

E10.21 Type 1 diabetes mellitus with diabetic nephropathy HCC

Type 1 diabetes mellitus with intercapillary glomerulosclerosis
Type 1 diabetes mellitus with intracapillary glomerulonephrosis
Type 1 diabetes mellitus with Kimmelstiel-Wilson disease

E10.22 Type 1 diabetes mellitus with diabetic chronic kidney disease HCC

Use additional code to identify stage of chronic kidney disease (N18.1-N18.6)

E10.29 Type 1 diabetes mellitus with other diabetic kidney complication HCC

Type 1 diabetes mellitus with renal tubular degeneration

AHA: 2016,1Q,13

E10.3 Type 1 diabetes mellitus with ophthalmic complications

AHA: 2016,4Q,11-13

One of the following 7th characters is to be assigned to codes in subcategories E10.32, E10.33, E10.34, E10.35, and E10.37 to designate laterality of the disease:
1 right eye
2 left eye
3 bilateral
9 unspecified eye

E10.31 Type 1 diabetes mellitus with unspecified diabetic retinopathy

DEF: Diabetic retinopathy: Diabetic complication from damage to the retinal vessels resulting in vision problems that can progress to blindness.

E10.311 Type 1 diabetes mellitus with unspecified diabetic retinopathy with macular edema HCC

E10.319 Type 1 diabetes mellitus with unspecified diabetic retinopathy without macular edema HCC

E10.32 Type 1 diabetes mellitus with mild nonproliferative diabetic retinopathy

Type 1 diabetes mellitus with nonproliferative diabetic retinopathy NOS

E10.321 Type 1 diabetes mellitus with mild nonproliferative diabetic retinopathy with macular edema HCC

E10.329 Type 1 diabetes mellitus with mild nonproliferative diabetic retinopathy without macular edema HCC

E10.33 Type 1 diabetes mellitus with moderate nonproliferative diabetic retinopathy

E10.331 Type 1 diabetes mellitus with moderate nonproliferative diabetic retinopathy with macular edema HCC

E10.339 Type 1 diabetes mellitus with moderate nonproliferative diabetic retinopathy without macular edema HCC

E10.34 Type 1 diabetes mellitus with severe nonproliferative diabetic retinopathy

E10.341 Type 1 diabetes mellitus with severe nonproliferative diabetic retinopathy with macular edema HCC

E10.349 Type 1 diabetes mellitus with severe nonproliferative diabetic retinopathy without macular edema HCC

E10.35 Type 1 diabetes mellitus with proliferative diabetic retinopathy

E10.351 Type 1 diabetes mellitus with proliferative diabetic retinopathy with macular edema HCC

E10.352 Type 1 diabetes mellitus with proliferative diabetic retinopathy with traction retinal detachment involving the macula HCC

E10.353 Type 1 diabetes mellitus with proliferative diabetic retinopathy with traction retinal detachment not involving the macula HCC

E10.354 Type 1 diabetes mellitus with proliferative diabetic retinopathy with combined traction retinal detachment and rhegmatogenous retinal detachment HCC

E10.355 Type 1 diabetes mellitus with stable proliferative diabetic retinopathy HCC

E10.359 Type 1 diabetes mellitus with proliferative diabetic retinopathy without macular edema HCC

E10.36 Type 1 diabetes mellitus with diabetic cataract HCC

AHA: 2019,2Q,30-31; 2016,4Q,142

E10.37 Type 1 diabetes mellitus with diabetic macular edema, resolved following treatment HCC

E10.39 Type 1 diabetes mellitus with other diabetic ophthalmic complication HCC

Use additional code to identify manifestation, such as:
diabetic glaucoma (H40-H42)

E10.4 Type 1 diabetes mellitus with neurological complications

E10.40 Type 1 diabetes mellitus with diabetic neuropathy, unspecified HCC

E10.41 Type 1 diabetes mellitus with diabetic mononeuropathy HCC

E10.42 Type 1 diabetes mellitus with diabetic polyneuropathy HCC

Type 1 diabetes mellitus with diabetic neuralgia

E10.43 Type 1 diabetes mellitus with diabetic autonomic (poly)neuropathy HCC

Type 1 diabetes mellitus with diabetic gastroparesis

AHA: 2013,4Q,114

E10.44 Type 1 diabetes mellitus with diabetic amyotrophy HCC

E10.49 Type 1 diabetes mellitus with other diabetic neurological complication HCC

E10.5 Type 1 diabetes mellitus with circulatory complications

E10.51 Type 1 diabetes mellitus with diabetic peripheral angiopathy without gangrene HCC

AHA: 2018,3Q,3-4; 2018,2Q,7

E10.52 Type 1 diabetes mellitus with diabetic peripheral angiopathy with gangrene CC HCC

Type 1 diabetes mellitus with diabetic gangrene

AHA: 2020,2Q,18; 2018,3Q,3; 2018,2Q,7; 2017,4Q,102

E10.59 Type 1 diabetes mellitus with other circulatory complications HCC

E10.6 Type 1 diabetes mellitus with other specified complications

E10.61 Type 1 diabetes mellitus with diabetic arthropathy

E10.610 Type 1 diabetes mellitus with diabetic neuropathic arthropathy HCC

Type 1 diabetes mellitus with Charcôt's joints

DEF: Charcot's joint: Progressive neurologic arthropathy in which chronic degeneration of joints in the weight-bearing areas with peripheral hypertrophy occurs as a complication of a neuropathy disorder. Supporting structures relax from a loss of sensation resulting in chronic joint instability.

E10.618 Type 1 diabetes mellitus with other diabetic arthropathy HCC

AHA: 2018,2Q,6

E10.62 Type 1 diabetes mellitus with skin complications

E10.620 Type 1 diabetes mellitus with diabetic dermatitis HCC

Type 1 diabetes mellitus with diabetic necrobiosis lipoidica

E10.621 Type 1 diabetes mellitus with foot ulcer HCC

Use additional code to identify site of ulcer (L97.4-, L97.5-)

AHA: 2020,2Q,19

E10.622 Type 1 diabetes mellitus with other skin ulcer HCC

Use additional code to identify site of ulcer (L97.1-L97.9, L98.41-L98.49)

AHA: 2021,1Q,7; 2017,4Q,17

E10.628 Type 1 diabetes mellitus with other skin complications HCC

E10.63 Type 1 diabetes mellitus with oral complications

E10.630 Type 1 diabetes mellitus with periodontal disease HCC

E10.638 Type 1 diabetes mellitus with other oral complications HCC

E10.64 Type 1 diabetes mellitus with hypoglycemia

AHA: 2017,1Q,42

E10.641 Type 1 diabetes mellitus with hypoglycemia with coma MCC HCC

E10.649 Type 1 diabetes mellitus with hypoglycemia without coma HCC

AHA: 2016,3Q,42; 2016,1Q,13; 2015,3Q,21

E10.65 Type 1 diabetes mellitus with hyperglycemia HCC

AHA: 2022,1Q,28; 2017,1Q,42; 2013,3Q,20

E10.69 Type 1 diabetes mellitus with other specified complication HCC

Use additional code to identify complication

AHA: 2022,1Q,28; 2016,4Q,141; 2016,1Q,13

E10.8 Type 1 diabetes mellitus with unspecified complications HCC

E10.9 Type 1 diabetes mellitus without complications HCC

AHA: 2020,2Q,18

E11 Type 2 diabetes mellitus

INCLUDES diabetes (mellitus) due to insulin secretory defect
diabetes NOS
insulin resistant diabetes (mellitus)

Use additional code to identify control using:
insulin (Z79.4)
oral antidiabetic drugs (Z79.84)
oral hypoglycemic drugs (Z79.84)

EXCLUDES 1 *diabetes mellitus due to underlying condition (E08.-)*
drug or chemical induced diabetes mellitus (E09.-)
gestational diabetes (O24.4-)
neonatal diabetes mellitus (P70.2)
postpancreatectomy diabetes mellitus (E13.-)
postprocedural diabetes mellitus (E13.-)
secondary diabetes mellitus NEC (E13.-)
type 1 diabetes mellitus (E10.-)

AHA: 2020,3Q,30; 2020,1Q,12; 2016,2Q,10; 2013,1Q,26

E11.0 Type 2 diabetes mellitus with hyperosmolarity

DEF: Diabetic hyperosmolarity: Extremely high levels of glucose in the blood without ketones.

E11.00 Type 2 diabetes mellitus with hyperosmolarity without nonketotic hyperglycemic-hyperosmolar coma (NKHHC) MCC H9 HCC

AHA: 2022,1Q,28

E11.01 Type 2 diabetes mellitus with hyperosmolarity with coma MCC H9 HCC

E11.1 Type 2 diabetes mellitus with ketoacidosis

AHA: 2017,4Q,6

DEF: Diabetic ketoacidosis: Potentially life-threatening complication due to a shortage of insulin in which the body switches to burning fatty acids and producing acidic ketone bodies.

E11.10 Type 2 diabetes mellitus with ketoacidosis without coma MCC H9 HCC

E11.11 Type 2 diabetes mellitus with ketoacidosis with coma MCC H9 HCC

E11.2 Type 2 diabetes mellitus with kidney complications

AHA: 2019,3Q,3; 2018,4Q,88

E11.21 Type 2 diabetes mellitus with diabetic nephropathy HCC

Type 2 diabetes mellitus with intercapillary glomerulosclerosis
Type 2 diabetes mellitus with intracapillary glomerulonephrosis
Type 2 diabetes mellitus with Kimmelstiel-Wilson disease

E11.22 Type 2 diabetes mellitus with diabetic chronic kidney disease HCC

Use additional code to identify stage of chronic kidney disease (N18.1-N18.6)

AHA: 2022,3Q,15

E11.29 Type 2 diabetes mellitus with other diabetic kidney complication HCC

Type 2 diabetes mellitus with renal tubular degeneration

E11.3 Type 2 diabetes mellitus with ophthalmic complications

AHA: 2016,4Q,11-13

One of the following 7th characters is to be assigned to codes in subcategories E11.32, E11.33, E11.34, E11.35, and E11.37 to designate laterality of the disease:
1 right eye
2 left eye
3 bilateral
9 unspecified eye

E11.31 Type 2 diabetes mellitus with unspecified diabetic retinopathy

DEF: Diabetic retinopathy: Diabetic complication from damage to the retinal vessels resulting in vision problems that can progress to blindness.

E11.311 Type 2 diabetes mellitus with unspecified diabetic retinopathy with macular edema HCC

E11.319 Type 2 diabetes mellitus with unspecified diabetic retinopathy without macular edema HCC

✓6th **E11.32 Type 2 diabetes mellitus with mild nonproliferative diabetic retinopathy**
Type 2 diabetes mellitus with nonproliferative diabetic retinopathy NOS

✓7th **E11.321 Type 2 diabetes mellitus with mild nonproliferative diabetic retinopathy with macular edema** HCC

✓7th **E11.329 Type 2 diabetes mellitus with mild nonproliferative diabetic retinopathy without macular edema** HCC

✓6th **E11.33 Type 2 diabetes mellitus with moderate nonproliferative diabetic retinopathy**

✓7th **E11.331 Type 2 diabetes mellitus with moderate nonproliferative diabetic retinopathy with macular edema** HCC

✓7th **E11.339 Type 2 diabetes mellitus with moderate nonproliferative diabetic retinopathy without macular edema** HCC

✓6th **E11.34 Type 2 diabetes mellitus with severe nonproliferative diabetic retinopathy**

✓7th **E11.341 Type 2 diabetes mellitus with severe nonproliferative diabetic retinopathy with macular edema** HCC

✓7th **E11.349 Type 2 diabetes mellitus with severe nonproliferative diabetic retinopathy without macular edema** HCC

✓6th **E11.35 Type 2 diabetes mellitus with proliferative diabetic retinopathy**

✓7th **E11.351 Type 2 diabetes mellitus with proliferative diabetic retinopathy with macular edema** HCC

✓7th **E11.352 Type 2 diabetes mellitus with proliferative diabetic retinopathy with traction retinal detachment involving the macula** HCC

✓7th **E11.353 Type 2 diabetes mellitus with proliferative diabetic retinopathy with traction retinal detachment not involving the macula** HCC

✓7th **E11.354 Type 2 diabetes mellitus with proliferative diabetic retinopathy with combined traction retinal detachment and rhegmatogenous retinal detachment** HCC

✓7th **E11.355 Type 2 diabetes mellitus with stable proliferative diabetic retinopathy** HCC

✓7th **E11.359 Type 2 diabetes mellitus with proliferative diabetic retinopathy without macular edema** HCC

E11.36 Type 2 diabetes mellitus with diabetic cataract HCC
AHA: 2019,2Q,30-31; 2016,4Q,142

✓x7th **E11.37 Type 2 diabetes mellitus with diabetic macular edema, resolved following treatment** HCC

E11.39 Type 2 diabetes mellitus with other diabetic ophthalmic complication HCC
Use additional code to identify manifestation, such as:
diabetic glaucoma (H40-H42)

✓5th **E11.4 Type 2 diabetes mellitus with neurological complications**
AHA: 2022,3Q,15

E11.40 Type 2 diabetes mellitus with diabetic neuropathy, unspecified HCC
AHA: 2013,4Q,129

E11.41 Type 2 diabetes mellitus with diabetic mononeuropathy HCC

E11.42 Type 2 diabetes mellitus with diabetic polyneuropathy HCC
Type 2 diabetes mellitus with diabetic neuralgia
AHA: 2020,1Q,12

E11.43 Type 2 diabetes mellitus with diabetic autonomic (poly)neuropathy HCC
Type 2 diabetes mellitus with diabetic gastroparesis
AHA: 2023,2Q,8; 2013,4Q,114

E11.44 Type 2 diabetes mellitus with diabetic amyotrophy HCC

E11.49 Type 2 diabetes mellitus with other diabetic neurological complication HCC

✓5th **E11.5 Type 2 diabetes mellitus with circulatory complications**

E11.51 Type 2 diabetes mellitus with diabetic peripheral angiopathy without gangrene HCC
AHA: 2018,3Q,3-4; 2018,2Q,7

E11.52 Type 2 diabetes mellitus with diabetic peripheral angiopathy with gangrene CC HCC
Type 2 diabetes mellitus with diabetic gangrene
AHA: 2020,2Q,18; 2018,3Q,3; 2018,2Q,7; 2017,4Q,102

E11.59 Type 2 diabetes mellitus with other circulatory complications HCC

✓5th **E11.6 Type 2 diabetes mellitus with other specified complications**

✓6th **E11.61 Type 2 diabetes mellitus with diabetic arthropathy**

E11.610 Type 2 diabetes mellitus with diabetic neuropathic arthropathy HCC
Type 2 diabetes mellitus with Charcôt's joints
DEF: Charcot's joint: Progressive neurologic arthropathy in which chronic degeneration of joints in the weight-bearing areas with peripheral hypertrophy occurs as a complication of a neuropathy disorder. Supporting structures relax from a loss of sensation resulting in chronic joint instability.

E11.618 Type 2 diabetes mellitus with other diabetic arthropathy HCC
AHA: 2018,2Q,6

✓6th **E11.62 Type 2 diabetes mellitus with skin complications**

E11.620 Type 2 diabetes mellitus with diabetic dermatitis HCC
Type 2 diabetes mellitus with diabetic necrobiosis lipoidica

E11.621 Type 2 diabetes mellitus with foot ulcer HCC
Use additional code to identify site of ulcer (L97.4-, L97.5-)
AHA: 2020,2Q,19; 2020,1Q,12

E11.622 Type 2 diabetes mellitus with other skin ulcer HCC
Use additional code to identify site of ulcer (L97.1-L97.9, L98.41-L98.49)
AHA: 2021,1Q,7; 2017,4Q,17

E11.628 Type 2 diabetes mellitus with other skin complications HCC

✓6th **E11.63 Type 2 diabetes mellitus with oral complications**

E11.630 Type 2 diabetes mellitus with periodontal disease HCC

E11.638 Type 2 diabetes mellitus with other oral complications HCC

✓6th **E11.64 Type 2 diabetes mellitus with hypoglycemia**
AHA: 2017,1Q,42

E11.641 Type 2 diabetes mellitus with hypoglycemia with coma MCC HCC

E11.649 Type 2 diabetes mellitus with hypoglycemia without coma HCC
AHA: 2016,3Q,42; 2015,3Q,21

E11.65 Type 2 diabetes mellitus with hyperglycemia HCC
AHA: 2023,2Q,10; 2022,1Q,28; 2017,1Q,42; 2013,3Q,20

E11.69 Type 2 diabetes mellitus with other specified complication HCC
Use additional code to identify complication
AHA: 2020,1Q,12; 2016,4Q,141; 2016,1Q,13

E11.8 Type 2 diabetes mellitus with unspecified complications HCC

E11.9 Type 2 diabetes mellitus without complications HCC
AHA: 2020,2Q,18

✓4th E13 Other specified diabetes mellitus

INCLUDES diabetes mellitus due to genetic defects of beta-cell function
diabetes mellitus due to genetic defects in insulin action
postpancreatectomy diabetes mellitus
postprocedural diabetes mellitus
secondary diabetes mellitus NEC

Use additional code to identify control using:
insulin (Z79.4)
oral antidiabetic drugs (Z79.84)
oral hypoglycemic drugs (Z79.84)

EXCLUDES 1 *diabetes (mellitus) due to autoimmune process (E10.-)*
diabetes (mellitus) due to immune mediated pancreatic islet beta-cell destruction (E10.-)
diabetes mellitus due to underlying condition (E08.-)
drug or chemical induced diabetes mellitus (E09.-)
gestational diabetes (O24.4-)
neonatal diabetes mellitus (P70.2)
type 1 diabetes mellitus (E10.-)

AHA: 2018,3Q,4; 2016,1Q,11-13

TIP: Use this category when the diabetes is documented as diabetes type 1.5. Synonymous terms used in the documentation may also include combined diabetes type 1 and type 2, latent autoimmune diabetes of adults (LADA), slow-progressing type 1 diabetes, or double diabetes.

TIP: When postprocedural or postpancreatectomy hypoinsulinemia (E89.1) is documented with postprocedural or postpancreatectomy diabetes mellitus (E13.-), code E89.1 should be sequenced first.

✓5th E13.0 Other specified diabetes mellitus with hyperosmolarity

DEF: Diabetic hyperosmolarity: Extremely high levels of glucose in the blood without ketones.

E13.00 Other specified diabetes mellitus with hyperosmolarity without nonketotic hyperglycemic-hyperosmolar coma (NKHHC) MCC H9 HCC

EXCLUDES 2 ~~*type 2 diabetes mellitus (E11.-)*~~

E13.01 Other specified diabetes mellitus with hyperosmolarity with coma MCC H9 HCC

✓5th E13.1 Other specified diabetes mellitus with ketoacidosis

AHA: 2016,2Q,10; 2013,1Q,26

DEF: Diabetic ketoacidosis: Potentially life-threatening complication due to a shortage of insulin in which the body switches to burning fatty acids and producing acidic ketone bodies.

E13.10 Other specified diabetes mellitus with ketoacidosis without coma MCC H9 HCC

E13.11 Other specified diabetes mellitus with ketoacidosis with coma MCC H9 HCC

✓5th E13.2 Other specified diabetes mellitus with kidney complications

AHA: 2019,3Q,3; 2018,4Q,88

E13.21 Other specified diabetes mellitus with diabetic nephropathy HCC

Other specified diabetes mellitus with intercapillary glomerulosclerosis
Other specified diabetes mellitus with intracapillary glomerulonephrosis
Other specified diabetes mellitus with Kimmelstiel-Wilson disease

E13.22 Other specified diabetes mellitus with diabetic chronic kidney disease HCC

Use additional code to identify stage of chronic kidney disease (N18.1-N18.6)

E13.29 Other specified diabetes mellitus with other diabetic kidney complication HCC

Other specified diabetes mellitus with renal tubular degeneration

✓5th E13.3 Other specified diabetes mellitus with ophthalmic complications

AHA: 2016,4Q,11-13

One of the following 7th characters is to be assigned to codes in subcategories E13.32, E13.33, E13.34, E13.35, and E13.37 to designate laterality of the disease:
1 right eye
2 left eye
3 bilateral
9 unspecified eye

✓6th E13.31 Other specified diabetes mellitus with unspecified diabetic retinopathy

DEF: Diabetic retinopathy: Diabetic complication from damage to the retinal vessels resulting in vision problems that can progress to blindness.

E13.311 Other specified diabetes mellitus with unspecified diabetic retinopathy with macular edema HCC

E13.319 Other specified diabetes mellitus with unspecified diabetic retinopathy without macular edema HCC

✓6th E13.32 Other specified diabetes mellitus with mild nonproliferative diabetic retinopathy

Other specified diabetes mellitus with nonproliferative diabetic retinopathy NOS

✓7th E13.321 Other specified diabetes mellitus with mild nonproliferative diabetic retinopathy with macular edema HCC

✓7th E13.329 Other specified diabetes mellitus with mild nonproliferative diabetic retinopathy without macular edema HCC

✓6th E13.33 Other specified diabetes mellitus with moderate nonproliferative diabetic retinopathy

✓7th E13.331 Other specified diabetes mellitus with moderate nonproliferative diabetic retinopathy with macular edema HCC

✓7th E13.339 Other specified diabetes mellitus with moderate nonproliferative diabetic retinopathy without macular edema HCC

✓6th E13.34 Other specified diabetes mellitus with severe nonproliferative diabetic retinopathy

✓7th E13.341 Other specified diabetes mellitus with severe nonproliferative diabetic retinopathy with macular edema HCC

✓7th E13.349 Other specified diabetes mellitus with severe nonproliferative diabetic retinopathy without macular edema HCC

✓6th E13.35 Other specified diabetes mellitus with proliferative diabetic retinopathy

✓7th E13.351 Other specified diabetes mellitus with proliferative diabetic retinopathy with macular edema HCC

✓7th E13.352 Other specified diabetes mellitus with proliferative diabetic retinopathy with traction retinal detachment involving the macula HCC

✓7th E13.353 Other specified diabetes mellitus with proliferative diabetic retinopathy with traction retinal detachment not involving the macula HCC

✓7th E13.354 Other specified diabetes mellitus with proliferative diabetic retinopathy with combined traction retinal detachment and rhegmatogenous retinal detachment HCC

✓7th E13.355 Other specified diabetes mellitus with stable proliferative diabetic retinopathy HCC

✓7th E13.359 Other specified diabetes mellitus with proliferative diabetic retinopathy without macular edema HCC

E13.36 Other specified diabetes mellitus with diabetic cataract HCC

AHA: 2019,2Q,30-31; 2016,4Q,142

✓x7th E13.37 Other specified diabetes mellitus with diabetic macular edema, resolved following treatment HCC

Chapter 4. Endocrine, Nutritional and Metabolic Diseases

E13.39 Other specified diabetes mellitus with other diabetic ophthalmic complication HCC
Use additional code to identify manifestation, such as:
diabetic glaucoma (H40-H42)

✓5th **E13.4 Other specified diabetes mellitus with neurological complications**

E13.40 Other specified diabetes mellitus with diabetic neuropathy, unspecified HCC

E13.41 Other specified diabetes mellitus with diabetic mononeuropathy HCC

E13.42 Other specified diabetes mellitus with diabetic polyneuropathy HCC
Other specified diabetes mellitus with diabetic neuralgia

E13.43 Other specified diabetes mellitus with diabetic autonomic (poly)neuropathy HCC
Other specified diabetes mellitus with diabetic gastroparesis
AHA: 2013,4Q,114

E13.44 Other specified diabetes mellitus with diabetic amyotrophy HCC

E13.49 Other specified diabetes mellitus with other diabetic neurological complication HCC

✓5th **E13.5 Other specified diabetes mellitus with circulatory complications**

E13.51 Other specified diabetes mellitus with diabetic peripheral angiopathy without gangrene HCC
AHA: 2018,3Q,3-4; 2018,2Q,7

E13.52 Other specified diabetes mellitus with diabetic peripheral angiopathy with gangrene CC HCC
Other specified diabetes mellitus with diabetic gangrene
AHA: 2020,2Q,18; 2018,3Q,3; 2018,2Q,7; 2017,4Q,102

E13.59 Other specified diabetes mellitus with other circulatory complications HCC

✓5th **E13.6 Other specified diabetes mellitus with other specified complications**

✓6th **E13.61 Other specified diabetes mellitus with diabetic arthropathy**

E13.610 Other specified diabetes mellitus with diabetic neuropathic arthropathy HCC
Other specified diabetes mellitus with Charcôt's joints
DEF: Charcot's joint: Progressive neurologic arthropathy in which chronic degeneration of joints in the weight-bearing areas with peripheral hypertrophy occurs as a complication of a neuropathy disorder. Supporting structures relax from a loss of sensation resulting in chronic joint instability.

E13.618 Other specified diabetes mellitus with other diabetic arthropathy HCC
AHA: 2018,2Q,6

✓6th **E13.62 Other specified diabetes mellitus with skin complications**

E13.620 Other specified diabetes mellitus with diabetic dermatitis HCC
Other specified diabetes mellitus with diabetic necrobiosis lipoidica

E13.621 Other specified diabetes mellitus with foot ulcer HCC
Use additional code to identify site of ulcer (L97.4-, L97.5-)
AHA: 2020,2Q,19

E13.622 Other specified diabetes mellitus with other skin ulcer HCC
Use additional code to identify site of ulcer (L97.1-L97.9, L98.41-L98.49)
AHA: 2021,1Q,7; 2017,4Q,17

E13.628 Other specified diabetes mellitus with other skin complications HCC

✓6th **E13.63 Other specified diabetes mellitus with oral complications**

E13.630 Other specified diabetes mellitus with periodontal disease HCC

E13.638 Other specified diabetes mellitus with other oral complications HCC

✓6th **E13.64 Other specified diabetes mellitus with hypoglycemia**
AHA: 2017,1Q,42

E13.641 Other specified diabetes mellitus with hypoglycemia with coma MCC HCC

E13.649 Other specified diabetes mellitus with hypoglycemia without coma HCC
AHA: 2016,3Q,42; 2015,3Q,21

E13.65 Other specified diabetes mellitus with hyperglycemia HCC
AHA: 2017,1Q,42; 2013,3Q,20

E13.69 Other specified diabetes mellitus with other specified complication HCC
Use additional code to identify complication
AHA: 2016,4Q,141; 2016,1Q,13

E13.8 Other specified diabetes mellitus with unspecified complications HCC

E13.9 Other specified diabetes mellitus without complications HCC
AHA: 2020,2Q,18

Other disorders of glucose regulation and pancreatic internal secretion (E15-E16)

E15 Nondiabetic hypoglycemic coma CC H9 HCC
INCLUDES drug-induced insulin coma in nondiabetic
hyperinsulinism with hypoglycemic coma
hypoglycemic coma NOS

✓4th **E16 Other disorders of pancreatic internal secretion**

E16.0 Drug-induced hypoglycemia without coma
EXCLUDES 1 *diabetes with hypoglycemia without coma (E09.649)*
Use additional code for adverse effect, if applicable, to identify drug (T36-T50 with fifth or sixth character 5)

E16.1 Other hypoglycemia
Functional hyperinsulinism
Functional nonhyperinsulinemic hypoglycemia
Hyperinsulinism NOS
Hyperplasia of pancreatic islet beta cells NOS
EXCLUDES 1 *diabetes with hypoglycemia (E08.649, E10.649, E11.649, E13.649)*
hypoglycemia in infant of diabetic mother (P70.1)
neonatal hypoglycemia (P70.4)

E16.2 Hypoglycemia, unspecified
EXCLUDES 1 *diabetes with hypoglycemia (E08.649, E10.649, E11.649, E13.649)*
AHA: 2016,3Q,42
TIP: Assign for nondiabetic hypoglycemic encephalopathy not further clarified in the documentation.

E16.3 Increased secretion of glucagon
Hyperplasia of pancreatic endocrine cells with glucagon excess

E16.4 Increased secretion of gastrin
Hypergastrinemia
Hyperplasia of pancreatic endocrine cells with gastrin excess
Zollinger-Ellison syndrome

E16.8 Other specified disorders of pancreatic internal secretion
Increased secretion from endocrine pancreas of growth hormone-releasing hormone
Increased secretion from endocrine pancreas of pancreatic polypeptide
Increased secretion from endocrine pancreas of somatostatin
Increased secretion from endocrine pancreas of vasoactive-intestinal polypeptide

E16.9 Disorder of pancreatic internal secretion, unspecified
Islet-cell hyperplasia NOS
Pancreatic endocrine cell hyperplasia NOS

Disorders of other endocrine glands (E2Ø-E35)

EXCLUDES 1 *galactorrhea (N64.3)*
gynecomastia (N62)

✓4th **E2Ø Hypoparathyroidism**

EXCLUDES 1 *Di George's syndrome (D82.1)*
postprocedural hypoparathyroidism (E89.2)
tetany NOS (R29.Ø)
transitory neonatal hypoparathyroidism (P71.4)

E2Ø.Ø Idiopathic hypoparathyroidism HCC
DEF: Abnormally low secretion of parathyroid hormones, with unknown cause, which triggers decreased calcium and increased phosphorus in the blood that can result in cataracts, muscle cramps, tetany, tingling, or burning in the lips, fingers, and toes.

E2Ø.1 Pseudohypoparathyroidism

▲ ✓5th **E2Ø.8 Other hypoparathyroidism**

● ✓6th **E2Ø.81 Hypoparathyroidism due to impaired parathyroid hormone secretion**

● **E2Ø.81Ø Autosomal dominant hypocalcemia**
Autosomal dominant hypocalcemia type 1 (ADH1)
Autosomal dominant hypocalcemia type 2 (ADH2)
Code also, if applicable, any associated conditions, such as:
calculus of kidney (N2Ø.Ø)
chronic kidney disease (N18.-)
respiratory distress (J8Ø, RØ6.-)
seizure disorder (G4Ø.-, R56.9)

● **E2Ø.811 Secondary hypoparathyroidism in diseases classified elsewhere**
Code first underlying condition, if known

● **E2Ø.812 Autoimmune hypoparathyroidism**
Code first, if applicable, underlying condition such as:
autoimmune polyglandular failure (E31.Ø)
Schmidt's syndrome (E31.Ø)

● **E2Ø.818 Other specified hypoparathyroidism due to impaired parathyroid hormone secretion**
Familial isolated hypoparathyroidism

● **E2Ø.819 Hypoparathyroidism due to impaired parathyroid hormone secretion, unspecified**

● **E2Ø.89 Other specified hypoparathyroidism**
Familial hypoparathyroidism

E2Ø.9 Hypoparathyroidism, unspecified HCC
Parathyroid tetany

✓4th **E21 Hyperparathyroidism and other disorders of parathyroid gland**

EXCLUDES 1 *adult osteomalacia (M83.-)*
ectopic hyperparathyroidism (E34.2)
hungry bone syndrome (E83.81)
infantile and juvenile osteomalacia (E55.Ø)

EXCLUDES 2 *familial hypocalciuric hypercalcemia (E83.52)*

E21.Ø Primary hyperparathyroidism HCC
Hyperplasia of parathyroid
Osteitis fibrosa cystica generalisata [von Recklinghausen's disease of bone]
DEF: Parathyroid dysfunction commonly caused by hyperplasia of two or more glands. Symptoms include hypercalcemia and increased parathyroid hormone levels.

E21.1 Secondary hyperparathyroidism, not elsewhere classified HCC
EXCLUDES 1 *secondary hyperparathyroidism of renal origin (N25.81)*

E21.2 Other hyperparathyroidism HCC
Tertiary hyperparathyroidism
EXCLUDES 1 *familial hypocalciuric hypercalcemia (E83.52)*

E21.3 Hyperparathyroidism, unspecified HCC

E21.4 Other specified disorders of parathyroid gland HCC

E21.5 Disorder of parathyroid gland, unspecified HCC

✓4th **E22 Hyperfunction of pituitary gland**

EXCLUDES 1 *Cushing's syndrome (E24.-)*
Nelson's syndrome (E24.1)
overproduction of ACTH not associated with Cushing's disease (E27.Ø)
overproduction of pituitary ACTH (E24.Ø)
overproduction of thyroid-stimulating hormone (EØ5.8-)

E22.Ø Acromegaly and pituitary gigantism HCC
Overproduction of growth hormone
EXCLUDES 1 *constitutional gigantism (E34.4)*
constitutional tall stature (E34.4)
increased secretion from endocrine pancreas of growth hormone-releasing hormone (E16.8)
DEF: Acromegaly: Chronic condition caused by overproduction of the pituitary growth hormone resulting in enlarged skeletal parts and facial features.

E22.1 Hyperprolactinemia CC HCC
Use additional code for adverse effect, if applicable, to identify drug (T36-T5Ø with fifth or sixth character 5)

E22.2 Syndrome of inappropriate secretion of antidiuretic hormone CC HCC

E22.8 Other hyperfunction of pituitary gland CC HCC
Central precocious puberty

E22.9 Hyperfunction of pituitary gland, unspecified CC HCC

✓4th **E23 Hypofunction and other disorders of the pituitary gland**

INCLUDES the listed conditions whether the disorder is in the pituitary or the hypothalamus

EXCLUDES 1 *postprocedural hypopituitarism (E89.3)*
short stature due to endocrine disorder (E34.3-)

E23.Ø Hypopituitarism CC HCC
Fertile eunuch syndrome
Hypogonadotropic hypogonadism
Idiopathic growth hormone deficiency
Isolated deficiency of gonadotropin
Isolated deficiency of growth hormone
Isolated deficiency of pituitary hormone
Kallmann's syndrome
Lorain-Levi short stature
Necrosis of pituitary gland (postpartum)
Panhypopituitarism
Pituitary cachexia
Pituitary insufficiency NOS
Pituitary short stature
Sheehan's syndrome
Simmonds' disease

E23.1 Drug-induced hypopituitarism HCC
Use additional code for adverse effect, if applicable, to identify drug (T36-T5Ø with fifth or sixth character 5)

E23.2 Diabetes insipidus CC HCC
EXCLUDES 1 *nephrogenic diabetes insipidus (N25.1)*

E23.3 Hypothalamic dysfunction, not elsewhere classified HCC
EXCLUDES 1 *Prader-Willi syndrome (Q87.11)*
Russell-Silver syndrome (Q87.19)

E23.6 Other disorders of pituitary gland HCC
Abscess of pituitary
Adiposogenital dystrophy

E23.7 Disorder of pituitary gland, unspecified HCC

✓4th **E24 Cushing's syndrome**

EXCLUDES 1 *congenital adrenal hyperplasia (E25.Ø)*

DEF: Abdominal striae, acne, hypertension, decreased carbohydrate tolerance, moon face, obesity, protein catabolism, and psychiatric disturbances resulting from increased adrenocortical secretion of cortisol caused by ACTH-dependent adrenocortical hyperplasia or tumor, or by steroid effects.

E24.Ø Pituitary-dependent Cushing's disease CC HCC
Overproduction of pituitary ACTH
Pituitary-dependent hypercorticalism

E24.1 Nelson's syndrome HCC

E24.2 Drug-induced Cushing's syndrome CC HCC
Use additional code for adverse effect, if applicable, to identify drug (T36-T5Ø with fifth or sixth character 5)

E24.3 Ectopic ACTH syndrome CC HCC

E24.4 Alcohol-induced pseudo-Cushing's syndrome CC HCC

E24.8 Other Cushing's syndrome CC HCC

E24.9 Cushing's syndrome, unspecified CC HCC

E25 Adrenogenital disorders

INCLUDES adrenogenital syndromes, virilizing or feminizing, whether acquired or due to adrenal hyperplasia
consequent on inborn enzyme defects in hormone synthesis
female adrenal pseudohermaphroditism
female heterosexual precocious pseudopuberty
male isosexual precocious pseudopuberty
male macrogenitosomia praecox
male sexual precocity with adrenal hyperplasia
male virilization (female)

EXCLUDES 1 *chromosomal abnormalities (Q90-Q99)*
indeterminate sex and pseudohermaphroditism (Q56)

E25.0 Congenital adrenogenital disorders associated with enzyme deficiency HCC
Congenital adrenal hyperplasia
21-Hydroxylase deficiency
Salt-losing congenital adrenal hyperplasia

E25.8 Other adrenogenital disorders HCC
Idiopathic adrenogenital disorder
Use additional code for adverse effect, if applicable, to identify drug (T36-T50 with fifth or sixth character 5)

E25.9 Adrenogenital disorder, unspecified HCC
Adrenogenital syndrome NOS

E26 Hyperaldosteronism

E26.0 Primary hyperaldosteronism

E26.01 Conn's syndrome HCC
Code also adrenal adenoma (D35.0-)

E26.02 Glucocorticoid-remediable aldosteronism HCC
Familial aldosteronism type I
DEF: Rare autosomal dominant familial form of primary aldosteronism in which the secretion of aldosterone is under the influence of adrenocorticotrophic hormone (ACTH) rather than the renin-angiotensin mechanism. Moderate hypersecretion of aldosterone and suppressed plasma renin activity that are rapidly reversed by administration of glucosteroids. Symptoms include hypertension and mild hypokalemia.

E26.09 Other primary hyperaldosteronism HCC
Primary aldosteronism due to adrenal hyperplasia (bilateral)

E26.1 Secondary hyperaldosteronism HCC

E26.8 Other hyperaldosteronism

E26.81 Bartter's syndrome HCC

E26.89 Other hyperaldosteronism HCC

E26.9 Hyperaldosteronism, unspecified HCC
Aldosteronism NOS
Hyperaldosteronism NOS

E27 Other disorders of adrenal gland

E27.0 Other adrenocortical overactivity CC HCC
Overproduction of ACTH, not associated with Cushing's disease
Premature adrenarche
EXCLUDES 1 *Cushing's syndrome (E24.-)*

E27.1 Primary adrenocortical insufficiency CC HCC
Addison's disease
Autoimmune adrenalitis
EXCLUDES 1 *Addison only phenotype adrenoleukodystrophy (E71.528)*
amyloidosis (E85.-)
tuberculous Addison's disease (A18.7)
Waterhouse-Friderichsen syndrome (A39.1)

E27.2 Addisonian crisis CC HCC
Adrenal crisis
Adrenocortical crisis
DEF: Life-threatening condition that occurs when there is not enough cortisol excreted from the adrenal glands. This condition may be due to injury to the adrenal glands or to the pituitary gland, which controls adrenal hormone secretion, or when a patient stops hydrocortisone treatment too quickly or too early.

E27.3 Drug-induced adrenocortical insufficiency CC HCC
Use additional code for adverse effect, if applicable, to identify drug (T36-T50 with fifth or sixth character 5)

E27.4 Other and unspecified adrenocortical insufficiency
EXCLUDES 1 *adrenoleukodystrophy [Addison-Schilder] (E71.528)*
Waterhouse-Friderichsen syndrome (A39.1)

E27.40 Unspecified adrenocortical insufficiency CC HCC
Adrenocortical insufficiency NOS
Hypoaldosteronism

E27.49 Other adrenocortical insufficiency CC HCC
Adrenal hemorrhage
Adrenal infarction

E27.5 Adrenomedullary hyperfunction CC HCC
Adrenomedullary hyperplasia
Catecholamine hypersecretion

E27.8 Other specified disorders of adrenal gland HCC
Abnormality of cortisol-binding globulin

E27.9 Disorder of adrenal gland, unspecified HCC

E28 Ovarian dysfunction
EXCLUDES 1 *isolated gonadotropin deficiency (E23.0)*
postprocedural ovarian failure (E89.4-)

E28.0 Estrogen excess ♀
Use additional code for adverse effect, if applicable, to identify drug (T36-T50 with fifth or sixth character 5)

E28.1 Androgen excess ♀
Hypersecretion of ovarian androgens
Use additional code for adverse effect, if applicable, to identify drug (T36-T50 with fifth or sixth character 5)

E28.2 Polycystic ovarian syndrome ♀
Sclerocystic ovary syndrome
Stein-Leventhal syndrome
AHA: 2022,2Q,16
DEF: Common hormonal disorder among women of reproductive age that involves enlarged ovaries with numerous small cysts located along the outer ovarian edge.

E28.3 Primary ovarian failure
EXCLUDES 1 *pure gonadal dysgenesis (Q99.1)*
Turner's syndrome (Q96.-)

E28.31 Premature menopause

E28.310 Symptomatic premature menopause A ♀
Symptoms such as flushing, sleeplessness, headache, lack of concentration, associated with premature menopause

E28.319 Asymptomatic premature menopause A ♀
Premature menopause NOS

E28.39 Other primary ovarian failure ♀
Decreased estrogen
Resistant ovary syndrome

E28.8 Other ovarian dysfunction ♀
Ovarian hyperfunction NOS
EXCLUDES 1 *postprocedural ovarian failure (E89.4-)*

E28.9 Ovarian dysfunction, unspecified ♀

E29 Testicular dysfunction
EXCLUDES 1 *androgen insensitivity syndrome (E34.5-)*
azoospermia or oligospermia NOS (N46.0-N46.1)
isolated gonadotropin deficiency (E23.0)
Klinefelter's syndrome (Q98.0-Q98.1, Q98.4)

E29.0 Testicular hyperfunction ♂
Hypersecretion of testicular hormones

E29.1 Testicular hypofunction ♂
Defective biosynthesis of testicular androgen NOS
5-delta-Reductase deficiency (with male pseudohermaphroditism)
Testicular hypogonadism NOS
Use additional code for adverse effect, if applicable, to identify drug (T36-T50 with fifth or sixth character 5)
EXCLUDES 1 *postprocedural testicular hypofunction (E89.5)*

E29.8 Other testicular dysfunction ♂

E29.9 Testicular dysfunction, unspecified ♂

E30 Disorders of puberty, not elsewhere classified

E30.0 Delayed puberty
Constitutional delay of puberty
Delayed sexual development

E3Ø.1 Precocious puberty P
Precocious menstruation
EXCLUDES 1 *Albright (-McCune) (-Sternberg) syndrome (Q78.1)*
central precocious puberty (E22.8)
congenital adrenal hyperplasia (E25.Ø)
female heterosexual precocious pseudopuberty (E25.-)
male isosexual precocious pseudopuberty (E25.-)

E3Ø.8 Other disorders of puberty P
Premature thelarche

E3Ø.9 Disorder of puberty, unspecified

✓4th **E31 Polyglandular dysfunction**
EXCLUDES 1 *ataxia telangiectasia [Louis-Bar] (G11.3)*
dystrophia myotonica [Steinert] (G71.11)
pseudohypoparathyroidism (E2Ø.1)

E31.Ø Autoimmune polyglandular failure HCC
Schmidt's syndrome

E31.1 Polyglandular hyperfunction HCC
EXCLUDES 1 *multiple endocrine adenomatosis (E31.2-)*
multiple endocrine neoplasia (E31.2-)

✓5th **E31.2 Multiple endocrine neoplasia [MEN] syndromes**
Multiple endocrine adenomatosis
Code also any associated malignancies and other conditions associated with the syndromes
DEF: Group of conditions in which several endocrine glands grow excessively (such as in adenomatous hyperplasia) and/or develop benign or malignant tumors. Tumors and hyperplasia associated with MEN often produce excess hormones, which impede normal physiology. There is no comprehensive cure known for MEN syndrome. Treatment is directed at the hyperplasia or tumors in each individual gland. Tumors are usually surgically removed and oral medications or hormonal injections are used to correct hormone imbalances.

E31.2Ø Multiple endocrine neoplasia [MEN] syndrome, unspecified HCC
Multiple endocrine adenomatosis NOS
Multiple endocrine neoplasia [MEN] syndrome NOS

E31.21 Multiple endocrine neoplasia [MEN] type I HCC
Wermer's syndrome

E31.22 Multiple endocrine neoplasia [MEN] type IIA HCC
Sipple's syndrome

E31.23 Multiple endocrine neoplasia [MEN] type IIB HCC

E31.8 Other polyglandular dysfunction HCC

E31.9 Polyglandular dysfunction, unspecified HCC

✓4th **E32 Diseases of thymus**
EXCLUDES 1 *aplasia or hypoplasia of thymus with immunodeficiency (D82.1)*
myasthenia gravis (G7Ø.Ø)

E32.Ø Persistent hyperplasia of thymus HCC
Hypertrophy of thymus

E32.1 Abscess of thymus CC HCC

E32.8 Other diseases of thymus HCC
EXCLUDES 1 *aplasia or hypoplasia with immunodeficiency (D82.1)*
thymoma (D15.Ø)

E32.9 Disease of thymus, unspecified HCC

✓4th **E34 Other endocrine disorders**
EXCLUDES 1 *pseudohypoparathyroidism (E2Ø.1)*

E34.Ø Carcinoid syndrome CC HCC
NOTE May be used as an additional code to identify functional activity associated with a carcinoid tumor.

E34.1 Other hypersecretion of intestinal hormones

E34.2 Ectopic hormone secretion, not elsewhere classified
EXCLUDES 1 *ectopic ACTH syndrome (E24.3)*

✓5th **E34.3 Short stature due to endocrine disorder**
EXCLUDES 1 *achondroplastic short stature (Q77.4)*
hypochondroplastic short stature (Q77.4)
nutritional short stature (E45)
pituitary short stature (E23.Ø)
progeria (E34.8)
renal short stature (N25.Ø)
Russell-Silver syndrome (Q87.19)
short-limbed stature with immunodeficiency (D82.2)
short stature (child) (R62.52)
short stature in specific dysmorphic syndromes - code to syndrome - see Alphabetical Index
short stature NOS (R62.52)
AHA: 2022,4Q,11-13

E34.3Ø Short stature due to endocrine disorder, unspecified

E34.31 Constitutional short stature
Constitutional delay of growth, puberty, or maturation

✓6th **E34.32 Genetic causes of short stature**

E34.321 Primary insulin-like growth factor-1 (IGF-1) deficiency
Acid-labile subunit gene (IGFALS) defect
Growth hormone gene 1 (GH1) defect with growth hormone neutralizing antibodies
Growth hormone insensitivity syndrome (GHIS)
Insulin-like growth factor 1 gene (IGF1) defect
Laron type short stature
Severe primary insulin-like growth factor-1 deficiency (SPIGFD)
Signal transducer and activator of transcription 5B gene (STAT5b) defect

E34.322 Insulin-like growth factor-1 (IGF-1) resistance
Genetic syndrome with resistance to insulin-like growth factor-1
Insulin-like growth factor-1 receptor (IGF-1R) defect
Post-insulin-like growth factor-1 receptor signaling defect

E34.328 Other genetic causes of short stature
Short stature due to ACAN gene variant
Short stature due to aggrecan deficiency
Short stature due to NPR-2 gene variant

E34.329 Unspecified genetic causes of short stature

E34.39 Other short stature due to endocrine disorder

E34.4 Constitutional tall stature HCC
Constitutional gigantism

✓5th **E34.5 Androgen insensitivity syndrome**
DEF: X-linked recessive condition in which individuals that are chromosomally male fail to develop normal male external genitalia due to an abnormality on the X chromosome that prohibits the body, completely or in part, from recognizing the androgens produced. ***Synonym(s):*** *AIS*

E34.5Ø Androgen insensitivity syndrome, unspecified
Androgen insensitivity NOS

E34.51 Complete androgen insensitivity syndrome
Complete androgen insensitivity
de Quervain syndrome
Goldberg-Maxwell syndrome

E34.52 Partial androgen insensitivity syndrome
Partial androgen insensitivity
Reifenstein syndrome

E34.8 Other specified endocrine disorders
Pineal gland dysfunction
Progeria
EXCLUDES 2 *pseudohypoparathyroidism (E2Ø.1)*

E34.9 Endocrine disorder, unspecified
Endocrine disturbance NOS
Hormone disturbance NOS

E35 Disorders of endocrine glands in diseases classified elsewhere
Code first underlying disease, such as:
late congenital syphilis of thymus gland [Dubois disease] ▶(A50.9)◀
Use additional code, if applicable, to identify:
sequelae of tuberculosis of other organs (B90.8)
EXCLUDES 1 *Echinococcus granulosus infection of thyroid gland (B67.3)*
meningococcal hemorrhagic adrenalitis (A39.1)
syphilis of endocrine gland (A52.79)
tuberculosis of adrenal gland, except calcification (A18.7)
tuberculosis of endocrine gland NEC (A18.82)
tuberculosis of thyroid gland (A18.81)
Waterhouse-Friderichsen syndrome (A39.1)

Intraoperative complications of endocrine system (E36)

E36 Intraoperative complications of endocrine system
EXCLUDES 2 *postprocedural endocrine and metabolic complications and disorders, not elsewhere classified (E89.-)*

E36.0 Intraoperative hemorrhage and hematoma of an endocrine system organ or structure complicating a procedure
EXCLUDES 1 *intraoperative hemorrhage and hematoma of an endocrine system organ or structure due to accidental puncture or laceration during a procedure (E36.1-)*

E36.01 Intraoperative hemorrhage and hematoma of an endocrine system organ or structure complicating an endocrine system procedure CC
AHA: 2020,1Q,19

E36.02 Intraoperative hemorrhage and hematoma of an endocrine system organ or structure complicating other procedure CC

E36.1 Accidental puncture and laceration of an endocrine system organ or structure during a procedure

E36.11 Accidental puncture and laceration of an endocrine system organ or structure during an endocrine system procedure CC

E36.12 Accidental puncture and laceration of an endocrine system organ or structure during other procedure CC

E36.8 Other intraoperative complications of endocrine system
Use additional code, if applicable, to further specify disorder

Malnutrition (E40-E46)

EXCLUDES 1 *intestinal malabsorption (K90.-)*
sequelae of protein-calorie malnutrition (E64.0)
EXCLUDES 2 *nutritional anemias (D50-D53)*
starvation (T73.0)
AHA: 2020,1Q,4-7; 2017,4Q,108; 2017,3Q,25
TIP: Assign additional code for BMI from category Z68, when documented. BMI can be based on documentation from clinicians who are not the patient's provider.
TIP: Malnutrition is not considered integral to cancer; assign the appropriate code in addition to the code for the specific type of cancer.

E40 Kwashiorkor MCC HCC
Severe malnutrition with nutritional edema with dyspigmentation of skin and hair
EXCLUDES 1 *marasmic kwashiorkor (E42)*

E41 Nutritional marasmus MCC HCC
Severe malnutrition with marasmus
EXCLUDES 1 *marasmic kwashiorkor (E42)*
AHA: 2017,3Q,24
DEF: Protein-calorie malabsorption or malnutrition in children characterized by tissue wasting, dehydration, and subcutaneous fat depletion. It may occur with infectious disease.

E42 Marasmic kwashiorkor MCC HCC
Intermediate form severe protein-calorie malnutrition
Severe protein-calorie malnutrition with signs of both kwashiorkor and marasmus

E43 Unspecified severe protein-calorie malnutrition MCC HCC
Starvation edema
AHA: 2022,1Q,13; 2020,1Q,5,6; 2017,4Q,108

E44 Protein-calorie malnutrition of moderate and mild degree
AHA: 2020,1Q,5
E44.0 Moderate protein-calorie malnutrition CC HCC
E44.1 Mild protein-calorie malnutrition CC HCC

E45 Retarded development following protein-calorie malnutrition CC HCC
Nutritional short stature
Nutritional stunting
Physical retardation due to malnutrition

E46 Unspecified protein-calorie malnutrition CC HCC
Malnutrition NOS
Protein-calorie imbalance NOS
EXCLUDES 1 *nutritional deficiency NOS (E63.9)*
AHA: 2018,4Q,82

Other nutritional deficiencies (E50-E64)

EXCLUDES 2 *nutritional anemias (D50-D53)*

E50 Vitamin A deficiency
EXCLUDES 1 *sequelae of vitamin A deficiency (E64.1)*
E50.0 Vitamin A deficiency with conjunctival xerosis
E50.1 Vitamin A deficiency with Bitot's spot and conjunctival xerosis
Bitot's spot in the young child
DEF: Vitamin A deficiency with conjunctival dryness and superficial spots of keratinized epithelium.
E50.2 Vitamin A deficiency with corneal xerosis
E50.3 Vitamin A deficiency with corneal ulceration and xerosis
E50.4 Vitamin A deficiency with keratomalacia
DEF: Vitamin A deficiency creating corneal dryness that progresses to corneal insensitivity, softness, and necrosis. It is usually bilateral.
E50.5 Vitamin A deficiency with night blindness
E50.6 Vitamin A deficiency with xerophthalmic scars of cornea
E50.7 Other ocular manifestations of vitamin A deficiency
Xerophthalmia NOS
E50.8 Other manifestations of vitamin A deficiency
Follicular keratosis
Xeroderma
E50.9 Vitamin A deficiency, unspecified
Hypovitaminosis A NOS

E51 Thiamine deficiency
EXCLUDES 1 *sequelae of thiamine deficiency (E64.8)*
E51.1 Beriberi
E51.11 Dry beriberi CC
Beriberi NOS
Beriberi with polyneuropathy
E51.12 Wet beriberi CC
Beriberi with cardiovascular manifestations
Cardiovascular beriberi
Shoshin disease
E51.2 Wernicke's encephalopathy CC
DEF: Deficiency of vitamin B1 resulting in a triad of acute mental confusion, ataxia, and ophthalmoplegia. The vast majority of affected patients are alcoholics.
E51.8 Other manifestations of thiamine deficiency CC
E51.9 Thiamine deficiency, unspecified CC

E52 Niacin deficiency [pellagra]
Niacin (-tryptophan) deficiency
Nicotinamide deficiency
Pellagra (alcoholic)
EXCLUDES 1 *sequelae of niacin deficiency (E64.8)*

E53 Deficiency of other B group vitamins
EXCLUDES 1 *sequelae of vitamin B deficiency (E64.8)*
E53.0 Riboflavin deficiency CC
Ariboflavinosis
Vitamin B2 deficiency
E53.1 Pyridoxine deficiency
Vitamin B6 deficiency
EXCLUDES 1 *pyridoxine-responsive sideroblastic anemia (D64.3)*
E53.8 Deficiency of other specified B group vitamins
Biotin deficiency
Cyanocobalamin deficiency
Folate deficiency
Folic acid deficiency
Pantothenic acid deficiency
Vitamin B12 deficiency
EXCLUDES 1 *folate deficiency anemia (D52.-)*
vitamin B12 deficiency anemia (D51.-)
E53.9 Vitamin B deficiency, unspecified

E54 Ascorbic acid deficiency
Deficiency of vitamin C
Scurvy
EXCLUDES 1 *scorbutic anemia (D53.2)*
sequelae of vitamin C deficiency (E64.2)
DEF: Vitamin C deficiency causing swollen gums, myalgia, weight loss, and weakness.

✓4th **E55 Vitamin D deficiency**
EXCLUDES 1 *adult osteomalacia (M83.-)*
osteoporosis (M8Ø.-)
sequelae of rickets (E64.3)

E55.Ø Rickets, active CC
Infantile osteomalacia
Juvenile osteomalacia
EXCLUDES 1 *celiac rickets (K9Ø.Ø)*
Crohn's rickets (K5Ø.-)
hereditary vitamin D-dependent rickets (E83.32)
inactive rickets (E64.3)
renal rickets (N25.Ø)
sequelae of rickets (E64.3)
vitamin D-resistant rickets (E83.31)
DEF: Rickets: Softening or weakening of the bones due to a lack of vitamin D, calcium, and phosphate.

E55.9 Vitamin D deficiency, unspecified
Avitaminosis D

✓4th **E56 Other vitamin deficiencies**
EXCLUDES 1 *sequelae of other vitamin deficiencies (E64.8)*

E56.Ø Deficiency of vitamin E
E56.1 Deficiency of vitamin K
EXCLUDES 1 *deficiency of coagulation factor due to vitamin K deficiency (D68.4)*
vitamin K deficiency of newborn (P53)

E56.8 Deficiency of other vitamins
E56.9 Vitamin deficiency, unspecified

E58 Dietary calcium deficiency
EXCLUDES 1 *disorders of calcium metabolism (E83.5-)*
sequelae of calcium deficiency (E64.8)

E59 Dietary selenium deficiency
Keshan disease
EXCLUDES 1 *sequelae of selenium deficiency (E64.8)*

E6Ø Dietary zinc deficiency

✓4th **E61 Deficiency of other nutrient elements**
Use additional code for adverse effect, if applicable, to identify drug (T36-T5Ø with fifth or sixth character 5)
EXCLUDES 1 *disorders of mineral metabolism (E83.-)*
iodine deficiency related thyroid disorders (EØØ-EØ2)
sequelae of malnutrition and other nutritional deficiencies (E64.-)

E61.Ø Copper deficiency
E61.1 Iron deficiency
EXCLUDES 1 *iron deficiency anemia (D5Ø.-)*

E61.2 Magnesium deficiency
E61.3 Manganese deficiency
E61.4 Chromium deficiency
E61.5 Molybdenum deficiency
E61.6 Vanadium deficiency
E61.7 Deficiency of multiple nutrient elements
E61.8 Deficiency of other specified nutrient elements
E61.9 Deficiency of nutrient element, unspecified

✓4th **E63 Other nutritional deficiencies**
EXCLUDES 2 *dehydration (E86.Ø)*
failure to thrive, adult (R62.7)
failure to thrive, child (R62.51)
feeding problems in newborn (P92.-)
sequelae of malnutrition and other nutritional deficiencies (E64.-)

E63.Ø Essential fatty acid [EFA] deficiency
E63.1 Imbalance of constituents of food intake
E63.8 Other specified nutritional deficiencies
E63.9 Nutritional deficiency, unspecified

✓4th **E64 Sequelae of malnutrition and other nutritional deficiencies**
NOTE This category is to be used to indicate conditions in categories E43, E44, E46, E5Ø-E63 as the cause of sequelae, which are themselves classified elsewhere. The 'sequelae' include conditions specified as such; they also include the late effects of diseases classifiable to the above categories if the disease itself is no longer present
Code first condition resulting from (sequela) of malnutrition and other nutritional deficiencies

E64.Ø Sequelae of protein-calorie malnutrition CC HCC
EXCLUDES 2 *retarded development following protein-calorie malnutrition (E45)*

E64.1 Sequelae of vitamin A deficiency
E64.2 Sequelae of vitamin C deficiency
E64.3 Sequelae of rickets
E64.8 Sequelae of other nutritional deficiencies
E64.9 Sequelae of unspecified nutritional deficiency

Overweight, obesity and other hyperalimentation (E65-E68)

E65 Localized adiposity
Fat pad

✓4th **E66 Overweight and obesity**
Code first obesity complicating pregnancy, childbirth and the puerperium, if applicable (O99.21-)
Use additional code to identify body mass index (BMI), if known (Z68.-)
EXCLUDES 1 *adiposogenital dystrophy (E23.6)*
lipomatosis NOS (E88.2)
lipomatosis dolorosa [Dercum] (E88.2)
Prader-Willi syndrome (Q87.11)
AHA: 2022,3Q,6; 2018,4Q,77,79-80
TIP: Do not assign a BMI code (Z68.-) when a pregnant patient is documented as being overweight or obese. Only a code from subcategory O99.21- and a code from this category should be assigned.

✓5th **E66.Ø Obesity due to excess calories**

E66.Ø1 Morbid (severe) obesity due to excess calories H11 HCC
EXCLUDES 1 *morbid (severe) obesity with alveolar hypoventilation (E66.2)*
AHA: 2022,3Q,6; 2022,2Q,9
TIP: Assign this code when Class 3 obesity is documented. Class 3 obesity is synonymous with morbid obesity.

E66.Ø9 Other obesity due to excess calories

E66.1 Drug-induced obesity
Use additional code for adverse effect, if applicable, to identify drug (T36-T5Ø with fifth or sixth character 5)

E66.2 Morbid (severe) obesity with alveolar hypoventilation CC HCC
Obesity hypoventilation syndrome (OHS)
Pickwickian syndrome

E66.3 Overweight
AHA: 2018,4Q,78

E66.8 Other obesity
E66.9 Obesity, unspecified
Obesity NOS
AHA: 2021,2Q,10

✓4th **E67 Other hyperalimentation**
EXCLUDES 1 *hyperalimentation NOS (R63.2)*
sequelae of hyperalimentation (E68)

E67.Ø Hypervitaminosis A
E67.1 Hypercarotenemia
DEF: Elevated blood carotene level as a result of excessive carotenoid ingestion or an inability to convert carotenoids to vitamin A. Characteristics often include yellow discoloration of the skin, which may follow overeating of carotenoid-rich foods such as carrots, sweet potatoes, or squash.

E67.2 Megavitamin-B6 syndrome
E67.3 Hypervitaminosis D
E67.8 Other specified hyperalimentation

E68 Sequelae of hyperalimentation
Code first condition resulting from (sequela) of hyperalimentation

Metabolic disorders (E70-E88)

EXCLUDES 1 *androgen insensitivity syndrome (E34.5-)*
congenital adrenal hyperplasia (E25.0)
hemolytic anemias attributable to enzyme disorders (D55.-)
▶Marfan syndrome (Q87.4-)◀
5-alpha-reductase deficiency (E29.1)

EXCLUDES 2 *Ehlers-Danlos syndromes (Q79.6-)*

AHA: 2018,2Q,6

4th **E70 Disorders of aromatic amino-acid metabolism**
- **E70.0 Classical phenylketonuria** CC HCC
- **E70.1 Other hyperphenylalaninemias** CC HCC
- 5th **E70.2 Disorders of tyrosine metabolism**
  - EXCLUDES 1 *transitory tyrosinemia of newborn (P74.5)*
  - **E70.20 Disorder of tyrosine metabolism, unspecified** CC HCC
  - **E70.21 Tyrosinemia** CC HCC
    - Hypertyrosinemia
  - **E70.29 Other disorders of tyrosine metabolism** CC HCC
    - Alkaptonuria
    - Ochronosis
- 5th **E70.3 Albinism**
  - **DEF:** Absence of pigment in skin, hair, and eyes. This genetic condition is often accompanied by astigmatism, photophobia, and nystagmus.
  - **E70.30 Albinism, unspecified** CC HCC
  - 6th **E70.31 Ocular albinism**
    - **E70.310 X-linked ocular albinism** CC HCC
    - **E70.311 Autosomal recessive ocular albinism** CC HCC
    - **E70.318 Other ocular albinism** CC HCC
    - **E70.319 Ocular albinism, unspecified** CC HCC
  - 6th **E70.32 Oculocutaneous albinism**
    - EXCLUDES 1 *Chediak-Higashi syndrome (E70.330)*
    Hermansky-Pudlak syndrome (E70.331)
    - **E70.320 Tyrosinase negative oculocutaneous albinism** CC HCC
      - Albinism I
      - Oculocutaneous albinism ty-neg
    - **E70.321 Tyrosinase positive oculocutaneous albinism** CC HCC
      - Albinism II
      - Oculocutaneous albinism ty-pos
    - **E70.328 Other oculocutaneous albinism** CC HCC
      - Cross syndrome
    - **E70.329 Oculocutaneous albinism, unspecified** CC HCC
  - 6th **E70.33 Albinism with hematologic abnormality**
    - **E70.330 Chediak-Higashi syndrome** CC HCC
    - **E70.331 Hermansky-Pudlak syndrome** CC HCC
    - **E70.338 Other albinism with hematologic abnormality** CC HCC
    - **E70.339 Albinism with hematologic abnormality, unspecified** CC HCC
  - **E70.39 Other specified albinism** CC HCC
    - Piebaldism
- 5th **E70.4 Disorders of histidine metabolism**
  - **E70.40 Disorders of histidine metabolism, unspecified** CC HCC
  - **E70.41 Histidinemia** CC HCC
  - **E70.49 Other disorders of histidine metabolism** CC HCC
- **E70.5 Disorders of tryptophan metabolism** CC HCC
- 5th **E70.8 Other disorders of aromatic amino-acid metabolism**
  - **AHA:** 2020,4Q,15-16
  - **E70.81 Aromatic L-amino acid decarboxylase deficiency** CC HCC
    - AADC deficiency
  - **E70.89 Other disorders of aromatic amino-acid metabolism** CC HCC
- **E70.9 Disorder of aromatic amino-acid metabolism, unspecified** CC HCC

4th **E71 Disorders of branched-chain amino-acid metabolism and fatty-acid metabolism**
- **E71.0 Maple-syrup-urine disease** CC HCC
- 5th **E71.1 Other disorders of branched-chain amino-acid metabolism**
  - 6th **E71.11 Branched-chain organic acidurias**
    - **E71.110 Isovaleric acidemia** CC HCC
    - **E71.111 3-methylglutaconic aciduria** CC HCC
    - **E71.118 Other branched-chain organic acidurias** CC HCC
  - 6th **E71.12 Disorders of propionate metabolism**
    - **E71.120 Methylmalonic acidemia** CC HCC
    - **E71.121 Propionic acidemia** CC HCC
    - **E71.128 Other disorders of propionate metabolism** CC HCC
  - **E71.19 Other disorders of branched-chain amino-acid metabolism** CC HCC
    - Hyperleucine-isoleucinemia
    - Hypervalinemia
- **E71.2 Disorder of branched-chain amino-acid metabolism, unspecified** CC HCC
- 5th **E71.3 Disorders of fatty-acid metabolism**
  - EXCLUDES 1 *peroxisomal disorders (E71.5)*
  Refsum's disease (G60.1)
  Schilder's disease (G37.0)
  - EXCLUDES 2 *carnitine deficiency due to inborn error of metabolism (E71.42)*
  - **E71.30 Disorder of fatty-acid metabolism, unspecified**
  - 6th **E71.31 Disorders of fatty-acid oxidation**
    - **E71.310 Long chain/very long chain acyl CoA dehydrogenase deficiency** CC HCC
      - ▶LCAD deficiency◀
      - ▶VLCAD deficiency◀
    - **E71.311 Medium chain acyl CoA dehydrogenase deficiency** CC HCC
      - ▶MCAD deficiency◀
    - **E71.312 Short chain acyl CoA dehydrogenase deficiency** CC HCC
      - ▶SCAD deficiency◀
    - **E71.313 Glutaric aciduria type II** CC HCC
      - Glutaric aciduria type II A
      - Glutaric aciduria type II B
      - Glutaric aciduria type II C
      - EXCLUDES 1 *glutaric aciduria (type 1) NOS (E72.3)*
    - **E71.314 Muscle carnitine palmitoyltransferase deficiency** CC HCC
    - **E71.318 Other disorders of fatty-acid oxidation** CC HCC
  - **E71.32 Disorders of ketone metabolism** CC HCC
  - **E71.39 Other disorders of fatty-acid metabolism** CC HCC
- 5th **E71.4 Disorders of carnitine metabolism**
  - EXCLUDES 1 *muscle carnitine palmitoyltransferase deficiency (E71.314)*
  - **E71.40 Disorder of carnitine metabolism, unspecified** HCC
  - **E71.41 Primary carnitine deficiency** HCC
  - **E71.42 Carnitine deficiency due to inborn errors of metabolism** HCC
    - Code also associated inborn error or metabolism
  - **E71.43 Iatrogenic carnitine deficiency** HCC
    - Carnitine deficiency due to hemodialysis
    - Carnitine deficiency due to Valproic acid therapy
  - 6th **E71.44 Other secondary carnitine deficiency**
    - **E71.440 Ruvalcaba-Myhre-Smith syndrome** HCC
    - **E71.448 Other secondary carnitine deficiency** HCC
- 5th **E71.5 Peroxisomal disorders**
  - EXCLUDES 1 *Schilder's disease (G37.0)*
  - **E71.50 Peroxisomal disorder, unspecified** CC HCC
  - 6th **E71.51 Disorders of peroxisome biogenesis**
    - Group 1 peroxisomal disorders
    - EXCLUDES 1 *Refsum's disease (G60.1)*
    - **E71.510 Zellweger syndrome** CC HCC
    - **E71.511 Neonatal adrenoleukodystrophy** CC HCC
      - EXCLUDES 1 *X-linked adrenoleukodystrophy (E71.42-)*
    - **E71.518 Other disorders of peroxisome biogenesis** CC HCC
  - 6th **E71.52 X-linked adrenoleukodystrophy**
    - **E71.520 Childhood cerebral X-linked adrenoleukodystrophy** CC HCC

E71.521 Adolescent X-linked adrenoleukodystrophy CC HCC

E71.522 Adrenomyeloneuropathy CC HCC

E71.528 Other X-linked adrenoleukodystrophy CC HCC
Addison only phenotype adrenoleukodystrophy
Addison-Schilder adrenoleukodystrophy

E71.529 X-linked adrenoleukodystrophy, unspecified type CC HCC

E71.53 Other group 2 peroxisomal disorders CC HCC

✓6th E71.54 Other peroxisomal disorders

E71.540 Rhizomelic chondrodysplasia punctata CC HCC
EXCLUDES 1 *chondrodysplasia punctata NOS (Q77.3)*

E71.541 Zellweger-like syndrome CC HCC

E71.542 Other group 3 peroxisomal disorders CC HCC

E71.548 Other peroxisomal disorders CC HCC

✓4th **E72 Other disorders of amino-acid metabolism**

EXCLUDES 1 *disorders of:*
aromatic amino-acid metabolism (E70.-)
branched-chain amino-acid metabolism (E71.0-E71.2)
fatty-acid metabolism (E71.3)
purine and pyrimidine metabolism (E79.-)
gout (M1A.-, M10.-)

✓5th E72.0 Disorders of amino-acid transport
EXCLUDES 1 *disorders of tryptophan metabolism (E70.5)*

E72.00 Disorders of amino-acid transport, unspecified CC HCC

E72.01 Cystinuria CC HCC

E72.02 Hartnup's disease CC HCC

E72.03 Lowe's syndrome CC HCC
Use additional code for associated glaucoma (H42)

E72.04 Cystinosis CC HCC
Fanconi (-de Toni) (-Debre) syndrome with cystinosis
EXCLUDES 1 *Fanconi (-de Toni) (-Debre) syndrome without cystinosis (E72.09)*

E72.09 Other disorders of amino-acid transport CC HCC
Fanconi (-de Toni) (-Debre) syndrome, unspecified

✓5th E72.1 Disorders of sulfur-bearing amino-acid metabolism
EXCLUDES 1 *cystinosis (E72.04)*
cystinuria (E72.01)
transcobalamin II deficiency (D51.2)

E72.10 Disorders of sulfur-bearing amino-acid metabolism, unspecified CC HCC

E72.11 Homocystinuria CC HCC
Cystathionine synthase deficiency
AHA: 2021,4Q,28

E72.12 Methylenetetrahydrofolate reductase deficiency CC HCC

E72.19 Other disorders of sulfur-bearing amino-acid metabolism CC HCC
Cystathioninuria
Methioninemia
Sulfite oxidase deficiency

✓5th E72.2 Disorders of urea cycle metabolism
EXCLUDES 1 *disorders of ornithine metabolism (E72.4)*

E72.20 Disorder of urea cycle metabolism, unspecified CC HCC
Hyperammonemia
EXCLUDES 1 *hyperammonemia- hyperornithinemia-homocitrullinemia syndrome E72.4*
transient hyperammonemia of newborn (P74.6)

E72.21 Argininemia CC HCC

E72.22 Arginosuccinic aciduria CC HCC

E72.23 Citrullinemia CC HCC

E72.29 Other disorders of urea cycle metabolism CC HCC

E72.3 Disorders of lysine and hydroxylysine metabolism CC HCC
Glutaric aciduria NOS
Glutaric aciduria (type I)
Hydroxylysinemia
Hyperlysinemia
EXCLUDES 1 *glutaric aciduria type II (E71.313)*
Refsum's disease (G60.1)
Zellweger syndrome (E71.510)

E72.4 Disorders of ornithine metabolism CC HCC
Hyperammonemia-Hyperornithinemia-Homocitrullinemia syndrome
Ornithinemia (types I, II)
Ornithine transcarbamylase deficiency
EXCLUDES 1 *hereditary choroidal dystrophy (H31.2-)*

✓5th E72.5 Disorders of glycine metabolism

E72.50 Disorder of glycine metabolism, unspecified CC HCC

E72.51 Non-ketotic hyperglycinemia CC HCC

E72.52 Trimethylaminuria CC HCC

E72.53 Primary hyperoxaluria CC HCC
Oxalosis
Oxaluria
AHA: 2018,4Q,29

E72.59 Other disorders of glycine metabolism CC HCC
D-glycericacidemia
Hyperhydroxyprolinemia
Hyperprolinemia (types I, II)
Sarcosinemia

✓5th E72.8 Other specified disorders of amino-acid metabolism
AHA: 2018,4Q,5

E72.81 Disorders of gamma aminobutyric acid metabolism CC HCC
4-hydroxybutyric aciduria
Disorders of GABA metabolism
GABA metabolic defect
GABA transaminase deficiency
GABA-T deficiency
Gamma-hydroxybutyric aciduria
SSADHD
Succinic semialdehyde dehydrogenase deficiency

E72.89 Other specified disorders of amino-acid metabolism CC HCC
Disorders of beta-amino-acid metabolism
Disorders of gamma-glutamyl cycle

E72.9 Disorder of amino-acid metabolism, unspecified CC HCC

✓4th **E73 Lactose intolerance**
DEF: Inability to break down sugar in dairy products due to a deficiency in the enzyme lactase.

E73.0 Congenital lactase deficiency

E73.1 Secondary lactase deficiency

E73.8 Other lactose intolerance

E73.9 Lactose intolerance, unspecified

✓4th **E74 Other disorders of carbohydrate metabolism**
EXCLUDES 1 *diabetes mellitus (E08-E13)*
hypoglycemia NOS (E16.2)
increased secretion of glucagon (E16.3)
mucopolysaccharidosis (E76.0-E76.3)

✓5th E74.0 Glycogen storage disease

E74.00 Glycogen storage disease, unspecified CC HCC

E74.01 von Gierke disease CC HCC
Type I glycogen storage disease

E74.02 Pompe disease CC HCC
Cardiac glycogenosis
Type II glycogen storage disease

E74.03 Cori disease CC HCC
Forbes disease
Type III glycogen storage disease

E74.04 McArdle disease CC HCC
Type V glycogen storage disease

● E74.05 Lysosome-associated membrane protein 2 [LAMP2] deficiency CC
Danon disease
Code also, if applicable, associated manifestations such as:
dilated cardiomyopathy (I42.0)
obstructive hypertrophic cardiomyopathy (I42.1)

E74.09 Other glycogen storage disease CC HCC
Andersen disease
Glycogen storage disease, types 0, IV, VI-XI
Hers disease
Liver phosphorylase deficiency
Muscle phosphofructokinase deficiency
Tauri disease

✓5th **E74.1 Disorders of fructose metabolism**
EXCLUDES 1 *muscle phosphofructokinase deficiency (E74.09)*

E74.10 Disorder of fructose metabolism, unspecified UNS
E74.11 Essential fructosuria
Fructokinase deficiency
E74.12 Hereditary fructose intolerance
Fructosemia
E74.19 Other disorders of fructose metabolism
Fructose-1, 6-diphosphatase deficiency

✓5th **E74.2 Disorders of galactose metabolism**
E74.20 Disorders of galactose metabolism, unspecified UNS CC HCC
E74.21 Galactosemia CC HCC
DEF: Any of three genetic disorders caused by a defective galactose metabolism. Symptoms include failure to thrive in infancy, jaundice, liver and spleen damage, cataracts, and mental retardation.
E74.29 Other disorders of galactose metabolism CC HCC
Galactokinase deficiency

✓5th **E74.3 Other disorders of intestinal carbohydrate absorption**
EXCLUDES 2 *lactose intolerance (E73.-)*
E74.31 Sucrase-isomaltase deficiency
E74.39 Other disorders of intestinal carbohydrate absorption
Disorder of intestinal carbohydrate absorption NOS
Glucose-galactose malabsorption
Sucrase deficiency

E74.4 Disorders of pyruvate metabolism and gluconeogenesis CC HCC
Deficiency of phosphoenolpyruvate carboxykinase
Deficiency of pyruvate carboxylase
Deficiency of pyruvate dehydrogenase
EXCLUDES 1 *disorders of pyruvate metabolism and gluconeogenesis with anemia (D55.-)*
Leigh's syndrome (G31.82)

✓5th **E74.8 Other specified disorders of carbohydrate metabolism**
AHA: 2020,4Q,16

✓6th **E74.81 Disorders of glucose transport, not elsewhere classified**
E74.810 Glucose transporter protein type 1 deficiency CC HCC
De Vivo syndrome
Glucose transport defect, blood-brain barrier
Glut1 deficiency
GLUT1 deficiency syndrome 1, infantile onset
GLUT1 deficiency syndrome 2, childhood onset
E74.818 Other disorders of glucose transport CC HCC
(Familial) renal glycosuria
E74.819 Disorders of glucose transport, unspecified UNS CC HCC
E74.89 Other specified disorders of carbohydrate metabolism CC HCC
Essential pentosuria

E74.9 Disorder of carbohydrate metabolism, unspecified UNS HCC

✓4th **E75 Disorders of sphingolipid metabolism and other lipid storage disorders**
EXCLUDES 1 *mucolipidosis, types I-III (E77.0-E77.1)*
Refsum's disease (G60.1)

✓5th **E75.0 GM2 gangliosidosis**
E75.00 GM2 gangliosidosis, unspecified UNS CC HCC
E75.01 Sandhoff disease CC HCC
E75.02 Tay-Sachs disease CC HCC
DEF: Genetic mutation of the HEXA gene that inhibits the breakdown of a toxic substance called ganglioside. The accumulation of ganglioside results in destruction of the neurons in the brain and spinal cord.

Tay-Sachs Disease

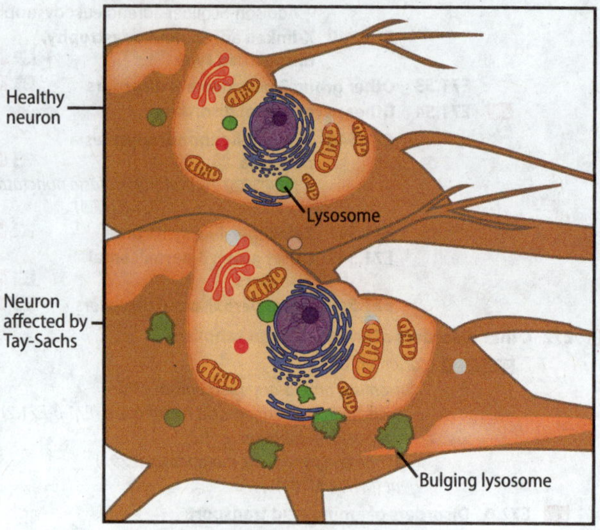

E75.09 Other GM2 gangliosidosis CC HCC
Adult GM2 gangliosidosis
Juvenile GM2 gangliosidosis

✓5th **E75.1 Other and unspecified gangliosidosis**
E75.10 Unspecified gangliosidosis UNS CC HCC
Gangliosidosis NOS
E75.11 Mucolipidosis IV CC HCC
E75.19 Other gangliosidosis CC HCC
GM1 gangliosidosis
GM3 gangliosidosis

✓5th **E75.2 Other sphingolipidosis**
EXCLUDES 1 *adrenoleukodystrophy [Addison-Schilder] (E71.528)*
E75.21 Fabry (-Anderson) disease HCC
E75.22 Gaucher disease HCC
E75.23 Krabbe disease CC HCC

✓6th **E75.24 Niemann-Pick disease**
Acid sphingomyelinase deficiency (ASMD)
E75.240 Niemann-Pick disease type A HCC
Acid sphingomyelinase deficiency type A (ASMD type A)
Infantile neurovisceral acid sphingomyelinase deficiency
E75.241 Niemann-Pick disease type B HCC
Acid sphingomyelinase deficiency type B (ASMD type B)
Chronic visceral acid sphingomyelinase deficiency
E75.242 Niemann-Pick disease type C HCC
E75.243 Niemann-Pick disease type D HCC
E75.244 Niemann-Pick disease type A/B HCC
Acid sphingomyelinase deficiency type A/B (ASMD type A/B)
Chronic neurovisceral acid sphingomyelinase deficiency
AHA: 2021,4Q,8-9
E75.248 Other Niemann-Pick disease HCC
E75.249 Niemann-Pick disease, unspecified UNS HCC
Acid sphingomyelinase deficiency (ASMD) NOS

E75.25 Metachromatic leukodystrophy CC HCC
E75.26 Sulfatase deficiency CC HCC
Multiple sulfatase deficiency (MSD)
AHA: 2018,4Q,5-6
● **E75.27 Pelizaeus-Merzbacher disease** CC
● **E75.28 Canavan disease** CC

E75.29 **Other sphingolipidosis** CC HCC
Farber's syndrome
Sulfatide lipidosis

E75.3 **Sphingolipidosis, unspecified** HCC

E75.4 **Neuronal ceroid lipofuscinosis** CC HCC
Batten disease
Bielschowsky-Jansky disease
Kufs disease
Spielmeyer-Vogt disease

E75.5 **Other lipid storage disorders**
Cerebrotendinous cholesterosis [van Bogaert-Scherer-Epstein]
Wolman's disease

E75.6 **Lipid storage disorder, unspecified**

E76 Disorders of glycosaminoglycan metabolism

E76.0 **Mucopolysaccharidosis, type I**

E76.01 **Hurler's syndrome** CC HCC

E76.02 **Hurler-Scheie syndrome** CC HCC

E76.03 **Scheie's syndrome** CC HCC

E76.1 **Mucopolysaccharidosis, type II** CC HCC
Hunter's syndrome

E76.2 **Other mucopolysaccharidoses**

E76.21 **Morquio mucopolysaccharidoses**

E76.210 **Morquio A mucopolysaccharidoses** CC HCC
Classic Morquio syndrome
Morquio syndrome A
Mucopolysaccharidosis, type IVA

E76.211 **Morquio B mucopolysaccharidoses** CC HCC
Morquio-like mucopolysaccharidoses
Morquio-like syndrome
Morquio syndrome B
Mucopolysaccharidosis, type IVB

E76.219 **Morquio mucopolysaccharidoses, unspecified** CC HCC
Morquio syndrome
Mucopolysaccharidosis, type IV

E76.22 **Sanfilippo mucopolysaccharidoses** CC HCC
Mucopolysaccharidosis, type III (A) (B) (C) (D)
Sanfilippo A syndrome
Sanfilippo B syndrome
Sanfilippo C syndrome
Sanfilippo D syndrome

E76.29 **Other mucopolysaccharidoses** CC HCC
beta-Glucuronidase deficiency
Maroteaux-Lamy (mild) (severe) syndrome
Mucopolysaccharidosis, types VI, VII

E76.3 **Mucopolysaccharidosis, unspecified** CC HCC

E76.8 **Other disorders of glucosaminoglycan metabolism** CC HCC

E76.9 **Glucosaminoglycan metabolism disorder, unspecified** CC HCC

E77 Disorders of glycoprotein metabolism

E77.0 **Defects in post-translational modification of lysosomal enzymes** HCC
Mucolipidosis II [I-cell disease]
Mucolipidosis III [pseudo-Hurler polydystrophy]

E77.1 **Defects in glycoprotein degradation** HCC
Aspartylglucosaminuria
Fucosidosis
Mannosidosis
Sialidosis [mucolipidosis I]

E77.8 **Other disorders of glycoprotein metabolism** HCC

E77.9 **Disorder of glycoprotein metabolism, unspecified** HCC

E78 Disorders of lipoprotein metabolism and other lipidemias
EXCLUDES 1 *sphingolipidosis (E75.0-E75.3)*

E78.0 **Pure hypercholesterolemia**
AHA: 2016,4Q,13-14

E78.00 **Pure hypercholesterolemia, unspecified**
Fredrickson's hyperlipoproteinemia, type IIa
Hyperbetalipoproteinemia
Low-density-lipoprotein-type [LDL] hyperlipoproteinemia
(Pure) hypercholesterolemia NOS
AHA: 2023,2Q,9; 2022,2Q,5-6

E78.01 **Familial hypercholesterolemia**

E78.1 **Pure hyperglyceridemia**
Elevated fasting triglycerides
Endogenous hyperglyceridemia
Fredrickson's hyperlipoproteinemia, type IV
Hyperlipidemia, group B
Hyperprebetalipoproteinemia
Very-low-density-lipoprotein-type [VLDL] hyperlipoproteinemia

E78.2 **Mixed hyperlipidemia**
Broad- or floating-betalipoproteinemia
Combined hyperlipidemia NOS
Elevated cholesterol with elevated triglycerides NEC
Fredrickson's hyperlipoproteinemia, type IIb or III
Hyperbetalipoproteinemia with prebetalipoproteinemia
Hypercholesteremia with endogenous hyperglyceridemia
Hyperlipidemia, group C
Tubo-eruptive xanthoma
Xanthoma tuberosum
EXCLUDES 1 *cerebrotendinous cholesterosis [van Bogaert-Scherer-Epstein] (E75.5)*
familial combined hyperlipidemia (E78.49)
AHA: 2023,2Q,9; 2022,2Q,6

E78.3 **Hyperchylomicronemia**
Chylomicron retention disease
Fredrickson's hyperlipoproteinemia, type I or V
Hyperlipidemia, group D
Mixed hyperglyceridemia

E78.4 **Other hyperlipidemia**
AHA: 2018,4Q,6

E78.41 **Elevated Lipoprotein(a)**
Elevated Lp(a)

E78.49 **Other hyperlipidemia**
Familial combined hyperlipidemia

E78.5 **Hyperlipidemia, unspecified**
AHA: 2022,2Q,5

E78.6 **Lipoprotein deficiency**
Abetalipoproteinemia
Depressed HDL cholesterol
High-density lipoprotein deficiency
Hypoalphalipoproteinemia
Hypobetalipoproteinemia (familial)
Lecithin cholesterol acyltransferase deficiency
Tangier disease

E78.7 **Disorders of bile acid and cholesterol metabolism**
EXCLUDES 1 *Niemann-Pick disease type C (E75.242)*

E78.70 **Disorder of bile acid and cholesterol metabolism, unspecified**

E78.71 **Barth syndrome** CC

E78.72 **Smith-Lemli-Opitz syndrome** CC

E78.79 **Other disorders of bile acid and cholesterol metabolism**
AHA: 2023,1Q,26

E78.8 **Other disorders of lipoprotein metabolism**

E78.81 **Lipoid dermatoarthritis**

E78.89 **Other lipoprotein metabolism disorders**

E78.9 **Disorder of lipoprotein metabolism, unspecified**

E79 Disorders of purine and pyrimidine metabolism
EXCLUDES 1 *Ataxia-telangiectasia (Q87.19)*
Bloom's syndrome (Q82.8)
Cockayne's syndrome (Q87.19)
calculus of kidney (N20.0)
combined immunodeficiency disorders (D81.-)
Fanconi's anemia (D61.09)
gout (M1A.-, M10.-)
orotaciduric anemia (D53.0)
progeria (E34.8)
Werner's syndrome (E34.8)
xeroderma pigmentosum (Q82.1)

E79.0 **Hyperuricemia without signs of inflammatory arthritis and tophaceous disease**
Asymptomatic hyperuricemia

E79.1 **Lesch-Nyhan syndrome** CC HCC
HGPRT deficiency

E79.2 **Myoadenylate deaminase deficiency** CC HCC

▲ E79.8 **Other disorders of purine and pyrimidine metabolism**
~~Hereditary xanthinuria~~

● E79.81 **Aicardi-Goutieres syndrome** CC

● E79.82 **Hereditary xanthinuria** CC

● E79.89 **Other specified disorders of purine and pyrimidine metabolism** CC

E79.9 **Disorder of purine and pyrimidine metabolism, unspecified** CC HCC

✓4th **E80 Disorders of porphyrin and bilirubin metabolism**

INCLUDES defects of catalase and peroxidase

E80.0 **Hereditary erythropoietic porphyria** CC HCC
Congenital erythropoietic porphyria
Erythropoietic protoporphyria

E80.1 **Porphyria cutanea tarda** CC HCC

✓5th E80.2 **Other and unspecified porphyria**

E80.20 **Unspecified porphyria** CC HCC
Porphyria NOS

E80.21 **Acute intermittent (hepatic) porphyria** CC HCC

E80.29 **Other porphyria** CC HCC
Hereditary coproporphyria

E80.3 **Defects of catalase and peroxidase** CC HCC
Acatalasia [Takahara]

E80.4 **Gilbert syndrome**

E80.5 **Crigler-Najjar syndrome**

E80.6 **Other disorders of bilirubin metabolism**
Dubin-Johnson syndrome
Rotor's syndrome
AHA: 2022,3Q,7
TIP: Assign codes E80.6 and K76.89 to report benign recurrent intrahepatic cholestasis (BRIC) or progressive familial intrahepatic cholestasis (PFIC).

E80.7 **Disorder of bilirubin metabolism, unspecified**

✓4th **E83 Disorders of mineral metabolism**

EXCLUDES 1 *dietary mineral deficiency (E58-E61)*
parathyroid disorders (E20-E21)
vitamin D deficiency (E55.-)

✓5th E83.0 **Disorders of copper metabolism**

E83.00 **Disorder of copper metabolism, unspecified**

E83.01 **Wilson's disease**
Code also associated Kayser Fleischer ring (H18.04-)

E83.09 **Other disorders of copper metabolism**
Menkes' (kinky hair) (steely hair) disease

✓5th E83.1 **Disorders of iron metabolism**

EXCLUDES 1 *iron deficiency anemia (D50.-)*
sideroblastic anemia (D64.0-D64.3)

E83.10 **Disorder of iron metabolism, unspecified**

✓6th E83.11 **Hemochromatosis**

EXCLUDES 1 *GALD (P78.84)*
gestational alloimmune liver disease (P78.84)
neonatal hemochromatosis (P78.84)

E83.110 **Hereditary hemochromatosis** HCC
Bronzed diabetes
Pigmentary cirrhosis (of liver)
Primary (hereditary) hemochromatosis

E83.111 **Hemochromatosis due to repeated red blood cell transfusions**
Iron overload due to repeated red blood cell transfusions
Transfusion (red blood cell) associated hemochromatosis

E83.118 **Other hemochromatosis**

E83.119 **Hemochromatosis, unspecified**

E83.19 **Other disorders of iron metabolism**
Use additional code, if applicable, for idiopathic pulmonary hemosiderosis (J84.03)

E83.2 **Disorders of zinc metabolism**
Acrodermatitis enteropathica

✓5th E83.3 **Disorders of phosphorus metabolism and phosphatases**

EXCLUDES 1 *adult osteomalacia (M83.-)*
osteoporosis (M80.-)

E83.30 **Disorder of phosphorus metabolism, unspecified**

E83.31 **Familial hypophosphatemia**
Vitamin D-resistant osteomalacia
Vitamin D-resistant rickets
EXCLUDES 1 *vitamin D-deficiency rickets (E55.0)*

E83.32 **Hereditary vitamin D-dependent rickets (type 1) (type 2)**
25-hydroxyvitamin D 1-alpha-hydroxylase deficiency
Pseudovitamin D deficiency
Vitamin D receptor defect

E83.39 **Other disorders of phosphorus metabolism**
Acid phosphatase deficiency
Hypophosphatasia

✓5th E83.4 **Disorders of magnesium metabolism**

E83.40 **Disorders of magnesium metabolism, unspecified**

E83.41 **Hypermagnesemia**
AHA: 2016,4Q,54

E83.42 **Hypomagnesemia**

E83.49 **Other disorders of magnesium metabolism**

✓5th E83.5 **Disorders of calcium metabolism**

EXCLUDES 1 ▶*autoimmune hypoparathyroidism (E20.812)*◀
▶*autosomal dominant hypocalcemia (E20.810)*◀
chondrocalcinosis (M11.1-M11.2)
hungry bone syndrome (E83.81)
hyperparathyroidism (E21.0-E21.3)
▶*secondary hypoparathyroidism in diseases classified elsewhere (E20.811)*◀

E83.50 **Unspecified disorder of calcium metabolism**

E83.51 **Hypocalcemia**

E83.52 **Hypercalcemia**
Familial hypocalciuric hypercalcemia

E83.59 **Other disorders of calcium metabolism**

✓5th E83.8 **Other disorders of mineral metabolism**

E83.81 **Hungry bone syndrome**

E83.89 **Other disorders of mineral metabolism**

E83.9 **Disorder of mineral metabolism, unspecified**

✓4th **E84 Cystic fibrosis**

INCLUDES mucoviscidosis

Code also exocrine pancreatic insufficiency (K86.81)

DEF: Genetic disorder affecting the respiratory, digestive, and reproductive systems in infants to young adults by disturbing exocrine gland function and causing chronic pulmonary disease with excess mucus production and pancreatic deficiency.

E84.0 **Cystic fibrosis with pulmonary manifestations** MCC HCC
Use additional code to identify any infectious organism present, such as:
Pseudomonas (B96.5)
AHA: 2021,1Q,23

✓5th E84.1 **Cystic fibrosis with intestinal manifestations**

E84.11 **Meconium ileus in cystic fibrosis** MCC HCC N
EXCLUDES 1 *meconium ileus not due to cystic fibrosis (P76.0)*

E84.19 **Cystic fibrosis with other intestinal manifestations** CC HCC
Distal intestinal obstruction syndrome

E84.8 **Cystic fibrosis with other manifestations** CC HCC

E84.9 **Cystic fibrosis, unspecified** CC HCC

✓4th **E85 Amyloidosis**

EXCLUDES 2 *Alzheimer's disease (G30.0-)*

DEF: Conditions of diverse etiologies characterized by the accumulation of insoluble fibrillar proteins (amyloid) in various organs and tissues of the body, compromising vital functions.

E85.0 **Non-neuropathic heredofamilial amyloidosis** CC HCC
Hereditary amyloid nephropathy
Code also associated disorders, such as:
autoinflammatory syndromes (M04.-)
EXCLUDES 2 *transthyretin-related (ATTR) familial amyloid cardiomyopathy (E85.4)*

E85.1 **Neuropathic heredofamilial amyloidosis** CC HCC
Amyloid polyneuropathy (Portuguese)
Transthyretin-related (ATTR) familial amyloid polyneuropathy
AHA: 2012,4Q,99

E85.2 **Heredofamilial amyloidosis, unspecified** CC HCC

E85.3 **Secondary systemic amyloidosis** CC HCC
Hemodialysis-associated amyloidosis

E85.4 **Organ-limited amyloidosis** CC HCC
Localized amyloidosis
Transthyretin-related (ATTR) familial amyloid cardiomyopathy

✓5th E85.8 **Other amyloidosis**
AHA: 2017,4Q,7

E85.81 **Light chain (AL) amyloidosis** CC HCC

E85.82 **Wild-type transthyretin-related (ATTR) amyloidosis** CC HCC
Senile systemic amyloidosis (SSA)

E85.89 **Other amyloidosis** CC HCC

E85.9 **Amyloidosis, unspecified** CC HCC

E86 Volume depletion
Use additional code(s) for any associated disorders of electrolyte and acid-base balance (E87.-)
EXCLUDES 1 *dehydration of newborn (P74.1)*
postprocedural hypovolemic shock (T81.19)
traumatic hypovolemic shock (T79.4)
EXCLUDES 2 *hypovolemic shock NOS (R57.1)*
AHA: 2019,2Q,7; 2018,2Q,6

E86.Ø **Dehydration**
AHA: 2019,2Q,7; 2019,1Q,12; 2014,1Q,7
TIP: Can be assigned in addition to hypernatremia (E87.0) or hyponatremia (E87.1), when documented.

E86.1 **Hypovolemia**
Depletion of volume of plasma

E86.9 **Volume depletion, unspecified**
DEF: Depletion of total body water (dehydration) and/or contraction of total intravascular plasma (hypovolemia).

E87 Other disorders of fluid, electrolyte and acid-base balance
EXCLUDES 1 *diabetes insipidus (E23.2)*
electrolyte imbalance associated with hyperemesis gravidarum (O21.1)
electrolyte imbalance following ectopic or molar pregnancy (OØ8.5)
familial periodic paralysis (G72.3)
▶*metabolic acidemia in newborn, unspecified (P19.9)*◀
AHA: 2018,2Q,6

E87.Ø **Hyperosmolality and hypernatremia** CC
Sodium [Na] excess
Sodium [Na] overload
EXCLUDES 1 ▶*diabetes with hyperosmolarity (EØ8, EØ9, E11, E13 with final characters .ØØ or .Ø1)*◀
AHA: 2022,1Q,28; 2014,1Q,7
TIP: Assign an additional code for dehydration (E86.0), when documented.

E87.1 **Hypo-osmolality and hyponatremia** CC
Sodium [Na] deficiency
EXCLUDES 1 *syndrome of inappropriate secretion of antidiuretic hormone (E22.2)*
AHA: 2014,1Q,7
TIP: Assign an additional code for dehydration (E86.0), when documented.

E87.2 **Acidosis**
EXCLUDES 1 *diabetic acidosis - see categories EØ8-E1Ø, E11, E13 with ketoacidosis*
AHA: 2022,4Q,13-14; 2020,3Q,30
DEF: Reduction of alkaline in the blood and tissues caused by an increase in acid and decrease in bicarbonate.

E87.2Ø **Acidosis, unspecified** CC
Lactic acidosis NOS
Metabolic acidosis NOS
Code also, if applicable, respiratory failure with hypercapnia (J96. with 5th character 2)

E87.21 **Acute metabolic acidosis** CC
Acute lactic acidosis

E87.22 **Chronic metabolic acidosis** CC
Chronic lactic acidosis
Code first underlying etiology, if applicable
AHA: 2022,4Q,14

E87.29 **Other acidosis** CC
Respiratory acidosis NOS
EXCLUDES 2 *acute respiratory acidosis (J96.Ø2)*
chronic respiratory acidosis (J96.12)

E87.3 **Alkalosis** CC
Alkalosis NOS
Metabolic alkalosis
Respiratory alkalosis

E87.4 **Mixed disorder of acid-base balance** CC

E87.5 **Hyperkalemia**
Potassium [K] excess
Potassium [K] overload

E87.6 **Hypokalemia**
Potassium [K] deficiency

E87.7 **Fluid overload**
EXCLUDES 1 *edema NOS (R6Ø.9)*
fluid retention (R6Ø.9)

E87.7Ø **Fluid overload, unspecified**
AHA: 2023,1Q,19

E87.71 **Transfusion associated circulatory overload**
Fluid overload due to transfusion (blood) (blood components)
TACO

E87.79 **Other fluid overload**

E87.8 **Other disorders of electrolyte and fluid balance, not elsewhere classified**
Electrolyte imbalance NOS
Hyperchloremia
Hypochloremia

E88 Other and unspecified metabolic disorders
Use additional codes for associated conditions
EXCLUDES 1 *histiocytosis X (chronic) (C96.6)*

E88.Ø **Disorders of plasma-protein metabolism, not elsewhere classified**
EXCLUDES 1 *monoclonal gammopathy (of undetermined significance) (D47.2)*
polyclonal hypergammaglobulinemia (D89.Ø)
Waldenstrom macroglobulinemia (C88.Ø)
EXCLUDES 2 *disorder of lipoprotein metabolism (E78.-)*

E88.Ø1 **Alpha-1-antitrypsin deficiency** HCC
AAT deficiency

E88.Ø2 **Plasminogen deficiency** CC
Dysplasminogenemia
Hypoplasminogenemia
Type 1 plasminogen deficiency
Type 2 plasminogen deficiency
Code also, if applicable, ligneous conjunctivitis (H1Ø.51)
Use additional code for associated findings, such as:
hydrocephalus (G91.4)
otitis media (H67.-)
respiratory disorder related to plasminogen deficiency (J99)
AHA: 2018,4Q,6-7

E88.Ø9 **Other disorders of plasma-protein metabolism, not elsewhere classified**
Bisalbuminemia

E88.1 **Lipodystrophy, not elsewhere classified**
Lipodystrophy NOS
EXCLUDES 1 *Whipple's disease (K9Ø.81)*

E88.2 **Lipomatosis, not elsewhere classified**
Lipomatosis NOS
Lipomatosis (Check) dolorosa [Dercum]

E88.3 **Tumor lysis syndrome** MCC
Tumor lysis syndrome (spontaneous)
Tumor lysis syndrome following antineoplastic drug chemotherapy
Use additional code for adverse effect, if applicable, to identify drug (T45.1X5)
AHA: 2020,1Q,37; 2019,2Q,24
DEF: Potentially fatal metabolic complication of tumor necrosis caused by spontaneous or treatment-related accumulation of byproducts from dying cancer cells. Symptoms include hyperkalemia, hyperphosphatemia, hypocalcemia, hyperuricemia, and hyperuricosuria.

E88.4 **Mitochondrial metabolism disorders**
EXCLUDES 1 *disorders of pyruvate metabolism (E74.4)*
Kearns-Sayre syndrome (H49.81)
Leber's disease (H47.22)
Leigh's encephalopathy (G31.82)
mitochondrial myopathy, NEC (G71.3)
Reye's syndrome (G93.7)

E88.4Ø **Mitochondrial metabolism disorder, unspecified** CC HCC

E88.41 **MELAS syndrome** CC HCC
Mitochondrial myopathy, encephalopathy, lactic acidosis and stroke-like episodes

E88.42 **MERRF syndrome** CC HCC
Myoclonic epilepsy associated with ragged-red fibers
Code also progressive myoclonic epilepsy (G4Ø.3-)

● E88.43 **Disorders of mitochondrial tRNA synthetases** CC

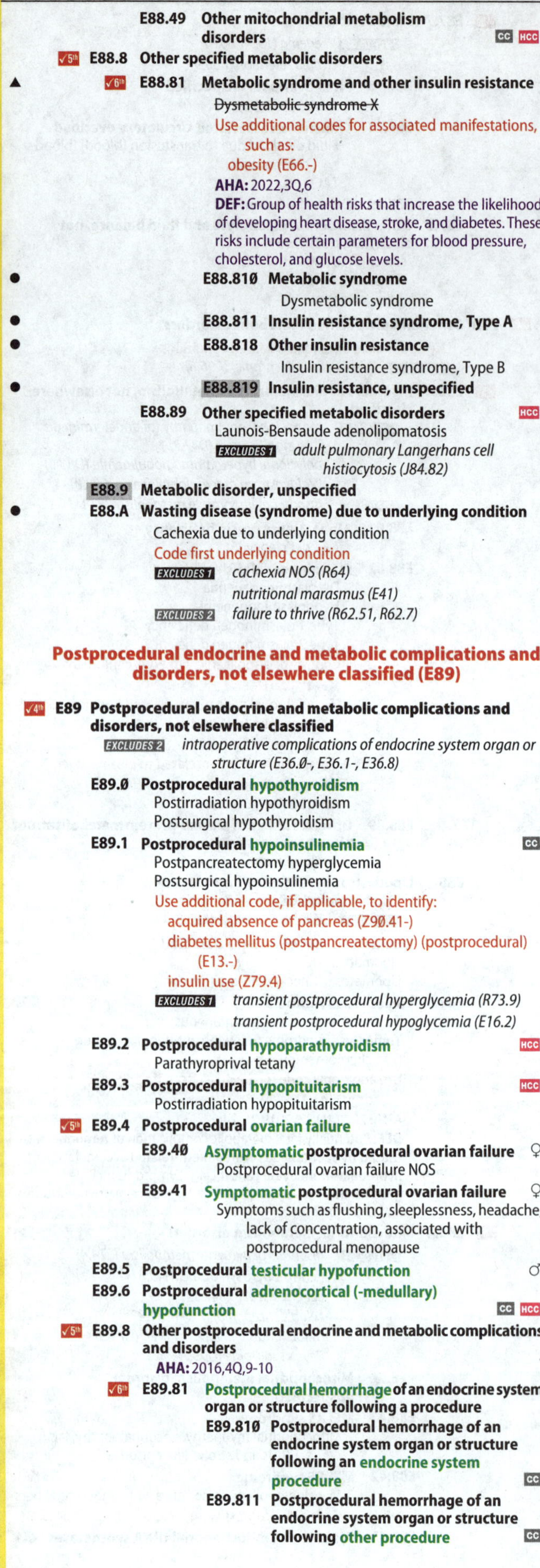

E88.49 Other mitochondrial metabolism disorders CC HCC

✓5th **E88.8 Other specified metabolic disorders**

▲ ✓6th **E88.81 Metabolic syndrome and other insulin resistance**

~~Dysmetabolic syndrome X~~

Use additional codes for associated manifestations, such as:

obesity (E66.-)

AHA: 2022,3Q,6

DEF: Group of health risks that increase the likelihood of developing heart disease, stroke, and diabetes. These risks include certain parameters for blood pressure, cholesterol, and glucose levels.

● **E88.810 Metabolic syndrome**

Dysmetabolic syndrome

● **E88.811 Insulin resistance syndrome, Type A**

● **E88.818 Other insulin resistance**

Insulin resistance syndrome, Type B

● **E88.819 Insulin resistance, unspecified**

E88.89 Other specified metabolic disorders HCC

Launois-Bensaude adenolipomatosis

EXCLUDES 1 *adult pulmonary Langerhans cell histiocytosis (J84.82)*

E88.9 Metabolic disorder, unspecified

● **E88.A Wasting disease (syndrome) due to underlying condition**

Cachexia due to underlying condition

Code first underlying condition

EXCLUDES 1 *cachexia NOS (R64)*

nutritional marasmus (E41)

EXCLUDES 2 *failure to thrive (R62.51, R62.7)*

Postprocedural endocrine and metabolic complications and disorders, not elsewhere classified (E89)

✓4th **E89 Postprocedural endocrine and metabolic complications and disorders, not elsewhere classified**

EXCLUDES 2 *intraoperative complications of endocrine system organ or structure (E36.0-, E36.1-, E36.8)*

E89.0 Postprocedural hypothyroidism

Postirradiation hypothyroidism

Postsurgical hypothyroidism

E89.1 Postprocedural hypoinsulinemia CC

Postpancreatectomy hyperglycemia

Postsurgical hypoinsulinemia

Use additional code, if applicable, to identify:

acquired absence of pancreas (Z90.41-)

diabetes mellitus (postpancreatectomy) (postprocedural) (E13.-)

insulin use (Z79.4)

EXCLUDES 1 *transient postprocedural hyperglycemia (R73.9)*

transient postprocedural hypoglycemia (E16.2)

E89.2 Postprocedural hypoparathyroidism HCC

Parathyroprival tetany

E89.3 Postprocedural hypopituitarism HCC

Postirradiation hypopituitarism

✓5th **E89.4 Postprocedural ovarian failure**

E89.40 Asymptomatic postprocedural ovarian failure ♀

Postprocedural ovarian failure NOS

E89.41 Symptomatic postprocedural ovarian failure ♀

Symptoms such as flushing, sleeplessness, headache, lack of concentration, associated with postprocedural menopause

E89.5 Postprocedural testicular hypofunction ♂

E89.6 Postprocedural adrenocortical (-medullary) hypofunction CC HCC

✓5th **E89.8 Other postprocedural endocrine and metabolic complications and disorders**

AHA: 2016,4Q,9-10

✓6th **E89.81 Postprocedural hemorrhage of an endocrine system organ or structure following a procedure**

E89.810 Postprocedural hemorrhage of an endocrine system organ or structure following an endocrine system procedure CC

E89.811 Postprocedural hemorrhage of an endocrine system organ or structure following other procedure CC

✓6th **E89.82 Postprocedural hematoma and seroma of an endocrine system organ or structure**

E89.820 Postprocedural hematoma of an endocrine system organ or structure following an endocrine system procedure CC

E89.821 Postprocedural hematoma of an endocrine system organ or structure following other procedure CC

E89.822 Postprocedural seroma of an endocrine system organ or structure following an endocrine system procedure CC

E89.823 Postprocedural seroma of an endocrine system organ or structure following other procedure CC

E89.89 Other postprocedural endocrine and metabolic complications and disorders CC

Use additional code, if applicable, to further specify disorder

Chapter 5. Mental, Behavioral and Neurodevelopmental Disorders (FØ1–F99)

Chapter-specific Guidelines with Coding Examples

The chapter-specific guidelines from the ICD-10-CM Official Guidelines for Coding and Reporting have been provided below. Along with these guidelines are coding examples, contained in the shaded boxes, that have been developed to help illustrate the coding and/or sequencing guidance found in these guidelines.

a. Pain disorders related to psychological factors

Assign code F45.41, for pain that is exclusively related to psychological disorders. As indicated by the Excludes 1 note under category G89, a code from category G89 should not be assigned with code F45.41.

> Perceived abdominal pain determined to be persistent somatoform pain disorder
>
> **F45.41 Pain disorder exclusively related to psychological factors**
>
> *Explanation*: This pain was diagnosed as being exclusively psychological; therefore, no code from category G89 is added.

Code F45.42, Pain disorders with related psychological factors, should be used with a code from category G89, Pain, not elsewhere classified, if there is documentation of a psychological component for a patient with acute or chronic pain.

See Section I.C.6. Pain

b. Mental and behavioral disorders due to psychoactive substance use

1) In remission

Selection of codes describing "in remission" for categories F1Ø–F19, Mental and behavioral disorders due to psychoactive substance use (categories F1Ø–F19 with -.11, -.21, -.91) requires the provider's clinical judgment and are assigned only on the basis of provider documentation (as defined in the Official Guidelines for Coding and Reporting), unless otherwise instructed by the classification.

Mild substance use disorders in early or sustained remission are classified to the appropriate codes for substance abuse in remission, and moderate or severe substance use disorders in early or sustained remission are classified to the appropriate codes for substance dependence in remission.

> Insomnia in patient with history of methamphetamine abuse; lab results indicate no current drug use
>
> **G47.ØØ Insomnia, unspecified**
>
> **F15.1Ø Other stimulant abuse, uncomplicated**
>
> *Explanation*: Insomnia is a common side-effect of stimulant use, such as methamphetamines. Although lab tests do not indicate that the patient is currently using methamphetamines, there is no specific documentation stating that the stimulant abuse is in remission. "History of" abuse does not equate to "in remission" in this instance.

2) Psychoactive substance use, abuse and dependence

When the provider documentation refers to use, abuse and dependence of the same substance (e.g. alcohol, opioid, cannabis, etc.), only one code should be assigned to identify the pattern of use based on the following hierarchy:

- If both use and abuse are documented, assign only the code for abuse
- If both abuse and dependence are documented, assign only the code for dependence
- If use, abuse and dependence are all documented, assign only the code for dependence
- If both use and dependence are documented, assign only the code for dependence.

> History and physical notes cannabis dependence; progress note says cannabis abuse
>
> **F12.2Ø Cannabis dependence, uncomplicated**
>
> *Explanation*: In the hierarchy, the dependence code is used if both abuse and dependence are documented.

> Discharge summary says cocaine abuse; progress notes list cocaine use
>
> **F14.1Ø Cocaine abuse, uncomplicated**
>
> *Explanation*: In the hierarchy, the abuse code is used if both abuse and use are documented.

3) Psychoactive substance use, unspecified

As with all other unspecified diagnoses, the codes for unspecified psychoactive substance use (F1Ø.9-, F11.9-, F12.9-, F13.9-, F14.9-, F15.9-, F16.9-, F18.9-, F19.9-) should only be assigned based on provider documentation and when they meet the definition of a reportable diagnosis (see Section III, Reporting Additional Diagnoses). These codes are to be used only when the psychoactive substance use is associated with a substance related disorder (chapter 5 disorders such as sexual dysfunction, sleep disorder, or a mental or behavioral disorder) or medical condition, and such a relationship is documented by the provider.

4) Medical conditions due to psychoactive substance use, abuse and dependence

Medical conditions due to substance use, abuse, and dependence are not classified as substance-induced disorders. Assign the diagnosis code for the medical condition as directed by the Alphabetical Index along with the appropriate psychoactive substance use, abuse or dependence code. For example, for alcoholic pancreatitis due to alcohol dependence, assign the appropriate code from subcategory K85.2, Alcohol induced acute pancreatitis, and the appropriate code from subcategory F1Ø.2, such as code F1Ø.2Ø, Alcohol dependence, uncomplicated. It would not be appropriate to assign code F1Ø.288, Alcohol dependence with other alcohol-induced disorder.

5) Blood alcohol level

A code from category Y9Ø, Evidence of alcohol involvement determined by blood alcohol level, may be assigned when this information is documented and the patient's provider has documented a condition classifiable to category F1Ø, Alcohol related disorders. The blood alcohol level does not need to be documented by the patient's provider in order for it to be coded.

See Section I.B.14. for blood alcohol level documentation by clinicians other than patient's provider.

c. Factitious disorder

Factitious disorder imposed on self or Munchausen's syndrome is a disorder in which a person falsely reports or causes his or her own physical or psychological signs or symptoms. For patients with documented factitious disorder on self or Munchausen's syndrome, assign the appropriate code from subcategory F68.1-, Factitious disorder imposed on self.

Munchausen's syndrome by proxy (MSBP) is a disorder in which a caregiver (perpetrator) falsely reports or causes an illness or injury in another person (victim) under his or her care, such as a child, an elderly adult, or a person who has a disability. The condition is also referred to as "factitious disorder imposed on another" or "factitious disorder by proxy." The perpetrator, not the victim, receives this diagnosis. Assign code F68.A, Factitious disorder imposed on another, to the perpetrator's record. For the victim of a patient suffering from MSBP, assign the appropriate code from categories T74, Adult and child abuse, neglect and other maltreatment, confirmed, or T76, Adult and child abuse, neglect and other maltreatment, suspected.

See Section I.C.19.f. Adult and child abuse, neglect and other maltreatment

d. Dementia

The ICD-10-CM classifies dementia (categories FØ1, FØ2, and FØ3) on the basis of the etiology and severity (unspecified, mild, moderate or severe). Selection of the appropriate severity level requires the provider's clinical judgment and codes should be assigned only on the basis of provider documentation (as defined in the *Official Guidelines for Coding and Reporting)*, unless otherwise instructed by the classification. If the documentation does not provide information about the severity of the dementia, assign the appropriate code for unspecified severity.

If a patient is admitted to an inpatient acute care hospital or other inpatient facility setting with dementia at one severity level and it progresses to a higher severity level, assign one code for the highest severity level reported during the stay.

Chapter 5. Mental, Behavioral and Neurodevelopmental Disorders (F01-F99)

INCLUDES disorders of psychological development

EXCLUDES 2 *symptoms, signs and abnormal clinical laboratory findings, not elsewhere classified (R00-R99)*

This chapter contains the following blocks:

- F01-F09 Mental disorders due to known physiological conditions
- F10-F19 Mental and behavioral disorders due to psychoactive substance use
- F20-F29 Schizophrenia, schizotypal, delusional, and other non-mood psychotic disorders
- F30-F39 Mood [affective] disorders
- F40-F48 Anxiety, dissociative, stress-related, somatoform and other nonpsychotic mental disorders
- F50-F59 Behavioral syndromes associated with physiological disturbances and physical factors
- F60-F69 Disorders of adult personality and behavior
- F70-F79 Intellectual disabilities
- F80-F89 Pervasive and specific developmental disorders
- F90-F98 Behavioral and emotional disorders with onset usually occurring in childhood and adolescence
- F99 Unspecified mental disorder

Mental disorders due to known physiological conditions (F01-F09)

NOTE This block comprises a range of mental disorders grouped together on the basis of their having in common a demonstrable etiology in cerebral disease, brain injury, or other insult leading to cerebral dysfunction. The dysfunction may be primary, as in diseases, injuries, and insults that affect the brain directly and selectively; or secondary, as in systemic diseases and disorders that attack the brain only as one of the multiple organs or systems of the body that are involved.

✓4th **F01 Vascular dementia**

Vascular dementia as a result of infarction of the brain due to vascular disease, including hypertensive cerebrovascular disease.

INCLUDES arteriosclerotic dementia
major neurocognitive disorder due to vascular disease
multi-infarct dementia

Code first the underlying physiological condition or sequelae of cerebrovascular disease.

AHA: 2022,4Q,14-15

✓5th **F01.5 Vascular dementia, unspecified severity**

F01.50 Vascular dementia, unspecified severity, without behavioral disturbance, psychotic disturbance, mood disturbance, and anxiety HCC A

Major neurocognitive disorder due to vascular disease NOS

Vascular dementia NOS

AHA: 2021,2Q,4

✓6th **F01.51 Vascular dementia, unspecified severity, with behavioral disturbance**

F01.511 Vascular dementia, unspecified severity, with agitation CC UPD HCC A

Major neurocognitive disorder due to vascular disease, unspecified severity, with aberrant motor behavior such as restlessness, rocking, pacing, or exit-seeking

Major neurocognitive disorder due to vascular disease, unspecified severity, with verbal or physical behaviors such as profanity, shouting, threatening, anger, aggression, combativeness, or violence

Vascular dementia, unspecified severity, with aberrant motor behavior such as restlessness, rocking, pacing, or exit-seeking

Vascular dementia, unspecified severity, with verbal or physical behaviors such as profanity, shouting, threatening, anger, aggression, combativeness, or violence

F01.518 Vascular dementia, unspecified severity, with other behavioral disturbance CC UPD HCC A

Major neurocognitive disorder due to vascular disease, unspecified severity, with behavioral disturbances such as sleep disturbance, social disinhibition, or sexual disinhibition

Vascular dementia, unspecified severity, with behavioral disturbances such as sleep disturbance, social disinhibition, or sexual disinhibition

Use additional code, if applicable, to identify wandering in vascular dementia (Z91.83)

F01.52 Vascular dementia, unspecified severity, with psychotic disturbance CC UPD HCC A

Major neurocognitive disorder due to vascular disease, unspecified severity, with psychotic disturbance such as hallucinations, paranoia, suspiciousness, or delusional state

Vascular dementia, unspecified severity, with psychotic disturbance such as hallucinations, paranoia, suspiciousness, or delusional state

F01.53 Vascular dementia, unspecified severity, with mood disturbance CC UPD HCC A

Major neurocognitive disorder due to vascular disease, unspecified severity, with mood disturbance such as depression, apathy, or anhedonia

Vascular dementia, unspecified severity, with mood disturbance such as depression, apathy, or anhedonia

F01.54 Vascular dementia, unspecified severity, with anxiety CC UPD HCC A

Major neurocognitive disorder due to vascular disease, unspecified severity, with anxiety

✓5th **F01.A Vascular dementia, mild**

EXCLUDES 1 *mild neurocognitive disorder due to known physiological condition with or without behavioral disturbance (F06.7-)*

F01.A0 Vascular dementia, mild, without behavioral disturbance, psychotic disturbance, mood disturbance, and anxiety UPD HCC A

Major neurocognitive disorder due to vascular disease, mild, NOS

Vascular dementia, mild, NOS

✓6th **F01.A1 Vascular dementia, mild, with behavioral disturbance**

F01.A11 Vascular dementia, mild, with agitation CC UPD HCC A

Major neurocognitive disorder due to vascular disease, mild, with aberrant motor behavior such as restlessness, rocking, pacing, or exit-seeking

Major neurocognitive disorder due to vascular disease, mild, with verbal or physical behaviors such as profanity, shouting, threatening, anger, aggression, combativeness, or violence

Vascular dementia, mild, with aberrant motor behavior such as restlessness, rocking, pacing, or exit-seeking

Vascular dementia, mild, with verbal or physical behaviors such as profanity, shouting, threatening, anger, aggression, combativeness, or violence

F01.A18 Vascular dementia, mild, with other behavioral disturbance CC UPD HCC A
Major neurocognitive disorder due to vascular disease, mild, with behavioral disturbances such as sleep disturbance, social disinhibition, or sexual disinhibition
Vascular dementia, mild, with behavioral disturbances such as sleep disturbance, social disinhibition, or sexual disinhibition
Use additional code, if applicable, to identify wandering in vascular dementia (Z91.83)

F01.A2 Vascular dementia, mild, with psychotic disturbance CC UPD HCC A
Major neurocognitive disorder due to vascular disease, mild, with psychotic disturbance such as hallucinations, paranoia, suspiciousness, or delusional state
Vascular dementia, mild, with psychotic disturbance such as hallucinations, paranoia, suspiciousness, or delusional state

F01.A3 Vascular dementia, mild, with mood disturbance CC UPD HCC A
Major neurocognitive disorder due to vascular disease, mild, with mood disturbance such as depression, apathy, or anhedonia
Vascular dementia, mild, with mood disturbance such as depression, apathy, or anhedonia

F01.A4 Vascular dementia, mild, with anxiety CC UPD HCC A
Major neurocognitive disorder due to vascular disease, mild, with anxiety

✓5th **F01.B Vascular dementia, moderate**

F01.B0 Vascular dementia, moderate, without behavioral disturbance, psychotic disturbance, mood disturbance, and anxiety UPD HCC A
Major neurocognitive disorder due to vascular disease, moderate, NOS
Vascular dementia, moderate, NOS

✓6th **F01.B1 Vascular dementia, moderate, with behavioral disturbance**

F01.B11 Vascular dementia, moderate, with agitation CC UPD HCC A
Major neurocognitive disorder due to vascular disease, moderate, with aberrant motor behavior such as restlessness, rocking, pacing, or exit-seeking
Major neurocognitive disorder due to vascular disease, moderate, with verbal or physical behaviors such as profanity, shouting, threatening, anger, aggression, combativeness, or violence
Vascular dementia, moderate, with aberrant motor behavior such as restlessness, rocking, pacing, or exit-seeking
Vascular dementia, moderate, with verbal or physical behaviors such as profanity, shouting, threatening, anger, aggression, combativeness, or violence

F01.B18 Vascular dementia, moderate, with other behavioral disturbance CC UPD HCC A
Major neurocognitive disorder due to vascular disease, moderate, with behavioral disturbances such as sleep disturbance, social disinhibition, or sexual disinhibition
Vascular dementia, moderate, with behavioral disturbances such as sleep disturbance, social disinhibition, or sexual disinhibition
Use additional code, if applicable, to identify wandering in vascular dementia (Z91.83)

F01.B2 Vascular dementia, moderate, with psychotic disturbance CC UPD HCC A
Major neurocognitive disorder due to vascular disease, moderate, with psychotic disturbance such as hallucinations, paranoia, suspiciousness, or delusional state
Vascular dementia, moderate, with psychotic disturbance such as hallucinations, paranoia, suspiciousness, or delusional state

F01.B3 Vascular dementia, moderate, with mood disturbance CC UPD HCC A
Major neurocognitive disorder due to vascular disease, moderate, with mood disturbance such as depression, apathy, or anhedonia
Vascular dementia, moderate, with mood disturbance such as depression, apathy, or anhedonia

F01.B4 Vascular dementia, moderate, with anxiety CC UPD HCC A
Major neurocognitive disorder due to vascular disease, moderate, with anxiety

✓5th **F01.C Vascular dementia, severe**

F01.C0 Vascular dementia, severe, without behavioral disturbance, psychotic disturbance, mood disturbance, and anxiety UPD HCC A
Major neurocognitive disorder due to vascular disease, severe, NOS
Vascular dementia, severe, NOS

✓6th **F01.C1 Vascular dementia, severe, with behavioral disturbance**

F01.C11 Vascular dementia, severe, with agitation CC UPD HCC A
Major neurocognitive disorder due to vascular disease, severe, with aberrant motor behavior such as restlessness, rocking, pacing, or exit-seeking
Major neurocognitive disorder due to vascular disease, severe, with verbal or physical behaviors such as profanity, shouting, threatening, anger, aggression, combativeness, or violence
Vascular dementia, severe, with aberrant motor behavior such as restlessness, rocking, pacing, or exit-seeking
Vascular dementia, severe, with verbal or physical behaviors such as profanity, shouting, threatening, anger, aggression, combativeness, or violence

F01.C18 Vascular dementia, severe, with other behavioral disturbance CC UPD HCC A
Major neurocognitive disorder due to vascular disease, severe, with behavioral disturbances such as sleep disturbance, social disinhibition, or sexual disinhibition
Vascular dementia, severe, with behavioral disturbances such as sleep disturbance, social disinhibition, or sexual disinhibition
Use additional code, if applicable, to identify wandering in vascular dementia (Z91.83)

F01.C2 Vascular dementia, severe, with psychotic disturbance CC UPD HCC A
Major neurocognitive disorder due to vascular disease, severe, with psychotic disturbance such as hallucinations, paranoia, suspiciousness, or delusional state
Vascular dementia, severe, with psychotic disturbance such as hallucinations, paranoia, suspiciousness, or delusional state

F01.C3 Vascular dementia, severe, with mood disturbance CC UPD HCC A
Major neurocognitive disorder due to vascular disease, severe, with mood disturbance such as depression, apathy, or anhedonia
Vascular dementia, severe, with mood disturbance such as depression, apathy, or anhedonia

FØ1.C4 Vascular dementia, severe, with anxiety CC UPD HCC A

Major neurocognitive disorder due to vascular disease, severe, with anxiety

✓4th FØ2 Dementia in other diseases classified elsewhere

INCLUDES major neurocognitive disorder in other diseases classified elsewhere

Code first the underlying physiological condition, such as:

- Alzheimer's (G3Ø.-)
- cerebral lipidosis (E75.4)
- Creutzfeldt-Jakob disease (A81.Ø-)
- dementia with Lewy bodies (G31.83)
- dementia with Parkinsonism (G31.83)
- epilepsy and recurrent seizures (G4Ø.-)
- frontotemporal dementia (G31.Ø9)
- hepatolenticular degeneration ▶(E83.Ø1)◀
- human immunodeficiency virus [HIV] disease (B2Ø)
- Huntington's disease (G1Ø)
- hypercalcemia (E83.52)
- hypothyroidism, acquired (EØØ-EØ3.-)
- intoxications (T36-T65)
- Jakob-Creutzfeldt disease (A81.Ø-)
- multiple sclerosis (G35)
- neurosyphilis (A52.17)
- niacin deficiency [pellagra] (E52)
- Parkinson's disease ▶(G2Ø.-)◀
- Pick's disease (G31.Ø1)
- polyarteritis nodosa (M3Ø.Ø)
- prion disease (A81.9)
- systemic lupus erythematosus (M32.-)
- traumatic brain injury (SØ6.-)
- trypanosomiasis (B56.-, B57.-)
- vitamin B deficiency (E53.8)

EXCLUDES 1 *mild neurocognitive disorder due to known physiological condition with or without behavioral disturbance (FØ6.7-)*

EXCLUDES 2 *dementia in alcohol and psychoactive substance disorders (F1Ø-F19, with .17, .27, .97)*
vascular dementia (FØ1.5-, FØ1.A-, FØ1.B-, FØ1.C-)

AHA: 2022,4Q,14-15

✓5th FØ2.8 Dementia in other diseases classified elsewhere, unspecified severity

AHA: 2022,4Q,15; 2022,1Q,25; 2017,2Q,7; 2016,4Q,141; 2016,2Q,6

TIP: A code from this subcategory should always be assigned with a code from category G30 when Alzheimer's disease is documented, even in the absence of documented dementia.

FØ2.8Ø *Dementia in other diseases classified elsewhere, unspecified severity, without behavioral disturbance, psychotic disturbance, mood disturbance, and anxiety* HCC

Dementia in other diseases classified elsewhere NOS

Major neurocognitive disorder in other diseases classified elsewhere NOS

✓6th FØ2.81 Dementia in other diseases classified elsewhere, unspecified severity, with behavioral disturbance

FØ2.811 *Dementia in other diseases classified elsewhere, unspecified severity, with agitation* CC HCC

Dementia in other diseases classified elsewhere, unspecified severity, with aberrant motor behavior such as restlessness, rocking, pacing, or exit-seeking

Dementia in other diseases classified elsewhere, unspecified severity, with verbal or physical behaviors such as profanity, shouting, threatening, anger, aggression, combativeness, or violence

Major neurocognitive disorder in other diseases classified elsewhere, unspecified severity, with aberrant motor behavior such as restlessness, rocking, pacing, or exit-seeking

Major neurocognitive disorder in other diseases classified elsewhere, unspecified severity, with verbal or physical behaviors such as profanity, shouting, threatening, anger, aggression, combativeness, or violence

FØ2.818 *Dementia in other diseases classified elsewhere, unspecified severity, with other behavioral disturbance* CC HCC

Dementia in other diseases classified elsewhere with sleep disturbance, social disinhibition, or sexual disinhibition

Major neurocognitive disorder in other diseases classified elsewhere with sleep disturbance, social disinhibition, or sexual disinhibition

Use additional code, if applicable, to identify wandering in dementia in conditions classified elsewhere (Z91.83)

FØ2.82 *Dementia in other diseases classified elsewhere, unspecified severity, with psychotic disturbance* CC HCC

Dementia in other diseases classified elsewhere, unspecified severity, with psychotic disturbance such as hallucinations, paranoia, suspiciousness, or delusional state

Major neurocognitive disorder in other diseases classified elsewhere, unspecified, with psychotic disturbance such as hallucinations, paranoia, suspiciousness, or delusional state

FØ2.83 *Dementia in other diseases classified elsewhere, unspecified severity, with mood disturbance* CC HCC

Dementia in other diseases classified elsewhere, unspecified severity, with mood disturbance such as depression, apathy, or anhedonia

Major neurocognitive disorder in other diseases classified elsewhere unspecified severity,with mood disturbance such as with depression, apathy, or anhedonia

FØ2.84 *Dementia in other diseases classified elsewhere, unspecified severity, with anxiety* CC HCC

Major neurocognitive disorder in other diseases classified elsewhere unspecified severity, with anxiety

✓5th FØ2.A Dementia in other diseases classified elsewhere, mild

EXCLUDES 1 *mild neurocognitive disorder due to known physiological condition with or without behavioral disturbance (FØ6.7-)*

FØ2.AØ *Dementia in other diseases classified elsewhere, mild, without behavioral disturbance, psychotic disturbance, mood disturbance, and anxiety* HCC

Dementia in other diseases classified elsewhere, mild, NOS

Major neurocognitive disorder in other diseases classified elsewhere, mild, NOS

FØ2.A1 Dementia in other diseases classified elsewhere, mild, with behavioral disturbance

FØ2.A11 Dementia in other diseases classified elsewhere, mild, with agitation CC HCC

Dementia in other diseases classified elsewhere, mild, with aberrant motor behavior such as restlessness, rocking, pacing, or exit-seeking

Dementia in other diseases classified elsewhere, mild, with verbal or physical behaviors such as profanity, shouting, threatening, anger, aggression, combativeness, or violence

Major neurocognitive disorder in other diseases classified elsewhere, mild, with aberrant motor behavior such as restlessness, rocking, pacing, or exit-seeking

Major neurocognitive disorder in other diseases classified elsewhere, mild, with verbal or physical behaviors such as profanity, shouting, threatening, anger, aggression, combativeness, or violence

FØ2.A18 Dementia in other diseases classified elsewhere, mild, with other behavioral disturbance CC HCC

Dementia in other diseases classified elsewhere, mild, with behavioral disturbances such as sleep disturbance, social disinhibition, or sexual disinhibition

Major neurocognitive disorder in other diseases classified elsewhere, mild, with behavioral disturbances such as sleep disturbance, social disinhibition, or sexual disinhibition

Use additional code, if applicable, to identify wandering in dementia in conditions classified elsewhere (Z91.83)

FØ2.A2 Dementia in other diseases classified elsewhere, mild, with psychotic disturbance CC HCC

Dementia in other diseases classified elsewhere, mild, with psychotic disturbance such as hallucinations, paranoia, suspiciousness, or delusional state

Major neurocognitive disorder in other diseases classified elsewhere, mild, with psychotic disturbance such as hallucinations, paranoia, suspiciousness, or delusional state

FØ2.A3 Dementia in other diseases classified elsewhere, mild, with mood disturbance CC HCC

Dementia in other diseases classified elsewhere, mild, with mood disturbance such as depression, apathy, or anhedonia

Major neurocognitive disorder in other diseases classified elsewhere, mild, with mood disturbance such as depression, apathy, or anhedonia

FØ2.A4 Dementia in other diseases classified elsewhere, mild, with anxiety CC HCC

Major neurocognitive disorder in other diseases classified elsewhere, mild, with anxiety

FØ2.B Dementia in other diseases classified elsewhere, moderate

FØ2.BØ Dementia in other diseases classified elsewhere, moderate, without behavioral disturbance, psychotic disturbance, mood disturbance, and anxiety HCC

Dementia in other diseases classified elsewhere, moderate, NOS

Major neurocognitive disorder in other diseases classified elsewhere, moderate, NOS

FØ2.B1 Dementia in other diseases classified elsewhere, moderate, with behavioral disturbance

FØ2.B11 Dementia in other diseases classified elsewhere, moderate, with agitation CC HCC

Dementia in other diseases classified elsewhere, moderate, with aberrant motor behavior such as restlessness, rocking, pacing, or exit-seeking

Dementia in other diseases classified elsewhere, moderate, with verbal or physical behaviors such as profanity, shouting, threatening, anger, aggression, combativeness, or violence

Major neurocognitive disorder in other diseases classified elsewhere, moderate, with aberrant motor behavior such as restlessness, rocking, pacing, or exit-seeking

Major neurocognitive disorder in other diseases classified elsewhere, moderate, with verbal or physical behaviors such as profanity, shouting, threatening, anger, aggression, combativeness, or violence

FØ2.B18 Dementia in other diseases classified elsewhere, moderate, with other behavioral disturbance CC HCC

Dementia in other diseases classified elsewhere, moderate, with behavioral disturbances such as sleep disturbance, social disinhibition, or sexual disinhibition

Major neurocognitive disorder in other diseases classified elsewhere, moderate, with behavioral disturbance such as sleep disturbance, social disinhibition, or sexual disinhibition

Use additional code, if applicable, to identify wandering in dementia in conditions classified elsewhere (Z91.83)

FØ2.B2 Dementia in other diseases classified elsewhere, moderate, with psychotic disturbance CC HCC

Dementia in other diseases classified elsewhere, moderate, with psychotic disturbance such as hallucinations, paranoia, suspiciousness, or delusional state

Major neurocognitive disorder in other diseases classified elsewhere, moderate, with psychotic disturbance such as hallucinations, paranoia, suspiciousness, or delusional state

FØ2.B3 Dementia in other diseases classified elsewhere, moderate, with mood disturbance CC HCC

Dementia in other diseases classified elsewhere, moderate, with mood disturbance such as depression, apathy, or anhedonia

Major neurocognitive disorder in other diseases classified elsewhere, moderate, with mood disturbance such as depression, apathy, or anhedonia

FØ2.B4 Dementia in other diseases classified elsewhere, moderate, with anxiety CC HCC

Major neurocognitive disorder in other diseases classified elsewhere, moderate, with anxiety

FØ2.C Dementia in other diseases classified elsewhere, severe

FØ2.CØ Dementia in other diseases classified elsewhere, severe, without behavioral disturbance, psychotic disturbance, mood disturbance, and anxiety HCC

Dementia in other diseases classified elsewhere, severe, NOS

Major neurocognitive disorder in other diseases classified elsewhere, severe, NOS

√6th FØ2.C1 Dementia in other diseases classified elsewhere, severe, with behavioral disturbance

FØ2.C11 Dementia in other diseases classified elsewhere, severe, with agitation CC HCC

Dementia in other diseases classified elsewhere, severe, with aberrant motor behavior such as restlessness, rocking, pacing, or exit-seeking

Dementia in other diseases classified elsewhere, severe, with verbal or physical behaviors such as profanity, shouting, threatening, anger, aggression, combativeness, or violence

Major neurocognitive disorder in other diseases classified elsewhere, severe, with aberrant motor behavior such as restlessness, rocking, pacing, or exit-seeking

Major neurocognitive disorder in other diseases classified elsewhere, severe, with verbal or physical behaviors such as profanity, shouting, threatening, anger, aggression, combativeness, or violence

FØ2.C18 Dementia in other diseases classified elsewhere, severe, with other behavioral disturbance CC HCC

Dementia in other diseases classified elsewhere, severe, with behavioral disturbances such as sleep disturbance, social disinhibition, or sexual disinhibition

Major neurocognitive disorder in other diseases classified elsewhere, severe, with behavioral disturbances such as sleep disturbance, social disinhibition, or sexual disinhibition

Use additional code, if applicable, to identify wandering in dementia in conditions classified elsewhere (Z91.83)

FØ2.C2 Dementia in other diseases classified elsewhere, severe, with psychotic disturbance CC HCC

Dementia in other diseases classified elsewhere, severe, with psychotic disturbance such as hallucinations, paranoia, suspiciousness, or delusional state

Major neurocognitive disorder in other diseases classified elsewhere, severe, with psychotic disturbance such as hallucinations, paranoia, suspiciousness, or delusional state

FØ2.C3 Dementia in other diseases classified elsewhere, severe, with mood disturbance CC HCC

Dementia in other diseases classified elsewhere, severe, with mood disturbance such as depression, apathy, or anhedonia

Major neurocognitive disorder in other diseases classified elsewhere, severe, with mood disturbance such as depression, apathy, or anhedonia

FØ2.C4 Dementia in other diseases classified elsewhere, severe, with anxiety CC HCC

Major neurocognitive disorder in other diseases classified elsewhere, severe, with anxiety

√4th FØ3 Unspecified dementia

Major neurocognitive disorder NOS
Presenile dementia NOS
Presenile psychosis NOS
Primary degenerative dementia NOS
Senile dementia NOS
Senile dementia depressed or paranoid type
Senile psychosis NOS

EXCLUDES 1 *senility NOS (R41.81)*

EXCLUDES 2 *mild memory disturbance due to known physiological condition (FØ6.8)*
senile dementia with delirium or acute confusional state (FØ5)

AHA: 2022,4Q,14-15

√5th FØ3.9 Unspecified dementia, unspecified severity

FØ3.90 Unspecified dementia, unspecified severity, without behavioral disturbance, psychotic disturbance, mood disturbance, and anxiety HIV HCC A

Dementia NOS

AHA: 2021,2Q,4; 2012,4Q,92

√6th FØ3.91 Unspecified dementia, unspecified severity, with behavioral disturbance

FØ3.911 Unspecified dementia, unspecified severity, with agitation CC HCC A

Unspecified dementia, unspecified severity, with aberrant motor behavior such as restlessness, rocking, pacing, or exit-seeking

Unspecified dementia, unspecified severity, with verbal or physical behaviors such as profanity, shouting, threatening, anger, aggression, combativeness, or violence

FØ3.918 Unspecified dementia, unspecified severity, with other behavioral disturbance CC HCC A

Unspecified dementia, unspecified severity, with behavioral disturbances such as sleep disturbance, social disinhibition, or sexual disinhibition

Use additional code, if applicable, to identify wandering in unspecified dementia (Z91.83)

FØ3.92 Unspecified dementia, unspecified severity, with psychotic disturbance CC HCC A

Unspecified dementia, unspecified severity, with psychotic disturbance such as hallucinations, paranoia, suspiciousness, or delusional state

FØ3.93 Unspecified dementia, unspecified severity, with mood disturbance CC HCC A

Unspecified dementia, unspecified severity, with mood disturbance such as depression, apathy, or anhedonia

FØ3.94 Unspecified dementia, unspecified severity, with anxiety CC HCC A

√5th FØ3.A Unspecified dementia, mild

EXCLUDES 1 *mild neurocognitive disorder due to known physiological condition with or without behavioral disturbance (FØ6.7-)*

FØ3.AØ Unspecified dementia, mild, without behavioral disturbance, psychotic disturbance, mood disturbance, and anxiety HCC A

Dementia, mild, NOS

√6th FØ3.A1 Unspecified dementia, mild, with behavioral disturbance

FØ3.A11 Unspecified dementia, mild, with agitation CC HCC A

Unspecified dementia, mild, with aberrant motor behavior such as restlessness, rocking, pacing, or exit-seeking

Unspecified dementia, mild, with verbal or physical behaviors such as profanity, shouting, threatening, anger, aggression, combativeness, or violence

F03.A18 **Unspecified dementia, mild, with other behavioral disturbance** CC HCC A
Unspecified dementia, mild, with behavioral disturbances such as sleep disturbance, social disinhibition, or sexual disinhibition
Use additional code, if applicable, to identify wandering in unspecified dementia (Z91.83)

F03.A2 **Unspecified dementia, mild, with psychotic disturbance** CC HCC A
Unspecified dementia, mild, with psychotic disturbance such as hallucinations, paranoia, suspiciousness, or delusional state

F03.A3 **Unspecified dementia, mild, with mood disturbance** CC HCC A
Unspecified dementia, mild, with mood disturbance such as depression, apathy, or anhedonia

F03.A4 **Unspecified dementia, mild, with anxiety** CC HCC A

✓5th F03.B **Unspecified dementia, moderate**

F03.B0 **Unspecified dementia, moderate, without behavioral disturbance, psychotic disturbance, mood disturbance, and anxiety** HCC A
Dementia, moderate, NOS

✓6th F03.B1 **Unspecified dementia, moderate, with behavioral disturbance**

F03.B11 **Unspecified dementia, moderate, with agitation** CC HCC A
Unspecified dementia, moderate, with aberrant motor behavior such as restlessness, rocking, pacing, or exit-seeking
Unspecified dementia, moderate, with verbal or physical behaviors such as profanity, shouting, threatening, anger, aggression, combativeness, or violence

F03.B18 **Unspecified dementia, moderate, with other behavioral disturbance** CC HCC A
Unspecified dementia, moderate, with behavioral disturbances such as sleep disturbance, social disinhibition, or sexual disinhibition
Use additional code, if applicable, to identify wandering in unspecified dementia (Z91.83)

F03.B2 **Unspecified dementia, moderate, with psychotic disturbance** CC HCC A
Unspecified dementia, moderate, with psychotic disturbance such as hallucinations, paranoia, suspiciousness, or delusional state

F03.B3 **Unspecified dementia, moderate, with mood disturbance** CC HCC A
Unspecified dementia, moderate, with mood disturbance such as depression, apathy, or anhedonia

F03.B4 **Unspecified dementia, moderate, with anxiety** CC HCC A

✓5th F03.C **Unspecified dementia, severe**

F03.C0 **Unspecified dementia, severe, without behavioral disturbance, psychotic disturbance, mood disturbance, and anxiety** HCC A
Dementia, severe, NOS

✓6th F03.C1 **Unspecified dementia, severe, with behavioral disturbance**

F03.C11 **Unspecified dementia, severe, with agitation** CC HCC A
Unspecified dementia, severe, with aberrant motor behavior such as restlessness, rocking, pacing, or exit-seeking
Unspecified dementia, severe, with verbal or physical behaviors such as profanity, shouting, threatening, anger, aggression, combativeness, or violence

F03.C18 **Unspecified dementia, severe, with other behavioral disturbance** CC HCC A
Unspecified dementia, severe, with behavioral disturbances such as sleep disturbance, social disinhibition, or sexual disinhibition
Use additional code, if applicable, to identify wandering in unspecified dementia (Z91.83)

F03.C2 **Unspecified dementia, severe, with psychotic disturbance** CC HCC A
Unspecified dementia, severe, with psychotic disturbance such as hallucinations, paranoia, suspiciousness, or delusional state

F03.C3 **Unspecified dementia, severe, with mood disturbance** CC HCC A
Unspecified dementia, severe, with mood disturbance such as depression, apathy, or anhedonia

F03.C4 **Unspecified dementia, severe, with anxiety** CC HCC A

F04 Amnestic disorder due to known physiological condition HCC
Korsakov's psychosis or syndrome, nonalcoholic
Code first the underlying physiological condition
EXCLUDES 1 *amnesia NOS (R41.3)*
anterograde amnesia (R41.1)
dissociative amnesia (F44.0)
retrograde amnesia (R41.2)
EXCLUDES 2 *alcohol-induced or unspecified Korsakov's syndrome (F10.26, F10.96)*
Korsakov's syndrome induced by other psychoactive substances (F13.26, F13.96, F19.16, F19.26, F19.96)

F05 Delirium due to known physiological condition CC
Acute or subacute brain syndrome
Acute or subacute confusional state (nonalcoholic)
Acute or subacute infective psychosis
Acute or subacute organic reaction
Acute or subacute psycho-organic syndrome
Delirium of mixed etiology
Delirium superimposed on dementia
Sundowning
▶Code first the underlying physiological condition, such as:◀
▶dementia (F03.9-)◀
EXCLUDES 1 *delirium NOS (R41.0)*
EXCLUDES 2 *delirium tremens alcohol-induced or unspecified (F10.231, F10.921)*
AHA: 2019,2Q,34

✓4th **F06 Other mental disorders due to known physiological condition**
INCLUDES mental disorders due to endocrine disorder
mental disorders due to exogenous hormone
mental disorders due to exogenous toxic substance
mental disorders due to primary cerebral disease
mental disorders due to somatic illness
mental disorders due to systemic disease affecting the brain
Code first the underlying physiological condition
EXCLUDES 1 *unspecified dementia (F03)*
EXCLUDES 2 *delirium due to known physiological condition (F05)*
dementia as classified in F01-F02
other mental disorders associated with alcohol and other psychoactive substances (F10-F19)

F06.0 **Psychotic disorder with hallucinations due to known physiological condition** CC
Organic hallucinatory state (nonalcoholic)
EXCLUDES 2 *hallucinations and perceptual disturbance induced by alcohol and other psychoactive substances (F10-F19 with .151, .251, .951)*
schizophrenia (F20.-)

F06.1 **Catatonic disorder due to known physiological condition**
Catatonia associated with another mental disorder
Catatonia NOS
EXCLUDES 1 *catatonic stupor (R40.1)*
stupor NOS (R40.1)
EXCLUDES 2 *catatonic schizophrenia (F20.2)*
dissociative stupor (F44.2)
DEF: Catatonic: Abnormal neuropsychiatric state characterized by stupor, immobility or purposeless movements, or unresponsiveness in a person who otherwise appears awake.

F06.2 Psychotic disorder with delusions due to known physiological condition CC
Paranoid and paranoid-hallucinatory organic states
Schizophrenia-like psychosis in epilepsy
EXCLUDES 2 *alcohol and drug-induced psychotic disorder (F10-F19 with .150, .250, .950)*
brief psychotic disorder (F23)
delusional disorder (F22)
schizophrenia (F20.-)

✓5th **F06.3 Mood disorder due to known physiological condition**
EXCLUDES 2 *mood disorders due to alcohol and other psychoactive substances (F10-F19 with .14, .24, .94)*
mood disorders, not due to known physiological condition or unspecified (F30-F39)

F06.30 Mood disorder due to known physiological condition, unspecified

F06.31 Mood disorder due to known physiological condition with depressive features
Depressive disorder due to known physiological condition, with depressive features

F06.32 Mood disorder due to known physiological condition with major depressive-like episode
Depressive disorder due to known physiological condition, with major depressive-like episode

F06.33 Mood disorder due to known physiological condition with manic features
Bipolar and related disorder due to a known physiological condition, with manic features
Bipolar and related disorder due to known physiological condition, with manic- or hypomanic-like episodes

F06.34 Mood disorder due to known physiological condition with mixed features
Bipolar and related disorder due to known physiological condition, with mixed features
Depressive disorder due to known physiological condition, with mixed features

F06.4 Anxiety disorder due to known physiological condition
EXCLUDES 2 *anxiety disorders due to alcohol and other psychoactive substances (F10-F19 with .180, .280, .980)*
anxiety disorders, not due to known physiological condition or unspecified (F40.-, F41.-)

✓5th **F06.7 Mild neurocognitive disorder due to known physiological condition**
Mild neurocognitive impairment due to a known physiological condition
Code first the underlying physiological condition, such as:
Alzheimer's disease (G30.-)
frontotemporal neurocognitive disorder (G31.09)
human immunodeficiency virus [HIV] disease (B20)
Huntington's disease (G10)
neurocognitive disorder with Lewy bodies (G31.83)
Parkinson's disease ▶(G20.-)◀
systemic lupus erythematosus (M32.-)
traumatic brain injury (S06.-)
vitamin B deficiency (E53-)
EXCLUDES 1 *age related cognitive decline (R41.81)*
altered mental status (R41.82)
cerebral degeneration (G31.9)
change in mental status (R41.82)
cognitive deficits following (sequelae of) cerebral hemorrhage or infarction (I69.01-I69.11-, I69.21-I69.31-, I69.81-I69.91-)
dementia (F01.-, F02.-, F03)
mild cognitive impairment due to unknown or unspecified etiology (G31.84)
neurologic neglect syndrome (R41.4)
personality change, nonpsychotic (F68.8)
AHA: 2022,4Q,16

F06.70 Mild neurocognitive disorder due to known physiological condition without behavioral disturbance HIV UPD
Mild neurocognitive disorder due to known physiological condition, NOS

F06.71 Mild neurocognitive disorder due to known physiological condition with behavioral disturbance HIV CC UPD

F06.8 Other specified mental disorders due to known physiological condition HIV
Epileptic psychosis NOS
Obsessive-compulsive and related disorder due to a known physiological condition
Organic dissociative disorder
Organic emotionally labile [asthenic] disorder

✓4th **F07 Personality and behavioral disorders due to known physiological condition**
Code first the underlying physiological condition

F07.0 Personality change due to known physiological condition
Frontal lobe syndrome
Limbic epilepsy personality syndrome
Lobotomy syndrome
Organic personality disorder
Organic pseudopsychopathic personality
Organic pseudoretarded personality
Postleucotomy syndrome
EXCLUDES 1 *mild cognitive impairment (G31.84)*
postconcussional syndrome (F07.81)
postencephalitic syndrome (F07.89)
signs and symptoms involving emotional state (R45.-)
EXCLUDES 2 *specific personality disorder (F60.-)*

✓5th **F07.8 Other personality and behavioral disorders due to known physiological condition**

F07.81 Postconcussional syndrome
Postcontusional syndrome (encephalopathy)
Post-traumatic brain syndrome, nonpsychotic
Use additional code to identify associated post-traumatic headache, if applicable (G44.3-)
EXCLUDES 1 *current concussion (brain) (S06.0-)*
postencephalitic syndrome (F07.89)
DEF: Concussion symptoms that persist for weeks or months after a head injury. These symptoms may include headache, giddiness, fatigue, insomnia, mood fluctuation, and a subjective feeling of impaired intellectual function with extreme reaction to normal stressors.

F07.89 Other personality and behavioral disorders due to known physiological condition UPD
Postencephalitic syndrome
Right hemispheric organic affective disorder

F07.9 Unspecified personality and behavioral disorder due to known physiological condition HIV
Organic psychosyndrome

F09 Unspecified mental disorder due to known physiological condition HIV
Mental disorder NOS due to known physiological condition
Organic brain syndrome NOS
Organic mental disorder NOS
Organic psychosis NOS
Symptomatic psychosis NOS
Code first the underlying physiological condition
EXCLUDES 1 *mild neurocognitive disorder due to known physiological condition (F06.7-)*
psychosis NOS (F29)

Mental and behavioral disorders due to psychoactive substance use (F10-F19)

AHA: 2022,4Q,16-17; 2022,1Q,34; 2020,1Q,9; 2018,4Q,69-70; 2017,4Q,8; 2017,2Q,27

TIP: Psychoactive substance withdrawal can occur in individuals who do not have a diagnosis of dependence but who use the substance regularly (i.e., use or abuse) and then reduce or cease the use.

✓4th **F10 Alcohol related disorders**
Use additional code for blood alcohol level, if applicable (Y90.-)
AHA: 2019,3Q,8

✓5th **F10.1 Alcohol abuse**
EXCLUDES 1 *alcohol dependence (F10.2-)*
alcohol use, unspecified (F10.9-)
AHA: 2018,1Q,16; 2015,2Q,15

F10.10 Alcohol abuse, uncomplicated
Alcohol use disorder, mild

F10.11 Alcohol abuse, in remission
Alcohol use disorder, mild, in early remission
Alcohol use disorder, mild, in sustained remission
AHA: 2022,1Q,25

✓6th **F10.12 Alcohol abuse with intoxication**

F10.120 Alcohol abuse with intoxication, uncomplicated HCC

F10.121 Alcohol abuse with intoxication delirium CC HCC

F10.129 Alcohol abuse with intoxication, unspecified HCC

✓6th F10.13 Alcohol abuse, with withdrawal

AHA: 2020,4Q,16-17

F10.130 Alcohol abuse with withdrawal, uncomplicated CC HCC

F10.131 Alcohol abuse with withdrawal delirium CC HCC

F10.132 Alcohol abuse with withdrawal with perceptual disturbance CC HCC

F10.139 Alcohol abuse with withdrawal, unspecified CC HCC

F10.14 Alcohol abuse with alcohol-induced mood disorder CC HCC

Alcohol use disorder, mild, with alcohol-induced bipolar or related disorder

Alcohol use disorder, mild, with alcohol-induced depressive disorder

✓6th F10.15 Alcohol abuse with alcohol-induced psychotic disorder

F10.150 Alcohol abuse with alcohol-induced psychotic disorder with delusions HCC

F10.151 Alcohol abuse with alcohol-induced psychotic disorder with hallucinations CC HCC

DEF: Psychosis lasting less than six months with slight or no clouding of consciousness in which auditory hallucinations predominate.

F10.159 Alcohol abuse with alcohol-induced psychotic disorder, unspecified CC HCC

✓6th F10.18 Alcohol abuse with other alcohol-induced disorders

AHA: 2022,1Q,33

F10.180 Alcohol abuse with alcohol-induced anxiety disorder CC HCC

AHA: 2022,1Q,25,33

F10.181 Alcohol abuse with alcohol-induced sexual dysfunction CC HCC

F10.182 Alcohol abuse with alcohol-induced sleep disorder HCC

F10.188 Alcohol abuse with other alcohol-induced disorder CC HCC

AHA: 2022,1Q,25

F10.19 Alcohol abuse with unspecified alcohol-induced disorder CC HCC

✓5th F10.2 Alcohol dependence

EXCLUDES 1 *alcohol abuse (F10.1-)*

alcohol use, unspecified (F10.9-)

EXCLUDES 2 *toxic effect of alcohol (T51.0-)*

F10.20 Alcohol dependence, uncomplicated HCC

Alcohol use disorder, moderate

Alcohol use disorder, severe

AHA: 2020,1Q,9

F10.21 Alcohol dependence, in remission HCC

Alcohol use disorder, moderate, in early remission

Alcohol use disorder, moderate, in sustained remission

Alcohol use disorder, severe, in early remission

Alcohol use disorder, severe, in sustained remission

✓6th F10.22 Alcohol dependence with intoxication

Acute drunkenness (in alcoholism)

EXCLUDES 2 *alcohol dependence with withdrawal (F10.23-)*

F10.220 Alcohol dependence with intoxication, uncomplicated HCC

F10.221 Alcohol dependence with intoxication delirium CC HCC

F10.229 Alcohol dependence with intoxication, unspecified HCC

✓6th F10.23 Alcohol dependence with withdrawal

EXCLUDES 2 *alcohol dependence with intoxication (F10.22-)*

AHA: 2018,1Q,16; 2015,2Q,15

F10.230 Alcohol dependence with withdrawal, uncomplicated CC HCC

F10.231 Alcohol dependence with withdrawal delirium CC HCC

F10.232 Alcohol dependence with withdrawal with perceptual disturbance CC HCC

F10.239 Alcohol dependence with withdrawal, unspecified CC HCC

F10.24 Alcohol dependence with alcohol-induced mood disorder CC HCC

Alcohol use disorder, moderate, with alcohol-induced bipolar or related disorder

Alcohol use disorder, moderate, with alcohol-induced depressive disorder

Alcohol use disorder, severe, with alcohol-induced bipolar or related disorder

Alcohol use disorder, severe, with alcohol-induced depressive disorder

✓6th F10.25 Alcohol dependence with alcohol-induced psychotic disorder

F10.250 Alcohol dependence with alcohol-induced psychotic disorder with delusions HCC

F10.251 Alcohol dependence with alcohol-induced psychotic disorder with hallucinations CC HCC

F10.259 Alcohol dependence with alcohol-induced psychotic disorder, unspecified CC HCC

F10.26 Alcohol dependence with alcohol-induced persisting amnestic disorder HCC

Alcohol use disorder, moderate, with alcohol-induced major neurocognitive disorder, amnestic-confabulatory type

Alcohol use disorder, severe, with alcohol-induced major neurocognitive disorder, amnestic-confabulatory type

DEF: Prominent and lasting reduced memory span and disordered time appreciation and confabulation that occurs in alcoholics as sequel to acute alcoholic psychosis.

F10.27 Alcohol dependence with alcohol-induced persisting dementia CC HCC

Alcohol use disorder, moderate, with alcohol-induced major neurocognitive disorder, nonamnestic-confabulatory type

Alcohol use disorder, severe, with alcohol-induced major neurocognitive disorder, nonamnestic-confabulatory type

✓6th F10.28 Alcohol dependence with other alcohol-induced disorders

F10.280 Alcohol dependence with alcohol-induced anxiety disorder CC HCC

F10.281 Alcohol dependence with alcohol-induced sexual dysfunction CC HCC

F10.282 Alcohol dependence with alcohol-induced sleep disorder HCC

F10.288 Alcohol dependence with other alcohol-induced disorder CC HCC

Alcohol use disorder, moderate, with alcohol-induced mild neurocognitive disorder

Alcohol use disorder, severe, with alcohol-induced mild neurocognitive disorder

AHA: 2020,1Q,9

F10.29 Alcohol dependence with unspecified alcohol-induced disorder CC HCC

✓5th F10.9 Alcohol use, unspecified

EXCLUDES 1 *alcohol abuse (F10.1-)*

alcohol dependence (F10.2-)

AHA: 2018,2Q,10-11

TIP: Assign a substance use code only when the provider documents a relationship between the use and an associated physical, mental, or behavioral disorder. As with all diagnoses, substance use codes must meet the definition of a reportable diagnosis.

F10.90 Alcohol use, unspecified, uncomplicated

F10.91 Alcohol use, unspecified, in remission

✓6th F10.92 Alcohol use, unspecified with intoxication

F10.920 Alcohol use, unspecified with intoxication, uncomplicated HCC

AHA: 2018,2Q,10-11

Chapter 5. Mental, Behavioral and Neurodevelopmental Disorders

F10.921 Alcohol use, unspecified with intoxication delirium CC HCC

F10.929 Alcohol use, unspecified with intoxication, unspecified HCC

F10.93 Alcohol use, unspecified with withdrawal

AHA: 2020,4Q,16-17

F10.930 Alcohol use, unspecified with withdrawal, uncomplicated CC HCC

F10.931 Alcohol use, unspecified with withdrawal delirium CC HCC

F10.932 Alcohol use, unspecified with withdrawal with perceptual disturbance CC HCC

F10.939 Alcohol use, unspecified with withdrawal, unspecified CC HCC

F10.94 Alcohol use, unspecified with alcohol-induced mood disorder CC HCC

Alcohol induced bipolar or related disorder, without use disorder

Alcohol induced depressive disorder, without use disorder

F10.95 Alcohol use, unspecified with alcohol-induced psychotic disorder

F10.950 Alcohol use, unspecified with alcohol-induced psychotic disorder with delusions HCC

F10.951 Alcohol use, unspecified with alcohol-induced psychotic disorder with hallucinations CC HCC

F10.959 Alcohol use, unspecified with alcohol-induced psychotic disorder, unspecified CC HCC

Alcohol-induced psychotic disorder without use disorder

F10.96 Alcohol use, unspecified with alcohol-induced persisting amnestic disorder HCC

Alcohol-induced major neurocognitive disorder, amnestic-confabulatory type, without use disorder

F10.97 Alcohol use, unspecified with alcohol-induced persisting dementia HCC

Alcohol-induced major neurocognitive disorder, nonamnestic-confabulatory type, without use disorder

F10.98 Alcohol use, unspecified with other alcohol-induced disorders

F10.980 Alcohol use, unspecified with alcohol-induced anxiety disorder CC HCC

Alcohol induced anxiety disorder, without use disorder

F10.981 Alcohol use, unspecified with alcohol-induced sexual dysfunction CC HCC

Alcohol induced sexual dysfunction, without use disorder

F10.982 Alcohol use, unspecified with alcohol-induced sleep disorder HCC

Alcohol induced sleep disorder, without use disorder

F10.988 Alcohol use, unspecified with other alcohol-induced disorder CC HCC

Alcohol induced mild neurocognitive disorder, without use disorder

F10.99 Alcohol use, unspecified with unspecified alcohol-induced disorder CC HCC

F11 Opioid related disorders

F11.1 Opioid abuse

EXCLUDES 1 *opioid dependence (F11.2-)*
opioid use, unspecified (F11.9-)

F11.10 Opioid abuse, uncomplicated HCC

Opioid use disorder, mild

F11.11 Opioid abuse, in remission HCC

Opioid use disorder, mild, in early remission

Opioid use disorder, mild, in sustained remission

F11.12 Opioid abuse with intoxication

F11.120 Opioid abuse with intoxication, uncomplicated HCC

F11.121 Opioid abuse with intoxication delirium CC HCC

F11.122 Opioid abuse with intoxication with perceptual disturbance HCC

F11.129 Opioid abuse with intoxication, unspecified HCC

F11.13 Opioid abuse with withdrawal CC HCC

AHA: 2020,4Q,16-17

F11.14 Opioid abuse with opioid-induced mood disorder HCC

Opioid use disorder, mild, with opioid-induced depressive disorder

F11.15 Opioid abuse with opioid-induced psychotic disorder

F11.150 Opioid abuse with opioid-induced psychotic disorder with delusions CC HCC

F11.151 Opioid abuse with opioid-induced psychotic disorder with hallucinations CC HCC

F11.159 Opioid abuse with opioid-induced psychotic disorder, unspecified HCC

F11.18 Opioid abuse with other opioid-induced disorder

F11.181 Opioid abuse with opioid-induced sexual dysfunction HCC

F11.182 Opioid abuse with opioid-induced sleep disorder HCC

F11.188 Opioid abuse with other opioid-induced disorder HCC

▶Opioid-associated amnestic syndrome with opioid abuse◀

F11.19 Opioid abuse with unspecified opioid-induced disorder HCC

F11.2 Opioid dependence

EXCLUDES 1 *opioid abuse (F11.1-)*
opioid use, unspecified (F11.9-)

EXCLUDES 2 *opioid poisoning (T40.0-T40.2-)*

F11.20 Opioid dependence, uncomplicated CC HCC

Opioid use disorder, moderate

Opioid use disorder, severe

F11.21 Opioid dependence, in remission HCC

Opioid use disorder, moderate, in early remission

Opioid use disorder, moderate, in sustained remission

Opioid use disorder, severe, in early remission

Opioid use disorder, severe, in sustained remission

F11.22 Opioid dependence with intoxication

EXCLUDES 1 *opioid dependence with withdrawal (F11.23)*

F11.220 Opioid dependence with intoxication, uncomplicated HCC

F11.221 Opioid dependence with intoxication delirium CC HCC

F11.222 Opioid dependence with intoxication with perceptual disturbance CC HCC

F11.229 Opioid dependence with intoxication, unspecified HCC

F11.23 Opioid dependence with withdrawal CC HCC

EXCLUDES 1 *opioid dependence with intoxication (F11.22-)*

F11.24 Opioid dependence with opioid-induced mood disorder HCC

Opioid use disorder, moderate, with opioid induced depressive disorder

F11.25 Opioid dependence with opioid-induced psychotic disorder

F11.250 Opioid dependence with opioid-induced psychotic disorder with delusions CC HCC

F11.251 Opioid dependence with opioid-induced psychotic disorder with hallucinations CC HCC

F11.259 Opioid dependence with opioid-induced psychotic disorder, unspecified CC HCC

F11.28 Opioid dependence with other opioid-induced disorder

F11.281 Opioid dependence with opioid-induced sexual dysfunction CC HCC

F11.282 Opioid dependence with opioid-induced sleep disorder CC HCC

F11.288 **Opioid dependence with other opioid-induced disorder** CC HCC
▶Opioid-associated amnestic syndrome with opioid dependence◀

F11.29 **Opioid dependence with unspecified opioid-induced disorder** HCC

✓5th F11.9 **Opioid use, unspecified**

EXCLUDES 1 *opioid abuse (F11.1-)*
opioid dependence (F11.2-)

TIP: Assign a substance use code only when the provider documents a relationship between the use and an associated physical, mental, or behavioral disorder. As with all diagnoses, substance use codes must meet the definition of a reportable diagnosis.

F11.90 **Opioid use, unspecified, uncomplicated**
AHA: 2018,2Q,10-11

F11.91 **Opioid use, unspecified, in remission**

✓6th F11.92 **Opioid use, unspecified with intoxication**

EXCLUDES 1 *opioid use, unspecified with withdrawal (F11.93)*

F11.920 **Opioid use, unspecified with intoxication, uncomplicated** HCC

F11.921 **Opioid use, unspecified with intoxication delirium** CC HCC
Opioid-induced delirium

F11.922 **Opioid use, unspecified with intoxication with perceptual disturbance** HCC

F11.929 **Opioid use, unspecified with intoxication, unspecified** HCC

F11.93 **Opioid use, unspecified with withdrawal** CC HCC

EXCLUDES 1 *opioid use, unspecified with intoxication (F11.92-)*

F11.94 **Opioid use, unspecified with opioid-induced mood disorder** HCC
Opioid induced depressive disorder, without use disorder

✓6th F11.95 **Opioid use, unspecified with opioid-induced psychotic disorder**

F11.950 **Opioid use, unspecified with opioid-induced psychotic disorder with delusions** CC HCC

F11.951 **Opioid use, unspecified with opioid-induced psychotic disorder with hallucinations** CC HCC

F11.959 **Opioid use, unspecified with opioid-induced psychotic disorder, unspecified** HCC

✓6th F11.98 **Opioid use, unspecified with other specified opioid-induced disorder**

F11.981 **Opioid use, unspecified with opioid-induced sexual dysfunction** HCC
Opioid induced sexual dysfunction, without use disorder

F11.982 **Opioid use, unspecified with opioid-induced sleep disorder** HCC
Opioid induced sleep disorder, without use disorder

F11.988 **Opioid use, unspecified with other opioid-induced disorder** HCC
▶Opioid-associated amnestic syndrome without use disorder◀
Opioid induced anxiety disorder, without use disorder

F11.99 **Opioid use, unspecified with unspecified opioid-induced disorder** HCC

✓4th F12 **Cannabis related disorders**

INCLUDES marijuana

AHA: 2020,1Q,8

✓5th F12.1 **Cannabis abuse**

EXCLUDES 1 *cannabis dependence (F12.2-)*
cannabis use, unspecified (F12.9-)

F12.10 **Cannabis abuse, uncomplicated**
Cannabis use disorder, mild

F12.11 **Cannabis abuse, in remission**
Cannabis use disorder, mild, in early remission
Cannabis use disorder, mild, in sustained remission

✓6th F12.12 **Cannabis abuse with intoxication**

F12.120 **Cannabis abuse with intoxication, uncomplicated** HCC

F12.121 **Cannabis abuse with intoxication delirium** CC HCC

F12.122 **Cannabis abuse with intoxication with perceptual disturbance** HCC

F12.129 **Cannabis abuse with intoxication, unspecified** HCC

F12.13 **Cannabis abuse with withdrawal** HCC
AHA: 2020,4Q,16-17

✓6th F12.15 **Cannabis abuse with psychotic disorder**

F12.150 **Cannabis abuse with psychotic disorder with delusions** CC HCC

F12.151 **Cannabis abuse with psychotic disorder with hallucinations** CC HCC

F12.159 **Cannabis abuse with psychotic disorder, unspecified** HCC

✓6th F12.18 **Cannabis abuse with other cannabis-induced disorder**

F12.180 **Cannabis abuse with cannabis-induced anxiety disorder** HCC

F12.188 **Cannabis abuse with other cannabis-induced disorder** HCC
Cannabis use disorder, mild, with cannabis-induced sleep disorder

F12.19 **Cannabis abuse with unspecified cannabis-induced disorder** HCC

✓5th F12.2 **Cannabis dependence**

EXCLUDES 1 *cannabis abuse (F12.1-)*
cannabis use, unspecified (F12.9-)

EXCLUDES 2 *cannabis poisoning (T40.7-)*

F12.20 **Cannabis dependence, uncomplicated** HCC
Cannabis use disorder, moderate
Cannabis use disorder, severe

F12.21 **Cannabis dependence, in remission** HCC
Cannabis use disorder, moderate, in early remission
Cannabis use disorder, moderate, in sustained remission
Cannabis use disorder, severe, in early remission
Cannabis use disorder, severe, in sustained remission

✓6th F12.22 **Cannabis dependence with intoxication**

F12.220 **Cannabis dependence with intoxication, uncomplicated** HCC

F12.221 **Cannabis dependence with intoxication delirium** CC HCC

F12.222 **Cannabis dependence with intoxication with perceptual disturbance** HCC

F12.229 **Cannabis dependence with intoxication, unspecified** HCC

F12.23 **Cannabis dependence with withdrawal** HCC
AHA: 2018,4Q,7

✓6th F12.25 **Cannabis dependence with psychotic disorder**

F12.250 **Cannabis dependence with psychotic disorder with delusions** CC HCC

F12.251 **Cannabis dependence with psychotic disorder with hallucinations** CC HCC

F12.259 **Cannabis dependence with psychotic disorder, unspecified** HCC

✓6th F12.28 **Cannabis dependence with other cannabis-induced disorder**

F12.280 **Cannabis dependence with cannabis-induced anxiety disorder** HCC

F12.288 **Cannabis dependence with other cannabis-induced disorder** HCC
Cannabis use disorder, moderate, with cannabis-induced sleep disorder
Cannabis use disorder, severe, with cannabis-induced sleep disorder

F12.29 **Cannabis dependence with unspecified cannabis-induced disorder** HCC

✓5th **F12.9 Cannabis use, unspecified**

EXCLUDES 1 *cannabis abuse (F12.1-)*
cannabis dependence (F12.2-)

TIP: Assign a substance use code only when the provider documents a relationship between the use and an associated physical, mental, or behavioral disorder. As with all diagnoses, substance use codes must meet the definition of a reportable diagnosis.

F12.90 Cannabis use, unspecified, uncomplicated
AHA: 2018,2Q,10-11

F12.91 Cannabis use, unspecified, in remission

✓6th **F12.92 Cannabis use, unspecified with intoxication**

F12.920 Cannabis use, unspecified with intoxication, uncomplicated HCC

F12.921 Cannabis use, unspecified with intoxication delirium CC HCC

F12.922 Cannabis use, unspecified with intoxication with perceptual disturbance HCC

F12.929 Cannabis use, unspecified with intoxication, unspecified HCC

F12.93 Cannabis use, unspecified with withdrawal HCC
AHA: 2018,4Q,7

✓6th **F12.95 Cannabis use, unspecified with psychotic disorder**

F12.950 Cannabis use, unspecified with psychotic disorder with delusions CC HCC

F12.951 Cannabis use, unspecified with psychotic disorder with hallucinations CC HCC

F12.959 Cannabis use, unspecified with psychotic disorder, unspecified HCC
Cannabis induced psychotic disorder, without use disorder

✓6th **F12.98 Cannabis use, unspecified with other cannabis-induced disorder**

F12.980 Cannabis use, unspecified with anxiety disorder HCC
Cannabis induced anxiety disorder, without use disorder

F12.988 Cannabis use, unspecified with other cannabis-induced disorder HCC
Cannabis induced sleep disorder, without use disorder

F12.99 Cannabis use, unspecified with unspecified cannabis-induced disorder HCC

✓4th **F13 Sedative, hypnotic, or anxiolytic related disorders**

✓5th **F13.1 Sedative, hypnotic or anxiolytic-related abuse**

EXCLUDES 1 *sedative, hypnotic or anxiolytic-related dependence (F13.2-)*
sedative, hypnotic, or anxiolytic use, unspecified (F13.9-)

F13.10 Sedative, hypnotic or anxiolytic abuse, uncomplicated HCC
Sedative, hypnotic, or anxiolytic use disorder, mild

F13.11 Sedative, hypnotic or anxiolytic abuse, in remission HCC
Sedative, hypnotic or anxiolytic use disorder, mild, in early remission
Sedative, hypnotic or anxiolytic use disorder, mild, in sustained remission

✓6th **F13.12 Sedative, hypnotic or anxiolytic abuse with intoxication**

F13.120 Sedative, hypnotic or anxiolytic abuse with intoxication, uncomplicated HCC

F13.121 Sedative, hypnotic or anxiolytic abuse with intoxication delirium CC HCC

F13.129 Sedative, hypnotic or anxiolytic abuse with intoxication, unspecified HCC

✓6th **F13.13 Sedative, hypnotic or anxiolytic abuse with withdrawal**
AHA: 2020,4Q,16-17

F13.130 Sedative, hypnotic or anxiolytic abuse with withdrawal, uncomplicated CC HCC

F13.131 Sedative, hypnotic or anxiolytic abuse with withdrawal delirium CC HCC

F13.132 Sedative, hypnotic or anxiolytic abuse with withdrawal with perceptual disturbance CC HCC

F13.139 Sedative, hypnotic or anxiolytic abuse with withdrawal, unspecified CC HCC

F13.14 Sedative, hypnotic or anxiolytic abuse with sedative, hypnotic or anxiolytic-induced mood disorder HCC
Sedative, hypnotic, or anxiolytic use disorder, mild, with sedative, hypnotic, or anxiolytic-induced bipolar or related disorder
Sedative, hypnotic, or anxiolytic use disorder, mild, with sedative, hypnotic, or anxiolytic-induced depressive disorder

✓6th **F13.15 Sedative, hypnotic or anxiolytic abuse with sedative, hypnotic or anxiolytic-induced psychotic disorder**

F13.150 Sedative, hypnotic or anxiolytic abuse with sedative, hypnotic or anxiolytic-induced psychotic disorder with delusions CC HCC

F13.151 Sedative, hypnotic or anxiolytic abuse with sedative, hypnotic or anxiolytic-induced psychotic disorder with hallucinations CC HCC

F13.159 Sedative, hypnotic or anxiolytic abuse with sedative, hypnotic or anxiolytic-induced psychotic disorder, unspecified HCC

✓6th **F13.18 Sedative, hypnotic or anxiolytic abuse with other sedative, hypnotic or anxiolytic-induced disorders**

F13.180 Sedative, hypnotic or anxiolytic abuse with sedative, hypnotic or anxiolytic-induced anxiety disorder HCC

F13.181 Sedative, hypnotic or anxiolytic abuse with sedative, hypnotic or anxiolytic-induced sexual dysfunction HCC

F13.182 Sedative, hypnotic or anxiolytic abuse with sedative, hypnotic or anxiolytic-induced sleep disorder HCC

F13.188 Sedative, hypnotic or anxiolytic abuse with other sedative, hypnotic or anxiolytic-induced disorder HCC

F13.19 Sedative, hypnotic or anxiolytic abuse with unspecified sedative, hypnotic or anxiolytic-induced disorder HCC

✓5th **F13.2 Sedative, hypnotic or anxiolytic-related dependence**

EXCLUDES 1 *sedative, hypnotic or anxiolytic-related abuse (F13.1-)*
sedative, hypnotic, or anxiolytic use, unspecified (F13.9-)

EXCLUDES 2 *sedative, hypnotic, or anxiolytic poisoning (T42.-)*

F13.20 Sedative, hypnotic or anxiolytic dependence, uncomplicated CC HCC

F13.21 Sedative, hypnotic or anxiolytic dependence, in remission HCC
Sedative, hypnotic or anxiolytic use disorder, moderate, in early remission
Sedative, hypnotic or anxiolytic use disorder, moderate, in sustained remission
Sedative, hypnotic or anxiolytic use disorder, severe, in early remission
Sedative, hypnotic or anxiolytic use disorder, severe, in sustained remission

✓6th **F13.22 Sedative, hypnotic or anxiolytic dependence with intoxication**

EXCLUDES 1 *sedative, hypnotic or anxiolytic dependence with withdrawal (F13.23-)*

F13.220 Sedative, hypnotic or anxiolytic dependence with intoxication, uncomplicated HCC

F13.221 Sedative, hypnotic or anxiolytic dependence with intoxication delirium CC HCC

F13.229 Sedative, hypnotic or anxiolytic dependence with intoxication, unspecified HCC

✓6th **F13.23 Sedative, hypnotic or anxiolytic dependence with withdrawal**
Sedative, hypnotic, or anxiolytic use disorder, moderate
Sedative, hypnotic, or anxiolytic use disorder, severe
EXCLUDES 1 *sedative, hypnotic or anxiolytic dependence with intoxication (F13.22-)*

F13.230 Sedative, hypnotic or anxiolytic dependence with withdrawal, uncomplicated CC HCC

F13.231 Sedative, hypnotic or anxiolytic dependence with withdrawal delirium CC HCC

F13.232 Sedative, hypnotic or anxiolytic dependence with withdrawal with perceptual disturbance CC HCC
Sedative, hypnotic, or anxiolytic withdrawal with perceptual disturbances

F13.239 Sedative, hypnotic or anxiolytic dependence with withdrawal, unspecified CC HCC
Sedative, hypnotic, or anxiolytic withdrawal without perceptual disturbances

F13.24 Sedative, hypnotic or anxiolytic dependence with sedative, hypnotic or anxiolytic-induced mood disorder HCC
Sedative, hypnotic, or anxiolytic use disorder, moderate, with sedative, hypnotic, or anxiolytic-induced bipolar or related disorder
Sedative, hypnotic, or anxiolytic use disorder, moderate, with sedative, hypnotic, or anxiolytic-induced depressive disorder
Sedative, hypnotic, or anxiolytic use disorder, severe, with sedative, hypnotic, or anxiolytic-induced bipolar or related disorder
Sedative, hypnotic, or anxiolytic use disorder, severe, with sedative, hypnotic, or anxiolytic-induced depressive disorder

✓6th **F13.25 Sedative, hypnotic or anxiolytic dependence with sedative, hypnotic or anxiolytic-induced psychotic disorder**

F13.250 Sedative, hypnotic or anxiolytic dependence with sedative, hypnotic or anxiolytic-induced psychotic disorder with delusions CC HCC

F13.251 Sedative, hypnotic or anxiolytic dependence with sedative, hypnotic or anxiolytic-induced psychotic disorder with hallucinations CC HCC

F13.259 Sedative, hypnotic or anxiolytic dependence with sedative, hypnotic or anxiolytic-induced psychotic disorder, unspecified CC HCC

F13.26 Sedative, hypnotic or anxiolytic dependence with sedative, hypnotic or anxiolytic-induced persisting amnestic disorder CC HCC

F13.27 Sedative, hypnotic or anxiolytic dependence with sedative, hypnotic or anxiolytic-induced persisting dementia CC HCC
Sedative, hypnotic, or anxiolytic use disorder, moderate, with sedative, hypnotic, or anxiolytic induced major neurocognitive disorder
Sedative, hypnotic, or anxiolytic use disorder, severe, with sedative, hypnotic, or anxiolytic-induced major neurocognitive disorder

✓6th **F13.28 Sedative, hypnotic or anxiolytic dependence with other sedative, hypnotic or anxiolytic-induced disorders**

F13.280 Sedative, hypnotic or anxiolytic dependence with sedative, hypnotic or anxiolytic-induced anxiety disorder CC HCC

F13.281 Sedative, hypnotic or anxiolytic dependence with sedative, hypnotic or anxiolytic-induced sexual dysfunction CC HCC

F13.282 Sedative, hypnotic or anxiolytic dependence with sedative, hypnotic or anxiolytic-induced sleep disorder CC HCC

F13.288 Sedative, hypnotic or anxiolytic dependence with other sedative, hypnotic or anxiolytic-induced disorder CC HCC
Sedative, hypnotic, or anxiolytic use disorder, moderate, with sedative, hypnotic, or anxiolytic-induced mild neurocognitive disorder
Sedative, hypnotic, or anxiolytic use disorder, severe, with sedative, hypnotic, or anxiolytic-induced mild neurocognitive disorder

F13.29 Sedative, hypnotic or anxiolytic dependence with unspecified sedative, hypnotic or anxiolytic-induced disorder HCC

✓5th **F13.9 Sedative, hypnotic or anxiolytic-related use, unspecified**
EXCLUDES 1 *sedative, hypnotic or anxiolytic-related abuse (F13.1-)*
sedative, hypnotic or anxiolytic-related dependence (F13.2-)

TIP: Assign a substance use code only when the provider documents a relationship between the use and an associated physical, mental, or behavioral disorder. As with all diagnoses, substance use codes must meet the definition of a reportable diagnosis.

F13.90 Sedative, hypnotic, or anxiolytic use, unspecified, uncomplicated
AHA: 2018,2Q,10-11

F13.91 Sedative, hypnotic or anxiolytic use, unspecified, in remission

✓6th **F13.92 Sedative, hypnotic or anxiolytic use, unspecified with intoxication**
EXCLUDES 1 *sedative, hypnotic or anxiolytic use, unspecified with withdrawal (F13.93-)*

F13.920 Sedative, hypnotic or anxiolytic use, unspecified with intoxication, uncomplicated HCC

F13.921 Sedative, hypnotic or anxiolytic use, unspecified with intoxication delirium CC HCC
Sedative, hypnotic, or anxiolytic-induced delirium

F13.929 Sedative, hypnotic or anxiolytic use, unspecified with intoxication, unspecified HCC

✓6th **F13.93 Sedative, hypnotic or anxiolytic use, unspecified with withdrawal**
EXCLUDES 1 *sedative, hypnotic or anxiolytic use, unspecified with intoxication (F13.92-)*

F13.930 Sedative, hypnotic or anxiolytic use, unspecified with withdrawal, uncomplicated CC HCC

F13.931 Sedative, hypnotic or anxiolytic use, unspecified with withdrawal delirium CC HCC

F13.932 Sedative, hypnotic or anxiolytic use, unspecified with withdrawal with perceptual disturbances CC HCC

F13.939 Sedative, hypnotic or anxiolytic use, unspecified with withdrawal, unspecified CC HCC

F13.94 Sedative, hypnotic or anxiolytic use, unspecified with sedative, hypnotic or anxiolytic-induced mood disorder HCC
Sedative, hypnotic, or anxiolytic-induced bipolar or related disorder, without use disorder
Sedative, hypnotic, or anxiolytic-induced depressive disorder, without use disorder

✓6th **F13.95 Sedative, hypnotic or anxiolytic use, unspecified with sedative, hypnotic or anxiolytic-induced psychotic disorder**

F13.950 Sedative, hypnotic or anxiolytic use, unspecified with sedative, hypnotic or anxiolytic-induced psychotic disorder with delusions CC HCC

F13.951 Sedative, hypnotic or anxiolytic use, unspecified with sedative, hypnotic or anxiolytic-induced psychotic disorder with hallucinations CC HCC

F13.959 **Sedative, hypnotic or anxiolytic use, unspecified with sedative, hypnotic or anxiolytic-induced psychotic disorder, unspecified** HCC
Sedative, hypnotic, or anxiolytic-induced psychotic disorder, without use disorder

F13.96 **Sedative, hypnotic or anxiolytic use, unspecified with sedative, hypnotic or anxiolytic-induced persisting amnestic disorder** HCC

F13.97 **Sedative, hypnotic or anxiolytic use, unspecified with sedative, hypnotic or anxiolytic-induced persisting dementia** CC HCC
Sedative, hypnotic, or anxiolytic-induced major neurocognitive disorder, without use disorder

✓6th **F13.98** **Sedative, hypnotic or anxiolytic use, unspecified with other sedative, hypnotic or anxiolytic-induced disorders**

F13.980 **Sedative, hypnotic or anxiolytic use, unspecified with sedative, hypnotic or anxiolytic-induced anxiety disorder** HCC
Sedative, hypnotic, or anxiolytic-induced anxiety disorder, without use disorder

F13.981 **Sedative, hypnotic or anxiolytic use, unspecified with sedative, hypnotic or anxiolytic-induced sexual dysfunction** HCC
Sedative, hypnotic, or anxiolytic-induced sexual dysfunction disorder, without use disorder

F13.982 **Sedative, hypnotic or anxiolytic use, unspecified with sedative, hypnotic or anxiolytic-induced sleep disorder** HCC
Sedative, hypnotic, or anxiolytic-induced sleep disorder, without use disorder

F13.988 **Sedative, hypnotic or anxiolytic use, unspecified with other sedative, hypnotic or anxiolytic-induced disorder** HCC
Sedative, hypnotic, or anxiolytic-induced mild neurocognitive disorder

F13.99 **Sedative, hypnotic or anxiolytic use, unspecified with unspecified sedative, hypnotic or anxiolytic-induced disorder** HCC

✓4th **F14 Cocaine related disorders**

EXCLUDES 2 *other stimulant-related disorders (F15.-)*

✓5th **F14.1 Cocaine abuse**

EXCLUDES 1 *cocaine dependence (F14.2-)*
cocaine use, unspecified (F14.9-)

F14.10 **Cocaine abuse, uncomplicated** HCC
Cocaine use disorder, mild

F14.11 **Cocaine abuse, in remission** HCC
Cocaine use disorder, mild, in early remission
Cocaine use disorder, mild, in sustained remission

✓6th **F14.12** **Cocaine abuse with intoxication**

F14.120 **Cocaine abuse with intoxication, uncomplicated** HCC

F14.121 **Cocaine abuse with intoxication with delirium** CC HCC

F14.122 **Cocaine abuse with intoxication with perceptual disturbance** HCC

F14.129 **Cocaine abuse with intoxication, unspecified** HCC

F14.13 **Cocaine abuse, unspecified with withdrawal** CC HCC
AHA: 2020,4Q,16-17

F14.14 **Cocaine abuse with cocaine-induced mood disorder** HCC
Cocaine use disorder, mild, with cocaine-induced bipolar or related disorder
Cocaine use disorder, mild, with cocaine-induced depressive disorder

✓6th **F14.15** **Cocaine abuse with cocaine-induced psychotic disorder**

F14.150 **Cocaine abuse with cocaine-induced psychotic disorder with delusions** CC HCC

F14.151 **Cocaine abuse with cocaine-induced psychotic disorder with hallucinations** CC HCC

F14.159 **Cocaine abuse with cocaine-induced psychotic disorder, unspecified** HCC

✓6th **F14.18** **Cocaine abuse with other cocaine-induced disorder**

F14.180 **Cocaine abuse with cocaine-induced anxiety disorder** HCC

F14.181 **Cocaine abuse with cocaine-induced sexual dysfunction** HCC

F14.182 **Cocaine abuse with cocaine-induced sleep disorder** HCC

F14.188 **Cocaine abuse with other cocaine-induced disorder** HCC
Cocaine use disorder, mild, with cocaine-induced obsessive compulsive or related disorder

F14.19 **Cocaine abuse with unspecified cocaine-induced disorder** HCC

✓5th **F14.2 Cocaine dependence**

EXCLUDES 1 *cocaine abuse (F14.1-)*
cocaine use, unspecified (F14.9-)

EXCLUDES 2 *cocaine poisoning (T40.5-)*

F14.20 **Cocaine dependence, uncomplicated** CC HCC
Cocaine use disorder, moderate
Cocaine use disorder, severe

F14.21 **Cocaine dependence, in remission** HCC
Cocaine use disorder, moderate, in early remission
Cocaine use disorder, moderate, in sustained remission
Cocaine use disorder, severe, in early remission
Cocaine use disorder, severe, in sustained remission

✓6th **F14.22** **Cocaine dependence with intoxication**

EXCLUDES 1 *cocaine dependence with withdrawal (F14.23)*

F14.220 **Cocaine dependence with intoxication, uncomplicated** HCC

F14.221 **Cocaine dependence with intoxication delirium** CC HCC

F14.222 **Cocaine dependence with intoxication with perceptual disturbance** CC HCC

F14.229 **Cocaine dependence with intoxication, unspecified** CC HCC

F14.23 **Cocaine dependence with withdrawal** CC HCC

EXCLUDES 1 *cocaine dependence with intoxication (F14.22-)*

F14.24 **Cocaine dependence with cocaine-induced mood disorder** HCC
Cocaine use disorder, moderate, with cocaine-induced bipolar or related disorder
Cocaine use disorder, moderate, with cocaine-induced depressive disorder
Cocaine use disorder, severe, with cocaine-induced bipolar or related disorder
Cocaine use disorder, severe, with cocaine-induced depressive disorder

✓6th **F14.25** **Cocaine dependence with cocaine-induced psychotic disorder**

F14.250 **Cocaine dependence with cocaine-induced psychotic disorder with delusions** CC HCC

F14.251 **Cocaine dependence with cocaine-induced psychotic disorder with hallucinations** CC HCC

F14.259 **Cocaine dependence with cocaine-induced psychotic disorder, unspecified** CC HCC

✓6th **F14.28** **Cocaine dependence with other cocaine-induced disorder**

F14.280 **Cocaine dependence with cocaine-induced anxiety disorder** CC HCC

F14.281 **Cocaine dependence with cocaine-induced sexual dysfunction** CC HCC

F14.282 **Cocaine dependence with cocaine-induced sleep disorder** CC HCC

F14.288 **Cocaine dependence with other cocaine-induced disorder** CC HCC
Cocaine use disorder, moderate, with cocaine-induced obsessive compulsive or related disorder
Cocaine use disorder, severe, with cocaine-induced obsessive compulsive or related disorder

F14.29 **Cocaine dependence with unspecified cocaine-induced disorder** HCC

✓5th F14.9 **Cocaine use, unspecified**
EXCLUDES 1 *cocaine abuse (F14.1-)*
cocaine dependence (F14.2-)

TIP: Assign a substance use code only when the provider documents a relationship between the use and an associated physical, mental, or behavioral disorder. As with all diagnoses, substance use codes must meet the definition of a reportable diagnosis.

F14.90 **Cocaine use, unspecified, uncomplicated**
AHA: 2018,2Q,10-11

F14.91 **Cocaine use, unspecified, in remission**

✓6th F14.92 **Cocaine use, unspecified with intoxication**

F14.920 **Cocaine use, unspecified with intoxication, uncomplicated** HCC

F14.921 **Cocaine use, unspecified with intoxication delirium** CC HCC

F14.922 **Cocaine use, unspecified with intoxication with perceptual disturbance** HCC

F14.929 **Cocaine use, unspecified with intoxication, unspecified** HCC

F14.93 **Cocaine use, unspecified with withdrawal** CC HCC
AHA: 2020,4Q,16-17

F14.94 **Cocaine use, unspecified with cocaine-induced mood disorder** HCC
Cocaine induced bipolar or related disorder, without use disorder
Cocaine induced depressive disorder, without use disorder

✓6th F14.95 **Cocaine use, unspecified with cocaine-induced psychotic disorder**

F14.950 **Cocaine use, unspecified with cocaine-induced psychotic disorder with delusions** CC HCC

F14.951 **Cocaine use, unspecified with cocaine-induced psychotic disorder with hallucinations** CC HCC

F14.959 **Cocaine use, unspecified with cocaine-induced psychotic disorder, unspecified** HCC
Cocaine induced psychotic disorder, without use disorder

✓6th F14.98 **Cocaine use, unspecified with other specified cocaine-induced disorder**

F14.980 **Cocaine use, unspecified with cocaine-induced anxiety disorder** HCC
Cocaine induced anxiety disorder, without use disorder

F14.981 **Cocaine use, unspecified with cocaine-induced sexual dysfunction** HCC
Cocaine induced sexual dysfunction, without use disorder

F14.982 **Cocaine use, unspecified with cocaine-induced sleep disorder** HCC
Cocaine induced sleep disorder, without use disorder

F14.988 **Cocaine use, unspecified with other cocaine-induced disorder** HCC
Cocaine induced obsessive compulsive or related disorder

F14.99 **Cocaine use, unspecified with unspecified cocaine-induced disorder** HCC

✓4th **F15 Other stimulant related disorders**
INCLUDES amphetamine-related disorders
caffeine
EXCLUDES 2 *cocaine-related disorders (F14.-)*

✓5th F15.1 **Other stimulant abuse**
EXCLUDES 1 *other stimulant dependence (F15.2-)*
other stimulant use, unspecified (F15.9-)

F15.10 **Other stimulant abuse, uncomplicated** HCC
Amphetamine type substance use disorder, mild
Other or unspecified stimulant use disorder, mild

F15.11 **Other stimulant abuse, in remission** HCC
Amphetamine type substance use disorder, mild, in early remission
Amphetamine type substance use disorder, mild, in sustained remission
Other or unspecified stimulant use disorder, mild, in early remission
Other or unspecified stimulant use disorder, mild, in sustained remission
AHA: 2021,3Q,8

✓6th F15.12 **Other stimulant abuse with intoxication**

F15.120 **Other stimulant abuse with intoxication, uncomplicated** HCC

F15.121 **Other stimulant abuse with intoxication delirium** CC HCC

F15.122 **Other stimulant abuse with intoxication with perceptual disturbance** HCC
Amphetamine or other stimulant use disorder, mild, with amphetamine or other stimulant intoxication, with perceptual disturbances

F15.129 **Other stimulant abuse with intoxication, unspecified** HCC
Amphetamine or other stimulant use disorder, mild, with amphetamine or other stimulant intoxication, without perceptual disturbances

F15.13 **Other stimulant abuse with withdrawal** CC HCC
AHA: 2020,4Q,16-17

F15.14 **Other stimulant abuse with stimulant-induced mood disorder** HCC
Amphetamine or other stimulant use disorder, mild, with amphetamine or other stimulant induced bipolar or related disorder
Amphetamine or other stimulant use disorder, mild, with amphetamine or other stimulant induced depressive disorder

✓6th F15.15 **Other stimulant abuse with stimulant-induced psychotic disorder**

F15.150 **Other stimulant abuse with stimulant-induced psychotic disorder with delusions** CC HCC

F15.151 **Other stimulant abuse with stimulant-induced psychotic disorder with hallucinations** CC HCC

F15.159 **Other stimulant abuse with stimulant-induced psychotic disorder, unspecified** HCC

✓6th F15.18 **Other stimulant abuse with other stimulant-induced disorder**

F15.180 **Other stimulant abuse with stimulant-induced anxiety disorder** HCC

F15.181 **Other stimulant abuse with stimulant-induced sexual dysfunction** HCC

F15.182 **Other stimulant abuse with stimulant-induced sleep disorder** HCC

F15.188 **Other stimulant abuse with other stimulant-induced disorder** HCC
Amphetamine or other stimulant use disorder, mild, with amphetamine or other stimulant induced obsessive-compulsive or related disorder

F15.19 **Other stimulant abuse with unspecified stimulant-induced disorder** HCC

✓5th **F15.2 Other stimulant dependence**

EXCLUDES 1 *other stimulant abuse (F15.1-)*
other stimulant use, unspecified (F15.9-)

F15.20 Other stimulant dependence, uncomplicated CC HCC
Amphetamine type substance use disorder, moderate
Amphetamine type substance use disorder, severe
Other or unspecified stimulant use disorder, moderate
Other or unspecified stimulant use disorder, severe

F15.21 Other stimulant dependence, in remission HCC
Amphetamine type substance use disorder, moderate, in early remission
Amphetamine type substance use disorder, moderate, in sustained remission
Amphetamine type substance use disorder, severe, in early remission
Amphetamine type substance use disorder, severe, in sustained remission
Other or unspecified stimulant use disorder, moderate, in early remission
Other or unspecified stimulant use disorder, moderate, in sustained remission
Other or unspecified stimulant use disorder, severe, in early remission
Other or unspecified stimulant use disorder, severe, in sustained remission

✓6th **F15.22 Other stimulant dependence with intoxication**

EXCLUDES 1 *other stimulant dependence with withdrawal (F15.23)*

F15.220 Other stimulant dependence with intoxication, uncomplicated HCC

F15.221 Other stimulant dependence with intoxication delirium CC HCC

F15.222 Other stimulant dependence with intoxication with perceptual disturbance CC HCC
Amphetamine or other stimulant use disorder, moderate, with amphetamine or other stimulant intoxication, with perceptual disturbances
Amphetamine or other stimulant use disorder, severe, with amphetamine or other stimulant intoxication, with perceptual disturbances

F15.229 Other stimulant dependence with intoxication, unspecified HCC
Amphetamine or other stimulant use disorder, moderate, with amphetamine or other stimulant intoxication, without perceptual disturbances
Amphetamine or other stimulant use disorder, severe, with amphetamine or other stimulant intoxication, without perceptual disturbances

F15.23 Other stimulant dependence with withdrawal CC HCC
Amphetamine or other stimulant withdrawal

EXCLUDES 1 *other stimulant dependence with intoxication (F15.22-)*

F15.24 Other stimulant dependence with stimulant-induced mood disorder HCC
Amphetamine or other stimulant use disorder, moderate, with amphetamine or other stimulant-induced bipolar or related disorder
Amphetamine or other stimulant use disorder, moderate, with amphetamine or other stimulant induced depressive disorder
Amphetamine or other stimulant use disorder, severe, with amphetamine or other stimulant-induced bipolar or related disorder
Amphetamine or other stimulant use disorder, severe, with amphetamine or other stimulant-induced depressive disorder

✓6th **F15.25 Other stimulant dependence with stimulant-induced psychotic disorder**

F15.250 Other stimulant dependence with stimulant-induced psychotic disorder with delusions CC HCC

F15.251 Other stimulant dependence with stimulant-induced psychotic disorder with hallucinations CC HCC

F15.259 Other stimulant dependence with stimulant-induced psychotic disorder, unspecified CC HCC

✓6th **F15.28 Other stimulant dependence with other stimulant-induced disorder**

F15.280 Other stimulant dependence with stimulant-induced anxiety disorder CC HCC

F15.281 Other stimulant dependence with stimulant-induced sexual dysfunction CC HCC

F15.282 Other stimulant dependence with stimulant-induced sleep disorder CC HCC

F15.288 Other stimulant dependence with other stimulant-induced disorder CC HCC
Amphetamine or other stimulant use disorder, moderate, with amphetamine orother stimulant induced obsessive compulsive or related disorder
Amphetamine or other stimulant use disorder, severe, with amphetamine or otherstimulant induced obsessive compulsive or related disorder

F15.29 Other stimulant dependence with unspecified stimulant-induced disorder HCC

✓5th **F15.9 Other stimulant use, unspecified**

EXCLUDES 1 *other stimulant abuse (F15.1-)*
other stimulant dependence (F15.2-)

TIP: Assign a substance use code only when the provider documents a relationship between the use and an associated physical, mental, or behavioral disorder. As with all diagnoses, substance use codes must meet the definition of a reportable diagnosis.

F15.90 Other stimulant use, unspecified, uncomplicated
AHA: 2018,2Q,10-11

F15.91 Other stimulant use, unspecified, in remission

✓6th **F15.92 Other stimulant use, unspecified with intoxication**

EXCLUDES 1 *other stimulant use, unspecified with withdrawal (F15.93)*

F15.920 Other stimulant use, unspecified with intoxication, uncomplicated HCC

F15.921 Other stimulant use, unspecified with intoxication delirium CC HCC
Amphetamine or other stimulant-induced delirium

F15.922 Other stimulant use, unspecified with intoxication with perceptual disturbance HCC

F15.929 Other stimulant use, unspecified with intoxication, unspecified HCC
Caffeine intoxication

F15.93 Other stimulant use, unspecified with withdrawal CC HCC
Caffeine withdrawal

EXCLUDES 1 *other stimulant use, unspecified with intoxication (F15.92-)*

F15.94 Other stimulant use, unspecified with stimulant-induced mood disorder HCC
Amphetamine or other stimulant-induced bipolar or related disorder, without use disorder
Amphetamine or other stimulant-induced depressive disorder, without use disorder

✓6th **F15.95 Other stimulant use, unspecified with stimulant-induced psychotic disorder**

F15.950 Other stimulant use, unspecified with stimulant-induced psychotic disorder with delusions CC HCC

F15.951 Other stimulant use, unspecified with stimulant-induced psychotic disorder with hallucinations CC HCC

F15.959 Other stimulant use, unspecified with stimulant-induced psychotic disorder, unspecified HCC
Amphetamine or other stimulant-induced psychotic disorder, without use disorder

√6th **F15.98 Other stimulant use, unspecified with other stimulant-induced disorder**

F15.980 Other stimulant use, unspecified with stimulant-induced anxiety disorder HCC
Amphetamine or other stimulant-induced anxiety disorder, without use disorder
Caffeine induced anxiety disorder, without use disorder

F15.981 Other stimulant use, unspecified with stimulant-induced sexual dysfunction HCC
Amphetamine or other stimulant-induced sexual dysfunction, without use disorder

F15.982 Other stimulant use, unspecified with stimulant-induced sleep disorder HCC
Amphetamine or other stimulant-induced sleep disorder, without use disorder
Caffeine induced sleep disorder, without use disorder

F15.988 Other stimulant use, unspecified with other stimulant-induced disorder HCC
Amphetamine or other stimulant-induced obsessive compulsive or related disorder, without use disorder

F15.99 Other stimulant use, unspecified with unspecified stimulant-induced disorder HCC

√4th **F16 Hallucinogen related disorders**

INCLUDES ecstasy
PCP
phencyclidine

AHA: 2018,4Q,31

√5th **F16.1 Hallucinogen abuse**

EXCLUDES 1 *hallucinogen dependence (F16.2-)*
hallucinogen use, unspecified (F16.9-)

F16.10 Hallucinogen abuse, uncomplicated HCC
Other hallucinogen use disorder, mild
Phencyclidine use disorder, mild

F16.11 Hallucinogen abuse, in remission HCC
Other hallucinogen use disorder, mild, in early remission
Other hallucinogen use disorder, mild, in sustained remission
Phencyclidine use disorder, mild, in early remission
Phencyclidine use disorder, mild, in sustained remission

√6th **F16.12 Hallucinogen abuse with intoxication**

F16.120 Hallucinogen abuse with intoxication, uncomplicated HCC

F16.121 Hallucinogen abuse with intoxication with delirium CC HCC

F16.122 Hallucinogen abuse with intoxication with perceptual disturbance HCC

F16.129 Hallucinogen abuse with intoxication, unspecified HCC

F16.14 Hallucinogen abuse with hallucinogen-induced mood disorder HCC
Other hallucinogen use disorder, mild, with other hallucinogen induced bipolar or related disorder
Other hallucinogen use disorder, mild, with other hallucinogen induced depressive disorder
Phencyclidine use disorder, mild, with phencyclidine induced bipolar or related disorder
Phencyclidine use disorder, mild, with phencyclidine induced depressive disorder

√6th **F16.15 Hallucinogen abuse with hallucinogen-induced psychotic disorder**

F16.150 Hallucinogen abuse with hallucinogen-induced psychotic disorder with delusions CC HCC

F16.151 Hallucinogen abuse with hallucinogen-induced psychotic disorder with hallucinations CC HCC

F16.159 Hallucinogen abuse with hallucinogen-induced psychotic disorder, unspecified HCC

√6th **F16.18 Hallucinogen abuse with other hallucinogen-induced disorder**

F16.180 Hallucinogen abuse with hallucinogen-induced anxiety disorder HCC

F16.183 Hallucinogen abuse with hallucinogen persisting perception disorder (flashbacks) HCC

F16.188 Hallucinogen abuse with other hallucinogen-induced disorder HCC

F16.19 Hallucinogen abuse with unspecified hallucinogen-induced disorder HCC

√5th **F16.2 Hallucinogen dependence**

EXCLUDES 1 *hallucinogen abuse (F16.1-)*
hallucinogen use, unspecified (F16.9-)

F16.20 Hallucinogen dependence, uncomplicated CC HCC
Other hallucinogen use disorder, moderate
Other hallucinogen use disorder, severe
Phencyclidine use disorder, moderate
Phencyclidine use disorder, severe

F16.21 Hallucinogen dependence, in remission HCC
Other hallucinogen use disorder, moderate, in early remission
Other hallucinogen use disorder, moderate, in sustained remission
Other hallucinogen use disorder, severe, in early remission
Other hallucinogen use disorder, severe, in sustained remission
Phencyclidine use disorder, moderate, in early remission
Phencyclidine use disorder, moderate, in sustained remission
Phencyclidine use disorder, severe, in early remission
Phencyclidine use disorder, severe, in sustained remission

√6th **F16.22 Hallucinogen dependence with intoxication**

F16.220 Hallucinogen dependence with intoxication, uncomplicated HCC

F16.221 Hallucinogen dependence with intoxication with delirium CC HCC

F16.229 Hallucinogen dependence with intoxication, unspecified HCC

F16.24 Hallucinogen dependence with hallucinogen-induced mood disorder HCC
Other hallucinogen use disorder, moderate, with other hallucinogen induced bipolar or related disorder
Other hallucinogen use disorder, moderate, with other hallucinogen induced depressive disorder
Other hallucinogen use disorder, severe, with other hallucinogen-induced bipolar or related disorder
Other hallucinogen use disorder, severe, with other hallucinogen-induced depressive disorder
Phencyclidine use disorder, moderate, with phencyclidine induced bipolar or related disorder
Phencyclidine use disorder, moderate, with phencyclidine induced depressive disorder
Phencyclidine use disorder, severe, with phencyclidine induced bipolar or related disorder
Phencyclidine use disorder, severe, with phencyclidine-induced depressive disorder

√6th **F16.25 Hallucinogen dependence with hallucinogen-induced psychotic disorder**

F16.250 Hallucinogen dependence with hallucinogen-induced psychotic disorder with delusions CC HCC

F16.251 Hallucinogen dependence with hallucinogen-induced psychotic disorder with hallucinations CC HCC

F16.259 Hallucinogen dependence with hallucinogen-induced psychotic disorder, unspecified CC HCC

√6th **F16.28 Hallucinogen dependence with other hallucinogen-induced disorder**

F16.280 Hallucinogen dependence with hallucinogen-induced anxiety disorder CC HCC

F16.283 Hallucinogen dependence with hallucinogen persisting perception disorder (flashbacks) CC HCC

F16.288 Hallucinogen dependence with other hallucinogen-induced disorder CC HCC

F16.29 Hallucinogen dependence with unspecified hallucinogen-induced disorder HCC

✓5th **F16.9 Hallucinogen use, unspecified**

EXCLUDES 1 *hallucinogen abuse (F16.1-)*
hallucinogen dependence (F16.2-)

TIP: Assign a substance use code only when the provider documents a relationship between the use and an associated physical, mental, or behavioral disorder. As with all diagnoses, substance use codes must meet the definition of a reportable diagnosis.

F16.90 Hallucinogen use, unspecified, uncomplicated
AHA: 2018,2Q,10-11

F16.91 Hallucinogen use, unspecified, in remission

✓6th **F16.92 Hallucinogen use, unspecified with intoxication**

F16.920 Hallucinogen use, unspecified with intoxication, uncomplicated HCC

F16.921 Hallucinogen use, unspecified with intoxication with delirium CC HCC
Other hallucinogen intoxication delirium

F16.929 Hallucinogen use, unspecified with intoxication, unspecified HCC

F16.94 Hallucinogen use, unspecified with hallucinogen-induced mood disorder HCC
Other hallucinogen induced bipolar or related disorder, without use disorder
Other hallucinogen induced depressive disorder, without use disorder
Phencyclidine induced bipolar or related disorder, without use disorder
Phencyclidine induced depressive disorder, without use disorder

✓6th **F16.95 Hallucinogen use, unspecified with hallucinogen-induced psychotic disorder**

F16.950 Hallucinogen use, unspecified with hallucinogen-induced psychotic disorder with delusions CC HCC

F16.951 Hallucinogen use, unspecified with hallucinogen-induced psychotic disorder with hallucinations CC HCC

F16.959 Hallucinogen use, unspecified with hallucinogen-induced psychotic disorder, unspecified HCC
Other hallucinogen induced psychotic disorder, without use disorder
Phencyclidine induced psychotic disorder, without use disorder

✓6th **F16.98 Hallucinogen use, unspecified with other specified hallucinogen-induced disorder**

F16.980 Hallucinogen use, unspecified with hallucinogen-induced anxiety disorder HCC
Other hallucinogen-induced anxiety disorder, without use disorder
Phencyclidine induced anxiety disorder, without use disorder

F16.983 Hallucinogen use, unspecified with hallucinogen persisting perception disorder (flashbacks) HCC

F16.988 Hallucinogen use, unspecified with other hallucinogen-induced disorder HCC

F16.99 Hallucinogen use, unspecified with unspecified hallucinogen-induced disorder HCC

✓4th **F17 Nicotine dependence**

EXCLUDES 1 *history of tobacco dependence (Z87.891)*
tobacco use NOS (Z72.0)

EXCLUDES 2 *tobacco use (smoking) during pregnancy, childbirth and the puerperium (O99.33-)*
toxic effect of nicotine (T65.2-)

AHA: 2013,4Q,108-109

✓5th **F17.2 Nicotine dependence**

✓6th **F17.20 Nicotine dependence, unspecified**

F17.200 Nicotine dependence, unspecified, uncomplicated UPD
Tobacco use disorder, mild
Tobacco use disorder, moderate
Tobacco use disorder, severe
AHA: 2016,1Q,36
TIP: Assign when provider documentation indicates "smoker" without further specification.

F17.201 Nicotine dependence, unspecified, in remission UPD
Tobacco use disorder, mild, in early remission
Tobacco use disorder, mild, in sustained remission
Tobacco use disorder, moderate, in early remission
Tobacco use disorder, moderate, in sustained remission
Tobacco use disorder, severe, in early remission
Tobacco use disorder, severe, in sustained remission

F17.203 Nicotine dependence unspecified, with withdrawal CC
Tobacco withdrawal

F17.208 Nicotine dependence, unspecified, with other nicotine-induced disorders

F17.209 Nicotine dependence, unspecified, with unspecified nicotine-induced disorders

✓6th **F17.21 Nicotine dependence, cigarettes**

F17.210 Nicotine dependence, cigarettes, uncomplicated UPD
AHA: 2017,2Q,28-29

F17.211 Nicotine dependence, cigarettes, in remission UPD
Tobacco use disorder, cigarettes, mild, in early remission
Tobacco use disorder, cigarettes, mild, in sustained remission
Tobacco use disorder, cigarettes, moderate, in early remission
Tobacco use disorder, cigarettes, moderate, in sustained remission
Tobacco use disorder, cigarettes, severe, in early remission
Tobacco use disorder, cigarettes, severe, in sustained remission

F17.213 Nicotine dependence, cigarettes, with withdrawal CC

F17.218 Nicotine dependence, cigarettes, with other nicotine-induced disorders

F17.219 Nicotine dependence, cigarettes, with unspecified nicotine-induced disorders

✓6th **F17.22 Nicotine dependence, chewing tobacco**

F17.220 Nicotine dependence, chewing tobacco, uncomplicated UPD

F17.221 Nicotine dependence, chewing tobacco, in remission UPD
Tobacco use disorder, chewing tobacco, mild, in early remission
Tobacco use disorder, chewing tobacco, mild, in sustained remission
Tobacco use disorder, chewing tobacco, moderate, in early remission
Tobacco use disorder, chewing tobacco, moderate, in sustained remission
Tobacco use disorder, chewing tobacco, severe, in early remission
Tobacco use disorder, chewing tobacco, severe, in sustained remission

F17.223 Nicotine dependence, chewing tobacco, with withdrawal CC

F17.228 Nicotine dependence, chewing tobacco, with other nicotine-induced disorders

F17.229 Nicotine dependence, chewing tobacco, with unspecified nicotine-induced disorders

✓6th **F17.29 Nicotine dependence, other tobacco product**

F17.290 Nicotine dependence, other tobacco product, uncomplicated UPD

AHA: 2017,2Q,28-29

F17.291 Nicotine dependence, other tobacco product, in remission UPD

Tobacco use disorder, other tobacco product, mild, in early remission

Tobacco use disorder, other tobacco product, mild, in sustained remission

Tobacco use disorder, other tobacco product, moderate, in early remission

Tobacco use disorder, other tobacco product, moderate, in sustained remission

Tobacco use disorder, other tobacco product, severe, in early remission

Tobacco use disorder, other tobacco product, severe, in sustained remission

F17.293 Nicotine dependence, other tobacco product, with withdrawal CC

F17.298 Nicotine dependence, other tobacco product, with other nicotine-induced disorders

F17.299 Nicotine dependence, other tobacco product, with unspecified nicotine-induced disorders

✓4th **F18 Inhalant related disorders**

INCLUDES volatile solvents

✓5th **F18.1 Inhalant abuse**

EXCLUDES 1 *inhalant dependence (F18.2-)*
inhalant use, unspecified (F18.9-)

F18.10 Inhalant abuse, uncomplicated HCC

Inhalant use disorder, mild

F18.11 Inhalant abuse, in remission HCC

Inhalant use disorder, mild, in early remission

Inhalant use disorder, mild, in sustained remission

✓6th **F18.12 Inhalant abuse with intoxication**

F18.120 Inhalant abuse with intoxication, uncomplicated HCC

F18.121 Inhalant abuse with intoxication delirium CC HCC

F18.129 Inhalant abuse with intoxication, unspecified HCC

F18.14 Inhalant abuse with inhalant-induced mood disorder HCC

Inhalant use disorder, mild, with inhalant induced depressive disorder

✓6th **F18.15 Inhalant abuse with inhalant-induced psychotic disorder**

F18.150 Inhalant abuse with inhalant-induced psychotic disorder with delusions CC HCC

F18.151 Inhalant abuse with inhalant-induced psychotic disorder with hallucinations CC HCC

F18.159 Inhalant abuse with inhalant-induced psychotic disorder, unspecified HCC

F18.17 Inhalant abuse with inhalant-induced dementia CC HCC

Inhalant use disorder, mild, with inhalant induced major neurocognitive disorder

✓6th **F18.18 Inhalant abuse with other inhalant-induced disorders**

F18.180 Inhalant abuse with inhalant-induced anxiety disorder HCC

F18.188 Inhalant abuse with other inhalant-induced disorder HCC

Inhalant use disorder, mild, with inhalant induced mild neurocognitive disorder

F18.19 Inhalant abuse with unspecified inhalant-induced disorder HCC

✓5th **F18.2 Inhalant dependence**

EXCLUDES 1 *inhalant abuse (F18.1-)*
inhalant use, unspecified (F18.9-)

F18.20 Inhalant dependence, uncomplicated CC HCC

Inhalant use disorder, moderate

Inhalant use disorder, severe

F18.21 Inhalant dependence, in remission HCC

Inhalant use disorder, moderate, in early remission

Inhalant use disorder, moderate, in sustained remission

Inhalant use disorder, severe, in early remission

Inhalant use disorder, severe, in sustained remission

✓6th **F18.22 Inhalant dependence with intoxication**

F18.220 Inhalant dependence with intoxication, uncomplicated HCC

F18.221 Inhalant dependence with intoxication delirium CC HCC

F18.229 Inhalant dependence with intoxication, unspecified HCC

F18.24 Inhalant dependence with inhalant-induced mood disorder HCC

Inhalant use disorder, moderate, with inhalant induced depressive disorder

Inhalant use disorder, severe, with inhalant induced depressive disorder

✓6th **F18.25 Inhalant dependence with inhalant-induced psychotic disorder**

F18.250 Inhalant dependence with inhalant-induced psychotic disorder with delusions CC HCC

F18.251 Inhalant dependence with inhalant-induced psychotic disorder with hallucinations CC HCC

F18.259 Inhalant dependence with inhalant-induced psychotic disorder, unspecified CC HCC

F18.27 Inhalant dependence with inhalant-induced dementia CC HCC

Inhalant use disorder, moderate, with inhalant induced major neurocognitive disorder

Inhalant use disorder, severe, with inhalant induced major neurocognitive disorder

✓6th **F18.28 Inhalant dependence with other inhalant-induced disorders**

F18.280 Inhalant dependence with inhalant-induced anxiety disorder CC HCC

F18.288 Inhalant dependence with other inhalant-induced disorder CC HCC

Inhalant use disorder, moderate, with inhalant-induced mild neurocognitive disorder

Inhalant use disorder, severe, with inhalant-induced mild neurocognitive disorder

F18.29 Inhalant dependence with unspecified inhalant-induced disorder HCC

✓5th **F18.9 Inhalant use, unspecified**

EXCLUDES 1 *inhalant abuse (F18.1-)*
inhalant dependence (F18.2-)

TIP: Assign a substance use code only when the provider documents a relationship between the use and an associated physical, mental, or behavioral disorder. As with all diagnoses, substance use codes must meet the definition of a reportable diagnosis.

F18.90 Inhalant use, unspecified, uncomplicated

AHA: 2018,2Q,10-11

F18.91 Inhalant use, unspecified, in remission

✓6th **F18.92 Inhalant use, unspecified with intoxication**

F18.920 Inhalant use, unspecified with intoxication, uncomplicated HCC

F18.921 Inhalant use, unspecified with intoxication with delirium CC HCC

F18.929 Inhalant use, unspecified with intoxication, unspecified HCC

F18.94 Inhalant use, unspecified with inhalant-induced mood disorder HCC

Inhalant induced depressive disorder

√6th **F18.95 Inhalant use, unspecified with inhalant-induced psychotic disorder**

F18.950 Inhalant use, unspecified with inhalant-induced psychotic disorder with delusions CC HCC

F18.951 Inhalant use, unspecified with inhalant-induced psychotic disorder with hallucinations CC HCC

F18.959 Inhalant use, unspecified with inhalant-induced psychotic disorder, unspecified HCC

F18.97 Inhalant use, unspecified with inhalant-induced persisting dementia CC HCC

Inhalant-induced major neurocognitive disorder

√6th **F18.98 Inhalant use, unspecified with other inhalant-induced disorders**

F18.980 Inhalant use, unspecified with inhalant-induced anxiety disorder HCC

F18.988 Inhalant use, unspecified with other inhalant-induced disorder HCC

Inhalant-induced mild neurocognitive disorder

F18.99 Inhalant use, unspecified with unspecified inhalant-induced disorder HCC

√4th **F19 Other psychoactive substance related disorders**

INCLUDES polysubstance drug use (indiscriminate drug use)

√5th **F19.1 Other psychoactive substance abuse**

EXCLUDES 1 *other psychoactive substance dependence (F19.2-)*
other psychoactive substance use, unspecified (F19.9-)

F19.10 Other psychoactive substance abuse, uncomplicated HCC

Other (or unknown) substance use disorder, mild

F19.11 Other psychoactive substance abuse, in remission HCC

Other (or unknown) substance use disorder, mild, in early remission

Other (or unknown) substance use disorder, mild, in sustained remission

√6th **F19.12 Other psychoactive substance abuse with intoxication**

F19.120 Other psychoactive substance abuse with intoxication, uncomplicated HCC

F19.121 Other psychoactive substance abuse with intoxication delirium CC HCC

F19.122 Other psychoactive substance abuse with intoxication with perceptual disturbances HCC

F19.129 Other psychoactive substance abuse with intoxication, unspecified HCC

√6th **F19.13 Other psychoactive substance abuse with withdrawal**

AHA: 2020,4Q,16-17

F19.130 Other psychoactive substance abuse with withdrawal, uncomplicated CC HCC

F19.131 Other psychoactive substance abuse with withdrawal delirium CC HCC

F19.132 Other psychoactive substance abuse with withdrawal with perceptual disturbance CC HCC

F19.139 Other psychoactive substance abuse with withdrawal, unspecified CC HCC

F19.14 Other psychoactive substance abuse with psychoactive substance-induced mood disorder HCC

Other (or unknown) substance use disorder, mild, with other (or unknown) substance-induced bipolar or related disorder

Other (or unknown) substance use disorder, mild, with other (or unknown) substance-induced depressive disorder

√6th **F19.15 Other psychoactive substance abuse with psychoactive substance-induced psychotic disorder**

F19.150 Other psychoactive substance abuse with psychoactive substance-induced psychotic disorder with delusions CC HCC

F19.151 Other psychoactive substance abuse with psychoactive substance-induced psychotic disorder with hallucinations CC HCC

F19.159 Other psychoactive substance abuse with psychoactive substance-induced psychotic disorder, unspecified HCC

F19.16 Other psychoactive substance abuse with psychoactive substance-induced persisting amnestic disorder HCC

F19.17 Other psychoactive substance abuse with psychoactive substance-induced persisting dementia CC HCC

Other (or unknown) substance use disorder, mild, with other (or unknown) substance-induced major neurocognitive disorder

√6th **F19.18 Other psychoactive substance abuse with other psychoactive substance-induced disorders**

F19.180 Other psychoactive substance abuse with psychoactive substance-induced anxiety disorder HCC

F19.181 Other psychoactive substance abuse with psychoactive substance-induced sexual dysfunction HCC

F19.182 Other psychoactive substance abuse with psychoactive substance-induced sleep disorder HCC

F19.188 Other psychoactive substance abuse with other psychoactive substance-induced disorder HCC

Other (or unknown) substance use disorder, mild, with other (or unknown) substance induced mild neurocognitive disorder

Other (or unknown) substance use disorder, mild, with other (or unknown) substance induced obsessive-compulsive or related disorder

F19.19 Other psychoactive substance abuse with unspecified psychoactive substance-induced disorder HCC

√5th **F19.2 Other psychoactive substance dependence**

EXCLUDES 1 *other psychoactive substance abuse (F19.1-)*
other psychoactive substance use, unspecified (F19.9-)

F19.20 Other psychoactive substance dependence, uncomplicated CC HCC

Other (or unknown) substance use disorder, moderate

Other (or unknown) substance use disorder, severe

F19.21 Other psychoactive substance dependence, in remission HCC

Other (or unknown) substance use disorder, moderate, in early remission

Other (or unknown) substance use disorder, moderate, in sustained remission

Other (or unknown) substance use disorder, severe, in early remission

Other (or unknown) substance use disorder, severe, in sustained remission

√6th **F19.22 Other psychoactive substance dependence with intoxication**

EXCLUDES 1 *other psychoactive substance dependence with withdrawal (F19.23-)*

F19.220 Other psychoactive substance dependence with intoxication, uncomplicated HCC

F19.221 Other psychoactive substance dependence with intoxication delirium CC HCC

F19.222 Other psychoactive substance dependence with intoxication with perceptual disturbance CC HCC

F19.229 Other psychoactive substance dependence with intoxication, unspecified HCC

√6th **F19.23 Other psychoactive substance dependence with withdrawal**

EXCLUDES 1 *other psychoactive substance dependence with intoxication (F19.22-)*

F19.230 Other psychoactive substance dependence with withdrawal, uncomplicated CC HCC

F19.231 Other psychoactive substance dependence with withdrawal delirium CC HCC

F19.232 Other psychoactive substance dependence with withdrawal with perceptual disturbance CC HCC

F19.239 Other psychoactive substance dependence with withdrawal, unspecified CC HCC

F19.24 Other psychoactive substance dependence with psychoactive substance-induced mood disorder HCC

Other (or unknown) substance use disorder, moderate, with other (or unknown) substance induced bipolar or related disorder

Other (or unknown) substance use disorder, moderate, with other (or unknown) substance induced depressive disorder

Other (or unknown) substance use disorder, severe, with other (or unknown) substance induced bipolar or related disorder

Other (or unknown) substance use disorder, severe, with other (or unknown) substance induced depressive disorder

✓6th **F19.25 Other psychoactive substance dependence with psychoactive substance-induced psychotic disorder**

F19.250 Other psychoactive substance dependence with psychoactive substance-induced psychotic disorder with delusions CC HCC

F19.251 Other psychoactive substance dependence with psychoactive substance-induced psychotic disorder with hallucinations CC HCC

F19.259 Other psychoactive substance dependence with psychoactive substance-induced psychotic disorder, unspecified CC HCC

F19.26 Other psychoactive substance dependence with psychoactive substance-induced persisting amnestic disorder CC HCC

F19.27 Other psychoactive substance dependence with psychoactive substance-induced persisting dementia CC HCC

Other (or unknown) substance use disorder, moderate, with other (or unknown) substance induced major neurocognitive disorder

Other (or unknown) substance use disorder, severe, with other (or unknown) substance induced major neurocognitive disorder

✓6th **F19.28 Other psychoactive substance dependence with other psychoactive substance-induced disorders**

F19.280 Other psychoactive substance dependence with psychoactive substance-induced anxiety disorder CC HCC

F19.281 Other psychoactive substance dependence with psychoactive substance-induced sexual dysfunction CC HCC

F19.282 Other psychoactive substance dependence with psychoactive substance-induced sleep disorder CC HCC

F19.288 Other psychoactive substance dependence with other psychoactive substance-induced disorder CC HCC

Other (or unknown) substance use disorder, moderate, with other (or unknown) substance induced mild neurocognitive disorder

Other (or unknown) substance use disorder, severe, with other (or unknown) substance induced mild neurocognitive disorder

Other (or unknown) substance use disorder, moderate, with other (or unknown) substance induced obsessive compulsive or related disorder

Other (or unknown) substance use disorder, severe, with other (or unknown) substance induced obsessive-compulsive or related disorder

F19.29 Other psychoactive substance dependence with unspecified psychoactive substance-induced disorder HCC

✓5th **F19.9 Other psychoactive substance use, unspecified**

EXCLUDES 1 *other psychoactive substance abuse (F19.1-)*
other psychoactive substance dependence (F19.2-)

TIP: Assign a substance use code only when the provider documents a relationship between the use and an associated physical, mental, or behavioral disorder. As with all diagnoses, substance use codes must meet the definition of a reportable diagnosis.

F19.90 Other psychoactive substance use, unspecified, uncomplicated

AHA: 2018,2Q,10-11

F19.91 Other psychoactive substance use, unspecified, in remission

✓6th **F19.92 Other psychoactive substance use, unspecified with intoxication**

EXCLUDES 1 *other psychoactive substance use, unspecified with withdrawal (F19.93)*

F19.920 Other psychoactive substance use, unspecified with intoxication, uncomplicated HCC

F19.921 Other psychoactive substance use, unspecified with intoxication with delirium CC HCC

Other (or unknown) substance-induced delirium

F19.922 Other psychoactive substance use, unspecified with intoxication with perceptual disturbance HCC

F19.929 Other psychoactive substance use, unspecified with intoxication, unspecified HCC

✓6th **F19.93 Other psychoactive substance use, unspecified with withdrawal**

EXCLUDES 1 *other psychoactive substance use, unspecified with intoxication (F19.92-)*

F19.930 Other psychoactive substance use, unspecified with withdrawal, uncomplicated CC HCC

F19.931 Other psychoactive substance use, unspecified with withdrawal delirium CC HCC

F19.932 Other psychoactive substance use, unspecified with withdrawal with perceptual disturbance CC HCC

F19.939 Other psychoactive substance use, unspecified with withdrawal, unspecified CC HCC

F19.94 Other psychoactive substance use, unspecified with psychoactive substance-induced mood disorder HCC

Other (or unknown) substance-induced bipolar or related disorder, without use disorder

Other (or unknown) substance-induced depressive disorder, without use disorder

✓6th **F19.95 Other psychoactive substance use, unspecified with psychoactive substance-induced psychotic disorder**

F19.950 Other psychoactive substance use, unspecified with psychoactive substance-induced psychotic disorder with delusions CC HCC

F19.951 Other psychoactive substance use, unspecified with psychoactive substance-induced psychotic disorder with hallucinations CC HCC

F19.959 Other psychoactive substance use, unspecified with psychoactive substance-induced psychotic disorder, unspecified HCC

Other or unknown substance-induced psychotic disorder, without use disorder

F19.96 Other psychoactive substance use, unspecified with psychoactive substance-induced persisting amnestic disorder HCC

F19.97 Other psychoactive substance use, unspecified with psychoactive substance-induced persisting dementia CC HCC
Other (or unknown) substance-induced major neurocognitive disorder, without use disorder

✓6th **F19.98 Other psychoactive substance use, unspecified with other psychoactive substance-induced disorders**

F19.980 Other psychoactive substance use, unspecified with psychoactive substance-induced anxiety disorder HCC
Other (or unknown) substance-induced anxiety disorder, without use disorder

F19.981 Other psychoactive substance use, unspecified with psychoactive substance-induced sexual dysfunction HCC
Other (or unknown) substance-induced sexual dysfunction, without use disorder

F19.982 Other psychoactive substance use, unspecified with psychoactive substance-induced sleep disorder HCC
Other (or unknown) substance-induced sleep disorder, without use disorder

F19.988 Other psychoactive substance use, unspecified with other psychoactive substance-induced disorder HCC
Other (or unknown) substance-induced mild neurocognitive disorder, without use disorder
Other (or unknown) substance-induced obsessive-compulsive or related disorder, without use disorder

F19.99 Other psychoactive substance use, unspecified with unspecified psychoactive substance-induced disorder HCC

Schizophrenia, schizotypal, delusional, and other non-mood psychotic disorders (F20-F29)

✓4th **F20 Schizophrenia**

EXCLUDES 1 *brief psychotic disorder (F23)*
cyclic schizophrenia (F25.0)
mood [affective] disorders with psychotic symptoms (F30.2, F31.2, F31.5, F31.64, F32.3, F33.3)
schizoaffective disorder (F25.-)
schizophrenic reaction NOS (F23)

EXCLUDES 2 *schizophrenic reaction in:*
alcoholism (F10.15-, F10.25-, F10.95-)
brain disease (F06.2)
epilepsy (F06.2)
psychoactive drug use (F11-F19 with .15, .25, .95)
schizotypal disorder (F21)

DEF: Group of disorders with disturbances in thought (delusions, hallucinations), mood (blunted, flattened, inappropriate affect), and sense of self. Schizophrenia also includes bizarre, purposeless behavior, repetitious activity, or inactivity.

F20.0 Paranoid schizophrenia CC HCC
Paraphrenic schizophrenia
EXCLUDES 1 *involutional paranoid state (F22)*
paranoia (F22)
DEF: Preoccupied with delusional suspicions and auditory hallucinations related to a single theme. This type of schizophrenia is usually hostile, grandiose, threatening, persecutory, and occasionally hypochondriacal.

F20.1 Disorganized schizophrenia CC HCC
Hebephrenic schizophrenia
Hebephrenia

F20.2 Catatonic schizophrenia CC HCC
Schizophrenic catalepsy
Schizophrenic catatonia
Schizophrenic flexibilitas cerea
EXCLUDES 1 *catatonic stupor (R40.1)*
DEF: Extreme changes in motor activity. One extreme is a decreased response or reaction to the environment and the other is spontaneous activity.

F20.3 Undifferentiated schizophrenia HCC
Atypical schizophrenia
EXCLUDES 1 *acute schizophrenia-like psychotic disorder (F23)*
EXCLUDES 2 *post-schizophrenic depression (F32.89)*

F20.5 Residual schizophrenia CC HCC
Restzustand (schizophrenic)
Schizophrenic residual state

✓5th **F20.8 Other schizophrenia**

F20.81 Schizophreniform disorder CC HCC
Schizophreniform psychosis NOS

F20.89 Other schizophrenia CC HCC
Cenesthopathic schizophrenia
Simple schizophrenia

F20.9 Schizophrenia, unspecified HCC
AHA: 2019,2Q,32

F21 Schizotypal disorder HCC
Borderline schizophrenia
Latent schizophrenia
Latent schizophrenic reaction
Prepsychotic schizophrenia
Prodromal schizophrenia
Pseudoneurotic schizophrenia
Pseudopsychopathic schizophrenia
Schizotypal personality disorder
EXCLUDES 2 *Asperger's syndrome (F84.5)*
schizoid personality disorder (F60.1)
DEF: Disorder characterized by various oddities of thinking, perception, communication, and behavior that may be manifested as magical thinking, ideas of reference, paranoid ideation, recurrent illusions and derealization (depersonalization), or social isolation.

F22 Delusional disorders HCC
Delusional dysmorphophobia
Involutional paranoid state
Paranoia
Paranoia querulans
Paranoid psychosis
Paranoid state
Paraphrenia (late)
Sensitiver Beziehungswahn
EXCLUDES 1 *mood [affective] disorders with psychotic symptoms (F30.2, F31.2, F31.5, F31.64, F32.3, F33.3)*
paranoid schizophrenia (F20.0)
EXCLUDES 2 *paranoid personality disorder (F60.0)*
paranoid psychosis, psychogenic (F23)
paranoid reaction (F23)

F23 Brief psychotic disorder CC HCC
Paranoid reaction
Psychogenic paranoid psychosis
EXCLUDES 2 *mood [affective] disorders with psychotic symptoms (F30.2, F31.2, F31.5, F31.64, F32.3, F33.3)*
AHA: 2019,2Q,32

F24 Shared psychotic disorder HCC
Folie a deux
Induced paranoid disorder
Induced psychotic disorder

✓4th **F25 Schizoaffective disorders**
EXCLUDES 1 *mood [affective] disorders with psychotic symptoms (F30.2, F31.2, F31.5, F31.64, F32.3, F33.3)*
schizophrenia (F20.-)

F25.0 Schizoaffective disorder, bipolar type HCC
Cyclic schizophrenia
Schizoaffective disorder, manic type
Schizoaffective disorder, mixed type
Schizoaffective psychosis, bipolar type

F25.1 Schizoaffective disorder, depressive type HCC
Schizoaffective psychosis, depressive type

F25.8 Other schizoaffective disorders HCC

F25.9 Schizoaffective disorder, unspecified HCC
Schizoaffective psychosis NOS

F28 Other psychotic disorder not due to a substance or known physiological condition HIV HCC
Chronic hallucinatory psychosis
Other specified schizophrenia spectrum and other psychotic disorder

F29 Unspecified psychosis not due to a substance or known physiological condition HIV HCC
Psychosis NOS
Unspecified schizophrenia spectrum and other psychotic disorder
EXCLUDES 1 *mental disorder NOS (F99)*
unspecified mental disorder due to known physiological condition (F09)

Mood [affective] disorders (F30-F39)

F30 Manic episode
INCLUDES bipolar disorder, single manic episode
mixed affective episode
EXCLUDES 1 *bipolar disorder (F31.-)*
major depressive disorder, recurrent (F33.-)
major depressive disorder, single episode (F32.-)
DEF: Mania: Characterized by abnormal states of elation or excitement out of keeping with the individual's circumstances and varying from enhanced liveliness (hypomania) to violent, almost uncontrollable, excitement. Aggression and anger, flight of ideas, distractibility, impaired judgment, and grandiose ideas are common.

F30.1 Manic episode without psychotic symptoms
F30.10 Manic episode without psychotic symptoms, unspecified CC HCC
F30.11 Manic episode without psychotic symptoms, mild CC HCC
F30.12 Manic episode without psychotic symptoms, moderate CC HCC
F30.13 Manic episode, severe, without psychotic symptoms CC HCC
F30.2 Manic episode, severe with psychotic symptoms CC HCC
Manic stupor
Mania with mood-congruent psychotic symptoms
Mania with mood-incongruent psychotic symptoms
F30.3 Manic episode in partial remission HCC
F30.4 Manic episode in full remission HCC
F30.8 Other manic episodes HCC
Hypomania
F30.9 Manic episode, unspecified CC HCC
Mania NOS

F31 Bipolar disorder
INCLUDES bipolar I disorder
bipolar type I disorder
manic-depressive illness
manic-depressive psychosis
manic-depressive reaction
seasonal bipolar disorder
EXCLUDES 1 *bipolar disorder, single manic episode (F30.-)*
major depressive disorder, recurrent (F33.-)
major depressive disorder, single episode (F32.-)
EXCLUDES 2 *cyclothymia (F34.0)*
AHA: 2020,1Q,23

F31.0 Bipolar disorder, current episode hypomanic CC HCC
F31.1 Bipolar disorder, current episode manic without psychotic features
F31.10 Bipolar disorder, current episode manic without psychotic features, unspecified CC HCC
F31.11 Bipolar disorder, current episode manic without psychotic features, mild CC HCC
F31.12 Bipolar disorder, current episode manic without psychotic features, moderate CC HCC
F31.13 Bipolar disorder, current episode manic without psychotic features, severe CC HCC
F31.2 Bipolar disorder, current episode manic severe with psychotic features CC HCC
Bipolar disorder, current episode manic with mood-congruent psychotic symptoms
Bipolar disorder, current episode manic with mood-incongruent psychotic symptoms
Bipolar I disorder, current or most recent episode manic with psychotic features
F31.3 Bipolar disorder, current episode depressed, mild or moderate severity
F31.30 Bipolar disorder, current episode depressed, mild or moderate severity, unspecified CC HCC
F31.31 Bipolar disorder, current episode depressed, mild CC HCC
F31.32 Bipolar disorder, current episode depressed, moderate CC HCC
F31.4 Bipolar disorder, current episode depressed, severe, without psychotic features CC HCC
F31.5 Bipolar disorder, current episode depressed, severe, with psychotic features CC HCC
Bipolar disorder, current episode depressed with mood-congruent psychotic symptoms
Bipolar disorder, current episode depressed with mood-incongruent psychotic symptoms
Bipolar I disorder, current or most recent episode depressed, with psychotic features
F31.6 Bipolar disorder, current episode mixed
F31.60 Bipolar disorder, current episode mixed, unspecified CC HCC
F31.61 Bipolar disorder, current episode mixed, mild CC HCC
F31.62 Bipolar disorder, current episode mixed, moderate CC HCC
F31.63 Bipolar disorder, current episode mixed, severe, without psychotic features CC HCC
F31.64 Bipolar disorder, current episode mixed, severe, with psychotic features CC HCC
Bipolar disorder, current episode mixed with mood-congruent psychotic symptoms
Bipolar disorder, current episode mixed with mood-incongruent psychotic symptoms
F31.7 Bipolar disorder, currently in remission
F31.70 Bipolar disorder, currently in remission, most recent episode unspecified HCC
F31.71 Bipolar disorder, in partial remission, most recent episode hypomanic HCC
F31.72 Bipolar disorder, in full remission, most recent episode hypomanic HCC
F31.73 Bipolar disorder, in partial remission, most recent episode manic HCC
F31.74 Bipolar disorder, in full remission, most recent episode manic HCC
F31.75 Bipolar disorder, in partial remission, most recent episode depressed HCC
F31.76 Bipolar disorder, in full remission, most recent episode depressed HCC
F31.77 Bipolar disorder, in partial remission, most recent episode mixed HCC
F31.78 Bipolar disorder, in full remission, most recent episode mixed HCC
F31.8 Other bipolar disorders
F31.81 Bipolar II disorder CC HCC
Bipolar disorder, type 2
F31.89 Other bipolar disorder CC HCC
Recurrent manic episodes NOS
F31.9 Bipolar disorder, unspecified HCC
Manic depression
AHA: 2020,1Q,23

F32 Depressive episode
INCLUDES single episode of agitated depression
single episode of depressive reaction
single episode of major depression
single episode of psychogenic depression
single episode of reactive depression
single episode of vital depression
EXCLUDES 1 *bipolar disorder (F31.-)*
manic episode (F30.-)
recurrent depressive disorder (F33.-)
EXCLUDES 2 *adjustment disorder (F43.2)*
AHA: 2020,1Q,23
DEF: Mood disorder that produces depression that may exhibit as sadness, low self-esteem, or guilt feelings. Other manifestations may be withdrawal from friends and family and interrupted sleep.
F32.0 Major depressive disorder, single episode, mild CC HCC
F32.1 Major depressive disorder, single episode, moderate CC HCC
F32.2 Major depressive disorder, single episode, severe without psychotic features CC HCC

F32.3 Major depressive disorder, single episode, severe with psychotic features CC HCC
- Single episode of major depression with mood-congruent psychotic symptoms
- Single episode of major depression with mood-incongruent psychotic symptoms
- Single episode of major depression with psychotic symptoms
- Single episode of psychogenic depressive psychosis
- Single episode of psychotic depression
- Single episode of reactive depressive psychosis

F32.4 Major depressive disorder, single episode, in partial remission HCC

F32.5 Major depressive disorder, single episode, in full remission HCC

✓5th **F32.8 Other depressive episodes**

AHA: 2016,4Q,14

F32.81 Premenstrual dysphoric disorder ♀

EXCLUDES 1 *premenstrual tension syndrome (N94.3)*

DEF: Severe manifestation of premenstrual syndrome (PMS) that can be disabling and destructive to day-to-day activities. It can exacerbate pre-existing emotional disorders, like depression and anxiety, and cause feelings of loss of control, fatigue, and irritability.

F32.89 Other specified depressive episodes
- Atypical depression
- Post-schizophrenic depression
- Single episode of 'masked' depression NOS

F32.9 Major depressive disorder, single episode, unspecified
- Major depression NOS

AHA: 2021,4Q,10; 2021,1Q,10; 2013,4Q,107

F32.A Depression, unspecified
- Depression NOS
- Depressive disorder NOS

AHA: 2021,4Q,9-10

✓4th **F33 Major depressive disorder, recurrent**

INCLUDES
- recurrent episodes of depressive reaction
- recurrent episodes of endogenous depression
- recurrent episodes of major depression
- recurrent episodes of psychogenic depression
- recurrent episodes of reactive depression
- recurrent episodes of seasonal affective disorder
- recurrent episodes of seasonal depressive disorder
- recurrent episodes of vital depression

EXCLUDES 1 *bipolar disorder (F31.-)*
manic episode (F30.-)

AHA: 2020,1Q,23

DEF: Mood disorder that produces depression that may exhibit as sadness, low self-esteem, or guilt feelings. Other manifestations may be withdrawal from friends and family and interrupted sleep.

F33.0 Major depressive disorder, recurrent, mild CC HCC

F33.1 Major depressive disorder, recurrent, moderate CC HCC

F33.2 Major depressive disorder, recurrent, severe without psychotic features CC HCC

F33.3 Major depressive disorder, recurrent, severe with psychotic symptoms CC HCC
- Endogenous depression with psychotic symptoms
- Major depressive disorder, recurrent, with psychotic features
- Recurrent severe episodes of major depression with mood-congruent psychotic symptoms
- Recurrent severe episodes of major depression with mood-incongruent psychotic symptoms
- Recurrent severe episodes of major depression with psychotic symptoms
- Recurrent severe episodes of psychogenic depressive psychosis
- Recurrent severe episodes of psychotic depression
- Recurrent severe episodes of reactive depressive psychosis

✓5th **F33.4 Major depressive disorder, recurrent, in remission**

F33.40 Major depressive disorder, recurrent, in remission, unspecified CC HCC

F33.41 Major depressive disorder, recurrent, in partial remission HCC

F33.42 Major depressive disorder, recurrent, in full remission HCC

F33.8 Other recurrent depressive disorders CC HCC
- Recurrent brief depressive episodes

F33.9 Major depressive disorder, recurrent, unspecified CC HCC
- Monopolar depression NOS

✓4th **F34 Persistent mood [affective] disorders**

F34.0 Cyclothymic disorder
- Affective personality disorder
- Cycloid personality
- Cyclothymia
- Cyclothymic personality

DEF: Mood disorder characterized by fast and repeated alterations between hypomanic and depressed moods.

F34.1 Dysthymic disorder
- Depressive neurosis
- Depressive personality disorder
- Dysthymia
- Neurotic depression
- Persistent anxiety depression
- Persistent depressive disorder

EXCLUDES 2 *anxiety depression (mild or not persistent) (F41.8)*

DEF: Depression without psychosis. It is a less severe but persistent depression and is considered a mild to moderate chronic form of depression.

✓5th **F34.8 Other persistent mood [affective] disorders**

AHA: 2016,4Q,14

F34.81 Disruptive mood dysregulation disorder CC HCC

F34.89 Other specified persistent mood disorders CC HCC

F34.9 Persistent mood [affective] disorder, unspecified CC HCC

F39 Unspecified mood [affective] disorder HCC
- Affective psychosis NOS

Anxiety, dissociative, stress-related, somatoform and other nonpsychotic mental disorders (F40-F48)

✓4th **F40 Phobic anxiety disorders**

DEF: Phobia: Broad-range anxiety with abnormally intense dread of certain objects or specific situations that would not normally have that effect.

✓5th **F40.0 Agoraphobia**

DEF: Profound anxiety or fear of leaving familiar settings like home, or being in unfamiliar locations or with strangers or crowds. Agoraphobia may or may not be preceded by recurrent panic attacks.

F40.00 Agoraphobia, unspecified

F40.01 Agoraphobia with panic disorder
- Panic disorder with agoraphobia

EXCLUDES 1 *panic disorder without agoraphobia (F41.0)*

F40.02 Agoraphobia without panic disorder

✓5th **F40.1 Social phobias**
- Anthropophobia
- Social anxiety disorder
- Social anxiety disorder of childhood
- Social neurosis

F40.10 Social phobia, unspecified

F40.11 Social phobia, generalized

✓5th **F40.2 Specific (isolated) phobias**

EXCLUDES 2 *dysmorphophobia (nondelusional) (F45.22)*
nosophobia (F45.22)

✓6th **F40.21 Animal type phobia**

F40.210 Arachnophobia
- Fear of spiders

F40.218 Other animal type phobia

✓6th **F40.22 Natural environment type phobia**

F40.220 Fear of thunderstorms

F40.228 Other natural environment type phobia

✓6th **F40.23 Blood, injection, injury type phobia**

F40.230 Fear of blood

F40.231 Fear of injections and transfusions

F40.232 Fear of other medical care

F40.233 Fear of injury

✓6th **F40.24 Situational type phobia**

F40.240 Claustrophobia

F40.241 Acrophobia

F40.242 Fear of bridges

F40.243 Fear of flying

F40.248 Other situational type phobia

✓6th **F40.29 Other specified phobia**

F40.290 Androphobia
- Fear of men

F40.291 **Gynephobia**
Fear of women

F40.298 **Other specified phobia**

F40.8 **Other phobic anxiety disorders**
Phobic anxiety disorder of childhood

F40.9 **Phobic anxiety disorder, unspecified**
Phobia NOS
Phobic state NOS

F41 Other anxiety disorders

EXCLUDES 2 *anxiety in:*
acute stress reaction (F43.0)
neurasthenia (F48.8)
psychophysiologic disorders (F45.-)
transient adjustment reaction (F43.2)
separation anxiety (F93.0)

F41.0 **Panic disorder [episodic paroxysmal anxiety]**
Panic attack
Panic state
EXCLUDES 1 *panic disorder with agoraphobia (F40.01)*
DEF: Neurotic disorder characterized by recurrent panic or anxiety, apprehension, fear, or terror. Symptoms include shortness of breath, palpitations, dizziness, and shakiness; fear of dying may persist.

F41.1 **Generalized anxiety disorder**
Anxiety neurosis
Anxiety reaction
Anxiety state
Overanxious disorder
EXCLUDES 2 *neurasthenia (F48.8)*

F41.3 **Other mixed anxiety disorders**

F41.8 **Other specified anxiety disorders**
Anxiety depression (mild or not persistent)
Anxiety hysteria
Mixed anxiety and depressive disorder
AHA: 2021,1Q,10

F41.9 **Anxiety disorder, unspecified**
Anxiety NOS
AHA: 2021,1Q,10

F42 Obsessive-compulsive disorder

EXCLUDES 2 *obsessive-compulsive personality (disorder) (F60.5)*
obsessive-compulsive symptoms occurring in depression (F32-F33)
obsessive-compulsive symptoms occurring in schizophrenia (F20.-)

AHA: 2016,4Q,14-15

F42.2 **Mixed obsessional thoughts and acts**

F42.3 **Hoarding disorder**

F42.4 **Excoriation (skin-picking) disorder**
EXCLUDES 1 *factitial dermatitis (L98.1)*
other specified behavioral and emotional disorders with onset usually occurring in early childhood and adolescence (F98.8)

F42.8 **Other obsessive-compulsive disorder**
Anancastic neurosis
Obsessive-compulsive neurosis

F42.9 **Obsessive-compulsive disorder, unspecified**

F43 Reaction to severe stress, and adjustment disorders

F43.0 **Acute stress reaction**
Acute crisis reaction
Acute reaction to stress
Combat and operational stress reaction
Combat fatigue
Crisis state
Psychic shock

F43.1 **Post-traumatic stress disorder (PTSD)**
Traumatic neurosis
DEF: Preoccupation with traumatic events beyond normal experience (i.e., rape, personal assault, etc.) that may also include recurring flashbacks of the trauma. Symptoms include difficulty remembering, sleeping, or concentrating, and guilt feelings for surviving.

F43.10 **Post-traumatic stress disorder, unspecified**

F43.11 **Post-traumatic stress disorder, acute**

F43.12 **Post-traumatic stress disorder, chronic**

F43.2 **Adjustment disorders**
Culture shock
Grief reaction
Hospitalism in children
EXCLUDES 2 *separation anxiety disorder of childhood (F93.0)*

F43.20 **Adjustment disorder, unspecified**

F43.21 **Adjustment disorder with depressed mood**
AHA: 2014,1Q,25

F43.22 **Adjustment disorder with anxiety**

F43.23 **Adjustment disorder with mixed anxiety and depressed mood**

F43.24 **Adjustment disorder with disturbance of conduct**

F43.25 **Adjustment disorder with mixed disturbance of emotions and conduct**

F43.29 **Adjustment disorder with other symptoms**

F43.8 **Other reactions to severe stress**
Other specified trauma and stressor-related disorder
AHA: 2022,4Q,17

F43.81 **Prolonged grief disorder**
Complicated grief
Complicated grief disorder
Persistent complex bereavement disorder

F43.89 **Other reactions to severe stress**

F43.9 **Reaction to severe stress, unspecified**
Trauma and stressor-related disorder, NOS
Unspecified trauma and stressor-related disorder

F44 Dissociative and conversion disorders

INCLUDES conversion hysteria
conversion reaction
hysteria
hysterical psychosis

EXCLUDES 2 *malingering [conscious simulation] (Z76.5)*

F44.0 **Dissociative amnesia** HCC
EXCLUDES 1 *amnesia NOS (R41.3)*
anterograde amnesia (R41.1)
dissociative amnesia with dissociative fugue (F44.1)
retrograde amnesia (R41.2)
EXCLUDES 2 *alcohol-or other psychoactive substance-induced amnestic disorder (F10, F13, F19 with .26, .96)*
amnestic disorder due to known physiological condition (F04)
postictal amnesia in epilepsy (G40.-)

F44.1 **Dissociative fugue** HCC
Dissociative amnesia with dissociative fugue
EXCLUDES 2 *postictal fugue in epilepsy (G40.-)*
DEF: Dissociative hysteria identified by memory loss and flight from familiar surroundings to a completely separate environment. Episodes may last hours or days. Conscious activity is not associated with perception of surroundings and there is no later memory of the episode.

F44.2 **Dissociative stupor**
EXCLUDES 1 *catatonic stupor (R40.1)*
stupor NOS (R40.1)
EXCLUDES 2 *catatonic disorder due to known physiological condition (F06.1)*
depressive stupor (F32, F33)
manic stupor (F30, F31)

F44.4 **Conversion disorder with motor symptom or deficit**
Conversion disorder with abnormal movement
Conversion disorder with speech symptoms
Conversion disorder with swallowing symptoms
Conversion disorder with weakness/paralysis
Dissociative motor disorders
Psychogenic aphonia
Psychogenic dysphonia

F44.5 **Conversion disorder with seizures or convulsions**
Conversion disorder with attacks or seizures
Dissociative convulsions
AHA: 2021,1Q,3; 2019,1Q,19

F44.6 **Conversion disorder with sensory symptom or deficit**
Conversion disorder with anesthesia or sensory loss
Conversion disorder with special sensory symptoms
Dissociative anesthesia and sensory loss
Psychogenic deafness

F44.7 **Conversion disorder with mixed symptom presentation**

✓5th **F44.8 Other dissociative and conversion disorders**

F44.81 Dissociative identity disorder HCC
Multiple personality disorder

F44.89 Other dissociative and conversion disorders
Ganser's syndrome
Psychogenic confusion
Psychogenic twilight state
Trance and possession disorders

F44.9 Dissociative and conversion disorder, unspecified
Dissociative disorder NOS

✓4th **F45 Somatoform disorders**

EXCLUDES 2 *dissociative and conversion disorders (F44.-)*
factitious disorders (F68.1-, F68.A)
hair-plucking (F63.3)
lalling (F80.0)
lisping (F80.0)
malingering [conscious simulation] (Z76.5)
nail-biting (F98.8)
psychological or behavioral factors associated with disorders or diseases classified elsewhere (F54)
sexual dysfunction, not due to a substance or known physiological condition (F52.-)
thumb-sucking (F98.8)
tic disorders (in childhood and adolescence) (F95.-)
Tourette's syndrome (F95.2)
trichotillomania (F63.3)

DEF: Types of disorders causing inconsistent physical symptoms that cannot be explained.

F45.0 Somatization disorder
Briquet's disorder
Multiple psychosomatic disorder

F45.1 Undifferentiated somatoform disorder
Somatic symptom disorder
Undifferentiated psychosomatic disorder

✓5th **F45.2 Hypochondriacal disorders**

EXCLUDES 2 *delusional dysmorphophobia (F22)*
fixed delusions about bodily functions or shape (F22)

F45.20 Hypochondriacal disorder, unspecified

F45.21 Hypochondriasis
Hypochondriacal neurosis
Illness anxiety disorder

F45.22 Body dysmorphic disorder
Dysmorphophobia (nondelusional)
Nosophobia

F45.29 Other hypochondriacal disorders

✓5th **F45.4 Pain disorders related to psychological factors**

EXCLUDES 1 *pain NOS (R52)*

F45.41 Pain disorder exclusively related to psychological factors
Somatoform pain disorder (persistent)

F45.42 Pain disorder with related psychological factors
Code also associated acute or chronic pain (G89.-)

F45.8 Other somatoform disorders
Psychogenic dysmenorrhea
Psychogenic dysphagia, including 'globus hystericus'
Psychogenic pruritus
Psychogenic torticollis
Somatoform autonomic dysfunction
Teeth grinding
EXCLUDES 1 *sleep related teeth grinding (G47.63)*

F45.9 Somatoform disorder, unspecified
Psychosomatic disorder NOS

✓4th **F48 Other nonpsychotic mental disorders**

F48.1 Depersonalization-derealization syndrome HCC

F48.2 Pseudobulbar affect
Involuntary emotional expression disorder
Code first underlying cause, if known, such as:
amyotrophic lateral sclerosis (G12.21)
multiple sclerosis (G35)
sequelae of cerebrovascular disease (I69.-)
sequelae of traumatic intracranial injury (S06.-)

F48.8 Other specified nonpsychotic mental disorders
Dhat syndrome
Neurasthenia
Occupational neurosis, including writer's cramp
Psychasthenia
Psychasthenic neurosis
Psychogenic syncope

F48.9 Nonpsychotic mental disorder, unspecified
Neurosis NOS

Behavioral syndromes associated with physiological disturbances and physical factors (F50-F59)

✓4th **F50 Eating disorders**

EXCLUDES 1 *anorexia NOS (R63.0)*
feeding problems of newborn (P92.-)
polyphagia (R63.2)

EXCLUDES 2 *feeding difficulties ►(R63.3-)◄*
feeding disorder in infancy or childhood (F98.2-)

AHA: 2022,1Q,13; 2018,4Q,82

TIP: Assign additional code for BMI from category Z68, when documented. BMI can be based on documentation from clinicians who are not the patient's provider.

✓5th **F50.0 Anorexia nervosa**

EXCLUDES 1 *loss of appetite (R63.0)*
psychogenic loss of appetite (F50.89)

DEF: Psychological eating disorder characterized by an intense fear of gaining weight and an unrealistic perception of body image that perpetuates the feeling of being fat or having too much fat. Avoidance of food and restrictive or unhealthy eating are common.

F50.00 Anorexia nervosa, unspecified CC

F50.01 Anorexia nervosa, restricting type CC

F50.02 Anorexia nervosa, binge eating/purging type CC
EXCLUDES 1 *bulimia nervosa (F50.2)*

F50.2 Bulimia nervosa CC
Bulimia NOS
Hyperorexia nervosa
EXCLUDES 1 *anorexia nervosa, binge eating/purging type (F50.02)*

DEF: Episodic pattern of overeating (binge eating) followed by purging or extreme exercise accompanied by an awareness of the abnormal eating pattern with a fear of not being able to stop eating.

✓5th **F50.8 Other eating disorders**

EXCLUDES 2 *pica of infancy and childhood (F98.3)*

AHA: 2017,4Q,9; 2016,4Q,15-16

F50.81 Binge eating disorder

F50.82 Avoidant/restrictive food intake disorder

F50.89 Other specified eating disorder
Pica in adults
Psychogenic loss of appetite

F50.9 Eating disorder, unspecified
Atypical anorexia nervosa
Atypical bulimia nervosa
Feeding or eating disorder, unspecified
Other specified feeding disorder

✓4th **F51 Sleep disorders not due to a substance or known physiological condition**

EXCLUDES 2 *organic sleep disorders (G47.-)*

✓5th **F51.0 Insomnia not due to a substance or known physiological condition**

EXCLUDES 2 *alcohol related insomnia (F10.182, F10.282, F10.982)*
drug-related insomnia (F11.182, F11.282, F11.982, F13.182, F13.282, F13.982, F14.182, F14.282, F14.982, F15.182, F15.282, F15.982, F19.182, F19.282, F19.982)
insomnia NOS (G47.0-)
insomnia due to known physiological condition (G47.0-)
organic insomnia (G47.0-)
sleep deprivation (Z72.820)

F51.01 Primary insomnia
Idiopathic insomnia

F51.02 Adjustment insomnia

F51.03 Paradoxical insomnia

F51.04 Psychophysiologic insomnia

F51.05 Insomnia due to other mental disorder
Code also associated mental disorder

F51.09 **Other insomnia not due to a substance or known physiological condition**

F51.1 **Hypersomnia not due to a substance or known physiological condition**
EXCLUDES 2 *alcohol related hypersomnia (F10.182, F10.282, F10.982)*
drug-related hypersomnia (F11.182, F11.282, F11.982, F13.182, F13.282, F13.982, F14.182, F14.282, F14.982, F15.182, F15.282, F15.982, F19.182, F19.282, F19.982)
hypersomnia NOS (G47.10)
hypersomnia due to known physiological condition (G47.10)
idiopathic hypersomnia (G47.11, G47.12)
narcolepsy (G47.4-)

F51.11 **Primary hypersomnia**

F51.12 **Insufficient sleep syndrome**
EXCLUDES 1 *sleep deprivation (Z72.820)*

F51.13 **Hypersomnia due to other mental disorder**
Code also associated mental disorder

F51.19 **Other hypersomnia not due to a substance or known physiological condition**

F51.3 **Sleepwalking [somnambulism]**
Non-rapid eye movement sleep arousal disorders, sleepwalking type

F51.4 **Sleep terrors [night terrors]**
Non-rapid eye movement sleep arousal disorders, sleep terror type

F51.5 **Nightmare disorder**
Dream anxiety disorder

F51.8 **Other sleep disorders not due to a substance or known physiological condition**

F51.9 **Sleep disorder not due to a substance or known physiological condition, unspecified**
Emotional sleep disorder NOS

F52 **Sexual dysfunction not due to a substance or known physiological condition**
EXCLUDES 2 *Dhat syndrome (F48.8)*

F52.0 **Hypoactive sexual desire disorder**
Lack or loss of sexual desire
Male hypoactive sexual desire disorder
Sexual anhedonia
EXCLUDES 1 *decreased libido (R68.82)*

F52.1 **Sexual aversion disorder**
Sexual aversion and lack of sexual enjoyment

F52.2 **Sexual arousal disorders**
Failure of genital response

F52.21 **Male erectile disorder** ♂
Erectile disorder
Psychogenic impotence
EXCLUDES 1 *impotence of organic origin (N52.-)*
impotence NOS (N52.-)

F52.22 **Female sexual arousal disorder** ♀
Female sexual interest/arousal disorder

F52.3 **Orgasmic disorder**
Inhibited orgasm
Psychogenic anorgasmy

F52.31 **Female orgasmic disorder** ♀

F52.32 **Male orgasmic disorder** ♂
Delayed ejaculation

F52.4 **Premature ejaculation** ♂

F52.5 **Vaginismus not due to a substance or known physiological condition** ♀
Psychogenic vaginismus
EXCLUDES 2 *vaginismus (due to a known physiological condition) (N94.2)*
DEF: Psychogenic response resulting in painful contractions of the vaginal canal muscles. This condition can be severe enough to prevent sexual intercourse.

F52.6 **Dyspareunia not due to a substance or known physiological condition**
Genito-pelvic pain penetration disorder
Psychogenic dyspareunia
EXCLUDES 2 *dyspareunia (due to a known physiological condition) (N94.1-)*

F52.8 **Other sexual dysfunction not due to a substance or known physiological condition**
Excessive sexual drive
Nymphomania
Satyriasis

F52.9 **Unspecified sexual dysfunction not due to a substance or known physiological condition** UPD
Sexual dysfunction NOS

F53 **Mental and behavioral disorders associated with the puerperium, not elsewhere classified**
EXCLUDES 1 *mood disorders with psychotic features (F30.2, F31.2, F31.5, F31.64, F32.3, F33.3)*
postpartum dysphoria (O90.6)
psychosis in schizophrenia, schizotypal, delusional, and other psychotic disorders (F20-F29)
AHA: 2018,4Q,8

F53.0 **Postpartum depression** M ♀
Postnatal depression, NOS
Postpartum depression, NOS

F53.1 **Puerperal psychosis** HCC M ♀
Postpartum psychosis
Puerperal psychosis, NOS

F54 ***Psychological and behavioral factors associated with disorders or diseases classified elsewhere***
Psychological factors affecting physical conditions
Code first the associated physical disorder, such as:
asthma (J45.-)
dermatitis (L23-L25)
gastric ulcer (K25.-)
mucous colitis (K58.-)
ulcerative colitis (K51.-)
urticaria (L50.-)
EXCLUDES 2 *tension-type headache (G44.2)*

F55 **Abuse of non-psychoactive substances**
EXCLUDES 2 *abuse of psychoactive substances (F10-F19)*

F55.0 **Abuse of antacids**

F55.1 **Abuse of herbal or folk remedies**

F55.2 **Abuse of laxatives**

F55.3 **Abuse of steroids or hormones**

F55.4 **Abuse of vitamins**

F55.8 **Abuse of other non-psychoactive substances**

F59 **Unspecified behavioral syndromes associated with physiological disturbances and physical factors**
Psychogenic physiological dysfunction NOS

Disorders of adult personality and behavior (F60-F69)

F60 **Specific personality disorders**

F60.0 **Paranoid personality disorder** HCC
Expansive paranoid personality (disorder)
Fanatic personality (disorder)
Paranoid personality (disorder)
Querulant personality (disorder)
Sensitive paranoid personality (disorder)
EXCLUDES 2 *paranoia (F22)*
paranoia querulans (F22)
paranoid psychosis (F22)
paranoid schizophrenia (F20.0)
paranoid state (F22)

F60.1 **Schizoid personality disorder** HCC
EXCLUDES 2 *Asperger's syndrome (F84.5)*
delusional disorder (F22)
schizoid disorder of childhood (F84.5)
schizophrenia (F20.-)
schizotypal disorder (F21)

F60.2 **Antisocial personality disorder** HCC
Amoral personality (disorder)
Asocial personality (disorder)
Dissocial personality disorder
Psychopathic personality (disorder)
Sociopathic personality (disorder)
EXCLUDES 1 *conduct disorders (F91.-)*
EXCLUDES 2 *borderline personality disorder (F60.3)*

F60.3 Borderline personality disorder HCC
Aggressive personality (disorder)
Emotionally unstable personality disorder
Explosive personality (disorder)
EXCLUDES 2 *antisocial personality disorder (F60.2)*

F60.4 Histrionic personality disorder HCC
Hysterical personality (disorder)
Psychoinfantile personality (disorder)

F60.5 Obsessive-compulsive personality disorder HCC
Anankastic personality (disorder)
Compulsive personality (disorder)
Obsessional personality (disorder)
EXCLUDES 2 *obsessive-compulsive disorder (F42.-)*

F60.6 Avoidant personality disorder HCC
Anxious personality disorder

F60.7 Dependent personality disorder HCC
Asthenic personality (disorder)
Inadequate personality (disorder)
Passive personality (disorder)
DEF: Lack of self-confidence, fear of abandonment, and an obsessive need to be taken care of.

✓5th **F60.8 Other specific personality disorders**

F60.81 Narcissistic personality disorder HCC

F60.89 Other specific personality disorders HCC
Eccentric personality disorder
"Haltlose" type personality disorder
Immature personality disorder
Passive-aggressive personality disorder
Psychoneurotic personality disorder
Self-defeating personality disorder

F60.9 Personality disorder, unspecified HCC
Character disorder NOS
Character neurosis NOS
Pathological personality NOS

✓4th **F63 Impulse disorders**
EXCLUDES 2 *habitual excessive use of alcohol or psychoactive substances (F10-F19)*
impulse disorders involving sexual behavior (F65.-)

F63.0 Pathological gambling
Compulsive gambling
Gambling disorder
EXCLUDES 1 *gambling and betting NOS (Z72.6)*
EXCLUDES 2 *excessive gambling by manic patients (F30, F31)*
gambling in antisocial personality disorder (F60.2)

F63.1 Pyromania
Pathological fire-setting
EXCLUDES 2 *fire-setting (by) (in):*
adult with antisocial personality disorder (F60.2)
alcohol or psychoactive substance intoxication (F10-F19)
conduct disorders (F91.-)
mental disorders due to known physiological condition (F01-F09)
schizophrenia (F20.-)

F63.2 Kleptomania
Pathological stealing
EXCLUDES 1 *shoplifting as the reason for observation for suspected mental disorder (Z03.8)*
EXCLUDES 2 *depressive disorder with stealing (F31-F33)*
stealing due to underlying mental condition - code to mental condition
stealing in mental disorders due to known physiological condition (F01-F09)

F63.3 Trichotillomania
Hair plucking
EXCLUDES 2 *other stereotyped movement disorder (F98.4)*

✓5th **F63.8 Other impulse disorders**

F63.81 Intermittent explosive disorder

F63.89 Other impulse disorders

F63.9 Impulse disorder, unspecified
Impulse control disorder NOS

✓4th **F64 Gender identity disorders**
AHA: 2016,4Q,16

F64.0 Transsexualism
Gender dysphoria in adolescents and adults
Gender identity disorder in adolescence and adulthood
▶Gender incongruence in adolescents and adults◀
▶Transgender◀
EXCLUDES 1 ▶*gender identity disorder of childhood (F64.2)*◀

F64.1 Dual role transvestism
Use additional code to identify sex reassignment status (Z87.890)
EXCLUDES 1 *gender identity disorder in childhood (F64.2)*
EXCLUDES 2 *fetishistic transvestism (F65.1)*

F64.2 Gender identity disorder of childhood P
Gender dysphoria in children
▶Gender incongruence of childhood◀
EXCLUDES 1 *gender identity disorder in adolescence and adulthood (F64.0)*
EXCLUDES 2 *sexual maturation disorder (F66)*

F64.8 Other gender identity disorders
Other specified gender dysphoria

F64.9 Gender identity disorder, unspecified
Gender dysphoria, unspecified
▶Gender incongruence, unspecified◀
Gender-role disorder NOS

✓4th **F65 Paraphilias**

F65.0 Fetishism
Fetishistic disorder

F65.1 Transvestic fetishism
Fetishistic transvestism
Transvestic disorder

F65.2 Exhibitionism
Exhibitionistic disorder

F65.3 Voyeurism
Voyeuristic disorder

F65.4 Pedophilia
Pedophilic disorder

✓5th **F65.5 Sadomasochism**

F65.50 Sadomasochism, unspecified

F65.51 Sexual masochism
Sexual masochism disorder

F65.52 Sexual sadism
Sexual sadism disorder

✓5th **F65.8 Other paraphilias**

F65.81 Frotteurism
Frotteuristic disorder

F65.89 Other paraphilias
Necrophilia
Other specified paraphilic disorder

F65.9 Paraphilia, unspecified
Paraphilic disorder, unspecified
Sexual deviation NOS

F66 Other sexual disorders
Sexual maturation disorder
Sexual relationship disorder

✓4th **F68 Other disorders of adult personality and behavior**
AHA: 2018,4Q,9,65

✓5th **F68.1 Factitious disorder imposed on self**
Compensation neurosis
Elaboration of physical symptoms for psychological reasons
Hospital hopper syndrome
Münchausen's syndrome
Peregrinating patient
EXCLUDES 2 *factitial dermatitis (L98.1)*
person feigning illness (with obvious motivation) (Z76.5)

F68.10 Factitious disorder imposed on self, unspecified CC

F68.11 Factitious disorder imposed on self, with predominantly psychological signs and symptoms

F68.12 Factitious disorder imposed on self, with predominantly physical signs and symptoms CC

F68.13 Factitious disorder imposed on self, with combined psychological and physical signs and symptoms

F68.A Factitious disorder imposed on another CC
Factitious disorder by proxy
Münchausen's by proxy

F68.8 Other specified disorders of adult personality and behavior

F69 Unspecified disorder of adult personality and behavior A

Intellectual disabilities (F70-F79)

Code first any associated physical or developmental disorders

EXCLUDES 1 *borderline intellectual functioning, IQ above 70 to 84 (R41.83)*

F70 Mild intellectual disabilities
IQ level 50-55 to approximately 70
Mild mental subnormality

F71 Moderate intellectual disabilities
IQ level 35-40 to 50-55
Moderate mental subnormality

F72 Severe intellectual disabilities CC
IQ 20-25 to 35-40
Severe mental subnormality

F73 Profound intellectual disabilities CC
IQ level below 20-25
Profound mental subnormality

4th **F78 Other intellectual disabilities**

5th **F78.A Other genetic related intellectual disabilities**
AHA: 2021,4Q,10-11

F78.A1 SYNGAP1-related intellectual disability
Code also, if applicable, any associated:
autism spectrum disorder (F84.0)
autistic disorder (F84.0)
encephalopathy (G93.4-)
epilepsy and recurrent seizures (G40.-)
other pervasive developmental disorders (F84.8)
pervasive developmental disorder, NOS (F84.9)

F78.A9 Other genetic related intellectual disability
Code also, if applicable, any associated disorders

F79 Unspecified intellectual disabilities
Mental deficiency NOS
Mental subnormality NOS

Pervasive and specific developmental disorders (F80-F89)

4th **F80 Specific developmental disorders of speech and language**

F80.0 Phonological disorder
Dyslalia
Functional speech articulation disorder
Lalling
Lisping
Phonological developmental disorder
Speech articulation developmental disorder
Speech-sound disorder
EXCLUDES 1 *speech articulation impairment due to aphasia NOS (R47.01)*
speech articulation impairment due to apraxia (R48.2)
EXCLUDES 2 *speech articulation impairment due to hearing loss (F80.4)*
speech articulation impairment due to intellectual disabilities (F70-F79)
speech articulation impairment with expressive language developmental disorder (F80.1)
speech articulation impairment with mixed receptive expressive language developmental disorder (F80.2)

F80.1 Expressive language disorder
Developmental dysphasia or aphasia, expressive type
EXCLUDES 1 *mixed receptive-expressive language disorder (F80.2)*
dysphasia and aphasia NOS (R47.-)
EXCLUDES 2 *acquired aphasia with epilepsy [Landau-Kleffner] (G40.80-)*
intellectual disabilities (F70-F79)
pervasive developmental disorders (F84.-)
selective mutism (F94.0)

F80.2 Mixed receptive-expressive language disorder
Developmental dysphasia or aphasia, receptive type
Developmental Wernicke's aphasia
EXCLUDES 1 *central auditory processing disorder (H93.25)*
dysphasia or aphasia NOS (R47.-)
expressive language disorder (F80.1)
expressive type dysphasia or aphasia (F80.1)
word deafness (H93.25)
EXCLUDES 2 *acquired aphasia with epilepsy [Landau-Kleffner] (G40.80-)*
intellectual disabilities (F70-F79)
pervasive developmental disorders (F84.-)
selective mutism (F94.0)

F80.4 Speech and language development delay due to hearing loss
Code also type of hearing loss (H90.-, H91.-)

5th **F80.8 Other developmental disorders of speech and language**
AHA: 2017,1Q,27

F80.81 Childhood onset fluency disorder
Cluttering NOS
Stuttering NOS
EXCLUDES 1 *adult onset fluency disorder (F98.5)*
fluency disorder in conditions classified elsewhere (R47.82)
fluency disorder (stuttering) following cerebrovascular disease (I69. with final characters -23)

F80.82 Social pragmatic communication disorder
EXCLUDES 1 *Asperger's syndrome (F84.5)*
autistic disorder (F84.0)
AHA: 2016,4Q,16

F80.89 Other developmental disorders of speech and language

F80.9 Developmental disorder of speech and language, unspecified
Communication disorder NOS
Language disorder NOS

4th **F81 Specific developmental disorders of scholastic skills**

F81.0 Specific reading disorder
"Backward reading"
Developmental dyslexia
Specific learning disorder, with impairment in reading
Specific reading retardation
EXCLUDES 1 *alexia NOS (R48.0)*
dyslexia NOS (R48.0)
DEF: Serious impairment of reading skills unexplained in relation to general intelligence and teaching processes.

F81.2 Mathematics disorder
Developmental acalculia
Developmental arithmetical disorder
Developmental Gerstmann's syndrome
Specific learning disorder, with impairment in mathematics
EXCLUDES 1 *acalculia NOS (R48.8)*
EXCLUDES 2 *arithmetical difficulties associated with a reading disorder (F81.0)*
arithmetical difficulties associated with a spelling disorder (F81.81)
arithmetical difficulties due to inadequate teaching (Z55.8)

5th **F81.8 Other developmental disorders of scholastic skills**

F81.81 Disorder of written expression
Specific learning disorder, with impairment in written expression
Specific spelling disorder

F81.89 Other developmental disorders of scholastic skills

F81.9 Developmental disorder of scholastic skills, unspecified UPD
Knowledge acquisition disability NOS
Learning disability NOS
Learning disorder NOS

F82 Specific developmental disorder of motor function
Clumsy child syndrome
Developmental coordination disorder
Developmental dyspraxia
EXCLUDES 1 *abnormalities of gait and mobility (R26.-)*
lack of coordination (R27.-)
EXCLUDES 2 *lack of coordination secondary to intellectual disabilities (F70-F79)*

F84 Pervasive developmental disorders
Code also any associated medical condition and intellectual disabilities

F84.Ø Autistic disorder CC
Autism spectrum disorder
Infantile autism
Infantile psychosis
Kanner's syndrome
EXCLUDES 1 *Asperger's syndrome (F84.5)*
AHA: 2017,1Q,27

F84.2 Rett's syndrome CC
EXCLUDES 1 *Asperger's syndrome (F84.5)*
autistic disorder (F84.Ø)
other childhood disintegrative disorder (F84.3)

F84.3 Other childhood disintegrative disorder CC P
Dementia infantilis
Disintegrative psychosis
Heller's syndrome
Symbiotic psychosis
Use additional code to identify any associated neurological condition
EXCLUDES 1 *Asperger's syndrome (F84.5)*
autistic disorder (F84.Ø)
Rett's syndrome (F84.2)

F84.5 Asperger's syndrome CC
Asperger's disorder
Autistic psychopathy
Schizoid disorder of childhood
DEF: High-functioning form of autism. Children with this syndrome usually develop speech on schedule, are generally very intelligent, and communicate well, but have considerable social shortcomings. ***Synonym(s):*** *AS.*

F84.8 Other pervasive developmental disorders CC
Overactive disorder associated with intellectual disabilities and stereotyped movements

F84.9 Pervasive developmental disorder, unspecified CC
Atypical autism

F88 Other disorders of psychological development
Developmental agnosia
Global developmental delay
Other specified neurodevelopmental disorder

F89 Unspecified disorder of psychological development
Developmental disorder NOS
Neurodevelopmental disorder NOS

Behavioral and emotional disorders with onset usually occurring in childhood and adolescence (F9Ø-F98)

NOTE Codes within categories F9Ø-F98 may be used regardless of the age of a patient. These disorders generally have onset within the childhood or adolescent years, but may continue throughout life or not be diagnosed until adulthood

F9Ø Attention-deficit hyperactivity disorders
INCLUDES attention deficit disorder with hyperactivity
attention deficit syndrome with hyperactivity
EXCLUDES 2 *anxiety disorders (F4Ø.-, F41.-)*
mood [affective] disorders (F3Ø-F39)
pervasive developmental disorders (F84.-)
schizophrenia (F2Ø.-)

F9Ø.Ø Attention-deficit hyperactivity disorder, predominantly inattentive type
Attention-deficit/hyperactivity disorder, predominantly inattentive presentation

F9Ø.1 Attention-deficit hyperactivity disorder, predominantly hyperactive type
Attention-deficit/hyperactivity disorder, predominantly hyperactive impulsive presentation

F9Ø.2 Attention-deficit hyperactivity disorder, combined type
Attention-deficit/hyperactivity disorder, combined presentation

F9Ø.8 Attention-deficit hyperactivity disorder, other type

F9Ø.9 Attention-deficit hyperactivity disorder, unspecified type
Attention-deficit hyperactivity disorder of childhood or adolescence NOS
Attention-deficit hyperactivity disorder NOS

F91 Conduct disorders
EXCLUDES 1 *antisocial behavior (Z72.81-)*
antisocial personality disorder (F6Ø.2)
EXCLUDES 2 *conduct problems associated with attention-deficit hyperactivity disorder (F9Ø.-)*
mood [affective] disorders (F3Ø-F39)
pervasive developmental disorders (F84.-)
schizophrenia (F2Ø.-)

F91.Ø Conduct disorder confined to family context

F91.1 Conduct disorder, childhood-onset type
Unsocialized conduct disorder
Conduct disorder, solitary aggressive type
Unsocialized aggressive disorder

F91.2 Conduct disorder, adolescent-onset type
Socialized conduct disorder
Conduct disorder, group type

F91.3 Oppositional defiant disorder

F91.8 Other conduct disorders
Other specified conduct disorder
Other specified disruptive disorder

F91.9 Conduct disorder, unspecified
Behavioral disorder NOS
Conduct disorder NOS
Disruptive behavior disorder NOS
Disruptive disorder NOS

F93 Emotional disorders with onset specific to childhood

F93.Ø Separation anxiety disorder of childhood
EXCLUDES 2 *mood [affective] disorders (F3Ø-F39)*
nonpsychotic mental disorders (F4Ø-F48)
phobic anxiety disorder of childhood (F4Ø.8)
social phobia (F4Ø.1)

F93.8 Other childhood emotional disorders
Identity disorder
EXCLUDES 2 *gender identity disorder of childhood (F64.2)*

F93.9 Childhood emotional disorder, unspecified

F94 Disorders of social functioning with onset specific to childhood and adolescence

F94.Ø Selective mutism
Elective mutism
EXCLUDES 2 *pervasive developmental disorders (F84.-)*
schizophrenia (F2Ø.-)
specific developmental disorders of speech and language (F8Ø.-)
transient mutism as part of separation anxiety in young children (F93.Ø)

F94.1 Reactive attachment disorder of childhood
Use additional code to identify any associated failure to thrive or growth retardation
EXCLUDES 1 *disinhibited attachment disorder of childhood (F94.2)*
normal variation in pattern of selective attachment
EXCLUDES 2 *Asperger's syndrome (F84.5)*
maltreatment syndromes (T74.-)
sexual or physical abuse in childhood, resulting in psychosocial problems (Z62.81-)

F94.2 Disinhibited attachment disorder of childhood
Affectionless psychopathy
Institutional syndrome
EXCLUDES 1 *reactive attachment disorder of childhood (F94.1)*
EXCLUDES 2 *Asperger's syndrome (F84.5)*
attention-deficit hyperactivity disorders (F9Ø.-)
hospitalism in children (F43.2-)

F94.8 Other childhood disorders of social functioning

F94.9 Childhood disorder of social functioning, unspecified

F95 Tic disorder

F95.Ø Transient tic disorder
Provisional tic disorder

F95.1 Chronic motor or vocal tic disorder

F95.2 Tourette's disorder
Combined vocal and multiple motor tic disorder [de la Tourette]
Tourette's syndrome

F95.8 Other tic disorders

F95.9 Tic disorder, unspecified
Tic NOS

F98 Other behavioral and emotional disorders with onset usually occurring in childhood and adolescence

EXCLUDES 2 *breath-holding spells (RØ6.89)*
gender identity disorder of childhood (F64.2)
Kleine-Levin syndrome (G47.13)
obsessive-compulsive disorder (F42.-)
sleep disorders not due to a substance or known physiological condition (F51.-)

F98.Ø Enuresis not due to a substance or known physiological condition

Enuresis (primary) (secondary) of nonorganic origin
Functional enuresis
Psychogenic enuresis
Urinary incontinence of nonorganic origin

EXCLUDES 1 *enuresis NOS (R32)*

F98.1 Encopresis not due to a substance or known physiological condition

Functional encopresis
Incontinence of feces of nonorganic origin
Psychogenic encopresis
Use additional code to identify the cause of any coexisting constipation

EXCLUDES 1 *encopresis NOS (R15.-)*

F98.2 Other feeding disorders of infancy and childhood

EXCLUDES 2 *anorexia nervosa and other eating disorders (F5Ø.-)*
feeding difficulties ▶(R63.3-)◀
feeding problems of newborn (P92.-)
pica of infancy or childhood (F98.3)

F98.21 Rumination disorder of infancy

F98.29 Other feeding disorders of infancy and early childhood

F98.3 Pica of infancy and childhood

F98.4 Stereotyped movement disorders

Stereotype/habit disorder

EXCLUDES 1 *abnormal involuntary movements (R25.-)*

EXCLUDES 2 *compulsions in obsessive-compulsive disorder (F42.-)*
hair plucking (F63.3)
movement disorders of organic origin (G2Ø-G25)
nail-biting (F98.8)
nose-picking (F98.8)
stereotypies that are part of a broader psychiatric condition (FØ1-F95)
thumb-sucking (F98.8)
tic disorders (F95.-)
trichotillomania (F63.3)

F98.5 Adult onset fluency disorder

EXCLUDES 1 *childhood onset fluency disorder (F8Ø.81)*
dysphasia (R47.Ø2)
fluency disorder in conditions classified elsewhere (R47.82)
fluency disorder (stuttering) following cerebrovascular disease (I69. with final characters -23)
tic disorders (F95.-)

F98.8 Other specified behavioral and emotional disorders with onset usually occurring in childhood and adolescence

Excessive masturbation
Nail-biting
Nose-picking
Thumb-sucking

F98.9 Unspecified behavioral and emotional disorders with onset usually occurring in childhood and adolescence

Unspecified mental disorder (F99)

F99 Mental disorder, not otherwise specified

Mental illness NOS

EXCLUDES 1 *unspecified mental disorder due to known physiological condition (FØ9)*

Chapter 6. Diseases of the Nervous System (GØØ–G99)

Chapter-specific Guidelines with Coding Examples

The chapter-specific guidelines from the ICD-10-CM Official Guidelines for Coding and Reporting have been provided below. Along with these guidelines are coding examples, contained in the shaded boxes, that have been developed to help illustrate the coding and/or sequencing guidance found in these guidelines.

a. Dominant/nondominant side

Codes from category G81, Hemiplegia and hemiparesis, and subcategories G83.1, Monoplegia of lower limb, G83.2, Monoplegia of upper limb, and G83.3, Monoplegia, unspecified, identify whether the dominant or nondominant side is affected. Should the affected side be documented, but not specified as dominant or nondominant, and the classification system does not indicate a default, code selection is as follows:

- For ambidextrous patients, the default should be dominant.
- If the left side is affected, the default is non-dominant.
- If the right side is affected, the default is dominant.

> Hemiplegia affecting left side of ambidextrous patient
>
> **G81.92 Hemiplegia, unspecified affecting left dominant side**
>
> *Explanation*: Documentation states that the left side is affected and dominant is used for ambidextrous persons.

> Right spastic hemiplegia, unknown whether patient is right- or left-handed
>
> **G81.11 Spastic hemiplegia affecting right dominant side**
>
> *Explanation*: Since it is unknown whether the patient is right- or left-handed, if the right side is affected, the default is dominant.

b. Pain—category G89

1) General coding information

Codes in category G89, Pain, not elsewhere classified, may be used in conjunction with codes from other categories and chapters to provide more detail about acute or chronic pain and neoplasm-related pain, unless otherwise indicated below.

If the pain is not specified as acute or chronic, post-thoracotomy, postprocedural, or neoplasm-related, do not assign codes from category G89.

A code from category G89 should not be assigned if the underlying (definitive) diagnosis is known, unless the reason for the encounter is pain control/ management and not management of the underlying condition.

When an admission or encounter is for a procedure aimed at treating the underlying condition (e.g., spinal fusion, kyphoplasty), a code for the underlying condition (e.g., vertebral fracture, spinal stenosis) should be assigned as the principal diagnosis. No code from category G89 should be assigned.

> Elderly patient with back pain is admitted for kyphoplasty for age-related osteopathic compression fracture at vertebra T3
>
> **M8Ø.Ø8XA Age-related osteoporosis with current pathological fracture, vertebra(e), initial encounter for fracture**
>
> *Explanation*: No code is assigned for the pain as it is inherent in the underlying condition being treated.

(a) Category G89 codes as principal or first-listed diagnosis

Category G89 codes are acceptable as principal diagnosis or the first-listed code:

- When pain control or pain management is the reason for the admission/encounter (e.g., a patient with displaced intervertebral disc, nerve impingement and severe back pain presents for injection of steroid into the spinal canal). The underlying cause of the pain should be reported as an additional diagnosis, if known.
- When a patient is admitted for the insertion of a neurostimulator for pain control, assign the appropriate pain code as the principal or first-listed diagnosis. When an admission or encounter is for a procedure aimed at treating the underlying condition and a neurostimulator is inserted for pain control during the same admission/encounter, a code for the underlying condition should be assigned as the principal diagnosis and the appropriate pain code should be assigned as a secondary diagnosis.

> Patient with chronic pain from lumbar spondylosis with radiculopathy not relieved by surgery is admitted for insertion of neurostimulator.
>
> **G89.29 Other chronic pain**
>
> **M47.26 Other spondylosis with radiculopathy, lumbar region**
>
> *Explanation*: Since the patient is admitted specifically for a neurostimulator implantation for pain management and not to treat the underlying spondylosis, the chronic pain code is sequenced first, followed by the underlying condition. Neither code M54.16 nor M54.5 is necessary because M47.26 describes the radiculopathy and the site.

(b) Use of category G89 codes in conjunction with site specific pain codes

(i) Assigning category G89 and site-specific pain codes

Codes from category G89 may be used in conjunction with codes that identify the site of pain (including codes from chapter 18) if the category G89 code provides additional information. For example, if the code describes the site of the pain, but does not fully describe whether the pain is acute or chronic, then both codes should be assigned.

> During hospital stay, patient is seen by orthopaedics to evaluate chronic left shoulder pain.
>
> **M25.512 Pain in left shoulder**
>
> **G89.29 Other chronic pain**
>
> *Explanation*: No underlying condition has been determined yet so the pain would be the reason for the visit. The M25 pain code in this instance does not fully describe the condition as it does not represent that the pain is chronic. The G89 chronic pain code is assigned to provide specificity.

(ii) Sequencing of category G89 codes with site-specific pain codes

The sequencing of category G89 codes with site-specific pain codes (including chapter 18 codes), is dependent on the circumstances of the encounter/admission as follows:

- If the encounter is for pain control or pain management, assign the code from category G89 followed by the code identifying the specific site of pain (e.g., encounter for pain management for acute neck pain from trauma is assigned code G89.11, Acute pain due to trauma, followed by code M54.2, Cervicalgia, to identify the site of pain).

> Management of acute, traumatic right knee pain
>
> **G89.11 Acute pain due to trauma**
>
> **M25.561 Pain in right knee**
>
> *Explanation*: The reason for the encounter is to manage or control the pain, not to treat or evaluate an underlying condition. The G89 pain code is assigned as the principal diagnosis but in this instance does not fully describe the condition as it does not include the site and laterality. The M25 pain code is added to provide this information.

- If the encounter is for any other reason except pain control or pain management, and a related definitive diagnosis has not been established (confirmed) by the provider, assign the code for the specific site of pain first, followed by the appropriate code from category G89.

> Tests are performed to investigate the source of the patient's chronic epigastric abdominal pain
>
> **R1Ø.13 Epigastric pain**
>
> **G89.29 Other chronic pain**
>
> *Explanation*: In this instance the patient's epigastric pain is not being treated; rather the source of the pain is being investigated. A code from chapter 18 for epigastric pain is sequenced before the additional specificity of the G89 code for the chronic pain.

2) Pain due to devices, implants and grafts

See Section I.C.19. Pain due to medical devices

3) Postoperative pain

The provider's documentation should be used to guide the coding of postoperative pain, as well as *Section III. Reporting Additional Diagnoses* and *Section IV. Diagnostic Coding and Reporting in the Outpatient Setting*.

The default for post-thoracotomy and other postoperative pain not specified as acute or chronic is the code for the acute form.

Routine or expected postoperative pain immediately after surgery should not be coded.

> Pain pump dose is increased for the patient's unexpected, extreme pain post-thoracotomy
>
> **G89.12 Acute post-thoracotomy pain**
>
> *Explanation*: When acute or chronic is not documented, default to acute. The use of "unexpected, extreme" and the increase of medication dosage indicate that the pain was more than routine or expected.

(a) Postoperative pain not associated with specific postoperative complication

Postoperative pain not associated with a specific postoperative complication is assigned to the appropriate postoperative pain code in category G89.

(b) Postoperative pain associated with specific postoperative complication

Postoperative pain associated with a specific postoperative complication (such as painful wire sutures) is assigned to the appropriate code(s) found in Chapter 19, Injury, poisoning, and certain other consequences of external causes. If appropriate, use additional code(s) from category G89 to identify acute or chronic pain (G89.18 or G89.28).

4) Chronic pain

Chronic pain is classified to subcategory G89.2. There is no time frame defining when pain becomes chronic pain. The provider's documentation should be used to guide use of these codes.

5) Neoplasm related pain

Code G89.3 is assigned to pain documented as being related, associated or due to cancer, primary or secondary malignancy, or tumor. This code is assigned regardless of whether the pain is acute or chronic.

This code may be assigned as the principal or first-listed code when the stated reason for the admission/encounter is documented as pain control/pain management. The underlying neoplasm should be reported as an additional diagnosis.

> Pain medication adjustment for chronic pain from bone metastasis
>
> **G89.3 Neoplasm related pain (acute)(chronic)**
>
> **C79.51 Secondary malignant neoplasm of bone**
>
> *Explanation*: Since the encounter was for pain medication management, the pain, rather than the neoplasm, was the reason for the encounter and is sequenced first. This "neoplasm-related pain" code includes both acute and chronic pain.

When the reason for the admission/encounter is management of the neoplasm and the pain associated with the neoplasm is also documented, code G89.3 may be assigned as an additional diagnosis. It is not necessary to assign an additional code for the site of the pain.

See Section I.C.2. for instructions on the sequencing of neoplasms for all other stated reasons for the admission/encounter (except for pain control/pain management).

> Patient with lung cancer presents with acute hip pain and is evaluated and found to have iliac bone metastasis
>
> **C79.51 Secondary malignant neoplasm of bone**
>
> **C34.9Ø Malignant neoplasm of unspecified part of unspecified bronchus or lung**
>
> **G89.3 Neoplasm related pain (acute)(chronic)**
>
> *Explanation*: The reason for the encounter was the evaluation and diagnosis of the bone metastasis, whose code would be assigned as first-listed, followed by codes for the primary neoplasm and the pain due to the iliac bone metastasis.

6) Chronic pain syndrome

Central pain syndrome (G89.Ø) and chronic pain syndrome (G89.4) are different than the term "chronic pain," and therefore codes should only be used when the provider has specifically documented this condition.

See Section I.C.5. Pain disorders related to psychological factors

Chapter 6. Diseases of the Nervous System (G00-G99)

EXCLUDES 2 *certain conditions originating in the perinatal period (P04-P96)*
certain infectious and parasitic diseases (A00-B99)
complications of pregnancy, childbirth and the puerperium (O00-O9A)
congenital malformations, deformations, and chromosomal abnormalities (Q00-Q99)
endocrine, nutritional and metabolic diseases (E00-E88)
injury, poisoning and certain other consequences of external causes (S00-T88)
neoplasms (C00-D49)
symptoms, signs and abnormal clinical and laboratory findings, not elsewhere classified (R00-R94)

This chapter contains the following blocks:

Inflammatory diseases of the central nervous system (G00-G09)

✓4th **G00 Bacterial meningitis, not elsewhere classified**

INCLUDES bacterial arachnoiditis
bacterial leptomeningitis
bacterial meningitis
bacterial pachymeningitis

EXCLUDES 1 *bacterial meningoencephalitis (G04.2)*
bacterial meningomyelitis (G04.2)

DEF: Inflammation of meningeal layers of the brain and spinal cord due to a bacterial infection.

G00.0 Hemophilus meningitis MCC
Meningitis due to Hemophilus influenzae

G00.1 Pneumococcal meningitis MCC
Meningtitis due to Streptococcal pneumoniae

G00.2 Streptococcal meningitis MCC
Use additional code to further identify organism (B95.0-B95.5)

G00.3 Staphylococcal meningitis MCC
Use additional code to further identify organism (B95.61-B95.8)

G00.8 Other bacterial meningitis MCC
Meningitis due to Escherichia coli
Meningitis due to Friedlander's bacillus
Meningitis due to Klebsiella
Use additional code to further identify organism (B96.-)

G00.9 Bacterial meningitis, unspecified MCC
Meningitis due to gram-negative bacteria, unspecified
Purulent meningitis NOS
Pyogenic meningitis NOS
Suppurative meningitis NOS

G01 Meningitis in bacterial diseases classified elsewhere MCC
Code first underlying disease

EXCLUDES 1 *meningitis (in):*
gonococcal (A54.81)
leptospirosis (A27.81)
listeriosis (A32.11)
Lyme disease (A69.21)
meningococcal (A39.0)
neurosyphilis (A52.13)
tuberculosis (A17.0)
meningoencephalitis and meningomyelitis in bacterial diseases classified elsewhere (G05)

G02 Meningitis in other infectious and parasitic diseases classified elsewhere MCC
Code first underlying disease, such as:
African trypanosomiasis (B56.-)
poliovirus infection (A80.-)

EXCLUDES 1 *candidal meningitis (B37.5)*
coccidioidomycosis meningitis (B38.4)
cryptococcal meningitis (B45.1)
herpesviral [herpes simplex] meningitis (B00.3)
infectious mononucleosis complicated by meningitis (B27.- with fifth character 2)
measles complicated by meningitis (B05.1)
meningoencephalitis and meningomyelitis in other infectious and parasitic diseases classified elsewhere (G05)
mumps meningitis (B26.1)
rubella meningitis (B06.02)
varicella [chickenpox] meningitis (B01.0)
zoster meningitis (B02.1)

✓4th **G03 Meningitis due to other and unspecified causes**

INCLUDES arachnoiditis NOS
leptomeningitis NOS
meningitis NOS
pachymeningitis NOS

EXCLUDES 1 *meningoencephalitis (G04.-)*
meningomyelitis (G04.-)

G03.0 Nonpyogenic meningitis MCC
Aseptic meningitis
Nonbacterial meningitis
DEF: Type of meningitis where no bacterial, viral, or other infectious source exists that explains the meningitis symptomology.

G03.1 Chronic meningitis CC

G03.2 Benign recurrent meningitis [Mollaret] CC
DEF: Aseptic or noninfectious inflammation of the meninges with the presence of Mollaret cells in the spinal fluid. The patient experiences recurrent bouts of inflammation, lasting anywhere from two to five days.

G03.8 Meningitis due to other specified causes MCC

G03.9 Meningitis, unspecified MCC
Arachnoiditis (spinal) NOS

✓4th **G04 Encephalitis, myelitis and encephalomyelitis**

INCLUDES acute ascending myelitis
meningoencephalitis
meningomyelitis

EXCLUDES 1 *encephalopathy NOS (G93.40)*

EXCLUDES 2 *acute transverse myelitis ▶(G37.3)◀*
alcoholic encephalopathy (G31.2)
multiple sclerosis (G35)
myalgic encephalomyelitis (G93.32)
subacute necrotizing myelitis (G37.4)
toxic encephalitis (G92.8)
toxic encephalopathy (G92.8)

DEF: Encephalitis: Inflammation of the brain, often caused by viral or bacterial infection.
DEF: Encephalomyelitis: Inflammatory disease, often viral in nature, that affects the brain and spinal cord.
DEF: Myelitis: Inflammation of the spinal cord.

✓5th **G04.0 Acute disseminated encephalitis and encephalomyelitis (ADEM)**

EXCLUDES 1 *acute necrotizing hemorrhagic encephalopathy (G04.3-)*
other noninfectious acute disseminated encephalomyelitis (noninfectious ADEM) (G04.81)

G04.00 Acute disseminated encephalitis and encephalomyelitis, unspecified MCC

G04.01 Postinfectious acute disseminated encephalitis and encephalomyelitis (postinfectious ADEM) MCC

EXCLUDES 1 *post chickenpox encephalitis (B01.1)*
post measles encephalitis (B05.0)
post measles myelitis (B05.1)

G04.02 Postimmunization acute disseminated encephalitis, myelitis and encephalomyelitis MCC
Encephalitis, post immunization
Encephalomyelitis, post immunization
Use additional code to identify the vaccine (T50.A-, T50.B-, T50.Z-)

G04.1 Tropical spastic paraplegia CC HCC

G04.2 Bacterial meningoencephalitis and meningomyelitis, not elsewhere classified MCC

✓5th **G04.3 Acute necrotizing hemorrhagic encephalopathy**

EXCLUDES 1 *acute disseminated encephalitis and encephalomyelitis (G04.0-)*

G04.30 Acute necrotizing hemorrhagic encephalopathy, unspecified MCC

G04.31 Postinfectious acute necrotizing hemorrhagic encephalopathy MCC

G04.32 Postimmunization acute necrotizing hemorrhagic encephalopathy MCC

Use additional code to identify the vaccine (T50.A-, T50.B-, T50.Z-)

G04.39 Other acute necrotizing hemorrhagic encephalopathy MCC

Code also underlying etiology, if applicable

✓5th **G04.8 Other encephalitis, myelitis and encephalomyelitis**

Code also any associated seizure (G40.-, R56.9)

G04.81 Other encephalitis and encephalomyelitis HIV MCC

Noninfectious acute disseminated encephalomyelitis (noninfectious ADEM)

G04.82 Acute flaccid myelitis MCC HCC

EXCLUDES 1 *transverse myelitis (G37.3)*

AHA: 2021,4Q,11

G04.89 Other myelitis HIV MCC HCC

AHA: 2020,1Q,14

✓5th **G04.9 Encephalitis, myelitis and encephalomyelitis, unspecified**

G04.90 Encephalitis and encephalomyelitis, unspecified HIV MCC

Ventriculitis (cerebral) NOS

G04.91 Myelitis, unspecified HIV MCC HCC

✓4th **G05 Encephalitis, myelitis and encephalomyelitis in diseases classified elsewhere**

Code first underlying disease, such as:
- congenital toxoplasmosis encephalitis, myelitis and encephalomyelitis (P37.1)
- cytomegaloviral encephalitis, myelitis and encephalomyelitis (B25.8)
- encephalitis, myelitis and encephalomyelitis (in) systemic lupus erythematosus (M32.19)
- eosinophilic meningoencephalitis (B83.2)
- human immunodeficiency virus [HIV] disease (B20)
- poliovirus (A80.-)
- suppurative otitis media (H66.01-H66.4)
- ▶systemic lupus erythematosus (M32.19)◀
- trichinellosis (B75)

EXCLUDES 1
- *adenoviral encephalitis, myelitis and encephalomyelitis (A85.1)*
- *encephalitis, myelitis and encephalomyelitis (in) measles (B05.0)*
- *enteroviral encephalitis, myelitis and encephalomyelitis (A85.0)*
- *herpesviral [herpes simplex] encephalitis, myelitis and encephalomyelitis (B00.4)*
- *listerial encephalitis, myelitis and encephalomyelitis (A32.12)*
- *meningococcal encephalitis, myelitis and encephalomyelitis (A39.81)*
- *mumps encephalitis, myelitis and encephalomyelitis (B26.2)*
- *postchickenpox encephalitis, myelitis and encephalomyelitis (B01.1-)*
- *rubella encephalitis, myelitis and encephalomyelitis (B06.01)*
- *toxoplasmosis encephalitis, myelitis and encephalomyelitis (B58.2)*
- *zoster encephalitis, myelitis and encephalomyelitis (B02.0)*

G05.3 Encephalitis and encephalomyelitis in diseases classified elsewhere MCC

Meningoencephalitis in diseases classified elsewhere

▶Code first underlying disease◀

G05.4 Myelitis in diseases classified elsewhere MCC HCC

Meningomyelitis in diseases classified elsewhere

✓4th **G06 Intracranial and intraspinal abscess and granuloma**

Use additional code (B95-B97) to identify infectious agent

DEF: Abscess: Circumscribed collection of pus resulting from bacteria, frequently associated with swelling and other signs of inflammation.

DEF: Granuloma: Abnormal, dense collections of cells forming a mass or nodule of chronically inflamed tissue with granulations that is usually associated with an infective process.

G06.0 Intracranial abscess and granuloma MCC

Brain [any part] abscess (embolic)
Cerebellar abscess (embolic)
Cerebral abscess (embolic)
Intracranial epidural abscess or granuloma
Intracranial extradural abscess or granuloma
Intracranial subdural abscess or granuloma
Otogenic abscess (embolic)

EXCLUDES 1 *tuberculous intracranial abscess and granuloma (A17.81)*

G06.1 Intraspinal abscess and granuloma MCC

Abscess (embolic) of spinal cord [any part]
Intraspinal epidural abscess or granuloma
Intraspinal extradural abscess or granuloma
Intraspinal subdural abscess or granuloma

EXCLUDES 1 *tuberculous intraspinal abscess and granuloma (A17.81)*

G06.2 Extradural and subdural abscess, unspecified MCC

G07 Intracranial and intraspinal abscess and granuloma in diseases classified elsewhere MCC

Code first underlying disease, such as:
- schistosomiasis granuloma of brain (B65.-)

EXCLUDES 1 *abscess of brain:*
- *amebic (A06.6)*
- *chromomycotic (B43.1)*
- *gonococcal (A54.82)*
- *tuberculous (A17.81)*

tuberculoma of meninges (A17.1)

G08 Intracranial and intraspinal phlebitis and thrombophlebitis MCC

Septic embolism of intracranial or intraspinal venous sinuses and veins
Septic endophlebitis of intracranial or intraspinal venous sinuses and veins
Septic phlebitis of intracranial or intraspinal venous sinuses and veins
Septic thrombophlebitis of intracranial or intraspinal venous sinuses and veins
Septic thrombosis of intracranial or intraspinal venous sinuses and veins

EXCLUDES 1 *intracranial phlebitis and thrombophlebitis complicating:*
- *abortion, ectopic or molar pregnancy (O00-O07, O08.7)*
- *pregnancy, childbirth and the puerperium (O22.5, O87.3)*

nonpyogenic intracranial phlebitis and thrombophlebitis (I67.6)

EXCLUDES 2 *intracranial phlebitis and thrombophlebitis complicating nonpyogenic intraspinal phlebitis and thrombophlebitis (G95.1)*

DEF: Inflammation and formation of a blood clot in a vein within the brain or spine, or their linings.

G09 Sequelae of inflammatory diseases of central nervous system

NOTE Category G09 is to be used to indicate conditions whose primary classification is to G00-G08 as the cause of sequelae, themselves classifiable elsewhere. The "sequelae" include conditions specified as residuals.

Code first condition resulting from (sequela) of inflammatory diseases of central nervous system

Systemic atrophies primarily affecting the central nervous system (G10-G14)

G10 Huntington's disease CC HCC
Huntington's chorea
Huntington's dementia
Use additional code, if applicable, to identify:
dementia with anxiety (F02.84, F02.A4, F02.B4, F02.C4)
dementia with behavioral disturbance (F02.81-, F02.A1-, F02.B1-, F02.C1-)
dementia with mood disturbance (F02.83, F02.A3, F02.B3, F02.C3)
dementia with psychotic disturbance (F02.82, F02.A2, F02.B2, F02.C2)
dementia without behavioral disturbance (F02.80, F02.A0, F02.B0, F02.C0)
mild neurocognitive disorder due to known physiological condition (F06.7-)
DEF: Genetic disease caused by degeneration of nerve cells in the brain, characterized by chronic progressive mental deterioration. Dementia and death occur within 15 to 20 years of onset.

G11 Hereditary ataxia
EXCLUDES 2 *cerebral palsy (G80.-)*
hereditary and idiopathic neuropathy (G60.-)
metabolic disorders (E70-E88)
DEF: Ataxia: Defect in muscular control or coordination due to a central nervous system disorder, particularly when voluntary muscular movements are attempted.

G11.0 Congenital nonprogressive ataxia CC HCC
G11.1 Early-onset cerebellar ataxia
AHA: 2020,4Q,17-18
G11.10 Early-onset cerebellar ataxia, unspecified CC HCC
G11.11 Friedreich ataxia CC HCC
Autosomal recessive Friedreich ataxia
Friedreich ataxia with retained reflexes
G11.19 Other early-onset cerebellar ataxia CC HCC
Early-onset cerebellar ataxia with essential tremor
Early-onset cerebellar ataxia with myoclonus [Hunt's ataxia]
Early-onset cerebellar ataxia with retained tendon reflexes
X-linked recessive spinocerebellar ataxia
G11.2 Late-onset cerebellar ataxia CC HCC A
G11.3 Cerebellar ataxia with defective DNA repair CC HCC
Ataxia telangiectasia [Louis-Bar]
EXCLUDES 2 *Cockayne's syndrome (Q87.19)*
other disorders of purine and pyrimidine metabolism (E79.-)
xeroderma pigmentosum (Q82.1)
G11.4 Hereditary spastic paraplegia CC HCC
● **G11.5 Hypomyelination - hypogonadotropic hypogonadism - hypodontia** CC
4H syndrome
Pol III-related leukodystrophy
● **G11.6 Leukodystrophy with vanishing white matter disease** CC
G11.8 Other hereditary ataxias CC HCC
G11.9 Hereditary ataxia, unspecified CC HCC
Hereditary cerebellar ataxia NOS
Hereditary cerebellar degeneration
Hereditary cerebellar disease
Hereditary cerebellar syndrome

G12 Spinal muscular atrophy and related syndromes
G12.0 Infantile spinal muscular atrophy, type I [Werdnig-Hoffman] CC HCC
G12.1 Other inherited spinal muscular atrophy CC HCC
Adult form spinal muscular atrophy
Childhood form, type II spinal muscular atrophy
Distal spinal muscular atrophy
Juvenile form, type III spinal muscular atrophy [Kugelberg-Welander]
Progressive bulbar palsy of childhood [Fazio-Londe]
Scapuloperoneal form spinal muscular atrophy
G12.2 Motor neuron disease
AHA: 2017,4Q,9-10
G12.20 Motor neuron disease, unspecified CC HCC
G12.21 Amyotrophic lateral sclerosis CC HCC A
G12.22 Progressive bulbar palsy CC HCC
G12.23 Primary lateral sclerosis CC HCC
G12.24 Familial motor neuron disease CC HCC
G12.25 Progressive spinal muscle atrophy CC HCC
G12.29 Other motor neuron disease CC HCC
G12.8 Other spinal muscular atrophies and related syndromes CC HCC
G12.9 Spinal muscular atrophy, unspecified CC HCC

G13 Systemic atrophies primarily affecting central nervous system in diseases classified elsewhere
G13.0 Paraneoplastic neuromyopathy and neuropathy HCC
Carcinomatous neuromyopathy
Sensorial paraneoplastic neuropathy [Denny Brown]
Code first underlying neoplasm (C00-D49)
G13.1 Other systemic atrophy primarily affecting central nervous system in neoplastic disease HCC
Paraneoplastic limbic encephalopathy
Code first underlying neoplasm (C00-D49)
G13.2 Systemic atrophy primarily affecting the central nervous system in myxedema HCC
Code first underlying disease, such as:
hypothyroidism (E03.-)
myxedematous congenital iodine deficiency (E00.1)
G13.8 Systemic atrophy primarily affecting central nervous system in other diseases classified elsewhere HCC
Code first underlying disease

G14 Postpolio syndrome
INCLUDES postpolio myelitic syndrome
EXCLUDES 1 *sequelae of poliomyelitis (B91)*

Extrapyramidal and movement disorders (G20-G26)

▲ **G20 Parkinson's disease**
Hemiparkinsonism
Idiopathic Parkinsonism or Parkinson's disease
Paralysis agitans
~~Parkinsonism or Parkinson's disease NOS~~
Primary Parkinsonism or Parkinson's disease
Use additional code, if applicable, to identify:
dementia with anxiety (F02.84, F02.A4, F02.B4, F02.C4)
dementia with behavioral disturbance (F02.81-, F02.A1-, F02.B1-, F02.C1-)
dementia with mood disturbance (F02.83, F02.A3, F02.B3, F02.C3)
dementia with psychotic disturbance (F02.82, F02.A2, F02.B2, F02.C2)
dementia without behavioral disturbance (F02.80, F02.A0, F02.B0, F02.C0)
mild neurocognitive disorder due to known physiological condition (F06.7-)
AHA: 2017,2Q,7; 2016,2Q,6
TIP: Repeated falls (R29.6) are not integral to Parkinson's disease and can be separately coded.

● **G20.A Parkinson's disease without dyskinesia**
● **G20.A1 Parkinson's disease without dyskinesia, without mention of fluctuations**
Parkinson's disease NOS
Parkinson's disease without dyskinesia, without mention of OFF episodes
● **G20.A2 Parkinson's disease without dyskinesia, with fluctuations**
Parkinson's disease without dyskinesia, with OFF episodes
● **G20.B Parkinson's disease with dyskinesia**
EXCLUDES 1 *drug induced dystonia (G24.0-)*
● **G20.B1 Parkinson's disease with dyskinesia, without mention of fluctuations**
Parkinson's disease with dyskinesia, without mention of OFF episodes
● **G20.B2 Parkinson's disease with dyskinesia, with fluctuations**
Parkinson's disease with dyskinesia, with OFF episodes
● **G20.C Parkinsonism, unspecified**
Parkinsonism, NOS
EXCLUDES 1 *Parkinson's disease NOS (G20.A1)*
Parkinson's disease with dyskinesia (G20.B-)
Parkinson's disease without dyskinesia (G20.A-)
secondary parkinsonism (G21-)

√4th G21 Secondary parkinsonism

EXCLUDES 1 *dementia with Parkinsonism (G31.83)*
Huntington's disease (G1Ø)
Shy-Drager syndrome (G9Ø.3)
syphilitic Parkinsonism (A52.19)

G21.Ø Malignant neuroleptic syndrome MCC
Use additional code for adverse effect, if applicable, to identify drug (T43.3X5, T43.4X5, T43.5Ø5, T43.595)
EXCLUDES 1 *neuroleptic induced parkinsonism (G21.11)*

√5th **G21.1 Other drug-induced secondary parkinsonism**

G21.11 Neuroleptic induced parkinsonism CC HCC
Use additional code for adverse effect, if applicable, to identify drug (T43.3X5, T43.4X5, T43.5Ø5, T43.595)
EXCLUDES 1 *malignant neuroleptic syndrome (G21.Ø)*

G21.19 Other drug induced secondary parkinsonism CC HCC
Other medication-induced parkinsonism
Use additional code for adverse effect, if applicable, to identify drug (T36-T5Ø with fifth or sixth character 5)

G21.2 Secondary parkinsonism due to other external agents CC HCC
Code first (T51-T65) to identify external agent

G21.3 Postencephalitic parkinsonism CC HCC

G21.4 Vascular parkinsonism HCC

G21.8 Other secondary parkinsonism CC HCC

G21.9 Secondary parkinsonism, unspecified CC HCC

√4th G23 Other degenerative diseases of basal ganglia

EXCLUDES 2 *multi-system degeneration of the autonomic nervous system (G9Ø.3)*

G23.Ø Hallervorden-Spatz disease CC HCC
Pigmentary pallidal degeneration

G23.1 Progressive supranuclear ophthalmoplegia [Steele-Richardson-Olszewski] CC HCC
Progressive supranuclear palsy

G23.2 Striatonigral degeneration CC HCC

● **G23.3 Hypomyelination with atrophy of the basal ganglia and cerebellum** CC
H-ABC

G23.8 Other specified degenerative diseases of basal ganglia CC HCC
Calcification of basal ganglia

G23.9 Degenerative disease of basal ganglia, unspecified CC HCC

√4th G24 Dystonia

INCLUDES dyskinesia
EXCLUDES 2 *athetoid cerebral palsy (G8Ø.3)*

DEF: Disorder of abnormal muscle tone, excessive or inadequate. Involuntary movements and prolonged muscle contractions result in tremors, abnormalities in posture, and twisting body motions that affect an isolated area or the whole body.

√5th **G24.Ø Drug induced dystonia**
Use additional code for adverse effect, if applicable, to identify drug (T36-T5Ø with fifth or sixth character 5)

G24.Ø1 Drug induced subacute dyskinesia
Drug induced blepharospasm
Drug induced orofacial dyskinesia
Neuroleptic induced tardive dyskinesia
Tardive dyskinesia

G24.Ø2 Drug induced acute dystonia CC
Acute dystonic reaction to drugs
Neuroleptic induced acute dystonia

G24.Ø9 Other drug induced dystonia CC

G24.1 Genetic torsion dystonia
Dystonia deformans progressiva
Dystonia musculorum deformans
Familial torsion dystonia
Idiopathic familial dystonia
Idiopathic (torsion) dystonia NOS
(Schwalbe-) Ziehen-Oppenheim disease

G24.2 Idiopathic nonfamilial dystonia CC

G24.3 Spasmodic torticollis
EXCLUDES 1 *congenital torticollis (Q68.Ø)*
hysterical torticollis (F44.4)
ocular torticollis (R29.891)
psychogenic torticollis (F45.8)
torticollis NOS (M43.6)
traumatic recurrent torticollis (S13.4)
DEF: Twisted, unnatural position of the neck due to contracted cervical muscles that pull the head to one side or cause involuntary shaking of the head.

G24.4 Idiopathic orofacial dystonia
Orofacial dyskinesia
EXCLUDES 1 *drug induced orofacial dyskinesia (G24.Ø1)*

G24.5 Blepharospasm
EXCLUDES 1 *drug induced blepharospasm (G24.Ø1)*
DEF: Involuntary contraction of the orbicularis oculi muscle, resulting in the eyelids being completely closed.

G24.8 Other dystonia CC
Acquired torsion dystonia NOS

G24.9 Dystonia, unspecified
Dyskinesia NOS

√4th G25 Other extrapyramidal and movement disorders

EXCLUDES 2 *sleep related movement disorders (G47.6-)*

G25.Ø Essential tremor
Familial tremor
EXCLUDES 1 *tremor NOS (R25.1)*

G25.1 Drug-induced tremor
Use additional code for adverse effect, if applicable, to identify drug (T36-T5Ø with fifth or sixth character 5)

G25.2 Other specified forms of tremor
Intention tremor

G25.3 Myoclonus
Drug-induced myoclonus
Palatal myoclonus
Use additional code for adverse effect, if applicable, to identify drug (T36-T5Ø with fifth or sixth character 5)
EXCLUDES 1 *facial myokymia (G51.4)*
myoclonic epilepsy (G4Ø.-)
DEF: Spasmodic, brief, involuntary muscle contractions that can be due to an undetermined etiology, drug-induced, or caused by a disease process.

G25.4 Drug-induced chorea
Use additional code for adverse effect, if applicable, to identify drug (T36-T5Ø with fifth or sixth character 5)

G25.5 Other chorea
Chorea NOS
EXCLUDES 1 *chorea NOS with heart involvement (IØ2.Ø)*
Huntington's chorea (G1Ø)
rheumatic chorea (IØ2.-)
Sydenham's chorea (IØ2.-)

√5th **G25.6 Drug induced tics and other tics of organic origin**

G25.61 Drug induced tics
Use additional code for adverse effect, if applicable, to identify drug (T36-T5Ø with fifth or sixth character 5)

G25.69 Other tics of organic origin
EXCLUDES 1 *habit spasm (F95.9)*
tic NOS (F95.9)
Tourette's syndrome (F95.2)

√5th **G25.7 Other and unspecified drug induced movement disorders**
Use additional code for adverse effect, if applicable, to identify drug (T36-T5Ø with fifth or sixth character 5)

G25.7Ø Drug induced movement disorder, unspecified

G25.71 Drug induced akathisia
Drug induced acathisia
Neuroleptic induced acute akathisia
Tardive akathisia

G25.79 Other drug induced movement disorders

√5th **G25.8 Other specified extrapyramidal and movement disorders**

G25.81 Restless legs syndrome
DEF: Neurological disorder of unknown etiology creating an irresistible urge to move the legs, which may temporarily relieve the symptoms. This syndrome is accompanied by motor restlessness and sensations of pain, burning, prickling, or tingling.

G25.82 Stiff-man syndrome CC

G25.83 Benign shuddering attacks

G25.89 **Other specified extrapyramidal and movement disorders**

G25.9 **Extrapyramidal and movement disorder, unspecified** CC

G26 ***Extrapyramidal and movement disorders in diseases classified elsewhere***
Code first underlying disease

Other degenerative diseases of the nervous system (G30-G32)

✓4th **G30 Alzheimer's disease**
INCLUDES Alzheimer's dementia senile and presenile forms
Use additional code, if applicable, to identify:
delirium, if applicable (F05)
dementia with anxiety (F02.84, F02.A4, F02.B4, F02.C4)
dementia with behavioral disturbance (F02.81-, F02.A1-, F02.B1-, F02.C1-)
dementia with mood disturbance (F02.83, F02.A3, F02.B3, F02.C3)
dementia with psychotic disturbance (F02.82, F02.A2, F02.B2, F02.C2)
dementia without behavioral disturbance (F02.80, F02.A0, F02.B0, F02.C0)
mild neurocognitive disorder due to known physiological condition (F06.7-)
EXCLUDES 1 *senile degeneration of brain NEC (G31.1)*
senile dementia NOS (F03)
senility NOS (R41.81)
AHA: 2022,4Q,15; 2017,1Q,43
TIP: A code from subcategory F02.8 should always be assigned with a code from this category, even in the absence of documented dementia.
TIP: Functional quadriplegia (R53.2) is not integral to Alzheimer's disease and can be coded in addition to codes from category G30.

G30.0 **Alzheimer's disease with early onset** HCC
G30.1 **Alzheimer's disease with late onset** HCC A
G30.8 **Other Alzheimer's disease** HCC
G30.9 **Alzheimer's disease, unspecified** HCC
AHA: 2016,2Q,6; 2012,4Q,95

✓4th **G31 Other degenerative diseases of nervous system, not elsewhere classified**
▶Use additional code, if applicable, for codes G31.0-G31.83, G31.85-G31.9, to identify:◀
dementia with anxiety (F02.84, F02.A4, F02.B4, F02.C4)
dementia with behavioral disturbance (F02.81-, F02.A1-, F02.B1-, F02.C1-)
dementia with mood disturbance (F02.83, F02.A3, F02.B3, F02.C3)
dementia with psychotic disturbance (F02.82, F02.A2, F02.B2, F02.C2)
dementia without behavioral disturbance (F02.80, F02.A0, F02.B0, F02.C0)
mild neurocognitive disorder due to known physiological condition (F06.7-)
EXCLUDES 2 *Reye's syndrome (G93.7)*

✓5th G31.0 **Frontotemporal dementia**

G31.01 **Pick's disease** HCC
Primary progressive aphasia
Progressive isolated aphasia
DEF: Progressive frontotemporal dementia with asymmetrical atrophy of the frontal and temporal regions of the cerebral cortex and abnormal rounded brain cells called Pick cells with the presence of abnormal staining of protein (called tau). Symptoms include prominent apathy, behavioral changes such as disinhibition and restlessness, echolalia, impairment of language, memory, and intellect, increased carelessness, poor personal hygiene, and decreased attention span.

G31.09 **Other frontotemporal neurocognitive disorder** HCC
Frontal dementia
Use additional code, if applicable, to identify mild neurocognitive disorders due to known physiological condition (F06.7-)

G31.1 **Senile degeneration of brain, not elsewhere classified** HCC
EXCLUDES 1 *Alzheimer's disease (G30.-)*
senility NOS (R41.81)

G31.2 **Degeneration of nervous system due to alcohol** HCC
Alcoholic cerebellar ataxia
Alcoholic cerebellar degeneration
Alcoholic cerebral degeneration
Alcoholic encephalopathy
Dysfunction of the autonomic nervous system due to alcohol
Code also associated alcoholism (F10.-)

✓5th G31.8 **Other specified degenerative diseases of nervous system**

● G31.80 **Leukodystrophy, unspecified**

G31.81 **Alpers disease** CC HCC
Grey-matter degeneration

G31.82 **Leigh's disease** CC HCC
Subacute necrotizing encephalopathy

G31.83 **Neurocognitive disorder with Lewy bodies** HCC
Lewy body dementia
Lewy body disease
Use additional code, if applicable, to identify mild neurocognitive disorders due to known physiological condition (F06.7-)
AHA: 2017,2Q,7; 2016,4Q,141
DEF: Cerebral dementia with neurophysiologic changes, increased hippocampal volume, hypoperfusion in the occipital lobes, beta amyloid deposits with neurofibrillary tangles, and atrophy of the cortex and brainstem. Hallmark neuropsychological characteristics include fluctuating cognition with pronounced variation in attention and alertness, recurrent hallucinations, and Parkinsonism.

G31.84 **Mild cognitive impairment of uncertain or unknown etiology**
Mild cognitive disorder NOS
Mild neurocognitive disorder of uncertain or unknown etiology
Use additional code to identify presence of:
alcohol abuse and dependence (F10.-)
exposure to environmental tobacco smoke (Z77.22)
history of tobacco dependence (Z87.891)
hypertension ▶(I10-I1A)◀
occupational exposure to environmental tobacco smoke (Z57.31)
tobacco dependence (F17.-)
tobacco use (Z72.0)
EXCLUDES 1 *age related cognitive decline (R41.81)*
altered mental status (R41.82)
cerebral degeneration (G31.9)
cerebrovascular diseases (I60-I69)
change in mental status (R41.82)
cognitive deficits following (sequelae of) cerebral hemorrhage or infarction (I69.01-, I69.11-, I69.21-, I69.31-, I69.81-, I69.91-)
cognitive impairment due to intracranial or head injury (S06.-)
dementia (F01.-, F02.-, F03)
mild neurocognitive disorder due to a known physiological condition (F06.7-)
neurologic neglect syndrome (R41.4)
personality change, nonpsychotic (F68.8)
AHA: 2021,3Q,3

G31.85 **Corticobasal degeneration** HCC

● G31.86 **Alexander disease**

G31.89 **Other specified degenerative diseases of nervous system** HCC

G31.9 **Degenerative disease of nervous system, unspecified** HCC
AHA: 2021,3Q,3

G32 Other degenerative disorders of nervous system in diseases classified elsewhere

G32.0 ***Subacute combined degeneration of spinal cord in diseases classified elsewhere*** CC HCC
Dana-Putnam syndrome
Sclerosis of spinal cord (combined) (dorsolateral) (posterolateral)
Code first underlying disease, such as:
~~anemia (D51.9)~~
▶other dietary vitamin B12 deficiency anemia◀ (D51.3)
▶vitamin B12 deficiency anemia due to intrinsic factor deficiency◀ (D51.0)
▶vitamin B12 deficiency anemia, unspecified (D51.8)◀
vitamin B12 deficiency (E53.8)
EXCLUDES 1 *syphilitic combined degeneration of spinal cord (A52.11)*

G32.8 Other specified degenerative disorders of nervous system in diseases classified elsewhere
Code first underlying disease, such as:
amyloidosis cerebral degeneration (E85.-)
cerebral degeneration (due to) hypothyroidism (E00.0-E03.9)
cerebral degeneration (due to) neoplasm (C00-D49)
cerebral degeneration (due to) vitamin B deficiency, except thiamine (E52-E53.-)
EXCLUDES 1 *superior hemorrhagic polioencephalitis [Wernicke's encephalopathy] (E51.2)*

G32.81 ***Cerebellar ataxia in diseases classified elsewhere*** CC HCC
Code first underlying disease, such as:
celiac disease (with gluten ataxia) (K90.0)
cerebellar ataxia (in) neoplastic disease (paraneoplastic cerebellar degeneration) (C00-D49)
non-celiac gluten ataxia (M35.9)
EXCLUDES 1 *systemic atrophy primarily affecting the central nervous system in alcoholic cerebellar ataxia (G31.2)*
systemic atrophy primarily affecting the central nervous system in myxedema (G13.2)

G32.89 ***Other specified degenerative disorders of nervous system in diseases classified elsewhere***
Degenerative encephalopathy in diseases classified elsewhere

Demyelinating diseases of the central nervous system (G35-G37)

G35 Multiple sclerosis HCC
Disseminated multiple sclerosis
Generalized multiple sclerosis
Multiple sclerosis NOS
Multiple sclerosis of brain stem
Multiple sclerosis of cord
AHA: 2021,1Q,7

G36 Other acute disseminated demyelination
EXCLUDES 1 *postinfectious encephalitis and encephalomyelitis NOS (G04.01)*
DEF: Demyelination: Abnormal loss of myelin, the protective white matter that insulates nerve endings and facilitates neuroreception and neurotransmission. When this substance is damaged, the nerve is short-circuited, resulting in impaired or loss of function.

G36.0 Neuromyelitis optica [Devic] CC HCC
Demyelination in optic neuritis
EXCLUDES 1 *optic neuritis NOS (H46)*

G36.1 Acute and subacute hemorrhagic leukoencephalitis [Hurst] CC HCC

G36.8 Other specified acute disseminated demyelination CC HCC

G36.9 Acute disseminated demyelination, unspecified HIV CC HCC

G37 Other demyelinating diseases of central nervous system

G37.0 Diffuse sclerosis of central nervous system CC HCC
Periaxial encephalitis
Schilder's disease
EXCLUDES 1 *X linked adrenoleukodystrophy (E71.52-)*

G37.1 Central demyelination of corpus callosum CC HCC

G37.2 Central pontine myelinolysis CC HCC
AHA: 2022,2Q,10

G37.3 Acute transverse myelitis in demyelinating disease of central nervous system CC HCC
Acute transverse myelitis NOS
Acute transverse myelopathy
EXCLUDES 1 *acute flaccid myelitis (G04.82)*
multiple sclerosis (G35)
neuromyelitis optica [Devic] (G36.0)

G37.4 Subacute necrotizing myelitis of central nervous system HIV MCC HCC

G37.5 Concentric sclerosis [Balo] of central nervous system CC HCC

▲ **G37.8 Other specified demyelinating diseases of central nervous system**

● **G37.81 Myelin oligodendrocyte glycoprotein antibody disease** CC
MOG antibody disease
Code also associated manifestations, if known, such as:
noninfectious acute disseminated encephalomyelitis (G04.81)
neuromyelitis optica (G36.0)

● **G37.89 Other specified demyelinating diseases of central nervous system** CC

G37.9 Demyelinating disease of central nervous system, unspecified HIV CC HCC

Episodic and paroxysmal disorders (G40-G47)

G40 Epilepsy and recurrent seizures
NOTE The following terms are to be considered equivalent to intractable: pharmacoresistant (pharmacologically resistant), treatment resistant, refractory (medically) and poorly controlled
EXCLUDES 1 *conversion disorder with seizures (F44.5)*
convulsions NOS (R56.9)
post traumatic seizures (R56.1)
seizure (convulsive) NOS (R56.9)
seizure of newborn (P90)
EXCLUDES 2 *hippocampal sclerosis (G93.81)*
mesial temporal sclerosis (G93.81)
temporal sclerosis (G93.81)
Todd's paralysis (G83.84)

G40.0 Localization-related (focal) (partial) idiopathic epilepsy and epileptic syndromes with seizures of localized onset
Benign childhood epilepsy with centrotemporal EEG spikes
Childhood epilepsy with occipital EEG paroxysms
EXCLUDES 1 *adult onset localization-related epilepsy (G40.1-, G40.2-)*

G40.00 Localization-related (focal) (partial) idiopathic epilepsy and epileptic syndromes with seizures of localized onset, not intractable
Localization-related (focal) (partial) idiopathic epilepsy and epileptic syndromes with seizures of localized onset without intractability

G40.001 Localization-related (focal) (partial) idiopathic epilepsy and epileptic syndromes with seizures of localized onset, not intractable, with status epilepticus CC HCC

G40.009 Localization-related (focal) (partial) idiopathic epilepsy and epileptic syndromes with seizures of localized onset, not intractable, without status epilepticus CC HCC
Localization-related (focal) (partial) idiopathic epilepsy and epileptic syndromes with seizures of localized onset NOS

G40.01 Localization-related (focal) (partial) idiopathic epilepsy and epileptic syndromes with seizures of localized onset, intractable

G40.011 Localization-related (focal) (partial) idiopathic epilepsy and epileptic syndromes with seizures of localized onset, intractable, with status epilepticus CC HCC

G40.019 Localization-related (focal) (partial) idiopathic epilepsy and epileptic syndromes with seizures of localized onset, intractable, without status epilepticus CC HCC

G40.1 Localization-related (focal) (partial) symptomatic epilepsy and epileptic syndromes with simple partial seizures
Attacks without alteration of consciousness
Epilepsia partialis continua [Kozhevnikof]
Simple partial seizures developing into secondarily generalized seizures

G40.10 Localization-related (focal) (partial) symptomatic epilepsy and epileptic syndromes with simple partial seizures, not intractable
Localization-related (focal) (partial) symptomatic epilepsy and epileptic syndromes with simple partial seizures without intractability

G40.101 Localization-related (focal) (partial) symptomatic epilepsy and epileptic syndromes with simple partial seizures, not intractable, with status epilepticus CC HCC

G40.109 Localization-related (focal) (partial) symptomatic epilepsy and epileptic syndromes with simple partial seizures, not intractable, without status epilepticus CC HCC
Localization-related (focal) (partial) symptomatic epilepsy and epileptic syndromes with simple partial seizures NOS

G40.11 Localization-related (focal) (partial) symptomatic epilepsy and epileptic syndromes with simple partial seizures, intractable

G40.111 Localization-related (focal) (partial) symptomatic epilepsy and epileptic syndromes with simple partial seizures, intractable, with status epilepticus CC HCC

G40.119 Localization-related (focal) (partial) symptomatic epilepsy and epileptic syndromes with simple partial seizures, intractable, without status epilepticus CC HCC

G40.2 Localization-related (focal) (partial) symptomatic epilepsy and epileptic syndromes with complex partial seizures
Attacks with alteration of consciousness, often with automatisms
Complex partial seizures developing into secondarily generalized seizures

G40.20 Localization-related (focal) (partial) symptomatic epilepsy and epileptic syndromes with complex partial seizures, not intractable
Localization-related (focal) (partial) symptomatic epilepsy and epileptic syndromes with complex partial seizures without intractability

G40.201 Localization-related (focal) (partial) symptomatic epilepsy and epileptic syndromes with complex partial seizures, not intractable, with status epilepticus CC HCC

G40.209 Localization-related (focal) (partial) symptomatic epilepsy and epileptic syndromes with complex partial seizures, not intractable, without status epilepticus CC HCC
Localization-related (focal) (partial) symptomatic epilepsy and epileptic syndromes with complex partial seizures NOS

G40.21 Localization-related (focal) (partial) symptomatic epilepsy and epileptic syndromes with complex partial seizures, intractable

G40.211 Localization-related (focal) (partial) symptomatic epilepsy and epileptic syndromes with complex partial seizures, intractable, with status epilepticus CC HCC

G40.219 Localization-related (focal) (partial) symptomatic epilepsy and epileptic syndromes with complex partial seizures, intractable, without status epilepticus CC HCC

G40.3 Generalized idiopathic epilepsy and epileptic syndromes
Code also MERRF syndrome, if applicable (E88.42)

G40.30 Generalized idiopathic epilepsy and epileptic syndromes, not intractable
Generalized idiopathic epilepsy and epileptic syndromes without intractability

G40.301 Generalized idiopathic epilepsy and epileptic syndromes, not intractable, with status epilepticus MCC HCC

G40.309 Generalized idiopathic epilepsy and epileptic syndromes, not intractable, without status epilepticus HCC
Generalized idiopathic epilepsy and epileptic syndromes NOS

G40.31 Generalized idiopathic epilepsy and epileptic syndromes, intractable

G40.311 Generalized idiopathic epilepsy and epileptic syndromes, intractable, with status epilepticus MCC HCC

G40.319 Generalized idiopathic epilepsy and epileptic syndromes, intractable, without status epilepticus MCC HCC

G40.A Absence epileptic syndrome
Childhood absence epilepsy [pyknolepsy]
Juvenile absence epilepsy
Absence epileptic syndrome, NOS

G40.A0 Absence epileptic syndrome, not intractable

G40.A01 Absence epileptic syndrome, not intractable, with status epilepticus HCC

G40.A09 Absence epileptic syndrome, not intractable, without status epilepticus HCC

G40.A1 Absence epileptic syndrome, intractable

G40.A11 Absence epileptic syndrome, intractable, with status epilepticus CC HCC

G40.A19 Absence epileptic syndrome, intractable, without status epilepticus CC HCC

G40.B Juvenile myoclonic epilepsy [impulsive petit mal]

G40.B0 Juvenile myoclonic epilepsy, not intractable

G40.B01 Juvenile myoclonic epilepsy, not intractable, with status epilepticus CC HCC

G40.B09 Juvenile myoclonic epilepsy, not intractable, without status epilepticus CC HCC

G40.B1 Juvenile myoclonic epilepsy, intractable

G40.B11 Juvenile myoclonic epilepsy, intractable, with status epilepticus CC HCC

G40.B19 Juvenile myoclonic epilepsy, intractable, without status epilepticus CC HCC

● **G40.C Lafora progressive myoclonus epilepsy**
Lafora body disease
Code also, if applicable, associated conditions such as dementia (F02.8-)

● **G40.C0 Lafora progressive myoclonus epilepsy, not intractable**

● **G40.C01 Lafora progressive myoclonus epilepsy, not intractable, with status epilepticus** CC

● **G40.C09 Lafora progressive myoclonus epilepsy, not intractable, without status epilepticus** CC
Lafora progressive myoclonus epilepsy NOS

● **G40.C1 Lafora progressive myoclonus epilepsy, intractable**

● **G40.C11 Lafora progressive myoclonus epilepsy, intractable, with status epilepticus** CC

● **G40.C19 Lafora progressive myoclonus epilepsy, intractable, without status epilepticus** CC

Chapter 6. Diseases of the Nervous System

G40.1–G40.C19

√5th **G40.4 Other generalized epilepsy and epileptic syndromes**
Epilepsy with grand mal seizures on awakening
Epilepsy with myoclonic absences
Epilepsy with myoclonic-astatic seizures
Grand mal seizure NOS
Nonspecific atonic epileptic seizures
Nonspecific clonic epileptic seizures
Nonspecific myoclonic epileptic seizures
Nonspecific tonic epileptic seizures
Nonspecific tonic-clonic epileptic seizures
Symptomatic early myoclonic encephalopathy

√6th **G40.40 Other generalized epilepsy and epileptic syndromes, not intractable**
Other generalized epilepsy and epileptic syndromes without intractability
Other generalized epilepsy and epileptic syndromes NOS

G40.401 Other generalized epilepsy and epileptic syndromes, not intractable, with status epilepticus HCC

G40.409 Other generalized epilepsy and epileptic syndromes, not intractable, without status epilepticus HCC

√6th **G40.41 Other generalized epilepsy and epileptic syndromes, intractable**

G40.411 Other generalized epilepsy and epileptic syndromes, intractable, with status epilepticus CC HCC

G40.419 Other generalized epilepsy and epileptic syndromes, intractable, without status epilepticus CC HCC

G40.42 Cyclin-Dependent Kinase-Like 5 Deficiency Disorder HCC
CDKL5
Use additional code, if known, to identify associated manifestations, such as:
cortical blindness (H47.61-)
global development delay (F88)
AHA: 2020,4Q,18-19

√5th **G40.5 Epileptic seizures related to external causes**
Epileptic seizures related to alcohol
Epileptic seizures related to drugs
Epileptic seizures related to hormonal changes
Epileptic seizures related to sleep deprivation
Epileptic seizures related to stress
Code also, if applicable, associated epilepsy and recurrent seizures (G40.-)
Use additional code for adverse effect, if applicable, to identify drug (T36-T50 with fifth or sixth character 5)

√6th **G40.50 Epileptic seizures related to external causes, not intractable**

G40.501 Epileptic seizures related to external causes, not intractable, with status epilepticus CC HCC

G40.509 Epileptic seizures related to external causes, not intractable, without status epilepticus CC HCC
Epileptic seizures related to external causes, NOS

√5th **G40.8 Other epilepsy and recurrent seizures**
Epilepsies and epileptic syndromes undetermined as to whether they are focal or generalized
Landau-Kleffner syndrome

√6th **G40.80 Other epilepsy**

G40.801 Other epilepsy, not intractable, with status epilepticus CC HCC
Other epilepsy without intractability with status epilepticus

G40.802 Other epilepsy, not intractable, without status epilepticus CC HCC
Other epilepsy NOS
Other epilepsy without intractability without status epilepticus

G40.803 Other epilepsy, intractable, with status epilepticus CC HCC

G40.804 Other epilepsy, intractable, without status epilepticus CC HCC

√6th **G40.81 Lennox-Gastaut syndrome**
DEF: Severe form of epilepsy with usual onset in early childhood. Seizures are frequent and difficult to treat, causing falls and intellectual impairment.

G40.811 Lennox-Gastaut syndrome, not intractable, with status epilepticus CC HCC

G40.812 Lennox-Gastaut syndrome, not intractable, without status epilepticus CC HCC

G40.813 Lennox-Gastaut syndrome, intractable, with status epilepticus CC HCC

G40.814 Lennox-Gastaut syndrome, intractable, without status epilepticus CC HCC

√6th **G40.82 Epileptic spasms**
Infantile spasms
Salaam attacks
West's syndrome

G40.821 Epileptic spasms, not intractable, with status epilepticus CC HCC

G40.822 Epileptic spasms, not intractable, without status epilepticus CC HCC

G40.823 Epileptic spasms, intractable, with status epilepticus CC HCC

G40.824 Epileptic spasms, intractable, without status epilepticus CC HCC

√6th **G40.83 Dravet syndrome**
Polymorphic epilepsy in infancy (PMEI)
Severe myoclonic epilepsy in infancy (SMEI)
AHA: 2020,4Q,19

G40.833 Dravet syndrome, intractable, with status epilepticus CC HCC

G40.834 Dravet syndrome, intractable, without status epilepticus CC HCC
Dravet syndrome NOS

G40.89 Other seizures CC HCC
EXCLUDES 1 *post traumatic seizures (R56.1)*
recurrent seizures NOS (G40.909)
seizure NOS (R56.9)

√5th **G40.9 Epilepsy, unspecified**
AHA: 2019,1Q,19

√6th **G40.90 Epilepsy, unspecified, not intractable**
Epilepsy, unspecified, without intractability

G40.901 Epilepsy, unspecified, not intractable, with status epilepticus HCC

G40.909 Epilepsy, unspecified, not intractable, without status epilepticus HCC
Epilepsy NOS
Epileptic convulsions NOS
Epileptic fits NOS
Epileptic seizures NOS
Recurrent seizures NOS
Seizure disorder NOS
AHA: 2021,2Q,3; 2021,1Q,3

√6th **G40.91 Epilepsy, unspecified, intractable**
Intractable seizure disorder NOS

G40.911 Epilepsy, unspecified, intractable, with status epilepticus CC HCC

G40.919 Epilepsy, unspecified, intractable, without status epilepticus CC HCC

✓4th G43 Migraine

NOTE The following terms are to be considered equivalent to intractable: pharmacoresistant (pharmacologically resistant), treatment resistant, refractory (medically) and poorly controlled

Use additional code for adverse effect, if applicable, to identify drug (T36-T5Ø with fifth or sixth character 5)

EXCLUDES 1 *headache NOS (R51.9)*
lower half migraine (G44.ØØ)

EXCLUDES 2 *headache syndromes (G44.-)*

DEF: Headaches that occur periodically on one or both sides of the head that may be associated with nausea and vomiting, sensitivity to light and sound, dizziness, distorted vision, and cognitive disturbances.

✓5th G43.Ø Migraine without aura
Common migraine
EXCLUDES 1 *chronic migraine without aura (G43.7-)*

✓6th G43.ØØ Migraine without aura, not intractable
Migraine without aura without mention of refractory migraine
G43.ØØ1 Migraine without aura, not intractable, with status migrainosus
G43.ØØ9 Migraine without aura, not intractable, without status migrainosus
Migraine without aura NOS

✓6th G43.Ø1 Migraine without aura, intractable
Migraine without aura with refractory migraine
G43.Ø11 Migraine without aura, intractable, with status migrainosus
G43.Ø19 Migraine without aura, intractable, without status migrainosus

✓5th G43.1 Migraine with aura
Basilar migraine
Classical migraine
Migraine equivalents
Migraine preceded or accompanied by transient focal neurological phenomena
Migraine triggered seizures
Migraine with acute-onset aura
Migraine with aura without headache (migraine equivalents)
Migraine with prolonged aura
Migraine with typical aura
Retinal migraine
Code also any associated seizure (G4Ø.-, R56.9)
EXCLUDES 1 ▶*chronic migraine with aura (G43.E-)*◀
persistent migraine aura (G43.5-, G43.6-)

✓6th G43.1Ø Migraine with aura, not intractable
Migraine with aura without mention of refractory migraine
G43.1Ø1 Migraine with aura, not intractable, with status migrainosus
G43.1Ø9 Migraine with aura, not intractable, without status migrainosus
Migraine with aura NOS

✓6th G43.11 Migraine with aura, intractable
Migraine with aura with refractory migraine
G43.111 Migraine with aura, intractable, with status migrainosus
G43.119 Migraine with aura, intractable, without status migrainosus

✓5th G43.4 Hemiplegic migraine
Familial migraine
Sporadic migraine

✓6th G43.4Ø Hemiplegic migraine, not intractable
Hemiplegic migraine without refractory migraine
G43.4Ø1 Hemiplegic migraine, not intractable, with status migrainosus
G43.4Ø9 Hemiplegic migraine, not intractable, without status migrainosus
Hemiplegic migraine NOS

✓6th G43.41 Hemiplegic migraine, intractable
Hemiplegic migraine with refractory migraine
G43.411 Hemiplegic migraine, intractable, with status migrainosus
G43.419 Hemiplegic migraine, intractable, without status migrainosus

✓5th G43.5 Persistent migraine aura without cerebral infarction

✓6th G43.5Ø Persistent migraine aura without cerebral infarction, not intractable
Persistent migraine aura without cerebral infarction, without refractory migraine
G43.5Ø1 Persistent migraine aura without cerebral infarction, not intractable, with status migrainosus
G43.5Ø9 Persistent migraine aura without cerebral infarction, not intractable, without status migrainosus
Persistent migraine aura NOS

✓6th G43.51 Persistent migraine aura without cerebral infarction, intractable
Persistent migraine aura without cerebral infarction, with refractory migraine
G43.511 Persistent migraine aura without cerebral infarction, intractable, with status migrainosus
G43.519 Persistent migraine aura without cerebral infarction, intractable, without status migrainosus

✓5th G43.6 Persistent migraine aura with cerebral infarction
Code also the type of cerebral infarction (I63.-)

✓6th G43.6Ø Persistent migraine aura with cerebral infarction, not intractable
Persistent migraine aura with cerebral infarction, without refractory migraine
G43.6Ø1 Persistent migraine aura with cerebral infarction, not intractable, with status migrainosus CC
G43.6Ø9 Persistent migraine aura with cerebral infarction, not intractable, without status migrainosus CC

✓6th G43.61 Persistent migraine aura with cerebral infarction, intractable
Persistent migraine aura with cerebral infarction, with refractory migraine
G43.611 Persistent migraine aura with cerebral infarction, intractable, with status migrainosus CC
G43.619 Persistent migraine aura with cerebral infarction, intractable, without status migrainosus CC

✓5th G43.7 Chronic migraine without aura
Transformed migraine
EXCLUDES 1 *migraine without aura (G43.Ø-)*

✓6th G43.7Ø Chronic migraine without aura, not intractable
Chronic migraine without aura, without refractory migraine
G43.7Ø1 Chronic migraine without aura, not intractable, with status migrainosus
G43.7Ø9 Chronic migraine without aura, not intractable, without status migrainosus
Chronic migraine without aura NOS

✓6th G43.71 Chronic migraine without aura, intractable
Chronic migraine without aura, with refractory migraine
G43.711 Chronic migraine without aura, intractable, with status migrainosus
G43.719 Chronic migraine without aura, intractable, without status migrainosus

✓5th G43.A Cyclical vomiting
EXCLUDES 1 *cyclical vomiting syndrome unrelated to migraine (R11.15)*
AHA: 2019,4Q,15
G43.AØ Cyclical vomiting, in migraine, not intractable
Cyclical vomiting, without refractory migraine
G43.A1 Cyclical vomiting, in migraine, intractable
Cyclical vomiting, with refractory migraine

✓5th G43.B Ophthalmoplegic migraine
G43.BØ Ophthalmoplegic migraine, not intractable
Ophthalmoplegic migraine, without refractory migraine
G43.B1 Ophthalmoplegic migraine, intractable
Ophthalmoplegic migraine, with refractory migraine

✓5th **G43.C Periodic headache syndromes in child or adult**

G43.CØ Periodic headache syndromes in child or adult, not intractable
Periodic headache syndromes in child or adult, without refractory migraine

G43.C1 Periodic headache syndromes in child or adult, intractable
Periodic headache syndromes in child or adult, with refractory migraine

✓5th **G43.D Abdominal migraine**

G43.DØ Abdominal migraine, not intractable
Abdominal migraine, without refractory migraine

G43.D1 Abdominal migraine, intractable
Abdominal migraine, with refractory migraine

✓5th **G43.8 Other migraine**

✓6th **G43.8Ø Other migraine, not intractable**
Other migraine, without refractory migraine

G43.8Ø1 Other migraine, not intractable, with status migrainosus

G43.8Ø9 Other migraine, not intractable, without status migrainosus

✓6th **G43.81 Other migraine, intractable**
Other migraine, with refractory migraine

G43.811 Other migraine, intractable, with status migrainosus

G43.819 Other migraine, intractable, without status migrainosus

✓6th **G43.82 Menstrual migraine, not intractable**
Menstrual headache, not intractable
Menstrual migraine, without refractory migraine
Menstrually related migraine, not intractable
Pre-menstrual headache, not intractable
Pre-menstrual migraine, not intractable
Pure menstrual migraine, not intractable
Code also associated premenstrual tension syndrome (N94.3)

G43.821 Menstrual migraine, not intractable, with status migrainosus ♀

G43.829 Menstrual migraine, not intractable, without status migrainosus ♀
Menstrual migraine NOS

✓6th **G43.83 Menstrual migraine, intractable**
Menstrual headache, intractable
Menstrual migraine, with refractory migraine
Menstrually related migraine, intractable
Pre-menstrual headache, intractable
Pre-menstrual migraine, intractable
Pure menstrual migraine, intractable
Code also associated premenstrual tension syndrome (N94.3)

G43.831 Menstrual migraine, intractable, with status migrainosus ♀

G43.839 Menstrual migraine, intractable, without status migrainosus ♀

✓5th **G43.9 Migraine, unspecified**

✓6th **G43.9Ø Migraine, unspecified, not intractable**
Migraine, unspecified, without refractory migraine

G43.9Ø1 Migraine, unspecified, not intractable, with status migrainosus
Status migrainosus NOS

G43.9Ø9 Migraine, unspecified, not intractable, without status migrainosus
Migraine NOS

✓6th **G43.91 Migraine, unspecified, intractable**
Migraine, unspecified, with refractory migraine

G43.911 Migraine, unspecified, intractable, with status migrainosus

G43.919 Migraine, unspecified, intractable, without status migrainosus

● ✓5th **G43.E Chronic migraine with aura**
EXCLUDES 1 *migraine with aura (G43.1-)*

● ✓6th **G43.EØ Chronic migraine with aura, not intractable**
Chronic migraine with aura, without refractory migraine

● **G43.EØ1 Chronic migraine with aura, not intractable, with status migrainosus**

● **G43.EØ9 Chronic migraine with aura, not intractable, without status migrainosus**
Chronic migraine with aura NOS

● ✓6th **G43.E1 Chronic migraine with aura, intractable**
Chronic migraine with aura, with refractory migraine

● **G43.E11 Chronic migraine with aura, intractable, with status migrainosus**

● **G43.E19 Chronic migraine with aura, intractable, without status migrainosus**

✓4th **G44 Other headache syndromes**
EXCLUDES 1 *headache NOS (R51.9)*
EXCLUDES 2 *atypical facial pain (G5Ø.1)*
headache due to lumbar puncture (G97.1)
migraines (G43.-)
trigeminal neuralgia (G5Ø.Ø)

✓5th **G44.Ø Cluster headaches and other trigeminal autonomic cephalgias (TAC)**
DEF: Cluster headache: Characteristic grouping or clustering of headaches that can last for a number of weeks or months and then completely disappear for months or years. They are typically not associated with gastrointestinal upset or light sensitivity as experienced in migraines.

✓6th **G44.ØØ Cluster headache syndrome, unspecified**
Ciliary neuralgia
Cluster headache NOS
Histamine cephalgia
Lower half migraine
Migrainous neuralgia

G44.ØØ1 Cluster headache syndrome, unspecified, intractable

G44.ØØ9 Cluster headache syndrome, unspecified, not intractable
Cluster headache syndrome NOS

✓6th **G44.Ø1 Episodic cluster headache**

G44.Ø11 Episodic cluster headache, intractable

G44.Ø19 Episodic cluster headache, not intractable
Episodic cluster headache NOS

✓6th **G44.Ø2 Chronic cluster headache**

G44.Ø21 Chronic cluster headache, intractable

G44.Ø29 Chronic cluster headache, not intractable
Chronic cluster headache NOS

✓6th **G44.Ø3 Episodic paroxysmal hemicrania**
Paroxysmal hemicrania NOS

G44.Ø31 Episodic paroxysmal hemicrania, intractable

G44.Ø39 Episodic paroxysmal hemicrania, not intractable
Episodic paroxysmal hemicrania NOS

✓6th **G44.Ø4 Chronic paroxysmal hemicrania**

G44.Ø41 Chronic paroxysmal hemicrania, intractable

G44.Ø49 Chronic paroxysmal hemicrania, not intractable
Chronic paroxysmal hemicrania NOS

✓6th **G44.Ø5 Short lasting unilateral neuralgiform headache with conjunctival injection and tearing (SUNCT)**

G44.Ø51 Short lasting unilateral neuralgiform headache with conjunctival injection and tearing (SUNCT), intractable

G44.Ø59 Short lasting unilateral neuralgiform headache with conjunctival injection and tearing (SUNCT), not intractable
Short lasting unilateral neuralgiform headache with conjunctival injection and tearing (SUNCT) NOS

✓6th **G44.Ø9 Other trigeminal autonomic cephalgias (TAC)**

G44.Ø91 Other trigeminal autonomic cephalgias (TAC), intractable

G44.Ø99 Other trigeminal autonomic cephalgias (TAC), not intractable

G44.1 Vascular headache, not elsewhere classified
EXCLUDES 2 *cluster headache (G44.Ø)*
complicated headache syndromes (G44.5-)
drug-induced headache (G44.4-)
migraine (G43.-)
other specified headache syndromes (G44.8-)
post-traumatic headache (G44.3-)
tension-type headache (G44.2-)

√5th **G44.2 Tension-type headache**

√6th **G44.2Ø Tension-type headache, unspecified**

G44.2Ø1 Tension-type headache, unspecified, intractable

G44.2Ø9 Tension-type headache, unspecified, not intractable
Tension headache NOS

√6th **G44.21 Episodic tension-type headache**

G44.211 Episodic tension-type headache, intractable

G44.219 Episodic tension-type headache, not intractable
Episodic tension-type headache NOS

√6th **G44.22 Chronic tension-type headache**

G44.221 Chronic tension-type headache, intractable

G44.229 Chronic tension-type headache, not intractable
Chronic tension-type headache NOS

√5th **G44.3 Post-traumatic headache**

√6th **G44.3Ø Post-traumatic headache, unspecified**

G44.3Ø1 Post-traumatic headache, unspecified, intractable

G44.3Ø9 Post-traumatic headache, unspecified, not intractable
Post-traumatic headache NOS

√6th **G44.31 Acute post-traumatic headache**

G44.311 Acute post-traumatic headache, intractable

G44.319 Acute post-traumatic headache, not intractable
Acute post-traumatic headache NOS

√6th **G44.32 Chronic post-traumatic headache**

G44.321 Chronic post-traumatic headache, intractable

G44.329 Chronic post-traumatic headache, not intractable
Chronic post-traumatic headache NOS

√5th **G44.4 Drug-induced headache, not elsewhere classified**
Medication overuse headache
Use additional code for adverse effect, if applicable, to identify drug (T36-T5Ø with fifth or sixth character 5)

G44.4Ø Drug-induced headache, not elsewhere classified, not intractable

G44.41 Drug-induced headache, not elsewhere classified, intractable

√5th **G44.5 Complicated headache syndromes**

G44.51 Hemicrania continua
DEF: Persistent primary headache of unknown causation occurring on one side of the face and head. May last for more than three months, with daily and continuous pain of moderate intensity with severe exacerbations.

G44.52 New daily persistent headache (NDPH)

G44.53 Primary thunderclap headache

G44.59 Other complicated headache syndrome

√5th **G44.8 Other specified headache syndromes**
EXCLUDES 2 *headache with orthostatic or positional component, not elsewhere classifed (R51.Ø)*

G44.81 Hypnic headache

G44.82 Headache associated with sexual activity
Orgasmic headache
Preorgasmic headache

G44.83 Primary cough headache

G44.84 Primary exertional headache

G44.85 Primary stabbing headache

G44.86 Cervicogenic headache
Code also associated cervical spinal condition, if known
AHA: 2021,4Q,11-12

G44.89 Other headache syndrome

√4th **G45 Transient cerebral ischemic attacks and related syndromes**
EXCLUDES 1 *neonatal cerebral ischemia (P91.Ø)*
transient retinal artery occlusion (H34.Ø-)
AHA: 2023,1Q,37; 2018,2Q,9
DEF: Transient cerebral ischemic attack: Intermittent or brief cerebral dysfunction from lack of oxygenation with no persistent neurological deficits associated with occlusive vascular disease. TIA may denote an impending cerebrovascular accident.

G45.Ø Vertebro-basilar artery syndrome CC

G45.1 Carotid artery syndrome (hemispheric) CC

G45.2 Multiple and bilateral precerebral artery syndromes CC

G45.3 Amaurosis fugax CC

G45.4 Transient global amnesia
EXCLUDES 1 *amnesia NOS (R41.3)*

G45.8 Other transient cerebral ischemic attacks and related syndromes CC

G45.9 Transient cerebral ischemic attack, unspecified CC
Spasm of cerebral artery
TIA
Transient cerebral ischemia NOS

√4th **G46 Vascular syndromes of brain in cerebrovascular diseases**
Code first underlying cerebrovascular disease (I6Ø-I69)

G46.Ø Middle cerebral artery syndrome CC

G46.1 Anterior cerebral artery syndrome CC

G46.2 Posterior cerebral artery syndrome CC

G46.3 Brain stem stroke syndrome
Benedikt syndrome
Claude syndrome
Foville syndrome
Millard-Gubler syndrome
Wallenberg syndrome
Weber syndrome

G46.4 Cerebellar stroke syndrome

G46.5 Pure motor lacunar syndrome

G46.6 Pure sensory lacunar syndrome

G46.7 Other lacunar syndromes

G46.8 Other vascular syndromes of brain in cerebrovascular diseases

√4th **G47 Sleep disorders**
EXCLUDES 2 *nightmares (F51.5)*
nonorganic sleep disorders (F51.-)
sleep terrors (F51.4)
sleepwalking (F51.3)

√5th **G47.Ø Insomnia**
EXCLUDES 2 *alcohol related insomnia (F1Ø.182, F1Ø.282, F1Ø.982)*
drug-related insomnia (F11.182, F11.282, F11.982, F13.182, F13.282, F13.982, F14.182, F14.282, F14.982, F15.182, F15.282, F15.982, F19.182, F19.282, F19.982)
idiopathic insomnia (F51.Ø1)
insomnia due to a mental disorder (F51.Ø5)
insomnia not due to a substance or known physiological condition (F51.Ø-)
nonorganic insomnia (F51.Ø-)
primary insomnia (F51.Ø1)
sleep apnea (G47.3-)

G47.ØØ Insomnia, unspecified
Insomnia NOS

G47.Ø1 Insomnia due to medical condition
Code also associated medical condition

G47.Ø9 Other insomnia

√5th **G47.1 Hypersomnia**
EXCLUDES 2 *alcohol-related hypersomnia (F1Ø.182, F1Ø.282, F1Ø.982)*
drug-related hypersomnia (F11.182, F11.282, F11.982, F13.182, F13.282, F13.982, F14.182, F14.282, F14.982, F15.182, F15.282, F15.982, F19.182, F19.282, F19.982)
hypersomnia due to a mental disorder (F51.13)
hypersomnia not due to a substance or known physiological condition (F51.1-)
primary hypersomnia (F51.11)
sleep apnea (G47.3-)

G47.1Ø Hypersomnia, unspecified
Hypersomnia NOS

G47.11 **Idiopathic hypersomnia with long sleep time**
Idiopathic hypersomnia NOS
G47.12 **Idiopathic hypersomnia without long sleep time**
G47.13 **Recurrent hypersomnia**
Kleine-Levin syndrome
Menstrual related hypersomnia
G47.14 **Hypersomnia due to medical condition**
Code also associated medical condition
G47.19 **Other hypersomnia**

√5th **G47.2** **Circadian rhythm sleep disorders**
Disorders of the sleep wake schedule
Inversion of nyctohemeral rhythm
Inversion of sleep rhythm
DEF: Circadian rhythm: Daily cycle (24-hour period) of physical, mental, and behavioral changes. It is largely influenced by environmental cues, such as changes in light or temperature.
Synonym(s): *sleep/wake cycle.*
G47.20 **Circadian rhythm sleep disorder, unspecified type**
Sleep wake schedule disorder NOS
G47.21 **Circadian rhythm sleep disorder, delayed sleep phase type**
Delayed sleep phase syndrome
G47.22 **Circadian rhythm sleep disorder, advanced sleep phase type**
G47.23 **Circadian rhythm sleep disorder, irregular sleep wake type**
Irregular sleep-wake pattern
G47.24 **Circadian rhythm sleep disorder, free running type**
Circadian rhythm sleep disorder, non-24-hour sleep-wake type
G47.25 **Circadian rhythm sleep disorder, jet lag type**
G47.26 **Circadian rhythm sleep disorder, shift work type**
G47.27 ***Circadian rhythm sleep disorder in conditions classified elsewhere***
Code first underlying condition
G47.29 **Other circadian rhythm sleep disorder**

√5th **G47.3** **Sleep apnea**
Code also any associated underlying condition
EXCLUDES 1 *apnea NOS (RØ6.81)*
Cheyne-Stokes breathing (RØ6.3)
pickwickian syndrome (E66.2)
sleep apnea of newborn (P28.3-)
G47.3Ø **Sleep apnea, unspecified**
Sleep apnea NOS
G47.31 **Primary central sleep apnea**
Idiopathic central sleep apnea
G47.32 **High altitude periodic breathing**
G47.33 **Obstructive sleep apnea (adult) (pediatric)**
Obstructive sleep apnea hypopnea
EXCLUDES 1 *obstructive sleep apnea of newborn (P28.3-)*
G47.34 **Idiopathic sleep related nonobstructive alveolar hypoventilation**
Sleep related hypoxia
G47.35 **Congenital central alveolar hypoventilation syndrome**
G47.36 ***Sleep related hypoventilation in conditions classified elsewhere***
Sleep related hypoxemia in conditions classified elsewhere
Code first underlying condition
G47.37 ***Central sleep apnea in conditions classified elsewhere***
Code first underlying condition
G47.39 **Other sleep apnea**

√5th **G47.4** **Narcolepsy and cataplexy**
√6th **G47.41** **Narcolepsy**
G47.411 **Narcolepsy with cataplexy**
G47.419 **Narcolepsy without cataplexy**
Narcolepsy NOS
√6th **G47.42** **Narcolepsy in conditions classified elsewhere**
Code first underlying condition
G47.421 ***Narcolepsy in conditions classified elsewhere with cataplexy***
G47.429 ***Narcolepsy in conditions classified elsewhere without cataplexy***

√5th **G47.5** **Parasomnia**
EXCLUDES 1 *alcohol induced parasomnia (F1Ø.182, F1Ø.282, F1Ø.982)*
drug induced parasomnia (F11.182, F11.282, F11.982, F13.182, F13.282, F13.982, F14.182, F14.282, F14.982, F15.182, F15.282, F15.982, F19.182, F19.282, F19.982)
parasomnia not due to a substance or known physiological condition (F51.8)
G47.5Ø **Parasomnia, unspecified**
Parasomnia NOS
G47.51 **Confusional arousals**
G47.52 **REM sleep behavior disorder**
G47.53 **Recurrent isolated sleep paralysis**
G47.54 ***Parasomnia in conditions classified elsewhere***
Code first underlying condition
G47.59 **Other parasomnia**

√5th **G47.6** **Sleep related movement disorders**
EXCLUDES 2 *restless legs syndrome (G25.81)*
G47.61 **Periodic limb movement disorder**
G47.62 **Sleep related leg cramps**
G47.63 **Sleep related bruxism**
EXCLUDES 1 *psychogenic bruxism (F45.8)*
G47.69 **Other sleep related movement disorders**

G47.8 **Other sleep disorders**
Other specified sleep-wake disorder
G47.9 **Sleep disorder, unspecified**
Sleep disorder NOS
Unspecified sleep-wake disorder

Nerve, nerve root and plexus disorders (G5Ø-G59)

EXCLUDES 1 *current traumatic nerve, nerve root and plexus disorders - see Injury, nerve by body region*
neuralgia NOS (M79.2)
neuritis NOS (M79.2)
peripheral neuritis in pregnancy (O26.82-)
radiculitis NOS (M54.1-)

√4th **G5Ø** **Disorders of trigeminal nerve**
INCLUDES disorders of 5th cranial nerve
G5Ø.Ø **Trigeminal neuralgia**
Syndrome of paroxysmal facial pain
Tic douloureux
G5Ø.1 **Atypical facial pain**
G5Ø.8 **Other disorders of trigeminal nerve**
G5Ø.9 **Disorder of trigeminal nerve, unspecified**

√4th **G51** **Facial nerve disorders**
INCLUDES disorders of 7th cranial nerve
G51.Ø **Bell's palsy**
Facial palsy
G51.1 **Geniculate ganglionitis**
EXCLUDES 1 *postherpetic geniculate ganglionitis (BØ2.21)*
G51.2 **Melkersson's syndrome**
Melkersson-Rosenthal syndrome
√5th **G51.3** **Clonic hemifacial spasm**
AHA: 2018,4Q,10
G51.31 **Clonic hemifacial spasm, right**
G51.32 **Clonic hemifacial spasm, left**
G51.33 **Clonic hemifacial spasm, bilateral**
G51.39 **Clonic hemifacial spasm, unspecified**
G51.4 **Facial myokymia**
G51.8 **Other disorders of facial nerve**
G51.9 **Disorder of facial nerve, unspecified**

√4th **G52** **Disorders of other cranial nerves**
EXCLUDES 2 *disorders of acoustic [8th] nerve (H93.3)*
disorders of optic [2nd] nerve (H46, H47.Ø)
paralytic strabismus due to nerve palsy (H49.Ø-H49.2)
G52.Ø **Disorders of olfactory nerve**
Disorders of 1st cranial nerve
G52.1 **Disorders of glossopharyngeal nerve**
Disorder of 9th cranial nerve
Glossopharyngeal neuralgia
G52.2 **Disorders of vagus nerve**
Disorders of pneumogastric [1Øth] nerve
G52.3 **Disorders of hypoglossal nerve**
Disorders of 12th cranial nerve

G52.7 **Disorders of multiple cranial nerves**
Polyneuritis cranialis

G52.8 **Disorders of other specified cranial nerves**

G52.9 **Cranial nerve disorder, unspecified**

G53 *Cranial nerve disorders in diseases classified elsewhere*
Code first underlying disease, such as:
neoplasm (CØØ-D49)

EXCLUDES 1 *multiple cranial nerve palsy in sarcoidosis (D86.82)*
multiple cranial nerve palsy in syphilis (A52.15)
postherpetic geniculate ganglionitis (BØ2.21)
postherpetic trigeminal neuralgia (BØ2.22)

✓4th **G54 Nerve root and plexus disorders**

EXCLUDES 1 *current traumatic nerve root and plexus disorders - see nerve injury by body region*
intervertebral disc disorders (M5Ø-M51)
neuralgia or neuritis NOS (M79.2)
neuritis or radiculitis brachial NOS (M54.13)
neuritis or radiculitis lumbar NOS (M54.16)
neuritis or radiculitis lumbosacral NOS (M54.17)
neuritis or radiculitis thoracic NOS (M54.14)
radiculitis NOS (M54.1Ø)
radiculopathy NOS (M54.1Ø)
spondylosis (M47.-)

G54.Ø **Brachial plexus disorders**
Thoracic outlet syndrome
AHA: 2023,2Q,8
DEF: Acquired disorder affecting the spinal nerves that send signals to the shoulder, arm, and hand, causing corresponding motor and sensory dysfunction. This disorder is characterized by regional paresthesia, pain, muscle weakness, and in severe cases paralysis.

G54.1 **Lumbosacral plexus disorders**

G54.2 **Cervical root disorders, not elsewhere classified**

G54.3 **Thoracic root disorders, not elsewhere classified**

G54.4 **Lumbosacral root disorders, not elsewhere classified**

G54.5 **Neuralgic amyotrophy**
Parsonage-Aldren-Turner syndrome
Shoulder-girdle neuritis

EXCLUDES 1 *neuralgic amyotrophy in diabetes mellitus (EØ8-E13 with .44)*

G54.6 **Phantom limb syndrome with pain** HCC

G54.7 **Phantom limb syndrome without pain** HCC
Phantom limb syndrome NOS

G54.8 **Other nerve root and plexus disorders**

G54.9 **Nerve root and plexus disorder, unspecified**

G55 *Nerve root and plexus compressions in diseases classified elsewhere*
Code first underlying disease, such as:
neoplasm (CØØ-D49)

EXCLUDES 1 *nerve root compression (due to) (in) ankylosing spondylitis (M45.-)*
nerve root compression (due to) (in) dorsopathies (M53.-, M54.-)
nerve root compression (due to) (in) intervertebral disc disorders (M5Ø.1.-, M51.1.-)
nerve root compression (due to) (in) spondylopathies (M46.-, M48.-)
nerve root compression (due to) (in) spondylosis (M47.Ø-, M47.2-)

✓4th **G56 Mononeuropathies of upper limb**

EXCLUDES 1 *current traumatic nerve disorder - see nerve injury by body region*

AHA: 2016,4Q,17-18

✓5th G56.Ø **Carpal tunnel syndrome**
DEF: Swelling and inflammation in the tendons or bursa surrounding the median nerve caused by repetitive activity. The resulting compression on the nerve causes pain, numbness, and tingling especially to the palm, index, middle finger, and thumb.

G56.ØØ **Carpal tunnel syndrome, unspecified upper limb**
G56.Ø1 **Carpal tunnel syndrome, right upper limb**
G56.Ø2 **Carpal tunnel syndrome, left upper limb**
G56.Ø3 **Carpal tunnel syndrome, bilateral upper limbs**

✓5th G56.1 **Other lesions of median nerve**

G56.1Ø **Other lesions of median nerve, unspecified upper limb**
G56.11 **Other lesions of median nerve, right upper limb**
G56.12 **Other lesions of median nerve, left upper limb**
G56.13 **Other lesions of median nerve, bilateral upper limbs**

✓5th G56.2 **Lesion of ulnar nerve**
Tardy ulnar nerve palsy

G56.2Ø **Lesion of ulnar nerve, unspecified upper limb**
G56.21 **Lesion of ulnar nerve, right upper limb**
G56.22 **Lesion of ulnar nerve, left upper limb**
G56.23 **Lesion of ulnar nerve, bilateral upper limbs**

✓5th G56.3 **Lesion of radial nerve**

G56.3Ø **Lesion of radial nerve, unspecified upper limb**
G56.31 **Lesion of radial nerve, right upper limb**
G56.32 **Lesion of radial nerve, left upper limb**
G56.33 **Lesion of radial nerve, bilateral upper limbs**

✓5th G56.4 **Causalgia of upper limb**
Complex regional pain syndrome II of upper limb

EXCLUDES 1 *complex regional pain syndrome I of lower limb (G9Ø.52-)*
complex regional pain syndrome I of upper limb (G9Ø.51-)
complex regional pain syndrome II of lower limb (G57.7-)
reflex sympathetic dystrophy of lower limb (G9Ø.52-)
reflex sympathetic dystrophy of upper limb (G9Ø.51-)

G56.4Ø **Causalgia of unspecified upper limb**
G56.41 **Causalgia of right upper limb**
G56.42 **Causalgia of left upper limb**
G56.43 **Causalgia of bilateral upper limbs**

✓5th G56.8 **Other specified mononeuropathies of upper limb**
Interdigital neuroma of upper limb

G56.8Ø **Other specified mononeuropathies of unspecified upper limb**
G56.81 **Other specified mononeuropathies of right upper limb**
G56.82 **Other specified mononeuropathies of left upper limb**
G56.83 **Other specified mononeuropathies of bilateral upper limbs**

✓5th G56.9 **Unspecified mononeuropathy of upper limb**

G56.9Ø **Unspecified mononeuropathy of unspecified upper limb**
G56.91 **Unspecified mononeuropathy of right upper limb**
G56.92 **Unspecified mononeuropathy of left upper limb**
G56.93 **Unspecified mononeuropathy of bilateral upper limbs**

✓4th **G57 Mononeuropathies of lower limb**

EXCLUDES 1 *current traumatic nerve disorder - see nerve injury by body region*

AHA: 2016,4Q,17-18

✓5th G57.Ø **Lesion of sciatic nerve**

EXCLUDES 1 *sciatica NOS (M54.3-)*

EXCLUDES 2 *sciatica attributed to intervertebral disc disorder (M51.1.-)*

G57.ØØ **Lesion of sciatic nerve, unspecified lower limb**
G57.Ø1 **Lesion of sciatic nerve, right lower limb**
G57.Ø2 **Lesion of sciatic nerve, left lower limb**
G57.Ø3 **Lesion of sciatic nerve, bilateral lower limbs**

✓5th G57.1 **Meralgia paresthetica**
Lateral cutaneous nerve of thigh syndrome

G57.1Ø **Meralgia paresthetica, unspecified lower limb**
G57.11 **Meralgia paresthetica, right lower limb**
G57.12 **Meralgia paresthetica, left lower limb**
G57.13 **Meralgia paresthetica, bilateral lower limbs**

✓5th G57.2 **Lesion of femoral nerve**

G57.2Ø **Lesion of femoral nerve, unspecified lower limb**
G57.21 **Lesion of femoral nerve, right lower limb**
G57.22 **Lesion of femoral nerve, left lower limb**
G57.23 **Lesion of femoral nerve, bilateral lower limbs**

✓5th G57.3 **Lesion of lateral popliteal nerve**
Peroneal nerve palsy
AHA: 2020,3Q,12

G57.3Ø **Lesion of lateral popliteal nerve, unspecified lower limb**
G57.31 **Lesion of lateral popliteal nerve, right lower limb**
G57.32 **Lesion of lateral popliteal nerve, left lower limb**
G57.33 **Lesion of lateral popliteal nerve, bilateral lower limbs**

5th G57.4 Lesion of medial popliteal nerve
- G57.40 Lesion of medial popliteal nerve, unspecified lower limb
- G57.41 Lesion of medial popliteal nerve, right lower limb
- G57.42 Lesion of medial popliteal nerve, left lower limb
- G57.43 Lesion of medial popliteal nerve, bilateral lower limbs

5th G57.5 Tarsal tunnel syndrome
- G57.50 Tarsal tunnel syndrome, unspecified lower limb
- G57.51 Tarsal tunnel syndrome, right lower limb
- G57.52 Tarsal tunnel syndrome, left lower limb
- G57.53 Tarsal tunnel syndrome, bilateral lower limbs

5th G57.6 Lesion of plantar nerve

Morton's metatarsalgia
- G57.60 Lesion of plantar nerve, unspecified lower limb
- G57.61 Lesion of plantar nerve, right lower limb
- G57.62 Lesion of plantar nerve, left lower limb
- G57.63 Lesion of plantar nerve, bilateral lower limbs

5th G57.7 Causalgia of lower limb

Complex regional pain syndrome II of lower limb

EXCLUDES 1 *complex regional pain syndrome I of lower limb (G90.52-)*
complex regional pain syndrome I of upper limb (G90.51-)
complex regional pain syndrome II of upper limb (G56.4-)
reflex sympathetic dystrophy of lower limb (G90.52-)
reflex sympathetic dystrophy of upper limb (G90.51-)
- G57.70 Causalgia of unspecified lower limb
- G57.71 Causalgia of right lower limb
- G57.72 Causalgia of left lower limb
- G57.73 Causalgia of bilateral lower limbs

5th G57.8 Other specified mononeuropathies of lower limb

Interdigital neuroma of lower limb
- G57.80 Other specified mononeuropathies of unspecified lower limb
- G57.81 Other specified mononeuropathies of right lower limb
- G57.82 Other specified mononeuropathies of left lower limb
- G57.83 Other specified mononeuropathies of bilateral lower limbs

5th G57.9 Unspecified mononeuropathy of lower limb
- G57.90 Unspecified mononeuropathy of unspecified lower limb
- G57.91 Unspecified mononeuropathy of right lower limb
- G57.92 Unspecified mononeuropathy of left lower limb
- G57.93 Unspecified mononeuropathy of bilateral lower limbs

4th **G58 Other mononeuropathies**
- G58.0 Intercostal neuropathy
- G58.7 Mononeuritis multiplex
- G58.8 Other specified mononeuropathies
- G58.9 Mononeuropathy, unspecified

G59 Mononeuropathy in diseases classified elsewhere

Code first underlying disease

EXCLUDES 1 *diabetic mononeuropathy (E08-E13 with .41)*
syphilitic nerve paralysis (A52.19)
syphilitic neuritis (A52.15)
tuberculous mononeuropathy (A17.83)

Polyneuropathies and other disorders of the peripheral nervous system (G60-G65)

EXCLUDES 1 *neuralgia NOS (M79.2)*
neuritis NOS (M79.2)
peripheral neuritis in pregnancy (O26.82-)
radiculitis NOS (M54.10)

4th **G60 Hereditary and idiopathic neuropathy**

G60.0 Hereditary motor and sensory neuropathy

Charcôt-Marie-Tooth disease
Dejerine-Sottas disease
Hereditary motor and sensory neuropathy, types I-IV
Hypertrophic neuropathy of infancy
Peroneal muscular atrophy (axonal type) (hypertrophic type)
Roussy-Levy syndrome

G60.1 Refsum's disease CC

Infantile Refsum disease

DEF: Genetic disorder of the lipid metabolism characterized by retinitis pigmentosa, degenerative nerve disease, ataxia, and dry, rough, scaly skin.

G60.2 Neuropathy in association with hereditary ataxia

G60.3 Idiopathic progressive neuropathy

G60.8 Other hereditary and idiopathic neuropathies

Dominantly inherited sensory neuropathy
Morvan's disease
Nelaton's syndrome
Recessively inherited sensory neuropathy

G60.9 Hereditary and idiopathic neuropathy, unspecified

4th **G61 Inflammatory polyneuropathy**

G61.0 Guillain-Barre syndrome CC HCC

Acute (post-)infective polyneuritis
Miller Fisher syndrome

AHA: 2020,3Q,12; 2014,2Q,4

DEF: Autoimmune disorder due to an immune response to foreign antigens with paraplegia of limbs, flaccid paralysis, ophthalmoplegia, ataxia, and areflexia. In most cases, this disorder is triggered by a mild viral infection, surgery, or following an immunization.

TIP: Guillain-Barre syndrome can occur as a sequela of *Campylobacter* enteritis. Assign code B94.8 for the sequelae as an additional diagnosis.

G61.1 Serum neuropathy HCC

Use additional code for adverse effect, if applicable, to identify serum (T50.-)

5th G61.8 Other inflammatory polyneuropathies
- G61.81 Chronic inflammatory demyelinating polyneuritis CC HCC
- G61.82 Multifocal motor neuropathy HCC
  MMN
  AHA: 2016,4Q,18
- G61.89 Other inflammatory polyneuropathies HCC

G61.9 Inflammatory polyneuropathy, unspecified HCC

4th **G62 Other and unspecified polyneuropathies**

G62.0 Drug-induced polyneuropathy HCC

Use additional code for adverse effect, if applicable, to identify drug (T36-T50 with fifth or sixth character 5)

G62.1 Alcoholic polyneuropathy HCC

AHA: 2019,3Q,8

G62.2 Polyneuropathy due to other toxic agents HCC

Code first (T51-T65) to identify toxic agent

5th G62.8 Other specified polyneuropathies
- G62.81 Critical illness polyneuropathy CC HCC
  Acute motor neuropathy
- G62.82 Radiation-induced polyneuropathy HCC
  Use additional external cause code (W88-W90, X39.0-) to identify cause
- G62.89 Other specified polyneuropathies
  AHA: 2016,2Q,11

G62.9 Polyneuropathy, unspecified

Neuropathy NOS

G63 Polyneuropathy in diseases classified elsewhere HCC

Code first underlying disease, such as:
- amyloidosis (E85.-)
- endocrine disease, except diabetes (E00-E07, E15-E16, E20-E34)
- metabolic diseases (E70-E88)
- neoplasm (C00-D49)
- nutritional deficiency (E40-E64)

EXCLUDES 1 *polyneuropathy (in):*
diabetes mellitus (E08-E13 with .42)
diphtheria (A36.83)
infectious mononucleosis complicated by polyneuropathy (B27.0-B27.9 with fifth character 1)
Lyme disease (A69.22)
mumps (B26.84)
postherpetic (B02.23)
rheumatoid arthritis (M05.5-)
scleroderma (M34.83)
systemic lupus erythematosus (M32.19)

AHA: 2021,1Q,7; 2012,4Q,99

G64 Other disorders of peripheral nervous system

Disorder of peripheral nervous system NOS

G65 Sequelae of inflammatory and toxic polyneuropathies
Code first condition resulting from (sequela) of inflammatory and toxic polyneuropathies

- **G65.0 Sequelae of Guillain-Barre syndrome** HCC
- **G65.1 Sequelae of other inflammatory polyneuropathy** HCC
- **G65.2 Sequelae of toxic polyneuropathy** HCC

Diseases of myoneural junction and muscle (G70-G73)

G70 Myasthenia gravis and other myoneural disorders
EXCLUDES 1 *botulism (A05.1, A48.51-A48.52)*
transient neonatal myasthenia gravis (P94.0)

G70.0 Myasthenia gravis
AHA: 2022,3Q,15
DEF: Autoimmune neuromuscular disorder caused by antibodies to the acetylcholine receptors at the neuromuscular junction, interfering with proper binding of the neurotransmitter from the neuron to the target muscle, causing muscle weakness, fatigue, and exhaustion, without pain or atrophy.

- **G70.00 Myasthenia gravis without (acute) exacerbation** HCC
  Myasthenia gravis NOS
- **G70.01 Myasthenia gravis with (acute) exacerbation** MCC HCC
  Myasthenia gravis in crisis

G70.1 Toxic myoneural disorders HCC
Code first (T51-T65) to identify toxic agent

G70.2 Congenital and developmental myasthenia HCC

G70.8 Other specified myoneural disorders

- **G70.80 Lambert-Eaton syndrome, unspecified** CC HCC
  Lambert-Eaton syndrome NOS
- ***G70.81 Lambert-Eaton syndrome in disease classified elsewhere*** CC HCC
  Code first underlying disease
  EXCLUDES 1 *Lambert-Eaton syndrome in neoplastic disease (G73.1)*
- **G70.89 Other specified myoneural disorders** HCC

G70.9 Myoneural disorder, unspecified HCC

G71 Primary disorders of muscles
EXCLUDES 2 *arthrogryposis multiplex congenita (Q74.3)*
metabolic disorders (E70-E88)
myositis (M60.-)

G71.0 Muscular dystrophy
AHA: 2022,4Q,17-18; 2018,4Q,11-12

- **G71.00 Muscular dystrophy, unspecified** HCC
- **G71.01 Duchenne or Becker muscular dystrophy** HCC
  Autosomal recessive, childhood type, muscular dystrophy resembling Duchenne or Becker muscular dystrophy
  Benign [Becker] muscular dystrophy
  Severe [Duchenne] muscular dystrophy
- **G71.02 Facioscapulohumeral muscular dystrophy** HCC
  Scapulohumeral muscular dystrophy
- **G71.03 Limb girdle muscular dystrophies**
  - **G71.031 Autosomal dominant limb girdle muscular dystrophy** HCC
    LGMD D4 calpain-3-related
    LGMD D5 collagen 6-related
    Limb girdle muscular dystrophy type 1
  - **G71.032 Autosomal recessive limb girdle muscular dystrophy due to calpain-3 dysfunction** HCC
    Limb girdle muscular dystrophy type 2A
    LGMD R1 calpain-3-related
    Primary calpainopathy
  - **G71.033 Limb girdle muscular dystrophy due to dysferlin dysfunction** HCC
    Dysferlinopathy
    LGMD R2 dysferlin-related
    Limb girdle muscular dystrophy type 2B
    Miyoshi Myopathy type 1
  - **G71.034 Limb girdle muscular dystrophy due to sarcoglycan dysfunction**
    - **G71.0340 Limb girdle muscular dystrophy due to sarcoglycan dysfunction, unspecified** HCC
      Sarcoglycanopathy, NOS
    - **G71.0341 Limb girdle muscular dystrophy due to alpha sarcoglycan dysfunction** HCC
      Alpha sarcoglycanopathy
      Limb-girdle muscular dystrophy due to alpha-sarcoglycan deficiency
      Limb girdle muscular dystrophy type 2D
    - **G71.0342 Limb girdle muscular dystrophy due to beta sarcoglycan dysfunction** HCC
      Beta sarcoglycanopathy
      Limb girdle muscular dystrophy due to beta-sarcoglycan deficiency
      Limb girdle muscular dystrophy type 2E
    - **G71.0349 Limb girdle muscular dystrophy due to other sarcoglycan dysfunction** HCC
      Delta sarcoglycanopathy
      Delta-sarcoglycan-related LGMD R6
      Gamma sarcoglycanopathy
      Gamma-sarcoglycan-related LGMD R5
      Limb girdle muscular dystrophy type 2C
      Limb girdle muscular dystrophy type 2F
  - **G71.035 Limb girdle muscular dystrophy due to anoctamin-5 dysfunction** HCC
    Anoctamin-5-related LGMD R12
    Anoctaminopathy
    Autosomal recessive limb girdle muscular dystrophy type 2L
    Miyoshi myopathy type 3
  - **G71.038 Other limb girdle muscular dystrophy** HCC
    LGMD R9 FKRP-related
    LGMD R22 collagen 6-related
    Limb girdle muscular dystrophy due to fukutin related protein dysfunction
    Limb girdle muscular dystrophy type 2I
    Other autosomal recessive limb girdle muscular dystrophy
  - **G71.039 Limb girdle muscular dystrophy, unspecified** HCC
- **G71.09 Other specified muscular dystrophies** HCC
  Benign scapuloperoneal muscular dystrophy with early contractures [Emery-Dreifuss]
  Congenital muscular dystrophy NOS
  Congenital muscular dystrophy with specific morphological abnormalities of the muscle fiber
  Distal muscular dystrophy
  Ocular muscular dystrophy
  Oculopharyngeal muscular dystrophy
  Scapuloperoneal muscular dystrophy

G71.1 Myotonic disorders

- **G71.11 Myotonic muscular dystrophy** HCC
  Dystrophia myotonica [Steinert]
  Myotonia atrophica
  Myotonic dystrophy
  Proximal myotonic myopathy (PROMM)
  Steinert disease
- **G71.12 Myotonia congenita**
  Acetazolamide responsive myotonia congenita
  Dominant myotonia congenita [Thomsen disease]
  Myotonia levior
  Recessive myotonia congenita [Becker disease]

G71.13 **Myotonic chondrodystrophy**
Chondrodystrophic myotonia
Congenital myotonic chondrodystrophy
Schwartz-Jampel disease

G71.14 **Drug induced myotonia**
Use additional code for adverse effect, if applicable, to identify drug (T36-T5Ø with fifth or sixth character 5)

G71.19 **Other specified myotonic disorders**
Myotonia fluctuans
Myotonia permanens
Neuromyotonia [Isaacs]
Paramyotonia congenita (of von Eulenburg)
Pseudomyotonia
Symptomatic myotonia

✓5th G71.2 **Congenital myopathies**
EXCLUDES 2 *arthrogryposis multiplex congenita (Q74.3)*
AHA: 2020,4Q,19-21

G71.2Ø **Congenital myopathy, unspecified** CC HCC

G71.21 **Nemaline myopathy** CC HCC

✓6th G71.22 **Centronuclear myopathy**

G71.22Ø **X-linked myotubular myopathy** CC HCC
Myotubular (centronuclear) myopathy

G71.228 **Other centronuclear myopathy** CC HCC
Autosomal centronuclear myopathy
Autosomal dominant centronuclear myopathy
Autosomal recessive centronuclear myopathy
Centronuclear myopathy, NOS

G71.29 **Other congenital myopathy** CC HCC
Central core disease
Minicore disease
Multicore disease
Multiminicore disease

G71.3 **Mitochondrial myopathy, not elsewhere classified**
EXCLUDES 1 *Kearns-Sayre syndrome (H49.81)*
Leber's disease (H47.21)
Leigh's encephalopathy (G31.82)
mitochondrial metabolism disorders (E88.4.-)
Reye's syndrome (G93.7)

G71.8 **Other primary disorders of muscles**

G71.9 **Primary disorder of muscle, unspecified**
Hereditary myopathy NOS

✓4th G72 **Other and unspecified myopathies**
EXCLUDES 1 *arthrogryposis multiplex congenita (Q74.3)*
dermatopolymyositis (M33.-)
ischemic infarction of muscle (M62.2-)
myositis (M6Ø.-)
polymyositis (M33.2.-)

G72.Ø **Drug-induced myopathy** CC
Use additional code for adverse effect, if applicable, to identify drug (T36-T5Ø with fifth or sixth character 5)

G72.1 **Alcoholic myopathy** CC
Use additional code to identify alcoholism (F1Ø.-)

G72.2 **Myopathy due to other toxic agents** CC
Code first (T51-T65) to identify toxic agent

G72.3 **Periodic paralysis**
Familial periodic paralysis
Hyperkalemic periodic paralysis (familial)
Hypokalemic periodic paralysis (familial)
Myotonic periodic paralysis (familial)
Normokalemic paralysis (familial)
Potassium sensitive periodic paralysis
EXCLUDES 1 *paramyotonia congenita (of von Eulenburg) (G71.19)*

✓5th G72.4 **Inflammatory and immune myopathies, not elsewhere classified**

G72.41 **Inclusion body myositis [IBM]**

G72.49 **Other inflammatory and immune myopathies, not elsewhere classified**
Inflammatory myopathy NOS

✓5th G72.8 **Other specified myopathies**

G72.81 **Critical illness myopathy** CC
Acute necrotizing myopathy
Acute quadriplegic myopathy
Intensive care (ICU) myopathy
Myopathy of critical illness
AHA: 2020,3Q,12

G72.89 **Other specified myopathies**

G72.9 **Myopathy, unspecified**

✓4th G73 **Disorders of myoneural junction and muscle in diseases classified elsewhere**

G73.1 ***Lambert-Eaton syndrome in neoplastic disease*** CC UPD HCC
Code first underlying neoplasm (CØØ-D49)
EXCLUDES 1 *Lambert-Eaton syndrome not associated with neoplasm (G7Ø.8Ø-G7Ø.81)*

G73.3 ***Myasthenic syndromes in other diseases classified elsewhere*** CC HCC
Code first underlying disease, such as:
neoplasm (CØØ-D49)
thyrotoxicosis (EØ5.-)

G73.7 ***Myopathy in diseases classified elsewhere***
Code first underlying disease, such as:
glycogen storage disease ▶(E74.Ø-)◀
hyperparathyroidism (E21.Ø, E21.3)
hypoparathyroidism (E2Ø.-)
lipid storage disorders (E75.-)
EXCLUDES 1 *myopathy in:*
rheumatoid arthritis (MØ5.32)
sarcoidosis (D86.87)
scleroderma (M34.82)
Sjogren syndrome (M35.Ø3)
systemic lupus erythematosus (M32.19)

Cerebral palsy and other paralytic syndromes (G8Ø-G83)

✓4th G8Ø **Cerebral palsy**
EXCLUDES 1 *hereditary spastic paraplegia (G11.4)*

G8Ø.Ø **Spastic quadriplegic cerebral palsy** MCC HCC
Congenital spastic paralysis (cerebral)

G8Ø.1 **Spastic diplegic cerebral palsy** CC HCC
Spastic cerebral palsy NOS

G8Ø.2 **Spastic hemiplegic cerebral palsy** CC HCC

G8Ø.3 **Athetoid cerebral palsy** CC HCC
Double athetosis (syndrome)
Dyskinetic cerebral palsy
Dystonic cerebral palsy
Vogt disease

G8Ø.4 **Ataxic cerebral palsy** HCC

G8Ø.8 **Other cerebral palsy** HCC
Mixed cerebral palsy syndromes

G8Ø.9 **Cerebral palsy, unspecified** HCC
Cerebral palsy NOS

✓4th G81 **Hemiplegia and hemiparesis**
NOTE This category is to be used only when hemiplegia (complete)(incomplete) is reported without further specification, or is stated to be old or longstanding but of unspecified cause. The category is also for use in multiple coding to identify these types of hemiplegia resulting from any cause.
EXCLUDES 1 *congenital cerebral palsy (G8Ø.-)*
hemiplegia and hemiparesis due to sequela of cerebrovascular disease (I69.Ø5-, I69.15-, I69.25-, I69.35-, I69.85-, I69.95-)
AHA: 2015,1Q,25
TIP: If the documentation specifies the affected side but not whether it is the dominant or nondominant side, the default is as follows: for ambidextrous patients, the default is dominant; when the left side is affected, the default is nondominant; and when the right side is affected, the default is dominant.

✓5th G81.Ø **Flaccid hemiplegia**

G81.ØØ **Flaccid hemiplegia affecting unspecified side** CC UNS HCC

G81.Ø1 **Flaccid hemiplegia affecting right dominant side** CC HCC

G81.Ø2 **Flaccid hemiplegia affecting left dominant side** CC HCC

G81.Ø3 **Flaccid hemiplegia affecting right nondominant side** CC HCC

G81.Ø4 Flaccid hemiplegia affecting left nondominant side CC HCC

✓5th G81.1 Spastic hemiplegia

G81.1Ø Spastic hemiplegia affecting unspecified side CC UNS HCC

G81.11 Spastic hemiplegia affecting right dominant side CC HCC

G81.12 Spastic hemiplegia affecting left dominant side CC HCC

G81.13 Spastic hemiplegia affecting right nondominant side CC HCC

G81.14 Spastic hemiplegia affecting left nondominant side CC HCC

✓5th G81.9 Hemiplegia, unspecified

AHA: 2014,1Q,23

G81.9Ø Hemiplegia, unspecified affecting unspecified side CC UNS HCC

G81.91 Hemiplegia, unspecified affecting right dominant side CC HCC

G81.92 Hemiplegia, unspecified affecting left dominant side CC HCC

G81.93 Hemiplegia, unspecified affecting right nondominant side CC HCC

G81.94 Hemiplegia, unspecified affecting left nondominant side CC HCC

✓4th G82 Paraplegia (paraparesis) and quadriplegia (quadriparesis)

NOTE This category is to be used only when the listed conditions are reported without further specification, or are stated to be old or longstanding but of unspecified cause. The category is also for use in multiple coding to identify these conditions resulting from any cause

EXCLUDES 1 *congenital cerebral palsy (G8Ø.-)*
functional quadriplegia (R53.2)
hysterical paralysis (F44.4)

✓5th G82.2 Paraplegia

Paralysis of both lower limbs NOS
Paraparesis (lower) NOS
Paraplegia (lower) NOS

AHA: 2017,3Q,3

G82.2Ø Paraplegia, unspecified CC HCC

G82.21 Paraplegia, complete CC HCC

G82.22 Paraplegia, incomplete CC HCC

✓5th G82.5 Quadriplegia

G82.5Ø Quadriplegia, unspecified MCC HCC

G82.51 Quadriplegia, C1-C4 complete MCC HCC

G82.52 Quadriplegia, C1-C4 incomplete MCC HCC

G82.53 Quadriplegia, C5-C7 complete MCC HCC

G82.54 Quadriplegia, C5-C7 incomplete MCC HCC

✓4th G83 Other paralytic syndromes

NOTE This category is to be used only when the listed conditions are reported without further specification, or are stated to be old or longstanding but of unspecified cause. The category is also for use in multiple coding to identify these conditions resulting from any cause.

INCLUDES paralysis (complete) (incomplete), except as in G8Ø-G82

G83.Ø Diplegia of upper limbs CC HCC

Diplegia (upper)
Paralysis of both upper limbs

✓5th G83.1 Monoplegia of lower limb

Paralysis of lower limb

EXCLUDES 1 *monoplegia of lower limbs due to sequela of cerebrovascular disease (I69.Ø4-, I69.14-, I69.24-, I69.34-, I69.84-, I69.94-)*

TIP: If the documentation specifies the affected side but not whether it is the dominant or nondominant side, the default is as follows: for ambidextrous patients, the default is dominant; when the left side is affected, the default is nondominant; and when the right side is affected, the default is dominant.

G83.1Ø Monoplegia of lower limb affecting unspecified side HCC

G83.11 Monoplegia of lower limb affecting right dominant side HCC

G83.12 Monoplegia of lower limb affecting left dominant side HCC

G83.13 Monoplegia of lower limb affecting right nondominant side HCC

G83.14 Monoplegia of lower limb affecting left nondominant side HCC

✓5th G83.2 Monoplegia of upper limb

Paralysis of upper limb

EXCLUDES 1 *monoplegia of upper limbs due to sequela of cerebrovascular disease (I69.Ø3-, I69.13-, I69.23-, I69.33-, I69.83-, I69.93-)*

TIP: If the documentation specifies the affected side but not whether it is the dominant or nondominant side, the default is as follows: for ambidextrous patients, the default is dominant; when the left side is affected, the default is nondominant; and when the right side is affected, the default is dominant.

G83.2Ø Monoplegia of upper limb affecting unspecified side HCC

G83.21 Monoplegia of upper limb affecting right dominant side HCC

G83.22 Monoplegia of upper limb affecting left dominant side HCC

G83.23 Monoplegia of upper limb affecting right nondominant side HCC

G83.24 Monoplegia of upper limb affecting left nondominant side HCC

✓5th G83.3 Monoplegia, unspecified

TIP: If the documentation specifies the affected side but not whether it is the dominant or nondominant side, the default is as follows: for ambidextrous patients, the default is dominant; when the left side is affected, the default is nondominant; and when the right side is affected, the default is dominant.

G83.3Ø Monoplegia, unspecified affecting unspecified side HCC

G83.31 Monoplegia, unspecified affecting right dominant side HCC

G83.32 Monoplegia, unspecified affecting left dominant side HCC

G83.33 Monoplegia, unspecified affecting right nondominant side HCC

G83.34 Monoplegia, unspecified affecting left nondominant side HCC

G83.4 Cauda equina syndrome CC HCC

Neurogenic bladder due to cauda equina syndrome

EXCLUDES 1 *cord bladder NOS (G95.89)*
neurogenic bladder NOS (N31.9)

AHA: 2020,3Q,24

DEF: Compression of the spinal nerve roots presenting with pain and tingling radiating down the buttocks, back of the thigh and calf, and into the foot in a sciatic manner with aching in the bladder, perineum, and sacrum. Loss of bowel and bladder control may also occur.

G83.5 Locked-in state MCC HCC

AHA: 2022,2Q,10

✓5th G83.8 Other specified paralytic syndromes

EXCLUDES 1 *paralytic syndromes due to current spinal cord injury - code to spinal cord injury (S14, S24, S34)*

G83.81 Brown-Sequard syndrome HCC

G83.82 Anterior cord syndrome HCC

G83.83 Posterior cord syndrome HCC

G83.84 Todd's paralysis (postepileptic) HCC

G83.89 Other specified paralytic syndromes HCC

G83.9 Paralytic syndrome, unspecified HCC

Other disorders of the nervous system (G89-G99)

G89 Pain, not elsewhere classified

Code also related psychological factors associated with pain (F45.42)

EXCLUDES 1 *generalized pain NOS (R52)*
pain disorders exclusively related to psychological factors (F45.41)
pain NOS (R52)

EXCLUDES 2 *atypical face pain (G50.1)*
headache syndromes (G44.-)
localized pain, unspecified type - code to pain by site, such as:
- *abdomen pain (R10.-)*
- *back pain (M54.9)*
- *breast pain (N64.4)*
- *chest pain (R07.1-R07.9)*
- *ear pain (H92.0-)*
- *eye pain (H57.1)*
- *headache (R51.9)*
- *joint pain (M25.5-)*
- *limb pain (M79.6-)*
- *lumbar region pain (M54.5-)*
- *painful urination (R30.9)*
- *pelvic and perineal pain (R10.2)*
- *renal colic (N23)*
- *shoulder pain (M25.51-)*
- *spine pain (M54.-)*
- *throat pain (R07.0)*
- *tongue pain (K14.6)*
- *tooth pain (K08.8)*

migraines (G43.-)
myalgia (M79.1-)
pain from prosthetic devices, implants, and grafts (T82.84, T83.84, T84.84, T85.84-)
phantom limb syndrome with pain (G54.6)
vulvar vestibulitis (N94.810)
vulvodynia (N94.81-)

G89.0 Central pain syndrome
Dejerine-Roussy syndrome
Myelopathic pain syndrome
Thalamic pain syndrome (hyperesthetic)

G89.1 Acute pain, not elsewhere classified

G89.11 Acute pain due to trauma

G89.12 Acute post-thoracotomy pain
Post-thoracotomy pain NOS

G89.18 Other acute postprocedural pain
Postoperative pain NOS
Postprocedural pain NOS

G89.2 Chronic pain, not elsewhere classified

EXCLUDES 1 *causalgia, lower limb (G57.7-)*
causalgia, upper limb (G56.4-)
central pain syndrome (G89.0)
chronic pain syndrome (G89.4)
complex regional pain syndrome II, lower limb (G57.7-)
complex regional pain syndrome II, upper limb (G56.4-)
neoplasm related chronic pain (G89.3)
reflex sympathetic dystrophy (G90.5-)

G89.21 Chronic pain due to trauma

G89.22 Chronic post-thoracotomy pain

G89.28 Other chronic postprocedural pain
Other chronic postoperative pain

G89.29 Other chronic pain

G89.3 Neoplasm related pain (acute) (chronic)
Cancer associated pain
Pain due to malignancy (primary) (secondary)
Tumor associated pain

G89.4 Chronic pain syndrome
Chronic pain associated with significant psychosocial dysfunction

G90 Disorders of autonomic nervous system

EXCLUDES 1 *dysfunction of the autonomic nervous system due to alcohol (G31.2)*

G90.0 Idiopathic peripheral autonomic neuropathy

G90.01 Carotid sinus syncope
Carotid sinus syndrome
DEF: Vagal activation caused by pressure on the carotid sinus baroreceptors. Sympathetic nerve impulses may cause sinus arrest or AV block.

G90.09 Other idiopathic peripheral autonomic neuropathy
Idiopathic peripheral autonomic neuropathy NOS

G90.1 Familial dysautonomia [Riley-Day] HCC

G90.2 Horner's syndrome
Bernard(-Horner) syndrome
Cervical sympathetic dystrophy or paralysis

G90.3 Multi-system degeneration of the autonomic nervous system CC HCC
Neurogenic orthostatic hypotension [Shy-Drager]
EXCLUDES 1 *orthostatic hypotension NOS (I95.1)*

G90.4 Autonomic dysreflexia
Use additional code to identify the cause, such as:
- fecal impaction (K56.41)
- pressure ulcer (pressure area) (L89.-)
- urinary tract infection (N39.0)

G90.5 Complex regional pain syndrome I (CRPS I)
Reflex sympathetic dystrophy
EXCLUDES 1 *causalgia of lower limb (G57.7-)*
causalgia of upper limb (G56.4-)
complex regional pain syndrome II of lower limb (G57.7-)
complex regional pain syndrome II of upper limb (G56.4-)

G90.50 Complex regional pain syndrome I, unspecified CC UNS

G90.51 Complex regional pain syndrome I of upper limb

G90.511 Complex regional pain syndrome I of right upper limb CC

G90.512 Complex regional pain syndrome I of left upper limb CC

G90.513 Complex regional pain syndrome I of upper limb, bilateral CC

G90.519 Complex regional pain syndrome I of unspecified upper limb CC UNS

G90.52 Complex regional pain syndrome I of lower limb

G90.521 Complex regional pain syndrome I of right lower limb CC

G90.522 Complex regional pain syndrome I of left lower limb CC

G90.523 Complex regional pain syndrome I of lower limb, bilateral CC

G90.529 Complex regional pain syndrome I of unspecified lower limb CC UNS

G90.59 Complex regional pain syndrome I of other specified site CC

G90.8 Other disorders of autonomic nervous system
AHA: 2023,2Q,8

G90.9 Disorder of the autonomic nervous system, unspecified

G90.A Postural orthostatic tachycardia syndrome [POTS]
Chronic orthostatic intolerance
Postural tachycardia syndrome
AHA: 2022,4Q,19-20

● **G90.B LMNB1-related autosomal dominant leukodystrophy**

G91 Hydrocephalus

INCLUDES acquired hydrocephalus

EXCLUDES 1 *Arnold-Chiari syndrome with hydrocephalus (Q07.-)*
congenital hydrocephalus (Q03.-)
spina bifida with hydrocephalus (Q05.-)

DEF: Abnormal buildup of cerebrospinal fluid in the brain causing dilation of the ventricles.

Hydrocephalus (Acquired)

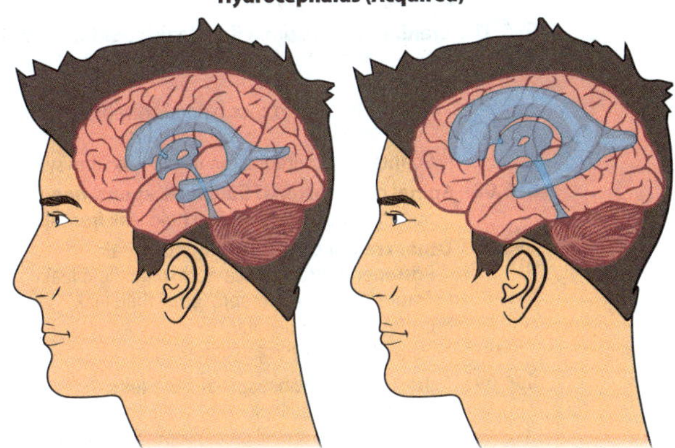

Normal ventricles — Hydrocephalic ventricles

G91.0 Communicating hydrocephalus CC HCC
Secondary normal pressure hydrocephalus

G91.1 Obstructive hydrocephalus CC HCC
DEF: Obstruction of the cerebrospinal fluid passage from the brain into the spinal canal characterized by headaches, drowsiness, poor coordination, urinary incontinence, nausea, vomiting, and papilledema.

G91.2 (Idiopathic) normal pressure hydrocephalus CC HCC
Normal pressure hydrocephalus NOS

G91.3 Post-traumatic hydrocephalus, unspecified CC HCC

G91.4 Hydrocephalus in diseases classified elsewhere HCC
Code first underlying condition, such as:
congenital syphilis (A50.4-)
neoplasm (C00-D49)
plasminogen deficiency (E88.02)
EXCLUDES 1 *hydrocephalus due to congenital toxoplasmosis (P37.1)*
AHA: 2014,3Q,3

G91.8 Other hydrocephalus CC HCC

G91.9 Hydrocephalus, unspecified CC HCC

G92 Toxic encephalopathy

AHA: 2022,1Q,52; 2021,4Q,12-14; 2021,1Q,13; 2017,1Q,39-40
DEF: Brain tissue degeneration due to a toxic substance.

G92.0 Immune effector cell-associated neurotoxicity syndrome
Code first underlying cause such as:
complications of immune effector cellular therapy (T80.82)
~~Code also associated signs and symptoms, such as seizures and cerebral edema~~
▶Code also, if applicable, associated signs and symptoms, such as:◀
cerebral edema (G93.6)
unspecified convulsions (R56.9)

G92.00 Immune effector cell-associated neurotoxicity syndrome, grade unspecified UPD
ICANS, grade unspecified

G92.01 Immune effector cell-associated neurotoxicity syndrome, grade 1 UPD
ICANS, grade 1

G92.02 Immune effector cell-associated neurotoxicity syndrome, grade 2 UPD
ICANS, grade 2

G92.03 Immune effector cell-associated neurotoxicity syndrome, grade 3 CC UPD
ICANS, grade 3

G92.04 Immune effector cell-associated neurotoxicity syndrome, grade 4 CC UPD
ICANS, grade 4

G92.05 Immune effector cell-associated neurotoxicity syndrome, grade 5 CC UPD
ICANS, grade 5

G92.8 Other toxic encephalopathy MCC
Toxic encephalitis
Toxic metabolic encephalopathy
Code first poisoning due to drug or toxin, if applicable, ▶(T36-T65 with fifth or sixth character 1-4)◀
Use additional code for adverse effect, if applicable, to identify drug (T36-T50 with fifth or sixth character 5)
AHA: 2022,1Q,52

G92.9 Unspecified toxic encephalopathy MCC
Code first poisoning due to drug or toxin, if applicable, ▶(T36-T65 with fifth or sixth character 1-4)◀
Use additional code for adverse effect, if applicable, to identify drug (T36-T50 with fifth or sixth character 5)

G93 Other disorders of brain

G93.0 Cerebral cysts
Arachnoid cyst
Porencephalic cyst, acquired
EXCLUDES 1 *acquired periventricular cysts of newborn (P91.1)*
congenital cerebral cysts (Q04.6)

G93.1 Anoxic brain damage, not elsewhere classified CC HCC
EXCLUDES 1 *cerebral anoxia due to anesthesia during labor and delivery (O74.3)*
cerebral anoxia due to anesthesia during the puerperium (O89.2)
neonatal anoxia (P84)
DEF: Brain injury not resulting from birth trauma that is due to lack of oxygen. Brain cells, when deprived of oxygen, begin to expire after four minutes.

G93.2 Benign intracranial hypertension
Pseudotumor
EXCLUDES 1 *hypertensive encephalopathy (I67.4)*
obstructive hydrocephalus (G91.1)

G93.3 Postviral and related fatigue syndromes
Use additional code, if applicable, for post COVID-19 condition, unspecified (U09.9)
EXCLUDES 1 *▶chronic fatigue NOS◀ (R53.82)*
neurasthenia (F48.8)
AHA: 2022,4Q,20

G93.31 Postviral fatigue syndrome

G93.32 Myalgic encephalomyelitis/chronic fatigue syndrome
Chronic fatigue syndrome
ME/CFS
Myalgic encephalomyelitis

G93.39 Other post infection and related fatigue syndromes

G93.4 Other and unspecified encephalopathy
EXCLUDES 1 ~~*alcoholic encephalopathy (G31.2)*~~
~~*encephalopathy in diseases classified elsewhere (G94)*~~
~~*hypertensive encephalopathy (I67.4)*~~
EXCLUDES 2 *▶alcoholic encephalopathy (G31.2)◀*
▶encephalopathy in diseases classified elsewhere (G94)◀
▶hypertensive encephalopathy (I67.4)◀
toxic (metabolic) encephalopathy (G92.8)

G93.40 Encephalopathy, unspecified HIV CC
AHA: 2017,2Q,8

G93.41 Metabolic encephalopathy HIV MCC
Septic encephalopathy
AHA: 2017,2Q,8; 2016,3Q,42; 2015,3Q,21
TIP: Assign separately when documented with diabetic hypoglycemia (E08.649, E09.649, E10.649, E11.649, E13.649).

● **G93.42 Megaloencephalic leukoencephalopathy with subcortical cysts** CC

● **G93.43 Leukoencephalopathy with calcifications and cysts** CC

● **G93.44 Adult-onset leukodystrophy with axonal spheroids** CC
Adult-onset leukoencephalopathy with axonal spheroids and pigmented glia

G93.49 Other encephalopathy HIV CC
Encephalopathy NEC
AHA: 2021,2Q,3; 2018,4Q,16; 2018,2Q,22,24; 2017,2Q,9

Chapter 6. Diseases of the Nervous System

G93.5 Compression of brain MCC HCC
Arnold-Chiari type 1 compression of brain
Compression of brain (stem)
Herniation of brain (stem)
EXCLUDES 1 *traumatic compression of brain (S06.A-)*
AHA: 2020,2Q,31

G93.6 Cerebral edema MCC HCC
EXCLUDES 1 *cerebral edema due to birth injury (P11.0)*
traumatic cerebral edema (S06.1-)
AHA: 2022,3Q,9-10

G93.7 Reye's syndrome MCC HCC P
Code first poisoning due to salicylates, if applicable (T39.0-, with sixth character 1-4)
Use additional code for adverse effect due to salicylates, if applicable (T39.0-, with sixth character 5)
DEF: Rare childhood illness often developed after a viral upper respiratory infection. Symptoms include vomiting, elevated serum transaminase, brain swelling, disturbances of consciousness, seizures, and changes in liver and other viscera; it can be fatal.

✓5th **G93.8 Other specified disorders of brain**

G93.81 Temporal sclerosis
Hippocampal sclerosis
Mesial temporal sclerosis

G93.82 Brain death MCC

G93.89 Other specified disorders of brain
Postradiation encephalopathy
AHA: 2020,2Q,24; 2019,3Q,8

G93.9 Disorder of brain, unspecified HIV

G94 Other disorders of brain in diseases classified elsewhere
Code first underlying disease
EXCLUDES 1 *encephalopathy in congenital syphilis (A50.49)*
encephalopathy in influenza (J09.X9, J10.81, J11.81)
encephalopathy in syphilis (A52.19)
hydrocephalus in diseases classified elsewhere (G91.4)
AHA: 2018,2Q,22; 2017,2Q,8-9

✓4th **G95 Other and unspecified diseases of spinal cord**
EXCLUDES 2 *myelitis (G04.-)*

G95.0 Syringomyelia and syringobulbia CC HCC

✓5th **G95.1 Vascular myelopathies**
EXCLUDES 2 *intraspinal phlebitis and thrombophlebitis, except non-pyogenic (G08)*

G95.11 Acute infarction of spinal cord (embolic) (nonembolic) MCC HCC
Anoxia of spinal cord
Arterial thrombosis of spinal cord

G95.19 Other vascular myelopathies MCC HCC
Edema of spinal cord
Hematomyelia
Nonpyogenic intraspinal phlebitis and thrombophlebitis
Subacute necrotic myelopathy

✓5th **G95.2 Other and unspecified cord compression**

G95.20 Unspecified cord compression HIV CC HCC

G95.29 Other cord compression HIV CC HCC

✓5th **G95.8 Other specified diseases of spinal cord**
EXCLUDES 1 *neurogenic bladder NOS (N31.9)*
neurogenic bladder due to cauda equina syndrome (G83.4)
neuromuscular dysfunction of bladder without spinal cord lesion (N31.-)

G95.81 Conus medullaris syndrome CC HCC

G95.89 Other specified diseases of spinal cord CC HCC
Cord bladder NOS
Drug-induced myelopathy
Radiation-induced myelopathy
EXCLUDES 1 *myelopathy NOS (G95.9)*

G95.9 Disease of spinal cord, unspecified HIV CC HCC
Myelopathy NOS

✓4th **G96 Other disorders of central nervous system**

✓5th **G96.0 Cerebrospinal fluid leak**
Code also if applicable:
intracranial hypotension (G96.81-)
EXCLUDES 1 *cerebrospinal fluid leak from spinal puncture (G97.0)*
AHA: 2020,4Q,21-22; 2018,2Q,13

G96.00 Cerebrospinal fluid leak, unspecified CC
Code also if applicable:
head injury (S00-S09)

G96.01 Cranial cerebrospinal fluid leak, spontaneous CC
Otorrhea due to spontaneous cerebrospinal fluid CSF leak
Rhinorrhea due to spontaneous cerebrospinal fluid CSF leak
Spontaneous cerebrospinal fluid leak from skull base

G96.02 Spinal cerebrospinal fluid leak, spontaneous CC
Spontaneous cerebrospinal fluid leak from spine

G96.08 Other cranial cerebrospinal fluid leak CC
Postoperative cranial cerebrospinal fluid leak
Traumatic cranial cerebrospinal fluid leak
Code also if applicable:
head injury ▶(S00 - S09)◀

G96.09 Other spinal cerebrospinal fluid leak CC
Other spinal CSF leak
Postoperative spinal cerebrospinal fluid leak
Traumatic spinal cerebrospinal fluid leak
Code also if applicable:
head injury ▶(S00 - S09)◀
AHA: 2022,3Q,24

✓5th **G96.1 Disorders of meninges, not elsewhere classified**

G96.11 Dural tear CC
Code also intracranial hypotension, if applicable (G96.81-)
EXCLUDES 1 *accidental puncture or laceration of dura during a procedure (G97.41)*
AHA: 2014,4Q,24

G96.12 Meningeal adhesions (cerebral) (spinal)

✓6th **G96.19 Other disorders of meninges, not elsewhere classified**
AHA: 2020,4Q,22

G96.191 Perineural cyst
Cervical nerve root cyst
Lumbar nerve root cyst
Sacral nerve root cyst
Tarlov cyst
Thoracic nerve root cyst

G96.198 Other disorders of meninges, not elsewhere classified

✓5th **G96.8 Other specified disorders of central nervous system**
AHA: 2020,4Q,21,23-24

✓6th **G96.81 Intracranial hypotension**
Code also any associated diagnoses, such as:
brachial amyotrophy (G54.5)
cerebrospinal fluid leak from spine (G96.02)
cranial nerve disorders in diseases classified elsewhere (G53)
nerve root and compressions in diseases classified elsewhere (G55)
nonpyogenic thrombosis of intracranial venous system (I67.6)
nontraumatic intracerebral hemorrhage (I61.-)
nontraumatic subdural hemorrhage (I62.0-)
other and unspecified cord compression (G95.2-)
other secondary parkinsonism (G21.8)
reversible cerebrovascular vasoconstriction syndrome (I67.841)
spinal cord herniation (G95.89)
stroke (I63.-)
syringomyelia (G95.0)
DEF: Central nervous system disorder resulting from a loss of cerebrospinal fluid (CSF) volume. More often associated with CSF leak at the level of the spine rather than the skull base, causes can be spontaneous, iatrogenic or traumatic spinal dura defects or holes, or overdrainage of CSF shunt devices. The most common symptom is headache.

G96.810 Intracranial hypotension, unspecified

G96.811 Intracranial hypotension, spontaneous

G96.819 Other intracranial hypotension

G96.89 Other specified disorders of central nervous system

G96.9 Disorder of central nervous system, unspecified HIV

√4th **G97 Intraoperative and postprocedural complications and disorders of nervous system, not elsewhere classified**

EXCLUDES 2 *intraoperative and postprocedural cerebrovascular infarction (I97.81-, I97.82-)*

AHA: 2016,4Q,9-10

G97.Ø Cerebrospinal fluid leak from spinal puncture CC

Code also any associated diagnoses or complications, such as:
intracranial hypotension following a procedure (G97.83-G97.84)

Spinal Puncture

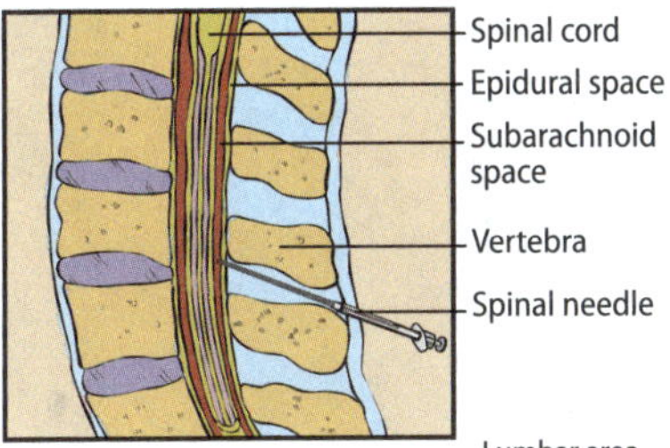

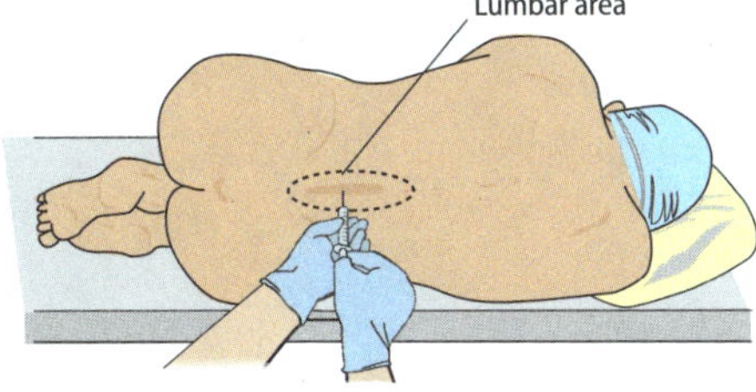

G97.1 Other reaction to spinal and lumbar puncture

Headache due to lumbar puncture
Other reaction to spinal dural puncture
Code also, if applicable, any associated headache with orthostatic component (R51.Ø)

G97.2 Intracranial hypotension following ventricular shunting CC

Code also any associated diagnoses or complications

√5th **G97.3 Intraoperative hemorrhage and hematoma of a nervous system organ or structure complicating a procedure**

EXCLUDES 1 *intraoperative hemorrhage and hematoma of a nervous system organ or structure due to accidental puncture and laceration during a procedure (G97.4-)*

G97.31 Intraoperative hemorrhage and hematoma of a nervous system organ or structure complicating a nervous system procedure CC

G97.32 Intraoperative hemorrhage and hematoma of a nervous system organ or structure complicating other procedure CC

√5th **G97.4 Accidental puncture and laceration of a nervous system organ or structure during a procedure**

G97.41 Accidental puncture or laceration of dura during a procedure CC

Incidental (inadvertent) durotomy
Code also any associated diagnoses or complications
AHA: 2014,4Q,24

G97.48 Accidental puncture and laceration of other nervous system organ or structure during a nervous system procedure CC

G97.49 Accidental puncture and laceration of other nervous system organ or structure during other procedure CC

√5th **G97.5 Postprocedural hemorrhage of a nervous system organ or structure following a procedure**

G97.51 Postprocedural hemorrhage of a nervous system organ or structure following a nervous system procedure CC

G97.52 Postprocedural hemorrhage of a nervous system organ or structure following other procedure CC

√5th **G97.6 Postprocedural hematoma and seroma of a nervous system organ or structure following a procedure**

G97.61 Postprocedural hematoma of a nervous system organ or structure following a nervous system procedure CC

AHA: 2020,3Q,24

G97.62 Postprocedural hematoma of a nervous system organ or structure following other procedure CC

G97.63 Postprocedural seroma of a nervous system organ or structure following a nervous system procedure CC

G97.64 Postprocedural seroma of a nervous system organ or structure following other procedure CC

√5th **G97.8 Other intraoperative and postprocedural complications and disorders of nervous system**

Use additional code to further specify disorder
AHA: 2020,4Q,23

G97.81 Other intraoperative complications of nervous system CC

G97.82 Other postprocedural complications and disorders of nervous system CC

AHA: 2022,1Q,34

G97.83 Intracranial hypotension following lumbar cerebrospinal fluid shunting CC

Code also any associated diagnoses or complications

G97.84 Intracranial hypotension following other procedure CC

Code also, if applicable:
accidental puncture or laceration of dura during a procedure (G97.41)
cerebrospinal fluid leak from spinal puncture (G97.Ø)

√4th **G98 Other disorders of nervous system not elsewhere classified**

INCLUDES nervous system disorder NOS

G98.Ø Neurogenic arthritis, not elsewhere classified

Nonsyphilitic neurogenic arthropathy NEC
Nonsyphilitic neurogenic spondylopathy NEC

EXCLUDES 1 *spondylopathy (in):*
syringomyelia and syringobulbia (G95.Ø)
tabes dorsalis (A52.11)

G98.8 Other disorders of nervous system HIV

Nervous system disorder NOS

√4th **G99 Other disorders of nervous system in diseases classified elsewhere**

G99.Ø Autonomic neuropathy in diseases classified elsewhere CC

Code first underlying disease, such as:
amyloidosis (E85.-)
gout (M1A.-, M1Ø.-)
hyperthyroidism (EØ5.-)

EXCLUDES 1 *diabetic autonomic neuropathy (EØ8-E13 with .43)*

G99.2 Myelopathy in diseases classified elsewhere CC HCC

Code first underlying disease, such as:
neoplasm (CØØ-D49)

EXCLUDES 1 *myelopathy in:*
intervertebral disease (M5Ø.Ø-, M51.Ø-)
spondylosis (M47.Ø-, M47.1-)

AHA: 2018,3Q,18-19

TIP: Use this code in addition to a spondylolisthesis code (M43.1-) or a spinal stenosis code (M48.0-) when either of these disorders is documented as the cause of the myelopathy.

G99.8 Other specified disorders of nervous system in diseases classified elsewhere

Code first underlying disorder, such as:
amyloidosis (E85.-)
avitaminosis ▶(E56.-)◀

EXCLUDES 1 *nervous system involvement in:*
cysticercosis (B69.Ø)
rubella (BØ6.Ø-)
syphilis (A52.1-)

Chapter 7. Diseases of the Eye and Adnexa (HØØ–H59)

Chapter-specific Guidelines with Coding Examples

The chapter-specific guidelines from the ICD-10-CM Official Guidelines for Coding and Reporting have been provided below. Along with these guidelines are coding examples, contained in the shaded boxes, that have been developed to help illustrate the coding and/or sequencing guidance found in these guidelines.

a. Glaucoma

1) Assigning glaucoma codes

Assign as many codes from category H4Ø, Glaucoma, as needed to identify the type of glaucoma, the affected eye, and the glaucoma stage.

2) Bilateral glaucoma with same type and stage

When a patient has bilateral glaucoma and both eyes are documented as being the same type and stage, and there is a code for bilateral glaucoma, report only the code for the type of glaucoma, bilateral, with the seventh character for the stage.

> Bilateral severe stage pigmentary glaucoma
>
> **H4Ø.1333 Pigmentary glaucoma, bilateral, severe stage**
>
> *Explanation*: In this scenario, the patient has the same type and stage of glaucoma in both eyes. As this type of glaucoma has a code for bilateral, assign only the code for the bilateral glaucoma with the seventh character for the stage.

When a patient has bilateral glaucoma and both eyes are documented as being the same type and stage, and the classification does not provide a code for bilateral glaucoma (i.e. subcategories H4Ø.1Ø and H4Ø.2Ø) report only one code for the type of glaucoma with the appropriate seventh character for the stage.

> Bilateral open-angle glaucoma; not specified as to type and stage indeterminate in both eyes
>
> **H4Ø.1ØX4 Unspecified open-angle glaucoma, indeterminate stage**
>
> *Explanation*: In this scenario, the patient has glaucoma of the same type and stage of both eyes, but there is no code specifically for bilateral glaucoma. Only one code is assigned with the appropriate seventh character for the stage.

3) Bilateral glaucoma stage with different types or stages

When a patient has bilateral glaucoma and each eye is documented as having a different type or stage, and the classification distinguishes laterality, assign the appropriate code for each eye rather than the code for bilateral glaucoma.

When a patient has bilateral glaucoma and each eye is documented as having a different type, and the classification does not distinguish laterality (i.e. subcategories H4Ø.1Ø and H4Ø.2Ø), assign one code for each type of glaucoma with the appropriate seventh character for the stage.

> Documentation relates mild, unspecified primary angle-closure glaucoma of the left eye with mild unspecified open-angle glaucoma of the right eye
>
> **H4Ø.2ØX1 Unspecified primary angle-closure glaucoma, mild stage**
>
> **H4Ø.1ØX1 Unspecified open-angle glaucoma, mild stage**
>
> *Explanation*: In this scenario the patient has a different type of glaucoma in each eye and the classification does not distinguish laterality. A code for each type of glaucoma is assigned, each with the appropriate seventh character for the stage.

When a patient has bilateral glaucoma and each eye is documented as having the same type, but different stage, and the classification does not distinguish laterality (i.e. subcategories H4Ø.1Ø and H4Ø.2Ø), assign a code for the type of glaucoma for each eye with the seventh character for the specific glaucoma stage documented for each eye.

> Bilateral open-angle glaucoma, not specified as to type; the right eye is documented to be in mild stage and the left eye as being in moderate stage
>
> **H4Ø.1ØX1 Unspecified open-angle glaucoma, mild stage**
>
> **H4Ø.1ØX2 Unspecified open-angle glaucoma, moderate stage**
>
> *Explanation*: In this scenario the patient has the same type of glaucoma in each eye but each eye is at a different stage, and the classification does not distinguish laterality at this subcategory level. Two codes are assigned; both codes represent the same type of glaucoma but each has a different seventh character identifying the appropriate stage for each eye.

4) Patient admitted with glaucoma and stage evolves during the admission

If a patient is admitted with glaucoma and the stage progresses during the admission, assign the code for highest stage documented.

> Patient admitted with mild low-tension glaucoma of the right eye, which progresses to moderate stage during the patient's stay
>
> **H4Ø.1212 Low-tension glaucoma, right eye, moderate stage**
>
> *Explanation*: When the glaucoma stage progresses during an admission, assign only the code for the highest stage documented.

5) Indeterminate stage glaucoma

Assignment of the seventh character "4" for "indeterminate stage" should be based on the clinical documentation. The seventh character "4" is used for glaucomas whose stage cannot be clinically determined. This seventh character should not be confused with the seventh character "Ø", unspecified, which should be assigned when there is no documentation regarding the stage of the glaucoma.

b. Blindness

If "blindness" or "low vision" of both eyes is documented but the visual impairment category is not documented, assign code H54.3, Unqualified visual loss, both eyes. If "blindness" or "low vision" in one eye is documented but the visual impairment category is not documented, assign a code from H54.6-, Unqualified visual loss, one eye. If "blindness" or "visual loss" is documented without any information about whether one or both eyes are affected, assign code H54.7, Unspecified visual loss.

> Blindness in 89-year-old male
>
> **H54.7 Unspecified visual loss**
>
> *Explanation*: Blindness is stated, but there is no mention of whether one or both eyes are affected or the severity of this visual impairment.

Chapter 7. Diseases of the Eye and Adnexa (HØØ-H59)

NOTE Use an external cause code following the code for the eye condition, if applicable, to identify the cause of the eye condition

EXCLUDES 2 *certain conditions originating in the perinatal period (PØ4-P96)*
certain infectious and parasitic diseases (AØØ-B99)
complications of pregnancy, childbirth and the puerperium (OØØ-O9A)
congenital malformations, deformations, and chromosomal abnormalities (QØØ-Q99)
diabetes mellitus related eye conditions (EØ9.3-, E1Ø.3-, E11.3-, E13.3-)
endocrine, nutritional and metabolic diseases (EØØ-E88)
injury (trauma) of eye and orbit (SØ5.-)
injury, poisoning and certain other consequences of external causes (SØØ-T88)
neoplasms (CØØ-D49)
symptoms, signs and abnormal clinical and laboratory findings, not elsewhere classified (RØØ-R94)
syphilis related eye disorders (A5Ø.Ø1, A5Ø.3-, A51.43, A52.71)

This chapter contains the following blocks:

HØØ-HØ5 Disorders of eyelid, lacrimal system and orbit
H1Ø-H11 Disorders of conjunctiva
H15-H22 Disorders of sclera, cornea, iris and ciliary body
H25-H28 Disorders of lens
H3Ø-H36 Disorders of choroid and retina
H4Ø-H42 Glaucoma
H43-H44 Disorders of vitreous body and globe
H46-H47 Disorders of optic nerve and visual pathways
H49-H52 Disorders of ocular muscles, binocular movement, accommodation and refraction
H53-H54 Visual disturbances and blindness
H55-H57 Other disorders of eye and adnexa
H59 Intraoperative and postprocedural complications and disorders of eye and adnexa, not elsewhere classified

Disorders of eyelid, lacrimal system and orbit (HØØ-HØ5)

EXCLUDES 2 *open wound of eyelid (SØ1.1-)*
superficial injury of eyelid (SØØ.1-, SØØ.2-)

✓4th HØØ Hordeolum and chalazion

✓5th HØØ.Ø Hordeolum (externum) (internum) of eyelid

DEF: Acute localized infection of the gland of Zeis (external hordeolum) or Molt or of the meibomian glands (internal hordeolum) of the orbit.

✓6th HØØ.Ø1 Hordeolum externum

Hordeolum NOS
Stye

HØØ.Ø11 Hordeolum externum right upper eyelid
HØØ.Ø12 Hordeolum externum right lower eyelid
HØØ.Ø13 Hordeolum externum right eye, unspecified eyelid
HØØ.Ø14 Hordeolum externum left upper eyelid
HØØ.Ø15 Hordeolum externum left lower eyelid
HØØ.Ø16 Hordeolum externum left eye, unspecified eyelid
HØØ.Ø19 Hordeolum externum unspecified eye, unspecified eyelid

✓6th HØØ.Ø2 Hordeolum internum

Infection of meibomian gland

HØØ.Ø21 Hordeolum internum right upper eyelid
HØØ.Ø22 Hordeolum internum right lower eyelid
HØØ.Ø23 Hordeolum internum right eye, unspecified eyelid
HØØ.Ø24 Hordeolum internum left upper eyelid
HØØ.Ø25 Hordeolum internum left lower eyelid
HØØ.Ø26 Hordeolum internum left eye, unspecified eyelid
HØØ.Ø29 Hordeolum internum unspecified eye, unspecified eyelid

✓6th HØØ.Ø3 Abscess of eyelid

Furuncle of eyelid

HØØ.Ø31 Abscess of right upper eyelid
HØØ.Ø32 Abscess of right lower eyelid
HØØ.Ø33 Abscess of eyelid right eye, unspecified eyelid
HØØ.Ø34 Abscess of left upper eyelid
HØØ.Ø35 Abscess of left lower eyelid
HØØ.Ø36 Abscess of eyelid left eye, unspecified eyelid
HØØ.Ø39 Abscess of eyelid unspecified eye, unspecified eyelid

✓5th HØØ.1 Chalazion

Meibomian (gland) cyst

EXCLUDES 2 *infected meibomian gland (HØØ.Ø2-)*

DEF: Noninfectious, obstructive mass in the oil gland of the eyelid that results in a small chronic lump or inflammation.

HØØ.11 Chalazion right upper eyelid
HØØ.12 Chalazion right lower eyelid
HØØ.13 Chalazion right eye, unspecified eyelid
HØØ.14 Chalazion left upper eyelid
HØØ.15 Chalazion left lower eyelid
HØØ.16 Chalazion left eye, unspecified eyelid
HØØ.19 Chalazion unspecified eye, unspecified eyelid

✓4th HØ1 Other inflammation of eyelid

✓5th HØ1.Ø Blepharitis

EXCLUDES 1 *blepharoconjunctivitis (H1Ø.5-)*

✓6th HØ1.ØØ Unspecified blepharitis

AHA: 2018,4Q,13

HØ1.ØØ1 Unspecified blepharitis right upper eyelid
HØ1.ØØ2 Unspecified blepharitis right lower eyelid
HØ1.ØØ3 Unspecified blepharitis right eye, unspecified eyelid
HØ1.ØØ4 Unspecified blepharitis left upper eyelid
HØ1.ØØ5 Unspecified blepharitis left lower eyelid
HØ1.ØØ6 Unspecified blepharitis left eye, unspecified eyelid
HØ1.ØØ9 Unspecified blepharitis unspecified eye, unspecified eyelid
HØ1.ØØA Unspecified blepharitis right eye, upper and lower eyelids
HØ1.ØØB Unspecified blepharitis left eye, upper and lower eyelids

✓6th HØ1.Ø1 Ulcerative blepharitis

AHA: 2018,4Q,13

HØ1.Ø11 Ulcerative blepharitis right upper eyelid
HØ1.Ø12 Ulcerative blepharitis right lower eyelid
HØ1.Ø13 Ulcerative blepharitis right eye, unspecified eyelid
HØ1.Ø14 Ulcerative blepharitis left upper eyelid
HØ1.Ø15 Ulcerative blepharitis left lower eyelid
HØ1.Ø16 Ulcerative blepharitis left eye, unspecified eyelid
HØ1.Ø19 Ulcerative blepharitis unspecified eye, unspecified eyelid
HØ1.Ø1A Ulcerative blepharitis right eye, upper and lower eyelids
HØ1.Ø1B Ulcerative blepharitis left eye, upper and lower eyelids

✓6th HØ1.Ø2 Squamous blepharitis

AHA: 2018,4Q,13

HØ1.Ø21 Squamous blepharitis right upper eyelid
HØ1.Ø22 Squamous blepharitis right lower eyelid
HØ1.Ø23 Squamous blepharitis right eye, unspecified eyelid
HØ1.Ø24 Squamous blepharitis left upper eyelid
HØ1.Ø25 Squamous blepharitis left lower eyelid
HØ1.Ø26 Squamous blepharitis left eye, unspecified eyelid
HØ1.Ø29 Squamous blepharitis unspecified eye, unspecified eyelid
HØ1.Ø2A Squamous blepharitis right eye, upper and lower eyelids
HØ1.Ø2B Squamous blepharitis left eye, upper and lower eyelids

✓5th HØ1.1 Noninfectious dermatoses of eyelid

✓6th HØ1.11 Allergic dermatitis of eyelid

Contact dermatitis of eyelid

HØ1.111 Allergic dermatitis of right upper eyelid
HØ1.112 Allergic dermatitis of right lower eyelid
HØ1.113 Allergic dermatitis of right eye, unspecified eyelid
HØ1.114 Allergic dermatitis of left upper eyelid
HØ1.115 Allergic dermatitis of left lower eyelid
HØ1.116 Allergic dermatitis of left eye, unspecified eyelid
HØ1.119 Allergic dermatitis of unspecified eye, unspecified eyelid

H01.12 Discoid lupus erythematosus of eyelid
- H01.121 Discoid lupus erythematosus of right upper eyelid
- H01.122 Discoid lupus erythematosus of right lower eyelid
- H01.123 Discoid lupus erythematosus of right eye, unspecified eyelid
- H01.124 Discoid lupus erythematosus of left upper eyelid
- H01.125 Discoid lupus erythematosus of left lower eyelid
- H01.126 Discoid lupus erythematosus of left eye, unspecified eyelid
- H01.129 Discoid lupus erythematosus of unspecified eye, unspecified eyelid

H01.13 Eczematous dermatitis of eyelid
- H01.131 Eczematous dermatitis of right upper eyelid
- H01.132 Eczematous dermatitis of right lower eyelid
- H01.133 Eczematous dermatitis of right eye, unspecified eyelid
- H01.134 Eczematous dermatitis of left upper eyelid
- H01.135 Eczematous dermatitis of left lower eyelid
- H01.136 Eczematous dermatitis of left eye, unspecified eyelid
- H01.139 Eczematous dermatitis of unspecified eye, unspecified eyelid

H01.14 Xeroderma of eyelid
- H01.141 Xeroderma of right upper eyelid
- H01.142 Xeroderma of right lower eyelid
- H01.143 Xeroderma of right eye, unspecified eyelid
- H01.144 Xeroderma of left upper eyelid
- H01.145 Xeroderma of left lower eyelid
- H01.146 Xeroderma of left eye, unspecified eyelid
- H01.149 Xeroderma of unspecified eye, unspecified eyelid

H01.8 Other specified inflammations of eyelid

H01.9 Unspecified inflammation of eyelid
Inflammation of eyelid NOS

H02 Other disorders of eyelid

EXCLUDES 1 *congenital malformations of eyelid (Q10.0-Q10.3)*

Entropion and Ectropion

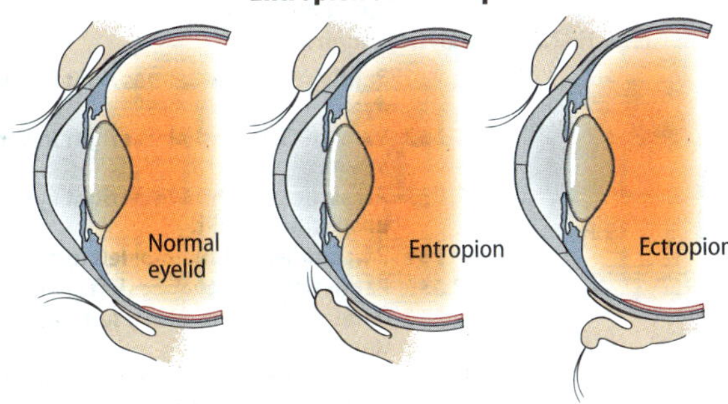

H02.0 Entropion and trichiasis of eyelid

DEF: Entropion: Inversion of the eyelid, turning the edge in toward the eyeball and causing irritation from contact of the lashes with the surface of the eye.

DEF: Trichiasis: Condition wherein the eyelid is in a normal position but lashes are ingrown or misdirected in their growth so that they irritate the tissues of the eye.

H02.00 Unspecified entropion of eyelid
- H02.001 Unspecified entropion of right upper eyelid
- H02.002 Unspecified entropion of right lower eyelid
- H02.003 Unspecified entropion of right eye, unspecified eyelid
- H02.004 Unspecified entropion of left upper eyelid
- H02.005 Unspecified entropion of left lower eyelid
- H02.006 Unspecified entropion of left eye, unspecified eyelid
- H02.009 Unspecified entropion of unspecified eye, unspecified eyelid

H02.01 Cicatricial entropion of eyelid
- H02.011 Cicatricial entropion of right upper eyelid
- H02.012 Cicatricial entropion of right lower eyelid
- H02.013 Cicatricial entropion of right eye, unspecified eyelid
- H02.014 Cicatricial entropion of left upper eyelid
- H02.015 Cicatricial entropion of left lower eyelid
- H02.016 Cicatricial entropion of left eye, unspecified eyelid
- H02.019 Cicatricial entropion of unspecified eye, unspecified eyelid

H02.02 Mechanical entropion of eyelid
- H02.021 Mechanical entropion of right upper eyelid
- H02.022 Mechanical entropion of right lower eyelid
- H02.023 Mechanical entropion of right eye, unspecified eyelid
- H02.024 Mechanical entropion of left upper eyelid
- H02.025 Mechanical entropion of left lower eyelid
- H02.026 Mechanical entropion of left eye, unspecified eyelid
- H02.029 Mechanical entropion of unspecified eye, unspecified eyelid

H02.03 Senile entropion of eyelid
- H02.031 Senile entropion of right upper eyelid A
- H02.032 Senile entropion of right lower eyelid A
- H02.033 Senile entropion of right eye, unspecified eyelid A
- H02.034 Senile entropion of left upper eyelid A
- H02.035 Senile entropion of left lower eyelid A
- H02.036 Senile entropion of left eye, unspecified eyelid A
- H02.039 Senile entropion of unspecified eye, unspecified eyelid A

H02.04 Spastic entropion of eyelid
- H02.041 Spastic entropion of right upper eyelid
- H02.042 Spastic entropion of right lower eyelid
- H02.043 Spastic entropion of right eye, unspecified eyelid
- H02.044 Spastic entropion of left upper eyelid
- H02.045 Spastic entropion of left lower eyelid
- H02.046 Spastic entropion of left eye, unspecified eyelid
- H02.049 Spastic entropion of unspecified eye, unspecified eyelid

H02.05 Trichiasis without entropion
- H02.051 Trichiasis without entropion right upper eyelid
- H02.052 Trichiasis without entropion right lower eyelid
- H02.053 Trichiasis without entropion right eye, unspecified eyelid
- H02.054 Trichiasis without entropion left upper eyelid
- H02.055 Trichiasis without entropion left lower eyelid
- H02.056 Trichiasis without entropion left eye, unspecified eyelid
- H02.059 Trichiasis without entropion unspecified eye, unspecified eyelid

H02.1 Ectropion of eyelid

DEF: Drooping of the lower eyelid away from the eye or outward turning or eversion of the edge of the eyelid, exposing the palpebral conjunctiva and causing irritation.

H02.10 Unspecified ectropion of eyelid
- H02.101 Unspecified ectropion of right upper eyelid
- H02.102 Unspecified ectropion of right lower eyelid
- H02.103 Unspecified ectropion of right eye, unspecified eyelid
- H02.104 Unspecified ectropion of left upper eyelid
- H02.105 Unspecified ectropion of left lower eyelid
- H02.106 Unspecified ectropion of left eye, unspecified eyelid

H02.109 Unspecified ectropion of unspecified eye, unspecified eyelid

√6th H02.11 Cicatricial ectropion of eyelid

H02.111 Cicatricial ectropion of right upper eyelid
H02.112 Cicatricial ectropion of right lower eyelid
H02.113 Cicatricial ectropion of right eye, unspecified eyelid
H02.114 Cicatricial ectropion of left upper eyelid
H02.115 Cicatricial ectropion of left lower eyelid
H02.116 Cicatricial ectropion of left eye, unspecified eyelid
H02.119 Cicatricial ectropion of unspecified eye, unspecified eyelid

√6th H02.12 Mechanical ectropion of eyelid

H02.121 Mechanical ectropion of right upper eyelid
H02.122 Mechanical ectropion of right lower eyelid
H02.123 Mechanical ectropion of right eye, unspecified eyelid
H02.124 Mechanical ectropion of left upper eyelid
H02.125 Mechanical ectropion of left lower eyelid
H02.126 Mechanical ectropion of left eye, unspecified eyelid
H02.129 Mechanical ectropion of unspecified eye, unspecified eyelid

√6th H02.13 Senile ectropion of eyelid

H02.131 Senile ectropion of right upper eyelid A
H02.132 Senile ectropion of right lower eyelid A
H02.133 Senile ectropion of right eye, unspecified eyelid A
H02.134 Senile ectropion of left upper eyelid A
H02.135 Senile ectropion of left lower eyelid A
H02.136 Senile ectropion of left eye, unspecified eyelid A
H02.139 Senile ectropion of unspecified eye, unspecified eyelid A

√6th H02.14 Spastic ectropion of eyelid

H02.141 Spastic ectropion of right upper eyelid
H02.142 Spastic ectropion of right lower eyelid
H02.143 Spastic ectropion of right eye, unspecified eyelid
H02.144 Spastic ectropion of left upper eyelid
H02.145 Spastic ectropion of left lower eyelid
H02.146 Spastic ectropion of left eye, unspecified eyelid
H02.149 Spastic ectropion of unspecified eye, unspecified eyelid

√6th H02.15 Paralytic ectropion of eyelid

AHA: 2018,4Q,13

H02.151 Paralytic ectropion of right upper eyelid
H02.152 Paralytic ectropion of right lower eyelid
H02.153 Paralytic ectropion of right eye, unspecified eyelid
H02.154 Paralytic ectropion of left upper eyelid
H02.155 Paralytic ectropion of left lower eyelid
H02.156 Paralytic ectropion of left eye, unspecified eyelid
H02.159 Paralytic ectropion of unspecified eye, unspecified eyelid

√5th H02.2 Lagophthalmos

AHA: 2018,4Q,14

DEF: Condition of the eye that prevents it from closing completely.

√6th H02.20 Unspecified lagophthalmos

H02.201 Unspecified lagophthalmos right upper eyelid
H02.202 Unspecified lagophthalmos right lower eyelid
H02.203 Unspecified lagophthalmos right eye, unspecified eyelid
H02.204 Unspecified lagophthalmos left upper eyelid
H02.205 Unspecified lagophthalmos left lower eyelid
H02.206 Unspecified lagophthalmos left eye, unspecified eyelid
H02.209 Unspecified lagophthalmos unspecified eye, unspecified eyelid
H02.20A Unspecified lagophthalmos right eye, upper and lower eyelids
H02.20B Unspecified lagophthalmos left eye, upper and lower eyelids
H02.20C Unspecified lagophthalmos, bilateral, upper and lower eyelids

√6th H02.21 Cicatricial lagophthalmos

H02.211 Cicatricial lagophthalmos right upper eyelid
H02.212 Cicatricial lagophthalmos right lower eyelid
H02.213 Cicatricial lagophthalmos right eye, unspecified eyelid
H02.214 Cicatricial lagophthalmos left upper eyelid
H02.215 Cicatricial lagophthalmos left lower eyelid
H02.216 Cicatricial lagophthalmos left eye, unspecified eyelid
H02.219 Cicatricial lagophthalmos unspecified eye, unspecified eyelid
H02.21A Cicatricial lagophthalmos right eye, upper and lower eyelids
H02.21B Cicatricial lagophthalmos left eye, upper and lower eyelids
H02.21C Cicatricial lagophthalmos, bilateral, upper and lower eyelids

√6th H02.22 Mechanical lagophthalmos

H02.221 Mechanical lagophthalmos right upper eyelid
H02.222 Mechanical lagophthalmos right lower eyelid
H02.223 Mechanical lagophthalmos right eye, unspecified eyelid
H02.224 Mechanical lagophthalmos left upper eyelid
H02.225 Mechanical lagophthalmos left lower eyelid
H02.226 Mechanical lagophthalmos left eye, unspecified eyelid
H02.229 Mechanical lagophthalmos unspecified eye, unspecified eyelid
H02.22A Mechanical lagophthalmos right eye, upper and lower eyelids
H02.22B Mechanical lagophthalmos left eye, upper and lower eyelids
H02.22C Mechanical lagophthalmos, bilateral, upper and lower eyelids

√6th H02.23 Paralytic lagophthalmos

H02.231 Paralytic lagophthalmos right upper eyelid
H02.232 Paralytic lagophthalmos right lower eyelid
H02.233 Paralytic lagophthalmos right eye, unspecified eyelid
H02.234 Paralytic lagophthalmos left upper eyelid
H02.235 Paralytic lagophthalmos left lower eyelid
H02.236 Paralytic lagophthalmos left eye, unspecified eyelid
H02.239 Paralytic lagophthalmos unspecified eye, unspecified eyelid
H02.23A Paralytic lagophthalmos right eye, upper and lower eyelids
H02.23B Paralytic lagophthalmos left eye, upper and lower eyelids
H02.23C Paralytic lagophthalmos, bilateral, upper and lower eyelids

√5th H02.3 Blepharochalasis

Pseudoptosis

DEF: Loss of elasticity and relaxation of skin of the eyelid, thickened or indurated skin on the eyelid associated with recurrent episodes of edema, and intracellular atrophy.

H02.30 Blepharochalasis unspecified eye, unspecified eyelid
H02.31 Blepharochalasis right upper eyelid
H02.32 Blepharochalasis right lower eyelid
H02.33 Blepharochalasis right eye, unspecified eyelid
H02.34 Blepharochalasis left upper eyelid
H02.35 Blepharochalasis left lower eyelid
H02.36 Blepharochalasis left eye, unspecified eyelid

H02.4 Ptosis of eyelid

H02.40 Unspecified ptosis of eyelid
- H02.401 Unspecified ptosis of right eyelid
- H02.402 Unspecified ptosis of left eyelid
- H02.403 Unspecified ptosis of bilateral eyelids
- H02.409 Unspecified ptosis of unspecified eyelid

H02.41 Mechanical ptosis of eyelid
- H02.411 Mechanical ptosis of right eyelid
- H02.412 Mechanical ptosis of left eyelid
- H02.413 Mechanical ptosis of bilateral eyelids
- H02.419 Mechanical ptosis of unspecified eyelid

H02.42 Myogenic ptosis of eyelid
- H02.421 Myogenic ptosis of right eyelid
- H02.422 Myogenic ptosis of left eyelid
- H02.423 Myogenic ptosis of bilateral eyelids
- H02.429 Myogenic ptosis of unspecified eyelid

H02.43 Paralytic ptosis of eyelid

Neurogenic ptosis of eyelid
- H02.431 Paralytic ptosis of right eyelid
- H02.432 Paralytic ptosis of left eyelid
- H02.433 Paralytic ptosis of bilateral eyelids
- H02.439 Paralytic ptosis unspecified eyelid

H02.5 Other disorders affecting eyelid function

EXCLUDES 2 *blepharospasm (G24.5)*
organic tic (G25.69)
psychogenic tic (F95.-)

H02.51 Abnormal innervation syndrome
- H02.511 Abnormal innervation syndrome right upper eyelid
- H02.512 Abnormal innervation syndrome right lower eyelid
- H02.513 Abnormal innervation syndrome right eye, unspecified eyelid
- H02.514 Abnormal innervation syndrome left upper eyelid
- H02.515 Abnormal innervation syndrome left lower eyelid
- H02.516 Abnormal innervation syndrome left eye, unspecified eyelid
- H02.519 Abnormal innervation syndrome unspecified eye, unspecified eyelid

H02.52 Blepharophimosis

Ankyloblepharon
- H02.521 Blepharophimosis right upper eyelid
- H02.522 Blepharophimosis right lower eyelid
- H02.523 Blepharophimosis right eye, unspecified eyelid
- H02.524 Blepharophimosis left upper eyelid
- H02.525 Blepharophimosis left lower eyelid
- H02.526 Blepharophimosis left eye, unspecified eyelid
- H02.529 Blepharophimosis unspecified eye, unspecified lid

H02.53 Eyelid retraction

Eyelid lag
- H02.531 Eyelid retraction right upper eyelid
- H02.532 Eyelid retraction right lower eyelid
- H02.533 Eyelid retraction right eye, unspecified eyelid
- H02.534 Eyelid retraction left upper eyelid
- H02.535 Eyelid retraction left lower eyelid
- H02.536 Eyelid retraction left eye, unspecified eyelid
- H02.539 Eyelid retraction unspecified eye, unspecified lid

H02.59 Other disorders affecting eyelid function

Deficient blink reflex
Sensory disorders

H02.6 Xanthelasma of eyelid

DEF: Condition in which there are small yellow tumors that occur on the eyelid, usually appearing near the nose.
- H02.60 Xanthelasma of unspecified eye, unspecified eyelid
- H02.61 Xanthelasma of right upper eyelid
- H02.62 Xanthelasma of right lower eyelid
- H02.63 Xanthelasma of right eye, unspecified eyelid
- H02.64 Xanthelasma of left upper eyelid
- H02.65 Xanthelasma of left lower eyelid
- H02.66 Xanthelasma of left eye, unspecified eyelid

H02.7 Other and unspecified degenerative disorders of eyelid and periocular area

H02.70 Unspecified degenerative disorders of eyelid and periocular area

H02.71 Chloasma of eyelid and periocular area

Dyspigmentation of eyelid
Hyperpigmentation of eyelid
- H02.711 Chloasma of right upper eyelid and periocular area
- H02.712 Chloasma of right lower eyelid and periocular area
- H02.713 Chloasma of right eye, unspecified eyelid and periocular area
- H02.714 Chloasma of left upper eyelid and periocular area
- H02.715 Chloasma of left lower eyelid and periocular area
- H02.716 Chloasma of left eye, unspecified eyelid and periocular area
- H02.719 Chloasma of unspecified eye, unspecified eyelid and periocular area

H02.72 Madarosis of eyelid and periocular area

Hypotrichosis of eyelid
- H02.721 Madarosis of right upper eyelid and periocular area
- H02.722 Madarosis of right lower eyelid and periocular area
- H02.723 Madarosis of right eye, unspecified eyelid and periocular area
- H02.724 Madarosis of left upper eyelid and periocular area
- H02.725 Madarosis of left lower eyelid and periocular area
- H02.726 Madarosis of left eye, unspecified eyelid and periocular area
- H02.729 Madarosis of unspecified eye, unspecified eyelid and periocular area

H02.73 Vitiligo of eyelid and periocular area

Hypopigmentation of eyelid
- H02.731 Vitiligo of right upper eyelid and periocular area
- H02.732 Vitiligo of right lower eyelid and periocular area
- H02.733 Vitiligo of right eye, unspecified eyelid and periocular area
- H02.734 Vitiligo of left upper eyelid and periocular area
- H02.735 Vitiligo of left lower eyelid and periocular area
- H02.736 Vitiligo of left eye, unspecified eyelid and periocular area
- H02.739 Vitiligo of unspecified eye, unspecified eyelid and periocular area

H02.79 Other degenerative disorders of eyelid and periocular area

H02.8 Other specified disorders of eyelid

H02.81 Retained foreign body in eyelid

Use additional code to identify the type of retained foreign body (Z18.-)

EXCLUDES 1 *laceration of eyelid with foreign body (S01.12-)*
retained intraocular foreign body (H44.6-, H44.7-)
superficial foreign body of eyelid and periocular area (S00.25-)
- H02.811 Retained foreign body in right upper eyelid
- H02.812 Retained foreign body in right lower eyelid
- H02.813 Retained foreign body in right eye, unspecified eyelid
- H02.814 Retained foreign body in left upper eyelid
- H02.815 Retained foreign body in left lower eyelid
- H02.816 Retained foreign body in left eye, unspecified eyelid
- H02.819 Retained foreign body in unspecified eye, unspecified eyelid

H02.82 Cysts of eyelid

Sebaceous cyst of eyelid
- H02.821 Cysts of right upper eyelid
- H02.822 Cysts of right lower eyelid

H02.823 Cysts of right eye, unspecified eyelid
H02.824 Cysts of left upper eyelid
H02.825 Cysts of left lower eyelid
H02.826 Cysts of left eye, unspecified eyelid
H02.829 Cysts of unspecified eye, unspecified eyelid

H02.83 Dermatochalasis of eyelid

DEF: Acquired form of connective tissue disorder associated with decreased elastic tissue and abnormal elastin formation, resulting in loss of elasticity of the skin of the eyelid. It is generally associated with aging.

H02.831 Dermatochalasis of right upper eyelid
H02.832 Dermatochalasis of right lower eyelid
H02.833 Dermatochalasis of right eye, unspecified eyelid
H02.834 Dermatochalasis of left upper eyelid
H02.835 Dermatochalasis of left lower eyelid
H02.836 Dermatochalasis of left eye, unspecified eyelid
H02.839 Dermatochalasis of unspecified eye, unspecified eyelid

H02.84 Edema of eyelid

Hyperemia of eyelid

H02.841 Edema of right upper eyelid
H02.842 Edema of right lower eyelid
H02.843 Edema of right eye, unspecified eyelid
H02.844 Edema of left upper eyelid
H02.845 Edema of left lower eyelid
H02.846 Edema of left eye, unspecified eyelid
H02.849 Edema of unspecified eye, unspecified eyelid

H02.85 Elephantiasis of eyelid

H02.851 Elephantiasis of right upper eyelid
H02.852 Elephantiasis of right lower eyelid
H02.853 Elephantiasis of right eye, unspecified eyelid
H02.854 Elephantiasis of left upper eyelid
H02.855 Elephantiasis of left lower eyelid
H02.856 Elephantiasis of left eye, unspecified eyelid
H02.859 Elephantiasis of unspecified eye, unspecified eyelid

H02.86 Hypertrichosis of eyelid

H02.861 Hypertrichosis of right upper eyelid
H02.862 Hypertrichosis of right lower eyelid
H02.863 Hypertrichosis of right eye, unspecified eyelid
H02.864 Hypertrichosis of left upper eyelid
H02.865 Hypertrichosis of left lower eyelid
H02.866 Hypertrichosis of left eye, unspecified eyelid
H02.869 Hypertrichosis of unspecified eye, unspecified eyelid

H02.87 Vascular anomalies of eyelid

H02.871 Vascular anomalies of right upper eyelid
H02.872 Vascular anomalies of right lower eyelid
H02.873 Vascular anomalies of right eye, unspecified eyelid
H02.874 Vascular anomalies of left upper eyelid
H02.875 Vascular anomalies of left lower eyelid
H02.876 Vascular anomalies of left eye, unspecified eyelid
H02.879 Vascular anomalies of unspecified eye, unspecified eyelid

H02.88 Meibomian gland dysfunction of eyelid

AHA: 2018,4Q,14-15

H02.881 Meibomian gland dysfunction right upper eyelid
H02.882 Meibomian gland dysfunction right lower eyelid
H02.883 Meibomian gland dysfunction of right eye, unspecified eyelid
H02.884 Meibomian gland dysfunction left upper eyelid
H02.885 Meibomian gland dysfunction left lower eyelid
H02.886 Meibomian gland dysfunction of left eye, unspecified eyelid
H02.889 Meibomian gland dysfunction of unspecified eye, unspecified eyelid
H02.88A Meibomian gland dysfunction right eye, upper and lower eyelids
H02.88B Meibomian gland dysfunction left eye, upper and lower eyelids

H02.89 Other specified disorders of eyelid

Hemorrhage of eyelid

H02.9 Unspecified disorder of eyelid

Disorder of eyelid NOS

H04 Disorders of lacrimal system

EXCLUDES 1 *congenital malformations of lacrimal system (Q10.4-Q10.6)*

H04.0 Dacryoadenitis

DEF: Inflammation of the lacrimal gland.

H04.00 Unspecified dacryoadenitis

H04.001 Unspecified dacryoadenitis, right lacrimal gland
H04.002 Unspecified dacryoadenitis, left lacrimal gland
H04.003 Unspecified dacryoadenitis, bilateral lacrimal glands
H04.009 Unspecified dacryoadenitis, unspecified lacrimal gland

H04.01 Acute dacryoadenitis

H04.011 Acute dacryoadenitis, right lacrimal gland
H04.012 Acute dacryoadenitis, left lacrimal gland
H04.013 Acute dacryoadenitis, bilateral lacrimal glands
H04.019 Acute dacryoadenitis, unspecified lacrimal gland

H04.02 Chronic dacryoadenitis

H04.021 Chronic dacryoadenitis, right lacrimal gland
H04.022 Chronic dacryoadenitis, left lacrimal gland
H04.023 Chronic dacryoadenitis, bilateral lacrimal gland
H04.029 Chronic dacryoadenitis, unspecified lacrimal gland

H04.03 Chronic enlargement of lacrimal gland

H04.031 Chronic enlargement of right lacrimal gland
H04.032 Chronic enlargement of left lacrimal gland
H04.033 Chronic enlargement of bilateral lacrimal glands
H04.039 Chronic enlargement of unspecified lacrimal gland

H04.1 Other disorders of lacrimal gland

H04.11 Dacryops

H04.111 Dacryops of right lacrimal gland
H04.112 Dacryops of left lacrimal gland
H04.113 Dacryops of bilateral lacrimal glands
H04.119 Dacryops of unspecified lacrimal gland

H04.12 Dry eye syndrome

Tear film insufficiency, NOS

H04.121 Dry eye syndrome of right lacrimal gland
H04.122 Dry eye syndrome of left lacrimal gland
H04.123 Dry eye syndrome of bilateral lacrimal glands
H04.129 Dry eye syndrome of unspecified lacrimal gland

H04.13 Lacrimal cyst

Lacrimal cystic degeneration

H04.131 Lacrimal cyst, right lacrimal gland
H04.132 Lacrimal cyst, left lacrimal gland
H04.133 Lacrimal cyst, bilateral lacrimal glands
H04.139 Lacrimal cyst, unspecified lacrimal gland

H04.14 Primary lacrimal gland atrophy

H04.141 Primary lacrimal gland atrophy, right lacrimal gland
H04.142 Primary lacrimal gland atrophy, left lacrimal gland
H04.143 Primary lacrimal gland atrophy, bilateral lacrimal glands
H04.149 Primary lacrimal gland atrophy, unspecified lacrimal gland

H04.15 Secondary lacrimal gland atrophy

H04.151 Secondary lacrimal gland atrophy, right lacrimal gland

H04.152 Secondary lacrimal gland atrophy, left lacrimal gland
H04.153 Secondary lacrimal gland atrophy, bilateral lacrimal glands
H04.159 Secondary lacrimal gland atrophy, unspecified lacrimal gland

H04.16 Lacrimal gland dislocation
H04.161 Lacrimal gland dislocation, right lacrimal gland
H04.162 Lacrimal gland dislocation, left lacrimal gland
H04.163 Lacrimal gland dislocation, bilateral lacrimal glands
H04.169 Lacrimal gland dislocation, unspecified lacrimal gland

H04.19 Other specified disorders of lacrimal gland

H04.2 Epiphora

DEF: Excessive tearing or overflow of tears down the cheeks often due to a stricture in the lacrimal passages but can be caused by other conditions.

H04.20 Unspecified epiphora
H04.201 Unspecified epiphora, right side
H04.202 Unspecified epiphora, left side
H04.203 Unspecified epiphora, bilateral
H04.209 Unspecified epiphora, unspecified side

H04.21 Epiphora due to excess lacrimation
H04.211 Epiphora due to excess lacrimation, right lacrimal gland
H04.212 Epiphora due to excess lacrimation, left lacrimal gland
H04.213 Epiphora due to excess lacrimation, bilateral lacrimal glands
H04.219 Epiphora due to excess lacrimation, unspecified lacrimal gland

H04.22 Epiphora due to insufficient drainage
H04.221 Epiphora due to insufficient drainage, right side
H04.222 Epiphora due to insufficient drainage, left side
H04.223 Epiphora due to insufficient drainage, bilateral
H04.229 Epiphora due to insufficient drainage, unspecified side

H04.3 Acute and unspecified inflammation of lacrimal passages

EXCLUDES 1 *neonatal dacryocystitis (P39.1)*

H04.30 Unspecified dacryocystitis
H04.301 Unspecified dacryocystitis of right lacrimal passage
H04.302 Unspecified dacryocystitis of left lacrimal passage
H04.303 Unspecified dacryocystitis of bilateral lacrimal passages
H04.309 Unspecified dacryocystitis of unspecified lacrimal passage

H04.31 Phlegmonous dacryocystitis
H04.311 Phlegmonous dacryocystitis of right lacrimal passage
H04.312 Phlegmonous dacryocystitis of left lacrimal passage
H04.313 Phlegmonous dacryocystitis of bilateral lacrimal passages
H04.319 Phlegmonous dacryocystitis of unspecified lacrimal passage

H04.32 Acute dacryocystitis
Acute dacryopericystitis
H04.321 Acute dacryocystitis of right lacrimal passage
H04.322 Acute dacryocystitis of left lacrimal passage
H04.323 Acute dacryocystitis of bilateral lacrimal passages
H04.329 Acute dacryocystitis of unspecified lacrimal passage

H04.33 Acute lacrimal canaliculitis
H04.331 Acute lacrimal canaliculitis of right lacrimal passage
H04.332 Acute lacrimal canaliculitis of left lacrimal passage
H04.333 Acute lacrimal canaliculitis of bilateral lacrimal passages
H04.339 Acute lacrimal canaliculitis of unspecified lacrimal passage

H04.4 Chronic inflammation of lacrimal passages

H04.41 Chronic dacryocystitis
H04.411 Chronic dacryocystitis of right lacrimal passage
H04.412 Chronic dacryocystitis of left lacrimal passage
H04.413 Chronic dacryocystitis of bilateral lacrimal passages
H04.419 Chronic dacryocystitis of unspecified lacrimal passage

H04.42 Chronic lacrimal canaliculitis
H04.421 Chronic lacrimal canaliculitis of right lacrimal passage
H04.422 Chronic lacrimal canaliculitis of left lacrimal passage
H04.423 Chronic lacrimal canaliculitis of bilateral lacrimal passages
H04.429 Chronic lacrimal canaliculitis of unspecified lacrimal passage

H04.43 Chronic lacrimal mucocele
H04.431 Chronic lacrimal mucocele of right lacrimal passage
H04.432 Chronic lacrimal mucocele of left lacrimal passage
H04.433 Chronic lacrimal mucocele of bilateral lacrimal passages
H04.439 Chronic lacrimal mucocele of unspecified lacrimal passage

H04.5 Stenosis and insufficiency of lacrimal passages

H04.51 Dacryolith
H04.511 Dacryolith of right lacrimal passage
H04.512 Dacryolith of left lacrimal passage
H04.513 Dacryolith of bilateral lacrimal passages
H04.519 Dacryolith of unspecified lacrimal passage

H04.52 Eversion of lacrimal punctum
H04.521 Eversion of right lacrimal punctum
H04.522 Eversion of left lacrimal punctum
H04.523 Eversion of bilateral lacrimal punctum
H04.529 Eversion of unspecified lacrimal punctum

H04.53 Neonatal obstruction of nasolacrimal duct

EXCLUDES 1 *congenital stenosis and stricture of lacrimal duct (Q10.5)*

H04.531 Neonatal obstruction of right nasolacrimal duct N
H04.532 Neonatal obstruction of left nasolacrimal duct N
H04.533 Neonatal obstruction of bilateral nasolacrimal duct N
H04.539 Neonatal obstruction of unspecified nasolacrimal duct N

H04.54 Stenosis of lacrimal canaliculi
H04.541 Stenosis of right lacrimal canaliculi
H04.542 Stenosis of left lacrimal canaliculi
H04.543 Stenosis of bilateral lacrimal canaliculi
H04.549 Stenosis of unspecified lacrimal canaliculi

H04.55 Acquired stenosis of nasolacrimal duct
H04.551 Acquired stenosis of right nasolacrimal duct
H04.552 Acquired stenosis of left nasolacrimal duct
H04.553 Acquired stenosis of bilateral nasolacrimal duct
H04.559 Acquired stenosis of unspecified nasolacrimal duct

H04.56 Stenosis of lacrimal punctum
H04.561 Stenosis of right lacrimal punctum
H04.562 Stenosis of left lacrimal punctum
H04.563 Stenosis of bilateral lacrimal punctum
H04.569 Stenosis of unspecified lacrimal punctum

H04.57 Stenosis of lacrimal sac
H04.571 Stenosis of right lacrimal sac
H04.572 Stenosis of left lacrimal sac
H04.573 Stenosis of bilateral lacrimal sac
H04.579 Stenosis of unspecified lacrimal sac

- ✓5th **HØ4.6 Other changes of lacrimal passages**
  - ✓6th **HØ4.61 Lacrimal fistula**
    - **HØ4.611 Lacrimal fistula right lacrimal passage**
    - **HØ4.612 Lacrimal fistula left lacrimal passage**
    - **HØ4.613 Lacrimal fistula bilateral lacrimal passages**
    - **HØ4.619 Lacrimal fistula unspecified lacrimal passage**
  - **HØ4.69 Other changes of lacrimal passages**
- ✓5th **HØ4.8 Other disorders of lacrimal system**
  - ✓6th **HØ4.81 Granuloma of lacrimal passages**
    - **HØ4.811 Granuloma of right lacrimal passage**
    - **HØ4.812 Granuloma of left lacrimal passage**
    - **HØ4.813 Granuloma of bilateral lacrimal passages**
    - **HØ4.819 Granuloma of unspecified lacrimal passage**
  - **HØ4.89 Other disorders of lacrimal system**
- **HØ4.9 Disorder of lacrimal system, unspecified**

✓4th **HØ5 Disorders of orbit**

EXCLUDES 1 *congenital malformation of orbit (Q1Ø.7)*

- ✓5th **HØ5.Ø Acute inflammation of orbit**
  - **HØ5.ØØ Unspecified acute inflammation of orbit**
  - ✓6th **HØ5.Ø1 Cellulitis of orbit**
    - Abscess of orbit
    - **HØ5.Ø11 Cellulitis of right orbit** CC
    - **HØ5.Ø12 Cellulitis of left orbit** CC
    - **HØ5.Ø13 Cellulitis of bilateral orbits** CC
    - **HØ5.Ø19 Cellulitis of unspecified orbit** CC UNS
  - ✓6th **HØ5.Ø2 Osteomyelitis of orbit**
    - **HØ5.Ø21 Osteomyelitis of right orbit** CC
    - **HØ5.Ø22 Osteomyelitis of left orbit** CC
    - **HØ5.Ø23 Osteomyelitis of bilateral orbits** CC
    - **HØ5.Ø29 Osteomyelitis of unspecified orbit** CC UNS
  - ✓6th **HØ5.Ø3 Periostitis of orbit**
    - **HØ5.Ø31 Periostitis of right orbit** CC
    - **HØ5.Ø32 Periostitis of left orbit** CC
    - **HØ5.Ø33 Periostitis of bilateral orbits** CC
    - **HØ5.Ø39 Periostitis of unspecified orbit** CC UNS
  - ✓6th **HØ5.Ø4 Tenonitis of orbit**
    - **HØ5.Ø41 Tenonitis of right orbit**
    - **HØ5.Ø42 Tenonitis of left orbit**
    - **HØ5.Ø43 Tenonitis of bilateral orbits**
    - **HØ5.Ø49 Tenonitis of unspecified orbit**
- ✓5th **HØ5.1 Chronic inflammatory disorders of orbit**
  - **HØ5.1Ø Unspecified chronic inflammatory disorders of orbit**
  - ✓6th **HØ5.11 Granuloma of orbit**
    - Pseudotumor (inflammatory) of orbit
    - **HØ5.111 Granuloma of right orbit**
    - **HØ5.112 Granuloma of left orbit**
    - **HØ5.113 Granuloma of bilateral orbits**
    - **HØ5.119 Granuloma of unspecified orbit**
  - ✓6th **HØ5.12 Orbital myositis**
    - **HØ5.121 Orbital myositis, right orbit**
    - **HØ5.122 Orbital myositis, left orbit**
    - **HØ5.123 Orbital myositis, bilateral**
    - **HØ5.129 Orbital myositis, unspecified orbit**
- ✓5th **HØ5.2 Exophthalmic conditions**
  - **HØ5.2Ø Unspecified exophthalmos**
  - ✓6th **HØ5.21 Displacement (lateral) of globe**
    - **HØ5.211 Displacement (lateral) of globe, right eye**
    - **HØ5.212 Displacement (lateral) of globe, left eye**
    - **HØ5.213 Displacement (lateral) of globe, bilateral**
    - **HØ5.219 Displacement (lateral) of globe, unspecified eye**
  - ✓6th **HØ5.22 Edema of orbit**
    - Orbital congestion
    - **HØ5.221 Edema of right orbit**
    - **HØ5.222 Edema of left orbit**
    - **HØ5.223 Edema of bilateral orbit**
    - **HØ5.229 Edema of unspecified orbit**
  - ✓6th **HØ5.23 Hemorrhage of orbit**
    - **HØ5.231 Hemorrhage of right orbit**
    - **HØ5.232 Hemorrhage of left orbit**
    - **HØ5.233 Hemorrhage of bilateral orbit**
    - **HØ5.239 Hemorrhage of unspecified orbit**
  - ✓6th **HØ5.24 Constant exophthalmos**
    - **HØ5.241 Constant exophthalmos, right eye**
    - **HØ5.242 Constant exophthalmos, left eye**
    - **HØ5.243 Constant exophthalmos, bilateral**
    - **HØ5.249 Constant exophthalmos, unspecified eye**
  - ✓6th **HØ5.25 Intermittent exophthalmos**
    - **HØ5.251 Intermittent exophthalmos, right eye**
    - **HØ5.252 Intermittent exophthalmos, left eye**
    - **HØ5.253 Intermittent exophthalmos, bilateral**
    - **HØ5.259 Intermittent exophthalmos, unspecified eye**
  - ✓6th **HØ5.26 Pulsating exophthalmos**
    - **HØ5.261 Pulsating exophthalmos, right eye**
    - **HØ5.262 Pulsating exophthalmos, left eye**
    - **HØ5.263 Pulsating exophthalmos, bilateral**
    - **HØ5.269 Pulsating exophthalmos, unspecified eye**
- ✓5th **HØ5.3 Deformity of orbit**
  - EXCLUDES 1 *congenital deformity of orbit (Q1Ø.7)*
    hypertelorism (Q75.2)
  - **HØ5.3Ø Unspecified deformity of orbit**
  - ✓6th **HØ5.31 Atrophy of orbit**
    - **HØ5.311 Atrophy of right orbit**
    - **HØ5.312 Atrophy of left orbit**
    - **HØ5.313 Atrophy of bilateral orbit**
    - **HØ5.319 Atrophy of unspecified orbit**
  - ✓6th **HØ5.32 Deformity of orbit due to bone disease**
    - Code also associated bone disease
    - **HØ5.321 Deformity of right orbit due to bone disease**
    - **HØ5.322 Deformity of left orbit due to bone disease**
    - **HØ5.323 Deformity of bilateral orbits due to bone disease**
    - **HØ5.329 Deformity of unspecified orbit due to bone disease**
  - ✓6th **HØ5.33 Deformity of orbit due to trauma or surgery**
    - **HØ5.331 Deformity of right orbit due to trauma or surgery**
    - **HØ5.332 Deformity of left orbit due to trauma or surgery**
    - **HØ5.333 Deformity of bilateral orbits due to trauma or surgery**
    - **HØ5.339 Deformity of unspecified orbit due to trauma or surgery**
  - ✓6th **HØ5.34 Enlargement of orbit**
    - **HØ5.341 Enlargement of right orbit**
    - **HØ5.342 Enlargement of left orbit**
    - **HØ5.343 Enlargement of bilateral orbits**
    - **HØ5.349 Enlargement of unspecified orbit**
  - ✓6th **HØ5.35 Exostosis of orbit**
    - **HØ5.351 Exostosis of right orbit**
    - **HØ5.352 Exostosis of left orbit**
    - **HØ5.353 Exostosis of bilateral orbits**
    - **HØ5.359 Exostosis of unspecified orbit**
- ✓5th **HØ5.4 Enophthalmos**
  - ✓6th **HØ5.4Ø Unspecified enophthalmos**
    - **HØ5.4Ø1 Unspecified enophthalmos, right eye**
    - **HØ5.4Ø2 Unspecified enophthalmos, left eye**
    - **HØ5.4Ø3 Unspecified enophthalmos, bilateral**
    - **HØ5.4Ø9 Unspecified enophthalmos, unspecified eye**
  - ✓6th **HØ5.41 Enophthalmos due to atrophy of orbital tissue**
    - **HØ5.411 Enophthalmos due to atrophy of orbital tissue, right eye**
    - **HØ5.412 Enophthalmos due to atrophy of orbital tissue, left eye**
    - **HØ5.413 Enophthalmos due to atrophy of orbital tissue, bilateral**
    - **HØ5.419 Enophthalmos due to atrophy of orbital tissue, unspecified eye**
  - ✓6th **HØ5.42 Enophthalmos due to trauma or surgery**
    - **HØ5.421 Enophthalmos due to trauma or surgery, right eye**
    - **HØ5.422 Enophthalmos due to trauma or surgery, left eye**

H05.423 Enophthalmos due to trauma or surgery, bilateral

H05.429 Enophthalmos due to trauma or surgery, unspecified eye

H05.5 Retained (old) foreign body following penetrating wound of orbit

Retrobulbar foreign body

Use additional code to identify the type of retained foreign body (Z18.-)

EXCLUDES 1 *current penetrating wound of orbit (S05.4-)*

EXCLUDES 2 *retained foreign body of eyelid (H02.81-)*

retained intraocular foreign body (H44.6-, H44.7-)

H05.50 Retained (old) foreign body following penetrating wound of unspecified orbit

H05.51 Retained (old) foreign body following penetrating wound of right orbit

H05.52 Retained (old) foreign body following penetrating wound of left orbit

H05.53 Retained (old) foreign body following penetrating wound of bilateral orbits

H05.8 Other disorders of orbit

H05.81 Cyst of orbit

Encephalocele of orbit

H05.811 Cyst of right orbit

H05.812 Cyst of left orbit

H05.813 Cyst of bilateral orbits

H05.819 Cyst of unspecified orbit

H05.82 Myopathy of extraocular muscles

H05.821 Myopathy of extraocular muscles, right orbit

H05.822 Myopathy of extraocular muscles, left orbit

H05.823 Myopathy of extraocular muscles, bilateral

H05.829 Myopathy of extraocular muscles, unspecified orbit

H05.89 Other disorders of orbit

H05.9 Unspecified disorder of orbit

Disorders of conjunctiva (H10-H11)

H10 Conjunctivitis

EXCLUDES 1 *keratoconjunctivitis (H16.2-)*

H10.0 Mucopurulent conjunctivitis

H10.01 Acute follicular conjunctivitis

H10.011 Acute follicular conjunctivitis, right eye

H10.012 Acute follicular conjunctivitis, left eye

H10.013 Acute follicular conjunctivitis, bilateral

H10.019 Acute follicular conjunctivitis, unspecified eye

H10.02 Other mucopurulent conjunctivitis

H10.021 Other mucopurulent conjunctivitis, right eye

H10.022 Other mucopurulent conjunctivitis, left eye

H10.023 Other mucopurulent conjunctivitis, bilateral

H10.029 Other mucopurulent conjunctivitis, unspecified eye

H10.1 Acute atopic conjunctivitis

Acute papillary conjunctivitis

H10.10 Acute atopic conjunctivitis, unspecified eye

H10.11 Acute atopic conjunctivitis, right eye

H10.12 Acute atopic conjunctivitis, left eye

H10.13 Acute atopic conjunctivitis, bilateral

H10.2 Other acute conjunctivitis

H10.21 Acute toxic conjunctivitis

Acute chemical conjunctivitis

Code first (T51-T65) to identify chemical and intent

EXCLUDES 1 *burn and corrosion of eye and adnexa (T26.-)*

H10.211 Acute toxic conjunctivitis, right eye

H10.212 Acute toxic conjunctivitis, left eye

H10.213 Acute toxic conjunctivitis, bilateral

H10.219 Acute toxic conjunctivitis, unspecified eye

H10.22 Pseudomembranous conjunctivitis

H10.221 Pseudomembranous conjunctivitis, right eye

H10.222 Pseudomembranous conjunctivitis, left eye

H10.223 Pseudomembranous conjunctivitis, bilateral

H10.229 Pseudomembranous conjunctivitis, unspecified eye

H10.23 Serous conjunctivitis, except viral

EXCLUDES 1 *viral conjunctivitis (B30.-)*

H10.231 Serous conjunctivitis, except viral, right eye

H10.232 Serous conjunctivitis, except viral, left eye

H10.233 Serous conjunctivitis, except viral, bilateral

H10.239 Serous conjunctivitis, except viral, unspecified eye

H10.3 Unspecified acute conjunctivitis

EXCLUDES 1 *ophthalmia neonatorum NOS (P39.1)*

H10.30 Unspecified acute conjunctivitis, unspecified eye

H10.31 Unspecified acute conjunctivitis, right eye

H10.32 Unspecified acute conjunctivitis, left eye

H10.33 Unspecified acute conjunctivitis, bilateral

H10.4 Chronic conjunctivitis

H10.40 Unspecified chronic conjunctivitis

H10.401 Unspecified chronic conjunctivitis, right eye

H10.402 Unspecified chronic conjunctivitis, left eye

H10.403 Unspecified chronic conjunctivitis, bilateral

H10.409 Unspecified chronic conjunctivitis, unspecified eye

H10.41 Chronic giant papillary conjunctivitis

H10.411 Chronic giant papillary conjunctivitis, right eye

H10.412 Chronic giant papillary conjunctivitis, left eye

H10.413 Chronic giant papillary conjunctivitis, bilateral

H10.419 Chronic giant papillary conjunctivitis, unspecified eye

H10.42 Simple chronic conjunctivitis

H10.421 Simple chronic conjunctivitis, right eye

H10.422 Simple chronic conjunctivitis, left eye

H10.423 Simple chronic conjunctivitis, bilateral

H10.429 Simple chronic conjunctivitis, unspecified eye

H10.43 Chronic follicular conjunctivitis

H10.431 Chronic follicular conjunctivitis, right eye

H10.432 Chronic follicular conjunctivitis, left eye

H10.433 Chronic follicular conjunctivitis, bilateral

H10.439 Chronic follicular conjunctivitis, unspecified eye

H10.44 Vernal conjunctivitis

EXCLUDES 1 *vernal keratoconjunctivitis with limbar and corneal involvement (H16.26-)*

H10.45 Other chronic allergic conjunctivitis

H10.5 Blepharoconjunctivitis

H10.50 Unspecified blepharoconjunctivitis

H10.501 Unspecified blepharoconjunctivitis, right eye

H10.502 Unspecified blepharoconjunctivitis, left eye

H10.503 Unspecified blepharoconjunctivitis, bilateral

H10.509 Unspecified blepharoconjunctivitis, unspecified eye

H10.51 Ligneous conjunctivitis

Code also underlying condition if known, such as: plasminogen deficiency (E88.02)

H10.511 Ligneous conjunctivitis, right eye

H10.512 Ligneous conjunctivitis, left eye

H10.513 Ligneous conjunctivitis, bilateral

H10.519 Ligneous conjunctivitis, unspecified eye

√6th **H10.52 Angular blepharoconjunctivitis**
- **H10.521 Angular blepharoconjunctivitis, right eye**
- **H10.522 Angular blepharoconjunctivitis, left eye**
- **H10.523 Angular blepharoconjunctivitis, bilateral**
- **H10.529 Angular blepharoconjunctivitis, unspecified eye**

√6th **H10.53 Contact blepharoconjunctivitis**
- **H10.531 Contact blepharoconjunctivitis, right eye**
- **H10.532 Contact blepharoconjunctivitis, left eye**
- **H10.533 Contact blepharoconjunctivitis, bilateral**
- **H10.539 Contact blepharoconjunctivitis, unspecified eye**

√5th **H10.8 Other conjunctivitis**

√6th **H10.81 Pingueculitis**

EXCLUDES 1 *pinguecula (H11.15-)*

- **H10.811 Pingueculitis, right eye**
- **H10.812 Pingueculitis, left eye**
- **H10.813 Pingueculitis, bilateral**
- **H10.819 Pingueculitis, unspecified eye**

√6th **H10.82 Rosacea conjunctivitis**

Code first underlying rosacea dermatitis (L71.-)

AHA: 2018,4Q,15

- **H10.821 Rosacea conjunctivitis, right eye**
- **H10.822 Rosacea conjunctivitis, left eye**
- **H10.823 Rosacea conjunctivitis, bilateral**
- **H10.829 Rosacea conjunctivitis, unspecified eye**

H10.89 Other conjunctivitis

H10.9 Unspecified conjunctivitis

√4th **H11 Other disorders of conjunctiva**

EXCLUDES 1 *keratoconjunctivitis (H16.2-)*

√5th **H11.0 Pterygium of eye**

EXCLUDES 1 *pseudopterygium (H11.81-)*

DEF: Benign, wedge-shaped, conjunctival thickening that advances from the inner corner of the eye toward the cornea.

Pterygium

Pterygium

√6th **H11.00 Unspecified pterygium of eye**
- **H11.001 Unspecified pterygium of right eye**
- **H11.002 Unspecified pterygium of left eye**
- **H11.003 Unspecified pterygium of eye, bilateral**
- **H11.009 Unspecified pterygium of unspecified eye**

√6th **H11.01 Amyloid pterygium**
- **H11.011 Amyloid pterygium of right eye**
- **H11.012 Amyloid pterygium of left eye**
- **H11.013 Amyloid pterygium of eye, bilateral**
- **H11.019 Amyloid pterygium of unspecified eye**

√6th **H11.02 Central pterygium of eye**
- **H11.021 Central pterygium of right eye**
- **H11.022 Central pterygium of left eye**
- **H11.023 Central pterygium of eye, bilateral**
- **H11.029 Central pterygium of unspecified eye**

√6th **H11.03 Double pterygium of eye**
- **H11.031 Double pterygium of right eye**
- **H11.032 Double pterygium of left eye**
- **H11.033 Double pterygium of eye, bilateral**
- **H11.039 Double pterygium of unspecified eye**

√6th **H11.04 Peripheral pterygium of eye, stationary**
- **H11.041 Peripheral pterygium, stationary, right eye**
- **H11.042 Peripheral pterygium, stationary, left eye**
- **H11.043 Peripheral pterygium, stationary, bilateral**
- **H11.049 Peripheral pterygium, stationary, unspecified eye**

√6th **H11.05 Peripheral pterygium of eye, progressive**
- **H11.051 Peripheral pterygium, progressive, right eye**
- **H11.052 Peripheral pterygium, progressive, left eye**
- **H11.053 Peripheral pterygium, progressive, bilateral**
- **H11.059 Peripheral pterygium, progressive, unspecified eye**

√6th **H11.06 Recurrent pterygium of eye**
- **H11.061 Recurrent pterygium of right eye**
- **H11.062 Recurrent pterygium of left eye**
- **H11.063 Recurrent pterygium of eye, bilateral**
- **H11.069 Recurrent pterygium of unspecified eye**

√5th **H11.1 Conjunctival degenerations and deposits**

EXCLUDES 2 *pseudopterygium (H11.81)*

H11.10 Unspecified conjunctival degenerations

√6th **H11.11 Conjunctival deposits**
- **H11.111 Conjunctival deposits, right eye**
- **H11.112 Conjunctival deposits, left eye**
- **H11.113 Conjunctival deposits, bilateral**
- **H11.119 Conjunctival deposits, unspecified eye**

√6th **H11.12 Conjunctival concretions**
- **H11.121 Conjunctival concretions, right eye**
- **H11.122 Conjunctival concretions, left eye**
- **H11.123 Conjunctival concretions, bilateral**
- **H11.129 Conjunctival concretions, unspecified eye**

√6th **H11.13 Conjunctival pigmentations**

Conjunctival argyrosis [argyria]

- **H11.131 Conjunctival pigmentations, right eye**
- **H11.132 Conjunctival pigmentations, left eye**
- **H11.133 Conjunctival pigmentations, bilateral**
- **H11.139 Conjunctival pigmentations, unspecified eye**

√6th **H11.14 Conjunctival xerosis, unspecified**

EXCLUDES 1 *xerosis of conjunctiva due to vitamin A deficiency (E50.0, E50.1)*

DEF: Abnormal dryness of the conjunctiva due to lack of sufficient tears or conjunctival secretions.

- **H11.141 Conjunctival xerosis, unspecified, right eye**
- **H11.142 Conjunctival xerosis, unspecified, left eye**
- **H11.143 Conjunctival xerosis, unspecified, bilateral**
- **H11.149 Conjunctival xerosis, unspecified, unspecified eye**

√6th **H11.15 Pinguecula**

EXCLUDES 1 *pingueculitis (H10.81-)*

DEF: Proliferation on the conjunctiva near the sclerocorneal junction, usually of the side of the nose and usually in older patients.

Pinguecula

Pinguecula

- **H11.151 Pinguecula, right eye**
- **H11.152 Pinguecula, left eye**
- **H11.153 Pinguecula, bilateral**
- **H11.159 Pinguecula, unspecified eye**

√5th **H11.2 Conjunctival scars**

√6th **H11.21 Conjunctival adhesions and strands (localized)**
- **H11.211 Conjunctival adhesions and strands (localized), right eye**
- **H11.212 Conjunctival adhesions and strands (localized), left eye**
- **H11.213 Conjunctival adhesions and strands (localized), bilateral**
- **H11.219 Conjunctival adhesions and strands (localized), unspecified eye**

H11.22 Conjunctival granuloma
H11.221 Conjunctival granuloma, right eye
H11.222 Conjunctival granuloma, left eye
H11.223 Conjunctival granuloma, bilateral
H11.229 Conjunctival granuloma, unspecified
H11.23 Symblepharon
H11.231 Symblepharon, right eye
H11.232 Symblepharon, left eye
H11.233 Symblepharon, bilateral
H11.239 Symblepharon, unspecified eye
H11.24 Scarring of conjunctiva
H11.241 Scarring of conjunctiva, right eye
H11.242 Scarring of conjunctiva, left eye
H11.243 Scarring of conjunctiva, bilateral
H11.249 Scarring of conjunctiva, unspecified eye
H11.3 Conjunctival hemorrhage
Subconjunctival hemorrhage
H11.30 Conjunctival hemorrhage, unspecified eye
H11.31 Conjunctival hemorrhage, right eye
H11.32 Conjunctival hemorrhage, left eye
H11.33 Conjunctival hemorrhage, bilateral
H11.4 Other conjunctival vascular disorders and cysts
H11.41 Vascular abnormalities of conjunctiva
Conjunctival aneurysm
H11.411 Vascular abnormalities of conjunctiva, right eye
H11.412 Vascular abnormalities of conjunctiva, left eye
H11.413 Vascular abnormalities of conjunctiva, bilateral
H11.419 Vascular abnormalities of conjunctiva, unspecified eye
H11.42 Conjunctival edema
H11.421 Conjunctival edema, right eye
H11.422 Conjunctival edema, left eye
H11.423 Conjunctival edema, bilateral
H11.429 Conjunctival edema, unspecified eye
H11.43 Conjunctival hyperemia
H11.431 Conjunctival hyperemia, right eye
H11.432 Conjunctival hyperemia, left eye
H11.433 Conjunctival hyperemia, bilateral
H11.439 Conjunctival hyperemia, unspecified eye
H11.44 Conjunctival cysts
H11.441 Conjunctival cysts, right eye
H11.442 Conjunctival cysts, left eye
H11.443 Conjunctival cysts, bilateral
H11.449 Conjunctival cysts, unspecified eye
H11.8 Other specified disorders of conjunctiva
H11.81 Pseudopterygium of conjunctiva
H11.811 Pseudopterygium of conjunctiva, right eye
H11.812 Pseudopterygium of conjunctiva, left eye
H11.813 Pseudopterygium of conjunctiva, bilateral
H11.819 Pseudopterygium of conjunctiva, unspecified eye
H11.82 Conjunctivochalasis
H11.821 Conjunctivochalasis, right eye
H11.822 Conjunctivochalasis, left eye
H11.823 Conjunctivochalasis, bilateral
H11.829 Conjunctivochalasis, unspecified eye
H11.89 Other specified disorders of conjunctiva
H11.9 Unspecified disorder of conjunctiva

Disorders of sclera, cornea, iris and ciliary body (H15-H22)

H15 Disorders of sclera

H15.0 Scleritis
H15.00 Unspecified scleritis
H15.001 Unspecified scleritis, right eye
H15.002 Unspecified scleritis, left eye
H15.003 Unspecified scleritis, bilateral
H15.009 Unspecified scleritis, unspecified eye
H15.01 Anterior scleritis
H15.011 Anterior scleritis, right eye
H15.012 Anterior scleritis, left eye
H15.013 Anterior scleritis, bilateral
H15.019 Anterior scleritis, unspecified eye
H15.02 Brawny scleritis
H15.021 Brawny scleritis, right eye
H15.022 Brawny scleritis, left eye
H15.023 Brawny scleritis, bilateral
H15.029 Brawny scleritis, unspecified eye
H15.03 Posterior scleritis
Sclerotenonitis
H15.031 Posterior scleritis, right eye
H15.032 Posterior scleritis, left eye
H15.033 Posterior scleritis, bilateral
H15.039 Posterior scleritis, unspecified eye
H15.04 Scleritis with corneal involvement
H15.041 Scleritis with corneal involvement, right eye
H15.042 Scleritis with corneal involvement, left eye
H15.043 Scleritis with corneal involvement, bilateral
H15.049 Scleritis with corneal involvement, unspecified eye
H15.05 Scleromalacia perforans
H15.051 Scleromalacia perforans, right eye
H15.052 Scleromalacia perforans, left eye
H15.053 Scleromalacia perforans, bilateral
H15.059 Scleromalacia perforans, unspecified eye
H15.09 Other scleritis
Scleral abscess
H15.091 Other scleritis, right eye
H15.092 Other scleritis, left eye
H15.093 Other scleritis, bilateral
H15.099 Other scleritis, unspecified eye
H15.1 Episcleritis
H15.10 Unspecified episcleritis
H15.101 Unspecified episcleritis, right eye
H15.102 Unspecified episcleritis, left eye
H15.103 Unspecified episcleritis, bilateral
H15.109 Unspecified episcleritis, unspecified eye
H15.11 Episcleritis periodica fugax
H15.111 Episcleritis periodica fugax, right eye
H15.112 Episcleritis periodica fugax, left eye
H15.113 Episcleritis periodica fugax, bilateral
H15.119 Episcleritis periodica fugax, unspecified eye
H15.12 Nodular episcleritis
H15.121 Nodular episcleritis, right eye
H15.122 Nodular episcleritis, left eye
H15.123 Nodular episcleritis, bilateral
H15.129 Nodular episcleritis, unspecified eye
H15.8 Other disorders of sclera
EXCLUDES 2 *blue sclera (Q13.5)*
degenerative myopia (H44.2-)
H15.81 Equatorial staphyloma
H15.811 Equatorial staphyloma, right eye
H15.812 Equatorial staphyloma, left eye
H15.813 Equatorial staphyloma, bilateral
H15.819 Equatorial staphyloma, unspecified eye
H15.82 Localized anterior staphyloma
H15.821 Localized anterior staphyloma, right eye
H15.822 Localized anterior staphyloma, left eye
H15.823 Localized anterior staphyloma, bilateral
H15.829 Localized anterior staphyloma, unspecified eye
H15.83 Staphyloma posticum
H15.831 Staphyloma posticum, right eye
H15.832 Staphyloma posticum, left eye
H15.833 Staphyloma posticum, bilateral
H15.839 Staphyloma posticum, unspecified eye
H15.84 Scleral ectasia
H15.841 Scleral ectasia, right eye
H15.842 Scleral ectasia, left eye
H15.843 Scleral ectasia, bilateral
H15.849 Scleral ectasia, unspecified eye
H15.85 Ring staphyloma
H15.851 Ring staphyloma, right eye

H15.852 Ring staphyloma, left eye
H15.853 Ring staphyloma, bilateral
H15.859 Ring staphyloma, unspecified eye
H15.89 Other disorders of sclera
H15.9 Unspecified disorder of sclera

H16 Keratitis

DEF: Condition in which the cornea becomes inflamed and irritated.

H16.0 Corneal ulcer

H16.00 Unspecified corneal ulcer
H16.001 Unspecified corneal ulcer, right eye
H16.002 Unspecified corneal ulcer, left eye
H16.003 Unspecified corneal ulcer, bilateral
H16.009 Unspecified corneal ulcer, unspecified eye

H16.01 Central corneal ulcer
H16.011 Central corneal ulcer, right eye
H16.012 Central corneal ulcer, left eye
H16.013 Central corneal ulcer, bilateral
H16.019 Central corneal ulcer, unspecified eye

H16.02 Ring corneal ulcer
H16.021 Ring corneal ulcer, right eye
H16.022 Ring corneal ulcer, left eye
H16.023 Ring corneal ulcer, bilateral
H16.029 Ring corneal ulcer, unspecified eye

H16.03 Corneal ulcer with hypopyon
H16.031 Corneal ulcer with hypopyon, right eye
H16.032 Corneal ulcer with hypopyon, left eye
H16.033 Corneal ulcer with hypopyon, bilateral
H16.039 Corneal ulcer with hypopyon, unspecified eye

H16.04 Marginal corneal ulcer
H16.041 Marginal corneal ulcer, right eye
H16.042 Marginal corneal ulcer, left eye
H16.043 Marginal corneal ulcer, bilateral
H16.049 Marginal corneal ulcer, unspecified eye

H16.05 Mooren's corneal ulcer
H16.051 Mooren's corneal ulcer, right eye
H16.052 Mooren's corneal ulcer, left eye
H16.053 Mooren's corneal ulcer, bilateral
H16.059 Mooren's corneal ulcer, unspecified eye

H16.06 Mycotic corneal ulcer
H16.061 Mycotic corneal ulcer, right eye
H16.062 Mycotic corneal ulcer, left eye
H16.063 Mycotic corneal ulcer, bilateral
H16.069 Mycotic corneal ulcer, unspecified eye

H16.07 Perforated corneal ulcer
H16.071 Perforated corneal ulcer, right eye
H16.072 Perforated corneal ulcer, left eye
H16.073 Perforated corneal ulcer, bilateral
H16.079 Perforated corneal ulcer, unspecified eye

H16.1 Other and unspecified superficial keratitis without conjunctivitis

H16.10 Unspecified superficial keratitis
H16.101 Unspecified superficial keratitis, right eye
H16.102 Unspecified superficial keratitis, left eye
H16.103 Unspecified superficial keratitis, bilateral
H16.109 Unspecified superficial keratitis, unspecified eye

H16.11 Macular keratitis
Areolar keratitis
Nummular keratitis
Stellate keratitis
Striate keratitis
H16.111 Macular keratitis, right eye
H16.112 Macular keratitis, left eye
H16.113 Macular keratitis, bilateral
H16.119 Macular keratitis, unspecified eye

H16.12 Filamentary keratitis
H16.121 Filamentary keratitis, right eye
H16.122 Filamentary keratitis, left eye
H16.123 Filamentary keratitis, bilateral
H16.129 Filamentary keratitis, unspecified eye

H16.13 Photokeratitis
Snow blindness
Welders keratitis
H16.131 Photokeratitis, right eye
H16.132 Photokeratitis, left eye
H16.133 Photokeratitis, bilateral
H16.139 Photokeratitis, unspecified eye

H16.14 Punctate keratitis
H16.141 Punctate keratitis, right eye
H16.142 Punctate keratitis, left eye
H16.143 Punctate keratitis, bilateral
H16.149 Punctate keratitis, unspecified eye

H16.2 Keratoconjunctivitis

H16.20 Unspecified keratoconjunctivitis
Superficial keratitis with conjunctivitis NOS
H16.201 Unspecified keratoconjunctivitis, right eye
H16.202 Unspecified keratoconjunctivitis, left eye
H16.203 Unspecified keratoconjunctivitis, bilateral
H16.209 Unspecified keratoconjunctivitis, unspecified eye

H16.21 Exposure keratoconjunctivitis
H16.211 Exposure keratoconjunctivitis, right eye
H16.212 Exposure keratoconjunctivitis, left eye
H16.213 Exposure keratoconjunctivitis, bilateral
H16.219 Exposure keratoconjunctivitis, unspecified eye

H16.22 Keratoconjunctivitis sicca, not specified as Sjögren's
EXCLUDES 1 *Sjögren's syndrome (M35.01)*
H16.221 Keratoconjunctivitis sicca, not specified as Sjögren's, right eye
H16.222 Keratoconjunctivitis sicca, not specified as Sjögren's, left eye
H16.223 Keratoconjunctivitis sicca, not specified as Sjögren's, bilateral
H16.229 Keratoconjunctivitis sicca, not specified as Sjögren's, unspecified eye

H16.23 Neurotrophic keratoconjunctivitis
H16.231 Neurotrophic keratoconjunctivitis, right eye
H16.232 Neurotrophic keratoconjunctivitis, left eye
H16.233 Neurotrophic keratoconjunctivitis, bilateral
H16.239 Neurotrophic keratoconjunctivitis, unspecified eye

H16.24 Ophthalmia nodosa
H16.241 Ophthalmia nodosa, right eye
H16.242 Ophthalmia nodosa, left eye
H16.243 Ophthalmia nodosa, bilateral
H16.249 Ophthalmia nodosa, unspecified eye

H16.25 Phlyctenular keratoconjunctivitis
H16.251 Phlyctenular keratoconjunctivitis, right eye
H16.252 Phlyctenular keratoconjunctivitis, left eye
H16.253 Phlyctenular keratoconjunctivitis, bilateral
H16.259 Phlyctenular keratoconjunctivitis, unspecified eye

H16.26 Vernal keratoconjunctivitis, with limbar and corneal involvement
EXCLUDES 1 *vernal conjunctivitis without limbar and corneal involvement (H10.44)*
H16.261 Vernal keratoconjunctivitis, with limbar and corneal involvement, right eye
H16.262 Vernal keratoconjunctivitis, with limbar and corneal involvement, left eye
H16.263 Vernal keratoconjunctivitis, with limbar and corneal involvement, bilateral
H16.269 Vernal keratoconjunctivitis, with limbar and corneal involvement, unspecified eye

H16.29 Other keratoconjunctivitis
H16.291 Other keratoconjunctivitis, right eye
H16.292 Other keratoconjunctivitis, left eye
H16.293 Other keratoconjunctivitis, bilateral
H16.299 Other keratoconjunctivitis, unspecified eye

H16.3 Interstitial and deep keratitis

H16.30 Unspecified interstitial keratitis
H16.301 Unspecified interstitial keratitis, right eye
H16.302 Unspecified interstitial keratitis, left eye

H16.303 Unspecified interstitial keratitis, bilateral
H16.309 Unspecified interstitial keratitis, unspecified eye

H16.31 Corneal abscess
H16.311 Corneal abscess, right eye
H16.312 Corneal abscess, left eye
H16.313 Corneal abscess, bilateral
H16.319 Corneal abscess, unspecified eye

H16.32 Diffuse interstitial keratitis
Cogan's syndrome
H16.321 Diffuse interstitial keratitis, right eye
H16.322 Diffuse interstitial keratitis, left eye
H16.323 Diffuse interstitial keratitis, bilateral
H16.329 Diffuse interstitial keratitis, unspecified eye

H16.33 Sclerosing keratitis
H16.331 Sclerosing keratitis, right eye
H16.332 Sclerosing keratitis, left eye
H16.333 Sclerosing keratitis, bilateral
H16.339 Sclerosing keratitis, unspecified eye

H16.39 Other interstitial and deep keratitis
H16.391 Other interstitial and deep keratitis, right eye
H16.392 Other interstitial and deep keratitis, left eye
H16.393 Other interstitial and deep keratitis, bilateral
H16.399 Other interstitial and deep keratitis, unspecified eye

H16.4 Corneal neovascularization

H16.40 Unspecified corneal neovascularization
H16.401 Unspecified corneal neovascularization, right eye
H16.402 Unspecified corneal neovascularization, left eye
H16.403 Unspecified corneal neovascularization, bilateral
H16.409 Unspecified corneal neovascularization, unspecified eye

H16.41 Ghost vessels (corneal)
H16.411 Ghost vessels (corneal), right eye
H16.412 Ghost vessels (corneal), left eye
H16.413 Ghost vessels (corneal), bilateral
H16.419 Ghost vessels (corneal), unspecified eye

H16.42 Pannus (corneal)
H16.421 Pannus (corneal), right eye
H16.422 Pannus (corneal), left eye
H16.423 Pannus (corneal), bilateral
H16.429 Pannus (corneal), unspecified eye

H16.43 Localized vascularization of cornea
H16.431 Localized vascularization of cornea, right eye
H16.432 Localized vascularization of cornea, left eye
H16.433 Localized vascularization of cornea, bilateral
H16.439 Localized vascularization of cornea, unspecified eye

H16.44 Deep vascularization of cornea
H16.441 Deep vascularization of cornea, right eye
H16.442 Deep vascularization of cornea, left eye
H16.443 Deep vascularization of cornea, bilateral
H16.449 Deep vascularization of cornea, unspecified eye

H16.8 Other keratitis UPD
H16.9 Unspecified keratitis

H17 Corneal scars and opacities

H17.0 Adherent leukoma
H17.00 Adherent leukoma, unspecified eye
H17.01 Adherent leukoma, right eye
H17.02 Adherent leukoma, left eye
H17.03 Adherent leukoma, bilateral

H17.1 Central corneal opacity
H17.10 Central corneal opacity, unspecified eye
H17.11 Central corneal opacity, right eye
H17.12 Central corneal opacity, left eye
H17.13 Central corneal opacity, bilateral

H17.8 Other corneal scars and opacities

H17.81 Minor opacity of cornea
Corneal nebula
H17.811 Minor opacity of cornea, right eye
H17.812 Minor opacity of cornea, left eye
H17.813 Minor opacity of cornea, bilateral
H17.819 Minor opacity of cornea, unspecified eye

H17.82 Peripheral opacity of cornea
H17.821 Peripheral opacity of cornea, right eye
H17.822 Peripheral opacity of cornea, left eye
H17.823 Peripheral opacity of cornea, bilateral
H17.829 Peripheral opacity of cornea, unspecified eye

H17.89 Other corneal scars and opacities
H17.9 Unspecified corneal scar and opacity

H18 Other disorders of cornea

H18.0 Corneal pigmentations and deposits

H18.00 Unspecified corneal deposit
H18.001 Unspecified corneal deposit, right eye
H18.002 Unspecified corneal deposit, left eye
H18.003 Unspecified corneal deposit, bilateral
H18.009 Unspecified corneal deposit, unspecified eye

H18.01 Anterior corneal pigmentations
Staehli's line
H18.011 Anterior corneal pigmentations, right eye
H18.012 Anterior corneal pigmentations, left eye
H18.013 Anterior corneal pigmentations, bilateral
H18.019 Anterior corneal pigmentations, unspecified eye

H18.02 Argentous corneal deposits
H18.021 Argentous corneal deposits, right eye
H18.022 Argentous corneal deposits, left eye
H18.023 Argentous corneal deposits, bilateral
H18.029 Argentous corneal deposits, unspecified eye

H18.03 Corneal deposits in metabolic disorders
Code also associated metabolic disorder
H18.031 Corneal deposits in metabolic disorders, right eye
H18.032 Corneal deposits in metabolic disorders, left eye
H18.033 Corneal deposits in metabolic disorders, bilateral
H18.039 Corneal deposits in metabolic disorders, unspecified eye

H18.04 Kayser-Fleischer ring
Code also associated Wilson's disease (E83.01)
H18.041 Kayser-Fleischer ring, right eye
H18.042 Kayser-Fleischer ring, left eye
H18.043 Kayser-Fleischer ring, bilateral
H18.049 Kayser-Fleischer ring, unspecified eye

H18.05 Posterior corneal pigmentations
Krukenberg's spindle
H18.051 Posterior corneal pigmentations, right eye
H18.052 Posterior corneal pigmentations, left eye
H18.053 Posterior corneal pigmentations, bilateral
H18.059 Posterior corneal pigmentations, unspecified eye

H18.06 Stromal corneal pigmentations
Hematocornea
H18.061 Stromal corneal pigmentations, right eye
H18.062 Stromal corneal pigmentations, left eye
H18.063 Stromal corneal pigmentations, bilateral
H18.069 Stromal corneal pigmentations, unspecified eye

H18.1 Bullous keratopathy
DEF: Corneal swelling due to a damaged corneal endothelium. Bullous keratopathy is characterized by recurring, rupturing epithelial blisters causing glaucoma, iridocyclitis, and Fuchs' dystrophy.
H18.10 Bullous keratopathy, unspecified eye
H18.11 Bullous keratopathy, right eye
H18.12 Bullous keratopathy, left eye
H18.13 Bullous keratopathy, bilateral

H18.2 Other and unspecified corneal edema
- **H18.20** Unspecified corneal edema
- **H18.21** Corneal edema secondary to contact lens
  - EXCLUDES 2 *other corneal disorders due to contact lens (H18.82-)*
  - **H18.211** Corneal edema secondary to contact lens, right eye
  - **H18.212** Corneal edema secondary to contact lens, left eye
  - **H18.213** Corneal edema secondary to contact lens, bilateral
  - **H18.219** Corneal edema secondary to contact lens, unspecified eye
- **H18.22** Idiopathic corneal edema
  - **H18.221** Idiopathic corneal edema, right eye
  - **H18.222** Idiopathic corneal edema, left eye
  - **H18.223** Idiopathic corneal edema, bilateral
  - **H18.229** Idiopathic corneal edema, unspecified eye
- **H18.23** Secondary corneal edema
  - **H18.231** Secondary corneal edema, right eye
  - **H18.232** Secondary corneal edema, left eye
  - **H18.233** Secondary corneal edema, bilateral
  - **H18.239** Secondary corneal edema, unspecified eye

H18.3 Changes of corneal membranes
- **H18.30** Unspecified corneal membrane change
- **H18.31** Folds and rupture in Bowman's membrane
  - **H18.311** Folds and rupture in Bowman's membrane, right eye
  - **H18.312** Folds and rupture in Bowman's membrane, left eye
  - **H18.313** Folds and rupture in Bowman's membrane, bilateral
  - **H18.319** Folds and rupture in Bowman's membrane, unspecified eye
- **H18.32** Folds in Descemet's membrane
  - **H18.321** Folds in Descemet's membrane, right eye
  - **H18.322** Folds in Descemet's membrane, left eye
  - **H18.323** Folds in Descemet's membrane, bilateral
  - **H18.329** Folds in Descemet's membrane, unspecified eye
- **H18.33** Rupture in Descemet's membrane
  - **H18.331** Rupture in Descemet's membrane, right eye
  - **H18.332** Rupture in Descemet's membrane, left eye
  - **H18.333** Rupture in Descemet's membrane, bilateral
  - **H18.339** Rupture in Descemet's membrane, unspecified eye

H18.4 Corneal degeneration
- EXCLUDES 1 *Mooren's ulcer (H16.0-)*
  recurrent erosion of cornea (H18.83-)
- **H18.40** Unspecified corneal degeneration
- **H18.41** Arcus senilis
  - Senile corneal changes
  - **H18.411** Arcus senilis, right eye
  - **H18.412** Arcus senilis, left eye
  - **H18.413** Arcus senilis, bilateral
  - **H18.419** Arcus senilis, unspecified eye
- **H18.42** Band keratopathy
  - **H18.421** Band keratopathy, right eye
  - **H18.422** Band keratopathy, left eye
  - **H18.423** Band keratopathy, bilateral
  - **H18.429** Band keratopathy, unspecified eye
- **H18.43** Other calcerous corneal degeneration
- **H18.44** Keratomalacia
  - EXCLUDES 1 *keratomalacia due to vitamin A deficiency (E50.4)*
  - **H18.441** Keratomalacia, right eye
  - **H18.442** Keratomalacia, left eye
  - **H18.443** Keratomalacia, bilateral
  - **H18.449** Keratomalacia, unspecified eye
- **H18.45** Nodular corneal degeneration
  - **H18.451** Nodular corneal degeneration, right eye
  - **H18.452** Nodular corneal degeneration, left eye
  - **H18.453** Nodular corneal degeneration, bilateral
  - **H18.459** Nodular corneal degeneration, unspecified eye
- **H18.46** Peripheral corneal degeneration
  - **H18.461** Peripheral corneal degeneration, right eye
  - **H18.462** Peripheral corneal degeneration, left eye
  - **H18.463** Peripheral corneal degeneration, bilateral
  - **H18.469** Peripheral corneal degeneration, unspecified eye
- **H18.49** Other corneal degeneration

H18.5 Hereditary corneal dystrophies
- AHA: 2020,4Q,24
- **H18.50** Unspecified hereditary corneal dystrophies
  - **H18.501** Unspecified hereditary corneal dystrophies, right eye
  - **H18.502** Unspecified hereditary corneal dystrophies, left eye
  - **H18.503** Unspecified hereditary corneal dystrophies, bilateral
  - **H18.509** Unspecified hereditary corneal dystrophies, unspecified eye
- **H18.51** Endothelial corneal dystrophy
  - Fuchs' dystrophy
  - **H18.511** Endothelial corneal dystrophy, right eye
  - **H18.512** Endothelial corneal dystrophy, left eye
  - **H18.513** Endothelial corneal dystrophy, bilateral
  - **H18.519** Endothelial corneal dystrophy, unspecified eye
- **H18.52** Epithelial (juvenile) corneal dystrophy
  - **H18.521** Epithelial (juvenile) corneal dystrophy, right eye
  - **H18.522** Epithelial (juvenile) corneal dystrophy, left eye
  - **H18.523** Epithelial (juvenile) corneal dystrophy, bilateral
  - **H18.529** Epithelial (juvenile) corneal dystrophy, unspecified eye
- **H18.53** Granular corneal dystrophy
  - **H18.531** Granular corneal dystrophy, right eye
  - **H18.532** Granular corneal dystrophy, left eye
  - **H18.533** Granular corneal dystrophy, bilateral
  - **H18.539** Granular corneal dystrophy, unspecified eye
- **H18.54** Lattice corneal dystrophy
  - **H18.541** Lattice corneal dystrophy, right eye
  - **H18.542** Lattice corneal dystrophy, left eye
  - **H18.543** Lattice corneal dystrophy, bilateral
  - **H18.549** Lattice corneal dystrophy, unspecified eye
- **H18.55** Macular corneal dystrophy
  - **H18.551** Macular corneal dystrophy, right eye
  - **H18.552** Macular corneal dystrophy, left eye
  - **H18.553** Macular corneal dystrophy, bilateral
  - **H18.559** Macular corneal dystrophy, unspecified eye
- **H18.59** Other hereditary corneal dystrophies
  - **H18.591** Other hereditary corneal dystrophies, right eye
  - **H18.592** Other hereditary corneal dystrophies, left eye
  - **H18.593** Other hereditary corneal dystrophies, bilateral
  - **H18.599** Other hereditary corneal dystrophies, unspecified eye

H18.6 Keratoconus
- **H18.60** Keratoconus, unspecified
  - **H18.601** Keratoconus, unspecified, right eye
  - **H18.602** Keratoconus, unspecified, left eye
  - **H18.603** Keratoconus, unspecified, bilateral
  - **H18.609** Keratoconus, unspecified, unspecified eye
- **H18.61** Keratoconus, stable
  - **H18.611** Keratoconus, stable, right eye
  - **H18.612** Keratoconus, stable, left eye
  - **H18.613** Keratoconus, stable, bilateral
  - **H18.619** Keratoconus, stable, unspecified eye

√6th H18.62 **Keratoconus, unstable**
Acute hydrops
H18.621 Keratoconus, unstable, right eye
H18.622 Keratoconus, unstable, left eye
H18.623 Keratoconus, unstable, bilateral
H18.629 Keratoconus, unstable, unspecified eye

√5th H18.7 **Other and unspecified corneal deformities**
EXCLUDES 1 *congenital malformations of cornea (Q13.3-Q13.4)*
H18.70 Unspecified corneal deformity
√6th H18.71 **Corneal ectasia**
H18.711 Corneal ectasia, right eye
H18.712 Corneal ectasia, left eye
H18.713 Corneal ectasia, bilateral
H18.719 Corneal ectasia, unspecified eye
√6th H18.72 **Corneal staphyloma**
H18.721 Corneal staphyloma, right eye
H18.722 Corneal staphyloma, left eye
H18.723 Corneal staphyloma, bilateral
H18.729 Corneal staphyloma, unspecified eye
√6th H18.73 **Descemetocele**
H18.731 Descemetocele, right eye
H18.732 Descemetocele, left eye
H18.733 Descemetocele, bilateral
H18.739 Descemetocele, unspecified eye
√6th H18.79 **Other corneal deformities**
H18.791 Other corneal deformities, right eye
H18.792 Other corneal deformities, left eye
H18.793 Other corneal deformities, bilateral
H18.799 Other corneal deformities, unspecified eye

√5th H18.8 **Other specified disorders of cornea**
√6th H18.81 **Anesthesia and hypoesthesia of cornea**
H18.811 Anesthesia and hypoesthesia of cornea, right eye
H18.812 Anesthesia and hypoesthesia of cornea, left eye
H18.813 Anesthesia and hypoesthesia of cornea, bilateral
H18.819 Anesthesia and hypoesthesia of cornea, unspecified eye
√6th H18.82 **Corneal disorder due to contact lens**
EXCLUDES 2 *corneal edema due to contact lens (H18.21-)*
H18.821 Corneal disorder due to contact lens, right eye
H18.822 Corneal disorder due to contact lens, left eye
H18.823 Corneal disorder due to contact lens, bilateral
H18.829 Corneal disorder due to contact lens, unspecified eye
√6th H18.83 **Recurrent erosion of cornea**
H18.831 Recurrent erosion of cornea, right eye
H18.832 Recurrent erosion of cornea, left eye
H18.833 Recurrent erosion of cornea, bilateral
H18.839 Recurrent erosion of cornea, unspecified eye
√6th H18.89 **Other specified disorders of cornea**
H18.891 Other specified disorders of cornea, right eye
H18.892 Other specified disorders of cornea, left eye
H18.893 Other specified disorders of cornea, bilateral
H18.899 Other specified disorders of cornea, unspecified eye

H18.9 **Unspecified disorder of cornea**

√4th **H20 Iridocyclitis**

√5th H20.0 **Acute and subacute iridocyclitis**
Acute anterior uveitis
Acute cyclitis
Acute iritis
Subacute anterior uveitis
Subacute cyclitis
Subacute iritis
EXCLUDES 1 *iridocyclitis, iritis, uveitis (due to) (in) diabetes mellitus (E08-E13 with .39)*
iridocyclitis, iritis, uveitis (due to) (in) diphtheria (A36.89)
iridocyclitis, iritis, uveitis (due to) (in) gonococcal (A54.32)
iridocyclitis, iritis, uveitis (due to) (in) herpes (simplex) (B00.51)
iridocyclitis, iritis, uveitis (due to) (in) herpes zoster (B02.32)
iridocyclitis, iritis, uveitis (due to) (in) late congenital syphilis (A50.39)
iridocyclitis, iritis, uveitis (due to) (in) late syphilis (A52.71)
iridocyclitis, iritis, uveitis (due to) (in) sarcoidosis (D86.83)
iridocyclitis, iritis, uveitis (due to) (in) syphilis (A51.43)
iridocyclitis, iritis, uveitis (due to) (in) toxoplasmosis (B58.09)
iridocyclitis, iritis, uveitis (due to) (in) tuberculosis (A18.54)
H20.00 Unspecified acute and subacute iridocyclitis CC
√6th H20.01 **Primary iridocyclitis**
H20.011 Primary iridocyclitis, right eye CC
H20.012 Primary iridocyclitis, left eye CC
H20.013 Primary iridocyclitis, bilateral CC
H20.019 Primary iridocyclitis, unspecified eye CC UNS
√6th H20.02 **Recurrent acute iridocyclitis**
H20.021 Recurrent acute iridocyclitis, right eye CC
H20.022 Recurrent acute iridocyclitis, left eye CC
H20.023 Recurrent acute iridocyclitis, bilateral CC
H20.029 Recurrent acute iridocyclitis, unspecified eye CC UNS
√6th H20.03 **Secondary infectious iridocyclitis**
H20.031 Secondary infectious iridocyclitis, right eye CC
H20.032 Secondary infectious iridocyclitis, left eye CC
H20.033 Secondary infectious iridocyclitis, bilateral CC
H20.039 Secondary infectious iridocyclitis, unspecified eye CC UNS
√6th H20.04 **Secondary noninfectious iridocyclitis**
H20.041 Secondary noninfectious iridocyclitis, right eye
H20.042 Secondary noninfectious iridocyclitis, left eye
H20.043 Secondary noninfectious iridocyclitis, bilateral
H20.049 Secondary noninfectious iridocyclitis, unspecified eye
√6th H20.05 **Hypopyon**
H20.051 Hypopyon, right eye
H20.052 Hypopyon, left eye
H20.053 Hypopyon, bilateral
H20.059 Hypopyon, unspecified eye

√5th H20.1 **Chronic iridocyclitis**
Use additional code for any associated cataract (H26.21-)
EXCLUDES 2 *posterior cyclitis (H30.2-)*
H20.10 Chronic iridocyclitis, unspecified eye
H20.11 Chronic iridocyclitis, right eye
H20.12 Chronic iridocyclitis, left eye
H20.13 Chronic iridocyclitis, bilateral

√5th H20.2 **Lens-induced iridocyclitis**
H20.20 Lens-induced iridocyclitis, unspecified eye
H20.21 Lens-induced iridocyclitis, right eye

H20.22 Lens-induced iridocyclitis, left eye
H20.23 Lens-induced iridocyclitis, bilateral

✓5th H20.8 Other iridocyclitis

EXCLUDES 2 *glaucomatocyclitis crises (H40.4-)*
posterior cyclitis (H30.2-)
sympathetic uveitis (H44.13-)

✓6th H20.81 Fuchs' heterochromic cyclitis
H20.811 Fuchs' heterochromic cyclitis, right eye
H20.812 Fuchs' heterochromic cyclitis, left eye
H20.813 Fuchs' heterochromic cyclitis, bilateral
H20.819 Fuchs' heterochromic cyclitis, unspecified eye

✓6th H20.82 Vogt-Koyanagi syndrome
H20.821 Vogt-Koyanagi syndrome, right eye
H20.822 Vogt-Koyanagi syndrome, left eye
H20.823 Vogt-Koyanagi syndrome, bilateral
H20.829 Vogt-Koyanagi syndrome, unspecified eye

H20.9 Unspecified iridocyclitis CC
Uveitis NOS

✓4th H21 Other disorders of iris and ciliary body

EXCLUDES 2 *sympathetic uveitis (H44.1-)*

✓5th H21.0 Hyphema

EXCLUDES 1 *traumatic hyphema (S05.1-)*

Hyphema

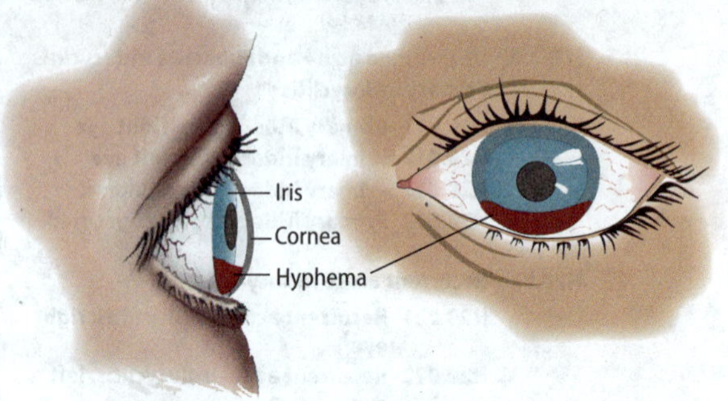

H21.00 Hyphema, unspecified eye
H21.01 Hyphema, right eye
H21.02 Hyphema, left eye
H21.03 Hyphema, bilateral

✓5th H21.1 Other vascular disorders of iris and ciliary body
Neovascularization of iris or ciliary body
Rubeosis iridis
Rubeosis of iris

✓6th H21.1X Other vascular disorders of iris and ciliary body
H21.1X1 Other vascular disorders of iris and ciliary body, right eye
H21.1X2 Other vascular disorders of iris and ciliary body, left eye
H21.1X3 Other vascular disorders of iris and ciliary body, bilateral
H21.1X9 Other vascular disorders of iris and ciliary body, unspecified eye

✓5th H21.2 Degeneration of iris and ciliary body

✓6th H21.21 Degeneration of chamber angle
H21.211 Degeneration of chamber angle, right eye
H21.212 Degeneration of chamber angle, left eye
H21.213 Degeneration of chamber angle, bilateral
H21.219 Degeneration of chamber angle, unspecified eye

✓6th H21.22 Degeneration of ciliary body
H21.221 Degeneration of ciliary body, right eye
H21.222 Degeneration of ciliary body, left eye
H21.223 Degeneration of ciliary body, bilateral
H21.229 Degeneration of ciliary body, unspecified eye

✓6th H21.23 Degeneration of iris (pigmentary)
Translucency of iris
H21.231 Degeneration of iris (pigmentary), right eye
H21.232 Degeneration of iris (pigmentary), left eye
H21.233 Degeneration of iris (pigmentary), bilateral
H21.239 Degeneration of iris (pigmentary), unspecified eye

✓6th H21.24 Degeneration of pupillary margin
H21.241 Degeneration of pupillary margin, right eye
H21.242 Degeneration of pupillary margin, left eye
H21.243 Degeneration of pupillary margin, bilateral
H21.249 Degeneration of pupillary margin, unspecified eye

✓6th H21.25 Iridoschisis
H21.251 Iridoschisis, right eye
H21.252 Iridoschisis, left eye
H21.253 Iridoschisis, bilateral
H21.259 Iridoschisis, unspecified eye

✓6th H21.26 Iris atrophy (essential) (progressive)
H21.261 Iris atrophy (essential) (progressive), right eye
H21.262 Iris atrophy (essential) (progressive), left eye
H21.263 Iris atrophy (essential) (progressive), bilateral
H21.269 Iris atrophy (essential) (progressive), unspecified eye

✓6th H21.27 Miotic pupillary cyst
H21.271 Miotic pupillary cyst, right eye
H21.272 Miotic pupillary cyst, left eye
H21.273 Miotic pupillary cyst, bilateral
H21.279 Miotic pupillary cyst, unspecified eye

H21.29 Other iris atrophy

✓5th H21.3 Cyst of iris, ciliary body and anterior chamber

EXCLUDES 2 *miotic pupillary cyst (H21.27-)*

✓6th H21.30 Idiopathic cysts of iris, ciliary body or anterior chamber
Cyst of iris, ciliary body or anterior chamber NOS
H21.301 Idiopathic cysts of iris, ciliary body or anterior chamber, right eye
H21.302 Idiopathic cysts of iris, ciliary body or anterior chamber, left eye
H21.303 Idiopathic cysts of iris, ciliary body or anterior chamber, bilateral
H21.309 Idiopathic cysts of iris, ciliary body or anterior chamber, unspecified eye

✓6th H21.31 Exudative cysts of iris or anterior chamber
H21.311 Exudative cysts of iris or anterior chamber, right eye
H21.312 Exudative cysts of iris or anterior chamber, left eye
H21.313 Exudative cysts of iris or anterior chamber, bilateral
H21.319 Exudative cysts of iris or anterior chamber, unspecified eye

✓6th H21.32 Implantation cysts of iris, ciliary body or anterior chamber
H21.321 Implantation cysts of iris, ciliary body or anterior chamber, right eye
H21.322 Implantation cysts of iris, ciliary body or anterior chamber, left eye
H21.323 Implantation cysts of iris, ciliary body or anterior chamber, bilateral
H21.329 Implantation cysts of iris, ciliary body or anterior chamber, unspecified eye

✓6th H21.33 Parasitic cyst of iris, ciliary body or anterior chamber
H21.331 Parasitic cyst of iris, ciliary body or anterior chamber, right eye CC
H21.332 Parasitic cyst of iris, ciliary body or anterior chamber, left eye CC
H21.333 Parasitic cyst of iris, ciliary body or anterior chamber, bilateral CC
H21.339 Parasitic cyst of iris, ciliary body or anterior chamber, unspecified eye CC UNS

✓6th H21.34 Primary cyst of pars plana
H21.341 Primary cyst of pars plana, right eye
H21.342 Primary cyst of pars plana, left eye
H21.343 Primary cyst of pars plana, bilateral

H21.349 Primary cyst of pars plana, unspecified eye

H21.35 Exudative cyst of pars plana
DEF: Protein, fatty-filled bullous elevation of the nonpigmented outermost ciliary epithelium of pars plana, due to fluid leak from blood vessels.
H21.351 Exudative cyst of pars plana, right eye
H21.352 Exudative cyst of pars plana, left eye
H21.353 Exudative cyst of pars plana, bilateral
H21.359 Exudative cyst of pars plana, unspecified eye

H21.4 Pupillary membranes
Iris bombé
Pupillary occlusion
Pupillary seclusion
EXCLUDES 1 *congenital pupillary membranes (Q13.8)*
H21.4Ø Pupillary membranes, unspecified eye
H21.41 Pupillary membranes, right eye
H21.42 Pupillary membranes, left eye
H21.43 Pupillary membranes, bilateral

H21.5 Other and unspecified adhesions and disruptions of iris and ciliary body
EXCLUDES 1 *corectopia (Q13.2)*

H21.5Ø Unspecified adhesions of iris
Synechia (iris) NOS
H21.5Ø1 Unspecified adhesions of iris, right eye
H21.5Ø2 Unspecified adhesions of iris, left eye
H21.5Ø3 Unspecified adhesions of iris, bilateral
H21.5Ø9 Unspecified adhesions of iris and ciliary body, unspecified eye

H21.51 Anterior synechiae (iris)
H21.511 Anterior synechiae (iris), right eye
H21.512 Anterior synechiae (iris), left eye
H21.513 Anterior synechiae (iris), bilateral
H21.519 Anterior synechiae (iris), unspecified eye

H21.52 Goniosynechiae
H21.521 Goniosynechiae, right eye
H21.522 Goniosynechiae, left eye
H21.523 Goniosynechiae, bilateral
H21.529 Goniosynechiae, unspecified eye

H21.53 Iridodialysis
H21.531 Iridodialysis, right eye
H21.532 Iridodialysis, left eye
H21.533 Iridodialysis, bilateral
H21.539 Iridodialysis, unspecified eye

H21.54 Posterior synechiae (iris)
H21.541 Posterior synechiae (iris), right eye
H21.542 Posterior synechiae (iris), left eye
H21.543 Posterior synechiae (iris), bilateral
H21.549 Posterior synechiae (iris), unspecified eye

H21.55 Recession of chamber angle
H21.551 Recession of chamber angle, right eye
H21.552 Recession of chamber angle, left eye
H21.553 Recession of chamber angle, bilateral
H21.559 Recession of chamber angle, unspecified eye

H21.56 Pupillary abnormalities
Deformed pupil
Ectopic pupil
Rupture of sphincter, pupil
EXCLUDES 1 *congenital deformity of pupil (Q13.2-)*
H21.561 Pupillary abnormality, right eye
H21.562 Pupillary abnormality, left eye
H21.563 Pupillary abnormality, bilateral
H21.569 Pupillary abnormality, unspecified eye

H21.8 Other specified disorders of iris and ciliary body
H21.81 Floppy iris syndrome
Intraoperative floppy iris syndrome (IFIS)
Use additional code for adverse effect, if applicable, to identify drug (T36-T5Ø with fifth or sixth character 5)
H21.82 Plateau iris syndrome (post-iridectomy) (postprocedural)
H21.89 Other specified disorders of iris and ciliary body

H21.9 Unspecified disorder of iris and ciliary body

H22 Disorders of iris and ciliary body in diseases classified elsewhere
Code first underlying disease, such as:
gout (M1A.-, M1Ø.-)
leprosy (A3Ø.-)
parasitic disease (B89)

Disorders of lens (H25-H28)

H25 Age-related cataract
Senile cataract
EXCLUDES 2 *capsular glaucoma with pseudoexfoliation of lens (H4Ø.1-)*

Cataracts

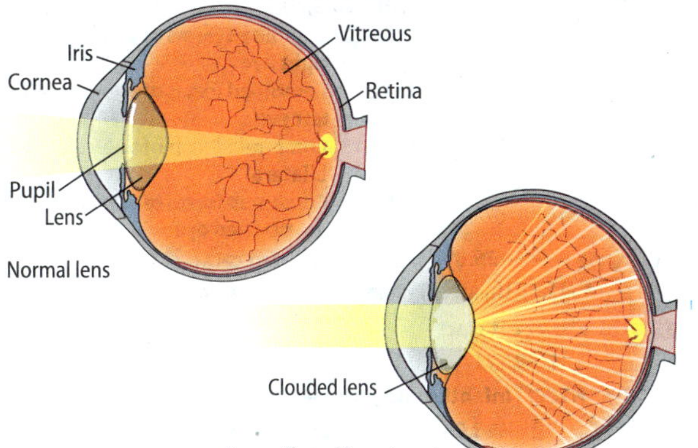

H25.Ø Age-related incipient cataract

H25.Ø1 Cortical age-related cataract
H25.Ø11 Cortical age-related cataract, right eye A
H25.Ø12 Cortical age-related cataract, left eye A
H25.Ø13 Cortical age-related cataract, bilateral A
H25.Ø19 Cortical age-related cataract, unspecified eye A

H25.Ø3 Anterior subcapsular polar age-related cataract
H25.Ø31 Anterior subcapsular polar age-related cataract, right eye A
H25.Ø32 Anterior subcapsular polar age-related cataract, left eye A
H25.Ø33 Anterior subcapsular polar age-related cataract, bilateral A
H25.Ø39 Anterior subcapsular polar age-related cataract, unspecified eye A

H25.Ø4 Posterior subcapsular polar age-related cataract
H25.Ø41 Posterior subcapsular polar age-related cataract, right eye A
H25.Ø42 Posterior subcapsular polar age-related cataract, left eye A
H25.Ø43 Posterior subcapsular polar age-related cataract, bilateral A
H25.Ø49 Posterior subcapsular polar age-related cataract, unspecified eye A

H25.Ø9 Other age-related incipient cataract
Coronary age-related cataract
Punctate age-related cataract
Water clefts
H25.Ø91 Other age-related incipient cataract, right eye A
H25.Ø92 Other age-related incipient cataract, left eye A
H25.Ø93 Other age-related incipient cataract, bilateral A
H25.Ø99 Other age-related incipient cataract, unspecified eye A

H25.1 Age-related nuclear cataract
Cataracta brunescens
Nuclear sclerosis cataract
AHA: 2019,2Q,31; 2016,1Q,32
H25.1Ø Age-related nuclear cataract, unspecified eye A
H25.11 Age-related nuclear cataract, right eye A
H25.12 Age-related nuclear cataract, left eye A
H25.13 Age-related nuclear cataract, bilateral A

√5th **H25.2 Age-related cataract, morgagnian type**
Age-related hypermature cataract
H25.20 Age-related cataract, morgagnian type, unspecified eye A
H25.21 Age-related cataract, morgagnian type, right eye A
H25.22 Age-related cataract, morgagnian type, left eye A
H25.23 Age-related cataract, morgagnian type, bilateral A
√5th **H25.8 Other age-related cataract**
√6th **H25.81 Combined forms of age-related cataract**
AHA: 2019,2Q,30
H25.811 Combined forms of age-related cataract, right eye A
H25.812 Combined forms of age-related cataract, left eye A
H25.813 Combined forms of age-related cataract, bilateral A
H25.819 Combined forms of age-related cataract, unspecified eye A
H25.89 Other age-related cataract A
H25.9 Unspecified age-related cataract A

√4th **H26 Other cataract**
EXCLUDES 1 *congenital cataract (Q12.0)*
√5th **H26.0 Infantile and juvenile cataract**
√6th **H26.00 Unspecified infantile and juvenile cataract**
H26.001 Unspecified infantile and juvenile cataract, right eye P
H26.002 Unspecified infantile and juvenile cataract, left eye P
H26.003 Unspecified infantile and juvenile cataract, bilateral P
H26.009 Unspecified infantile and juvenile cataract, unspecified eye P
√6th **H26.01 Infantile and juvenile cortical, lamellar, or zonular cataract**
H26.011 Infantile and juvenile cortical, lamellar, or zonular cataract, right eye P
H26.012 Infantile and juvenile cortical, lamellar, or zonular cataract, left eye P
H26.013 Infantile and juvenile cortical, lamellar, or zonular cataract, bilateral P
H26.019 Infantile and juvenile cortical, lamellar, or zonular cataract, unspecified eye P
√6th **H26.03 Infantile and juvenile nuclear cataract**
H26.031 Infantile and juvenile nuclear cataract, right eye P
H26.032 Infantile and juvenile nuclear cataract, left eye P
H26.033 Infantile and juvenile nuclear cataract, bilateral P
H26.039 Infantile and juvenile nuclear cataract, unspecified eye P
√6th **H26.04 Anterior subcapsular polar infantile and juvenile cataract**
H26.041 Anterior subcapsular polar infantile and juvenile cataract, right eye P
H26.042 Anterior subcapsular polar infantile and juvenile cataract, left eye P
H26.043 Anterior subcapsular polar infantile and juvenile cataract, bilateral P
H26.049 Anterior subcapsular polar infantile and juvenile cataract, unspecified eye P
√6th **H26.05 Posterior subcapsular polar infantile and juvenile cataract**
H26.051 Posterior subcapsular polar infantile and juvenile cataract, right eye P
H26.052 Posterior subcapsular polar infantile and juvenile cataract, left eye P
H26.053 Posterior subcapsular polar infantile and juvenile cataract, bilateral P
H26.059 Posterior subcapsular polar infantile and juvenile cataract, unspecified eye P
√6th **H26.06 Combined forms of infantile and juvenile cataract**
H26.061 Combined forms of infantile and juvenile cataract, right eye P
H26.062 Combined forms of infantile and juvenile cataract, left eye P
H26.063 Combined forms of infantile and juvenile cataract, bilateral P
H26.069 Combined forms of infantile and juvenile cataract, unspecified eye P
H26.09 Other infantile and juvenile cataract P
√5th **H26.1 Traumatic cataract**
Use additional code (Chapter 20) to identify external cause
√6th **H26.10 Unspecified traumatic cataract**
H26.101 Unspecified traumatic cataract, right eye
H26.102 Unspecified traumatic cataract, left eye
H26.103 Unspecified traumatic cataract, bilateral
H26.109 Unspecified traumatic cataract, unspecified eye
√6th **H26.11 Localized traumatic opacities**
H26.111 Localized traumatic opacities, right eye
H26.112 Localized traumatic opacities, left eye
H26.113 Localized traumatic opacities, bilateral
H26.119 Localized traumatic opacities, unspecified eye
√6th **H26.12 Partially resolved traumatic cataract**
H26.121 Partially resolved traumatic cataract, right eye
H26.122 Partially resolved traumatic cataract, left eye
H26.123 Partially resolved traumatic cataract, bilateral
H26.129 Partially resolved traumatic cataract, unspecified eye
√6th **H26.13 Total traumatic cataract**
H26.131 Total traumatic cataract, right eye
H26.132 Total traumatic cataract, left eye
H26.133 Total traumatic cataract, bilateral
H26.139 Total traumatic cataract, unspecified eye
√5th **H26.2 Complicated cataract**
H26.20 Unspecified complicated cataract
Cataracta complicata NOS
√6th **H26.21 Cataract with neovascularization**
▶Code also, if applicable, associated condition, such as:◀
chronic iridocyclitis (H20.1-)
H26.211 Cataract with neovascularization, right eye
H26.212 Cataract with neovascularization, left eye
H26.213 Cataract with neovascularization, bilateral
H26.219 Cataract with neovascularization, unspecified eye
√6th **H26.22 Cataract secondary to ocular disorders (degenerative) (inflammatory)**
Code also associated ocular disorder
H26.221 Cataract secondary to ocular disorders (degenerative) (inflammatory), right eye
H26.222 Cataract secondary to ocular disorders (degenerative) (inflammatory), left eye
H26.223 Cataract secondary to ocular disorders (degenerative) (inflammatory), bilateral
H26.229 Cataract secondary to ocular disorders (degenerative) (inflammatory), unspecified eye
√6th **H26.23 Glaucomatous flecks (subcapsular)**
Code first underlying glaucoma (H40-H42)
H26.231 Glaucomatous flecks (subcapsular), right eye
H26.232 Glaucomatous flecks (subcapsular), left eye
H26.233 Glaucomatous flecks (subcapsular), bilateral
H26.239 Glaucomatous flecks (subcapsular), unspecified eye
√5th **H26.3 Drug-induced cataract**
Toxic cataract
Use additional code for adverse effect, if applicable, to identify drug (T36-T50 with fifth or sixth character 5)
H26.30 Drug-induced cataract, unspecified eye
H26.31 Drug-induced cataract, right eye
H26.32 Drug-induced cataract, left eye
H26.33 Drug-induced cataract, bilateral

H26.4 Secondary cataract
H26.40 Unspecified secondary cataract
H26.41 Soemmering's ring
H26.411 Soemmering's ring, right eye
H26.412 Soemmering's ring, left eye
H26.413 Soemmering's ring, bilateral
H26.419 Soemmering's ring, unspecified eye
H26.49 Other secondary cataract
AHA: 2018,2Q,14
H26.491 Other secondary cataract, right eye
H26.492 Other secondary cataract, left eye
H26.493 Other secondary cataract, bilateral
H26.499 Other secondary cataract, unspecified eye
H26.8 Other specified cataract
H26.9 Unspecified cataract

H27 Other disorders of lens
EXCLUDES 1 *congenital lens malformations (Q12.-)*
mechanical complications of intraocular lens implant (T85.2)
pseudophakia (Z96.1)

H27.0 Aphakia
Acquired absence of lens
Acquired aphakia
Aphakia due to trauma
EXCLUDES 1 *cataract extraction status (Z98.4-)*
congenital absence of lens (Q12.3)
congenital aphakia (Q12.3)
H27.00 Aphakia, unspecified eye
H27.01 Aphakia, right eye
H27.02 Aphakia, left eye
H27.03 Aphakia, bilateral
H27.1 Dislocation of lens
H27.10 Unspecified dislocation of lens
H27.11 Subluxation of lens
H27.111 Subluxation of lens, right eye
H27.112 Subluxation of lens, left eye
H27.113 Subluxation of lens, bilateral
H27.119 Subluxation of lens, unspecified eye
H27.12 Anterior dislocation of lens
H27.121 Anterior dislocation of lens, right eye
H27.122 Anterior dislocation of lens, left eye
H27.123 Anterior dislocation of lens, bilateral
H27.129 Anterior dislocation of lens, unspecified eye
H27.13 Posterior dislocation of lens
H27.131 Posterior dislocation of lens, right eye
H27.132 Posterior dislocation of lens, left eye
H27.133 Posterior dislocation of lens, bilateral
H27.139 Posterior dislocation of lens, unspecified eye
H27.8 Other specified disorders of lens
H27.9 Unspecified disorder of lens

H28 Cataract in diseases classified elsewhere
Code first underlying disease, such as:
hypoparathyroidism (E20.-)
myotonia (G71.1-)
myxedema (E03.-)
protein-calorie malnutrition (E40-E46)
EXCLUDES 1 *cataract in diabetes mellitus (E08.36, E09.36, E10.36, E11.36, E13.36)*

Disorders of choroid and retina (H30-H36)

H30 Chorioretinal inflammation
H30.0 Focal chorioretinal inflammation
Focal chorioretinitis
Focal choroiditis
Focal retinitis
Focal retinochoroiditis
H30.00 Unspecified focal chorioretinal inflammation
Focal chorioretinitis NOS
Focal choroiditis NOS
Focal retinitis NOS
Focal retinochoroiditis NOS
H30.001 Unspecified focal chorioretinal inflammation, right eye
H30.002 Unspecified focal chorioretinal inflammation, left eye
H30.003 Unspecified focal chorioretinal inflammation, bilateral
H30.009 Unspecified focal chorioretinal inflammation, unspecified eye
H30.01 Focal chorioretinal inflammation, juxtapapillary
H30.011 Focal chorioretinal inflammation, juxtapapillary, right eye
H30.012 Focal chorioretinal inflammation, juxtapapillary, left eye
H30.013 Focal chorioretinal inflammation, juxtapapillary, bilateral
H30.019 Focal chorioretinal inflammation, juxtapapillary, unspecified eye
H30.02 Focal chorioretinal inflammation of posterior pole
H30.021 Focal chorioretinal inflammation of posterior pole, right eye
H30.022 Focal chorioretinal inflammation of posterior pole, left eye
H30.023 Focal chorioretinal inflammation of posterior pole, bilateral
H30.029 Focal chorioretinal inflammation of posterior pole, unspecified eye
H30.03 Focal chorioretinal inflammation, peripheral
H30.031 Focal chorioretinal inflammation, peripheral, right eye
H30.032 Focal chorioretinal inflammation, peripheral, left eye
H30.033 Focal chorioretinal inflammation, peripheral, bilateral
H30.039 Focal chorioretinal inflammation, peripheral, unspecified eye
H30.04 Focal chorioretinal inflammation, macular or paramacular
H30.041 Focal chorioretinal inflammation, macular or paramacular, right eye
H30.042 Focal chorioretinal inflammation, macular or paramacular, left eye
H30.043 Focal chorioretinal inflammation, macular or paramacular, bilateral
H30.049 Focal chorioretinal inflammation, macular or paramacular, unspecified eye
H30.1 Disseminated chorioretinal inflammation
Disseminated chorioretinitis
Disseminated choroiditis
Disseminated retinitis
Disseminated retinochoroiditis
EXCLUDES 2 *exudative retinopathy (H35.02-)*
H30.10 Unspecified disseminated chorioretinal inflammation
Disseminated chorioretinitis NOS
Disseminated choroiditis NOS
Disseminated retinitis NOS
Disseminated retinochoroiditis NOS
H30.101 Unspecified disseminated chorioretinal inflammation, right eye CC
H30.102 Unspecified disseminated chorioretinal inflammation, left eye CC
H30.103 Unspecified disseminated chorioretinal inflammation, bilateral CC
H30.109 Unspecified disseminated chorioretinal inflammation, unspecified eye CC UNS
H30.11 Disseminated chorioretinal inflammation of posterior pole
H30.111 Disseminated chorioretinal inflammation of posterior pole, right eye CC
H30.112 Disseminated chorioretinal inflammation of posterior pole, left eye CC
H30.113 Disseminated chorioretinal inflammation of posterior pole, bilateral CC
H30.119 Disseminated chorioretinal inflammation of posterior pole, unspecified eye CC UNS
H30.12 Disseminated chorioretinal inflammation, peripheral
H30.121 Disseminated chorioretinal inflammation, peripheral right eye CC
H30.122 Disseminated chorioretinal inflammation, peripheral, left eye CC

H30.123 Disseminated chorioretinal inflammation, peripheral, bilateral CC
H30.129 Disseminated chorioretinal inflammation, peripheral, unspecified eye CC UNS
√6th H30.13 Disseminated chorioretinal inflammation, generalized
H30.131 Disseminated chorioretinal inflammation, generalized, right eye CC
H30.132 Disseminated chorioretinal inflammation, generalized, left eye CC
H30.133 Disseminated chorioretinal inflammation, generalized, bilateral CC
H30.139 Disseminated chorioretinal inflammation, generalized, unspecified eye CC UNS
√6th H30.14 Acute posterior multifocal placoid pigment epitheliopathy
H30.141 Acute posterior multifocal placoid pigment epitheliopathy, right eye CC
H30.142 Acute posterior multifocal placoid pigment epitheliopathy, left eye CC
H30.143 Acute posterior multifocal placoid pigment epitheliopathy, bilateral CC
H30.149 Acute posterior multifocal placoid pigment epitheliopathy, unspecified eye CC UNS
√5th H30.2 Posterior cyclitis
Pars planitis
H30.20 Posterior cyclitis, unspecified eye
H30.21 Posterior cyclitis, right eye
H30.22 Posterior cyclitis, left eye
H30.23 Posterior cyclitis, bilateral
√5th H30.8 Other chorioretinal inflammations
√6th H30.81 Harada's disease
H30.811 Harada's disease, right eye
H30.812 Harada's disease, left eye
H30.813 Harada's disease, bilateral
H30.819 Harada's disease, unspecified eye
√6th H30.89 Other chorioretinal inflammations
H30.891 Other chorioretinal inflammations, right eye CC
H30.892 Other chorioretinal inflammations, left eye CC
H30.893 Other chorioretinal inflammations, bilateral CC
H30.899 Other chorioretinal inflammations, unspecified eye CC UNS
√5th H30.9 Unspecified chorioretinal inflammation
Chorioretinitis NOS
Choroiditis NOS
Neuroretinitis NOS
Retinitis NOS
Retinochoroiditis NOS
H30.90 Unspecified chorioretinal inflammation, unspecified eye CC UNS
H30.91 Unspecified chorioretinal inflammation, right eye CC
H30.92 Unspecified chorioretinal inflammation, left eye CC
H30.93 Unspecified chorioretinal inflammation, bilateral CC
√4th H31 Other disorders of choroid
√5th H31.0 Chorioretinal scars
EXCLUDES 2 *postsurgical chorioretinal scars (H59.81-)*
√6th H31.00 Unspecified chorioretinal scars
H31.001 Unspecified chorioretinal scars, right eye
H31.002 Unspecified chorioretinal scars, left eye
H31.003 Unspecified chorioretinal scars, bilateral
H31.009 Unspecified chorioretinal scars, unspecified eye
√6th H31.01 Macula scars of posterior pole (postinflammatory) (post-traumatic)
EXCLUDES 1 *postprocedural choriorentinal scar (H59.81-)*
H31.011 Macula scars of posterior pole (postinflammatory) (post-traumatic), right eye
H31.012 Macula scars of posterior pole (postinflammatory) (post-traumatic), left eye
H31.013 Macula scars of posterior pole (postinflammatory) (post-traumatic), bilateral
H31.019 Macula scars of posterior pole (postinflammatory) (post-traumatic), unspecified eye
√6th H31.02 Solar retinopathy
H31.021 Solar retinopathy, right eye
H31.022 Solar retinopathy, left eye
H31.023 Solar retinopathy, bilateral
H31.029 Solar retinopathy, unspecified eye
√6th H31.09 Other chorioretinal scars
H31.091 Other chorioretinal scars, right eye
H31.092 Other chorioretinal scars, left eye
H31.093 Other chorioretinal scars, bilateral
H31.099 Other chorioretinal scars, unspecified eye
√5th H31.1 Choroidal degeneration
EXCLUDES 2 *angioid streaks of macula (H35.33)*
√6th H31.10 Unspecified choroidal degeneration
Choroidal sclerosis NOS
H31.101 Choroidal degeneration, unspecified, right eye
H31.102 Choroidal degeneration, unspecified, left eye
H31.103 Choroidal degeneration, unspecified, bilateral
H31.109 Choroidal degeneration, unspecified, unspecified eye
√6th H31.11 Age-related choroidal atrophy
H31.111 Age-related choroidal atrophy, right eye A
H31.112 Age-related choroidal atrophy, left eye A
H31.113 Age-related choroidal atrophy, bilateral A
H31.119 Age-related choroidal atrophy, unspecified eye A
√6th H31.12 Diffuse secondary atrophy of choroid
H31.121 Diffuse secondary atrophy of choroid, right eye
H31.122 Diffuse secondary atrophy of choroid, left eye
H31.123 Diffuse secondary atrophy of choroid, bilateral
H31.129 Diffuse secondary atrophy of choroid, unspecified eye
√5th H31.2 Hereditary choroidal dystrophy
EXCLUDES 2 *hyperornithinemia (E72.4)*
ornithinemia (E72.4)
H31.20 Hereditary choroidal dystrophy, unspecified
H31.21 Choroideremia
H31.22 Choroidal dystrophy (central areolar) (generalized) (peripapillary)
H31.23 Gyrate atrophy, choroid
H31.29 Other hereditary choroidal dystrophy
√5th H31.3 Choroidal hemorrhage and rupture
√6th H31.30 Unspecified choroidal hemorrhage
H31.301 Unspecified choroidal hemorrhage, right eye
H31.302 Unspecified choroidal hemorrhage, left eye
H31.303 Unspecified choroidal hemorrhage, bilateral
H31.309 Unspecified choroidal hemorrhage, unspecified eye
√6th H31.31 Expulsive choroidal hemorrhage
H31.311 Expulsive choroidal hemorrhage, right eye
H31.312 Expulsive choroidal hemorrhage, left eye
H31.313 Expulsive choroidal hemorrhage, bilateral
H31.319 Expulsive choroidal hemorrhage, unspecified eye
√6th H31.32 Choroidal rupture
H31.321 Choroidal rupture, right eye CC
H31.322 Choroidal rupture, left eye CC
H31.323 Choroidal rupture, bilateral CC

H31.329 Choroidal rupture, unspecified eye CC UNS

✓5th H31.4 Choroidal detachment

✓6th H31.4Ø Unspecified choroidal detachment

H31.4Ø1 Unspecified choroidal detachment, right eye CC

H31.4Ø2 Unspecified choroidal detachment, left eye CC

H31.4Ø3 Unspecified choroidal detachment, bilateral CC

H31.4Ø9 Unspecified choroidal detachment, unspecified eye CC UNS

✓6th H31.41 Hemorrhagic choroidal detachment

H31.411 Hemorrhagic choroidal detachment, right eye CC

H31.412 Hemorrhagic choroidal detachment, left eye CC

H31.413 Hemorrhagic choroidal detachment, bilateral CC

H31.419 Hemorrhagic choroidal detachment, unspecified eye CC UNS

✓6th H31.42 Serous choroidal detachment

H31.421 Serous choroidal detachment, right eye CC

H31.422 Serous choroidal detachment, left eye CC

H31.423 Serous choroidal detachment, bilateral CC

H31.429 Serous choroidal detachment, unspecified eye CC UNS

H31.8 Other specified disorders of choroid

H31.9 Unspecified disorder of choroid

H32 Chorioretinal disorders in diseases classified elsewhere

Code first underlying disease, such as:

congenital toxoplasmosis (P37.1)

histoplasmosis (B39.-)

leprosy (A3Ø.-)

EXCLUDES 1 *chorioretinitis (in):*

toxoplasmosis (acquired) (B58.Ø1)

tuberculosis (A18.53)

✓4th **H33 Retinal detachments and breaks**

EXCLUDES 1 *detachment of retinal pigment epithelium (H35.72-, H35.73-)*

Retinal Detachment

✓5th H33.Ø Retinal detachment with retinal break

Rhegmatogenous retinal detachment

EXCLUDES 1 *serous retinal detachment (without retinal break) (H33.2-)*

✓6th H33.ØØ Unspecified retinal detachment with retinal break

H33.ØØ1 Unspecified retinal detachment with retinal break, right eye

H33.ØØ2 Unspecified retinal detachment with retinal break, left eye

H33.ØØ3 Unspecified retinal detachment with retinal break, bilateral

H33.ØØ9 Unspecified retinal detachment with retinal break, unspecified eye

✓6th H33.Ø1 Retinal detachment with single break

H33.Ø11 Retinal detachment with single break, right eye

H33.Ø12 Retinal detachment with single break, left eye

H33.Ø13 Retinal detachment with single break, bilateral

H33.Ø19 Retinal detachment with single break, unspecified eye

✓6th H33.Ø2 Retinal detachment with multiple breaks

H33.Ø21 Retinal detachment with multiple breaks, right eye

H33.Ø22 Retinal detachment with multiple breaks, left eye

H33.Ø23 Retinal detachment with multiple breaks, bilateral

H33.Ø29 Retinal detachment with multiple breaks, unspecified eye

✓6th H33.Ø3 Retinal detachment with giant retinal tear

H33.Ø31 Retinal detachment with giant retinal tear, right eye

H33.Ø32 Retinal detachment with giant retinal tear, left eye

H33.Ø33 Retinal detachment with giant retinal tear, bilateral

H33.Ø39 Retinal detachment with giant retinal tear, unspecified eye

✓6th H33.Ø4 Retinal detachment with retinal dialysis

H33.Ø41 Retinal detachment with retinal dialysis, right eye

H33.Ø42 Retinal detachment with retinal dialysis, left eye

H33.Ø43 Retinal detachment with retinal dialysis, bilateral

H33.Ø49 Retinal detachment with retinal dialysis, unspecified eye

✓6th H33.Ø5 Total retinal detachment

H33.Ø51 Total retinal detachment, right eye

H33.Ø52 Total retinal detachment, left eye

H33.Ø53 Total retinal detachment, bilateral

H33.Ø59 Total retinal detachment, unspecified eye

✓5th H33.1 Retinoschisis and retinal cysts

EXCLUDES 1 *congenital retinoschisis (Q14.1)*

microcystoid degeneration of retina (H35.42-)

✓6th H33.1Ø Unspecified retinoschisis

H33.1Ø1 Unspecified retinoschisis, right eye

H33.1Ø2 Unspecified retinoschisis, left eye

H33.1Ø3 Unspecified retinoschisis, bilateral

H33.1Ø9 Unspecified retinoschisis, unspecified eye

✓6th H33.11 Cyst of ora serrata

H33.111 Cyst of ora serrata, right eye

H33.112 Cyst of ora serrata, left eye

H33.113 Cyst of ora serrata, bilateral

H33.119 Cyst of ora serrata, unspecified eye

✓6th H33.12 Parasitic cyst of retina

H33.121 Parasitic cyst of retina, right eye CC

H33.122 Parasitic cyst of retina, left eye CC

H33.123 Parasitic cyst of retina, bilateral CC

H33.129 Parasitic cyst of retina, unspecified eye CC UNS

✓6th H33.19 Other retinoschisis and retinal cysts

Pseudocyst of retina

H33.191 Other retinoschisis and retinal cysts, right eye

H33.192 Other retinoschisis and retinal cysts, left eye

H33.193 Other retinoschisis and retinal cysts, bilateral

H33.199 Other retinoschisis and retinal cysts, unspecified eye

✓5th H33.2 Serous retinal detachment

Retinal detachment NOS

Retinal detachment without retinal break

EXCLUDES 1 *central serous chorioretinopathy (H35.71-)*

H33.2Ø Serous retinal detachment, unspecified eye CC UNS

H33.21 Serous retinal detachment, right eye CC

H33.22 Serous retinal detachment, left eye CC

H33.23 Serous retinal detachment, bilateral CC

✓5th **H33.3 Retinal breaks without detachment**

EXCLUDES 1 *chorioretinal scars after surgery for detachment (H59.81-)*
peripheral retinal degeneration without break (H35.4-)

✓6th **H33.30 Unspecified retinal break**

H33.301 Unspecified retinal break, right eye
H33.302 Unspecified retinal break, left eye
H33.303 Unspecified retinal break, bilateral
H33.309 Unspecified retinal break, unspecified eye

✓6th **H33.31 Horseshoe tear of retina without detachment**

Operculum of retina without detachment

H33.311 Horseshoe tear of retina without detachment, right eye
H33.312 Horseshoe tear of retina without detachment, left eye
H33.313 Horseshoe tear of retina without detachment, bilateral
H33.319 Horseshoe tear of retina without detachment, unspecified eye

✓6th **H33.32 Round hole of retina without detachment**

H33.321 Round hole, right eye
H33.322 Round hole, left eye
H33.323 Round hole, bilateral
H33.329 Round hole, unspecified eye

✓6th **H33.33 Multiple defects of retina without detachment**

H33.331 Multiple defects of retina without detachment, right eye
H33.332 Multiple defects of retina without detachment, left eye
H33.333 Multiple defects of retina without detachment, bilateral
H33.339 Multiple defects of retina without detachment, unspecified eye

✓5th **H33.4 Traction detachment of retina**

Proliferative vitreo-retinopathy with retinal detachment

H33.40 Traction detachment of retina, unspecified eye CC UNS
H33.41 Traction detachment of retina, right eye CC
H33.42 Traction detachment of retina, left eye CC
H33.43 Traction detachment of retina, bilateral CC

H33.8 Other retinal detachments CC

✓4th **H34 Retinal vascular occlusions**

EXCLUDES 1 *amaurosis fugax (G45.3)*

✓5th **H34.0 Transient retinal artery occlusion**

H34.00 Transient retinal artery occlusion, unspecified eye CC UNS
H34.01 Transient retinal artery occlusion, right eye CC
H34.02 Transient retinal artery occlusion, left eye CC
H34.03 Transient retinal artery occlusion, bilateral CC

✓5th **H34.1 Central retinal artery occlusion**

H34.10 Central retinal artery occlusion, unspecified eye CC UNS
H34.11 Central retinal artery occlusion, right eye CC
H34.12 Central retinal artery occlusion, left eye CC
H34.13 Central retinal artery occlusion, bilateral CC

✓5th **H34.2 Other retinal artery occlusions**

✓6th **H34.21 Partial retinal artery occlusion**

Hollenhorst's plaque
Retinal microembolism

H34.211 Partial retinal artery occlusion, right eye CC
H34.212 Partial retinal artery occlusion, left eye CC
H34.213 Partial retinal artery occlusion, bilateral CC
H34.219 Partial retinal artery occlusion, unspecified eye CC UNS

✓6th **H34.23 Retinal artery branch occlusion**

H34.231 Retinal artery branch occlusion, right eye CC
H34.232 Retinal artery branch occlusion, left eye CC
H34.233 Retinal artery branch occlusion, bilateral CC
H34.239 Retinal artery branch occlusion, unspecified eye CC UNS

✓5th **H34.8 Other retinal vascular occlusions**

AHA: 2016,4Q,19

✓6th **H34.81 Central retinal vein occlusion**

One of the following 7th characters is to be assigned to codes in subcategory H34.81 to designate the severity of the occlusion:
0 with macular edema
1 with retinal neovascularization
2 stable
old central retinal vein occlusion

✓7th **H34.811 Central retinal vein occlusion, right eye** CC
✓7th **H34.812 Central retinal vein occlusion, left eye** CC
✓7th **H34.813 Central retinal vein occlusion, bilateral** CC
✓7th **H34.819 Central retinal vein occlusion, unspecified eye** CC UNS

✓6th **H34.82 Venous engorgement**

Incipient retinal vein occlusion
Partial retinal vein occlusion

H34.821 Venous engorgement, right eye
H34.822 Venous engorgement, left eye
H34.823 Venous engorgement, bilateral
H34.829 Venous engorgement, unspecified eye

✓6th **H34.83 Tributary (branch) retinal vein occlusion**

One of the following 7th characters is to be assigned to codes in subcategory H34.83 to designate the severity of the occlusion:
0 with macular edema
1 with retinal neovascularization
2 stable
old tributary (branch) retinal vein occlusion

✓7th **H34.831 Tributary (branch) retinal vein occlusion, right eye**
✓7th **H34.832 Tributary (branch) retinal vein occlusion, left eye**
✓7th **H34.833 Tributary (branch) retinal vein occlusion, bilateral**
✓7th **H34.839 Tributary (branch) retinal vein occlusion, unspecified eye**

H34.9 Unspecified retinal vascular occlusion CC

✓4th **H35 Other retinal disorders**

EXCLUDES 2 *diabetic retinal disorders (E08.311-E08.359, E09.311-E09.359, E10.311-E10.359, E11.311-E11.359, E13.311-E13.359)*

✓5th **H35.0 Background retinopathy and retinal vascular changes**

Code also any associated hypertension (I10)

H35.00 Unspecified background retinopathy

✓6th **H35.01 Changes in retinal vascular appearance**

Retinal vascular sheathing

H35.011 Changes in retinal vascular appearance, right eye
H35.012 Changes in retinal vascular appearance, left eye
H35.013 Changes in retinal vascular appearance, bilateral
H35.019 Changes in retinal vascular appearance, unspecified eye

✓6th **H35.02 Exudative retinopathy**

Coats retinopathy

H35.021 Exudative retinopathy, right eye
H35.022 Exudative retinopathy, left eye
H35.023 Exudative retinopathy, bilateral
H35.029 Exudative retinopathy, unspecified eye

✓6th **H35.03 Hypertensive retinopathy**

H35.031 Hypertensive retinopathy, right eye
H35.032 Hypertensive retinopathy, left eye
H35.033 Hypertensive retinopathy, bilateral
H35.039 Hypertensive retinopathy, unspecified eye

✓6th **H35.04 Retinal micro-aneurysms, unspecified**

H35.041 Retinal micro-aneurysms, unspecified, right eye
H35.042 Retinal micro-aneurysms, unspecified, left eye

H35.043 Retinal micro-aneurysms, unspecified, bilateral
H35.049 Retinal micro-aneurysms, unspecified, unspecified eye

H35.05 Retinal neovascularization, unspecified
H35.051 Retinal neovascularization, unspecified, right eye
H35.052 Retinal neovascularization, unspecified, left eye
H35.053 Retinal neovascularization, unspecified, bilateral
H35.059 Retinal neovascularization, unspecified, unspecified eye

H35.06 Retinal vasculitis
Eales disease
Retinal perivasculitis
DEF: Sight-threatening intraocular inflammation of the retinal blood vessels that causes minimal, partial, or even complete blindness.
H35.061 Retinal vasculitis, right eye
H35.062 Retinal vasculitis, left eye
H35.063 Retinal vasculitis, bilateral
H35.069 Retinal vasculitis, unspecified eye

H35.07 Retinal telangiectasis
H35.071 Retinal telangiectasis, right eye
H35.072 Retinal telangiectasis, left eye
H35.073 Retinal telangiectasis, bilateral
H35.079 Retinal telangiectasis, unspecified eye

H35.09 Other intraretinal microvascular abnormalities
Retinal varices

H35.1 Retinopathy of prematurity

H35.10 Retinopathy of prematurity, unspecified
Retinopathy of prematurity NOS
H35.101 Retinopathy of prematurity, unspecified, right eye
H35.102 Retinopathy of prematurity, unspecified, left eye
H35.103 Retinopathy of prematurity, unspecified, bilateral
H35.109 Retinopathy of prematurity, unspecified, unspecified eye

H35.11 Retinopathy of prematurity, stage 0
H35.111 Retinopathy of prematurity, stage 0, right eye
H35.112 Retinopathy of prematurity, stage 0, left eye
H35.113 Retinopathy of prematurity, stage 0, bilateral
H35.119 Retinopathy of prematurity, stage 0, unspecified eye

H35.12 Retinopathy of prematurity, stage 1
H35.121 Retinopathy of prematurity, stage 1, right eye
H35.122 Retinopathy of prematurity, stage 1, left eye
H35.123 Retinopathy of prematurity, stage 1, bilateral
H35.129 Retinopathy of prematurity, stage 1, unspecified eye

H35.13 Retinopathy of prematurity, stage 2
H35.131 Retinopathy of prematurity, stage 2, right eye
H35.132 Retinopathy of prematurity, stage 2, left eye
H35.133 Retinopathy of prematurity, stage 2, bilateral
H35.139 Retinopathy of prematurity, stage 2, unspecified eye

H35.14 Retinopathy of prematurity, stage 3
H35.141 Retinopathy of prematurity, stage 3, right eye
H35.142 Retinopathy of prematurity, stage 3, left eye
H35.143 Retinopathy of prematurity, stage 3, bilateral
H35.149 Retinopathy of prematurity, stage 3, unspecified eye

H35.15 Retinopathy of prematurity, stage 4
H35.151 Retinopathy of prematurity, stage 4, right eye
H35.152 Retinopathy of prematurity, stage 4, left eye
H35.153 Retinopathy of prematurity, stage 4, bilateral
H35.159 Retinopathy of prematurity, stage 4, unspecified eye

H35.16 Retinopathy of prematurity, stage 5
H35.161 Retinopathy of prematurity, stage 5, right eye
H35.162 Retinopathy of prematurity, stage 5, left eye
H35.163 Retinopathy of prematurity, stage 5, bilateral
H35.169 Retinopathy of prematurity, stage 5, unspecified eye

H35.17 Retrolental fibroplasia
H35.171 Retrolental fibroplasia, right eye
H35.172 Retrolental fibroplasia, left eye
H35.173 Retrolental fibroplasia, bilateral
H35.179 Retrolental fibroplasia, unspecified eye

H35.2 Other non-diabetic proliferative retinopathy
Proliferative vitreo-retinopathy
▶Thaslassemia proliferative retinopathy◀
EXCLUDES 1 *proliferative vitreo-retinopathy with retinal detachment (H33.4-)*
EXCLUDES 2 ▶*proliferative sickle-cell retinopathy (H36.82-)*◀
H35.20 Other non-diabetic proliferative retinopathy, unspecified eye
H35.21 Other non-diabetic proliferative retinopathy, right eye
H35.22 Other non-diabetic proliferative retinopathy, left eye
H35.23 Other non-diabetic proliferative retinopathy, bilateral

H35.3 Degeneration of macula and posterior pole
H35.30 Unspecified macular degeneration A
Age-related macular degeneration

H35.31 Nonexudative age-related macular degeneration
Atrophic age-related macular degeneration
Dry age-related macular degeneration
AHA: 2016,4Q,20-21

One of the following 7th characters is to be assigned to each code in subcategory H35.31 to designate the stage of the disease:
0 stage unspecified
1 early dry stage
2 intermediate dry stage
3 advanced atrophic without subfoveal involvement
advanced dry stage
4 advanced atrophic with subfoveal involvement

H35.311 Nonexudative age-related macular degeneration, right eye A
H35.312 Nonexudative age-related macular degeneration, left eye A
H35.313 Nonexudative age-related macular degeneration, bilateral A
H35.319 Nonexudative age-related macular degeneration, unspecified eye A

H35.32 Exudative age-related macular degeneration
Wet age-related macular degeneration
AHA: 2016,4Q,20-21

One of the following 7th characters is to be assigned to each code in subcategory H35.32 to designate the stage of the disease:
0 stage unspecified
1 with active choroidal neovascularization
2 with inactive choroidal neovascularization
with involuted or regressed neovascularization
3 with inactive scar

H35.321 Exudative age-related macular degeneration, right eye HCC A
H35.322 Exudative age-related macular degeneration, left eye HCC A
H35.323 Exudative age-related macular degeneration, bilateral HCC A
H35.329 Exudative age-related macular degeneration, unspecified eye HCC A

H35.33 Angioid streaks of macula
DEF: Degeneration of the choroid, characterized by broad, irregular, dark brown streaks radiating from the optic disc; occurs with pseudoxanthoma elasticum or Paget's disease.

6th **H35.34 Macular cyst, hole, or pseudohole**
- **H35.341 Macular cyst, hole, or pseudohole, right eye**
- **H35.342 Macular cyst, hole, or pseudohole, left eye**
- **H35.343 Macular cyst, hole, or pseudohole, bilateral**
- **H35.349 Macular cyst, hole, or pseudohole, unspecified eye**

6th **H35.35 Cystoid macular degeneration**
EXCLUDES 1 *cystoid macular edema following cataract surgery (H59.Ø3-)*
- **H35.351 Cystoid macular degeneration, right eye**
- **H35.352 Cystoid macular degeneration, left eye**
- **H35.353 Cystoid macular degeneration, bilateral**
- **H35.359 Cystoid macular degeneration, unspecified eye**

6th **H35.36 Drusen (degenerative) of macula**
AHA: 2017,1Q,51; 2016,4Q,21
- **H35.361 Drusen (degenerative) of macula, right eye**
- **H35.362 Drusen (degenerative) of macula, left eye**
- **H35.363 Drusen (degenerative) of macula, bilateral**
- **H35.369 Drusen (degenerative) of macula, unspecified eye**

6th **H35.37 Puckering of macula**
- **H35.371 Puckering of macula, right eye**
- **H35.372 Puckering of macula, left eye**
- **H35.373 Puckering of macula, bilateral**
- **H35.379 Puckering of macula, unspecified eye**

6th **H35.38 Toxic maculopathy**
Code first poisoning due to drug or toxin, if applicable ▶(T36-T65 with fifth or sixth character 1-4)◀
Use additional code for adverse effect, if applicable, to identify drug (T36-T5Ø with fifth or sixth character 5)
- **H35.381 Toxic maculopathy, right eye**
- **H35.382 Toxic maculopathy, left eye**
- **H35.383 Toxic maculopathy, bilateral**
- **H35.389 Toxic maculopathy, unspecified eye**

5th **H35.4 Peripheral retinal degeneration**
EXCLUDES 1 *hereditary retinal degeneration (dystrophy) (H35.5-)*
peripheral retinal degeneration with retinal break (H33.3-)

H35.4Ø Unspecified peripheral retinal degeneration

6th **H35.41 Lattice degeneration of retina**
Palisade degeneration of retina
DEF: Degeneration of the retina, often bilateral, that is usually benign. It is characterized by lines intersecting at irregular intervals in the peripheral retina. Retinal thinning and retinal holes may occur.
- **H35.411 Lattice degeneration of retina, right eye**
- **H35.412 Lattice degeneration of retina, left eye**
- **H35.413 Lattice degeneration of retina, bilateral**
- **H35.419 Lattice degeneration of retina, unspecified eye**

6th **H35.42 Microcystoid degeneration of retina**
- **H35.421 Microcystoid degeneration of retina, right eye**
- **H35.422 Microcystoid degeneration of retina, left eye**
- **H35.423 Microcystoid degeneration of retina, bilateral**
- **H35.429 Microcystoid degeneration of retina, unspecified eye**

6th **H35.43 Paving stone degeneration of retina**
- **H35.431 Paving stone degeneration of retina, right eye**
- **H35.432 Paving stone degeneration of retina, left eye**
- **H35.433 Paving stone degeneration of retina, bilateral**
- **H35.439 Paving stone degeneration of retina, unspecified eye**

6th **H35.44 Age-related reticular degeneration of retina**
- **H35.441 Age-related reticular degeneration of retina, right eye** A
- **H35.442 Age-related reticular degeneration of retina, left eye** A
- **H35.443 Age-related reticular degeneration of retina, bilateral** A
- **H35.449 Age-related reticular degeneration of retina, unspecified eye** A

6th **H35.45 Secondary pigmentary degeneration**
- **H35.451 Secondary pigmentary degeneration, right eye**
- **H35.452 Secondary pigmentary degeneration, left eye**
- **H35.453 Secondary pigmentary degeneration, bilateral**
- **H35.459 Secondary pigmentary degeneration, unspecified eye**

6th **H35.46 Secondary vitreoretinal degeneration**
- **H35.461 Secondary vitreoretinal degeneration, right eye**
- **H35.462 Secondary vitreoretinal degeneration, left eye**
- **H35.463 Secondary vitreoretinal degeneration, bilateral**
- **H35.469 Secondary vitreoretinal degeneration, unspecified eye**

5th **H35.5 Hereditary retinal dystrophy**
EXCLUDES 1 *dystrophies primarily involving Bruch's membrane (H31.1-)*

H35.5Ø Unspecified hereditary retinal dystrophy

H35.51 Vitreoretinal dystrophy

H35.52 Pigmentary retinal dystrophy
Albipunctate retinal dystrophy
Retinitis pigmentosa
Tapetoretinal dystrophy

H35.53 Other dystrophies primarily involving the sensory retina
Stargardt's disease

H35.54 Dystrophies primarily involving the retinal pigment epithelium
Vitelliform retinal dystrophy

5th **H35.6 Retinal hemorrhage**
- **H35.6Ø Retinal hemorrhage, unspecified eye**
- **H35.61 Retinal hemorrhage, right eye**
- **H35.62 Retinal hemorrhage, left eye**
- **H35.63 Retinal hemorrhage, bilateral**

5th **H35.7 Separation of retinal layers**
EXCLUDES 1 *retinal detachment (serous) (H33.2-)*
rhegmatogenous retinal detachment (H33.Ø-)

H35.7Ø Unspecified separation of retinal layers CC

6th **H35.71 Central serous chorioretinopathy**
- **H35.711 Central serous chorioretinopathy, right eye**
- **H35.712 Central serous chorioretinopathy, left eye**
- **H35.713 Central serous chorioretinopathy, bilateral**
- **H35.719 Central serous chorioretinopathy, unspecified eye**

6th **H35.72 Serous detachment of retinal pigment epithelium**
- **H35.721 Serous detachment of retinal pigment epithelium, right eye** CC
- **H35.722 Serous detachment of retinal pigment epithelium, left eye** CC
- **H35.723 Serous detachment of retinal pigment epithelium, bilateral** CC
- **H35.729 Serous detachment of retinal pigment epithelium, unspecified eye** CC UNS

6th **H35.73 Hemorrhagic detachment of retinal pigment epithelium**
- **H35.731 Hemorrhagic detachment of retinal pigment epithelium, right eye** CC
- **H35.732 Hemorrhagic detachment of retinal pigment epithelium, left eye** CC
- **H35.733 Hemorrhagic detachment of retinal pigment epithelium, bilateral** CC

H35.739 Hemorrhagic detachment of retinal pigment epithelium, unspecified eye CC UNS

✓5th H35.8 Other specified retinal disorders

EXCLUDES 2 *retinal hemorrhage (H35.6-)*

H35.81 Retinal edema
Retinal cotton wool spots

H35.82 Retinal ischemia CC

H35.89 Other specified retinal disorders

H35.9 Unspecified retinal disorder

▲✓4th H36 Retinal disorders in diseases classified elsewhere

Code first underlying disease, such as:
lipid storage disorders (E75.-)
sickle-cell disorders (D57.-)

EXCLUDES 1 *arteriosclerotic retinopathy (H35.0-)*
diabetic retinopathy (E08.3-, E09.3-, E10.3-, E11.3-, E13.3-)

● ✓5th H36.8 Other retinal disorders in diseases classified elsewhere

● ✓6th H36.81 Nonproliferative sickle-cell retinopathy

● H36.811 Nonproliferative sickle-cell retinopathy, right eye

● H36.812 Nonproliferative sickle-cell retinopathy, left eye

● H36.813 Nonproliferative sickle-cell retinopathy, bilateral

● H36.819 Nonproliferative sickle-cell retinopathy, unspecified eye

● ✓6th H36.82 Proliferative sickle-cell retinopathy

● H36.821 Proliferative sickle-cell retinopathy, right eye

● H36.822 Proliferative sickle-cell retinopathy, left eye

● H36.823 Proliferative sickle-cell retinopathy, bilateral

● H36.829 Proliferative sickle-cell retinopathy, unspecified eye

● H36.89 Other retinal disorders in diseases classified elsewhere
Retinal dystrophy in lipid storage disorders

Glaucoma (H40-H42)

✓4th H40 Glaucoma

EXCLUDES 1 *absolute glaucoma (H44.51-)*
congenital glaucoma (Q15.0)
traumatic glaucoma due to birth injury (P15.3)

Open Angle/Angle Closure Glaucoma

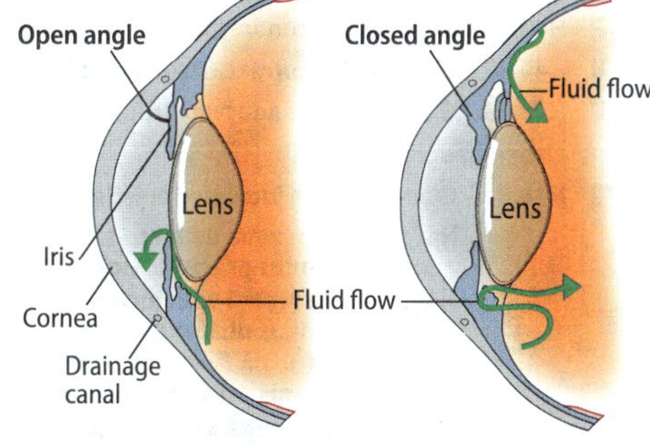

✓5th H40.0 Glaucoma suspect

✓6th H40.00 Preglaucoma, unspecified

H40.001 Preglaucoma, unspecified, right eye

H40.002 Preglaucoma, unspecified, left eye

H40.003 Preglaucoma, unspecified, bilateral

H40.009 Preglaucoma, unspecified, unspecified eye

✓6th H40.01 Open angle with borderline findings, low risk
Open angle, low risk

H40.011 Open angle with borderline findings, low risk, right eye

H40.012 Open angle with borderline findings, low risk, left eye

H40.013 Open angle with borderline findings, low risk, bilateral

H40.019 Open angle with borderline findings, low risk, unspecified eye

✓6th H40.02 Open angle with borderline findings, high risk
Open angle, high risk

H40.021 Open angle with borderline findings, high risk, right eye

H40.022 Open angle with borderline findings, high risk, left eye

H40.023 Open angle with borderline findings, high risk, bilateral

H40.029 Open angle with borderline findings, high risk, unspecified eye

✓6th H40.03 Anatomical narrow angle
Primary angle closure suspect

H40.031 Anatomical narrow angle, right eye

H40.032 Anatomical narrow angle, left eye

H40.033 Anatomical narrow angle, bilateral

H40.039 Anatomical narrow angle, unspecified eye

✓6th H40.04 Steroid responder

H40.041 Steroid responder, right eye

H40.042 Steroid responder, left eye

H40.043 Steroid responder, bilateral

H40.049 Steroid responder, unspecified eye

✓6th H40.05 Ocular hypertension

H40.051 Ocular hypertension, right eye

H40.052 Ocular hypertension, left eye

H40.053 Ocular hypertension, bilateral

H40.059 Ocular hypertension, unspecified eye

✓6th H40.06 Primary angle closure without glaucoma damage

H40.061 Primary angle closure without glaucoma damage, right eye

H40.062 Primary angle closure without glaucoma damage, left eye

H40.063 Primary angle closure without glaucoma damage, bilateral

H40.069 Primary angle closure without glaucoma damage, unspecified eye

✓5th H40.1 Open-angle glaucoma

One of the following 7th characters is to be assigned to each code in subcategories H40.10, H40.11, H40.12, H40.13, and H40.14 to designate the stage of glaucoma.
0 stage unspecified
1 mild stage
2 moderate stage
3 severe stage
4 indeterminate stage

✓x7th H40.10 Unspecified open-angle glaucoma
TIP: Only one code from this subcategory should be assigned when both left and right eyes are the same stage.

✓6th H40.11 Primary open-angle glaucoma
Chronic simple glaucoma
AHA: 2016,4Q,22

✓7th H40.111 Primary open-angle glaucoma, right eye

✓7th H40.112 Primary open-angle glaucoma, left eye

✓7th H40.113 Primary open-angle glaucoma, bilateral

✓7th H40.119 Primary open-angle glaucoma, unspecified eye

✓6th H40.12 Low-tension glaucoma

✓7th H40.121 Low-tension glaucoma, right eye UPD

✓7th H40.122 Low-tension glaucoma, left eye UPD

✓7th H40.123 Low-tension glaucoma, bilateral UPD

✓7th H40.129 Low-tension glaucoma, unspecified eye UPD

✓6th H40.13 Pigmentary glaucoma

✓7th H40.131 Pigmentary glaucoma, right eye UPD

✓7th H40.132 Pigmentary glaucoma, left eye UPD

✓7th H40.133 Pigmentary glaucoma, bilateral UPD

✓7th H40.139 Pigmentary glaucoma, unspecified eye UPD

✓6th H40.14 Capsular glaucoma with pseudoexfoliation of lens

✓7th H40.141 Capsular glaucoma with pseudoexfoliation of lens, right eye

✓7th H40.142 Capsular glaucoma with pseudoexfoliation of lens, left eye

✓7th H40.143 Capsular glaucoma with pseudoexfoliation of lens, bilateral

√7th **H40.149** Capsular glaucoma with pseudoexfoliation of lens, unspecified eye

√6th **H40.15** Residual stage of open-angle glaucoma

H40.151 Residual stage of open-angle glaucoma, right eye UPD

H40.152 Residual stage of open-angle glaucoma, left eye UPD

H40.153 Residual stage of open-angle glaucoma, bilateral UPD

H40.159 Residual stage of open-angle glaucoma, unspecified eye UPD

√5th **H40.2** Primary angle-closure glaucoma

EXCLUDES 1 *aqueous misdirection (H40.83-)*
malignant glaucoma (H40.83-)

One of the following 7th characters is to be assigned to code H40.20 and H40.22 to designate the stage of glaucoma.
- 0 stage unspecified
- 1 mild stage
- 2 moderate stage
- 3 severe stage
- 4 indeterminate stage

√x7th **H40.20** Unspecified primary angle-closure glaucoma

TIP: Only one code from this subcategory should be assigned when both left and right eyes are the same stage.

√6th **H40.21** Acute angle-closure glaucoma

Acute angle-closure glaucoma attack
Acute angle-closure glaucoma crisis

H40.211 Acute angle-closure glaucoma, right eye CC

H40.212 Acute angle-closure glaucoma, left eye CC

H40.213 Acute angle-closure glaucoma, bilateral CC

H40.219 Acute angle-closure glaucoma, unspecified eye CC UNS

√6th **H40.22** Chronic angle-closure glaucoma

Chronic primary angle closure glaucoma

√7th **H40.221** Chronic angle-closure glaucoma, right eye

√7th **H40.222** Chronic angle-closure glaucoma, left eye

√7th **H40.223** Chronic angle-closure glaucoma, bilateral

√7th **H40.229** Chronic angle-closure glaucoma, unspecified eye

√6th **H40.23** Intermittent angle-closure glaucoma

H40.231 Intermittent angle-closure glaucoma, right eye

H40.232 Intermittent angle-closure glaucoma, left eye

H40.233 Intermittent angle-closure glaucoma, bilateral

H40.239 Intermittent angle-closure glaucoma, unspecified eye

√6th **H40.24** Residual stage of angle-closure glaucoma

H40.241 Residual stage of angle-closure glaucoma, right eye

H40.242 Residual stage of angle-closure glaucoma, left eye

H40.243 Residual stage of angle-closure glaucoma, bilateral

H40.249 Residual stage of angle-closure glaucoma, unspecified eye

√5th **H40.3** Glaucoma secondary to eye trauma

Code also underlying condition

One of the following 7th characters is to be assigned to each code in subcategory H40.3 to designate the stage of glaucoma.
- 0 stage unspecified
- 1 mild stage
- 2 moderate stage
- 3 severe stage
- 4 indeterminate stage

√x7th **H40.30** Glaucoma secondary to eye trauma, unspecified eye

√x7th **H40.31** Glaucoma secondary to eye trauma, right eye

√x7th **H40.32** Glaucoma secondary to eye trauma, left eye

√x7th **H40.33** Glaucoma secondary to eye trauma, bilateral

√5th **H40.4** Glaucoma secondary to eye inflammation

Code also underlying condition

One of the following 7th characters is to be assigned to each code in subcategory H40.4 to designate the stage of glaucoma.
- 0 stage unspecified
- 1 mild stage
- 2 moderate stage
- 3 severe stage
- 4 indeterminate stage

√x7th **H40.40** Glaucoma secondary to eye inflammation, unspecified eye

√x7th **H40.41** Glaucoma secondary to eye inflammation, right eye

√x7th **H40.42** Glaucoma secondary to eye inflammation, left eye

√x7th **H40.43** Glaucoma secondary to eye inflammation, bilateral

√5th **H40.5** Glaucoma secondary to other eye disorders

Code also underlying eye disorder

One of the following 7th characters is to be assigned to each code in subcategory H40.5 to designate the stage of glaucoma.
- 0 stage unspecified
- 1 mild stage
- 2 moderate stage
- 3 severe stage
- 4 indeterminate stage

√x7th **H40.50** Glaucoma secondary to other eye disorders, unspecified eye

√x7th **H40.51** Glaucoma secondary to other eye disorders, right eye

√x7th **H40.52** Glaucoma secondary to other eye disorders, left eye

√x7th **H40.53** Glaucoma secondary to other eye disorders, bilateral

√5th **H40.6** Glaucoma secondary to drugs

Use additional code for adverse effect, if applicable, to identify drug (T36-T50 with fifth or sixth character 5)

One of the following 7th characters is to be assigned to each code in subcategory H40.6 to designate the stage of glaucoma
- 0 stage unspecified
- 1 mild stage
- 2 moderate stage
- 3 severe stage
- 4 indeterminate stage

√x7th **H40.60** Glaucoma secondary to drugs, unspecified eye

√x7th **H40.61** Glaucoma secondary to drugs, right eye

√x7th **H40.62** Glaucoma secondary to drugs, left eye

√x7th **H40.63** Glaucoma secondary to drugs, bilateral

√5th **H40.8** Other glaucoma

√6th **H40.81** Glaucoma with increased episcleral venous pressure

H40.811 Glaucoma with increased episcleral venous pressure, right eye

H40.812 Glaucoma with increased episcleral venous pressure, left eye

H40.813 Glaucoma with increased episcleral venous pressure, bilateral

H40.819 Glaucoma with increased episcleral venous pressure, unspecified eye

√6th **H40.82** Hypersecretion glaucoma

H40.821 Hypersecretion glaucoma, right eye

H40.822 Hypersecretion glaucoma, left eye

H40.823 Hypersecretion glaucoma, bilateral

H40.829 Hypersecretion glaucoma, unspecified eye

√6th **H40.83** Aqueous misdirection

Malignant glaucoma

H40.831 Aqueous misdirection, right eye

H40.832 Aqueous misdirection, left eye

H40.833 Aqueous misdirection, bilateral

H40.839 Aqueous misdirection, unspecified eye

H40.89 Other specified glaucoma

H40.9 Unspecified glaucoma

H42 Glaucoma in diseases classified elsewhere
Code first underlying condition, such as:
amyloidosis (E85.-)
aniridia (Q13.1)
glaucoma (in) diabetes mellitus (E08.39, E09.39, E10.39, E11.39, E13.39)
Lowe's syndrome (E72.03)
Reiger's anomaly (Q13.81)
specified metabolic disorder (E70-E88)
EXCLUDES 1 *glaucoma (in) onchocerciasis (B73.02)*
glaucoma (in) syphilis (A52.71)
glaucoma (in) tuberculous (A18.59)

Disorders of vitreous body and globe (H43-H44)

H43 Disorders of vitreous body
H43.0 Vitreous prolapse
EXCLUDES 1 *traumatic vitreous prolapse (S05.2-)*
vitreous syndrome following cataract surgery (H59.0-)
H43.00 Vitreous prolapse, unspecified eye
H43.01 Vitreous prolapse, right eye
H43.02 Vitreous prolapse, left eye
H43.03 Vitreous prolapse, bilateral
H43.1 Vitreous hemorrhage
H43.10 Vitreous hemorrhage, unspecified eye HCC
H43.11 Vitreous hemorrhage, right eye HCC
H43.12 Vitreous hemorrhage, left eye HCC
H43.13 Vitreous hemorrhage, bilateral HCC
H43.2 Crystalline deposits in vitreous body
H43.20 Crystalline deposits in vitreous body, unspecified eye
H43.21 Crystalline deposits in vitreous body, right eye
H43.22 Crystalline deposits in vitreous body, left eye
H43.23 Crystalline deposits in vitreous body, bilateral
H43.3 Other vitreous opacities
H43.31 Vitreous membranes and strands
H43.311 Vitreous membranes and strands, right eye
H43.312 Vitreous membranes and strands, left eye
H43.313 Vitreous membranes and strands, bilateral
H43.319 Vitreous membranes and strands, unspecified eye
H43.39 Other vitreous opacities
Vitreous floaters
H43.391 Other vitreous opacities, right eye
H43.392 Other vitreous opacities, left eye
H43.393 Other vitreous opacities, bilateral
H43.399 Other vitreous opacities, unspecified eye
H43.8 Other disorders of vitreous body
EXCLUDES 1 *proliferative vitreo-retinopathy with retinal detachment (H33.4-)*
EXCLUDES 2 *vitreous abscess (H44.02-)*
H43.81 Vitreous degeneration
Vitreous detachment
H43.811 Vitreous degeneration, right eye
H43.812 Vitreous degeneration, left eye
H43.813 Vitreous degeneration, bilateral
H43.819 Vitreous degeneration, unspecified eye
H43.82 Vitreomacular adhesion
Vitreomacular traction
H43.821 Vitreomacular adhesion, right eye A
H43.822 Vitreomacular adhesion, left eye A
H43.823 Vitreomacular adhesion, bilateral A
H43.829 Vitreomacular adhesion, unspecified eye A
H43.89 Other disorders of vitreous body
H43.9 Unspecified disorder of vitreous body

H44 Disorders of globe
INCLUDES disorders affecting multiple structures of eye
H44.0 Purulent endophthalmitis
Use additional code to identify organism
EXCLUDES 1 *bleb associated endophthalmitis (H59.4-)*
H44.00 Unspecified purulent endophthalmitis
H44.001 Unspecified purulent endophthalmitis, right eye CC
H44.002 Unspecified purulent endophthalmitis, left eye CC
H44.003 Unspecified purulent endophthalmitis, bilateral CC
H44.009 Unspecified purulent endophthalmitis, unspecified eye CC UNS
H44.01 Panophthalmitis (acute)
H44.011 Panophthalmitis (acute), right eye CC
H44.012 Panophthalmitis (acute), left eye CC
H44.013 Panophthalmitis (acute), bilateral CC
H44.019 Panophthalmitis (acute), unspecified eye CC UNS
H44.02 Vitreous abscess (chronic)
H44.021 Vitreous abscess (chronic), right eye CC
H44.022 Vitreous abscess (chronic), left eye CC
H44.023 Vitreous abscess (chronic), bilateral CC
H44.029 Vitreous abscess (chronic), unspecified eye CC UNS
H44.1 Other endophthalmitis
EXCLUDES 1 *bleb associated endophthalmitis (H59.4-)*
EXCLUDES 2 *ophthalmia nodosa (H16.2-)*
H44.11 Panuveitis
DEF: Inflammation of all layers of the uvea of the eye, including the choroid, iris, and ciliary body. It also typically involves the lens, retina, optic nerve, and vitreous and causes reduced vision or blindness.
H44.111 Panuveitis, right eye CC
H44.112 Panuveitis, left eye CC
H44.113 Panuveitis, bilateral CC
H44.119 Panuveitis, unspecified eye CC UNS
H44.12 Parasitic endophthalmitis, unspecified
H44.121 Parasitic endophthalmitis, unspecified, right eye CC
H44.122 Parasitic endophthalmitis, unspecified, left eye CC
H44.123 Parasitic endophthalmitis, unspecified, bilateral CC
H44.129 Parasitic endophthalmitis, unspecified, unspecified eye CC UNS
H44.13 Sympathetic uveitis
H44.131 Sympathetic uveitis, right eye CC
H44.132 Sympathetic uveitis, left eye CC
H44.133 Sympathetic uveitis, bilateral CC
H44.139 Sympathetic uveitis, unspecified eye CC UNS
H44.19 Other endophthalmitis CC
H44.2 Degenerative myopia
Malignant myopia
AHA: 2017,4Q,10-11
H44.20 Degenerative myopia, unspecified eye
H44.21 Degenerative myopia, right eye
H44.22 Degenerative myopia, left eye
H44.23 Degenerative myopia, bilateral
H44.2A Degenerative myopia with choroidal neovascularization
Use additional code for any associated choroid disorders (H31.-)
H44.2A1 Degenerative myopia with choroidal neovascularization, right eye
H44.2A2 Degenerative myopia with choroidal neovascularization, left eye
H44.2A3 Degenerative myopia with choroidal neovascularization, bilateral eye
H44.2A9 Degenerative myopia with choroidal neovascularization, unspecified eye
H44.2B Degenerative myopia with macular hole
H44.2B1 Degenerative myopia with macular hole, right eye
H44.2B2 Degenerative myopia with macular hole, left eye
H44.2B3 Degenerative myopia with macular hole, bilateral eye
H44.2B9 Degenerative myopia with macular hole, unspecified eye

Chapter 7. Diseases of the Eye and Adnexa H42–H44.2B9

√6th H44.2C Degenerative myopia with retinal detachment
Use additional code to identify the retinal detachment (H33.-)
H44.2C1 Degenerative myopia with retinal detachment, right eye
H44.2C2 Degenerative myopia with retinal detachment, left eye
H44.2C3 Degenerative myopia with retinal detachment, bilateral eye
H44.2C9 Degenerative myopia with retinal detachment, unspecified eye
√6th H44.2D Degenerative myopia with foveoschisis
H44.2D1 Degenerative myopia with foveoschisis, right eye
H44.2D2 Degenerative myopia with foveoschisis, left eye
H44.2D3 Degenerative myopia with foveoschisis, bilateral eye
H44.2D9 Degenerative myopia with foveoschisis, unspecified eye
√6th H44.2E Degenerative myopia with other maculopathy
H44.2E1 Degenerative myopia with other maculopathy, right eye
H44.2E2 Degenerative myopia with other maculopathy, left eye
H44.2E3 Degenerative myopia with other maculopathy, bilateral eye
H44.2E9 Degenerative myopia with other maculopathy, unspecified eye
√5th H44.3 Other and unspecified degenerative disorders of globe
H44.30 Unspecified degenerative disorder of globe
√6th H44.31 Chalcosis
H44.311 Chalcosis, right eye
H44.312 Chalcosis, left eye
H44.313 Chalcosis, bilateral
H44.319 Chalcosis, unspecified eye
√6th H44.32 Siderosis of eye
DEF: Iron pigment deposits within tissue of the eyeball caused by high iron content of the blood. Symptoms include cataracts, rust-colored anterior subcapsular deposits, iris heterochromia, pupillary mydriasis, and depressed electroretinogram amplitudes.
H44.321 Siderosis of eye, right eye
H44.322 Siderosis of eye, left eye
H44.323 Siderosis of eye, bilateral
H44.329 Siderosis of eye, unspecified eye
√6th H44.39 Other degenerative disorders of globe
H44.391 Other degenerative disorders of globe, right eye
H44.392 Other degenerative disorders of globe, left eye
H44.393 Other degenerative disorders of globe, bilateral
H44.399 Other degenerative disorders of globe, unspecified eye
√5th H44.4 Hypotony of eye
H44.40 Unspecified hypotony of eye
√6th H44.41 Flat anterior chamber hypotony of eye
H44.411 Flat anterior chamber hypotony of right eye
H44.412 Flat anterior chamber hypotony of left eye
H44.413 Flat anterior chamber hypotony of eye, bilateral
H44.419 Flat anterior chamber hypotony of unspecified eye
√6th H44.42 Hypotony of eye due to ocular fistula
H44.421 Hypotony of right eye due to ocular fistula
H44.422 Hypotony of left eye due to ocular fistula
H44.423 Hypotony of eye due to ocular fistula, bilateral
H44.429 Hypotony of unspecified eye due to ocular fistula
√6th H44.43 Hypotony of eye due to other ocular disorders
H44.431 Hypotony of eye due to other ocular disorders, right eye
H44.432 Hypotony of eye due to other ocular disorders, left eye
H44.433 Hypotony of eye due to other ocular disorders, bilateral
H44.439 Hypotony of eye due to other ocular disorders, unspecified eye
√6th H44.44 Primary hypotony of eye
H44.441 Primary hypotony of right eye
H44.442 Primary hypotony of left eye
H44.443 Primary hypotony of eye, bilateral
H44.449 Primary hypotony of unspecified eye
√5th H44.5 Degenerated conditions of globe
H44.50 Unspecified degenerated conditions of globe
√6th H44.51 Absolute glaucoma
H44.511 Absolute glaucoma, right eye
H44.512 Absolute glaucoma, left eye
H44.513 Absolute glaucoma, bilateral
H44.519 Absolute glaucoma, unspecified eye
√6th H44.52 Atrophy of globe
Phthisis bulbi
H44.521 Atrophy of globe, right eye
H44.522 Atrophy of globe, left eye
H44.523 Atrophy of globe, bilateral
H44.529 Atrophy of globe, unspecified eye
√6th H44.53 Leucocoria
H44.531 Leucocoria, right eye
H44.532 Leucocoria, left eye
H44.533 Leucocoria, bilateral
H44.539 Leucocoria, unspecified eye
√5th H44.6 Retained (old) intraocular foreign body, magnetic
Use additional code to identify magnetic foreign body (Z18.11)
EXCLUDES 1 *current intraocular foreign body (S05.-)*
EXCLUDES 2 *retained foreign body in eyelid (H02.81-)*
retained (old) foreign body following penetrating wound of orbit (H05.5-)
retained (old) intraocular foreign body, nonmagnetic (H44.7-)
√6th H44.60 Unspecified retained (old) intraocular foreign body, magnetic
H44.601 Unspecified retained (old) intraocular foreign body, magnetic, right eye
H44.602 Unspecified retained (old) intraocular foreign body, magnetic, left eye
H44.603 Unspecified retained (old) intraocular foreign body, magnetic, bilateral
H44.609 Unspecified retained (old) intraocular foreign body, magnetic, unspecified eye
√6th H44.61 Retained (old) magnetic foreign body in anterior chamber
H44.611 Retained (old) magnetic foreign body in anterior chamber, right eye
H44.612 Retained (old) magnetic foreign body in anterior chamber, left eye
H44.613 Retained (old) magnetic foreign body in anterior chamber, bilateral
H44.619 Retained (old) magnetic foreign body in anterior chamber, unspecified eye
√6th H44.62 Retained (old) magnetic foreign body in iris or ciliary body
H44.621 Retained (old) magnetic foreign body in iris or ciliary body, right eye
H44.622 Retained (old) magnetic foreign body in iris or ciliary body, left eye
H44.623 Retained (old) magnetic foreign body in iris or ciliary body, bilateral
H44.629 Retained (old) magnetic foreign body in iris or ciliary body, unspecified eye
√6th H44.63 Retained (old) magnetic foreign body in lens
H44.631 Retained (old) magnetic foreign body in lens, right eye
H44.632 Retained (old) magnetic foreign body in lens, left eye
H44.633 Retained (old) magnetic foreign body in lens, bilateral
H44.639 Retained (old) magnetic foreign body in lens, unspecified eye
√6th H44.64 Retained (old) magnetic foreign body in posterior wall of globe
H44.641 Retained (old) magnetic foreign body in posterior wall of globe, right eye
H44.642 Retained (old) magnetic foreign body in posterior wall of globe, left eye

H44.643 Retained (old) magnetic foreign body in posterior wall of globe, bilateral

H44.649 Retained (old) magnetic foreign body in posterior wall of globe, unspecified eye

H44.65 Retained (old) magnetic foreign body in vitreous body

H44.651 Retained (old) magnetic foreign body in vitreous body, right eye

H44.652 Retained (old) magnetic foreign body in vitreous body, left eye

H44.653 Retained (old) magnetic foreign body in vitreous body, bilateral

H44.659 Retained (old) magnetic foreign body in vitreous body, unspecified eye

H44.69 Retained (old) intraocular foreign body, magnetic, in other or multiple sites

H44.691 Retained (old) intraocular foreign body, magnetic, in other or multiple sites, right eye

H44.692 Retained (old) intraocular foreign body, magnetic, in other or multiple sites, left eye

H44.693 Retained (old) intraocular foreign body, magnetic, in other or multiple sites, bilateral

H44.699 Retained (old) intraocular foreign body, magnetic, in other or multiple sites, unspecified eye

H44.7 Retained (old) intraocular foreign body, nonmagnetic

Use additional code to identify nonmagnetic foreign body (Z18.01-Z18.10, Z18.12, Z18.2-Z18.9)

EXCLUDES 1 *current intraocular foreign body (S05.-)*

EXCLUDES 2 *retained foreign body in eyelid (H02.81-)*

retained (old) foreign body following penetrating wound of orbit (H05.5-)

retained (old) intraocular foreign body, magnetic (H44.6-)

H44.70 Unspecified retained (old) intraocular foreign body, nonmagnetic

H44.701 Unspecified retained (old) intraocular foreign body, nonmagnetic, right eye

H44.702 Unspecified retained (old) intraocular foreign body, nonmagnetic, left eye

H44.703 Unspecified retained (old) intraocular foreign body, nonmagnetic, bilateral

H44.709 Unspecified retained (old) intraocular foreign body, nonmagnetic, unspecified eye

Retained (old) intraocular foreign body NOS

H44.71 Retained (nonmagnetic) (old) foreign body in anterior chamber

H44.711 Retained (nonmagnetic) (old) foreign body in anterior chamber, right eye

H44.712 Retained (nonmagnetic) (old) foreign body in anterior chamber, left eye

H44.713 Retained (nonmagnetic) (old) foreign body in anterior chamber, bilateral

H44.719 Retained (nonmagnetic) (old) foreign body in anterior chamber, unspecified eye

H44.72 Retained (nonmagnetic) (old) foreign body in iris or ciliary body

H44.721 Retained (nonmagnetic) (old) foreign body in iris or ciliary body, right eye

H44.722 Retained (nonmagnetic) (old) foreign body in iris or ciliary body, left eye

H44.723 Retained (nonmagnetic) (old) foreign body in iris or ciliary body, bilateral

H44.729 Retained (nonmagnetic) (old) foreign body in iris or ciliary body, unspecified eye

H44.73 Retained (nonmagnetic) (old) foreign body in lens

H44.731 Retained (nonmagnetic) (old) foreign body in lens, right eye

H44.732 Retained (nonmagnetic) (old) foreign body in lens, left eye

H44.733 Retained (nonmagnetic) (old) foreign body in lens, bilateral

H44.739 Retained (nonmagnetic) (old) foreign body in lens, unspecified eye

H44.74 Retained (nonmagnetic) (old) foreign body in posterior wall of globe

H44.741 Retained (nonmagnetic) (old) foreign body in posterior wall of globe, right eye

H44.742 Retained (nonmagnetic) (old) foreign body in posterior wall of globe, left eye

H44.743 Retained (nonmagnetic) (old) foreign body in posterior wall of globe, bilateral

H44.749 Retained (nonmagnetic) (old) foreign body in posterior wall of globe, unspecified eye

H44.75 Retained (nonmagnetic) (old) foreign body in vitreous body

H44.751 Retained (nonmagnetic) (old) foreign body in vitreous body, right eye

H44.752 Retained (nonmagnetic) (old) foreign body in vitreous body, left eye

H44.753 Retained (nonmagnetic) (old) foreign body in vitreous body, bilateral

H44.759 Retained (nonmagnetic) (old) foreign body in vitreous body, unspecified eye

H44.79 Retained (old) intraocular foreign body, nonmagnetic, in other or multiple sites

H44.791 Retained (old) intraocular foreign body, nonmagnetic, in other or multiple sites, right eye

H44.792 Retained (old) intraocular foreign body, nonmagnetic, in other or multiple sites, left eye

H44.793 Retained (old) intraocular foreign body, nonmagnetic, in other or multiple sites, bilateral

H44.799 Retained (old) intraocular foreign body, nonmagnetic, in other or multiple sites, unspecified eye

H44.8 Other disorders of globe

H44.81 Hemophthalmos

DEF: Pool of blood within the eyeball, not from a current injury.

H44.811 Hemophthalmos, right eye

H44.812 Hemophthalmos, left eye

H44.813 Hemophthalmos, bilateral

H44.819 Hemophthalmos, unspecified eye

H44.82 Luxation of globe

H44.821 Luxation of globe, right eye

H44.822 Luxation of globe, left eye

H44.823 Luxation of globe, bilateral

H44.829 Luxation of globe, unspecified eye

H44.89 Other disorders of globe

AHA: 2022,1Q,33

H44.9 Unspecified disorder of globe

Disorders of optic nerve and visual pathways (H46-H47)

H46 Optic neuritis

EXCLUDES 2 *ischemic optic neuropathy (H47.01-)*

neuromyelitis optica [Devic] (G36.0)

H46.0 Optic papillitis

H46.00 Optic papillitis, unspecified eye CC UNS

H46.01 Optic papillitis, right eye CC

H46.02 Optic papillitis, left eye CC

H46.03 Optic papillitis, bilateral CC

H46.1 Retrobulbar neuritis

Retrobulbar neuritis NOS

EXCLUDES 1 *syphilitic retrobulbar neuritis (A52.15)*

H46.10 Retrobulbar neuritis, unspecified eye CC UNS

H46.11 Retrobulbar neuritis, right eye CC

H46.12 Retrobulbar neuritis, left eye CC

H46.13 Retrobulbar neuritis, bilateral CC

H46.2 Nutritional optic neuropathy

H46.3 Toxic optic neuropathy

Code first (T51-T65) to identify cause

H46.8 Other optic neuritis CC

H46.9 Unspecified optic neuritis CC

H47 Other disorders of optic [2nd] nerve and visual pathways

H47.0 Disorders of optic nerve, not elsewhere classified

H47.01 Ischemic optic neuropathy

H47.011 Ischemic optic neuropathy, right eye

H47.012 Ischemic optic neuropathy, left eye
H47.013 Ischemic optic neuropathy, bilateral
H47.019 Ischemic optic neuropathy, unspecified eye

✓6th H47.02 Hemorrhage in optic nerve sheath
H47.021 Hemorrhage in optic nerve sheath, right eye
H47.022 Hemorrhage in optic nerve sheath, left eye
H47.023 Hemorrhage in optic nerve sheath, bilateral
H47.029 Hemorrhage in optic nerve sheath, unspecified eye

✓6th H47.03 Optic nerve hypoplasia
H47.031 Optic nerve hypoplasia, right eye
H47.032 Optic nerve hypoplasia, left eye
H47.033 Optic nerve hypoplasia, bilateral
H47.039 Optic nerve hypoplasia, unspecified eye

✓6th H47.09 Other disorders of optic nerve, not elsewhere classified
Compression of optic nerve
H47.091 Other disorders of optic nerve, not elsewhere classified, right eye
H47.092 Other disorders of optic nerve, not elsewhere classified, left eye
H47.093 Other disorders of optic nerve, not elsewhere classified, bilateral
H47.099 Other disorders of optic nerve, not elsewhere classified, unspecified eye

✓5th H47.1 Papilledema
DEF: Swelling of the optic papilla, the raised area connected to the optic disk made up of nerves that enter the eyeball. It may be caused by increased intracranial pressure, decreased ocular pressure, or a retinal disorder.
H47.10 Unspecified papilledema CC
H47.11 Papilledema associated with increased intracranial pressure CC
H47.12 Papilledema associated with decreased ocular pressure
H47.13 Papilledema associated with retinal disorder

✓6th H47.14 Foster-Kennedy syndrome
H47.141 Foster-Kennedy syndrome, right eye
H47.142 Foster-Kennedy syndrome, left eye
H47.143 Foster-Kennedy syndrome, bilateral
H47.149 Foster-Kennedy syndrome, unspecified eye

✓5th H47.2 Optic atrophy
H47.20 Unspecified optic atrophy

✓6th H47.21 Primary optic atrophy
H47.211 Primary optic atrophy, right eye
H47.212 Primary optic atrophy, left eye
H47.213 Primary optic atrophy, bilateral
H47.219 Primary optic atrophy, unspecified eye

H47.22 Hereditary optic atrophy
Leber's optic atrophy

✓6th H47.23 Glaucomatous optic atrophy
H47.231 Glaucomatous optic atrophy, right eye
H47.232 Glaucomatous optic atrophy, left eye
H47.233 Glaucomatous optic atrophy, bilateral
H47.239 Glaucomatous optic atrophy, unspecified eye

✓6th H47.29 Other optic atrophy
Temporal pallor of optic disc
H47.291 Other optic atrophy, right eye
H47.292 Other optic atrophy, left eye
H47.293 Other optic atrophy, bilateral
H47.299 Other optic atrophy, unspecified eye

✓5th H47.3 Other disorders of optic disc

✓6th H47.31 Coloboma of optic disc
H47.311 Coloboma of optic disc, right eye
H47.312 Coloboma of optic disc, left eye
H47.313 Coloboma of optic disc, bilateral
H47.319 Coloboma of optic disc, unspecified eye

✓6th H47.32 Drusen of optic disc
H47.321 Drusen of optic disc, right eye
H47.322 Drusen of optic disc, left eye
H47.323 Drusen of optic disc, bilateral
H47.329 Drusen of optic disc, unspecified eye

✓6th H47.33 Pseudopapilledema of optic disc
H47.331 Pseudopapilledema of optic disc, right eye
H47.332 Pseudopapilledema of optic disc, left eye
H47.333 Pseudopapilledema of optic disc, bilateral
H47.339 Pseudopapilledema of optic disc, unspecified eye

✓6th H47.39 Other disorders of optic disc
H47.391 Other disorders of optic disc, right eye
H47.392 Other disorders of optic disc, left eye
H47.393 Other disorders of optic disc, bilateral
H47.399 Other disorders of optic disc, unspecified eye

✓5th H47.4 Disorders of optic chiasm
Code also underlying condition
H47.41 Disorders of optic chiasm in (due to) inflammatory disorders CC
H47.42 Disorders of optic chiasm in (due to) neoplasm CC
H47.43 Disorders of optic chiasm in (due to) vascular disorders CC
H47.49 Disorders of optic chiasm in (due to) other disorders CC

✓5th H47.5 Disorders of other visual pathways
Disorders of optic tracts, geniculate nuclei and optic radiations
Code also underlying condition

✓6th H47.51 Disorders of visual pathways in (due to) inflammatory disorders
H47.511 Disorders of visual pathways in (due to) inflammatory disorders, right side CC
H47.512 Disorders of visual pathways in (due to) inflammatory disorders, left side CC
H47.519 Disorders of visual pathways in (due to) inflammatory disorders, unspecified side CC UNS

✓6th H47.52 Disorders of visual pathways in (due to) neoplasm
H47.521 Disorders of visual pathways in (due to) neoplasm, right side CC
H47.522 Disorders of visual pathways in (due to) neoplasm, left side CC
H47.529 Disorders of visual pathways in (due to) neoplasm, unspecified side CC UNS

✓6th H47.53 Disorders of visual pathways in (due to) vascular disorders
H47.531 Disorders of visual pathways in (due to) vascular disorders, right side CC
H47.532 Disorders of visual pathways in (due to) vascular disorders, left side CC
H47.539 Disorders of visual pathways in (due to) vascular disorders, unspecified side CC UNS

✓5th H47.6 Disorders of visual cortex
Code also underlying condition
EXCLUDES 1 *injury to visual cortex S04.04-*

✓6th H47.61 Cortical blindness
H47.611 Cortical blindness, right side of brain
H47.612 Cortical blindness, left side of brain
H47.619 Cortical blindness, unspecified side of brain

✓6th H47.62 Disorders of visual cortex in (due to) inflammatory disorders
H47.621 Disorders of visual cortex in (due to) inflammatory disorders, right side of brain CC
H47.622 Disorders of visual cortex in (due to) inflammatory disorders, left side of brain CC
H47.629 Disorders of visual cortex in (due to) inflammatory disorders, unspecified side of brain CC UNS

✓6th H47.63 Disorders of visual cortex in (due to) neoplasm
H47.631 Disorders of visual cortex in (due to) neoplasm, right side of brain CC
H47.632 Disorders of visual cortex in (due to) neoplasm, left side of brain CC
H47.639 Disorders of visual cortex in (due to) neoplasm, unspecified side of brain CC UNS

✓6th **H47.64 Disorders of visual cortex in (due to) vascular disorders**
- **H47.641 Disorders of visual cortex in (due to) vascular disorders, right side of brain** CC
- **H47.642 Disorders of visual cortex in (due to) vascular disorders, left side of brain** CC
- **H47.649 Disorders of visual cortex in (due to) vascular disorders, unspecified side of brain** CC UNS

H47.9 Unspecified disorder of visual pathways

Disorders of ocular muscles, binocular movement, accommodation and refraction (H49-H52)

EXCLUDES 2 *nystagmus and other irregular eye movements (H55)*

✓4th **H49 Paralytic strabismus**

EXCLUDES 2 *internal ophthalmoplegia (H52.51-)*
internuclear ophthalmoplegia (H51.2-)
progressive supranuclear ophthalmoplegia (G23.1)

DEF: Strabismus: Misalignment of the eyes with the inability to move and focus in the same direction due to conditions affecting the muscles controlling them.

✓5th **H49.Ø Third [oculomotor] nerve palsy**
- **H49.ØØ Third [oculomotor] nerve palsy, unspecified eye**
- **H49.Ø1 Third [oculomotor] nerve palsy, right eye**
- **H49.Ø2 Third [oculomotor] nerve palsy, left eye**
- **H49.Ø3 Third [oculomotor] nerve palsy, bilateral**

✓5th **H49.1 Fourth [trochlear] nerve palsy**
- **H49.1Ø Fourth [trochlear] nerve palsy, unspecified eye**
- **H49.11 Fourth [trochlear] nerve palsy, right eye**
- **H49.12 Fourth [trochlear] nerve palsy, left eye**
- **H49.13 Fourth [trochlear] nerve palsy, bilateral**

✓5th **H49.2 Sixth [abducent] nerve palsy**
- **H49.2Ø Sixth [abducent] nerve palsy, unspecified eye**
- **H49.21 Sixth [abducent] nerve palsy, right eye**
- **H49.22 Sixth [abducent] nerve palsy, left eye**
- **H49.23 Sixth [abducent] nerve palsy, bilateral**

✓5th **H49.3 Total (external) ophthalmoplegia**
- **H49.3Ø Total (external) ophthalmoplegia, unspecified eye**
- **H49.31 Total (external) ophthalmoplegia, right eye**
- **H49.32 Total (external) ophthalmoplegia, left eye**
- **H49.33 Total (external) ophthalmoplegia, bilateral**

✓5th **H49.4 Progressive external ophthalmoplegia**

EXCLUDES 1 *Kearns-Sayre syndrome (H49.81-)*

- **H49.4Ø Progressive external ophthalmoplegia, unspecified eye**
- **H49.41 Progressive external ophthalmoplegia, right eye**
- **H49.42 Progressive external ophthalmoplegia, left eye**
- **H49.43 Progressive external ophthalmoplegia, bilateral**

✓5th **H49.8 Other paralytic strabismus**

✓6th **H49.81 Kearns-Sayre syndrome**

Progressive external ophthalmoplegia with pigmentary retinopathy

~~Use additional code for other manifestation, such as: heart block (I45.9)~~

▶Code also, if applicable, other manifestations, such as:◀
▶heart block (I45.9)◀

- **H49.811 Kearns-Sayre syndrome, right eye** CC HCC
- **H49.812 Kearns-Sayre syndrome, left eye** CC HCC
- **H49.813 Kearns-Sayre syndrome, bilateral** CC HCC
- **H49.819 Kearns-Sayre syndrome, unspecified eye** CC UNS HCC

✓6th **H49.88 Other paralytic strabismus**

External ophthalmoplegia NOS

- **H49.881 Other paralytic strabismus, right eye**
- **H49.882 Other paralytic strabismus, left eye**
- **H49.883 Other paralytic strabismus, bilateral**
- **H49.889 Other paralytic strabismus, unspecified eye**

H49.9 Unspecified paralytic strabismus

✓4th **H5Ø Other strabismus**

DEF: Strabismus: Misalignment of the eyes with the inability to move and focus in the same direction due to conditions affecting the muscles controlling them.

✓5th **H5Ø.Ø Esotropia**

Convergent concomitant strabismus

EXCLUDES 1 *intermittent esotropia (H5Ø.31-, H5Ø.32)*

H5Ø.ØØ Unspecified esotropia

✓6th **H5Ø.Ø1 Monocular esotropia**
- **H5Ø.Ø11 Monocular esotropia, right eye**
- **H5Ø.Ø12 Monocular esotropia, left eye**

✓6th **H5Ø.Ø2 Monocular esotropia with A pattern**
- **H5Ø.Ø21 Monocular esotropia with A pattern, right eye**
- **H5Ø.Ø22 Monocular esotropia with A pattern, left eye**

✓6th **H5Ø.Ø3 Monocular esotropia with V pattern**
- **H5Ø.Ø31 Monocular esotropia with V pattern, right eye**
- **H5Ø.Ø32 Monocular esotropia with V pattern, left eye**

✓6th **H5Ø.Ø4 Monocular esotropia with other noncomitancies**
- **H5Ø.Ø41 Monocular esotropia with other noncomitancies, right eye**
- **H5Ø.Ø42 Monocular esotropia with other noncomitancies, left eye**

H5Ø.Ø5 Alternating esotropia
H5Ø.Ø6 Alternating esotropia with A pattern
H5Ø.Ø7 Alternating esotropia with V pattern
H5Ø.Ø8 Alternating esotropia with other noncomitancies

Eye Muscle Diseases

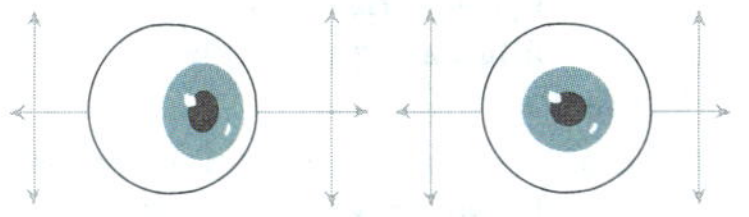

R. L.
Monocular (one eye only) esotropia (inward)

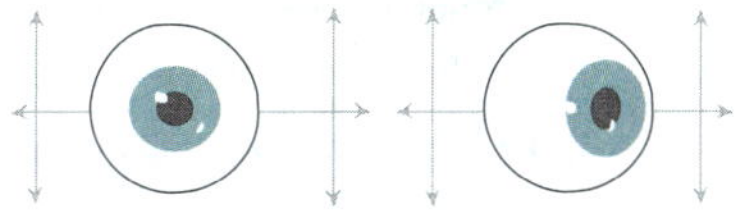

Monocular exotropia (outward)

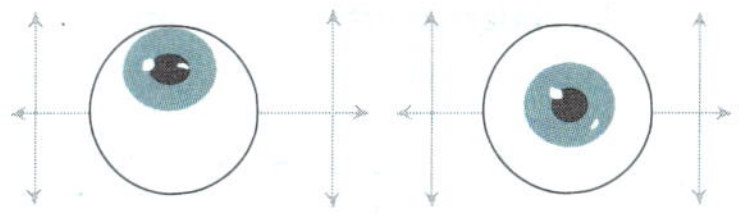

Monocular hypertropia (upward)

✓5th **H5Ø.1 Exotropia**

Divergent concomitant strabismus

EXCLUDES 1 *intermittent exotropia (H5Ø.33-, H5Ø.34)*

H5Ø.1Ø Unspecified exotropia

✓6th **H5Ø.11 Monocular exotropia**
- **H5Ø.111 Monocular exotropia, right eye**
- **H5Ø.112 Monocular exotropia, left eye**

✓6th **H5Ø.12 Monocular exotropia with A pattern**
- **H5Ø.121 Monocular exotropia with A pattern, right eye**
- **H5Ø.122 Monocular exotropia with A pattern, left eye**

✓6th **H5Ø.13 Monocular exotropia with V pattern**
- **H5Ø.131 Monocular exotropia with V pattern, right eye**
- **H5Ø.132 Monocular exotropia with V pattern, left eye**

✓6th **H5Ø.14 Monocular exotropia with other noncomitancies**
- **H5Ø.141 Monocular exotropia with other noncomitancies, right eye**
- **H5Ø.142 Monocular exotropia with other noncomitancies, left eye**

H5Ø.15 Alternating exotropia
H5Ø.16 Alternating exotropia with A pattern
H5Ø.17 Alternating exotropia with V pattern

Chapter 7. Diseases of the Eye and Adnexa
H47.64–H5Ø.17

H5Ø.18 Alternating exotropia with other noncomitancies

H5Ø.2 Vertical strabismus
Hypertropia
H5Ø.21 Vertical strabismus, right eye
H5Ø.22 Vertical strabismus, left eye

H5Ø.3 Intermittent heterotropia
H5Ø.3Ø Unspecified intermittent heterotropia
H5Ø.31 Intermittent monocular esotropia
H5Ø.311 Intermittent monocular esotropia, right eye
H5Ø.312 Intermittent monocular esotropia, left eye
H5Ø.32 Intermittent alternating esotropia
H5Ø.33 Intermittent monocular exotropia
H5Ø.331 Intermittent monocular exotropia, right eye
H5Ø.332 Intermittent monocular exotropia, left eye
H5Ø.34 Intermittent alternating exotropia

H5Ø.4 Other and unspecified heterotropia
H5Ø.4Ø Unspecified heterotropia
H5Ø.41 Cyclotropia
H5Ø.411 Cyclotropia, right eye
H5Ø.412 Cyclotropia, left eye
H5Ø.42 Monofixation syndrome
H5Ø.43 Accommodative component in esotropia

H5Ø.5 Heterophoria
H5Ø.5Ø Unspecified heterophoria
H5Ø.51 Esophoria
H5Ø.52 Exophoria
H5Ø.53 Vertical heterophoria
H5Ø.54 Cyclophoria
H5Ø.55 Alternating heterophoria

H5Ø.6 Mechanical strabismus
H5Ø.6Ø Mechanical strabismus, unspecified
H5Ø.61 Brown's sheath syndrome
H5Ø.611 Brown's sheath syndrome, right eye
H5Ø.612 Brown's sheath syndrome, left eye
● H5Ø.62 Inferior oblique muscle entrapment
● H5Ø.621 Inferior oblique muscle entrapment, right eye
● H5Ø.622 Inferior oblique muscle entrapment, left eye
● H5Ø.629 Inferior oblique muscle entrapment, unspecified eye
● H5Ø.63 Inferior rectus muscle entrapment
● H5Ø.631 Inferior rectus muscle entrapment, right eye
● H5Ø.632 Inferior rectus muscle entrapment, left eye
● H5Ø.639 Inferior rectus muscle entrapment, unspecified eye
● H5Ø.64 Lateral rectus muscle entrapment
● H5Ø.641 Lateral rectus muscle entrapment, right eye
● H5Ø.642 Lateral rectus muscle entrapment, left eye
● H5Ø.649 Lateral rectus muscle entrapment, unspecified eye
● H5Ø.65 Medial rectus muscle entrapment
● H5Ø.651 Medial rectus muscle entrapment, right eye
● H5Ø.652 Medial rectus muscle entrapment, left eye
● H5Ø.659 Medial rectus muscle entrapment, unspecified eye
● H5Ø.66 Superior oblique muscle entrapment
● H5Ø.661 Superior oblique muscle entrapment, right eye
● H5Ø.662 Superior oblique muscle entrapment, left eye
● H5Ø.669 Superior oblique muscle entrapment, unspecified eye
● H5Ø.67 Superior rectus muscle entrapment
● H5Ø.671 Superior rectus muscle entrapment, right eye
● H5Ø.672 Superior rectus muscle entrapment, left eye
● H5Ø.679 Superior rectus muscle entrapment, unspecified eye
● H5Ø.68 Extraocular muscle entrapment, unspecified
● H5Ø.681 Extraocular muscle entrapment, unspecified, right eye
● H5Ø.682 Extraocular muscle entrapment, unspecified, left eye
● H5Ø.689 Extraocular muscle entrapment, unspecified, unspecified eye
H5Ø.69 Other mechanical strabismus
Strabismus due to adhesions
Traumatic limitation of duction of eye muscle

H5Ø.8 Other specified strabismus
H5Ø.81 Duane's syndrome
H5Ø.811 Duane's syndrome, right eye
H5Ø.812 Duane's syndrome, left eye
H5Ø.89 Other specified strabismus

H5Ø.9 Unspecified strabismus

H51 Other disorders of binocular movement
H51.Ø Palsy (spasm) of conjugate gaze
H51.1 Convergence insufficiency and excess
H51.11 Convergence insufficiency
H51.12 Convergence excess
H51.2 Internuclear ophthalmoplegia
H51.2Ø Internuclear ophthalmoplegia, unspecified eye
H51.21 Internuclear ophthalmoplegia, right eye
H51.22 Internuclear ophthalmoplegia, left eye
H51.23 Internuclear ophthalmoplegia, bilateral
H51.8 Other specified disorders of binocular movement
H51.9 Unspecified disorder of binocular movement

H52 Disorders of refraction and accommodation
H52.Ø Hypermetropia
H52.ØØ Hypermetropia, unspecified eye
H52.Ø1 Hypermetropia, right eye
H52.Ø2 Hypermetropia, left eye
H52.Ø3 Hypermetropia, bilateral

H52.1 Myopia
EXCLUDES 1 *degenerative myopia (H44.2-)*
H52.1Ø Myopia, unspecified eye
H52.11 Myopia, right eye
H52.12 Myopia, left eye
H52.13 Myopia, bilateral

H52.2 Astigmatism
H52.2Ø Unspecified astigmatism
H52.2Ø1 Unspecified astigmatism, right eye
H52.2Ø2 Unspecified astigmatism, left eye
H52.2Ø3 Unspecified astigmatism, bilateral
H52.2Ø9 Unspecified astigmatism, unspecified eye
H52.21 Irregular astigmatism
H52.211 Irregular astigmatism, right eye
H52.212 Irregular astigmatism, left eye
H52.213 Irregular astigmatism, bilateral
H52.219 Irregular astigmatism, unspecified eye
H52.22 Regular astigmatism
H52.221 Regular astigmatism, right eye
H52.222 Regular astigmatism, left eye
H52.223 Regular astigmatism, bilateral
H52.229 Regular astigmatism, unspecified eye

H52.3 Anisometropia and aniseikonia
H52.31 Anisometropia
H52.32 Aniseikonia

H52.4 Presbyopia

H52.5 Disorders of accommodation
H52.51 Internal ophthalmoplegia (complete) (total)
H52.511 Internal ophthalmoplegia (complete) (total), right eye
H52.512 Internal ophthalmoplegia (complete) (total), left eye
H52.513 Internal ophthalmoplegia (complete) (total), bilateral
H52.519 Internal ophthalmoplegia (complete) (total), unspecified eye

H52.52 Paresis of accommodation
- H52.521 Paresis of accommodation, right eye
- H52.522 Paresis of accommodation, left eye
- H52.523 Paresis of accommodation, bilateral
- H52.529 Paresis of accommodation, unspecified eye

H52.53 Spasm of accommodation
- H52.531 Spasm of accommodation, right eye
- H52.532 Spasm of accommodation, left eye
- H52.533 Spasm of accommodation, bilateral
- H52.539 Spasm of accommodation, unspecified eye

H52.6 Other disorders of refraction

H52.7 Unspecified disorder of refraction

Visual disturbances and blindness (H53-H54)

H53 Visual disturbances

H53.0 Amblyopia ex anopsia

EXCLUDES 1 *amblyopia due to vitamin A deficiency (E50.5)*

H53.00 Unspecified amblyopia
- H53.001 Unspecified amblyopia, right eye
- H53.002 Unspecified amblyopia, left eye
- H53.003 Unspecified amblyopia, bilateral
- H53.009 Unspecified amblyopia, unspecified eye

H53.01 Deprivation amblyopia
- H53.011 Deprivation amblyopia, right eye
- H53.012 Deprivation amblyopia, left eye
- H53.013 Deprivation amblyopia, bilateral
- H53.019 Deprivation amblyopia, unspecified eye

H53.02 Refractive amblyopia
- H53.021 Refractive amblyopia, right eye
- H53.022 Refractive amblyopia, left eye
- H53.023 Refractive amblyopia, bilateral
- H53.029 Refractive amblyopia, unspecified eye

H53.03 Strabismic amblyopia

EXCLUDES 1 *strabismus (H50.-)*

- H53.031 Strabismic amblyopia, right eye
- H53.032 Strabismic amblyopia, left eye
- H53.033 Strabismic amblyopia, bilateral
- H53.039 Strabismic amblyopia, unspecified eye

H53.04 Amblyopia suspect

AHA: 2016,4Q,22-23

- H53.041 Amblyopia suspect, right eye
- H53.042 Amblyopia suspect, left eye
- H53.043 Amblyopia suspect, bilateral
- H53.049 Amblyopia suspect, unspecified eye

H53.1 Subjective visual disturbances

EXCLUDES 1 *subjective visual disturbances due to vitamin A deficiency (E50.5)*
visual hallucinations (R44.1)

H53.10 Unspecified subjective visual disturbances

H53.11 Day blindness

Hemeralopia

H53.12 Transient visual loss

Scintillating scotoma

EXCLUDES 1 *amaurosis fugax (G45.3-)*
transient retinal artery occlusion (H34.0-)

AHA: 2022,1Q,30

- H53.121 Transient visual loss, right eye CC
- H53.122 Transient visual loss, left eye CC
- H53.123 Transient visual loss, bilateral CC
- H53.129 Transient visual loss, unspecified eye CC UNS

H53.13 Sudden visual loss
- H53.131 Sudden visual loss, right eye CC
- H53.132 Sudden visual loss, left eye CC
- H53.133 Sudden visual loss, bilateral CC
- H53.139 Sudden visual loss, unspecified eye CC UNS

H53.14 Visual discomfort

Asthenopia
Photophobia

- H53.141 Visual discomfort, right eye
- H53.142 Visual discomfort, left eye
- H53.143 Visual discomfort, bilateral
- H53.149 Visual discomfort, unspecified

H53.15 Visual distortions of shape and size

Metamorphopsia

H53.16 Psychophysical visual disturbances

H53.19 Other subjective visual disturbances

Visual halos

AHA: 2022,1Q,30

H53.2 Diplopia

Double vision

H53.3 Other and unspecified disorders of binocular vision
- H53.30 Unspecified disorder of binocular vision
- H53.31 Abnormal retinal correspondence
- H53.32 Fusion with defective stereopsis
- H53.33 Simultaneous visual perception without fusion
- H53.34 Suppression of binocular vision

H53.4 Visual field defects

H53.40 Unspecified visual field defects

H53.41 Scotoma involving central area

Central scotoma

AHA: 2022,1Q,30

- H53.411 Scotoma involving central area, right eye
- H53.412 Scotoma involving central area, left eye
- H53.413 Scotoma involving central area, bilateral
- H53.419 Scotoma involving central area, unspecified eye

H53.42 Scotoma of blind spot area

Enlarged blind spot

- H53.421 Scotoma of blind spot area, right eye
- H53.422 Scotoma of blind spot area, left eye
- H53.423 Scotoma of blind spot area, bilateral
- H53.429 Scotoma of blind spot area, unspecified eye

H53.43 Sector or arcuate defects

Arcuate scotoma
Bjerrum scotoma

- H53.431 Sector or arcuate defects, right eye
- H53.432 Sector or arcuate defects, left eye
- H53.433 Sector or arcuate defects, bilateral
- H53.439 Sector or arcuate defects, unspecified eye

H53.45 Other localized visual field defect

Peripheral visual field defect
Ring scotoma NOS
Scotoma NOS

- H53.451 Other localized visual field defect, right eye
- H53.452 Other localized visual field defect, left eye
- H53.453 Other localized visual field defect, bilateral
- H53.459 Other localized visual field defect, unspecified eye

H53.46 Homonymous bilateral field defects

Homonymous hemianopia
Homonymous hemianopsia
Quadrant anopia
Quadrant anopsia

- H53.461 Homonymous bilateral field defects, right side
- H53.462 Homonymous bilateral field defects, left side
- H53.469 Homonymous bilateral field defects, unspecified side
  Homonymous bilateral field defects NOS

H53.47 Heteronymous bilateral field defects

Heteronymous hemianop(s)ia

H53.48 Generalized contraction of visual field
- H53.481 Generalized contraction of visual field, right eye
- H53.482 Generalized contraction of visual field, left eye
- H53.483 Generalized contraction of visual field, bilateral
- H53.489 Generalized contraction of visual field, unspecified eye

H53.5 Color vision deficiencies
Color blindness
EXCLUDES 2 *day blindness (H53.11)*
H53.50 Unspecified color vision deficiencies
Color blindness NOS
H53.51 Achromatopsia
DEF: Nonprogressive genetic visual disorder characterized by complete color blindness, decreased vision, and light sensitivity.
H53.52 Acquired color vision deficiency
H53.53 Deuteranomaly
Deuteranopia
DEF: Male-only genetic disorder causing difficulty in distinguishing green and red; no shortened spectrum.
H53.54 Protanomaly
Protanopia
H53.55 Tritanomaly
Tritanopia
H53.59 Other color vision deficiencies
H53.6 Night blindness
EXCLUDES 1 *night blindness due to vitamin A deficiency (E50.5)*
H53.60 Unspecified night blindness
H53.61 Abnormal dark adaptation curve
H53.62 Acquired night blindness
H53.63 Congenital night blindness
H53.69 Other night blindness
H53.7 Vision sensitivity deficiencies
H53.71 Glare sensitivity
H53.72 Impaired contrast sensitivity
H53.8 Other visual disturbances
H53.9 Unspecified visual disturbance

H54 Blindness and low vision
NOTE For definition of visual impairment categories see table below
Code first any associated underlying cause of the blindness
EXCLUDES 1 *amaurosis fugax (G45.3)*
AHA: 2017,4Q,11-12
H54.0 Blindness, both eyes
Visual impairment categories 3, 4, 5 in both eyes.
H54.0X Blindness, both eyes, different category levels
H54.0X3 Blindness right eye, category 3
H54.0X33 Blindness right eye category 3, blindness left eye category 3
H54.0X34 Blindness right eye category 3, blindness left eye category 4
H54.0X35 Blindness right eye category 3, blindness left eye category 5
H54.0X4 Blindness right eye, category 4
H54.0X43 Blindness right eye category 4, blindness left eye category 3
H54.0X44 Blindness right eye category 4, blindness left eye category 4
H54.0X45 Blindness right eye category 4, blindness left eye category 5
H54.0X5 Blindness right eye, category 5
H54.0X53 Blindness right eye category 5, blindness left eye category 3
H54.0X54 Blindness right eye category 5, blindness left eye category 4
H54.0X55 Blindness right eye category 5, blindness left eye category 5
H54.1 Blindness, one eye, low vision other eye
Visual impairment categories 3, 4, 5 in one eye, with categories 1 or 2 in the other eye.
H54.10 Blindness, one eye, low vision other eye, unspecified eyes
H54.11 Blindness, right eye, low vision left eye
H54.113 Blindness right eye category 3, low vision left eye
H54.1131 Blindness right eye category 3, low vision left eye category 1
H54.1132 Blindness right eye category 3, low vision left eye category 2
H54.114 Blindness right eye category 4, low vision left eye
H54.1141 Blindness right eye category 4, low vision left eye category 1
H54.1142 Blindness right eye category 4, low vision left eye category 2
H54.115 Blindness right eye category 5, low vision left eye
H54.1151 Blindness right eye category 5, low vision left eye category 1
H54.1152 Blindness right eye category 5, low vision left eye category 2
H54.12 Blindness, left eye, low vision right eye
H54.121 Low vision right eye category 1, blindness left eye
H54.1213 Low vision right eye category 1, blindness left eye category 3
H54.1214 Low vision right eye category 1, blindness left eye category 4
H54.1215 Low vision right eye category 1, blindness left eye category 5
H54.122 Low vision right eye category 2, blindness left eye
H54.1223 Low vision right eye category 2, blindness left eye category 3
H54.1224 Low vision right eye category 2, blindness left eye category 4
H54.1225 Low vision right eye category 2, blindness left eye category 5
H54.2 Low vision, both eyes
Visual impairment categories 1 or 2 in both eyes.
H54.2X Low vision, both eyes, different category levels
H54.2X1 Low vision, right eye, category 1
H54.2X11 Low vision right eye category 1, low vision left eye category 1
H54.2X12 Low vision right eye category 1, low vision left eye category 2
H54.2X2 Low vision, right eye, category 2
H54.2X21 Low vision right eye category 2, low vision left eye category 1
H54.2X22 Low vision right eye category 2, low vision left eye category 2
H54.3 Unqualified visual loss, both eyes
Visual impairment category 9 in both eyes.
TIP: Assign only when both eyes are documented as affected by blindness or low vision but the visual impairment category is not documented.
H54.4 Blindness, one eye
Visual impairment categories 3, 4, 5 in one eye [normal vision in other eye]
H54.40 Blindness, one eye, unspecified eye
H54.41 Blindness, right eye, normal vision left eye
H54.413 Blindness, right eye, category 3
H54.413A Blindness right eye category 3, normal vision left eye
H54.414 Blindness, right eye, category 4
H54.414A Blindness right eye category 4, normal vision left eye
H54.415 Blindness, right eye, category 5
H54.415A Blindness right eye category 5, normal vision left eye
H54.42 Blindness, left eye, normal vision right eye
H54.42A Blindness, left eye, category 3-5
H54.42A3 Blindness left eye category 3, normal vision right eye
H54.42A4 Blindness left eye category 4, normal vision right eye
H54.42A5 Blindness left eye category 5, normal vision right eye
H54.5 Low vision, one eye
Visual impairment categories 1 or 2 in one eye [normal vision in other eye].
H54.50 Low vision, one eye, unspecified eye

✓6th **H54.51 Low vision, right eye, normal vision left eye**

▲ ✓7th **H54.511 Low vision, right eye, category 1**

H54.511A Low vision right eye category 1, normal vision left eye

● ✓7th **H54.512 Low vision, right eye, category 2**

H54.512A Low vision right eye category 2, normal vision left eye

✓7th **H54.52 Low vision, left eye, normal vision right eye**

✓7th **H54.52A Low vision, left eye, category 1-2**

H54.52A1 Low vision left eye category 1, normal vision right eye

H54.52A2 Low vision left eye category 2, normal vision right eye

✓5th **H54.6 Unqualified visual loss, one eye**

Visual impairment category 9 in one eye [normal vision in other eye].

TIP: Assign a code from this category only when one eye is documented as affected by blindness or low vision but the visual impairment category is not documented.

H54.60 Unqualified visual loss, one eye, unspecified

H54.61 Unqualified visual loss, right eye, normal vision left eye

H54.62 Unqualified visual loss, left eye, normal vision right eye

H54.7 Unspecified visual loss UPD

Visual impairment category 9 NOS

TIP: Assign only when documentation specifies blindness, visual loss, or low vision but not whether one or both eyes are affected or the visual impairment category.

H54.8 Legal blindness, as defined in USA

Blindness NOS according to USA definition

EXCLUDES 1 *legal blindness with specification of impairment level (H54.0-H54.7)*

NOTE The table below gives a classification of severity of visual impairment recommended by a WHO Study Group on the Prevention of Blindness, Geneva, 6-10 November 1972.

The term "low vision" in category H54 comprises categories 1 and 2 of the table, the term "blindness" categories 3, 4 and 5, and the term "unqualified visual loss" category 9.

If the extent of the visual field is taken into account, patients with a field no greater than 10 but greater than 5 around central fixation should be placed in category 3 and patients with a field no greater than 5 around central fixation should be placed in category 4, even if the central acuity is not impaired.

Category of visual impairment	Visual acuity with best possible correction	
	Maximum less than:	Minimum equal to or better than:
1	6/18 3/10 (0.3) 20/70	6/60 1/10 (0.1) 20/200
2	6/60 1/10 (0.1) 20/200	3/60 1/20 (0.05) 20/400
3	3/60 1/200 (0.05) 20/400	1/60 (finger counting at one meter) 1/50 (0.02) 5/300 (20/1200)
4	1/60 (finger counting at one meter) 1/50 (0.02) 5/300	Light perception
5	No light perception	
9	Undetermined or unspecified	

Other disorders of eye and adnexa (H55-H57)

✓4th **H55 Nystagmus and other irregular eye movements**

✓5th **H55.0 Nystagmus**

DEF: Rapid, rhythmic, involuntary movements of the eyeball in vertical, horizontal, rotational, or mixed directions.

H55.00 Unspecified nystagmus

H55.01 Congenital nystagmus

H55.02 Latent nystagmus

H55.03 Visual deprivation nystagmus

H55.04 Dissociated nystagmus

H55.09 Other forms of nystagmus

✓5th **H55.8 Other irregular eye movements**

AHA: 2020,4Q,25

H55.81 Deficient saccadic eye movements

H55.82 Deficient smooth pursuit eye movements

H55.89 Other irregular eye movements

✓4th **H57 Other disorders of eye and adnexa**

✓5th **H57.0 Anomalies of pupillary function**

H57.00 Unspecified anomaly of pupillary function

H57.01 Argyll Robertson pupil, atypical

EXCLUDES 1 *syphilitic Argyll Robertson pupil (A52.19)*

H57.02 Anisocoria

H57.03 Miosis

H57.04 Mydriasis

✓6th **H57.05 Tonic pupil**

H57.051 Tonic pupil, right eye

H57.052 Tonic pupil, left eye

H57.053 Tonic pupil, bilateral

H57.059 Tonic pupil, unspecified eye

H57.09 Other anomalies of pupillary function

✓5th **H57.1 Ocular pain**

H57.10 Ocular pain, unspecified eye

H57.11 Ocular pain, right eye

H57.12 Ocular pain, left eye

H57.13 Ocular pain, bilateral

✓5th **H57.8 Other specified disorders of eye and adnexa**

AHA: 2018,4Q,15-16

✓6th **H57.81 Brow ptosis**

H57.811 Brow ptosis, right

H57.812 Brow ptosis, left

H57.813 Brow ptosis, bilateral

H57.819 Brow ptosis, unspecified

H57.89 Other specified disorders of eye and adnexa

● ✓6th **H57.8A Foreign body sensation eye (ocular)**

● **H57.8A1 Foreign body sensation, right eye**

● **H57.8A2 Foreign body sensation, left eye**

● **H57.8A3 Foreign body sensation, bilateral eyes**

● **H57.8A9 Foreign body sensation, unspecified eye**

H57.9 Unspecified disorder of eye and adnexa UPD

Intraoperative and postprocedural complications and disorders of eye and adnexa, not elsewhere classified (H59)

✓4th **H59 Intraoperative and postprocedural complications and disorders of eye and adnexa, not elsewhere classified**

EXCLUDES 1 *mechanical complication of intraocular lens (T85.2)*
mechanical complication of other ocular prosthetic devices, implants and grafts (T85.3)
pseudophakia (Z96.1)
secondary cataracts (H26.4-)

✓5th **H59.0 Disorders of the eye following cataract surgery**

✓6th **H59.01 Keratopathy (bullous aphakic) following cataract surgery**

Vitreal corneal syndrome

Vitreous (touch) syndrome

H59.011 Keratopathy (bullous aphakic) following cataract surgery, right eye CC

H59.012 Keratopathy (bullous aphakic) following cataract surgery, left eye CC

H59.013 Keratopathy (bullous aphakic) following cataract surgery, bilateral CC

H59.019 Keratopathy (bullous aphakic) following cataract surgery, unspecified eye CC UNS

√6th H59.02 Cataract (lens) fragments in eye following cataract surgery
H59.021 Cataract (lens) fragments in eye following cataract surgery, right eye
H59.022 Cataract (lens) fragments in eye following cataract surgery, left eye
H59.023 Cataract (lens) fragments in eye following cataract surgery, bilateral
H59.029 Cataract (lens) fragments in eye following cataract surgery, unspecified eye

√6th H59.03 Cystoid macular edema following cataract surgery
H59.031 Cystoid macular edema following cataract surgery, right eye CC
H59.032 Cystoid macular edema following cataract surgery, left eye CC
H59.033 Cystoid macular edema following cataract surgery, bilateral CC
H59.039 Cystoid macular edema following cataract surgery, unspecified eye CC UNS

√6th H59.09 Other disorders of the eye following cataract surgery
H59.091 Other disorders of the right eye following cataract surgery CC
H59.092 Other disorders of the left eye following cataract surgery CC
H59.093 Other disorders of the eye following cataract surgery, bilateral CC
H59.099 Other disorders of unspecified eye following cataract surgery CC UNS

√5th H59.1 Intraoperative hemorrhage and hematoma of eye and adnexa complicating a procedure
EXCLUDES 1 *intraoperative hemorrhage and hematoma of eye and adnexa due to accidental puncture or laceration during a procedure (H59.2-)*

√6th H59.11 Intraoperative hemorrhage and hematoma of eye and adnexa complicating an ophthalmic procedure
H59.111 Intraoperative hemorrhage and hematoma of right eye and adnexa complicating an ophthalmic procedure CC
H59.112 Intraoperative hemorrhage and hematoma of left eye and adnexa complicating an ophthalmic procedure CC
H59.113 Intraoperative hemorrhage and hematoma of eye and adnexa complicating an ophthalmic procedure, bilateral CC
H59.119 Intraoperative hemorrhage and hematoma of unspecified eye and adnexa complicating an ophthalmic procedure CC UNS

√6th H59.12 Intraoperative hemorrhage and hematoma of eye and adnexa complicating other procedure
H59.121 Intraoperative hemorrhage and hematoma of right eye and adnexa complicating other procedure CC
H59.122 Intraoperative hemorrhage and hematoma of left eye and adnexa complicating other procedure CC
H59.123 Intraoperative hemorrhage and hematoma of eye and adnexa complicating other procedure, bilateral CC
H59.129 Intraoperative hemorrhage and hematoma of unspecified eye and adnexa complicating other procedure CC UNS

√5th H59.2 Accidental puncture and laceration of eye and adnexa during a procedure

√6th H59.21 Accidental puncture and laceration of eye and adnexa during an ophthalmic procedure
H59.211 Accidental puncture and laceration of right eye and adnexa during an ophthalmic procedure CC
H59.212 Accidental puncture and laceration of left eye and adnexa during an ophthalmic procedure CC
H59.213 Accidental puncture and laceration of eye and adnexa during an ophthalmic procedure, bilateral CC
H59.219 Accidental puncture and laceration of unspecified eye and adnexa during an ophthalmic procedure CC UNS

√6th H59.22 Accidental puncture and laceration of eye and adnexa during other procedure
H59.221 Accidental puncture and laceration of right eye and adnexa during other procedure CC
H59.222 Accidental puncture and laceration of left eye and adnexa during other procedure CC
H59.223 Accidental puncture and laceration of eye and adnexa during other procedure, bilateral CC
H59.229 Accidental puncture and laceration of unspecified eye and adnexa during other procedure CC UNS

√5th H59.3 Postprocedural hemorrhage, hematoma, and seroma of eye and adnexa following a procedure
AHA: 2016,4Q,9-10

√6th H59.31 Postprocedural hemorrhage of eye and adnexa following an ophthalmic procedure
H59.311 Postprocedural hemorrhage of right eye and adnexa following an ophthalmic procedure CC
H59.312 Postprocedural hemorrhage of left eye and adnexa following an ophthalmic procedure CC
H59.313 Postprocedural hemorrhage of eye and adnexa following an ophthalmic procedure, bilateral CC
H59.319 Postprocedural hemorrhage of unspecified eye and adnexa following an ophthalmic procedure CC UNS

√6th H59.32 Postprocedural hemorrhage of eye and adnexa following other procedure
H59.321 Postprocedural hemorrhage of right eye and adnexa following other procedure CC
H59.322 Postprocedural hemorrhage of left eye and adnexa following other procedure CC
H59.323 Postprocedural hemorrhage of eye and adnexa following other procedure, bilateral CC
H59.329 Postprocedural hemorrhage of unspecified eye and adnexa following other procedure CC UNS

√6th H59.33 Postprocedural hematoma of eye and adnexa following an ophthalmic procedure
H59.331 Postprocedural hematoma of right eye and adnexa following an ophthalmic procedure CC
H59.332 Postprocedural hematoma of left eye and adnexa following an ophthalmic procedure CC
H59.333 Postprocedural hematoma of eye and adnexa following an ophthalmic procedure, bilateral CC
H59.339 Postprocedural hematoma of unspecified eye and adnexa following an ophthalmic procedure CC UNS

√6th H59.34 Postprocedural hematoma of eye and adnexa following other procedure
H59.341 Postprocedural hematoma of right eye and adnexa following other procedure CC
H59.342 Postprocedural hematoma of left eye and adnexa following other procedure CC
H59.343 Postprocedural hematoma of eye and adnexa following other procedure, bilateral CC
H59.349 Postprocedural hematoma of unspecified eye and adnexa following other procedure CC UNS

√6th H59.35 Postprocedural seroma of eye and adnexa following an ophthalmic procedure
H59.351 Postprocedural seroma of right eye and adnexa following an ophthalmic procedure CC
H59.352 Postprocedural seroma of left eye and adnexa following an ophthalmic procedure CC
H59.353 Postprocedural seroma of eye and adnexa following an ophthalmic procedure, bilateral CC

H59.359 **Postprocedural seroma of unspecified eye and adnexa following an ophthalmic procedure** CC UNS

✓6th **H59.36** **Postprocedural seroma of eye and adnexa following other procedure**

H59.361 **Postprocedural seroma of right eye and adnexa following other procedure** CC

H59.362 **Postprocedural seroma of left eye and adnexa following other procedure** CC

H59.363 **Postprocedural seroma of eye and adnexa following other procedure, bilateral** CC

H59.369 **Postprocedural seroma of unspecified eye and adnexa following other procedure** CC UNS

✓5th **H59.4** **Inflammation (infection) of postprocedural bleb**

Postprocedural blebitis

EXCLUDES 1 *filtering (vitreous) bleb after glaucoma surgery status (Z98.83)*

H59.40 **Inflammation (infection) of postprocedural bleb, unspecified**

H59.41 **Inflammation (infection) of postprocedural bleb, stage 1**

H59.42 **Inflammation (infection) of postprocedural bleb, stage 2**

H59.43 **Inflammation (infection) of postprocedural bleb, stage 3**

Bleb endophthalmitis

✓5th **H59.8** **Other intraoperative and postprocedural complications and disorders of eye and adnexa, not elsewhere classified**

✓6th **H59.81** **Chorioretinal scars after surgery for detachment**

H59.811 **Chorioretinal scars after surgery for detachment, right eye** CC

H59.812 **Chorioretinal scars after surgery for detachment, left eye** CC

H59.813 **Chorioretinal scars after surgery for detachment, bilateral** CC

H59.819 **Chorioretinal scars after surgery for detachment, unspecified eye** CC UNS

H59.88 **Other intraoperative complications of eye and adnexa, not elsewhere classified** CC

H59.89 **Other postprocedural complications and disorders of eye and adnexa, not elsewhere classified** CC

AHA: 2020,3Q,29

Chapter 8. Diseases of the Ear and Mastoid Process (H60–H95)

Chapter-specific Guidelines with Coding Examples
Reserved for future guideline expansion.

Chapter 8. Diseases of the Ear and Mastoid Process (H6Ø-H95)

NOTE Use an external cause code following the code for the ear condition, if applicable, to identify the cause of the ear condition

EXCLUDES 2 *certain conditions originating in the perinatal period (PØ4-P96)*
certain infectious and parasitic diseases (AØØ-B99)
complications of pregnancy, childbirth and the puerperium (OØØ-O9A)
congenital malformations, deformations and chromosomal abnormalities (QØØ-Q99)
endocrine, nutritional and metabolic diseases (EØØ-E88)
injury, poisoning and certain other consequences of external causes (SØØ-T88)
neoplasms (CØØ-D49)
symptoms, signs and abnormal clinical and laboratory findings, not elsewhere classified (RØØ-R94)

This chapter contains the following blocks:

H6Ø-H62 Diseases of external ear
H65-H75 Diseases of middle ear and mastoid
H8Ø-H83 Diseases of inner ear
H9Ø-H94 Other disorders of ear
H95 Intraoperative and postprocedural complications and disorders of ear and mastoid process, not elsewhere classified

Diseases of external ear (H6Ø-H62)

4th H6Ø Otitis externa

TIP: When the specific infectious agent is identified, a code from Chapter 1 is assigned instead of a code from this category.

5th H6Ø.Ø Abscess of external ear

Boil of external ear
Carbuncle of auricle or external auditory canal
Furuncle of external ear

H6Ø.ØØ Abscess of external ear, unspecified ear
H6Ø.Ø1 Abscess of right external ear
H6Ø.Ø2 Abscess of left external ear
H6Ø.Ø3 Abscess of external ear, bilateral

5th H6Ø.1 Cellulitis of external ear

Cellulitis of auricle
Cellulitis of external auditory canal

H6Ø.1Ø Cellulitis of external ear, unspecified ear
H6Ø.11 Cellulitis of right external ear
H6Ø.12 Cellulitis of left external ear
H6Ø.13 Cellulitis of external ear, bilateral

5th H6Ø.2 Malignant otitis externa

H6Ø.2Ø Malignant otitis externa, unspecified ear CC UNS
H6Ø.21 Malignant otitis externa, right ear CC
H6Ø.22 Malignant otitis externa, left ear CC
H6Ø.23 Malignant otitis externa, bilateral CC

5th H6Ø.3 Other infective otitis externa

6th H6Ø.31 Diffuse otitis externa

H6Ø.311 Diffuse otitis externa, right ear
H6Ø.312 Diffuse otitis externa, left ear
H6Ø.313 Diffuse otitis externa, bilateral
H6Ø.319 Diffuse otitis externa, unspecified ear

6th H6Ø.32 Hemorrhagic otitis externa

H6Ø.321 Hemorrhagic otitis externa, right ear
H6Ø.322 Hemorrhagic otitis externa, left ear
H6Ø.323 Hemorrhagic otitis externa, bilateral
H6Ø.329 Hemorrhagic otitis externa, unspecified ear

6th H6Ø.33 Swimmer's ear

DEF: Commonly occurs when water gets trapped in the ear after swimming.

H6Ø.331 Swimmer's ear, right ear
H6Ø.332 Swimmer's ear, left ear
H6Ø.333 Swimmer's ear, bilateral
H6Ø.339 Swimmer's ear, unspecified ear

6th H6Ø.39 Other infective otitis externa

H6Ø.391 Other infective otitis externa, right ear
H6Ø.392 Other infective otitis externa, left ear
H6Ø.393 Other infective otitis externa, bilateral
H6Ø.399 Other infective otitis externa, unspecified ear

5th H6Ø.4 Cholesteatoma of external ear

Keratosis obturans of external ear (canal)

EXCLUDES 2 *cholesteatoma of middle ear (H71.-)*
recurrent cholesteatoma of postmastoidectomy cavity (H95.Ø-)

DEF: Cholesteatoma: Noncancerous cyst-like mass of cell debris, including cholesterol and epithelial cells resulting from trauma, repeated or improperly healed infections, and congenital enclosure of epidermal cells.

H6Ø.4Ø Cholesteatoma of external ear, unspecified ear
H6Ø.41 Cholesteatoma of right external ear
H6Ø.42 Cholesteatoma of left external ear
H6Ø.43 Cholesteatoma of external ear, bilateral

5th H6Ø.5 Acute noninfective otitis externa

6th H6Ø.5Ø Unspecified acute noninfective otitis externa

Acute otitis externa NOS

H6Ø.5Ø1 Unspecified acute noninfective otitis externa, right ear
H6Ø.5Ø2 Unspecified acute noninfective otitis externa, left ear
H6Ø.5Ø3 Unspecified acute noninfective otitis externa, bilateral
H6Ø.5Ø9 Unspecified acute noninfective otitis externa, unspecified ear

6th H6Ø.51 Acute actinic otitis externa

H6Ø.511 Acute actinic otitis externa, right ear
H6Ø.512 Acute actinic otitis externa, left ear
H6Ø.513 Acute actinic otitis externa, bilateral
H6Ø.519 Acute actinic otitis externa, unspecified ear

6th H6Ø.52 Acute chemical otitis externa

H6Ø.521 Acute chemical otitis externa, right ear
H6Ø.522 Acute chemical otitis externa, left ear
H6Ø.523 Acute chemical otitis externa, bilateral
H6Ø.529 Acute chemical otitis externa, unspecified ear

6th H6Ø.53 Acute contact otitis externa

H6Ø.531 Acute contact otitis externa, right ear
H6Ø.532 Acute contact otitis externa, left ear
H6Ø.533 Acute contact otitis externa, bilateral
H6Ø.539 Acute contact otitis externa, unspecified ear

6th H6Ø.54 Acute eczematoid otitis externa

H6Ø.541 Acute eczematoid otitis externa, right ear
H6Ø.542 Acute eczematoid otitis externa, left ear
H6Ø.543 Acute eczematoid otitis externa, bilateral
H6Ø.549 Acute eczematoid otitis externa, unspecified ear

6th H6Ø.55 Acute reactive otitis externa

H6Ø.551 Acute reactive otitis externa, right ear
H6Ø.552 Acute reactive otitis externa, left ear
H6Ø.553 Acute reactive otitis externa, bilateral
H6Ø.559 Acute reactive otitis externa, unspecified ear

6th H6Ø.59 Other noninfective acute otitis externa

H6Ø.591 Other noninfective acute otitis externa, right ear
H6Ø.592 Other noninfective acute otitis externa, left ear
H6Ø.593 Other noninfective acute otitis externa, bilateral
H6Ø.599 Other noninfective acute otitis externa, unspecified ear

5th H6Ø.6 Unspecified chronic otitis externa

H6Ø.6Ø Unspecified chronic otitis externa, unspecified ear
H6Ø.61 Unspecified chronic otitis externa, right ear
H6Ø.62 Unspecified chronic otitis externa, left ear
H6Ø.63 Unspecified chronic otitis externa, bilateral

5th H6Ø.8 Other otitis externa

6th H6Ø.8X Other otitis externa

H6Ø.8X1 Other otitis externa, right ear
H6Ø.8X2 Other otitis externa, left ear
H6Ø.8X3 Other otitis externa, bilateral
H6Ø.8X9 Other otitis externa, unspecified ear

5th H6Ø.9 Unspecified otitis externa

H6Ø.9Ø Unspecified otitis externa, unspecified ear
H6Ø.91 Unspecified otitis externa, right ear

H60.92 Unspecified otitis externa, left ear
H60.93 Unspecified otitis externa, bilateral

H61 Other disorders of external ear

H61.0 Chondritis and perichondritis of external ear
Chondrodermatitis nodularis chronica helicis
Perichondritis of auricle
Perichondritis of pinna

H61.00 Unspecified perichondritis of external ear
H61.001 Unspecified perichondritis of right external ear
H61.002 Unspecified perichondritis of left external ear
H61.003 Unspecified perichondritis of external ear, bilateral
H61.009 Unspecified perichondritis of external ear, unspecified ear

H61.01 Acute perichondritis of external ear
H61.011 Acute perichondritis of right external ear
H61.012 Acute perichondritis of left external ear
H61.013 Acute perichondritis of external ear, bilateral
H61.019 Acute perichondritis of external ear, unspecified ear

H61.02 Chronic perichondritis of external ear
H61.021 Chronic perichondritis of right external ear
H61.022 Chronic perichondritis of left external ear
H61.023 Chronic perichondritis of external ear, bilateral
H61.029 Chronic perichondritis of external ear, unspecified ear

H61.03 Chondritis of external ear
Chondritis of auricle
Chondritis of pinna
AHA: 2015,1Q,18
DEF: Infection that has progressed into the cartilage and presents as indurated and edematous skin over the pinna. Vascular compromise occurs with tissue necrosis and deformity.
H61.031 Chondritis of right external ear
H61.032 Chondritis of left external ear
H61.033 Chondritis of external ear, bilateral
H61.039 Chondritis of external ear, unspecified ear

H61.1 Noninfective disorders of pinna
EXCLUDES 2 *cauliflower ear (M95.1-)*
gouty tophi of ear (M1A.-)

H61.10 Unspecified noninfective disorders of pinna
Disorder of pinna NOS
H61.101 Unspecified noninfective disorders of pinna, right ear
H61.102 Unspecified noninfective disorders of pinna, left ear
H61.103 Unspecified noninfective disorders of pinna, bilateral
H61.109 Unspecified noninfective disorders of pinna, unspecified ear

H61.11 Acquired deformity of pinna
Acquired deformity of auricle
EXCLUDES 2 *cauliflower ear (M95.1-)*
H61.111 Acquired deformity of pinna, right ear
H61.112 Acquired deformity of pinna, left ear
H61.113 Acquired deformity of pinna, bilateral
H61.119 Acquired deformity of pinna, unspecified ear

H61.12 Hematoma of pinna
Hematoma of auricle
H61.121 Hematoma of pinna, right ear
H61.122 Hematoma of pinna, left ear
H61.123 Hematoma of pinna, bilateral
H61.129 Hematoma of pinna, unspecified ear

H61.19 Other noninfective disorders of pinna
H61.191 Noninfective disorders of pinna, right ear
H61.192 Noninfective disorders of pinna, left ear
H61.193 Noninfective disorders of pinna, bilateral
H61.199 Noninfective disorders of pinna, unspecified ear

H61.2 Impacted cerumen
Wax in ear
H61.20 Impacted cerumen, unspecified ear
H61.21 Impacted cerumen, right ear
H61.22 Impacted cerumen, left ear
H61.23 Impacted cerumen, bilateral

H61.3 Acquired stenosis of external ear canal
Collapse of external ear canal
EXCLUDES 1 *postprocedural stenosis of external ear canal (H95.81-)*

H61.30 Acquired stenosis of external ear canal, unspecified
H61.301 Acquired stenosis of right external ear canal, unspecified
H61.302 Acquired stenosis of left external ear canal, unspecified
H61.303 Acquired stenosis of external ear canal, unspecified, bilateral
H61.309 Acquired stenosis of external ear canal, unspecified, unspecified ear

H61.31 Acquired stenosis of external ear canal secondary to trauma
H61.311 Acquired stenosis of right external ear canal secondary to trauma
H61.312 Acquired stenosis of left external ear canal secondary to trauma
H61.313 Acquired stenosis of external ear canal secondary to trauma, bilateral
H61.319 Acquired stenosis of external ear canal secondary to trauma, unspecified ear

H61.32 Acquired stenosis of external ear canal secondary to inflammation and infection
DEF: Narrowing of the external ear canal due to chronic inflammation or infection.
H61.321 Acquired stenosis of right external ear canal secondary to inflammation and infection
H61.322 Acquired stenosis of left external ear canal secondary to inflammation and infection
H61.323 Acquired stenosis of external ear canal secondary to inflammation and infection, bilateral
H61.329 Acquired stenosis of external ear canal secondary to inflammation and infection, unspecified ear

H61.39 Other acquired stenosis of external ear canal
H61.391 Other acquired stenosis of right external ear canal
H61.392 Other acquired stenosis of left external ear canal
H61.393 Other acquired stenosis of external ear canal, bilateral
H61.399 Other acquired stenosis of external ear canal, unspecified ear

H61.8 Other specified disorders of external ear

H61.81 Exostosis of external canal
H61.811 Exostosis of right external canal
H61.812 Exostosis of left external canal
H61.813 Exostosis of external canal, bilateral
H61.819 Exostosis of external canal, unspecified ear

H61.89 Other specified disorders of external ear
H61.891 Other specified disorders of right external ear
H61.892 Other specified disorders of left external ear
H61.893 Other specified disorders of external ear, bilateral
H61.899 Other specified disorders of external ear, unspecified ear

H61.9 Disorder of external ear, unspecified
H61.90 Disorder of external ear, unspecified, unspecified ear
H61.91 Disorder of right external ear, unspecified
H61.92 Disorder of left external ear, unspecified
H61.93 Disorder of external ear, unspecified, bilateral

4th **H62 Disorders of external ear in diseases classified elsewhere**

5th **H62.4 Otitis externa in other diseases classified elsewhere**

Code first underlying disease, such as:
erysipelas (A46)
impetigo ▶(LØ1.Ø-)◀

EXCLUDES 1 *otitis externa (in):*
candidiasis (B37.84)
herpes viral [herpes simplex] (BØØ.1)
herpes zoster (BØ2.8)

H62.4Ø Otitis externa in other diseases classified elsewhere, unspecified ear
H62.41 Otitis externa in other diseases classified elsewhere, right ear
H62.42 Otitis externa in other diseases classified elsewhere, left ear
H62.43 Otitis externa in other diseases classified elsewhere, bilateral

5th **H62.8 Other disorders of external ear in diseases classified elsewhere**

Code first underlying disease, such as:
gout (M1A.-, M1Ø.-)

6th **H62.8X Other disorders of external ear in diseases classified elsewhere**

H62.8X1 Other disorders of right external ear in diseases classified elsewhere
H62.8X2 Other disorders of left external ear in diseases classified elsewhere
H62.8X3 Other disorders of external ear in diseases classified elsewhere, bilateral
H62.8X9 Other disorders of external ear in diseases classified elsewhere, unspecified ear

Diseases of middle ear and mastoid (H65-H75)

4th **H65 Nonsuppurative otitis media**

INCLUDES nonsuppurative otitis media with myringitis

Use additional code for any associated perforated tympanic membrane (H72.-)

Use additional code, if applicable, to identify:
exposure to environmental tobacco smoke (Z77.22)
exposure to tobacco smoke in the perinatal period (P96.81)
history of tobacco dependence (Z87.891)
infectious agent (B95-B97)
occupational exposure to environmental tobacco smoke (Z57.31)
tobacco dependence (F17.-)
tobacco use (Z72.Ø)

5th **H65.Ø Acute serous otitis media**

Acute and subacute secretory otitis

H65.ØØ Acute serous otitis media, unspecified ear
H65.Ø1 Acute serous otitis media, right ear
H65.Ø2 Acute serous otitis media, left ear
H65.Ø3 Acute serous otitis media, bilateral
H65.Ø4 Acute serous otitis media, recurrent, right ear
H65.Ø5 Acute serous otitis media, recurrent, left ear
H65.Ø6 Acute serous otitis media, recurrent, bilateral
H65.Ø7 Acute serous otitis media, recurrent, unspecified ear

5th **H65.1 Other acute nonsuppurative otitis media**

EXCLUDES 1 *otitic barotrauma (T7Ø.Ø)*
otitis media (acute) NOS (H66.9)

6th **H65.11 Acute and subacute allergic otitis media (mucoid) (sanguinous) (serous)**

H65.111 Acute and subacute allergic otitis media (mucoid) (sanguinous) (serous), right ear
H65.112 Acute and subacute allergic otitis media (mucoid) (sanguinous) (serous), left ear
H65.113 Acute and subacute allergic otitis media (mucoid) (sanguinous) (serous), bilateral
H65.114 Acute and subacute allergic otitis media (mucoid) (sanguinous) (serous), recurrent, right ear
H65.115 Acute and subacute allergic otitis media (mucoid) (sanguinous) (serous), recurrent, left ear
H65.116 Acute and subacute allergic otitis media (mucoid) (sanguinous) (serous), recurrent, bilateral
H65.117 Acute and subacute allergic otitis media (mucoid) (sanguinous) (serous), recurrent, unspecified ear
H65.119 Acute and subacute allergic otitis media (mucoid) (sanguinous) (serous), unspecified ear

6th **H65.19 Other acute nonsuppurative otitis media**

Acute and subacute mucoid otitis media
Acute and subacute nonsuppurative otitis media NOS
Acute and subacute sanguinous otitis media
Acute and subacute seromucinous otitis media

H65.191 Other acute nonsuppurative otitis media, right ear
H65.192 Other acute nonsuppurative otitis media, left ear
H65.193 Other acute nonsuppurative otitis media, bilateral
H65.194 Other acute nonsuppurative otitis media, recurrent, right ear
H65.195 Other acute nonsuppurative otitis media, recurrent, left ear
H65.196 Other acute nonsuppurative otitis media, recurrent, bilateral
H65.197 Other acute nonsuppurative otitis media recurrent, unspecified ear
H65.199 Other acute nonsuppurative otitis media, unspecified ear

5th **H65.2 Chronic serous otitis media**

Chronic tubotympanal catarrh

H65.2Ø Chronic serous otitis media, unspecified ear
H65.21 Chronic serous otitis media, right ear
H65.22 Chronic serous otitis media, left ear
H65.23 Chronic serous otitis media, bilateral

5th **H65.3 Chronic mucoid otitis media**

Chronic mucinous otitis media
Chronic secretory otitis media
Chronic transudative otitis media
Glue ear

EXCLUDES 1 *adhesive middle ear disease (H74.1)*

H65.3Ø Chronic mucoid otitis media, unspecified ear
H65.31 Chronic mucoid otitis media, right ear
H65.32 Chronic mucoid otitis media, left ear
H65.33 Chronic mucoid otitis media, bilateral

5th **H65.4 Other chronic nonsuppurative otitis media**

6th **H65.41 Chronic allergic otitis media**

H65.411 Chronic allergic otitis media, right ear
H65.412 Chronic allergic otitis media, left ear
H65.413 Chronic allergic otitis media, bilateral
H65.419 Chronic allergic otitis media, unspecified ear

6th **H65.49 Other chronic nonsuppurative otitis media**

Chronic exudative otitis media
Chronic nonsuppurative otitis media NOS
Chronic otitis media with effusion (nonpurulent)
Chronic seromucinous otitis media

H65.491 Other chronic nonsuppurative otitis media, right ear
H65.492 Other chronic nonsuppurative otitis media, left ear
H65.493 Other chronic nonsuppurative otitis media, bilateral
H65.499 Other chronic nonsuppurative otitis media, unspecified ear

5th **H65.9 Unspecified nonsuppurative otitis media**

Allergic otitis media NOS
Catarrhal otitis media NOS
Exudative otitis media NOS
Mucoid otitis media NOS
Otitis media with effusion (nonpurulent) NOS
Secretory otitis media NOS
Seromucinous otitis media NOS
Serous otitis media NOS
Transudative otitis media NOS

H65.9Ø Unspecified nonsuppurative otitis media, unspecified ear
H65.91 Unspecified nonsuppurative otitis media, right ear
H65.92 Unspecified nonsuppurative otitis media, left ear
H65.93 Unspecified nonsuppurative otitis media, bilateral

H66 Suppurative and unspecified otitis media

INCLUDES suppurative and unspecified otitis media with myringitis

Use additional code to identify:
- exposure to environmental tobacco smoke (Z77.22)
- exposure to tobacco smoke in the perinatal period (P96.81)
- history of tobacco dependence (Z87.891)
- occupational exposure to environmental tobacco smoke (Z57.31)
- tobacco dependence (F17.-)
- tobacco use (Z72.0)

AHA: 2016,1Q,34

H66.0 Acute suppurative otitis media

H66.00 Acute suppurative otitis media without spontaneous rupture of ear drum
- **H66.001** Acute suppurative otitis media without spontaneous rupture of ear drum, right ear
- **H66.002** Acute suppurative otitis media without spontaneous rupture of ear drum, left ear
- **H66.003** Acute suppurative otitis media without spontaneous rupture of ear drum, bilateral
- **H66.004** Acute suppurative otitis media without spontaneous rupture of ear drum, recurrent, right ear
- **H66.005** Acute suppurative otitis media without spontaneous rupture of ear drum, recurrent, left ear
- **H66.006** Acute suppurative otitis media without spontaneous rupture of ear drum, recurrent, bilateral
- **H66.007** Acute suppurative otitis media without spontaneous rupture of ear drum, recurrent, unspecified ear
- **H66.009** Acute suppurative otitis media without spontaneous rupture of ear drum, unspecified ear

H66.01 Acute suppurative otitis media with spontaneous rupture of ear drum

DEF: Sudden, severe inflammation of the middle ear, causing pressure that perforates the ear drum tissue.
- **H66.011** Acute suppurative otitis media with spontaneous rupture of ear drum, right ear
- **H66.012** Acute suppurative otitis media with spontaneous rupture of ear drum, left ear
- **H66.013** Acute suppurative otitis media with spontaneous rupture of ear drum, bilateral
- **H66.014** Acute suppurative otitis media with spontaneous rupture of ear drum, recurrent, right ear
- **H66.015** Acute suppurative otitis media with spontaneous rupture of ear drum, recurrent, left ear
- **H66.016** Acute suppurative otitis media with spontaneous rupture of ear drum, recurrent, bilateral
- **H66.017** Acute suppurative otitis media with spontaneous rupture of ear drum, recurrent, unspecified ear
- **H66.019** Acute suppurative otitis media with spontaneous rupture of ear drum, unspecified ear

H66.1 Chronic tubotympanic suppurative otitis media

Benign chronic suppurative otitis media
Chronic tubotympanic disease

Use additional code for any associated perforated tympanic membrane (H72.-)
- **H66.10** Chronic tubotympanic suppurative otitis media, unspecified
- **H66.11** Chronic tubotympanic suppurative otitis media, right ear
- **H66.12** Chronic tubotympanic suppurative otitis media, left ear
- **H66.13** Chronic tubotympanic suppurative otitis media, bilateral

H66.2 Chronic atticoantral suppurative otitis media

Chronic atticoantral disease

Use additional code for any associated perforated tympanic membrane (H72.-)
- **H66.20** Chronic atticoantral suppurative otitis media, unspecified ear
- **H66.21** Chronic atticoantral suppurative otitis media, right ear
- **H66.22** Chronic atticoantral suppurative otitis media, left ear
- **H66.23** Chronic atticoantral suppurative otitis media, bilateral

H66.3 Other chronic suppurative otitis media

Chronic suppurative otitis media NOS

Use additional code for any associated perforated tympanic membrane (H72.-)

EXCLUDES 1 *tuberculous otitis media (A18.6)*

H66.3X Other chronic suppurative otitis media
- **H66.3X1** Other chronic suppurative otitis media, right ear
- **H66.3X2** Other chronic suppurative otitis media, left ear
- **H66.3X3** Other chronic suppurative otitis media, bilateral
- **H66.3X9** Other chronic suppurative otitis media, unspecified ear

H66.4 Suppurative otitis media, unspecified

Purulent otitis media NOS

Use additional code for any associated perforated tympanic membrane (H72.-)
- **H66.40** Suppurative otitis media, unspecified, unspecified ear
- **H66.41** Suppurative otitis media, unspecified, right ear
- **H66.42** Suppurative otitis media, unspecified, left ear
- **H66.43** Suppurative otitis media, unspecified, bilateral

H66.9 Otitis media, unspecified

Otitis media NOS
Acute otitis media NOS
Chronic otitis media NOS

Use additional code for any associated perforated tympanic membrane (H72.-)
- **H66.90** Otitis media, unspecified, unspecified ear
- **H66.91** Otitis media, unspecified, right ear
- **H66.92** Otitis media, unspecified, left ear
- **H66.93** Otitis media, unspecified, bilateral

H67 Otitis media in diseases classified elsewhere

Code first underlying disease, such as:
- plasminogen deficiency (E88.02)
- viral disease NEC (B00-B34)

Use additional code for any associated perforated tympanic membrane (H72.-)

EXCLUDES 1 *otitis media in:*
- *influenza (J09.X9, J10.83, J11.83)*
- *measles (B05.3)*
- *scarlet fever (A38.0)*
- *tuberculosis (A18.6)*

- *H67.1 Otitis media in diseases classified elsewhere, right ear*
- *H67.2 Otitis media in diseases classified elsewhere, left ear*
- *H67.3 Otitis media in diseases classified elsewhere, bilateral*
- *H67.9 Otitis media in diseases classified elsewhere, unspecified ear*

H68 Eustachian salpingitis and obstruction

DEF: Eustachian tube: Internal channel between the tympanic cavity and the nasopharynx that equalizes internal pressure to the outside pressure and drains mucous production from the middle ear.

H68.0 Eustachian salpingitis

H68.00 Unspecified Eustachian salpingitis
- **H68.001** Unspecified Eustachian salpingitis, right ear
- **H68.002** Unspecified Eustachian salpingitis, left ear
- **H68.003** Unspecified Eustachian salpingitis, bilateral
- **H68.009** Unspecified Eustachian salpingitis, unspecified ear

H68.01 Acute Eustachian salpingitis
- **H68.011** Acute Eustachian salpingitis, right ear
- **H68.012** Acute Eustachian salpingitis, left ear
- **H68.013** Acute Eustachian salpingitis, bilateral
- **H68.019** Acute Eustachian salpingitis, unspecified ear

H68.02 Chronic Eustachian salpingitis
- **H68.021** Chronic Eustachian salpingitis, right ear
- **H68.022** Chronic Eustachian salpingitis, left ear

H68.023 Chronic Eustachian salpingitis, bilateral
H68.029 Chronic Eustachian salpingitis, unspecified ear

H68.1 Obstruction of Eustachian tube
Stenosis of Eustachian tube
Stricture of Eustachian tube

H68.10 Unspecified obstruction of Eustachian tube
H68.101 Unspecified obstruction of Eustachian tube, right ear
H68.102 Unspecified obstruction of Eustachian tube, left ear
H68.103 Unspecified obstruction of Eustachian tube, bilateral
H68.109 Unspecified obstruction of Eustachian tube, unspecified ear

H68.11 Osseous obstruction of Eustachian tube
H68.111 Osseous obstruction of Eustachian tube, right ear
H68.112 Osseous obstruction of Eustachian tube, left ear
H68.113 Osseous obstruction of Eustachian tube, bilateral
H68.119 Osseous obstruction of Eustachian tube, unspecified ear

H68.12 Intrinsic cartilagenous obstruction of Eustachian tube
H68.121 Intrinsic cartilagenous obstruction of Eustachian tube, right ear
H68.122 Intrinsic cartilagenous obstruction of Eustachian tube, left ear
H68.123 Intrinsic cartilagenous obstruction of Eustachian tube, bilateral
H68.129 Intrinsic cartilagenous obstruction of Eustachian tube, unspecified ear

H68.13 Extrinsic cartilagenous obstruction of Eustachian tube
Compression of Eustachian tube
H68.131 Extrinsic cartilagenous obstruction of Eustachian tube, right ear
H68.132 Extrinsic cartilagenous obstruction of Eustachian tube, left ear
H68.133 Extrinsic cartilagenous obstruction of Eustachian tube, bilateral
H68.139 Extrinsic cartilagenous obstruction of Eustachian tube, unspecified ear

H69 Other and unspecified disorders of Eustachian tube

DEF: Eustachian tube: Internal channel between the tympanic cavity and the nasopharynx that equalizes internal pressure to the outside pressure and drains mucous production from the middle ear.

H69.0 Patulous Eustachian tube
H69.00 Patulous Eustachian tube, unspecified ear
H69.01 Patulous Eustachian tube, right ear
H69.02 Patulous Eustachian tube, left ear
H69.03 Patulous Eustachian tube, bilateral

H69.8 Other specified disorders of Eustachian tube
H69.80 Other specified disorders of Eustachian tube, unspecified ear
H69.81 Other specified disorders of Eustachian tube, right ear
H69.82 Other specified disorders of Eustachian tube, left ear
H69.83 Other specified disorders of Eustachian tube, bilateral

H69.9 Unspecified Eustachian tube disorder
H69.90 Unspecified Eustachian tube disorder, unspecified ear
H69.91 Unspecified Eustachian tube disorder, right ear
H69.92 Unspecified Eustachian tube disorder, left ear
H69.93 Unspecified Eustachian tube disorder, bilateral

H70 Mastoiditis and related conditions

H70.0 Acute mastoiditis
Abscess of mastoid
Empyema of mastoid

H70.00 Acute mastoiditis without complications
H70.001 Acute mastoiditis without complications, right ear CC
H70.002 Acute mastoiditis without complications, left ear CC
H70.003 Acute mastoiditis without complications, bilateral CC
H70.009 Acute mastoiditis without complications, unspecified ear CC UNS

H70.01 Subperiosteal abscess of mastoid
H70.011 Subperiosteal abscess of mastoid, right ear CC
H70.012 Subperiosteal abscess of mastoid, left ear CC
H70.013 Subperiosteal abscess of mastoid, bilateral CC
H70.019 Subperiosteal abscess of mastoid, unspecified ear CC UNS

H70.09 Acute mastoiditis with other complications
H70.091 Acute mastoiditis with other complications, right ear CC
H70.092 Acute mastoiditis with other complications, left ear CC
H70.093 Acute mastoiditis with other complications, bilateral CC
H70.099 Acute mastoiditis with other complications, unspecified ear CC UNS

H70.1 Chronic mastoiditis
Caries of mastoid
Fistula of mastoid
EXCLUDES 1 *tuberculous mastoiditis (A18.03)*
H70.10 Chronic mastoiditis, unspecified ear
H70.11 Chronic mastoiditis, right ear
H70.12 Chronic mastoiditis, left ear
H70.13 Chronic mastoiditis, bilateral

H70.2 Petrositis
Inflammation of petrous bone

H70.20 Unspecified petrositis
H70.201 Unspecified petrositis, right ear
H70.202 Unspecified petrositis, left ear
H70.203 Unspecified petrositis, bilateral
H70.209 Unspecified petrositis, unspecified ear

H70.21 Acute petrositis
DEF: Sudden, severe inflammation of the petrous temporal bone behind the ear, associated with a middle ear infection.
H70.211 Acute petrositis, right ear
H70.212 Acute petrositis, left ear
H70.213 Acute petrositis, bilateral
H70.219 Acute petrositis, unspecified ear

H70.22 Chronic petrositis
H70.221 Chronic petrositis, right ear
H70.222 Chronic petrositis, left ear
H70.223 Chronic petrositis, bilateral
H70.229 Chronic petrositis, unspecified ear

H70.8 Other mastoiditis and related conditions
EXCLUDES 1 *preauricular sinus and cyst (Q18.1)*
sinus, fistula, and cyst of branchial cleft (Q18.0)

H70.81 Postauricular fistula
H70.811 Postauricular fistula, right ear
H70.812 Postauricular fistula, left ear
H70.813 Postauricular fistula, bilateral
H70.819 Postauricular fistula, unspecified ear

H70.89 Other mastoiditis and related conditions
H70.891 Other mastoiditis and related conditions, right ear
H70.892 Other mastoiditis and related conditions, left ear
H70.893 Other mastoiditis and related conditions, bilateral
H70.899 Other mastoiditis and related conditions, unspecified ear

H70.9 Unspecified mastoiditis
H70.90 Unspecified mastoiditis, unspecified ear
H70.91 Unspecified mastoiditis, right ear
H70.92 Unspecified mastoiditis, left ear
H70.93 Unspecified mastoiditis, bilateral

H71 Cholesteatoma of middle ear

EXCLUDES 2 *cholesteatoma of external ear (H60.4-)*
recurrent cholesteatoma of postmastoidectomy cavity (H95.0-)

AHA: 2021,3Q,8

DEF: Cholesteatoma: Noncancerous cyst-like mass of cell debris, including cholesterol and epithelial cells resulting from trauma, repeated or improperly healed infections, and congenital enclosure of epidermal cells.

Cholesteatoma of Middle Ear

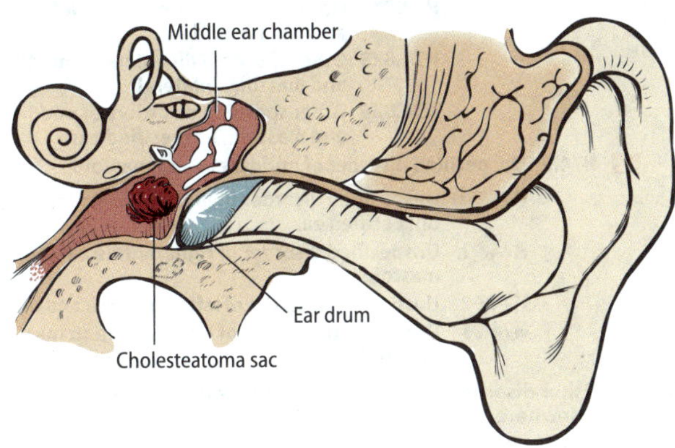

H71.0 Cholesteatoma of attic
- **H71.00** Cholesteatoma of attic, unspecified ear
- **H71.01** Cholesteatoma of attic, right ear
- **H71.02** Cholesteatoma of attic, left ear
- **H71.03** Cholesteatoma of attic, bilateral

H71.1 Cholesteatoma of tympanum
- **H71.10** Cholesteatoma of tympanum, unspecified ear
- **H71.11** Cholesteatoma of tympanum, right ear
- **H71.12** Cholesteatoma of tympanum, left ear
- **H71.13** Cholesteatoma of tympanum, bilateral

H71.2 Cholesteatoma of mastoid
- **H71.20** Cholesteatoma of mastoid, unspecified ear
- **H71.21** Cholesteatoma of mastoid, right ear
- **H71.22** Cholesteatoma of mastoid, left ear
- **H71.23** Cholesteatoma of mastoid, bilateral

H71.3 Diffuse cholesteatosis

AHA: 2021,3Q,8
- **H71.30** Diffuse cholesteatosis, unspecified ear
- **H71.31** Diffuse cholesteatosis, right ear
- **H71.32** Diffuse cholesteatosis, left ear
- **H71.33** Diffuse cholesteatosis, bilateral

H71.9 Unspecified cholesteatoma
- **H71.90** Unspecified cholesteatoma, unspecified ear
- **H71.91** Unspecified cholesteatoma, right ear
- **H71.92** Unspecified cholesteatoma, left ear
- **H71.93** Unspecified cholesteatoma, bilateral

H72 Perforation of tympanic membrane

INCLUDES persistent post-traumatic perforation of ear drum
postinflammatory perforation of ear drum

Code first any associated otitis media (H65.-, H66.1-, H66.2-, H66.3-, H66.4-, H66.9-, H67.-)

EXCLUDES 1 *acute suppurative otitis media with rupture of the tympanic membrane (H66.01-)*
traumatic rupture of ear drum (S09.2-)

H72.0 Central perforation of tympanic membrane
- **H72.00** Central perforation of tympanic membrane, unspecified ear
- **H72.01** Central perforation of tympanic membrane, right ear
- **H72.02** Central perforation of tympanic membrane, left ear
- **H72.03** Central perforation of tympanic membrane, bilateral

H72.1 Attic perforation of tympanic membrane

Perforation of pars flaccida
- **H72.10** Attic perforation of tympanic membrane, unspecified ear
- **H72.11** Attic perforation of tympanic membrane, right ear
- **H72.12** Attic perforation of tympanic membrane, left ear
- **H72.13** Attic perforation of tympanic membrane, bilateral

H72.2 Other marginal perforations of tympanic membrane

H72.2X Other marginal perforations of tympanic membrane
- **H72.2X1** Other marginal perforations of tympanic membrane, right ear
- **H72.2X2** Other marginal perforations of tympanic membrane, left ear
- **H72.2X3** Other marginal perforations of tympanic membrane, bilateral
- **H72.2X9** Other marginal perforations of tympanic membrane, unspecified ear

H72.8 Other perforations of tympanic membrane

H72.81 Multiple perforations of tympanic membrane
- **H72.811** Multiple perforations of tympanic membrane, right ear
- **H72.812** Multiple perforations of tympanic membrane, left ear
- **H72.813** Multiple perforations of tympanic membrane, bilateral
- **H72.819** Multiple perforations of tympanic membrane, unspecified ear

H72.82 Total perforations of tympanic membrane
- **H72.821** Total perforations of tympanic membrane, right ear
- **H72.822** Total perforations of tympanic membrane, left ear
- **H72.823** Total perforations of tympanic membrane, bilateral
- **H72.829** Total perforations of tympanic membrane, unspecified ear

H72.9 Unspecified perforation of tympanic membrane
- **H72.90** Unspecified perforation of tympanic membrane, unspecified ear
- **H72.91** Unspecified perforation of tympanic membrane, right ear
- **H72.92** Unspecified perforation of tympanic membrane, left ear
- **H72.93** Unspecified perforation of tympanic membrane, bilateral

H73 Other disorders of tympanic membrane

H73.0 Acute myringitis

EXCLUDES 1 *acute myringitis with otitis media (H65, H66)*

H73.00 Unspecified acute myringitis

Acute tympanitis NOS
- **H73.001** Acute myringitis, right ear
- **H73.002** Acute myringitis, left ear
- **H73.003** Acute myringitis, bilateral
- **H73.009** Acute myringitis, unspecified ear

H73.01 Bullous myringitis

DEF: Bacterial or viral otitis media that is characterized by the appearance of serous or hemorrhagic blebs on the ear drum and sudden onset of severe pain in ear.
- **H73.011** Bullous myringitis, right ear
- **H73.012** Bullous myringitis, left ear
- **H73.013** Bullous myringitis, bilateral
- **H73.019** Bullous myringitis, unspecified ear

H73.09 Other acute myringitis
- **H73.091** Other acute myringitis, right ear
- **H73.092** Other acute myringitis, left ear
- **H73.093** Other acute myringitis, bilateral
- **H73.099** Other acute myringitis, unspecified ear

H73.1 Chronic myringitis

Chronic tympanitis

EXCLUDES 1 *chronic myringitis with otitis media (H65, H66)*
- **H73.10** Chronic myringitis, unspecified ear
- **H73.11** Chronic myringitis, right ear
- **H73.12** Chronic myringitis, left ear
- **H73.13** Chronic myringitis, bilateral

H73.2 Unspecified myringitis
- **H73.20** Unspecified myringitis, unspecified ear
- **H73.21** Unspecified myringitis, right ear
- **H73.22** Unspecified myringitis, left ear
- **H73.23** Unspecified myringitis, bilateral

H73.8 Other specified disorders of tympanic membrane

H73.81 Atrophic flaccid tympanic membrane
- **H73.811** Atrophic flaccid tympanic membrane, right ear

H73.812 Atrophic flaccid tympanic membrane, left ear
H73.813 Atrophic flaccid tympanic membrane, bilateral
H73.819 Atrophic flaccid tympanic membrane, unspecified ear

6th H73.82 Atrophic nonflaccid tympanic membrane
H73.821 Atrophic nonflaccid tympanic membrane, right ear
H73.822 Atrophic nonflaccid tympanic membrane, left ear
H73.823 Atrophic nonflaccid tympanic membrane, bilateral
H73.829 Atrophic nonflaccid tympanic membrane, unspecified ear

6th H73.89 Other specified disorders of tympanic membrane
H73.891 Other specified disorders of tympanic membrane, right ear
H73.892 Other specified disorders of tympanic membrane, left ear
H73.893 Other specified disorders of tympanic membrane, bilateral
H73.899 Other specified disorders of tympanic membrane, unspecified ear

5th H73.9 Unspecified disorder of tympanic membrane
H73.90 Unspecified disorder of tympanic membrane, unspecified ear
H73.91 Unspecified disorder of tympanic membrane, right ear
H73.92 Unspecified disorder of tympanic membrane, left ear
H73.93 Unspecified disorder of tympanic membrane, bilateral

4th **H74 Other disorders of middle ear mastoid**

EXCLUDES 2 mastoiditis (H70.-)

5th H74.0 Tympanosclerosis

DEF: Calcification of tissue in the ear drum, middle ear bones, and middle ear canal.

H74.01 Tympanosclerosis, right ear
H74.02 Tympanosclerosis, left ear
H74.03 Tympanosclerosis, bilateral
H74.09 Tympanosclerosis, unspecified ear

5th H74.1 Adhesive middle ear disease

Adhesive otitis

EXCLUDES 1 glue ear (H65.3-)

H74.11 Adhesive right middle ear disease
H74.12 Adhesive left middle ear disease
H74.13 Adhesive middle ear disease, bilateral
H74.19 Adhesive middle ear disease, unspecified ear

5th H74.2 Discontinuity and dislocation of ear ossicles
H74.20 Discontinuity and dislocation of ear ossicles, unspecified ear
H74.21 Discontinuity and dislocation of right ear ossicles
H74.22 Discontinuity and dislocation of left ear ossicles
H74.23 Discontinuity and dislocation of ear ossicles, bilateral

5th H74.3 Other acquired abnormalities of ear ossicles

6th H74.31 Ankylosis of ear ossicles
H74.311 Ankylosis of ear ossicles, right ear
H74.312 Ankylosis of ear ossicles, left ear
H74.313 Ankylosis of ear ossicles, bilateral
H74.319 Ankylosis of ear ossicles, unspecified ear

6th H74.32 Partial loss of ear ossicles
H74.321 Partial loss of ear ossicles, right ear
H74.322 Partial loss of ear ossicles, left ear
H74.323 Partial loss of ear ossicles, bilateral
H74.329 Partial loss of ear ossicles, unspecified ear

6th H74.39 Other acquired abnormalities of ear ossicles
H74.391 Other acquired abnormalities of right ear ossicles
H74.392 Other acquired abnormalities of left ear ossicles
H74.393 Other acquired abnormalities of ear ossicles, bilateral
H74.399 Other acquired abnormalities of ear ossicles, unspecified ear

5th H74.4 Polyp of middle ear
H74.40 Polyp of middle ear, unspecified ear
H74.41 Polyp of right middle ear
H74.42 Polyp of left middle ear
H74.43 Polyp of middle ear, bilateral

5th H74.8 Other specified disorders of middle ear and mastoid

6th H74.8X Other specified disorders of middle ear and mastoid
H74.8X1 Other specified disorders of right middle ear and mastoid
H74.8X2 Other specified disorders of left middle ear and mastoid
H74.8X3 Other specified disorders of middle ear and mastoid, bilateral
H74.8X9 Other specified disorders of middle ear and mastoid, unspecified ear

5th H74.9 Unspecified disorder of middle ear and mastoid
H74.90 Unspecified disorder of middle ear and mastoid, unspecified ear
H74.91 Unspecified disorder of right middle ear and mastoid
H74.92 Unspecified disorder of left middle ear and mastoid
H74.93 Unspecified disorder of middle ear and mastoid, bilateral

4th **H75 Other disorders of middle ear and mastoid in diseases classified elsewhere**

Code first underlying disease

5th H75.0 Mastoiditis in infectious and parasitic diseases classified elsewhere

EXCLUDES 1 mastoiditis (in):
syphilis (A52.77)
tuberculosis (A18.03)

H75.00 Mastoiditis in infectious and parasitic diseases classified elsewhere, unspecified ear
H75.01 Mastoiditis in infectious and parasitic diseases classified elsewhere, right ear
H75.02 Mastoiditis in infectious and parasitic diseases classified elsewhere, left ear
H75.03 Mastoiditis in infectious and parasitic diseases classified elsewhere, bilateral

5th H75.8 Other specified disorders of middle ear and mastoid in diseases classified elsewhere
H75.80 Other specified disorders of middle ear and mastoid in diseases classified elsewhere, unspecified ear
H75.81 Other specified disorders of right middle ear and mastoid in diseases classified elsewhere
H75.82 Other specified disorders of left middle ear and mastoid in diseases classified elsewhere
H75.83 Other specified disorders of middle ear and mastoid in diseases classified elsewhere, bilateral

Diseases of inner ear (H80-H83)

4th **H80 Otosclerosis**

INCLUDES otospongiosis

5th H80.0 Otosclerosis involving oval window, nonobliterative
H80.00 Otosclerosis involving oval window, nonobliterative, unspecified ear
H80.01 Otosclerosis involving oval window, nonobliterative, right ear
H80.02 Otosclerosis involving oval window, nonobliterative, left ear
H80.03 Otosclerosis involving oval window, nonobliterative, bilateral

5th H80.1 Otosclerosis involving oval window, obliterative
H80.10 Otosclerosis involving oval window, obliterative, unspecified ear
H80.11 Otosclerosis involving oval window, obliterative, right ear
H80.12 Otosclerosis involving oval window, obliterative, left ear
H80.13 Otosclerosis involving oval window, obliterative, bilateral

5th H80.2 Cochlear otosclerosis

Otosclerosis involving otic capsule
Otosclerosis involving round window

H80.20 Cochlear otosclerosis, unspecified ear
H80.21 Cochlear otosclerosis, right ear
H80.22 Cochlear otosclerosis, left ear
H80.23 Cochlear otosclerosis, bilateral

✓5th **H80.8 Other otosclerosis**
- **H80.80 Other otosclerosis, unspecified ear**
- **H80.81 Other otosclerosis, right ear**
- **H80.82 Other otosclerosis, left ear**
- **H80.83 Other otosclerosis, bilateral**

✓5th **H80.9 Unspecified otosclerosis**
- **H80.90 Unspecified otosclerosis, unspecified ear**
- **H80.91 Unspecified otosclerosis, right ear**
- **H80.92 Unspecified otosclerosis, left ear**
- **H80.93 Unspecified otosclerosis, bilateral**

✓4th **H81 Disorders of vestibular function**

EXCLUDES 1 *epidemic vertigo (A88.1)*
vertigo NOS (R42)

✓5th **H81.0 Meniere's disease**

Labyrinthine hydrops
Meniere's syndrome or vertigo
DEF: Distended membranous labyrinth of the middle ear from fluctuating pressure of fluid (hydrops) that causes vertigo, tinnitus, pressure, and hearing loss that may last on and off for several hours. Episodes may occur in clusters or may subside for weeks, months, or even years.
- **H81.01 Meniere's disease, right ear**
- **H81.02 Meniere's disease, left ear**
- **H81.03 Meniere's disease, bilateral**
- **H81.09 Meniere's disease, unspecified ear**

✓5th **H81.1 Benign paroxysmal vertigo**
- **H81.10 Benign paroxysmal vertigo, unspecified ear**
- **H81.11 Benign paroxysmal vertigo, right ear**
- **H81.12 Benign paroxysmal vertigo, left ear**
- **H81.13 Benign paroxysmal vertigo, bilateral**

✓5th **H81.2 Vestibular neuronitis**

DEF: Transient benign vertigo caused by inflammation of the vestibular nerve. It is characterized by response to caloric stimulation on one side and nystagmus with rhythmic movement of the eyes. Normal auditory function is present.
- **H81.20 Vestibular neuronitis, unspecified ear**
- **H81.21 Vestibular neuronitis, right ear**
- **H81.22 Vestibular neuronitis, left ear**
- **H81.23 Vestibular neuronitis, bilateral**

✓5th **H81.3 Other peripheral vertigo**

✓6th **H81.31 Aural vertigo**
- **H81.311 Aural vertigo, right ear**
- **H81.312 Aural vertigo, left ear**
- **H81.313 Aural vertigo, bilateral**
- **H81.319 Aural vertigo, unspecified ear**

✓6th **H81.39 Other peripheral vertigo**

Lermoyez' syndrome
Otogenic vertigo
Peripheral vertigo NOS
- **H81.391 Other peripheral vertigo, right ear**
- **H81.392 Other peripheral vertigo, left ear**
- **H81.393 Other peripheral vertigo, bilateral**
- **H81.399 Other peripheral vertigo, unspecified ear**

H81.4 Vertigo of central origin

Central positional nystagmus

✓5th **H81.8 Other disorders of vestibular function**

✓6th **H81.8X Other disorders of vestibular function**
- **H81.8X1 Other disorders of vestibular function, right ear**
- **H81.8X2 Other disorders of vestibular function, left ear**
- **H81.8X3 Other disorders of vestibular function, bilateral**
- **H81.8X9 Other disorders of vestibular function, unspecified ear**

  AHA: 2022,2Q,12

✓5th **H81.9 Unspecified disorder of vestibular function**

Vertiginous syndrome NOS
- **H81.90 Unspecified disorder of vestibular function, unspecified ear**
- **H81.91 Unspecified disorder of vestibular function, right ear**
- **H81.92 Unspecified disorder of vestibular function, left ear**
- **H81.93 Unspecified disorder of vestibular function, bilateral**

✓4th **H82 Vertiginous syndromes in diseases classified elsewhere**

Code first underlying disease

EXCLUDES 1 *epidemic vertigo (A88.1)*
- *H82.1* ***Vertiginous syndromes in diseases classified elsewhere, right ear***
- *H82.2* ***Vertiginous syndromes in diseases classified elsewhere, left ear***
- *H82.3* ***Vertiginous syndromes in diseases classified elsewhere, bilateral***
- *H82.9* ***Vertiginous syndromes in diseases classified elsewhere, unspecified ear***

✓4th **H83 Other diseases of inner ear**

✓5th **H83.0 Labyrinthitis**

DEF: Inflammation of the inner ear, or labyrinth, characterized by pus, vertigo, dizziness, nausea, and hearing loss.
- **H83.01 Labyrinthitis, right ear**
- **H83.02 Labyrinthitis, left ear**
- **H83.03 Labyrinthitis, bilateral**
- **H83.09 Labyrinthitis, unspecified ear**

✓5th **H83.1 Labyrinthine fistula**
- **H83.11 Labyrinthine fistula, right ear**
- **H83.12 Labyrinthine fistula, left ear**
- **H83.13 Labyrinthine fistula, bilateral**
- **H83.19 Labyrinthine fistula, unspecified ear**

✓5th **H83.2 Labyrinthine dysfunction**

Labyrinthine hypersensitivity
Labyrinthine hypofunction
Labyrinthine loss of function
DEF: Decreased function of the labyrinth sensors.

✓6th **H83.2X Labyrinthine dysfunction**
- **H83.2X1 Labyrinthine dysfunction, right ear**
- **H83.2X2 Labyrinthine dysfunction, left ear**
- **H83.2X3 Labyrinthine dysfunction, bilateral**
- **H83.2X9 Labyrinthine dysfunction, unspecified ear**

✓5th **H83.3 Noise effects on inner ear**

Acoustic trauma of inner ear
Noise-induced hearing loss of inner ear

✓6th **H83.3X Noise effects on inner ear**
- **H83.3X1 Noise effects on right inner ear**
- **H83.3X2 Noise effects on left inner ear**
- **H83.3X3 Noise effects on inner ear, bilateral**
- **H83.3X9 Noise effects on inner ear, unspecified ear**

✓5th **H83.8 Other specified diseases of inner ear**

✓6th **H83.8X Other specified diseases of inner ear**
- **H83.8X1 Other specified diseases of right inner ear**
- **H83.8X2 Other specified diseases of left inner ear**
- **H83.8X3 Other specified diseases of inner ear, bilateral**
- **H83.8X9 Other specified diseases of inner ear, unspecified ear**

✓5th **H83.9 Unspecified disease of inner ear**
- **H83.90 Unspecified disease of inner ear, unspecified ear**
- **H83.91 Unspecified disease of right inner ear**
- **H83.92 Unspecified disease of left inner ear**
- **H83.93 Unspecified disease of inner ear, bilateral**

Other disorders of ear (H90-H94)

✓4th **H90 Conductive and sensorineural hearing loss**

EXCLUDES 1 *deaf nonspeaking NEC (H91.3)*
deafness NOS (H91.9-)
hearing loss NOS (H91.9-)
noise-induced hearing loss (H83.3-)
ototoxic hearing loss (H91.0-)
sudden (idiopathic) hearing loss (H91.2-)

AHA: 2015,2Q,7
DEF: Conductive hearing loss: Hearing loss due to the inability of soundwaves to move from the outer (external) ear to the inner ear.
DEF: Sensorineural hearing loss: Hearing loss that occurs from damage to the hair cells of the inner ear or problems with the nerve pathways from the inner ear to the brain.

H90.0 Conductive hearing loss, bilateral

Chapter 8. Diseases of the Ear and Mastoid Process

H80.8–H90.0

5th H90.1 Conductive hearing loss, unilateral with unrestricted hearing on the contralateral side
- H90.11 Conductive hearing loss, unilateral, right ear, with unrestricted hearing on the contralateral side
- H90.12 Conductive hearing loss, unilateral, left ear, with unrestricted hearing on the contralateral side

H90.2 Conductive hearing loss, unspecified
Conductive deafness NOS

H90.3 Sensorineural hearing loss, bilateral

5th H90.4 Sensorineural hearing loss, unilateral with unrestricted hearing on the contralateral side
- H90.41 Sensorineural hearing loss, unilateral, right ear, with unrestricted hearing on the contralateral side
- H90.42 Sensorineural hearing loss, unilateral, left ear, with unrestricted hearing on the contralateral side

H90.5 Unspecified sensorineural hearing loss
Central hearing loss NOS
Congenital deafness NOS
Neural hearing loss NOS
Perceptive hearing loss NOS
Sensorineural deafness NOS
Sensory hearing loss NOS
EXCLUDES 1 *abnormal auditory perception (H93.2-)*
psychogenic deafness (F44.6)

H90.6 Mixed conductive and sensorineural hearing loss, bilateral
AHA: 2015,2Q,7

5th H90.7 Mixed conductive and sensorineural hearing loss, unilateral with unrestricted hearing on the contralateral side
- H90.71 Mixed conductive and sensorineural hearing loss, unilateral, right ear, with unrestricted hearing on the contralateral side
- H90.72 Mixed conductive and sensorineural hearing loss, unilateral, left ear, with unrestricted hearing on the contralateral side

H90.8 Mixed conductive and sensorineural hearing loss, unspecified

5th H90.A Conductive and sensorineural hearing loss with restricted hearing on the contralateral side
AHA: 2016,4Q,23-25

6th H90.A1 Conductive hearing loss, unilateral, with restricted hearing on the contralateral side
- H90.A11 Conductive hearing loss, unilateral, right ear with restricted hearing on the contralateral side
- H90.A12 Conductive hearing loss, unilateral, left ear with restricted hearing on the contralateral side

6th H90.A2 Sensorineural hearing loss, unilateral, with restricted hearing on the contralateral side
- H90.A21 Sensorineural hearing loss, unilateral, right ear, with restricted hearing on the contralateral side
- H90.A22 Sensorineural hearing loss, unilateral, left ear, with restricted hearing on the contralateral side

6th H90.A3 Mixed conductive and sensorineural hearing loss, unilateral with restricted hearing on the contralateral side
- H90.A31 Mixed conductive and sensorineural hearing loss, unilateral, right ear with restricted hearing on the contralateral side
- H90.A32 Mixed conductive and sensorineural hearing, unilateral, left ear with restricted hearing on the contralateral side

4th H91 Other and unspecified hearing loss
EXCLUDES 1 *abnormal auditory perception (H93.2-)*
hearing loss as classified in H90.-
impacted cerumen (H61.2-)
noise-induced hearing loss (H83.3-)
psychogenic deafness (F44.6)
transient ischemic deafness (H93.01-)

5th H91.0 Ototoxic hearing loss
Code first poisoning due to drug or toxin, if applicable ►(T36-T65 with fifth or sixth character 1-4)◄
Use additional code for adverse effect, if applicable, to identify drug (T36-T50 with fifth or sixth character 5)
- H91.01 Ototoxic hearing loss, right ear
- H91.02 Ototoxic hearing loss, left ear
- H91.03 Ototoxic hearing loss, bilateral
- H91.09 Ototoxic hearing loss, unspecified ear

5th H91.1 Presbycusis
Presbyacusia
- H91.10 Presbycusis, unspecified ear
- H91.11 Presbycusis, right ear
- H91.12 Presbycusis, left ear
- H91.13 Presbycusis, bilateral

5th H91.2 Sudden idiopathic hearing loss
Sudden hearing loss NOS
- H91.20 Sudden idiopathic hearing loss, unspecified ear
- H91.21 Sudden idiopathic hearing loss, right ear
- H91.22 Sudden idiopathic hearing loss, left ear
- H91.23 Sudden idiopathic hearing loss, bilateral

H91.3 Deaf nonspeaking, not elsewhere classified

5th H91.8 Other specified hearing loss

6th H91.8X Other specified hearing loss
- H91.8X1 Other specified hearing loss, right ear
- H91.8X2 Other specified hearing loss, left ear
- H91.8X3 Other specified hearing loss, bilateral
- H91.8X9 Other specified hearing loss, unspecified ear

5th H91.9 Unspecified hearing loss
Deafness NOS
High frequency deafness
Low frequency deafness
- H91.90 Unspecified hearing loss, unspecified ear
- H91.91 Unspecified hearing loss, right ear
- H91.92 Unspecified hearing loss, left ear
- H91.93 Unspecified hearing loss, bilateral

4th H92 Otalgia and effusion of ear

5th H92.0 Otalgia
- H92.01 Otalgia, right ear
- H92.02 Otalgia, left ear
- H92.03 Otalgia, bilateral
- H92.09 Otalgia, unspecified ear

5th H92.1 Otorrhea
EXCLUDES 1 *leakage of cerebrospinal fluid through ear (G96.0)*
- H92.10 Otorrhea, unspecified ear
- H92.11 Otorrhea, right ear
- H92.12 Otorrhea, left ear
- H92.13 Otorrhea, bilateral

5th H92.2 Otorrhagia
EXCLUDES 1 *traumatic otorrhagia - code to injury*
- H92.20 Otorrhagia, unspecified ear
- H92.21 Otorrhagia, right ear
- H92.22 Otorrhagia, left ear
- H92.23 Otorrhagia, bilateral

4th H93 Other disorders of ear, not elsewhere classified

5th H93.0 Degenerative and vascular disorders of ear
EXCLUDES 1 *presbycusis (H91.1)*

6th H93.01 Transient ischemic deafness
- H93.011 Transient ischemic deafness, right ear
- H93.012 Transient ischemic deafness, left ear
- H93.013 Transient ischemic deafness, bilateral
- H93.019 Transient ischemic deafness, unspecified ear

6th H93.09 Unspecified degenerative and vascular disorders of ear
- H93.091 Unspecified degenerative and vascular disorders of right ear
- H93.092 Unspecified degenerative and vascular disorders of left ear
- H93.093 Unspecified degenerative and vascular disorders of ear, bilateral
- H93.099 Unspecified degenerative and vascular disorders of unspecified ear

5th H93.1 Tinnitus
- H93.11 Tinnitus, right ear
- H93.12 Tinnitus, left ear
- H93.13 Tinnitus, bilateral
- H93.19 Tinnitus, unspecified ear

5th H93.A Pulsatile tinnitus
AHA: 2023,2Q,18; 2016,4Q,25-26
- H93.A1 Pulsatile tinnitus, right ear
- H93.A2 Pulsatile tinnitus, left ear
- H93.A3 Pulsatile tinnitus, bilateral

H93.A9 Pulsatile tinnitus, unspecified ear

H93.2 Other abnormal auditory perceptions

EXCLUDES 2 *auditory hallucinations (R44.Ø)*

H93.21 Auditory recruitment

H93.211 Auditory recruitment, right ear

H93.212 Auditory recruitment, left ear

H93.213 Auditory recruitment, bilateral

H93.219 Auditory recruitment, unspecified ear

H93.22 Diplacusis

H93.221 Diplacusis, right ear

H93.222 Diplacusis, left ear

H93.223 Diplacusis, bilateral

H93.229 Diplacusis, unspecified ear

H93.23 Hyperacusis

DEF: Exceptionally acute sense of hearing caused by such conditions as Bell's palsy. This term may also refer to painful sensitivity to sounds.

H93.231 Hyperacusis, right ear

H93.232 Hyperacusis, left ear

H93.233 Hyperacusis, bilateral

H93.239 Hyperacusis, unspecified ear

H93.24 Temporary auditory threshold shift

H93.241 Temporary auditory threshold shift, right ear

H93.242 Temporary auditory threshold shift, left ear

H93.243 Temporary auditory threshold shift, bilateral

H93.249 Temporary auditory threshold shift, unspecified ear

H93.25 Central auditory processing disorder

Congenital auditory imperception

Word deafness

EXCLUDES 1 *mixed receptive-expressive language disorder (F8Ø.2)*

H93.29 Other abnormal auditory perceptions

H93.291 Other abnormal auditory perceptions, right ear

H93.292 Other abnormal auditory perceptions, left ear

H93.293 Other abnormal auditory perceptions, bilateral

H93.299 Other abnormal auditory perceptions, unspecified ear

H93.3 Disorders of acoustic nerve

Disorder of 8th cranial nerve

EXCLUDES 1 *acoustic neuroma (D33.3)*

syphilitic acoustic neuritis (A52.15)

H93.3X Disorders of acoustic nerve

H93.3X1 Disorders of right acoustic nerve

H93.3X2 Disorders of left acoustic nerve

H93.3X3 Disorders of bilateral acoustic nerves

H93.3X9 Disorders of unspecified acoustic nerve

H93.8 Other specified disorders of ear

H93.8X Other specified disorders of ear

H93.8X1 Other specified disorders of right ear

H93.8X2 Other specified disorders of left ear

H93.8X3 Other specified disorders of ear, bilateral

H93.8X9 Other specified disorders of ear, unspecified ear

H93.9 Unspecified disorder of ear

H93.9Ø Unspecified disorder of ear, unspecified ear UPD

H93.91 Unspecified disorder of right ear UPD

H93.92 Unspecified disorder of left ear UPD

H93.93 Unspecified disorder of ear, bilateral UPD

H94 Other disorders of ear in diseases classified elsewhere

H94.Ø Acoustic neuritis in infectious and parasitic diseases classified elsewhere

Code first underlying disease, such as:

parasitic disease (B65-B89)

EXCLUDES 1 *acoustic neuritis (in):*

herpes zoster (BØ2.29)

syphilis (A52.15)

H94.ØØ Acoustic neuritis in infectious and parasitic diseases classified elsewhere, unspecified ear

H94.Ø1 Acoustic neuritis in infectious and parasitic diseases classified elsewhere, right ear

H94.Ø2 Acoustic neuritis in infectious and parasitic diseases classified elsewhere, left ear

H94.Ø3 Acoustic neuritis in infectious and parasitic diseases classified elsewhere, bilateral

H94.8 Other specified disorders of ear in diseases classified elsewhere

Code first underlying disease, such as:

congenital syphilis (A5Ø.Ø)

EXCLUDES 1 *aural myiasis (B87.4)*

syphilitic labyrinthitis (A52.79)

H94.8Ø Other specified disorders of ear in diseases classified elsewhere, unspecified ear

H94.81 Other specified disorders of right ear in diseases classified elsewhere

H94.82 Other specified disorders of left ear in diseases classified elsewhere

H94.83 Other specified disorders of ear in diseases classified elsewhere, bilateral

Intraoperative and postprocedural complications and disorders of ear and mastoid process, not elsewhere classified (H95)

H95 Intraoperative and postprocedural complications and disorders of ear and mastoid process, not elsewhere classified

AHA: 2016,4Q,9-10

H95.Ø Recurrent cholesteatoma of postmastoidectomy cavity

H95.ØØ Recurrent cholesteatoma of postmastoidectomy cavity, unspecified ear

H95.Ø1 Recurrent cholesteatoma of postmastoidectomy cavity, right ear

H95.Ø2 Recurrent cholesteatoma of postmastoidectomy cavity, left ear

H95.Ø3 Recurrent cholesteatoma of postmastoidectomy cavity, bilateral ears

H95.1 Other disorders of ear and mastoid process following mastoidectomy

H95.11 Chronic inflammation of postmastoidectomy cavity

H95.111 Chronic inflammation of postmastoidectomy cavity, right ear

H95.112 Chronic inflammation of postmastoidectomy cavity, left ear

H95.113 Chronic inflammation of postmastoidectomy cavity, bilateral ears

H95.119 Chronic inflammation of postmastoidectomy cavity, unspecified ear

H95.12 Granulation of postmastoidectomy cavity

H95.121 Granulation of postmastoidectomy cavity, right ear

H95.122 Granulation of postmastoidectomy cavity, left ear

H95.123 Granulation of postmastoidectomy cavity, bilateral ears

H95.129 Granulation of postmastoidectomy cavity, unspecified ear

H95.13 Mucosal cyst of postmastoidectomy cavity

H95.131 Mucosal cyst of postmastoidectomy cavity, right ear

H95.132 Mucosal cyst of postmastoidectomy cavity, left ear

H95.133 Mucosal cyst of postmastoidectomy cavity, bilateral ears

H95.139 Mucosal cyst of postmastoidectomy cavity, unspecified ear

H95.19 Other disorders following mastoidectomy

H95.191 Other disorders following mastoidectomy, right ear

H95.192 Other disorders following mastoidectomy, left ear

H95.193 Other disorders following mastoidectomy, bilateral ears

H95.199 Other disorders following mastoidectomy, unspecified ear

H95.2 Intraoperative hemorrhage and hematoma of ear and mastoid process complicating a procedure ✓5th

EXCLUDES 1 *intraoperative hemorrhage and hematoma of ear and mastoid process due to accidental puncture or laceration during a procedure (H95.3-)*

H95.21 Intraoperative hemorrhage and hematoma of ear and mastoid process complicating a procedure on the ear and mastoid process CC

H95.22 Intraoperative hemorrhage and hematoma of ear and mastoid process complicating other procedure CC

H95.3 Accidental puncture and laceration of ear and mastoid process during a procedure ✓5th

H95.31 Accidental puncture and laceration of the ear and mastoid process during a procedure on the ear and mastoid process CC

H95.32 Accidental puncture and laceration of the ear and mastoid process during other procedure CC

H95.4 Postprocedural hemorrhage of ear and mastoid process following a procedure ✓5th

H95.41 Postprocedural hemorrhage of ear and mastoid process following a procedure on the ear and mastoid process CC

H95.42 Postprocedural hemorrhage of ear and mastoid process following other procedure CC

H95.5 Postprocedural hematoma and seroma of ear and mastoid process following a procedure ✓5th

H95.51 Postprocedural hematoma of ear and mastoid process following a procedure on the ear and mastoid process CC

H95.52 Postprocedural hematoma of ear and mastoid process following other procedure CC

H95.53 Postprocedural seroma of ear and mastoid process following a procedure on the ear and mastoid process CC

H95.54 Postprocedural seroma of ear and mastoid process following other procedure CC

H95.8 Other intraoperative and postprocedural complications and disorders of the ear and mastoid process, not elsewhere classified ✓5th

EXCLUDES 2 *postprocedural complications and disorders following mastoidectomy (H95.Ø-, H95.1-)*

H95.81 Postprocedural stenosis of external ear canal ✓6th

H95.811 Postprocedural stenosis of right external ear canal CC

H95.812 Postprocedural stenosis of left external ear canal CC

H95.813 Postprocedural stenosis of external ear canal, bilateral CC

H95.819 Postprocedural stenosis of unspecified external ear canal CC UNS

H95.88 Other intraoperative complications and disorders of the ear and mastoid process, not elsewhere classified CC

Use additional code, if applicable, to further specify disorder

H95.89 Other postprocedural complications and disorders of the ear and mastoid process, not elsewhere classified CC

Use additional code, if applicable, to further specify disorder

Chapter 9. Diseases of the Circulatory System (I00–I99)

Chapter-specific Guidelines with Coding Examples

The chapter-specific guidelines from the ICD-10-CM Official Guidelines for Coding and Reporting have been provided below. Along with these guidelines are coding examples, contained in the shaded boxes, that have been developed to help illustrate the coding and/or sequencing guidance found in these guidelines.

a. Hypertension

The classification presumes a causal relationship between hypertension and heart involvement and between hypertension and kidney involvement, as the two conditions are linked by the term "with" in the Alphabetic Index. These conditions should be coded as related even in the absence of provider documentation explicitly linking them, unless the documentation clearly states the conditions are unrelated.

For hypertension and conditions not specifically linked by relational terms such as "with," "associated with" or "due to" in the classification, provider documentation must link the conditions in order to code them as related.

1) Hypertension with heart disease

Hypertension with heart conditions classified to I50.- or I51.4–I51.7, I51.89, I51.9, are assigned to a code from category I11, Hypertensive heart disease. Use additional code(s) from category I50, Heart failure, to identify the type(s) of heart failure in those patients with heart failure.

The same heart conditions (I50.-, I51.4–I51.7, I51.89, I51.9) with hypertension are coded separately if the provider has documented they are unrelated to the hypertension. Sequence according to the circumstances of the admission/encounter.

2) Hypertensive chronic kidney disease

Assign codes from category I12, Hypertensive chronic kidney disease, when both hypertension and a condition classifiable to category N18, Chronic kidney disease (CKD), are present. CKD should not be coded as hypertensive if the provider indicates the CKD is not related to the hypertension.

The appropriate code from category N18 should be used as a secondary code with a code from category I12 to identify the stage of chronic kidney disease.

See Section I.C.14. Chronic kidney disease.

If a patient has hypertensive chronic kidney disease and acute renal failure, the acute renal failure should also be coded. Sequence according to the circumstances of the admission/encounter.

Patient is admitted with stage IV chronic kidney disease (CKD) due to polycystic kidney disease. Patient also is on lisinopril for hypertension.

N18.4	**Chronic kidney disease, stage 4 (severe)**
Q61.3	**Polycystic kidney, unspecified**
I10	**Essential (primary) hypertension**

Explanation: A combination code describing a relationship between hypertension and CKD is not used because the physician documentation identifies the polycystic kidney disease as the cause for the CKD.

3) Hypertensive heart and chronic kidney disease

Assign codes from combination category I13, Hypertensive heart and chronic kidney disease, when there is hypertension with both heart and kidney involvement. If heart failure is present, assign an additional code from category I50 to identify the type of heart failure.

The appropriate code from category N18, Chronic kidney disease, should be used as a secondary code with a code from category I13 to identify the stage of chronic kidney disease.

See Section I.C.14. Chronic kidney disease.

The codes in category I13, Hypertensive heart and chronic kidney disease, are combination codes that include hypertension, heart disease and chronic kidney disease. The Includes note at I13 specifies that the conditions included at I11 and I12 are included together in I13. If a patient has hypertension, heart disease and chronic kidney disease, then a code from I13 should be used, not individual codes for hypertension, heart disease and chronic kidney disease, or codes from I11 or I12.

For patients with both acute renal failure and chronic kidney disease, the acute renal failure should also be coded. Sequence according to the circumstances of the admission/encounter.

Patient admitted with acute tubular necrosis, history of hypertensive heart and kidney disease with congestive heart failure and stage 3a chronic kidney disease

N17.0	**Acute kidney failure with tubular necrosis**
I13.0	**Hypertensive heart and chronic kidney disease with heart failure and stage 1 through stage 4 chronic kidney disease, or unspecified chronic kidney disease**
I50.9	**Heart failure, unspecified**
N18.31	**Chronic kidney disease, stage 3a**

Explanation: It is appropriate to report an acute kidney failure code and a chronic kidney failure code when both conditions are treated during an encounter. In this instance, the acute renal failure was the focus of treatment and therefore sequenced as principal diagnosis. Combination codes in category I13 are used to report conditions classifiable to *both* categories I11 and I12. Do not report conditions classifiable to I11 and I12 separately. Use additional codes to report the type of heart failure and stage of CKD.

4) Hypertensive cerebrovascular disease

For hypertensive cerebrovascular disease, first assign the appropriate code from categories I60–I69, followed by the appropriate hypertension code.

Rupture of cerebral aneurysm caused by malignant hypertension

I60.7	**Nontraumatic subarachnoid hemorrhage from unspecified intracranial artery**
I10	**Essential (primary) hypertension**

Explanation: Hypertensive cerebrovascular disease requires two codes: the appropriate I60–I69 code followed by the appropriate hypertension code.

5) Hypertensive retinopathy

Subcategory H35.0, Background retinopathy and retinal vascular changes, should be used along with a code from categories I10–I15, in the Hypertensive diseases section, to include the systemic hypertension. The sequencing is based on the reason for the encounter.

6) Hypertension, secondary

Secondary hypertension is due to an underlying condition. Two codes are required: one to identify the underlying etiology and one from category I15 to identify the hypertension. Sequencing of codes is determined by the reason for admission/encounter.

Renovascular hypertension due to renal artery atherosclerosis

I15.0	**Renovascular hypertension**
I70.1	**Atherosclerosis of renal artery**

Explanation: Secondary hypertension requires two codes: a code to identify the etiology and the appropriate I15 code.

7) Hypertension, transient

Assign code R03.0, Elevated blood pressure reading without diagnosis of hypertension, unless patient has an established diagnosis of hypertension. Assign code O13.-, Gestational [pregnancy-induced] hypertension without significant proteinuria, or O14.-, Pre-eclampsia, for transient hypertension of pregnancy.

8) Hypertension, controlled

This diagnostic statement usually refers to an existing state of hypertension under control by therapy. Assign the appropriate code from categories I10–I15, Hypertensive diseases.

9) Hypertension, uncontrolled

Uncontrolled hypertension may refer to untreated hypertension or hypertension not responding to current therapeutic regimen. In either case, assign the appropriate code from categories I10–I15, Hypertensive diseases.

10) Hypertensive crisis

Assign a code from category I16, Hypertensive crisis, for documented hypertensive urgency, hypertensive emergency or unspecified hypertensive crisis. Code also any identified hypertensive disease (I10–I15). The sequencing is based on the reason for the encounter.

11) Pulmonary hypertension

Pulmonary hypertension is classified to category I27, Other pulmonary heart diseases. For secondary pulmonary hypertension (I27.1, I27.2-), code also any associated conditions or adverse effects of drugs or toxins.

The sequencing is based on the reason for the encounter, except for adverse effects of drugs (See Section I.C.19.e.).

12)Hypertension, Resistant

Resistant hypertension refers to blood pressure of a patient with hypertension that remains above goal in spite of the use of antihypertensive medications. Assign code I1A.Ø, Resistant hypertension, as an additional code when apparent treatment resistant hypertension, treatment resistant hypertension, or true resistant hypertension is documented by the provider. A code for the specific type of existing hypertension is sequenced first, if known.

b. Atherosclerotic coronary artery disease and angina

ICD-10-CM has combination codes for atherosclerotic heart disease with angina pectoris. The subcategories for these codes are I25.11, Atherosclerotic heart disease of native coronary artery with angina pectoris and I25.7, Atherosclerosis of coronary artery bypass graft(s) and coronary artery of transplanted heart with angina pectoris.

When using one of these combination codes it is not necessary to use an additional code for angina pectoris. A causal relationship can be assumed in a patient with both atherosclerosis and angina pectoris, unless the documentation indicates the angina is due to something other than the atherosclerosis.

If a patient with coronary artery disease is admitted due to an acute myocardial infarction (AMI), the AMI should be sequenced before the coronary artery disease.

See Section I.C.9. Acute myocardial infarction (AMI)

c. Intraoperative and postprocedural cerebrovascular accident

Medical record documentation should clearly specify the cause- and- effect relationship between the medical intervention and the cerebrovascular accident in order to assign a code for intraoperative or postprocedural cerebrovascular accident.

Proper code assignment depends on whether it was an infarction or hemorrhage and whether it occurred intraoperatively or postoperatively. If it was a cerebral hemorrhage, code assignment depends on the type of procedure performed.

d. Sequelae of cerebrovascular disease

1) Category I69, Sequelae of cerebrovascular disease

Category I69 is used to indicate conditions classifiable to categories I6Ø–I67 as the causes of sequela (neurologic deficits), themselves classified elsewhere. These "late effects" include neurologic deficits that persist after initial onset of conditions classifiable to categories I6Ø–I67. The neurologic deficits caused by cerebrovascular disease may be present from the onset or may arise at any time after the onset of the condition classifiable to categories I6Ø–I67.

Codes from category I69, Sequelae of cerebrovascular disease, that specify hemiplegia, hemiparesis and monoplegia identify whether the dominant or nondominant side is affected. Should the affected side be documented, but not specified as dominant or nondominant, and the classification system does not indicate a default, code selection is as follows:

- For ambidextrous patients, the default should be dominant.
- If the left side is affected, the default is non-dominant.
- If the right side is affected, the default is dominant.

2) Codes from category I69 with codes from I6Ø–I67

Codes from category I69 may be assigned on a health care record with codes from I6Ø–I67, if the patient has a current cerebrovascular disease and deficits from an old cerebrovascular disease.

3) Codes from category I69 and personal history of transient ischemic attack (TIA) and cerebral infarction (Z86.73)

Codes from category I69 should not be assigned if the patient does not have neurologic deficits.

See Section I.C.21.4. History (of) for use of personal history codes

e. Acute myocardial infarction (AMI)

1) Type 1 ST elevation myocardial infarction (STEMI) and non ST elevation myocardial infarction (NSTEMI)

The ICD-10-CM codes for type 1 acute myocardial infarction (AMI) identify the site, such as anterolateral wall or true posterior wall. Subcategories I21.Ø-I21.2 and code I21.3 are used for type 1 ST elevation myocardial infarction (STEMI). Code I21.4, Non-ST elevation (NSTEMI) myocardial infarction, is used for type 1 non-ST elevation myocardial infarction (NSTEMI) and nontransmural MIs.

If a type 1 NSTEMI evolves to STEMI, assign the STEMI code. If a type 1 STEMI converts to NSTEMI due to thrombolytic therapy, it is still coded as STEMI.

For encounters occurring while the myocardial infarction is equal to, or less than, four weeks old, including transfers to another acute setting or a postacute setting, and the myocardial infarction meets the definition for "other diagnoses" (see Section III, Reporting Additional Diagnoses), codes from category I21 may continue to be reported. For encounters after the 4-week time frame and the patient is still receiving care related to the myocardial infarction, the appropriate aftercare code should be assigned, rather than a code from category I21. For old or healed myocardial infarctions not requiring further care, code I25.2, Old myocardial infarction, may be assigned.

2) Acute myocardial infarction, unspecified

Code I21.9, Acute myocardial infarction, unspecified, is the default for unspecified acute myocardial infarction or unspecified type. If only type 1 STEMI or transmural MI without the site is documented, assign code I21.3, ST elevation (STEMI) myocardial infarction of unspecified site.

3) AMI documented as nontransmural or subendocardial but site provided

If an AMI is documented as nontransmural or subendocardial, but the site is provided, it is still coded as a subendocardial AMI.

See Section I.C.21.3. for information on coding status post administration of tPA in a different facility within the last 24 hours.

4) Subsequent acute myocardial infarction

A code from category I22, Subsequent ST elevation (STEMI) and non-ST elevation (NSTEMI) myocardial infarction, is to be used when a patient who has suffered a type 1 or unspecified AMI has a new AMI within the 4-week time frame of the initial AMI. A code from category I22 must be used in conjunction with a code from category I21. The sequencing of the I22 and I21 codes depends on the circumstances of the encounter.

Do not assign code I22 for subsequent myocardial infarctions other than type 1 or unspecified. For subsequent type 2 AMI assign only code I21.A1. For subsequent type 4 or type 5 AMI, assign only code I21.A9.

If a subsequent myocardial infarction of one type occurs within 4 weeks of a myocardial infarction of a different type, assign the appropriate codes from category I21 to identify each type. Do not assign a code from I22. Codes from category I22 should only be assigned if both the initial and subsequent myocardial infarctions are type 1 or unspecified.

5) Other types of myocardial infarction

The ICD-10-CM provides codes for different types of myocardial infarction. Type 1 myocardial infarctions are assigned to codes I21.Ø–I21.4.

Type 2 myocardial infarction (myocardial infarction due to demand ischemia or secondary to ischemic imbalance) is assigned to code I21.A1, Myocardial infarction type 2 with the underlying cause coded first. Do not assign code I24.8, Other forms of acute ischemic heart disease, for the demand ischemia. If a type 2 AMI is described as NSTEMI or STEMI, only assign code I21.A1. Codes I21.Ø1–I21.4 should only be assigned for type 1 AMIs.

Acute myocardial infarctions type 3, 4a, 4b, 4c and 5 are assigned to code I21.A9, Other myocardial infarction type.

The "Code also" and "Code first" notes should be followed related to complications, and for coding of postprocedural myocardial infarctions during or following cardiac surgery.

Myocardial infarction involving the left circumflex artery occurring during PTCA with stent insertion to treat coronary artery disease

I25.1Ø	**Atherosclerotic heart disease of native coronary artery without angina pectoris**
I97.79Ø	**Other intraoperative cardiac functional disturbances during cardiac surgery**
I21.A9	**Other myocardial infarction type**

Explanation: A myocardial infarction occurring during a revascularization procedure is not considered a type 1 myocardial infarction (MI) and should not be coded to a type 1 MI code (I21.Ø-, I21.1-, I21.2-, I21.3) even when the specific site of the MI is documented. According to the code first instruction at I21.A9, the complication code (I97.79Ø) should be sequenced before code I21.A9.

6) Myocardial Infarction with Coronary Microvascular Dysfunction

Coronary microvascular dysfunction (CMD) is a condition that impacts the microvasculature by restricting microvascular flow and increasing microvascular resistance. Code I21.B, Myocardial infarction with coronary microvascular dysfunction, is assigned for myocardial infarction with coronary microvascular disease, myocardial infarction with coronary microvascular dysfunction, and myocardial infarction with non-obstructive coronary arteries (MINOCA) with microvascular disease.

Chapter 9. Diseases of the Circulatory System (I00-I99)

EXCLUDES 2 *certain conditions originating in the perinatal period (P04-P96)*
certain infectious and parasitic diseases (A00-B99)
complications of pregnancy, childbirth and the puerperium (O00-O9A)
congenital malformations, deformations, and chromosomal abnormalities (Q00-Q99)
endocrine, nutritional and metabolic diseases (E00-E88)
injury, poisoning and certain other consequences of external causes (S00-T88)
neoplasms (C00-D49)
symptoms, signs and abnormal clinical and laboratory findings, not elsewhere classified (R00-R94)
systemic connective tissue disorders (M30-M36)
transient cerebral ischemic attacks and related syndromes (G45.-)

This chapter contains the following blocks:

Acute rheumatic fever (I00-I02)

DEF: Rheumatic fever: Inflammatory disease that can follow a throat infection by group A *streptococci*. Complications can involve the joints (arthritis), subcutaneous tissue (nodules), skin (erythema marginatum), heart (carditis), or brain (chorea).

I00 Rheumatic fever without heart involvement
INCLUDES arthritis, rheumatic, acute or subacute
EXCLUDES 1 *rheumatic fever with heart involvement (I01.0-I01.9)*

✓4th **I01 Rheumatic fever with heart involvement**
EXCLUDES 1 *chronic diseases of rheumatic origin (I05-I09) unless rheumatic fever is also present or there is evidence of reactivation or activity of the rheumatic process*

I01.0 Acute rheumatic pericarditis CC
Any condition in I00 with pericarditis
Rheumatic pericarditis (acute)
EXCLUDES 1 *acute pericarditis not specified as rheumatic (I30.-)*

I01.1 Acute rheumatic endocarditis CC
Any condition in I00 with endocarditis or valvulitis
Acute rheumatic valvulitis

I01.2 Acute rheumatic myocarditis CC
Any condition in I00 with myocarditis

I01.8 Other acute rheumatic heart disease CC
Any condition in I00 with other or multiple types of heart involvement
Acute rheumatic pancarditis

I01.9 Acute rheumatic heart disease, unspecified CC
Any condition in I00 with unspecified type of heart involvement
Rheumatic carditis, acute
Rheumatic heart disease, active or acute

✓4th **I02 Rheumatic chorea**
INCLUDES Sydenham's chorea
EXCLUDES 1 *chorea NOS (G25.5)*
Huntington's chorea (G10)

I02.0 Rheumatic chorea with heart involvement CC
Chorea NOS with heart involvement
Rheumatic chorea with heart involvement of any type classifiable under I01.-

I02.9 Rheumatic chorea without heart involvement CC
Rheumatic chorea NOS

Chronic rheumatic heart diseases (I05-I09)

✓4th **I05 Rheumatic mitral valve diseases**
INCLUDES conditions classifiable to both I05.0 and I05.2-I05.9, whether specified as rheumatic or not
EXCLUDES 1 *mitral valve disease specified as nonrheumatic (I34.-)*
mitral valve disease with aortic and/or tricuspid valve involvement (I08.-)

I05.0 Rheumatic mitral stenosis
Mitral (valve) obstruction (rheumatic)

I05.1 Rheumatic mitral insufficiency
Rheumatic mitral incompetence
Rheumatic mitral regurgitation
EXCLUDES 1 *mitral insufficiency not specified as rheumatic (I34.0)*

I05.2 Rheumatic mitral stenosis with insufficiency
Rheumatic mitral stenosis with incompetence or regurgitation

I05.8 Other rheumatic mitral valve diseases
Rheumatic mitral (valve) failure

I05.9 Rheumatic mitral valve disease, unspecified
Rheumatic mitral (valve) disorder (chronic) NOS

✓4th **I06 Rheumatic aortic valve diseases**
EXCLUDES 1 *aortic valve disease not specified as rheumatic (I35.-)*
aortic valve disease with mitral and/or tricuspid valve involvement (I08.-)

I06.0 Rheumatic aortic stenosis
Rheumatic aortic (valve) obstruction

I06.1 Rheumatic aortic insufficiency
Rheumatic aortic incompetence
Rheumatic aortic regurgitation

I06.2 Rheumatic aortic stenosis with insufficiency
Rheumatic aortic stenosis with incompetence or regurgitation

I06.8 Other rheumatic aortic valve diseases

I06.9 Rheumatic aortic valve disease, unspecified
Rheumatic aortic (valve) disease NOS

✓4th **I07 Rheumatic tricuspid valve diseases**
INCLUDES rheumatic tricuspid valve diseases specified as rheumatic or unspecified
EXCLUDES 1 *tricuspid valve disease specified as nonrheumatic (I36.-)*
tricuspid valve disease with aortic and/or mitral valve involvement (I08.-)

I07.0 Rheumatic tricuspid stenosis
Tricuspid (valve) stenosis (rheumatic)

I07.1 Rheumatic tricuspid insufficiency
Tricuspid (valve) insufficiency (rheumatic)

I07.2 Rheumatic tricuspid stenosis and insufficiency

I07.8 Other rheumatic tricuspid valve diseases

I07.9 Rheumatic tricuspid valve disease, unspecified
Rheumatic tricuspid valve disorder NOS

✓4th **I08 Multiple valve diseases**
INCLUDES multiple valve diseases specified as rheumatic or unspecified
EXCLUDES 1 *endocarditis, valve unspecified (I38)*
multiple valve disease specified a nonrheumatic (I34.-, I35.-, I36.-, I37.-, I38.-, Q22.-, Q23.-, Q24.8-)
rheumatic valve disease NOS (I09.1)

I08.0 Rheumatic disorders of both mitral and aortic valves
Involvement of both mitral and aortic valves specified as rheumatic or unspecified
AHA: 2019,2Q,5

I08.1 Rheumatic disorders of both mitral and tricuspid valves

I08.2 Rheumatic disorders of both aortic and tricuspid valves

I08.3 Combined rheumatic disorders of mitral, aortic and tricuspid valves

I08.8 Other rheumatic multiple valve diseases

I08.9 Rheumatic multiple valve disease, unspecified

✓4th **I09 Other rheumatic heart diseases**

I09.0 Rheumatic myocarditis CC
EXCLUDES 1 *myocarditis not specified as rheumatic (I51.4)*

I09.1 Rheumatic diseases of endocardium, valve unspecified
Rheumatic endocarditis (chronic)
Rheumatic valvulitis (chronic)
EXCLUDES 1 *endocarditis, valve unspecified (I38)*

I09.2 Chronic rheumatic pericarditis CC
Adherent pericardium, rheumatic
Chronic rheumatic mediastinopericarditis
Chronic rheumatic myopericarditis
EXCLUDES 1 *chronic pericarditis not specified as rheumatic (I31.-)*

✓5th **I09.8 Other specified rheumatic heart diseases**

I09.81 Rheumatic heart failure CC HCC
Use additional code to identify type of heart failure (I50.-)

I09.89 Other specified rheumatic heart diseases
Rheumatic disease of pulmonary valve

I09.9 Rheumatic heart disease, unspecified
Rheumatic carditis
EXCLUDES 1 *rheumatoid carditis (M05.31)*

Hypertensive diseases (I1Ø-I1A)

Use additional code to identify:
- exposure to environmental tobacco smoke (Z77.22)
- history of tobacco dependence (Z87.891)
- occupational exposure to environmental tobacco smoke (Z57.31)
- tobacco dependence (F17.-)
- tobacco use (Z72.Ø)

EXCLUDES 1 *neonatal hypertension (P29.2)*
primary pulmonary hypertension (I27.Ø)

EXCLUDES 2 *hypertensive disease complicating pregnancy, childbirth and the puerperium (O1Ø-O11, O13-O16)*

I1Ø Essential (primary) hypertension

INCLUDES high blood pressure
hypertension (arterial) (benign) (essential) (malignant) (primary) (systemic)

EXCLUDES 1 *hypertensive disease complicating pregnancy, childbirth and the puerperium (O1Ø-O11, O13-O16)*

EXCLUDES 2 *essential (primary) hypertension involving vessels of brain (I6Ø-I69)*
essential (primary) hypertension involving vessels of eye (H35.Ø-)

AHA: 2022,1Q,36; 2020,1Q,12; 2018,2Q,9; 2016,4Q,27

✓4th **I11 Hypertensive heart disease**

INCLUDES any condition in I5Ø.- or I51.4-I51.7, I51.89, I51.9 due to hypertension

AHA: 2018,2Q,9

TIP: Do not assign a code from this category when provider documentation indicates the heart disease is attributable to another cause.

I11.Ø Hypertensive heart disease with heart failure HCC
Hypertensive heart failure
Use additional code to identify type of heart failure (I5Ø.-)
AHA: 2017,1Q,47

I11.9 Hypertensive heart disease without heart failure
Hypertensive heart disease NOS

✓4th **I12 Hypertensive chronic kidney disease**

INCLUDES any condition in N18 and N26 — due to hypertension
arteriosclerosis of kidney
arteriosclerotic nephritis (chronic) (interstitial)
hypertensive nephropathy
nephrosclerosis

EXCLUDES 1 *hypertension due to kidney disease (I15.Ø, I15.1)*
renovascular hypertension (I15.Ø)
secondary hypertension (I15.-)

EXCLUDES 2 *acute kidney failure (N17.-)*

AHA: 2019,3Q,3; 2018,4Q,88; 2016,3Q,22

TIP: Do not assign a code from this category when provider documentation indicates the chronic kidney disease (CKD) is attributable to another cause.

I12.Ø Hypertensive chronic kidney disease with stage 5 chronic kidney disease or end stage renal disease CC HCC
Use additional code to identify the stage of chronic kidney disease (N18.5, N18.6)

I12.9 Hypertensive chronic kidney disease with stage 1 through stage 4 chronic kidney disease, or unspecified chronic kidney disease
Hypertensive chronic kidney disease NOS
Hypertensive renal disease NOS
Use additional code to identify the stage of chronic kidney disease (N18.1-N18.4, N18.9)

✓4th **I13 Hypertensive heart and chronic kidney disease**

INCLUDES any condition in I11.- with any condition in I12.-
cardiorenal disease
cardiovascular renal disease

TIP: Do not assign a code from this category when provider documentation indicates the heart and/or chronic kidney disease is attributable to another cause.

I13.Ø Hypertensive heart and chronic kidney disease with heart failure and stage 1 through stage 4 chronic kidney disease, or unspecified chronic kidney disease CC HCC
Use additional code to identify type of heart failure (I5Ø.-)
Use additional code to identify stage of chronic kidney disease (N18.1-N18.4, N18.9)

✓5th **I13.1 Hypertensive heart and chronic kidney disease without heart failure**

I13.1Ø Hypertensive heart and chronic kidney disease without heart failure, with stage 1 through stage 4 chronic kidney disease, or unspecified chronic kidney disease
Hypertensive heart disease and hypertensive chronic kidney disease NOS
Use additional code to identify the stage of chronic kidney disease (N18.1-N18.4, N18.9)

I13.11 Hypertensive heart and chronic kidney disease without heart failure, with stage 5 chronic kidney disease, or end stage renal disease CC HCC
Use additional code to identify the stage of chronic kidney disease (N18.5, N18.6)

I13.2 Hypertensive heart and chronic kidney disease with heart failure and with stage 5 chronic kidney disease, or end stage renal disease CC HCC
Use additional code to identify type of heart failure (I5Ø.-)
Use additional code to identify the stage of chronic kidney disease (N18.5, N18.6)

✓4th **I15 Secondary hypertension**

Code also underlying condition

EXCLUDES 1 *postprocedural hypertension (I97.3)*

EXCLUDES 2 *secondary hypertension involving vessels of brain (I6Ø-I69)*
secondary hypertension involving vessels of eye (H35.Ø-)

I15.Ø Renovascular hypertension

I15.1 Hypertension secondary to other renal disorders
AHA: 2016,3Q,22

I15.2 Hypertension secondary to endocrine disorders
AHA: 2023,2Q,16

I15.8 Other secondary hypertension

I15.9 Secondary hypertension, unspecified

✓4th **I16 Hypertensive crisis**

Code also any identified hypertensive disease ▶(I1Ø-I15, I1A)◀

AHA: 2016,4Q,26-28

I16.Ø Hypertensive urgency

I16.1 Hypertensive emergency CC

I16.9 Hypertensive crisis, unspecified CC

● ✓4th **I1A Other hypertension**

● **I1A.Ø Resistant hypertension**
Apparent treatment resistant hypertension
Treatment resistant hypertension
True resistant hypertension
Code first specific type of existing hypertension, if known, such as:
- essential hypertension (I1Ø)
- secondary hypertension (I15.-)

Ischemic heart diseases (I2Ø-I25)

Code also the presence of hypertension ▶(I1Ø-I1A)◀

✓4th **I2Ø Angina pectoris**

Use additional code to identify:
- exposure to environmental tobacco smoke (Z77.22)
- history of tobacco dependence (Z87.891)
- occupational exposure to environmental tobacco smoke (Z57.31)
- tobacco dependence (F17.-)
- tobacco use (Z72.Ø)

EXCLUDES 1 *angina pectoris with atherosclerotic heart disease of native coronary arteries (I25.1-)*
atherosclerosis of coronary artery bypass graft(s) and coronary artery of transplanted heart with angina pectoris (I25.7-)
postinfarction angina (I23.7)

DEF: Chest pain due to reduced blood flow resulting in a lack of oxygen to the heart muscles.

I2Ø.Ø Unstable angina CC HCC
Accelerated angina
Crescendo angina
De novo effort angina
Intermediate coronary syndrome
Preinfarction syndrome
Worsening effort angina

I2Ø.1 Angina pectoris with documented spasm CC HCC
Angiospastic angina
Prinzmetal angina
Spasm-induced angina
Variant angina

I2Ø.2 Refractory angina pectoris CC HCC
AHA: 2022,4Q,20-21

▲ ✓5th **I2Ø.8 Other forms of angina pectoris**
~~Angina equivalent~~
~~Angina of effort~~
~~Coronary slow flow syndrome~~
~~Stenocardia~~
~~Stable angina~~
Use additional code(s) for symptoms associated with angina equivalent

● **I2Ø.81 Angina pectoris with coronary microvascular dysfunction**
Angina pectoris with coronary microvascular disease

● **I2Ø.89 Other forms of angina pectoris**
Angina equivalent
Angina of effort
Coronary slow flow syndrome
Stable angina
Stenocardia

I2Ø.9 Angina pectoris, unspecified HCC
Angina NOS
Anginal syndrome
Cardiac angina
Ischemic chest pain

✓4th **I21 Acute myocardial infarction**
INCLUDES cardiac infarction
coronary (artery) embolism
coronary (artery) occlusion
coronary (artery) rupture
coronary (artery) thrombosis
infarction of heart, myocardium, or ventricle
myocardial infarction specified as acute or with a stated duration of 4 weeks (28 days) or less from onset

Use additional code, if applicable, to identify:
exposure to environmental tobacco smoke (Z77.22)
history of tobacco dependence (Z87.891)
occupational exposure to environmental tobacco smoke (Z57.31)
status post administration of tPA (rtPA) in a different facility within the last 24 hours prior to admission to current facility (Z92.82)
tobacco dependence (F17.-)
tobacco use (Z72.Ø)

EXCLUDES 2 *old myocardial infarction (I25.2)*
postmyocardial infarction syndrome (I24.1)
subsequent type 1 myocardial infarction (I22.-)

AHA: 2019,2Q,5; 2018,4Q,68; 2018,3Q,5; 2017,4Q,12-14; 2017,1Q,44-45; 2016,4Q,140; 2015,2Q,16; 2013,1Q,25; 2012,4Q,96,102-103

TIP: When chronic total occlusion and myocardial infarction are documented as being in different vessels, assign code I25.82 Chronic total occlusion of coronary artery, in addition to the myocardial infarction code.

✓5th **I21.Ø ST elevation (STEMI) myocardial infarction of anterior wall**
Type 1 ST elevation myocardial infarction of anterior wall
DEF: ST elevation myocardial infarction: Complete obstruction of one or more coronary arteries causing decreased blood flow (ischemia) and necrosis of myocardial muscle cells.

I21.Ø1 ST elevation (STEMI) myocardial infarction involving left main coronary artery MCC HCC

I21.Ø2 ST elevation (STEMI) myocardial infarction involving left anterior descending coronary artery MCC HCC
ST elevation (STEMI) myocardial infarction involving diagonal coronary artery
AHA: 2013,1Q,25

I21.Ø9 ST elevation (STEMI) myocardial infarction involving other coronary artery of anterior wall MCC HCC
Acute transmural myocardial infarction of anterior wall
Anteroapical transmural (Q wave) infarction (acute)
Anterolateral transmural (Q wave) infarction (acute)
Anteroseptal transmural (Q wave) infarction (acute)
Transmural (Q wave) infarction (acute) (of) anterior (wall) NOS
AHA: 2012,4Q,102-103

✓5th **I21.1 ST elevation (STEMI) myocardial infarction of inferior wall**
Type 1 ST elevation myocardial infarction of inferior wall
DEF: ST elevation myocardial infarction: Complete obstruction of one or more coronary arteries causing decreased blood flow (ischemia) and necrosis of myocardial muscle cells.

I21.11 ST elevation (STEMI) myocardial infarction involving right coronary artery MCC HCC
Inferoposterior transmural (Q wave) infarction (acute)

I21.19 ST elevation (STEMI) myocardial infarction involving other coronary artery of inferior wall MCC HCC
Acute transmural myocardial infarction of inferior wall
Inferolateral transmural (Q wave) infarction (acute)
Transmural (Q wave) infarction (acute) (of) diaphragmatic wall
Transmural (Q wave) infarction (acute) (of) inferior (wall) NOS
EXCLUDES 2 *ST elevation (STEMI) myocardial infarction involving left circumflex coronary artery (I21.21)*
AHA: 2012,4Q,96

✓5th **I21.2 ST elevation (STEMI) myocardial infarction of other sites**
Type 1 ST elevation myocardial infarction of other sites
DEF: ST elevation myocardial infarction: Complete obstruction of one or more coronary arteries causing decreased blood flow (ischemia) and necrosis of myocardial muscle cells.

I21.21 ST elevation (STEMI) myocardial infarction involving left circumflex coronary artery MCC HCC
ST elevation (STEMI) myocardial infarction involving oblique marginal coronary artery

I21.29 ST elevation (STEMI) myocardial infarction involving other sites MCC HCC
Acute transmural myocardial infarction of other sites
Apical-lateral transmural (Q wave) infarction (acute)
Basal-lateral transmural (Q wave) infarction (acute)
High lateral transmural (Q wave) infarction (acute)
Lateral (wall) NOS transmural (Q wave) infarction (acute)
Posterior (true) transmural (Q wave) infarction (acute)
Posterobasal transmural (Q wave) infarction (acute)
Posterolateral transmural (Q wave) infarction (acute)
Posteroseptal transmural (Q wave) infarction (acute)
Septal transmural (Q wave) infarction (acute) NOS

I21.3 ST elevation (STEMI) myocardial infarction of unspecified site MCC HCC
Acute transmural myocardial infarction of unspecified site
Transmural (Q wave) myocardial infarction NOS
Type 1 ST elevation myocardial infarction of unspecified site
DEF: ST elevation myocardial infarction: Complete obstruction of one or more coronary arteries causing decreased blood flow (ischemia) and necrosis of myocardial muscle cells.

I21.4 Non-ST elevation (NSTEMI) myocardial infarction MCC HCC
Acute subendocardial myocardial infarction
Non-Q wave myocardial infarction NOS
Nontransmural myocardial infarction NOS
Type 1 non-ST elevation myocardial infarction
AHA: 2023,2Q,29; 2021,3Q,6; 2019,2Q,33; 2017,1Q,44-45
DEF: Partial obstruction of one or more coronary arteries that causes decreased blood flow (ischemia) and may cause partial thickness necrosis of myocardial muscle cells.

I21.9 Acute myocardial infarction, unspecified MCC HCC
Myocardial infarction (acute) NOS

√5th **I21.A Other type of myocardial infarction**

AHA: 2019,2Q,5

I21.A1 Myocardial infarction type 2 MCC HCC

Myocardial infarction due to demand ischemia
Myocardial infarction secondary to ischemic imbalance

Code first the underlying cause, such as:
anemia (D50.0-D64.9)
chronic obstructive pulmonary disease (J44.-)
paroxysmal tachycardia (I47.0-I47.9)
shock (R57.0-R57.9)

AHA: 2019,4Q,53; 2017,4Q,13-14

DEF: Often referred to as due to demand ischemia, myocardial infarction (MI) type 2 refers to an MI due to ischemia and necrosis resulting from an oxygen imbalance to the heart. This mismatch between oxygen decreased supply and increased demand is caused by conditions other than coronary artery disease such as vasospasm, embolism, anemia, hypertension, hypotension, or arrhythmias.

I21.A9 Other myocardial infarction type MCC HCC

Myocardial infarction associated with revascularization procedure
Myocardial infarction type 3
Myocardial infarction type 4a
Myocardial infarction type 4b
Myocardial infarction type 4c
Myocardial infarction type 5

Code first, if applicable, postprocedural myocardial infarction following cardiac surgery (I97.190), or postprocedural myocardial infarction during cardiac surgery (I97.790)

Code also complication, if known and applicable, such as:
(acute) stent occlusion (T82.897-)
(acute) stent stenosis (T82.855-)
(acute) stent thrombosis (T82.867-)
cardiac arrest due to underlying cardiac condition (I46.2)
complication of percutaneous coronary intervention (PCI) (I97.89)
occlusion of coronary artery bypass graft (T82.218-)

AHA: 2021,3Q,6; 2019,2Q,33

● **I21.B Myocardial infarction with coronary microvascular dysfunction** MCC

Myocardial infarction with coronary microvascular disease
Myocardial infarction with nonobstructive coronary arteries [MINOCA] with microvascular disease

√4th **I22 Subsequent ST elevation (STEMI) and non-ST elevation (NSTEMI) myocardial infarction**

INCLUDES acute myocardial infarction occurring within four weeks (28 days) of a previous acute myocardial infarction, regardless of site
cardiac infarction
coronary (artery) embolism
coronary (artery) occlusion
coronary (artery) rupture
coronary (artery) thrombosis
infarction of heart, myocardium, or ventricle
recurrent myocardial infarction
reinfarction of myocardium
rupture of heart, myocardium, or ventricle
subsequent type 1 myocardial infarction

Use additional code, if applicable, to identify:
exposure to environmental tobacco smoke (Z77.22)
history of tobacco dependence (Z87.891)
occupational exposure to environmental tobacco smoke (Z57.31)
status post administration of tPA (rtPA) in a different facility within the last 24 hours prior to admission to current facility (Z92.82)
tobacco dependence (F17.-)
tobacco use (Z72.0)

EXCLUDES 1 *subsequent myocardial infarction, type 2 (I21.A1)*
subsequent myocardial infarction of other type (type 3) (type 4) (type 5) (I21.A9)

AHA: 2018,4Q,68; 2018,3Q,5; 2017,4Q,12-13; 2017,2Q,11; 2013,1Q,25; 2012,4Q,97,102-103

DEF: Non-ST elevation myocardial infarction: Partial obstruction of one or more coronary arteries that causes decreased blood flow (ischemia) and may cause partial thickness necrosis of myocardial muscle cells.

DEF: ST elevation myocardial infarction: Complete obstruction of one or more coronary arteries causing decreased blood flow (ischemia) and necrosis of myocardial muscle cells.

TIP: When chronic total occlusion and myocardial infarction are documented as being in different vessels, assign code I25.82 Chronic total occlusion of coronary artery, in addition to the myocardial infarction code.

I22.0 Subsequent ST elevation (STEMI) myocardial infarction of anterior wall MCC HCC

Subsequent acute transmural myocardial infarction of anterior wall
Subsequent transmural (Q wave) infarction (acute)(of) anterior (wall) NOS
Subsequent anteroapical transmural (Q wave) infarction (acute)
Subsequent anterolateral transmural (Q wave) infarction (acute)
Subsequent anteroseptal transmural (Q wave) infarction (acute)

I22.1 Subsequent ST elevation (STEMI) myocardial infarction of inferior wall MCC HCC

Subsequent acute transmural myocardial infarction of inferior wall
Subsequent transmural (Q wave) infarction (acute)(of) diaphragmatic wall
Subsequent transmural (Q wave) infarction (acute)(of) inferior (wall) NOS
Subsequent inferolateral transmural (Q wave) infarction (acute)
Subsequent inferoposterior transmural (Q wave) infarction (acute)

AHA: 2012,4Q,102

I22.2 Subsequent non-ST elevation (NSTEMI) myocardial infarction MCC HCC

Subsequent acute subendocardial myocardial infarction
Subsequent non-Q wave myocardial infarction NOS
Subsequent nontransmural myocardial infarction NOS

I22.8 Subsequent ST elevation (STEMI) myocardial infarction of other sites MCC HCC
Subsequent acute transmural myocardial infarction of other sites
Subsequent apical-lateral transmural (Q wave) myocardial infarction (acute)
Subsequent basal-lateral transmural (Q wave) myocardial infarction (acute)
Subsequent high lateral transmural (Q wave) myocardial infarction (acute)
Subsequent posterior (true) transmural (Q wave) myocardial infarction (acute)
Subsequent posterobasal transmural (Q wave) myocardial infarction (acute)
Subsequent posterolateral transmural (Q wave) myocardial infarction (acute)
Subsequent posteroseptal transmural (Q wave) myocardial infarction (acute)
Subsequent septal NOS transmural (Q wave) myocardial infarction (acute)
Subsequent transmural (Q wave) myocardial infarction (acute)(of) lateral (wall) NOS

I22.9 Subsequent ST elevation (STEMI) myocardial infarction of unspecified site MCC HCC
Subsequent acute myocardial infarction of unspecified site
Subsequent myocardial infarction (acute) NOS

✓4th **I23 Certain current complications following ST elevation (STEMI) and non-ST elevation (NSTEMI) myocardial infarction (within the 28 day period)**
AHA: 2017,2Q,11
DEF: ST elevation myocardial infarction: Complete obstruction of one or more coronary arteries causing decreased blood flow (ischemia) and necrosis of myocardial muscle cells.
DEF: Non-ST elevation myocardial infarction: Partial obstruction of one or more coronary arteries that causes decreased blood flow (ischemia) and may cause partial thickness necrosis of myocardial muscle cells.

I23.Ø Hemopericardium as current complication following acute myocardial infarction CC HCC A
EXCLUDES 1 *hemopericardium not specified as current complication following acute myocardial infarction (I31.2)*

I23.1 Atrial septal defect as current complication following acute myocardial infarction CC HCC A
EXCLUDES 1 *acquired atrial septal defect not specified as current complication following acute myocardial infarction (I51.Ø)*

I23.2 Ventricular septal defect as current complication following acute myocardial infarction CC HCC A
EXCLUDES 1 *acquired ventricular septal defect not specified as current complication following acute myocardial infarction (I51.Ø)*

I23.3 Rupture of cardiac wall without hemopericardium as current complication following acute myocardial infarction CC HCC A

I23.4 Rupture of chordae tendineae as current complication following acute myocardial infarction MCC HCC
EXCLUDES 1 *rupture of chordae tendineae not specified as current complication following acute myocardial infarction (I51.1)*

I23.5 Rupture of papillary muscle as current complication following acute myocardial infarction MCC HCC
EXCLUDES 1 *rupture of papillary muscle not specified as current complication following acute myocardial infarction (I51.2)*

I23.6 Thrombosis of atrium, auricular appendage, and ventricle as current complications following acute myocardial infarction CC HCC A
EXCLUDES 1 *thrombosis of atrium, auricular appendage, and ventricle not specified as current complication following acute myocardial infarction (I51.3)*

I23.7 Postinfarction angina CC HCC A
AHA: 2015,2Q,16
TIP: When postinfarction angina occurs with atherosclerotic coronary artery disease, code both I23.7 and I25.118 for atherosclerotic disease with other forms of angina pectoris.

I23.8 Other current complications following acute myocardial infarction CC HCC A

✓4th **I24 Other acute ischemic heart diseases**
EXCLUDES 1 *angina pectoris (I2Ø.-)*
transient myocardial ischemia in newborn (P29.4)
EXCLUDES 2 *non-ischemic myocardial injury (I5A)*

I24.Ø Acute coronary thrombosis not resulting in myocardial infarction CC HCC
Acute coronary (artery) (vein) embolism not resulting in myocardial infarction
Acute coronary (artery) (vein) occlusion not resulting in myocardial infarction
Acute coronary (artery) (vein) thromboembolism not resulting in myocardial infarction
EXCLUDES 1 *atherosclerotic heart disease (I25.1-)*
AHA: 2013,1Q,24

I24.1 Dressler's syndrome CC HCC
Postmyocardial infarction syndrome
EXCLUDES 1 *postinfarction angina (I23.7)*
DEF: Fever, leukocytosis, chest pain, evidence of pericarditis, pleurisy, and pneumonia occurring days or weeks after a myocardial infarction.

▲ ✓5th **I24.8 Other forms of acute ischemic heart disease**
EXCLUDES 1 *myocardial infarction due to demand ischemia (I21.A1)*
AHA: 2019,4Q,53; 2017,4Q,13

● **I24.81 Acute coronary microvascular dysfunction** CC
Acute (presentation of) coronary microvascular disease

● **I24.89 Other forms of acute ischemic heart disease** CC

I24.9 Acute ischemic heart disease, unspecified CC HCC
EXCLUDES 1 *ischemic heart disease (chronic) NOS (I25.9)*

✓4th **I25 Chronic ischemic heart disease**
Use additional code to identify:
chronic total occlusion of coronary artery (I25.82)
exposure to environmental tobacco smoke (Z77.22)
history of tobacco dependence (Z87.891)
occupational exposure to environmental tobacco smoke (Z57.31)
tobacco dependence (F17.-)
tobacco use (Z72.Ø)
EXCLUDES 2 *non-ischemic myocardial injury (I5A)*
AHA: 2022,4Q,20-21

✓5th **I25.1 Atherosclerotic heart disease of native coronary artery**
Atherosclerotic cardiovascular disease
Coronary (artery) atheroma
Coronary (artery) atherosclerosis
Coronary (artery) disease
Coronary (artery) sclerosis
Use additional code, if applicable, to identify:
coronary atherosclerosis due to calcified coronary lesion (I25.84)
coronary atherosclerosis due to lipid rich plaque (I25.83)
EXCLUDES 2 *atheroembolism (I75.-)*
atherosclerosis of coronary artery bypass graft(s) and transplanted heart (I25.7-)

Atheromas

Atheromas (fatty tissue and/or plaque)
Lumen

I25.1Ø Atherosclerotic heart disease of native coronary artery without angina pectoris A
Atherosclerotic heart disease NOS
AHA: 2021,3Q,6-7; 2015,2Q,16; 2012,4Q,92

✓6th **I25.11 Atherosclerotic heart disease of native coronary artery with angina pectoris**

I25.11Ø Atherosclerotic heart disease of native coronary artery with unstable angina pectoris CC HCC A
EXCLUDES 1 *unstable angina without atherosclerotic heart disease (I2Ø.Ø)*

I25.111 Atherosclerotic heart disease of native coronary artery with angina pectoris with documented spasm HCC A

EXCLUDES 1 *angina pectoris with documented spasm without atherosclerotic heart disease (I2Ø.1)*

▲ **I25.112 Atherosclerotic heart disease of native coronary artery with refractory angina pectoris** CC HCC A

I25.118 Atherosclerotic heart disease of native coronary artery with other forms of angina pectoris HCC A

EXCLUDES 1 *other forms of angina pectoris without atherosclerotic heart disease ►(I2Ø.8-)◄*

AHA: 2015,2Q,16

TIP: When postinfarction angina occurs with atherosclerotic coronary artery disease, code both I23.7 and I25.118 for atherosclerotic disease with other forms of angina pectoris.

I25.119 Atherosclerotic heart disease of native coronary artery with unspecified angina pectoris HCC A

Atherosclerotic heart disease with angina NOS

Atherosclerotic heart disease with ischemic chest pain

EXCLUDES 1 *unspecified angina pectoris without atherosclerotic heart disease (I2Ø.9)*

I25.2 Old myocardial infarction

Healed myocardial infarction

Past myocardial infarction diagnosed by ECG or other investigation, but currently presenting no symptoms

I25.3 Aneurysm of heart CC

Mural aneurysm

Ventricular aneurysm

✓5th **I25.4 Coronary artery aneurysm and dissection**

I25.41 Coronary artery aneurysm

Coronary arteriovenous fistula, acquired

EXCLUDES 1 *congenital coronary (artery) aneurysm (Q24.5)*

I25.42 Coronary artery dissection MCC

DEF: Tear in the intimal arterial wall of a coronary artery resulting in the sudden intrusion of blood within the layers of the wall.

I25.5 Ischemic cardiomyopathy

EXCLUDES 2 *coronary atherosclerosis (I25.1-, I25.7-)*

AHA: 2022,3Q,17

I25.6 Silent myocardial ischemia

✓5th **I25.7 Atherosclerosis of coronary artery bypass graft(s) and coronary artery of transplanted heart with angina pectoris**

Use additional code, if applicable, to identify:

coronary atherosclerosis due to calcified coronary lesion (I25.84)

coronary atherosclerosis due to lipid rich plaque (I25.83)

EXCLUDES 1 *atherosclerosis of bypass graft(s) of transplanted heart without angina pectoris (I25.812)*

atherosclerosis of coronary artery bypass graft(s) without angina pectoris (I25.81Ø)

atherosclerosis of native coronary artery of transplanted heart without angina pectoris (I25.811)

✓6th **I25.7Ø Atherosclerosis of coronary artery bypass graft(s), unspecified, with angina pectoris**

I25.7ØØ Atherosclerosis of coronary artery bypass graft(s), unspecified, with unstable angina pectoris CC HCC A

EXCLUDES 1 *unstable angina pectoris without atherosclerosis of coronary artery bypass graft (I2Ø.Ø)*

I25.7Ø1 Atherosclerosis of coronary artery bypass graft(s), unspecified, with angina pectoris with documented spasm HCC A

EXCLUDES 1 *angina pectoris with documented spasm without atherosclerosis of coronary artery bypass graft (I2Ø.1)*

I25.7Ø2 Atherosclerosis of coronary artery bypass graft(s), unspecified, with refractory angina pectoris CC HCC A

AHA: 2022,4Q,21

I25.7Ø8 Atherosclerosis of coronary artery bypass graft(s), unspecified, with other forms of angina pectoris HCC A

EXCLUDES 1 *other forms of angina pectoris without atherosclerosis of coronary artery bypass graft ►(I2Ø.8-)◄*

I25.7Ø9 Atherosclerosis of coronary artery bypass graft(s), unspecified, with unspecified angina pectoris HCC A

EXCLUDES 1 *unspecified angina pectoris without atherosclerosis of coronary artery bypass graft (I2Ø.9)*

✓6th **I25.71 Atherosclerosis of autologous vein coronary artery bypass graft(s) with angina pectoris**

I25.71Ø Atherosclerosis of autologous vein coronary artery bypass graft(s) with unstable angina pectoris CC HCC A

EXCLUDES 1 *unstable angina without atherosclerosis of autologous vein coronary artery bypass graft(s) (I2Ø.Ø)*

EXCLUDES 2 *embolism or thrombus of coronary artery bypass graft(s) (T82.8-)*

I25.711 Atherosclerosis of autologous vein coronary artery bypass graft(s) with angina pectoris with documented spasm CC HCC A

EXCLUDES 1 *angina pectoris with documented spasm without atherosclerosis of autologous vein coronary artery bypass graft(s) (I2Ø.1)*

I25.712 Atherosclerosis of autologous vein coronary artery bypass graft(s) with refractory angina pectoris CC HCC A

I25.718 Atherosclerosis of autologous vein coronary artery bypass graft(s) with other forms of angina pectoris CC HCC A

EXCLUDES 1 *other forms of angina pectoris without atherosclerosis of autologous vein coronary artery bypass graft(s) ►(I2Ø.8-)◄*

I25.719 Atherosclerosis of autologous vein coronary artery bypass graft(s) with unspecified angina pectoris CC HCC A

EXCLUDES 1 *unspecified angina pectoris without atherosclerosis of autologous vein coronary artery bypass graft(s) (I2Ø.9)*

✓6th **I25.72 Atherosclerosis of autologous artery coronary artery bypass graft(s) with angina pectoris**

Atherosclerosis of internal mammary artery graft with angina pectoris

I25.72Ø Atherosclerosis of autologous artery coronary artery bypass graft(s) with unstable angina pectoris CC HCC A

EXCLUDES 1 *unstable angina without atherosclerosis of autologous artery coronary artery bypass graft(s) (I2Ø.Ø)*

I25.721 Atherosclerosis of autologous artery coronary artery bypass graft(s) with angina pectoris with documented spasm CC HCC A

EXCLUDES 1 *angina pectoris with documented spasm without atherosclerosis of autologous artery coronary artery bypass graft(s) (I20.1)*

I25.722 Atherosclerosis of autologous artery coronary artery bypass graft(s) with refractory angina pectoris CC HCC A

I25.728 Atherosclerosis of autologous artery coronary artery bypass graft(s) with other forms of angina pectoris CC HCC A

EXCLUDES 1 *other forms of angina pectoris without atherosclerosis of autologous artery coronary artery bypass graft(s) ▶(I20.8-)◀*

I25.729 Atherosclerosis of autologous artery coronary artery bypass graft(s) with unspecified angina pectoris CC HCC A

EXCLUDES 1 *unspecified angina pectoris without atherosclerosis of autologous artery coronary artery bypass graft(s) (I20.9)*

√6th **I25.73 Atherosclerosis of nonautologous biological coronary artery bypass graft(s) with angina pectoris**

I25.730 Atherosclerosis of nonautologous biological coronary artery bypass graft(s) with unstable angina pectoris CC HCC A

EXCLUDES 1 *unstable angina without atherosclerosis of nonautologous biological coronary artery bypass graft(s) (I20.0)*

I25.731 Atherosclerosis of nonautologous biological coronary artery bypass graft(s) with angina pectoris with documented spasm CC HCC A

EXCLUDES 1 *angina pectoris with documented spasm without atherosclerosis of nonautologous biological coronary artery bypass graft(s) (I20.1)*

I25.732 Atherosclerosis of nonautologous biological coronary artery bypass graft(s) with refractory angina pectoris CC HCC A

I25.738 Atherosclerosis of nonautologous biological coronary artery bypass graft(s) with other forms of angina pectoris CC HCC A

EXCLUDES 1 *other forms of angina pectoris without atherosclerosis of nonautologous biological coronary artery bypass graft(s) ▶(I20.8-)◀*

I25.739 Atherosclerosis of nonautologous biological coronary artery bypass graft(s) with unspecified angina pectoris CC HCC A

EXCLUDES 1 *unspecified angina pectoris without atherosclerosis of nonautologous biological coronary artery bypass graft(s) (I20.9)*

√6th **I25.75 Atherosclerosis of native coronary artery of transplanted heart with angina pectoris**

EXCLUDES 1 *atherosclerosis of native coronary artery of transplanted heart without angina pectoris (I25.811)*

I25.750 Atherosclerosis of native coronary artery of transplanted heart with unstable angina CC HCC

I25.751 Atherosclerosis of native coronary artery of transplanted heart with angina pectoris with documented spasm CC HCC

I25.752 Atherosclerosis of native coronary artery of transplanted heart with refractory angina pectoris CC HCC A

I25.758 Atherosclerosis of native coronary artery of transplanted heart with other forms of angina pectoris CC HCC

I25.759 Atherosclerosis of native coronary artery of transplanted heart with unspecified angina pectoris CC HCC

√6th **I25.76 Atherosclerosis of bypass graft of coronary artery of transplanted heart with angina pectoris**

EXCLUDES 1 *atherosclerosis of bypass graft of coronary artery of transplanted heart without angina pectoris (I25.812)*

I25.760 Atherosclerosis of bypass graft of coronary artery of transplanted heart with unstable angina CC HCC A

I25.761 Atherosclerosis of bypass graft of coronary artery of transplanted heart with angina pectoris with documented spasm CC HCC A

I25.762 Atherosclerosis of bypass graft of coronary artery of transplanted heart with refractory angina pectoris CC HCC A

I25.768 Atherosclerosis of bypass graft of coronary artery of transplanted heart with other forms of angina pectoris CC HCC A

I25.769 Atherosclerosis of bypass graft of coronary artery of transplanted heart with unspecified angina pectoris CC HCC A

√6th **I25.79 Atherosclerosis of other coronary artery bypass graft(s) with angina pectoris**

I25.790 Atherosclerosis of other coronary artery bypass graft(s) with unstable angina pectoris CC HCC A

EXCLUDES 1 *unstable angina without atherosclerosis of other coronary artery bypass graft(s) (I20.0)*

I25.791 Atherosclerosis of other coronary artery bypass graft(s) with angina pectoris with documented spasm CC HCC A

EXCLUDES 1 *angina pectoris with documented spasm without atherosclerosis of other coronary artery bypass graft(s) (I20.1)*

I25.792 Atherosclerosis of other coronary artery bypass graft(s) with refractory angina pectoris CC HCC A

I25.798 Atherosclerosis of other coronary artery bypass graft(s) with other forms of angina pectoris CC HCC A

EXCLUDES 1 *other forms of angina pectoris without atherosclerosis of other coronary artery bypass graft(s) ▶(I20.8-)◀*

I25.799 Atherosclerosis of other coronary artery bypass graft(s) with unspecified angina pectoris CC HCC A

EXCLUDES 1 *unspecified angina pectoris without atherosclerosis of other coronary artery bypass graft(s) (I20.9)*

I25.8 Other forms of chronic ischemic heart disease

I25.81 Atherosclerosis of other coronary vessels without angina pectoris
Use additional code, if applicable, to identify:
coronary atherosclerosis due to calcified coronary lesion (I25.84)
coronary atherosclerosis due to lipid rich plaque (I25.83)
EXCLUDES 2 *atherosclerotic heart disease of native coronary artery without angina pectoris (I25.10)*

I25.810 Atherosclerosis of coronary artery bypass graft(s) without angina pectoris CC A
Atherosclerosis of coronary artery bypass graft NOS
EXCLUDES 1 *atherosclerosis of coronary bypass graft(s) with angina pectoris (I25.70-I25.73-, I25.79-)*

I25.811 Atherosclerosis of native coronary artery of transplanted heart without angina pectoris CC
Atherosclerosis of native coronary artery of transplanted heart NOS
EXCLUDES 1 *atherosclerosis of native coronary artery of transplanted heart with angina pectoris (I25.75-)*

I25.812 Atherosclerosis of bypass graft of coronary artery of transplanted heart without angina pectoris CC A
Atherosclerosis of bypass graft of transplanted heart NOS
EXCLUDES 1 *atherosclerosis of bypass graft of transplanted heart with angina pectoris (I25.76)*

I25.82 Chronic total occlusion of coronary artery UPD
Complete occlusion of coronary artery
Total occlusion of coronary artery
Code first coronary atherosclerosis (I25.1-, I25.7-, I25.81-)
EXCLUDES 1 *acute coronary occulsion with myocardial infarction ▶(I21.0-I21.B, I22.-)◀*
acute coronary occlusion without myocardial infarction (I24.0)
AHA: 2018,3Q,5
DEF: Complete blockage of the coronary artery due to plaque accumulation over an extended period of time, resulting in substantial reduction of blood flow. Symptoms include angina or chest pain.
TIP: Report this code in addition to a code from category I21 or I22 when the chronic total occlusion and the myocardial infarction are documented as being in different vessels.

I25.83 Coronary atherosclerosis due to lipid rich plaque UPD A
Code first coronary atherosclerosis (I25.1-, I25.7-, I25.81-)

I25.84 Coronary atherosclerosis due to calcified coronary lesion UPD
Coronary atherosclerosis due to severely calcified coronary lesion
Code first coronary atherosclerosis (I25.1-, I25.7-, I25.81-)

● **I25.85 Chronic coronary microvascular dysfunction**
Chronic (presentation of) coronary microvascular disease
Coronary microvascular dysfunction NOS

I25.89 Other forms of chronic ischemic heart disease

I25.9 Chronic ischemic heart disease, unspecified
Ischemic heart disease (chronic) NOS

Pulmonary heart disease and diseases of pulmonary circulation (I26-I28)

I26 Pulmonary embolism
INCLUDES pulmonary (acute)(artery)(vein) infarction
pulmonary (acute) (artery)(vein) thromboembolism
pulmonary (acute)(artery)(vein) thrombosis
EXCLUDES 1 ▶*cor pulmonale without embolism (I27.81)*◀
EXCLUDES 2 *chronic pulmonary embolism (I27.82)*
personal history of pulmonary embolism (Z86.711)
pulmonary embolism complicating abortion, ectopic or molar pregnancy (O00-O07, O08.2)
pulmonary embolism complicating pregnancy, childbirth and the puerperium (O88.-)
pulmonary embolism due to trauma (T79.0, T79.1)
pulmonary embolism due to complications of surgical and medical care (T80.0, T81.7-, T82.8-)
septic (non-pulmonary) arterial embolism (I76)
AHA: 2022,3Q,8

I26.0 Pulmonary embolism with acute cor pulmonale
DEF: Cor pulmonale: Heart-lung disease appearing in identifiable forms as chronic or acute. The chronic form of this heart-lung disease is marked by dilation, hypertrophy and failure of the right ventricle due to a disease that has affected the function of the lungs, excluding congenital or left heart diseases and is also called chronic cardiopulmonary disease. The acute form is an overload of the right ventricle from a rapid onset of pulmonary hypertension, usually arising from a pulmonary embolism.

I26.01 Septic pulmonary embolism with acute cor pulmonale MCC UPD HCC
Code first underlying infection

I26.02 Saddle embolus of pulmonary artery with acute cor pulmonale MCC H10 HCC

I26.09 Other pulmonary embolism with acute cor pulmonale MCC H10 HCC
Acute cor pulmonale NOS
AHA: 2014,4Q,21

I26.9 Pulmonary embolism without acute cor pulmonale

I26.90 Septic pulmonary embolism without acute cor pulmonale MCC UPD HCC
Code first underlying infection

I26.92 Saddle embolus of pulmonary artery without acute cor pulmonale MCC H10 HCC

I26.93 Single subsegmental pulmonary embolism without acute cor pulmonale MCC H10 HCC
Subsegmental pulmonary embolism NOS
AHA: 2021,2Q,9; 2019,4Q,6-7

I26.94 Multiple subsegmental pulmonary emboli without acute cor pulmonale MCC H10 HCC
AHA: 2022,2Q,13; 2021,2Q,9; 2019,4Q,6-7

I26.99 Other pulmonary embolism without acute cor pulmonale MCC H10 HCC
Acute pulmonary embolism NOS
Pulmonary embolism NOS
AHA: 2022,2Q,13; 2020,3Q,10-11; 2019,2Q,22

I27 Other pulmonary heart diseases

I27.0 Primary pulmonary hypertension CC HCC
Heritable pulmonary arterial hypertension
Idiopathic pulmonary arterial hypertension
Primary group 1 pulmonary hypertension
Primary pulmonary arterial hypertension
EXCLUDES 1 *persistent pulmonary hypertension of newborn (P29.30)*
pulmonary hypertension NOS (I27.20)
secondary pulmonary arterial hypertension (I27.21)
secondary pulmonary hypertension (I27.29)
DEF: Condition that occurs when pressure within the pulmonary artery is elevated and vascular resistance is observed in the lungs.

I27.1 Kyphoscoliotic heart disease CC HCC

I27.2 Other secondary pulmonary hypertension
Code also associated underlying condition
EXCLUDES 1 *Eisenmenger's syndrome (I27.83)*
AHA: 2017,4Q,14-15; 2014,4Q,21
DEF: Condition that occurs when pressure within the pulmonary artery is elevated and vascular resistance is observed in the lungs.

I27.20 Pulmonary hypertension, unspecified HCC
Pulmonary hypertension NOS

I27.21 Secondary pulmonary arterial hypertension HCC

(Associated) (drug-induced) (toxin-induced) pulmonary arterial hypertension NOS

(Associated) (drug-induced) (toxin-induced) (secondary) group 1 pulmonary hypertension

Code also associated conditions if applicable, or adverse effects of drugs or toxins, such as:

- adverse effect of appetite depressants (T50.5X5)
- congenital heart disease (Q20-Q28)
- human immunodeficiency virus [HIV] disease (B20)
- polymyositis (M33.2-)
- portal hypertension (K76.6)
- rheumatoid arthritis (M05.-)
- schistosomiasis (B65.-)
- Sjogren syndrome (M35.0-)
- systemic sclerosis (M34.-)

I27.22 Pulmonary hypertension due to left heart disease HCC

Group 2 pulmonary hypertension

Code also associated left heart disease, if known, such as:

- multiple valve disease (I08.-)
- rheumatic aortic valve diseases (I06.-)
- rheumatic mitral valve diseases (I05.-)

I27.23 Pulmonary hypertension due to lung diseases and hypoxia HCC

Group 3 pulmonary hypertension

Code also associated lung disease, if known, such as:

- bronchiectasis (J47.-)
- cystic fibrosis with pulmonary manifestations (E84.0)
- interstitial lung disease (J84.-)
- pleural effusion (J90)
- sleep apnea (G47.3-)

I27.24 Chronic thromboembolic pulmonary hypertension HCC

Group 4 pulmonary hypertension

Code also associated pulmonary embolism, if applicable (I26.-, I27.82)

I27.29 Other secondary pulmonary hypertension HCC

Group 5 pulmonary hypertension

Pulmonary hypertension with unclear multifactorial mechanisms

Pulmonary hypertension due to hematologic disorders

Pulmonary hypertension due to metabolic disorders

Pulmonary hypertension due to other systemic disorders

Code also other associated disorders, if known, such as:

- chronic myeloid leukemia (C92.10-C92.22)
- essential thrombocythemia (D47.3)
- Gaucher disease (E75.22)
- hypertensive chronic kidney disease with end stage renal disease (I12.0, I13.11, I13.2)
- hyperthyroidism (E05.-)
- hypothyroidism (E00-E03)
- polycythemia vera (D45)
- sarcoidosis (D86.-)

AHA: 2016,2Q,8

✓5th **I27.8 Other specified pulmonary heart diseases**

I27.81 Cor pulmonale (chronic) HCC

Cor pulmonale NOS

▶Code also, if applicable, right heart failure (I50.81-)◀

EXCLUDES 1 *acute cor pulmonale (I26.0-)*

AHA: 2014,4Q,21

DEF: Heart-lung disease appearing in identifiable forms as chronic or acute. The chronic form of this heart-lung disease is marked by dilation, hypertrophy and failure of the right ventricle due to a disease that has affected the function of the lungs, excluding congenital or left heart diseases and is also called chronic cardiopulmonary disease. The acute form is an overload of the right ventricle from a rapid onset of pulmonary hypertension, usually arising from a pulmonary embolism.

I27.82 Chronic pulmonary embolism CC HCC

Use additional code, if applicable, for associated long-term (current) use of anticoagulants (Z79.01)

EXCLUDES 1 *personal history of pulmonary embolism (Z86.711)*

AHA: 2021,2Q,9

DEF: Long-standing condition commonly associated with pulmonary hypertension in which small blood clots travel to the lungs repeatedly over many weeks, months, or years, requiring continuation of established anticoagulant or thrombolytic therapy.

I27.83 Eisenmenger's syndrome HCC

Eisenmenger's complex

(Irreversible) Eisenmenger's disease

Pulmonary hypertension with right to left shunt related to congenital heart disease

Code also underlying heart defect, if known, such as:

- atrial septal defect (Q21.1-)
- Eisenmenger's defect (Q21.8)
- patent ductus arteriosus (Q25.0)
- ventricular septal defect (Q21.0)

DEF: Pulmonary hypertension with congenital communication between two circulations resulting in a right to left shunt. This causes reduced oxygen saturation in the arterial blood, leading to cyanosis and organ damage. Once it develops, this life-threating condition is irreversible.

I27.89 Other specified pulmonary heart diseases HCC

I27.9 Pulmonary heart disease, unspecified HCC

Chronic cardiopulmonary disease

✓4th **I28 Other diseases of pulmonary vessels**

I28.0 Arteriovenous fistula of pulmonary vessels CC HCC

EXCLUDES 1 *congenital arteriovenous fistula (Q25.72)*

I28.1 Aneurysm of pulmonary artery CC HCC

EXCLUDES 1 *congenital aneurysm (Q25.79)*

congenital arteriovenous aneurysm (Q25.72)

I28.8 Other diseases of pulmonary vessels HCC

Pulmonary arteritis

Pulmonary endarteritis

Rupture of pulmonary vessels

Stenosis of pulmonary vessels

Stricture of pulmonary vessels

I28.9 Disease of pulmonary vessels, unspecified HCC

Other forms of heart disease (I30-I5A)

✓4th **I30 Acute pericarditis**

INCLUDES acute mediastinopericarditis

acute myopericarditis

acute pericardial effusion

acute pleuropericarditis

acute pneumopericarditis

EXCLUDES 1 *Dressler's syndrome (I24.1)*

rheumatic pericarditis (acute) (I01.0)

viral pericarditis due to Coxsakie virus (B33.23)

DEF: Pericarditis: Inflammation affecting the pericardium, the fibroserous membrane that surrounds the heart.

I30.0 Acute nonspecific idiopathic pericarditis CC

I30.1 Infective pericarditis CC

Pneumococcal pericarditis

Pneumopyopericardium

Purulent pericarditis

Pyopericarditis

Pyopericardium

Pyopneumopericardium

Staphylococcal pericarditis

Streptococcal pericarditis

Suppurative pericarditis

Viral pericarditis

Use additional code (B95-B97) to identify infectious agent

I30.8 Other forms of acute pericarditis CC

I30.9 Acute pericarditis, unspecified CC

✓4th **I31 Other diseases of pericardium**

EXCLUDES 1 *diseases of pericardium specified as rheumatic (IØ9.2)*
postcardiotomy syndrome (I97.Ø)
traumatic injury to pericardium (S26.-)

I31.Ø Chronic adhesive pericarditis CC
Accretio cordis
Adherent pericardium
Adhesive mediastinopericarditis

I31.1 Chronic constrictive pericarditis CC
Concretio cordis
Pericardial calcification

I31.2 Hemopericardium, not elsewhere classified CC
EXCLUDES 1 *hemopericardium as current complication following acute myocardial infarction (I23.Ø)*
malignant pericardial effusion (I31.31)

DEF: Presence of blood in the pericardial sac (pericardium). It can lead to potentially fatal cardiac tamponade if enough blood enters the pericardial cavity.

✓5th **I31.3 Pericardial effusion (noninflammatory)**
EXCLUDES 1 *acute pericardial effusion (I3Ø.9)*
AHA: 2022,4Q,22; 2019,1Q,16

I31.31 Malignant pericardial effusion in diseases classified elsewhere CC
Code first underlying neoplasm (CØØ-D49)
AHA: 2022,4Q,22

I31.39 Other pericardial effusion (noninflammatory) CC
Chylopericardium

I31.4 Cardiac tamponade CC UPD
Code first underlying cause
DEF: Life-threatening condition in which fluid or blood accumulates in the space between the muscle of the heart (myocardium) and the outer sac that covers the heart (pericardium), resulting in compression of the heart.

Cardiac Tamponade

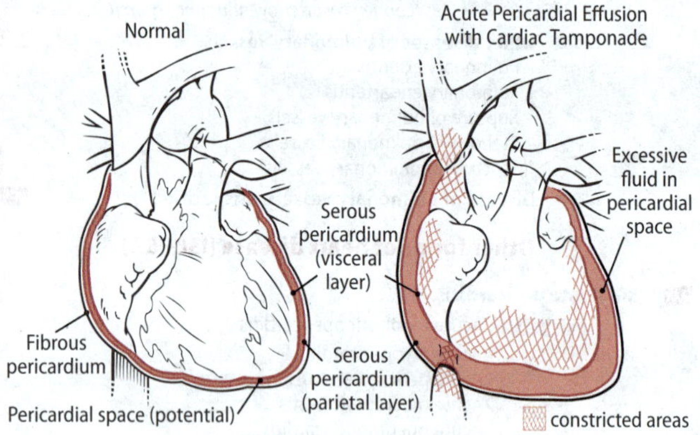

I31.8 Other specified diseases of pericardium CC
Epicardial plaques
Focal pericardial adhesions

I31.9 Disease of pericardium, unspecified CC
Pericarditis (chronic) NOS

I32 Pericarditis in diseases classified elsewhere CC
Code first underlying disease
EXCLUDES 1 *pericarditis (in):*
coxsackie (virus) (B33.23)
gonococcal (A54.83)
meningococcal (A39.53)
rheumatoid (arthritis) (MØ5.31)
syphilitic (A52.Ø6)
systemic lupus erythematosus (M32.12)
tuberculosis (A18.84)

DEF: Pericarditis: Inflammation affecting the pericardium, the fibroserous membrane that surrounds the heart.

✓4th **I33 Acute and subacute endocarditis**
EXCLUDES 1 *acute rheumatic endocarditis (IØ1.1)*
endocarditis NOS (I38)

DEF: Endocarditis: Inflammatory disease of the interior lining of the heart chamber and heart valves.

I33.Ø Acute and subacute infective endocarditis HIV MCC
Bacterial endocarditis (acute) (subacute)
Infective endocarditis (acute) (subacute) NOS
Endocarditis lenta (acute) (subacute)
Malignant endocarditis (acute) (subacute)
Purulent endocarditis (acute) (subacute)
Septic endocarditis (acute) (subacute)
Ulcerative endocarditis (acute) (subacute)
Vegetative endocarditis (acute) (subacute)
Use additional code (B95-B97) to identify infectious agent

I33.9 Acute and subacute endocarditis, unspecified HIV MCC
Acute endocarditis NOS
Acute myoendocarditis NOS
Acute periendocarditis NOS
Subacute endocarditis NOS
Subacute myoendocarditis NOS
Subacute periendocarditis NOS

✓4th **I34 Nonrheumatic mitral valve disorders**
EXCLUDES 1 *mitral valve disease (IØ5.9)*
mitral valve failure (IØ5.8)
mitral valve stenosis (IØ5.Ø)
mitral valve disorder of unspecified cause with diseases of aortic and/or tricuspid valve(s) (IØ8.-)
mitral valve disorder of unspecified cause with mitral stenosis or obstruction (IØ5.Ø)
mitral valve disorder specified as congenital (Q23.2, Q23.9)
mitral valve disorder specified as rheumatic (IØ5.-)

I34.Ø Nonrheumatic mitral (valve) insufficiency
Nonrheumatic mitral (valve) incompetence NOS
Nonrheumatic mitral (valve) regurgitation NOS
Code also, if applicable:
nonrheumatic mitral (valve) annulus calcification (I34.81)

I34.1 Nonrheumatic mitral (valve) prolapse
Floppy nonrheumatic mitral valve syndrome
EXCLUDES 1 *Marfan's syndrome (Q87.4-)*

I34.2 Nonrheumatic mitral (valve) stenosis
Code also, if applicable:
nonrheumatic mitral (valve) annulus calcification (I34.81)

✓5th **I34.8 Other nonrheumatic mitral valve disorders**
AHA: 2022,4Q,23

I34.81 Nonrheumatic mitral (valve) annulus calcification
Nonrheumatic mitral (valve) annular calcification
Mitral (valve) annulus calcification NOS
Code also, if applicable:
nonrheumatic mitral (valve) insufficiency (I34.Ø)
nonrheumatic mitral (valve) stenosis (I34.2)

I34.89 Other nonrheumatic mitral valve disorders

I34.9 Nonrheumatic mitral valve disorder, unspecified

✓4th **I35 Nonrheumatic aortic valve disorders**
EXCLUDES 1 *aortic valve disorder of unspecified cause but with diseases of mitral and/or tricuspid valve(s) (IØ8.-)*
aortic valve disorder specified as congenital (Q23.Ø, Q23.1)
aortic valve disorder specified as rheumatic (IØ6.-)
hypertrophic subaortic stenosis (I42.1)

I35.Ø Nonrheumatic aortic (valve) stenosis

I35.1 Nonrheumatic aortic (valve) insufficiency
Nonrheumatic aortic (valve) incompetence NOS
Nonrheumatic aortic (valve) regurgitation NOS

I35.2 Nonrheumatic aortic (valve) stenosis with insufficiency

I35.8 Other nonrheumatic aortic valve disorders

I35.9 Nonrheumatic aortic valve disorder, unspecified

✓4th **I36 Nonrheumatic tricuspid valve disorders**
EXCLUDES 1 *tricuspid valve disorders of unspecified cause (IØ7.-)*
tricuspid valve disorders specified as congenital (Q22.4, Q22.8, Q22.9)
tricuspid valve disorders specified as rheumatic (IØ7.-)
tricuspid valve disorders with aortic and/or mitral valve involvement (IØ8.-)

I36.Ø Nonrheumatic tricuspid (valve) stenosis

I36.1 Nonrheumatic tricuspid (valve) insufficiency
Nonrheumatic tricuspid (valve) incompetence
Nonrheumatic tricuspid (valve) regurgitation

I36.2 Nonrheumatic tricuspid (valve) stenosis with insufficiency

I36.8 Other nonrheumatic tricuspid valve disorders

I36.9 Nonrheumatic tricuspid valve disorder, unspecified

I37 Nonrheumatic pulmonary valve disorders

EXCLUDES 1 *pulmonary valve disorder specified as congenital (Q22.1, Q22.2, Q22.3)*
pulmonary valve disorder specified as rheumatic (I09.89)

I37.0 Nonrheumatic pulmonary valve stenosis

I37.1 Nonrheumatic pulmonary valve insufficiency
Nonrheumatic pulmonary valve incompetence
Nonrheumatic pulmonary valve regurgitation

I37.2 Nonrheumatic pulmonary valve stenosis with insufficiency

I37.8 Other nonrheumatic pulmonary valve disorders

I37.9 Nonrheumatic pulmonary valve disorder, unspecified

I38 Endocarditis, valve unspecified CC

INCLUDES endocarditis (chronic) NOS
valvular incompetence NOS
valvular insufficiency NOS
valvular regurgitation NOS
valvular stenosis NOS
valvulitis (chronic) NOS

EXCLUDES 1 *congenital insufficiency of cardiac valve NOS (Q24.8)*
congenital stenosis of cardiac valve NOS (Q24.8)
endocardial fibroelastosis (I42.4)
endocarditis specified as rheumatic (I09.1)

DEF: Endocarditis: Inflammatory disease of the interior lining of the heart chamber and heart valves.

I39 Endocarditis and heart valve disorders in diseases classified elsewhere CC

Code first underlying disease, such as:
Q fever (A78)

EXCLUDES 1 *endocardial involvement in:*
candidiasis (B37.6)
gonococcal infection (A54.83)
Libman-Sacks disease (M32.11)
listerosis (A32.82)
meningococcal infection (A39.51)
rheumatoid arthritis (M05.31)
syphilis (A52.03)
tuberculosis (A18.84)
typhoid fever (A01.02)

DEF: Endocarditis: Inflammatory disease of the interior lining of the heart chamber and heart valves.

I40 Acute myocarditis

INCLUDES subacute myocarditis

EXCLUDES 1 *acute rheumatic myocarditis (I01.2)*

DEF: Myocarditis: Inflammation of the middle layer of the heart, which is composed of muscle tissue.

I40.0 Infective myocarditis HIV MCC
Septic myocarditis
Use additional code (B95-B97) to identify infectious agent

I40.1 Isolated myocarditis HIV MCC
Fiedler's myocarditis
Giant cell myocarditis
Idiopathic myocarditis

I40.8 Other acute myocarditis HIV MCC

I40.9 Acute myocarditis, unspecified HIV MCC

I41 Myocarditis in diseases classified elsewhere MCC

Code first underlying disease, such as:
typhus (A75.0-A75.9)

EXCLUDES 1 *myocarditis (in):*
Chagas' disease (chronic) (B57.2)
acute (B57.0)
coxsackie (virus) infection (B33.22)
diphtheritic (A36.81)
gonococcal (A54.83)
influenzal (J09.X9, J10.82, J11.82)
meningococcal (A39.52)
mumps (B26.82)
rheumatoid arthritis (M05.31)
sarcoid (D86.85)
syphilis (A52.06)
toxoplasmosis (B58.81)
tuberculous (A18.84)

DEF: Myocarditis: Inflammation of the middle layer of the heart, which is composed of muscle tissue.

I42 Cardiomyopathy

INCLUDES myocardiopathy

Code first pre-existing cardiomyopathy complicating pregnancy and puerperium (O99.4)

EXCLUDES 2 *ischemic cardiomyopathy (I25.5)*
peripartum cardiomyopathy (O90.3)
ventricular hypertrophy (I51.7)

I42.0 Dilated cardiomyopathy CC HCC
Congestive cardiomyopathy

I42.1 Obstructive hypertrophic cardiomyopathy CC HCC
Hypertrophic subaortic stenosis (idiopathic)
DEF: Cardiomyopathy marked by left ventricle hypertrophy and an enlarged septum that result in obstructed blood flow, arrhythmias, mitral regurgitation, and sudden cardiac death.
TIP: When this condition is described as inherited, assign code Q24.8.

I42.2 Other hypertrophic cardiomyopathy CC HCC
Nonobstructive hypertrophic cardiomyopathy

I42.3 Endomyocardial (eosinophilic) disease CC HCC
Endomyocardial (tropical) fibrosis
Loffler's endocarditis

I42.4 Endocardial fibroelastosis CC HCC
Congenital cardiomyopathy
Elastomyofibrosis

I42.5 Other restrictive cardiomyopathy CC HCC
Constrictive cardiomyopathy NOS

I42.6 Alcoholic cardiomyopathy CC HCC
Code also presence of alcoholism (F10.-)

I42.7 Cardiomyopathy due to drug and external agent CC HCC
Code first poisoning due to drug or toxin, if applicable ▶(T36-T65 with fifth or sixth character 1-4)◀
Use additional code for adverse effect, if applicable, to identify drug (T36-T50 with fifth or sixth character 5)
AHA: 2021,3Q,8

I42.8 Other cardiomyopathies CC HCC

I42.9 Cardiomyopathy, unspecified CC HCC
Cardiomyopathy (primary) (secondary) NOS

I43 Cardiomyopathy in diseases classified elsewhere CC HCC

Code first underlying disease, such as:
amyloidosis (E85.-)
glycogen storage disease ▶(E74.0-)◀
gout (M10.0-)
thyrotoxicosis (E05.0-E05.9-)

EXCLUDES 1 *cardiomyopathy (in):*
coxsackie (virus) (B33.24)
diphtheria (A36.81)
sarcoidosis (D86.85)
tuberculosis (A18.84)

I44 Atrioventricular and left bundle-branch block

I44.0 Atrioventricular block, first degree

I44.1 Atrioventricular block, second degree
Atrioventricular block, type I and II
Möbitz block, type I and II
Second degree block, type I and II
Wenckebach's block

I44.2 Atrioventricular block, complete CC HCC
Complete heart block NOS
Third degree block
AHA: 2019,2Q,4

✓5th **I44.3 Other and unspecified atrioventricular block**
Atrioventricular block NOS

I44.30 Unspecified atrioventricular block
I44.39 Other atrioventricular block

I44.4 Left anterior fascicular block
I44.5 Left posterior fascicular block

✓5th **I44.6 Other and unspecified fascicular block**

I44.60 Unspecified fascicular block
Left bundle-branch hemiblock NOS
I44.69 Other fascicular block

I44.7 Left bundle-branch block, unspecified

Conduction Disorders

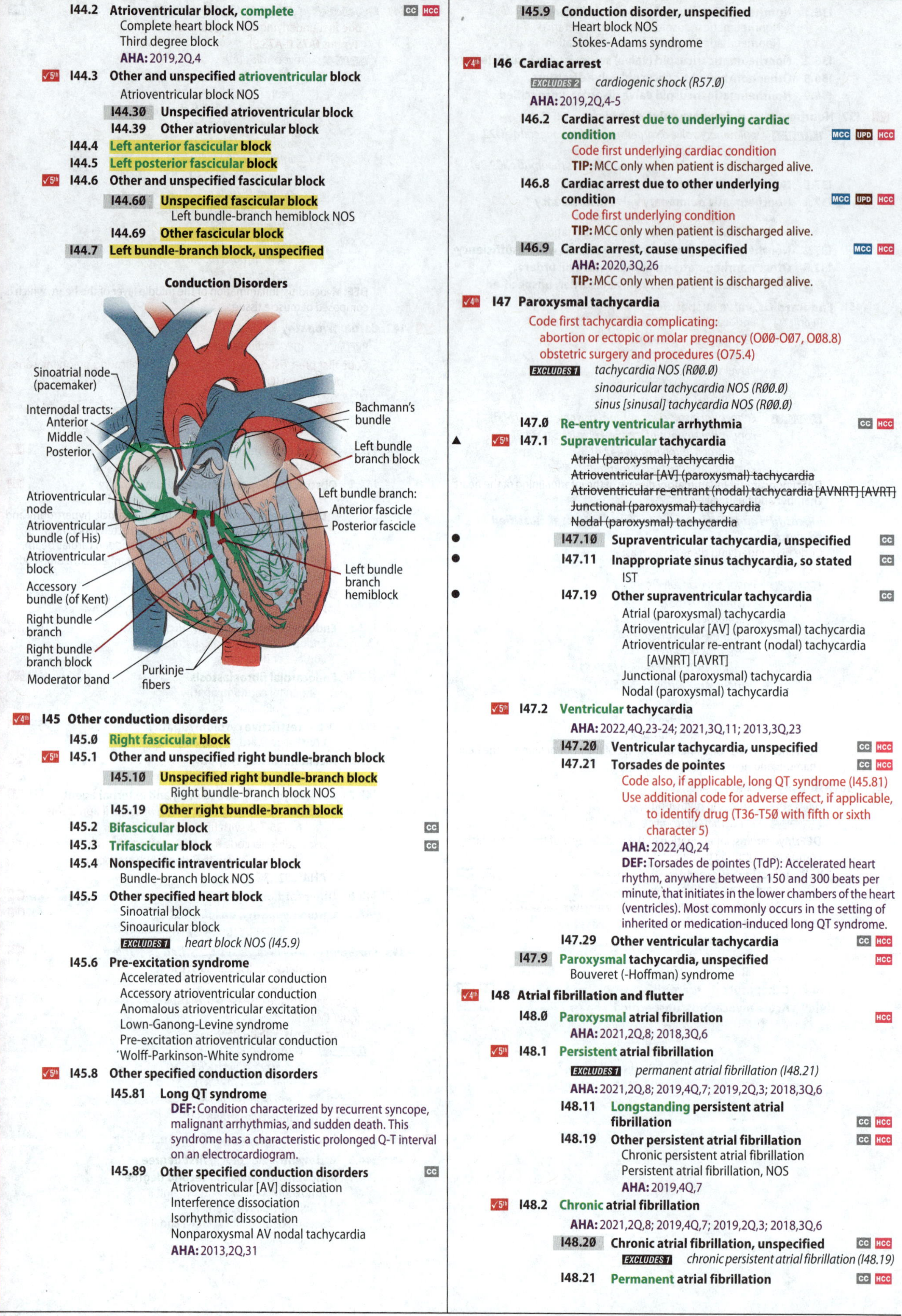

✓4th **I45 Other conduction disorders**

I45.0 Right fascicular block

✓5th **I45.1 Other and unspecified right bundle-branch block**

I45.10 Unspecified right bundle-branch block
Right bundle-branch block NOS
I45.19 Other right bundle-branch block

I45.2 Bifascicular block CC
I45.3 Trifascicular block CC
I45.4 Nonspecific intraventricular block
Bundle-branch block NOS
I45.5 Other specified heart block
Sinoatrial block
Sinoauricular block
EXCLUDES 1 *heart block NOS (I45.9)*
I45.6 Pre-excitation syndrome
Accelerated atrioventricular conduction
Accessory atrioventricular conduction
Anomalous atrioventricular excitation
Lown-Ganong-Levine syndrome
Pre-excitation atrioventricular conduction
Wolff-Parkinson-White syndrome

✓5th **I45.8 Other specified conduction disorders**

I45.81 Long QT syndrome
DEF: Condition characterized by recurrent syncope, malignant arrhythmias, and sudden death. This syndrome has a characteristic prolonged Q-T interval on an electrocardiogram.
I45.89 Other specified conduction disorders CC
Atrioventricular [AV] dissociation
Interference dissociation
Isorhythmic dissociation
Nonparoxysmal AV nodal tachycardia
AHA: 2013,2Q,31

I45.9 Conduction disorder, unspecified
Heart block NOS
Stokes-Adams syndrome

✓4th **I46 Cardiac arrest**
EXCLUDES 2 *cardiogenic shock (R57.0)*
AHA: 2019,2Q,4-5

I46.2 Cardiac arrest due to underlying cardiac condition MCC UPD HCC
Code first underlying cardiac condition
TIP: MCC only when patient is discharged alive.
I46.8 Cardiac arrest due to other underlying condition MCC UPD HCC
Code first underlying condition
TIP: MCC only when patient is discharged alive.
I46.9 Cardiac arrest, cause unspecified MCC HCC
AHA: 2020,3Q,26
TIP: MCC only when patient is discharged alive.

✓4th **I47 Paroxysmal tachycardia**
Code first tachycardia complicating:
abortion or ectopic or molar pregnancy (O00-O07, O08.8)
obstetric surgery and procedures (O75.4)
EXCLUDES 1 *tachycardia NOS (R00.0)*
sinoauricular tachycardia NOS (R00.0)
sinus [sinusal] tachycardia NOS (R00.0)

I47.0 Re-entry ventricular arrhythmia CC HCC

▲ ✓5th **I47.1 Supraventricular tachycardia**
~~Atrial (paroxysmal) tachycardia~~
~~Atrioventricular [AV] (paroxysmal) tachycardia~~
~~Atrioventricular re-entrant (nodal) tachycardia [AVNRT] [AVRT]~~
~~Junctional (paroxysmal) tachycardia~~
~~Nodal (paroxysmal) tachycardia~~

● **I47.10 Supraventricular tachycardia, unspecified** CC
● **I47.11 Inappropriate sinus tachycardia, so stated** CC
IST
● **I47.19 Other supraventricular tachycardia** CC
Atrial (paroxysmal) tachycardia
Atrioventricular [AV] (paroxysmal) tachycardia
Atrioventricular re-entrant (nodal) tachycardia [AVNRT] [AVRT]
Junctional (paroxysmal) tachycardia
Nodal (paroxysmal) tachycardia

✓5th **I47.2 Ventricular tachycardia**
AHA: 2022,4Q,23-24; 2021,3Q,11; 2013,3Q,23

I47.20 Ventricular tachycardia, unspecified CC HCC
I47.21 Torsades de pointes CC HCC
Code also, if applicable, long QT syndrome (I45.81)
Use additional code for adverse effect, if applicable, to identify drug (T36-T50 with fifth or sixth character 5)
AHA: 2022,4Q,24
DEF: Torsades de pointes (TdP): Accelerated heart rhythm, anywhere between 150 and 300 beats per minute, that initiates in the lower chambers of the heart (ventricles). Most commonly occurs in the setting of inherited or medication-induced long QT syndrome.
I47.29 Other ventricular tachycardia CC HCC

I47.9 Paroxysmal tachycardia, unspecified HCC
Bouveret (-Hoffman) syndrome

✓4th **I48 Atrial fibrillation and flutter**

I48.0 Paroxysmal atrial fibrillation HCC
AHA: 2021,2Q,8; 2018,3Q,6

✓5th **I48.1 Persistent atrial fibrillation**
EXCLUDES 1 *permanent atrial fibrillation (I48.21)*
AHA: 2021,2Q,8; 2019,4Q,7; 2019,2Q,3; 2018,3Q,6

I48.11 Longstanding persistent atrial fibrillation CC HCC
I48.19 Other persistent atrial fibrillation CC HCC
Chronic persistent atrial fibrillation
Persistent atrial fibrillation, NOS
AHA: 2019,4Q,7

✓5th **I48.2 Chronic atrial fibrillation**
AHA: 2021,2Q,8; 2019,4Q,7; 2019,2Q,3; 2018,3Q,6

I48.20 Chronic atrial fibrillation, unspecified CC HCC
EXCLUDES 1 *chronic persistent atrial fibrillation (I48.19)*
I48.21 Permanent atrial fibrillation CC HCC

I48.3 **Typical atrial flutter** CC HCC
Type I atrial flutter

I48.4 **Atypical atrial flutter** CC HCC
Type II atrial flutter

✓5th **I48.9** **Unspecified atrial fibrillation and atrial flutter**

I48.91 **Unspecified atrial fibrillation** HCC

I48.92 **Unspecified atrial flutter** CC HCC

✓4th **I49 Other cardiac arrhythmias**

Code first cardiac arrhythmia complicating:
abortion or ectopic or molar pregnancy (OØØ-OØ7, OØ8.8)
obstetric surgery and procedures (O75.4)

EXCLUDES 1 *neonatal dysrhythmia (P29.1-)*
sinoatrial bradycardia (RØØ.1)
sinus bradycardia (RØØ.1)
vagal bradycardia (RØØ.1)

EXCLUDES 2 *bradycardia NOS (RØØ.1)*

✓5th **I49.Ø** **Ventricular fibrillation and flutter**

I49.Ø1 **Ventricular fibrillation** MCC HCC
AHA: 2022,2Q,14
TIP: MCC only when patient is discharged alive.

I49.Ø2 **Ventricular flutter** MCC HCC

I49.1 **Atrial premature depolarization**
Atrial premature beats

I49.2 **Junctional premature depolarization** CC HCC

I49.3 **Ventricular premature depolarization**
AHA: 2020,2Q,23

✓5th **I49.4** **Other and unspecified premature depolarization**

I49.4Ø **Unspecified premature depolarization**
Premature beats NOS

I49.49 **Other premature depolarization**
Ectopic beats
Extrasystoles
Extrasystolic arrhythmias
Premature contractions

I49.5 **Sick sinus syndrome** HCC
Tachycardia-bradycardia syndrome
AHA: 2019,1Q,33
TIP: The presence of a pacemaker controls but does not cure sick sinus syndrome and therefore is considered a reportable chronic condition. When a pacemaker is evaluated by a provider, this code and code Z95.0 Presence of cardiac pacemaker, should be reported, even in the absence of any notable changes or management.

I49.8 **Other specified cardiac arrhythmias**
Brugada syndrome
Coronary sinus rhythm disorder
Ectopic rhythm disorder
Nodal rhythm disorder

I49.9 **Cardiac arrhythmia, unspecified**
Arrhythmia (cardiac) NOS

✓4th **I5Ø Heart failure**

Code first:
heart failure complicating abortion or ectopic or molar pregnancy (OØØ-OØ7, OØ8.8)
heart failure due to hypertension (I11.Ø)
heart failure due to hypertension with chronic kidney disease (I13.-)
heart failure following surgery (I97.13-)
obstetric surgery and procedures (O75.4)
rheumatic heart failure (IØ9.81)

EXCLUDES 2 *cardiac arrest (I46.-)*
neonatal cardiac failure (P29.Ø)

AHA: 2018,4Q,67; 2018,2Q,9; 2017,1Q,47; 2014,1Q,25; 2013,2Q,33

I5Ø.1 **Left ventricular failure, unspecified** CC HCC
Cardiac asthma
Edema of lung with heart disease NOS
Edema of lung with heart failure
Left heart failure
Pulmonary edema with heart disease NOS
Pulmonary edema with heart failure

EXCLUDES 1 *edema of lung without heart disease or heart failure (J81.-)*
pulmonary edema without heart disease or failure (J81.-)

✓5th **I5Ø.2** **Systolic (congestive) heart failure**
Heart failure with reduced ejection fraction [HFrEF]
Systolic left ventricular heart failure
Code also end stage heart failure, if applicable (I5Ø.84)

EXCLUDES 1 *combined systolic (congestive) and diastolic (congestive) heart failure (I5Ø.4-)*

AHA: 2020,3Q,32; 2017,1Q,46; 2016,1Q,10

I5Ø.2Ø **Unspecified systolic (congestive) heart failure** CC HCC

I5Ø.21 **Acute systolic (congestive) heart failure** MCC HCC

I5Ø.22 **Chronic systolic (congestive) heart failure** CC HCC

I5Ø.23 **Acute on chronic systolic (congestive) heart failure** MCC HCC

✓5th **I5Ø.3** **Diastolic (congestive) heart failure**
Diastolic left ventricular heart failure
Heart failure with normal ejection fraction
Heart failure with preserved ejection fraction [HFpEF]
Code also end stage heart failure, if applicable (I5Ø.84)

EXCLUDES 1 *combined systolic (congestive) and diastolic (congestive) heart failure (I5Ø.4-)*

AHA: 2020,3Q,32; 2017,1Q,46; 2016,1Q,10

I5Ø.3Ø **Unspecified diastolic (congestive) heart failure** CC HCC

I5Ø.31 **Acute diastolic (congestive) heart failure** MCC HCC

I5Ø.32 **Chronic diastolic (congestive) heart failure** CC HCC

I5Ø.33 **Acute on chronic diastolic (congestive) heart failure** MCC HCC

✓5th **I5Ø.4** **Combined systolic (congestive) and diastolic (congestive) heart failure**
Combined systolic and diastolic left ventricular heart failure
Heart failure with reduced ejection fraction and diastolic dysfunction
Code also end stage heart failure, if applicable (I5Ø.84)
AHA: 2017,1Q,46; 2016,1Q,10

I5Ø.4Ø **Unspecified combined systolic (congestive) and diastolic (congestive) heart failure** CC HCC

I5Ø.41 **Acute combined systolic (congestive) and diastolic (congestive) heart failure** MCC HCC

I5Ø.42 **Chronic combined systolic (congestive) and diastolic (congestive) heart failure** CC HCC

I5Ø.43 **Acute on chronic combined systolic (congestive) and diastolic (congestive) heart failure** MCC HCC

✓5th **I5Ø.8** **Other heart failure**
AHA: 2022,3Q,16; 2017,4Q,15-16

✓6th **I5Ø.81** **Right heart failure**
Right ventricular failure

I5Ø.81Ø **Right heart failure, unspecified** HCC
Right heart failure without mention of left heart failure
Right ventricular failure NOS

I5Ø.811 **Acute right heart failure** HCC
Acute isolated right heart failure
Acute (isolated) right ventricular failure

I5Ø.812 **Chronic right heart failure** HCC
Chronic isolated right heart failure
Chronic (isolated) right ventricular failure

I5Ø.813 **Acute on chronic right heart failure** HCC
Acute on chronic isolated right heart failure
Acute on chronic (isolated) right ventricular failure
Acute decompensation of chronic (isolated) right ventricular failure
Acute exacerbation of chronic (isolated) right ventricular failure

I5Ø.814 **Right heart failure due to left heart failure** HCC
Right ventricular failure secondary to left ventricular failure
Code also the type of left ventricular failure, if known (I5Ø.2-I5Ø.43)

EXCLUDES 1 *right heart failure with but not due to left heart failure (I5Ø.82)*

I50.82 Biventricular heart failure HCC
Code also the type of left ventricular failure as systolic, diastolic, or combined, if known (I50.2-I50.43)

I50.83 High output heart failure HCC
DEF: Occurs when the high demand for blood exceeds the capacity of a normally functioning heart to meet the demand.

I50.84 End stage heart failure HCC
Stage D heart failure
Code also the type of heart failure as systolic, diastolic, or combined, if known (I50.2-I50.43)

I50.89 Other heart failure HCC

I50.9 Heart failure, unspecified HCC
Cardiac, heart or myocardial failure NOS
Congestive heart disease
Congestive heart failure NOS
EXCLUDES 2 *fluid overload unrelated to congestive heart failure (E87.70)*
AHA: 2017,4Q,15-16; 2017,1Q,45-46; 2014,4Q,21; 2012,4Q,92

4th I51 Complications and ill-defined descriptions of heart disease
EXCLUDES 1 *any condition in I51.4-I51.9 due to hypertension (I11.-)*
any condition in I51.4-I51.9 due to hypertension and chronic kidney disease (I13.-)
heart disease specified as rheumatic (I00-I09)

I51.0 Cardiac septal defect, acquired CC A
Acquired septal atrial defect (old)
Acquired septal auricular defect (old)
Acquired septal ventricular defect (old)
EXCLUDES 1 *cardiac septal defect as current complication following acute myocardial infarction (I23.1, I23.2)*
DEF: Abnormal communication between opposite heart chambers due to a defect of the septum. It is not present at birth.

I51.1 Rupture of chordae tendineae, not elsewhere classified MCC HCC
EXCLUDES 1 *rupture of chordae tendineae as current complication following acute myocardial infarction (I23.4)*

I51.2 Rupture of papillary muscle, not elsewhere classified MCC HCC
EXCLUDES 1 *rupture of papillary muscle as current complication following acute myocardial infarction (I23.5)*

I51.3 Intracardiac thrombosis, not elsewhere classified
Apical thrombosis (old)
Atrial thrombosis (old)
Auricular thrombosis (old)
Mural thrombosis (old)
Ventricular thrombosis (old)
EXCLUDES 1 *intracardiac thrombosis as current complication following acute myocardial infarction (I23.6)*
AHA: 2013,1Q,24

I51.4 Myocarditis, unspecified HCC
Chronic (interstitial) myocarditis
Myocardial fibrosis
Myocarditis NOS
EXCLUDES 1 *acute or subacute myocarditis (I40.-)*
AHA: 2018,4Q,67; 2018,2Q,9

I51.5 Myocardial degeneration HCC
Fatty degeneration of heart or myocardium
Myocardial disease
Senile degeneration of heart or myocardium
AHA: 2018,4Q,67; 2018,2Q,9

I51.7 Cardiomegaly
Cardiac dilatation
Cardiac hypertrophy
Ventricular dilatation
AHA: 2018,4Q,67; 2018,2Q,9

5th I51.8 Other ill-defined heart diseases
AHA: 2018,2Q,9

I51.81 Takotsubo syndrome CC
Reversible left ventricular dysfunction following sudden emotional stress
Stress induced cardiomyopathy
Takotsubo cardiomyopathy
Transient left ventricular apical ballooning syndrome
DEF: Complex of symptoms mimicking myocardial infarct in absence of heart disease, with the majority of cases occurring in postmenopausal women. Heart muscles are temporarily weakened, and a sudden, massive surge of adrenalin stuns the heart, greatly reducing the ability to pump blood.

I51.89 Other ill-defined heart diseases
Carditis (acute)(chronic)
Pancarditis (acute)(chronic)
AHA: 2019,2Q,5; 2018,4Q,67

I51.9 Heart disease, unspecified
AHA: 2018,4Q,67; 2018,2Q,9

I52 Other heart disorders in diseases classified elsewhere
Code first underlying disease, such as:
congenital syphilis (A50.5)
mucopolysaccharidosis (E76.3)
schistosomiasis (B65.0-B65.9)
EXCLUDES 1 *heart disease (in):*
gonococcal infection (A54.83)
meningococcal infection (A39.50)
rheumatoid arthritis (M05.31)
syphilis (A52.06)

I5A Non-ischemic myocardial injury (non-traumatic) CC
Acute (non-ischemic) myocardial injury
Chronic (non-ischemic) myocardial injury
Unspecified (non-ischemic) myocardial injury
Code first the underlying cause, if known and applicable, such as:
acute kidney failure (N17.-)
acute myocarditis (I40.-)
cardiomyopathy (I42.-)
chronic kidney disease (CKD) (N18.-)
heart failure (I50.-)
hypertensive urgency (I16.0)
nonrheumatic aortic valve disorders (I35.-)
paroxysmal tachycardia (I47.-)
pulmonary embolism (I26.-)
pulmonary hypertension (I27.0, I27.2-)
sepsis (A41.-)
takotsubo syndrome (I51.81)
EXCLUDES 1 *acute myocardial infarction (I21.-)*
injury of heart (S26.-)
EXCLUDES 2 *other acute ischemic heart diseases (I24.-)*
AHA: 2021,4Q,14-15

Cerebrovascular diseases (I60-I69)

Use additional code to identify presence of:
alcohol abuse and dependence (F10.-)
exposure to environmental tobacco smoke (Z77.22)
history of tobacco dependence (Z87.891)
hypertension ▶(I10-I1A)◀
occupational exposure to environmental tobacco smoke (Z57.31)
tobacco dependence (F17.-)
tobacco use (Z72.0)
EXCLUDES 1 *traumatic intracranial hemorrhage (S06.-)*
AHA: 2014,3Q,5; 2012,4Q,91-92

4th I60 Nontraumatic subarachnoid hemorrhage
▶Use additional code, if known, to indicate National Institutes of Health Stroke Scale (NIHSS) score (R29.7-)◀
EXCLUDES 1 *syphilitic ruptured cerebral aneurysm (A52.05)*
EXCLUDES 2 *sequelae of subarachnoid hemorrhage (I69.0-)*

5th I60.0 Nontraumatic subarachnoid hemorrhage from carotid siphon and bifurcation

I60.00 Nontraumatic subarachnoid hemorrhage from unspecified carotid siphon and bifurcation MCC HCC

I60.01 Nontraumatic subarachnoid hemorrhage from right carotid siphon and bifurcation MCC HCC

I60.02 Nontraumatic subarachnoid hemorrhage from left carotid siphon and bifurcation MCC HCC

I60.1 Nontraumatic subarachnoid hemorrhage from middle cerebral artery
- I60.10 Nontraumatic subarachnoid hemorrhage from unspecified middle cerebral artery MCC HCC
- I60.11 Nontraumatic subarachnoid hemorrhage from right middle cerebral artery MCC HCC
- I60.12 Nontraumatic subarachnoid hemorrhage from left middle cerebral artery MCC HCC

I60.2 Nontraumatic subarachnoid hemorrhage from anterior communicating artery MCC HCC

I60.3 Nontraumatic subarachnoid hemorrhage from posterior communicating artery
- I60.30 Nontraumatic subarachnoid hemorrhage from unspecified posterior communicating artery MCC HCC
- I60.31 Nontraumatic subarachnoid hemorrhage from right posterior communicating artery MCC HCC
- I60.32 Nontraumatic subarachnoid hemorrhage from left posterior communicating artery MCC HCC

I60.4 Nontraumatic subarachnoid hemorrhage from basilar artery MCC HCC

I60.5 Nontraumatic subarachnoid hemorrhage from vertebral artery
- I60.50 Nontraumatic subarachnoid hemorrhage from unspecified vertebral artery MCC HCC
- I60.51 Nontraumatic subarachnoid hemorrhage from right vertebral artery MCC HCC
- I60.52 Nontraumatic subarachnoid hemorrhage from left vertebral artery MCC HCC

I60.6 Nontraumatic subarachnoid hemorrhage from other intracranial arteries MCC HCC

I60.7 Nontraumatic subarachnoid hemorrhage from unspecified intracranial artery MCC HCC
- Ruptured (congenital) berry aneurysm
- Ruptured (congenital) cerebral aneurysm
- Subarachnoid hemorrhage (nontraumatic) from cerebral artery NOS
- Subarachnoid hemorrhage (nontraumatic) from communicating artery NOS

EXCLUDES 1 *berry aneurysm, nonruptured (I67.1)*

I60.8 Other nontraumatic subarachnoid hemorrhage MCC HCC
- Meningeal hemorrhage
- Rupture of cerebral arteriovenous malformation

I60.9 Nontraumatic subarachnoid hemorrhage, unspecified MCC HCC

I61 Nontraumatic intracerebral hemorrhage

▶Use additional code, if known, to indicate National Institutes of Health Stroke Scale (NIHSS) score (R29.7-)◀

EXCLUDES 2 *sequelae of intracerebral hemorrhage (I69.1-)*

AHA: 2022,3Q,9-10; 2017,2Q,9-10

I61.0 Nontraumatic intracerebral hemorrhage in hemisphere, subcortical MCC HCC
- Deep intracerebral hemorrhage (nontraumatic)
- **AHA:** 2016,4Q,27

I61.1 Nontraumatic intracerebral hemorrhage in hemisphere, cortical MCC HCC
- Cerebral lobe hemorrhage (nontraumatic)
- Superficial intracerebral hemorrhage (nontraumatic)

I61.2 Nontraumatic intracerebral hemorrhage in hemisphere, unspecified MCC HCC

I61.3 Nontraumatic intracerebral hemorrhage in brain stem MCC HCC

I61.4 Nontraumatic intracerebral hemorrhage in cerebellum MCC HCC

I61.5 Nontraumatic intracerebral hemorrhage, intraventricular MCC HCC

I61.6 Nontraumatic intracerebral hemorrhage, multiple localized MCC HCC

I61.8 Other nontraumatic intracerebral hemorrhage MCC HCC

I61.9 Nontraumatic intracerebral hemorrhage, unspecified MCC HCC

I62 Other and unspecified nontraumatic intracranial hemorrhage

▶Use additional code, if known, to indicate National Institutes of Health Stroke Scale (NIHSS) score (R29.7-)◀

EXCLUDES 2 *sequelae of intracranial hemorrhage (I69.2)*

I62.0 Nontraumatic subdural hemorrhage
- I62.00 Nontraumatic subdural hemorrhage, unspecified MCC HCC
- I62.01 Nontraumatic acute subdural hemorrhage MCC HCC
- I62.02 Nontraumatic subacute subdural hemorrhage MCC HCC
- I62.03 Nontraumatic chronic subdural hemorrhage MCC HCC

I62.1 Nontraumatic extradural hemorrhage MCC HCC
- Nontraumatic epidural hemorrhage

I62.9 Nontraumatic intracranial hemorrhage, unspecified CC HCC

I63 Cerebral infarction

INCLUDES occlusion and stenosis of cerebral and precerebral arteries, resulting in cerebral infarction

Use additional code, if applicable, to identify status post administration of tPA (rtPA) in a different facility within the last 24 hours prior to admission to current facility (Z92.82)

Use additional code, if known, to indicate National Institutes of Health Stroke Scale (NIHSS) score (R29.7-)

EXCLUDES 1 *neonatal cerebral infarction (P91.82-)*

EXCLUDES 2 *▶chronic, without residual deficits (sequelae) (Z86.73)◀*
sequelae of cerebral infarction (I69.3-)

AHA: 2017,2Q,9-10; 2016,4Q,28,61-62; 2015,1Q,25; 2014,1Q,23

TIP: Weakness on one side of the body documented as secondary to stroke is synonymous with hemiparesis/hemiplegia (G81.-). Weakness of one limb documented as secondary to stroke is synonymous with monoplegia (G83.1-, G83.2-, G83.3-).

I63.0 Cerebral infarction due to thrombosis of precerebral arteries
- I63.00 Cerebral infarction due to thrombosis of unspecified precerebral artery MCC HCC
- I63.01 Cerebral infarction due to thrombosis of vertebral artery
  - I63.011 Cerebral infarction due to thrombosis of right vertebral artery MCC HCC
  - I63.012 Cerebral infarction due to thrombosis of left vertebral artery MCC HCC
  - I63.013 Cerebral infarction due to thrombosis of bilateral vertebral arteries MCC HCC
  - I63.019 Cerebral infarction due to thrombosis of unspecified vertebral artery MCC HCC
- I63.02 Cerebral infarction due to thrombosis of basilar artery MCC HCC
- I63.03 Cerebral infarction due to thrombosis of carotid artery
  - I63.031 Cerebral infarction due to thrombosis of right carotid artery MCC HCC
  - I63.032 Cerebral infarction due to thrombosis of left carotid artery MCC HCC
  - I63.033 Cerebral infarction due to thrombosis of bilateral carotid arteries MCC HCC
  - I63.039 Cerebral infarction due to thrombosis of unspecified carotid artery MCC HCC
- I63.09 Cerebral infarction due to thrombosis of other precerebral artery MCC HCC

I63.1 Cerebral infarction due to embolism of precerebral arteries
- I63.10 Cerebral infarction due to embolism of unspecified precerebral artery MCC HCC
- I63.11 Cerebral infarction due to embolism of vertebral artery
  - I63.111 Cerebral infarction due to embolism of right vertebral artery MCC HCC
  - I63.112 Cerebral infarction due to embolism of left vertebral artery MCC HCC
  - I63.113 Cerebral infarction due to embolism of bilateral vertebral arteries MCC HCC
  - I63.119 Cerebral infarction due to embolism of unspecified vertebral artery MCC HCC
- I63.12 Cerebral infarction due to embolism of basilar artery MCC HCC
- I63.13 Cerebral infarction due to embolism of carotid artery
  - I63.131 Cerebral infarction due to embolism of right carotid artery MCC HCC
  - I63.132 Cerebral infarction due to embolism of left carotid artery MCC HCC
  - I63.133 Cerebral infarction due to embolism of bilateral carotid arteries MCC HCC
  - I63.139 Cerebral infarction due to embolism of unspecified carotid artery MCC HCC
- I63.19 Cerebral infarction due to embolism of other precerebral artery MCC HCC

Chapter 9. Diseases of the Circulatory System I60.1–I63.19

5th I63.2 Cerebral infarction due to unspecified occlusion or stenosis of precerebral arteries
AHA: 2020,3Q,27-28
- I63.20 Cerebral infarction due to unspecified occlusion or stenosis of unspecified precerebral arteries MCC HCC
- 6th I63.21 Cerebral infarction due to unspecified occlusion or stenosis of vertebral arteries
  - I63.211 Cerebral infarction due to unspecified occlusion or stenosis of right vertebral artery MCC HCC
  - I63.212 Cerebral infarction due to unspecified occlusion or stenosis of left vertebral artery MCC HCC
  - I63.213 Cerebral infarction due to unspecified occlusion or stenosis of bilateral vertebral arteries MCC HCC
  - I63.219 Cerebral infarction due to unspecified occlusion or stenosis of unspecified vertebral artery MCC HCC
- I63.22 Cerebral infarction due to unspecified occlusion or stenosis of basilar artery MCC HCC
- 6th I63.23 Cerebral infarction due to unspecified occlusion or stenosis of carotid arteries
  - I63.231 Cerebral infarction due to unspecified occlusion or stenosis of right carotid arteries MCC HCC
  - I63.232 Cerebral infarction due to unspecified occlusion or stenosis of left carotid arteries MCC HCC
  - I63.233 Cerebral infarction due to unspecified occlusion or stenosis of bilateral carotid arteries MCC HCC
  - I63.239 Cerebral infarction due to unspecified occlusion or stenosis of unspecified carotid artery MCC HCC
- I63.29 Cerebral infarction due to unspecified occlusion or stenosis of other precerebral arteries MCC HCC

5th I63.3 Cerebral infarction due to thrombosis of cerebral arteries
- I63.30 Cerebral infarction due to thrombosis of unspecified cerebral artery MCC HCC
- 6th I63.31 Cerebral infarction due to thrombosis of middle cerebral artery
  - I63.311 Cerebral infarction due to thrombosis of right middle cerebral artery MCC HCC
  - I63.312 Cerebral infarction due to thrombosis of left middle cerebral artery MCC HCC
  - I63.313 Cerebral infarction due to thrombosis of bilateral middle cerebral arteries MCC HCC
  - I63.319 Cerebral infarction due to thrombosis of unspecified middle cerebral artery MCC HCC
- 6th I63.32 Cerebral infarction due to thrombosis of anterior cerebral artery
  - I63.321 Cerebral infarction due to thrombosis of right anterior cerebral artery MCC HCC
  - I63.322 Cerebral infarction due to thrombosis of left anterior cerebral artery MCC HCC
  - I63.323 Cerebral infarction due to thrombosis of bilateral anterior cerebral arteries MCC HCC
  - I63.329 Cerebral infarction due to thrombosis of unspecified anterior cerebral artery MCC HCC
- 6th I63.33 Cerebral infarction due to thrombosis of posterior cerebral artery
  - I63.331 Cerebral infarction due to thrombosis of right posterior cerebral artery MCC HCC
  - I63.332 Cerebral infarction due to thrombosis of left posterior cerebral artery MCC HCC
  - I63.333 Cerebral infarction due to thrombosis of bilateral posterior cerebral arteries MCC HCC
  - I63.339 Cerebral infarction due to thrombosis of unspecified posterior cerebral artery MCC HCC
- 6th I63.34 Cerebral infarction due to thrombosis of cerebellar artery
  - I63.341 Cerebral infarction due to thrombosis of right cerebellar artery MCC HCC
  - I63.342 Cerebral infarction due to thrombosis of left cerebellar artery MCC HCC
  - I63.343 Cerebral infarction due to thrombosis of bilateral cerebellar arteries MCC HCC
  - I63.349 Cerebral infarction due to thrombosis of unspecified cerebellar artery MCC HCC
- I63.39 Cerebral infarction due to thrombosis of other cerebral artery MCC HCC

5th I63.4 Cerebral infarction due to embolism of cerebral arteries
- I63.40 Cerebral infarction due to embolism of unspecified cerebral artery MCC HCC
- 6th I63.41 Cerebral infarction due to embolism of middle cerebral artery
  - I63.411 Cerebral infarction due to embolism of right middle cerebral artery MCC HCC
  - I63.412 Cerebral infarction due to embolism of left middle cerebral artery MCC HCC
  - I63.413 Cerebral infarction due to embolism of bilateral middle cerebral arteries MCC HCC
  - I63.419 Cerebral infarction due to embolism of unspecified middle cerebral artery MCC HCC
- 6th I63.42 Cerebral infarction due to embolism of anterior cerebral artery
  - I63.421 Cerebral infarction due to embolism of right anterior cerebral artery MCC HCC
  - I63.422 Cerebral infarction due to embolism of left anterior cerebral artery MCC HCC
  - I63.423 Cerebral infarction due to embolism of bilateral anterior cerebral arteries MCC HCC
  - I63.429 Cerebral infarction due to embolism of unspecified anterior cerebral artery MCC HCC
- 6th I63.43 Cerebral infarction due to embolism of posterior cerebral artery
  - I63.431 Cerebral infarction due to embolism of right posterior cerebral artery MCC HCC
  - I63.432 Cerebral infarction due to embolism of left posterior cerebral artery MCC HCC
  - I63.433 Cerebral infarction due to embolism of bilateral posterior cerebral arteries MCC HCC
  - I63.439 Cerebral infarction due to embolism of unspecified posterior cerebral artery MCC HCC
- 6th I63.44 Cerebral infarction due to embolism of cerebellar artery
  - I63.441 Cerebral infarction due to embolism of right cerebellar artery MCC HCC
  - I63.442 Cerebral infarction due to embolism of left cerebellar artery MCC HCC
  - I63.443 Cerebral infarction due to embolism of bilateral cerebellar arteries MCC HCC
  - I63.449 Cerebral infarction due to embolism of unspecified cerebellar artery MCC HCC
- I63.49 Cerebral infarction due to embolism of other cerebral artery MCC HCC

5th I63.5 Cerebral infarction due to unspecified occlusion or stenosis of cerebral arteries
- I63.50 Cerebral infarction due to unspecified occlusion or stenosis of unspecified cerebral artery MCC HCC
- 6th I63.51 Cerebral infarction due to unspecified occlusion or stenosis of middle cerebral artery
  - I63.511 Cerebral infarction due to unspecified occlusion or stenosis of right middle cerebral artery MCC HCC
  - I63.512 Cerebral infarction due to unspecified occlusion or stenosis of left middle cerebral artery MCC HCC
  - I63.513 Cerebral infarction due to unspecified occlusion or stenosis of bilateral middle cerebral arteries MCC HCC
  - I63.519 Cerebral infarction due to unspecified occlusion or stenosis of unspecified middle cerebral artery MCC HCC
- 6th I63.52 Cerebral infarction due to unspecified occlusion or stenosis of anterior cerebral artery
  - I63.521 Cerebral infarction due to unspecified occlusion or stenosis of right anterior cerebral artery MCC HCC

I63.522 Cerebral infarction due to unspecified occlusion or stenosis of left anterior cerebral artery MCC HCC

I63.523 Cerebral infarction due to unspecified occlusion or stenosis of bilateral anterior cerebral arteries MCC HCC

I63.529 Cerebral infarction due to unspecified occlusion or stenosis of unspecified anterior cerebral artery MCC HCC

I63.53 Cerebral infarction due to unspecified occlusion or stenosis of posterior cerebral artery

I63.531 Cerebral infarction due to unspecified occlusion or stenosis of right posterior cerebral artery MCC HCC

I63.532 Cerebral infarction due to unspecified occlusion or stenosis of left posterior cerebral artery MCC HCC

I63.533 Cerebral infarction due to unspecified occlusion or stenosis of bilateral posterior cerebral arteries MCC HCC

I63.539 Cerebral infarction due to unspecified occlusion or stenosis of unspecified posterior cerebral artery MCC HCC

I63.54 Cerebral infarction due to unspecified occlusion or stenosis of cerebellar artery

I63.541 Cerebral infarction due to unspecified occlusion or stenosis of right cerebellar artery MCC HCC

I63.542 Cerebral infarction due to unspecified occlusion or stenosis of left cerebellar artery MCC HCC

I63.543 Cerebral infarction due to unspecified occlusion or stenosis of bilateral cerebellar arteries MCC HCC

I63.549 Cerebral infarction due to unspecified occlusion or stenosis of unspecified cerebellar artery MCC HCC

I63.59 Cerebral infarction due to unspecified occlusion or stenosis of other cerebral artery MCC HCC

I63.6 Cerebral infarction due to cerebral venous thrombosis, nonpyogenic MCC HCC

I63.8 Other cerebral infarction

AHA: 2018,4Q,16

I63.81 Other cerebral infarction due to occlusion or stenosis of small artery MCC HCC

Lacunar infarction

AHA: 2020,3Q,27

I63.89 Other cerebral infarction MCC HCC

AHA: 2022,1Q,25

I63.9 Cerebral infarction, unspecified MCC HCC

Stroke NOS

EXCLUDES 2 *transient cerebral ischemic attacks and related syndromes (G45.-)*

AHA: 2020,2Q,29

TIP: When provider documentation does not identify the location of an infarction, imaging reports can be used to pinpoint the location and lead to a more specific infarction code.

I65 Occlusion and stenosis of precerebral arteries, not resulting in cerebral infarction

INCLUDES embolism of precerebral artery
narrowing of precerebral artery
obstruction (complete) (partial) of precerebral artery
thrombosis of precerebral artery

EXCLUDES 1 *insufficiency, NOS, of precerebral artery (G45.-)*
insufficiency of precerebral arteries causing cerebral infarction (I63.Ø-I63.2)

AHA: 2018,2Q,9

I65.Ø Occlusion and stenosis of vertebral artery

I65.Ø1 Occlusion and stenosis of right vertebral artery

I65.Ø2 Occlusion and stenosis of left vertebral artery

I65.Ø3 Occlusion and stenosis of bilateral vertebral arteries

I65.Ø9 Occlusion and stenosis of unspecified vertebral artery

I65.1 Occlusion and stenosis of basilar artery

I65.2 Occlusion and stenosis of carotid artery

AHA: 2021,1Q,4; 2020,3Q,28

I65.21 Occlusion and stenosis of right carotid artery

I65.22 Occlusion and stenosis of left carotid artery

I65.23 Occlusion and stenosis of bilateral carotid arteries

I65.29 Occlusion and stenosis of unspecified carotid artery

I65.8 Occlusion and stenosis of other precerebral arteries

I65.9 Occlusion and stenosis of unspecified precerebral artery

Occlusion and stenosis of precerebral artery NOS

I66 Occlusion and stenosis of cerebral arteries, not resulting in cerebral infarction

INCLUDES embolism of cerebral artery
narrowing of cerebral artery
obstruction (complete) (partial) of cerebral artery
thrombosis of cerebral artery

EXCLUDES 1 *occlusion and stenosis of cerebral artery causing cerebral infarction (I63.3-I63.5)*

I66.Ø Occlusion and stenosis of middle cerebral artery

I66.Ø1 Occlusion and stenosis of right middle cerebral artery

I66.Ø2 Occlusion and stenosis of left middle cerebral artery

I66.Ø3 Occlusion and stenosis of bilateral middle cerebral arteries

I66.Ø9 Occlusion and stenosis of unspecified middle cerebral artery

I66.1 Occlusion and stenosis of anterior cerebral artery

I66.11 Occlusion and stenosis of right anterior cerebral artery

I66.12 Occlusion and stenosis of left anterior cerebral artery

I66.13 Occlusion and stenosis of bilateral anterior cerebral arteries

I66.19 Occlusion and stenosis of unspecified anterior cerebral artery

I66.2 Occlusion and stenosis of posterior cerebral artery

I66.21 Occlusion and stenosis of right posterior cerebral artery

I66.22 Occlusion and stenosis of left posterior cerebral artery

I66.23 Occlusion and stenosis of bilateral posterior cerebral arteries

I66.29 Occlusion and stenosis of unspecified posterior cerebral artery

I66.3 Occlusion and stenosis of cerebellar arteries

I66.8 Occlusion and stenosis of other cerebral arteries

Occlusion and stenosis of perforating arteries

I66.9 Occlusion and stenosis of unspecified cerebral artery

I67 Other cerebrovascular diseases

EXCLUDES 1 ▶*occlusion and stenosis of cerebral artery causing cerebral infarction (I63.3-I63.5-)*◀
▶*occlusion and stenosis of precerebral artery causing cerebral infarction (I63.2-)*◀

EXCLUDES 2 *sequelae of the listed conditions (I69.8)*

I67.Ø Dissection of cerebral arteries, nonruptured MCC HCC

EXCLUDES 1 *ruptured cerebral arteries (I6Ø.7)*

AHA: 2021,3Q,5

DEF: Dissecting aneurysm: Tear within an arterial wall that allows blood to accumulate between the outer and middle layers, creating a false lumen.

I67.1 Cerebral aneurysm, nonruptured
Cerebral aneurysm NOS
Cerebral arteriovenous fistula, acquired
Internal carotid artery aneurysm, intracranial portion
Internal carotid artery aneurysm, NOS
EXCLUDES 1 *congenital cerebral aneurysm, nonruptured (Q28.-)*
ruptured cerebral aneurysm (I60.7)
AHA: 2021,3Q,5
TIP: A diagnosis of dissecting aneurysm should be coded to the dissection code, I67.0. The bulging/aneurysm, although present, occurred secondary to the dissection. The dissection represents the most significant problem.

Berry Aneurysm

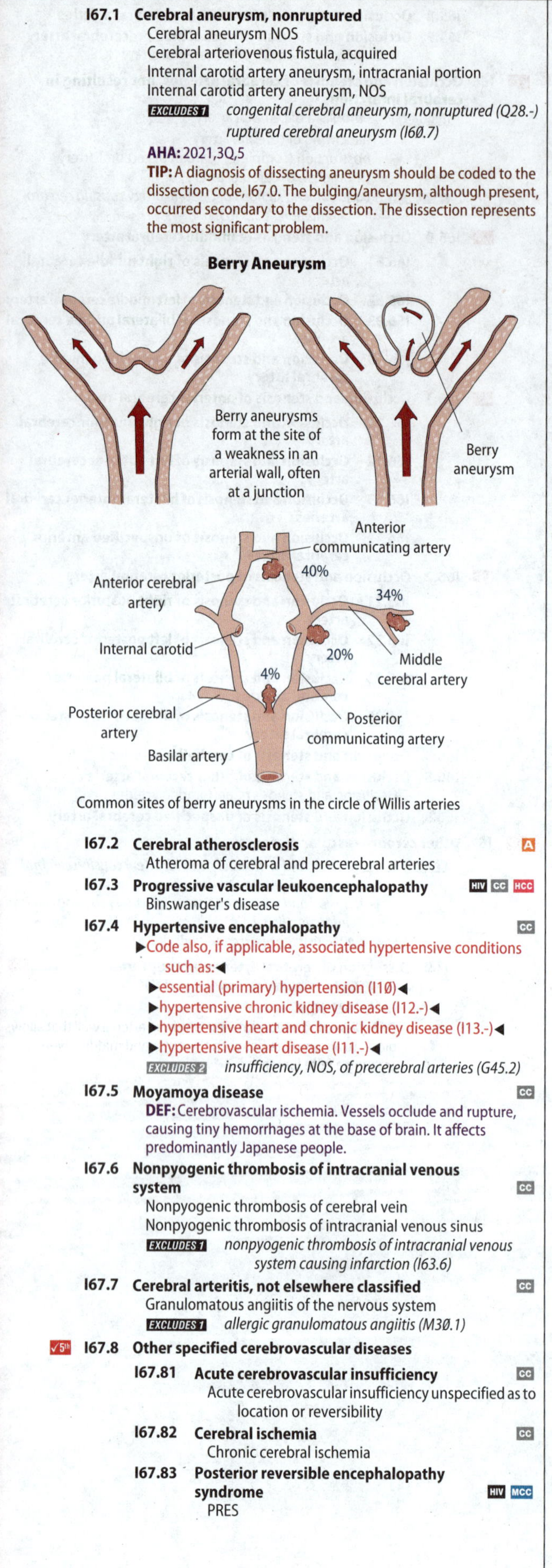

Common sites of berry aneurysms in the circle of Willis arteries

I67.2 Cerebral atherosclerosis A
Atheroma of cerebral and precerebral arteries
I67.3 Progressive vascular leukoencephalopathy HIV CC HCC
Binswanger's disease
I67.4 Hypertensive encephalopathy CC
▶Code also, if applicable, associated hypertensive conditions such as:◀
▶essential (primary) hypertension (I10)◀
▶hypertensive chronic kidney disease (I12.-)◀
▶hypertensive heart and chronic kidney disease (I13.-)◀
▶hypertensive heart disease (I11.-)◀
EXCLUDES 2 *insufficiency, NOS, of precerebral arteries (G45.2)*
I67.5 Moyamoya disease CC
DEF: Cerebrovascular ischemia. Vessels occlude and rupture, causing tiny hemorrhages at the base of brain. It affects predominantly Japanese people.
I67.6 Nonpyogenic thrombosis of intracranial venous system CC
Nonpyogenic thrombosis of cerebral vein
Nonpyogenic thrombosis of intracranial venous sinus
EXCLUDES 1 *nonpyogenic thrombosis of intracranial venous system causing infarction (I63.6)*
I67.7 Cerebral arteritis, not elsewhere classified CC
Granulomatous angiitis of the nervous system
EXCLUDES 1 *allergic granulomatous angiitis (M30.1)*
✓5th **I67.8 Other specified cerebrovascular diseases**
I67.81 Acute cerebrovascular insufficiency CC
Acute cerebrovascular insufficiency unspecified as to location or reversibility
I67.82 Cerebral ischemia CC
Chronic cerebral ischemia
I67.83 Posterior reversible encephalopathy syndrome HIV MCC
PRES

✓6th **I67.84 Cerebral vasospasm and vasoconstriction**
I67.841 Reversible cerebrovascular vasoconstriction syndrome CC
Call-Fleming syndrome
Code first underlying condition, if applicable, such as eclampsia (O15.00-O15.9)
I67.848 Other cerebrovascular vasospasm and vasoconstriction CC
✓6th **I67.85 Hereditary cerebrovascular diseases**
AHA: 2018,4Q,17
I67.850 Cerebral autosomal dominant arteriopathy with subcortical infarcts and leukoencephalopathy CC
CADASIL
Code also any associated diagnoses, such as:
epilepsy (G40.-)
stroke (I63.-)
vascular dementia (F01.-)
I67.858 Other hereditary cerebrovascular disease CC
I67.89 Other cerebrovascular disease CC
AHA: 2023,2Q,18
I67.9 Cerebrovascular disease, unspecified
✓4th **I68 Cerebrovascular disorders in diseases classified elsewhere**
I68.0 Cerebral amyloid angiopathy
Code first underlying amyloidosis (E85.-)
I68.2 Cerebral arteritis in other diseases classified elsewhere CC
Code first underlying disease
EXCLUDES 1 *cerebral arteritis (in):*
listerosis (A32.89)
syphilis (A52.04)
systemic lupus erythematosus (M32.19)
tuberculosis (A18.89)
I68.8 Other cerebrovascular disorders in diseases classified elsewhere
Code first underlying disease
EXCLUDES 1 *syphilitic cerebral aneurysm (A52.05)*
✓4th **I69 Sequelae of cerebrovascular disease**
NOTE Category I69 is to be used to indicate conditions in I60-I67 as the cause of sequelae. The "sequelae" include conditions specified as such or as residuals which may occur at any time after the onset of the causal condition
EXCLUDES 1 *personal history of cerebral infarction without residual deficit (Z86.73)*
personal history of prolonged reversible ischemic neurologic deficit (PRIND) (Z86.73)
personal history of reversible ischemic neurologcial deficit (RIND) (Z86.73)
sequelae of traumatic intracranial injury (S06.-)
AHA: 2023,1Q,37; 2020,2Q,29; 2017,1Q,47; 2016,4Q,28; 2015,1Q,25; 2012,4Q,106
TIP: Weakness on one side of the body (unilateral weakness) documented as secondary to old cerebrovascular disease is synonymous with hemiparesis/hemiplegia. Weakness of one limb documented as secondary to old cerebrovascular disease is synonymous with monoplegia.
TIP: For codes describing hemiplegia, hemiparesis, and monoplegia; if the documentation identifies the affected side but not whether it is the dominant or nondominant side, the default is as follows: for ambidextrous patients, the default is dominant; when the left side is affected, the default is nondominant; and when the right side is affected, the default is dominant.
✓5th **I69.0 Sequelae of nontraumatic subarachnoid hemorrhage**
I69.00 Unspecified sequelae of nontraumatic subarachnoid hemorrhage
✓6th **I69.01 Cognitive deficits following nontraumatic subarachnoid hemorrhage**
I69.010 Attention and concentration deficit following nontraumatic subarachnoid hemorrhage
I69.011 Memory deficit following nontraumatic subarachnoid hemorrhage
I69.012 Visuospatial deficit and spatial neglect following nontraumatic subarachnoid hemorrhage
I69.013 Psychomotor deficit following nontraumatic subarachnoid hemorrhage

I69.014 Frontal lobe and executive function deficit following nontraumatic subarachnoid hemorrhage

I69.015 Cognitive social or emotional deficit following nontraumatic subarachnoid hemorrhage

I69.018 Other symptoms and signs involving cognitive functions following nontraumatic subarachnoid hemorrhage

I69.019 Unspecified symptoms and signs involving cognitive functions following nontraumatic subarachnoid hemorrhage

I69.02 Speech and language deficits following nontraumatic subarachnoid hemorrhage

I69.020 Aphasia following nontraumatic subarachnoid hemorrhage

I69.021 Dysphasia following nontraumatic subarachnoid hemorrhage

I69.022 Dysarthria following nontraumatic subarachnoid hemorrhage

I69.023 Fluency disorder following nontraumatic subarachnoid hemorrhage

Stuttering following nontraumatic subarachnoid hemorrhage

I69.028 Other speech and language deficits following nontraumatic subarachnoid hemorrhage

I69.03 Monoplegia of upper limb following nontraumatic subarachnoid hemorrhage

AHA: 2017,1Q,47

I69.031 Monoplegia of upper limb following nontraumatic subarachnoid hemorrhage affecting right dominant side HCC

I69.032 Monoplegia of upper limb following nontraumatic subarachnoid hemorrhage affecting left dominant side HCC

I69.033 Monoplegia of upper limb following nontraumatic subarachnoid hemorrhage affecting right non-dominant side HCC

I69.034 Monoplegia of upper limb following nontraumatic subarachnoid hemorrhage affecting left non-dominant side HCC

I69.039 Monoplegia of upper limb following nontraumatic subarachnoid hemorrhage affecting unspecified side HCC

I69.04 Monoplegia of lower limb following nontraumatic subarachnoid hemorrhage

AHA: 2017,1Q,47

I69.041 Monoplegia of lower limb following nontraumatic subarachnoid hemorrhage affecting right dominant side HCC

I69.042 Monoplegia of lower limb following nontraumatic subarachnoid hemorrhage affecting left dominant side HCC

I69.043 Monoplegia of lower limb following nontraumatic subarachnoid hemorrhage affecting right non-dominant side HCC

I69.044 Monoplegia of lower limb following nontraumatic subarachnoid hemorrhage affecting left non-dominant side HCC

I69.049 Monoplegia of lower limb following nontraumatic subarachnoid hemorrhage affecting unspecified side HCC

I69.05 Hemiplegia and hemiparesis following nontraumatic subarachnoid hemorrhage

AHA: 2015,1Q,25

I69.051 Hemiplegia and hemiparesis following nontraumatic subarachnoid hemorrhage affecting right dominant side CC HCC

I69.052 Hemiplegia and hemiparesis following nontraumatic subarachnoid hemorrhage affecting left dominant side CC HCC

I69.053 Hemiplegia and hemiparesis following nontraumatic subarachnoid hemorrhage affecting right non-dominant side CC HCC

I69.054 Hemiplegia and hemiparesis following nontraumatic subarachnoid hemorrhage affecting left non-dominant side CC HCC

I69.059 Hemiplegia and hemiparesis following nontraumatic subarachnoid hemorrhage affecting unspecified side CC UNS HCC

I69.06 Other paralytic syndrome following nontraumatic subarachnoid hemorrhage

Use additional code to identify type of paralytic syndrome, such as:
locked-in state (G83.5)
quadriplegia (G82.5-)

EXCLUDES 1 *hemiplegia/hemiparesis following nontraumatic subarachnoid hemorrhage (I69.05-)*
monoplegia of lower limb following nontraumatic subarachnoid hemorrhage (I69.04-)
monoplegia of upper limb following nontraumatic subarachnoid hemorrhage (I69.03-)

I69.061 Other paralytic syndrome following nontraumatic subarachnoid hemorrhage affecting right dominant side HCC

I69.062 Other paralytic syndrome following nontraumatic subarachnoid hemorrhage affecting left dominant side HCC

I69.063 Other paralytic syndrome following nontraumatic subarachnoid hemorrhage affecting right non-dominant side HCC

I69.064 Other paralytic syndrome following nontraumatic subarachnoid hemorrhage affecting left non-dominant side HCC

I69.065 Other paralytic syndrome following nontraumatic subarachnoid hemorrhage, bilateral HCC

I69.069 Other paralytic syndrome following nontraumatic subarachnoid hemorrhage affecting unspecified side HCC

I69.09 Other sequelae of nontraumatic subarachnoid hemorrhage

I69.090 Apraxia following nontraumatic subarachnoid hemorrhage

I69.091 Dysphagia following nontraumatic subarachnoid hemorrhage

Use additional code to identify the type of dysphagia, if known (R13.11-R13.19)

I69.092 Facial weakness following nontraumatic subarachnoid hemorrhage

Facial droop following nontraumatic subarachnoid hemorrhage

I69.093 Ataxia following nontraumatic subarachnoid hemorrhage

I69.098 Other sequelae following nontraumatic subarachnoid hemorrhage

Alterations of sensation following nontraumatic subarachnoid hemorrhage
Disturbance of vision following nontraumatic subarachnoid hemorrhage

Use additional code to identify the sequelae

I69.1 Sequelae of nontraumatic intracerebral hemorrhage

I69.10 Unspecified sequelae of nontraumatic intracerebral hemorrhage

I69.11 Cognitive deficits following nontraumatic intracerebral hemorrhage

I69.110 Attention and concentration deficit following nontraumatic intracerebral hemorrhage

I69.111 Memory deficit following nontraumatic intracerebral hemorrhage

I69.112 Visuospatial deficit and spatial neglect following nontraumatic intracerebral hemorrhage

I69.113 Psychomotor deficit following nontraumatic intracerebral hemorrhage

I69.114 Frontal lobe and executive function deficit following nontraumatic intracerebral hemorrhage

I69.115 Cognitive social or emotional deficit following nontraumatic intracerebral hemorrhage

I69.118 Other symptoms and signs involving cognitive functions following nontraumatic intracerebral hemorrhage

I69.119 Unspecified symptoms and signs involving cognitive functions following nontraumatic intracerebral hemorrhage

✓6th **I69.12 Speech and language deficits following nontraumatic intracerebral hemorrhage**

I69.120 Aphasia following nontraumatic intracerebral hemorrhage

I69.121 Dysphasia following nontraumatic intracerebral hemorrhage

I69.122 Dysarthria following nontraumatic intracerebral hemorrhage

I69.123 Fluency disorder following nontraumatic intracerebral hemorrhage

Stuttering following nontraumatic intracerebral hemorrhage

I69.128 Other speech and language deficits following nontraumatic intracerebral hemorrhage

✓6th **I69.13 Monoplegia of upper limb following nontraumatic intracerebral hemorrhage**

AHA: 2017,1Q,47

I69.131 Monoplegia of upper limb following nontraumatic intracerebral hemorrhage affecting right dominant side HCC

I69.132 Monoplegia of upper limb following nontraumatic intracerebral hemorrhage affecting left dominant side HCC

I69.133 Monoplegia of upper limb following nontraumatic intracerebral hemorrhage affecting right non-dominant side HCC

I69.134 Monoplegia of upper limb following nontraumatic intracerebral hemorrhage affecting left non-dominant side HCC

I69.139 Monoplegia of upper limb following nontraumatic intracerebral hemorrhage affecting unspecified side HCC

✓6th **I69.14 Monoplegia of lower limb following nontraumatic intracerebral hemorrhage**

AHA: 2017,1Q,47

I69.141 Monoplegia of lower limb following nontraumatic intracerebral hemorrhage affecting right dominant side HCC

I69.142 Monoplegia of lower limb following nontraumatic intracerebral hemorrhage affecting left dominant side HCC

I69.143 Monoplegia of lower limb following nontraumatic intracerebral hemorrhage affecting right non-dominant side HCC

I69.144 Monoplegia of lower limb following nontraumatic intracerebral hemorrhage affecting left non-dominant side HCC

I69.149 Monoplegia of lower limb following nontraumatic intracerebral hemorrhage affecting unspecified side HCC

✓6th **I69.15 Hemiplegia and hemiparesis following nontraumatic intracerebral hemorrhage**

AHA: 2015,1Q,25

I69.151 Hemiplegia and hemiparesis following nontraumatic intracerebral hemorrhage affecting right dominant side CC HCC

I69.152 Hemiplegia and hemiparesis following nontraumatic intracerebral hemorrhage affecting left dominant side CC HCC

I69.153 Hemiplegia and hemiparesis following nontraumatic intracerebral hemorrhage affecting right non-dominant side CC HCC

I69.154 Hemiplegia and hemiparesis following nontraumatic intracerebral hemorrhage affecting left non-dominant side CC HCC

I69.159 Hemiplegia and hemiparesis following nontraumatic intracerebral hemorrhage affecting unspecified side CC UNS HCC

✓6th **I69.16 Other paralytic syndrome following nontraumatic intracerebral hemorrhage**

Use additional code to identify type of paralytic syndrome, such as:
- locked-in state (G83.5)
- quadriplegia (G82.5-)

EXCLUDES 1 *hemiplegia/hemiparesis following nontraumatic intracerebral hemorrhage (I69.15-)*
monoplegia of lower limb following nontraumatic intracerebral hemorrhage (I69.14-)
monoplegia of upper limb following nontraumatic intracerebral hemorrhage (I69.13-)

I69.161 Other paralytic syndrome following nontraumatic intracerebral hemorrhage affecting right dominant side HCC

I69.162 Other paralytic syndrome following nontraumatic intracerebral hemorrhage affecting left dominant side HCC

I69.163 Other paralytic syndrome following nontraumatic intracerebral hemorrhage affecting right non-dominant side HCC

I69.164 Other paralytic syndrome following nontraumatic intracerebral hemorrhage affecting left non-dominant side HCC

I69.165 Other paralytic syndrome following nontraumatic intracerebral hemorrhage, bilateral HCC

I69.169 Other paralytic syndrome following nontraumatic intracerebral hemorrhage affecting unspecified side HCC

✓6th **I69.19 Other sequelae of nontraumatic intracerebral hemorrhage**

I69.190 Apraxia following nontraumatic intracerebral hemorrhage

I69.191 Dysphagia following nontraumatic intracerebral hemorrhage

Use additional code to identify the type of dysphagia, if known (R13.11-R13.19)

I69.192 Facial weakness following nontraumatic intracerebral hemorrhage

Facial droop following nontraumatic intracerebral hemorrhage

I69.193 Ataxia following nontraumatic intracerebral hemorrhage

I69.198 Other sequelae of nontraumatic intracerebral hemorrhage

Alteration of sensations following nontraumatic intracerebral hemorrhage

Disturbance of vision following nontraumatic intracerebral hemorrhage

Use additional code to identify the sequelae

✓5th **I69.2 Sequelae of other nontraumatic intracranial hemorrhage**

I69.20 Unspecified sequelae of other nontraumatic intracranial hemorrhage

✓6th **I69.21 Cognitive deficits following other nontraumatic intracranial hemorrhage**

I69.210 Attention and concentration deficit following other nontraumatic intracranial hemorrhage

I69.211 Memory deficit following other nontraumatic intracranial hemorrhage

I69.212 Visuospatial deficit and spatial neglect following other nontraumatic intracranial hemorrhage

I69.213 Psychomotor deficit following other nontraumatic intracranial hemorrhage

I69.214 Frontal lobe and executive function deficit following other nontraumatic intracranial hemorrhage

I69.215 Cognitive social or emotional deficit following other nontraumatic intracranial hemorrhage

I69.218 Other symptoms and signs involving cognitive functions following other nontraumatic intracranial hemorrhage

I69.219 Unspecified symptoms and signs involving cognitive functions following other nontraumatic intracranial hemorrhage

✓6th I69.22 Speech and language deficits following other nontraumatic intracranial hemorrhage

I69.220 Aphasia following other nontraumatic intracranial hemorrhage

I69.221 Dysphasia following other nontraumatic intracranial hemorrhage

I69.222 Dysarthria following other nontraumatic intracranial hemorrhage

I69.223 Fluency disorder following other nontraumatic intracranial hemorrhage
Stuttering following other nontraumatic intracranial hemorrhage

I69.228 Other speech and language deficits following other nontraumatic intracranial hemorrhage

✓6th I69.23 Monoplegia of upper limb following other nontraumatic intracranial hemorrhage
AHA: 2017,1Q,47

I69.231 Monoplegia of upper limb following other nontraumatic intracranial hemorrhage affecting right dominant side HCC

I69.232 Monoplegia of upper limb following other nontraumatic intracranial hemorrhage affecting left dominant side HCC

I69.233 Monoplegia of upper limb following other nontraumatic intracranial hemorrhage affecting right non-dominant side HCC

I69.234 Monoplegia of upper limb following other nontraumatic intracranial hemorrhage affecting left non-dominant side HCC

I69.239 Monoplegia of upper limb following other nontraumatic intracranial hemorrhage affecting unspecified side HCC

✓6th I69.24 Monoplegia of lower limb following other nontraumatic intracranial hemorrhage
AHA: 2017,1Q,47

I69.241 Monoplegia of lower limb following other nontraumatic intracranial hemorrhage affecting right dominant side HCC

I69.242 Monoplegia of lower limb following other nontraumatic intracranial hemorrhage affecting left dominant side HCC

I69.243 Monoplegia of lower limb following other nontraumatic intracranial hemorrhage affecting right non-dominant side HCC

I69.244 Monoplegia of lower limb following other nontraumatic intracranial hemorrhage affecting left non-dominant side HCC

I69.249 Monoplegia of lower limb following other nontraumatic intracranial hemorrhage affecting unspecified side HCC

✓6th I69.25 Hemiplegia and hemiparesis following other nontraumatic intracranial hemorrhage
AHA: 2015,1Q,25

I69.251 Hemiplegia and hemiparesis following other nontraumatic intracranial hemorrhage affecting right dominant side CC HCC

I69.252 Hemiplegia and hemiparesis following other nontraumatic intracranial hemorrhage affecting left dominant side CC HCC

I69.253 Hemiplegia and hemiparesis following other nontraumatic intracranial hemorrhage affecting right non-dominant side CC HCC

I69.254 Hemiplegia and hemiparesis following other nontraumatic intracranial hemorrhage affecting left non-dominant side CC HCC

I69.259 Hemiplegia and hemiparesis following other nontraumatic intracranial hemorrhage affecting unspecified side CC UNS HCC

✓6th I69.26 Other paralytic syndrome following other nontraumatic intracranial hemorrhage
Use additional code to identify type of paralytic syndrome, such as:
locked-in state (G83.5)
quadriplegia (G82.5-)

EXCLUDES 1 *hemiplegia/hemiparesis following other nontraumatic intracranial hemorrhage (I69.25-)*
monoplegia of lower limb following other nontraumatic intracranial hemorrhage (I69.24-)
monoplegia of upper limb following other nontraumatic intracranial hemorrhage (I69.23-)

I69.261 Other paralytic syndrome following other nontraumatic intracranial hemorrhage affecting right dominant side HCC

I69.262 Other paralytic syndrome following other nontraumatic intracranial hemorrhage affecting left dominant side HCC

I69.263 Other paralytic syndrome following other nontraumatic intracranial hemorrhage affecting right non-dominant side HCC

I69.264 Other paralytic syndrome following other nontraumatic intracranial hemorrhage affecting left non-dominant side HCC

I69.265 Other paralytic syndrome following other nontraumatic intracranial hemorrhage, bilateral HCC

I69.269 Other paralytic syndrome following other nontraumatic intracranial hemorrhage affecting unspecified side HCC

✓6th I69.29 Other sequelae of other nontraumatic intracranial hemorrhage

I69.290 Apraxia following other nontraumatic intracranial hemorrhage

I69.291 Dysphagia following other nontraumatic intracranial hemorrhage
Use additional code to identify the type of dysphagia, if known (R13.11-R13.19)

I69.292 Facial weakness following other nontraumatic intracranial hemorrhage
Facial droop following other nontraumatic intracranial hemorrhage

I69.293 Ataxia following other nontraumatic intracranial hemorrhage

I69.298 Other sequelae of other nontraumatic intracranial hemorrhage
Alteration of sensation following other nontraumatic intracranial hemorrhage
Disturbance of vision following other nontraumatic intracranial hemorrhage
Use additional code to identify the sequelae

✓5th I69.3 Sequelae of cerebral infarction
Sequelae of stroke NOS
AHA: 2013,4Q,127-128; 2012,4Q,92,94

I69.30 Unspecified sequelae of cerebral infarction

✓6th I69.31 Cognitive deficits following cerebral infarction

I69.310 Attention and concentration deficit following cerebral infarction

I69.311 Memory deficit following cerebral infarction

I69.312 Visuospatial deficit and spatial neglect following cerebral infarction

I69.313 Psychomotor deficit following cerebral infarction

I69.314 Frontal lobe and executive function deficit following cerebral infarction

I69.315 Cognitive social or emotional deficit following cerebral infarction

I69.318 Other symptoms and signs involving cognitive functions following cerebral infarction

I69.319 Unspecified symptoms and signs involving cognitive functions following cerebral infarction

I69.32 Speech and language deficits following cerebral infarction

I69.320 Aphasia following cerebral infarction

I69.321 Dysphasia following cerebral infarction

AHA: 2012,4Q,91

I69.322 Dysarthria following cerebral infarction

EXCLUDES 2 *transient ischemic attack (TIA) (G45.9)*

I69.323 Fluency disorder following cerebral infarction

Stuttering following cerebral infarction

I69.328 Other speech and language deficits following cerebral infarction

I69.33 Monoplegia of upper limb following cerebral infarction

AHA: 2017,1Q,47

I69.331 Monoplegia of upper limb following cerebral infarction affecting right dominant side HCC

I69.332 Monoplegia of upper limb following cerebral infarction affecting left dominant side HCC

I69.333 Monoplegia of upper limb following cerebral infarction affecting right non-dominant side HCC

I69.334 Monoplegia of upper limb following cerebral infarction affecting left non-dominant side HCC

I69.339 Monoplegia of upper limb following cerebral infarction affecting unspecified side HCC

I69.34 Monoplegia of lower limb following cerebral infarction

AHA: 2017,1Q,47

I69.341 Monoplegia of lower limb following cerebral infarction affecting right dominant side HCC

I69.342 Monoplegia of lower limb following cerebral infarction affecting left dominant side HCC

I69.343 Monoplegia of lower limb following cerebral infarction affecting right non-dominant side HCC

I69.344 Monoplegia of lower limb following cerebral infarction affecting left non-dominant side HCC

I69.349 Monoplegia of lower limb following cerebral infarction affecting unspecified side HCC

I69.35 Hemiplegia and hemiparesis following cerebral infarction

AHA: 2015,1Q,25

I69.351 Hemiplegia and hemiparesis following cerebral infarction affecting right dominant side CC HCC

EXCLUDES 2 *transient ischemic attack (TIA) (G45.9)*

I69.352 Hemiplegia and hemiparesis following cerebral infarction affecting left dominant side CC HCC

I69.353 Hemiplegia and hemiparesis following cerebral infarction affecting right non-dominant side CC HCC

I69.354 Hemiplegia and hemiparesis following cerebral infarction affecting left non-dominant side CC HCC

AHA: 2012,4Q,91

I69.359 Hemiplegia and hemiparesis following cerebral infarction affecting unspecified side CC UNS HCC

I69.36 Other paralytic syndrome following cerebral infarction

Use additional code to identify type of paralytic syndrome, such as:
locked-in state (G83.5)
quadriplegia (G82.5-)

EXCLUDES 1 *hemiplegia/hemiparesis following cerebral infarction (I69.35-)*
monoplegia of lower limb following cerebral infarction (I69.34-)
monoplegia of upper limb following cerebral infarction (I69.33-)

I69.361 Other paralytic syndrome following cerebral infarction affecting right dominant side HCC

I69.362 Other paralytic syndrome following cerebral infarction affecting left dominant side HCC

I69.363 Other paralytic syndrome following cerebral infarction affecting right non-dominant side HCC

I69.364 Other paralytic syndrome following cerebral infarction affecting left non-dominant side HCC

I69.365 Other paralytic syndrome following cerebral infarction, bilateral HCC

I69.369 Other paralytic syndrome following cerebral infarction affecting unspecified side HCC

I69.39 Other sequelae of cerebral infarction

I69.390 Apraxia following cerebral infarction

I69.391 Dysphagia following cerebral infarction

Use additional code to identify the type of dysphagia, if known (R13.11-R13.19)

I69.392 Facial weakness following cerebral infarction

Facial droop following cerebral infarction

I69.393 Ataxia following cerebral infarction

I69.398 Other sequelae of cerebral infarction

Alteration of sensation following cerebral infarction
Disturbance of vision following cerebral infarction

Use additional code to identify the sequelae

AHA: 2020,2Q,29

I69.8 Sequelae of other cerebrovascular diseases

EXCLUDES 1 *sequelae of traumatic intracranial injury (S06.-)*

I69.80 Unspecified sequelae of other cerebrovascular disease

I69.81 Cognitive deficits following other cerebrovascular disease

I69.810 Attention and concentration deficit following other cerebrovascular disease

I69.811 Memory deficit following other cerebrovascular disease

I69.812 Visuospatial deficit and spatial neglect following other cerebrovascular disease

I69.813 Psychomotor deficit following other cerebrovascular disease

I69.814 Frontal lobe and executive function deficit following other cerebrovascular disease

I69.815 Cognitive social or emotional deficit following other cerebrovascular disease

I69.818 Other symptoms and signs involving cognitive functions following other cerebrovascular disease

I69.819 Unspecified symptoms and signs involving cognitive functions following other cerebrovascular disease

I69.82 Speech and language deficits following other cerebrovascular disease

I69.820 Aphasia following other cerebrovascular disease

I69.821 Dysphasia following other cerebrovascular disease

I69.822 Dysarthria following other cerebrovascular disease

I69.823 Fluency disorder following other cerebrovascular disease
Stuttering following other cerebrovascular disease

I69.828 Other speech and language deficits following other cerebrovascular disease
AHA: 2019,3Q,8

✓6th I69.83 Monoplegia of upper limb following other cerebrovascular disease
AHA: 2017,1Q,47

I69.831 Monoplegia of upper limb following other cerebrovascular disease affecting right dominant side HCC

I69.832 Monoplegia of upper limb following other cerebrovascular disease affecting left dominant side HCC

I69.833 Monoplegia of upper limb following other cerebrovascular disease affecting right non-dominant side HCC

I69.834 Monoplegia of upper limb following other cerebrovascular disease affecting left non-dominant side HCC

I69.839 Monoplegia of upper limb following other cerebrovascular disease affecting unspecified side HCC

✓6th I69.84 Monoplegia of lower limb following other cerebrovascular disease
AHA: 2017,1Q,47

I69.841 Monoplegia of lower limb following other cerebrovascular disease affecting right dominant side HCC

I69.842 Monoplegia of lower limb following other cerebrovascular disease affecting left dominant side HCC

I69.843 Monoplegia of lower limb following other cerebrovascular disease affecting right non-dominant side HCC

I69.844 Monoplegia of lower limb following other cerebrovascular disease affecting left non-dominant side HCC

I69.849 Monoplegia of lower limb following other cerebrovascular disease affecting unspecified side HCC

✓6th I69.85 Hemiplegia and hemiparesis following other cerebrovascular disease
AHA: 2015,1Q,25

I69.851 Hemiplegia and hemiparesis following other cerebrovascular disease affecting right dominant side CC HCC

I69.852 Hemiplegia and hemiparesis following other cerebrovascular disease affecting left dominant side CC HCC

I69.853 Hemiplegia and hemiparesis following other cerebrovascular disease affecting right non-dominant side CC HCC

I69.854 Hemiplegia and hemiparesis following other cerebrovascular disease affecting left non-dominant side CC HCC

I69.859 Hemiplegia and hemiparesis following other cerebrovascular disease affecting unspecified side CC UNS HCC

✓6th I69.86 Other paralytic syndrome following other cerebrovascular disease
Use additional code to identify type of paralytic syndrome, such as:
locked-in state (G83.5)
quadriplegia (G82.5-)

EXCLUDES 1 *hemiplegia/hemiparesis following other cerebrovascular disease (I69.85-)*
monoplegia of lower limb following other cerebrovascular disease (I69.84-)
monoplegia of upper limb following other cerebrovascular disease (I69.83-)

I69.861 Other paralytic syndrome following other cerebrovascular disease affecting right dominant side HCC

I69.862 Other paralytic syndrome following other cerebrovascular disease affecting left dominant side HCC

I69.863 Other paralytic syndrome following other cerebrovascular disease affecting right non-dominant side HCC

I69.864 Other paralytic syndrome following other cerebrovascular disease affecting left non-dominant side HCC

I69.865 Other paralytic syndrome following other cerebrovascular disease, bilateral HCC

I69.869 Other paralytic syndrome following other cerebrovascular disease affecting unspecified side HCC

✓6th I69.89 Other sequelae of other cerebrovascular disease

I69.890 Apraxia following other cerebrovascular disease

I69.891 Dysphagia following other cerebrovascular disease
Use additional code to identify the type of dysphagia, if known (R13.11-R13.19)

I69.892 Facial weakness following other cerebrovascular disease
Facial droop following other cerebrovascular disease

I69.893 Ataxia following other cerebrovascular disease

I69.898 Other sequelae of other cerebrovascular disease
Alteration of sensation following other cerebrovascular disease
Disturbance of vision following other cerebrovascular disease
Use additional code to identify the sequelae

✓5th I69.9 Sequelae of unspecified cerebrovascular diseases

EXCLUDES 1 *sequelae of stroke (I69.3)*
sequelae of traumatic intracranial injury (S06.-)

I69.90 Unspecified sequelae of unspecified cerebrovascular disease

✓6th I69.91 Cognitive deficits following unspecified cerebrovascular disease

I69.910 Attention and concentration deficit following unspecified cerebrovascular disease

I69.911 Memory deficit following unspecified cerebrovascular disease

I69.912 Visuospatial deficit and spatial neglect following unspecified cerebrovascular disease

I69.913 Psychomotor deficit following unspecified cerebrovascular disease

I69.914 Frontal lobe and executive function deficit following unspecified cerebrovascular disease

I69.915 Cognitive social or emotional deficit following unspecified cerebrovascular disease

I69.918 Other symptoms and signs involving cognitive functions following unspecified cerebrovascular disease

I69.919 Unspecified symptoms and signs involving cognitive functions following unspecified cerebrovascular disease

✓6th I69.92 Speech and language deficits following unspecified cerebrovascular disease

I69.920 Aphasia following unspecified cerebrovascular disease

I69.921 Dysphasia following unspecified cerebrovascular disease

I69.922 Dysarthria following unspecified cerebrovascular disease

I69.923 Fluency disorder following unspecified cerebrovascular disease
Stuttering following unspecified cerebrovascular disease

I69.928 Other speech and language deficits following unspecified cerebrovascular disease

✓6th I69.93 Monoplegia of upper limb following unspecified cerebrovascular disease
AHA: 2017,1Q,47

I69.931 Monoplegia of upper limb following unspecified cerebrovascular disease affecting right dominant side HCC

I69.932 Monoplegia of upper limb following unspecified cerebrovascular disease affecting left dominant side HCC

I69.933 **Monoplegia of upper limb following unspecified cerebrovascular disease affecting right non-dominant side** HCC

I69.934 **Monoplegia of upper limb following unspecified cerebrovascular disease affecting left non-dominant side** HCC

I69.939 **Monoplegia of upper limb following unspecified cerebrovascular disease affecting unspecified side** HCC

6th I69.94 **Monoplegia of lower limb following unspecified cerebrovascular disease**

AHA: 2017,1Q,47

I69.941 **Monoplegia of lower limb following unspecified cerebrovascular disease affecting right dominant side** HCC

I69.942 **Monoplegia of lower limb following unspecified cerebrovascular disease affecting left dominant side** HCC

I69.943 **Monoplegia of lower limb following unspecified cerebrovascular disease affecting right non-dominant side** HCC

I69.944 **Monoplegia of lower limb following unspecified cerebrovascular disease affecting left non-dominant side** HCC

I69.949 **Monoplegia of lower limb following unspecified cerebrovascular disease affecting unspecified side** HCC

6th I69.95 **Hemiplegia and hemiparesis following unspecified cerebrovascular disease**

AHA: 2015,1Q,25

I69.951 **Hemiplegia and hemiparesis following unspecified cerebrovascular disease affecting right dominant side** CC HCC

I69.952 **Hemiplegia and hemiparesis following unspecified cerebrovascular disease affecting left dominant side** CC HCC

I69.953 **Hemiplegia and hemiparesis following unspecified cerebrovascular disease affecting right non-dominant side** CC HCC

I69.954 **Hemiplegia and hemiparesis following unspecified cerebrovascular disease affecting left non-dominant side** CC HCC

I69.959 **Hemiplegia and hemiparesis following unspecified cerebrovascular disease affecting unspecified side** CC UNS HCC

6th I69.96 **Other paralytic syndrome following unspecified cerebrovascular disease**

Use additional code to identify type of paralytic syndrome, such as:
- locked-in state (G83.5)
- quadriplegia (G82.5-)

EXCLUDES 1 *hemiplegia/hemiparesis following unspecified cerebrovascular disease (I69.95-)*
monoplegia of lower limb following unspecified cerebrovascular disease (I69.94-)
monoplegia of upper limb following unspecified cerebrovascular disease (I69.93-)

I69.961 **Other paralytic syndrome following unspecified cerebrovascular disease affecting right dominant side** HCC

I69.962 **Other paralytic syndrome following unspecified cerebrovascular disease affecting left dominant side** HCC

I69.963 **Other paralytic syndrome following unspecified cerebrovascular disease affecting right non-dominant side** HCC

I69.964 **Other paralytic syndrome following unspecified cerebrovascular disease affecting left non-dominant side** HCC

I69.965 **Other paralytic syndrome following unspecified cerebrovascular disease, bilateral** HCC

I69.969 **Other paralytic syndrome following unspecified cerebrovascular disease affecting unspecified side** HCC

6th I69.99 **Other sequelae of unspecified cerebrovascular disease**

I69.990 **Apraxia following unspecified cerebrovascular disease**

I69.991 **Dysphagia following unspecified cerebrovascular disease**

Use additional code to identify the type of dysphagia, if known (R13.11-R13.19)

I69.992 **Facial weakness following unspecified cerebrovascular disease**

Facial droop following unspecified cerebrovascular disease

I69.993 **Ataxia following unspecified cerebrovascular disease**

I69.998 **Other sequelae following unspecified cerebrovascular disease**

Alteration in sensation following unspecified cerebrovascular disease
Disturbance of vision following unspecified cerebrovascular disease

Use additional code to identify the sequelae

Diseases of arteries, arterioles and capillaries (I7Ø-I79)

4th I7Ø **Atherosclerosis**

INCLUDES arterial degeneration
arteriolosclerosis
arteriosclerosis
arteriosclerotic vascular disease
arteriovascular degeneration
atheroma
endarteritis deformans or obliterans
senile arteritis
senile endarteritis
vascular degeneration

Use additional code to identify:
- exposure to environmental tobacco smoke (Z77.22)
- history of tobacco dependence (Z87.891)
- occupational exposure to environmental tobacco smoke (Z57.31)
- tobacco dependence (F17.-)
- tobacco use (Z72.Ø)

EXCLUDES 2 *arteriosclerotic cardiovascular disease (I25.1-)*
arteriosclerotic heart disease (I25.1-)
atheroembolism (I75.-)
cerebral atherosclerosis (I67.2)
coronary atherosclerosis (I25.1-)
mesenteric atherosclerosis (K55.1)
precerebral atherosclerosis (I67.2)
primary pulmonary atherosclerosis (I27.Ø)

I7Ø.Ø **Atherosclerosis of aorta** HCC A

I7Ø.1 **Atherosclerosis of renal artery** HCC A

Goldblatt's kidney

EXCLUDES 2 *atherosclerosis of renal arterioles (I12.-)*

5th I7Ø.2 **Atherosclerosis of native arteries of the extremities**

Monckeberg's (medial) sclerosis

Use additional code, if applicable, to identify chronic total occlusion of artery of extremity (I7Ø.92)

EXCLUDES 2 *atherosclerosis of bypass graft of extremities (I7Ø.3Ø-I7Ø.79)*

AHA: 2020,4Q,98; 2018,3Q,4; 2018,2Q,7

6th I7Ø.2Ø **Unspecified atherosclerosis of native arteries of extremities**

I7Ø.2Ø1 **Unspecified atherosclerosis of native arteries of extremities, right leg** HCC A

I7Ø.2Ø2 **Unspecified atherosclerosis of native arteries of extremities, left leg** HCC A

I7Ø.2Ø3 **Unspecified atherosclerosis of native arteries of extremities, bilateral legs** HCC A

I7Ø.2Ø8 **Unspecified atherosclerosis of native arteries of extremities, other extremity** HCC A

I7Ø.2Ø9 **Unspecified atherosclerosis of native arteries of extremities, unspecified extremity** HCC A

6th I7Ø.21 **Atherosclerosis of native arteries of extremities with intermittent claudication**

I7Ø.211 **Atherosclerosis of native arteries of extremities with intermittent claudication, right leg** HCC A

I70.212 Atherosclerosis of native arteries of extremities with intermittent claudication, left leg HCC A

I70.213 Atherosclerosis of native arteries of extremities with intermittent claudication, bilateral legs HCC A

I70.218 Atherosclerosis of native arteries of extremities with intermittent claudication, other extremity HCC A

I70.219 Atherosclerosis of native arteries of extremities with intermittent claudication, unspecified extremity HCC A

I70.22 Atherosclerosis of native arteries of extremities with rest pain

INCLUDES any condition classifiable to I70.21-
chronic limb-threatening ischemia NOS of native arteries of extremities
chronic limb-threatening ischemia of native arteries of extremities with rest pain
critical limb ischemia NOS of native arteries of extremities
critical limb ischemia of native arteries of extremities with rest pain

I70.221 Atherosclerosis of native arteries of extremities with rest pain, right leg HCC A

I70.222 Atherosclerosis of native arteries of extremities with rest pain, left leg HCC A

I70.223 Atherosclerosis of native arteries of extremities with rest pain, bilateral legs HCC A

I70.228 Atherosclerosis of native arteries of extremities with rest pain, other extremity HCC A

I70.229 Atherosclerosis of native arteries of extremities with rest pain, unspecified extremity HCC A

I70.23 Atherosclerosis of native arteries of right leg with ulceration

INCLUDES any condition classifiable to I70.211 and I70.221
chronic limb-threatening ischemia of native arteries of right leg with ulceration
critical limb ischemia of native arteries of right leg with ulceration

Use additional code to identify severity of ulcer (L97.-)

I70.231 Atherosclerosis of native arteries of right leg with ulceration of thigh HCC A

I70.232 Atherosclerosis of native arteries of right leg with ulceration of calf HCC A

I70.233 Atherosclerosis of native arteries of right leg with ulceration of ankle HCC A

I70.234 Atherosclerosis of native arteries of right leg with ulceration of heel and midfoot HCC A

Atherosclerosis of native arteries of right leg with ulceration of plantar surface of midfoot

I70.235 Atherosclerosis of native arteries of right leg with ulceration of other part of foot HCC A

Atherosclerosis of native arteries of right leg extremities with ulceration of toe

I70.238 Atherosclerosis of native arteries of right leg with ulceration of other part of lower leg HCC A

I70.239 Atherosclerosis of native arteries of right leg with ulceration of unspecified site HCC A

I70.24 Atherosclerosis of native arteries of left leg with ulceration

INCLUDES any condition classifiable to I70.212 and I70.222
chronic limb-threatening ischemia of native arteries of left leg with ulceration
critical limb ischemia of native arteries of left leg with ulceration

Use additional code to identify severity of ulcer (L97.-)

I70.241 Atherosclerosis of native arteries of left leg with ulceration of thigh HCC A

I70.242 Atherosclerosis of native arteries of left leg with ulceration of calf HCC A

I70.243 Atherosclerosis of native arteries of left leg with ulceration of ankle HCC A

I70.244 Atherosclerosis of native arteries of left leg with ulceration of heel and midfoot HCC A

Atherosclerosis of native arteries of left leg with ulceration of plantar surface of midfoot

I70.245 Atherosclerosis of native arteries of left leg with ulceration of other part of foot HCC A

Atherosclerosis of native arteries of left leg extremities with ulceration of toe

I70.248 Atherosclerosis of native arteries of left leg with ulceration of other part of lower leg HCC A

I70.249 Atherosclerosis of native arteries of left leg with ulceration of unspecified site HCC A

I70.25 Atherosclerosis of native arteries of other extremities with ulceration HCC A

INCLUDES any condition classifiable to I70.218 and I70.228

Use additional code to identify the severity of the ulcer (L98.49-)

I70.26 Atherosclerosis of native arteries of extremities with gangrene

INCLUDES any condition classifiable to I70.21-, I70.22-, I70.23-, I70.24-, and I70.25-
chronic limb-threatening ischemia of native arteries of extremities with gangrene
critical limb ischemia of native arteries of extremities with gangrene

Use additional code to identify the severity of any ulcer (L97.-, L98.49-), if applicable

I70.261 Atherosclerosis of native arteries of extremities with gangrene, right leg CC HCC A

I70.262 Atherosclerosis of native arteries of extremities with gangrene, left leg CC HCC A

I70.263 Atherosclerosis of native arteries of extremities with gangrene, bilateral legs CC HCC A

I70.268 Atherosclerosis of native arteries of extremities with gangrene, other extremity CC HCC A

I70.269 Atherosclerosis of native arteries of extremities with gangrene, unspecified extremity CC UNS HCC A

I70.29 Other atherosclerosis of native arteries of extremities

I70.291 Other atherosclerosis of native arteries of extremities, right leg HCC A

I70.292 Other atherosclerosis of native arteries of extremities, left leg HCC A

I70.293 Other atherosclerosis of native arteries of extremities, bilateral legs HCC A

I70.298 Other atherosclerosis of native arteries of extremities, other extremity HCC A

I70.299 Other atherosclerosis of native arteries of extremities, unspecified extremity HCC A

√5th **I70.3 Atherosclerosis of unspecified type of bypass graft(s) of the extremities**
Use additional code, if applicable, to identify chronic total occlusion of artery of extremity (I70.92)
EXCLUDES 1 *embolism or thrombus of bypass graft(s) of extremities (T82.8-)*
AHA: 2020,4Q,98

√6th **I70.30 Unspecified atherosclerosis of unspecified type of bypass graft(s) of the extremities**
I70.301 Unspecified atherosclerosis of unspecified type of bypass graft(s) of the extremities, right leg HCC A
I70.302 Unspecified atherosclerosis of unspecified type of bypass graft(s) of the extremities, left leg HCC A
I70.303 Unspecified atherosclerosis of unspecified type of bypass graft(s) of the extremities, bilateral legs HCC A
I70.308 Unspecified atherosclerosis of unspecified type of bypass graft(s) of the extremities, other extremity HCC A
I70.309 Unspecified atherosclerosis of unspecified type of bypass graft(s) of the extremities, unspecified extremity HCC A

√6th **I70.31 Atherosclerosis of unspecified type of bypass graft(s) of the extremities with intermittent claudication**
I70.311 Atherosclerosis of unspecified type of bypass graft(s) of the extremities with intermittent claudication, right leg HCC A
I70.312 Atherosclerosis of unspecified type of bypass graft(s) of the extremities with intermittent claudication, left leg HCC A
I70.313 Atherosclerosis of unspecified type of bypass graft(s) of the extremities with intermittent claudication, bilateral legs HCC A
I70.318 Atherosclerosis of unspecified type of bypass graft(s) of the extremities with intermittent claudication, other extremity HCC A
I70.319 Atherosclerosis of unspecified type of bypass graft(s) of the extremities with intermittent claudication, unspecified extremity HCC A

√6th **I70.32 Atherosclerosis of unspecified type of bypass graft(s) of the extremities with rest pain**
INCLUDES any condition classifiable to I70.31-
chronic limb-threatening ischemia NOS of unspecified type of bypass graft(s) of the extremities
chronic limb-threatening ischemia of unspecified type of bypass graft(s) of the extremities with rest pain
critical limb ischemia NOS of unspecified type of bypass graft(s) of the extremities
critical limb ischemia of unspecified type of bypass graft(s) of the extremities with rest pain
I70.321 Atherosclerosis of unspecified type of bypass graft(s) of the extremities with rest pain, right leg HCC A
I70.322 Atherosclerosis of unspecified type of bypass graft(s) of the extremities with rest pain, left leg HCC A
I70.323 Atherosclerosis of unspecified type of bypass graft(s) of the extremities with rest pain, bilateral legs HCC A
I70.328 Atherosclerosis of unspecified type of bypass graft(s) of the extremities with rest pain, other extremity HCC A
I70.329 Atherosclerosis of unspecified type of bypass graft(s) of the extremities with rest pain, unspecified extremity HCC A

√6th **I70.33 Atherosclerosis of unspecified type of bypass graft(s) of the right leg with ulceration**
INCLUDES any condition classifiable to I70.311 and I70.321
chronic limb-threatening ischemia of unspecified type of bypass graft(s) of the right leg with ulceration
critical limb ischemia of unspecified type of bypass graft(s) of the right leg with ulceration
Use additional code to identify severity of ulcer (L97.-)
I70.331 Atherosclerosis of unspecified type of bypass graft(s) of the right leg with ulceration of thigh CC HCC A
I70.332 Atherosclerosis of unspecified type of bypass graft(s) of the right leg with ulceration of calf CC HCC A
I70.333 Atherosclerosis of unspecified type of bypass graft(s) of the right leg with ulceration of ankle CC HCC A
I70.334 Atherosclerosis of unspecified type of bypass graft(s) of the right leg with ulceration of heel and midfoot CC HCC A
Atherosclerosis of unspecified type of bypass graft(s) of right leg with ulceration of plantar surface of midfoot
I70.335 Atherosclerosis of unspecified type of bypass graft(s) of the right leg with ulceration of other part of foot HCC A
Atherosclerosis of unspecified type of bypass graft(s) of the right leg with ulceration of toe
I70.338 Atherosclerosis of unspecified type of bypass graft(s) of the right leg with ulceration of other part of lower leg CC HCC A
I70.339 Atherosclerosis of unspecified type of bypass graft(s) of the right leg with ulceration of unspecified site CC HCC A

√6th **I70.34 Atherosclerosis of unspecified type of bypass graft(s) of the left leg with ulceration**
INCLUDES any condition classifiable to I70.312 and I70.322
chronic limb-threatening ischemia of unspecified type of bypass graft(s) of the left leg with ulceration
critical limb ischemia of unspecified type of bypass graft(s) of the left leg with ulceration
Use additional code to identify severity of ulcer (L97.-)
I70.341 Atherosclerosis of unspecified type of bypass graft(s) of the left leg with ulceration of thigh CC HCC A
I70.342 Atherosclerosis of unspecified type of bypass graft(s) of the left leg with ulceration of calf CC HCC A
I70.343 Atherosclerosis of unspecified type of bypass graft(s) of the left leg with ulceration of ankle CC HCC A
I70.344 Atherosclerosis of unspecified type of bypass graft(s) of the left leg with ulceration of heel and midfoot CC HCC A
Atherosclerosis of unspecified type of bypass graft(s) of left leg with ulceration of plantar surface of midfoot
I70.345 Atherosclerosis of unspecified type of bypass graft(s) of the left leg with ulceration of other part of foot HCC A
Atherosclerosis of unspecified type of bypass graft(s) of the left leg with ulceration of toe
I70.348 Atherosclerosis of unspecified type of bypass graft(s) of the left leg with ulceration of other part of lower leg CC HCC A
I70.349 Atherosclerosis of unspecified type of bypass graft(s) of the left leg with ulceration of unspecified site CC HCC A

I70.35 Atherosclerosis of unspecified type of bypass graft(s) of other extremity with ulceration HCC A
INCLUDES any condition classifiable to I70.318 and I70.328
Use additional code to identify severity of ulcer (L98.49-)

✓6th I70.36 Atherosclerosis of unspecified type of bypass graft(s) of the extremities with gangrene
INCLUDES any condition classifiable to I70.31-, I70.32-, I70.33-, I70.34-, I70.35
chronic limb-threatening ischemia of unspecified type of bypass graft(s) of the extremities with gangrene
critical limb ischemia of unspecified type of bypass graft(s) of the extremities with gangrene
Use additional code to identify the severity of any ulcer (L97.-, L98.49-), if applicable

I70.361 Atherosclerosis of unspecified type of bypass graft(s) of the extremities with gangrene, right leg CC HCC A
I70.362 Atherosclerosis of unspecified type of bypass graft(s) of the extremities with gangrene, left leg CC HCC A
I70.363 Atherosclerosis of unspecified type of bypass graft(s) of the extremities with gangrene, bilateral legs CC HCC A
I70.368 Atherosclerosis of unspecified type of bypass graft(s) of the extremities with gangrene, other extremity CC HCC A
I70.369 Atherosclerosis of unspecified type of bypass graft(s) of the extremities with gangrene, unspecified extremity CC UNS HCC A

✓6th I70.39 Other atherosclerosis of unspecified type of bypass graft(s) of the extremities

I70.391 Other atherosclerosis of unspecified type of bypass graft(s) of the extremities, right leg HCC A
I70.392 Other atherosclerosis of unspecified type of bypass graft(s) of the extremities, left leg HCC A
I70.393 Other atherosclerosis of unspecified type of bypass graft(s) of the extremities, bilateral legs HCC A
I70.398 Other atherosclerosis of unspecified type of bypass graft(s) of the extremities, other extremity HCC A
I70.399 Other atherosclerosis of unspecified type of bypass graft(s) of the extremities, unspecified extremity HCC A

✓5th I70.4 Atherosclerosis of autologous vein bypass graft(s) of the extremities
Use additional code, if applicable, to identify chronic total occlusion of artery of extremity (I70.92)
AHA: 2020,4Q,98

✓6th I70.40 Unspecified atherosclerosis of autologous vein bypass graft(s) of the extremities

I70.401 Unspecified atherosclerosis of autologous vein bypass graft(s) of the extremities, right leg HCC A
I70.402 Unspecified atherosclerosis of autologous vein bypass graft(s) of the extremities, left leg HCC A
I70.403 Unspecified atherosclerosis of autologous vein bypass graft(s) of the extremities, bilateral legs HCC A
I70.408 Unspecified atherosclerosis of autologous vein bypass graft(s) of the extremities, other extremity HCC A
I70.409 Unspecified atherosclerosis of autologous vein bypass graft(s) of the extremities, unspecified extremity HCC A

✓6th I70.41 Atherosclerosis of autologous vein bypass graft(s) of the extremities with intermittent claudication

I70.411 Atherosclerosis of autologous vein bypass graft(s) of the extremities with intermittent claudication, right leg HCC A
I70.412 Atherosclerosis of autologous vein bypass graft(s) of the extremities with intermittent claudication, left leg HCC A
I70.413 Atherosclerosis of autologous vein bypass graft(s) of the extremities with intermittent claudication, bilateral legs HCC A
I70.418 Atherosclerosis of autologous vein bypass graft(s) of the extremities with intermittent claudication, other extremity HCC A
I70.419 Atherosclerosis of autologous vein bypass graft(s) of the extremities with intermittent claudication, unspecified extremity HCC A

✓6th I70.42 Atherosclerosis of autologous vein bypass graft(s) of the extremities with rest pain
INCLUDES any condition classifiable to I70.41-
chronic limb-threatening ischemia NOS of autologous vein bypass graft(s) of the extremities
chronic limb-threatening ischemia of autologous vein bypass graft(s) of the extremities with rest pain
critical limb ischemia NOS of autologous vein bypass graft(s) of the extremities
critical limb ischemia of autologous vein bypass graft(s) of the extremities with rest pain

I70.421 Atherosclerosis of autologous vein bypass graft(s) of the extremities with rest pain, right leg HCC A
I70.422 Atherosclerosis of autologous vein bypass graft(s) of the extremities with rest pain, left leg HCC A
I70.423 Atherosclerosis of autologous vein bypass graft(s) of the extremities with rest pain, bilateral legs HCC A
I70.428 Atherosclerosis of autologous vein bypass graft(s) of the extremities with rest pain, other extremity HCC A
I70.429 Atherosclerosis of autologous vein bypass graft(s) of the extremities with rest pain, unspecified extremity HCC A

✓6th I70.43 Atherosclerosis of autologous vein bypass graft(s) of the right leg with ulceration
INCLUDES any condition classifiable to I70.411 and I70.421
chronic limb-threatening ischemia of autologous vein bypass graft(s) of the right leg with ulceration
critical limb ischemia of autologous vein bypass graft(s) of the right leg with ulceration
Use additional code to identify severity of ulcer (L97.-)

I70.431 Atherosclerosis of autologous vein bypass graft(s) of the right leg with ulceration of thigh CC HCC A
I70.432 Atherosclerosis of autologous vein bypass graft(s) of the right leg with ulceration of calf CC HCC A
I70.433 Atherosclerosis of autologous vein bypass graft(s) of the right leg with ulceration of ankle CC HCC A
I70.434 Atherosclerosis of autologous vein bypass graft(s) of the right leg with ulceration of heel and midfoot CC HCC A
Atherosclerosis of autologous vein bypass graft(s) of right leg with ulceration of plantar surface of midfoot
I70.435 Atherosclerosis of autologous vein bypass graft(s) of the right leg with ulceration of other part of foot HCC A
Atherosclerosis of autologous vein bypass graft(s) of right leg with ulceration of toe
I70.438 Atherosclerosis of autologous vein bypass graft(s) of the right leg with ulceration of other part of lower leg CC HCC A
I70.439 Atherosclerosis of autologous vein bypass graft(s) of the right leg with ulceration of unspecified site CC HCC A

√6th **I7Ø.44 Atherosclerosis of autologous vein bypass graft(s) of the left leg with ulceration**
INCLUDES any condition classifiable to I7Ø.412 and I7Ø.422
chronic limb-threatening ischemia of autologous vein bypass graft(s) of the left leg with ulceration
critical limb ischemia of autologous vein bypass graft(s) of the left leg with ulceration
Use additional code to identify severity of ulcer (L97.-)

I7Ø.441 Atherosclerosis of autologous vein bypass graft(s) of the left leg with ulceration of thigh CC HCC A

I7Ø.442 Atherosclerosis of autologous vein bypass graft(s) of the left leg with ulceration of calf CC HCC A

I7Ø.443 Atherosclerosis of autologous vein bypass graft(s) of the left leg with ulceration of ankle CC HCC A

I7Ø.444 Atherosclerosis of autologous vein bypass graft(s) of the left leg with ulceration of heel and midfoot CC HCC A
Atherosclerosis of autologous vein bypass graft(s) of left leg with ulceration of plantar surface of midfoot

I7Ø.445 Atherosclerosis of autologous vein bypass graft(s) of the left leg with ulceration of other part of foot HCC A
Atherosclerosis of autologous vein bypass graft(s) of left leg with ulceration of toe

I7Ø.448 Atherosclerosis of autologous vein bypass graft(s) of the left leg with ulceration of other part of lower leg CC HCC A

I7Ø.449 Atherosclerosis of autologous vein bypass graft(s) of the left leg with ulceration of unspecified site CC HCC A

I7Ø.45 Atherosclerosis of autologous vein bypass graft(s) of other extremity with ulceration HCC A
INCLUDES any condition classifiable to I7Ø.418, I7Ø.428, and I7Ø.438
Use additional code to identify severity of ulcer (L98.49)

√6th **I7Ø.46 Atherosclerosis of autologous vein bypass graft(s) of the extremities with gangrene**
INCLUDES any condition classifiable to I7Ø.41-, I7Ø.42-, and I7Ø.43-, I7Ø.44-, I7Ø.45
chronic limb-threatening ischemia of autologous vein bypass graft(s) of the extremities with gangrene
critical limb ischemia of autologous vein bypass graft(s) of the extremities with gangrene
Use additional code to identify the severity of any ulcer (L97.-, L98.49-), if applicable

I7Ø.461 Atherosclerosis of autologous vein bypass graft(s) of the extremities with gangrene, right leg CC HCC A

I7Ø.462 Atherosclerosis of autologous vein bypass graft(s) of the extremities with gangrene, left leg CC HCC A

I7Ø.463 Atherosclerosis of autologous vein bypass graft(s) of the extremities with gangrene, bilateral legs CC HCC A

I7Ø.468 Atherosclerosis of autologous vein bypass graft(s) of the extremities with gangrene, other extremity CC HCC A

I7Ø.469 Atherosclerosis of autologous vein bypass graft(s) of the extremities with gangrene, unspecified extremity CC UNS HCC A

√6th **I7Ø.49 Other atherosclerosis of autologous vein bypass graft(s) of the extremities**

I7Ø.491 Other atherosclerosis of autologous vein bypass graft(s) of the extremities, right leg HCC A

I7Ø.492 Other atherosclerosis of autologous vein bypass graft(s) of the extremities, left leg HCC A

I7Ø.493 Other atherosclerosis of autologous vein bypass graft(s) of the extremities, bilateral legs HCC A

I7Ø.498 Other atherosclerosis of autologous vein bypass graft(s) of the extremities, other extremity HCC A

I7Ø.499 Other atherosclerosis of autologous vein bypass graft(s) of the extremities, unspecified extremity HCC A

√5th **I7Ø.5 Atherosclerosis of nonautologous biological bypass graft(s) of the extremities**
Use additional code, if applicable, to identify chronic total occlusion of artery of extremity (I7Ø.92)
AHA: 2020,4Q,98

√6th **I7Ø.5Ø Unspecified atherosclerosis of nonautologous biological bypass graft(s) of the extremities**

I7Ø.5Ø1 Unspecified atherosclerosis of nonautologous biological bypass graft(s) of the extremities, right leg HCC A

I7Ø.5Ø2 Unspecified atherosclerosis of nonautologous biological bypass graft(s) of the extremities, left leg HCC A

I7Ø.5Ø3 Unspecified atherosclerosis of nonautologous biological bypass graft(s) of the extremities, bilateral legs HCC A

I7Ø.5Ø8 Unspecified atherosclerosis of nonautologous biological bypass graft(s) of the extremities, other extremity HCC A

I7Ø.5Ø9 Unspecified atherosclerosis of nonautologous biological bypass graft(s) of the extremities, unspecified extremity HCC A

√6th **I7Ø.51 Atherosclerosis of nonautologous biological bypass graft(s) of the extremities intermittent claudication**

I7Ø.511 Atherosclerosis of nonautologous biological bypass graft(s) of the extremities with intermittent claudication, right leg HCC A

I7Ø.512 Atherosclerosis of nonautologous biological bypass graft(s) of the extremities with intermittent claudication, left leg HCC A

I7Ø.513 Atherosclerosis of nonautologous biological bypass graft(s) of the extremities with intermittent claudication, bilateral legs HCC A

I7Ø.518 Atherosclerosis of nonautologous biological bypass graft(s) of the extremities with intermittent claudication, other extremity HCC A

I7Ø.519 Atherosclerosis of nonautologous biological bypass graft(s) of the extremities with intermittent claudication, unspecified extremity HCC A

√6th **I7Ø.52 Atherosclerosis of nonautologous biological bypass graft(s) of the extremities with rest pain**
INCLUDES any condition classifiable to I7Ø.51-
chronic limb-threatening ischemia NOS of nonautologous biological bypass graft(s) of the extremities
chronic limb-threatening ischemia of nonautologous biological bypass graft(s) of the extremities with rest pain
critical limb ischemia NOS of nonautologous biological bypass graft(s) of the extremities
critical limb ischemia of nonautologous biological bypass graft(s) of the extremities with rest pain

I7Ø.521 Atherosclerosis of nonautologous biological bypass graft(s) of the extremities with rest pain, right leg HCC A

I7Ø.522 Atherosclerosis of nonautologous biological bypass graft(s) of the extremities with rest pain, left leg HCC A

I7Ø.523 Atherosclerosis of nonautologous biological bypass graft(s) of the extremities with rest pain, bilateral legs HCC A

I70.528 Atherosclerosis of nonautologous biological bypass graft(s) of the extremities with rest pain, other extremity HCC A

I70.529 Atherosclerosis of nonautologous biological bypass graft(s) of the extremities with rest pain, unspecified extremity HCC A

√6th **I70.53 Atherosclerosis of nonautologous biological bypass graft(s) of the right leg with ulceration**

INCLUDES any condition classifiable to I70.511 and I70.521
chronic limb-threatening ischemia of nonautologous biological bypass graft(s) of the right leg with ulceration
critical limb ischemia of nonautologous biological bypass graft(s) of the right leg with ulceration

Use additional code to identify severity of ulcer (L97.-)

I70.531 Atherosclerosis of nonautologous biological bypass graft(s) of the right leg with ulceration of thigh CC HCC A

I70.532 Atherosclerosis of nonautologous biological bypass graft(s) of the right leg with ulceration of calf CC HCC A

I70.533 Atherosclerosis of nonautologous biological bypass graft(s) of the right leg with ulceration of ankle CC HCC A

I70.534 Atherosclerosis of nonautologous biological bypass graft(s) of the right leg with ulceration of heel and midfoot CC HCC A

Atherosclerosis of nonautologous biological bypass graft(s) of right leg with ulceration of plantar surface of midfoot

I70.535 Atherosclerosis of nonautologous biological bypass graft(s) of the right leg with ulceration of other part of foot HCC A

Atherosclerosis of nonautologous biological bypass graft(s) of the right leg with ulceration of toe

I70.538 Atherosclerosis of nonautologous biological bypass graft(s) of the right leg with ulceration of other part of lower leg CC HCC A

I70.539 Atherosclerosis of nonautologous biological bypass graft(s) of the right leg with ulceration of unspecified site CC HCC A

√6th **I70.54 Atherosclerosis of nonautologous biological bypass graft(s) of the left leg with ulceration**

INCLUDES any condition classifiable to I70.512 and I70.522
chronic limb-threatening ischemia of nonautologous biological bypass graft(s) of the left leg with ulceration
critical limb ischemia of nonautologous biological bypass graft(s) of the left leg with ulceration

Use additional code to identify severity of ulcer (L97.-)

I70.541 Atherosclerosis of nonautologous biological bypass graft(s) of the left leg with ulceration of thigh CC HCC A

I70.542 Atherosclerosis of nonautologous biological bypass graft(s) of the left leg with ulceration of calf CC HCC A

I70.543 Atherosclerosis of nonautologous biological bypass graft(s) of the left leg with ulceration of ankle CC HCC A

I70.544 Atherosclerosis of nonautologous biological bypass graft(s) of the left leg with ulceration of heel and midfoot CC HCC A

Atherosclerosis of nonautologous biological bypass graft(s) of left leg with ulceration of plantar surface of midfoot

I70.545 Atherosclerosis of nonautologous biological bypass graft(s) of the left leg with ulceration of other part of foot HCC A

Atherosclerosis of nonautologous biological bypass graft(s) of the left leg with ulceration of toe

I70.548 Atherosclerosis of nonautologous biological bypass graft(s) of the left leg with ulceration of other part of lower leg CC HCC A

I70.549 Atherosclerosis of nonautologous biological bypass graft(s) of the left leg with ulceration of unspecified site CC HCC A

I70.55 Atherosclerosis of nonautologous biological bypass graft(s) of other extremity with ulceration HCC A

INCLUDES any condition classifiable to I70.518, I70.528, and I70.538

Use additional code to identify severity of ulcer (L98.49)

√6th **I70.56 Atherosclerosis of nonautologous biological bypass graft(s) of the extremities with gangrene**

INCLUDES any condition classifiable to I70.51-, I70.52-, and I70.53-, I70.54-, I70.55
chronic limb-threatening ischemia of nonautologous biological bypass graft(s) of the extremities with gangrene
critical limb ischemia of nonautologous biological bypass graft(s) of the extremities with gangrene

Use additional code to identify the severity of any ulcer (L97.-, L98.49-), if applicable

I70.561 Atherosclerosis of nonautologous biological bypass graft(s) of the extremities with gangrene, right leg CC HCC A

I70.562 Atherosclerosis of nonautologous biological bypass graft(s) of the extremities with gangrene, left leg CC HCC A

I70.563 Atherosclerosis of nonautologous biological bypass graft(s) of the extremities with gangrene, bilateral legs CC HCC A

I70.568 Atherosclerosis of nonautologous biological bypass graft(s) of the extremities with gangrene, other extremity CC HCC A

I70.569 Atherosclerosis of nonautologous biological bypass graft(s) of the extremities with gangrene, unspecified extremity CC UNS HCC A

√6th **I70.59 Other atherosclerosis of nonautologous biological bypass graft(s) of the extremities**

I70.591 Other atherosclerosis of nonautologous biological bypass graft(s) of the extremities, right leg HCC A

I70.592 Other atherosclerosis of nonautologous biological bypass graft(s) of the extremities, left leg HCC A

I70.593 Other atherosclerosis of nonautologous biological bypass graft(s) of the extremities, bilateral legs HCC A

I70.598 Other atherosclerosis of nonautologous biological bypass graft(s) of the extremities, other extremity HCC A

I70.599 Other atherosclerosis of nonautologous biological bypass graft(s) of the extremities, unspecified extremity HCC A

√5th **I70.6 Atherosclerosis of nonbiological bypass graft(s) of the extremities**

Use additional code, if applicable, to identify chronic total occlusion of artery of extremity (I70.92)

AHA: 2020,4Q,98

√6th **I70.60 Unspecified atherosclerosis of nonbiological bypass graft(s) of the extremities**

I70.601 Unspecified atherosclerosis of nonbiological bypass graft(s) of the extremities, right leg HCC A

I70.602 Unspecified atherosclerosis of nonbiological bypass graft(s) of the extremities, left leg HCC A

I70.603 Unspecified atherosclerosis of nonbiological bypass graft(s) of the extremities, bilateral legs HCC A

I70.608 Unspecified atherosclerosis of nonbiological bypass graft(s) of the extremities, other extremity HCC A

I70.609 Unspecified atherosclerosis of nonbiological bypass graft(s) of the extremities, unspecified extremity HCC A

✓6th **I70.61** Atherosclerosis of nonbiological bypass graft(s) of the extremities with intermittent claudication

I70.611 Atherosclerosis of nonbiological bypass graft(s) of the extremities with intermittent claudication, right leg HCC A

I70.612 Atherosclerosis of nonbiological bypass graft(s) of the extremities with intermittent claudication, left leg HCC A

I70.613 Atherosclerosis of nonbiological bypass graft(s) of the extremities with intermittent claudication, bilateral legs HCC A

I70.618 Atherosclerosis of nonbiological bypass graft(s) of the extremities with intermittent claudication, other extremity HCC A

I70.619 Atherosclerosis of nonbiological bypass graft(s) of the extremities with intermittent claudication, unspecified extremity HCC A

✓6th **I70.62** Atherosclerosis of nonbiological bypass graft(s) of the extremities with rest pain

INCLUDES any condition classifiable to I70.61-

chronic limb-threatening ischemia NOS of nonbiological bypass graft(s) of the extremities

chronic limb-threatening ischemia of nonbiological bypass graft(s) of the extremities with rest pain

critical limb ischemia NOS of nonbiological bypass graft(s) of the extremities

critical limb ischemia of nonbiological bypass graft(s) of the extremities with rest pain

I70.621 Atherosclerosis of nonbiological bypass graft(s) of the extremities with rest pain, right leg HCC A

I70.622 Atherosclerosis of nonbiological bypass graft(s) of the extremities with rest pain, left leg HCC A

I70.623 Atherosclerosis of nonbiological bypass graft(s) of the extremities with rest pain, bilateral legs HCC A

I70.628 Atherosclerosis of nonbiological bypass graft(s) of the extremities with rest pain, other extremity HCC A

I70.629 Atherosclerosis of nonbiological bypass graft(s) of the extremities with rest pain, unspecified extremity HCC A

✓6th **I70.63** Atherosclerosis of nonbiological bypass graft(s) of the right leg with ulceration

INCLUDES any condition classifiable to I70.611 and I70.621

chronic limb-threatening ischemia of nonbiological bypass graft(s) of the right leg with ulceration

critical limb ischemia of nonbiological bypass graft(s) of the right leg with ulceration

Use additional code to identify severity of ulcer (L97.-)

I70.631 Atherosclerosis of nonbiological bypass graft(s) of the right leg with ulceration of thigh CC HCC A

I70.632 Atherosclerosis of nonbiological bypass graft(s) of the right leg with ulceration of calf CC HCC A

I70.633 Atherosclerosis of nonbiological bypass graft(s) of the right leg with ulceration of ankle CC HCC A

I70.634 Atherosclerosis of nonbiological bypass graft(s) of the right leg with ulceration of heel and midfoot CC HCC A

Atherosclerosis of nonbiological bypass graft(s) of right leg with ulceration of plantar surface of midfoot

I70.635 Atherosclerosis of nonbiological bypass graft(s) of the right leg with ulceration of other part of foot HCC A

Atherosclerosis of nonbiological bypass graft(s) of the right leg with ulceration of toe

I70.638 Atherosclerosis of nonbiological bypass graft(s) of the right leg with ulceration of other part of lower leg CC HCC A

I70.639 Atherosclerosis of nonbiological bypass graft(s) of the right leg with ulceration of unspecified site CC HCC A

✓6th **I70.64** Atherosclerosis of nonbiological bypass graft(s) of the left leg with ulceration

INCLUDES any condition classifiable to I70.612 and I70.622

chronic limb-threatening ischemia of nonbiological bypass graft(s) of the left leg with ulceration

critical limb ischemia of nonbiological bypass graft(s) of the left leg with ulceration

Use additional code to identify severity of ulcer (L97.-)

I70.641 Atherosclerosis of nonbiological bypass graft(s) of the left leg with ulceration of thigh CC HCC A

I70.642 Atherosclerosis of nonbiological bypass graft(s) of the left leg with ulceration of calf CC HCC A

I70.643 Atherosclerosis of nonbiological bypass graft(s) of the left leg with ulceration of ankle CC HCC A

I70.644 Atherosclerosis of nonbiological bypass graft(s) of the left leg with ulceration of heel and midfoot CC HCC A

Atherosclerosis of nonbiological bypass graft(s) of left leg with ulceration of plantar surface of midfoot

I70.645 Atherosclerosis of nonbiological bypass graft(s) of the left leg with ulceration of other part of foot HCC A

Atherosclerosis of nonbiological bypass graft(s) of the left leg with ulceration of toe

I70.648 Atherosclerosis of nonbiological bypass graft(s) of the left leg with ulceration of other part of lower leg CC HCC A

I70.649 Atherosclerosis of nonbiological bypass graft(s) of the left leg with ulceration of unspecified site CC HCC A

I70.65 Atherosclerosis of nonbiological bypass graft(s) of other extremity with ulceration HCC A

INCLUDES any condition classifiable to I70.618 and I70.628

Use additional code to identify severity of ulcer (L98.49)

✓6th **I70.66** Atherosclerosis of nonbiological bypass graft(s) of the extremities with gangrene

INCLUDES any condition classifiable to I70.61-, I70.62-, I70.63-, I70.64-, I70.65

chronic limb-threatening ischemia of nonbiological bypass graft(s) of the extremities with gangrene

critical limb ischemia of nonbiological bypass graft(s) of the extremities with gangrene

Use additional code to identify the severity of any ulcer (L97.-, L98.49-), if applicable

I70.661 Atherosclerosis of nonbiological bypass graft(s) of the extremities with gangrene, right leg CC HCC A

I70.662 Atherosclerosis of nonbiological bypass graft(s) of the extremities with gangrene, left leg CC HCC A

I70.663 Atherosclerosis of nonbiological bypass graft(s) of the extremities with gangrene, bilateral legs CC HCC A

I70.668 Atherosclerosis of nonbiological bypass graft(s) of the extremities with gangrene, other extremity CC HCC A

I70.669 Atherosclerosis of nonbiological bypass graft(s) of the extremities with gangrene, unspecified extremity CC UNS HCC A

✓6th I70.69 Other atherosclerosis of nonbiological bypass graft(s) of the extremities

I70.691 Other atherosclerosis of nonbiological bypass graft(s) of the extremities, right leg HCC A

I70.692 Other atherosclerosis of nonbiological bypass graft(s) of the extremities, left leg HCC A

I70.693 Other atherosclerosis of nonbiological bypass graft(s) of the extremities, bilateral legs HCC A

I70.698 Other atherosclerosis of nonbiological bypass graft(s) of the extremities, other extremity HCC A

I70.699 Other atherosclerosis of nonbiological bypass graft(s) of the extremities, unspecified extremity HCC A

✓5th I70.7 Atherosclerosis of other type of bypass graft(s) of the extremities

Use additional code, if applicable, to identify chronic total occlusion of artery of extremity (I70.92)

AHA: 2020,4Q,98

✓6th I70.70 Unspecified atherosclerosis of other type of bypass graft(s) of the extremities

I70.701 Unspecified atherosclerosis of other type of bypass graft(s) of the extremities, right leg HCC A

I70.702 Unspecified atherosclerosis of other type of bypass graft(s) of the extremities, left leg HCC A

I70.703 Unspecified atherosclerosis of other type of bypass graft(s) of the extremities, bilateral legs HCC A

I70.708 Unspecified atherosclerosis of other type of bypass graft(s) of the extremities, other extremity HCC A

I70.709 Unspecified atherosclerosis of other type of bypass graft(s) of the extremities, unspecified extremity HCC A

✓6th I70.71 Atherosclerosis of other type of bypass graft(s) of the extremities with intermittent claudication

I70.711 Atherosclerosis of other type of bypass graft(s) of the extremities with intermittent claudication, right leg HCC A

I70.712 Atherosclerosis of other type of bypass graft(s) of the extremities with intermittent claudication, left leg HCC A

I70.713 Atherosclerosis of other type of bypass graft(s) of the extremities with intermittent claudication, bilateral legs HCC A

I70.718 Atherosclerosis of other type of bypass graft(s) of the extremities with intermittent claudication, other extremity HCC A

I70.719 Atherosclerosis of other type of bypass graft(s) of the extremities with intermittent claudication, unspecified extremity HCC A

✓6th I70.72 Atherosclerosis of other type of bypass graft(s) of the extremities with rest pain

INCLUDES any condition classifiable to I70.71-
chronic limb-threatening ischemia NOS of other type of bypass graft(s) of the extremities
chronic limb-threatening ischemia of other type of bypass graft(s) of the extremities with rest pain
critical limb ischemia NOS of other type of bypass graft(s) of the extremities
critical limb ischemia of other type of bypass graft(s) of the extremities with rest pain

I70.721 Atherosclerosis of other type of bypass graft(s) of the extremities with rest pain, right leg HCC A

I70.722 Atherosclerosis of other type of bypass graft(s) of the extremities with rest pain, left leg HCC A

I70.723 Atherosclerosis of other type of bypass graft(s) of the extremities with rest pain, bilateral legs HCC A

I70.728 Atherosclerosis of other type of bypass graft(s) of the extremities with rest pain, other extremity HCC A

I70.729 Atherosclerosis of other type of bypass graft(s) of the extremities with rest pain, unspecified extremity HCC A

✓6th I70.73 Atherosclerosis of other type of bypass graft(s) of the right leg with ulceration

INCLUDES any condition classifiable to I70.711 and I70.721
chronic limb-threatening ischemia of other type of bypass graft(s) of the right leg with ulceration
critical limb ischemia of other type of bypass graft(s) of the right leg with ulceration

Use additional code to identify severity of ulcer (L97.-)

I70.731 Atherosclerosis of other type of bypass graft(s) of the right leg with ulceration of thigh CC HCC A

I70.732 Atherosclerosis of other type of bypass graft(s) of the right leg with ulceration of calf CC HCC A

I70.733 Atherosclerosis of other type of bypass graft(s) of the right leg with ulceration of ankle CC HCC A

I70.734 Atherosclerosis of other type of bypass graft(s) of the right leg with ulceration of heel and midfoot CC HCC A

Atherosclerosis of other type of bypass graft(s) of right leg with ulceration of plantar surface of midfoot

I70.735 Atherosclerosis of other type of bypass graft(s) of the right leg with ulceration of other part of foot HCC A

Atherosclerosis of other type of bypass graft(s) of right leg with ulceration of toe

I70.738 Atherosclerosis of other type of bypass graft(s) of the right leg with ulceration of other part of lower leg CC HCC A

I70.739 Atherosclerosis of other type of bypass graft(s) of the right leg with ulceration of unspecified site CC HCC A

✓6th I70.74 Atherosclerosis of other type of bypass graft(s) of the left leg with ulceration

INCLUDES any condition classifiable to I70.712 and I70.722
chronic limb-threatening ischemia of other type of bypass graft(s) of the left leg with ulceration
critical limb ischemia of other type of bypass graft(s) of the left leg with ulceration

Use additional code to identify severity of ulcer (L97.-)

I70.741 Atherosclerosis of other type of bypass graft(s) of the left leg with ulceration of thigh CC HCC A

I70.742 Atherosclerosis of other type of bypass graft(s) of the left leg with ulceration of calf CC HCC A

I70.743 Atherosclerosis of other type of bypass graft(s) of the left leg with ulceration of ankle CC HCC A

I70.744 Atherosclerosis of other type of bypass graft(s) of the left leg with ulceration of heel and midfoot CC HCC A
Atherosclerosis of other type of bypass graft(s) of left leg with ulceration of plantar surface of midfoot

I70.745 Atherosclerosis of other type of bypass graft(s) of the left leg with ulceration of other part of foot HCC A
Atherosclerosis of other type of bypass graft(s) of left leg with ulceration of toe

I70.748 Atherosclerosis of other type of bypass graft(s) of the left leg with ulceration of other part of lower leg CC HCC A

I70.749 Atherosclerosis of other type of bypass graft(s) of the left leg with ulceration of unspecified site CC HCC A

I70.75 Atherosclerosis of other type of bypass graft(s) of other extremity with ulceration HCC A
INCLUDES any condition classifiable to I70.718 and I70.728
Use additional code to identify severity of ulcer (L98.49)

6th I70.76 Atherosclerosis of other type of bypass graft(s) of the extremities with gangrene
INCLUDES any condition classifiable to I70.71-, I70.72-, I70.73-, I70.74-, I70.75
chronic limb-threatening ischemia of other type of bypass graft(s) of the extremities with gangrene
critical limb ischemia of other type of bypass graft(s) of the extremities with gangrene
Use additional code to identify the severity of any ulcer (L97.-, L98.49-), if applicable

I70.761 Atherosclerosis of other type of bypass graft(s) of the extremities with gangrene, right leg CC HCC A

I70.762 Atherosclerosis of other type of bypass graft(s) of the extremities with gangrene, left leg CC HCC A

I70.763 Atherosclerosis of other type of bypass graft(s) of the extremities with gangrene, bilateral legs CC HCC A

I70.768 Atherosclerosis of other type of bypass graft(s) of the extremities with gangrene, other extremity CC HCC A

I70.769 Atherosclerosis of other type of bypass graft(s) of the extremities with gangrene, unspecified extremity CC UNS HCC A

6th I70.79 Other atherosclerosis of other type of bypass graft(s) of the extremities

I70.791 Other atherosclerosis of other type of bypass graft(s) of the extremities, right leg HCC A

I70.792 Other atherosclerosis of other type of bypass graft(s) of the extremities, left leg HCC A

I70.793 Other atherosclerosis of other type of bypass graft(s) of the extremities, bilateral legs HCC A

I70.798 Other atherosclerosis of other type of bypass graft(s) of the extremities, other extremity HCC A

I70.799 Other atherosclerosis of other type of bypass graft(s) of the extremities, unspecified extremity HCC A

I70.8 Atherosclerosis of other arteries A
TIP: Arteriosclerosis of the iliac arteries is coded here.

5th I70.9 Other and unspecified atherosclerosis

I70.90 Unspecified atherosclerosis A

I70.91 Generalized atherosclerosis A

I70.92 Chronic total occlusion of artery of the extremities CC UPD HCC A
Complete occlusion of artery of the extremities
Total occlusion of artery of the extremities
Code first atherosclerosis of arteries of the extremities (I70.2-, I70.3-, I70.4-, I70.5-, I70.6-, I70.7-)

4th **I71 Aortic aneurysm and dissection**
Code first, if applicable:
syphilitic aortic aneurysm (A52.01)
traumatic aortic aneurysm (S25.09, S35.09)
AHA: 2022,4Q,24-26
TIP: A diagnosis of dissecting aneurysm should be coded to subcategory I71.0 only. The bulging/aneurysm, although present, occurred secondary to the dissection. The dissection represents the most significant problem.

5th I71.0 Dissection of aorta

I71.00 Dissection of unspecified site of aorta MCC HCC

6th I71.01 Dissection of thoracic aorta

I71.010 Dissection of ascending aorta MCC HCC

I71.011 Dissection of aortic arch MCC HCC

I71.012 Dissection of descending thoracic aorta MCC HCC

I71.019 Dissection of thoracic aorta, unspecified MCC HCC

I71.02 Dissection of abdominal aorta MCC HCC

I71.03 Dissection of thoracoabdominal aorta MCC HCC

5th I71.1 Thoracic aortic aneurysm, ruptured

I71.10 Thoracic aortic aneurysm, ruptured, unspecified MCC HCC

I71.11 Aneurysm of the ascending aorta, ruptured MCC HCC

I71.12 Aneurysm of the aortic arch, ruptured MCC HCC

I71.13 Aneurysm of the descending thoracic aorta, ruptured MCC HCC

5th I71.2 Thoracic aortic aneurysm, without rupture

I71.20 Thoracic aortic aneurysm, without rupture, unspecified HCC

I71.21 Aneurysm of the ascending aorta, without rupture HCC

I71.22 Aneurysm of the aortic arch, without rupture HCC

I71.23 Aneurysm of the descending thoracic aorta, without rupture HCC

5th I71.3 Abdominal aortic aneurysm, ruptured

I71.30 Abdominal aortic aneurysm, ruptured, unspecified MCC HCC

I71.31 Pararenal abdominal aortic aneurysm, ruptured MCC HCC

I71.32 Juxtarenal abdominal aortic aneurysm, ruptured MCC HCC

I71.33 Infrarenal abdominal aortic aneurysm, ruptured MCC HCC

5th I71.4 Abdominal aortic aneurysm, without rupture

I71.40 Abdominal aortic aneurysm, without rupture, unspecified HCC

I71.41 Pararenal abdominal aortic aneurysm, without rupture HCC

I71.42 Juxtarenal abdominal aortic aneurysm, without rupture HCC

I71.43 Infrarenal abdominal aortic aneurysm, without rupture HCC

5th I71.5 Thoracoabdominal aortic aneurysm, ruptured

I71.50 Thoracoabdominal aortic aneurysm, ruptured, unspecified MCC HCC

▲ I71.51 Supraceliac aneurysm of the thoracoabdominal aorta, ruptured MCC HCC

▲ I71.52 Paravisceral aneurysm of the thoracoabdominal aorta, ruptured MCC HCC

5th I71.6 Thoracoabdominal aortic aneurysm, without rupture

I71.60 Thoracoabdominal aortic aneurysm, without rupture, unspecified HCC

▲ I71.61 Supraceliac aneurysm of the thoracoabdominal aorta, without rupture HCC

▲ I71.62 Paravisceral aneurysm of the thoracoabdominal aorta, without rupture HCC

I71.8 Aortic aneurysm of unspecified site, ruptured MCC HCC
Rupture of aorta NOS

I71.9 Aortic aneurysm of unspecified site, without rupture HCC
Aneurysm of aorta
Dilatation of aorta
Hyaline necrosis of aorta

I72 Other aneurysm

INCLUDES aneurysm (cirsoid) (false) (ruptured)

EXCLUDES 2 *acquired aneurysm (I77.Ø)*
aneurysm (of) aorta (I71.-)
aneurysm (of) arteriovenous NOS (Q27.3-)
carotid artery dissection (I77.71)
cerebral (nonruptured) aneurysm (I67.1)
coronary aneurysm (I25.4)
coronary artery dissection (I25.42)
dissection of artery NEC (I77.79)
dissection of precerebral artery, congenital (nonruptured) (Q28.1)
heart aneurysm (I25.3)
iliac artery dissection (I77.72)
precerebral artery, congential (nonruptured) (Q28.1)
pulmonary artery aneurysm (I28.1)
renal artery dissection (I77.73)
retinal aneurysm (H35.Ø)
ruptured cerebral aneurysm (I6Ø.7)
varicose aneurysm (I77.Ø)
vertebral artery dissection (I77.74)

AHA: 2016,4Q,28-29

I72.Ø Aneurysm of carotid artery HCC
Aneurysm of common carotid artery
Aneurysm of external carotid artery
Aneurysm of internal carotid artery, extracranial portion
EXCLUDES 1 *aneurysm of internal carotid artery, intracranial portion (I67.1)*
aneurysm of internal carotid artery NOS (I67.1)

I72.1 Aneurysm of artery of upper extremity HCC

I72.2 Aneurysm of renal artery HCC

I72.3 Aneurysm of iliac artery HCC

I72.4 Aneurysm of artery of lower extremity HCC
AHA: 2019,2Q,21

I72.5 Aneurysm of other precerebral arteries HCC
Aneurysm of basilar artery (trunk)
EXCLUDES 2 *aneurysm of carotid artery (I72.Ø)*
aneurysm of vertebral artery (I72.6)
dissection of carotid artery (I77.71)
dissection of other precerebral arteries (I77.75)
dissection of vertebral artery (I77.74)

I72.6 Aneurysm of vertebral artery HCC
EXCLUDES 2 *dissection of vertebral artery (I77.74)*

I72.8 Aneurysm of other specified arteries HCC

I72.9 Aneurysm of unspecified site HCC

Aneurysm

I73 Other peripheral vascular diseases

EXCLUDES 2 *chilblains (T69.1)*
frostbite (T33-T34)
immersion hand or foot (T69.Ø-)
spasm of cerebral artery (G45.9)

AHA: 2018,4Q,87

I73.Ø Raynaud's syndrome
Raynaud's disease
Raynaud's phenomenon (secondary)
DEF: Constriction of the arteries of the digits caused by cold or by nerve or arterial damage and can be prompted by stress or emotion. Blood cannot reach the skin and soft tissues and the skin turns white with blue mottling.

I73.ØØ Raynaud's syndrome without gangrene

I73.Ø1 Raynaud's syndrome with gangrene CC HCC

I73.1 Thromboangiitis obliterans [Buerger's disease] HCC
DEF: Inflammatory disease of the extremity blood vessels, mainly the lower blood vessels. This disease is associated with heavy tobacco use. The arteries are more affected than veins. It occurs primarily in young men and leads to tissue ischemia and gangrene.

I73.8 Other specified peripheral vascular diseases
EXCLUDES 1 *diabetic (peripheral) angiopathy (EØ8-E13 with .51-.52)*

I73.81 Erythromelalgia HCC

I73.89 Other specified peripheral vascular diseases HCC
Acrocyanosis
Erythrocyanosis
Simple acroparesthesia [Schultze's type]
Vasomotor acroparesthesia [Nothnagel's type]

I73.9 Peripheral vascular disease, unspecified HCC
Intermittent claudication
Peripheral angiopathy NOS
Spasm of artery
EXCLUDES 1 *atherosclerosis of the extremities (I7Ø.2-I7Ø.7-)*
AHA: 2018,2Q,7

I74 Arterial embolism and thrombosis

INCLUDES embolic infarction
embolic occlusion
thrombotic infarction
thrombotic occlusion

Code first:
embolism and thrombosis complicating abortion or ectopic or molar pregnancy (OØØ-OØ7, OØ8.2)
embolism and thrombosis complicating pregnancy, childbirth and the puerperium (O88.-)

EXCLUDES 2 *atheroembolism (I75.-)*
basilar embolism and thrombosis (I63.Ø-I63.2, I65.1)
carotid embolism and thrombosis (I63.Ø-I63.2, I65.2)
cerebral embolism and thrombosis (I63.3-I63.5, I66.-)
coronary embolism and thrombosis (I21-I25)
mesenteric embolism and thrombosis (K55.Ø-)
ophthalmic embolism and thrombosis (H34.-)
precerebral embolism and thrombosis NOS (I63.Ø-I63.2, I65.9)
pulmonary embolism and thrombosis (I26.-)
renal embolism and thrombosis (N28.Ø)
retinal embolism and thrombosis (H34.-)
septic embolism and thrombosis (I76)
vertebral embolism and thrombosis (I63.Ø-I63.2, I65.Ø)

AHA: 2023,2Q,7

I74.Ø Embolism and thrombosis of abdominal aorta

I74.Ø1 Saddle embolus of abdominal aorta MCC HCC

I74.Ø9 Other arterial embolism and thrombosis of abdominal aorta CC HCC
Aortic bifurcation syndrome
Aortoiliac obstruction
Leriche's syndrome

I74.1 Embolism and thrombosis of other and unspecified parts of aorta

I74.1Ø Embolism and thrombosis of unspecified parts of aorta CC HCC

I74.11 Embolism and thrombosis of thoracic aorta CC HCC

I74.19 Embolism and thrombosis of other parts of aorta CC HCC

I74.2 Embolism and thrombosis of arteries of the upper extremities CC HCC

I74.3 Embolism and thrombosis of arteries of the lower extremities CC HCC

I74.4 Embolism and thrombosis of arteries of extremities, unspecified CC HCC
Peripheral arterial embolism NOS

I74.5 Embolism and thrombosis of iliac artery CC HCC

I74.8 Embolism and thrombosis of other arteries CC HCC

I74.9 Embolism and thrombosis of unspecified artery CC HCC

4th I75 Atheroembolism
INCLUDES atherothrombotic microembolism
cholesterol embolism

5th I75.Ø Atheroembolism of extremities

6th I75.Ø1 Atheroembolism of upper extremity

I75.Ø11 Atheroembolism of right upper extremity CC HCC

I75.Ø12 Atheroembolism of left upper extremity CC HCC

I75.Ø13 Atheroembolism of bilateral upper extremities CC HCC

I75.Ø19 Atheroembolism of unspecified upper extremity CC UNS HCC

6th I75.Ø2 Atheroembolism of lower extremity

I75.Ø21 Atheroembolism of right lower extremity CC HCC

I75.Ø22 Atheroembolism of left lower extremity CC HCC

I75.Ø23 Atheroembolism of bilateral lower extremities CC HCC

I75.Ø29 Atheroembolism of unspecified lower extremity CC UNS HCC

5th I75.8 Atheroembolism of other sites

I75.81 Atheroembolism of kidney CC HCC
Use additional code for any associated acute kidney failure and chronic kidney disease (N17.-, N18.-)

I75.89 Atheroembolism of other site CC HCC

I76 Septic arterial embolism CC UPD HCC
Code first underlying infection, such as:
infective endocarditis (I33.Ø)
lung abscess (J85.-)
Use additional code to identify the site of the embolism (I74.-)
EXCLUDES 2 *septic pulmonary embolism (I26.Ø1, I26.9Ø)*

4th I77 Other disorders of arteries and arterioles
EXCLUDES 2 *collagen (vascular) diseases (M3Ø-M36)*
hypersensitivity angiitis (M31.Ø)
pulmonary artery (I28.-)

I77.Ø Arteriovenous fistula, acquired HCC
Aneurysmal varix
Arteriovenous aneurysm, acquired
EXCLUDES 1 *arteriovenous aneurysm NOS (Q27.3-)*
presence of arteriovenous shunt (fistula) for dialysis (Z99.2)
traumatic - see injury of blood vessel by body region
EXCLUDES 2 *cerebral (I67.1)*
coronary (I25.4)
DEF: Communication between an artery and vein caused by trauma or invasive procedures.

I77.1 Stricture of artery HCC
Narrowing of artery
AHA: 2021,3Q,12

I77.2 Rupture of artery CC HCC
Erosion of artery
Fistula of artery
Ulcer of artery
EXCLUDES 1 *traumatic rupture of artery - see injury of blood vessel by body region*

I77.3 Arterial fibromuscular dysplasia HCC
Fibromuscular hyperplasia (of) carotid artery
Fibromuscular hyperplasia (of) renal artery

I77.4 Celiac artery compression syndrome CC HCC
AHA: 2021,3Q,12

I77.5 Necrosis of artery CC HCC

I77.6 Arteritis, unspecified HCC
Aortitis NOS
Endarteritis NOS
EXCLUDES 1 *arteritis or endarteritis:*
aortic arch (M31.4)
cerebral NEC (I67.7)
coronary (I25.89)
deformans (I7Ø.-)
giant cell (M31.5, M31.6)
obliterans (I7Ø.-)
senile (I7Ø.-)

5th I77.7 Other arterial dissection
EXCLUDES 2 *dissection of aorta (I71.Ø-)*
dissection of coronary artery (I25.42)
AHA: 2016,4Q,28-29

I77.7Ø Dissection of unspecified artery MCC HCC

I77.71 Dissection of carotid artery MCC HCC

I77.72 Dissection of iliac artery MCC HCC

I77.73 Dissection of renal artery MCC HCC

I77.74 Dissection of vertebral artery MCC HCC
EXCLUDES 2 *aneurysm of vertebral artery (I72.6)*

I77.75 Dissection of other precerebral arteries MCC HCC
Dissection of basilar artery (trunk)
EXCLUDES 2 *aneurysm of carotid artery (I72.Ø)*
aneurysm of other precerebral arteries (I72.5)
aneurysm of vertebral artery (I72.6)
dissection of carotid artery (I77.71)
dissection of vertebral artery (I77.74)

I77.76 Dissection of artery of upper extremity MCC HCC

I77.77 Dissection of artery of lower extremity MCC HCC

I77.79 Dissection of other specified artery MCC HCC

5th I77.8 Other specified disorders of arteries and arterioles

6th I77.81 Aortic ectasia
Ectasis aorta
EXCLUDES 1 *aortic aneurysm and dissection (I71.-)*

I77.81Ø Thoracic aortic ectasia HCC

I77.811 Abdominal aortic ectasia HCC

I77.812 Thoracoabdominal aortic ectasia HCC

I77.819 Aortic ectasia, unspecified site HCC

I77.82 Antineutrophilic cytoplasmic antibody [ANCA] vasculitis HCC
ANCA associated vasculitis
ANCA positive vasculitis
EXCLUDES 2 *eosinophilic granulomatosis with polyangiitis (M3Ø.1)*
granulomatosis with polyangiitis (M31.3-)
microscopic polyangiitis (M31.7)
AHA: 2022,4Q,26-27

I77.89 Other specified disorders of arteries and arterioles HCC
AHA: 2021,1Q,23

I77.9 Disorder of arteries and arterioles, unspecified HCC
AHA: 2021,1Q,4; 2018,2Q,7

4th I78 Diseases of capillaries

I78.Ø Hereditary hemorrhagic telangiectasia HCC
Rendu-Osler-Weber disease

I78.1 Nevus, non-neoplastic
Araneus nevus
Senile nevus
Spider nevus
Stellar nevus
EXCLUDES 1 *nevus NOS (D22.-)*
vascular NOS (Q82.5)
EXCLUDES 2 *blue nevus (D22.-)*
flammeus nevus (Q82.5)
hairy nevus (D22.-)
melanocytic nevus (D22.-)
pigmented nevus (D22.-)
portwine nevus (Q82.5)
sanguineous nevus (Q82.5)
strawberry nevus (Q82.5)
verrucous nevus (Q82.5)
AHA: 2019,1Q,21

I78.8 Other diseases of capillaries

I78.9 Disease of capillaries, unspecified

✓4th I79 Disorders of arteries, arterioles and capillaries in diseases classified elsewhere

I79.Ø ***Aneurysm of aorta in diseases classified elsewhere*** HCC
Code first underlying disease
EXCLUDES 1 *syphilitic aneurysm (A52.Ø1)*

I79.1 ***Aortitis in diseases classified elsewhere*** HCC
Code first underlying disease
EXCLUDES 1 *syphilitic aortitis (A52.Ø2)*

I79.8 ***Other disorders of arteries, arterioles and capillaries in diseases classified elsewhere*** HCC
Code first underlying disease, such as:
amyloidosis (E85.-)
EXCLUDES 1 *diabetic (peripheral) angiopathy (EØ8-E13 with .51-.52)*
syphilitic endarteritis (A52.Ø9)
tuberculous endarteritis (A18.89)

Diseases of veins, lymphatic vessels and lymph nodes, not elsewhere classified (I8Ø-I89)

✓4th I8Ø Phlebitis and thrombophlebitis

INCLUDES endophlebitis
inflammation, vein
periphlebitis
suppurative phlebitis

Code first:
phlebitis and thrombophlebitis complicating abortion, ectopic or molar pregnancy (OØØ-OØ7, OØ8.7)
phlebitis and thrombophlebitis complicating pregnancy, childbirth and the puerperium (O22.-, O87.-)

EXCLUDES 1 *venous embolism and thrombosis of lower extremities (I82.4-, I82.5-, I82.81-)*

✓5th I8Ø.Ø Phlebitis and thrombophlebitis of superficial vessels of lower extremities
Phlebitis and thrombophlebitis of femoropopliteal vein

I8Ø.ØØ Phlebitis and thrombophlebitis of superficial vessels of unspecified lower extremity

I8Ø.Ø1 Phlebitis and thrombophlebitis of superficial vessels of right lower extremity

I8Ø.Ø2 Phlebitis and thrombophlebitis of superficial vessels of left lower extremity

I8Ø.Ø3 Phlebitis and thrombophlebitis of superficial vessels of lower extremities, bilateral

✓5th I8Ø.1 Phlebitis and thrombophlebitis of femoral vein
Phlebitis and thrombophlebitis of common femoral vein
Phlebitis and thrombophlebitis of deep femoral vein

I8Ø.1Ø Phlebitis and thrombophlebitis of unspecified femoral vein CC UNS HCC

I8Ø.11 Phlebitis and thrombophlebitis of right femoral vein CC HCC

I8Ø.12 Phlebitis and thrombophlebitis of left femoral vein CC HCC

I8Ø.13 Phlebitis and thrombophlebitis of femoral vein, bilateral CC HCC

✓5th I8Ø.2 Phlebitis and thrombophlebitis of other and unspecified deep vessels of lower extremities

✓6th I8Ø.2Ø Phlebitis and thrombophlebitis of unspecified deep vessels of lower extremities

I8Ø.2Ø1 Phlebitis and thrombophlebitis of unspecified deep vessels of right lower extremity CC HCC

I8Ø.2Ø2 Phlebitis and thrombophlebitis of unspecified deep vessels of left lower extremity CC HCC

I8Ø.2Ø3 Phlebitis and thrombophlebitis of unspecified deep vessels of lower extremities, bilateral CC HCC

I8Ø.2Ø9 Phlebitis and thrombophlebitis of unspecified deep vessels of unspecified lower extremity CC UNS HCC

✓6th I8Ø.21 Phlebitis and thrombophlebitis of iliac vein
Phlebitis and thrombophlebitis of common iliac vein
Phlebitis and thrombophlebitis of external iliac vein
Phlebitis and thrombophlebitis of internal iliac vein

I8Ø.211 Phlebitis and thrombophlebitis of right iliac vein CC HCC

I8Ø.212 Phlebitis and thrombophlebitis of left iliac vein CC HCC

I8Ø.213 Phlebitis and thrombophlebitis of iliac vein, bilateral CC HCC

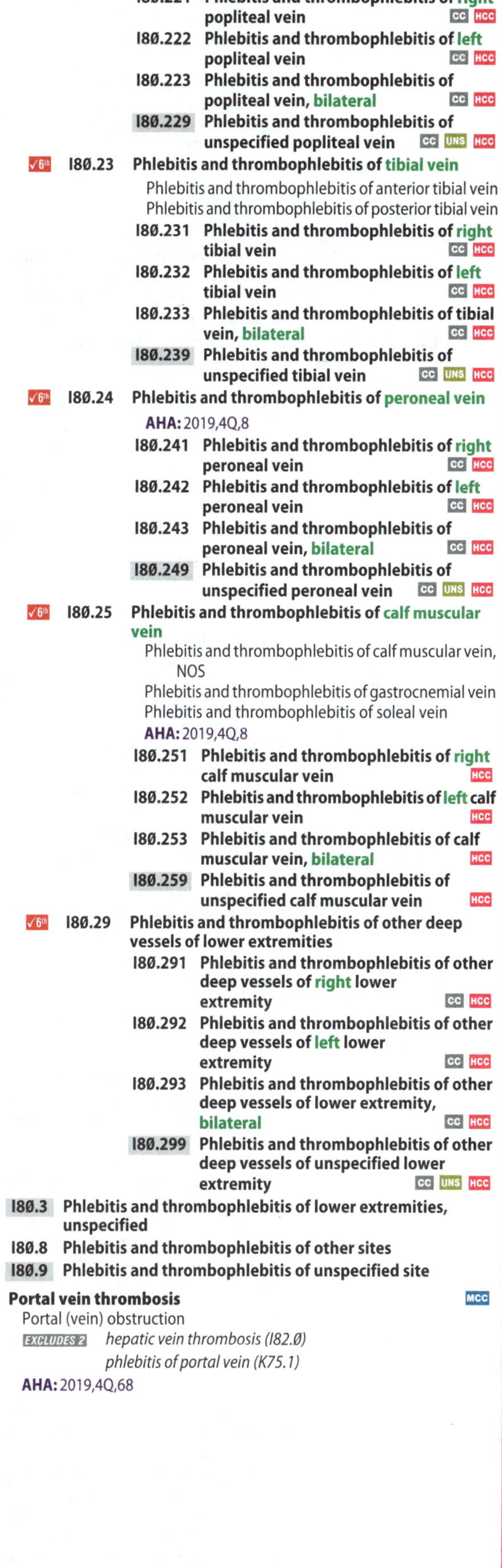

I8Ø.219 Phlebitis and thrombophlebitis of unspecified iliac vein CC UNS HCC

✓6th I8Ø.22 Phlebitis and thrombophlebitis of popliteal vein

I8Ø.221 Phlebitis and thrombophlebitis of right popliteal vein CC HCC

I8Ø.222 Phlebitis and thrombophlebitis of left popliteal vein CC HCC

I8Ø.223 Phlebitis and thrombophlebitis of popliteal vein, bilateral CC HCC

I8Ø.229 Phlebitis and thrombophlebitis of unspecified popliteal vein CC UNS HCC

✓6th I8Ø.23 Phlebitis and thrombophlebitis of tibial vein
Phlebitis and thrombophlebitis of anterior tibial vein
Phlebitis and thrombophlebitis of posterior tibial vein

I8Ø.231 Phlebitis and thrombophlebitis of right tibial vein CC HCC

I8Ø.232 Phlebitis and thrombophlebitis of left tibial vein CC HCC

I8Ø.233 Phlebitis and thrombophlebitis of tibial vein, bilateral CC HCC

I8Ø.239 Phlebitis and thrombophlebitis of unspecified tibial vein CC UNS HCC

✓6th I8Ø.24 Phlebitis and thrombophlebitis of peroneal vein
AHA: 2019,4Q,8

I8Ø.241 Phlebitis and thrombophlebitis of right peroneal vein CC HCC

I8Ø.242 Phlebitis and thrombophlebitis of left peroneal vein CC HCC

I8Ø.243 Phlebitis and thrombophlebitis of peroneal vein, bilateral CC HCC

I8Ø.249 Phlebitis and thrombophlebitis of unspecified peroneal vein CC UNS HCC

✓6th I8Ø.25 Phlebitis and thrombophlebitis of calf muscular vein
Phlebitis and thrombophlebitis of calf muscular vein, NOS
Phlebitis and thrombophlebitis of gastrocnemial vein
Phlebitis and thrombophlebitis of soleal vein
AHA: 2019,4Q,8

I8Ø.251 Phlebitis and thrombophlebitis of right calf muscular vein HCC

I8Ø.252 Phlebitis and thrombophlebitis of left calf muscular vein HCC

I8Ø.253 Phlebitis and thrombophlebitis of calf muscular vein, bilateral HCC

I8Ø.259 Phlebitis and thrombophlebitis of unspecified calf muscular vein HCC

✓6th I8Ø.29 Phlebitis and thrombophlebitis of other deep vessels of lower extremities

I8Ø.291 Phlebitis and thrombophlebitis of other deep vessels of right lower extremity CC HCC

I8Ø.292 Phlebitis and thrombophlebitis of other deep vessels of left lower extremity CC HCC

I8Ø.293 Phlebitis and thrombophlebitis of other deep vessels of lower extremity, bilateral CC HCC

I8Ø.299 Phlebitis and thrombophlebitis of other deep vessels of unspecified lower extremity CC UNS HCC

I8Ø.3 Phlebitis and thrombophlebitis of lower extremities, unspecified

I8Ø.8 Phlebitis and thrombophlebitis of other sites

I8Ø.9 Phlebitis and thrombophlebitis of unspecified site

I81 Portal vein thrombosis MCC
Portal (vein) obstruction
EXCLUDES 2 *hepatic vein thrombosis (I82.Ø)*
phlebitis of portal vein (K75.1)
AHA: 2019,4Q,68

✓4th **I82 Other venous embolism and thrombosis**

Code first venous embolism and thrombosis complicating:
abortion, ectopic or molar pregnancy (O00-O07, O08.7)
pregnancy, childbirth and the puerperium (O22.-, O87.-)

EXCLUDES 2 *venous embolism and thrombosis (of):*
cerebral (I63.6, I67.6)
coronary (I21-I25)
intracranial and intraspinal, septic or NOS (G08)
intracranial, nonpyogenic (I67.6)
intraspinal, nonpyogenic (G95.1)
mesenteric (K55.0-)
portal (I81)
pulmonary (I26.-)

I82.0 Budd-Chiari syndrome MCC HCC
Hepatic vein thrombosis
DEF: Thrombosis or other obstruction of the hepatic veins. Symptoms include an enlarged liver, extensive collateral vessels, intractable ascites, and severe portal hypertension.

I82.1 Thrombophlebitis migrans CC

✓5th **I82.2 Embolism and thrombosis of vena cava and other thoracic veins**

✓6th **I82.21 Embolism and thrombosis of superior vena cava**

I82.210 Acute embolism and thrombosis of superior vena cava CC HCC
Embolism and thrombosis of superior vena cava NOS

I82.211 Chronic embolism and thrombosis of superior vena cava CC HCC

✓6th **I82.22 Embolism and thrombosis of inferior vena cava**

I82.220 Acute embolism and thrombosis of inferior vena cava MCC HCC
Embolism and thrombosis of inferior vena cava NOS

I82.221 Chronic embolism and thrombosis of inferior vena cava MCC HCC

✓6th **I82.29 Embolism and thrombosis of other thoracic veins**
Embolism and thrombosis of brachiocephalic (innominate) vein

I82.290 Acute embolism and thrombosis of other thoracic veins CC HCC

I82.291 Chronic embolism and thrombosis of other thoracic veins CC HCC

I82.3 Embolism and thrombosis of renal vein CC HCC

✓5th **I82.4 Acute embolism and thrombosis of deep veins of lower extremity**

✓6th **I82.40 Acute embolism and thrombosis of unspecified deep veins of lower extremity**
Deep vein thrombosis NOS
DVT NOS

EXCLUDES 1 *acute embolism and thrombosis of unspecified deep veins of distal lower extremity (I82.4Z-)*
acute embolism and thrombosis of unspecified deep veins of proximal lower extremity (I82.4Y-)

I82.401 Acute embolism and thrombosis of unspecified deep veins of right lower extremity CC H10 HCC

I82.402 Acute embolism and thrombosis of unspecified deep veins of left lower extremity CC H10 HCC

I82.403 Acute embolism and thrombosis of unspecified deep veins of lower extremity, bilateral CC H10 HCC

I82.409 Acute embolism and thrombosis of unspecified deep veins of unspecified lower extremity CC H10 UNS HCC

✓6th **I82.41 Acute embolism and thrombosis of femoral vein**
Acute embolism and thrombosis of common femoral vein
Acute embolism and thrombosis of deep femoral vein

I82.411 Acute embolism and thrombosis of right femoral vein CC H10 HCC

I82.412 Acute embolism and thrombosis of left femoral vein CC H10 HCC

I82.413 Acute embolism and thrombosis of femoral vein, bilateral CC H10 HCC

I82.419 Acute embolism and thrombosis of unspecified femoral vein CC H10 UNS HCC

✓6th **I82.42 Acute embolism and thrombosis of iliac vein**
Acute embolism and thrombosis of common iliac vein
Acute embolism and thrombosis of external iliac vein
Acute embolism and thrombosis of internal iliac vein

I82.421 Acute embolism and thrombosis of right iliac vein CC H10 HCC

I82.422 Acute embolism and thrombosis of left iliac vein CC H10 HCC

I82.423 Acute embolism and thrombosis of iliac vein, bilateral CC H10 HCC

I82.429 Acute embolism and thrombosis of unspecified iliac vein CC H10 UNS HCC

✓6th **I82.43 Acute embolism and thrombosis of popliteal vein**

I82.431 Acute embolism and thrombosis of right popliteal vein CC H10 HCC

I82.432 Acute embolism and thrombosis of left popliteal vein CC H10 HCC

I82.433 Acute embolism and thrombosis of popliteal vein, bilateral CC H10 HCC

I82.439 Acute embolism and thrombosis of unspecified popliteal vein CC H10 UNS HCC

✓6th **I82.44 Acute embolism and thrombosis of tibial vein**
Acute embolism and thrombosis of anterior tibial vein
Acute embolism and thrombosis of posterior tibial vein

I82.441 Acute embolism and thrombosis of right tibial vein CC H10 HCC

I82.442 Acute embolism and thrombosis of left tibial vein CC H10 HCC

I82.443 Acute embolism and thrombosis of tibial vein, bilateral CC H10 HCC

I82.449 Acute embolism and thrombosis of unspecified tibial vein CC H10 UNS HCC

✓6th **I82.45 Acute embolism and thrombosis of peroneal vein**
AHA: 2019,4Q,8-10

I82.451 Acute embolism and thrombosis of right peroneal vein CC H10 HCC

I82.452 Acute embolism and thrombosis of left peroneal vein CC H10 HCC

I82.453 Acute embolism and thrombosis of peroneal vein, bilateral CC H10 HCC

I82.459 Acute embolism and thrombosis of unspecified peroneal vein CC H10 UNS HCC

✓6th **I82.46 Acute embolism and thrombosis of calf muscular vein**
Acute embolism and thrombosis of calf muscular vein, NOS
Acute embolism and thrombosis of gastrocnemial vein
Acute embolism and thrombosis of soleal vein
AHA: 2019,4Q,8-10

I82.461 Acute embolism and thrombosis of right calf muscular vein HCC

I82.462 Acute embolism and thrombosis of left calf muscular vein HCC

I82.463 Acute embolism and thrombosis of calf muscular vein, bilateral HCC

I82.469 Acute embolism and thrombosis of unspecified calf muscular vein HCC

✓6th **I82.49 Acute embolism and thrombosis of other specified deep vein of lower extremity**

I82.491 Acute embolism and thrombosis of other specified deep vein of right lower extremity CC H10 HCC

I82.492 Acute embolism and thrombosis of other specified deep vein of left lower extremity CC H10 HCC

I82.493 Acute embolism and thrombosis of other specified deep vein of lower extremity, bilateral CC H10 HCC

I82.499 Acute embolism and thrombosis of other specified deep vein of unspecified lower extremity CC H10 UNS HCC

✓6th **I82.4Y Acute embolism and thrombosis of unspecified deep veins of proximal lower extremity**
Acute embolism and thrombosis of deep vein of thigh NOS
Acute embolism and thrombosis of deep vein of upper leg NOS

I82.4Y1 Acute embolism and thrombosis of unspecified deep veins of right proximal lower extremity CC H10 HCC

I82.4Y2 Acute embolism and thrombosis of unspecified deep veins of left proximal lower extremity CC H10 HCC

I82.4Y3 Acute embolism and thrombosis of unspecified deep veins of proximal lower extremity, bilateral CC H10 HCC

I82.4Y9 Acute embolism and thrombosis of unspecified deep veins of unspecified proximal lower extremity CC H10 UNS HCC

✓6th **I82.4Z Acute embolism and thrombosis of unspecified deep veins of distal lower extremity**
Acute embolism and thrombosis of deep vein of calf NOS
Acute embolism and thrombosis of deep vein of lower leg NOS

I82.4Z1 Acute embolism and thrombosis of unspecified deep veins of right distal lower extremity CC H10 HCC

I82.4Z2 Acute embolism and thrombosis of unspecified deep veins of left distal lower extremity CC H10 HCC

I82.4Z3 Acute embolism and thrombosis of unspecified deep veins of distal lower extremity, bilateral CC H10 HCC

I82.4Z9 Acute embolism and thrombosis of unspecified deep veins of unspecified distal lower extremity CC H10 UNS HCC

✓5th **I82.5 Chronic embolism and thrombosis of deep veins of lower extremity**
Use additional code, if applicable, for associated long-term (current) use of anticoagulants (Z79.01)
EXCLUDES 1 *personal history of venous embolism and thrombosis (Z86.718)*
AHA: 2020,2Q,20

✓6th **I82.50 Chronic embolism and thrombosis of unspecified deep veins of lower extremity**
EXCLUDES 1 *chronic embolism and thrombosis of unspecified deep veins of distal lower extremity (I82.5Z-)*
chronic embolism and thrombosis of unspecified deep veins of proximal lower extremity (I82.5Y-)

I82.501 Chronic embolism and thrombosis of unspecified deep veins of right lower extremity CC HCC

I82.502 Chronic embolism and thrombosis of unspecified deep veins of left lower extremity CC HCC

I82.503 Chronic embolism and thrombosis of unspecified deep veins of lower extremity, bilateral CC HCC

I82.509 Chronic embolism and thrombosis of unspecified deep veins of unspecified lower extremity CC UNS HCC

✓6th **I82.51 Chronic embolism and thrombosis of femoral vein**
Chronic embolism and thrombosis of common femoral vein
Chronic embolism and thrombosis of deep femoral vein

I82.511 Chronic embolism and thrombosis of right femoral vein CC HCC

I82.512 Chronic embolism and thrombosis of left femoral vein CC HCC

I82.513 Chronic embolism and thrombosis of femoral vein, bilateral CC HCC

I82.519 Chronic embolism and thrombosis of unspecified femoral vein CC UNS HCC

✓6th **I82.52 Chronic embolism and thrombosis of iliac vein**
Chronic embolism and thrombosis of common iliac vein
Chronic embolism and thrombosis of external iliac vein
Chronic embolism and thrombosis of internal iliac vein

I82.521 Chronic embolism and thrombosis of right iliac vein CC HCC

I82.522 Chronic embolism and thrombosis of left iliac vein CC HCC

I82.523 Chronic embolism and thrombosis of iliac vein, bilateral CC HCC

I82.529 Chronic embolism and thrombosis of unspecified iliac vein CC UNS HCC

✓6th **I82.53 Chronic embolism and thrombosis of popliteal vein**

I82.531 Chronic embolism and thrombosis of right popliteal vein CC HCC

I82.532 Chronic embolism and thrombosis of left popliteal vein CC HCC

I82.533 Chronic embolism and thrombosis of popliteal vein, bilateral CC HCC

I82.539 Chronic embolism and thrombosis of unspecified popliteal vein CC UNS HCC

✓6th **I82.54 Chronic embolism and thrombosis of tibial vein**
Chronic embolism and thrombosis of anterior tibial vein
Chronic embolism and thrombosis of posterior tibial vein

I82.541 Chronic embolism and thrombosis of right tibial vein CC HCC

I82.542 Chronic embolism and thrombosis of left tibial vein CC HCC

I82.543 Chronic embolism and thrombosis of tibial vein, bilateral CC HCC

I82.549 Chronic embolism and thrombosis of unspecified tibial vein CC UNS HCC

✓6th **I82.55 Chronic embolism and thrombosis of peroneal vein**
AHA: 2019,4Q,8-10

I82.551 Chronic embolism and thrombosis of right peroneal vein CC HCC

I82.552 Chronic embolism and thrombosis of left peroneal vein CC HCC

I82.553 Chronic embolism and thrombosis of peroneal vein, bilateral CC HCC

I82.559 Chronic embolism and thrombosis of unspecified peroneal vein CC UNS HCC

✓6th **I82.56 Chronic embolism and thrombosis of calf muscular vein**
Chronic embolism and thrombosis of calf muscular vein NOS
Chronic embolism and thrombosis of gastrocnemial vein
Chronic embolism and thrombosis of soleal vein
AHA: 2019,4Q,8-10

I82.561 Chronic embolism and thrombosis of right calf muscular vein HCC

I82.562 Chronic embolism and thrombosis of left calf muscular vein HCC

I82.563 Chronic embolism and thrombosis of calf muscular vein, bilateral HCC

I82.569 Chronic embolism and thrombosis of unspecified calf muscular vein HCC

✓6th **I82.59 Chronic embolism and thrombosis of other specified deep vein of lower extremity**

I82.591 Chronic embolism and thrombosis of other specified deep vein of right lower extremity CC HCC

I82.592 Chronic embolism and thrombosis of other specified deep vein of left lower extremity CC HCC

I82.593 Chronic embolism and thrombosis of other specified deep vein of lower extremity, bilateral CC HCC

I82.599 Chronic embolism and thrombosis of other specified deep vein of unspecified lower extremity CC UNS HCC

✓6th **I82.5Y Chronic embolism and thrombosis of unspecified deep veins of proximal lower extremity**
Chronic embolism and thrombosis of deep veins of thigh NOS
Chronic embolism and thrombosis of deep veins of upper leg NOS

I82.5Y1 Chronic embolism and thrombosis of unspecified deep veins of right proximal lower extremity CC HCC

I82.5Y2 Chronic embolism and thrombosis of unspecified deep veins of left proximal lower extremity CC HCC

I82.5Y3 Chronic embolism and thrombosis of unspecified deep veins of proximal lower extremity, bilateral CC HCC

I82.5Y9 Chronic embolism and thrombosis of unspecified deep veins of unspecified proximal lower extremity CC UNS HCC

✓6th **I82.5Z Chronic embolism and thrombosis of unspecified deep veins of distal lower extremity**
Chronic embolism and thrombosis of deep veins of calf NOS
Chronic embolism and thrombosis of deep veins of lower leg NOS

I82.5Z1 Chronic embolism and thrombosis of unspecified deep veins of right distal lower extremity CC HCC

I82.5Z2 Chronic embolism and thrombosis of unspecified deep veins of left distal lower extremity CC HCC

I82.5Z3 Chronic embolism and thrombosis of unspecified deep veins of distal lower extremity, bilateral CC HCC

I82.5Z9 Chronic embolism and thrombosis of unspecified deep veins of unspecified distal lower extremity CC UNS HCC

✓5th **I82.6 Acute embolism and thrombosis of veins of upper extremity**

✓6th **I82.60 Acute embolism and thrombosis of unspecified veins of upper extremity**

I82.601 Acute embolism and thrombosis of unspecified veins of right upper extremity CC

I82.602 Acute embolism and thrombosis of unspecified veins of left upper extremity CC

I82.603 Acute embolism and thrombosis of unspecified veins of upper extremity, bilateral CC

I82.609 Acute embolism and thrombosis of unspecified veins of unspecified upper extremity CC UNS

✓6th **I82.61 Acute embolism and thrombosis of superficial veins of upper extremity**
Acute embolism and thrombosis of antecubital vein
Acute embolism and thrombosis of basilic vein
Acute embolism and thrombosis of cephalic vein

I82.611 Acute embolism and thrombosis of superficial veins of right upper extremity CC

I82.612 Acute embolism and thrombosis of superficial veins of left upper extremity CC

I82.613 Acute embolism and thrombosis of superficial veins of upper extremity, bilateral CC

I82.619 Acute embolism and thrombosis of superficial veins of unspecified upper extremity CC UNS

✓6th **I82.62 Acute embolism and thrombosis of deep veins of upper extremity**
Acute embolism and thrombosis of brachial vein
Acute embolism and thrombosis of radial vein
Acute embolism and thrombosis of ulnar vein

I82.621 Acute embolism and thrombosis of deep veins of right upper extremity CC HCC

I82.622 Acute embolism and thrombosis of deep veins of left upper extremity CC HCC

I82.623 Acute embolism and thrombosis of deep veins of upper extremity, bilateral CC HCC

I82.629 Acute embolism and thrombosis of deep veins of unspecified upper extremity CC UNS HCC

✓5th **I82.7 Chronic embolism and thrombosis of veins of upper extremity**
Use additional code, if applicable, for associated long-term (current) use of anticoagulants (Z79.01)
EXCLUDES 1 *personal history of venous embolism and thrombosis (Z86.718)*

✓6th **I82.70 Chronic embolism and thrombosis of unspecified veins of upper extremity**

I82.701 Chronic embolism and thrombosis of unspecified veins of right upper extremity CC

I82.702 Chronic embolism and thrombosis of unspecified veins of left upper extremity CC

I82.703 Chronic embolism and thrombosis of unspecified veins of upper extremity, bilateral CC

I82.709 Chronic embolism and thrombosis of unspecified veins of unspecified upper extremity CC UNS

✓6th **I82.71 Chronic embolism and thrombosis of superficial veins of upper extremity**
Chronic embolism and thrombosis of antecubital vein
Chronic embolism and thrombosis of basilic vein
Chronic embolism and thrombosis of cephalic vein

I82.711 Chronic embolism and thrombosis of superficial veins of right upper extremity CC

I82.712 Chronic embolism and thrombosis of superficial veins of left upper extremity CC

I82.713 Chronic embolism and thrombosis of superficial veins of upper extremity, bilateral CC

I82.719 Chronic embolism and thrombosis of superficial veins of unspecified upper extremity CC UNS

✓6th **I82.72 Chronic embolism and thrombosis of deep veins of upper extremity**
Chronic embolism and thrombosis of brachial vein
Chronic embolism and thrombosis of radial vein
Chronic embolism and thrombosis of ulnar vein

I82.721 Chronic embolism and thrombosis of deep veins of right upper extremity CC HCC

I82.722 Chronic embolism and thrombosis of deep veins of left upper extremity CC HCC

I82.723 Chronic embolism and thrombosis of deep veins of upper extremity, bilateral CC HCC

I82.729 Chronic embolism and thrombosis of deep veins of unspecified upper extremity CC UNS HCC

✓5th **I82.A Embolism and thrombosis of axillary vein**

✓6th **I82.A1 Acute embolism and thrombosis of axillary vein**

I82.A11 Acute embolism and thrombosis of right axillary vein CC HCC

I82.A12 Acute embolism and thrombosis of left axillary vein CC HCC

I82.A13 Acute embolism and thrombosis of axillary vein, bilateral CC HCC

I82.A19 Acute embolism and thrombosis of unspecified axillary vein CC UNS HCC

✓6th **I82.A2 Chronic embolism and thrombosis of axillary vein**

I82.A21 Chronic embolism and thrombosis of right axillary vein CC HCC

I82.A22 Chronic embolism and thrombosis of left axillary vein CC HCC

I82.A23 Chronic embolism and thrombosis of axillary vein, bilateral CC HCC

I82.A29 Chronic embolism and thrombosis of unspecified axillary vein CC UNS HCC

✓5th **I82.B Embolism and thrombosis of subclavian vein**

✓6th **I82.B1 Acute embolism and thrombosis of subclavian vein**

I82.B11 Acute embolism and thrombosis of right subclavian vein CC HCC

I82.B12 Acute embolism and thrombosis of left subclavian vein CC HCC

I82.B13 Acute embolism and thrombosis of subclavian vein, bilateral CC HCC

I82.B19 Acute embolism and thrombosis of unspecified subclavian vein CC UNS HCC

✓6th I82.B2 Chronic embolism and thrombosis of subclavian vein

I82.B21 Chronic embolism and thrombosis of right subclavian vein CC HCC

I82.B22 Chronic embolism and thrombosis of left subclavian vein CC HCC

I82.B23 Chronic embolism and thrombosis of subclavian vein, bilateral CC HCC

I82.B29 Chronic embolism and thrombosis of unspecified subclavian vein CC UNS HCC

✓5th I82.C Embolism and thrombosis of internal jugular vein

✓6th I82.C1 Acute embolism and thrombosis of internal jugular vein

I82.C11 Acute embolism and thrombosis of right internal jugular vein CC HCC

I82.C12 Acute embolism and thrombosis of left internal jugular vein CC HCC

I82.C13 Acute embolism and thrombosis of internal jugular vein, bilateral CC HCC

I82.C19 Acute embolism and thrombosis of unspecified internal jugular vein CC UNS HCC

✓6th I82.C2 Chronic embolism and thrombosis of internal jugular vein

I82.C21 Chronic embolism and thrombosis of right internal jugular vein CC HCC

I82.C22 Chronic embolism and thrombosis of left internal jugular vein CC HCC

I82.C23 Chronic embolism and thrombosis of internal jugular vein, bilateral CC HCC

I82.C29 Chronic embolism and thrombosis of unspecified internal jugular vein CC UNS HCC

✓5th I82.8 Embolism and thrombosis of other specified veins

Use additional code, if applicable, for associated long-term (current) use of anticoagulants (Z79.01)

✓6th I82.81 Embolism and thrombosis of superficial veins of lower extremities

Embolism and thrombosis of saphenous vein (greater) (lesser)

I82.811 Embolism and thrombosis of superficial veins of right lower extremity CC

I82.812 Embolism and thrombosis of superficial veins of left lower extremity CC

I82.813 Embolism and thrombosis of superficial veins of lower extremities, bilateral CC

I82.819 Embolism and thrombosis of superficial veins of unspecified lower extremity CC UNS

✓6th I82.89 Embolism and thrombosis of other specified veins

I82.890 Acute embolism and thrombosis of other specified veins CC

I82.891 Chronic embolism and thrombosis of other specified veins CC

✓5th I82.9 Embolism and thrombosis of unspecified vein

I82.90 Acute embolism and thrombosis of unspecified vein CC UNS

Embolism of vein NOS
Thrombosis (vein) NOS

I82.91 Chronic embolism and thrombosis of unspecified vein CC UNS

✓4th **I83 Varicose veins of lower extremities**

EXCLUDES 2 *varicose veins complicating pregnancy (O22.0-)*
varicose veins complicating the puerperium (O87.4)

✓5th I83.0 Varicose veins of lower extremities with ulcer

Use additional code to identify severity of ulcer (L97.-)

✓6th I83.00 Varicose veins of unspecified lower extremity with ulcer

I83.001 Varicose veins of unspecified lower extremity with ulcer of thigh HCC A

I83.002 Varicose veins of unspecified lower extremity with ulcer of calf HCC A

I83.003 Varicose veins of unspecified lower extremity with ulcer of ankle HCC A

I83.004 Varicose veins of unspecified lower extremity with ulcer of heel and midfoot HCC A

Varicose veins of unspecified lower extremity with ulcer of plantar surface of midfoot

I83.005 Varicose veins of unspecified lower extremity with ulcer other part of foot HCC A

Varicose veins of unspecified lower extremity with ulcer of toe

I83.008 Varicose veins of unspecified lower extremity with ulcer other part of lower leg HCC A

I83.009 Varicose veins of unspecified lower extremity with ulcer of unspecified site HCC A

✓6th I83.01 Varicose veins of right lower extremity with ulcer

I83.011 Varicose veins of right lower extremity with ulcer of thigh HCC A

I83.012 Varicose veins of right lower extremity with ulcer of calf HCC A

I83.013 Varicose veins of right lower extremity with ulcer of ankle HCC A

I83.014 Varicose veins of right lower extremity with ulcer of heel and midfoot HCC A

Varicose veins of right lower extremity with ulcer of plantar surface of midfoot

I83.015 Varicose veins of right lower extremity with ulcer other part of foot HCC A

Varicose veins of right lower extremity with ulcer of toe

I83.018 Varicose veins of right lower extremity with ulcer other part of lower leg HCC A

I83.019 Varicose veins of right lower extremity with ulcer of unspecified site HCC A

✓6th I83.02 Varicose veins of left lower extremity with ulcer

I83.021 Varicose veins of left lower extremity with ulcer of thigh HCC A

I83.022 Varicose veins of left lower extremity with ulcer of calf HCC A

I83.023 Varicose veins of left lower extremity with ulcer of ankle HCC A

I83.024 Varicose veins of left lower extremity with ulcer of heel and midfoot HCC A

Varicose veins of left lower extremity with ulcer of plantar surface of midfoot

I83.025 Varicose veins of left lower extremity with ulcer other part of foot HCC A

Varicose veins of left lower extremity with ulcer of toe

I83.028 Varicose veins of left lower extremity with ulcer other part of lower leg HCC A

I83.029 Varicose veins of left lower extremity with ulcer of unspecified site HCC A

✓5th I83.1 Varicose veins of lower extremities with inflammation

I83.10 Varicose veins of unspecified lower extremity with inflammation A

I83.11 Varicose veins of right lower extremity with inflammation A

I83.12 Varicose veins of left lower extremity with inflammation A

✓5th I83.2 Varicose veins of lower extremities with both ulcer and inflammation

Use additional code to identify severity of ulcer (L97.-)

✓6th I83.20 Varicose veins of unspecified lower extremity with both ulcer and inflammation

I83.201 Varicose veins of unspecified lower extremity with both ulcer of thigh and inflammation CC HCC A

I83.202 Varicose veins of unspecified lower extremity with both ulcer of calf and inflammation CC HCC A

I83.203 Varicose veins of unspecified lower extremity with both ulcer of ankle and inflammation CC HCC A

I83.204 Varicose veins of unspecified lower extremity with both ulcer of heel and midfoot and inflammation CC HCC A
Varicose veins of unspecified lower extremity with both ulcer of plantar surface of midfoot and inflammation

I83.205 Varicose veins of unspecified lower extremity with both ulcer of other part of foot and inflammation CC HCC A
Varicose veins of unspecified lower extremity with both ulcer of toe and inflammation

I83.208 Varicose veins of unspecified lower extremity with both ulcer of other part of lower extremity and inflammation CC HCC A

I83.209 Varicose veins of unspecified lower extremity with both ulcer of unspecified site and inflammation CC HCC A

✓6th **I83.21 Varicose veins of right lower extremity with both ulcer and inflammation**

I83.211 Varicose veins of right lower extremity with both ulcer of thigh and inflammation CC HCC A

I83.212 Varicose veins of right lower extremity with both ulcer of calf and inflammation CC HCC A

I83.213 Varicose veins of right lower extremity with both ulcer of ankle and inflammation CC HCC A

I83.214 Varicose veins of right lower extremity with both ulcer of heel and midfoot and inflammation CC HCC A
Varicose veins of right lower extremity with both ulcer of plantar surface of midfoot and inflammation

I83.215 Varicose veins of right lower extremity with both ulcer other part of foot and inflammation CC HCC A
Varicose veins of right lower extremity with both ulcer of toe and inflammation

I83.218 Varicose veins of right lower extremity with both ulcer of other part of lower extremity and inflammation CC HCC A

I83.219 Varicose veins of right lower extremity with both ulcer of unspecified site and inflammation CC HCC A

✓6th **I83.22 Varicose veins of left lower extremity with both ulcer and inflammation**

I83.221 Varicose veins of left lower extremity with both ulcer of thigh and inflammation CC HCC A

I83.222 Varicose veins of left lower extremity with both ulcer of calf and inflammation CC HCC A

I83.223 Varicose veins of left lower extremity with both ulcer of ankle and inflammation CC HCC A

I83.224 Varicose veins of left lower extremity with both ulcer of heel and midfoot and inflammation CC HCC A
Varicose veins of left lower extremity with both ulcer of plantar surface of midfoot and inflammation

I83.225 Varicose veins of left lower extremity with both ulcer other part of foot and inflammation CC HCC A
Varicose veins of left lower extremity with both ulcer of toe and inflammation

I83.228 Varicose veins of left lower extremity with both ulcer of other part of lower extremity and inflammation CC HCC A

I83.229 Varicose veins of left lower extremity with both ulcer of unspecified site and inflammation CC HCC A

✓5th **I83.8 Varicose veins of lower extremities with other complications**

✓6th **I83.81 Varicose veins of lower extremities with pain**

I83.811 Varicose veins of right lower extremity with pain A

I83.812 Varicose veins of left lower extremity with pain A

I83.813 Varicose veins of bilateral lower extremities with pain A

I83.819 Varicose veins of unspecified lower extremity with pain A

✓6th **I83.89 Varicose veins of lower extremities with other complications**
Varicose veins of lower extremities with edema
Varicose veins of lower extremities with swelling

I83.891 Varicose veins of right lower extremity with other complications A

I83.892 Varicose veins of left lower extremity with other complications A

I83.893 Varicose veins of bilateral lower extremities with other complications A

I83.899 Varicose veins of unspecified lower extremity with other complications A

✓5th **I83.9 Asymptomatic varicose veins of lower extremities**
Phlebectasia of lower extremities
Varicose veins of lower extremities
Varix of lower extremities

I83.90 Asymptomatic varicose veins of unspecified lower extremity A
Varicose veins NOS

I83.91 Asymptomatic varicose veins of right lower extremity A

I83.92 Asymptomatic varicose veins of left lower extremity A

I83.93 Asymptomatic varicose veins of bilateral lower extremities A

✓4th **I85 Esophageal varices**
Use additional code to identify:
alcohol abuse and dependence (F10.-)

✓5th **I85.0 Esophageal varices**
Idiopathic esophageal varices
Primary esophageal varices

I85.00 Esophageal varices without bleeding CC HCC
Esophageal varices NOS

I85.01 Esophageal varices with bleeding MCC HCC

✓5th **I85.1 Secondary esophageal varices**
Esophageal varices secondary to alcoholic liver disease
Esophageal varices secondary to cirrhosis of liver
Esophageal varices secondary to schistosomiasis
Esophageal varices secondary to toxic liver disease
Code first underlying disease

I85.10 Secondary esophageal varices without bleeding CC HCC

I85.11 Secondary esophageal varices with bleeding MCC HCC

✓4th **I86 Varicose veins of other sites**
EXCLUDES 1 *varicose veins of unspecified site (I83.9-)*
EXCLUDES 2 *retinal varices (H35.0-)*

I86.0 Sublingual varices
DEF: Distended, tortuous veins beneath the tongue.

I86.1 Scrotal varices ♂
Varicocele

I86.2 Pelvic varices

I86.3 Vulval varices ♀
EXCLUDES 1 *vulval varices complicating childbirth and the puerperium (O87.8)*
vulval varices complicating pregnancy (O22.1-)

I86.4 Gastric varices

I86.8 Varicose veins of other specified sites A
Varicose ulcer of nasal septum

✓4th **I87 Other disorders of veins**

✓5th **I87.0 Postthrombotic syndrome**
Chronic venous hypertension due to deep vein thrombosis
Postphlebitic syndrome
EXCLUDES 1 *chronic venous hypertension without deep vein thrombosis (I87.3-)*

✓6th **I87.00 Postthrombotic syndrome without complications**
Asymptomatic postthrombotic syndrome

I87.001 Postthrombotic syndrome without complications of right lower extremity

I87.002 Postthrombotic syndrome without complications of left lower extremity

I87.003 Postthrombotic syndrome without complications of bilateral lower extremity

I87.009 **Postthrombotic syndrome without complications of unspecified extremity**
Postthrombotic syndrome NOS

✓6th I87.01 **Postthrombotic syndrome with ulcer**
Use additional code to specify site and severity of ulcer (L97.-)

I87.011 **Postthrombotic syndrome with ulcer of right lower extremity** CC HCC

I87.012 **Postthrombotic syndrome with ulcer of left lower extremity** CC HCC

I87.013 **Postthrombotic syndrome with ulcer of bilateral lower extremity** CC HCC

I87.019 **Postthrombotic syndrome with ulcer of unspecified lower extremity** CC UNS HCC

✓6th I87.02 **Postthrombotic syndrome with inflammation**

I87.021 **Postthrombotic syndrome with inflammation of right lower extremity**

I87.022 **Postthrombotic syndrome with inflammation of left lower extremity**

I87.023 **Postthrombotic syndrome with inflammation of bilateral lower extremity**

I87.029 **Postthrombotic syndrome with inflammation of unspecified lower extremity**

✓6th I87.03 **Postthrombotic syndrome with ulcer and inflammation**
Use additional code to specify site and severity of ulcer (L97.-)

I87.031 **Postthrombotic syndrome with ulcer and inflammation of right lower extremity** CC HCC

I87.032 **Postthrombotic syndrome with ulcer and inflammation of left lower extremity** CC HCC

I87.033 **Postthrombotic syndrome with ulcer and inflammation of bilateral lower extremity** CC HCC

I87.039 **Postthrombotic syndrome with ulcer and inflammation of unspecified lower extremity** CC UNS HCC

✓6th I87.09 **Postthrombotic syndrome with other complications**

I87.091 **Postthrombotic syndrome with other complications of right lower extremity**

I87.092 **Postthrombotic syndrome with other complications of left lower extremity**

I87.093 **Postthrombotic syndrome with other complications of bilateral lower extremity**

I87.099 **Postthrombotic syndrome with other complications of unspecified lower extremity**

I87.1 **Compression of vein** CC
Stricture of vein
Vena cava syndrome (inferior) (superior)
EXCLUDES 2 *compression of pulmonary vein (I28.8)*
AHA: 2023,2Q,8

I87.2 **Venous insufficiency (chronic) (peripheral)**
Stasis dermatitis
▶Use additional code, if applicable, to specify site and severity of ulcer (L97.-)◀
▶Code also, if applicable, associated hypertensive conditions such as:◀
▶essential (primary) hypertension (I10)◀
▶hypertensive chronic kidney disease (I12.-)◀
▶hypertensive heart and chronic kidney disease (I13.-)◀
▶hypertensive heart disease (I11.-)◀
EXCLUDES 1 *stasis dermatitis with varicose veins of lower extremities (I83.1-, I83.2-)*
DEF: Insufficient drainage of venous blood in any part of the body that results in edema or dermatosis.

✓5th I87.3 **Chronic venous hypertension (idiopathic)**
Stasis edema
EXCLUDES 1 *chronic venous hypertension due to deep vein thrombosis (I87.0-)*
varicose veins of lower extremities (I83.-)

✓6th I87.30 **Chronic venous hypertension (idiopathic) without complications**
Asymptomatic chronic venous hypertension (idiopathic)

I87.301 **Chronic venous hypertension (idiopathic) without complications of right lower extremity**

I87.302 **Chronic venous hypertension (idiopathic) without complications of left lower extremity**

I87.303 **Chronic venous hypertension (idiopathic) without complications of bilateral lower extremity**

I87.309 **Chronic venous hypertension (idiopathic) without complications of unspecified lower extremity**
Chronic venous hypertension NOS

✓6th I87.31 **Chronic venous hypertension (idiopathic) with ulcer**
Use additional code to specify site and severity of ulcer (L97.-)

I87.311 **Chronic venous hypertension (idiopathic) with ulcer of right lower extremity** CC HCC

I87.312 **Chronic venous hypertension (idiopathic) with ulcer of left lower extremity** CC HCC

I87.313 **Chronic venous hypertension (idiopathic) with ulcer of bilateral lower extremity** CC HCC

I87.319 **Chronic venous hypertension (idiopathic) with ulcer of unspecified lower extremity** CC UNS HCC

✓6th I87.32 **Chronic venous hypertension (idiopathic) with inflammation**

I87.321 **Chronic venous hypertension (idiopathic) with inflammation of right lower extremity**

I87.322 **Chronic venous hypertension (idiopathic) with inflammation of left lower extremity**

I87.323 **Chronic venous hypertension (idiopathic) with inflammation of bilateral lower extremity**

I87.329 **Chronic venous hypertension (idiopathic) with inflammation of unspecified lower extremity**

✓6th I87.33 **Chronic venous hypertension (idiopathic) with ulcer and inflammation**
Use additional code to specify site and severity of ulcer (L97.-)

I87.331 **Chronic venous hypertension (idiopathic) with ulcer and inflammation of right lower extremity** CC HCC

I87.332 **Chronic venous hypertension (idiopathic) with ulcer and inflammation of left lower extremity** CC HCC

I87.333 **Chronic venous hypertension (idiopathic) with ulcer and inflammation of bilateral lower extremity** CC HCC

I87.339 **Chronic venous hypertension (idiopathic) with ulcer and inflammation of unspecified lower extremity** CC UNS HCC

✓6th I87.39 **Chronic venous hypertension (idiopathic) with other complications**

I87.391 **Chronic venous hypertension (idiopathic) with other complications of right lower extremity**

I87.392 **Chronic venous hypertension (idiopathic) with other complications of left lower extremity**

I87.393 **Chronic venous hypertension (idiopathic) with other complications of bilateral lower extremity**

I87.399 **Chronic venous hypertension (idiopathic) with other complications of unspecified lower extremity**

I87.8 Other specified disorders of veins
Phlebosclerosis
Venofibrosis

I87.9 Disorder of vein, unspecified

✓4th **I88 Nonspecific lymphadenitis**
EXCLUDES 1 *acute lymphadenitis, except mesenteric (LØ4.-)*
enlarged lymph nodes NOS (R59.-)
human immunodeficiency virus [HIV] disease resulting in generalized lymphadenopathy (B2Ø)

I88.Ø Nonspecific mesenteric lymphadenitis
Mesenteric lymphadenitis (acute)(chronic)

I88.1 Chronic lymphadenitis, except mesenteric
Adenitis
Lymphadenitis

I88.8 Other nonspecific lymphadenitis

I88.9 Nonspecific lymphadenitis, unspecified
Lymphadenitis NOS

✓4th **I89 Other noninfective disorders of lymphatic vessels and lymph nodes**
EXCLUDES 1 *chylocele, tunica vaginalis (nonfilarial) NOS (N5Ø.89)*
enlarged lymph nodes NOS (R59.-)
filarial chylocele (B74.-)
hereditary lymphedema (Q82.Ø)

I89.Ø Lymphedema, not elsewhere classified
Elephantiasis (nonfilarial) NOS
Lymphangiectasis
Obliteration, lymphatic vessel
Praecox lymphedema
Secondary lymphedema
EXCLUDES 1 *postmastectomy lymphedema (I97.2)*

I89.1 Lymphangitis
Chronic lymphangitis
Lymphangitis NOS
Subacute lymphangitis
EXCLUDES 1 *acute lymphangitis (LØ3.-)*

I89.8 Other specified noninfective disorders of lymphatic vessels and lymph nodes
Chylocele (nonfilarial)
Chylous ascites
Chylous cyst
Lipomelanotic reticulosis
Lymph node or vessel fistula
Lymph node or vessel infarction
Lymph node or vessel rupture

I89.9 Noninfective disorder of lymphatic vessels and lymph nodes, unspecified
Disease of lymphatic vessels NOS

Other and unspecified disorders of the circulatory system (I95-I99)

✓4th **I95 Hypotension**
EXCLUDES 1 *cardiovascular collapse (R57.9) (~R57.9)*
maternal hypotension syndrome (O26.5-)
nonspecific low blood pressure reading NOS (RØ3.1)

I95.Ø Idiopathic hypotension

I95.1 Orthostatic hypotension
Hypotension, postural
EXCLUDES 1 *neurogenic orthostatic hypotension [Shy-Drager] (G9Ø.3)*
orthostatic hypotension due to drugs (I95.2)
AHA: 2023,2Q,8

I95.2 Hypotension due to drugs
Orthostatic hypotension due to drugs
Use additional code for adverse effect, if applicable, to identify drug (T36-T5Ø with fifth or sixth character 5)

I95.3 Hypotension of hemodialysis
Intra-dialytic hypotension

✓5th **I95.8 Other hypotension**

I95.81 Postprocedural hypotension

I95.89 Other hypotension
Chronic hypotension

I95.9 Hypotension, unspecified

I96 Gangrene, not elsewhere classified CC HCC
Gangrenous cellulitis
EXCLUDES 1 *gangrene in atherosclerosis of native arteries of the extremities (I7Ø.26)*
gangrene in hernia (K4Ø.1, K4Ø.4, K41.1, K41.4, K42.1, K43.1-, K44.1, K45.1, K46.1)
gangrene in other peripheral vascular diseases (I73.-)
gangrene of certain specified sites - see Alphabetical Index
gas gangrene (A48.Ø)
pyoderma gangrenosum (L88)
EXCLUDES 2 *gangrene in diabetes mellitus (EØ8-E13 with .52)*
AHA: 2022,3Q,13; 2018,4Q,87; 2018,3Q,3; 2017,3Q,6; 2013,2Q,34

✓4th **I97 Intraoperative and postprocedural complications and disorders of circulatory system, not elsewhere classified**
EXCLUDES 2 *postprocedural shock (T81.1-)*
AHA: 2021,1Q,13; 2019,2Q,21

I97.Ø Postcardiotomy syndrome

✓5th **I97.1 Other postprocedural cardiac functional disturbances**
EXCLUDES 2 *acute pulmonary insufficiency following thoracic surgery (J95.1)*
intraoperative cardiac functional disturbances (I97.7-)

✓6th **I97.11 Postprocedural cardiac insufficiency**

I97.11Ø Postprocedural cardiac insufficiency following cardiac surgery CC

I97.111 Postprocedural cardiac insufficiency following other surgery CC

✓6th **I97.12 Postprocedural cardiac arrest**

I97.12Ø Postprocedural cardiac arrest following cardiac surgery CC

I97.121 Postprocedural cardiac arrest following other surgery CC

✓6th **I97.13 Postprocedural heart failure**
Use additional code to identify the heart failure (I5Ø.-)

I97.13Ø Postprocedural heart failure following cardiac surgery CC

I97.131 Postprocedural heart failure following other surgery CC

✓6th **I97.19 Other postprocedural cardiac functional disturbances**
Use additional code, if applicable, to further specify disorder

I97.19Ø Other postprocedural cardiac functional disturbances following cardiac surgery CC
Use additional code, if applicable, for type 4 or type 5 myocardial infarction, to further specify disorder
AHA: 2019,2Q,33

I97.191 Other postprocedural cardiac functional disturbances following other surgery CC

I97.2 Postmastectomy lymphedema syndrome A
Elephantiasis due to mastectomy
Obliteration of lymphatic vessels

I97.3 Postprocedural hypertension

✓5th **I97.4 Intraoperative hemorrhage and hematoma of a circulatory system organ or structure complicating a procedure**
EXCLUDES 1 *intraoperative hemorrhage and hematoma of a circulatory system organ or structure due to accidental puncture and laceration during a procedure (I97.5-)*
EXCLUDES 2 *intraoperative cerebrovascular hemorrhage complicating a procedure (G97.3-)*

✓6th **I97.41 Intraoperative hemorrhage and hematoma of a circulatory system organ or structure complicating a circulatory system procedure**

I97.41Ø Intraoperative hemorrhage and hematoma of a circulatory system organ or structure complicating a cardiac catheterization CC

I97.411 Intraoperative hemorrhage and hematoma of a circulatory system organ or structure complicating a cardiac bypass CC

I97.418 Intraoperative hemorrhage and hematoma of a circulatory system organ or structure complicating other circulatory system procedure CC

I97.42 Intraoperative hemorrhage and hematoma of a circulatory system organ or structure complicating other procedure CC
AHA: 2020,1Q,19

✓5th **I97.5 Accidental puncture and laceration of a circulatory system organ or structure during a procedure**
EXCLUDES 2 *accidental puncture and laceration of brain during a procedure (G97.4-)*

I97.51 Accidental puncture and laceration of a circulatory system organ or structure during a circulatory system procedure CC
AHA: 2019,2Q,24

I97.52 Accidental puncture and laceration of a circulatory system organ or structure during other procedure CC

✓5th **I97.6 Postprocedural hemorrhage, hematoma and seroma of a circulatory system organ or structure following a procedure**
EXCLUDES 2 *postprocedural cerebrovascular hemorrhage complicating a procedure (G97.5-)*
AHA: 2016,4Q,9-10

✓6th **I97.61 Postprocedural hemorrhage of a circulatory system organ or structure following a circulatory system procedure**

I97.610 Postprocedural hemorrhage of a circulatory system organ or structure following a cardiac catheterization CC

I97.611 Postprocedural hemorrhage of a circulatory system organ or structure following cardiac bypass CC

I97.618 Postprocedural hemorrhage of a circulatory system organ or structure following other circulatory system procedure CC

✓6th **I97.62 Postprocedural hemorrhage, hematoma and seroma of a circulatory system organ or structure following other procedure**

I97.620 Postprocedural hemorrhage of a circulatory system organ or structure following other procedure CC

I97.621 Postprocedural hematoma of a circulatory system organ or structure following other procedure CC

I97.622 Postprocedural seroma of a circulatory system organ or structure following other procedure CC

✓6th **I97.63 Postprocedural hematoma of a circulatory system organ or structure following a circulatory system procedure**

I97.630 Postprocedural hematoma of a circulatory system organ or structure following a cardiac catheterization CC

I97.631 Postprocedural hematoma of a circulatory system organ or structure following cardiac bypass CC

I97.638 Postprocedural hematoma of a circulatory system organ or structure following other circulatory system procedure CC

✓6th **I97.64 Postprocedural seroma of a circulatory system organ or structure following a circulatory system procedure**

I97.640 Postprocedural seroma of a circulatory system organ or structure following a cardiac catheterization CC

I97.641 Postprocedural seroma of a circulatory system organ or structure following cardiac bypass CC

I97.648 Postprocedural seroma of a circulatory system organ or structure following other circulatory system procedure CC

✓5th **I97.7 Intraoperative cardiac functional disturbances**
EXCLUDES 2 *acute pulmonary insufficiency following thoracic surgery (J95.1)*
postprocedural cardiac functional disturbances (I97.1-)

✓6th **I97.71 Intraoperative cardiac arrest**

I97.710 Intraoperative cardiac arrest during cardiac surgery CC

I97.711 Intraoperative cardiac arrest during other surgery CC

✓6th **I97.79 Other intraoperative cardiac functional disturbances**
Use additional code, if applicable, to further specify disorder

I97.790 Other intraoperative cardiac functional disturbances during cardiac surgery CC

I97.791 Other intraoperative cardiac functional disturbances during other surgery CC

✓5th **I97.8 Other intraoperative and postprocedural complications and disorders of the circulatory system, not elsewhere classified**
Use additional code, if applicable, to further specify disorder

✓6th **I97.81 Intraoperative cerebrovascular infarction**

I97.810 Intraoperative cerebrovascular infarction during cardiac surgery CC HCC

I97.811 Intraoperative cerebrovascular infarction during other surgery CC HCC

✓6th **I97.82 Postprocedural cerebrovascular infarction**

I97.820 Postprocedural cerebrovascular infarction following cardiac surgery CC HCC

I97.821 Postprocedural cerebrovascular infarction following other surgery CC HCC

I97.88 Other intraoperative complications of the circulatory system, not elsewhere classified CC

I97.89 Other postprocedural complications and disorders of the circulatory system, not elsewhere classified CC
AHA: 2021,3Q,33; 2020,3Q,3-8; 2019,2Q,33

✓4th **I99 Other and unspecified disorders of circulatory system**

I99.8 Other disorder of circulatory system
AHA: 2020,4Q,98

I99.9 Unspecified disorder of circulatory system

I97.4 Intraoperative hemorrhage and hematoma of a circulatory system organ or structure complicating a procedure
AHA: 2020,1Q,19

I97.5 Accidental puncture and laceration of a circulatory system organ or structure during a procedure
[illegible]

I97.51 Accidental puncture and laceration of a circulatory system organ or structure during a circulatory system procedure
AHA: 2019,1Q,36

I97.52 Accidental puncture and laceration of a circulatory system organ or structure during other procedure

I97.6 Postprocedural hemorrhage, hematoma and seroma of a circulatory system organ or structure following a procedure
[illegible]
AHA: 2016,4Q,9-10

I97.61 Postprocedural hemorrhage of a circulatory system organ or structure following a circulatory system procedure

I97.610 Postprocedural hemorrhage of a circulatory system organ or structure following a cardiac catheterization

I97.611 Postprocedural hemorrhage of a circulatory system organ or structure following cardiac bypass

I97.618 Postprocedural hemorrhage of a circulatory system organ or structure following other circulatory system procedure

I97.62 Postprocedural hemorrhage, hematoma and seroma of a circulatory system organ or structure following other procedure

I97.620 Postprocedural hemorrhage of a circulatory system organ or structure following other procedure

I97.621 Postprocedural hematoma of a circulatory system organ or structure following other procedure

I97.622 Postprocedural seroma of a circulatory system organ or structure following other procedure

I97.63 Postprocedural hematoma of a circulatory system organ or structure following a circulatory system procedure
[illegible]

I97.64 Postprocedural seroma of a circulatory system organ or structure following a circulatory system procedure
[illegible]

I97.7 Intraoperative cardiac functional disturbances
[illegible]

I97.71 Intraoperative cardiac arrest

I97.710 Intraoperative cardiac arrest during cardiac surgery

I97.711 Intraoperative cardiac arrest during other surgery

I97.79 Other intraoperative cardiac functional disturbances
Use additional code, if applicable, to further specify disorder

I97.790 Other intraoperative cardiac functional disturbances during cardiac surgery

I97.791 Other intraoperative cardiac functional disturbances during other surgery

I97.8 Other intraoperative and postprocedural complications and disorders of the circulatory system, not elsewhere classified
Use additional code, if applicable, to further specify disorder

I97.81 Intraoperative cerebrovascular infarction

I97.810 Intraoperative cerebrovascular infarction during cardiac surgery

I97.811 Intraoperative cerebrovascular infarction during other surgery

I97.82 Postprocedural cerebrovascular infarction

I97.820 Postprocedural cerebrovascular infarction following cardiac surgery

I97.821 Postprocedural cerebrovascular infarction following other surgery

I97.88 Other intraoperative complications of the circulatory system, not elsewhere classified

I97.89 Other postprocedural complications and disorders of the circulatory system, not elsewhere classified
AHA: 2021,1Q,37; 2020,2Q,18; 2019,2Q,35

I99 Other and unspecified disorders of circulatory system

I99.8 Other disorder of circulatory system
AHA: 2021,3Q,9

I99.9 Unspecified disorder of circulatory system

Chapter 10. Diseases of the Respiratory System (JØØ–J99), UØ7.Ø

Chapter-specific Guidelines with Coding Examples

The chapter-specific guidelines from the ICD-10-CM Official Guidelines for Coding and Reporting have been provided below. Along with these guidelines are coding examples, contained in the shaded boxes, that have been developed to help illustrate the coding and/or sequencing guidance found in these guidelines.

a. Chronic obstructive pulmonary disease [COPD] and asthma

1) Acute exacerbation of chronic obstructive bronchitis and asthma

The codes in categories J44 and J45 distinguish between uncomplicated cases and those in acute exacerbation. An acute exacerbation is a worsening or a decompensation of a chronic condition. An acute exacerbation is not equivalent to an infection superimposed on a chronic condition, though an exacerbation may be triggered by an infection.

Vancomycin IV was started to treat a patient with acute pneumonia due to *Streptococcus pneumoniae*. Patient also with acute exacerbation of COPD continued on home meds.

J13 **Pneumonia due to Streptococcus pneumoniae**

J44.Ø **Chronic obstructive pulmonary disease with (acute) lower respiratory infection**

J44.1 **Chronic obstructive pulmonary disease with (acute) exacerbation**

Explanation: ICD-10-CM uses combination codes to create organism-specific classifications for acute pneumonia. Category J44 codes include combination codes with severity components, which differentiate between COPD with acute lower respiratory infection (acute pneumonia), COPD with acute exacerbation, and COPD without mention of a complication (unspecified).

An acute exacerbation is a worsening or a decompensation of a chronic condition. An acute exacerbation is not equivalent to an infection superimposed on a chronic condition, though an exacerbation may be triggered by an infection, as in this example. Treatment of the pneumonia necessitated the inpatient admission. Instructional notes at J44.Ø say to "code also to identify the infection," which informs the coder that another code must be assigned if applicable. Sequencing of the pneumonia and COPD exacerbation are governed by the Section II, "Selection of Principal Diagnosis," guidelines. In this case it was the pneumonia that was "chiefly responsible for occasioning the admission" with the IV vancomycin treatment.

Exacerbation of moderate persistent asthma with status asthmaticus

J45.42 **Moderate persistent asthma with status asthmaticus**

Explanation: Category J45 Asthma includes severity-specific subcategories and fifth-character codes to distinguish between uncomplicated cases, those in acute exacerbation, and those with status asthmaticus.

b. Acute respiratory failure

1) Acute respiratory failure as principal diagnosis

A code from subcategory J96.Ø, Acute respiratory failure, or subcategory J96.2, Acute and chronic respiratory failure, may be assigned as a principal diagnosis when it is the condition established after study to be chiefly responsible for occasioning the admission to the hospital, and the selection is supported by the Alphabetic Index and Tabular List. However, chapter-specific coding guidelines (such as obstetrics, poisoning, HIV, newborn) that provide sequencing direction take precedence.

Acute hypoxic respiratory failure due to COPD exacerbation

J96.Ø1 **Acute respiratory failure with hypoxia**

J44.1 **Chronic obstructive pulmonary disease with (acute) exacerbation**

Explanation: Category J96 classifies respiratory failure with combination codes that designate the severity and the presence of hypoxia and hypercapnia. Code J96.Ø1 is sequenced as the first-listed diagnosis, as the reason for the admission. Respiratory failure may be assigned as a principal diagnosis when it is the condition established after study to be chiefly responsible for occasioning the admission to the hospital and the selection is supported by the Alphabetic Index and Tabular List.

2) Acute respiratory failure as secondary diagnosis

Respiratory failure may be listed as a secondary diagnosis if it occurs after admission, or if it is present on admission, but does not meet the definition of principal diagnosis.

Acute respiratory failure due to accidental oxycodone overdose

T4Ø.2X1A **Poisoning by other opioids, accidental (unintentional), initial encounter**

J96.ØØ **Acute respiratory failure, unspecified whether with hypoxia or hypercapnia**

Explanation: Respiratory failure may be assigned as a principal diagnosis when it is the condition established after study to be chiefly responsible for occasioning the admission to the hospital, and the selection is supported by the Alphabetic Index and Tabular List. However, chapter-specific coding guidelines, such as poisoning, that provide sequencing direction take precedence. When coding a poisoning or reaction to the improper use of a medication (e.g., overdose, wrong substance given or taken in error, wrong route of administration), first assign the appropriate code from categories T36–T5Ø. Use additional code(s) for all manifestations of the poisoning. In this instance, the respiratory failure is a manifestation of the poisoning and is sequenced as a secondary diagnosis.

Acute pneumococcal pneumonia with subsequent development of acute respiratory failure

J13 **Pneumonia due to Streptococcus pneumoniae**

J96.ØØ **Acute respiratory failure, unspecified whether with hypoxia or hypercapnia**

Explanation: Acute respiratory failure may be listed as a secondary diagnosis if it occurs after admission, or if it is present on admission but does not meet the definition of principal diagnosis.

3) Sequencing of acute respiratory failure and another acute condition

When a patient is admitted with respiratory failure and another acute condition, (e.g., myocardial infarction, cerebrovascular accident, aspiration pneumonia), the principal diagnosis will not be the same in every situation. This applies whether the other acute condition is a respiratory or nonrespiratory condition. Selection of the principal diagnosis will be dependent on the circumstances of admission. If both the respiratory failure and the other acute condition are equally responsible for occasioning the admission to the hospital, and there are no chapter-specific sequencing rules, the guideline regarding two or more diagnoses that equally meet the definition for principal diagnosis (*Section II, C.*) may be applied in these situations.

If the documentation is not clear as to whether acute respiratory failure and another condition are equally responsible for occasioning the admission, query the provider for clarification.

Acute pneumococcal pneumonia and acute respiratory failure, both present on admission

J96.ØØ **Acute respiratory failure, unspecified whether with hypoxia or hypercapnia**

J13 **Pneumonia due to Streptococcus pneumoniae**

Explanation: When a patient is admitted with respiratory failure and another acute condition, such as a bacterial pneumonia, the principal diagnosis is not the same in every situation. This applies whether the other acute condition is a respiratory or nonrespiratory condition. The principal diagnosis depends on the circumstances of admission.

c. Influenza due to certain identified influenza viruses

Code only confirmed cases of influenza due to certain identified influenza viruses (category JØ9), and due to other identified influenza virus (category J1Ø). This is an exception to the hospital inpatient guideline Section II, H. (Uncertain Diagnosis).

In this context, "confirmation" does not require documentation of positive laboratory testing specific for avian or other novel influenza A or other identified influenza virus. However, coding should be based on the provider's diagnostic statement that the patient has avian influenza, or other novel influenza A, for category JØ9, or has another particular identified strain of influenza, such as H1N1 or H3N2, but not identified as novel or variant, for category J1Ø.

If the provider records "suspected" or "possible" or "probable" avian influenza, or novel influenza, or other identified influenza, then the appropriate influenza code from category J11, Influenza due to unidentified influenza virus, should be assigned. A code from category JØ9, Influenza due to certain identified influenza viruses, should not be assigned nor should a code from category J1Ø, Influenza due to other identified influenza virus.

Influenza due to avian influenza virus with pneumonia

JØ9.X1 **Influenza due to identified novel influenza A virus with pneumonia**

Explanation: Codes in category JØ9 Influenza due to certain identified influenza viruses should be assigned only for confirmed cases. "Confirmation" does not require positive laboratory testing of a specific influenza virus but does need to be based on the provider's diagnostic statement, which should not include terms such as "possible," "probable," or "suspected."

d. Ventilator associated pneumonia

1) Documentation of ventilator associated pneumonia

As with all procedural or postprocedural complications, code assignment is based on the provider's documentation of the relationship between the condition and the procedure.

Code J95.851, Ventilator associated pneumonia, should be assigned only when the provider has documented ventilator associated pneumonia (VAP). An additional code to identify the organism (e.g., Pseudomonas aeruginosa, code B96.5) should also be assigned. Do not assign an additional code from categories J12–J18 to identify the type of pneumonia.

Code J95.851 should not be assigned for cases where the patient has pneumonia and is on a mechanical ventilator and the provider has not specifically stated that the pneumonia is ventilator-associated pneumonia. If the documentation is unclear as to whether the patient has a pneumonia that is a complication attributable to the mechanical ventilator, query the provider.

2) Ventilator associated pneumonia develops after admission

A patient may be admitted with one type of pneumonia (e.g., code J13, Pneumonia due to Streptococcus pneumonia) and subsequently develop VAP. In this instance, the principal diagnosis would be the appropriate code from categories J12–J18 for the pneumonia diagnosed at the time of admission. Code J95.851, Ventilator associated pneumonia, would be assigned as an additional diagnosis when the provider has also documented the presence of ventilator associated pneumonia.

Patient with pneumonia due to *Klebsiella pneumoniae* develops superimposed MRSA ventilator-associated pneumonia

J15.Ø **Pneumonia due to Klebsiella pneumoniae**

J95.851 **Ventilator associated pneumonia**

B95.62 **Methicillin resistant Staphylococcus aureus infection as the cause of diseases classified elsewhere**

Explanation: Code assignment for ventilator-associated pneumonia is based on the provider's documentation of the relationship between the condition and the procedure and is reported only when the provider has documented ventilator-associated pneumonia (VAP).

A patient may be admitted with one type of pneumonia and subsequently develop VAP. In this example, the principal diagnosis code describes the pneumonia diagnosed at the time of admission, with code J95.851 Ventilator associated pneumonia, assigned as secondary.

e. Vaping-related disorders

For patients presenting with condition(s) related to vaping, assign code UØ7.Ø, Vaping-related disorder, as the principal diagnosis. For lung injury due to vaping, assign only code UØ7.Ø. Assign additional codes for other manifestations, such as acute respiratory failure (subcategory J96.Ø-) or pneumonitis (code J68.Ø).

Associated respiratory signs and symptoms due to vaping, such as cough, shortness of breath, etc., are not coded separately, when a definitive diagnosis has been established. However, it would be appropriate to code separately any gastrointestinal symptoms, such as diarrhea and abdominal pain.

See Section I.C.1.g.1.c.i. for Pneumonia confirmed as due to COVID-19

23-year-old patient with history of anxiety disorder admitted with fever, dyspnea and nonproductive cough. Patient's respiratory function continued to clinically worsen, requiring intubation for suspected ARDS and required OGT suction for coffee ground hematemesis. Following extubating, patient confirmed the use of THC vaping cartridge preceding development of symptoms. Discharge diagnosis is ARDS due to EVALI and anxiety disorder.

UØ7.Ø **Vaping related disorder**

J8Ø **Acute respiratory distress syndrome**

K92.Ø **Hematemesis**

F41.9 **Anxiety disorder, unspecified**

Explanation: Codes UØ7.Ø and J8Ø represent the vaping-related disorder and its associated manifestation, the acute respiratory distress syndrome (ARDS). The symptoms that brought the patient in are not coded separately because these are integral to the vaping disorder and the ARDS, unlike the hematemesis (vomiting blood) a gastrointestinal symptom that is not integral to either of these conditions.

Chapter 10. Diseases of the Respiratory System (J00-J99)

NOTE When a respiratory condition is described as occurring in more than one site and is not specifically indexed, it should be classified to the lower anatomic site (e.g., tracheobronchitis to bronchitis in J40).

Use additional code, where applicable, to identify:
- exposure to environmental tobacco smoke (Z77.22)
- exposure to tobacco smoke in the perinatal period (P96.81)
- history of tobacco dependence (Z87.891)
- occupational exposure to environmental tobacco smoke (Z57.31)
- tobacco dependence (F17.-)
- tobacco use (Z72.0)

EXCLUDES 2 *certain conditions originating in the perinatal period (P04-P96)*
certain infectious and parasitic diseases (A00-B99)
complications of pregnancy, childbirth and the puerperium (O00-O9A)
congenital malformations, deformations and chromosomal abnormalities (Q00-Q99)
endocrine, nutritional and metabolic diseases (E00-E88)
injury, poisoning and certain other consequences of external causes (S00-T88)
neoplasms (C00-D49)
smoke inhalation (T59.81-)
symptoms, signs and abnormal clinical and laboratory findings, not elsewhere classified (R00-R94)

This chapter contains the following blocks:

- J00-J06 Acute upper respiratory infections
- J09-J18 Influenza and pneumonia
- J20-J22 Other acute lower respiratory infections
- J30-J39 Other diseases of upper respiratory tract
- J40-J4A Chronic lower respiratory diseases
- J60-J70 Lung diseases due to external agents
- J80-J84 Other respiratory diseases principally affecting the interstitium
- J85-J86 Suppurative and necrotic conditions of the lower respiratory tract
- J90-J94 Other diseases of the pleura
- J95 Intraoperative and postprocedural complications and disorders of respiratory system, not elsewhere classified
- J96-J99 Other diseases of the respiratory system

Acute upper respiratory infections (J00-J06)

EXCLUDES 1 *chronic obstructive pulmonary disease with acute lower respiratory infection (J44.0)*

J00 Acute nasopharyngitis [common cold]
Acute rhinitis
Coryza (acute)
Infective nasopharyngitis NOS
Infective rhinitis
Nasal catarrh, acute
Nasopharyngitis NOS
EXCLUDES 1 *acute pharyngitis (J02.-)*
acute sore throat NOS (J02.9)
influenza virus with other respiratory manifestations (J09.X2, J10.1, J11.1)
pharyngitis NOS (J02.9)
rhinitis NOS (J31.0)
sore throat NOS (J02.9)
EXCLUDES 2 *allergic rhinitis (J30.1-J30.9)*
chronic pharyngitis (J31.2)
chronic rhinitis (J31.0)
chronic sore throat (J31.2)
nasopharyngitis, chronic (J31.1)
vasomotor rhinitis (J30.0)

✓4th **J01 Acute sinusitis**
INCLUDES acute abscess of sinus
acute empyema of sinus
acute infection of sinus
acute inflammation of sinus
acute suppuration of sinus
Use additional code (B95-B97) to identify infectious agent
EXCLUDES 1 *sinusitis NOS (J32.9)*
EXCLUDES 2 *chronic sinusitis (J32.0-J32.8)*

✓5th **J01.0 Acute maxillary sinusitis**
Acute antritis
J01.00 Acute maxillary sinusitis, unspecified
J01.01 Acute recurrent maxillary sinusitis

✓5th **J01.1 Acute frontal sinusitis**
J01.10 Acute frontal sinusitis, unspecified
J01.11 Acute recurrent frontal sinusitis

✓5th **J01.2 Acute ethmoidal sinusitis**
J01.20 Acute ethmoidal sinusitis, unspecified
J01.21 Acute recurrent ethmoidal sinusitis

✓5th **J01.3 Acute sphenoidal sinusitis**
J01.30 Acute sphenoidal sinusitis, unspecified
J01.31 Acute recurrent sphenoidal sinusitis

✓5th **J01.4 Acute pansinusitis**
J01.40 Acute pansinusitis, unspecified
J01.41 Acute recurrent pansinusitis

✓5th **J01.8 Other acute sinusitis**
J01.80 Other acute sinusitis
Acute sinusitis involving more than one sinus but not pansinusitis
J01.81 Other acute recurrent sinusitis
Acute recurrent sinusitis involving more than one sinus but not pansinusitis

✓5th **J01.9 Acute sinusitis, unspecified**
J01.90 Acute sinusitis, unspecified
J01.91 Acute recurrent sinusitis, unspecified

✓4th **J02 Acute pharyngitis**
INCLUDES acute sore throat
EXCLUDES 1 *acute laryngopharyngitis (J06.0)*
peritonsillar abscess (J36)
pharyngeal abscess (J39.1)
retropharyngeal abscess (J39.0)
EXCLUDES 2 *chronic pharyngitis (J31.2)*

J02.0 Streptococcal pharyngitis
Septic pharyngitis
Streptococcal sore throat
EXCLUDES 2 *scarlet fever (A38.-)*

J02.8 Acute pharyngitis due to other specified organisms
Use additional code (B95-B97) to identify infectious agent
EXCLUDES 1 *acute pharyngitis due to coxsackie virus (B08.5)*
acute pharyngitis due to gonococcus (A54.5)
acute pharyngitis due to herpes [simplex] virus (B00.2)
acute pharyngitis due to infectious mononucleosis (B27.-)
enteroviral vesicular pharyngitis (B08.5)

J02.9 Acute pharyngitis, unspecified
Gangrenous pharyngitis (acute)
Infective pharyngitis (acute) NOS
Pharyngitis (acute) NOS
Sore throat (acute) NOS
Suppurative pharyngitis (acute)
Ulcerative pharyngitis (acute)
EXCLUDES 1 *influenza virus with other respiratory manifestations (J09.X2, J10.1, J11.1)*

✓4th **J03 Acute tonsillitis**
EXCLUDES 1 *acute sore throat (J02.-)*
hypertrophy of tonsils (J35.1)
peritonsillar abscess (J36)
sore throat NOS (J02.9)
streptococcal sore throat (J02.0)
EXCLUDES 2 *chronic tonsillitis (J35.0)*

✓5th **J03.0 Streptococcal tonsillitis**
J03.00 Acute streptococcal tonsillitis, unspecified
J03.01 Acute recurrent streptococcal tonsillitis

✓5th **J03.8 Acute tonsillitis due to other specified organisms**
Use additional code (B95-B97) to identify infectious agent
EXCLUDES 1 *diphtheritic tonsillitis (A36.0)*
herpesviral pharyngotonsillitis (B00.2)
streptococcal tonsillitis (J03.0)
tuberculous tonsillitis (A15.8)
Vincent's tonsillitis (A69.1)
J03.80 Acute tonsillitis due to other specified organisms
J03.81 Acute recurrent tonsillitis due to other specified organisms

✓5th **J03.9 Acute tonsillitis, unspecified**
Follicular tonsillitis (acute)
Gangrenous tonsillitis (acute)
Infective tonsillitis (acute)
Tonsillitis (acute) NOS
Ulcerative tonsillitis (acute)
EXCLUDES 1 *influenza virus with other respiratory manifestations (J09.X2, J10.1, J11.1)*
J03.90 Acute tonsillitis, unspecified
J03.91 Acute recurrent tonsillitis, unspecified

J04 Acute laryngitis and tracheitis

Code also influenza, if present, such as:
influenza due to identified novel influenza A virus with other respiratory manifestations (J09.X2)
influenza due to other identified influenza virus with other respiratory manifestations (J10.1)
influenza due to unidentified influenza virus with other respiratory manifestations (J11.1)
Use additional code (B95-B97) to identify infectious agent

EXCLUDES 1 *acute obstructive laryngitis [croup] and epiglottitis (J05.-)*
EXCLUDES 2 *laryngismus (stridulus) (J38.5)*

J04.0 Acute laryngitis
Edematous laryngitis (acute)
Laryngitis (acute) NOS
Subglottic laryngitis (acute)
Suppurative laryngitis (acute)
Ulcerative laryngitis (acute)
EXCLUDES 1 *acute obstructive laryngitis (J05.0)*
EXCLUDES 2 *chronic laryngitis (J37.0)*

J04.1 Acute tracheitis
Acute viral tracheitis
Catarrhal tracheitis (acute)
Tracheitis (acute) NOS
EXCLUDES 2 *chronic tracheitis (J42)*

J04.10 Acute tracheitis without obstruction

J04.11 Acute tracheitis with obstruction MCC

J04.2 Acute laryngotracheitis
Laryngotracheitis NOS
Tracheitis (acute) with laryngitis (acute)
EXCLUDES 1 *acute obstructive laryngotracheitis (J05.0)*
EXCLUDES 2 *chronic laryngotracheitis (J37.1)*

J04.3 Supraglottitis, unspecified

J04.30 Supraglottitis, unspecified, without obstruction

J04.31 Supraglottitis, unspecified, with obstruction MCC

J05 Acute obstructive laryngitis [croup] and epiglottitis

Code also, influenza, if present, such as:
influenza due to identified novel influenza A virus with other respiratory manifestations (J09.X2)
influenza due to other identified influenza virus with other respiratory manifestations (J10.1)
influenza due to unidentified influenza virus with other respiratory manifestations (J11.1)
Use additional code (B95-B97) to identify infectious agent

J05.0 Acute obstructive laryngitis [croup]
Obstructive laryngitis (acute) NOS
Obstructive laryngotracheitis NOS
DEF: Acute laryngeal obstruction due to allergies, foreign bodies, or in the majority of cases a viral infection. Symptoms include a harsh, barking cough, hoarseness, and a persistent, high-pitched respiratory sound (stridor).

J05.1 Acute epiglottitis
EXCLUDES 2 *epiglottitis, chronic (J37.0)*

J05.10 Acute epiglottitis without obstruction CC
Epiglottitis NOS

J05.11 Acute epiglottitis with obstruction MCC

J06 Acute upper respiratory infections of multiple and unspecified sites

EXCLUDES 1 *acute respiratory infection NOS (J22)*
influenza virus with other respiratory manifestations (J09.X2, J10.1, J11.1)
streptococcal pharyngitis (J02.0)

J06.0 Acute laryngopharyngitis

J06.9 Acute upper respiratory infection, unspecified
Upper respiratory disease, acute
Upper respiratory infection NOS
Use additional code (B95-B97) to identify infectious agent, if known, such as:
respiratory syncytial virus (RSV) (B97.4)
AHA: 2020,1Q,22

Influenza and pneumonia (J09-J18)

▶Use additional code, if applicable, to identify resistance to antimicrobial drugs (Z16.-)◀

EXCLUDES 2 *allergic or eosinophilic pneumonia (J82)*
aspiration pneumonia NOS (J69.0)
meconium pneumonia (P24.01)
neonatal aspiration pneumonia (P24.-)
pneumonia due to solids and liquids (J69.-)
congenital pneumonia (P23.9)
lipid pneumonia (J69.1)
rheumatic pneumonia (I00)
ventilator associated pneumonia (J95.851)

AHA: 2017,4Q,96
TIP: Hemoptysis (R04.2) is not customarily associated with pneumonia and may be reported separately.

J09 Influenza due to certain identified influenza viruses

EXCLUDES 1 *influenza A/H1N1 (J10.-)*
influenza due to other identified influenza virus (J10.-)
influenza due to unidentified influenza virus (J11.-)
seasonal influenza due to other identified influenza virus (J10.-)
seasonal influenza due to unidentified influenza virus (J11.-)

J09.X Influenza due to identified novel influenza A virus
Avian influenza
Bird influenza
Influenza A/H5N1
Influenza of other animal origin, not bird or swine
Swine influenza virus (viruses that normally cause infections in pigs)
AHA: 2016,3Q,10

J09.X1 Influenza due to identified novel influenza A virus with pneumonia HIV MCC
Code also, if applicable, associated:
lung abscess (J85.1)
other specified type of pneumonia

J09.X2 Influenza due to identified novel influenza A virus with other respiratory manifestations
Influenza due to identified novel influenza A virus NOS
Influenza due to identified novel influenza A virus with laryngitis
Influenza due to identified novel influenza A virus with pharyngitis
Influenza due to identified novel influenza A virus with upper respiratory symptoms
Use additional code, if applicable, for associated:
pleural effusion (J91.8)
sinusitis (J01.-)

J09.X3 Influenza due to identified novel influenza A virus with gastrointestinal manifestations
Influenza due to identified novel influenza A virus gastroenteritis
EXCLUDES 1 *'intestinal flu' [viral gastroenteritis] (A08.-)*

J09.X9 Influenza due to identified novel influenza A virus with other manifestations
Influenza due to identified novel influenza A virus with encephalopathy
Influenza due to identified novel influenza A virus with myocarditis
Influenza due to identified novel influenza A virus with otitis media
Use additional code to identify manifestation

J10 Influenza due to other identified influenza virus

INCLUDES influenza A (non-novel)
influenza B
influenza C
EXCLUDES 1 *influenza due to avian influenza virus (J09.X-)*
influenza due to swine flu (J09.X-)
influenza due to unidentifed influenza virus (J11.-)

J10.0 Influenza due to other identified influenza virus with pneumonia
Code also associated lung abscess, if applicable (J85.1)

J10.00 Influenza due to other identified influenza virus with unspecified type of pneumonia MCC

J10.01 Influenza due to other identified influenza virus with the same other identified influenza virus pneumonia MCC

J10.08 Influenza due to other identified influenza virus with other specified pneumonia HIV MCC
Code also other specified type of pneumonia

J10.1 Influenza due to other identified influenza virus with other respiratory manifestations
Influenza due to other identified influenza virus NOS
Influenza due to other identified influenza virus with laryngitis
Influenza due to other identified influenza virus with pharyngitis
Influenza due to other identified influenza virus with upper respiratory symptoms
Use additional code for associated pleural effusion, if applicable (J91.8)
Use additional code for associated sinusitis, if applicable (J01.-)
AHA: 2016,3Q,10-11

J10.2 Influenza due to other identified influenza virus with gastrointestinal manifestations
Influenza due to other identified influenza virus gastroenteritis
EXCLUDES 1 *"intestinal flu" [viral gastroenteritis] (A08.-)*

✓5th **J10.8 Influenza due to other identified influenza virus with other manifestations**

J10.81 Influenza due to other identified influenza virus with encephalopathy

J10.82 Influenza due to other identified influenza virus with myocarditis

J10.83 Influenza due to other identified influenza virus with otitis media
Use additional code for any associated perforated tympanic membrane (H72.-)

J10.89 Influenza due to other identified influenza virus with other manifestations
Use additional codes to identify the manifestations

✓4th **J11 Influenza due to unidentified influenza virus**

✓5th **J11.0 Influenza due to unidentified influenza virus with pneumonia**
Code also associated lung abscess, if applicable (J85.1)
AHA: 2016,3Q,11

J11.00 Influenza due to unidentified influenza virus with unspecified type of pneumonia MCC
Influenza with pneumonia NOS

J11.08 Influenza due to unidentified influenza virus with specified pneumonia MCC
Code also other specified type of pneumonia

J11.1 Influenza due to unidentified influenza virus with other respiratory manifestations
Influenza NOS
Influenzal laryngitis NOS
Influenzal pharyngitis NOS
Influenza with upper respiratory symptoms NOS
Use additional code for associated pleural effusion, if applicable (J91.8)
Use additional code for associated sinusitis, if applicable (J01.-)

J11.2 Influenza due to unidentified influenza virus with gastrointestinal manifestations
Influenza gastroenteritis NOS
EXCLUDES 1 *"intestinal flu" [viral gastroenteritis] (A08.-)*

✓5th **J11.8 Influenza due to unidentified influenza virus with other manifestations**

J11.81 Influenza due to unidentified influenza virus with encephalopathy
Influenzal encephalopathy NOS

J11.82 Influenza due to unidentified influenza virus with myocarditis
Influenzal myocarditis NOS

J11.83 Influenza due to unidentified influenza virus with otitis media
Influenzal otitis media NOS
Use additional code for any associated perforated tympanic membrane (H72.-)

J11.89 Influenza due to unidentified influenza virus with other manifestations
Use additional codes to identify the manifestations

✓4th **J12 Viral pneumonia, not elsewhere classified**
INCLUDES bronchopneumonia due to viruses other than influenza viruses
Code first associated influenza, if applicable (J09.X1, J10.0-, J11.0)
Code also associated abscess, if applicable (J85.1)
EXCLUDES 1 *aspiration pneumonia due to anesthesia during labor and delivery (O74.0)*
aspiration pneumonia due to anesthesia during pregnancy (O29)
aspiration pneumonia due to anesthesia during puerperium (O89.0)
aspiration pneumonia due to solids and liquids (J69.-)
aspiration pneumonia NOS (J69.0)
congenital pneumonia (P23.0)
congenital rubella pneumonitis (P35.0)
interstitial pneumonia NOS (J84.9)
lipid pneumonia (J69.1)
neonatal aspiration pneumonia (P24.-)
AHA: 2020,2Q,28; 2019,1Q,35; 2018,3Q,24; 2016,3Q,15; 2013,4Q,118

J12.0 Adenoviral pneumonia MCC

J12.1 Respiratory syncytial virus pneumonia MCC
RSV pneumonia

J12.2 Parainfluenza virus pneumonia MCC

J12.3 Human metapneumovirus pneumonia HIV MCC

✓5th **J12.8 Other viral pneumonia**

J12.81 Pneumonia due to SARS-associated coronavirus HIV MCC
Severe acute respiratory syndrome NOS
DEF: Inflammation of the lungs with consolidation, caused by the severe adult respiratory syndrome (SARS)-associated coronavirus or SARS-CoV. This pneumonia should not be confused with that caused by SARS-CoV-2 (COVID-19).

J12.82 Pneumonia due to coronavirus disease 2019 HIV MCC UPD
Pneumonia due to 2019 novel coronavirus (SARS-CoV-2)
Pneumonia due to COVID-19
Code first COVID-19 (U07.1)
AHA: 2021,1Q,25-30,31-49

J12.89 Other viral pneumonia HIV MCC
AHA: 2021,1Q,33-34; 2020,2Q,8,11; 2020,1Q,34-36

J12.9 Viral pneumonia, unspecified HIV MCC

J13 Pneumonia due to Streptococcus pneumoniae HIV MCC HCC
Bronchopneumonia due to S. pneumoniae
Code first associated influenza, if applicable (J09.X1, J10.0-, J11.0-)
Code also associated abscess, if applicable (J85.1)
EXCLUDES 1 *congenital pneumonia due to S. pneumoniae (P23.6)*
lobar pneumonia, unspecified organism (J18.1)
pneumonia due to other streptococci (J15.3-J15.4)
AHA: 2020,2Q,28; 2019,1Q,35; 2018,3Q,24; 2016,3Q,15; 2013,4Q,118

J14 Pneumonia due to Hemophilus influenzae HIV MCC HCC
Bronchopneumonia due to H. influenzae
Code first associated influenza, if applicable (J09.X1, J10.0-, J11.0-)
Code also associated abscess, if applicable (J85.1)
EXCLUDES 1 *congenital pneumonia due to H. influenzae (P23.6)*
AHA: 2020,2Q,28; 2019,1Q,35; 2018,3Q,24; 2016,3Q,15; 2013,4Q,118

✓4th **J15 Bacterial pneumonia, not elsewhere classified**
INCLUDES Bronchopneumonia due to bacteria other than S. pneumoniae and H. influenzae
Code first associated influenza, if applicable (J09.X1, J10.0-, -J11.0-)
Code also associated abscess, if applicable (J85.1)
EXCLUDES 1 *chlamydial pneumonia (J16.0)*
congenital pneumonia (P23.-)
Legionnaires' disease (A48.1)
spirochetal pneumonia (A69.8)
AHA: 2020,2Q,28; 2019,1Q,35; 2018,3Q,24; 2016,3Q,15; 2013,4Q,118

J15.0 Pneumonia due to Klebsiella pneumoniae HIV MCC HCC

J15.1 Pneumonia due to Pseudomonas HIV MCC HCC

✓5th **J15.2 Pneumonia due to staphylococcus**

J15.20 Pneumonia due to staphylococcus, unspecified HIV MCC HCC

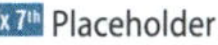

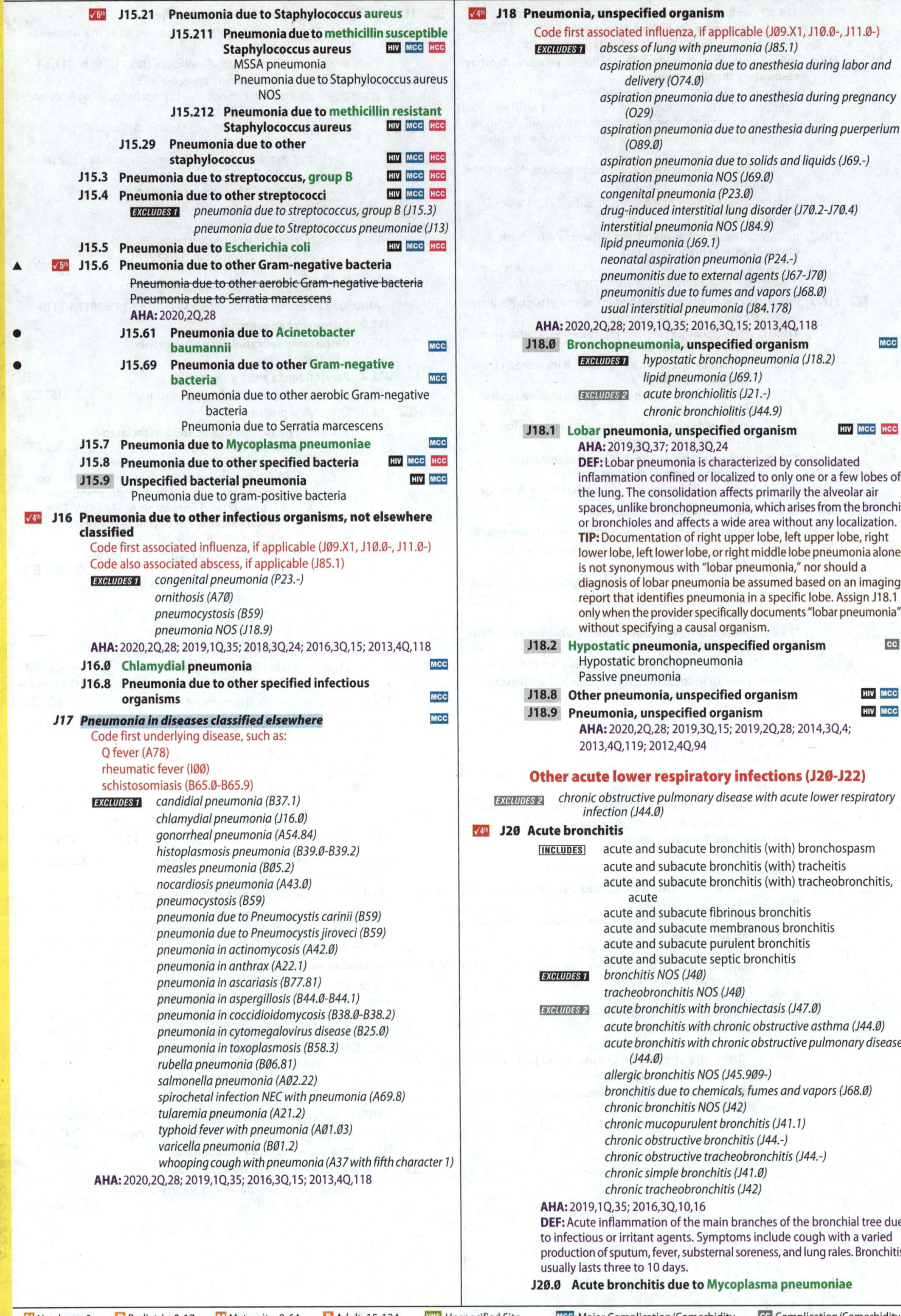

✓6th **J15.21 Pneumonia due to Staphylococcus aureus**

J15.211 Pneumonia due to methicillin susceptible Staphylococcus aureus HIV MCC HCC

MSSA pneumonia

Pneumonia due to Staphylococcus aureus NOS

J15.212 Pneumonia due to methicillin resistant Staphylococcus aureus HIV MCC HCC

J15.29 Pneumonia due to other staphylococcus HIV MCC HCC

J15.3 Pneumonia due to streptococcus, group B HIV MCC HCC

J15.4 Pneumonia due to other streptococci HIV MCC HCC

EXCLUDES 1 *pneumonia due to streptococcus, group B (J15.3)*

pneumonia due to Streptococcus pneumoniae (J13)

J15.5 Pneumonia due to Escherichia coli HIV MCC HCC

▲ ✓5th **J15.6 Pneumonia due to other Gram-negative bacteria**

~~Pneumonia due to other aerobic Gram-negative bacteria~~

~~Pneumonia due to Serratia marcescens~~

AHA: 2020,2Q,28

● **J15.61 Pneumonia due to Acinetobacter baumannii** MCC

● **J15.69 Pneumonia due to other Gram-negative bacteria** MCC

Pneumonia due to other aerobic Gram-negative bacteria

Pneumonia due to Serratia marcescens

J15.7 Pneumonia due to Mycoplasma pneumoniae MCC

J15.8 Pneumonia due to other specified bacteria HIV MCC HCC

J15.9 Unspecified bacterial pneumonia HIV MCC

Pneumonia due to gram-positive bacteria

✓4th **J16 Pneumonia due to other infectious organisms, not elsewhere classified**

Code first associated influenza, if applicable (J09.X1, J10.0-, J11.0-)

Code also associated abscess, if applicable (J85.1)

EXCLUDES 1 *congenital pneumonia (P23.-)*

ornithosis (A70)

pneumocystosis (B59)

pneumonia NOS (J18.9)

AHA: 2020,2Q,28; 2019,1Q,35; 2018,3Q,24; 2016,3Q,15; 2013,4Q,118

J16.0 Chlamydial pneumonia MCC

J16.8 Pneumonia due to other specified infectious organisms MCC

J17 Pneumonia in diseases classified elsewhere MCC

Code first underlying disease, such as:

Q fever (A78)

rheumatic fever (I00)

schistosomiasis (B65.0-B65.9)

EXCLUDES 1 *candidial pneumonia (B37.1)*

chlamydial pneumonia (J16.0)

gonorrheal pneumonia (A54.84)

histoplasmosis pneumonia (B39.0-B39.2)

measles pneumonia (B05.2)

nocardiosis pneumonia (A43.0)

pneumocystosis (B59)

pneumonia due to Pneumocystis carinii (B59)

pneumonia due to Pneumocystis jiroveci (B59)

pneumonia in actinomycosis (A42.0)

pneumonia in anthrax (A22.1)

pneumonia in ascariasis (B77.81)

pneumonia in aspergillosis (B44.0-B44.1)

pneumonia in coccidioidomycosis (B38.0-B38.2)

pneumonia in cytomegalovirus disease (B25.0)

pneumonia in toxoplasmosis (B58.3)

rubella pneumonia (B06.81)

salmonella pneumonia (A02.22)

spirochetal infection NEC with pneumonia (A69.8)

tularemia pneumonia (A21.2)

typhoid fever with pneumonia (A01.03)

varicella pneumonia (B01.2)

whooping cough with pneumonia (A37 with fifth character 1)

AHA: 2020,2Q,28; 2019,1Q,35; 2016,3Q,15; 2013,4Q,118

✓4th **J18 Pneumonia, unspecified organism**

Code first associated influenza, if applicable (J09.X1, J10.0-, J11.0-)

EXCLUDES 1 *abscess of lung with pneumonia (J85.1)*

aspiration pneumonia due to anesthesia during labor and delivery (O74.0)

aspiration pneumonia due to anesthesia during pregnancy (O29)

aspiration pneumonia due to anesthesia during puerperium (O89.0)

aspiration pneumonia due to solids and liquids (J69.-)

aspiration pneumonia NOS (J69.0)

congenital pneumonia (P23.0)

drug-induced interstitial lung disorder (J70.2-J70.4)

interstitial pneumonia NOS (J84.9)

lipid pneumonia (J69.1)

neonatal aspiration pneumonia (P24.-)

pneumonitis due to external agents (J67-J70)

pneumonitis due to fumes and vapors (J68.0)

usual interstitial pneumonia (J84.178)

AHA: 2020,2Q,28; 2019,1Q,35; 2016,3Q,15; 2013,4Q,118

J18.0 Bronchopneumonia, unspecified organism MCC

EXCLUDES 1 *hypostatic bronchopneumonia (J18.2)*

lipid pneumonia (J69.1)

EXCLUDES 2 *acute bronchiolitis (J21.-)*

chronic bronchiolitis (J44.9)

J18.1 Lobar pneumonia, unspecified organism HIV MCC HCC

AHA: 2019,3Q,37; 2018,3Q,24

DEF: Lobar pneumonia is characterized by consolidated inflammation confined or localized to only one or a few lobes of the lung. The consolidation affects primarily the alveolar air spaces, unlike bronchopneumonia, which arises from the bronchi or bronchioles and affects a wide area without any localization.

TIP: Documentation of right upper lobe, left upper lobe, right lower lobe, left lower lobe, or right middle lobe pneumonia alone is not synonymous with "lobar pneumonia," nor should a diagnosis of lobar pneumonia be assumed based on an imaging report that identifies pneumonia in a specific lobe. Assign J18.1 only when the provider specifically documents "lobar pneumonia" without specifying a causal organism.

J18.2 Hypostatic pneumonia, unspecified organism CC

Hypostatic bronchopneumonia

Passive pneumonia

J18.8 Other pneumonia, unspecified organism HIV MCC

J18.9 Pneumonia, unspecified organism HIV MCC

AHA: 2020,2Q,28; 2019,3Q,15; 2019,2Q,28; 2014,3Q,4; 2013,4Q,119; 2012,4Q,94

Other acute lower respiratory infections (J20-J22)

EXCLUDES 2 *chronic obstructive pulmonary disease with acute lower respiratory infection (J44.0)*

✓4th **J20 Acute bronchitis**

INCLUDES acute and subacute bronchitis (with) bronchospasm

acute and subacute bronchitis (with) tracheitis

acute and subacute bronchitis (with) tracheobronchitis, acute

acute and subacute fibrinous bronchitis

acute and subacute membranous bronchitis

acute and subacute purulent bronchitis

acute and subacute septic bronchitis

EXCLUDES 1 *bronchitis NOS (J40)*

tracheobronchitis NOS (J40)

EXCLUDES 2 *acute bronchitis with bronchiectasis (J47.0)*

acute bronchitis with chronic obstructive asthma (J44.0)

acute bronchitis with chronic obstructive pulmonary disease (J44.0)

allergic bronchitis NOS (J45.909-)

bronchitis due to chemicals, fumes and vapors (J68.0)

chronic bronchitis NOS (J42)

chronic mucopurulent bronchitis (J41.1)

chronic obstructive bronchitis (J44.-)

chronic obstructive tracheobronchitis (J44.-)

chronic simple bronchitis (J41.0)

chronic tracheobronchitis (J42)

AHA: 2019,1Q,35; 2016,3Q,10,16

DEF: Acute inflammation of the main branches of the bronchial tree due to infectious or irritant agents. Symptoms include cough with a varied production of sputum, fever, substernal soreness, and lung rales. Bronchitis usually lasts three to 10 days.

J20.0 Acute bronchitis due to Mycoplasma pneumoniae

J2Ø.1 Acute bronchitis due to Hemophilus influenzae

J2Ø.2 Acute bronchitis due to streptococcus

J2Ø.3 Acute bronchitis due to coxsackievirus

J2Ø.4 Acute bronchitis due to parainfluenza virus

J2Ø.5 Acute bronchitis due to respiratory syncytial virus
Acute bronchitis due to RSV

J2Ø.6 Acute bronchitis due to rhinovirus

J2Ø.7 Acute bronchitis due to echovirus

J2Ø.8 Acute bronchitis due to other specified organisms
AHA: 2020,1Q,34-36
TIP: Assign as a secondary code for a patient with acute bronchitis confirmed as due to COVID-19; assign U07.1 as the principal or first-listed code.

J2Ø.9 Acute bronchitis, unspecified

✓4th **J21 Acute bronchiolitis**
INCLUDES acute bronchiolitis with bronchospasm
EXCLUDES 2 *respiratory bronchiolitis interstitial lung disease (J84.115)*

J21.Ø Acute bronchiolitis due to respiratory syncytial virus CC
Acute bronchiolitis due to RSV

J21.1 Acute bronchiolitis due to human metapneumovirus CC

J21.8 Acute bronchiolitis due to other specified organisms CC

J21.9 Acute bronchiolitis, unspecified CC
Bronchiolitis (acute)
EXCLUDES 1 *chronic bronchiolitis (J44.-)*

J22 Unspecified acute lower respiratory infection
Acute (lower) respiratory (tract) infection NOS
EXCLUDES 1 *upper respiratory infection (acute) (JØ6.9)*
AHA: 2020,1Q,22,34-36
TIP: Assign as a secondary code for a patient with a respiratory infection specified as acute or lower that is documented as being associated with COVID-19; assign U07.1 as the principal or first-listed code. If the respiratory infection documentation does not specify acute or lower, assign J98.8.

Other diseases of upper respiratory tract (J3Ø-J39)

✓4th **J3Ø Vasomotor and allergic rhinitis**
INCLUDES spasmodic rhinorrhea
EXCLUDES 1 *allergic rhinitis with asthma (bronchial) (J45.9Ø9)*
rhinitis NOS (J31.Ø)

J3Ø.Ø Vasomotor rhinitis
DEF: Noninfectious and nonallergic type of rhinitis for which the cause is often unknown. Symptoms often mimic those of allergic rhinitis with a diagnosis of vasomotor rhinitis typically made after ruling out allergens as the cause.

J3Ø.1 Allergic rhinitis due to pollen
Allergy NOS due to pollen
Hay fever
Pollinosis

J3Ø.2 Other seasonal allergic rhinitis

J3Ø.5 Allergic rhinitis due to food

✓5th **J3Ø.8 Other allergic rhinitis**

J3Ø.81 Allergic rhinitis due to animal (cat) (dog) hair and dander

J3Ø.89 Other allergic rhinitis
Perennial allergic rhinitis

J3Ø.9 Allergic rhinitis, unspecified

✓4th **J31 Chronic rhinitis, nasopharyngitis and pharyngitis**
~~Use additional code to identify:~~
~~exposure to environmental tobacco smoke (Z77.22)~~
~~exposure to tobacco smoke in the perinatal period (P96.81)~~
~~history of tobacco dependence (Z87.891)~~
~~occupational exposure to environmental tobacco smoke (Z57.31)~~
~~tobacco dependence (F17.-)~~
~~tobacco use (Z72.Ø)~~

J31.Ø Chronic rhinitis
Atrophic rhinitis (chronic)
Granulomatous rhinitis (chronic)
Hypertrophic rhinitis (chronic)
Obstructive rhinitis (chronic)
Ozena
Purulent rhinitis (chronic)
Rhinitis (chronic) NOS
Ulcerative rhinitis (chronic)
EXCLUDES 1 *allergic rhinitis (J3Ø.1-J3Ø.9)*
vasomotor rhinitis (J3Ø.Ø)
DEF: Persistent inflammation of the mucous membranes of the nose, characterized by a postnasal drip.

J31.1 Chronic nasopharyngitis
EXCLUDES 2 *acute nasopharyngitis (JØØ)*
DEF: Persistent inflammation of the mucous membranes extending from the nares to the pharynx. It is characterized by constant irritation in the nasopharynx and postnasal drip.

J31.2 Chronic pharyngitis
Atrophic pharyngitis (chronic)
Chronic sore throat
Granular pharyngitis (chronic)
Hypertrophic pharyngitis (chronic)
EXCLUDES 2 *acute pharyngitis (JØ2.9)*

✓4th **J32 Chronic sinusitis**
INCLUDES sinus abscess
sinus empyema
sinus infection
sinus suppuration
Use additional code to identify:
~~exposure to environmental tobacco smoke (Z77.22)~~
~~exposure to tobacco smoke in the perinatal period (P96.81)~~
~~history of tobacco dependence (Z87.891)~~
infectious agent (B95-B97)
~~occupational exposure to environmental tobacco smoke (Z57.31)~~
~~tobacco dependence (F17.-)~~
~~tobacco use (Z72.Ø)~~
EXCLUDES 2 *acute sinusitis (JØ1.-)*

J32.Ø Chronic maxillary sinusitis
Antritis (chronic)
Maxillary sinusitis NOS

J32.1 Chronic frontal sinusitis
Frontal sinusitis NOS

J32.2 Chronic ethmoidal sinusitis
Ethmoidal sinusitis NOS
EXCLUDES 1 *Woakes' ethmoiditis (J33.1)*

J32.3 Chronic sphenoidal sinusitis
Sphenoidal sinusitis NOS

J32.4 Chronic pansinusitis
Pansinusitis NOS

J32.8 Other chronic sinusitis
Sinusitis (chronic) involving more than one sinus but not pansinusitis

J32.9 Chronic sinusitis, unspecified
Sinusitis (chronic) NOS

✓4th **J33 Nasal polyp**
~~Use additional code to identify:~~
~~exposure to environmental tobacco smoke (Z77.22)~~
~~exposure to tobacco smoke in the perinatal period (P96.81)~~
~~history of tobacco dependence (Z87.891)~~
~~occupational exposure to environmental tobacco smoke (Z57.31)~~
~~tobacco dependence (F17.-)~~
~~tobacco use (Z72.Ø)~~
EXCLUDES 1 *adenomatous polyps (D14.Ø)*

J33.Ø Polyp of nasal cavity
Choanal polyp
Nasopharyngeal polyp

J33.1 Polypoid sinus degeneration
Woakes' syndrome or ethmoiditis

J33.8 **Other polyp of sinus**
Accessory polyp of sinus
Ethmoidal polyp of sinus
Maxillary polyp of sinus
Sphenoidal polyp of sinus

UNS J33.9 **Nasal polyp, unspecified**

4th **J34 Other and unspecified disorders of nose and nasal sinuses**
EXCLUDES 2 *varicose ulcer of nasal septum (I86.8)*

J34.Ø **Abscess, furuncle and carbuncle of nose**
Cellulitis of nose
Necrosis of nose
Ulceration of nose

J34.1 **Cyst and mucocele of nose and nasal sinus**

J34.2 **Deviated nasal septum**
Deflection or deviation of septum (nasal) (acquired)
EXCLUDES 1 *congenital deviated nasal septum (Q67.4)*
DEF: Condition in which the nasal septum, a thin wall composed of cartilage and bone that separates the two nostrils, is crooked or displaced from the midline.

J34.3 **Hypertrophy of nasal turbinates**
DEF: Overgrowth of bones within the nasal turbinate, which are ridges of bone and soft tissue that project from the sidewalls of the nasal passages. Hypertrophy can cause obstruction of the nasal passages.

5th J34.8 **Other specified disorders of nose and nasal sinuses**

J34.81 **Nasal mucositis (ulcerative)**
Code also type of associated therapy, such as:
antineoplastic and immunosuppressive drugs (T45.1X-)
radiological procedure and radiotherapy (Y84.2)
EXCLUDES 2 *gastrointestinal mucositis (ulcerative) (K92.81)*
mucositis (ulcerative) of vagina and vulva (N76.81)
oral mucositis (ulcerative) (K12.3-)

J34.89 **Other specified disorders of nose and nasal sinuses**
Perforation of nasal septum NOS
Rhinolith

UNS J34.9 **Unspecified disorder of nose and nasal sinuses**

4th **J35 Chronic diseases of tonsils and adenoids**
~~Use additional code to identify:~~
~~exposure to environmental tobacco smoke (Z77.22)~~
~~exposure to tobacco smoke in the perinatal period (P96.81)~~
~~history of tobacco dependence (Z87.891)~~
~~occupational exposure to environmental tobacco smoke (Z57.31)~~
~~tobacco dependence (F17.-)~~
~~tobacco use (Z72.Ø)~~

5th J35.Ø **Chronic tonsillitis and adenoiditis**
EXCLUDES 2 *acute tonsillitis (JØ3.-)*

J35.Ø1 **Chronic tonsillitis**
J35.Ø2 **Chronic adenoiditis**
J35.Ø3 **Chronic tonsillitis and adenoiditis**

J35.1 **Hypertrophy of tonsils**
Enlargement of tonsils
EXCLUDES 1 *hypertrophy of tonsils with tonsillitis (J35.Ø-)*

J35.2 **Hypertrophy of adenoids**
Enlargement of adenoids
EXCLUDES 1 *hypertrophy of adenoids with adenoiditis (J35.Ø-)*

J35.3 **Hypertrophy of tonsils with hypertrophy of adenoids**
EXCLUDES 1 *hypertrophy of tonsils and adenoids with tonsillitis and adenoiditis (J35.Ø3)*

J35.8 **Other chronic diseases of tonsils and adenoids**
Adenoid vegetations
Amygdalolith
Calculus, tonsil
Cicatrix of tonsil (and adenoid)
Tonsillar tag
Ulcer of tonsil

UNS J35.9 **Chronic disease of tonsils and adenoids, unspecified**
Disease (chronic) of tonsils and adenoids NOS

J36 Peritonsillar abscess CC
INCLUDES abscess of tonsil
peritonsillar cellulitis
quinsy
Use additional code (B95-B97) to identify infectious agent
EXCLUDES 1 *acute tonsillitis (JØ3.-)*
chronic tonsillitis (J35.Ø)
retropharyngeal abscess (J39.Ø)
tonsillitis NOS (JØ3.9-)

4th **J37 Chronic laryngitis and laryngotracheitis**
Use additional code to identify:
exposure to environmental tobacco smoke (Z77.22)
exposure to tobacco smoke in the perinatal period (P96.81)
history of tobacco dependence (Z87.891)
infectious agent (B95-B97)
occupational exposure to environmental tobacco smoke (Z57.31)
tobacco dependence (F17.-)
tobacco use (Z72.Ø)

J37.Ø **Chronic laryngitis**
Catarrhal laryngitis
Hypertrophic laryngitis
Sicca laryngitis
EXCLUDES 2 *acute laryngitis (JØ4.Ø)*
obstructive (acute) laryngitis (JØ5.Ø)

J37.1 **Chronic laryngotracheitis**
Laryngitis, chronic, with tracheitis (chronic)
Tracheitis, chronic, with laryngitis
EXCLUDES 1 *chronic tracheitis (J42)*
EXCLUDES 2 *acute laryngotracheitis (JØ4.2)*
acute tracheitis (JØ4.1)

4th **J38 Diseases of vocal cords and larynx, not elsewhere classified**
~~Use additional code to identify:~~
~~exposure to environmental tobacco smoke (Z77.22)~~
~~exposure to tobacco smoke in the perinatal period (P96.81)~~
~~history of tobacco dependence (Z87.891)~~
~~occupational exposure to environmental tobacco smoke (Z57.31)~~
~~tobacco dependence (F17.-)~~
~~tobacco use (Z72.Ø)~~
EXCLUDES 1 *congenital laryngeal stridor (P28.89)*
obstructive laryngitis (acute) (JØ5.Ø)
postprocedural subglottic stenosis (J95.5)
stridor (RØ6.1)
ulcerative laryngitis (JØ4.Ø)

5th J38.Ø **Paralysis of vocal cords and larynx**
Laryngoplegia
Paralysis of glottis

UNS J38.ØØ **Paralysis of vocal cords and larynx, unspecified**
J38.Ø1 **Paralysis of vocal cords and larynx, unilateral**
J38.Ø2 **Paralysis of vocal cords and larynx, bilateral**

J38.1 **Polyp of vocal cord and larynx**
EXCLUDES 1 *adenomatous polyps (D14.1)*

J38.2 **Nodules of vocal cords**
Chorditis (fibrinous)(nodosa)(tuberosa)
Singer's nodes
Teacher's nodes

J38.3 **Other diseases of vocal cords**
Abscess of vocal cords
Cellulitis of vocal cords
Granuloma of vocal cords
Leukokeratosis of vocal cords
Leukoplakia of vocal cords

J38.4 **Edema of larynx**
Edema (of) glottis
Subglottic edema
Supraglottic edema
EXCLUDES 1 *acute obstructive laryngitis [croup] (JØ5.Ø)*
edematous laryngitis (JØ4.Ø)

J38.5 **Laryngeal spasm**
Laryngismus (stridulus)

J38.6 **Stenosis of larynx**

J38.7 Other diseases of larynx
Abscess of larynx
Cellulitis of larynx
Disease of larynx NOS
Necrosis of larynx
Pachyderma of larynx
Perichondritis of larynx
Ulcer of larynx

√4th J39 Other diseases of upper respiratory tract
EXCLUDES 1 *acute respiratory infection NOS (J22)*
acute upper respiratory infection (JØ6.9)
upper respiratory inflammation due to chemicals, gases, fumes or vapors (J68.2)

J39.Ø Retropharyngeal and parapharyngeal abscess CC
Peripharyngeal abscess
EXCLUDES 1 *peritonsillar abscess (J36)*
DEF: Purulent infection behind the pharynx and the front of the precerebral fascia, characterized by neck stiffness, cervical lymphadenopathy, sore throat, fever, and stridor.

J39.1 Other abscess of pharynx CC
Cellulitis of pharynx
Nasopharyngeal abscess

J39.2 Other diseases of pharynx
Cyst of pharynx
Edema of pharynx
EXCLUDES 2 *chronic pharyngitis (J31.2)*
ulcerative pharyngitis (JØ2.9)

J39.3 Upper respiratory tract hypersensitivity reaction, site unspecified
EXCLUDES 1 *hypersensitivity reaction of upper respiratory tract, such as:*
extrinsic allergic alveolitis (J67.9)
pneumoconiosis (J6Ø-J67.9)

J39.8 Other specified diseases of upper respiratory tract
AHA: 2023,1Q,30

J39.9 Disease of upper respiratory tract, unspecified

Chronic lower respiratory diseases (J4Ø-J4A)

EXCLUDES 1 *bronchitis due to chemicals, gases, fumes and vapors (J68.Ø)*
EXCLUDES 2 *cystic fibrosis (E84.-)*

J4Ø Bronchitis, not specified as acute or chronic
Bronchitis NOS
Bronchitis with tracheitis NOS
Catarrhal bronchitis
Tracheobronchitis NOS
Use additional code to identify:
exposure to environmental tobacco smoke (Z77.22)
exposure to tobacco smoke in the perinatal period (P96.81)
history of tobacco dependence (Z87.891)
occupational exposure to environmental tobacco smoke (Z57.31)
tobacco dependence (F17.-)
tobacco use (Z72.Ø)
EXCLUDES 1 *acute bronchitis (J2Ø.-)*
allergic bronchitis NOS (J45.9Ø9-)
asthmatic bronchitis NOS (J45.9-)
bronchitis due to chemicals, gases, fumes and vapors (J68.Ø)
AHA: 2020,1Q,34-36
TIP: Assign as a secondary code for a patient with bronchitis of unspecified acuity due to COVID-19; assign U07.1 as the principal or first-listed code.

√4th J41 Simple and mucopurulent chronic bronchitis
Use additional code to identify:
exposure to environmental tobacco smoke (Z77.22)
exposure to tobacco smoke in the perinatal period (P96.81)
history of tobacco dependence (Z87.891)
occupational exposure to environmental tobacco smoke (Z57.31)
tobacco dependence (F17.-)
tobacco use (Z72.Ø)
EXCLUDES 1 ~~*chronic bronchitis NOS (J42)*~~
~~*chronic obstructive bronchitis (J44.-)*~~
EXCLUDES 2 ▶*chronic bronchitis NOS (J42)*◀
▶*chronic obstructive bronchitis (J44.-)*◀

J41.Ø Simple chronic bronchitis HCC
J41.1 Mucopurulent chronic bronchitis HCC
J41.8 Mixed simple and mucopurulent chronic bronchitis HCC

J42 Unspecified chronic bronchitis HCC
Chronic bronchitis NOS
Chronic tracheitis
Chronic tracheobronchitis
Use additional code to identify:
exposure to environmental tobacco smoke (Z77.22)
exposure to tobacco smoke in the perinatal period (P96.81)
history of tobacco dependence (Z87.891)
occupational exposure to environmental tobacco smoke (Z57.31)
tobacco dependence (F17.-)
tobacco use (Z72.Ø)
EXCLUDES 1 ▶*bronchiolitis obliterans and bronchiolitis obliterans syndrome (J44.81)*◀
chronic asthmatic bronchitis (J44.-)
chronic bronchitis with airways obstruction (J44.-)
chronic emphysematous bronchitis (J44.-)
chronic obstructive pulmonary disease NOS (J44.9)
simple and mucopurulent chronic bronchitis (J41.-)

√4th J43 Emphysema
~~Use additional code to identify:~~
~~exposure to environmental tobacco smoke (Z77.22)~~
~~history of tobacco dependence (Z87.891)~~
~~occupational exposure to environmental tobacco smoke (Z57.31)~~
~~tobacco dependence (F17.-)~~
~~tobacco use (Z72.Ø)~~
EXCLUDES 1 *compensatory emphysema (J98.3)*
emphysema due to inhalation of chemicals, gases, fumes or vapors (J68.4)
~~*emphysema with chronic (obstructive) bronchitis (J44.-)*~~
~~*emphysematous (obstructive) bronchitis (J44.-)*~~
interstitial emphysema (J98.2)
mediastinal emphysema (J98.2)
neonatal interstitial emphysema (P25.Ø)
surgical (subcutaneous) emphysema (T81.82)
EXCLUDES 2 ▶*emphysema with chronic (obstructive) bronchitis (J44.-)*◀
▶*emphysematous (obstructive) bronchitis (J44.-)*◀
traumatic subcutaneous emphysema (T79.7)
DEF: Pathological condition in which there is destructive enlargement of the air sacs in the lungs resulting in damage and lack of elasticity to the alveolar walls, commonly seen in long-term smokers.

Emphysema

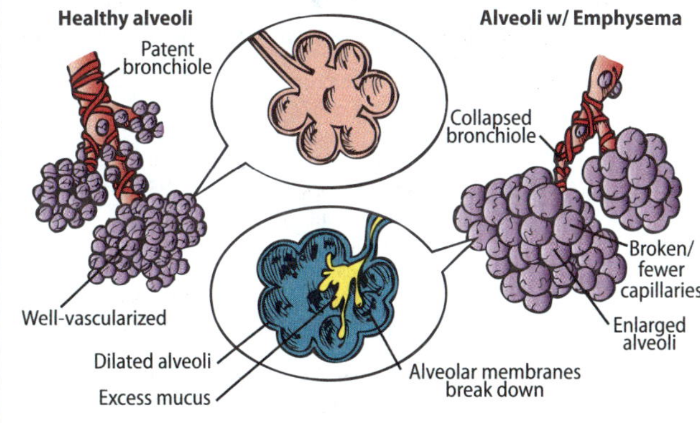

J43.Ø Unilateral pulmonary emphysema [MacLeod's syndrome] HCC
Swyer-James syndrome
Unilateral emphysema
Unilateral hyperlucent lung
Unilateral pulmonary artery functional hypoplasia
Unilateral transparency of lung

J43.1 Panlobular emphysema HCC
Panacinar emphysema

J43.2 Centrilobular emphysema HCC
J43.8 Other emphysema HCC
J43.9 Emphysema, unspecified HCC
Bullous emphysema (lung)(pulmonary)
Emphysema (lung)(pulmonary) NOS
Emphysematous bleb
Vesicular emphysema (lung)(pulmonary)
AHA: 2019,1Q,34-36; 2017,4Q,97-98

J44 Other chronic obstructive pulmonary disease

INCLUDES asthma with chronic obstructive pulmonary disease
chronic asthmatic (obstructive) bronchitis
chronic bronchitis with airway obstruction
chronic bronchitis with emphysema
chronic emphysematous bronchitis
chronic obstructive asthma
chronic obstructive bronchitis
chronic obstructive tracheobronchitis

Code also type of asthma, if applicable (J45.-)

~~Use additional code to identify:~~
~~exposure to environmental tobacco smoke (Z77.22)~~
~~history of tobacco dependence (Z87.891)~~
~~occupational exposure to environmental tobacco smoke (Z57.31)~~
~~tobacco dependence (F17.-)~~
~~tobacco use (Z72.Ø)~~

EXCLUDES 1 *~~bronchiectasis (J47.-)~~*
chronic bronchitis NOS (J42)
chronic simple and mucopurulent bronchitis (J41.-)
chronic tracheitis (J42)
chronic tracheobronchitis (J42)
~~emphysema without chronic bronchitis (J43.-)~~

EXCLUDES 2 ▶*bronchiectasis (J47.-)*◀
▶*emphysema without chronic bronchitis (J43.-)*◀

AHA: 2019,1Q,34-36; 2017,4Q,97-98; 2017,1Q,25-26; 2016,3Q,15-16; 2013,4Q,109

J44.Ø Chronic obstructive pulmonary disease with (acute) lower respiratory infection CC HCC

Code also to identify the infection

AHA: 2019,1Q,35; 2017,4Q,96; 2017,1Q,24-25

TIP: Do not assign when only aspiration pneumonia is present. Aspiration pneumonia is not classified as a respiratory infection.

J44.1 Chronic obstructive pulmonary disease with (acute) exacerbation CC HCC

Decompensated COPD
Decompensated COPD with (acute) exacerbation

EXCLUDES 2 *chronic obstructive pulmonary disease [COPD] with acute bronchitis (J44.Ø)*
lung diseases due to external agents (J6Ø-J7Ø)

AHA: 2019,1Q,34; 2017,4Q,96; 2017,1Q,26; 2016,1Q,36

TIP: Exacerbation of COPD should not be assumed based upon worsening of a concomitant respiratory disease or when COPD is described as end-stage.

● **J44.8 Other specified chronic obstructive pulmonary disease**

● **J44.81 Bronchiolitis obliterans and bronchiolitis obliterans syndrome**

Obliterative bronchiolitis

Code first, if applicable:
complication of bone marrow transplant (T86.Ø9)
complication of stem cell transplant (T86.5)
heart-lung transplant rejection (T86.31)
lung transplant rejection (T86.81Ø)
other complications of heart-lung transplant (T86.39)
other complications of lung transplant (T86.818)

Code also, if applicable, associated conditions, such as:
chronic graft-versus-host disease (D89.811)
chronic lung allograft dysfunction (J4A.-)
chronic respiratory conditions due to chemicals, gases, fumes and vapors (J68.4)

● **J44.89 Other specified chronic obstructive pulmonary disease**

Chronic asthmatic (obstructive) bronchitis
Chronic emphysematous bronchitis

J44.9 Chronic obstructive pulmonary disease, unspecified HCC

Chronic obstructive airway disease NOS
Chronic obstructive lung disease NOS

EXCLUDES 2 *lung diseases due to external agents (J6Ø-J7Ø)*

AHA: 2019,1Q,36; 2017,4Q,96-97; 2016,1Q,36; 2014,4Q,21; 2013,4Q,109

● **J4A Chronic lung allograft dysfunction**

Code first, if applicable:
heart-lung transplant rejection (T86.31)
lung transplant rejection (T86.81Ø)
other complications of heart-lung transplant (T86.39)
other complications of lung transplant (T86.818)

Code also, if applicable, bronchiolitis obliterans syndrome (J44.81)

● **J4A.Ø Restrictive allograft syndrome**

Code also, if applicable, for mixed chronic lung allograft dysfunction, bronchiolitis obliterans syndrome (J44.81)

● **J4A.8 Other chronic lung allograft dysfunction**

● **J4A.9 Chronic lung allograft dysfunction, unspecified**

J45 Asthma

INCLUDES allergic (predominantly) asthma
allergic bronchitis NOS
allergic rhinitis with asthma
atopic asthma
extrinsic allergic asthma
hay fever with asthma
idiosyncratic asthma
intrinsic nonallergic asthma
nonallergic asthma

Use additional code to identify:
eosinophilic asthma (J82.83)
exposure to environmental tobacco smoke (Z77.22)
exposure to tobacco smoke in the perinatal period (P96.81)
history of tobacco dependence (Z87.891)
occupational exposure to environmental tobacco smoke (Z57.31)
tobacco dependence (F17.-)
tobacco use (Z72.Ø)

EXCLUDES 1 *detergent asthma (J69.8)*
miner's asthma (J6Ø)
wheezing NOS (RØ6.2)
wood asthma (J67.8)

EXCLUDES 2 *asthma with chronic obstructive pulmonary disease (J44.9)*
chronic asthmatic (obstructive) bronchitis (J44.9)
chronic obstructive asthma (J44.9)

AHA: 2023,1Q,17; 2019,1Q,36; 2017,1Q,25-26; 2012,4Q,99

DEF: Status asthmaticus: Severe, intractable episode of asthma that is unresponsive to normal therapeutic measures.

J45.2 Mild intermittent asthma

J45.2Ø Mild intermittent asthma, uncomplicated

Mild intermittent asthma NOS

J45.21 Mild intermittent asthma with (acute) exacerbation CC

J45.22 Mild intermittent asthma with status asthmaticus CC

J45.3 Mild persistent asthma

J45.3Ø Mild persistent asthma, uncomplicated

Mild persistent asthma NOS

J45.31 Mild persistent asthma with (acute) exacerbation CC

AHA: 2016,1Q,35

J45.32 Mild persistent asthma with status asthmaticus CC

J45.4 Moderate persistent asthma

J45.4Ø Moderate persistent asthma, uncomplicated

Moderate persistent asthma NOS

J45.41 Moderate persistent asthma with (acute) exacerbation CC

AHA: 2017,1Q,26

J45.42 Moderate persistent asthma with status asthmaticus CC

J45.5 Severe persistent asthma

J45.5Ø Severe persistent asthma, uncomplicated

Severe persistent asthma NOS

J45.51 Severe persistent asthma with (acute) exacerbation CC

J45.52 Severe persistent asthma with status asthmaticus CC

✓5th **J45.9 Other and unspecified asthma**

✓6th **J45.90 Unspecified asthma**

Asthmatic bronchitis NOS
Childhood asthma NOS
Late onset asthma
AHA: 2017,4Q,96; 2017,1Q,25

J45.901 Unspecified asthma with (acute) exacerbation CC

J45.902 Unspecified asthma with status asthmaticus CC

J45.909 Unspecified asthma, uncomplicated

Asthma NOS
EXCLUDES 2 *lung diseases due to external agents (J60-J70)*
AHA: 2017,1Q,25

✓6th **J45.99 Other asthma**

J45.990 Exercise induced bronchospasm
J45.991 Cough variant asthma
J45.998 Other asthma

✓4th **J47 Bronchiectasis**

INCLUDES bronchiolectasis
Use additional code to identify:
exposure to environmental tobacco smoke (Z77.22)
exposure to tobacco smoke in the perinatal period (P96.81)
history of tobacco dependence (Z87.891)
occupational exposure to environmental tobacco smoke (Z57.31)
tobacco dependence (F17.-)
tobacco use (Z72.0)
EXCLUDES 1 *congenital bronchiectasis (Q33.4)*
tuberculous bronchiectasis (current disease) (A15.0)

DEF: Dilation of the bronchi with mucus production and persistent cough due to infection or chronic conditions that causes diminished lung capacity and frequent infections of the lung.

J47.0 Bronchiectasis with acute lower respiratory infection CC HCC

Bronchiectasis with acute bronchitis
Code also to identify infection, if applicable

J47.1 Bronchiectasis with (acute) exacerbation CC HCC

AHA: 2021,1Q,23

J47.9 Bronchiectasis, uncomplicated HCC

Bronchiectasis NOS

Lung diseases due to external agents (J60-J70)

EXCLUDES 2 *asthma (J45.-)*
malignant neoplasm of bronchus and lung (C34.-)

DEF: Pneumoconiosis: Condition caused by inhaling inorganic dust particles, typically associated with occupations that require regular exposure to mineral dusts. A form of interstitial lung disease that contributes to the inflammation of the air sacs, causing the lung tissue to harden.

J60 Coalworker's pneumoconiosis HCC A

Anthracosilicosis
Anthracosis
Black lung disease
Coalworker's lung
EXCLUDES 1 *coalworker pneumoconiosis with tuberculosis, any type in A15 (J65)*

J61 Pneumoconiosis due to asbestos and other mineral fibers HCC A

Asbestosis
EXCLUDES 1 *pleural plaque with asbestosis (J92.0)*
pneumoconiosis with tuberculosis, any type in A15 (J65)

✓4th **J62 Pneumoconiosis due to dust containing silica**

INCLUDES silicotic fibrosis (massive) of lung
EXCLUDES 1 *pneumoconiosis with tuberculosis, any type in A15 (J65)*

J62.0 Pneumoconiosis due to talc dust HCC

J62.8 Pneumoconiosis due to other dust containing silica HCC

Silicosis NOS

✓4th **J63 Pneumoconiosis due to other inorganic dusts**

EXCLUDES 1 *pneumoconiosis with tuberculosis, any type in A15 (J65)*

J63.0 Aluminosis (of lung) HCC
J63.1 Bauxite fibrosis (of lung) HCC
J63.2 Berylliosis HCC
J63.3 Graphite fibrosis (of lung) HCC
J63.4 Siderosis HCC

AHA: 2019,3Q,8

J63.5 Stannosis HCC

J63.6 Pneumoconiosis due to other specified inorganic dusts HCC

J64 Unspecified pneumoconiosis HCC

EXCLUDES 1 *pneumonoconiosis with tuberculosis, any type in A15 (J65)*

J65 Pneumoconiosis associated with tuberculosis HCC

Any condition in J60-J64 with tuberculosis, any type in A15
Silicotuberculosis

✓4th **J66 Airway disease due to specific organic dust**

EXCLUDES 2 *allergic alveolitis (J67.-)*
asbestosis (J61)
bagassosis (J67.1)
farmer's lung (J67.0)
hypersensitivity pneumonitis due to organic dust (J67.-)
reactive airways dysfunction syndrome (J68.3)

J66.0 Byssinosis HCC

Airway disease due to cotton dust

J66.1 Flax-dressers' disease HCC
J66.2 Cannabinosis HCC
J66.8 Airway disease due to other specific organic dusts HCC

✓4th **J67 Hypersensitivity pneumonitis due to organic dust**

INCLUDES allergic alveolitis and pneumonitis due to inhaled organic dust and particles of fungal, actinomycetic or other origin
EXCLUDES 1 *pneumonitis due to inhalation of chemicals, gases, fumes or vapors (J68.0)*

J67.0 Farmer's lung HCC

Harvester's lung
Haymaker's lung
Moldy hay disease

J67.1 Bagassosis HCC

Bagasse disease
Bagasse pneumonitis

J67.2 Bird fancier's lung HCC

Budgerigar fancier's disease or lung
Pigeon fancier's disease or lung

J67.3 Suberosis HCC

Corkhandler's disease or lung
Corkworker's disease or lung

J67.4 Maltworker's lung HCC

Alveolitis due to Aspergillus clavatus

J67.5 Mushroom-worker's lung HCC

J67.6 Maple-bark-stripper's lung HCC

Alveolitis due to Cryptostroma corticale
Cryptostromosis

J67.7 Air conditioner and humidifier lung CC HCC

Allergic alveolitis due to fungal, thermophilic actinomycetes and other organisms growing in ventilation [air conditioning] systems

J67.8 Hypersensitivity pneumonitis due to other organic dusts CC HCC

Cheese-washer's lung
Coffee-worker's lung
Fish-meal worker's lung
Furrier's lung
Sequoiosis

J67.9 Hypersensitivity pneumonitis due to unspecified organic dust CC HCC

Allergic alveolitis (extrinsic) NOS
Hypersensitivity pneumonitis NOS

✓4th **J68 Respiratory conditions due to inhalation of chemicals, gases, fumes and vapors**

Code first (T51-T65) to identify cause
Use additional code to identify associated respiratory conditions, such as:
acute respiratory failure (J96.0-)

J68.0 Bronchitis and pneumonitis due to chemicals, gases, fumes and vapors CC HCC

Chemical bronchitis (acute)
AHA: 2019,2Q,31

J68.1 Pulmonary edema due to chemicals, gases, fumes and vapors MCC HCC

Chemical pulmonary edema (acute) (chronic)
EXCLUDES 1 *pulmonary edema (acute) (chronic) NOS (J81.-)*

J68.2 Upper respiratory inflammation due to chemicals, gases, fumes and vapors, not elsewhere classified HCC

Chapter 10. Diseases of the Respiratory System

J45.9–J68.2

J68.3 Other acute and subacute respiratory conditions due to chemicals, gases, fumes and vapors HCC
Reactive airways dysfunction syndrome

J68.4 Chronic respiratory conditions due to chemicals, gases, fumes and vapors HCC
~~Emphysema (diffuse) (chronic) due to inhalation of chemicals, gases, fumes and vapors~~
~~Obliterative bronchiolitis (chronic) (subacute) due to inhalation of chemicals, gases, fumes and vapors~~
~~Pulmonary fibrosis (chronic) due to inhalation of chemicals, gases, fumes and vapors~~
▶Code also, if applicable, chronic conditions, such as:◀
▶emphysema (J43.-)◀
▶obliterative bronchiolitis (J44.81)◀
▶pulmonary fibrosis (J84.10)◀
EXCLUDES 1 *chronic pulmonary edema due to chemicals, gases, fumes and vapors (J68.1)*

J68.8 Other respiratory conditions due to chemicals, gases, fumes and vapors HCC

J68.9 Unspecified respiratory condition due to chemicals, gases, fumes and vapors HCC

J69 Pneumonitis due to solids and liquids
EXCLUDES 1 *neonatal aspiration syndromes (P24.-)*
postprocedural pneumonitis (J95.4)
AHA: 2017,1Q,24
DEF: Pneumonitis: Noninfectious inflammation of the walls of the alveoli in the lung tissue due to inhalation of food, vomit, oils, essences, or other solids or liquids.

J69.0 Pneumonitis due to inhalation of food and vomit MCC HCC
Aspiration pneumonia NOS
Aspiration pneumonia (due to) food (regurgitated)
Aspiration pneumonia (due to) gastric secretions
Aspiration pneumonia (due to) milk
Aspiration pneumonia (due to) vomit
Code also any associated foreign body in respiratory tract (T17.-)
EXCLUDES 1 *chemical pneumonitis due to anesthesia (J95.4)*
obstetric aspiration pneumonitis (O74.0)
AHA: 2020,2Q,11,28; 2019,3Q,17; 2019,2Q,6,31

J69.1 Pneumonitis due to inhalation of oils and essences MCC HCC
Exogenous lipoid pneumonia
Lipid pneumonia NOS
Code first (T51-T65) to identify substance
EXCLUDES 1 *endogenous lipoid pneumonia (J84.89)*

J69.8 Pneumonitis due to inhalation of other solids and liquids MCC HCC
Pneumonitis due to aspiration of blood
Pneumonitis due to aspiration of detergent
Code first (T51-T65) to identify substance

J70 Respiratory conditions due to other external agents

J70.0 Acute pulmonary manifestations due to radiation CC HCC
Radiation pneumonitis
Use additional code (W88-W90, X39.0-) to identify the external cause

J70.1 Chronic and other pulmonary manifestations due to radiation CC HCC
Fibrosis of lung following radiation
Use additional code (W88-W90, X39.0-) to identify the external cause

J70.2 Acute drug-induced interstitial lung disorders HCC
Use additional code for adverse effect, if applicable, to identify drug (T36-T50 with fifth or sixth character 5)
EXCLUDES 1 *interstitial pneumonia NOS (J84.9)*
lymphoid interstitial pneumonia (J84.2)
AHA: 2019,2Q,28

J70.3 Chronic drug-induced interstitial lung disorders HCC
Use additional code for adverse effect, if applicable, to identify drug (T36-T50 with fifth or sixth character 5)
EXCLUDES 1 *interstitial pneumonia NOS (J84.9)*
lymphoid interstitial pneumonia (J84.2)

J70.4 Drug-induced interstitial lung disorders, unspecified HCC
Use additional code for adverse effect, if applicable, to identify drug (T36-T50 with fifth or sixth character 5)
EXCLUDES 1 *interstitial pneumonia NOS (J84.9)*
lymphoid interstitial pneumonia (J84.2)
AHA: 2019,2Q,28

J70.5 Respiratory conditions due to smoke inhalation HCC
Code first smoke inhalation (T59.81-)
EXCLUDES 2 *smoke inhalation due to chemicals, gases, fumes and vapors (J68.9)*
AHA: 2013,4Q,121

J70.8 Respiratory conditions due to other specified external agents HCC
Code first (T51-T65) to identify the external agent

J70.9 Respiratory conditions due to unspecified external agent HCC
Code first (T51-T65) to identify the external agent

Other respiratory diseases principally affecting the interstitium (J80-J84)

J80 Acute respiratory distress syndrome MCC HCC
Acute respiratory distress syndrome in adult or child
Adult hyaline membrane disease
EXCLUDES 1 *respiratory distress syndrome in newborn (perinatal) (P22.0)*
AHA: 2021,1Q,23; 2020,4Q,96; 2020,1Q,34-36; 2017,1Q,26
DEF: Lung inflammation or injury resulting in a build-up of fluid in the air sacs, preventing the passage of oxygen from the air into the bloodstream.
TIP: Assign as a secondary code for a patient with acute respiratory distress syndrome (ARDS) due to COVID-19; assign code U07.1 as the principal or first-listed code.

J81 Pulmonary edema
Use additional code to identify:
exposure to environmental tobacco smoke (Z77.22)
history of tobacco dependence (Z87.891)
occupational exposure to environmental tobacco smoke (Z57.31)
tobacco dependence (F17.-)
tobacco use (Z72.0)
EXCLUDES 1 *chemical (acute) pulmonary edema (J68.1)*
hypostatic pneumonia (J18.2)
passive pneumonia (J18.2)
pulmonary edema due to external agents (J60-J70)
pulmonary edema with heart disease NOS (I50.1)
pulmonary edema with heart failure (I50.1)
DEF: Accumulation of fluid in the air sacs of the lungs, making it difficult to breathe.

J81.0 Acute pulmonary edema MCC HCC
Acute edema of lung
AHA: 2023,1Q,25; 2020,3Q,27

J81.1 Chronic pulmonary edema CC
Pulmonary congestion (chronic) (passive)
Pulmonary edema NOS

J82 Pulmonary eosinophilia, not elsewhere classified
EXCLUDES 2 *pulmonary eosinophilia due to aspergillosis (B44.-)*
pulmonary eosinophilia due to drugs (J70.2-J70.4)
pulmonary eosinophilia due to specified parasitic infection (B50-B83)
pulmonary eosinophilia due to systemic connective tissue disorders (M30-M36)
pulmonary infiltrate NOS (R91.8)
DEF: Infiltration of eosinophils (white blood cells of the immune system) into the parenchyma of the lungs, resulting in cough, fever, and dyspnea.

J82.8 Pulmonary eosinophilia, not elsewhere classified
AHA: 2020,4Q,25-27

J82.81 Chronic eosinophilic pneumonia CC HCC
Eosinophilic pneumonia, NOS

J82.82 Acute eosinophilic pneumonia CC

J82.83 Eosinophilic asthma CC
Code first asthma, by type, such as:
mild intermittent asthma (J45.2-)
mild persistent asthma (J45.3-)
moderate persistent asthma (J45.4-)
severe persistent asthma (J45.5-)

J82.89 Other pulmonary eosinophilia, not elsewhere classified CC HCC
Allergic pneumonia
Loffler's pneumonia
Tropical (pulmonary) eosinophilia NOS

J84 Other interstitial pulmonary diseases

EXCLUDES 1 *drug-induced interstitial lung disorders (J70.2-J70.4)*
interstitial emphysema (J98.2)

EXCLUDES 2 *lung diseases due to external agents (J60-J70)*

DEF: Interstitial: Within the small spaces or gaps occurring in tissue or organs.

J84.0 Alveolar and parieto-alveolar conditions

J84.01 Alveolar proteinosis CC HCC

DEF: Reduced ventilation due to proteinaceous deposits on alveoli. Symptoms include dyspnea, cough, chest pain, weakness, weight loss, and hemoptysis.

J84.02 Pulmonary alveolar microlithiasis CC HCC

J84.03 Idiopathic pulmonary hemosiderosis CC HCC

Essential brown induration of lung

Code first underlying disease, such as:
disorders of iron metabolism (E83.1-)

EXCLUDES 1 *acute idiopathic pulmonary hemorrhage in infants [AIPHI] (R04.81)*

DEF: Fibrosis of the alveolar walls marked by abnormal accumulation of iron as hemosiderin in the lungs. It primarily affects children and symptoms include anemia, fluid in the lungs, and blood in the sputum. Etiology is unknown.

J84.09 Other alveolar and parieto-alveolar conditions CC HCC

J84.1 Other interstitial pulmonary diseases with fibrosis

EXCLUDES 1 *pulmonary fibrosis (chronic) due to inhalation of chemicals, gases, fumes or vapors (J68.4)*
pulmonary fibrosis (chronic) following radiation (J70.1)

J84.10 Pulmonary fibrosis, unspecified HCC

Capillary fibrosis of lung
Cirrhosis of lung (chronic) NOS
Fibrosis of lung (atrophic) (chronic) (confluent) (massive) (perialveolar) (peribronchial) NOS
Induration of lung (chronic) NOS
Postinflammatory pulmonary fibrosis

J84.11 Idiopathic interstitial pneumonia

EXCLUDES 1 *lymphoid interstitial pneumonia (J84.2)*
pneumocystis pneumonia (B59)

J84.111 Idiopathic interstitial pneumonia, not otherwise specified HCC

J84.112 Idiopathic pulmonary fibrosis HCC

Cryptogenic fibrosing alveolitis
Idiopathic fibrosing alveolitis

J84.113 Idiopathic non-specific interstitial pneumonitis HCC

EXCLUDES 1 *non-specific interstitial pneumonia NOS, or due to known underlying cause (J84.89)*

J84.114 Acute interstitial pneumonitis CC HCC

Hamman-Rich syndrome

EXCLUDES 1 *pneumocystis pneumonia (B59)*

J84.115 Respiratory bronchiolitis interstitial lung disease HCC

J84.116 Cryptogenic organizing pneumonia CC HCC

EXCLUDES 1 *organizing pneumonia NOS, or due to known underlying cause (J84.89)*

J84.117 Desquamative interstitial pneumonia CC HCC

J84.17 Other interstitial pulmonary diseases with fibrosis in diseases classified elsewhere

AHA: 2020,4Q,27-28

J84.170 Interstitial lung disease with progressive fibrotic phenotype in diseases classified elsewhere HCC

Progressive fibrotic interstitial lung disease

Code first underlying disease, such as:
lung diseases due to external agents (J60-J70)
rheumatoid arthritis (M05.00-M06.9)
sarcoidosis ▶(D86.-)◀
systemic connective tissue disorders (M30-M36)

J84.178 Other interstitial pulmonary diseases with fibrosis in diseases classified elsewhere HCC

Interstitial pneumonia (nonspecific) (usual) due to collagen vascular disease
Interstitial pneumonia (nonspecific) (usual) in diseases classified elsewhere
Organizing pneumonia due to collagen vascular disease
Organizing pneumonia in diseases classified elsewhere

Code first underlying disease, such as:
progressive systemic sclerosis (M34.0)
rheumatoid arthritis (M05.00-M06.9)
systemic lupus erythematosis (M32.0-M32.9)

J84.2 Lymphoid interstitial pneumonia CC HCC

Lymphoid interstitial pneumonitis

J84.8 Other specified interstitial pulmonary diseases

EXCLUDES 1 *exogenous lipoid pneumonia (J69.1)*
unspecified lipoid pneumonia (J69.1)

J84.81 Lymphangioleiomyomatosis MCC HCC

Lymphangiomyomatosis

J84.82 Adult pulmonary Langerhans cell histiocytosis CC HCC A

Adult PLCH

J84.83 Surfactant mutations of the lung MCC HCC

DEF: Genetic disorder resulting in insufficient secretion of a complex mixture of phospholipids and proteins that reduce surface tension in the alveoli following the onset of breathing to facilitate lung expansion in the newborn. It is the leading indication for pediatric lung transplantation.

J84.84 Other interstitial lung diseases of childhood

J84.841 Neuroendocrine cell hyperplasia of infancy MCC HCC

J84.842 Pulmonary interstitial glycogenosis MCC HCC

J84.843 Alveolar capillary dysplasia with vein misalignment MCC HCC

J84.848 Other interstitial lung diseases of childhood MCC HCC

J84.89 Other specified interstitial pulmonary diseases HCC

Endogenous lipoid pneumonia
Interstitial pneumonitis
Non-specific interstitial pneumonitis NOS
Organizing pneumonia NOS

Code first, if applicable:
poisoning due to drug or toxin (T51-T65 with fifth or sixth character to indicate intent), for toxic pneumonopathy
underlying cause of pneumonopathy, if known

Use additional code, for adverse effect, to identify drug (T36-T50 with fifth or sixth character 5), if drug-induced

EXCLUDES 1 *cryptogenic organizing pneumonia (J84.116)*
idiopathic non-specific interstitial pneumonitis (J84.113)
lymphoid interstitial pneumonia (J84.2)
lipoid pneumonia, exogenous or unspecified (J69.1)

AHA: 2021,4Q,106; 2021,1Q,48; 2019,2Q,28

J84.9 Interstitial pulmonary disease, unspecified CC HCC

Interstitial pneumonia NOS

Suppurative and necrotic conditions of the lower respiratory tract (J85-J86)

J85 Abscess of lung and mediastinum

Use additional code (B95-B97) to identify infectious agent

J85.0 Gangrene and necrosis of lung MCC HCC

J85.1 Abscess of lung with pneumonia MCC HCC

Code also the type of pneumonia

J85.2 Abscess of lung without pneumonia MCC HCC

Abscess of lung NOS

J85.3 Abscess of mediastinum MCC HCC

√4th **J86 Pyothorax**

Use additional code (B95-B97) to identify infectious agent

EXCLUDES 1 *abscess of lung (J85.-)*
pyothorax due to tuberculosis (A15.6)

DEF: Collection of pus in the pleural space that is commonly caused by an infection that spreads from the lung, such as bacterial pneumonia or a lung abscess.

J86.Ø Pyothorax with fistula MCC HCC
Bronchocutaneous fistula
Bronchopleural fistula
Hepatopleural fistula
Mediastinal fistula
Pleural fistula
Thoracic fistula
Any condition classifiable to J86.9 with fistula
DEF: Purulent infection of the respiratory cavity, with communication from a cavity to another structure.

J86.9 Pyothorax without fistula MCC HCC
Abscess of pleura
Abscess of thorax
Empyema (chest) (lung) (pleura)
Fibrinopurulent pleurisy
Purulent pleurisy
Pyopneumothorax
Septic pleurisy
Seropurulent pleurisy
Suppurative pleurisy

Other diseases of the pleura (J9Ø-J94)

J9Ø Pleural effusion, not elsewhere classified CC
Encysted pleurisy
Pleural effusion NOS
Pleurisy with effusion (exudative) (serous)

EXCLUDES 1 *chylous (pleural) effusion (J94.Ø)*
malignant pleural effusion (J91.Ø)
pleurisy NOS (RØ9.1)
tuberculous pleural effusion (A15.6)

DEF: Collection of lymph and other fluid within the pleural space.

√4th **J91 Pleural effusion in conditions classified elsewhere**

EXCLUDES 2 *pleural effusion in heart failure (I5Ø.-)*
pleural effusion in systemic lupus erythematosus (M32.13)

DEF: Collection of lymph and other fluid within the pleural space.

J91.Ø Malignant pleural effusion CC
Code first underlying neoplasm (CØØ-D49)
AHA: 2022,3Q,14

J91.8 Pleural effusion in other conditions classified elsewhere CC
Code first underlying disease, such as:
filariasis (B74.Ø-B74.9)
influenza (JØ9.X2, J1Ø.1, J11.1)
AHA: 2015,2Q,15
TIP: Assign this code as a secondary diagnosis to congestive heart failure (I5Ø.-) only if pleural effusion is specifically evaluated or treated.

Pleural Effusion

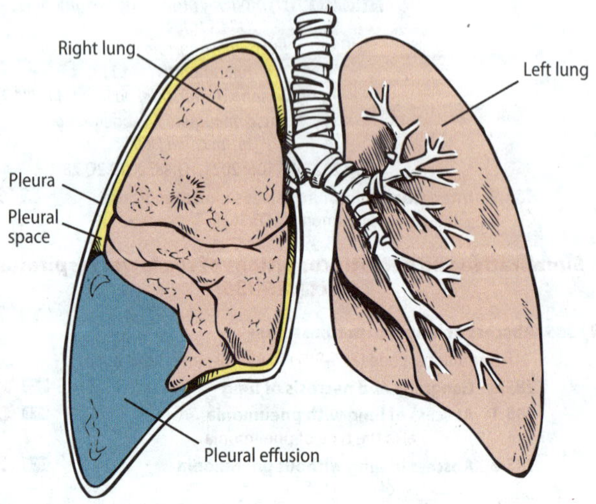

√4th **J92 Pleural plaque**

INCLUDES pleural thickening

DEF: Areas of fibrous thickening that form on the parietal or visceral pleura, the membranes that line the ribs and lungs.

J92.Ø Pleural plaque with presence of asbestos

J92.9 Pleural plaque without asbestos
Pleural plaque NOS

√4th **J93 Pneumothorax and air leak**

EXCLUDES 1 *congenital or perinatal pneumothorax (P25.1)*
postprocedural air leak (J95.812)
postprocedural pneumothorax (J95.811)
pyopneumothorax (J86.-)
traumatic pneumothorax (S27.Ø)
tuberculous (current disease) pneumothorax (A15.-)

DEF: Pneumothorax: Lung displacement due to abnormal leakage of air or gas that is trapped in the pleural space formed by the membrane that encloses the lungs and lines the thoracic cavity.

J93.Ø Spontaneous tension pneumothorax MCC
DEF: Leaking air from the lung into the lining, causing collapse.

√5th **J93.1 Other spontaneous pneumothorax**

J93.11 Primary spontaneous pneumothorax CC

J93.12 Secondary spontaneous pneumothorax CC UPD
Code first underlying condition, such as:
catamenial pneumothorax due to endometriosis (N8Ø.B-)
cystic fibrosis (E84.-)
eosinophilic pneumonia ▶(J82.81-J82.82)◀
lymphangioleiomyomatosis (J84.81)
malignant neoplasm of bronchus and lung (C34.-)
▶Marfan syndrome (Q87.4-)◀
pneumonia due to Pneumocystis carinii (B59)
secondary malignant neoplasm of lung (C78.Ø-)
spontaneous rupture of the esophagus (K22.3)

√5th **J93.8 Other pneumothorax and air leak**

J93.81 Chronic pneumothorax CC

J93.82 Other air leak CC
Persistent air leak

J93.83 Other pneumothorax CC
Acute pneumothorax
Spontaneous pneumothorax NOS
AHA: 2020,3Q,9-10

J93.9 Pneumothorax, unspecified CC
Pneumothorax NOS

√4th **J94 Other pleural conditions**

EXCLUDES 1 *pleurisy NOS (RØ9.1)*
traumatic hemopneumothorax (S27.2)
traumatic hemothorax (S27.1)
tuberculous pleural conditions (current disease) (A15.-)

J94.Ø Chylous effusion CC
Chyliform effusion
DEF: Fluid within the pleural space due to the leaking of lymph contents into the space, usually as a result of thoracic duct damage or injury or mediastinal lymphoma.

J94.1 Fibrothorax
DEF: Fibrosis within the pleural lining of the lungs commonly seen as a stiff layer surrounding the lung typically attributed to traumatic hemothorax or pleural effusion.

J94.2 Hemothorax CC
Hemopneumothorax

J94.8 Other specified pleural conditions CC
Hydropneumothorax
Hydrothorax
AHA: 2021,1Q,48

J94.9 Pleural condition, unspecified

Intraoperative and postprocedural complications and disorders of respiratory system, not elsewhere classified (J95)

✓4th **J95 Intraoperative and postprocedural complications and disorders of respiratory system, not elsewhere classified**

EXCLUDES 2 *aspiration pneumonia (J69.-)*
emphysema (subcutaneous) resulting from a procedure (T81.82)
hypostatic pneumonia (J18.2)
pulmonary manifestations due to radiation (J70.0-J70.1)

✓5th **J95.0 Tracheostomy complications**

DEF: Tracheostomy: Formation of a tracheal opening on the neck surface with tube insertion to allow for respiration in cases of obstruction or decreased patency. A tracheostomy may be planned or performed on an emergency basis for temporary or long-term use.

J95.00 Unspecified tracheostomy complication CC HCC

J95.01 Hemorrhage from tracheostomy stoma CC HCC

J95.02 Infection of tracheostomy stoma CC HCC

Use additional code to identify type of infection, such as:
cellulitis of neck (L03.221)
sepsis (A40, A41.-)

J95.03 Malfunction of tracheostomy stoma CC HCC

Mechanical complication of tracheostomy stoma
Obstruction of tracheostomy airway
Tracheal stenosis due to tracheostomy

J95.04 Tracheo-esophageal fistula following tracheostomy CC HCC

J95.09 Other tracheostomy complication CC HCC

J95.1 Acute pulmonary insufficiency following thoracic surgery MCC HCC

EXCLUDES 2 *functional disturbances following cardiac surgery (I97.0, I97.1-)*

J95.2 Acute pulmonary insufficiency following nonthoracic surgery MCC HCC

EXCLUDES 2 *functional disturbances following cardiac surgery (I97.0, I97.1-)*

J95.3 Chronic pulmonary insufficiency following surgery MCC HCC

EXCLUDES 2 *functional disturbances following cardiac surgery (I97.0, I97.1-)*

J95.4 Chemical pneumonitis due to anesthesia CC

Mendelson's syndrome
Postprocedural aspiration pneumonia
Use additional code for adverse effect, if applicable, to identify drug (T41.- with fifth or sixth character 5)

EXCLUDES 1 *aspiration pneumonitis due to anesthesia complicating labor and delivery (O74.0)*
aspiration pneumonitis due to anesthesia complicating pregnancy (O29)
aspiration pneumonitis due to anesthesia complicating the puerperium (O89.01)

J95.5 Postprocedural subglottic stenosis CC

✓5th **J95.6 Intraoperative hemorrhage and hematoma of a respiratory system organ or structure complicating a procedure**

EXCLUDES 1 *intraoperative hemorrhage and hematoma of a respiratory system organ or structure due to accidental puncture and laceration during procedure (J95.7-)*

J95.61 Intraoperative hemorrhage and hematoma of a respiratory system organ or structure complicating a respiratory system procedure CC

J95.62 Intraoperative hemorrhage and hematoma of a respiratory system organ or structure complicating other procedure CC

✓5th **J95.7 Accidental puncture and laceration of a respiratory system organ or structure during a procedure**

EXCLUDES 2 *postprocedural pneumothorax (J95.811)*

J95.71 Accidental puncture and laceration of a respiratory system organ or structure during a respiratory system procedure CC

J95.72 Accidental puncture and laceration of a respiratory system organ or structure during other procedure CC

✓5th **J95.8 Other intraoperative and postprocedural complications and disorders of respiratory system, not elsewhere classified**

AHA: 2016,4Q,9-10

✓6th **J95.81 Postprocedural pneumothorax and air leak**

J95.811 Postprocedural pneumothorax CC H14

AHA: 2021,1Q,48

J95.812 Postprocedural air leak CC

✓6th **J95.82 Postprocedural respiratory failure**

EXCLUDES 1 *respiratory failure in other conditions (J96.-)*

J95.821 Acute postprocedural respiratory failure MCC HCC

Postprocedural respiratory failure NOS

J95.822 Acute and chronic postprocedural respiratory failure MCC HCC

✓6th **J95.83 Postprocedural hemorrhage of a respiratory system organ or structure following a procedure**

AHA: 2023,2Q,28

J95.830 Postprocedural hemorrhage of a respiratory system organ or structure following a respiratory system procedure CC

J95.831 Postprocedural hemorrhage of a respiratory system organ or structure following other procedure CC

J95.84 Transfusion-related acute lung injury (TRALI) CC

DEF: Relatively rare, but serious, pulmonary complication of blood transfusion, with acute respiratory distress, noncardiogenic pulmonary edema, cyanosis, hypoxemia, hypotension, fever, and chills.

✓6th **J95.85 Complication of respirator [ventilator]**

J95.850 Mechanical complication of respirator CC HCC

EXCLUDES 1 *encounter for respirator [ventilator] dependence during power failure (Z99.12)*

J95.851 Ventilator associated pneumonia CC HCC

Ventilator associated pneumonitis
Use additional code to identify the organism, if known (B95.-, B96.-, B97.-)

EXCLUDES 1 *ventilator lung in newborn (P27.8)*

AHA: 2020,2Q,17; 2017,1Q,25

J95.859 Other complication of respirator [ventilator] CC HCC

AHA: 2021,1Q,48

✓6th **J95.86 Postprocedural hematoma and seroma of a respiratory system organ or structure following a procedure**

J95.860 Postprocedural hematoma of a respiratory system organ or structure following a respiratory system procedure CC

J95.861 Postprocedural hematoma of a respiratory system organ or structure following other procedure CC

J95.862 Postprocedural seroma of a respiratory system organ or structure following a respiratory system procedure CC

J95.863 Postprocedural seroma of a respiratory system organ or structure following other procedure CC

J95.87 Transfusion-associated dyspnea (TAD) CC

EXCLUDES 1 *transfusion associated circulatory overload (TACO) (E87.71)*
transfusion-related acute lung injury (TRALI) (J95.84)

AHA: 2022,4Q,27

J95.88 Other intraoperative complications of respiratory system, not elsewhere classified CC

J95.89 Other postprocedural complications and disorders of respiratory system, not elsewhere classified CC

Use additional code to identify disorder, such as:
aspiration pneumonia (J69.-)
bacterial or viral pneumonia (J12-J18)

EXCLUDES 2 *acute pulmonary insufficiency following thoracic surgery (J95.1)*
postprocedural subglottic stenosis (J95.5)

Other diseases of the respiratory system (J96-J99)

✓4th J96 Respiratory failure, not elsewhere classified

EXCLUDES 1 *acute respiratory distress syndrome (J8Ø)*
cardiorespiratory failure (RØ9.2)
newborn respiratory distress syndrome (P22.Ø)
postprocedural respiratory failure (J95.82-)
respiratory arrest (RØ9.2)
respiratory arrest of newborn (P28.81)
respiratory failure of newborn (P28.5)

AHA: 2021,1Q,27,44-45; 2020,4Q,96

✓5th J96.Ø Acute respiratory failure

J96.ØØ Acute respiratory failure, unspecified whether with hypoxia or hypercapnia MCC HCC
AHA: 2016,3Q,14; 2013,4Q,121

J96.Ø1 Acute respiratory failure with hypoxia MCC HCC
AHA: 2020,3Q,12

J96.Ø2 Acute respiratory failure with hypercapnia MCC HCC
Acute respiratory acidosis

✓5th J96.1 Chronic respiratory failure

J96.1Ø Chronic respiratory failure, unspecified whether with hypoxia or hypercapnia CC HCC
AHA: 2016,1Q,38; 2015,1Q,21

J96.11 Chronic respiratory failure with hypoxia CC HCC
AHA: 2013,4Q,129

J96.12 Chronic respiratory failure with hypercapnia CC HCC
Chronic respiratory acidosis

✓5th J96.2 Acute and chronic respiratory failure
Acute on chronic respiratory failure

J96.2Ø Acute and chronic respiratory failure, unspecified whether with hypoxia or hypercapnia MCC HCC

J96.21 Acute and chronic respiratory failure with hypoxia MCC HCC

J96.22 Acute and chronic respiratory failure with hypercapnia MCC HCC

✓5th J96.9 Respiratory failure, unspecified

J96.9Ø Respiratory failure, unspecified, unspecified whether with hypoxia or hypercapnia MCC HCC

J96.91 Respiratory failure, unspecified with hypoxia MCC HCC

J96.92 Respiratory failure, unspecified with hypercapnia MCC HCC

✓4th J98 Other respiratory disorders

Use additional code to identify:
exposure to environmental tobacco smoke (Z77.22)
exposure to tobacco smoke in the perinatal period (P96.81)
history of tobacco dependence (Z87.891)
occupational exposure to environmental tobacco smoke (Z57.31)
tobacco dependence (F17.-)
tobacco use (Z72.Ø)

EXCLUDES 1 *newborn apnea (P28.4-)*
newborn sleep apnea (P28.3-)

EXCLUDES 2 *apnea NOS (RØ6.81)*
sleep apnea (G47.3-)

✓5th J98.Ø Diseases of bronchus, not elsewhere classified

J98.Ø1 Acute bronchospasm

EXCLUDES 1 *acute bronchiolitis with bronchospasm (J21.-)*
acute bronchitis with bronchospasm (J2Ø.-)
asthma (J45.-)
exercise induced bronchospasm (J45.99Ø)

J98.Ø9 Other diseases of bronchus, not elsewhere classified
Broncholithiasis
Calcification of bronchus
Stenosis of bronchus
Tracheobronchial collapse
Tracheobronchial dyskinesia
Ulcer of bronchus
AHA: 2022,3Q,8

✓5th J98.1 Pulmonary collapse

EXCLUDES 1 *therapeutic collapse of lung status (Z98.3)*

J98.11 Atelectasis CC

EXCLUDES 1 *newborn atelectasis*
tuberculous atelectasis (current disease) (A15)

DEF: Collapse of lung tissue affecting part or all of one lung, preventing normal oxygen absorption to healthy tissues.

J98.19 Other pulmonary collapse CC

J98.2 Interstitial emphysema HCC
Mediastinal emphysema

EXCLUDES 1 *emphysema NOS (J43.9)*
emphysema in newborn (P25.Ø)
surgical emphysema (subcutaneous) (T81.82)
traumatic subcutaneous emphysema (T79.7)

J98.3 Compensatory emphysema HCC

DEF: Distention of all or part of the lung caused by disease processes or surgical intervention that decreased volume in another part of the lung, causing an overcompensation reaction. Compensatory emphysema occurs in association with pneumonias, pleural effusions, atelectasis, empyema, and pneumothorax.

J98.4 Other disorders of lung
Calcification of lung
Cystic lung disease (acquired)
Lung disease NOS
Pulmolithiasis

EXCLUDES 1 *acute interstitial pneumonitis (J84.114)*
pulmonary insufficiency following surgery (J95.1-J95.2)

✓5th J98.5 Diseases of mediastinum, not elsewhere classified

EXCLUDES 2 *abscess of mediastinum (J85.3)*

AHA: 2016,4Q,29

J98.51 Mediastinitis MCC H8
Code first underlying condition, if applicable, such as postoperative mediastinitis (T81.-)

J98.59 Other diseases of mediastinum, not elsewhere classified MCC H8
Fibrosis of mediastinum
Hernia of mediastinum
Retraction of mediastinum

J98.6 Disorders of diaphragm
Diaphragmatitis
Paralysis of diaphragm
Relaxation of diaphragm

EXCLUDES 1 *congenital malformation of diaphragm NEC (Q79.1)*
congenital diaphragmatic hernia (Q79.Ø)

EXCLUDES 2 *diaphragmatic hernia (K44.-)*

J98.8 Other specified respiratory disorders
AHA: 2020,1Q,34-36

TIP: Assign as a secondary code for a patient with a respiratory infection that is not further specified but is documented as being associated with COVID-19; assign U07.1 as the principal or first-listed code. If the respiratory infection documentation specifies acute or lower respiratory infection (NOS), assign J22 instead.

J98.9 Respiratory disorder, unspecified
Respiratory disease (chronic) NOS

J99 Respiratory disorders in diseases classified elsewhere HCC

Code first underlying disease, such as:
- amyloidosis (E85.-)
- ankylosing spondylitis ▶(M45.-)◀
- congenital syphilis ▶(A5Ø.-)◀
- cryoglobulinemia (D89.1)
- early congenital syphilis ▶(A5Ø.Ø-)◀
- plasminogen deficiency (E88.Ø2)
- schistosomiasis (B65.Ø-B65.9)

EXCLUDES 1 *respiratory disorders in:*
- *amebiasis (AØ6.5)*
- *blastomycosis (B4Ø.Ø-B4Ø.2)*
- *candidiasis (B37.1)*
- *coccidioidomycosis (B38.Ø-B38.2)*
- *cystic fibrosis with pulmonary manifestations (E84.Ø)*
- *dermatomyositis (M33.Ø1, M33.11)*
- *histoplasmosis (B39.Ø-B39.2)*
- *late syphilis (A52.72, A52.73)*
- *polymyositis (M33.21)*
- *Sjogren syndrome (M35.Ø2)*
- *systemic lupus erythematosus (M32.13)*
- *systemic sclerosis (M34.81)*
- *Wegener's granulomatosis (M31.3Ø-M31.31)*

Chapter 10. Diseases of the Respiratory System

J99–J99

Chapter 11. Diseases of the Digestive System (KØØ–K95)

Chapter-specific Guidelines with Coding Examples
Reserved for future guideline expansion.

Chapter 11. Diseases of the Digestive System (K00-K95)

EXCLUDES 2 *certain conditions originating in the perinatal period (P04-P96)*
certain infectious and parasitic diseases (A00-B99)
complications of pregnancy, childbirth and the puerperium (O00-O9A)
congenital malformations, deformations and chromosomal abnormalities (Q00-Q99)
endocrine, nutritional and metabolic diseases (E00-E88)
injury, poisoning and certain other consequences of external causes (S00-T88)
neoplasms (C00-D49)
symptoms, signs and abnormal clinical and laboratory findings, not elsewhere classified (R00-R94)

This chapter contains the following blocks:

K00-K14 Diseases of oral cavity and salivary glands
K20-K31 Diseases of esophagus, stomach and duodenum
K35-K38 Diseases of appendix
K40-K46 Hernia
K50-K52 Noninfective enteritis and colitis
K55-K64 Other diseases of intestines
K65-K68 Diseases of peritoneum and retroperitoneum
K70-K77 Diseases of liver
K80-K87 Disorders of gallbladder, biliary tract and pancreas
K90-K95 Other diseases of the digestive system

Diseases of oral cavity and salivary glands (K00-K14)

✓4th **K00 Disorders of tooth development and eruption**

EXCLUDES 2 *embedded and impacted teeth (K01.-)*

K00.0 Anodontia
Hypodontia
Oligodontia
EXCLUDES 1 *acquired absence of teeth (K08.1-)*
DEF: Partial or complete absence of teeth due to a congenital defect involving the tooth bud.

K00.1 Supernumerary teeth
Distomolar
Fourth molar
Mesiodens
Paramolar
Supplementary teeth
EXCLUDES 2 *supernumerary roots (K00.2)*

K00.2 Abnormalities of size and form of teeth
Concrescence of teeth
Fusion of teeth
Gemination of teeth
Dens evaginatus
Dens in dente
Dens invaginatus
Enamel pearls
Macrodontia
Microdontia
Peg-shaped [conical] teeth
Supernumerary roots
Taurodontism
Tuberculum paramolare
EXCLUDES 1 *abnormalities of teeth due to congenital syphilis (A50.5)*
tuberculum Carabelli, which is regarded as a normal variation and should not be coded

K00.3 Mottled teeth
Dental fluorosis
Mottling of enamel
Nonfluoride enamel opacities
EXCLUDES 2 *deposits [accretions] on teeth (K03.6)*

K00.4 Disturbances in tooth formation
Aplasia and hypoplasia of cementum
Dilaceration of tooth
Enamel hypoplasia (neonatal) (postnatal) (prenatal)
Regional odontodysplasia
Turner's tooth
EXCLUDES 1 *Hutchinson's teeth and mulberry molars in congenital syphilis (A50.5)*
EXCLUDES 2 *mottled teeth (K00.3)*

K00.5 Hereditary disturbances in tooth structure, not elsewhere classified
Amelogenesis imperfecta
Dentinogenesis imperfecta
Odontogenesis imperfecta
Dentinal dysplasia
Shell teeth

K00.6 Disturbances in tooth eruption
Dentia praecox
Natal tooth
Neonatal tooth
Premature eruption of tooth
Premature shedding of primary [deciduous] tooth
Prenatal teeth
Retained [persistent] primary tooth
EXCLUDES 2 *embedded and impacted teeth (K01.-)*

K00.7 Teething syndrome

K00.8 Other disorders of tooth development
Color changes during tooth formation
Intrinsic staining of teeth NOS
EXCLUDES 2 *posteruptive color changes (K03.7)*

K00.9 Disorder of tooth development, unspecified
Disorder of odontogenesis NOS

✓4th **K01 Embedded and impacted teeth**

EXCLUDES 1 *abnormal position of fully erupted teeth (M26.3-)*

K01.0 Embedded teeth

K01.1 Impacted teeth

✓4th **K02 Dental caries**

INCLUDES caries of dentine
dental cavities
early childhood caries
pre-eruptive caries
recurrent caries (dentino enamel junction) (enamel) (to the pulp)
tooth decay

Tooth Anatomy

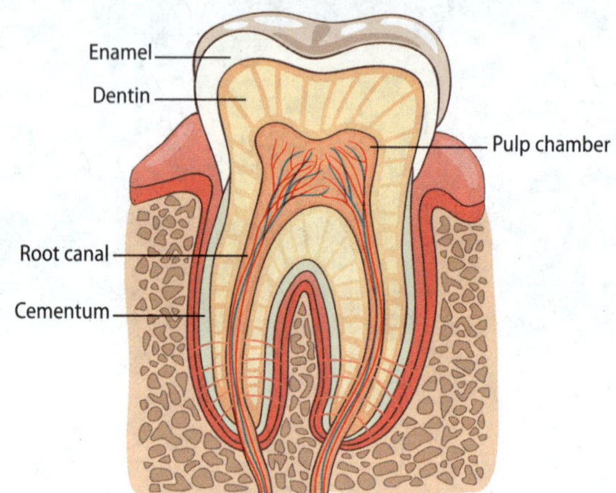

K02.3 Arrested dental caries
Arrested coronal and root caries

✓5th **K02.5 Dental caries on pit and fissure surface**
Dental caries on chewing surface of tooth

K02.51 Dental caries on pit and fissure surface limited to enamel
White spot lesions [initial caries] on pit and fissure surface of tooth

K02.52 Dental caries on pit and fissure surface penetrating into dentin
Primary dental caries, cervical origin

K02.53 Dental caries on pit and fissure surface penetrating into pulp

✓5th **K02.6 Dental caries on smooth surface**

K02.61 Dental caries on smooth surface limited to enamel
White spot lesions [initial caries] on smooth surface of tooth

K02.62 Dental caries on smooth surface penetrating into dentin

K02.63 Dental caries on smooth surface penetrating into pulp

K02.7 Dental root caries

K02.9 Dental caries, unspecified

K03 Other diseases of hard tissues of teeth

EXCLUDES 2 *bruxism (F45.8)*
dental caries (K02.-)
teeth-grinding NOS (F45.8)

K03.0 Excessive attrition of teeth
Approximal wear of teeth
Occlusal wear of teeth
DEF: Attrition: In dentistry, wearing away or erosion of tooth surface from abrasive food or grinding teeth.

K03.1 Abrasion of teeth
Dentifrice abrasion of teeth
Habitual abrasion of teeth
Occupational abrasion of teeth
Ritual abrasion of teeth
Traditional abrasion of teeth
Wedge defect NOS

K03.2 Erosion of teeth
Erosion of teeth due to diet
Erosion of teeth due to drugs and medicaments
Erosion of teeth due to persistent vomiting
Erosion of teeth NOS
Idiopathic erosion of teeth
Occupational erosion of teeth

K03.3 Pathological resorption of teeth
Internal granuloma of pulp
Resorption of teeth (external)

K03.4 Hypercementosis
Cementation hyperplasia

K03.5 Ankylosis of teeth

K03.6 Deposits [accretions] on teeth
Betel deposits [accretions] on teeth
Black deposits [accretions] on teeth
Extrinsic staining of teeth NOS
Green deposits [accretions] on teeth
Materia alba deposits [accretions] on teeth
Orange deposits [accretions] on teeth
Staining of teeth NOS
Subgingival dental calculus
Supragingival dental calculus
Tobacco deposits [accretions] on teeth

K03.7 Posteruptive color changes of dental hard tissues
EXCLUDES 2 *deposits [accretions] on teeth (K03.6)*

K03.8 Other specified diseases of hard tissues of teeth

K03.81 Cracked tooth
EXCLUDES 1 *asymptomatic craze lines in enamel - omit code*
broken or fractured tooth due to trauma (S02.5)

K03.89 Other specified diseases of hard tissues of teeth

K03.9 Disease of hard tissues of teeth, unspecified

K04 Diseases of pulp and periapical tissues
AHA: 2016,4Q,29-30

K04.0 Pulpitis
Acute pulpitis
Chronic (hyperplastic) (ulcerative) pulpitis

K04.01 Reversible pulpitis CC

K04.02 Irreversible pulpitis CC

K04.1 Necrosis of pulp
Pulpal gangrene

K04.2 Pulp degeneration
Denticles
Pulpal calcifications
Pulpal stones

K04.3 Abnormal hard tissue formation in pulp
Secondary or irregular dentine

K04.4 Acute apical periodontitis of pulpal origin CC
Acute apical periodontitis NOS
EXCLUDES 1 *acute periodontitis (K05.2-)*
DEF: Severe inflammation of the area surrounding the tip of a tooth's root that is often secondary to infection or trauma.

K04.5 Chronic apical periodontitis
Apical or periapical granuloma
Apical periodontitis NOS
EXCLUDES 1 *chronic periodontitis (K05.3-)*

K04.6 Periapical abscess with sinus
Dental abscess with sinus
Dentoalveolar abscess with sinus

K04.7 Periapical abscess without sinus
Dental abscess without sinus
Dentoalveolar abscess without sinus

K04.8 Radicular cyst
Apical (periodontal) cyst
Periapical cyst
Residual radicular cyst
EXCLUDES 2 *lateral periodontal cyst (K09.0)*
DEF: Most common odontogenic cyst in tissue around the tooth apex due to chronic inflammation of dental pulp.

K04.9 Other and unspecified diseases of pulp and periapical tissues

K04.90 Unspecified diseases of pulp and periapical tissues

K04.99 Other diseases of pulp and periapical tissues

K05 Gingivitis and periodontal diseases
Use additional code to identify:
alcohol abuse and dependence (F10.-)
exposure to environmental tobacco smoke (Z77.22)
exposure to tobacco smoke in the perinatal period (P96.81)
history of tobacco dependence (Z87.891)
occupational exposure to environmental tobacco smoke (Z57.31)
tobacco dependence (F17.-)
tobacco use (Z72.0)
AHA: 2016,4Q,29-30

K05.0 Acute gingivitis
EXCLUDES 1 *acute necrotizing ulcerative gingivitis (A69.1)*
herpesviral [herpes simplex] gingivostomatitis (B00.2)

K05.00 Acute gingivitis, plaque induced
Acute gingivitis NOS
Plaque induced gingival disease

K05.01 Acute gingivitis, non-plaque induced

K05.1 Chronic gingivitis
Desquamative gingivitis (chronic)
Gingivitis (chronic) NOS
Hyperplastic gingivitis (chronic)
Pregnancy associated gingivitis
Simple marginal gingivitis (chronic)
Ulcerative gingivitis (chronic)
Code first, if applicable, diseases of the digestive system complicating pregnacy (O99.61-)

K05.10 Chronic gingivitis, plaque induced
Chronic gingivitis NOS
Gingivitis NOS

K05.11 Chronic gingivitis, non-plaque induced

K05.2 Aggressive periodontitis
Acute pericoronitis
EXCLUDES 1 *acute apical periodontitis (K04.4)*
periapical abscess (K04.7)
periapical abscess with sinus (K04.6)

K05.20 Aggressive periodontitis, unspecified

K05.21 Aggressive periodontitis, localized
Periodontal abscess

K05.211 Aggressive periodontitis, localized, slight

K05.212 Aggressive periodontitis, localized, moderate

K05.213 Aggressive periodontitis, localized, severe

K05.219 Aggressive periodontitis, localized, unspecified severity

K05.22 Aggressive periodontitis, generalized

K05.221 Aggressive periodontitis, generalized, slight

K05.222 Aggressive periodontitis, generalized, moderate

K05.223 Aggressive periodontitis, generalized, severe

K05.229 Aggressive periodontitis, generalized, unspecified severity

K05.3 Chronic periodontitis
Chronic pericoronitis
Complex periodontitis
Periodontitis NOS
Simplex periodontitis
EXCLUDES 1 *chronic apical periodontitis (K04.5)*

K05.30 Chronic periodontitis, unspecified

K05.31 Chronic periodontitis, localized

K05.311 Chronic periodontitis, localized, slight

K05.312 Chronic periodontitis, localized, moderate

KØ5.313 Chronic periodontitis, localized, severe
KØ5.319 Chronic periodontitis, localized, unspecified severity

✓6th KØ5.32 Chronic periodontitis, generalized
KØ5.321 Chronic periodontitis, generalized, slight
KØ5.322 Chronic periodontitis, generalized, moderate
KØ5.323 Chronic periodontitis, generalized, severe
KØ5.329 Chronic periodontitis, generalized, unspecified

KØ5.4 Periodontosis
Juvenile periodontosis

KØ5.5 Other periodontal diseases
Combined periodontic-endodontic lesion
Narrow gingival width (of periodontal soft tissue)
EXCLUDES 2 *leukoplakia of gingiva (K13.21)*

KØ5.6 Periodontal disease, unspecified

✓4th KØ6 Other disorders of gingiva and edentulous alveolar ridge
EXCLUDES 2 *acute gingivitis (KØ5.Ø)*
atrophy of edentulous alveolar ridge (KØ8.2)
chronic gingivitis (KØ5.1)
gingivitis NOS (KØ5.1)
AHA: 2016,4Q,29-30

✓5th KØ6.Ø Gingival recession
Gingival recession (postinfective) (postprocedural)
AHA: 2017,4Q,16

✓6th KØ6.Ø1 Gingival recession, localized
KØ6.Ø1Ø Localized gingival recession, unspecified
Localized gingival recession, NOS
KØ6.Ø11 Localized gingival recession, minimal
KØ6.Ø12 Localized gingival recession, moderate
KØ6.Ø13 Localized gingival recession, severe

✓6th KØ6.Ø2 Gingival recession, generalized
KØ6.Ø2Ø Generalized gingival recession, unspecified
Generalized gingival recession, NOS
KØ6.Ø21 Generalized gingival recession, minimal
KØ6.Ø22 Generalized gingival recession, moderate
KØ6.Ø23 Generalized gingival recession, severe

KØ6.1 Gingival enlargement
Gingival fibromatosis

KØ6.2 Gingival and edentulous alveolar ridge lesions associated with trauma
Irritative hyperplasia of edentulous ridge [denture hyperplasia]
Use additional code (Chapter 2Ø) to identify external cause or denture status (Z97.2)

KØ6.3 Horizontal alveolar bone loss

KØ6.8 Other specified disorders of gingiva and edentulous alveolar ridge
Fibrous epulis
Flabby alveolar ridge
Giant cell epulis
Peripheral giant cell granuloma of gingiva
Pyogenic granuloma of gingiva
Vertical ridge deficiency
EXCLUDES 2 *gingival cyst (KØ9.Ø)*

KØ6.9 Disorder of gingiva and edentulous alveolar ridge, unspecified

✓4th KØ8 Other disorders of teeth and supporting structures
EXCLUDES 2 *dentofacial anomalies [including malocclusion] (M26.-)*
disorders of jaw (M27.-)
AHA: 2016,4Q,29-30

KØ8.Ø Exfoliation of teeth due to systemic causes
Code also underlying systemic condition

✓5th KØ8.1 Complete loss of teeth
Acquired loss of teeth, complete
EXCLUDES 1 *congenital absence of teeth (KØØ.Ø)*
exfoliation of teeth due to systemic causes (KØ8.Ø)
partial loss of teeth (KØ8.4-)

✓6th KØ8.1Ø Complete loss of teeth, unspecified cause
KØ8.1Ø1 Complete loss of teeth, unspecified cause, class I
KØ8.1Ø2 Complete loss of teeth, unspecified cause, class II
KØ8.1Ø3 Complete loss of teeth, unspecified cause, class III
KØ8.1Ø4 Complete loss of teeth, unspecified cause, class IV
KØ8.1Ø9 Complete loss of teeth, unspecified cause, unspecified class
Edentulism NOS

✓6th KØ8.11 Complete loss of teeth due to trauma
KØ8.111 Complete loss of teeth due to trauma, class I
KØ8.112 Complete loss of teeth due to trauma, class II
KØ8.113 Complete loss of teeth due to trauma, class III
KØ8.114 Complete loss of teeth due to trauma, class IV
KØ8.119 Complete loss of teeth due to trauma, unspecified class

✓6th KØ8.12 Complete loss of teeth due to periodontal diseases
KØ8.121 Complete loss of teeth due to periodontal diseases, class I
KØ8.122 Complete loss of teeth due to periodontal diseases, class II
KØ8.123 Complete loss of teeth due to periodontal diseases, class III
KØ8.124 Complete loss of teeth due to periodontal diseases, class IV
KØ8.129 Complete loss of teeth due to periodontal diseases, unspecified class

✓6th KØ8.13 Complete loss of teeth due to caries
KØ8.131 Complete loss of teeth due to caries, class I
KØ8.132 Complete loss of teeth due to caries, class II
KØ8.133 Complete loss of teeth due to caries, class III
KØ8.134 Complete loss of teeth due to caries, class IV
KØ8.139 Complete loss of teeth due to caries, unspecified class

✓6th KØ8.19 Complete loss of teeth due to other specified cause
KØ8.191 Complete loss of teeth due to other specified cause, class I
KØ8.192 Complete loss of teeth due to other specified cause, class II
KØ8.193 Complete loss of teeth due to other specified cause, class III
KØ8.194 Complete loss of teeth due to other specified cause, class IV
KØ8.199 Complete loss of teeth due to other specified cause, unspecified class

✓5th KØ8.2 Atrophy of edentulous alveolar ridge
KØ8.2Ø Unspecified atrophy of edentulous alveolar ridge
Atrophy of the mandible NOS
Atrophy of the maxilla NOS
KØ8.21 Minimal atrophy of the mandible
Minimal atrophy of the edentulous mandible
KØ8.22 Moderate atrophy of the mandible
Moderate atrophy of the edentulous mandible
KØ8.23 Severe atrophy of the mandible
Severe atrophy of the edentulous mandible
KØ8.24 Minimal atrophy of maxilla
Minimal atrophy of the edentulous maxilla
KØ8.25 Moderate atrophy of the maxilla
Moderate atrophy of the edentulous maxilla
KØ8.26 Severe atrophy of the maxilla
Severe atrophy of the edentulous maxilla

KØ8.3 Retained dental root

✓5th KØ8.4 Partial loss of teeth
Acquired loss of teeth, partial
EXCLUDES 1 *complete loss of teeth (KØ8.1-)*
congenital absence of teeth (KØØ.Ø)
EXCLUDES 2 *exfoliation of teeth due to systemic causes (KØ8.Ø)*

✓6th KØ8.4Ø Partial loss of teeth, unspecified cause
KØ8.4Ø1 Partial loss of teeth, unspecified cause, class I
KØ8.4Ø2 Partial loss of teeth, unspecified cause, class II
KØ8.4Ø3 Partial loss of teeth, unspecified cause, class III
KØ8.4Ø4 Partial loss of teeth, unspecified cause, class IV

K08.409 Partial loss of teeth, unspecified cause, unspecified class
Tooth extraction status NOS

K08.41 Partial loss of teeth due to trauma

K08.411 Partial loss of teeth due to trauma, class I

K08.412 Partial loss of teeth due to trauma, class II

K08.413 Partial loss of teeth due to trauma, class III

K08.414 Partial loss of teeth due to trauma, class IV

K08.419 Partial loss of teeth due to trauma, unspecified class

K08.42 Partial loss of teeth due to periodontal diseases

K08.421 Partial loss of teeth due to periodontal diseases, class I

K08.422 Partial loss of teeth due to periodontal diseases, class II

K08.423 Partial loss of teeth due to periodontal diseases, class III

K08.424 Partial loss of teeth due to periodontal diseases, class IV

K08.429 Partial loss of teeth due to periodontal diseases, unspecified class

K08.43 Partial loss of teeth due to caries

K08.431 Partial loss of teeth due to caries, class I

K08.432 Partial loss of teeth due to caries, class II

K08.433 Partial loss of teeth due to caries, class III

K08.434 Partial loss of teeth due to caries, class IV

K08.439 Partial loss of teeth due to caries, unspecified class

K08.49 Partial loss of teeth due to other specified cause

K08.491 Partial loss of teeth due to other specified cause, class I

K08.492 Partial loss of teeth due to other specified cause, class II

K08.493 Partial loss of teeth due to other specified cause, class III

K08.494 Partial loss of teeth due to other specified cause, class IV

K08.499 Partial loss of teeth due to other specified cause, unspecified class

K08.5 Unsatisfactory restoration of tooth
Defective bridge, crown, filling
Defective dental restoration
EXCLUDES 1 *dental restoration status (Z98.811)*
EXCLUDES 2 *endosseous dental implant failure (M27.6-)*
unsatisfactory endodontic treatment (M27.5-)

K08.50 Unsatisfactory restoration of tooth, unspecified
Defective dental restoration NOS

K08.51 Open restoration margins of tooth
Dental restoration failure of marginal integrity
Open margin on tooth restoration
Poor gingival margin to tooth restoration

K08.52 Unrepairable overhanging of dental restorative materials
Overhanging of tooth restoration

K08.53 Fractured dental restorative material
EXCLUDES 1 *cracked tooth (K03.81)*
traumatic fracture of tooth (S02.5)

K08.530 Fractured dental restorative material without loss of material

K08.531 Fractured dental restorative material with loss of material

K08.539 Fractured dental restorative material, unspecified

K08.54 Contour of existing restoration of tooth biologically incompatible with oral health
Dental restoration failure of periodontal anatomical integrity
Unacceptable contours of existing restoration of tooth
Unacceptable morphology of existing restoration of tooth

K08.55 Allergy to existing dental restorative material
Use additional code to identify the specific type of allergy

K08.56 Poor aesthetic of existing restoration of tooth
Dental restoration aesthetically inadequate or displeasing

K08.59 Other unsatisfactory restoration of tooth
Other defective dental restoration

K08.8 Other specified disorders of teeth and supporting structures

K08.81 Primary occlusal trauma

K08.82 Secondary occlusal trauma

K08.89 Other specified disorders of teeth and supporting structures
Enlargement of alveolar ridge NOS
Insufficient anatomic crown height
Insufficient clinical crown length
Irregular alveolar process
Toothache NOS

K08.9 Disorder of teeth and supporting structures, unspecified

K09 Cysts of oral region, not elsewhere classified
INCLUDES lesions showing histological features both of aneurysmal cyst and of another fibro-osseous lesion
EXCLUDES 2 *cysts of jaw (M27.0-, M27.4-)*
radicular cyst (K04.8)

K09.0 Developmental odontogenic cysts
Dentigerous cyst
Eruption cyst
Follicular cyst
Gingival cyst
Lateral periodontal cyst
Primordial cyst
EXCLUDES 2 *keratocysts (D16.4, D16.5)*
odontogenic keratocystic tumors (D16.4, D16.5)

K09.1 Developmental (nonodontogenic) cysts of oral region
Cyst (of) incisive canal
Cyst (of) palatine of papilla
Globulomaxillary cyst
Median palatal cyst
Nasoalveolar cyst
Nasolabial cyst
Nasopalatine duct cyst

K09.8 Other cysts of oral region, not elsewhere classified
Dermoid cyst
Epidermoid cyst
Epstein's pearl
Lymphoepithelial cyst

K09.9 Cyst of oral region, unspecified

K11 Diseases of salivary glands
Use additional code to identify:
alcohol abuse and dependence (F10.-)
exposure to environmental tobacco smoke (Z77.22)
exposure to tobacco smoke in the perinatal period (P96.81)
history of tobacco dependence (Z87.891)
occupational exposure to environmental tobacco smoke (Z57.31)
tobacco dependence (F17.-)
tobacco use (Z72.0)

K11.0 Atrophy of salivary gland

K11.1 Hypertrophy of salivary gland
DEF: Overgrowth of or enlarged salivary gland tissue caused by infection, salivary duct blockage, autoimmune diseases, and benign and malignant tumors.

K11.2 Sialoadenitis
Parotitis
EXCLUDES 1 *epidemic parotitis (B26.-)*
mumps (B26.-)
uveoparotid fever [Heerfordt] (D86.89)
DEF: Inflammation of the salivary gland.

K11.20 Sialoadenitis, unspecified

K11.21 Acute sialoadenitis
EXCLUDES 1 *acute recurrent sialoadenitis (K11.22)*

K11.22 Acute recurrent sialoadenitis

K11.23 Chronic sialoadenitis

K11.3 Abscess of salivary gland CC

K11.4 Fistula of salivary gland CC
EXCLUDES 1 *congenital fistula of salivary gland (Q38.4)*

K11.5 Sialolithiasis
Calculus of salivary gland or duct
Stone of salivary gland or duct

K11.6 Mucocele of salivary gland
Mucous extravasation cyst of salivary gland
Mucous retention cyst of salivary gland
Ranula

K11.7 Disturbances of salivary secretion
Hypoptyalism
Ptyalism
Xerostomia
EXCLUDES 2 *dry mouth NOS (R68.2)*

K11.8 Other diseases of salivary glands
Benign lymphoepithelial lesion of salivary gland
Mikulicz' disease
Necrotizing sialometaplasia
Sialectasia
Stenosis of salivary duct
Stricture of salivary duct
EXCLUDES 1 *Sjogren syndrome (M35.Ø-)*

K11.9 Disease of salivary gland, unspecified
Sialoadenopathy NOS

✓4th K12 Stomatitis and related lesions
Use additional code to identify:
alcohol abuse and dependence (F1Ø.-)
exposure to environmental tobacco smoke (Z77.22)
exposure to tobacco smoke in the perinatal period (P96.81)
history of tobacco dependence (Z87.891)
occupational exposure to environmental tobacco smoke (Z57.31)
tobacco dependence (F17.-)
tobacco use (Z72.Ø)
EXCLUDES 1 *cancrum oris (A69.Ø)*
cheilitis (K13.Ø)
gangrenous stomatitis (A69.Ø)
herpesviral [herpes simplex] gingivostomatitis (BØØ.2)
noma (A69.Ø)

K12.Ø Recurrent oral aphthae
Aphthous stomatitis (major) (minor)
Bednar's aphthae
Periadenitis mucosa necrotica recurrens
Recurrent aphthous ulcer
Stomatitis herpetiformis
DEF: Disorder of unknown etiology with small oval or round painful ulcers of the mouth marked by a grayish exudate and a red halo effect.

K12.1 Other forms of stomatitis
Stomatitis NOS
Denture stomatitis
Ulcerative stomatitis
Vesicular stomatitis
EXCLUDES 1 *acute necrotizing ulcerative stomatitis (A69.1)*
Vincent's stomatitis (A69.1)

K12.2 Cellulitis and abscess of mouth CC
Cellulitis of mouth (floor)
Submandibular abscess
EXCLUDES 2 *abscess of salivary gland (K11.3)*
abscess of tongue (K14.Ø)
periapical abscess (KØ4.6-KØ4.7)
periodontal abscess (KØ5.21)
peritonsillar abscess (J36)

✓5th K12.3 Oral mucositis (ulcerative)
Mucositis (oral) (oropharyneal)
EXCLUDES 2 *gastrointestinal mucositis (ulcerative) (K92.81)*
mucositis (ulcerative) of vagina and vulva (N76.81)
nasal mucositis (ulcerative) (J34.81)

K12.3Ø Oral mucositis (ulcerative), unspecified

K12.31 Oral mucositis (ulcerative) due to antineoplastic therapy
Use additional code for adverse effect, if applicable, to identify antineoplastic and immunosuppressive drugs (T45.1X5)
Use additional code for other antineoplastic therapy, such as:
radiological procedure and radiotherapy (Y84.2)

K12.32 Oral mucositis (ulcerative) due to other drugs
Use additional code for adverse effect, if applicable, to identify drug (T36-T5Ø with fifth or sixth character 5)

K12.33 Oral mucositis (ulcerative) due to radiation
Use additional external cause code (W88-W9Ø, X39.Ø-) to identify cause

K12.39 Other oral mucositis (ulcerative)
Viral oral mucositis (ulcerative)

✓4th K13 Other diseases of lip and oral mucosa
INCLUDES epithelial disturbances of tongue
Use additional code to identify:
alcohol abuse and dependence (F1Ø.-)
exposure to environmental tobacco smoke (Z77.22)
exposure to tobacco smoke in the perinatal period (P96.81)
history of tobacco dependence (Z87.891)
occupational exposure to environmental tobacco smoke (Z57.31)
tobacco dependence (F17.-)
tobacco use (Z72.Ø)
EXCLUDES 2 *certain disorders of gingiva and edentulous alveolar ridge (KØ5-KØ6)*
cysts of oral region (KØ9.-)
diseases of tongue (K14.-)
stomatitis and related lesions (K12.-)

K13.Ø Diseases of lips
Abscess of lips
Angular cheilitis
Cellulitis of lips
Cheilitis NOS
Cheilodynia
Cheilosis
Exfoliative cheilitis
Fistula of lips
Glandular cheilitis
Hypertrophy of lips
Perlèche NEC
EXCLUDES 1 *ariboflavinosis (E53.Ø)*
cheilitis due to radiation-related disorders (L55-L59)
congenital fistula of lips (Q38.Ø)
congenital hypertrophy of lips (Q18.6)
perlèche due to candidiasis (B37.83)
perlèche due to riboflavin deficiency (E53.Ø)

K13.1 Cheek and lip biting

✓5th K13.2 Leukoplakia and other disturbances of oral epithelium, including tongue
EXCLUDES 1 *carcinoma in situ of oral epithelium (DØØ.Ø-)*
hairy leukoplakia (K13.3)
DEF: Leukoplakia: Thickened white patches or lesions appearing on a mucous membrane, such as oral mucosa or tongue.

K13.21 Leukoplakia of oral mucosa, including tongue
Leukokeratosis of oral mucosa
Leukoplakia of gingiva, lips, tongue
EXCLUDES 1 *hairy leukoplakia (K13.3)*
leukokeratosis nicotina palati (K13.24)

K13.22 Minimal keratinized residual ridge mucosa
Minimal keratinization of alveolar ridge mucosa

K13.23 Excessive keratinized residual ridge mucosa
Excessive keratinization of alveolar ridge mucosa

K13.24 Leukokeratosis nicotina palati
Smoker's palate

K13.29 Other disturbances of oral epithelium, including tongue
Erythroplakia of mouth or tongue
Focal epithelial hyperplasia of mouth or tongue
Leukoedema of mouth or tongue
Other oral epithelium disturbances

K13.3 Hairy leukoplakia

K13.4 Granuloma and granuloma-like lesions of oral mucosa
Eosinophilic granuloma
Granuloma pyogenicum
Verrucous xanthoma

K13.5 Oral submucous fibrosis
Submucous fibrosis of tongue

K13.6 Irritative hyperplasia of oral mucosa
EXCLUDES 2 *irritative hyperplasia of edentulous ridge [denture hyperplasia] (KØ6.2)*

✓5th K13.7 Other and unspecified lesions of oral mucosa

K13.7Ø Unspecified lesions of oral mucosa

K13.79 Other lesions of oral mucosa
Focal oral mucinosis
AHA: 2022,2Q,7

K14 Diseases of tongue

Use additional code to identify:
alcohol abuse and dependence (F1Ø.-)
exposure to environmental tobacco smoke (Z77.22)
history of tobacco dependence (Z87.891)
occupational exposure to environmental tobacco smoke (Z57.31)
tobacco dependence (F17.-)
tobacco use (Z72.Ø)

EXCLUDES 2 *erythroplakia (K13.29)*
focal epithelial hyperplasia (K13.29)
leukedema of tongue (K13.29)
leukoplakia of tongue (K13.21)
hairy leukoplakia (K13.3)
macroglossia (congenital) (Q38.2)
submucous fibrosis of tongue (K13.5)

K14.Ø Glossitis
Abscess of tongue
Ulceration (traumatic) of tongue
EXCLUDES 1 *atrophic glossitis (K14.4)*
DEF: Inflammation and swelling of the tongue that may be associated with infection, adverse drug reactions, smoking, or injury.

K14.1 Geographic tongue
Benign migratory glossitis
Glossitis areata exfoliativa

K14.2 Median rhomboid glossitis

K14.3 Hypertrophy of tongue papillae
Black hairy tongue
Coated tongue
Hypertrophy of foliate papillae
Lingua villosa nigra

K14.4 Atrophy of tongue papillae
Atrophic glossitis

K14.5 Plicated tongue
Fissured tongue
Furrowed tongue
Scrotal tongue
EXCLUDES 1 *fissured tongue, congenital (Q38.3)*

K14.6 Glossodynia
Glossopyrosis
Painful tongue

K14.8 Other diseases of tongue
Atrophy of tongue
Crenated tongue
Enlargement of tongue
Glossocele
Glossoptosis
Hypertrophy of tongue

K14.9 Disease of tongue, unspecified
Glossopathy NOS

Diseases of esophagus, stomach and duodenum (K2Ø-K31)

EXCLUDES 2 *hiatus hernia (K44.-)*

K2Ø Esophagitis

Use additional code to identify:
alcohol abuse and dependence (F1Ø.-)

EXCLUDES 1 *erosion of esophagus (K22.1-)*
esophagitis with gastro-esophageal reflux disease (K21.Ø-)
reflux esophagitis (K21.Ø-)
ulcerative esophagitis (K22.1-)

EXCLUDES 2 *eosinophilic gastritis or gastroenteritis (K52.81)*

AHA: 2023,1Q,20

K2Ø.Ø Eosinophilic esophagitis
AHA: 2020,4Q,9

K2Ø.8 Other esophagitis
AHA: 2020,4Q,28-29

K2Ø.8Ø Other esophagitis without bleeding
Abscess of esophagus
Other esophagitis NOS

K2Ø.81 Other esophagitis with bleeding MCC

K2Ø.9 Esophagitis, unspecified
AHA: 2020,4Q,28-29

K2Ø.9Ø Esophagitis, unspecified without bleeding
Esophagitis NOS

K2Ø.91 Esophagitis, unspecified with bleeding MCC

K21 Gastro-esophageal reflux disease
EXCLUDES 1 *newborn esophageal reflux (P78.83)*

K21.Ø Gastro-esophageal reflux disease with esophagitis
AHA: 2020,4Q,28-29

K21.ØØ Gastro-esophageal reflux disease with esophagitis, without bleeding
Reflux esophagitis

K21.Ø1 Gastro-esophageal reflux disease with esophagitis, with bleeding MCC

K21.9 Gastro-esophageal reflux disease without esophagitis
Esophageal reflux NOS
AHA: 2016,1Q,18

K22 Other diseases of esophagus
EXCLUDES 2 *esophageal varices (I85.-)*

K22.Ø Achalasia of cardia
Achalasia NOS
Cardiospasm
EXCLUDES 1 *congenital cardiospasm (Q39.5)*
DEF: Esophageal motility disorder that is caused by absence of the esophageal peristalsis and impaired relaxation of the lower esophageal sphincter. It is characterized by dysphagia, regurgitation, and heartburn.

K22.1 Ulcer of esophagus
Barrett's ulcer
Erosion of esophagus
Fungal ulcer of esophagus
Peptic ulcer of esophagus
Ulcer of esophagus due to ingestion of chemicals
Ulcer of esophagus due to ingestion of drugs and medicaments
Ulcerative esophagitis
Code first poisoning due to drug or toxin, if applicable ▶(T36-T65 with fifth or sixth character 1-4)◀
Use additional code for adverse effect, if applicable, to identify drug (T36-T5Ø with fifth or sixth character 5)
EXCLUDES 1 *Barrett's esophagus (K22.7-)*
AHA: 2018,3Q,22; 2017,3Q,27
TIP: Assign a code for "with bleeding" when an esophageal ulcer and bleeding (hematemesis) are documented. The ICD-10-CM classification assumes the two are related without the provider linking the two conditions. Evidence of bleeding during a procedure is not required.

K22.1Ø Ulcer of esophagus without bleeding CC
Ulcer of esophagus NOS

K22.11 Ulcer of esophagus with bleeding MCC
EXCLUDES 2 *bleeding esophageal varices (I85.Ø1, I85.11)*
AHA: 2023,1Q,20
TIP: For bleeding esophageal ulcers resulting from anticoagulant therapy, assign this code, code D68.32 Hemorrhagic disorder due to extrinsic circulating anticoagulant, and adverse effect code T45.515- with the appropriate seventh character. Either code K22.11 or D68.32 may be sequenced first, depending on the circumstances of admission.

K22.2 Esophageal obstruction
Compression of esophagus
Constriction of esophagus
Stenosis of esophagus
Stricture of esophagus
EXCLUDES 1 *congenital stenosis or stricture of esophagus (Q39.3)*

K22.3 Perforation of esophagus MCC
Rupture of esophagus
EXCLUDES 1 *traumatic perforation of (thoracic) esophagus (S27.8-)*

K22.4 Dyskinesia of esophagus
Corkscrew esophagus
Diffuse esophageal spasm
Spasm of esophagus
EXCLUDES 1 *cardiospasm (K22.Ø)*

K22.5 Diverticulum of esophagus, acquired
Esophageal pouch, acquired
EXCLUDES 1 *diverticulum of esophagus (congenital) (Q39.6)*

K22.6 Gastro-esophageal laceration-hemorrhage syndrome MCC
Mallory-Weiss syndrome

√5th **K22.7 Barrett's esophagus**
Barrett's disease
Barrett's syndrome
EXCLUDES 1 *Barrett's ulcer (K22.1)*
malignant neoplasm of esophagus (C15.-)
DEF: Metaplastic disorder in which specialized columnar epithelial cells replace the normal squamous epithelial cells. Secondary to chronic gastroesophageal reflux damage to the mucosa, this disorder increases the risk of developing adenocarcinoma.

K22.70 Barrett's esophagus without dysplasia
Barrett's esophagus NOS

√6th **K22.71 Barrett's esophagus with dysplasia**
K22.710 Barrett's esophagus with low grade dysplasia
K22.711 Barrett's esophagus with high grade dysplasia
K22.719 Barrett's esophagus with dysplasia, unspecified

√5th **K22.8 Other specified diseases of esophagus**
EXCLUDES 2 *esophageal varices (I85.-)*
Paterson-Kelly syndrome (D50.1)
AHA: 2021,4Q,15; 2020,1Q,16

K22.81 Esophageal polyp
EXCLUDES 1 *benign neoplasm of esophagus (D13.0)*

K22.82 Esophagogastric junction polyp
EXCLUDES 1 *benign neoplasm of stomach (D13.1)*

K22.89 Other specified disease of esophagus
Hemorrhage of esophagus NOS

K22.9 Disease of esophagus, unspecified

K23 Disorders of esophagus in diseases classified elsewhere
Code first underlying disease, such as:
congenital syphilis (A50.5)
EXCLUDES 1 *late syphilis (A52.79)*
megaesophagus due to Chagas' disease (B57.31)
tuberculosis (A18.83)

√4th **K25 Gastric ulcer**
INCLUDES erosion (acute) of stomach
pylorus ulcer (peptic)
stomach ulcer (peptic)
Use additional code to identify:
alcohol abuse and dependence (F10.-)
EXCLUDES 1 *acute gastritis (K29.0-)*
peptic ulcer NOS (K27.-)
AHA: 2021,1Q,9,11; 2017,3Q,27
TIP: Assign a code for "with hemorrhage" when a gastric ulcer and GI bleeding are documented. The ICD-10-CM classification assumes the two are related without the provider linking the two conditions. Evidence of bleeding during a procedure is not required.
TIP: For bleeding ulcers resulting from anticoagulant therapy, assign the appropriate "with hemorrhage" ulcer code from this category, code D68.32 Hemorrhagic disorder due to extrinsic circulating anticoagulant, and adverse effect code T45.515- with the appropriate seventh character. Either the bleeding ulcer code or code D68.32 may be sequenced first, depending on the circumstances of admission.

K25.0 Acute gastric ulcer with hemorrhage MCC
AHA: 2023,1Q,16
K25.1 Acute gastric ulcer with perforation MCC HCC
K25.2 Acute gastric ulcer with both hemorrhage and perforation MCC HCC
K25.3 Acute gastric ulcer without hemorrhage or perforation CC
K25.4 Chronic or unspecified gastric ulcer with hemorrhage MCC
K25.5 Chronic or unspecified gastric ulcer with perforation MCC HCC
K25.6 Chronic or unspecified gastric ulcer with both hemorrhage and perforation MCC HCC
K25.7 Chronic gastric ulcer without hemorrhage or perforation
K25.9 Gastric ulcer, unspecified as acute or chronic, without hemorrhage or perforation

Gastrointestinal Ulcers

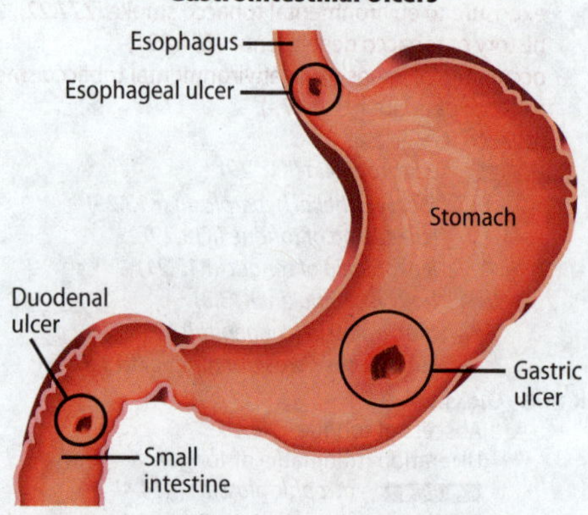

√4th **K26 Duodenal ulcer**
INCLUDES duodenum ulcer (peptic)
erosion (acute) of duodenum
postpyloric ulcer (peptic)
Use additional code to identify:
alcohol abuse and dependence (F10.-)
EXCLUDES 1 *peptic ulcer NOS (K27.-)*
AHA: 2023,2Q,11; 2017,3Q,27
TIP: Assign a code for "with hemorrhage" when a duodenal ulcer and GI bleeding are documented. The ICD-10-CM classification assumes the two are related without the provider linking the two conditions. Evidence of bleeding during a procedure is not required.
TIP: For bleeding ulcers resulting from anticoagulant therapy, assign the appropriate "with hemorrhage" ulcer code from this category, code D68.32 Hemorrhagic disorder due to extrinsic circulating anticoagulant, and adverse effect code T45.515- with the appropriate seventh character. Either the bleeding ulcer code or code D68.32 may be sequenced first, depending on the circumstances of admission.

K26.0 Acute duodenal ulcer with hemorrhage MCC
K26.1 Acute duodenal ulcer with perforation MCC HCC
K26.2 Acute duodenal ulcer with both hemorrhage and perforation MCC HCC
K26.3 Acute duodenal ulcer without hemorrhage or perforation CC
K26.4 Chronic or unspecified duodenal ulcer with hemorrhage MCC
AHA: 2016,1Q,14
K26.5 Chronic or unspecified duodenal ulcer with perforation MCC HCC
K26.6 Chronic or unspecified duodenal ulcer with both hemorrhage and perforation MCC HCC
K26.7 Chronic duodenal ulcer without hemorrhage or perforation
K26.9 Duodenal ulcer, unspecified as acute or chronic, without hemorrhage or perforation

√4th **K27 Peptic ulcer, site unspecified**
INCLUDES gastroduodenal ulcer NOS
peptic ulcer NOS
Use additional code to identify:
alcohol abuse and dependence (F10.-)
EXCLUDES 1 *peptic ulcer of newborn (P78.82)*
AHA: 2017,3Q,27
TIP: Assign a code for "with hemorrhage" when a peptic ulcer and GI bleeding are documented. The ICD-10-CM classification assumes the two are related without the provider linking the two conditions. Evidence of bleeding during a procedure is not required.
TIP: For bleeding ulcers resulting from anticoagulant therapy, assign the appropriate "with hemorrhage" ulcer code from this category, code D68.32 Hemorrhagic disorder due to extrinsic circulating anticoagulant, and adverse effect code T45.515- with the appropriate seventh character. Either the bleeding ulcer code or code D68.32 may be sequenced first, depending on the circumstances of admission.

K27.0 Acute peptic ulcer, site unspecified, with hemorrhage MCC
K27.1 Acute peptic ulcer, site unspecified, with perforation MCC HCC
K27.2 Acute peptic ulcer, site unspecified, with both hemorrhage and perforation MCC HCC
K27.3 Acute peptic ulcer, site unspecified, without hemorrhage or perforation CC

K27.4 Chronic or unspecified peptic ulcer, site unspecified, with hemorrhage MCC

K27.5 Chronic or unspecified peptic ulcer, site unspecified, with perforation MCC HCC

K27.6 Chronic or unspecified peptic ulcer, site unspecified, with both hemorrhage and perforation MCC HCC

K27.7 Chronic peptic ulcer, site unspecified, without hemorrhage or perforation

K27.9 Peptic ulcer, site unspecified, unspecified as acute or chronic, without hemorrhage or perforation

K28 Gastrojejunal ulcer

INCLUDES anastomotic ulcer (peptic) or erosion
gastrocolic ulcer (peptic) or erosion
gastrointestinal ulcer (peptic) or erosion
gastrojejunal ulcer (peptic) or erosion
jejunal ulcer (peptic) or erosion
marginal ulcer (peptic) or erosion
stomal ulcer (peptic) or erosion

Use additional code to identify:
alcohol abuse and dependence (F10.-)

EXCLUDES 1 *primary ulcer of small intestine (K63.3)*

AHA: 2017,3Q,27

TIP: Assign a code for "with hemorrhage" when a gastrojejunal ulcer and GI bleeding are documented. The ICD-10-CM classification assumes the two are related without the provider linking the two conditions. Evidence of bleeding during a procedure is not required.

TIP: For bleeding ulcers resulting from anticoagulant therapy, assign the appropriate "with hemorrhage" ulcer code from this category, code D68.32 Hemorrhagic disorder due to extrinsic circulating anticoagulant, and adverse effect code T45.515- with the appropriate seventh character. Either the bleeding ulcer code or code D68.32 may be sequenced first, depending on the circumstances of admission.

K28.0 Acute gastrojejunal ulcer with hemorrhage MCC

K28.1 Acute gastrojejunal ulcer with perforation MCC HCC

K28.2 Acute gastrojejunal ulcer with both hemorrhage and perforation MCC HCC

K28.3 Acute gastrojejunal ulcer without hemorrhage or perforation CC

K28.4 Chronic or unspecified gastrojejunal ulcer with hemorrhage MCC

K28.5 Chronic or unspecified gastrojejunal ulcer with perforation MCC HCC

K28.6 Chronic or unspecified gastrojejunal ulcer with both hemorrhage and perforation MCC HCC

K28.7 Chronic gastrojejunal ulcer without hemorrhage or perforation

K28.9 Gastrojejunal ulcer, unspecified as acute or chronic, without hemorrhage or perforation

K29 Gastritis and duodenitis

EXCLUDES 1 *eosinophilic gastritis or gastroenteritis (K52.81)*
Zollinger-Ellison syndrome (E16.4)

AHA: 2018,3Q,22

TIP: Assign a code for "with bleeding" when gastritis or duodenitis and GI bleeding are documented. The ICD-10-CM classification assumes the two are related without the provider linking the two conditions. Evidence of bleeding during a procedure is not required.

TIP: For bleeding ulcers resulting from anticoagulant therapy, assign the appropriate "with hemorrhage" ulcer code from this category, code D68.32 Hemorrhagic disorder due to extrinsic circulating anticoagulant, and adverse effect code T45.515- with the appropriate seventh character. Either the bleeding ulcer code or code D68.32 may be sequenced first, depending on the circumstances of admission.

K29.0 Acute gastritis

Use additional code to identify:
alcohol abuse and dependence (F10.-)

EXCLUDES 1 *erosion (acute) of stomach (K25.-)*

K29.00 Acute gastritis without bleeding

K29.01 Acute gastritis with bleeding MCC

K29.2 Alcoholic gastritis

Use additional code to identify:
alcohol abuse and dependence (F10.-)

K29.20 Alcoholic gastritis without bleeding

K29.21 Alcoholic gastritis with bleeding MCC

K29.3 Chronic superficial gastritis

K29.30 Chronic superficial gastritis without bleeding

K29.31 Chronic superficial gastritis with bleeding MCC

K29.4 Chronic atrophic gastritis

Gastric atrophy

K29.40 Chronic atrophic gastritis without bleeding

K29.41 Chronic atrophic gastritis with bleeding MCC

K29.5 Unspecified chronic gastritis

Chronic antral gastritis
Chronic fundal gastritis

K29.50 Unspecified chronic gastritis without bleeding

K29.51 Unspecified chronic gastritis with bleeding MCC

K29.6 Other gastritis

Giant hypertrophic gastritis
Granulomatous gastritis
Menetrier's disease

K29.60 Other gastritis without bleeding

K29.61 Other gastritis with bleeding MCC

K29.7 Gastritis, unspecified

K29.70 Gastritis, unspecified, without bleeding

K29.71 Gastritis, unspecified, with bleeding MCC

K29.8 Duodenitis

K29.80 Duodenitis without bleeding

K29.81 Duodenitis with bleeding MCC

K29.9 Gastroduodenitis, unspecified

K29.90 Gastroduodenitis, unspecified, without bleeding

K29.91 Gastroduodenitis, unspecified, with bleeding MCC

K30 Functional dyspepsia

Indigestion

EXCLUDES 1 *dyspepsia NOS (R10.13)*
heartburn (R12)
nervous dyspepsia (F45.8)
neurotic dyspepsia (F45.8)
psychogenic dyspepsia (F45.8)

K31 Other diseases of stomach and duodenum

INCLUDES functional disorders of stomach

EXCLUDES 2 *diabetic gastroparesis (E08.43, E09.43, E10.43, E11.43, E13.43)*
diverticulum of duodenum (K57.00-K57.13)

K31.0 Acute dilatation of stomach CC

Acute distention of stomach

K31.1 Adult hypertrophic pyloric stenosis CC A

Pyloric stenosis NOS

EXCLUDES 1 *congenital or infantile pyloric stenosis (Q40.0)*

K31.2 Hourglass stricture and stenosis of stomach

EXCLUDES 1 *congenital hourglass stomach (Q40.2)*
hourglass contraction of stomach (K31.89)

K31.3 Pylorospasm, not elsewhere classified

EXCLUDES 1 *congenital or infantile pylorospasm (Q40.0)*
neurotic pylorospasm (F45.8)
psychogenic pylorospasm (F45.8)

K31.4 Gastric diverticulum

EXCLUDES 1 *congenital diverticulum of stomach (Q40.2)*

K31.5 Obstruction of duodenum CC

Constriction of duodenum
Duodenal ileus (chronic)
Stenosis of duodenum
Stricture of duodenum
Volvulus of duodenum

EXCLUDES 1 *congenital stenosis of duodenum (Q41.0)*

K31.6 Fistula of stomach and duodenum CC

Gastrocolic fistula
Gastrojejunocolic fistula

K31.7 Polyp of stomach and duodenum

EXCLUDES 1 *adenomatous polyp of stomach (D13.1)*

AHA: 2020,1Q,16

K31.8 Other specified diseases of stomach and duodenum

K31.81 Angiodysplasia of stomach and duodenum

TIP: Assign a code for "with bleeding" when angiodysplasia of the stomach or the duodenum and GI bleeding are documented. The ICD-10-CM classification assumes the two are related without the provider linking the two conditions. Evidence of bleeding during a procedure is not required.

K31.811 Angiodysplasia of stomach and duodenum with bleeding MCC

AHA: 2023,1Q,16

K31.819 **Angiodysplasia of stomach and duodenum without bleeding**
Angiodysplasia of stomach and duodenum NOS

K31.82 **Dieulafoy lesion (hemorrhagic) of stomach and duodenum** MCC
EXCLUDES 2 *Dieulafoy lesion of intestine (K63.81)*
DEF: Abnormally large submucosal artery protruding through a defect in the stomach mucosa or intestines that can cause massive and life-threatening hemorrhaging.

K31.83 **Achlorhydria**
DEF: Absence of hydrochloric acid in gastric secretions due to gastric mucosa atrophy. Achlorhydria is unresponsive to histamines.

K31.84 **Gastroparesis**
Gastroparalysis
Code first underlying disease, if known, such as:
anorexia nervosa (F50.0-)
diabetes mellitus (E08.43, E09.43, E10.43, E11.43, E13.43)
scleroderma (M34.-)
AHA: 2013,4Q,114

K31.89 **Other diseases of stomach and duodenum**
AHA: 2020,1Q,15; 2017,1Q,28

K31.9 **Disease of stomach and duodenum, unspecified**

✓5th K31.A **Gastric intestinal metaplasia**
AHA: 2021,4Q,15-16

K31.A0 **Gastric intestinal metaplasia, unspecified**
Gastric intestinal metaplasia indefinite for dysplasia
Gastric intestinal metaplasia NOS

✓6th K31.A1 **Gastric intestinal metaplasia without dysplasia**

K31.A11 **Gastric intestinal metaplasia without dysplasia, involving the antrum**

K31.A12 **Gastric intestinal metaplasia without dysplasia, involving the body (corpus)**

K31.A13 **Gastric intestinal metaplasia without dysplasia, involving the fundus**

K31.A14 **Gastric intestinal metaplasia without dysplasia, involving the cardia**

K31.A15 **Gastric intestinal metaplasia without dysplasia, involving multiple sites**

K31.A19 **Gastric intestinal metaplasia without dysplasia, unspecified site**

✓6th K31.A2 **Gastric intestinal metaplasia with dysplasia**

K31.A21 **Gastric intestinal metaplasia with low grade dysplasia**

K31.A22 **Gastric intestinal metaplasia with high grade dysplasia**

K31.A29 **Gastric intestinal metaplasia with dysplasia, unspecified**

Diseases of appendix (K35-K38)

✓4th K35 **Acute appendicitis**
AHA: 2018,4Q,17-18

✓5th K35.2 **Acute appendicitis with generalized peritonitis**
~~Appendicitis (acute) with generalized (diffuse) peritonitis following rupture or perforation of appendix~~

▲ ✓6th K35.20 **Acute appendicitis with generalized peritonitis, without abscess**
~~(Acute) appendicitis with generalized peritonitis NOS~~

● K35.200 **Acute appendicitis with generalized peritonitis, without perforation or abscess** CC
(Acute) appendicitis with generalized peritonitis without rupture or perforation of appendix NOS

● K35.201 **Acute appendicitis with generalized peritonitis, with perforation, without abscess** CC
Appendicitis (acute) with generalized (diffuse) peritonitis following rupture or perforation of appendix NOS

● K35.209 **Acute appendicitis with generalized peritonitis, without abscess, unspecified as to perforation** CC
(Acute) appendicitis with generalized peritonitis NOS

▲ ✓6th K35.21 **Acute appendicitis with generalized peritonitis, with abscess**

● K35.210 **Acute appendicitis with generalized peritonitis, without perforation, with abscess** MCC
(Acute) appendicitis with generalized peritonitis without rupture or perforation of appendix, with abscess

● K35.211 **Acute appendicitis with generalized peritonitis, with perforation and abscess** MCC
Appendicitis (acute) with generalized (diffuse) peritonitis following rupture or perforation of appendix, with abscess

● K35.219 **Acute appendicitis with generalized peritonitis, with abscess, unspecified as to perforation** MCC
(Acute) appendicitis with generalized peritonitis and abscess NOS

✓5th K35.3 **Acute appendicitis with localized peritonitis**

K35.30 **Acute appendicitis with localized peritonitis, without perforation or gangrene** CC
Acute appendicitis with localized peritonitis NOS

K35.31 **Acute appendicitis with localized peritonitis and gangrene, without perforation** CC

K35.32 **Acute appendicitis with perforation, localized peritonitis, and gangrene, without abscess** MCC
(Acute) appendicitis with perforation NOS
Perforated appendix NOS
Ruptured appendix (with localized peritonitis) NOS
AHA: 2020,1Q,16

K35.33 **Acute appendicitis with perforation, localized peritonitis, and gangrene, with abscess** MCC
(Acute) appendicitis with (peritoneal) abscess NOS
Ruptured appendix with localized peritonitis and abscess

✓5th K35.8 **Other and unspecified acute appendicitis**

K35.80 **Unspecified acute appendicitis** CC
Acute appendicitis NOS
Acute appendicitis without (localized) (generalized) peritonitis

✓6th K35.89 **Other acute appendicitis**
AHA: 2020,1Q,16

K35.890 **Other acute appendicitis without perforation or gangrene** CC

K35.891 **Other acute appendicitis without perforation, with gangrene** CC
(Acute) appendicitis with gangrene NOS

K36 **Other appendicitis**
Chronic appendicitis
Recurrent appendicitis

K37 **Unspecified appendicitis**
EXCLUDES 1 *unspecified appendicitis with peritonitis (K35.2-, K35.3-)*

✓4th K38 **Other diseases of appendix**

K38.0 **Hyperplasia of appendix**

K38.1 **Appendicular concretions**
Fecalith of appendix
Stercolith of appendix

K38.2 **Diverticulum of appendix**

K38.3 **Fistula of appendix**

K38.8 **Other specified diseases of appendix**
Intussusception of appendix

K38.9 **Disease of appendix, unspecified**

Hernia (K40-K46)

NOTE Hernia with both gangrene and obstruction is classified to hernia with gangrene.

INCLUDES acquired hernia
congenital [except diaphragmatic or hiatus] hernia
recurrent hernia

AHA: 2021,3Q,30-31

TIP: Do not assign a code for bilateral hernia when the right and left sides have differing pathology. For example, two codes would be assigned for bilateral femoral hernia in which the left side is incarcerated (with obstruction) but the right side is not incarcerated; the code for bilateral would not apply in this case.

K40 Inguinal hernia

INCLUDES bubonocele
direct inguinal hernia
double inguinal hernia
indirect inguinal hernia
inguinal hernia NOS
oblique inguinal hernia
scrotal hernia

DEF: Within the groin region.

K40.0 Bilateral inguinal hernia, with obstruction, without gangrene

Inguinal hernia (bilateral) causing obstruction without gangrene
Incarcerated inguinal hernia (bilateral) without gangrene
Irreducible inguinal hernia (bilateral) without gangrene
Strangulated inguinal hernia (bilateral) without gangrene

K40.00 Bilateral inguinal hernia, with obstruction, without gangrene, not specified as recurrent CC
Bilateral inguinal hernia, with obstruction, without gangrene NOS

K40.01 Bilateral inguinal hernia, with obstruction, without gangrene, recurrent CC

K40.1 Bilateral inguinal hernia, with gangrene

K40.10 Bilateral inguinal hernia, with gangrene, not specified as recurrent MCC
Bilateral inguinal hernia, with gangrene NOS

K40.11 Bilateral inguinal hernia, with gangrene, recurrent MCC

K40.2 Bilateral inguinal hernia, without obstruction or gangrene

K40.20 Bilateral inguinal hernia, without obstruction or gangrene, not specified as recurrent
Bilateral inguinal hernia NOS

K40.21 Bilateral inguinal hernia, without obstruction or gangrene, recurrent

K40.3 Unilateral inguinal hernia, with obstruction, without gangrene

Inguinal hernia (unilateral) causing obstruction without gangrene
Incarcerated inguinal hernia (unilateral) without gangrene
Irreducible inguinal hernia (unilateral) without gangrene
Strangulated inguinal hernia (unilateral) without gangrene

K40.30 Unilateral inguinal hernia, with obstruction, without gangrene, not specified as recurrent CC
Inguinal hernia, with obstruction NOS
Unilateral inguinal hernia, with obstruction, without gangrene NOS

K40.31 Unilateral inguinal hernia, with obstruction, without gangrene, recurrent CC

K40.4 Unilateral inguinal hernia, with gangrene

K40.40 Unilateral inguinal hernia, with gangrene, not specified as recurrent MCC
Inguinal hernia with gangrene NOS
Unilateral inguinal hernia with gangrene NOS

K40.41 Unilateral inguinal hernia, with gangrene, recurrent MCC

K40.9 Unilateral inguinal hernia, without obstruction or gangrene

K40.90 Unilateral inguinal hernia, without obstruction or gangrene, not specified as recurrent
Inguinal hernia NOS
Unilateral inguinal hernia NOS

K40.91 Unilateral inguinal hernia, without obstruction or gangrene, recurrent

Hernia Sites

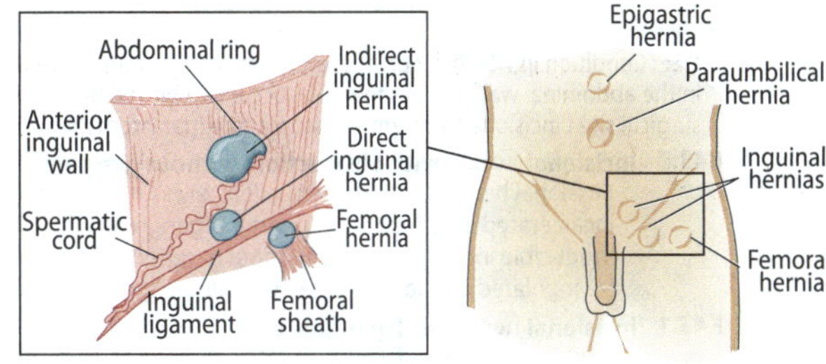

K41 Femoral hernia

K41.0 Bilateral femoral hernia, with obstruction, without gangrene

Femoral hernia (bilateral) causing obstruction, without gangrene
Incarcerated femoral hernia (bilateral), without gangrene
Irreducible femoral hernia (bilateral), without gangrene
Strangulated femoral hernia (bilateral), without gangrene

K41.00 Bilateral femoral hernia, with obstruction, without gangrene, not specified as recurrent CC
Bilateral femoral hernia, with obstruction, without gangrene NOS

K41.01 Bilateral femoral hernia, with obstruction, without gangrene, recurrent CC

K41.1 Bilateral femoral hernia, with gangrene

K41.10 Bilateral femoral hernia, with gangrene, not specified as recurrent MCC
Bilateral femoral hernia, with gangrene NOS

K41.11 Bilateral femoral hernia, with gangrene, recurrent MCC

K41.2 Bilateral femoral hernia, without obstruction or gangrene

K41.20 Bilateral femoral hernia, without obstruction or gangrene, not specified as recurrent
Bilateral femoral hernia NOS

K41.21 Bilateral femoral hernia, without obstruction or gangrene, recurrent

K41.3 Unilateral femoral hernia, with obstruction, without gangrene

Femoral hernia (unilateral) causing obstruction, without gangrene
Incarcerated femoral hernia (unilateral), without gangrene
Irreducible femoral hernia (unilateral), without gangrene
Strangulated femoral hernia (unilateral), without gangrene

K41.30 Unilateral femoral hernia, with obstruction, without gangrene, not specified as recurrent CC
Femoral hernia, with obstruction NOS
Unilateral femoral hernia, with obstruction NOS

K41.31 Unilateral femoral hernia, with obstruction, without gangrene, recurrent CC

K41.4 Unilateral femoral hernia, with gangrene

K41.40 Unilateral femoral hernia, with gangrene, not specified as recurrent MCC
Femoral hernia, with gangrene NOS
Unilateral femoral hernia, with gangrene NOS

K41.41 Unilateral femoral hernia, with gangrene, recurrent MCC

K41.9 Unilateral femoral hernia, without obstruction or gangrene

K41.90 Unilateral femoral hernia, without obstruction or gangrene, not specified as recurrent
Femoral hernia NOS
Unilateral femoral hernia NOS

K41.91 Unilateral femoral hernia, without obstruction or gangrene, recurrent

K42 Umbilical hernia

INCLUDES paraumbilical hernia

EXCLUDES 1 *omphalocele (Q79.2)*

K42.0 Umbilical hernia with obstruction, without gangrene CC
Umbilical hernia causing obstruction, without gangrene
Incarcerated umbilical hernia, without gangrene
Irreducible umbilical hernia, without gangrene
Strangulated umbilical hernia, without gangrene

K42.1 Umbilical hernia with gangrene MCC
Gangrenous umbilical hernia

K42.9 Umbilical hernia without obstruction or gangrene
Umbilical hernia NOS

✓4th K43 Ventral hernia

DEF: Condition in which a loop of bowel protrudes through a weakness in the abdominal wall muscles that may occur as a birth defect, past surgical site (incisional), or form at a stomal site (parastomal).

K43.Ø Incisional hernia with obstruction, without gangrene CC
Incisional hernia causing obstruction, without gangrene
Incarcerated incisional hernia, without gangrene
Irreducible incisional hernia, without gangrene
Strangulated incisional hernia, without gangrene

K43.1 Incisional hernia with gangrene MCC
Gangrenous incisional hernia
AHA: 2020,2Q,22

K43.2 Incisional hernia without obstruction or gangrene
Incisional hernia NOS

K43.3 Parastomal hernia with obstruction, without gangrene CC
Incarcerated parastomal hernia, without gangrene
Irreducible parastomal hernia, without gangrene
Parastomal hernia causing obstruction, without gangrene
Strangulated parastomal hernia, without gangrene

K43.4 Parastomal hernia with gangrene MCC
Gangrenous parastomal hernia

K43.5 Parastomal hernia without obstruction or gangrene
Parastomal hernia NOS

K43.6 Other and unspecified ventral hernia with obstruction, without gangrene CC
Epigastric hernia causing obstruction, without gangrene
Hypogastric hernia causing obstruction, without gangrene
Incarcerated epigastric hernia without gangrene
Incarcerated hypogastric hernia without gangrene
Incarcerated midline hernia without gangrene
Incarcerated spigelian hernia without gangrene
Incarcerated subxiphoid hernia without gangrene
Irreducible epigastric hernia without gangrene
Irreducible hypogastric hernia without gangrene
Irreducible midline hernia without gangrene
Irreducible spigelian hernia without gangrene
Irreducible subxiphoid hernia without gangrene
Midline hernia causing obstruction, without gangrene
Spigelian hernia causing obstruction, without gangrene
Strangulated epigastric hernia without gangrene
Strangulated hypogastric hernia without gangrene
Strangulated midline hernia without gangrene
Strangulated spigelian hernia without gangrene
Strangulated subxiphoid hernia without gangrene
Subxiphoid hernia causing obstruction, without gangrene

K43.7 Other and unspecified ventral hernia with gangrene MCC
Any condition listed under K43.6 specified as gangrenous

K43.9 Ventral hernia without obstruction or gangrene
Epigastric hernia
Ventral hernia NOS

✓4th K44 Diaphragmatic hernia

INCLUDES hiatus hernia (esophageal) (sliding)
paraesophageal hernia

EXCLUDES 1 *congenital diaphragmatic hernia (Q79.Ø)*
congenital hiatus hernia (Q4Ø.1)

DEF: Protrusion of an abdominal organ, usually the stomach, through the esophageal opening within the diaphragm and occurring in two types: the sliding hiatal hernia and the paraesophageal hernia.

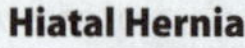
Hiatal Hernia

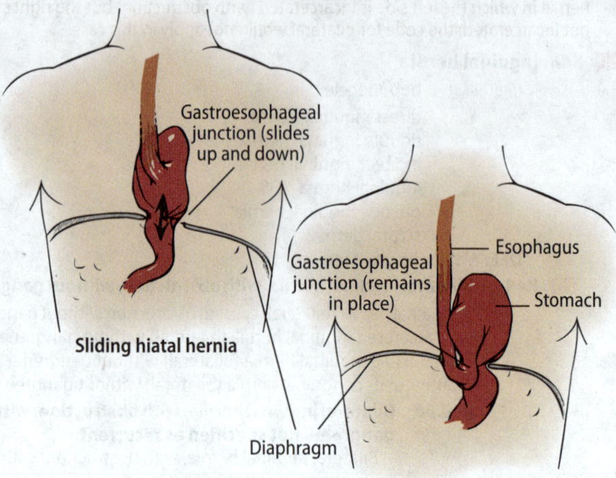

K44.Ø Diaphragmatic hernia with obstruction, without gangrene CC
Diaphragmatic hernia causing obstruction
Incarcerated diaphragmatic hernia
Irreducible diaphragmatic hernia
Strangulated diaphragmatic hernia
AHA: 2022,2Q,13

K44.1 Diaphragmatic hernia with gangrene MCC
Gangrenous diaphragmatic hernia

K44.9 Diaphragmatic hernia without obstruction or gangrene
Diaphragmatic hernia NOS

✓4th K45 Other abdominal hernia

INCLUDES abdominal hernia, specified site NEC
lumbar hernia
obturator hernia
pudendal hernia
retroperitoneal hernia
sciatic hernia

K45.Ø Other specified abdominal hernia with obstruction, without gangrene CC
Other specified abdominal hernia causing obstruction
Other specified incarcerated abdominal hernia
Other specified irreducible abdominal hernia
Other specified strangulated abdominal hernia

K45.1 Other specified abdominal hernia with gangrene MCC
Any condition listed under K45 specified as gangrenous

K45.8 Other specified abdominal hernia without obstruction or gangrene

✓4th K46 Unspecified abdominal hernia

INCLUDES enterocele
epiplocele
hernia NOS
interstitial hernia
intestinal hernia
intra-abdominal hernia

EXCLUDES 1 *vaginal enterocele (N81.5)*

K46.Ø Unspecified abdominal hernia with obstruction, without gangrene CC
Unspecified abdominal hernia causing obstruction
Unspecified incarcerated abdominal hernia
Unspecified irreducible abdominal hernia
Unspecified strangulated abdominal hernia

K46.1 Unspecified abdominal hernia with gangrene MCC
Any condition listed under K46 specified as gangrenous

K46.9 **Unspecified abdominal hernia without obstruction or gangrene**
Abdominal hernia NOS

Noninfective enteritis and colitis (K50-K52)

INCLUDES noninfective inflammatory bowel disease
EXCLUDES 1 *irritable bowel syndrome (K58.-)*
megacolon (K59.3-)

K50 Crohn's disease [regional enteritis]
INCLUDES granulomatous enteritis
Use additional code to identify manifestations, such as:
pyoderma gangrenosum (L88)
EXCLUDES 1 *ulcerative colitis (K51.-)*
AHA: 2019,3Q,5; 2012,4Q,104
DEF: Chronic inflammation of the gastrointestinal tract characterized by chronic granulomatous disease, most commonly affecting the intestines and the terminal ileum.

K50.0 Crohn's disease of small intestine
Crohn's disease [regional enteritis] of duodenum
Crohn's disease [regional enteritis] of ileum
Crohn's disease [regional enteritis] of jejunum
Regional ileitis
Terminal ileitis
EXCLUDES 1 *Crohn's disease of both small and large intestine (K50.8-)*

K50.00 Crohn's disease of small intestine without complications CC HCC
K50.01 Crohn's disease of small intestine with complications
K50.011 Crohn's disease of small intestine with rectal bleeding CC HCC
K50.012 Crohn's disease of small intestine with intestinal obstruction CC HCC
K50.013 Crohn's disease of small intestine with fistula CC HCC
K50.014 Crohn's disease of small intestine with abscess CC HCC
AHA: 2012,4Q,104
K50.018 Crohn's disease of small intestine with other complication CC HCC
K50.019 Crohn's disease of small intestine with unspecified complications CC HCC

K50.1 Crohn's disease of large intestine
Crohn's disease [regional enteritis] of colon
Crohn's disease [regional enteritis] of large bowel
Crohn's disease [regional enteritis] of rectum
Granulomatous colitis
Regional colitis
EXCLUDES 1 *Crohn's disease of both small and large intestine (K50.8)*

K50.10 Crohn's disease of large intestine without complications CC HCC
K50.11 Crohn's disease of large intestine with complications
K50.111 Crohn's disease of large intestine with rectal bleeding CC HCC
K50.112 Crohn's disease of large intestine with intestinal obstruction CC HCC
K50.113 Crohn's disease of large intestine with fistula CC HCC
K50.114 Crohn's disease of large intestine with abscess CC HCC
K50.118 Crohn's disease of large intestine with other complication CC HCC
K50.119 Crohn's disease of large intestine with unspecified complications CC HCC

K50.8 Crohn's disease of both small and large intestine
K50.80 Crohn's disease of both small and large intestine without complications CC HCC
K50.81 Crohn's disease of both small and large intestine with complications
K50.811 Crohn's disease of both small and large intestine with rectal bleeding CC HCC
K50.812 Crohn's disease of both small and large intestine with intestinal obstruction CC HCC
K50.813 Crohn's disease of both small and large intestine with fistula CC HCC
K50.814 Crohn's disease of both small and large intestine with abscess CC HCC
K50.818 Crohn's disease of both small and large intestine with other complication CC HCC
K50.819 Crohn's disease of both small and large intestine with unspecified complications CC HCC

K50.9 Crohn's disease, unspecified
K50.90 Crohn's disease, unspecified, without complications CC HCC
Crohn's disease NOS
Regional enteritis NOS
K50.91 Crohn's disease, unspecified, with complications
K50.911 Crohn's disease, unspecified, with rectal bleeding CC HCC
K50.912 Crohn's disease, unspecified, with intestinal obstruction CC HCC
K50.913 Crohn's disease, unspecified, with fistula CC HCC
K50.914 Crohn's disease, unspecified, with abscess CC HCC
K50.918 Crohn's disease, unspecified, with other complication CC HCC
K50.919 Crohn's disease, unspecified, with unspecified complications CC HCC

K51 Ulcerative colitis
Use additional code to identify manifestations, such as:
pyoderma gangrenosum (L88)
EXCLUDES 1 *Crohn's disease [regional enteritis] (K50.-)*

K51.0 Ulcerative (chronic) pancolitis
Backwash ileitis
K51.00 Ulcerative (chronic) pancolitis without complications CC HCC
Ulcerative (chronic) pancolitis NOS
K51.01 Ulcerative (chronic) pancolitis with complications
K51.011 Ulcerative (chronic) pancolitis with rectal bleeding CC HCC
K51.012 Ulcerative (chronic) pancolitis with intestinal obstruction CC HCC
K51.013 Ulcerative (chronic) pancolitis with fistula CC HCC
K51.014 Ulcerative (chronic) pancolitis with abscess CC HCC
K51.018 Ulcerative (chronic) pancolitis with other complication CC HCC
K51.019 Ulcerative (chronic) pancolitis with unspecified complications CC HCC

K51.2 Ulcerative (chronic) proctitis
K51.20 Ulcerative (chronic) proctitis without complications CC HCC
Ulcerative (chronic) proctitis NOS
K51.21 Ulcerative (chronic) proctitis with complications
K51.211 Ulcerative (chronic) proctitis with rectal bleeding CC HCC
K51.212 Ulcerative (chronic) proctitis with intestinal obstruction CC HCC
K51.213 Ulcerative (chronic) proctitis with fistula CC HCC
K51.214 Ulcerative (chronic) proctitis with abscess CC HCC
K51.218 Ulcerative (chronic) proctitis with other complication CC HCC
K51.219 Ulcerative (chronic) proctitis with unspecified complications CC HCC

K51.3 Ulcerative (chronic) rectosigmoiditis
K51.30 Ulcerative (chronic) rectosigmoiditis without complications CC HCC
Ulcerative (chronic) rectosigmoiditis NOS
K51.31 Ulcerative (chronic) rectosigmoiditis with complications
K51.311 Ulcerative (chronic) rectosigmoiditis with rectal bleeding CC HCC
K51.312 Ulcerative (chronic) rectosigmoiditis with intestinal obstruction CC HCC
K51.313 Ulcerative (chronic) rectosigmoiditis with fistula CC HCC
K51.314 Ulcerative (chronic) rectosigmoiditis with abscess CC HCC
K51.318 Ulcerative (chronic) rectosigmoiditis with other complication CC HCC

K51.319 Ulcerative (chronic) rectosigmoiditis with unspecified complications CC HCC

✓5th K51.4 Inflammatory polyps of colon

EXCLUDES 1 ~~adenomatous polyp of colon (D12.6)~~
~~polyposis of colon (D12.6)~~
~~polyps of colon NOS (K63.5)~~

EXCLUDES 2 ▶*adenomatous polyp of colon (D12.6)*◀
▶*polyposis of colon (D12.6)*◀
▶*polyps of colon NOS (K63.5)*◀

K51.40 Inflammatory polyps of colon without complications CC HCC
Inflammatory polyps of colon NOS

✓6th K51.41 Inflammatory polyps of colon with complications

K51.411 Inflammatory polyps of colon with rectal bleeding CC HCC

K51.412 Inflammatory polyps of colon with intestinal obstruction CC HCC

K51.413 Inflammatory polyps of colon with fistula CC HCC

K51.414 Inflammatory polyps of colon with abscess CC HCC

K51.418 Inflammatory polyps of colon with other complication CC HCC

K51.419 Inflammatory polyps of colon with unspecified complications CC HCC

✓5th K51.5 Left sided colitis
Left hemicolitis

K51.50 Left sided colitis without complications CC HCC
Left sided colitis NOS

✓6th K51.51 Left sided colitis with complications

K51.511 Left sided colitis with rectal bleeding CC HCC

K51.512 Left sided colitis with intestinal obstruction CC HCC

K51.513 Left sided colitis with fistula CC HCC

K51.514 Left sided colitis with abscess CC HCC

K51.518 Left sided colitis with other complication CC HCC

K51.519 Left sided colitis with unspecified complications CC HCC

✓5th K51.8 Other ulcerative colitis

K51.80 Other ulcerative colitis without complications CC HCC

✓6th K51.81 Other ulcerative colitis with complications

K51.811 Other ulcerative colitis with rectal bleeding CC HCC

K51.812 Other ulcerative colitis with intestinal obstruction CC HCC

K51.813 Other ulcerative colitis with fistula CC HCC

K51.814 Other ulcerative colitis with abscess CC HCC

K51.818 Other ulcerative colitis with other complication CC HCC

K51.819 Other ulcerative colitis with unspecified complications CC HCC

✓5th K51.9 Ulcerative colitis, unspecified

K51.90 Ulcerative colitis, unspecified, without complications CC HCC

✓6th K51.91 Ulcerative colitis, unspecified, with complications

K51.911 Ulcerative colitis, unspecified with rectal bleeding CC HCC

K51.912 Ulcerative colitis, unspecified with intestinal obstruction CC HCC

K51.913 Ulcerative colitis, unspecified with fistula CC HCC

K51.914 Ulcerative colitis, unspecified with abscess CC HCC

K51.918 Ulcerative colitis, unspecified with other complication CC HCC

K51.919 Ulcerative colitis, unspecified with unspecified complications CC HCC

✓4th **K52 Other and unspecified noninfective gastroenteritis and colitis**
AHA: 2016,4Q,30-31

K52.0 Gastroenteritis and colitis due to radiation CC

K52.1 Toxic gastroenteritis and colitis CC
Drug-induced gastroenteritis and colitis
Code first (T51-T65) to identify toxic agent
Use additional code for adverse effect, if applicable, to identify drug (T36-T50 with fifth or sixth character 5)
AHA: 2019,1Q,17

✓5th K52.2 Allergic and dietetic gastroenteritis and colitis
Food hypersensitivity gastroenteritis or colitis
Use additional code to identify type of food allergy (Z91.01-, Z91.02-)

EXCLUDES 2 *allergic eosinophilic colitis (K52.82)*
allergic eosinophilic esophagitis (K20.0)
allergic eosinophilic gastritis (K52.81)
allergic eosinophilic gastroenteritis (K52.81)

DEF: True immunoglobulin E (IgE)-mediated allergic reaction of the lining of the stomach, intestines, or colon to food proteins. It causes nausea, vomiting, diarrhea, and abdominal cramping.

K52.21 Food protein-induced enterocolitis syndrome
FPIES
Use additional code for hypovolemic shock, if present (R57.1)

K52.22 Food protein-induced enteropathy

K52.29 Other allergic and dietetic gastroenteritis and colitis
Allergic proctocolitis
Food hypersensitivity gastroenteritis or colitis
Food-induced eosinophilic proctocolitis
Food protein-induced proctocolitis
Immediate gastrointestinal hypersensitivity
Milk protein-induced proctocolitis

K52.3 Indeterminate colitis
Colonic inflammatory bowel disease unclassified (IBDU)
EXCLUDES 1 *unspecified colitis (K52.9)*

✓5th K52.8 Other specified noninfective gastroenteritis and colitis

K52.81 Eosinophilic gastritis or gastroenteritis
Eosinophilic enteritis
EXCLUDES 2 *eosinophilic esophagitis (K20.0)*
DEF: Disorder involving the accumulation of eosinophil in the lining of the stomach or multiple levels of the gastrointestinal tract, but without a known cause such as connective tissue disease, drug reaction, malignancy, or parasitic infection.

K52.82 Eosinophilic colitis
EXCLUDES 2 *allergic proctocolitis (K52.29)*
food-induced eosinophilic proctocolitis (K52.29)
food protein-induced enterocolitis syndrome (FPIES) (K52.21)
food protein-induced proctocolitis (K52.29)
milk protein-induced proctocolitis (K52.29)
DEF: Disorder involving the accumulation of eosinophil in the tissues lining the colon, but without a known cause such as connective tissue disease, drug reaction, malignancy, or parasitic infection. The resultant inflammation may cause extreme abdominal pain, diarrhea, or bloody stool.

✓6th K52.83 Microscopic colitis

K52.831 Collagenous colitis

K52.832 Lymphocytic colitis

K52.838 Other microscopic colitis

K52.839 Microscopic colitis, unspecified

K52.89 Other specified noninfective gastroenteritis and colitis
AHA: 2019,1Q,20

K52.9 Noninfective gastroenteritis and colitis, unspecified
Colitis NOS
Enteritis NOS
Gastroenteritis NOS
Ileitis NOS
Jejunitis NOS
Sigmoiditis NOS
EXCLUDES 1 *diarrhea NOS (R19.7)*
functional diarrhea (K59.1)
infectious gastroenteritis and colitis NOS (A09)
neonatal diarrhea (noninfective) (P78.3)
psychogenic diarrhea (F45.8)
AHA: 2021,3Q,3

Other diseases of intestines (K55-K64)

K55 Vascular disorders of intestine

EXCLUDES 1 *necrotizing enterocolitis of newborn (P77.-)*

EXCLUDES 2 *▶angioectasia (angiodysplasia) duodenum (K31.81-)◀*

AHA: 2016,4Q,32

K55.0 Acute vascular disorders of intestine

Infarction of appendices epiploicae
Mesenteric (artery) (vein) embolism
Mesenteric (artery) (vein) infarction
Mesenteric (artery) (vein) thrombosis

AHA: 2019,4Q,68

K55.01 Acute (reversible) ischemia of small intestine

K55.011 Focal (segmental) acute (reversible) ischemia of small intestine MCC HCC

K55.012 Diffuse acute (reversible) ischemia of small intestine MCC HCC

K55.019 Acute (reversible) ischemia of small intestine, extent unspecified MCC HCC

K55.02 Acute infarction of small intestine

Gangrene of small intestine
Necrosis of small intestine

K55.021 Focal (segmental) acute infarction of small intestine MCC HCC

K55.022 Diffuse acute infarction of small intestine MCC HCC

K55.029 Acute infarction of small intestine, extent unspecified MCC HCC

K55.03 Acute (reversible) ischemia of large intestine

Acute fulminant ischemic colitis
Subacute ischemic colitis

K55.031 Focal (segmental) acute (reversible) ischemia of large intestine MCC HCC

K55.032 Diffuse acute (reversible) ischemia of large intestine MCC HCC

K55.039 Acute (reversible) ischemia of large intestine, extent unspecified MCC HCC

AHA: 2019,4Q,68

K55.04 Acute infarction of large intestine

Gangrene of large intestine
Necrosis of large intestine

K55.041 Focal (segmental) acute infarction of large intestine MCC HCC

K55.042 Diffuse acute infarction of large intestine MCC HCC

K55.049 Acute infarction of large intestine, extent unspecified MCC HCC

K55.05 Acute (reversible) ischemia of intestine, part unspecified

K55.051 Focal (segmental) acute (reversible) ischemia of intestine, part unspecified MCC HCC

K55.052 Diffuse acute (reversible) ischemia of intestine, part unspecified MCC HCC

K55.059 Acute (reversible) ischemia of intestine, part and extent unspecified MCC HCC

K55.06 Acute infarction of intestine, part unspecified

Acute intestinal infarction
Gangrene of intestine
Necrosis of intestine

K55.061 Focal (segmental) acute infarction of intestine, part unspecified MCC HCC

K55.062 Diffuse acute infarction of intestine, part unspecified MCC HCC

K55.069 Acute infarction of intestine, part and extent unspecified MCC HCC

K55.1 Chronic vascular disorders of intestine CC HCC

Chronic ischemic colitis
Chronic ischemic enteritis
Chronic ischemic enterocolitis
Ischemic stricture of intestine
Mesenteric atherosclerosis
Mesenteric vascular insufficiency

K55.2 Angiodysplasia of colon

AHA: 2018,3Q,21

TIP: Assign a code for "with hemorrhage" when angiodysplasia and GI bleeding are documented. The ICD-10-CM classification assumes the two are related without the provider linking the two conditions. Evidence of bleeding during a procedure is not required.

K55.20 Angiodysplasia of colon without hemorrhage

K55.21 Angiodysplasia of colon with hemorrhage MCC

DEF: Small vascular abnormalities due to fragile blood vessels in the colon, resulting in blood loss from the gastrointestinal (GI) tract.

K55.3 Necrotizing enterocolitis

EXCLUDES 1 *necrotizing enterocolitis of newborn (P77.-)*

EXCLUDES 2 *necrotizing enterocolitis due to Clostridium difficile (A04.7-)*

K55.30 Necrotizing enterocolitis, unspecified MCC HCC

Necrotizing enterocolitis, NOS

K55.31 Stage 1 necrotizing enterocolitis MCC HCC

Necrotizing enterocolitis without pneumatosis, without perforation

K55.32 Stage 2 necrotizing enterocolitis MCC HCC

Necrotizing enterocolitis with pneumatosis, without perforation

K55.33 Stage 3 necrotizing enterocolitis MCC HCC

Necrotizing enterocolitis with perforation
Necrotizing enterocolitis with pneumatosis and perforation

K55.8 Other vascular disorders of intestine CC HCC

K55.9 Vascular disorder of intestine, unspecified CC HCC

Ischemic colitis
Ischemic enteritis
Ischemic enterocolitis

K56 Paralytic ileus and intestinal obstruction without hernia

EXCLUDES 1 *congenital stricture or stenosis of intestine (Q41-Q42)*
cystic fibrosis with meconium ileus (E84.11)
ischemic stricture of intestine (K55.1)
meconium ileus NOS (P76.0)
neonatal intestinal obstructions classifiable to P76.-
obstruction of duodenum (K31.5)
postprocedural intestinal obstruction (K91.3-)

EXCLUDES 2 *stenosis of anus or rectum (K62.4)*

K56.0 Paralytic ileus CC HCC

Paralysis of bowel
Paralysis of colon
Paralysis of intestine

EXCLUDES 1 *gallstone ileus (K56.3)*
ileus NOS (K56.7)
obstructive ileus NOS (K56.69-)

DEF: Intestinal obstruction due to paralysis of bowel motility or peristalsis.

K56.1 Intussusception CC HCC

Intussusception or invagination of bowel
Intussusception or invagination of colon
Intussusception or invagination of intestine
Intussusception or invagination of rectum

EXCLUDES 2 *intussusception of appendix (K38.8)*

DEF: Intestinal obstruction due to prolapse of a bowel section into an adjacent section. It occurs primarily in children and symptoms include acute abdominal pain, vomiting, and passage of blood and mucus from the rectum.

K56.2 Volvulus MCC HCC
Strangulation of colon or intestine
Torsion of colon or intestine
Twist of colon or intestine
EXCLUDES 2 *volvulus of duodenum (K31.5)*
DEF: Twisting, knotting, or entanglement of the bowel on itself that may quickly compromise oxygen supply to the intestinal tissues. A volvulus usually occurs at the sigmoid and ileocecal areas of the intestines.

Volvulus

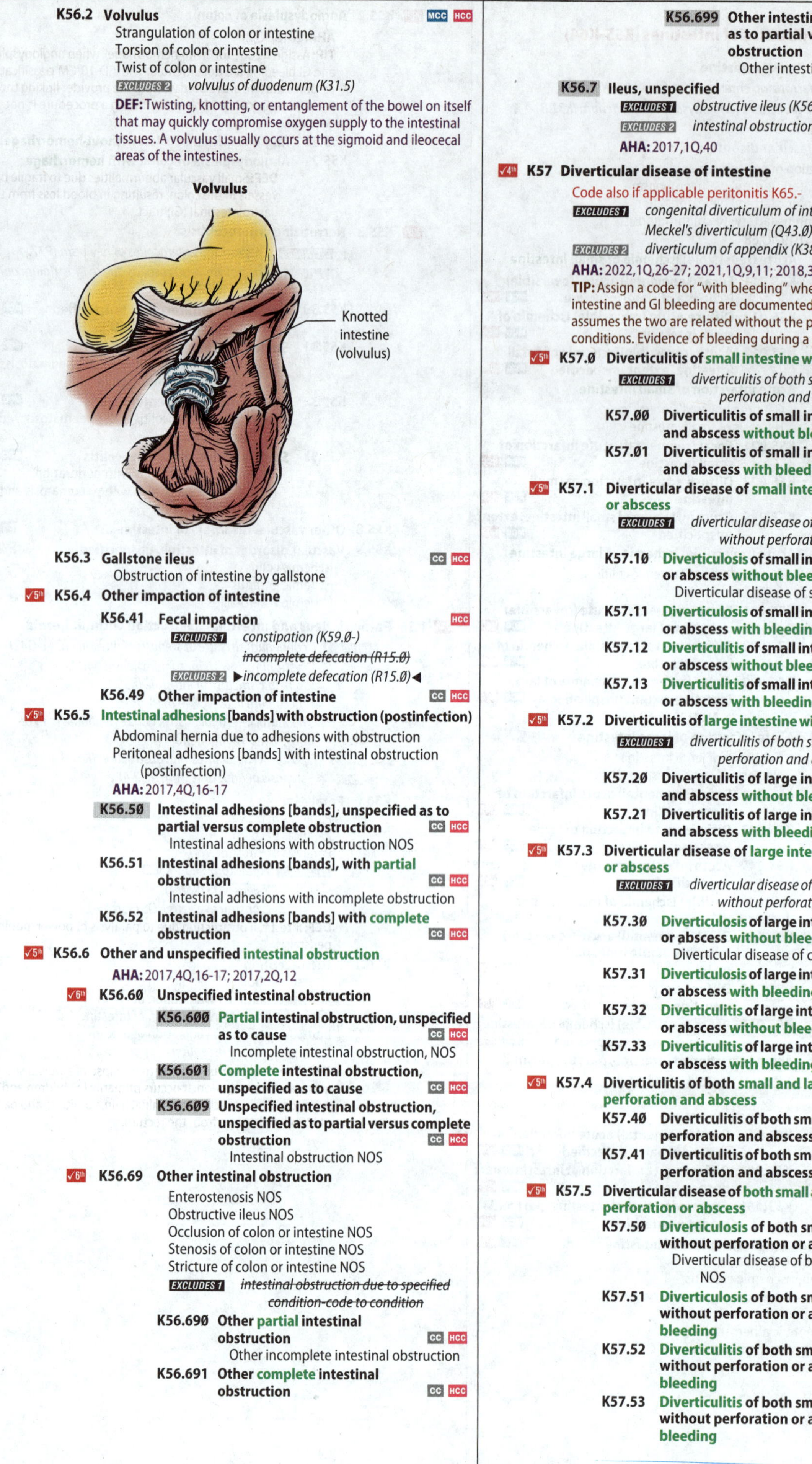

K56.3 Gallstone ileus CC HCC
Obstruction of intestine by gallstone

✓5th **K56.4 Other impaction of intestine**

K56.41 Fecal impaction HCC
EXCLUDES 1 *constipation (K59.Ø-)*
~~*incomplete defecation (R15.Ø)*~~
EXCLUDES 2 ▶*incomplete defecation (R15.Ø)*◀

K56.49 Other impaction of intestine CC HCC

✓5th **K56.5 Intestinal adhesions [bands] with obstruction (postinfection)**
Abdominal hernia due to adhesions with obstruction
Peritoneal adhesions [bands] with intestinal obstruction (postinfection)
AHA: 2017,4Q,16-17

K56.5Ø Intestinal adhesions [bands], unspecified as to partial versus complete obstruction CC HCC
Intestinal adhesions with obstruction NOS

K56.51 Intestinal adhesions [bands], with partial obstruction CC HCC
Intestinal adhesions with incomplete obstruction

K56.52 Intestinal adhesions [bands] with complete obstruction CC HCC

✓5th **K56.6 Other and unspecified intestinal obstruction**
AHA: 2017,4Q,16-17; 2017,2Q,12

✓6th **K56.6Ø Unspecified intestinal obstruction**

K56.6ØØ Partial intestinal obstruction, unspecified as to cause CC HCC
Incomplete intestinal obstruction, NOS

K56.6Ø1 Complete intestinal obstruction, unspecified as to cause CC HCC

K56.6Ø9 Unspecified intestinal obstruction, unspecified as to partial versus complete obstruction CC HCC
Intestinal obstruction NOS

✓6th **K56.69 Other intestinal obstruction**
Enterostenosis NOS
Obstructive ileus NOS
Occlusion of colon or intestine NOS
Stenosis of colon or intestine NOS
Stricture of colon or intestine NOS
EXCLUDES 1 ~~*intestinal obstruction due to specified condition-code to condition*~~

K56.69Ø Other partial intestinal obstruction CC HCC
Other incomplete intestinal obstruction

K56.691 Other complete intestinal obstruction CC HCC

K56.699 Other intestinal obstruction unspecified as to partial versus complete obstruction CC HCC
Other intestinal obstruction, NEC

K56.7 Ileus, unspecified CC HCC
EXCLUDES 1 *obstructive ileus (K56.69-)*
EXCLUDES 2 *intestinal obstruction with hernia (K4Ø-K46)*
AHA: 2017,1Q,40

✓4th **K57 Diverticular disease of intestine**
Code also if applicable peritonitis K65.-
EXCLUDES 1 *congenital diverticulum of intestine (Q43.8)*
Meckel's diverticulum (Q43.Ø)
EXCLUDES 2 *diverticulum of appendix (K38.2)*
AHA: 2022,1Q,26-27; 2021,1Q,9,11; 2018,3Q,21
TIP: Assign a code for "with bleeding" when diverticular disease of the intestine and GI bleeding are documented. The ICD-10-CM classification assumes the two are related without the provider linking the two conditions. Evidence of bleeding during a procedure is not required.

✓5th **K57.Ø Diverticulitis of small intestine with perforation and abscess**
EXCLUDES 1 *diverticulitis of both small and large intestine with perforation and abscess (K57.4-)*

K57.ØØ Diverticulitis of small intestine with perforation and abscess without bleeding CC

K57.Ø1 Diverticulitis of small intestine with perforation and abscess with bleeding MCC

✓5th **K57.1 Diverticular disease of small intestine without perforation or abscess**
EXCLUDES 1 *diverticular disease of both small and large intestine without perforation or abscess (K57.5-)*

K57.1Ø Diverticulosis of small intestine without perforation or abscess without bleeding
Diverticular disease of small intestine NOS

K57.11 Diverticulosis of small intestine without perforation or abscess with bleeding MCC

K57.12 Diverticulitis of small intestine without perforation or abscess without bleeding CC

K57.13 Diverticulitis of small intestine without perforation or abscess with bleeding MCC

✓5th **K57.2 Diverticulitis of large intestine with perforation and abscess**
EXCLUDES 1 *diverticulitis of both small and large intestine with perforation and abscess (K57.4-)*

K57.2Ø Diverticulitis of large intestine with perforation and abscess without bleeding CC

K57.21 Diverticulitis of large intestine with perforation and abscess with bleeding MCC

✓5th **K57.3 Diverticular disease of large intestine without perforation or abscess**
EXCLUDES 1 *diverticular disease of both small and large intestine without perforation or abscess (K57.5-)*

K57.3Ø Diverticulosis of large intestine without perforation or abscess without bleeding
Diverticular disease of colon NOS

K57.31 Diverticulosis of large intestine without perforation or abscess with bleeding MCC

K57.32 Diverticulitis of large intestine without perforation or abscess without bleeding CC

K57.33 Diverticulitis of large intestine without perforation or abscess with bleeding MCC

✓5th **K57.4 Diverticulitis of both small and large intestine with perforation and abscess**

K57.4Ø Diverticulitis of both small and large intestine with perforation and abscess without bleeding CC

K57.41 Diverticulitis of both small and large intestine with perforation and abscess with bleeding MCC

✓5th **K57.5 Diverticular disease of both small and large intestine without perforation or abscess**

K57.5Ø Diverticulosis of both small and large intestine without perforation or abscess without bleeding
Diverticular disease of both small and large intestine NOS

K57.51 Diverticulosis of both small and large intestine without perforation or abscess with bleeding MCC

K57.52 Diverticulitis of both small and large intestine without perforation or abscess without bleeding CC

K57.53 Diverticulitis of both small and large intestine without perforation or abscess with bleeding MCC

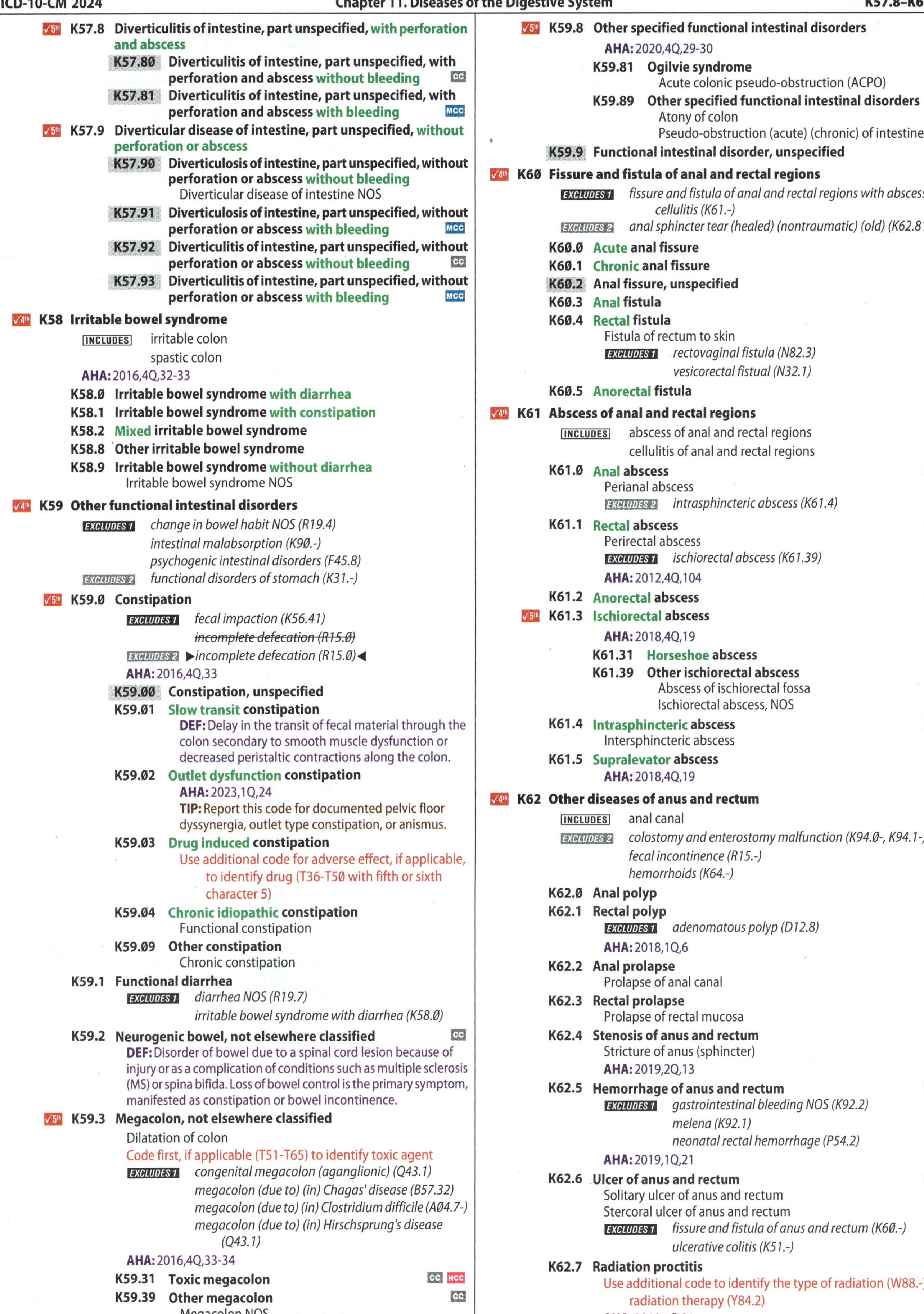

K57.8 Diverticulitis of intestine, part unspecified, with perforation and abscess
- K57.80 Diverticulitis of intestine, part unspecified, with perforation and abscess without bleeding CC
- K57.81 Diverticulitis of intestine, part unspecified, with perforation and abscess with bleeding MCC

K57.9 Diverticular disease of intestine, part unspecified, without perforation or abscess
- K57.90 Diverticulosis of intestine, part unspecified, without perforation or abscess without bleeding
  - Diverticular disease of intestine NOS
- K57.91 Diverticulosis of intestine, part unspecified, without perforation or abscess with bleeding MCC
- K57.92 Diverticulitis of intestine, part unspecified, without perforation or abscess without bleeding CC
- K57.93 Diverticulitis of intestine, part unspecified, without perforation or abscess with bleeding MCC

K58 Irritable bowel syndrome

INCLUDES irritable colon
spastic colon

AHA: 2016,4Q,32-33

- K58.0 Irritable bowel syndrome with diarrhea
- K58.1 Irritable bowel syndrome with constipation
- K58.2 Mixed irritable bowel syndrome
- K58.8 Other irritable bowel syndrome
- K58.9 Irritable bowel syndrome without diarrhea
  - Irritable bowel syndrome NOS

K59 Other functional intestinal disorders

EXCLUDES 1 *change in bowel habit NOS (R19.4)*
intestinal malabsorption (K90.-)
psychogenic intestinal disorders (F45.8)

EXCLUDES 2 *functional disorders of stomach (K31.-)*

K59.0 Constipation

EXCLUDES 1 *fecal impaction (K56.41)*
~~*incomplete defecation (R15.0)*~~

EXCLUDES 2 ▶*incomplete defecation (R15.0)*◀

AHA: 2016,4Q,33

- K59.00 Constipation, unspecified
- K59.01 Slow transit constipation
  - DEF: Delay in the transit of fecal material through the colon secondary to smooth muscle dysfunction or decreased peristaltic contractions along the colon.
- K59.02 Outlet dysfunction constipation
  - AHA: 2023,1Q,24
  - TIP: Report this code for documented pelvic floor dyssynergia, outlet type constipation, or anismus.
- K59.03 Drug induced constipation
  - Use additional code for adverse effect, if applicable, to identify drug (T36-T50 with fifth or sixth character 5)
- K59.04 Chronic idiopathic constipation
  - Functional constipation
- K59.09 Other constipation
  - Chronic constipation

K59.1 Functional diarrhea

EXCLUDES 1 *diarrhea NOS (R19.7)*
irritable bowel syndrome with diarrhea (K58.0)

K59.2 Neurogenic bowel, not elsewhere classified CC

DEF: Disorder of bowel due to a spinal cord lesion because of injury or as a complication of conditions such as multiple sclerosis (MS) or spina bifida. Loss of bowel control is the primary symptom, manifested as constipation or bowel incontinence.

K59.3 Megacolon, not elsewhere classified

Dilatation of colon

Code first, if applicable (T51-T65) to identify toxic agent

EXCLUDES 1 *congenital megacolon (aganglionic) (Q43.1)*
megacolon (due to) (in) Chagas' disease (B57.32)
megacolon (due to) (in) Clostridium difficile (A04.7-)
megacolon (due to) (in) Hirschsprung's disease (Q43.1)

AHA: 2016,4Q,33-34

- K59.31 Toxic megacolon CC HCC
- K59.39 Other megacolon CC
  - Megacolon NOS

K59.4 Anal spasm

Proctalgia fugax

K59.8 Other specified functional intestinal disorders

AHA: 2020,4Q,29-30

- K59.81 Ogilvie syndrome
  - Acute colonic pseudo-obstruction (ACPO)
- K59.89 Other specified functional intestinal disorders
  - Atony of colon
  - Pseudo-obstruction (acute) (chronic) of intestine

K59.9 Functional intestinal disorder, unspecified

K60 Fissure and fistula of anal and rectal regions

EXCLUDES 1 *fissure and fistula of anal and rectal regions with abscess or cellulitis (K61.-)*

EXCLUDES 2 *anal sphincter tear (healed) (nontraumatic) (old) (K62.81)*

- K60.0 Acute anal fissure
- K60.1 Chronic anal fissure
- K60.2 Anal fissure, unspecified
- K60.3 Anal fistula
- K60.4 Rectal fistula
  - Fistula of rectum to skin
  - EXCLUDES 1 *rectovaginal fistula (N82.3)* *vesicorectal fistual (N32.1)*
- K60.5 Anorectal fistula

K61 Abscess of anal and rectal regions

INCLUDES abscess of anal and rectal regions
cellulitis of anal and rectal regions

- K61.0 Anal abscess CC
  - Perianal abscess
  - EXCLUDES 2 *intrasphincteric abscess (K61.4)*
- K61.1 Rectal abscess CC
  - Perirectal abscess
  - EXCLUDES 1 *ischiorectal abscess (K61.39)*
  - AHA: 2012,4Q,104
- K61.2 Anorectal abscess CC
- K61.3 Ischiorectal abscess
  - AHA: 2018,4Q,19
  - K61.31 Horseshoe abscess
  - K61.39 Other ischiorectal abscess
    - Abscess of ischiorectal fossa
    - Ischiorectal abscess, NOS
- K61.4 Intrasphincteric abscess CC
  - Intersphincteric abscess
- K61.5 Supralevator abscess
  - AHA: 2018,4Q,19

K62 Other diseases of anus and rectum

INCLUDES anal canal

EXCLUDES 2 *colostomy and enterostomy malfunction (K94.0-, K94.1-)*
fecal incontinence (R15.-)
hemorrhoids (K64.-)

- K62.0 Anal polyp
- K62.1 Rectal polyp
  - EXCLUDES 1 *adenomatous polyp (D12.8)*
  - AHA: 2018,1Q,6
- K62.2 Anal prolapse
  - Prolapse of anal canal
- K62.3 Rectal prolapse
  - Prolapse of rectal mucosa
- K62.4 Stenosis of anus and rectum
  - Stricture of anus (sphincter)
  - AHA: 2019,2Q,13
- K62.5 Hemorrhage of anus and rectum CC
  - EXCLUDES 1 *gastrointestinal bleeding NOS (K92.2)* *melena (K92.1)* *neonatal rectal hemorrhage (P54.2)*
  - AHA: 2019,1Q,21
- K62.6 Ulcer of anus and rectum CC
  - Solitary ulcer of anus and rectum
  - Stercoral ulcer of anus and rectum
  - EXCLUDES 1 *fissure and fistula of anus and rectum (K60.-)* *ulcerative colitis (K51.-)*
- K62.7 Radiation proctitis
  - Use additional code to identify the type of radiation (W88.-) or radiation therapy (Y84.2)
  - AHA: 2019,1Q,21

✓5th K62.8 Other specified diseases of anus and rectum

EXCLUDES 2 *ulcerative proctitis (K51.2)*

K62.81 Anal sphincter tear (healed) (nontraumatic) (old)
Tear of anus, nontraumatic
Use additional code for any associated fecal incontinence (R15.-)
EXCLUDES 2 *anal fissure (K6Ø.-)*
anal sphincter tear (healed) (old) complicating delivery (O34.7-)
traumatic tear of anal sphincter (S31.831)

K62.82 Dysplasia of anus
Anal intraepithelial neoplasia I and II (AIN I and II) (histologically confirmed)
Dysplasia of anus NOS
Mild and moderate dysplasia of anus (histologically confirmed)
EXCLUDES 1 *abnormal results from anal cytologic examination without histologic confirmation (R85.61-)*
anal intraepithelial neoplasia III (DØ1.3)
carcinoma in situ of anus (DØ1.3)
HGSIL of anus (R85.613)
severe dysplasia of anus (DØ1.3)

K62.89 Other specified diseases of anus and rectum
Proctitis NOS
Use additional code for any associated fecal incontinence (R15.-)

K62.9 Disease of anus and rectum, unspecified

✓4th K63 Other diseases of intestine

K63.Ø Abscess of intestine CC
EXCLUDES 1 *abscess of intestine with Crohn's disease (K5Ø.Ø14, K5Ø.114, K5Ø.814, K5Ø.914)*
abscess of intestine with diverticular disease (K57.Ø, K57.2, K57.4, K57.8)
abscess of intestine with ulcerative colitis (K51.Ø14, K51.214, K51.314, K51.414, K51.514, K51.814, K51.914)
EXCLUDES 2 *abscess of anal and rectal regions (K61.-)*
abscess of appendix (K35.3-)

K63.1 Perforation of intestine (nontraumatic) MCC HCC
Perforation (nontraumatic) of rectum
EXCLUDES 1 *perforation (nontraumatic) of duodenum (K26.-)*
perforation (nontraumatic) of intestine with diverticular disease (K57.Ø, K57.2, K57.4, K57.8)
EXCLUDES 2 *perforation (nontraumatic) of appendix (K35.2-, K35.3-)*
AHA: 2020,2Q,22

K63.2 Fistula of intestine CC
EXCLUDES 1 *fistula of duodenum (K31.6)*
fistula of intestine with Crohn's disease (K5Ø.Ø13, K5Ø.113, K5Ø.813, K5Ø.913)
fistula of intestine with ulcerative colitis (K51.Ø13, K51.213, K51.313, K51.413, K51.513, K51.813, K51.913)
EXCLUDES 2 *fistula of anal and rectal regions (K6Ø.-)*
fistula of appendix (K38.3)
intestinal-genital fistula, female (N82.2-N82.4)
vesicointestinal fistula (N32.1)
AHA: 2017,3Q,4

K63.3 Ulcer of intestine CC
Primary ulcer of small intestine
EXCLUDES 1 *duodenal ulcer (K26.-)*
gastrointestinal ulcer (K28.-)
gastrojejunal ulcer (K28.-)
jejunal ulcer (K28.-)
peptic ulcer, site unspecified (K27.-)
ulcer of intestine with perforation (K63.1)
ulcer of anus or rectum (K62.6)
ulcerative colitis (K51.-)

K63.4 Enteroptosis

K63.5 Polyp of colon
EXCLUDES 1 ~~*adenomatous polyp of colon (D12.-)*~~
~~*inflammatory polyp of colon (K51.4-)*~~
~~*polyposis of colon (D12.6)*~~
EXCLUDES 2 ►*adenomatous polyp of colon (D12.-)*◄
►*inflammatory polyp of colon (K51.4-)*◄
►*polyposis of colon (D12.6)*◄
AHA: 2019,1Q,33; 2018,2Q,14; 2017,1Q,15; 2015,2Q,14
TIP: Assign this code when documentation states hyperplastic colon polyp regardless of the site in the colon. Slow-growing, hyperplastic polyps are not precancerous and are classified differently from benign or adenomatous polyps.

✓5th K63.8 Other specified diseases of intestine

K63.81 Dieulafoy lesion of intestine MCC
EXCLUDES 2 *Dieulafoy lesion of stomach and duodenum (K31.82)*
DEF: Abnormally large submucosal artery protruding through a defect in the stomach mucosa or intestines that can cause massive and life-threatening hemorrhaging.

● **✓6th K63.82 Intestinal microbial overgrowth**
● **✓7th K63.821 Small intestinal bacterial overgrowth**
● **K63.8211 Small intestinal bacterial overgrowth, hydrogen-subtype**
● **K63.8212 Small intestinal bacterial overgrowth, hydrogen sulfide-subtype**
● **K63.8219 Small intestinal bacterial overgrowth, unspecified**
● **K63.822 Small intestinal fungal overgrowth**
● **K63.829 Intestinal methanogen overgrowth, unspecified**

K63.89 Other specified diseases of intestine
AHA: 2013,2Q,31

K63.9 Disease of intestine, unspecified

✓4th K64 Hemorrhoids and perianal venous thrombosis
INCLUDES piles
EXCLUDES 1 *hemorrhoids complicating childbirth and the puerperium (O87.2)*
hemorrhoids complicating pregnancy (O22.4)

Hemorrhoids

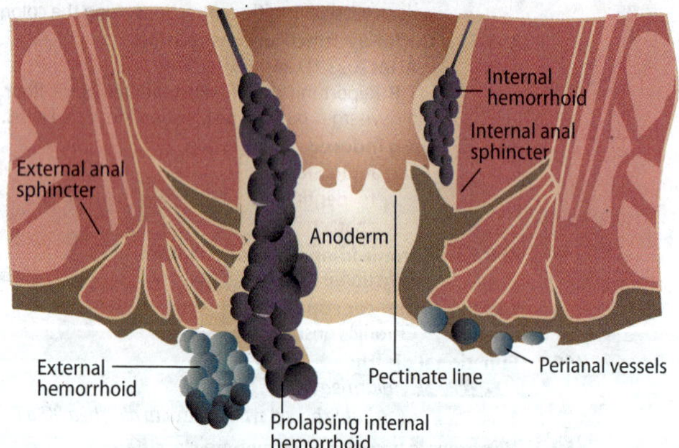

K64.Ø First degree hemorrhoids
Grade/stage I hemorrhoids
Hemorrhoids (bleeding) without prolapse outside of anal canal

K64.1 Second degree hemorrhoids
Grade/stage II hemorrhoids
Hemorrhoids (bleeding) that prolapse with straining, but retract spontaneously

K64.2 Third degree hemorrhoids
Grade/stage III hemorrhoids
Hemorrhoids (bleeding) that prolapse with straining and require manual replacement back inside anal canal

K64.3 Fourth degree hemorrhoids
Grade/stage IV hemorrhoids
Hemorrhoids (bleeding) with prolapsed tissue that cannot be manually replaced

K64.4 Residual hemorrhoidal skin tags
External hemorrhoids, NOS
Skin tags of anus

K64.5 Perianal venous thrombosis
External hemorrhoids with thrombosis
Perianal hematoma
Thrombosed hemorrhoids NOS

K64.8 Other hemorrhoids
Internal hemorrhoids, without mention of degree
Prolapsed hemorrhoids, degree not specified

K64.9 Unspecified hemorrhoids
Hemorrhoids (bleeding) NOS
Hemorrhoids (bleeding) without mention of degree

Diseases of peritoneum and retroperitoneum (K65-K68)

✓4th **K65 Peritonitis**
Use additional code (B95-B97), to identify infectious agent, if known
Code also if applicable diverticular disease of intestine (K57.-)
EXCLUDES 1 *acute appendicitis with generalized peritonitis (K35.2-)*
aseptic peritonitis (T81.6)
benign paroxysmal peritonitis (E85.Ø)
chemical peritonitis (T81.6)
gonococcal peritonitis (A54.85)
neonatal peritonitis (P78.Ø-P78.1)
pelvic peritonitis, female (N73.3-N73.5)
periodic familial peritonitis (E85.Ø)
peritonitis due to talc or other foreign substance (T81.6)
peritonitis in chlamydia (A74.81)
peritonitis in diphtheria (A36.89)
peritonitis in syphilis (late) (A52.74)
peritonitis in tuberculosis (A18.31)
peritonitis with or following abortion or ectopic or molar pregnancy (OØØ-OØ7, OØ8.Ø)
peritonitis with or following appendicitis (K35.-)
puerperal peritonitis (O85)
retroperitoneal infections (K68.-)

K65.Ø Generalized (acute) peritonitis MCC HCC
Pelvic peritonitis (acute), male
Subphrenic peritonitis (acute)
Suppurative peritonitis (acute)

K65.1 Peritoneal abscess MCC HCC
Abdominopelvic abscess
Abscess (of) omentum
Abscess (of) peritoneum
Mesenteric abscess
Retrocecal abscess
Subdiaphragmatic abscess
Subhepatic abscess
Subphrenic abscess
AHA: 2022,1Q,26; 2019,1Q,15

K65.2 Spontaneous bacterial peritonitis MCC HCC
EXCLUDES 1 *bacterial peritonitis NOS (K65.9)*

K65.3 Choleperitonitis MCC HCC
Peritonitis due to bile
DEF: Inflammation of the peritoneum due to leakage of bile into the peritoneal cavity resulting from rupture of the bile passages or gallbladder.

K65.4 Sclerosing mesenteritis CC HCC
Fat necrosis of peritoneum
(Idiopathic) sclerosing mesenteric fibrosis
Mesenteric lipodystrophy
Mesenteric panniculitis
Retractile mesenteritis

K65.8 Other peritonitis MCC HCC
Chronic proliferative peritonitis
Peritonitis due to urine

K65.9 Peritonitis, unspecified MCC HCC
Bacterial peritonitis NOS
AHA: 2022,1Q,27; 2013,2Q,31

✓4th **K66 Other disorders of peritoneum**
EXCLUDES 2 *ascites (R18.-)*
peritoneal effusion (chronic) (R18.8)

K66.Ø Peritoneal adhesions (postprocedural) (postinfection)
Adhesions (of) abdominal (wall)
Adhesions (of) diaphragm
Adhesions (of) intestine
Adhesions (of) male pelvis
Adhesions (of) omentum
Adhesions (of) stomach
Adhesive bands
Mesenteric adhesions
EXCLUDES 1 *female pelvic adhesions [bands] (N73.6)*
peritoneal adhesions with intestinal obstruction (K56.5-)

K66.1 Hemoperitoneum MCC
▶Peritoneal hematoma◀
▶Peritoneal hemorrhage◀
EXCLUDES 1 *traumatic hemoperitoneum (S36.8-)*
EXCLUDES 2 ▶*retroperitoneal hematoma (K68.3)*◀
▶*retroperitoneal hemorrhage (K68.3)*◀
AHA: 2022,1Q,22-23

K66.8 Other specified disorders of peritoneum

K66.9 Disorder of peritoneum, unspecified

K67 ***Disorders of peritoneum in infectious diseases classified elsewhere*** MCC HCC
Code first underlying disease, such as:
congenital syphilis (A5Ø.Ø)
helminthiasis (B65.Ø-B83.9)
EXCLUDES 1 *peritonitis in chlamydia (A74.81)*
peritonitis in diphtheria (A36.89)
peritonitis in gonococcal (A54.85)
peritonitis in syphilis (late) (A52.74)
peritonitis in tuberculosis (A18.31)

✓4th **K68 Disorders of retroperitoneum**

✓5th **K68.1 Retroperitoneal abscess**

K68.11 Postprocedural retroperitoneal abscess CC H11 H12 H13
EXCLUDES 2 *infection following procedure (T81.4-)*

K68.12 Psoas muscle abscess MCC HCC

K68.19 Other retroperitoneal abscess MCC HCC
AHA: 2023,2Q,27; 2019,1Q,15
TIP: This code should be used for a diagnosis of internal presacral abscess. If an intra-abdominal abscess is also present, code K65.1 can also be assigned; sequencing depends on the circumstances of admission.

● **K68.2 Retroperitoneal fibrosis** MCC
Code also, if applicable, associated obstruction of ureter (N13.5)

● **K68.3 Retroperitoneal hematoma** MCC
Retroperitoneal hemorrhage

K68.9 Other disorders of retroperitoneum MCC

Diseases of liver (K7Ø-K77)

EXCLUDES 1 *jaundice NOS (R17)*
EXCLUDES 2 *hemochromatosis (E83.11-)*
Reye's syndrome (G93.7)
viral hepatitis (B15-B19)
Wilson's disease ▶*(E83.Ø1)*◀

✓4th **K7Ø Alcoholic liver disease**
Use additional code to identify:
alcohol abuse and dependence (F1Ø.-)

K7Ø.Ø Alcoholic fatty liver A

✓5th **K7Ø.1 Alcoholic hepatitis**

K7Ø.1Ø Alcoholic hepatitis without ascites A

K7Ø.11 Alcoholic hepatitis with ascites A

K7Ø.2 Alcoholic fibrosis and sclerosis of liver A

✓5th **K7Ø.3 Alcoholic cirrhosis of liver**
Alcoholic cirrhosis NOS

K7Ø.3Ø Alcoholic cirrhosis of liver without ascites HCC A

K7Ø.31 Alcoholic cirrhosis of liver with ascites HCC A
AHA: 2018,1Q,4

K70.4 Alcoholic hepatic failure
Acute alcoholic hepatic failure
Alcoholic hepatic failure NOS
Chronic alcoholic hepatic failure
Subacute alcoholic hepatic failure

K70.40 Alcoholic hepatic failure without coma HCC A

K70.41 Alcoholic hepatic failure with coma MCC HCC A

K70.9 Alcoholic liver disease, unspecified HCC A

K71 Toxic liver disease
INCLUDES drug-induced idiosyncratic (unpredictable) liver disease
drug-induced toxic (predictable) liver disease
Code first poisoning due to drug or toxin, if applicable ▶(T36-T65 with fifth or sixth character 1-4)◀
Use additional code for adverse effect, if applicable, to identify drug (T36-T50 with fifth or sixth character 5)
EXCLUDES 2 *alcoholic liver disease (K70.-)*
Budd-Chiari syndrome (I82.0)

K71.0 Toxic liver disease with cholestasis
Cholestasis with hepatocyte injury
"Pure" cholestasis

K71.1 Toxic liver disease with hepatic necrosis
Hepatic failure (acute) (chronic) due to drugs

K71.10 Toxic liver disease with hepatic necrosis, without coma

K71.11 Toxic liver disease with hepatic necrosis, with coma MCC HCC

K71.2 Toxic liver disease with acute hepatitis

K71.3 Toxic liver disease with chronic persistent hepatitis

K71.4 Toxic liver disease with chronic lobular hepatitis

K71.5 Toxic liver disease with chronic active hepatitis
Toxic liver disease with lupoid hepatitis

K71.50 Toxic liver disease with chronic active hepatitis without ascites

K71.51 Toxic liver disease with chronic active hepatitis with ascites
AHA: 2018,1Q,4

K71.6 Toxic liver disease with hepatitis, not elsewhere classified

K71.7 Toxic liver disease with fibrosis and cirrhosis of liver

K71.8 Toxic liver disease with other disorders of liver
Toxic liver disease with focal nodular hyperplasia
Toxic liver disease with hepatic granulomas
Toxic liver disease with peliosis hepatis
Toxic liver disease with veno-occlusive disease of liver

K71.9 Toxic liver disease, unspecified

K72 Hepatic failure, not elsewhere classified
INCLUDES fulminant hepatitis NEC, with hepatic failure
liver (cell) necrosis with hepatic failure
malignant hepatitis NEC, with hepatic failure
yellow liver atrophy or dystrophy
EXCLUDES 1 *alcoholic hepatic failure (K70.4)*
hepatic failure with toxic liver disease (K71.1-)
icterus of newborn (P55-P59)
postprocedural hepatic failure (K91.82)
EXCLUDES 2 *hepatic failure complicating abortion or ectopic or molar pregnancy (O00-O07, O08.8)*
hepatic failure complicating pregnancy, childbirth and the puerperium (O26.6-)
viral hepatitis with hepatic coma (B15-B19)
AHA: 2017,1Q,41

K72.0 Acute and subacute hepatic failure
Acute non-viral hepatitis NOS
AHA: 2015,2Q,17; 2014,2Q,13

K72.00 Acute and subacute hepatic failure without coma MCC
AHA: 2021,1Q,13

K72.01 Acute and subacute hepatic failure with coma MCC HCC

K72.1 Chronic hepatic failure
End stage liver disease

K72.10 Chronic hepatic failure without coma HCC
AHA: 2021,1Q,13

K72.11 Chronic hepatic failure with coma MCC HCC

K72.9 Hepatic failure, unspecified

K72.90 Hepatic failure, unspecified without coma HCC
AHA: 2022,1Q,52; 2018,4Q,20; 2016,2Q,35

K72.91 Hepatic failure, unspecified with coma MCC HCC
Hepatic coma NOS

K73 Chronic hepatitis, not elsewhere classified
EXCLUDES 1 *alcoholic hepatitis (chronic) (K70.1-)*
drug-induced hepatitis (chronic) (K71.-)
granulomatous hepatitis (chronic) NEC (K75.3)
reactive, nonspecific hepatitis (chronic) (K75.2)
viral hepatitis (chronic) (B15-B19)

K73.0 Chronic persistent hepatitis, not elsewhere classified HCC

K73.1 Chronic lobular hepatitis, not elsewhere classified HCC

K73.2 Chronic active hepatitis, not elsewhere classified HCC

K73.8 Other chronic hepatitis, not elsewhere classified HCC

K73.9 Chronic hepatitis, unspecified HCC

K74 Fibrosis and cirrhosis of liver
Code also, if applicable, viral hepatitis (acute) (chronic) (B15-B19)
EXCLUDES 1 *alcoholic cirrhosis (of liver) (K70.3)*
alcoholic fibrosis of liver (K70.2)
cardiac sclerosis of liver (K76.1)
cirrhosis (of liver) with toxic liver disease (K71.7)
congenital cirrhosis (of liver) (P78.81)
pigmentary cirrhosis (of liver) (E83.110)

K74.0 Hepatic fibrosis
Code first underlying liver disease, such as:
nonalcoholic steatohepatitis (NASH) (K75.81)
AHA: 2020,4Q,30-31

K74.00 Hepatic fibrosis, unspecified UPD

K74.01 Hepatic fibrosis, early fibrosis UPD
Hepatic fibrosis, stage F1 or stage F2

K74.02 Hepatic fibrosis, advanced fibrosis UPD
Hepatic fibrosis, stage F3
EXCLUDES 1 *cirrhosis of liver (K74.6-)*
hepatic fibrosis, stage F4 (K74.6-)

K74.1 Hepatic sclerosis

K74.2 Hepatic fibrosis with hepatic sclerosis

K74.3 Primary biliary cirrhosis HCC
Chronic nonsuppurative destructive cholangitis
Primary biliary cholangitis
EXCLUDES 2 *primary sclerosing cholangitis (K83.01)*

K74.4 Secondary biliary cirrhosis HCC

K74.5 Biliary cirrhosis, unspecified HCC

K74.6 Other and unspecified cirrhosis of liver
AHA: 2020,4Q,30-31

K74.60 Unspecified cirrhosis of liver HCC
Cirrhosis (of liver) NOS
AHA: 2018,1Q,4

K74.69 Other cirrhosis of liver HCC
Cryptogenic cirrhosis (of liver)
Macronodular cirrhosis (of liver)
Micronodular cirrhosis (of liver)
Mixed type cirrhosis (of liver)
Portal cirrhosis (of liver)
Postnecrotic cirrhosis (of liver)

K75 Other inflammatory liver diseases
EXCLUDES 2 *toxic liver disease (K71.-)*

K75.0 Abscess of liver MCC
Cholangitic hepatic abscess
Hematogenic hepatic abscess
Hepatic abscess NOS
Lymphogenic hepatic abscess
Pylephlebitic hepatic abscess
EXCLUDES 1 *amebic liver abscess (A06.4)*
cholangitis without liver abscess (K83.09)
pylephlebitis without liver abscess (K75.1)
EXCLUDES 2 *acute or subacute hepatitis NOS (B17.9)*
acute or subacute non-viral hepatitis (K72.0)
chronic hepatitis NEC (K73.8)

K75.1 Phlebitis of portal vein MCC
Pylephlebitis
EXCLUDES 1 *pylephlebitic liver abscess (K75.0)*
DEF: Inflammation of the portal vein or branches due to diverticulitis, perforated appendicitis, or peritonitis. Symptoms include fever, chills, jaundice, sweating, and abscess in various body parts.

K75.2 Nonspecific reactive hepatitis
EXCLUDES 1 *acute or subacute hepatitis (K72.Ø-)*
chronic hepatitis NEC (K73.-)
viral hepatitis (B15-B19)

K75.3 Granulomatous hepatitis, not elsewhere classified
EXCLUDES 1 *acute or subacute hepatitis (K72.Ø-)*
chronic hepatitis NEC (K73.-)
viral hepatitis (B15-B19)

K75.4 Autoimmune hepatitis HCC
Lupoid hepatitis NEC

✓5th **K75.8 Other specified inflammatory liver diseases**

K75.81 Nonalcoholic steatohepatitis (NASH)
Use additional code, if applicable, hepatic fibrosis (K74.Ø-)

K75.89 Other specified inflammatory liver diseases

K75.9 Inflammatory liver disease, unspecified
Hepatitis NOS
EXCLUDES 1 *acute or subacute hepatitis (K72.Ø-)*
chronic hepatitis NEC (K73.-)
viral hepatitis (B15-B19)
AHA: 2015,2Q,17

✓4th **K76 Other diseases of liver**
EXCLUDES 2 *alcoholic liver disease (K7Ø.-)*
amyloid degeneration of liver (E85.-)
cystic disease of liver (congenital) (Q44.6)
hepatic vein thrombosis (I82.Ø)
hepatomegaly NOS (R16.Ø)
pigmentary cirrhosis (of liver) (E83.11Ø)
portal vein thrombosis (I81)
toxic liver disease (K71.-)

K76.Ø Fatty (change of) liver, not elsewhere classified
Nonalcoholic fatty liver disease (NAFLD)
EXCLUDES 1 *nonalcoholic steatohepatitis (NASH) (K75.81)*

K76.1 Chronic passive congestion of liver
Cardiac cirrhosis
Cardiac sclerosis

K76.2 Central hemorrhagic necrosis of liver MCC
EXCLUDES 1 *liver necrosis with hepatic failure (K72.-)*

K76.3 Infarction of liver MCC

K76.4 Peliosis hepatis
Hepatic angiomatosis

K76.5 Hepatic veno-occlusive disease
EXCLUDES 1 *Budd-Chiari syndrome (I82.Ø)*

K76.6 Portal hypertension CC HCC
Use additional code for any associated complications, such as:
portal hypertensive gastropathy (K31.89)
AHA: 2020,1Q,15

K76.7 Hepatorenal syndrome MCC HCC
EXCLUDES 1 *hepatorenal syndrome following labor and delivery ▶(O9Ø.41)◀*
postprocedural hepatorenal syndrome (K91.83)

✓5th **K76.8 Other specified diseases of liver**

K76.81 Hepatopulmonary syndrome UPD HCC
Code first underlying liver disease, such as:
alcoholic cirrhosis of liver (K7Ø.3-)
cirrhosis of liver without mention of alcohol (K74.6-)

K76.82 Hepatic encephalopathy HCC
Hepatic encephalopathy, NOS
Hepatic encephalopathy without coma
Hepatocerebral intoxication
Portal-systemic encephalopathy
Code also underlying liver disease, such as:
acute and subacute hepatic failure without coma (K72.ØØ)
alcoholic hepatic failure without coma (K7Ø.4Ø)
chronic hepatic failure without coma (K72.1Ø)
hepatic failure with toxic liver disease without coma (K71.1Ø)
hepatic failure without coma (K72.9Ø)
icterus of newborn (P55-P59)
postprocedural hepatic failure (K91.82)
viral hepatitis without hepatic coma (B15.9, B16.1, B16.9, B17.1Ø, B19.1Ø, B19.2Ø, B19.9)
EXCLUDES 1 *acute and subacute hepatic failure with coma (K72.Ø1)*
alcoholic hepatic failure with coma (K7Ø.41)
chronic hepatic failure with coma (K72.11)
hepatic failure with coma (K72.91)
AHA: 2022,4Q,27-28

K76.89 Other specified diseases of liver
Cyst (simple) of liver
Focal nodular hyperplasia of liver
Hepatoptosis
AHA: 2023,1Q,26; 2022,3Q,7
TIP: Assign codes E80.6 and K76.89 to report benign recurrent intrahepatic cholestasis (BRIC) or progressive familial intrahepatic cholestasis (PFIC).

K76.9 Liver disease, unspecified

K77 Liver disorders in diseases classified elsewhere CC
Code first underlying disease, such as:
amyloidosis (E85.-)
congenital syphilis (A5Ø.Ø, A5Ø.5)
congenital toxoplasmosis (P37.1)
infectious mononucleosis with liver disease (B27.Ø-B27.9 with fifth character 9)
schistosomiasis (B65.Ø-B65.9)
EXCLUDES 1 *alcoholic hepatitis (K7Ø.1-)*
alcoholic liver disease (K7Ø.-)
cytomegaloviral hepatitis (B25.1)
herpesviral [herpes simplex] hepatitis (BØØ.81)
mumps hepatitis (B26.81)
sarcoidosis with liver disease (D86.89)
secondary syphilis with liver disease (A51.45)
syphilis (late) with liver disease (A52.74)
toxoplasmosis (acquired) hepatitis (B58.1)
tuberculosis with liver disease (A18.83)

Disorders of gallbladder, biliary tract and pancreas (K80-K87)

K80 Cholelithiasis

EXCLUDES 1 *retained cholelithiasis following cholecystectomy (K91.86)*

AHA: 2018,4Q,20

DEF: Presence or formation of concretions (calculi or "gallstones") in the gallbladder. The stones contain cholesterol, calcium carbonate, or calcium bilirubinate in pure forms or in various combinations.

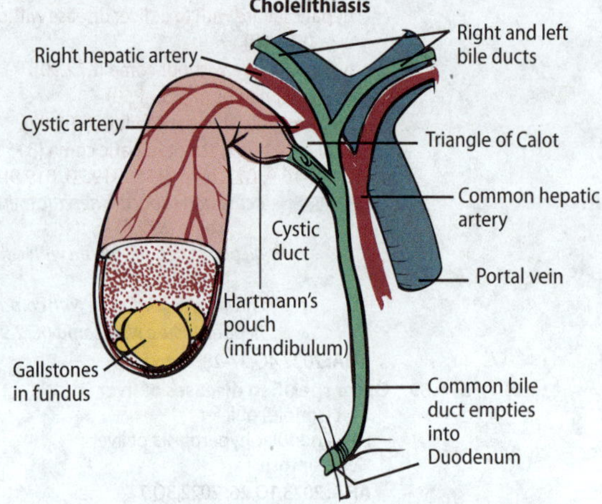

K80.0 Calculus of gallbladder with acute cholecystitis

Any condition listed in K80.2 with acute cholecystitis

Use additional code if applicable for associated gangrene of gallbladder (K82.A1), or perforation of gallbladder (K82.A2)

- **K80.00 Calculus of gallbladder with acute cholecystitis without obstruction** CC
  - **AHA:** 2023,2Q,11
- **K80.01 Calculus of gallbladder with acute cholecystitis with obstruction** CC

K80.1 Calculus of gallbladder with other cholecystitis

Use additional code if applicable for associated gangrene of gallbladder (K82.A1), or perforation of gallbladder (K82.A2)

- **K80.10 Calculus of gallbladder with chronic cholecystitis without obstruction** CC
  - Cholelithiasis with cholecystitis NOS
- **K80.11 Calculus of gallbladder with chronic cholecystitis with obstruction** CC
- **K80.12 Calculus of gallbladder with acute and chronic cholecystitis without obstruction** CC
- **K80.13 Calculus of gallbladder with acute and chronic cholecystitis with obstruction** CC
- **K80.18 Calculus of gallbladder with other cholecystitis without obstruction** CC
- **K80.19 Calculus of gallbladder with other cholecystitis with obstruction** CC

K80.2 Calculus of gallbladder without cholecystitis

Cholecystolithiasis without cholecystitis
Cholelithiasis (without cholecystitis)
Colic (recurrent) of gallbladder (without cholecystitis)
Gallstone (impacted) of cystic duct (without cholecystitis)
Gallstone (impacted) of gallbladder (without cholecystitis)

- **K80.20 Calculus of gallbladder without cholecystitis without obstruction**
- **K80.21 Calculus of gallbladder without cholecystitis with obstruction** CC

K80.3 Calculus of bile duct with cholangitis

Any condition listed in K80.5 with cholangitis

DEF: Cholangitis: Inflammation of the bile ducts.

- **K80.30 Calculus of bile duct with cholangitis, unspecified, without obstruction** CC
- **K80.31 Calculus of bile duct with cholangitis, unspecified, with obstruction** CC
- **K80.32 Calculus of bile duct with acute cholangitis without obstruction** CC
- **K80.33 Calculus of bile duct with acute cholangitis with obstruction** CC
- **K80.34 Calculus of bile duct with chronic cholangitis without obstruction** CC
- **K80.35 Calculus of bile duct with chronic cholangitis with obstruction** CC
- **K80.36 Calculus of bile duct with acute and chronic cholangitis without obstruction** CC
- **K80.37 Calculus of bile duct with acute and chronic cholangitis with obstruction** CC

K80.4 Calculus of bile duct with cholecystitis

Any condition listed in K80.5 with cholecystitis (with cholangitis)

▶Code also, if applicable, fistula of bile duct◀ (K83.3)

Use additional code if applicable for associated gangrene of gallbladder (K82.A1), or perforation of gallbladder (K82.A2)

AHA: 2019,1Q,17

- **K80.40 Calculus of bile duct with cholecystitis, unspecified, without obstruction** CC
- **K80.41 Calculus of bile duct with cholecystitis, unspecified, with obstruction** CC
  - **AHA:** 2019,1Q,17
- **K80.42 Calculus of bile duct with acute cholecystitis without obstruction** CC
- **K80.43 Calculus of bile duct with acute cholecystitis with obstruction** CC
- **K80.44 Calculus of bile duct with chronic cholecystitis without obstruction** CC
- **K80.45 Calculus of bile duct with chronic cholecystitis with obstruction** CC
- **K80.46 Calculus of bile duct with acute and chronic cholecystitis without obstruction** CC
- **K80.47 Calculus of bile duct with acute and chronic cholecystitis with obstruction** CC

K80.5 Calculus of bile duct without cholangitis or cholecystitis

Choledocholithiasis (without cholangitis or cholecystitis)
Gallstone (impacted) of bile duct NOS (without cholangitis or cholecystitis)
Gallstone (impacted) of common duct (without cholangitis or cholecystitis)
Gallstone (impacted) of hepatic duct (without cholangitis or cholecystitis)
Hepatic cholelithiasis (without cholangitis or cholecystitis)
Hepatic colic (recurrent) (without cholangitis or cholecystitis)

DEF: Cholangitis: Inflammation of the bile ducts.

- **K80.50 Calculus of bile duct without cholangitis or cholecystitis without obstruction**
- **K80.51 Calculus of bile duct without cholangitis or cholecystitis with obstruction** CC

K80.6 Calculus of gallbladder and bile duct with cholecystitis

Use additional code if applicable for associated gangrene of gallbladder (K82.A1), or perforation of gallbladder (K82.A2)

- **K80.60 Calculus of gallbladder and bile duct with cholecystitis, unspecified, without obstruction** CC
- **K80.61 Calculus of gallbladder and bile duct with cholecystitis, unspecified, with obstruction** CC
- **K80.62 Calculus of gallbladder and bile duct with acute cholecystitis without obstruction** CC
- **K80.63 Calculus of gallbladder and bile duct with acute cholecystitis with obstruction** CC
- **K80.64 Calculus of gallbladder and bile duct with chronic cholecystitis without obstruction** CC
- **K80.65 Calculus of gallbladder and bile duct with chronic cholecystitis with obstruction** CC
- **K80.66 Calculus of gallbladder and bile duct with acute and chronic cholecystitis without obstruction** CC
- **K80.67 Calculus of gallbladder and bile duct with acute and chronic cholecystitis with obstruction** MCC

K80.7 Calculus of gallbladder and bile duct without cholecystitis

- **K80.70 Calculus of gallbladder and bile duct without cholecystitis without obstruction**
- **K80.71 Calculus of gallbladder and bile duct without cholecystitis with obstruction** CC

K80.8 Other cholelithiasis

- **K80.80 Other cholelithiasis without obstruction**
- **K80.81 Other cholelithiasis with obstruction** CC

K81 Cholecystitis

Use additional code if applicable for associated gangrene of gallbladder (K82.A1), or perforation of gallbladder (K82.A2)

EXCLUDES 1 *cholecystitis with cholelithiasis (K8Ø.-)*

AHA: 2018,4Q,20

K81.Ø Acute cholecystitis CC

Abscess of gallbladder
Angiocholecystitis
Emphysematous (acute) cholecystitis
Empyema of gallbladder
Gangrene of gallbladder
Gangrenous cholecystitis
Suppurative cholecystitis

K81.1 Chronic cholecystitis

K81.2 Acute cholecystitis with chronic cholecystitis CC

K81.9 Cholecystitis, unspecified

K82 Other diseases of gallbladder

EXCLUDES 1 *nonvisualization of gallbladder (R93.2)*
postcholecystectomy syndrome (K91.5)

K82.Ø Obstruction of gallbladder CC

Occlusion of cystic duct or gallbladder without cholelithiasis
Stenosis of cystic duct or gallbladder without cholelithiasis
Stricture of cystic duct or gallbladder without cholelithiasis

EXCLUDES 1 *obstruction of gallbladder with cholelithiasis (K8Ø.-)*

K82.1 Hydrops of gallbladder CC

Mucocele of gallbladder

K82.2 Perforation of gallbladder MCC

Rupture of cystic duct or gallbladder

EXCLUDES 1 *perforation of gallbladder in cholecystitis (K82.A2)*

K82.3 Fistula of gallbladder CC

Cholecystocolic fistula
Cholecystoduodenal fistula

K82.4 Cholesterolosis of gallbladder

Strawberry gallbladder

EXCLUDES 1 *cholesterolosis of gallbladder with cholecystitis (K81.-)*
cholesterolosis of gallbladder with cholelithiasis (K8Ø.-)

K82.8 Other specified diseases of gallbladder

Adhesions of cystic duct or gallbladder
Atrophy of cystic duct or gallbladder
Cyst of cystic duct or gallbladder
Dyskinesia of cystic duct or gallbladder
Hypertrophy of cystic duct or gallbladder
Nonfunctioning of cystic duct or gallbladder
Ulcer of cystic duct or gallbladder

K82.9 Disease of gallbladder, unspecified

K82.A Disorders of gallbladder in diseases classified elsewhere

Code first the type of cholecystitis (K81.-), or cholelithiasis with cholecystitis (K8Ø.ØØ-K8Ø.19, K8Ø.4Ø-K8Ø.47, K8Ø.6Ø-K8Ø.67)

AHA: 2018,4Q,19-20

K82.A1 Gangrene of gallbladder in cholecystitis

K82.A2 Perforation of gallbladder in cholecystitis CC

K83 Other diseases of biliary tract

EXCLUDES 1 *postcholecystectomy syndrome (K91.5)*

EXCLUDES 2 *conditions involving the cystic duct (K81-K82)*
conditions involving the gallbladder (K81-K82)

K83.Ø Cholangitis

EXCLUDES 1 *cholangitic liver abscess (K75.Ø)*
cholangitis with choledocholithiasis (K8Ø.3-, K8Ø.4-)

EXCLUDES 2 *chronic nonsuppurative destructive cholangitis (K74.3)*
primary biliary cholangitis (K74.3)
primary biliary cirrhosis (K74.3)

AHA: 2018,4Q,20

K83.Ø1 Primary sclerosing cholangitis CC

K83.Ø9 Other cholangitis CC

Ascending cholangitis
Cholangitis NOS
Primary cholangitis
Recurrent cholangitis
Sclerosing cholangitis
Secondary cholangitis
Stenosing cholangitis
Suppurative cholangitis

K83.1 Obstruction of bile duct MCC

Occlusion of bile duct without cholelithiasis
Stenosis of bile duct without cholelithiasis
Stricture of bile duct without cholelithiasis

EXCLUDES 1 *congenital obstruction of bile duct (Q44.3)*
obstruction of bile duct with cholelithiasis (K8Ø.-)

AHA: 2023,1Q,26; 2016,1Q,18

K83.2 Perforation of bile duct MCC

Rupture of bile duct

K83.3 Fistula of bile duct CC

Choledochoduodenal fistula

AHA: 2019,1Q,17

K83.4 Spasm of sphincter of Oddi

K83.5 Biliary cyst

K83.8 Other specified diseases of biliary tract

Adhesions of biliary tract
Atrophy of biliary tract
Hypertrophy of biliary tract
Ulcer of biliary tract

K83.9 Disease of biliary tract, unspecified

K85 Acute pancreatitis

INCLUDES acute (recurrent) pancreatitis
subacute pancreatitis

AHA: 2016,4Q,34

K85.Ø Idiopathic acute pancreatitis

K85.ØØ Idiopathic acute pancreatitis without necrosis or infection MCC

K85.Ø1 Idiopathic acute pancreatitis with uninfected necrosis MCC

K85.Ø2 Idiopathic acute pancreatitis with infected necrosis MCC

K85.1 Biliary acute pancreatitis

Gallstone pancreatitis

AHA: 2023,2Q,11

K85.1Ø Biliary acute pancreatitis without necrosis or infection MCC

K85.11 Biliary acute pancreatitis with uninfected necrosis MCC

K85.12 Biliary acute pancreatitis with infected necrosis MCC

K85.2 Alcohol induced acute pancreatitis

EXCLUDES 2 *alcohol induced chronic pancreatitis (K86.Ø)*

K85.2Ø Alcohol induced acute pancreatitis without necrosis or infection MCC

AHA: 2020,1Q,9

K85.21 Alcohol induced acute pancreatitis with uninfected necrosis MCC

K85.22 Alcohol induced acute pancreatitis with infected necrosis MCC

K85.3 Drug induced acute pancreatitis

Use additional code for adverse effect, if applicable, to identify drug (T36-T5Ø with fifth or sixth character 5)

Use additional code to identify drug abuse and dependence (F11.- F17.-)

K85.3Ø Drug induced acute pancreatitis without necrosis or infection MCC

K85.31 Drug induced acute pancreatitis with uninfected necrosis MCC

K85.32 Drug induced acute pancreatitis with infected necrosis MCC

K85.8 Other acute pancreatitis

K85.8Ø Other acute pancreatitis without necrosis or infection MCC

K85.81 Other acute pancreatitis with uninfected necrosis MCC

K85.82 Other acute pancreatitis with infected necrosis MCC

K85.9 Acute pancreatitis, unspecified

Pancreatitis NOS

K85.9Ø Acute pancreatitis without necrosis or infection, unspecified MCC

K85.91 Acute pancreatitis with uninfected necrosis, unspecified MCC

K85.92 Acute pancreatitis with infected necrosis, unspecified MCC

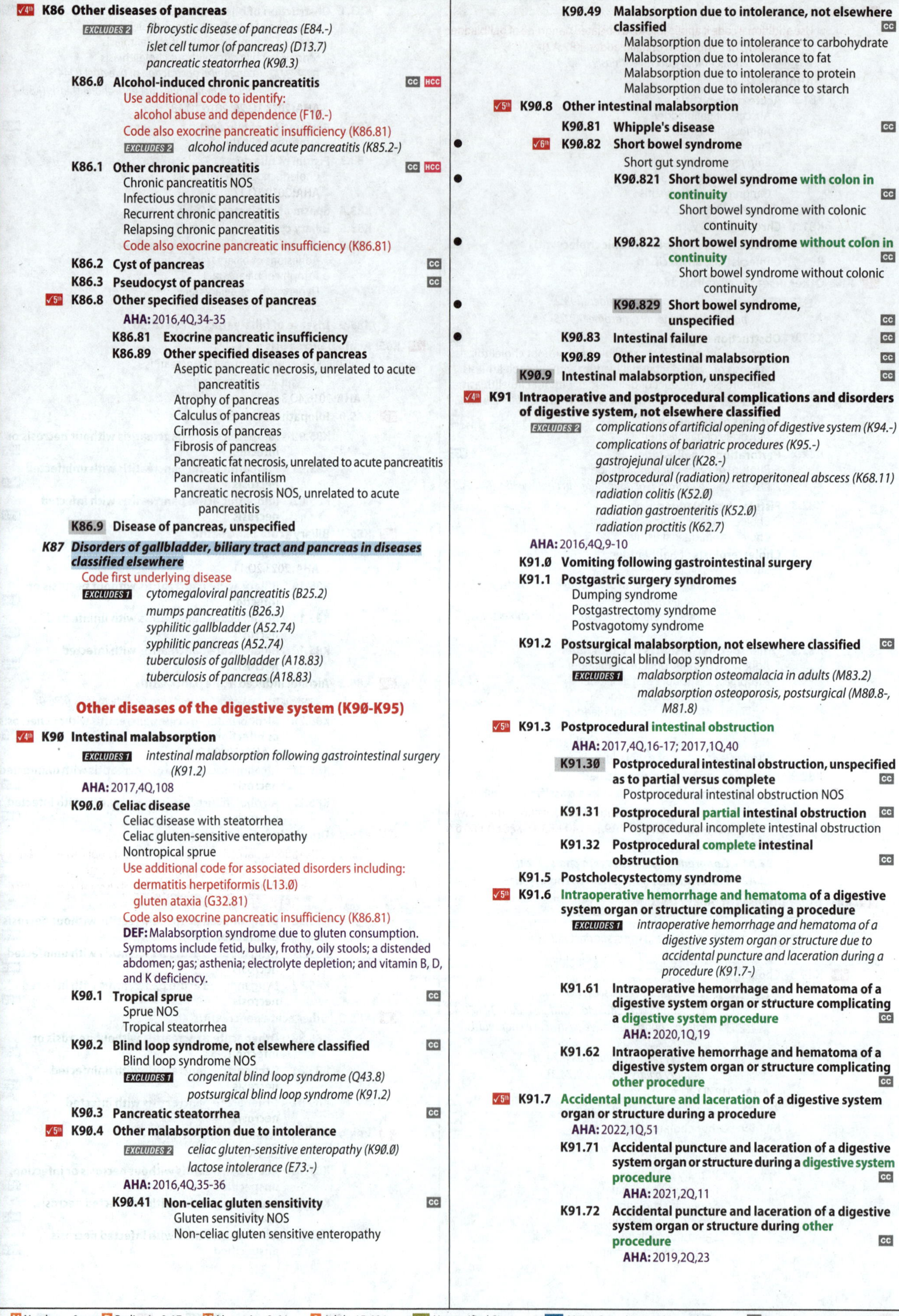

K86 Other diseases of pancreas

EXCLUDES 2 *fibrocystic disease of pancreas (E84.-)*
islet cell tumor (of pancreas) (D13.7)
pancreatic steatorrhea (K90.3)

K86.0 Alcohol-induced chronic pancreatitis CC HCC
Use additional code to identify:
alcohol abuse and dependence (F10.-)
Code also exocrine pancreatic insufficiency (K86.81)
EXCLUDES 2 *alcohol induced acute pancreatitis (K85.2-)*

K86.1 Other chronic pancreatitis CC HCC
Chronic pancreatitis NOS
Infectious chronic pancreatitis
Recurrent chronic pancreatitis
Relapsing chronic pancreatitis
Code also exocrine pancreatic insufficiency (K86.81)

K86.2 Cyst of pancreas CC

K86.3 Pseudocyst of pancreas CC

K86.8 Other specified diseases of pancreas
AHA: 2016,4Q,34-35

K86.81 Exocrine pancreatic insufficiency

K86.89 Other specified diseases of pancreas
Aseptic pancreatic necrosis, unrelated to acute pancreatitis
Atrophy of pancreas
Calculus of pancreas
Cirrhosis of pancreas
Fibrosis of pancreas
Pancreatic fat necrosis, unrelated to acute pancreatitis
Pancreatic infantilism
Pancreatic necrosis NOS, unrelated to acute pancreatitis

K86.9 Disease of pancreas, unspecified

K87 Disorders of gallbladder, biliary tract and pancreas in diseases classified elsewhere
Code first underlying disease
EXCLUDES 1 *cytomegaloviral pancreatitis (B25.2)*
mumps pancreatitis (B26.3)
syphilitic gallbladder (A52.74)
syphilitic pancreas (A52.74)
tuberculosis of gallbladder (A18.83)
tuberculosis of pancreas (A18.83)

Other diseases of the digestive system (K90-K95)

K90 Intestinal malabsorption
EXCLUDES 1 *intestinal malabsorption following gastrointestinal surgery (K91.2)*
AHA: 2017,4Q,108

K90.0 Celiac disease
Celiac disease with steatorrhea
Celiac gluten-sensitive enteropathy
Nontropical sprue
Use additional code for associated disorders including:
dermatitis herpetiformis (L13.0)
gluten ataxia (G32.81)
Code also exocrine pancreatic insufficiency (K86.81)
DEF: Malabsorption syndrome due to gluten consumption. Symptoms include fetid, bulky, frothy, oily stools; a distended abdomen; gas; asthenia; electrolyte depletion; and vitamin B, D, and K deficiency.

K90.1 Tropical sprue CC
Sprue NOS
Tropical steatorrhea

K90.2 Blind loop syndrome, not elsewhere classified CC
Blind loop syndrome NOS
EXCLUDES 1 *congenital blind loop syndrome (Q43.8)*
postsurgical blind loop syndrome (K91.2)

K90.3 Pancreatic steatorrhea CC

K90.4 Other malabsorption due to intolerance
EXCLUDES 2 *celiac gluten-sensitive enteropathy (K90.0)*
lactose intolerance (E73.-)
AHA: 2016,4Q,35-36

K90.41 Non-celiac gluten sensitivity CC
Gluten sensitivity NOS
Non-celiac gluten sensitive enteropathy

K90.49 Malabsorption due to intolerance, not elsewhere classified CC
Malabsorption due to intolerance to carbohydrate
Malabsorption due to intolerance to fat
Malabsorption due to intolerance to protein
Malabsorption due to intolerance to starch

K90.8 Other intestinal malabsorption

K90.81 Whipple's disease CC

● **K90.82 Short bowel syndrome**
Short gut syndrome

● **K90.821 Short bowel syndrome with colon in continuity** CC
Short bowel syndrome with colonic continuity

● **K90.822 Short bowel syndrome without colon in continuity** CC
Short bowel syndrome without colonic continuity

● **K90.829 Short bowel syndrome, unspecified** CC

● **K90.83 Intestinal failure** CC

K90.89 Other intestinal malabsorption CC

K90.9 Intestinal malabsorption, unspecified CC

K91 Intraoperative and postprocedural complications and disorders of digestive system, not elsewhere classified
EXCLUDES 2 *complications of artificial opening of digestive system (K94.-)*
complications of bariatric procedures (K95.-)
gastrojejunal ulcer (K28.-)
postprocedural (radiation) retroperitoneal abscess (K68.11)
radiation colitis (K52.0)
radiation gastroenteritis (K52.0)
radiation proctitis (K62.7)
AHA: 2016,4Q,9-10

K91.0 Vomiting following gastrointestinal surgery

K91.1 Postgastric surgery syndromes
Dumping syndrome
Postgastrectomy syndrome
Postvagotomy syndrome

K91.2 Postsurgical malabsorption, not elsewhere classified CC
Postsurgical blind loop syndrome
EXCLUDES 1 *malabsorption osteomalacia in adults (M83.2)*
malabsorption osteoporosis, postsurgical (M80.8-, M81.8)

K91.3 Postprocedural intestinal obstruction
AHA: 2017,4Q,16-17; 2017,1Q,40

K91.30 Postprocedural intestinal obstruction, unspecified as to partial versus complete CC
Postprocedural intestinal obstruction NOS

K91.31 Postprocedural partial intestinal obstruction CC
Postprocedural incomplete intestinal obstruction

K91.32 Postprocedural complete intestinal obstruction CC

K91.5 Postcholecystectomy syndrome

K91.6 Intraoperative hemorrhage and hematoma of a digestive system organ or structure complicating a procedure
EXCLUDES 1 *intraoperative hemorrhage and hematoma of a digestive system organ or structure due to accidental puncture and laceration during a procedure (K91.7-)*

K91.61 Intraoperative hemorrhage and hematoma of a digestive system organ or structure complicating a digestive system procedure CC
AHA: 2020,1Q,19

K91.62 Intraoperative hemorrhage and hematoma of a digestive system organ or structure complicating other procedure CC

K91.7 Accidental puncture and laceration of a digestive system organ or structure during a procedure
AHA: 2022,1Q,51

K91.71 Accidental puncture and laceration of a digestive system organ or structure during a digestive system procedure CC
AHA: 2021,2Q,11

K91.72 Accidental puncture and laceration of a digestive system organ or structure during other procedure CC
AHA: 2019,2Q,23

K91.8 Other intraoperative and postprocedural complications and disorders of digestive system

- **K91.81** Other intraoperative complications of digestive system — CC
- **K91.82** Postprocedural hepatic failure — CC
- **K91.83** Postprocedural hepatorenal syndrome — CC
- **K91.84** Postprocedural hemorrhage of a digestive system organ or structure following a procedure
  - **K91.840** Postprocedural hemorrhage of a digestive system organ or structure following a digestive system procedure — CC
    AHA: 2016,1Q,15
  - **K91.841** Postprocedural hemorrhage of a digestive system organ or structure following other procedure — CC
- **K91.85** Complications of intestinal pouch
  - **K91.850** Pouchitis — CC HCC
    Inflammation of internal ileoanal pouch
    DEF: Inflammatory complication of an existing surgically created ileoanal pouch, resulting in multiple GI complaints, including diarrhea, abdominal pain, rectal bleeding, fecal urgency, or incontinence.
  - **K91.858** Other complications of intestinal pouch — CC HCC
    AHA: 2019,2Q,13
- **K91.86** Retained cholelithiasis following cholecystectomy — CC
- **K91.87** Postprocedural hematoma and seroma of a digestive system organ or structure following a procedure
  - **K91.870** Postprocedural hematoma of a digestive system organ or structure following a digestive system procedure — CC
    AHA: 2022,1Q,24
  - **K91.871** Postprocedural hematoma of a digestive system organ or structure following other procedure — CC
  - **K91.872** Postprocedural seroma of a digestive system organ or structure following a digestive system procedure — CC
  - **K91.873** Postprocedural seroma of a digestive system organ or structure following other procedure — CC
- **K91.89** Other postprocedural complications and disorders of digestive system — CC
  Use additional code, if applicable, to further specify disorder
  EXCLUDES 2 *postprocedural retroperitoneal abscess (K68.11)*
  AHA: 2020,2Q,22; 2017,1Q,40

K92 Other diseases of digestive system

EXCLUDES 1 *neonatal gastrointestinal hemorrhage (P54.0-P54.3)*

- **K92.0 Hematemesis** — CC
- **K92.1 Melena** — CC
  EXCLUDES 1 *occult blood in feces (R19.5)*
- **K92.2 Gastrointestinal hemorrhage, unspecified** — CC
  Gastric hemorrhage NOS
  Intestinal hemorrhage NOS
  EXCLUDES 1 *acute hemorrhagic gastritis (K29.01)*
  hemorrhage of anus and rectum (K62.5)
  angiodysplasia of stomach with hemorrhage (K31.811)
  diverticular disease with hemorrhage (K57.-)
  gastritis and duodenitis with hemorrhage (K29.-)
  peptic ulcer with hemorrhage (K25-K28)
  AHA: 2021,1Q,11
- **K92.8 Other specified diseases of the digestive system**
  - **K92.81** Gastrointestinal mucositis (ulcerative) — CC
    Code also type of associated therapy, such as:
    antineoplastic and immunosuppressive drugs (T45.1X-)
    radiological procedure and radiotherapy (Y84.2)
    EXCLUDES 2 *mucositis (ulcerative) of vagina and vulva (N76.81)*
    nasal mucositis (ulcerative) (J34.81)
    oral mucositis (ulcerative) (K12.3-)
  - **K92.89** Other specified diseases of the digestive system
- **K92.9 Disease of digestive system, unspecified**

K94 Complications of artificial openings of the digestive system

- **K94.0 Colostomy complications**
  - **K94.00** Colostomy complication, unspecified — HCC
  - **K94.01** Colostomy hemorrhage — CC HCC
  - **K94.02** Colostomy infection — CC HCC
    Use additional code to specify type of infection, such as:
    cellulitis of abdominal wall (L03.311)
    sepsis (A40.-, A41.-)
  - **K94.03** Colostomy malfunction — CC HCC
    Mechanical complication of colostomy
  - **K94.09** Other complications of colostomy — CC HCC
- **K94.1 Enterostomy complications**
  - **K94.10** Enterostomy complication, unspecified — HCC
  - **K94.11** Enterostomy hemorrhage — CC HCC
  - **K94.12** Enterostomy infection — CC HCC
    Use additional code to specify type of infection, such as:
    cellulitis of abdominal wall (L03.311)
    sepsis (A40.-, A41.-)
  - **K94.13** Enterostomy malfunction — CC HCC
    Mechanical complication of enterostomy
  - **K94.19** Other complications of enterostomy — CC HCC
- **K94.2 Gastrostomy complications**
  - **K94.20** Gastrostomy complication, unspecified — HCC
  - **K94.21** Gastrostomy hemorrhage — HCC
  - **K94.22** Gastrostomy infection — CC HCC
    Use additional code to specify type of infection, such as:
    cellulitis of abdominal wall (L03.311)
    sepsis (A40.-, A41.-)
  - **K94.23** Gastrostomy malfunction — CC HCC
    Mechanical complication of gastrostomy
    AHA: 2019,1Q,26
  - **K94.29** Other complications of gastrostomy — HCC
- **K94.3 Esophagostomy complications**
  - **K94.30** Esophagostomy complications, unspecified — CC HCC
  - **K94.31** Esophagostomy hemorrhage — CC HCC
  - **K94.32** Esophagostomy infection — CC HCC
    Use additional code to identify the infection
  - **K94.33** Esophagostomy malfunction — CC HCC
    Mechanical complication of esophagostomy
  - **K94.39** Other complications of esophagostomy — CC HCC

K95 Complications of bariatric procedures

- **K95.0 Complications of gastric band procedure**
  - **K95.01** Infection due to gastric band procedure — CC H11
    Use additional code to specify type of infection or organism, such as:
    bacterial and viral infectious agents (B95.-, B96.-)
    cellulitis of abdominal wall (L03.311)
    sepsis (A40.-, A41.-)
  - **K95.09** Other complications of gastric band procedure — CC
    Use additional code, if applicable, to further specify complication
- **K95.8 Complications of other bariatric procedure**
  EXCLUDES 1 *complications of gastric band surgery (K95.0-)*
  - **K95.81** Infection due to other bariatric procedure — CC H11
    Use additional code to specify type of infection or organism, such as:
    bacterial and viral infectious agents (B95.-, B96.-)
    cellulitis of abdominal wall (L03.311)
    sepsis (A40.-, A41.-)
  - **K95.89** Other complications of other bariatric procedure — CC
    Use additional code, if applicable, to further specify complication

Additional Character Required | Placeholder | Questionable PDx | Manifestation | Unspecified | UPD Unacceptable PDx | H1-H14 HAC | HCC CMS-HCC Dx | HIV HIV Dx

Chapter 12. Diseases of the Skin and Subcutaneous Tissue (LØØ–L99)

Chapter-specific Guidelines with Coding Examples

The chapter-specific guidelines from the ICD-10-CM Official Guidelines for Coding and Reporting have been provided below. Along with these guidelines are coding examples, contained in the shaded boxes, that have been developed to help illustrate the coding and/or sequencing guidance found in these guidelines.

a. Pressure ulcer stage codes

1) Pressure ulcer stages

Codes in category L89, Pressure ulcer, identify the site and stage of the pressure ulcer.

The ICD-10-CM classifies pressure ulcer stages based on severity, which is designated by stages 1-4, deep tissue pressure injury, unspecified stage, and unstageable.

Assign as many codes from category L89 as needed to identify all the pressure ulcers the patient has, if applicable.

See Section I.B.14. for pressure ulcer stage documentation by clinicians other than patient's provider

> Nursing notes: Dressings changed daily on stage 4 ulcer on heel and stage 2 ulcer on elbow
>
> Discharge summary: Pressure ulcers on right heel and left elbow
>
> **L89.614 Pressure ulcer of right heel, stage 4**
>
> **L89.Ø22 Pressure ulcer of left elbow, stage 2**
>
> *Explanation:* Right heel and left elbow pressure ulcers were documented by the patient's provider in the discharge summary. Although the stage of these ulcers was not included in the provider's diagnostic statement, it is appropriate to code the stage from documentation from other clinicians involved in the patient's care, such as the nurse's notes, according to section I.B.14. Combination codes from category L89 Pressure ulcer, identify the site of the pressure ulcer as well as the stage. Assign as many codes from category L89 as needed to identify all the pressure ulcers the patient has.

2) Unstageable pressure ulcers

Assignment of the code for unstageable pressure ulcer (L89.--Ø) should be based on the clinical documentation. These codes are used for pressure ulcers whose stage cannot be clinically determined (e.g., the ulcer is covered by eschar or has been treated with a skin or muscle graft). This code should not be confused with the codes for unspecified stage (L89.--9). When there is no documentation regarding the stage of the pressure ulcer, assign the appropriate code for unspecified stage (L89.--9).

> Pressure ulcer of the right lower back documented as unstageable due to the presence of thick eschar covering the ulcer
>
> **L89.13Ø Pressure ulcer of right lower back, unstageable**
>
> *Explanation:* Codes for unstageable pressure ulcers are assigned when the stage cannot be clinically determined (e.g., the ulcer is covered by eschar or has been treated with a skin or muscle graft).

If during an encounter, the stage of an unstageable pressure ulcer is revealed after debridement, assign only the code for the stage revealed following debridement.

3) Documented pressure ulcer stage

Assignment of the pressure ulcer stage code should be guided by clinical documentation of the stage or documentation of the terms found in the Alphabetic Index. For clinical terms describing the stage that are not found in the Alphabetic Index, and there is no documentation of the stage, the provider should be queried.

> Left heel pressure ulcer with partial thickness skin loss involving the dermis
>
> **L89.622 Pressure ulcer of left heel, stage 2**
>
> *Explanation:* Code assignment for the pressure ulcer stage should be guided by either the clinical documentation of the stage or the documentation of terms found in the Alphabetic Index. The clinical documentation describing the left heel pressure ulcer "partial thickness skin loss involving the dermis" matches the ICD-10-CM index parenthetical description for stage 2 "(abrasion, blister, partial thickness skin loss involving epidermis and/or dermis)."

4) Patients admitted with pressure ulcers documented as healed

No code is assigned if the documentation states that the pressure ulcer is completely healed at the time of admission.

5) Pressure ulcers documented as healing

Pressure ulcers described as healing should be assigned the appropriate pressure ulcer stage code based on the documentation in the medical record. If the documentation does not provide information about the stage of the healing pressure ulcer, assign the appropriate code for unspecified stage.

If the documentation is unclear as to whether the patient has a current (new) pressure ulcer or if the patient is being treated for a healing pressure ulcer, query the provider.

For ulcers that were present on admission but healed at the time of discharge, assign the code for the site and stage of the pressure ulcer at the time of admission.

> H & P noted healing stage 2 sacral pressure ulcer. Resolved at time of discharge summary.
>
> **L89.152 Pressure ulcer of sacral region, stage 2**
>
> *Explanation:* Although completely healed upon discharge, the pressure ulcer required observation and/or treatment and should be coded based on the site and stage upon admission.

6) Patient admitted with pressure ulcer evolving into another stage during the admission

If a patient is admitted to an inpatient hospital with a pressure ulcer at one stage and it progresses to a higher stage, two separate codes should be assigned: one code for the site and stage of the ulcer on admission and a second code for the same ulcer site and the highest stage reported during the stay.

> Stage 3 right hip pressure ulcer worsened during admission to a stage 4
>
> **L89.213 Pressure ulcer of right hip, stage 3**
>
> **L89.214 Pressure ulcer of right hip, stage 4**
>
> *Explanation:* A pressure ulcer that progresses from a lower stage to a higher stage is assigned two codes, one for the documented stage upon admission and one for the documented stage at discharge.

7) Pressure-induced deep tissue damage

For pressure-induced deep tissue damage or deep tissue pressure injury, assign only the appropriate code for pressure-induced deep tissue damage (L89.--6).

b. Non-pressure chronic ulcers

1) Patients admitted with non-pressure ulcers documented as healed

No code is assigned if the documentation states that the non-pressure ulcer is completely healed at the time of admission.

2) Non-pressure ulcers documented as healing

Non-pressure ulcers described as healing should be assigned the appropriate non-pressure ulcer code based on the documentation in the medical record. If the documentation does not provide information about the severity of the healing non-pressure ulcer, assign the appropriate code for unspecified severity.

If the documentation is unclear as to whether the patient has a current (new) non-pressure ulcer or if the patient is being treated for a healing non-pressure ulcer, query the provider.

For ulcers that were present on admission but healed at the time of discharge, assign the code for the site and severity of the non-pressure ulcer at the time of admission.

> Admission diagnosis: Chronic ulcer, fat layer exposed, on left ankle
>
> Discharge diagnosis: Resolution of ulcer on the left ankle
>
> **L97.322 Non-pressure chronic ulcer of left ankle with fat layer exposed**
>
> *Explanation:* Although the ulcer was documented as resolved (healed) at discharge, a code representing the site and severity of the ulcer upon admission should be appended.

3) Patient admitted with non-pressure ulcer that progresses to another severity level during the admission

If a patient is admitted to an inpatient hospital with a non-pressure ulcer at one severity level and it progresses to a higher severity level, two separate codes should be assigned: one code for the site and severity level of the ulcer on admission and a second code for the same ulcer site and the highest severity level reported during the stay.

See Section I.B.14. for pressure ulcer stage documentation by clinicians other than patient's provider

Chapter 12. Diseases of the Skin and Subcutaneous Tissue (L00-L99)

EXCLUDES 2 *certain conditions originating in the perinatal period (P04-P96)*
certain infectious and parasitic diseases (A00-B99)
complications of pregnancy, childbirth and the puerperium (O00-O9A)
congenital malformations, deformations, and chromosomal abnormalities (Q00-Q99)
endocrine, nutritional and metabolic diseases (E00-E88)
lipomelanotic reticulosis (I89.8)
neoplasms (C00-D49)
symptoms, signs and abnormal clinical and laboratory findings, not elsewhere classified (R00-R94)
systemic connective tissue disorders (M30-M36)
viral warts (B07.-)

AHA: 2022,2Q,7

This chapter contains the following blocks:

L00-L08 Infections of the skin and subcutaneous tissue
L10-L14 Bullous disorders
L20-L30 Dermatitis and eczema
L40-L45 Papulosquamous disorders
L49-L54 Urticaria and erythema
L55-L59 Radiation-related disorders of the skin and subcutaneous tissue
L60-L75 Disorders of skin appendages
L76 Intraoperative and postprocedural complications of skin and subcutaneous tissue
L80-L99 Other disorders of the skin and subcutaneous tissue

Infections of the skin and subcutaneous tissue (L00-L08)

Use additional code (B95-B97) to identify infectious agent

EXCLUDES 2 *hordeolum (H00.0)*
infective dermatitis (L30.3)
local infections of skin classified in Chapter 1
lupus panniculitis (L93.2)
panniculitis NOS (M79.3)
panniculitis of neck and back (M54.0-)
perlèche NOS (K13.0)
perlèche due to candidiasis (B37.0)
perlèche due to riboflavin deficiency (E53.0)
pyogenic granuloma (L98.0)
relapsing panniculitis [Weber-Christian] (M35.6)
viral warts (B07.-)
zoster (B02.-)

L00 Staphylococcal scalded skin syndrome
Ritter's disease
Use additional code to identify percentage of skin exfoliation (L49.-)
EXCLUDES 1 *bullous impetigo (L01.03)*
pemphigus neonatorum (L01.03)
toxic epidermal necrolysis [Lyell] (L51.2)
DEF: Infectious skin disease of children younger than 5 years marked by eruptions ranging from a few localized blisters to widespread, easily ruptured, fine vesicles and bullae affecting almost the entire body. It results in exfoliation of large planes of skin and leaves raw areas.

✓4th **L01 Impetigo**
EXCLUDES 1 *impetigo herpetiformis (L40.1)*
DEF: Acute, superficial, highly contagious skin infection commonly occurring in children. Skin lesions usually appear on the face and consist of vesicles and bullae that burst and form yellow crusts.

✓5th **L01.0 Impetigo**
Impetigo contagiosa
Impetigo vulgaris

L01.00 Impetigo, unspecified
Impetigo NOS

L01.01 Non-bullous impetigo

L01.02 Bockhart's impetigo
Impetigo follicularis
Perifolliculitis NOS
Superficial pustular perifolliculitis
DEF: Superficial inflammation of the hair follicles commonly caused by *Staphylococcus aureus* that manifests as rounded, sphere-shaped, pustular eruptions in the areas of the scalp, beard, underarms, extremities, and buttocks.

L01.03 Bullous impetigo
Impetigo neonatorum
Pemphigus neonatorum

L01.09 Other impetigo
Ulcerative impetigo

L01.1 Impetiginization of other dermatoses

✓4th **L02 Cutaneous abscess, furuncle and carbuncle**
Use additional code to identify organism (B95-B96)
EXCLUDES 2 *abscess of anus and rectal regions (K61.-)*
abscess of female genital organs (external) (N76.4)
abscess of male genital organs (external) (N48.2, N49.-)
DEF: Carbuncle: Infection of the skin that arises from a collection of interconnected infected boils or furuncles, usually from hair follicles infected by *Staphylococcus*. This condition can produce pus and form drainage cavities.
DEF: Furuncle: Inflamed, painful abscess, cyst, or nodule on the skin caused by bacteria, often *Staphylococcus*, entering along the hair follicle.

✓5th **L02.0 Cutaneous abscess, furuncle and carbuncle of face**
EXCLUDES 2 *abscess of ear, external (H60.0)*
abscess of eyelid (H00.0)
abscess of head [any part, except face] (L02.8)
abscess of lacrimal gland (H04.0)
abscess of lacrimal passages (H04.3)
abscess of mouth (K12.2)
abscess of nose (J34.0)
abscess of orbit (H05.0)
submandibular abscess (K12.2)

L02.01 Cutaneous abscess of face CC
L02.02 Furuncle of face
Boil of face
Folliculitis of face
L02.03 Carbuncle of face

✓5th **L02.1 Cutaneous abscess, furuncle and carbuncle of neck**
L02.11 Cutaneous abscess of neck CC
L02.12 Furuncle of neck
Boil of neck
Folliculitis of neck
L02.13 Carbuncle of neck

✓5th **L02.2 Cutaneous abscess, furuncle and carbuncle of trunk**
EXCLUDES 1 *non-newborn omphalitis (L08.82)*
omphalitis of newborn (P38.-)
EXCLUDES 2 *abscess of breast (N61.1)*
abscess of buttocks (L02.3)
abscess of female external genital organs (N76.4)
abscess of hip (L02.4)
abscess of male external genital organs (N48.2, N49.-)

✓6th **L02.21 Cutaneous abscess of trunk**
L02.211 Cutaneous abscess of abdominal wall CC
L02.212 Cutaneous abscess of back [any part, except buttock] CC
L02.213 Cutaneous abscess of chest wall CC
L02.214 Cutaneous abscess of groin CC
L02.215 Cutaneous abscess of perineum CC
L02.216 Cutaneous abscess of umbilicus CC
L02.219 Cutaneous abscess of trunk, unspecified CC

✓6th **L02.22 Furuncle of trunk**
Boil of trunk
Folliculitis of trunk
L02.221 Furuncle of abdominal wall
L02.222 Furuncle of back [any part, except buttock]
L02.223 Furuncle of chest wall
L02.224 Furuncle of groin
L02.225 Furuncle of perineum
L02.226 Furuncle of umbilicus
L02.229 Furuncle of trunk, unspecified

✓6th **L02.23 Carbuncle of trunk**
L02.231 Carbuncle of abdominal wall
L02.232 Carbuncle of back [any part, except buttock]
L02.233 Carbuncle of chest wall
L02.234 Carbuncle of groin
L02.235 Carbuncle of perineum
L02.236 Carbuncle of umbilicus
L02.239 Carbuncle of trunk, unspecified

✓5th **L02.3 Cutaneous abscess, furuncle and carbuncle of buttock**
EXCLUDES 1 *pilonidal cyst with abscess (L05.01)*
L02.31 Cutaneous abscess of buttock CC
Cutaneous abscess of gluteal region

L02.32 **Furuncle of buttock**
Boil of buttock
Folliculitis of buttock
Furuncle of gluteal region

L02.33 **Carbuncle of buttock**
Carbuncle of gluteal region

✓5th **L02.4 Cutaneous abscess, furuncle and carbuncle of limb**
EXCLUDES 2 *cutaneous abscess, furuncle and carbuncle of foot (L02.6-)*
cutaneous abscess, furuncle and carbuncle of groin (L02.214, L02.224, L02.234)
cutaneous abscess, furuncle and carbuncle of hand (L02.5-)

✓6th **L02.41 Cutaneous abscess of limb**
- **L02.411 Cutaneous abscess of right axilla** CC
- **L02.412 Cutaneous abscess of left axilla** CC
- **L02.413 Cutaneous abscess of right upper limb** CC
- **L02.414 Cutaneous abscess of left upper limb** CC
- **L02.415 Cutaneous abscess of right lower limb** CC
- **L02.416 Cutaneous abscess of left lower limb** CC
- **L02.419 Cutaneous abscess of limb, unspecified** CC UNS

✓6th **L02.42 Furuncle of limb**
Boil of limb
Folliculitis of limb
- **L02.421 Furuncle of right axilla**
- **L02.422 Furuncle of left axilla**
- **L02.423 Furuncle of right upper limb**
- **L02.424 Furuncle of left upper limb**
- **L02.425 Furuncle of right lower limb**
- **L02.426 Furuncle of left lower limb**
- **L02.429 Furuncle of limb, unspecified**

✓6th **L02.43 Carbuncle of limb**
- **L02.431 Carbuncle of right axilla**
- **L02.432 Carbuncle of left axilla**
- **L02.433 Carbuncle of right upper limb**
- **L02.434 Carbuncle of left upper limb**
- **L02.435 Carbuncle of right lower limb**
- **L02.436 Carbuncle of left lower limb**
- **L02.439 Carbuncle of limb, unspecified**

✓5th **L02.5 Cutaneous abscess, furuncle and carbuncle of hand**

✓6th **L02.51 Cutaneous abscess of hand**
- **L02.511 Cutaneous abscess of right hand** CC
- **L02.512 Cutaneous abscess of left hand** CC
- **L02.519 Cutaneous abscess of unspecified hand** CC UNS

✓6th **L02.52 Furuncle hand**
Boil of hand
Folliculitis of hand
- **L02.521 Furuncle right hand**
- **L02.522 Furuncle left hand**
- **L02.529 Furuncle unspecified hand**

✓6th **L02.53 Carbuncle of hand**
- **L02.531 Carbuncle of right hand**
- **L02.532 Carbuncle of left hand**
- **L02.539 Carbuncle of unspecified hand**

✓5th **L02.6 Cutaneous abscess, furuncle and carbuncle of foot**

✓6th **L02.61 Cutaneous abscess of foot**
- **L02.611 Cutaneous abscess of right foot** CC
- **L02.612 Cutaneous abscess of left foot** CC
- **L02.619 Cutaneous abscess of unspecified foot** CC UNS

✓6th **L02.62 Furuncle of foot**
Boil of foot
Folliculitis of foot
- **L02.621 Furuncle of right foot**
- **L02.622 Furuncle of left foot**
- **L02.629 Furuncle of unspecified foot**

✓6th **L02.63 Carbuncle of foot**
- **L02.631 Carbuncle of right foot**
- **L02.632 Carbuncle of left foot**
- **L02.639 Carbuncle of unspecified foot**

✓5th **L02.8 Cutaneous abscess, furuncle and carbuncle of other sites**

✓6th **L02.81 Cutaneous abscess of other sites**
- **L02.811 Cutaneous abscess of head [any part, except face]** CC
- **L02.818 Cutaneous abscess of other sites** CC

✓6th **L02.82 Furuncle of other sites**
Boil of other sites
Folliculitis of other sites
- **L02.821 Furuncle of head [any part, except face]**
- **L02.828 Furuncle of other sites**

✓6th **L02.83 Carbuncle of other sites**
- **L02.831 Carbuncle of head [any part, except face]**
- **L02.838 Carbuncle of other sites**

✓5th **L02.9 Cutaneous abscess, furuncle and carbuncle, unspecified**
- **L02.91 Cutaneous abscess, unspecified** CC
- **L02.92 Furuncle, unspecified**
  Boil NOS
  Furunculosis NOS
- **L02.93 Carbuncle, unspecified**

✓4th **L03 Cellulitis and acute lymphangitis**
EXCLUDES 2 *cellulitis of anal and rectal region (K61.-)*
cellulitis of external auditory canal (H60.1)
cellulitis of eyelid (H00.0)
cellulitis of female external genital organs (N76.4)
cellulitis of lacrimal apparatus (H04.3)
cellulitis of male external genital organs (N48.2, N49.-)
cellulitis of mouth (K12.2)
cellulitis of nose (J34.0)
eosinophilic cellulitis [Wells] (L98.3)
febrile neutrophilic dermatosis [Sweet] (L98.2)
lymphangitis (chronic) (subacute) (I89.1)

AHA: 2017,4Q,100

DEF: Cellulitis: Infection of the skin and subcutaneous tissues, most often caused by *Staphylococcus* or *Streptococcus* bacteria secondary to a cutaneous lesion. Progression of the inflammation may lead to abscess and tissue death, or even systemic infection-like bacteremia.

DEF: Lymphangitis: Inflammation of the lymph channels most often caused by *Streptococcus.*

✓5th **L03.0 Cellulitis and acute lymphangitis of finger and toe**
Infection of nail
Onychia
Paronychia
Perionychia

✓6th **L03.01 Cellulitis of finger**
Felon
Whitlow
EXCLUDES 1 *herpetic whitlow (B00.89)*
DEF: Felon: Superficial bacterial skin infection at the tip of the finger.
- **L03.011 Cellulitis of right finger**
- **L03.012 Cellulitis of left finger**
- **L03.019 Cellulitis of unspecified finger**

✓6th **L03.02 Acute lymphangitis of finger**
Hangnail with lymphangitis of finger
- **L03.021 Acute lymphangitis of right finger**
- **L03.022 Acute lymphangitis of left finger**
- **L03.029 Acute lymphangitis of unspecified finger**

✓6th **L03.03 Cellulitis of toe**
- **L03.031 Cellulitis of right toe**
- **L03.032 Cellulitis of left toe**
- **L03.039 Cellulitis of unspecified toe**

✓6th **L03.04 Acute lymphangitis of toe**
Hangnail with lymphangitis of toe
- **L03.041 Acute lymphangitis of right toe**
- **L03.042 Acute lymphangitis of left toe**
- **L03.049 Acute lymphangitis of unspecified toe**

✓5th **L03.1 Cellulitis and acute lymphangitis of other parts of limb**

✓6th **L03.11 Cellulitis of other parts of limb**
EXCLUDES 2 *cellulitis of fingers (L03.01-)*
cellulitis of toes (L03.03-)
groin (L03.314)
- **L03.111 Cellulitis of right axilla** CC
- **L03.112 Cellulitis of left axilla** CC
- **L03.113 Cellulitis of right upper limb** CC
- **L03.114 Cellulitis of left upper limb** CC
- **L03.115 Cellulitis of right lower limb** CC

LØ3.116 Cellulitis of left lower limb CC
LØ3.119 Cellulitis of unspecified part of limb CC UNS

✓6th LØ3.12 Acute lymphangitis of other parts of limb

EXCLUDES 2 *acute lymphangitis of fingers (LØ3.2-)*
acute lymphangitis of groin (LØ3.324)
acute lymphangitis of toes (LØ3.Ø4-)

LØ3.121 Acute lymphangitis of right axilla CC
LØ3.122 Acute lymphangitis of left axilla CC
LØ3.123 Acute lymphangitis of right upper limb CC
LØ3.124 Acute lymphangitis of left upper limb CC
LØ3.125 Acute lymphangitis of right lower limb CC
LØ3.126 Acute lymphangitis of left lower limb CC
LØ3.129 Acute lymphangitis of unspecified part of limb CC UNS

✓5th LØ3.2 Cellulitis and acute lymphangitis of face and neck

✓6th LØ3.21 Cellulitis and acute lymphangitis of face

LØ3.211 Cellulitis of face CC

EXCLUDES 2 *abscess of orbit (HØ5.Ø1-)*
cellulitis of ear (H6Ø.1-)
cellulitis of eyelid (HØØ.Ø-)
cellulitis of head (LØ3.81)
cellulitis of lacrimal apparatus (HØ4.3)
cellulitis of lip (K13.Ø)
cellulitis of mouth (K12.2)
cellulitis of nose (internal) (J34.Ø)
cellulitis of orbit (HØ5.Ø1-)
cellulitis of scalp (LØ3.81)

AHA: 2013,4Q,123

LØ3.212 Acute lymphangitis of face CC
LØ3.213 Periorbital cellulitis CC
Preseptal cellulitis

AHA: 2016,4Q,36

✓6th LØ3.22 Cellulitis and acute lymphangitis of neck

LØ3.221 Cellulitis of neck CC
LØ3.222 Acute lymphangitis of neck CC

✓5th LØ3.3 Cellulitis and acute lymphangitis of trunk

✓6th LØ3.31 Cellulitis of trunk

EXCLUDES 2 *cellulitis of anal and rectal regions (K61.-)*
cellulitis of breast NOS (N61.Ø)
cellulitis of female external genital organs (N76.4)
cellulitis of male external genital organs (N48.2, N49.-)
omphalitis of newborn (P38.-)
puerperal cellulitis of breast (O91.2)

LØ3.311 Cellulitis of abdominal wall CC

EXCLUDES 2 *cellulitis of umbilicus (LØ3.316)*
cellulitis of groin (LØ3.314)

LØ3.312 Cellulitis of back [any part except buttock] CC
LØ3.313 Cellulitis of chest wall CC
LØ3.314 Cellulitis of groin CC
LØ3.315 Cellulitis of perineum CC
LØ3.316 Cellulitis of umbilicus CC
LØ3.317 Cellulitis of buttock CC
LØ3.319 Cellulitis of trunk, unspecified CC

✓6th LØ3.32 Acute lymphangitis of trunk

LØ3.321 Acute lymphangitis of abdominal wall CC
LØ3.322 Acute lymphangitis of back [any part except buttock] CC
LØ3.323 Acute lymphangitis of chest wall CC
LØ3.324 Acute lymphangitis of groin CC
LØ3.325 Acute lymphangitis of perineum CC
LØ3.326 Acute lymphangitis of umbilicus CC
LØ3.327 Acute lymphangitis of buttock CC
LØ3.329 Acute lymphangitis of trunk, unspecified CC

✓5th LØ3.8 Cellulitis and acute lymphangitis of other sites

✓6th LØ3.81 Cellulitis of other sites

LØ3.811 Cellulitis of head [any part, except face] CC
Cellulitis of scalp

EXCLUDES 2 *cellulitis of face (LØ3.211)*

LØ3.818 Cellulitis of other sites CC

✓6th LØ3.89 Acute lymphangitis of other sites

LØ3.891 Acute lymphangitis of head [any part, except face] CC
LØ3.898 Acute lymphangitis of other sites CC

✓5th LØ3.9 Cellulitis and acute lymphangitis, unspecified

LØ3.9Ø Cellulitis, unspecified CC
LØ3.91 Acute lymphangitis, unspecified CC

EXCLUDES 1 *lymphangitis NOS (I89.1)*

✓4th **LØ4 Acute lymphadenitis**

INCLUDES abscess (acute) of lymph nodes, except mesenteric
acute lymphadenitis, except mesenteric

EXCLUDES 1 *chronic or subacute lymphadenitis, except mesenteric (I88.1)*
enlarged lymph nodes (R59.-)
human immunodeficiency virus [HIV] disease resulting in generalized lymphadenopathy (B2Ø)
lymphadenitis NOS (I88.9)
nonspecific mesenteric lymphadenitis (I88.Ø)

DEF: Inflammation or enlargement of the lymph nodes.

LØ4.Ø Acute lymphadenitis of face, head and neck
LØ4.1 Acute lymphadenitis of trunk
LØ4.2 Acute lymphadenitis of upper limb
Acute lymphadenitis of axilla
Acute lymphadenitis of shoulder
LØ4.3 Acute lymphadenitis of lower limb
Acute lymphadenitis of hip

EXCLUDES 2 *acute lymphadenitis of groin (LØ4.1)*

LØ4.8 Acute lymphadenitis of other sites
LØ4.9 Acute lymphadenitis, unspecified

✓4th **LØ5 Pilonidal cyst and sinus**

DEF: Pilonidal cyst: Sac or sinus cavity of trapped epithelial tissues in the sacrococcygeal region, usually associated with ingrown hair.

DEF: Pilonidal sinus: Fistula, tract, or channel that extends from an infected area of ingrown hair to another site within the skin or out to the skin surface.

Pilonidal Cyst

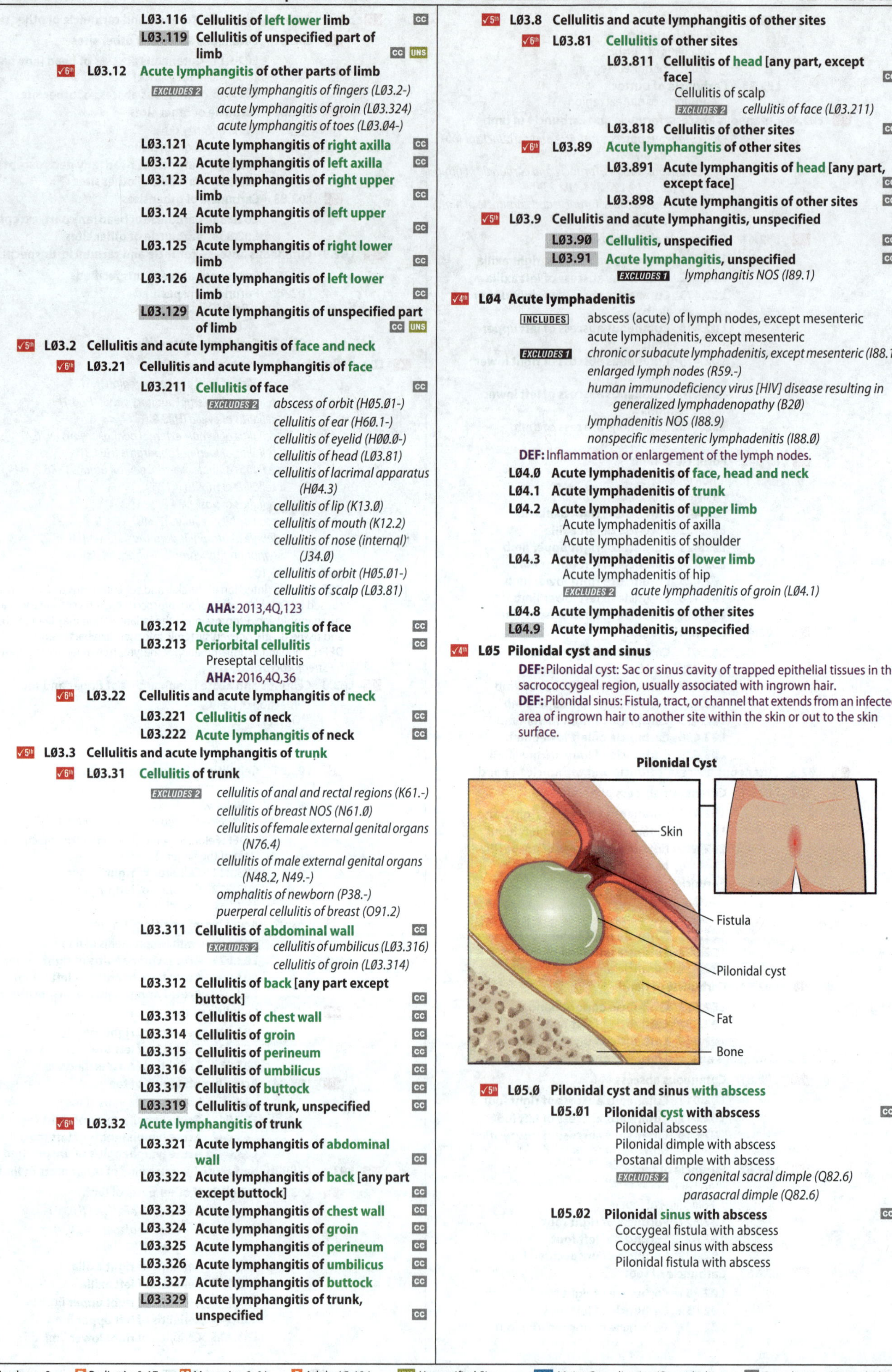

✓5th LØ5.Ø Pilonidal cyst and sinus with abscess

LØ5.Ø1 Pilonidal cyst with abscess CC
Pilonidal abscess
Pilonidal dimple with abscess
Postanal dimple with abscess

EXCLUDES 2 *congenital sacral dimple (Q82.6)*
parasacral dimple (Q82.6)

LØ5.Ø2 Pilonidal sinus with abscess CC
Coccygeal fistula with abscess
Coccygeal sinus with abscess
Pilonidal fistula with abscess

L05.9 Pilonidal cyst and sinus without abscess

L05.91 Pilonidal cyst without abscess
Pilonidal dimple
Postanal dimple
Pilonidal cyst NOS
EXCLUDES 2 *congenital sacral dimple (Q82.6)*
parasacral dimple (Q82.6)

L05.92 Pilonidal sinus without abscess
Coccygeal fistula
Coccygeal sinus without abscess
Pilonidal fistula

L08 Other local infections of skin and subcutaneous tissue

L08.0 Pyoderma
Dermatitis gangrenosa
Purulent dermatitis
Septic dermatitis
Suppurative dermatitis
EXCLUDES 1 *pyoderma gangrenosum (L88)*
pyoderma vegetans (L08.81)
DEF: Any superficial skin disease commonly characterized by the discharging of pus not attributed to another condition.

L08.1 Erythrasma HIV CC
DEF: Chronic, superficial skin infection of brown scaly patches, commonly found in skin folds most prevalent in the overweight or diabetic population.

L08.8 Other specified local infections of the skin and subcutaneous tissue

L08.81 Pyoderma vegetans
EXCLUDES 1 *pyoderma gangrenosum (L88)*
pyoderma NOS (L08.0)

L08.82 Omphalitis not of newborn
EXCLUDES 1 *omphalitis of newborn (P38.-)*

L08.89 Other specified local infections of the skin and subcutaneous tissue

L08.9 Local infection of the skin and subcutaneous tissue, unspecified

Bullous disorders (L10-L14)

EXCLUDES 1 *benign familial pemphigus [Hailey-Hailey] (Q82.8)*
staphylococcal scalded skin syndrome (L00)
toxic epidermal necrolysis [Lyell] (L51.2)

L10 Pemphigus
EXCLUDES 1 *pemphigus neonatorum (L01.03)*

L10.0 Pemphigus vulgaris CC
L10.1 Pemphigus vegetans CC
L10.2 Pemphigus foliaceous CC
L10.3 Brazilian pemphigus [fogo selvagem] CC
L10.4 Pemphigus erythematosus CC
Senear-Usher syndrome
L10.5 Drug-induced pemphigus CC
Use additional code for adverse effect, if applicable, to identify drug (T36-T50 with fifth or sixth character 5)

L10.8 Other pemphigus
L10.81 Paraneoplastic pemphigus CC
L10.89 Other pemphigus CC

L10.9 Pemphigus, unspecified CC

L11 Other acantholytic disorders

L11.0 Acquired keratosis follicularis
EXCLUDES 1 *keratosis follicularis (congenital) [Darier-White] (Q82.8)*
AHA: 2021,3Q,10

L11.1 Transient acantholytic dermatosis [Grover]
L11.8 Other specified acantholytic disorders
L11.9 Acantholytic disorder, unspecified

L12 Pemphigoid
EXCLUDES 1 *herpes gestationis (O26.4-)*
impetigo herpetiformis (L40.1)

L12.0 Bullous pemphigoid CC
L12.1 Cicatricial pemphigoid
Benign mucous membrane pemphigoid
DEF: Chronic autoimmune disease characterized by subepidermal blistering lesions of the mucosa, including the conjunctiva. It is seen predominantly in the elderly and produces adhesions and scarring.

L12.2 Chronic bullous disease of childhood P
Juvenile dermatitis herpetiformis

L12.3 Acquired epidermolysis bullosa
EXCLUDES 1 *epidermolysis bullosa (congenital) (Q81.-)*

L12.30 Acquired epidermolysis bullosa, unspecified CC HCC
L12.31 Epidermolysis bullosa due to drug CC HCC
Use additional code for adverse effect, if applicable, to identify drug (T36-T50 with fifth or sixth character 5)
L12.35 Other acquired epidermolysis bullosa CC HCC

L12.8 Other pemphigoid CC
L12.9 Pemphigoid, unspecified CC

L13 Other bullous disorders

L13.0 Dermatitis herpetiformis
Duhring's disease
Hydroa herpetiformis
EXCLUDES 1 *juvenile dermatitis herpetiformis (L12.2)*
senile dermatitis herpetiformis (L12.0)
DEF: Skin disease to which people are genetically predisposed resulting from an immunological response to gluten. Dermatitis herpetiformis is an extremely pruritic eruption of various lesions that frequently heal, leaving hyperpigmentation or hypopigmentation and occasionally scarring. It is usually associated with asymptomatic gluten-sensitive enteropathy.

L13.1 Subcorneal pustular dermatitis
Sneddon-Wilkinson disease
L13.8 Other specified bullous disorders
L13.9 Bullous disorder, unspecified

L14 Bullous disorders in diseases classified elsewhere
Code first underlying disease

Dermatitis and eczema (L20-L30)

NOTE In this block the terms dermatitis and eczema are used synonymously and interchangeably.

EXCLUDES 2 *chronic (childhood) granulomatous disease (D71)*
dermatitis gangrenosa (L08.0)
dermatitis herpetiformis (L13.0)
dry skin dermatitis (L85.3)
factitial dermatitis (L98.1)
perioral dermatitis (L71.0)
radiation-related disorders of the skin and subcutaneous tissue (L55-L59)
stasis dermatitis (I87.2)

L20 Atopic dermatitis

L20.0 Besnier's prurigo
L20.8 Other atopic dermatitis
EXCLUDES 2 *circumscribed neurodermatitis (L28.0)*

L20.81 Atopic neurodermatitis
Diffuse neurodermatitis
L20.82 Flexural eczema
L20.83 Infantile (acute) (chronic) eczema P
L20.84 Intrinsic (allergic) eczema
L20.89 Other atopic dermatitis

L20.9 Atopic dermatitis, unspecified

L21 Seborrheic dermatitis
EXCLUDES 2 *infective dermatitis (L30.3)*
seborrheic keratosis (L82.-)

L21.0 Seborrhea capitis
Cradle cap
AHA: 2018,1Q,6
TIP: Assign for dandruff in an adult patient.
L21.1 Seborrheic infantile dermatitis P
L21.8 Other seborrheic dermatitis
L21.9 Seborrheic dermatitis, unspecified
Seborrhea NOS

L22 Diaper dermatitis
Diaper erythema
Diaper rash
Psoriasiform diaper rash
AHA: 2021,4Q,18

✓4th **L23 Allergic contact dermatitis**

EXCLUDES 1 *allergy NOS (T78.40)*
contact dermatitis NOS (L25.9)
dermatitis NOS (L30.9)

EXCLUDES 2 *dermatitis due to substances taken internally (L27.-)*
dermatitis of eyelid (H01.1-)
diaper dermatitis (L22)
eczema of external ear (H60.5-)
irritant contact dermatitis (L24.-)
perioral dermatitis (L71.0)
radiation-related disorders of the skin and subcutaneous tissue (L55-L59)

L23.0 Allergic contact dermatitis due to metals
Allergic contact dermatitis due to chromium
Allergic contact dermatitis due to nickel

L23.1 Allergic contact dermatitis due to adhesives

L23.2 Allergic contact dermatitis due to cosmetics

L23.3 Allergic contact dermatitis due to drugs in contact with skin
Use additional code for adverse effect, if applicable, to identify drug (T36-T50 with fifth or sixth character 5)
EXCLUDES 2 *dermatitis due to ingested drugs and medicaments (L27.0-L27.1)*

L23.4 Allergic contact dermatitis due to dyes

L23.5 Allergic contact dermatitis due to other chemical products
Allergic contact dermatitis due to cement
Allergic contact dermatitis due to insecticide
Allergic contact dermatitis due to plastic
Allergic contact dermatitis due to rubber

L23.6 Allergic contact dermatitis due to food in contact with the skin
EXCLUDES 2 *dermatitis due to ingested food (L27.2)*

L23.7 Allergic contact dermatitis due to plants, except food
EXCLUDES 2 *allergy NOS due to pollen (J30.1)*

✓5th **L23.8 Allergic contact dermatitis due to other agents**

L23.81 Allergic contact dermatitis due to animal (cat) (dog) dander
Allergic contact dermatitis due to animal (cat) (dog) hair

L23.89 Allergic contact dermatitis due to other agents

UNS **L23.9 Allergic contact dermatitis, unspecified cause**
Allergic contact eczema NOS

✓4th **L24 Irritant contact dermatitis**

EXCLUDES 1 *allergy NOS (T78.40)*
contact dermatitis NOS (L25.9)
dermatitis NOS (L30.9)

EXCLUDES 2 *allergic contact dermatitis (L23.-)*
dermatitis due to substances taken internally (L27.-)
dermatitis of eyelid (H01.1-)
diaper dermatitis (L22)
eczema of external ear (H60.5-)
perioral dermatitis (L71.0)
radiation-related disorders of the skin and subcutaneous tissue (L55-L59)

L24.0 Irritant contact dermatitis due to detergents

L24.1 Irritant contact dermatitis due to oils and greases

L24.2 Irritant contact dermatitis due to solvents
Irritant contact dermatitis due to chlorocompound
Irritant contact dermatitis due to cyclohexane
Irritant contact dermatitis due to ester
Irritant contact dermatitis due to glycol
Irritant contact dermatitis due to hydrocarbon
Irritant contact dermatitis due to ketone

L24.3 Irritant contact dermatitis due to cosmetics

L24.4 Irritant contact dermatitis due to drugs in contact with skin
Use additional code for adverse effect, if applicable, to identify drug (T36-T50 with fifth or sixth character 5)

L24.5 Irritant contact dermatitis due to other chemical products
Irritant contact dermatitis due to cement
Irritant contact dermatitis due to insecticide
Irritant contact dermatitis due to plastic
Irritant contact dermatitis due to rubber

L24.6 Irritant contact dermatitis due to food in contact with skin
EXCLUDES 2 *dermatitis due to ingested food (L27.2)*

L24.7 Irritant contact dermatitis due to plants, except food
EXCLUDES 2 *allergy NOS to pollen (J30.1)*

✓5th **L24.8 Irritant contact dermatitis due to other agents**

L24.81 Irritant contact dermatitis due to metals
Irritant contact dermatitis due to chromium
Irritant contact dermatitis due to nickel

L24.89 Irritant contact dermatitis due to other agents
Irritant contact dermatitis due to dyes

UNS **L24.9 Irritant contact dermatitis, unspecified cause**
Irritant contact eczema NOS

✓5th **L24.A Irritant contact dermatitis due to friction or contact with body fluids**
EXCLUDES 1 *irritant contact dermatitis related to stoma or fistula (L24.B-)*
EXCLUDES 2 *erythema intertrigo (L30.4)*
AHA: 2021,4Q,16-18

UNS **L24.A0 Irritant contact dermatitis due to friction or contact with body fluids, unspecified**

L24.A1 Irritant contact dermatitis due to saliva

L24.A2 Irritant contact dermatitis due to fecal, urinary or dual incontinence
EXCLUDES 1 *diaper dermatitis (L22)*

L24.A9 Irritant contact dermatitis due friction or contact with other specified body fluids
Irritant contact dermatitis related to endotracheal tube
Wound fluids, exudate

✓5th **L24.B Irritant contact dermatitis related to stoma or fistula**
Use additional code to identify any artificial opening status (Z93.-), if applicable, for contact dermatitis related to stoma secretions
AHA: 2021,4Q,16-18

UNS **L24.B0 Irritant contact dermatitis related to unspecified stoma or fistula**
Irritant contact dermatitis related to fistula NOS
Irritant contact dermatitis related to stoma NOS

L24.B1 Irritant contact dermatitis related to digestive stoma or fistula
Irritant contact dermatitis related to gastrostomy
Irritant contact dermatitis related to jejunostomy
Irritant contact dermatitis related to saliva or spit fistula

L24.B2 Irritant contact dermatitis related to respiratory stoma or fistula
Irritant contact dermatitis related to tracheostomy

L24.B3 Irritant contact dermatitis related to fecal or urinary stoma or fistula
Irritant contact dermatitis related to colostomy
Irritant contact dermatitis related to enterocutaneous fistula
Irritant contact dermatitis related to ileostomy

✓4th **L25 Unspecified contact dermatitis**

EXCLUDES 1 *allergic contact dermatitis (L23.-)*
allergy NOS (T78.40)
dermatitis NOS (L30.9)
irritant contact dermatitis (L24.-)

EXCLUDES 2 *dermatitis due to ingested substances (L27.-)*
dermatitis of eyelid (H01.1-)
eczema of external ear (H60.5-)
perioral dermatitis (L71.0)
radiation-related disorders of the skin and subcutaneous tissue (L55-L59)

UNS **L25.0 Unspecified contact dermatitis due to cosmetics**

UNS **L25.1 Unspecified contact dermatitis due to drugs in contact with skin**
Use additional code for adverse effect, if applicable, to identify drug (T36-T50 with fifth or sixth character 5)
EXCLUDES 2 *dermatitis due to ingested drugs and medicaments (L27.0-L27.1)*

UNS **L25.2 Unspecified contact dermatitis due to dyes**

UNS **L25.3 Unspecified contact dermatitis due to other chemical products**
Unspecified contact dermatitis due to cement
Unspecified contact dermatitis due to insecticide

UNS **L25.4 Unspecified contact dermatitis due to food in contact with skin**
EXCLUDES 2 *dermatitis due to ingested food (L27.2)*

UNS **L25.5 Unspecified contact dermatitis due to plants, except food**
EXCLUDES 1 *nettle rash (L50.9)*
EXCLUDES 2 *allergy NOS due to pollen (J30.1)*

UNS **L25.8 Unspecified contact dermatitis due to other agents**

L25.9 Unspecified contact dermatitis, unspecified cause
Contact dermatitis (occupational) NOS
Contact eczema (occupational) NOS

L26 Exfoliative dermatitis
Hebra's pityriasis
EXCLUDES 1 *Ritter's disease (L00)*

✓4th **L27 Dermatitis due to substances taken internally**
EXCLUDES 1 *allergy NOS (T78.40)*
EXCLUDES 2 *adverse food reaction, except dermatitis (T78.0-T78.1)*
contact dermatitis (L23-L25)
drug photoallergic response (L56.1)
drug phototoxic response (L56.0)
urticaria (L50.-)

L27.0 Generalized skin eruption due to drugs and medicaments taken internally
Use additional code for adverse effect, if applicable, to identify drug (T36-T50 with fifth or sixth character 5)

L27.1 Localized skin eruption due to drugs and medicaments taken internally
Use additional code for adverse effect, if applicable, to identify drug (T36-T50 with fifth or sixth character 5)

L27.2 Dermatitis due to ingested food
EXCLUDES 2 *dermatitis due to food in contact with skin (L23.6, L24.6, L25.4)*

L27.8 Dermatitis due to other substances taken internally
L27.9 Dermatitis due to unspecified substance taken internally

✓4th **L28 Lichen simplex chronicus and prurigo**
L28.0 Lichen simplex chronicus
Circumscribed neurodermatitis
Lichen NOS
L28.1 Prurigo nodularis
L28.2 Other prurigo
Prurigo NOS
Prurigo Hebra
Prurigo mitis
Urticaria papulosa

✓4th **L29 Pruritus**
EXCLUDES 1 *neurotic excoriation (L98.1)*
psychogenic pruritus (F45.8)
L29.0 Pruritus ani
L29.1 Pruritus scroti ♂
L29.2 Pruritus vulvae ♀
L29.3 Anogenital pruritus, unspecified
L29.8 Other pruritus
L29.9 Pruritus, unspecified
Itch NOS

✓4th **L30 Other and unspecified dermatitis**
EXCLUDES 2 *contact dermatitis (L23-L25)*
dry skin dermatitis (L85.3)
small plaque parapsoriasis (L41.3)
stasis dermatitis (I87.2)
L30.0 Nummular dermatitis
L30.1 Dyshidrosis [pompholyx]
L30.2 Cutaneous autosensitization
Candidid [levurid]
Dermatophytid
Eczematid
L30.3 Infective dermatitis
Infectious eczematoid dermatitis
L30.4 Erythema intertrigo
L30.5 Pityriasis alba
AHA: 2018,1Q,6
L30.8 Other specified dermatitis
L30.9 Dermatitis, unspecified
Eczema NOS

Papulosquamous disorders (L40-L45)

✓4th **L40 Psoriasis**
DEF: Chronic autoimmune condition that speeds up skin cell growth, causing excessive immature skin cells to form raised, rounded erythematous lesions covered by dry, silvery scaling patches. Most commonly found on the scalp, elbows, knees, hands, feet, and genitals, it can also affect the joints with stiffness and swelling.
L40.0 Psoriasis vulgaris
Nummular psoriasis
Plaque psoriasis
L40.1 Generalized pustular psoriasis
Impetigo herpetiformis
Von Zumbusch's disease
L40.2 Acrodermatitis continua
L40.3 Pustulosis palmaris et plantaris
L40.4 Guttate psoriasis
✓5th **L40.5 Arthropathic psoriasis**
L40.50 Arthropathic psoriasis, unspecified HCC
L40.51 Distal interphalangeal psoriatic arthropathy HCC
L40.52 Psoriatic arthritis mutilans HCC
L40.53 Psoriatic spondylitis HCC
L40.54 Psoriatic juvenile arthropathy HCC
L40.59 Other psoriatic arthropathy HCC
L40.8 Other psoriasis
Flexural psoriasis
L40.9 Psoriasis, unspecified

✓4th **L41 Parapsoriasis**
EXCLUDES 1 *poikiloderma vasculare atrophicans (L94.5)*
L41.0 Pityriasis lichenoides et varioliformis acuta
Mucha-Habermann disease
L41.1 Pityriasis lichenoides chronica
L41.3 Small plaque parapsoriasis
L41.4 Large plaque parapsoriasis
L41.5 Retiform parapsoriasis
L41.8 Other parapsoriasis
L41.9 Parapsoriasis, unspecified

L42 Pityriasis rosea

✓4th **L43 Lichen planus**
EXCLUDES 1 *lichen planopilaris (L66.1)*
L43.0 Hypertrophic lichen planus
L43.1 Bullous lichen planus
L43.2 Lichenoid drug reaction
Use additional code for adverse effect, if applicable, to identify drug (T36-T50 with fifth or sixth character 5)
L43.3 Subacute (active) lichen planus
Lichen planus tropicus
L43.8 Other lichen planus
L43.9 Lichen planus, unspecified

✓4th **L44 Other papulosquamous disorders**
L44.0 Pityriasis rubra pilaris
L44.1 Lichen nitidus
DEF: Chronic, inflammatory, asymptomatic skin disorder, characterized by numerous glistening, flat-topped, discrete, skin-colored micropapules, most often on the penis, lower abdomen, inner thighs, wrists, forearms, breasts, and buttocks.
L44.2 Lichen striatus
L44.3 Lichen ruber moniliformis
L44.4 Infantile papular acrodermatitis [Gianotti-Crosti] P
L44.8 Other specified papulosquamous disorders
L44.9 Papulosquamous disorder, unspecified

L45 Papulosquamous disorders in diseases classified elsewhere
Code first underlying disease

Urticaria and erythema (L49-L54)

EXCLUDES 1 *Lyme disease (A69.2-)*
rosacea (L71.-)

L49 Exfoliation due to erythematous conditions according to extent of body surface involved

Code first erythematous condition causing exfoliation, such as:
- Ritter's disease (LØØ)
- (Staphylococcal) scalded skin syndrome (LØØ)
- Stevens-Johnson syndrome (L51.1)
- Stevens-Johnson syndrome-toxic epidermal necrolysis overlap syndrome (L51.3)
- toxic epidermal necrolysis (L51.2)

DEF: Exfoliation: Falling or sloughing off skin in layers.

L49.Ø Exfoliation due to erythematous condition involving less than 1Ø percent of body surface UPD
Exfoliation due to erythematous condition NOS

L49.1 Exfoliation due to erythematous condition involving 1Ø-19 percent of body surface UPD

L49.2 Exfoliation due to erythematous condition involving 2Ø-29 percent of body surface UPD

L49.3 Exfoliation due to erythematous condition involving 3Ø-39 percent of body surface CC UPD

L49.4 Exfoliation due to erythematous condition involving 4Ø-49 percent of body surface CC UPD

L49.5 Exfoliation due to erythematous condition involving 5Ø-59 percent of body surface CC UPD

L49.6 Exfoliation due to erythematous condition involving 6Ø-69 percent of body surface CC UPD

L49.7 Exfoliation due to erythematous condition involving 7Ø-79 percent of body surface CC UPD

L49.8 Exfoliation due to erythematous condition involving 8Ø-89 percent of body surface CC UPD

L49.9 Exfoliation due to erythematous condition involving 9Ø or more percent of body surface CC UPD

L5Ø Urticaria

EXCLUDES 1 *allergic contact dermatitis (L23.-)*
angioneurotic edema (T78.3)
giant urticaria (T78.3)
hereditary angio-edema (D84.1)
Quincke's edema (T78.3)
serum urticaria (T8Ø.6-)
solar urticaria (L56.3)
urticaria neonatorum (P83.8)
urticaria papulosa (L28.2)
urticaria pigmentosa (D47.Ø1)

DEF: Eruption of itching edema of the skin. ***Synonym(s):*** *hives.*

L5Ø.Ø Allergic urticaria

L5Ø.1 Idiopathic urticaria

L5Ø.2 Urticaria due to cold and heat
EXCLUDES 2 *familial cold urticaria (MØ4.2)*

L5Ø.3 Dermatographic urticaria

L5Ø.4 Vibratory urticaria

L5Ø.5 Cholinergic urticaria

L5Ø.6 Contact urticaria

L5Ø.8 Other urticaria
Chronic urticaria
Recurrent periodic urticaria

L5Ø.9 Urticaria, unspecified

L51 Erythema multiforme

Use additional code for adverse effect, if applicable, to identify drug (T36-T5Ø with fifth or sixth character 5)

Use additional code to identify associated manifestations, such as:
- arthropathy associated with dermatological disorders (M14.8-)
- conjunctival edema (H11.42)
- conjunctivitis (H1Ø.22-)
- corneal scars and opacities (H17.-)
- corneal ulcer (H16.Ø-)
- edema of eyelid (HØ2.84-)
- inflammation of eyelid (HØ1.8)
- keratoconjunctivitis sicca (H16.22-)
- mechanical lagophthalmos (HØ2.22-)
- stomatitis (K12.-)
- symblepharon (H11.23-)

Use additional code to identify percentage of skin exfoliation (L49.-)

EXCLUDES 1 *staphylococcal scalded skin syndrome (LØØ)*
Ritter's disease (LØØ)

DEF: Acute complex of symptoms with a varied pattern of skin eruptions, such as macular, bullous, papular, nodose, or vesicular lesions on the neck, face, and legs. Erythema (redness of skin and mucous membranes) multiforme (multiple forms) is a hypersensitivity (allergic) reaction that can occur at any age but primarily affects children or young adults.

L51.Ø Nonbullous erythema multiforme

L51.1 Stevens-Johnson syndrome CC HCC

L51.2 Toxic epidermal necrolysis [Lyell] CC HCC

L51.3 Stevens-Johnson syndrome-toxic epidermal necrolysis overlap syndrome CC HCC
SJS-TEN overlap syndrome

L51.8 Other erythema multiforme

L51.9 Erythema multiforme, unspecified
Erythema iris
Erythema multiforme major NOS
Erythema multiforme minor NOS
Herpes iris

L52 Erythema nodosum

EXCLUDES 1 *tuberculous erythema nodosum (A18.4)*

DEF: Form of panniculitis (inflammation of the fat layer beneath the skin) most often occurring in women. Commonly seen as a hypersensitivity reaction to infections, drugs, sarcoidosis, and specific enteropathies. The acute stage is associated with fever, malaise, and arthralgia. The lesions are pink to blue in color as tender nodules and are found on the front of the legs below the knees.

L53 Other erythematous conditions

EXCLUDES 1 *erythema ab igne (L59.Ø)*
erythema due to external agents in contact with skin (L23-L25)
erythema intertrigo (L3Ø.4)

L53.Ø Toxic erythema CC
Code first poisoning due to drug or toxin, if applicable ▶(T36-T65 with fifth or sixth character 1-4)◀
Use additional code for adverse effect, if applicable, to identify drug (T36-T5Ø with fifth or sixth character 5)
EXCLUDES 1 *neonatal erythema toxicum (P83.1)*

L53.1 Erythema annulare centrifugum CC

L53.2 Erythema marginatum CC

L53.3 Other chronic figurate erythema CC

L53.8 Other specified erythematous conditions

L53.9 Erythematous condition, unspecified
Erythema NOS
Erythroderma NOS

L54 Erythema in diseases classified elsewhere
Code first underlying disease

Radiation-related disorders of the skin and subcutaneous tissue (L55-L59)

L55 Sunburn

L55.Ø Sunburn of first degree

L55.1 Sunburn of second degree

L55.2 Sunburn of third degree

L55.9 Sunburn, unspecified

✓4th L56 Other acute skin changes due to ultraviolet radiation

Use additional code to identify the source of the ultraviolet radiation (W89, X32)

L56.Ø Drug phototoxic response

Use additional code for adverse effect, if applicable, to identify drug (T36-T5Ø with fifth or sixth character 5)

L56.1 Drug photoallergic response

Use additional code for adverse effect, if applicable, to identify drug (T36-T5Ø with fifth or sixth character 5)

L56.2 Photocontact dermatitis [berloque dermatitis]

L56.3 Solar urticaria

L56.4 Polymorphous light eruption

L56.5 Disseminated superficial actinic porokeratosis (DSAP)

DEF: Autosomal dominant skin condition occurring in sun-exposed areas of the skin (particularly the arms and legs), characterized by superficial annular, keratotic, brownish-red spots or thickenings with depressed centers and sharp, ridged borders. It may evolve into squamous cell carcinoma.

L56.8 Other specified acute skin changes due to ultraviolet radiation

L56.9 Acute skin change due to ultraviolet radiation, unspecified

✓4th L57 Skin changes due to chronic exposure to nonionizing radiation

Use additional code to identify the source of the ultraviolet radiation (W89), or other nonionizing radiation (W9Ø)

L57.Ø Actinic keratosis

Keratosis NOS
Senile keratosis
Solar keratosis

L57.1 Actinic reticuloid

L57.2 Cutis rhomboidalis nuchae

L57.3 Poikiloderma of Civatte

L57.4 Cutis laxa senilis

Elastosis senilis

L57.5 Actinic granuloma

L57.8 Other skin changes due to chronic exposure to nonionizing radiation

Farmer's skin
Sailor's skin
Solar dermatitis

L57.9 Skin changes due to chronic exposure to nonionizing radiation, unspecified

✓4th L58 Radiodermatitis

Use additional code to identify the source of the radiation (W88, W9Ø)

L58.Ø Acute radiodermatitis

L58.1 Chronic radiodermatitis

L58.9 Radiodermatitis, unspecified

✓4th L59 Other disorders of skin and subcutaneous tissue related to radiation

L59.Ø Erythema ab igne [dermatitis ab igne]

L59.8 Other specified disorders of the skin and subcutaneous tissue related to radiation

AHA: 2017,1Q,33

L59.9 Disorder of the skin and subcutaneous tissue related to radiation, unspecified

Disorders of skin appendages (L6Ø-L75)

EXCLUDES 1 *congenital malformations of integument (Q84.-)*

✓4th L6Ø Nail disorders

EXCLUDES 2 *clubbing of nails (R68.3)*
onychia and paronychia (LØ3.Ø-)

Nail Disorders

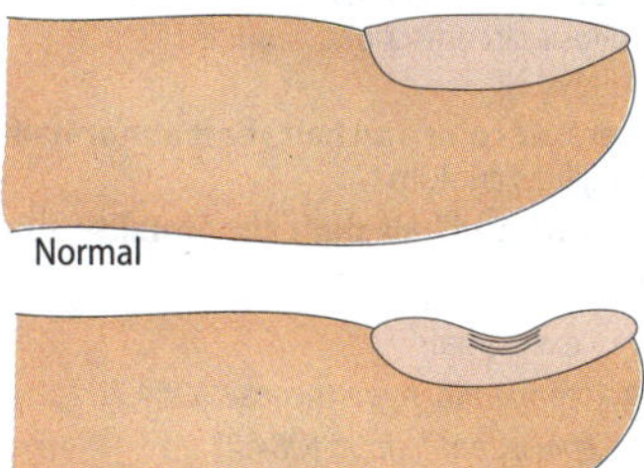

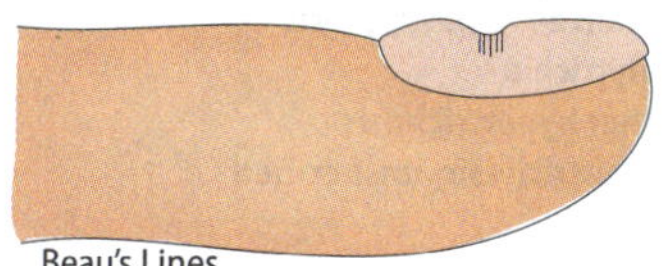

L6Ø.Ø Ingrowing nail

L6Ø.1 Onycholysis

L6Ø.2 Onychogryphosis

L6Ø.3 Nail dystrophy

L6Ø.4 Beau's lines

L6Ø.5 Yellow nail syndrome

L6Ø.8 Other nail disorders

L6Ø.9 Nail disorder, unspecified

L62 Nail disorders in diseases classified elsewhere

Code first underlying disease, such as:
pachydermoperiostosis (M89.4-)

✓4th L63 Alopecia areata

L63.Ø Alopecia (capitis) totalis

L63.1 Alopecia universalis

L63.2 Ophiasis

L63.8 Other alopecia areata

L63.9 Alopecia areata, unspecified

✓4th L64 Androgenic alopecia

INCLUDES male-pattern baldness

L64.Ø Drug-induced androgenic alopecia

Use additional code for adverse effect, if applicable, to identify drug (T36-T5Ø with fifth or sixth character 5)

L64.8 Other androgenic alopecia

L64.9 Androgenic alopecia, unspecified

✓4th L65 Other nonscarring hair loss

Use additional code for adverse effect, if applicable, to identify drug (T36-T5Ø with fifth or sixth character 5)

EXCLUDES 1 *trichotillomania (F63.3)*

L65.Ø Telogen effluvium

DEF: Form of nonscarring alopecia characterized by shedding of hair from premature telogen development in follicles due to stress, including shock, childbirth, surgery, drugs, or weight loss.

L65.1 Anagen effluvium

L65.2 Alopecia mucinosa

L65.8 Other specified nonscarring hair loss

L65.9 Nonscarring hair loss, unspecified

Alopecia NOS

✓4th L66 Cicatricial alopecia [scarring hair loss]

L66.Ø Pseudopelade

L66.1 Lichen planopilaris

Follicular lichen planus

L66.2 Folliculitis decalvans

L66.3 Perifolliculitis capitis abscedens

L66.4 Folliculitis ulerythematosa reticulata

L66.8 Other cicatricial alopecia

AHA: 2015,1Q,19

L66.9 Cicatricial alopecia, unspecified

✓4th L67 Hair color and hair shaft abnormalities

EXCLUDES 1 *monilethrix (Q84.1)*
pili annulati (Q84.1)
telogen effluvium (L65.Ø)

L67.Ø Trichorrhexis nodosa

L67.1 Variations in hair color
Canities
Greyness, hair (premature)
Heterochromia of hair
Poliosis circumscripta, acquired
Poliosis NOS

L67.8 Other hair color and hair shaft abnormalities
Fragilitas crinium

L67.9 Hair color and hair shaft abnormality, unspecified

✓4th L68 Hypertrichosis

INCLUDES excess hair
EXCLUDES 1 *congenital hypertrichosis (Q84.2)*
persistent lanugo (Q84.2)

L68.Ø Hirsutism
L68.1 Acquired hypertrichosis lanuginosa
L68.2 Localized hypertrichosis
L68.3 Polytrichia
L68.8 Other hypertrichosis
L68.9 Hypertrichosis, unspecified

✓4th L7Ø Acne

EXCLUDES 2 *acne keloid (L73.Ø)*

L7Ø.Ø Acne vulgaris
L7Ø.1 Acne conglobata
L7Ø.2 Acne varioliformis
Acne necrotica miliaris
DEF: Rare form of acne characterized by development of persistent brown papulopustules followed by scar formation. This type of acne usually presents on the brow and temporoparietal part of the scalp.

L7Ø.3 Acne tropica
L7Ø.4 Infantile acne P
L7Ø.5 Acné excoriée
Acné excoriée des jeunes filles
Picker's acne
L7Ø.8 Other acne
L7Ø.9 Acne, unspecified

✓4th L71 Rosacea

Use additional code for adverse effect, if applicable, to identify drug (T36-T5Ø with fifth or sixth character 5)

L71.Ø Perioral dermatitis
L71.1 Rhinophyma
L71.8 Other rosacea
AHA: 2018,4Q,15
L71.9 Rosacea, unspecified

✓4th L72 Follicular cysts of skin and subcutaneous tissue

L72.Ø Epidermal cyst

✓5th L72.1 Pilar and trichodermal cyst
L72.11 Pilar cyst
L72.12 Trichodermal cyst
Trichilemmal (proliferating) cyst

L72.2 Steatocystoma multiplex
L72.3 Sebaceous cyst
EXCLUDES 2 *pilar cyst (L72.11)*
trichilemmal (proliferating) cyst (L72.12)
L72.8 Other follicular cysts of the skin and subcutaneous tissue
L72.9 Follicular cyst of the skin and subcutaneous tissue, unspecified

✓4th L73 Other follicular disorders

L73.Ø Acne keloid
L73.1 Pseudofolliculitis barbae
L73.2 Hidradenitis suppurativa
L73.8 Other specified follicular disorders
Sycosis barbae
L73.9 Follicular disorder, unspecified

✓4th L74 Eccrine sweat disorders

EXCLUDES 2 *generalized hyperhidrosis (R61)*

DEF: Eccrine sweat glands: Glands found in the dermal and hypodermal layer of the skin throughout the body, particularly on the forehead, scalp, axillae, palms, and soles. These glands produce watery and neutral or slightly acidic sweat.

L74.Ø Miliaria rubra
L74.1 Miliaria crystallina
L74.2 Miliaria profunda
Miliaria tropicalis
L74.3 Miliaria, unspecified
L74.4 Anhidrosis
Hypohidrosis
DEF: Inability to sweat normally. When the body can't cool itself through perspiration it can lead to heatstroke, a life-threatening condition.

✓5th L74.5 Focal hyperhidrosis

✓6th L74.51 Primary focal hyperhidrosis
L74.51Ø Primary focal hyperhidrosis, axilla
L74.511 Primary focal hyperhidrosis, face
L74.512 Primary focal hyperhidrosis, palms
L74.513 Primary focal hyperhidrosis, soles
L74.519 Primary focal hyperhidrosis, unspecified

L74.52 Secondary focal hyperhidrosis
Frey's syndrome

L74.8 Other eccrine sweat disorders
L74.9 Eccrine sweat disorder, unspecified
Sweat gland disorder NOS

✓4th L75 Apocrine sweat disorders

EXCLUDES 1 *dyshidrosis (L3Ø.1)*
hidradenitis suppurativa (L73.2)

DEF: Apocrine sweat glands: Found in the axilla, areola, and circumanal region, these glands begin to function in puberty and produce viscid milky secretions in response to external stimuli.

L75.Ø Bromhidrosis
L75.1 Chromhidrosis
L75.2 Apocrine miliaria
Fox-Fordyce disease
DEF: Chronic, usually pruritic disease evidenced by small follicular papular eruptions, especially in the axillary and pubic areas. Apocrine miliaria develops from the closure and rupture of the affected apocrine glands' intraepidermal portion of the ducts.
L75.8 Other apocrine sweat disorders
L75.9 Apocrine sweat disorder, unspecified

Intraoperative and postprocedural complications of skin and subcutaneous tissue (L76)

✓4th L76 Intraoperative and postprocedural complications of skin and subcutaneous tissue

AHA: 2016,4Q,9-10

✓5th L76.Ø Intraoperative hemorrhage and hematoma of skin and subcutaneous tissue complicating a procedure

EXCLUDES 1 *intraoperative hemorrhage and hematoma of skin and subcutaneous tissue due to accidental puncture and laceration during a procedure (L76.1-)*

L76.Ø1 Intraoperative hemorrhage and hematoma of skin and subcutaneous tissue complicating a dermatologic procedure CC
L76.Ø2 Intraoperative hemorrhage and hematoma of skin and subcutaneous tissue complicating other procedure CC

✓5th L76.1 Accidental puncture and laceration of skin and subcutaneous tissue during a procedure

L76.11 Accidental puncture and laceration of skin and subcutaneous tissue during a dermatologic procedure CC
L76.12 Accidental puncture and laceration of skin and subcutaneous tissue during other procedure CC

✓5th L76.2 Postprocedural hemorrhage of skin and subcutaneous tissue following a procedure

L76.21 Postprocedural hemorrhage of skin and subcutaneous tissue following a dermatologic procedure CC
L76.22 Postprocedural hemorrhage of skin and subcutaneous tissue following other procedure CC

✓5th **L76.3 Postprocedural hematoma and seroma of skin and subcutaneous tissue following a procedure**

L76.31 Postprocedural hematoma of skin and subcutaneous tissue following a dermatologic procedure CC

L76.32 Postprocedural hematoma of skin and subcutaneous tissue following other procedure CC

L76.33 Postprocedural seroma of skin and subcutaneous tissue following a dermatologic procedure CC

L76.34 Postprocedural seroma of skin and subcutaneous tissue following other procedure CC

✓5th **L76.8 Other intraoperative and postprocedural complications of skin and subcutaneous tissue**

Use additional code, if applicable, to further specify disorder

L76.81 Other intraoperative complications of skin and subcutaneous tissue

L76.82 Other postprocedural complications of skin and subcutaneous tissue

AHA: 2017,3Q,6

Other disorders of the skin and subcutaneous tissue (L8Ø-L99)

L8Ø Vitiligo

EXCLUDES 2 *vitiligo of eyelids (H02.73-)*
vitiligo of vulva (N90.89)

DEF: Persistent, progressive development of nonpigmented white patches on otherwise normal skin.

✓4th **L81 Other disorders of pigmentation**

EXCLUDES 1 *birthmark NOS (Q82.5)*
Peutz-Jeghers syndrome (Q85.89)

EXCLUDES 2 *nevus - see Alphabetical Index*

L81.Ø Postinflammatory hyperpigmentation

L81.1 Chloasma

L81.2 Freckles

L81.3 Cafe au lait spots

L81.4 Other melanin hyperpigmentation
Lentigo

L81.5 Leukoderma, not elsewhere classified

L81.6 Other disorders of diminished melanin formation

L81.7 Pigmented purpuric dermatosis
Angioma serpiginosum

L81.8 Other specified disorders of pigmentation
Iron pigmentation
Tattoo pigmentation

L81.9 Disorder of pigmentation, unspecified

✓4th **L82 Seborrheic keratosis**

INCLUDES basal cell papilloma
dermatosis papulosa nigra
Leser-Trélat disease

EXCLUDES 2 *seborrheic dermatitis (L21.-)*

DEF: Common, benign, noninvasive, lightly pigmented, warty growth composed of basaloid cells that usually appear at middle age as soft, easily crumbling plaques on the face, trunk, and extremities.

L82.Ø Inflamed seborrheic keratosis

AHA: 2023,2Q,12; 2021,3Q,10

L82.1 Other seborrheic keratosis
Seborrheic keratosis NOS

L83 Acanthosis nigricans
Confluent and reticulated papillomatosis

DEF: Diffuse, velvety hyperplasia of the spinous skin layer of the axilla and other body folds marked by gray, brown, or black pigmentation. In adult form, it is often associated with malignant acanthosis nigricans in a benign, nevoid form relatively generalized.

L84 Corns and callosities
Callus
Clavus

✓4th **L85 Other epidermal thickening**

EXCLUDES 2 *hypertrophic disorders of the skin (L91.-)*

L85.Ø Acquired ichthyosis

EXCLUDES 1 *congenital ichthyosis (Q80.-)*

L85.1 Acquired keratosis [keratoderma] palmaris et plantaris

EXCLUDES 1 *inherited keratosis palmaris et plantaris (Q82.8)*

L85.2 Keratosis punctata (palmaris et plantaris)

L85.3 Xerosis cutis
Dry skin dermatitis

L85.8 Other specified epidermal thickening
Cutaneous horn

L85.9 Epidermal thickening, unspecified

L86 Keratoderma in diseases classified elsewhere

Code first underlying disease, such as:
Reiter's disease (MØ2.3-)

EXCLUDES 1 *gonococcal keratoderma (A54.89)*
gonococcal keratosis (A54.89)
keratoderma due to vitamin A deficiency (E5Ø.8)
keratosis due to vitamin A deficiency (E5Ø.8)
xeroderma due to vitamin A deficiency (E5Ø.8)

✓4th **L87 Transepidermal elimination disorders**

EXCLUDES 1 *granuloma annulare (perforating) (L92.Ø)*

L87.Ø Keratosis follicularis et parafollicularis in cutem penetrans
Hyperkeratosis follicularis penetrans
Kyrle disease

L87.1 Reactive perforating collagenosis

L87.2 Elastosis perforans serpiginosa

L87.8 Other transepidermal elimination disorders

L87.9 Transepidermal elimination disorder, unspecified

L88 Pyoderma gangrenosum CC
Phagedenic pyoderma

EXCLUDES 1 *dermatitis gangrenosa (LØ8.Ø)*

DEF: Persistent debilitating skin disease characterized by irregular, boggy, blue-red ulcerations, with central healing and undermined edges.

✓4th **L89 Pressure ulcer**

INCLUDES bed sore
decubitus ulcer
plaster ulcer
pressure area
pressure sore

Code first any associated gangrene (I96)

EXCLUDES 2 *decubitus (trophic) ulcer of cervix (uteri) (N86)*
diabetic ulcers (EØ8.621, EØ8.622, EØ9.621, EØ9.622, E1Ø.621, E1Ø.622, E11.621, E11.622, E13.621, E13.622)
non-pressure chronic ulcer of skin (L97.-)
skin infections (LØØ-LØ8)
varicose ulcer (I83.Ø, I83.2)

AHA: 2022,2Q,8; 2021,1Q,24; 2019,4Q,10-11,54; 2018,4Q,69; 2018,3Q,3; 2018,2Q,21; 2017,4Q,109; 2017,1Q,49; 2016,4Q,143

TIP: The stage of a diagnosed pressure ulcer can be based on documentation from clinicians who are not the patient's provider.

Four Stages of Pressure Ulcer

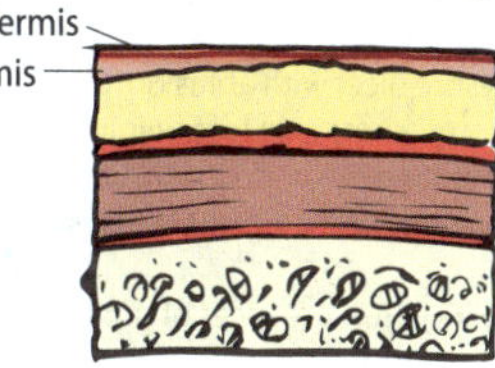

Stage 1
Persistent focal edema

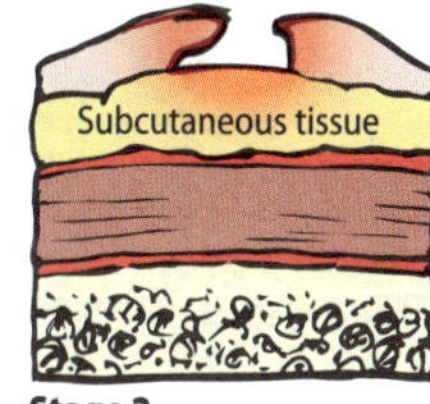

Stage 2
Abrasion, blister, partial thickness skin loss involving epidermis and/or dermis

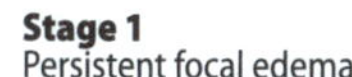

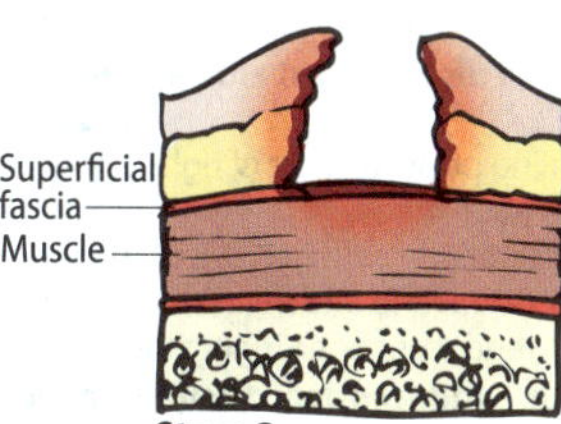

Stage 3
Full thickness skin loss involving damage or necrosis of subcutaneous tissue

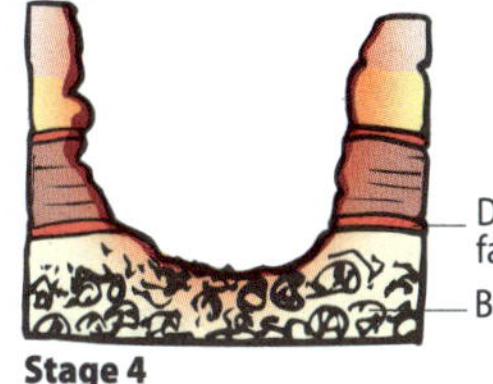

Stage 4
Necrosis of soft tissues through to underlying muscle, tendon, or bone

✓5th **L89.Ø Pressure ulcer of elbow**

✓6th **L89.ØØ Pressure ulcer of unspecified elbow**

L89.ØØØ Pressure ulcer of unspecified elbow, unstageable HCC

L89.001 Pressure ulcer of unspecified elbow, stage 1
Healing pressure ulcer of unspecified elbow, stage 1
Pressure pre-ulcer skin changes limited to persistent focal edema, unspecified elbow

L89.002 Pressure ulcer of unspecified elbow, stage 2 HCC
Healing pressure ulcer of unspecified elbow, stage 2
Pressure ulcer with abrasion, blister, partial thickness skin loss involving epidermis and/or dermis, unspecified elbow

L89.003 Pressure ulcer of unspecified elbow, stage 3 MCC H4 UNS HCC
Healing pressure ulcer of unspecified elbow, stage 3
Pressure ulcer with full thickness skin loss involving damage or necrosis of subcutaneous tissue, unspecified elbow

L89.004 Pressure ulcer of unspecified elbow, stage 4 MCC H4 UNS HCC
Healing pressure ulcer of unspecified elbow, stage 4
Pressure ulcer with necrosis of soft tissues through to underlying muscle, tendon, or bone, unspecified elbow

L89.006 Pressure-induced deep tissue damage of unspecified elbow

L89.009 Pressure ulcer of unspecified elbow, unspecified stage
Healing pressure ulcer of elbow NOS
Healing pressure ulcer of unspecified elbow, unspecified stage

✓6th **L89.01 Pressure ulcer of right elbow**

L89.010 Pressure ulcer of right elbow, unstageable HCC

L89.011 Pressure ulcer of right elbow, stage 1
Healing pressure ulcer of right elbow, stage 1
Pressure pre-ulcer skin changes limited to persistent focal edema, right elbow

L89.012 Pressure ulcer of right elbow, stage 2 HCC
Healing pressure ulcer of right elbow, stage 2
Pressure ulcer with abrasion, blister, partial thickness skin loss involving epidermis and/or dermis, right elbow

L89.013 Pressure ulcer of right elbow, stage 3 MCC H4 HCC
Healing pressure ulcer of right elbow, stage 3
Pressure ulcer with full thickness skin loss involving damage or necrosis of subcutaneous tissue, right elbow

L89.014 Pressure ulcer of right elbow, stage 4 MCC H4 HCC
Healing pressure ulcer of right elbow, stage 4
Pressure ulcer with necrosis of soft tissues through to underlying muscle, tendon, or bone, right elbow

L89.016 Pressure-induced deep tissue damage of right elbow

L89.019 Pressure ulcer of right elbow, unspecified stage
Healing pressure ulcer of right elbow NOS

✓6th **L89.02 Pressure ulcer of left elbow**

L89.020 Pressure ulcer of left elbow, unstageable HCC

L89.021 Pressure ulcer of left elbow, stage 1
Healing pressure ulcer of left elbow, stage 1
Pressure pre-ulcer skin changes limited to persistent focal edema, left elbow

L89.022 Pressure ulcer of left elbow, stage 2 HCC
Healing pressure ulcer of left elbow, stage 2
Pressure ulcer with abrasion, blister, partial thickness skin loss involving epidermis and/or dermis, left elbow

L89.023 Pressure ulcer of left elbow, stage 3 MCC H4 HCC
Healing pressure ulcer of left elbow, stage 3
Pressure ulcer with full thickness skin loss involving damage or necrosis of subcutaneous tissue, left elbow

L89.024 Pressure ulcer of left elbow, stage 4 MCC H4 HCC
Healing pressure ulcer of left elbow, stage 4
Pressure ulcer with necrosis of soft tissues through to underlying muscle, tendon, or bone, left elbow

L89.026 Pressure-induced deep tissue damage of left elbow

L89.029 Pressure ulcer of left elbow, unspecified stage
Healing pressure ulcer of left elbow NOS

✓5th **L89.1 Pressure ulcer of back**

✓6th **L89.10 Pressure ulcer of unspecified part of back**

L89.100 Pressure ulcer of unspecified part of back, unstageable HCC

L89.101 Pressure ulcer of unspecified part of back, stage 1
Healing pressure ulcer of unspecified part of back, stage 1
Pressure pre-ulcer skin changes limited to persistent focal edema, unspecified part of back

L89.102 Pressure ulcer of unspecified part of back, stage 2 HCC
Healing pressure ulcer of unspecified part of back, stage 2
Pressure ulcer with abrasion, blister, partial thickness skin loss involving epidermis and/or dermis, unspecified part of back

L89.103 Pressure ulcer of unspecified part of back, stage 3 MCC H4 HCC
Healing pressure ulcer of unspecified part of back, stage 3
Pressure ulcer with full thickness skin loss involving damage or necrosis of subcutaneous tissue, unspecified part of back

L89.104 Pressure ulcer of unspecified part of back, stage 4 MCC H4 HCC
Healing pressure ulcer of unspecified part of back, stage 4
Pressure ulcer with necrosis of soft tissues through to underlying muscle, tendon, or bone, unspecified part of back

L89.106 Pressure-induced deep tissue damage of unspecified part of back

L89.109 Pressure ulcer of unspecified part of back, unspecified stage
Healing pressure ulcer of unspecified part of back NOS
Healing pressure ulcer of unspecified part of back, unspecified stage

✓6th **L89.11 Pressure ulcer of right upper back**
Pressure ulcer of right shoulder blade

L89.110 Pressure ulcer of right upper back, unstageable HCC

L89.111 Pressure ulcer of right upper back, stage 1
Healing pressure ulcer of right upper back, stage 1
Pressure pre-ulcer skin changes limited to persistent focal edema, right upper back

L89.112 Pressure ulcer of right upper back, stage 2 HCC
- Healing pressure ulcer of right upper back, stage 2
- Pressure ulcer with abrasion, blister, partial thickness skin loss involving epidermis and/or dermis, right upper back

L89.113 Pressure ulcer of right upper back, stage 3 MCC H4 HCC
- Healing pressure ulcer of right upper back, stage 3
- Pressure ulcer with full thickness skin loss involving damage or necrosis of subcutaneous tissue, right upper back

L89.114 Pressure ulcer of right upper back, stage 4 MCC H4 HCC
- Healing pressure ulcer of right upper back, stage 4
- Pressure ulcer with necrosis of soft tissues through to underlying muscle, tendon, or bone, right upper back

L89.116 Pressure-induced deep tissue damage of right upper back

L89.119 Pressure ulcer of right upper back, unspecified stage
- Healing pressure ulcer of right upper back NOS
- Healing pressure ulcer of right upper back, unspecified stage

√6th **L89.12 Pressure ulcer of left upper back**
- Pressure ulcer of left shoulder blade

L89.120 Pressure ulcer of left upper back, unstageable HCC

L89.121 Pressure ulcer of left upper back, stage 1
- Healing pressure ulcer of left upper back, stage 1
- Pressure pre-ulcer skin changes limited to persistent focal edema, left upper back

L89.122 Pressure ulcer of left upper back, stage 2 HCC
- Healing pressure ulcer of left upper back, stage 2
- Pressure ulcer with abrasion, blister, partial thickness skin loss involving epidermis and/or dermis, left upper back

L89.123 Pressure ulcer of left upper back, stage 3 MCC H4 HCC
- Healing pressure ulcer of left upper back, stage 3
- Pressure ulcer with full thickness skin loss involving damage or necrosis of subcutaneous tissue, left upper back

L89.124 Pressure ulcer of left upper back, stage 4 MCC H4 HCC
- Healing pressure ulcer of left upper back, stage 4
- Pressure ulcer with necrosis of soft tissues through to underlying muscle, tendon, or bone, left upper back

L89.126 Pressure-induced deep tissue damage of left upper back

L89.129 Pressure ulcer of left upper back, unspecified stage
- Healing pressure ulcer of left upper back NOS
- Healing pressure ulcer of left upper back, unspecified stage

√6th **L89.13 Pressure ulcer of right lower back**

L89.130 Pressure ulcer of right lower back, unstageable HCC

L89.131 Pressure ulcer of right lower back, stage 1
- Healing pressure ulcer of right lower back, stage 1
- Pressure pre-ulcer skin changes limited to persistent focal edema, right lower back

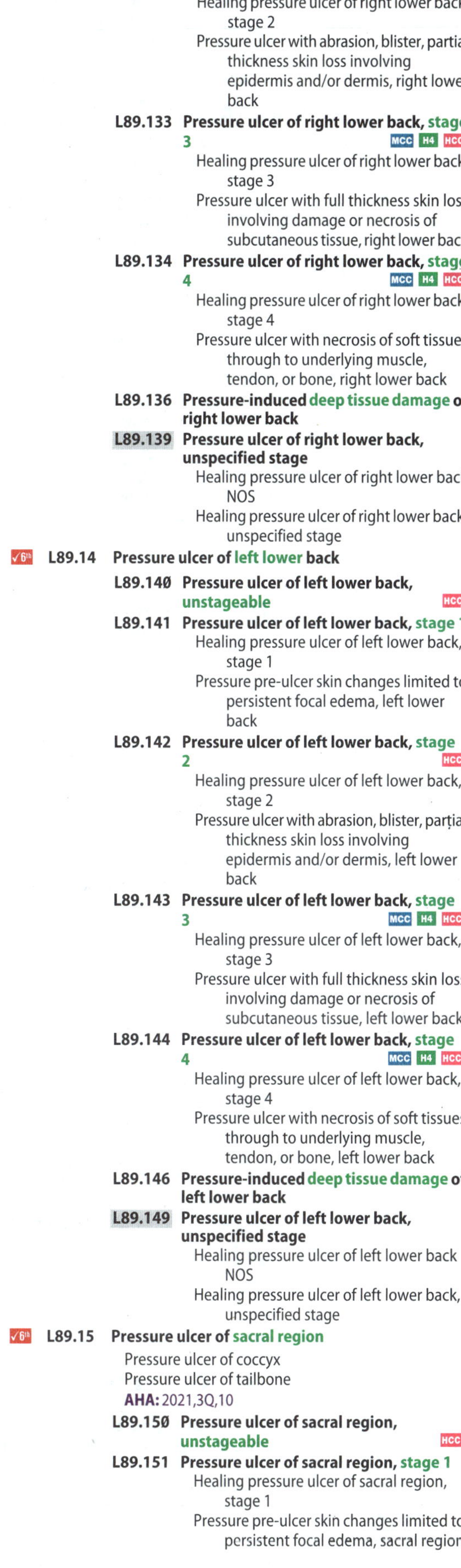

L89.132 Pressure ulcer of right lower back, stage 2 HCC
- Healing pressure ulcer of right lower back, stage 2
- Pressure ulcer with abrasion, blister, partial thickness skin loss involving epidermis and/or dermis, right lower back

L89.133 Pressure ulcer of right lower back, stage 3 MCC H4 HCC
- Healing pressure ulcer of right lower back, stage 3
- Pressure ulcer with full thickness skin loss involving damage or necrosis of subcutaneous tissue, right lower back

L89.134 Pressure ulcer of right lower back, stage 4 MCC H4 HCC
- Healing pressure ulcer of right lower back, stage 4
- Pressure ulcer with necrosis of soft tissues through to underlying muscle, tendon, or bone, right lower back

L89.136 Pressure-induced deep tissue damage of right lower back

L89.139 Pressure ulcer of right lower back, unspecified stage
- Healing pressure ulcer of right lower back NOS
- Healing pressure ulcer of right lower back, unspecified stage

√6th **L89.14 Pressure ulcer of left lower back**

L89.140 Pressure ulcer of left lower back, unstageable HCC

L89.141 Pressure ulcer of left lower back, stage 1
- Healing pressure ulcer of left lower back, stage 1
- Pressure pre-ulcer skin changes limited to persistent focal edema, left lower back

L89.142 Pressure ulcer of left lower back, stage 2 HCC
- Healing pressure ulcer of left lower back, stage 2
- Pressure ulcer with abrasion, blister, partial thickness skin loss involving epidermis and/or dermis, left lower back

L89.143 Pressure ulcer of left lower back, stage 3 MCC H4 HCC
- Healing pressure ulcer of left lower back, stage 3
- Pressure ulcer with full thickness skin loss involving damage or necrosis of subcutaneous tissue, left lower back

L89.144 Pressure ulcer of left lower back, stage 4 MCC H4 HCC
- Healing pressure ulcer of left lower back, stage 4
- Pressure ulcer with necrosis of soft tissues through to underlying muscle, tendon, or bone, left lower back

L89.146 Pressure-induced deep tissue damage of left lower back

L89.149 Pressure ulcer of left lower back, unspecified stage
- Healing pressure ulcer of left lower back NOS
- Healing pressure ulcer of left lower back, unspecified stage

√6th **L89.15 Pressure ulcer of sacral region**
- Pressure ulcer of coccyx
- Pressure ulcer of tailbone

AHA: 2021,3Q,10

L89.150 Pressure ulcer of sacral region, unstageable HCC

L89.151 Pressure ulcer of sacral region, stage 1
- Healing pressure ulcer of sacral region, stage 1
- Pressure pre-ulcer skin changes limited to persistent focal edema, sacral region

L89.152 Pressure ulcer of sacral region, stage 2 HCC
Healing pressure ulcer of sacral region, stage 2
Pressure ulcer with abrasion, blister, partial thickness skin loss involving epidermis and/or dermis, sacral region

L89.153 Pressure ulcer of sacral region, stage 3 MCC H4 HCC
Healing pressure ulcer of sacral region, stage 3
Pressure ulcer with full thickness skin loss involving damage or necrosis of subcutaneous tissue, sacral region

L89.154 Pressure ulcer of sacral region, stage 4 MCC H4 HCC
Healing pressure ulcer of sacral region, stage 4
Pressure ulcer with necrosis of soft tissues through to underlying muscle, tendon, or bone, sacral region
AHA: 2022,2Q,8

L89.156 Pressure-induced deep tissue damage of sacral region

L89.159 Pressure ulcer of sacral region, unspecified stage
Healing pressure ulcer of sacral region NOS
Healing pressure ulcer of sacral region, unspecified stage

✓5th **L89.2 Pressure ulcer of hip**

✓6th **L89.20 Pressure ulcer of unspecified hip**

L89.200 Pressure ulcer of unspecified hip, unstageable HCC

L89.201 Pressure ulcer of unspecified hip, stage 1
Healing pressure ulcer of unspecified hip back, stage 1
Pressure pre-ulcer skin changes limited to persistent focal edema, unspecified hip

L89.202 Pressure ulcer of unspecified hip, stage 2 HCC
Healing pressure ulcer of unspecified hip, stage 2
Pressure ulcer with abrasion, blister, partial thickness skin loss involving epidermis and/or dermis, unspecified hip

L89.203 Pressure ulcer of unspecified hip, stage 3 MCC H4 UNS HCC
Healing pressure ulcer of unspecified hip, stage 3
Pressure ulcer with full thickness skin loss involving damage or necrosis of subcutaneous tissue, unspecified hip

L89.204 Pressure ulcer of unspecified hip, stage 4 MCC H4 UNS HCC
Healing pressure ulcer of unspecified hip, stage 4
Pressure ulcer with necrosis of soft tissues through to underlying muscle, tendon, or bone, unspecified hip

L89.206 Pressure-induced deep tissue damage of unspecified hip

L89.209 Pressure ulcer of unspecified hip, unspecified stage
Healing pressure ulcer of unspecified hip NOS
Healing pressure ulcer of unspecified hip, unspecified stage

✓6th **L89.21 Pressure ulcer of right hip**

L89.210 Pressure ulcer of right hip, unstageable HCC

L89.211 Pressure ulcer of right hip, stage 1
Healing pressure ulcer of right hip back, stage 1
Pressure pre-ulcer skin changes limited to persistent focal edema, right hip

L89.212 Pressure ulcer of right hip, stage 2 HCC
Healing pressure ulcer of right hip, stage 2
Pressure ulcer with abrasion, blister, partial thickness skin loss involving epidermis and/or dermis, right hip

L89.213 Pressure ulcer of right hip, stage 3 MCC H4 HCC
Healing pressure ulcer of right hip, stage 3
Pressure ulcer with full thickness skin loss involving damage or necrosis of subcutaneous tissue, right hip

L89.214 Pressure ulcer of right hip, stage 4 MCC H4 HCC
Healing pressure ulcer of right hip, stage 4
Pressure ulcer with necrosis of soft tissues through to underlying muscle, tendon, or bone, right hip

L89.216 Pressure-induced deep tissue damage of right hip

L89.219 Pressure ulcer of right hip, unspecified stage
Healing pressure ulcer of right hip NOS
Healing pressure ulcer of right hip, unspecified stage

✓6th **L89.22 Pressure ulcer of left hip**

L89.220 Pressure ulcer of left hip, unstageable HCC

L89.221 Pressure ulcer of left hip, stage 1
Healing pressure ulcer of left hip back, stage 1
Pressure pre-ulcer skin changes limited to persistent focal edema, left hip

L89.222 Pressure ulcer of left hip, stage 2 HCC
Healing pressure ulcer of left hip, stage 2
Pressure ulcer with abrasion, blister, partial thickness skin loss involving epidermis and/or dermis, left hip

L89.223 Pressure ulcer of left hip, stage 3 MCC H4 HCC
Healing pressure ulcer of left hip, stage 3
Pressure ulcer with full thickness skin loss involving damage or necrosis of subcutaneous tissue, left hip

L89.224 Pressure ulcer of left hip, stage 4 MCC H4 HCC
Healing pressure ulcer of left hip, stage 4
Pressure ulcer with necrosis of soft tissues through to underlying muscle, tendon, or bone, left hip

L89.226 Pressure-induced deep tissue damage of left hip

L89.229 Pressure ulcer of left hip, unspecified stage
Healing pressure ulcer of left hip NOS
Healing pressure ulcer of left hip, unspecified stage

✓5th **L89.3 Pressure ulcer of buttock**
AHA: 2021,3Q,10

✓6th **L89.30 Pressure ulcer of unspecified buttock**

L89.300 Pressure ulcer of unspecified buttock, unstageable HCC

L89.301 Pressure ulcer of unspecified buttock, stage 1
Healing pressure ulcer of unspecified buttock, stage 1
Pressure pre-ulcer skin changes limited to persistent focal edema, unspecified buttock

L89.302 Pressure ulcer of unspecified buttock, stage 2 HCC
Healing pressure ulcer of unspecified buttock, stage 2
Pressure ulcer with abrasion, blister, partial thickness skin loss involving epidermis and/or dermis, unspecified buttock

L89.303 Pressure ulcer of unspecified buttock, stage 3 MCC H4 UNS HCC
Healing pressure ulcer of unspecified buttock, stage 3
Pressure ulcer with full thickness skin loss involving damage or necrosis of subcutaneous tissue, unspecified buttock

L89.304 Pressure ulcer of unspecified buttock, stage 4 MCC H4 UNS HCC
Healing pressure ulcer of unspecified buttock, stage 4
Pressure ulcer with necrosis of soft tissues through to underlying muscle, tendon, or bone, unspecified buttock

L89.306 Pressure-induced deep tissue damage of unspecified buttock

L89.309 Pressure ulcer of unspecified buttock, unspecified stage
Healing pressure ulcer of unspecified buttock NOS
Healing pressure ulcer of unspecified buttock, unspecified stage

✓6th **L89.31 Pressure ulcer of right buttock**

L89.310 Pressure ulcer of right buttock, unstageable HCC

L89.311 Pressure ulcer of right buttock, stage 1
Healing pressure ulcer of right buttock, stage 1
Pressure pre-ulcer skin changes limited to persistent focal edema, right buttock

L89.312 Pressure ulcer of right buttock, stage 2 HCC
Healing pressure ulcer of right buttock, stage 2
Pressure ulcer with abrasion, blister, partial thickness skin loss involving epidermis and/or dermis, right buttock

L89.313 Pressure ulcer of right buttock, stage 3 MCC H4 HCC
Healing pressure ulcer of right buttock, stage 3
Pressure ulcer with full thickness skin loss involving damage or necrosis of subcutaneous tissue, right buttock

L89.314 Pressure ulcer of right buttock, stage 4 MCC H4 HCC
Healing pressure ulcer of right buttock, stage 4
Pressure ulcer with necrosis of soft tissues through to underlying muscle, tendon, or bone, right buttock

L89.316 Pressure-induced deep tissue damage of right buttock

L89.319 Pressure ulcer of right buttock, unspecified stage
Healing pressure ulcer of right buttock NOS
Healing pressure ulcer of right buttock, unspecified stage

✓6th **L89.32 Pressure ulcer of left buttock**

L89.320 Pressure ulcer of left buttock, unstageable HCC

L89.321 Pressure ulcer of left buttock, stage 1
Healing pressure ulcer of left buttock, stage 1
Pressure pre-ulcer skin changes limited to persistent focal edema, left buttock

L89.322 Pressure ulcer of left buttock, stage 2 HCC
Healing pressure ulcer of left buttock, stage 2
Pressure ulcer with abrasion, blister, partial thickness skin loss involving epidermis and/or dermis, left buttock

L89.323 Pressure ulcer of left buttock, stage 3 MCC H4 HCC
Healing pressure ulcer of left buttock, stage 3
Pressure ulcer with full thickness skin loss involving damage or necrosis of subcutaneous tissue, left buttock

L89.324 Pressure ulcer of left buttock, stage 4 MCC H4 HCC
Healing pressure ulcer of left buttock, stage 4
Pressure ulcer with necrosis of soft tissues through to underlying muscle, tendon, or bone, left buttock

L89.326 Pressure-induced deep tissue damage of left buttock

L89.329 Pressure ulcer of left buttock, unspecified stage
Healing pressure ulcer of left buttock NOS
Healing pressure ulcer of left buttock, unspecified stage

✓5th **L89.4 Pressure ulcer of contiguous site of back, buttock and hip**

L89.40 Pressure ulcer of contiguous site of back, buttock and hip, unspecified stage
Healing pressure ulcer of contiguous site of back, buttock and hip NOS
Healing pressure ulcer of contiguous site of back, buttock and hip, unspecified stage

L89.41 Pressure ulcer of contiguous site of back, buttock and hip, stage 1
Healing pressure ulcer of contiguous site of back, buttock and hip, stage 1
Pressure pre-ulcer skin changes limited to persistent focal edema, contiguous site of back, buttock and hip

L89.42 Pressure ulcer of contiguous site of back, buttock and hip, stage 2 HCC
Healing pressure ulcer of contiguous site of back, buttock and hip, stage 2
Pressure ulcer with abrasion, blister, partial thickness skin loss involving epidermis and/or dermis, contiguous site of back, buttock and hip

L89.43 Pressure ulcer of contiguous site of back, buttock and hip, stage 3 MCC H4 HCC
Healing pressure ulcer of contiguous site of back, buttock and hip, stage 3
Pressure ulcer with full thickness skin loss involving damage or necrosis of subcutaneous tissue, contiguous site of back, buttock and hip

L89.44 Pressure ulcer of contiguous site of back, buttock and hip, stage 4 MCC H4 HCC
Healing pressure ulcer of contiguous site of back, buttock and hip, stage 4
Pressure ulcer with necrosis of soft tissues through to underlying muscle, tendon, or bone, contiguous site of back, buttock and hip

L89.45 Pressure ulcer of contiguous site of back, buttock and hip, unstageable HCC

L89.46 Pressure-induced deep tissue damage of contiguous site of back, buttock and hip

✓5th **L89.5 Pressure ulcer of ankle**

✓6th **L89.50 Pressure ulcer of unspecified ankle**

L89.500 Pressure ulcer of unspecified ankle, unstageable HCC

L89.501 Pressure ulcer of unspecified ankle, stage 1
Healing pressure ulcer of unspecified ankle, stage 1
Pressure pre-ulcer skin changes limited to persistent focal edema, unspecified ankle

L89.502 Pressure ulcer of unspecified ankle, stage 2 HCC
Healing pressure ulcer of unspecified ankle, stage 2
Pressure ulcer with abrasion, blister, partial thickness skin loss involving epidermis and/or dermis, unspecified ankle

L89.503 **Pressure ulcer of unspecified ankle, stage 3** MCC H4 UNS HCC
Healing pressure ulcer of unspecified ankle, stage 3
Pressure ulcer with full thickness skin loss involving damage or necrosis of subcutaneous tissue, unspecified ankle

L89.504 **Pressure ulcer of unspecified ankle, stage 4** MCC H4 UNS HCC
Healing pressure ulcer of unspecified ankle, stage 4
Pressure ulcer with necrosis of soft tissues through to underlying muscle, tendon, or bone, unspecified ankle

L89.506 **Pressure-induced deep tissue damage of unspecified ankle**

L89.509 **Pressure ulcer of unspecified ankle, unspecified stage**
Healing pressure ulcer of unspecified ankle NOS
Healing pressure ulcer of unspecified ankle, unspecified stage

✓6th L89.51 **Pressure ulcer of right ankle**

L89.510 **Pressure ulcer of right ankle, unstageable** HCC

L89.511 **Pressure ulcer of right ankle, stage 1**
Healing pressure ulcer of right ankle, stage 1
Pressure pre-ulcer skin changes limited to persistent focal edema, right ankle

L89.512 **Pressure ulcer of right ankle, stage 2** HCC
Healing pressure ulcer of right ankle, stage 2
Pressure ulcer with abrasion, blister, partial thickness skin loss involving epidermis and/or dermis, right ankle

L89.513 **Pressure ulcer of right ankle, stage 3** MCC H4 HCC
Healing pressure ulcer of right ankle, stage 3
Pressure ulcer with full thickness skin loss involving damage or necrosis of subcutaneous tissue, right ankle

L89.514 **Pressure ulcer of right ankle, stage 4** MCC H4 HCC
Healing pressure ulcer of right ankle, stage 4
Pressure ulcer with necrosis of soft tissues through to underlying muscle, tendon, or bone, right ankle

L89.516 **Pressure-induced deep tissue damage of right ankle**

L89.519 **Pressure ulcer of right ankle, unspecified stage**
Healing pressure ulcer of right ankle NOS
Healing pressure ulcer of right ankle, unspecified stage

✓6th L89.52 **Pressure ulcer of left ankle**

L89.520 **Pressure ulcer of left ankle, unstageable** HCC

L89.521 **Pressure ulcer of left ankle, stage 1**
Healing pressure ulcer of left ankle, stage 1
Pressure pre-ulcer skin changes limited to persistent focal edema, left ankle

L89.522 **Pressure ulcer of left ankle, stage 2** HCC
Healing pressure ulcer of left ankle, stage 2
Pressure ulcer with abrasion, blister, partial thickness skin loss involving epidermis and/or dermis, left ankle

L89.523 **Pressure ulcer of left ankle, stage 3** MCC H4 HCC
Healing pressure ulcer of left ankle, stage 3
Pressure ulcer with full thickness skin loss involving damage or necrosis of subcutaneous tissue, left ankle

L89.524 **Pressure ulcer of left ankle, stage 4** MCC H4 HCC
Healing pressure ulcer of left ankle, stage 4
Pressure ulcer with necrosis of soft tissues through to underlying muscle, tendon, or bone, left ankle

L89.526 **Pressure-induced deep tissue damage of left ankle**

L89.529 **Pressure ulcer of left ankle, unspecified stage**
Healing pressure ulcer of left ankle NOS
Healing pressure ulcer of left ankle, unspecified stage

✓5th L89.6 **Pressure ulcer of heel**

✓6th L89.60 **Pressure ulcer of unspecified heel**

L89.600 **Pressure ulcer of unspecified heel, unstageable** HCC

L89.601 **Pressure ulcer of unspecified heel, stage 1**
Healing pressure ulcer of unspecified heel, stage 1
Pressure pre-ulcer skin changes limited to persistent focal edema, unspecified heel

L89.602 **Pressure ulcer of unspecified heel, stage 2** HCC
Healing pressure ulcer of unspecified heel, stage 2
Pressure ulcer with abrasion, blister, partial thickness skin loss involving epidermis and/or dermis, unspecified heel

L89.603 **Pressure ulcer of unspecified heel, stage 3** MCC H4 UNS HCC
Healing pressure ulcer of unspecified heel, stage 3
Pressure ulcer with full thickness skin loss involving damage or necrosis of subcutaneous tissue, unspecified heel

L89.604 **Pressure ulcer of unspecified heel, stage 4** MCC H4 UNS HCC
Healing pressure ulcer of unspecified heel, stage 4
Pressure ulcer with necrosis of soft tissues through to underlying muscle, tendon, or bone, unspecified heel

L89.606 **Pressure-induced deep tissue damage of unspecified heel**

L89.609 **Pressure ulcer of unspecified heel, unspecified stage**
Healing pressure ulcer of unspecified heel NOS
Healing pressure ulcer of unspecified heel, unspecified stage

✓6th L89.61 **Pressure ulcer of right heel**

L89.610 **Pressure ulcer of right heel, unstageable** HCC

L89.611 **Pressure ulcer of right heel, stage 1**
Healing pressure ulcer of right heel, stage 1
Pressure pre-ulcer skin changes limited to persistent focal edema, right heel

L89.612 **Pressure ulcer of right heel, stage 2** HCC
Healing pressure ulcer of right heel, stage 2
Pressure ulcer with abrasion, blister, partial thickness skin loss involving epidermis and/or dermis, right heel

L89.613 **Pressure ulcer of right heel, stage 3** MCC H4 HCC
Healing pressure ulcer of right heel, stage 3
Pressure ulcer with full thickness skin loss involving damage or necrosis of subcutaneous tissue, right heel

L89.614 **Pressure ulcer of right heel, stage 4** MCC H4 HCC
Healing pressure ulcer of right heel, stage 4
Pressure ulcer with necrosis of soft tissues through to underlying muscle, tendon, or bone, right heel

L89.616 **Pressure-induced deep tissue damage of right heel**

L89.619 Pressure ulcer of right heel, unspecified stage
Healing pressure ulcer of right heel NOS
Healing pressure ulcer of right heel, unspecified stage

L89.62 Pressure ulcer of left heel

L89.620 Pressure ulcer of left heel, unstageable HCC

L89.621 Pressure ulcer of left heel, stage 1
Healing pressure ulcer of left heel, stage 1
Pressure pre-ulcer skin changes limited to persistent focal edema, left heel

L89.622 Pressure ulcer of left heel, stage 2 HCC
Healing pressure ulcer of left heel, stage 2
Pressure ulcer with abrasion, blister, partial thickness skin loss involving epidermis and/or dermis, left heel

L89.623 Pressure ulcer of left heel, stage 3 MCC H4 HCC
Healing pressure ulcer of left heel, stage 3
Pressure ulcer with full thickness skin loss involving damage or necrosis of subcutaneous tissue, left heel

L89.624 Pressure ulcer of left heel, stage 4 MCC H4 HCC
Healing pressure ulcer of left heel, stage 4
Pressure ulcer with necrosis of soft tissues through to underlying muscle, tendon, or bone, left heel

L89.626 Pressure-induced deep tissue damage of left heel

L89.629 Pressure ulcer of left heel, unspecified stage
Healing pressure ulcer of left heel NOS
Healing pressure ulcer of left heel, unspecified stage

L89.8 Pressure ulcer of other site

L89.81 Pressure ulcer of head
Pressure ulcer of face

L89.810 Pressure ulcer of head, unstageable HCC

L89.811 Pressure ulcer of head, stage 1
Healing pressure ulcer of head, stage 1
Pressure pre-ulcer skin changes limited to persistent focal edema, head

L89.812 Pressure ulcer of head, stage 2 HCC
Healing pressure ulcer of head, stage 2
Pressure ulcer with abrasion, blister, partial thickness skin loss involving epidermis and/or dermis, head

L89.813 Pressure ulcer of head, stage 3 MCC H4 HCC
Healing pressure ulcer of head, stage 3
Pressure ulcer with full thickness skin loss involving damage or necrosis of subcutaneous tissue, head

L89.814 Pressure ulcer of head, stage 4 MCC H4 HCC
Healing pressure ulcer of head, stage 4
Pressure ulcer with necrosis of soft tissues through to underlying muscle, tendon, or bone, head

L89.816 Pressure-induced deep tissue damage of head

L89.819 Pressure ulcer of head, unspecified stage
Healing pressure ulcer of head NOS
Healing pressure ulcer of head, unspecified stage

L89.89 Pressure ulcer of other site

L89.890 Pressure ulcer of other site, unstageable HCC

L89.891 Pressure ulcer of other site, stage 1
Healing pressure ulcer of other site, stage 1
Pressure pre-ulcer skin changes limited to persistent focal edema, other site

L89.892 Pressure ulcer of other site, stage 2 HCC
Healing pressure ulcer of other site, stage 2
Pressure ulcer with abrasion, blister, partial thickness skin loss involving epidermis and/or dermis, other site

L89.893 Pressure ulcer of other site, stage 3 MCC H4 HCC
Healing pressure ulcer of other site, stage 3
Pressure ulcer with full thickness skin loss involving damage or necrosis of subcutaneous tissue, other site

L89.894 Pressure ulcer of other site, stage 4 MCC H4 HCC
Healing pressure ulcer of other site, stage 4
Pressure ulcer with necrosis of soft tissues through to underlying muscle, tendon, or bone, other site

L89.896 Pressure-induced deep tissue damage of other site

L89.899 Pressure ulcer of other site, unspecified stage
Healing pressure ulcer of other site NOS
Healing pressure ulcer of other site, unspecified stage

L89.9 Pressure ulcer of unspecified site

L89.90 Pressure ulcer of unspecified site, unspecified stage
Healing pressure ulcer of unspecified site NOS
Healing pressure ulcer of unspecified site, unspecified stage

L89.91 Pressure ulcer of unspecified site, stage 1
Healing pressure ulcer of unspecified site, stage 1
Pressure pre-ulcer skin changes limited to persistent focal edema, unspecified site

L89.92 Pressure ulcer of unspecified site, stage 2 HCC
Healing pressure ulcer of unspecified site, stage 2
Pressure ulcer with abrasion, blister, partial thickness skin loss involving epidermis and/or dermis, unspecified site

L89.93 Pressure ulcer of unspecified site, stage 3 MCC H4 HCC
Healing pressure ulcer of unspecified site, stage 3
Pressure ulcer with full thickness skin loss involving damage or necrosis of subcutaneous tissue, unspecified site

L89.94 Pressure ulcer of unspecified site, stage 4 MCC H4 HCC
Healing pressure ulcer of unspecified site, stage 4
Pressure ulcer with necrosis of soft tissues through to underlying muscle, tendon, or bone, unspecified site

L89.95 Pressure ulcer of unspecified site, unstageable HCC

L89.96 Pressure-induced deep tissue damage of unspecified site

L90 Atrophic disorders of skin

L90.0 Lichen sclerosus et atrophicus
EXCLUDES 2 *lichen sclerosus of external female genital organs (N90.4)*
lichen sclerosus of external male genital organs (N48.0)

L90.1 Anetoderma of Schweninger-Buzzi

L90.2 Anetoderma of Jadassohn-Pellizzari

L90.3 Atrophoderma of Pasini and Pierini

L90.4 Acrodermatitis chronica atrophicans

L90.5 Scar conditions and fibrosis of skin
Adherent scar (skin)
Cicatrix
Disfigurement of skin due to scar
Fibrosis of skin NOS
Scar NOS
EXCLUDES 2 *hypertrophic scar (L91.0)*
keloid scar (L91.0)
AHA: 2016,2Q,5; 2015,1Q,19

L90.6 Striae atrophicae

L90.8 Other atrophic disorders of skin

L90.9 Atrophic disorder of skin, unspecified

L91 Hypertrophic disorders of skin

L91.Ø Hypertrophic scar
Keloid
Keloid scar
EXCLUDES 2 *acne keloid (L73.Ø)*
scar NOS (L9Ø.5)
DEF: Overgrowth of scar tissue due to excess amounts of collagen during connective tissue repair, occurring mainly on the upper trunk and face.

L91.8 Other hypertrophic disorders of the skin

L91.9 Hypertrophic disorder of the skin, unspecified

L92 Granulomatous disorders of skin and subcutaneous tissue
EXCLUDES 2 *actinic granuloma (L57.5)*

L92.Ø Granuloma annulare
Perforating granuloma annulare

L92.1 Necrobiosis lipoidica, not elsewhere classified
EXCLUDES 1 *necrobiosis lipoidica associated with diabetes mellitus (EØ8-E13 with .62Ø)*

L92.2 Granuloma faciale [eosinophilic granuloma of skin]

L92.3 Foreign body granuloma of the skin and subcutaneous tissue
Use additional code to identify the type of retained foreign body (Z18.-)

L92.8 Other granulomatous disorders of the skin and subcutaneous tissue

L92.9 Granulomatous disorder of the skin and subcutaneous tissue, unspecified
EXCLUDES 2 *umbilical granuloma (P83.81)*
AHA: 2017,4Q,21-22

L93 Lupus erythematosus
Use additional code for adverse effect, if applicable, to identify drug (T36-T5Ø with fifth or sixth character 5)
EXCLUDES 1 *lupus exedens (A18.4)*
lupus vulgaris (A18.4)
scleroderma (M34.-)
systemic lupus erythematosus (M32.-)
DEF: Inflammatory, autoimmune skin condition in which the body's autoimmune system attacks healthy tissue of the integumentary system.

L93.Ø Discoid lupus erythematosus
Lupus erythematosus NOS

L93.1 Subacute cutaneous lupus erythematosus

L93.2 Other local lupus erythematosus
Lupus erythematosus profundus
Lupus panniculitis

L94 Other localized connective tissue disorders
EXCLUDES 1 *systemic connective tissue disorders (M3Ø-M36)*

L94.Ø Localized scleroderma [morphea]
Circumscribed scleroderma

L94.1 Linear scleroderma
En coup de sabre lesion

L94.2 Calcinosis cutis

L94.3 Sclerodactyly

L94.4 Gottron's papules

L94.5 Poikiloderma vasculare atrophicans

L94.6 Ainhum

L94.8 Other specified localized connective tissue disorders

L94.9 Localized connective tissue disorder, unspecified

L95 Vasculitis limited to skin, not elsewhere classified
EXCLUDES 1 *angioma serpiginosum (L81.7)*
Henoch(-Schonlein) purpura (D69.Ø)
hypersensitivity angiitis (M31.Ø)
lupus panniculitis (L93.2)
panniculitis NOS (M79.3)
panniculitis of neck and back (M54.Ø-)
polyarteritis nodosa (M3Ø.Ø)
relapsing panniculitis (M35.6)
rheumatoid vasculitis (MØ5.2)
serum sickness (T8Ø.6-)
urticaria (L5Ø.-)
Wegener's granulomatosis (M31.3-)

L95.Ø Livedoid vasculitis
Atrophie blanche (en plaque)

L95.1 Erythema elevatum diutinum

L95.8 Other vasculitis limited to the skin

L95.9 Vasculitis limited to the skin, unspecified

L97 Non-pressure chronic ulcer of lower limb, not elsewhere classified
INCLUDES chronic ulcer of skin of lower limb NOS
non-healing ulcer of skin
non-infected sinus of skin
trophic ulcer NOS
tropical ulcer NOS
ulcer of skin of lower limb NOS
Code first any associated underlying condition, such as:
any associated gangrene (I96)
atherosclerosis of the lower extremities (I7Ø.23-, I7Ø.24-, I7Ø.33-, I7Ø.34-, I7Ø.43-, I7Ø.44-, I7Ø.53-, I7Ø.54-, I7Ø.63-, I7Ø.64-, I7Ø.73-, I7Ø.74-)
chronic venous hypertension (I87.31-, I87.33-)
diabetic ulcers (EØ8.621, EØ8.622, EØ9.621, EØ9.622, E1Ø.621, E1Ø.622, E11.621, E11.622, E13.621, E13.622)
postphlebitic syndrome (I87.Ø1-, I87.Ø3-)
postthrombotic syndrome (I87.Ø1-, I87.Ø3-)
varicose ulcer (I83.Ø-, I83.2-)
EXCLUDES 2 *pressure ulcer (pressure area) (L89.-)*
skin infections (LØØ-LØ8)
specific infections classified to AØØ-B99
AHA: 2021,1Q,7; 2020,2Q,19; 2018,4Q,69; 2017,4Q,17
TIP: The depth and/or severity of a diagnosed nonpressure ulcer can be determined based on medical record documentation from clinicians who are not the patient's provider.
TIP: Assign a code from this category/subcategory for nonpressure ulcers documented as acute.

L97.1 Non-pressure chronic ulcer of thigh

L97.1Ø Non-pressure chronic ulcer of unspecified thigh

L97.1Ø1 Non-pressure chronic ulcer of unspecified thigh limited to breakdown of skin CC UNS HCC

L97.1Ø2 Non-pressure chronic ulcer of unspecified thigh with fat layer exposed CC UNS HCC

L97.1Ø3 Non-pressure chronic ulcer of unspecified thigh with necrosis of muscle CC UNS HCC

L97.1Ø4 Non-pressure chronic ulcer of unspecified thigh with necrosis of bone CC UNS HCC

L97.1Ø5 Non-pressure chronic ulcer of unspecified thigh with muscle involvement without evidence of necrosis CC UNS HCC

L97.1Ø6 Non-pressure chronic ulcer of unspecified thigh with bone involvement without evidence of necrosis CC UNS HCC

L97.1Ø8 Non-pressure chronic ulcer of unspecified thigh with other specified severity CC UNS HCC

L97.1Ø9 Non-pressure chronic ulcer of unspecified thigh with unspecified severity CC UNS HCC

L97.11 Non-pressure chronic ulcer of right thigh

L97.111 Non-pressure chronic ulcer of right thigh limited to breakdown of skin CC HCC

L97.112 Non-pressure chronic ulcer of right thigh with fat layer exposed CC HCC

L97.113 Non-pressure chronic ulcer of right thigh with necrosis of muscle CC HCC

L97.114 Non-pressure chronic ulcer of right thigh with necrosis of bone CC HCC

L97.115 Non-pressure chronic ulcer of right thigh with muscle involvement without evidence of necrosis CC HCC

L97.116 Non-pressure chronic ulcer of right thigh with bone involvement without evidence of necrosis CC HCC

L97.118 Non-pressure chronic ulcer of right thigh with other specified severity CC HCC

L97.119 Non-pressure chronic ulcer of right thigh with unspecified severity CC HCC

L97.12 Non-pressure chronic ulcer of left thigh

L97.121 Non-pressure chronic ulcer of left thigh limited to breakdown of skin CC HCC

L97.122 Non-pressure chronic ulcer of left thigh with fat layer exposed CC HCC

L97.123 Non-pressure chronic ulcer of left thigh with necrosis of muscle CC HCC

L97.124 Non-pressure chronic ulcer of left thigh with necrosis of bone CC HCC

L97.125 Non-pressure chronic ulcer of left thigh with muscle involvement without evidence of necrosis CC HCC

L97.126 Non-pressure chronic ulcer of left thigh with bone involvement without evidence of necrosis CC HCC

L97.128 Non-pressure chronic ulcer of left thigh with other specified severity CC HCC

L97.129 Non-pressure chronic ulcer of left thigh with unspecified severity CC HCC

✓5th L97.2 Non-pressure chronic ulcer of calf

✓6th L97.20 Non-pressure chronic ulcer of unspecified calf

L97.201 Non-pressure chronic ulcer of unspecified calf limited to breakdown of skin CC UNS HCC

L97.202 Non-pressure chronic ulcer of unspecified calf with fat layer exposed CC UNS HCC

L97.203 Non-pressure chronic ulcer of unspecified calf with necrosis of muscle CC UNS HCC

L97.204 Non-pressure chronic ulcer of unspecified calf with necrosis of bone CC UNS HCC

L97.205 Non-pressure chronic ulcer of unspecified calf with muscle involvement without evidence of necrosis CC UNS HCC

L97.206 Non-pressure chronic ulcer of unspecified calf with bone involvement without evidence of necrosis CC UNS HCC

L97.208 Non-pressure chronic ulcer of unspecified calf with other specified severity CC UNS HCC

L97.209 Non-pressure chronic ulcer of unspecified calf with unspecified severity CC UNS HCC

✓6th L97.21 Non-pressure chronic ulcer of right calf

L97.211 Non-pressure chronic ulcer of right calf limited to breakdown of skin CC HCC

L97.212 Non-pressure chronic ulcer of right calf with fat layer exposed CC HCC

L97.213 Non-pressure chronic ulcer of right calf with necrosis of muscle CC HCC

L97.214 Non-pressure chronic ulcer of right calf with necrosis of bone CC HCC

L97.215 Non-pressure chronic ulcer of right calf with muscle involvement without evidence of necrosis CC HCC

L97.216 Non-pressure chronic ulcer of right calf with bone involvement without evidence of necrosis CC HCC

L97.218 Non-pressure chronic ulcer of right calf with other specified severity CC HCC

L97.219 Non-pressure chronic ulcer of right calf with unspecified severity CC HCC

✓6th L97.22 Non-pressure chronic ulcer of left calf

L97.221 Non-pressure chronic ulcer of left calf limited to breakdown of skin CC HCC

L97.222 Non-pressure chronic ulcer of left calf with fat layer exposed CC HCC

L97.223 Non-pressure chronic ulcer of left calf with necrosis of muscle CC HCC

L97.224 Non-pressure chronic ulcer of left calf with necrosis of bone CC HCC

L97.225 Non-pressure chronic ulcer of left calf with muscle involvement without evidence of necrosis CC HCC

L97.226 Non-pressure chronic ulcer of left calf with bone involvement without evidence of necrosis CC HCC

L97.228 Non-pressure chronic ulcer of left calf with other specified severity CC HCC

L97.229 Non-pressure chronic ulcer of left calf with unspecified severity CC HCC

✓5th L97.3 Non-pressure chronic ulcer of ankle

✓6th L97.30 Non-pressure chronic ulcer of unspecified ankle

L97.301 Non-pressure chronic ulcer of unspecified ankle limited to breakdown of skin CC UNS HCC

L97.302 Non-pressure chronic ulcer of unspecified ankle with fat layer exposed CC UNS HCC

L97.303 Non-pressure chronic ulcer of unspecified ankle with necrosis of muscle CC UNS HCC

L97.304 Non-pressure chronic ulcer of unspecified ankle with necrosis of bone CC UNS HCC

L97.305 Non-pressure chronic ulcer of unspecified ankle with muscle involvement without evidence of necrosis CC UNS HCC

L97.306 Non-pressure chronic ulcer of unspecified ankle with bone involvement without evidence of necrosis CC UNS HCC

L97.308 Non-pressure chronic ulcer of unspecified ankle with other specified severity CC UNS HCC

L97.309 Non-pressure chronic ulcer of unspecified ankle with unspecified severity CC UNS HCC

✓6th L97.31 Non-pressure chronic ulcer of right ankle

L97.311 Non-pressure chronic ulcer of right ankle limited to breakdown of skin CC HCC

L97.312 Non-pressure chronic ulcer of right ankle with fat layer exposed CC HCC

L97.313 Non-pressure chronic ulcer of right ankle with necrosis of muscle CC HCC

L97.314 Non-pressure chronic ulcer of right ankle with necrosis of bone CC HCC

L97.315 Non-pressure chronic ulcer of right ankle with muscle involvement without evidence of necrosis CC HCC

L97.316 Non-pressure chronic ulcer of right ankle with bone involvement without evidence of necrosis CC HCC

L97.318 Non-pressure chronic ulcer of right ankle with other specified severity CC HCC

L97.319 Non-pressure chronic ulcer of right ankle with unspecified severity CC HCC

✓6th L97.32 Non-pressure chronic ulcer of left ankle

L97.321 Non-pressure chronic ulcer of left ankle limited to breakdown of skin CC HCC

L97.322 Non-pressure chronic ulcer of left ankle with fat layer exposed CC HCC

L97.323 Non-pressure chronic ulcer of left ankle with necrosis of muscle CC HCC

L97.324 Non-pressure chronic ulcer of left ankle with necrosis of bone CC HCC

L97.325 Non-pressure chronic ulcer of left ankle with muscle involvement without evidence of necrosis CC HCC

L97.326 Non-pressure chronic ulcer of left ankle with bone involvement without evidence of necrosis CC HCC

L97.328 Non-pressure chronic ulcer of left ankle with other specified severity CC HCC

L97.329 Non-pressure chronic ulcer of left ankle with unspecified severity CC HCC

✓5th L97.4 Non-pressure chronic ulcer of heel and midfoot

Non-pressure chronic ulcer of plantar surface of midfoot

✓6th L97.40 Non-pressure chronic ulcer of unspecified heel and midfoot

L97.401 Non-pressure chronic ulcer of unspecified heel and midfoot limited to breakdown of skin CC UNS HCC

L97.402 Non-pressure chronic ulcer of unspecified heel and midfoot with fat layer exposed CC UNS HCC

L97.403 Non-pressure chronic ulcer of unspecified heel and midfoot with necrosis of muscle CC UNS HCC

L97.404 Non-pressure chronic ulcer of unspecified heel and midfoot with necrosis of bone CC UNS HCC

L97.405 Non-pressure chronic ulcer of unspecified heel and midfoot with muscle involvement without evidence of necrosis CC UNS HCC

L97.406 Non-pressure chronic ulcer of unspecified heel and midfoot with bone involvement without evidence of necrosis CC UNS HCC

L97.408 Non-pressure chronic ulcer of unspecified heel and midfoot with other specified severity CC UNS HCC

L97.409 Non-pressure chronic ulcer of unspecified heel and midfoot with unspecified severity CC UNS HCC

✓6th L97.41 Non-pressure chronic ulcer of right heel and midfoot

L97.411 Non-pressure chronic ulcer of right heel and midfoot limited to breakdown of skin CC HCC

L97.412 Non-pressure chronic ulcer of right heel and midfoot with fat layer exposed CC HCC
AHA: 2020,2Q,19

L97.413 Non-pressure chronic ulcer of right heel and midfoot with necrosis of muscle CC HCC

L97.414 Non-pressure chronic ulcer of right heel and midfoot with necrosis of bone CC HCC

L97.415 Non-pressure chronic ulcer of right heel and midfoot with muscle involvement without evidence of necrosis CC HCC

L97.416 Non-pressure chronic ulcer of right heel and midfoot with bone involvement without evidence of necrosis CC HCC

L97.418 Non-pressure chronic ulcer of right heel and midfoot with other specified severity CC HCC

L97.419 Non-pressure chronic ulcer of right heel and midfoot with unspecified severity CC HCC

✓6th L97.42 Non-pressure chronic ulcer of left heel and midfoot

L97.421 Non-pressure chronic ulcer of left heel and midfoot limited to breakdown of skin CC HCC
AHA: 2016,1Q,12

L97.422 Non-pressure chronic ulcer of left heel and midfoot with fat layer exposed CC HCC
AHA: 2020,2Q,19

L97.423 Non-pressure chronic ulcer of left heel and midfoot with necrosis of muscle CC HCC

L97.424 Non-pressure chronic ulcer of left heel and midfoot with necrosis of bone CC HCC

L97.425 Non-pressure chronic ulcer of left heel and midfoot with muscle involvement without evidence of necrosis CC HCC

L97.426 Non-pressure chronic ulcer of left heel and midfoot with bone involvement without evidence of necrosis CC HCC

L97.428 Non-pressure chronic ulcer of left heel and midfoot with other specified severity CC HCC

L97.429 Non-pressure chronic ulcer of left heel and midfoot with unspecified severity CC HCC

✓5th L97.5 Non-pressure chronic ulcer of other part of foot
Non-pressure chronic ulcer of toe

✓6th L97.50 Non-pressure chronic ulcer of other part of unspecified foot

L97.501 Non-pressure chronic ulcer of other part of unspecified foot limited to breakdown of skin HCC

L97.502 Non-pressure chronic ulcer of other part of unspecified foot with fat layer exposed HCC

L97.503 Non-pressure chronic ulcer of other part of unspecified foot with necrosis of muscle HCC

L97.504 Non-pressure chronic ulcer of other part of unspecified foot with necrosis of bone HCC

L97.505 Non-pressure chronic ulcer of other part of unspecified foot with muscle involvement without evidence of necrosis CC HCC

L97.506 Non-pressure chronic ulcer of other part of unspecified foot with bone involvement without evidence of necrosis CC HCC

L97.508 Non-pressure chronic ulcer of other part of unspecified foot with other specified severity CC HCC

L97.509 Non-pressure chronic ulcer of other part of unspecified foot with unspecified severity HCC

✓6th L97.51 Non-pressure chronic ulcer of other part of right foot
AHA: 2020,1Q,12

L97.511 Non-pressure chronic ulcer of other part of right foot limited to breakdown of skin HCC

L97.512 Non-pressure chronic ulcer of other part of right foot with fat layer exposed HCC
AHA: 2020,2Q,19

L97.513 Non-pressure chronic ulcer of other part of right foot with necrosis of muscle HCC

L97.514 Non-pressure chronic ulcer of other part of right foot with necrosis of bone HCC

L97.515 Non-pressure chronic ulcer of other part of right foot with muscle involvement without evidence of necrosis CC HCC

L97.516 Non-pressure chronic ulcer of other part of right foot with bone involvement without evidence of necrosis CC HCC

L97.518 Non-pressure chronic ulcer of other part of right foot with other specified severity CC HCC

L97.519 Non-pressure chronic ulcer of other part of right foot with unspecified severity HCC

✓6th L97.52 Non-pressure chronic ulcer of other part of left foot
AHA: 2020,1Q,12

L97.521 Non-pressure chronic ulcer of other part of left foot limited to breakdown of skin HCC

L97.522 Non-pressure chronic ulcer of other part of left foot with fat layer exposed HCC
AHA: 2020,2Q,19

L97.523 Non-pressure chronic ulcer of other part of left foot with necrosis of muscle HCC

L97.524 Non-pressure chronic ulcer of other part of left foot with necrosis of bone HCC

L97.525 Non-pressure chronic ulcer of other part of left foot with muscle involvement without evidence of necrosis CC HCC

L97.526 Non-pressure chronic ulcer of other part of left foot with bone involvement without evidence of necrosis CC HCC

L97.528 Non-pressure chronic ulcer of other part of left foot with other specified severity CC HCC

L97.529 Non-pressure chronic ulcer of other part of left foot with unspecified severity HCC

✓5th L97.8 Non-pressure chronic ulcer of other part of lower leg

✓6th L97.80 Non-pressure chronic ulcer of other part of unspecified lower leg

L97.801 Non-pressure chronic ulcer of other part of unspecified lower leg limited to breakdown of skin CC HCC

L97.802 Non-pressure chronic ulcer of other part of unspecified lower leg with fat layer exposed CC HCC

L97.803 Non-pressure chronic ulcer of other part of unspecified lower leg with necrosis of muscle CC HCC

L97.804 Non-pressure chronic ulcer of other part of unspecified lower leg with necrosis of bone CC HCC

L97.805 Non-pressure chronic ulcer of other part of unspecified lower leg with muscle involvement without evidence of necrosis CC HCC

L97.806 Non-pressure chronic ulcer of other part of unspecified lower leg with bone involvement without evidence of necrosis CC HCC

L97.808 Non-pressure chronic ulcer of other part of unspecified lower leg with other specified severity CC HCC

L97.809 Non-pressure chronic ulcer of other part of unspecified lower leg with unspecified severity CC HCC

✓6th L97.81 Non-pressure chronic ulcer of other part of right lower leg

L97.811 Non-pressure chronic ulcer of other part of right lower leg limited to breakdown of skin CC HCC

L97.812 Non-pressure chronic ulcer of other part of right lower leg with fat layer exposed CC HCC

L97.813 Non-pressure chronic ulcer of other part of right lower leg with necrosis of muscle CC HCC

L97.814 Non-pressure chronic ulcer of other part of right lower leg with necrosis of bone CC HCC

L97.815 Non-pressure chronic ulcer of other part of right lower leg with muscle involvement without evidence of necrosis CC HCC

L97.816 Non-pressure chronic ulcer of other part of right lower leg with bone involvement without evidence of necrosis CC HCC

L97.818 Non-pressure chronic ulcer of other part of right lower leg with other specified severity CC HCC

L97.819 Non-pressure chronic ulcer of other part of right lower leg with unspecified severity CC HCC

✓6th L97.82 Non-pressure chronic ulcer of other part of left lower leg

L97.821 Non-pressure chronic ulcer of other part of left lower leg limited to breakdown of skin CC HCC

L97.822 Non-pressure chronic ulcer of other part of left lower leg with fat layer exposed CC HCC

L97.823 Non-pressure chronic ulcer of other part of left lower leg with necrosis of muscle CC HCC

L97.824 Non-pressure chronic ulcer of other part of left lower leg with necrosis of bone CC HCC

L97.825 Non-pressure chronic ulcer of other part of left lower leg with muscle involvement without evidence of necrosis CC HCC

L97.826 Non-pressure chronic ulcer of other part of left lower leg with bone involvement without evidence of necrosis CC HCC

L97.828 Non-pressure chronic ulcer of other part of left lower leg with other specified severity CC HCC

L97.829 Non-pressure chronic ulcer of other part of left lower leg with unspecified severity CC HCC

✓5th L97.9 Non-pressure chronic ulcer of unspecified part of lower leg

✓6th L97.90 Non-pressure chronic ulcer of unspecified part of unspecified lower leg

L97.901 Non-pressure chronic ulcer of unspecified part of unspecified lower leg limited to breakdown of skin CC UNS HCC

L97.902 Non-pressure chronic ulcer of unspecified part of unspecified lower leg with fat layer exposed CC UNS HCC

L97.903 Non-pressure chronic ulcer of unspecified part of unspecified lower leg with necrosis of muscle CC UNS HCC

L97.904 Non-pressure chronic ulcer of unspecified part of unspecified lower leg with necrosis of bone CC UNS HCC

L97.905 Non-pressure chronic ulcer of unspecified part of unspecified lower leg with muscle involvement without evidence of necrosis CC UNS HCC

L97.906 Non-pressure chronic ulcer of unspecified part of unspecified lower leg with bone involvement without evidence of necrosis CC UNS HCC

L97.908 Non-pressure chronic ulcer of unspecified part of unspecified lower leg with other specified severity CC UNS HCC

L97.909 Non-pressure chronic ulcer of unspecified part of unspecified lower leg with unspecified severity CC UNS HCC

✓6th L97.91 Non-pressure chronic ulcer of unspecified part of right lower leg

L97.911 Non-pressure chronic ulcer of unspecified part of right lower leg limited to breakdown of skin CC HCC

L97.912 Non-pressure chronic ulcer of unspecified part of right lower leg with fat layer exposed CC HCC

L97.913 Non-pressure chronic ulcer of unspecified part of right lower leg with necrosis of muscle CC HCC

L97.914 Non-pressure chronic ulcer of unspecified part of right lower leg with necrosis of bone CC HCC

L97.915 Non-pressure chronic ulcer of unspecified part of right lower leg with muscle involvement without evidence of necrosis CC HCC

L97.916 Non-pressure chronic ulcer of unspecified part of right lower leg with bone involvement without evidence of necrosis CC HCC

L97.918 Non-pressure chronic ulcer of unspecified part of right lower leg with other specified severity CC HCC

L97.919 Non-pressure chronic ulcer of unspecified part of right lower leg with unspecified severity CC HCC

✓6th L97.92 Non-pressure chronic ulcer of unspecified part of left lower leg

L97.921 Non-pressure chronic ulcer of unspecified part of left lower leg limited to breakdown of skin CC HCC

L97.922 Non-pressure chronic ulcer of unspecified part of left lower leg with fat layer exposed CC HCC

L97.923 Non-pressure chronic ulcer of unspecified part of left lower leg with necrosis of muscle CC HCC

L97.924 Non-pressure chronic ulcer of unspecified part of left lower leg with necrosis of bone CC HCC

L97.925 Non-pressure chronic ulcer of unspecified part of left lower leg with muscle involvement without evidence of necrosis CC HCC

L97.926 Non-pressure chronic ulcer of unspecified part of left lower leg with bone involvement without evidence of necrosis CC HCC

L97.928 Non-pressure chronic ulcer of unspecified part of left lower leg with other specified severity CC HCC

L97.929 Non-pressure chronic ulcer of unspecified part of left lower leg with unspecified severity CC HCC

✓4th **L98 Other disorders of skin and subcutaneous tissue, not elsewhere classified**

L98.0 Pyogenic granuloma

EXCLUDES 2 *pyogenic granuloma of gingiva (K06.8)*
pyogenic granuloma of maxillary alveolar ridge (K04.5)
pyogenic granuloma of oral mucosa (K13.4)

DEF: Solitary polypoid capillary hemangioma often associated with local irritation, trauma, and superimposed inflammation. Located on the skin and gingival or oral mucosa, they bleed easily and may ulcerate and form crusted sores.

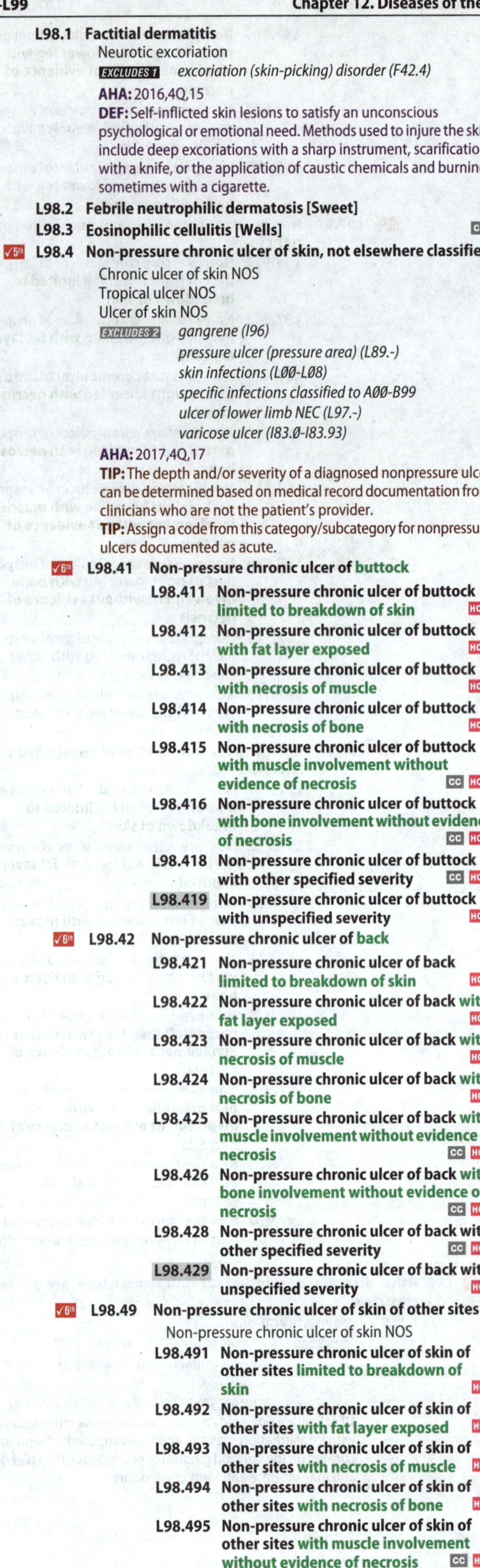

L98.1 Factitial dermatitis
Neurotic excoriation
EXCLUDES 1 *excoriation (skin-picking) disorder (F42.4)*
AHA: 2016,4Q,15
DEF: Self-inflicted skin lesions to satisfy an unconscious psychological or emotional need. Methods used to injure the skin include deep excoriations with a sharp instrument, scarification with a knife, or the application of caustic chemicals and burning, sometimes with a cigarette.

L98.2 Febrile neutrophilic dermatosis [Sweet]

L98.3 Eosinophilic cellulitis [Wells] CC

✓5th **L98.4 Non-pressure chronic ulcer of skin, not elsewhere classified**
Chronic ulcer of skin NOS
Tropical ulcer NOS
Ulcer of skin NOS
EXCLUDES 2 *gangrene (I96)*
pressure ulcer (pressure area) (L89.-)
skin infections (LØØ-LØ8)
specific infections classified to AØØ-B99
ulcer of lower limb NEC (L97.-)
varicose ulcer (I83.Ø-I83.93)
AHA: 2017,4Q,17
TIP: The depth and/or severity of a diagnosed nonpressure ulcer can be determined based on medical record documentation from clinicians who are not the patient's provider.
TIP: Assign a code from this category/subcategory for nonpressure ulcers documented as acute.

✓6th **L98.41 Non-pressure chronic ulcer of buttock**
L98.411 Non-pressure chronic ulcer of buttock limited to breakdown of skin HCC
L98.412 Non-pressure chronic ulcer of buttock with fat layer exposed HCC
L98.413 Non-pressure chronic ulcer of buttock with necrosis of muscle HCC
L98.414 Non-pressure chronic ulcer of buttock with necrosis of bone HCC
L98.415 Non-pressure chronic ulcer of buttock with muscle involvement without evidence of necrosis CC HCC
L98.416 Non-pressure chronic ulcer of buttock with bone involvement without evidence of necrosis CC HCC
L98.418 Non-pressure chronic ulcer of buttock with other specified severity CC HCC
L98.419 Non-pressure chronic ulcer of buttock with unspecified severity HCC

✓6th **L98.42 Non-pressure chronic ulcer of back**
L98.421 Non-pressure chronic ulcer of back limited to breakdown of skin HCC
L98.422 Non-pressure chronic ulcer of back with fat layer exposed HCC
L98.423 Non-pressure chronic ulcer of back with necrosis of muscle HCC
L98.424 Non-pressure chronic ulcer of back with necrosis of bone HCC
L98.425 Non-pressure chronic ulcer of back with muscle involvement without evidence of necrosis CC HCC
L98.426 Non-pressure chronic ulcer of back with bone involvement without evidence of necrosis CC HCC
L98.428 Non-pressure chronic ulcer of back with other specified severity CC HCC
L98.429 Non-pressure chronic ulcer of back with unspecified severity HCC

✓6th **L98.49 Non-pressure chronic ulcer of skin of other sites**
Non-pressure chronic ulcer of skin NOS
L98.491 Non-pressure chronic ulcer of skin of other sites limited to breakdown of skin HCC
L98.492 Non-pressure chronic ulcer of skin of other sites with fat layer exposed HCC
L98.493 Non-pressure chronic ulcer of skin of other sites with necrosis of muscle HCC
L98.494 Non-pressure chronic ulcer of skin of other sites with necrosis of bone HCC
L98.495 Non-pressure chronic ulcer of skin of other sites with muscle involvement without evidence of necrosis CC HCC
L98.496 Non-pressure chronic ulcer of skin of other sites with bone involvement without evidence of necrosis CC HCC
L98.498 Non-pressure chronic ulcer of skin of other sites with other specified severity CC HCC
L98.499 Non-pressure chronic ulcer of skin of other sites with unspecified severity HCC

L98.5 Mucinosis of the skin
Focal mucinosis
Lichen myxedematosus
Reticular erythematous mucinosis
EXCLUDES 1 *focal oral mucinosis (K13.79)*
myxedema (EØ3.9)

L98.6 Other infiltrative disorders of the skin and subcutaneous tissue
EXCLUDES 1 *hyalinosis cutis et mucosae (E78.89)*

L98.7 Excessive and redundant skin and subcutaneous tissue
Loose or sagging skin, following bariatric surgery weight loss
Loose or sagging skin following dietary weight loss
Loose or sagging skin, NOS
EXCLUDES 2 *acquired excess or redundant skin of eyelid (HØ2.3-)*
congenital excess or redundant skin of eyelid (Q1Ø.3)
skin changes due to chronic exposure to nonionizing radiation (L57.-)
AHA: 2022,3Q,11; 2016,4Q,36

L98.8 Other specified disorders of the skin and subcutaneous tissue
AHA: 2013,2Q,32

L98.9 Disorder of the skin and subcutaneous tissue, unspecified

L99 Other disorders of skin and subcutaneous tissue in diseases classified elsewhere
Code first underlying disease, such as:
amyloidosis (E85.-)
EXCLUDES 1 *skin disorders in diabetes (EØ8-E13 with .62-)*
skin disorders in gonorrhea (A54.89)
skin disorders in syphilis (A51.31, A52.79)
AHA: 2021,1Q,39

Chapter 13. Diseases of the Musculoskeletal System and Connective Tissue (MØØ–M99)

Chapter-specific Guidelines with Coding Examples

The chapter-specific guidelines from the ICD-10-CM Official Guidelines for Coding and Reporting have been provided below. Along with these guidelines are coding examples, contained in the shaded boxes, that have been developed to help illustrate the coding and/or sequencing guidance found in these guidelines.

a. Site and laterality

Most of the codes within Chapter 13 have site and laterality designations. The site represents the bone, joint or the muscle involved. For some conditions where more than one bone, joint or muscle is usually involved, such as osteoarthritis, there is a "multiple sites" code available. For categories where no multiple site code is provided and more than one bone, joint or muscle is involved, multiple codes should be used to indicate the different sites involved.

Rheumatoid arthritis of multiple sites without rheumatoid factor

MØ6.Ø9 Rheumatoid arthritis without rheumatoid factor, multiple sites

Explanation: For some conditions where more than one bone, joint or muscle is usually involved, such as rheumatoid arthritis, there is a "multiple sites" code available.

Osteomyelitis of the fourth thoracic and second lumbar vertebrae

M46.24 Osteomyelitis of vertebra, thoracic region

M46.26 Osteomyelitis of vertebra, lumbar region

Explanation: For categories without a multiple site code and more than one bone, joint, or muscle is involved, multiple codes should be used to indicate the different sites involved.

1) Bone versus joint

For certain conditions, the bone may be affected at the upper or lower end, (e.g., avascular necrosis of bone, M87, Osteoporosis, M8Ø, M81). Though the portion of the bone affected may be at the joint, the site designation will be the bone, not the joint.

Idiopathic avascular necrosis of the femoral head of the left hip joint

M87.Ø52 Idiopathic aseptic necrosis of left femur

Explanation: For certain conditions such as avascular necrosis, the bone may be affected at the joint, but the site designation is the bone, not the joint.

b. Acute traumatic versus chronic or recurrent musculoskeletal conditions

Many musculoskeletal conditions are a result of previous injury or trauma to a site, or are recurrent conditions. Bone, joint or muscle conditions that are the result of a healed injury are usually found in chapter 13. Recurrent bone, joint or muscle conditions are also usually found in chapter 13. Any current, acute injury should be coded to the appropriate injury code from chapter 19. Chronic or recurrent conditions should generally be coded with a code from chapter 13. If it is difficult to determine from the documentation in the record which code is best to describe a condition, query the provider.

Acute traumatic bucket-handle tear of right medial meniscus

S83.211A Bucket-handle tear of medial meniscus, current injury, right knee, initial encounter

Explanation: Any current, acute injury is not coded in chapter 13. It should instead be coded to the appropriate injury code from chapter 19.

Old bucket-handle tear of right medial meniscus

M23.2Ø3 Derangement of unspecified medial meniscus due to old tear or injury, right knee

Explanation: Chronic or recurrent conditions should generally be coded with a code from chapter 13.

c. Coding of pathologic fractures

7th character A is for use as long as the patient is receiving active treatment for the fracture. Examples of active treatment are: surgical treatment, emergency department encounter, evaluation and continuing treatment by the same or a different physician. While the patient may be seen by a new or different provider over the course of treatment for a pathological fracture, assignment of the 7th character is based on whether the patient is undergoing active treatment and not whether the provider is seeing the patient for the first time.

Patient admitted for repair of pathologic fracture of left foot, unknown cause. The surgery will be performed by his orthopedic specialist who he has been seeing for this fracture for the past month.

M84.475A Pathological fracture, left foot, initial encounter for fracture

Explanation: Seventh character A is for use as long as the patient is receiving active treatment for a pathologic fracture. Examples of active treatment are surgical treatment, emergency department encounter, evaluation, and continuing treatment by the same or a different physician.

The seventh character is based on whether the patient is undergoing active treatment such as surgery, and not whether the provider is seeing the patient for the first time.

7th character D is to be used for encounters after the patient has completed active treatment for the fracture and is receiving routine care for the fracture during the healing or recovery phase. The other 7th characters, listed under each subcategory in the Tabular List, are to be used for subsequent encounters for treatment of problems associated with the healing, such as malunions, nonunions, and sequelae.

Care for complications of surgical treatment for fracture repairs during the healing or recovery phase should be coded with the appropriate complication codes.

See Section I.C.19. Coding of traumatic fractures.

d. Osteoporosis

Osteoporosis is a systemic condition, meaning that all bones of the musculoskeletal system are affected. Therefore, site is not a component of the codes under category M81, Osteoporosis without current pathological fracture. The site codes under category M8Ø, Osteoporosis with current pathological fracture, identify the site of the fracture, not the osteoporosis.

1) Osteoporosis without pathological fracture

Category M81, Osteoporosis without current pathological fracture, is for use for patients with osteoporosis who do not currently have a pathologic fracture due to the osteoporosis, even if they have had a fracture in the past. For patients with a history of osteoporosis fractures, status code Z87.31Ø, Personal history of (healed) osteoporosis fracture, should follow the code from M81.

Age-related osteoporosis with healed osteoporotic fracture of the lumbar vertebra

M81.Ø Age-related osteoporosis without current pathological fracture

Z87.31Ø Personal history of (healed) osteoporosis fracture

Explanation: Category M81 is used for patients with osteoporosis who do not currently have a pathologic fracture due to the osteoporosis. To report a previous (healed) fracture, status code Z87.310 Personal history of (healed) osteoporosis fracture, should follow the code from M81.

2) Osteoporosis with current pathological fracture

Category M8Ø, Osteoporosis with current pathological fracture, is for patients who have a current pathologic fracture at the time of an encounter. The codes under M8Ø identify the site of the fracture. A code from category M8Ø, not a traumatic fracture code, should be used for any patient with known osteoporosis who suffers a fracture, even if the patient had a minor fall or trauma, if that fall or trauma would not usually break a normal, healthy bone.

Disuse osteoporosis with current fracture of right shoulder sustained lifting a grocery bag, initial encounter

M8Ø.811A Other osteoporosis with current pathological fracture, right shoulder, initial encounter for fracture

Explanation: A code from category M80, not a traumatic fracture code, should be used for any patient with known osteoporosis who suffers a fracture, even if the patient had a minor fall or trauma, if that fall or trauma would not usually break a normal, healthy bone.

e. Multisystem inflammatory syndrome

See Section I.C.1.g.1.l. for Multisystem Inflammatory Syndrome

Muscle/Tendon Table

ICD-10-CM categorizes certain muscles and tendons in the upper and lower extremities by their action (e.g., extension, flexion), their anatomical location (e.g., posterior, anterior), and/or whether they are intrinsic or extrinsic to a certain anatomical area. The Muscle/Tendon Table is provided at the beginning of chapters 13 and 19 as a resource to help users when code selection depends on one or more of these characteristics. Please note that this table is not all-inclusive, and proper code assignment should be based on the provider's documentation.

Body Region	Muscle	Extensor Tendon	Flexor Tendon	Other Tendon
Shoulder				
	Deltoid	Posterior deltoid	Anterior deltoid	
	Rotator cuff			
	Infraspinatus			Infraspinatus
	Subscapularis			Subscapularis
	Supraspinatus			Supraspinatus
	Teres minor			Teres minor
	Teres major	Teres major		
Upper arm				
	Anterior muscles			
	Biceps brachii — long head		Biceps brachii — long head	
	Biceps brachii — short head		Biceps brachii — short head	
	Brachialis		Brachialis	
	Coracobrachialis		Coracobrachialis	
	Posterior muscles			
	Triceps brachii	Triceps brachii		
Forearm				
	Anterior muscles			
	Flexors			
	Deep			
	Flexor digitorum profundus		Flexor digitorum profundus	
	Flexor pollicis longus		Flexor pollicis longus	
	Intermediate			
	Flexor digitorum superficialis		Flexor digitorum superficialis	
	Superficial			
	Flexor carpi radialis		Flexor carpi radialis	
	Flexor carpi ulnaris		Flexor carpi ulnaris	
	Palmaris longus		Palmaris longus	
	Pronators			
	Pronator quadratus			Pronator quadratus
	Pronator teres			Pronator teres
	Posterior muscles			
	Extensors			
	Deep			
	Abductor pollicis longus			Abductor pollicis longus
	Extensor indicis	Extensor indicis		
	Extensor pollicis brevis	Extensor pollicis brevis		
	Extensor pollicis longus	Extensor pollicis longus		
	Superficial			
	Brachioradialis			Brachioradialis
	Extensor carpi radialis brevis	Extensor carpi radialis brevis		
	Extensor carpi radialis longus	Extensor carpi radialis longus		
	Extensor carpi ulnaris	Extensor carpi ulnaris		
	Extensor digiti minimi	Extensor digiti minimi		
	Extensor digitorum	Extensor digitorum		
	Anconeus	Anconeus		
	Supinator			Supinator

Body Region	Muscle	Extensor Tendon	Flexor Tendon	Other Tendon
Hand				
Extrinsic — attach to a site in the forearm as well as a site in the hand with action related to hand movement at the wrist				
	Extensor carpi radialis brevis	Extensor carpi radialis brevis		
	Extensor carpi radialis longus	Extensor carpi radialis longus		
	Extensor carpi ulnaris	Extensor carpi ulnaris		
	Flexor carpi radialis		Flexor carpi radialis	
	Flexor carpi ulnaris		Flexor carpi ulnaris	
	Flexor digitorum superficialis		Flexor digitorum superficialis	
	Palmaris longus		Palmaris longus	
Extrinsic — attach to a site in the forearm as well as a site in the hand with action in the hand related to finger movement				
	Adductor pollicis longus			Adductor pollicis longus
	Extensor digiti minimi	Extensor digiti minimi		
	Extensor digitorum	Extensor digitorum		
	Extensor indicis	Extensor indicis		
	Flexor digitorum profundus		Flexor digitorum profundus	
	Flexor digitorum superficialis		Flexor digitorum superficialis	
Extrinsic — attach to a site in the forearm as well as a site in the hand with action in the hand related to thumb movement				
	Extensor pollicis brevis	Extensor pollicis brevis		
	Extensor pollicis longus	Extensor pollicis longus		
	Flexor pollicis longus		Flexor pollicis longus	
Intrinsic — found within the hand only				
	Adductor pollicis			Adductor pollicis
	Dorsal interossei	Dorsal interossei	Dorsal interossei	
	Lumbricals	Lumbricals	Lumbricals	
	Palmaris brevis			Palmaris brevis
	Palmar interossei	Palmar interossei	Palmar interossei	
	Hypothenar muscles			
	Abductor digiti minimi			Abductor digiti minimi
	Flexor digiti minimi brevis		Flexor digiti minimi brevis	
	Opponens digiti minimi		Opponens digiti minimi	
	Thenar muscles			
	Abductor pollicis brevis			Abductor pollicis brevis
	Flexor pollicis brevis		Flexor pollicis brevis	
	Opponens pollicis		Opponens pollicis	
Thigh				
	Anterior muscles			
	Iliopsoas		Iliopsoas	
	Pectineus		Pectineus	
	Quadriceps	Quadriceps		
	Rectus femoris	Rectus femoris — Extends knee	Rectus femoris — Flexes hip	
	Vastus intermedius	Vastus intermedius		
	Vastus lateralis	Vastus lateralis		
	Vastus medialis	Vastus medialis		
	Sartorius		Sartorius	
	Medial muscles			
	Adductor brevis			Adductor brevis
	Adductor longus			Adductor longus
	Adductor magnus			Adductor magnus
	Gracilis			Gracilis
	Obturator externus			Obturator externus
	Posterior muscles			
	Hamstring	Hamstring — Extends hip	Hamstring — Flexes knee	
	Biceps femoris	Biceps femoris	Biceps femoris	
	Semimembranosus	Semimembranosus	Semimembranosus	
	Semitendinosus	Semitendinosus	Semitendinosus	

Body Region	Muscle	Extensor Tendon	Flexor Tendon	Other Tendon
Lower leg				
	Anterior muscles			
	Extensor digitorum longus	Extensor digitorum longus		
	Extensor hallucis longus	Extensor hallucis longus		
	Fibularis (peroneus) tertius	Fibularis (peroneus) tertius		
	Tibialis anterior	Tibialis anterior		Tibialis anterior
	Lateral muscles			
	Fibularis (peroneus) brevis		Fibularis (peroneus) brevis	
	Fibularis (peroneus) longus		Fibularis (peroneus) longus	
	Posterior muscles			
	Deep			
	Flexor digitorum longus		Flexor digitorum longus	
	Flexor hallucis longus		Flexor hallucis longus	
	Popliteus		Popliteus	
	Tibialis posterior		Tibialis posterior	
	Superficial			
	Gastrocnemius		Gastrocnemius	
	Plantaris		Plantaris	
	Soleus		Soleus	
				Calcaneal (Achilles)
Ankle/Foot				
Extrinsic — attach to a site in the lower leg as well as a site in the foot with action related to foot movement at the ankle				
	Plantaris		Plantaris	
	Soleus		Soleus	
	Tibialis anterior	Tibialis anterior		
	Tibialis posterior		Tibialis posterior	
Extrinsic — attach to a site in the lower leg as well as a site in the foot with action in the foot related to toe movement				
	Extensor digitorum longus	Extensor digitorum longus		
	Extensor hallucis longus	Extensor hallucis longus		
	Flexor digitorum longus		Flexor digitorum longus	
	Flexor hallucis longus		Flexor hallucis longus	
Intrinsic — found within the ankle/foot only				
	Dorsal muscles			
	Extensor digitorum brevis	Extensor digitorum brevis		
	Extensor hallucis brevis	Extensor hallucis brevis		
	Plantar muscles			
	Abductor digiti minimi		Abductor digiti minimi	
	Abductor hallucis		Abductor hallucis	
	Dorsal interossei	Dorsal interossei	Dorsal interossei	
	Flexor digiti minimi brevis		Flexor digiti minimi brevis	
	Flexor digitorum brevis		Flexor digitorum brevis	
	Flexor hallucis brevis		Flexor hallucis brevis	
	Lumbricals	Lumbricals	Lumbricals	
	Quadratus plantae		Quadratus plantae	
	Plantar interossei	Plantar interossei	Plantar interossei	

Chapter 13. Diseases of the Musculoskeletal System and Connective Tissue (M00-M99)

NOTE Use an external cause code following the code for the musculoskeletal condition, if applicable, to identify the cause of the musculoskeletal condition

EXCLUDES 2 *arthropathic psoriasis (L40.5-)*
certain conditions originating in the perinatal period (P04-P96)
certain infectious and parasitic diseases (A00-B99)
compartment syndrome (traumatic) (T79.A-)
complications of pregnancy, childbirth and the puerperium (O00-O9A)
congenital malformations, deformations, and chromosomal abnormalities (Q00-Q99)
endocrine, nutritional and metabolic diseases (E00-E88)
injury, poisoning and certain other consequences of external causes (S00-T88)
neoplasms (C00-D49)
symptoms, signs and abnormal clinical and laboratory findings, not elsewhere classified (R00-R94)

This chapter contains the following blocks:

ARTHROPATHIES (M00-M25)

INCLUDES disorders affecting predominantly peripheral (limb) joints

Infectious arthropathies (M00-M02)

NOTE This block comprises arthropathies due to microbiological agents. Distinction is made between the following types of etiological relationship:

a) direct infection of joint, where organisms invade synovial tissue and microbial antigen is present in the joint;

b) indirect infection, which may be of two types: a reactive arthropathy, where microbial infection of the body is established but neither organisms nor antigens can be identified in the joint, and a postinfective arthropathy, where microbial antigen is present but recovery of an organism is inconstant and evidence of local multiplication is lacking.

AHA: 2019,3Q,16

✓4th **M00 Pyogenic arthritis**

EXCLUDES 2 *infection and inflammatory reaction due to internal joint prosthesis (T84.5-)*

AHA: 2022,1Q,31

DEF: Pyogenic: Relating to or involving pus production, often referred to as suppurative or purulent.

✓5th **M00.0 Staphylococcal arthritis and polyarthritis**

Use additional code (B95.61-B95.8) to identify bacterial agent

M00.00 Staphylococcal arthritis, unspecified joint CC UNS HCC

✓6th **M00.01 Staphylococcal arthritis, shoulder**

M00.011 Staphylococcal arthritis, right shoulder CC HCC

M00.012 Staphylococcal arthritis, left shoulder CC HCC

M00.019 Staphylococcal arthritis, unspecified shoulder CC UNS HCC

✓6th **M00.02 Staphylococcal arthritis, elbow**

M00.021 Staphylococcal arthritis, right elbow CC HCC

M00.022 Staphylococcal arthritis, left elbow CC HCC

M00.029 Staphylococcal arthritis, unspecified elbow CC UNS HCC

✓6th **M00.03 Staphylococcal arthritis, wrist**

Staphylococcal arthritis of carpal bones

M00.031 Staphylococcal arthritis, right wrist CC HCC

M00.032 Staphylococcal arthritis, left wrist CC HCC

M00.039 Staphylococcal arthritis, unspecified wrist CC UNS HCC

✓6th **M00.04 Staphylococcal arthritis, hand**

Staphylococcal arthritis of metacarpus and phalanges

M00.041 Staphylococcal arthritis, right hand CC HCC

M00.042 Staphylococcal arthritis, left hand CC HCC

M00.049 Staphylococcal arthritis, unspecified hand CC UNS HCC

✓6th **M00.05 Staphylococcal arthritis, hip**

M00.051 Staphylococcal arthritis, right hip CC HCC

M00.052 Staphylococcal arthritis, left hip CC HCC

M00.059 Staphylococcal arthritis, unspecified hip CC UNS HCC

✓6th **M00.06 Staphylococcal arthritis, knee**

M00.061 Staphylococcal arthritis, right knee CC HCC

M00.062 Staphylococcal arthritis, left knee CC HCC

M00.069 Staphylococcal arthritis, unspecified knee CC UNS HCC

✓6th **M00.07 Staphylococcal arthritis, ankle and foot**

Staphylococcal arthritis, tarsus, metatarsus and phalanges

M00.071 Staphylococcal arthritis, right ankle and foot CC HCC

M00.072 Staphylococcal arthritis, left ankle and foot CC HCC

M00.079 Staphylococcal arthritis, unspecified ankle and foot CC UNS HCC

M00.08 Staphylococcal arthritis, vertebrae CC HCC

M00.09 Staphylococcal polyarthritis CC HCC

✓5th **M00.1 Pneumococcal arthritis and polyarthritis**

M00.10 Pneumococcal arthritis, unspecified joint CC UNS HCC

✓6th **M00.11 Pneumococcal arthritis, shoulder**

M00.111 Pneumococcal arthritis, right shoulder CC HCC

M00.112 Pneumococcal arthritis, left shoulder CC HCC

M00.119 Pneumococcal arthritis, unspecified shoulder CC UNS HCC

✓6th **M00.12 Pneumococcal arthritis, elbow**

M00.121 Pneumococcal arthritis, right elbow CC HCC

M00.122 Pneumococcal arthritis, left elbow CC HCC

M00.129 Pneumococcal arthritis, unspecified elbow CC UNS HCC

✓6th **M00.13 Pneumococcal arthritis, wrist**

Pneumococcal arthritis of carpal bones

M00.131 Pneumococcal arthritis, right wrist CC HCC

M00.132 Pneumococcal arthritis, left wrist CC HCC

M00.139 Pneumococcal arthritis, unspecified wrist CC UNS HCC

✓6th **M00.14 Pneumococcal arthritis, hand**

Pneumococcal arthritis of metacarpus and phalanges

M00.141 Pneumococcal arthritis, right hand CC HCC

M00.142 Pneumococcal arthritis, left hand CC HCC

M00.149 Pneumococcal arthritis, unspecified hand CC UNS HCC

✓6th **M00.15 Pneumococcal arthritis, hip**

M00.151 Pneumococcal arthritis, right hip CC HCC

M00.152 Pneumococcal arthritis, left hip CC HCC
M00.159 Pneumococcal arthritis, unspecified hip CC UNS HCC
6th **M00.16** Pneumococcal arthritis, knee
M00.161 Pneumococcal arthritis, right knee CC HCC
M00.162 Pneumococcal arthritis, left knee CC HCC
M00.169 Pneumococcal arthritis, unspecified knee CC UNS HCC
6th **M00.17** Pneumococcal arthritis, ankle and foot
Pneumococcal arthritis, tarsus, metatarsus and phalanges
M00.171 Pneumococcal arthritis, right ankle and foot CC HCC
M00.172 Pneumococcal arthritis, left ankle and foot CC HCC
M00.179 Pneumococcal arthritis, unspecified ankle and foot CC UNS HCC
M00.18 Pneumococcal arthritis, vertebrae CC HCC
M00.19 Pneumococcal polyarthritis CC HCC
5th **M00.2** Other streptococcal arthritis and polyarthritis
Use additional code (B95.0-B95.2, B95.4-B95.5) to identify bacterial agent
M00.20 Other streptococcal arthritis, unspecified joint CC UNS HCC
6th **M00.21** Other streptococcal arthritis, shoulder
M00.211 Other streptococcal arthritis, right shoulder CC HCC
M00.212 Other streptococcal arthritis, left shoulder CC HCC
M00.219 Other streptococcal arthritis, unspecified shoulder CC UNS HCC
6th **M00.22** Other streptococcal arthritis, elbow
M00.221 Other streptococcal arthritis, right elbow CC HCC
M00.222 Other streptococcal arthritis, left elbow CC HCC
M00.229 Other streptococcal arthritis, unspecified elbow CC UNS HCC
6th **M00.23** Other streptococcal arthritis, wrist
Other streptococcal arthritis of carpal bones
M00.231 Other streptococcal arthritis, right wrist CC HCC
M00.232 Other streptococcal arthritis, left wrist CC HCC
M00.239 Other streptococcal arthritis, unspecified wrist CC UNS HCC
6th **M00.24** Other streptococcal arthritis, hand
Other streptococcal arthritis metacarpus and phalanges
M00.241 Other streptococcal arthritis, right hand CC HCC
M00.242 Other streptococcal arthritis, left hand CC HCC
M00.249 Other streptococcal arthritis, unspecified hand CC UNS HCC
6th **M00.25** Other streptococcal arthritis, hip
M00.251 Other streptococcal arthritis, right hip CC HCC
M00.252 Other streptococcal arthritis, left hip CC HCC
M00.259 Other streptococcal arthritis, unspecified hip CC UNS HCC
6th **M00.26** Other streptococcal arthritis, knee
M00.261 Other streptococcal arthritis, right knee CC HCC
M00.262 Other streptococcal arthritis, left knee CC HCC
M00.269 Other streptococcal arthritis, unspecified knee CC UNS HCC
6th **M00.27** Other streptococcal arthritis, ankle and foot
Other streptococcal arthritis, tarsus, metatarsus and phalanges
M00.271 Other streptococcal arthritis, right ankle and foot CC HCC
M00.272 Other streptococcal arthritis, left ankle and foot CC HCC
M00.279 Other streptococcal arthritis, unspecified ankle and foot CC UNS HCC
M00.28 Other streptococcal arthritis, vertebrae CC HCC
M00.29 Other streptococcal polyarthritis CC HCC
5th **M00.8** Arthritis and polyarthritis due to other bacteria
Use additional code (B96) to identify bacteria
M00.80 Arthritis due to other bacteria, unspecified joint CC UNS HCC
6th **M00.81** Arthritis due to other bacteria, shoulder
M00.811 Arthritis due to other bacteria, right shoulder CC HCC
M00.812 Arthritis due to other bacteria, left shoulder CC HCC
M00.819 Arthritis due to other bacteria, unspecified shoulder CC UNS HCC
6th **M00.82** Arthritis due to other bacteria, elbow
M00.821 Arthritis due to other bacteria, right elbow CC HCC
M00.822 Arthritis due to other bacteria, left elbow CC HCC
M00.829 Arthritis due to other bacteria, unspecified elbow CC UNS HCC
6th **M00.83** Arthritis due to other bacteria, wrist
Arthritis due to other bacteria, carpal bones
M00.831 Arthritis due to other bacteria, right wrist CC HCC
M00.832 Arthritis due to other bacteria, left wrist CC HCC
M00.839 Arthritis due to other bacteria, unspecified wrist CC UNS HCC
6th **M00.84** Arthritis due to other bacteria, hand
Arthritis due to other bacteria, metacarpus and phalanges
M00.841 Arthritis due to other bacteria, right hand CC HCC
M00.842 Arthritis due to other bacteria, left hand CC HCC
M00.849 Arthritis due to other bacteria, unspecified hand CC UNS HCC
6th **M00.85** Arthritis due to other bacteria, hip
M00.851 Arthritis due to other bacteria, right hip CC HCC
M00.852 Arthritis due to other bacteria, left hip CC HCC
M00.859 Arthritis due to other bacteria, unspecified hip CC UNS HCC
6th **M00.86** Arthritis due to other bacteria, knee
AHA: 2019,3Q,16
M00.861 Arthritis due to other bacteria, right knee CC HCC
M00.862 Arthritis due to other bacteria, left knee CC HCC
M00.869 Arthritis due to other bacteria, unspecified knee CC UNS HCC
6th **M00.87** Arthritis due to other bacteria, ankle and foot
Arthritis due to other bacteria, tarsus, metatarsus, and phalanges
M00.871 Arthritis due to other bacteria, right ankle and foot CC HCC
M00.872 Arthritis due to other bacteria, left ankle and foot CC HCC
M00.879 Arthritis due to other bacteria, unspecified ankle and foot CC UNS HCC
M00.88 Arthritis due to other bacteria, vertebrae CC HCC
M00.89 Polyarthritis due to other bacteria CC HCC
M00.9 Pyogenic arthritis, unspecified CC HCC
Infective arthritis NOS

MØ1 Direct infections of joint in infectious and parasitic diseases classified elsewhere

Code first underlying disease, such as:
leprosy [Hansen's disease] (A3Ø.-)
mycoses (B35-B49)
O'nyong-nyong fever (A92.1)
paratyphoid fever (AØ1.1-AØ1.4)

EXCLUDES 1
arthropathy in Lyme disease (A69.23)
gonococcal arthritis (A54.42)
meningococcal arthritis (A39.83)
mumps arthritis (B26.85)
postinfective arthropathy (MØ2.-)
postmeningococcal arthritis (A39.84)
reactive arthritis (MØ2.3)
rubella arthritis (BØ6.82)
sarcoidosis arthritis (D86.86)
tuberculosis arthritis (A18.Ø1-A18.Ø2)
typhoid fever arthritis (AØ1.Ø4)

MØ1.X Direct infection of joint in infectious and parasitic diseases classified elsewhere

MØ1.XØ Direct infection of unspecified joint in infectious and parasitic diseases classified elsewhere CC UNS HCC

MØ1.X1 Direct infection of shoulder joint in infectious and parasitic diseases classified elsewhere

MØ1.X11 Direct infection of right shoulder in infectious and parasitic diseases classified elsewhere CC HCC

MØ1.X12 Direct infection of left shoulder in infectious and parasitic diseases classified elsewhere CC HCC

MØ1.X19 Direct infection of unspecified shoulder in infectious and parasitic diseases classified elsewhere CC UNS HCC

MØ1.X2 Direct infection of elbow in infectious and parasitic diseases classified elsewhere

MØ1.X21 Direct infection of right elbow in infectious and parasitic diseases classified elsewhere CC HCC

MØ1.X22 Direct infection of left elbow in infectious and parasitic diseases classified elsewhere CC HCC

MØ1.X29 Direct infection of unspecified elbow in infectious and parasitic diseases classified elsewhere CC UNS HCC

MØ1.X3 Direct infection of wrist in infectious and parasitic diseases classified elsewhere

Direct infection of carpal bones in infectious and parasitic diseases classified elsewhere

MØ1.X31 Direct infection of right wrist in infectious and parasitic diseases classified elsewhere CC HCC

MØ1.X32 Direct infection of left wrist in infectious and parasitic diseases classified elsewhere CC HCC

MØ1.X39 Direct infection of unspecified wrist in infectious and parasitic diseases classified elsewhere CC UNS HCC

MØ1.X4 Direct infection of hand in infectious and parasitic diseases classified elsewhere

Direct infection of metacarpus and phalanges in infectious and parasitic diseases classified elsewhere

MØ1.X41 Direct infection of right hand in infectious and parasitic diseases classified elsewhere CC HCC

MØ1.X42 Direct infection of left hand in infectious and parasitic diseases classified elsewhere CC HCC

MØ1.X49 Direct infection of unspecified hand in infectious and parasitic diseases classified elsewhere CC UNS HCC

MØ1.X5 Direct infection of hip in infectious and parasitic diseases classified elsewhere

MØ1.X51 Direct infection of right hip in infectious and parasitic diseases classified elsewhere CC HCC

MØ1.X52 Direct infection of left hip in infectious and parasitic diseases classified elsewhere CC HCC

MØ1.X59 Direct infection of unspecified hip in infectious and parasitic diseases classified elsewhere CC UNS HCC

MØ1.X6 Direct infection of knee in infectious and parasitic diseases classified elsewhere

MØ1.X61 Direct infection of right knee in infectious and parasitic diseases classified elsewhere CC HCC

MØ1.X62 Direct infection of left knee in infectious and parasitic diseases classified elsewhere CC HCC

MØ1.X69 Direct infection of unspecified knee in infectious and parasitic diseases classified elsewhere CC UNS HCC

MØ1.X7 Direct infection of ankle and foot in infectious and parasitic diseases classified elsewhere

Direct infection of tarsus, metatarsus and phalanges in infectious and parasitic diseases classified elsewhere

MØ1.X71 Direct infection of right ankle and foot in infectious and parasitic diseases classified elsewhere CC HCC

MØ1.X72 Direct infection of left ankle and foot in infectious and parasitic diseases classified elsewhere CC HCC

MØ1.X79 Direct infection of unspecified ankle and foot in infectious and parasitic diseases classified elsewhere CC UNS HCC

MØ1.X8 Direct infection of vertebrae in infectious and parasitic diseases classified elsewhere CC HCC

MØ1.X9 Direct infection of multiple joints in infectious and parasitic diseases classified elsewhere CC HCC

MØ2 Postinfective and reactive arthropathies

Code first underlying disease, such as:
congenital syphilis [Clutton's joints] (A5Ø.5)
enteritis due to Yersinia enterocolitica (AØ4.6)
infective endocarditis (I33.Ø)
viral hepatitis (B15-B19)

EXCLUDES 1
Behcet's disease (M35.2)
direct infections of joint in infectious and parasitic diseases classified elsewhere (MØ1.-)
mumps arthritis (B26.85)
postmeningococcal arthritis (A39.84)
rheumatic fever (IØØ)
rubella arthritis (BØ6.82)
syphilis arthritis (late) (A52.77)
tabetic arthropathy [Charcôt's] (A52.16)

MØ2.Ø Arthropathy following intestinal bypass

MØ2.ØØ Arthropathy following intestinal bypass, unspecified site

MØ2.Ø1 Arthropathy following intestinal bypass, shoulder

MØ2.Ø11 Arthropathy following intestinal bypass, right shoulder

MØ2.Ø12 Arthropathy following intestinal bypass, left shoulder

MØ2.Ø19 Arthropathy following intestinal bypass, unspecified shoulder

MØ2.Ø2 Arthropathy following intestinal bypass, elbow

MØ2.Ø21 Arthropathy following intestinal bypass, right elbow

MØ2.Ø22 Arthropathy following intestinal bypass, left elbow

MØ2.Ø29 Arthropathy following intestinal bypass, unspecified elbow

MØ2.Ø3 Arthropathy following intestinal bypass, wrist

Arthropathy following intestinal bypass, carpal bones

MØ2.Ø31 Arthropathy following intestinal bypass, right wrist

MØ2.Ø32 Arthropathy following intestinal bypass, left wrist

MØ2.Ø39 Arthropathy following intestinal bypass, unspecified wrist

MØ2.Ø4 Arthropathy following intestinal bypass, hand

Arthropathy following intestinal bypass, metacarpals and phalanges

MØ2.Ø41 Arthropathy following intestinal bypass, right hand

MØ2.Ø42 Arthropathy following intestinal bypass, left hand

MØ2.Ø49 Arthropathy following intestinal bypass, unspecified hand

√6th MØ2.Ø5 **Arthropathy following intestinal bypass, hip**
- MØ2.Ø51 **Arthropathy following intestinal bypass, right hip**
- MØ2.Ø52 **Arthropathy following intestinal bypass, left hip**
- MØ2.Ø59 **Arthropathy following intestinal bypass, unspecified hip**

√6th MØ2.Ø6 **Arthropathy following intestinal bypass, knee**
- MØ2.Ø61 **Arthropathy following intestinal bypass, right knee**
- MØ2.Ø62 **Arthropathy following intestinal bypass, left knee**
- MØ2.Ø69 **Arthropathy following intestinal bypass, unspecified knee**

√6th MØ2.Ø7 **Arthropathy following intestinal bypass, ankle and foot**
Arthropathy following intestinal bypass, tarsus, metatarsus and phalanges
- MØ2.Ø71 **Arthropathy following intestinal bypass, right ankle and foot**
- MØ2.Ø72 **Arthropathy following intestinal bypass, left ankle and foot**
- MØ2.Ø79 **Arthropathy following intestinal bypass, unspecified ankle and foot**

MØ2.Ø8 **Arthropathy following intestinal bypass, vertebrae**
MØ2.Ø9 **Arthropathy following intestinal bypass, multiple sites**

√5th MØ2.1 **Postdysenteric arthropathy**

MØ2.1Ø **Postdysenteric arthropathy, unspecified site** CC UNS HCC

√6th MØ2.11 **Postdysenteric arthropathy, shoulder**
- MØ2.111 **Postdysenteric arthropathy, right shoulder** CC HCC
- MØ2.112 **Postdysenteric arthropathy, left shoulder** CC HCC
- MØ2.119 **Postdysenteric arthropathy, unspecified shoulder** CC UNS HCC

√6th MØ2.12 **Postdysenteric arthropathy, elbow**
- MØ2.121 **Postdysenteric arthropathy, right elbow** CC HCC
- MØ2.122 **Postdysenteric arthropathy, left elbow** CC HCC
- MØ2.129 **Postdysenteric arthropathy, unspecified elbow** CC UNS HCC

√6th MØ2.13 **Postdysenteric arthropathy, wrist**
Postdysenteric arthropathy, carpal bones
- MØ2.131 **Postdysenteric arthropathy, right wrist** CC HCC
- MØ2.132 **Postdysenteric arthropathy, left wrist** CC HCC
- MØ2.139 **Postdysenteric arthropathy, unspecified wrist** CC UNS HCC

√6th MØ2.14 **Postdysenteric arthropathy, hand**
Postdysenteric arthropathy, metacarpus and phalanges
- MØ2.141 **Postdysenteric arthropathy, right hand** CC HCC
- MØ2.142 **Postdysenteric arthropathy, left hand** CC HCC
- MØ2.149 **Postdysenteric arthropathy, unspecified hand** CC UNS HCC

√6th MØ2.15 **Postdysenteric arthropathy, hip**
- MØ2.151 **Postdysenteric arthropathy, right hip** CC HCC
- MØ2.152 **Postdysenteric arthropathy, left hip** CC HCC
- MØ2.159 **Postdysenteric arthropathy, unspecified hip** CC UNS HCC

√6th MØ2.16 **Postdysenteric arthropathy, knee**
- MØ2.161 **Postdysenteric arthropathy, right knee** CC HCC
- MØ2.162 **Postdysenteric arthropathy, left knee** CC HCC
- MØ2.169 **Postdysenteric arthropathy, unspecified knee** CC UNS HCC

√6th MØ2.17 **Postdysenteric arthropathy, ankle and foot**
Postdysenteric arthropathy, tarsus, metatarsus and phalanges
- MØ2.171 **Postdysenteric arthropathy, right ankle and foot** CC HCC
- MØ2.172 **Postdysenteric arthropathy, left ankle and foot** CC HCC
- MØ2.179 **Postdysenteric arthropathy, unspecified ankle and foot** CC UNS HCC

MØ2.18 **Postdysenteric arthropathy, vertebrae** CC HCC
MØ2.19 **Postdysenteric arthropathy, multiple sites** CC HCC

√5th MØ2.2 **Postimmunization arthropathy**

MØ2.2Ø **Postimmunization arthropathy, unspecified site**

√6th MØ2.21 **Postimmunization arthropathy, shoulder**
- MØ2.211 **Postimmunization arthropathy, right shoulder**
- MØ2.212 **Postimmunization arthropathy, left shoulder**
- MØ2.219 **Postimmunization arthropathy, unspecified shoulder**

√6th MØ2.22 **Postimmunization arthropathy, elbow**
- MØ2.221 **Postimmunization arthropathy, right elbow**
- MØ2.222 **Postimmunization arthropathy, left elbow**
- MØ2.229 **Postimmunization arthropathy, unspecified elbow**

√6th MØ2.23 **Postimmunization arthropathy, wrist**
Postimmunization arthropathy, carpal bones
- MØ2.231 **Postimmunization arthropathy, right wrist**
- MØ2.232 **Postimmunization arthropathy, left wrist**
- MØ2.239 **Postimmunization arthropathy, unspecified wrist**

√6th MØ2.24 **Postimmunization arthropathy, hand**
Postimmunization arthropathy, metacarpus and phalanges
- MØ2.241 **Postimmunization arthropathy, right hand**
- MØ2.242 **Postimmunization arthropathy, left hand**
- MØ2.249 **Postimmunization arthropathy, unspecified hand**

√6th MØ2.25 **Postimmunization arthropathy, hip**
- MØ2.251 **Postimmunization arthropathy, right hip**
- MØ2.252 **Postimmunization arthropathy, left hip**
- MØ2.259 **Postimmunization arthropathy, unspecified hip**

√6th MØ2.26 **Postimmunization arthropathy, knee**
- MØ2.261 **Postimmunization arthropathy, right knee**
- MØ2.262 **Postimmunization arthropathy, left knee**
- MØ2.269 **Postimmunization arthropathy, unspecified knee**

√6th MØ2.27 **Postimmunization arthropathy, ankle and foot**
Postimmunization arthropathy, tarsus, metatarsus and phalanges
- MØ2.271 **Postimmunization arthropathy, right ankle and foot**
- MØ2.272 **Postimmunization arthropathy, left ankle and foot**
- MØ2.279 **Postimmunization arthropathy, unspecified ankle and foot**

MØ2.28 **Postimmunization arthropathy, vertebrae**
MØ2.29 **Postimmunization arthropathy, multiple sites**

√5th MØ2.3 **Reiter's disease**
Reactive arthritis
DEF: Arthritis, iridocyclitis, and urethritis, sometimes with diarrhea. While symptoms may recur, arthritis is constant.

MØ2.3Ø **Reiter's disease, unspecified site** CC UNS HCC

√6th MØ2.31 **Reiter's disease, shoulder**
- MØ2.311 **Reiter's disease, right shoulder** CC HCC
- MØ2.312 **Reiter's disease, left shoulder** CC HCC
- MØ2.319 **Reiter's disease, unspecified shoulder** CC UNS HCC

√6th MØ2.32 **Reiter's disease, elbow**
- MØ2.321 **Reiter's disease, right elbow** CC HCC
- MØ2.322 **Reiter's disease, left elbow** CC HCC

M02.329 Reiter's disease, unspecified elbow CC UNS HCC

M02.33 Reiter's disease, wrist
Reiter's disease, carpal bones
M02.331 Reiter's disease, right wrist CC HCC
M02.332 Reiter's disease, left wrist CC HCC
M02.339 Reiter's disease, unspecified wrist CC UNS HCC

M02.34 Reiter's disease, hand
Reiter's disease, metacarpus and phalanges
M02.341 Reiter's disease, right hand CC HCC
M02.342 Reiter's disease, left hand CC HCC
M02.349 Reiter's disease, unspecified hand CC UNS HCC

M02.35 Reiter's disease, hip
M02.351 Reiter's disease, right hip CC HCC
M02.352 Reiter's disease, left hip CC HCC
M02.359 Reiter's disease, unspecified hip CC UNS HCC

M02.36 Reiter's disease, knee
M02.361 Reiter's disease, right knee CC HCC
M02.362 Reiter's disease, left knee CC HCC
M02.369 Reiter's disease, unspecified knee CC UNS HCC

M02.37 Reiter's disease, ankle and foot
Reiter's disease, tarsus, metatarsus and phalanges
M02.371 Reiter's disease, right ankle and foot CC HCC
M02.372 Reiter's disease, left ankle and foot CC HCC
M02.379 Reiter's disease, unspecified ankle and foot CC UNS HCC

M02.38 Reiter's disease, vertebrae CC HCC
M02.39 Reiter's disease, multiple sites CC HCC

M02.8 Other reactive arthropathies
M02.80 Other reactive arthropathies, unspecified site CC UNS HCC

M02.81 Other reactive arthropathies, shoulder
M02.811 Other reactive arthropathies, right shoulder CC HCC
M02.812 Other reactive arthropathies, left shoulder CC HCC
M02.819 Other reactive arthropathies, unspecified shoulder CC UNS HCC

M02.82 Other reactive arthropathies, elbow
M02.821 Other reactive arthropathies, right elbow CC HCC
M02.822 Other reactive arthropathies, left elbow CC HCC
M02.829 Other reactive arthropathies, unspecified elbow CC UNS HCC

M02.83 Other reactive arthropathies, wrist
Other reactive arthropathies, carpal bones
M02.831 Other reactive arthropathies, right wrist CC HCC
M02.832 Other reactive arthropathies, left wrist CC HCC
M02.839 Other reactive arthropathies, unspecified wrist CC UNS HCC

M02.84 Other reactive arthropathies, hand
Other reactive arthropathies, metacarpus and phalanges
M02.841 Other reactive arthropathies, right hand CC HCC
M02.842 Other reactive arthropathies, left hand CC HCC
M02.849 Other reactive arthropathies, unspecified hand CC UNS HCC

M02.85 Other reactive arthropathies, hip
M02.851 Other reactive arthropathies, right hip CC HCC
M02.852 Other reactive arthropathies, left hip CC HCC
M02.859 Other reactive arthropathies, unspecified hip CC UNS HCC

M02.86 Other reactive arthropathies, knee
M02.861 Other reactive arthropathies, right knee CC HCC
M02.862 Other reactive arthropathies, left knee CC HCC
M02.869 Other reactive arthropathies, unspecified knee CC UNS HCC

M02.87 Other reactive arthropathies, ankle and foot
Other reactive arthropathies, tarsus, metatarsus and phalanges
M02.871 Other reactive arthropathies, right ankle and foot CC HCC
M02.872 Other reactive arthropathies, left ankle and foot CC HCC
M02.879 Other reactive arthropathies, unspecified ankle and foot CC UNS HCC

M02.88 Other reactive arthropathies, vertebrae CC HCC
M02.89 Other reactive arthropathies, multiple sites CC HCC

M02.9 Reactive arthropathy, unspecified HCC

Autoinflammatory syndromes (M04)

M04 Autoinflammatory syndromes
EXCLUDES 2 *Crohn's disease (K50.-)*
AHA: 2016,4Q,37

M04.1 Periodic fever syndromes HCC
Familial Mediterranean fever
Hyperimmunoglobin D syndrome
Mevalonate kinase deficiency
Tumor necrosis factor receptor associated periodic syndrome [TRAPS]

M04.2 Cryopyrin-associated periodic syndromes HCC
Chronic infantile neurological, cutaneous and articular syndrome [CINCA]
Familial cold autoinflammatory syndrome
Familial cold urticaria
Muckle-Wells syndrome
Neonatal onset multisystemic inflammatory disorder [NOMID]

M04.8 Other autoinflammatory syndromes HCC
Blau syndrome
Deficiency of interleukin 1 receptor antagonist [DIRA]
Majeed syndrome
Periodic fever, aphthous stomatitis, pharyngitis, and adenopathy syndrome [PFAPA]
Pyogenic arthritis, pyoderma gangrenosum, and acne syndrome [PAPA]

M04.9 Autoinflammatory syndrome, unspecified HCC

Inflammatory polyarthropathies (M05-M14)

M05 Rheumatoid arthritis with rheumatoid factor
EXCLUDES 1 *juvenile rheumatoid arthritis (M08.-)*
rheumatic fever (I00)
rheumatoid arthritis of spine (M45.-)
AHA: 2020,4Q,31-32
DEF: Rheumatoid arthritis: Autoimmune systemic disease that causes chronic inflammation of the joints and other areas of the body, manifested by inflammatory changes in articular structures and synovial membranes, atrophy, and loss in bone density.

M05.0 Felty's syndrome
Rheumatoid arthritis with splenoadenomegaly and leukopenia
M05.00 Felty's syndrome, unspecified site HCC

M05.01 Felty's syndrome, shoulder
M05.011 Felty's syndrome, right shoulder HCC
M05.012 Felty's syndrome, left shoulder HCC
M05.019 Felty's syndrome, unspecified shoulder HCC

M05.02 Felty's syndrome, elbow
M05.021 Felty's syndrome, right elbow HCC
M05.022 Felty's syndrome, left elbow HCC
M05.029 Felty's syndrome, unspecified elbow HCC

M05.03 Felty's syndrome, wrist
Felty's syndrome, carpal bones
M05.031 Felty's syndrome, right wrist HCC
M05.032 Felty's syndrome, left wrist HCC
M05.039 Felty's syndrome, unspecified wrist HCC

Chapter 13. Diseases of the Musculoskeletal System and Connective Tissue
M02.329–M05.039

✓6th **MØ5.Ø4 Felty's syndrome, hand**
Felty's syndrome, metacarpus and phalanges
MØ5.Ø41 Felty's syndrome, right hand HCC
MØ5.Ø42 Felty's syndrome, left hand HCC
MØ5.Ø49 Felty's syndrome, unspecified hand HCC

✓6th **MØ5.Ø5 Felty's syndrome, hip**
MØ5.Ø51 Felty's syndrome, right hip HCC
MØ5.Ø52 Felty's syndrome, left hip HCC
MØ5.Ø59 Felty's syndrome, unspecified hip HCC

✓6th **MØ5.Ø6 Felty's syndrome, knee**
MØ5.Ø61 Felty's syndrome, right knee HCC
MØ5.Ø62 Felty's syndrome, left knee HCC
MØ5.Ø69 Felty's syndrome, unspecified knee HCC

✓6th **MØ5.Ø7 Felty's syndrome, ankle and foot**
Felty's syndrome, tarsus, metatarsus and phalanges
MØ5.Ø71 Felty's syndrome, right ankle and foot HCC
MØ5.Ø72 Felty's syndrome, left ankle and foot HCC
MØ5.Ø79 Felty's syndrome, unspecified ankle and foot HCC

MØ5.Ø9 Felty's syndrome, multiple sites HCC

✓5th **MØ5.1 Rheumatoid lung disease with rheumatoid arthritis**
MØ5.1Ø Rheumatoid lung disease with rheumatoid arthritis of unspecified site HCC

✓6th **MØ5.11 Rheumatoid lung disease with rheumatoid arthritis of shoulder**
MØ5.111 Rheumatoid lung disease with rheumatoid arthritis of right shoulder HCC
MØ5.112 Rheumatoid lung disease with rheumatoid arthritis of left shoulder HCC
MØ5.119 Rheumatoid lung disease with rheumatoid arthritis of unspecified shoulder HCC

✓6th **MØ5.12 Rheumatoid lung disease with rheumatoid arthritis of elbow**
MØ5.121 Rheumatoid lung disease with rheumatoid arthritis of right elbow HCC
MØ5.122 Rheumatoid lung disease with rheumatoid arthritis of left elbow HCC
MØ5.129 Rheumatoid lung disease with rheumatoid arthritis of unspecified elbow HCC

✓6th **MØ5.13 Rheumatoid lung disease with rheumatoid arthritis of wrist**
Rheumatoid lung disease with rheumatoid arthritis, carpal bones
MØ5.131 Rheumatoid lung disease with rheumatoid arthritis of right wrist HCC
MØ5.132 Rheumatoid lung disease with rheumatoid arthritis of left wrist HCC
MØ5.139 Rheumatoid lung disease with rheumatoid arthritis of unspecified wrist HCC

✓6th **MØ5.14 Rheumatoid lung disease with rheumatoid arthritis of hand**
Rheumatoid lung disease with rheumatoid arthritis, metacarpus and phalanges
MØ5.141 Rheumatoid lung disease with rheumatoid arthritis of right hand HCC
MØ5.142 Rheumatoid lung disease with rheumatoid arthritis of left hand HCC
MØ5.149 Rheumatoid lung disease with rheumatoid arthritis of unspecified hand HCC

✓6th **MØ5.15 Rheumatoid lung disease with rheumatoid arthritis of hip**
MØ5.151 Rheumatoid lung disease with rheumatoid arthritis of right hip HCC
MØ5.152 Rheumatoid lung disease with rheumatoid arthritis of left hip HCC
MØ5.159 Rheumatoid lung disease with rheumatoid arthritis of unspecified hip HCC

✓6th **MØ5.16 Rheumatoid lung disease with rheumatoid arthritis of knee**
MØ5.161 Rheumatoid lung disease with rheumatoid arthritis of right knee HCC
MØ5.162 Rheumatoid lung disease with rheumatoid arthritis of left knee HCC
MØ5.169 Rheumatoid lung disease with rheumatoid arthritis of unspecified knee HCC

✓6th **MØ5.17 Rheumatoid lung disease with rheumatoid arthritis of ankle and foot**
Rheumatoid lung disease with rheumatoid arthritis, tarsus, metatarsus and phalanges
MØ5.171 Rheumatoid lung disease with rheumatoid arthritis of right ankle and foot HCC
MØ5.172 Rheumatoid lung disease with rheumatoid arthritis of left ankle and foot HCC
MØ5.179 Rheumatoid lung disease with rheumatoid arthritis of unspecified ankle and foot HCC

MØ5.19 Rheumatoid lung disease with rheumatoid arthritis of multiple sites HCC

✓5th **MØ5.2 Rheumatoid vasculitis with rheumatoid arthritis**
MØ5.2Ø Rheumatoid vasculitis with rheumatoid arthritis of unspecified site HCC

✓6th **MØ5.21 Rheumatoid vasculitis with rheumatoid arthritis of shoulder**
MØ5.211 Rheumatoid vasculitis with rheumatoid arthritis of right shoulder HCC
MØ5.212 Rheumatoid vasculitis with rheumatoid arthritis of left shoulder HCC
MØ5.219 Rheumatoid vasculitis with rheumatoid arthritis of unspecified shoulder HCC

✓6th **MØ5.22 Rheumatoid vasculitis with rheumatoid arthritis of elbow**
MØ5.221 Rheumatoid vasculitis with rheumatoid arthritis of right elbow HCC
MØ5.222 Rheumatoid vasculitis with rheumatoid arthritis of left elbow HCC
MØ5.229 Rheumatoid vasculitis with rheumatoid arthritis of unspecified elbow HCC

✓6th **MØ5.23 Rheumatoid vasculitis with rheumatoid arthritis of wrist**
Rheumatoid vasculitis with rheumatoid arthritis, carpal bones
MØ5.231 Rheumatoid vasculitis with rheumatoid arthritis of right wrist HCC
MØ5.232 Rheumatoid vasculitis with rheumatoid arthritis of left wrist HCC
MØ5.239 Rheumatoid vasculitis with rheumatoid arthritis of unspecified wrist HCC

✓6th **MØ5.24 Rheumatoid vasculitis with rheumatoid arthritis of hand**
Rheumatoid vasculitis with rheumatoid arthritis, metacarpus and phalanges
MØ5.241 Rheumatoid vasculitis with rheumatoid arthritis of right hand HCC
MØ5.242 Rheumatoid vasculitis with rheumatoid arthritis of left hand HCC
MØ5.249 Rheumatoid vasculitis with rheumatoid arthritis of unspecified hand HCC

✓6th **MØ5.25 Rheumatoid vasculitis with rheumatoid arthritis of hip**
MØ5.251 Rheumatoid vasculitis with rheumatoid arthritis of right hip HCC
MØ5.252 Rheumatoid vasculitis with rheumatoid arthritis of left hip HCC
MØ5.259 Rheumatoid vasculitis with rheumatoid arthritis of unspecified hip HCC

✓6th **MØ5.26 Rheumatoid vasculitis with rheumatoid arthritis of knee**
MØ5.261 Rheumatoid vasculitis with rheumatoid arthritis of right knee HCC
MØ5.262 Rheumatoid vasculitis with rheumatoid arthritis of left knee HCC
MØ5.269 Rheumatoid vasculitis with rheumatoid arthritis of unspecified knee HCC

M05.27 Rheumatoid vasculitis with rheumatoid arthritis of ankle and foot
Rheumatoid vasculitis with rheumatoid arthritis, tarsus, metatarsus and phalanges
M05.271 Rheumatoid vasculitis with rheumatoid arthritis of right ankle and foot HCC
M05.272 Rheumatoid vasculitis with rheumatoid arthritis of left ankle and foot HCC
M05.279 Rheumatoid vasculitis with rheumatoid arthritis of unspecified ankle and foot HCC
M05.29 Rheumatoid vasculitis with rheumatoid arthritis of multiple sites HCC

M05.3 Rheumatoid heart disease with rheumatoid arthritis
Rheumatoid carditis
Rheumatoid endocarditis
Rheumatoid myocarditis
Rheumatoid pericarditis
M05.30 Rheumatoid heart disease with rheumatoid arthritis of unspecified site HCC
M05.31 Rheumatoid heart disease with rheumatoid arthritis of shoulder
M05.311 Rheumatoid heart disease with rheumatoid arthritis of right shoulder HCC
M05.312 Rheumatoid heart disease with rheumatoid arthritis of left shoulder HCC
M05.319 Rheumatoid heart disease with rheumatoid arthritis of unspecified shoulder HCC
M05.32 Rheumatoid heart disease with rheumatoid arthritis of elbow
M05.321 Rheumatoid heart disease with rheumatoid arthritis of right elbow HCC
M05.322 Rheumatoid heart disease with rheumatoid arthritis of left elbow HCC
M05.329 Rheumatoid heart disease with rheumatoid arthritis of unspecified elbow HCC
M05.33 Rheumatoid heart disease with rheumatoid arthritis of wrist
Rheumatoid heart disease with rheumatoid arthritis, carpal bones
M05.331 Rheumatoid heart disease with rheumatoid arthritis of right wrist HCC
M05.332 Rheumatoid heart disease with rheumatoid arthritis of left wrist HCC
M05.339 Rheumatoid heart disease with rheumatoid arthritis of unspecified wrist HCC
M05.34 Rheumatoid heart disease with rheumatoid arthritis of hand
Rheumatoid heart disease with rheumatoid arthritis, metacarpus and phalanges
M05.341 Rheumatoid heart disease with rheumatoid arthritis of right hand HCC
M05.342 Rheumatoid heart disease with rheumatoid arthritis of left hand HCC
M05.349 Rheumatoid heart disease with rheumatoid arthritis of unspecified hand HCC
M05.35 Rheumatoid heart disease with rheumatoid arthritis of hip
M05.351 Rheumatoid heart disease with rheumatoid arthritis of right hip HCC
M05.352 Rheumatoid heart disease with rheumatoid arthritis of left hip HCC
M05.359 Rheumatoid heart disease with rheumatoid arthritis of unspecified hip HCC
M05.36 Rheumatoid heart disease with rheumatoid arthritis of knee
M05.361 Rheumatoid heart disease with rheumatoid arthritis of right knee HCC
M05.362 Rheumatoid heart disease with rheumatoid arthritis of left knee HCC
M05.369 Rheumatoid heart disease with rheumatoid arthritis of unspecified knee HCC
M05.37 Rheumatoid heart disease with rheumatoid arthritis of ankle and foot
Rheumatoid heart disease with rheumatoid arthritis, tarsus, metatarsus and phalanges
M05.371 Rheumatoid heart disease with rheumatoid arthritis of right ankle and foot HCC
M05.372 Rheumatoid heart disease with rheumatoid arthritis of left ankle and foot HCC
M05.379 Rheumatoid heart disease with rheumatoid arthritis of unspecified ankle and foot HCC
M05.39 Rheumatoid heart disease with rheumatoid arthritis of multiple sites HCC

M05.4 Rheumatoid myopathy with rheumatoid arthritis
M05.40 Rheumatoid myopathy with rheumatoid arthritis of unspecified site CC UNS HCC
M05.41 Rheumatoid myopathy with rheumatoid arthritis of shoulder
M05.411 Rheumatoid myopathy with rheumatoid arthritis of right shoulder CC HCC
M05.412 Rheumatoid myopathy with rheumatoid arthritis of left shoulder CC HCC
M05.419 Rheumatoid myopathy with rheumatoid arthritis of unspecified shoulder CC UNS HCC
M05.42 Rheumatoid myopathy with rheumatoid arthritis of elbow
M05.421 Rheumatoid myopathy with rheumatoid arthritis of right elbow CC HCC
M05.422 Rheumatoid myopathy with rheumatoid arthritis of left elbow CC HCC
M05.429 Rheumatoid myopathy with rheumatoid arthritis of unspecified elbow CC UNS HCC
M05.43 Rheumatoid myopathy with rheumatoid arthritis of wrist
Rheumatoid myopathy with rheumatoid arthritis, carpal bones
M05.431 Rheumatoid myopathy with rheumatoid arthritis of right wrist CC HCC
M05.432 Rheumatoid myopathy with rheumatoid arthritis of left wrist CC HCC
M05.439 Rheumatoid myopathy with rheumatoid arthritis of unspecified wrist CC UNS HCC
M05.44 Rheumatoid myopathy with rheumatoid arthritis of hand
Rheumatoid myopathy with rheumatoid arthritis, metacarpus and phalanges
M05.441 Rheumatoid myopathy with rheumatoid arthritis of right hand CC HCC
M05.442 Rheumatoid myopathy with rheumatoid arthritis of left hand CC HCC
M05.449 Rheumatoid myopathy with rheumatoid arthritis of unspecified hand CC UNS HCC
M05.45 Rheumatoid myopathy with rheumatoid arthritis of hip
M05.451 Rheumatoid myopathy with rheumatoid arthritis of right hip CC HCC
M05.452 Rheumatoid myopathy with rheumatoid arthritis of left hip CC HCC
M05.459 Rheumatoid myopathy with rheumatoid arthritis of unspecified hip CC UNS HCC
M05.46 Rheumatoid myopathy with rheumatoid arthritis of knee
M05.461 Rheumatoid myopathy with rheumatoid arthritis of right knee CC HCC
M05.462 Rheumatoid myopathy with rheumatoid arthritis of left knee CC HCC
M05.469 Rheumatoid myopathy with rheumatoid arthritis of unspecified knee CC UNS HCC
M05.47 Rheumatoid myopathy with rheumatoid arthritis of ankle and foot
Rheumatoid myopathy with rheumatoid arthritis, tarsus, metatarsus and phalanges
M05.471 Rheumatoid myopathy with rheumatoid arthritis of right ankle and foot CC HCC

MØ5.472 Rheumatoid myopathy with rheumatoid arthritis of left ankle and foot CC HCC

MØ5.479 Rheumatoid myopathy with rheumatoid arthritis of unspecified ankle and foot CC UNS HCC

MØ5.49 Rheumatoid myopathy with rheumatoid arthritis of multiple sites CC HCC

✓5th MØ5.5 Rheumatoid polyneuropathy with rheumatoid arthritis

MØ5.5Ø Rheumatoid polyneuropathy with rheumatoid arthritis of unspecified site HCC

✓6th MØ5.51 Rheumatoid polyneuropathy with rheumatoid arthritis of shoulder

MØ5.511 Rheumatoid polyneuropathy with rheumatoid arthritis of right shoulder HCC

MØ5.512 Rheumatoid polyneuropathy with rheumatoid arthritis of left shoulder HCC

MØ5.519 Rheumatoid polyneuropathy with rheumatoid arthritis of unspecified shoulder HCC

✓6th MØ5.52 Rheumatoid polyneuropathy with rheumatoid arthritis of elbow

MØ5.521 Rheumatoid polyneuropathy with rheumatoid arthritis of right elbow HCC

MØ5.522 Rheumatoid polyneuropathy with rheumatoid arthritis of left elbow HCC

MØ5.529 Rheumatoid polyneuropathy with rheumatoid arthritis of unspecified elbow HCC

✓6th MØ5.53 Rheumatoid polyneuropathy with rheumatoid arthritis of wrist

Rheumatoid polyneuropathy with rheumatoid arthritis, carpal bones

MØ5.531 Rheumatoid polyneuropathy with rheumatoid arthritis of right wrist HCC

MØ5.532 Rheumatoid polyneuropathy with rheumatoid arthritis of left wrist HCC

MØ5.539 Rheumatoid polyneuropathy with rheumatoid arthritis of unspecified wrist HCC

✓6th MØ5.54 Rheumatoid polyneuropathy with rheumatoid arthritis of hand

Rheumatoid polyneuropathy with rheumatoid arthritis, metacarpus and phalanges

MØ5.541 Rheumatoid polyneuropathy with rheumatoid arthritis of right hand HCC

MØ5.542 Rheumatoid polyneuropathy with rheumatoid arthritis of left hand HCC

MØ5.549 Rheumatoid polyneuropathy with rheumatoid arthritis of unspecified hand HCC

✓6th MØ5.55 Rheumatoid polyneuropathy with rheumatoid arthritis of hip

MØ5.551 Rheumatoid polyneuropathy with rheumatoid arthritis of right hip HCC

MØ5.552 Rheumatoid polyneuropathy with rheumatoid arthritis of left hip HCC

MØ5.559 Rheumatoid polyneuropathy with rheumatoid arthritis of unspecified hip HCC

✓6th MØ5.56 Rheumatoid polyneuropathy with rheumatoid arthritis of knee

MØ5.561 Rheumatoid polyneuropathy with rheumatoid arthritis of right knee HCC

MØ5.562 Rheumatoid polyneuropathy with rheumatoid arthritis of left knee HCC

MØ5.569 Rheumatoid polyneuropathy with rheumatoid arthritis of unspecified knee HCC

✓6th MØ5.57 Rheumatoid polyneuropathy with rheumatoid arthritis of ankle and foot

Rheumatoid polyneuropathy with rheumatoid arthritis, tarsus, metatarsus and phalanges

MØ5.571 Rheumatoid polyneuropathy with rheumatoid arthritis of right ankle and foot HCC

MØ5.572 Rheumatoid polyneuropathy with rheumatoid arthritis of left ankle and foot HCC

MØ5.579 Rheumatoid polyneuropathy with rheumatoid arthritis of unspecified ankle and foot HCC

MØ5.59 Rheumatoid polyneuropathy with rheumatoid arthritis of multiple sites HCC

✓5th MØ5.6 Rheumatoid arthritis with involvement of other organs and systems

MØ5.6Ø Rheumatoid arthritis of unspecified site with involvement of other organs and systems HCC

✓6th MØ5.61 Rheumatoid arthritis of shoulder with involvement of other organs and systems

MØ5.611 Rheumatoid arthritis of right shoulder with involvement of other organs and systems HCC

MØ5.612 Rheumatoid arthritis of left shoulder with involvement of other organs and systems HCC

MØ5.619 Rheumatoid arthritis of unspecified shoulder with involvement of other organs and systems HCC

✓6th MØ5.62 Rheumatoid arthritis of elbow with involvement of other organs and systems

MØ5.621 Rheumatoid arthritis of right elbow with involvement of other organs and systems HCC

MØ5.622 Rheumatoid arthritis of left elbow with involvement of other organs and systems HCC

MØ5.629 Rheumatoid arthritis of unspecified elbow with involvement of other organs and systems HCC

✓6th MØ5.63 Rheumatoid arthritis of wrist with involvement of other organs and systems

Rheumatoid arthritis of carpal bones with involvement of other organs and systems

MØ5.631 Rheumatoid arthritis of right wrist with involvement of other organs and systems HCC

MØ5.632 Rheumatoid arthritis of left wrist with involvement of other organs and systems HCC

MØ5.639 Rheumatoid arthritis of unspecified wrist with involvement of other organs and systems HCC

✓6th MØ5.64 Rheumatoid arthritis of hand with involvement of other organs and systems

Rheumatoid arthritis of metacarpus and phalanges with involvement of other organs and systems

MØ5.641 Rheumatoid arthritis of right hand with involvement of other organs and systems HCC

MØ5.642 Rheumatoid arthritis of left hand with involvement of other organs and systems HCC

MØ5.649 Rheumatoid arthritis of unspecified hand with involvement of other organs and systems HCC

✓6th MØ5.65 Rheumatoid arthritis of hip with involvement of other organs and systems

MØ5.651 Rheumatoid arthritis of right hip with involvement of other organs and systems HCC

MØ5.652 Rheumatoid arthritis of left hip with involvement of other organs and systems HCC

MØ5.659 Rheumatoid arthritis of unspecified hip with involvement of other organs and systems HCC

✓6th MØ5.66 Rheumatoid arthritis of knee with involvement of other organs and systems

MØ5.661 Rheumatoid arthritis of right knee with involvement of other organs and systems HCC

MØ5.662 Rheumatoid arthritis of left knee with involvement of other organs and systems HCC

MØ5.669 Rheumatoid arthritis of unspecified knee with involvement of other organs and systems HCC

✓6th M05.67 Rheumatoid arthritis of ankle and foot with involvement of other organs and systems
Rheumatoid arthritis of tarsus, metatarsus and phalanges with involvement of other organs and systems

M05.671 Rheumatoid arthritis of right ankle and foot with involvement of other organs and systems HCC

M05.672 Rheumatoid arthritis of left ankle and foot with involvement of other organs and systems HCC

M05.679 Rheumatoid arthritis of unspecified ankle and foot with involvement of other organs and systems HCC

M05.69 Rheumatoid arthritis of multiple sites with involvement of other organs and systems HCC

✓5th M05.7 Rheumatoid arthritis with rheumatoid factor without organ or systems involvement

M05.70 Rheumatoid arthritis with rheumatoid factor of unspecified site without organ or systems involvement HCC

✓6th M05.71 Rheumatoid arthritis with rheumatoid factor of shoulder without organ or systems involvement

M05.711 Rheumatoid arthritis with rheumatoid factor of right shoulder without organ or systems involvement HCC

M05.712 Rheumatoid arthritis with rheumatoid factor of left shoulder without organ or systems involvement HCC

M05.719 Rheumatoid arthritis with rheumatoid factor of unspecified shoulder without organ or systems involvement HCC

✓6th M05.72 Rheumatoid arthritis with rheumatoid factor of elbow without organ or systems involvement

M05.721 Rheumatoid arthritis with rheumatoid factor of right elbow without organ or systems involvement HCC

M05.722 Rheumatoid arthritis with rheumatoid factor of left elbow without organ or systems involvement HCC

M05.729 Rheumatoid arthritis with rheumatoid factor of unspecified elbow without organ or systems involvement HCC

✓6th M05.73 Rheumatoid arthritis with rheumatoid factor of wrist without organ or systems involvement

M05.731 Rheumatoid arthritis with rheumatoid factor of right wrist without organ or systems involvement HCC

M05.732 Rheumatoid arthritis with rheumatoid factor of left wrist without organ or systems involvement HCC

M05.739 Rheumatoid arthritis with rheumatoid factor of unspecified wrist without organ or systems involvement HCC

✓6th M05.74 Rheumatoid arthritis with rheumatoid factor of hand without organ or systems involvement

M05.741 Rheumatoid arthritis with rheumatoid factor of right hand without organ or systems involvement HCC

M05.742 Rheumatoid arthritis with rheumatoid factor of left hand without organ or systems involvement HCC

M05.749 Rheumatoid arthritis with rheumatoid factor of unspecified hand without organ or systems involvement HCC

✓6th M05.75 Rheumatoid arthritis with rheumatoid factor of hip without organ or systems involvement

M05.751 Rheumatoid arthritis with rheumatoid factor of right hip without organ or systems involvement HCC

M05.752 Rheumatoid arthritis with rheumatoid factor of left hip without organ or systems involvement HCC

M05.759 Rheumatoid arthritis with rheumatoid factor of unspecified hip without organ or systems involvement HCC

✓6th M05.76 Rheumatoid arthritis with rheumatoid factor of knee without organ or systems involvement

M05.761 Rheumatoid arthritis with rheumatoid factor of right knee without organ or systems involvement HCC

M05.762 Rheumatoid arthritis with rheumatoid factor of left knee without organ or systems involvement HCC

M05.769 Rheumatoid arthritis with rheumatoid factor of unspecified knee without organ or systems involvement HCC

✓6th M05.77 Rheumatoid arthritis with rheumatoid factor of ankle and foot without organ or systems involvement

M05.771 Rheumatoid arthritis with rheumatoid factor of right ankle and foot without organ or systems involvement HCC

M05.772 Rheumatoid arthritis with rheumatoid factor of left ankle and foot without organ or systems involvement HCC

M05.779 Rheumatoid arthritis with rheumatoid factor of unspecified ankle and foot without organ or systems involvement HCC

M05.79 Rheumatoid arthritis with rheumatoid factor of multiple sites without organ or systems involvement HCC

M05.7A Rheumatoid arthritis with rheumatoid factor of other specified site without organ or systems involvement HCC

✓5th M05.8 Other rheumatoid arthritis with rheumatoid factor

M05.80 Other rheumatoid arthritis with rheumatoid factor of unspecified site HCC

✓6th M05.81 Other rheumatoid arthritis with rheumatoid factor of shoulder

M05.811 Other rheumatoid arthritis with rheumatoid factor of right shoulder HCC

M05.812 Other rheumatoid arthritis with rheumatoid factor of left shoulder HCC

M05.819 Other rheumatoid arthritis with rheumatoid factor of unspecified shoulder HCC

✓6th M05.82 Other rheumatoid arthritis with rheumatoid factor of elbow

M05.821 Other rheumatoid arthritis with rheumatoid factor of right elbow HCC

M05.822 Other rheumatoid arthritis with rheumatoid factor of left elbow HCC

M05.829 Other rheumatoid arthritis with rheumatoid factor of unspecified elbow HCC

✓6th M05.83 Other rheumatoid arthritis with rheumatoid factor of wrist

M05.831 Other rheumatoid arthritis with rheumatoid factor of right wrist HCC

M05.832 Other rheumatoid arthritis with rheumatoid factor of left wrist HCC

M05.839 Other rheumatoid arthritis with rheumatoid factor of unspecified wrist HCC

✓6th M05.84 Other rheumatoid arthritis with rheumatoid factor of hand

M05.841 Other rheumatoid arthritis with rheumatoid factor of right hand HCC

M05.842 Other rheumatoid arthritis with rheumatoid factor of left hand HCC

M05.849 Other rheumatoid arthritis with rheumatoid factor of unspecified hand HCC

✓6th M05.85 Other rheumatoid arthritis with rheumatoid factor of hip

M05.851 Other rheumatoid arthritis with rheumatoid factor of right hip HCC

M05.852 Other rheumatoid arthritis with rheumatoid factor of left hip HCC

M05.859 Other rheumatoid arthritis with rheumatoid factor of unspecified hip HCC

✓6th M05.86 Other rheumatoid arthritis with rheumatoid factor of knee

M05.861 Other rheumatoid arthritis with rheumatoid factor of right knee HCC

M05.862 Other rheumatoid arthritis with rheumatoid factor of left knee HCC

MØ5.869 Other rheumatoid arthritis with rheumatoid factor of unspecified knee HCC

MØ5.87 Other rheumatoid arthritis with rheumatoid factor of ankle and foot
- MØ5.871 Other rheumatoid arthritis with rheumatoid factor of right ankle and foot HCC
- MØ5.872 Other rheumatoid arthritis with rheumatoid factor of left ankle and foot HCC
- MØ5.879 Other rheumatoid arthritis with rheumatoid factor of unspecified ankle and foot HCC

MØ5.89 Other rheumatoid arthritis with rheumatoid factor of multiple sites HCC

MØ5.8A Other rheumatoid arthritis with rheumatoid factor of other specified site HCC

MØ5.9 Rheumatoid arthritis with rheumatoid factor, unspecified HCC

MØ6 Other rheumatoid arthritis

AHA: 2020,4Q,31-32

DEF: Rheumatoid arthritis: Autoimmune systemic disease that causes chronic inflammation of the joints and other areas of the body, manifested by inflammatory changes in articular structures and synovial membranes, atrophy, and loss in bone density.

MØ6.Ø Rheumatoid arthritis without rheumatoid factor

MØ6.ØØ Rheumatoid arthritis without rheumatoid factor, unspecified site HCC

MØ6.Ø1 Rheumatoid arthritis without rheumatoid factor, shoulder
- MØ6.Ø11 Rheumatoid arthritis without rheumatoid factor, right shoulder HCC
- MØ6.Ø12 Rheumatoid arthritis without rheumatoid factor, left shoulder HCC
- MØ6.Ø19 Rheumatoid arthritis without rheumatoid factor, unspecified shoulder HCC

MØ6.Ø2 Rheumatoid arthritis without rheumatoid factor, elbow
- MØ6.Ø21 Rheumatoid arthritis without rheumatoid factor, right elbow HCC
- MØ6.Ø22 Rheumatoid arthritis without rheumatoid factor, left elbow HCC
- MØ6.Ø29 Rheumatoid arthritis without rheumatoid factor, unspecified elbow HCC

MØ6.Ø3 Rheumatoid arthritis without rheumatoid factor, wrist
- MØ6.Ø31 Rheumatoid arthritis without rheumatoid factor, right wrist HCC
- MØ6.Ø32 Rheumatoid arthritis without rheumatoid factor, left wrist HCC
- MØ6.Ø39 Rheumatoid arthritis without rheumatoid factor, unspecified wrist HCC

MØ6.Ø4 Rheumatoid arthritis without rheumatoid factor, hand
- MØ6.Ø41 Rheumatoid arthritis without rheumatoid factor, right hand HCC
- MØ6.Ø42 Rheumatoid arthritis without rheumatoid factor, left hand HCC
- MØ6.Ø49 Rheumatoid arthritis without rheumatoid factor, unspecified hand HCC

MØ6.Ø5 Rheumatoid arthritis without rheumatoid factor, hip
- MØ6.Ø51 Rheumatoid arthritis without rheumatoid factor, right hip HCC
- MØ6.Ø52 Rheumatoid arthritis without rheumatoid factor, left hip HCC
- MØ6.Ø59 Rheumatoid arthritis without rheumatoid factor, unspecified hip HCC

MØ6.Ø6 Rheumatoid arthritis without rheumatoid factor, knee
- MØ6.Ø61 Rheumatoid arthritis without rheumatoid factor, right knee HCC
- MØ6.Ø62 Rheumatoid arthritis without rheumatoid factor, left knee HCC
- MØ6.Ø69 Rheumatoid arthritis without rheumatoid factor, unspecified knee HCC

MØ6.Ø7 Rheumatoid arthritis without rheumatoid factor, ankle and foot
- MØ6.Ø71 Rheumatoid arthritis without rheumatoid factor, right ankle and foot HCC
- MØ6.Ø72 Rheumatoid arthritis without rheumatoid factor, left ankle and foot HCC
- MØ6.Ø79 Rheumatoid arthritis without rheumatoid factor, unspecified ankle and foot HCC

MØ6.Ø8 Rheumatoid arthritis without rheumatoid factor, vertebrae HCC

MØ6.Ø9 Rheumatoid arthritis without rheumatoid factor, multiple sites HCC

MØ6.ØA Rheumatoid arthritis without rheumatoid factor, other specified site HCC

MØ6.1 Adult-onset Still's disease HCC A

EXCLUDES 1 *Still's disease NOS (MØ8.2-)*

DEF: Type of systemic arthritis characterized by a transient rash and spiking fevers. This condition may resolve or develop into a chronic condition and may affect internal organs, as well as joints.

Synonym(s): *AOSD*

MØ6.2 Rheumatoid bursitis

MØ6.2Ø Rheumatoid bursitis, unspecified site HCC

MØ6.21 Rheumatoid bursitis, shoulder
- MØ6.211 Rheumatoid bursitis, right shoulder HCC
- MØ6.212 Rheumatoid bursitis, left shoulder HCC
- MØ6.219 Rheumatoid bursitis, unspecified shoulder HCC

MØ6.22 Rheumatoid bursitis, elbow
- MØ6.221 Rheumatoid bursitis, right elbow HCC
- MØ6.222 Rheumatoid bursitis, left elbow HCC
- MØ6.229 Rheumatoid bursitis, unspecified elbow HCC

MØ6.23 Rheumatoid bursitis, wrist
- MØ6.231 Rheumatoid bursitis, right wrist HCC
- MØ6.232 Rheumatoid bursitis, left wrist HCC
- MØ6.239 Rheumatoid bursitis, unspecified wrist HCC

MØ6.24 Rheumatoid bursitis, hand
- MØ6.241 Rheumatoid bursitis, right hand HCC
- MØ6.242 Rheumatoid bursitis, left hand HCC
- MØ6.249 Rheumatoid bursitis, unspecified hand HCC

MØ6.25 Rheumatoid bursitis, hip
- MØ6.251 Rheumatoid bursitis, right hip HCC
- MØ6.252 Rheumatoid bursitis, left hip HCC
- MØ6.259 Rheumatoid bursitis, unspecified hip HCC

MØ6.26 Rheumatoid bursitis, knee
- MØ6.261 Rheumatoid bursitis, right knee HCC
- MØ6.262 Rheumatoid bursitis, left knee HCC
- MØ6.269 Rheumatoid bursitis, unspecified knee HCC

MØ6.27 Rheumatoid bursitis, ankle and foot
- MØ6.271 Rheumatoid bursitis, right ankle and foot HCC
- MØ6.272 Rheumatoid bursitis, left ankle and foot HCC
- MØ6.279 Rheumatoid bursitis, unspecified ankle and foot HCC

MØ6.28 Rheumatoid bursitis, vertebrae HCC

MØ6.29 Rheumatoid bursitis, multiple sites HCC

MØ6.3 Rheumatoid nodule

MØ6.3Ø Rheumatoid nodule, unspecified site HCC

MØ6.31 Rheumatoid nodule, shoulder
- MØ6.311 Rheumatoid nodule, right shoulder HCC
- MØ6.312 Rheumatoid nodule, left shoulder HCC
- MØ6.319 Rheumatoid nodule, unspecified shoulder HCC

MØ6.32 Rheumatoid nodule, elbow
- MØ6.321 Rheumatoid nodule, right elbow HCC
- MØ6.322 Rheumatoid nodule, left elbow HCC
- MØ6.329 Rheumatoid nodule, unspecified elbow HCC

MØ6.33 Rheumatoid nodule, wrist
- MØ6.331 Rheumatoid nodule, right wrist HCC
- MØ6.332 Rheumatoid nodule, left wrist HCC
- MØ6.339 Rheumatoid nodule, unspecified wrist HCC

M06.34 Rheumatoid nodule, hand
- M06.341 Rheumatoid nodule, right hand HCC
- M06.342 Rheumatoid nodule, left hand HCC
- M06.349 Rheumatoid nodule, unspecified hand HCC

M06.35 Rheumatoid nodule, hip
- M06.351 Rheumatoid nodule, right hip HCC
- M06.352 Rheumatoid nodule, left hip HCC
- M06.359 Rheumatoid nodule, unspecified hip HCC

M06.36 Rheumatoid nodule, knee
- M06.361 Rheumatoid nodule, right knee HCC
- M06.362 Rheumatoid nodule, left knee HCC
- M06.369 Rheumatoid nodule, unspecified knee HCC

M06.37 Rheumatoid nodule, ankle and foot
- M06.371 Rheumatoid nodule, right ankle and foot HCC
- M06.372 Rheumatoid nodule, left ankle and foot HCC
- M06.379 Rheumatoid nodule, unspecified ankle and foot HCC

M06.38 Rheumatoid nodule, vertebrae HCC

M06.39 Rheumatoid nodule, multiple sites HCC

M06.4 Inflammatory polyarthropathy HCC

EXCLUDES 1 *polyarthritis NOS (M13.0)*

M06.8 Other specified rheumatoid arthritis

M06.80 Other specified rheumatoid arthritis, unspecified site HCC

M06.81 Other specified rheumatoid arthritis, shoulder
- M06.811 Other specified rheumatoid arthritis, right shoulder HCC
- M06.812 Other specified rheumatoid arthritis, left shoulder HCC
- M06.819 Other specified rheumatoid arthritis, unspecified shoulder HCC

M06.82 Other specified rheumatoid arthritis, elbow
- M06.821 Other specified rheumatoid arthritis, right elbow HCC
- M06.822 Other specified rheumatoid arthritis, left elbow HCC
- M06.829 Other specified rheumatoid arthritis, unspecified elbow HCC

M06.83 Other specified rheumatoid arthritis, wrist
- M06.831 Other specified rheumatoid arthritis, right wrist HCC
- M06.832 Other specified rheumatoid arthritis, left wrist HCC
- M06.839 Other specified rheumatoid arthritis, unspecified wrist HCC

M06.84 Other specified rheumatoid arthritis, hand
- M06.841 Other specified rheumatoid arthritis, right hand HCC
- M06.842 Other specified rheumatoid arthritis, left hand HCC
- M06.849 Other specified rheumatoid arthritis, unspecified hand HCC

M06.85 Other specified rheumatoid arthritis, hip
- M06.851 Other specified rheumatoid arthritis, right hip HCC
- M06.852 Other specified rheumatoid arthritis, left hip HCC
- M06.859 Other specified rheumatoid arthritis, unspecified hip HCC

M06.86 Other specified rheumatoid arthritis, knee
- M06.861 Other specified rheumatoid arthritis, right knee HCC
- M06.862 Other specified rheumatoid arthritis, left knee HCC
- M06.869 Other specified rheumatoid arthritis, unspecified knee HCC

M06.87 Other specified rheumatoid arthritis, ankle and foot
- M06.871 Other specified rheumatoid arthritis, right ankle and foot HCC
- M06.872 Other specified rheumatoid arthritis, left ankle and foot HCC
- M06.879 Other specified rheumatoid arthritis, unspecified ankle and foot HCC

M06.88 Other specified rheumatoid arthritis, vertebrae HCC

M06.89 Other specified rheumatoid arthritis, multiple sites HCC

M06.8A Other specified rheumatoid arthritis, other specified site HCC

M06.9 Rheumatoid arthritis, unspecified HCC

M07 Enteropathic arthropathies

Code also associated enteropathy, such as:
- regional enteritis [Crohn's disease] (K50.-)
- ulcerative colitis (K51.-)

EXCLUDES 1 *psoriatic arthropathies (L40.5-)*

M07.6 Enteropathic arthropathies

M07.60 Enteropathic arthropathies, unspecified site

M07.61 Enteropathic arthropathies, shoulder
- M07.611 Enteropathic arthropathies, right shoulder
- M07.612 Enteropathic arthropathies, left shoulder
- M07.619 Enteropathic arthropathies, unspecified shoulder

M07.62 Enteropathic arthropathies, elbow
- M07.621 Enteropathic arthropathies, right elbow
- M07.622 Enteropathic arthropathies, left elbow
- M07.629 Enteropathic arthropathies, unspecified elbow

M07.63 Enteropathic arthropathies, wrist
- M07.631 Enteropathic arthropathies, right wrist
- M07.632 Enteropathic arthropathies, left wrist
- M07.639 Enteropathic arthropathies, unspecified wrist

M07.64 Enteropathic arthropathies, hand
- M07.641 Enteropathic arthropathies, right hand
- M07.642 Enteropathic arthropathies, left hand
- M07.649 Enteropathic arthropathies, unspecified hand

M07.65 Enteropathic arthropathies, hip
- M07.651 Enteropathic arthropathies, right hip
- M07.652 Enteropathic arthropathies, left hip
- M07.659 Enteropathic arthropathies, unspecified hip

M07.66 Enteropathic arthropathies, knee
- M07.661 Enteropathic arthropathies, right knee
- M07.662 Enteropathic arthropathies, left knee
- M07.669 Enteropathic arthropathies, unspecified knee

M07.67 Enteropathic arthropathies, ankle and foot
- M07.671 Enteropathic arthropathies, right ankle and foot
- M07.672 Enteropathic arthropathies, left ankle and foot
- M07.679 Enteropathic arthropathies, unspecified ankle and foot

M07.68 Enteropathic arthropathies, vertebrae

M07.69 Enteropathic arthropathies, multiple sites

M08 Juvenile arthritis

Code also any associated underlying condition, such as:
- regional enteritis [Crohn's disease] (K50.-)
- ulcerative colitis (K51.-)

EXCLUDES 1 *arthropathy in Whipple's disease (M14.8)*
Felty's syndrome (M05.0)
juvenile dermatomyositis (M33.0-)
psoriatic juvenile arthropathy (L40.54)

AHA: 2020,4Q,31-32

M08.0 Unspecified juvenile rheumatoid arthritis

Juvenile rheumatoid arthritis with or without rheumatoid factor

M08.00 Unspecified juvenile rheumatoid arthritis of unspecified site HCC

M08.01 Unspecified juvenile rheumatoid arthritis, shoulder
- M08.011 Unspecified juvenile rheumatoid arthritis, right shoulder HCC
- M08.012 Unspecified juvenile rheumatoid arthritis, left shoulder HCC
- M08.019 Unspecified juvenile rheumatoid arthritis, unspecified shoulder HCC

MØ8.Ø2 Unspecified juvenile rheumatoid arthritis of elbow
- **MØ8.Ø21 Unspecified juvenile rheumatoid arthritis, right elbow** HCC
- **MØ8.Ø22 Unspecified juvenile rheumatoid arthritis, left elbow** HCC
- **MØ8.Ø29 Unspecified juvenile rheumatoid arthritis, unspecified elbow** HCC

MØ8.Ø3 Unspecified juvenile rheumatoid arthritis, wrist
- **MØ8.Ø31 Unspecified juvenile rheumatoid arthritis, right wrist** HCC
- **MØ8.Ø32 Unspecified juvenile rheumatoid arthritis, left wrist** HCC
- **MØ8.Ø39 Unspecified juvenile rheumatoid arthritis, unspecified wrist** HCC

MØ8.Ø4 Unspecified juvenile rheumatoid arthritis, hand
- **MØ8.Ø41 Unspecified juvenile rheumatoid arthritis, right hand** HCC
- **MØ8.Ø42 Unspecified juvenile rheumatoid arthritis, left hand** HCC
- **MØ8.Ø49 Unspecified juvenile rheumatoid arthritis, unspecified hand** HCC

MØ8.Ø5 Unspecified juvenile rheumatoid arthritis, hip
- **MØ8.Ø51 Unspecified juvenile rheumatoid arthritis, right hip** HCC
- **MØ8.Ø52 Unspecified juvenile rheumatoid arthritis, left hip** HCC
- **MØ8.Ø59 Unspecified juvenile rheumatoid arthritis, unspecified hip** HCC

MØ8.Ø6 Unspecified juvenile rheumatoid arthritis, knee
- **MØ8.Ø61 Unspecified juvenile rheumatoid arthritis, right knee** HCC
- **MØ8.Ø62 Unspecified juvenile rheumatoid arthritis, left knee** HCC
- **MØ8.Ø69 Unspecified juvenile rheumatoid arthritis, unspecified knee** HCC

MØ8.Ø7 Unspecified juvenile rheumatoid arthritis, ankle and foot
- **MØ8.Ø71 Unspecified juvenile rheumatoid arthritis, right ankle and foot** HCC
- **MØ8.Ø72 Unspecified juvenile rheumatoid arthritis, left ankle and foot** HCC
- **MØ8.Ø79 Unspecified juvenile rheumatoid arthritis, unspecified ankle and foot** HCC

MØ8.Ø8 Unspecified juvenile rheumatoid arthritis, vertebrae HCC

MØ8.Ø9 Unspecified juvenile rheumatoid arthritis, multiple sites HCC

MØ8.ØA Unspecified juvenile rheumatoid arthritis, other specified site HCC

MØ8.1 Juvenile ankylosing spondylitis HCC

EXCLUDES 1 *ankylosing spondylitis in adults (M45.Ø-)*

MØ8.2 Juvenile rheumatoid arthritis with systemic onset

Still's disease NOS

EXCLUDES 1 *adult-onset Still's disease (MØ6.1-)*

DEF: Systemic juvenile rheumatoid arthritis characterized by a transient rash and spiking fevers that may affect internal organs, as well as joints.

MØ8.2Ø Juvenile rheumatoid arthritis with systemic onset, unspecified site HCC

MØ8.21 Juvenile rheumatoid arthritis with systemic onset, shoulder
- **MØ8.211 Juvenile rheumatoid arthritis with systemic onset, right shoulder** HCC
- **MØ8.212 Juvenile rheumatoid arthritis with systemic onset, left shoulder** HCC
- **MØ8.219 Juvenile rheumatoid arthritis with systemic onset, unspecified shoulder** HCC

MØ8.22 Juvenile rheumatoid arthritis with systemic onset, elbow
- **MØ8.221 Juvenile rheumatoid arthritis with systemic onset, right elbow** HCC
- **MØ8.222 Juvenile rheumatoid arthritis with systemic onset, left elbow** HCC
- **MØ8.229 Juvenile rheumatoid arthritis with systemic onset, unspecified elbow** HCC

MØ8.23 Juvenile rheumatoid arthritis with systemic onset, wrist
- **MØ8.231 Juvenile rheumatoid arthritis with systemic onset, right wrist** HCC
- **MØ8.232 Juvenile rheumatoid arthritis with systemic onset, left wrist** HCC
- **MØ8.239 Juvenile rheumatoid arthritis with systemic onset, unspecified wrist** HCC

MØ8.24 Juvenile rheumatoid arthritis with systemic onset, hand
- **MØ8.241 Juvenile rheumatoid arthritis with systemic onset, right hand** HCC
- **MØ8.242 Juvenile rheumatoid arthritis with systemic onset, left hand** HCC
- **MØ8.249 Juvenile rheumatoid arthritis with systemic onset, unspecified hand** HCC

MØ8.25 Juvenile rheumatoid arthritis with systemic onset, hip
- **MØ8.251 Juvenile rheumatoid arthritis with systemic onset, right hip** HCC
- **MØ8.252 Juvenile rheumatoid arthritis with systemic onset, left hip** HCC
- **MØ8.259 Juvenile rheumatoid arthritis with systemic onset, unspecified hip** HCC

MØ8.26 Juvenile rheumatoid arthritis with systemic onset, knee
- **MØ8.261 Juvenile rheumatoid arthritis with systemic onset, right knee** HCC
- **MØ8.262 Juvenile rheumatoid arthritis with systemic onset, left knee** HCC
- **MØ8.269 Juvenile rheumatoid arthritis with systemic onset, unspecified knee** HCC

MØ8.27 Juvenile rheumatoid arthritis with systemic onset, ankle and foot
- **MØ8.271 Juvenile rheumatoid arthritis with systemic onset, right ankle and foot** HCC
- **MØ8.272 Juvenile rheumatoid arthritis with systemic onset, left ankle and foot** HCC
- **MØ8.279 Juvenile rheumatoid arthritis with systemic onset, unspecified ankle and foot** HCC

MØ8.28 Juvenile rheumatoid arthritis with systemic onset, vertebrae HCC

MØ8.29 Juvenile rheumatoid arthritis with systemic onset, multiple sites HCC

MØ8.2A Juvenile rheumatoid arthritis with systemic onset, other specified site HCC

MØ8.3 Juvenile rheumatoid polyarthritis (seronegative) HCC

MØ8.4 Pauciarticular juvenile rheumatoid arthritis

MØ8.4Ø Pauciarticular juvenile rheumatoid arthritis, unspecified site HCC

MØ8.41 Pauciarticular juvenile rheumatoid arthritis, shoulder
- **MØ8.411 Pauciarticular juvenile rheumatoid arthritis, right shoulder** HCC
- **MØ8.412 Pauciarticular juvenile rheumatoid arthritis, left shoulder** HCC
- **MØ8.419 Pauciarticular juvenile rheumatoid arthritis, unspecified shoulder** HCC

MØ8.42 Pauciarticular juvenile rheumatoid arthritis, elbow
- **MØ8.421 Pauciarticular juvenile rheumatoid arthritis, right elbow** HCC
- **MØ8.422 Pauciarticular juvenile rheumatoid arthritis, left elbow** HCC
- **MØ8.429 Pauciarticular juvenile rheumatoid arthritis, unspecified elbow** HCC

MØ8.43 Pauciarticular juvenile rheumatoid arthritis, wrist
- **MØ8.431 Pauciarticular juvenile rheumatoid arthritis, right wrist** HCC
- **MØ8.432 Pauciarticular juvenile rheumatoid arthritis, left wrist** HCC
- **MØ8.439 Pauciarticular juvenile rheumatoid arthritis, unspecified wrist** HCC

MØ8.44 Pauciarticular juvenile rheumatoid arthritis, hand
- **MØ8.441 Pauciarticular juvenile rheumatoid arthritis, right hand** HCC
- **MØ8.442 Pauciarticular juvenile rheumatoid arthritis, left hand** HCC
- **MØ8.449 Pauciarticular juvenile rheumatoid arthritis, unspecified hand** HCC

MØ8.45 Pauciarticular juvenile rheumatoid arthritis, hip
- **MØ8.451 Pauciarticular juvenile rheumatoid arthritis, right hip** HCC

M08.452 Pauciarticular juvenile rheumatoid arthritis, left hip HCC
M08.459 Pauciarticular juvenile rheumatoid arthritis, unspecified hip HCC
✓6th M08.46 Pauciarticular juvenile rheumatoid arthritis, knee
M08.461 Pauciarticular juvenile rheumatoid arthritis, right knee HCC
M08.462 Pauciarticular juvenile rheumatoid arthritis, left knee HCC
M08.469 Pauciarticular juvenile rheumatoid arthritis, unspecified knee HCC
✓6th M08.47 Pauciarticular juvenile rheumatoid arthritis, ankle and foot
M08.471 Pauciarticular juvenile rheumatoid arthritis, right ankle and foot HCC
M08.472 Pauciarticular juvenile rheumatoid arthritis, left ankle and foot HCC
M08.479 Pauciarticular juvenile rheumatoid arthritis, unspecified ankle and foot HCC
M08.48 Pauciarticular juvenile rheumatoid arthritis, vertebrae HCC
M08.4A Pauciarticular juvenile rheumatoid arthritis, other specified site HCC
✓5th M08.8 Other juvenile arthritis
M08.80 Other juvenile arthritis, unspecified site HCC
✓6th M08.81 Other juvenile arthritis, shoulder
M08.811 Other juvenile arthritis, right shoulder HCC
M08.812 Other juvenile arthritis, left shoulder HCC
M08.819 Other juvenile arthritis, unspecified shoulder HCC
✓6th M08.82 Other juvenile arthritis, elbow
M08.821 Other juvenile arthritis, right elbow HCC
M08.822 Other juvenile arthritis, left elbow HCC
M08.829 Other juvenile arthritis, unspecified elbow HCC
✓6th M08.83 Other juvenile arthritis, wrist
M08.831 Other juvenile arthritis, right wrist HCC
M08.832 Other juvenile arthritis, left wrist HCC
M08.839 Other juvenile arthritis, unspecified wrist HCC
✓6th M08.84 Other juvenile arthritis, hand
M08.841 Other juvenile arthritis, right hand HCC
M08.842 Other juvenile arthritis, left hand HCC
M08.849 Other juvenile arthritis, unspecified hand HCC
✓6th M08.85 Other juvenile arthritis, hip
M08.851 Other juvenile arthritis, right hip HCC
M08.852 Other juvenile arthritis, left hip HCC
M08.859 Other juvenile arthritis, unspecified hip HCC
✓6th M08.86 Other juvenile arthritis, knee
M08.861 Other juvenile arthritis, right knee HCC
M08.862 Other juvenile arthritis, left knee HCC
M08.869 Other juvenile arthritis, unspecified knee HCC
✓6th M08.87 Other juvenile arthritis, ankle and foot
M08.871 Other juvenile arthritis, right ankle and foot HCC
M08.872 Other juvenile arthritis, left ankle and foot HCC
M08.879 Other juvenile arthritis, unspecified ankle and foot HCC
M08.88 Other juvenile arthritis, other specified site HCC
Other juvenile arthritis, vertebrae
M08.89 Other juvenile arthritis, multiple sites HCC
✓5th M08.9 Juvenile arthritis, unspecified
EXCLUDES 1 *juvenile rheumatoid arthritis, unspecified (M08.0-)*
M08.90 Juvenile arthritis, unspecified, unspecified site HCC
✓6th M08.91 Juvenile arthritis, unspecified, shoulder
M08.911 Juvenile arthritis, unspecified, right shoulder HCC
M08.912 Juvenile arthritis, unspecified, left shoulder HCC
M08.919 Juvenile arthritis, unspecified, unspecified shoulder HCC
✓6th M08.92 Juvenile arthritis, unspecified, elbow
M08.921 Juvenile arthritis, unspecified, right elbow HCC
M08.922 Juvenile arthritis, unspecified, left elbow HCC
M08.929 Juvenile arthritis, unspecified, unspecified elbow HCC
✓6th M08.93 Juvenile arthritis, unspecified, wrist
M08.931 Juvenile arthritis, unspecified, right wrist HCC
M08.932 Juvenile arthritis, unspecified, left wrist HCC
M08.939 Juvenile arthritis, unspecified, unspecified wrist HCC
✓6th M08.94 Juvenile arthritis, unspecified, hand
M08.941 Juvenile arthritis, unspecified, right hand HCC
M08.942 Juvenile arthritis, unspecified, left hand HCC
M08.949 Juvenile arthritis, unspecified, unspecified hand HCC
✓6th M08.95 Juvenile arthritis, unspecified, hip
M08.951 Juvenile arthritis, unspecified, right hip HCC
M08.952 Juvenile arthritis, unspecified, left hip HCC
M08.959 Juvenile arthritis, unspecified, unspecified hip HCC
✓6th M08.96 Juvenile arthritis, unspecified, knee
M08.961 Juvenile arthritis, unspecified, right knee HCC
M08.962 Juvenile arthritis, unspecified, left knee HCC
M08.969 Juvenile arthritis, unspecified, unspecified knee HCC
✓6th M08.97 Juvenile arthritis, unspecified, ankle and foot
M08.971 Juvenile arthritis, unspecified, right ankle and foot HCC
M08.972 Juvenile arthritis, unspecified, left ankle and foot HCC
M08.979 Juvenile arthritis, unspecified, unspecified ankle and foot HCC
M08.98 Juvenile arthritis, unspecified, vertebrae HCC
M08.99 Juvenile arthritis, unspecified, multiple sites HCC
M08.9A Juvenile arthritis, unspecified, other specified site HCC

✓4th **M1A Chronic gout**

Use additional code to identify:
autonomic neuropathy in diseases classified elsewhere (G99.0)
calculus of urinary tract in diseases classified elsewhere (N22)
cardiomyopathy in diseases classified elsewhere (I43)
disorders of external ear in diseases classified elsewhere (H61.1-, H62.8-)
disorders of iris and ciliary body in diseases classified elsewhere (H22)
glomerular disorders in diseases classified elsewhere (N08)

EXCLUDES 1 *gout NOS (M10.-)*
EXCLUDES 2 *acute gout (M10.-)*

The appropriate 7th character is to be added to each code from category M1A.
0 without tophus (tophi)
1 with tophus (tophi)

✓5th M1A.0 Idiopathic chronic gout
Chronic gouty bursitis
Primary chronic gout
✓x7th M1A.00 Idiopathic chronic gout, unspecified site
✓6th M1A.01 Idiopathic chronic gout, shoulder
✓7th M1A.011 Idiopathic chronic gout, right shoulder
✓7th M1A.012 Idiopathic chronic gout, left shoulder
✓7th M1A.019 Idiopathic chronic gout, unspecified shoulder
✓6th M1A.02 Idiopathic chronic gout, elbow
✓7th M1A.021 Idiopathic chronic gout, right elbow

√7th M1A.022 Idiopathic chronic gout, left elbow
√7th M1A.029 Idiopathic chronic gout, unspecified elbow
√6th M1A.03 Idiopathic chronic gout, wrist
√7th M1A.031 Idiopathic chronic gout, right wrist
√7th M1A.032 Idiopathic chronic gout, left wrist
√7th M1A.039 Idiopathic chronic gout, unspecified wrist
√6th M1A.04 Idiopathic chronic gout, hand
√7th M1A.041 Idiopathic chronic gout, right hand
√7th M1A.042 Idiopathic chronic gout, left hand
√7th M1A.049 Idiopathic chronic gout, unspecified hand
√6th M1A.05 Idiopathic chronic gout, hip
√7th M1A.051 Idiopathic chronic gout, right hip
√7th M1A.052 Idiopathic chronic gout, left hip
√7th M1A.059 Idiopathic chronic gout, unspecified hip
√6th M1A.06 Idiopathic chronic gout, knee
√7th M1A.061 Idiopathic chronic gout, right knee
√7th M1A.062 Idiopathic chronic gout, left knee
√7th M1A.069 Idiopathic chronic gout, unspecified knee
√6th M1A.07 Idiopathic chronic gout, ankle and foot
√7th M1A.071 Idiopathic chronic gout, right ankle and foot
√7th M1A.072 Idiopathic chronic gout, left ankle and foot
√7th M1A.079 Idiopathic chronic gout, unspecified ankle and foot
√x7th M1A.08 Idiopathic chronic gout, vertebrae
√x7th M1A.09 Idiopathic chronic gout, multiple sites

√5th M1A.1 Lead-induced chronic gout
Code first toxic effects of lead and its compounds (T56.0-)
√x7th M1A.10 Lead-induced chronic gout, unspecified site
√6th M1A.11 Lead-induced chronic gout, shoulder
√7th M1A.111 Lead-induced chronic gout, right shoulder
√7th M1A.112 Lead-induced chronic gout, left shoulder
√7th M1A.119 Lead-induced chronic gout, unspecified shoulder
√6th M1A.12 Lead-induced chronic gout, elbow
√7th M1A.121 Lead-induced chronic gout, right elbow
√7th M1A.122 Lead-induced chronic gout, left elbow
√7th M1A.129 Lead-induced chronic gout, unspecified elbow
√6th M1A.13 Lead-induced chronic gout, wrist
√7th M1A.131 Lead-induced chronic gout, right wrist
√7th M1A.132 Lead-induced chronic gout, left wrist
√7th M1A.139 Lead-induced chronic gout, unspecified wrist
√6th M1A.14 Lead-induced chronic gout, hand
√7th M1A.141 Lead-induced chronic gout, right hand
√7th M1A.142 Lead-induced chronic gout, left hand
√7th M1A.149 Lead-induced chronic gout, unspecified hand
√6th M1A.15 Lead-induced chronic gout, hip
√7th M1A.151 Lead-induced chronic gout, right hip
√7th M1A.152 Lead-induced chronic gout, left hip
√7th M1A.159 Lead-induced chronic gout, unspecified hip
√6th M1A.16 Lead-induced chronic gout, knee
√7th M1A.161 Lead-induced chronic gout, right knee
√7th M1A.162 Lead-induced chronic gout, left knee
√7th M1A.169 Lead-induced chronic gout, unspecified knee
√6th M1A.17 Lead-induced chronic gout, ankle and foot
√7th M1A.171 Lead-induced chronic gout, right ankle and foot
√7th M1A.172 Lead-induced chronic gout, left ankle and foot
√7th M1A.179 Lead-induced chronic gout, unspecified ankle and foot
√x7th M1A.18 Lead-induced chronic gout, vertebrae
√x7th M1A.19 Lead-induced chronic gout, multiple sites

√5th M1A.2 Drug-induced chronic gout
Use additional code for adverse effect, if applicable, to identify drug (T36-T50 with fifth or sixth character 5)
√x7th M1A.20 Drug-induced chronic gout, unspecified site
√6th M1A.21 Drug-induced chronic gout, shoulder
√7th M1A.211 Drug-induced chronic gout, right shoulder
√7th M1A.212 Drug-induced chronic gout, left shoulder
√7th M1A.219 Drug-induced chronic gout, unspecified shoulder
√6th M1A.22 Drug-induced chronic gout, elbow
√7th M1A.221 Drug-induced chronic gout, right elbow
√7th M1A.222 Drug-induced chronic gout, left elbow
√7th M1A.229 Drug-induced chronic gout, unspecified elbow
√6th M1A.23 Drug-induced chronic gout, wrist
√7th M1A.231 Drug-induced chronic gout, right wrist
√7th M1A.232 Drug-induced chronic gout, left wrist
√7th M1A.239 Drug-induced chronic gout, unspecified wrist
√6th M1A.24 Drug-induced chronic gout, hand
√7th M1A.241 Drug-induced chronic gout, right hand
√7th M1A.242 Drug-induced chronic gout, left hand
√7th M1A.249 Drug-induced chronic gout, unspecified hand
√6th M1A.25 Drug-induced chronic gout, hip
√7th M1A.251 Drug-induced chronic gout, right hip
√7th M1A.252 Drug-induced chronic gout, left hip
√7th M1A.259 Drug-induced chronic gout, unspecified hip
√6th M1A.26 Drug-induced chronic gout, knee
√7th M1A.261 Drug-induced chronic gout, right knee
√7th M1A.262 Drug-induced chronic gout, left knee
√7th M1A.269 Drug-induced chronic gout, unspecified knee
√6th M1A.27 Drug-induced chronic gout, ankle and foot
√7th M1A.271 Drug-induced chronic gout, right ankle and foot
√7th M1A.272 Drug-induced chronic gout, left ankle and foot
√7th M1A.279 Drug-induced chronic gout, unspecified ankle and foot
√x7th M1A.28 Drug-induced chronic gout, vertebrae
√x7th M1A.29 Drug-induced chronic gout, multiple sites

√5th M1A.3 Chronic gout due to renal impairment
Code first associated renal disease
√x7th M1A.30 Chronic gout due to renal impairment, unspecified site
√6th M1A.31 Chronic gout due to renal impairment, shoulder
√7th M1A.311 Chronic gout due to renal impairment, right shoulder
√7th M1A.312 Chronic gout due to renal impairment, left shoulder
√7th M1A.319 Chronic gout due to renal impairment, unspecified shoulder
√6th M1A.32 Chronic gout due to renal impairment, elbow
√7th M1A.321 Chronic gout due to renal impairment, right elbow
√7th M1A.322 Chronic gout due to renal impairment, left elbow
√7th M1A.329 Chronic gout due to renal impairment, unspecified elbow
√6th M1A.33 Chronic gout due to renal impairment, wrist
√7th M1A.331 Chronic gout due to renal impairment, right wrist
√7th M1A.332 Chronic gout due to renal impairment, left wrist
√7th M1A.339 Chronic gout due to renal impairment, unspecified wrist
√6th M1A.34 Chronic gout due to renal impairment, hand
√7th M1A.341 Chronic gout due to renal impairment, right hand
√7th M1A.342 Chronic gout due to renal impairment, left hand
√7th M1A.349 Chronic gout due to renal impairment, unspecified hand

M1A.35 **Chronic gout due to renal impairment, hip**
- M1A.351 Chronic gout due to renal impairment, right hip
- M1A.352 Chronic gout due to renal impairment, left hip
- M1A.359 Chronic gout due to renal impairment, unspecified hip

M1A.36 **Chronic gout due to renal impairment, knee**
- M1A.361 Chronic gout due to renal impairment, right knee
- M1A.362 Chronic gout due to renal impairment, left knee
- M1A.369 Chronic gout due to renal impairment, unspecified knee

M1A.37 **Chronic gout due to renal impairment, ankle and foot**
- M1A.371 Chronic gout due to renal impairment, right ankle and foot
- M1A.372 Chronic gout due to renal impairment, left ankle and foot
- M1A.379 Chronic gout due to renal impairment, unspecified ankle and foot

M1A.38 **Chronic gout due to renal impairment, vertebrae**

M1A.39 **Chronic gout due to renal impairment, multiple sites**

M1A.4 **Other secondary chronic gout**

Code first associated condition

M1A.40 **Other secondary chronic gout, unspecified site**

M1A.41 **Other secondary chronic gout, shoulder**
- M1A.411 Other secondary chronic gout, right shoulder
- M1A.412 Other secondary chronic gout, left shoulder
- M1A.419 Other secondary chronic gout, unspecified shoulder

M1A.42 **Other secondary chronic gout, elbow**
- M1A.421 Other secondary chronic gout, right elbow
- M1A.422 Other secondary chronic gout, left elbow
- M1A.429 Other secondary chronic gout, unspecified elbow

M1A.43 **Other secondary chronic gout, wrist**
- M1A.431 Other secondary chronic gout, right wrist
- M1A.432 Other secondary chronic gout, left wrist
- M1A.439 Other secondary chronic gout, unspecified wrist

M1A.44 **Other secondary chronic gout, hand**
- M1A.441 Other secondary chronic gout, right hand
- M1A.442 Other secondary chronic gout, left hand
- M1A.449 Other secondary chronic gout, unspecified hand

M1A.45 **Other secondary chronic gout, hip**
- M1A.451 Other secondary chronic gout, right hip
- M1A.452 Other secondary chronic gout, left hip
- M1A.459 Other secondary chronic gout, unspecified hip

M1A.46 **Other secondary chronic gout, knee**
- M1A.461 Other secondary chronic gout, right knee
- M1A.462 Other secondary chronic gout, left knee
- M1A.469 Other secondary chronic gout, unspecified knee

M1A.47 **Other secondary chronic gout, ankle and foot**
- M1A.471 Other secondary chronic gout, right ankle and foot
- M1A.472 Other secondary chronic gout, left ankle and foot
- M1A.479 Other secondary chronic gout, unspecified ankle and foot

M1A.48 **Other secondary chronic gout, vertebrae**

M1A.49 **Other secondary chronic gout, multiple sites**

M1A.9 **Chronic gout, unspecified**

M10 Gout

Acute gout
Gout attack
Gout flare
Podagra

Use additional code to identify:
- autonomic neuropathy in diseases classified elsewhere (G99.0)
- calculus of urinary tract in diseases classified elsewhere (N22)
- cardiomyopathy in diseases classified elsewhere (I43)
- disorders of external ear in diseases classified elsewhere (H61.1-, H62.8-)
- disorders of iris and ciliary body in diseases classified elsewhere (H22)
- glomerular disorders in diseases classified elsewhere (N08)

EXCLUDES 2 *chronic gout (M1A.-)*

DEF: Purine and pyrimidine metabolic disorders, manifested by hyperuricemia and recurrent acute inflammatory arthritis. Monosodium urate or monohydrate crystals may be deposited in and around the joints, leading to joint destruction and severe crippling.

M10.0 **Idiopathic gout**

Gouty bursitis
Primary gout

M10.00 **Idiopathic gout, unspecified site**

M10.01 **Idiopathic gout, shoulder**
- M10.011 Idiopathic gout, right shoulder
- M10.012 Idiopathic gout, left shoulder
- M10.019 Idiopathic gout, unspecified shoulder

M10.02 **Idiopathic gout, elbow**
- M10.021 Idiopathic gout, right elbow
- M10.022 Idiopathic gout, left elbow
- M10.029 Idiopathic gout, unspecified elbow

M10.03 **Idiopathic gout, wrist**
- M10.031 Idiopathic gout, right wrist
- M10.032 Idiopathic gout, left wrist
- M10.039 Idiopathic gout, unspecified wrist

M10.04 **Idiopathic gout, hand**
- M10.041 Idiopathic gout, right hand
- M10.042 Idiopathic gout, left hand
- M10.049 Idiopathic gout, unspecified hand

M10.05 **Idiopathic gout, hip**
- M10.051 Idiopathic gout, right hip
- M10.052 Idiopathic gout, left hip
- M10.059 Idiopathic gout, unspecified hip

M10.06 **Idiopathic gout, knee**
- M10.061 Idiopathic gout, right knee
- M10.062 Idiopathic gout, left knee
- M10.069 Idiopathic gout, unspecified knee

M10.07 **Idiopathic gout, ankle and foot**
- M10.071 Idiopathic gout, right ankle and foot
- M10.072 Idiopathic gout, left ankle and foot
- M10.079 Idiopathic gout, unspecified ankle and foot

M10.08 **Idiopathic gout, vertebrae**

M10.09 **Idiopathic gout, multiple sites**

M10.1 **Lead-induced gout**

Code first toxic effects of lead and its compounds (T56.0-)

M10.10 **Lead-induced gout, unspecified site**

M10.11 **Lead-induced gout, shoulder**
- M10.111 Lead-induced gout, right shoulder
- M10.112 Lead-induced gout, left shoulder
- M10.119 Lead-induced gout, unspecified shoulder

M10.12 **Lead-induced gout, elbow**
- M10.121 Lead-induced gout, right elbow
- M10.122 Lead-induced gout, left elbow
- M10.129 Lead-induced gout, unspecified elbow

M10.13 **Lead-induced gout, wrist**
- M10.131 Lead-induced gout, right wrist
- M10.132 Lead-induced gout, left wrist
- M10.139 Lead-induced gout, unspecified wrist

M10.14 **Lead-induced gout, hand**
- M10.141 Lead-induced gout, right hand
- M10.142 Lead-induced gout, left hand
- M10.149 Lead-induced gout, unspecified hand

M10.15 **Lead-induced gout, hip**
- M10.151 Lead-induced gout, right hip
- M10.152 Lead-induced gout, left hip
- M10.159 Lead-induced gout, unspecified hip

M10.16 Lead-induced gout, knee
M10.161 Lead-induced gout, right knee
M10.162 Lead-induced gout, left knee
M10.169 Lead-induced gout, unspecified knee
M10.17 Lead-induced gout, ankle and foot
M10.171 Lead-induced gout, right ankle and foot
M10.172 Lead-induced gout, left ankle and foot
M10.179 Lead-induced gout, unspecified ankle and foot
M10.18 Lead-induced gout, vertebrae
M10.19 Lead-induced gout, multiple sites
M10.2 Drug-induced gout
Use additional code for adverse effect, if applicable, to identify drug (T36-T50 with fifth or sixth character 5)
M10.20 Drug-induced gout, unspecified site
M10.21 Drug-induced gout, shoulder
M10.211 Drug-induced gout, right shoulder
M10.212 Drug-induced gout, left shoulder
M10.219 Drug-induced gout, unspecified shoulder
M10.22 Drug-induced gout, elbow
M10.221 Drug-induced gout, right elbow
M10.222 Drug-induced gout, left elbow
M10.229 Drug-induced gout, unspecified elbow
M10.23 Drug-induced gout, wrist
M10.231 Drug-induced gout, right wrist
M10.232 Drug-induced gout, left wrist
M10.239 Drug-induced gout, unspecified wrist
M10.24 Drug-induced gout, hand
M10.241 Drug-induced gout, right hand
M10.242 Drug-induced gout, left hand
M10.249 Drug-induced gout, unspecified hand
M10.25 Drug-induced gout, hip
M10.251 Drug-induced gout, right hip
M10.252 Drug-induced gout, left hip
M10.259 Drug-induced gout, unspecified hip
M10.26 Drug-induced gout, knee
M10.261 Drug-induced gout, right knee
M10.262 Drug-induced gout, left knee
M10.269 Drug-induced gout, unspecified knee
M10.27 Drug-induced gout, ankle and foot
M10.271 Drug-induced gout, right ankle and foot
M10.272 Drug-induced gout, left ankle and foot
M10.279 Drug-induced gout, unspecified ankle and foot
M10.28 Drug-induced gout, vertebrae
M10.29 Drug-induced gout, multiple sites
M10.3 Gout due to renal impairment
Code first associated renal disease
M10.30 Gout due to renal impairment, unspecified site
M10.31 Gout due to renal impairment, shoulder
M10.311 Gout due to renal impairment, right shoulder
M10.312 Gout due to renal impairment, left shoulder
M10.319 Gout due to renal impairment, unspecified shoulder
M10.32 Gout due to renal impairment, elbow
M10.321 Gout due to renal impairment, right elbow
M10.322 Gout due to renal impairment, left elbow
M10.329 Gout due to renal impairment, unspecified elbow
M10.33 Gout due to renal impairment, wrist
M10.331 Gout due to renal impairment, right wrist
M10.332 Gout due to renal impairment, left wrist
M10.339 Gout due to renal impairment, unspecified wrist
M10.34 Gout due to renal impairment, hand
M10.341 Gout due to renal impairment, right hand
M10.342 Gout due to renal impairment, left hand
M10.349 Gout due to renal impairment, unspecified hand
M10.35 Gout due to renal impairment, hip
M10.351 Gout due to renal impairment, right hip
M10.352 Gout due to renal impairment, left hip
M10.359 Gout due to renal impairment, unspecified hip
M10.36 Gout due to renal impairment, knee
M10.361 Gout due to renal impairment, right knee
M10.362 Gout due to renal impairment, left knee
M10.369 Gout due to renal impairment, unspecified knee
M10.37 Gout due to renal impairment, ankle and foot
M10.371 Gout due to renal impairment, right ankle and foot
M10.372 Gout due to renal impairment, left ankle and foot
M10.379 Gout due to renal impairment, unspecified ankle and foot
M10.38 Gout due to renal impairment, vertebrae
M10.39 Gout due to renal impairment, multiple sites
M10.4 Other secondary gout
Code first associated condition
M10.40 Other secondary gout, unspecified site
M10.41 Other secondary gout, shoulder
M10.411 Other secondary gout, right shoulder
M10.412 Other secondary gout, left shoulder
M10.419 Other secondary gout, unspecified shoulder
M10.42 Other secondary gout, elbow
M10.421 Other secondary gout, right elbow
M10.422 Other secondary gout, left elbow
M10.429 Other secondary gout, unspecified elbow
M10.43 Other secondary gout, wrist
M10.431 Other secondary gout, right wrist
M10.432 Other secondary gout, left wrist
M10.439 Other secondary gout, unspecified wrist
M10.44 Other secondary gout, hand
M10.441 Other secondary gout, right hand
M10.442 Other secondary gout, left hand
M10.449 Other secondary gout, unspecified hand
M10.45 Other secondary gout, hip
M10.451 Other secondary gout, right hip
M10.452 Other secondary gout, left hip
M10.459 Other secondary gout, unspecified hip
M10.46 Other secondary gout, knee
M10.461 Other secondary gout, right knee
M10.462 Other secondary gout, left knee
M10.469 Other secondary gout, unspecified knee
M10.47 Other secondary gout, ankle and foot
M10.471 Other secondary gout, right ankle and foot
M10.472 Other secondary gout, left ankle and foot
M10.479 Other secondary gout, unspecified ankle and foot
M10.48 Other secondary gout, vertebrae
M10.49 Other secondary gout, multiple sites
M10.9 Gout, unspecified
Gout NOS

M11 Other crystal arthropathies

M11.0 Hydroxyapatite deposition disease
DEF: Disease caused by deposits of calcium phosphate crystals in the soft tissues close to the joint (especially tendons) or in the joints. These calcifications can be mono or polyarticular and can cause destruction of the joint involved.
M11.00 Hydroxyapatite deposition disease, unspecified site
M11.01 Hydroxyapatite deposition disease, shoulder
M11.011 Hydroxyapatite deposition disease, right shoulder
M11.012 Hydroxyapatite deposition disease, left shoulder
M11.019 Hydroxyapatite deposition disease, unspecified shoulder
M11.02 Hydroxyapatite deposition disease, elbow
M11.021 Hydroxyapatite deposition disease, right elbow
M11.022 Hydroxyapatite deposition disease, left elbow
M11.029 Hydroxyapatite deposition disease, unspecified elbow

M11.03 Hydroxyapatite deposition disease, wrist
M11.031 Hydroxyapatite deposition disease, right wrist
M11.032 Hydroxyapatite deposition disease, left wrist
M11.039 Hydroxyapatite deposition disease, unspecified wrist
M11.04 Hydroxyapatite deposition disease, hand
M11.041 Hydroxyapatite deposition disease, right hand
M11.042 Hydroxyapatite deposition disease, left hand
M11.049 Hydroxyapatite deposition disease, unspecified hand
M11.05 Hydroxyapatite deposition disease, hip
M11.051 Hydroxyapatite deposition disease, right hip
M11.052 Hydroxyapatite deposition disease, left hip
M11.059 Hydroxyapatite deposition disease, unspecified hip
M11.06 Hydroxyapatite deposition disease, knee
M11.061 Hydroxyapatite deposition disease, right knee
M11.062 Hydroxyapatite deposition disease, left knee
M11.069 Hydroxyapatite deposition disease, unspecified knee
M11.07 Hydroxyapatite deposition disease, ankle and foot
M11.071 Hydroxyapatite deposition disease, right ankle and foot
M11.072 Hydroxyapatite deposition disease, left ankle and foot
M11.079 Hydroxyapatite deposition disease, unspecified ankle and foot
M11.08 Hydroxyapatite deposition disease, vertebrae
M11.09 Hydroxyapatite deposition disease, multiple sites
M11.1 Familial chondrocalcinosis
M11.10 Familial chondrocalcinosis, unspecified site
M11.11 Familial chondrocalcinosis, shoulder
M11.111 Familial chondrocalcinosis, right shoulder
M11.112 Familial chondrocalcinosis, left shoulder
M11.119 Familial chondrocalcinosis, unspecified shoulder
M11.12 Familial chondrocalcinosis, elbow
M11.121 Familial chondrocalcinosis, right elbow
M11.122 Familial chondrocalcinosis, left elbow
M11.129 Familial chondrocalcinosis, unspecified elbow
M11.13 Familial chondrocalcinosis, wrist
M11.131 Familial chondrocalcinosis, right wrist
M11.132 Familial chondrocalcinosis, left wrist
M11.139 Familial chondrocalcinosis, unspecified wrist
M11.14 Familial chondrocalcinosis, hand
M11.141 Familial chondrocalcinosis, right hand
M11.142 Familial chondrocalcinosis, left hand
M11.149 Familial chondrocalcinosis, unspecified hand
M11.15 Familial chondrocalcinosis, hip
M11.151 Familial chondrocalcinosis, right hip
M11.152 Familial chondrocalcinosis, left hip
M11.159 Familial chondrocalcinosis, unspecified hip
M11.16 Familial chondrocalcinosis, knee
M11.161 Familial chondrocalcinosis, right knee
M11.162 Familial chondrocalcinosis, left knee
M11.169 Familial chondrocalcinosis, unspecified knee
M11.17 Familial chondrocalcinosis, ankle and foot
M11.171 Familial chondrocalcinosis, right ankle and foot
M11.172 Familial chondrocalcinosis, left ankle and foot
M11.179 Familial chondrocalcinosis, unspecified ankle and foot
M11.18 Familial chondrocalcinosis, vertebrae
M11.19 Familial chondrocalcinosis, multiple sites
M11.2 Other chondrocalcinosis
Chondrocalcinosis NOS
AHA: 2018,3Q,20
TIP: Pseudogout is captured with codes in this subcategory.
M11.20 Other chondrocalcinosis, unspecified site
M11.21 Other chondrocalcinosis, shoulder
M11.211 Other chondrocalcinosis, right shoulder
M11.212 Other chondrocalcinosis, left shoulder
M11.219 Other chondrocalcinosis, unspecified shoulder
M11.22 Other chondrocalcinosis, elbow
M11.221 Other chondrocalcinosis, right elbow
M11.222 Other chondrocalcinosis, left elbow
M11.229 Other chondrocalcinosis, unspecified elbow
M11.23 Other chondrocalcinosis, wrist
M11.231 Other chondrocalcinosis, right wrist
M11.232 Other chondrocalcinosis, left wrist
M11.239 Other chondrocalcinosis, unspecified wrist
M11.24 Other chondrocalcinosis, hand
M11.241 Other chondrocalcinosis, right hand
M11.242 Other chondrocalcinosis, left hand
M11.249 Other chondrocalcinosis, unspecified hand
M11.25 Other chondrocalcinosis, hip
M11.251 Other chondrocalcinosis, right hip
M11.252 Other chondrocalcinosis, left hip
M11.259 Other chondrocalcinosis, unspecified hip
M11.26 Other chondrocalcinosis, knee
M11.261 Other chondrocalcinosis, right knee
M11.262 Other chondrocalcinosis, left knee
M11.269 Other chondrocalcinosis, unspecified knee
M11.27 Other chondrocalcinosis, ankle and foot
M11.271 Other chondrocalcinosis, right ankle and foot
M11.272 Other chondrocalcinosis, left ankle and foot
M11.279 Other chondrocalcinosis, unspecified ankle and foot
M11.28 Other chondrocalcinosis, vertebrae
M11.29 Other chondrocalcinosis, multiple sites
M11.8 Other specified crystal arthropathies
M11.80 Other specified crystal arthropathies, unspecified site
M11.81 Other specified crystal arthropathies, shoulder
M11.811 Other specified crystal arthropathies, right shoulder
M11.812 Other specified crystal arthropathies, left shoulder
M11.819 Other specified crystal arthropathies, unspecified shoulder
M11.82 Other specified crystal arthropathies, elbow
M11.821 Other specified crystal arthropathies, right elbow
M11.822 Other specified crystal arthropathies, left elbow
M11.829 Other specified crystal arthropathies, unspecified elbow
M11.83 Other specified crystal arthropathies, wrist
M11.831 Other specified crystal arthropathies, right wrist
M11.832 Other specified crystal arthropathies, left wrist
M11.839 Other specified crystal arthropathies, unspecified wrist
M11.84 Other specified crystal arthropathies, hand
M11.841 Other specified crystal arthropathies, right hand
M11.842 Other specified crystal arthropathies, left hand
M11.849 Other specified crystal arthropathies, unspecified hand
M11.85 Other specified crystal arthropathies, hip
M11.851 Other specified crystal arthropathies, right hip

M11.852 Other specified crystal arthropathies, left hip
M11.859 Other specified crystal arthropathies, unspecified hip
M11.86 Other specified crystal arthropathies, knee
M11.861 Other specified crystal arthropathies, right knee
M11.862 Other specified crystal arthropathies, left knee
M11.869 Other specified crystal arthropathies, unspecified knee
M11.87 Other specified crystal arthropathies, ankle and foot
M11.871 Other specified crystal arthropathies, right ankle and foot
M11.872 Other specified crystal arthropathies, left ankle and foot
M11.879 Other specified crystal arthropathies, unspecified ankle and foot
M11.88 Other specified crystal arthropathies, vertebrae
M11.89 Other specified crystal arthropathies, multiple sites
M11.9 Crystal arthropathy, unspecified

M12 Other and unspecified arthropathy

EXCLUDES 1 *arthrosis (M15-M19)*
cricoarytenoid arthropathy (J38.7)

M12.0 Chronic postrheumatic arthropathy [Jaccoud]
M12.00 Chronic postrheumatic arthropathy [Jaccoud], unspecified site HCC
M12.01 Chronic postrheumatic arthropathy [Jaccoud], shoulder
M12.011 Chronic postrheumatic arthropathy [Jaccoud], right shoulder HCC
M12.012 Chronic postrheumatic arthropathy [Jaccoud], left shoulder HCC
M12.019 Chronic postrheumatic arthropathy [Jaccoud], unspecified shoulder HCC
M12.02 Chronic postrheumatic arthropathy [Jaccoud], elbow
M12.021 Chronic postrheumatic arthropathy [Jaccoud], right elbow HCC
M12.022 Chronic postrheumatic arthropathy [Jaccoud], left elbow HCC
M12.029 Chronic postrheumatic arthropathy [Jaccoud], unspecified elbow HCC
M12.03 Chronic postrheumatic arthropathy [Jaccoud], wrist
M12.031 Chronic postrheumatic arthropathy [Jaccoud], right wrist HCC
M12.032 Chronic postrheumatic arthropathy [Jaccoud], left wrist HCC
M12.039 Chronic postrheumatic arthropathy [Jaccoud], unspecified wrist HCC
M12.04 Chronic postrheumatic arthropathy [Jaccoud], hand
M12.041 Chronic postrheumatic arthropathy [Jaccoud], right hand HCC
M12.042 Chronic postrheumatic arthropathy [Jaccoud], left hand HCC
M12.049 Chronic postrheumatic arthropathy [Jaccoud], unspecified hand HCC
M12.05 Chronic postrheumatic arthropathy [Jaccoud], hip
M12.051 Chronic postrheumatic arthropathy [Jaccoud], right hip HCC
M12.052 Chronic postrheumatic arthropathy [Jaccoud], left hip HCC
M12.059 Chronic postrheumatic arthropathy [Jaccoud], unspecified hip HCC
M12.06 Chronic postrheumatic arthropathy [Jaccoud], knee
M12.061 Chronic postrheumatic arthropathy [Jaccoud], right knee HCC
M12.062 Chronic postrheumatic arthropathy [Jaccoud], left knee HCC
M12.069 Chronic postrheumatic arthropathy [Jaccoud], unspecified knee HCC
M12.07 Chronic postrheumatic arthropathy [Jaccoud], ankle and foot
M12.071 Chronic postrheumatic arthropathy [Jaccoud], right ankle and foot HCC
M12.072 Chronic postrheumatic arthropathy [Jaccoud], left ankle and foot HCC
M12.079 Chronic postrheumatic arthropathy [Jaccoud], unspecified ankle and foot HCC
M12.08 Chronic postrheumatic arthropathy [Jaccoud], other specified site HCC
Chronic postrheumatic arthropathy [Jaccoud], vertebrae
M12.09 Chronic postrheumatic arthropathy [Jaccoud], multiple sites HCC

M12.1 Kaschin-Beck disease
Osteochondroarthrosis deformans endemica
M12.10 Kaschin-Beck disease, unspecified site
M12.11 Kaschin-Beck disease, shoulder
M12.111 Kaschin-Beck disease, right shoulder
M12.112 Kaschin-Beck disease, left shoulder
M12.119 Kaschin-Beck disease, unspecified shoulder
M12.12 Kaschin-Beck disease, elbow
M12.121 Kaschin-Beck disease, right elbow
M12.122 Kaschin-Beck disease, left elbow
M12.129 Kaschin-Beck disease, unspecified elbow
M12.13 Kaschin-Beck disease, wrist
M12.131 Kaschin-Beck disease, right wrist
M12.132 Kaschin-Beck disease, left wrist
M12.139 Kaschin-Beck disease, unspecified wrist
M12.14 Kaschin-Beck disease, hand
M12.141 Kaschin-Beck disease, right hand
M12.142 Kaschin-Beck disease, left hand
M12.149 Kaschin-Beck disease, unspecified hand
M12.15 Kaschin-Beck disease, hip
M12.151 Kaschin-Beck disease, right hip
M12.152 Kaschin-Beck disease, left hip
M12.159 Kaschin-Beck disease, unspecified hip
M12.16 Kaschin-Beck disease, knee
M12.161 Kaschin-Beck disease, right knee
M12.162 Kaschin-Beck disease, left knee
M12.169 Kaschin-Beck disease, unspecified knee
M12.17 Kaschin-Beck disease, ankle and foot
M12.171 Kaschin-Beck disease, right ankle and foot
M12.172 Kaschin-Beck disease, left ankle and foot
M12.179 Kaschin-Beck disease, unspecified ankle and foot
M12.18 Kaschin-Beck disease, vertebrae
M12.19 Kaschin-Beck disease, multiple sites

M12.2 Villonodular synovitis (pigmented)
M12.20 Villonodular synovitis (pigmented), unspecified site
M12.21 Villonodular synovitis (pigmented), shoulder
M12.211 Villonodular synovitis (pigmented), right shoulder
M12.212 Villonodular synovitis (pigmented), left shoulder
M12.219 Villonodular synovitis (pigmented), unspecified shoulder
M12.22 Villonodular synovitis (pigmented), elbow
M12.221 Villonodular synovitis (pigmented), right elbow
M12.222 Villonodular synovitis (pigmented), left elbow
M12.229 Villonodular synovitis (pigmented), unspecified elbow
M12.23 Villonodular synovitis (pigmented), wrist
M12.231 Villonodular synovitis (pigmented), right wrist
M12.232 Villonodular synovitis (pigmented), left wrist
M12.239 Villonodular synovitis (pigmented), unspecified wrist
M12.24 Villonodular synovitis (pigmented), hand
M12.241 Villonodular synovitis (pigmented), right hand
M12.242 Villonodular synovitis (pigmented), left hand
M12.249 Villonodular synovitis (pigmented), unspecified hand

✓6th M12.25 Villonodular synovitis (pigmented), hip
M12.251 Villonodular synovitis (pigmented), right hip
M12.252 Villonodular synovitis (pigmented), left hip
M12.259 Villonodular synovitis (pigmented), unspecified hip
✓6th M12.26 Villonodular synovitis (pigmented), knee
M12.261 Villonodular synovitis (pigmented), right knee
M12.262 Villonodular synovitis (pigmented), left knee
M12.269 Villonodular synovitis (pigmented), unspecified knee
✓6th M12.27 Villonodular synovitis (pigmented), ankle and foot
M12.271 Villonodular synovitis (pigmented), right ankle and foot
M12.272 Villonodular synovitis (pigmented), left ankle and foot
M12.279 Villonodular synovitis (pigmented), unspecified ankle and foot
M12.28 Villonodular synovitis (pigmented), other specified site
Villonodular synovitis (pigmented), vertebrae
M12.29 Villonodular synovitis (pigmented), multiple sites
✓5th M12.3 Palindromic rheumatism
DEF: Sudden and recurring attacks of moderate to severe joint pain and swelling generally occurring in the hands or feet of unknown etiology. After the attack subsides, the joints appear normal again.
M12.30 Palindromic rheumatism, unspecified site
✓6th M12.31 Palindromic rheumatism, shoulder
M12.311 Palindromic rheumatism, right shoulder
M12.312 Palindromic rheumatism, left shoulder
M12.319 Palindromic rheumatism, unspecified shoulder
✓6th M12.32 Palindromic rheumatism, elbow
M12.321 Palindromic rheumatism, right elbow
M12.322 Palindromic rheumatism, left elbow
M12.329 Palindromic rheumatism, unspecified elbow
✓6th M12.33 Palindromic rheumatism, wrist
M12.331 Palindromic rheumatism, right wrist
M12.332 Palindromic rheumatism, left wrist
M12.339 Palindromic rheumatism, unspecified wrist
✓6th M12.34 Palindromic rheumatism, hand
M12.341 Palindromic rheumatism, right hand
M12.342 Palindromic rheumatism, left hand
M12.349 Palindromic rheumatism, unspecified hand
✓6th M12.35 Palindromic rheumatism, hip
M12.351 Palindromic rheumatism, right hip
M12.352 Palindromic rheumatism, left hip
M12.359 Palindromic rheumatism, unspecified hip
✓6th M12.36 Palindromic rheumatism, knee
M12.361 Palindromic rheumatism, right knee
M12.362 Palindromic rheumatism, left knee
M12.369 Palindromic rheumatism, unspecified knee
✓6th M12.37 Palindromic rheumatism, ankle and foot
M12.371 Palindromic rheumatism, right ankle and foot
M12.372 Palindromic rheumatism, left ankle and foot
M12.379 Palindromic rheumatism, unspecified ankle and foot
M12.38 Palindromic rheumatism, other specified site
Palindromic rheumatism, vertebrae
M12.39 Palindromic rheumatism, multiple sites
✓5th M12.4 Intermittent hydrarthrosis
M12.40 Intermittent hydrarthrosis, unspecified site
✓6th M12.41 Intermittent hydrarthrosis, shoulder
M12.411 Intermittent hydrarthrosis, right shoulder
M12.412 Intermittent hydrarthrosis, left shoulder
M12.419 Intermittent hydrarthrosis, unspecified shoulder
✓6th M12.42 Intermittent hydrarthrosis, elbow
M12.421 Intermittent hydrarthrosis, right elbow
M12.422 Intermittent hydrarthrosis, left elbow
M12.429 Intermittent hydrarthrosis, unspecified elbow
✓6th M12.43 Intermittent hydrarthrosis, wrist
M12.431 Intermittent hydrarthrosis, right wrist
M12.432 Intermittent hydrarthrosis, left wrist
M12.439 Intermittent hydrarthrosis, unspecified wrist
✓6th M12.44 Intermittent hydrarthrosis, hand
M12.441 Intermittent hydrarthrosis, right hand
M12.442 Intermittent hydrarthrosis, left hand
M12.449 Intermittent hydrarthrosis, unspecified hand
✓6th M12.45 Intermittent hydrarthrosis, hip
M12.451 Intermittent hydrarthrosis, right hip
M12.452 Intermittent hydrarthrosis, left hip
M12.459 Intermittent hydrarthrosis, unspecified hip
✓6th M12.46 Intermittent hydrarthrosis, knee
M12.461 Intermittent hydrarthrosis, right knee
M12.462 Intermittent hydrarthrosis, left knee
M12.469 Intermittent hydrarthrosis, unspecified knee
✓6th M12.47 Intermittent hydrarthrosis, ankle and foot
M12.471 Intermittent hydrarthrosis, right ankle and foot
M12.472 Intermittent hydrarthrosis, left ankle and foot
M12.479 Intermittent hydrarthrosis, unspecified ankle and foot
M12.48 Intermittent hydrarthrosis, other site
M12.49 Intermittent hydrarthrosis, multiple sites
✓5th M12.5 Traumatic arthropathy
EXCLUDES 1 *current injury-see Alphabetic Index*
post-traumatic osteoarthritis of first carpometacarpal joint (M18.2-M18.3)
post-traumatic osteoarthritis of hip (M16.4-M16.5)
post-traumatic osteoarthritis of knee (M17.2-M17.3)
post-traumatic osteoarthritis NOS (M19.1-)
post-traumatic osteoarthritis of other single joints (M19.1-)
AHA: 2015,1Q,17
M12.50 Traumatic arthropathy, unspecified site
✓6th M12.51 Traumatic arthropathy, shoulder
M12.511 Traumatic arthropathy, right shoulder
M12.512 Traumatic arthropathy, left shoulder
M12.519 Traumatic arthropathy, unspecified shoulder
✓6th M12.52 Traumatic arthropathy, elbow
M12.521 Traumatic arthropathy, right elbow
M12.522 Traumatic arthropathy, left elbow
M12.529 Traumatic arthropathy, unspecified elbow
✓6th M12.53 Traumatic arthropathy, wrist
M12.531 Traumatic arthropathy, right wrist
M12.532 Traumatic arthropathy, left wrist
M12.539 Traumatic arthropathy, unspecified wrist
✓6th M12.54 Traumatic arthropathy, hand
M12.541 Traumatic arthropathy, right hand
M12.542 Traumatic arthropathy, left hand
M12.549 Traumatic arthropathy, unspecified hand
✓6th M12.55 Traumatic arthropathy, hip
M12.551 Traumatic arthropathy, right hip
M12.552 Traumatic arthropathy, left hip
M12.559 Traumatic arthropathy, unspecified hip
✓6th M12.56 Traumatic arthropathy, knee
M12.561 Traumatic arthropathy, right knee
M12.562 Traumatic arthropathy, left knee
M12.569 Traumatic arthropathy, unspecified knee
✓6th M12.57 Traumatic arthropathy, ankle and foot
M12.571 Traumatic arthropathy, right ankle and foot
M12.572 Traumatic arthropathy, left ankle and foot

M12.579 Traumatic arthropathy, unspecified ankle and foot

M12.58 Traumatic arthropathy, other specified site
Traumatic arthropathy, vertebrae

M12.59 Traumatic arthropathy, multiple sites

M12.8 Other specific arthropathies, not elsewhere classified
Transient arthropathy

M12.80 Other specific arthropathies, not elsewhere classified, unspecified site

M12.81 Other specific arthropathies, not elsewhere classified, shoulder
M12.811 Other specific arthropathies, not elsewhere classified, right shoulder
M12.812 Other specific arthropathies, not elsewhere classified, left shoulder
M12.819 Other specific arthropathies, not elsewhere classified, unspecified shoulder

M12.82 Other specific arthropathies, not elsewhere classified, elbow
M12.821 Other specific arthropathies, not elsewhere classified, right elbow
M12.822 Other specific arthropathies, not elsewhere classified, left elbow
M12.829 Other specific arthropathies, not elsewhere classified, unspecified elbow

M12.83 Other specific arthropathies, not elsewhere classified, wrist
M12.831 Other specific arthropathies, not elsewhere classified, right wrist
M12.832 Other specific arthropathies, not elsewhere classified, left wrist
M12.839 Other specific arthropathies, not elsewhere classified, unspecified wrist

M12.84 Other specific arthropathies, not elsewhere classified, hand
M12.841 Other specific arthropathies, not elsewhere classified, right hand
M12.842 Other specific arthropathies, not elsewhere classified, left hand
M12.849 Other specific arthropathies, not elsewhere classified, unspecified hand

M12.85 Other specific arthropathies, not elsewhere classified, hip
M12.851 Other specific arthropathies, not elsewhere classified, right hip
M12.852 Other specific arthropathies, not elsewhere classified, left hip
M12.859 Other specific arthropathies, not elsewhere classified, unspecified hip

M12.86 Other specific arthropathies, not elsewhere classified, knee
M12.861 Other specific arthropathies, not elsewhere classified, right knee
M12.862 Other specific arthropathies, not elsewhere classified, left knee
M12.869 Other specific arthropathies, not elsewhere classified, unspecified knee

M12.87 Other specific arthropathies, not elsewhere classified, ankle and foot
M12.871 Other specific arthropathies, not elsewhere classified, right ankle and foot
M12.872 Other specific arthropathies, not elsewhere classified, left ankle and foot
M12.879 Other specific arthropathies, not elsewhere classified, unspecified ankle and foot

M12.88 Other specific arthropathies, not elsewhere classified, other specified site
Other specific arthropathies, not elsewhere classified, vertebrae

M12.89 Other specific arthropathies, not elsewhere classified, multiple sites

M12.9 Arthropathy, unspecified

M13 Other arthritis
EXCLUDES 1 *arthrosis (M15-M19)*
osteoarthritis (M15-M19)

M13.0 Polyarthritis, unspecified

M13.1 Monoarthritis, not elsewhere classified

M13.10 Monoarthritis, not elsewhere classified, unspecified site

M13.11 Monoarthritis, not elsewhere classified, shoulder
M13.111 Monoarthritis, not elsewhere classified, right shoulder
M13.112 Monoarthritis, not elsewhere classified, left shoulder
M13.119 Monoarthritis, not elsewhere classified, unspecified shoulder

M13.12 Monoarthritis, not elsewhere classified, elbow
M13.121 Monoarthritis, not elsewhere classified, right elbow
M13.122 Monoarthritis, not elsewhere classified, left elbow
M13.129 Monoarthritis, not elsewhere classified, unspecified elbow

M13.13 Monoarthritis, not elsewhere classified, wrist
M13.131 Monoarthritis, not elsewhere classified, right wrist
M13.132 Monoarthritis, not elsewhere classified, left wrist
M13.139 Monoarthritis, not elsewhere classified, unspecified wrist

M13.14 Monoarthritis, not elsewhere classified, hand
M13.141 Monoarthritis, not elsewhere classified, right hand
M13.142 Monoarthritis, not elsewhere classified, left hand
M13.149 Monoarthritis, not elsewhere classified, unspecified hand

M13.15 Monoarthritis, not elsewhere classified, hip
M13.151 Monoarthritis, not elsewhere classified, right hip
M13.152 Monoarthritis, not elsewhere classified, left hip
M13.159 Monoarthritis, not elsewhere classified, unspecified hip

M13.16 Monoarthritis, not elsewhere classified, knee
M13.161 Monoarthritis, not elsewhere classified, right knee
M13.162 Monoarthritis, not elsewhere classified, left knee
M13.169 Monoarthritis, not elsewhere classified, unspecified knee

M13.17 Monoarthritis, not elsewhere classified, ankle and foot
M13.171 Monoarthritis, not elsewhere classified, right ankle and foot
M13.172 Monoarthritis, not elsewhere classified, left ankle and foot
M13.179 Monoarthritis, not elsewhere classified, unspecified ankle and foot

M13.8 Other specified arthritis
Allergic arthritis
EXCLUDES 1 *osteoarthritis (M15-M19)*

M13.80 Other specified arthritis, unspecified site

M13.81 Other specified arthritis, shoulder
M13.811 Other specified arthritis, right shoulder
M13.812 Other specified arthritis, left shoulder
M13.819 Other specified arthritis, unspecified shoulder

M13.82 Other specified arthritis, elbow
M13.821 Other specified arthritis, right elbow
M13.822 Other specified arthritis, left elbow
M13.829 Other specified arthritis, unspecified elbow

M13.83 Other specified arthritis, wrist
M13.831 Other specified arthritis, right wrist
M13.832 Other specified arthritis, left wrist
M13.839 Other specified arthritis, unspecified wrist

M13.84 Other specified arthritis, hand
M13.841 Other specified arthritis, right hand
M13.842 Other specified arthritis, left hand
M13.849 Other specified arthritis, unspecified hand

M13.85 Other specified arthritis, hip
M13.851 Other specified arthritis, right hip
M13.852 Other specified arthritis, left hip
M13.859 Other specified arthritis, unspecified hip

M13.86 Other specified arthritis, knee
- **M13.861 Other specified arthritis, right knee**
- **M13.862 Other specified arthritis, left knee**
- **M13.869 Other specified arthritis, unspecified knee**

M13.87 Other specified arthritis, ankle and foot
- **M13.871 Other specified arthritis, right ankle and foot**
- **M13.872 Other specified arthritis, left ankle and foot**
- **M13.879 Other specified arthritis, unspecified ankle and foot**

M13.88 Other specified arthritis, other site

M13.89 Other specified arthritis, multiple sites

M14 Arthropathies in other diseases classified elsewhere

EXCLUDES 1 *arthropathy in:*
- *diabetes mellitus (EØ8-E13 with .61-)*
- *hematological disorders (M36.2-M36.3)*
- *hypersensitivity reactions (M36.4)*
- *neoplastic disease (M36.1)*
- *neurosyphillis (A52.16)*
- *sarcoidosis (D86.86)*

enteropathic arthropathies (MØ7.-)
juvenile psoriatic arthropathy (L4Ø.54)
lipoid dermatoarthritis (E78.81)

M14.6 Charcôt's joint

Neuropathic arthropathy

EXCLUDES 1 *Charcôt's joint in diabetes mellitus (EØ8-E13 with .61Ø)*
Charcôt's joint in tabes dorsalis (A52.16)

DEF: Progressive neurologic arthropathy in which chronic degeneration of joints in the weight-bearing areas with peripheral hypertrophy occurs as a complication of a neuropathy disorder. Supporting structures relax from a loss of sensation resulting in chronic joint instability.

M14.6Ø Charcôt's joint, unspecified site

M14.61 Charcôt's joint, shoulder
- **M14.611 Charcôt's joint, right shoulder**
- **M14.612 Charcôt's joint, left shoulder**
- **M14.619 Charcôt's joint, unspecified shoulder**

M14.62 Charcôt's joint, elbow
- **M14.621 Charcôt's joint, right elbow**
- **M14.622 Charcôt's joint, left elbow**
- **M14.629 Charcôt's joint, unspecified elbow**

M14.63 Charcôt's joint, wrist
- **M14.631 Charcôt's joint, right wrist**
- **M14.632 Charcôt's joint, left wrist**
- **M14.639 Charcôt's joint, unspecified wrist**

M14.64 Charcôt's joint, hand
- **M14.641 Charcôt's joint, right hand**
- **M14.642 Charcôt's joint, left hand**
- **M14.649 Charcôt's joint, unspecified hand**

M14.65 Charcôt's joint, hip
- **M14.651 Charcôt's joint, right hip**
- **M14.652 Charcôt's joint, left hip**
- **M14.659 Charcôt's joint, unspecified hip**

M14.66 Charcôt's joint, knee
- **M14.661 Charcôt's joint, right knee**
- **M14.662 Charcôt's joint, left knee**
- **M14.669 Charcôt's joint, unspecified knee**

M14.67 Charcôt's joint, ankle and foot
- **M14.671 Charcôt's joint, right ankle and foot**
- **M14.672 Charcôt's joint, left ankle and foot**
- **M14.679 Charcôt's joint, unspecified ankle and foot**

M14.68 Charcôt's joint, vertebrae

M14.69 Charcôt's joint, multiple sites

M14.8 Arthropathies in other specified diseases classified elsewhere

Code first underlying disease, such as:
- amyloidosis (E85.-)
- erythema multiforme (L51.-)
- erythema nodosum (L52)
- hemochromatosis (E83.11-)
- hyperparathyroidism (E21.-)
- hypothyroidism (EØØ-EØ3)
- sickle-cell disorders (D57.-)
- thyrotoxicosis [hyperthyroidism] (EØ5.-)
- Whipple's disease (K9Ø.81)

M14.8Ø Arthropathies in other specified diseases classified elsewhere, unspecified site

M14.81 Arthropathies in other specified diseases classified elsewhere, shoulder
- ***M14.811 Arthropathies in other specified diseases classified elsewhere, right shoulder***
- ***M14.812 Arthropathies in other specified diseases classified elsewhere, left shoulder***
- ***M14.819 Arthropathies in other specified diseases classified elsewhere, unspecified shoulder***

M14.82 Arthropathies in other specified diseases classified elsewhere, elbow
- ***M14.821 Arthropathies in other specified diseases classified elsewhere, right elbow***
- ***M14.822 Arthropathies in other specified diseases classified elsewhere, left elbow***
- ***M14.829 Arthropathies in other specified diseases classified elsewhere, unspecified elbow***

M14.83 Arthropathies in other specified diseases classified elsewhere, wrist
- ***M14.831 Arthropathies in other specified diseases classified elsewhere, right wrist***
- ***M14.832 Arthropathies in other specified diseases classified elsewhere, left wrist***
- ***M14.839 Arthropathies in other specified diseases classified elsewhere, unspecified wrist***

M14.84 Arthropathies in other specified diseases classified elsewhere, hand
- ***M14.841 Arthropathies in other specified diseases classified elsewhere, right hand***
- ***M14.842 Arthropathies in other specified diseases classified elsewhere, left hand***
- ***M14.849 Arthropathies in other specified diseases classified elsewhere, unspecified hand***

M14.85 Arthropathies in other specified diseases classified elsewhere, hip
- ***M14.851 Arthropathies in other specified diseases classified elsewhere, right hip***
- ***M14.852 Arthropathies in other specified diseases classified elsewhere, left hip***
- ***M14.859 Arthropathies in other specified diseases classified elsewhere, unspecified hip***

M14.86 Arthropathies in other specified diseases classified elsewhere, knee
- ***M14.861 Arthropathies in other specified diseases classified elsewhere, right knee***
- ***M14.862 Arthropathies in other specified diseases classified elsewhere, left knee***
- ***M14.869 Arthropathies in other specified diseases classified elsewhere, unspecified knee***

M14.87 Arthropathies in other specified diseases classified elsewhere, ankle and foot
- ***M14.871 Arthropathies in other specified diseases classified elsewhere, right ankle and foot***
- ***M14.872 Arthropathies in other specified diseases classified elsewhere, left ankle and foot***
- ***M14.879 Arthropathies in other specified diseases classified elsewhere, unspecified ankle and foot***

M14.88 Arthropathies in other specified diseases classified elsewhere, vertebrae

M14.89 Arthropathies in other specified diseases classified elsewhere, multiple sites

Osteoarthritis (M15-M19)

EXCLUDES 2 *osteoarthritis of spine (M47.-)*

AHA: 2020,2Q,14; 2016,4Q,147

TIP: Assign a primary osteoarthritis code when the site of the osteoarthritis is documented but the type of osteoarthritis — primary, secondary, generalized, or post-traumatic — is not documented. Primary is considered the default.

M15 Polyosteoarthritis
INCLUDES arthritis of multiple sites
EXCLUDES 1 *bilateral involvement of single joint (M16-M19)*

M15.0 Primary generalized (osteo)arthritis
M15.1 Heberden's nodes (with arthropathy)
Interphalangeal distal osteoarthritis
M15.2 Bouchard's nodes (with arthropathy)
Juxtaphalangeal distal osteoarthritis
M15.3 Secondary multiple arthritis
Post-traumatic polyosteoarthritis
M15.4 Erosive (osteo)arthritis
M15.8 Other polyosteoarthritis
M15.9 Polyosteoarthritis, unspecified
Generalized osteoarthritis NOS

M16 Osteoarthritis of hip
AHA: 2016,4Q,146
M16.0 Bilateral primary osteoarthritis of hip
AHA: 2018,2Q,15
M16.1 Unilateral primary osteoarthritis of hip
Primary osteoarthritis of hip NOS
AHA: 2018,2Q,15
M16.10 Unilateral primary osteoarthritis, unspecified hip
M16.11 Unilateral primary osteoarthritis, right hip
M16.12 Unilateral primary osteoarthritis, left hip
M16.2 Bilateral osteoarthritis resulting from hip dysplasia
M16.3 Unilateral osteoarthritis resulting from hip dysplasia
Dysplastic osteoarthritis of hip NOS
M16.30 Unilateral osteoarthritis resulting from hip dysplasia, unspecified hip
M16.31 Unilateral osteoarthritis resulting from hip dysplasia, right hip
M16.32 Unilateral osteoarthritis resulting from hip dysplasia, left hip
M16.4 Bilateral post-traumatic osteoarthritis of hip
M16.5 Unilateral post-traumatic osteoarthritis of hip
Post-traumatic osteoarthritis of hip NOS
M16.50 Unilateral post-traumatic osteoarthritis, unspecified hip
M16.51 Unilateral post-traumatic osteoarthritis, right hip
M16.52 Unilateral post-traumatic osteoarthritis, left hip
M16.6 Other bilateral secondary osteoarthritis of hip
M16.7 Other unilateral secondary osteoarthritis of hip
Secondary osteoarthritis of hip NOS
M16.9 Osteoarthritis of hip, unspecified

M17 Osteoarthritis of knee
AHA: 2016,4Q,146-147
M17.0 Bilateral primary osteoarthritis of knee
AHA: 2018,2Q,15
M17.1 Unilateral primary osteoarthritis of knee
Primary osteoarthritis of knee NOS
AHA: 2018,2Q,15
M17.10 Unilateral primary osteoarthritis, unspecified knee
M17.11 Unilateral primary osteoarthritis, right knee
M17.12 Unilateral primary osteoarthritis, left knee
M17.2 Bilateral post-traumatic osteoarthritis of knee
M17.3 Unilateral post-traumatic osteoarthritis of knee
Post-traumatic osteoarthritis of knee NOS
M17.30 Unilateral post-traumatic osteoarthritis, unspecified knee
M17.31 Unilateral post-traumatic osteoarthritis, right knee
M17.32 Unilateral post-traumatic osteoarthritis, left knee
M17.4 Other bilateral secondary osteoarthritis of knee
M17.5 Other unilateral secondary osteoarthritis of knee
Secondary osteoarthritis of knee NOS
M17.9 Osteoarthritis of knee, unspecified

M18 Osteoarthritis of first carpometacarpal joint
M18.0 Bilateral primary osteoarthritis of first carpometacarpal joints
M18.1 Unilateral primary osteoarthritis of first carpometacarpal joint
Primary osteoarthritis of first carpometacarpal joint NOS
M18.10 Unilateral primary osteoarthritis of first carpometacarpal joint, unspecified hand
M18.11 Unilateral primary osteoarthritis of first carpometacarpal joint, right hand
M18.12 Unilateral primary osteoarthritis of first carpometacarpal joint, left hand
M18.2 Bilateral post-traumatic osteoarthritis of first carpometacarpal joints
M18.3 Unilateral post-traumatic osteoarthritis of first carpometacarpal joint
Post-traumatic osteoarthritis of first carpometacarpal joint NOS
M18.30 Unilateral post-traumatic osteoarthritis of first carpometacarpal joint, unspecified hand
M18.31 Unilateral post-traumatic osteoarthritis of first carpometacarpal joint, right hand
M18.32 Unilateral post-traumatic osteoarthritis of first carpometacarpal joint, left hand
M18.4 Other bilateral secondary osteoarthritis of first carpometacarpal joints
M18.5 Other unilateral secondary osteoarthritis of first carpometacarpal joint
Secondary osteoarthritis of first carpometacarpal joint NOS
M18.50 Other unilateral secondary osteoarthritis of first carpometacarpal joint, unspecified hand
M18.51 Other unilateral secondary osteoarthritis of first carpometacarpal joint, right hand
M18.52 Other unilateral secondary osteoarthritis of first carpometacarpal joint, left hand
M18.9 Osteoarthritis of first carpometacarpal joint, unspecified

M19 Other and unspecified osteoarthritis
EXCLUDES 1 *polyarthritis (M15.-)*
EXCLUDES 2 *arthrosis of spine (M47.-)*
hallux rigidus (M20.2)
osteoarthritis of spine (M47.-)
AHA: 2020,4Q,31-32
M19.0 Primary osteoarthritis of other joints
AHA: 2018,2Q,15; 2016,4Q,145
M19.01 Primary osteoarthritis, shoulder
M19.011 Primary osteoarthritis, right shoulder
M19.012 Primary osteoarthritis, left shoulder
M19.019 Primary osteoarthritis, unspecified shoulder
M19.02 Primary osteoarthritis, elbow
M19.021 Primary osteoarthritis, right elbow
M19.022 Primary osteoarthritis, left elbow
M19.029 Primary osteoarthritis, unspecified elbow
M19.03 Primary osteoarthritis, wrist
M19.031 Primary osteoarthritis, right wrist
M19.032 Primary osteoarthritis, left wrist
M19.039 Primary osteoarthritis, unspecified wrist
M19.04 Primary osteoarthritis, hand
EXCLUDES 2 *primary osteoarthritis of first carpometacarpal joint (M18.0-, M18.1-)*
M19.041 Primary osteoarthritis, right hand
M19.042 Primary osteoarthritis, left hand
M19.049 Primary osteoarthritis, unspecified hand
M19.07 Primary osteoarthritis ankle and foot
M19.071 Primary osteoarthritis, right ankle and foot
M19.072 Primary osteoarthritis, left ankle and foot
M19.079 Primary osteoarthritis, unspecified ankle and foot
M19.09 Primary osteoarthritis, other specified site
M19.1 Post-traumatic osteoarthritis of other joints
M19.11 Post-traumatic osteoarthritis, shoulder
M19.111 Post-traumatic osteoarthritis, right shoulder
M19.112 Post-traumatic osteoarthritis, left shoulder
M19.119 Post-traumatic osteoarthritis, unspecified shoulder
M19.12 Post-traumatic osteoarthritis, elbow
M19.121 Post-traumatic osteoarthritis, right elbow
M19.122 Post-traumatic osteoarthritis, left elbow

M19.129 Post-traumatic osteoarthritis, unspecified elbow

M19.13 Post-traumatic osteoarthritis, wrist

M19.131 Post-traumatic osteoarthritis, right wrist

M19.132 Post-traumatic osteoarthritis, left wrist

M19.139 Post-traumatic osteoarthritis, unspecified wrist

M19.14 Post-traumatic osteoarthritis, hand

EXCLUDES 2 *post-traumatic osteoarthritis of first carpometacarpal joint (M18.2-, M18.3-)*

M19.141 Post-traumatic osteoarthritis, right hand

M19.142 Post-traumatic osteoarthritis, left hand

M19.149 Post-traumatic osteoarthritis, unspecified hand

M19.17 Post-traumatic osteoarthritis, ankle and foot

M19.171 Post-traumatic osteoarthritis, right ankle and foot

M19.172 Post-traumatic osteoarthritis, left ankle and foot

M19.179 Post-traumatic osteoarthritis, unspecified ankle and foot

M19.19 Post-traumatic osteoarthritis, other specified site

M19.2 Secondary osteoarthritis of other joints

M19.21 Secondary osteoarthritis, shoulder

M19.211 Secondary osteoarthritis, right shoulder

M19.212 Secondary osteoarthritis, left shoulder

M19.219 Secondary osteoarthritis, unspecified shoulder

M19.22 Secondary osteoarthritis, elbow

M19.221 Secondary osteoarthritis, right elbow

M19.222 Secondary osteoarthritis, left elbow

M19.229 Secondary osteoarthritis, unspecified elbow

M19.23 Secondary osteoarthritis, wrist

M19.231 Secondary osteoarthritis, right wrist

M19.232 Secondary osteoarthritis, left wrist

M19.239 Secondary osteoarthritis, unspecified wrist

M19.24 Secondary osteoarthritis, hand

M19.241 Secondary osteoarthritis, right hand

M19.242 Secondary osteoarthritis, left hand

M19.249 Secondary osteoarthritis, unspecified hand

M19.27 Secondary osteoarthritis, ankle and foot

M19.271 Secondary osteoarthritis, right ankle and foot

M19.272 Secondary osteoarthritis, left ankle and foot

M19.279 Secondary osteoarthritis, unspecified ankle and foot

M19.29 Secondary osteoarthritis, other specified site

M19.9 Osteoarthritis, unspecified site

TIP: Assign M19.90 when neither the site nor the type of osteoarthritis — primary, secondary, or post-traumatic — is documented.

M19.90 Unspecified osteoarthritis, unspecified site
Arthritis NOS
Arthrosis NOS
Osteoarthritis NOS
AHA: 2016,4Q,145-147

M19.91 Primary osteoarthritis, unspecified site
Primary osteoarthritis NOS

M19.92 Post-traumatic osteoarthritis, unspecified site
Post-traumatic osteoarthritis NOS

M19.93 Secondary osteoarthritis, unspecified site
Secondary osteoarthritis NOS

Other joint disorders (M20-M25)

EXCLUDES 2 *joints of the spine (M40-M54)*

M20 Acquired deformities of fingers and toes

EXCLUDES 1 *acquired absence of fingers and toes (Z89.-)*
congenital absence of fingers and toes (Q71.3-, Q72.3-)
congenital deformities and malformations of fingers and toes (Q66.-, Q68-Q70, Q74.-)

M20.0 Deformity of finger(s)

EXCLUDES 1 *clubbing of fingers (R68.3)*
palmar fascial fibromatosis [Dupuytren] (M72.0)
trigger finger (M65.3)

M20.00 Unspecified deformity of finger(s)

M20.001 Unspecified deformity of right finger(s)

M20.002 Unspecified deformity of left finger(s)

M20.009 Unspecified deformity of unspecified finger(s)

M20.01 Mallet finger

M20.011 Mallet finger of right finger(s)

M20.012 Mallet finger of left finger(s)

M20.019 Mallet finger of unspecified finger(s)

M20.02 Boutonnière deformity

DEF: Deformity of the finger caused by flexion of the proximal interphalangeal joint and hyperextension of the distal joint. The deformity results from rheumatoid arthritis, osteoarthritis, or injury.

M20.021 Boutonnière deformity of right finger(s)

M20.022 Boutonnière deformity of left finger(s)

M20.029 Boutonnière deformity of unspecified finger(s)

M20.03 Swan-neck deformity

DEF: Flexed distal and hyperextended proximal interphalangeal joint most commonly caused by rheumatoid arthritis.

M20.031 Swan-neck deformity of right finger(s)

M20.032 Swan-neck deformity of left finger(s)

M20.039 Swan-neck deformity of unspecified finger(s)

M20.09 Other deformity of finger(s)

M20.091 Other deformity of right finger(s)

M20.092 Other deformity of left finger(s)

M20.099 Other deformity of finger(s), unspecified finger(s)

M20.1 Hallux valgus (acquired)

EXCLUDES 2 *bunion (M21.6-)*

AHA: 2016,4Q,38

DEF: Deformity in which the great toe deviates toward the other toes and may even be positioned over or under the second toe.

Hallux Valgus

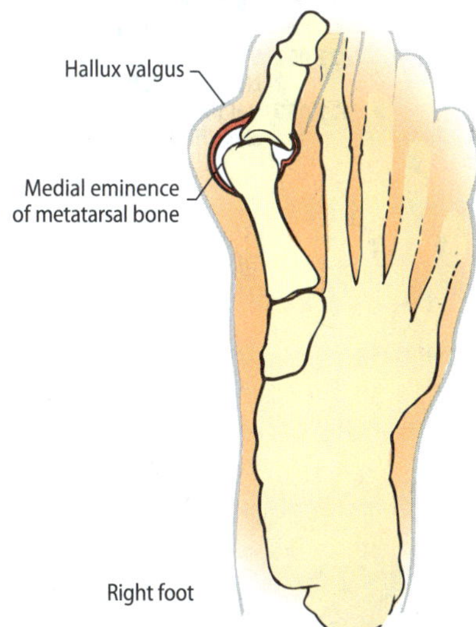

M20.10 Hallux valgus (acquired), unspecified foot

M20.11 Hallux valgus (acquired), right foot

M20.12 Hallux valgus (acquired), left foot

✓5th **M20.2 Hallux rigidus**
- **M20.20 Hallux rigidus, unspecified foot**
- **M20.21 Hallux rigidus, right foot**
- **M20.22 Hallux rigidus, left foot**

✓5th **M20.3 Hallux varus (acquired)**

DEF: Deformity in which the great toe deviates away from the other toes.

- **M20.30 Hallux varus (acquired), unspecified foot**
- **M20.31 Hallux varus (acquired), right foot**
- **M20.32 Hallux varus (acquired), left foot**

✓5th **M20.4 Other hammer toe(s) (acquired)**
- **M20.40 Other hammer toe(s) (acquired), unspecified foot**
- **M20.41 Other hammer toe(s) (acquired), right foot**
- **M20.42 Other hammer toe(s) (acquired), left foot**

✓5th **M20.5 Other deformities of toe(s) (acquired)**

✓6th **M20.5X Other deformities of toe(s) (acquired)**
- **M20.5X1 Other deformities of toe(s) (acquired), right foot**
- **M20.5X2 Other deformities of toe(s) (acquired), left foot**
- **M20.5X9 Other deformities of toe(s) (acquired), unspecified foot**

✓5th **M20.6 Acquired deformities of toe(s), unspecified**
- **M20.60 Acquired deformities of toe(s), unspecified, unspecified foot**
- **M20.61 Acquired deformities of toe(s), unspecified, right foot**
- **M20.62 Acquired deformities of toe(s), unspecified, left foot**

✓4th **M21 Other acquired deformities of limbs**

EXCLUDES 1 *acquired absence of limb (Z89.-)*
congenital absence of limbs (Q71-Q73)
congenital deformities and malformations of limbs (Q65-Q66, Q68-Q74)

EXCLUDES 2 *acquired deformities of fingers or toes (M20.-)*
coxa plana (M91.2)

✓5th **M21.0 Valgus deformity, not elsewhere classified**

EXCLUDES 1 *metatarsus valgus (Q66.6)*
talipes calcaneovalgus (Q66.4-)

- **M21.00 Valgus deformity, not elsewhere classified, unspecified site**

✓6th **M21.02 Valgus deformity, not elsewhere classified, elbow**

Cubitus valgus

- **M21.021 Valgus deformity, not elsewhere classified, right elbow**
- **M21.022 Valgus deformity, not elsewhere classified, left elbow**
- **M21.029 Valgus deformity, not elsewhere classified, unspecified elbow**

✓6th **M21.05 Valgus deformity, not elsewhere classified, hip**
- **M21.051 Valgus deformity, not elsewhere classified, right hip**
- **M21.052 Valgus deformity, not elsewhere classified, left hip**
- **M21.059 Valgus deformity, not elsewhere classified, unspecified hip**

✓6th **M21.06 Valgus deformity, not elsewhere classified, knee**

Genu valgum
Knock knee

DEF: Genu valga/valgum: Condition in which the thighs slant inward, causing the knees to be angled abnormally close together, leaving the space between the ankles wider than normal.

Genu Valga (knock-knee)

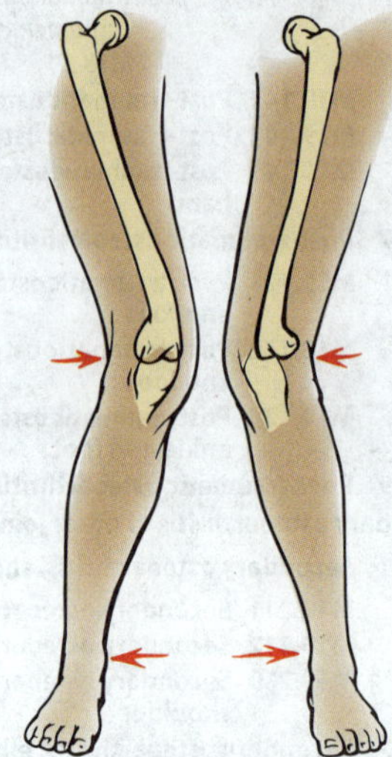

- **M21.061 Valgus deformity, not elsewhere classified, right knee**
- **M21.062 Valgus deformity, not elsewhere classified, left knee**
- **M21.069 Valgus deformity, not elsewhere classified, unspecified knee**

✓6th **M21.07 Valgus deformity, not elsewhere classified, ankle**
- **M21.071 Valgus deformity, not elsewhere classified, right ankle**
- **M21.072 Valgus deformity, not elsewhere classified, left ankle**
- **M21.079 Valgus deformity, not elsewhere classified, unspecified ankle**

✓5th **M21.1 Varus deformity, not elsewhere classified**

EXCLUDES 1 *metatarsus varus (Q66.22-)*
tibia vara (M92.51-)

- **M21.10 Varus deformity, not elsewhere classified, unspecified site**

✓6th **M21.12 Varus deformity, not elsewhere classified, elbow**

Cubitus varus, elbow

- **M21.121 Varus deformity, not elsewhere classified, right elbow**
- **M21.122 Varus deformity, not elsewhere classified, left elbow**
- **M21.129 Varus deformity, not elsewhere classified, unspecified elbow**

✓6th **M21.15 Varus deformity, not elsewhere classified, hip**
- **M21.151 Varus deformity, not elsewhere classified, right hip**
- **M21.152 Varus deformity, not elsewhere classified, left hip**
- **M21.159 Varus deformity, not elsewhere classified, unspecified**

✓6th **M21.16 Varus deformity, not elsewhere classified, knee**

Bow leg

Genu varum

DEF: Genu varus/varum: Condition in which the thighs and/or legs are bowed in an outward curve with an abnormally increased space between the knees.

Genu Varus (bowleg)

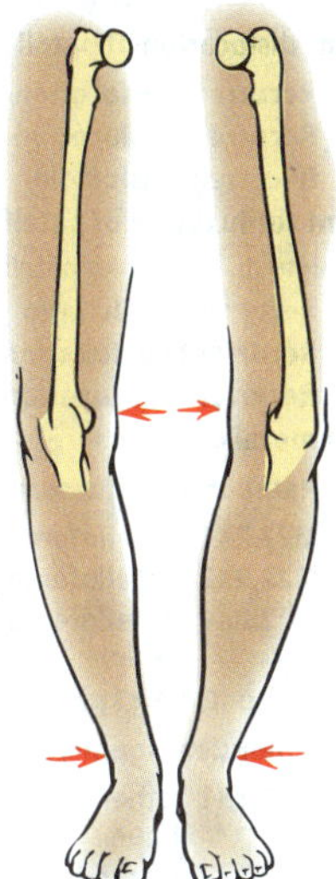

M21.161 Varus deformity, not elsewhere classified, right knee

M21.162 Varus deformity, not elsewhere classified, left knee

M21.169 Varus deformity, not elsewhere classified, unspecified knee

✓6th **M21.17 Varus deformity, not elsewhere classified, ankle**

M21.171 Varus deformity, not elsewhere classified, right ankle

M21.172 Varus deformity, not elsewhere classified, left ankle

M21.179 Varus deformity, not elsewhere classified, unspecified ankle

✓5th **M21.2 Flexion deformity**

M21.20 Flexion deformity, unspecified site

✓6th **M21.21 Flexion deformity, shoulder**

M21.211 Flexion deformity, right shoulder

M21.212 Flexion deformity, left shoulder

M21.219 Flexion deformity, unspecified shoulder

✓6th **M21.22 Flexion deformity, elbow**

M21.221 Flexion deformity, right elbow

M21.222 Flexion deformity, left elbow

M21.229 Flexion deformity, unspecified elbow

✓6th **M21.23 Flexion deformity, wrist**

M21.231 Flexion deformity, right wrist

M21.232 Flexion deformity, left wrist

M21.239 Flexion deformity, unspecified wrist

✓6th **M21.24 Flexion deformity, finger joints**

M21.241 Flexion deformity, right finger joints

M21.242 Flexion deformity, left finger joints

M21.249 Flexion deformity, unspecified finger joints

✓6th **M21.25 Flexion deformity, hip**

M21.251 Flexion deformity, right hip

M21.252 Flexion deformity, left hip

M21.259 Flexion deformity, unspecified hip

✓6th **M21.26 Flexion deformity, knee**

M21.261 Flexion deformity, right knee

M21.262 Flexion deformity, left knee

M21.269 Flexion deformity, unspecified knee

✓6th **M21.27 Flexion deformity, ankle and toes**

M21.271 Flexion deformity, right ankle and toes

M21.272 Flexion deformity, left ankle and toes

M21.279 Flexion deformity, unspecified ankle and toes

✓5th **M21.3 Wrist or foot drop (acquired)**

✓6th **M21.33 Wrist drop (acquired)**

M21.331 Wrist drop, right wrist

M21.332 Wrist drop, left wrist

M21.339 Wrist drop, unspecified wrist

✓6th **M21.37 Foot drop (acquired)**

M21.371 Foot drop, right foot

M21.372 Foot drop, left foot

M21.379 Foot drop, unspecified foot

✓5th **M21.4 Flat foot [pes planus] (acquired)**

EXCLUDES 1 *congenital pes planus (Q66.5-)*

M21.40 Flat foot [pes planus] (acquired), unspecified foot

M21.41 Flat foot [pes planus] (acquired), right foot

M21.42 Flat foot [pes planus] (acquired), left foot

✓5th **M21.5 Acquired clawhand, clubhand, clawfoot and clubfoot**

EXCLUDES 1 *clubfoot, not specified as acquired (Q66.89)*

✓6th **M21.51 Acquired clawhand**

M21.511 Acquired clawhand, right hand

M21.512 Acquired clawhand, left hand

M21.519 Acquired clawhand, unspecified hand

✓6th **M21.52 Acquired clubhand**

M21.521 Acquired clubhand, right hand

M21.522 Acquired clubhand, left hand

M21.529 Acquired clubhand, unspecified hand

✓6th **M21.53 Acquired clawfoot**

DEF: High foot arch with hyperextended toes at the metatarsophalangeal joint and flexed toes at the distal joints.

M21.531 Acquired clawfoot, right foot

M21.532 Acquired clawfoot, left foot

M21.539 Acquired clawfoot, unspecified foot

✓6th **M21.54 Acquired clubfoot**

DEF: Acquired anomaly of the foot with the heel elevated and rotated outward and the toes pointing inward.

M21.541 Acquired clubfoot, right foot

M21.542 Acquired clubfoot, left foot

M21.549 Acquired clubfoot, unspecified foot

✓5th **M21.6 Other acquired deformities of foot**

EXCLUDES 2 *deformities of toe (acquired) (M20.1-M20.6-)*

AHA: 2016,4Q,38

✓6th **M21.61 Bunion**

M21.611 Bunion of right foot

M21.612 Bunion of left foot

M21.619 Bunion of unspecified foot

✓6th **M21.62 Bunionette**

M21.621 Bunionette of right foot

M21.622 Bunionette of left foot

M21.629 Bunionette of unspecified foot

✓6th **M21.6X Other acquired deformities of foot**

M21.6X1 Other acquired deformities of right foot

M21.6X2 Other acquired deformities of left foot

M21.6X9 Other acquired deformities of unspecified foot

✓5th **M21.7 Unequal limb length (acquired)**

NOTE The site used should correspond to the shorter limb

M21.70 Unequal limb length (acquired), unspecified site

✓6th **M21.72 Unequal limb length (acquired), humerus**

M21.721 Unequal limb length (acquired), right humerus

M21.722 Unequal limb length (acquired), left humerus

M21.729 Unequal limb length (acquired), unspecified humerus

✓6th **M21.73 Unequal limb length (acquired), ulna and radius**

M21.731 Unequal limb length (acquired), right ulna

M21.732 Unequal limb length (acquired), left ulna

M21.733 Unequal limb length (acquired), right radius

M21.734 Unequal limb length (acquired), left radius

M21.739 Unequal limb length (acquired), unspecified ulna and radius

M21.75 Unequal limb length (acquired), femur
- M21.751 Unequal limb length (acquired), right femur
- M21.752 Unequal limb length (acquired), left femur
- M21.759 Unequal limb length (acquired), unspecified femur

M21.76 Unequal limb length (acquired), tibia and fibula
- M21.761 Unequal limb length (acquired), right tibia
- M21.762 Unequal limb length (acquired), left tibia
- M21.763 Unequal limb length (acquired), right fibula
- M21.764 Unequal limb length (acquired), left fibula
- M21.769 Unequal limb length (acquired), unspecified tibia and fibula

M21.8 Other specified acquired deformities of limbs

EXCLUDES 2 *coxa plana (M91.2)*

- M21.80 Other specified acquired deformities of unspecified limb

M21.82 Other specified acquired deformities of upper arm
- M21.821 Other specified acquired deformities of right upper arm
- M21.822 Other specified acquired deformities of left upper arm
- M21.829 Other specified acquired deformities of unspecified upper arm

M21.83 Other specified acquired deformities of forearm
- M21.831 Other specified acquired deformities of right forearm
- M21.832 Other specified acquired deformities of left forearm
- M21.839 Other specified acquired deformities of unspecified forearm

M21.85 Other specified acquired deformities of thigh
- M21.851 Other specified acquired deformities of right thigh
- M21.852 Other specified acquired deformities of left thigh
- M21.859 Other specified acquired deformities of unspecified thigh

M21.86 Other specified acquired deformities of lower leg
- M21.861 Other specified acquired deformities of right lower leg
- M21.862 Other specified acquired deformities of left lower leg
- M21.869 Other specified acquired deformities of unspecified lower leg

M21.9 Unspecified acquired deformity of limb and hand
- M21.90 Unspecified acquired deformity of unspecified limb

M21.92 Unspecified acquired deformity of upper arm
- M21.921 Unspecified acquired deformity of right upper arm
- M21.922 Unspecified acquired deformity of left upper arm
- M21.929 Unspecified acquired deformity of unspecified upper arm

M21.93 Unspecified acquired deformity of forearm
- M21.931 Unspecified acquired deformity of right forearm
- M21.932 Unspecified acquired deformity of left forearm
- M21.939 Unspecified acquired deformity of unspecified forearm

M21.94 Unspecified acquired deformity of hand
- M21.941 Unspecified acquired deformity of hand, right hand
- M21.942 Unspecified acquired deformity of hand, left hand
- M21.949 Unspecified acquired deformity of hand, unspecified hand

M21.95 Unspecified acquired deformity of thigh
- M21.951 Unspecified acquired deformity of right thigh
- M21.952 Unspecified acquired deformity of left thigh
- M21.959 Unspecified acquired deformity of unspecified thigh

M21.96 Unspecified acquired deformity of lower leg
- M21.961 Unspecified acquired deformity of right lower leg
- M21.962 Unspecified acquired deformity of left lower leg
- M21.969 Unspecified acquired deformity of unspecified lower leg

M22 Disorder of patella

EXCLUDES 2 *traumatic dislocation of patella (S83.0-)*

M22.0 Recurrent dislocation of patella
- M22.00 Recurrent dislocation of patella, unspecified knee
- M22.01 Recurrent dislocation of patella, right knee
- M22.02 Recurrent dislocation of patella, left knee

M22.1 Recurrent subluxation of patella

Incomplete dislocation of patella

- M22.10 Recurrent subluxation of patella, unspecified knee
- M22.11 Recurrent subluxation of patella, right knee
- M22.12 Recurrent subluxation of patella, left knee

M22.2 Patellofemoral disorders

M22.2X Patellofemoral disorders
- M22.2X1 Patellofemoral disorders, right knee
- M22.2X2 Patellofemoral disorders, left knee
- M22.2X9 Patellofemoral disorders, unspecified knee

M22.3 Other derangements of patella

M22.3X Other derangements of patella
- M22.3X1 Other derangements of patella, right knee
- M22.3X2 Other derangements of patella, left knee
- M22.3X9 Other derangements of patella, unspecified knee

M22.4 Chondromalacia patellae
- M22.40 Chondromalacia patellae, unspecified knee
- M22.41 Chondromalacia patellae, right knee
- M22.42 Chondromalacia patellae, left knee

M22.8 Other disorders of patella

M22.8X Other disorders of patella
- M22.8X1 Other disorders of patella, right knee
- M22.8X2 Other disorders of patella, left knee
- M22.8X9 Other disorders of patella, unspecified knee

M22.9 Unspecified disorder of patella
- M22.90 Unspecified disorder of patella, unspecified knee
- M22.91 Unspecified disorder of patella, right knee
- M22.92 Unspecified disorder of patella, left knee

M23 Internal derangement of knee

EXCLUDES 1 *ankylosis (M24.66)*
deformity of knee (M21.-)
osteochondritis dissecans (M93.2)

EXCLUDES 2 *current injury - see injury of knee and lower leg (S80-S89)*
recurrent dislocation or subluxation of joints (M24.4)
recurrent dislocation or subluxation of patella (M22.0-M22.1)

M23.0 Cystic meniscus

M23.00 Cystic meniscus, unspecified meniscus

Cystic meniscus, unspecified lateral meniscus
Cystic meniscus, unspecified medial meniscus

- M23.000 Cystic meniscus, unspecified lateral meniscus, right knee
- M23.001 Cystic meniscus, unspecified lateral meniscus, left knee
- M23.002 Cystic meniscus, unspecified lateral meniscus, unspecified knee
- M23.003 Cystic meniscus, unspecified medial meniscus, right knee
- M23.004 Cystic meniscus, unspecified medial meniscus, left knee
- M23.005 Cystic meniscus, unspecified medial meniscus, unspecified knee
- M23.006 Cystic meniscus, unspecified meniscus, right knee
- M23.007 Cystic meniscus, unspecified meniscus, left knee
- M23.009 Cystic meniscus, unspecified meniscus, unspecified knee

√6th M23.01 Cystic meniscus, anterior horn of medial meniscus
M23.011 Cystic meniscus, anterior horn of medial meniscus, right knee
M23.012 Cystic meniscus, anterior horn of medial meniscus, left knee
M23.019 Cystic meniscus, anterior horn of medial meniscus, unspecified knee
√6th M23.02 Cystic meniscus, posterior horn of medial meniscus
M23.021 Cystic meniscus, posterior horn of medial meniscus, right knee
M23.022 Cystic meniscus, posterior horn of medial meniscus, left knee
M23.029 Cystic meniscus, posterior horn of medial meniscus, unspecified knee
√6th M23.03 Cystic meniscus, other medial meniscus
M23.031 Cystic meniscus, other medial meniscus, right knee
M23.032 Cystic meniscus, other medial meniscus, left knee
M23.039 Cystic meniscus, other medial meniscus, unspecified knee
√6th M23.04 Cystic meniscus, anterior horn of lateral meniscus
M23.041 Cystic meniscus, anterior horn of lateral meniscus, right knee
M23.042 Cystic meniscus, anterior horn of lateral meniscus, left knee
M23.049 Cystic meniscus, anterior horn of lateral meniscus, unspecified knee
√6th M23.05 Cystic meniscus, posterior horn of lateral meniscus
M23.051 Cystic meniscus, posterior horn of lateral meniscus, right knee
M23.052 Cystic meniscus, posterior horn of lateral meniscus, left knee
M23.059 Cystic meniscus, posterior horn of lateral meniscus, unspecified knee
√6th M23.06 Cystic meniscus, other lateral meniscus
M23.061 Cystic meniscus, other lateral meniscus, right knee
M23.062 Cystic meniscus, other lateral meniscus, left knee
M23.069 Cystic meniscus, other lateral meniscus, unspecified knee

√5th M23.2 Derangement of meniscus due to old tear or injury
Old bucket-handle tear
AHA: 2019,2Q,26

Derangement of Meniscus

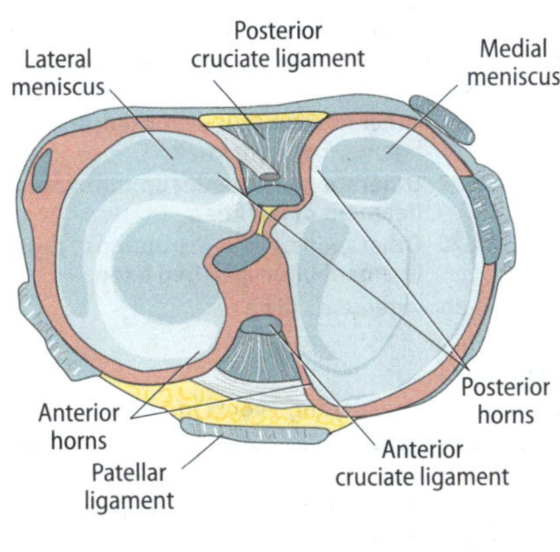

Overhead view of right knee

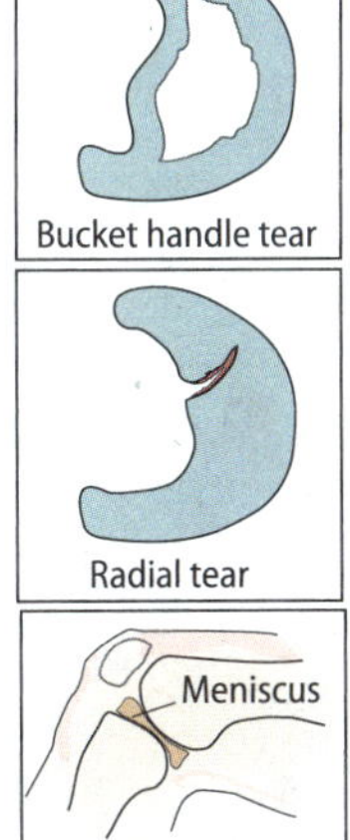

√6th M23.20 Derangement of unspecified meniscus due to old tear or injury
Derangement of unspecified lateral meniscus due to old tear or injury
Derangement of unspecified medial meniscus due to old tear or injury
M23.200 Derangement of unspecified lateral meniscus due to old tear or injury, right knee
M23.201 Derangement of unspecified lateral meniscus due to old tear or injury, left knee
M23.202 Derangement of unspecified lateral meniscus due to old tear or injury, unspecified knee
M23.203 Derangement of unspecified medial meniscus due to old tear or injury, right knee
M23.204 Derangement of unspecified medial meniscus due to old tear or injury, left knee
M23.205 Derangement of unspecified medial meniscus due to old tear or injury, unspecified knee
M23.206 Derangement of unspecified meniscus due to old tear or injury, right knee
M23.207 Derangement of unspecified meniscus due to old tear or injury, left knee
M23.209 Derangement of unspecified meniscus due to old tear or injury, unspecified knee
√6th M23.21 Derangement of anterior horn of medial meniscus due to old tear or injury
M23.211 Derangement of anterior horn of medial meniscus due to old tear or injury, right knee
M23.212 Derangement of anterior horn of medial meniscus due to old tear or injury, left knee
M23.219 Derangement of anterior horn of medial meniscus due to old tear or injury, unspecified knee
√6th M23.22 Derangement of posterior horn of medial meniscus due to old tear or injury
M23.221 Derangement of posterior horn of medial meniscus due to old tear or injury, right knee
M23.222 Derangement of posterior horn of medial meniscus due to old tear or injury, left knee
M23.229 Derangement of posterior horn of medial meniscus due to old tear or injury, unspecified knee
√6th M23.23 Derangement of other medial meniscus due to old tear or injury
M23.231 Derangement of other medial meniscus due to old tear or injury, right knee
M23.232 Derangement of other medial meniscus due to old tear or injury, left knee
M23.239 Derangement of other medial meniscus due to old tear or injury, unspecified knee
√6th M23.24 Derangement of anterior horn of lateral meniscus due to old tear or injury
M23.241 Derangement of anterior horn of lateral meniscus due to old tear or injury, right knee
M23.242 Derangement of anterior horn of lateral meniscus due to old tear or injury, left knee
M23.249 Derangement of anterior horn of lateral meniscus due to old tear or injury, unspecified knee
√6th M23.25 Derangement of posterior horn of lateral meniscus due to old tear or injury
M23.251 Derangement of posterior horn of lateral meniscus due to old tear or injury, right knee
M23.252 Derangement of posterior horn of lateral meniscus due to old tear or injury, left knee
M23.259 Derangement of posterior horn of lateral meniscus due to old tear or injury, unspecified knee
√6th M23.26 Derangement of other lateral meniscus due to old tear or injury
M23.261 Derangement of other lateral meniscus due to old tear or injury, right knee
M23.262 Derangement of other lateral meniscus due to old tear or injury, left knee
M23.269 Derangement of other lateral meniscus due to old tear or injury, unspecified knee

5th M23.3 Other meniscus derangements
Degenerate meniscus
Detached meniscus
Retained meniscus

6th M23.30 Other meniscus derangements, unspecified meniscus
Other meniscus derangements, unspecified lateral meniscus
Other meniscus derangements, unspecified medial meniscus

M23.300 Other meniscus derangements, unspecified lateral meniscus, right knee
M23.301 Other meniscus derangements, unspecified lateral meniscus, left knee
M23.302 Other meniscus derangements, unspecified lateral meniscus, unspecified knee
M23.303 Other meniscus derangements, unspecified medial meniscus, right knee
M23.304 Other meniscus derangements, unspecified medial meniscus, left knee
M23.305 Other meniscus derangements, unspecified medial meniscus, unspecified knee
M23.306 Other meniscus derangements, unspecified meniscus, right knee
M23.307 Other meniscus derangements, unspecified meniscus, left knee
M23.309 Other meniscus derangements, unspecified meniscus, unspecified knee

6th M23.31 Other meniscus derangements, anterior horn of medial meniscus
M23.311 Other meniscus derangements, anterior horn of medial meniscus, right knee
M23.312 Other meniscus derangements, anterior horn of medial meniscus, left knee
M23.319 Other meniscus derangements, anterior horn of medial meniscus, unspecified knee

6th M23.32 Other meniscus derangements, posterior horn of medial meniscus
M23.321 Other meniscus derangements, posterior horn of medial meniscus, right knee
M23.322 Other meniscus derangements, posterior horn of medial meniscus, left knee
M23.329 Other meniscus derangements, posterior horn of medial meniscus, unspecified knee

6th M23.33 Other meniscus derangements, other medial meniscus
M23.331 Other meniscus derangements, other medial meniscus, right knee
M23.332 Other meniscus derangements, other medial meniscus, left knee
M23.339 Other meniscus derangements, other medial meniscus, unspecified knee

6th M23.34 Other meniscus derangements, anterior horn of lateral meniscus
M23.341 Other meniscus derangements, anterior horn of lateral meniscus, right knee
M23.342 Other meniscus derangements, anterior horn of lateral meniscus, left knee
M23.349 Other meniscus derangements, anterior horn of lateral meniscus, unspecified knee

6th M23.35 Other meniscus derangements, posterior horn of lateral meniscus
M23.351 Other meniscus derangements, posterior horn of lateral meniscus, right knee
M23.352 Other meniscus derangements, posterior horn of lateral meniscus, left knee
M23.359 Other meniscus derangements, posterior horn of lateral meniscus, unspecified knee

6th M23.36 Other meniscus derangements, other lateral meniscus
M23.361 Other meniscus derangements, other lateral meniscus, right knee
M23.362 Other meniscus derangements, other lateral meniscus, left knee
M23.369 Other meniscus derangements, other lateral meniscus, unspecified knee

5th M23.4 Loose body in knee
M23.40 Loose body in knee, unspecified knee
M23.41 Loose body in knee, right knee
M23.42 Loose body in knee, left knee

5th M23.5 Chronic instability of knee
M23.50 Chronic instability of knee, unspecified knee
M23.51 Chronic instability of knee, right knee
M23.52 Chronic instability of knee, left knee

5th M23.6 Other spontaneous disruption of ligament(s) of knee

6th M23.60 Other spontaneous disruption of unspecified ligament of knee
M23.601 Other spontaneous disruption of unspecified ligament of right knee
M23.602 Other spontaneous disruption of unspecified ligament of left knee
M23.609 Other spontaneous disruption of unspecified ligament of unspecified knee

6th M23.61 Other spontaneous disruption of anterior cruciate ligament of knee
M23.611 Other spontaneous disruption of anterior cruciate ligament of right knee
M23.612 Other spontaneous disruption of anterior cruciate ligament of left knee
M23.619 Other spontaneous disruption of anterior cruciate ligament of unspecified knee

6th M23.62 Other spontaneous disruption of posterior cruciate ligament of knee
M23.621 Other spontaneous disruption of posterior cruciate ligament of right knee
M23.622 Other spontaneous disruption of posterior cruciate ligament of left knee
M23.629 Other spontaneous disruption of posterior cruciate ligament of unspecified knee

6th M23.63 Other spontaneous disruption of medial collateral ligament of knee
M23.631 Other spontaneous disruption of medial collateral ligament of right knee
M23.632 Other spontaneous disruption of medial collateral ligament of left knee
M23.639 Other spontaneous disruption of medial collateral ligament of unspecified knee

6th M23.64 Other spontaneous disruption of lateral collateral ligament of knee
M23.641 Other spontaneous disruption of lateral collateral ligament of right knee
M23.642 Other spontaneous disruption of lateral collateral ligament of left knee
M23.649 Other spontaneous disruption of lateral collateral ligament of unspecified knee

6th M23.67 Other spontaneous disruption of capsular ligament of knee
M23.671 Other spontaneous disruption of capsular ligament of right knee
M23.672 Other spontaneous disruption of capsular ligament of left knee
M23.679 Other spontaneous disruption of capsular ligament of unspecified knee

5th M23.8 Other internal derangements of knee
Laxity of ligament of knee
Snapping knee

6th M23.8X Other internal derangements of knee
M23.8X1 Other internal derangements of right knee
M23.8X2 Other internal derangements of left knee
M23.8X9 Other internal derangements of unspecified knee

5th M23.9 Unspecified internal derangement of knee
M23.90 Unspecified internal derangement of unspecified knee
M23.91 Unspecified internal derangement of right knee
M23.92 Unspecified internal derangement of left knee

✓4th M24 Other specific joint derangements

EXCLUDES 1 *current injury - see injury of joint by body region*

EXCLUDES 2 *ganglion (M67.4)*
snapping knee (M23.8-)
temporomandibular joint disorders (M26.6-)

AHA: 2020,4Q,31-32

✓5th M24.Ø Loose body in joint

EXCLUDES 2 *loose body in knee (M23.4)*

M24.ØØ Loose body in unspecified joint

✓6th M24.Ø1 Loose body in shoulder
- **M24.Ø11 Loose body in right shoulder**
- **M24.Ø12 Loose body in left shoulder**
- **M24.Ø19 Loose body in unspecified shoulder**

✓6th M24.Ø2 Loose body in elbow
- **M24.Ø21 Loose body in right elbow**
- **M24.Ø22 Loose body in left elbow**
- **M24.Ø29 Loose body in unspecified elbow**

✓6th M24.Ø3 Loose body in wrist
- **M24.Ø31 Loose body in right wrist**
- **M24.Ø32 Loose body in left wrist**
- **M24.Ø39 Loose body in unspecified wrist**

✓6th M24.Ø4 Loose body in finger joints
- **M24.Ø41 Loose body in right finger joint(s)**
- **M24.Ø42 Loose body in left finger joint(s)**
- **M24.Ø49 Loose body in unspecified finger joint(s)**

✓6th M24.Ø5 Loose body in hip
- **M24.Ø51 Loose body in right hip**
- **M24.Ø52 Loose body in left hip**
- **M24.Ø59 Loose body in unspecified hip**

✓6th M24.Ø7 Loose body in ankle and toe joints
- **M24.Ø71 Loose body in right ankle**
- **M24.Ø72 Loose body in left ankle**
- **M24.Ø73 Loose body in unspecified ankle**
- **M24.Ø74 Loose body in right toe joint(s)**
- **M24.Ø75 Loose body in left toe joint(s)**
- **M24.Ø76 Loose body in unspecified toe joints**

M24.Ø8 Loose body, other site

✓5th M24.1 Other articular cartilage disorders

EXCLUDES 2 *chondrocalcinosis ▶(M11.1-, M11.2-)◀*
internal derangement of knee (M23.-)
metastatic calcification ▶(E83.59)◀
ochronosis ▶(E7Ø.29)◀

M24.1Ø Other articular cartilage disorders, unspecified site

✓6th M24.11 Other articular cartilage disorders, shoulder
- **M24.111 Other articular cartilage disorders, right shoulder**
- **M24.112 Other articular cartilage disorders, left shoulder**
- **M24.119 Other articular cartilage disorders, unspecified shoulder**

✓6th M24.12 Other articular cartilage disorders, elbow
- **M24.121 Other articular cartilage disorders, right elbow**
- **M24.122 Other articular cartilage disorders, left elbow**
- **M24.129 Other articular cartilage disorders, unspecified elbow**

✓6th M24.13 Other articular cartilage disorders, wrist
- **M24.131 Other articular cartilage disorders, right wrist**
- **M24.132 Other articular cartilage disorders, left wrist**
- **M24.139 Other articular cartilage disorders, unspecified wrist**

✓6th M24.14 Other articular cartilage disorders, hand
- **M24.141 Other articular cartilage disorders, right hand**
- **M24.142 Other articular cartilage disorders, left hand**
- **M24.149 Other articular cartilage disorders, unspecified hand**

✓6th M24.15 Other articular cartilage disorders, hip
- **M24.151 Other articular cartilage disorders, right hip**
- **M24.152 Other articular cartilage disorders, left hip**
- **M24.159 Other articular cartilage disorders, unspecified hip**

✓6th M24.17 Other articular cartilage disorders, ankle and foot
- **M24.171 Other articular cartilage disorders, right ankle**
- **M24.172 Other articular cartilage disorders, left ankle**
- **M24.173 Other articular cartilage disorders, unspecified ankle**
- **M24.174 Other articular cartilage disorders, right foot**
- **M24.175 Other articular cartilage disorders, left foot**
- **M24.176 Other articular cartilage disorders, unspecified foot**

M24.19 Other articular cartilage disorders, other specified site

✓5th M24.2 Disorder of ligament

Instability secondary to old ligament injury
Ligamentous laxity NOS

EXCLUDES 1 *familial ligamentous laxity (M35.7)*

EXCLUDES 2 *internal derangement of knee (M23.5-M23.8X9)*

M24.2Ø Disorder of ligament, unspecified site

✓6th M24.21 Disorder of ligament, shoulder
- **M24.211 Disorder of ligament, right shoulder**
- **M24.212 Disorder of ligament, left shoulder**
- **M24.219 Disorder of ligament, unspecified shoulder**

✓6th M24.22 Disorder of ligament, elbow
- **M24.221 Disorder of ligament, right elbow**
- **M24.222 Disorder of ligament, left elbow**
- **M24.229 Disorder of ligament, unspecified elbow**

✓6th M24.23 Disorder of ligament, wrist
- **M24.231 Disorder of ligament, right wrist**
- **M24.232 Disorder of ligament, left wrist**
- **M24.239 Disorder of ligament, unspecified wrist**

✓6th M24.24 Disorder of ligament, hand
- **M24.241 Disorder of ligament, right hand**
- **M24.242 Disorder of ligament, left hand**
- **M24.249 Disorder of ligament, unspecified hand**

✓6th M24.25 Disorder of ligament, hip
- **M24.251 Disorder of ligament, right hip**
- **M24.252 Disorder of ligament, left hip**
- **M24.259 Disorder of ligament, unspecified hip**

✓6th M24.27 Disorder of ligament, ankle and foot
- **M24.271 Disorder of ligament, right ankle**
- **M24.272 Disorder of ligament, left ankle**
- **M24.273 Disorder of ligament, unspecified ankle**
- **M24.274 Disorder of ligament, right foot**
- **M24.275 Disorder of ligament, left foot**
- **M24.276 Disorder of ligament, unspecified foot**

M24.28 Disorder of ligament, vertebrae

AHA: 2023,2Q,13

M24.29 Disorder of ligament, other specified site

✓5th M24.3 Pathological dislocation of joint, not elsewhere classified

EXCLUDES 1 *congenital dislocation or displacement of joint - see congenital malformations and deformations of the musculoskeletal system (Q65-Q79)*
current injury - see injury of joints and ligaments by body region
recurrent dislocation of joint (M24.4-)

M24.3Ø Pathological dislocation of unspecified joint, not elsewhere classified

✓6th M24.31 Pathological dislocation of shoulder, not elsewhere classified
- **M24.311 Pathological dislocation of right shoulder, not elsewhere classified**
- **M24.312 Pathological dislocation of left shoulder, not elsewhere classified**
- **M24.319 Pathological dislocation of unspecified shoulder, not elsewhere classified**

✓6th M24.32 Pathological dislocation of elbow, not elsewhere classified
- **M24.321 Pathological dislocation of right elbow, not elsewhere classified**
- **M24.322 Pathological dislocation of left elbow, not elsewhere classified**
- **M24.329 Pathological dislocation of unspecified elbow, not elsewhere classified**

✓6th **M24.33 Pathological dislocation of wrist, not elsewhere classified**
- **M24.331 Pathological dislocation of right wrist, not elsewhere classified**
- **M24.332 Pathological dislocation of left wrist, not elsewhere classified**
- **M24.339 Pathological dislocation of unspecified wrist, not elsewhere classified**

✓6th **M24.34 Pathological dislocation of hand, not elsewhere classified**
- **M24.341 Pathological dislocation of right hand, not elsewhere classified**
- **M24.342 Pathological dislocation of left hand, not elsewhere classified**
- **M24.349 Pathological dislocation of unspecified hand, not elsewhere classified**

✓6th **M24.35 Pathological dislocation of hip, not elsewhere classified**

AHA: 2022,1Q,32
- **M24.351 Pathological dislocation of right hip, not elsewhere classified**
- **M24.352 Pathological dislocation of left hip, not elsewhere classified**
- **M24.359 Pathological dislocation of unspecified hip, not elsewhere classified**

✓6th **M24.36 Pathological dislocation of knee, not elsewhere classified**
- **M24.361 Pathological dislocation of right knee, not elsewhere classified**
- **M24.362 Pathological dislocation of left knee, not elsewhere classified**
- **M24.369 Pathological dislocation of unspecified knee, not elsewhere classified**

✓6th **M24.37 Pathological dislocation of ankle and foot, not elsewhere classified**
- **M24.371 Pathological dislocation of right ankle, not elsewhere classified**
- **M24.372 Pathological dislocation of left ankle, not elsewhere classified**
- **M24.373 Pathological dislocation of unspecified ankle, not elsewhere classified**
- **M24.374 Pathological dislocation of right foot, not elsewhere classified**
- **M24.375 Pathological dislocation of left foot, not elsewhere classified**
- **M24.376 Pathological dislocation of unspecified foot, not elsewhere classified**

M24.39 Pathological dislocation of other specified joint, not elsewhere classified

✓5th **M24.4 Recurrent dislocation of joint**

Recurrent subluxation of joint

EXCLUDES 2 *recurrent dislocation of patella (M22.Ø-M22.1)*
recurrent vertebral dislocation (M43.3-, M43.4, M43.5-)

M24.4Ø Recurrent dislocation, unspecified joint

✓6th **M24.41 Recurrent dislocation, shoulder**
- **M24.411 Recurrent dislocation, right shoulder**
- **M24.412 Recurrent dislocation, left shoulder**
- **M24.419 Recurrent dislocation, unspecified shoulder**

✓6th **M24.42 Recurrent dislocation, elbow**
- **M24.421 Recurrent dislocation, right elbow**
- **M24.422 Recurrent dislocation, left elbow**
- **M24.429 Recurrent dislocation, unspecified elbow**

✓6th **M24.43 Recurrent dislocation, wrist**
- **M24.431 Recurrent dislocation, right wrist**
- **M24.432 Recurrent dislocation, left wrist**
- **M24.439 Recurrent dislocation, unspecified wrist**

✓6th **M24.44 Recurrent dislocation, hand and finger(s)**
- **M24.441 Recurrent dislocation, right hand**
- **M24.442 Recurrent dislocation, left hand**
- **M24.443 Recurrent dislocation, unspecified hand**
- **M24.444 Recurrent dislocation, right finger**
- **M24.445 Recurrent dislocation, left finger**
- **M24.446 Recurrent dislocation, unspecified finger**

✓6th **M24.45 Recurrent dislocation, hip**
- **M24.451 Recurrent dislocation, right hip**
- **M24.452 Recurrent dislocation, left hip**
- **M24.459 Recurrent dislocation, unspecified hip**

✓6th **M24.46 Recurrent dislocation, knee**
- **M24.461 Recurrent dislocation, right knee**
- **M24.462 Recurrent dislocation, left knee**
- **M24.469 Recurrent dislocation, unspecified knee**

✓6th **M24.47 Recurrent dislocation, ankle, foot and toes**
- **M24.471 Recurrent dislocation, right ankle**
- **M24.472 Recurrent dislocation, left ankle**
- **M24.473 Recurrent dislocation, unspecified ankle**
- **M24.474 Recurrent dislocation, right foot**
- **M24.475 Recurrent dislocation, left foot**
- **M24.476 Recurrent dislocation, unspecified foot**
- **M24.477 Recurrent dislocation, right toe(s)**
- **M24.478 Recurrent dislocation, left toe(s)**
- **M24.479 Recurrent dislocation, unspecified toe(s)**

M24.49 Recurrent dislocation, other specified joint

✓5th **M24.5 Contracture of joint**

EXCLUDES 1 *contracture of muscle without contracture of joint (M62.4-)*
contracture of tendon (sheath) without contracture of joint (M62.4-)
Dupuytren's contracture (M72.Ø)

EXCLUDES 2 *acquired deformities of limbs (M2Ø-M21)*

AHA: 2016,2Q,6

M24.5Ø Contracture, unspecified joint

✓6th **M24.51 Contracture, shoulder**
- **M24.511 Contracture, right shoulder**
- **M24.512 Contracture, left shoulder**
- **M24.519 Contracture, unspecified shoulder**

✓6th **M24.52 Contracture, elbow**
- **M24.521 Contracture, right elbow**
- **M24.522 Contracture, left elbow**
- **M24.529 Contracture, unspecified elbow**

✓6th **M24.53 Contracture, wrist**
- **M24.531 Contracture, right wrist**
- **M24.532 Contracture, left wrist**
- **M24.539 Contracture, unspecified wrist**

✓6th **M24.54 Contracture, hand**
- **M24.541 Contracture, right hand**
- **M24.542 Contracture, left hand**
- **M24.549 Contracture, unspecified hand**

✓6th **M24.55 Contracture, hip**
- **M24.551 Contracture, right hip**
- **M24.552 Contracture, left hip**
- **M24.559 Contracture, unspecified hip**

✓6th **M24.56 Contracture, knee**
- **M24.561 Contracture, right knee**
- **M24.562 Contracture, left knee**
- **M24.569 Contracture, unspecified knee**

✓6th **M24.57 Contracture, ankle and foot**
- **M24.571 Contracture, right ankle**
- **M24.572 Contracture, left ankle**
- **M24.573 Contracture, unspecified ankle**
- **M24.574 Contracture, right foot**
- **M24.575 Contracture, left foot**
- **M24.576 Contracture, unspecified foot**

M24.59 Contracture, other specified joint

✓5th **M24.6 Ankylosis of joint**

EXCLUDES 1 *stiffness of joint without ankylosis (M25.6-)*

EXCLUDES 2 *spine (M43.2-)*

DEF: Ankylosis: Abnormal union or fusion of bones in a joint, which is normally moveable.

M24.6Ø Ankylosis, unspecified joint

✓6th **M24.61 Ankylosis, shoulder**
- **M24.611 Ankylosis, right shoulder**
- **M24.612 Ankylosis, left shoulder**
- **M24.619 Ankylosis, unspecified shoulder**

✓6th **M24.62 Ankylosis, elbow**
- **M24.621 Ankylosis, right elbow**
- **M24.622 Ankylosis, left elbow**
- **M24.629 Ankylosis, unspecified elbow**

✓6th **M24.63 Ankylosis, wrist**
- **M24.631 Ankylosis, right wrist**
- **M24.632 Ankylosis, left wrist**
- **M24.639 Ankylosis, unspecified wrist**

- M24.64 Ankylosis, hand
  - M24.641 Ankylosis, right hand
  - M24.642 Ankylosis, left hand
  - M24.649 Ankylosis, unspecified hand
- M24.65 Ankylosis, hip
  - M24.651 Ankylosis, right hip
  - M24.652 Ankylosis, left hip
  - M24.659 Ankylosis, unspecified hip
- M24.66 Ankylosis, knee
  - M24.661 Ankylosis, right knee
  - M24.662 Ankylosis, left knee
  - M24.669 Ankylosis, unspecified knee
- M24.67 Ankylosis, ankle and foot
  - M24.671 Ankylosis, right ankle
  - M24.672 Ankylosis, left ankle
  - M24.673 Ankylosis, unspecified ankle
  - M24.674 Ankylosis, right foot
  - M24.675 Ankylosis, left foot
  - M24.676 Ankylosis, unspecified foot
- M24.69 Ankylosis, other specified joint

M24.7 Protrusio acetabuli

DEF: Intrapelvic protrusion of the acetabulum characterized by the sinking of the floor of the acetabulum, causing the femoral head to protrude. It limits hip movement and is of unknown etiology. ***Synonym(s):*** *Otto's pelvis.*

M24.8 Other specific joint derangements, not elsewhere classified

EXCLUDES 2 *iliotibial band syndrome (M76.3)*

- M24.80 Other specific joint derangements of unspecified joint, not elsewhere classified
- M24.81 Other specific joint derangements of shoulder, not elsewhere classified
  - M24.811 Other specific joint derangements of right shoulder, not elsewhere classified
  - M24.812 Other specific joint derangements of left shoulder, not elsewhere classified
  - M24.819 Other specific joint derangements of unspecified shoulder, not elsewhere classified
- M24.82 Other specific joint derangements of elbow, not elsewhere classified
  - M24.821 Other specific joint derangements of right elbow, not elsewhere classified
  - M24.822 Other specific joint derangements of left elbow, not elsewhere classified
  - M24.829 Other specific joint derangements of unspecified elbow, not elsewhere classified
- M24.83 Other specific joint derangements of wrist, not elsewhere classified
  - M24.831 Other specific joint derangements of right wrist, not elsewhere classified
  - M24.832 Other specific joint derangements of left wrist, not elsewhere classified
  - M24.839 Other specific joint derangements of unspecified wrist, not elsewhere classified
- M24.84 Other specific joint derangements of hand, not elsewhere classified
  - M24.841 Other specific joint derangements of right hand, not elsewhere classified
  - M24.842 Other specific joint derangements of left hand, not elsewhere classified
  - M24.849 Other specific joint derangements of unspecified hand, not elsewhere classified
- M24.85 Other specific joint derangements of hip, not elsewhere classified

  Irritable hip
  - M24.851 Other specific joint derangements of right hip, not elsewhere classified
  - M24.852 Other specific joint derangements of left hip, not elsewhere classified
  - M24.859 Other specific joint derangements of unspecified hip, not elsewhere classified
- M24.87 Other specific joint derangements of ankle and foot, not elsewhere classified
  - M24.871 Other specific joint derangements of right ankle, not elsewhere classified
  - M24.872 Other specific joint derangements of left ankle, not elsewhere classified
  - M24.873 Other specific joint derangements of unspecified ankle, not elsewhere classified
  - M24.874 Other specific joint derangements of right foot, not elsewhere classified
  - M24.875 Other specific joint derangements left foot, not elsewhere classified
  - M24.876 Other specific joint derangements of unspecified foot, not elsewhere classified
- M24.89 Other specific joint derangement of other specified joint, not elsewhere classified

M24.9 Joint derangement, unspecified

M25 Other joint disorder, not elsewhere classified

EXCLUDES 2
abnormality of gait and mobility (R26.-)
acquired deformities of limb (M20-M21)
calcification of bursa (M71.4-)
calcification of shoulder (joint) (M75.3)
calcification of tendon (M65.2-)
difficulty in walking (R26.2)
temporomandibular joint disorder (M26.6-)

AHA: 2020,4Q,31-32

M25.0 Hemarthrosis

EXCLUDES 1
current injury - see injury of joint by body region
hemophilic arthropathy (M36.2)

- M25.00 Hemarthrosis, unspecified joint CC UNS
- M25.01 Hemarthrosis, shoulder
  - M25.011 Hemarthrosis, right shoulder CC
  - M25.012 Hemarthrosis, left shoulder CC
  - M25.019 Hemarthrosis, unspecified shoulder CC UNS
- M25.02 Hemarthrosis, elbow
  - M25.021 Hemarthrosis, right elbow CC
  - M25.022 Hemarthrosis, left elbow CC
  - M25.029 Hemarthrosis, unspecified elbow CC UNS
- M25.03 Hemarthrosis, wrist
  - M25.031 Hemarthrosis, right wrist CC
  - M25.032 Hemarthrosis, left wrist CC
  - M25.039 Hemarthrosis, unspecified wrist CC UNS
- M25.04 Hemarthrosis, hand
  - M25.041 Hemarthrosis, right hand CC
  - M25.042 Hemarthrosis, left hand CC
  - M25.049 Hemarthrosis, unspecified hand CC UNS
- M25.05 Hemarthrosis, hip
  - M25.051 Hemarthrosis, right hip CC
  - M25.052 Hemarthrosis, left hip CC
  - M25.059 Hemarthrosis, unspecified hip CC UNS
- M25.06 Hemarthrosis, knee
  - M25.061 Hemarthrosis, right knee CC
  - M25.062 Hemarthrosis, left knee CC
  - M25.069 Hemarthrosis, unspecified knee CC UNS
- M25.07 Hemarthrosis, ankle and foot
  - M25.071 Hemarthrosis, right ankle CC
  - M25.072 Hemarthrosis, left ankle CC
  - M25.073 Hemarthrosis, unspecified ankle CC UNS
  - M25.074 Hemarthrosis, right foot CC
  - M25.075 Hemarthrosis, left foot CC
  - M25.076 Hemarthrosis, unspecified foot CC UNS
- M25.08 Hemarthrosis, other specified site CC

  Hemarthrosis, vertebrae

M25.1 Fistula of joint

- M25.10 Fistula, unspecified joint
- M25.11 Fistula, shoulder
  - M25.111 Fistula, right shoulder
  - M25.112 Fistula, left shoulder
  - M25.119 Fistula, unspecified shoulder
- M25.12 Fistula, elbow
  - M25.121 Fistula, right elbow
  - M25.122 Fistula, left elbow
  - M25.129 Fistula, unspecified elbow

M25.13 Fistula, wrist
M25.131 Fistula, right wrist
M25.132 Fistula, left wrist
M25.139 Fistula, unspecified wrist
M25.14 Fistula, hand
M25.141 Fistula, right hand
M25.142 Fistula, left hand
M25.149 Fistula, unspecified hand
M25.15 Fistula, hip
M25.151 Fistula, right hip
M25.152 Fistula, left hip
M25.159 Fistula, unspecified hip
M25.16 Fistula, knee
M25.161 Fistula, right knee
M25.162 Fistula, left knee
M25.169 Fistula, unspecified knee
M25.17 Fistula, ankle and foot
M25.171 Fistula, right ankle
M25.172 Fistula, left ankle
M25.173 Fistula, unspecified ankle
M25.174 Fistula, right foot
M25.175 Fistula, left foot
M25.176 Fistula, unspecified foot
M25.18 Fistula, other specified site
Fistula, vertebrae

M25.2 Flail joint
DEF: Hinged joint that exhibits an abnormal or excessive degree of range and mobility.
M25.20 Flail joint, unspecified joint
M25.21 Flail joint, shoulder
M25.211 Flail joint, right shoulder
M25.212 Flail joint, left shoulder
M25.219 Flail joint, unspecified shoulder
M25.22 Flail joint, elbow
M25.221 Flail joint, right elbow
M25.222 Flail joint, left elbow
M25.229 Flail joint, unspecified elbow
M25.23 Flail joint, wrist
M25.231 Flail joint, right wrist
M25.232 Flail joint, left wrist
M25.239 Flail joint, unspecified wrist
M25.24 Flail joint, hand
M25.241 Flail joint, right hand
M25.242 Flail joint, left hand
M25.249 Flail joint, unspecified hand
M25.25 Flail joint, hip
M25.251 Flail joint, right hip
M25.252 Flail joint, left hip
M25.259 Flail joint, unspecified hip
M25.26 Flail joint, knee
M25.261 Flail joint, right knee
M25.262 Flail joint, left knee
M25.269 Flail joint, unspecified knee
M25.27 Flail joint, ankle and foot
M25.271 Flail joint, right ankle and foot
M25.272 Flail joint, left ankle and foot
M25.279 Flail joint, unspecified ankle and foot
M25.28 Flail joint, other site

M25.3 Other instability of joint
EXCLUDES 1 *instability of joint secondary to old ligament injury (M24.2-)*
instability of joint secondary to removal of joint prosthesis (M96.8-)
EXCLUDES 2 *spinal instabilities (M53.2-)*
M25.30 Other instability, unspecified joint
M25.31 Other instability, shoulder
M25.311 Other instability, right shoulder
M25.312 Other instability, left shoulder
M25.319 Other instability, unspecified shoulder
M25.32 Other instability, elbow
M25.321 Other instability, right elbow
M25.322 Other instability, left elbow
M25.329 Other instability, unspecified elbow
M25.33 Other instability, wrist
M25.331 Other instability, right wrist
M25.332 Other instability, left wrist
M25.339 Other instability, unspecified wrist
M25.34 Other instability, hand
M25.341 Other instability, right hand
M25.342 Other instability, left hand
M25.349 Other instability, unspecified hand
M25.35 Other instability, hip
M25.351 Other instability, right hip
M25.352 Other instability, left hip
M25.359 Other instability, unspecified hip
M25.36 Other instability, knee
M25.361 Other instability, right knee
M25.362 Other instability, left knee
M25.369 Other instability, unspecified knee
M25.37 Other instability, ankle and foot
M25.371 Other instability, right ankle
M25.372 Other instability, left ankle
M25.373 Other instability, unspecified ankle
M25.374 Other instability, right foot
M25.375 Other instability, left foot
M25.376 Other instability, unspecified foot
M25.39 Other instability, other specified joint

M25.4 Effusion of joint
EXCLUDES 1 *hydrarthrosis in yaws (A66.6)*
intermittent hydrarthrosis (M12.4-)
other infective (teno)synovitis (M65.1-)
M25.40 Effusion, unspecified joint
M25.41 Effusion, shoulder
M25.411 Effusion, right shoulder
M25.412 Effusion, left shoulder
M25.419 Effusion, unspecified shoulder
M25.42 Effusion, elbow
M25.421 Effusion, right elbow
M25.422 Effusion, left elbow
M25.429 Effusion, unspecified elbow
M25.43 Effusion, wrist
M25.431 Effusion, right wrist
M25.432 Effusion, left wrist
M25.439 Effusion, unspecified wrist
M25.44 Effusion, hand
M25.441 Effusion, right hand
M25.442 Effusion, left hand
M25.449 Effusion, unspecified hand
M25.45 Effusion, hip
M25.451 Effusion, right hip
M25.452 Effusion, left hip
M25.459 Effusion, unspecified hip
M25.46 Effusion, knee
M25.461 Effusion, right knee
M25.462 Effusion, left knee
M25.469 Effusion, unspecified knee
M25.47 Effusion, ankle and foot
M25.471 Effusion, right ankle
M25.472 Effusion, left ankle
M25.473 Effusion, unspecified ankle
M25.474 Effusion, right foot
M25.475 Effusion, left foot
M25.476 Effusion, unspecified foot
M25.48 Effusion, other site

M25.5 Pain in joint
EXCLUDES 2 *pain in fingers (M79.64-)*
pain in foot (M79.67-)
pain in hand (M79.64-)
pain in limb (M79.6-)
pain in toes (M79.67-)
M25.50 Pain in unspecified joint
M25.51 Pain in shoulder
M25.511 Pain in right shoulder
M25.512 Pain in left shoulder
M25.519 Pain in unspecified shoulder
M25.52 Pain in elbow
M25.521 Pain in right elbow
M25.522 Pain in left elbow
M25.529 Pain in unspecified elbow

✓6th M25.53 Pain in wrist
M25.531 Pain in right wrist
M25.532 Pain in left wrist
M25.539 Pain in unspecified wrist
✓6th M25.54 Pain in joints of hand
AHA: 2016,4Q,38
M25.541 Pain in joints of right hand
M25.542 Pain in joints of left hand
M25.549 Pain in joints of unspecified hand
Pain in joints of hand NOS
✓6th M25.55 Pain in hip
M25.551 Pain in right hip
M25.552 Pain in left hip
M25.559 Pain in unspecified hip
✓6th M25.56 Pain in knee
M25.561 Pain in right knee
M25.562 Pain in left knee
M25.569 Pain in unspecified knee
✓6th M25.57 Pain in ankle and joints of foot
M25.571 Pain in right ankle and joints of right foot
M25.572 Pain in left ankle and joints of left foot
M25.579 Pain in unspecified ankle and joints of unspecified foot
M25.59 Pain in other specified joint
✓5th M25.6 Stiffness of joint, not elsewhere classified
EXCLUDES 1 *ankylosis of joint (M24.6-)*
contracture of joint (M24.5-)
M25.60 Stiffness of unspecified joint, not elsewhere classified
✓6th M25.61 Stiffness of shoulder, not elsewhere classified
M25.611 Stiffness of right shoulder, not elsewhere classified
M25.612 Stiffness of left shoulder, not elsewhere classified
M25.619 Stiffness of unspecified shoulder, not elsewhere classified
✓6th M25.62 Stiffness of elbow, not elsewhere classified
M25.621 Stiffness of right elbow, not elsewhere classified
M25.622 Stiffness of left elbow, not elsewhere classified
M25.629 Stiffness of unspecified elbow, not elsewhere classified
✓6th M25.63 Stiffness of wrist, not elsewhere classified
M25.631 Stiffness of right wrist, not elsewhere classified
M25.632 Stiffness of left wrist, not elsewhere classified
M25.639 Stiffness of unspecified wrist, not elsewhere classified
✓6th M25.64 Stiffness of hand, not elsewhere classified
M25.641 Stiffness of right hand, not elsewhere classified
M25.642 Stiffness of left hand, not elsewhere classified
M25.649 Stiffness of unspecified hand, not elsewhere classified
✓6th M25.65 Stiffness of hip, not elsewhere classified
M25.651 Stiffness of right hip, not elsewhere classified
M25.652 Stiffness of left hip, not elsewhere classified
M25.659 Stiffness of unspecified hip, not elsewhere classified
✓6th M25.66 Stiffness of knee, not elsewhere classified
M25.661 Stiffness of right knee, not elsewhere classified
M25.662 Stiffness of left knee, not elsewhere classified
M25.669 Stiffness of unspecified knee, not elsewhere classified
✓6th M25.67 Stiffness of ankle and foot, not elsewhere classified
M25.671 Stiffness of right ankle, not elsewhere classified
M25.672 Stiffness of left ankle, not elsewhere classified
M25.673 Stiffness of unspecified ankle, not elsewhere classified
M25.674 Stiffness of right foot, not elsewhere classified
M25.675 Stiffness of left foot, not elsewhere classified
M25.676 Stiffness of unspecified foot, not elsewhere classified
M25.69 Stiffness of other specified joint, not elsewhere classified
✓5th M25.7 Osteophyte
M25.70 Osteophyte, unspecified joint
✓6th M25.71 Osteophyte, shoulder
M25.711 Osteophyte, right shoulder
M25.712 Osteophyte, left shoulder
M25.719 Osteophyte, unspecified shoulder
✓6th M25.72 Osteophyte, elbow
M25.721 Osteophyte, right elbow
M25.722 Osteophyte, left elbow
M25.729 Osteophyte, unspecified elbow
✓6th M25.73 Osteophyte, wrist
M25.731 Osteophyte, right wrist
M25.732 Osteophyte, left wrist
M25.739 Osteophyte, unspecified wrist
✓6th M25.74 Osteophyte, hand
M25.741 Osteophyte, right hand
M25.742 Osteophyte, left hand
M25.749 Osteophyte, unspecified hand
✓6th M25.75 Osteophyte, hip
M25.751 Osteophyte, right hip
M25.752 Osteophyte, left hip
M25.759 Osteophyte, unspecified hip
✓6th M25.76 Osteophyte, knee
M25.761 Osteophyte, right knee
M25.762 Osteophyte, left knee
M25.769 Osteophyte, unspecified knee
✓6th M25.77 Osteophyte, ankle and foot
M25.771 Osteophyte, right ankle
M25.772 Osteophyte, left ankle
M25.773 Osteophyte, unspecified ankle
M25.774 Osteophyte, right foot
M25.775 Osteophyte, left foot
M25.776 Osteophyte, unspecified foot
M25.78 Osteophyte, vertebrae
✓5th M25.8 Other specified joint disorders
M25.80 Other specified joint disorders, unspecified joint
✓6th M25.81 Other specified joint disorders, shoulder
AHA: 2022,3Q,18
M25.811 Other specified joint disorders, right shoulder
M25.812 Other specified joint disorders, left shoulder
M25.819 Other specified joint disorders, unspecified shoulder
✓6th M25.82 Other specified joint disorders, elbow
M25.821 Other specified joint disorders, right elbow
M25.822 Other specified joint disorders, left elbow
M25.829 Other specified joint disorders, unspecified elbow
✓6th M25.83 Other specified joint disorders, wrist
M25.831 Other specified joint disorders, right wrist
M25.832 Other specified joint disorders, left wrist
M25.839 Other specified joint disorders, unspecified wrist
✓6th M25.84 Other specified joint disorders, hand
M25.841 Other specified joint disorders, right hand
M25.842 Other specified joint disorders, left hand
M25.849 Other specified joint disorders, unspecified hand
✓6th M25.85 Other specified joint disorders, hip
AHA: 2014,4Q,25
M25.851 Other specified joint disorders, right hip
M25.852 Other specified joint disorders, left hip
M25.859 Other specified joint disorders, unspecified hip
✓6th M25.86 Other specified joint disorders, knee
M25.861 Other specified joint disorders, right knee
M25.862 Other specified joint disorders, left knee

M25.869 **Other specified joint disorders, unspecified knee**

✓6th M25.87 **Other specified joint disorders, ankle and foot**

M25.871 **Other specified joint disorders, right ankle and foot**

M25.872 **Other specified joint disorders, left ankle and foot**

M25.879 **Other specified joint disorders, unspecified ankle and foot**

M25.9 **Joint disorder, unspecified**

Dentofacial anomalies [including malocclusion] and other disorders of jaw (M26-M27)

EXCLUDES 1 *hemifacial atrophy or hypertrophy (Q67.4)*
unilateral condylar hyperplasia or hypoplasia (M27.8)

✓4th M26 **Dentofacial anomalies [including malocclusion]**

✓5th M26.Ø **Major anomalies of jaw size**

EXCLUDES 1 *acromegaly (E22.Ø)*
Robin's syndrome (Q87.Ø)

M26.ØØ **Unspecified anomaly of jaw size**

M26.Ø1 **Maxillary hyperplasia**

M26.Ø2 **Maxillary hypoplasia**
AHA: 2014,3Q,23

M26.Ø3 **Mandibular hyperplasia**

M26.Ø4 **Mandibular hypoplasia**

M26.Ø5 **Macrogenia**

M26.Ø6 **Microgenia**

M26.Ø7 **Excessive tuberosity of jaw**
Entire maxillary tuberosity

M26.Ø9 **Other specified anomalies of jaw size**

✓5th M26.1 **Anomalies of jaw-cranial base relationship**

M26.1Ø **Unspecified anomaly of jaw-cranial base relationship**

M26.11 **Maxillary asymmetry**

M26.12 **Other jaw asymmetry**

M26.19 **Other specified anomalies of jaw-cranial base relationship**
AHA: 2020,1Q,21

✓5th M26.2 **Anomalies of dental arch relationship**

M26.2Ø **Unspecified anomaly of dental arch relationship**

✓6th M26.21 **Malocclusion, Angle's class**

M26.211 **Malocclusion, Angle's class I**
Neutro-occlusion

M26.212 **Malocclusion, Angle's class II**
Disto-occlusion Division I
Disto-occlusion Division II

M26.213 **Malocclusion, Angle's class III**
Mesio-occlusion

M26.219 **Malocclusion, Angle's class, unspecified**

✓6th M26.22 **Open occlusal relationship**

M26.22Ø **Open anterior occlusal relationship**
Anterior open bite

M26.221 **Open posterior occlusal relationship**
Posterior open bite

M26.23 **Excessive horizontal overlap**
Excessive horizontal overjet

M26.24 **Reverse articulation**
Crossbite (anterior) (posterior)

M26.25 **Anomalies of interarch distance**

M26.29 **Other anomalies of dental arch relationship**
Midline deviation of dental arch
Overbite (excessive) deep
Overbite (excessive) horizontal
Overbite (excessive) vertical
Posterior lingual occlusion of mandibular teeth

✓5th M26.3 **Anomalies of tooth position of fully erupted tooth or teeth**

EXCLUDES 2 *embedded and impacted teeth (KØ1.-)*

M26.3Ø **Unspecified anomaly of tooth position of fully erupted tooth or teeth**
Abnormal spacing of fully erupted tooth or teeth NOS
Displacement of fully erupted tooth or teeth NOS
Transposition of fully erupted tooth or teeth NOS

M26.31 **Crowding of fully erupted teeth**

M26.32 **Excessive spacing of fully erupted teeth**
Diastema of fully erupted tooth or teeth NOS

M26.33 **Horizontal displacement of fully erupted tooth or teeth**
Tipped tooth or teeth
Tipping of fully erupted tooth

M26.34 **Vertical displacement of fully erupted tooth or teeth**
Extruded tooth
Infraeruption of tooth or teeth
Supraeruption of tooth or teeth

M26.35 **Rotation of fully erupted tooth or teeth**

M26.36 **Insufficient interocclusal distance of fully erupted teeth (ridge)**
Lack of adequate intermaxillary vertical dimension of fully erupted teeth

M26.37 **Excessive interocclusal distance of fully erupted teeth**
Excessive intermaxillary vertical dimension of fully erupted teeth
Loss of occlusal vertical dimension of fully erupted teeth

M26.39 **Other anomalies of tooth position of fully erupted tooth or teeth**

M26.4 **Malocclusion, unspecified**

✓5th M26.5 **Dentofacial functional abnormalities**

EXCLUDES 1 *bruxism (F45.8)*
teeth-grinding NOS (F45.8)

M26.5Ø **Dentofacial functional abnormalities, unspecified**

M26.51 **Abnormal jaw closure**

M26.52 **Limited mandibular range of motion**

M26.53 **Deviation in opening and closing of the mandible**

M26.54 **Insufficient anterior guidance**
Insufficient anterior occlusal guidance

M26.55 **Centric occlusion maximum intercuspation discrepancy**
EXCLUDES 1 *centric occlusion NOS (M26.59)*

M26.56 **Non-working side interference**
Balancing side interference

M26.57 **Lack of posterior occlusal support**

M26.59 **Other dentofacial functional abnormalities**
Centric occlusion (of teeth) NOS
Malocclusion due to abnormal swallowing
Malocclusion due to mouth breathing
Malocclusion due to tongue, lip or finger habits

✓5th M26.6 **Temporomandibular joint disorders**

EXCLUDES 2 *current temporomandibular joint dislocation (SØ3.Ø)*
current temporomandibular joint sprain (SØ3.4)

AHA: 2016,4Q,38-39

Temporomandibular Joint

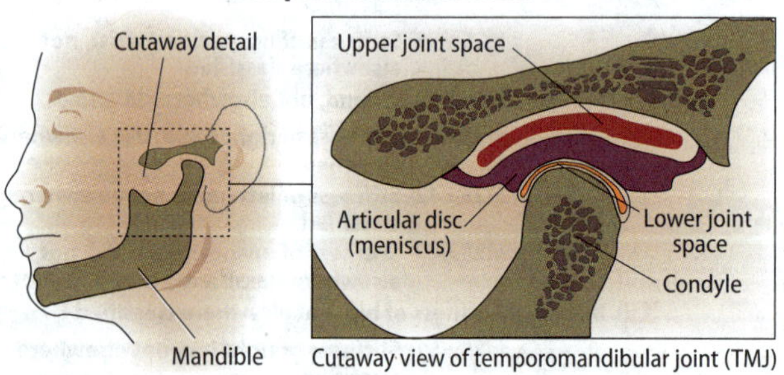

Cutaway view of temporomandibular joint (TMJ)

✓6th M26.6Ø **Temporomandibular joint disorder, unspecified**

M26.6Ø1 **Right temporomandibular joint disorder, unspecified**

M26.6Ø2 **Left temporomandibular joint disorder, unspecified**

M26.6Ø3 **Bilateral temporomandibular joint disorder, unspecified**

M26.6Ø9 **Unspecified temporomandibular joint disorder, unspecified side**
Temporomandibular joint disorder NOS

✓6th M26.61 **Adhesions and ankylosis of temporomandibular joint**

M26.611 **Adhesions and ankylosis of right temporomandibular joint**

M26.612 **Adhesions and ankylosis of left temporomandibular joint**

M26.613 **Adhesions and ankylosis of bilateral temporomandibular joint**

M26.619 Adhesions and ankylosis of temporomandibular joint, unspecified side

M26.62 Arthralgia of temporomandibular joint
- M26.621 Arthralgia of right temporomandibular joint
- M26.622 Arthralgia of left temporomandibular joint
- M26.623 Arthralgia of bilateral temporomandibular joint
- M26.629 Arthralgia of temporomandibular joint, unspecified side

M26.63 Articular disc disorder of temporomandibular joint
- M26.631 Articular disc disorder of right temporomandibular joint
- M26.632 Articular disc disorder of left temporomandibular joint
- M26.633 Articular disc disorder of bilateral temporomandibular joint
- M26.639 Articular disc disorder of temporomandibular joint, unspecified side

M26.64 Arthritis of temporomandibular joint

AHA: 2020,4Q,32
- M26.641 Arthritis of right temporomandibular joint
- M26.642 Arthritis of left temporomandibular joint
- M26.643 Arthritis of bilateral temporomandibular joint
- M26.649 Arthritis of unspecified temporomandibular joint

M26.65 Arthropathy of temporomandibular joint

AHA: 2020,4Q,32
- M26.651 Arthropathy of right temporomandibular joint
- M26.652 Arthropathy of left temporomandibular joint
- M26.653 Arthropathy of bilateral temporomandibular joint
- M26.659 Arthropathy of unspecified temporomandibular joint

M26.69 Other specified disorders of temporomandibular joint

M26.7 Dental alveolar anomalies
- M26.70 Unspecified alveolar anomaly
- M26.71 Alveolar maxillary hyperplasia
- M26.72 Alveolar mandibular hyperplasia
- M26.73 Alveolar maxillary hypoplasia
- M26.74 Alveolar mandibular hypoplasia
- M26.79 Other specified alveolar anomalies

M26.8 Other dentofacial anomalies
- M26.81 Anterior soft tissue impingement
  - Anterior soft tissue impingement on teeth
- M26.82 Posterior soft tissue impingement
  - Posterior soft tissue impingement on teeth
- M26.89 Other dentofacial anomalies

M26.9 Dentofacial anomaly, unspecified

M27 Other diseases of jaws

M27.0 Developmental disorders of jaws
- Latent bone cyst of jaw
- Stafne's cyst
- Torus mandibularis
- Torus palatinus

M27.1 Giant cell granuloma, central
- Giant cell granuloma NOS

EXCLUDES 1 *peripheral giant cell granuloma (K06.8)*

M27.2 Inflammatory conditions of jaws
- Osteitis of jaw(s)
- Osteomyelitis (neonatal) jaw(s)
- Osteoradionecrosis jaw(s)
- Periostitis jaw(s)
- Sequestrum of jaw bone

Use additional code (W88-W90, X39.0) to identify radiation, if radiation-induced

EXCLUDES 2 *osteonecrosis of jaw due to drug (M87.180)*

M27.3 Alveolitis of jaws
- Alveolar osteitis
- Dry socket

M27.4 Other and unspecified cysts of jaw

EXCLUDES 1 *cysts of oral region (K09.-)*
latent bone cyst of jaw (M27.0)
Stafne's cyst (M27.0)

- M27.40 Unspecified cyst of jaw
  - Cyst of jaw NOS
- M27.49 Other cysts of jaw
  - Aneurysmal cyst of jaw
  - Hemorrhagic cyst of jaw
  - Traumatic cyst of jaw

M27.5 Periradicular pathology associated with previous endodontic treatment
- M27.51 Perforation of root canal space due to endodontic treatment
- M27.52 Endodontic overfill
- M27.53 Endodontic underfill
- M27.59 Other periradicular pathology associated with previous endodontic treatment

M27.6 Endosseous dental implant failure
- M27.61 Osseointegration failure of dental implant
  - Hemorrhagic complications of dental implant placement
  - Iatrogenic osseointegration failure of dental implant
  - Osseointegration failure of dental implant due to complications of systemic disease
  - Osseointegration failure of dental implant due to poor bone quality
  - Pre-integration failure of dental implant NOS
  - Pre-osseointegration failure of dental implant
- M27.62 Post-osseointegration biological failure of dental implant
  - Failure of dental implant due to lack of attached gingiva
  - Failure of dental implant due to occlusal trauma (caused by poor prosthetic design)
  - Failure of dental implant due to parafunctional habits
  - Failure of dental implant due to periodontal infection (peri-implantitis)
  - Failure of dental implant due to poor oral hygiene
  - Iatrogenic post-osseointegration failure of dental implant
  - Post-osseointegration failure of dental implant due to complications of systemic disease
- M27.63 Post-osseointegration mechanical failure of dental implant
  - Failure of dental prosthesis causing loss of dental implant
  - Fracture of dental implant

  EXCLUDES 2 *cracked tooth (K03.81)*
  fractured dental restorative material with loss of material (K08.531)
  fractured dental restorative material without loss of material (K08.530)
  fractured tooth (S02.5)
- M27.69 Other endosseous dental implant failure
  - Dental implant failure NOS

M27.8 Other specified diseases of jaws
- Cherubism
- Exostosis
- Fibrous dysplasia
- Unilateral condylar hyperplasia
- Unilateral condylar hypoplasia

EXCLUDES 1 *jaw pain (R68.84)*

M27.9 Disease of jaws, unspecified

Systemic connective tissue disorders (M30-M36)

INCLUDES autoimmune disease NOS
collagen (vascular) disease NOS
systemic autoimmune disease
systemic collagen (vascular) disease

EXCLUDES 1 *autoimmune disease, single organ or single cell-type -code to relevant condition category*

M30 Polyarteritis nodosa and related conditions

EXCLUDES 1 *microscopic polyarteritis (M31.7)*

M30.0 Polyarteritis nodosa CC HCC

M30.1 Polyarteritis with lung involvement [Churg-Strauss] CC HCC
Allergic granulomatous angiitis
Eosinophilic granulomatosis with polyangiitis [EGPA]
AHA: 2021,1Q,23

M30.2 Juvenile polyarteritis CC HCC

M30.3 Mucocutaneous lymph node syndrome [Kawasaki] CC HCC

M30.8 Other conditions related to polyarteritis nodosa CC HCC
Polyangiitis overlap syndrome

4th M31 Other necrotizing vasculopathies

M31.0 Hypersensitivity angiitis CC HCC
Goodpasture's syndrome

5th **M31.1 Thrombotic microangiopathy**
AHA: 2021,4Q,19

M31.10 Thrombotic microangiopathy, unspecified MCC HCC

M31.11 Hematopoietic stem cell transplantation-associated thrombotic microangiopathy [HSCT-TMA] MCC HCC
Transplant-associated thrombotic microangiopathy [TA-TMA]
Code first if applicable:
complications of bone marrow transplant (T86.0-)
complications of stem cell transplant (T86.5)
Use additional code to identify specific organ dysfunction, such as:
acute kidney failure (N17.-)
acute respiratory distress syndrome (J80)
capillary leak syndrome (I78.8)
diffuse alveolar hemorrhage (R04.89)
encephalopathy (metabolic) (septic) (G93.41)
fluid overload, unspecified (E87.70)
graft versus host disease (D89.81-)
hemolytic uremic syndrome (D59.3-)
hepatic failure (K72.-)
hepatic veno-occlusive disease (K76.5)
idiopathic interstitial pneumonia (J84.11-)
sinusoidal obstruction syndrome (K76.5)

M31.19 Other thrombotic microangiopathy MCC HCC
Thrombotic thrombocytopenic purpura

M31.2 Lethal midline granuloma CC HCC

5th **M31.3 Wegener's granulomatosis**
Granulomatosis with polyangiitis
Necrotizing respiratory granulomatosis
AHA: 2021,1Q,23

M31.30 Wegener's granulomatosis without renal involvement CC HCC
Wegener's granulomatosis NOS
AHA: 2021,2Q,10

M31.31 Wegener's granulomatosis with renal involvement CC HCC

M31.4 Aortic arch syndrome [Takayasu] CC HCC

M31.5 Giant cell arteritis with polymyalgia rheumatica HCC

M31.6 Other giant cell arteritis HCC

M31.7 Microscopic polyangiitis CC HCC
Microscopic polyarteritis
EXCLUDES 1 *polyarteritis nodosa (M30.0)*
AHA: 2021,1Q,23

M31.8 Other specified necrotizing vasculopathies CC HCC
Hypocomplementemic vasculitis
Septic vasculitis

M31.9 Necrotizing vasculopathy, unspecified CC HCC

4th M32 Systemic lupus erythematosus (SLE)

EXCLUDES 1 *lupus erythematosus (discoid) (NOS) (L93.0)*
AHA: 2020,4Q,11; 2018,3Q,14
TIP: There is no default code for "lupus NOS." Query the provider for the specific type of lupus in order to assign the appropriate code.

M32.0 Drug-induced systemic lupus erythematosus HCC
Use additional code for adverse effect, if applicable, to identify drug (T36-T50 with fifth or sixth character 5)

5th **M32.1 Systemic lupus erythematosus with organ or system involvement**

M32.10 Systemic lupus erythematosus, organ or system involvement unspecified HCC

M32.11 Endocarditis in systemic lupus erythematosus CC HCC
Libman-Sacks disease

M32.12 Pericarditis in systemic lupus erythematosus CC HCC
Lupus pericarditis

M32.13 Lung involvement in systemic lupus erythematosus HCC
Pleural effusion due to systemic lupus erythematosus

M32.14 Glomerular disease in systemic lupus erythematosus HCC
Lupus renal disease NOS
AHA: 2013,4Q,125

M32.15 Tubulo-interstitial nephropathy in systemic lupus erythematosus HCC

M32.19 Other organ or system involvement in systemic lupus erythematosus HCC
▶Use additional code(s) to identify organ or system involvement, such as encephalitis (G05.3)◀

M32.8 Other forms of systemic lupus erythematosus HCC

M32.9 Systemic lupus erythematosus, unspecified HCC
SLE NOS
Systemic lupus erythematosus NOS
Systemic lupus erythematosus without organ involvement

4th M33 Dermatopolymyositis

AHA: 2017,4Q,18

5th **M33.0 Juvenile dermatomyositis**

M33.00 Juvenile dermatomyositis, organ involvement unspecified CC HCC

M33.01 Juvenile dermatomyositis with respiratory involvement CC HCC

M33.02 Juvenile dermatomyositis with myopathy CC HCC

M33.03 Juvenile dermatomyositis without myopathy CC HCC

M33.09 Juvenile dermatomyositis with other organ involvement CC HCC

5th **M33.1 Other dermatomyositis**
Adult dermatomyositis

M33.10 Other dermatomyositis, organ involvement unspecified CC HCC

M33.11 Other dermatomyositis with respiratory involvement CC HCC

M33.12 Other dermatomyositis with myopathy CC HCC

M33.13 Other dermatomyositis without myopathy CC HCC
Dermatomyositis NOS

M33.19 Other dermatomyositis with other organ involvement CC HCC

5th **M33.2 Polymyositis**

M33.20 Polymyositis, organ involvement unspecified CC HCC

M33.21 Polymyositis with respiratory involvement CC HCC

M33.22 Polymyositis with myopathy CC HCC

M33.29 Polymyositis with other organ involvement CC HCC

5th **M33.9 Dermatopolymyositis, unspecified**

M33.90 Dermatopolymyositis, unspecified, organ involvement unspecified CC HCC

M33.91 Dermatopolymyositis, unspecified with respiratory involvement CC HCC

M33.92 Dermatopolymyositis, unspecified with myopathy CC HCC

M33.93 Dermatopolymyositis, unspecified without myopathy CC HCC

M33.99 Dermatopolymyositis, unspecified with other organ involvement CC HCC

4th M34 Systemic sclerosis [scleroderma]

EXCLUDES 1 *circumscribed scleroderma (L94.0)*
neonatal scleroderma (P83.88)

M34.0 Progressive systemic sclerosis HCC

M34.1 CR(E)ST syndrome HCC
Combination of calcinosis, Raynaud's phenomenon, esophageal dysfunction, sclerodactyly, telangiectasia

M34.2 **Systemic sclerosis induced by drug and chemical** HCC
Code first poisoning due to drug or toxin, if applicable ▶(T36-T65 with fifth or sixth character 1-4)◀
Use additional code for adverse effect, if applicable, to identify drug (T36-T50 with fifth or sixth character 5)

✓5th M34.8 **Other forms of systemic sclerosis**

M34.81 **Systemic sclerosis with lung involvement** CC HCC
Code also if applicable:
other interstitial pulmonary diseases (J84.89)
secondary pulmonary arterial hypertension (I27.21)

M34.82 **Systemic sclerosis with myopathy** CC HCC

M34.83 **Systemic sclerosis with polyneuropathy** HCC

M34.89 **Other systemic sclerosis** HCC

M34.9 **Systemic sclerosis, unspecified** HCC

✓4th **M35 Other systemic involvement of connective tissue**
EXCLUDES 1 *reactive perforating collagenosis (L87.1)*

✓5th M35.0 **Sjogren syndrome**
Sicca syndrome
Use additional code to identify associated manifestations
EXCLUDES 1 *dry mouth, unspecified (R68.2)*
AHA: 2021,4Q,20
DEF: Autoimmune disease associated with keratoconjunctivitis, laryngopharyngitis, rhinitis, dry mouth, enlarged parotid gland, and chronic polyarthritis.

M35.00 **Sjogren syndrome, unspecified** HCC

M35.01 **Sjogren syndrome with keratoconjunctivitis** HCC

M35.02 **Sjogren syndrome with lung involvement** HCC

M35.03 **Sjogren syndrome with myopathy** CC HCC

M35.04 **Sjogren syndrome with tubulo-interstitial nephropathy** HCC
Renal tubular acidosis in sicca syndrome

M35.05 **Sjogren syndrome with inflammatory arthritis** HCC

M35.06 **Sjogren syndrome with peripheral nervous system involvement** HCC

M35.07 **Sjogren syndrome with central nervous system involvement** CC HCC

M35.08 **Sjogren syndrome with gastrointestinal involvement** HCC

M35.0A **Sjogren syndrome with glomerular disease** HCC

M35.0B **Sjogren syndrome with vasculitis** HCC

M35.0C **Sjogren syndrome with dental involvement** HCC

M35.09 **Sjogren syndrome with other organ involvement** HCC

M35.1 **Other overlap syndromes** CC HCC
Mixed connective tissue disease
EXCLUDES 1 *polyangiitis overlap syndrome (M30.8)*

M35.2 **Behcet's disease** CC HCC

M35.3 **Polymyalgia rheumatica** HCC
EXCLUDES 1 *polymyalgia rheumatica with giant cell arteritis (M31.5)*

M35.4 **Diffuse (eosinophilic) fasciitis**

M35.5 **Multifocal fibrosclerosis** CC HCC

M35.6 **Relapsing panniculitis [Weber-Christian]**
EXCLUDES 1 *lupus panniculitis (L93.2)*
panniculitis NOS (M79.3-)

M35.7 **Hypermobility syndrome**
Familial ligamentous laxity
EXCLUDES 1 *ligamentous laxity, NOS (M24.2-)*
EXCLUDES 2 *Ehlers-Danlos syndromes (Q79.6-)*

✓5th M35.8 **Other specified systemic involvement of connective tissue**
AHA: 2021,1Q,36; 2020,3Q,13-14

M35.81 **Multisystem inflammatory syndrome** CC HCC
MIS-A
MIS-C
Multisystem inflammatory syndrome in adults
Multisystem inflammatory syndrome in children
Pediatric inflammatory multisystem syndrome
PIMS
Code first, if applicable, COVID-19 (U07.1)
Code also any associated complications such as:
acute hepatic failure (K72.0-)
acute kidney failure (N17.-)
acute myocarditis (I40.-)
acute respiratory distress syndrome (J80)
cardiac arrhythmia (I47-I49.-)
pneumonia due to COVID-19 (J12.82)
severe sepsis (R65.2-)
viral cardiomyopathy (B33.24)
viral pericarditis (B33.23)
Use additional code, if applicable, for:
exposure to COVID-19 or SARS-CoV-2 infection (Z20.822)
personal history of COVID-19 (Z86.16)
post COVID-19 condition (U09.9)
AHA: 2021,4Q,102; 2021,1Q,29,36,41
DEF: Hyperinflammatory condition that seems to be largely associated with past or present coronavirus disease 2019 (COVID-19) infection. Predominantly occurring in children, with less frequent occurrences in adults, symptoms often include fever, laboratory evidence of inflammation, and evidence of clinically severe illness requiring hospitalization with multisystem (two or more) organ involvement. ***Synonym(s):*** *MIS, MIS-C.*

M35.89 **Other specified systemic involvement of connective tissue** CC HCC

M35.9 **Systemic involvement of connective tissue, unspecified** HCC
Autoimmune disease (systemic) NOS
Collagen (vascular) disease NOS

✓4th **M36 Systemic disorders of connective tissue in diseases classified elsewhere**
EXCLUDES 2 *arthropathies in diseases classified elsewhere (M14.-)*

M36.0 ***Dermato(poly)myositis in neoplastic disease*** CC HCC
Code first underlying neoplasm (C00-D49)

M36.1 ***Arthropathy in neoplastic disease***
Code first underlying neoplasm, such as:
leukemia (C91-C95)
malignant histiocytosis (C96.A)
multiple myeloma (C90.0)

M36.2 ***Hemophilic arthropathy***
Hemarthrosis in hemophilic arthropathy
Code first underlying disease, such as:
factor VIII deficiency (D66)
with vascular defect (D68.0-)
factor IX deficiency (D67)
hemophilia (classical) (D66)
hemophilia B (D67)
hemophilia C (D68.1)

M36.3 ***Arthropathy in other blood disorders***

M36.4 ***Arthropathy in hypersensitivity reactions classified elsewhere***
Code first underlying disease, such as:
Henoch (-Schonlein) purpura (D69.0)
serum sickness (T80.6-)

M36.8 ***Systemic disorders of connective tissue in other diseases classified elsewhere*** HCC
Code first underlying disease, such as:
alkaptonuria ▶(E70.29)◀
hypogammaglobulinemia (D80.-)
ochronosis ▶(E70.29)◀

DORSOPATHIES (M40-M54)

Deforming dorsopathies (M40-M43)

M40 Kyphosis and lordosis

Code first underlying disease

EXCLUDES 1 *congenital kyphosis and lordosis (Q76.4)*
kyphoscoliosis (M41.-)
postprocedural kyphosis and lordosis (M96.-)

Kyphosis and Lordosis

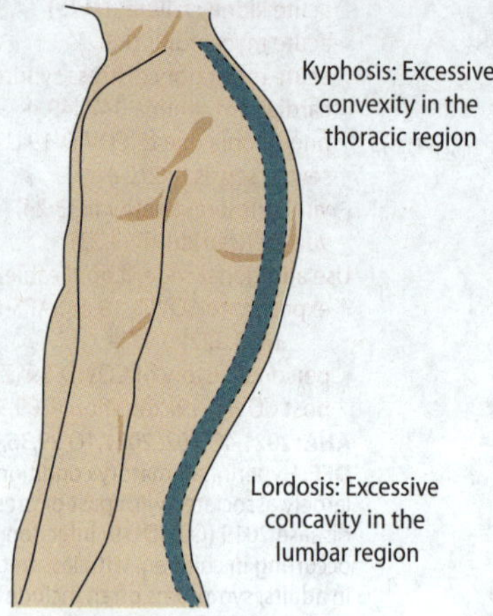

M40.0 Postural kyphosis

EXCLUDES 1 *osteochondrosis of spine (M42.-)*

- **M40.00** Postural kyphosis, site unspecified
- **M40.03** Postural kyphosis, cervicothoracic region
- **M40.04** Postural kyphosis, thoracic region
- **M40.05** Postural kyphosis, thoracolumbar region

M40.1 Other secondary kyphosis

- **M40.10** Other secondary kyphosis, site unspecified UPD
- **M40.12** Other secondary kyphosis, cervical region UPD
- **M40.13** Other secondary kyphosis, cervicothoracic region UPD
- **M40.14** Other secondary kyphosis, thoracic region UPD
- **M40.15** Other secondary kyphosis, thoracolumbar region UPD

M40.2 Other and unspecified kyphosis

M40.20 Unspecified kyphosis

- **M40.202** Unspecified kyphosis, cervical region
- **M40.203** Unspecified kyphosis, cervicothoracic region
- **M40.204** Unspecified kyphosis, thoracic region
- **M40.205** Unspecified kyphosis, thoracolumbar region
- **M40.209** Unspecified kyphosis, site unspecified

M40.29 Other kyphosis

- **M40.292** Other kyphosis, cervical region
- **M40.293** Other kyphosis, cervicothoracic region
- **M40.294** Other kyphosis, thoracic region
- **M40.295** Other kyphosis, thoracolumbar region
- **M40.299** Other kyphosis, site unspecified

M40.3 Flatback syndrome

- **M40.30** Flatback syndrome, site unspecified
- **M40.35** Flatback syndrome, thoracolumbar region
- **M40.36** Flatback syndrome, lumbar region
- **M40.37** Flatback syndrome, lumbosacral region

M40.4 Postural lordosis

Acquired lordosis

- **M40.40** Postural lordosis, site unspecified
- **M40.45** Postural lordosis, thoracolumbar region
- **M40.46** Postural lordosis, lumbar region
- **M40.47** Postural lordosis, lumbosacral region

M40.5 Lordosis, unspecified

- **M40.50** Lordosis, unspecified, site unspecified
- **M40.55** Lordosis, unspecified, thoracolumbar region
- **M40.56** Lordosis, unspecified, lumbar region
- **M40.57** Lordosis, unspecified, lumbosacral region

M41 Scoliosis

INCLUDES kyphoscoliosis

EXCLUDES 1 *congenital scoliosis due to bony malformation (Q76.3)*
congenital scoliosis NOS (Q67.5)
kyphoscoliotic heart disease (I27.1)
postural congenital scoliosis (Q67.5)

EXCLUDES 2 *postprocedural scoliosis ▶(M96.89)◀*
▶postradiation scoliosis (M96.5)◀

Scoliosis

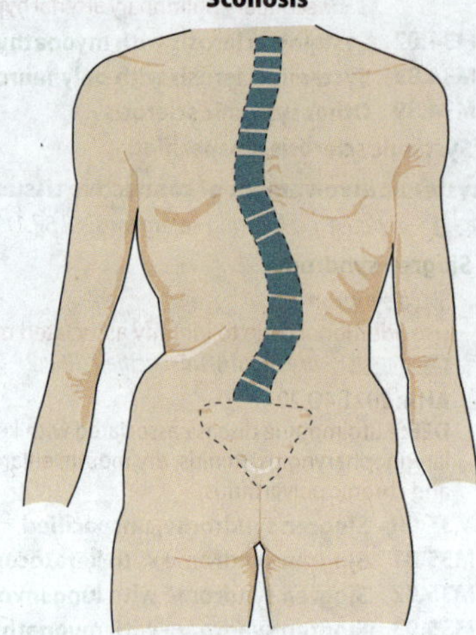

Lateral curvature of spine

AHA: 2022,1Q,30

M41.0 Infantile idiopathic scoliosis

AHA: 2014,4Q,26

- **M41.00** Infantile idiopathic scoliosis, site unspecified
- **M41.02** Infantile idiopathic scoliosis, cervical region
- **M41.03** Infantile idiopathic scoliosis, cervicothoracic region
- **M41.04** Infantile idiopathic scoliosis, thoracic region
- **M41.05** Infantile idiopathic scoliosis, thoracolumbar region
- **M41.06** Infantile idiopathic scoliosis, lumbar region
- **M41.07** Infantile idiopathic scoliosis, lumbosacral region
- **M41.08** Infantile idiopathic scoliosis, sacral and sacrococcygeal region

M41.1 Juvenile and adolescent idiopathic scoliosis

M41.11 Juvenile idiopathic scoliosis

AHA: 2014,4Q,28

- **M41.112** Juvenile idiopathic scoliosis, cervical region
- **M41.113** Juvenile idiopathic scoliosis, cervicothoracic region
- **M41.114** Juvenile idiopathic scoliosis, thoracic region
- **M41.115** Juvenile idiopathic scoliosis, thoracolumbar region
- **M41.116** Juvenile idiopathic scoliosis, lumbar region
- **M41.117** Juvenile idiopathic scoliosis, lumbosacral region
- **M41.119** Juvenile idiopathic scoliosis, site unspecified

▲ **M41.12 Adolescent idiopathic scoliosis**

- **M41.122** Adolescent idiopathic scoliosis, cervical region
- **M41.123** Adolescent idiopathic scoliosis, cervicothoracic region
- **M41.124** Adolescent idiopathic scoliosis, thoracic region
- **M41.125** Adolescent idiopathic scoliosis, thoracolumbar region
- **M41.126** Adolescent idiopathic scoliosis, lumbar region
- **M41.127** Adolescent idiopathic scoliosis, lumbosacral region
- **M41.129** Adolescent idiopathic scoliosis, site unspecified

M41.2 Other idiopathic scoliosis

- **M41.20** Other idiopathic scoliosis, site unspecified
- **M41.22** Other idiopathic scoliosis, cervical region

M41.23 Other idiopathic scoliosis, cervicothoracic region
M41.24 Other idiopathic scoliosis, thoracic region
M41.25 Other idiopathic scoliosis, thoracolumbar region
M41.26 Other idiopathic scoliosis, lumbar region
M41.27 Other idiopathic scoliosis, lumbosacral region

5th M41.3 Thoracogenic scoliosis

M41.30 Thoracogenic scoliosis, site unspecified
M41.34 Thoracogenic scoliosis, thoracic region
M41.35 Thoracogenic scoliosis, thoracolumbar region

5th M41.4 Neuromuscular scoliosis

Scoliosis secondary to cerebral palsy, Friedreich's ataxia, poliomyelitis and other neuromuscular disorders
Code also underlying condition
AHA: 2014,4Q,27

M41.40 Neuromuscular scoliosis, site unspecified
M41.41 Neuromuscular scoliosis, occipito-atlanto-axial region
M41.42 Neuromuscular scoliosis, cervical region
M41.43 Neuromuscular scoliosis, cervicothoracic region
M41.44 Neuromuscular scoliosis, thoracic region
M41.45 Neuromuscular scoliosis, thoracolumbar region
M41.46 Neuromuscular scoliosis, lumbar region
M41.47 Neuromuscular scoliosis, lumbosacral region

5th M41.5 Other secondary scoliosis

Code first underlying disease
AHA: 2019,1Q,19

M41.50 Other secondary scoliosis, site unspecified UPD
M41.52 Other secondary scoliosis, cervical region UPD
M41.53 Other secondary scoliosis, cervicothoracic region UPD
M41.54 Other secondary scoliosis, thoracic region UPD
M41.55 Other secondary scoliosis, thoracolumbar region UPD
M41.56 Other secondary scoliosis, lumbar region UPD
M41.57 Other secondary scoliosis, lumbosacral region UPD

5th M41.8 Other forms of scoliosis

AHA: 2022,1Q,30

M41.80 Other forms of scoliosis, site unspecified
M41.82 Other forms of scoliosis, cervical region
M41.83 Other forms of scoliosis, cervicothoracic region
M41.84 Other forms of scoliosis, thoracic region
M41.85 Other forms of scoliosis, thoracolumbar region
M41.86 Other forms of scoliosis, lumbar region
M41.87 Other forms of scoliosis, lumbosacral region

M41.9 Scoliosis, unspecified

AHA: 2022,1Q,30

4th M42 Spinal osteochondrosis

5th M42.0 Juvenile osteochondrosis of spine

Calve's disease
Scheuermann's disease
EXCLUDES 1 *postural kyphosis (M40.0)*

M42.00 Juvenile osteochondrosis of spine, site unspecified
M42.01 Juvenile osteochondrosis of spine, occipito-atlanto-axial region
M42.02 Juvenile osteochondrosis of spine, cervical region
M42.03 Juvenile osteochondrosis of spine, cervicothoracic region
M42.04 Juvenile osteochondrosis of spine, thoracic region
M42.05 Juvenile osteochondrosis of spine, thoracolumbar region
M42.06 Juvenile osteochondrosis of spine, lumbar region
M42.07 Juvenile osteochondrosis of spine, lumbosacral region
M42.08 Juvenile osteochondrosis of spine, sacral and sacrococcygeal region
M42.09 Juvenile osteochondrosis of spine, multiple sites in spine

5th M42.1 Adult osteochondrosis of spine

M42.10 Adult osteochondrosis of spine, site unspecified A
M42.11 Adult osteochondrosis of spine, occipito-atlanto-axial region A
M42.12 Adult osteochondrosis of spine, cervical region A
M42.13 Adult osteochondrosis of spine, cervicothoracic region A
M42.14 Adult osteochondrosis of spine, thoracic region A
M42.15 Adult osteochondrosis of spine, thoracolumbar region A
M42.16 Adult osteochondrosis of spine, lumbar region A
M42.17 Adult osteochondrosis of spine, lumbosacral region A
M42.18 Adult osteochondrosis of spine, sacral and sacrococcygeal region A
M42.19 Adult osteochondrosis of spine, multiple sites in spine A

M42.9 Spinal osteochondrosis, unspecified

4th M43 Other deforming dorsopathies

EXCLUDES 1 *congenital spondylolysis and spondylolisthesis (Q76.2)*
hemivertebra (Q76.3-Q76.4)
Klippel-Feil syndrome (Q76.1)
lumbarization and sacralization (Q76.4)
platyspondylisis (Q76.4)
spina bifida occulta (Q76.0)
spinal curvature in osteoporosis (M80.-)
spinal curvature in Paget's disease of bone [osteitis deformans] (M88.-)

5th M43.0 Spondylolysis

EXCLUDES 1 *congenital spondylolysis (Q76.2)*
spondylolisthesis (M43.1)

M43.00 Spondylolysis, site unspecified
M43.01 Spondylolysis, occipito-atlanto-axial region
M43.02 Spondylolysis, cervical region
M43.03 Spondylolysis, cervicothoracic region
M43.04 Spondylolysis, thoracic region
M43.05 Spondylolysis, thoracolumbar region
M43.06 Spondylolysis, lumbar region
M43.07 Spondylolysis, lumbosacral region
M43.08 Spondylolysis, sacral and sacrococcygeal region
M43.09 Spondylolysis, multiple sites in spine

5th M43.1 Spondylolisthesis

EXCLUDES 1 *acute traumatic of lumbosacral region (S33.1)*
acute traumatic of sites other than lumbosacral - code to Fracture, vertebra, by region
congenital spondylolisthesis (Q76.2)
AHA: 2020,2Q,21; 2018,3Q,18
TIP: Code also any associated radiculopathy (M54.1-) and/or myelopathy (G99.2).

M43.10 Spondylolisthesis, site unspecified
M43.11 Spondylolisthesis, occipito-atlanto-axial region
M43.12 Spondylolisthesis, cervical region
M43.13 Spondylolisthesis, cervicothoracic region
M43.14 Spondylolisthesis, thoracic region
M43.15 Spondylolisthesis, thoracolumbar region
M43.16 Spondylolisthesis, lumbar region
M43.17 Spondylolisthesis, lumbosacral region
M43.18 Spondylolisthesis, sacral and sacrococcygeal region
M43.19 Spondylolisthesis, multiple sites in spine

5th M43.2 Fusion of spine

Ankylosis of spinal joint
EXCLUDES 1 *ankylosing spondylitis (M45.0-)*
congenital fusion of spine (Q76.4)
EXCLUDES 2 *arthrodesis status (Z98.1)*
pseudoarthrosis after fusion or arthrodesis (M96.0)

M43.20 Fusion of spine, site unspecified
M43.21 Fusion of spine, occipito-atlanto-axial region
M43.22 Fusion of spine, cervical region
M43.23 Fusion of spine, cervicothoracic region
M43.24 Fusion of spine, thoracic region
M43.25 Fusion of spine, thoracolumbar region
M43.26 Fusion of spine, lumbar region
M43.27 Fusion of spine, lumbosacral region
M43.28 Fusion of spine, sacral and sacrococcygeal region

M43.3 Recurrent atlantoaxial dislocation with myelopathy
M43.4 Other recurrent atlantoaxial dislocation

5th M43.5 Other recurrent vertebral dislocation

EXCLUDES 1 *biomechanical lesions NEC (M99.-)*

6th M43.5X Other recurrent vertebral dislocation

M43.5X2 Other recurrent vertebral dislocation, cervical region

M43.5X3 Other recurrent vertebral dislocation, cervicothoracic region

M43.5X4 Other recurrent vertebral dislocation, thoracic region

M43.5X5 Other recurrent vertebral dislocation, thoracolumbar region

M43.5X6 Other recurrent vertebral dislocation, lumbar region

M43.5X7 Other recurrent vertebral dislocation, lumbosacral region

M43.5X8 Other recurrent vertebral dislocation, sacral and sacrococcygeal region

M43.5X9 Other recurrent vertebral dislocation, site unspecified

M43.6 Torticollis

EXCLUDES 1 *congenital (sternomastoid) torticollis (Q68.Ø)*
current injury - see Injury, of spine, by body region
ocular torticollis (R29.891)
psychogenic torticollis (F45.8)
spasmodic torticollis (G24.3)
torticollis due to birth injury (P15.2)

DEF: Twisted, unnatural position of the neck due to contracted cervical muscles that pull the head to one side.

5th **M43.8 Other specified deforming dorsopathies**

EXCLUDES 2 *kyphosis and lordosis (M4Ø.-)*
scoliosis (M41.-)

6th **M43.8X Other specified deforming dorsopathies**

M43.8X1 Other specified deforming dorsopathies, occipito-atlanto-axial region

M43.8X2 Other specified deforming dorsopathies, cervical region

M43.8X3 Other specified deforming dorsopathies, cervicothoracic region

M43.8X4 Other specified deforming dorsopathies, thoracic region

M43.8X5 Other specified deforming dorsopathies, thoracolumbar region

M43.8X6 Other specified deforming dorsopathies, lumbar region

M43.8X7 Other specified deforming dorsopathies, lumbosacral region

M43.8X8 Other specified deforming dorsopathies, sacral and sacrococcygeal region

M43.8X9 Other specified deforming dorsopathies, site unspecified

M43.9 Deforming dorsopathy, unspecified

Curvature of spine NOS

Spondylopathies (M45-M49)

4th **M45 Ankylosing spondylitis**

Rheumatoid arthritis of spine

EXCLUDES 1 *arthropathy in Reiter's disease (MØ2.3-)*
juvenile (ankylosing) spondylitis (MØ8.1)

EXCLUDES 2 *Behcet's disease (M35.2)*

M45.Ø Ankylosing spondylitis of multiple sites in spine HCC

M45.1 Ankylosing spondylitis of occipito-atlanto-axial region HCC

M45.2 Ankylosing spondylitis of cervical region HCC

M45.3 Ankylosing spondylitis of cervicothoracic region HCC

M45.4 Ankylosing spondylitis of thoracic region HCC

M45.5 Ankylosing spondylitis of thoracolumbar region HCC

M45.6 Ankylosing spondylitis lumbar region HCC

M45.7 Ankylosing spondylitis of lumbosacral region HCC

M45.8 Ankylosing spondylitis sacral and sacrococcygeal region HCC

M45.9 Ankylosing spondylitis of unspecified sites in spine HCC

5th **M45.A Non-radiographic axial spondyloarthritis**

AHA: 2021,4Q,21-22

M45.AØ Non-radiographic axial spondyloarthritis of unspecified sites in spine HCC

M45.A1 Non-radiographic axial spondyloarthritis of occipito-atlanto-axial region HCC

M45.A2 Non-radiographic axial spondyloarthritis of cervical region HCC

M45.A3 Non-radiographic axial spondyloarthritis of cervicothoracic region HCC

M45.A4 Non-radiographic axial spondyloarthritis of thoracic region HCC

M45.A5 Non-radiographic axial spondyloarthritis of thoracolumbar region HCC

M45.A6 Non-radiographic axial spondyloarthritis of lumbar region HCC

M45.A7 Non-radiographic axial spondyloarthritis of lumbosacral region HCC

M45.A8 Non-radiographic axial spondyloarthritis of sacral and sacrococcygeal region HCC

M45.AB Non-radiographic axial spondyloarthritis of multiple sites in spine HCC

4th **M46 Other inflammatory spondylopathies**

5th **M46.Ø Spinal enthesopathy**

Disorder of ligamentous or muscular attachments of spine

M46.ØØ Spinal enthesopathy, site unspecified HCC

M46.Ø1 Spinal enthesopathy, occipito-atlanto-axial region HCC

M46.Ø2 Spinal enthesopathy, cervical region HCC

M46.Ø3 Spinal enthesopathy, cervicothoracic region HCC

M46.Ø4 Spinal enthesopathy, thoracic region HCC

M46.Ø5 Spinal enthesopathy, thoracolumbar region HCC

M46.Ø6 Spinal enthesopathy, lumbar region HCC

M46.Ø7 Spinal enthesopathy, lumbosacral region HCC

M46.Ø8 Spinal enthesopathy, sacral and sacrococcygeal region HCC

M46.Ø9 Spinal enthesopathy, multiple sites in spine HCC

M46.1 Sacroiliitis, not elsewhere classified HCC

AHA: 2020,2Q,14

DEF: Inflammation of the sacroiliac joint (situated at the juncture of the sacrum and hip). Symptoms include pain in the buttocks or lower back that can extend down one or both legs.

5th **M46.2 Osteomyelitis of vertebra**

M46.2Ø Osteomyelitis of vertebra, site unspecified CC UNS HCC

M46.21 Osteomyelitis of vertebra, occipito-atlanto-axial region CC HCC

M46.22 Osteomyelitis of vertebra, cervical region CC HCC

M46.23 Osteomyelitis of vertebra, cervicothoracic region CC HCC

M46.24 Osteomyelitis of vertebra, thoracic region CC HCC

M46.25 Osteomyelitis of vertebra, thoracolumbar region CC HCC

M46.26 Osteomyelitis of vertebra, lumbar region CC HCC

M46.27 Osteomyelitis of vertebra, lumbosacral region CC HCC

M46.28 Osteomyelitis of vertebra, sacral and sacrococcygeal region CC HCC

5th **M46.3 Infection of intervertebral disc (pyogenic)**

Use additional code (B95-B97) to identify infectious agent

M46.3Ø Infection of intervertebral disc (pyogenic), site unspecified CC UNS HCC

M46.31 Infection of intervertebral disc (pyogenic), occipito-atlanto-axial region CC HCC

M46.32 Infection of intervertebral disc (pyogenic), cervical region CC HCC

M46.33 Infection of intervertebral disc (pyogenic), cervicothoracic region CC HCC

M46.34 Infection of intervertebral disc (pyogenic), thoracic region CC HCC

M46.35 Infection of intervertebral disc (pyogenic), thoracolumbar region CC HCC

M46.36 Infection of intervertebral disc (pyogenic), lumbar region CC HCC

M46.37 Infection of intervertebral disc (pyogenic), lumbosacral region CC HCC

M46.38 Infection of intervertebral disc (pyogenic), sacral and sacrococcygeal region CC HCC

M46.39 Infection of intervertebral disc (pyogenic), multiple sites in spine CC HCC

5th **M46.4 Discitis, unspecified**

M46.4Ø Discitis, unspecified, site unspecified

M46.41 Discitis, unspecified, occipito-atlanto-axial region

M46.42 Discitis, unspecified, cervical region

M46.43 Discitis, unspecified, cervicothoracic region

M46.44 Discitis, unspecified, thoracic region

M46.45 Discitis, unspecified, thoracolumbar region

M46.46 Discitis, unspecified, lumbar region

M46.47 Discitis, unspecified, lumbosacral region

M46.48 Discitis, unspecified, sacral and sacrococcygeal region

M46.49 Discitis, unspecified, multiple sites in spine

M46.5 Other infective spondylopathies

M46.50 Other infective spondylopathies, site unspecified HCC

M46.51 Other infective spondylopathies, occipito-atlanto-axial region HCC

M46.52 Other infective spondylopathies, cervical region HCC

M46.53 Other infective spondylopathies, cervicothoracic region HCC

M46.54 Other infective spondylopathies, thoracic region HCC

M46.55 Other infective spondylopathies, thoracolumbar region HCC

M46.56 Other infective spondylopathies, lumbar region HCC

M46.57 Other infective spondylopathies, lumbosacral region HCC

M46.58 Other infective spondylopathies, sacral and sacrococcygeal region HCC

M46.59 Other infective spondylopathies, multiple sites in spine HCC

M46.8 Other specified inflammatory spondylopathies

M46.80 Other specified inflammatory spondylopathies, site unspecified HCC

M46.81 Other specified inflammatory spondylopathies, occipito-atlanto-axial region HCC

M46.82 Other specified inflammatory spondylopathies, cervical region HCC

M46.83 Other specified inflammatory spondylopathies, cervicothoracic region HCC

M46.84 Other specified inflammatory spondylopathies, thoracic region HCC

M46.85 Other specified inflammatory spondylopathies, thoracolumbar region HCC

M46.86 Other specified inflammatory spondylopathies, lumbar region HCC

M46.87 Other specified inflammatory spondylopathies, lumbosacral region HCC

M46.88 Other specified inflammatory spondylopathies, sacral and sacrococcygeal region HCC

M46.89 Other specified inflammatory spondylopathies, multiple sites in spine HCC

M46.9 Unspecified inflammatory spondylopathy

M46.90 Unspecified inflammatory spondylopathy, site unspecified HCC

M46.91 Unspecified inflammatory spondylopathy, occipito-atlanto-axial region HCC

M46.92 Unspecified inflammatory spondylopathy, cervical region HCC
AHA: 2019,3Q,10

M46.93 Unspecified inflammatory spondylopathy, cervicothoracic region HCC

M46.94 Unspecified inflammatory spondylopathy, thoracic region HCC

M46.95 Unspecified inflammatory spondylopathy, thoracolumbar region HCC

M46.96 Unspecified inflammatory spondylopathy, lumbar region HCC

M46.97 Unspecified inflammatory spondylopathy, lumbosacral region HCC

M46.98 Unspecified inflammatory spondylopathy, sacral and sacrococcygeal region HCC

M46.99 Unspecified inflammatory spondylopathy, multiple sites in spine HCC

M47 Spondylosis

INCLUDES arthrosis or osteoarthritis of spine
degeneration of facet joints

AHA: 2020,1Q,17; 2019,3Q,10-11; 2016,4Q,147

M47.0 Anterior spinal and vertebral artery compression syndromes

M47.01 Anterior spinal artery compression syndromes

M47.011 Anterior spinal artery compression syndromes, occipito-atlanto-axial region CC

M47.012 Anterior spinal artery compression syndromes, cervical region CC
AHA: 2023,1Q,37

M47.013 Anterior spinal artery compression syndromes, cervicothoracic region CC

M47.014 Anterior spinal artery compression syndromes, thoracic region CC

M47.015 Anterior spinal artery compression syndromes, thoracolumbar region CC

M47.016 Anterior spinal artery compression syndromes, lumbar region CC

M47.019 Anterior spinal artery compression syndromes, site unspecified CC UNS

M47.02 Vertebral artery compression syndromes

M47.021 Vertebral artery compression syndromes, occipito-atlanto-axial region CC

M47.022 Vertebral artery compression syndromes, cervical region CC
AHA: 2023,1Q,37

M47.029 Vertebral artery compression syndromes, site unspecified CC UNS

M47.1 Other spondylosis with myelopathy

Spondylogenic compression of spinal cord

EXCLUDES 1 *vertebral subluxation (M43.3-M43.5X9)*

AHA: 2020,1Q,17

M47.10 Other spondylosis with myelopathy, site unspecified CC UNS

M47.11 Other spondylosis with myelopathy, occipito-atlanto-axial region CC

M47.12 Other spondylosis with myelopathy, cervical region CC

M47.13 Other spondylosis with myelopathy, cervicothoracic region CC

M47.14 Other spondylosis with myelopathy, thoracic region CC

M47.15 Other spondylosis with myelopathy, thoracolumbar region CC

M47.16 Other spondylosis with myelopathy, lumbar region CC

M47.2 Other spondylosis with radiculopathy

AHA: 2020,1Q,17

M47.20 Other spondylosis with radiculopathy, site unspecified

M47.21 Other spondylosis with radiculopathy, occipito-atlanto-axial region

M47.22 Other spondylosis with radiculopathy, cervical region

M47.23 Other spondylosis with radiculopathy, cervicothoracic region

M47.24 Other spondylosis with radiculopathy, thoracic region

M47.25 Other spondylosis with radiculopathy, thoracolumbar region

M47.26 Other spondylosis with radiculopathy, lumbar region

M47.27 Other spondylosis with radiculopathy, lumbosacral region

M47.28 Other spondylosis with radiculopathy, sacral and sacrococcygeal region

M47.8 Other spondylosis

M47.81 Spondylosis without myelopathy or radiculopathy

AHA: 2019,3Q,10-11; 2018,2Q,14

M47.811 Spondylosis without myelopathy or radiculopathy, occipito-atlanto-axial region

M47.812 Spondylosis without myelopathy or radiculopathy, cervical region

M47.813 Spondylosis without myelopathy or radiculopathy, cervicothoracic region

M47.814 Spondylosis without myelopathy or radiculopathy, thoracic region

M47.815 Spondylosis without myelopathy or radiculopathy, thoracolumbar region

M47.816 Spondylosis without myelopathy or radiculopathy, lumbar region

M47.817 Spondylosis without myelopathy or radiculopathy, lumbosacral region

M47.818 Spondylosis without myelopathy or radiculopathy, sacral and sacrococcygeal region

M47.819 **Spondylosis without myelopathy or radiculopathy, site unspecified**

✓6th **M47.89** **Other spondylosis**

M47.891 **Other spondylosis, occipito-atlanto-axial region**

M47.892 **Other spondylosis, cervical region**

M47.893 **Other spondylosis, cervicothoracic region**

M47.894 **Other spondylosis, thoracic region**

M47.895 **Other spondylosis, thoracolumbar region**

M47.896 **Other spondylosis, lumbar region**

M47.897 **Other spondylosis, lumbosacral region**

M47.898 **Other spondylosis, sacral and sacrococcygeal region**

M47.899 **Other spondylosis, site unspecified**

M47.9 **Spondylosis, unspecified**

✓4th **M48** **Other spondylopathies**

✓5th **M48.Ø** **Spinal stenosis**

Caudal stenosis

AHA: 2020,1Q,17; 2018,3Q,18-19

TIP: Code also any associated radiculopathy (M54.1-) and/or myelopathy (G99.2).

M48.ØØ **Spinal stenosis, site unspecified**

M48.Ø1 **Spinal stenosis, occipito-atlanto-axial region**

M48.Ø2 **Spinal stenosis, cervical region**

M48.Ø3 **Spinal stenosis, cervicothoracic region**

M48.Ø4 **Spinal stenosis, thoracic region**

M48.Ø5 **Spinal stenosis, thoracolumbar region**

✓6th **M48.Ø6** **Spinal stenosis, lumbar region**

AHA: 2018,3Q,19; 2017,4Q,18-19

M48.Ø61 **Spinal stenosis, lumbar region without neurogenic claudication**

Spinal stenosis, lumbar region NOS

M48.Ø62 **Spinal stenosis, lumbar region with neurogenic claudication**

M48.Ø7 **Spinal stenosis, lumbosacral region**

M48.Ø8 **Spinal stenosis, sacral and sacrococcygeal region**

✓5th **M48.1** **Ankylosing hyperostosis [Forestier]**

Diffuse idiopathic skeletal hyperostosis [DISH]

M48.1Ø **Ankylosing hyperostosis [Forestier], site unspecified**

M48.11 **Ankylosing hyperostosis [Forestier], occipito-atlanto-axial region**

M48.12 **Ankylosing hyperostosis [Forestier], cervical region**

M48.13 **Ankylosing hyperostosis [Forestier], cervicothoracic region**

M48.14 **Ankylosing hyperostosis [Forestier], thoracic region**

M48.15 **Ankylosing hyperostosis [Forestier], thoracolumbar region**

M48.16 **Ankylosing hyperostosis [Forestier], lumbar region**

M48.17 **Ankylosing hyperostosis [Forestier], lumbosacral region**

M48.18 **Ankylosing hyperostosis [Forestier], sacral and sacrococcygeal region**

M48.19 **Ankylosing hyperostosis [Forestier], multiple sites in spine**

✓5th **M48.2** **Kissing spine**

M48.2Ø **Kissing spine, site unspecified**

M48.21 **Kissing spine, occipito-atlanto-axial region**

M48.22 **Kissing spine, cervical region**

M48.23 **Kissing spine, cervicothoracic region**

M48.24 **Kissing spine, thoracic region**

M48.25 **Kissing spine, thoracolumbar region**

M48.26 **Kissing spine, lumbar region**

M48.27 **Kissing spine, lumbosacral region**

✓5th **M48.3** **Traumatic spondylopathy**

M48.3Ø **Traumatic spondylopathy, site unspecified** CC UNS

M48.31 **Traumatic spondylopathy, occipito-atlanto-axial region** CC

M48.32 **Traumatic spondylopathy, cervical region** CC

M48.33 **Traumatic spondylopathy, cervicothoracic region** CC

M48.34 **Traumatic spondylopathy, thoracic region** CC

M48.35 **Traumatic spondylopathy, thoracolumbar region** CC

M48.36 **Traumatic spondylopathy, lumbar region** CC

M48.37 **Traumatic spondylopathy, lumbosacral region** CC

M48.38 **Traumatic spondylopathy, sacral and sacrococcygeal region** CC

✓5th **M48.4** **Fatigue fracture of vertebra**

Stress fracture of vertebra

EXCLUDES 1 *pathological fracture NOS (M84.4-)*
pathological fracture of vertebra due to neoplasm (M84.58)
pathological fracture of vertebra due to osteoporosis (M8Ø.-)
pathological fracture of vertebra due to other diagnosis (M84.68)
traumatic fracture of vertebrae (S12.Ø-S12.3-, S22.Ø-, S32.Ø-)

The appropriate 7th character is to be added to each code from subcategory M48.4.
A initial encounter for fracture
D subsequent encounter for fracture with routine healing
G subsequent encounter for fracture with delayed healing
S sequela of fracture

✓x7th **M48.4Ø** **Fatigue fracture of vertebra, site unspecified**

✓x7th **M48.41** **Fatigue fracture of vertebra, occipito-atlanto-axial region**

✓x7th **M48.42** **Fatigue fracture of vertebra, cervical region**

✓x7th **M48.43** **Fatigue fracture of vertebra, cervicothoracic region**

✓x7th **M48.44** **Fatigue fracture of vertebra, thoracic region**

✓x7th **M48.45** **Fatigue fracture of vertebra, thoracolumbar region**

✓x7th **M48.46** **Fatigue fracture of vertebra, lumbar region**

✓x7th **M48.47** **Fatigue fracture of vertebra, lumbosacral region**

✓x7th **M48.48** **Fatigue fracture of vertebra, sacral and sacrococcygeal region**

✓5th **M48.5** **Collapsed vertebra, not elsewhere classified**

Collapsed vertebra NOS
Compression fracture of vertebra NOS
Wedging of vertebra NOS

EXCLUDES 1 *current injury - see Injury of spine, by body region*
fatigue fracture of vertebra (M48.4)
pathological fracture NOS (M84.4-)
pathological fracture of vertebra due to neoplasm (M84.58)
pathological fracture of vertebra due to osteoporosis (M8Ø.-)
pathological fracture of vertebra due to other diagnosis (M84.68)
stress fracture of vertebra (M48.4-)
traumatic fracture of vertebra (S12.-, S22.-, S32.-)

The appropriate 7th character is to be added to each code from subcategory M48.5.
A initial encounter for fracture
D subsequent encounter for fracture with routine healing
G subsequent encounter for fracture with delayed healing
S sequela of fracture

✓x7th **M48.5Ø** **Collapsed vertebra, not elsewhere classified, site unspecified** CC UNS HCC

✓x7th **M48.51** **Collapsed vertebra, not elsewhere classified, occipito-atlanto-axial region** CC HCC

✓x7th **M48.52** **Collapsed vertebra, not elsewhere classified, cervical region** CC HCC

✓x7th **M48.53** **Collapsed vertebra, not elsewhere classified, cervicothoracic region** CC HCC

✓x7th **M48.54** **Collapsed vertebra, not elsewhere classified, thoracic region** CC HCC

✓x7th **M48.55** **Collapsed vertebra, not elsewhere classified, thoracolumbar region** CC HCC

✓x7th **M48.56** **Collapsed vertebra, not elsewhere classified, lumbar region** CC HCC

✓x7th **M48.57** **Collapsed vertebra, not elsewhere classified, lumbosacral region** CC HCC

✓x7th **M48.58** **Collapsed vertebra, not elsewhere classified, sacral and sacrococcygeal region** CC HCC

✓5th **M48.8** **Other specified spondylopathies**

Ossification of posterior longitudinal ligament

✓6th **M48.8X** **Other specified spondylopathies**

M48.8X1 **Other specified spondylopathies, occipito-atlanto-axial region** HCC

M48.8X2 **Other specified spondylopathies, cervical region** HCC

M48.8X3 Other specified spondylopathies, cervicothoracic region HCC

M48.8X4 Other specified spondylopathies, thoracic region HCC

M48.8X5 Other specified spondylopathies, thoracolumbar region HCC

M48.8X6 Other specified spondylopathies, lumbar region HCC

M48.8X7 Other specified spondylopathies, lumbosacral region HCC

M48.8X8 Other specified spondylopathies, sacral and sacrococcygeal region HCC

M48.8X9 Other specified spondylopathies, site unspecified HCC

M48.9 Spondylopathy, unspecified

M49 Spondylopathies in diseases classified elsewhere

INCLUDES curvature of spine in diseases classified elsewhere
deformity of spine in diseases classified elsewhere
kyphosis in diseases classified elsewhere
scoliosis in diseases classified elsewhere
spondylopathy in diseases classified elsewhere

Code first underlying disease, such as:
brucellosis (A23.-)
Charcôt-Marie-Tooth disease (G60.0)
enterobacterial infections (A01-A04)
osteitis fibrosa cystica (E21.0)

EXCLUDES 1 *curvature of spine in tuberculosis [Pott's] (A18.01)*
enteropathic arthropathies (M07.-)
gonococcal spondylitis (A54.41)
neuropathic spondylopathy in syringomyelia (G95.0)
neuropathic spondylopathy in tabes dorsalis (A52.11)
neuropathic [tabes dorsalis] spondylitis (A52.11)
nonsyphilitic neuropathic spondylopathy NEC (G98.0)
spondylitis in syphilis (acquired) (A52.77)
tuberculous spondylitis (A18.01)
typhoid fever spondylitis (A01.05)

M49.8 Spondylopathy in diseases classified elsewhere

M49.80 Spondylopathy in diseases classified elsewhere, site unspecified HCC

M49.81 Spondylopathy in diseases classified elsewhere, occipito-atlanto-axial region HCC

M49.82 Spondylopathy in diseases classified elsewhere, cervical region HCC

M49.83 Spondylopathy in diseases classified elsewhere, cervicothoracic region HCC

M49.84 Spondylopathy in diseases classified elsewhere, thoracic region HCC

M49.85 Spondylopathy in diseases classified elsewhere, thoracolumbar region HCC

M49.86 Spondylopathy in diseases classified elsewhere, lumbar region HCC

M49.87 Spondylopathy in diseases classified elsewhere, lumbosacral region HCC

M49.88 Spondylopathy in diseases classified elsewhere, sacral and sacrococcygeal region HCC

M49.89 Spondylopathy in diseases classified elsewhere, multiple sites in spine HCC

Other dorsopathies (M50-M54)

EXCLUDES 1 *current injury - see injury of spine by body region*
discitis NOS (M46.4-)

M50 Cervical disc disorders

INCLUDES cervicothoracic disc disorders
cervicothoracic disc disorders with cervicalgia

AHA: 2016,4Q,39-40; 2016,1Q,17

M50.0 Cervical disc disorder with myelopathy

AHA: 2018,3Q,19

M50.00 Cervical disc disorder with myelopathy, unspecified cervical region CC UNS

M50.01 Cervical disc disorder with myelopathy, high cervical region CC
C2-C3 disc disorder with myelopathy
C3-C4 disc disorder with myelopathy

M50.02 Cervical disc disorder with myelopathy, mid-cervical region

M50.020 Cervical disc disorder with myelopathy, mid-cervical region, unspecified level CC UNS

M50.021 Cervical disc disorder at C4-C5 level with myelopathy CC
C4-C5 disc disorder with myelopathy

M50.022 Cervical disc disorder at C5-C6 level with myelopathy CC
C5-C6 disc disorder with myelopathy

M50.023 Cervical disc disorder at C6-C7 level with myelopathy CC
C6-C7 disc disorder with myelopathy

M50.03 Cervical disc disorder with myelopathy, cervicothoracic region CC
C7-T1 disc disorder with myelopathy

M50.1 Cervical disc disorder with radiculopathy

EXCLUDES 2 *brachial radiculitis NOS (M54.13)*

AHA: 2018,3Q,19

M50.10 Cervical disc disorder with radiculopathy, unspecified cervical region

M50.11 Cervical disc disorder with radiculopathy, high cervical region
C2-C3 disc disorder with radiculopathy
C3 radiculopathy due to disc disorder
C3-C4 disc disorder with radiculopathy
C4 radiculopathy due to disc disorder

M50.12 Cervical disc disorder with radiculopathy, mid-cervical region

M50.120 Mid-cervical disc disorder, unspecified level

M50.121 Cervical disc disorder at C4-C5 level with radiculopathy
C4-C5 disc disorder with radiculopathy
C5 radiculopathy due to disc disorder

M50.122 Cervical disc disorder at C5-C6 level with radiculopathy
C5-C6 disc disorder with radiculopathy
C6 radiculopathy due to disc disorder

M50.123 Cervical disc disorder at C6-C7 level with radiculopathy
C6-C7 disc disorder with radiculopathy
C7 radiculopathy due to disc disorder

M50.13 Cervical disc disorder with radiculopathy, cervicothoracic region
C7-T1 disc disorder with radiculopathy
C8 radiculopathy due to disc disorder

M50.2 Other cervical disc displacement

M50.20 Other cervical disc displacement, unspecified cervical region

M50.21 Other cervical disc displacement, high cervical region
Other C2-C3 cervical disc displacement
Other C3-C4 cervical disc displacement

M50.22 Other cervical disc displacement, mid-cervical region

M50.220 Other cervical disc displacement, mid-cervical region, unspecified level

M50.221 Other cervical disc displacement at C4-C5 level
Other C4-C5 cervical disc displacement

M50.222 Other cervical disc displacement at C5-C6 level
Other C5-C6 cervical disc displacement

M50.223 Other cervical disc displacement at C6-C7 level
Other C6-C7 cervical disc displacement

M50.23 Other cervical disc displacement, cervicothoracic region
Other C7-T1 cervical disc displacement

M50.3 Other cervical disc degeneration

M50.30 Other cervical disc degeneration, unspecified cervical region

M50.31 Other cervical disc degeneration, high cervical region
Other C2-C3 cervical disc degeneration
Other C3-C4 cervical disc degeneration

M50.32 Other cervical disc degeneration, mid-cervical region

M50.320 Other cervical disc degeneration, mid-cervical region, unspecified level

M50.321 Other cervical disc degeneration at C4-C5 level
Other C4-C5 cervical disc degeneration

M5Ø.322 Other cervical disc degeneration at C5-C6 level
Other C5-C6 cervical disc degeneration

M5Ø.323 Other cervical disc degeneration at C6-C7 level
Other C6-C7 cervical disc degeneration

M5Ø.33 Other cervical disc degeneration, cervicothoracic region
Other C7-T1 cervical disc degeneration

✓5th M5Ø.8 Other cervical disc disorders

M5Ø.8Ø Other cervical disc disorders, unspecified cervical region

M5Ø.81 Other cervical disc disorders, high cervical region
Other C2-C3 cervical disc disorders
Other C3-C4 cervical disc disorders

✓6th M5Ø.82 Other cervical disc disorders, mid-cervical region

M5Ø.82Ø Other cervical disc disorders, mid-cervical region, unspecified level

M5Ø.821 Other cervical disc disorders at C4-C5 level
Other C4-C5 cervical disc disorders

M5Ø.822 Other cervical disc disorders at C5-C6 level
Other C5-C6 cervical disc disorders

M5Ø.823 Other cervical disc disorders at C6-C7 level
Other C6-C7 cervical disc disorders

M5Ø.83 Other cervical disc disorders, cervicothoracic region
Other C7-T1 cervical disc disorders

✓5th M5Ø.9 Cervical disc disorder, unspecified

M5Ø.9Ø Cervical disc disorder, unspecified, unspecified cervical region

M5Ø.91 Cervical disc disorder, unspecified, high cervical region
C2-C3 cervical disc disorder, unspecified
C3-C4 cervical disc disorder, unspecified

✓6th M5Ø.92 Cervical disc disorder, unspecified, mid-cervical region

M5Ø.92Ø Unspecified cervical disc disorder, mid-cervical region, unspecified level

M5Ø.921 Unspecified cervical disc disorder at C4-C5 level
Unspecified C4-C5 cervical disc disorder

M5Ø.922 Unspecified cervical disc disorder at C5-C6 level
Unspecified C5-C6 cervical disc disorder

M5Ø.923 Unspecified cervical disc disorder at C6-C7 level
Unspecified C6-C7 cervical disc disorder

M5Ø.93 Cervical disc disorder, unspecified, cervicothoracic region
C7-T1 cervical disc disorder, unspecified

✓4th M51 Thoracic, thoracolumbar, and lumbosacral intervertebral disc disorders

EXCLUDES 2 *cervical and cervicothoracic disc disorders (M5Ø.-)*
sacral and sacrococcygeal disorders (M53.3)

✓5th M51.Ø Thoracic, thoracolumbar and lumbosacral intervertebral disc disorders with myelopathy

M51.Ø4 Intervertebral disc disorders with myelopathy, thoracic region CC

M51.Ø5 Intervertebral disc disorders with myelopathy, thoracolumbar region CC

M51.Ø6 Intervertebral disc disorders with myelopathy, lumbar region CC

✓5th M51.1 Thoracic, thoracolumbar and lumbosacral intervertebral disc disorders with radiculopathy
Sciatica due to intervertebral disc disorder

EXCLUDES 1 *lumbar radiculitis NOS (M54.16)*
sciatica NOS (M54.3)

AHA: 2018,3Q,18

M51.14 Intervertebral disc disorders with radiculopathy, thoracic region

M51.15 Intervertebral disc disorders with radiculopathy, thoracolumbar region

M51.16 Intervertebral disc disorders with radiculopathy, lumbar region

M51.17 Intervertebral disc disorders with radiculopathy, lumbosacral region

✓5th M51.2 Other thoracic, thoracolumbar and lumbosacral intervertebral disc displacement
Lumbago due to displacement of intervertebral disc

AHA: 2022,1Q,26

Displacement Intervertebral Disc

Normal Top View   Herniated Top View

M51.24 Other intervertebral disc displacement, thoracic region

M51.25 Other intervertebral disc displacement, thoracolumbar region

M51.26 Other intervertebral disc displacement, lumbar region

M51.27 Other intervertebral disc displacement, lumbosacral region

✓5th M51.3 Other thoracic, thoracolumbar and lumbosacral intervertebral disc degeneration

AHA: 2022,1Q,26; 2018,2Q,15; 2013,3Q,22

M51.34 Other intervertebral disc degeneration, thoracic region

M51.35 Other intervertebral disc degeneration, thoracolumbar region

M51.36 Other intervertebral disc degeneration, lumbar region

M51.37 Other intervertebral disc degeneration, lumbosacral region

✓5th M51.4 Schmorl's nodes

DEF: Irregular bone defect in the margin of the vertebral body that causes herniation into the end plate of the vertebral body.

M51.44 Schmorl's nodes, thoracic region

M51.45 Schmorl's nodes, thoracolumbar region

M51.46 Schmorl's nodes, lumbar region

M51.47 Schmorl's nodes, lumbosacral region

✓5th M51.8 Other thoracic, thoracolumbar and lumbosacral intervertebral disc disorders

M51.84 Other intervertebral disc disorders, thoracic region

M51.85 Other intervertebral disc disorders, thoracolumbar region

M51.86 Other intervertebral disc disorders, lumbar region

M51.87 Other intervertebral disc disorders, lumbosacral region

M51.9 Unspecified thoracic, thoracolumbar and lumbosacral intervertebral disc disorder

✓5th M51.A Other lumbar and lumbosacral annulus fibrosus disc defects

AHA: 2022,4Q,28-29

M51.AØ Intervertebral annulus fibrosus defect, lumbar region, unspecified size
Code first, if applicable, lumbar disc herniation (M51.Ø6, M51.16, M51.26)

M51.A1 Intervertebral annulus fibrosus defect, small, lumbar region
Code first, if applicable, lumbar disc herniation (M51.Ø6, M51.16, M51.26)

M51.A2 Intervertebral annulus fibrosus defect, large, lumbar region
Code first, if applicable, lumbar disc herniation (M51.Ø6, M51.16, M51.26)

M51.A3 Intervertebral annulus fibrosus defect, lumbosacral region, unspecified size
Code first, if applicable, lumbosacral disc herniation (M51.17, M51.27)

M51.A4 Intervertebral annulus fibrosus defect, small, lumbosacral region
Code first, if applicable, lumbosacral disc herniation (M51.17, M51.27)

M51.A5 **Intervertebral annulus fibrosus defect, large, lumbosacral region**
Code first, if applicable, lumbosacral disc herniation (M51.17, M51.27)

M53 Other and unspecified dorsopathies, not elsewhere classified

M53.Ø Cervicocranial syndrome
Posterior cervical sympathetic syndrome

M53.1 Cervicobrachial syndrome
EXCLUDES 2 *cervical disc disorder (M5Ø.-)*
thoracic outlet syndrome (G54.Ø)

M53.2 Spinal instabilities

M53.2X Spinal instabilities
M53.2X1 Spinal instabilities, occipito-atlanto-axial region
M53.2X2 Spinal instabilities, cervical region
M53.2X3 Spinal instabilities, cervicothoracic region
M53.2X4 Spinal instabilities, thoracic region
M53.2X5 Spinal instabilities, thoracolumbar region
M53.2X6 Spinal instabilities, lumbar region
M53.2X7 Spinal instabilities, lumbosacral region
M53.2X8 Spinal instabilities, sacral and sacrococcygeal region
M53.2X9 Spinal instabilities, site unspecified

M53.3 Sacrococcygeal disorders, not elsewhere classified
Coccygodynia

M53.8 Other specified dorsopathies
M53.8Ø Other specified dorsopathies, site unspecified
M53.81 Other specified dorsopathies, occipito-atlanto-axial region
M53.82 Other specified dorsopathies, cervical region
M53.83 Other specified dorsopathies, cervicothoracic region
M53.84 Other specified dorsopathies, thoracic region
M53.85 Other specified dorsopathies, thoracolumbar region
M53.86 Other specified dorsopathies, lumbar region
M53.87 Other specified dorsopathies, lumbosacral region
M53.88 Other specified dorsopathies, sacral and sacrococcygeal region

M53.9 Dorsopathy, unspecified

M54 Dorsalgia
EXCLUDES 1 *psychogenic dorsalgia (F45.41)*

M54.Ø Panniculitis affecting regions of neck and back
EXCLUDES 1 *lupus panniculitis (L93.2)*
panniculitis NOS (M79.3)
relapsing [Weber-Christian] panniculitis (M35.6)

M54.ØØ Panniculitis affecting regions of neck and back, site unspecified
M54.Ø1 Panniculitis affecting regions of neck and back, occipito-atlanto-axial region
M54.Ø2 Panniculitis affecting regions of neck and back, cervical region
M54.Ø3 Panniculitis affecting regions of neck and back, cervicothoracic region
M54.Ø4 Panniculitis affecting regions of neck and back, thoracic region
M54.Ø5 Panniculitis affecting regions of neck and back, thoracolumbar region
M54.Ø6 Panniculitis affecting regions of neck and back, lumbar region
M54.Ø7 Panniculitis affecting regions of neck and back, lumbosacral region
M54.Ø8 Panniculitis affecting regions of neck and back, sacral and sacrococcygeal region
M54.Ø9 Panniculitis affecting regions, neck and back, multiple sites in spine

M54.1 Radiculopathy
Brachial neuritis or radiculitis NOS
Lumbar neuritis or radiculitis NOS
Lumbosacral neuritis or radiculitis NOS
Radiculitis NOS
Thoracic neuritis or radiculitis NOS
EXCLUDES 1 *neuralgia and neuritis NOS (M79.2)*
radiculopathy with cervical disc disorder (M5Ø.1)
radiculopathy with lumbar and other intervertebral disc disorder (M51.1-)
radiculopathy with spondylosis (M47.2-)

AHA: 2018,3Q,18

TIP: A code from this subcategory can be used in addition to a spondylolisthesis code (M43.1-) or a spinal stenosis code (M48.0-) when either condition is documented as the cause of the radiculopathy.

M54.1Ø Radiculopathy, site unspecified
M54.11 Radiculopathy, occipito-atlanto-axial region
M54.12 Radiculopathy, cervical region
M54.13 Radiculopathy, cervicothoracic region
M54.14 Radiculopathy, thoracic region
M54.15 Radiculopathy, thoracolumbar region
M54.16 Radiculopathy, lumbar region
M54.17 Radiculopathy, lumbosacral region
M54.18 Radiculopathy, sacral and sacrococcygeal region

M54.2 Cervicalgia
EXCLUDES 1 *cervicalgia due to intervertebral cervical disc disorder (M5Ø.-)*

M54.3 Sciatica
EXCLUDES 1 *lesion of sciatic nerve (G57.Ø)*
sciatica due to intervertebral disc disorder (M51.1-)
sciatica with lumbago (M54.4-)

M54.3Ø Sciatica, unspecified side
M54.31 Sciatica, right side
M54.32 Sciatica, left side

M54.4 Lumbago with sciatica
EXCLUDES 1 *lumbago with sciatica due to intervertebral disc disorder (M51.1-)*

AHA: 2016,2Q,7

M54.4Ø Lumbago with sciatica, unspecified side
M54.41 Lumbago with sciatica, right side
M54.42 Lumbago with sciatica, left side

M54.5 Low back pain
EXCLUDES 1 *low back strain (S39.Ø12)*
lumbago due to intervertebral disc displacement (M51.2-)
lumbago with sciatica (M54.4-)

AHA: 2021,4Q,22

M54.5Ø Low back pain, unspecified
Loin pain
Lumbago NOS
M54.51 Vertebrogenic low back pain
Low back vertebral endplate pain
M54.59 Other low back pain

M54.6 Pain in thoracic spine
EXCLUDES 1 *pain in thoracic spine due to intervertebral disc disorder (M51.-)*

M54.8 Other dorsalgia
EXCLUDES 1 *dorsalgia in thoracic region (M54.6)*
low back pain (M54.5-)

M54.81 Occipital neuralgia
M54.89 Other dorsalgia

M54.9 Dorsalgia, unspecified
Backache NOS
Back pain NOS

SOFT TISSUE DISORDERS (M60-M79)

Disorders of muscles (M60-M63)

EXCLUDES 1 *dermatopolymyositis (M33.-)*
myopathy in amyloidosis (E85.-)
myopathy in polyarteritis nodosa (M30.0)
myopathy in rheumatoid arthritis (M05.32)
myopathy in scleroderma (M34.-)
myopathy in Sjögren's syndrome (M35.03)
myopathy in systemic lupus erythematosus (M32.-)

EXCLUDES 2 *muscular dystrophies and myopathies (G71-G72)*

M60 Myositis
EXCLUDES 2 *inclusion body myositis [IBM] (G72.41)*

M60.0 Infective myositis
Tropical pyomyositis
Use additional code (B95-B97) to identify infectious agent

M60.00 Infective myositis, unspecified site
M60.000 Infective myositis, unspecified right arm CC
Infective myositis, right upper limb NOS
M60.001 Infective myositis, unspecified left arm CC
Infective myositis, left upper limb NOS
M60.002 Infective myositis, unspecified arm CC UNS
Infective myositis, upper limb NOS
M60.003 Infective myositis, unspecified right leg CC
Infective myositis, right lower limb NOS
M60.004 Infective myositis, unspecified left leg CC
Infective myositis, left lower limb NOS
M60.005 Infective myositis, unspecified leg CC UNS
Infective myositis, lower limb NOS
M60.009 Infective myositis, unspecified site CC UNS

M60.01 Infective myositis, shoulder
M60.011 Infective myositis, right shoulder CC
M60.012 Infective myositis, left shoulder CC
M60.019 Infective myositis, unspecified shoulder CC UNS

M60.02 Infective myositis, upper arm
M60.021 Infective myositis, right upper arm CC
M60.022 Infective myositis, left upper arm CC
M60.029 Infective myositis, unspecified upper arm CC UNS

M60.03 Infective myositis, forearm
M60.031 Infective myositis, right forearm CC
M60.032 Infective myositis, left forearm CC
M60.039 Infective myositis, unspecified forearm CC UNS

M60.04 Infective myositis, hand and fingers
M60.041 Infective myositis, right hand CC
M60.042 Infective myositis, left hand CC
M60.043 Infective myositis, unspecified hand CC UNS
M60.044 Infective myositis, right finger(s) CC
M60.045 Infective myositis, left finger(s) CC
M60.046 Infective myositis, unspecified finger(s) CC UNS

M60.05 Infective myositis, thigh
M60.051 Infective myositis, right thigh CC
M60.052 Infective myositis, left thigh CC
M60.059 Infective myositis, unspecified thigh CC UNS

M60.06 Infective myositis, lower leg
M60.061 Infective myositis, right lower leg CC
M60.062 Infective myositis, left lower leg CC
M60.069 Infective myositis, unspecified lower leg CC UNS

M60.07 Infective myositis, ankle, foot and toes
M60.070 Infective myositis, right ankle CC
M60.071 Infective myositis, left ankle CC
M60.072 Infective myositis, unspecified ankle CC UNS
M60.073 Infective myositis, right foot CC
M60.074 Infective myositis, left foot CC
M60.075 Infective myositis, unspecified foot CC UNS
M60.076 Infective myositis, right toe(s) CC
M60.077 Infective myositis, left toe(s) CC
M60.078 Infective myositis, unspecified toe(s) CC UNS

M60.08 Infective myositis, other site CC
M60.09 Infective myositis, multiple sites CC

M60.1 Interstitial myositis
M60.10 Interstitial myositis of unspecified site

M60.11 Interstitial myositis, shoulder
M60.111 Interstitial myositis, right shoulder
M60.112 Interstitial myositis, left shoulder
M60.119 Interstitial myositis, unspecified shoulder

M60.12 Interstitial myositis, upper arm
M60.121 Interstitial myositis, right upper arm
M60.122 Interstitial myositis, left upper arm
M60.129 Interstitial myositis, unspecified upper arm

M60.13 Interstitial myositis, forearm
M60.131 Interstitial myositis, right forearm
M60.132 Interstitial myositis, left forearm
M60.139 Interstitial myositis, unspecified forearm

M60.14 Interstitial myositis, hand
M60.141 Interstitial myositis, right hand
M60.142 Interstitial myositis, left hand
M60.149 Interstitial myositis, unspecified hand

M60.15 Interstitial myositis, thigh
M60.151 Interstitial myositis, right thigh
M60.152 Interstitial myositis, left thigh
M60.159 Interstitial myositis, unspecified thigh

M60.16 Interstitial myositis, lower leg
M60.161 Interstitial myositis, right lower leg
M60.162 Interstitial myositis, left lower leg
M60.169 Interstitial myositis, unspecified lower leg

M60.17 Interstitial myositis, ankle and foot
M60.171 Interstitial myositis, right ankle and foot
M60.172 Interstitial myositis, left ankle and foot
M60.179 Interstitial myositis, unspecified ankle and foot

M60.18 Interstitial myositis, other site
M60.19 Interstitial myositis, multiple sites

M60.2 Foreign body granuloma of soft tissue, not elsewhere classified
Use additional code to identify the type of retained foreign body (Z18.-)
EXCLUDES 1 *foreign body granuloma of skin and subcutaneous tissue (L92.3)*

M60.20 Foreign body granuloma of soft tissue, not elsewhere classified, unspecified site

M60.21 Foreign body granuloma of soft tissue, not elsewhere classified, shoulder
M60.211 Foreign body granuloma of soft tissue, not elsewhere classified, right shoulder
M60.212 Foreign body granuloma of soft tissue, not elsewhere classified, left shoulder
M60.219 Foreign body granuloma of soft tissue, not elsewhere classified, unspecified shoulder

M60.22 Foreign body granuloma of soft tissue, not elsewhere classified, upper arm
M60.221 Foreign body granuloma of soft tissue, not elsewhere classified, right upper arm
M60.222 Foreign body granuloma of soft tissue, not elsewhere classified, left upper arm
M60.229 Foreign body granuloma of soft tissue, not elsewhere classified, unspecified upper arm

M60.23 Foreign body granuloma of soft tissue, not elsewhere classified, forearm
M60.231 Foreign body granuloma of soft tissue, not elsewhere classified, right forearm
M60.232 Foreign body granuloma of soft tissue, not elsewhere classified, left forearm

M60.239 Foreign body granuloma of soft tissue, not elsewhere classified, unspecified forearm

M60.24 Foreign body granuloma of soft tissue, not elsewhere classified, hand
- M60.241 Foreign body granuloma of soft tissue, not elsewhere classified, right hand
- M60.242 Foreign body granuloma of soft tissue, not elsewhere classified, left hand
- M60.249 Foreign body granuloma of soft tissue, not elsewhere classified, unspecified hand

M60.25 Foreign body granuloma of soft tissue, not elsewhere classified, thigh
- M60.251 Foreign body granuloma of soft tissue, not elsewhere classified, right thigh
- M60.252 Foreign body granuloma of soft tissue, not elsewhere classified, left thigh
- M60.259 Foreign body granuloma of soft tissue, not elsewhere classified, unspecified thigh

M60.26 Foreign body granuloma of soft tissue, not elsewhere classified, lower leg
- M60.261 Foreign body granuloma of soft tissue, not elsewhere classified, right lower leg
- M60.262 Foreign body granuloma of soft tissue, not elsewhere classified, left lower leg
- M60.269 Foreign body granuloma of soft tissue, not elsewhere classified, unspecified lower leg

M60.27 Foreign body granuloma of soft tissue, not elsewhere classified, ankle and foot
- M60.271 Foreign body granuloma of soft tissue, not elsewhere classified, right ankle and foot
- M60.272 Foreign body granuloma of soft tissue, not elsewhere classified, left ankle and foot
- M60.279 Foreign body granuloma of soft tissue, not elsewhere classified, unspecified ankle and foot

M60.28 Foreign body granuloma of soft tissue, not elsewhere classified, other site

M60.8 Other myositis

M60.80 Other myositis, unspecified site

M60.81 Other myositis shoulder
- M60.811 Other myositis, right shoulder
- M60.812 Other myositis, left shoulder
- M60.819 Other myositis, unspecified shoulder

M60.82 Other myositis, upper arm
- M60.821 Other myositis, right upper arm
- M60.822 Other myositis, left upper arm
- M60.829 Other myositis, unspecified upper arm

M60.83 Other myositis, forearm
- M60.831 Other myositis, right forearm
- M60.832 Other myositis, left forearm
- M60.839 Other myositis, unspecified forearm

M60.84 Other myositis, hand
- M60.841 Other myositis, right hand
- M60.842 Other myositis, left hand
- M60.849 Other myositis, unspecified hand

M60.85 Other myositis, thigh
- M60.851 Other myositis, right thigh
- M60.852 Other myositis, left thigh
- M60.859 Other myositis, unspecified thigh

M60.86 Other myositis, lower leg
- M60.861 Other myositis, right lower leg
- M60.862 Other myositis, left lower leg
- M60.869 Other myositis, unspecified lower leg

M60.87 Other myositis, ankle and foot
- M60.871 Other myositis, right ankle and foot
- M60.872 Other myositis, left ankle and foot
- M60.879 Other myositis, unspecified ankle and foot

M60.88 Other myositis, other site

M60.89 Other myositis, multiple sites

M60.9 Myositis, unspecified

M61 Calcification and ossification of muscle

M61.0 Myositis ossificans traumatica

M61.00 Myositis ossificans traumatica, unspecified site

M61.01 Myositis ossificans traumatica, shoulder
- M61.011 Myositis ossificans traumatica, right shoulder
- M61.012 Myositis ossificans traumatica, left shoulder
- M61.019 Myositis ossificans traumatica, unspecified shoulder

M61.02 Myositis ossificans traumatica, upper arm
- M61.021 Myositis ossificans traumatica, right upper arm
- M61.022 Myositis ossificans traumatica, left upper arm
- M61.029 Myositis ossificans traumatica, unspecified upper arm

M61.03 Myositis ossificans traumatica, forearm
- M61.031 Myositis ossificans traumatica, right forearm
- M61.032 Myositis ossificans traumatica, left forearm
- M61.039 Myositis ossificans traumatica, unspecified forearm

M61.04 Myositis ossificans traumatica, hand
- M61.041 Myositis ossificans traumatica, right hand
- M61.042 Myositis ossificans traumatica, left hand
- M61.049 Myositis ossificans traumatica, unspecified hand

M61.05 Myositis ossificans traumatica, thigh
- M61.051 Myositis ossificans traumatica, right thigh
- M61.052 Myositis ossificans traumatica, left thigh
- M61.059 Myositis ossificans traumatica, unspecified thigh

M61.06 Myositis ossificans traumatica, lower leg
- M61.061 Myositis ossificans traumatica, right lower leg
- M61.062 Myositis ossificans traumatica, left lower leg
- M61.069 Myositis ossificans traumatica, unspecified lower leg

M61.07 Myositis ossificans traumatica, ankle and foot
- M61.071 Myositis ossificans traumatica, right ankle and foot
- M61.072 Myositis ossificans traumatica, left ankle and foot
- M61.079 Myositis ossificans traumatica, unspecified ankle and foot

M61.08 Myositis ossificans traumatica, other site

M61.09 Myositis ossificans traumatica, multiple sites

M61.1 Myositis ossificans progressiva

Fibrodysplasia ossificans progressiva

M61.10 Myositis ossificans progressiva, unspecified site

M61.11 Myositis ossificans progressiva, shoulder
- M61.111 Myositis ossificans progressiva, right shoulder
- M61.112 Myositis ossificans progressiva, left shoulder
- M61.119 Myositis ossificans progressiva, unspecified shoulder

M61.12 Myositis ossificans progressiva, upper arm
- M61.121 Myositis ossificans progressiva, right upper arm
- M61.122 Myositis ossificans progressiva, left upper arm
- M61.129 Myositis ossificans progressiva, unspecified arm

M61.13 Myositis ossificans progressiva, forearm
- M61.131 Myositis ossificans progressiva, right forearm
- M61.132 Myositis ossificans progressiva, left forearm
- M61.139 Myositis ossificans progressiva, unspecified forearm

M61.14 Myositis ossificans progressiva, hand and finger(s)
- M61.141 Myositis ossificans progressiva, right hand
- M61.142 Myositis ossificans progressiva, left hand

M61.143 Myositis ossificans progressiva, unspecified hand
M61.144 Myositis ossificans progressiva, right finger(s)
M61.145 Myositis ossificans progressiva, left finger(s)
M61.146 Myositis ossificans progressiva, unspecified finger(s)

√6th M61.15 Myositis ossificans progressiva, thigh
M61.151 Myositis ossificans progressiva, right thigh
M61.152 Myositis ossificans progressiva, left thigh
M61.159 Myositis ossificans progressiva, unspecified thigh

√6th M61.16 Myositis ossificans progressiva, lower leg
M61.161 Myositis ossificans progressiva, right lower leg
M61.162 Myositis ossificans progressiva, left lower leg
M61.169 Myositis ossificans progressiva, unspecified lower leg

√6th M61.17 Myositis ossificans progressiva, ankle, foot and toe(s)
M61.171 Myositis ossificans progressiva, right ankle
M61.172 Myositis ossificans progressiva, left ankle
M61.173 Myositis ossificans progressiva, unspecified ankle
M61.174 Myositis ossificans progressiva, right foot
M61.175 Myositis ossificans progressiva, left foot
M61.176 Myositis ossificans progressiva, unspecified foot
M61.177 Myositis ossificans progressiva, right toe(s)
M61.178 Myositis ossificans progressiva, left toe(s)
M61.179 Myositis ossificans progressiva, unspecified toe(s)

M61.18 Myositis ossificans progressiva, other site
M61.19 Myositis ossificans progressiva, multiple sites

√5th M61.2 Paralytic calcification and ossification of muscle
Myositis ossificans associated with quadriplegia or paraplegia

M61.20 Paralytic calcification and ossification of muscle, unspecified site

√6th M61.21 Paralytic calcification and ossification of muscle, shoulder
M61.211 Paralytic calcification and ossification of muscle, right shoulder
M61.212 Paralytic calcification and ossification of muscle, left shoulder
M61.219 Paralytic calcification and ossification of muscle, unspecified shoulder

√6th M61.22 Paralytic calcification and ossification of muscle, upper arm
M61.221 Paralytic calcification and ossification of muscle, right upper arm
M61.222 Paralytic calcification and ossification of muscle, left upper arm
M61.229 Paralytic calcification and ossification of muscle, unspecified upper arm

√6th M61.23 Paralytic calcification and ossification of muscle, forearm
M61.231 Paralytic calcification and ossification of muscle, right forearm
M61.232 Paralytic calcification and ossification of muscle, left forearm
M61.239 Paralytic calcification and ossification of muscle, unspecified forearm

√6th M61.24 Paralytic calcification and ossification of muscle, hand
M61.241 Paralytic calcification and ossification of muscle, right hand
M61.242 Paralytic calcification and ossification of muscle, left hand
M61.249 Paralytic calcification and ossification of muscle, unspecified hand

√6th M61.25 Paralytic calcification and ossification of muscle, thigh
M61.251 Paralytic calcification and ossification of muscle, right thigh
M61.252 Paralytic calcification and ossification of muscle, left thigh
M61.259 Paralytic calcification and ossification of muscle, unspecified thigh

√6th M61.26 Paralytic calcification and ossification of muscle, lower leg
M61.261 Paralytic calcification and ossification of muscle, right lower leg
M61.262 Paralytic calcification and ossification of muscle, left lower leg
M61.269 Paralytic calcification and ossification of muscle, unspecified lower leg

√6th M61.27 Paralytic calcification and ossification of muscle, ankle and foot
M61.271 Paralytic calcification and ossification of muscle, right ankle and foot
M61.272 Paralytic calcification and ossification of muscle, left ankle and foot
M61.279 Paralytic calcification and ossification of muscle, unspecified ankle and foot

M61.28 Paralytic calcification and ossification of muscle, other site
M61.29 Paralytic calcification and ossification of muscle, multiple sites

√5th M61.3 Calcification and ossification of muscles associated with burns
Myositis ossificans associated with burns

M61.30 Calcification and ossification of muscles associated with burns, unspecified site

√6th M61.31 Calcification and ossification of muscles associated with burns, shoulder
M61.311 Calcification and ossification of muscles associated with burns, right shoulder
M61.312 Calcification and ossification of muscles associated with burns, left shoulder
M61.319 Calcification and ossification of muscles associated with burns, unspecified shoulder

√6th M61.32 Calcification and ossification of muscles associated with burns, upper arm
M61.321 Calcification and ossification of muscles associated with burns, right upper arm
M61.322 Calcification and ossification of muscles associated with burns, left upper arm
M61.329 Calcification and ossification of muscles associated with burns, unspecified upper arm

√6th M61.33 Calcification and ossification of muscles associated with burns, forearm
M61.331 Calcification and ossification of muscles associated with burns, right forearm
M61.332 Calcification and ossification of muscles associated with burns, left forearm
M61.339 Calcification and ossification of muscles associated with burns, unspecified forearm

√6th M61.34 Calcification and ossification of muscles associated with burns, hand
M61.341 Calcification and ossification of muscles associated with burns, right hand
M61.342 Calcification and ossification of muscles associated with burns, left hand
M61.349 Calcification and ossification of muscles associated with burns, unspecified hand

√6th M61.35 Calcification and ossification of muscles associated with burns, thigh
M61.351 Calcification and ossification of muscles associated with burns, right thigh
M61.352 Calcification and ossification of muscles associated with burns, left thigh
M61.359 Calcification and ossification of muscles associated with burns, unspecified thigh

√6th M61.36 Calcification and ossification of muscles associated with burns, lower leg
M61.361 Calcification and ossification of muscles associated with burns, right lower leg
M61.362 Calcification and ossification of muscles associated with burns, left lower leg
M61.369 Calcification and ossification of muscles associated with burns, unspecified lower leg

M61.37 Calcification and ossification of muscles associated with burns, ankle and foot
- M61.371 Calcification and ossification of muscles associated with burns, right ankle and foot
- M61.372 Calcification and ossification of muscles associated with burns, left ankle and foot
- M61.379 Calcification and ossification of muscles associated with burns, unspecified ankle and foot

M61.38 Calcification and ossification of muscles associated with burns, other site

M61.39 Calcification and ossification of muscles associated with burns, multiple sites

M61.4 Other calcification of muscle

EXCLUDES 1 *calcific tendinitis NOS (M65.2-)*
calcific tendinitis of shoulder (M75.3)

M61.40 Other calcification of muscle, unspecified site

M61.41 Other calcification of muscle, shoulder
- M61.411 Other calcification of muscle, right shoulder
- M61.412 Other calcification of muscle, left shoulder
- M61.419 Other calcification of muscle, unspecified shoulder

M61.42 Other calcification of muscle, upper arm
- M61.421 Other calcification of muscle, right upper arm
- M61.422 Other calcification of muscle, left upper arm
- M61.429 Other calcification of muscle, unspecified upper arm

M61.43 Other calcification of muscle, forearm
- M61.431 Other calcification of muscle, right forearm
- M61.432 Other calcification of muscle, left forearm
- M61.439 Other calcification of muscle, unspecified forearm

M61.44 Other calcification of muscle, hand
- M61.441 Other calcification of muscle, right hand
- M61.442 Other calcification of muscle, left hand
- M61.449 Other calcification of muscle, unspecified hand

M61.45 Other calcification of muscle, thigh
- M61.451 Other calcification of muscle, right thigh
- M61.452 Other calcification of muscle, left thigh
- M61.459 Other calcification of muscle, unspecified thigh

M61.46 Other calcification of muscle, lower leg
- M61.461 Other calcification of muscle, right lower leg
- M61.462 Other calcification of muscle, left lower leg
- M61.469 Other calcification of muscle, unspecified lower leg

M61.47 Other calcification of muscle, ankle and foot
- M61.471 Other calcification of muscle, right ankle and foot
- M61.472 Other calcification of muscle, left ankle and foot
- M61.479 Other calcification of muscle, unspecified ankle and foot

M61.48 Other calcification of muscle, other site

M61.49 Other calcification of muscle, multiple sites

M61.5 Other ossification of muscle

M61.50 Other ossification of muscle, unspecified site

M61.51 Other ossification of muscle, shoulder
- M61.511 Other ossification of muscle, right shoulder
- M61.512 Other ossification of muscle, left shoulder
- M61.519 Other ossification of muscle, unspecified shoulder

M61.52 Other ossification of muscle, upper arm
- M61.521 Other ossification of muscle, right upper arm
- M61.522 Other ossification of muscle, left upper arm
- M61.529 Other ossification of muscle, unspecified upper arm

M61.53 Other ossification of muscle, forearm
- M61.531 Other ossification of muscle, right forearm
- M61.532 Other ossification of muscle, left forearm
- M61.539 Other ossification of muscle, unspecified forearm

M61.54 Other ossification of muscle, hand
- M61.541 Other ossification of muscle, right hand
- M61.542 Other ossification of muscle, left hand
- M61.549 Other ossification of muscle, unspecified hand

M61.55 Other ossification of muscle, thigh
- M61.551 Other ossification of muscle, right thigh
- M61.552 Other ossification of muscle, left thigh
- M61.559 Other ossification of muscle, unspecified thigh

M61.56 Other ossification of muscle, lower leg
- M61.561 Other ossification of muscle, right lower leg
- M61.562 Other ossification of muscle, left lower leg
- M61.569 Other ossification of muscle, unspecified lower leg

M61.57 Other ossification of muscle, ankle and foot
- M61.571 Other ossification of muscle, right ankle and foot
- M61.572 Other ossification of muscle, left ankle and foot
- M61.579 Other ossification of muscle, unspecified ankle and foot

M61.58 Other ossification of muscle, other site

M61.59 Other ossification of muscle, multiple sites

M61.9 Calcification and ossification of muscle, unspecified

M62 Other disorders of muscle

EXCLUDES 1 *alcoholic myopathy (G72.1)*
cramp and spasm (R25.2)
drug-induced myopathy (G72.Ø)
myalgia (M79.1-)
stiff-man syndrome (G25.82)

EXCLUDES 2 *nontraumatic hematoma of muscle (M79.81)*

M62.Ø Separation of muscle (nontraumatic)

Diastasis of muscle

EXCLUDES 1 *diastasis recti complicating pregnancy, labor and delivery (O71.8)*
traumatic separation of muscle - see strain of muscle by body region

M62.ØØ Separation of muscle (nontraumatic), unspecified site

M62.Ø1 Separation of muscle (nontraumatic), shoulder
- M62.Ø11 Separation of muscle (nontraumatic), right shoulder
- M62.Ø12 Separation of muscle (nontraumatic), left shoulder
- M62.Ø19 Separation of muscle (nontraumatic), unspecified shoulder

M62.Ø2 Separation of muscle (nontraumatic), upper arm
- M62.Ø21 Separation of muscle (nontraumatic), right upper arm
- M62.Ø22 Separation of muscle (nontraumatic), left upper arm
- M62.Ø29 Separation of muscle (nontraumatic), unspecified upper arm

M62.Ø3 Separation of muscle (nontraumatic), forearm
- M62.Ø31 Separation of muscle (nontraumatic), right forearm
- M62.Ø32 Separation of muscle (nontraumatic), left forearm
- M62.Ø39 Separation of muscle (nontraumatic), unspecified forearm

M62.Ø4 Separation of muscle (nontraumatic), hand
- M62.Ø41 Separation of muscle (nontraumatic), right hand
- M62.Ø42 Separation of muscle (nontraumatic), left hand
- M62.Ø49 Separation of muscle (nontraumatic), unspecified hand

√6th **M62.Ø5 Separation of muscle (nontraumatic), thigh**
- **M62.Ø51 Separation of muscle (nontraumatic), right thigh**
- **M62.Ø52 Separation of muscle (nontraumatic), left thigh**
- **M62.Ø59 Separation of muscle (nontraumatic), unspecified thigh**

√6th **M62.Ø6 Separation of muscle (nontraumatic), lower leg**
- **M62.Ø61 Separation of muscle (nontraumatic), right lower leg**
- **M62.Ø62 Separation of muscle (nontraumatic), left lower leg**
- **M62.Ø69 Separation of muscle (nontraumatic), unspecified lower leg**

√6th **M62.Ø7 Separation of muscle (nontraumatic), ankle and foot**
- **M62.Ø71 Separation of muscle (nontraumatic), right ankle and foot**
- **M62.Ø72 Separation of muscle (nontraumatic), left ankle and foot**
- **M62.Ø79 Separation of muscle (nontraumatic), unspecified ankle and foot**

M62.Ø8 Separation of muscle (nontraumatic), other site

√5th **M62.1 Other rupture of muscle (nontraumatic)**

EXCLUDES 1 *traumatic rupture of muscle - see strain of muscle by body region*

EXCLUDES 2 *rupture of tendon (M66.-)*

M62.1Ø Other rupture of muscle (nontraumatic), unspecified site

√6th **M62.11 Other rupture of muscle (nontraumatic), shoulder**
- **M62.111 Other rupture of muscle (nontraumatic), right shoulder**
- **M62.112 Other rupture of muscle (nontraumatic), left shoulder**
- **M62.119 Other rupture of muscle (nontraumatic), unspecified shoulder**

√6th **M62.12 Other rupture of muscle (nontraumatic), upper arm**
- **M62.121 Other rupture of muscle (nontraumatic), right upper arm**
- **M62.122 Other rupture of muscle (nontraumatic), left upper arm**
- **M62.129 Other rupture of muscle (nontraumatic), unspecified upper arm**

√6th **M62.13 Other rupture of muscle (nontraumatic), forearm**
- **M62.131 Other rupture of muscle (nontraumatic), right forearm**
- **M62.132 Other rupture of muscle (nontraumatic), left forearm**
- **M62.139 Other rupture of muscle (nontraumatic), unspecified forearm**

√6th **M62.14 Other rupture of muscle (nontraumatic), hand**
- **M62.141 Other rupture of muscle (nontraumatic), right hand**
- **M62.142 Other rupture of muscle (nontraumatic), left hand**
- **M62.149 Other rupture of muscle (nontraumatic), unspecified hand**

√6th **M62.15 Other rupture of muscle (nontraumatic), thigh**
- **M62.151 Other rupture of muscle (nontraumatic), right thigh**
- **M62.152 Other rupture of muscle (nontraumatic), left thigh**
- **M62.159 Other rupture of muscle (nontraumatic), unspecified thigh**

√6th **M62.16 Other rupture of muscle (nontraumatic), lower leg**
- **M62.161 Other rupture of muscle (nontraumatic), right lower leg**
- **M62.162 Other rupture of muscle (nontraumatic), left lower leg**
- **M62.169 Other rupture of muscle (nontraumatic), unspecified lower leg**

√6th **M62.17 Other rupture of muscle (nontraumatic), ankle and foot**
- **M62.171 Other rupture of muscle (nontraumatic), right ankle and foot**
- **M62.172 Other rupture of muscle (nontraumatic), left ankle and foot**
- **M62.179 Other rupture of muscle (nontraumatic), unspecified ankle and foot**

M62.18 Other rupture of muscle (nontraumatic), other site

√5th **M62.2 Nontraumatic ischemic infarction of muscle**

EXCLUDES 1 *compartment syndrome (traumatic) (T79.A-)*
nontraumatic compartment syndrome (M79.A-)
rhabdomyolysis (M62.82)
traumatic ischemia of muscle (T79.6)
Volkmann's ischemic contracture (T79.6)

M62.2Ø Nontraumatic ischemic infarction of muscle, unspecified site

√6th **M62.21 Nontraumatic ischemic infarction of muscle, shoulder**
- **M62.211 Nontraumatic ischemic infarction of muscle, right shoulder**
- **M62.212 Nontraumatic ischemic infarction of muscle, left shoulder**
- **M62.219 Nontraumatic ischemic infarction of muscle, unspecified shoulder**

√6th **M62.22 Nontraumatic ischemic infarction of muscle, upper arm**
- **M62.221 Nontraumatic ischemic infarction of muscle, right upper arm**
- **M62.222 Nontraumatic ischemic infarction of muscle, left upper arm**
- **M62.229 Nontraumatic ischemic infarction of muscle, unspecified upper arm**

√6th **M62.23 Nontraumatic ischemic infarction of muscle, forearm**
- **M62.231 Nontraumatic ischemic infarction of muscle, right forearm**
- **M62.232 Nontraumatic ischemic infarction of muscle, left forearm**
- **M62.239 Nontraumatic ischemic infarction of muscle, unspecified forearm**

√6th **M62.24 Nontraumatic ischemic infarction of muscle, hand**
- **M62.241 Nontraumatic ischemic infarction of muscle, right hand**
- **M62.242 Nontraumatic ischemic infarction of muscle, left hand**
- **M62.249 Nontraumatic ischemic infarction of muscle, unspecified hand**

√6th **M62.25 Nontraumatic ischemic infarction of muscle, thigh**
- **M62.251 Nontraumatic ischemic infarction of muscle, right thigh**
- **M62.252 Nontraumatic ischemic infarction of muscle, left thigh**
- **M62.259 Nontraumatic ischemic infarction of muscle, unspecified thigh**

√6th **M62.26 Nontraumatic ischemic infarction of muscle, lower leg**
- **M62.261 Nontraumatic ischemic infarction of muscle, right lower leg**
- **M62.262 Nontraumatic ischemic infarction of muscle, left lower leg**
- **M62.269 Nontraumatic ischemic infarction of muscle, unspecified lower leg**

√6th **M62.27 Nontraumatic ischemic infarction of muscle, ankle and foot**
- **M62.271 Nontraumatic ischemic infarction of muscle, right ankle and foot**
- **M62.272 Nontraumatic ischemic infarction of muscle, left ankle and foot**
- **M62.279 Nontraumatic ischemic infarction of muscle, unspecified ankle and foot**

M62.28 Nontraumatic ischemic infarction of muscle, other site

M62.3 Immobility syndrome (paraplegic)

√5th **M62.4 Contracture of muscle**

Contracture of tendon (sheath)

EXCLUDES 1 *contracture of joint (M24.5-)*

M62.4Ø Contracture of muscle, unspecified site

√6th **M62.41 Contracture of muscle, shoulder**
- **M62.411 Contracture of muscle, right shoulder**
- **M62.412 Contracture of muscle, left shoulder**
- **M62.419 Contracture of muscle, unspecified shoulder**

√6th **M62.42 Contracture of muscle, upper arm**
- **M62.421 Contracture of muscle, right upper arm**
- **M62.422 Contracture of muscle, left upper arm**
- **M62.429 Contracture of muscle, unspecified upper arm**

6th M62.43 Contracture of muscle, forearm
M62.431 Contracture of muscle, right forearm
M62.432 Contracture of muscle, left forearm
M62.439 Contracture of muscle, unspecified forearm

6th M62.44 Contracture of muscle, hand
M62.441 Contracture of muscle, right hand
M62.442 Contracture of muscle, left hand
M62.449 Contracture of muscle, unspecified hand

6th M62.45 Contracture of muscle, thigh
M62.451 Contracture of muscle, right thigh
M62.452 Contracture of muscle, left thigh
M62.459 Contracture of muscle, unspecified thigh

6th M62.46 Contracture of muscle, lower leg
AHA: 2023,2Q,14
M62.461 Contracture of muscle, right lower leg
M62.462 Contracture of muscle, left lower leg
M62.469 Contracture of muscle, unspecified lower leg

6th M62.47 Contracture of muscle, ankle and foot
M62.471 Contracture of muscle, right ankle and foot
M62.472 Contracture of muscle, left ankle and foot
M62.479 Contracture of muscle, unspecified ankle and foot

M62.48 Contracture of muscle, other site
M62.49 Contracture of muscle, multiple sites

5th M62.5 Muscle wasting and atrophy, not elsewhere classified
Disuse atrophy NEC
EXCLUDES 1 *neuralgic amyotrophy (G54.5)*
progressive muscular atrophy (G12.21)
sarcopenia (M62.84)
EXCLUDES 2 *pelvic muscle wasting (N81.84)*

M62.50 Muscle wasting and atrophy, not elsewhere classified, unspecified site

6th M62.51 Muscle wasting and atrophy, not elsewhere classified, shoulder
M62.511 Muscle wasting and atrophy, not elsewhere classified, right shoulder
M62.512 Muscle wasting and atrophy, not elsewhere classified, left shoulder
M62.519 Muscle wasting and atrophy, not elsewhere classified, unspecified shoulder

6th M62.52 Muscle wasting and atrophy, not elsewhere classified, upper arm
M62.521 Muscle wasting and atrophy, not elsewhere classified, right upper arm
M62.522 Muscle wasting and atrophy, not elsewhere classified, left upper arm
M62.529 Muscle wasting and atrophy, not elsewhere classified, unspecified upper arm

6th M62.53 Muscle wasting and atrophy, not elsewhere classified, forearm
M62.531 Muscle wasting and atrophy, not elsewhere classified, right forearm
M62.532 Muscle wasting and atrophy, not elsewhere classified, left forearm
M62.539 Muscle wasting and atrophy, not elsewhere classified, unspecified forearm

6th M62.54 Muscle wasting and atrophy, not elsewhere classified, hand
M62.541 Muscle wasting and atrophy, not elsewhere classified, right hand
M62.542 Muscle wasting and atrophy, not elsewhere classified, left hand
M62.549 Muscle wasting and atrophy, not elsewhere classified, unspecified hand

6th M62.55 Muscle wasting and atrophy, not elsewhere classified, thigh
M62.551 Muscle wasting and atrophy, not elsewhere classified, right thigh
M62.552 Muscle wasting and atrophy, not elsewhere classified, left thigh
M62.559 Muscle wasting and atrophy, not elsewhere classified, unspecified thigh

6th M62.56 Muscle wasting and atrophy, not elsewhere classified, lower leg
M62.561 Muscle wasting and atrophy, not elsewhere classified, right lower leg
M62.562 Muscle wasting and atrophy, not elsewhere classified, left lower leg
M62.569 Muscle wasting and atrophy, not elsewhere classified, unspecified lower leg

6th M62.57 Muscle wasting and atrophy, not elsewhere classified, ankle and foot
M62.571 Muscle wasting and atrophy, not elsewhere classified, right ankle and foot
M62.572 Muscle wasting and atrophy, not elsewhere classified, left ankle and foot
M62.579 Muscle wasting and atrophy, not elsewhere classified, unspecified ankle and foot

M62.58 Muscle wasting and atrophy, not elsewhere classified, other site
M62.59 Muscle wasting and atrophy, not elsewhere classified, multiple sites

6th M62.5A Muscle wasting and atrophy, not elsewhere classified, back
AHA: 2022,4Q,29
M62.5A0 Muscle wasting and atrophy, not elsewhere classified, back, cervical
M62.5A1 Muscle wasting and atrophy, not elsewhere classified, back, thoracic
M62.5A2 Muscle wasting and atrophy, not elsewhere classified, back, lumbosacral
M62.5A9 Muscle wasting and atrophy, not elsewhere classified, back, unspecified level

5th M62.8 Other specified disorders of muscle
EXCLUDES 2 *nontraumatic hematoma of muscle (M79.81)*

M62.81 Muscle weakness (generalized)
EXCLUDES 1 *muscle weakness in sarcopenia (M62.84)*

M62.82 Rhabdomyolysis CC
EXCLUDES 1 *traumatic rhabdomyolysis (T79.6)*
AHA: 2019,2Q,12
DEF: Rapid disintegration or destruction of skeletal muscle caused by direct or indirect injury, resulting in the excretion of muscle protein myoglobin into the urine.

6th M62.83 Muscle spasm
M62.830 Muscle spasm of back
M62.831 Muscle spasm of calf
Charley-horse
M62.838 Other muscle spasm

M62.84 Sarcopenia
Age-related sarcopenia
Code first underlying disease, if applicable, such as:
disorders of myoneural junction and muscle disease in diseases classified elsewhere (G73.-)
other and unspecified myopathies (G72.-)
primary disorders of muscles (G71.-)
AHA: 2016,4Q,41

M62.89 Other specified disorders of muscle
Muscle (sheath) hernia

M62.9 Disorder of muscle, unspecified

4th M63 Disorders of muscle in diseases classified elsewhere
Code first underlying disease, such as:
leprosy (A30.-)
neoplasm ▶(C49.-, C79.89, D21.-, D48.1-)◀
schistosomiasis (B65.-)
trichinellosis (B75)
EXCLUDES 1 *myopathy in cysticercosis (B69.81)*
myopathy in endocrine diseases (G73.7)
myopathy in metabolic diseases (G73.7)
myopathy in sarcoidosis (D86.87)
myopathy in secondary syphilis (A51.49)
myopathy in syphilis (late) (A52.78)
myopathy in toxoplasmosis (B58.82)
myopathy in tuberculosis (A18.09)

5th M63.8 Disorders of muscle in diseases classified elsewhere
M63.80 Disorders of muscle in diseases classified elsewhere, unspecified site

M63.81 Disorders of muscle in diseases classified elsewhere, shoulder
M63.811 *Disorders of muscle in diseases classified elsewhere, right shoulder*
M63.812 *Disorders of muscle in diseases classified elsewhere, left shoulder*
M63.819 *Disorders of muscle in diseases classified elsewhere, unspecified shoulder*

M63.82 Disorders of muscle in diseases classified elsewhere, upper arm
M63.821 *Disorders of muscle in diseases classified elsewhere, right upper arm*
M63.822 *Disorders of muscle in diseases classified elsewhere, left upper arm*
M63.829 *Disorders of muscle in diseases classified elsewhere, unspecified upper arm*

M63.83 Disorders of muscle in diseases classified elsewhere, forearm
M63.831 *Disorders of muscle in diseases classified elsewhere, right forearm*
M63.832 *Disorders of muscle in diseases classified elsewhere, left forearm*
M63.839 *Disorders of muscle in diseases classified elsewhere, unspecified forearm*

M63.84 Disorders of muscle in diseases classified elsewhere, hand
M63.841 *Disorders of muscle in diseases classified elsewhere, right hand*
M63.842 *Disorders of muscle in diseases classified elsewhere, left hand*
M63.849 *Disorders of muscle in diseases classified elsewhere, unspecified hand*

M63.85 Disorders of muscle in diseases classified elsewhere, thigh
M63.851 *Disorders of muscle in diseases classified elsewhere, right thigh*
M63.852 *Disorders of muscle in diseases classified elsewhere, left thigh*
M63.859 *Disorders of muscle in diseases classified elsewhere, unspecified thigh*

M63.86 Disorders of muscle in diseases classified elsewhere, lower leg
M63.861 *Disorders of muscle in diseases classified elsewhere, right lower leg*
M63.862 *Disorders of muscle in diseases classified elsewhere, left lower leg*
M63.869 *Disorders of muscle in diseases classified elsewhere, unspecified lower leg*

M63.87 Disorders of muscle in diseases classified elsewhere, ankle and foot
M63.871 *Disorders of muscle in diseases classified elsewhere, right ankle and foot*
M63.872 *Disorders of muscle in diseases classified elsewhere, left ankle and foot*
M63.879 *Disorders of muscle in diseases classified elsewhere, unspecified ankle and foot*

M63.88 *Disorders of muscle in diseases classified elsewhere, other site*
M63.89 *Disorders of muscle in diseases classified elsewhere, multiple sites*

Disorders of synovium and tendon (M65-M67)

M65 Synovitis and tenosynovitis

EXCLUDES 1 *chronic crepitant synovitis of hand and wrist (M70.0-)*
current injury - see injury of ligament or tendon by body region
soft tissue disorders related to use, overuse and pressure (M70.-)

M65.0 Abscess of tendon sheath

Use additional code (B95-B96) to identify bacterial agent.

M65.00 Abscess of tendon sheath, unspecified site

M65.01 Abscess of tendon sheath, shoulder
M65.011 Abscess of tendon sheath, right shoulder
M65.012 Abscess of tendon sheath, left shoulder
M65.019 Abscess of tendon sheath, unspecified shoulder

M65.02 Abscess of tendon sheath, upper arm
M65.021 Abscess of tendon sheath, right upper arm
M65.022 Abscess of tendon sheath, left upper arm
M65.029 Abscess of tendon sheath, unspecified upper arm

M65.03 Abscess of tendon sheath, forearm
M65.031 Abscess of tendon sheath, right forearm
M65.032 Abscess of tendon sheath, left forearm
M65.039 Abscess of tendon sheath, unspecified forearm

M65.04 Abscess of tendon sheath, hand
M65.041 Abscess of tendon sheath, right hand
M65.042 Abscess of tendon sheath, left hand
M65.049 Abscess of tendon sheath, unspecified hand

M65.05 Abscess of tendon sheath, thigh
M65.051 Abscess of tendon sheath, right thigh
M65.052 Abscess of tendon sheath, left thigh
M65.059 Abscess of tendon sheath, unspecified thigh

M65.06 Abscess of tendon sheath, lower leg
M65.061 Abscess of tendon sheath, right lower leg
M65.062 Abscess of tendon sheath, left lower leg
M65.069 Abscess of tendon sheath, unspecified lower leg

M65.07 Abscess of tendon sheath, ankle and foot
M65.071 Abscess of tendon sheath, right ankle and foot
M65.072 Abscess of tendon sheath, left ankle and foot
M65.079 Abscess of tendon sheath, unspecified ankle and foot

M65.08 Abscess of tendon sheath, other site

M65.1 Other infective (teno)synovitis

M65.10 Other infective (teno)synovitis, unspecified site

M65.11 Other infective (teno)synovitis, shoulder
M65.111 Other infective (teno)synovitis, right shoulder
M65.112 Other infective (teno)synovitis, left shoulder
M65.119 Other infective (teno)synovitis, unspecified shoulder

M65.12 Other infective (teno)synovitis, elbow
M65.121 Other infective (teno)synovitis, right elbow
M65.122 Other infective (teno)synovitis, left elbow
M65.129 Other infective (teno)synovitis, unspecified elbow

M65.13 Other infective (teno)synovitis, wrist
M65.131 Other infective (teno)synovitis, right wrist
M65.132 Other infective (teno)synovitis, left wrist
M65.139 Other infective (teno)synovitis, unspecified wrist

M65.14 Other infective (teno)synovitis, hand
M65.141 Other infective (teno)synovitis, right hand
M65.142 Other infective (teno)synovitis, left hand
M65.149 Other infective (teno)synovitis, unspecified hand

M65.15 Other infective (teno)synovitis, hip
M65.151 Other infective (teno)synovitis, right hip
M65.152 Other infective (teno)synovitis, left hip
M65.159 Other infective (teno)synovitis, unspecified hip

M65.16 Other infective (teno)synovitis, knee
M65.161 Other infective (teno)synovitis, right knee
M65.162 Other infective (teno)synovitis, left knee
M65.169 Other infective (teno)synovitis, unspecified knee

M65.17 Other infective (teno)synovitis, ankle and foot
M65.171 Other infective (teno)synovitis, right ankle and foot
M65.172 Other infective (teno)synovitis, left ankle and foot
M65.179 Other infective (teno)synovitis, unspecified ankle and foot

M65.18 Other infective (teno)synovitis, other site
M65.19 Other infective (teno)synovitis, multiple sites

M65.2 Calcific tendinitis

EXCLUDES 1 *tendinitis as classified in M75-M77*
calcified tendinitis of shoulder (M75.3)

M65.20 Calcific tendinitis, unspecified site

M65.22 Calcific tendinitis, upper arm
M65.221 Calcific tendinitis, right upper arm
M65.222 Calcific tendinitis, left upper arm
M65.229 Calcific tendinitis, unspecified upper arm
M65.23 Calcific tendinitis, forearm
M65.231 Calcific tendinitis, right forearm
M65.232 Calcific tendinitis, left forearm
M65.239 Calcific tendinitis, unspecified forearm
M65.24 Calcific tendinitis, hand
M65.241 Calcific tendinitis, right hand
M65.242 Calcific tendinitis, left hand
M65.249 Calcific tendinitis, unspecified hand
M65.25 Calcific tendinitis, thigh
M65.251 Calcific tendinitis, right thigh
M65.252 Calcific tendinitis, left thigh
M65.259 Calcific tendinitis, unspecified thigh
M65.26 Calcific tendinitis, lower leg
M65.261 Calcific tendinitis, right lower leg
M65.262 Calcific tendinitis, left lower leg
M65.269 Calcific tendinitis, unspecified lower leg
M65.27 Calcific tendinitis, ankle and foot
M65.271 Calcific tendinitis, right ankle and foot
M65.272 Calcific tendinitis, left ankle and foot
M65.279 Calcific tendinitis, unspecified ankle and foot
M65.28 Calcific tendinitis, other site
M65.29 Calcific tendinitis, multiple sites
M65.3 Trigger finger
Nodular tendinous disease
M65.30 Trigger finger, unspecified finger
M65.31 Trigger thumb
M65.311 Trigger thumb, right thumb
M65.312 Trigger thumb, left thumb
M65.319 Trigger thumb, unspecified thumb
M65.32 Trigger finger, index finger
M65.321 Trigger finger, right index finger
M65.322 Trigger finger, left index finger
M65.329 Trigger finger, unspecified index finger
M65.33 Trigger finger, middle finger
M65.331 Trigger finger, right middle finger
M65.332 Trigger finger, left middle finger
M65.339 Trigger finger, unspecified middle finger
M65.34 Trigger finger, ring finger
M65.341 Trigger finger, right ring finger
M65.342 Trigger finger, left ring finger
M65.349 Trigger finger, unspecified ring finger
M65.35 Trigger finger, little finger
M65.351 Trigger finger, right little finger
M65.352 Trigger finger, left little finger
M65.359 Trigger finger, unspecified little finger
M65.4 Radial styloid tenosynovitis [de Quervain]
M65.8 Other synovitis and tenosynovitis
M65.80 Other synovitis and tenosynovitis, unspecified site
M65.81 Other synovitis and tenosynovitis, shoulder
M65.811 Other synovitis and tenosynovitis, right shoulder
M65.812 Other synovitis and tenosynovitis, left shoulder
M65.819 Other synovitis and tenosynovitis, unspecified shoulder
M65.82 Other synovitis and tenosynovitis, upper arm
M65.821 Other synovitis and tenosynovitis, right upper arm
M65.822 Other synovitis and tenosynovitis, left upper arm
M65.829 Other synovitis and tenosynovitis, unspecified upper arm
M65.83 Other synovitis and tenosynovitis, forearm
M65.831 Other synovitis and tenosynovitis, right forearm
M65.832 Other synovitis and tenosynovitis, left forearm
M65.839 Other synovitis and tenosynovitis, unspecified forearm
M65.84 Other synovitis and tenosynovitis, hand
M65.841 Other synovitis and tenosynovitis, right hand
M65.842 Other synovitis and tenosynovitis, left hand
M65.849 Other synovitis and tenosynovitis, unspecified hand
M65.85 Other synovitis and tenosynovitis, thigh
M65.851 Other synovitis and tenosynovitis, right thigh
M65.852 Other synovitis and tenosynovitis, left thigh
M65.859 Other synovitis and tenosynovitis, unspecified thigh
M65.86 Other synovitis and tenosynovitis, lower leg
M65.861 Other synovitis and tenosynovitis, right lower leg
M65.862 Other synovitis and tenosynovitis, left lower leg
M65.869 Other synovitis and tenosynovitis, unspecified lower leg
M65.87 Other synovitis and tenosynovitis, ankle and foot
M65.871 Other synovitis and tenosynovitis, right ankle and foot
M65.872 Other synovitis and tenosynovitis, left ankle and foot
M65.879 Other synovitis and tenosynovitis, unspecified ankle and foot
M65.88 Other synovitis and tenosynovitis, other site
M65.89 Other synovitis and tenosynovitis, multiple sites
M65.9 Synovitis and tenosynovitis, unspecified

M66 Spontaneous rupture of synovium and tendon

INCLUDES rupture that occurs when a normal force is applied to tissues that are inferred to have less than normal strength

EXCLUDES 2 *rotator cuff syndrome (M75.1-)*
rupture where an abnormal force is applied to normal tissue - see injury of tendon by body region

M66.0 Rupture of popliteal cyst
M66.1 Rupture of synovium
Rupture of synovial cyst
EXCLUDES 2 *rupture of popliteal cyst (M66.0)*
M66.10 Rupture of synovium, unspecified joint
M66.11 Rupture of synovium, shoulder
M66.111 Rupture of synovium, right shoulder
M66.112 Rupture of synovium, left shoulder
M66.119 Rupture of synovium, unspecified shoulder
M66.12 Rupture of synovium, elbow
M66.121 Rupture of synovium, right elbow
M66.122 Rupture of synovium, left elbow
M66.129 Rupture of synovium, unspecified elbow
M66.13 Rupture of synovium, wrist
M66.131 Rupture of synovium, right wrist
M66.132 Rupture of synovium, left wrist
M66.139 Rupture of synovium, unspecified wrist
M66.14 Rupture of synovium, hand and fingers
M66.141 Rupture of synovium, right hand
M66.142 Rupture of synovium, left hand
M66.143 Rupture of synovium, unspecified hand
M66.144 Rupture of synovium, right finger(s)
M66.145 Rupture of synovium, left finger(s)
M66.146 Rupture of synovium, unspecified finger(s)
M66.15 Rupture of synovium, hip
M66.151 Rupture of synovium, right hip
M66.152 Rupture of synovium, left hip
M66.159 Rupture of synovium, unspecified hip
M66.17 Rupture of synovium, ankle, foot and toes
M66.171 Rupture of synovium, right ankle
M66.172 Rupture of synovium, left ankle
M66.173 Rupture of synovium, unspecified ankle
M66.174 Rupture of synovium, right foot
M66.175 Rupture of synovium, left foot
M66.176 Rupture of synovium, unspecified foot
M66.177 Rupture of synovium, right toe(s)
M66.178 Rupture of synovium, left toe(s)

M66.179 Rupture of synovium, unspecified toe(s)
M66.18 Rupture of synovium, other site
✓5th M66.2 Spontaneous rupture of extensor tendons
TIP: Refer to the Muscle/Tendon table at the beginning of this chapter.
M66.20 Spontaneous rupture of extensor tendons, unspecified site
✓6th M66.21 Spontaneous rupture of extensor tendons, shoulder
M66.211 Spontaneous rupture of extensor tendons, right shoulder
M66.212 Spontaneous rupture of extensor tendons, left shoulder
M66.219 Spontaneous rupture of extensor tendons, unspecified shoulder
✓6th M66.22 Spontaneous rupture of extensor tendons, upper arm
M66.221 Spontaneous rupture of extensor tendons, right upper arm
M66.222 Spontaneous rupture of extensor tendons, left upper arm
M66.229 Spontaneous rupture of extensor tendons, unspecified upper arm
✓6th M66.23 Spontaneous rupture of extensor tendons, forearm
M66.231 Spontaneous rupture of extensor tendons, right forearm
M66.232 Spontaneous rupture of extensor tendons, left forearm
M66.239 Spontaneous rupture of extensor tendons, unspecified forearm
✓6th M66.24 Spontaneous rupture of extensor tendons, hand
M66.241 Spontaneous rupture of extensor tendons, right hand
M66.242 Spontaneous rupture of extensor tendons, left hand
M66.249 Spontaneous rupture of extensor tendons, unspecified hand
✓6th M66.25 Spontaneous rupture of extensor tendons, thigh
M66.251 Spontaneous rupture of extensor tendons, right thigh
M66.252 Spontaneous rupture of extensor tendons, left thigh
M66.259 Spontaneous rupture of extensor tendons, unspecified thigh
✓6th M66.26 Spontaneous rupture of extensor tendons, lower leg
M66.261 Spontaneous rupture of extensor tendons, right lower leg
M66.262 Spontaneous rupture of extensor tendons, left lower leg
M66.269 Spontaneous rupture of extensor tendons, unspecified lower leg
✓6th M66.27 Spontaneous rupture of extensor tendons, ankle and foot
M66.271 Spontaneous rupture of extensor tendons, right ankle and foot
M66.272 Spontaneous rupture of extensor tendons, left ankle and foot
M66.279 Spontaneous rupture of extensor tendons, unspecified ankle and foot
M66.28 Spontaneous rupture of extensor tendons, other site
M66.29 Spontaneous rupture of extensor tendons, multiple sites
✓5th M66.3 Spontaneous rupture of flexor tendons
TIP: Refer to the Muscle/Tendon table at the beginning of this chapter.
M66.30 Spontaneous rupture of flexor tendons, unspecified site
✓6th M66.31 Spontaneous rupture of flexor tendons, shoulder
M66.311 Spontaneous rupture of flexor tendons, right shoulder
M66.312 Spontaneous rupture of flexor tendons, left shoulder
M66.319 Spontaneous rupture of flexor tendons, unspecified shoulder
✓6th M66.32 Spontaneous rupture of flexor tendons, upper arm
M66.321 Spontaneous rupture of flexor tendons, right upper arm
M66.322 Spontaneous rupture of flexor tendons, left upper arm
M66.329 Spontaneous rupture of flexor tendons, unspecified upper arm
✓6th M66.33 Spontaneous rupture of flexor tendons, forearm
M66.331 Spontaneous rupture of flexor tendons, right forearm
M66.332 Spontaneous rupture of flexor tendons, left forearm
M66.339 Spontaneous rupture of flexor tendons, unspecified forearm
✓6th M66.34 Spontaneous rupture of flexor tendons, hand
M66.341 Spontaneous rupture of flexor tendons, right hand
M66.342 Spontaneous rupture of flexor tendons, left hand
M66.349 Spontaneous rupture of flexor tendons, unspecified hand
✓6th M66.35 Spontaneous rupture of flexor tendons, thigh
M66.351 Spontaneous rupture of flexor tendons, right thigh
M66.352 Spontaneous rupture of flexor tendons, left thigh
M66.359 Spontaneous rupture of flexor tendons, unspecified thigh
✓6th M66.36 Spontaneous rupture of flexor tendons, lower leg
M66.361 Spontaneous rupture of flexor tendons, right lower leg
M66.362 Spontaneous rupture of flexor tendons, left lower leg
M66.369 Spontaneous rupture of flexor tendons, unspecified lower leg
✓6th M66.37 Spontaneous rupture of flexor tendons, ankle and foot
M66.371 Spontaneous rupture of flexor tendons, right ankle and foot
M66.372 Spontaneous rupture of flexor tendons, left ankle and foot
M66.379 Spontaneous rupture of flexor tendons, unspecified ankle and foot
M66.38 Spontaneous rupture of flexor tendons, other site
M66.39 Spontaneous rupture of flexor tendons, multiple sites
✓5th M66.8 Spontaneous rupture of other tendons
TIP: Refer to the Muscle/Tendon table at the beginning of this chapter.
M66.80 Spontaneous rupture of other tendons, unspecified site
✓6th M66.81 Spontaneous rupture of other tendons, shoulder
M66.811 Spontaneous rupture of other tendons, right shoulder
M66.812 Spontaneous rupture of other tendons, left shoulder
M66.819 Spontaneous rupture of other tendons, unspecified shoulder
✓6th M66.82 Spontaneous rupture of other tendons, upper arm
M66.821 Spontaneous rupture of other tendons, right upper arm
M66.822 Spontaneous rupture of other tendons, left upper arm
M66.829 Spontaneous rupture of other tendons, unspecified upper arm
✓6th M66.83 Spontaneous rupture of other tendons, forearm
M66.831 Spontaneous rupture of other tendons, right forearm
M66.832 Spontaneous rupture of other tendons, left forearm
M66.839 Spontaneous rupture of other tendons, unspecified forearm
✓6th M66.84 Spontaneous rupture of other tendons, hand
M66.841 Spontaneous rupture of other tendons, right hand
M66.842 Spontaneous rupture of other tendons, left hand
M66.849 Spontaneous rupture of other tendons, unspecified hand
✓6th M66.85 Spontaneous rupture of other tendons, thigh
M66.851 Spontaneous rupture of other tendons, right thigh
M66.852 Spontaneous rupture of other tendons, left thigh

M66.859 Spontaneous rupture of other tendons, unspecified thigh

✓6th M66.86 Spontaneous rupture of other tendons, lower leg

M66.861 Spontaneous rupture of other tendons, right lower leg

M66.862 Spontaneous rupture of other tendons, left lower leg

M66.869 Spontaneous rupture of other tendons, unspecified lower leg

✓6th M66.87 Spontaneous rupture of other tendons, ankle and foot

M66.871 Spontaneous rupture of other tendons, right ankle and foot

M66.872 Spontaneous rupture of other tendons, left ankle and foot

M66.879 Spontaneous rupture of other tendons, unspecified ankle and foot

M66.88 Spontaneous rupture of other tendons, other sites

M66.89 Spontaneous rupture of other tendons, multiple sites

M66.9 Spontaneous rupture of unspecified tendon

Rupture at musculotendinous junction, nontraumatic

✓4th **M67 Other disorders of synovium and tendon**

EXCLUDES 1 *palmar fascial fibromatosis [Dupuytren] (M72.Ø)*
tendinitis NOS (M77.9-)
xanthomatosis localized to tendons (E78.2)

✓5th **M67.Ø Short Achilles tendon (acquired)**

M67.ØØ Short Achilles tendon (acquired), unspecified ankle

M67.Ø1 Short Achilles tendon (acquired), right ankle

M67.Ø2 Short Achilles tendon (acquired), left ankle

✓5th **M67.2 Synovial hypertrophy, not elsewhere classified**

EXCLUDES 1 *villonodular synovitis (pigmented) (M12.2-)*

M67.2Ø Synovial hypertrophy, not elsewhere classified, unspecified site

✓6th M67.21 Synovial hypertrophy, not elsewhere classified, shoulder

M67.211 Synovial hypertrophy, not elsewhere classified, right shoulder

M67.212 Synovial hypertrophy, not elsewhere classified, left shoulder

M67.219 Synovial hypertrophy, not elsewhere classified, unspecified shoulder

✓6th M67.22 Synovial hypertrophy, not elsewhere classified, upper arm

M67.221 Synovial hypertrophy, not elsewhere classified, right upper arm

M67.222 Synovial hypertrophy, not elsewhere classified, left upper arm

M67.229 Synovial hypertrophy, not elsewhere classified, unspecified upper arm

✓6th M67.23 Synovial hypertrophy, not elsewhere classified, forearm

M67.231 Synovial hypertrophy, not elsewhere classified, right forearm

M67.232 Synovial hypertrophy, not elsewhere classified, left forearm

M67.239 Synovial hypertrophy, not elsewhere classified, unspecified forearm

✓6th M67.24 Synovial hypertrophy, not elsewhere classified, hand

M67.241 Synovial hypertrophy, not elsewhere classified, right hand

M67.242 Synovial hypertrophy, not elsewhere classified, left hand

M67.249 Synovial hypertrophy, not elsewhere classified, unspecified hand

✓6th M67.25 Synovial hypertrophy, not elsewhere classified, thigh

M67.251 Synovial hypertrophy, not elsewhere classified, right thigh

M67.252 Synovial hypertrophy, not elsewhere classified, left thigh

M67.259 Synovial hypertrophy, not elsewhere classified, unspecified thigh

✓6th M67.26 Synovial hypertrophy, not elsewhere classified, lower leg

M67.261 Synovial hypertrophy, not elsewhere classified, right lower leg

M67.262 Synovial hypertrophy, not elsewhere classified, left lower leg

M67.269 Synovial hypertrophy, not elsewhere classified, unspecified lower leg

✓6th M67.27 Synovial hypertrophy, not elsewhere classified, ankle and foot

M67.271 Synovial hypertrophy, not elsewhere classified, right ankle and foot

M67.272 Synovial hypertrophy, not elsewhere classified, left ankle and foot

M67.279 Synovial hypertrophy, not elsewhere classified, unspecified ankle and foot

M67.28 Synovial hypertrophy, not elsewhere classified, other site

M67.29 Synovial hypertrophy, not elsewhere classified, multiple sites

✓5th **M67.3 Transient synovitis**

Toxic synovitis

EXCLUDES 1 *palindromic rheumatism (M12.3-)*

M67.3Ø Transient synovitis, unspecified site

✓6th M67.31 Transient synovitis, shoulder

M67.311 Transient synovitis, right shoulder

M67.312 Transient synovitis, left shoulder

M67.319 Transient synovitis, unspecified shoulder

✓6th M67.32 Transient synovitis, elbow

M67.321 Transient synovitis, right elbow

M67.322 Transient synovitis, left elbow

M67.329 Transient synovitis, unspecified elbow

✓6th M67.33 Transient synovitis, wrist

M67.331 Transient synovitis, right wrist

M67.332 Transient synovitis, left wrist

M67.339 Transient synovitis, unspecified wrist

✓6th M67.34 Transient synovitis, hand

M67.341 Transient synovitis, right hand

M67.342 Transient synovitis, left hand

M67.349 Transient synovitis, unspecified hand

✓6th M67.35 Transient synovitis, hip

M67.351 Transient synovitis, right hip

M67.352 Transient synovitis, left hip

M67.359 Transient synovitis, unspecified hip

✓6th M67.36 Transient synovitis, knee

M67.361 Transient synovitis, right knee

M67.362 Transient synovitis, left knee

M67.369 Transient synovitis, unspecified knee

✓6th M67.37 Transient synovitis, ankle and foot

M67.371 Transient synovitis, right ankle and foot

M67.372 Transient synovitis, left ankle and foot

M67.379 Transient synovitis, unspecified ankle and foot

M67.38 Transient synovitis, other site

M67.39 Transient synovitis, multiple sites

✓5th **M67.4 Ganglion**

Ganglion of joint or tendon (sheath)

EXCLUDES 1 *ganglion in yaws (A66.6)*

EXCLUDES 2 *cyst of bursa (M71.2-M71.3)*
cyst of synovium (M71.2-M71.3)

DEF: Fluid-filled, benign cyst appearing on a tendon sheath or aponeurosis, frequently connecting to an underlying joint.

M67.4Ø Ganglion, unspecified site

✓6th M67.41 Ganglion, shoulder

M67.411 Ganglion, right shoulder

M67.412 Ganglion, left shoulder

M67.419 Ganglion, unspecified shoulder

✓6th M67.42 Ganglion, elbow

M67.421 Ganglion, right elbow

M67.422 Ganglion, left elbow

M67.429 Ganglion, unspecified elbow

✓6th **M67.43 Ganglion, wrist**

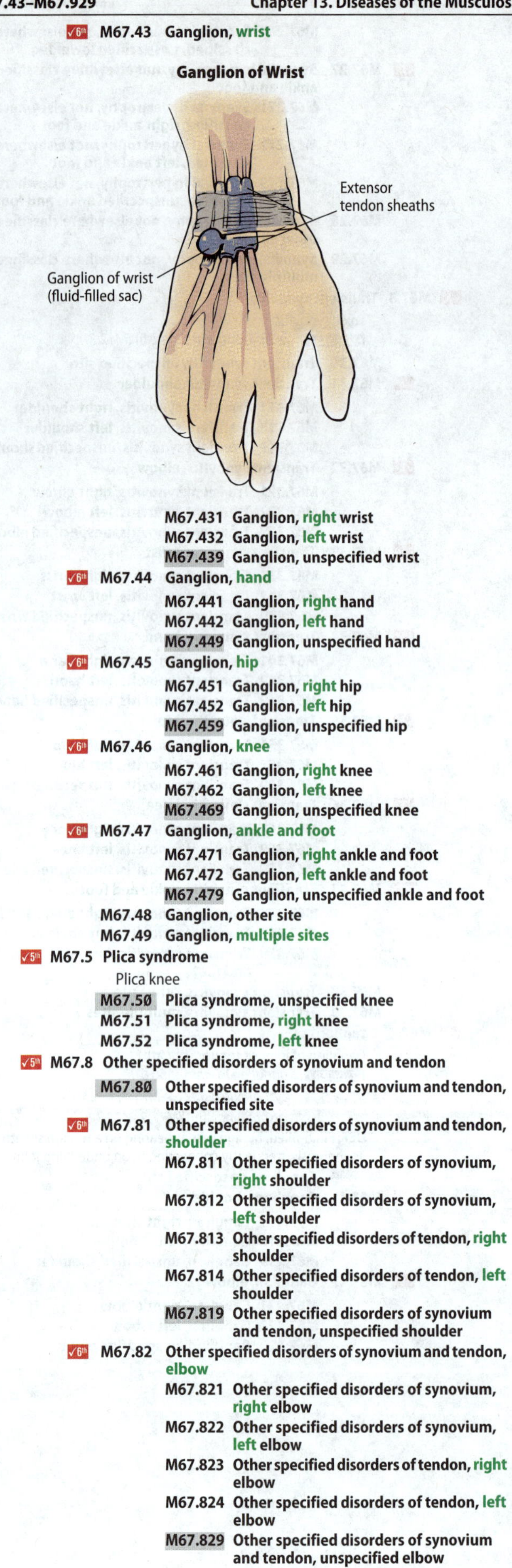

M67.431 Ganglion, right wrist
M67.432 Ganglion, left wrist
M67.439 Ganglion, unspecified wrist

✓6th **M67.44 Ganglion, hand**
M67.441 Ganglion, right hand
M67.442 Ganglion, left hand
M67.449 Ganglion, unspecified hand

✓6th **M67.45 Ganglion, hip**
M67.451 Ganglion, right hip
M67.452 Ganglion, left hip
M67.459 Ganglion, unspecified hip

✓6th **M67.46 Ganglion, knee**
M67.461 Ganglion, right knee
M67.462 Ganglion, left knee
M67.469 Ganglion, unspecified knee

✓6th **M67.47 Ganglion, ankle and foot**
M67.471 Ganglion, right ankle and foot
M67.472 Ganglion, left ankle and foot
M67.479 Ganglion, unspecified ankle and foot

M67.48 Ganglion, other site
M67.49 Ganglion, multiple sites

✓5th **M67.5 Plica syndrome**
Plica knee
M67.50 Plica syndrome, unspecified knee
M67.51 Plica syndrome, right knee
M67.52 Plica syndrome, left knee

✓5th **M67.8 Other specified disorders of synovium and tendon**
M67.80 Other specified disorders of synovium and tendon, unspecified site

✓6th **M67.81 Other specified disorders of synovium and tendon, shoulder**
M67.811 Other specified disorders of synovium, right shoulder
M67.812 Other specified disorders of synovium, left shoulder
M67.813 Other specified disorders of tendon, right shoulder
M67.814 Other specified disorders of tendon, left shoulder
M67.819 Other specified disorders of synovium and tendon, unspecified shoulder

✓6th **M67.82 Other specified disorders of synovium and tendon, elbow**
M67.821 Other specified disorders of synovium, right elbow
M67.822 Other specified disorders of synovium, left elbow
M67.823 Other specified disorders of tendon, right elbow
M67.824 Other specified disorders of tendon, left elbow
M67.829 Other specified disorders of synovium and tendon, unspecified elbow

✓6th **M67.83 Other specified disorders of synovium and tendon, wrist**
M67.831 Other specified disorders of synovium, right wrist
M67.832 Other specified disorders of synovium, left wrist
M67.833 Other specified disorders of tendon, right wrist
M67.834 Other specified disorders of tendon, left wrist
M67.839 Other specified disorders of synovium and tendon, unspecified wrist

✓6th **M67.84 Other specified disorders of synovium and tendon, hand**
M67.841 Other specified disorders of synovium, right hand
M67.842 Other specified disorders of synovium, left hand
M67.843 Other specified disorders of tendon, right hand
M67.844 Other specified disorders of tendon, left hand
M67.849 Other specified disorders of synovium and tendon, unspecified hand

✓6th **M67.85 Other specified disorders of synovium and tendon, hip**
M67.851 Other specified disorders of synovium, right hip
M67.852 Other specified disorders of synovium, left hip
M67.853 Other specified disorders of tendon, right hip
M67.854 Other specified disorders of tendon, left hip
M67.859 Other specified disorders of synovium and tendon, unspecified hip

✓6th **M67.86 Other specified disorders of synovium and tendon, knee**
M67.861 Other specified disorders of synovium, right knee
M67.862 Other specified disorders of synovium, left knee
M67.863 Other specified disorders of tendon, right knee
M67.864 Other specified disorders of tendon, left knee
M67.869 Other specified disorders of synovium and tendon, unspecified knee

✓6th **M67.87 Other specified disorders of synovium and tendon, ankle and foot**
M67.871 Other specified disorders of synovium, right ankle and foot
M67.872 Other specified disorders of synovium, left ankle and foot
M67.873 Other specified disorders of tendon, right ankle and foot
M67.874 Other specified disorders of tendon, left ankle and foot
M67.879 Other specified disorders of synovium and tendon, unspecified ankle and foot

M67.88 Other specified disorders of synovium and tendon, other site
M67.89 Other specified disorders of synovium and tendon, multiple sites

✓5th **M67.9 Unspecified disorder of synovium and tendon**
M67.90 Unspecified disorder of synovium and tendon, unspecified site

✓6th **M67.91 Unspecified disorder of synovium and tendon, shoulder**
M67.911 Unspecified disorder of synovium and tendon, right shoulder
M67.912 Unspecified disorder of synovium and tendon, left shoulder
M67.919 Unspecified disorder of synovium and tendon, unspecified shoulder

✓6th **M67.92 Unspecified disorder of synovium and tendon, upper arm**
M67.921 Unspecified disorder of synovium and tendon, right upper arm
M67.922 Unspecified disorder of synovium and tendon, left upper arm
M67.929 Unspecified disorder of synovium and tendon, unspecified upper arm

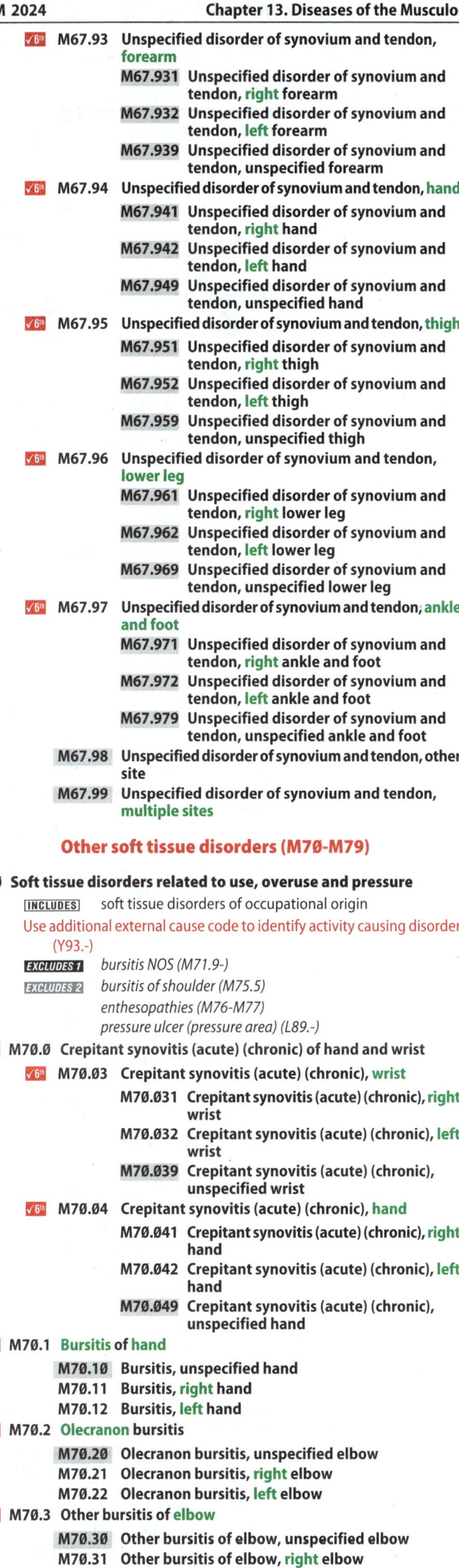

√6th **M67.93** Unspecified disorder of synovium and tendon, forearm
- **M67.931** Unspecified disorder of synovium and tendon, right forearm
- **M67.932** Unspecified disorder of synovium and tendon, left forearm
- **M67.939** Unspecified disorder of synovium and tendon, unspecified forearm

√6th **M67.94** Unspecified disorder of synovium and tendon, hand
- **M67.941** Unspecified disorder of synovium and tendon, right hand
- **M67.942** Unspecified disorder of synovium and tendon, left hand
- **M67.949** Unspecified disorder of synovium and tendon, unspecified hand

√6th **M67.95** Unspecified disorder of synovium and tendon, thigh
- **M67.951** Unspecified disorder of synovium and tendon, right thigh
- **M67.952** Unspecified disorder of synovium and tendon, left thigh
- **M67.959** Unspecified disorder of synovium and tendon, unspecified thigh

√6th **M67.96** Unspecified disorder of synovium and tendon, lower leg
- **M67.961** Unspecified disorder of synovium and tendon, right lower leg
- **M67.962** Unspecified disorder of synovium and tendon, left lower leg
- **M67.969** Unspecified disorder of synovium and tendon, unspecified lower leg

√6th **M67.97** Unspecified disorder of synovium and tendon, ankle and foot
- **M67.971** Unspecified disorder of synovium and tendon, right ankle and foot
- **M67.972** Unspecified disorder of synovium and tendon, left ankle and foot
- **M67.979** Unspecified disorder of synovium and tendon, unspecified ankle and foot

M67.98 Unspecified disorder of synovium and tendon, other site

M67.99 Unspecified disorder of synovium and tendon, multiple sites

Other soft tissue disorders (M7Ø-M79)

√4th **M7Ø Soft tissue disorders related to use, overuse and pressure**

INCLUDES soft tissue disorders of occupational origin

Use additional external cause code to identify activity causing disorder (Y93.-)

EXCLUDES 1 *bursitis NOS (M71.9-)*

EXCLUDES 2 *bursitis of shoulder (M75.5)*
enthesopathies (M76-M77)
pressure ulcer (pressure area) (L89.-)

√5th **M7Ø.Ø** Crepitant synovitis (acute) (chronic) of hand and wrist

√6th **M7Ø.Ø3** Crepitant synovitis (acute) (chronic), wrist
- **M7Ø.Ø31** Crepitant synovitis (acute) (chronic), right wrist
- **M7Ø.Ø32** Crepitant synovitis (acute) (chronic), left wrist
- **M7Ø.Ø39** Crepitant synovitis (acute) (chronic), unspecified wrist

√6th **M7Ø.Ø4** Crepitant synovitis (acute) (chronic), hand
- **M7Ø.Ø41** Crepitant synovitis (acute) (chronic), right hand
- **M7Ø.Ø42** Crepitant synovitis (acute) (chronic), left hand
- **M7Ø.Ø49** Crepitant synovitis (acute) (chronic), unspecified hand

√5th **M7Ø.1** Bursitis of hand
- **M7Ø.1Ø** Bursitis, unspecified hand
- **M7Ø.11** Bursitis, right hand
- **M7Ø.12** Bursitis, left hand

√5th **M7Ø.2** Olecranon bursitis
- **M7Ø.2Ø** Olecranon bursitis, unspecified elbow
- **M7Ø.21** Olecranon bursitis, right elbow
- **M7Ø.22** Olecranon bursitis, left elbow

√5th **M7Ø.3** Other bursitis of elbow
- **M7Ø.3Ø** Other bursitis of elbow, unspecified elbow
- **M7Ø.31** Other bursitis of elbow, right elbow
- **M7Ø.32** Other bursitis of elbow, left elbow

√5th **M7Ø.4** Prepatellar bursitis
- **M7Ø.4Ø** Prepatellar bursitis, unspecified knee
- **M7Ø.41** Prepatellar bursitis, right knee
- **M7Ø.42** Prepatellar bursitis, left knee

Knee Bursae

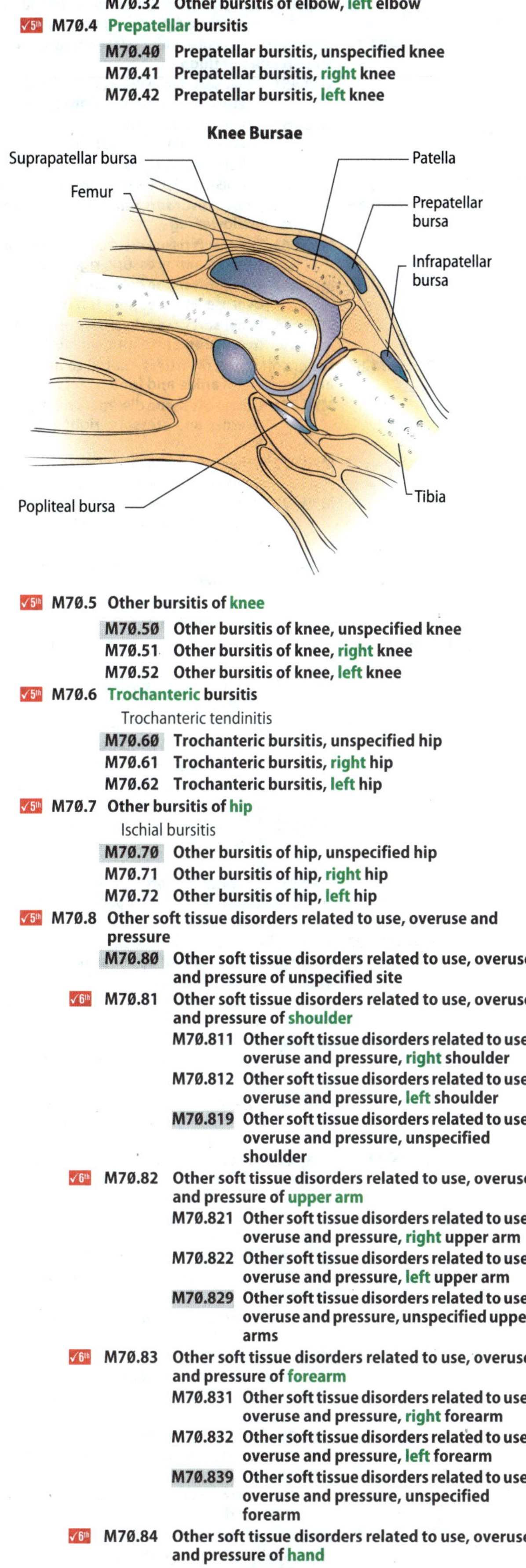

√5th **M7Ø.5** Other bursitis of knee
- **M7Ø.5Ø** Other bursitis of knee, unspecified knee
- **M7Ø.51** Other bursitis of knee, right knee
- **M7Ø.52** Other bursitis of knee, left knee

√5th **M7Ø.6** Trochanteric bursitis

Trochanteric tendinitis
- **M7Ø.6Ø** Trochanteric bursitis, unspecified hip
- **M7Ø.61** Trochanteric bursitis, right hip
- **M7Ø.62** Trochanteric bursitis, left hip

√5th **M7Ø.7** Other bursitis of hip

Ischial bursitis
- **M7Ø.7Ø** Other bursitis of hip, unspecified hip
- **M7Ø.71** Other bursitis of hip, right hip
- **M7Ø.72** Other bursitis of hip, left hip

√5th **M7Ø.8** Other soft tissue disorders related to use, overuse and pressure

M7Ø.8Ø Other soft tissue disorders related to use, overuse and pressure of unspecified site

√6th **M7Ø.81** Other soft tissue disorders related to use, overuse and pressure of shoulder
- **M7Ø.811** Other soft tissue disorders related to use, overuse and pressure, right shoulder
- **M7Ø.812** Other soft tissue disorders related to use, overuse and pressure, left shoulder
- **M7Ø.819** Other soft tissue disorders related to use, overuse and pressure, unspecified shoulder

√6th **M7Ø.82** Other soft tissue disorders related to use, overuse and pressure of upper arm
- **M7Ø.821** Other soft tissue disorders related to use, overuse and pressure, right upper arm
- **M7Ø.822** Other soft tissue disorders related to use, overuse and pressure, left upper arm
- **M7Ø.829** Other soft tissue disorders related to use, overuse and pressure, unspecified upper arms

√6th **M7Ø.83** Other soft tissue disorders related to use, overuse and pressure of forearm
- **M7Ø.831** Other soft tissue disorders related to use, overuse and pressure, right forearm
- **M7Ø.832** Other soft tissue disorders related to use, overuse and pressure, left forearm
- **M7Ø.839** Other soft tissue disorders related to use, overuse and pressure, unspecified forearm

√6th **M7Ø.84** Other soft tissue disorders related to use, overuse and pressure of hand
- **M7Ø.841** Other soft tissue disorders related to use, overuse and pressure, right hand
- **M7Ø.842** Other soft tissue disorders related to use, overuse and pressure, left hand

M70.849 Other soft tissue disorders related to use, overuse and pressure, unspecified hand

M70.85 Other soft tissue disorders related to use, overuse and pressure of thigh

- **M70.851** Other soft tissue disorders related to use, overuse and pressure, right thigh
- **M70.852** Other soft tissue disorders related to use, overuse and pressure, left thigh
- **M70.859** Other soft tissue disorders related to use, overuse and pressure, unspecified thigh

M70.86 Other soft tissue disorders related to use, overuse and pressure lower leg

- **M70.861** Other soft tissue disorders related to use, overuse and pressure, right lower leg
- **M70.862** Other soft tissue disorders related to use, overuse and pressure, left lower leg
- **M70.869** Other soft tissue disorders related to use, overuse and pressure, unspecified leg

M70.87 Other soft tissue disorders related to use, overuse and pressure of ankle and foot

- **M70.871** Other soft tissue disorders related to use, overuse and pressure, right ankle and foot
- **M70.872** Other soft tissue disorders related to use, overuse and pressure, left ankle and foot
- **M70.879** Other soft tissue disorders related to use, overuse and pressure, unspecified ankle and foot

M70.88 Other soft tissue disorders related to use, overuse and pressure other site

M70.89 Other soft tissue disorders related to use, overuse and pressure multiple sites

M70.9 Unspecified soft tissue disorder related to use, overuse and pressure

M70.90 Unspecified soft tissue disorder related to use, overuse and pressure of unspecified site

M70.91 Unspecified soft tissue disorder related to use, overuse and pressure of shoulder

- **M70.911** Unspecified soft tissue disorder related to use, overuse and pressure, right shoulder
- **M70.912** Unspecified soft tissue disorder related to use, overuse and pressure, left shoulder
- **M70.919** Unspecified soft tissue disorder related to use, overuse and pressure, unspecified shoulder

M70.92 Unspecified soft tissue disorder related to use, overuse and pressure of upper arm

- **M70.921** Unspecified soft tissue disorder related to use, overuse and pressure, right upper arm
- **M70.922** Unspecified soft tissue disorder related to use, overuse and pressure, left upper arm
- **M70.929** Unspecified soft tissue disorder related to use, overuse and pressure, unspecified upper arm

M70.93 Unspecified soft tissue disorder related to use, overuse and pressure of forearm

- **M70.931** Unspecified soft tissue disorder related to use, overuse and pressure, right forearm
- **M70.932** Unspecified soft tissue disorder related to use, overuse and pressure, left forearm
- **M70.939** Unspecified soft tissue disorder related to use, overuse and pressure, unspecified forearm

M70.94 Unspecified soft tissue disorder related to use, overuse and pressure of hand

- **M70.941** Unspecified soft tissue disorder related to use, overuse and pressure, right hand
- **M70.942** Unspecified soft tissue disorder related to use, overuse and pressure, left hand
- **M70.949** Unspecified soft tissue disorder related to use, overuse and pressure, unspecified hand

M70.95 Unspecified soft tissue disorder related to use, overuse and pressure of thigh

- **M70.951** Unspecified soft tissue disorder related to use, overuse and pressure, right thigh
- **M70.952** Unspecified soft tissue disorder related to use, overuse and pressure, left thigh
- **M70.959** Unspecified soft tissue disorder related to use, overuse and pressure, unspecified thigh

M70.96 Unspecified soft tissue disorder related to use, overuse and pressure lower leg

- **M70.961** Unspecified soft tissue disorder related to use, overuse and pressure, right lower leg
- **M70.962** Unspecified soft tissue disorder related to use, overuse and pressure, left lower leg
- **M70.969** Unspecified soft tissue disorder related to use, overuse and pressure, unspecified lower leg

M70.97 Unspecified soft tissue disorder related to use, overuse and pressure of ankle and foot

- **M70.971** Unspecified soft tissue disorder related to use, overuse and pressure, right ankle and foot
- **M70.972** Unspecified soft tissue disorder related to use, overuse and pressure, left ankle and foot
- **M70.979** Unspecified soft tissue disorder related to use, overuse and pressure, unspecified ankle and foot

M70.98 Unspecified soft tissue disorder related to use, overuse and pressure other

M70.99 Unspecified soft tissue disorder related to use, overuse and pressure multiple sites

M71 Other bursopathies

EXCLUDES 1 *bunion (M20.1)*
bursitis related to use, overuse or pressure (M70.-)
enthesopathies (M76-M77)

M71.0 Abscess of bursa

Use additional code (B95.-, B96.-) to identify causative organism

M71.00 Abscess of bursa, unspecified site

M71.01 Abscess of bursa, shoulder

- **M71.011** Abscess of bursa, right shoulder
- **M71.012** Abscess of bursa, left shoulder
- **M71.019** Abscess of bursa, unspecified shoulder

M71.02 Abscess of bursa, elbow

- **M71.021** Abscess of bursa, right elbow
- **M71.022** Abscess of bursa, left elbow
- **M71.029** Abscess of bursa, unspecified elbow

M71.03 Abscess of bursa, wrist

- **M71.031** Abscess of bursa, right wrist
- **M71.032** Abscess of bursa, left wrist
- **M71.039** Abscess of bursa, unspecified wrist

M71.04 Abscess of bursa, hand

- **M71.041** Abscess of bursa, right hand
- **M71.042** Abscess of bursa, left hand
- **M71.049** Abscess of bursa, unspecified hand

M71.05 Abscess of bursa, hip

- **M71.051** Abscess of bursa, right hip
- **M71.052** Abscess of bursa, left hip
- **M71.059** Abscess of bursa, unspecified hip

M71.06 Abscess of bursa, knee

- **M71.061** Abscess of bursa, right knee
- **M71.062** Abscess of bursa, left knee
- **M71.069** Abscess of bursa, unspecified knee

M71.07 Abscess of bursa, ankle and foot

- **M71.071** Abscess of bursa, right ankle and foot
- **M71.072** Abscess of bursa, left ankle and foot
- **M71.079** Abscess of bursa, unspecified ankle and foot

M71.08 Abscess of bursa, other site

M71.09 Abscess of bursa, multiple sites

M71.1 Other infective bursitis

Use additional code (B95.-, B96.-) to identify causative organism

M71.10 Other infective bursitis, unspecified site

M71.11 Other infective bursitis, shoulder

- **M71.111** Other infective bursitis, right shoulder
- **M71.112** Other infective bursitis, left shoulder
- **M71.119** Other infective bursitis, unspecified shoulder

M71.12 Other infective bursitis, elbow

- **M71.121** Other infective bursitis, right elbow
- **M71.122** Other infective bursitis, left elbow

M71.129 Other infective bursitis, unspecified elbow

✓6th M71.13 Other infective bursitis, wrist

M71.131 Other infective bursitis, right wrist
M71.132 Other infective bursitis, left wrist
M71.139 Other infective bursitis, unspecified wrist

✓6th M71.14 Other infective bursitis, hand

M71.141 Other infective bursitis, right hand
M71.142 Other infective bursitis, left hand
M71.149 Other infective bursitis, unspecified hand

✓6th M71.15 Other infective bursitis, hip

M71.151 Other infective bursitis, right hip
M71.152 Other infective bursitis, left hip
M71.159 Other infective bursitis, unspecified hip

✓6th M71.16 Other infective bursitis, knee

M71.161 Other infective bursitis, right knee
M71.162 Other infective bursitis, left knee
M71.169 Other infective bursitis, unspecified knee

✓6th M71.17 Other infective bursitis, ankle and foot

M71.171 Other infective bursitis, right ankle and foot
M71.172 Other infective bursitis, left ankle and foot
M71.179 Other infective bursitis, unspecified ankle and foot

M71.18 Other infective bursitis, other site
M71.19 Other infective bursitis, multiple sites

✓5th M71.2 Synovial cyst of popliteal space [Baker]

EXCLUDES 1 *synovial cyst of popliteal space with rupture (M66.0)*

DEF: Sac filled with clear synovial fluid in adults, usually secondary to disease inside the joint, located on the back of the knee in the popliteal fossa area. In children, the cyst usually represents a ganglion of one of the tendons in the knee.

Baker's Cyst

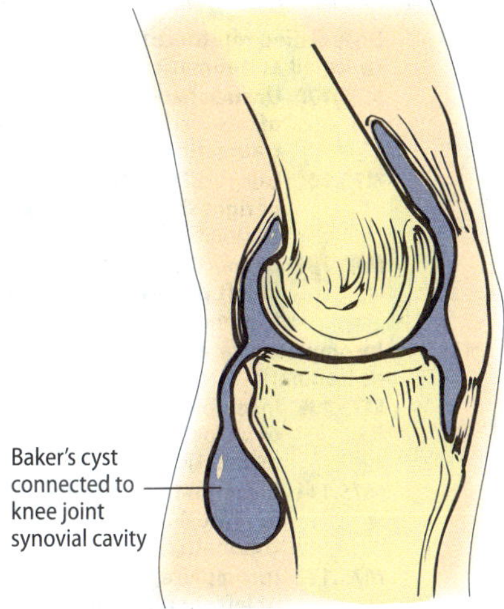

M71.20 Synovial cyst of popliteal space [Baker], unspecified knee
M71.21 Synovial cyst of popliteal space [Baker], right knee
M71.22 Synovial cyst of popliteal space [Baker], left knee

✓5th M71.3 Other bursal cyst

Synovial cyst NOS

EXCLUDES 1 *synovial cyst with rupture (M66.1-)*

M71.30 Other bursal cyst, unspecified site

✓6th M71.31 Other bursal cyst, shoulder

M71.311 Other bursal cyst, right shoulder
M71.312 Other bursal cyst, left shoulder
M71.319 Other bursal cyst, unspecified shoulder

✓6th M71.32 Other bursal cyst, elbow

M71.321 Other bursal cyst, right elbow
M71.322 Other bursal cyst, left elbow
M71.329 Other bursal cyst, unspecified elbow

✓6th M71.33 Other bursal cyst, wrist

M71.331 Other bursal cyst, right wrist
M71.332 Other bursal cyst, left wrist
M71.339 Other bursal cyst, unspecified wrist

✓6th M71.34 Other bursal cyst, hand

M71.341 Other bursal cyst, right hand
M71.342 Other bursal cyst, left hand
M71.349 Other bursal cyst, unspecified hand

✓6th M71.35 Other bursal cyst, hip

M71.351 Other bursal cyst, right hip
M71.352 Other bursal cyst, left hip
M71.359 Other bursal cyst, unspecified hip

✓6th M71.37 Other bursal cyst, ankle and foot

M71.371 Other bursal cyst, right ankle and foot
M71.372 Other bursal cyst, left ankle and foot
M71.379 Other bursal cyst, unspecified ankle and foot

M71.38 Other bursal cyst, other site
M71.39 Other bursal cyst, multiple sites

✓5th M71.4 Calcium deposit in bursa

EXCLUDES 2 *calcium deposit in bursa of shoulder (M75.3)*

M71.40 Calcium deposit in bursa, unspecified site

✓6th M71.42 Calcium deposit in bursa, elbow

M71.421 Calcium deposit in bursa, right elbow
M71.422 Calcium deposit in bursa, left elbow
M71.429 Calcium deposit in bursa, unspecified elbow

✓6th M71.43 Calcium deposit in bursa, wrist

M71.431 Calcium deposit in bursa, right wrist
M71.432 Calcium deposit in bursa, left wrist
M71.439 Calcium deposit in bursa, unspecified wrist

✓6th M71.44 Calcium deposit in bursa, hand

M71.441 Calcium deposit in bursa, right hand
M71.442 Calcium deposit in bursa, left hand
M71.449 Calcium deposit in bursa, unspecified hand

✓6th M71.45 Calcium deposit in bursa, hip

M71.451 Calcium deposit in bursa, right hip
M71.452 Calcium deposit in bursa, left hip
M71.459 Calcium deposit in bursa, unspecified hip

✓6th M71.46 Calcium deposit in bursa, knee

M71.461 Calcium deposit in bursa, right knee
M71.462 Calcium deposit in bursa, left knee
M71.469 Calcium deposit in bursa, unspecified knee

✓6th M71.47 Calcium deposit in bursa, ankle and foot

M71.471 Calcium deposit in bursa, right ankle and foot
M71.472 Calcium deposit in bursa, left ankle and foot
M71.479 Calcium deposit in bursa, unspecified ankle and foot

M71.48 Calcium deposit in bursa, other site
M71.49 Calcium deposit in bursa, multiple sites

✓5th M71.5 Other bursitis, not elsewhere classified

EXCLUDES 1 *bursitis NOS (M71.9-)*

EXCLUDES 2 *bursitis of shoulder (M75.5)*
bursitis of tibial collateral [Pellegrini-Stieda] (M76.4-)

M71.50 Other bursitis, not elsewhere classified, unspecified site

✓6th M71.52 Other bursitis, not elsewhere classified, elbow

M71.521 Other bursitis, not elsewhere classified, right elbow
M71.522 Other bursitis, not elsewhere classified, left elbow
M71.529 Other bursitis, not elsewhere classified, unspecified elbow

✓6th M71.53 Other bursitis, not elsewhere classified, wrist

M71.531 Other bursitis, not elsewhere classified, right wrist
M71.532 Other bursitis, not elsewhere classified, left wrist
M71.539 Other bursitis, not elsewhere classified, unspecified wrist

✓6th M71.54 Other bursitis, not elsewhere classified, hand

M71.541 Other bursitis, not elsewhere classified, right hand
M71.542 Other bursitis, not elsewhere classified, left hand

M71.549 Other bursitis, not elsewhere classified, unspecified hand

√6th M71.55 Other bursitis, not elsewhere classified, hip
- M71.551 Other bursitis, not elsewhere classified, right hip
- M71.552 Other bursitis, not elsewhere classified, left hip
- M71.559 Other bursitis, not elsewhere classified, unspecified hip

√6th M71.56 Other bursitis, not elsewhere classified, knee
- M71.561 Other bursitis, not elsewhere classified, right knee
- M71.562 Other bursitis, not elsewhere classified, left knee
- M71.569 Other bursitis, not elsewhere classified, unspecified knee

√6th M71.57 Other bursitis, not elsewhere classified, ankle and foot
- M71.571 Other bursitis, not elsewhere classified, right ankle and foot
- M71.572 Other bursitis, not elsewhere classified, left ankle and foot
- M71.579 Other bursitis, not elsewhere classified, unspecified ankle and foot

M71.58 Other bursitis, not elsewhere classified, other site

√5th M71.8 Other specified bursopathies

M71.80 Other specified bursopathies, unspecified site

√6th M71.81 Other specified bursopathies, shoulder
- M71.811 Other specified bursopathies, right shoulder
- M71.812 Other specified bursopathies, left shoulder
- M71.819 Other specified bursopathies, unspecified shoulder

√6th M71.82 Other specified bursopathies, elbow
- M71.821 Other specified bursopathies, right elbow
- M71.822 Other specified bursopathies, left elbow
- M71.829 Other specified bursopathies, unspecified elbow

√6th M71.83 Other specified bursopathies, wrist
- M71.831 Other specified bursopathies, right wrist
- M71.832 Other specified bursopathies, left wrist
- M71.839 Other specified bursopathies, unspecified wrist

√6th M71.84 Other specified bursopathies, hand
- M71.841 Other specified bursopathies, right hand
- M71.842 Other specified bursopathies, left hand
- M71.849 Other specified bursopathies, unspecified hand

√6th M71.85 Other specified bursopathies, hip
- M71.851 Other specified bursopathies, right hip
- M71.852 Other specified bursopathies, left hip
- M71.859 Other specified bursopathies, unspecified hip

√6th M71.86 Other specified bursopathies, knee
- M71.861 Other specified bursopathies, right knee
- M71.862 Other specified bursopathies, left knee
- M71.869 Other specified bursopathies, unspecified knee

√6th M71.87 Other specified bursopathies, ankle and foot
- M71.871 Other specified bursopathies, right ankle and foot
- M71.872 Other specified bursopathies, left ankle and foot
- M71.879 Other specified bursopathies, unspecified ankle and foot

M71.88 Other specified bursopathies, other site

M71.89 Other specified bursopathies, multiple sites

M71.9 Bursopathy, unspecified
Bursitis NOS

√4th M72 Fibroblastic disorders

EXCLUDES 2 *retroperitoneal fibromatosis (D48.3)*

M72.0 Palmar fascial fibromatosis [Dupuytren] A
DEF: Dupuytren's contracture: Flexion deformity of a finger, due to shortened, thickened fibrosing of palmar fascia. The cause is unknown, but it is associated with long-standing epilepsy.

M72.1 Knuckle pads

M72.2 Plantar fascial fibromatosis
Plantar fasciitis
DEF: Rapid-growing and multiplanar nodular swellings and pain in the foot that is not associated with contractures.

M72.4 Pseudosarcomatous fibromatosis
Nodular fasciitis

M72.6 Necrotizing fasciitis MCC HCC
Use additional code (B95.-, B96.-) to identify causative organism

M72.8 Other fibroblastic disorders
Abscess of fascia
Fasciitis NEC
Other infective fasciitis
Use additional code to (B95.-, B96.-) identify causative organism
EXCLUDES 1 *diffuse (eosinophilic) fasciitis (M35.4)*
necrotizing fasciitis (M72.6)
nodular fasciitis (M72.4)
perirenal fasciitis NOS (N13.5)
perirenal fasciitis with infection (N13.6)
plantar fasciitis (M72.2)

M72.9 Fibroblastic disorder, unspecified
Fasciitis NOS
Fibromatosis NOS

√4th M75 Shoulder lesions

EXCLUDES 2 *shoulder-hand syndrome (M89.0-)*

√5th M75.0 Adhesive capsulitis of shoulder
Frozen shoulder
Periarthritis of shoulder
AHA: 2015,2Q,23
- M75.00 Adhesive capsulitis of unspecified shoulder
- M75.01 Adhesive capsulitis of right shoulder
- M75.02 Adhesive capsulitis of left shoulder

√5th M75.1 Rotator cuff tear or rupture, not specified as traumatic
Rotator cuff syndrome
Supraspinatus syndrome
Supraspinatus tear or rupture, not specified as traumatic
EXCLUDES 1 *tear of rotator cuff, traumatic (S46.01-)*

√6th M75.10 Unspecified rotator cuff tear or rupture, not specified as traumatic
- M75.100 Unspecified rotator cuff tear or rupture of unspecified shoulder, not specified as traumatic
- M75.101 Unspecified rotator cuff tear or rupture of right shoulder, not specified as traumatic
- M75.102 Unspecified rotator cuff tear or rupture of left shoulder, not specified as traumatic

√6th M75.11 Incomplete rotator cuff tear or rupture not specified as traumatic
- M75.110 Incomplete rotator cuff tear or rupture of unspecified shoulder, not specified as traumatic
- M75.111 Incomplete rotator cuff tear or rupture of right shoulder, not specified as traumatic
- M75.112 Incomplete rotator cuff tear or rupture of left shoulder, not specified as traumatic

√6th M75.12 Complete rotator cuff tear or rupture not specified as traumatic
- M75.120 Complete rotator cuff tear or rupture of unspecified shoulder, not specified as traumatic
- M75.121 Complete rotator cuff tear or rupture of right shoulder, not specified as traumatic
- M75.122 Complete rotator cuff tear or rupture of left shoulder, not specified as traumatic

√5th M75.2 Bicipital tendinitis
- M75.20 Bicipital tendinitis, unspecified shoulder
- M75.21 Bicipital tendinitis, right shoulder
- M75.22 Bicipital tendinitis, left shoulder

√5th M75.3 Calcific tendinitis of shoulder
Calcified bursa of shoulder
- M75.30 Calcific tendinitis of unspecified shoulder
- M75.31 Calcific tendinitis of right shoulder
- M75.32 Calcific tendinitis of left shoulder

√5th M75.4 Impingement syndrome of shoulder
AHA: 2022,3Q,18
- M75.40 Impingement syndrome of unspecified shoulder

M75.41 Impingement syndrome of right shoulder
M75.42 Impingement syndrome of left shoulder
M75.5 Bursitis of shoulder
M75.50 Bursitis of unspecified shoulder
M75.51 Bursitis of right shoulder
M75.52 Bursitis of left shoulder
M75.8 Other shoulder lesions
M75.80 Other shoulder lesions, unspecified shoulder
M75.81 Other shoulder lesions, right shoulder
M75.82 Other shoulder lesions, left shoulder
M75.9 Shoulder lesion, unspecified
M75.90 Shoulder lesion, unspecified, unspecified shoulder
M75.91 Shoulder lesion, unspecified, right shoulder
M75.92 Shoulder lesion, unspecified, left shoulder

M76 Enthesopathies, lower limb, excluding foot
EXCLUDES 2 *bursitis due to use, overuse and pressure (M70.-)*
enthesopathies of ankle and foot (M77.5-)
M76.0 Gluteal tendinitis
M76.00 Gluteal tendinitis, unspecified hip
M76.01 Gluteal tendinitis, right hip
M76.02 Gluteal tendinitis, left hip
M76.1 Psoas tendinitis
M76.10 Psoas tendinitis, unspecified hip
M76.11 Psoas tendinitis, right hip
M76.12 Psoas tendinitis, left hip
M76.2 Iliac crest spur
M76.20 Iliac crest spur, unspecified hip
M76.21 Iliac crest spur, right hip
M76.22 Iliac crest spur, left hip
M76.3 Iliotibial band syndrome
M76.30 Iliotibial band syndrome, unspecified leg
M76.31 Iliotibial band syndrome, right leg
M76.32 Iliotibial band syndrome, left leg
M76.4 Tibial collateral bursitis [Pellegrini-Stieda]
M76.40 Tibial collateral bursitis [Pellegrini-Stieda], unspecified leg
M76.41 Tibial collateral bursitis [Pellegrini-Stieda], right leg
M76.42 Tibial collateral bursitis [Pellegrini-Stieda], left leg
M76.5 Patellar tendinitis
M76.50 Patellar tendinitis, unspecified knee
M76.51 Patellar tendinitis, right knee
M76.52 Patellar tendinitis, left knee
M76.6 Achilles tendinitis
Achilles bursitis
M76.60 Achilles tendinitis, unspecified leg
M76.61 Achilles tendinitis, right leg
M76.62 Achilles tendinitis, left leg
M76.7 Peroneal tendinitis
M76.70 Peroneal tendinitis, unspecified leg
M76.71 Peroneal tendinitis, right leg
M76.72 Peroneal tendinitis, left leg
M76.8 Other specified enthesopathies of lower limb, excluding foot
M76.81 Anterior tibial syndrome
M76.811 Anterior tibial syndrome, right leg
M76.812 Anterior tibial syndrome, left leg
M76.819 Anterior tibial syndrome, unspecified leg
M76.82 Posterior tibial tendinitis
M76.821 Posterior tibial tendinitis, right leg
M76.822 Posterior tibial tendinitis, left leg
M76.829 Posterior tibial tendinitis, unspecified leg
M76.89 Other specified enthesopathies of lower limb, excluding foot
M76.891 Other specified enthesopathies of right lower limb, excluding foot
M76.892 Other specified enthesopathies of left lower limb, excluding foot
M76.899 Other specified enthesopathies of unspecified lower limb, excluding foot
M76.9 Unspecified enthesopathy, lower limb, excluding foot

M77 Other enthesopathies
EXCLUDES 1 *bursitis NOS (M71.9-)*
EXCLUDES 2 *bursitis due to use, overuse and pressure (M70.-)*
osteophyte (M25.7)
spinal enthesopathy (M46.0-)
M77.0 Medial epicondylitis
M77.00 Medial epicondylitis, unspecified elbow
M77.01 Medial epicondylitis, right elbow
M77.02 Medial epicondylitis, left elbow
M77.1 Lateral epicondylitis
Tennis elbow
M77.10 Lateral epicondylitis, unspecified elbow
M77.11 Lateral epicondylitis, right elbow
M77.12 Lateral epicondylitis, left elbow
M77.2 Periarthritis of wrist
M77.20 Periarthritis, unspecified wrist
M77.21 Periarthritis, right wrist
M77.22 Periarthritis, left wrist
M77.3 Calcaneal spur
DEF: Overgrowth of calcaneus bone on the underside of the heel that causes pain on walking. Calcaneal spur is due to a chronic avulsion injury of the plantar fascia from the calcaneus.
M77.30 Calcaneal spur, unspecified foot
M77.31 Calcaneal spur, right foot
M77.32 Calcaneal spur, left foot
M77.4 Metatarsalgia
EXCLUDES 1 *Morton's metatarsalgia (G57.6)*
M77.40 Metatarsalgia, unspecified foot
M77.41 Metatarsalgia, right foot
M77.42 Metatarsalgia, left foot
M77.5 Other enthesopathy of foot and ankle
M77.50 Other enthesopathy of unspecified foot and ankle
M77.51 Other enthesopathy of right foot and ankle
M77.52 Other enthesopathy of left foot and ankle
M77.8 Other enthesopathies, not elsewhere classified
M77.9 Enthesopathy, unspecified
Bone spur NOS
Capsulitis NOS
Periarthritis NOS
Tendinitis NOS

M79 Other and unspecified soft tissue disorders, not elsewhere classified
EXCLUDES 1 *psychogenic rheumatism (F45.8)*
soft tissue pain, psychogenic (F45.41)
M79.0 Rheumatism, unspecified
EXCLUDES 1 *fibromyalgia (M79.7)*
palindromic rheumatism (M12.3-)
M79.1 Myalgia
Myofascial pain syndrome
EXCLUDES 1 *fibromyalgia (M79.7)*
myositis (M60.-)
AHA: 2018,4Q,21
M79.10 Myalgia, unspecified site
M79.11 Myalgia of mastication muscle
M79.12 Myalgia of auxiliary muscles, head and neck
M79.18 Myalgia, other site
M79.2 Neuralgia and neuritis, unspecified
EXCLUDES 1 *brachial radiculitis NOS (M54.1)*
lumbosacral radiculitis NOS (M54.1)
mononeuropathies (G56-G58)
radiculitis NOS (M54.1)
sciatica (M54.3-M54.4)
TIP: Assign for documented neuropathic pain.
M79.3 Panniculitis, unspecified
EXCLUDES 1 *lupus panniculitis (L93.2)*
neck and back panniculitis (M54.0-)
relapsing [Weber-Christian] panniculitis (M35.6)
M79.4 Hypertrophy of (infrapatellar) fat pad
M79.5 Residual foreign body in soft tissue
EXCLUDES 1 *foreign body granuloma of skin and subcutaneous tissue (L92.3)*
foreign body granuloma of soft tissue (M60.2-)
AHA: 2023,2Q,27

M79.6 Pain in limb, hand, foot, fingers and toes
EXCLUDES 2 *pain in joint (M25.5-)*

M79.6Ø Pain in limb, unspecified
- **M79.6Ø1 Pain in right arm**
  Pain in right upper limb NOS
- **M79.6Ø2 Pain in left arm**
  Pain in left upper limb NOS
- **M79.6Ø3 Pain in arm, unspecified**
  Pain in upper limb NOS
- **M79.6Ø4 Pain in right leg**
  Pain in right lower limb NOS
- **M79.6Ø5 Pain in left leg**
  Pain in left lower limb NOS
- **M79.6Ø6 Pain in leg, unspecified**
  Pain in lower limb NOS
- **M79.6Ø9 Pain in unspecified limb**
  Pain in limb NOS

M79.62 Pain in upper arm
Pain in axillary region
- **M79.621 Pain in right upper arm**
- **M79.622 Pain in left upper arm**
- **M79.629 Pain in unspecified upper arm**

M79.63 Pain in forearm
- **M79.631 Pain in right forearm**
- **M79.632 Pain in left forearm**
- **M79.639 Pain in unspecified forearm**

M79.64 Pain in hand and fingers
- **M79.641 Pain in right hand**
- **M79.642 Pain in left hand**
- **M79.643 Pain in unspecified hand**
- **M79.644 Pain in right finger(s)**
- **M79.645 Pain in left finger(s)**
- **M79.646 Pain in unspecified finger(s)**

M79.65 Pain in thigh
- **M79.651 Pain in right thigh**
- **M79.652 Pain in left thigh**
- **M79.659 Pain in unspecified thigh**

M79.66 Pain in lower leg
- **M79.661 Pain in right lower leg**
- **M79.662 Pain in left lower leg**
- **M79.669 Pain in unspecified lower leg**

M79.67 Pain in foot and toes
- **M79.671 Pain in right foot**
- **M79.672 Pain in left foot**
- **M79.673 Pain in unspecified foot**
- **M79.674 Pain in right toe(s)**
- **M79.675 Pain in left toe(s)**
- **M79.676 Pain in unspecified toe(s)**

M79.7 Fibromyalgia
Fibromyositis
Fibrositis
Myofibrositis

M79.A Nontraumatic compartment syndrome
Code first, if applicable, associated postprocedural complication
EXCLUDES 1 *compartment syndrome NOS (T79.A-)*
fibromyalgia (M79.7)
nontraumatic ischemic infarction of muscle (M62.2-)
traumatic compartment syndrome (T79.A-)

M79.A1 Nontraumatic compartment syndrome of upper extremity
Nontraumatic compartment syndrome of shoulder, arm, forearm, wrist, hand, and fingers
- **M79.A11 Nontraumatic compartment syndrome of right upper extremity** CC
- **M79.A12 Nontraumatic compartment syndrome of left upper extremity** CC
- **M79.A19 Nontraumatic compartment syndrome of unspecified upper extremity** CC UNS

M79.A2 Nontraumatic compartment syndrome of lower extremity
Nontraumatic compartment syndrome of hip, buttock, thigh, leg, foot, and toes
- **M79.A21 Nontraumatic compartment syndrome of right lower extremity** CC
- **M79.A22 Nontraumatic compartment syndrome of left lower extremity** CC
- **M79.A29 Nontraumatic compartment syndrome of unspecified lower extremity** CC UNS

- **M79.A3 Nontraumatic compartment syndrome of abdomen** CC
- **M79.A9 Nontraumatic compartment syndrome of other sites** CC

M79.8 Other specified soft tissue disorders
- **M79.81 Nontraumatic hematoma of soft tissue**
  Nontraumatic hematoma of muscle
  Nontraumatic seroma of muscle and soft tissue
- **M79.89 Other specified soft tissue disorders**
  Polyalgia

M79.9 Soft tissue disorder, unspecified

OSTEOPATHIES AND CHONDROPATHIES (M8Ø-M94)

Disorders of bone density and structure (M8Ø-M85)

M8Ø Osteoporosis with current pathological fracture
INCLUDES osteoporosis with current fragility fracture
Use additional code to identify major osseous defect, if applicable (M89.7-)
EXCLUDES 1 *collapsed vertebra NOS (M48.5)*
pathological fracture NOS (M84.4)
wedging of vertebra NOS (M48.5)
EXCLUDES 2 *personal history of (healed) osteoporosis fracture (Z87.31Ø)*
AHA: 2018,2Q,12
TIP: The site codes in this category identify the site of the fracture, not the site of the osteoporosis.

The appropriate 7th character is to be added to each code from category M8Ø:
- A initial encounter for fracture
- D subsequent encounter for fracture with routine healing
- G subsequent encounter for fracture with delayed healing
- K subsequent encounter for fracture with nonunion
- P subsequent encounter for fracture with malunion
- S sequela

M8Ø.Ø Age-related osteoporosis with current pathological fracture
Involutional osteoporosis with current pathological fracture
Osteoporosis NOS with current pathological fracture
Postmenopausal osteoporosis with current pathological fracture
Senile osteoporosis with current pathological fracture

M8Ø.ØØ Age-related osteoporosis with current pathological fracture, unspecified site CC UNS A

M8Ø.Ø1 Age-related osteoporosis with current pathological fracture, shoulder
- **M8Ø.Ø11 Age-related osteoporosis with current pathological fracture, right shoulder** CC A
- **M8Ø.Ø12 Age-related osteoporosis with current pathological fracture, left shoulder** CC A
- **M8Ø.Ø19 Age-related osteoporosis with current pathological fracture, unspecified shoulder** CC UNS A

M8Ø.Ø2 Age-related osteoporosis with current pathological fracture, humerus
- **M8Ø.Ø21 Age-related osteoporosis with current pathological fracture, right humerus** CC A
- **M8Ø.Ø22 Age-related osteoporosis with current pathological fracture, left humerus** CC A
- **M8Ø.Ø29 Age-related osteoporosis with current pathological fracture, unspecified humerus** CC UNS A

M8Ø.Ø3 Age-related osteoporosis with current pathological fracture, forearm
Age-related osteoporosis with current pathological fracture of wrist
- **M8Ø.Ø31 Age-related osteoporosis with current pathological fracture, right forearm** CC A
- **M8Ø.Ø32 Age-related osteoporosis with current pathological fracture, left forearm** CC A
- **M8Ø.Ø39 Age-related osteoporosis with current pathological fracture, unspecified forearm** CC UNS A

M80.04 Age-related osteoporosis with current pathological fracture, hand
M80.041 Age-related osteoporosis with current pathological fracture, right hand CC A
M80.042 Age-related osteoporosis with current pathological fracture, left hand CC A
M80.049 Age-related osteoporosis with current pathological fracture, unspecified hand CC UNS A
M80.05 Age-related osteoporosis with current pathological fracture, femur
Age-related osteoporosis with current pathological fracture of hip
M80.051 Age-related osteoporosis with current pathological fracture, right femur CC HCC A
M80.052 Age-related osteoporosis with current pathological fracture, left femur CC HCC A
M80.059 Age-related osteoporosis with current pathological fracture, unspecified femur CC UNS HCC A
M80.06 Age-related osteoporosis with current pathological fracture, lower leg
M80.061 Age-related osteoporosis with current pathological fracture, right lower leg CC A
M80.062 Age-related osteoporosis with current pathological fracture, left lower leg CC A
M80.069 Age-related osteoporosis with current pathological fracture, unspecified lower leg CC UNS A
M80.07 Age-related osteoporosis with current pathological fracture, ankle and foot
M80.071 Age-related osteoporosis with current pathological fracture, right ankle and foot CC A
M80.072 Age-related osteoporosis with current pathological fracture, left ankle and foot CC A
M80.079 Age-related osteoporosis with current pathological fracture, unspecified ankle and foot CC UNS A
M80.08 Age-related osteoporosis with current pathological fracture, vertebra(e) CC HCC A
M80.0A Age-related osteoporosis with current pathological fracture, other site CC A
AHA: 2020,4Q,32-33
● M80.0B Age-related osteoporosis with current pathological fracture, pelvis
● M80.0B1 Age-related osteoporosis with current pathological fracture, right pelvis CC
● M80.0B2 Age-related osteoporosis with current pathological fracture, left pelvis CC
● M80.0B9 Age-related osteoporosis with current pathological fracture, unspecified pelvis CC

M80.8 Other osteoporosis with current pathological fracture
Drug-induced osteoporosis with current pathological fracture
Idiopathic osteoporosis with current pathological fracture
Osteoporosis of disuse with current pathological fracture
Postoophorectomy osteoporosis with current pathological fracture
Postsurgical malabsorption osteoporosis with current pathological fracture
Post-traumatic osteoporosis with current pathological fracture
Use additional code for adverse effect, if applicable, to identify drug (T36-T50 with fifth or sixth character 5)
M80.80 Other osteoporosis with current pathological fracture, unspecified site CC UNS
M80.81 Other osteoporosis with pathological fracture, shoulder
M80.811 Other osteoporosis with current pathological fracture, right shoulder CC
M80.812 Other osteoporosis with current pathological fracture, left shoulder CC
M80.819 Other osteoporosis with current pathological fracture, unspecified shoulder CC UNS
M80.82 Other osteoporosis with current pathological fracture, humerus
M80.821 Other osteoporosis with current pathological fracture, right humerus CC
M80.822 Other osteoporosis with current pathological fracture, left humerus CC
M80.829 Other osteoporosis with current pathological fracture, unspecified humerus CC UNS
M80.83 Other osteoporosis with current pathological fracture, forearm
Other osteoporosis with current pathological fracture of wrist
M80.831 Other osteoporosis with current pathological fracture, right forearm CC
M80.832 Other osteoporosis with current pathological fracture, left forearm CC
M80.839 Other osteoporosis with current pathological fracture, unspecified forearm CC UNS
M80.84 Other osteoporosis with current pathological fracture, hand
M80.841 Other osteoporosis with current pathological fracture, right hand CC
M80.842 Other osteoporosis with current pathological fracture, left hand CC
M80.849 Other osteoporosis with current pathological fracture, unspecified hand CC UNS
M80.85 Other osteoporosis with current pathological fracture, femur
Other osteoporosis with current pathological fracture of hip
M80.851 Other osteoporosis with current pathological fracture, right femur CC HCC
M80.852 Other osteoporosis with current pathological fracture, left femur CC HCC
M80.859 Other osteoporosis with current pathological fracture, unspecified femur CC UNS HCC
M80.86 Other osteoporosis with current pathological fracture, lower leg
M80.861 Other osteoporosis with current pathological fracture, right lower leg CC
M80.862 Other osteoporosis with current pathological fracture, left lower leg CC
M80.869 Other osteoporosis with current pathological fracture, unspecified lower leg CC UNS
M80.87 Other osteoporosis with current pathological fracture, ankle and foot
M80.871 Other osteoporosis with current pathological fracture, right ankle and foot CC
M80.872 Other osteoporosis with current pathological fracture, left ankle and foot CC
M80.879 Other osteoporosis with current pathological fracture, unspecified ankle and foot CC UNS
M80.88 Other osteoporosis with current pathological fracture, vertebra(e) CC HCC
M80.8A Other osteoporosis with current pathological fracture, other site CC
AHA: 2020,4Q,32
● M80.8B Other osteoporosis with current pathological fracture, pelvis
● M80.8B1 Other osteoporosis with current pathological fracture, right pelvis CC
● M80.8B2 Other osteoporosis with current pathological fracture, left pelvis CC
● M80.8B9 Other osteoporosis with current pathological fracture, unspecified pelvis CC

✓4th **M81 Osteoporosis without current pathological fracture**
Use additional code to identify:
major osseous defect, if applicable (M89.7-)
personal history of (healed) osteoporosis fracture, if applicable (Z87.31Ø)
EXCLUDES 1 *osteoporosis with current pathological fracture (M8Ø.-)*
Sudeck's atrophy (M89.Ø)

M81.Ø Age-related osteoporosis without current pathological fracture A
Involutional osteoporosis without current pathological fracture
Osteoporosis NOS
Postmenopausal osteoporosis without current pathological fracture
Senile osteoporosis without current pathological fracture

M81.6 Localized osteoporosis [Lequesne]
EXCLUDES 1 *Sudeck's atrophy (M89.Ø)*

M81.8 Other osteoporosis without current pathological fracture
Drug-induced osteoporosis without current pathological fracture
Idiopathic osteoporosis without current pathological fracture
Osteoporosis of disuse without current pathological fracture
Postoophorectomy osteoporosis without current pathological fracture
Postsurgical malabsorption osteoporosis without current pathological fracture
Post-traumatic osteoporosis without current pathological fracture
Use additional code for adverse effect, if applicable, to identify drug (T36-T5Ø with fifth or sixth character 5)

✓4th **M83 Adult osteomalacia**
EXCLUDES 1 *infantile and juvenile osteomalacia (E55.Ø)*
renal osteodystrophy (N25.Ø)
rickets (active) (E55.Ø)
rickets (active) sequelae (E64.3)
vitamin D-resistant osteomalacia ▶(E83.31)◀
vitamin D-resistant rickets (active) ▶(E83.31)◀

M83.Ø Puerperal osteomalacia M ♀
M83.1 Senile osteomalacia A
M83.2 Adult osteomalacia due to malabsorption A
Postsurgical malabsorption osteomalacia in adults
M83.3 Adult osteomalacia due to malnutrition A
M83.4 Aluminum bone disease
M83.5 Other drug-induced osteomalacia in adults A
Use additional code for adverse effect, if applicable, to identify drug (T36-T5Ø with fifth or sixth character 5)
M83.8 Other adult osteomalacia A
M83.9 Adult osteomalacia, unspecified A

✓4th **M84 Disorder of continuity of bone**
EXCLUDES 2 *traumatic fracture of bone-see fracture, by site*

✓5th **M84.3 Stress fracture**
Fatigue fracture
March fracture
Stress fracture NOS
Stress reaction
Use additional external cause code(s) to identify the cause of the stress fracture
EXCLUDES 1 *pathological fracture due to osteoporosis (M8Ø.-)*
pathological fracture NOS (M84.4.-)
traumatic fracture (S12.-, S22.-, S32.-, S42.-, S52.-, S62.-, S72.-, S82.-, S92.-)
EXCLUDES 2 *personal history of (healed) stress (fatigue) fracture (Z87.312)*
stress fracture of vertebra (M48.4-)

The appropriate 7th character is to be added to each code from subcategory M84.3.
A initial encounter for fracture
D subsequent encounter for fracture with routine healing
G subsequent encounter for fracture with delayed healing
K subsequent encounter for fracture with nonunion
P subsequent encounter for fracture with malunion
S sequela

✓x7th **M84.3Ø Stress fracture, unspecified site** CC UNS
✓6th **M84.31 Stress fracture, shoulder**
✓7th **M84.311 Stress fracture, right shoulder** CC
✓7th **M84.312 Stress fracture, left shoulder** CC
✓7th **M84.319 Stress fracture, unspecified shoulder** CC UNS
✓6th **M84.32 Stress fracture, humerus**
✓7th **M84.321 Stress fracture, right humerus** CC
✓7th **M84.322 Stress fracture, left humerus** CC
✓7th **M84.329 Stress fracture, unspecified humerus** CC UNS
✓6th **M84.33 Stress fracture, ulna and radius**
✓7th **M84.331 Stress fracture, right ulna** CC
✓7th **M84.332 Stress fracture, left ulna** CC
✓7th **M84.333 Stress fracture, right radius** CC
✓7th **M84.334 Stress fracture, left radius** CC
✓7th **M84.339 Stress fracture, unspecified ulna and radius** CC UNS
✓6th **M84.34 Stress fracture, hand and fingers**
✓7th **M84.341 Stress fracture, right hand** CC
✓7th **M84.342 Stress fracture, left hand** CC
✓7th **M84.343 Stress fracture, unspecified hand** CC UNS
✓7th **M84.344 Stress fracture, right finger(s)** CC
✓7th **M84.345 Stress fracture, left finger(s)** CC
✓7th **M84.346 Stress fracture, unspecified finger(s)** CC UNS
✓6th **M84.35 Stress fracture, pelvis and femur**
Stress fracture, hip
✓7th **M84.35Ø Stress fracture, pelvis** CC
✓7th **M84.351 Stress fracture, right femur** CC
✓7th **M84.352 Stress fracture, left femur** CC
✓7th **M84.353 Stress fracture, unspecified femur** CC UNS
✓7th **M84.359 Stress fracture, hip, unspecified** CC
✓6th **M84.36 Stress fracture, tibia and fibula**
✓7th **M84.361 Stress fracture, right tibia** CC
✓7th **M84.362 Stress fracture, left tibia** CC
✓7th **M84.363 Stress fracture, right fibula** CC
✓7th **M84.364 Stress fracture, left fibula** CC
✓7th **M84.369 Stress fracture, unspecified tibia and fibula** CC UNS
✓6th **M84.37 Stress fracture, ankle, foot and toes**
✓7th **M84.371 Stress fracture, right ankle** CC
✓7th **M84.372 Stress fracture, left ankle** CC
✓7th **M84.373 Stress fracture, unspecified ankle** CC UNS
✓7th **M84.374 Stress fracture, right foot** CC
✓7th **M84.375 Stress fracture, left foot** CC
✓7th **M84.376 Stress fracture, unspecified foot** CC UNS
✓7th **M84.377 Stress fracture, right toe(s)** CC
✓7th **M84.378 Stress fracture, left toe(s)** CC
✓7th **M84.379 Stress fracture, unspecified toe(s)** CC UNS
✓x7th **M84.38 Stress fracture, other site** CC
EXCLUDES 2 *stress fracture of vertebra (M48.4-)*

M84.4 Pathological fracture, not elsewhere classified

Chronic fracture
Pathological fracture NOS

EXCLUDES 1 *collapsed vertebra NEC (M48.5)*
pathological fracture in neoplastic disease (M84.5-)
pathological fracture in osteoporosis (M80.-)
pathological fracture in other disease (M84.6-)
stress fracture (M84.3-)
traumatic fracture (S12.-, S22.-, S32.-, S42.-, S52.-, S62.-, S72.-, S82.-, S92.-)

EXCLUDES 2 *personal history of (healed) pathological fracture (Z87.311)*

The appropriate 7th character is to be added to each code from subcategory M84.4.
A initial encounter for fracture
D subsequent encounter for fracture with routine healing
G subsequent encounter for fracture with delayed healing
K subsequent encounter for fracture with nonunion
P subsequent encounter for fracture with malunion
S sequela

M84.40 Pathological fracture, unspecified site CC UNS
M84.41 Pathological fracture, shoulder
- **M84.411 Pathological fracture, right shoulder** CC
- **M84.412 Pathological fracture, left shoulder** CC
- **M84.419 Pathological fracture, unspecified shoulder** CC UNS

M84.42 Pathological fracture, humerus
- **M84.421 Pathological fracture, right humerus** CC
- **M84.422 Pathological fracture, left humerus** CC
- **M84.429 Pathological fracture, unspecified humerus** CC UNS

M84.43 Pathological fracture, ulna and radius
- **M84.431 Pathological fracture, right ulna** CC
- **M84.432 Pathological fracture, left ulna** CC
- **M84.433 Pathological fracture, right radius** CC
- **M84.434 Pathological fracture, left radius** CC
- **M84.439 Pathological fracture, unspecified ulna and radius** CC UNS

M84.44 Pathological fracture, hand and fingers
- **M84.441 Pathological fracture, right hand** CC
- **M84.442 Pathological fracture, left hand** CC
- **M84.443 Pathological fracture, unspecified hand** CC UNS
- **M84.444 Pathological fracture, right finger(s)** CC
- **M84.445 Pathological fracture, left finger(s)** CC
- **M84.446 Pathological fracture, unspecified finger(s)** CC UNS

M84.45 Pathological fracture, femur and pelvis

AHA: 2016,4Q,43
- **M84.451 Pathological fracture, right femur** CC HCC
- **M84.452 Pathological fracture, left femur** CC HCC
- **M84.453 Pathological fracture, unspecified femur** CC UNS HCC
- **M84.454 Pathological fracture, pelvis** CC
- **M84.459 Pathological fracture, hip, unspecified** CC HCC

M84.46 Pathological fracture, tibia and fibula
- **M84.461 Pathological fracture, right tibia** CC
- **M84.462 Pathological fracture, left tibia** CC
- **M84.463 Pathological fracture, right fibula** CC
- **M84.464 Pathological fracture, left fibula** CC
- **M84.469 Pathological fracture, unspecified tibia and fibula** CC UNS

M84.47 Pathological fracture, ankle, foot and toes
- **M84.471 Pathological fracture, right ankle** CC
- **M84.472 Pathological fracture, left ankle** CC
- **M84.473 Pathological fracture, unspecified ankle** CC UNS
- **M84.474 Pathological fracture, right foot** CC
- **M84.475 Pathological fracture, left foot** CC
- **M84.476 Pathological fracture, unspecified foot** CC UNS
- **M84.477 Pathological fracture, right toe(s)** CC
- **M84.478 Pathological fracture, left toe(s)** CC
- **M84.479 Pathological fracture, unspecified toe(s)** CC UNS

M84.48 Pathological fracture, other site CC

M84.5 Pathological fracture in neoplastic disease

Code also underlying neoplasm

The appropriate 7th character is to be added to each code from subcategory M84.5.
A initial encounter for fracture
D subsequent encounter for fracture with routine healing
G subsequent encounter for fracture with delayed healing
K subsequent encounter for fracture with nonunion
P subsequent encounter for fracture with malunion
S sequela

M84.50 Pathological fracture in neoplastic disease, unspecified site CC UNS
M84.51 Pathological fracture in neoplastic disease, shoulder
- **M84.511 Pathological fracture in neoplastic disease, right shoulder** CC
- **M84.512 Pathological fracture in neoplastic disease, left shoulder** CC
- **M84.519 Pathological fracture in neoplastic disease, unspecified shoulder** CC UNS

M84.52 Pathological fracture in neoplastic disease, humerus
- **M84.521 Pathological fracture in neoplastic disease, right humerus** CC
- **M84.522 Pathological fracture in neoplastic disease, left humerus** CC
- **M84.529 Pathological fracture in neoplastic disease, unspecified humerus** CC UNS

M84.53 Pathological fracture in neoplastic disease, ulna and radius
- **M84.531 Pathological fracture in neoplastic disease, right ulna** CC
- **M84.532 Pathological fracture in neoplastic disease, left ulna** CC
- **M84.533 Pathological fracture in neoplastic disease, right radius** CC
- **M84.534 Pathological fracture in neoplastic disease, left radius** CC
- **M84.539 Pathological fracture in neoplastic disease, unspecified ulna and radius** CC UNS

M84.54 Pathological fracture in neoplastic disease, hand
- **M84.541 Pathological fracture in neoplastic disease, right hand** CC
- **M84.542 Pathological fracture in neoplastic disease, left hand** CC
- **M84.549 Pathological fracture in neoplastic disease, unspecified hand** CC UNS

M84.55 Pathological fracture in neoplastic disease, pelvis and femur
- **M84.550 Pathological fracture in neoplastic disease, pelvis** CC
- **M84.551 Pathological fracture in neoplastic disease, right femur** CC HCC
- **M84.552 Pathological fracture in neoplastic disease, left femur** CC HCC
- **M84.553 Pathological fracture in neoplastic disease, unspecified femur** CC UNS HCC
- **M84.559 Pathological fracture in neoplastic disease, hip, unspecified** CC UNS HCC

M84.56 Pathological fracture in neoplastic disease, tibia and fibula
- **M84.561 Pathological fracture in neoplastic disease, right tibia** CC
- **M84.562 Pathological fracture in neoplastic disease, left tibia** CC
- **M84.563 Pathological fracture in neoplastic disease, right fibula** CC
- **M84.564 Pathological fracture in neoplastic disease, left fibula** CC

√7th **M84.569 Pathological fracture in neoplastic disease, unspecified tibia and fibula** CC UNS

√6th **M84.57 Pathological fracture in neoplastic disease, ankle and foot**

√7th **M84.571 Pathological fracture in neoplastic disease, right ankle** CC

√7th **M84.572 Pathological fracture in neoplastic disease, left ankle** CC

√7th **M84.573 Pathological fracture in neoplastic disease, unspecified ankle** CC UNS

√7th **M84.574 Pathological fracture in neoplastic disease, right foot** CC

√7th **M84.575 Pathological fracture in neoplastic disease, left foot** CC

√7th **M84.576 Pathological fracture in neoplastic disease, unspecified foot** CC UNS

√x7th **M84.58 Pathological fracture in neoplastic disease, other specified site** CC

Pathological fracture in neoplastic disease, vertebrae

√5th **M84.6 Pathological fracture in other disease**

Code also underlying condition

EXCLUDES 1 *pathological fracture in osteoporosis (M8Ø.-)*

The appropriate 7th character is to be added to each code from subcategory M84.6.
A initial encounter for fracture
D subsequent encounter for fracture with routine healing
G subsequent encounter for fracture with delayed healing
K subsequent encounter for fracture with nonunion
P subsequent encounter for fracture with malunion
S sequela

√x7th **M84.6Ø Pathological fracture in other disease, unspecified site** CC UNS

√6th **M84.61 Pathological fracture in other disease, shoulder**

√7th **M84.611 Pathological fracture in other disease, right shoulder** CC

√7th **M84.612 Pathological fracture in other disease, left shoulder** CC

√7th **M84.619 Pathological fracture in other disease, unspecified shoulder** CC UNS

√6th **M84.62 Pathological fracture in other disease, humerus**

√7th **M84.621 Pathological fracture in other disease, right humerus** CC

√7th **M84.622 Pathological fracture in other disease, left humerus** CC

√7th **M84.629 Pathological fracture in other disease, unspecified humerus** CC UNS

√6th **M84.63 Pathological fracture in other disease, ulna and radius**

√7th **M84.631 Pathological fracture in other disease, right ulna** CC

√7th **M84.632 Pathological fracture in other disease, left ulna** CC

√7th **M84.633 Pathological fracture in other disease, right radius** CC

√7th **M84.634 Pathological fracture in other disease, left radius** CC

√7th **M84.639 Pathological fracture in other disease, unspecified ulna and radius** CC UNS

√6th **M84.64 Pathological fracture in other disease, hand**

√7th **M84.641 Pathological fracture in other disease, right hand** CC

√7th **M84.642 Pathological fracture in other disease, left hand** CC

√7th **M84.649 Pathological fracture in other disease, unspecified hand** CC UNS

√6th **M84.65 Pathological fracture in other disease, pelvis and femur**

√7th **M84.65Ø Pathological fracture in other disease, pelvis** CC

√7th **M84.651 Pathological fracture in other disease, right femur** CC HCC

√7th **M84.652 Pathological fracture in other disease, left femur** CC HCC

√7th **M84.653 Pathological fracture in other disease, unspecified femur** CC UNS HCC

√7th **M84.659 Pathological fracture in other disease, hip, unspecified** CC HCC

√6th **M84.66 Pathological fracture in other disease, tibia and fibula**

√7th **M84.661 Pathological fracture in other disease, right tibia** CC

√7th **M84.662 Pathological fracture in other disease, left tibia** CC

√7th **M84.663 Pathological fracture in other disease, right fibula** CC

√7th **M84.664 Pathological fracture in other disease, left fibula** CC

√7th **M84.669 Pathological fracture in other disease, unspecified tibia and fibula** CC UNS

√6th **M84.67 Pathological fracture in other disease, ankle and foot**

√7th **M84.671 Pathological fracture in other disease, right ankle** CC

√7th **M84.672 Pathological fracture in other disease, left ankle** CC

√7th **M84.673 Pathological fracture in other disease, unspecified ankle** CC UNS

√7th **M84.674 Pathological fracture in other disease, right foot** CC

√7th **M84.675 Pathological fracture in other disease, left foot** CC

√7th **M84.676 Pathological fracture in other disease, unspecified foot** CC UNS

√x7th **M84.68 Pathological fracture in other disease, other site** CC

√5th **M84.7 Nontraumatic fracture, not elsewhere classified**

√6th **M84.75 Atypical femoral fracture**

AHA: 2016,4Q,41-42

The appropriate 7th character is to be added to each code from M84.75.
A initial encounter for fracture
D subsequent encounter for fracture with routine healing
G subsequent encounter for fracture with delayed healing
K subsequent encounter for fracture with nonunion
P subsequent encounter for fracture with malunion
S sequela

√7th **M84.75Ø Atypical femoral fracture, unspecified** CC

√7th **M84.751 Incomplete atypical femoral fracture, right leg** CC

√7th **M84.752 Incomplete atypical femoral fracture, left leg** CC

√7th **M84.753 Incomplete atypical femoral fracture, unspecified leg** CC UNS

√7th **M84.754 Complete transverse atypical femoral fracture, right leg** CC HCC

√7th **M84.755 Complete transverse atypical femoral fracture, left leg** CC HCC

√7th **M84.756 Complete transverse atypical femoral fracture, unspecified leg** CC UNS HCC

√7th **M84.757 Complete oblique atypical femoral fracture, right leg** CC HCC

√7th **M84.758 Complete oblique atypical femoral fracture, left leg** CC HCC

√7th **M84.759 Complete oblique atypical femoral fracture, unspecified leg** CC UNS HCC

√5th **M84.8 Other disorders of continuity of bone**

M84.8Ø Other disorders of continuity of bone, unspecified site

√6th **M84.81 Other disorders of continuity of bone, shoulder**

M84.811 Other disorders of continuity of bone, right shoulder

M84.812 Other disorders of continuity of bone, left shoulder

M84.819 Other disorders of continuity of bone, unspecified shoulder

√6th **M84.82 Other disorders of continuity of bone, humerus**

M84.821 Other disorders of continuity of bone, right humerus

M84.822 Other disorders of continuity of bone, left humerus

M84.829 Other disorders of continuity of bone, unspecified humerus

M84.83 Other disorders of continuity of bone, ulna and radius
M84.831 Other disorders of continuity of bone, right ulna
M84.832 Other disorders of continuity of bone, left ulna
M84.833 Other disorders of continuity of bone, right radius
M84.834 Other disorders of continuity of bone, left radius
M84.839 Other disorders of continuity of bone, unspecified ulna and radius

M84.84 Other disorders of continuity of bone, hand
M84.841 Other disorders of continuity of bone, right hand
M84.842 Other disorders of continuity of bone, left hand
M84.849 Other disorders of continuity of bone, unspecified hand

M84.85 Other disorders of continuity of bone, pelvic region and thigh
M84.851 Other disorders of continuity of bone, right pelvic region and thigh
M84.852 Other disorders of continuity of bone, left pelvic region and thigh
M84.859 Other disorders of continuity of bone, unspecified pelvic region and thigh

M84.86 Other disorders of continuity of bone, tibia and fibula
M84.861 Other disorders of continuity of bone, right tibia
M84.862 Other disorders of continuity of bone, left tibia
M84.863 Other disorders of continuity of bone, right fibula
M84.864 Other disorders of continuity of bone, left fibula
M84.869 Other disorders of continuity of bone, unspecified tibia and fibula

M84.87 Other disorders of continuity of bone, ankle and foot
M84.871 Other disorders of continuity of bone, right ankle and foot
M84.872 Other disorders of continuity of bone, left ankle and foot
M84.879 Other disorders of continuity of bone, unspecified ankle and foot

M84.88 Other disorders of continuity of bone, other site

M84.9 Disorder of continuity of bone, unspecified

M85 Other disorders of bone density and structure

EXCLUDES 1 *osteogenesis imperfecta (Q78.0)*
osteopetrosis (Q78.2)
osteopoikilosis (Q78.8)
polyostotic fibrous dysplasia (Q78.1)

M85.0 Fibrous dysplasia (monostotic)
EXCLUDES 2 *fibrous dysplasia of jaw (M27.8)*

M85.00 Fibrous dysplasia (monostotic), unspecified site

M85.01 Fibrous dysplasia (monostotic), shoulder
M85.011 Fibrous dysplasia (monostotic), right shoulder
M85.012 Fibrous dysplasia (monostotic), left shoulder
M85.019 Fibrous dysplasia (monostotic), unspecified shoulder

M85.02 Fibrous dysplasia (monostotic), upper arm
M85.021 Fibrous dysplasia (monostotic), right upper arm
M85.022 Fibrous dysplasia (monostotic), left upper arm
M85.029 Fibrous dysplasia (monostotic), unspecified upper arm

M85.03 Fibrous dysplasia (monostotic), forearm
M85.031 Fibrous dysplasia (monostotic), right forearm
M85.032 Fibrous dysplasia (monostotic), left forearm
M85.039 Fibrous dysplasia (monostotic), unspecified forearm

M85.04 Fibrous dysplasia (monostotic), hand
M85.041 Fibrous dysplasia (monostotic), right hand
M85.042 Fibrous dysplasia (monostotic), left hand
M85.049 Fibrous dysplasia (monostotic), unspecified hand

M85.05 Fibrous dysplasia (monostotic), thigh
M85.051 Fibrous dysplasia (monostotic), right thigh
M85.052 Fibrous dysplasia (monostotic), left thigh
M85.059 Fibrous dysplasia (monostotic), unspecified thigh

M85.06 Fibrous dysplasia (monostotic), lower leg
M85.061 Fibrous dysplasia (monostotic), right lower leg
M85.062 Fibrous dysplasia (monostotic), left lower leg
M85.069 Fibrous dysplasia (monostotic), unspecified lower leg

M85.07 Fibrous dysplasia (monostotic), ankle and foot
M85.071 Fibrous dysplasia (monostotic), right ankle and foot
M85.072 Fibrous dysplasia (monostotic), left ankle and foot
M85.079 Fibrous dysplasia (monostotic), unspecified ankle and foot

M85.08 Fibrous dysplasia (monostotic), other site
M85.09 Fibrous dysplasia (monostotic), multiple sites

M85.1 Skeletal fluorosis

M85.10 Skeletal fluorosis, unspecified site

M85.11 Skeletal fluorosis, shoulder
M85.111 Skeletal fluorosis, right shoulder
M85.112 Skeletal fluorosis, left shoulder
M85.119 Skeletal fluorosis, unspecified shoulder

M85.12 Skeletal fluorosis, upper arm
M85.121 Skeletal fluorosis, right upper arm
M85.122 Skeletal fluorosis, left upper arm
M85.129 Skeletal fluorosis, unspecified upper arm

M85.13 Skeletal fluorosis, forearm
M85.131 Skeletal fluorosis, right forearm
M85.132 Skeletal fluorosis, left forearm
M85.139 Skeletal fluorosis, unspecified forearm

M85.14 Skeletal fluorosis, hand
M85.141 Skeletal fluorosis, right hand
M85.142 Skeletal fluorosis, left hand
M85.149 Skeletal fluorosis, unspecified hand

M85.15 Skeletal fluorosis, thigh
M85.151 Skeletal fluorosis, right thigh
M85.152 Skeletal fluorosis, left thigh
M85.159 Skeletal fluorosis, unspecified thigh

M85.16 Skeletal fluorosis, lower leg
M85.161 Skeletal fluorosis, right lower leg
M85.162 Skeletal fluorosis, left lower leg
M85.169 Skeletal fluorosis, unspecified lower leg

M85.17 Skeletal fluorosis, ankle and foot
M85.171 Skeletal fluorosis, right ankle and foot
M85.172 Skeletal fluorosis, left ankle and foot
M85.179 Skeletal fluorosis, unspecified ankle and foot

M85.18 Skeletal fluorosis, other site
M85.19 Skeletal fluorosis, multiple sites

M85.2 Hyperostosis of skull
DEF: Abnormal bone growth on the inner aspect of the cranial bones.

M85.3 Osteitis condensans

M85.30 Osteitis condensans, unspecified site

M85.31 Osteitis condensans, shoulder
M85.311 Osteitis condensans, right shoulder
M85.312 Osteitis condensans, left shoulder
M85.319 Osteitis condensans, unspecified shoulder

M85.32 Osteitis condensans, upper arm
M85.321 Osteitis condensans, right upper arm
M85.322 Osteitis condensans, left upper arm
M85.329 Osteitis condensans, unspecified upper arm

6th M85.33 Osteitis condensans, forearm
M85.331 Osteitis condensans, right forearm
M85.332 Osteitis condensans, left forearm
M85.339 Osteitis condensans, unspecified forearm
6th M85.34 Osteitis condensans, hand
M85.341 Osteitis condensans, right hand
M85.342 Osteitis condensans, left hand
M85.349 Osteitis condensans, unspecified hand
6th M85.35 Osteitis condensans, thigh
M85.351 Osteitis condensans, right thigh
M85.352 Osteitis condensans, left thigh
M85.359 Osteitis condensans, unspecified thigh
6th M85.36 Osteitis condensans, lower leg
M85.361 Osteitis condensans, right lower leg
M85.362 Osteitis condensans, left lower leg
M85.369 Osteitis condensans, unspecified lower leg
6th M85.37 Osteitis condensans, ankle and foot
M85.371 Osteitis condensans, right ankle and foot
M85.372 Osteitis condensans, left ankle and foot
M85.379 Osteitis condensans, unspecified ankle and foot
M85.38 Osteitis condensans, other site
M85.39 Osteitis condensans, multiple sites
5th M85.4 Solitary bone cyst
EXCLUDES 2 *solitary cyst of jaw (M27.4)*
M85.40 Solitary bone cyst, unspecified site
6th M85.41 Solitary bone cyst, shoulder
M85.411 Solitary bone cyst, right shoulder
M85.412 Solitary bone cyst, left shoulder
M85.419 Solitary bone cyst, unspecified shoulder
6th M85.42 Solitary bone cyst, humerus
M85.421 Solitary bone cyst, right humerus
M85.422 Solitary bone cyst, left humerus
M85.429 Solitary bone cyst, unspecified humerus
6th M85.43 Solitary bone cyst, ulna and radius
M85.431 Solitary bone cyst, right ulna and radius
M85.432 Solitary bone cyst, left ulna and radius
M85.439 Solitary bone cyst, unspecified ulna and radius
6th M85.44 Solitary bone cyst, hand
M85.441 Solitary bone cyst, right hand
M85.442 Solitary bone cyst, left hand
M85.449 Solitary bone cyst, unspecified hand
6th M85.45 Solitary bone cyst, pelvis
M85.451 Solitary bone cyst, right pelvis
M85.452 Solitary bone cyst, left pelvis
M85.459 Solitary bone cyst, unspecified pelvis
6th M85.46 Solitary bone cyst, tibia and fibula
M85.461 Solitary bone cyst, right tibia and fibula
M85.462 Solitary bone cyst, left tibia and fibula
M85.469 Solitary bone cyst, unspecified tibia and fibula
6th M85.47 Solitary bone cyst, ankle and foot
M85.471 Solitary bone cyst, right ankle and foot
M85.472 Solitary bone cyst, left ankle and foot
M85.479 Solitary bone cyst, unspecified ankle and foot
M85.48 Solitary bone cyst, other site
5th M85.5 Aneurysmal bone cyst
EXCLUDES 2 *aneurysmal cyst of jaw (M27.4)*
DEF: Solitary bone lesion that bulges into the periosteum and is marked by a calcified rim.
M85.50 Aneurysmal bone cyst, unspecified site
6th M85.51 Aneurysmal bone cyst, shoulder
M85.511 Aneurysmal bone cyst, right shoulder
M85.512 Aneurysmal bone cyst, left shoulder
M85.519 Aneurysmal bone cyst, unspecified shoulder
6th M85.52 Aneurysmal bone cyst, upper arm
M85.521 Aneurysmal bone cyst, right upper arm
M85.522 Aneurysmal bone cyst, left upper arm
M85.529 Aneurysmal bone cyst, unspecified upper arm
6th M85.53 Aneurysmal bone cyst, forearm
M85.531 Aneurysmal bone cyst, right forearm
M85.532 Aneurysmal bone cyst, left forearm
M85.539 Aneurysmal bone cyst, unspecified forearm
6th M85.54 Aneurysmal bone cyst, hand
M85.541 Aneurysmal bone cyst, right hand
M85.542 Aneurysmal bone cyst, left hand
M85.549 Aneurysmal bone cyst, unspecified hand
6th M85.55 Aneurysmal bone cyst, thigh
M85.551 Aneurysmal bone cyst, right thigh
M85.552 Aneurysmal bone cyst, left thigh
M85.559 Aneurysmal bone cyst, unspecified thigh
6th M85.56 Aneurysmal bone cyst, lower leg
M85.561 Aneurysmal bone cyst, right lower leg
M85.562 Aneurysmal bone cyst, left lower leg
M85.569 Aneurysmal bone cyst, unspecified lower leg
6th M85.57 Aneurysmal bone cyst, ankle and foot
M85.571 Aneurysmal bone cyst, right ankle and foot
M85.572 Aneurysmal bone cyst, left ankle and foot
M85.579 Aneurysmal bone cyst, unspecified ankle and foot
M85.58 Aneurysmal bone cyst, other site
M85.59 Aneurysmal bone cyst, multiple sites
5th M85.6 Other cyst of bone
EXCLUDES 1 *cyst of jaw NEC (M27.4)*
osteitis fibrosa cystica generalisata [von Recklinghausen's disease of bone] (E21.0)
M85.60 Other cyst of bone, unspecified site
6th M85.61 Other cyst of bone, shoulder
M85.611 Other cyst of bone, right shoulder
M85.612 Other cyst of bone, left shoulder
M85.619 Other cyst of bone, unspecified shoulder
6th M85.62 Other cyst of bone, upper arm
M85.621 Other cyst of bone, right upper arm
M85.622 Other cyst of bone, left upper arm
M85.629 Other cyst of bone, unspecified upper arm
6th M85.63 Other cyst of bone, forearm
M85.631 Other cyst of bone, right forearm
M85.632 Other cyst of bone, left forearm
M85.639 Other cyst of bone, unspecified forearm
6th M85.64 Other cyst of bone, hand
M85.641 Other cyst of bone, right hand
M85.642 Other cyst of bone, left hand
M85.649 Other cyst of bone, unspecified hand
6th M85.65 Other cyst of bone, thigh
M85.651 Other cyst of bone, right thigh
M85.652 Other cyst of bone, left thigh
M85.659 Other cyst of bone, unspecified thigh
6th M85.66 Other cyst of bone, lower leg
M85.661 Other cyst of bone, right lower leg
M85.662 Other cyst of bone, left lower leg
M85.669 Other cyst of bone, unspecified lower leg
6th M85.67 Other cyst of bone, ankle and foot
M85.671 Other cyst of bone, right ankle and foot
M85.672 Other cyst of bone, left ankle and foot
M85.679 Other cyst of bone, unspecified ankle and foot
M85.68 Other cyst of bone, other site
M85.69 Other cyst of bone, multiple sites
5th M85.8 Other specified disorders of bone density and structure
Hyperostosis of bones, except skull
Osteosclerosis, acquired
EXCLUDES 1 *diffuse idiopathic skeletal hyperostosis [DISH] (M48.1)*
osteosclerosis congenita (Q77.4)
osteosclerosis fragilitas (generalista) (Q78.2)
osteosclerosis myelofibrosis (D75.81)
M85.80 Other specified disorders of bone density and structure, unspecified site
6th M85.81 Other specified disorders of bone density and structure, shoulder
M85.811 Other specified disorders of bone density and structure, right shoulder
M85.812 Other specified disorders of bone density and structure, left shoulder
M85.819 Other specified disorders of bone density and structure, unspecified shoulder

√6th M85.82 Other specified disorders of bone density and structure, upper arm
M85.821 Other specified disorders of bone density and structure, right upper arm
M85.822 Other specified disorders of bone density and structure, left upper arm
M85.829 Other specified disorders of bone density and structure, unspecified upper arm

√6th M85.83 Other specified disorders of bone density and structure, forearm
M85.831 Other specified disorders of bone density and structure, right forearm
M85.832 Other specified disorders of bone density and structure, left forearm
M85.839 Other specified disorders of bone density and structure, unspecified forearm

√6th M85.84 Other specified disorders of bone density and structure, hand
M85.841 Other specified disorders of bone density and structure, right hand
M85.842 Other specified disorders of bone density and structure, left hand
M85.849 Other specified disorders of bone density and structure, unspecified hand

√6th M85.85 Other specified disorders of bone density and structure, thigh
M85.851 Other specified disorders of bone density and structure, right thigh
M85.852 Other specified disorders of bone density and structure, left thigh
M85.859 Other specified disorders of bone density and structure, unspecified thigh

√6th M85.86 Other specified disorders of bone density and structure, lower leg
M85.861 Other specified disorders of bone density and structure, right lower leg
M85.862 Other specified disorders of bone density and structure, left lower leg
M85.869 Other specified disorders of bone density and structure, unspecified lower leg

√6th M85.87 Other specified disorders of bone density and structure, ankle and foot
M85.871 Other specified disorders of bone density and structure, right ankle and foot
M85.872 Other specified disorders of bone density and structure, left ankle and foot
M85.879 Other specified disorders of bone density and structure, unspecified ankle and foot

M85.88 Other specified disorders of bone density and structure, other site

M85.89 Other specified disorders of bone density and structure, multiple sites

M85.9 Disorder of bone density and structure, unspecified
AHA: 2021,3Q,11

Other osteopathies (M86-M9Ø)

EXCLUDES 1 *postprocedural osteopathies (M96.-)*

√4th **M86 Osteomyelitis**

Use additional code (B95-B97) to identify infectious agent
Use additional code to identify major osseous defect, if applicable (M89.7-)

EXCLUDES 1 *osteomyelitis due to:*
echinococcus (B67.2)
gonococcus (A54.43)
salmonella (AØ2.24)

EXCLUDES 2 *ostemyelitis of:*
orbit (HØ5.Ø-)
petrous bone (H7Ø.2-)
vertebra (M46.2-)

√5th M86.Ø Acute hematogenous osteomyelitis
M86.ØØ Acute hematogenous osteomyelitis, unspecified site CC UNS HCC

√6th M86.Ø1 Acute hematogenous osteomyelitis, shoulder
M86.Ø11 Acute hematogenous osteomyelitis, right shoulder CC HCC
M86.Ø12 Acute hematogenous osteomyelitis, left shoulder CC HCC
M86.Ø19 Acute hematogenous osteomyelitis, unspecified shoulder CC UNS HCC

√6th M86.Ø2 Acute hematogenous osteomyelitis, humerus
M86.Ø21 Acute hematogenous osteomyelitis, right humerus CC HCC
M86.Ø22 Acute hematogenous osteomyelitis, left humerus CC HCC
M86.Ø29 Acute hematogenous osteomyelitis, unspecified humerus CC UNS HCC

√6th M86.Ø3 Acute hematogenous osteomyelitis, radius and ulna
M86.Ø31 Acute hematogenous osteomyelitis, right radius and ulna CC HCC
M86.Ø32 Acute hematogenous osteomyelitis, left radius and ulna CC HCC
M86.Ø39 Acute hematogenous osteomyelitis, unspecified radius and ulna CC UNS HCC

√6th M86.Ø4 Acute hematogenous osteomyelitis, hand
M86.Ø41 Acute hematogenous osteomyelitis, right hand CC HCC
M86.Ø42 Acute hematogenous osteomyelitis, left hand CC HCC
M86.Ø49 Acute hematogenous osteomyelitis, unspecified hand CC UNS HCC

√6th M86.Ø5 Acute hematogenous osteomyelitis, femur
M86.Ø51 Acute hematogenous osteomyelitis, right femur CC HCC
M86.Ø52 Acute hematogenous osteomyelitis, left femur CC HCC
M86.Ø59 Acute hematogenous osteomyelitis, unspecified femur CC UNS HCC

√6th M86.Ø6 Acute hematogenous osteomyelitis, tibia and fibula
M86.Ø61 Acute hematogenous osteomyelitis, right tibia and fibula CC HCC
M86.Ø62 Acute hematogenous osteomyelitis, left tibia and fibula CC HCC
M86.Ø69 Acute hematogenous osteomyelitis, unspecified tibia and fibula CC UNS HCC

√6th M86.Ø7 Acute hematogenous osteomyelitis, ankle and foot
M86.Ø71 Acute hematogenous osteomyelitis, right ankle and foot CC HCC
M86.Ø72 Acute hematogenous osteomyelitis, left ankle and foot CC HCC
M86.Ø79 Acute hematogenous osteomyelitis, unspecified ankle and foot CC UNS HCC

M86.Ø8 Acute hematogenous osteomyelitis, other sites CC HCC

M86.Ø9 Acute hematogenous osteomyelitis, multiple sites CC HCC

√5th M86.1 Other acute osteomyelitis
M86.1Ø Other acute osteomyelitis, unspecified site CC UNS HCC

√6th M86.11 Other acute osteomyelitis, shoulder
M86.111 Other acute osteomyelitis, right shoulder CC HCC
M86.112 Other acute osteomyelitis, left shoulder CC HCC
M86.119 Other acute osteomyelitis, unspecified shoulder CC UNS HCC

√6th M86.12 Other acute osteomyelitis, humerus
M86.121 Other acute osteomyelitis, right humerus CC HCC
M86.122 Other acute osteomyelitis, left humerus CC HCC
M86.129 Other acute osteomyelitis, unspecified humerus CC UNS HCC

√6th M86.13 Other acute osteomyelitis, radius and ulna
M86.131 Other acute osteomyelitis, right radius and ulna CC HCC
M86.132 Other acute osteomyelitis, left radius and ulna CC HCC
M86.139 Other acute osteomyelitis, unspecified radius and ulna CC UNS HCC

√6th M86.14 Other acute osteomyelitis, hand
M86.141 Other acute osteomyelitis, right hand CC HCC
M86.142 Other acute osteomyelitis, left hand CC HCC

M86.149 Other acute osteomyelitis, unspecified hand CC UNS HCC

✓6th M86.15 Other acute osteomyelitis, femur

M86.151 Other acute osteomyelitis, right femur CC HCC

M86.152 Other acute osteomyelitis, left femur CC HCC

M86.159 Other acute osteomyelitis, unspecified femur CC UNS HCC

✓6th M86.16 Other acute osteomyelitis, tibia and fibula

M86.161 Other acute osteomyelitis, right tibia and fibula CC HCC

M86.162 Other acute osteomyelitis, left tibia and fibula CC HCC

M86.169 Other acute osteomyelitis, unspecified tibia and fibula CC UNS HCC

✓6th M86.17 Other acute osteomyelitis, ankle and foot

AHA: 2020,1Q,12

M86.171 Other acute osteomyelitis, right ankle and foot CC HCC

M86.172 Other acute osteomyelitis, left ankle and foot CC HCC

M86.179 Other acute osteomyelitis, unspecified ankle and foot CC UNS HCC

M86.18 Other acute osteomyelitis, other site CC HCC

M86.19 Other acute osteomyelitis, multiple sites CC HCC

✓5th M86.2 Subacute osteomyelitis

M86.2Ø Subacute osteomyelitis, unspecified site CC UNS HCC

✓6th M86.21 Subacute osteomyelitis, shoulder

M86.211 Subacute osteomyelitis, right shoulder CC HCC

M86.212 Subacute osteomyelitis, left shoulder CC HCC

M86.219 Subacute osteomyelitis, unspecified shoulder CC UNS HCC

✓6th M86.22 Subacute osteomyelitis, humerus

M86.221 Subacute osteomyelitis, right humerus CC HCC

M86.222 Subacute osteomyelitis, left humerus CC HCC

M86.229 Subacute osteomyelitis, unspecified humerus CC UNS HCC

✓6th M86.23 Subacute osteomyelitis, radius and ulna

M86.231 Subacute osteomyelitis, right radius and ulna CC HCC

M86.232 Subacute osteomyelitis, left radius and ulna CC HCC

M86.239 Subacute osteomyelitis, unspecified radius and ulna CC UNS HCC

✓6th M86.24 Subacute osteomyelitis, hand

M86.241 Subacute osteomyelitis, right hand CC HCC

M86.242 Subacute osteomyelitis, left hand CC HCC

M86.249 Subacute osteomyelitis, unspecified hand CC UNS HCC

✓6th M86.25 Subacute osteomyelitis, femur

M86.251 Subacute osteomyelitis, right femur CC HCC

M86.252 Subacute osteomyelitis, left femur CC HCC

M86.259 Subacute osteomyelitis, unspecified femur CC UNS HCC

✓6th M86.26 Subacute osteomyelitis, tibia and fibula

M86.261 Subacute osteomyelitis, right tibia and fibula CC HCC

M86.262 Subacute osteomyelitis, left tibia and fibula CC HCC

M86.269 Subacute osteomyelitis, unspecified tibia and fibula CC UNS HCC

✓6th M86.27 Subacute osteomyelitis, ankle and foot

M86.271 Subacute osteomyelitis, right ankle and foot CC HCC

M86.272 Subacute osteomyelitis, left ankle and foot CC HCC

M86.279 Subacute osteomyelitis, unspecified ankle and foot CC UNS HCC

M86.28 Subacute osteomyelitis, other site CC HCC

M86.29 Subacute osteomyelitis, multiple sites CC HCC

✓5th M86.3 Chronic multifocal osteomyelitis

M86.3Ø Chronic multifocal osteomyelitis, unspecified site CC UNS HCC

✓6th M86.31 Chronic multifocal osteomyelitis, shoulder

M86.311 Chronic multifocal osteomyelitis, right shoulder CC HCC

M86.312 Chronic multifocal osteomyelitis, left shoulder CC HCC

M86.319 Chronic multifocal osteomyelitis, unspecified shoulder CC UNS HCC

✓6th M86.32 Chronic multifocal osteomyelitis, humerus

M86.321 Chronic multifocal osteomyelitis, right humerus CC HCC

M86.322 Chronic multifocal osteomyelitis, left humerus CC HCC

M86.329 Chronic multifocal osteomyelitis, unspecified humerus CC UNS HCC

✓6th M86.33 Chronic multifocal osteomyelitis, radius and ulna

M86.331 Chronic multifocal osteomyelitis, right radius and ulna CC HCC

M86.332 Chronic multifocal osteomyelitis, left radius and ulna CC HCC

M86.339 Chronic multifocal osteomyelitis, unspecified radius and ulna CC UNS HCC

✓6th M86.34 Chronic multifocal osteomyelitis, hand

M86.341 Chronic multifocal osteomyelitis, right hand CC HCC

M86.342 Chronic multifocal osteomyelitis, left hand CC HCC

M86.349 Chronic multifocal osteomyelitis, unspecified hand CC UNS HCC

✓6th M86.35 Chronic multifocal osteomyelitis, femur

M86.351 Chronic multifocal osteomyelitis, right femur CC HCC

M86.352 Chronic multifocal osteomyelitis, left femur CC HCC

M86.359 Chronic multifocal osteomyelitis, unspecified femur CC UNS HCC

✓6th M86.36 Chronic multifocal osteomyelitis, tibia and fibula

M86.361 Chronic multifocal osteomyelitis, right tibia and fibula CC HCC

M86.362 Chronic multifocal osteomyelitis, left tibia and fibula CC HCC

M86.369 Chronic multifocal osteomyelitis, unspecified tibia and fibula CC UNS HCC

✓6th M86.37 Chronic multifocal osteomyelitis, ankle and foot

M86.371 Chronic multifocal osteomyelitis, right ankle and foot CC HCC

M86.372 Chronic multifocal osteomyelitis, left ankle and foot CC HCC

M86.379 Chronic multifocal osteomyelitis, unspecified ankle and foot CC UNS HCC

M86.38 Chronic multifocal osteomyelitis, other site CC HCC

M86.39 Chronic multifocal osteomyelitis, multiple sites CC HCC

✓5th M86.4 Chronic osteomyelitis with draining sinus

M86.4Ø Chronic osteomyelitis with draining sinus, unspecified site CC UNS HCC

✓6th M86.41 Chronic osteomyelitis with draining sinus, shoulder

M86.411 Chronic osteomyelitis with draining sinus, right shoulder CC HCC

M86.412 Chronic osteomyelitis with draining sinus, left shoulder CC HCC

M86.419 Chronic osteomyelitis with draining sinus, unspecified shoulder CC UNS HCC

✓6th M86.42 Chronic osteomyelitis with draining sinus, humerus

M86.421 Chronic osteomyelitis with draining sinus, right humerus CC HCC

M86.422 Chronic osteomyelitis with draining sinus, left humerus CC HCC

M86.429 Chronic osteomyelitis with draining sinus, unspecified humerus CC UNS HCC

M86.43 Chronic osteomyelitis with draining sinus, radius and ulna
M86.431 Chronic osteomyelitis with draining sinus, right radius and ulna CC HCC
M86.432 Chronic osteomyelitis with draining sinus, left radius and ulna CC HCC
M86.439 Chronic osteomyelitis with draining sinus, unspecified radius and ulna CC UNS HCC
M86.44 Chronic osteomyelitis with draining sinus, hand
M86.441 Chronic osteomyelitis with draining sinus, right hand CC HCC
M86.442 Chronic osteomyelitis with draining sinus, left hand CC HCC
M86.449 Chronic osteomyelitis with draining sinus, unspecified hand CC UNS HCC
M86.45 Chronic osteomyelitis with draining sinus, femur
M86.451 Chronic osteomyelitis with draining sinus, right femur CC HCC
M86.452 Chronic osteomyelitis with draining sinus, left femur CC HCC
M86.459 Chronic osteomyelitis with draining sinus, unspecified femur CC UNS HCC
M86.46 Chronic osteomyelitis with draining sinus, tibia and fibula
M86.461 Chronic osteomyelitis with draining sinus, right tibia and fibula CC HCC
M86.462 Chronic osteomyelitis with draining sinus, left tibia and fibula CC HCC
M86.469 Chronic osteomyelitis with draining sinus, unspecified tibia and fibula CC UNS HCC
M86.47 Chronic osteomyelitis with draining sinus, ankle and foot
M86.471 Chronic osteomyelitis with draining sinus, right ankle and foot CC HCC
M86.472 Chronic osteomyelitis with draining sinus, left ankle and foot CC HCC
M86.479 Chronic osteomyelitis with draining sinus, unspecified ankle and foot CC UNS HCC
M86.48 Chronic osteomyelitis with draining sinus, other site CC HCC
M86.49 Chronic osteomyelitis with draining sinus, multiple sites CC HCC
M86.5 Other chronic hematogenous osteomyelitis
M86.50 Other chronic hematogenous osteomyelitis, unspecified site CC UNS HCC
M86.51 Other chronic hematogenous osteomyelitis, shoulder
M86.511 Other chronic hematogenous osteomyelitis, right shoulder CC HCC
M86.512 Other chronic hematogenous osteomyelitis, left shoulder CC HCC
M86.519 Other chronic hematogenous osteomyelitis, unspecified shoulder CC UNS HCC
M86.52 Other chronic hematogenous osteomyelitis, humerus
M86.521 Other chronic hematogenous osteomyelitis, right humerus CC HCC
M86.522 Other chronic hematogenous osteomyelitis, left humerus CC HCC
M86.529 Other chronic hematogenous osteomyelitis, unspecified humerus CC UNS HCC
M86.53 Other chronic hematogenous osteomyelitis, radius and ulna
M86.531 Other chronic hematogenous osteomyelitis, right radius and ulna CC HCC
M86.532 Other chronic hematogenous osteomyelitis, left radius and ulna CC HCC
M86.539 Other chronic hematogenous osteomyelitis, unspecified radius and ulna CC UNS HCC
M86.54 Other chronic hematogenous osteomyelitis, hand
M86.541 Other chronic hematogenous osteomyelitis, right hand CC HCC
M86.542 Other chronic hematogenous osteomyelitis, left hand CC HCC
M86.549 Other chronic hematogenous osteomyelitis, unspecified hand CC UNS HCC
M86.55 Other chronic hematogenous osteomyelitis, femur
M86.551 Other chronic hematogenous osteomyelitis, right femur CC HCC
M86.552 Other chronic hematogenous osteomyelitis, left femur CC HCC
M86.559 Other chronic hematogenous osteomyelitis, unspecified femur CC UNS HCC
M86.56 Other chronic hematogenous osteomyelitis, tibia and fibula
M86.561 Other chronic hematogenous osteomyelitis, right tibia and fibula CC HCC
M86.562 Other chronic hematogenous osteomyelitis, left tibia and fibula CC HCC
M86.569 Other chronic hematogenous osteomyelitis, unspecified tibia and fibula CC UNS HCC
M86.57 Other chronic hematogenous osteomyelitis, ankle and foot
M86.571 Other chronic hematogenous osteomyelitis, right ankle and foot CC HCC
M86.572 Other chronic hematogenous osteomyelitis, left ankle and foot CC HCC
M86.579 Other chronic hematogenous osteomyelitis, unspecified ankle and foot CC UNS HCC
M86.58 Other chronic hematogenous osteomyelitis, other site CC HCC
M86.59 Other chronic hematogenous osteomyelitis, multiple sites CC HCC
M86.6 Other chronic osteomyelitis
M86.60 Other chronic osteomyelitis, unspecified site CC UNS HCC
M86.61 Other chronic osteomyelitis, shoulder
M86.611 Other chronic osteomyelitis, right shoulder CC HCC
M86.612 Other chronic osteomyelitis, left shoulder CC HCC
M86.619 Other chronic osteomyelitis, unspecified shoulder CC UNS HCC
M86.62 Other chronic osteomyelitis, humerus
M86.621 Other chronic osteomyelitis, right humerus CC HCC
M86.622 Other chronic osteomyelitis, left humerus CC HCC
M86.629 Other chronic osteomyelitis, unspecified humerus CC UNS HCC
M86.63 Other chronic osteomyelitis, radius and ulna
M86.631 Other chronic osteomyelitis, right radius and ulna CC HCC
M86.632 Other chronic osteomyelitis, left radius and ulna CC HCC
M86.639 Other chronic osteomyelitis, unspecified radius and ulna CC UNS HCC
M86.64 Other chronic osteomyelitis, hand
M86.641 Other chronic osteomyelitis, right hand CC HCC
M86.642 Other chronic osteomyelitis, left hand CC HCC
M86.649 Other chronic osteomyelitis, unspecified hand CC UNS HCC
M86.65 Other chronic osteomyelitis, thigh
M86.651 Other chronic osteomyelitis, right thigh CC HCC
M86.652 Other chronic osteomyelitis, left thigh CC HCC
M86.659 Other chronic osteomyelitis, unspecified thigh CC UNS HCC
M86.66 Other chronic osteomyelitis, tibia and fibula
M86.661 Other chronic osteomyelitis, right tibia and fibula CC HCC

M86.662 Other chronic osteomyelitis, left tibia and fibula CC HCC

M86.669 Other chronic osteomyelitis, unspecified tibia and fibula CC UNS HCC

✓6th M86.67 Other chronic osteomyelitis, ankle and foot

M86.671 Other chronic osteomyelitis, right ankle and foot CC HCC

AHA: 2016,1Q,13

M86.672 Other chronic osteomyelitis, left ankle and foot CC HCC

M86.679 Other chronic osteomyelitis, unspecified ankle and foot CC UNS HCC

M86.68 Other chronic osteomyelitis, other site CC HCC

M86.69 Other chronic osteomyelitis, multiple sites CC HCC

✓5th M86.8 Other osteomyelitis

Brodie's abscess

AHA: 2022,1Q,31

✓6th M86.8X Other osteomyelitis

M86.8X0 Other osteomyelitis, multiple sites CC HCC

M86.8X1 Other osteomyelitis, shoulder CC HCC

M86.8X2 Other osteomyelitis, upper arm CC HCC

M86.8X3 Other osteomyelitis, forearm CC HCC

M86.8X4 Other osteomyelitis, hand CC HCC

M86.8X5 Other osteomyelitis, thigh CC HCC

M86.8X6 Other osteomyelitis, lower leg CC HCC

M86.8X7 Other osteomyelitis, ankle and foot CC HCC

M86.8X8 Other osteomyelitis, other site CC HCC

M86.8X9 Other osteomyelitis, unspecified sites CC UNS HCC

M86.9 Osteomyelitis, unspecified CC HCC

Infection of bone NOS

Periostitis without osteomyelitis

✓4th M87 Osteonecrosis

INCLUDES avascular necrosis of bone

Use additional code to identify major osseous defect, if applicable (M89.7-)

EXCLUDES 1 *juvenile osteonecrosis (M91-M92)*

osteochondropathies (M90-M93)

✓5th M87.0 Idiopathic aseptic necrosis of bone

M87.00 Idiopathic aseptic necrosis of unspecified bone CC UNS HCC

✓6th M87.01 Idiopathic aseptic necrosis of shoulder

Idiopathic aseptic necrosis of clavicle and scapula

M87.011 Idiopathic aseptic necrosis of right shoulder CC HCC

M87.012 Idiopathic aseptic necrosis of left shoulder CC HCC

M87.019 Idiopathic aseptic necrosis of unspecified shoulder CC UNS HCC

✓6th M87.02 Idiopathic aseptic necrosis of humerus

M87.021 Idiopathic aseptic necrosis of right humerus CC HCC

M87.022 Idiopathic aseptic necrosis of left humerus CC HCC

M87.029 Idiopathic aseptic necrosis of unspecified humerus CC UNS HCC

✓6th M87.03 Idiopathic aseptic necrosis of radius, ulna and carpus

M87.031 Idiopathic aseptic necrosis of right radius CC HCC

M87.032 Idiopathic aseptic necrosis of left radius CC HCC

M87.033 Idiopathic aseptic necrosis of unspecified radius CC UNS HCC

M87.034 Idiopathic aseptic necrosis of right ulna CC HCC

M87.035 Idiopathic aseptic necrosis of left ulna CC HCC

M87.036 Idiopathic aseptic necrosis of unspecified ulna CC UNS HCC

M87.037 Idiopathic aseptic necrosis of right carpus CC HCC

M87.038 Idiopathic aseptic necrosis of left carpus CC HCC

M87.039 Idiopathic aseptic necrosis of unspecified carpus CC UNS HCC

✓6th M87.04 Idiopathic aseptic necrosis of hand and fingers

Idiopathic aseptic necrosis of metacarpals and phalanges of hands

M87.041 Idiopathic aseptic necrosis of right hand CC HCC

M87.042 Idiopathic aseptic necrosis of left hand CC HCC

M87.043 Idiopathic aseptic necrosis of unspecified hand CC UNS HCC

M87.044 Idiopathic aseptic necrosis of right finger(s) CC HCC

M87.045 Idiopathic aseptic necrosis of left finger(s) CC HCC

M87.046 Idiopathic aseptic necrosis of unspecified finger(s) CC UNS HCC

✓6th M87.05 Idiopathic aseptic necrosis of pelvis and femur

M87.050 Idiopathic aseptic necrosis of pelvis CC HCC

M87.051 Idiopathic aseptic necrosis of right femur CC HCC

M87.052 Idiopathic aseptic necrosis of left femur CC HCC

M87.059 Idiopathic aseptic necrosis of unspecified femur CC UNS HCC

✓6th M87.06 Idiopathic aseptic necrosis of tibia and fibula

M87.061 Idiopathic aseptic necrosis of right tibia CC HCC

M87.062 Idiopathic aseptic necrosis of left tibia CC HCC

M87.063 Idiopathic aseptic necrosis of unspecified tibia CC UNS HCC

M87.064 Idiopathic aseptic necrosis of right fibula CC HCC

M87.065 Idiopathic aseptic necrosis of left fibula CC HCC

M87.066 Idiopathic aseptic necrosis of unspecified fibula CC UNS HCC

✓6th M87.07 Idiopathic aseptic necrosis of ankle, foot and toes

Idiopathic aseptic necrosis of metatarsus, tarsus, and phalanges of toes

M87.071 Idiopathic aseptic necrosis of right ankle CC HCC

M87.072 Idiopathic aseptic necrosis of left ankle CC HCC

M87.073 Idiopathic aseptic necrosis of unspecified ankle CC UNS HCC

M87.074 Idiopathic aseptic necrosis of right foot CC HCC

M87.075 Idiopathic aseptic necrosis of left foot CC HCC

M87.076 Idiopathic aseptic necrosis of unspecified foot CC UNS HCC

M87.077 Idiopathic aseptic necrosis of right toe(s) CC HCC

M87.078 Idiopathic aseptic necrosis of left toe(s) CC HCC

M87.079 Idiopathic aseptic necrosis of unspecified toe(s) CC UNS HCC

M87.08 Idiopathic aseptic necrosis of bone, other site CC HCC

M87.09 Idiopathic aseptic necrosis of bone, multiple sites CC HCC

✓5th M87.1 Osteonecrosis due to drugs

Use additional code for adverse effect, if applicable, to identify drug (T36-T50 with fifth or sixth character 5)

M87.10 Osteonecrosis due to drugs, unspecified bone CC UNS HCC

✓6th M87.11 Osteonecrosis due to drugs, shoulder

M87.111 Osteonecrosis due to drugs, right shoulder CC HCC

M87.112 Osteonecrosis due to drugs, left shoulder CC HCC

M87.119 Osteonecrosis due to drugs, unspecified shoulder CC UNS HCC

✓6th M87.12 Osteonecrosis due to drugs, humerus

M87.121 Osteonecrosis due to drugs, right humerus CC HCC

M87.122 Osteonecrosis due to drugs, left humerus CC HCC
M87.129 Osteonecrosis due to drugs, unspecified humerus CC UNS HCC
✓6th M87.13 Osteonecrosis due to drugs of radius, ulna and carpus
M87.131 Osteonecrosis due to drugs of right radius CC HCC
M87.132 Osteonecrosis due to drugs of left radius CC HCC
M87.133 Osteonecrosis due to drugs of unspecified radius CC UNS HCC
M87.134 Osteonecrosis due to drugs of right ulna CC HCC
M87.135 Osteonecrosis due to drugs of left ulna CC HCC
M87.136 Osteonecrosis due to drugs of unspecified ulna CC UNS HCC
M87.137 Osteonecrosis due to drugs of right carpus CC HCC
M87.138 Osteonecrosis due to drugs of left carpus CC HCC
M87.139 Osteonecrosis due to drugs of unspecified carpus CC UNS HCC
✓6th M87.14 Osteonecrosis due to drugs, hand and fingers
M87.141 Osteonecrosis due to drugs, right hand CC HCC
M87.142 Osteonecrosis due to drugs, left hand CC HCC
M87.143 Osteonecrosis due to drugs, unspecified hand CC UNS HCC
M87.144 Osteonecrosis due to drugs, right finger(s) CC HCC
M87.145 Osteonecrosis due to drugs, left finger(s) CC HCC
M87.146 Osteonecrosis due to drugs, unspecified finger(s) CC UNS HCC
✓6th M87.15 Osteonecrosis due to drugs, pelvis and femur
M87.150 Osteonecrosis due to drugs, pelvis CC HCC
M87.151 Osteonecrosis due to drugs, right femur CC HCC
M87.152 Osteonecrosis due to drugs, left femur CC HCC
M87.159 Osteonecrosis due to drugs, unspecified femur CC UNS HCC
✓6th M87.16 Osteonecrosis due to drugs, tibia and fibula
M87.161 Osteonecrosis due to drugs, right tibia CC HCC
M87.162 Osteonecrosis due to drugs, left tibia CC HCC
M87.163 Osteonecrosis due to drugs, unspecified tibia CC UNS HCC
M87.164 Osteonecrosis due to drugs, right fibula CC HCC
M87.165 Osteonecrosis due to drugs, left fibula CC HCC
M87.166 Osteonecrosis due to drugs, unspecified fibula CC UNS HCC
✓6th M87.17 Osteonecrosis due to drugs, ankle, foot and toes
M87.171 Osteonecrosis due to drugs, right ankle CC HCC
M87.172 Osteonecrosis due to drugs, left ankle CC HCC
M87.173 Osteonecrosis due to drugs, unspecified ankle CC UNS HCC
M87.174 Osteonecrosis due to drugs, right foot CC HCC
M87.175 Osteonecrosis due to drugs, left foot CC HCC
M87.176 Osteonecrosis due to drugs, unspecified foot CC UNS HCC
M87.177 Osteonecrosis due to drugs, right toe(s) CC HCC
M87.178 Osteonecrosis due to drugs, left toe(s) CC HCC
M87.179 Osteonecrosis due to drugs, unspecified toe(s) CC UNS HCC
✓6th M87.18 Osteonecrosis due to drugs, other site
M87.180 Osteonecrosis due to drugs, jaw CC HCC
M87.188 Osteonecrosis due to drugs, other site CC HCC
M87.19 Osteonecrosis due to drugs, multiple sites CC HCC
✓5th M87.2 Osteonecrosis due to previous trauma
M87.20 Osteonecrosis due to previous trauma, unspecified bone CC UNS HCC
✓6th M87.21 Osteonecrosis due to previous trauma, shoulder
M87.211 Osteonecrosis due to previous trauma, right shoulder CC HCC
M87.212 Osteonecrosis due to previous trauma, left shoulder CC HCC
M87.219 Osteonecrosis due to previous trauma, unspecified shoulder CC UNS HCC
✓6th M87.22 Osteonecrosis due to previous trauma, humerus
M87.221 Osteonecrosis due to previous trauma, right humerus CC HCC
M87.222 Osteonecrosis due to previous trauma, left humerus CC HCC
M87.229 Osteonecrosis due to previous trauma, unspecified humerus CC UNS HCC
✓6th M87.23 Osteonecrosis due to previous trauma of radius, ulna and carpus
M87.231 Osteonecrosis due to previous trauma of right radius CC HCC
M87.232 Osteonecrosis due to previous trauma of left radius CC HCC
M87.233 Osteonecrosis due to previous trauma of unspecified radius CC UNS HCC
M87.234 Osteonecrosis due to previous trauma of right ulna CC HCC
M87.235 Osteonecrosis due to previous trauma of left ulna CC HCC
M87.236 Osteonecrosis due to previous trauma of unspecified ulna CC UNS HCC
M87.237 Osteonecrosis due to previous trauma of right carpus CC HCC
M87.238 Osteonecrosis due to previous trauma of left carpus CC HCC
M87.239 Osteonecrosis due to previous trauma of unspecified carpus CC UNS HCC
✓6th M87.24 Osteonecrosis due to previous trauma, hand and fingers
M87.241 Osteonecrosis due to previous trauma, right hand CC HCC
M87.242 Osteonecrosis due to previous trauma, left hand CC HCC
M87.243 Osteonecrosis due to previous trauma, unspecified hand CC UNS HCC
M87.244 Osteonecrosis due to previous trauma, right finger(s) CC HCC
M87.245 Osteonecrosis due to previous trauma, left finger(s) CC HCC
M87.246 Osteonecrosis due to previous trauma, unspecified finger(s) CC UNS HCC
✓6th M87.25 Osteonecrosis due to previous trauma, pelvis and femur
M87.250 Osteonecrosis due to previous trauma, pelvis CC HCC
M87.251 Osteonecrosis due to previous trauma, right femur CC HCC
M87.252 Osteonecrosis due to previous trauma, left femur CC HCC
M87.256 Osteonecrosis due to previous trauma, unspecified femur CC UNS HCC
✓6th M87.26 Osteonecrosis due to previous trauma, tibia and fibula
M87.261 Osteonecrosis due to previous trauma, right tibia CC HCC
M87.262 Osteonecrosis due to previous trauma, left tibia CC HCC
M87.263 Osteonecrosis due to previous trauma, unspecified tibia CC UNS HCC
M87.264 Osteonecrosis due to previous trauma, right fibula CC HCC
M87.265 Osteonecrosis due to previous trauma, left fibula CC HCC

M87.266 Osteonecrosis due to previous trauma, unspecified fibula CC UNS HCC

✓6th M87.27 Osteonecrosis due to previous trauma, ankle, foot and toes

M87.271 Osteonecrosis due to previous trauma, right ankle CC HCC

M87.272 Osteonecrosis due to previous trauma, left ankle CC HCC

M87.273 Osteonecrosis due to previous trauma, unspecified ankle CC UNS HCC

M87.274 Osteonecrosis due to previous trauma, right foot CC HCC

M87.275 Osteonecrosis due to previous trauma, left foot CC HCC

M87.276 Osteonecrosis due to previous trauma, unspecified foot CC UNS HCC

M87.277 Osteonecrosis due to previous trauma, right toe(s) CC HCC

M87.278 Osteonecrosis due to previous trauma, left toe(s) CC HCC

M87.279 Osteonecrosis due to previous trauma, unspecified toe(s) CC UNS HCC

M87.28 Osteonecrosis due to previous trauma, other site CC HCC

M87.29 Osteonecrosis due to previous trauma, multiple sites CC HCC

✓5th M87.3 Other secondary osteonecrosis

M87.30 Other secondary osteonecrosis, unspecified bone CC UNS HCC

✓6th M87.31 Other secondary osteonecrosis, shoulder

M87.311 Other secondary osteonecrosis, right shoulder CC HCC

M87.312 Other secondary osteonecrosis, left shoulder CC HCC

M87.319 Other secondary osteonecrosis, unspecified shoulder CC UNS HCC

✓6th M87.32 Other secondary osteonecrosis, humerus

M87.321 Other secondary osteonecrosis, right humerus CC HCC

M87.322 Other secondary osteonecrosis, left humerus CC HCC

M87.329 Other secondary osteonecrosis, unspecified humerus CC UNS HCC

✓6th M87.33 Other secondary osteonecrosis of radius, ulna and carpus

M87.331 Other secondary osteonecrosis of right radius CC HCC

M87.332 Other secondary osteonecrosis of left radius CC HCC

M87.333 Other secondary osteonecrosis of unspecified radius CC UNS HCC

M87.334 Other secondary osteonecrosis of right ulna CC HCC

M87.335 Other secondary osteonecrosis of left ulna CC HCC

M87.336 Other secondary osteonecrosis of unspecified ulna CC UNS HCC

M87.337 Other secondary osteonecrosis of right carpus CC HCC

M87.338 Other secondary osteonecrosis of left carpus CC HCC

M87.339 Other secondary osteonecrosis of unspecified carpus CC UNS HCC

✓6th M87.34 Other secondary osteonecrosis, hand and fingers

M87.341 Other secondary osteonecrosis, right hand CC HCC

M87.342 Other secondary osteonecrosis, left hand CC HCC

M87.343 Other secondary osteonecrosis, unspecified hand CC UNS HCC

M87.344 Other secondary osteonecrosis, right finger(s) CC HCC

M87.345 Other secondary osteonecrosis, left finger(s) CC HCC

M87.346 Other secondary osteonecrosis, unspecified finger(s) CC UNS HCC

✓6th M87.35 Other secondary osteonecrosis, pelvis and femur

M87.350 Other secondary osteonecrosis, pelvis CC HCC

M87.351 Other secondary osteonecrosis, right femur CC HCC

M87.352 Other secondary osteonecrosis, left femur CC HCC

M87.353 Other secondary osteonecrosis, unspecified femur CC UNS HCC

✓6th M87.36 Other secondary osteonecrosis, tibia and fibula

M87.361 Other secondary osteonecrosis, right tibia CC HCC

M87.362 Other secondary osteonecrosis, left tibia CC HCC

M87.363 Other secondary osteonecrosis, unspecified tibia CC UNS HCC

M87.364 Other secondary osteonecrosis, right fibula CC HCC

M87.365 Other secondary osteonecrosis, left fibula CC HCC

M87.366 Other secondary osteonecrosis, unspecified fibula CC UNS HCC

✓6th M87.37 Other secondary osteonecrosis, ankle and foot

M87.371 Other secondary osteonecrosis, right ankle CC HCC

M87.372 Other secondary osteonecrosis, left ankle CC HCC

M87.373 Other secondary osteonecrosis, unspecified ankle CC UNS HCC

M87.374 Other secondary osteonecrosis, right foot CC HCC

M87.375 Other secondary osteonecrosis, left foot CC HCC

M87.376 Other secondary osteonecrosis, unspecified foot CC UNS HCC

M87.377 Other secondary osteonecrosis, right toe(s) CC HCC

M87.378 Other secondary osteonecrosis, left toe(s) CC HCC

M87.379 Other secondary osteonecrosis, unspecified toe(s) CC UNS HCC

M87.38 Other secondary osteonecrosis, other site CC HCC

M87.39 Other secondary osteonecrosis, multiple sites CC HCC

✓5th M87.8 Other osteonecrosis

M87.80 Other osteonecrosis, unspecified bone CC UNS HCC

✓6th M87.81 Other osteonecrosis, shoulder

M87.811 Other osteonecrosis, right shoulder CC HCC

M87.812 Other osteonecrosis, left shoulder CC HCC

M87.819 Other osteonecrosis, unspecified shoulder CC UNS HCC

✓6th M87.82 Other osteonecrosis, humerus

M87.821 Other osteonecrosis, right humerus CC HCC

M87.822 Other osteonecrosis, left humerus CC HCC

M87.829 Other osteonecrosis, unspecified humerus CC UNS HCC

✓6th M87.83 Other osteonecrosis of radius, ulna and carpus

M87.831 Other osteonecrosis of right radius CC HCC

M87.832 Other osteonecrosis of left radius CC HCC

M87.833 Other osteonecrosis of unspecified radius CC UNS HCC

M87.834 Other osteonecrosis of right ulna CC HCC

M87.835 Other osteonecrosis of left ulna CC HCC

M87.836 Other osteonecrosis of unspecified ulna CC UNS HCC

M87.837 Other osteonecrosis of right carpus CC HCC

M87.838 Other osteonecrosis of left carpus CC HCC

M87.839 Other osteonecrosis of unspecified carpus CC UNS HCC

M87.84 Other osteonecrosis, hand and fingers
M87.841 Other osteonecrosis, right hand CC HCC
M87.842 Other osteonecrosis, left hand CC HCC
M87.843 Other osteonecrosis, unspecified hand CC UNS HCC
M87.844 Other osteonecrosis, right finger(s) CC HCC
M87.845 Other osteonecrosis, left finger(s) CC HCC
M87.849 Other osteonecrosis, unspecified finger(s) CC UNS HCC
M87.85 Other osteonecrosis, pelvis and femur
M87.850 Other osteonecrosis, pelvis CC HCC
M87.851 Other osteonecrosis, right femur CC HCC
M87.852 Other osteonecrosis, left femur CC HCC
M87.859 Other osteonecrosis, unspecified femur CC UNS HCC
M87.86 Other osteonecrosis, tibia and fibula
M87.861 Other osteonecrosis, right tibia CC HCC
M87.862 Other osteonecrosis, left tibia CC HCC
M87.863 Other osteonecrosis, unspecified tibia CC UNS HCC
M87.864 Other osteonecrosis, right fibula CC HCC
M87.865 Other osteonecrosis, left fibula CC HCC
M87.869 Other osteonecrosis, unspecified fibula CC UNS HCC
M87.87 Other osteonecrosis, ankle, foot and toes
M87.871 Other osteonecrosis, right ankle CC HCC
M87.872 Other osteonecrosis, left ankle CC HCC
M87.873 Other osteonecrosis, unspecified ankle CC UNS HCC
M87.874 Other osteonecrosis, right foot CC HCC
M87.875 Other osteonecrosis, left foot CC HCC
M87.876 Other osteonecrosis, unspecified foot CC UNS HCC
M87.877 Other osteonecrosis, right toe(s) CC HCC
M87.878 Other osteonecrosis, left toe(s) CC HCC
M87.879 Other osteonecrosis, unspecified toe(s) CC UNS HCC
M87.88 Other osteonecrosis, other site CC HCC
M87.89 Other osteonecrosis, multiple sites CC HCC
M87.9 Osteonecrosis, unspecified CC HCC
Necrosis of bone NOS

M88 Osteitis deformans [Paget's disease of bone]
EXCLUDES 1 *osteitis deformans in neoplastic disease (M9Ø.6)*
DEF: Bone disease characterized by numerous cycles of bone resorption by the body. Resorption is followed by accelerated repair attempts, causing bone deformities and bowing, with associated fractures and pain.
M88.Ø Osteitis deformans of skull
M88.1 Osteitis deformans of vertebrae
M88.8 Osteitis deformans of other bones
M88.81 Osteitis deformans of shoulder
M88.811 Osteitis deformans of right shoulder
M88.812 Osteitis deformans of left shoulder
M88.819 Osteitis deformans of unspecified shoulder
M88.82 Osteitis deformans of upper arm
M88.821 Osteitis deformans of right upper arm
M88.822 Osteitis deformans of left upper arm
M88.829 Osteitis deformans of unspecified upper arm
M88.83 Osteitis deformans of forearm
M88.831 Osteitis deformans of right forearm
M88.832 Osteitis deformans of left forearm
M88.839 Osteitis deformans of unspecified forearm
M88.84 Osteitis deformans of hand
M88.841 Osteitis deformans of right hand
M88.842 Osteitis deformans of left hand
M88.849 Osteitis deformans of unspecified hand
M88.85 Osteitis deformans of thigh
M88.851 Osteitis deformans of right thigh
M88.852 Osteitis deformans of left thigh
M88.859 Osteitis deformans of unspecified thigh
M88.86 Osteitis deformans of lower leg
M88.861 Osteitis deformans of right lower leg
M88.862 Osteitis deformans of left lower leg
M88.869 Osteitis deformans of unspecified lower leg
M88.87 Osteitis deformans of ankle and foot
M88.871 Osteitis deformans of right ankle and foot
M88.872 Osteitis deformans of left ankle and foot
M88.879 Osteitis deformans of unspecified ankle and foot
M88.88 Osteitis deformans of other bones
EXCLUDES 2 *osteitis deformans of skull (M88.Ø)*
osteitis deformans of vertebrae (M88.1)
M88.89 Osteitis deformans of multiple sites
M88.9 Osteitis deformans of unspecified bone

M89 Other disorders of bone
M89.Ø Algoneurodystrophy
Shoulder-hand syndrome
Sudeck's atrophy
EXCLUDES 1 *causalgia, lower limb (G57.7-)*
causalgia, upper limb (G56.4-)
complex regional pain syndrome II, lower limb (G57.7-)
complex regional pain syndrome II, upper limb (G56.4-)
reflex sympathetic dystrophy (G9Ø.5-)
M89.ØØ Algoneurodystrophy, unspecified site
M89.Ø1 Algoneurodystrophy, shoulder
M89.Ø11 Algoneurodystrophy, right shoulder
M89.Ø12 Algoneurodystrophy, left shoulder
M89.Ø19 Algoneurodystrophy, unspecified shoulder
M89.Ø2 Algoneurodystrophy, upper arm
M89.Ø21 Algoneurodystrophy, right upper arm
M89.Ø22 Algoneurodystrophy, left upper arm
M89.Ø29 Algoneurodystrophy, unspecified upper arm
M89.Ø3 Algoneurodystrophy, forearm
M89.Ø31 Algoneurodystrophy, right forearm
M89.Ø32 Algoneurodystrophy, left forearm
M89.Ø39 Algoneurodystrophy, unspecified forearm
M89.Ø4 Algoneurodystrophy, hand
M89.Ø41 Algoneurodystrophy, right hand
M89.Ø42 Algoneurodystrophy, left hand
M89.Ø49 Algoneurodystrophy, unspecified hand
M89.Ø5 Algoneurodystrophy, thigh
M89.Ø51 Algoneurodystrophy, right thigh
M89.Ø52 Algoneurodystrophy, left thigh
M89.Ø59 Algoneurodystrophy, unspecified thigh
M89.Ø6 Algoneurodystrophy, lower leg
M89.Ø61 Algoneurodystrophy, right lower leg
M89.Ø62 Algoneurodystrophy, left lower leg
M89.Ø69 Algoneurodystrophy, unspecified lower leg
M89.Ø7 Algoneurodystrophy, ankle and foot
M89.Ø71 Algoneurodystrophy, right ankle and foot
M89.Ø72 Algoneurodystrophy, left ankle and foot
M89.Ø79 Algoneurodystrophy, unspecified ankle and foot
M89.Ø8 Algoneurodystrophy, other site
M89.Ø9 Algoneurodystrophy, multiple sites
M89.1 Physeal arrest
Arrest of growth plate
Epiphyseal arrest
Growth plate arrest
M89.12 Physeal arrest, humerus
M89.121 Complete physeal arrest, right proximal humerus
M89.122 Complete physeal arrest, left proximal humerus
M89.123 Partial physeal arrest, right proximal humerus

M89.124 Partial physeal arrest, left proximal humerus
M89.125 Complete physeal arrest, right distal humerus
M89.126 Complete physeal arrest, left distal humerus
M89.127 Partial physeal arrest, right distal humerus
M89.128 Partial physeal arrest, left distal humerus
M89.129 Physeal arrest, humerus, unspecified

M89.13 Physeal arrest, forearm
M89.131 Complete physeal arrest, right distal radius
M89.132 Complete physeal arrest, left distal radius
M89.133 Partial physeal arrest, right distal radius
M89.134 Partial physeal arrest, left distal radius
M89.138 Other physeal arrest of forearm
M89.139 Physeal arrest, forearm, unspecified

M89.15 Physeal arrest, femur
M89.151 Complete physeal arrest, right proximal femur
M89.152 Complete physeal arrest, left proximal femur
M89.153 Partial physeal arrest, right proximal femur
M89.154 Partial physeal arrest, left proximal femur
M89.155 Complete physeal arrest, right distal femur
M89.156 Complete physeal arrest, left distal femur
M89.157 Partial physeal arrest, right distal femur
M89.158 Partial physeal arrest, left distal femur
M89.159 Physeal arrest, femur, unspecified

M89.16 Physeal arrest, lower leg
M89.160 Complete physeal arrest, right proximal tibia
M89.161 Complete physeal arrest, left proximal tibia
M89.162 Partial physeal arrest, right proximal tibia
M89.163 Partial physeal arrest, left proximal tibia
M89.164 Complete physeal arrest, right distal tibia
M89.165 Complete physeal arrest, left distal tibia
M89.166 Partial physeal arrest, right distal tibia
M89.167 Partial physeal arrest, left distal tibia
M89.168 Other physeal arrest of lower leg
M89.169 Physeal arrest, lower leg, unspecified

M89.18 Physeal arrest, other site

M89.2 Other disorders of bone development and growth

M89.20 Other disorders of bone development and growth, unspecified site

M89.21 Other disorders of bone development and growth, shoulder
M89.211 Other disorders of bone development and growth, right shoulder
M89.212 Other disorders of bone development and growth, left shoulder
M89.219 Other disorders of bone development and growth, unspecified shoulder

M89.22 Other disorders of bone development and growth, humerus
M89.221 Other disorders of bone development and growth, right humerus
M89.222 Other disorders of bone development and growth, left humerus
M89.229 Other disorders of bone development and growth, unspecified humerus

M89.23 Other disorders of bone development and growth, ulna and radius
M89.231 Other disorders of bone development and growth, right ulna
M89.232 Other disorders of bone development and growth, left ulna
M89.233 Other disorders of bone development and growth, right radius
M89.234 Other disorders of bone development and growth, left radius
M89.239 Other disorders of bone development and growth, unspecified ulna and radius

M89.24 Other disorders of bone development and growth, hand
M89.241 Other disorders of bone development and growth, right hand
M89.242 Other disorders of bone development and growth, left hand
M89.249 Other disorders of bone development and growth, unspecified hand

M89.25 Other disorders of bone development and growth, femur
M89.251 Other disorders of bone development and growth, right femur
M89.252 Other disorders of bone development and growth, left femur
M89.259 Other disorders of bone development and growth, unspecified femur

M89.26 Other disorders of bone development and growth, tibia and fibula
M89.261 Other disorders of bone development and growth, right tibia
M89.262 Other disorders of bone development and growth, left tibia
M89.263 Other disorders of bone development and growth, right fibula
M89.264 Other disorders of bone development and growth, left fibula
M89.269 Other disorders of bone development and growth, unspecified lower leg

M89.27 Other disorders of bone development and growth, ankle and foot
M89.271 Other disorders of bone development and growth, right ankle and foot
M89.272 Other disorders of bone development and growth, left ankle and foot
M89.279 Other disorders of bone development and growth, unspecified ankle and foot

M89.28 Other disorders of bone development and growth, other site

M89.29 Other disorders of bone development and growth, multiple sites

M89.3 Hypertrophy of bone

M89.30 Hypertrophy of bone, unspecified site

M89.31 Hypertrophy of bone, shoulder
M89.311 Hypertrophy of bone, right shoulder
M89.312 Hypertrophy of bone, left shoulder
M89.319 Hypertrophy of bone, unspecified shoulder

M89.32 Hypertrophy of bone, humerus
M89.321 Hypertrophy of bone, right humerus
M89.322 Hypertrophy of bone, left humerus
M89.329 Hypertrophy of bone, unspecified humerus

M89.33 Hypertrophy of bone, ulna and radius
M89.331 Hypertrophy of bone, right ulna
M89.332 Hypertrophy of bone, left ulna
M89.333 Hypertrophy of bone, right radius
M89.334 Hypertrophy of bone, left radius
M89.339 Hypertrophy of bone, unspecified ulna and radius

M89.34 Hypertrophy of bone, hand
M89.341 Hypertrophy of bone, right hand
M89.342 Hypertrophy of bone, left hand
M89.349 Hypertrophy of bone, unspecified hand

M89.35 Hypertrophy of bone, femur
M89.351 Hypertrophy of bone, right femur
M89.352 Hypertrophy of bone, left femur
M89.359 Hypertrophy of bone, unspecified femur

M89.36 Hypertrophy of bone, tibia and fibula
M89.361 Hypertrophy of bone, right tibia
M89.362 Hypertrophy of bone, left tibia
M89.363 Hypertrophy of bone, right fibula
M89.364 Hypertrophy of bone, left fibula
M89.369 Hypertrophy of bone, unspecified tibia and fibula

M89.37 Hypertrophy of bone, ankle and foot
M89.371 Hypertrophy of bone, right ankle and foot
M89.372 Hypertrophy of bone, left ankle and foot
M89.379 Hypertrophy of bone, unspecified ankle and foot

M89.38 Hypertrophy of bone, other site
M89.39 Hypertrophy of bone, multiple sites

✓5th **M89.4 Other hypertrophic osteoarthropathy**
Marie-Bamberger disease
Pachydermoperiostosis
M89.40 Other hypertrophic osteoarthropathy, unspecified site
✓6th **M89.41 Other hypertrophic osteoarthropathy, shoulder**
M89.411 Other hypertrophic osteoarthropathy, right shoulder
M89.412 Other hypertrophic osteoarthropathy, left shoulder
M89.419 Other hypertrophic osteoarthropathy, unspecified shoulder
✓6th **M89.42 Other hypertrophic osteoarthropathy, upper arm**
M89.421 Other hypertrophic osteoarthropathy, right upper arm
M89.422 Other hypertrophic osteoarthropathy, left upper arm
M89.429 Other hypertrophic osteoarthropathy, unspecified upper arm
✓6th **M89.43 Other hypertrophic osteoarthropathy, forearm**
M89.431 Other hypertrophic osteoarthropathy, right forearm
M89.432 Other hypertrophic osteoarthropathy, left forearm
M89.439 Other hypertrophic osteoarthropathy, unspecified forearm
✓6th **M89.44 Other hypertrophic osteoarthropathy, hand**
M89.441 Other hypertrophic osteoarthropathy, right hand
M89.442 Other hypertrophic osteoarthropathy, left hand
M89.449 Other hypertrophic osteoarthropathy, unspecified hand
✓6th **M89.45 Other hypertrophic osteoarthropathy, thigh**
M89.451 Other hypertrophic osteoarthropathy, right thigh
M89.452 Other hypertrophic osteoarthropathy, left thigh
M89.459 Other hypertrophic osteoarthropathy, unspecified thigh
✓6th **M89.46 Other hypertrophic osteoarthropathy, lower leg**
M89.461 Other hypertrophic osteoarthropathy, right lower leg
M89.462 Other hypertrophic osteoarthropathy, left lower leg
M89.469 Other hypertrophic osteoarthropathy, unspecified lower leg
✓6th **M89.47 Other hypertrophic osteoarthropathy, ankle and foot**
M89.471 Other hypertrophic osteoarthropathy, right ankle and foot
M89.472 Other hypertrophic osteoarthropathy, left ankle and foot
M89.479 Other hypertrophic osteoarthropathy, unspecified ankle and foot
M89.48 Other hypertrophic osteoarthropathy, other site
M89.49 Other hypertrophic osteoarthropathy, multiple sites

✓5th **M89.5 Osteolysis**
Use additional code to identify major osseous defect, if applicable (M89.7-)
EXCLUDES 2 *periprosthetic osteolysis of internal prosthetic joint (T84.05-)*
M89.50 Osteolysis, unspecified site
✓6th **M89.51 Osteolysis, shoulder**
M89.511 Osteolysis, right shoulder
M89.512 Osteolysis, left shoulder
M89.519 Osteolysis, unspecified shoulder
✓6th **M89.52 Osteolysis, upper arm**
M89.521 Osteolysis, right upper arm
M89.522 Osteolysis, left upper arm
M89.529 Osteolysis, unspecified upper arm
✓6th **M89.53 Osteolysis, forearm**
M89.531 Osteolysis, right forearm
M89.532 Osteolysis, left forearm
M89.539 Osteolysis, unspecified forearm
✓6th **M89.54 Osteolysis, hand**
M89.541 Osteolysis, right hand
M89.542 Osteolysis, left hand
M89.549 Osteolysis, unspecified hand
✓6th **M89.55 Osteolysis, thigh**
M89.551 Osteolysis, right thigh
M89.552 Osteolysis, left thigh
M89.559 Osteolysis, unspecified thigh
✓6th **M89.56 Osteolysis, lower leg**
M89.561 Osteolysis, right lower leg
M89.562 Osteolysis, left lower leg
M89.569 Osteolysis, unspecified lower leg
✓6th **M89.57 Osteolysis, ankle and foot**
M89.571 Osteolysis, right ankle and foot
M89.572 Osteolysis, left ankle and foot
M89.579 Osteolysis, unspecified ankle and foot
M89.58 Osteolysis, other site
M89.59 Osteolysis, multiple sites

✓5th **M89.6 Osteopathy after poliomyelitis**
Use additional code (B91) to identify previous poliomyelitis
EXCLUDES 1 *postpolio syndrome (G14)*
M89.60 Osteopathy after poliomyelitis, unspecified site HCC
✓6th **M89.61 Osteopathy after poliomyelitis, shoulder**
M89.611 Osteopathy after poliomyelitis, right shoulder HCC
M89.612 Osteopathy after poliomyelitis, left shoulder HCC
M89.619 Osteopathy after poliomyelitis, unspecified shoulder HCC
✓6th **M89.62 Osteopathy after poliomyelitis, upper arm**
M89.621 Osteopathy after poliomyelitis, right upper arm HCC
M89.622 Osteopathy after poliomyelitis, left upper arm HCC
M89.629 Osteopathy after poliomyelitis, unspecified upper arm HCC
✓6th **M89.63 Osteopathy after poliomyelitis, forearm**
M89.631 Osteopathy after poliomyelitis, right forearm HCC
M89.632 Osteopathy after poliomyelitis, left forearm HCC
M89.639 Osteopathy after poliomyelitis, unspecified forearm HCC
✓6th **M89.64 Osteopathy after poliomyelitis, hand**
M89.641 Osteopathy after poliomyelitis, right hand HCC
M89.642 Osteopathy after poliomyelitis, left hand HCC
M89.649 Osteopathy after poliomyelitis, unspecified hand HCC
✓6th **M89.65 Osteopathy after poliomyelitis, thigh**
M89.651 Osteopathy after poliomyelitis, right thigh HCC
M89.652 Osteopathy after poliomyelitis, left thigh HCC
M89.659 Osteopathy after poliomyelitis, unspecified thigh HCC
✓6th **M89.66 Osteopathy after poliomyelitis, lower leg**
M89.661 Osteopathy after poliomyelitis, right lower leg HCC
M89.662 Osteopathy after poliomyelitis, left lower leg HCC
M89.669 Osteopathy after poliomyelitis, unspecified lower leg HCC
✓6th **M89.67 Osteopathy after poliomyelitis, ankle and foot**
M89.671 Osteopathy after poliomyelitis, right ankle and foot HCC
M89.672 Osteopathy after poliomyelitis, left ankle and foot HCC
M89.679 Osteopathy after poliomyelitis, unspecified ankle and foot HCC
M89.68 Osteopathy after poliomyelitis, other site HCC
M89.69 Osteopathy after poliomyelitis, multiple sites HCC

M89.7 Major osseous defect

Code first underlying disease, if known, such as:
- aseptic necrosis of bone (M87.-)
- malignant neoplasm of bone (C4Ø.-)
- osteolysis ►(M89.5-)◄
- osteomyelitis (M86.-)
- osteonecrosis (M87.-)
- osteoporosis (M8Ø.-, M81.-)
- periprosthetic osteolysis (T84.Ø5-)

M89.7Ø Major osseous defect, unspecified site

M89.71 Major osseous defect, shoulder region

Major osseous defect clavicle or scapula

M89.711 Major osseous defect, right shoulder region
M89.712 Major osseous defect, left shoulder region
M89.719 Major osseous defect, unspecified shoulder region

M89.72 Major osseous defect, humerus

M89.721 Major osseous defect, right humerus
M89.722 Major osseous defect, left humerus
M89.729 Major osseous defect, unspecified humerus

M89.73 Major osseous defect, forearm

Major osseous defect of radius and ulna

M89.731 Major osseous defect, right forearm
M89.732 Major osseous defect, left forearm
M89.739 Major osseous defect, unspecified forearm

M89.74 Major osseous defect, hand

Major osseous defect of carpus, fingers, metacarpus

M89.741 Major osseous defect, right hand
M89.742 Major osseous defect, left hand
M89.749 Major osseous defect, unspecified hand

M89.75 Major osseous defect, pelvic region and thigh

Major osseous defect of femur and pelvis

M89.751 Major osseous defect, right pelvic region and thigh
M89.752 Major osseous defect, left pelvic region and thigh
M89.759 Major osseous defect, unspecified pelvic region and thigh

M89.76 Major osseous defect, lower leg

Major osseous defect of fibula and tibia

M89.761 Major osseous defect, right lower leg
M89.762 Major osseous defect, left lower leg
M89.769 Major osseous defect, unspecified lower leg

M89.77 Major osseous defect, ankle and foot

Major osseous defect of metatarsus, tarsus, toes

M89.771 Major osseous defect, right ankle and foot
M89.772 Major osseous defect, left ankle and foot
M89.779 Major osseous defect, unspecified ankle and foot

M89.78 Major osseous defect, other site
M89.79 Major osseous defect, multiple sites

M89.8 Other specified disorders of bone

Infantile cortical hyperostoses
Post-traumatic subperiosteal ossification
AHA: 2022,2Q,10

M89.8X Other specified disorders of bone

M89.8XØ Other specified disorders of bone, multiple sites
M89.8X1 Other specified disorders of bone, shoulder
M89.8X2 Other specified disorders of bone, upper arm
M89.8X3 Other specified disorders of bone, forearm
AHA: 2019,3Q,9
M89.8X4 Other specified disorders of bone, hand
M89.8X5 Other specified disorders of bone, thigh
M89.8X6 Other specified disorders of bone, lower leg
M89.8X7 Other specified disorders of bone, ankle and foot
M89.8X8 Other specified disorders of bone, other site
AHA: 2023,2Q,18
M89.8X9 Other specified disorders of bone, unspecified site

M89.9 Disorder of bone, unspecified

M9Ø Osteopathies in diseases classified elsewhere

EXCLUDES 1 *osteochondritis, osteomyelitis, and osteopathy (in):*
- *cryptococcosis (B45.3)*
- *diabetes mellitus (EØ8-E13 with .69-)*
- *gonococcal (A54.43)*
- *neurogenic syphilis (A52.11)*
- *renal osteodystrophy (N25.Ø)*
- *salmonellosis (AØ2.24)*
- *secondary syphilis (A51.46)*
- *syphilis (late) (A52.77)*

M9Ø.5 Osteonecrosis in diseases classified elsewhere

Code first underlying disease, such as:
- caisson disease (T7Ø.3)
- hemoglobinopathy (D5Ø-D64)

M9Ø.5Ø Osteonecrosis in diseases classified elsewhere, unspecified site CC UNS HCC

M9Ø.51 Osteonecrosis in diseases classified elsewhere, shoulder

M9Ø.511 Osteonecrosis in diseases classified elsewhere, right shoulder CC HCC
M9Ø.512 Osteonecrosis in diseases classified elsewhere, left shoulder CC HCC
M9Ø.519 Osteonecrosis in diseases classified elsewhere, unspecified shoulder CC UNS HCC

M9Ø.52 Osteonecrosis in diseases classified elsewhere, upper arm

M9Ø.521 Osteonecrosis in diseases classified elsewhere, right upper arm CC HCC
M9Ø.522 Osteonecrosis in diseases classified elsewhere, left upper arm CC HCC
M9Ø.529 Osteonecrosis in diseases classified elsewhere, unspecified upper arm CC UNS HCC

M9Ø.53 Osteonecrosis in diseases classified elsewhere, forearm

M9Ø.531 Osteonecrosis in diseases classified elsewhere, right forearm CC HCC
M9Ø.532 Osteonecrosis in diseases classified elsewhere, left forearm CC HCC
M9Ø.539 Osteonecrosis in diseases classified elsewhere, unspecified forearm CC UNS HCC

M9Ø.54 Osteonecrosis in diseases classified elsewhere, hand

M9Ø.541 Osteonecrosis in diseases classified elsewhere, right hand CC HCC
M9Ø.542 Osteonecrosis in diseases classified elsewhere, left hand CC HCC
M9Ø.549 Osteonecrosis in diseases classified elsewhere, unspecified hand CC UNS HCC

M9Ø.55 Osteonecrosis in diseases classified elsewhere, thigh

M9Ø.551 Osteonecrosis in diseases classified elsewhere, right thigh CC HCC
M9Ø.552 Osteonecrosis in diseases classified elsewhere, left thigh CC HCC
M9Ø.559 Osteonecrosis in diseases classified elsewhere, unspecified thigh CC UNS HCC

M9Ø.56 Osteonecrosis in diseases classified elsewhere, lower leg

M9Ø.561 Osteonecrosis in diseases classified elsewhere, right lower leg CC HCC
M9Ø.562 Osteonecrosis in diseases classified elsewhere, left lower leg CC HCC
M9Ø.569 Osteonecrosis in diseases classified elsewhere, unspecified lower leg CC UNS HCC

M9Ø.57 Osteonecrosis in diseases classified elsewhere, ankle and foot

M9Ø.571 Osteonecrosis in diseases classified elsewhere, right ankle and foot CC HCC

M90.572 Osteonecrosis in diseases classified elsewhere, left ankle and foot CC HCC

M90.579 Osteonecrosis in diseases classified elsewhere, unspecified ankle and foot CC UNS HCC

M90.58 Osteonecrosis in diseases classified elsewhere, other site CC HCC

M90.59 Osteonecrosis in diseases classified elsewhere, multiple sites CC HCC

M90.6 Osteitis deformans in neoplastic diseases

Osteitis deformans in malignant neoplasm of bone

Code first the neoplasm (C40.-, C41.-)

EXCLUDES 1 *osteitis deformans [Paget's disease of bone] (M88.-)*

M90.60 Osteitis deformans in neoplastic diseases, unspecified site

M90.61 Osteitis deformans in neoplastic diseases, shoulder

M90.611 Osteitis deformans in neoplastic diseases, right shoulder

M90.612 Osteitis deformans in neoplastic diseases, left shoulder

M90.619 Osteitis deformans in neoplastic diseases, unspecified shoulder

M90.62 Osteitis deformans in neoplastic diseases, upper arm

M90.621 Osteitis deformans in neoplastic diseases, right upper arm

M90.622 Osteitis deformans in neoplastic diseases, left upper arm

M90.629 Osteitis deformans in neoplastic diseases, unspecified upper arm

M90.63 Osteitis deformans in neoplastic diseases, forearm

M90.631 Osteitis deformans in neoplastic diseases, right forearm

M90.632 Osteitis deformans in neoplastic diseases, left forearm

M90.639 Osteitis deformans in neoplastic diseases, unspecified forearm

M90.64 Osteitis deformans in neoplastic diseases, hand

M90.641 Osteitis deformans in neoplastic diseases, right hand

M90.642 Osteitis deformans in neoplastic diseases, left hand

M90.649 Osteitis deformans in neoplastic diseases, unspecified hand

M90.65 Osteitis deformans in neoplastic diseases, thigh

M90.651 Osteitis deformans in neoplastic diseases, right thigh

M90.652 Osteitis deformans in neoplastic diseases, left thigh

M90.659 Osteitis deformans in neoplastic diseases, unspecified thigh

M90.66 Osteitis deformans in neoplastic diseases, lower leg

M90.661 Osteitis deformans in neoplastic diseases, right lower leg

M90.662 Osteitis deformans in neoplastic diseases, left lower leg

M90.669 Osteitis deformans in neoplastic diseases, unspecified lower leg

M90.67 Osteitis deformans in neoplastic diseases, ankle and foot

M90.671 Osteitis deformans in neoplastic diseases, right ankle and foot

M90.672 Osteitis deformans in neoplastic diseases, left ankle and foot

M90.679 Osteitis deformans in neoplastic diseases, unspecified ankle and foot

M90.68 Osteitis deformans in neoplastic diseases, other site

M90.69 Osteitis deformans in neoplastic diseases, multiple sites

M90.8 Osteopathy in diseases classified elsewhere

Code first underlying disease, such as:
- rickets (E55.0)
- vitamin-D-resistant rickets ▶(E83.31)◀

M90.80 Osteopathy in diseases classified elsewhere, unspecified site

M90.81 Osteopathy in diseases classified elsewhere, shoulder

M90.811 Osteopathy in diseases classified elsewhere, right shoulder

M90.812 Osteopathy in diseases classified elsewhere, left shoulder

M90.819 Osteopathy in diseases classified elsewhere, unspecified shoulder

M90.82 Osteopathy in diseases classified elsewhere, upper arm

M90.821 Osteopathy in diseases classified elsewhere, right upper arm

M90.822 Osteopathy in diseases classified elsewhere, left upper arm

M90.829 Osteopathy in diseases classified elsewhere, unspecified upper arm

M90.83 Osteopathy in diseases classified elsewhere, forearm

M90.831 Osteopathy in diseases classified elsewhere, right forearm

M90.832 Osteopathy in diseases classified elsewhere, left forearm

M90.839 Osteopathy in diseases classified elsewhere, unspecified forearm

M90.84 Osteopathy in diseases classified elsewhere, hand

M90.841 Osteopathy in diseases classified elsewhere, right hand

M90.842 Osteopathy in diseases classified elsewhere, left hand

M90.849 Osteopathy in diseases classified elsewhere, unspecified hand

M90.85 Osteopathy in diseases classified elsewhere, thigh

M90.851 Osteopathy in diseases classified elsewhere, right thigh

M90.852 Osteopathy in diseases classified elsewhere, left thigh

M90.859 Osteopathy in diseases classified elsewhere, unspecified thigh

M90.86 Osteopathy in diseases classified elsewhere, lower leg

M90.861 Osteopathy in diseases classified elsewhere, right lower leg

M90.862 Osteopathy in diseases classified elsewhere, left lower leg

M90.869 Osteopathy in diseases classified elsewhere, unspecified lower leg

M90.87 Osteopathy in diseases classified elsewhere, ankle and foot

M90.871 Osteopathy in diseases classified elsewhere, right ankle and foot

M90.872 Osteopathy in diseases classified elsewhere, left ankle and foot

M90.879 Osteopathy in diseases classified elsewhere, unspecified ankle and foot

M90.88 Osteopathy in diseases classified elsewhere, other site

M90.89 Osteopathy in diseases classified elsewhere, multiple sites

Chondropathies (M91-M94)

EXCLUDES 1 *postprocedural chondropathies (M96.-)*

M91 Juvenile osteochondrosis of hip and pelvis

EXCLUDES 1 *slipped upper femoral epiphysis (nontraumatic) (M93.0-)*

M91.0 Juvenile osteochondrosis of pelvis

Osteochondrosis (juvenile) of acetabulum
Osteochondrosis (juvenile) of iliac crest [Buchanan]
Osteochondrosis (juvenile) of ischiopubic synchondrosis [van Neck]
Osteochondrosis (juvenile) of symphysis pubis [Pierson]

M91.1 Juvenile osteochondrosis of head of femur [Legg-Calve-Perthes]

M91.10 Juvenile osteochondrosis of head of femur [Legg-Calve-Perthes], unspecified leg

M91.11 Juvenile osteochondrosis of head of femur [Legg-Calve-Perthes], right leg

M91.12 Juvenile osteochondrosis of head of femur [Legg-Calve-Perthes], left leg

M91.2 Coxa plana

Hip deformity due to previous juvenile osteochondrosis

M91.20 Coxa plana, unspecified hip

M91.21 Coxa plana, right hip

M91.22 Coxa plana, left hip

M91.3 Pseudocoxalgia

M91.30 Pseudocoxalgia, unspecified hip

M91.31 Pseudocoxalgia, right hip
M91.32 Pseudocoxalgia, left hip

5th **M91.4 Coxa magna**
M91.40 Coxa magna, unspecified hip
M91.41 Coxa magna, right hip
M91.42 Coxa magna, left hip

5th **M91.8 Other juvenile osteochondrosis of hip and pelvis**
Juvenile osteochondrosis after reduction of congenital dislocation of hip
M91.80 Other juvenile osteochondrosis of hip and pelvis, unspecified leg
M91.81 Other juvenile osteochondrosis of hip and pelvis, right leg
M91.82 Other juvenile osteochondrosis of hip and pelvis, left leg

5th **M91.9 Juvenile osteochondrosis of hip and pelvis, unspecified**
M91.90 Juvenile osteochondrosis of hip and pelvis, unspecified, unspecified leg
M91.91 Juvenile osteochondrosis of hip and pelvis, unspecified, right leg
M91.92 Juvenile osteochondrosis of hip and pelvis, unspecified, left leg

4th **M92 Other juvenile osteochondrosis**

5th **M92.0 Juvenile osteochondrosis of humerus**
Osteochondrosis (juvenile) of capitulum of humerus [Panner]
Osteochondrosis (juvenile) of head of humerus [Haas]
M92.00 Juvenile osteochondrosis of humerus, unspecified arm
M92.01 Juvenile osteochondrosis of humerus, right arm
M92.02 Juvenile osteochondrosis of humerus, left arm

5th **M92.1 Juvenile osteochondrosis of radius and ulna**
Osteochondrosis (juvenile) of lower ulna [Burns]
Osteochondrosis (juvenile) of radial head [Brailsford]
M92.10 Juvenile osteochondrosis of radius and ulna, unspecified arm
M92.11 Juvenile osteochondrosis of radius and ulna, right arm
M92.12 Juvenile osteochondrosis of radius and ulna, left arm

5th **M92.2 Juvenile osteochondrosis, hand**
6th **M92.20 Unspecified juvenile osteochondrosis, hand**
M92.201 Unspecified juvenile osteochondrosis, right hand
M92.202 Unspecified juvenile osteochondrosis, left hand
M92.209 Unspecified juvenile osteochondrosis, unspecified hand
6th **M92.21 Osteochondrosis (juvenile) of carpal lunate [Kienbock]**
M92.211 Osteochondrosis (juvenile) of carpal lunate [Kienbock], right hand
M92.212 Osteochondrosis (juvenile) of carpal lunate [Kienbock], left hand
M92.219 Osteochondrosis (juvenile) of carpal lunate [Kienbock], unspecified hand
6th **M92.22 Osteochondrosis (juvenile) of metacarpal heads [Mauclaire]**
M92.221 Osteochondrosis (juvenile) of metacarpal heads [Mauclaire], right hand
M92.222 Osteochondrosis (juvenile) of metacarpal heads [Mauclaire], left hand
M92.229 Osteochondrosis (juvenile) of metacarpal heads [Mauclaire], unspecified hand
6th **M92.29 Other juvenile osteochondrosis, hand**
M92.291 Other juvenile osteochondrosis, right hand
M92.292 Other juvenile osteochondrosis, left hand
M92.299 Other juvenile osteochondrosis, unspecified hand

5th **M92.3 Other juvenile osteochondrosis, upper limb**
M92.30 Other juvenile osteochondrosis, unspecified upper limb
M92.31 Other juvenile osteochondrosis, right upper limb
M92.32 Other juvenile osteochondrosis, left upper limb

5th **M92.4 Juvenile osteochondrosis of patella**
Osteochondrosis (juvenile) of primary patellar center [Kohler]
Osteochondrosis (juvenile) of secondary patellar centre [Sinding Larsen]
M92.40 Juvenile osteochondrosis of patella, unspecified knee
M92.41 Juvenile osteochondrosis of patella, right knee
M92.42 Juvenile osteochondrosis of patella, left knee

5th **M92.5 Juvenile osteochondrosis of tibia and fibula**
AHA: 2020,4Q,33-34
6th **M92.50 Unspecified juvenile osteochondrosis of tibia and fibula**
M92.501 Unspecified juvenile osteochondrosis, right leg
M92.502 Unspecified juvenile osteochondrosis, left leg
M92.503 Unspecified juvenile osteochondrosis, bilateral leg
M92.509 Unspecified juvenile osteochondrosis, unspecified leg
6th **M92.51 Juvenile osteochondrosis of proximal tibia**
Blount disease
Tibia vara
M92.511 Juvenile osteochondrosis of proximal tibia, right leg
M92.512 Juvenile osteochondrosis of proximal tibia,left leg
M92.513 Juvenile osteochondrosis of proximal tibia, bilateral
M92.519 Juvenile osteochondrosis of proximal tibia, unspecified leg
6th **M92.52 Juvenile osteochondrosis of tibia tubercle**
Osgood-Schlatter disease
M92.521 Juvenile osteochondrosis of tibia tubercle, right leg
M92.522 Juvenile osteochondrosis of tibia tubercle, left leg
M92.523 Juvenile osteochondrosis of tibia tubercle, bilateral
M92.529 Juvenile osteochondrosis of tibia tubercle, unspecified leg
6th **M92.59 Other juvenile osteochondrosis of tibia and fibula**
M92.591 Other juvenile osteochondrosis of tibia and fibula, right leg
M92.592 Other juvenile osteochondrosis of tibia and fibula, left leg
M92.593 Other juvenile osteochondrosis of tibia and fibula, bilateral
M92.599 Other juvenile osteochondrosis of tibia and fibula, unspecified leg

5th **M92.6 Juvenile osteochondrosis of tarsus**
Osteochondrosis (juvenile) of calcaneum [Sever]
Osteochondrosis (juvenile) of os tibiale externum [Haglund]
Osteochondrosis (juvenile) of talus [Diaz]
Osteochondrosis (juvenile) of tarsal navicular [Kohler]
M92.60 Juvenile osteochondrosis of tarsus, unspecified ankle
M92.61 Juvenile osteochondrosis of tarsus, right ankle
M92.62 Juvenile osteochondrosis of tarsus, left ankle

5th **M92.7 Juvenile osteochondrosis of metatarsus**
Osteochondrosis (juvenile) of fifth metatarsus [Iselin]
Osteochondrosis (juvenile) of second metatarsus [Freiberg]
M92.70 Juvenile osteochondrosis of metatarsus, unspecified foot
M92.71 Juvenile osteochondrosis of metatarsus, right foot
M92.72 Juvenile osteochondrosis of metatarsus, left foot

M92.8 Other specified juvenile osteochondrosis
Calcaneal apophysitis
DEF: Calcaneal apophysitis: Inflammation of the calcaneus at the point of Achilles tendon insertion usually occurring in boys ages 8 to 14. Pain, tenderness, and localized swelling are present.

M92.9 Juvenile osteochondrosis, unspecified
Juvenile apophysitis NOS
Juvenile epiphysitis NOS
Juvenile osteochondritis NOS
Juvenile osteochondrosis NOS

M93 Other osteochondropathies

EXCLUDES 2 *osteochondrosis of spine (M42.-)*

M93.0 Slipped upper femoral epiphysis (nontraumatic)

Slipped capital femoral epiphysis (SCFE)
Slipped upper femoral epiphysis (SUFE)
Use additional code for associated chondrolysis (M94.3)
AHA: 2022,4Q,30-31

M93.00 Unspecified slipped upper femoral epiphysis (nontraumatic)

- **M93.001** Unspecified slipped upper femoral epiphysis (nontraumatic), right hip
- **M93.002** Unspecified slipped upper femoral epiphysis (nontraumatic), left hip
- **M93.003** Unspecified slipped upper femoral epiphysis (nontraumatic), unspecified hip
- **M93.004** Unspecified slipped upper femoral epiphysis (nontraumatic), bilateral hips

M93.01 Acute slipped upper femoral epiphysis, stable (nontraumatic)

- **M93.011** Acute slipped upper femoral epiphysis, stable (nontraumatic), right hip
- **M93.012** Acute slipped upper femoral epiphysis, stable (nontraumatic), left hip
- **M93.013** Acute slipped upper femoral epiphysis, stable (nontraumatic), unspecified hip
- **M93.014** Acute slipped upper femoral epiphysis, stable (nontraumatic), bilateral hips

M93.02 Chronic slipped upper femoral epiphysis, stable (nontraumatic)

- **M93.021** Chronic slipped upper femoral epiphysis, stable (nontraumatic), right hip
- **M93.022** Chronic slipped upper femoral epiphysis, stable (nontraumatic), left hip
- **M93.023** Chronic slipped upper femoral epiphysis, stable (nontraumatic), unspecified hip
- **M93.024** Chronic slipped upper femoral epiphysis, stable (nontraumatic), bilateral hips

M93.03 Acute on chronic slipped upper femoral epiphysis, stable (nontraumatic)

- **M93.031** Acute on chronic slipped upper femoral epiphysis, stable (nontraumatic), right hip
- **M93.032** Acute on chronic slipped upper femoral epiphysis, stable (nontraumatic), left hip
- **M93.033** Acute on chronic slipped upper femoral epiphysis, stable (nontraumatic), unspecified hip
- **M93.034** Acute on chronic slipped upper femoral epiphysis, stable (nontraumatic), bilateral hips

M93.04 Acute slipped upper femoral epiphysis, unstable (nontraumatic)

- **M93.041** Acute slipped upper femoral epiphysis, unstable (nontraumatic), right hip
- **M93.042** Acute slipped upper femoral epiphysis, unstable (nontraumatic), left hip
- **M93.043** Acute slipped upper femoral epiphysis, unstable (nontraumatic), unspecified hip
- **M93.044** Acute slipped upper femoral epiphysis, unstable (nontraumatic), bilateral hips

M93.05 Acute on chronic slipped upper femoral epiphysis, unstable (nontraumatic)

- **M93.051** Acute on chronic slipped upper femoral epiphysis, unstable (nontraumatic), right hip
- **M93.052** Acute on chronic slipped upper femoral epiphysis, unstable (nontraumatic), left hip
- **M93.053** Acute on chronic slipped upper femoral epiphysis, unstable (nontraumatic), unspecified hip
- **M93.054** Acute on chronic slipped upper femoral epiphysis, unstable (nontraumatic), bilateral hips

M93.06 Acute slipped upper femoral epiphysis, unspecified stability (nontraumatic)

- **M93.061** Acute slipped upper femoral epiphysis, unspecified stability (nontraumatic), right hip
- **M93.062** Acute slipped upper femoral epiphysis, unspecified stability (nontraumatic), left hip
- **M93.063** Acute slipped upper femoral epiphysis, unspecified stability (nontraumatic), unspecified hip
- **M93.064** Acute slipped upper femoral epiphysis, unspecified stability (nontraumatic), bilateral hips

M93.07 Acute on chronic slipped upper femoral epiphysis, unspecified stability (nontraumatic)

- **M93.071** Acute on chronic slipped upper femoral epiphysis, unspecified stability (nontraumatic), right hip
- **M93.072** Acute on chronic slipped upper femoral epiphysis, unspecified stability (nontraumatic), left hip
- **M93.073** Acute on chronic slipped upper femoral epiphysis, unspecified stability (nontraumatic), unspecified hip
- **M93.074** Acute on chronic slipped upper femoral epiphysis, unspecified stability (nontraumatic), bilateral hips

M93.1 Kienbock's disease of adults A

Adult osteochondrosis of carpal lunates

M93.2 Osteochondritis dissecans

DEF: Avascular necrosis caused by lack of blood flow to the bone and cartilage of a joint causing the bone to die. This can result in splinters or pieces of cartilage breaking off in the joint.

M93.20 Osteochondritis dissecans of unspecified site

M93.21 Osteochondritis dissecans of shoulder

- **M93.211** Osteochondritis dissecans, right shoulder
- **M93.212** Osteochondritis dissecans, left shoulder
- **M93.219** Osteochondritis dissecans, unspecified shoulder

M93.22 Osteochondritis dissecans of elbow

- **M93.221** Osteochondritis dissecans, right elbow
- **M93.222** Osteochondritis dissecans, left elbow
- **M93.229** Osteochondritis dissecans, unspecified elbow

M93.23 Osteochondritis dissecans of wrist

- **M93.231** Osteochondritis dissecans, right wrist
- **M93.232** Osteochondritis dissecans, left wrist
- **M93.239** Osteochondritis dissecans, unspecified wrist

M93.24 Osteochondritis dissecans of joints of hand

- **M93.241** Osteochondritis dissecans, joints of right hand
- **M93.242** Osteochondritis dissecans, joints of left hand
- **M93.249** Osteochondritis dissecans, joints of unspecified hand

M93.25 Osteochondritis dissecans of hip

- **M93.251** Osteochondritis dissecans, right hip
- **M93.252** Osteochondritis dissecans, left hip
- **M93.259** Osteochondritis dissecans, unspecified hip

M93.26 Osteochondritis dissecans knee

- **M93.261** Osteochondritis dissecans, right knee
- **M93.262** Osteochondritis dissecans, left knee
- **M93.269** Osteochondritis dissecans, unspecified knee

M93.27 Osteochondritis dissecans of ankle and joints of foot

- **M93.271** Osteochondritis dissecans, right ankle and joints of right foot
- **M93.272** Osteochondritis dissecans, left ankle and joints of left foot
- **M93.279** Osteochondritis dissecans, unspecified ankle and joints of foot

M93.28 Osteochondritis dissecans other site

M93.29 Osteochondritis dissecans multiple sites

M93.8 Other specified osteochondropathies

M93.80 Other specified osteochondropathies of unspecified site

M93.81 Other specified osteochondropathies of shoulder

- **M93.811** Other specified osteochondropathies, right shoulder
- **M93.812** Other specified osteochondropathies, left shoulder
- **M93.819** Other specified osteochondropathies, unspecified shoulder

Chapter 13. Diseases of the Musculoskeletal System and Connective Tissue
M93–M93.819

6th M93.82 Other specified osteochondropathies of upper arm
M93.821 Other specified osteochondropathies, right upper arm
M93.822 Other specified osteochondropathies, left upper arm
M93.829 Other specified osteochondropathies, unspecified upper arm
6th M93.83 Other specified osteochondropathies of forearm
M93.831 Other specified osteochondropathies, right forearm
M93.832 Other specified osteochondropathies, left forearm
M93.839 Other specified osteochondropathies, unspecified forearm
6th M93.84 Other specified osteochondropathies of hand
M93.841 Other specified osteochondropathies, right hand
M93.842 Other specified osteochondropathies, left hand
M93.849 Other specified osteochondropathies, unspecified hand
6th M93.85 Other specified osteochondropathies of thigh
M93.851 Other specified osteochondropathies, right thigh
M93.852 Other specified osteochondropathies, left thigh
M93.859 Other specified osteochondropathies, unspecified thigh
6th M93.86 Other specified osteochondropathies lower leg
M93.861 Other specified osteochondropathies, right lower leg
M93.862 Other specified osteochondropathies, left lower leg
M93.869 Other specified osteochondropathies, unspecified lower leg
6th M93.87 Other specified osteochondropathies of ankle and foot
M93.871 Other specified osteochondropathies, right ankle and foot
M93.872 Other specified osteochondropathies, left ankle and foot
M93.879 Other specified osteochondropathies, unspecified ankle and foot
M93.88 Other specified osteochondropathies other site
M93.89 Other specified osteochondropathies multiple sites
5th M93.9 Osteochondropathy, unspecified
Apophysitis NOS
Epiphysitis NOS
Osteochondritis NOS
Osteochondrosis NOS
M93.9Ø Osteochondropathy, unspecified of unspecified site
6th M93.91 Osteochondropathy, unspecified of shoulder
M93.911 Osteochondropathy, unspecified, right shoulder
M93.912 Osteochondropathy, unspecified, left shoulder
M93.919 Osteochondropathy, unspecified, unspecified shoulder
6th M93.92 Osteochondropathy, unspecified of upper arm
M93.921 Osteochondropathy, unspecified, right upper arm
M93.922 Osteochondropathy, unspecified, left upper arm
M93.929 Osteochondropathy, unspecified, unspecified upper arm
6th M93.93 Osteochondropathy, unspecified of forearm
M93.931 Osteochondropathy, unspecified, right forearm
M93.932 Osteochondropathy, unspecified, left forearm
M93.939 Osteochondropathy, unspecified, unspecified forearm
6th M93.94 Osteochondropathy, unspecified of hand
M93.941 Osteochondropathy, unspecified, right hand
M93.942 Osteochondropathy, unspecified, left hand
M93.949 Osteochondropathy, unspecified, unspecified hand
6th M93.95 Osteochondropathy, unspecified of thigh
M93.951 Osteochondropathy, unspecified, right thigh
M93.952 Osteochondropathy, unspecified, left thigh
M93.959 Osteochondropathy, unspecified, unspecified thigh
6th M93.96 Osteochondropathy, unspecified lower leg
M93.961 Osteochondropathy, unspecified, right lower leg
M93.962 Osteochondropathy, unspecified, left lower leg
M93.969 Osteochondropathy, unspecified, unspecified lower leg
6th M93.97 Osteochondropathy, unspecified of ankle and foot
M93.971 Osteochondropathy, unspecified, right ankle and foot
M93.972 Osteochondropathy, unspecified, left ankle and foot
M93.979 Osteochondropathy, unspecified, unspecified ankle and foot
M93.98 Osteochondropathy, unspecified other site
M93.99 Osteochondropathy, unspecified multiple sites

4th M94 Other disorders of cartilage
M94.Ø Chondrocostal junction syndrome [Tietze]
Costochondritis
M94.1 Relapsing polychondritis
5th M94.2 Chondromalacia
EXCLUDES 1 *chondromalacia patellae (M22.4)*
M94.2Ø Chondromalacia, unspecified site
6th M94.21 Chondromalacia, shoulder
M94.211 Chondromalacia, right shoulder
M94.212 Chondromalacia, left shoulder
M94.219 Chondromalacia, unspecified shoulder
6th M94.22 Chondromalacia, elbow
M94.221 Chondromalacia, right elbow
M94.222 Chondromalacia, left elbow
M94.229 Chondromalacia, unspecified elbow
6th M94.23 Chondromalacia, wrist
M94.231 Chondromalacia, right wrist
M94.232 Chondromalacia, left wrist
M94.239 Chondromalacia, unspecified wrist
6th M94.24 Chondromalacia, joints of hand
M94.241 Chondromalacia, joints of right hand
M94.242 Chondromalacia, joints of left hand
M94.249 Chondromalacia, joints of unspecified hand
6th M94.25 Chondromalacia, hip
M94.251 Chondromalacia, right hip
M94.252 Chondromalacia, left hip
M94.259 Chondromalacia, unspecified hip
6th M94.26 Chondromalacia, knee
M94.261 Chondromalacia, right knee
M94.262 Chondromalacia, left knee
M94.269 Chondromalacia, unspecified knee
6th M94.27 Chondromalacia, ankle and joints of foot
M94.271 Chondromalacia, right ankle and joints of right foot
M94.272 Chondromalacia, left ankle and joints of left foot
M94.279 Chondromalacia, unspecified ankle and joints of foot
M94.28 Chondromalacia, other site
M94.29 Chondromalacia, multiple sites
5th M94.3 Chondrolysis
Code first any associated slipped upper femoral epiphysis (nontraumatic) (M93.Ø-)
6th M94.35 Chondrolysis, hip
M94.351 Chondrolysis, right hip
M94.352 Chondrolysis, left hip
M94.359 Chondrolysis, unspecified hip
5th M94.8 Other specified disorders of cartilage
6th M94.8X Other specified disorders of cartilage
M94.8XØ Other specified disorders of cartilage, multiple sites

M94.8X1 Other specified disorders of cartilage, shoulder

M94.8X2 Other specified disorders of cartilage, upper arm

M94.8X3 Other specified disorders of cartilage, forearm

M94.8X4 Other specified disorders of cartilage, hand

M94.8X5 Other specified disorders of cartilage, thigh

M94.8X6 Other specified disorders of cartilage, lower leg

M94.8X7 Other specified disorders of cartilage, ankle and foot

M94.8X8 Other specified disorders of cartilage, other site

M94.8X9 Other specified disorders of cartilage, unspecified sites

M94.9 Disorder of cartilage, unspecified

Other disorders of the musculoskeletal system and connective tissue (M95)

✓4th **M95 Other acquired deformities of musculoskeletal system and connective tissue**

EXCLUDES 2 *acquired absence of limbs and organs (Z89-Z90)*
acquired deformities of limbs (M20-M21)
congenital malformations and deformations of the musculoskeletal system (Q65-Q79)
deforming dorsopathies (M40-M43)
dentofacial anomalies [including malocclusion] (M26.-)
postprocedural musculoskeletal disorders (M96.-)

M95.0 Acquired deformity of nose
EXCLUDES 2 *deviated nasal septum (J34.2)*

✓5th M95.1 Cauliflower ear
EXCLUDES 2 *other acquired deformities of ear (H61.1)*
DEF: Acquired deformity of the external ear due to injury or subsequent perichondritis.

M95.10 Cauliflower ear, unspecified ear

M95.11 Cauliflower ear, right ear

M95.12 Cauliflower ear, left ear

M95.2 Other acquired deformity of head
AHA: 2023,1Q,30; 2022,1Q,34

M95.3 Acquired deformity of neck

M95.4 Acquired deformity of chest and rib
AHA: 2022,2Q,14; 2014,4Q,26-27

M95.5 Acquired deformity of pelvis
EXCLUDES 1 *maternal care for known or suspected disproportion (O33.-)*

M95.8 Other specified acquired deformities of musculoskeletal system

M95.9 Acquired deformity of musculoskeletal system, unspecified

Intraoperative and postprocedural complications and disorders of musculoskeletal system, not elsewhere classified (M96)

✓4th **M96 Intraoperative and postprocedural complications and disorders of musculoskeletal system, not elsewhere classified**

EXCLUDES 2 *arthropathy following intestinal bypass (M02.0-)*
complications of internal orthopedic prosthetic devices, implants and grafts (T84.-)
disorders associated with osteoporosis (M80)
periprosthetic fracture around internal prosthetic joint (M97.-)
presence of functional implants and other devices (Z96-Z97)

M96.0 Pseudarthrosis after fusion or arthrodesis CC

M96.1 Postlaminectomy syndrome, not elsewhere classified

M96.2 Postradiation kyphosis

M96.3 Postlaminectomy kyphosis

M96.4 Postsurgical lordosis

M96.5 Postradiation scoliosis

✓5th M96.6 Fracture of bone following insertion of orthopedic implant, joint prosthesis, or bone plate
Intraoperative fracture of bone during insertion of orthopedic implant, joint prosthesis, or bone plate
EXCLUDES 2 *complication of internal orthopedic devices, implants or grafts (T84.-)*

✓6th M96.62 Fracture of humerus following insertion of orthopedic implant, joint prosthesis, or bone plate

M96.621 Fracture of humerus following insertion of orthopedic implant, joint prosthesis, or bone plate, right arm CC HCC

M96.622 Fracture of humerus following insertion of orthopedic implant, joint prosthesis, or bone plate, left arm CC HCC

M96.629 Fracture of humerus following insertion of orthopedic implant, joint prosthesis, or bone plate, unspecified arm CC UNS HCC

✓6th M96.63 Fracture of radius or ulna following insertion of orthopedic implant, joint prosthesis, or bone plate

M96.631 Fracture of radius or ulna following insertion of orthopedic implant, joint prosthesis, or bone plate, right arm CC HCC

M96.632 Fracture of radius or ulna following insertion of orthopedic implant, joint prosthesis, or bone plate, left arm CC HCC

M96.639 Fracture of radius or ulna following insertion of orthopedic implant, joint prosthesis, or bone plate, unspecified arm CC UNS HCC

M96.65 Fracture of pelvis following insertion of orthopedic implant, joint prosthesis, or bone plate CC HCC

✓6th M96.66 Fracture of femur following insertion of orthopedic implant, joint prosthesis, or bone plate

M96.661 Fracture of femur following insertion of orthopedic implant, joint prosthesis, or bone plate, right leg CC HCC

M96.662 Fracture of femur following insertion of orthopedic implant, joint prosthesis, or bone plate, left leg CC HCC

M96.669 Fracture of femur following insertion of orthopedic implant, joint prosthesis, or bone plate, unspecified leg CC UNS HCC

✓6th M96.67 Fracture of tibia or fibula following insertion of orthopedic implant, joint prosthesis, or bone plate

M96.671 Fracture of tibia or fibula following insertion of orthopedic implant, joint prosthesis, or bone plate, right leg CC HCC

M96.672 Fracture of tibia or fibula following insertion of orthopedic implant, joint prosthesis, or bone plate, left leg CC HCC

M96.679 Fracture of tibia or fibula following insertion of orthopedic implant, joint prosthesis, or bone plate, unspecified leg CC UNS HCC

M96.69 Fracture of other bone following insertion of orthopedic implant, joint prosthesis, or bone plate CC HCC

✓5th M96.8 Other intraoperative and postprocedural complications and disorders of musculoskeletal system, not elsewhere classified
AHA: 2016,4Q,9-10

✓6th M96.81 Intraoperative hemorrhage and hematoma of a musculoskeletal structure complicating a procedure
EXCLUDES 1 *intraoperative hemorrhage and hematoma of a musculoskeletal structure due to accidental puncture and laceration during a procedure (M96.82-)*

M96.810 Intraoperative hemorrhage and hematoma of a musculoskeletal structure complicating a musculoskeletal system procedure CC

M96.811 Intraoperative hemorrhage and hematoma of a musculoskeletal structure complicating other procedure CC

6th **M96.82 Accidental puncture and laceration of a musculoskeletal structure during a procedure**

M96.820 Accidental puncture and laceration of a musculoskeletal structure during a musculoskeletal system procedure CC

M96.821 Accidental puncture and laceration of a musculoskeletal structure during other procedure CC

6th **M96.83 Postprocedural hemorrhage of a musculoskeletal structure following a procedure**

M96.830 Postprocedural hemorrhage of a musculoskeletal structure following a musculoskeletal system procedure CC

M96.831 Postprocedural hemorrhage of a musculoskeletal structure following other procedure CC

6th **M96.84 Postprocedural hematoma and seroma of a musculoskeletal structure following a procedure**

M96.840 Postprocedural hematoma of a musculoskeletal structure following a musculoskeletal system procedure CC

M96.841 Postprocedural hematoma of a musculoskeletal structure following other procedure CC

AHA: 2016,4Q,10

M96.842 Postprocedural seroma of a musculoskeletal structure following a musculoskeletal system procedure CC

M96.843 Postprocedural seroma of a musculoskeletal structure following other procedure CC

AHA: 2023,2Q,13; 2018,3Q,6

M96.89 Other intraoperative and postprocedural complications and disorders of the musculoskeletal system CC

Instability of joint secondary to removal of joint prosthesis

Use additional code, if applicable, to further specify disorder

AHA: 2023,2Q,14; 2022,2Q,14; 2021,1Q,5

5th **M96.A Fracture of ribs, sternum and thorax associated with compression of the chest and cardiopulmonary resuscitation**

AHA: 2022,4Q,31-33

M96.A1 Fracture of sternum associated with chest compression and cardiopulmonary resuscitation CC

Fracture of xiphoid process associated with chest compression and cardiopulmonary resuscitation

M96.A2 Fracture of one rib associated with chest compression and cardiopulmonary resuscitation CC

M96.A3 Multiple fractures of ribs associated with chest compression and cardiopulmonary resuscitation CC

AHA: 2022,4Q,32

M96.A4 Flail chest associated with chest compression and cardiopulmonary resuscitation MCC

M96.A9 Other fracture associated with chest compression and cardiopulmonary resuscitation CC

Periprosthetic fractures around internal prosthetic joint (M97)

4th **M97 Periprosthetic fracture around internal prosthetic joint**

▶Code first, if known, the specific type and cause of fracture, such as traumatic or pathological◀

EXCLUDES 2 *fracture of bone following insertion of orthopedic implant, joint prosthesis or bone plate (M96.6-)*
breakage (fracture) of prosthetic joint (T84.01-)

AHA: 2016,4Q,42-43

The appropriate 7th character is to be added to each code from category M97.
A initial encounter
D subsequent encounter
S sequela

5th **M97.0 Periprosthetic fracture around internal prosthetic hip joint**

AHA: 2018,1Q,21; 2016,4Q,42

x7th **M97.01 Periprosthetic fracture around internal prosthetic right hip joint** CC HCC

x7th **M97.02 Periprosthetic fracture around internal prosthetic left hip joint** CC HCC

5th **M97.1 Periprosthetic fracture around internal prosthetic knee joint**

x7th **M97.11 Periprosthetic fracture around internal prosthetic right knee joint** CC

x7th **M97.12 Periprosthetic fracture around internal prosthetic left knee joint** CC

5th **M97.2 Periprosthetic fracture around internal prosthetic ankle joint**

x7th **M97.21 Periprosthetic fracture around internal prosthetic right ankle joint** CC

x7th **M97.22 Periprosthetic fracture around internal prosthetic left ankle joint** CC

5th **M97.3 Periprosthetic fracture around internal prosthetic shoulder joint**

x7th **M97.31 Periprosthetic fracture around internal prosthetic right shoulder joint** CC

x7th **M97.32 Periprosthetic fracture around internal prosthetic left shoulder joint** CC

5th **M97.4 Periprosthetic fracture around internal prosthetic elbow joint**

x7th **M97.41 Periprosthetic fracture around internal prosthetic right elbow joint** CC

x7th **M97.42 Periprosthetic fracture around internal prosthetic left elbow joint** CC

x7th **M97.8 Periprosthetic fracture around other internal prosthetic joint** CC

Periprosthetic fracture around internal prosthetic finger joint
Periprosthetic fracture around internal prosthetic spinal joint
Periprosthetic fracture around internal prosthetic toe joint
Periprosthetic fracture around internal prosthetic wrist joint
Use additional code to identify the joint (Z96.6-)

x7th UNS **M97.9 Periprosthetic fracture around unspecified internal prosthetic joint** CC

Biomechanical lesions, not elsewhere classified (M99)

4th **M99 Biomechanical lesions, not elsewhere classified**

NOTE This category should not be used if the condition can be classified elsewhere.

DEF: Biomechanical lesion: Term used by osteopathic and chiropractic physicians to describe musculoskeletal conditions treated that are not more appropriately classified elsewhere.

5th **M99.0 Segmental and somatic dysfunction**

M99.00 Segmental and somatic dysfunction of head region

M99.01 Segmental and somatic dysfunction of cervical region

M99.02 Segmental and somatic dysfunction of thoracic region

M99.03 Segmental and somatic dysfunction of lumbar region

M99.04 Segmental and somatic dysfunction of sacral region

M99.05 Segmental and somatic dysfunction of pelvic region

M99.06 Segmental and somatic dysfunction of lower extremity

M99.07 Segmental and somatic dysfunction of upper extremity

M99.08 Segmental and somatic dysfunction of rib cage

M99.09 Segmental and somatic dysfunction of abdomen and other regions

5th **M99.1 Subluxation complex (vertebral)**

M99.10 Subluxation complex (vertebral) of head region CC HS

M99.11 Subluxation complex (vertebral) of cervical region CC HS

M99.12 Subluxation complex (vertebral) of thoracic region

M99.13 Subluxation complex (vertebral) of lumbar region

M99.14 Subluxation complex (vertebral) of sacral region

M99.15 Subluxation complex (vertebral) of pelvic region

M99.16 Subluxation complex (vertebral) of lower extremity

M99.17 Subluxation complex (vertebral) of upper extremity

M99.18 Subluxation complex (vertebral) of rib cage CC HS

M99.19 Subluxation complex (vertebral) of abdomen and other regions

5th **M99.2 Subluxation stenosis of neural canal**

M99.20 Subluxation stenosis of neural canal of head region

M99.21 Subluxation stenosis of neural canal of cervical region

M99.22 Subluxation stenosis of neural canal of thoracic region

M99.23 Subluxation stenosis of neural canal of lumbar region
M99.24 Subluxation stenosis of neural canal of sacral region
M99.25 Subluxation stenosis of neural canal of pelvic region
M99.26 Subluxation stenosis of neural canal of lower extremity
M99.27 Subluxation stenosis of neural canal of upper extremity
M99.28 Subluxation stenosis of neural canal of rib cage
M99.29 Subluxation stenosis of neural canal of abdomen and other regions

✓5th M99.3 Osseous stenosis of neural canal
M99.30 Osseous stenosis of neural canal of head region
M99.31 Osseous stenosis of neural canal of cervical region
M99.32 Osseous stenosis of neural canal of thoracic region
M99.33 Osseous stenosis of neural canal of lumbar region
M99.34 Osseous stenosis of neural canal of sacral region
M99.35 Osseous stenosis of neural canal of pelvic region
M99.36 Osseous stenosis of neural canal of lower extremity
M99.37 Osseous stenosis of neural canal of upper extremity
M99.38 Osseous stenosis of neural canal of rib cage
M99.39 Osseous stenosis of neural canal of abdomen and other regions

✓5th M99.4 Connective tissue stenosis of neural canal
M99.40 Connective tissue stenosis of neural canal of head region
M99.41 Connective tissue stenosis of neural canal of cervical region
M99.42 Connective tissue stenosis of neural canal of thoracic region
M99.43 Connective tissue stenosis of neural canal of lumbar region
M99.44 Connective tissue stenosis of neural canal of sacral region
M99.45 Connective tissue stenosis of neural canal of pelvic region
M99.46 Connective tissue stenosis of neural canal of lower extremity
M99.47 Connective tissue stenosis of neural canal of upper extremity
M99.48 Connective tissue stenosis of neural canal of rib cage
M99.49 Connective tissue stenosis of neural canal of abdomen and other regions

✓5th M99.5 Intervertebral disc stenosis of neural canal
M99.50 Intervertebral disc stenosis of neural canal of head region
M99.51 Intervertebral disc stenosis of neural canal of cervical region
M99.52 Intervertebral disc stenosis of neural canal of thoracic region
M99.53 Intervertebral disc stenosis of neural canal of lumbar region
M99.54 Intervertebral disc stenosis of neural canal of sacral region
M99.55 Intervertebral disc stenosis of neural canal of pelvic region
M99.56 Intervertebral disc stenosis of neural canal of lower extremity
M99.57 Intervertebral disc stenosis of neural canal of upper extremity
M99.58 Intervertebral disc stenosis of neural canal of rib cage
M99.59 Intervertebral disc stenosis of neural canal of abdomen and other regions

✓5th M99.6 Osseous and subluxation stenosis of intervertebral foramina
M99.60 Osseous and subluxation stenosis of intervertebral foramina of head region
M99.61 Osseous and subluxation stenosis of intervertebral foramina of cervical region
M99.62 Osseous and subluxation stenosis of intervertebral foramina of thoracic region
M99.63 Osseous and subluxation stenosis of intervertebral foramina of lumbar region
M99.64 Osseous and subluxation stenosis of intervertebral foramina of sacral region
M99.65 Osseous and subluxation stenosis of intervertebral foramina of pelvic region
M99.66 Osseous and subluxation stenosis of intervertebral foramina of lower extremity
M99.67 Osseous and subluxation stenosis of intervertebral foramina of upper extremity
M99.68 Osseous and subluxation stenosis of intervertebral foramina of rib cage
M99.69 Osseous and subluxation stenosis of intervertebral foramina of abdomen and other regions

✓5th M99.7 Connective tissue and disc stenosis of intervertebral foramina
M99.70 Connective tissue and disc stenosis of intervertebral foramina of head region
M99.71 Connective tissue and disc stenosis of intervertebral foramina of cervical region
M99.72 Connective tissue and disc stenosis of intervertebral foramina of thoracic region
M99.73 Connective tissue and disc stenosis of intervertebral foramina of lumbar region
M99.74 Connective tissue and disc stenosis of intervertebral foramina of sacral region
M99.75 Connective tissue and disc stenosis of intervertebral foramina of pelvic region
M99.76 Connective tissue and disc stenosis of intervertebral foramina of lower extremity
M99.77 Connective tissue and disc stenosis of intervertebral foramina of upper extremity
M99.78 Connective tissue and disc stenosis of intervertebral foramina of rib cage
M99.79 Connective tissue and disc stenosis of intervertebral foramina of abdomen and other regions

✓5th M99.8 Other biomechanical lesions
M99.80 Other biomechanical lesions of head region
M99.81 Other biomechanical lesions of cervical region
M99.82 Other biomechanical lesions of thoracic region
M99.83 Other biomechanical lesions of lumbar region
M99.84 Other biomechanical lesions of sacral region
M99.85 Other biomechanical lesions of pelvic region
M99.86 Other biomechanical lesions of lower extremity
M99.87 Other biomechanical lesions of upper extremity
M99.88 Other biomechanical lesions of rib cage
M99.89 Other biomechanical lesions of abdomen and other regions

M99.9 Biomechanical lesion, unspecified

Chapter 14. Diseases of Genitourinary System (NØØ–N99)

Chapter-specific Guidelines with Coding Examples

The chapter-specific guidelines from the ICD-10-CM Official Guidelines for Coding and Reporting have been provided below. Along with these guidelines are coding examples, contained in the shaded boxes, that have been developed to help illustrate the coding and/or sequencing guidance found in these guidelines.

a. Chronic kidney disease

1) Stages of chronic kidney disease (CKD)

The ICD-10-CM classifies CKD based on severity. The severity of CKD is designated by stages 1-5. Stage 2, code N18.2, equates to mild CKD; stage 3, codes N18.3Ø-N18.32, equate to moderate CKD; and stage 4, code N18.4, equates to severe CKD. Code N18.6, End stage renal disease (ESRD), is assigned when the provider has documented end-stage renal disease (ESRD).

If both a stage of CKD and ESRD are documented, assign code N18.6 only.

Stage 5 chronic kidney disease with ESRD requiring chronic dialysis

N18.6 **End stage renal disease**

Z99.2 **Dependence on renal dialysis**

Explanation: The diagnostic statement indicates the patient has chronic kidney disease, documented both as stage 5 and as ESRD requiring chronic dialysis. Code N18.6 End stage renal disease (ESRD), is assigned when the provider has documented end-stage-renal disease (ESRD). If both a stage of CKD and ESRD are documented, assign code N18.6 only.

2) Chronic kidney disease and kidney transplant status

Patients who have undergone kidney transplant may still have some form of chronic kidney disease (CKD) because the kidney transplant may not fully restore kidney function. Therefore, the presence of CKD alone does not constitute a transplant complication. Assign the appropriate N18 code for the patient's stage of CKD and code Z94.Ø, Kidney transplant status. If a transplant complication such as failure or rejection or other transplant complication is documented, see section I.C.19.g for information on coding complications of a kidney transplant. If the documentation is unclear as to whether the patient has a complication of the transplant, query the provider.

Patient with residual chronic kidney disease stage 1 after kidney transplant

N18.1 **Chronic kidney disease, stage 1**

Z94.Ø **Kidney transplant status**

Explanation: Patients who have undergone kidney transplant may still have some form of chronic kidney disease (CKD) because the kidney transplant may not fully restore kidney function. The presence of CKD alone does not constitute a transplant complication. Assign the appropriate N18 code for the patient's stage of CKD and code Z94.Ø Kidney transplant status.

3) Chronic kidney disease with other conditions

Patients with CKD may also suffer from other serious conditions, most commonly diabetes mellitus and hypertension. The sequencing of the CKD code in relationship to codes for other contributing conditions is based on the conventions in the Tabular List.

See I.C.9. Hypertensive chronic kidney disease.

See I.C.19. Chronic kidney disease and kidney transplant complications.

Type 1 diabetic chronic kidney disease, stage 2

E1Ø.22 **Type 1 diabetes mellitus with diabetic chronic kidney disease**

N18.2 **Chronic kidney disease, stage 2 (mild)**

Explanation: Patients with CKD may also suffer from other serious conditions such as diabetes mellitus. The sequencing of the CKD code in relationship to codes for other contributing conditions is based on the conventions in the Tabular List. Diabetic CKD code E1Ø.22 includes an instructional note to "Use additional code to identify stage of chronic kidney disease (N18.1–N18.6)," thus providing sequencing direction.

Chapter 14. Diseases of the Genitourinary System (NØØ-N99)

EXCLUDES 2 *certain conditions originating in the perinatal period (PØ4-P96)*
certain infectious and parasitic diseases (AØØ-B99)
complications of pregnancy, childbirth and the puerperium (OØØ-O9A)
congenital malformations, deformations and chromosomal abnormalities (QØØ-Q99)
endocrine, nutritional and metabolic diseases (EØØ-E88)
injury, poisoning and certain other consequences of external causes (SØØ-T88)
neoplasms (CØØ-D49)
symptoms, signs and abnormal clinical and laboratory findings, not elsewhere classified (RØØ-R94)

This chapter contains the following blocks:

NØØ-NØ8 Glomerular diseases
N1Ø-N16 Renal tubulo-interstitial diseases
N17-N19 Acute kidney failure and chronic kidney disease
N2Ø-N23 Urolithiasis
N25-N29 Other disorders of kidney and ureter
N3Ø-N39 Other diseases of the urinary system
N4Ø-N53 Diseases of male genital organs
N6Ø-N65 Disorders of breast
N7Ø-N77 Inflammatory diseases of female pelvic organs
N8Ø-N98 Noninflammatory disorders of female genital tract
N99 Intraoperative and postprocedural complications and disorders of genitourinary system, not elsewhere classified

Glomerular diseases (NØØ-NØ8)

Code also any associated kidney failure (N17-N19).

EXCLUDES 1 *hypertensive chronic kidney disease (I12.-)*

AHA: 2020,4Q,34-35

DEF: Glomeruli: Clusters of microscopic blood vessels located within the kidneys containing small pores through which waste products are filtered from the blood and urine is formed.

DEF: Glomerulonephritis: Disease of the kidney with diffuse inflammation of the capillary loops of the glomeruli.

✓4th **NØØ Acute nephritic syndrome**

INCLUDES acute glomerular disease
acute glomerulonephritis
acute nephritis

EXCLUDES 1 *acute tubulo-interstitial nephritis (N1Ø)*
nephritic syndrome NOS (NØ5.-)

AHA: 2021,1Q,23

NØØ.Ø Acute nephritic syndrome with minor glomerular abnormality MCC
Acute nephritic syndrome with minimal change lesion

NØØ.1 Acute nephritic syndrome with focal and segmental glomerular lesions MCC
Acute nephritic syndrome with focal and segmental hyalinosis
Acute nephritic syndrome with focal and segmental sclerosis
Acute nephritic syndrome with focal glomerulonephritis

NØØ.2 Acute nephritic syndrome with diffuse membranous glomerulonephritis MCC

NØØ.3 Acute nephritic syndrome with diffuse mesangial proliferative glomerulonephritis MCC

NØØ.4 Acute nephritic syndrome with diffuse endocapillary proliferative glomerulonephritis MCC

NØØ.5 Acute nephritic syndrome with diffuse mesangiocapillary glomerulonephritis MCC
Acute nephritic syndrome with membranoproliferative glomerulonephritis, types 1 and 3, or NOS
EXCLUDES 1 *acute nephritic syndrome with C3 glomerulonephritis (NØØ.A)*
acute nephritic syndrome with C3 glomerulopathy (NØØ.A)

NØØ.6 Acute nephritic syndrome with dense deposit disease MCC
Acute nephritic syndrome with C3 glomerulopathy with dense deposit disease
Acute nephritic syndrome with membranoproliferative glomerulonephritis, type 2

NØØ.7 Acute nephritic syndrome with diffuse crescentic glomerulonephritis MCC
Acute nephritic syndrome with extracapillary glomerulonephritis

NØØ.8 Acute nephritic syndrome with other morphologic changes MCC
Acute nephritic syndrome with proliferative glomerulonephritis NOS

NØØ.9 Acute nephritic syndrome with unspecified morphologic changes MCC

NØØ.A Acute nephritic syndrome with C3 glomerulonephritis MCC
Acute nephritic syndrome with C3 glomerulopathy, NOS
EXCLUDES 1 *acute nephritic syndrome (with C3 glomerulopathy) with dense deposit disease (NØØ.6)*

✓4th **NØ1 Rapidly progressive nephritic syndrome**

INCLUDES rapidly progressive glomerular disease
rapidly progressive glomerulonephritis
rapidly progressive nephritis

EXCLUDES 1 *nephritic syndrome NOS (NØ5.-)*

AHA: 2021,1Q,23

NØ1.Ø Rapidly progressive nephritic syndrome with minor glomerular abnormality MCC
Rapidly progressive nephritic syndrome with minimal change lesion

NØ1.1 Rapidly progressive nephritic syndrome with focal and segmental glomerular lesions MCC
Rapidly progressive nephritic syndrome with focal and segmental hyalinosis
Rapidly progressive nephritic syndrome with focal and segmental sclerosis
Rapidly progressive nephritic syndrome with focal glomerulonephritis

NØ1.2 Rapidly progressive nephritic syndrome with diffuse membranous glomerulonephritis MCC

NØ1.3 Rapidly progressive nephritic syndrome with diffuse mesangial proliferative glomerulonephritis MCC

NØ1.4 Rapidly progressive nephritic syndrome with diffuse endocapillary proliferative glomerulonephritis MCC

NØ1.5 Rapidly progressive nephritic syndrome with diffuse mesangiocapillary glomerulonephritis MCC
Rapidly progressive nephritic syndrome with membranoproliferative glomerulonephritis, types 1 and 3, or NOS
EXCLUDES 1 *rapidly progressive nephritic syndrome with C3 glomerulonephritis (NØ1.A)*
rapidly progressive nephritic syndrome with C3 glomerulopathy (NØ1.A)

NØ1.6 Rapidly progressive nephritic syndrome with dense deposit disease MCC
Rapidly progressive nephritic syndrome with C3 glomerulopathy with dense deposit disease
Rapidly progressive nephritic syndrome with membranoproliferative glomerulonephritis, type 2

NØ1.7 Rapidly progressive nephritic syndrome with diffuse crescentic glomerulonephritis MCC
Rapidly progressive nephritic syndrome with extracapillary glomerulonephritis

NØ1.8 Rapidly progressive nephritic syndrome with other morphologic changes MCC
Rapidly progressive nephritic syndrome with proliferative glomerulonephritis NOS

NØ1.9 Rapidly progressive nephritic syndrome with unspecified morphologic changes MCC

NØ1.A Rapidly progressive nephritic syndrome with C3 glomerulonephritis MCC
Rapidly progressive nephritic syndrome with C3 glomerulopathy, NOS
EXCLUDES 1 *rapidly progressive nephritic syndrome (with C3 glomerulopathy) with dense deposit disease (NØ1.6)*

✓4th **NØ2 Recurrent and persistent hematuria**

EXCLUDES 1 *acute cystitis with hematuria (N3Ø.Ø1)*
hematuria NOS (R31.9)
hematuria not associated with specified morphologic lesions (R31.-)

NØ2.Ø Recurrent and persistent hematuria with minor glomerular abnormality CC
Recurrent and persistent hematuria with minimal change lesion

NØ2.1 Recurrent and persistent hematuria with focal and segmental glomerular lesions CC
Recurrent and persistent hematuria with focal and segmental hyalinosis
Recurrent and persistent hematuria with focal and segmental sclerosis
Recurrent and persistent hematuria with focal glomerulonephritis

NØ2.2 Recurrent and persistent hematuria with diffuse membranous glomerulonephritis CC

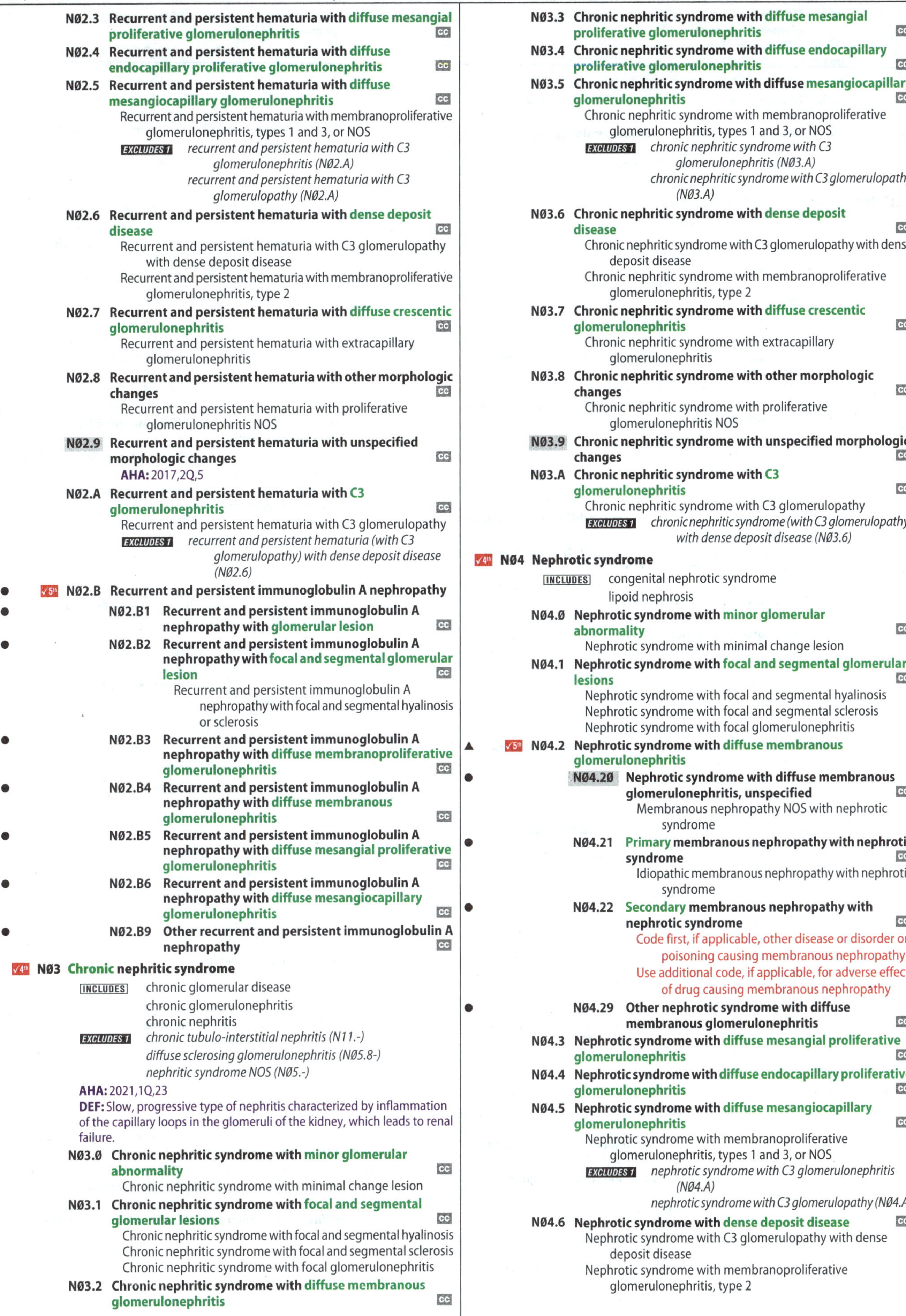

N02.3 Recurrent and persistent hematuria with diffuse mesangial proliferative glomerulonephritis CC

N02.4 Recurrent and persistent hematuria with diffuse endocapillary proliferative glomerulonephritis CC

N02.5 Recurrent and persistent hematuria with diffuse mesangiocapillary glomerulonephritis CC

Recurrent and persistent hematuria with membranoproliferative glomerulonephritis, types 1 and 3, or NOS

EXCLUDES 1 *recurrent and persistent hematuria with C3 glomerulonephritis (N02.A)*
recurrent and persistent hematuria with C3 glomerulopathy (N02.A)

N02.6 Recurrent and persistent hematuria with dense deposit disease CC

Recurrent and persistent hematuria with C3 glomerulopathy with dense deposit disease
Recurrent and persistent hematuria with membranoproliferative glomerulonephritis, type 2

N02.7 Recurrent and persistent hematuria with diffuse crescentic glomerulonephritis CC

Recurrent and persistent hematuria with extracapillary glomerulonephritis

N02.8 Recurrent and persistent hematuria with other morphologic changes CC

Recurrent and persistent hematuria with proliferative glomerulonephritis NOS

N02.9 Recurrent and persistent hematuria with unspecified morphologic changes CC

AHA: 2017,2Q,5

N02.A Recurrent and persistent hematuria with C3 glomerulonephritis CC

Recurrent and persistent hematuria with C3 glomerulopathy

EXCLUDES 1 *recurrent and persistent hematuria (with C3 glomerulopathy) with dense deposit disease (N02.6)*

● ✓5th **N02.B Recurrent and persistent immunoglobulin A nephropathy**

● **N02.B1 Recurrent and persistent immunoglobulin A nephropathy with glomerular lesion** CC

● **N02.B2 Recurrent and persistent immunoglobulin A nephropathy with focal and segmental glomerular lesion** CC

Recurrent and persistent immunoglobulin A nephropathy with focal and segmental hyalinosis or sclerosis

● **N02.B3 Recurrent and persistent immunoglobulin A nephropathy with diffuse membranoproliferative glomerulonephritis** CC

● **N02.B4 Recurrent and persistent immunoglobulin A nephropathy with diffuse membranous glomerulonephritis** CC

● **N02.B5 Recurrent and persistent immunoglobulin A nephropathy with diffuse mesangial proliferative glomerulonephritis** CC

● **N02.B6 Recurrent and persistent immunoglobulin A nephropathy with diffuse mesangiocapillary glomerulonephritis** CC

● **N02.B9 Other recurrent and persistent immunoglobulin A nephropathy** CC

✓4th **N03 Chronic nephritic syndrome**

INCLUDES chronic glomerular disease
chronic glomerulonephritis
chronic nephritis

EXCLUDES 1 *chronic tubulo-interstitial nephritis (N11.-)*
diffuse sclerosing glomerulonephritis (N05.8-)
nephritic syndrome NOS (N05.-)

AHA: 2021,1Q,23

DEF: Slow, progressive type of nephritis characterized by inflammation of the capillary loops in the glomeruli of the kidney, which leads to renal failure.

N03.0 Chronic nephritic syndrome with minor glomerular abnormality CC

Chronic nephritic syndrome with minimal change lesion

N03.1 Chronic nephritic syndrome with focal and segmental glomerular lesions CC

Chronic nephritic syndrome with focal and segmental hyalinosis
Chronic nephritic syndrome with focal and segmental sclerosis
Chronic nephritic syndrome with focal glomerulonephritis

N03.2 Chronic nephritic syndrome with diffuse membranous glomerulonephritis CC

N03.3 Chronic nephritic syndrome with diffuse mesangial proliferative glomerulonephritis CC

N03.4 Chronic nephritic syndrome with diffuse endocapillary proliferative glomerulonephritis CC

N03.5 Chronic nephritic syndrome with diffuse mesangiocapillary glomerulonephritis CC

Chronic nephritic syndrome with membranoproliferative glomerulonephritis, types 1 and 3, or NOS

EXCLUDES 1 *chronic nephritic syndrome with C3 glomerulonephritis (N03.A)*
chronic nephritic syndrome with C3 glomerulopathy (N03.A)

N03.6 Chronic nephritic syndrome with dense deposit disease CC

Chronic nephritic syndrome with C3 glomerulopathy with dense deposit disease
Chronic nephritic syndrome with membranoproliferative glomerulonephritis, type 2

N03.7 Chronic nephritic syndrome with diffuse crescentic glomerulonephritis CC

Chronic nephritic syndrome with extracapillary glomerulonephritis

N03.8 Chronic nephritic syndrome with other morphologic changes CC

Chronic nephritic syndrome with proliferative glomerulonephritis NOS

N03.9 Chronic nephritic syndrome with unspecified morphologic changes CC

N03.A Chronic nephritic syndrome with C3 glomerulonephritis CC

Chronic nephritic syndrome with C3 glomerulopathy

EXCLUDES 1 *chronic nephritic syndrome (with C3 glomerulopathy) with dense deposit disease (N03.6)*

✓4th **N04 Nephrotic syndrome**

INCLUDES congenital nephrotic syndrome
lipoid nephrosis

N04.0 Nephrotic syndrome with minor glomerular abnormality CC

Nephrotic syndrome with minimal change lesion

N04.1 Nephrotic syndrome with focal and segmental glomerular lesions CC

Nephrotic syndrome with focal and segmental hyalinosis
Nephrotic syndrome with focal and segmental sclerosis
Nephrotic syndrome with focal glomerulonephritis

▲ ✓5th **N04.2 Nephrotic syndrome with diffuse membranous glomerulonephritis**

● **N04.20 Nephrotic syndrome with diffuse membranous glomerulonephritis, unspecified** CC

Membranous nephropathy NOS with nephrotic syndrome

● **N04.21 Primary membranous nephropathy with nephrotic syndrome** CC

Idiopathic membranous nephropathy with nephrotic syndrome

● **N04.22 Secondary membranous nephropathy with nephrotic syndrome** CC

Code first, if applicable, other disease or disorder or poisoning causing membranous nephropathy
Use additional code, if applicable, for adverse effect of drug causing membranous nephropathy

● **N04.29 Other nephrotic syndrome with diffuse membranous glomerulonephritis** CC

N04.3 Nephrotic syndrome with diffuse mesangial proliferative glomerulonephritis CC

N04.4 Nephrotic syndrome with diffuse endocapillary proliferative glomerulonephritis CC

N04.5 Nephrotic syndrome with diffuse mesangiocapillary glomerulonephritis CC

Nephrotic syndrome with membranoproliferative glomerulonephritis, types 1 and 3, or NOS

EXCLUDES 1 *nephrotic syndrome with C3 glomerulonephritis (N04.A)*
nephrotic syndrome with C3 glomerulopathy (N04.A)

N04.6 Nephrotic syndrome with dense deposit disease CC

Nephrotic syndrome with C3 glomerulopathy with dense deposit disease
Nephrotic syndrome with membranoproliferative glomerulonephritis, type 2

NØ4.7 Nephrotic syndrome with diffuse crescentic glomerulonephritis CC
Nephrotic syndrome with extracapillary glomerulonephritis

NØ4.8 Nephrotic syndrome with other morphologic changes CC
Nephrotic syndrome with proliferative glomerulonephritis NOS

NØ4.9 Nephrotic syndrome with unspecified morphologic changes CC

NØ4.A Nephrotic syndrome with C3 glomerulonephritis CC
Nephrotic syndrome with C3 glomerulopathy
EXCLUDES 1 *nephrotic syndrome (with C3 glomerulopathy) with dense deposit disease (NØ4.6)*

NØ5 Unspecified nephritic syndrome
INCLUDES glomerular disease NOS
glomerulonephritis NOS
nephritis NOS
nephropathy NOS and renal disease NOS with morphological lesion specified in .Ø-.8
EXCLUDES 1 *nephropathy NOS with no stated morphological lesion (N28.9)*
renal disease NOS with no stated morphological lesion (N28.9)
tubulo-interstitial nephritis NOS (N12)

NØ5.Ø Unspecified nephritic syndrome with minor glomerular abnormality
Unspecified nephritic syndrome with minimal change lesion

NØ5.1 Unspecified nephritic syndrome with focal and segmental glomerular lesions
Unspecified nephritic syndrome with focal and segmental hyalinosis
Unspecified nephritic syndrome with focal and segmental sclerosis
Unspecified nephritic syndrome with focal glomerulonephritis

NØ5.2 Unspecified nephritic syndrome with diffuse membranous glomerulonephritis CC

NØ5.3 Unspecified nephritic syndrome with diffuse mesangial proliferative glomerulonephritis CC

NØ5.4 Unspecified nephritic syndrome with diffuse endocapillary proliferative glomerulonephritis CC

NØ5.5 Unspecified nephritic syndrome with diffuse mesangiocapillary glomerulonephritis CC
Unspecified nephritic syndrome with membranoproliferative glomerulonephritis, types 1 and 3, or NOS
EXCLUDES 1 *unspecified nephritic syndrome with C3 glomerulonephritis (NØ5.A)*
unspecified nephritic syndrome with C3 glomerulopathy (NØ5.A)

NØ5.6 Unspecified nephritic syndrome with dense deposit disease
Unspecified nephritic syndrome with C3 glomerulopathy with dense deposit disease
Unspecified nephritic syndrome with membranoproliferative glomerulonephritis, type 2

NØ5.7 Unspecified nephritic syndrome with diffuse crescentic glomerulonephritis
Unspecified nephritic syndrome with extracapillary glomerulonephritis

NØ5.8 Unspecified nephritic syndrome with other morphologic changes
Unspecified nephritic syndrome with proliferative glomerulonephritis NOS

NØ5.9 Unspecified nephritic syndrome with unspecified morphologic changes

NØ5.A Unspecified nephritic syndrome with C3 glomerulonephritis CC
Unspecified nephritic syndrome with C3 glomerulopathy
EXCLUDES 1 *unspecified nephritic syndrome (with C3 glomerulopathy) with dense deposit disease (NØ5.6)*

NØ6 Isolated proteinuria with specified morphological lesion
EXCLUDES 1 *proteinuria not associated with specific morphologic lesions (R8Ø.Ø)*

NØ6.Ø Isolated proteinuria with minor glomerular abnormality
Isolated proteinuria with minimal change lesion

NØ6.1 Isolated proteinuria with focal and segmental glomerular lesions
Isolated proteinuria with focal and segmental hyalinosis
Isolated proteinuria with focal and segmental sclerosis
Isolated proteinuria with focal glomerulonephritis

▲ **NØ6.2 Isolated proteinuria with diffuse membranous glomerulonephritis**

● **NØ6.2Ø Isolated proteinuria with diffuse membranous glomerulonephritis, unspecified** CC
Membranous nephropathy, NOS
EXCLUDES 1 *membranous nephropathy NOS with nephrotic syndrome (NØ4.2Ø)*

● **NØ6.21 Primary membranous nephropathy with isolated proteinuria** CC
Idiopathic membranous nephropathy (with isolated proteinuria)
Primary membranous nephropathy, NOS
EXCLUDES 1 *primary membranous nephropathy with nephrotic syndrome (NØ4.21)*

● **NØ6.22 Secondary membranous nephropathy with isolated proteinuria** CC
Secondary membranous nephropathy, NOS
Code first, if applicable, other disease or disorder or poisoning causing membranous nephropathy
Use additional code, if applicable, for adverse effect of drug causing membranous nephropathy
EXCLUDES 1 *secondary membranous nephropathy with nephrotic syndrome (NØ4.22)*

● **NØ6.29 Other isolated proteinuria with diffuse membranous glomerulonephritis** CC

NØ6.3 Isolated proteinuria with diffuse mesangial proliferative glomerulonephritis CC

NØ6.4 Isolated proteinuria with diffuse endocapillary proliferative glomerulonephritis CC

NØ6.5 Isolated proteinuria with diffuse mesangiocapillary glomerulonephritis CC
Isolated proteinuria with membranoproliferative glomerulonephritis, types 1 and 3, or NOS
EXCLUDES 1 *isolated proteinuria with C3 glomerulonephritis (NØ6.A)*
isolated proteinuria with C3 glomerulopathy (NØ6.A)

NØ6.6 Isolated proteinuria with dense deposit disease
Isolated proteinuria with C3 glomerulopathy with dense deposit disease
Isolated proteinuria with membranoproliferative glomerulonephritis, type 2

NØ6.7 Isolated proteinuria with diffuse crescentic glomerulonephritis
Isolated proteinuria with extracapillary glomerulonephritis

NØ6.8 Isolated proteinuria with other morphologic lesion
Isolated proteinuria with proliferative glomerulonephritis NOS

NØ6.9 Isolated proteinuria with unspecified morphologic lesion

NØ6.A Isolated proteinuria with C3 glomerulonephritis CC
Isolated proteinuria with C3 glomerulopathy
EXCLUDES 1 *isolated proteinuria (with C3 glomerulopathy) with dense deposit disease (NØ6.6)*

NØ7 Hereditary nephropathy, not elsewhere classified
EXCLUDES 2 *Alport's syndrome (Q87.81-)*
hereditary amyloid nephropathy (E85.-)
nail patella syndrome (Q87.2)
non-neuropathic heredofamilial amyloidosis (E85.-)

NØ7.Ø Hereditary nephropathy, not elsewhere classified with minor glomerular abnormality
Hereditary nephropathy, not elsewhere classified with minimal change lesion

NØ7.1 Hereditary nephropathy, not elsewhere classified with focal and segmental glomerular lesions
Hereditary nephropathy, not elsewhere classified with focal and segmental hyalinosis
Hereditary nephropathy, not elsewhere classified with focal and segmental sclerosis
Hereditary nephropathy, not elsewhere classified with focal glomerulonephritis

NØ7.2 Hereditary nephropathy, not elsewhere classified with diffuse membranous glomerulonephritis CC

NØ7.3 Hereditary nephropathy, not elsewhere classified with diffuse mesangial proliferative glomerulonephritis CC

NØ7.4 Hereditary nephropathy, not elsewhere classified with diffuse endocapillary proliferative glomerulonephritis CC

N07.5 Hereditary nephropathy, not elsewhere classified with diffuse mesangiocapillary glomerulonephritis CC

Hereditary nephropathy, not elsewhere classified with membranoproliferative glomerulonephritis, types 1 and 3, or NOS

EXCLUDES 1 *hereditary nephropathy, not elsewhere classified with C3 glomerulonephritis (N07.A)*
hereditary nephropathy, not elsewhere classified with C3 glomerulopathy (N07.A)

N07.6 Hereditary nephropathy, not elsewhere classified with dense deposit disease

Hereditary nephropathy, not elsewhere classified with C3 glomerulopathy with dense deposit disease
Hereditary nephropathy, not elsewhere classified with membranoproliferative glomerulonephritis, type 2

N07.7 Hereditary nephropathy, not elsewhere classified with diffuse crescentic glomerulonephritis

Hereditary nephropathy, not elsewhere classified with extracapillary glomerulonephritis

N07.8 Hereditary nephropathy, not elsewhere classified with other morphologic lesions

Hereditary nephropathy, not elsewhere classified with proliferative glomerulonephritis NOS

N07.9 Hereditary nephropathy, not elsewhere classified with unspecified morphologic lesions

N07.A Hereditary nephropathy, not elsewhere classified with C3 glomerulonephritis CC

Hereditary nephropathy, not elsewhere classified with C3 glomerulopathy

EXCLUDES 1 *hereditary nephropathy, not elsewhere classified (with C3 glomerulopathy) with dense deposit disease (N07.6)*

N08 Glomerular disorders in diseases classified elsewhere

Glomerulonephritis
Nephritis
Nephropathy
Code first underlying disease, such as:
amyloidosis (E85.-)
congenital syphilis (A50.5)
cryoglobulinemia (D89.1)
disseminated intravascular coagulation (D65)
gout (M1A.-, M10.-)
microscopic polyangiitis (M31.7)
multiple myeloma (C90.0-)
sepsis (A40.0-A41.9)
sickle-cell disease (D57.0-D57.8)

EXCLUDES 1 *glomerulonephritis, nephritis and nephropathy (in):*
antiglomerular basement membrane disease (M31.0)
diabetes (E08-E13 with .21)
gonococcal (A54.21)
Goodpasture's syndrome (M31.0)
hemolytic-uremic syndrome (D59.3-)
lupus (M32.14)
mumps (B26.83)
syphilis (A52.75)
systemic lupus erythematosus (M32.14)
Wegener's granulomatosis (M31.31)
pyelonephritis in diseases classified elsewhere (N16)
renal tubulo-interstitial disorders classified elsewhere (N16)

Renal tubulo-interstitial diseases (N10-N16)

INCLUDES pyelonephritis
EXCLUDES 1 *pyeloureteritis cystica (N28.85)*

N10 Acute pyelonephritis CC HG

Acute infectious interstitial nephritis
Acute pyelitis
Acute tubulo-interstitial nephritis
Hemoglobin nephrosis
Myoglobin nephrosis
Use additional code (B95-B97), to identify infectious agent
AHA: 2020,3Q,25; 2019,3Q,13

✓4th **N11 Chronic tubulo-interstitial nephritis**

INCLUDES chronic infectious interstitial nephritis
chronic pyelitis
chronic pyelonephritis
Use additional code (B95-B97), to identify infectious agent

N11.0 Nonobstructive reflux-associated chronic pyelonephritis

Pyelonephritis (chronic) associated with (vesicoureteral) reflux

EXCLUDES 1 *vesicoureteral reflux NOS (N13.70)*

N11.1 Chronic obstructive pyelonephritis CC

Pyelonephritis (chronic) associated with anomaly of pelviureteric junction
Pyelonephritis (chronic) associated with anomaly of pyeloureteric junction
Pyelonephritis (chronic) associated with crossing of vessel
Pyelonephritis (chronic) associated with kinking of ureter
Pyelonephritis (chronic) associated with obstruction of ureter
Pyelonephritis (chronic) associated with stricture of pelviureteric junction
Pyelonephritis (chronic) associated with stricture of ureter

EXCLUDES 1 *calculous pyelonephritis (N20.9)*
obstructive uropathy (N13.-)

N11.8 Other chronic tubulo-interstitial nephritis CC

Nonobstructive chronic pyelonephritis NOS

N11.9 Chronic tubulo-interstitial nephritis, unspecified CC HG

Chronic interstitial nephritis NOS
Chronic pyelitis NOS
Chronic pyelonephritis NOS

N12 Tubulo-interstitial nephritis, not specified as acute or chronic CC HG

Interstitial nephritis NOS
Pyelitis NOS
Pyelonephritis NOS

EXCLUDES 1 *calculous pyelonephritis (N20.9)*

✓4th **N13 Obstructive and reflux uropathy**

EXCLUDES 2 *calculus of kidney and ureter without hydronephrosis (N20.-)*
congenital obstructive defects of renal pelvis and ureter (Q62.0-Q62.3)
hydronephrosis with ureteropelvic junction obstruction (Q62.11)
obstructive pyelonephritis (N11.1)

DEF: Hydronephrosis: Distension of the kidney caused by an accumulation of urine that cannot flow out due to an obstruction that may be caused by conditions such as kidney stones or vesicoureteral reflux.

N13.0 Hydronephrosis with ureteropelvic junction obstruction CC

Hydronephrosis due to acquired occlusion of ureteropelvic junction

EXCLUDES 2 *hydronephrosis with ureteropelvic junction obstruction due to calculus (N13.2)*

AHA: 2016,4Q,43

Hydronephrosis/UPJ Obstruction

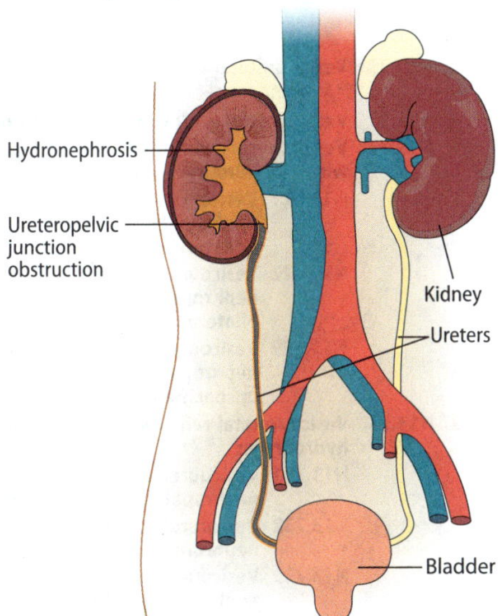

N13.1 Hydronephrosis with ureteral stricture, not elsewhere classified CC
EXCLUDES 1 *hydronephrosis with ureteral stricture with infection (N13.6)*

N13.2 Hydronephrosis with renal and ureteral calculous obstruction CC
EXCLUDES 1 *hydronephrosis with renal and ureteral calculous obstruction with infection (N13.6)*

✓5th **N13.3 Other and unspecified hydronephrosis**
EXCLUDES 1 *hydronephrosis with infection (N13.6)*

N13.30 Unspecified hydronephrosis CC

N13.39 Other hydronephrosis CC

N13.4 Hydroureter CC
EXCLUDES 1 *congenital hydroureter (Q62.3-)*
hydroureter with infection (N13.6)
vesicoureteral-reflux with hydroureter (N13.73-)
DEF: Abnormal enlargement or distension of the ureter with water or urine caused by an obstruction.

N13.5 Crossing vessel and stricture of ureter without hydronephrosis
Kinking and stricture of ureter without hydronephrosis
EXCLUDES 1 *crossing vessel and stricture of ureter without hydronephrosis with infection (N13.6)*

N13.6 Pyonephrosis CC H6
Conditions in N13.0-N13.5 with infection
Obstructive uropathy with infection
Use additional code (B95-B97), to identify infectious agent
AHA: 2018,2Q,21

✓5th **N13.7 Vesicoureteral-reflux**
EXCLUDES 1 *reflux-associated pyelonephritis (N11.0)*
DEF: Urine passage from the bladder flows backward up into the ureter and kidneys that can lead to bacterial infection and an increase in hydrostatic pressure, causing kidney damage.

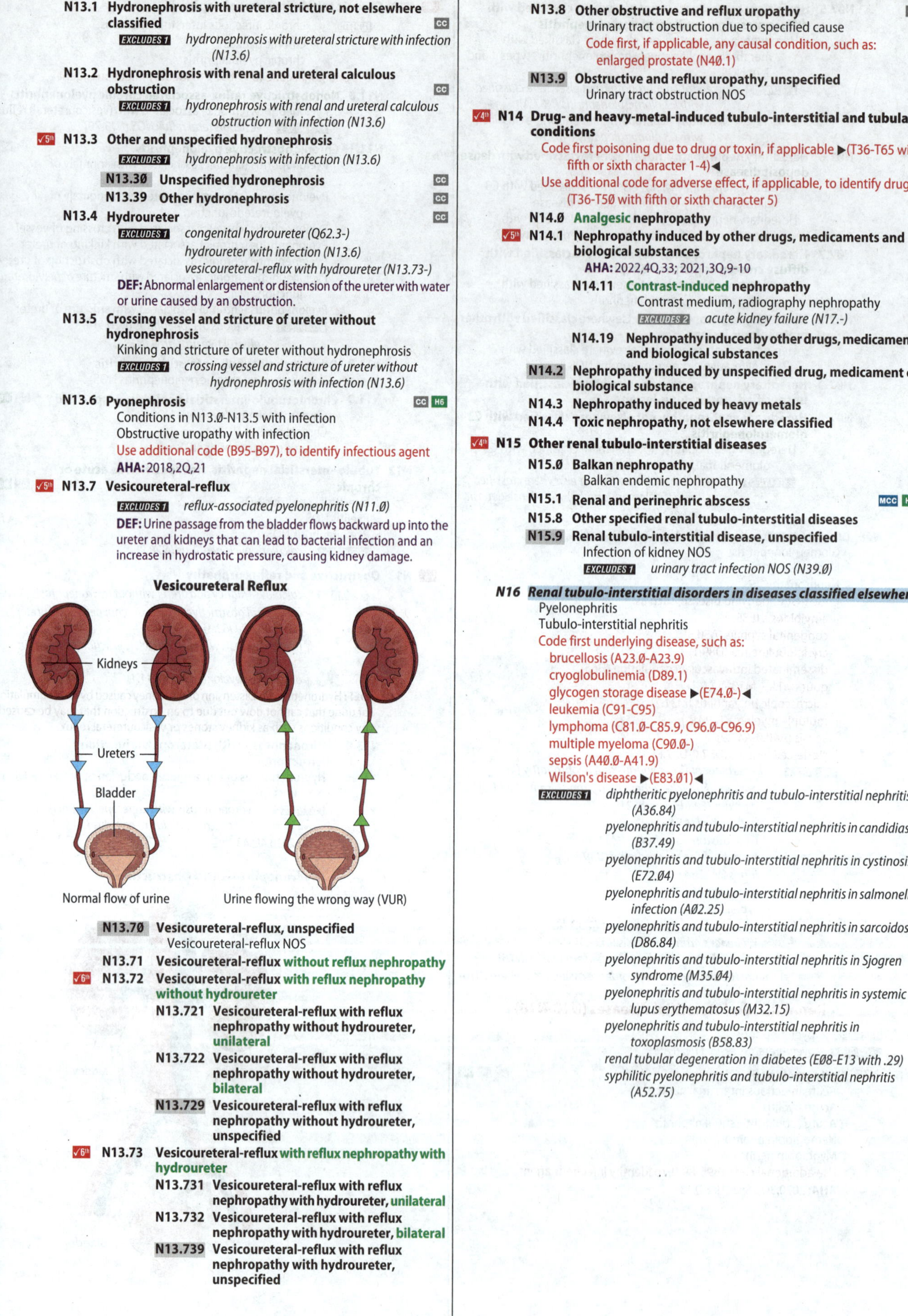

N13.70 Vesicoureteral-reflux, unspecified
Vesicoureteral-reflux NOS

N13.71 Vesicoureteral-reflux without reflux nephropathy

✓6th **N13.72 Vesicoureteral-reflux with reflux nephropathy without hydroureter**

N13.721 Vesicoureteral-reflux with reflux nephropathy without hydroureter, unilateral

N13.722 Vesicoureteral-reflux with reflux nephropathy without hydroureter, bilateral

N13.729 Vesicoureteral-reflux with reflux nephropathy without hydroureter, unspecified

✓6th **N13.73 Vesicoureteral-reflux with reflux nephropathy with hydroureter**

N13.731 Vesicoureteral-reflux with reflux nephropathy with hydroureter, unilateral

N13.732 Vesicoureteral-reflux with reflux nephropathy with hydroureter, bilateral

N13.739 Vesicoureteral-reflux with reflux nephropathy with hydroureter, unspecified

N13.8 Other obstructive and reflux uropathy CC
Urinary tract obstruction due to specified cause
Code first, if applicable, any causal condition, such as:
enlarged prostate (N40.1)

N13.9 Obstructive and reflux uropathy, unspecified
Urinary tract obstruction NOS

✓4th **N14 Drug- and heavy-metal-induced tubulo-interstitial and tubular conditions**
Code first poisoning due to drug or toxin, if applicable ▶(T36-T65 with fifth or sixth character 1-4)◀
Use additional code for adverse effect, if applicable, to identify drug (T36-T50 with fifth or sixth character 5)

N14.0 Analgesic nephropathy

✓5th **N14.1 Nephropathy induced by other drugs, medicaments and biological substances**
AHA: 2022,4Q,33; 2021,3Q,9-10

N14.11 Contrast-induced nephropathy
Contrast medium, radiography nephropathy
EXCLUDES 2 *acute kidney failure (N17.-)*

N14.19 Nephropathy induced by other drugs, medicaments and biological substances

N14.2 Nephropathy induced by unspecified drug, medicament or biological substance

N14.3 Nephropathy induced by heavy metals

N14.4 Toxic nephropathy, not elsewhere classified

✓4th **N15 Other renal tubulo-interstitial diseases**

N15.0 Balkan nephropathy
Balkan endemic nephropathy

N15.1 Renal and perinephric abscess MCC H6

N15.8 Other specified renal tubulo-interstitial diseases

N15.9 Renal tubulo-interstitial disease, unspecified
Infection of kidney NOS
EXCLUDES 1 *urinary tract infection NOS (N39.0)*

N16 Renal tubulo-interstitial disorders in diseases classified elsewhere
Pyelonephritis
Tubulo-interstitial nephritis
Code first underlying disease, such as:
brucellosis (A23.0-A23.9)
cryoglobulinemia (D89.1)
glycogen storage disease ▶(E74.0-)◀
leukemia (C91-C95)
lymphoma (C81.0-C85.9, C96.0-C96.9)
multiple myeloma (C90.0-)
sepsis (A40.0-A41.9)
Wilson's disease ▶(E83.01)◀
EXCLUDES 1 *diphtheritic pyelonephritis and tubulo-interstitial nephritis (A36.84)*
pyelonephritis and tubulo-interstitial nephritis in candidiasis (B37.49)
pyelonephritis and tubulo-interstitial nephritis in cystinosis (E72.04)
pyelonephritis and tubulo-interstitial nephritis in salmonella infection (A02.25)
pyelonephritis and tubulo-interstitial nephritis in sarcoidosis (D86.84)
pyelonephritis and tubulo-interstitial nephritis in Sjogren syndrome (M35.04)
pyelonephritis and tubulo-interstitial nephritis in systemic lupus erythematosus (M32.15)
pyelonephritis and tubulo-interstitial nephritis in toxoplasmosis (B58.83)
renal tubular degeneration in diabetes (E08-E13 with .29)
syphilitic pyelonephritis and tubulo-interstitial nephritis (A52.75)

Acute kidney failure and chronic kidney disease (N17-N19)

EXCLUDES 2 *congenital renal failure (P96.Ø)*
drug- and heavy-metal-induced tubulo-interstitial and tubular conditions (N14.-)
extrarenal uremia (R39.2)
hemolytic-uremic syndrome (D59.3-)
hepatorenal syndrome (K76.7)
postpartum hepatorenal syndrome ▶(O9Ø.41)◀
posttraumatic renal failure (T79.5)
prerenal uremia (R39.2)
renal failure complicating abortion or ectopic or molar pregnancy (OØØ-OØ7, OØ8.4)
renal failure following labor and delivery ▶(O9Ø.41)◀
renal failure postprocedural (N99.Ø)

✓4th **N17 Acute kidney failure**
Code also associated underlying condition
EXCLUDES 1 *posttraumatic renal failure (T79.5)*
AHA: 2020,3Q,22; 2019,2Q,7; 2019,1Q,12; 2013,4Q,124

N17.Ø Acute kidney failure with tubular necrosis MCC HCC
Acute tubular necrosis
Renal tubular necrosis
Tubular necrosis NOS
AHA: 2022,4Q,33; 2021,3Q,10

N17.1 Acute kidney failure with acute cortical necrosis MCC HCC
Acute cortical necrosis
Cortical necrosis NOS
Renal cortical necrosis

N17.2 Acute kidney failure with medullary necrosis MCC HCC
Medullary [papillary] necrosis NOS
Acute medullary [papillary] necrosis
Renal medullary [papillary] necrosis

N17.8 Other acute kidney failure CC HCC

N17.9 Acute kidney failure, unspecified CC HCC
Acute kidney injury (nontraumatic)
EXCLUDES 2 *traumatic kidney injury (S37.Ø-)*

✓4th **N18 Chronic kidney disease (CKD)**
Code first any associated:
diabetic chronic kidney disease (EØ8.22, EØ9.22, E1Ø.22, E11.22, E13.22)
hypertensive chronic kidney disease (I12.-, I13.-)
Use additional code to identify kidney transplant status, if applicable, (Z94.Ø)
AHA: 2023,1Q,17; 2022,4Q,14; 2019,3Q,3; 2018,4Q,88; 2013,1Q,24

N18.1 Chronic kidney disease, stage 1

N18.2 Chronic kidney disease, stage 2 (mild)

✓5th **N18.3 Chronic kidney disease, stage 3 (moderate)**
AHA: 2020,4Q,35

N18.3Ø Chronic kidney disease, stage 3 unspecified HCC

N18.31 Chronic kidney disease, stage 3a HCC

N18.32 Chronic kidney disease, stage 3b HCC

N18.4 Chronic kidney disease, stage 4 (severe) CC HCC

N18.5 Chronic kidney disease, stage 5 CC HCC
EXCLUDES 1 *chronic kidney disease, stage 5 requiring chronic dialysis (N18.6)*
DEF: End-stage renal disease (ESRD) with a GFR value of 15 ml/min or less not yet requiring chronic dialysis.
TIP: When both ESRD and CKD 5 are documented, code only for ESRD.

N18.6 End stage renal disease MCC HCC
Chronic kidney disease requiring chronic dialysis
Use additional code to identify dialysis status (Z99.2)
AHA: 2023,1Q,19; 2022,3Q,15; 2016,3Q,22; 2016,1Q,12; 2013,4Q,124-125
TIP: When both ESRD and CKD 5 are documented, code only for ESRD.

N18.9 Chronic kidney disease, unspecified
Chronic renal disease
Chronic renal failure NOS
Chronic renal insufficiency
Chronic uremia NOS
Diffuse sclerosing glomerulonephritis NOS

N19 Unspecified kidney failure
Uremia NOS
EXCLUDES 1 *acute kidney failure (N17.-)*
chronic kidney disease (N18.-)
chronic uremia (N18.9)
extrarenal uremia (R39.2)
prerenal uremia (R39.2)
renal insufficiency (acute) (N28.9)
uremia of newborn (P96.Ø)

Urolithiasis (N2Ø-N23)

AHA: 2017,1Q,5; 2015,2Q,8
TIP: Codes from this code block can be assigned based on the diagnosis listed in a radiology report when authenticated by a radiologist and available at the time of code assignment.

✓4th **N2Ø Calculus of kidney and ureter**
Calculous pyelonephritis
EXCLUDES 1 *nephrocalcinosis ▶(E83.59)◀*
that with hydronephrosis (N13.2)
AHA: 2019,3Q,13

N2Ø.Ø Calculus of kidney
Nephrolithiasis NOS
Renal calculus
Renal stone
Staghorn calculus
Stone in kidney
AHA: 2019,3Q,13

N2Ø.1 Calculus of ureter CC
Calculus of the ureteropelvic junction
Ureteric stone
AHA: 2016,3Q,22

N2Ø.2 Calculus of kidney with calculus of ureter CC

N2Ø.9 Urinary calculus, unspecified

✓4th **N21 Calculus of lower urinary tract**
INCLUDES calculus of lower urinary tract with cystitis and urethritis

N21.Ø Calculus in bladder
Calculus in diverticulum of bladder
Urinary bladder stone
EXCLUDES 2 *staghorn calculus (N2Ø.Ø)*

N21.1 Calculus in urethra
EXCLUDES 2 *calculus of prostate (N42.Ø)*

N21.8 Other lower urinary tract calculus

N21.9 Calculus of lower urinary tract, unspecified
EXCLUDES 1 *calculus of urinary tract NOS (N2Ø.9)*

N22 Calculus of urinary tract in diseases classified elsewhere
Code first underlying disease, such as:
gout (M1A.-, M1Ø.-)
schistosomiasis (B65.Ø-B65.9)

N23 Unspecified renal colic

Other disorders of kidney and ureter (N25-N29)

EXCLUDES 2 *disorders of kidney and ureter with urolithiasis (N2Ø-N23)*

✓4th **N25 Disorders resulting from impaired renal tubular function**

N25.Ø Renal osteodystrophy
Azotemic osteodystrophy
Phosphate-losing tubular disorders
Renal rickets
Renal short stature
EXCLUDES 2 *metabolic disorders classifiable to E7Ø-E88*
DEF: Various bone diseases occurring when kidney function is impaired or fails. Abnormal levels of phosphorous and calcium can lead to osteomalacia, osteoporosis, or osteosclerosis.

N25.1 Nephrogenic diabetes insipidus CC HCC
EXCLUDES 1 *diabetes insipidus NOS (E23.2)*
DEF: Type of diabetes due to the inability of renal tubules to reabsorb water back into the body. It is not responsive to vasopressin (antidiuretic hormone) and it is characterized by excessive thirst and excessive urine production. It may develop into chronic renal insufficiency.

N25.8 Other disorders resulting from impaired renal tubular function

N25.81 Secondary hyperparathyroidism of renal origin CC HCC

EXCLUDES 1 *secondary hyperparathyroidism, non-renal (E21.1)*

EXCLUDES 2 *metabolic disorders classifiable to E70-E88*

DEF: Parathyroid dysfunction caused by chronic renal failure. Phosphate clearance and vitamin D production is impaired resulting in lowered calcium blood levels and an excessive production of parathyroid hormone.

N25.89 Other disorders resulting from impaired renal tubular function

Hypokalemic nephropathy
Lightwood-Albright syndrome
Renal tubular acidosis NOS

N25.9 Disorder resulting from impaired renal tubular function, unspecified

N26 Unspecified contracted kidney

EXCLUDES 1 *contracted kidney due to hypertension (I12.-)*
diffuse sclerosing glomerulonephritis (N05.8.-)
hypertensive nephrosclerosis (arteriolar) (arteriosclerotic) (I12.-)
small kidney of unknown cause (N27.-)

N26.1 Atrophy of kidney (terminal)

N26.2 Page kidney

N26.9 Renal sclerosis, unspecified

N27 Small kidney of unknown cause

INCLUDES oligonephronia

N27.0 Small kidney, unilateral

N27.1 Small kidney, bilateral

N27.9 Small kidney, unspecified

N28 Other disorders of kidney and ureter, not elsewhere classified

N28.0 Ischemia and infarction of kidney CC HCC

Renal artery embolism
Renal artery obstruction
Renal artery occlusion
Renal artery thrombosis
Renal infarct

EXCLUDES 1 *atherosclerosis of renal artery (extrarenal part) (I70.1)*
congenital stenosis of renal artery (Q27.1)
Goldblatt's kidney (I70.1)

N28.1 Cyst of kidney, acquired

Cyst (multiple) (solitary) of kidney (acquired)

EXCLUDES 1 *cystic kidney disease (congenital) (Q61.-)*

N28.8 Other specified disorders of kidney and ureter

EXCLUDES 1 *hydroureter (N13.4)*
ureteric stricture with hydronephrosis (N13.1)
ureteric stricture without hydronephrosis (N13.5)

N28.81 Hypertrophy of kidney

N28.82 Megaloureter

N28.83 Nephroptosis

N28.84 Pyelitis cystica CC H6

N28.85 Pyeloureteritis cystica CC H6

N28.86 Ureteritis cystica CC H6

N28.89 Other specified disorders of kidney and ureter

N28.9 Disorder of kidney and ureter, unspecified

Nephropathy NOS
Renal disease (acute) NOS
Renal insufficiency (acute)

EXCLUDES 1 *chronic renal insufficiency (N18.9)*
unspecified nephritic syndrome (N05.-)

AHA: 2016,1Q,13

N29 Other disorders of kidney and ureter in diseases classified elsewhere

Code first underlying disease, such as:
amyloidosis (E85.-)
nephrocalcinosis ►(E83.59)◄
schistosomiasis (B65.0-B65.9)

EXCLUDES 1 *disorders of kidney and ureter in:*
cystinosis (E72.0)
gonorrhea (A54.21)
syphilis (A52.75)
tuberculosis (A18.11)

Other diseases of the urinary system (N30-N39)

EXCLUDES 2 *urinary infection (complicating):*
abortion or ectopic or molar pregnancy (O00-O07, O08.8)
pregnancy, childbirth and the puerperium (O23.-, O75.3, O86.2-)

N30 Cystitis

Use additional code to identify infectious agent (B95-B97)

EXCLUDES 1 *prostatocystitis (N41.3)*

AHA: 2017,1Q,6

DEF: Inflammation of the urinary bladder. Symptoms include dysuria, frequency of urination, urgency, and hematuria.

N30.0 Acute cystitis

EXCLUDES 1 *irradiation cystitis (N30.4-)*
trigonitis (N30.3-)

N30.00 Acute cystitis without hematuria CC H6

N30.01 Acute cystitis with hematuria CC H6

N30.1 Interstitial cystitis (chronic)

N30.10 Interstitial cystitis (chronic) without hematuria

N30.11 Interstitial cystitis (chronic) with hematuria

N30.2 Other chronic cystitis

N30.20 Other chronic cystitis without hematuria

N30.21 Other chronic cystitis with hematuria

N30.3 Trigonitis

Urethrotrigonitis

N30.30 Trigonitis without hematuria

N30.31 Trigonitis with hematuria

N30.4 Irradiation cystitis

N30.40 Irradiation cystitis without hematuria CC

N30.41 Irradiation cystitis with hematuria CC

N30.8 Other cystitis

Abscess of bladder

N30.80 Other cystitis without hematuria

N30.81 Other cystitis with hematuria

N30.9 Cystitis, unspecified

N30.90 Cystitis, unspecified without hematuria

N30.91 Cystitis, unspecified with hematuria

N31 Neuromuscular dysfunction of bladder, not elsewhere classified

Use additional code to identify any associated urinary incontinence (N39.3-N39.4-)

EXCLUDES 1 *cord bladder NOS (G95.89)*
neurogenic bladder due to cauda equina syndrome (G83.4)
neuromuscular dysfunction due to spinal cord lesion (G95.89)

N31.0 Uninhibited neuropathic bladder, not elsewhere classified

N31.1 Reflex neuropathic bladder, not elsewhere classified

N31.2 Flaccid neuropathic bladder, not elsewhere classified

Atonic (motor) (sensory) neuropathic bladder
Autonomous neuropathic bladder
Nonreflex neuropathic bladder

N31.8 Other neuromuscular dysfunction of bladder

N31.9 Neuromuscular dysfunction of bladder, unspecified

Neurogenic bladder dysfunction NOS

N32 Other disorders of bladder

EXCLUDES 2 *calculus of bladder (N21.0)*
cystocele (N81.1-)
hernia or prolapse of bladder, female (N81.1-)

N32.0 Bladder-neck obstruction

Bladder-neck stenosis (acquired)

EXCLUDES 1 *congenital bladder-neck obstruction (Q64.3-)*

DEF: Bladder outlet and vesicourethral obstruction that occurs as a consequence of benign prostatic hypertrophy or prostatic cancer. It may also occur in either sex due to strictures, radiation, cystoscopy, catheterization, injury, infection, blood clots, bladder cancer, impaction, or other disease that compresses the bladder neck.

N32.1 Vesicointestinal fistula CC

Vesicorectal fistula

N32.2 Vesical fistula, not elsewhere classified CC

EXCLUDES 1 *fistula between bladder and female genital tract (N82.0-N82.1)*

N32.3 Diverticulum of bladder

EXCLUDES 1 *congenital diverticulum of bladder (Q64.6)*
diverticulitis of bladder (N30.8-)

✓5th N32.8 Other specified disorders of bladder

N32.81 Overactive bladder

Detrusor muscle hyperactivity

EXCLUDES 1 *frequent urination due to specified bladder condition — code to condition*

DEF: Sudden involuntary contractions of the muscular wall of the bladder that results in a sudden, strong urge to urinate.

N32.89 Other specified disorders of bladder

Bladder hemorrhage
Bladder hypertrophy
Calcified bladder
Contracted bladder

N32.9 Bladder disorder, unspecified

N33 Bladder disorders in diseases classified elsewhere

Code first underlying disease, such as:
schistosomiasis (B65.Ø-B65.9)

EXCLUDES 1 *bladder disorder in syphilis (A52.76)*
bladder disorder in tuberculosis (A18.12)
candidal cystitis (B37.41)
chlamydial cystitis (A56.Ø1)
cystitis in gonorrhea (A54.Ø1)
cystitis in neurogenic bladder (N31.-)
diphtheritic cystitis (A36.85)
neurogenic bladder (N31.-)
syphilitic cystitis (A52.76)
trichomonal cystitis (A59.Ø3)

✓4th N34 Urethritis and urethral syndrome

Use additional code (B95-B97), to identify infectious agent

EXCLUDES 2 *Reiter's disease (MØ2.3-)*
urethritis in diseases with a predominantly sexual mode of transmission (A5Ø-A64)
urethrotrigonitis (N3Ø.3-)

AHA: 2017,1Q,6

N34.Ø Urethral abscess CC H6

Abscess (of) Cowper's gland
Abscess (of) Littre's gland
Abscess (of) urethral (gland)
Periurethral abscess

EXCLUDES 1 *urethral caruncle (N36.2)*

N34.1 Nonspecific urethritis

Nongonococcal urethritis
Nonvenereal urethritis

N34.2 Other urethritis

Meatitis, urethral
Postmenopausal urethritis
Ulcer of urethra (meatus)
Urethritis NOS

N34.3 Urethral syndrome, unspecified

✓4th N35 Urethral stricture

EXCLUDES 1 *congenital urethral stricture (Q64.3-)*
postprocedural urethral stricture (N99.1-)

AHA: 2018,4Q,21-22

✓5th N35.Ø Post-traumatic urethral stricture

Urethral stricture due to injury

EXCLUDES 1 *postprocedural urethral stricture (N99.1-)*

✓6th N35.Ø1 Post-traumatic urethral stricture, male

N35.Ø1Ø Post-traumatic urethral stricture, male, meatal ♂

N35.Ø11 Post-traumatic bulbous urethral stricture ♂

N35.Ø12 Post-traumatic membranous urethral stricture ♂

N35.Ø13 Post-traumatic anterior urethral stricture ♂

N35.Ø14 Post-traumatic urethral stricture, male, unspecified ♂

N35.Ø16 Post-traumatic urethral stricture, male, overlapping sites ♂

✓6th N35.Ø2 Post-traumatic urethral stricture, female

N35.Ø21 Urethral stricture due to childbirth ♀

N35.Ø28 Other post-traumatic urethral stricture, female ♀

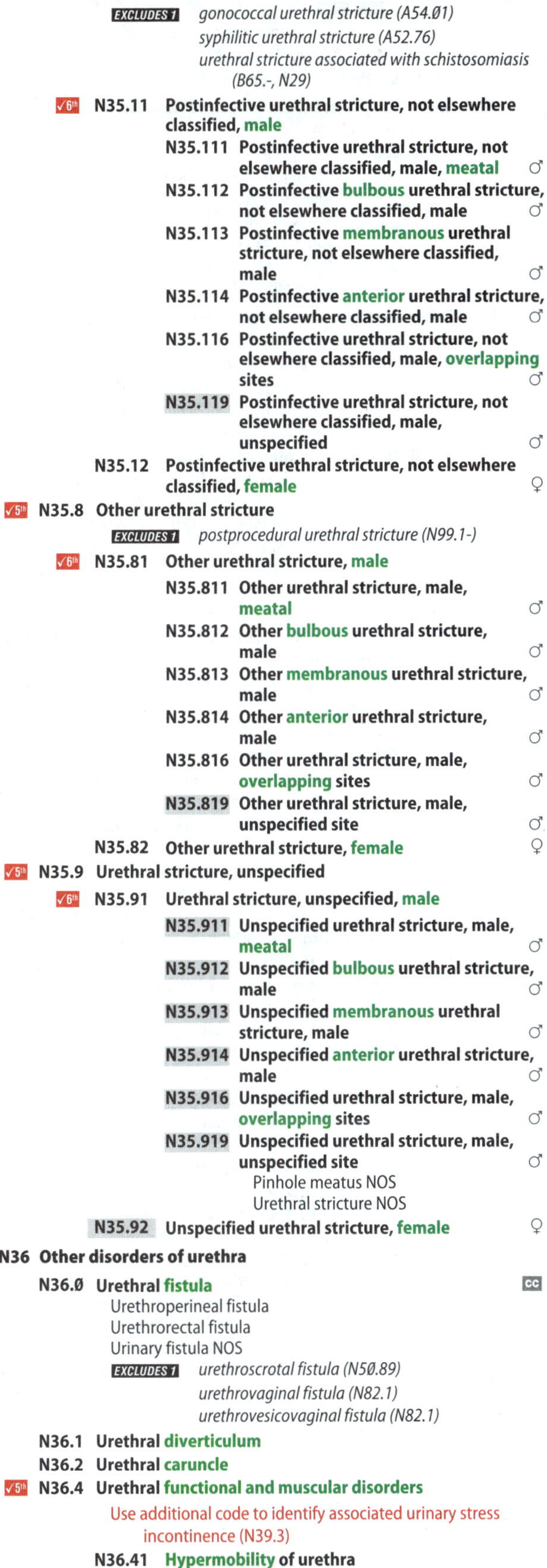

✓5th N35.1 Postinfective urethral stricture, not elsewhere classified

EXCLUDES 1 *gonococcal urethral stricture (A54.Ø1)*
syphilitic urethral stricture (A52.76)
urethral stricture associated with schistosomiasis (B65.-, N29)

✓6th N35.11 Postinfective urethral stricture, not elsewhere classified, male

N35.111 Postinfective urethral stricture, not elsewhere classified, male, meatal ♂

N35.112 Postinfective bulbous urethral stricture, not elsewhere classified, male ♂

N35.113 Postinfective membranous urethral stricture, not elsewhere classified, male ♂

N35.114 Postinfective anterior urethral stricture, not elsewhere classified, male ♂

N35.116 Postinfective urethral stricture, not elsewhere classified, male, overlapping sites ♂

N35.119 Postinfective urethral stricture, not elsewhere classified, male, unspecified ♂

N35.12 Postinfective urethral stricture, not elsewhere classified, female ♀

✓5th N35.8 Other urethral stricture

EXCLUDES 1 *postprocedural urethral stricture (N99.1-)*

✓6th N35.81 Other urethral stricture, male

N35.811 Other urethral stricture, male, meatal ♂

▲ **N35.812 Other bulbous urethral stricture, male** ♂

N35.813 Other membranous urethral stricture, male ♂

N35.814 Other anterior urethral stricture, male ♂

N35.816 Other urethral stricture, male, overlapping sites ♂

N35.819 Other urethral stricture, male, unspecified site ♂

N35.82 Other urethral stricture, female ♀

✓5th N35.9 Urethral stricture, unspecified

✓6th N35.91 Urethral stricture, unspecified, male

N35.911 Unspecified urethral stricture, male, meatal ♂

N35.912 Unspecified bulbous urethral stricture, male ♂

N35.913 Unspecified membranous urethral stricture, male ♂

N35.914 Unspecified anterior urethral stricture, male ♂

N35.916 Unspecified urethral stricture, male, overlapping sites ♂

N35.919 Unspecified urethral stricture, male, unspecified site ♂

Pinhole meatus NOS
Urethral stricture NOS

N35.92 Unspecified urethral stricture, female ♀

✓4th N36 Other disorders of urethra

N36.Ø Urethral fistula CC

Urethroperineal fistula
Urethrorectal fistula
Urinary fistula NOS

EXCLUDES 1 *urethroscrotal fistula (N5Ø.89)*
urethrovaginal fistula (N82.1)
urethrovesicovaginal fistula (N82.1)

N36.1 Urethral diverticulum

N36.2 Urethral caruncle

✓5th N36.4 Urethral functional and muscular disorders

Use additional code to identify associated urinary stress incontinence (N39.3)

N36.41 Hypermobility of urethra

N36.42 Intrinsic sphincter deficiency (ISD)

N36.43 Combined hypermobility of urethra and intrinsic sphincter deficiency

N36.44 Muscular disorders of urethra

Bladder sphincter dyssynergy

N36.5 Urethral false passage

N36.8 Other specified disorders of urethra
EXCLUDES 1 *congenital urethrocele (Q64.7)*
female urethrocele (N81.Ø)
AHA: 2022,2Q,7

N36.9 Urethral disorder, unspecified

N37 *Urethral disorders in diseases classified elsewhere*
Code first underlying disease
EXCLUDES 1 *urethritis (in):*
candidal infection (B37.41)
chlamydial (A56.Ø1)
gonorrhea (A54.Ø1)
syphilis (A52.76)
trichomonal infection (A59.Ø3)
tuberculosis (A18.13)

✓4th **N39 Other disorders of urinary system**
EXCLUDES 2 *hematuria NOS (R31.-)*
proteinuria NOS (R8Ø.-)
recurrent or persistent hematuria (NØ2.-)
recurrent or persistent hematuria with specified morphological lesion (NØ2.-)

N39.Ø Urinary tract infection, site not specified CC H6
Use additional code (B95-B97), to identify infectious agent
EXCLUDES 1 *candidiasis of urinary tract (B37.4-)*
neonatal urinary tract infection (P39.3)
pyuria (R82.81)
urinary tract infection of specified site, such as:
cystitis (N3Ø.-)
urethritis (N34.-)
AHA: 2019,3Q,17; 2018,2Q,21,22; 2018,1Q,16; 2017,1Q,6; 2012,4Q,94

N39.3 Stress incontinence (female) (male)
Code also any associated overactive bladder (N32.81)
EXCLUDES 1 *mixed incontinence (N39.46)*

✓5th **N39.4 Other specified urinary incontinence**
Code also any associated overactive bladder (N32.81)
EXCLUDES 1 *enuresis NOS (R32)*
functional urinary incontinence (R39.81)
urinary incontinence associated with cognitive impairment (R39.81)
urinary incontinence NOS (R32)
urinary incontinence of nonorganic origin (F98.Ø)

N39.41 Urge incontinence
EXCLUDES 1 *mixed incontinence (N39.46)*

N39.42 Incontinence without sensory awareness
Insensible (urinary) incontinence

N39.43 Post-void dribbling

N39.44 Nocturnal enuresis
EXCLUDES 2 *nocturnal polyuria (R35.81)*

N39.45 Continuous leakage

N39.46 Mixed incontinence
Urge and stress incontinence

✓6th **N39.49 Other specified urinary incontinence**
AHA: 2016,4Q,44

N39.49Ø Overflow incontinence

N39.491 Coital incontinence

N39.492 Postural (urinary) incontinence

N39.498 Other specified urinary incontinence
Reflex incontinence
Total incontinence

N39.8 Other specified disorders of urinary system

N39.9 Disorder of urinary system, unspecified

Diseases of male genital organs (N4Ø-N53)

✓4th **N4Ø Benign prostatic hyperplasia**
INCLUDES adenofibromatous hypertrophy of prostate
benign hypertrophy of the prostate
benign prostatic hypertrophy
BPH
enlarged prostate
nodular prostate
polyp of prostate
EXCLUDES 1 *benign neoplasms of prostate (adenoma, benign) (fibroadenoma) (fibroma) (myoma) (D29.1)*
EXCLUDES 2 *malignant neoplasm of prostate (C61)*
DEF: Enlargement of the prostate gland due to an abnormal proliferation of fibrostromal tissue in the paraurethral glands. This condition causes impingement of the urethra resulting in obstructed urinary flow.

N4Ø.Ø Benign prostatic hyperplasia without lower urinary tract symptoms A ♂
Enlarged prostate NOS
Enlarged prostate without LUTS

N4Ø.1 Benign prostatic hyperplasia with lower urinary tract symptoms A ♂
Enlarged prostate with LUTS
Use additional code for associated symptoms, when specified:
incomplete bladder emptying (R39.14)
nocturia (R35.1)
straining on urination (R39.16)
urinary frequency (R35.Ø)
urinary hesitancy (R39.11)
urinary incontinence (N39.4-)
urinary obstruction (N13.8)
urinary retention (R33.8)
urinary urgency (R39.15)
weak urinary stream (R39.12)
AHA: 2018,4Q,55

N4Ø.2 Nodular prostate without lower urinary tract symptoms A ♂
Nodular prostate without LUTS

N4Ø.3 Nodular prostate with lower urinary tract symptoms A ♂
Use additional code for associated symptoms, when specified:
incomplete bladder emptying (R39.14)
nocturia (R35.1)
straining on urination (R39.16)
urinary frequency (R35.Ø)
urinary hesitancy (R39.11)
urinary incontinence (N39.4-)
urinary obstruction (N13.8)
urinary retention (R33.8)
urinary urgency (R39.15)
weak urinary stream (R39.12)

✓4th **N41 Inflammatory diseases of prostate**
Use additional code (B95-B97), to identify infectious agent

N41.Ø Acute prostatitis CC A ♂

N41.1 Chronic prostatitis A ♂

N41.2 Abscess of prostate CC A ♂

N41.3 Prostatocystitis A ♂

N41.4 Granulomatous prostatitis A ♂

N41.8 Other inflammatory diseases of prostate A ♂

N41.9 Inflammatory disease of prostate, unspecified A ♂
Prostatitis NOS

✓4th **N42 Other and unspecified disorders of prostate**

N42.Ø Calculus of prostate A ♂
Prostatic stone
DEF: Formation of a small, solid stone often composed of calcium carbonate or calcium phosphate in the prostate gland.

N42.1 Congestion and hemorrhage of prostate A ♂
EXCLUDES 1 *enlarged prostate (N4Ø.-)*
hematuria (R31.-)
hyperplasia of prostate (N4Ø.-)
inflammatory diseases of prostate (N41.-)

✓5th **N42.3 Dysplasia of prostate**
AHA: 2016,4Q,44

N42.3Ø Unspecified dysplasia of prostate ♂

N42.31 **Prostatic intraepithelial neoplasia** ♂
PIN
Prostatic intraepithelial neoplasia I (PIN I)
Prostatic intraepithelial neoplasia II (PIN II)
EXCLUDES 1 *prostatic intraepithelial neoplasia III (PIN III) (D07.5)*
DEF: Abnormality of shape and size of the intraepithelial tissues of the prostate. It is a premalignant condition characterized by stalks and absence of a basilar cell layer.

N42.32 **Atypical small acinar proliferation of prostate** ♂

N42.39 **Other dysplasia of prostate** ♂

✓5th N42.8 **Other specified disorders of prostate**

N42.81 **Prostatodynia syndrome** A ♂
Painful prostate syndrome

N42.82 **Prostatosis syndrome** A ♂

N42.83 **Cyst of prostate** A ♂

N42.89 **Other specified disorders of prostate** A ♂

N42.9 **Disorder of prostate, unspecified** A ♂

✓4th N43 **Hydrocele and spermatocele**
INCLUDES hydrocele of spermatic cord, testis or tunica vaginalis
EXCLUDES 1 *congenital hydrocele (P83.5)*
DEF: Hydrocele: Serous fluid that collects in the tunica vaginalis of the scrotum along the spermatic cord in males.

N43.0 **Encysted hydrocele** ♂

N43.1 **Infected hydrocele** CC ♂
Use additional code (B95-B97), to identify infectious agent

N43.2 **Other hydrocele** ♂

Hydrocele

N43.3 **Hydrocele, unspecified** ♂

✓5th N43.4 **Spermatocele of epididymis**
Spermatic cyst
DEF: Spermatocele: Noncancerous accumulation of fluid and dead sperm cells normally located at the head of the epididymis that exhibits itself as a hard, smooth scrotal mass and do not normally require treatment unless they become enlarged or cause pain.

N43.40 **Spermatocele of epididymis, unspecified** ♂

N43.41 **Spermatocele of epididymis, single** ♂

N43.42 **Spermatocele of epididymis, multiple** ♂

✓4th N44 **Noninflammatory disorders of testis**

✓5th N44.0 **Torsion of testis**

N44.00 **Torsion of testis, unspecified** CC ♂

N44.01 **Extravaginal torsion of spermatic cord** CC ♂
DEF: Torsion of the spermatic cord just below the tunica vaginalis attachments.

N44.02 **Intravaginal torsion of spermatic cord** CC ♂
Torsion of spermatic cord NOS

N44.03 **Torsion of appendix testis** CC ♂

N44.04 **Torsion of appendix epididymis** CC ♂

N44.1 **Cyst of tunica albuginea testis** ♂

N44.2 **Benign cyst of testis** ♂

N44.8 **Other noninflammatory disorders of the testis** ♂

✓4th N45 **Orchitis and epididymitis**
Use additional code (B95-B97), to identify infectious agent

N45.1 **Epididymitis** ♂

N45.2 **Orchitis** ♂

N45.3 **Epididymo-orchitis** ♂

N45.4 **Abscess of epididymis or testis** CC ♂

✓4th N46 **Male infertility**
EXCLUDES 1 *vasectomy status (Z98.52)*

✓5th N46.0 **Azoospermia**
Absolute male infertility
Male infertility due to germinal (cell) aplasia
Male infertility due to spermatogenic arrest (complete)
DEF: Failure of the development of sperm or the absence of sperm in semen.

N46.01 **Organic azoospermia** A ♂
Azoospermia NOS

✓6th N46.02 **Azoospermia due to extratesticular causes**
Code also associated cause

N46.021 **Azoospermia due to drug therapy** A ♂

N46.022 **Azoospermia due to infection** A ♂

N46.023 **Azoospermia due to obstruction of efferent ducts** A ♂

N46.024 **Azoospermia due to radiation** A ♂

N46.025 **Azoospermia due to systemic disease** A ♂

N46.029 **Azoospermia due to other extratesticular causes** A ♂

✓5th N46.1 **Oligospermia**
Male infertility due to germinal cell desquamation
Male infertility due to hypospermatogenesis
Male infertility due to incomplete spermatogenic arrest
DEF: Insufficient production of sperm in semen.

N46.11 **Organic oligospermia** A ♂
Oligospermia NOS

✓6th N46.12 **Oligospermia due to extratesticular causes**
Code also associated cause

N46.121 **Oligospermia due to drug therapy** A ♂

N46.122 **Oligospermia due to infection** A ♂

N46.123 **Oligospermia due to obstruction of efferent ducts** A ♂

N46.124 **Oligospermia due to radiation** A ♂

N46.125 **Oligospermia due to systemic disease** A ♂

N46.129 **Oligospermia due to other extratesticular causes** A ♂

N46.8 **Other male infertility** A ♂

N46.9 **Male infertility, unspecified** A ♂

✓4th N47 **Disorders of prepuce**

N47.0 **Adherent prepuce, newborn** N ♂

N47.1 **Phimosis** ♂
DEF: Condition in which the foreskin is contracted and cannot be drawn back behind the glans penis.

N47.2 **Paraphimosis** ♂

N47.3 **Deficient foreskin** ♂

N47.4 **Benign cyst of prepuce** ♂

N47.5 **Adhesions of prepuce and glans penis** ♂

N47.6 **Balanoposthitis** ♂
Use additional code (B95-B97), to identify infectious agent
EXCLUDES 1 *balanitis (N48.1)*

N47.7 **Other inflammatory diseases of prepuce** ♂
Use additional code (B95-B97), to identify infectious agent

N47.8 **Other disorders of prepuce** ♂

✓4th N48 **Other disorders of penis**

N48.0 **Leukoplakia of penis** ♂
Balanitis xerotica obliterans
Kraurosis of penis
Lichen sclerosus of external male genital organs
EXCLUDES 1 *carcinoma in situ of penis (D07.4)*

N48.1 **Balanitis** ♂
Use additional code (B95-B97), to identify infectious agent
EXCLUDES 1 *amebic balanitis (A06.8)*
balanitis xerotica obliterans (N48.0)
candidal balanitis (B37.42)
gonococcal balanitis (A54.23)
herpesviral [herpes simplex] balanitis (A60.01)
DEF: Inflammation of the glans penis, most often affecting uncircumcised males.

N48.2 Other inflammatory disorders of penis
Use additional code (B95-B97), to identify infectious agent
EXCLUDES 1 *balanitis (N48.1)*
balanitis xerotica obliterans (N48.Ø)
balanoposthitis (N47.6)

N48.21 Abscess of corpus cavernosum and penis ♂
N48.22 Cellulitis of corpus cavernosum and penis ♂
N48.29 Other inflammatory disorders of penis ♂

N48.3 Priapism
Painful erection
Code first underlying cause

N48.3Ø Priapism, unspecified CC ♂
N48.31 Priapism due to trauma CC ♂
N48.32 Priapism due to disease classified elsewhere CC ♂
N48.33 Priapism, drug-induced CC ♂
N48.39 Other priapism CC ♂

N48.5 Ulcer of penis ♂
N48.6 Induration penis plastica ♂
Peyronie's disease
Plastic induration of penis

N48.8 Other specified disorders of penis

N48.81 Thrombosis of superficial vein of penis ♂
N48.82 Acquired torsion of penis ♂
Acquired torsion of penis NOS
EXCLUDES 1 *congenital torsion of penis (Q55.63)*
N48.83 Acquired buried penis ♂
EXCLUDES 1 *congenital hidden penis (Q55.64)*
N48.89 Other specified disorders of penis ♂

N48.9 Disorder of penis, unspecified ♂

N49 Inflammatory disorders of male genital organs, not elsewhere classified
Use additional code (B95-B97), to identify infectious agent
EXCLUDES 1 *inflammation of penis (N48.1, N48.2-)*
orchitis and epididymitis (N45.-)

N49.Ø Inflammatory disorders of seminal vesicle ♂
Vesiculitis NOS
N49.1 Inflammatory disorders of spermatic cord, tunica vaginalis and vas deferens ♂
Vasitis
N49.2 Inflammatory disorders of scrotum ♂
N49.3 Fournier gangrene ♂
AHA: 2020,2Q,18
N49.8 Inflammatory disorders of other specified male genital organs ♂
Inflammation of multiple sites in male genital organs
N49.9 Inflammatory disorder of unspecified male genital organ ♂
Abscess of unspecified male genital organ
Boil of unspecified male genital organ
Carbuncle of unspecified male genital organ
Cellulitis of unspecified male genital organ

N5Ø Other and unspecified disorders of male genital organs
EXCLUDES 2 *torsion of testis (N44.Ø-)*

N5Ø.Ø Atrophy of testis ♂
N5Ø.1 Vascular disorders of male genital organs ♂
Hematocele, NOS, of male genital organs
Hemorrhage of male genital organs
Thrombosis of male genital organs
N5Ø.3 Cyst of epididymis ♂
N5Ø.8 Other specified disorders of male genital organs
AHA: 2016,4Q,45

N5Ø.81 Testicular pain
N5Ø.811 Right testicular pain ♂
N5Ø.812 Left testicular pain ♂
N5Ø.819 Testicular pain, unspecified ♂
N5Ø.82 Scrotal pain ♂
N5Ø.89 Other specified disorders of the male genital organs ♂
Atrophy of scrotum, seminal vesicle, spermatic cord, tunica vaginalis and vas deferens
Chylocele, tunica vaginalis (nonfilarial) NOS
Edema of scrotum, seminal vesicle, spermatic cord, tunica vaginalis and vas deferens
Hypertrophy of scrotum, seminal vesicle, spermatic cord, tunica vaginalis and vas deferens
Stricture of spermatic cord, tunica vaginalis, and vas deferens
Ulcer of scrotum, seminal vesicle, spermatic cord, testis, tunica vaginalis and vas deferens
Urethroscrotal fistula

N5Ø.9 Disorder of male genital organs, unspecified ♂

N51 Disorders of male genital organs in diseases classified elsewhere ♂
Code first underlying disease, such as:
filariasis (B74.Ø-B74.9)
EXCLUDES 1 *amebic balanitis (AØ6.8)*
candidal balanitis (B37.42)
gonococcal balanitis (A54.23)
gonococcal prostatitis (A54.22)
herpesviral [herpes simplex] balanitis (A6Ø.Ø1)
trichomonal prostatitis (A59.Ø2)
tuberculous prostatitis (A18.14)

N52 Male erectile dysfunction
EXCLUDES 1 *psychogenic impotence (F52.21)*

N52.Ø Vasculogenic erectile dysfunction
N52.Ø1 Erectile dysfunction due to arterial insufficiency A ♂
N52.Ø2 Corporo-venous occlusive erectile dysfunction A ♂
N52.Ø3 Combined arterial insufficiency and corporo-venous occlusive erectile dysfunction A ♂
N52.1 Erectile dysfunction due to diseases classified elsewhere A ♂
Code first underlying disease
N52.2 Drug-induced erectile dysfunction A ♂
N52.3 Postprocedural erectile dysfunction
AHA: 2016,4Q,45
N52.31 Erectile dysfunction following radical prostatectomy A ♂
N52.32 Erectile dysfunction following radical cystectomy A ♂
N52.33 Erectile dysfunction following urethral surgery A ♂
N52.34 Erectile dysfunction following simple prostatectomy A ♂
N52.35 Erectile dysfunction following radiation therapy A ♂
N52.36 Erectile dysfunction following interstitial seed therapy A ♂
N52.37 Erectile dysfunction following prostate ablative therapy A ♂
Erectile dysfunction following cryotherapy
Erectile dysfunction following other prostate ablative therapies
Erectile dysfunction following ultrasound ablative therapies
N52.39 Other and unspecified postprocedural erectile dysfunction A ♂
N52.8 Other male erectile dysfunction A ♂
N52.9 Male erectile dysfunction, unspecified A ♂
Impotence NOS

N53 Other male sexual dysfunction
EXCLUDES 1 *psychogenic sexual dysfunction (F52.-)*

N53.1 Ejaculatory dysfunction
EXCLUDES 1 *premature ejaculation (F52.4)*
N53.11 Retarded ejaculation ♂
N53.12 Painful ejaculation ♂
N53.13 Anejaculatory orgasm ♂
N53.14 Retrograde ejaculation ♂
DEF: Form of male sexual dysfunction in which the semen enters the bladder instead of going out through the urethra during ejaculation.

N53.19 Other ejaculatory dysfunction ♂
Ejaculatory dysfunction NOS
N53.8 Other male sexual dysfunction ♂
N53.9 Unspecified male sexual dysfunction ♂

Disorders of breast (N60-N65)

EXCLUDES 1 *disorders of breast associated with childbirth (O91-O92)*

N60 Benign mammary dysplasia
INCLUDES fibrocystic mastopathy
N60.0 Solitary cyst of breast
Cyst of breast
N60.01 Solitary cyst of right breast
N60.02 Solitary cyst of left breast
N60.09 Solitary cyst of unspecified breast
N60.1 Diffuse cystic mastopathy
Cystic breast
Fibrocystic disease of breast
EXCLUDES 1 *diffuse cystic mastopathy with epithelial proliferation (N60.3-)*
N60.11 Diffuse cystic mastopathy of right breast A
N60.12 Diffuse cystic mastopathy of left breast A
N60.19 Diffuse cystic mastopathy of unspecified breast A
N60.2 Fibroadenosis of breast
Adenofibrosis of breast
EXCLUDES 2 *fibroadenoma of breast (D24.-)*
N60.21 Fibroadenosis of right breast
N60.22 Fibroadenosis of left breast
N60.29 Fibroadenosis of unspecified breast
N60.3 Fibrosclerosis of breast
Cystic mastopathy with epithelial proliferation
N60.31 Fibrosclerosis of right breast
N60.32 Fibrosclerosis of left breast
N60.39 Fibrosclerosis of unspecified breast
N60.4 Mammary duct ectasia
N60.41 Mammary duct ectasia of right breast
N60.42 Mammary duct ectasia of left breast
N60.49 Mammary duct ectasia of unspecified breast
N60.8 Other benign mammary dysplasias
N60.81 Other benign mammary dysplasias of right breast
N60.82 Other benign mammary dysplasias of left breast
N60.89 Other benign mammary dysplasias of unspecified breast
N60.9 Unspecified benign mammary dysplasia
N60.91 Unspecified benign mammary dysplasia of right breast
N60.92 Unspecified benign mammary dysplasia of left breast
N60.99 Unspecified benign mammary dysplasia of unspecified breast

N61 Inflammatory disorders of breast
EXCLUDES 1 *inflammatory carcinoma of breast (C50.9)*
inflammatory disorder of breast associated with childbirth (O91.-)
neonatal infective mastitis (P39.0)
thrombophlebitis of breast [Mondor's disease] (I80.8)
N61.0 Mastitis without abscess
Infective mastitis (acute) (nonpuerperal) (subacute)
Mastitis (acute) (nonpuerperal) (subacute) NOS
Cellulitis (acute) (nonpuerperal) (subacute) of breast NOS
Cellulitis (acute) (nonpuerperal) (subacute) of nipple NOS
N61.1 Abscess of the breast and nipple
Abscess (acute) (chronic) (nonpuerperal) of areola
Abscess (acute) (chronic) (nonpuerperal) of breast
Carbuncle of breast
Mastitis with abscess
N61.2 Granulomatous mastitis
AHA: 2020,4Q,35
N61.20 Granulomatous mastitis, unspecified breast
N61.21 Granulomatous mastitis, right breast
N61.22 Granulomatous mastitis, left breast
N61.23 Granulomatous mastitis, bilateral breast

N62 Hypertrophy of breast
Gynecomastia
Hypertrophy of breast NOS
Massive pubertal hypertrophy of breast
EXCLUDES 1 *breast engorgement of newborn (P83.4)*
disproportion of reconstructed breast (N65.1)

N63 Unspecified lump in breast
Nodule(s) NOS in breast
AHA: 2022,3Q,8; 2019,4Q,12; 2017,4Q,19
N63.0 Unspecified lump in unspecified breast
N63.1 Unspecified lump in the right breast
N63.10 Unspecified lump in the right breast, unspecified quadrant
N63.11 Unspecified lump in the right breast, upper outer quadrant
N63.12 Unspecified lump in the right breast, upper inner quadrant
N63.13 Unspecified lump in the right breast, lower outer quadrant
N63.14 Unspecified lump in the right breast, lower inner quadrant
N63.15 Unspecified lump in the right breast, overlapping quadrants
N63.2 Unspecified lump in the left breast
N63.20 Unspecified lump in the left breast, unspecified quadrant
N63.21 Unspecified lump in the left breast, upper outer quadrant
N63.22 Unspecified lump in the left breast, upper inner quadrant
N63.23 Unspecified lump in the left breast, lower outer quadrant
N63.24 Unspecified lump in the left breast, lower inner quadrant
N63.25 Unspecified lump in the left breast, overlapping quadrants
N63.3 Unspecified lump in axillary tail
N63.31 Unspecified lump in axillary tail of the right breast
N63.32 Unspecified lump in axillary tail of the left breast
N63.4 Unspecified lump in breast, subareolar
N63.41 Unspecified lump in right breast, subareolar
N63.42 Unspecified lump in left breast, subareolar

N64 Other disorders of breast
EXCLUDES 2 *mechanical complication of breast prosthesis and implant (T85.4-)*
N64.0 Fissure and fistula of nipple
N64.1 Fat necrosis of breast UPD
Fat necrosis (segmental) of breast
Code first breast necrosis due to breast graft (T85.898)
N64.2 Atrophy of breast
N64.3 Galactorrhea not associated with childbirth
N64.4 Mastodynia
N64.5 Other signs and symptoms in breast
EXCLUDES 2 *abnormal findings on diagnostic imaging of breast (R92.-)*
N64.51 Induration of breast
N64.52 Nipple discharge
EXCLUDES 1 *abnormal findings in nipple discharge (R89.-)*
N64.53 Retraction of nipple
N64.59 Other signs and symptoms in breast
N64.8 Other specified disorders of breast
N64.81 Ptosis of breast A
EXCLUDES 1 *ptosis of native breast in relation to reconstructed breast (N65.1)*
N64.82 Hypoplasia of breast A
Micromastia
EXCLUDES 1 *congenital absence of breast (Q83.0)*
hypoplasia of native breast in relation to reconstructed breast (N65.1)
N64.89 Other specified disorders of breast
Galactocele
Subinvolution of breast (postlactational)
AHA: 2019,1Q,32; 2018,1Q,3
N64.9 Disorder of breast, unspecified

N65 Deformity and disproportion of reconstructed breast

N65.Ø Deformity of reconstructed breast A
Contour irregularity in reconstructed breast
Excess tissue in reconstructed breast
Misshapen reconstructed breast

N65.1 Disproportion of reconstructed breast A
Breast asymmetry between native breast and reconstructed breast
Disproportion between native breast and reconstructed breast

Inflammatory diseases of female pelvic organs (N7Ø-N77)

EXCLUDES 1 *inflammatory diseases of female pelvic organs complicating:*
abortion or ectopic or molar pregnancy (OØØ-OØ7, OØ8.Ø)
pregnancy, childbirth and the puerperium (O23.-, O75.3, O85, O86.-)

N7Ø Salpingitis and oophoritis
INCLUDES abscess (of) fallopian tube
abscess (of) ovary
pyosalpinx
salpingo-oophoritis
tubo-ovarian abscess
tubo-ovarian inflammatory disease
Use additional code (B95-B97), to identify infectious agent
EXCLUDES 1 *gonococcal infection (A54.24)*
tuberculous infection (A18.17)

N7Ø.Ø Acute salpingitis and oophoritis
N7Ø.Ø1 Acute salpingitis CC ♀
N7Ø.Ø2 Acute oophoritis CC ♀
N7Ø.Ø3 Acute salpingitis and oophoritis CC ♀

N7Ø.1 Chronic salpingitis and oophoritis
Hydrosalpinx
N7Ø.11 Chronic salpingitis ♀
N7Ø.12 Chronic oophoritis ♀
N7Ø.13 Chronic salpingitis and oophoritis ♀

N7Ø.9 Salpingitis and oophoritis, unspecified
N7Ø.91 Salpingitis, unspecified ♀
N7Ø.92 Oophoritis, unspecified ♀
N7Ø.93 Salpingitis and oophoritis, unspecified ♀

N71 Inflammatory disease of uterus, except cervix
INCLUDES endo (myo) metritis
metritis
myometritis
pyometra
uterine abscess
Use additional code (B95-B97), to identify infectious agent
EXCLUDES 1 *hyperplastic endometritis (N85.Ø-)*
infection of uterus following delivery (O85, O86.-)

N71.Ø Acute inflammatory disease of uterus CC ♀
N71.1 Chronic inflammatory disease of uterus ♀
N71.9 Inflammatory disease of uterus, unspecified ♀

N72 Inflammatory disease of cervix uteri ♀
INCLUDES cervicitis (with or without erosion or ectropion)
endocervicitis (with or without erosion or ectropion)
exocervicitis (with or without erosion or ectropion)
Use additional code (B95-B97), to identify infectious agent
EXCLUDES 1 *erosion and ectropion of cervix without cervicitis (N86)*

N73 Other female pelvic inflammatory diseases
Use additional code (B95-B97), to identify infectious agent

N73.Ø Acute parametritis and pelvic cellulitis CC ♀
Abscess of broad ligament
Abscess of parametrium
Pelvic cellulitis, female
DEF: Parametritis: Inflammation of the parametrium.

N73.1 Chronic parametritis and pelvic cellulitis ♀
Any condition in N73.Ø specified as chronic
EXCLUDES 1 *tuberculous parametritis and pelvic cellutlis (A18.17)*

N73.2 Unspecified parametritis and pelvic cellulitis ♀
Any condition in N73.Ø unspecified whether acute or chronic

N73.3 Female acute pelvic peritonitis MCC ♀
N73.4 Female chronic pelvic peritonitis CC ♀
EXCLUDES 1 *tuberculous pelvic (female) peritonitis (A18.17)*
N73.5 Female pelvic peritonitis, unspecified ♀
N73.6 Female pelvic peritoneal adhesions (postinfective) ♀
EXCLUDES 2 *postprocedural pelvic peritoneal adhesions (N99.4)*
AHA: 2014,1Q,6
N73.8 Other specified female pelvic inflammatory diseases ♀
N73.9 Female pelvic inflammatory disease, unspecified ♀
Female pelvic infection or inflammation NOS

N74 Female pelvic inflammatory disorders in diseases classified elsewhere ♀
Code first underlying disease
EXCLUDES 1 *chlamydial cervicitis (A56.Ø2)*
chlamydial pelvic inflammatory disease (A56.11)
gonococcal cervicitis (A54.Ø3)
gonococcal pelvic inflammatory disease (A54.24)
herpesviral [herpes simplex] cervicitis (A6Ø.Ø3)
herpesviral [herpes simplex] pelvic inflammatory disease (A6Ø.Ø9)
syphilitic cervicitis (A52.76)
syphilitic pelvic inflammatory disease (A52.76)
trichomonal cervicitis (A59.Ø9)
tuberculous cervicitis (A18.16)
tuberculous pelvic inflammatory disease (A18.17)

N75 Diseases of Bartholin's gland
DEF: Bartholin's gland: Mucous-producing gland found in the vestibular bulbs on either side of the vaginal orifice and connected to the mucosal membrane at the opening by a duct.
N75.Ø Cyst of Bartholin's gland ♀
N75.1 Abscess of Bartholin's gland CC ♀
N75.8 Other diseases of Bartholin's gland ♀
Bartholinitis
N75.9 Disease of Bartholin's gland, unspecified ♀

N76 Other inflammation of vagina and vulva
Use additional code (B95-B97), to identify infectious agent
EXCLUDES 2 *senile (atrophic) vaginitis (N95.2)*
vulvar vestibulitis (N94.81Ø)

N76.Ø Acute vaginitis ♀
Acute vulvovaginitis
Vaginitis NOS
Vulvovaginitis NOS
N76.1 Subacute and chronic vaginitis ♀
Chronic vulvovaginitis
Subacute vulvovaginitis
N76.2 Acute vulvitis ♀
Vulvitis NOS
N76.3 Subacute and chronic vulvitis ♀
N76.4 Abscess of vulva CC ♀
Furuncle of vulva
N76.5 Ulceration of vagina ♀
N76.6 Ulceration of vulva ♀
N76.8 Other specified inflammation of vagina and vulva
N76.81 Mucositis (ulcerative) of vagina and vulva CC ♀
Code also type of associated therapy, such as:
antineoplastic and immunosuppressive drugs (T45.1X-)
radiological procedure and radiotherapy (Y84.2)
EXCLUDES 2 *gastrointestinal mucositis (ulcerative) (K92.81)*
nasal mucositis (ulcerative) (J34.81)
oral mucositis (ulcerative) (K12.3-)
N76.82 Fournier disease of vagina and vulva HCC ♀
Fournier gangrene of vagina and vulva
Code also, if applicable, diabetes mellitus (EØ8-E13 with .9)
EXCLUDES 1 *gangrene in diabetes mellitus (EØ8-E13 with .52)*
AHA: 2022,4Q,34
N76.89 Other specified inflammation of vagina and vulva ♀

N77 Vulvovaginal ulceration and inflammation in diseases classified elsewhere
N77.Ø Ulceration of vulva in diseases classified elsewhere ♀
Code first underlying disease, such as:
Behcet's disease (M35.2)
EXCLUDES 1 *ulceration of vulva in gonococcal infection (A54.Ø2)*
ulceration of vulva in herpesviral [herpes simplex] infection (A6Ø.Ø4)
ulceration of vulva in syphilis (A51.Ø)
ulceration of vulva in tuberculosis (A18.18)

N77.1 ***Vaginitis, vulvitis and vulvovaginitis in diseases classified elsewhere*** ♀

Code first underlying disease, such as:

pinworm (B8Ø)

EXCLUDES 1 *candidal vulvovaginitis (B37.3-)*

chlamydial vulvovaginitis (A56.Ø2)

gonococcal vulvovaginitis (A54.Ø2)

herpesviral [herpes simplex] vulvovaginitis (A6Ø.Ø4)

trichomonal vulvovaginitis (A59.Ø1)

tuberculous vulvovaginitis (A18.18)

vulvovaginitis in early syphilis (A51.Ø)

vulvovaginitis in late syphilis (A52.76)

Noninflammatory disorders of female genital tract (N8Ø-N98)

N8Ø Endometriosis

AHA: 2022,4Q,34-36

DEF: Aberrant uterine mucosal tissue appearing in areas of the pelvic cavity outside of its normal location, lining the uterus, and inflaming surrounding tissues often resulting in infertility or spontaneous abortion.

N8Ø.Ø Endometriosis of uterus

Endometriosis of the cervix

EXCLUDES 1 *stromal endometriosis (D39.Ø)*

N8Ø.ØØ Endometriosis of the uterus, unspecified ♀

N8Ø.Ø1 Superficial endometriosis of the uterus ♀

N8Ø.Ø2 Deep endometriosis of the uterus ♀

Deep retrocervical endometriosis

N8Ø.Ø3 Adenomyosis of the uterus ♀

Adenomyosis NOS

N8Ø.1 Endometriosis of ovary

N8Ø.1Ø Endometriosis of ovary, unspecified depth

N8Ø.1Ø1 Endometriosis of right ovary, unspecified depth ♀

N8Ø.1Ø2 Endometriosis of left ovary, unspecified depth ♀

N8Ø.1Ø3 Endometriosis of bilateral ovaries, unspecified depth ♀

N8Ø.1Ø9 Endometriosis of ovary, unspecified side, unspecified depth ♀

Endometriosis of ovary NOS

N8Ø.11 Superficial endometriosis of the ovary

N8Ø.111 Superficial endometriosis of right ovary ♀

AHA: 2022,4Q,35

N8Ø.112 Superficial endometriosis of left ovary ♀

N8Ø.113 Superficial endometriosis of bilateral ovaries ♀

N8Ø.119 Superficial endometriosis of ovary, unspecified ovary ♀

N8Ø.12 Deep endometriosis of ovary

Deep ovarian endometriosis

Endometrioma

N8Ø.121 Deep endometriosis of right ovary ♀

N8Ø.122 Deep endometriosis of left ovary ♀

N8Ø.123 Deep endometriosis of bilateral ovaries ♀

N8Ø.129 Deep endometriosis of ovary, unspecified ovary ♀

N8Ø.2 Endometriosis of fallopian tube

N8Ø.2Ø Endometriosis of fallopian tube, unspecified depth

N8Ø.2Ø1 Endometriosis of right fallopian tube, unspecified depth ♀

N8Ø.2Ø2 Endometriosis of left fallopian tube, unspecified depth ♀

N8Ø.2Ø3 Endometriosis of bilateral fallopian tubes, unspecified depth ♀

N8Ø.2Ø9 Endometriosis of unspecified fallopian tube, unspecified depth ♀

Endometriosis fallopian tube NOS

N8Ø.21 Superficial endometriosis of fallopian tube

N8Ø.211 Superficial endometriosis of right fallopian tube ♀

N8Ø.212 Superficial endometriosis of left fallopian tube ♀

N8Ø.213 Superficial endometriosis of bilateral fallopian tubes ♀

N8Ø.219 Superficial endometriosis of unspecified fallopian tube ♀

N8Ø.22 Deep endometriosis of the fallopian tube

Deep endometriosis involving muscular wall of fallopian tube

N8Ø.221 Deep endometriosis of right fallopian tube ♀

N8Ø.222 Deep endometriosis of left fallopian tube ♀

N8Ø.223 Deep endometriosis of bilateral fallopian tubes ♀

N8Ø.229 Deep endometriosis of unspecified fallopian tube ♀

N8Ø.3 Endometriosis of pelvic peritoneum

N8Ø.3Ø Endometriosis of pelvic peritoneum, unspecified ♀

Endometriosis of the retroperitoneum NOS

N8Ø.31 Endometriosis of the anterior cul-de-sac

N8Ø.311 Superficial endometriosis of the anterior cul-de-sac ♀

N8Ø.312 Deep endometriosis of the anterior cul-de-sac ♀

N8Ø.319 Endometriosis of the anterior cul-de-sac, unspecified depth ♀

Endometriosis of the anterior cul-de-sac NOS

N8Ø.32 Endometriosis of the posterior cul-de-sac

N8Ø.321 Superficial endometriosis of the posterior cul-de-sac ♀

N8Ø.322 Deep endometriosis of the posterior cul-de-sac ♀

N8Ø.329 Endometriosis of the posterior cul-de-sac, unspecified depth ♀

Endometriosis of the posterior cul-de-sac NOS

N8Ø.33 Superficial endometriosis of the pelvic sidewall

N8Ø.331 Superficial endometriosis of the right pelvic sidewall ♀

N8Ø.332 Superficial endometriosis of the left pelvic sidewall ♀

N8Ø.333 Superficial endometriosis of bilateral pelvic sidewall ♀

N8Ø.339 Superficial endometriosis of pelvic sidewall, unspecified side ♀

N8Ø.34 Deep endometriosis of the pelvic sidewall

N8Ø.341 Deep endometriosis of the right pelvic sidewall ♀

N8Ø.342 Deep endometriosis of the left pelvic sidewall ♀

N8Ø.343 Deep endometriosis of the bilateral pelvic sidewall ♀

N8Ø.349 Deep endometriosis of the pelvic sidewall, unspecified side ♀

AHA: 2022,4Q,36

N8Ø.35 Endometriosis of the pelvic sidewall, unspecified depth

N8Ø.351 Endometriosis of the right pelvic sidewall, unspecified depth ♀

N8Ø.352 Endometriosis of the left pelvic sidewall, unspecified depth ♀

N8Ø.353 Endometriosis of bilateral pelvic sidewall, unspecified depth ♀

N8Ø.359 Endometriosis of pelvic sidewall, unspecified side, unspecified depth ♀

Endometriosis of the pelvic sidewall NOS

N8Ø.36 Superficial endometriosis of the pelvic brim

N8Ø.361 Superficial endometriosis of the right pelvic brim ♀

N8Ø.362 Superficial endometriosis of the left pelvic brim ♀

N8Ø.363 Superficial endometriosis of bilateral pelvic brim ♀

N8Ø.369 Superficial endometriosis of the pelvic brim, unspecified side ♀

N8Ø.37 Deep endometriosis of the pelvic brim

N8Ø.371 Deep endometriosis of the right pelvic brim ♀

N8Ø.372 Deep endometriosis of the left pelvic brim ♀

N8Ø.373 Deep endometriosis of bilateral pelvic brim ♀
N8Ø.379 Deep endometriosis of the pelvic brim, unspecified side ♀
N8Ø.38 Endometriosis of the pelvic brim, unspecified depth
N8Ø.381 Endometriosis of the right pelvic brim, unspecified depth ♀
N8Ø.382 Endometriosis of the left pelvic brim, unspecified depth ♀
N8Ø.383 Endometriosis of bilateral pelvic brim, unspecified depth ♀
N8Ø.389 Endometriosis of the pelvic brim, unspecified side, unspecified depth ♀
Endometriosis of the pelvic brim NOS
N8Ø.3A Superficial endometriosis of the uterosacral ligament(s)
N8Ø.3A1 Superficial endometriosis of the right uterosacral ligament ♀
N8Ø.3A2 Superficial endometriosis of the left uterosacral ligament ♀
N8Ø.3A3 Superficial endometriosis of the bilateral uterosacral ligament(s) ♀
N8Ø.3A9 Superficial endometriosis of the uterosacral ligament(s), unspecified side ♀
N8Ø.3B Deep endometriosis of the uterosacral ligament(s)
N8Ø.3B1 Deep endometriosis of the right uterosacral ligament ♀
N8Ø.3B2 Deep endometriosis of the left uterosacral ligament ♀
N8Ø.3B3 Deep endometriosis of bilateral uterosacral ligament(s) ♀
N8Ø.3B9 Deep endometriosis of the uterosacral ligament(s), unspecified side ♀
N8Ø.3C Endometriosis of the uterosacral ligament(s), unspecified depth
N8Ø.3C1 Endometriosis of the right uterosacral ligament, unspecified depth ♀
N8Ø.3C2 Endometriosis of the left uterosacral ligament, unspecified depth ♀
N8Ø.3C3 Endometriosis of bilateral uterosacral ligament(s), unspecified depth ♀
N8Ø.3C9 Endometriosis of the uterosacral ligament(s), unspecified side, unspecified depth ♀
Endometriosis of the uterosacral ligament(s) NOS
N8Ø.39 Endometriosis of other pelvic peritoneum
N8Ø.391 Superficial endometriosis of the pelvic peritoneum, other specified sites ♀
N8Ø.392 Deep endometriosis of the pelvic peritoneum, other specified sites ♀
N8Ø.399 Endometriosis of the pelvic peritoneum, other specified sites, unspecified depth ♀
N8Ø.4 Endometriosis of rectovaginal septum and vagina
N8Ø.4Ø Endometriosis of rectovaginal septum, unspecified involvement of vagina ♀
Endometriosis of the rectovaginal septum, NOS
N8Ø.41 Endometriosis of rectovaginal septum without involvement of vagina ♀
N8Ø.42 Endometriosis of rectovaginal septum with involvement of vagina ♀
N8Ø.5 Endometriosis of intestine
N8Ø.5Ø Endometriosis of intestine, unspecified ♀
N8Ø.51 Endometriosis of the rectum
N8Ø.511 Superficial endometriosis of the rectum ♀
N8Ø.512 Deep endometriosis of the rectum ♀
Deep endometriosis of the rectum, multifocal
N8Ø.519 Endometriosis of the rectum, unspecified depth ♀
Endometriosis of the rectum NOS
N8Ø.52 Endometriosis of the sigmoid colon
N8Ø.521 Superficial endometriosis of the sigmoid colon ♀
N8Ø.522 Deep endometriosis of the sigmoid colon ♀
N8Ø.529 Endometriosis of the sigmoid colon, unspecified depth ♀
Endometriosis of the sigmoid colon NOS
N8Ø.53 Endometriosis of the cecum
N8Ø.531 Superficial endometriosis of the cecum ♀
N8Ø.532 Deep endometriosis of the cecum ♀
N8Ø.539 Endometriosis of the cecum, unspecified depth ♀
Endometriosis of the cecum NOS
N8Ø.54 Endometriosis of the appendix
N8Ø.541 Superficial endometriosis of the appendix ♀
N8Ø.542 Deep endometriosis of the appendix ♀
N8Ø.549 Endometriosis of the appendix, unspecified depth ♀
Endometriosis of the appendix NOS
N8Ø.55 Endometriosis of other parts of the colon
Endometriosis of descending colon
Endometriosis of transverse colon
N8Ø.551 Superficial endometriosis of other parts of the colon ♀
N8Ø.552 Deep endometriosis of other parts of the colon ♀
N8Ø.559 Endometriosis of other parts of the colon, unspecified depth ♀
Endometriosis of colon NOS
N8Ø.56 Endometriosis of the small intestine
N8Ø.561 Superficial endometriosis of the small intestine ♀
N8Ø.562 Deep endometriosis of the small intestine ♀
Deep endometriosis of the small intestine, multifocal
N8Ø.569 Endometriosis of the small intestine, unspecified depth ♀
Endometriosis of the small intestine NOS
N8Ø.6 Endometriosis in cutaneous scar ♀
N8Ø.A Endometriosis of bladder and ureters
N8Ø.AØ Endometriosis of bladder, unspecified depth ♀
Endometriosis of bladder NOS
N8Ø.A1 Superficial endometriosis of bladder ♀
N8Ø.A2 Deep endometriosis of bladder ♀
N8Ø.A4 Superficial endometriosis of ureter
Extrinsic endometriosis of ureter
Code also, if applicable, obstructive and reflux uropathy (N13.-)
N8Ø.A41 Superficial endometriosis of right ureter ♀
N8Ø.A42 Superficial endometriosis of left ureter ♀
N8Ø.A43 Superficial endometriosis of bilateral ureters ♀
N8Ø.A49 Superficial endometriosis of unspecified ureter ♀
N8Ø.A5 Deep endometriosis of ureter
Intrinsic endometriosis of ureter
Code also, if applicable, obstructive and reflux uropathy (N13.-)
N8Ø.A51 Deep endometriosis of right ureter ♀
N8Ø.A52 Deep endometriosis of left ureter ♀
N8Ø.A53 Deep endometriosis of bilateral ureters ♀
N8Ø.A59 Deep endometriosis of unspecified ureter ♀
N8Ø.A6 Endometriosis of ureter, unspecified depth
Code also, if applicable, obstructive and reflux uropathy (N13.-)
N8Ø.A61 Endometriosis of right ureter, unspecified depth ♀
N8Ø.A62 Endometriosis of left ureter, unspecified depth ♀
N8Ø.A63 Endometriosis of bilateral ureters, unspecified depth ♀
N8Ø.A69 Endometriosis of unspecified ureter, unspecified depth ♀

✓5th **N8Ø.B Endometriosis of cardiothoracic space**
Endometriosis of thorax
Code also, if applicable:
catamenial hemothorax (J94.2)
catamenial pneumothorax (J93.12)

N8Ø.B1 Endometriosis of pleura ♀
N8Ø.B2 Endometriosis of lung ♀
✓6th **N8Ø.B3 Endometriosis of diaphragm**
N8Ø.B31 Superficial endometriosis of diaphragm ♀
N8Ø.B32 Deep endometriosis of diaphragm ♀
N8Ø.B39 Endometriosis of diaphragm, unspecified depth ♀
Endometriosis of the diaphragm NOS
N8Ø.B4 Endometriosis of the pericardial space ♀
N8Ø.B5 Endometriosis of the mediastinal space ♀
N8Ø.B6 Endometriosis of cardiothoracic space ♀

✓5th **N8Ø.C Endometriosis of the abdomen**
N8Ø.CØ Endometriosis of the abdomen, unspecified ♀
Endometriosis of the abdomen NOS
✓6th **N8Ø.C1 Endometriosis of the anterior abdominal wall**
N8Ø.C1Ø Endometriosis of the anterior abdominal wall, subcutaneous tissue ♀
N8Ø.C11 Endometriosis of the anterior abdominal wall, fascia and muscular layers ♀
N8Ø.C19 Endometriosis of the anterior abdominal wall, unspecified depth ♀
Endometriosis of the anterior abdominal wall NOS
N8Ø.C2 Endometriosis of the umbilicus ♀
N8Ø.C3 Endometriosis of the inguinal canal ♀
N8Ø.C4 Endometriosis of extra-pelvic abdominal peritoneum ♀
N8Ø.C9 Endometriosis of other site of abdomen ♀

✓5th **N8Ø.D Endometriosis of the pelvic nerves**
Endometriosis of the nerves of the retroperitoneum
N8Ø.DØ Endometriosis of the pelvic nerves, unspecified ♀
Endometriosis of nerve of the retroperitoneum, NOS
N8Ø.D1 Endometriosis of the sacral splanchnic nerves ♀
Endometriosis of the pelvic splanchnic nerves
N8Ø.D2 Endometriosis of the sacral nerve roots ♀
N8Ø.D3 Endometriosis of the obturator nerve ♀
N8Ø.D4 Endometriosis of the sciatic nerve ♀
N8Ø.D5 Endometriosis of the pudendal nerve ♀
N8Ø.D6 Endometriosis of the femoral nerve ♀
N8Ø.D9 Endometriosis of other pelvic nerve ♀
Endometriosis of the other nerves of the retroperitoneum

N8Ø.8 Other endometriosis ♀
Endometriosis of other site

N8Ø.9 Endometriosis, unspecified ♀

✓4th **N81 Female genital prolapse**
EXCLUDES 1 *genital prolapse complicating pregnancy, labor or delivery (O34.5-)*
prolapse and hernia of ovary and fallopian tube (N83.4-)
prolapse of vaginal vault after hysterectomy (N99.3)

Types of Pelvic Organ Prolapse

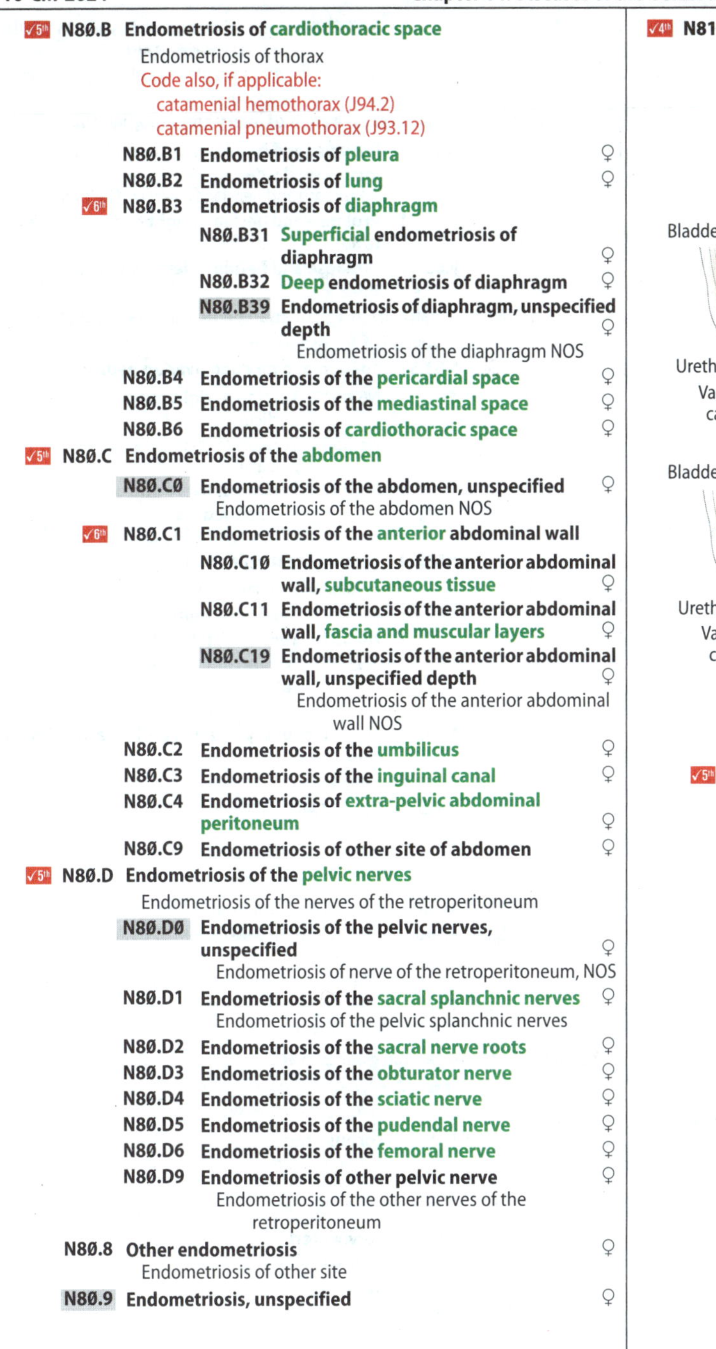

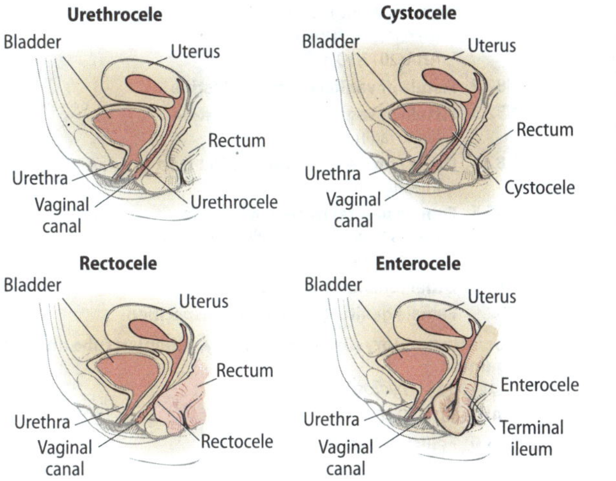

N81.Ø Urethrocele ♀
EXCLUDES 1 *urethrocele with cystocele (N81.1-)*
urethrocele with prolapse of uterus (N81.2-N81.4)

✓5th **N81.1 Cystocele**
Cystocele with urethrocele
Cystourethrocele
EXCLUDES 1 *cystocele with prolapse of uterus (N81.2-N81.4)*
N81.1Ø Cystocele, unspecified ♀
Prolapse of (anterior) vaginal wall NOS
N81.11 Cystocele, midline ♀
N81.12 Cystocele, lateral ♀
Paravaginal cystocele
DEF: Detachment of the lateral support connections of the vagina at the arcus tendineus fasciae pelvis (ATFP) that results in bladder drop. The bladder herniates into the vagina laterally.

N81.2 Incomplete uterovaginal prolapse ♀
First degree uterine prolapse
Prolapse of cervix NOS
Second degree uterine prolapse
EXCLUDES 1 *cervical stump prolapse (N81.85)*

N81.3 Complete uterovaginal prolapse ♀
Procidentia (uteri) NOS
Third degree uterine prolapse

N81.4 Uterovaginal prolapse, unspecified ♀
Prolapse of uterus NOS

N81.5 Vaginal enterocele ♀
EXCLUDES 1 *enterocele with prolapse of uterus (N81.2-N81.4)*

N81.6 Rectocele ♀
Prolapse of posterior vaginal wall
Use additional code for any associated fecal incontinence, if applicable (R15.-)
EXCLUDES 1 ▶*rectocele with prolapse of uterus (N81.2-N81.4)*◀
EXCLUDES 2 *perineocele (N81.81)*
rectal prolapse (K62.3)
~~*rectocele with prolapse of uterus (N81.2-N81.4)*~~

✓5th **N81.8 Other female genital prolapse**
N81.81 Perineocele ♀
N81.82 Incompetence or weakening of pubocervical tissue ♀
N81.83 Incompetence or weakening of rectovaginal tissue ♀
N81.84 Pelvic muscle wasting ♀
Disuse atrophy of pelvic muscles and anal sphincter
N81.85 Cervical stump prolapse ♀
N81.89 Other female genital prolapse ♀
Deficient perineum
Old laceration of muscles of pelvic floor

N81.9 Female genital prolapse, unspecified ♀

N82 Fistulae involving female genital tract
EXCLUDES 1 *vesicointestinal fistulae (N32.1)*

N82.Ø Vesicovaginal fistula CC ♀

N82.1 Other female urinary-genital tract fistulae CC ♀
Cervicovesical fistula
Ureterovaginal fistula
Urethrovaginal fistula
Uteroureteric fistula
Uterovesical fistula
AHA: 2017,3Q,3

N82.2 Fistula of vagina to small intestine CC ♀

N82.3 Fistula of vagina to large intestine CC ♀
Rectovaginal fistula

N82.4 Other female intestinal-genital tract fistulae CC ♀
Intestinouterine fistula

N82.5 Female genital tract-skin fistulae CC ♀
Uterus to abdominal wall fistula
Vaginoperineal fistula

N82.8 Other female genital tract fistulae CC ♀

N82.9 Female genital tract fistula, unspecified CC ♀

N83 Noninflammatory disorders of ovary, fallopian tube and broad ligament
EXCLUDES 2 *hydrosalpinx (N7Ø.1-)*
AHA: 2016,4Q,46

N83.Ø Follicular cyst of ovary
Cyst of graafian follicle
Hemorrhagic follicular cyst (of ovary)

N83.ØØ Follicular cyst of ovary, unspecified side ♀

N83.Ø1 Follicular cyst of right ovary ♀

N83.Ø2 Follicular cyst of left ovary ♀

N83.1 Corpus luteum cyst
Hemorrhagic corpus luteum cyst
AHA: 2022,1Q,23

N83.1Ø Corpus luteum cyst of ovary, unspecified side ♀

N83.11 Corpus luteum cyst of right ovary ♀

N83.12 Corpus luteum cyst of left ovary ♀

N83.2 Other and unspecified ovarian cysts
EXCLUDES 1 *developmental ovarian cyst (Q5Ø.1)*
neoplastic ovarian cyst (D27.-)
polycystic ovarian syndrome (E28.2)
Stein-Leventhal syndrome (E28.2)
AHA: 2022,1Q,23

N83.2Ø Unspecified ovarian cysts

N83.2Ø1 Unspecified ovarian cyst, right side ♀

N83.2Ø2 Unspecified ovarian cyst, left side ♀

N83.2Ø9 Unspecified ovarian cyst, unspecified side ♀
Ovarian cyst, NOS

N83.29 Other ovarian cysts
Retention cyst of ovary
Simple cyst of ovary

N83.291 Other ovarian cyst, right side ♀

N83.292 Other ovarian cyst, left side ♀

N83.299 Other ovarian cyst, unspecified side ♀

N83.3 Acquired atrophy of ovary and fallopian tube

N83.31 Acquired atrophy of ovary

N83.311 Acquired atrophy of right ovary ♀

N83.312 Acquired atrophy of left ovary ♀

N83.319 Acquired atrophy of ovary, unspecified side ♀
Acquired atrophy of ovary, NOS

N83.32 Acquired atrophy of fallopian tube

N83.321 Acquired atrophy of right fallopian tube ♀

N83.322 Acquired atrophy of left fallopian tube ♀

N83.329 Acquired atrophy of fallopian tube, unspecified side ♀
Acquired atrophy of fallopian tube, NOS

N83.33 Acquired atrophy of ovary and fallopian tube

N83.331 Acquired atrophy of right ovary and fallopian tube ♀

N83.332 Acquired atrophy of left ovary and fallopian tube ♀

N83.339 Acquired atrophy of ovary and fallopian tube, unspecified side ♀
Acquired atrophy of ovary and fallopian tube, NOS

N83.4 Prolapse and hernia of ovary and fallopian tube

N83.4Ø Prolapse and hernia of ovary and fallopian tube, unspecified side ♀
Prolapse and hernia of ovary and fallopian tube, NOS

N83.41 Prolapse and hernia of right ovary and fallopian tube ♀

N83.42 Prolapse and hernia of left ovary and fallopian tube ♀

N83.5 Torsion of ovary, ovarian pedicle and fallopian tube
Torsion of accessory tube

N83.51 Torsion of ovary and ovarian pedicle

N83.511 Torsion of right ovary and ovarian pedicle CC ♀

N83.512 Torsion of left ovary and ovarian pedicle CC ♀

N83.519 Torsion of ovary and ovarian pedicle, unspecified side CC UNS ♀
Torsion of ovary and ovarian pedicle, NOS

N83.52 Torsion of fallopian tube
Torsion of hydatid of Morgagni

N83.521 Torsion of right fallopian tube CC ♀

N83.522 Torsion of left fallopian tube CC ♀

N83.529 Torsion of fallopian tube, unspecified side CC UNS ♀
Torsion of fallopian tube, NOS

N83.53 Torsion of ovary, ovarian pedicle and fallopian tube CC ♀

N83.6 Hematosalpinx ♀
EXCLUDES 1 *hematosalpinx (with) (in):*
hematocolpos (N89.7)
hematometra (N85.7)
tubal pregnancy (OØØ.1-)

N83.7 Hematoma of broad ligament ♀

N83.8 Other noninflammatory disorders of ovary, fallopian tube and broad ligament ♀
Broad ligament laceration syndrome [Allen-Masters]

N83.9 Noninflammatory disorder of ovary, fallopian tube and broad ligament, unspecified ♀

N84 Polyp of female genital tract
EXCLUDES 1 *adenomatous polyp (D28.-)*
placental polyp (O9Ø.89)

N84.Ø Polyp of corpus uteri ♀
Polyp of endometrium
Polyp of uterus NOS
EXCLUDES 1 *polypoid endometrial hyperplasia (N85.Ø-)*

N84.1 Polyp of cervix uteri ♀
Mucous polyp of cervix

N84.2 Polyp of vagina ♀

N84.3 Polyp of vulva ♀
Polyp of labia

N84.8 Polyp of other parts of female genital tract ♀

N84.9 Polyp of female genital tract, unspecified ♀

N85 Other noninflammatory disorders of uterus, except cervix
EXCLUDES 1 *endometriosis (N8Ø.-)*
inflammatory diseases of uterus (N71.-)
noninflammatory disorders of cervix, except malposition (N86-N88)
polyp of corpus uteri (N84.Ø)
uterine prolapse (N81.-)

N85.Ø Endometrial hyperplasia

N85.ØØ Endometrial hyperplasia, unspecified ♀
Hyperplasia (adenomatous) (cystic) (glandular) of endometrium
Hyperplastic endometritis

N85.Ø1 Benign endometrial hyperplasia ♀
Endometrial hyperplasia (complex) (simple) without atypia

N85.Ø2 Endometrial intraepithelial neoplasia [EIN] ♀
Endometrial hyperplasia with atypia
EXCLUDES 1 *malignant neoplasm of endometrium (with endometrial intraepithelial neoplasia [EIN]) (C54.1)*

N85.2 **Hypertrophy of uterus** ♀
Bulky or enlarged uterus
EXCLUDES 1 *puerperal hypertrophy of uterus (O9Ø.89)*

N85.3 **Subinvolution of uterus** ♀
EXCLUDES 1 *puerperal subinvolution of uterus (O9Ø.89)*

N85.4 **Malposition of uterus** ♀
Anteversion of uterus
Retroflexion of uterus
Retroversion of uterus
EXCLUDES 1 *malposition of uterus complicating pregnancy, labor or delivery (O34.5-, O65.5)*

N85.5 **Inversion of uterus** ♀
EXCLUDES 1 *current obstetric trauma (O71.2)*
postpartum inversion of uterus (O71.2)
DEF: Abnormality in which the uterus turns inside out.

Inversion of Uterus

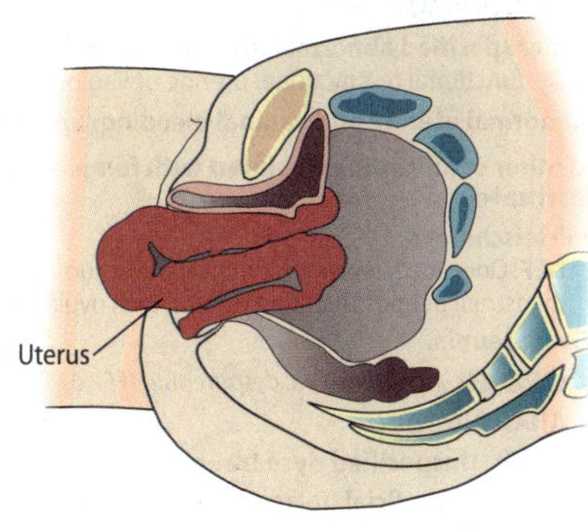

N85.6 **Intrauterine synechiae** ♀

N85.7 **Hematometra** ♀
Hematosalpinx with hematometra
EXCLUDES 1 *hematometra with hematocolpos (N89.7)*
DEF: Accumulation of blood within the uterus.

N85.8 **Other specified noninflammatory disorders of uterus** ♀
Atrophy of uterus, acquired
Fibrosis of uterus NOS

N85.9 **Noninflammatory disorder of uterus, unspecified** ♀
Disorder of uterus NOS

N85.A **Isthmocele**
Isthmocele (non-pregnant state)
Code also any associated conditions such as:
abnormal uterine and vaginal bleeding, unspecified (N93.9)
female infertility of uterine origin (N97.2)
pelvic and perineal pain (R1Ø.2)
EXCLUDES 1 *maternal care for cesarean scar defect (isthmocele) (O34.22)*
AHA: 2022,4Q,36-37

N86 **Erosion and ectropion of cervix uteri** ♀
Decubitus (trophic) ulcer of cervix
Eversion of cervix
EXCLUDES 1 *erosion and ectropion of cervix with cervicitis (N72)*

✓4th N87 **Dysplasia of cervix uteri**
EXCLUDES 1 *abnormal results from cervical cytologic examination without histologic confirmation (R87.61-)*
carcinoma in situ of cervix uteri (DØ6.-)
cervical intraepithelial neoplasia III [CIN III] (DØ6.-)
HGSIL of cervix (R87.613)
severe dysplasia of cervix uteri (DØ6.-)

N87.Ø **Mild cervical dysplasia** ♀
Cervical intraepithelial neoplasia I [CIN I]

N87.1 **Moderate cervical dysplasia** ♀
Cervical intraepithelial neoplasia II [CIN II]

N87.9 **Dysplasia of cervix uteri, unspecified** ♀
Anaplasia of cervix
Cervical atypism
Cervical dysplasia NOS

✓4th N88 **Other noninflammatory disorders of cervix uteri**
EXCLUDES 2 *inflammatory disease of cervix (N72)*
polyp of cervix (N84.1)

N88.Ø **Leukoplakia of cervix uteri** ♀

N88.1 **Old laceration of cervix uteri** ♀
Adhesions of cervix
EXCLUDES 1 *current obstetric trauma (O71.3)*

N88.2 **Stricture and stenosis of cervix uteri** ♀
EXCLUDES 1 *stricture and stenosis of cervix uteri complicating labor (O65.5)*

N88.3 **Incompetence of cervix uteri** ♀
Investigation and management of (suspected) cervical incompetence in a nonpregnant woman
EXCLUDES 1 *cervical incompetence complicating pregnancy (O34.3-)*
DEF: Inadequate functioning of the cervix marked by abnormal widening during pregnancy and causing premature birth or miscarriage.

N88.4 **Hypertrophic elongation of cervix uteri** ♀

N88.8 **Other specified noninflammatory disorders of cervix uteri** ♀
EXCLUDES 1 *current obstetric trauma (O71.3)*

N88.9 **Noninflammatory disorder of cervix uteri, unspecified** ♀

✓4th N89 **Other noninflammatory disorders of vagina**
EXCLUDES 1 *abnormal results from vaginal cytologic examination without histologic confirmation (R87.62-)*
carcinoma in situ of vagina (DØ7.2)
HGSIL of vagina (R87.623)
inflammation of vagina (N76.-)
senile (atrophic) vaginitis (N95.2)
severe dysplasia of vagina (DØ7.2)
trichomonal leukorrhea (A59.ØØ)
vaginal intraepithelial neoplasia [VAIN], grade III (DØ7.2)

N89.Ø **Mild vaginal dysplasia** ♀
Vaginal intraepithelial neoplasia [VAIN], grade I

N89.1 **Moderate vaginal dysplasia** ♀
Vaginal intraepithelial neoplasia [VAIN], grade II

N89.3 **Dysplasia of vagina, unspecified** ♀

N89.4 **Leukoplakia of vagina** ♀

N89.5 **Stricture and atresia of vagina** ♀
Vaginal adhesions
Vaginal stenosis
EXCLUDES 1 *congenital atresia or stricture (Q52.4)*
postprocedural adhesions of vagina (N99.2)

N89.6 **Tight hymenal ring** ♀
Rigid hymen
Tight introitus
EXCLUDES 1 *imperforate hymen (Q52.3)*

N89.7 **Hematocolpos** ♀
Hematocolpos with hematometra or hematosalpinx
AHA: 2016,4Q,58

N89.8 **Other specified noninflammatory disorders of vagina** ♀
Leukorrhea NOS
Old vaginal laceration
Pessary ulcer of vagina
EXCLUDES 1 *current obstetric trauma (O7Ø.-, O71.4, O71.7-O71.8)*
old laceration involving muscles of pelvic floor (N81.8)

N89.9 **Noninflammatory disorder of vagina, unspecified** ♀

✓4th N9Ø **Other noninflammatory disorders of vulva and perineum**
EXCLUDES 1 *anogenital (venereal) warts (A63.Ø)*
carcinoma in situ of vulva (DØ7.1)
condyloma acuminatum (A63.Ø)
current obstetric trauma (O7Ø.-, O71.7-O71.8)
inflammation of vulva (N76.-)
severe dysplasia of vulva (DØ7.1)
vulvar intraepithelial neoplasm III [VIN III] (DØ7.1)

N9Ø.Ø **Mild vulvar dysplasia** ♀
Vulvar intraepithelial neoplasia [VIN], grade I

N9Ø.1 **Moderate vulvar dysplasia** ♀
Vulvar intraepithelial neoplasia [VIN], grade II

N9Ø.3 **Dysplasia of vulva, unspecified** ♀

N90.4 Leukoplakia of vulva ♀
Dystrophy of vulva
Kraurosis of vulva
Lichen sclerosus of external female genital organs

N90.5 Atrophy of vulva ♀
Stenosis of vulva

✓5th **N90.6 Hypertrophy of vulva**
AHA: 2016,4Q,46

N90.60 Unspecified hypertrophy of vulva ♀
Unspecified hypertrophy of labia

N90.61 Childhood asymmetric labium majus enlargement ♀
CALME

N90.69 Other specified hypertrophy of vulva ♀
Other specified hypertrophy of labia

N90.7 Vulvar cyst ♀

✓5th **N90.8 Other specified noninflammatory disorders of vulva and perineum**

✓6th **N90.81 Female genital mutilation status**
Female genital cutting status

N90.810 Female genital mutilation status, unspecified ♀
Female genital cutting status, unspecified
Female genital mutilation status NOS

N90.811 Female genital mutilation Type I status ♀
Clitorectomy status
Female genital cutting Type I status

N90.812 Female genital mutilation Type II status ♀
Clitorectomy with excision of labia minora status
Female genital cutting Type II status

N90.813 Female genital mutilation Type III status ♀
Female genital cutting Type III status
Infibulation status

N90.818 Other female genital mutilation status ♀
Female genital cutting Type IV status
Female genital mutilation Type IV status
Other female genital cutting status

N90.89 Other specified noninflammatory disorders of vulva and perineum ♀
Adhesions of vulva
Hypertrophy of clitoris

N90.9 Noninflammatory disorder of vulva and perineum, unspecified ♀

✓4th **N91 Absent, scanty and rare menstruation**
EXCLUDES 1 *ovarian dysfunction (E28.-)*

N91.0 Primary amenorrhea ♀
N91.1 Secondary amenorrhea ♀
N91.2 Amenorrhea, unspecified ♀
N91.3 Primary oligomenorrhea ♀
N91.4 Secondary oligomenorrhea ♀
N91.5 Oligomenorrhea, unspecified ♀
Hypomenorrhea NOS

✓4th **N92 Excessive, frequent and irregular menstruation**
EXCLUDES 1 *postmenopausal bleeding (N95.0)*
precocious puberty (menstruation) (E30.1)

N92.0 Excessive and frequent menstruation with regular cycle ♀
Heavy periods NOS
Menorrhagia NOS
Polymenorrhea

N92.1 Excessive and frequent menstruation with irregular cycle ♀
Irregular intermenstrual bleeding
Irregular, shortened intervals between menstrual bleeding
Menometrorrhagia
Metrorrhagia

N92.2 Excessive menstruation at puberty P ♀
Excessive bleeding associated with onset of menstrual periods
Pubertal menorrhagia
Puberty bleeding

N92.3 Ovulation bleeding ♀
Regular intermenstrual bleeding

N92.4 Excessive bleeding in the premenopausal period ♀
Climacteric menorrhagia or metrorrhagia
Menopausal menorrhagia or metrorrhagia
Perimenopausal bleeding
Perimenopausal menorrhagia or metrorrhagia
Preclimacteric menorrhagia or metrorrhagia
Premenopausal menorrhagia or metrorrhagia

N92.5 Other specified irregular menstruation ♀

N92.6 Irregular menstruation, unspecified ♀
Irregular bleeding NOS
Irregular periods NOS
EXCLUDES 1 *irregular menstruation with:*
lengthened intervals or scanty bleeding (N91.3-N91.5)
shortened intervals or excessive bleeding (N92.1)

✓4th **N93 Other abnormal uterine and vaginal bleeding**
EXCLUDES 1 *neonatal vaginal hemorrhage (P54.6)*
precocious puberty (menstruation) (E30.1)
pseudomenses (P54.6)

N93.0 Postcoital and contact bleeding ♀

N93.1 Pre-pubertal vaginal bleeding ♀
AHA: 2016,4Q,47

N93.8 Other specified abnormal uterine and vaginal bleeding ♀
Dysfunctional or functional uterine or vaginal bleeding NOS

N93.9 Abnormal uterine and vaginal bleeding, unspecified ♀

✓4th **N94 Pain and other conditions associated with female genital organs and menstrual cycle**

N94.0 Mittelschmerz ♀
DEF: One-sided, lower abdominal pain occurring between menstrual periods that is associated with ovulation.

✓5th **N94.1 Dyspareunia**
EXCLUDES 1 *psychogenic dyspareunia (F52.6)*
AHA: 2016,4Q,47

N94.10 Unspecified dyspareunia ♀
N94.11 Superficial (introital) dyspareunia ♀
N94.12 Deep dyspareunia ♀
N94.19 Other specified dyspareunia ♀

N94.2 Vaginismus ♀
EXCLUDES 1 *psychogenic vaginismus (F52.5)*
DEF: Spontaneous contractions of the muscles surrounding the vagina, causing it to constrict or close.

N94.3 Premenstrual tension syndrome ♀
Code also associated menstrual migraine (G43.82-, G43.83-)
EXCLUDES 1 *premenstrual dysphoric disorder (F32.81)*

N94.4 Primary dysmenorrhea ♀
N94.5 Secondary dysmenorrhea ♀
N94.6 Dysmenorrhea, unspecified ♀
EXCLUDES 1 *psychogenic dysmenorrhea (F45.8)*

✓5th **N94.8 Other specified conditions associated with female genital organs and menstrual cycle**

✓6th **N94.81 Vulvodynia**

N94.810 Vulvar vestibulitis ♀
N94.818 Other vulvodynia ♀
N94.819 Vulvodynia, unspecified ♀
Vulvodynia NOS

N94.89 Other specified conditions associated with female genital organs and menstrual cycle ♀
DEF: Hydrocele: Serous fluid that collects in the canal of Nuck in females.

N94.9 Unspecified condition associated with female genital organs and menstrual cycle ♀

✓4th **N95 Menopausal and other perimenopausal disorders**
Menopausal and other perimenopausal disorders due to naturally occurring (age-related) menopause and perimenopause
EXCLUDES 1 *excessive bleeding in the premenopausal period (N92.4)*
menopausal and perimenopausal disorders due to artificial or premature menopause (E89.4-, E28.31-)
premature menopause (E28.31-)
EXCLUDES 2 *postmenopausal osteoporosis (M81.0-)*
postmenopausal osteoporosis with current pathological fracture (M80.0-)
postmenopausal urethritis (N34.2)

N95.0 Postmenopausal bleeding ♀

N95.1 **Menopausal and female climacteric states** ♀
Symptoms such as flushing, sleeplessness, headache, lack of concentration, associated with natural (age-related) menopause
Use additional code for associated symptoms
EXCLUDES 1 *asymptomatic menopausal state (Z78.Ø)*
symptoms associated with artificial menopause (E89.41)
symptoms associated with premature menopause (E28.31Ø)

N95.2 **Postmenopausal atrophic vaginitis** ♀
Senile (atrophic) vaginitis

N95.8 **Other specified menopausal and perimenopausal disorders** ♀

N95.9 **Unspecified menopausal and perimenopausal disorder** ♀

N96 **Recurrent pregnancy loss** ♀
Investigation or care in a nonpregnant woman with history of recurrent pregnancy loss
EXCLUDES 1 *recurrent pregnancy loss with current pregnancy (O26.2-)*

4th N97 **Female infertility**
INCLUDES inability to achieve a pregnancy
sterility, female NOS
EXCLUDES 2 *female infertility associated with:*
hypopituitarism (E23.Ø)
incompetence of cervix uteri (N88.3)
Stein-Leventhal syndrome (E28.2)
DEF: Infertility: Inability to conceive for at least one year with regular intercourse.
DEF: Primary infertility: Infertility occurring in patients who have never conceived.
DEF: Secondary infertility: Infertility occurring in patients who have previously conceived.

N97.Ø **Female infertility associated with anovulation** ♀
AHA: 2022,2Q,16

N97.1 **Female infertility of tubal origin** ♀
Female infertility associated with congenital anomaly of tube
Female infertility due to tubal block
Female infertility due to tubal occlusion
Female infertility due to tubal stenosis

N97.2 **Female infertility of uterine origin** ♀
Female infertility associated with congenital anomaly of uterus
Female infertility due to nonimplantation of ovum

N97.8 **Female infertility of other origin** ♀
AHA: 2022,2Q,15

N97.9 **Female infertility, unspecified** ♀

4th N98 **Complications associated with artificial fertilization**

N98.Ø **Infection associated with artificial insemination** CC ♀

N98.1 **Hyperstimulation of ovaries** CC ♀
Hyperstimulation of ovaries NOS
Hyperstimulation of ovaries associated with induced ovulation

N98.2 **Complications of attempted introduction of fertilized ovum following in vitro fertilization** CC ♀

N98.3 **Complications of attempted introduction of embryo in embryo transfer** CC ♀

N98.8 **Other complications associated with artificial fertilization** CC ♀

N98.9 **Complication associated with artificial fertilization, unspecified** CC ♀

Intraoperative and postprocedural complications and disorders of genitourinary system, not elsewhere classified (N99)

4th N99 **Intraoperative and postprocedural complications and disorders of genitourinary system, not elsewhere classified**
EXCLUDES 2 *irradiation cystitis (N3Ø.4-)*
postoophorectomy osteoporosis with current pathological fracture (M8Ø.8-)
postoophorectomy osteoporosis without current pathological fracture (M81.8)

N99.Ø **Postprocedural (acute) (chronic) kidney failure**
Use additional code to type of kidney disease

5th N99.1 **Postprocedural urethral stricture**
Postcatheterization urethral stricture

6th N99.11 **Postprocedural urethral stricture, male**
AHA: 2016,4Q,47-48

N99.11Ø **Postprocedural urethral stricture, male, meatal** ♂
N99.111 **Postprocedural bulbous urethral stricture, male** ♂
N99.112 **Postprocedural membranous urethral stricture, male** ♂
N99.113 **Postprocedural anterior bulbous urethral stricture, male** ♂
N99.114 **Postprocedural urethral stricture, male, unspecified** ♂
N99.115 **Postprocedural fossa navicularis urethral stricture** ♂
N99.116 **Postprocedural urethral stricture, male, overlapping sites** ♂

N99.12 **Postprocedural urethral stricture, female** ♀

N99.2 **Postprocedural adhesions of vagina** ♀

N99.3 **Prolapse of vaginal vault after hysterectomy** ♀

N99.4 **Postprocedural pelvic peritoneal adhesions**
EXCLUDES 2 *pelvic peritoneal adhesions NOS (N73.6)*
postinfective pelvic peritoneal adhesions (N73.6)

5th N99.5 **Complications of stoma of urinary tract**
EXCLUDES 2 *mechanical complication of urinary catheter (T83.Ø-)*
AHA: 2016,4Q,48

6th N99.51 **Complication of cystostomy**

N99.51Ø **Cystostomy hemorrhage** CC HCC
N99.511 **Cystostomy infection** CC HCC
N99.512 **Cystostomy malfunction** CC HCC
N99.518 **Other cystostomy complication** CC HCC

6th N99.52 **Complication of incontinent external stoma of urinary tract**

N99.52Ø **Hemorrhage of incontinent external stoma of urinary tract** HCC
N99.521 **Infection of incontinent external stoma of urinary tract** HCC
N99.522 **Malfunction of incontinent external stoma of urinary tract** HCC
N99.523 **Herniation of incontinent stoma of urinary tract** HCC
N99.524 **Stenosis of incontinent stoma of urinary tract** HCC
N99.528 **Other complication of incontinent external stoma of urinary tract** HCC

6th N99.53 **Complication of continent stoma of urinary tract**

N99.53Ø **Hemorrhage of continent stoma of urinary tract** HCC
N99.531 **Infection of continent stoma of urinary tract** HCC
N99.532 **Malfunction of continent stoma of urinary tract** HCC
N99.533 **Herniation of continent stoma of urinary tract** HCC
N99.534 **Stenosis of continent stoma of urinary tract** HCC
N99.538 **Other complication of continent stoma of urinary tract** HCC

5th N99.6 **Intraoperative hemorrhage and hematoma of a genitourinary system organ or structure complicating a procedure**
EXCLUDES 1 *intraoperative hemorrhage and hematoma of a genitourinary system organ or structure due to accidental puncture or laceration during a procedure (N99.7-)*

N99.61 **Intraoperative hemorrhage and hematoma of a genitourinary system organ or structure complicating a genitourinary system procedure** CC

N99.62 **Intraoperative hemorrhage and hematoma of a genitourinary system organ or structure complicating other procedure** CC

5th N99.7 **Accidental puncture and laceration of a genitourinary system organ or structure during a procedure**

N99.71 **Accidental puncture and laceration of a genitourinary system organ or structure during a genitourinary system procedure** CC

N99.72 Accidental puncture and laceration of a genitourinary system organ or structure during other procedure CC

✓5th N99.8 Other intraoperative and postprocedural complications and disorders of genitourinary system

AHA: 2016,4Q,9-10

N99.81 Other intraoperative complications of genitourinary system

✓6th N99.82 Postprocedural hemorrhage of a genitourinary system organ or structure following a procedure

N99.820 Postprocedural hemorrhage of a genitourinary system organ or structure following a genitourinary system procedure CC

N99.821 Postprocedural hemorrhage of a genitourinary system organ or structure following other procedure CC

N99.83 Residual ovary syndrome ♀

✓6th N99.84 Postprocedural hematoma and seroma of a genitourinary system organ or structure following a procedure

N99.840 Postprocedural hematoma of a genitourinary system organ or structure following a genitourinary system procedure CC

N99.841 Postprocedural hematoma of a genitourinary system organ or structure following other procedure CC

N99.842 Postprocedural seroma of a genitourinary system organ or structure following a genitourinary system procedure CC

N99.843 Postprocedural seroma of a genitourinary system organ or structure following other procedure CC

N99.85 Post endometrial ablation syndrome ♀

AHA: 2019,4Q,12

N99.89 Other postprocedural complications and disorders of genitourinary system

Chapter 15. Pregnancy, Childbirth, and the Puerperium (O00–O9A)

Chapter-specific Guidelines with Coding Examples

The chapter-specific guidelines from the ICD-10-CM Official Guidelines for Coding and Reporting have been provided below. Along with these guidelines are coding examples, contained in the shaded boxes, that have been developed to help illustrate the coding and/or sequencing guidance found in these guidelines.

a. General rules for obstetric cases

1) Codes from Chapter 15 and sequencing priority

Obstetric cases require codes from chapter 15, codes in the range O00–O9A, Pregnancy, Childbirth, and the Puerperium. Chapter 15 codes have sequencing priority over codes from other chapters. Additional codes from other chapters may be used in conjunction with chapter 15 codes to further specify conditions. Should the provider document that the pregnancy is incidental to the encounter, then code Z33.1, Pregnant state, incidental, should be used in place of any chapter 15 codes. It is the provider's responsibility to state that the condition being treated is not affecting the pregnancy.

Pregnant patient at 25 weeks' gestation admitted for bladder abscess

O23.12	**Infections of bladder in pregnancy, second trimester**
N30.80	**Other cystitis without hematuria**
Z3A.25	**25 weeks gestation of pregnancy**

Explanation: The documentation does not indicate that the pregnancy is incidental or in any way unaffected by the bladder abscess; therefore, an obstetrics code should be sequenced first. An additional code was provided to identify the specific bladder condition as this information is not called out specifically in the obstetrics code.

2) Chapter 15 codes used only on the maternal record

Chapter 15 codes are to be used only on the maternal record, never on the record of the newborn.

3) Final character for trimester

The majority of codes in Chapter 15 have a final character indicating the trimester of pregnancy. The timeframes for the trimesters are indicated at the beginning of the chapter. If trimester is not a component of a code, it is because the condition always occurs in a specific trimester, or the concept of trimester of pregnancy is not applicable. Certain codes have characters for only certain trimesters because the condition does not occur in all trimesters, but it may occur in more than just one.

Assignment of the final character for trimester should be based on the provider's documentation of the trimester (or number of weeks) for the current admission/encounter. This applies to the assignment of trimester for pre-existing conditions as well as those that develop during or are due to the pregnancy. The provider's documentation of the number of weeks may be used to assign the appropriate code identifying the trimester.

Whenever delivery occurs during the current admission, and there is an "in childbirth" option for the obstetric complication being coded, the "in childbirth" code should be assigned. When the classification does not provide an obstetric code with an "in childbirth" option, it is appropriate to assign a code describing the current trimester.

Pregnant patient at 21 weeks' gestation admitted with excessive vomiting

O21.2	**Late vomiting of pregnancy**
Z3A.21	**21 weeks gestation of pregnancy**

Explanation: Category O21 classifies vomiting in pregnancy. Although code selection is based on whether the vomiting is before or after 20 completed weeks, these codes are not further classified by trimester. If vomiting only in the second trimester was documented, the provider should be queried for the specific week of gestation, as this will affect code selection.

4) Selection of trimester for inpatient admissions that encompass more than one trimester

In instances when a patient is admitted to a hospital for complications of pregnancy during one trimester and remains in the hospital into a subsequent trimester, the trimester character for the antepartum complication code should be assigned on the basis of the trimester when the complication developed, not the trimester of the discharge. If the condition developed prior to the current admission/encounter or represents a pre-existing condition, the trimester character for the trimester at the time of the admission/encounter should be assigned.

Patient admitted at 27 6/7 weeks' gestation for hemorrhaging from partial placenta previa; three days after admission at 28 1/7 weeks' gestation, she developed gestational hypertension

O44.32	**Partial placenta previa with hemorrhage, second trimester**
O13.3	**Gestational [pregnancy-induced] hypertension without significant proteinuria, third trimester**
Z3A.27	**27 weeks gestation of pregnancy**

Explanation: The patient presented with hemorrhaging from partial placenta previa while still in her 27th week, which falls within the second trimester. The gestational hypertension did not occur until three days after admission, putting the patient in her 28th week of pregnancy or what is considered to be the third trimester. The weeks of gestation captured by a code from category Z3A should represent only the gestational weeks upon admission.

5) Unspecified trimester

Each category that includes codes for trimester has a code for "unspecified trimester." The "unspecified trimester" code should rarely be used, such as when the documentation in the record is insufficient to determine the trimester and it is not possible to obtain clarification.

6) 7th character for fetus identification

Where applicable, a 7th character is to be assigned for certain categories (O31, O32, O33.3–O33.6, O35, O36, O40, O41, O60.1, O60.2, O64, and O69) to identify the fetus for which the complication code applies.

Assign 7th character "0":

- For single gestations
- When the documentation in the record is insufficient to determine the fetus affected and it is not possible to obtain clarification.
- When it is not possible to clinically determine which fetus is affected.

7) Completed weeks of gestation

In ICD-10-CM, "completed" weeks of gestation refers to full weeks. For example, if the provider documents gestation at 39 weeks and 6 days, the code for 39 weeks of gestation should be assigned, as the patient has not yet reached 40 completed weeks.

b. Selection of OB principal or first-listed diagnosis

1) Routine outpatient prenatal visits

For routine outpatient prenatal visits when no complications are present, a code from category Z34, Encounter for supervision of normal pregnancy, should be used as the first-listed diagnosis. These codes should not be used in conjunction with chapter 15 codes.

2) Supervision of high-risk pregnancy

Codes from category O09, Supervision of high-risk pregnancy, are intended for use only during the prenatal period. For complications during the labor or delivery episode as a result of a high-risk pregnancy, assign the applicable complication codes from Chapter 15. If there are no complications during the labor or delivery episode, assign code O80, Encounter for full-term uncomplicated delivery.

For routine prenatal outpatient visits for patients with high-risk pregnancies, a code from category O09, Supervision of high-risk pregnancy, should be used as the first-listed diagnosis. Secondary chapter 15 codes may be used in conjunction with these codes if appropriate.

36-year-old with history of preterm labor admitted in labor with second child at 39 weeks' gestation, delivered healthy baby without complications

O80	**Encounter for full-term uncomplicated delivery**
Z3A.39	**39 weeks gestation of pregnancy**
Z37.0	**Single live birth**

Explanation: Although this patient is over 35 and having her second child (elderly multigravida) and has a history of preterm labor with her first child, no codes from category O09.- should be appended. In the absence of any other complications noted during the encounter, code O80 is the most appropriate code to describe the principal diagnosis.

3) Episodes when no delivery occurs

In episodes when no delivery occurs, the principal diagnosis should correspond to the principal complication of the pregnancy which necessitated the encounter. Should more than one complication exist, all of which are treated or monitored, any of the complication codes may be sequenced first.

4) When a delivery occurs

When an obstetric patient is admitted and delivers during that admission, the condition that prompted the admission should be sequenced as the principal diagnosis. If multiple conditions prompted the admission, sequence the one most related to the delivery as the principal diagnosis. A code for any complication of the delivery should be assigned as an additional diagnosis. In cases of cesarean delivery, if the patient was admitted with a condition that resulted in the performance of a cesarean procedure, that condition should be selected as the principal diagnosis. If the reason for the admission was unrelated to the condition resulting in the cesarean delivery, the condition related to the reason for the admission should be selected as the principal diagnosis.

Maternal patient with diet-controlled gestational diabetes was admitted at 38 weeks' gestation in obstructed labor due to footling presentation; cesarean performed for the malpresentation

O64.8XXØ Obstructed labor due to other malposition and malpresentation, not applicable or unspecified

O24.42Ø Gestational diabetes mellitus in childbirth, diet controlled

Z3A.38 38 weeks gestation of pregnancy

Z37.Ø Single live birth

Explanation: The obstructed labor necessitated the cesarean procedure.

At 39 weeks' gestation, a maternal patient presents with hemorrhage with coagulation defect; the next day the patient goes into labor and eventually delivers via cesarean section due to arrested active phase of labor

O46.ØØ3 Antepartum hemorrhage with coagulation defect, unspecified, third trimester

O62.1 Secondary uterine inertia

Z3A.39 39 weeks gestation of pregnancy

Z37.Ø Single live birth

Explanation: The patient was admitted because of the antepartum hemorrhage with coagulation defect. The arrested active phase, although the reason for the cesarean delivery, did not develop until later into the stay.

5) Outcome of delivery

A code from category Z37, Outcome of delivery, should be included on every maternal record when a delivery has occurred. These codes are not to be used on subsequent records or on the newborn record.

c. Pre-existing conditions versus conditions due to the pregnancy

Certain categories in Chapter 15 distinguish between conditions of the mother that existed prior to pregnancy (pre-existing) and those that are a direct result of pregnancy. When assigning codes from Chapter 15, it is important to assess if a condition was pre-existing prior to pregnancy or developed during or due to the pregnancy in order to assign the correct code.

Categories that do not distinguish between pre-existing and pregnancy-related conditions may be used for either. It is acceptable to use codes specifically for the puerperium with codes complicating pregnancy and childbirth if a condition arises postpartum during the delivery encounter.

d. Pre-existing hypertension in pregnancy

Category O1Ø, Pre-existing hypertension complicating pregnancy, childbirth and the puerperium, includes codes for hypertensive heart and hypertensive chronic kidney disease. When assigning one of the O1Ø codes that includes hypertensive heart disease or hypertensive chronic kidney disease, it is necessary to add a secondary code from the appropriate hypertension category to specify the type of heart failure or chronic kidney disease.

See Section I.C.9. Hypertension.

e. Fetal conditions affecting the management of the mother

1) Codes from categories O35 and O36

Codes from categories O35, Maternal care for known or suspected fetal abnormality and damage, and O36, Maternal care for other fetal problems, are assigned only when the fetal condition is actually responsible for modifying the management of the mother, i.e., by requiring diagnostic studies, additional observation, special care, or termination of pregnancy. The fact that the fetal condition exists does not justify assigning a code from this series to the mother's record.

A patient is seen in ED for spotting 15 weeks into her pregnancy; the doctors also suspect fetal hydrocephalus.

O26.852 Spotting complicating pregnancy, second trimester

Z3A.15 15 weeks gestation of pregnancy

Explanation: Whether the fetal hydrocephalus was suspected or confirmed, an additional code is not warranted for this condition as the documentation does not indicate that this fetal condition is in any way altering the management of the mother or complicating her pregnancy.

2) In utero surgery

In cases when surgery is performed on the fetus, a diagnosis code from category O35, Maternal care for known or suspected fetal abnormality and damage, should be assigned identifying the fetal condition. Assign the appropriate procedure code for the procedure performed.

No code from Chapter 16, the perinatal codes, should be used on the mother's record to identify fetal conditions. Surgery performed in utero on a fetus is still to be coded as an obstetric encounter.

f. HIV infection in pregnancy, childbirth and the puerperium

During pregnancy, childbirth or the puerperium, a patient admitted because of an HIV-related illness should receive a principal diagnosis from subcategory O98.7-, Human immunodeficiency [HIV] disease complicating pregnancy, childbirth and the puerperium, followed by the code(s) for the HIV-related illness(es).

Patients with asymptomatic HIV infection status admitted during pregnancy, childbirth, or the puerperium should receive codes of O98.7- and Z21, Asymptomatic human immunodeficiency virus [HIV] infection status.

A previously asymptomatic HIV patient who is 13 weeks pregnant is admitted with oral thrush.

O98.711 Human immunodeficiency virus [HIV] disease complicating pregnancy, first trimester

B2Ø Human immunodeficiency virus [HIV] disease

B37.Ø Candidal stomatitis

Z3A.13 13 weeks gestation of pregnancy

Explanation: Because oral thrush is an HIV-related condition, this patient is now considered to have HIV disease. An obstetrics code indicating that HIV is complicating the pregnancy is coded first, followed by B2Ø for HIV disease as well as a code for the oral thrush.

g. Diabetes mellitus in pregnancy

Diabetes mellitus is a significant complicating factor in pregnancy. Pregnant patients who are diabetic should be assigned a code from category O24, Diabetes mellitus in pregnancy, childbirth, and the puerperium, first, followed by the appropriate diabetes code(s) (EØ8–E13) from Chapter 4.

h. Long term use of insulin and oral hypoglycemics

See section I.C.4.a.3 for information on the long-term use of insulin and oral hypoglycemics.

i. Gestational (pregnancy induced) diabetes

Gestational (pregnancy induced) diabetes can occur during the second and third trimester of pregnancy in patients who were not diabetic prior to pregnancy. Gestational diabetes can cause complications in the pregnancy similar to those of pre-existing diabetes mellitus. It also puts the patient at greater risk of developing diabetes after the pregnancy.

Codes for gestational diabetes are in subcategory O24.4, Gestational diabetes mellitus. No other code from category O24, Diabetes mellitus in pregnancy, childbirth, and the puerperium, should be used with a code from O24.4.

The codes under subcategory O24.4 include diet controlled, insulin controlled, and controlled by oral hypoglycemic drugs. If a patient with gestational diabetes is treated with both diet and insulin, only the code for insulin-controlled is required. If a patient with gestational diabetes is treated with both diet and oral hypoglycemic medications, only the code for "controlled by oral hypoglycemic drugs" is required. Codes Z79.4, Long-term (current) use of insulin, Z79.84, Long-term (current) use of oral hypoglycemic drugs, and Z79.85, Long-term (current) use of injectable non-insulin antidiabetic drugs, should not be assigned with codes from subcategory O24.4.

An abnormal glucose tolerance in pregnancy is assigned a code from subcategory O99.81, Abnormal glucose complicating pregnancy, childbirth, and the puerperium.

> Patient at 39 weeks term pregnancy with gestational diabetes was admitted in labor and delivered a healthy newborn. Patient is on a diabetic diet with daily metformin.
>
> **O24.425** **Gestational diabetes mellitus in childbirth, controlled by oral hypoglycemic drugs**
>
> **Z3A.39** **39 weeks gestation of pregnancy**
>
> **Z37.Ø** **Single live birth**
>
> *Explanation:* When the patient is admitted for delivery and the patient's gestational diabetes is controlled by both diet and oral hypoglycemic medications, only the combination code in subcategory O24.4- Gestational diabetes mellitus, is reported. No code is added for diet controlled diabetes, and no Z code for long-term use of oral hypoglycemics is reported with the O24.4 combination codes.

j. Sepsis and septic shock complicating abortion, pregnancy, childbirth and the puerperium

When assigning a chapter 15 code for sepsis complicating abortion, pregnancy, childbirth, and the puerperium, a code for the specific type of infection should be assigned as an additional diagnosis. If severe sepsis is present, a code from subcategory R65.2, Severe sepsis, and code(s) for associated organ dysfunction(s) should also be assigned as additional diagnoses.

> Patient is seen several days after a miscarriage with sepsis; cultures return MSSA
>
> **OØ3.87** **Sepsis following complete or unspecified spontaneous abortion**
>
> **B95.61** **Methicillin susceptible Staphylococcus aureus infection as the cause of diseases classified elsewhere**
>
> *Explanation:* The type of infection that caused this patient to become septic was methicillin susceptible *Staphylococcus aureus* (MSSA), which as a secondary code helps capture all aspects related to this patient's septic condition.

k. Puerperal sepsis

Code O85, Puerperal sepsis, should be assigned with a secondary code to identify the causal organism (e.g., for a bacterial infection, assign a code from category B95–B96, Bacterial infections in conditions classified elsewhere). A code from category A4Ø, Streptococcal sepsis, or A41, Other sepsis, should not be used for puerperal sepsis. If applicable, use additional codes to identify severe sepsis (R65.2-) and any associated acute organ dysfunction.

Code O85 should not be assigned for sepsis following an obstetrical procedure (See Section I.C.1.d.5.b., Sepsis due to a postprocedural infection).

l. Alcohol, tobacco and drug use during pregnancy, childbirth and the puerperium

1) Alcohol use during pregnancy, childbirth and the puerperium

Codes under subcategory O99.31, Alcohol use complicating pregnancy, childbirth, and the puerperium, should be assigned for any pregnancy case when a patient uses alcohol during the pregnancy or postpartum. A secondary code from category F1Ø, Alcohol related disorders, should also be assigned to identify manifestations of the alcohol use.

2) Tobacco use during pregnancy, childbirth and the puerperium

Codes under subcategory O99.33, Smoking (tobacco) complicating pregnancy, childbirth, and the puerperium, should be assigned for any pregnancy case when a patient uses any type of tobacco product during the pregnancy or postpartum.

A secondary code from category F17, Nicotine dependence, should also be assigned to identify the type of nicotine dependence.

3) Drug use during pregnancy, childbirth and the puerperium

Codes under subcategory O99.32, Drug use complicating pregnancy, childbirth, and the puerperium, should be assigned for any pregnancy case when a patient uses drugs during the pregnancy or postpartum. This can involve illegal drugs, or inappropriate use or abuse of prescription drugs. Secondary code(s) from categories F11–F16 and F18–F19 should also be assigned to identify manifestations of the drug use.

m. Poisoning, toxic effects, adverse effects and underdosing in a pregnant patient

A code from subcategory O9A.2, Injury, poisoning and certain other consequences of external causes complicating pregnancy, childbirth, and the puerperium, should be sequenced first, followed by the appropriate injury, poisoning, toxic effect, adverse effect or underdosing code, and then the additional code(s) that specifies the condition caused by the poisoning, toxic effect, adverse effect or underdosing.

See Section I.C.19. Adverse effects, poisoning, underdosing and toxic effects.

> Patient admitted with accidental carbon monoxide poisoning from a gas heating implement; the patient is 18 weeks pregnant
>
> **O9A.212** **Injury, poisoning and certain other consequences of external causes complicating pregnancy, second trimester**
>
> **T58.11XA** **Toxic effect of carbon monoxide from utility gas, accidental (unintentional), initial encounter**
>
> **Z3A.18** **18 weeks gestation of pregnancy**
>
> *Explanation:* Although the carbon monoxide poisoning is the reason the patient was admitted, a code from the obstetrics chapter must be sequenced first. Chapter 15 codes have sequencing priority over codes from other chapters.

n. Normal delivery, code O8Ø

1) Encounter for full term uncomplicated delivery

Code O8Ø should be assigned when a patient is admitted for a full-term normal delivery and delivers a single, healthy infant without any complications antepartum, during the delivery, or postpartum during the delivery episode. Code O8Ø is always a principal diagnosis. It is not to be used if any other code from chapter 15 is needed to describe a current complication of the antenatal, delivery, or postnatal period. Additional codes from other chapters may be used with code O8Ø if they are not related to or are in any way complicating the pregnancy.

2) Uncomplicated delivery with resolved antepartum complication

Code O8Ø may be used if the patient had a complication at some point during the pregnancy, but the complication is not present at the time of the admission for delivery.

> Patient presents in labor at 39 weeks' gestation and delivers a healthy newborn; patient had abnormal glucose levels in her first trimester, which have since resolved
>
> **O8Ø** **Encounter for full-term uncomplicated delivery**
>
> **Z37.Ø** **Single live birth**
>
> *Explanation:* The abnormal glucose levels during the first trimester cannot be coded if they are not affecting the patient's current trimester. Without additional complications associated with the pregnancy, fetus, or mother, code O8Ø is appropriate.

3) Outcome of delivery for O8Ø

Z37.Ø, Single live birth, is the only outcome of delivery code appropriate for use with O8Ø.

o. The peripartum and postpartum periods

1) Peripartum and postpartum periods

The postpartum period begins immediately after delivery and continues for six weeks following delivery. The peripartum period is defined as the last month of pregnancy to five months postpartum.

2) Peripartum and postpartum complication

A postpartum complication is any complication occurring within the six-week period.

3) Pregnancy-related complications after 6-week period

Chapter 15 codes may also be used to describe pregnancy-related complications after the peripartum or postpartum period if the provider documents that a condition is pregnancy related.

> Patient admitted for varicose veins. She had a baby boy three months ago; the varicose veins started to appear one month ago. The doctor attributes the patient's pregnancy as the cause of the varicose veins, which continue to be painful and bother the patient. She is seeking surgical relief.
>
> **O87.4** **Varicose veins of the lower extremity in the puerperium**
>
> *Explanation:* Although the varicose veins occurred several months after the delivery of the newborn, the doctor attributed the varicose veins to pregnancy and therefore a code from chapter 15 is appropriate.

4) Admission for routine postpartum care following delivery outside hospital

When the mother delivers outside the hospital prior to admission and is admitted for routine postpartum care and no complications are noted, code Z39.Ø, Encounter for care and examination of mother immediately after delivery, should be assigned as the principal diagnosis.

5) Pregnancy associated cardiomyopathy

Pregnancy associated cardiomyopathy, code O9Ø.3, is unique in that it may be diagnosed in the third trimester of pregnancy but may continue to progress months after delivery. For this reason, it is referred to as peripartum cardiomyopathy. Code O9Ø.3 is only for use when the cardiomyopathy develops as a result of pregnancy in a patient who did not have pre-existing heart disease.

p. Code O94, Sequelae of complication of pregnancy, childbirth, and the puerperium

1) Code O94

Code O94, Sequelae of complication of pregnancy, childbirth, and the puerperium, is for use in those cases when an initial complication of a pregnancy develops a sequela or sequelae requiring care or treatment at a future date.

2) After the initial postpartum period

This code may be used at any time after the initial postpartum period.

3) Sequencing of code O94

This code, like all sequela codes, is to be sequenced following the code describing the sequelae of the complication.

q. Termination of pregnancy and spontaneous abortions

1) Abortion with liveborn fetus

When an attempted termination of pregnancy results in a liveborn fetus, assign code Z33.2, Encounter for elective termination of pregnancy and a code from category Z37, Outcome of Delivery.

2) Retained products of conception following an abortion

Subsequent encounters for retained products of conception following a spontaneous abortion or elective termination of pregnancy, without complications are assigned OØ3.4, Incomplete spontaneous, abortion without complication, or code OØ7.4, Failed attempted termination of pregnancy without complication. This advice is appropriate even when the patient was discharged previously with a discharge diagnosis of complete abortion. If the patient has a specific complication associated with the spontaneous abortion or elective termination of pregnancy in addition to retained products of conception, assign the appropriate complication code (e.g., OØ3.-, OØ4.-, OØ7.-) instead of code OØ3.4 or OØ7.4.

Patient was seen two days ago for complete spontaneous abortion but returns today for urinary tract infection (UTI) with ultrasound showing retained products of conception

OØ3.38	**Urinary tract infection following incomplete spontaneous abortion**

Explanation: Although the diagnosis from the patient's previous stay indicated that the patient had a complete abortion, it is now determined that there were actually retained products of conception (POC). An abortion with retained POC is considered incomplete and in this case resulted in the patient developing a UTI.

3) Complications leading to abortion

Codes from Chapter 15 may be used as additional codes to identify any documented complications of the pregnancy in conjunction with codes in categories in OØ4, OØ7 and OØ8.

4) Hemorrhage following elective abortion

For hemorrhage post elective abortion, assign code OØ4.6, Delayed or excessive hemorrhage following (induced) termination of pregnancy. Do not assign code O72.1, Other immediate postpartum hemorrhage, as this code should not be assigned for post abortion conditions.

r. Abuse in a pregnant patient

For suspected or confirmed cases of abuse of a pregnant patient, a code(s) from subcategories O9A.3, Physical abuse complicating pregnancy, childbirth, and the puerperium, O9A.4, Sexual abuse complicating pregnancy, childbirth, and the puerperium, and O9A.5, Psychological abuse complicating pregnancy, childbirth, and the puerperium, should be sequenced first, followed by the appropriate codes (if applicable) to identify any associated current injury due to physical abuse, sexual abuse, and the perpetrator of abuse.

See Section I.C.19. Adult and child abuse, neglect and other maltreatment.

s. COVID-19 infection in pregnancy, childbirth, and the puerperium

During pregnancy, childbirth or the puerperium, when COVID-19 is the reason for admission/encounter , code O98.5-, Other viral diseases complicating pregnancy, childbirth and the puerperium, should be sequenced as the principal/first-listed diagnosis, and code UØ7.1, COVID-19, and the appropriate codes for associated manifestation(s) should be assigned as additional diagnoses. Codes from Chapter 15 always take sequencing priority.

If the reason for admission/encounter is unrelated to COVID-19 but the patient tests positive for COVID-19 during the admission/encounter, the appropriate code for the reason for admission/encounter should be sequenced as the principal/first-listed diagnosis, and codes O98.5- and UØ7.1, as well as the appropriate codes for associated COVID-19 manifestations, should be assigned as additional diagnoses.

Patient admitted in labor at 39 weeks' gestation and delivered a healthy newborn. Prenatal care consisted of some hyperemesis early in the pregnancy that has since resolved. No complications encountered during or following delivery. As per hospital protocol, during the pandemic, all patients are to be screened for COVID-19, and the patient tested positive. She remains asymptomatic, will be sent home to quarantine for 14 days.

O98.52	**Other viral diseases complicating childbirth**
UØ7.1	**COVID-19**
Z3A.39	**39 weeks gestation of pregnancy**
Z37.Ø	**Single live birth**

Explanation: No code is assigned for the hyperemesis as it resolved prior to this admission. Per guideline I.C.1.g.1.f, a screening code is generally not appropriate during the pandemic phase of COVID-19. Most hospitals screen their patients upon admission to the hospital to ensure proper protocols are in place for monitoring and treating those patients who do test positive for the disease. A positive test result alone is confirmation of the disease, according to guideline I.C.1.g.1.a, and code UØ7.1 should be assigned. A claim for any patient admitted during pregnancy, childbirth, or the puerperium and who tests positive or is treated for COVID-19 should have a code from subcategory O98.5- sequenced first, followed by code UØ7.1. As the patient was asymptomatic, no additional codes are assigned to represent any manifestation of the COVID-19 infection.

Chapter 15. Pregnancy, Childbirth and the Puerperium (O00-O9A)

NOTE CODES FROM THIS CHAPTER ARE FOR USE ONLY ON MATERNAL RECORDS, NEVER ON NEWBORN RECORDS

Codes from this chapter are for use for conditions related to or aggravated by the pregnancy, childbirth, or by the puerperium (maternal causes or obstetric causes)

NOTE Trimesters are counted from the first day of the last menstrual period. They are defined as follows:

1st trimester- less than 14 weeks 0 days

2nd trimester- 14 weeks 0 days to less than 28 weeks 0 days

3rd trimester- 28 weeks 0 days until delivery

▶Use additional code, if applicable, from category Z3A, Weeks of gestation, to identify the specific week of the pregnancy, if known.◀

EXCLUDES 1 *supervision of normal pregnancy (Z34.-)*

EXCLUDES 2 *mental and behavioral disorders associated with the puerperium (F53.-)*
obstetrical tetanus (A34)
postpartum necrosis of pituitary gland (E23.0)
puerperal osteomalacia (M83.0)

AHA: 2016,1Q,3-5; 2014,3Q,17

This chapter contains the following blocks:

Pregnancy with abortive outcome (O00-O08)

EXCLUDES 1 *continuing pregnancy in multiple gestation after abortion of one fetus or more (O31.1-, O31.3-)*

TIP: Do not assign a code from category Z3A with codes in this code block.

✓4th **O00 Ectopic pregnancy**

INCLUDES ruptured ectopic pregnancy

Use additional code from category O08 to identify any associated complication

AHA: 2016,4Q,48-50; 2014,3Q,17

DEF: Implantation of a fertilized egg outside the uterus, usually in the fallopian tube or abdomen that requires emergency treatment.

✓5th **O00.0 Abdominal pregnancy**

EXCLUDES 1 *maternal care for viable fetus in abdominal pregnancy (O36.7-)*

O00.00 Abdominal pregnancy without intrauterine pregnancy CC M ♀
Abdominal pregnancy NOS

O00.01 Abdominal pregnancy with intrauterine pregnancy CC M ♀

✓5th **O00.1 Tubal pregnancy**
Fallopian pregnancy
Rupture of (fallopian) tube due to pregnancy
Tubal abortion
AHA: 2017,4Q,20

✓6th **O00.10 Tubal pregnancy without intrauterine pregnancy**
Tubal pregnancy NOS

O00.101 Right tubal pregnancy without intrauterine pregnancy CC M ♀

O00.102 Left tubal pregnancy without intrauterine pregnancy CC M ♀

O00.109 Unspecified tubal pregnancy without intrauterine pregnancy CC UNS M ♀

✓6th **O00.11 Tubal pregnancy with intrauterine pregnancy**

O00.111 Right tubal pregnancy with intrauterine pregnancy CC M ♀

O00.112 Left tubal pregnancy with intrauterine pregnancy CC M ♀

O00.119 Unspecified tubal pregnancy with intrauterine pregnancy CC UNS M ♀

✓5th **O00.2 Ovarian pregnancy**
AHA: 2017,4Q,20

✓6th **O00.20 Ovarian pregnancy without intrauterine pregnancy**
Ovarian pregnancy NOS

O00.201 Right ovarian pregnancy without intrauterine pregnancy CC M ♀

O00.202 Left ovarian pregnancy without intrauterine pregnancy CC M ♀

O00.209 Unspecified ovarian pregnancy without intrauterine pregnancy CC UNS M ♀

✓6th **O00.21 Ovarian pregnancy with intrauterine pregnancy**

O00.211 Right ovarian pregnancy with intrauterine pregnancy CC M ♀

O00.212 Left ovarian pregnancy with intrauterine pregnancy CC M ♀

O00.219 Unspecified ovarian pregnancy with intrauterine pregnancy CC UNS M ♀

✓5th **O00.8 Other ectopic pregnancy**
Cervical pregnancy
Cornual pregnancy
Intraligamentous pregnancy
Mural pregnancy

O00.80 Other ectopic pregnancy without intrauterine pregnancy CC M ♀
Other ectopic pregnancy NOS

O00.81 Other ectopic pregnancy with intrauterine pregnancy CC M ♀

✓5th **O00.9 Ectopic pregnancy, unspecified**

O00.90 Unspecified ectopic pregnancy without intrauterine pregnancy CC M ♀
Ectopic pregnancy NOS

O00.91 Unspecified ectopic pregnancy with intrauterine pregnancy CC M ♀

✓4th **O01 Hydatidiform mole**

Use additional code from category O08 to identify any associated complication

EXCLUDES 1 *chorioadenoma (destruens) (D39.2)*
malignant hydatidiform mole (D39.2)

AHA: 2014,3Q,17

DEF: Abnormal product of pregnancy, marked by a mass of cysts resembling a bunch of grapes due to chorionic villi proliferation and dissolution. It must be surgically removed.

O01.0 Classical hydatidiform mole M ♀
Complete hydatidiform mole

O01.1 Incomplete and partial hydatidiform mole M ♀

O01.9 Hydatidiform mole, unspecified M ♀
Trophoblastic disease NOS
Vesicular mole NOS

✓4th **O02 Other abnormal products of conception**

Use additional code from category O08 to identify any associated complication

EXCLUDES 1 *papyraceous fetus (O31.0-)*

AHA: 2014,3Q,17

O02.0 Blighted ovum and nonhydatidiform mole M ♀
Carneous mole
Fleshy mole
Intrauterine mole NOS
Molar pregnancy NEC
Pathological ovum

O02.1 Missed abortion M ♀
Early fetal death, before completion of 20 weeks of gestation, with retention of dead fetus

EXCLUDES 1 *failed induced abortion (O07.-)*
fetal death (intrauterine) (late) (O36.4)
missed abortion with blighted ovum (O02.0)
missed abortion with hydatidiform mole (O01.-)
missed abortion with nonhydatidiform (O02.0)
missed abortion with other abnormal products of conception (O02.8-)
missed delivery (O36.4)
stillbirth (P95)

AHA: 2022,2Q,3; 2019,3Q,11

√5th **O02.8 Other specified abnormal products of conception**

EXCLUDES 1 *abnormal products of conception with blighted ovum (O02.0)*
abnormal products of conception with hydatidiform mole (O01.-)
abnormal products of conception with nonhydatidiform mole (O02.0)

O02.81 Inappropriate change in quantitative human chorionic gonadotropin (hCG) in early pregnancy M ♀
Biochemical pregnancy
Chemical pregnancy
Inappropriate level of quantitative human chorionic gonadotropin (hCG) for gestational age in early pregnancy

O02.89 Other abnormal products of conception M ♀

O02.9 Abnormal product of conception, unspecified M ♀

√4th **O03 Spontaneous abortion**

NOTE Incomplete abortion includes retained products of conception following spontaneous abortion

INCLUDES miscarriage

AHA: 2023,1Q,17

O03.0 Genital tract and pelvic infection following incomplete spontaneous abortion CC M ♀
Endometritis following incomplete spontaneous abortion
Oophoritis following incomplete spontaneous abortion
Parametritis following incomplete spontaneous abortion
Pelvic peritonitis following incomplete spontaneous abortion
Salpingitis following incomplete spontaneous abortion
Salpingo-oophoritis following incomplete spontaneous abortion

EXCLUDES 1 *sepsis following incomplete spontaneous abortion (O03.37)*
urinary tract infection following incomplete spontaneous abortion (O03.38)

O03.1 Delayed or excessive hemorrhage following incomplete spontaneous abortion M ♀
Afibrinogenemia following incomplete spontaneous abortion
Defibrination syndrome following incomplete spontaneous abortion
Hemolysis following incomplete spontaneous abortion
Intravascular coagulation following incomplete spontaneous abortion

AHA: 2022,1Q,19

O03.2 Embolism following incomplete spontaneous abortion MCC M ♀
Air embolism following incomplete spontaneous abortion
Amniotic fluid embolism following incomplete spontaneous abortion
Blood-clot embolism following incomplete spontaneous abortion
Embolism NOS following incomplete spontaneous abortion
Fat embolism following incomplete spontaneous abortion
Pulmonary embolism following incomplete spontaneous abortion
Pyemic embolism following incomplete spontaneous abortion
Septic or septicopyemic embolism following incomplete spontaneous abortion
Soap embolism following incomplete spontaneous abortion

√5th **O03.3 Other and unspecified complications following incomplete spontaneous abortion**

O03.30 Unspecified complication following incomplete spontaneous abortion CC M ♀

O03.31 Shock following incomplete spontaneous abortion MCC M ♀
Circulatory collapse following incomplete spontaneous abortion
Shock (postprocedural) following incomplete spontaneous abortion

EXCLUDES 1 *shock due to infection following incomplete spontaneous abortion (O03.37)*

O03.32 Renal failure following incomplete spontaneous abortion MCC M ♀
Kidney failure (acute) following incomplete spontaneous abortion
Oliguria following incomplete spontaneous abortion
Renal shutdown following incomplete spontaneous abortion
Renal tubular necrosis following incomplete spontaneous abortion
Uremia following incomplete spontaneous abortion

O03.33 Metabolic disorder following incomplete spontaneous abortion CC M ♀

O03.34 Damage to pelvic organs following incomplete spontaneous abortion CC M ♀
Laceration, perforation, tear or chemical damage of bladder following incomplete spontaneous abortion
Laceration, perforation, tear or chemical damage of bowel following incomplete spontaneous abortion
Laceration, perforation, tear or chemical damage of broad ligament following incomplete spontaneous abortion
Laceration, perforation, tear or chemical damage of cervix following incomplete spontaneous abortion
Laceration, perforation, tear or chemical damage of periurethral tissue following incomplete spontaneous abortion
Laceration, perforation, tear or chemical damage of uterus following incomplete spontaneous abortion
Laceration, perforation, tear or chemical damage of vagina following incomplete spontaneous abortion

O03.35 Other venous complications following incomplete spontaneous abortion CC M ♀

O03.36 Cardiac arrest following incomplete spontaneous abortion CC M ♀

O03.37 Sepsis following incomplete spontaneous abortion CC M ♀
Use additional code to identify infectious agent (B95-B97)
Use additional code to identify severe sepsis, if applicable (R65.2-)

EXCLUDES 1 *septic or septicopyemic embolism following incomplete spontaneous abortion (O03.2)*

O03.38 Urinary tract infection following incomplete spontaneous abortion CC M ♀
Cystitis following incomplete spontaneous abortion

O03.39 Incomplete spontaneous abortion with other complications CC M ♀

O03.4 Incomplete spontaneous abortion without complication M ♀

O03.5 Genital tract and pelvic infection following complete or unspecified spontaneous abortion CC M ♀
Endometritis following complete or unspecified spontaneous abortion
Oophoritis following complete or unspecified spontaneous abortion
Parametritis following complete or unspecified spontaneous abortion
Pelvic peritonitis following complete or unspecified spontaneous abortion
Salpingitis following complete or unspecified spontaneous abortion
Salpingo-oophoritis following complete or unspecified spontaneous abortion

EXCLUDES 1 *sepsis following complete or unspecified spontaneous abortion (O03.87)*
urinary tract infection following complete or unspecified spontaneous abortion (O03.88)

O03.6 Delayed or excessive hemorrhage following complete or unspecified spontaneous abortion M ♀
Afibrinogenemia following complete or unspecified spontaneous abortion
Defibrination syndrome following complete or unspecified spontaneous abortion
Hemolysis following complete or unspecified spontaneous abortion
Intravascular coagulation following complete or unspecified spontaneous abortion
AHA: 2022,1Q,19

O03.7 Embolism following complete or unspecified spontaneous abortion CC M ♀
Air embolism following complete or unspecified spontaneous abortion
Amniotic fluid embolism following complete or unspecified spontaneous abortion
Blood-clot embolism following complete or unspecified spontaneous abortion
Embolism NOS following complete or unspecified spontaneous abortion
Fat embolism following complete or unspecified spontaneous abortion
Pulmonary embolism following complete or unspecified spontaneous abortion
Pyemic embolism following complete or unspecified spontaneous abortion
Septic or septicopyemic embolism following complete or unspecified spontaneous abortion
Soap embolism following complete or unspecified spontaneous abortion

✓5th **O03.8 Other and unspecified complications following complete or unspecified spontaneous abortion**

O03.80 Unspecified complication following complete or unspecified spontaneous abortion CC M ♀

O03.81 Shock following complete or unspecified spontaneous abortion MCC M ♀
Circulatory collapse following complete or unspecified spontaneous abortion
Shock (postprocedural) following complete or unspecified spontaneous abortion
EXCLUDES 1 *shock due to infection following complete or unspecified spontaneous abortion (O03.87)*

O03.82 Renal failure following complete or unspecified spontaneous abortion MCC M ♀
Kidney failure (acute) following complete or unspecified spontaneous abortion
Oliguria following complete or unspecified spontaneous abortion
Renal shutdown following complete or unspecified spontaneous abortion
Renal tubular necrosis following complete or unspecified spontaneous abortion
Uremia following complete or unspecified spontaneous abortion

O03.83 Metabolic disorder following complete or unspecified spontaneous abortion CC M ♀

O03.84 Damage to pelvic organs following complete or unspecified spontaneous abortion CC M ♀
Laceration, perforation, tear or chemical damage of bladder following complete or unspecified spontaneous abortion
Laceration, perforation, tear or chemical damage of bowel following complete or unspecified spontaneous abortion
Laceration, perforation, tear or chemical damage of broad ligament following complete or unspecified spontaneous abortion
Laceration, perforation, tear or chemical damage of cervix following complete or unspecified spontaneous abortion
Laceration, perforation, tear or chemical damage of periurethral tissue following complete or unspecified spontaneous abortion
Laceration, perforation, tear or chemical damage of uterus following complete or unspecified spontaneous abortion
Laceration, perforation, tear or chemical damage of vagina following complete or unspecified spontaneous abortion

O03.85 Other venous complications following complete or unspecified spontaneous abortion CC M ♀

O03.86 Cardiac arrest following complete or unspecified spontaneous abortion CC M ♀

O03.87 Sepsis following complete or unspecified spontaneous abortion CC M ♀
Use additional code to identify infectious agent (B95-B97)
Use additional code to identify severe sepsis, if applicable (R65.2-)
EXCLUDES 1 *septic or septicopyemic embolism following complete or unspecified spontaneous abortion (O03.7)*

O03.88 Urinary tract infection following complete or unspecified spontaneous abortion CC M ♀
Cystitis following complete or unspecified spontaneous abortion

O03.89 Complete or unspecified spontaneous abortion with other complications CC M ♀

O03.9 Complete or unspecified spontaneous abortion without complication M ♀
Miscarriage NOS
Spontaneous abortion NOS

✓4th **O04 Complications following (induced) termination of pregnancy**
INCLUDES complications following (induced) termination of pregnancy
EXCLUDES 1 ~~*encounter for elective termination of pregnancy, uncomplicated (Z33.2)*~~
~~*failed attempted termination of pregnancy (O07.-)*~~
EXCLUDES 2 ▶*encounter for elective termination of pregnancy, uncomplicated (Z33.2)*◀
▶*failed attempted termination of pregnancy (O07.-)*◀

O04.5 Genital tract and pelvic infection following (induced) termination of pregnancy CC M ♀
Endometritis following (induced) termination of pregnancy
Oophoritis following (induced) termination of pregnancy
Parametritis following (induced) termination of pregnancy
Pelvic peritonitis following (induced) termination of pregnancy
Salpingitis following (induced) termination of pregnancy
Salpingo-oophoritis following (induced) termination of pregnancy
EXCLUDES 1 *sepsis following (induced) termination of pregnancy (O04.87)*
urinary tract infection following (induced) termination of pregnancy (O04.88)

O04.6 Delayed or excessive hemorrhage following (induced) termination of pregnancy M ♀
Afibrinogenemia following (induced) termination of pregnancy
Defibrination syndrome following (induced) termination of pregnancy
Hemolysis following (induced) termination of pregnancy
Intravascular coagulation following (induced) termination of pregnancy
AHA: 2023,2Q,15; 2019,3Q,11

O04.7 Embolism following (induced) termination of pregnancy MCC M ♀
Air embolism following (induced) termination of pregnancy
Amniotic fluid embolism following (induced) termination of pregnancy
Blood-clot embolism following (induced) termination of pregnancy
Embolism NOS following (induced) termination of pregnancy
Fat embolism following (induced) termination of pregnancy
Pulmonary embolism following (induced) termination of pregnancy
Pyemic embolism following (induced) termination of pregnancy
Septic or septicopyemic embolism following (induced) termination of pregnancy
Soap embolism following (induced) termination of pregnancy

✓5th **O04.8 (Induced) termination of pregnancy with other and unspecified complications**

O04.80 (Induced) termination of pregnancy with unspecified complications CC M ♀

Chapter 15. Pregnancy, Childbirth and the Puerperium

O03.6–O04.80

O04.81 Shock following (induced) termination of pregnancy MCC M ♀
Circulatory collapse following (induced) termination of pregnancy
Shock (postprocedural) following (induced) termination of pregnancy
EXCLUDES 1 *shock due to infection following (induced) termination of pregnancy (O04.87)*

O04.82 Renal failure following (induced) termination of pregnancy MCC M ♀
Kidney failure (acute) following (induced) termination of pregnancy
Oliguria following (induced) termination of pregnancy
Renal shutdown following (induced) termination of pregnancy
Renal tubular necrosis following (induced) termination of pregnancy
Uremia following (induced) termination of pregnancy

O04.83 Metabolic disorder following (induced) termination of pregnancy CC M ♀

O04.84 Damage to pelvic organs following (induced) termination of pregnancy CC M ♀
Laceration, perforation, tear or chemical damage of bladder following (induced) termination of pregnancy
Laceration, perforation, tear or chemical damage of bowel following (induced) termination of pregnancy
Laceration, perforation, tear or chemical damage of broad ligament following (induced) termination of pregnancy
Laceration, perforation, tear or chemical damage of cervix following (induced) termination of pregnancy
Laceration, perforation, tear or chemical damage of periurethral tissue following (induced) termination of pregnancy
Laceration, perforation, tear or chemical damage of uterus following (induced) termination of pregnancy
Laceration, perforation, tear or chemical damage of vagina following (induced) termination of pregnancy

O04.85 Other venous complications following (induced) termination of pregnancy CC M ♀

O04.86 Cardiac arrest following (induced) termination of pregnancy CC M ♀

O04.87 Sepsis following (induced) termination of pregnancy CC M ♀
Use additional code to identify infectious agent (B95-B97)
Use additional code to identify severe sepsis, if applicable (R65.2-)
EXCLUDES 1 *septic or septicopyemic embolism following (induced) termination of pregnancy (O04.7)*

O04.88 Urinary tract infection following (induced) termination of pregnancy CC M ♀
Cystitis following (induced) termination of pregnancy

O04.89 (Induced) termination of pregnancy with other complications CC M ♀

✓4th **O07 Failed attempted termination of pregnancy**
INCLUDES failure of attempted induction of termination of pregnancy
incomplete elective abortion
EXCLUDES 1 *incomplete spontaneous abortion (O03.0-)*

O07.0 Genital tract and pelvic infection following failed attempted termination of pregnancy CC M ♀
Endometritis following failed attempted termination of pregnancy
Oophoritis following failed attempted termination of pregnancy
Parametritis following failed attempted termination of pregnancy
Pelvic peritonitis following failed attempted termination of pregnancy
Salpingitis following failed attempted termination of pregnancy
Salpingo-oophoritis following failed attempted termination of pregnancy
EXCLUDES 1 *sepsis following failed attempted termination of pregnancy (O07.37)*
urinary tract infection following failed attempted termination of pregnancy (O07.38)

O07.1 Delayed or excessive hemorrhage following failed attempted termination of pregnancy CC M ♀
Afibrinogenemia following failed attempted termination of pregnancy
Defibrination syndrome following failed attempted termination of pregnancy
Hemolysis following failed attempted termination of pregnancy
Intravascular coagulation following failed attempted termination of pregnancy

O07.2 Embolism following failed attempted termination of pregnancy MCC M ♀
Air embolism following failed attempted termination of pregnancy
Amniotic fluid embolism following failed attempted termination of pregnancy
Blood-clot embolism following failed attempted termination of pregnancy
Embolism NOS following failed attempted termination of pregnancy
Fat embolism following failed attempted termination of pregnancy
Pulmonary embolism following failed attempted termination of pregnancy
Pyemic embolism following failed attempted termination of pregnancy
Septic or septicopyemic embolism following failed attempted termination of pregnancy
Soap embolism following failed attempted termination of pregnancy

✓5th **O07.3 Failed attempted termination of pregnancy with other and unspecified complications**

O07.30 Failed attempted termination of pregnancy with unspecified complications CC M ♀

O07.31 Shock following failed attempted termination of pregnancy MCC M ♀
Circulatory collapse following failed attempted termination of pregnancy
Shock (postprocedural) following failed attempted termination of pregnancy
EXCLUDES 1 *shock due to infection following failed attempted termination of pregnancy (O07.37)*

O07.32 Renal failure following failed attempted termination of pregnancy MCC M ♀
Kidney failure (acute) following failed attempted termination of pregnancy
Oliguria following failed attempted termination of pregnancy
Renal shutdown following failed attempted termination of pregnancy
Renal tubular necrosis following failed attempted termination of pregnancy
Uremia following failed attempted termination of pregnancy

O07.33 Metabolic disorder following failed attempted termination of pregnancy CC M ♀

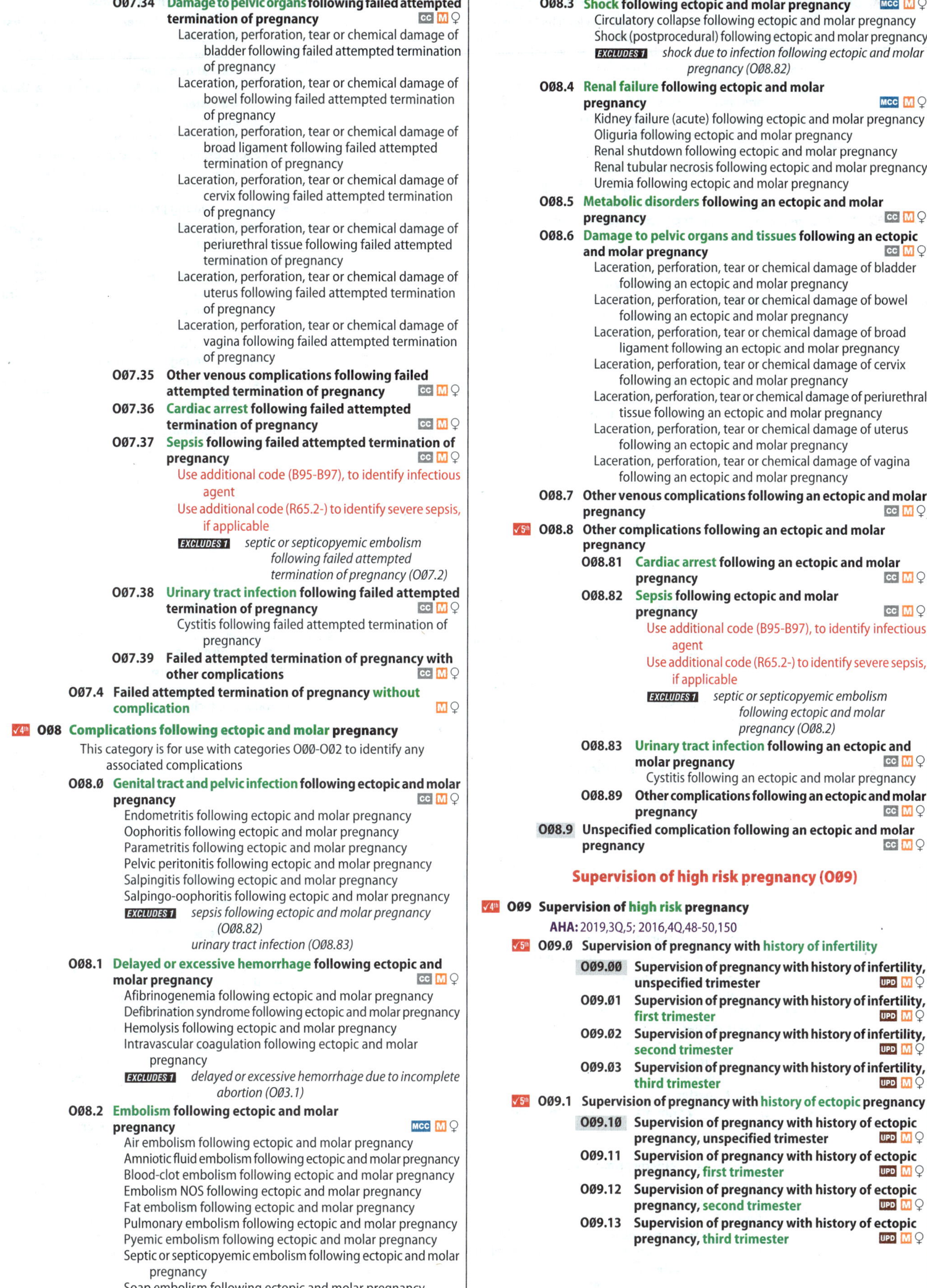

O07.34 **Damage to pelvic organs following failed attempted termination of pregnancy** CC M ♀
Laceration, perforation, tear or chemical damage of bladder following failed attempted termination of pregnancy
Laceration, perforation, tear or chemical damage of bowel following failed attempted termination of pregnancy
Laceration, perforation, tear or chemical damage of broad ligament following failed attempted termination of pregnancy
Laceration, perforation, tear or chemical damage of cervix following failed attempted termination of pregnancy
Laceration, perforation, tear or chemical damage of periurethral tissue following failed attempted termination of pregnancy
Laceration, perforation, tear or chemical damage of uterus following failed attempted termination of pregnancy
Laceration, perforation, tear or chemical damage of vagina following failed attempted termination of pregnancy

O07.35 **Other venous complications following failed attempted termination of pregnancy** CC M ♀

O07.36 **Cardiac arrest following failed attempted termination of pregnancy** CC M ♀

O07.37 **Sepsis following failed attempted termination of pregnancy** CC M ♀
Use additional code (B95-B97), to identify infectious agent
Use additional code (R65.2-) to identify severe sepsis, if applicable
EXCLUDES 1 *septic or septicopyemic embolism following failed attempted termination of pregnancy (O07.2)*

O07.38 **Urinary tract infection following failed attempted termination of pregnancy** CC M ♀
Cystitis following failed attempted termination of pregnancy

O07.39 **Failed attempted termination of pregnancy with other complications** CC M ♀

O07.4 **Failed attempted termination of pregnancy without complication** M ♀

✓4th O08 **Complications following ectopic and molar pregnancy**
This category is for use with categories O00-O02 to identify any associated complications

O08.0 **Genital tract and pelvic infection following ectopic and molar pregnancy** CC M ♀
Endometritis following ectopic and molar pregnancy
Oophoritis following ectopic and molar pregnancy
Parametritis following ectopic and molar pregnancy
Pelvic peritonitis following ectopic and molar pregnancy
Salpingitis following ectopic and molar pregnancy
Salpingo-oophoritis following ectopic and molar pregnancy
EXCLUDES 1 *sepsis following ectopic and molar pregnancy (O08.82)*
urinary tract infection (O08.83)

O08.1 **Delayed or excessive hemorrhage following ectopic and molar pregnancy** CC M ♀
Afibrinogenemia following ectopic and molar pregnancy
Defibrination syndrome following ectopic and molar pregnancy
Hemolysis following ectopic and molar pregnancy
Intravascular coagulation following ectopic and molar pregnancy
EXCLUDES 1 *delayed or excessive hemorrhage due to incomplete abortion (O03.1)*

O08.2 **Embolism following ectopic and molar pregnancy** MCC M ♀
Air embolism following ectopic and molar pregnancy
Amniotic fluid embolism following ectopic and molar pregnancy
Blood-clot embolism following ectopic and molar pregnancy
Embolism NOS following ectopic and molar pregnancy
Fat embolism following ectopic and molar pregnancy
Pulmonary embolism following ectopic and molar pregnancy
Pyemic embolism following ectopic and molar pregnancy
Septic or septicopyemic embolism following ectopic and molar pregnancy
Soap embolism following ectopic and molar pregnancy

O08.3 **Shock following ectopic and molar pregnancy** MCC M ♀
Circulatory collapse following ectopic and molar pregnancy
Shock (postprocedural) following ectopic and molar pregnancy
EXCLUDES 1 *shock due to infection following ectopic and molar pregnancy (O08.82)*

O08.4 **Renal failure following ectopic and molar pregnancy** MCC M ♀
Kidney failure (acute) following ectopic and molar pregnancy
Oliguria following ectopic and molar pregnancy
Renal shutdown following ectopic and molar pregnancy
Renal tubular necrosis following ectopic and molar pregnancy
Uremia following ectopic and molar pregnancy

O08.5 **Metabolic disorders following an ectopic and molar pregnancy** CC M ♀

O08.6 **Damage to pelvic organs and tissues following an ectopic and molar pregnancy** CC M ♀
Laceration, perforation, tear or chemical damage of bladder following an ectopic and molar pregnancy
Laceration, perforation, tear or chemical damage of bowel following an ectopic and molar pregnancy
Laceration, perforation, tear or chemical damage of broad ligament following an ectopic and molar pregnancy
Laceration, perforation, tear or chemical damage of cervix following an ectopic and molar pregnancy
Laceration, perforation, tear or chemical damage of periurethral tissue following an ectopic and molar pregnancy
Laceration, perforation, tear or chemical damage of uterus following an ectopic and molar pregnancy
Laceration, perforation, tear or chemical damage of vagina following an ectopic and molar pregnancy

O08.7 **Other venous complications following an ectopic and molar pregnancy** CC M ♀

✓5th O08.8 **Other complications following an ectopic and molar pregnancy**

O08.81 **Cardiac arrest following an ectopic and molar pregnancy** CC M ♀

O08.82 **Sepsis following ectopic and molar pregnancy** CC M ♀
Use additional code (B95-B97), to identify infectious agent
Use additional code (R65.2-) to identify severe sepsis, if applicable
EXCLUDES 1 *septic or septicopyemic embolism following ectopic and molar pregnancy (O08.2)*

O08.83 **Urinary tract infection following an ectopic and molar pregnancy** CC M ♀
Cystitis following an ectopic and molar pregnancy

O08.89 **Other complications following an ectopic and molar pregnancy** CC M ♀

O08.9 **Unspecified complication following an ectopic and molar pregnancy** CC M ♀

Supervision of high risk pregnancy (O09)

✓4th O09 **Supervision of high risk pregnancy**
AHA: 2019,3Q,5; 2016,4Q,48-50,150

✓5th O09.0 **Supervision of pregnancy with history of infertility**

O09.00 **Supervision of pregnancy with history of infertility, unspecified trimester** UPD M ♀

O09.01 **Supervision of pregnancy with history of infertility, first trimester** UPD M ♀

O09.02 **Supervision of pregnancy with history of infertility, second trimester** UPD M ♀

O09.03 **Supervision of pregnancy with history of infertility, third trimester** UPD M ♀

✓5th O09.1 **Supervision of pregnancy with history of ectopic pregnancy**

O09.10 **Supervision of pregnancy with history of ectopic pregnancy, unspecified trimester** UPD M ♀

O09.11 **Supervision of pregnancy with history of ectopic pregnancy, first trimester** UPD M ♀

O09.12 **Supervision of pregnancy with history of ectopic pregnancy, second trimester** UPD M ♀

O09.13 **Supervision of pregnancy with history of ectopic pregnancy, third trimester** UPD M ♀

5th O09.A Supervision of pregnancy with history of molar pregnancy

DEF: Molar pregnancy: Trophoblastic neoplasm that mimics pregnancy by proliferating from a pathologic ovum and resulting only in a mass of cysts resembling grapes, 80 percent of which are benign, but require surgical removal.

O09.A0 Supervision of pregnancy with history of molar pregnancy, unspecified trimester UPD M ♀

O09.A1 Supervision of pregnancy with history of molar pregnancy, first trimester UPD M ♀

O09.A2 Supervision of pregnancy with history of molar pregnancy, second trimester UPD M ♀

O09.A3 Supervision of pregnancy with history of molar pregnancy, third trimester UPD M ♀

5th O09.2 Supervision of pregnancy with other poor reproductive or obstetric history

EXCLUDES 2 *pregnancy care for patient with history of recurrent pregnancy loss (O26.2-)*

6th O09.21 Supervision of pregnancy with history of pre-term labor

O09.211 Supervision of pregnancy with history of pre-term labor, first trimester UPD M ♀

O09.212 Supervision of pregnancy with history of pre-term labor, second trimester UPD M ♀

O09.213 Supervision of pregnancy with history of pre-term labor, third trimester UPD M ♀

O09.219 Supervision of pregnancy with history of pre-term labor, unspecified trimester UPD M ♀

6th O09.29 Supervision of pregnancy with other poor reproductive or obstetric history

Supervision of pregnancy with history of neonatal death

Supervision of pregnancy with history of stillbirth

O09.291 Supervision of pregnancy with other poor reproductive or obstetric history, first trimester UPD M ♀

O09.292 Supervision of pregnancy with other poor reproductive or obstetric history, second trimester UPD M ♀

O09.293 Supervision of pregnancy with other poor reproductive or obstetric history, third trimester UPD M ♀

O09.299 Supervision of pregnancy with other poor reproductive or obstetric history, unspecified trimester UPD M ♀

5th O09.3 Supervision of pregnancy with insufficient antenatal care

Supervision of concealed pregnancy

Supervision of hidden pregnancy

O09.30 Supervision of pregnancy with insufficient antenatal care, unspecified trimester UPD M ♀

O09.31 Supervision of pregnancy with insufficient antenatal care, first trimester UPD M ♀

O09.32 Supervision of pregnancy with insufficient antenatal care, second trimester UPD M ♀

O09.33 Supervision of pregnancy with insufficient antenatal care, third trimester UPD M ♀

5th O09.4 Supervision of pregnancy with grand multiparity

O09.40 Supervision of pregnancy with grand multiparity, unspecified trimester UPD M ♀

O09.41 Supervision of pregnancy with grand multiparity, first trimester UPD M ♀

O09.42 Supervision of pregnancy with grand multiparity, second trimester UPD M ♀

O09.43 Supervision of pregnancy with grand multiparity, third trimester UPD M ♀

5th O09.5 Supervision of elderly primigravida and multigravida

Pregnancy for a female 35 years and older at expected date of delivery

6th O09.51 Supervision of elderly primigravida

O09.511 Supervision of elderly primigravida, first trimester UPD M ♀

O09.512 Supervision of elderly primigravida, second trimester UPD M ♀

O09.513 Supervision of elderly primigravida, third trimester UPD M ♀

O09.519 Supervision of elderly primigravida, unspecified trimester UPD M ♀

6th O09.52 Supervision of elderly multigravida

O09.521 Supervision of elderly multigravida, first trimester UPD M ♀

O09.522 Supervision of elderly multigravida, second trimester UPD M ♀

O09.523 Supervision of elderly multigravida, third trimester UPD M ♀

O09.529 Supervision of elderly multigravida, unspecified trimester UPD M ♀

5th O09.6 Supervision of young primigravida and multigravida

Supervision of pregnancy for a female less than 16 years old at expected date of delivery

6th O09.61 Supervision of young primigravida

O09.611 Supervision of young primigravida, first trimester UPD M ♀

O09.612 Supervision of young primigravida, second trimester UPD M ♀

O09.613 Supervision of young primigravida, third trimester UPD M ♀

O09.619 Supervision of young primigravida, unspecified trimester UPD M ♀

6th O09.62 Supervision of young multigravida

O09.621 Supervision of young multigravida, first trimester UPD M ♀

O09.622 Supervision of young multigravida, second trimester UPD M ♀

O09.623 Supervision of young multigravida, third trimester UPD M ♀

O09.629 Supervision of young multigravida, unspecified trimester UPD M ♀

5th O09.7 Supervision of high risk pregnancy due to social problems

O09.70 Supervision of high risk pregnancy due to social problems, unspecified trimester UPD M ♀

O09.71 Supervision of high risk pregnancy due to social problems, first trimester UPD M ♀

O09.72 Supervision of high risk pregnancy due to social problems, second trimester UPD M ♀

O09.73 Supervision of high risk pregnancy due to social problems, third trimester UPD M ♀

5th O09.8 Supervision of other high risk pregnancies

6th O09.81 Supervision of pregnancy resulting from assisted reproductive technology

Supervision of pregnancy resulting from in-vitro fertilization

EXCLUDES 2 *gestational carrier status (Z33.3)*

O09.811 Supervision of pregnancy resulting from assisted reproductive technology, first trimester UPD M ♀

O09.812 Supervision of pregnancy resulting from assisted reproductive technology, second trimester UPD M ♀

O09.813 Supervision of pregnancy resulting from assisted reproductive technology, third trimester UPD M ♀

O09.819 Supervision of pregnancy resulting from assisted reproductive technology, unspecified trimester UPD M ♀

6th O09.82 Supervision of pregnancy with history of in utero procedure during previous pregnancy

O09.821 Supervision of pregnancy with history of in utero procedure during previous pregnancy, first trimester UPD M ♀

O09.822 Supervision of pregnancy with history of in utero procedure during previous pregnancy, second trimester UPD M ♀

O09.823 Supervision of pregnancy with history of in utero procedure during previous pregnancy, third trimester UPD M ♀

O09.829 Supervision of pregnancy with history of in utero procedure during previous pregnancy, unspecified trimester UPD M ♀

EXCLUDES 1 *supervision of pregnancy affected by in utero procedure during current pregnancy (O35.7)*

6th O09.89 Supervision of other high risk pregnancies

O09.891 Supervision of other high risk pregnancies, first trimester UPD M ♀

O09.892 Supervision of other high risk pregnancies, second trimester UPD M ♀

O09.893 Supervision of other high risk pregnancies, third trimester UPD M ♀

O09.899 Supervision of other high risk pregnancies, unspecified trimester UPD M ♀

✓5th O09.9 Supervision of high risk pregnancy, unspecified

O09.90 Supervision of high risk pregnancy, unspecified, unspecified trimester UPD M ♀

O09.91 Supervision of high risk pregnancy, unspecified, first trimester UPD M ♀

O09.92 Supervision of high risk pregnancy, unspecified, second trimester UPD M ♀

O09.93 Supervision of high risk pregnancy, unspecified, third trimester UPD M ♀

Edema, proteinuria and hypertensive disorders in pregnancy, childbirth and the puerperium (O10-O16)

AHA: 2016,4Q,50

✓4th **O10 Pre-existing hypertension complicating pregnancy, childbirth and the puerperium**

INCLUDES pre-existing hypertension with pre-existing proteinuria complicating pregnancy, childbirth and the puerperium

EXCLUDES 2 *pre-existing hypertension with superimposed pre-eclampsia complicating pregnancy, childbirth and the puerperium (O11.-)*

✓5th O10.0 Pre-existing essential hypertension complicating pregnancy, childbirth and the puerperium

Any condition in I10 specified as a reason for obstetric care during pregnancy, childbirth or the puerperium

✓6th O10.01 Pre-existing essential hypertension complicating pregnancy

O10.011 Pre-existing essential hypertension complicating pregnancy, first trimester CC M ♀

O10.012 Pre-existing essential hypertension complicating pregnancy, second trimester CC M ♀

O10.013 Pre-existing essential hypertension complicating pregnancy, third trimester CC M ♀

O10.019 Pre-existing essential hypertension complicating pregnancy, unspecified trimester M ♀

O10.02 Pre-existing essential hypertension complicating childbirth CC M ♀

O10.03 Pre-existing essential hypertension complicating the puerperium M ♀

✓5th O10.1 Pre-existing hypertensive heart disease complicating pregnancy, childbirth and the puerperium

Any condition in I11 specified as a reason for obstetric care during pregnancy, childbirth or the puerperium

Use additional code from I11 to identify the type of hypertensive heart disease

✓6th O10.11 Pre-existing hypertensive heart disease complicating pregnancy

O10.111 Pre-existing hypertensive heart disease complicating pregnancy, first trimester M ♀

O10.112 Pre-existing hypertensive heart disease complicating pregnancy, second trimester M ♀

O10.113 Pre-existing hypertensive heart disease complicating pregnancy, third trimester M ♀

O10.119 Pre-existing hypertensive heart disease complicating pregnancy, unspecified trimester M ♀

O10.12 Pre-existing hypertensive heart disease complicating childbirth M ♀

O10.13 Pre-existing hypertensive heart disease complicating the puerperium M ♀

✓5th O10.2 Pre-existing hypertensive chronic kidney disease complicating pregnancy, childbirth and the puerperium

Any condition in I12 specified as a reason for obstetric care during pregnancy, childbirth or the puerperium

Use additional code from I12 to identify the type of hypertensive chronic kidney disease

✓6th O10.21 Pre-existing hypertensive chronic kidney disease complicating pregnancy

O10.211 Pre-existing hypertensive chronic kidney disease complicating pregnancy, first trimester M ♀

O10.212 Pre-existing hypertensive chronic kidney disease complicating pregnancy, second trimester M ♀

O10.213 Pre-existing hypertensive chronic kidney disease complicating pregnancy, third trimester M ♀

O10.219 Pre-existing hypertensive chronic kidney disease complicating pregnancy, unspecified trimester M ♀

O10.22 Pre-existing hypertensive chronic kidney disease complicating childbirth M ♀

O10.23 Pre-existing hypertensive chronic kidney disease complicating the puerperium M ♀

✓5th O10.3 Pre-existing hypertensive heart and chronic kidney disease complicating pregnancy, childbirth and the puerperium

Any condition in I13 specified as a reason for obstetric care during pregnancy, childbirth or the puerperium

Use additional code from I13 to identify the type of hypertensive heart and chronic kidney disease

✓6th O10.31 Pre-existing hypertensive heart and chronic kidney disease complicating pregnancy

O10.311 Pre-existing hypertensive heart and chronic kidney disease complicating pregnancy, first trimester M ♀

O10.312 Pre-existing hypertensive heart and chronic kidney disease complicating pregnancy, second trimester M ♀

O10.313 Pre-existing hypertensive heart and chronic kidney disease complicating pregnancy, third trimester M ♀

O10.319 Pre-existing hypertensive heart and chronic kidney disease complicating pregnancy, unspecified trimester M ♀

O10.32 Pre-existing hypertensive heart and chronic kidney disease complicating childbirth M ♀

O10.33 Pre-existing hypertensive heart and chronic kidney disease complicating the puerperium M ♀

✓5th O10.4 Pre-existing secondary hypertension complicating pregnancy, childbirth and the puerperium

Any condition in I15 specified as a reason for obstetric care during pregnancy, childbirth or the puerperium

Use additional code from I15 to identify the type of secondary hypertension

✓6th O10.41 Pre-existing secondary hypertension complicating pregnancy

O10.411 Pre-existing secondary hypertension complicating pregnancy, first trimester CC M ♀

O10.412 Pre-existing secondary hypertension complicating pregnancy, second trimester CC M ♀

O10.413 Pre-existing secondary hypertension complicating pregnancy, third trimester CC M ♀

O10.419 Pre-existing secondary hypertension complicating pregnancy, unspecified trimester M ♀

O10.42 Pre-existing secondary hypertension complicating childbirth MCC M ♀

O10.43 Pre-existing secondary hypertension complicating the puerperium CC M ♀

✓5th O10.9 Unspecified pre-existing hypertension complicating pregnancy, childbirth and the puerperium

✓6th O10.91 Unspecified pre-existing hypertension complicating pregnancy

O10.911 Unspecified pre-existing hypertension complicating pregnancy, first trimester CC M ♀

O10.912 Unspecified pre-existing hypertension complicating pregnancy, second trimester CC M ♀

O10.913 Unspecified pre-existing hypertension complicating pregnancy, third trimester CC M ♀

O10.919 Unspecified pre-existing hypertension complicating pregnancy, unspecified trimester M ♀

O10.92 Unspecified pre-existing hypertension complicating childbirth CC M ♀

O10.93 Unspecified pre-existing hypertension complicating the puerperium M ♀

✓4th O11 Pre-existing hypertension with pre-eclampsia

INCLUDES ▶conditions in O10 complicated by pre-eclampsia◀
pre-eclampsia superimposed pre-existing in hypertension

Use additional code from O10 to identify the type of hypertension

DEF: Complication of pregnancy manifesting in the development of borderline hypertension, protein in the urine, and unresponsive swelling between the 20th week of pregnancy and the end of the first week following birth in mild to moderate cases. Severe preeclampsia presents with hypertension, associated with marked swelling, proteinuria, abdominal pain, and/or visual changes.

O11.1 Pre-existing hypertension with pre-eclampsia, first trimester MCC M ♀

O11.2 Pre-existing hypertension with pre-eclampsia, second trimester MCC M ♀

O11.3 Pre-existing hypertension with pre-eclampsia, third trimester MCC M ♀

O11.4 Pre-existing hypertension with pre-eclampsia, complicating childbirth M ♀

O11.5 Pre-existing hypertension with pre-eclampsia, complicating the puerperium M ♀

O11.9 Pre-existing hypertension with pre-eclampsia, unspecified trimester M ♀

✓4th O12 Gestational [pregnancy-induced] edema and proteinuria without hypertension

✓5th O12.0 Gestational edema

O12.00 Gestational edema, unspecified trimester M ♀

O12.01 Gestational edema, first trimester M ♀

O12.02 Gestational edema, second trimester M ♀

O12.03 Gestational edema, third trimester M ♀

O12.04 Gestational edema, complicating childbirth M ♀

O12.05 Gestational edema, complicating the puerperium M ♀

✓5th O12.1 Gestational proteinuria

O12.10 Gestational proteinuria, unspecified trimester M ♀

O12.11 Gestational proteinuria, first trimester CC M ♀

O12.12 Gestational proteinuria, second trimester CC M ♀

O12.13 Gestational proteinuria, third trimester CC M ♀

O12.14 Gestational proteinuria, complicating childbirth M ♀

O12.15 Gestational proteinuria, complicating the puerperium M ♀

✓5th O12.2 Gestational edema with proteinuria

O12.20 Gestational edema with proteinuria, unspecified trimester M ♀

O12.21 Gestational edema with proteinuria, first trimester CC M ♀

O12.22 Gestational edema with proteinuria, second trimester CC M ♀

O12.23 Gestational edema with proteinuria, third trimester CC M ♀

O12.24 Gestational edema with proteinuria, complicating childbirth M ♀

O12.25 Gestational edema with proteinuria, complicating the puerperium M ♀

✓4th O13 Gestational [pregnancy-induced] hypertension without significant proteinuria

INCLUDES gestational hypertension NOS
transient hypertension of pregnancy

AHA: 2016,1Q,5

O13.1 Gestational [pregnancy-induced] hypertension without significant proteinuria, first trimester M ♀

O13.2 Gestational [pregnancy-induced] hypertension without significant proteinuria, second trimester M ♀

O13.3 Gestational [pregnancy-induced] hypertension without significant proteinuria, third trimester M ♀

O13.4 Gestational [pregnancy-induced] hypertension without significant proteinuria, complicating childbirth M ♀

O13.5 Gestational [pregnancy-induced] hypertension without significant proteinuria, complicating the puerperium M ♀

O13.9 Gestational [pregnancy-induced] hypertension without significant proteinuria, unspecified trimester M ♀

✓4th O14 Pre-eclampsia

EXCLUDES 1 *pre-existing hypertension with pre-eclampsia (O11)*

DEF: Complication of pregnancy manifesting in the development of borderline hypertension, protein in the urine, and unresponsive swelling between the 20th week of pregnancy and the end of the first week following birth in mild to moderate cases. Severe preeclampsia presents with hypertension, associated with marked swelling, proteinuria, abdominal pain, and/or visual changes.

✓5th O14.0 Mild to moderate pre-eclampsia

AHA: 2019,3Q,12; 2019,2Q,8

O14.00 Mild to moderate pre-eclampsia, unspecified trimester M ♀

O14.02 Mild to moderate pre-eclampsia, second trimester CC M ♀

O14.03 Mild to moderate pre-eclampsia, third trimester CC M ♀

O14.04 Mild to moderate pre-eclampsia, complicating childbirth M ♀

AHA: 2019,2Q,8

O14.05 Mild to moderate pre-eclampsia, complicating the puerperium M ♀

✓5th O14.1 Severe pre-eclampsia

EXCLUDES 1 *HELLP syndrome (O14.2-)*

AHA: 2019,3Q,12

O14.10 Severe pre-eclampsia, unspecified trimester M ♀

O14.12 Severe pre-eclampsia, second trimester MCC M ♀

O14.13 Severe pre-eclampsia, third trimester MCC M ♀

O14.14 Severe pre-eclampsia complicating childbirth M ♀

O14.15 Severe pre-eclampsia, complicating the puerperium M ♀

✓5th O14.2 HELLP syndrome

Severe pre-eclampsia with hemolysis, elevated liver enzymes and low platelet count (HELLP)

AHA: 2019,3Q,12

O14.20 HELLP syndrome (HELLP), unspecified trimester M ♀

O14.22 HELLP syndrome (HELLP), second trimester MCC M ♀

O14.23 HELLP syndrome (HELLP), third trimester MCC M ♀

O14.24 HELLP syndrome, complicating childbirth M ♀

O14.25 HELLP syndrome, complicating the puerperium M ♀

✓5th O14.9 Unspecified pre-eclampsia

O14.90 Unspecified pre-eclampsia, unspecified trimester M ♀

O14.92 Unspecified pre-eclampsia, second trimester CC M ♀

O14.93 Unspecified pre-eclampsia, third trimester CC M ♀

O14.94 Unspecified pre-eclampsia, complicating childbirth M ♀

O14.95 Unspecified pre-eclampsia, complicating the puerperium M ♀

✓4th O15 Eclampsia

INCLUDES convulsions following conditions in O10-O14 and O16

DEF: Tetany and toxemia producing seizure activity or coma in a pregnant patient who most often has presented with prior preeclampsia (i.e., hypertension, albuminuria, and edema).

✓5th O15.0 Eclampsia complicating pregnancy

O15.00 Eclampsia complicating pregnancy, unspecified trimester M ♀

O15.02 Eclampsia complicating pregnancy, second trimester MCC M ♀

O15.03 Eclampsia complicating pregnancy, third trimester MCC M ♀

O15.1 Eclampsia complicating labor MCC M ♀

O15.2 Eclampsia complicating the puerperium MCC M ♀

O15.9 Eclampsia, unspecified as to time period M ♀
Eclampsia NOS

O16 Unspecified maternal hypertension

O16.1 Unspecified maternal hypertension, first trimester CC M ♀
O16.2 Unspecified maternal hypertension, second trimester CC M ♀
O16.3 Unspecified maternal hypertension, third trimester CC M ♀
O16.4 Unspecified maternal hypertension, complicating childbirth M ♀
O16.5 Unspecified maternal hypertension, complicating the puerperium M ♀
O16.9 Unspecified maternal hypertension, unspecified trimester M ♀

Other maternal disorders predominantly related to pregnancy (O20-O29)

EXCLUDES 2 *maternal care related to the fetus and amniotic cavity and possible delivery problems (O30-O48)*
maternal diseases classifiable elsewhere but complicating pregnancy, labor and delivery, and the puerperium (O98-O99)

O20 Hemorrhage in early pregnancy

INCLUDES hemorrhage before completion of 20 weeks gestation
EXCLUDES 1 *pregnancy with abortive outcome (O00-O08)*

O20.0 Threatened abortion CC M ♀
Hemorrhage specified as due to threatened abortion
DEF: Bloody discharge during pregnancy. The cervix may be dilated and pregnancy threatened, but the pregnancy is not terminated.

O20.8 Other hemorrhage in early pregnancy M ♀
O20.9 Hemorrhage in early pregnancy, unspecified CC M ♀

O21 Excessive vomiting in pregnancy

O21.0 Mild hyperemesis gravidarum M ♀
Hyperemesis gravidarum, mild or unspecified, starting before the end of the 20th week of gestation

O21.1 Hyperemesis gravidarum with metabolic disturbance M ♀
Hyperemesis gravidarum, starting before the end of the 20th week of gestation, with metabolic disturbance such as carbohydrate depletion
Hyperemesis gravidarum, starting before the end of the 20th week of gestation, with metabolic disturbance such as dehydration
Hyperemesis gravidarum, starting before the end of the 20th week of gestation, with metabolic disturbance such as electrolyte imbalance

O21.2 Late vomiting of pregnancy M ♀
Excessive vomiting starting after 20 completed weeks of gestation

O21.8 Other vomiting complicating pregnancy M ♀
Vomiting due to diseases classified elsewhere, complicating pregnancy
Use additional code, to identify cause

O21.9 Vomiting of pregnancy, unspecified M ♀

O22 Venous complications and hemorrhoids in pregnancy

EXCLUDES 1 *venous complications of:*
abortion NOS (O03.9)
ectopic or molar pregnancy (O08.7)
failed attempted abortion (O07.35)
induced abortion (O04.85)
spontaneous abortion (O03.89)
EXCLUDES 2 *obstetric pulmonary embolism (O88.-)*
venous complications and hemorrhoids of childbirth and the puerperium (O87.-)

O22.0 Varicose veins of lower extremity in pregnancy
Varicose veins NOS in pregnancy
DEF: Distended, tortuous veins of the lower extremities associated with pregnancy.

O22.00 Varicose veins of lower extremity in pregnancy, unspecified trimester M ♀
O22.01 Varicose veins of lower extremity in pregnancy, first trimester M ♀
O22.02 Varicose veins of lower extremity in pregnancy, second trimester M ♀
O22.03 Varicose veins of lower extremity in pregnancy, third trimester M ♀

O22.1 Genital varices in pregnancy
Perineal varices in pregnancy
Vaginal varices in pregnancy
Vulval varices in pregnancy

O22.10 Genital varices in pregnancy, unspecified trimester M ♀
O22.11 Genital varices in pregnancy, first trimester M ♀
O22.12 Genital varices in pregnancy, second trimester M ♀
O22.13 Genital varices in pregnancy, third trimester M ♀

O22.2 Superficial thrombophlebitis in pregnancy
Phlebitis in pregnancy NOS
Thrombophlebitis of legs in pregnancy
Thrombosis in pregnancy NOS
Use additional code to identify the superficial thrombophlebitis (I80.0-)

O22.20 Superficial thrombophlebitis in pregnancy, unspecified trimester CC M ♀
O22.21 Superficial thrombophlebitis in pregnancy, first trimester CC M ♀
O22.22 Superficial thrombophlebitis in pregnancy, second trimester CC M ♀
O22.23 Superficial thrombophlebitis in pregnancy, third trimester CC M ♀

O22.3 Deep phlebothrombosis in pregnancy
Deep vein thrombosis, antepartum
Use additional code to identify the deep vein thrombosis (I82.4-, I82.5-, I82.62-, I82.72-)
Use additional code, if applicable, for associated long-term (current) use of anticoagulants (Z79.01)

O22.30 Deep phlebothrombosis in pregnancy, unspecified trimester CC M ♀
O22.31 Deep phlebothrombosis in pregnancy, first trimester MCC M ♀
O22.32 Deep phlebothrombosis in pregnancy, second trimester MCC M ♀
O22.33 Deep phlebothrombosis in pregnancy, third trimester MCC M ♀

O22.4 Hemorrhoids in pregnancy

O22.40 Hemorrhoids in pregnancy, unspecified trimester CC M ♀
O22.41 Hemorrhoids in pregnancy, first trimester CC M ♀
O22.42 Hemorrhoids in pregnancy, second trimester CC M ♀
O22.43 Hemorrhoids in pregnancy, third trimester CC M ♀

O22.5 Cerebral venous thrombosis in pregnancy
Cerebrovenous sinus thrombosis in pregnancy

O22.50 Cerebral venous thrombosis in pregnancy, unspecified trimester CC M ♀
O22.51 Cerebral venous thrombosis in pregnancy, first trimester CC M ♀
O22.52 Cerebral venous thrombosis in pregnancy, second trimester CC M ♀
O22.53 Cerebral venous thrombosis in pregnancy, third trimester CC M ♀

O22.8 Other venous complications in pregnancy

O22.8X Other venous complications in pregnancy

O22.8X1 Other venous complications in pregnancy, first trimester CC M ♀
O22.8X2 Other venous complications in pregnancy, second trimester CC M ♀
O22.8X3 Other venous complications in pregnancy, third trimester CC M ♀
O22.8X9 Other venous complications in pregnancy, unspecified trimester CC M ♀

O22.9 Venous complication in pregnancy, unspecified
Gestational phlebitis NOS
Gestational phlebopathy NOS
Gestational thrombosis NOS

O22.90 Venous complication in pregnancy, unspecified, unspecified trimester CC M ♀
O22.91 Venous complication in pregnancy, unspecified, first trimester M ♀

O22.92 Venous complication in pregnancy, unspecified, second trimester M ♀

O22.93 Venous complication in pregnancy, unspecified, third trimester M ♀

✓4th O23 Infections of genitourinary tract in pregnancy

Use additional code to identify organism (B95.-, B96.-)

EXCLUDES 2 *gonococcal infections complicating pregnancy, childbirth and the puerperium (O98.2)*
infections with a predominantly sexual mode of transmission NOS complicating pregnancy, childbirth and the puerperium (O98.3)
syphilis complicating pregnancy, childbirth and the puerperium (O98.1)
tuberculosis of genitourinary system complicating pregnancy, childbirth and the puerperium (O98.0)
venereal disease NOS complicating pregnancy, childbirth and the puerperium (O98.3)

AHA: 2018,2Q,20

✓5th O23.0 Infections of kidney in pregnancy

Pyelonephritis in pregnancy

O23.00 Infections of kidney in pregnancy, unspecified trimester M ♀

O23.01 Infections of kidney in pregnancy, first trimester CC M ♀

O23.02 Infections of kidney in pregnancy, second trimester CC M ♀

O23.03 Infections of kidney in pregnancy, third trimester CC M ♀

✓5th O23.1 Infections of bladder in pregnancy

O23.10 Infections of bladder in pregnancy, unspecified trimester M ♀

O23.11 Infections of bladder in pregnancy, first trimester CC M ♀

O23.12 Infections of bladder in pregnancy, second trimester CC M ♀

O23.13 Infections of bladder in pregnancy, third trimester CC M ♀

✓5th O23.2 Infections of urethra in pregnancy

O23.20 Infections of urethra in pregnancy, unspecified trimester M ♀

O23.21 Infections of urethra in pregnancy, first trimester CC M ♀

O23.22 Infections of urethra in pregnancy, second trimester CC M ♀

O23.23 Infections of urethra in pregnancy, third trimester CC M ♀

✓5th O23.3 Infections of other parts of urinary tract in pregnancy

O23.30 Infections of other parts of urinary tract in pregnancy, unspecified trimester M ♀

O23.31 Infections of other parts of urinary tract in pregnancy, first trimester CC M ♀

O23.32 Infections of other parts of urinary tract in pregnancy, second trimester CC M ♀

O23.33 Infections of other parts of urinary tract in pregnancy, third trimester CC M ♀

✓5th O23.4 Unspecified infection of urinary tract in pregnancy

O23.40 Unspecified infection of urinary tract in pregnancy, unspecified trimester M ♀

O23.41 Unspecified infection of urinary tract in pregnancy, first trimester CC M ♀

O23.42 Unspecified infection of urinary tract in pregnancy, second trimester CC M ♀

O23.43 Unspecified infection of urinary tract in pregnancy, third trimester CC M ♀

✓5th O23.5 Infections of the genital tract in pregnancy

✓6th O23.51 Infection of cervix in pregnancy

O23.511 Infections of cervix in pregnancy, first trimester CC M ♀

O23.512 Infections of cervix in pregnancy, second trimester CC M ♀

O23.513 Infections of cervix in pregnancy, third trimester CC M ♀

O23.519 Infections of cervix in pregnancy, unspecified trimester M ♀

✓6th O23.52 Salpingo-oophoritis in pregnancy

Oophoritis in pregnancy
Salpingitis in pregnancy

O23.521 Salpingo-oophoritis in pregnancy, first trimester CC M ♀

O23.522 Salpingo-oophoritis in pregnancy, second trimester CC M ♀

O23.523 Salpingo-oophoritis in pregnancy, third trimester CC M ♀

O23.529 Salpingo-oophoritis in pregnancy, unspecified trimester M ♀

✓6th O23.59 Infection of other part of genital tract in pregnancy

AHA: 2022,1Q,20

O23.591 Infection of other part of genital tract in pregnancy, first trimester CC M ♀

O23.592 Infection of other part of genital tract in pregnancy, second trimester CC M ♀

O23.593 Infection of other part of genital tract in pregnancy, third trimester CC M ♀

O23.599 Infection of other part of genital tract in pregnancy, unspecified trimester M ♀

✓5th O23.9 Unspecified genitourinary tract infection in pregnancy

Genitourinary tract infection in pregnancy NOS

O23.90 Unspecified genitourinary tract infection in pregnancy, unspecified trimester M ♀

O23.91 Unspecified genitourinary tract infection in pregnancy, first trimester CC M ♀

O23.92 Unspecified genitourinary tract infection in pregnancy, second trimester CC M ♀

O23.93 Unspecified genitourinary tract infection in pregnancy, third trimester CC M ♀

✓4th O24 Diabetes mellitus in pregnancy, childbirth and the puerperium

✓5th O24.0 Pre-existing type 1 diabetes mellitus, in pregnancy, childbirth and the puerperium

Juvenile onset diabetes mellitus, in pregnancy, childbirth and the puerperium
Ketosis-prone diabetes mellitus in pregnancy, childbirth and the puerperium

Use additional code from category E10 to further identify any manifestations

✓6th O24.01 Pre-existing type 1 diabetes mellitus, in pregnancy

O24.011 Pre-existing type 1 diabetes mellitus, in pregnancy, first trimester CC M ♀

O24.012 Pre-existing type 1 diabetes mellitus, in pregnancy, second trimester CC M ♀

O24.013 Pre-existing type 1 diabetes mellitus, in pregnancy, third trimester CC M ♀

O24.019 Pre-existing type 1 diabetes mellitus, in pregnancy, unspecified trimester CC M ♀

O24.02 Pre-existing type 1 diabetes mellitus, in childbirth MCC M ♀

O24.03 Pre-existing type 1 diabetes mellitus, in the puerperium CC M ♀

✓5th O24.1 Pre-existing type 2 diabetes mellitus, in pregnancy, childbirth and the puerperium

Insulin-resistant diabetes mellitus in pregnancy, childbirth and the puerperium

Use additional code (for):
from category E11 to further identify any manifestations
long-term (current) use of insulin (Z79.4)

✓6th O24.11 Pre-existing type 2 diabetes mellitus, in pregnancy

O24.111 Pre-existing type 2 diabetes mellitus, in pregnancy, first trimester CC M ♀

O24.112 Pre-existing type 2 diabetes mellitus, in pregnancy, second trimester CC M ♀

O24.113 Pre-existing type 2 diabetes mellitus, in pregnancy, third trimester CC M ♀

O24.119 Pre-existing type 2 diabetes mellitus, in pregnancy, unspecified trimester CC M ♀

O24.12 Pre-existing type 2 diabetes mellitus, in childbirth MCC M ♀

O24.13 Pre-existing type 2 diabetes mellitus, in the puerperium CC M ♀

O24.3 Unspecified pre-existing diabetes mellitus in pregnancy, childbirth and the puerperium
Use additional code (for):
from category E11 to further identify any manifestation
long-term (current) use of insulin (Z79.4)

O24.31 Unspecified pre-existing diabetes mellitus in pregnancy

O24.311 Unspecified pre-existing diabetes mellitus in pregnancy, first trimester CC M ♀

O24.312 Unspecified pre-existing diabetes mellitus in pregnancy, second trimester CC M ♀

O24.313 Unspecified pre-existing diabetes mellitus in pregnancy, third trimester CC M ♀

O24.319 Unspecified pre-existing diabetes mellitus in pregnancy, unspecified trimester CC M ♀

O24.32 Unspecified pre-existing diabetes mellitus in childbirth MCC M ♀

O24.33 Unspecified pre-existing diabetes mellitus in the puerperium CC M ♀

O24.4 Gestational diabetes mellitus
Diabetes mellitus arising in pregnancy
Gestational diabetes mellitus NOS
AHA: 2020,3Q,30; 2016,4Q,50; 2015,4Q,34

O24.41 Gestational diabetes mellitus in pregnancy

O24.410 Gestational diabetes mellitus in pregnancy, diet controlled M ♀

O24.414 Gestational diabetes mellitus in pregnancy, insulin controlled M ♀

O24.415 Gestational diabetes mellitus in pregnancy, controlled by oral hypoglycemic drugs M ♀
Gestational diabetes mellitus in pregnancy, controlled by oral antidiabetic drugs

O24.419 Gestational diabetes mellitus in pregnancy, unspecified control M ♀

O24.42 Gestational diabetes mellitus in childbirth
AHA: 2016,1Q,5

O24.420 Gestational diabetes mellitus in childbirth, diet controlled M ♀

O24.424 Gestational diabetes mellitus in childbirth, insulin controlled M ♀

O24.425 Gestational diabetes mellitus in childbirth, controlled by oral hypoglycemic drugs M ♀
Gestational diabetes mellitus in childbirth, controlled by oral antidiabetic drugs

O24.429 Gestational diabetes mellitus in childbirth, unspecified control M ♀

O24.43 Gestational diabetes mellitus in the puerperium

O24.430 Gestational diabetes mellitus in the puerperium, diet controlled M ♀

O24.434 Gestational diabetes mellitus in the puerperium, insulin controlled M ♀

O24.435 Gestational diabetes mellitus in puerperium, controlled by oral hypoglycemic drugs M ♀
Gestational diabetes mellitus in puerperium, controlled by oral antidiabetic drugs

O24.439 Gestational diabetes mellitus in the puerperium, unspecified control M ♀

O24.8 Other pre-existing diabetes mellitus in pregnancy, childbirth, and the puerperium
Use additional code (for):
from categories E08, E09 and E13 to further identify any manifestation
long-term (current) use of insulin (Z79.4)

O24.81 Other pre-existing diabetes mellitus in pregnancy

O24.811 Other pre-existing diabetes mellitus in pregnancy, first trimester CC M ♀

O24.812 Other pre-existing diabetes mellitus in pregnancy, second trimester CC M ♀

O24.813 Other pre-existing diabetes mellitus in pregnancy, third trimester CC M ♀

O24.819 Other pre-existing diabetes mellitus in pregnancy, unspecified trimester CC M ♀

O24.82 Other pre-existing diabetes mellitus in childbirth MCC M ♀

O24.83 Other pre-existing diabetes mellitus in the puerperium CC M ♀

O24.9 Unspecified diabetes mellitus in pregnancy, childbirth and the puerperium
Use additional code for long-term (current) use of insulin (Z79.4)

O24.91 Unspecified diabetes mellitus in pregnancy

O24.911 Unspecified diabetes mellitus in pregnancy, first trimester CC M ♀

O24.912 Unspecified diabetes mellitus in pregnancy, second trimester CC M ♀

O24.913 Unspecified diabetes mellitus in pregnancy, third trimester CC M ♀

O24.919 Unspecified diabetes mellitus in pregnancy, unspecified trimester CC M ♀

O24.92 Unspecified diabetes mellitus in childbirth M ♀

O24.93 Unspecified diabetes mellitus in the puerperium CC M ♀

O25 Malnutrition in pregnancy, childbirth and the puerperium

O25.1 Malnutrition in pregnancy

O25.10 Malnutrition in pregnancy, unspecified trimester M ♀

O25.11 Malnutrition in pregnancy, first trimester M ♀

O25.12 Malnutrition in pregnancy, second trimester M ♀

O25.13 Malnutrition in pregnancy, third trimester M ♀

O25.2 Malnutrition in childbirth M ♀

O25.3 Malnutrition in the puerperium M ♀

O26 Maternal care for other conditions predominantly related to pregnancy

O26.0 Excessive weight gain in pregnancy
EXCLUDES 2 *gestational edema (O12.0, O12.2)*

O26.00 Excessive weight gain in pregnancy, unspecified trimester M ♀

O26.01 Excessive weight gain in pregnancy, first trimester M ♀

O26.02 Excessive weight gain in pregnancy, second trimester M ♀

O26.03 Excessive weight gain in pregnancy, third trimester M ♀

O26.1 Low weight gain in pregnancy

O26.10 Low weight gain in pregnancy, unspecified trimester M ♀

O26.11 Low weight gain in pregnancy, first trimester M ♀

O26.12 Low weight gain in pregnancy, second trimester M ♀

O26.13 Low weight gain in pregnancy, third trimester M ♀

O26.2 Pregnancy care for patient with recurrent pregnancy loss

O26.20 Pregnancy care for patient with recurrent pregnancy loss, unspecified trimester M ♀

O26.21 Pregnancy care for patient with recurrent pregnancy loss, first trimester M ♀

O26.22 Pregnancy care for patient with recurrent pregnancy loss, second trimester M ♀

O26.23 Pregnancy care for patient with recurrent pregnancy loss, third trimester M ♀

O26.3 Retained intrauterine contraceptive device in pregnancy

O26.30 Retained intrauterine contraceptive device in pregnancy, unspecified trimester M ♀

O26.31 Retained intrauterine contraceptive device in pregnancy, first trimester M ♀

O26.32 Retained intrauterine contraceptive device in pregnancy, second trimester M ♀

O26.33 Retained intrauterine contraceptive device in pregnancy, third trimester M ♀

O26.4 Herpes gestationis
DEF: Rare skin disorder of unknown origin that appears on the abdomen in the second and third trimester as intensely itchy blisters that spread to other sites.

O26.40 Herpes gestationis, unspecified trimester M ♀

O26.41 Herpes gestationis, first trimester M♀
O26.42 Herpes gestationis, second trimester M♀
O26.43 Herpes gestationis, third trimester M♀

✓5th O26.5 Maternal hypotension syndrome
Supine hypotensive syndrome
O26.50 Maternal hypotension syndrome, unspecified trimester M♀
O26.51 Maternal hypotension syndrome, first trimester M♀
O26.52 Maternal hypotension syndrome, second trimester M♀
O26.53 Maternal hypotension syndrome, third trimester M♀

✓5th O26.6 Liver and biliary tract disorders in pregnancy, childbirth and the puerperium
Use additional code to identify the specific disorder
EXCLUDES 2 *hepatorenal syndrome following labor and delivery ▶(O90.41)◀*
✓6th O26.61 Liver and biliary tract disorders in pregnancy
O26.611 Liver and biliary tract disorders in pregnancy, first trimester CC M♀
O26.612 Liver and biliary tract disorders in pregnancy, second trimester CC M♀
O26.613 Liver and biliary tract disorders in pregnancy, third trimester CC M♀
O26.619 Liver and biliary tract disorders in pregnancy, unspecified trimester M♀
O26.62 Liver and biliary tract disorders in childbirth CC M♀
AHA: 2023,1Q,26
O26.63 Liver and biliary tract disorders in the puerperium M♀
● ✓6th O26.64 Intrahepatic cholestasis of pregnancy
● O26.641 Intrahepatic cholestasis of pregnancy, first trimester CC
● O26.642 Intrahepatic cholestasis of pregnancy, second trimester CC
● O26.643 Intrahepatic cholestasis of pregnancy, third trimester CC
● O26.649 Intrahepatic cholestasis of pregnancy, unspecified trimester

✓5th O26.7 Subluxation of symphysis (pubis) in pregnancy, childbirth and the puerperium
EXCLUDES 1 *traumatic separation of symphysis (pubis) during childbirth (O71.6)*
✓6th O26.71 Subluxation of symphysis (pubis) in pregnancy
O26.711 Subluxation of symphysis (pubis) in pregnancy, first trimester M♀
O26.712 Subluxation of symphysis (pubis) in pregnancy, second trimester M♀
O26.713 Subluxation of symphysis (pubis) in pregnancy, third trimester M♀
O26.719 Subluxation of symphysis (pubis) in pregnancy, unspecified trimester M♀
O26.72 Subluxation of symphysis (pubis) in childbirth M♀
O26.73 Subluxation of symphysis (pubis) in the puerperium M♀

✓5th O26.8 Other specified pregnancy related conditions
✓6th O26.81 Pregnancy related exhaustion and fatigue
O26.811 Pregnancy related exhaustion and fatigue, first trimester M♀
O26.812 Pregnancy related exhaustion and fatigue, second trimester M♀
O26.813 Pregnancy related exhaustion and fatigue, third trimester M♀
O26.819 Pregnancy related exhaustion and fatigue, unspecified trimester M♀
✓6th O26.82 Pregnancy related peripheral neuritis
O26.821 Pregnancy related peripheral neuritis, first trimester M♀
O26.822 Pregnancy related peripheral neuritis, second trimester M♀
O26.823 Pregnancy related peripheral neuritis, third trimester M♀
O26.829 Pregnancy related peripheral neuritis, unspecified trimester M♀
✓6th O26.83 Pregnancy related renal disease
Use additional code to identify the specific disorder
O26.831 Pregnancy related renal disease, first trimester CC M♀
O26.832 Pregnancy related renal disease, second trimester CC M♀
O26.833 Pregnancy related renal disease, third trimester CC M♀
O26.839 Pregnancy related renal disease, unspecified trimester M♀
✓6th O26.84 Uterine size-date discrepancy complicating pregnancy
EXCLUDES 1 *encounter for suspected problem with fetal growth ruled out (Z03.74)*
O26.841 Uterine size-date discrepancy, first trimester M♀
O26.842 Uterine size-date discrepancy, second trimester M♀
O26.843 Uterine size-date discrepancy, third trimester M♀
O26.849 Uterine size-date discrepancy, unspecified trimester M♀
✓6th O26.85 Spotting complicating pregnancy
O26.851 Spotting complicating pregnancy, first trimester M♀
O26.852 Spotting complicating pregnancy, second trimester M♀
O26.853 Spotting complicating pregnancy, third trimester M♀
O26.859 Spotting complicating pregnancy, unspecified trimester M♀
O26.86 Pruritic urticarial papules and plaques of pregnancy (PUPPP) M♀
Polymorphic eruption of pregnancy
✓6th O26.87 Cervical shortening
EXCLUDES 1 *encounter for suspected cervical shortening ruled out (Z03.75)*
DEF: Cervix that has shortened to less than 25 mm before the 24th week of pregnancy. A shortened cervix is a warning sign for impending premature delivery and is treated by cervical cerclage placement or progesterone.
O26.872 Cervical shortening, second trimester CC M♀
O26.873 Cervical shortening, third trimester CC M♀
O26.879 Cervical shortening, unspecified trimester CC M♀
✓6th O26.89 Other specified pregnancy related conditions
▶Use additional code, if applicable, to identify specific condition such as insulin resistance (E88.81-)◀
AHA: 2015,3Q,40
O26.891 Other specified pregnancy related conditions, first trimester M♀
O26.892 Other specified pregnancy related conditions, second trimester M♀
O26.893 Other specified pregnancy related conditions, third trimester M♀
O26.899 Other specified pregnancy related conditions, unspecified trimester M♀

✓5th O26.9 Pregnancy related conditions, unspecified
O26.90 Pregnancy related conditions, unspecified, unspecified trimester M♀
O26.91 Pregnancy related conditions, unspecified, first trimester M♀
O26.92 Pregnancy related conditions, unspecified, second trimester M♀
O26.93 Pregnancy related conditions, unspecified, third trimester M♀

✓4th O28 Abnormal findings on antenatal screening of mother
EXCLUDES 1 *diagnostic findings classified elsewhere - see Alphabetical Index*
O28.0 Abnormal hematological finding on antenatal screening of mother M♀
O28.1 Abnormal biochemical finding on antenatal screening of mother M♀
O28.2 Abnormal cytological finding on antenatal screening of mother M♀

O28.3 Abnormal ultrasonic finding on antenatal screening of mother M ♀

O28.4 Abnormal radiological finding on antenatal screening of mother M ♀

O28.5 Abnormal chromosomal and genetic finding on antenatal screening of mother M ♀

O28.8 Other abnormal findings on antenatal screening of mother M ♀

O28.9 Unspecified abnormal findings on antenatal screening of mother M ♀

✓4th O29 Complications of anesthesia during pregnancy

INCLUDES maternal complications arising from the administration of a general, regional or local anesthetic, analgesic or other sedation during pregnancy

Use additional code, if necessary, to identify the complication

EXCLUDES 2 *complications of anesthesia during labor and delivery (O74.-)*
complications of anesthesia during the puerperium (O89.-)

✓5th O29.0 Pulmonary complications of anesthesia during pregnancy

✓6th O29.01 Aspiration pneumonitis due to anesthesia during pregnancy

Inhalation of stomach contents or secretions NOS due to anesthesia during pregnancy
Mendelson's syndrome due to anesthesia during pregnancy

O29.011 Aspiration pneumonitis due to anesthesia during pregnancy, first trimester M ♀

O29.012 Aspiration pneumonitis due to anesthesia during pregnancy, second trimester M ♀

O29.013 Aspiration pneumonitis due to anesthesia during pregnancy, third trimester M ♀

O29.019 Aspiration pneumonitis due to anesthesia during pregnancy, unspecified trimester M ♀

✓6th O29.02 Pressure collapse of lung due to anesthesia during pregnancy

O29.021 Pressure collapse of lung due to anesthesia during pregnancy, first trimester M ♀

O29.022 Pressure collapse of lung due to anesthesia during pregnancy, second trimester M ♀

O29.023 Pressure collapse of lung due to anesthesia during pregnancy, third trimester M ♀

O29.029 Pressure collapse of lung due to anesthesia during pregnancy, unspecified trimester M ♀

✓6th O29.09 Other pulmonary complications of anesthesia during pregnancy

O29.091 Other pulmonary complications of anesthesia during pregnancy, first trimester M ♀

O29.092 Other pulmonary complications of anesthesia during pregnancy, second trimester M ♀

O29.093 Other pulmonary complications of anesthesia during pregnancy, third trimester M ♀

O29.099 Other pulmonary complications of anesthesia during pregnancy, unspecified trimester M ♀

✓5th O29.1 Cardiac complications of anesthesia during pregnancy

✓6th O29.11 Cardiac arrest due to anesthesia during pregnancy

O29.111 Cardiac arrest due to anesthesia during pregnancy, first trimester M ♀

O29.112 Cardiac arrest due to anesthesia during pregnancy, second trimester M ♀

O29.113 Cardiac arrest due to anesthesia during pregnancy, third trimester M ♀

O29.119 Cardiac arrest due to anesthesia during pregnancy, unspecified trimester M ♀

✓6th O29.12 Cardiac failure due to anesthesia during pregnancy

O29.121 Cardiac failure due to anesthesia during pregnancy, first trimester M ♀

O29.122 Cardiac failure due to anesthesia during pregnancy, second trimester M ♀

O29.123 Cardiac failure due to anesthesia during pregnancy, third trimester M ♀

O29.129 Cardiac failure due to anesthesia during pregnancy, unspecified trimester M ♀

✓6th O29.19 Other cardiac complications of anesthesia during pregnancy

O29.191 Other cardiac complications of anesthesia during pregnancy, first trimester M ♀

O29.192 Other cardiac complications of anesthesia during pregnancy, second trimester M ♀

O29.193 Other cardiac complications of anesthesia during pregnancy, third trimester M ♀

O29.199 Other cardiac complications of anesthesia during pregnancy, unspecified trimester M ♀

✓5th O29.2 Central nervous system complications of anesthesia during pregnancy

✓6th O29.21 Cerebral anoxia due to anesthesia during pregnancy

O29.211 Cerebral anoxia due to anesthesia during pregnancy, first trimester M ♀

O29.212 Cerebral anoxia due to anesthesia during pregnancy, second trimester M ♀

O29.213 Cerebral anoxia due to anesthesia during pregnancy, third trimester M ♀

O29.219 Cerebral anoxia due to anesthesia during pregnancy, unspecified trimester M ♀

✓6th O29.29 Other central nervous system complications of anesthesia during pregnancy

O29.291 Other central nervous system complications of anesthesia during pregnancy, first trimester M ♀

O29.292 Other central nervous system complications of anesthesia during pregnancy, second trimester M ♀

O29.293 Other central nervous system complications of anesthesia during pregnancy, third trimester M ♀

O29.299 Other central nervous system complications of anesthesia during pregnancy, unspecified trimester M ♀

✓5th O29.3 Toxic reaction to local anesthesia during pregnancy

✓6th O29.3X Toxic reaction to local anesthesia during pregnancy

O29.3X1 Toxic reaction to local anesthesia during pregnancy, first trimester M ♀

O29.3X2 Toxic reaction to local anesthesia during pregnancy, second trimester M ♀

O29.3X3 Toxic reaction to local anesthesia during pregnancy, third trimester M ♀

O29.3X9 Toxic reaction to local anesthesia during pregnancy, unspecified trimester M ♀

✓5th O29.4 Spinal and epidural anesthesia induced headache during pregnancy

O29.40 Spinal and epidural anesthesia induced headache during pregnancy, unspecified trimester M ♀

O29.41 Spinal and epidural anesthesia induced headache during pregnancy, first trimester M ♀

O29.42 Spinal and epidural anesthesia induced headache during pregnancy, second trimester M ♀

O29.43 Spinal and epidural anesthesia induced headache during pregnancy, third trimester M ♀

✓5th O29.5 Other complications of spinal and epidural anesthesia during pregnancy

✓6th O29.5X Other complications of spinal and epidural anesthesia during pregnancy

O29.5X1 Other complications of spinal and epidural anesthesia during pregnancy, first trimester M ♀

O29.5X2 Other complications of spinal and epidural anesthesia during pregnancy, second trimester M ♀

O29.5X3 Other complications of spinal and epidural anesthesia during pregnancy, third trimester M ♀

O29.5X9 Other complications of spinal and epidural anesthesia during pregnancy, unspecified trimester M ♀

✓5th O29.6 Failed or difficult intubation for anesthesia during pregnancy

O29.60 Failed or difficult intubation for anesthesia during pregnancy, unspecified trimester M ♀

O29.61 Failed or difficult intubation for anesthesia during pregnancy, first trimester M ♀

Chapter 15. Pregnancy, Childbirth and the Puerperium

O28.3–O29.61

O29.62 Failed or difficult intubation for anesthesia during pregnancy, second trimester M ♀

O29.63 Failed or difficult intubation for anesthesia during pregnancy, third trimester M ♀

5th O29.8 Other complications of anesthesia during pregnancy

6th O29.8X Other complications of anesthesia during pregnancy

O29.8X1 Other complications of anesthesia during pregnancy, first trimester M ♀

O29.8X2 Other complications of anesthesia during pregnancy, second trimester M ♀

O29.8X3 Other complications of anesthesia during pregnancy, third trimester M ♀

O29.8X9 Other complications of anesthesia during pregnancy, unspecified trimester M ♀

5th O29.9 Unspecified complication of anesthesia during pregnancy

O29.90 Unspecified complication of anesthesia during pregnancy, unspecified trimester M ♀

O29.91 Unspecified complication of anesthesia during pregnancy, first trimester M ♀

O29.92 Unspecified complication of anesthesia during pregnancy, second trimester M ♀

O29.93 Unspecified complication of anesthesia during pregnancy, third trimester M ♀

Maternal care related to the fetus and amniotic cavity and possible delivery problems (O30-O48)

4th O30 Multiple gestation

Code also any complications specific to multiple gestation

AHA: 2016,4Q,51

5th O30.0 Twin pregnancy

6th O30.00 Twin pregnancy, unspecified number of placenta and unspecified number of amniotic sacs

O30.001 Twin pregnancy, unspecified number of placenta and unspecified number of amniotic sacs, first trimester M ♀

O30.002 Twin pregnancy, unspecified number of placenta and unspecified number of amniotic sacs, second trimester M ♀

O30.003 Twin pregnancy, unspecified number of placenta and unspecified number of amniotic sacs, third trimester M ♀

O30.009 Twin pregnancy, unspecified number of placenta and unspecified number of amniotic sacs, unspecified trimester M ♀

6th O30.01 Twin pregnancy, monochorionic/monoamniotic

Twin pregnancy, one placenta, one amniotic sac

EXCLUDES 1 *conjoined twins (O30.02-)*

O30.011 Twin pregnancy, monochorionic/monoamniotic, first trimester M ♀

O30.012 Twin pregnancy, monochorionic/monoamniotic, second trimester M ♀

O30.013 Twin pregnancy, monochorionic/monoamniotic, third trimester M ♀

O30.019 Twin pregnancy, monochorionic/monoamniotic, unspecified trimester M ♀

6th O30.02 Conjoined twin pregnancy

O30.021 Conjoined twin pregnancy, first trimester M ♀

O30.022 Conjoined twin pregnancy, second trimester M ♀

O30.023 Conjoined twin pregnancy, third trimester M ♀

O30.029 Conjoined twin pregnancy, unspecified trimester M ♀

6th O30.03 Twin pregnancy, monochorionic/diamniotic

Twin pregnancy, one placenta, two amniotic sacs

O30.031 Twin pregnancy, monochorionic/diamniotic, first trimester M ♀

O30.032 Twin pregnancy, monochorionic/diamniotic, second trimester M ♀

O30.033 Twin pregnancy, monochorionic/diamniotic, third trimester M ♀

O30.039 Twin pregnancy, monochorionic/diamniotic, unspecified trimester M ♀

6th O30.04 Twin pregnancy, dichorionic/diamniotic

Twin pregnancy, two placentae, two amniotic sacs

O30.041 Twin pregnancy, dichorionic/diamniotic, first trimester M ♀

O30.042 Twin pregnancy, dichorionic/diamniotic, second trimester M ♀

O30.043 Twin pregnancy, dichorionic/diamniotic, third trimester M ♀

O30.049 Twin pregnancy, dichorionic/diamniotic, unspecified trimester M ♀

6th O30.09 Twin pregnancy, unable to determine number of placenta and number of amniotic sacs

O30.091 Twin pregnancy, unable to determine number of placenta and number of amniotic sacs, first trimester M ♀

O30.092 Twin pregnancy, unable to determine number of placenta and number of amniotic sacs, second trimester M ♀

O30.093 Twin pregnancy, unable to determine number of placenta and number of amniotic sacs, third trimester M ♀

O30.099 Twin pregnancy, unable to determine number of placenta and number of amniotic sacs, unspecified trimester M ♀

5th O30.1 Triplet pregnancy

6th O30.10 Triplet pregnancy, unspecified number of placenta and unspecified number of amniotic sacs

AHA: 2016,2Q,8

O30.101 Triplet pregnancy, unspecified number of placenta and unspecified number of amniotic sacs, first trimester CC M ♀

O30.102 Triplet pregnancy, unspecified number of placenta and unspecified number of amniotic sacs, second trimester CC M ♀

O30.103 Triplet pregnancy, unspecified number of placenta and unspecified number of amniotic sacs, third trimester CC M ♀

O30.109 Triplet pregnancy, unspecified number of placenta and unspecified number of amniotic sacs, unspecified trimester M ♀

6th O30.11 Triplet pregnancy with two or more monochorionic fetuses

O30.111 Triplet pregnancy with two or more monochorionic fetuses, first trimester CC M ♀

O30.112 Triplet pregnancy with two or more monochorionic fetuses, second trimester CC M ♀

O30.113 Triplet pregnancy with two or more monochorionic fetuses, third trimester CC M ♀

O30.119 Triplet pregnancy with two or more monochorionic fetuses, unspecified trimester M ♀

6th O30.12 Triplet pregnancy with two or more monoamniotic fetuses

O30.121 Triplet pregnancy with two or more monoamniotic fetuses, first trimester CC M ♀

O30.122 Triplet pregnancy with two or more monoamniotic fetuses, second trimester CC M ♀

O30.123 Triplet pregnancy with two or more monoamniotic fetuses, third trimester CC M ♀

O30.129 Triplet pregnancy with two or more monoamniotic fetuses, unspecified trimester M ♀

6th O30.13 Triplet pregnancy, trichorionic/triamniotic

AHA: 2018,4Q,22

O30.131 Triplet pregnancy, trichorionic/triamniotic, first trimester CC M ♀

O30.132 Triplet pregnancy, trichorionic/triamniotic, second trimester CC M ♀

O30.133 Triplet pregnancy, trichorionic/triamniotic, third trimester CC M ♀

O30.139 Triplet pregnancy, trichorionic/triamniotic, unspecified trimester M ♀

✓6th O30.19 Triplet pregnancy, unable to determine number of placenta and number of amniotic sacs

O30.191 Triplet pregnancy, unable to determine number of placenta and number of amniotic sacs, first trimester CC M ♀

O30.192 Triplet pregnancy, unable to determine number of placenta and number of amniotic sacs, second trimester CC M ♀

O30.193 Triplet pregnancy, unable to determine number of placenta and number of amniotic sacs, third trimester CC M ♀

O30.199 Triplet pregnancy, unable to determine number of placenta and number of amniotic sacs, unspecified trimester M ♀

✓5th O30.2 Quadruplet pregnancy

✓6th O30.20 Quadruplet pregnancy, unspecified number of placenta and unspecified number of amniotic sacs

O30.201 Quadruplet pregnancy, unspecified number of placenta and unspecified number of amniotic sacs, first trimester CC M ♀

O30.202 Quadruplet pregnancy, unspecified number of placenta and unspecified number of amniotic sacs, second trimester CC M ♀

O30.203 Quadruplet pregnancy, unspecified number of placenta and unspecified number of amniotic sacs, third trimester CC M ♀

O30.209 Quadruplet pregnancy, unspecified number of placenta and unspecified number of amniotic sacs, unspecified trimester M ♀

✓6th O30.21 Quadruplet pregnancy with two or more monochorionic fetuses

O30.211 Quadruplet pregnancy with two or more monochorionic fetuses, first trimester CC M ♀

O30.212 Quadruplet pregnancy with two or more monochorionic fetuses, second trimester CC M ♀

O30.213 Quadruplet pregnancy with two or more monochorionic fetuses, third trimester CC M ♀

O30.219 Quadruplet pregnancy with two or more monochorionic fetuses, unspecified trimester M ♀

✓6th O30.22 Quadruplet pregnancy with two or more monoamniotic fetuses

O30.221 Quadruplet pregnancy with two or more monoamniotic fetuses, first trimester CC M ♀

O30.222 Quadruplet pregnancy with two or more monoamniotic fetuses, second trimester CC M ♀

O30.223 Quadruplet pregnancy with two or more monoamniotic fetuses, third trimester CC M ♀

O30.229 Quadruplet pregnancy with two or more monoamniotic fetuses, unspecified trimester M ♀

✓6th O30.23 Quadruplet pregnancy, quadrachorionic/quadra-amniotic

AHA: 2018,4Q,22

O30.231 Quadruplet pregnancy, quadrachorionic/quadra-amniotic, first trimester CC M ♀

O30.232 Quadruplet pregnancy, quadrachorionic/quadra-amniotic, second trimester CC M ♀

O30.233 Quadruplet pregnancy, quadrachorionic/quadra-amniotic, third trimester CC M ♀

O30.239 Quadruplet pregnancy, quadrachorionic/quadra-amniotic, unspecified trimester M ♀

✓6th O30.29 Quadruplet pregnancy, unable to determine number of placenta and number of amniotic sacs

O30.291 Quadruplet pregnancy, unable to determine number of placenta and number of amniotic sacs, first trimester CC M ♀

O30.292 Quadruplet pregnancy, unable to determine number of placenta and number of amniotic sacs, second trimester CC M ♀

O30.293 Quadruplet pregnancy, unable to determine number of placenta and number of amniotic sacs, third trimester CC M ♀

O30.299 Quadruplet pregnancy, unable to determine number of placenta and number of amniotic sacs, unspecified trimester M ♀

✓5th O30.8 Other specified multiple gestation

Multiple gestation pregnancy greater then quadruplets

✓6th O30.80 Other specified multiple gestation, unspecified number of placenta and unspecified number of amniotic sacs

O30.801 Other specified multiple gestation, unspecified number of placenta and unspecified number of amniotic sacs, first trimester CC M ♀

O30.802 Other specified multiple gestation, unspecified number of placenta and unspecified number of amniotic sacs, second trimester CC M ♀

O30.803 Other specified multiple gestation, unspecified number of placenta and unspecified number of amniotic sacs, third trimester CC M ♀

O30.809 Other specified multiple gestation, unspecified number of placenta and unspecified number of amniotic sacs, unspecified trimester M ♀

✓6th O30.81 Other specified multiple gestation with two or more monochorionic fetuses

O30.811 Other specified multiple gestation with two or more monochorionic fetuses, first trimester CC M ♀

O30.812 Other specified multiple gestation with two or more monochorionic fetuses, second trimester CC M ♀

O30.813 Other specified multiple gestation with two or more monochorionic fetuses, third trimester CC M ♀

O30.819 Other specified multiple gestation with two or more monochorionic fetuses, unspecified trimester M ♀

✓6th O30.82 Other specified multiple gestation with two or more monoamniotic fetuses

O30.821 Other specified multiple gestation with two or more monoamniotic fetuses, first trimester CC M ♀

O30.822 Other specified multiple gestation with two or more monoamniotic fetuses, second trimester CC M ♀

O30.823 Other specified multiple gestation with two or more monoamniotic fetuses, third trimester CC M ♀

O30.829 Other specified multiple gestation with two or more monoamniotic fetuses, unspecified trimester M ♀

√6th **O30.83 Other specified multiple gestation, number of chorions and amnions are both equal to the number of fetuses**
Pentachorionic, penta-amniotic pregnancy (quintuplets)
Hexachorionic, hexa-amniotic pregnancy (sextuplets)
Heptachorionic, hepta-amniotic pregnancy (septuplets)
AHA: 2018,4Q,22

O30.831 Other specified multiple gestation, number of chorions and amnions are both equal to the number of fetuses, first trimester CC M ♀

O30.832 Other specified multiple gestation, number of chorions and amnions are both equal to the number of fetuses, second trimester CC M ♀

O30.833 Other specified multiple gestation, number of chorions and amnions are both equal to the number of fetuses, third trimester CC M ♀

O30.839 Other specified multiple gestation, number of chorions and amnions are both equal to the number of fetuses, unspecified trimester M ♀

√6th **O30.89 Other specified multiple gestation, unable to determine number of placenta and number of amniotic sacs**

O30.891 Other specified multiple gestation, unable to determine number of placenta and number of amniotic sacs, first trimester CC M ♀

O30.892 Other specified multiple gestation, unable to determine number of placenta and number of amniotic sacs, second trimester CC M ♀

O30.893 Other specified multiple gestation, unable to determine number of placenta and number of amniotic sacs, third trimester CC M ♀

O30.899 Other specified multiple gestation, unable to determine number of placenta and number of amniotic sacs, unspecified trimester M ♀

√5th **O30.9 Multiple gestation, unspecified**
Multiple pregnancy NOS

O30.90 Multiple gestation, unspecified, unspecified trimester M ♀

O30.91 Multiple gestation, unspecified, first trimester M ♀

O30.92 Multiple gestation, unspecified, second trimester M ♀

O30.93 Multiple gestation, unspecified, third trimester M ♀

√4th **O31 Complications specific to multiple gestation**

EXCLUDES 2 *delayed delivery of second twin, triplet, etc. (O63.2)*
malpresentation of one fetus or more (O32.9)
placental transfusion syndromes (O43.0-)

AHA: 2012,4Q,107

One of the following 7th characters is to be assigned to each code under category O31. 7th character 0 is for single gestations and multiple gestations where the fetus is unspecified. 7th characters 1 through 9 are for cases of multiple gestations to identify the fetus for which the code applies. The appropriate code from category O30, Multiple gestation, must also be assigned when assigning a code from category O31 that has a 7th character of 1 through 9.

- 0 not applicable or unspecified
- 1 fetus 1
- 2 fetus 2
- 3 fetus 3
- 4 fetus 4
- 5 fetus 5
- 9 other fetus

√5th **O31.0 Papyraceous fetus**
Fetus compressus
DEF: Fetus that has died, but remains in utero for weeks before delivery, becoming compacted and mummified in appearance, with skin resembling parchment. Occurs most commonly in multigestational pregnancies. ***Synonym(s):*** *paper doll fetus.*

√x7th **O31.00 Papyraceous fetus, unspecified trimester** M ♀

√x7th **O31.01 Papyraceous fetus, first trimester** M ♀

√x7th **O31.02 Papyraceous fetus, second trimester** M ♀

√x7th **O31.03 Papyraceous fetus, third trimester** M ♀

√5th **O31.1 Continuing pregnancy after spontaneous abortion of one fetus or more**

√x7th **O31.10 Continuing pregnancy after spontaneous abortion of one fetus or more, unspecified trimester** M ♀

√x7th **O31.11 Continuing pregnancy after spontaneous abortion of one fetus or more, first trimester** M ♀

√x7th **O31.12 Continuing pregnancy after spontaneous abortion of one fetus or more, second trimester** M ♀

√x7th **O31.13 Continuing pregnancy after spontaneous abortion of one fetus or more, third trimester** M ♀

√5th **O31.2 Continuing pregnancy after intrauterine death of one fetus or more**

√x7th **O31.20 Continuing pregnancy after intrauterine death of one fetus or more, unspecified trimester** M ♀

√x7th **O31.21 Continuing pregnancy after intrauterine death of one fetus or more, first trimester** M ♀

√x7th **O31.22 Continuing pregnancy after intrauterine death of one fetus or more, second trimester** M ♀

√x7th **O31.23 Continuing pregnancy after intrauterine death of one fetus or more, third trimester** M ♀

√5th **O31.3 Continuing pregnancy after elective fetal reduction of one fetus or more**
Continuing pregnancy after selective termination of one fetus or more

√x7th **O31.30 Continuing pregnancy after elective fetal reduction of one fetus or more, unspecified trimester** M ♀

√x7th **O31.31 Continuing pregnancy after elective fetal reduction of one fetus or more, first trimester** M ♀

√x7th **O31.32 Continuing pregnancy after elective fetal reduction of one fetus or more, second trimester** M ♀

√x7th **O31.33 Continuing pregnancy after elective fetal reduction of one fetus or more, third trimester** M ♀

√5th **O31.8 Other complications specific to multiple gestation**

√6th **O31.8X Other complications specific to multiple gestation**

√7th **O31.8X1 Other complications specific to multiple gestation, first trimester** CC M ♀

√7th **O31.8X2 Other complications specific to multiple gestation, second trimester** CC M ♀

√7th **O31.8X3 Other complications specific to multiple gestation, third trimester** CC M ♀

√7th **O31.8X9 Other complications specific to multiple gestation, unspecified trimester** CC M ♀

O32 Maternal care for malpresentation of fetus

INCLUDES the listed conditions as a reason for observation, hospitalization or other obstetric care of the mother, or for cesarean delivery before onset of labor

EXCLUDES 1 *malpresentation of fetus with obstructed labor (O64.-)*

AHA: 2012,4Q,107

One of the following 7th characters is to be assigned to each code under category O32. 7th character Ø is for single gestations and multiple gestations where the fetus is unspecified. 7th characters 1 through 9 are for cases of multiple gestations to identify the fetus for which the code applies. The appropriate code from category O3Ø, Multiple gestation, must also be assigned when assigning a code from category O32 that has a 7th character of 1 through 9.
Ø not applicable or unspecified
1 fetus 1
2 fetus 2
3 fetus 3
4 fetus 4
5 fetus 5
9 other fetus

Fetal Malpresentation

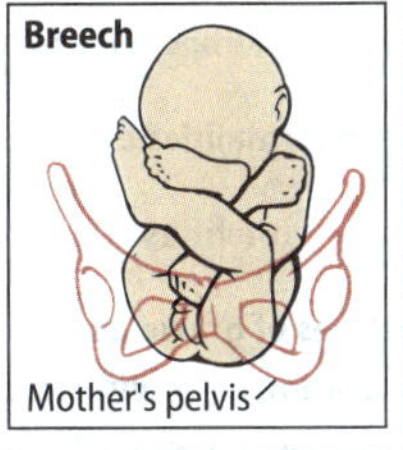

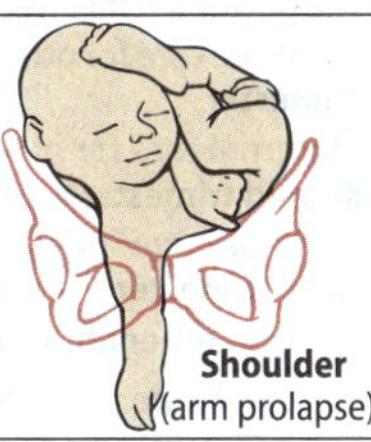

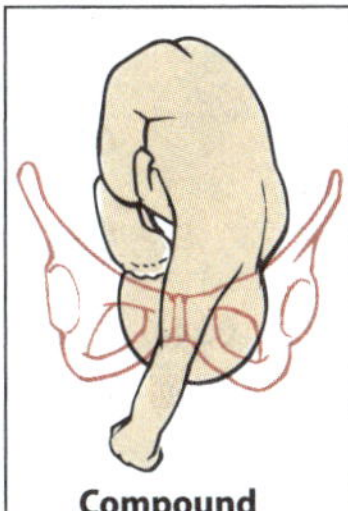
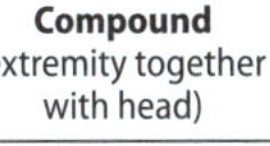

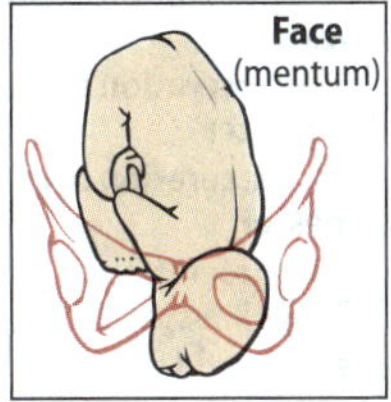

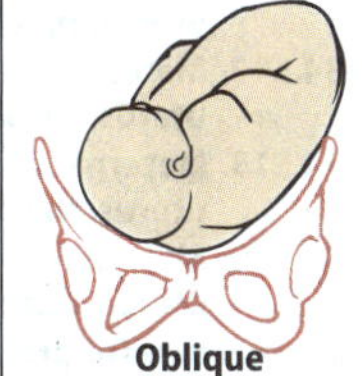

O32.Ø **Maternal care for unstable lie** M ♀

O32.1 **Maternal care for breech presentation** M ♀
Maternal care for buttocks presentation
Maternal care for complete breech
Maternal care for frank breech
EXCLUDES 1 *footling presentation (O32.8)*
incomplete breech (O32.8)
DEF: Fetus presentation in a longitudinal lie with the buttocks or feet closest to birth canal that may require external cephalic version or cesarean delivery.

O32.2 **Maternal care for transverse and oblique lie** M ♀
Maternal care for oblique presentation
Maternal care for transverse presentation

O32.3 **Maternal care for face, brow and chin presentation** M ♀

O32.4 **Maternal care for high head at term** M ♀
Maternal care for failure of head to enter pelvic brim

O32.6 **Maternal care for compound presentation** M ♀

O32.8 **Maternal care for other malpresentation of fetus** M ♀
Maternal care for footling presentation
Maternal care for incomplete breech

O32.9 **Maternal care for malpresentation of fetus, unspecified** M ♀

O33 Maternal care for disproportion

INCLUDES the listed conditions as a reason for observation, hospitalization or other obstetric care of the mother, or for cesarean delivery before onset of labor

EXCLUDES 1 *disproportion with obstructed labor (O65-O66)*

O33.Ø **Maternal care for disproportion due to deformity of maternal pelvic bones** CC M ♀
Maternal care for disproportion due to pelvic deformity causing disproportion NOS

O33.1 **Maternal care for disproportion due to generally contracted pelvis** M ♀
Maternal care for disproportion due to contracted pelvis NOS causing disproportion

O33.2 **Maternal care for disproportion due to inlet contraction of pelvis** M ♀
Maternal care for disproportion due to inlet contraction (pelvis) causing disproportion

O33.3 **Maternal care for disproportion due to outlet contraction of pelvis** M ♀
Maternal care for disproportion due to mid-cavity contraction (pelvis)
Maternal care for disproportion due to outlet contraction (pelvis)

One of the following 7th characters is to be assigned to code O33.3. 7th character Ø is for single gestations and multiple gestations where the fetus is unspecified. 7th characters 1 through 9 are for cases of multiple gestations to identify the fetus for which the code applies. The appropriate code from category O3Ø, Multiple gestation, must also be assigned when assigning code O33.3 with a 7th character of 1 through 9.
Ø not applicable or unspecified
1 fetus 1
2 fetus 2
3 fetus 3
4 fetus 4
5 fetus 5
9 other fetus

O33.4 **Maternal care for disproportion of mixed maternal and fetal origin** M ♀

One of the following 7th characters is to be assigned to code O33.4. 7th character Ø is for single gestations and multiple gestations where the fetus is unspecified. 7th characters 1 through 9 are for cases of multiple gestations to identify the fetus for which the code applies. The appropriate code from category O3Ø, Multiple gestation, must also be assigned when assigning code O33.4 with a 7th character of 1 through 9.
Ø not applicable or unspecified
1 fetus 1
2 fetus 2
3 fetus 3
4 fetus 4
5 fetus 5
9 other fetus

O33.5 **Maternal care for disproportion due to unusually large fetus** M ♀
Maternal care for disproportion due to disproportion of fetal origin with normally formed fetus
Maternal care for disproportion due to fetal disproportion NOS

One of the following 7th characters is to be assigned to code O33.5. 7th character Ø is for single gestations and multiple gestations where the fetus is unspecified. 7th characters 1 through 9 are for cases of multiple gestations to identify the fetus for which the code applies. The appropriate code from category O3Ø, Multiple gestation, must also be assigned when assigning code O33.5 with a 7th character of 1 through 9.
Ø not applicable or unspecified
1 fetus 1
2 fetus 2
3 fetus 3
4 fetus 4
5 fetus 5
9 other fetus

O33.6 **Maternal care for disproportion due to hydrocephalic fetus** M ♀

One of the following 7th characters is to be assigned to code O33.6. 7th character Ø is for single gestations and multiple gestations where the fetus is unspecified. 7th characters 1 through 9 are for cases of multiple gestations to identify the fetus for which the code applies. The appropriate code from category O3Ø, Multiple gestation, must also be assigned when assigning code O33.6 with a 7th character of 1 through 9.
Ø not applicable or unspecified
1 fetus 1
2 fetus 2
3 fetus 3
4 fetus 4
5 fetus 5
9 other fetus

Chapter 15. Pregnancy, Childbirth and the Puerperium

O32–O33.6

√x7th **O33.7 Maternal care for disproportion due to other fetal deformities** M ♀
Maternal care for disproportion due to fetal ascites
Maternal care for disproportion due to fetal hydrops
Maternal care for disproportion due to fetal meningomyelocele
Maternal care for disproportion due to fetal sacral teratoma
Maternal care for disproportion due to fetal tumor
EXCLUDES 1 *obstructed labor due to other fetal deformities (O66.3)*
AHA: 2016,4Q,51

One of the following 7th characters is to be assigned to code O33.7. 7th character Ø is for single gestations and multiple gestations where the fetus is unspecified. 7th characters 1 through 9 are for cases of multiple gestations to identify the fetus for which the code applies. The appropriate code from category O3Ø, Multiple gestation, must also be assigned when assigning code O33.7 with a 7th character of 1 through 9.
Ø not applicable or unspecified
1 fetus 1
2 fetus 2
3 fetus 3
4 fetus 4
5 fetus 5
9 other fetus

O33.8 Maternal care for disproportion of other origin M ♀
O33.9 Maternal care for disproportion, unspecified M ♀
Maternal care for disproportion due to cephalopelvic disproportion NOS
Maternal care for disproportion due to fetopelvic disproportion NOS

√4th **O34 Maternal care for abnormality of pelvic organs**
INCLUDES the listed conditions as a reason for hospitalization or other obstetric care of the mother, or for cesarean delivery before onset of labor
Code first any associated obstructed labor (O65.5)
Use additional code for specific condition

√5th **O34.Ø Maternal care for congenital malformation of uterus**
Maternal care for double uterus
Maternal care for uterus bicornis
O34.ØØ Maternal care for unspecified congenital malformation of uterus, unspecified trimester M ♀
O34.Ø1 Maternal care for unspecified congenital malformation of uterus, first trimester M ♀
O34.Ø2 Maternal care for unspecified congenital malformation of uterus, second trimester M ♀
O34.Ø3 Maternal care for unspecified congenital malformation of uterus, third trimester M ♀

√5th **O34.1 Maternal care for benign tumor of corpus uteri**
EXCLUDES 2 *maternal care for benign tumor of cervix (O34.4-)*
maternal care for malignant neoplasm of uterus (O9A.1-)
O34.1Ø Maternal care for benign tumor of corpus uteri, unspecified trimester M ♀
O34.11 Maternal care for benign tumor of corpus uteri, first trimester M ♀
O34.12 Maternal care for benign tumor of corpus uteri, second trimester M ♀
O34.13 Maternal care for benign tumor of corpus uteri, third trimester M ♀

√5th **O34.2 Maternal care due to uterine scar from previous surgery**
AHA: 2020,4Q,36; 2016,4Q,76
√6th **O34.21 Maternal care for scar from previous cesarean delivery**
AHA: 2018,3Q,23; 2016,4Q,51-52
O34.211 Maternal care for low transverse scar from previous cesarean delivery M ♀
O34.212 Maternal care for vertical scar from previous cesarean delivery M ♀
Maternal care for classical scar from previous cesarean delivery
O34.218 Maternal care for other type scar from previous cesarean delivery M ♀
Mid-transverse T incision
O34.219 Maternal care for unspecified type scar from previous cesarean delivery M ♀
O34.22 Maternal care for cesarean scar defect (isthmocele) M ♀
O34.29 Maternal care due to uterine scar from other previous surgery M ♀
Maternal care due to uterine scar from other transmural uterine incision

√5th **O34.3 Maternal care for cervical incompetence**
Maternal care for cerclage with or without cervical incompetence
Maternal care for Shirodkar suture with or without cervical incompetence
DEF: Inadequate functioning of the cervix marked by abnormal widening during pregnancy and causing premature birth or miscarriage.
O34.3Ø Maternal care for cervical incompetence, unspecified trimester M ♀
O34.31 Maternal care for cervical incompetence, first trimester MCC M ♀
O34.32 Maternal care for cervical incompetence, second trimester MCC M ♀
O34.33 Maternal care for cervical incompetence, third trimester MCC M ♀

√5th **O34.4 Maternal care for other abnormalities of cervix**
O34.4Ø Maternal care for other abnormalities of cervix, unspecified trimester M ♀
O34.41 Maternal care for other abnormalities of cervix, first trimester M ♀
O34.42 Maternal care for other abnormalities of cervix, second trimester M ♀
O34.43 Maternal care for other abnormalities of cervix, third trimester M ♀

√5th **O34.5 Maternal care for other abnormalities of gravid uterus**
√6th **O34.51 Maternal care for incarceration of gravid uterus**
O34.511 Maternal care for incarceration of gravid uterus, first trimester M ♀
O34.512 Maternal care for incarceration of gravid uterus, second trimester M ♀
O34.513 Maternal care for incarceration of gravid uterus, third trimester M ♀
O34.519 Maternal care for incarceration of gravid uterus, unspecified trimester M ♀
√6th **O34.52 Maternal care for prolapse of gravid uterus**
O34.521 Maternal care for prolapse of gravid uterus, first trimester M ♀
O34.522 Maternal care for prolapse of gravid uterus, second trimester M ♀
O34.523 Maternal care for prolapse of gravid uterus, third trimester M ♀
O34.529 Maternal care for prolapse of gravid uterus, unspecified trimester M ♀
√6th **O34.53 Maternal care for retroversion of gravid uterus**
O34.531 Maternal care for retroversion of gravid uterus, first trimester M ♀
O34.532 Maternal care for retroversion of gravid uterus, second trimester M ♀
O34.533 Maternal care for retroversion of gravid uterus, third trimester M ♀
O34.539 Maternal care for retroversion of gravid uterus, unspecified trimester M ♀
√6th **O34.59 Maternal care for other abnormalities of gravid uterus**
O34.591 Maternal care for other abnormalities of gravid uterus, first trimester M ♀
O34.592 Maternal care for other abnormalities of gravid uterus, second trimester M ♀
O34.593 Maternal care for other abnormalities of gravid uterus, third trimester M ♀
O34.599 Maternal care for other abnormalities of gravid uterus, unspecified trimester M ♀

√5th **O34.6 Maternal care for abnormality of vagina**
EXCLUDES 2 *maternal care for vaginal varices in pregnancy (O22.1-)*
O34.6Ø Maternal care for abnormality of vagina, unspecified trimester M ♀
O34.61 Maternal care for abnormality of vagina, first trimester M ♀
O34.62 Maternal care for abnormality of vagina, second trimester M ♀
O34.63 Maternal care for abnormality of vagina, third trimester M ♀

O34.7 Maternal care for abnormality of vulva and perineum

EXCLUDES 2 *maternal care for perineal and vulval varices in pregnancy (O22.1-)*

O34.70 Maternal care for abnormality of vulva and perineum, unspecified trimester M ♀

O34.71 Maternal care for abnormality of vulva and perineum, first trimester M ♀

O34.72 Maternal care for abnormality of vulva and perineum, second trimester M ♀

O34.73 Maternal care for abnormality of vulva and perineum, third trimester M ♀

O34.8 Maternal care for other abnormalities of pelvic organs

O34.80 Maternal care for other abnormalities of pelvic organs, unspecified trimester M ♀

O34.81 Maternal care for other abnormalities of pelvic organs, first trimester M ♀

O34.82 Maternal care for other abnormalities of pelvic organs, second trimester M ♀

O34.83 Maternal care for other abnormalities of pelvic organs, third trimester M ♀

O34.9 Maternal care for abnormality of pelvic organ, unspecified

O34.90 Maternal care for abnormality of pelvic organ, unspecified, unspecified trimester M ♀

O34.91 Maternal care for abnormality of pelvic organ, unspecified, first trimester M ♀

O34.92 Maternal care for abnormality of pelvic organ, unspecified, second trimester M ♀

O34.93 Maternal care for abnormality of pelvic organ, unspecified, third trimester M ♀

O35 Maternal care for known or suspected fetal abnormality and damage

INCLUDES the listed conditions in the fetus as a reason for hospitalization or other obstetric care to the mother, or for termination of pregnancy

Code also any associated maternal condition

EXCLUDES 1 *encounter for suspected maternal and fetal conditions ruled out (Z03.7-)*

AHA: 2022,4Q,37

One of the following 7th characters is to be assigned to each code under category O35. 7th character Ø is for single gestations and multiple gestations where the fetus is unspecified. 7th characters 1 through 9 are for cases of multiple gestations to identify the fetus for which the code applies. The appropriate code from category O30, Multiple gestation, must also be assigned when assigning a code from category O35 that has a 7th character of 1 through 9.

- Ø not applicable or unspecified
- 1 fetus 1
- 2 fetus 2
- 3 fetus 3
- 4 fetus 4
- 5 fetus 5
- 9 other fetus

O35.Ø Maternal care for (suspected) central nervous system malformation in fetus

EXCLUDES 2 *chromosomal abnormality in fetus (O35.1-)*

O35.ØØ Maternal care for (suspected) central nervous system malformation or damage in fetus, unspecified M ♀

O35.Ø1 Maternal care for (suspected) central nervous system malformation or damage in fetus, agenesis of the corpus callosum M ♀

O35.Ø2 Maternal care for (suspected) central nervous system malformation or damage in fetus, anencephaly M ♀

O35.Ø3 Maternal care for (suspected) central nervous system malformation or damage in fetus, choroid plexus cysts M ♀

O35.Ø4 Maternal care for (suspected) central nervous system malformation or damage in fetus, encephalocele M ♀

O35.Ø5 Maternal care for (suspected) central nervous system malformation or damage in fetus, holoprosencephaly M ♀

O35.Ø6 Maternal care for (suspected) central nervous system malformation or damage in fetus, hydrocephaly M ♀
Maternal care for fetal hydrocephalus

O35.Ø7 Maternal care for (suspected) central nervous system malformation or damage in fetus, microcephaly M ♀

O35.Ø8 Maternal care for (suspected) central nervous system malformation or damage in fetus, spina bifida M ♀

O35.Ø9 Maternal care for (suspected) other central nervous system malformation or damage in fetus M ♀

O35.1 Maternal care for (suspected) chromosomal abnormality in fetus

AHA: 2023,2Q,15

O35.1Ø Maternal care for (suspected) chromosomal abnormality in fetus, unspecified M ♀

O35.11 Maternal care for (suspected) chromosomal abnormality in fetus, Trisomy 13 M ♀

O35.12 Maternal care for (suspected) chromosomal abnormality in fetus, Trisomy 18 M ♀

O35.13 Maternal care for (suspected) chromosomal abnormality in fetus, Trisomy 21 M ♀

O35.14 Maternal care for (suspected) chromosomal abnormality in fetus, Turner Syndrome M ♀

O35.15 Maternal care for (suspected) chromosomal abnormality in fetus, sex chromosome abnormality M ♀

O35.19 Maternal care for (suspected) chromosomal abnormality in fetus, other chromosomal abnormality M ♀

O35.A Maternal care for other (suspected) fetal abnormality and damage, fetal facial anomalies M ♀

O35.B Maternal care for other (suspected) fetal abnormality and damage, fetal cardiac anomalies M ♀

O35.C Maternal care for other (suspected) fetal abnormality and damage, fetal pulmonary anomalies M ♀

O35.D Maternal care for other (suspected) fetal abnormality and damage, fetal gastrointestinal anomalies M ♀

O35.E Maternal care for other (suspected) fetal abnormality and damage, fetal genitourinary anomalies M ♀

O35.F Maternal care for other (suspected) fetal abnormality and damage, fetal musculoskeletal anomalies of trunk M ♀

EXCLUDES 2 *maternal care for other (suspected) fetal abnormality and damage, fetal lower extremities anomalies (O35.H)*
maternal care for other (suspected) fetal abnormality and damage, fetal upper extremities anomalies (O35.G)

O35.G Maternal care for other (suspected) fetal abnormality and damage, fetal upper extremities anomalies M ♀

O35.H Maternal care for other (suspected) fetal abnormality and damage, fetal lower extremities anomalies M ♀

O35.2 Maternal care for (suspected) hereditary disease in fetus M ♀

EXCLUDES 2 *chromosomal abnormality in fetus (O35.1-)*

O35.3 Maternal care for (suspected) damage to fetus from viral disease in mother M ♀
Maternal care for damage to fetus from maternal cytomegalovirus infection
Maternal care for damage to fetus from maternal rubella

O35.4 Maternal care for (suspected) damage to fetus from alcohol M ♀

O35.5 Maternal care for (suspected) damage to fetus by drugs M ♀
Maternal care for damage to fetus from drug addiction

O35.6 Maternal care for (suspected) damage to fetus by radiation M ♀

O35.7 Maternal care for (suspected) damage to fetus by other medical procedures M ♀
Maternal care for damage to fetus by amniocentesis
Maternal care for damage to fetus by biopsy procedures
Maternal care for damage to fetus by hematological investigation
Maternal care for damage to fetus by intrauterine contraceptive device
Maternal care for damage to fetus by intrauterine surgery

O35.8 Maternal care for other (suspected) fetal abnormality and damage M ♀
Maternal care for damage to fetus from maternal listeriosis
Maternal care for damage to fetus from maternal toxoplasmosis

O35.9 Maternal care for (suspected) fetal abnormality and damage, unspecified M ♀

O36 Maternal care for other fetal problems

INCLUDES the listed conditions in the fetus as a reason for hospitalization or other obstetric care of the mother, or for termination of pregnancy

EXCLUDES 1 *encounter for suspected maternal and fetal conditions ruled out (Z03.7-)*

placental transfusion syndromes (O43.0-)

EXCLUDES 2 *labor and delivery complicated by fetal stress (O77.-)*

AHA: 2015,3Q,40

One of the following 7th characters is to be assigned to each code under category O36. 7th character 0 is for single gestations and multiple gestations where the fetus is unspecified. 7th characters 1 through 9 are for cases of multiple gestations to identify the fetus for which the code applies. The appropriate code from category O30, Multiple gestation, must also be assigned when assigning a code from category O36 that has a 7th character of 1 through 9.

- 0 not applicable or unspecified
- 1 fetus 1
- 2 fetus 2
- 3 fetus 3
- 4 fetus 4
- 5 fetus 5
- 9 other fetus

O36.0 Maternal care for rhesus isoimmunization

Maternal care for Rh incompatibility (with hydrops fetalis)

O36.01 Maternal care for anti-D [Rh] antibodies

AHA: 2014,4Q,17

O36.011 Maternal care for anti-D [Rh] antibodies, first trimester CC M ♀

O36.012 Maternal care for anti-D [Rh] antibodies, second trimester CC M ♀

O36.013 Maternal care for anti-D [Rh] antibodies, third trimester CC M ♀

O36.019 Maternal care for anti-D [Rh] antibodies, unspecified trimester M ♀

O36.09 Maternal care for other rhesus isoimmunization

O36.091 Maternal care for other rhesus isoimmunization, first trimester CC M ♀

O36.092 Maternal care for other rhesus isoimmunization, second trimester CC M ♀

O36.093 Maternal care for other rhesus isoimmunization, third trimester CC M ♀

O36.099 Maternal care for other rhesus isoimmunization, unspecified trimester M ♀

O36.1 Maternal care for other isoimmunization

Maternal care for ABO isoimmunization

O36.11 Maternal care for Anti-A sensitization

Maternal care for isoimmunization NOS (with hydrops fetalis)

O36.111 Maternal care for Anti-A sensitization, first trimester M ♀

O36.112 Maternal care for Anti-A sensitization, second trimester M ♀

O36.113 Maternal care for Anti-A sensitization, third trimester M ♀

O36.119 Maternal care for Anti-A sensitization, unspecified trimester M ♀

O36.19 Maternal care for other isoimmunization

Maternal care for Anti-B sensitization

O36.191 Maternal care for other isoimmunization, first trimester M ♀

O36.192 Maternal care for other isoimmunization, second trimester M ♀

O36.193 Maternal care for other isoimmunization, third trimester M ♀

O36.199 Maternal care for other isoimmunization, unspecified trimester M ♀

O36.2 Maternal care for hydrops fetalis

Maternal care for hydrops fetalis NOS

Maternal care for hydrops fetalis not associated with isoimmunization

EXCLUDES 1 *hydrops fetalis associated with ABO isoimmunization (O36.1-)*

hydrops fetalis associated with rhesus isoimmunization (O36.0-)

DEF: Hydrops fetalis: Abnormal fluid buildup in at least two of the following fetal organ spaces: the skin (edema), abdomen (ascites), around the heart (pericardia effusion), and around the lung (pleural effusion). Fluid accumulation may also occur in the mother as polyhydramnios and edema of the placenta.

O36.20 Maternal care for hydrops fetalis, unspecified trimester M ♀

O36.21 Maternal care for hydrops fetalis, first trimester M ♀

O36.22 Maternal care for hydrops fetalis, second trimester M ♀

O36.23 Maternal care for hydrops fetalis, third trimester M ♀

O36.4 Maternal care for intrauterine death CC M ♀

Maternal care for intrauterine fetal death NOS

Maternal care for intrauterine fetal death after completion of 20 weeks of gestation

Maternal care for late fetal death

Maternal care for missed delivery

EXCLUDES 1 *missed abortion (O02.1)*

stillbirth (P95)

AHA: 2022,2Q,3

O36.5 Maternal care for known or suspected poor fetal growth

O36.51 Maternal care for known or suspected placental insufficiency

O36.511 Maternal care for known or suspected placental insufficiency, first trimester M ♀

O36.512 Maternal care for known or suspected placental insufficiency, second trimester M ♀

O36.513 Maternal care for known or suspected placental insufficiency, third trimester M ♀

O36.519 Maternal care for known or suspected placental insufficiency, unspecified trimester M ♀

O36.59 Maternal care for other known or suspected poor fetal growth

Maternal care for known or suspected light-for-dates NOS

Maternal care for known or suspected small-for-dates NOS

O36.591 Maternal care for other known or suspected poor fetal growth, first trimester M ♀

O36.592 Maternal care for other known or suspected poor fetal growth, second trimester M ♀

O36.593 Maternal care for other known or suspected poor fetal growth, third trimester M ♀

O36.599 Maternal care for other known or suspected poor fetal growth, unspecified trimester M ♀

O36.6 Maternal care for excessive fetal growth

Maternal care for known or suspected large-for-dates

O36.60 Maternal care for excessive fetal growth, unspecified trimester M ♀

O36.61 Maternal care for excessive fetal growth, first trimester M ♀

O36.62 Maternal care for excessive fetal growth, second trimester M ♀

O36.63 Maternal care for excessive fetal growth, third trimester M ♀

O36.7 Maternal care for viable fetus in abdominal pregnancy

O36.70 Maternal care for viable fetus in abdominal pregnancy, unspecified trimester M ♀

O36.71 Maternal care for viable fetus in abdominal pregnancy, first trimester M ♀

O36.72 Maternal care for viable fetus in abdominal pregnancy, second trimester M ♀

✓x7th O36.73 **Maternal care for viable fetus in abdominal pregnancy, third trimester** M ♀

✓5th **O36.8 Maternal care for other specified fetal problems**

✓x7th O36.80 **Pregnancy with inconclusive fetal viability** UPD M ♀

Encounter to determine fetal viability of pregnancy

AHA: 2019,2Q,29

✓6th O36.81 **Decreased fetal movements**

✓7th O36.812 **Decreased fetal movements, second trimester** M ♀

✓7th O36.813 **Decreased fetal movements, third trimester** M ♀

✓7th O36.819 **Decreased fetal movements, unspecified trimester** M ♀

✓6th O36.82 **Fetal anemia and thrombocytopenia**

✓7th O36.821 **Fetal anemia and thrombocytopenia, first trimester** M ♀

✓7th O36.822 **Fetal anemia and thrombocytopenia, second trimester** M ♀

✓7th O36.823 **Fetal anemia and thrombocytopenia, third trimester** M ♀

✓7th O36.829 **Fetal anemia and thrombocytopenia, unspecified trimester** M ♀

✓6th O36.83 **Maternal care for abnormalities of the fetal heart rate or rhythm**

Maternal care for depressed fetal heart rate tones
Maternal care for fetal bradycardia
Maternal care for fetal heart rate abnormal variability
Maternal care for fetal heart rate decelerations
Maternal care for fetal heart rate irregularity
Maternal care for fetal tachycardia
Maternal care for non-reassuring fetal heart rate or rhythm

AHA: 2017,4Q,20

TIP: Assign for documented fetal tachycardia, bradycardia, decelerations, or loss of variability detected during antenatal testing.

✓7th O36.831 **Maternal care for abnormalities of the fetal heart rate or rhythm, first trimester** M ♀

✓7th O36.832 **Maternal care for abnormalities of the fetal heart rate or rhythm, second trimester** M ♀

✓7th O36.833 **Maternal care for abnormalities of the fetal heart rate or rhythm, third trimester** M ♀

✓7th O36.839 **Maternal care for abnormalities of the fetal heart rate or rhythm, unspecified trimester** M ♀

✓6th O36.89 **Maternal care for other specified fetal problems**

✓7th O36.891 **Maternal care for other specified fetal problems, first trimester** M ♀

✓7th O36.892 **Maternal care for other specified fetal problems, second trimester** M ♀

✓7th O36.893 **Maternal care for other specified fetal problems, third trimester** M ♀

✓7th O36.899 **Maternal care for other specified fetal problems, unspecified trimester** M ♀

✓5th **O36.9 Maternal care for fetal problem, unspecified**

✓x7th O36.90 **Maternal care for fetal problem, unspecified, unspecified trimester** M ♀

✓x7th O36.91 **Maternal care for fetal problem, unspecified, first trimester** M ♀

✓x7th O36.92 **Maternal care for fetal problem, unspecified, second trimester** M ♀

✓x7th O36.93 **Maternal care for fetal problem, unspecified, third trimester** M ♀

✓4th **O40 Polyhydramnios**

INCLUDES hydramnios

EXCLUDES 1 *encounter for suspected maternal and fetal conditions ruled out (Z03.7-)*

AHA: 2016,1Q,4

DEF: Excess amniotic fluid surrounding the fetus, typically defined as a total fluid volume of greater than 24 cm.

One of the following 7th characters is to be assigned to each code under category O40. 7th character 0 is for single gestations and multiple gestations where the fetus is unspecified. 7th characters 1 through 9 are for cases of multiple gestations to identify the fetus for which the code applies. The appropriate code from category O30, Multiple gestation, must also be assigned when assigning a code from category O40 that has a 7th character of 1 through 9.

0 not applicable or unspecified
1 fetus 1
2 fetus 2
3 fetus 3
4 fetus 4
5 fetus 5
9 other fetus

✓x7th O40.1 **Polyhydramnios, first trimester** M ♀

✓x7th O40.2 **Polyhydramnios, second trimester** M ♀

✓x7th O40.3 **Polyhydramnios, third trimester** M ♀

✓x7th O40.9 **Polyhydramnios, unspecified trimester** M ♀

✓4th **O41 Other disorders of amniotic fluid and membranes**

EXCLUDES 1 *encounter for suspected maternal and fetal conditions ruled out (Z03.7-)*

One of the following 7th characters is to be assigned to each code under category O41. 7th character 0 is for single gestations and multiple gestations where the fetus is unspecified. 7th characters 1 through 9 are for cases of multiple gestations to identify the fetus for which the code applies. The appropriate code from category O30, Multiple gestation, must also be assigned when assigning a code from category O41 that has a 7th character of 1 through 9.

0 not applicable or unspecified
1 fetus 1
2 fetus 2
3 fetus 3
4 fetus 4
5 fetus 5
9 other fetus

✓5th O41.0 **Oligohydramnios**

Oligohydramnios without rupture of membranes

DEF: Low amniotic fluid, occurring most frequently in the last trimester.

✓x7th O41.00 **Oligohydramnios, unspecified trimester** M ♀

✓x7th O41.01 **Oligohydramnios, first trimester** CC M ♀

✓x7th O41.02 **Oligohydramnios, second trimester** CC M ♀

✓x7th O41.03 **Oligohydramnios, third trimester** CC M ♀

✓5th O41.1 **Infection of amniotic sac and membranes**

✓6th O41.10 **Infection of amniotic sac and membranes, unspecified**

✓7th O41.101 **Infection of amniotic sac and membranes, unspecified, first trimester** MCC M ♀

✓7th O41.102 **Infection of amniotic sac and membranes, unspecified, second trimester** MCC M ♀

✓7th O41.103 **Infection of amniotic sac and membranes, unspecified, third trimester** MCC M ♀

✓7th O41.109 **Infection of amniotic sac and membranes, unspecified, unspecified trimester** M ♀

✓6th O41.12 **Chorioamnionitis**

AHA: 2019,2Q,34

✓7th O41.121 **Chorioamnionitis, first trimester** MCC M ♀

✓7th O41.122 **Chorioamnionitis, second trimester** MCC M ♀

✓7th O41.123 **Chorioamnionitis, third trimester** MCC M ♀

✓7th O41.129 **Chorioamnionitis, unspecified trimester** M ♀

✓6th O41.14 **Placentitis**

✓7th O41.141 **Placentitis, first trimester** MCC M ♀

✓7th O41.142 **Placentitis, second trimester** MCC M ♀

O41.143 Placentitis, third trimester MCC M ♀

O41.149 Placentitis, unspecified trimester M ♀

O41.8 Other specified disorders of amniotic fluid and membranes

O41.8X Other specified disorders of amniotic fluid and membranes

O41.8X1 Other specified disorders of amniotic fluid and membranes, first trimester M ♀

O41.8X2 Other specified disorders of amniotic fluid and membranes, second trimester M ♀

O41.8X3 Other specified disorders of amniotic fluid and membranes, third trimester M ♀

O41.8X9 Other specified disorders of amniotic fluid and membranes, unspecified trimester M ♀

O41.9 Disorder of amniotic fluid and membranes, unspecified

O41.90 Disorder of amniotic fluid and membranes, unspecified, unspecified trimester M ♀

O41.91 Disorder of amniotic fluid and membranes, unspecified, first trimester M ♀

O41.92 Disorder of amniotic fluid and membranes, unspecified, second trimester M ♀

O41.93 Disorder of amniotic fluid and membranes, unspecified, third trimester M ♀

O42 Premature rupture of membranes

AHA: 2016,1Q,3

O42.0 Premature rupture of membranes, onset of labor within 24 hours of rupture

O42.00 Premature rupture of membranes, onset of labor within 24 hours of rupture, unspecified weeks of gestation M ♀

O42.01 Preterm premature rupture of membranes, onset of labor within 24 hours of rupture

Premature rupture of membranes before 37 completed weeks of gestation

O42.011 Preterm premature rupture of membranes, onset of labor within 24 hours of rupture, first trimester M ♀

O42.012 Preterm premature rupture of membranes, onset of labor within 24 hours of rupture, second trimester M ♀

O42.013 Preterm premature rupture of membranes, onset of labor within 24 hours of rupture, third trimester M ♀

O42.019 Preterm premature rupture of membranes, onset of labor within 24 hours of rupture, unspecified trimester M ♀

O42.02 Full-term premature rupture of membranes, onset of labor within 24 hours of rupture M ♀

Premature rupture of membranes at or after 37 completed weeks of gestation, onset of labor within 24 hours of rupture

O42.1 Premature rupture of membranes, onset of labor more than 24 hours following rupture

AHA: 2016,1Q,5

O42.10 Premature rupture of membranes, onset of labor more than 24 hours following rupture, unspecified weeks of gestation M ♀

O42.11 Preterm premature rupture of membranes, onset of labor more than 24 hours following rupture

Premature rupture of membranes before 37 completed weeks of gestation

O42.111 Preterm premature rupture of membranes, onset of labor more than 24 hours following rupture, first trimester M ♀

O42.112 Preterm premature rupture of membranes, onset of labor more than 24 hours following rupture, second trimester M ♀

O42.113 Preterm premature rupture of membranes, onset of labor more than 24 hours following rupture, third trimester M ♀

O42.119 Preterm premature rupture of membranes, onset of labor more than 24 hours following rupture, unspecified trimester M ♀

O42.12 Full-term premature rupture of membranes, onset of labor more than 24 hours following rupture M ♀

Premature rupture of membranes at or after 37 completed weeks of gestation, onset of labor more than 24 hours following rupture

O42.9 Premature rupture of membranes, unspecified as to length of time between rupture and onset of labor

O42.90 Premature rupture of membranes, unspecified as to length of time between rupture and onset of labor, unspecified weeks of gestation M ♀

O42.91 Preterm premature rupture of membranes, unspecified as to length of time between rupture and onset of labor

Premature rupture of membranes before 37 completed weeks of gestation

O42.911 Preterm premature rupture of membranes, unspecified as to length of time between rupture and onset of labor, first trimester M ♀

O42.912 Preterm premature rupture of membranes, unspecified as to length of time between rupture and onset of labor, second trimester M ♀

O42.913 Preterm premature rupture of membranes, unspecified as to length of time between rupture and onset of labor, third trimester M ♀

O42.919 Preterm premature rupture of membranes, unspecified as to length of time between rupture and onset of labor, unspecified trimester M ♀

O42.92 Full-term premature rupture of membranes, unspecified as to length of time between rupture and onset of labor M ♀

Premature rupture of membranes at or after 37 completed weeks of gestation, unspecified as to length of time between rupture and onset of labor

O43 Placental disorders

EXCLUDES 2 *maternal care for poor fetal growth due to placental insufficiency (O36.5-)*
placenta previa (O44.-)
placental polyp (O90.89)
placentitis (O41.14-)
premature separation of placenta [abruptio placentae] (O45.-)

O43.0 Placental transfusion syndromes

O43.01 Fetomaternal placental transfusion syndrome

Maternofetal placental transfusion syndrome

O43.011 Fetomaternal placental transfusion syndrome, first trimester M ♀

O43.012 Fetomaternal placental transfusion syndrome, second trimester M ♀

O43.013 Fetomaternal placental transfusion syndrome, third trimester M ♀

O43.019 Fetomaternal placental transfusion syndrome, unspecified trimester M ♀

√6th **O43.02 Fetus-to-fetus placental transfusion syndrome**

DEF: Condition in which an imbalance in amniotic fluid occurs due to uneven blood flow between twins sharing a placenta.

Twin to Twin Transfusion Syndrome (TTTS)

Healthy twins Twins with TTTS

O43.021 Fetus-to-fetus placental transfusion syndrome, first trimester M ♀

O43.022 Fetus-to-fetus placental transfusion syndrome, second trimester M ♀

O43.023 Fetus-to-fetus placental transfusion syndrome, third trimester M ♀

O43.029 Fetus-to-fetus placental transfusion syndrome, unspecified trimester M ♀

√5th **O43.1 Malformation of placenta**

√6th **O43.10 Malformation of placenta, unspecified**

Abnormal placenta NOS

O43.101 Malformation of placenta, unspecified, first trimester M ♀

O43.102 Malformation of placenta, unspecified, second trimester M ♀

O43.103 Malformation of placenta, unspecified, third trimester M ♀

O43.109 Malformation of placenta, unspecified, unspecified trimester M ♀

√6th **O43.11 Circumvallate placenta**

O43.111 Circumvallate placenta, first trimester M ♀

O43.112 Circumvallate placenta, second trimester M ♀

O43.113 Circumvallate placenta, third trimester M ♀

O43.119 Circumvallate placenta, unspecified trimester M ♀

√6th **O43.12 Velamentous insertion of umbilical cord**

O43.121 Velamentous insertion of umbilical cord, first trimester M ♀

O43.122 Velamentous insertion of umbilical cord, second trimester M ♀

O43.123 Velamentous insertion of umbilical cord, third trimester M ♀

O43.129 Velamentous insertion of umbilical cord, unspecified trimester M ♀

√6th **O43.19 Other malformation of placenta**

O43.191 Other malformation of placenta, first trimester M ♀

O43.192 Other malformation of placenta, second trimester M ♀

O43.193 Other malformation of placenta, third trimester M ♀

O43.199 Other malformation of placenta, unspecified trimester M ♀

√5th **O43.2 Morbidly adherent placenta**

Code also associated third stage postpartum hemorrhage, if applicable (O72.0)

EXCLUDES 1 *retained placenta (O73.-)*

√6th **O43.21 Placenta accreta**

DEF: Condition where the placenta adheres too deeply to the uterine wall; often associated with placenta previa.

O43.211 Placenta accreta, first trimester M ♀

O43.212 Placenta accreta, second trimester M ♀

O43.213 Placenta accreta, third trimester M ♀

O43.219 Placenta accreta, unspecified trimester M ♀

√6th **O43.22 Placenta increta**

AHA: 2022,1Q,20

DEF: Condition where the placenta adheres too deeply to the uterine wall and penetrates the muscle; often associated with placenta previa.

O43.221 Placenta increta, first trimester M ♀

O43.222 Placenta increta, second trimester M ♀

O43.223 Placenta increta, third trimester M ♀

O43.229 Placenta increta, unspecified trimester M ♀

√6th **O43.23 Placenta percreta**

DEF: Condition where the placenta attaches through the uterine muscle and may invade other organs, resulting in antenatal complications, premature delivery, retention of all or a portion of the placenta, or postpartum bleeding.

O43.231 Placenta percreta, first trimester M ♀

O43.232 Placenta percreta, second trimester M ♀

O43.233 Placenta percreta, third trimester M ♀

O43.239 Placenta percreta, unspecified trimester M ♀

√5th **O43.8 Other placental disorders**

√6th **O43.81 Placental infarction**

O43.811 Placental infarction, first trimester M ♀

O43.812 Placental infarction, second trimester M ♀

O43.813 Placental infarction, third trimester M ♀

O43.819 Placental infarction, unspecified trimester M ♀

√6th **O43.89 Other placental disorders**

Placental dysfunction

O43.891 Other placental disorders, first trimester M ♀

O43.892 Other placental disorders, second trimester M ♀

O43.893 Other placental disorders, third trimester M ♀

O43.899 Other placental disorders, unspecified trimester M ♀

√5th **O43.9 Unspecified placental disorder**

O43.90 Unspecified placental disorder, unspecified trimester M ♀

O43.91 Unspecified placental disorder, first trimester M ♀

O43.92 Unspecified placental disorder, second trimester M ♀

O43.93 Unspecified placental disorder, third trimester M ♀

√4th **O44 Placenta previa**

AHA: 2016,4Q,52-53

DEF: Placenta implanted in the lower segment of the uterus, which commonly causes hemorrhage in the last trimester of pregnancy.

√5th **O44.0 Complete placenta previa NOS or without hemorrhage**

Placenta previa NOS

O44.00 Complete placenta previa NOS or without hemorrhage, unspecified trimester M ♀

O44.01 Complete placenta previa NOS or without hemorrhage, first trimester CC M ♀

O44.02 Complete placenta previa NOS or without hemorrhage, second trimester CC M ♀

O44.03 Complete placenta previa NOS or without hemorrhage, third trimester CC M ♀

√5th **O44.1 Complete placenta previa with hemorrhage**

EXCLUDES 1 *labor and delivery complicated by hemorrhage from vasa previa (O69.4)*

O44.10 Complete placenta previa with hemorrhage, unspecified trimester M ♀

O44.11 Complete placenta previa with hemorrhage, first trimester MCC M ♀

Chapter 15. Pregnancy, Childbirth and the Puerperium

O43.02–O44.11

O44.12 Complete placenta previa with hemorrhage, second trimester MCC M ♀

O44.13 Complete placenta previa with hemorrhage, third trimester MCC M ♀

√5th O44.2 Partial placenta previa without hemorrhage

Marginal placenta previa, NOS or without hemorrhage

O44.2Ø Partial placenta previa NOS or without hemorrhage, unspecified trimester M ♀

O44.21 Partial placenta previa NOS or without hemorrhage, first trimester CC M ♀

O44.22 Partial placenta previa NOS or without hemorrhage, second trimester CC M ♀

O44.23 Partial placenta previa NOS or without hemorrhage, third trimester CC M ♀

√5th O44.3 Partial placenta previa with hemorrhage

Marginal placenta previa with hemorrhage

O44.3Ø Partial placenta previa with hemorrhage, unspecified trimester M ♀

O44.31 Partial placenta previa with hemorrhage, first trimester MCC M ♀

O44.32 Partial placenta previa with hemorrhage, second trimester MCC M ♀

O44.33 Partial placenta previa with hemorrhage, third trimester MCC M ♀

√5th O44.4 Low lying placenta NOS or without hemorrhage

Low implantation of placenta NOS or without hemorrhage

O44.4Ø Low lying placenta NOS or without hemorrhage, unspecified trimester M ♀

O44.41 Low lying placenta NOS or without hemorrhage, first trimester CC M ♀

O44.42 Low lying placenta NOS or without hemorrhage, second trimester CC M ♀

O44.43 Low lying placenta NOS or without hemorrhage, third trimester CC M ♀

√5th O44.5 Low lying placenta with hemorrhage

Low implantation of placenta with hemorrhage

O44.5Ø Low lying placenta with hemorrhage, unspecified trimester M ♀

O44.51 Low lying placenta with hemorrhage, first trimester MCC M ♀

O44.52 Low lying placenta with hemorrhage, second trimester MCC M ♀

O44.53 Low lying placenta with hemorrhage, third trimester MCC M ♀

√4th O45 Premature separation of placenta [abruptio placentae]

√5th O45.Ø Premature separation of placenta with coagulation defect

√6th O45.ØØ Premature separation of placenta with coagulation defect, unspecified

O45.ØØ1 Premature separation of placenta with coagulation defect, unspecified, first trimester MCC M ♀

O45.ØØ2 Premature separation of placenta with coagulation defect, unspecified, second trimester MCC M ♀

O45.ØØ3 Premature separation of placenta with coagulation defect, unspecified, third trimester MCC M ♀

O45.ØØ9 Premature separation of placenta with coagulation defect, unspecified, unspecified trimester M ♀

√6th O45.Ø1 Premature separation of placenta with afibrinogenemia

Premature separation of placenta with hypofibrinogenemia

O45.Ø11 Premature separation of placenta with afibrinogenemia, first trimester MCC M ♀

O45.Ø12 Premature separation of placenta with afibrinogenemia, second trimester MCC M ♀

O45.Ø13 Premature separation of placenta with afibrinogenemia, third trimester MCC M ♀

O45.Ø19 Premature separation of placenta with afibrinogenemia, unspecified trimester M ♀

√6th O45.Ø2 Premature separation of placenta with disseminated intravascular coagulation

O45.Ø21 Premature separation of placenta with disseminated intravascular coagulation, first trimester MCC M ♀

O45.Ø22 Premature separation of placenta with disseminated intravascular coagulation, second trimester MCC M ♀

O45.Ø23 Premature separation of placenta with disseminated intravascular coagulation, third trimester MCC M ♀

O45.Ø29 Premature separation of placenta with disseminated intravascular coagulation, unspecified trimester M ♀

√6th O45.Ø9 Premature separation of placenta with other coagulation defect

O45.Ø91 Premature separation of placenta with other coagulation defect, first trimester MCC M ♀

O45.Ø92 Premature separation of placenta with other coagulation defect, second trimester MCC M ♀

O45.Ø93 Premature separation of placenta with other coagulation defect, third trimester MCC M ♀

O45.Ø99 Premature separation of placenta with other coagulation defect, unspecified trimester M ♀

√5th O45.8 Other premature separation of placenta

√6th O45.8X Other premature separation of placenta

O45.8X1 Other premature separation of placenta, first trimester MCC M ♀

O45.8X2 Other premature separation of placenta, second trimester MCC M ♀

O45.8X3 Other premature separation of placenta, third trimester MCC M ♀

O45.8X9 Other premature separation of placenta, unspecified trimester M ♀

√5th O45.9 Premature separation of placenta, unspecified

Abruptio placentae NOS

O45.9Ø Premature separation of placenta, unspecified, unspecified trimester M ♀

O45.91 Premature separation of placenta, unspecified, first trimester MCC M ♀

O45.92 Premature separation of placenta, unspecified, second trimester MCC M ♀

O45.93 Premature separation of placenta, unspecified, third trimester MCC M ♀

√4th O46 Antepartum hemorrhage, not elsewhere classified

EXCLUDES 1 *hemorrhage in early pregnancy (O2Ø.-)*
intrapartum hemorrhage NEC (O67.-)
placenta previa (O44.-)
premature separation of placenta [abruptio placentae] (O45.-)

DEF: Uterine hemorrhage prior to delivery that is not related to placenta previa or abruptio placentae.

√5th O46.Ø Antepartum hemorrhage with coagulation defect

√6th O46.ØØ Antepartum hemorrhage with coagulation defect, unspecified

O46.ØØ1 Antepartum hemorrhage with coagulation defect, unspecified, first trimester MCC M ♀

O46.ØØ2 Antepartum hemorrhage with coagulation defect, unspecified, second trimester MCC M ♀

O46.ØØ3 Antepartum hemorrhage with coagulation defect, unspecified, third trimester MCC M ♀

O46.ØØ9 Antepartum hemorrhage with coagulation defect, unspecified, unspecified trimester M ♀

√6th O46.Ø1 Antepartum hemorrhage with afibrinogenemia

Antepartum hemorrhage with hypofibrinogenemia

O46.Ø11 Antepartum hemorrhage with afibrinogenemia, first trimester MCC M ♀

O46.Ø12 Antepartum hemorrhage with afibrinogenemia, second trimester MCC M ♀

O46.013 Antepartum hemorrhage with afibrinogenemia, third trimester MCC M ♀

O46.019 Antepartum hemorrhage with afibrinogenemia, unspecified trimester M ♀

✓6th O46.02 Antepartum hemorrhage with disseminated intravascular coagulation

O46.021 Antepartum hemorrhage with disseminated intravascular coagulation, first trimester MCC M ♀

O46.022 Antepartum hemorrhage with disseminated intravascular coagulation, second trimester MCC M ♀

O46.023 Antepartum hemorrhage with disseminated intravascular coagulation, third trimester MCC M ♀

O46.029 Antepartum hemorrhage with disseminated intravascular coagulation, unspecified trimester M ♀

✓6th O46.09 Antepartum hemorrhage with other coagulation defect

O46.091 Antepartum hemorrhage with other coagulation defect, first trimester MCC M ♀

O46.092 Antepartum hemorrhage with other coagulation defect, second trimester MCC M ♀

O46.093 Antepartum hemorrhage with other coagulation defect, third trimester MCC M ♀

O46.099 Antepartum hemorrhage with other coagulation defect, unspecified trimester M ♀

✓5th O46.8 Other antepartum hemorrhage

✓6th O46.8X Other antepartum hemorrhage

O46.8X1 Other antepartum hemorrhage, first trimester M ♀

O46.8X2 Other antepartum hemorrhage, second trimester M ♀

O46.8X3 Other antepartum hemorrhage, third trimester M ♀

O46.8X9 Other antepartum hemorrhage, unspecified trimester M ♀

✓5th O46.9 Antepartum hemorrhage, unspecified

O46.90 Antepartum hemorrhage, unspecified, unspecified trimester M ♀

O46.91 Antepartum hemorrhage, unspecified, first trimester M ♀

O46.92 Antepartum hemorrhage, unspecified, second trimester M ♀

O46.93 Antepartum hemorrhage, unspecified, third trimester M ♀

✓4th O47 False labor

INCLUDES Braxton Hicks contractions
threatened labor

EXCLUDES 1 *preterm labor (O60.-)*

AHA: 2021,1Q,10

✓5th O47.0 False labor before 37 completed weeks of gestation

O47.00 False labor before 37 completed weeks of gestation, unspecified trimester M ♀

O47.02 False labor before 37 completed weeks of gestation, second trimester CC M ♀

O47.03 False labor before 37 completed weeks of gestation, third trimester CC M ♀

O47.1 False labor at or after 37 completed weeks of gestation CC M ♀

O47.9 False labor, unspecified M ♀

✓4th O48 Late pregnancy

AHA: 2022,2Q,3

O48.0 Post-term pregnancy M ♀
Pregnancy over 40 completed weeks to 42 completed weeks gestation

O48.1 Prolonged pregnancy M ♀
Pregnancy which has advanced beyond 42 completed weeks gestation
AHA: 2016,1Q,5

Complications of labor and delivery (O60-O77)

✓4th O60 Preterm labor

INCLUDES onset (spontaneous) of labor before 37 completed weeks of gestation

EXCLUDES 1 *false labor (O47.0-)*
threatened labor NOS (O47.0-)

✓5th O60.0 Preterm labor without delivery

O60.00 Preterm labor without delivery, unspecified trimester M ♀

O60.02 Preterm labor without delivery, second trimester MCC M ♀

O60.03 Preterm labor without delivery, third trimester MCC M ♀

✓5th O60.1 Preterm labor with preterm delivery

AHA: 2016,2Q,10

One of the following 7th characters is to be assigned to each code under subcategory O60.1. 7th character 0 is for single gestations and multiple gestations where the fetus is unspecified. 7th characters 1 through 9 are for cases of multiple gestations to identify the fetus for which the code applies. The appropriate code from category O30, Multiple gestation, must also be assigned when assigning a code from subcategory O60.1 that has a 7th character of 1 through 9.
0 not applicable or unspecified
1 fetus 1
2 fetus 2
3 fetus 3
4 fetus 4
5 fetus 5
9 other fetus

✓x7th O60.10 Preterm labor with preterm delivery, unspecified trimester CC M ♀
Preterm labor with delivery NOS

✓x7th O60.12 Preterm labor second trimester with preterm delivery second trimester MCC M ♀

✓x7th O60.13 Preterm labor second trimester with preterm delivery third trimester MCC M ♀

✓x7th O60.14 Preterm labor third trimester with preterm delivery third trimester MCC M ♀

✓5th O60.2 Term delivery with preterm labor

One of the following 7th characters is to be assigned to each code under subcategory O60.2. 7th character 0 is for single gestations and multiple gestations where the fetus is unspecified. 7th characters 1 through 9 are for cases of multiple gestations to identify the fetus for which the code applies. The appropriate code from category O30, Multiple gestation, must also be assigned when assigning a code from subcategory O60.2 that has a 7th character of 1 through 9.
0 not applicable or unspecified
1 fetus 1
2 fetus 2
3 fetus 3
4 fetus 4
5 fetus 5
9 other fetus

✓x7th O60.20 Term delivery with preterm labor, unspecified trimester CC M ♀

✓x7th O60.22 Term delivery with preterm labor, second trimester MCC M ♀

✓x7th O60.23 Term delivery with preterm labor, third trimester MCC M ♀

✓4th O61 Failed induction of labor

O61.0 Failed medical induction of labor M ♀
Failed induction (of labor) by oxytocin
Failed induction (of labor) by prostaglandins

O61.1 Failed instrumental induction of labor M ♀
Failed mechanical induction (of labor)
Failed surgical induction (of labor)

O61.8 Other failed induction of labor M ♀

O61.9 Failed induction of labor, unspecified M ♀

✓4th O62 Abnormalities of forces of labor

DEF: Uterine inertia: Weak or poorly coordinated contractions of the uterus during labor.

O62.Ø Primary inadequate contractions M ♀
Failure of cervical dilatation
Primary hypotonic uterine dysfunction
Uterine inertia during latent phase of labor

O62.1 Secondary uterine inertia M ♀
Arrested active phase of labor
Secondary hypotonic uterine dysfunction

O62.2 Other uterine inertia M ♀
Atony of uterus without hemorrhage
Atony of uterus NOS
Desultory labor
Hypotonic uterine dysfunction NOS
Irregular labor
Poor contractions
Slow slope active phase of labor
Uterine inertia NOS

EXCLUDES 1 *atony of uterus with hemorrhage (postpartum) (O72.1)*
postpartum atony of uterus without hemorrhage (O75.89)

DEF: Uterine atony: Failure of the uterine muscles to contract after the fetus and placenta are delivered.

O62.3 Precipitate labor M ♀
DEF: Rapid labor with delivery occurring in three hours or less from the onset of contractions.

O62.4 Hypertonic, incoordinate, and prolonged uterine contractions M ♀
Cervical spasm
Contraction ring dystocia
Dyscoordinate labor
Hour-glass contraction of uterus
Hypertonic uterine dysfunction
Incoordinate uterine action
Tetanic contractions
Uterine dystocia NOS
Uterine spasm

EXCLUDES 1 *dystocia (fetal) (maternal) NOS (O66.9)*

O62.8 Other abnormalities of forces of labor M ♀

O62.9 Abnormality of forces of labor, unspecified M ♀

✓4th O63 Long labor

O63.Ø Prolonged first stage (of labor) M ♀

O63.1 Prolonged second stage (of labor) M ♀

O63.2 Delayed delivery of second twin, triplet, etc. M ♀

O63.9 Long labor, unspecified CC M ♀
Prolonged labor NOS

✓4th O64 Obstructed labor due to malposition and malpresentation of fetus

One of the following 7th characters is to be assigned to each code under category O64. 7th character Ø is for single gestations and multiple gestations where the fetus is unspecified. 7th characters 1 through 9 are for cases of multiple gestations to identify the fetus for which the code applies. The appropriate code from category O3Ø, Multiple gestation, must also be assigned when assigning a code from category O64 that has a 7th character of 1 through 9.

Ø not applicable or unspecified
1 fetus 1
2 fetus 2
3 fetus 3
4 fetus 4
5 fetus 5
9 other fetus

Fetal Malposition

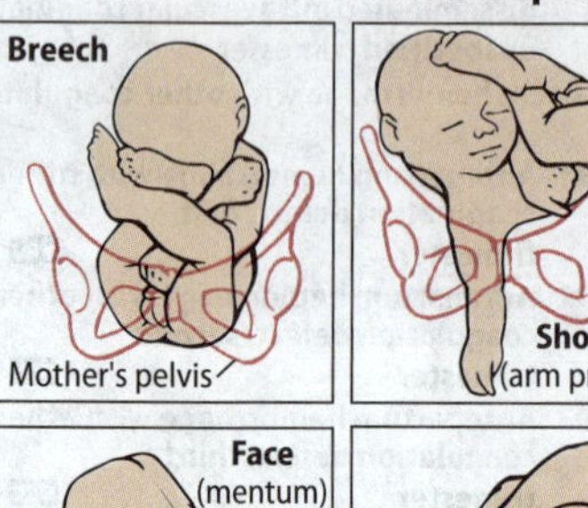

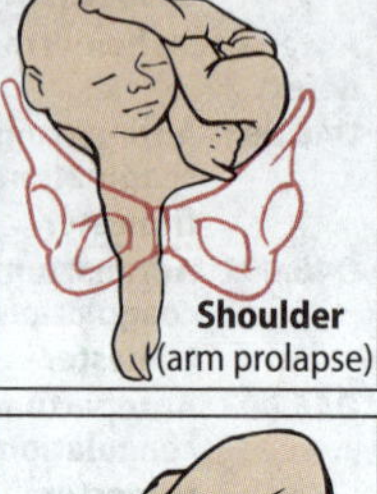

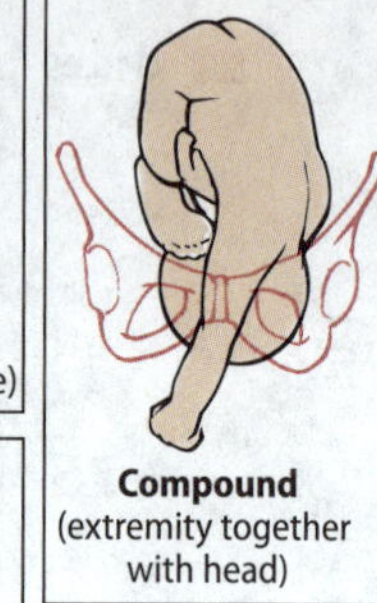

✓x7th O64.Ø Obstructed labor due to incomplete rotation of fetal head M ♀
Deep transverse arrest
Obstructed labor due to persistent occipitoiliac (position)
Obstructed labor due to persistent occipitoposterior (position)
Obstructed labor due to persistent occipitosacral (position)
Obstructed labor due to persistent occipitotransverse (position)

✓x7th O64.1 Obstructed labor due to breech presentation M ♀
Obstructed labor due to buttocks presentation
Obstructed labor due to complete breech presentation
Obstructed labor due to frank breech presentation

✓x7th O64.2 Obstructed labor due to face presentation M ♀
Obstructed labor due to chin presentation

✓x7th O64.3 Obstructed labor due to brow presentation M ♀

✓x7th O64.4 Obstructed labor due to shoulder presentation M ♀
Prolapsed arm

EXCLUDES 1 *impacted shoulders (O66.Ø)*
shoulder dystocia (O66.Ø)

✓x7th O64.5 Obstructed labor due to compound presentation M ♀

✓x7th O64.8 Obstructed labor due to other malposition and malpresentation M ♀
Obstructed labor due to footling presentation
Obstructed labor due to incomplete breech presentation

✓x7th O64.9 Obstructed labor due to malposition and malpresentation, unspecified M ♀

✓4th O65 Obstructed labor due to maternal pelvic abnormality

O65.Ø Obstructed labor due to deformed pelvis M ♀

O65.1 Obstructed labor due to generally contracted pelvis M ♀

O65.2 Obstructed labor due to pelvic inlet contraction M ♀

O65.3 Obstructed labor due to pelvic outlet and mid-cavity contraction M ♀

O65.4 Obstructed labor due to fetopelvic disproportion, unspecified M ♀
EXCLUDES 1 *dystocia due to abnormality of fetus (O66.2-O66.3)*

O65.5 Obstructed labor due to abnormality of maternal pelvic organs M ♀
Obstructed labor due to conditions listed in O34.-
Use additional code to identify abnormality of pelvic organs O34.-

O65.8 Obstructed labor due to other maternal pelvic abnormalities M ♀

O65.9 Obstructed labor due to maternal pelvic abnormality, unspecified M ♀

✓4th **O66 Other obstructed labor**

O66.Ø Obstructed labor due to shoulder dystocia M ♀
Impacted shoulders
DEF: Obstructed labor due to impacted fetal shoulders. It is an emergency condition that may require cesarean section, forceps delivery, vacuum extraction, or symphysiotomy.

O66.1 Obstructed labor due to locked twins M ♀

O66.2 Obstructed labor due to unusually large fetus M ♀

O66.3 Obstructed labor due to other abnormalities of fetus M ♀
Dystocia due to fetal ascites
Dystocia due to fetal hydrops
Dystocia due to fetal meningomyelocele
Dystocia due to fetal sacral teratoma
Dystocia due to fetal tumor
Dystocia due to hydrocephalic fetus
Use additional code to identify cause of obstruction

✓5th **O66.4 Failed trial of labor**

O66.4Ø Failed trial of labor, unspecified M ♀

O66.41 Failed attempted vaginal birth after previous cesarean delivery M ♀
Code first rupture of uterus, if applicable (O71.Ø-, O71.1)

O66.5 Attempted application of vacuum extractor and forceps M ♀
Attempted application of vacuum or forceps, with subsequent delivery by forceps or cesarean delivery

O66.6 Obstructed labor due to other multiple fetuses M ♀

O66.8 Other specified obstructed labor M ♀
Use additional code to identify cause of obstruction

O66.9 Obstructed labor, unspecified M ♀
Dystocia NOS
Fetal dystocia NOS
Maternal dystocia NOS

✓4th **O67 Labor and delivery complicated by intrapartum hemorrhage, not elsewhere classified**
EXCLUDES 1 *antepartum hemorrhage NEC (O46.-)*
placenta previa (O44.-)
premature separation of placenta [abruptio placentae] (O45.-)
EXCLUDES 2 *postpartum hemorrhage (O72.-)*

O67.Ø Intrapartum hemorrhage with coagulation defect MCC M ♀
Intrapartum hemorrhage (excessive) associated with afibrinogenemia
Intrapartum hemorrhage (excessive) associated with disseminated intravascular coagulation
Intrapartum hemorrhage (excessive) associated with hyperfibrinolysis
Intrapartum hemorrhage (excessive) associated with hypofibrinogenemia

O67.8 Other intrapartum hemorrhage M ♀
Excessive intrapartum hemorrhage

O67.9 Intrapartum hemorrhage, unspecified M ♀

O68 Labor and delivery complicated by abnormality of fetal acid-base balance CC M ♀
Fetal acidemia complicating labor and delivery
Fetal acidosis complicating labor and delivery
Fetal alkalosis complicating labor and delivery
Fetal metabolic acidemia complicating labor and delivery
EXCLUDES 1 *fetal stress NOS (O77.9)*
labor and delivery complicated by electrocardiographic evidence of fetal stress (O77.8)
labor and delivery complicated by ultrasonic evidence of fetal stress (O77.8)
EXCLUDES 2 *abnormality in fetal heart rate or rhythm (O76)*
labor and delivery complicated by meconium in amniotic fluid (O77.Ø)

✓4th **O69 Labor and delivery complicated by umbilical cord complications**
AHA: 2016,1Q,5

One of the following 7th characters is to be assigned to each code under category O69. 7th character Ø is for single gestations and multiple gestations where the fetus is unspecified. 7th characters 1 through 9 are for cases of multiple gestations to identify the fetus for which the code applies. The appropriate code from category O3Ø, Multiple gestation, must also be assigned when assigning a code from category O69 that has a 7th character of 1 through 9.
Ø not applicable or unspecified
1 fetus 1
2 fetus 2
3 fetus 3
4 fetus 4
5 fetus 5
9 other fetus

✓x7th **O69.Ø Labor and delivery complicated by prolapse of cord** M ♀
DEF: Abnormal presentation of the fetus marked by a protruding umbilical cord during labor. It can cause fetal death.

✓x7th **O69.1 Labor and delivery complicated by cord around neck, with compression** M ♀
EXCLUDES 1 *labor and delivery complicated by cord around neck, without compression (O69.81)*

✓x7th **O69.2 Labor and delivery complicated by other cord entanglement, with compression** M ♀
Labor and delivery complicated by compression of cord NOS
Labor and delivery complicated by entanglement of cords of twins in monoamniotic sac
Labor and delivery complicated by knot in cord
EXCLUDES 1 *labor and delivery complicated by other cord entanglement, without compression (O69.82)*

✓x7th **O69.3 Labor and delivery complicated by short cord** M ♀

✓x7th **O69.4 Labor and delivery complicated by vasa previa** M ♀
Labor and delivery complicated by hemorrhage from vasa previa

✓x7th **O69.5 Labor and delivery complicated by vascular lesion of cord** M ♀
Labor and delivery complicated by cord bruising
Labor and delivery complicated by cord hematoma
Labor and delivery complicated by thrombosis of umbilical vessels

✓5th **O69.8 Labor and delivery complicated by other cord complications**

✓x7th **O69.81 Labor and delivery complicated by cord around neck, without compression** M ♀
AHA: 2016,1Q,5

✓x7th **O69.82 Labor and delivery complicated by other cord entanglement, without compression** M ♀

✓x7th **O69.89 Labor and delivery complicated by other cord complications** M ♀
AHA: 2023,2Q,29

✓x7th **O69.9 Labor and delivery complicated by cord complication, unspecified** M ♀

✓4th **O7Ø Perineal laceration during delivery**
INCLUDES episiotomy extended by laceration
EXCLUDES 1 *obstetric high vaginal laceration alone (O71.4)*
AHA: 2016,2Q,34; 2016,1Q,3-4,5

O7Ø.Ø First degree perineal laceration during delivery M ♀
Perineal laceration, rupture or tear involving fourchette during delivery
Perineal laceration, rupture or tear involving labia during delivery
Perineal laceration, rupture or tear involving skin during delivery
Perineal laceration, rupture or tear involving vagina during delivery
Perineal laceration, rupture or tear involving vulva during delivery
Slight perineal laceration, rupture or tear during delivery

O7Ø.1 Second degree perineal laceration during delivery M ♀
Perineal laceration, rupture or tear during delivery as in O7Ø.Ø, also involving pelvic floor
Perineal laceration, rupture or tear during delivery as in O7Ø.Ø, also involving perineal muscles
Perineal laceration, rupture or tear during delivery as in O7Ø.Ø, also involving vaginal muscles
EXCLUDES 1 *perineal laceration involving anal sphincter (O7Ø.2)*

Chapter 15. Pregnancy, Childbirth and the Puerperium

O65.9–O7Ø.1

O70.2 Third degree perineal laceration during delivery

Perineal laceration, rupture or tear during delivery as in O70.1, also involving anal sphincter

Perineal laceration, rupture or tear during delivery as in O70.1, also involving rectovaginal septum

Perineal laceration, rupture or tear during delivery as in O70.1, also involving sphincter NOS

EXCLUDES 1 *anal sphincter tear during delivery without third degree perineal laceration (O70.4)*

perineal laceration involving anal or rectal mucosa (O70.3)

AHA: 2016,4Q,53-54

O70.20 Third degree perineal laceration during delivery, unspecified CC M ♀

O70.21 Third degree perineal laceration during delivery, IIIa CC M ♀

Third degree perineal laceration during delivery with less than 50% of external anal sphincter (EAS) thickness torn

O70.22 Third degree perineal laceration during delivery, IIIb CC M ♀

Third degree perineal laceration during delivery with more than 50% external anal sphincter (EAS) thickness torn

O70.23 Third degree perineal laceration during delivery, IIIc CC M ♀

Third degree perineal laceration during delivery with both external anal sphincter (EAS) and internal anal sphincter (IAS) torn

O70.3 Fourth degree perineal laceration during delivery CC M ♀

Perineal laceration, rupture or tear during delivery as in O70.2, also involving anal mucosa

Perineal laceration, rupture or tear during delivery as in O70.2, also involving rectal mucosa

O70.4 Anal sphincter tear complicating delivery, not associated with third degree laceration CC M ♀

EXCLUDES 1 *anal sphincter tear with third degree perineal laceration (O70.2)*

O70.9 Perineal laceration during delivery, unspecified M ♀

O71 Other obstetric trauma

INCLUDES obstetric damage from instruments

O71.0 Rupture of uterus (spontaneous) before onset of labor

EXCLUDES 1 *disruption of (current) cesarean delivery wound (O90.0)*

laceration of uterus, NEC (O71.81)

O71.00 Rupture of uterus before onset of labor, unspecified trimester M ♀

O71.02 Rupture of uterus before onset of labor, second trimester MCC M ♀

O71.03 Rupture of uterus before onset of labor, third trimester MCC M ♀

O71.1 Rupture of uterus during labor MCC M ♀

Rupture of uterus not stated as occurring before onset of labor

EXCLUDES 1 *disruption of cesarean delivery wound (O90.0)*

laceration of uterus, NEC (O71.81)

O71.2 Postpartum inversion of uterus CC M ♀

O71.3 Obstetric laceration of cervix CC M ♀

Annular detachment of cervix

O71.4 Obstetric high vaginal laceration alone CC M ♀

Laceration of vaginal wall without perineal laceration

EXCLUDES 1 *obstetric high vaginal laceration with perineal laceration (O70.-)*

AHA: 2016,1Q,5

O71.5 Other obstetric injury to pelvic organs CC M ♀

Obstetric injury to bladder

Obstetric injury to urethra

EXCLUDES 2 *obstetric periurethral trauma (O71.82)*

AHA: 2014,4Q,18

O71.6 Obstetric damage to pelvic joints and ligaments CC M ♀

Obstetric avulsion of inner symphyseal cartilage

Obstetric damage to coccyx

Obstetric traumatic separation of symphysis (pubis)

O71.7 Obstetric hematoma of pelvis CC M ♀

Obstetric hematoma of perineum

Obstetric hematoma of vagina

Obstetric hematoma of vulva

O71.8 Other specified obstetric trauma

O71.81 Laceration of uterus, not elsewhere classified M ♀

O71.82 Other specified trauma to perineum and vulva M ♀

Obstetric periurethral trauma

AHA: 2016,1Q,4; 2014,4Q,18

O71.89 Other specified obstetric trauma M ♀

O71.9 Obstetric trauma, unspecified M ♀

O72 Postpartum hemorrhage

INCLUDES hemorrhage after delivery of fetus or infant

O72.0 Third-stage hemorrhage CC M ♀

Hemorrhage associated with retained, trapped or adherent placenta

Retained placenta NOS

Code also type of adherent placenta (O43.2-)

AHA: 2019,3Q,11

O72.1 Other immediate postpartum hemorrhage CC M ♀

Hemorrhage following delivery of placenta

Postpartum hemorrhage (atonic) NOS

Uterine atony with hemorrhage

EXCLUDES 1 *uterine atony NOS (O62.2)*

uterine atony without hemorrhage (O62.2)

postpartum atony of uterus without hemorrhage (O75.89)

AHA: 2023,2Q,15; 2016,1Q,4

DEF: Uterine atony: Failure of the uterine muscles to contract after the fetus and placenta are delivered.

O72.2 Delayed and secondary postpartum hemorrhage CC M ♀

Hemorrhage associated with retained portions of placenta or membranes after the first 24 hours following delivery of placenta

Retained products of conception NOS, following delivery

O72.3 Postpartum coagulation defects M ♀

Postpartum afibrinogenemia

Postpartum fibrinolysis

O73 Retained placenta and membranes, without hemorrhage

EXCLUDES 1 *placenta accreta (O43.21-)*

placenta increta (O43.22-)

placenta percreta (O43.23-)

DEF: Postpartum condition resulting from failure to expel placental membrane tissues due to failed contractions of the uterine wall.

O73.0 Retained placenta without hemorrhage M ♀

Adherent placenta, without hemorrhage

Trapped placenta without hemorrhage

O73.1 Retained portions of placenta and membranes, without hemorrhage M ♀

Retained products of conception following delivery, without hemorrhage

O74 Complications of anesthesia during labor and delivery

INCLUDES maternal complications arising from the administration of a general, regional or local anesthetic, analgesic or other sedation during labor and delivery

Use additional code, if applicable, to identify specific complication

O74.0 Aspiration pneumonitis due to anesthesia during labor and delivery M ♀

Inhalation of stomach contents or secretions NOS due to anesthesia during labor and delivery

Mendelson's syndrome due to anesthesia during labor and delivery

O74.1 Other pulmonary complications of anesthesia during labor and delivery M ♀

O74.2 Cardiac complications of anesthesia during labor and delivery M ♀

O74.3 Central nervous system complications of anesthesia during labor and delivery M ♀

O74.4 Toxic reaction to local anesthesia during labor and delivery M ♀

O74.5 Spinal and epidural anesthesia-induced headache during labor and delivery M ♀

O74.6 Other complications of spinal and epidural anesthesia during labor and delivery M ♀

O74.7 Failed or difficult intubation for anesthesia during labor and delivery M ♀

O74.8 Other complications of anesthesia during labor and delivery M ♀

O74.9 Complication of anesthesia during labor and delivery, unspecified M ♀

O75 Other complications of labor and delivery, not elsewhere classified

EXCLUDES 2 *puerperal (postpartum) infection (O86.-)*
puerperal (postpartum) sepsis (O85)

O75.Ø Maternal distress during labor and delivery M ♀

O75.1 Shock during or following labor and delivery MCC M ♀
Obstetric shock following labor and delivery

O75.2 Pyrexia during labor, not elsewhere classified CC M ♀

O75.3 Other infection during labor MCC M ♀
Sepsis during labor
Use additional code (B95-B97), to identify infectious agent

O75.4 Other complications of obstetric surgery and procedures M ♀
Cardiac arrest following obstetric surgery or procedures
Cardiac failure following obstetric surgery or procedures
Cerebral anoxia following obstetric surgery or procedures
Pulmonary edema following obstetric surgery or procedures
Use additional code to identify specific complication
EXCLUDES 2 *complications of anesthesia during labor and delivery (O74.-)*
disruption of obstetrical (surgical) wound (O9Ø.Ø-O9Ø.1)
hematoma of obstetrical (surgical) wound (O9Ø.2)
infection of obstetrical (surgical) wound (O86.Ø-)

O75.5 Delayed delivery after artificial rupture of membranes M ♀

O75.8 Other specified complications of labor and delivery

O75.81 Maternal exhaustion complicating labor and delivery M ♀

O75.82 Onset (spontaneous) of labor after 37 completed weeks of gestation but before 39 completed weeks gestation, with delivery by (planned) cesarean section M ♀
Delivery by (planned) cesarean section occurring after 37 completed weeks of gestation but before 39 completed weeks gestation due to (spontaneous) onset of labor
Code first to specify reason for planned cesarean section such as:
cephalopelvic disproportion (normally formed fetus) (O33.9)
previous cesarean delivery ▶(O34.21-)◀
AHA: 2022,2Q,3

O75.89 Other specified complications of labor and delivery M ♀

O75.9 Complication of labor and delivery, unspecified M ♀

O76 Abnormality in fetal heart rate and rhythm complicating labor and delivery M ♀
Depressed fetal heart rate tones complicating labor and delivery
Fetal bradycardia complicating labor and delivery
Fetal heart rate decelerations complicating labor and delivery
Fetal heart rate irregularity complicating labor and delivery
Fetal heart rate abnormal variability complicating labor and delivery
Fetal tachycardia complicating labor and delivery
Non-reassuring fetal heart rate or rhythm complicating labor and delivery
EXCLUDES 1 *fetal stress NOS (O77.9)*
labor and delivery complicated by electrocardiographic evidence of fetal stress (O77.8)
labor and delivery complicated by ultrasonic evidence of fetal stress (O77.8)
EXCLUDES 2 *fetal metabolic acidemia (O68)*
other fetal stress (O77.Ø-O77.1)
AHA: 2013,4Q,118

O77 Other fetal stress complicating labor and delivery

O77.Ø Labor and delivery complicated by meconium in amniotic fluid M ♀
AHA: 2022,2Q,16; 2013,4Q,117-118

O77.1 Fetal stress in labor or delivery due to drug administration M ♀

O77.8 Labor and delivery complicated by other evidence of fetal stress M ♀
Labor and delivery complicated by electrocardiographic evidence of fetal stress
Labor and delivery complicated by ultrasonic evidence of fetal stress
EXCLUDES 1 *abnormality of fetal acid-base balance (O68)*
abnormality in fetal heart rate or rhythm (O76)
fetal metabolic acidemia (O68)

O77.9 Labor and delivery complicated by fetal stress, unspecified M ♀
EXCLUDES 1 *abnormality of fetal acid-base balance (O68)*
abnormality in fetal heart rate or rhythm (O76)
fetal metabolic acidemia (O68)

Encounter for delivery (O8Ø-O82)

O8Ø Encounter for full-term uncomplicated delivery M ♀
NOTE Delivery requiring minimal or no assistance, with or without episiotomy, without fetal manipulation [e.g., rotation version] or instrumentation [forceps] of a spontaneous, cephalic, vaginal, full-term, single, live-born infant. This code is for use as a single diagnosis code and is not to be used with any other code from chapter 15.
Use additional code to indicate outcome of delivery (Z37.Ø)
AHA: 2016,4Q,150; 2014,2Q,9

O82 Encounter for cesarean delivery without indication M ♀
Use additional code to indicate outcome of delivery (Z37.Ø)

Complications predominantly related to the puerperium (O85-O92)

EXCLUDES 2 *mental and behavioral disorders associated with the puerperium (F53.-)*
obstetrical tetanus (A34)
puerperal osteomalacia (M83.Ø)

O85 Puerperal sepsis MCC M ♀
Postpartum sepsis
Puerperal peritonitis
Puerperal pyemia
Use additional code (B95-B97), to identify infectious agent
Use additional code (R65.2-) to identify severe sepsis, if applicable
EXCLUDES 1 *fever of unknown origin following delivery (O86.4)*
genital tract infection following delivery (O86.1-)
obstetric pyemic and septic embolism (O88.3-)
puerperal septic thrombophlebitis (O86.81)
urinary tract infection following delivery (O86.2-)
EXCLUDES 2 *sepsis during labor (O75.3)*
AHA: 2022,2Q,5; 2020,2Q,32; 2019,2Q,39; 2018,4Q,23

O86 Other puerperal infections
Use additional code (B95-B97), to identify infectious agent
EXCLUDES 2 *infection during labor (O75.3)*
obstetrical tetanus (A34)

O86.Ø Infection of obstetric surgical wound
Infected cesarean delivery wound following delivery
Infected perineal repair following delivery
EXCLUDES 1 *complications of procedures, not elsewhere classified (T81.4-)*
postprocedural fever NOS (R5Ø.82)
postprocedural retroperitoneal abscess (K68.11)
AHA: 2020,2Q,32; 2018,4Q,22-23,62

O86.ØØ Infection of obstetric surgical wound, unspecified M ♀

O86.Ø1 Infection of obstetric surgical wound, superficial incisional site M ♀
Subcutaneous abscess following an obstetrical procedure
Stitch abscess following an obstetrical procedure

O86.Ø2 Infection of obstetric surgical wound, deep incisional site M ♀
Intramuscular abscess following an obstetrical procedure
Sub-fascial abscess following an obstetrical procedure
AHA: 2020,2Q,32

O86.03 Infection of obstetric surgical wound, organ and space site M ♀
Intraabdominal abscess following an obstetrical procedure
Subphrenic abscess following an obstetrical procedure

O86.04 Sepsis following an obstetrical procedure MCC M ♀
Use additional code to identify the sepsis
AHA: 2020,2Q,32; 2019,2Q,39

O86.09 Infection of obstetric surgical wound, other surgical site M ♀

✓5th **O86.1 Other infection of genital tract following delivery**

O86.11 Cervicitis following delivery CC M ♀
O86.12 Endometritis following delivery CC M ♀
O86.13 Vaginitis following delivery CC M ♀
O86.19 Other infection of genital tract following delivery CC M ♀

✓5th **O86.2 Urinary tract infection following delivery**

O86.20 Urinary tract infection following delivery, unspecified CC M ♀
Puerperal urinary tract infection NOS
AHA: 2022,2Q,5

O86.21 Infection of kidney following delivery CC M ♀
O86.22 Infection of bladder following delivery CC M ♀
Infection of urethra following delivery
O86.29 Other urinary tract infection following delivery CC M ♀

O86.4 Pyrexia of unknown origin following delivery CC M ♀
Puerperal infection NOS following delivery
Puerperal pyrexia NOS following delivery
EXCLUDES 2 *pyrexia during labor (O75.2)*
DEF: Fever of unknown origin experienced by the mother after childbirth.

✓5th **O86.8 Other specified puerperal infections**

O86.81 Puerperal septic thrombophlebitis MCC M ♀
O86.89 Other specified puerperal infections MCC M ♀

✓4th **O87 Venous complications and hemorrhoids in the puerperium**

INCLUDES venous complications in labor, delivery and the puerperium
EXCLUDES 2 *obstetric embolism (O88.-)*
puerperal septic thrombophlebitis (O86.81)
venous complications in pregnancy (O22.-)

O87.0 Superficial thrombophlebitis in the puerperium CC M ♀
Puerperal phlebitis NOS
Puerperal thrombosis NOS
▶Use additional code, if applicable, to identify the superficial vein thrombosis, such as thrombosis of superficial vessels of lower extremities (I80.0-)◀

O87.1 Deep phlebothrombosis in the puerperium MCC M ♀
Deep vein thrombosis, postpartum
Pelvic thrombophlebitis, postpartum
Use additional code to identify the deep vein thrombosis (I82.4-, I82.5-, I82.62-, I82.72-)
Use additional code, if applicable, for associated long-term (current) use of anticoagulants (Z79.01)

O87.2 Hemorrhoids in the puerperium CC M ♀
O87.3 Cerebral venous thrombosis in the puerperium CC M ♀
Cerebrovenous sinus thrombosis in the puerperium
O87.4 Varicose veins of lower extremity in the puerperium M ♀
O87.8 Other venous complications in the puerperium CC M ♀
Genital varices in the puerperium
O87.9 Venous complication in the puerperium, unspecified M ♀
Puerperal phlebopathy NOS

✓4th **O88 Obstetric embolism**

EXCLUDES 1 *embolism complicating abortion NOS (O03.2)*
embolism complicating ectopic or molar pregnancy (O08.2)
embolism complicating failed attempted abortion (O07.2)
embolism complicating induced abortion (O04.7)
embolism complicating spontaneous abortion (O03.2, O03.7)

✓5th **O88.0 Obstetric air embolism**
DEF: Sudden blocking of the pulmonary artery or right ventricle with air or nitrogen bubbles.

✓6th **O88.01 Obstetric air embolism in pregnancy**

O88.011 Air embolism in pregnancy, first trimester MCC M ♀
O88.012 Air embolism in pregnancy, second trimester MCC M ♀
O88.013 Air embolism in pregnancy, third trimester MCC M ♀
O88.019 Air embolism in pregnancy, unspecified trimester M ♀

O88.02 Air embolism in childbirth MCC M ♀
O88.03 Air embolism in the puerperium MCC M ♀

✓5th **O88.1 Amniotic fluid embolism**
Anaphylactoid syndrome in pregnancy

✓6th **O88.11 Amniotic fluid embolism in pregnancy**

O88.111 Amniotic fluid embolism in pregnancy, first trimester MCC M ♀
O88.112 Amniotic fluid embolism in pregnancy, second trimester MCC M ♀
O88.113 Amniotic fluid embolism in pregnancy, third trimester MCC M ♀
O88.119 Amniotic fluid embolism in pregnancy, unspecified trimester M ♀

O88.12 Amniotic fluid embolism in childbirth MCC M ♀
O88.13 Amniotic fluid embolism in the puerperium MCC M ♀

✓5th **O88.2 Obstetric thromboembolism**

✓6th **O88.21 Thromboembolism in pregnancy**
Obstetric (pulmonary) embolism NOS

O88.211 Thromboembolism in pregnancy, first trimester MCC M ♀
O88.212 Thromboembolism in pregnancy, second trimester MCC M ♀
O88.213 Thromboembolism in pregnancy, third trimester MCC M ♀
O88.219 Thromboembolism in pregnancy, unspecified trimester M ♀

O88.22 Thromboembolism in childbirth MCC M ♀
O88.23 Thromboembolism in the puerperium MCC M ♀
Puerperal (pulmonary) embolism NOS

✓5th **O88.3 Obstetric pyemic and septic embolism**

✓6th **O88.31 Pyemic and septic embolism in pregnancy**

O88.311 Pyemic and septic embolism in pregnancy, first trimester MCC M ♀
O88.312 Pyemic and septic embolism in pregnancy, second trimester MCC M ♀
O88.313 Pyemic and septic embolism in pregnancy, third trimester MCC M ♀
O88.319 Pyemic and septic embolism in pregnancy, unspecified trimester CC M ♀

O88.32 Pyemic and septic embolism in childbirth MCC M ♀
O88.33 Pyemic and septic embolism in the puerperium MCC M ♀

✓5th **O88.8 Other obstetric embolism**
Obstetric fat embolism

✓6th **O88.81 Other embolism in pregnancy**

O88.811 Other embolism in pregnancy, first trimester MCC M ♀
O88.812 Other embolism in pregnancy, second trimester MCC M ♀
O88.813 Other embolism in pregnancy, third trimester MCC M ♀
O88.819 Other embolism in pregnancy, unspecified trimester M ♀

O88.82 Other embolism in childbirth MCC M ♀
O88.83 Other embolism in the puerperium MCC M ♀

✓4th **O89 Complications of anesthesia during the puerperium**

INCLUDES maternal complications arising from the administration of a general, regional or local anesthetic, analgesic or other sedation during the puerperium
Use additional code, if applicable, to identify specific complication

✓5th **O89.0 Pulmonary complications of anesthesia during the puerperium**

O89.01 Aspiration pneumonitis due to anesthesia during the puerperium M ♀
Inhalation of stomach contents or secretions NOS due to anesthesia during the puerperium
Mendelson's syndrome due to anesthesia during the puerperium

N Newborn: 0 P Pediatric: 0-17 M Maternity: 9-64 A Adult: 15-124 UNS Unspecified Site MCC Major Complication/Comorbidity CC Complication/Comorbidity

O89.Ø9 Other pulmonary complications of anesthesia during the puerperium M ♀

O89.1 Cardiac complications of anesthesia during the puerperium M ♀

O89.2 Central nervous system complications of anesthesia during the puerperium M ♀

O89.3 Toxic reaction to local anesthesia during the puerperium M ♀

O89.4 Spinal and epidural anesthesia-induced headache during the puerperium M ♀

O89.5 Other complications of spinal and epidural anesthesia during the puerperium M ♀

O89.6 Failed or difficult intubation for anesthesia during the puerperium M ♀

O89.8 Other complications of anesthesia during the puerperium M ♀

O89.9 Complication of anesthesia during the puerperium, unspecified M ♀

✓4th **O9Ø Complications of the puerperium, not elsewhere classified**

O9Ø.Ø Disruption of cesarean delivery wound M ♀
Dehiscence of cesarean delivery wound
EXCLUDES 1 *rupture of uterus (spontaneous) before onset of labor (O71.Ø-)*
rupture of uterus during labor (O71.1)

O9Ø.1 Disruption of perineal obstetric wound M ♀
Disruption of wound of episiotomy
Disruption of wound of perineal laceration
Secondary perineal tear

O9Ø.2 Hematoma of obstetric wound M ♀

O9Ø.3 Peripartum cardiomyopathy MCC M ♀
Conditions in I42- arising during pregnancy and the puerperium
EXCLUDES 1 *pre-existing heart disease complicating pregnancy and the puerperium (O99.4-)*
AHA: 2022,3Q,16-17
DEF: Any structural or functional abnormality of the ventricular myocardium. It is a noninflammatory disease of obscure or unknown etiology with onset during the postpartum period.

▲ ✓5th O9Ø.4 Postpartum acute kidney failure
~~Hepatorenal syndrome following labor and delivery~~
EXCLUDES 1 ▶*non-anuria and oliguria (R34)*◀

● O9Ø.41 Hepatorenal syndrome following labor and delivery MCC

● O9Ø.49 Other postpartum acute kidney failure MCC
Postpartum acute kidney failure
Puerperal anuria
Puerperal oliguria

O9Ø.5 Postpartum thyroiditis M ♀

O9Ø.6 Postpartum mood disturbance M ♀
Postpartum blues
Postpartum dysphoria
Postpartum sadness
EXCLUDES 1 *postpartum depression (F53.Ø)*
puerperal psychosis (F53.1)

✓5th O9Ø.8 Other complications of the puerperium, not elsewhere classified

O9Ø.81 Anemia of the puerperium M ♀
Postpartum anemia NOS
EXCLUDES 1 *pre-existing anemia complicating the puerperium (O99.Ø3)*
AHA: 2019,3Q,11

O9Ø.89 Other complications of the puerperium, not elsewhere classified M ♀
Placental polyp

O9Ø.9 Complication of the puerperium, unspecified M ♀

✓4th **O91 Infections of breast associated with pregnancy, the puerperium and lactation**
Use additional code to identify infection

✓5th O91.Ø Infection of nipple associated with pregnancy, the puerperium and lactation

✓6th O91.Ø1 Infection of nipple associated with pregnancy
Gestational abscess of nipple

O91.Ø11 Infection of nipple associated with pregnancy, first trimester M ♀

O91.Ø12 Infection of nipple associated with pregnancy, second trimester M ♀

O91.Ø13 Infection of nipple associated with pregnancy, third trimester M ♀

O91.Ø19 Infection of nipple associated with pregnancy, unspecified trimester M ♀

O91.Ø2 Infection of nipple associated with the puerperium M ♀
Puerperal abscess of nipple

O91.Ø3 Infection of nipple associated with lactation M ♀
Abscess of nipple associated with lactation

✓5th O91.1 Abscess of breast associated with pregnancy, the puerperium and lactation

✓6th O91.11 Abscess of breast associated with pregnancy
Gestational mammary abscess
Gestational purulent mastitis
Gestational subareolar abscess

O91.111 Abscess of breast associated with pregnancy, first trimester M ♀

O91.112 Abscess of breast associated with pregnancy, second trimester M ♀

O91.113 Abscess of breast associated with pregnancy, third trimester M ♀

O91.119 Abscess of breast associated with pregnancy, unspecified trimester M ♀

O91.12 Abscess of breast associated with the puerperium M ♀
Puerperal mammary abscess
Puerperal purulent mastitis
Puerperal subareolar abscess

O91.13 Abscess of breast associated with lactation M ♀
Mammary abscess associated with lactation
Purulent mastitis associated with lactation
Subareolar abscess associated with lactation

✓5th O91.2 Nonpurulent mastitis associated with pregnancy, the puerperium and lactation

✓6th O91.21 Nonpurulent mastitis associated with pregnancy
Gestational interstitial mastitis
Gestational lymphangitis of breast
Gestational mastitis NOS
Gestational parenchymatous mastitis

O91.211 Nonpurulent mastitis associated with pregnancy, first trimester M ♀

O91.212 Nonpurulent mastitis associated with pregnancy, second trimester M ♀

O91.213 Nonpurulent mastitis associated with pregnancy, third trimester M ♀

O91.219 Nonpurulent mastitis associated with pregnancy, unspecified trimester M ♀

O91.22 Nonpurulent mastitis associated with the puerperium M ♀
Puerperal interstitial mastitis
Puerperal lymphangitis of breast
Puerperal mastitis NOS
Puerperal parenchymatous mastitis

O91.23 Nonpurulent mastitis associated with lactation M ♀
Interstitial mastitis associated with lactation
Lymphangitis of breast associated with lactation
Mastitis NOS associated with lactation
Parenchymatous mastitis associated with lactation

✓4th **O92 Other disorders of breast and disorders of lactation associated with pregnancy and the puerperium**

✓5th O92.Ø Retracted nipple associated with pregnancy, the puerperium, and lactation

✓6th O92.Ø1 Retracted nipple associated with pregnancy

O92.Ø11 Retracted nipple associated with pregnancy, first trimester M ♀

O92.Ø12 Retracted nipple associated with pregnancy, second trimester M ♀

O92.Ø13 Retracted nipple associated with pregnancy, third trimester M ♀

O92.Ø19 Retracted nipple associated with pregnancy, unspecified trimester M ♀

O92.Ø2 Retracted nipple associated with the puerperium M ♀

O92.Ø3 Retracted nipple associated with lactation M ♀

✓5th O92.1 Cracked nipple associated with pregnancy, the puerperium, and lactation
Fissure of nipple, gestational or puerperal

✓6th O92.11 Cracked nipple associated with pregnancy

O92.111 Cracked nipple associated with pregnancy, first trimester M ♀

Chapter 15. Pregnancy, Childbirth and the Puerperium

O92.112 Cracked nipple associated with pregnancy, second trimester M♀

O92.113 Cracked nipple associated with pregnancy, third trimester M♀

O92.119 Cracked nipple associated with pregnancy, unspecified trimester M♀

O92.12 Cracked nipple associated with the puerperium M♀

O92.13 Cracked nipple associated with lactation M♀

✓5th O92.2 Other and unspecified disorders of breast associated with pregnancy and the puerperium

O92.20 Unspecified disorder of breast associated with pregnancy and the puerperium M♀

O92.29 Other disorders of breast associated with pregnancy and the puerperium M♀

O92.3 Agalactia M♀

Primary agalactia

EXCLUDES 1 *elective agalactia (O92.5)*
secondary agalactia (O92.5)
therapeutic agalactia (O92.5)

DEF: Absence of milk secretion in a female after delivery.

O92.4 Hypogalactia M♀

O92.5 Suppressed lactation M♀

Elective agalactia
Secondary agalactia
Therapeutic agalactia

EXCLUDES 1 *primary agalactia (O92.3)*

O92.6 Galactorrhea M♀

DEF: Excessive or persistent milk secretion by the breast that may occur in the absence of nursing.

✓5th O92.7 Other and unspecified disorders of lactation

O92.70 Unspecified disorders of lactation M♀

O92.79 Other disorders of lactation M♀

Puerperal galactocele

Other obstetric conditions, not elsewhere classified (O94-O9A)

O94 Sequelae of complication of pregnancy, childbirth, and the puerperium UPD M♀

NOTE This category is to be used to indicate conditions in O00-O77.-, O85-O94 and O98-O9A.- as the cause of late effects. The sequelae include conditions specified as such, or as late effects, which may occur at any time after the puerperium

Code first condition resulting from (sequela) of complication of pregnancy, childbirth, and the puerperium

AHA: 2022,3Q,16-17

✓4th **O98 Maternal infectious and parasitic diseases classifiable elsewhere but complicating pregnancy, childbirth and the puerperium**

INCLUDES the listed conditions when complicating the pregnant state, when aggravated by the pregnancy, or as a reason for obstetric care

Use additional code (Chapter 1), to identify specific infectious or parasitic disease

EXCLUDES 2 *herpes gestationis (O26.4-)*
infectious carrier state (O99.82-, O99.83-)
obstetrical tetanus (A34)
puerperal infection (O86.-)
puerperal sepsis (O85)
when the reason for maternal care is that the disease is known or suspected to have affected the fetus (O35-O36)

✓5th O98.0 Tuberculosis complicating pregnancy, childbirth and the puerperium

Conditions in A15-A19

✓6th O98.01 Tuberculosis complicating pregnancy

O98.011 Tuberculosis complicating pregnancy, first trimester CC M♀

O98.012 Tuberculosis complicating pregnancy, second trimester CC M♀

O98.013 Tuberculosis complicating pregnancy, third trimester CC M♀

O98.019 Tuberculosis complicating pregnancy, unspecified trimester M♀

O98.02 Tuberculosis complicating childbirth CC M♀

O98.03 Tuberculosis complicating the puerperium CC M♀

✓5th O98.1 Syphilis complicating pregnancy, childbirth and the puerperium

Conditions in A50-A53

✓6th O98.11 Syphilis complicating pregnancy

O98.111 Syphilis complicating pregnancy, first trimester CC M♀

O98.112 Syphilis complicating pregnancy, second trimester CC M♀

O98.113 Syphilis complicating pregnancy, third trimester CC M♀

O98.119 Syphilis complicating pregnancy, unspecified trimester M♀

O98.12 Syphilis complicating childbirth CC M♀

O98.13 Syphilis complicating the puerperium CC M♀

✓5th O98.2 Gonorrhea complicating pregnancy, childbirth and the puerperium

Conditions in A54.-

✓6th O98.21 Gonorrhea complicating pregnancy

O98.211 Gonorrhea complicating pregnancy, first trimester CC M♀

O98.212 Gonorrhea complicating pregnancy, second trimester CC M♀

O98.213 Gonorrhea complicating pregnancy, third trimester CC M♀

O98.219 Gonorrhea complicating pregnancy, unspecified trimester M♀

O98.22 Gonorrhea complicating childbirth CC M♀

O98.23 Gonorrhea complicating the puerperium CC M♀

✓5th O98.3 Other infections with a predominantly sexual mode of transmission complicating pregnancy, childbirth and the puerperium

Conditions in A55-A64

AHA: 2020,1Q,20

✓6th O98.31 Other infections with a predominantly sexual mode of transmission complicating pregnancy

O98.311 Other infections with a predominantly sexual mode of transmission complicating pregnancy, first trimester CC M♀

O98.312 Other infections with a predominantly sexual mode of transmission complicating pregnancy, second trimester CC M♀

O98.313 Other infections with a predominantly sexual mode of transmission complicating pregnancy, third trimester CC M♀

O98.319 Other infections with a predominantly sexual mode of transmission complicating pregnancy, unspecified trimester M♀

O98.32 Other infections with a predominantly sexual mode of transmission complicating childbirth CC M♀

O98.33 Other infections with a predominantly sexual mode of transmission complicating the puerperium CC M♀

✓5th O98.4 Viral hepatitis complicating pregnancy, childbirth and the puerperium

Conditions in B15-B19

✓6th O98.41 Viral hepatitis complicating pregnancy

O98.411 Viral hepatitis complicating pregnancy, first trimester CC M♀

O98.412 Viral hepatitis complicating pregnancy, second trimester CC M♀

O98.413 Viral hepatitis complicating pregnancy, third trimester CC M♀

O98.419 Viral hepatitis complicating pregnancy, unspecified trimester M♀

O98.42 Viral hepatitis complicating childbirth CC M♀

O98.43 Viral hepatitis complicating the puerperium CC M♀

O98.5 Other viral diseases complicating pregnancy, childbirth and the puerperium
Conditions in A8Ø-BØ9, B25-B34, R87.81-, R87.82-
EXCLUDES 1 *human immunodeficiency virus [HIV] disease complicating pregnancy, childbirth and the puerperium (O98.7-)*
TIP: Assign a code from this subcategory as the principal or first-listed diagnosis for a patient admitted/presenting during pregnancy, childbirth, or the puerperium because of COVID-19; assign U07.1 and codes for associated manifestations as secondary codes.

O98.51 Other viral diseases complicating pregnancy
O98.511 Other viral diseases complicating pregnancy, first trimester CC M ♀
O98.512 Other viral diseases complicating pregnancy, second trimester CC M ♀
O98.513 Other viral diseases complicating pregnancy, third trimester CC M ♀
O98.519 Other viral diseases complicating pregnancy, unspecified trimester M ♀
O98.52 Other viral diseases complicating childbirth CC M ♀
O98.53 Other viral diseases complicating the puerperium CC M ♀

O98.6 Protozoal diseases complicating pregnancy, childbirth and the puerperium
Conditions in B5Ø-B64
O98.61 Protozoal diseases complicating pregnancy
O98.611 Protozoal diseases complicating pregnancy, first trimester CC M ♀
O98.612 Protozoal diseases complicating pregnancy, second trimester CC M ♀
O98.613 Protozoal diseases complicating pregnancy, third trimester CC M ♀
O98.619 Protozoal diseases complicating pregnancy, unspecified trimester M ♀
O98.62 Protozoal diseases complicating childbirth CC M ♀
O98.63 Protozoal diseases complicating the puerperium CC M ♀

O98.7 Human immunodeficiency virus [HIV] disease complicating pregnancy, childbirth and the puerperium
Use additional code to identify the type of HIV disease:
acquired immune deficiency syndrome (AIDS) (B2Ø)
asymptomatic HIV status (Z21)
HIV positive NOS (Z21)
symptomatic HIV disease (B2Ø)
O98.71 Human immunodeficiency virus [HIV] disease complicating pregnancy
O98.711 Human immunodeficiency virus [HIV] disease complicating pregnancy, first trimester CC M ♀
O98.712 Human immunodeficiency virus [HIV] disease complicating pregnancy, second trimester CC M ♀
O98.713 Human immunodeficiency virus [HIV] disease complicating pregnancy, third trimester CC M ♀
O98.719 Human immunodeficiency virus [HIV] disease complicating pregnancy, unspecified trimester M ♀
O98.72 Human immunodeficiency virus [HIV] disease complicating childbirth CC M ♀
O98.73 Human immunodeficiency virus [HIV] disease complicating the puerperium CC M ♀

O98.8 Other maternal infectious and parasitic diseases complicating pregnancy, childbirth and the puerperium
AHA: 2020,1Q,10
O98.81 Other maternal infectious and parasitic diseases complicating pregnancy
O98.811 Other maternal infectious and parasitic diseases complicating pregnancy, first trimester CC M ♀
O98.812 Other maternal infectious and parasitic diseases complicating pregnancy, second trimester CC M ♀
O98.813 Other maternal infectious and parasitic diseases complicating pregnancy, third trimester CC M ♀
O98.819 Other maternal infectious and parasitic diseases complicating pregnancy, unspecified trimester M ♀
O98.82 Other maternal infectious and parasitic diseases complicating childbirth CC M ♀
O98.83 Other maternal infectious and parasitic diseases complicating the puerperium CC M ♀
AHA: 2022,2Q,5

O98.9 Unspecified maternal infectious and parasitic disease complicating pregnancy, childbirth and the puerperium
O98.91 Unspecified maternal infectious and parasitic disease complicating pregnancy
O98.911 Unspecified maternal infectious and parasitic disease complicating pregnancy, first trimester CC M ♀
O98.912 Unspecified maternal infectious and parasitic disease complicating pregnancy, second trimester CC M ♀
O98.913 Unspecified maternal infectious and parasitic disease complicating pregnancy, third trimester CC M ♀
O98.919 Unspecified maternal infectious and parasitic disease complicating pregnancy, unspecified trimester M ♀
O98.92 Unspecified maternal infectious and parasitic disease complicating childbirth CC M ♀
O98.93 Unspecified maternal infectious and parasitic disease complicating the puerperium CC M ♀

O99 Other maternal diseases classifiable elsewhere but complicating pregnancy, childbirth and the puerperium
INCLUDES conditions which complicate the pregnant state, are aggravated by the pregnancy or are a main reason for obstetric care
Use additional code to identify specific condition
EXCLUDES 2 *when the reason for maternal care is that the condition is known or suspected to have affected the fetus (O35-O36)*

O99.Ø Anemia complicating pregnancy, childbirth and the puerperium
Conditions in D5Ø-D64
EXCLUDES 1 *anemia arising in the puerperium (O9Ø.81)*
postpartum anemia NOS (O9Ø.81)
AHA: 2019,3Q,11
O99.Ø1 Anemia complicating pregnancy
AHA: 2016,1Q,4
O99.Ø11 Anemia complicating pregnancy, first trimester M ♀
O99.Ø12 Anemia complicating pregnancy, second trimester M ♀
O99.Ø13 Anemia complicating pregnancy, third trimester M ♀
O99.Ø19 Anemia complicating pregnancy, unspecified trimester M ♀
O99.Ø2 Anemia complicating childbirth M ♀
O99.Ø3 Anemia complicating the puerperium M ♀
EXCLUDES 1 *postpartum anemia not pre-existing prior to delivery (O9Ø.81)*

O99.1 Other diseases of the blood and blood-forming organs and certain disorders involving the immune mechanism complicating pregnancy, childbirth and the puerperium
Conditions in D65-D89
EXCLUDES 1 *hemorrhage with coagulation defects (O45.-, O46.Ø-, O67.Ø, O72.3)*
O99.11 Other diseases of the blood and blood-forming organs and certain disorders involving the immune mechanism complicating pregnancy
O99.111 Other diseases of the blood and blood-forming organs and certain disorders involving the immune mechanism complicating pregnancy, first trimester CC M ♀
O99.112 Other diseases of the blood and blood-forming organs and certain disorders involving the immune mechanism complicating pregnancy, second trimester CC M ♀
O99.113 Other diseases of the blood and blood-forming organs and certain disorders involving the immune mechanism complicating pregnancy, third trimester CC M ♀

O99.119 Other diseases of the blood and blood-forming organs and certain disorders involving the immune mechanism complicating pregnancy, unspecified trimester CC M ♀

O99.12 Other diseases of the blood and blood-forming organs and certain disorders involving the immune mechanism complicating childbirth CC M ♀

O99.13 Other diseases of the blood and blood-forming organs and certain disorders involving the immune mechanism complicating the puerperium CC M ♀

✓5th **O99.2 Endocrine, nutritional and metabolic diseases complicating pregnancy, childbirth and the puerperium**

Conditions in E00-E89

EXCLUDES 2 *diabetes mellitus (O24.-)*
malnutrition (O25.-)
postpartum thyroiditis (O90.5)

✓6th **O99.21 Obesity complicating pregnancy, childbirth, and the puerperium**

Use additional code to identify the type of obesity (E66.-)

AHA: 2021,2Q,10; 2018,4Q,80

TIP: Do not assign a BMI code (Z68.-) for obese or overweight patients who are pregnant.

O99.210 Obesity complicating pregnancy, unspecified trimester M ♀

O99.211 Obesity complicating pregnancy, first trimester M ♀

O99.212 Obesity complicating pregnancy, second trimester M ♀

O99.213 Obesity complicating pregnancy, third trimester M ♀

O99.214 Obesity complicating childbirth M ♀

O99.215 Obesity complicating the puerperium M ♀

✓6th **O99.28 Other endocrine, nutritional and metabolic diseases complicating pregnancy, childbirth and the puerperium**

AHA: 2021,1Q,8

O99.280 Endocrine, nutritional and metabolic diseases complicating pregnancy, unspecified trimester M ♀

O99.281 Endocrine, nutritional and metabolic diseases complicating pregnancy, first trimester M ♀

O99.282 Endocrine, nutritional and metabolic diseases complicating pregnancy, second trimester M ♀

O99.283 Endocrine, nutritional and metabolic diseases complicating pregnancy, third trimester M ♀

O99.284 Endocrine, nutritional and metabolic diseases complicating childbirth M ♀

O99.285 Endocrine, nutritional and metabolic diseases complicating the puerperium M ♀

✓5th **O99.3 Mental disorders and diseases of the nervous system complicating pregnancy, childbirth and the puerperium**

✓6th **O99.31 Alcohol use complicating pregnancy, childbirth, and the puerperium**

Use additional code(s) from F10 to identify manifestations of the alcohol use

O99.310 Alcohol use complicating pregnancy, unspecified trimester M ♀

O99.311 Alcohol use complicating pregnancy, first trimester M ♀

O99.312 Alcohol use complicating pregnancy, second trimester M ♀

O99.313 Alcohol use complicating pregnancy, third trimester M ♀

O99.314 Alcohol use complicating childbirth M ♀

O99.315 Alcohol use complicating the puerperium M ♀

✓6th **O99.32 Drug use complicating pregnancy, childbirth, and the puerperium**

Use additional code(s) from F11-F16 and F18-F19 to identify manifestations of the drug use

AHA: 2018,4Q,69-70; 2018,2Q,10

TIP: When drug use is documented during pregnancy, assign first a code from this subcategory followed by an additional code from F11-F16 and F18-F19 identifying the specific drug use even if not documented as associated with a physical, mental, or behavioral disorder. According to chapter 15 guidelines, it is the provider's responsibility to state that the condition being treated is *not* affecting the pregnancy.

O99.320 Drug use complicating pregnancy, unspecified trimester M ♀

O99.321 Drug use complicating pregnancy, first trimester CC M ♀

O99.322 Drug use complicating pregnancy, second trimester CC M ♀

O99.323 Drug use complicating pregnancy, third trimester CC M ♀

O99.324 Drug use complicating childbirth CC M ♀

O99.325 Drug use complicating the puerperium CC M ♀

✓6th **O99.33 Tobacco use disorder complicating pregnancy, childbirth, and the puerperium**

Smoking complicating pregnancy, childbirth, and the puerperium

Use additional code from category F17 to identify type of tobacco nicotine dependence

O99.330 Smoking (tobacco) complicating pregnancy, unspecified trimester M ♀

O99.331 Smoking (tobacco) complicating pregnancy, first trimester M ♀

O99.332 Smoking (tobacco) complicating pregnancy, second trimester M ♀

O99.333 Smoking (tobacco) complicating pregnancy, third trimester M ♀

O99.334 Smoking (tobacco) complicating childbirth M ♀

O99.335 Smoking (tobacco) complicating the puerperium M ♀

✓6th **O99.34 Other mental disorders complicating pregnancy, childbirth, and the puerperium**

Conditions in F01-F09, F20-F52 and F54-F99

EXCLUDES 2 *postpartum mood disturbance (O90.6)*
postnatal psychosis (F53.1)
puerperal psychosis (F53.1)

O99.340 Other mental disorders complicating pregnancy, unspecified trimester M ♀

O99.341 Other mental disorders complicating pregnancy, first trimester M ♀

O99.342 Other mental disorders complicating pregnancy, second trimester M ♀

O99.343 Other mental disorders complicating pregnancy, third trimester M ♀

O99.344 Other mental disorders complicating childbirth M ♀

O99.345 Other mental disorders complicating the puerperium M ♀

AHA: 2018,4Q,8

✓6th **O99.35 Diseases of the nervous system complicating pregnancy, childbirth, and the puerperium**

Conditions in G00-G99

EXCLUDES 2 *pregnancy related peripheral neuritis (O26.8-)*

O99.350 Diseases of the nervous system complicating pregnancy, unspecified trimester M ♀

O99.351 Diseases of the nervous system complicating pregnancy, first trimester M ♀

O99.352 Diseases of the nervous system complicating pregnancy, second trimester M ♀

O99.353 Diseases of the nervous system complicating pregnancy, third trimester M ♀

O99.354 Diseases of the nervous system complicating childbirth CC M ♀

O99.355 Diseases of the nervous system complicating the puerperium CC M ♀

O99.4 Diseases of the circulatory system complicating pregnancy, childbirth and the puerperium
Conditions in I00-I99
EXCLUDES 1 *peripartum cardiomyopathy (O90.3)*
EXCLUDES 2 *hypertensive disorders (O10-O16)*
obstetric embolism (O88.-)
venous complications and cerebrovenous sinus thrombosis in labor, childbirth and the puerperium (O87.-)
venous complications and cerebrovenous sinus thrombosis in pregnancy (O22.-)
AHA: 2016,2Q,8

O99.41 Diseases of the circulatory system complicating pregnancy
O99.411 Diseases of the circulatory system complicating pregnancy, first trimester CC M ♀
O99.412 Diseases of the circulatory system complicating pregnancy, second trimester CC M ♀
O99.413 Diseases of the circulatory system complicating pregnancy, third trimester CC M ♀
O99.419 Diseases of the circulatory system complicating pregnancy, unspecified trimester M ♀
O99.42 Diseases of the circulatory system complicating childbirth MCC M ♀
O99.43 Diseases of the circulatory system complicating the puerperium CC M ♀

O99.5 Diseases of the respiratory system complicating pregnancy, childbirth and the puerperium
Conditions in J00-J99

O99.51 Diseases of the respiratory system complicating pregnancy
O99.511 Diseases of the respiratory system complicating pregnancy, first trimester M ♀
O99.512 Diseases of the respiratory system complicating pregnancy, second trimester M ♀
O99.513 Diseases of the respiratory system complicating pregnancy, third trimester M ♀
O99.519 Diseases of the respiratory system complicating pregnancy, unspecified trimester M ♀
O99.52 Diseases of the respiratory system complicating childbirth M ♀
O99.53 Diseases of the respiratory system complicating the puerperium M ♀

O99.6 Diseases of the digestive system complicating pregnancy, childbirth and the puerperium
Conditions in K00-K93
EXCLUDES 2 *hemorrhoids in pregnancy (O22.4-)*
liver and biliary tract disorders in pregnancy, childbirth and the puerperium (O26.6-)

O99.61 Diseases of the digestive system complicating pregnancy
AHA: 2016,1Q,4
O99.611 Diseases of the digestive system complicating pregnancy, first trimester M ♀
O99.612 Diseases of the digestive system complicating pregnancy, second trimester M ♀
O99.613 Diseases of the digestive system complicating pregnancy, third trimester M ♀
O99.619 Diseases of the digestive system complicating pregnancy, unspecified trimester M ♀
O99.62 Diseases of the digestive system complicating childbirth M ♀
O99.63 Diseases of the digestive system complicating the puerperium M ♀

O99.7 Diseases of the skin and subcutaneous tissue complicating pregnancy, childbirth and the puerperium
Conditions in L00-L99
EXCLUDES 2 *herpes gestationis (O26.4)*
pruritic urticarial papules and plaques of pregnancy (PUPPP) (O26.86)

O99.71 Diseases of the skin and subcutaneous tissue complicating pregnancy
O99.711 Diseases of the skin and subcutaneous tissue complicating pregnancy, first trimester M ♀
O99.712 Diseases of the skin and subcutaneous tissue complicating pregnancy, second trimester M ♀
O99.713 Diseases of the skin and subcutaneous tissue complicating pregnancy, third trimester M ♀
O99.719 Diseases of the skin and subcutaneous tissue complicating pregnancy, unspecified trimester M ♀
O99.72 Diseases of the skin and subcutaneous tissue complicating childbirth M ♀
O99.73 Diseases of the skin and subcutaneous tissue complicating the puerperium M ♀

O99.8 Other specified diseases and conditions complicating pregnancy, childbirth and the puerperium
Conditions in D00-D48, H00-H95, M00-N99, and Q00-Q99
Use additional code to identify condition
EXCLUDES 2 *genitourinary infections in pregnancy (O23.-)*
infection of genitourinary tract following delivery (O86.1-O86.4)
malignant neoplasm complicating pregnancy, childbirth and the puerperium (O9A.1-)
maternal care for known or suspected abnormality of maternal pelvic organs (O34.-)
postpartum acute kidney failure ▶(O90.49)◀
traumatic injuries in pregnancy (O9A.2-)

O99.81 Abnormal glucose complicating pregnancy, childbirth and the puerperium
EXCLUDES 1 *gestational diabetes (O24.4-)*
O99.810 Abnormal glucose complicating pregnancy M ♀
O99.814 Abnormal glucose complicating childbirth M ♀
O99.815 Abnormal glucose complicating the puerperium M ♀

O99.82 Streptococcus B carrier state complicating pregnancy, childbirth and the puerperium
EXCLUDES 1 *carrier of streptococcus group B (GBS) in a nonpregnant woman (Z22.330)*
DEF: *Streptococcus* group B colonization: Bacteria normally found in the vagina or lower intestine of many healthy adult women that may infect the fetus during childbirth, causing mental or physical handicaps or death. Women who test positive for *Streptococcus* group B during pregnancy are considered a "colonized" status and are treated with IV antibiotics at the time of delivery and may also be treated with oral antibiotics during the pregnancy.
O99.820 Streptococcus B carrier state complicating pregnancy UPD M ♀
O99.824 Streptococcus B carrier state complicating childbirth M ♀
AHA: 2019,2Q,8
O99.825 Streptococcus B carrier state complicating the puerperium UPD M ♀

O99.83 Other infection carrier state complicating pregnancy, childbirth and the puerperium
Use additional code to identify the carrier state (Z22.-)
O99.830 Other infection carrier state complicating pregnancy CC M ♀
O99.834 Other infection carrier state complicating childbirth CC M ♀
O99.835 Other infection carrier state complicating the puerperium CC M ♀

Additional Character Required | x7th Placeholder | Questionable PDx | Manifestation | Unspecified | UPD Unacceptable PDx | H1-H14 HAC | HCC CMS-HCC Dx | HIV HIV Dx

√6th **O99.84 Bariatric surgery status complicating pregnancy, childbirth and the puerperium**
Gastric banding status complicating pregnancy, childbirth and the puerperium
Gastric bypass status for obesity complicating pregnancy, childbirth and the puerperium
Obesity surgery status complicating pregnancy, childbirth and the puerperium

O99.840 Bariatric surgery status complicating pregnancy, unspecified trimester M ♀
O99.841 Bariatric surgery status complicating pregnancy, first trimester M ♀
O99.842 Bariatric surgery status complicating pregnancy, second trimester M ♀
O99.843 Bariatric surgery status complicating pregnancy, third trimester M ♀
O99.844 Bariatric surgery status complicating childbirth M ♀
O99.845 Bariatric surgery status complicating the puerperium M ♀

√6th **O99.89 Other specified diseases and conditions complicating pregnancy, childbirth and the puerperium**
AHA: 2020,4Q,36-37

O99.891 Other specified diseases and conditions complicating pregnancy M ♀
O99.892 Other specified diseases and conditions complicating childbirth M ♀
O99.893 Other specified diseases and conditions complicating puerperium M ♀

√4th **O9A Maternal malignant neoplasms, traumatic injuries and abuse classifiable elsewhere but complicating pregnancy, childbirth and the puerperium**

√5th **O9A.1 Malignant neoplasm complicating pregnancy, childbirth and the puerperium**
Conditions in CØØ-C96
Use additional code to identify neoplasm
EXCLUDES 2 *maternal care for benign tumor of corpus uteri (O34.1-)*
maternal care for benign tumor of cervix (O34.4-)
AHA: 2015,3Q,19

√6th **O9A.11 Malignant neoplasm complicating pregnancy**
O9A.111 Malignant neoplasm complicating pregnancy, first trimester M ♀
O9A.112 Malignant neoplasm complicating pregnancy, second trimester M ♀
O9A.113 Malignant neoplasm complicating pregnancy, third trimester M ♀
O9A.119 Malignant neoplasm complicating pregnancy, unspecified trimester M ♀

O9A.12 Malignant neoplasm complicating childbirth M ♀
O9A.13 Malignant neoplasm complicating the puerperium M ♀

√5th **O9A.2 Injury, poisoning and certain other consequences of external causes complicating pregnancy, childbirth and the puerperium**
Conditions in SØØ-T88, except T74 and T76
Use additional code(s) to identify the injury or poisoning
EXCLUDES 2 *physical, sexual and psychological abuse complicating pregnancy, childbirth and the puerperium (O9A.3-, O9A.4-, O9A.5-)*

√6th **O9A.21 Injury, poisoning and certain other consequences of external causes complicating pregnancy**
O9A.211 Injury, poisoning and certain other consequences of external causes complicating pregnancy, first trimester M ♀
O9A.212 Injury, poisoning and certain other consequences of external causes complicating pregnancy, second trimester M ♀
O9A.213 Injury, poisoning and certain other consequences of external causes complicating pregnancy, third trimester M ♀
O9A.219 Injury, poisoning and certain other consequences of external causes complicating pregnancy, unspecified trimester M ♀

O9A.22 Injury, poisoning and certain other consequences of external causes complicating childbirth M ♀
O9A.23 Injury, poisoning and certain other consequences of external causes complicating the puerperium M ♀

√5th **O9A.3 Physical abuse complicating pregnancy, childbirth and the puerperium**
Conditions in T74.11 or T76.11
Use additional code (if applicable):
to identify any associated current injury due to physical abuse
to identify the perpetrator of abuse (YØ7.-)
EXCLUDES 2 *sexual abuse complicating pregnancy, childbirth and the puerperium (O9A.4)*

√6th **O9A.31 Physical abuse complicating pregnancy**
O9A.311 Physical abuse complicating pregnancy, first trimester M ♀
O9A.312 Physical abuse complicating pregnancy, second trimester M ♀
O9A.313 Physical abuse complicating pregnancy, third trimester M ♀
O9A.319 Physical abuse complicating pregnancy, unspecified trimester M ♀

O9A.32 Physical abuse complicating childbirth M ♀
O9A.33 Physical abuse complicating the puerperium M ♀

√5th **O9A.4 Sexual abuse complicating pregnancy, childbirth and the puerperium**
Conditions in T74.21 or T76.21
Use additional code (if applicable):
to identify any associated current injury due to sexual abuse
to identify the perpetrator of abuse (YØ7.-)

√6th **O9A.41 Sexual abuse complicating pregnancy**
O9A.411 Sexual abuse complicating pregnancy, first trimester M ♀
O9A.412 Sexual abuse complicating pregnancy, second trimester M ♀
O9A.413 Sexual abuse complicating pregnancy, third trimester M ♀
O9A.419 Sexual abuse complicating pregnancy, unspecified trimester M ♀

O9A.42 Sexual abuse complicating childbirth M ♀
O9A.43 Sexual abuse complicating the puerperium M ♀

√5th **O9A.5 Psychological abuse complicating pregnancy, childbirth and the puerperium**
Conditions in T74.31 or T76.31
Use additional code to identify the perpetrator of abuse (YØ7.-)

√6th **O9A.51 Psychological abuse complicating pregnancy**
O9A.511 Psychological abuse complicating pregnancy, first trimester M ♀
O9A.512 Psychological abuse complicating pregnancy, second trimester M ♀
O9A.513 Psychological abuse complicating pregnancy, third trimester M ♀
O9A.519 Psychological abuse complicating pregnancy, unspecified trimester M ♀

O9A.52 Psychological abuse complicating childbirth M ♀
O9A.53 Psychological abuse complicating the puerperium M ♀

Chapter 16. Certain Conditions Originating in the Perinatal Period (PØØ–P96)

Chapter-specific Guidelines with Coding Examples

The chapter-specific guidelines from the ICD-10-CM Official Guidelines for Coding and Reporting have been provided below. Along with these guidelines are coding examples, contained in the shaded boxes, that have been developed to help illustrate the coding and/or sequencing guidance found in these guidelines.

For coding and reporting purposes the perinatal period is defined as before birth through the 28th day following birth. The following guidelines are provided for reporting purposes

a. General perinatal rules

1) Use of Chapter 16 codes

Codes in this chapter are never for use on the maternal record. Codes from Chapter 15, the obstetric chapter, are never permitted on the newborn record. Chapter 16 codes may be used throughout the life of the patient if the condition is still present.

2) Principal diagnosis for birth record

When coding the birth episode in a newborn record, assign a code from category Z38, Liveborn infants according to place of birth and type of delivery, as the principal diagnosis. A code from category Z38 is assigned only once, to a newborn at the time of birth. If a newborn is transferred to another institution, a code from category Z38 should not be used at the receiving hospital.

A code from category Z38 is used only on the newborn record, not on the mother's record.

> Newborn delivered via vaginal delivery in Rural Hospital A, experienced meconium aspiration resulting in pneumonia. Rural Hospital A is not equipped to handle the extensive respiratory therapy this baby needs and transfers the patient to Metropolis Hospital B, where the pneumonia resolves and the newborn is eventually discharged.
>
> *Rural Hospital A*
>
> **Z38.ØØ Single liveborn infant, delivered vaginally**
>
> **P24.Ø1 Meconium aspiration with respiratory symptoms**
>
> Metropolis Hospital B
>
> **P24.Ø1 Meconium aspiration with respiratory symptoms**
>
> *Explanation:* A code from category Z38 is a one-time use only code. The hospital that actually delivered the newborn, in this case Rural Hospital A, can append a code from category Z38 but for the delivery admission only. Once the patient is transferred or discharged, the Z38 category no longer applies for that patient.
>
> The reason for the transfer to Metropolis Hospital B was for the respiratory symptoms (pneumonia) the newborn was exhibiting secondary to aspirating meconium.

3) Use of codes from other chapters with codes from Chapter 16

Codes from other chapters may be used with codes from chapter 16 if the codes from the other chapters provide more specific detail. Codes for signs and symptoms may be assigned when a definitive diagnosis has not been established. If the reason for the encounter is a perinatal condition, the code from chapter 16 should be sequenced first.

4) Use of Chapter 16 codes after the perinatal period

Should a condition originate in the perinatal period, and continue throughout the life of the patient, the perinatal code should continue to be used regardless of the patient's age.

> A 7-year-old patient with history of birth injury that resulted in Erb's palsy is seen for subscapularis release
>
> **P14.Ø Erb's paralysis due to birth injury**
>
> *Explanation:* Although in this instance Erb's palsy is specifically related to a birth injury, it has not resolved and continues to be a health concern. A perinatal code is appropriate even though this patient is beyond the perinatal period.

5) Birth process or community acquired conditions

If a newborn has a condition that may be either due to the birth process or community acquired and the documentation does not indicate which it is, the default is due to the birth process and the code from Chapter 16 should be used. If the condition is community-acquired, a code from Chapter 16 should not be assigned.

For COVID-19 infection in a newborn, see guideline I.C.16.h.

6) Code all clinically significant conditions

All clinically significant conditions noted on routine newborn examination should be coded. A condition is clinically significant if it requires:

clinical evaluation; or

therapeutic treatment; or

diagnostic procedures; or

extended length of hospital stay; or

increased nursing care and/or monitoring; or

has implications for future health care needs

Note: The perinatal guidelines listed above are the same as the general coding guidelines for "additional diagnoses", except for the final point regarding implications for future health care needs. Codes should be assigned for conditions that have been specified by the provider as having implications for future health care needs.

b. Observation and evaluation of newborns for suspected conditions not found

1) Use of ZØ5 codes

Assign a code from category ZØ5, Observation and evaluation of newborn for suspected diseases and conditions ruled out, to identify those instances when a healthy newborn is evaluated for a suspected condition/disease that is determined after study not to be present. Do not use a code from category ZØ5 when the patient is documented to have signs or symptoms of a suspected problem; in such cases code the sign or symptom.

2) ZØ5 on other than the birth record

A code from category ZØ5 may also be assigned as a principal or first-listed code for readmissions or encounters when the code from category Z38 code no longer applies. Codes from category ZØ5 are for use only for healthy newborns and infants for which no condition after study is found to be present.

3) ZØ5 on a birth record

A code from category ZØ5 is to be used as a secondary code after the code from category Z38, Liveborn infants according to place of birth and type of delivery.

> Newborn delivered via vaginal delivery; previous ultrasounds showed what appeared to be an abnormality of the right kidney. Kidney function tests were performed and ultrasounds taken and any genitourinary conditions ruled out.
>
> **Z38.ØØ Single liveborn infant, delivered vaginally**
>
> **ZØ5.6 Observation and evaluation of newborn for suspected genitourinary condition ruled out**
>
> Explanation: The newborn had no signs or symptoms of kidney or other genitourinary condition but was evaluated after delivery due to the abnormal prenatal ultrasound findings. A Z code describing the type and place of birth should be coded first, followed by a Z05 category code for the work performed to rule out a suspected genitourinary condition.

c. Coding additional perinatal diagnoses

1) Assigning codes for conditions that require treatment

Assign codes for conditions that require treatment or further investigation, prolong the length of stay, or require resource utilization.

2) Codes for conditions specified as having implications for future health care needs

Assign codes for conditions that have been specified by the provider as having implications for future health care needs.

Note: This guideline should not be used for adult patients.

An abnormal noise was heard in the left hip of a post-term newborn during a physical examination. The pediatrician would like to follow the patient after discharge as a hip click can be an early sign of hip dysplasia. The newborn was delivered via cesarean at 41 weeks.

Z38.Ø1	**Single liveborn infant, delivered by cesarean**
PØ8.21	**Post-term newborn**
R29.4	**Clicking hip**

Explanation: The abnormal hip noise or click is appended as a secondary diagnosis not only because it is an abnormal finding upon examination, but also due to its potential to be part of a bigger health issue. The hip dysplasia has not yet been diagnosed and does not warrant a code at this time.

d. Prematurity and fetal growth retardation

Providers utilize different criteria in determining prematurity. A code for prematurity should not be assigned unless it is documented. Assignment of codes in categories PØ5, Disorders of newborn related to slow fetal growth and fetal malnutrition, and PØ7, Disorders of newborn related to short gestation and low birth weight, not elsewhere classified, should be based on the recorded birth weight and estimated gestational age.

When both birth weight and gestational age are available, two codes from category PØ7 should be assigned, with the code for birth weight sequenced before the code for gestational age.

e. Low birth weight and immaturity status

Codes from category PØ7, Disorders of newborn related to short gestation and low birth weight, not elsewhere classified, are for use for a child or adult who was premature or had a low birth weight as a newborn and this is affecting the patient's current health status.

See Section I.C.21. Factors influencing health status and contact with health services, Status.

A 35-year-old patient, who weighed 659 grams at birth, is seen for heart disease documented as being a consequence of the low birth weight

I51.9	**Heart disease, unspecified**
PØ7.Ø2	**Extremely low birth weight newborn, 5ØØ–749 grams**

Explanation: A code from subcategories PØ7.Ø- and PØ7.1- is appropriate, regardless of the age of the patient, as long as the documentation provides a clear link between the patient's current illness and the low birth weight.

f. Bacterial sepsis of newborn

Category P36, Bacterial sepsis of newborn, includes congenital sepsis. If a perinate is documented as having sepsis without documentation of congenital or community acquired, the default is congenital and a code from category P36 should be assigned. If the P36 code includes the causal organism, an additional code from category B95, Streptococcus, Staphylococcus, and Enterococcus as the cause of diseases classified elsewhere, or B96, Other bacterial agents as the cause of diseases classified elsewhere, should not be assigned. If the P36 code does not include the causal organism, assign an additional code from category B96. If applicable, use additional codes to identify severe sepsis (R65.2-) and any associated acute organ dysfunction.

A full-term infant develops severe sepsis 24 hours after discharge from the hospital and is readmitted; cultures identified *E. coli* as the infective agent

P36.4	**Sepsis of newborn due to Escherichia coli**
R65.2Ø	**Severe sepsis without septic shock**

Explanation: Even though this newborn was discharged and could have acquired *E. coli* from his/her external environment, due to the lack of documentation specifying specifically how this pathogen was acquired, the default is to code the *E. coli* sepsis as congenital. A code from chapter 1, "Certain Infectious and Parasitic Diseases," is not required because the perinatal sepsis code identifies both the sepsis and the bacteria causing the sepsis.

g. Stillbirth

Code P95, Stillbirth, is only for use in institutions that maintain separate records for stillbirths. No other code should be used with P95. Code P95 should not be used on the mother's record.

h. COVID-19 infection in newborn

For a newborn that tests positive for COVID-19, assign code UØ7.1, COVID-19, and the appropriate codes for associated manifestation(s) in neonates/newborns in the absence of documentation indicating a specific type of transmission. For a newborn that tests positive for COVID-19 and the provider documents the condition was contracted in utero or during the birth process, assign codes P35.8, Other congenital viral diseases, and UØ7.1, COVID-19. When coding the birth episode in a newborn record, the appropriate code from category Z38, Liveborn infants according to place of birth and type of delivery, should be assigned as the principal diagnosis.

Chapter 16. Certain Conditions Originating in the Perinatal Period (P00-P96)

NOTE Codes from this chapter are for use on newborn records only, never on maternal records

INCLUDES conditions that have their origin in the fetal or perinatal period (before birth through the first 28 days after birth) even if morbidity occurs later

EXCLUDES 2 *congenital malformations, deformations and chromosomal abnormalities (Q00-Q99)*
endocrine, nutritional and metabolic diseases (E00-E88)
injury, poisoning and certain other consequences of external causes (S00-T88)
neoplasms (C00-D49)
tetanus neonatorum (A33)

This chapter contains the following blocks:

P00-P04 Newborn affected by maternal factors and by complications of pregnancy, labor, and delivery
P05-P08 Disorders of newborn related to length of gestation and fetal growth
P09 Abnormal findings on neonatal screening
P10-P15 Birth trauma
P19-P29 Respiratory and cardiovascular disorders specific to the perinatal period
P35-P39 Infections specific to the perinatal period
P50-P61 Hemorrhagic and hematological disorders of newborn
P70-P74 Transitory endocrine and metabolic disorders specific to newborn
P76-P78 Digestive system disorders of newborn
P80-P83 Conditions involving the integument and temperature regulation of newborn
P84 Other problems with newborn
P90-P96 Other disorders originating in the perinatal period

Newborn affected by maternal factors and by complications of pregnancy, labor, and delivery (P00-P04)

NOTE These codes are for use when the listed maternal conditions are specified as the cause of confirmed morbidity or potential morbidity which have their origin in the perinatal period (before birth through the first 28 days after birth).

AHA: 2016,4Q,54-55

✓4th **P00 Newborn affected by maternal conditions that may be unrelated to present pregnancy**
Code first any current condition in newborn
EXCLUDES 2 *encounter for observation of newborn for suspected diseases and conditions ruled out (Z05.-)*
newborn affected by maternal complications of pregnancy (P01.-)
newborn affected by maternal endocrine and metabolic disorders (P70-P74)
newborn affected by noxious substances transmitted via placenta or breast milk (P04.-)

P00.0 Newborn affected by maternal hypertensive disorders
Newborn affected by maternal conditions classifiable to O10-O11, O13-O16

P00.1 Newborn affected by maternal renal and urinary tract diseases
Newborn affected by maternal conditions classifiable to N00-N39

P00.2 Newborn affected by maternal infectious and parasitic diseases
Newborn affected by maternal infectious disease classifiable to A00-B99, J09 and J10
EXCLUDES 1 *maternal genital tract or other localized infections (P00.8)*
EXCLUDES 2 *infections specific to the perinatal period (P35-P39)*
newborn affected by (positive) maternal group B streptococcus (GBS) colonization (P00.82)
AHA: 2019,2Q,10; 2015,3Q,20

P00.3 Newborn affected by other maternal circulatory and respiratory diseases
Newborn affected by maternal conditions classifiable to I00-I99, J00-J99, Q20-Q34 and not included in P00.0, P00.2

P00.4 Newborn affected by maternal nutritional disorders
Newborn affected by maternal disorders classifiable to E40-E64
Maternal malnutrition NOS

P00.5 Newborn affected by maternal injury
Newborn affected by maternal conditions classifiable to O9A.2-

P00.6 Newborn affected by surgical procedure on mother
Newborn affected by amniocentesis
EXCLUDES 1 *Cesarean delivery for present delivery (P03.4)*
damage to placenta from amniocentesis, Cesarean delivery or surgical induction (P02.1)
previous surgery to uterus or pelvic organs (P03.89)
EXCLUDES 2 *newborn affected by complication of (fetal) intrauterine procedure (P96.5)*

P00.7 Newborn affected by other medical procedures on mother, not elsewhere classified
Newborn affected by radiation to mother
EXCLUDES 1 *damage to placenta from amniocentesis, cesarean delivery or surgical induction (P02.1)*
newborn affected by other complications of labor and delivery (P03.-)

✓5th **P00.8 Newborn affected by other maternal conditions**

P00.81 Newborn affected by periodontal disease in mother

P00.82 Newborn affected by (positive) maternal group B streptococcus (GBS) colonization
Contact with positive maternal group B streptococcus
AHA: 2021,4Q,23

P00.89 Newborn affected by other maternal conditions
Newborn affected by conditions classifiable to T80-T88
Newborn affected by maternal genital tract or other localized infections
Newborn affected by maternal systemic lupus erythematosus
Use additional code to identify infectious agent, if known
EXCLUDES 2 *newborn affected by positive maternal group B streptococcus (GBS) colonization (P00.82)*
AHA: 2019,2Q,9

P00.9 Newborn affected by unspecified maternal condition

✓4th **P01 Newborn affected by maternal complications of pregnancy**
Code first any current condition in newborn
EXCLUDES 2 *encounter for observation of newborn for suspected diseases and conditions ruled out (Z05.-)*

P01.0 Newborn affected by incompetent cervix

P01.1 Newborn affected by premature rupture of membranes

P01.2 Newborn affected by oligohydramnios
EXCLUDES 1 *oligohydramnios due to premature rupture of membranes (P01.1)*
DEF: Low amniotic fluid level, resulting in underdeveloped organs in the fetus.

P01.3 Newborn affected by polyhydramnios
Newborn affected by hydramnios
DEF: Excess amniotic fluid surrounding the fetus, typically defined as a total fluid volume of greater than 24 cm.

P01.4 Newborn affected by ectopic pregnancy
Newborn affected by abdominal pregnancy

P01.5 Newborn affected by multiple pregnancy
Newborn affected by triplet (pregnancy)
Newborn affected by twin (pregnancy)

P01.6 Newborn affected by maternal death

P01.7 Newborn affected by malpresentation before labor
Newborn affected by breech presentation before labor
Newborn affected by external version before labor
Newborn affected by face presentation before labor
Newborn affected by transverse lie before labor
Newborn affected by unstable lie before labor

P01.8 Newborn affected by other maternal complications of pregnancy

P01.9 Newborn affected by maternal complication of pregnancy, unspecified

✓4th **P02 Newborn affected by complications of placenta, cord and membranes**
Code first any current condition in newborn
EXCLUDES 2 *encounter for observation of newborn for suspected diseases and conditions ruled out (Z05.-)*

P02.0 Newborn affected by placenta previa
DEF: Placenta developed in the lower segment of the uterus that can cause hemorrhaging leading to preterm delivery.

P02.1 Newborn affected by other forms of placental separation and hemorrhage
Newborn affected by abruptio placenta
Newborn affected by accidental hemorrhage
Newborn affected by antepartum hemorrhage
Newborn affected by damage to placenta from amniocentesis, cesarean delivery or surgical induction
Newborn affected by maternal blood loss
Newborn affected by premature separation of placenta

✓5th **P02.2 Newborn affected by other and unspecified morphological and functional abnormalities of placenta**

P02.20 Newborn affected by unspecified morphological and functional abnormalities of placenta

P02.29 Newborn affected by other morphological and functional abnormalities of placenta
Newborn affected by placental dysfunction
Newborn affected by placental infarction
Newborn affected by placental insufficiency

P02.3 Newborn affected by placental transfusion syndromes
Newborn affected by placental and cord abnormalities resulting in twin-to-twin or other transplacental transfusion

P02.4 Newborn affected by prolapsed cord

P02.5 Newborn affected by other compression of umbilical cord
Newborn affected by entanglement of umbilical cord
Newborn affected by knot in umbilical cord
Newborn affected by umbilical cord (tightly) around neck
AHA: 2022,1Q,22

✓5th **P02.6 Newborn affected by other and unspecified conditions of umbilical cord**

P02.60 Newborn affected by unspecified conditions of umbilical cord

P02.69 Newborn affected by other conditions of umbilical cord
Newborn affected by short umbilical cord
Newborn affected by vasa previa
EXCLUDES 1 *newborn affected by single umbilical artery (Q27.0)*

✓5th **P02.7 Newborn affected by chorioamnionitis**
AHA: 2018,4Q,23-24
DEF: Inflammation of the fetal membranes due to maternal infection characterized by fetal tachycardia, respiratory distress, apnea, weak cries, and poor sucking.

P02.70 Newborn affected by fetal inflammatory response syndrome HCC
Newborn affected by FIRS

P02.78 Newborn affected by other conditions from chorioamnionitis
Newborn affected by amnionitis
Newborn affected by membranitis
Newborn affected by placentitis

P02.8 Newborn affected by other abnormalities of membranes

P02.9 Newborn affected by abnormality of membranes, unspecified

✓4th **P03 Newborn affected by other complications of labor and delivery**
Code first any current condition in newborn
EXCLUDES 2 *encounter for observation of newborn for suspected diseases and conditions ruled out (Z05.-)*

P03.0 Newborn affected by breech delivery and extraction

P03.1 Newborn affected by other malpresentation, malposition and disproportion during labor and delivery
Newborn affected by contracted pelvis
Newborn affected by conditions classifiable to O64-O66
Newborn affected by persistent occipitoposterior
Newborn affected by transverse lie

P03.2 Newborn affected by forceps delivery

Forceps Assisted Birth

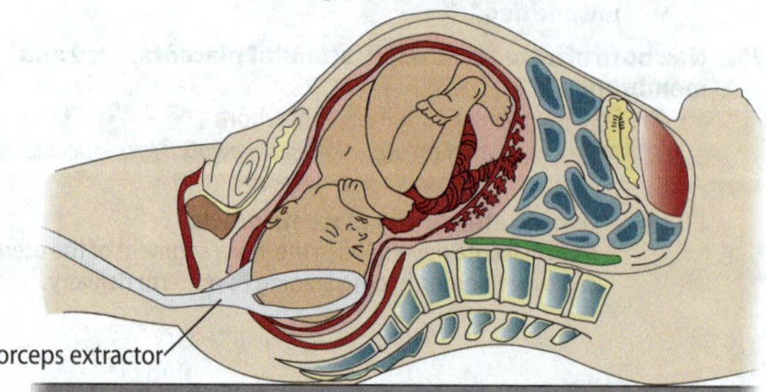

P03.3 Newborn affected by delivery by vacuum extractor [ventouse]

Vacuum Assisted Birth

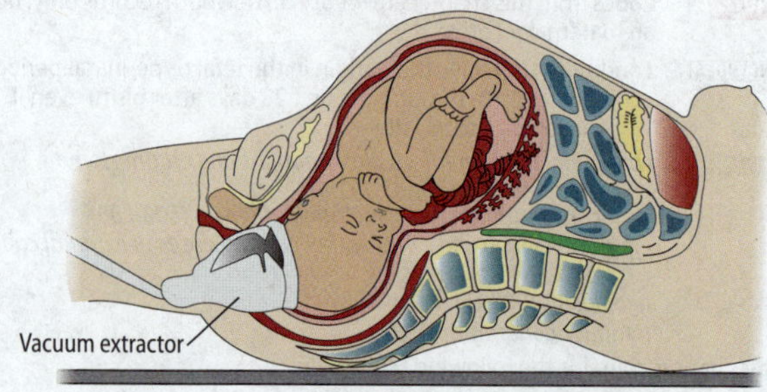

P03.4 Newborn affected by Cesarean delivery

P03.5 Newborn affected by precipitate delivery
Newborn affected by rapid second stage

P03.6 Newborn affected by abnormal uterine contractions
Newborn affected by conditions classifiable to O62.-, except O62.3
Newborn affected by hypertonic labor
Newborn affected by uterine inertia

✓5th **P03.8 Newborn affected by other specified complications of labor and delivery**

✓6th **P03.81 Newborn affected by abnormality in fetal (intrauterine) heart rate or rhythm**
EXCLUDES 1 *neonatal cardiac dysrhythmia (P29.1-)*

P03.810 Newborn affected by abnormality in fetal (intrauterine) heart rate or rhythm before the onset of labor

P03.811 Newborn affected by abnormality in fetal (intrauterine) heart rate or rhythm during labor

P03.819 Newborn affected by abnormality in fetal (intrauterine) heart rate or rhythm, unspecified as to time of onset

P03.82 Meconium passage during delivery
EXCLUDES 1 *meconium aspiration (P24.00, P24.01)*
meconium staining (P96.83)
DEF: Fetal intestinal activity that increases in response to a fetomaternal distressed state during delivery. The anal sphincter relaxes and meconium is passed into the amniotic fluid.

P03.89 Newborn affected by other specified complications of labor and delivery
Newborn affected by abnormality of maternal soft tissues
Newborn affected by conditions classifiable to O60-O75 and by procedures used in labor and delivery not included in P02.- and P03.0-P03.6
Newborn affected by induction of labor

P03.9 Newborn affected by complication of labor and delivery, unspecified

✓4th **P04 Newborn affected by noxious substances transmitted via placenta or breast milk**
INCLUDES nonteratogenic effects of substances transmitted via placenta
Code first any current condition in newborn, if applicable
EXCLUDES 2 *congenital malformations (Q00-Q99)*
encounter for observation of newborn for suspected diseases and conditions ruled out (Z05.-)
neonatal jaundice from excessive hemolysis due to drugs or toxins transmitted from mother (P58.4)
newborn in contact with and (suspected) exposures hazardous to health not transmitted via placenta or breast milk (Z77.-)

P04.0 Newborn affected by maternal anesthesia and analgesia in pregnancy, labor and delivery
Newborn affected by reactions and intoxications from maternal opiates and tranquilizers administered for procedures during pregnancy or labor and delivery
EXCLUDES 2 *newborn affected by other maternal medication (P04.1-)*

P04.1 Newborn affected by other maternal medication

▶Code first, if applicable, withdrawal symptoms from maternal use of drugs of addiction◀ (P96.1)
▶withdrawal symptoms from therapeutic use of drugs in newborn (P96.2)◀

EXCLUDES 1 *dysmorphism due to warfarin (Q86.2)*
fetal hydantoin syndrome (Q86.1)

EXCLUDES 2 *maternal anesthesia and analgesia in pregnancy, labor and delivery (P04.0)*
maternal use of drugs of addiction (P04.4-)

AHA: 2018,4Q,24-25

P04.11 Newborn affected by maternal antineoplastic chemotherapy
P04.12 Newborn affected by maternal cytotoxic drugs
P04.13 Newborn affected by maternal use of anticonvulsants
P04.14 Newborn affected by maternal use of opiates
P04.15 Newborn affected by maternal use of antidepressants
P04.16 Newborn affected by maternal use of amphetamines
P04.17 Newborn affected by maternal use of sedative-hypnotics
P04.1A Newborn affected by maternal use of anxiolytics
P04.18 Newborn affected by other maternal medication
P04.19 Newborn affected by maternal use of unspecified medication

P04.2 Newborn affected by maternal use of tobacco

Newborn affected by exposure in utero to tobacco smoke

EXCLUDES 2 *newborn exposure to environmental tobacco smoke (P96.81)*

P04.3 Newborn affected by maternal use of alcohol

EXCLUDES 1 *fetal alcohol syndrome (Q86.0)*

P04.4 Newborn affected by maternal use of drugs of addiction

AHA: 2018,4Q,25

P04.40 Newborn affected by maternal use of unspecified drugs of addiction
P04.41 Newborn affected by maternal use of cocaine
P04.42 Newborn affected by maternal use of hallucinogens

EXCLUDES 2 *newborn affected by other maternal medication (P04.1-)*

P04.49 Newborn affected by maternal use of other drugs of addiction

EXCLUDES 2 *newborn affected by maternal anesthesia and analgesia (P04.0)*
withdrawal symptoms from maternal use of drugs of addiction (P96.1)

P04.5 Newborn affected by maternal use of nutritional chemical substances

P04.6 Newborn affected by maternal exposure to environmental chemical substances

P04.8 Newborn affected by other maternal noxious substances

AHA: 2018,4Q,25

P04.81 Newborn affected by maternal use of cannabis
P04.89 Newborn affected by other maternal noxious substances

P04.9 Newborn affected by maternal noxious substance, unspecified

Disorders of newborn related to length of gestation and fetal growth (P05-P08)

P05 Disorders of newborn related to slow fetal growth and fetal malnutrition

AHA: 2016,4Q,55-56

P05.0 Newborn light for gestational age

Newborn light-for-dates
Weight below but length above 10th percentile for gestational age

P05.00 Newborn light for gestational age, unspecified weight
P05.01 Newborn light for gestational age, less than 500 grams
P05.02 Newborn light for gestational age, 500-749 grams
P05.03 Newborn light for gestational age, 750-999 grams
P05.04 Newborn light for gestational age, 1000-1249 grams
P05.05 Newborn light for gestational age, 1250-1499 grams
P05.06 Newborn light for gestational age, 1500-1749 grams
P05.07 Newborn light for gestational age, 1750-1999 grams
P05.08 Newborn light for gestational age, 2000-2499 grams
P05.09 Newborn light for gestational age, 2500 grams and over

Newborn light for gestational age, other

P05.1 Newborn small for gestational age

Newborn small-and-light-for-dates
Newborn small-for-dates
Weight and length below 10th percentile for gestational age

P05.10 Newborn small for gestational age, unspecified weight
P05.11 Newborn small for gestational age, less than 500 grams
P05.12 Newborn small for gestational age, 500-749 grams
P05.13 Newborn small for gestational age, 750-999 grams
P05.14 Newborn small for gestational age, 1000-1249 grams
P05.15 Newborn small for gestational age, 1250-1499 grams
P05.16 Newborn small for gestational age, 1500-1749 grams
P05.17 Newborn small for gestational age, 1750-1999 grams
P05.18 Newborn small for gestational age, 2000-2499 grams
P05.19 Newborn small for gestational age, other

Newborn small for gestational age, 2500 grams and over

P05.2 Newborn affected by fetal (intrauterine) malnutrition not light or small for gestational age

Infant, not light or small for gestational age, showing signs of fetal malnutrition, such as dry, peeling skin and loss of subcutaneous tissue

EXCLUDES 1 *newborn affected by fetal malnutrition with light for gestational age (P05.0-)*
newborn affected by fetal malnutrition with small for gestational age (P05.1-)

P05.9 Newborn affected by slow intrauterine growth, unspecified

Newborn affected by fetal growth retardation NOS

P07 Disorders of newborn related to short gestation and low birth weight, not elsewhere classified

NOTE When both birth weight and gestational age of the newborn are available, both should be coded with birth weight sequenced before gestational age

INCLUDES the listed conditions, without further specification, as the cause of morbidity or additional care, in newborn

P07.0 Extremely low birth weight newborn

Newborn birth weight 999 g. or less

EXCLUDES 1 *low birth weight due to slow fetal growth and fetal malnutrition (P05.-)*

P07.00 Extremely low birth weight newborn, unspecified weight
P07.01 Extremely low birth weight newborn, less than 500 grams
P07.02 Extremely low birth weight newborn, 500-749 grams
P07.03 Extremely low birth weight newborn, 750-999 grams

P07.1 Other low birth weight newborn

Newborn birth weight 1000-2499 g.

EXCLUDES 1 *low birth weight due to slow fetal growth and fetal malnutrition (P05.-)*

P07.10 Other low birth weight newborn, unspecified weight
P07.14 Other low birth weight newborn, 1000-1249 grams
P07.15 Other low birth weight newborn, 1250-1499 grams
P07.16 Other low birth weight newborn, 1500-1749 grams
P07.17 Other low birth weight newborn, 1750-1999 grams
P07.18 Other low birth weight newborn, 2000-2499 grams

P07.2 Extreme immaturity of newborn

Less than 28 completed weeks (less than 196 completed days) of gestation.

P07.20 Extreme immaturity of newborn, unspecified weeks of gestation

Gestational age less than 28 completed weeks NOS

P07.21 Extreme immaturity of newborn, gestational age less than 23 completed weeks
Extreme immaturity of newborn, gestational age less than 23 weeks, 0 days

P07.22 Extreme immaturity of newborn, gestational age 23 completed weeks
Extreme immaturity of newborn, gestational age 23 weeks, 0 days through 23 weeks, 6 days

P07.23 Extreme immaturity of newborn, gestational age 24 completed weeks
Extreme immaturity of newborn, gestational age 24 weeks, 0 days through 24 weeks, 6 days

P07.24 Extreme immaturity of newborn, gestational age 25 completed weeks
Extreme immaturity of newborn, gestational age 25 weeks, 0 days through 25 weeks, 6 days

P07.25 Extreme immaturity of newborn, gestational age 26 completed weeks
Extreme immaturity of newborn, gestational age 26 weeks, 0 days through 26 weeks, 6 days

P07.26 Extreme immaturity of newborn, gestational age 27 completed weeks
Extreme immaturity of newborn, gestational age 27 weeks, 0 days through 27 weeks, 6 days

√5th **P07.3 Preterm [premature] newborn [other]**
28 completed weeks or more but less than 37 completed weeks (196 completed days but less than 259 completed days) of gestation
Prematurity NOS
AHA: 2017,3Q,26

P07.30 Preterm newborn, unspecified weeks of gestation

P07.31 Preterm newborn, gestational age 28 completed weeks
Preterm newborn, gestational age 28 weeks, 0 days through 28 weeks, 6 days

P07.32 Preterm newborn, gestational age 29 completed weeks
Preterm newborn, gestational age 29 weeks, 0 days through 29 weeks, 6 days

P07.33 Preterm newborn, gestational age 30 completed weeks
Preterm newborn, gestational age 30 weeks, 0 days through 30 weeks, 6 days

P07.34 Preterm newborn, gestational age 31 completed weeks
Preterm newborn, gestational age 31 weeks, 0 days through 31 weeks, 6 days

P07.35 Preterm newborn, gestational age 32 completed weeks
Preterm newborn, gestational age 32 weeks, 0 days through 32 weeks, 6 days

P07.36 Preterm newborn, gestational age 33 completed weeks
Preterm newborn, gestational age 33 weeks, 0 days through 33 weeks, 6 days

P07.37 Preterm newborn, gestational age 34 completed weeks
Preterm newborn, gestational age 34 weeks, 0 days through 34 weeks, 6 days

P07.38 Preterm newborn, gestational age 35 completed weeks
Preterm newborn, gestational age 35 weeks, 0 days through 35 weeks, 6 days

P07.39 Preterm newborn, gestational age 36 completed weeks
Preterm newborn, gestational age 36 weeks, 0 days through 36 weeks, 6 days

√4th **P08 Disorders of newborn related to long gestation and high birth weight**

NOTE When both birth weight and gestational age of the newborn are available, priority of assignment should be given to birth weight

INCLUDES the listed conditions, without further specification, as causes of morbidity or additional care, in newborn

P08.0 Exceptionally large newborn baby
Usually implies a birth weight of 4500 g. or more
EXCLUDES 1 *syndrome of infant of diabetic mother (P70.1)*
syndrome of infant of mother with gestational diabetes (P70.0)

P08.1 Other heavy for gestational age newborn
Other newborn heavy- or large-for-dates regardless of period of gestation
Usually implies a birth weight of 4000 g. to 4499 g.
EXCLUDES 1 *newborn with a birth weight of 4500 or more (P08.0)*
syndrome of infant of diabetic mother (P70.1)
syndrome of infant of mother with gestational diabetes (P70.0)

√5th **P08.2 Late newborn, not heavy for gestational age**
AHA: 2014,1Q,14

P08.21 Post-term newborn
Newborn with gestation period over 40 completed weeks to 42 completed weeks

P08.22 Prolonged gestation of newborn
Newborn with gestation period over 42 completed weeks (294 days or more), not heavy- or large-for-dates.
Postmaturity NOS

Abnormal findings on neonatal screening (P09)

√4th **P09 Abnormal findings on neonatal screening**
INCLUDES abnormal findings on state mandated newborn screens
failed newborn screening
EXCLUDES 2 *nonspecific serologic evidence of human immunodeficiency virus [HIV] (R75)*
AHA: 2021,4Q,24

P09.1 Abnormal findings on neonatal screening for inborn errors of metabolism

P09.2 Abnormal findings on neonatal screening for congenital endocrine disease
Abnormal findings on neonatal screening for congenital adrenal hyperplasia
Abnormal findings on neonatal screening for hypothyroidism screen

P09.3 Abnormal findings on neonatal screening for congenital hematologic disorders
▶Abnormal findings for hemoglobinopathy screening◀
Abnormal findings on red cell membrane defects screen
Abnormal findings on sickle cell screen

P09.4 Abnormal findings on neonatal screening for cystic fibrosis

P09.5 Abnormal findings on neonatal screening for critical congenital heart disease
Neonatal congenital heart disease screening failure

P09.6 Abnormal findings on neonatal screening for neonatal hearing loss
EXCLUDES 2 *encounter for hearing examination following failed hearing screening (Z01.110)*

P09.8 Other abnormal findings on neonatal screening

P09.9 Abnormal findings on neonatal screening, unspecified

Birth trauma (P10-P15)

√4th **P10 Intracranial laceration and hemorrhage due to birth injury**
EXCLUDES 1 *intracranial hemorrhage of newborn NOS (P52.9)*
intracranial hemorrhage of newborn due to anoxia or hypoxia (P52.-)
nontraumatic intracranial hemorrhage of newborn (P52.-)

P10.0 Subdural hemorrhage due to birth injury MCC
Subdural hematoma (localized) due to birth injury
EXCLUDES 1 *subdural hemorrhage accompanying tentorial tear (P10.4)*

P10.1 Cerebral hemorrhage due to birth injury MCC

P10.2 Intraventricular hemorrhage due to birth injury CC

P10.3 Subarachnoid hemorrhage due to birth injury MCC

P10.4 Tentorial tear due to birth injury MCC

P10.8 Other intracranial lacerations and hemorrhages due to birth injury MCC

P10.9 Unspecified intracranial laceration and hemorrhage due to birth injury MCC

√4th **P11 Other birth injuries to central nervous system**

P11.0 Cerebral edema due to birth injury MCC

P11.1 Other specified brain damage due to birth injury

P11.2 Unspecified brain damage due to birth injury MCC

P11.3 Birth injury to facial nerve
Facial palsy due to birth injury

P11.4 Birth injury to other cranial nerves

P11.5 **Birth injury to spine and spinal cord**
Fracture of spine due to birth injury

P11.9 **Birth injury to central nervous system, unspecified** MCC

P12 Birth injury to scalp

Birth Injuries to Scalp

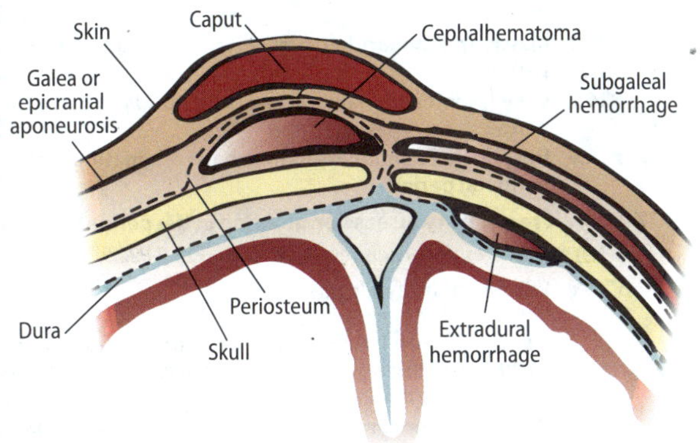

P12.0 **Cephalhematoma due to birth injury**
DEF: Condition that occurs in a neonate when blood vessels between the skull and periosteum rupture and blood collects in the subperiosteal space (below the periosteum). It is typically caused by prolonged labor or trauma due to instrument-assisted delivery (e.g., forceps, vacuum extraction), although in rare circumstances, it may indicate a linear skull fracture with intracranial hemorrhage.

P12.1 **Chignon (from vacuum extraction) due to birth injury**
DEF: Artificial swelling of the scalp that occurs when a collection of interstitial fluid and blood forms in the area of the scalp where the suction cup was applied during a vacuum-assisted delivery.

P12.2 **Epicranial subaponeurotic hemorrhage due to birth injury** CC
Subgaleal hemorrhage

P12.3 **Bruising of scalp due to birth injury**

P12.4 **Injury of scalp of newborn due to monitoring equipment**
Sampling incision of scalp of newborn
Scalp clip (electrode) injury of newborn

P12.8 **Other birth injuries to scalp**

P12.81 **Caput succedaneum**
DEF: Swelling of the scalp as a result of pressure being exerted on the head from the vaginal walls, uterus, or instrumentation used in assisting a delivery (e.g., vacuum).

P12.89 **Other birth injuries to scalp**

P12.9 **Birth injury to scalp, unspecified**

P13 Birth injury to skeleton
EXCLUDES 2 *birth injury to spine (P11.5)*

P13.0 **Fracture of skull due to birth injury**

P13.1 **Other birth injuries to skull**
EXCLUDES 1 *cephalhematoma (P12.0)*

P13.2 **Birth injury to femur**

P13.3 **Birth injury to other long bones**

P13.4 **Fracture of clavicle due to birth injury**

P13.8 **Birth injuries to other parts of skeleton**

P13.9 **Birth injury to skeleton, unspecified**

P14 Birth injury to peripheral nervous system

P14.0 **Erb's paralysis due to birth injury**
DEF: Erb's paralysis: Most common type of brachial plexus (peripheral nerve) injury in a neonate that involves nerve damage at the level of C5-C6. ***Synonym(s):*** *Erb's palsy*

P14.1 **Klumpke's paralysis due to birth injury**

P14.2 **Phrenic nerve paralysis due to birth injury**

P14.3 **Other brachial plexus birth injuries**

P14.8 **Birth injuries to other parts of peripheral nervous system**

P14.9 **Birth injury to peripheral nervous system, unspecified**

P15 Other birth injuries

P15.0 **Birth injury to liver**
Rupture of liver due to birth injury

P15.1 **Birth injury to spleen**
Rupture of spleen due to birth injury

P15.2 **Sternomastoid injury due to birth injury**

P15.3 **Birth injury to eye**
Subconjunctival hemorrhage due to birth injury
Traumatic glaucoma due to birth injury

P15.4 **Birth injury to face**
Facial congestion due to birth injury

P15.5 **Birth injury to external genitalia**

P15.6 **Subcutaneous fat necrosis due to birth injury**

P15.8 **Other specified birth injuries**

P15.9 **Birth injury, unspecified**

Respiratory and cardiovascular disorders specific to the perinatal period (P19-P29)

P19 Metabolic acidemia in newborn
INCLUDES metabolic acidemia in newborn

P19.0 **Metabolic acidemia in newborn first noted before onset of labor**

P19.1 **Metabolic acidemia in newborn first noted during labor**

P19.2 **Metabolic acidemia noted at birth**

▲ **P19.9** **Metabolic acidemia in newborn, unspecified**

P22 Respiratory distress of newborn
AHA: 2019,2Q,29

P22.0 **Respiratory distress syndrome of newborn** MCC
Cardiorespiratory distress syndrome of newborn
Hyaline membrane disease
Idiopathic respiratory distress syndrome [IRDS or RDS] of newborn
Pulmonary hypoperfusion syndrome
Respiratory distress syndrome, type I
EXCLUDES 2 *respiratory arrest of newborn (P28.81)*
respiratory failure of newborn NOS (P28.5)
AHA: 2019,2Q,29
DEF: Severe chest contractions upon air intake and expiratory grunting. The infant appears blue due to oxygen deficiency and has a rapid respiratory rate, formerly called hyaline membrane disease.

P22.1 **Transient tachypnea of newborn**
Idiopathic tachypnea of newborn
Respiratory distress syndrome, type II
Wet lung syndrome
DEF: Rapid, labored breathing of a newborn. It is a short-term problem that begins after birth and lasts about three days.

P22.8 **Other respiratory distress of newborn**
EXCLUDES 1 *respiratory arrest of newborn (P28.81)*
respiratory failure of newborn NOS (P28.5)

P22.9 **Respiratory distress of newborn, unspecified**
EXCLUDES 1 *respiratory arrest of newborn (P28.81)*
respiratory failure of newborn NOS (P28.5)

P23 Congenital pneumonia
INCLUDES infective pneumonia acquired in utero or during birth
EXCLUDES 1 *neonatal pneumonia resulting from aspiration (P24.-)*

P23.0 **Congenital pneumonia due to viral agent** MCC
Use additional code (B97) to identify organism
EXCLUDES 1 *congenital rubella pneumonitis (P35.0)*

P23.1 **Congenital pneumonia due to Chlamydia** MCC

P23.2 **Congenital pneumonia due to staphylococcus** MCC

P23.3 **Congenital pneumonia due to streptococcus, group B** MCC

P23.4 **Congenital pneumonia due to Escherichia coli** MCC

P23.5 **Congenital pneumonia due to Pseudomonas** MCC

P23.6 **Congenital pneumonia due to other bacterial agents** MCC
Congenital pneumonia due to Hemophilus influenzae
Congenital pneumonia due to Klebsiella pneumoniae
Congenital pneumonia due to Mycoplasma
Congenital pneumonia due to Streptococcus, except group B
Use additional code (B95-B96) to identify organism

P23.8 **Congenital pneumonia due to other organisms** MCC

P23.9 **Congenital pneumonia, unspecified** MCC

P24 Neonatal aspiration

INCLUDES aspiration in utero and during delivery

P24.Ø Meconium aspiration

EXCLUDES 1 *meconium passage (without aspiration) during delivery (PØ3.82)*
meconium staining (P96.83)

DEF: Meconium in the trachea or seen on chest x-ray after birth.

P24.ØØ Meconium aspiration without respiratory symptoms
Meconium aspiration NOS

P24.Ø1 Meconium aspiration with respiratory symptoms MCC
Meconium aspiration pneumonia
Meconium aspiration pneumonitis
Meconium aspiration syndrome NOS
Use additional code to identify any secondary pulmonary hypertension, if applicable (I27.2-)
DEF: Aspiration of fetal intestinal material during or prior to delivery. It is usually a complication of placental insufficiency, causing pneumonitis and bronchial obstruction (inflammatory reaction of lungs).

P24.1 Neonatal aspiration of (clear) amniotic fluid and mucus
Neonatal aspiration of liquor (amnii)

P24.1Ø Neonatal aspiration of (clear) amniotic fluid and mucus without respiratory symptoms
Neonatal aspiration of amniotic fluid and mucus NOS

P24.11 Neonatal aspiration of (clear) amniotic fluid and mucus with respiratory symptoms MCC
Neonatal aspiration of amniotic fluid and mucus with pneumonia
Neonatal aspiration of amniotic fluid and mucus with pneumonitis
Use additional code to identify any secondary pulmonary hypertension, if applicable (I27.2-)

P24.2 Neonatal aspiration of blood

P24.2Ø Neonatal aspiration of blood without respiratory symptoms
Neonatal aspiration of blood NOS

P24.21 Neonatal aspiration of blood with respiratory symptoms MCC
Neonatal aspiration of blood with pneumonia
Neonatal aspiration of blood with pneumonitis
Use additional code to identify any secondary pulmonary hypertension, if applicable (I27.2-)

P24.3 Neonatal aspiration of milk and regurgitated food
Neonatal aspiration of stomach contents

P24.3Ø Neonatal aspiration of milk and regurgitated food without respiratory symptoms
Neonatal aspiration of milk and regurgitated food NOS

P24.31 Neonatal aspiration of milk and regurgitated food with respiratory symptoms MCC
Neonatal aspiration of milk and regurgitated food with pneumonia
Neonatal aspiration of milk and regurgitated food with pneumonitis
Use additional code to identify any secondary pulmonary hypertension, if applicable (I27.2-)

P24.8 Other neonatal aspiration

P24.8Ø Other neonatal aspiration without respiratory symptoms
Neonatal aspiration NEC

P24.81 Other neonatal aspiration with respiratory symptoms MCC
Neonatal aspiration pneumonia NEC
Neonatal aspiration with pneumonitis NEC
Neonatal aspiration with pneumonia NOS
Neonatal aspiration with pneumonitis NOS
Use additional code to identify any secondary pulmonary hypertension, if applicable (I27.2-)

P24.9 Neonatal aspiration, unspecified

P25 Interstitial emphysema and related conditions originating in the perinatal period

P25.Ø Interstitial emphysema originating in the perinatal period MCC

P25.1 Pneumothorax originating in the perinatal period MCC

P25.2 Pneumomediastinum originating in the perinatal period MCC

P25.3 Pneumopericardium originating in the perinatal period MCC

P25.8 Other conditions related to interstitial emphysema originating in the perinatal period MCC

P26 Pulmonary hemorrhage originating in the perinatal period

EXCLUDES 1 *acute idiopathic hemorrhage in infants over 28 days old (RØ4.81)*

P26.Ø Tracheobronchial hemorrhage originating in the perinatal period MCC

P26.1 Massive pulmonary hemorrhage originating in the perinatal period MCC

P26.8 Other pulmonary hemorrhages originating in the perinatal period MCC

P26.9 Unspecified pulmonary hemorrhage originating in the perinatal period MCC

P27 Chronic respiratory disease originating in the perinatal period

EXCLUDES 2 *respiratory distress of newborn (P22.Ø-P22.9)*

P27.Ø Wilson-Mikity syndrome MCC
Pulmonary dysmaturity
DEF: Pulmonary insufficiency in newborn babies, especially those with low birth weight. Rapid onset of hypercapnia and cyanosis occur during the first month of life frequently resulting in death.

P27.1 Bronchopulmonary dysplasia originating in the perinatal period MCC

P27.8 Other chronic respiratory diseases originating in the perinatal period MCC
Congenital pulmonary fibrosis
Ventilator lung in newborn

P27.9 Unspecified chronic respiratory disease originating in the perinatal period MCC

P28 Other respiratory conditions originating in the perinatal period

Code also, if applicable, congenital malformations of the respiratory system (Q3Ø-Q34)

P28.Ø Primary atelectasis of newborn CC
Primary failure to expand terminal respiratory units
Pulmonary hypoplasia associated with short gestation
Pulmonary immaturity NOS

P28.1 Other and unspecified atelectasis of newborn

P28.1Ø Unspecified atelectasis of newborn CC
Atelectasis of newborn NOS

P28.11 Resorption atelectasis without respiratory distress syndrome CC
EXCLUDES 1 *resorption atelectasis with respiratory distress syndrome (P22.Ø)*

P28.19 Other atelectasis of newborn CC
Partial atelectasis of newborn
Secondary atelectasis of newborn

P28.2 Cyanotic attacks of newborn CC
EXCLUDES 1 *apnea of newborn (P28.3- - P28.4-)*

P28.3 Primary sleep apnea of newborn
Sleep apnea of newborn NOS
EXCLUDES 2 *other apnea of newborn (P28.4-)*
AHA: 2022,4Q,38-39
DEF: Unexplained cessation of breathing when a neonate makes no respiratory effort for 20 seconds or longer or when a neonate's breathing cessation is accompanied by cyanosis, bradycardia, or hypotonia.

P28.3Ø Primary sleep apnea of newborn, unspecified CC
Transient oxygen desaturation spells of newborn during sleep

P28.31 Primary central sleep apnea of newborn CC

P28.32 Primary obstructive sleep apnea of newborn CC

P28.33 Primary mixed sleep apnea of newborn CC

P28.39 Other primary sleep apnea of newborn CC

P28.4 Other apnea of newborn
EXCLUDES 2 *primary sleep apnea of newborn (P28.3-)*
AHA: 2022,4Q,38-39

P28.4Ø Unspecified apnea of newborn CC
Apnea of newborn, NOS
Transient oxygen desaturation spells of newborn

P28.41 Central neonatal apnea of newborn CC

P28.42 Obstructive apnea of newborn CC

P28.43 Mixed neonatal apnea of newborn CC

P28.49 Other apnea of newborn CC
Apnea of prematurity

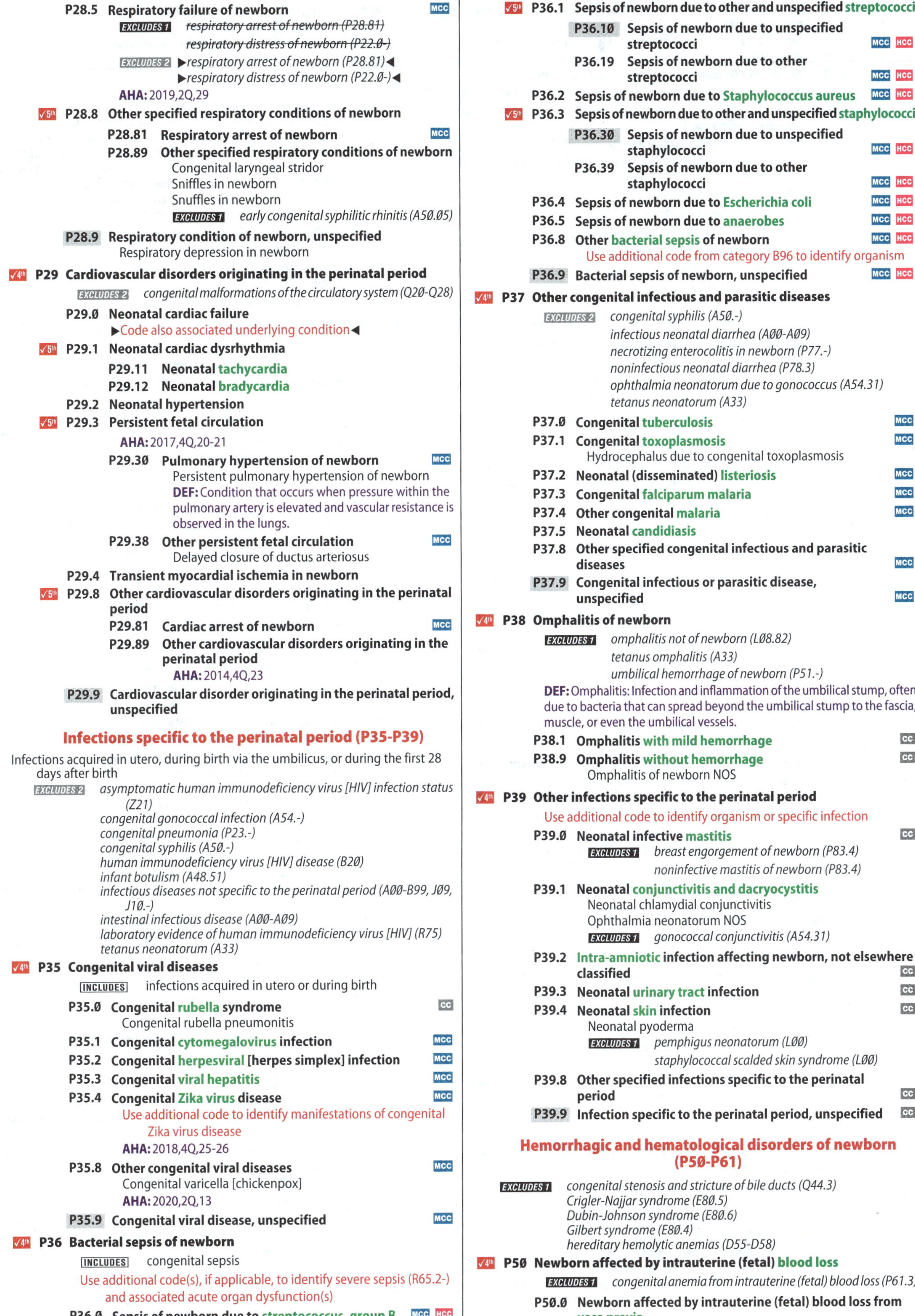

P28.5 **Respiratory failure of newborn** MCC
EXCLUDES 1 ~~respiratory arrest of newborn (P28.81)~~
~~respiratory distress of newborn (P22.0-)~~
EXCLUDES 2 ▶*respiratory arrest of newborn (P28.81)*◀
▶*respiratory distress of newborn (P22.0-)*◀
AHA: 2019,2Q,29

✓5th P28.8 **Other specified respiratory conditions of newborn**
P28.81 **Respiratory arrest of newborn** MCC
P28.89 **Other specified respiratory conditions of newborn**
Congenital laryngeal stridor
Sniffles in newborn
Snuffles in newborn
EXCLUDES 1 *early congenital syphilitic rhinitis (A50.05)*

P28.9 **Respiratory condition of newborn, unspecified**
Respiratory depression in newborn

✓4th **P29 Cardiovascular disorders originating in the perinatal period**
EXCLUDES 2 *congenital malformations of the circulatory system (Q20-Q28)*
P29.0 **Neonatal cardiac failure**
▶Code also associated underlying condition◀
✓5th P29.1 **Neonatal cardiac dysrhythmia**
P29.11 **Neonatal tachycardia**
P29.12 **Neonatal bradycardia**
P29.2 **Neonatal hypertension**
✓5th P29.3 **Persistent fetal circulation**
AHA: 2017,4Q,20-21
P29.30 **Pulmonary hypertension of newborn** MCC
Persistent pulmonary hypertension of newborn
DEF: Condition that occurs when pressure within the pulmonary artery is elevated and vascular resistance is observed in the lungs.
P29.38 **Other persistent fetal circulation** MCC
Delayed closure of ductus arteriosus
P29.4 **Transient myocardial ischemia in newborn**
✓5th P29.8 **Other cardiovascular disorders originating in the perinatal period**
P29.81 **Cardiac arrest of newborn** MCC
P29.89 **Other cardiovascular disorders originating in the perinatal period**
AHA: 2014,4Q,23
P29.9 **Cardiovascular disorder originating in the perinatal period, unspecified**

Infections specific to the perinatal period (P35-P39)

Infections acquired in utero, during birth via the umbilicus, or during the first 28 days after birth

EXCLUDES 2 *asymptomatic human immunodeficiency virus [HIV] infection status (Z21)*
congenital gonococcal infection (A54.-)
congenital pneumonia (P23.-)
congenital syphilis (A50.-)
human immunodeficiency virus [HIV] disease (B20)
infant botulism (A48.51)
infectious diseases not specific to the perinatal period (A00-B99, J09, J10.-)
intestinal infectious disease (A00-A09)
laboratory evidence of human immunodeficiency virus [HIV] (R75)
tetanus neonatorum (A33)

✓4th **P35 Congenital viral diseases**
INCLUDES infections acquired in utero or during birth
P35.0 **Congenital rubella syndrome** CC
Congenital rubella pneumonitis
P35.1 **Congenital cytomegalovirus infection** MCC
P35.2 **Congenital herpesviral [herpes simplex] infection** MCC
P35.3 **Congenital viral hepatitis** MCC
P35.4 **Congenital Zika virus disease** MCC
Use additional code to identify manifestations of congenital Zika virus disease
AHA: 2018,4Q,25-26
P35.8 **Other congenital viral diseases** MCC
Congenital varicella [chickenpox]
AHA: 2020,2Q,13
P35.9 **Congenital viral disease, unspecified** MCC

✓4th **P36 Bacterial sepsis of newborn**
INCLUDES congenital sepsis
Use additional code(s), if applicable, to identify severe sepsis (R65.2-) and associated acute organ dysfunction(s)
P36.0 **Sepsis of newborn due to streptococcus, group B** MCC HCC
✓5th P36.1 **Sepsis of newborn due to other and unspecified streptococci**
P36.10 **Sepsis of newborn due to unspecified streptococci** MCC HCC
P36.19 **Sepsis of newborn due to other streptococci** MCC HCC
P36.2 **Sepsis of newborn due to Staphylococcus aureus** MCC HCC
✓5th P36.3 **Sepsis of newborn due to other and unspecified staphylococci**
P36.30 **Sepsis of newborn due to unspecified staphylococci** MCC HCC
P36.39 **Sepsis of newborn due to other staphylococci** MCC HCC
P36.4 **Sepsis of newborn due to Escherichia coli** MCC HCC
P36.5 **Sepsis of newborn due to anaerobes** MCC HCC
P36.8 **Other bacterial sepsis of newborn** MCC HCC
Use additional code from category B96 to identify organism
P36.9 **Bacterial sepsis of newborn, unspecified** MCC HCC

✓4th **P37 Other congenital infectious and parasitic diseases**
EXCLUDES 2 *congenital syphilis (A50.-)*
infectious neonatal diarrhea (A00-A09)
necrotizing enterocolitis in newborn (P77.-)
noninfectious neonatal diarrhea (P78.3)
ophthalmia neonatorum due to gonococcus (A54.31)
tetanus neonatorum (A33)
P37.0 **Congenital tuberculosis** MCC
P37.1 **Congenital toxoplasmosis** MCC
Hydrocephalus due to congenital toxoplasmosis
P37.2 **Neonatal (disseminated) listeriosis** MCC
P37.3 **Congenital falciparum malaria** MCC
P37.4 **Other congenital malaria** MCC
P37.5 **Neonatal candidiasis**
P37.8 **Other specified congenital infectious and parasitic diseases** MCC
P37.9 **Congenital infectious or parasitic disease, unspecified** MCC

✓4th **P38 Omphalitis of newborn**
EXCLUDES 1 *omphalitis not of newborn (L08.82)*
tetanus omphalitis (A33)
umbilical hemorrhage of newborn (P51.-)
DEF: Omphalitis: Infection and inflammation of the umbilical stump, often due to bacteria that can spread beyond the umbilical stump to the fascia, muscle, or even the umbilical vessels.
P38.1 **Omphalitis with mild hemorrhage** CC
P38.9 **Omphalitis without hemorrhage** CC
Omphalitis of newborn NOS

✓4th **P39 Other infections specific to the perinatal period**
Use additional code to identify organism or specific infection
P39.0 **Neonatal infective mastitis** CC
EXCLUDES 1 *breast engorgement of newborn (P83.4)*
noninfective mastitis of newborn (P83.4)
P39.1 **Neonatal conjunctivitis and dacryocystitis**
Neonatal chlamydial conjunctivitis
Ophthalmia neonatorum NOS
EXCLUDES 1 *gonococcal conjunctivitis (A54.31)*
P39.2 **Intra-amniotic infection affecting newborn, not elsewhere classified** CC
P39.3 **Neonatal urinary tract infection** CC
P39.4 **Neonatal skin infection** CC
Neonatal pyoderma
EXCLUDES 1 *pemphigus neonatorum (L00)*
staphylococcal scalded skin syndrome (L00)
P39.8 **Other specified infections specific to the perinatal period** CC
P39.9 **Infection specific to the perinatal period, unspecified** CC

Hemorrhagic and hematological disorders of newborn (P50-P61)

EXCLUDES 1 *congenital stenosis and stricture of bile ducts (Q44.3)*
Crigler-Najjar syndrome (E80.5)
Dubin-Johnson syndrome (E80.6)
Gilbert syndrome (E80.4)
hereditary hemolytic anemias (D55-D58)

✓4th **P50 Newborn affected by intrauterine (fetal) blood loss**
EXCLUDES 1 *congenital anemia from intrauterine (fetal) blood loss (P61.3)*
P50.0 **Newborn affected by intrauterine (fetal) blood loss from vasa previa**

P5Ø.1 Newborn affected by intrauterine (fetal) blood loss from ruptured cord

P5Ø.2 Newborn affected by intrauterine (fetal) blood loss from placenta

P5Ø.3 Newborn affected by hemorrhage into co-twin

P5Ø.4 Newborn affected by hemorrhage into maternal circulation

P5Ø.5 Newborn affected by intrauterine (fetal) blood loss from cut end of co-twin's cord

P5Ø.8 Newborn affected by other intrauterine (fetal) blood loss

P5Ø.9 Newborn affected by intrauterine (fetal) blood loss, unspecified
Newborn affected by fetal hemorrhage NOS

✓4th P51 Umbilical hemorrhage of newborn

EXCLUDES 1 *omphalitis with mild hemorrhage (P38.1)*
umbilical hemorrhage from cut end of co-twins cord (P5Ø.5)

P51.Ø Massive umbilical hemorrhage of newborn

P51.8 Other umbilical hemorrhages of newborn
Slipped umbilical ligature NOS

P51.9 Umbilical hemorrhage of newborn, unspecified

✓4th P52 Intracranial nontraumatic hemorrhage of newborn

INCLUDES intracranial hemorrhage due to anoxia or hypoxia

EXCLUDES 1 *intracranial hemorrhage due to birth injury (P1Ø.-)*
intracranial hemorrhage due to other injury (SØ6.-)

P52.Ø Intraventricular (nontraumatic) hemorrhage, grade 1, of newborn CC
Bleeding into germinal matrix
Subependymal hemorrhage (without intraventricular extension)

P52.1 Intraventricular (nontraumatic) hemorrhage, grade 2, of newborn CC
Bleeding into ventricle
Subependymal hemorrhage with intraventricular extension

✓5th P52.2 Intraventricular (nontraumatic) hemorrhage, grade 3 and grade 4, of newborn

P52.21 Intraventricular (nontraumatic) hemorrhage, grade 3, of newborn MCC
Subependymal hemorrhage with intraventricular extension with enlargement of ventricle

P52.22 Intraventricular (nontraumatic) hemorrhage, grade 4, of newborn MCC
Bleeding into cerebral cortex
Subependymal hemorrhage with intracerebral extension

P52.3 Unspecified intraventricular (nontraumatic) hemorrhage of newborn CC

P52.4 Intracerebral (nontraumatic) hemorrhage of newborn MCC

P52.5 Subarachnoid (nontraumatic) hemorrhage of newborn MCC

P52.6 Cerebellar (nontraumatic) and posterior fossa hemorrhage of newborn MCC

P52.8 Other intracranial (nontraumatic) hemorrhages of newborn MCC

P52.9 Intracranial (nontraumatic) hemorrhage of newborn, unspecified MCC

P53 Hemorrhagic disease of newborn CC
Vitamin K deficiency of newborn

✓4th P54 Other neonatal hemorrhages

EXCLUDES 1 *newborn affected by (intrauterine) blood loss (P5Ø.-)*
pulmonary hemorrhage originating in the perinatal period (P26.-)

P54.Ø Neonatal hematemesis

EXCLUDES 1 *neonatal hematemesis due to swallowed maternal blood (P78.2)*

P54.1 Neonatal melena MCC

EXCLUDES 1 *neonatal melena due to swallowed maternal blood (P78.2)*

P54.2 Neonatal rectal hemorrhage MCC

P54.3 Other neonatal gastrointestinal hemorrhage MCC

P54.4 Neonatal adrenal hemorrhage CC

P54.5 Neonatal cutaneous hemorrhage
Neonatal bruising
Neonatal ecchymoses
Neonatal petechiae
Neonatal superficial hematomata

EXCLUDES 2 *bruising of scalp due to birth injury (P12.3)*
cephalhematoma due to birth injury (P12.Ø)

P54.6 Neonatal vaginal hemorrhage ♀
Neonatal pseudomenses

P54.8 Other specified neonatal hemorrhages

P54.9 Neonatal hemorrhage, unspecified

✓4th P55 Hemolytic disease of newborn

P55.Ø Rh isoimmunization of newborn

DEF: Incompatible Rh fetal-maternal blood grouping that prematurely destroys red blood cells. Symptoms include jaundice, asphyxia, pulmonary hypertension, edema, respiratory distress, kernicterus, and coagulopathies. It is detected by a Coombs test.

TIP: A positive Coombs test without documentation of associated Rh isoimmunization should be coded to R79.89 Other specified abnormal findings of blood chemistry.

P55.1 ABO isoimmunization of newborn
AHA: 2015,3Q,20

P55.8 Other hemolytic diseases of newborn
AHA: 2018,3Q,24

P55.9 Hemolytic disease of newborn, unspecified

✓4th P56 Hydrops fetalis due to hemolytic disease

EXCLUDES 1 *hydrops fetalis NOS (P83.2)*

P56.Ø Hydrops fetalis due to isoimmunization MCC

✓5th P56.9 Hydrops fetalis due to other and unspecified hemolytic disease

P56.9Ø Hydrops fetalis due to unspecified hemolytic disease MCC

P56.99 Hydrops fetalis due to other hemolytic disease MCC

✓4th P57 Kernicterus

P57.Ø Kernicterus due to isoimmunization MCC

DEF: Complication of erythroblastosis fetalis associated with severe neural symptoms, high blood bilirubin levels, and nerve cell destruction. It results in bilirubin-pigmented gray matter of the central nervous system.

P57.8 Other specified kernicterus MCC

EXCLUDES 1 *Crigler-Najjar syndrome (E8Ø.5)*

P57.9 Kernicterus, unspecified MCC

✓4th P58 Neonatal jaundice due to other excessive hemolysis

EXCLUDES 1 *jaundice due to isoimmunization (P55-P57)*

P58.Ø Neonatal jaundice due to bruising

P58.1 Neonatal jaundice due to bleeding

P58.2 Neonatal jaundice due to infection

P58.3 Neonatal jaundice due to polycythemia

✓5th P58.4 Neonatal jaundice due to drugs or toxins transmitted from mother or given to newborn

Code first poisoning due to drug or toxin, if applicable ▶(T36-T65 with fifth or sixth character 1-4)◀

Use additional code for adverse effect, if applicable, to identify drug (T36-T5Ø with fifth or sixth character 5)

P58.41 Neonatal jaundice due to drugs or toxins transmitted from mother

P58.42 Neonatal jaundice due to drugs or toxins given to newborn

P58.5 Neonatal jaundice due to swallowed maternal blood

P58.8 Neonatal jaundice due to other specified excessive hemolysis

P58.9 Neonatal jaundice due to excessive hemolysis, unspecified

✓4th P59 Neonatal jaundice from other and unspecified causes

EXCLUDES 1 *jaundice due to inborn errors of metabolism (E7Ø-E88)*
kernicterus (P57.-)

P59.Ø Neonatal jaundice associated with preterm delivery
Hyperbilirubinemia of prematurity
Jaundice due to delayed conjugation associated with preterm delivery

P59.1 Inspissated bile syndrome MCC

DEF: Biliary obstruction in newborn resulting from obstruction of outflow tract.

✓5th P59.2 Neonatal jaundice from other and unspecified hepatocellular damage

EXCLUDES 1 *congenital viral hepatitis (P35.3)*

P59.2Ø Neonatal jaundice from unspecified hepatocellular damage MCC

P59.29 Neonatal jaundice from other hepatocellular damage MCC
Neonatal giant cell hepatitis
Neonatal (idiopathic) hepatitis

P59.3 Neonatal jaundice from breast milk inhibitor

P59.8 Neonatal jaundice from other specified causes

P59.9 Neonatal jaundice, unspecified
Neonatal physiological jaundice (intense)(prolonged) NOS
AHA: 2015,3Q,20

P60 Disseminated intravascular coagulation of newborn MCC
Defibrination syndrome of newborn

✓4th **P61 Other perinatal hematological disorders**
EXCLUDES 1 *transient hypogammaglobulinemia of infancy (D80.7)*

P61.0 Transient neonatal thrombocytopenia MCC
Neonatal thrombocytopenia due to exchange transfusion
Neonatal thrombocytopenia due to idiopathic maternal thrombocytopenia
Neonatal thrombocytopenia due to isoimmunization
DEF: Temporary decrease in blood platelets of a newborn that is secondary to placental insufficiency.

P61.1 Polycythemia neonatorum
DEF: Abnormal increase of total red blood cells of a newborn that results in hyperviscosity, which slows the flow of blood through small blood vessels.

P61.2 Anemia of prematurity CC
P61.3 Congenital anemia from fetal blood loss CC
P61.4 Other congenital anemias, not elsewhere classified CC
Congenital anemia NOS

P61.5 Transient neonatal neutropenia MCC
EXCLUDES 1 *congenital neutropenia (nontransient) (D70.0)*
DEF: Low blood neutrophil counts of newborn that occurs due to maternal hypertension, sepsis, twin-twin transfusion, alloimmunization, and hemolytic disease.

P61.6 Other transient neonatal disorders of coagulation CC
P61.8 Other specified perinatal hematological disorders
P61.9 Perinatal hematological disorder, unspecified

Transitory endocrine and metabolic disorders specific to newborn (P70-P74)

INCLUDES transitory endocrine and metabolic disturbances caused by the infant's response to maternal endocrine and metabolic factors, or its adjustment to extrauterine environment
AHA: 2018,2Q,6

✓4th **P70 Transitory disorders of carbohydrate metabolism specific to newborn**

P70.0 Syndrome of infant of mother with gestational diabetes
Newborn (with hypoglycemia) affected by maternal gestational diabetes
EXCLUDES 1 *newborn (with hypoglycemia) affected by maternal (pre-existing) diabetes mellitus (P70.1)*
syndrome of infant of a diabetic mother (P70.1)

P70.1 Syndrome of infant of a diabetic mother
Newborn (with hypoglycemia) affected by maternal (pre-existing) diabetes mellitus
EXCLUDES 1 *newborn (with hypoglycemia) affected by maternal gestational diabetes (P70.0)*
syndrome of infant of mother with gestational diabetes (P70.0)

P70.2 Neonatal diabetes mellitus CC
P70.3 Iatrogenic neonatal hypoglycemia
P70.4 Other neonatal hypoglycemia
Transitory neonatal hypoglycemia
P70.8 Other transitory disorders of carbohydrate metabolism of newborn CC
P70.9 Transitory disorder of carbohydrate metabolism of newborn, unspecified

✓4th **P71 Transitory neonatal disorders of calcium and magnesium metabolism**

P71.0 Cow's milk hypocalcemia in newborn CC
P71.1 Other neonatal hypocalcemia CC
EXCLUDES 1 *neonatal hypoparathyroidism (P71.4)*
P71.2 Neonatal hypomagnesemia CC
P71.3 Neonatal tetany without calcium or magnesium deficiency CC
Neonatal tetany NOS
P71.4 Transitory neonatal hypoparathyroidism CC
P71.8 Other transitory neonatal disorders of calcium and magnesium metabolism CC
AHA: 2016,4Q,54
P71.9 Transitory neonatal disorder of calcium and magnesium metabolism, unspecified CC

✓4th **P72 Other transitory neonatal endocrine disorders**
EXCLUDES 1 *congenital hypothyroidism with or without goiter (E03.0-E03.1)*
dyshormogenetic goiter (E07.1)
Pendred's syndrome (E07.1)

P72.0 Neonatal goiter, not elsewhere classified CC
Transitory congenital goiter with normal functioning
P72.1 Transitory neonatal hyperthyroidism CC
Neonatal thyrotoxicosis
P72.2 Other transitory neonatal disorders of thyroid function, not elsewhere classified CC
Transitory neonatal hypothyroidism
P72.8 Other specified transitory neonatal endocrine disorders CC
P72.9 Transitory neonatal endocrine disorder, unspecified

✓4th **P74 Other transitory neonatal electrolyte and metabolic disturbances**
AHA: 2018,4Q,26-27

P74.0 Late metabolic acidosis of newborn MCC
EXCLUDES 1 *(fetal) metabolic acidosis of newborn (P19)*
P74.1 Dehydration of newborn
✓5th **P74.2 Disturbances of sodium balance of newborn**
P74.21 Hypernatremia of newborn
P74.22 Hyponatremia of newborn
✓5th **P74.3 Disturbances of potassium balance of newborn**
P74.31 Hyperkalemia of newborn
P74.32 Hypokalemia of newborn
✓5th **P74.4 Other transitory electrolyte disturbances of newborn**
P74.41 Alkalosis of newborn CC
Hyperbicarbonatemia
✓6th **P74.42 Disturbances of chlorine balance of newborn**
P74.421 Hyperchloremia of newborn
Hyperchloremic metabolic acidosis
EXCLUDES 2 *late metabolic acidosis of the newborn (P74.0)*
P74.422 Hypochloremia of newborn
P74.49 Other transitory electrolyte disturbance of newborn
P74.5 Transitory tyrosinemia of newborn CC
P74.6 Transitory hyperammonemia of newborn CC
P74.8 Other transitory metabolic disturbances of newborn CC
Amino-acid metabolic disorders described as transitory
P74.9 Transitory metabolic disturbance of newborn, unspecified

Digestive system disorders of newborn (P76-P78)

✓4th **P76 Other intestinal obstruction of newborn**

P76.0 Meconium plug syndrome
Meconium ileus NOS
EXCLUDES 1 *meconium ileus in cystic fibrosis (E84.11)*
DEF: Meconium obstruction of a newborn's intestines, resulting from unusually thick or hard meconium.
P76.1 Transitory ileus of newborn CC
EXCLUDES 1 *Hirschsprung's disease (Q43.1)*
P76.2 Intestinal obstruction due to inspissated milk
P76.8 Other specified intestinal obstruction of newborn
EXCLUDES 1 *intestinal obstruction classifiable to K56.-*
P76.9 Intestinal obstruction of newborn, unspecified

✓4th **P77 Necrotizing enterocolitis of newborn**
DEF: Serious intestinal infection and inflammation in preterm infants. Severity is measured by stages and may progress to life-threatening perforation or peritonitis. Resection surgical treatment may be necessary.

P77.1 Stage 1 necrotizing enterocolitis in newborn MCC
Necrotizing enterocolitis without pneumatosis, without perforation
DEF: Broad-spectrum symptoms with nonspecific signs, including feeding intolerance, abdominal distention, bradycardia, and metabolic abnormalities.

P77.2 Stage 2 necrotizing enterocolitis in newborn MCC
Necrotizing enterocolitis with pneumatosis, without perforation
DEF: Radiographic confirmation of necrotizing enterocolitis showing intestinal dilatation, fixed loops of bowels, pneumatosis intestinalis, metabolic acidosis, and thrombocytopenia.

P77.3 Stage 3 necrotizing enterocolitis in newborn MCC
Necrotizing enterocolitis with perforation
Necrotizing enterocolitis with pneumatosis and perforation
DEF: Advanced stage in which an infant demonstrates signs of bowel perforation, septic shock, metabolic acidosis, ascites, disseminated intravascular coagulopathy, and neutropenia.

P77.9 Necrotizing enterocolitis in newborn, unspecified MCC
Necrotizing enterocolitis in newborn, NOS

4th **P78 Other perinatal digestive system disorders**
EXCLUDES 1 *cystic fibrosis (E84.0-E84.9)*
neonatal gastrointestinal hemorrhages (P54.0-P54.3)

P78.0 Perinatal intestinal perforation MCC
Meconium peritonitis

P78.1 Other neonatal peritonitis
Neonatal peritonitis NOS

P78.2 Neonatal hematemesis and melena due to swallowed maternal blood

P78.3 Noninfective neonatal diarrhea
Neonatal diarrhea NOS

5th **P78.8 Other specified perinatal digestive system disorders**

P78.81 Congenital cirrhosis (of liver)

P78.82 Peptic ulcer of newborn

P78.83 Newborn esophageal reflux
Neonatal esophageal reflux

P78.84 Gestational alloimmune liver disease
GALD
Neonatal hemochromatosis
EXCLUDES 1 *hemochromatosis (E83.11-)*
AHA: 2017,4Q,21
DEF: Severe hepatic injury with onset during fetal development with manifestations beginning during fetal life. It is due to maternal antibodies to fetal hepatic cells (hepatocytes) that cross the placenta into the fetal circulation, causing hepatic cell necrosis.

P78.89 Other specified perinatal digestive system disorders

P78.9 Perinatal digestive system disorder, unspecified

Conditions involving the integument and temperature regulation of newborn (P80-P83)

4th **P80 Hypothermia of newborn**
DEF: Decrease in newborn body temperature due to their larger ratio of surface area to body weight, thin skin with blood vessels close to the surface, and a limited amount of subcutaneous fat.

P80.0 Cold injury syndrome
Severe and usually chronic hypothermia associated with a pink flushed appearance, edema and neurological and biochemical abnormalities.
EXCLUDES 1 *mild hypothermia of newborn (P80.8)*

P80.8 Other hypothermia of newborn
Mild hypothermia of newborn

P80.9 Hypothermia of newborn, unspecified

4th **P81 Other disturbances of temperature regulation of newborn**

P81.0 Environmental hyperthermia of newborn

P81.8 Other specified disturbances of temperature regulation of newborn

P81.9 Disturbance of temperature regulation of newborn, unspecified
Fever of newborn NOS

4th **P83 Other conditions of integument specific to newborn**
EXCLUDES 1 *congenital malformations of skin and integument (Q80-Q84)*
hydrops fetalis due to hemolytic disease (P56.-)
neonatal skin infection (P39.4)
staphylococcal scalded skin syndrome (L00)
EXCLUDES 2 *cradle cap (L21.0)*
diaper [napkin] dermatitis (L22)

P83.0 Sclerema neonatorum CC
DEF: Diffuse, rapidly progressing white, waxy, nonpitting hardening of tissue, usually of legs and feet that is life-threatening. It is found in preterm or debilitated infants. Etiology is unknown.

P83.1 Neonatal erythema toxicum

P83.2 Hydrops fetalis not due to hemolytic disease MCC
Hydrops fetalis NOS
DEF: Severe, life-threatening problem of a newborn characterized by severe edema of the entire body. It is unrelated to immune response.

5th **P83.3 Other and unspecified edema specific to newborn**

P83.30 Unspecified edema specific to newborn CC

P83.39 Other edema specific to newborn CC

P83.4 Breast engorgement of newborn
Noninfective mastitis of newborn

P83.5 Congenital hydrocele ♂
DEF: Hydrocele: Serous fluid that collects in the tunica vaginalis of the scrotum along the spermatic cord in males.

P83.6 Umbilical polyp of newborn

5th **P83.8 Other specified conditions of integument specific to newborn**
AHA: 2017,4Q,21-22

P83.81 Umbilical granuloma
EXCLUDES 2 *granulomatous disorder of the skin and subcutaneous tissue, unspecified (L92.9)*

P83.88 Other specified conditions of integument specific to newborn
Bronze baby syndrome
Neonatal scleroderma
Urticaria neonatorum

P83.9 Condition of the integument specific to newborn, unspecified

Other problems with newborn (P84)

P84 Other problems with newborn
Acidemia of newborn
Acidosis of newborn
Anoxia of newborn NOS
Asphyxia of newborn NOS
Hypercapnia of newborn
Hypoxemia of newborn
Hypoxia of newborn NOS
Mixed metabolic and respiratory acidosis of newborn
EXCLUDES 1 *intracranial hemorrhage due to anoxia or hypoxia (P52.-)*
hypoxic ischemic encephalopathy [HIE] (P91.6-)
late metabolic acidosis of newborn (P74.0)

Other disorders originating in the perinatal period (P90-P96)

P90 Convulsions of newborn MCC
EXCLUDES 1 *benign myoclonic epilepsy in infancy (G40.3-)*
benign neonatal convulsions (familial) (G40.3-)

4th **P91 Other disturbances of cerebral status of newborn**

P91.0 Neonatal cerebral ischemia MCC
EXCLUDES 1 *neonatal cerebral infarction (P91.82-)*

P91.1 Acquired periventricular cysts of newborn MCC

P91.2 Neonatal cerebral leukomalacia MCC
Periventricular leukomalacia

P91.3 Neonatal cerebral irritability MCC

P91.4 Neonatal cerebral depression MCC

P91.5 Neonatal coma MCC

5th **P91.6 Hypoxic ischemic encephalopathy [HIE]**
EXCLUDES 1 *neonatal cerebral depression (P91.4)*
neonatal cerebral irritability (P91.3)
neonatal coma (P91.5)
AHA: 2017,4Q,22

P91.60 Hypoxic ischemic encephalopathy [HIE], unspecified CC

P91.61 Mild hypoxic ischemic encephalopathy [HIE] CC

P91.62 Moderate hypoxic ischemic encephalopathy [HIE] CC

P91.63 Severe hypoxic ischemic encephalopathy [HIE] MCC

5th **P91.8 Other specified disturbances of cerebral status of newborn**
AHA: 2017,4Q,22

6th **P91.81 Neonatal encephalopathy**

P91.811 Neonatal encephalopathy in diseases classified elsewhere
Code first underlying condition, if known, such as:
congenital cirrhosis (of liver) (P78.81)
intracranial nontraumatic hemorrhage of newborn (P52.-)
kernicterus (P57.-)

P91.819 Neonatal encephalopathy, unspecified

P91.82 Neonatal cerebral infarction
Neonatal stroke
Perinatal arterial ischemic stroke
Perinatal cerebral infarction
EXCLUDES 1 *cerebral infarction (I63.-)*
EXCLUDES 2 *intracranial hemorrhage of newborn (P52.-)*
AHA: 2020,4Q,37-38

P91.821 Neonatal cerebral infarction, right side of brain MCC HCC

P91.822 Neonatal cerebral infarction, left side of brain MCC HCC

P91.823 Neonatal cerebral infarction, bilateral MCC HCC

P91.829 Neonatal cerebral infarction, unspecified side MCC HCC

P91.88 Other specified disturbances of cerebral status of newborn

P91.9 Disturbance of cerebral status of newborn, unspecified

P92 Feeding problems of newborn
EXCLUDES 1 *eating disorders (F50.-)*
EXCLUDES 2 *feeding problems in child over 28 days old ▶(R63.3-)◀*
AHA: 2016,3Q,19

P92.0 Vomiting of newborn
EXCLUDES 1 *vomiting of child over 28 days old (R11.-)*

P92.01 Bilious vomiting of newborn MCC
EXCLUDES 1 *bilious vomiting in child over 28 days old (R11.14)*

P92.09 Other vomiting of newborn
EXCLUDES 1 *regurgitation of food in newborn (P92.1)*

P92.1 Regurgitation and rumination of newborn

P92.2 Slow feeding of newborn

P92.3 Underfeeding of newborn

P92.4 Overfeeding of newborn

P92.5 Neonatal difficulty in feeding at breast
AHA: 2017,1Q,28

P92.6 Failure to thrive in newborn
EXCLUDES 1 *failure to thrive in child over 28 days old (R62.51)*

P92.8 Other feeding problems of newborn

P92.9 Feeding problem of newborn, unspecified

P93 Reactions and intoxications due to drugs administered to newborn
INCLUDES reactions and intoxications due to drugs administered to fetus affecting newborn
EXCLUDES 1 *jaundice due to drugs or toxins transmitted from mother or given to newborn (P58.4-)*
reactions and intoxications from maternal opiates, tranquilizers and other medication (P04.0-P04.1, P04.4-)
withdrawal symptoms from maternal use of drugs of addiction (P96.1)
withdrawal symptoms from therapeutic use of drugs in newborn (P96.2)

P93.0 Grey baby syndrome CC
Grey syndrome from chloramphenicol administration in newborn

P93.8 Other reactions and intoxications due to drugs administered to newborn CC
Use additional code for adverse effect, if applicable, to identify drug (T36-T50 with fifth or sixth character 5)

P94 Disorders of muscle tone of newborn

P94.0 Transient neonatal myasthenia gravis CC
EXCLUDES 1 *myasthenia gravis (G70.0)*

P94.1 Congenital hypertonia

P94.2 Congenital hypotonia
Floppy baby syndrome, unspecified

P94.8 Other disorders of muscle tone of newborn

P94.9 Disorder of muscle tone of newborn, unspecified

P95 Stillbirth
Deadborn fetus NOS
Fetal death of unspecified cause
Stillbirth NOS
EXCLUDES 1 *maternal care for intrauterine death (O36.4)*
missed abortion (O02.1)
outcome of delivery, stillbirth (Z37.1, Z37.3, Z37.4, Z37.7)

P96 Other conditions originating in the perinatal period

P96.0 Congenital renal failure
Uremia of newborn

P96.1 Neonatal withdrawal symptoms from maternal use of drugs of addiction CC
Drug withdrawal syndrome in infant of dependent mother
Neonatal abstinence syndrome
EXCLUDES 1 *reactions and intoxications from maternal opiates and tranquilizers administered during labor and delivery (P04.0)*
AHA: 2018,4Q,24-25

P96.2 Withdrawal symptoms from therapeutic use of drugs in newborn CC

P96.3 Wide cranial sutures of newborn
Neonatal craniotabes

P96.5 Complication to newborn due to (fetal) intrauterine procedure
EXCLUDES 2 *newborn affected by amniocentesis (P00.6)*

P96.8 Other specified conditions originating in the perinatal period

P96.81 Exposure to (parental) (environmental) tobacco smoke in the perinatal period
EXCLUDES 2 *exposure to environmental tobacco smoke after the perinatal period (Z77.22)*
newborn affected by in utero exposure to tobacco (P04.2)

P96.82 Delayed separation of umbilical cord

P96.83 Meconium staining
EXCLUDES 1 *meconium aspiration (P24.00, P24.01)*
meconium passage during delivery (P03.82)
DEF: Meconium passed in utero causing discoloration on the fetal skin and nails or on the umbilicus. This staining may be incidental or may be an indicator of significant fetal stress that could affect outcomes.

P96.89 Other specified conditions originating in the perinatal period
Use additional code to specify condition

P96.9 Condition originating in the perinatal period, unspecified
Congenital debility NOS

Chapter 17. Congenital Malformations, Deformations, and Chromosomal Abnormalities (QØØ–Q99)

Chapter-specific Guidelines with Coding Examples

The chapter-specific guidelines from the ICD-10-CM Official Guidelines for Coding and Reporting have been provided below. Along with these guidelines are coding examples, contained in the shaded boxes, that have been developed to help illustrate the coding and/or sequencing guidance found in these guidelines.

Assign an appropriate code(s) from categories QØØ–Q99, Congenital malformations, deformations, and chromosomal abnormalities when a malformation/deformation or chromosomal abnormality is documented. A malformation/deformation/or chromosomal abnormality may be the principal/first-listed diagnosis on a record or a secondary diagnosis.

When a malformation/deformation/or chromosomal abnormality does not have a unique code assignment, assign additional code(s) for any manifestations that may be present.

When the code assignment specifically identifies the malformation/deformation/or chromosomal abnormality, manifestations that are an inherent component of the anomaly should not be coded separately. Additional codes should be assigned for manifestations that are not an inherent component.

8-day-old infant with tetralogy of Fallot and pulmonary stenosis

Q21.3 **Tetralogy of Fallot**

Explanation: Pulmonary stenosis is inherent in the disease process of tetralogy of Fallot. When the code assignment specifically identifies the malformation/deformation/or chromosomal abnormality, manifestations that are inherent components of the anomaly should not be coded separately.

7-month-old infant with Down syndrome and common atrioventricular canal

Q9Ø.9 **Down syndrome, unspecified**

Q21.23 **Complete atrioventricular septal defect**

Explanation: While a common atrioventricular canal is often associated with patients with Down syndrome, this manifestation is not an inherent component and may be reported separately. When the code assignment specifically identifies the anomaly, manifestations that are inherent components of the condition should not be coded separately. Additional codes should be assigned for manifestations that are not inherent components.

Codes from Chapter 17 may be used throughout the life of the patient. If a congenital malformation or deformity has been corrected, a personal history code should be used to identify the history of the malformation or deformity. Although present at birth, a malformation/deformation/or chromosomal abnormality may not be identified until later in life. Whenever the condition is diagnosed by the provider, it is appropriate to assign a code from codes QØØ–Q99. For the birth admission, the appropriate code from category Z38, Liveborn infants, according to place of birth and type of delivery, should be sequenced as the principal diagnosis, followed by any congenital anomaly codes, QØØ–Q99.

Three-year-old with history of corrected ventricular septal defect

Z87.74 **Personal history of (corrected) congenital malformations of heart and circulatory system**

Explanation: If a congenital malformation or deformity has been corrected, a personal history code should be used to identify the history of the malformation or deformity.

Forty-year-old man with headaches diagnosed with congenital arteriovenous malformation of cerebral vessels by brain scan

Q28.2 **Arteriovenous malformation of cerebral vessels**

Explanation: Although present at birth, malformations may not be identified until later in life. Whenever a congenital condition is diagnosed by the physician, it is appropriate to assign a code from the range QØØ–Q99.

Newborn with anencephaly delivered vaginally in hospital

Z38.ØØ **Single liveborn infant, delivered vaginally**

QØØ.Ø **Anencephaly**

Explanation: For the birth admission, the appropriate code from category Z38 Liveborn infants, according to place of birth and type of delivery, should be sequenced as the principal diagnosis, followed by any congenital anomaly codes, QØØ–Q99.

Chapter 17. Congenital Malformations, Deformations and Chromosomal Abnormalities (QØØ-Q99)

NOTE Codes from this chapter are not for use on maternal records

EXCLUDES 2 *inborn errors of metabolism (E7Ø-E88)*

This chapter contains the following blocks:

QØØ-QØ7 Congenital malformations of the nervous system
Q1Ø-Q18 Congenital malformations of eye, ear, face and neck
Q2Ø-Q28 Congenital malformations of the circulatory system
Q3Ø-Q34 Congenital malformations of the respiratory system
Q35-Q37 Cleft lip and cleft palate
Q38-Q45 Other congenital malformations of the digestive system
Q5Ø-Q56 Congenital malformations of genital organs
Q6Ø-Q64 Congenital malformations of the urinary system
Q65-Q79 Congenital malformations and deformations of the musculoskeletal system
Q8Ø-Q89 Other congenital malformations
Q9Ø-Q99 Chromosomal abnormalities, not elsewhere classified

Congenital malformations of the nervous system (QØØ-QØ7)

✓4th **QØØ Anencephaly and similar malformations**

QØØ.Ø Anencephaly MCC HCC
Acephaly
Acrania
Amyelencephaly
Hemianencephaly
Hemicephaly

QØØ.1 Craniorachischisis MCC HCC

QØØ.2 Iniencephaly MCC HCC

✓4th **QØ1 Encephalocele**

INCLUDES Arnold-Chiari syndrome, type III
encephalocystocele
encephalomyelocele
hydroencephalocele
hydromeningocele, cranial
meningocele, cerebral
meningoencephalocele

EXCLUDES 1 *Meckel-Gruber syndrome (Q61.9)*

DEF: Congenital protrusion of brain tissue through a defect in the skull.

QØ1.Ø Frontal encephalocele CC HCC

QØ1.1 Nasofrontal encephalocele CC HCC

QØ1.2 Occipital encephalocele CC HCC

QØ1.8 Encephalocele of other sites CC HCC

QØ1.9 Encephalocele, unspecified CC HCC

QØ2 Microcephaly HCC

INCLUDES hydromicrocephaly
micrencephalon

Code first, if applicable, congenital Zika virus disease

EXCLUDES 1 *Meckel-Gruber syndrome (Q61.9)*

AHA: 2018,4Q,26

DEF: Congenital disorder in which the head circumference is more than two standard deviations below the mean for age, sex, race, and gestation and associated with a decreased life expectancy.

✓4th **QØ3 Congenital hydrocephalus**

INCLUDES hydrocephalus in newborn

EXCLUDES 1 *acquired hydrocephalus (G91.-)*
Arnold-Chiari syndrome, type II (QØ7.Ø-)
hydrocephalus due to congenital toxoplasmosis (P37.1)
hydrocephalus with spina bifida (QØ5.Ø-QØ5.4)

DEF: Hydrocephalus: Abnormal buildup of cerebrospinal fluid in the brain causing dilation of the ventricles.

Congenital Hydrocephalus

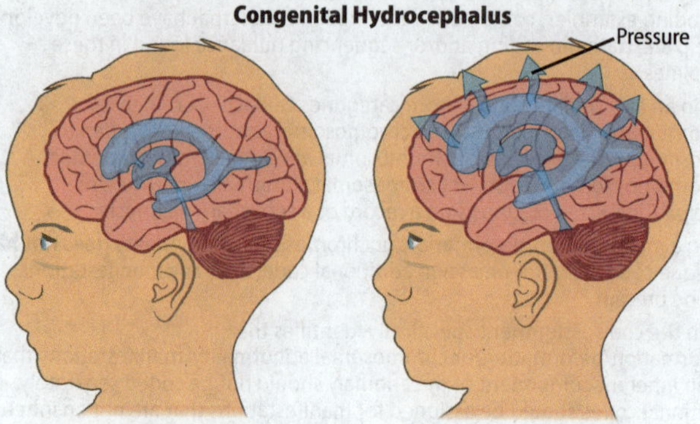

Pressure

Normal ventricles

Hydrocephalic ventricles

QØ3.Ø Malformations of aqueduct of Sylvius HCC
Anomaly of aqueduct of Sylvius
Obstruction of aqueduct of Sylvius, congenital
Stenosis of aqueduct of Sylvius

QØ3.1 Atresia of foramina of Magendie and Luschka HCC
Dandy-Walker syndrome

QØ3.8 Other congenital hydrocephalus HCC

QØ3.9 Congenital hydrocephalus, unspecified HCC

✓4th **QØ4 Other congenital malformations of brain**

EXCLUDES 1 *cyclopia (Q87.Ø)*
macrocephaly (Q75.3)

QØ4.Ø Congenital malformations of corpus callosum MCC HCC
Agenesis of corpus callosum

QØ4.1 Arhinencephaly MCC HCC

QØ4.2 Holoprosencephaly MCC HCC

QØ4.3 Other reduction deformities of brain MCC HCC
Absence of part of brain
Agenesis of part of brain
Agyria
Aplasia of part of brain
Hydranencephaly
Hypoplasia of part of brain
Lissencephaly
Microgyria
Pachygyria

EXCLUDES 1 *congenital malformations of corpus callosum (QØ4.Ø)*

QØ4.4 Septo-optic dysplasia of brain CC HCC

QØ4.5 Megalencephaly CC HCC

QØ4.6 Congenital cerebral cysts CC HCC
Porencephaly
Schizencephaly

EXCLUDES 1 *acquired porencephalic cyst (G93.Ø)*

QØ4.8 Other specified congenital malformations of brain CC HCC
Arnold-Chiari syndrome, type IV
Macrogyria

QØ4.9 Congenital malformation of brain, unspecified HCC
Congenital anomaly NOS of brain
Congenital deformity NOS of brain
Congenital disease or lesion NOS of brain
Multiple anomalies NOS of brain, congenital

Q05 Spina bifida

INCLUDES hydromeningocele (spinal)
meningocele (spinal)
meningomyelocele
myelocele
myelomeningocele
rachischisis
spina bifida (aperta)(cystica)
syringomyelocele

Use additional code for any associated paraplegia (paraparesis) (G82.2-)

EXCLUDES 1 *Arnold-Chiari syndrome, type II (Q07.0-)*
spina bifida occulta (Q76.0)

DEF: Lack of closure in the vertebral column with protrusion of the spinal cord through the defect, often in the lumbosacral area. This condition can be recognized by the presence of alpha-fetoproteins in the amniotic fluid.

Spina Bifida

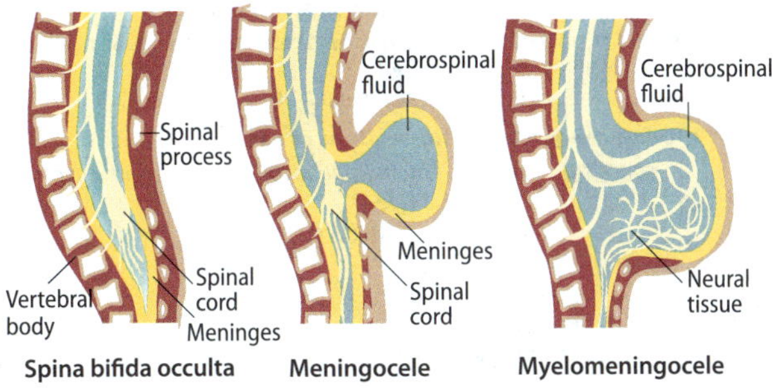

Q05.0 Cervical spina bifida with hydrocephalus CC HCC
Q05.1 Thoracic spina bifida with hydrocephalus CC HCC
Dorsal spina bifida with hydrocephalus
Thoracolumbar spina bifida with hydrocephalus
Q05.2 Lumbar spina bifida with hydrocephalus CC HCC
Lumbosacral spina bifida with hydrocephalus
Q05.3 Sacral spina bifida with hydrocephalus CC HCC
Q05.4 Unspecified spina bifida with hydrocephalus CC HCC
Q05.5 Cervical spina bifida without hydrocephalus HCC
Q05.6 Thoracic spina bifida without hydrocephalus HCC
Dorsal spina bifida NOS
Thoracolumbar spina bifida NOS
Q05.7 Lumbar spina bifida without hydrocephalus HCC
Lumbosacral spina bifida NOS
Q05.8 Sacral spina bifida without hydrocephalus HCC
Q05.9 Spina bifida, unspecified HCC

Q06 Other congenital malformations of spinal cord

Q06.0 Amyelia HCC
Q06.1 Hypoplasia and dysplasia of spinal cord HCC
Atelomyelia
Myelatelia
Myelodysplasia of spinal cord
Q06.2 Diastematomyelia HCC
DEF: Rare congenital anomaly often associated with spina bifida. The spinal cord is separated into longitudinal halves by a bony, cartilaginous or fibrous septum, each half surrounded by a dural sac.
Q06.3 Other congenital cauda equina malformations HCC
Q06.4 Hydromyelia HCC
Hydrorachis
Q06.8 Other specified congenital malformations of spinal cord HCC
Q06.9 Congenital malformation of spinal cord, unspecified HCC
Congenital anomaly NOS of spinal cord
Congenital deformity NOS of spinal cord
Congenital disease or lesion NOS of spinal cord

Q07 Other congenital malformations of nervous system

EXCLUDES 2 *congenital central alveolar hypoventilation syndrome (G47.35)*
familial dysautonomia [Riley-Day] (G90.1)
neurofibromatosis (nonmalignant) (Q85.0-)

Q07.0 Arnold-Chiari syndrome
Arnold-Chiari syndrome, type II
EXCLUDES 1 *Arnold-Chiari syndrome, type III (Q01.-)*
Arnold-Chiari syndrome, type IV (Q04.8)
DEF: Congenital malformation of the brain in which the cerebellum protrudes through the foramen magnum into the spinal canal.
Q07.00 Arnold-Chiari syndrome without spina bifida or hydrocephalus HCC
Q07.01 Arnold-Chiari syndrome with spina bifida HCC
Q07.02 Arnold-Chiari syndrome with hydrocephalus CC HCC
Q07.03 Arnold-Chiari syndrome with spina bifida and hydrocephalus CC HCC
Q07.8 Other specified congenital malformations of nervous system HCC
Agenesis of nerve
Displacement of brachial plexus
Jaw-winking syndrome
Marcus Gunn's syndrome
Q07.9 Congenital malformation of nervous system, unspecified HCC
Congenital anomaly NOS of nervous system
Congenital deformity NOS of nervous system
Congenital disease or lesion NOS of nervous system

Congenital malformations of eye, ear, face and neck (Q10-Q18)

EXCLUDES 2 *cleft lip and cleft palate (Q35-Q37)*
congenital malformation of cervical spine (Q05.0, Q05.5, Q67.5, Q76.0-Q76.4)
congenital malformation of larynx (Q31.-)
congenital malformation of lip NEC (Q38.0)
congenital malformation of nose (Q30.-)
congenital malformation of parathyroid gland (Q89.2)
congenital malformation of thyroid gland (Q89.2)

Q10 Congenital malformations of eyelid, lacrimal apparatus and orbit

EXCLUDES 1 *cryptophthalmos NOS (Q11.2)*
cryptophthalmos syndrome (Q87.0)

Q10.0 Congenital ptosis
DEF: Congenital drooping of the eyelid. Ptosis is mostly idiopathic, but may occur genetically.
Q10.1 Congenital ectropion
Q10.2 Congenital entropion
Q10.3 Other congenital malformations of eyelid
Ablepharon
Blepharophimosis, congenital
Coloboma of eyelid
Congenital absence or agenesis of cilia
Congenital absence or agenesis of eyelid
Congenital accessory eyelid
Congenital accessory eye muscle
Congenital malformation of eyelid NOS
Q10.4 Absence and agenesis of lacrimal apparatus
Congenital absence of punctum lacrimale
Q10.5 Congenital stenosis and stricture of lacrimal duct
Q10.6 Other congenital malformations of lacrimal apparatus
Congenital malformation of lacrimal apparatus NOS
Q10.7 Congenital malformation of orbit

Q11 Anophthalmos, microphthalmos and macrophthalmos

Q11.0 Cystic eyeball
Q11.1 Other anophthalmos
Anophthalmos NOS
Agenesis of eye
Aplasia of eye
Q11.2 Microphthalmos
Cryptophthalmos NOS
Dysplasia of eye
Hypoplasia of eye
Rudimentary eye
EXCLUDES 1 *cryptophthalmos syndrome (Q87.0)*
Q11.3 Macrophthalmos
EXCLUDES 1 *macrophthalmos in congenital glaucoma (Q15.0)*

Q12 Congenital lens malformations

Q12.0 Congenital cataract

Q12.1 Congenital displaced lens

Q12.2 Coloboma of lens

Coloboma of Lens

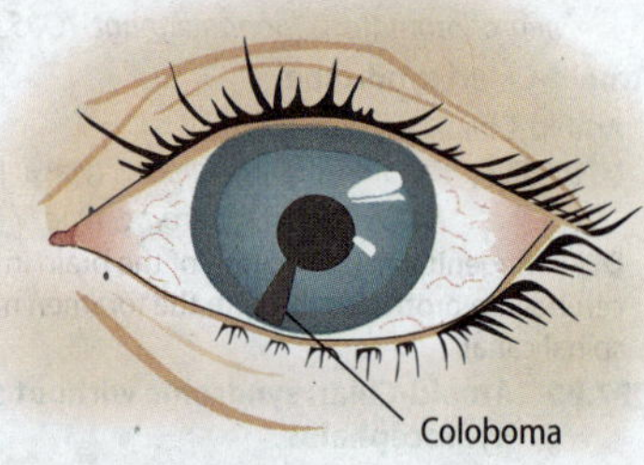

Q12.3 Congenital aphakia

Q12.4 Spherophakia

Q12.8 Other congenital lens malformations
Microphakia

Q12.9 Congenital lens malformation, unspecified

√4th Q13 Congenital malformations of anterior segment of eye

Q13.0 Coloboma of iris
Coloboma NOS
DEF: Defective or absent section of ocular tissue that may present as mild cupping or a small pit in the ocular disc due to extensive defects in the iris, ciliary body, choroids, and retina.

Q13.1 Absence of iris
Aniridia
Use additional code for associated glaucoma (H42)
DEF: Incompletely formed or absent iris. It affects both eyes and is a dominant trait.

Q13.2 Other congenital malformations of iris
Anisocoria, congenital
Atresia of pupil
Congenital malformation of iris NOS
Corectopia

Q13.3 Congenital corneal opacity

Q13.4 Other congenital corneal malformations
Congenital malformation of cornea NOS
Microcornea
Peter's anomaly

Q13.5 Blue sclera

√5th **Q13.8 Other congenital malformations of anterior segment of eye**

Q13.81 Rieger's anomaly
Use additional code for associated glaucoma (H42)

Q13.89 Other congenital malformations of anterior segment of eye

Q13.9 Congenital malformation of anterior segment of eye, unspecified

√4th Q14 Congenital malformations of posterior segment of eye

EXCLUDES 2 *optic nerve hypoplasia (H47.03-)*

Q14.0 Congenital malformation of vitreous humor
Congenital vitreous opacity

Q14.1 Congenital malformation of retina
Congenital retinal aneurysm

Q14.2 Congenital malformation of optic disc
Coloboma of optic disc

Q14.3 Congenital malformation of choroid

Q14.8 Other congenital malformations of posterior segment of eye
Coloboma of the fundus

Q14.9 Congenital malformation of posterior segment of eye, unspecified

√4th Q15 Other congenital malformations of eye

EXCLUDES 1 *congenital nystagmus (H55.01)*
ocular albinism (E70.31-)
optic nerve hypoplasia (H47.03-)
retinitis pigmentosa (H35.52)

Q15.0 Congenital glaucoma
Axenfeld's anomaly
Buphthalmos
Glaucoma of childhood
Glaucoma of newborn
Hydrophthalmos
Keratoglobus, congenital, with glaucoma
Macrocornea with glaucoma
Macrophthalmos in congenital glaucoma
Megalocornea with glaucoma

Q15.8 Other specified congenital malformations of eye

Q15.9 Congenital malformation of eye, unspecified
Congenital anomaly of eye
Congenital deformity of eye

√4th Q16 Congenital malformations of ear causing impairment of hearing

EXCLUDES 1 *congenital deafness (H90.-)*

Q16.0 Congenital absence of (ear) auricle

Q16.1 Congenital absence, atresia and stricture of auditory canal (external)
Congenital atresia or stricture of osseous meatus

Q16.2 Absence of eustachian tube

Q16.3 Congenital malformation of ear ossicles
Congenital fusion of ear ossicles

Q16.4 Other congenital malformations of middle ear
Congenital malformation of middle ear NOS

Q16.5 Congenital malformation of inner ear
Congenital anomaly of membranous labyrinth
Congenital anomaly of organ of Corti

Q16.9 Congenital malformation of ear causing impairment of hearing, unspecified
Congenital absence of ear NOS

√4th Q17 Other congenital malformations of ear

EXCLUDES 1 *congenital malformations of ear with impairment of hearing (Q16.0-Q16.9)*
preauricular sinus (Q18.1)

Q17.0 Accessory auricle
Accessory tragus
Polyotia
Preauricular appendage or tag
Supernumerary ear
Supernumerary lobule

Q17.1 Macrotia
DEF: Birth defect characterized by abnormal enlargement of the pinna of the ear.

Q17.2 Microtia

Q17.3 Other misshapen ear
Pointed ear

Q17.4 Misplaced ear
Low-set ears
EXCLUDES 1 *cervical auricle (Q18.2)*

Q17.5 Prominent ear
Bat ear

Q17.8 Other specified congenital malformations of ear
Congenital absence of lobe of ear

Q17.9 Congenital malformation of ear, unspecified
Congenital anomaly of ear NOS

√4th Q18 Other congenital malformations of face and neck

EXCLUDES 1 *cleft lip and cleft palate (Q35-Q37)*
conditions classified to Q67.0-Q67.4
congenital malformations of skull and face bones (Q75.-)
cyclopia (Q87.0)
dentofacial anomalies [including malocclusion] (M26.-)
malformation syndromes affecting facial appearance (Q87.0)
persistent thyroglossal duct (Q89.2)

Q18.0 Sinus, fistula and cyst of branchial cleft
Branchial vestige

Q18.1 Preauricular sinus and cyst
Cervicoaural fistula
Fistula of auricle, congenital

Q18.2 Other branchial cleft malformations
Branchial cleft malformation NOS
Cervical auricle
Otocephaly

Q18.3 Webbing of neck
Pterygium colli
DEF: Congenital malformation characterized by a thick, triangular skinfold that stretches from the lateral side of the neck across the shoulder. It is associated with genetic conditions such as Turner's and Noonan's syndromes.

Q18.4 Macrostomia
DEF: Rare congenital craniofacial bilateral or unilateral anomaly of the mouth due to malformed maxillary and mandibular processes. It results in an abnormally large mouth extending toward the ear.

Q18.5 Microstomia

Q18.6 Macrocheilia
Hypertrophy of lip, congenital

Q18.7 Microcheilia

Q18.8 Other specified congenital malformations of face and neck
Medial cyst of face and neck
Medial fistula of face and neck
Medial sinus of face and neck

Q18.9 Congenital malformation of face and neck, unspecified
Congenital anomaly NOS of face and neck

Congenital malformations of the circulatory system (Q2Ø-Q28)

Q2Ø Congenital malformations of cardiac chambers and connections
EXCLUDES 1 *dextrocardia with situs inversus (Q89.3)*
mirror-image atrial arrangement with situs inversus (Q89.3)

Q2Ø.Ø Common arterial trunk MCC
Persistent truncus arteriosus
EXCLUDES 1 *aortic septal defect (Q21.4)*

Q2Ø.1 Double outlet right ventricle MCC
Taussig-Bing syndrome

Q2Ø.2 Double outlet left ventricle MCC

Q2Ø.3 Discordant ventriculoarterial connection MCC
Dextrotransposition of aorta
Transposition of great vessels (complete)

Q2Ø.4 Double inlet ventricle MCC
Common ventricle
Cor triloculare biatriatum
Single ventricle

Q2Ø.5 Discordant atrioventricular connection CC
Corrected transposition
Levotransposition
Ventricular inversion

Q2Ø.6 Isomerism of atrial appendages
Isomerism of atrial appendages with asplenia or polysplenia

Q2Ø.8 Other congenital malformations of cardiac chambers and connections
Cor binoculare

Q2Ø.9 Congenital malformation of cardiac chambers and connections, unspecified

Q21 Congenital malformations of cardiac septa
EXCLUDES 1 *acquired cardiac septal defect (I51.Ø)*

Q21.Ø Ventricular septal defect CC
Roger's disease

Ventricular Septal Defect

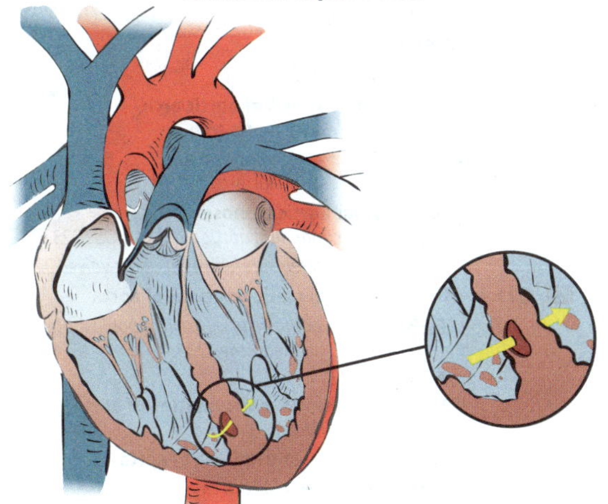

Q21.1 Atrial septal defect
EXCLUDES 2 *ostium primum atrial septal defect (type I) (Q21.2Ø)*
AHA: 2022,4Q,39-40

Atrial Septal Defect

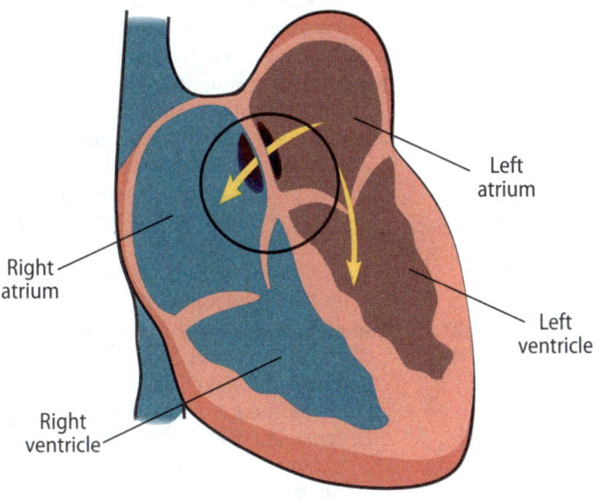

Q21.1Ø Atrial septal defect, unspecified CC

Q21.11 Secundum atrial septal defect CC
Fenestrated atrial septum
Patent or persistent ostium secundum defect (type II)

Q21.12 Patent foramen ovale CC
Persistent foramen ovale

Q21.13 Coronary sinus atrial septal defect CC
Coronary sinus defect
Unroofed coronary sinus

Q21.14 Superior sinus venosus atrial septal defect CC
Superior vena cava type atrial septal defect

Q21.15 Inferior sinus venosus atrial septal defect CC
Inferior vena cava type atrial septal defect

Q21.16 Sinus venosus atrial septal defect, unspecified CC
Sinus venosus defect, NOS

Q21.19 Other specified atrial septal defect CC
Common atrium
Other specified atrial septal abnormality

Q21.2 Atrioventricular septal defect
Atrioventricular canal defect
Endocardial cushion defect
Ostium primum atrial septal defect (type I)
AHA: 2022,4Q,39-40

Atrioventricular Septal Defect

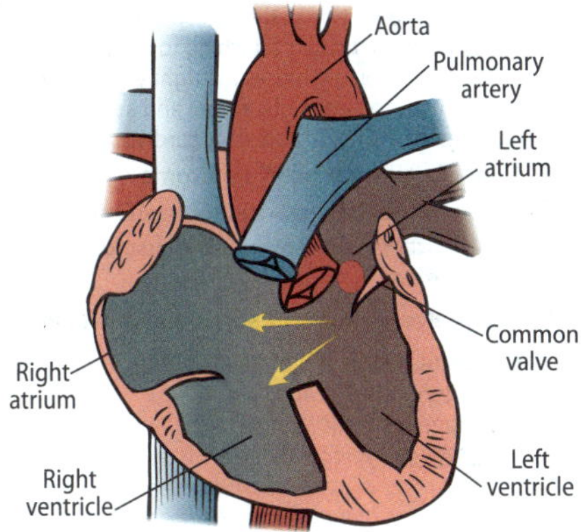

Q21.2Ø Atrioventricular septal defect, unspecified as to partial or complete CC
Atrioventricular canal, NOS
Endocardial cushion defect NOS
Ostium primum atrial septal defect (type I) NOS

Q21.21 Partial atrioventricular septal defect CC
Incomplete atrioventricular canal
Incomplete atrioventricular septal defect
Incomplete endocardial cushion defect
Ostium primum atrial septal defect (type I) with separate atrioventricular valves
Partial atrioventricular canal
Partial endocardial cushion defect

Q21.22 Transitional atrioventricular septal defect CC
Intermediate atrioventricular canal
Intermediate atrioventricular septal defect
Intermediate endocardial cushion defect
Ostium primum atrial septal defect (type I) with separate atrioventricular valves and a small or restrictive inlet VSD
Transitional atrioventricular canal
Transitional endocardial cushion defect

Q21.23 Complete atrioventricular septal defect CC
Common atrioventricular canal
Common atrioventricular septal defect
Common endocardial cushion defect
Ostium primum atrial septal defect (type I) with common atrioventricular valve and a moderate or larger inlet VSD

Q21.3 Tetralogy of Fallot MCC
Ventricular septal defect with pulmonary stenosis or atresia, dextroposition of aorta and hypertrophy of right ventricle.
AHA: 2014,3Q,16

Q21.4 Aortopulmonary septal defect
Aortic septal defect
Aortopulmonary window

Q21.8 Other congenital malformations of cardiac septa
Eisenmenger's defect
Pentalogy of Fallot
Code also, if applicable:
Eisenmenger's complex (I27.83)
Eisenmenger's syndrome (I27.83)

Q21.9 Congenital malformation of cardiac septum, unspecified
Septal (heart) defect NOS

✓4th Q22 Congenital malformations of pulmonary and tricuspid valves

Q22.Ø Pulmonary valve atresia MCC

Q22.1 Congenital pulmonary valve stenosis CC

Q22.2 Congenital pulmonary valve insufficiency CC
Congenital pulmonary valve regurgitation
AHA: 2022,4Q,39-40

Q22.3 Other congenital malformations of pulmonary valve CC
Congenital malformation of pulmonary valve NOS
Supernumerary cusps of pulmonary valve

Q22.4 Congenital tricuspid stenosis MCC
Congenital tricuspid atresia

Q22.5 Ebstein's anomaly MCC
DEF: Malformation of the tricuspid valve characterized by septal and posterior leaflets attaching to the wall of the right ventricle. Ebstein's anomaly causes the right ventricle to fuse with the atrium into a large right atrium and a small ventricle and leads to heart failure and abnormal cardiac rhythm.

Q22.6 Hypoplastic right heart syndrome MCC

Q22.8 Other congenital malformations of tricuspid valve MCC

Q22.9 Congenital malformation of tricuspid valve, unspecified MCC

✓4th Q23 Congenital malformations of aortic and mitral valves

Q23.Ø Congenital stenosis of aortic valve CC
Congenital aortic atresia
Congenital aortic stenosis NOS
EXCLUDES 1 *congenital stenosis of aortic valve in hypoplastic left heart syndrome (Q23.4)*
congenital subaortic stenosis (Q24.4)
supravalvular aortic stenosis (congenital) (Q25.3)

Q23.1 Congenital insufficiency of aortic valve CC
Bicuspid aortic valve
Congenital aortic insufficiency

Q23.2 Congenital mitral stenosis CC
Congenital mitral atresia

Q23.3 Congenital mitral insufficiency CC

Q23.4 Hypoplastic left heart syndrome MCC

Q23.8 Other congenital malformations of aortic and mitral valves

Q23.9 Congenital malformation of aortic and mitral valves, unspecified

✓4th Q24 Other congenital malformations of heart

EXCLUDES 1 *endocardial fibroelastosis (I42.4)*

Q24.Ø Dextrocardia CC
EXCLUDES 1 *dextrocardia with situs inversus (Q89.3)*
isomerism of atrial appendages (with asplenia or polysplenia) (Q2Ø.6)
mirror-image atrial arrangement with situs inversus (Q89.3)
DEF: Congenital condition in which the heart is located on the right side of the chest rather than in its normal position on the left.

Q24.1 Levocardia CC

Q24.2 Cor triatriatum MCC

Q24.3 Pulmonary infundibular stenosis CC
Subvalvular pulmonic stenosis

Q24.4 Congenital subaortic stenosis MCC
DEF: Congenital heart defect characterized by stenosis of the left ventricular outflow tract due to a fibrous tissue ring or septal hypertrophy below the aortic valve.

Q24.5 Malformation of coronary vessels CC
Congenital coronary (artery) aneurysm

Q24.6 Congenital heart block MCC

Q24.8 Other specified congenital malformations of heart
Congenital diverticulum of left ventricle
Congenital malformation of myocardium
Congenital malformation of pericardium
Malposition of heart
Uhl's disease

Q24.9 Congenital malformation of heart, unspecified
Congenital anomaly of heart
Congenital disease of heart

✓4th Q25 Congenital malformations of great arteries

Q25.Ø Patent ductus arteriosus CC
Patent ductus Botallo
Persistent ductus arteriosus
DEF: Condition in which the normal channel between the pulmonary artery and the aorta fails to close at birth, causing arterial blood to recirculate in the lungs and inhibiting the blood supply to the aorta. ***Synonym(s):*** *PDA.*

Q25.1 Coarctation of aorta CC
Coarctation of aorta (preductal) (postductal)
Stenosis of aorta
AHA: 2016,4Q,56-57

✓5th **Q25.2 Atresia of aorta**
AHA: 2016,4Q,56-57

Q25.21 Interruption of aortic arch CC
Atresia of aortic arch

Q25.29 Other atresia of aorta CC
Atresia of aorta

Q25.3 Supravalvular aortic stenosis CC
EXCLUDES 1 *congenital aortic stenosis NOS (Q23.Ø)*
congenital stenosis of aortic valve (Q23.Ø)

✓5th **Q25.4 Other congenital malformations of aorta**
EXCLUDES 1 *hypoplasia of aorta in hypoplastic left heart syndrome (Q23.4)*
AHA: 2016,4Q,57

Q25.40 Congenital malformation of aorta unspecified CC

Q25.41 Absence and aplasia of aorta CC

Q25.42 Hypoplasia of aorta CC

Q25.43 Congenital aneurysm of aorta CC
Congenital aneurysm of aortic root
Congenital aneurysm of aortic sinus

Q25.44 Congenital dilation of aorta CC

Q25.45 Double aortic arch CC
Vascular ring of aorta

Aortic Arch Anomalies

Normal aortic arch

Double aortic arch

Right aortic arch

Q25.46 Tortuous aortic arch CC
Persistent convolutions of aortic arch

Q25.47 Right aortic arch CC
Persistent right aortic arch

Q25.48 Anomalous origin of subclavian artery CC

Q25.49 Other congenital malformations of aorta CC
Aortic arch
Bovine arch

Q25.5 Atresia of pulmonary artery MCC

Q25.6 Stenosis of pulmonary artery MCC
Supravalvular pulmonary stenosis

✓5th **Q25.7 Other congenital malformations of pulmonary artery**

Q25.71 Coarctation of pulmonary artery MCC

Q25.72 Congenital pulmonary arteriovenous malformation MCC
Congenital pulmonary arteriovenous aneurysm

Q25.79 Other congenital malformations of pulmonary artery MCC
Aberrant pulmonary artery
Agenesis of pulmonary artery
Congenital aneurysm of pulmonary artery
Congenital anomaly of pulmonary artery
Hypoplasia of pulmonary artery

Q25.8 Other congenital malformations of other great arteries CC

Q25.9 Congenital malformation of great arteries, unspecified CC

✓4th **Q26 Congenital malformations of great veins**

Q26.Ø Congenital stenosis of vena cava CC
Congenital stenosis of vena cava (inferior)(superior)

Q26.1 Persistent left superior vena cava CC

Q26.2 Total anomalous pulmonary venous connection CC
Total anomalous pulmonary venous return [TAPVR], subdiaphragmatic
Total anomalous pulmonary venous return [TAPVR], supradiaphragmatic

Q26.3 Partial anomalous pulmonary venous connection CC
Partial anomalous pulmonary venous return

Q26.4 Anomalous pulmonary venous connection, unspecified CC

Q26.5 Anomalous portal venous connection

Q26.6 Portal vein-hepatic artery fistula

Q26.8 Other congenital malformations of great veins CC
Absence of vena cava (inferior) (superior)
Azygos continuation of inferior vena cava
Persistent left posterior cardinal vein
Scimitar syndrome

Q26.9 Congenital malformation of great vein, unspecified CC
Congenital anomaly of vena cava (inferior) (superior) NOS

✓4th **Q27 Other congenital malformations of peripheral vascular system**

EXCLUDES 2 *anomalies of cerebral and precerebral vessels (Q28.Ø-Q28.3)*
anomalies of coronary vessels (Q24.5)
anomalies of pulmonary artery (Q25.5-Q25.7)
congenital retinal aneurysm (Q14.1)
hemangioma and lymphangioma (D18.-)

Q27.Ø Congenital absence and hypoplasia of umbilical artery
Single umbilical artery

Q27.1 Congenital renal artery stenosis

Q27.2 Other congenital malformations of renal artery
Congenital malformation of renal artery NOS
Multiple renal arteries

✓5th **Q27.3 Arteriovenous malformation (peripheral)**
Arteriovenous aneurysm
EXCLUDES 1 *acquired arteriovenous aneurysm (I77.Ø)*
EXCLUDES 2 *arteriovenous malformation of cerebral vessels (Q28.2)*
arteriovenous malformation of precerebral vessels (Q28.Ø)

DEF: Arteriovenous malformation: Connecting passage between an artery and a vein.

Q27.3Ø Arteriovenous malformation, site unspecified CC

Q27.31 Arteriovenous malformation of vessel of upper limb

Q27.32 Arteriovenous malformation of vessel of lower limb

Q27.33 Arteriovenous malformation of digestive system vessel
AHA: 2018,3Q,21

Q27.34 Arteriovenous malformation of renal vessel

Q27.39 Arteriovenous malformation, other site

Q27.4 Congenital phlebectasia CC

Q27.8 Other specified congenital malformations of peripheral vascular system
Absence of peripheral vascular system
Atresia of peripheral vascular system
Congenital aneurysm (peripheral)
Congenital stricture, artery
Congenital varix
EXCLUDES 1 *arteriovenous malformation (Q27.3-)*

Q27.9 Congenital malformation of peripheral vascular system, unspecified
Anomaly of artery or vein NOS

✓4th **Q28 Other congenital malformations of circulatory system**

EXCLUDES 1 *congenital aneurysm NOS (Q27.8)*
congenital coronary aneurysm (Q24.5)
ruptured cerebral arteriovenous malformation (I6Ø.8)
ruptured malformation of precerebral vessels (I72.Ø)
EXCLUDES 2 *congenital peripheral aneurysm (Q27.8)*
congenital pulmonary aneurysm (Q25.79)
congenital retinal aneurysm (Q14.1)

Q28.Ø Arteriovenous malformation of precerebral vessels CC
Congenital arteriovenous precerebral aneurysm (nonruptured)

Q28.1 Other malformations of precerebral vessels CC
Congenital malformation of precerebral vessels NOS
Congenital precerebral aneurysm (nonruptured)

Q28.2 Arteriovenous malformation of cerebral vessels MCC
Arteriovenous malformation of brain NOS
Congenital arteriovenous cerebral aneurysm (nonruptured)

Q28.3 Other malformations of cerebral vessels MCC
Congenital cerebral aneurysm (nonruptured)
Congenital malformation of cerebral vessels NOS
Developmental venous anomaly

Q28.8 Other specified congenital malformations of circulatory system CC
Congenital aneurysm, specified site NEC
Spinal vessel anomaly

Q28.9 Congenital malformation of circulatory system, unspecified CC

Congenital malformations of the respiratory system (Q3Ø-Q34)

✓4th **Q3Ø Congenital malformations of nose**

EXCLUDES 1 *congenital deviation of nasal septum (Q67.4)*

Q3Ø.Ø Choanal atresia
Atresia of nares (anterior) (posterior)
Congenital stenosis of nares (anterior) (posterior)

Q3Ø.1 Agenesis and underdevelopment of nose
Congenital absent of nose

Q3Ø.2 Fissured, notched and cleft nose

Q3Ø.3 Congenital perforated nasal septum

Q3Ø.8 Other congenital malformations of nose
Accessory nose
Congenital anomaly of nasal sinus wall
AHA: 2022,2Q,17

Q3Ø.9 Congenital malformation of nose, unspecified

✓4th Q31 Congenital malformations of larynx
EXCLUDES 1 *congenital laryngeal stridor NOS (P28.89)*

Q31.Ø Web of larynx
Glottic web of larynx
Subglottic web of larynx
Web of larynx NOS
DEF: Congenital malformation of the larynx marked by thin, translucent, or thick fibrotic membrane-like structure between the vocal folds. It is characterized by shortness of breath and stridor.

Q31.1 Congenital subglottic stenosis CC

Q31.2 Laryngeal hypoplasia CC

Q31.3 Laryngocele CC

Q31.5 Congenital laryngomalacia CC

Q31.8 Other congenital malformations of larynx CC
Absence of larynx
Agenesis of larynx
Atresia of larynx
Congenital cleft thyroid cartilage
Congenital fissure of epiglottis
Congenital stenosis of larynx NEC
Posterior cleft of cricoid cartilage

Q31.9 Congenital malformation of larynx, unspecified CC

✓4th Q32 Congenital malformations of trachea and bronchus
EXCLUDES 1 *congenital bronchiectasis (Q33.4)*

Q32.Ø Congenital tracheomalacia CC

Q32.1 Other congenital malformations of trachea CC
Atresia of trachea
Congenital anomaly of tracheal cartilage
Congenital dilatation of trachea
Congenital malformation of trachea
Congenital stenosis of trachea
Congenital tracheocele

Q32.2 Congenital bronchomalacia CC

Q32.3 Congenital stenosis of bronchus CC

Q32.4 Other congenital malformations of bronchus CC
Absence of bronchus
Agenesis of bronchus
Atresia of bronchus
Congenital diverticulum of bronchus
Congenital malformation of bronchus NOS

✓4th Q33 Congenital malformations of lung

Q33.Ø Congenital cystic lung CC
Congenital cystic lung disease
Congenital honeycomb lung
Congenital polycystic lung disease
EXCLUDES 1 *cystic fibrosis (E84.Ø)*
cystic lung disease, acquired or unspecified (J98.4)

Q33.1 Accessory lobe of lung
Azygos lobe (fissured), lung

Q33.2 Sequestration of lung MCC

Q33.3 Agenesis of lung MCC
Congenital absence of lung (lobe)

Q33.4 Congenital bronchiectasis CC

Q33.5 Ectopic tissue in lung

Q33.6 Congenital hypoplasia and dysplasia of lung MCC
EXCLUDES 1 *pulmonary hypoplasia associated with short gestation (P28.Ø)*

Q33.8 Other congenital malformations of lung

Q33.9 Congenital malformation of lung, unspecified

✓4th Q34 Other congenital malformations of respiratory system
EXCLUDES 2 *congenital central alveolar hypoventilation syndrome (G47.35)*

Q34.Ø Anomaly of pleura

Q34.1 Congenital cyst of mediastinum

Q34.8 Other specified congenital malformations of respiratory system
Atresia of nasopharynx

Q34.9 Congenital malformation of respiratory system, unspecified
Congenital absence of respiratory system
Congenital anomaly of respiratory system NOS

Cleft lip and cleft palate (Q35-Q37)

Use additional code to identify associated malformation of the nose (Q3Ø.2)

EXCLUDES 2 *Robin's syndrome (Q87.Ø)*

✓4th Q35 Cleft palate
INCLUDES fissure of palate
palatoschisis
EXCLUDES 1 *cleft palate with cleft lip (Q37.-)*
DEF: Congenital fissure or defect of the roof of the mouth opening to the nasal cavity due to failure of embryonic cells to fuse completely.

Cleft Palate

Cleft in soft palate — Cleft in hard and soft palate

Q35.1 Cleft hard palate

Q35.3 Cleft soft palate

Q35.5 Cleft hard palate with cleft soft palate

Q35.7 Cleft uvula

Q35.9 Cleft palate, unspecified
Cleft palate NOS

✓4th Q36 Cleft lip
INCLUDES cheiloschisis
congenital fissure of lip
harelip
labium leporinum
EXCLUDES 1 *cleft lip with cleft palate (Q37.-)*
DEF: Congenital fissure or opening in the upper lip due to failure of embryonic cells to fuse completely.

Cleft Lip

Unilateral incomplete — Unilateral complete — Bilateral complete

Q36.Ø Cleft lip, bilateral

Q36.1 Cleft lip, median

Q36.9 Cleft lip, unilateral
Cleft lip NOS

✓4th Q37 Cleft palate with cleft lip
INCLUDES cheilopalatoschisis

Q37.Ø Cleft hard palate with bilateral cleft lip

Q37.1 Cleft hard palate with unilateral cleft lip
Cleft hard palate with cleft lip NOS

Q37.2 Cleft soft palate with bilateral cleft lip

Q37.3 Cleft soft palate with unilateral cleft lip
Cleft soft palate with cleft lip NOS

Q37.4 Cleft hard and soft palate with bilateral cleft lip

Q37.5 Cleft hard and soft palate with unilateral cleft lip
Cleft hard and soft palate with cleft lip NOS

Q37.8 Unspecified cleft palate with bilateral cleft lip

Q37.9 Unspecified cleft palate with unilateral cleft lip
Cleft palate with cleft lip NOS

Other congenital malformations of the digestive system (Q38-Q45)

Q38 Other congenital malformations of tongue, mouth and pharynx

EXCLUDES 1 *dentofacial anomalies (M26.-)*
macrostomia (Q18.4)
microstomia (Q18.5)

Q38.Ø Congenital malformations of lips, not elsewhere classified
Congenital fistula of lip
Congenital malformation of lip NOS
Van der Woude's syndrome
EXCLUDES 1 *cleft lip (Q36.-)*
cleft lip with cleft palate (Q37.-)
macrocheilia (Q18.6)
microcheilia (Q18.7)

Q38.1 Ankyloglossia
Tongue tie

Q38.2 Macroglossia
Congenital hypertrophy of tongue

Q38.3 Other congenital malformations of tongue
Aglossia
Bifid tongue
Congenital adhesion of tongue
Congenital fissure of tongue
Congenital malformation of tongue NOS
Double tongue
Hypoglossia
Hypoplasia of tongue
Microglossia

Q38.4 Congenital malformations of salivary glands and ducts
Atresia of salivary glands and ducts
Congenital absence of salivary glands and ducts
Congenital accessory salivary glands and ducts
Congenital fistula of salivary gland

Q38.5 Congenital malformations of palate, not elsewhere classified
Congenital absence of uvula
Congenital high arched palate
Congenital malformation of palate NOS
EXCLUDES 1 *cleft palate (Q35.-)*
cleft palate with cleft lip (Q37.-)

Q38.6 Other congenital malformations of mouth
Congenital malformation of mouth NOS

Q38.7 Congenital pharyngeal pouch
Congenital diverticulum of pharynx
EXCLUDES 1 *pharyngeal pouch syndrome (D82.1)*

Q38.8 Other congenital malformations of pharynx
Congenital malformation of pharynx NOS
Imperforate pharynx

Q39 Congenital malformations of esophagus

Q39.Ø Atresia of esophagus without fistula MCC
Atresia of esophagus NOS

Q39.1 Atresia of esophagus with tracheo-esophageal fistula MCC
Atresia of esophagus with broncho-esophageal fistula

Q39.2 Congenital tracheo-esophageal fistula without atresia MCC
Congenital tracheo-esophageal fistula NOS

Q39.3 Congenital stenosis and stricture of esophagus MCC

Q39.4 Esophageal web MCC

Q39.5 Congenital dilatation of esophagus CC
Congenital cardiospasm

Q39.6 Congenital diverticulum of esophagus CC
Congenital esophageal pouch

Q39.8 Other congenital malformations of esophagus CC
Congenital absence of esophagus
Congenital displacement of esophagus
Congenital duplication of esophagus

Q39.9 Congenital malformation of esophagus, unspecified CC

Q4Ø Other congenital malformations of upper alimentary tract

Q4Ø.Ø Congenital hypertrophic pyloric stenosis
Congenital or infantile constriction
Congenital or infantile hypertrophy
Congenital or infantile spasm
Congenital or infantile stenosis
Congenital or infantile stricture

Q4Ø.1 Congenital hiatus hernia
Congenital displacement of cardia through esophageal hiatus
EXCLUDES 1 *congenital diaphragmatic hernia (Q79.Ø)*

Q4Ø.2 Other specified congenital malformations of stomach
Congenital displacement of stomach
Congenital diverticulum of stomach
Congenital hourglass stomach
Congenital duplication of stomach
Megalogastria
Microgastria

Q4Ø.3 Congenital malformation of stomach, unspecified

Q4Ø.8 Other specified congenital malformations of upper alimentary tract

Q4Ø.9 Congenital malformation of upper alimentary tract, unspecified
Congenital anomaly of upper alimentary tract
Congenital deformity of upper alimentary tract

Q41 Congenital absence, atresia and stenosis of small intestine

INCLUDES congenital obstruction, occlusion or stricture of small intestine or intestine NOS
EXCLUDES 1 *cystic fibrosis with intestinal manifestation (E84.11)*
meconium ileus NOS (without cystic fibrosis) (P76.Ø)

Q41.Ø Congenital absence, atresia and stenosis of duodenum CC

Q41.1 Congenital absence, atresia and stenosis of jejunum CC
Apple peel syndrome
Imperforate jejunum

Q41.2 Congenital absence, atresia and stenosis of ileum CC

Q41.8 Congenital absence, atresia and stenosis of other specified parts of small intestine CC

Q41.9 Congenital absence, atresia and stenosis of small intestine, part unspecified CC
Congenital absence, atresia and stenosis of intestine NOS

Q42 Congenital absence, atresia and stenosis of large intestine

INCLUDES congenital obstruction, occlusion and stricture of large intestine

Q42.Ø Congenital absence, atresia and stenosis of rectum with fistula CC

Q42.1 Congenital absence, atresia and stenosis of rectum without fistula CC
Imperforate rectum

Q42.2 Congenital absence, atresia and stenosis of anus with fistula CC

Q42.3 Congenital absence, atresia and stenosis of anus without fistula CC
Imperforate anus

Q42.8 Congenital absence, atresia and stenosis of other parts of large intestine CC

Q42.9 Congenital absence, atresia and stenosis of large intestine, part unspecified CC

Q43 Other congenital malformations of intestine

Q43.Ø Meckel's diverticulum (displaced) (hypertrophic)
Persistent omphalomesenteric duct
Persistent vitelline duct
DEF: Congenital, abnormal remnant of embryonic digestive system development that leaves a sacculation or outpouching from the wall of the small intestine near the terminal part of the ileum made of acid-secreting tissue as in the stomach.

Q43.1 Hirschsprung's disease CC
Aganglionosis
Congenital (aganglionic) megacolon
DEF: Congenital enlargement or dilation of the colon, with the absence of nerve cells in a segment of colon distally that causes the inability to defecate.

Q43.2 Other congenital functional disorders of colon CC
Congenital dilatation of colon

Q43.3 Congenital malformations of intestinal fixation CC
Congenital omental, anomalous adhesions [bands]
Congenital peritoneal adhesions [bands]
Incomplete rotation of cecum and colon
Insufficient rotation of cecum and colon
Jackson's membrane
Malrotation of colon
Rotation failure of cecum and colon
Universal mesentery

Q43.4 Duplication of intestine CC

Q43.5 Ectopic anus CC

Q43.6 Congenital fistula of rectum and anus CC
EXCLUDES 1 *congenital fistula of anus with absence, atresia and stenosis (Q42.2)*
congenital fistula of rectum with absence, atresia and stenosis (Q42.0)
congenital rectovaginal fistula (Q52.2)
congenital urethrorectal fistula (Q64.73)
pilonidal fistula or sinus (L05.-)

Q43.7 Persistent cloaca CC
Cloaca NOS

Q43.8 Other specified congenital malformations of intestine CC
Congenital blind loop syndrome
Congenital diverticulitis, colon
Congenital diverticulum, intestine
Dolichocolon
Megaloappendix
Megaloduodenum
Microcolon
Transposition of appendix
Transposition of colon
Transposition of intestine
AHA: 2013,2Q,31

Q43.9 Congenital malformation of intestine, unspecified CC

Q44 Congenital malformations of gallbladder, bile ducts and liver

Q44.0 Agenesis, aplasia and hypoplasia of gallbladder CC
Congenital absence of gallbladder

Q44.1 Other congenital malformations of gallbladder CC
Congenital malformation of gallbladder NOS
Intrahepatic gallbladder

Q44.2 Atresia of bile ducts MCC

Q44.3 Congenital stenosis and stricture of bile ducts MCC

Q44.4 Choledochal cyst CC

Q44.5 Other congenital malformations of bile ducts CC
Accessory hepatic duct
Biliary duct duplication
Congenital malformation of bile duct NOS
Cystic duct duplication

Q44.6 Cystic disease of liver CC
Fibrocystic disease of liver

▲ **Q44.7 Other congenital malformations of liver**
~~Accessory liver~~
~~Alagille's syndrome~~
~~Congenital absence of liver~~
~~Congenital hepatomegaly~~
~~Congenital malformation of liver NOS~~
▶Code also, if applicable, associated malformations affecting other systems◀

● **Q44.70 Other congenital malformation of liver, unspecified** CC
Congenital malformation of liver, NOS

● **Q44.71 Alagille syndrome** CC
Alagille-Watson syndrome

● **Q44.79 Other congenital malformations of liver** CC
Accessory liver
Congenital absence of liver
Congenital hepatomegaly

Q45 Other congenital malformations of digestive system
EXCLUDES 2 *congenital diaphragmatic hernia (Q79.0)*
congenital hiatus hernia (Q40.1)

Q45.0 Agenesis, aplasia and hypoplasia of pancreas CC
Congenital absence of pancreas

Q45.1 Annular pancreas CC

Q45.2 Congenital pancreatic cyst CC

Q45.3 Other congenital malformations of pancreas and pancreatic duct CC
Accessory pancreas
Congenital malformation of pancreas or pancreatic duct NOS
EXCLUDES 1 *congenital diabetes mellitus (E10.-)*
cystic fibrosis (E84.0-E84.9)
fibrocystic disease of pancreas (E84.-)
neonatal diabetes mellitus (P70.2)

Q45.8 Other specified congenital malformations of digestive system
Absence (complete) (partial) of alimentary tract NOS
Duplication of digestive system
Malposition, congenital of digestive system

Q45.9 Congenital malformation of digestive system, unspecified
Congenital anomaly of digestive system
Congenital deformity of digestive system

Congenital malformations of genital organs (Q50-Q56)

EXCLUDES 1 *androgen insensitivity syndrome (E34.5-)*
syndromes associated with anomalies in the number and form of chromosomes (Q90-Q99)

Q50 Congenital malformations of ovaries, fallopian tubes and broad ligaments

Q50.0 Congenital absence of ovary
EXCLUDES 1 *Turner's syndrome (Q96.-)*

Q50.01 Congenital absence of ovary, unilateral ♀

Q50.02 Congenital absence of ovary, bilateral ♀

Q50.1 Developmental ovarian cyst ♀

Q50.2 Congenital torsion of ovary ♀

Q50.3 Other congenital malformations of ovary

Q50.31 Accessory ovary ♀

Q50.32 Ovarian streak ♀
46, XX with streak gonads

Q50.39 Other congenital malformation of ovary ♀
Congenital malformation of ovary NOS

Q50.4 Embryonic cyst of fallopian tube ♀
Fimbrial cyst

Q50.5 Embryonic cyst of broad ligament ♀
Epoophoron cyst
Parovarian cyst

Q50.6 Other congenital malformations of fallopian tube and broad ligament ♀
Absence of fallopian tube and broad ligament
Accessory fallopian tube and broad ligament
Atresia of fallopian tube and broad ligament
Congenital malformation of fallopian tube or broad ligament NOS

Q51 Congenital malformations of uterus and cervix

Q51.0 Agenesis and aplasia of uterus ♀
Congenital absence of uterus

Q51.1 Doubling of uterus with doubling of cervix and vagina

Q51.10 Doubling of uterus with doubling of cervix and vagina without obstruction ♀
Doubling of uterus with doubling of cervix and vagina NOS

Q51.11 Doubling of uterus with doubling of cervix and vagina with obstruction ♀

Q51.2 Other doubling of uterus
Doubling of uterus NOS
Septate uterus
AHA: 2018,4Q,27

Q51.21 Complete doubling of uterus ♀
Complete septate uterus

Q51.22 Partial doubling of uterus ♀
Partial septate uterus

Q51.28 Other and unspecified doubling of uterus ♀
Septate uterus NOS

Q51.3 Bicornate uterus ♀
Bicornate uterus, complete or partial

Q51.4 Unicornate uterus ♀
Unicornate uterus with or without a separate uterine horn
Uterus with only one functioning horn

Q51.5 Agenesis and aplasia of cervix ♀
Congenital absence of cervix

Q51.6 Embryonic cyst of cervix ♀

Q51.7 Congenital fistulae between uterus and digestive and urinary tracts ♀

Q51.8 Other congenital malformations of uterus and cervix

Q51.81 Other congenital malformations of uterus

Q51.810 Arcuate uterus ♀
Arcuatus uterus

Q51.811 Hypoplasia of uterus ♀

Q51.818 Other congenital malformations of uterus ♀
Mullerian anomaly of uterus NEC

Q51.82 Other congenital malformations of cervix

Q51.820 Cervical duplication ♀

Q51.821 Hypoplasia of cervix ♀

Q51.828 Other congenital malformations of cervix ♀

Q51.9 Congenital malformation of uterus and cervix, unspecified ♀

✓4th **Q52 Other congenital malformations of female genitalia**

Q52.0 Congenital absence of vagina ♀
Vaginal agenesis, total or partial

✓5th **Q52.1 Doubling of vagina**
EXCLUDES 1 *doubling of vagina with doubling of uterus and cervix (Q51.1-)*

Q52.10 Doubling of vagina, unspecified ♀
Septate vagina NOS

Q52.11 Transverse vaginal septum ♀

✓6th **Q52.12 Longitudinal vaginal septum**
AHA: 2016,4Q,58-59

Q52.120 Longitudinal vaginal septum, nonobstructing ♀

Q52.121 Longitudinal vaginal septum, obstructing, right side ♀

Q52.122 Longitudinal vaginal septum, obstructing, left side ♀

Q52.123 Longitudinal vaginal septum, microperforate, right side ♀

Q52.124 Longitudinal vaginal septum, microperforate, left side ♀

Q52.129 Other and unspecified longitudinal vaginal septum ♀

Q52.2 Congenital rectovaginal fistula ♀
EXCLUDES 1 *cloaca (Q43.7)*

Q52.3 Imperforate hymen ♀
DEF: Obstructive anomaly of vagina, characterized by complete closure of the membranous fold around the external opening of the vagina, obstructing the vaginal introitus.

Q52.4 Other congenital malformations of vagina ♀
Canal of Nuck cyst, congenital
Congenital malformation of vagina NOS
Embryonic vaginal cyst
Gartner's duct cyst
AHA: 2022,2Q,15

Q52.5 Fusion of labia ♀

Q52.6 Congenital malformation of clitoris ♀

✓5th **Q52.7 Other and unspecified congenital malformations of vulva**

Q52.70 Unspecified congenital malformations of vulva ♀
Congenital malformation of vulva NOS

Q52.71 Congenital absence of vulva ♀

Q52.79 Other congenital malformations of vulva ♀
Congenital cyst of vulva

Q52.8 Other specified congenital malformations of female genitalia ♀

Q52.9 Congenital malformation of female genitalia, unspecified ♀

✓4th **Q53 Undescended and ectopic testicle**

✓5th **Q53.0 Ectopic testis**

Q53.00 Ectopic testis, unspecified ♂

Q53.01 Ectopic testis, unilateral ♂

Q53.02 Ectopic testes, bilateral ♂

✓5th **Q53.1 Undescended testicle, unilateral**
AHA: 2017,4Q,22-23

Q53.10 Unspecified undescended testicle, unilateral ♂

✓6th **Q53.11 Abdominal testis, unilateral**

Q53.111 Unilateral intraabdominal testis ♂

Q53.112 Unilateral inguinal testis ♂

Q53.12 Ectopic perineal testis, unilateral ♂

Q53.13 Unilateral high scrotal testis ♂

✓5th **Q53.2 Undescended testicle, bilateral**
AHA: 2017,4Q,22-23

Q53.20 Undescended testicle, unspecified, bilateral ♂

✓6th **Q53.21 Abdominal testis, bilateral**

Q53.211 Bilateral intraabdominal testes ♂

Q53.212 Bilateral inguinal testes ♂

Q53.22 Ectopic perineal testis, bilateral ♂

Q53.23 Bilateral high scrotal testes ♂

Q53.9 Undescended testicle, unspecified ♂
Cryptorchism NOS

✓4th **Q54 Hypospadias**
EXCLUDES 1 *epispadias (Q64.0)*
DEF: Abnormal opening of the urethra on the ventral (underside) surface of the penis.

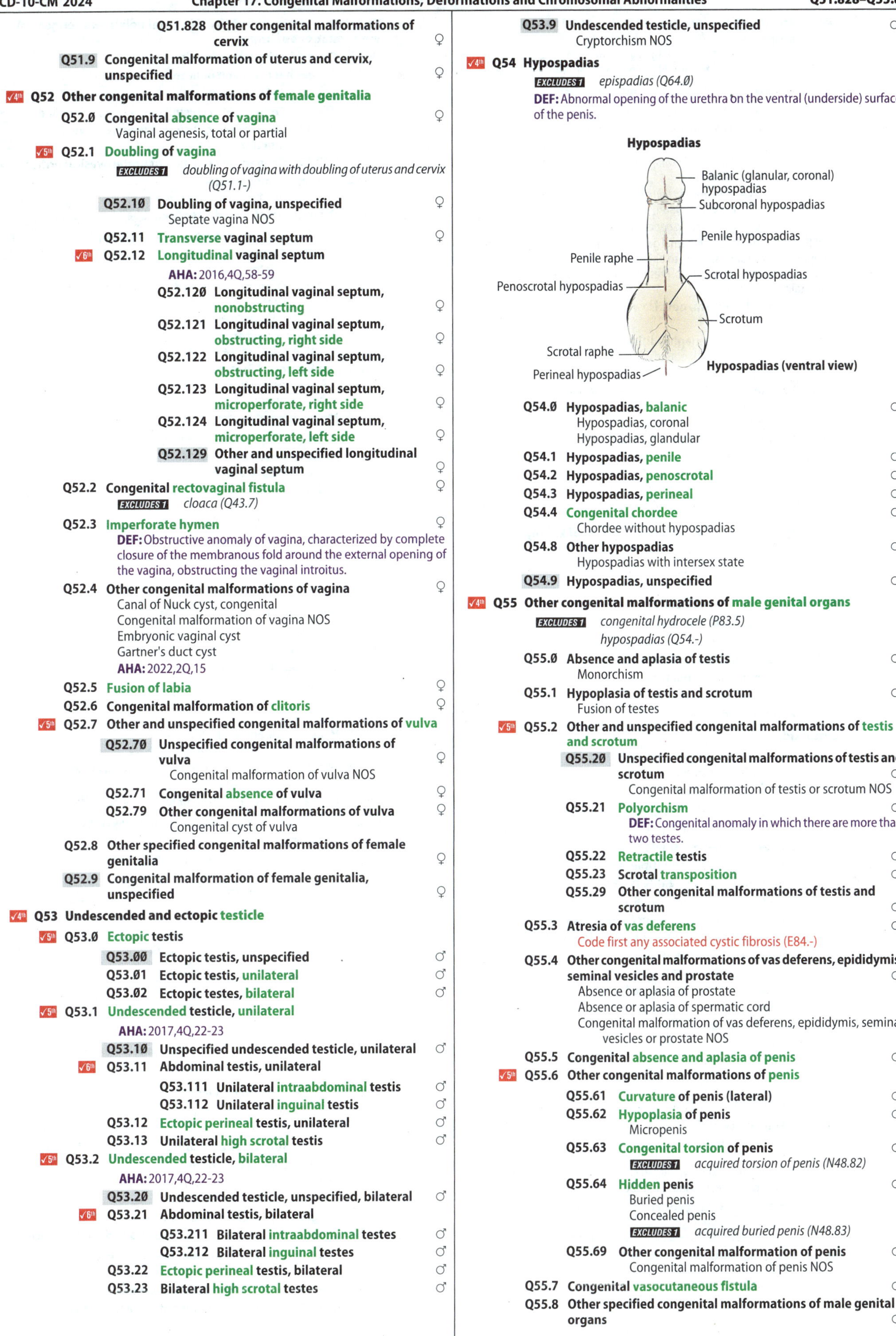

Q54.0 Hypospadias, balanic ♂
Hypospadias, coronal
Hypospadias, glandular

Q54.1 Hypospadias, penile ♂

Q54.2 Hypospadias, penoscrotal ♂

Q54.3 Hypospadias, perineal ♂

Q54.4 Congenital chordee ♂
Chordee without hypospadias

Q54.8 Other hypospadias ♂
Hypospadias with intersex state

Q54.9 Hypospadias, unspecified ♂

✓4th **Q55 Other congenital malformations of male genital organs**
EXCLUDES 1 *congenital hydrocele (P83.5)*
hypospadias (Q54.-)

Q55.0 Absence and aplasia of testis ♂
Monorchism

Q55.1 Hypoplasia of testis and scrotum ♂
Fusion of testes

✓5th **Q55.2 Other and unspecified congenital malformations of testis and scrotum**

Q55.20 Unspecified congenital malformations of testis and scrotum ♂
Congenital malformation of testis or scrotum NOS

Q55.21 Polyorchism ♂
DEF: Congenital anomaly in which there are more than two testes.

Q55.22 Retractile testis ♂

Q55.23 Scrotal transposition ♂

Q55.29 Other congenital malformations of testis and scrotum ♂

Q55.3 Atresia of vas deferens ♂
Code first any associated cystic fibrosis (E84.-)

Q55.4 Other congenital malformations of vas deferens, epididymis, seminal vesicles and prostate ♂
Absence or aplasia of prostate
Absence or aplasia of spermatic cord
Congenital malformation of vas deferens, epididymis, seminal vesicles or prostate NOS

Q55.5 Congenital absence and aplasia of penis ♂

✓5th **Q55.6 Other congenital malformations of penis**

Q55.61 Curvature of penis (lateral) ♂

Q55.62 Hypoplasia of penis ♂
Micropenis

Q55.63 Congenital torsion of penis ♂
EXCLUDES 1 *acquired torsion of penis (N48.82)*

Q55.64 Hidden penis ♂
Buried penis
Concealed penis
EXCLUDES 1 *acquired buried penis (N48.83)*

Q55.69 Other congenital malformation of penis ♂
Congenital malformation of penis NOS

Q55.7 Congenital vasocutaneous fistula ♂

Q55.8 Other specified congenital malformations of male genital organs ♂

Q55.9 Congenital malformation of male genital organ, unspecified ♂
Congenital anomaly of male genital organ
Congenital deformity of male genital organ

Q56 Indeterminate sex and pseudohermaphroditism
EXCLUDES 1 *46, XX true hermaphrodite (Q99.1)*
androgen insensitivity syndrome (E34.5-)
chimera 46, XX/46, XY true hermaphrodite (Q99.Ø)
female pseudohermaphroditism with adrenocortical disorder (E25.-)
pseudohermaphroditism with specified chromosomal anomaly (Q96-Q99)
pure gonadal dysgenesis (Q99.1)
DEF: Indeterminate sex: External genitalia that is nondescript, lacking the physical appearance specific to either sex.
DEF: Pseudohermaphroditism: Presence of gonads of one sex and external genitalia of another sex.

Q56.Ø Hermaphroditism, not elsewhere classified
Ovotestis
Q56.1 Male pseudohermaphroditism, not elsewhere classified ♂
46, XY with streak gonads
Male pseudohermaphroditism NOS
Q56.2 Female pseudohermaphroditism, not elsewhere classified ♀
Female pseudohermaphroditism NOS
Q56.3 Pseudohermaphroditism, unspecified
Q56.4 Indeterminate sex, unspecified
Ambiguous genitalia

Congenital malformations of the urinary system (Q6Ø-Q64)

Q6Ø Renal agenesis and other reduction defects of kidney
INCLUDES congenital absence of kidney
congenital atrophy of kidney
infantile atrophy of kidney

Q6Ø.Ø Renal agenesis, unilateral CC
Q6Ø.1 Renal agenesis, bilateral CC
Q6Ø.2 Renal agenesis, unspecified CC
Q6Ø.3 Renal hypoplasia, unilateral CC
Q6Ø.4 Renal hypoplasia, bilateral CC
Q6Ø.5 Renal hypoplasia, unspecified CC
Q6Ø.6 Potter's syndrome CC

Q61 Cystic kidney disease
EXCLUDES 1 *acquired cyst of kidney (N28.1)*
Potter's syndrome (Q6Ø.6)

Q61.Ø Congenital renal cyst
Q61.ØØ Congenital renal cyst, unspecified CC
Cyst of kidney NOS (congenital)
Q61.Ø1 Congenital single renal cyst CC
Q61.Ø2 Congenital multiple renal cysts CC
Q61.1 Polycystic kidney, infantile type
Polycystic kidney, autosomal recessive
Q61.11 Cystic dilatation of collecting ducts CC
Q61.19 Other polycystic kidney, infantile type CC
Q61.2 Polycystic kidney, adult type CC
Polycystic kidney, autosomal dominant
Q61.3 Polycystic kidney, unspecified CC
AHA: 2016,3Q,22
Q61.4 Renal dysplasia CC
Multicystic dysplastic kidney
Multicystic kidney (development)
Multicystic kidney disease
Multicystic renal dysplasia
EXCLUDES 1 *polycystic kidney disease (Q61.11-Q61.3)*
Q61.5 Medullary cystic kidney CC
Nephronophthisis
Sponge kidney NOS
DEF: Sponge kidney: Dilated collecting tubules that are usually asymptomatic. Calcinosis in tubules may cause renal insufficiency.
Q61.8 Other cystic kidney diseases CC
Fibrocystic kidney
Fibrocystic renal degeneration or disease
Q61.9 Cystic kidney disease, unspecified CC
Meckel-Gruber syndrome

Q62 Congenital obstructive defects of renal pelvis and congenital malformations of ureter
Q62.Ø Congenital hydronephrosis CC
Q62.1 Congenital occlusion of ureter
Atresia and stenosis of ureter
Q62.1Ø Congenital occlusion of ureter, unspecified CC
Q62.11 Congenital occlusion of ureteropelvic junction CC
Q62.12 Congenital occlusion of ureterovesical orifice CC
Q62.2 Congenital megaureter CC
Congenital dilatation of ureter
Q62.3 Other obstructive defects of renal pelvis and ureter
Q62.31 Congenital ureterocele, orthotopic CC
Q62.32 Cecoureterocele CC
Ectopic ureterocele
Q62.39 Other obstructive defects of renal pelvis and ureter CC
Ureteropelvic junction obstruction NOS
Q62.4 Agenesis of ureter
Congenital absence ureter
Q62.5 Duplication of ureter
Accessory ureter
Double ureter
Q62.6 Malposition of ureter
Q62.6Ø Malposition of ureter, unspecified
Q62.61 Deviation of ureter
Q62.62 Displacement of ureter
Q62.63 Anomalous implantation of ureter
Ectopia of ureter
Ectopic ureter
Q62.69 Other malposition of ureter
Q62.7 Congenital vesico-uretero-renal reflux
Q62.8 Other congenital malformations of ureter
Anomaly of ureter NOS

Q63 Other congenital malformations of kidney
EXCLUDES 1 *congenital nephrotic syndrome (NØ4.-)*
Q63.Ø Accessory kidney
Q63.1 Lobulated, fused and horseshoe kidney
Q63.2 Ectopic kidney
Congenital displaced kidney
Malrotation of kidney
Q63.3 Hyperplastic and giant kidney
Compensatory hypertrophy of kidney
Q63.8 Other specified congenital malformations of kidney
Congenital renal calculi
Q63.9 Congenital malformation of kidney, unspecified

Q64 Other congenital malformations of urinary system
Q64.Ø Epispadias
EXCLUDES 1 *hypospadias (Q54.-)*

Epispadias

Normal external urethral orifice
Glans penis
Foreskin (retracted)
Epispadias
Epispadias (dorsal view)

Q64.1 Exstrophy of urinary bladder
Q64.1Ø Exstrophy of urinary bladder, unspecified CC
Ectopia vesicae
Q64.11 Supravesical fissure of urinary bladder CC
Q64.12 Cloacal exstrophy of urinary bladder CC
Q64.19 Other exstrophy of urinary bladder CC
Extroversion of bladder
Q64.2 Congenital posterior urethral valves CC
Q64.3 Other atresia and stenosis of urethra and bladder neck
Q64.31 Congenital bladder neck obstruction CC
Congenital obstruction of vesicourethral orifice
Q64.32 Congenital stricture of urethra CC
Q64.33 Congenital stricture of urinary meatus CC

Q64.39 **Other atresia and stenosis of urethra and bladder neck** CC
Atresia and stenosis of urethra and bladder neck NOS

Q64.4 **Malformation of urachus**
Cyst of urachus
Patent urachus
Prolapse of urachus

Q64.5 **Congenital absence of bladder and urethra**

Q64.6 **Congenital diverticulum of bladder**

Q64.7 **Other and unspecified congenital malformations of bladder and urethra**
EXCLUDES 1 *congenital prolapse of bladder (mucosa) (Q79.4)*

Q64.70 **Unspecified congenital malformation of bladder and urethra**
Malformation of bladder or urethra NOS

Q64.71 **Congenital prolapse of urethra**

Q64.72 **Congenital prolapse of urinary meatus**

Q64.73 **Congenital urethrorectal fistula**

Q64.74 **Double urethra**

Q64.75 **Double urinary meatus**

Q64.79 **Other congenital malformations of bladder and urethra**

Q64.8 **Other specified congenital malformations of urinary system**

Q64.9 **Congenital malformation of urinary system, unspecified**
Congenital anomaly NOS of urinary system
Congenital deformity NOS of urinary system

Congenital malformations and deformations of the musculoskeletal system (Q65-Q79)

Q65 **Congenital deformities of hip**
EXCLUDES 1 *clicking hip (R29.4)*

Q65.0 **Congenital dislocation of hip, unilateral**

Q65.00 **Congenital dislocation of unspecified hip, unilateral**

Q65.01 **Congenital dislocation of right hip, unilateral**

Q65.02 **Congenital dislocation of left hip, unilateral**

Q65.1 **Congenital dislocation of hip, bilateral**

Q65.2 **Congenital dislocation of hip, unspecified**

Q65.3 **Congenital partial dislocation of hip, unilateral**

Q65.30 **Congenital partial dislocation of unspecified hip, unilateral**

Q65.31 **Congenital partial dislocation of right hip, unilateral**

Q65.32 **Congenital partial dislocation of left hip, unilateral**

Q65.4 **Congenital partial dislocation of hip, bilateral**

Q65.5 **Congenital partial dislocation of hip, unspecified**

Q65.6 **Congenital unstable hip**
Congenital dislocatable hip

Q65.8 **Other congenital deformities of hip**

Q65.81 **Congenital coxa valga**

Q65.82 **Congenital coxa vara**

Q65.89 **Other specified congenital deformities of hip**
Anteversion of femoral neck
Congenital acetabular dysplasia

Q65.9 **Congenital deformity of hip, unspecified**

Q66 **Congenital deformities of feet**
EXCLUDES 1 *reduction defects of feet (Q72.-)*
valgus deformities (acquired) (M21.0-)
varus deformities (acquired) (M21.1-)

AHA: 2019,4Q,13

Q66.0 **Congenital talipes equinovarus**

Q66.00 **Congenital talipes equinovarus, unspecified foot**

Q66.01 **Congenital talipes equinovarus, right foot**

Q66.02 **Congenital talipes equinovarus, left foot**

Q66.1 **Congenital talipes calcaneovarus**

Q66.10 **Congenital talipes calcaneovarus, unspecified foot**

Q66.11 **Congenital talipes calcaneovarus, right foot**

Q66.12 **Congenital talipes calcaneovarus, left foot**

Q66.2 **Congenital metatarsus (primus) varus**
AHA: 2016,4Q,59

Q66.21 **Congenital metatarsus primus varus**

Q66.211 **Congenital metatarsus primus varus, right foot**

Q66.212 **Congenital metatarsus primus varus, left foot**

Q66.219 **Congenital metatarsus primus varus, unspecified foot**

Q66.22 **Congenital metatarsus adductus**
Congenital metatarsus varus

Q66.221 **Congenital metatarsus adductus, right foot**

Q66.222 **Congenital metatarsus adductus, left foot**

Q66.229 **Congenital metatarsus adductus, unspecified foot**

Q66.3 **Other congenital varus deformities of feet**
Hallux varus, congenital

Q66.30 **Other congenital varus deformities of feet, unspecified foot**

Q66.31 **Other congenital varus deformities of feet, right foot**

Q66.32 **Other congenital varus deformities of feet, left foot**

Q66.4 **Congenital talipes calcaneovalgus**

Q66.40 **Congenital talipes calcaneovalgus, unspecified foot**

Q66.41 **Congenital talipes calcaneovalgus, right foot**

Q66.42 **Congenital talipes calcaneovalgus, left foot**

Q66.5 **Congenital pes planus**
Congenital flat foot
Congenital rigid flat foot
Congenital spastic (everted) flat foot
EXCLUDES 1 *pes planus, acquired (M21.4)*

Q66.50 **Congenital pes planus, unspecified foot**

Q66.51 **Congenital pes planus, right foot**

Q66.52 **Congenital pes planus, left foot**

Q66.6 **Other congenital valgus deformities of feet**
Congenital metatarsus valgus

Q66.7 **Congenital pes cavus**

Q66.70 **Congenital pes cavus, unspecified foot**

Q66.71 **Congenital pes cavus, right foot**

Q66.72 **Congenital pes cavus, left foot**

Q66.8 **Other congenital deformities of feet**

Q66.80 **Congenital vertical talus deformity, unspecified foot**

Q66.81 **Congenital vertical talus deformity, right foot**

Q66.82 **Congenital vertical talus deformity, left foot**

Q66.89 **Other specified congenital deformities of feet**
Congenital asymmetric talipes
Congenital clubfoot NOS
Congenital talipes NOS
Congenital tarsal coalition
Hammer toe, congenital
DEF: Clubfoot: Congenital anomaly of the foot with the heel elevated and rotated outward and the toes pointing inward.

Q66.9 **Congenital deformity of feet, unspecified**

Q66.90 **Congenital deformity of feet, unspecified, unspecified foot**

Q66.91 **Congenital deformity of feet, unspecified, right foot**

Q66.92 **Congenital deformity of feet, unspecified, left foot**

Q67 **Congenital musculoskeletal deformities of head, face, spine and chest**
EXCLUDES 1 *congenital malformation syndromes classified to Q87.-*
Potter's syndrome (Q60.6)

Q67.0 **Congenital facial asymmetry**

Q67.1 **Congenital compression facies**

Q67.2 **Dolichocephaly**
EXCLUDES 1 ▶*sagittal craniosynostosis (Q75.01)*◀

Q67.3 **Plagiocephaly**
EXCLUDES 1 ▶*coronal craniosynostosis (Q75.02-)*◀
▶*lambdoid craniosynostosis (Q75.04-)*◀

Q67.4 **Other congenital deformities of skull, face and jaw**
Congenital depressions in skull
Congenital hemifacial atrophy or hypertrophy
Deviation of nasal septum, congenital
Squashed or bent nose, congenital
EXCLUDES 1 *dentofacial anomalies [including malocclusion] (M26.-)*
syphilitic saddle nose (A50.5)
DEF: Deviated septum: Condition in which the nasal septum, a thin wall composed of cartilage and bone that separates the two nostrils, is crooked or displaced from the midline.

Q67.5 Congenital deformity of spine CC
Congenital postural scoliosis
Congenital scoliosis NOS
EXCLUDES 1 *infantile idiopathic scoliosis (M41.Ø)*
scoliosis due to congenital bony malformation (Q76.3)
AHA: 2014,4Q,26

Q67.6 Pectus excavatum
Congenital funnel chest

Q67.7 Pectus carinatum
Congenital pigeon chest

Q67.8 Other congenital deformities of chest CC
Congenital deformity of chest wall NOS

Q68 Other congenital musculoskeletal deformities
EXCLUDES 1 *reduction defects of limb(s) (Q71-Q73)*
EXCLUDES 2 *congenital myotonic chondrodystrophy (G71.13)*

Q68.Ø Congenital deformity of sternocleidomastoid muscle
Congenital contracture of sternocleidomastoid (muscle)
Congenital (sternomastoid) torticollis
Sternomastoid tumor (congenital)

Q68.1 Congenital deformity of finger(s) and hand CC
Congenital clubfinger
Spade-like hand (congenital)

Q68.2 Congenital deformity of knee
Congenital dislocation of knee
Congenital genu recurvatum

Q68.3 Congenital bowing of femur
EXCLUDES 1 *anteversion of femur (neck) (Q65.89)*

Q68.4 Congenital bowing of tibia and fibula

Q68.5 Congenital bowing of long bones of leg, unspecified

Q68.6 Discoid meniscus

Q68.8 Other specified congenital musculoskeletal deformities
Congenital deformity of clavicle
Congenital deformity of elbow
Congenital deformity of forearm
Congenital deformity of scapula
Congenital deformity of wrist
Congenital dislocation of elbow
Congenital dislocation of shoulder
Congenital dislocation of wrist

Q69 Polydactyly

Q69.Ø Accessory finger(s)

Q69.1 Accessory thumb(s)

Q69.2 Accessory toe(s)
Accessory hallux

Q69.9 Polydactyly, unspecified
Supernumerary digit(s) NOS

Q7Ø Syndactyly

Q7Ø.Ø Fused fingers
Complex syndactyly of fingers with synostosis
Q7Ø.ØØ Fused fingers, unspecified hand
Q7Ø.Ø1 Fused fingers, right hand
Q7Ø.Ø2 Fused fingers, left hand
Q7Ø.Ø3 Fused fingers, bilateral

Q7Ø.1 Webbed fingers
Simple syndactyly of fingers without synostosis
Q7Ø.1Ø Webbed fingers, unspecified hand
Q7Ø.11 Webbed fingers, right hand
Q7Ø.12 Webbed fingers, left hand
Q7Ø.13 Webbed fingers, bilateral

Q7Ø.2 Fused toes
Complex syndactyly of toes with synostosis
Q7Ø.2Ø Fused toes, unspecified foot
Q7Ø.21 Fused toes, right foot
Q7Ø.22 Fused toes, left foot
Q7Ø.23 Fused toes, bilateral

Q7Ø.3 Webbed toes
Simple syndactyly of toes without synostosis
Q7Ø.3Ø Webbed toes, unspecified foot
Q7Ø.31 Webbed toes, right foot
Q7Ø.32 Webbed toes, left foot
Q7Ø.33 Webbed toes, bilateral

Q7Ø.4 Polysyndactyly, unspecified
EXCLUDES 1 *specified syndactyly of hand and feet - code to specified conditions (Q7Ø.Ø-Q7Ø.3-)*

Q7Ø.9 Syndactyly, unspecified
Symphalangy NOS

Q71 Reduction defects of upper limb

Q71.Ø Congenital complete absence of upper limb
Q71.ØØ Congenital complete absence of unspecified upper limb
Q71.Ø1 Congenital complete absence of right upper limb
Q71.Ø2 Congenital complete absence of left upper limb
Q71.Ø3 Congenital complete absence of upper limb, bilateral

Q71.1 Congenital absence of upper arm and forearm with hand present
Q71.1Ø Congenital absence of unspecified upper arm and forearm with hand present
Q71.11 Congenital absence of right upper arm and forearm with hand present
Q71.12 Congenital absence of left upper arm and forearm with hand present
Q71.13 Congenital absence of upper arm and forearm with hand present, bilateral

Q71.2 Congenital absence of both forearm and hand
Q71.2Ø Congenital absence of both forearm and hand, unspecified upper limb
Q71.21 Congenital absence of both forearm and hand, right upper limb
Q71.22 Congenital absence of both forearm and hand, left upper limb
Q71.23 Congenital absence of both forearm and hand, bilateral

Q71.3 Congenital absence of hand and finger
Q71.3Ø Congenital absence of unspecified hand and finger
Q71.31 Congenital absence of right hand and finger
Q71.32 Congenital absence of left hand and finger
Q71.33 Congenital absence of hand and finger, bilateral

Q71.4 Longitudinal reduction defect of radius
Clubhand (congenital)
Radial clubhand
Q71.4Ø Longitudinal reduction defect of unspecified radius
Q71.41 Longitudinal reduction defect of right radius
Q71.42 Longitudinal reduction defect of left radius
Q71.43 Longitudinal reduction defect of radius, bilateral

Q71.5 Longitudinal reduction defect of ulna
Q71.5Ø Longitudinal reduction defect of unspecified ulna
Q71.51 Longitudinal reduction defect of right ulna
Q71.52 Longitudinal reduction defect of left ulna
Q71.53 Longitudinal reduction defect of ulna, bilateral

Q71.6 Lobster-claw hand
Q71.6Ø Lobster-claw hand, unspecified hand
Q71.61 Lobster-claw right hand
Q71.62 Lobster-claw left hand
Q71.63 Lobster-claw hand, bilateral

Q71.8 Other reduction defects of upper limb

Q71.81 Congenital shortening of upper limb
Q71.811 Congenital shortening of right upper limb
Q71.812 Congenital shortening of left upper limb
Q71.813 Congenital shortening of upper limb, bilateral
Q71.819 Congenital shortening of unspecified upper limb

Q71.89 Other reduction defects of upper limb
Q71.891 Other reduction defects of right upper limb
Q71.892 Other reduction defects of left upper limb
Q71.893 Other reduction defects of upper limb, bilateral
Q71.899 Other reduction defects of unspecified upper limb

Q71.9 Unspecified reduction defect of upper limb
Q71.9Ø Unspecified reduction defect of unspecified upper limb
Q71.91 Unspecified reduction defect of right upper limb
Q71.92 Unspecified reduction defect of left upper limb
Q71.93 Unspecified reduction defect of upper limb, bilateral

Q72 Reduction defects of lower limb

Q72.Ø Congenital complete absence of lower limb
- **Q72.ØØ Congenital complete absence of unspecified lower limb**
- **Q72.Ø1 Congenital complete absence of right lower limb**
- **Q72.Ø2 Congenital complete absence of left lower limb**
- **Q72.Ø3 Congenital complete absence of lower limb, bilateral**

Q72.1 Congenital absence of thigh and lower leg with foot present
- **Q72.1Ø Congenital absence of unspecified thigh and lower leg with foot present**
- **Q72.11 Congenital absence of right thigh and lower leg with foot present**
- **Q72.12 Congenital absence of left thigh and lower leg with foot present**
- **Q72.13 Congenital absence of thigh and lower leg with foot present, bilateral**

Q72.2 Congenital absence of both lower leg and foot
- **Q72.2Ø Congenital absence of both lower leg and foot, unspecified lower limb**
- **Q72.21 Congenital absence of both lower leg and foot, right lower limb**
- **Q72.22 Congenital absence of both lower leg and foot, left lower limb**
- **Q72.23 Congenital absence of both lower leg and foot, bilateral**

Q72.3 Congenital absence of foot and toe(s)
- **Q72.3Ø Congenital absence of unspecified foot and toe(s)**
- **Q72.31 Congenital absence of right foot and toe(s)**
- **Q72.32 Congenital absence of left foot and toe(s)**
- **Q72.33 Congenital absence of foot and toe(s), bilateral**

Q72.4 Longitudinal reduction defect of femur

Proximal femoral focal deficiency
- **Q72.4Ø Longitudinal reduction defect of unspecified femur**
- **Q72.41 Longitudinal reduction defect of right femur**
- **Q72.42 Longitudinal reduction defect of left femur**
- **Q72.43 Longitudinal reduction defect of femur, bilateral**

Q72.5 Longitudinal reduction defect of tibia
- **Q72.5Ø Longitudinal reduction defect of unspecified tibia**
- **Q72.51 Longitudinal reduction defect of right tibia**
- **Q72.52 Longitudinal reduction defect of left tibia**
- **Q72.53 Longitudinal reduction defect of tibia, bilateral**

Q72.6 Longitudinal reduction defect of fibula
- **Q72.6Ø Longitudinal reduction defect of unspecified fibula**
- **Q72.61 Longitudinal reduction defect of right fibula**
- **Q72.62 Longitudinal reduction defect of left fibula**
- **Q72.63 Longitudinal reduction defect of fibula, bilateral**

Q72.7 Split foot
- **Q72.7Ø Split foot, unspecified lower limb**
- **Q72.71 Split foot, right lower limb**
- **Q72.72 Split foot, left lower limb**
- **Q72.73 Split foot, bilateral**

Q72.8 Other reduction defects of lower limb
- **Q72.81 Congenital shortening of lower limb**
  - **Q72.811 Congenital shortening of right lower limb**
  - **Q72.812 Congenital shortening of left lower limb**
  - **Q72.813 Congenital shortening of lower limb, bilateral**
  - **Q72.819 Congenital shortening of unspecified lower limb**
- **Q72.89 Other reduction defects of lower limb**
  - **Q72.891 Other reduction defects of right lower limb**
  - **Q72.892 Other reduction defects of left lower limb**
  - **Q72.893 Other reduction defects of lower limb, bilateral**
  - **Q72.899 Other reduction defects of unspecified lower limb**

Q72.9 Unspecified reduction defect of lower limb
- **Q72.9Ø Unspecified reduction defect of unspecified lower limb**
- **Q72.91 Unspecified reduction defect of right lower limb**
- **Q72.92 Unspecified reduction defect of left lower limb**
- **Q72.93 Unspecified reduction defect of lower limb, bilateral**

Q73 Reduction defects of unspecified limb

Q73.Ø Congenital absence of unspecified limb(s)

Amelia NOS

Q73.1 Phocomelia, unspecified limb(s)

Phocomelia NOS

Q73.8 Other reduction defects of unspecified limb(s)

Longitudinal reduction deformity of unspecified limb(s)
Ectromelia of limb NOS
Hemimelia of limb NOS
Reduction defect of limb NOS

Q74 Other congenital malformations of limb(s)

EXCLUDES 1 *polydactyly (Q69.-)*
reduction defect of limb (Q71-Q73)
syndactyly (Q7Ø.-)

Q74.Ø Other congenital malformations of upper limb(s), including shoulder girdle

Accessory carpal bones
Cleidocranial dysostosis
Congenital pseudarthrosis of clavicle
Macrodactylia (fingers)
Madelung's deformity
Radioulnar synostosis
Sprengel's deformity
Triphalangeal thumb

Q74.1 Congenital malformation of knee

Congenital absence of patella
Congenital dislocation of patella
Congenital genu valgum
Congenital genu varum
Rudimentary patella

EXCLUDES 1 *congenital dislocation of knee (Q68.2)*
congenital genu recurvatum (Q68.2)
nail patella syndrome (Q87.2)

Q74.2 Other congenital malformations of lower limb(s), including pelvic girdle

Congenital fusion of sacroiliac joint
Congenital malformation of ankle joint
Congenital malformation of sacroiliac joint

EXCLUDES 1 *anteversion of femur (neck) (Q65.89)*

Q74.3 Arthrogryposis multiplex congenita CC

Q74.8 Other specified congenital malformations of limb(s)

Q74.9 Unspecified congenital malformation of limb(s)

Congenital anomaly of limb(s) NOS

Q75 Other congenital malformations of skull and face bones

EXCLUDES 1 *congenital malformation of face NOS (Q18.-)*
congenital malformation syndromes classified to Q87.-
dentofacial anomalies [including malocclusion] (M26.-)
musculoskeletal deformities of head and face (Q67.Ø-Q67.4)
skull defects associated with congenital anomalies of brain such as:
anencephaly (QØØ.Ø)
encephalocele (QØ1.-)
hydrocephalus (QØ3.-)
microcephaly (QØ2)

▲ **Q75.Ø Craniosynostosis**

~~Acrocephaly~~
~~Imperfect fusion of skull~~
~~Oxycephaly~~
~~Trigonocephaly~~

DEF: Congenital condition in which one or more of the cranial sutures fuse prematurely, creating a deformed or aberrant head shape.

● **Q75.ØØ Craniosynostosis unspecified**

Craniosynostosis NOS
- ● **Q75.ØØ1 Craniosynostosis unspecified, unilateral**
- ● **Q75.ØØ2 Craniosynostosis unspecified, bilateral**
- ● **Q75.ØØ9 Craniosynostosis unspecified**

  Imperfect fusion of skull

● **Q75.Ø1 Sagittal craniosynostosis**

Non-deformational dolichocephaly
Non-deformational scaphocephaly

EXCLUDES 1 *plagiocephaly (Q67.3)*

● ✓6th Q75.02 Coronal craniosynostosis
Non-deformational anterior plagiocephaly
EXCLUDES 1 *dolichocephaly (Q67.2)*

● Q75.021 Coronal craniosynostosis unilateral
Non-deformational anterior plagiocephaly

● Q75.022 Coronal craniosynostosis bilateral
Non-deformational brachycephaly

● Q75.029 Coronal craniosynostosis unspecified

● Q75.03 Metopic craniosynostosis
Trigonocephaly

● ✓6th Q75.04 Lambdoid craniosynostosis
Non-deformational posterior plagiocephaly
EXCLUDES 1 *dolichocephaly (Q67.2)*

● Q75.041 Lambdoid craniosynostosis, unilateral

● Q75.042 Lambdoid craniosynostosis, bilateral

● Q75.049 Lambdoid craniosynostosis, unspecified

● ✓6th Q75.05 Multi-suture craniosynostosis

● Q75.051 Cloverleaf skull
Kleeblattschaedel skull

● Q75.052 Pansynostosis

● Q75.058 Other multi-suture craniosynostosis
EXCLUDES 1 *coronal craniosynostosis, bilateral (Q75.022)*
lambdoid craniosynostosis, bilateral (Q75.042)

● Q75.08 Other single-suture craniosynostosis

Q75.1 Craniofacial dysostosis
Crouzon's disease

Q75.2 Hypertelorism

Q75.3 Macrocephaly

Q75.4 Mandibulofacial dysostosis
Franceschetti syndrome
Treacher Collins syndrome

Q75.5 Oculomandibular dysostosis

Q75.8 Other specified congenital malformations of skull and face bones
Absence of skull bone, congenital
Congenital deformity of forehead
Platybasia

Q75.9 Congenital malformation of skull and face bones, unspecified
Congenital anomaly of face bones NOS
Congenital anomaly of skull NOS

✓4th Q76 Congenital malformations of spine and bony thorax
EXCLUDES 1 *congenital musculoskeletal deformities of spine and chest (Q67.5-Q67.8)*

Q76.0 Spina bifida occulta
EXCLUDES 1 *meningocele (spinal) (Q05.-)*
spina bifida (aperta) (cystica) (Q05.-)

Q76.1 Klippel-Feil syndrome
Cervical fusion syndrome

Q76.2 Congenital spondylolisthesis
Congenital spondylolysis
EXCLUDES 1 *spondylolisthesis (acquired) (M43.1-)*
spondylolysis (acquired) (M43.0-)

Q76.3 Congenital scoliosis due to congenital bony malformation CC
Hemivertebra fusion or failure of segmentation with scoliosis

✓5th Q76.4 Other congenital malformations of spine, not associated with scoliosis

✓6th Q76.41 Congenital kyphosis

Q76.411 Congenital kyphosis, occipito-atlanto-axial region

Q76.412 Congenital kyphosis, cervical region

Q76.413 Congenital kyphosis, cervicothoracic region

Q76.414 Congenital kyphosis, thoracic region

Q76.415 Congenital kyphosis, thoracolumbar region

Q76.419 Congenital kyphosis, unspecified region

✓6th Q76.42 Congenital lordosis

Q76.425 Congenital lordosis, thoracolumbar region CC

Q76.426 Congenital lordosis, lumbar region CC

Q76.427 Congenital lordosis, lumbosacral region CC

Q76.428 Congenital lordosis, sacral and sacrococcygeal region CC

Q76.429 Congenital lordosis, unspecified region CC

Q76.49 Other congenital malformations of spine, not associated with scoliosis
Congenital absence of vertebra NOS
Congenital fusion of spine NOS
Congenital malformation of lumbosacral (joint) (region) NOS
Congenital malformation of spine NOS
Hemivertebra NOS
Malformation of spine NOS
Platyspondylisis NOS
Supernumerary vertebra NOS

Q76.5 Cervical rib
Supernumerary rib in cervical region

Q76.6 Other congenital malformations of ribs CC
Accessory rib
Congenital absence of rib
Congenital fusion of ribs
Congenital malformation of ribs NOS
EXCLUDES 1 *short rib syndrome (Q77.2)*

Q76.7 Congenital malformation of sternum CC
Congenital absence of sternum
Sternum bifidum

Q76.8 Other congenital malformations of bony thorax CC

Q76.9 Congenital malformation of bony thorax, unspecified CC

✓4th Q77 Osteochondrodysplasia with defects of growth of tubular bones and spine
EXCLUDES 1 *mucopolysaccharidosis (E76.0-E76.3)*
EXCLUDES 2 *congenital myotonic chondrodystrophy (G71.13)*

Q77.0 Achondrogenesis
Hypochondrogenesis

Q77.1 Thanatophoric short stature

Q77.2 Short rib syndrome CC
Asphyxiating thoracic dysplasia [Jeune]

Q77.3 Chondrodysplasia punctata
EXCLUDES 1 *Rhizomelic chondrodysplasia punctata (E71.43)*

Q77.4 Achondroplasia
Hypochondroplasia
Osteosclerosis congenita

Q77.5 Diastrophic dysplasia

Q77.6 Chondroectodermal dysplasia
Ellis-van Creveld syndrome

Q77.7 Spondyloepiphyseal dysplasia

Q77.8 Other osteochondrodysplasia with defects of growth of tubular bones and spine

Q77.9 Osteochondrodysplasia with defects of growth of tubular bones and spine, unspecified

✓4th Q78 Other osteochondrodysplasias
EXCLUDES 2 *congenital myotonic chondrodystrophy (G71.13)*

Q78.0 Osteogenesis imperfecta CC
Fragilitas ossium
Osteopsathyrosis

Q78.1 Polyostotic fibrous dysplasia
Albright(-McCune)(-Sternberg) syndrome

Q78.2 Osteopetrosis CC
Albers-Schonberg syndrome
Osteosclerosis NOS
DEF: Rare congenital condition in which the bones are excessively dense, resulting from a discrepancy in the formation and breakdown of bone.

Q78.3 Progressive diaphyseal dysplasia
Camurati-Engelmann syndrome

Q78.4 Enchondromatosis
Maffucci's syndrome
Ollier's disease

Q78.5 Metaphyseal dysplasia
Pyle's syndrome

Q78.6 Multiple congenital exostoses
Diaphyseal aclasis

Q78.8 Other specified osteochondrodysplasias
Osteopoikilosis

Q78.9 Osteochondrodysplasia, unspecified
Chondrodystrophy NOS
Osteodystrophy NOS

Q79 Congenital malformations of musculoskeletal system, not elsewhere classified

EXCLUDES 2 *congenital (sternomastoid) torticollis (Q68.Ø)*

Q79.Ø Congenital diaphragmatic hernia MCC

EXCLUDES 1 *congenital hiatus hernia (Q4Ø.1)*

Q79.1 Other congenital malformations of diaphragm MCC

Absence of diaphragm
Congenital malformation of diaphragm NOS
Eventration of diaphragm

Q79.2 Exomphalos MCC

Omphalocele

EXCLUDES 1 *umbilical hernia (K42.-)*

Q79.3 Gastroschisis MCC

Gastroschisis

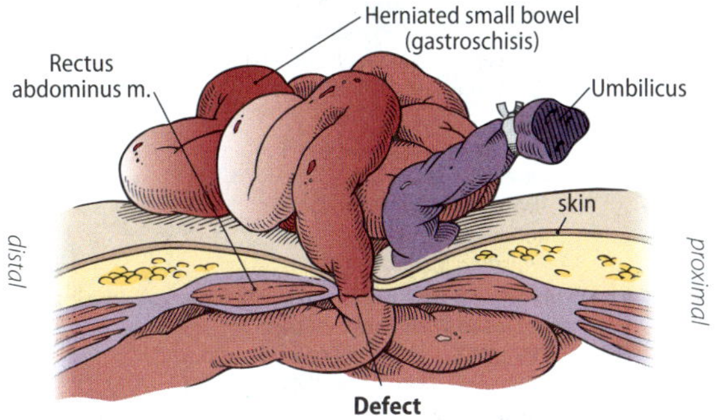

Q79.4 Prune belly syndrome MCC

Congenital prolapse of bladder mucosa
Eagle-Barrett syndrome

Q79.5 Other congenital malformations of abdominal wall

EXCLUDES 1 *umbilical hernia (K42.-)*

Q79.51 Congenital hernia of bladder MCC

Q79.59 Other congenital malformations of abdominal wall MCC

Q79.6 Ehlers-Danlos syndromes

AHA: 2019,4Q,13-14

DEF: Connective tissue disorder that causes hyperextended skin and joints and results in fragile blood vessels with bleeding, poor wound healing, and subcutaneous pseudotumors.

Q79.6Ø Ehlers-Danlos syndrome, unspecified CC

Q79.61 Classical Ehlers-Danlos syndrome CC

Classical EDS (cEDS)

Q79.62 Hypermobile Ehlers-Danlos syndrome CC

Hypermobile EDS (hEDS)

Q79.63 Vascular Ehlers-Danlos syndrome CC

Vascular EDS (vEDS)

Q79.69 Other Ehlers-Danlos syndromes CC

Q79.8 Other congenital malformations of musculoskeletal system

Absence of muscle
Absence of tendon
Accessory muscle
Amyotrophia congenita
Congenital constricting bands
Congenital shortening of tendon
Poland syndrome

Q79.9 Congenital malformation of musculoskeletal system, unspecified

Congenital anomaly of musculoskeletal system NOS
Congenital deformity of musculoskeletal system NOS

Other congenital malformations (Q8Ø-Q89)

Q8Ø Congenital ichthyosis

EXCLUDES 1 *Refsum's disease (G6Ø.1)*

DEF: Excessive production of skin cells resulting in red, dry, scaly skin.

Q8Ø.Ø Ichthyosis vulgaris

Q8Ø.1 X-linked ichthyosis

Q8Ø.2 Lamellar ichthyosis

Collodion baby

Q8Ø.3 Congenital bullous ichthyosiform erythroderma

Q8Ø.4 Harlequin fetus

Q8Ø.8 Other congenital ichthyosis

Q8Ø.9 Congenital ichthyosis, unspecified

Q81 Epidermolysis bullosa

Q81.Ø Epidermolysis bullosa simplex

EXCLUDES 1 *Cockayne's syndrome (Q87.19)*

Q81.1 Epidermolysis bullosa letalis

Herlitz' syndrome

Q81.2 Epidermolysis bullosa dystrophica

Q81.8 Other epidermolysis bullosa

Q81.9 Epidermolysis bullosa, unspecified

Q82 Other congenital malformations of skin

EXCLUDES 1 *acrodermatitis enteropathica (E83.2)*
congenital erythropoietic porphyria (E8Ø.Ø)
pilonidal cyst or sinus (LØ5.-)
Sturge-Weber (-Dimitri) syndrome (Q85.89)

Q82.Ø Hereditary lymphedema

Q82.1 Xeroderma pigmentosum

Q82.2 Congenital cutaneous mastocytosis

Congenital diffuse cutaneous mastocytosis
Congenital maculopapular cutaneous mastocytosis
Congenital urticaria pigmentosa

EXCLUDES 1 *cutaneous mastocytosis NOS (D47.Ø1)*
diffuse cutaneous mastocytosis (with onset after newborn period) (D47.Ø1)
malignant mastocytosis (C96.2-)
systemic mastocytosis (D47.Ø2)
urticaria pigmentosa (non-congenital) (with onset after newborn period) (D47.Ø1)

AHA: 2017,4Q,5

Q82.3 Incontinentia pigmenti

Q82.4 Ectodermal dysplasia (anhidrotic)

EXCLUDES 1 *Ellis-van Creveld syndrome (Q77.6)*

Q82.5 Congenital non-neoplastic nevus

Birthmark NOS
Flammeus Nevus
Portwine Nevus
Sanguineous Nevus
Strawberry Nevus
Vascular Nevus NOS
Verrucous Nevus

EXCLUDES 2 *araneus nevus (I78.1)*
Cafe au lait spots (L81.3)
lentigo (L81.4)
melanocytic nevus (D22.-)
nevus NOS (D22.-)
pigmented nevus (D22.-)
spider nevus (I78.1)
stellar nevus (I78.1)

Q82.6 Congenital sacral dimple

Parasacral dimple

EXCLUDES 2 *pilonidal cyst with abscess (LØ5.Ø1)*
pilonidal cyst without abscess (LØ5.91)

AHA: 2016,4Q,60

Q82.8 Other specified congenital malformations of skin

Abnormal palmar creases
Accessory skin tags
Benign familial pemphigus [Hailey-Hailey]
Congenital poikiloderma
Cutis laxa (hyperelastica)
Dermatoglyphic anomalies
Inherited keratosis palmaris et plantaris
Keratosis follicularis [Darier-White]

EXCLUDES 1 *Ehlers-Danlos syndromes (Q79.6-)*

AHA: 2021,3Q,10; 2016,1Q,17

Q82.9 Congenital malformation of skin, unspecified

Q83 Congenital malformations of breast

EXCLUDES 2 *absence of pectoral muscle (Q79.8)*
hypoplasia of breast (N64.82)
micromastia (N64.82)

Q83.Ø Congenital absence of breast with absent nipple

Q83.1 Accessory breast

Supernumerary breast

Q83.2 Absent nipple

Q83.3 Accessory nipple

Supernumerary nipple

Q83.8 Other congenital malformations of breast

Q83.9 Congenital malformation of breast, unspecified

Q84 Other congenital malformations of integument

Q84.0 Congenital alopecia
Congenital atrichosis

Q84.1 Congenital morphological disturbances of hair, not elsewhere classified
Beaded hair
Monilethrix
Pili annulati
EXCLUDES 1 *Menkes' kinky hair syndrome ▶(E83.09)◀*

Q84.2 Other congenital malformations of hair
Congenital hypertrichosis
Congenital malformation of hair NOS
Persistent lanugo

Q84.3 Anonychia
EXCLUDES 1 *nail patella syndrome (Q87.2)*

Q84.4 Congenital leukonychia

Q84.5 Enlarged and hypertrophic nails
Congenital onychauxis
Pachyonychia

Q84.6 Other congenital malformations of nails
Congenital clubnail
Congenital koilonychia
Congenital malformation of nail NOS

Q84.8 Other specified congenital malformations of integument
Aplasia cutis congenita

Q84.9 Congenital malformation of integument, unspecified
Congenital anomaly of integument NOS
Congenital deformity of integument NOS

Q85 Phakomatoses, not elsewhere classified
EXCLUDES 1 *ataxia telangiectasia [Louis-Bar] (G11.3)*
familial dysautonomia [Riley-Day] (G90.1)

Q85.0 Neurofibromatosis (nonmalignant)

Q85.00 Neurofibromatosis, unspecified HCC

Q85.01 Neurofibromatosis, type 1 HCC
Von Recklinghausen disease

Q85.02 Neurofibromatosis, type 2 HCC
Acoustic neurofibromatosis
DEF: Inherited condition with cutaneous lesions, benign tumors of peripheral nerves, and bilateral 8th nerve masses.

Q85.03 Schwannomatosis HCC
DEF: Genetic mutation (SMARCB1/INI1) causing multiple benign tumors along the nerve pathways, except on the 8th cranial (vestibular) nerve.

Q85.09 Other neurofibromatosis HCC

Q85.1 Tuberous sclerosis CC HCC
Bourneville's disease
Epiloia

Q85.8 Other phakomatoses, not elsewhere classified
EXCLUDES 1 *Meckel-Gruber syndrome (Q61.9)*
AHA: 2022,4Q,40-41; 2021,3Q,12

▲ **Q85.81 PTEN hamartoma tumor syndrome** CC HCC
PHTS
~~PTEN hamartoma tumor syndrome~~
PTEN related Cowden syndrome
Code also, if applicable, genetic susceptibility to malignant neoplasm (Z15.0-)
AHA: 2022,4Q,41
TIP: PTEN hamartoma tumor syndrome (PHTS) manifests differently in each patient. Separate codes should be assigned in addition to code Q85.81 for any manifestations of PHTS, such as macrocephaly, autism, or learning delays.

Q85.82 Other Cowden syndrome CC HCC

Q85.83 Von Hippel-Lindau syndrome CC HCC
Code also manifestations
AHA: 2023,2Q,16

Q85.89 Other phakomatoses, not elsewhere classified CC HCC
Peutz-Jeghers syndrome
Sturge-Weber(-Dimitri) syndrome

Q85.9 Phakomatosis, unspecified CC HCC
Hamartosis NOS

Q86 Congenital malformation syndromes due to known exogenous causes, not elsewhere classified
EXCLUDES 2 *iodine-deficiency-related hypothyroidism (E00-E02)*
nonteratogenic effects of substances transmitted via placenta or breast milk (P04.-)

Q86.0 Fetal alcohol syndrome (dysmorphic)

Q86.1 Fetal hydantoin syndrome
Meadow's syndrome

Q86.2 Dysmorphism due to warfarin

Q86.8 Other congenital malformation syndromes due to known exogenous causes

Q87 Other specified congenital malformation syndromes affecting multiple systems
Use additional code(s) to identify all associated manifestations

Q87.0 Congenital malformation syndromes predominantly affecting facial appearance
Acrocephalopolysyndactyly
Acrocephalosyndactyly [Apert]
Cryptophthalmos syndrome
Cyclopia
Goldenhar syndrome
Moebius syndrome
Oro-facial-digital syndrome
Robin syndrome
Whistling face

Q87.1 Congenital malformation syndromes predominantly associated with short stature
EXCLUDES 1 *Ellis-van Creveld syndrome (Q77.6)*
Smith-Lemli-Opitz syndrome (E78.72)
AHA: 2019,4Q,14-15

Q87.11 Prader-Willi syndrome CC

Q87.19 Other congenital malformation syndromes predominantly associated with short stature CC
Aarskog syndrome
Cockayne syndrome
De Lange syndrome
Dubowitz syndrome
Noonan syndrome
Robinow-Silverman-Smith syndrome
Russell-Silver syndrome
Seckel syndrome

Q87.2 Congenital malformation syndromes predominantly involving limbs CC
Holt-Oram syndrome
Klippel-Trenaunay-Weber syndrome
Nail patella syndrome
Rubinstein-Taybi syndrome
Sirenomelia syndrome
Thrombocytopenia with absent radius [TAR] syndrome
VATER syndrome

Q87.3 Congenital malformation syndromes involving early overgrowth CC
Beckwith-Wiedemann syndrome
Sotos syndrome
Weaver syndrome

▲ **Q87.4 Marfan syndrome**
DEF: Disorder that affects the connective tissue of multiple systems, including disproportionally long or abnormal bone structure and eye and cardiovascular complications.

▲ **Q87.40 Marfan syndrome, unspecified** CC

▲ **Q87.41 Marfan syndrome with cardiovascular manifestations**

▲ **Q87.410 Marfan syndrome with aortic dilation** CC

▲ **Q87.418 Marfan syndrome with other cardiovascular manifestations** CC

▲ **Q87.42 Marfan syndrome with ocular manifestations** CC

▲ **Q87.43 Marfan syndrome with skeletal manifestation** CC

Q87.5 Other congenital malformation syndromes with other skeletal changes CC

Q87.8 Other specified congenital malformation syndromes, not elsewhere classified
EXCLUDES 1 *Zellweger syndrome (E71.510)*

Q87.81 Alport syndrome CC
Use additional code to identify stage of chronic kidney disease (N18.1-N18.6)

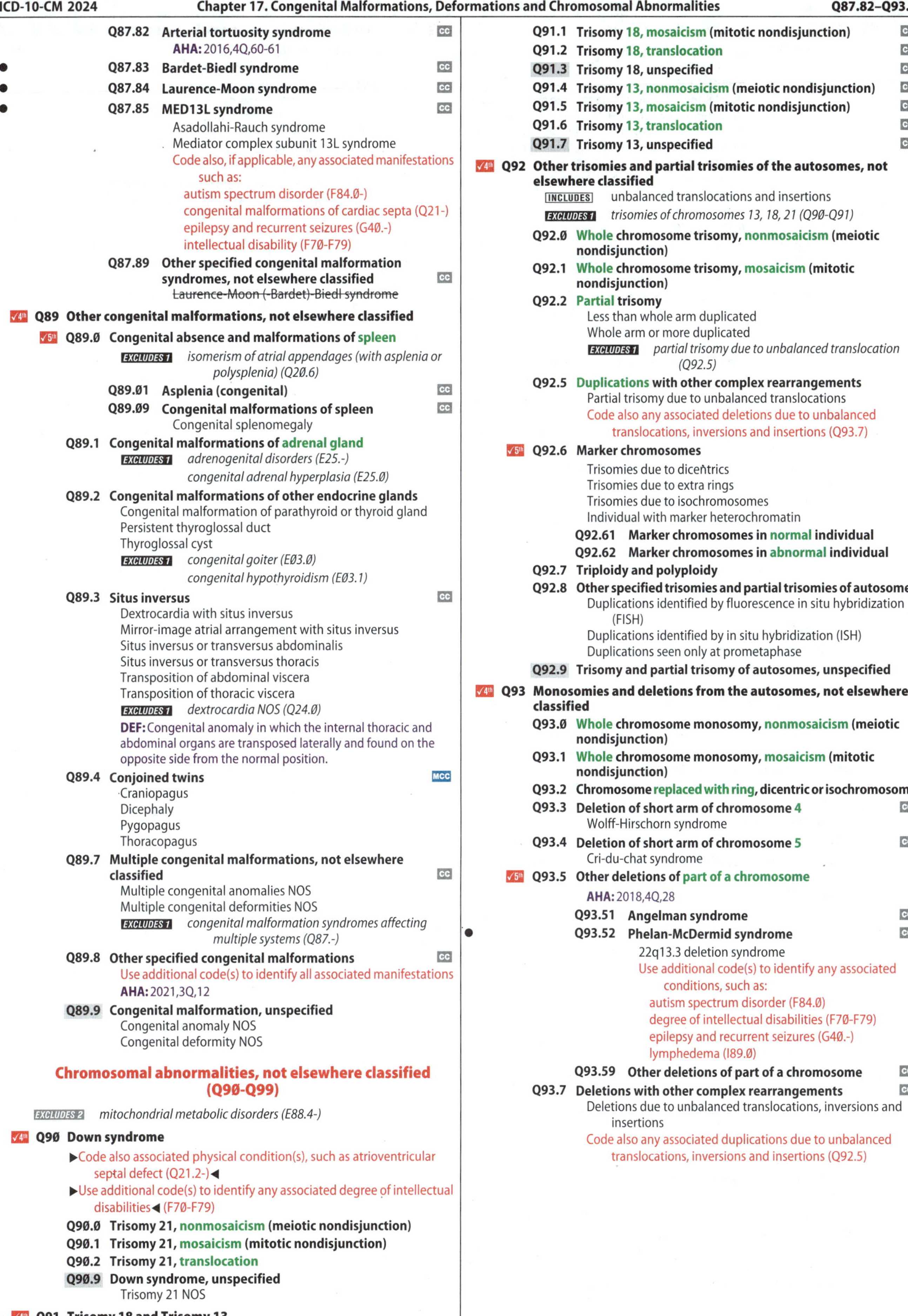

Q87.82 **Arterial tortuosity syndrome** CC
AHA: 2016,4Q,60-61

● Q87.83 **Bardet-Biedl syndrome** CC

● Q87.84 **Laurence-Moon syndrome** CC

● Q87.85 **MED13L syndrome** CC
Asadollahi-Rauch syndrome
Mediator complex subunit 13L syndrome
Code also, if applicable, any associated manifestations such as:
autism spectrum disorder (F84.Ø-)
congenital malformations of cardiac septa (Q21-)
epilepsy and recurrent seizures (G4Ø.-)
intellectual disability (F7Ø-F79)

Q87.89 **Other specified congenital malformation syndromes, not elsewhere classified** CC
~~Laurence-Moon (-Bardet)-Biedl syndrome~~

√4th **Q89 Other congenital malformations, not elsewhere classified**

√5th **Q89.Ø Congenital absence and malformations of spleen**
EXCLUDES 1 *isomerism of atrial appendages (with asplenia or polysplenia) (Q2Ø.6)*

Q89.Ø1 **Asplenia (congenital)** CC

Q89.Ø9 **Congenital malformations of spleen** CC
Congenital splenomegaly

Q89.1 Congenital malformations of adrenal gland
EXCLUDES 1 *adrenogenital disorders (E25.-)*
congenital adrenal hyperplasia (E25.Ø)

Q89.2 Congenital malformations of other endocrine glands
Congenital malformation of parathyroid or thyroid gland
Persistent thyroglossal duct
Thyroglossal cyst
EXCLUDES 1 *congenital goiter (EØ3.Ø)*
congenital hypothyroidism (EØ3.1)

Q89.3 Situs inversus CC
Dextrocardia with situs inversus
Mirror-image atrial arrangement with situs inversus
Situs inversus or transversus abdominalis
Situs inversus or transversus thoracis
Transposition of abdominal viscera
Transposition of thoracic viscera
EXCLUDES 1 *dextrocardia NOS (Q24.Ø)*
DEF: Congenital anomaly in which the internal thoracic and abdominal organs are transposed laterally and found on the opposite side from the normal position.

Q89.4 Conjoined twins MCC
Craniopagus
Dicephaly
Pygopagus
Thoracopagus

Q89.7 Multiple congenital malformations, not elsewhere classified CC
Multiple congenital anomalies NOS
Multiple congenital deformities NOS
EXCLUDES 1 *congenital malformation syndromes affecting multiple systems (Q87.-)*

Q89.8 Other specified congenital malformations CC
Use additional code(s) to identify all associated manifestations
AHA: 2021,3Q,12

Q89.9 Congenital malformation, unspecified
Congenital anomaly NOS
Congenital deformity NOS

Chromosomal abnormalities, not elsewhere classified (Q9Ø-Q99)

EXCLUDES 2 *mitochondrial metabolic disorders (E88.4-)*

√4th **Q9Ø Down syndrome**
▶Code also associated physical condition(s), such as atrioventricular septal defect (Q21.2-)◀
▶Use additional code(s) to identify any associated degree of intellectual disabilities◀ (F7Ø-F79)

Q9Ø.Ø Trisomy 21, nonmosaicism (meiotic nondisjunction)
Q9Ø.1 Trisomy 21, mosaicism (mitotic nondisjunction)
Q9Ø.2 Trisomy 21, translocation
Q9Ø.9 Down syndrome, unspecified
Trisomy 21 NOS

√4th **Q91 Trisomy 18 and Trisomy 13**

Q91.Ø Trisomy 18, nonmosaicism (meiotic nondisjunction) CC
Q91.1 Trisomy 18, mosaicism (mitotic nondisjunction) CC
Q91.2 Trisomy 18, translocation CC
Q91.3 Trisomy 18, unspecified CC
Q91.4 Trisomy 13, nonmosaicism (meiotic nondisjunction) CC
Q91.5 Trisomy 13, mosaicism (mitotic nondisjunction) CC
Q91.6 Trisomy 13, translocation CC
Q91.7 Trisomy 13, unspecified CC

√4th **Q92 Other trisomies and partial trisomies of the autosomes, not elsewhere classified**
INCLUDES unbalanced translocations and insertions
EXCLUDES 1 *trisomies of chromosomes 13, 18, 21 (Q9Ø-Q91)*

Q92.Ø Whole chromosome trisomy, nonmosaicism (meiotic nondisjunction)
Q92.1 Whole chromosome trisomy, mosaicism (mitotic nondisjunction)
Q92.2 Partial trisomy
Less than whole arm duplicated
Whole arm or more duplicated
EXCLUDES 1 *partial trisomy due to unbalanced translocation (Q92.5)*

Q92.5 Duplications with other complex rearrangements
Partial trisomy due to unbalanced translocations
Code also any associated deletions due to unbalanced translocations, inversions and insertions (Q93.7)

√5th **Q92.6 Marker chromosomes**
Trisomies due to dicentrics
Trisomies due to extra rings
Trisomies due to isochromosomes
Individual with marker heterochromatin

Q92.61 **Marker chromosomes in normal individual**
Q92.62 **Marker chromosomes in abnormal individual**

Q92.7 Triploidy and polyploidy
Q92.8 Other specified trisomies and partial trisomies of autosomes
Duplications identified by fluorescence in situ hybridization (FISH)
Duplications identified by in situ hybridization (ISH)
Duplications seen only at prometaphase
Q92.9 Trisomy and partial trisomy of autosomes, unspecified

√4th **Q93 Monosomies and deletions from the autosomes, not elsewhere classified**

Q93.Ø Whole chromosome monosomy, nonmosaicism (meiotic nondisjunction)
Q93.1 Whole chromosome monosomy, mosaicism (mitotic nondisjunction)
Q93.2 Chromosome replaced with ring, dicentric or isochromosome
Q93.3 Deletion of short arm of chromosome 4 CC
Wolff-Hirschorn syndrome
Q93.4 Deletion of short arm of chromosome 5 CC
Cri-du-chat syndrome

√5th **Q93.5 Other deletions of part of a chromosome**
AHA: 2018,4Q,28

Q93.51 **Angelman syndrome** CC

● Q93.52 **Phelan-McDermid syndrome** CC
22q13.3 deletion syndrome
Use additional code(s) to identify any associated conditions, such as:
autism spectrum disorder (F84.Ø)
degree of intellectual disabilities (F7Ø-F79)
epilepsy and recurrent seizures (G4Ø.-)
lymphedema (I89.Ø)

Q93.59 **Other deletions of part of a chromosome** CC

Q93.7 Deletions with other complex rearrangements CC
Deletions due to unbalanced translocations, inversions and insertions
Code also any associated duplications due to unbalanced translocations, inversions and insertions (Q92.5)

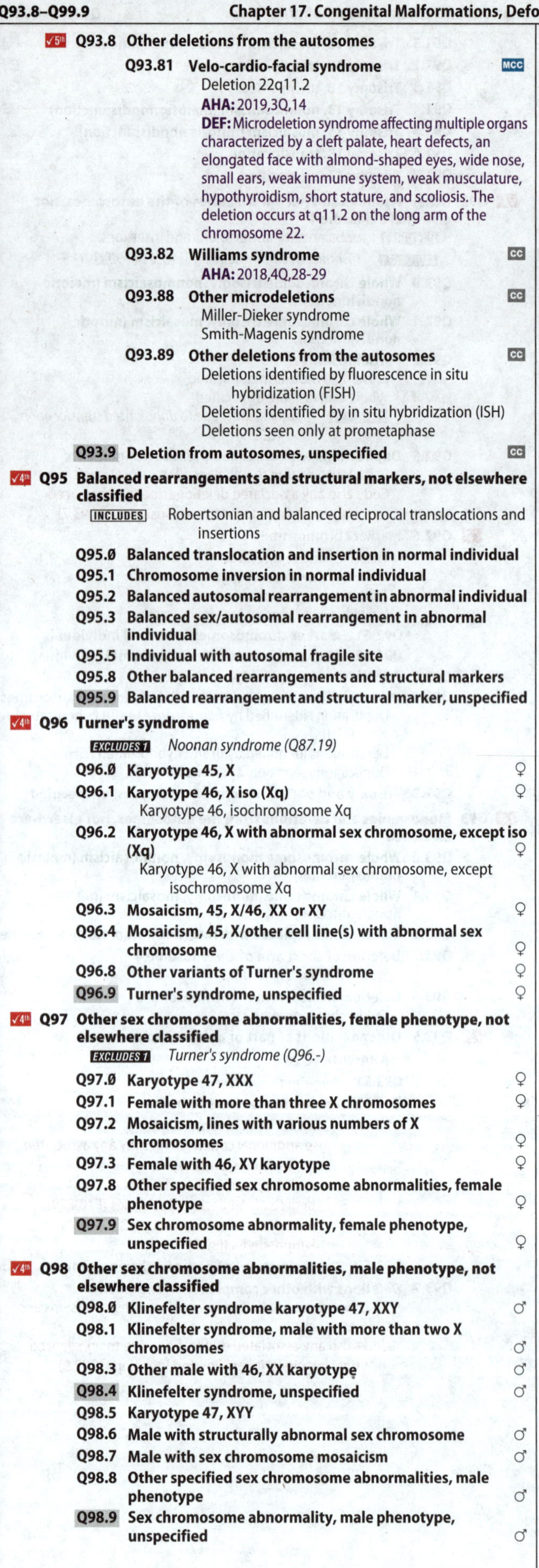

✓5th **Q93.8 Other deletions from the autosomes**

Q93.81 Velo-cardio-facial syndrome MCC
Deletion 22q11.2
AHA: 2019,3Q,14
DEF: Microdeletion syndrome affecting multiple organs characterized by a cleft palate, heart defects, an elongated face with almond-shaped eyes, wide nose, small ears, weak immune system, weak musculature, hypothyroidism, short stature, and scoliosis. The deletion occurs at q11.2 on the long arm of the chromosome 22.

Q93.82 Williams syndrome CC
AHA: 2018,4Q,28-29

Q93.88 Other microdeletions CC
Miller-Dieker syndrome
Smith-Magenis syndrome

Q93.89 Other deletions from the autosomes CC
Deletions identified by fluorescence in situ hybridization (FISH)
Deletions identified by in situ hybridization (ISH)
Deletions seen only at prometaphase

Q93.9 Deletion from autosomes, unspecified CC

✓4th **Q95 Balanced rearrangements and structural markers, not elsewhere classified**

INCLUDES Robertsonian and balanced reciprocal translocations and insertions

Q95.Ø Balanced translocation and insertion in normal individual
Q95.1 Chromosome inversion in normal individual
Q95.2 Balanced autosomal rearrangement in abnormal individual
Q95.3 Balanced sex/autosomal rearrangement in abnormal individual
Q95.5 Individual with autosomal fragile site
Q95.8 Other balanced rearrangements and structural markers
Q95.9 Balanced rearrangement and structural marker, unspecified

✓4th **Q96 Turner's syndrome**

EXCLUDES 1 *Noonan syndrome (Q87.19)*

Q96.Ø Karyotype 45, X ♀
Q96.1 Karyotype 46, X iso (Xq) ♀
Karyotype 46, isochromosome Xq
Q96.2 Karyotype 46, X with abnormal sex chromosome, except iso (Xq) ♀
Karyotype 46, X with abnormal sex chromosome, except isochromosome Xq
Q96.3 Mosaicism, 45, X/46, XX or XY ♀
Q96.4 Mosaicism, 45, X/other cell line(s) with abnormal sex chromosome ♀
Q96.8 Other variants of Turner's syndrome ♀
Q96.9 Turner's syndrome, unspecified ♀

✓4th **Q97 Other sex chromosome abnormalities, female phenotype, not elsewhere classified**

EXCLUDES 1 *Turner's syndrome (Q96.-)*

Q97.Ø Karyotype 47, XXX ♀
Q97.1 Female with more than three X chromosomes ♀
Q97.2 Mosaicism, lines with various numbers of X chromosomes ♀
Q97.3 Female with 46, XY karyotype ♀
Q97.8 Other specified sex chromosome abnormalities, female phenotype ♀
Q97.9 Sex chromosome abnormality, female phenotype, unspecified ♀

✓4th **Q98 Other sex chromosome abnormalities, male phenotype, not elsewhere classified**

Q98.Ø Klinefelter syndrome karyotype 47, XXY ♂
Q98.1 Klinefelter syndrome, male with more than two X chromosomes ♂
Q98.3 Other male with 46, XX karyotype ♂
Q98.4 Klinefelter syndrome, unspecified ♂
Q98.5 Karyotype 47, XYY ♂
Q98.6 Male with structurally abnormal sex chromosome ♂
Q98.7 Male with sex chromosome mosaicism ♂
Q98.8 Other specified sex chromosome abnormalities, male phenotype ♂
Q98.9 Sex chromosome abnormality, male phenotype, unspecified ♂

✓4th **Q99 Other chromosome abnormalities, not elsewhere classified**

Q99.Ø Chimera 46, XX/46, XY
Chimera 46, XX/46, XY true hermaphrodite

Q99.1 46, XX true hermaphrodite
46, XX with streak gonads
46, XY with streak gonads
Pure gonadal dysgenesis

Q99.2 Fragile X chromosome
Fragile X syndrome

Q99.8 Other specified chromosome abnormalities

Q99.9 Chromosomal abnormality, unspecified

Chapter 18. Symptoms, Signs, and Abnormal Clinical and Laboratory Findings, Not Elsewhere Classified (RØØ–R99)

Chapter-specific Guidelines with Coding Examples

The chapter-specific guidelines from the ICD-10-CM Official Guidelines for Coding and Reporting have been provided below. Along with these guidelines are coding examples, contained in the shaded boxes, that have been developed to help illustrate the coding and/or sequencing guidance found in these guidelines.

Chapter 18 includes symptoms, signs, abnormal results of clinical or other investigative procedures, and ill-defined conditions regarding which no diagnosis classifiable elsewhere is recorded. Signs and symptoms that point to a specific diagnosis have been assigned to a category in other chapters of the classification.

a. Use of symptom codes

Codes that describe symptoms and signs are acceptable for reporting purposes when a related definitive diagnosis has not been established (confirmed) by the provider.

Chest pain of unknown origin

RØ7.9 **Chest pain, unspecified**

Explanation: Codes that describe symptoms such as chest pain are acceptable for reporting purposes when the provider has not established (confirmed) a related definitive diagnosis.

b. Use of a symptom code with a definitive diagnosis code

Codes for signs and symptoms may be reported in addition to a related definitive diagnosis when the sign or symptom is not routinely associated with that diagnosis, such as the various signs and symptoms associated with complex syndromes. The definitive diagnosis code should be sequenced before the symptom code.

Signs or symptoms that are associated routinely with a disease process should not be assigned as additional codes, unless otherwise instructed by the classification.

Pneumonia with hemoptysis

J18.9 **Pneumonia, unspecified organism**

RØ4.2 **Hemoptysis**

Explanation: Codes for signs and symptoms may be reported in addition to a related definitive diagnosis when the sign or symptom is not routinely associated with that diagnosis.

Abdominal pain due to acute appendicitis

K35.8Ø **Unspecified acute appendicitis**

Explanation: Codes for signs or symptoms routinely associated with a disease process should not be assigned unless the classification instructs otherwise.

c. Combination codes that include symptoms

ICD-10-CM contains a number of combination codes that identify both the definitive diagnosis and common symptoms of that diagnosis. When using one of these combination codes, an additional code should not be assigned for the symptom.

Acute gastritis with hemorrhage

K29.Ø1 **Acute gastritis with bleeding**

Explanation: When a combination code identifies both the definitive diagnosis and the symptom, an additional code should not be assigned for the symptom.

d. Repeated falls

Code R29.6, Repeated falls, is for use for encounters when a patient has recently fallen and the reason for the fall is being investigated.

Code Z91.81, History of falling, is for use when a patient has fallen in the past and is at risk for future falls. When appropriate, both codes R29.6 and Z91.81 may be assigned together.

e. Coma

Code R4Ø.2Ø, Unspecified coma, **should** be assigned **when the underlying cause of the coma is not known, or the cause is a traumatic brain injury and the coma scale is not documented in the medical record**.

Do not report codes for unspecified coma, individual or total Glasgow coma scale scores for a patient with a medically induced coma or a sedated patient.

1) Coma scale

The coma scale codes (R4Ø.21- to R4Ø.24-) can be used in conjunction with traumatic brain injury codes. These codes **cannot be used with R4Ø.2A, Nontraumatic coma due to underlying condition. They** are primarily for use by trauma registries, but they may be used in any setting where this information is collected. The coma scale codes should be sequenced after the diagnosis code(s).

These codes, one from each subcategory, are needed to complete the scale. The 7th character indicates when the scale was recorded. The 7th character should match for all three codes.

At a minimum, report the initial score documented on presentation at your facility. This may be a score from the emergency medicine technician (EMT) or in the emergency department. If desired, a facility may choose to capture multiple coma scale scores.

Assign code R4Ø.24-, Glasgow coma scale, total score, when only the total score is documented in the medical record and not the individual score(s).

If multiple coma scores are captured within the first 24 hours after hospital admission, assign only the code for the score at the time of admission. ICD-10-CM does not classify coma scores that are reported after admission but less than 24 hours later.

See Section I.B.14. for coma scale documentation by clinicians other than patient's provider

23-year-old man found down after unknown injury with skull fracture and with concussion and loss of consciousness of unknown duration. EMS evaluated the patient in the field and reported the individual Glasgow coma scores:

Eye opening response—3: eyes open to speech

Verbal response—4: confused but coherent speech

Motor response—6: obeys commands fully

SØ2.ØXXA **Fracture of vault of skull, initial encounter for closed fracture**

SØ6.ØX9A **Concussion with loss of consciousness of unspecified duration, initial encounter**

R4Ø.2131 **Coma scale, eyes open, to sound, in the field [EMT or ambulance]**

R4Ø.2241 **Coma scale, best verbal response, confused conversation, in the field [EMT or ambulance]**

R4Ø.2361 **Coma scale, best motor response, obeys commands, in the field [EMT or ambulance]**

Explanation: When individual scores for the Glasgow coma scale are documented, one code from each category is needed to complete the scale. The seventh character indicates when the scale was recorded and should match for all three codes. Assign a code from subcategory R4Ø.24- Glasgow coma scale, total score, when only the total and not the individual score(s) is documented.

f. Functional quadriplegia

GUIDELINE HAS BEEN DELETED EFFECTIVE OCTOBER 1, 2017

g. SIRS due to non-infectious process

The systemic inflammatory response syndrome (SIRS) can develop as a result of certain non-infectious disease processes, such as trauma, malignant neoplasm, or pancreatitis. When SIRS is documented with a noninfectious condition, and no subsequent infection is documented, the code for the underlying condition, such as an injury, should be assigned, followed by code R65.1Ø, Systemic inflammatory response syndrome (SIRS) of non-infectious origin without acute organ dysfunction, or code R65.11, Systemic inflammatory response syndrome (SIRS) of non-infectious origin with acute organ dysfunction. If an associated acute organ dysfunction is documented, the appropriate code(s) for the specific type of organ dysfunction(s) should be assigned in addition to code R65.11. If acute organ dysfunction is documented, but it cannot be determined if the acute organ dysfunction is associated with SIRS or due to another condition (e.g., directly due to the trauma), the provider should be queried.

Systemic inflammatory response syndrome (SIRS) due to acute gallstone pancreatitis

K85.1Ø **Biliary acute pancreatitis without necrosis or infection**

R65.1Ø **Systemic inflammatory response syndrome [SIRS] of non-infectious origin without acute organ dysfunction**

Explanation: When SIRS is documented with a non-infectious condition without subsequent infection documented, the code for the underlying condition such as pancreatitis should be assigned followed by the appropriate code for SIRS of noninfectious origin, either with or without associated organ dysfunction.

h. Death NOS

Code R99, Ill-defined and unknown cause of mortality, is only for use in the very limited circumstance when a patient who has already died is brought into an emergency department or other healthcare facility and is pronounced dead upon arrival. It does not represent the discharge disposition of death.

i. NIHSS stroke scale

The NIH stroke scale (NIHSS) codes (R29.7- -) can be used in conjunction with acute stroke codes (**I6Ø**-I63) to identify the patient's neurological status and the severity of the stroke. The stroke scale codes should be sequenced after the acute stroke diagnosis code(s).

At a minimum, report the initial score documented. If desired, a facility may choose to capture multiple stroke scale scores.

See Section I.B.14. for NIHSS stroke scale documentation by clinicians other than patient's provider

Patient admitted with CVA seen by neurology consult who documents moderate to severe stroke, 17 on NIHSS stroke scale.

I63.9 **Cerebral infarction, unspecified**

R29.717 **NIHSS score 17**

Explanation: Unspecified cerebral vascular accident (CVA) is sequenced before the NIHSS stroke scale score code. The stroke scale is an assessment tool to help measure stroke-related neurological deficits. Fifteen items are evaluated by trained observers and include such conditions as levels of consciousness, language, dysarthria, ataxia, and sensory loss. A facility may report multiple stroke scale scores if it wants to.

Chapter 18. Symptoms, Signs and Abnormal Clinical and Laboratory Findings, Not Elsewhere Classified (R00-R99)

NOTE This chapter includes symptoms, signs, abnormal results of clinical or other investigative procedures, and ill-defined conditions regarding which no diagnosis classifiable elsewhere is recorded.

Signs and symptoms that point rather definitely to a given diagnosis have been assigned to a category in other chapters of the classification. In general, categories in this chapter include the less well-defined conditions and symptoms that, without the necessary study of the case to establish a final diagnosis, point perhaps equally to two or more diseases or to two or more systems of the body. Practically all categories in the chapter could be designated 'not otherwise specified', 'unknown etiology' or 'transient'. The Alphabetical Index should be consulted to determine which symptoms and signs are to be allocated here and which to other chapters. The residual subcategories, numbered .8, are generally provided for other relevant symptoms that cannot be allocated elsewhere in the classification.

The conditions and signs or symptoms included in categories R00-R94 consist of:

(a) cases for which no more specific diagnosis can be made even after all the facts bearing on the case have been investigated;

(b) signs or symptoms existing at the time of initial encounter that proved to be transient and whose causes could not be determined;

(c) provisional diagnosis in a patient who failed to return for further investigation or care;

(d) cases referred elsewhere for investigation or treatment before the diagnosis was made;

(e) cases in which a more precise diagnosis was not available for any other reason;

(f) certain symptoms, for which supplementary information is provided, that represent important problems in medical care in their own right.

EXCLUDES 2 *abnormal findings on antenatal screening of mother (O28.-)*
certain conditions originating in the perinatal period (P04-P96)
signs and symptoms classified in the body system chapters
signs and symptoms of breast (N63, N64.5)

AHA: 2017,1Q,6,7

This chapter contains the following blocks:

R00-R09 Symptoms and signs involving the circulatory and respiratory systems
R10-R19 Symptoms and signs involving the digestive system and abdomen
R20-R23 Symptoms and signs involving the skin and subcutaneous tissue
R25-R29 Symptoms and signs involving the nervous and musculoskeletal systems
R30-R39 Symptoms and signs involving the genitourinary system
R40-R46 Symptoms and signs involving cognition, perception, emotional state and behavior
R47-R49 Symptoms and signs involving speech and voice
R50-R69 General symptoms and signs
R70-R79 Abnormal findings on examination of blood, without diagnosis
R80-R82 Abnormal findings on examination of urine, without diagnosis
R83-R89 Abnormal findings on examination of other body fluids, substances and tissues, without diagnosis
R90-R94 Abnormal findings on diagnostic imaging and in function studies, without diagnosis
R97 Abnormal tumor markers
R99 Ill-defined and unknown cause of mortality

Symptoms and signs involving the circulatory and respiratory systems (R00-R09)

R00 Abnormalities of heart beat
EXCLUDES 1 *abnormalities originating in the perinatal period (P29.1-)*
EXCLUDES 2 *specified arrhythmias (I47-I49)*

R00.0 Tachycardia, unspecified
Rapid heart beat
Sinoauricular tachycardia NOS
Sinus [sinusal] tachycardia NOS
EXCLUDES 1 ▶*inappropriate sinus tachycardia, so stated (I47.11)*◀
neonatal tachycardia (P29.11)
paroxysmal tachycardia (I47.-)
AHA: 2022,4Q,46
DEF: Excessively rapid heart rate of more than 100 beats per minute.

R00.1 Bradycardia, unspecified
Sinoatrial bradycardia
Sinus bradycardia
Slow heart beat
Vagal bradycardia
Use additional code for adverse effect, if applicable, to identify drug (T36-T50 with fifth or sixth character 5)
EXCLUDES 1 *neonatal bradycardia (P29.12)*
AHA: 2020,2Q,23
DEF: Slowed heartbeat, usually defined as a rate fewer than 60 beats per minute. Heart rhythm may be slow as a result of a congenital defect or an acquired problem.

R00.2 Palpitations
Awareness of heart beat

R00.8 Other abnormalities of heart beat

R00.9 Unspecified abnormalities of heart beat

R01 Cardiac murmurs and other cardiac sounds
EXCLUDES 1 *cardiac murmurs and sounds originating in the perinatal period (P29.8)*

R01.0 Benign and innocent cardiac murmurs
Functional cardiac murmur

R01.1 Cardiac murmur, unspecified
Cardiac bruit NOS
Heart murmur NOS
Systolic murmur NOS

R01.2 Other cardiac sounds
Cardiac dullness, increased or decreased
Precordial friction

R03 Abnormal blood-pressure reading, without diagnosis

R03.0 Elevated blood-pressure reading, without diagnosis of hypertension
NOTE This category is to be used to record an episode of elevated blood pressure in a patient in whom no formal diagnosis of hypertension has been made, or as an isolated incidental finding.

R03.1 Nonspecific low blood-pressure reading
EXCLUDES 1 *hypotension (I95.-)*
maternal hypotension syndrome (O26.5-)
neurogenic orthostatic hypotension (G90.3)

R04 Hemorrhage from respiratory passages

R04.0 Epistaxis
Hemorrhage from nose
Nosebleed
AHA: 2023,2Q,28

R04.1 Hemorrhage from throat
EXCLUDES 2 *hemoptysis (R04.2)*

R04.2 Hemoptysis CC
Blood-stained sputum
Cough with hemorrhage
AHA: 2013,4Q,118

R04.8 Hemorrhage from other sites in respiratory passages

R04.81 Acute idiopathic pulmonary hemorrhage in infants CC P
AIPHI
Acute idiopathic hemorrhage in infants over 28 days old
EXCLUDES 1 *perinatal pulmonary hemorrhage (P26.-)*
von Willebrand disease (D68.0-)

R04.89 Hemorrhage from other sites in respiratory passages CC
Pulmonary hemorrhage NOS

R04.9 Hemorrhage from respiratory passages, unspecified CC

R05 Cough
EXCLUDES 1 *paroxysmal cough due to Bordetella pertussis (A37.0-)*
smoker's cough (J41.0)
EXCLUDES 2 *cough with hemorrhage (R04.2)*
AHA: 2021,4Q,24-25; 2016,2Q,33

R05.1 Acute cough

R05.2 Subacute cough

R05.3 Chronic cough
Persistent cough
Refractory cough
Unexplained cough

R05.4 Cough syncope UPD
Code first syncope and collapse (R55)

R05.8 Other specified cough

Chapter 18. Symptoms, Signs and Abnormal Clinical and Laboratory Findings
R00–R05.8

RØ5.9 Cough, unspecified

RØ6 Abnormalities of breathing

EXCLUDES 1 *acute respiratory distress syndrome (J8Ø)*
respiratory arrest (RØ9.2)
respiratory arrest of newborn (P28.81)
respiratory distress syndrome of newborn (P22.-)
respiratory failure (J96.-)
respiratory failure of newborn (P28.5)

RØ6.Ø Dyspnea

EXCLUDES 1 *tachypnea NOS (RØ6.82)*
transient tachypnea of newborn (P22.1)

RØ6.ØØ Dyspnea, unspecified
AHA: 2017,1Q,26

RØ6.Ø1 Orthopnea

RØ6.Ø2 Shortness of breath

RØ6.Ø3 Acute respiratory distress
AHA: 2017,4Q,23

RØ6.Ø9 Other forms of dyspnea

RØ6.1 Stridor

EXCLUDES 1 *congenital laryngeal stridor (P28.89)*
laryngismus (stridulus) (J38.5)

DEF: Certain type of wheezing described as a loud, constant, musical sound produced when breathing with an obstructed airway, like the inspiratory sound heard when laryngeal or esophageal obstruction is present.

RØ6.2 Wheezing

EXCLUDES 1 *asthma (J45.-)*

AHA: 2016,2Q,33
DEF: High-pitched whistling sound during breathing due to stenosis of the respiratory passageway. Wheezing is associated with asthma, sleep apnea, bronchiectasis, bronchiolitis, COPD, and pleural effusion.

RØ6.3 Periodic breathing CC
Cheyne-Stokes breathing

RØ6.4 Hyperventilation

EXCLUDES 1 *psychogenic hyperventilation (F45.8)*

RØ6.5 Mouth breathing

EXCLUDES 2 *dry mouth NOS (R68.2)*

RØ6.6 Hiccough

EXCLUDES 1 *psychogenic hiccough (F45.8)*

RØ6.7 Sneezing

RØ6.8 Other abnormalities of breathing

RØ6.81 Apnea, not elsewhere classified
Apnea NOS

EXCLUDES 1 *apnea (of) newborn (P28.4-)*
sleep apnea (G47.3-)
sleep apnea of newborn (primary) (P28.3-)

RØ6.82 Tachypnea, not elsewhere classified
Tachypnea NOS

EXCLUDES 1 *transitory tachypnea of newborn (P22.1)*

RØ6.83 Snoring

RØ6.89 Other abnormalities of breathing
Breath-holding (spells)
Sighing

RØ6.9 Unspecified abnormalities of breathing

RØ7 Pain in throat and chest

EXCLUDES 1 *epidemic myalgia (B33.Ø)*

EXCLUDES 2 *jaw pain R68.84*
pain in breast (N64.4)

RØ7.Ø Pain in throat

EXCLUDES 1 *chronic sore throat (J31.2)*
sore throat (acute) NOS (JØ2.9)

EXCLUDES 2 *dysphagia (R13.1-)*
pain in neck (M54.2)

RØ7.1 Chest pain on breathing
Painful respiration

RØ7.2 Precordial pain
DEF: Pain felt in the anterior (front) chest wall over the region of the heart. This type of pain is generally felt slightly to the left of the sternum, but may also extend into the surrounding chest wall region.

RØ7.8 Other chest pain

RØ7.81 Pleurodynia
Pleurodynia NOS

EXCLUDES 1 *epidemic pleurodynia (B33.Ø)*

RØ7.82 Intercostal pain

RØ7.89 Other chest pain
Anterior chest-wall pain NOS
AHA: 2021,1Q,42

RØ7.9 Chest pain, unspecified

RØ9 Other symptoms and signs involving the circulatory and respiratory system

EXCLUDES 1 *acute respiratory distress syndrome (J8Ø)*
respiratory arrest of newborn (P28.81)
respiratory distress syndrome of newborn (P22.Ø)
respiratory failure (J96.-)
respiratory failure of newborn (P28.5)

RØ9.Ø Asphyxia and hypoxemia

EXCLUDES 1 *asphyxia due to carbon monoxide (T58.-)*
asphyxia due to foreign body in respiratory tract (T17.-)
birth (intrauterine) asphyxia (P84)
hyperventilation (RØ6.4)
traumatic asphyxia (T71.-)

EXCLUDES 2 *hypercapnia (RØ6.89)*

RØ9.Ø1 Asphyxia CC
DEF: Interference of oxygen intake due to obstruction or injury of airways resulting in a lack of oxygen perfusion to the tissues or excessive carbon dioxide in the blood. Can cause unconsciousness or death.

RØ9.Ø2 Hypoxemia
AHA: 2019,3Q,15
DEF: Insufficient oxygen in the arterial blood resulting in inadequate delivery of oxygen to the body tissues.

RØ9.1 Pleurisy

EXCLUDES 1 *pleurisy with effusion (J9Ø)*

RØ9.2 Respiratory arrest MCC HCC
Cardiorespiratory failure

EXCLUDES 1 *cardiac arrest (I46.-)*
respiratory arrest of newborn (P28.81)
respiratory distress of newborn (P22.Ø)
respiratory failure (J96.-)
respiratory failure of newborn (P28.5)
respiratory insufficiency (RØ6.89)
respiratory insufficiency of newborn (P28.5)

TIP: MCC only when patient is discharged alive.

RØ9.3 Abnormal sputum
Abnormal amount of sputum
Abnormal color of sputum
Abnormal odor of sputum
Excessive sputum

EXCLUDES 1 *blood-stained sputum (RØ4.2)*

RØ9.8 Other specified symptoms and signs involving the circulatory and respiratory systems

RØ9.81 Nasal congestion

RØ9.82 Postnasal drip

RØ9.89 Other specified symptoms and signs involving the circulatory and respiratory systems
Abnormal chest percussion
Bruit (arterial)
Chest tympany
Choking sensation
~~Feeling of foreign body in throat~~
Friction sounds in chest
Rales
Weak pulse

EXCLUDES 2 *foreign body in throat (T17.2-)*
wheezing (RØ6.2)

AHA: 2021,1Q,42

● **RØ9.A Foreign body sensation of the circulatory and respiratory system**

● **RØ9.AØ Foreign body sensation, unspecified**

● **RØ9.A1 Foreign body sensation, nose**

● **RØ9.A2 Foreign body sensation, throat**
Foreign body sensation globus

● **RØ9.A9 Foreign body sensation, other site**

Symptoms and signs involving the digestive system and abdomen (R1Ø-R19)

EXCLUDES 2 *congenital or infantile pylorospasm (Q4Ø.Ø)*
gastrointestinal hemorrhage (K92.Ø-K92.2)
intestinal obstruction (K56.-)
newborn gastrointestinal hemorrhage (P54.Ø-P54.3)
newborn intestinal obstruction (P76.-)
pylorospasm (K31.3)
signs and symptoms involving the urinary system (R3Ø-R39)
symptoms referable to female genital organs (N94.-)
symptoms referable to male genital organs (N48-N5Ø)

R1Ø Abdominal and pelvic pain
EXCLUDES 1 *renal colic (N23)*
EXCLUDES 2 *dorsalgia (M54.-)*
flatulence and related conditions (R14.-)

R1Ø.Ø Acute abdomen
Severe abdominal pain (generalized) (with abdominal rigidity)
EXCLUDES 1 *abdominal rigidity NOS (R19.3)*
generalized abdominal pain NOS (R1Ø.84)
localized abdominal pain (R1Ø.1-R1Ø.3-)

R1Ø.1 Pain localized to upper abdomen
R1Ø.1Ø Upper abdominal pain, unspecified
R1Ø.11 Right upper quadrant pain
R1Ø.12 Left upper quadrant pain
R1Ø.13 Epigastric pain
Dyspepsia
EXCLUDES 1 *functional dyspepsia (K3Ø)*

Abdominal Pain

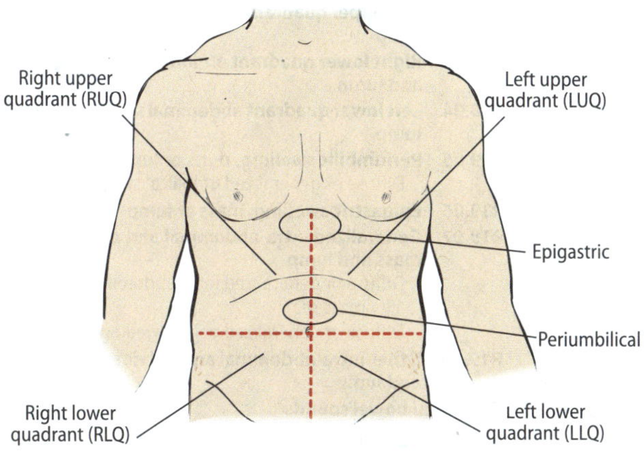

R1Ø.2 Pelvic and perineal pain
EXCLUDES 1 *vulvodynia (N94.81)*

R1Ø.3 Pain localized to other parts of lower abdomen
R1Ø.3Ø Lower abdominal pain, unspecified
R1Ø.31 Right lower quadrant pain
R1Ø.32 Left lower quadrant pain
R1Ø.33 Periumbilical pain

R1Ø.8 Other abdominal pain
R1Ø.81 Abdominal tenderness
Abdominal tenderness NOS
R1Ø.811 Right upper quadrant abdominal tenderness
R1Ø.812 Left upper quadrant abdominal tenderness
R1Ø.813 Right lower quadrant abdominal tenderness
R1Ø.814 Left lower quadrant abdominal tenderness
R1Ø.815 Periumbilic abdominal tenderness
R1Ø.816 Epigastric abdominal tenderness
R1Ø.817 Generalized abdominal tenderness
R1Ø.819 Abdominal tenderness, unspecified site
R1Ø.82 Rebound abdominal tenderness
R1Ø.821 Right upper quadrant rebound abdominal tenderness
R1Ø.822 Left upper quadrant rebound abdominal tenderness
R1Ø.823 Right lower quadrant rebound abdominal tenderness
R1Ø.824 Left lower quadrant rebound abdominal tenderness
R1Ø.825 Periumbilic rebound abdominal tenderness
R1Ø.826 Epigastric rebound abdominal tenderness
R1Ø.827 Generalized rebound abdominal tenderness
R1Ø.829 Rebound abdominal tenderness, unspecified site
R1Ø.83 Colic P
Colic NOS
Infantile colic
EXCLUDES 1 *colic in adult and child over 12 months old (R1Ø.84)*
DEF: Inconsolable crying in an otherwise well-fed and healthy infant for more than three hours a day, three days a week, for more than three weeks.
R1Ø.84 Generalized abdominal pain
EXCLUDES 1 *generalized abdominal pain associated with acute abdomen (R1Ø.Ø)*

R1Ø.9 Unspecified abdominal pain

R11 Nausea and vomiting
EXCLUDES 1 *cyclical vomiting associated with migraine (G43.A-)*
excessive vomiting in pregnancy (O21.-)
hematemesis (K92.Ø)
neonatal hematemesis (P54.Ø)
newborn vomiting (P92.Ø-)
psychogenic vomiting (F5Ø.89)
vomiting associated with bulimia nervosa (F5Ø.2)
vomiting following gastrointestinal surgery (K91.Ø)
AHA: 2017,1Q,28

R11.Ø Nausea
Nausea NOS
Nausea without vomiting

R11.1 Vomiting
R11.1Ø Vomiting, unspecified
Vomiting NOS
R11.11 Vomiting without nausea
R11.12 Projectile vomiting
R11.13 Vomiting of fecal matter
R11.14 Bilious vomiting
Bilious emesis
R11.15 Cyclical vomiting syndrome unrelated to migraine
Cyclic vomiting syndrome NOS
Persistent vomiting
EXCLUDES 1 *cyclical vomiting in migraine (G43.A-)*
EXCLUDES 2 *bulimia nervosa (F5Ø.2)*
diabetes mellitus due to underlying condition (EØ8.-)
AHA: 2019,4Q,15

R11.2 Nausea with vomiting, unspecified
Persistent nausea with vomiting NOS
AHA: 2020,1Q,8

R12 Heartburn
EXCLUDES 1 *dyspepsia NOS (R1Ø.13)*
functional dyspepsia (K3Ø)

R13 Aphagia and dysphagia
R13.Ø Aphagia
Inability to swallow
EXCLUDES 1 *psychogenic aphagia (F5Ø.9)*

✓5th **R13.1 Dysphagia**

Code first, if applicable, dysphagia following cerebrovascular disease (I69. with final characters -91)

EXCLUDES 1 *psychogenic dysphagia (F45.8)*

Swallowing Function

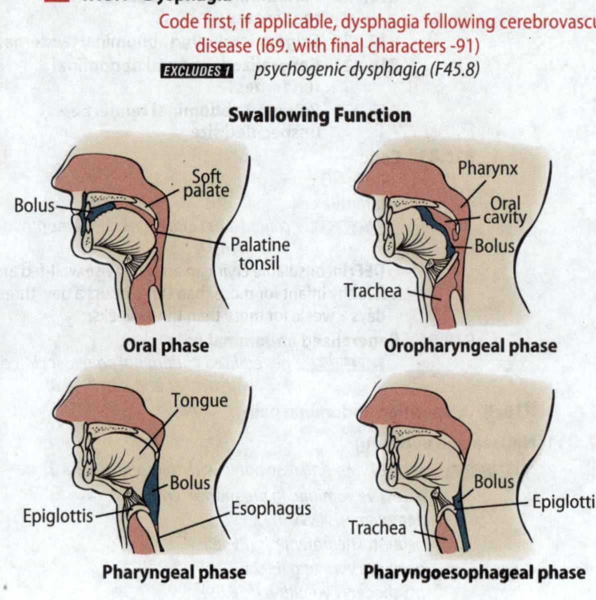

R13.10 Dysphagia, unspecified
Difficulty in swallowing NOS

R13.11 Dysphagia, oral phase

R13.12 Dysphagia, oropharyngeal phase

R13.13 Dysphagia, pharyngeal phase

R13.14 Dysphagia, pharyngoesophageal phase

R13.19 Other dysphagia
Cervical dysphagia
Neurogenic dysphagia

✓4th **R14 Flatulence and related conditions**

EXCLUDES 1 *psychogenic aerophagy (F45.8)*

R14.0 Abdominal distension (gaseous)
Bloating
Tympanites (abdominal) (intestinal)

R14.1 Gas pain

R14.2 Eructation

R14.3 Flatulence

✓4th **R15 Fecal incontinence**

INCLUDES encopresis NOS

EXCLUDES 1 *fecal incontinence of nonorganic origin (F98.1)*

R15.0 Incomplete defecation

EXCLUDES 1 *constipation (K59.0-)*
fecal impaction (K56.41)

R15.1 Fecal smearing
Fecal soiling

R15.2 Fecal urgency

R15.9 Full incontinence of feces
Fecal incontinence NOS

✓4th **R16 Hepatomegaly and splenomegaly, not elsewhere classified**

R16.0 Hepatomegaly, not elsewhere classified
Hepatomegaly NOS

R16.1 Splenomegaly, not elsewhere classified
Splenomegaly NOS

R16.2 Hepatomegaly with splenomegaly, not elsewhere classified
Hepatosplenomegaly NOS

R17 Unspecified jaundice CC

EXCLUDES 1 *neonatal jaundice (P55, P57-P59)*

✓4th **R18 Ascites**

INCLUDES fluid in peritoneal cavity

EXCLUDES 1 *ascites in alcoholic cirrhosis (K70.31)*
ascites in alcoholic hepatitis (K70.11)
ascites in toxic liver disease with chronic active hepatitis (K71.51)

DEF: Abnormal accumulation of free fluid in the abdominal cavity, causing distention and tightness in addition to shortness of breath as the fluid accumulates. Ascites is usually an underlying disorder and can be a manifestation of any number of diseases.

R18.0 Malignant ascites CC UPD

Code first malignancy, such as:
malignant neoplasm of ovary (C56.-)
secondary malignant neoplasm of retroperitoneum and peritoneum (C78.6)

R18.8 Other ascites CC
Ascites NOS
Peritoneal effusion (chronic)
AHA: 2018,1Q,4

✓4th **R19 Other symptoms and signs involving the digestive system and abdomen**

EXCLUDES 1 *acute abdomen (R10.0)*

✓5th **R19.0 Intra-abdominal and pelvic swelling, mass and lump**

EXCLUDES 1 *abdominal distension (gaseous) (R14.-)*
ascites (R18.-)

R19.00 Intra-abdominal and pelvic swelling, mass and lump, unspecified site

R19.01 Right upper quadrant abdominal swelling, mass and lump

R19.02 Left upper quadrant abdominal swelling, mass and lump

R19.03 Right lower quadrant abdominal swelling, mass and lump

R19.04 Left lower quadrant abdominal swelling, mass and lump

R19.05 Periumbilic swelling, mass or lump
Diffuse or generalized umbilical swelling or mass

R19.06 Epigastric swelling, mass or lump

R19.07 Generalized intra-abdominal and pelvic swelling, mass and lump
Diffuse or generalized intra-abdominal swelling or mass NOS
Diffuse or generalized pelvic swelling or mass NOS

R19.09 Other intra-abdominal and pelvic swelling, mass and lump

✓5th **R19.1 Abnormal bowel sounds**

R19.11 Absent bowel sounds

R19.12 Hyperactive bowel sounds

R19.15 Other abnormal bowel sounds
Abnormal bowel sounds NOS

R19.2 Visible peristalsis
Hyperperistalsis
DEF: Visible movements of muscular attempts to move food through the digestive tract due to pyloric obstruction, stomach obstruction, or intestinal obstruction.

✓5th **R19.3 Abdominal rigidity**

EXCLUDES 1 *abdominal rigidity with severe abdominal pain (R10.0)*

R19.30 Abdominal rigidity, unspecified site

R19.31 Right upper quadrant abdominal rigidity

R19.32 Left upper quadrant abdominal rigidity

R19.33 Right lower quadrant abdominal rigidity

R19.34 Left lower quadrant abdominal rigidity

R19.35 Periumbilic abdominal rigidity

R19.36 Epigastric abdominal rigidity

R19.37 Generalized abdominal rigidity

R19.4 Change in bowel habit

EXCLUDES 1 *constipation (K59.0-)*
functional diarrhea (K59.1)

R19.5 Other fecal abnormalities
Abnormal stool color
Bulky stools
Mucus in stools
Occult blood in feces
Occult blood in stools
EXCLUDES 1 *melena (K92.1)*
neonatal melena (P54.1)
AHA: 2021,1Q,9; 2019,1Q,32

R19.6 Halitosis

R19.7 Diarrhea, unspecified
Diarrhea NOS
EXCLUDES 1 *functional diarrhea (K59.1)*
neonatal diarrhea (P78.3)
psychogenic diarrhea (F45.8)
AHA: 2021,3Q,3

R19.8 Other specified symptoms and signs involving the digestive system and abdomen

Symptoms and signs involving the skin and subcutaneous tissue (R20-R23)

EXCLUDES 2 *symptoms relating to breast (N64.4-N64.5)*

R20 Disturbances of skin sensation
EXCLUDES 1 *dissociative anesthesia and sensory loss (F44.6)*
psychogenic disturbances (F45.8)

R20.0 Anesthesia of skin

R20.1 Hypoesthesia of skin

R20.2 Paresthesia of skin
Formication
Pins and needles
Tingling skin
EXCLUDES 1 *acroparesthesia (I73.8)*

R20.3 Hyperesthesia

R20.8 Other disturbances of skin sensation

R20.9 Unspecified disturbances of skin sensation

R21 Rash and other nonspecific skin eruption
INCLUDES rash NOS
EXCLUDES 1 *specified type of rash - code to condition*
vesicular eruption (R23.8)

R22 Localized swelling, mass and lump of skin and subcutaneous tissue
INCLUDES subcutaneous nodules (localized)(superficial)
EXCLUDES 1 *abnormal findings on diagnostic imaging (R90-R93)*
edema (R60.-)
enlarged lymph nodes (R59.-)
localized adiposity (E65)
swelling of joint (M25.4-)

R22.0 Localized swelling, mass and lump, head

R22.1 Localized swelling, mass and lump, neck

R22.2 Localized swelling, mass and lump, trunk
EXCLUDES 1 *intra-abdominal or pelvic mass and lump (R19.0-)*
intra-abdominal or pelvic swelling (R19.0-)
EXCLUDES 2 *breast mass and lump (N63)*
AHA: 2022,3Q,8

R22.3 Localized swelling, mass and lump, upper limb

R22.30 Localized swelling, mass and lump, unspecified upper limb

R22.31 Localized swelling, mass and lump, right upper limb

R22.32 Localized swelling, mass and lump, left upper limb

R22.33 Localized swelling, mass and lump, upper limb, bilateral

R22.4 Localized swelling, mass and lump, lower limb

R22.40 Localized swelling, mass and lump, unspecified lower limb

R22.41 Localized swelling, mass and lump, right lower limb

R22.42 Localized swelling, mass and lump, left lower limb

R22.43 Localized swelling, mass and lump, lower limb, bilateral

R22.9 Localized swelling, mass and lump, unspecified

R23 Other skin changes

R23.0 Cyanosis
EXCLUDES 1 *acrocyanosis (I73.8)*
cyanotic attacks of newborn (P28.2)
DEF: Bluish or purplish discoloration of the skin due to an inadequate oxygen blood level.

R23.1 Pallor
Clammy skin

R23.2 Flushing
Excessive blushing
Code first, if applicable, menopausal and female climacteric states (N95.1)

R23.3 Spontaneous ecchymoses
Petechiae
EXCLUDES 1 *ecchymoses of newborn (P54.5)*
purpura (D69.-)

R23.4 Changes in skin texture
Desquamation of skin
Induration of skin
Scaling of skin
EXCLUDES 1 *epidermal thickening NOS (L85.9)*

R23.8 Other skin changes

R23.9 Unspecified skin changes

Symptoms and signs involving the nervous and musculoskeletal systems (R25-R29)

R25 Abnormal involuntary movements
EXCLUDES 1 *specific movement disorders (G20-G26)*
stereotyped movement disorders (F98.4)
tic disorders (F95.-)

R25.0 Abnormal head movements

R25.1 Tremor, unspecified
EXCLUDES 1 *chorea NOS (G25.5)*
essential tremor (G25.0)
hysterical tremor (F44.4)
intention tremor (G25.2)

R25.2 Cramp and spasm
EXCLUDES 2 *carpopedal spasm (R29.0)*
charley-horse (M62.831)
infantile spasms (G40.4-)
muscle spasm of back (M62.830)
muscle spasm of calf (M62.831)

R25.3 Fasciculation
Twitching NOS

R25.8 Other abnormal involuntary movements

R25.9 Unspecified abnormal involuntary movements

R26 Abnormalities of gait and mobility
EXCLUDES 1 *ataxia NOS (R27.0)*
hereditary ataxia (G11.-)
locomotor (syphilitic) ataxia (A52.11)
immobility syndrome (paraplegic) (M62.3)

R26.0 Ataxic gait
Staggering gait
AHA: 2022,2Q,12

R26.1 Paralytic gait
Spastic gait

R26.2 Difficulty in walking, not elsewhere classified
EXCLUDES 1 *falling (R29.6)*
unsteadiness on feet (R26.81)
AHA: 2016,2Q,7

R26.8 Other abnormalities of gait and mobility

R26.81 Unsteadiness on feet

R26.89 Other abnormalities of gait and mobility
AHA: 2020,2Q,29

R26.9 Unspecified abnormalities of gait and mobility

R27 Other lack of coordination
EXCLUDES 1 *ataxic gait (R26.0)*
hereditary ataxia (G11.-)
vertigo NOS (R42)

R27.0 Ataxia, unspecified
EXCLUDES 1 *ataxia following cerebrovascular disease (I69. with final characters -93)*

R27.8 Other lack of coordination

R27.9 Unspecified lack of coordination

R29 Other symptoms and signs involving the nervous and musculoskeletal systems

R29.0 Tetany CC
Carpopedal spasm
EXCLUDES 1 *hysterical tetany (F44.5)*
neonatal tetany (P71.3)
parathyroid tetany (E20.9)
post-thyroidectomy tetany (E89.2)
DEF: Calcium or other mineral imbalance causing voluntary muscles such as hands, feet, or larynx to spasm rhythmically.

R29.1 Meningismus CC

R29.2 Abnormal reflex
EXCLUDES 2 *abnormal pupillary reflex (H57.0)*
hyperactive gag reflex (J39.2)
vasovagal reaction or syncope (R55)

R29.3 Abnormal posture

R29.4 Clicking hip
EXCLUDES 1 *congenital deformities of hip (Q65.-)*

R29.5 Transient paralysis CC
Code first any associated spinal cord injury (S14.0, S14.1-, S24.0, S24.1-, S34.0-, S34.1-)
EXCLUDES 1 *transient ischemic attack (G45.9)*

R29.6 Repeated falls
Falling
Tendency to fall
EXCLUDES 2 *at risk for falling (Z91.81)*
history of falling (Z91.81)
AHA: 2016,2Q,6

R29.7 National Institutes of Health Stroke Scale (NIHSS) score
Code first the type of cerebral infarction (I63.-)
AHA: 2016,4Q,61-62
TIP: Codes from this subcategory may be assigned based on medical record documentation from clinicians who are not the patient's provider.

R29.70 NIHSS score 0-9
R29.700 NIHSS score 0 UPD
R29.701 NIHSS score 1 UPD
R29.702 NIHSS score 2 UPD
R29.703 NIHSS score 3 UPD
R29.704 NIHSS score 4 UPD
R29.705 NIHSS score 5 UPD
R29.706 NIHSS score 6 UPD
R29.707 NIHSS score 7 UPD
R29.708 NIHSS score 8 UPD
R29.709 NIHSS score 9 UPD

R29.71 NIHSS score 10-19
R29.710 NIHSS score 10 UPD
R29.711 NIHSS score 11 UPD
R29.712 NIHSS score 12 UPD
R29.713 NIHSS score 13 UPD
R29.714 NIHSS score 14 UPD
R29.715 NIHSS score 15 UPD
R29.716 NIHSS score 16 UPD
R29.717 NIHSS score 17 UPD
R29.718 NIHSS score 18 UPD
R29.719 NIHSS score 19 UPD

R29.72 NIHSS score 20-29
R29.720 NIHSS score 20 UPD
R29.721 NIHSS score 21 UPD
R29.722 NIHSS score 22 UPD
R29.723 NIHSS score 23 UPD
R29.724 NIHSS score 24 UPD
R29.725 NIHSS score 25 UPD
R29.726 NIHSS score 26 UPD
R29.727 NIHSS score 27 UPD
R29.728 NIHSS score 28 UPD
R29.729 NIHSS score 29 UPD

R29.73 NIHSS score 30-39
R29.730 NIHSS score 30 UPD
R29.731 NIHSS score 31 UPD
R29.732 NIHSS score 32 UPD
R29.733 NIHSS score 33 UPD
R29.734 NIHSS score 34 UPD
R29.735 NIHSS score 35 UPD
R29.736 NIHSS score 36 UPD
R29.737 NIHSS score 37 UPD
R29.738 NIHSS score 38 UPD
R29.739 NIHSS score 39 UPD

R29.74 NIHSS score 40-42
R29.740 NIHSS score 40 UPD
R29.741 NIHSS score 41 UPD
R29.742 NIHSS score 42 UPD

R29.8 Other symptoms and signs involving the nervous and musculoskeletal systems

R29.81 Other symptoms and signs involving the nervous system

R29.810 Facial weakness
Facial droop
EXCLUDES 1 *Bell's palsy (G51.0)*
facial weakness following cerebrovascular disease (I69. with final characters -92)

R29.818 Other symptoms and signs involving the nervous system

R29.89 Other symptoms and signs involving the musculoskeletal system
EXCLUDES 2 *pain in limb (M79.6-)*

R29.890 Loss of height
EXCLUDES 1 *osteoporosis (M80-M81)*

R29.891 Ocular torticollis
EXCLUDES 1 *congenital (sternomastoid) torticollis Q68.0*
psychogenic torticollis (F45.8)
spasmodic torticollis (G24.3)
torticollis due to birth injury (P15.8)
torticollis NOS M43.6
DEF: Abnormal head posture as a result of a contracted state of cervical muscles to correct a visual disturbance, either double vision or a visual field defect.

R29.898 Other symptoms and signs involving the musculoskeletal system

R29.9 Unspecified symptoms and signs involving the nervous and musculoskeletal systems

R29.90 Unspecified symptoms and signs involving the nervous system

R29.91 Unspecified symptoms and signs involving the musculoskeletal system

Symptoms and signs involving the genitourinary system (R30-R39)

R30 Pain associated with micturition
EXCLUDES 1 *psychogenic pain associated with micturition (F45.8)*

R30.0 Dysuria
Strangury

R30.1 Vesical tenesmus
DEF: Feeling of a full bladder even when there is little or no urine in the bladder.

R30.9 Painful micturition, unspecified
Painful urination NOS

R31 Hematuria
EXCLUDES 1 *hematuria included with underlying conditions, such as:*
acute cystitis with hematuria (N30.01)
recurrent and persistent hematuria in glomerular diseases (N02.-)
AHA: 2017,1Q,17

R31.0 Gross hematuria

R31.1 Benign essential microscopic hematuria

R31.2 Other microscopic hematuria
AHA: 2016,4Q,62

R31.21 Asymptomatic microscopic hematuria
AMH

R31.29 Other microscopic hematuria

R31.9 Hematuria, unspecified

R32 Unspecified urinary incontinence
Enuresis NOS
EXCLUDES 1 *functional urinary incontinence (R39.81)*
nonorganic enuresis (F98.Ø)
stress incontinence and other specified urinary incontinence (N39.3-N39.4-)
urinary incontinence associated with cognitive impairment (R39.81)

✓4th **R33 Retention of urine**
EXCLUDES 1 *psychogenic retention of urine (F45.8)*

R33.Ø Drug induced retention of urine
Use additional code for adverse effect, if applicable, to identify drug (T36-T5Ø with fifth or sixth character 5)

R33.8 Other retention of urine
Code first, if applicable, any causal condition, such as:
enlarged prostate (N4Ø.1)
AHA: 2018,4Q,55

R33.9 Retention of urine, unspecified

R34 Anuria and oliguria
EXCLUDES 1 *anuria and oliguria complicating abortion or ectopic or molar pregnancy (OØØ-OØ7, OØ8.4)*
anuria and oliguria complicating pregnancy (O26.83-)
anuria and oliguria complicating the puerperium ▶(O9Ø.49)◀

✓4th **R35 Polyuria**
Code first, if applicable, any causal condition, such as:
enlarged prostate (N4Ø.1)
EXCLUDES 1 *psychogenic polyuria (F45.8)*

R35.Ø Frequency of micturition
R35.1 Nocturia
✓5th **R35.8 Other polyuria**
AHA: 2021,4Q,26
R35.81 Nocturnal polyuria
EXCLUDES 2 *nocturnal enuresis (N39.44)*
R35.89 Other polyuria
Polyuria NOS

✓4th **R36 Urethral discharge**
R36.Ø Urethral discharge without blood
R36.1 Hematospermia ♂
R36.9 Urethral discharge, unspecified
Penile discharge NOS
Urethrorrhea

R37 Sexual dysfunction, unspecified

✓4th **R39 Other and unspecified symptoms and signs involving the genitourinary system**
R39.Ø Extravasation of urine CC
✓5th **R39.1 Other difficulties with micturition**
Code first, if applicable, any causal condition, such as:
enlarged prostate (N4Ø.1)
R39.11 Hesitancy of micturition
R39.12 Poor urinary stream
Weak urinary steam
R39.13 Splitting of urinary stream
R39.14 Feeling of incomplete bladder emptying
R39.15 Urgency of urination
EXCLUDES 1 *urge incontinence (N39.41, N39.46)*
R39.16 Straining to void
✓6th **R39.19 Other difficulties with micturition**
AHA: 2016,4Q,63
R39.191 Need to immediately re-void
R39.192 Position dependent micturition
R39.198 Other difficulties with micturition
R39.2 Extrarenal uremia
Prerenal uremia
EXCLUDES 1 *uremia NOS (N19)*
✓5th **R39.8 Other symptoms and signs involving the genitourinary system**
AHA: 2017,4Q,22-23
R39.81 Functional urinary incontinence
Urinary incontinence due to cognitive impairment, or severe physical disability or immobility
EXCLUDES 1 *stress incontinence and other specified urinary incontinence (N39.3-N39.4-)*
urinary incontinence NOS (R32)
R39.82 Chronic bladder pain
AHA: 2016,4Q,64
R39.83 Unilateral non-palpable testicle ♂
R39.84 Bilateral non-palpable testicles ♂
R39.89 Other symptoms and signs involving the genitourinary system
R39.9 Unspecified symptoms and signs involving the genitourinary system

Symptoms and signs involving cognition, perception, emotional state and behavior (R4Ø-R46)

EXCLUDES 2 *symptoms and signs constituting part of a pattern of mental disorder (FØ1-F99)*

✓4th **R4Ø Somnolence, stupor and coma**
EXCLUDES 1 *neonatal coma (P91.5)*
somnolence, stupor and coma in diabetes (EØ8-E13)
somnolence, stupor and coma in hepatic failure (K72.-)
somnolence, stupor and coma in hypoglycemia (nondiabetic) (E15)

R4Ø.Ø Somnolence
Drowsiness
EXCLUDES 1 *coma (R4Ø.2-)*

R4Ø.1 Stupor
Catatonic stupor
Semicoma
EXCLUDES 1 *catatonic schizophrenia (F2Ø.2)*
coma (R4Ø.2-)
depressive stupor (F31-F33)
dissociative stupor (F44.2)
manic stupor (F3Ø.2)

✓5th **R4Ø.2 Coma**
Code first any associated:
fracture of skull (SØ2.-)
intracranial injury (SØ6.-)
NOTE One code from each subcategory, R4Ø.21-R4Ø.23, is required to complete the coma scale
AHA: 2020,3Q,46; 2019,2Q,12; 2018,4Q,70; 2017,4Q,23-25,95; 2015,2Q,17; 2014,1Q,19
TIP: The codes for individual (R40.21-, R40.22-, R40.23-) or total (R40.24-) coma scale scores are only assigned as secondary diagnoses with traumatic brain injury (TBI) codes (S06.2X-, S06.30-, S06.9X-). While individual or total coma scale scores may be useful to providers in their clinical decision making when trying to establish a diagnosis, the codes reflecting these scores may not be assigned in conjunction with conditions other than TBIs.
TIP: Codes for individual (R40.21-, R40.22-, R40.23-) or total (R40.24-) coma scale scores may be assigned based on medical record documentation from clinicians who are not the patient's provider.
TIP: It is not appropriate to assign individual (R40.21- , R40.22-, R40.23-) or total (R40.24-) coma scale score codes for patients who are sedated or in medically induced comas.

R4Ø.2Ø Unspecified coma MCC HCC
Coma NOS
Unconsciousness NOS
AHA: 2021,4Q,112-113; 2021,2Q,5

✓6th **R4Ø.21 Coma scale, eyes open**

The following appropriate 7th character is to be added to subcategory R4Ø.21-, R4Ø.22-, R4Ø.23-, and R4Ø.24-.
Ø unspecified time
1 in the field [EMT or ambulance]
2 at arrival to emergency department
3 at hospital admission
4 24 hours or more after hospital admission

✓7th **R4Ø.211 Coma scale, eyes open, never** MCC UPD HCC
Coma scale eye opening score of 1
✓7th **R4Ø.212 Coma scale, eyes open, to pain** MCC UPD HCC
Coma scale eye opening score of 2
✓7th **R4Ø.213 Coma scale, eyes open, to sound** UPD
Coma scale eye opening score of 3
✓7th **R4Ø.214 Coma scale, eyes open, spontaneous** UPD
Coma scale eye opening score of 4

√6th **R40.22 Coma scale, best verbal response**

√7th **R40.221 Coma scale, best verbal response, none** MCC UPD HCC
Coma scale verbal score of 1

√7th **R40.222 Coma scale, best verbal response, incomprehensible words** MCC UPD HCC
Coma scale verbal score of 2
Incomprehensible sounds (2-5 years of age)
Moans/grunts to pain; restless (< 2 years old)

√7th **R40.223 Coma scale, best verbal response, inappropriate words** UPD
Coma scale verbal score of 3
Inappropriate crying or screaming (< 2 years of age)
Screaming (2-5 years of age)

√7th **R40.224 Coma scale, best verbal response, confused conversation** UPD
Coma scale verbal score of 4
Inappropriate words (2-5 years of age)
Irritable cries (< 2 years of age)

√7th **R40.225 Coma scale, best verbal response, oriented** UPD
Coma scale verbal score of 5
Cooing or babbling or crying appropriately (< 2 years of age)
Uses appropriate words (2-5 years of age)

√6th **R40.23 Coma scale, best motor response**

√7th **R40.231 Coma scale, best motor response, none** MCC UPD HCC
Coma scale motor score of 1

√7th **R40.232 Coma scale, best motor response, extension** MCC UPD HCC
Abnormal extensor posturing to pain or noxious stimuli (< 2 years of age)
Coma scale motor score of 2
Extensor posturing to pain or noxious stimuli (2-5 years of age)

√7th **R40.233 Coma scale, best motor response, abnormal flexion** UPD
Abnormal flexure posturing to pain or noxious stimuli (2-5 years of age)
Coma scale motor score of 3
Flexion/decorticate posturing (< 2 years of age)

√7th **R40.234 Coma scale, best motor response, flexion withdrawal** MCC UPD HCC
Coma scale motor score of 4
Withdraws from pain or noxious stimuli (2-5 years of age)

√7th **R40.235 Coma scale, best motor response, localizes pain** UPD
Coma scale motor score of 5
Localizes pain (2-5 years of age)
Withdraws to touch (< 2 years of age)

√7th **R40.236 Coma scale, best motor response, obeys commands** UPD
Coma scale motor score of 6
Normal or spontaneous movement (< 2 years of age)
Obeys commands (2-5 years of age)

√6th **R40.24 Glasgow coma scale, total score**
NOTE Assign a code from subcategory R40.24, when only the total coma score is documented
AHA: 2021,2Q,4; 2016,4Q,64-65

√7th **R40.241 Glasgow coma scale score 13-15** UPD
√7th **R40.242 Glasgow coma scale score 9-12** UPD
√7th **R40.243 Glasgow coma scale score 3-8** UPD HCC
√7th **R40.244 Other coma, without documented Glasgow coma scale score, or with partial score reported** UPD HCC

● **R40.2A Nontraumatic coma due to underlying condition** MCC
Secondary coma
Code first underlying condition

R40.3 Persistent vegetative state CC HCC
DEF: Persistent wakefulness without consciousness due to a nonfunctioning cerebral cortex.

R40.4 Transient alteration of awareness
AHA: 2020,2Q,24

√4th **R41 Other symptoms and signs involving cognitive functions and awareness**
EXCLUDES 1 *dissociative [conversion] disorders (F44.-)*
▶mild cognitive impairment of uncertain or unknown etiology)◀ (G31.84)

R41.0 Disorientation, unspecified
Confusion NOS
Delirium NOS
AHA: 2022,2Q,11; 2019,2Q,34

R41.1 Anterograde amnesia

R41.2 Retrograde amnesia

R41.3 Other amnesia
Amnesia NOS
Memory loss NOS
EXCLUDES 1 *amnestic disorder due to known physiologic condition (F04)*
amnestic syndrome due to psychoactive substance use (F10-F19 with 5th character .6)
mild memory disturbance due to known physiological condition (F06.8)
transient global amnesia (G45.4)

R41.4 Neurologic neglect syndrome CC
Asomatognosia
Hemi-akinesia
Hemi-inattention
Hemispatial neglect
Left-sided neglect
Sensory neglect
Visuospatial neglect
EXCLUDES 1 *visuospatial deficit (R41.842)*

√5th **R41.8 Other symptoms and signs involving cognitive functions and awareness**

R41.81 Age-related cognitive decline A
Senility NOS

R41.82 Altered mental status, unspecified
Change in mental status NOS
EXCLUDES 1 *altered level of consciousness (R40.-)*
altered mental status due to known condition - code to condition
delirium NOS (R41.0)
AHA: 2012,4Q,97

R41.83 Borderline intellectual functioning UPD
IQ level 71 to 84
EXCLUDES 1 *intellectual disabilities (F70-F79)*

√6th **R41.84 Other specified cognitive deficit**
EXCLUDES 1 *cognitive deficits as sequelae of cerebrovascular disease (I69.01-, I69.11-, I69.21-, I69.31-, I69.81-, I69.91-)*

R41.840 Attention and concentration deficit
EXCLUDES 1 *attention-deficit hyperactivity disorders (F90.-)*

R41.841 Cognitive communication deficit

R41.842 Visuospatial deficit

R41.843 Psychomotor deficit

R41.844 Frontal lobe and executive function deficit

R41.89 Other symptoms and signs involving cognitive functions and awareness
Anosognosia

R41.9 Unspecified symptoms and signs involving cognitive functions and awareness
Unspecified neurocognitive disorder

R42 Dizziness and giddiness
Light-headedness
Vertigo NOS
EXCLUDES 1 *vertiginous syndromes (H81.-)*
vertigo from infrasound (T75.23)

√4th **R43 Disturbances of smell and taste**

R43.0 Anosmia
DEF: Permanent or transient absence of smell that may be congenital or acquired.

R43.1 Parosmia
DEF: Abnormal perception of smell usually triggered by environmental odors.

R43.2 Parageusia
DEF: Abnormal perception of taste.

R43.8 Other disturbances of smell and taste
Mixed disturbance of smell and taste

R43.9 Unspecified disturbances of smell and taste

R44 Other symptoms and signs involving general sensations and perceptions
EXCLUDES 1 *alcoholic hallucinations (F10.151, F10.251, F10.951)*
hallucinations in drug psychosis (F11-F19 with fifth to sixth characters 51)
hallucinations in mood disorders with psychotic symptoms (F30.2, F31.5, F32.3, F33.3)
hallucinations in schizophrenia, schizotypal and delusional disorders (F20-F29)
EXCLUDES 2 *disturbances of skin sensation (R20.-)*

R44.0 Auditory hallucinations CC
R44.1 Visual hallucinations
R44.2 Other hallucinations CC
R44.3 Hallucinations, unspecified CC
AHA: 2022,2Q,11
R44.8 Other symptoms and signs involving general sensations and perceptions
R44.9 Unspecified symptoms and signs involving general sensations and perceptions

R45 Symptoms and signs involving emotional state

R45.0 Nervousness
Nervous tension
R45.1 Restlessness and agitation
R45.2 Unhappiness
R45.3 Demoralization and apathy
EXCLUDES 1 *anhedonia (R45.84)*
R45.4 Irritability and anger
R45.5 Hostility
R45.6 Violent behavior
R45.7 State of emotional shock and stress, unspecified
R45.8 Other symptoms and signs involving emotional state
R45.81 Low self-esteem
R45.82 Worries
R45.83 Excessive crying of child, adolescent or adult
EXCLUDES 1 *excessive crying of infant (baby) R68.11*
R45.84 Anhedonia
R45.85 Homicidal and suicidal ideations
EXCLUDES 1 *suicide attempt (T14.91)*
R45.850 Homicidal ideations UPD
R45.851 Suicidal ideations CC
AHA: 2022,1Q,29
DEF: Thoughts of committing suicide but no actual attempt of suicide has been made.
R45.86 Emotional lability
R45.87 Impulsiveness
R45.88 Nonsuicidal self-harm HCC
Nonsuicidal self-injury
Nonsuicidal self-mutilation
Self-inflicted injury without suicidal intent
Code also injury, if known
AHA: 2021,4Q,26-27
R45.89 Other symptoms and signs involving emotional state
▶Flat affect◀
▶Loneliness◀

R46 Symptoms and signs involving appearance and behavior
EXCLUDES 1 *appearance and behavior in schizophrenia, schizotypal and delusional disorders (F20-F29)*
mental and behavioral disorders (F01-F99)

R46.0 Very low level of personal hygiene
R46.1 Bizarre personal appearance
R46.2 Strange and inexplicable behavior
R46.3 Overactivity
R46.4 Slowness and poor responsiveness
EXCLUDES 1 *stupor (R40.1)*
R46.5 Suspiciousness and marked evasiveness
R46.6 Undue concern and preoccupation with stressful events
R46.7 Verbosity and circumstantial detail obscuring reason for contact
R46.8 Other symptoms and signs involving appearance and behavior
R46.81 Obsessive-compulsive behavior UPD
EXCLUDES 1 *obsessive-compulsive disorder (F42.-)*
R46.89 Other symptoms and signs involving appearance and behavior UPD

Symptoms and signs involving speech and voice (R47-R49)

R47 Speech disturbances, not elsewhere classified
EXCLUDES 1 *autism (F84.0)*
cluttering (F80.81)
specific developmental disorders of speech and language (F80.-)
stuttering (F80.81)

R47.0 Dysphasia and aphasia
R47.01 Aphasia CC
EXCLUDES 1 *aphasia following cerebrovascular disease (I69. with final characters -20)*
progressive isolated aphasia (G31.01)
R47.02 Dysphasia
EXCLUDES 1 *dysphasia following cerebrovascular disease (I69. with final characters -21)*
R47.1 Dysarthria and anarthria
EXCLUDES 1 *dysarthria following cerebrovascular disease (I69. with final characters -22)*
R47.8 Other speech disturbances
EXCLUDES 1 *dysarthria following cerebrovascular disease (I69. with final characters -28)*
R47.81 Slurred speech
R47.82 Fluency disorder in conditions classified elsewhere
Stuttering in conditions classified elsewhere
Code first underlying disease or condition, such as:
Parkinson's disease ▶(G20.-)◀
EXCLUDES 1 *adult onset fluency disorder (F98.5)*
childhood onset fluency disorder (F80.81)
fluency disorder (stuttering) following cerebrovascular disease (I69. with final characters -23)
R47.89 Other speech disturbances
R47.9 Unspecified speech disturbances

R48 Dyslexia and other symbolic dysfunctions, not elsewhere classified
EXCLUDES 1 *specific developmental disorders of scholastic skills (F81.-)*

R48.0 Dyslexia and alexia
R48.1 Agnosia
Astereognosia (astereognosis)
Autotopagnosia
EXCLUDES 1 *visual object agnosia (R48.3)*
DEF: Inability to recognize common things such as faces, objects, smells, or voices.
R48.2 Apraxia
EXCLUDES 1 *apraxia following cerebrovascular disease (I69. with final characters -90)*
R48.3 Visual agnosia
Prosopagnosia
Simultanagnosia (asimultagnosia)
R48.8 Other symbolic dysfunctions
Acalculia
Agraphia
AHA: 2017,1Q,27
R48.9 Unspecified symbolic dysfunctions

R49 Voice and resonance disorders
EXCLUDES 1 *psychogenic voice and resonance disorders (F44.4)*

R49.0 Dysphonia
Hoarseness
R49.1 Aphonia
Loss of voice
R49.2 Hypernasality and hyponasality
R49.21 Hypernasality
R49.22 Hyponasality
R49.8 Other voice and resonance disorders
R49.9 Unspecified voice and resonance disorder
Change in voice NOS
Resonance disorder NOS

General symptoms and signs (R50-R69)

R50 Fever of other and unknown origin

EXCLUDES 1 *chills without fever (R68.83)*
febrile convulsions (R56.0-)
fever of unknown origin during labor (O75.2)
fever of unknown origin in newborn (P81.9)
hypothermia due to illness (R68.0)
malignant hyperthermia due to anesthesia (T88.3)
puerperal pyrexia NOS (O86.4)

R50.2 Drug induced fever
Use additional code for adverse effect, if applicable, to identify drug (T36-T50 with fifth or sixth character 5)
EXCLUDES 1 *postvaccination (postimmunization) fever (R50.83)*

R50.8 Other specified fever

R50.81 Fever presenting with conditions classified elsewhere
Code first underlying condition when associated fever is present, such as with:
leukemia (C91-C95)
neutropenia (D70.-)
sickle-cell disease (D57.-)
AHA: 2020,3Q,22; 2014,4Q,22

R50.82 Postprocedural fever
EXCLUDES 1 *postprocedural infection (T81.4-)*
posttransfusion fever (R50.84)
postvaccination (postimmunization) fever (R50.83)

R50.83 Postvaccination fever
Postimmunization fever

R50.84 Febrile nonhemolytic transfusion reaction
FNHTR
Posttransfusion fever

R50.9 Fever, unspecified
Fever NOS
Fever of unknown origin [FUO]
Fever with chills
Fever with rigors
Hyperpyrexia NOS
Persistent fever
Pyrexia NOS

R51 Headache

EXCLUDES 2 *atypical face pain (G50.1)*
migraine and other headache syndromes (G43-G44)
trigeminal neuralgia (G50.0)
AHA: 2020,4Q,38-39

R51.0 Headache with orthostatic component, not elsewhere classified
Headache with positional component, not elsewhere classified

R51.9 Headache, unspecified
Facial pain NOS

R52 Pain, unspecified
Acute pain NOS
Generalized pain NOS
Pain NOS
EXCLUDES 1 *acute and chronic pain, not elsewhere classified (G89.-)*
localized pain, unspecified type - code to pain by site, such as:
abdomen pain (R10.-)
back pain (M54.9)
breast pain (N64.4)
chest pain (R07.1-R07.9)
ear pain (H92.0-)
eye pain (H57.1)
headache (R51.9)
joint pain (M25.5-)
limb pain (M79.6-)
lumbar region pain (M54.5-)
pelvic and perineal pain (R10.2)
renal colic (N23)
shoulder pain (M25.51-)
spine pain (M54.-)
throat pain (R07.0)
tongue pain (K14.6)
tooth pain (K08.8)
pain disorders exclusively related to psychological factors (F45.41)

R53 Malaise and fatigue

R53.0 Neoplastic (malignant) related fatigue
Code first associated neoplasm

R53.1 Weakness
Asthenia NOS
EXCLUDES 1 *age-related weakness (R54)*
muscle weakness (generalized) (M62.81)
sarcopenia (M62.84)
senile asthenia (R54)
AHA: 2017,1Q,7; 2015,1Q,25

R53.2 Functional quadriplegia MCC HCC
Complete immobility due to severe physical disability or frailty
EXCLUDES 1 *frailty NOS (R54)*
hysterical paralysis (F44.4)
immobility syndrome (M62.3)
neurologic quadriplegia (G82.5-)
quadriplegia (G82.50)
AHA: 2022,4Q,15; 2016,2Q,6
DEF: Inability to move due to a nonphysiological condition, such as dementia. The patient has no mental ability to move independently.

R53.8 Other malaise and fatigue
EXCLUDES 1 *combat exhaustion and fatigue (F43.0)*
congenital debility (P96.9)
exhaustion and fatigue due to excessive exertion (T73.3)
exhaustion and fatigue due to exposure (T73.2)
exhaustion and fatigue due to heat (T67.-)
exhaustion and fatigue due to pregnancy (O26.8-)
exhaustion and fatigue due to recurrent depressive episode (F33)
exhaustion and fatigue due to senile debility (R54)

R53.81 Other malaise
Chronic debility
Debility NOS
General physical deterioration
Malaise NOS
Nervous debility
EXCLUDES 1 *age-related physical debility (R54)*
AHA: 2021,1Q,43

R53.82 Chronic fatigue, unspecified
EXCLUDES 1 *chronic fatigue syndrome (G93.32)*
myalgic encephalomyelitis (G93.32)
►other post infection and related fatigue syndromes◄ (G93.39)
postviral fatigue syndrome (G93.31)

R53.83 Other fatigue
Fatigue NOS
Lack of energy
Lethargy
Tiredness
EXCLUDES 2 *exhaustion and fatigue due to depressive episode (F32.-)*

R54 Age-related physical debility A
Frailty
Old age
Senescence
Senile asthenia
Senile debility
EXCLUDES 1 *age-related cognitive decline (R41.81)*
sarcopenia (M62.84)
senile psychosis (F03)
senility NOS (R41.81)

R55 Syncope and collapse
Blackout
Fainting
Vasovagal attack
EXCLUDES 1 *cardiogenic shock (R57.Ø)*
carotid sinus syncope (G9Ø.Ø1)
heat syncope (T67.1)
neurocirculatory asthenia (F45.8)
neurogenic orthostatic hypotension (G9Ø.3)
orthostatic hypotension (I95.1)
postprocedural shock (T81.1-)
psychogenic syncope (F48.8)
shock NOS (R57.9)
shock complicating or following abortion or ectopic or molar pregnancy (OØØ-OØ7, OØ8.3)
shock complicating or following labor and delivery (O75.1)
Stokes-Adams attack (I45.9)
unconsciousness NOS (R4Ø.2-)

✓4th **R56 Convulsions, not elsewhere classified**
EXCLUDES 1 *dissociative convulsions and seizures (F44.5)*
epileptic convulsions and seizures (G4Ø.-)
newborn convulsions and seizures (P9Ø)

✓5th **R56.Ø Febrile convulsions**

R56.ØØ Simple febrile convulsions CC HCC
Febrile convulsion NOS
Febrile seizure NOS

R56.Ø1 Complex febrile convulsions CC HCC
Atypical febrile seizure
Complex febrile seizure
Complicated febrile seizure
EXCLUDES 1 *status epilepticus (G4Ø.9Ø1)*

R56.1 Post traumatic seizures CC HCC
EXCLUDES 1 *post traumatic epilepsy (G4Ø.-)*

R56.9 Unspecified convulsions HCC
Convulsion disorder
Fit NOS
Recurrent convulsions
Seizure(s) (convulsive) NOS
AHA: 2022,4Q,46; 2021,1Q,3; 2019,1Q,19

✓4th **R57 Shock, not elsewhere classified**
EXCLUDES 1 *anaphylactic shock NOS (T78.2)*
anaphylactic reaction or shock due to adverse food reaction (T78.Ø-)
anaphylactic shock due to adverse effect of correct drug or medicament properly administered (T88.6)
anaphylactic shock due to serum (T8Ø.5-)
electric shock (T75.4)
obstetric shock (O75.1)
postprocedural shock (T81.1-)
psychic shock (F43.Ø)
shock complicating or following ectopic or molar pregnancy (OØØ-OØ7, OØ8.3)
shock due to anesthesia (T88.2)
shock due to lightning (T75.Ø1)
toxic shock syndrome (A48.3)
traumatic shock (T79.4)

R57.Ø Cardiogenic shock MCC HCC
EXCLUDES 2 *septic shock (R65.21)*
AHA: 2020,3Q,26
DEF: Associated with myocardial infarction, cardiac tamponade, and massive pulmonary embolism. Symptoms include mental confusion, reduced blood pressure, tachycardia, pallor, and cold, clammy skin.
TIP: MCC only when patient is discharged alive.

R57.1 Hypovolemic shock MCC HCC
AHA: 2019,2Q,7
TIP: MCC only when patient is discharged alive.

R57.8 Other shock MCC HCC
TIP: MCC only when patient is discharged alive.

R57.9 Shock, unspecified CC HCC
Failure of peripheral circulation NOS

R58 Hemorrhage, not elsewhere classified
Hemorrhage NOS
EXCLUDES 1 *hemorrhage included with underlying conditions, such as:*
acute duodenal ulcer with hemorrhage (K26.Ø)
acute gastritis with bleeding (K29.Ø1)
ulcerative enterocolitis with rectal bleeding (K51.Ø1)

✓4th **R59 Enlarged lymph nodes**
INCLUDES swollen glands
EXCLUDES 1 *acute lymphadenitis (LØ4.-)*
chronic lymphadenitis (I88.1)
lymphadenitis NOS (I88.9)
mesenteric (acute) (chronic) lymphadenitis (I88.Ø)

R59.Ø Localized enlarged lymph nodes

R59.1 Generalized enlarged lymph nodes
Lymphadenopathy NOS

R59.9 Enlarged lymph nodes, unspecified

✓4th **R6Ø Edema, not elsewhere classified**
EXCLUDES 1 *angioneurotic edema (T78.3)*
ascites (R18.-)
cerebral edema (G93.6)
cerebral edema due to birth injury (P11.Ø)
edema of larynx (J38.4)
edema of nasopharynx (J39.2)
edema of pharynx (J39.2)
gestational edema (O12.Ø-)
hereditary edema (Q82.Ø)
hydrops fetalis NOS (P83.2)
hydrothorax (J94.8)
newborn edema (P83.3)
pulmonary edema (J81.-)

R6Ø.Ø Localized edema

R6Ø.1 Generalized edema
EXCLUDES 2 *nutritional edema (E4Ø-E46)*

R6Ø.9 Edema, unspecified
Fluid retention NOS

R61 Generalized hyperhidrosis
Excessive sweating
Night sweats
Secondary hyperhidrosis
Code first, if applicable, menopausal and female climacteric states (N95.1)
EXCLUDES 1 *focal (primary) (secondary) hyperhidrosis (L74.5-)*
Frey's syndrome (L74.52)
localized (primary) (secondary) hyperhidrosis (L74.5-)

✓4th **R62 Lack of expected normal physiological development in childhood and adults**
EXCLUDES 1 *delayed puberty (E3Ø.Ø)*
gonadal dysgenesis (Q99.1)
hypopituitarism (E23.Ø)

R62.Ø Delayed milestone in childhood P
Delayed attainment of expected physiological developmental stage
Late talker
Late walker

✓5th **R62.5 Other and unspecified lack of expected normal physiological development in childhood**
EXCLUDES 1 *HIV disease resulting in failure to thrive (B2Ø)*
physical retardation due to malnutrition (E45)

R62.5Ø Unspecified lack of expected normal physiological development in childhood
Infantilism NOS

R62.51 Failure to thrive (child) P
Failure to gain weight
EXCLUDES 1 *failure to thrive in child under 28 days old (P92.6)*
AHA: 2018,4Q,82
DEF: Organic failure to thrive (FTT): Acute or chronic illness that interferes with nutritional intake, absorption, metabolism excretion, and energy requirements.
DEF: Nonorganic failure to thrive (FTT): Symptom of neglect or abuse.

R62.52 Short stature (child)
Lack of growth
Physical retardation
Short stature NOS
EXCLUDES 1 *short stature due to endocrine disorder (E34.3-)*

R62.59 **Other lack of expected normal physiological development in childhood**

R62.7 **Adult failure to thrive** A

✓4th **R63 Symptoms and signs concerning food and fluid intake**

EXCLUDES 1 *bulimia NOS (F5Ø.2)*

R63.Ø **Anorexia**

Loss of appetite

EXCLUDES 1 *anorexia nervosa (F5Ø.Ø-)*
loss of appetite of nonorganic origin (F5Ø.89)

AHA: 2018,4Q,82

TIP: Assign an additional code from category Z68 when BMI is documented. BMI can be based on documentation from clinicians who are not the patient's provider.

R63.1 **Polydipsia**

Excessive thirst

R63.2 **Polyphagia**

Excessive eating
Hyperalimentation NOS

✓5th R63.3 **Feeding difficulties**

EXCLUDES 2 *eating disorders (F5Ø.-)*
feeding problems of newborn (P92.-)
infant feeding disorder of nonorganic origin (F98.2-)

AHA: 2021,4Q,27-28; 2017,1Q,28; 2016,3Q,19

R63.3Ø **Feeding difficulties, unspecified**

R63.31 **Pediatric feeding disorder, acute** P

Pediatric feeding dysfunction, acute

Code also, if applicable, associated conditions such as:
aspiration pneumonia (J69.Ø)
dysphagia (R13.1-)
gastro-esophageal reflux disease (K21.-)
malnutrition (E4Ø-E46)

R63.32 **Pediatric feeding disorder, chronic** P

Pediatric feeding dysfunction, chronic

Code also, if applicable, associated conditions such as:
aspiration pneumonia (J69.Ø)
dysphagia (R13.1-)
gastro-esophageal reflux disease (K21.-)
malnutrition (E4Ø-E46)

R63.39 **Other feeding difficulties**

Feeding problem (elderly) (infant) NOS
Picky eater

R63.4 **Abnormal weight loss**

AHA: 2018,4Q,82

TIP: Assign an additional code from category Z68 when BMI is documented. BMI can be based on documentation from clinicians who are not the patient's provider.

R63.5 **Abnormal weight gain**

EXCLUDES 1 *excessive weight gain in pregnancy (O26.Ø-)*
obesity (E66.-)

AHA: 2018,4Q,82

TIP: Assign an additional code from category Z68 when BMI is documented. BMI can be based on documentation from clinicians who are not the patient's provider.

R63.6 **Underweight**

Use additional code to identify body mass index (BMI), if known (Z68.-)

EXCLUDES 1 *abnormal weight loss (R63.4)*
anorexia nervosa (F5Ø.Ø-)
malnutrition (E4Ø-E46)

AHA: 2018,4Q,82

R63.8 **Other symptoms and signs concerning food and fluid intake**

R64 Cachexia CC HCC

~~Wasting syndrome~~
~~Code first underlying condition, if known~~

EXCLUDES 1 *abnormal weight loss (R63.4)*
▶*cachexia due to underlying condition (E88.A)*◀
nutritional marasmus (E41)

AHA: 2018,4Q,82; 2017,3Q,24

✓4th **R65 Symptoms and signs specifically associated with systemic inflammation and infection**

AHA: 2019,2Q,38

TIP: When documentation states SIRS with an infection, assign only a code for the infection. ICD-10-CM does not offer a code for SIRS due to infectious process. If sepsis is suspected, query the provider.

✓5th R65.1 **Systemic inflammatory response syndrome [SIRS] of non-infectious origin**

Code first underlying condition, such as:
heatstroke (T67.Ø-)
injury and trauma (SØØ-T88)

EXCLUDES 1 *sepsis - code to infection*
severe sepsis (R65.2)

R65.1Ø **Systemic inflammatory response syndrome [SIRS] of non-infectious origin without acute organ dysfunction** CC UPD HCC

Systemic inflammatory response syndrome (SIRS) NOS

AHA: 2019,2Q,24

R65.11 **Systemic inflammatory response syndrome [SIRS] of non-infectious origin with acute organ dysfunction** MCC UPD HCC

Use additional code to identify specific acute organ dysfunction, such as:
acute kidney failure (N17.-)
acute respiratory failure (J96.Ø-)
critical illness myopathy (G72.81)
critical illness polyneuropathy (G62.81)
disseminated intravascular coagulopathy [DIC] (D65)
encephalopathy (metabolic) (septic) (G93.41)
hepatic failure (K72.Ø-)

✓5th R65.2 **Severe sepsis**

Infection with associated acute organ dysfunction
Sepsis with acute organ dysfunction
Sepsis with multiple organ dysfunction
Systemic inflammatory response syndrome due to infectious process with acute organ dysfunction

Code first underlying infection, such as:
infection following a procedure (T81.4-)
infections following infusion, transfusion and therapeutic injection (T8Ø.2-)
puerperal sepsis (O85)
sepsis following complete or unspecified spontaneous abortion (OØ3.87)
sepsis following ectopic and molar pregnancy (OØ8.82)
sepsis following incomplete spontaneous abortion (OØ3.37)
sepsis following (induced) termination of pregnancy (OØ4.87)
sepsis NOS (A41.9)

Use additional code to identify specific acute organ dysfunction, such as:
acute kidney failure (N17.-)
acute respiratory failure (J96.Ø-)
critical illness myopathy (G72.81)
critical illness polyneuropathy (G62.81)
disseminated intravascular coagulopathy [DIC] (D65)
encephalopathy (metabolic) (septic) (G93.41)
hepatic failure (K72.Ø-)

AHA: 2020,2Q,17; 2018,4Q,62-63; 2017,4Q,98-99; 2016,3Q,8

R65.2Ø **Severe sepsis without septic shock** MCC UPD HCC

Severe sepsis NOS

AHA: 2020,2Q,17; 2016,3Q,14; 2013,4Q,119

R65.21 **Severe sepsis with septic shock** MCC UPD HCC

AHA: 2018,4Q,63

✓4th **R68 Other general symptoms and signs**

R68.Ø **Hypothermia, not associated with low environmental temperature**

EXCLUDES 1 *hypothermia NOS (accidental) (T68)*
hypothermia due to anesthesia (T88.51)
hypothermia due to low environmental temperature (T68)
newborn hypothermia (P8Ø.-)

R68.1 Nonspecific symptoms peculiar to infancy
EXCLUDES 1 *colic, infantile (R10.83)*
neonatal cerebral irritability (P91.3)
teething syndrome (K00.7)

R68.11 Excessive crying of infant (baby)
EXCLUDES 1 *excessive crying of child, adolescent, or adult (R45.83)*

R68.12 Fussy infant (baby)
Irritable infant

R68.13 Apparent life threatening event in infant (ALTE)
Apparent life threatening event in newborn
Brief resolved unexplained event (BRUE)
Code first confirmed diagnosis, if known
Use additional code(s) for associated signs and symptoms if no confirmed diagnosis established, or if signs and symptoms are not associated routinely with confirmed diagnosis, or provide additional information for cause of ALTE

R68.19 Other nonspecific symptoms peculiar to infancy

R68.2 Dry mouth, unspecified
EXCLUDES 1 *dry mouth due to dehydration (E86.0)*
dry mouth due to Sjogren syndrome (M35.0-)
salivary gland hyposecretion (K11.7)

R68.3 Clubbing of fingers
Clubbing of nails
EXCLUDES 1 *congenital clubfinger (Q68.1)*
DEF: Enlarged soft tissue of the distal fingers that usually occurs in heart and lung diseases.

R68.8 Other general symptoms and signs

R68.81 Early satiety
DEF: Premature feeling of being full after eating only a small amount of food. The mechanism of satiety is multifactorial.

R68.82 Decreased libido
Decreased sexual desire

R68.83 Chills (without fever)
Chills NOS
EXCLUDES 1 *chills with fever (R50.9)*

R68.84 Jaw pain
Mandibular pain
Maxilla pain
EXCLUDES 1 *temporomandibular joint arthralgia (M26.62-)*

R68.89 Other general symptoms and signs

R69 Illness, unspecified
Unknown and unspecified cases of morbidity

Abnormal findings on examination of blood, without diagnosis (R70-R79)

EXCLUDES 2 *abnormal findings on antenatal screening of mother (O28.-)*
abnormalities of lipids (E78.-)
abnormalities of platelets and thrombocytes (D69.-)
abnormalities of white blood cells classified elsewhere (D70-D72)
coagulation hemorrhagic disorders (D65-D68)
diagnostic abnormal findings classified elsewhere - see Alphabetical Index
hemorrhagic and hematological disorders of newborn (P50-P61)

R70 Elevated erythrocyte sedimentation rate and abnormality of plasma viscosity

R70.0 Elevated erythrocyte sedimentation rate

R70.1 Abnormal plasma viscosity

R71 Abnormality of red blood cells
EXCLUDES 1 *anemias (D50-D64)*
anemia of premature infant (P61.2)
benign (familial) polycythemia (D75.0)
congenital anemias (P61.2-P61.4)
newborn anemia due to isoimmunization (P55.-)
polycythemia neonatorum (P61.1)
polycythemia NOS (D75.1)
polycythemia vera (D45)
secondary polycythemia (D75.1)

R71.0 Precipitous drop in hematocrit
Drop (precipitous) in hemoglobin
Drop in hematocrit

R71.8 Other abnormality of red blood cells
Abnormal red-cell morphology NOS
Abnormal red-cell volume NOS
Anisocytosis
Poikilocytosis

R73 Elevated blood glucose level
EXCLUDES 1 *diabetes mellitus (E08-E13)*
diabetes mellitus in pregnancy, childbirth and the puerperium (O24.-)
neonatal disorders (P70.0-P70.2)
postsurgical hypoinsulinemia (E89.1)

R73.0 Abnormal glucose
EXCLUDES 1 *abnormal glucose in pregnancy (O99.81-)*
diabetes mellitus (E08-E13)
dysmetabolic syndrome X ▶(E88.81-)◀
gestational diabetes (O24.4-)
glycosuria (R81)
hypoglycemia (E16.2)

R73.01 Impaired fasting glucose
Elevated fasting glucose

R73.02 Impaired glucose tolerance (oral)
Elevated glucose tolerance

R73.03 Prediabetes
Latent diabetes
AHA: 2016,4Q,65

R73.09 Other abnormal glucose
Abnormal glucose NOS
Abnormal non-fasting glucose tolerance

R73.9 Hyperglycemia, unspecified

R74 Abnormal serum enzyme levels

R74.0 Nonspecific elevation of levels of transaminase and lactic acid dehydrogenase [LDH]
AHA: 2020,4Q,39

R74.01 Elevation of levels of liver transaminase levels
Elevation of levels of alanine transaminase (ALT)
Elevation of levels of aspartate transaminase (AST)

R74.02 Elevation of levels of lactic acid dehydrogenase [LDH]

R74.8 Abnormal levels of other serum enzymes
Abnormal level of acid phosphatase
Abnormal level of alkaline phosphatase
Abnormal level of amylase
Abnormal level of lipase [triacylglycerol lipase]
AHA: 2019,2Q,6

R74.9 Abnormal serum enzyme level, unspecified

R75 Inconclusive laboratory evidence of human immunodeficiency virus [HIV]
Nonconclusive HIV-test finding in infants
EXCLUDES 1 *asymptomatic human immunodeficiency virus [HIV] infection status (Z21)*
human immunodeficiency virus [HIV] disease (B20)

R76 Other abnormal immunological findings in serum

R76.0 Raised antibody titer
EXCLUDES 1 *isoimmunization in pregnancy (O36.0-O36.1)*
isoimmunization affecting newborn (P55.-)
AHA: 2021,1Q,6

R76.1 Nonspecific reaction to test for tuberculosis

R76.11 Nonspecific reaction to tuberculin skin test without active tuberculosis
Abnormal result of Mantoux test
PPD positive
Tuberculin (skin test) positive
Tuberculin (skin test) reactor
EXCLUDES 1 *nonspecific reaction to cell mediated immunity measurement of gamma interferon antigen response without active tuberculosis (R76.12)*

R76.12 Nonspecific reaction to cell mediated immunity measurement of gamma interferon antigen response without active tuberculosis
Nonspecific reaction to QuantiFERON-TB test (QFT) without active tuberculosis
EXCLUDES 1 *nonspecific reaction to tuberculin skin test without active tuberculosis (R76.11)*
positive tuberculin skin test (R76.11)

R76.8 Other specified abnormal immunological findings in serum
Raised level of immunoglobulins NOS
AHA: 2021,1Q,6

R76.9 Abnormal immunological finding in serum, unspecified

R77 Other abnormalities of plasma proteins
EXCLUDES 1 *disorders of plasma-protein metabolism (E88.Ø-)*

R77.Ø Abnormality of albumin

R77.1 Abnormality of globulin
Hyperglobulinemia NOS

R77.2 Abnormality of alphafetoprotein

R77.8 Other specified abnormalities of plasma proteins

R77.9 Abnormality of plasma protein, unspecified
AHA: 2019,2Q,6

R78 Findings of drugs and other substances, not normally found in blood
Use additional code to identify the any retained foreign body, if applicable (Z18.-)
EXCLUDES 1 ~~*mental or behavioral disorders due to psychoactive substance use (F1Ø-F19)*~~
EXCLUDES 2 ▶*mental or behavioral disorders due to psychoactive substance use (F1Ø-F19)*◀

R78.Ø Finding of alcohol in blood
Use additional external cause code (Y9Ø.-), for detail regarding alcohol level

R78.1 Finding of opiate drug in blood

R78.2 Finding of cocaine in blood

R78.3 Finding of hallucinogen in blood

R78.4 Finding of other drugs of addictive potential in blood

R78.5 Finding of other psychotropic drug in blood

R78.6 Finding of steroid agent in blood

R78.7 Finding of abnormal level of heavy metals in blood

R78.71 Abnormal lead level in blood
EXCLUDES 1 *lead poisoning (T56.Ø-)*

R78.79 Finding of abnormal level of heavy metals in blood

R78.8 Finding of other specified substances, not normally found in blood

R78.81 Bacteremia CC
EXCLUDES 1 *sepsis — code to specified infection*
DEF: Laboratory finding of bacteria in the blood in the absence of two or more signs of sepsis. Transient in nature, it can progress to septicemia with a severe infectious process.

R78.89 Finding of other specified substances, not normally found in blood
Finding of abnormal level of lithium in blood

R78.9 Finding of unspecified substance, not normally found in blood

R79 Other abnormal findings of blood chemistry
Use additional code to identify any retained foreign body, if applicable (Z18.-)
EXCLUDES 1 *asymptomatic hyperuricemia (E79.Ø)*
hyperglycemia NOS (R73.9)
hypoglycemia NOS (E16.2)
neonatal hypoglycemia (P7Ø.3-P7Ø.4)
specific findings indicating disorder of amino-acid metabolism (E7Ø-E72)
specific findings indicating disorder of carbohydrate metabolism (E73-E74)
specific findings indicating disorder of lipid metabolism (E75.-)

R79.Ø Abnormal level of blood mineral
Abnormal blood level of cobalt
Abnormal blood level of copper
Abnormal blood level of iron
Abnormal blood level of magnesium
Abnormal blood level of mineral NEC
Abnormal blood level of zinc
EXCLUDES 1 *abnormal level of lithium (R78.89)*
disorders of mineral metabolism (E83.-)
neonatal hypomagnesemia (P71.2)
nutritional mineral deficiency (E58-E61)

R79.1 Abnormal coagulation profile
Abnormal or prolonged bleeding time
Abnormal or prolonged coagulation time
Abnormal or prolonged partial thromboplastin time [PTT]
Abnormal or prolonged prothrombin time [PT]
Low von Willebrand factor
EXCLUDES 1 *coagulation defects (D68.-)*
EXCLUDES 2 *abnormality of fluid, electrolyte or acid-base balance (E86-E87)*

R79.8 Other specified abnormal findings of blood chemistry

R79.81 Abnormal blood-gas level

R79.82 Elevated C-reactive protein [CRP]

R79.83 Abnormal findings of blood amino-acid level
Homocysteinemia
EXCLUDES 1 *disorders of amino-acid metabolism (E7Ø-E72)*
AHA: 2021,4Q,28

R79.89 Other specified abnormal findings of blood chemistry
AHA: 2019,2Q,6
TIP: Assign for positive Coombs test when not further clarified in the documentation.

R79.9 Abnormal finding of blood chemistry, unspecified

Abnormal findings on examination of urine, without diagnosis (R8Ø-R82)

EXCLUDES 1 *abnormal findings on antenatal screening of mother (O28.-)*
diagnostic abnormal findings classified elsewhere - see Alphabetical Index
specific findings indicating disorder of amino-acid metabolism (E7Ø-E72)
specific findings indicating disorder of carbohydrate metabolism (E73-E74)

R8Ø Proteinuria
EXCLUDES 1 *gestational proteinuria (O12.1-)*

R8Ø.Ø Isolated proteinuria
Idiopathic proteinuria
EXCLUDES 1 *isolated proteinuria with specific morphological lesion (NØ6.-)*

R8Ø.1 Persistent proteinuria, unspecified

R8Ø.2 Orthostatic proteinuria, unspecified
Postural proteinuria

R8Ø.3 Bence Jones proteinuria

R8Ø.8 Other proteinuria

R8Ø.9 Proteinuria, unspecified
Albuminuria NOS

R81 Glycosuria
EXCLUDES 1 *renal glycosuria (E74.818)*

R82 Other and unspecified abnormal findings in urine
INCLUDES chromoabnormalities in urine
Use additional code to identify any retained foreign body, if applicable (Z18.-)
EXCLUDES 2 *hematuria (R31.-)*

R82.Ø Chyluria CC
EXCLUDES 1 *filarial chyluria (B74.-)*

R82.1 Myoglobinuria CC

R82.2 Biliuria

R82.3 Hemoglobinuria
EXCLUDES 1 *hemoglobinuria due to hemolysis from external causes NEC (D59.6)*
hemoglobinuria due to paroxysmal nocturnal [Marchiafava-Micheli] (D59.5)
DEF: Free hemoglobin in blood due to rapid hemolysis of red blood cells. Causes include burns, crushed injury, sickle cell anemia, thalassemia, parasitic infections, or kidney infections.

R82.4 Acetonuria
Ketonuria
DEF: Excessive excretion of acetone in urine that commonly occurs in diabetic acidosis.

R82.5 Elevated urine levels of drugs, medicaments and biological substances
Elevated urine levels of catecholamines
Elevated urine levels of indoleacetic acid
Elevated urine levels of 17-ketosteroids
Elevated urine levels of steroids

R82.6 Abnormal urine levels of substances chiefly nonmedicinal as to source
Abnormal urine level of heavy metals

√5th **R82.7 Abnormal findings on microbiological examination of urine**
EXCLUDES 1 *colonization status (Z22.-)*
AHA: 2016,4Q,65
R82.71 Bacteriuria
R82.79 Other abnormal findings on microbiological examination of urine
Positive culture findings of urine

√5th **R82.8 Abnormal findings on cytological and histological examination of urine**
AHA: 2019,4Q,16
R82.81 Pyuria
Sterile pyuria
R82.89 Other abnormal findings on cytological and histological examination of urine

√5th **R82.9 Other and unspecified abnormal findings in urine**
R82.90 Unspecified abnormal findings in urine
R82.91 Other chromoabnormalities of urine
Chromoconversion (dipstick)
Idiopathic dipstick converts positive for blood with no cellular forms in sediment
EXCLUDES 1 *hemoglobinuria (R82.3)*
myoglobinuria (R82.1)
√6th **R82.99 Other abnormal findings in urine**
AHA: 2018,4Q,29-30
R82.991 Hypocitraturia
R82.992 Hyperoxaluria
EXCLUDES 1 *primary hyperoxaluria (E72.53)*
R82.993 Hyperuricosuria
R82.994 Hypercalciuria
Idiopathic hypercalciuria
R82.998 Other abnormal findings in urine
Cells and casts in urine
Crystalluria
Melanuria

Abnormal findings on examination of other body fluids, substances and tissues, without diagnosis (R83-R89)

EXCLUDES 1 *abnormal findings on antenatal screening of mother (O28.-)*
diagnostic abnormal findings classified elsewhere - see Alphabetical Index
EXCLUDES 2 *abnormal findings on examination of blood, without diagnosis (R70-R79)*
abnormal findings on examination of urine, without diagnosis (R80-R82)
abnormal tumor markers (R97.-)

√4th **R83 Abnormal findings in cerebrospinal fluid**
R83.0 Abnormal level of enzymes in cerebrospinal fluid
R83.1 Abnormal level of hormones in cerebrospinal fluid
R83.2 Abnormal level of other drugs, medicaments and biological substances in cerebrospinal fluid
R83.3 Abnormal level of substances chiefly nonmedicinal as to source in cerebrospinal fluid
R83.4 Abnormal immunological findings in cerebrospinal fluid
R83.5 Abnormal microbiological findings in cerebrospinal fluid
Positive culture findings in cerebrospinal fluid
EXCLUDES 1 *colonization status (Z22.-)*
R83.6 Abnormal cytological findings in cerebrospinal fluid
R83.8 Other abnormal findings in cerebrospinal fluid
Abnormal chromosomal findings in cerebrospinal fluid
R83.9 Unspecified abnormal finding in cerebrospinal fluid

√4th **R84 Abnormal findings in specimens from respiratory organs and thorax**
INCLUDES abnormal findings in bronchial washings
abnormal findings in nasal secretions
abnormal findings in pleural fluid
abnormal findings in sputum
abnormal findings in throat scrapings
EXCLUDES 1 *blood-stained sputum (R04.2)*
R84.0 Abnormal level of enzymes in specimens from respiratory organs and thorax
R84.1 Abnormal level of hormones in specimens from respiratory organs and thorax
R84.2 Abnormal level of other drugs, medicaments and biological substances in specimens from respiratory organs and thorax
R84.3 Abnormal level of substances chiefly nonmedicinal as to source in specimens from respiratory organs and thorax
R84.4 Abnormal immunological findings in specimens from respiratory organs and thorax
R84.5 Abnormal microbiological findings in specimens from respiratory organs and thorax
Positive culture findings in specimens from respiratory organs and thorax
EXCLUDES 1 *colonization status (Z22.-)*
R84.6 Abnormal cytological findings in specimens from respiratory organs and thorax
R84.7 Abnormal histological findings in specimens from respiratory organs and thorax
R84.8 Other abnormal findings in specimens from respiratory organs and thorax
Abnormal chromosomal findings in specimens from respiratory organs and thorax
R84.9 Unspecified abnormal finding in specimens from respiratory organs and thorax

√4th **R85 Abnormal findings in specimens from digestive organs and abdominal cavity**
INCLUDES abnormal findings in peritoneal fluid
abnormal findings in saliva
EXCLUDES 1 *cloudy peritoneal dialysis effluent (R88.0)*
fecal abnormalities (R19.5)
R85.0 Abnormal level of enzymes in specimens from digestive organs and abdominal cavity
R85.1 Abnormal level of hormones in specimens from digestive organs and abdominal cavity
R85.2 Abnormal level of other drugs, medicaments and biological substances in specimens from digestive organs and abdominal cavity
R85.3 Abnormal level of substances chiefly nonmedicinal as to source in specimens from digestive organs and abdominal cavity
R85.4 Abnormal immunological findings in specimens from digestive organs and abdominal cavity
R85.5 Abnormal microbiological findings in specimens from digestive organs and abdominal cavity
Positive culture findings in specimens from digestive organs and abdominal cavity
EXCLUDES 1 *colonization status (Z22.-)*
√5th **R85.6 Abnormal cytological findings in specimens from digestive organs and abdominal cavity**
√6th **R85.61 Abnormal cytologic smear of anus**
EXCLUDES 1 *abnormal cytological findings in specimens from other digestive organs and abdominal cavity (R85.69)*
anal intraepithelial neoplasia I [AIN I] (K62.82)
anal intraepithelial neoplasia II [AIN II] (K62.82)
anal intraepithelial neoplasia III [AIN III] (D01.3)
carcinoma in situ of anus (histologically confirmed) (D01.3)
dysplasia (mild) (moderate) of anus (histologically confirmed) (K62.82)
severe dysplasia of anus (histologically confirmed) (D01.3)
EXCLUDES 2 *anal high risk human papillomavirus (HPV) DNA test positive (R85.81)*
anal low risk human papillomavirus (HPV) DNA test positive (R85.82)
R85.610 Atypical squamous cells of undetermined significance on cytologic smear of anus [ASC-US]
R85.611 Atypical squamous cells cannot exclude high grade squamous intraepithelial lesion on cytologic smear of anus [ASC-H]
R85.612 Low grade squamous intraepithelial lesion on cytologic smear of anus [LGSIL]
R85.613 High grade squamous intraepithelial lesion on cytologic smear of anus [HGSIL]
R85.614 Cytologic evidence of malignancy on smear of anus
R85.615 Unsatisfactory cytologic smear of anus
Inadequate sample of cytologic smear of anus
R85.616 Satisfactory anal smear but lacking transformation zone
R85.618 Other abnormal cytological findings on specimens from anus

R85.619 Unspecified abnormal cytological findings in specimens from anus
Abnormal anal cytology NOS
Atypical glandular cells of anus NOS

R85.69 Abnormal cytological findings in specimens from other digestive organs and abdominal cavity

R85.7 Abnormal histological findings in specimens from digestive organs and abdominal cavity

✓5th **R85.8 Other abnormal findings in specimens from digestive organs and abdominal cavity**

R85.81 Anal high risk human papillomavirus [HPV] DNA test positive
EXCLUDES 1 *anogenital warts due to human papillomavirus (HPV) (A63.Ø)*
condyloma acuminatum (A63.Ø)

R85.82 Anal low risk human papillomavirus [HPV] DNA test positive
Use additional code for associated human papillomavirus (B97.7)

R85.89 Other abnormal findings in specimens from digestive organs and abdominal cavity
Abnormal chromosomal findings in specimens from digestive organs and abdominal cavity

R85.9 Unspecified abnormal finding in specimens from digestive organs and abdominal cavity

✓4th **R86 Abnormal findings in specimens from male genital organs**
INCLUDES abnormal findings in prostatic secretions
abnormal findings in semen, seminal fluid
abnormal spermatozoa
EXCLUDES 1 *azoospermia (N46.Ø-)*
oligospermia (N46.1-)

R86.Ø Abnormal level of enzymes in specimens from male genital organs ♂

R86.1 Abnormal level of hormones in specimens from male genital organs ♂

R86.2 Abnormal level of other drugs, medicaments and biological substances in specimens from male genital organs ♂

R86.3 Abnormal level of substances chiefly nonmedicinal as to source in specimens from male genital organs ♂

R86.4 Abnormal immunological findings in specimens from male genital organs ♂

R86.5 Abnormal microbiological findings in specimens from male genital organs ♂
Positive culture findings in specimens from male genital organs
EXCLUDES 1 *colonization status (Z22.-)*

R86.6 Abnormal cytological findings in specimens from male genital organs ♂

R86.7 Abnormal histological findings in specimens from male genital organs ♂

R86.8 Other abnormal findings in specimens from male genital organs ♂
Abnormal chromosomal findings in specimens from male genital organs

R86.9 Unspecified abnormal finding in specimens from male genital organs ♂

✓4th **R87 Abnormal findings in specimens from female genital organs**
INCLUDES abnormal findings in secretion and smears from cervix uteri
abnormal findings in secretion and smears from vagina
abnormal findings in secretion and smears from vulva

R87.Ø Abnormal level of enzymes in specimens from female genital organs ♀

R87.1 Abnormal level of hormones in specimens from female genital organs ♀

R87.2 Abnormal level of other drugs, medicaments and biological substances in specimens from female genital organs ♀

R87.3 Abnormal level of substances chiefly nonmedicinal as to source in specimens from female genital organs ♀

R87.4 Abnormal immunological findings in specimens from female genital organs ♀

R87.5 Abnormal microbiological findings in specimens from female genital organs ♀
Positive culture findings in specimens from female genital organs
EXCLUDES 1 *colonization status (Z22.-)*

✓5th **R87.6 Abnormal cytological findings in specimens from female genital organs**

✓6th **R87.61 Abnormal cytological findings in specimens from cervix uteri**
EXCLUDES 1 *abnormal cytological findings in specimens from other female genital organs (R87.69)*
abnormal cytological findings in specimens from vagina (R87.62-)
carcinoma in situ of cervix uteri (histologically confirmed) (DØ6.-)
cervical intraepithelial neoplasia I [CIN I] (N87.Ø)
cervical intraepithelial neoplasia II [CIN II] (N87.1)
cervical intraepithelial neoplasia III [CIN III] (DØ6.-)
dysplasia (mild) (moderate) of cervix uteri (histologically confirmed) (N87.-)
severe dysplasia of cervix uteri (histologically confirmed) (DØ6.-)
EXCLUDES 2 *cervical high risk human papillomavirus (HPV) DNA test positive (R87.81Ø)*
cervical low risk human papillomavirus (HPV) DNA test positive (R87.82Ø)

R87.61Ø Atypical squamous cells of undetermined significance on cytologic smear of cervix [ASC-US] ♀

R87.611 Atypical squamous cells cannot exclude high grade squamous intraepithelial lesion on cytologic smear of cervix [ASC-H] ♀

R87.612 Low grade squamous intraepithelial lesion on cytologic smear of cervix [LGSIL] ♀

R87.613 High grade squamous intraepithelial lesion on cytologic smear of cervix [HGSIL] ♀

R87.614 Cytologic evidence of malignancy on smear of cervix ♀

R87.615 Unsatisfactory cytologic smear of cervix ♀
Inadequate sample of cytologic smear of cervix

R87.616 Satisfactory cervical smear but lacking transformation zone ♀

R87.618 Other abnormal cytological findings on specimens from cervix uteri ♀

R87.619 Unspecified abnormal cytological findings in specimens from cervix uteri ♀
Abnormal cervical cytology NOS
Abnormal Papanicolaou smear of cervix NOS
Abnormal thin preparation smear of cervix NOS
Atypical endocervical cells of cervix NOS
Atypical endometrial cells of cervix NOS
Atypical glandular cells of cervix NOS

R87.62 Abnormal cytological findings in specimens from vagina

Use additional code to identify acquired absence of uterus and cervix, if applicable (Z90.71-)

EXCLUDES 1 *abnormal cytological findings in specimens from cervix uteri (R87.61-)*
abnormal cytological findings in specimens from other female genital organs (R87.69)
carcinoma in situ of vagina (histologically confirmed) (DØ7.2)
dysplasia (mild) (moderate) of vagina (histologically confirmed) (N89.-)
severe dysplasia of vagina (histologically confirmed) (DØ7.2)
vaginal intraepithelial neoplasia I [VAIN I] (N89.Ø)
vaginal intraepithelial neoplasia II [VAIN II] (N89.1)
vaginal intraepithelial neoplasia III [VAIN III] (DØ7.2)

EXCLUDES 2 *vaginal high risk human papillomavirus (HPV) DNA test positive (R87.811)*
vaginal low risk human papillomavirus (HPV) DNA test positive (R87.821)

R87.62Ø Atypical squamous cells of undetermined significance on cytologic smear of vagina [ASC-US] ♀

R87.621 Atypical squamous cells cannot exclude high grade squamous intraepithelial lesion on cytologic smear of vagina [ASC-H] ♀

R87.622 Low grade squamous intraepithelial lesion on cytologic smear of vagina [LGSIL] ♀

R87.623 High grade squamous intraepithelial lesion on cytologic smear of vagina [HGSIL] ♀

R87.624 Cytologic evidence of malignancy on smear of vagina ♀

R87.625 Unsatisfactory cytologic smear of vagina ♀

Inadequate sample of cytologic smear of vagina

R87.628 Other abnormal cytological findings on specimens from vagina ♀

R87.629 Unspecified abnormal cytological findings in specimens from vagina ♀

Abnormal Papanicolaou smear of vagina NOS
Abnormal thin preparation smear of vagina NOS
Abnormal vaginal cytology NOS
Atypical endocervical cells of vagina NOS
Atypical endometrial cells of vagina NOS
Atypical glandular cells of vagina NOS

R87.69 Abnormal cytological findings in specimens from other female genital organs ♀

Abnormal cytological findings in specimens from female genital organs NOS

EXCLUDES 1 *dysplasia of vulva (histologically confirmed) (N9Ø.Ø-N9Ø.3)*

R87.7 Abnormal histological findings in specimens from female genital organs ♀

EXCLUDES 1 *carcinoma in situ (histologically confirmed) of female genital organs (DØ6-DØ7.3)*
cervical intraepithelial neoplasia I [CIN I] (N87.Ø)
cervical intraepithelial neoplasia II [CIN II] (N87.1)
cervical intraepithelial neoplasia III [CIN III] (DØ6.-)
dysplasia (mild) (moderate) of cervix uteri (histologically confirmed) (N87.-)
dysplasia (mild) (moderate) of vagina (histologically confirmed) (N89.-)
severe dysplasia of cervix uteri (histologically confirmed) (DØ6.-)
severe dysplasia of vagina (histologically confirmed) (DØ7.2)
vaginal intraepithelial neoplasia I [VAIN I] (N89.Ø)
vaginal intraepithelial neoplasia II [VAIN II] (N89.1)
vaginal intraepithelial neoplasia III [VAIN III] (DØ7.2)

R87.8 Other abnormal findings in specimens from female genital organs

R87.81 High risk human papillomavirus [HPV] DNA test positive from female genital organs

EXCLUDES 1 *anogenital warts due to human papillomavirus (HPV) (A63.Ø)*
condyloma acuminatum (A63.Ø)

R87.81Ø Cervical high risk human papillomavirus [HPV] DNA test positive ♀

R87.811 Vaginal high risk human papillomavirus [HPV] DNA test positive ♀

R87.82 Low risk human papillomavirus [HPV] DNA test positive from female genital organs

Use additional code for associated human papillomavirus (B97.7)

R87.82Ø Cervical low risk human papillomavirus [HPV] DNA test positive ♀

R87.821 Vaginal low risk human papillomavirus [HPV] DNA test positive ♀

R87.89 Other abnormal findings in specimens from female genital organs ♀

Abnormal chromosomal findings in specimens from female genital organs

R87.9 Unspecified abnormal finding in specimens from female genital organs ♀

R88 Abnormal findings in other body fluids and substances

R88.Ø Cloudy (hemodialysis) (peritoneal) dialysis effluent

R88.8 Abnormal findings in other body fluids and substances

R89 Abnormal findings in specimens from other organs, systems and tissues

INCLUDES abnormal findings in nipple discharge
abnormal findings in synovial fluid
abnormal findings in wound secretions

R89.Ø Abnormal level of enzymes in specimens from other organs, systems and tissues

R89.1 Abnormal level of hormones in specimens from other organs, systems and tissues

R89.2 Abnormal level of other drugs, medicaments and biological substances in specimens from other organs, systems and tissues

R89.3 Abnormal level of substances chiefly nonmedicinal as to source in specimens from other organs, systems and tissues

R89.4 Abnormal immunological findings in specimens from other organs, systems and tissues

R89.5 Abnormal microbiological findings in specimens from other organs, systems and tissues

Positive culture findings in specimens from other organs, systems and tissues

EXCLUDES 1 *colonization status (Z22.-)*

R89.6 Abnormal cytological findings in specimens from other organs, systems and tissues

R89.7 Abnormal histological findings in specimens from other organs, systems and tissues

R89.8 Other abnormal findings in specimens from other organs, systems and tissues

Abnormal chromosomal findings in specimens from other organs, systems and tissues

R89.9 Unspecified abnormal finding in specimens from other organs, systems and tissues

Abnormal findings on diagnostic imaging and in function studies, without diagnosis (R9Ø-R94)

INCLUDES nonspecific abnormal findings on diagnostic imaging by computerized axial tomography [CAT scan]
nonspecific abnormal findings on diagnostic imaging by magnetic resonance imaging [MRI][NMR]
nonspecific abnormal findings on diagnostic imaging by positron emission tomography [PET scan]
nonspecific abnormal findings on diagnostic imaging by thermography
nonspecific abnormal findings on diagnostic imaging by ultrasound [echogram]
nonspecific abnormal findings on diagnostic imaging by X-ray examination

EXCLUDES 1 *abnormal findings on antenatal screening of mother (O28.-)*
diagnostic abnormal findings classified elsewhere - see Alphabetical Index

R9Ø Abnormal findings on diagnostic imaging of central nervous system

R9Ø.Ø Intracranial space-occupying lesion found on diagnostic imaging of central nervous system

✓5th **R90.8 Other abnormal findings on diagnostic imaging of central nervous system**

R90.81 Abnormal echoencephalogram

R90.82 White matter disease, unspecified

R90.89 Other abnormal findings on diagnostic imaging of central nervous system

Other cerebrovascular abnormality found on diagnostic imaging of central nervous system

✓4th **R91 Abnormal findings on diagnostic imaging of lung**

R91.1 Solitary pulmonary nodule

Coin lesion lung

Solitary pulmonary nodule, subsegmental branch of the bronchial tree

R91.8 Other nonspecific abnormal finding of lung field

Lung mass NOS found on diagnostic imaging of lung

Pulmonary infiltrate NOS

Shadow, lung

✓4th **R92 Abnormal and inconclusive findings on diagnostic imaging of breast**

R92.0 Mammographic microcalcification found on diagnostic imaging of breast

EXCLUDES 2 *mammographic calcification (calculus) found on diagnostic imaging of breast (R92.1)*

DEF: Calcium and cellular debris deposits in the breast that cannot be felt but can be detected on a mammogram. The deposits can be a sign of cancer, benign conditions, or changes in the breast tissue as a result of inflammation, injury, or an obstructed duct.

R92.1 Mammographic calcification found on diagnostic imaging of breast

Mammographic calculus found on diagnostic imaging of breast

R92.2 Inconclusive mammogram

~~Dense breasts NOS~~

Inconclusive mammogram NEC

~~Inconclusive mammography due to dense breasts~~

Inconclusive mammography NEC

AHA: 2015,1Q,24

● ✓5th **R92.3 Mammographic density found on imaging of breast**

Code also, if applicable, inconclusive mammogram (R92.2)

● **R92.30 Dense breasts, unspecified**

Dense breasts NOS

Low density

● ✓6th **R92.31 Mammographic fatty tissue density of breast**

Breast Imaging Reporting and Data System (BI-RADS): A

Breast Imaging Reporting and Data System (BI-RADS): 1

● **R92.311 Mammographic fatty tissue density, right breast**

● **R92.312 Mammographic fatty tissue density, left breast**

● **R92.313 Mammographic fatty tissue density, bilateral breasts**

● ✓6th **R92.32 Mammographic fibroglandular density of breast**

Breast Imaging Reporting and Data System (BI-RADS): B

Breast Imaging Reporting and Data System (BI-RADS): 2

● **R92.321 Mammographic fibroglandular density, right breast**

● **R92.322 Mammographic fibroglandular density, left breast**

● **R92.323 Mammographic fibroglandular density, bilateral breasts**

● ✓6th **R92.33 Mammographic heterogeneous density of breast**

Breast Imaging Reporting and Data System (BI-RADS): C

Breast Imaging Reporting and Data System (BI-RADS): 3

● **R92.331 Mammographic heterogeneous density, right breast**

● **R92.332 Mammographic heterogeneous density, left breast**

● **R92.333 Mammographic heterogeneous density, bilateral breasts**

● ✓6th **R92.34 Mammographic extreme density of breast**

Breast Imaging Reporting and Data System (BI-RADS): D

Breast Imaging Reporting and Data System (BI-RADS): 4

● **R92.341 Mammographic extreme density, right breast**

● **R92.342 Mammographic extreme density, left breast**

● **R92.343 Mammographic extreme density, bilateral breasts**

R92.8 Other abnormal and inconclusive findings on diagnostic imaging of breast

✓4th **R93 Abnormal findings on diagnostic imaging of other body structures**

R93.0 Abnormal findings on diagnostic imaging of skull and head, not elsewhere classified

EXCLUDES 1 *intracranial space-occupying lesion found on diagnostic imaging (R90.0)*

R93.1 Abnormal findings on diagnostic imaging of heart and coronary circulation

Abnormal echocardiogram NOS

Abnormal heart shadow

R93.2 Abnormal findings on diagnostic imaging of liver and biliary tract

Nonvisualization of gallbladder

R93.3 Abnormal findings on diagnostic imaging of other parts of digestive tract

✓5th **R93.4 Abnormal findings on diagnostic imaging of urinary organs**

EXCLUDES 2 *hypertrophy of kidney (N28.81)*

AHA: 2016,4Q,66

R93.41 Abnormal radiologic findings on diagnostic imaging of renal pelvis, ureter, or bladder

Filling defect of bladder found on diagnostic imaging

Filling defect of renal pelvis found on diagnostic imaging

Filling defect of ureter found on diagnostic imaging

✓6th **R93.42 Abnormal radiologic findings on diagnostic imaging of kidney**

R93.421 Abnormal radiologic findings on diagnostic imaging of right kidney

R93.422 Abnormal radiologic findings on diagnostic imaging of left kidney

R93.429 Abnormal radiologic findings on diagnostic imaging of unspecified kidney

R93.49 Abnormal radiologic findings on diagnostic imaging of other urinary organs

R93.5 Abnormal findings on diagnostic imaging of other abdominal regions, including retroperitoneum

R93.6 Abnormal findings on diagnostic imaging of limbs

EXCLUDES 2 *abnormal finding in skin and subcutaneous tissue (R93.8-)*

AHA: 2020,1Q,14

R93.7 Abnormal findings on diagnostic imaging of other parts of musculoskeletal system

EXCLUDES 2 *abnormal findings on diagnostic imaging of skull (R93.0)*

✓5th **R93.8 Abnormal findings on diagnostic imaging of other specified body structures**

AHA: 2018,4Q,30

✓6th **R93.81 Abnormal radiologic findings on diagnostic imaging of testis**

R93.811 Abnormal radiologic findings on diagnostic imaging of right testicle ♂

R93.812 Abnormal radiologic findings on diagnostic imaging of left testicle ♂

R93.813 Abnormal radiologic findings on diagnostic imaging of testicles, bilateral ♂

R93.819 Abnormal radiologic findings on diagnostic imaging of unspecified testicle ♂

R93.89 Abnormal findings on diagnostic imaging of other specified body structures

Abnormal finding by radioisotope localization of placenta

Abnormal radiological finding in skin and subcutaneous tissue

Mediastinal shift

R93.9 Diagnostic imaging inconclusive due to excess body fat of patient

R94 Abnormal results of function studies

INCLUDES abnormal results of radionuclide [radioisotope] uptake studies
abnormal results of scintigraphy

R94.0 Abnormal results of function studies of central nervous system

R94.01 Abnormal electroencephalogram [EEG]

R94.02 Abnormal brain scan

R94.09 Abnormal results of other function studies of central nervous system

R94.1 Abnormal results of function studies of peripheral nervous system and special senses

R94.11 Abnormal results of function studies of eye

R94.110 Abnormal electro-oculogram [EOG]

R94.111 Abnormal electroretinogram [ERG]
Abnormal retinal function study

R94.112 Abnormal visually evoked potential [VEP]

R94.113 Abnormal oculomotor study

R94.118 Abnormal results of other function studies of eye

R94.12 Abnormal results of function studies of ear and other special senses
AHA: 2016,3Q,17

R94.120 Abnormal auditory function study

R94.121 Abnormal vestibular function study

R94.128 Abnormal results of other function studies of ear and other special senses

R94.13 Abnormal results of function studies of peripheral nervous system

R94.130 Abnormal response to nerve stimulation, unspecified

R94.131 Abnormal electromyogram [EMG]
EXCLUDES 1 *electromyogram of eye (R94.113)*

R94.138 Abnormal results of other function studies of peripheral nervous system

R94.2 Abnormal results of pulmonary function studies
Reduced ventilatory capacity
Reduced vital capacity

R94.3 Abnormal results of cardiovascular function studies

R94.30 Abnormal result of cardiovascular function study, unspecified

R94.31 Abnormal electrocardiogram [ECG] [EKG]
EXCLUDES 1 *long QT syndrome (I45.81)*

R94.39 Abnormal result of other cardiovascular function study
Abnormal electrophysiological intracardiac studies
Abnormal phonocardiogram
Abnormal vectorcardiogram
AHA: 2023,1Q,25

R94.4 Abnormal results of kidney function studies
Abnormal renal function test

R94.5 Abnormal results of liver function studies

R94.6 Abnormal results of thyroid function studies

R94.7 Abnormal results of other endocrine function studies
EXCLUDES 2 *abnormal glucose (R73.0-)*

R94.8 Abnormal results of function studies of other organs and systems
Abnormal basal metabolic rate [BMR]
Abnormal bladder function test
Abnormal splenic function test

Abnormal tumor markers (R97)

R97 Abnormal tumor markers
Elevated tumor associated antigens [TAA]
Elevated tumor specific antigens [TSA]

R97.0 Elevated carcinoembryonic antigen [CEA]

R97.1 Elevated cancer antigen 125 [CA 125]

R97.2 Elevated prostate specific antigen [PSA]
AHA: 2016,4Q,66

R97.20 Elevated prostate specific antigen [PSA] A ♂

R97.21 Rising PSA following treatment for malignant neoplasm of prostate A ♂
AHA: 2023,2Q,5

R97.8 Other abnormal tumor markers

Ill-defined and unknown cause of mortality (R99)

R99 Ill-defined and unknown cause of mortality
Death (unexplained) NOS
Unspecified cause of mortality

Chapter 19. Injury, Poisoning, and Certain Other Consequences of External Causes (SØØ–T88)

Chapter-specific Guidelines with Coding Examples

The chapter-specific guidelines from the ICD-10-CM Official Guidelines for Coding and Reporting have been provided below. Along with these guidelines are coding examples, contained in the shaded boxes, that have been developed to help illustrate the coding and/or sequencing guidance found in these guidelines.

a. Application of 7th characters in Chapter 19

Most categories in chapter 19 have a 7th character requirement for each applicable code. Most categories in this chapter have three 7th character values (with the exception of fractures): A, initial encounter, D, subsequent encounter and S, sequela. Categories for traumatic fractures have additional 7th character values. While the patient may be seen by a new or different provider over the course of treatment for an injury, assignment of the 7th character is based on whether the patient is undergoing active treatment and not whether the provider is seeing the patient for the first time.

For complication codes, active treatment refers to treatment for the condition described by the code, even though it may be related to an earlier precipitating problem. For example, code T84.5ØXA, Infection and inflammatory reaction due to unspecified internal joint prosthesis, initial encounter, is used when active treatment is provided for the infection, even though the condition relates to the prosthetic device, implant or graft that was placed at a previous encounter.

7th character "A", initial encounter is used for each encounter where the patient is receiving active treatment for the condition.

Patient admitted after fall from a skateboard onto the sidewalk, x-rays identify a nondisplaced fracture to the distal pole of the right scaphoid bone. The patient is placed in a cast.

S62.Ø14A	**Nondisplaced fracture of distal pole of navicular [scaphoid] bone of right wrist, initial encounter for closed fracture**
VØØ.131A	**Fall from skateboard, initial encounter**
Y92.48Ø	**Sidewalk as the place of occurrence of the external cause**
Y93.51	**Activity, roller skating (inline) and skateboarding**
Y99.8	**Other external cause status**

Explanation: This fracture would be coded with a seventh character A for initial encounter because the patient received x-rays to identify the site of the fracture and treatment was rendered; this would be considered active treatment.

7th character "D" subsequent encounter is used for encounters after the patient has completed active treatment of the condition and is receiving routine care for the condition during the healing or recovery phase.

Patient admitted after fall from a skateboard onto the sidewalk resulted in casting of the right arm. X-rays are taken to evaluate how well the nondisplaced fracture to the distal pole of the right scaphoid bone is healing. The physician feels the fracture is healing appropriately; no adjustments to the cast are made.

S62.Ø14D	**Nondisplaced fracture of distal pole of navicular [scaphoid] bone of right wrist, subsequent encounter for fracture with routine healing**
VØØ.131D	**Fall from skateboard, subsequent encounter**

Explanation: This fracture would be coded with a seventh character D for subsequent encounter, whether the same physician who provided the initial cast application or a different physician is now seeing the patient. Although the patient received x-rays, the intent of the x-rays was to assess how the fracture was healing. There was no active treatment rendered and the visit is therefore considered a subsequent encounter.

The aftercare Z codes should not be used for aftercare for conditions such as injuries or poisonings, where 7th characters are provided to identify subsequent care. For example, for aftercare of an injury, assign the acute injury code with the 7th character "D" (subsequent encounter).

7th character "S", sequela, is for use for complications or conditions that arise as a direct result of a condition, such as scar formation after a burn. The scars are sequelae of the burn. When using 7th character "S", it is necessary to use both the injury code that precipitated the sequela and the code for the sequela itself. The "S" is added only to the injury code, not the sequela code. The 7th character "S" identifies the injury responsible for the sequela. The specific type of sequela (e.g. scar) is sequenced first, followed by the injury code.

See Section I.B.10. Sequelae, (Late Effects)

Patient with a history of a nondisplaced fracture to the distal pole of the right scaphoid bone due to a fall from a skateboard is admitted for evaluation of arthritis to the right wrist that has developed as a consequence of the traumatic fracture.

M12.531	**Traumatic arthropathy, right wrist**
S62.Ø14S	**Nondisplaced fracture of distal pole of navicular [scaphoid] bone of right wrist, sequela**
VØØ.131S	**Fall from skateboard, sequela**

Explanation: The code identifying the specific sequela condition (traumatic arthritis) should be coded first followed by the injury that instigated the development of the sequela (fracture). The scaphoid fracture injury code is given a 7th character S for sequela to represent its role as the inciting injury. The fracture has healed and is not being managed or treated on this admit and therefore is not applicable as a first listed or principal diagnosis. However, it is directly related to the development of the arthritis and should be appended as a secondary code to signify this cause and effect relationship.

b. Coding of injuries

When coding injuries, assign separate codes for each injury unless a combination code is provided, in which case the combination code is assigned. Codes from category TØ7, Unspecified multiple injuries should not be assigned in the inpatient setting unless information for a more specific code is not available. Traumatic injury codes (SØØ–T14.9) are not to be used for normal, healing surgical wounds or to identify complications of surgical wounds.

The code for the most serious injury, as determined by the provider and the focus of treatment, is sequenced first.

1) Superficial injuries

Superficial injuries such as abrasions or contusions are not coded when associated with more severe injuries of the same site.

2) Primary injury with damage to nerves/blood vessels

When a primary injury results in minor damage to peripheral nerves or blood vessels, the primary injury is sequenced first with additional code(s) for injuries to nerves and spinal cord (such as category SØ4), and/or injury to blood vessels (such as category S15). When the primary injury is to the blood vessels or nerves, that injury should be sequenced first.

3) Iatrogenic injuries

Injury codes from Chapter 19 should not be assigned for injuries that occur during, or as a result of, a medical intervention. Assign the appropriate complication code(s).

c. Coding of traumatic fractures

The principles of multiple coding of injuries should be followed in coding fractures. Fractures of specified sites are coded individually by site in accordance with both the provisions within categories SØ2, S12, S22, S32, S42, S49, S52, S59, S62, S72, S79, S82, S89, S92 and the level of detail furnished by medical record content.

A fracture not indicated as open or closed should be coded to closed. A fracture not indicated whether displaced or not displaced should be coded to displaced.

More specific guidelines are as follows:

1) Initial vs. subsequent encounter for fractures

Traumatic fractures are coded using the appropriate 7th character for initial encounter (A, B, C) for each encounter where the patient is receiving active treatment for the fracture. The appropriate 7th character for initial encounter should also be assigned for a patient who delayed seeking treatment for the fracture or nonunion.

Fractures are coded using the appropriate 7th character for subsequent care for encounters after the patient has completed active treatment of the fracture and is receiving routine care for the fracture during the healing or recovery phase.

Care for complications of surgical treatment for fracture repairs during the healing or recovery phase should be coded with the appropriate complication codes.

Care of complications of fractures, such as malunion and nonunion, should be reported with the appropriate 7th character for subsequent care with nonunion (K, M, N,) or subsequent care with malunion (P, Q, R).

Malunion/nonunion: The appropriate 7th character for initial encounter should also be assigned for a patient who delayed seeking treatment for the fracture or nonunion.

Female patient fell during a forest hiking excursion almost six months ago and until recently did not feel she needed to seek medical attention for her left ankle pain; x-rays show nonunion of lateral malleolus and surgery has been scheduled

S82.62XA	**Displaced fracture of lateral malleolus of left fibula, initial encounter for closed fracture**
W01.0XXA	**Fall on same level from slipping, tripping and stumbling without subsequent striking against object, initial encounter**
Y92.821	**Forest as place of occurrence of the external cause**
Y93.01	**Activity, walking, marching and hiking**
Y99.8	**Other external cause status**

Explanation: A seventh character of A is used for the lateral malleolus nonunion fracture to signify that the fracture is receiving active treatment. The delayed care for the fracture has resulted in a nonunion, but capturing the nonunion in the seventh character is trumped by the provision of active care.

The open fracture designations in the assignment of the 7th character for fractures of the forearm, femur and lower leg, including ankle are based on the Gustilo open fracture classification. When the Gustilo classification type is not specified for an open fracture, the 7th character for open fracture type I or II should be assigned (B, E, H, M, Q).

A 17-year-old arrives at the trauma center with open, displaced right forearm fracture with extensive soft tissue damage. He fell while being tackled playing football for his high school team. On-call orthopaedic specialist documents segmental type IIIA fracture of radial shaft with no need for plastic consult.

S52.361C	**Displaced segmental fracture of shaft of radius, right arm, initial encounter for open fracture type IIIA, IIIB, or IIIC**
W03.XXXA	**Other fall on same level due to collision with another person, initial encounter**
Y92.321	**Football field as the place of occurrence of the external cause**
Y93.61	**Activity, American tackle football**

Explanation: The seventh character for forearm fractures capture the type of encounter and whether the fracture is open or closed; open fractures are broken down further by the type of fracture based on the Gustilo classification. The Gustilo classification describes the severity of open fracture and soft tissue injury. Type IIIA describes an open fracture with extensive soft tissue injury but adequate soft tissue remaining for wound coverage. A segmental fracture means that the bone is broken in two places, leaving at least one segment unattached to the bone. There is no need to report an additional code for the soft tissue injury as it is captured in the fracture code.

A code from category M80, not a traumatic fracture code, should be used for any patient with known osteoporosis who suffers a fracture, even if the patient had a minor fall or trauma, if that fall or trauma would not usually break a normal, healthy bone.

See Section I.C.13. Osteoporosis.

The aftercare Z codes should not be used for aftercare for traumatic fractures. For aftercare of a traumatic fracture, assign the acute fracture code with the appropriate 7th character.

2) Multiple fractures sequencing

Multiple fractures are sequenced in accordance with the severity of the fracture.

3) Physeal fractures

For physeal fractures, assign only the code identifying the type of physeal fracture. Do not assign a separate code to identify the specific bone that is fractured.

d. Coding of burns and corrosions

The ICD-10-CM makes a distinction between burns and corrosions. The burn codes are for thermal burns, except sunburns, that come from a heat source, such as a fire or hot appliance. The burn codes are also for burns resulting from electricity and radiation. Corrosions are burns due to chemicals. The guidelines are the same for burns and corrosions.

Current burns (T20–T25) are classified by depth, extent and by agent (X code). Burns are classified by depth as first degree (erythema), second degree (blistering), and third degree (full-thickness involvement). Burns of the eye and internal organs (T26–T28) are classified by site, but not by degree.

1) Sequencing of burn and related condition codes

Sequence first the code that reflects the highest degree of burn when more than one burn is present.

a. When the reason for the admission or encounter is for treatment of external multiple burns, sequence first the code that reflects the burn of the highest degree.

b. When a patient has both internal and external burns, the circumstances of admission govern the selection of the principal diagnosis or first-listed diagnosis.

c. When a patient is admitted for burn injuries and other related conditions such as smoke inhalation and/or respiratory failure, the circumstances of admission govern the selection of the principal or first-listed diagnosis.

Patient admitted with minor first-degree burns to multiple sites of her right and left hands as well as severe smoke inhalation. While she was sleeping at home, a candle on her dresser lit the bedroom curtains on fire.

T59.811A	**Toxic effect of smoke, accidental (unintentional), initial encounter**
J70.5	**Respiratory conditions due to smoke inhalation**
T23.191A	**Burn of first degree of multiple sites of right wrist and hand, initial encounter**
T23.192A	**Burn of first degree of multiple sites of left wrist and hand, initial encounter**
X08.8XXA	**Exposure to other specified smoke, fire and flames, initial encounter**
Y92.003	**Bedroom of unspecified non-institutional (private) residence as the place of occurrence of the external cause**
Y93.84	**Activity, sleeping**

Explanation: Based on the documentation, the inhalation injury is more severe than the first-degree burns and is sequenced first. The burns to the hands are appended as secondary diagnoses.

2) Burns of the same anatomic site

Classify burns of the same anatomic site and on the same side but of different degrees to the subcategory identifying the highest degree recorded in the diagnosis (e.g., for second and third degree burns of right thigh, assign only code T24.311-).

3) Non-healing burns

Non-healing burns are coded as acute burns.

Necrosis of burned skin should be coded as a non-healed burn.

4) Infected burn

For any documented infected burn site, use an additional code for the infection.

5) Assign separate codes for each burn site

When coding burns, assign separate codes for each burn site. Category T30, Burn and corrosion, body region unspecified is extremely vague and should rarely be used.

Codes for burns of "multiple sites" should only be assigned when the medical record documentation does not specify the individual sites.

Patient is admitted with third-degree burns of the scalp as well as second-degree burns to the back of the right hand

T20.35XA	**Burn of third degree of scalp [any part], initial encounter**
T23.261A	**Burn of second degree of back of right hand, initial encounter**

Explanation: Two codes may be reported as the hand and face represent distinct burn sites.

6) Burns and corrosions classified according to extent of body surface involved

Assign codes from category T31, Burns classified according to extent of body surface involved, or T32, Corrosions classified according to extent of body surface involved, for acute burns or corrosions when the site of the burn or corrosion is not specified or when there is a need for additional data. It is advisable to use category T31 as additional coding when needed to provide data for evaluating burn mortality, such as that needed by burn units. It is also advisable to use category T31 as an additional code for reporting purposes when there is mention of a third-degree burn involving 20 percent or more of the body surface. Codes from categories T31 and T32 should not be used for sequelae of burns or corrosions.

Categories T31 and T32 are based on the classic "rule of nines" in estimating body surface involved: head and neck are assigned nine percent, each arm nine percent, each leg 18 percent, the anterior trunk 18 percent, posterior trunk 18 percent, and genitalia one percent. Providers may change these percentage assignments where necessary to accommodate infants and children who have proportionately larger heads than adults, and patients who have large buttocks, thighs, or abdomen that involve burns.

Patient seen in burn unit for dressing change after he accidentally spilled acetic acid on himself two days ago. The second-degree burns to his right thigh, covering about 3 percent of his body surface, are healing appropriately.

T54.2X1D **Toxic effect of corrosive acids and acid-like substances, accidental (unintentional), subsequent encounter**

T24.611D **Corrosion of second degree of right thigh, subsequent encounter**

T32.Ø **Corrosions involving less than 1Ø% of body surface**

Explanation: Code T32.Ø provides additional information as to how much of the patient's body was affected by the corrosive substance.

7) Encounters for treatment of sequela of burns

Encounters for the treatment of the late effects of burns or corrosions (i.e., scars or joint contractures) should be coded with a burn or corrosion code with the 7th character "S" for sequela.

8) Sequelae with a late effect code and current burn

When appropriate, both a code for a current burn or corrosion with 7th character "A" or "D" and a burn or corrosion code with 7th character "S" may be assigned on the same record (when both a current burn and sequelae of an old burn exist). Burns and corrosions do not heal at the same rate and a current healing wound may still exist with sequela of a healed burn or corrosion.

See Section I.B.10. Sequela (Late Effects)

Female patient seen in ED for second-degree burn to the left ear; she also has significant scarring on her left elbow from a third-degree burn from childhood

T2Ø.212A **Burn of second degree of left ear [any part, except ear drum], initial encounter**

L9Ø.5 **Scar conditions and fibrosis of skin**

T22.322S **Burn of third degree of left elbow, sequela**

Explanation: The patient is being seen for management of a current second-degree burn, which is reflected in the code by appending the seventh character of A, indicating active treatment or management of this burn. The elbow scarring is a sequela of a previous third-degree burn. The sequela condition precedes the original burn injury, which is appended with a seventh character of S.

9) Use of an external cause code with burns and corrosions

An external cause code should be used with burns and corrosions to identify the source and intent of the burn, as well as the place where it occurred.

e. Adverse effects, poisoning, and toxic effects

Codes in categories T36–T65 are combination codes that include the substance that was taken as well as the intent. No additional external cause code is required for poisonings, toxic effects, adverse effects and underdosing codes.

1) Do not code directly from the Table of Drugs

Do not code directly from the Table of Drugs and Chemicals. Always refer back to the Tabular List.

2) Use as many codes as necessary to describe

Use as many codes as necessary to describe completely all drugs, medicinal or biological substances.

3) If the same code would describe the causative agent

If the same code would describe the causative agent for more than one adverse reaction, poisoning, toxic effect or underdosing, assign the code only once.

4) If two or more drugs, medicinal or biological substances

If two or more drugs, medicinal or biological substances are taken, code each individually unless a combination code is listed in the Table of Drugs and Chemicals.

If multiple unspecified drugs, medicinal or biological substances were taken, assign the appropriate code from subcategory T5Ø.91, Poisoning by, adverse effect of and underdosing of multiple unspecified drugs, medicaments and biological substances.

5) The occurrence of drug toxicity is classified in ICD-10-CM as follows:

(a) Adverse effect

When coding an adverse effect of a drug that has been correctly prescribed and properly administered, assign the appropriate code for the nature of the adverse effect followed by the appropriate code for the adverse effect of the drug (T36–T5Ø). The code for the drug should have a 5th or 6th character "5" (for example T36.ØX5-) Examples of the nature of an adverse effect are tachycardia, delirium, gastrointestinal hemorrhaging, vomiting, hypokalemia, hepatitis, renal failure, or respiratory failure.

Patient admitted for stomach pain and jaundice, indicated by physician as possible side-effects of Inderal, recently started for hypertension. Inderal was discontinued and the patient switched to Atenolol instead.

R1Ø.9 **Unspecified abdominal pain**

R17 **Unspecified jaundice**

T44.7X5A **Adverse effect of beta-adrenoreceptor antagonists, initial encounter**

I1Ø **Essential (primary) hypertension**

Explanation: The side-effects caused by the drug are listed first, followed by the code for the adverse effect of the drug to capture the specific drug that was used.

(b) Poisoning

When coding a poisoning or reaction to the improper use of a medication (e.g., overdose, wrong substance given or taken in error, wrong route of administration), first assign the appropriate code from categories T36–T5Ø. The poisoning codes have an associated intent as their 5th or 6th character (accidental, intentional self-harm, assault and undetermined). If the intent of the poisoning is unknown or unspecified, code the intent as accidental intent. The undetermined intent is only for use if the documentation in the record specifies that the intent cannot be determined. Use additional code(s) for all manifestations of poisonings.

A 55-year-old female status post recent left knee replacement is admitted due to confusion, dizziness, and nausea. Her spouse brought in her prescribed Xanax, Ambien, and Percocet bottles but has no idea how many she took. It is suspected that her symptoms are due to an overdose of these medications.

T42.4X1A **Poisoning by benzodiazepines, accidental (unintentional), initial encounter**

T42.6X1A **Poisoning by other antiepileptic and sedative-hypnotic drugs, accidental (unintentional), initial encounter**

T4Ø.2X1A **Poisoning by other opioids, accidental (unintentional), initial encounter**

R41.Ø **Disorientation, unspecified**

R42 **Dizziness and giddiness**

R11.Ø **Nausea**

Explanation: It was not documented whether the overdose of the drugs was accidental or intentional; therefore the correct reporting of the poisoning codes is accidental intent. The poisoning codes are sequenced first, followed by manifestations of the poisoning.

If there is also a diagnosis of abuse or dependence of the substance, the abuse or dependence is assigned as an additional code.

Examples of poisoning include:

(i) Error was made in drug prescription
Errors made in drug prescription or in the administration of the drug by provider, nurse, patient, or other person.

(ii Overdose of a drug intentionally taken
If an overdose of a drug was intentionally taken or administered and resulted in drug toxicity, it would be coded as a poisoning.

(iii) Nonprescribed drug taken with correctly prescribed and properly administered drug
If a nonprescribed drug or medicinal agent was taken in combination with a correctly prescribed and properly administered drug, any drug toxicity or other reaction resulting from the interaction of the two drugs would be classified as a poisoning.

(iv) Interaction of drug(s) and alcohol
When a reaction results from the interaction of a drug(s) and alcohol, this would be classified as poisoning.
See Section I.C.4. if poisoning is the result of insulin pump malfunctions.
For Sequela (Late Effects) see Section I.B.1Ø.

(c) Underdosing

Underdosing refers to taking less of a medication than is prescribed by a provider or a manufacturer's instruction. Discontinuing the use of a prescribed medication on the patient's own initiative (not directed by the patient's provider) is also classified as an underdosing. For underdosing, assign the code from categories T36–T5Ø (fifth or sixth character "6"). Documentation of a change in the patient's condition is not required in order to assign an underdosing code. Documentation that the patient is taking less of a medication than is prescribed or discontinued the prescribed medication is sufficient for code assignment.

Codes for underdosing should never be assigned as principal or first-listed codes. If a patient has a relapse or exacerbation of the medical condition for which the drug is prescribed because of the reduction in dose, then the medical condition itself should be coded.

Noncompliance (Z91.12-, Z91.13-, Z91.14- and **Z91.A4-**) or complication of care (Y63.6-Y63.9) codes are to be used with an underdosing code to indicate intent, if known.

> Patient admitted for atrial fibrillation with history of chronic atrial fibrillation for which she is prescribed amiodarone. Financial concerns have left the patient unable to pay for her prescriptions and she has been skipping her amiodarone dose every other day to offset the cost.
>
> **I48.2Ø** **Chronic atrial fibrillation, unspecified**
>
> **T46.2X6A** **Underdosing of other antidysrhythmic drugs, initial encounter**
>
> **Z91.12Ø** **Patient's intentional underdosing of medication regimen due to financial hardship**
>
> *Explanation:* By skipping her amiodarone pill every other day, the patient's atrial fibrillation returned. The condition for which the drug was being taken is reported first, followed by an underdosing code to show that the patient was not adhering to her prescription regimen. The Z code helps elaborate on the patient's social and/or economic circumstances that led to the patient taking less then what she was prescribed.

(d) Toxic effects

When a harmful substance is ingested or comes in contact with a person, this is classified as a toxic effect. The toxic effect codes are in categories T51–T65. **When coding a toxic effect, assign the toxic effect code first, followed by codes for all associated manifestations of the toxic effect.**

Toxic effect codes have an associated intent: accidental, intentional self-harm, assault and undetermined.

For Sequela (Late Effects) see Section I.B.1Ø. Sequela

f. Adult and child abuse, neglect and other maltreatment

Sequence first the appropriate code from categories T74.- (Adult and child abuse, neglect and other maltreatment, confirmed) or T76.- (Adult and child abuse, neglect and other maltreatment, suspected) for abuse, neglect and other maltreatment, followed by any accompanying mental health or injury code(s).

If the documentation in the medical record states abuse or neglect it is coded as confirmed (T74.-). It is coded as suspected if it is documented as suspected (T76.-).

For cases of confirmed abuse or neglect an external cause code from the assault section (X92–YØ9) should be added to identify the cause of any physical injuries. A perpetrator code (YØ7) should be added when the perpetrator of the abuse is known. For suspected cases of abuse or neglect, do not report external cause or perpetrator code.

If a suspected case of abuse, neglect or mistreatment is ruled out during an encounter code ZØ4.71, Encounter for examination and observation following alleged physical adult abuse, ruled out, or code ZØ4.72, Encounter for examination and observation following alleged child physical abuse, ruled out, should be used, not a code from T76.

If a suspected case of alleged rape or sexual abuse is ruled out during an encounter code ZØ4.41, Encounter for examination and observation following alleged adult rape or code ZØ4.42, Encounter for examination and observation following alleged child rape, should be used, not a code from T76.

If a suspected case of forced sexual exploitation or forced labor exploitation is ruled out during an encounter, code ZØ4.81, Encounter for examination and observation of victim following forced sexual exploitation, or code ZØ4.82, Encounter for examination and observation of victim following forced labor exploitation, should be used, not a code from T76.

See Section I.C.15. Abuse in a pregnant patient.

g. Complications of care

1) General guidelines for complications of care

(a) Documentation of complications of care

See Section I.B.16. for information on documentation of complications of care.

2) Pain due to medical devices

Pain associated with devices, implants or grafts left in a surgical site (for example painful hip prosthesis) is assigned to the appropriate code(s) found in Chapter 19, Injury, poisoning, and certain other consequences of external causes. Specific codes for pain due to medical devices are found in the T code section of the ICD-10-CM. Use additional code(s) from category G89 to identify acute or chronic pain due to presence of the device, implant or graft (G89.18 or G89.28).

3) Transplant complications

(a) Transplant complications other than kidney

Codes under category T86, Complications of transplanted organs and tissues, are for use for both complications and rejection of transplanted organs. A transplant complication code is only assigned if the complication affects the function of the transplanted organ. Two codes are required to fully describe a transplant complication: the appropriate code from category T86 and a secondary code that identifies the complication.

Pre-existing conditions or conditions that develop after the transplant are not coded as complications unless they affect the function of the transplanted organs.

See I.C.21. for transplant organ removal status

See I.C.2. for malignant neoplasm associated with transplanted organ.

<u>See I.C.1.d.4. for sequencing of sepsis due to infection in transplanted organ</u>

(b) Kidney transplant complications

Patients who have undergone kidney transplant may still have some form of chronic kidney disease (CKD) because the kidney transplant may not fully restore kidney function. Code T86.1- should be assigned for documented complications of a kidney transplant, such as transplant failure or rejection or other transplant complication. Code T86.1- should not be assigned for post kidney transplant patients who have chronic kidney (CKD) unless a transplant complication such as transplant failure or rejection is documented. If the documentation is unclear as to whether the patient has a complication of the transplant, query the provider.

Conditions that affect the function of the transplanted kidney, other than CKD, should be assigned a code from subcategory T86.1, Complications of transplanted organ, Kidney, and a secondary code that identifies the complication.

For patients with CKD following a kidney transplant, but who do not have a complication such as failure or rejection, *see section I.C.14. Chronic kidney disease and kidney transplant status.*

<u>See I.C.1.d.4. for sequencing of sepsis due to infection in transplanted organ</u>

> Patient with chronic kidney disease stage 2; history of successful kidney transplant with no complications identified
>
> **N18.2** **Chronic kidney disease, stage 2 (mild)**
>
> **Z94.Ø** **Kidney transplant status**
>
> *Explanation:* This patient's stage 2 CKD is not indicated as being due to the transplanted kidney but instead is just the residual disease the patient had prior to the transplant.

4) Complication codes that include the external cause

As with certain other T codes, some of the complications of care codes have the external cause included in the code. The code includes the nature of the complication as well as the type of procedure that caused the complication. No external cause code indicating the type of procedure is necessary for these codes.

5) Complications of care codes within the body system chapters

Intraoperative and postprocedural complication codes are found within the body system chapters with codes specific to the organs and structures of that body system. These codes should be sequenced first, followed by a code(s) for the specific complication, if applicable.

Complication codes from the body system chapters should be assigned for intraoperative and postprocedural complications (e.g., the appropriate complication code from chapter 9 would be assigned for a vascular intraoperative or postprocedural complication) unless the complication is specifically indexed to a T code in chapter 19.

> During a spinal fusion procedure, the surgeon inadvertently punctured the dura. The midline durotomy was repaired, and the fusion procedure was completed.
>
> **G97.41** **Accidental puncture or laceration of dura during a procedure**
>
> *Explanation:* The accidental durotomy is not coded to an injury code in chapter 19 but instead is categorized to the nervous system chapter.

Muscle/Tendon Table

ICD-10-CM categorizes certain muscles and tendons in the upper and lower extremities by their action (e.g., extension, flexion), their anatomical location (e.g., posterior, anterior), and/or whether they are intrinsic or extrinsic to a certain anatomical area. The Muscle/Tendon Table is provided at the beginning of chapters 13 and 19 as a resource to help users when code selection depends on one or more of these characteristics. Please note that this table is not all-inclusive, and proper code assignment should be based on the provider's documentation.

Body Region	Muscle	Extensor Tendon	Flexor Tendon	Other Tendon
Shoulder				
	Deltoid	Posterior deltoid	Anterior deltoid	
	Rotator cuff			
	Infraspinatus			Infraspinatus
	Subscapularis			Subscapularis
	Supraspinatus			Supraspinatus
	Teres minor			Teres minor
	Teres major	Teres major		
Upper arm				
	Anterior muscles			
	Biceps brachii — long head		Biceps brachii — long head	
	Biceps brachii — short head		Biceps brachii — short head	
	Brachialis		Brachialis	
	Coracobrachialis		Coracobrachialis	
	Posterior muscles			
	Triceps brachii	Triceps brachii		
Forearm				
	Anterior muscles			
	Flexors			
	Deep			
	Flexor digitorum profundus		Flexor digitorum profundus	
	Flexor pollicis longus		Flexor pollicis longus	
	Intermediate			
	Flexor digitorum superficialis		Flexor digitorum superficialis	
	Superficial			
	Flexor carpi radialis		Flexor carpi radialis	
	Flexor carpi ulnaris		Flexor carpi ulnaris	
	Palmaris longus		Palmaris longus	
	Pronators			
	Pronator quadratus			Pronator quadratus
	Pronator teres			Pronator teres
	Posterior muscles			
	Extensors			
	Deep			
	Abductor pollicis longus			Abductor pollicis longus
	Extensor indicis	Extensor indicis		
	Extensor pollicis brevis	Extensor pollicis brevis		
	Extensor pollicis longus	Extensor pollicis longus		
	Superficial			
	Brachioradialis			Brachioradialis
	Extensor carpi radialis brevis	Extensor carpi radialis brevis		
	Extensor carpi radialis longus	Extensor carpi radialis longus		
	Extensor carpi ulnaris	Extensor carpi ulnaris		
	Extensor digiti minimi	Extensor digiti minimi		
	Extensor digitorum	Extensor digitorum		
	Anconeus	Anconeus		
	Supinator			Supinator

Body Region	Muscle	Extensor Tendon	Flexor Tendon	Other Tendon
Hand				
Extrinsic — attach to a site in the forearm as well as a site in the hand with action related to hand movement at the wrist				
	Extensor carpi radialis brevis	Extensor carpi radialis brevis		
	Extensor carpi radialis longus	Extensor carpi radialis longus		
	Extensor carpi ulnaris	Extensor carpi ulnaris		
	Flexor carpi radialis		Flexor carpi radialis	
	Flexor carpi ulnaris		Flexor carpi ulnaris	
	Flexor digitorum superficialis		Flexor digitorum superficialis	
	Palmaris longus		Palmaris longus	
Extrinsic — attach to a site in the forearm as well as a site in the hand with action in the hand related to finger movement				
	Adductor pollicis longus			Adductor pollicis longus
	Extensor digiti minimi	Extensor digiti minimi		
	Extensor digitorum	Extensor digitorum		
	Extensor indicis	Extensor indicis		
	Flexor digitorum profundus		Flexor digitorum profundus	
	Flexor digitorum superficialis		Flexor digitorum superficialis	
Extrinsic — attach to a site in the forearm as well as a site in the hand with action in the hand related to thumb movement				
	Extensor pollicis brevis	Extensor pollicis brevis		
	Extensor pollicis longus	Extensor pollicis longus		
	Flexor pollicis longus		Flexor pollicis longus	
Intrinsic — found within the hand only				
	Adductor pollicis			Adductor pollicis
	Dorsal interossei	Dorsal interossei	Dorsal interossei	
	Lumbricals	Lumbricals	Lumbricals	
	Palmaris brevis			Palmaris brevis
	Palmar interossei	Palmar interossei	Palmar interossei	
	Hypothenar muscles			
	Abductor digiti minimi			Abductor digiti minimi
	Flexor digiti minimi brevis		Flexor digiti minimi brevis	
	Opponens digiti minimi		Opponens digiti minimi	
	Thenar muscles			
	Abductor pollicis brevis			Abductor pollicis brevis
	Flexor pollicis brevis		Flexor pollicis brevis	
	Opponens pollicis		Opponens pollicis	
Thigh				
	Anterior muscles			
	Iliopsoas		Iliopsoas	
	Pectineus		Pectineus	
	Quadriceps	Quadriceps		
	Rectus femoris	Rectus femoris — Extends knee	Rectus femoris — Flexes hip	
	Vastus intermedius	Vastus intermedius		
	Vastus lateralis	Vastus lateralis		
	Vastus medialis	Vastus medialis		
	Sartorius		Sartorius	
	Medial muscles			
	Adductor brevis			Adductor brevis
	Adductor longus			Adductor longus
	Adductor magnus			Adductor magnus
	Gracilis			Gracilis
	Obturator externus			Obturator externus
	Posterior muscles			
	Hamstring	Hamstring — Extends hip	Hamstring — Flexes knee	
	Biceps femoris	Biceps femoris	Biceps femoris	
	Semimembranosus	Semimembranosus	Semimembranosus	
	Semitendinosus	Semitendinosus	Semitendinosus	

Body Region	Muscle	Extensor Tendon	Flexor Tendon	Other Tendon
Lower leg				
	Anterior muscles			
	Extensor digitorum longus	Extensor digitorum longus		
	Extensor hallucis longus	Extensor hallucis longus		
	Fibularis (peroneus) tertius	Fibularis (peroneus) tertius		
	Tibialis anterior	Tibialis anterior		Tibialis anterior
	Lateral muscles			
	Fibularis (peroneus) brevis		Fibularis (peroneus) brevis	
	Fibularis (peroneus) longus		Fibularis (peroneus) longus	
	Posterior muscles			
	Deep			
	Flexor digitorum longus		Flexor digitorum longus	
	Flexor hallucis longus		Flexor hallucis longus	
	Popliteus		Popliteus	
	Tibialis posterior		Tibialis posterior	
	Superficial			
	Gastrocnemius		Gastrocnemius	
	Plantaris		Plantaris	
	Soleus		Soleus	
				Calcaneal (Achilles)
Ankle/Foot				
Extrinsic — attach to a site in the lower leg as well as a site in the foot with action related to foot movement at the ankle				
	Plantaris		Plantaris	
	Soleus		Soleus	
	Tibialis anterior	Tibialis anterior		
	Tibialis posterior		Tibialis posterior	
Extrinsic — attach to a site in the lower leg as well as a site in the foot with action in the foot related to toe movement				
	Extensor digitorum longus	Extensor digitorum longus		
	Extensor hallucis longus	Extensor hallucis longus		
	Flexor digitorum longus		Flexor digitorum longus	
	Flexor hallucis longus		Flexor hallucis longus	
Intrinsic — found within the ankle/foot only				
	Dorsal muscles			
	Extensor digitorum brevis	Extensor digitorum brevis		
	Extensor hallucis brevis	Extensor hallucis brevis		
	Plantar muscles			
	Abductor digiti minimi		Abductor digiti minimi	
	Abductor hallucis		Abductor hallucis	
	Dorsal interossei	Dorsal interossei	Dorsal interossei	
	Flexor digiti minimi brevis		Flexor digiti minimi brevis	
	Flexor digitorum brevis		Flexor digitorum brevis	
	Flexor hallucis brevis		Flexor hallucis brevis	
	Lumbricals	Lumbricals	Lumbricals	
	Quadratus plantae		Quadratus plantae	
	Plantar interossei	Plantar interossei	Plantar interossei	

Chapter 19. Injury, Poisoning and Certain Other Consequences of External Causes (S00-T88)

NOTE Use secondary code(s) from Chapter 20, External causes of morbidity, to indicate cause of injury. Codes within the T section that include the external cause do not require an additional external cause code.

Use additional code to identify any retained foreign body, if applicable (Z18.-)

EXCLUDES 1 *birth trauma (P10-P15)*
obstetric trauma (O70-O71)

NOTE The chapter uses the S-section for coding different types of injuries related to single body regions and the T-section to cover injuries to unspecified body regions as well as poisoning and certain other consequences of external causes.

AHA: 2016,2Q,3-7; 2015,4Q,35-38; 2015,3Q,37-39,40; 2015,2Q,6; 2015,1Q,3-21

TIP: The specific site of an injury can be determined from the radiology report when authenticated by a radiologist and available at the time of code assignment.

This chapter contains the following blocks:

S00-S09 Injuries to the head
S10-S19 Injuries to the neck
S20-S29 Injuries to the thorax
S30-S39 Injuries to the abdomen, lower back, lumbar spine, pelvis and external genitals
S40-S49 Injuries to the shoulder and upper arm
S50-S59 Injuries to the elbow and forearm
S60-S69 Injuries to the wrist, hand and fingers
S70-S79 Injuries to the hip and thigh
S80-S89 Injuries to the knee and lower leg
S90-S99 Injuries to the ankle and foot
T07 Injuries involving multiple body regions
T14 Injury of unspecified body region
T15-T19 Effects of foreign body entering through natural orifice
T20-T25 Burns and corrosions of external body surface, specified by site
T26-T28 Burns and corrosions confined to eye and internal organs
T30-T32 Burns and corrosions of multiple and unspecified body regions
T33-T34 Frostbite
T36-T50 Poisoning by, adverse effect of and underdosing of drugs, medicaments and biological substances
T51-T65 Toxic effects of substances chiefly nonmedicinal as to source
T66-T78 Other and unspecified effects of external causes
T79 Certain early complications of trauma
T80-T88 Complications of surgical and medical care, not elsewhere classified

Injuries to the head (S00-S09)

INCLUDES injuries of ear
injuries of eye
injuries of face [any part]
injuries of gum
injuries of jaw
injuries of oral cavity
injuries of palate
injuries of periocular area
injuries of scalp
injuries of temporomandibular joint area
injuries of tongue
injuries of tooth

Code also for any associated infection

EXCLUDES 2 *burns and corrosions (T20-T32)*
effects of foreign body in ear (T16)
effects of foreign body in larynx (T17.3)
effects of foreign body in mouth NOS (T18.0)
effects of foreign body in nose (T17.0-T17.1)
effects of foreign body in pharynx (T17.2)
effects of foreign body on external eye (T15.-)
frostbite (T33-T34)
insect bite or sting, venomous (T63.4)

√4th **S00 Superficial injury of head**

EXCLUDES 1 *diffuse cerebral contusion (S06.2-)*
focal cerebral contusion (S06.3-)
injury of eye and orbit (S05.-)
open wound of head (S01.-)

The appropriate 7th character is to be added to each code from category S00.
A initial encounter
D subsequent encounter
S sequela

√5th **S00.0 Superficial injury of scalp**

√x7th **S00.00 Unspecified superficial injury of scalp**
√x7th **S00.01 Abrasion of scalp**
√x7th **S00.02 Blister (nonthermal) of scalp**
√x7th **S00.03 Contusion of scalp**
Bruise of scalp
Hematoma of scalp
√x7th **S00.04 External constriction of part of scalp**
√x7th **S00.05 Superficial foreign body of scalp**
Splinter in the scalp
√x7th **S00.06 Insect bite (nonvenomous) of scalp**
√x7th **S00.07 Other superficial bite of scalp**
EXCLUDES 1 *open bite of scalp (S01.05)*

√5th **S00.1 Contusion of eyelid and periocular area**
Black eye
EXCLUDES 2 *contusion of eyeball and orbital tissues (S05.1-)*

√x7th **S00.10 Contusion of unspecified eyelid and periocular area**
√x7th **S00.11 Contusion of right eyelid and periocular area**
√x7th **S00.12 Contusion of left eyelid and periocular area**

√5th **S00.2 Other and unspecified superficial injuries of eyelid and periocular area**
EXCLUDES 2 *superficial injury of conjunctiva and cornea (S05.0-)*

√6th **S00.20 Unspecified superficial injury of eyelid and periocular area**
√7th **S00.201 Unspecified superficial injury of right eyelid and periocular area**
√7th **S00.202 Unspecified superficial injury of left eyelid and periocular area**
√7th **S00.209 Unspecified superficial injury of unspecified eyelid and periocular area**

√6th **S00.21 Abrasion of eyelid and periocular area**
√7th **S00.211 Abrasion of right eyelid and periocular area**
√7th **S00.212 Abrasion of left eyelid and periocular area**
√7th **S00.219 Abrasion of unspecified eyelid and periocular area**

√6th **S00.22 Blister (nonthermal) of eyelid and periocular area**
√7th **S00.221 Blister (nonthermal) of right eyelid and periocular area**
√7th **S00.222 Blister (nonthermal) of left eyelid and periocular area**
√7th **S00.229 Blister (nonthermal) of unspecified eyelid and periocular area**

√6th **S00.24 External constriction of eyelid and periocular area**
√7th **S00.241 External constriction of right eyelid and periocular area**
√7th **S00.242 External constriction of left eyelid and periocular area**
√7th **S00.249 External constriction of unspecified eyelid and periocular area**

√6th **S00.25 Superficial foreign body of eyelid and periocular area**
Splinter of eyelid and periocular area
EXCLUDES 2 *retained foreign body in eyelid (H02.81-)*
√7th **S00.251 Superficial foreign body of right eyelid and periocular area**
√7th **S00.252 Superficial foreign body of left eyelid and periocular area**
√7th **S00.259 Superficial foreign body of unspecified eyelid and periocular area**

√6th **S00.26 Insect bite (nonvenomous) of eyelid and periocular area**
√7th **S00.261 Insect bite (nonvenomous) of right eyelid and periocular area**
√7th **S00.262 Insect bite (nonvenomous) of left eyelid and periocular area**
√7th **S00.269 Insect bite (nonvenomous) of unspecified eyelid and periocular area**

√6th **S00.27 Other superficial bite of eyelid and periocular area**
EXCLUDES 1 *open bite of eyelid and periocular area (S01.15)*
√7th **S00.271 Other superficial bite of right eyelid and periocular area**
√7th **S00.272 Other superficial bite of left eyelid and periocular area**
√7th **S00.279 Other superficial bite of unspecified eyelid and periocular area**

√5th **S00.3 Superficial injury of nose**

√x7th **S00.30 Unspecified superficial injury of nose**
√x7th **S00.31 Abrasion of nose**
√x7th **S00.32 Blister (nonthermal) of nose**
√x7th **S00.33 Contusion of nose**
Bruise of nose
Hematoma of nose
√x7th **S00.34 External constriction of nose**

√x7th S00.35 Superficial foreign body of nose
Splinter in the nose
√x7th S00.36 Insect bite (nonvenomous) of nose
√x7th S00.37 Other superficial bite of nose
EXCLUDES 1 *open bite of nose (S01.25)*
√5th S00.4 Superficial injury of ear
√6th S00.40 Unspecified superficial injury of ear
√7th S00.401 Unspecified superficial injury of right ear
√7th S00.402 Unspecified superficial injury of left ear
√7th S00.409 Unspecified superficial injury of unspecified ear
√6th S00.41 Abrasion of ear
√7th S00.411 Abrasion of right ear
√7th S00.412 Abrasion of left ear
√7th S00.419 Abrasion of unspecified ear
√6th S00.42 Blister (nonthermal) of ear
√7th S00.421 Blister (nonthermal) of right ear
√7th S00.422 Blister (nonthermal) of left ear
√7th S00.429 Blister (nonthermal) of unspecified ear
√6th S00.43 Contusion of ear
Bruise of ear
Hematoma of ear
√7th S00.431 Contusion of right ear
√7th S00.432 Contusion of left ear
√7th S00.439 Contusion of unspecified ear
√6th S00.44 External constriction of ear
√7th S00.441 External constriction of right ear
√7th S00.442 External constriction of left ear
√7th S00.449 External constriction of unspecified ear
√6th S00.45 Superficial foreign body of ear
Splinter in the ear
√7th S00.451 Superficial foreign body of right ear
√7th S00.452 Superficial foreign body of left ear
√7th S00.459 Superficial foreign body of unspecified ear
√6th S00.46 Insect bite (nonvenomous) of ear
√7th S00.461 Insect bite (nonvenomous) of right ear
√7th S00.462 Insect bite (nonvenomous) of left ear
√7th S00.469 Insect bite (nonvenomous) of unspecified ear
√6th S00.47 Other superficial bite of ear
EXCLUDES 1 *open bite of ear (S01.35)*
√7th S00.471 Other superficial bite of right ear
√7th S00.472 Other superficial bite of left ear
√7th S00.479 Other superficial bite of unspecified ear
√5th S00.5 Superficial injury of lip and oral cavity
√6th S00.50 Unspecified superficial injury of lip and oral cavity
√7th S00.501 Unspecified superficial injury of lip
√7th S00.502 Unspecified superficial injury of oral cavity
√6th S00.51 Abrasion of lip and oral cavity
√7th S00.511 Abrasion of lip
√7th S00.512 Abrasion of oral cavity
√6th S00.52 Blister (nonthermal) of lip and oral cavity
√7th S00.521 Blister (nonthermal) of lip
√7th S00.522 Blister (nonthermal) of oral cavity
√6th S00.53 Contusion of lip and oral cavity
√7th S00.531 Contusion of lip
Bruise of lip
Hematoma of lip
√7th S00.532 Contusion of oral cavity
Bruise of oral cavity
Hematoma of oral cavity
√6th S00.54 External constriction of lip and oral cavity
√7th S00.541 External constriction of lip
√7th S00.542 External constriction of oral cavity
√6th S00.55 Superficial foreign body of lip and oral cavity
√7th S00.551 Superficial foreign body of lip
Splinter of lip and oral cavity
√7th S00.552 Superficial foreign body of oral cavity
Splinter of lip and oral cavity
√6th S00.56 Insect bite (nonvenomous) of lip and oral cavity
√7th S00.561 Insect bite (nonvenomous) of lip
√7th S00.562 Insect bite (nonvenomous) of oral cavity
√6th S00.57 Other superficial bite of lip and oral cavity
√7th S00.571 Other superficial bite of lip
EXCLUDES 1 *open bite of lip (S01.551)*
√7th S00.572 Other superficial bite of oral cavity
EXCLUDES 1 *open bite of oral cavity (S01.552)*
√5th S00.8 Superficial injury of other parts of head
Superficial injuries of face [any part]
√x7th S00.80 Unspecified superficial injury of other part of head
√x7th S00.81 Abrasion of other part of head
√x7th S00.82 Blister (nonthermal) of other part of head
√x7th S00.83 Contusion of other part of head
Bruise of other part of head
Hematoma of other part of head
√x7th S00.84 External constriction of other part of head
√x7th S00.85 Superficial foreign body of other part of head
Splinter in other part of head
√x7th S00.86 Insect bite (nonvenomous) of other part of head
√x7th S00.87 Other superficial bite of other part of head
EXCLUDES 1 *open bite of other part of head (S01.85)*
√5th S00.9 Superficial injury of unspecified part of head
√x7th S00.90 Unspecified superficial injury of unspecified part of head
√x7th S00.91 Abrasion of unspecified part of head
√x7th S00.92 Blister (nonthermal) of unspecified part of head
√x7th S00.93 Contusion of unspecified part of head
Bruise of head
Hematoma of head
√x7th S00.94 External constriction of unspecified part of head
√x7th S00.95 Superficial foreign body of unspecified part of head
Splinter of head
√x7th S00.96 Insect bite (nonvenomous) of unspecified part of head
√x7th S00.97 Other superficial bite of unspecified part of head
EXCLUDES 1 *open bite of head (S01.95)*

√4th **S01 Open wound of head**
Code also any associated:
injury of cranial nerve (S04.-)
injury of muscle and tendon of head (S09.1-)
intracranial injury (S06.-)
wound infection
EXCLUDES 1 *open skull fracture (S02.- with 7th character B)*
EXCLUDES 2 *injury of eye and orbit (S05.-)*
traumatic amputation of part of head (S08.-)

The appropriate 7th character is to be added to each code from category S01.
A initial encounter
D subsequent encounter
S sequela

√5th S01.0 Open wound of scalp
EXCLUDES 1 *avulsion of scalp (S08.0-)*
√x7th S01.00 Unspecified open wound of scalp
√x7th S01.01 Laceration without foreign body of scalp
√x7th S01.02 Laceration with foreign body of scalp
√x7th S01.03 Puncture wound without foreign body of scalp
√x7th S01.04 Puncture wound with foreign body of scalp
√x7th S01.05 Open bite of scalp
Bite of scalp NOS
EXCLUDES 1 *superficial bite of scalp (S00.06, S00.07-)*

√5th **S01.1 Open wound of eyelid and periocular area**
Open wound of eyelid and periocular area with or without involvement of lacrimal passages

√6th **S01.10 Unspecified open wound of eyelid and periocular area**
√7th **S01.101 Unspecified open wound of right eyelid and periocular area** CC
√7th **S01.102 Unspecified open wound of left eyelid and periocular area** CC
√7th **S01.109 Unspecified open wound of unspecified eyelid and periocular area** CC UNS

√6th **S01.11 Laceration without foreign body of eyelid and periocular area**
√7th **S01.111 Laceration without foreign body of right eyelid and periocular area**
√7th **S01.112 Laceration without foreign body of left eyelid and periocular area**
√7th **S01.119 Laceration without foreign body of unspecified eyelid and periocular area**

√6th **S01.12 Laceration with foreign body of eyelid and periocular area**
√7th **S01.121 Laceration with foreign body of right eyelid and periocular area**
√7th **S01.122 Laceration with foreign body of left eyelid and periocular area**
√7th **S01.129 Laceration with foreign body of unspecified eyelid and periocular area**

√6th **S01.13 Puncture wound without foreign body of eyelid and periocular area**
√7th **S01.131 Puncture wound without foreign body of right eyelid and periocular area**
√7th **S01.132 Puncture wound without foreign body of left eyelid and periocular area**
√7th **S01.139 Puncture wound without foreign body of unspecified eyelid and periocular area**

√6th **S01.14 Puncture wound with foreign body of eyelid and periocular area**
√7th **S01.141 Puncture wound with foreign body of right eyelid and periocular area**
√7th **S01.142 Puncture wound with foreign body of left eyelid and periocular area**
√7th **S01.149 Puncture wound with foreign body of unspecified eyelid and periocular area**

√6th **S01.15 Open bite of eyelid and periocular area**
Bite of eyelid and periocular area NOS
EXCLUDES 1 *superficial bite of eyelid and periocular area (S00.26, S00.27)*
√7th **S01.151 Open bite of right eyelid and periocular area**
√7th **S01.152 Open bite of left eyelid and periocular area**
√7th **S01.159 Open bite of unspecified eyelid and periocular area**

√5th **S01.2 Open wound of nose**
√x7th **S01.20 Unspecified open wound of nose**
√x7th **S01.21 Laceration without foreign body of nose**
√x7th **S01.22 Laceration with foreign body of nose**
√x7th **S01.23 Puncture wound without foreign body of nose**
√x7th **S01.24 Puncture wound with foreign body of nose**
√x7th **S01.25 Open bite of nose**
Bite of nose NOS
EXCLUDES 1 *superficial bite of nose (S00.36, S00.37)*

√5th **S01.3 Open wound of ear**
√6th **S01.30 Unspecified open wound of ear**
√7th **S01.301 Unspecified open wound of right ear**
√7th **S01.302 Unspecified open wound of left ear**
√7th **S01.309 Unspecified open wound of unspecified ear**

√6th **S01.31 Laceration without foreign body of ear**
√7th **S01.311 Laceration without foreign body of right ear**
√7th **S01.312 Laceration without foreign body of left ear**
√7th **S01.319 Laceration without foreign body of unspecified ear**

√6th **S01.32 Laceration with foreign body of ear**
√7th **S01.321 Laceration with foreign body of right ear**
√7th **S01.322 Laceration with foreign body of left ear**
√7th **S01.329 Laceration with foreign body of unspecified ear**

√6th **S01.33 Puncture wound without foreign body of ear**
√7th **S01.331 Puncture wound without foreign body of right ear**
√7th **S01.332 Puncture wound without foreign body of left ear**
√7th **S01.339 Puncture wound without foreign body of unspecified ear**

√6th **S01.34 Puncture wound with foreign body of ear**
√7th **S01.341 Puncture wound with foreign body of right ear**
√7th **S01.342 Puncture wound with foreign body of left ear**
√7th **S01.349 Puncture wound with foreign body of unspecified ear**

√6th **S01.35 Open bite of ear**
Bite of ear NOS
EXCLUDES 1 *superficial bite of ear (S00.46, S00.47)*
√7th **S01.351 Open bite of right ear**
√7th **S01.352 Open bite of left ear**
√7th **S01.359 Open bite of unspecified ear**

√5th **S01.4 Open wound of cheek and temporomandibular area**
√6th **S01.40 Unspecified open wound of cheek and temporomandibular area**
√7th **S01.401 Unspecified open wound of right cheek and temporomandibular area**
√7th **S01.402 Unspecified open wound of left cheek and temporomandibular area**
√7th **S01.409 Unspecified open wound of unspecified cheek and temporomandibular area**

√6th **S01.41 Laceration without foreign body of cheek and temporomandibular area**
√7th **S01.411 Laceration without foreign body of right cheek and temporomandibular area**
√7th **S01.412 Laceration without foreign body of left cheek and temporomandibular area**
√7th **S01.419 Laceration without foreign body of unspecified cheek and temporomandibular area**

√6th **S01.42 Laceration with foreign body of cheek and temporomandibular area**
√7th **S01.421 Laceration with foreign body of right cheek and temporomandibular area**
√7th **S01.422 Laceration with foreign body of left cheek and temporomandibular area**
√7th **S01.429 Laceration with foreign body of unspecified cheek and temporomandibular area**

√6th **S01.43 Puncture wound without foreign body of cheek and temporomandibular area**
√7th **S01.431 Puncture wound without foreign body of right cheek and temporomandibular area**
√7th **S01.432 Puncture wound without foreign body of left cheek and temporomandibular area**
√7th **S01.439 Puncture wound without foreign body of unspecified cheek and temporomandibular area**

√6th **S01.44 Puncture wound with foreign body of cheek and temporomandibular area**
√7th **S01.441 Puncture wound with foreign body of right cheek and temporomandibular area**
√7th **S01.442 Puncture wound with foreign body of left cheek and temporomandibular area**
√7th **S01.449 Puncture wound with foreign body of unspecified cheek and temporomandibular area**

√6th **S01.45 Open bite of cheek and temporomandibular area**
Bite of cheek and temporomandibular area NOS
EXCLUDES 2 *superficial bite of cheek and temporomandibular area (S00.86, S00.87)*
√7th **S01.451 Open bite of right cheek and temporomandibular area**
√7th **S01.452 Open bite of left cheek and temporomandibular area**
√7th **S01.459 Open bite of unspecified cheek and temporomandibular area**

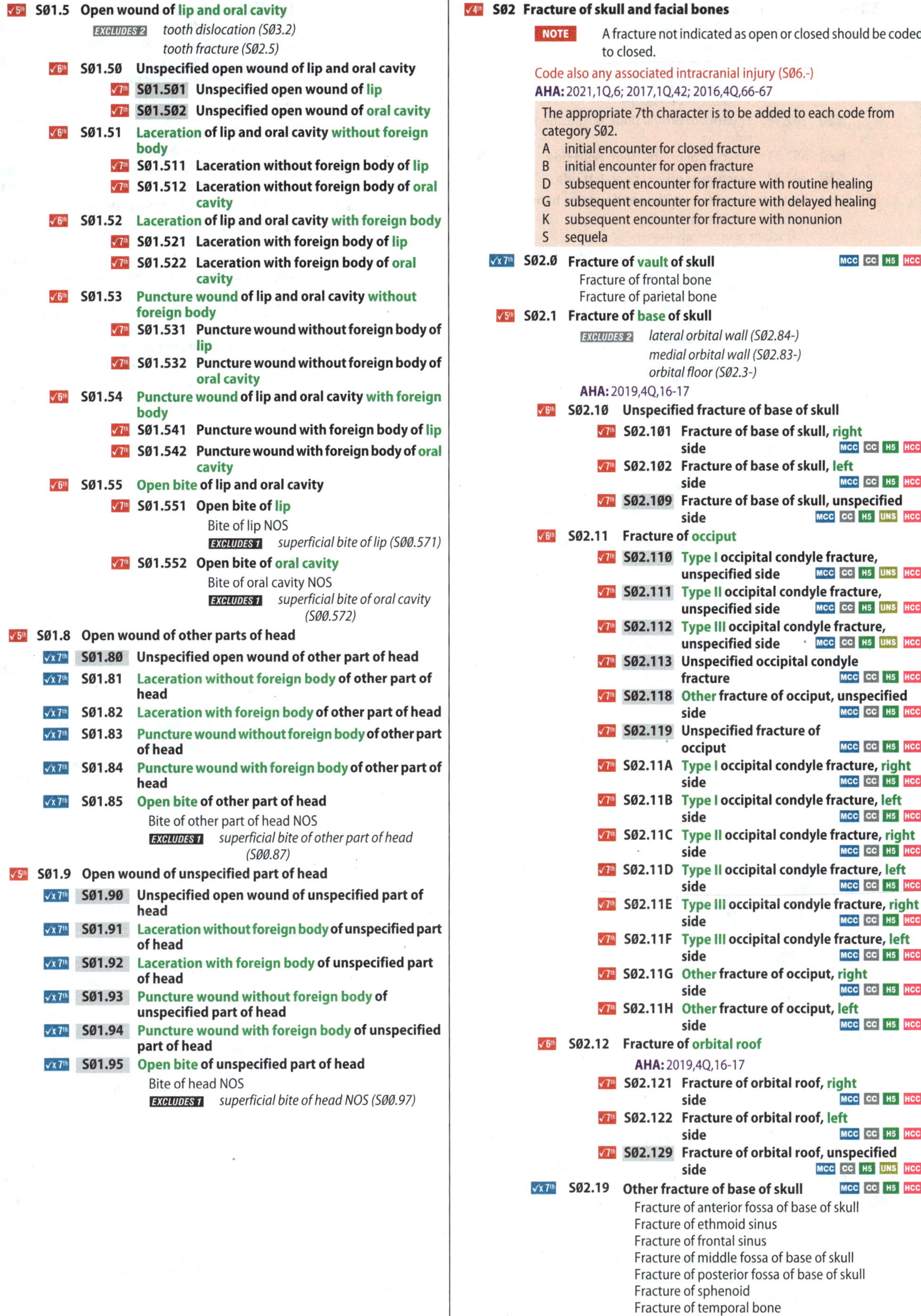

SØ1.5 Open wound of lip and oral cavity
EXCLUDES 2 *tooth dislocation (SØ3.2)*
tooth fracture (SØ2.5)

SØ1.5Ø Unspecified open wound of lip and oral cavity
SØ1.5Ø1 Unspecified open wound of lip
SØ1.5Ø2 Unspecified open wound of oral cavity

SØ1.51 Laceration of lip and oral cavity without foreign body
SØ1.511 Laceration without foreign body of lip
SØ1.512 Laceration without foreign body of oral cavity

SØ1.52 Laceration of lip and oral cavity with foreign body
SØ1.521 Laceration with foreign body of lip
SØ1.522 Laceration with foreign body of oral cavity

SØ1.53 Puncture wound of lip and oral cavity without foreign body
SØ1.531 Puncture wound without foreign body of lip
SØ1.532 Puncture wound without foreign body of oral cavity

SØ1.54 Puncture wound of lip and oral cavity with foreign body
SØ1.541 Puncture wound with foreign body of lip
SØ1.542 Puncture wound with foreign body of oral cavity

SØ1.55 Open bite of lip and oral cavity
SØ1.551 Open bite of lip
Bite of lip NOS
EXCLUDES 1 *superficial bite of lip (SØØ.571)*
SØ1.552 Open bite of oral cavity
Bite of oral cavity NOS
EXCLUDES 1 *superficial bite of oral cavity (SØØ.572)*

SØ1.8 Open wound of other parts of head
SØ1.8Ø Unspecified open wound of other part of head
SØ1.81 Laceration without foreign body of other part of head
SØ1.82 Laceration with foreign body of other part of head
SØ1.83 Puncture wound without foreign body of other part of head
SØ1.84 Puncture wound with foreign body of other part of head
SØ1.85 Open bite of other part of head
Bite of other part of head NOS
EXCLUDES 1 *superficial bite of other part of head (SØØ.87)*

SØ1.9 Open wound of unspecified part of head
SØ1.9Ø Unspecified open wound of unspecified part of head
SØ1.91 Laceration without foreign body of unspecified part of head
SØ1.92 Laceration with foreign body of unspecified part of head
SØ1.93 Puncture wound without foreign body of unspecified part of head
SØ1.94 Puncture wound with foreign body of unspecified part of head
SØ1.95 Open bite of unspecified part of head
Bite of head NOS
EXCLUDES 1 *superficial bite of head NOS (SØØ.97)*

SØ2 Fracture of skull and facial bones
NOTE A fracture not indicated as open or closed should be coded to closed.
Code also any associated intracranial injury (SØ6.-)
AHA: 2021,1Q,6; 2017,1Q,42; 2016,4Q,66-67

The appropriate 7th character is to be added to each code from category SØ2.
A initial encounter for closed fracture
B initial encounter for open fracture
D subsequent encounter for fracture with routine healing
G subsequent encounter for fracture with delayed healing
K subsequent encounter for fracture with nonunion
S sequela

SØ2.Ø Fracture of vault of skull MCC CC H5 HCC
Fracture of frontal bone
Fracture of parietal bone

SØ2.1 Fracture of base of skull
EXCLUDES 2 *lateral orbital wall (SØ2.84-)*
medial orbital wall (SØ2.83-)
orbital floor (SØ2.3-)
AHA: 2019,4Q,16-17

SØ2.1Ø Unspecified fracture of base of skull
SØ2.1Ø1 Fracture of base of skull, right side MCC CC H5 HCC
SØ2.1Ø2 Fracture of base of skull, left side MCC CC H5 HCC
SØ2.1Ø9 Fracture of base of skull, unspecified side MCC CC H5 UNS HCC

SØ2.11 Fracture of occiput
SØ2.11Ø Type I occipital condyle fracture, unspecified side MCC CC H5 UNS HCC
SØ2.111 Type II occipital condyle fracture, unspecified side MCC CC H5 UNS HCC
SØ2.112 Type III occipital condyle fracture, unspecified side MCC CC H5 UNS HCC
SØ2.113 Unspecified occipital condyle fracture MCC CC H5 HCC
SØ2.118 Other fracture of occiput, unspecified side MCC CC H5 HCC
SØ2.119 Unspecified fracture of occiput MCC CC H5 HCC
SØ2.11A Type I occipital condyle fracture, right side MCC CC H5 HCC
SØ2.11B Type I occipital condyle fracture, left side MCC CC H5 HCC
SØ2.11C Type II occipital condyle fracture, right side MCC CC H5 HCC
SØ2.11D Type II occipital condyle fracture, left side MCC CC H5 HCC
SØ2.11E Type III occipital condyle fracture, right side MCC CC H5 HCC
SØ2.11F Type III occipital condyle fracture, left side MCC CC H5 HCC
SØ2.11G Other fracture of occiput, right side MCC CC H5 HCC
SØ2.11H Other fracture of occiput, left side MCC CC H5 HCC

SØ2.12 Fracture of orbital roof
AHA: 2019,4Q,16-17
SØ2.121 Fracture of orbital roof, right side MCC CC H5 HCC
SØ2.122 Fracture of orbital roof, left side MCC CC H5 HCC
SØ2.129 Fracture of orbital roof, unspecified side MCC CC H5 UNS HCC

SØ2.19 Other fracture of base of skull MCC CC H5 HCC
Fracture of anterior fossa of base of skull
Fracture of ethmoid sinus
Fracture of frontal sinus
Fracture of middle fossa of base of skull
Fracture of posterior fossa of base of skull
Fracture of sphenoid
Fracture of temporal bone

SØ2.2 Fracture of nasal bones CC H5

√5th **SØ2.3 Fracture of orbital floor**

Fracture of inferior orbital wall

EXCLUDES 1 *orbit NOS (SØ2.85)*

EXCLUDES 2 *lateral orbital wall (SØ2.84-)*
medial orbital wall (SØ2.83-)
orbital roof (SØ2.1-)

√x7th **SØ2.3Ø Fracture of orbital floor, unspecified side** CC H5 UNS HCC

√x7th **SØ2.31 Fracture of orbital floor, right side** CC H5 HCC

√x7th **SØ2.32 Fracture of orbital floor, left side** CC H5 HCC

√5th **SØ2.4 Fracture of malar, maxillary and zygoma bones**

Fracture of superior maxilla
Fracture of upper jaw (bone)
Fracture of zygomatic process of temporal bone

√6th **SØ2.4Ø Fracture of malar, maxillary and zygoma bones, unspecified**

√7th **SØ2.4ØØ Malar fracture, unspecified side** CC H5 UNS HCC

√7th **SØ2.4Ø1 Maxillary fracture, unspecified side** CC H5 UNS HCC

√7th **SØ2.4Ø2 Zygomatic fracture, unspecified side** CC H5 UNS HCC

√7th **SØ2.4ØA Malar fracture, right side** CC H5 HCC

√7th **SØ2.4ØB Malar fracture, left side** CC H5 HCC

√7th **SØ2.4ØC Maxillary fracture, right side** CC H5 HCC

√7th **SØ2.4ØD Maxillary fracture, left side** CC H5 HCC

√7th **SØ2.4ØE Zygomatic fracture, right side** CC H5 HCC

√7th **SØ2.4ØF Zygomatic fracture, left side** CC H5 HCC

√6th **SØ2.41 LeFort fracture**

DEF: Named for Rene Le Fort, these fractures describe different combinations of multiple fractures that occur from significant force to the midface. A common denominator in all three types of LeFort fractures is fracture of the pterygoid processes, which are two bony plates resembling wings that extend downward from the sphenoid bone.

LeFort Fracture Types

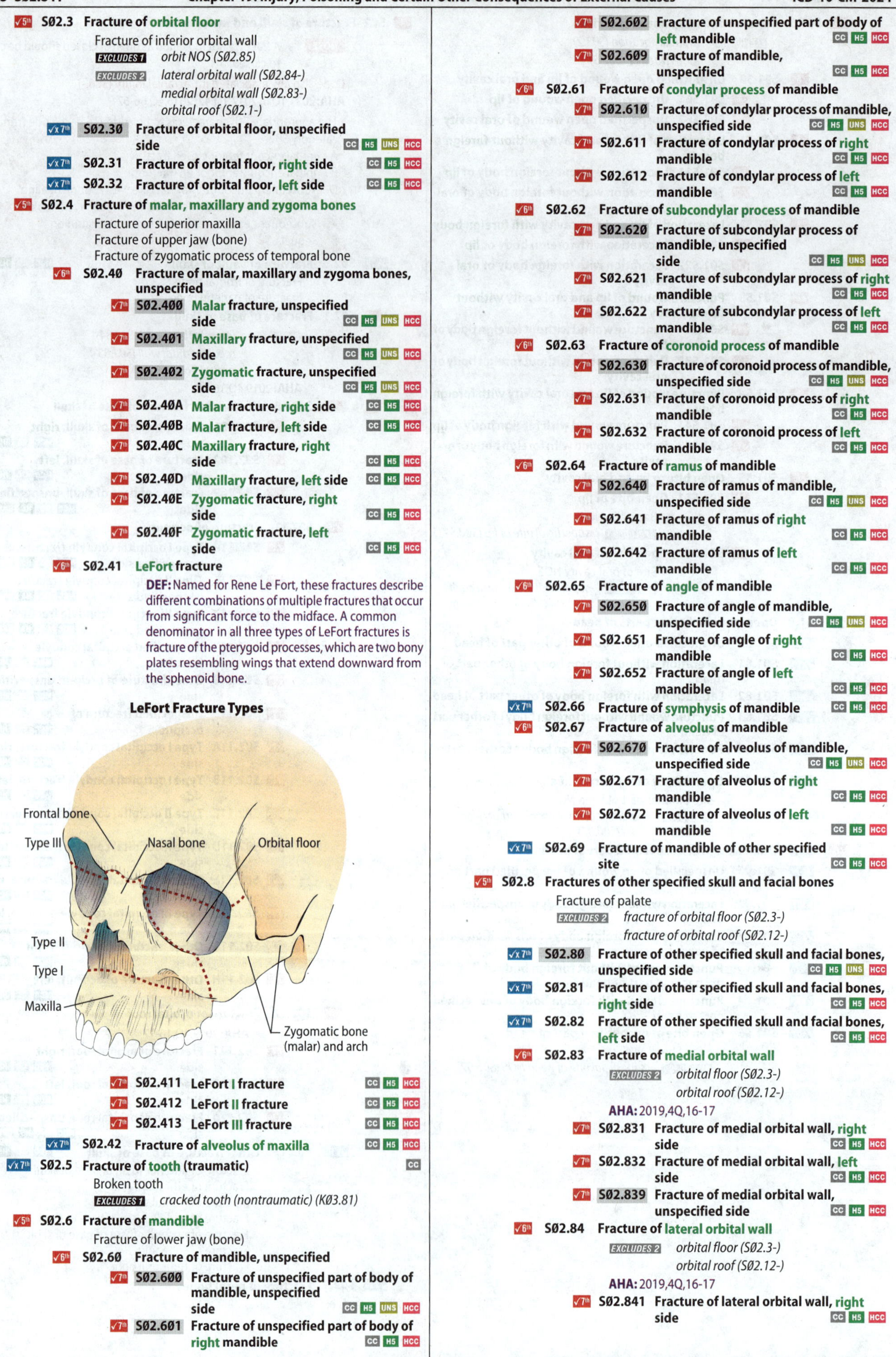

√7th **SØ2.411 LeFort I fracture** CC H5 HCC

√7th **SØ2.412 LeFort II fracture** CC H5 HCC

√7th **SØ2.413 LeFort III fracture** CC H5 HCC

√x7th **SØ2.42 Fracture of alveolus of maxilla** CC H5 HCC

√x7th **SØ2.5 Fracture of tooth (traumatic)** CC

Broken tooth

EXCLUDES 1 *cracked tooth (nontraumatic) (KØ3.81)*

√5th **SØ2.6 Fracture of mandible**

Fracture of lower jaw (bone)

√6th **SØ2.6Ø Fracture of mandible, unspecified**

√7th **SØ2.6ØØ Fracture of unspecified part of body of mandible, unspecified side** CC H5 UNS HCC

√7th **SØ2.6Ø1 Fracture of unspecified part of body of right mandible** CC H5 HCC

√7th **SØ2.6Ø2 Fracture of unspecified part of body of left mandible** CC H5 HCC

√7th **SØ2.6Ø9 Fracture of mandible, unspecified** CC H5 HCC

√6th **SØ2.61 Fracture of condylar process of mandible**

√7th **SØ2.61Ø Fracture of condylar process of mandible, unspecified side** CC H5 UNS HCC

√7th **SØ2.611 Fracture of condylar process of right mandible** CC H5 HCC

√7th **SØ2.612 Fracture of condylar process of left mandible** CC H5 HCC

√6th **SØ2.62 Fracture of subcondylar process of mandible**

√7th **SØ2.62Ø Fracture of subcondylar process of mandible, unspecified side** CC H5 UNS HCC

√7th **SØ2.621 Fracture of subcondylar process of right mandible** CC H5 HCC

√7th **SØ2.622 Fracture of subcondylar process of left mandible** CC H5 HCC

√6th **SØ2.63 Fracture of coronoid process of mandible**

√7th **SØ2.63Ø Fracture of coronoid process of mandible, unspecified side** CC H5 UNS HCC

√7th **SØ2.631 Fracture of coronoid process of right mandible** CC H5 HCC

√7th **SØ2.632 Fracture of coronoid process of left mandible** CC H5 HCC

√6th **SØ2.64 Fracture of ramus of mandible**

√7th **SØ2.64Ø Fracture of ramus of mandible, unspecified side** CC H5 UNS HCC

√7th **SØ2.641 Fracture of ramus of right mandible** CC H5 HCC

√7th **SØ2.642 Fracture of ramus of left mandible** CC H5 HCC

√6th **SØ2.65 Fracture of angle of mandible**

√7th **SØ2.65Ø Fracture of angle of mandible, unspecified side** CC H5 UNS HCC

√7th **SØ2.651 Fracture of angle of right mandible** CC H5 HCC

√7th **SØ2.652 Fracture of angle of left mandible** CC H5 HCC

√x7th **SØ2.66 Fracture of symphysis of mandible** CC H5 HCC

√6th **SØ2.67 Fracture of alveolus of mandible**

√7th **SØ2.67Ø Fracture of alveolus of mandible, unspecified side** CC H5 UNS HCC

√7th **SØ2.671 Fracture of alveolus of right mandible** CC H5 HCC

√7th **SØ2.672 Fracture of alveolus of left mandible** CC H5 HCC

√x7th **SØ2.69 Fracture of mandible of other specified site** CC H5 HCC

√5th **SØ2.8 Fractures of other specified skull and facial bones**

Fracture of palate

EXCLUDES 2 *fracture of orbital floor (SØ2.3-)*
fracture of orbital roof (SØ2.12-)

√x7th **SØ2.8Ø Fracture of other specified skull and facial bones, unspecified side** CC H5 UNS HCC

√x7th **SØ2.81 Fracture of other specified skull and facial bones, right side** CC H5 HCC

√x7th **SØ2.82 Fracture of other specified skull and facial bones, left side** CC H5 HCC

√6th **SØ2.83 Fracture of medial orbital wall**

EXCLUDES 2 *orbital floor (SØ2.3-)*
orbital roof (SØ2.12-)

AHA: 2019,4Q,16-17

√7th **SØ2.831 Fracture of medial orbital wall, right side** CC H5 HCC

√7th **SØ2.832 Fracture of medial orbital wall, left side** CC H5 HCC

√7th **SØ2.839 Fracture of medial orbital wall, unspecified side** CC H5 HCC

√6th **SØ2.84 Fracture of lateral orbital wall**

EXCLUDES 2 *orbital floor (SØ2.3-)*
orbital roof (SØ2.12-)

AHA: 2019,4Q,16-17

√7th **SØ2.841 Fracture of lateral orbital wall, right side** CC H5 HCC

S02.842 **Fracture of lateral orbital wall, left side** CC H5 HCC

S02.849 **Fracture of lateral orbital wall, unspecified side** CC H5 HCC

S02.85 **Fracture of orbit, unspecified** CC H5 HCC
Fracture of orbit NOS
Fracture of orbit wall NOS
EXCLUDES 1 *lateral orbital wall (S02.84-)*
medial orbital wall (S02.83-)
orbital floor (S02.3-)
orbital roof (S02.12-)

S02.9 **Fracture of unspecified skull and facial bones**

S02.91 **Unspecified fracture of skull** MCC CC H5 HCC
AHA: 2020,2Q,24

S02.92 **Unspecified fracture of facial bones** CC H5 HCC

S03 Dislocation and sprain of joints and ligaments of head

INCLUDES avulsion of joint (capsule) or ligament of head
laceration of cartilage, joint (capsule) or ligament of head
sprain of cartilage, joint (capsule) or ligament of head
traumatic hemarthrosis of joint or ligament of head
traumatic rupture of joint or ligament of head
traumatic subluxation of joint or ligament of head
traumatic tear of joint or ligament of head

Code also any associated open wound

EXCLUDES 2 *strain of muscle or tendon of head (S09.1)*

The appropriate 7th character is to be added to each code from category S03.
A initial encounter
D subsequent encounter
S sequela

S03.0 **Dislocation of jaw**
Dislocation of jaw (cartilage) (meniscus)
Dislocation of mandible
Dislocation of temporomandibular (joint)
AHA: 2016,4Q,67

S03.00 **Dislocation of jaw, unspecified side**

S03.01 **Dislocation of jaw, right side**

S03.02 **Dislocation of jaw, left side**

S03.03 **Dislocation of jaw, bilateral**

S03.1 **Dislocation of septal cartilage of nose**

S03.2 **Dislocation of tooth**

S03.4 **Sprain of jaw**
Sprain of temporomandibular (joint) (ligament)
AHA: 2016,4Q,67

S03.40 **Sprain of jaw, unspecified side**

S03.41 **Sprain of jaw, right side**

S03.42 **Sprain of jaw, left side**

S03.43 **Sprain of jaw, bilateral**

S03.8 **Sprain of joints and ligaments of other parts of head**

S03.9 **Sprain of joints and ligaments of unspecified parts of head**

S04 Injury of cranial nerve

The selection of side should be based on the side of the body being affected

Code first any associated intracranial injury (S06.-)

Code also any associated:
open wound of head (S01.-)
skull fracture (S02.-)

The appropriate 7th character is to be added to each code from category S04.
A initial encounter
D subsequent encounter
S sequela

S04.0 **Injury of optic nerve and pathways**
Use additional code to identify any visual field defect or blindness (H53.4-, H54.-)

S04.01 **Injury of optic nerve**
Injury of 2nd cranial nerve

S04.011 **Injury of optic nerve, right eye** CC

S04.012 **Injury of optic nerve, left eye** CC

S04.019 **Injury of optic nerve, unspecified eye** CC UNS
Injury of optic nerve NOS

S04.02 **Injury of optic chiasm** CC

S04.03 **Injury of optic tract and pathways**
Injury of optic radiation

S04.031 **Injury of optic tract and pathways, right side** CC

S04.032 **Injury of optic tract and pathways, left side** CC

S04.039 **Injury of optic tract and pathways, unspecified side** CC UNS
Injury of optic tract and pathways NOS

S04.04 **Injury of visual cortex**

S04.041 **Injury of visual cortex, right side** CC

S04.042 **Injury of visual cortex, left side** CC

S04.049 **Injury of visual cortex, unspecified side** CC UNS
Injury of visual cortex NOS

S04.1 **Injury of oculomotor nerve**
Injury of 3rd cranial nerve

S04.10 **Injury of oculomotor nerve, unspecified side** CC UNS

S04.11 **Injury of oculomotor nerve, right side** CC

S04.12 **Injury of oculomotor nerve, left side** CC

S04.2 **Injury of trochlear nerve**
Injury of 4th cranial nerve

S04.20 **Injury of trochlear nerve, unspecified side** CC UNS

S04.21 **Injury of trochlear nerve, right side** CC

S04.22 **Injury of trochlear nerve, left side** CC

S04.3 **Injury of trigeminal nerve**
Injury of 5th cranial nerve

S04.30 **Injury of trigeminal nerve, unspecified side** CC UNS

S04.31 **Injury of trigeminal nerve, right side** CC

S04.32 **Injury of trigeminal nerve, left side** CC

S04.4 **Injury of abducent nerve**
Injury of 6th cranial nerve

S04.40 **Injury of abducent nerve, unspecified side** CC UNS

S04.41 **Injury of abducent nerve, right side** CC

S04.42 **Injury of abducent nerve, left side** CC

S04.5 **Injury of facial nerve**
Injury of 7th cranial nerve

S04.50 **Injury of facial nerve, unspecified side** CC UNS

S04.51 **Injury of facial nerve, right side** CC

S04.52 **Injury of facial nerve, left side** CC

S04.6 **Injury of acoustic nerve**
Injury of auditory nerve
Injury of 8th cranial nerve

S04.60 **Injury of acoustic nerve, unspecified side** CC UNS

S04.61 **Injury of acoustic nerve, right side** CC

S04.62 **Injury of acoustic nerve, left side** CC

S04.7 **Injury of accessory nerve**
Injury of 11th cranial nerve

S04.70 **Injury of accessory nerve, unspecified side** CC UNS

S04.71 **Injury of accessory nerve, right side** CC

S04.72 **Injury of accessory nerve, left side** CC

S04.8 **Injury of other cranial nerves**

S04.81 **Injury of olfactory [1st] nerve**

S04.811 **Injury of olfactory [1st] nerve, right side** CC

S04.812 **Injury of olfactory [1st] nerve, left side** CC

S04.819 **Injury of olfactory [1st] nerve, unspecified side** CC

S04.89 **Injury of other cranial nerves**
Injury of vagus [10th] nerve

S04.891 **Injury of other cranial nerves, right side** CC

S04.892 Injury of other cranial nerves, left side CC

S04.899 Injury of other cranial nerves, unspecified side CC UNS

S04.9 Injury of unspecified cranial nerve CC

S05 Injury of eye and orbit

INCLUDES open wound of eye and orbit

EXCLUDES 2 *2nd cranial [optic] nerve injury (S04.0-)*
3rd cranial [oculomotor] nerve injury (S04.1-)
open wound of eyelid and periocular area (S01.1-)
orbital bone fracture (S02.1-, S02.3-, S02.8-)
superficial injury of eyelid (S00.1-S00.2)

The appropriate 7th character is to be added to each code from category S05.
A initial encounter
D subsequent encounter
S sequela

S05.0 Injury of conjunctiva and corneal abrasion without foreign body

EXCLUDES 1 *foreign body in conjunctival sac (T15.1)*
foreign body in cornea (T15.0)

S05.00 Injury of conjunctiva and corneal abrasion without foreign body, unspecified eye

S05.01 Injury of conjunctiva and corneal abrasion without foreign body, right eye

S05.02 Injury of conjunctiva and corneal abrasion without foreign body, left eye

S05.1 Contusion of eyeball and orbital tissues

Traumatic hyphema

EXCLUDES 2 *black eye NOS (S00.1)*
contusion of eyelid and periocular area (S00.1)

S05.10 Contusion of eyeball and orbital tissues, unspecified eye

S05.11 Contusion of eyeball and orbital tissues, right eye

S05.12 Contusion of eyeball and orbital tissues, left eye

S05.2 Ocular laceration and rupture with prolapse or loss of intraocular tissue

S05.20 Ocular laceration and rupture with prolapse or loss of intraocular tissue, unspecified eye CC UNS

S05.21 Ocular laceration and rupture with prolapse or loss of intraocular tissue, right eye CC

S05.22 Ocular laceration and rupture with prolapse or loss of intraocular tissue, left eye CC

S05.3 Ocular laceration without prolapse or loss of intraocular tissue

Laceration of eye NOS

AHA: 2022,1Q,33

DEF: Tear in ocular tissue without displacing structures that is due to blunt trauma. It is characterized by pain, redness, and decreased vision.

S05.30 Ocular laceration without prolapse or loss of intraocular tissue, unspecified eye CC UNS

S05.31 Ocular laceration without prolapse or loss of intraocular tissue, right eye CC

S05.32 Ocular laceration without prolapse or loss of intraocular tissue, left eye CC

S05.4 Penetrating wound of orbit with or without foreign body

EXCLUDES 2 *retained (old) foreign body following penetrating wound in orbit (H05.5-)*

S05.40 Penetrating wound of orbit with or without foreign body, unspecified eye CC UNS

S05.41 Penetrating wound of orbit with or without foreign body, right eye CC

S05.42 Penetrating wound of orbit with or without foreign body, left eye CC

S05.5 Penetrating wound with foreign body of eyeball

EXCLUDES 2 *retained (old) intraocular foreign body (H44.6-, H44.7)*

S05.50 Penetrating wound with foreign body of unspecified eyeball CC UNS

S05.51 Penetrating wound with foreign body of right eyeball CC

S05.52 Penetrating wound with foreign body of left eyeball CC

S05.6 Penetrating wound without foreign body of eyeball

Ocular penetration NOS

S05.60 Penetrating wound without foreign body of unspecified eyeball

S05.61 Penetrating wound without foreign body of right eyeball

S05.62 Penetrating wound without foreign body of left eyeball

S05.7 Avulsion of eye

Traumatic enucleation

S05.70 Avulsion of unspecified eye CC UNS

S05.71 Avulsion of right eye CC

S05.72 Avulsion of left eye CC

S05.8 Other injuries of eye and orbit

Lacrimal duct injury

S05.8X Other injuries of eye and orbit

S05.8X1 Other injuries of right eye and orbit CC

S05.8X2 Other injuries of left eye and orbit CC

S05.8X9 Other injuries of unspecified eye and orbit CC UNS

S05.9 Unspecified injury of eye and orbit

Injury of eye NOS

S05.90 Unspecified injury of unspecified eye and orbit

S05.91 Unspecified injury of right eye and orbit CC

S05.92 Unspecified injury of left eye and orbit CC

S06 Intracranial injury

NOTE 7th characters D and S do not apply to codes in category S06 with 6th character 7 – death due to brain injury prior to regaining consciousness, or 8 – death due to other cause prior to regaining consciousness.

INCLUDES traumatic brain injury

Code also any associated:
open wound of head (S01.-)
skull fracture (S02.-)

Use additional code, if applicable, to identify mild neurocognitive disorders due to known physiological condition (F06.7-)

EXCLUDES 1 *head injury NOS (S09.90)*

AHA: 2022,4Q,42-45; 2017,4Q,25; 2017,1Q,42; 2015,3Q,37

TIP: Do not assign Z87.820 Personal history of traumatic brain injury, when residual conditions persist after an intracranial injury. The codes for the residual conditions should be first listed, followed by a code from category S06 using seventh character S to identify sequelae.

The appropriate 7th character is to be added to each code from category S06.
A initial encounter
D subsequent encounter
S sequela

S06.0 Concussion

Commotio cerebri

EXCLUDES 1 *concussion with other intracranial injuries classified in subcategories S06.1- to S06.6-, and S06.81- to S06.89-, code to specified intracranial injury*

AHA: 2016,4Q,67-68

S06.0X Concussion

S06.0X0 Concussion without loss of consciousness CC HCC

S06.0X1 Concussion with loss of consciousness of 30 minutes or less CC HS HCC
Concussion with brief loss of consciousness

S06.0XA Concussion with loss of consciousness status unknown CC HS HCC
Concussion NOS

S06.0X9 Concussion with loss of consciousness of unspecified duration CC HS HCC

S06.1 Traumatic cerebral edema

Diffuse traumatic cerebral edema
Focal traumatic cerebral edema

AHA: 2019,3Q,35; 2015,1Q,12-13

S06.1X Traumatic cerebral edema

S06.1X0 Traumatic cerebral edema without loss of consciousness MCC HCC

S06.1X1 Traumatic cerebral edema with loss of consciousness of 30 minutes or less MCC H5 HCC
Traumatic cerebral edema with brief loss of consciousness

S06.1X2 Traumatic cerebral edema with loss of consciousness of 31 minutes to 59 minutes MCC H5 HCC

S06.1X3 Traumatic cerebral edema with loss of consciousness of 1 hour to 5 hours 59 minutes MCC H5 HCC

S06.1X4 Traumatic cerebral edema with loss of consciousness of 6 hours to 24 hours MCC H5 HCC

S06.1X5 Traumatic cerebral edema with loss of consciousness greater than 24 hours with return to pre-existing conscious level MCC H5 HCC

S06.1X6 Traumatic cerebral edema with loss of consciousness greater than 24 hours without return to pre-existing conscious level with patient surviving MCC H5 HCC

S06.1X7 Traumatic cerebral edema with loss of consciousness of any duration with death due to brain injury prior to regaining consciousness MCC H5

S06.1X8 Traumatic cerebral edema with loss of consciousness of any duration with death due to other cause prior to regaining consciousness MCC H5

S06.1XA Traumatic cerebral edema with loss of consciousness status unknown MCC H5 HCC
Traumatic cerebral edema NOS

S06.1X9 Traumatic cerebral edema with loss of consciousness of unspecified duration MCC H5 HCC

S06.2 Diffuse traumatic brain injury
Diffuse axonal brain injury
Use additional code, if applicable, for traumatic brain compression or herniation (S06.A-)
EXCLUDES 1 *traumatic diffuse cerebral edema (S06.1X-)*
AHA: 2020,3Q,46
TIP: Assign additional code(s) for individual (R40.21-, R40.22-, R40.23-) or total (R40.24-) coma scale scores. It is appropriate to code the coma scale scores based on documentation provided by clinicians who are not the patient's provider (such as emergency medical technician).

S06.2X Diffuse traumatic brain injury

S06.2X0 Diffuse traumatic brain injury without loss of consciousness HCC

S06.2X1 Diffuse traumatic brain injury with loss of consciousness of 30 minutes or less CC H5 HCC
Diffuse traumatic brain injury with brief loss of consciousness

S06.2X2 Diffuse traumatic brain injury with loss of consciousness of 31 minutes to 59 minutes CC H5 HCC

S06.2X3 Diffuse traumatic brain injury with loss of consciousness of 1 hour to 5 hours 59 minutes CC H5 HCC

S06.2X4 Diffuse traumatic brain injury with loss of consciousness of 6 hours to 24 hours CC H5 HCC

S06.2X5 Diffuse traumatic brain injury with loss of consciousness greater than 24 hours with return to pre-existing conscious levels CC H5 HCC

S06.2X6 Diffuse traumatic brain injury with loss of consciousness greater than 24 hours without return to pre-existing conscious level with patient surviving MCC H5 HCC

S06.2X7 Diffuse traumatic brain injury with loss of consciousness of any duration with death due to brain injury prior to regaining consciousness MCC H5

S06.2X8 Diffuse traumatic brain injury with loss of consciousness of any duration with death due to other cause prior to regaining consciousness MCC H5

S06.2XA Diffuse traumatic brain injury with loss of consciousness status unknown CC H5 HCC
Diffuse traumatic brain injury NOS

S06.2X9 Diffuse traumatic brain injury with loss of consciousness of unspecified duration CC H5 HCC

S06.3 Focal traumatic brain injury
Use additional code, if applicable, for traumatic brain compression or herniation (S06.A-)
EXCLUDES 1 ~~*any condition classifiable to S06.4-S06.6*~~
EXCLUDES 2 ▶*any condition classifiable to S06.4-S06.6*◀
focal cerebral edema (S06.1)
AHA: 2020,3Q,46; 2019,3Q,35; 2015,1Q,12-13
TIP: Assign additional code(s) for individual (R40.21-, R40.22-, R40.23-) or total (R40.24-) coma scale scores. It is appropriate to code the coma scale scores based on documentation provided by clinicians who are not the patient's provider (such as emergency medical technician).

S06.30 Unspecified focal traumatic brain injury

S06.300 Unspecified focal traumatic brain injury without loss of consciousness HCC

S06.301 Unspecified focal traumatic brain injury with loss of consciousness of 30 minutes or less CC H5 HCC
Unspecified focal traumatic brain injury with brief loss of consciousness

S06.302 Unspecified focal traumatic brain injury with loss of consciousness of 31 minutes to 59 minutes CC H5 HCC

S06.303 Unspecified focal traumatic brain injury with loss of consciousness of 1 hour to 5 hours 59 minutes CC H5 HCC

S06.304 Unspecified focal traumatic brain injury with loss of consciousness of 6 hours to 24 hours CC H5 HCC

S06.305 Unspecified focal traumatic brain injury with loss of consciousness greater than 24 hours with return to pre-existing conscious level CC H5 HCC

S06.306 Unspecified focal traumatic brain injury with loss of consciousness greater than 24 hours without return to pre-existing conscious level with patient surviving MCC H5 HCC

S06.307 Unspecified focal traumatic brain injury with loss of consciousness of any duration with death due to brain injury prior to regaining consciousness MCC H5

S06.308 Unspecified focal traumatic brain injury with loss of consciousness of any duration with death due to other cause prior to regaining consciousness MCC H5

S06.30A Unspecified focal traumatic brain injury with loss of consciousness status unknown CC H5 HCC
Unspecified focal traumatic brain injury NOS

S06.309 Unspecified focal traumatic brain injury with loss of consciousness of unspecified duration CC H5 HCC

S06.31 Contusion and laceration of right cerebrum

S06.310 Contusion and laceration of right cerebrum without loss of consciousness MCC H5 HCC

S06.311 Contusion and laceration of right cerebrum with loss of consciousness of 30 minutes or less MCC H5 HCC
Contusion and laceration of right cerebrum with brief loss of consciousness

S06.312 Contusion and laceration of right cerebrum with loss of consciousness of 31 minutes to 59 minutes MCC H5 HCC

S06.313 Contusion and laceration of right cerebrum with loss of consciousness of 1 hour to 5 hours 59 minutes MCC H5 HCC

S06.314 Contusion and laceration of right cerebrum with loss of consciousness of 6 hours to 24 hours MCC H5 HCC

7th **S06.315 Contusion and laceration of right cerebrum with loss of consciousness greater than 24 hours with return to pre-existing conscious level** MCC HS HCC

7th **S06.316 Contusion and laceration of right cerebrum with loss of consciousness greater than 24 hours without return to pre-existing conscious level with patient surviving** MCC HS HCC

7th **S06.317 Contusion and laceration of right cerebrum with loss of consciousness of any duration with death due to brain injury prior to regaining consciousness** MCC HS

7th **S06.318 Contusion and laceration of right cerebrum with loss of consciousness of any duration with death due to other cause prior to regaining consciousness** MCC HS

7th **S06.31A Contusion and laceration of right cerebrum with loss of consciousness status unknown** MCC HS HCC

Contusion and laceration of right cerebrum NOS

7th **S06.319 Contusion and laceration of right cerebrum with loss of consciousness of unspecified duration** MCC HS HCC

6th **S06.32 Contusion and laceration of left cerebrum**

7th **S06.320 Contusion and laceration of left cerebrum without loss of consciousness** MCC HS HCC

7th **S06.321 Contusion and laceration of left cerebrum with loss of consciousness of 30 minutes or less** MCC HS HCC

Contusion and laceration of left cerebrum with brief loss of consciousness

7th **S06.322 Contusion and laceration of left cerebrum with loss of consciousness of 31 minutes to 59 minutes** MCC HS HCC

7th **S06.323 Contusion and laceration of left cerebrum with loss of consciousness of 1 hour to 5 hours 59 minutes** MCC HS HCC

7th **S06.324 Contusion and laceration of left cerebrum with loss of consciousness of 6 hours to 24 hours** MCC HS HCC

7th **S06.325 Contusion and laceration of left cerebrum with loss of consciousness greater than 24 hours with return to pre-existing conscious level** MCC HS HCC

7th **S06.326 Contusion and laceration of left cerebrum with loss of consciousness greater than 24 hours without return to pre-existing conscious level with patient surviving** MCC HS HCC

7th **S06.327 Contusion and laceration of left cerebrum with loss of consciousness of any duration with death due to brain injury prior to regaining consciousness** MCC HS

7th **S06.328 Contusion and laceration of left cerebrum with loss of consciousness of any duration with death due to other cause prior to regaining consciousness** MCC HS

7th **S06.32A Contusion and laceration of left cerebrum with loss of consciousness status unknown** MCC HS HCC

Contusion and laceration of left cerebrum NOS

7th **S06.329 Contusion and laceration of left cerebrum with loss of consciousness of unspecified duration** MCC HS HCC

6th **S06.33 Contusion and laceration of cerebrum, unspecified**

7th **S06.330 Contusion and laceration of cerebrum, unspecified, without loss of consciousness** MCC HS HCC

7th **S06.331 Contusion and laceration of cerebrum, unspecified, with loss of consciousness of 30 minutes or less** MCC HS HCC

Contusion and laceration of cerebrum, unspecified, with brief loss of consciousness

7th **S06.332 Contusion and laceration of cerebrum, unspecified, with loss of consciousness of 31 minutes to 59 minutes** MCC HS HCC

7th **S06.333 Contusion and laceration of cerebrum, unspecified, with loss of consciousness of 1 hour to 5 hours 59 minutes** MCC HS HCC

7th **S06.334 Contusion and laceration of cerebrum, unspecified, with loss of consciousness of 6 hours to 24 hours** MCC HS HCC

7th **S06.335 Contusion and laceration of cerebrum, unspecified, with loss of consciousness greater than 24 hours with return to pre-existing conscious level** MCC HS HCC

7th **S06.336 Contusion and laceration of cerebrum, unspecified, with loss of consciousness greater than 24 hours without return to pre-existing conscious level with patient surviving** MCC HS HCC

7th **S06.337 Contusion and laceration of cerebrum, unspecified, with loss of consciousness of any duration with death due to brain injury prior to regaining consciousness** MCC HS

7th **S06.338 Contusion and laceration of cerebrum, unspecified, with loss of consciousness of any duration with death due to other cause prior to regaining consciousness** MCC HS

7th **S06.33A Contusion and laceration of cerebrum, unspecified, with loss of consciousness status unknown** MCC HS UNS HCC

Contusion and laceration of cerebrum NOS

7th **S06.339 Contusion and laceration of cerebrum, unspecified, with loss of consciousness of unspecified duration** MCC HS HCC

6th **S06.34 Traumatic hemorrhage of right cerebrum**

Traumatic intracerebral hemorrhage and hematoma of right cerebrum

7th **S06.340 Traumatic hemorrhage of right cerebrum without loss of consciousness** MCC HS HCC

7th **S06.341 Traumatic hemorrhage of right cerebrum with loss of consciousness of 30 minutes or less** MCC HS HCC

Traumatic hemorrhage of right cerebrum with loss of consciousness

7th **S06.342 Traumatic hemorrhage of right cerebrum with loss of consciousness of 31 minutes to 59 minutes** MCC HS HCC

7th **S06.343 Traumatic hemorrhage of right cerebrum with loss of consciousness of 1 hours to 5 hours 59 minutes** MCC HS HCC

7th **S06.344 Traumatic hemorrhage of right cerebrum with loss of consciousness of 6 hours to 24 hours** MCC HS HCC

7th **S06.345 Traumatic hemorrhage of right cerebrum with loss of consciousness greater than 24 hours with return to pre-existing conscious level** MCC HS HCC

7th **S06.346 Traumatic hemorrhage of right cerebrum with loss of consciousness greater than 24 hours without return to pre-existing conscious level with patient surviving** MCC HS HCC

7th **S06.347 Traumatic hemorrhage of right cerebrum with loss of consciousness of any duration with death due to brain injury prior to regaining consciousness** MCC HS

7th **S06.348 Traumatic hemorrhage of right cerebrum with loss of consciousness of any duration with death due to other cause prior to regaining consciousness** MCC HS

7th **S06.34A Traumatic hemorrhage of right cerebrum with loss of consciousness status unknown** MCC HS HCC

Traumatic hemorrhage of right cerebrum NOS

7th **S06.349 Traumatic hemorrhage of right cerebrum with loss of consciousness of unspecified duration** MCC HS HCC

S06.35 Traumatic hemorrhage of left cerebrum
Traumatic intracerebral hemorrhage and hematoma of left cerebrum
S06.350 Traumatic hemorrhage of left cerebrum without loss of consciousness MCC H5 HCC
S06.351 Traumatic hemorrhage of left cerebrum with loss of consciousness of 30 minutes or less MCC H5 HCC
Traumatic hemorrhage of left cerebrum with brief loss of consciousness
S06.352 Traumatic hemorrhage of left cerebrum with loss of consciousness of 31 minutes to 59 minutes MCC H5 HCC
S06.353 Traumatic hemorrhage of left cerebrum with loss of consciousness of 1 hours to 5 hours 59 minutes MCC H5 HCC
S06.354 Traumatic hemorrhage of left cerebrum with loss of consciousness of 6 hours to 24 hours MCC H5 HCC
S06.355 Traumatic hemorrhage of left cerebrum with loss of consciousness greater than 24 hours with return to pre-existing conscious level MCC H5 HCC
S06.356 Traumatic hemorrhage of left cerebrum with loss of consciousness greater than 24 hours without return to pre-existing conscious level with patient surviving MCC H5 HCC
S06.357 Traumatic hemorrhage of left cerebrum with loss of consciousness of any duration with death due to brain injury prior to regaining consciousness MCC H5
S06.358 Traumatic hemorrhage of left cerebrum with loss of consciousness of any duration with death due to other cause prior to regaining consciousness MCC H5
S06.35A Traumatic hemorrhage of left cerebrum with loss of consciousness status unknown MCC H5 HCC
Traumatic hemorrhage of left cerebrum NOS
S06.359 Traumatic hemorrhage of left cerebrum with loss of consciousness of unspecified duration MCC H5 HCC

S06.36 Traumatic hemorrhage of cerebrum, unspecified
Traumatic intracerebral hemorrhage and hematoma, unspecified
S06.360 Traumatic hemorrhage of cerebrum, unspecified, without loss of consciousness MCC H5 HCC
S06.361 Traumatic hemorrhage of cerebrum, unspecified, with loss of consciousness of 30 minutes or less MCC H5 HCC
Traumatic hemorrhage of cerebrum, unspecified, with brief loss of consciousness
S06.362 Traumatic hemorrhage of cerebrum, unspecified, with loss of consciousness of 31 minutes to 59 minutes MCC H5 HCC
S06.363 Traumatic hemorrhage of cerebrum, unspecified, with loss of consciousness of 1 hours to 5 hours 59 minutes MCC H5 HCC
S06.364 Traumatic hemorrhage of cerebrum, unspecified, with loss of consciousness of 6 hours to 24 hours MCC H5 HCC
S06.365 Traumatic hemorrhage of cerebrum, unspecified, with loss of consciousness greater than 24 hours with return to pre-existing conscious level MCC H5 HCC
S06.366 Traumatic hemorrhage of cerebrum, unspecified, with loss of consciousness greater than 24 hours without return to pre-existing conscious level with patient surviving MCC H5 HCC
S06.367 Traumatic hemorrhage of cerebrum, unspecified, with loss of consciousness of any duration with death due to brain injury prior to regaining consciousness MCC H5
S06.368 Traumatic hemorrhage of cerebrum, unspecified, with loss of consciousness of any duration with death due to other cause prior to regaining consciousness MCC H5
S06.36A Traumatic hemorrhage of cerebrum, unspecified, with loss of consciousness status unknown MCC H5 UNS HCC
Traumatic hemorrhage of cerebrum NOS
S06.369 Traumatic hemorrhage of cerebrum, unspecified, with loss of consciousness of unspecified duration MCC H5 HCC

S06.37 Contusion, laceration, and hemorrhage of cerebellum
S06.370 Contusion, laceration, and hemorrhage of cerebellum without loss of consciousness MCC H5 HCC
S06.371 Contusion, laceration, and hemorrhage of cerebellum with loss of consciousness of 30 minutes or less CC H5 HCC
Contusion, laceration, and hemorrhage of cerebellum with brief loss of consciousness
S06.372 Contusion, laceration, and hemorrhage of cerebellum with loss of consciousness of 31 minutes to 59 minutes CC H5 HCC
S06.373 Contusion, laceration, and hemorrhage of cerebellum with loss of consciousness of 1 hour to 5 hours 59 minutes CC H5 HCC
S06.374 Contusion, laceration, and hemorrhage of cerebellum with loss of consciousness of 6 hours to 24 hours CC H5 HCC
S06.375 Contusion, laceration, and hemorrhage of cerebellum with loss of consciousness greater than 24 hours with return to pre-existing conscious level CC H5 HCC
S06.376 Contusion, laceration, and hemorrhage of cerebellum with loss of consciousness greater than 24 hours without return to pre-existing conscious level with patient surviving MCC H5 HCC
S06.377 Contusion, laceration, and hemorrhage of cerebellum with loss of consciousness of any duration with death due to brain injury prior to regaining consciousness MCC H5
S06.378 Contusion, laceration, and hemorrhage of cerebellum with loss of consciousness of any duration with death due to other cause prior to regaining consciousness MCC H5
S06.37A Contusion, laceration, and hemorrhage of cerebellum with loss of consciousness status unknown MCC H5 HCC
Contusion, laceration, and hemorrhage of cerebellum NOS
S06.379 Contusion, laceration, and hemorrhage of cerebellum with loss of consciousness of unspecified duration CC H5 HCC

S06.38 Contusion, laceration, and hemorrhage of brainstem
S06.380 Contusion, laceration, and hemorrhage of brainstem without loss of consciousness MCC H5 HCC
S06.381 Contusion, laceration, and hemorrhage of brainstem with loss of consciousness of 30 minutes or less CC H5 HCC
Contusion, laceration, and hemorrhage of brainstem with brief loss of consciousness
S06.382 Contusion, laceration, and hemorrhage of brainstem with loss of consciousness of 31 minutes to 59 minutes CC H5 HCC
S06.383 Contusion, laceration, and hemorrhage of brainstem with loss of consciousness of 1 hour to 5 hours 59 minutes CC H5 HCC
S06.384 Contusion, laceration, and hemorrhage of brainstem with loss of consciousness of 6 hours to 24 hours CC H5 HCC

√7th **S06.385 Contusion, laceration, and hemorrhage of brainstem with loss of consciousness greater than 24 hours with return to pre-existing conscious level** CC H5 HCC

√7th **S06.386 Contusion, laceration, and hemorrhage of brainstem with loss of consciousness greater than 24 hours without return to pre-existing conscious level with patient surviving** MCC H5 HCC

√7th **S06.387 Contusion, laceration, and hemorrhage of brainstem with loss of consciousness of any duration with death due to brain injury prior to regaining consciousness** MCC H5

√7th **S06.388 Contusion, laceration, and hemorrhage of brainstem with loss of consciousness of any duration with death due to other cause prior to regaining consciousness** MCC H5

√7th **S06.38A Contusion, laceration, and hemorrhage of brainstem with loss of consciousness status unknown** MCC H5 HCC

Contusion, laceration, and hemorrhage of brainstem NOS

√7th **S06.389 Contusion, laceration, and hemorrhage of brainstem with loss of consciousness of unspecified duration** CC H5 HCC

√5th **S06.4 Epidural hemorrhage**

Extradural hemorrhage NOS

Extradural hemorrhage (traumatic)

DEF: Epidural space: Space between the endosteum of the cranium (skull) and the dura mater, the outermost layer of a three-layer membrane that covers the brain.

√6th **S06.4X Epidural hemorrhage**

√7th **S06.4X0 Epidural hemorrhage without loss of consciousness** MCC H5 HCC

√7th **S06.4X1 Epidural hemorrhage with loss of consciousness of 30 minutes or less** MCC H5 HCC

Epidural hemorrhage with brief loss of consciousness

√7th **S06.4X2 Epidural hemorrhage with loss of consciousness of 31 minutes to 59 minutes** MCC H5 HCC

√7th **S06.4X3 Epidural hemorrhage with loss of consciousness of 1 hour to 5 hours 59 minutes** MCC H5 HCC

√7th **S06.4X4 Epidural hemorrhage with loss of consciousness of 6 hours to 24 hours** MCC H5 HCC

√7th **S06.4X5 Epidural hemorrhage with loss of consciousness greater than 24 hours with return to pre-existing conscious level** MCC H5 HCC

√7th **S06.4X6 Epidural hemorrhage with loss of consciousness greater than 24 hours without return to pre-existing conscious level with patient surviving** MCC H5 HCC

√7th **S06.4X7 Epidural hemorrhage with loss of consciousness of any duration with death due to brain injury prior to regaining consciousness** MCC H5

√7th **S06.4X8 Epidural hemorrhage with loss of consciousness of any duration with death due to other causes prior to regaining consciousness** MCC H5

√7th **S06.4XA Epidural hemorrhage with loss of consciousness status unknown** MCC H5 HCC

Epidural hemorrhage NOS

√7th **S06.4X9 Epidural hemorrhage with loss of consciousness of unspecified duration** MCC H5 HCC

√5th **S06.5 Traumatic subdural hemorrhage**

Use additional code, if applicable, for traumatic brain compression or herniation (S06.A-)

AHA: 2021,2Q,5; 2021,1Q,4

DEF: Subdural: Potential space between the dura mater and arachnoid membrane around the brain.

√6th **S06.5X Traumatic subdural hemorrhage**

√7th **S06.5X0 Traumatic subdural hemorrhage without loss of consciousness** MCC H5 HCC

√7th **S06.5X1 Traumatic subdural hemorrhage with loss of consciousness of 30 minutes or less** MCC H5 HCC

Traumatic subdural hemorrhage with brief loss of consciousness

√7th **S06.5X2 Traumatic subdural hemorrhage with loss of consciousness of 31 minutes to 59 minutes** MCC H5 HCC

√7th **S06.5X3 Traumatic subdural hemorrhage with loss of consciousness of 1 hour to 5 hours 59 minutes** MCC H5 HCC

√7th **S06.5X4 Traumatic subdural hemorrhage with loss of consciousness of 6 hours to 24 hours** MCC H5 HCC

√7th **S06.5X5 Traumatic subdural hemorrhage with loss of consciousness greater than 24 hours with return to pre-existing conscious level** MCC H5 HCC

√7th **S06.5X6 Traumatic subdural hemorrhage with loss of consciousness greater than 24 hours without return to pre-existing conscious level with patient surviving** MCC H5 HCC

√7th **S06.5X7 Traumatic subdural hemorrhage with loss of consciousness of any duration with death due to brain injury before regaining consciousness** MCC H5

√7th **S06.5X8 Traumatic subdural hemorrhage with loss of consciousness of any duration with death due to other cause before regaining consciousness** MCC H5

√7th **S06.5XA Traumatic subdural hemorrhage with loss of consciousness status unknown** MCC H5 HCC

Traumatic subdural hemorrhage NOS

AHA: 2022,4Q,44

√7th **S06.5X9 Traumatic subdural hemorrhage with loss of consciousness of unspecified duration** MCC H5 HCC

√5th **S06.6 Traumatic subarachnoid hemorrhage**

Use additional code, if applicable, for traumatic brain compression or herniation (S06.A-)

AHA: 2021,2Q,5; 2021,1Q,4

DEF: Subarachnoid: Space located between the arachnoid membrane and the pia mater that contains cerebrospinal fluid.

√6th **S06.6X Traumatic subarachnoid hemorrhage**

√7th **S06.6X0 Traumatic subarachnoid hemorrhage without loss of consciousness** MCC H5 HCC

√7th **S06.6X1 Traumatic subarachnoid hemorrhage with loss of consciousness of 30 minutes or less** MCC H5 HCC

Traumatic subarachnoid hemorrhage with brief loss of consciousness

√7th **S06.6X2 Traumatic subarachnoid hemorrhage with loss of consciousness of 31 minutes to 59 minutes** MCC H5 HCC

√7th **S06.6X3 Traumatic subarachnoid hemorrhage with loss of consciousness of 1 hour to 5 hours 59 minutes** MCC H5 HCC

√7th **S06.6X4 Traumatic subarachnoid hemorrhage with loss of consciousness of 6 hours to 24 hours** MCC H5 HCC

√7th **S06.6X5 Traumatic subarachnoid hemorrhage with loss of consciousness greater than 24 hours with return to pre-existing conscious level** MCC H5 HCC

√7th **S06.6X6 Traumatic subarachnoid hemorrhage with loss of consciousness greater than 24 hours without return to pre-existing conscious level with patient surviving** MCC H5 HCC

S06.6X7 Traumatic subarachnoid hemorrhage with loss of consciousness of any duration with death due to brain injury prior to regaining consciousness MCC H5

S06.6X8 Traumatic subarachnoid hemorrhage with loss of consciousness of any duration with death due to other cause prior to regaining consciousness MCC H5

S06.6XA Traumatic subarachnoid hemorrhage with loss of consciousness status unknown MCC H5 HCC
Traumatic subarachnoid hemorrhage NOS
AHA: 2022,4Q,44

S06.6X9 Traumatic subarachnoid hemorrhage with loss of consciousness of unspecified duration MCC H5 HCC

S06.8 Other specified intracranial injuries

S06.81 Injury of right internal carotid artery, intracranial portion, not elsewhere classified

S06.810 Injury of right internal carotid artery, intracranial portion, not elsewhere classified without loss of consciousness HCC

S06.811 Injury of right internal carotid artery, intracranial portion, not elsewhere classified with loss of consciousness of 30 minutes or less CC H5 HCC
Injury of right internal carotid artery, intracranial portion, not elsewhere classified with brief loss of consciousness

S06.812 Injury of right internal carotid artery, intracranial portion, not elsewhere classified with loss of consciousness of 31 minutes to 59 minutes CC H5 HCC

S06.813 Injury of right internal carotid artery, intracranial portion, not elsewhere classified with loss of consciousness of 1 hour to 5 hours 59 minutes CC H5 HCC

S06.814 Injury of right internal carotid artery, intracranial portion, not elsewhere classified with loss of consciousness of 6 hours to 24 hours CC H5 HCC

S06.815 Injury of right internal carotid artery, intracranial portion, not elsewhere classified with loss of consciousness greater than 24 hours with return to pre-existing conscious level CC H5 HCC

S06.816 Injury of right internal carotid artery, intracranial portion, not elsewhere classified with loss of consciousness greater than 24 hours without return to pre-existing conscious level with patient surviving MCC H5 HCC

S06.817 Injury of right internal carotid artery, intracranial portion, not elsewhere classified with loss of consciousness of any duration with death due to brain injury prior to regaining consciousness MCC H5

S06.818 Injury of right internal carotid artery, intracranial portion, not elsewhere classified with loss of consciousness of any duration with death due to other cause prior to regaining consciousness MCC H5

S06.81A Injury of right internal carotid artery, intracranial portion, not elsewhere classified with loss of consciousness status unknown CC H5 HCC
Injury of right internal carotid artery, intracranial portion, not elsewhere classified NOS

S06.819 Injury of right internal carotid artery, intracranial portion, not elsewhere classified with loss of consciousness of unspecified duration CC H5 HCC

S06.82 Injury of left internal carotid artery, intracranial portion, not elsewhere classified

S06.820 Injury of left internal carotid artery, intracranial portion, not elsewhere classified without loss of consciousness HCC

S06.821 Injury of left internal carotid artery, intracranial portion, not elsewhere classified with loss of consciousness of 30 minutes or less CC H5 HCC
Injury of left internal carotid artery, intracranial portion, not elsewhere classified with brief loss of consciousness

S06.822 Injury of left internal carotid artery, intracranial portion, not elsewhere classified with loss of consciousness of 31 minutes to 59 minutes CC H5 HCC

S06.823 Injury of left internal carotid artery, intracranial portion, not elsewhere classified with loss of consciousness of 1 hour to 5 hours 59 minutes CC H5 HCC

S06.824 Injury of left internal carotid artery, intracranial portion, not elsewhere classified with loss of consciousness of 6 hours to 24 hours CC H5 HCC

S06.825 Injury of left internal carotid artery, intracranial portion, not elsewhere classified with loss of consciousness greater than 24 hours with return to pre-existing conscious level CC H5 HCC

S06.826 Injury of left internal carotid artery, intracranial portion, not elsewhere classified with loss of consciousness greater than 24 hours without return to pre-existing conscious level with patient surviving MCC H5 HCC

S06.827 Injury of left internal carotid artery, intracranial portion, not elsewhere classified with loss of consciousness of any duration with death due to brain injury prior to regaining consciousness MCC H5

S06.828 Injury of left internal carotid artery, intracranial portion, not elsewhere classified with loss of consciousness of any duration with death due to other cause prior to regaining consciousness MCC H5

S06.82A Injury of left internal carotid artery, intracranial portion, not elsewhere classified with loss of consciousness status unknown CC H5 HCC
Injury of left internal carotid artery, intracranial portion, not elsewhere classified NOS

S06.829 Injury of left internal carotid artery, intracranial portion, not elsewhere classified with loss of consciousness of unspecified duration CC H5 HCC

S06.8A Primary blast injury of brain, not elsewhere classified
Code also, if applicable, focal traumatic brain injury (S06.3-)
EXCLUDES 2 *traumatic cerebral edema (S06.1)*

S06.8A0 Primary blast injury of brain, not elsewhere classified without loss of consciousness CC H5 HCC

S06.8A1 Primary blast injury of brain, not elsewhere classified with loss of consciousness of 30 minutes or less CC H5 HCC
Primary blast injury of brain, not elsewhere classified with brief loss of consciousness

S06.8A2 Primary blast injury of brain, not elsewhere classified with loss of consciousness of 31 minutes to 59 minutes CC H5 HCC

S06.8A3 Primary blast injury of brain, not elsewhere classified with loss of consciousness of 1 hour to 5 hours 59 minutes CC H5 HCC

S06.8A4 Primary blast injury of brain, not elsewhere classified with loss of consciousness of 6 hours to 24 hours CC H5 HCC

√7th **S06.8A5 Primary blast injury of brain, not elsewhere classified with loss of consciousness greater than 24 hours with return to pre-existing conscious level** CC H5 HCC

√7th **S06.8A6 Primary blast injury of brain, not elsewhere classified with loss of consciousness greater than 24 hours without return to pre-existing conscious level with patient surviving** MCC H5 HCC

√7th **S06.8A7 Primary blast injury of brain, not elsewhere classified with loss of consciousness of any duration with death due to brain injury prior to regaining consciousness** MCC H5

√7th **S06.8A8 Primary blast injury of brain, not elsewhere classified with loss of consciousness of any duration with death due to other cause prior to regaining consciousness** MCC H5

√7th **S06.8AA Primary blast injury of brain, not elsewhere classified with loss of consciousness status unknown** CC H5 HCC
Primary blast injury of brain NOS

√7th **S06.8A9 Primary blast injury of brain, not elsewhere classified with loss of consciousness of unspecified duration** CC H5 HCC

√6th **S06.89 Other specified intracranial injury**
EXCLUDES 1 *concussion (S06.0X-)*

√7th **S06.890 Other specified intracranial injury without loss of consciousness** HCC

√7th **S06.891 Other specified intracranial injury with loss of consciousness of 30 minutes or less** CC H5 HCC
Other specified intracranial injury with brief loss of consciousness

√7th **S06.892 Other specified intracranial injury with loss of consciousness of 31 minutes to 59 minutes** CC H5 HCC

√7th **S06.893 Other specified intracranial injury with loss of consciousness of 1 hour to 5 hours 59 minutes** CC H5 HCC

√7th **S06.894 Other specified intracranial injury with loss of consciousness of 6 hours to 24 hours** CC H5 HCC

√7th **S06.895 Other specified intracranial injury with loss of consciousness greater than 24 hours with return to pre-existing conscious level** CC H5 HCC

√7th **S06.896 Other specified intracranial injury with loss of consciousness greater than 24 hours without return to pre-existing conscious level with patient surviving** MCC H5 HCC

√7th **S06.897 Other specified intracranial injury with loss of consciousness of any duration with death due to brain injury prior to regaining consciousness** MCC H5

√7th **S06.898 Other specified intracranial injury with loss of consciousness of any duration with death due to other cause prior to regaining consciousness** MCC H5

√7th **S06.89A Other specified intracranial injury with loss of consciousness status unknown** CC H5 HCC

√7th **S06.899 Other specified intracranial injury with loss of consciousness of unspecified duration** CC H5 HCC

√5th **S06.9 Unspecified intracranial injury**
Brain injury NOS
Head injury NOS with loss of consciousness
Traumatic brain injury NOS
EXCLUDES 1 *conditions classifiable to S06.0- to S06.8- code to specified intracranial injury*
head injury NOS (S09.90)
AHA: 2020,3Q,46; 2020,2Q,31
TIP: Assign additional code(s) for individual (R40.21-, R40.22-, R40.23-) or total (R40.24-) coma scale scores. It is appropriate to code the coma scale scores based on documentation provided by clinicians who are not the patient's provider (such as emergency medical technician).

√6th **S06.9X Unspecified intracranial injury**

√7th **S06.9X0 Unspecified intracranial injury without loss of consciousness** HCC

√7th **S06.9X1 Unspecified intracranial injury with loss of consciousness of 30 minutes or less** CC H5 HCC
Unspecified intracranial injury with brief loss of consciousness

√7th **S06.9X2 Unspecified intracranial injury with loss of consciousness of 31 minutes to 59 minutes** CC H5 HCC

√7th **S06.9X3 Unspecified intracranial injury with loss of consciousness of 1 hour to 5 hours 59 minutes** CC H5 HCC

√7th **S06.9X4 Unspecified intracranial injury with loss of consciousness of 6 hours to 24 hours** CC H5 HCC

√7th **S06.9X5 Unspecified intracranial injury with loss of consciousness greater than 24 hours with return to pre-existing conscious level** CC H5 HCC

√7th **S06.9X6 Unspecified intracranial injury with loss of consciousness greater than 24 hours without return to pre-existing conscious level with patient surviving** MCC H5 HCC

√7th **S06.9X7 Unspecified intracranial injury with loss of consciousness of any duration with death due to brain injury prior to regaining consciousness** MCC H5

√7th **S06.9X8 Unspecified intracranial injury with loss of consciousness of any duration with death due to other cause prior to regaining consciousness** MCC H5

√7th **S06.9XA Unspecified intracranial injury with loss of consciousness status unknown** CC H5 HCC

√7th **S06.9X9 Unspecified intracranial injury with loss of consciousness of unspecified duration** CC H5 HCC

√5th **S06.A Traumatic brain compression and herniation**
Traumatic cerebral compression
Code first the underlying traumatic brain injury, such as:
diffuse traumatic brain injury (S06.2-)
focal traumatic brain injury (S06.3-)
traumatic subarachnoid hemorrhage (S06.6-)
traumatic subdural hemorrhage (S06.5-)
AHA: 2021,4Q,29

√x7th **S06.A0 Traumatic brain compression without herniation** MCC UPD HCC
Traumatic brain compression NOS
Traumatic cerebral compression NOS

√x7th **S06.A1 Traumatic brain compression with herniation** MCC UPD HCC
Traumatic brain herniation
Traumatic brainstem compression with herniation
Traumatic cerebellar compression with herniation
Traumatic cerebral compression with herniation

S07 Crushing injury of head

Use additional code for all associated injuries, such as:
intracranial injuries (S06.-)
skull fractures (S02.-)

The appropriate 7th character is to be added to each code from category S07.
A initial encounter
D subsequent encounter
S sequela

S07.0 Crushing injury of face CC HS

S07.1 Crushing injury of skull CC HS

S07.8 Crushing injury of other parts of head CC HS

S07.9 Crushing injury of head, part unspecified CC HS

S08 Avulsion and traumatic amputation of part of head

An amputation not identified as partial or complete should be coded to complete

The appropriate 7th character is to be added to each code from category S08.
A initial encounter
D subsequent encounter
S sequela

S08.0 Avulsion of scalp

S08.1 Traumatic amputation of ear

S08.11 Complete traumatic amputation of ear

S08.111 Complete traumatic amputation of right ear

S08.112 Complete traumatic amputation of left ear

S08.119 Complete traumatic amputation of unspecified ear

S08.12 Partial traumatic amputation of ear

S08.121 Partial traumatic amputation of right ear

S08.122 Partial traumatic amputation of left ear

S08.129 Partial traumatic amputation of unspecified ear

S08.8 Traumatic amputation of other parts of head

S08.81 Traumatic amputation of nose

S08.811 Complete traumatic amputation of nose

S08.812 Partial traumatic amputation of nose

S08.89 Traumatic amputation of other parts of head

S09 Other and unspecified injuries of head

The appropriate 7th character is to be added to each code from category S09.
A initial encounter
D subsequent encounter
S sequela

S09.0 Injury of blood vessels of head, not elsewhere classified CC

EXCLUDES 1 *injury of cerebral blood vessels (S06.-)*
injury of precerebral blood vessels (S15.-)

S09.1 Injury of muscle and tendon of head

Code also any associated open wound (S01.-)

EXCLUDES 2 *sprain to joints and ligament of head (S03.9)*

S09.10 Unspecified injury of muscle and tendon of head

Injury of muscle and tendon of head NOS

S09.11 Strain of muscle and tendon of head

S09.12 Laceration of muscle and tendon of head

S09.19 Other specified injury of muscle and tendon of head

S09.2 Traumatic rupture of ear drum

EXCLUDES 1 *traumatic rupture of ear drum due to blast injury (S09.31-)*

S09.20 Traumatic rupture of unspecified ear drum CC UNS

S09.21 Traumatic rupture of right ear drum CC

S09.22 Traumatic rupture of left ear drum CC

S09.3 Other specified and unspecified injury of middle and inner ear

EXCLUDES 1 *injury to ear NOS (S09.91-)*

EXCLUDES 2 *injury to external ear (S00.4-, S01.3-, S08.1-)*

S09.30 Unspecified injury of middle and inner ear

S09.301 Unspecified injury of right middle and inner ear CC

S09.302 Unspecified injury of left middle and inner ear CC

S09.309 Unspecified injury of unspecified middle and inner ear CC UNS

S09.31 Primary blast injury of ear

Blast injury of ear NOS

S09.311 Primary blast injury of right ear CC

S09.312 Primary blast injury of left ear CC

S09.313 Primary blast injury of ear, bilateral CC

S09.319 Primary blast injury of unspecified ear CC UNS

S09.39 Other specified injury of middle and inner ear

Secondary blast injury to ear

S09.391 Other specified injury of right middle and inner ear CC

S09.392 Other specified injury of left middle and inner ear CC

S09.399 Other specified injury of unspecified middle and inner ear CC UNS

S09.8 Other specified injuries of head

S09.9 Unspecified injury of face and head

S09.90 Unspecified injury of head

Head injury NOS

EXCLUDES 1 *brain injury NOS (S06.9-)*
head injury NOS with loss of consciousness (S06.9-)
intracranial injury NOS (S06.9-)

S09.91 Unspecified injury of ear

Injury of ear NOS

S09.92 Unspecified injury of nose

Injury of nose NOS

S09.93 Unspecified injury of face

Injury of face NOS

AHA: 2019,2Q,23

Injuries to the neck (S10-S19)

INCLUDES injuries of nape
injuries of supraclavicular region
injuries of throat

EXCLUDES 2 *burns and corrosions (T20-T32)*
effects of foreign body in esophagus (T18.1)
effects of foreign body in larynx (T17.3)
effects of foreign body in pharynx (T17.2)
effects of foreign body in trachea (T17.4)
frostbite (T33-T34)
insect bite or sting, venomous (T63.4)

S10 Superficial injury of neck

The appropriate 7th character is to be added to each code from category S10.
A initial encounter
D subsequent encounter
S sequela

S10.0 Contusion of throat

Contusion of cervical esophagus
Contusion of larynx
Contusion of pharynx
Contusion of trachea

S10.1 Other and unspecified superficial injuries of throat

S10.10 Unspecified superficial injuries of throat

S10.11 Abrasion of throat

S10.12 Blister (nonthermal) of throat

S10.14 External constriction of part of throat

S10.15 Superficial foreign body of throat

Splinter in the throat

S10.16 Insect bite (nonvenomous) of throat

S10.17 Other superficial bite of throat

EXCLUDES 1 *open bite of throat (S11.85)*

✓5th **S10.8 Superficial injury of other specified parts of neck**
- ✓x7th **S10.80 Unspecified superficial injury of other specified part of neck**
- ✓x7th **S10.81 Abrasion of other specified part of neck**
- ✓x7th **S10.82 Blister (nonthermal) of other specified part of neck**
- ✓x7th **S10.83 Contusion of other specified part of neck**
- ✓x7th **S10.84 External constriction of other specified part of neck**
- ✓x7th **S10.85 Superficial foreign body of other specified part of neck**
  - Splinter in other specified part of neck
- ✓x7th **S10.86 Insect bite of other specified part of neck**
- ✓x7th **S10.87 Other superficial bite of other specified part of neck**
  - EXCLUDES 1 *open bite of other specified parts of neck (S11.85)*

✓5th **S10.9 Superficial injury of unspecified part of neck**
- ✓x7th **S10.90 Unspecified superficial injury of unspecified part of neck**
- ✓x7th **S10.91 Abrasion of unspecified part of neck**
- ✓x7th **S10.92 Blister (nonthermal) of unspecified part of neck**
- ✓x7th **S10.93 Contusion of unspecified part of neck**
- ✓x7th **S10.94 External constriction of unspecified part of neck**
- ✓x7th **S10.95 Superficial foreign body of unspecified part of neck**
- ✓x7th **S10.96 Insect bite of unspecified part of neck**
- ✓x7th **S10.97 Other superficial bite of unspecified part of neck**

✓4th **S11 Open wound of neck**

Code also any associated:
- spinal cord injury (S14.0, S14.1-)
- wound infection

EXCLUDES 2 *open fracture of vertebra (S12.- with 7th character B)*

The appropriate 7th character is to be added to each code from category S11.
- A initial encounter
- D subsequent encounter
- S sequela

✓5th **S11.0 Open wound of larynx and trachea**
- ✓6th **S11.01 Open wound of larynx**
  - EXCLUDES 2 *open wound of vocal cord (S11.03)*
  - ✓7th **S11.011 Laceration without foreign body of larynx** MCC
  - ✓7th **S11.012 Laceration with foreign body of larynx** MCC
  - ✓7th **S11.013 Puncture wound without foreign body of larynx** MCC
  - ✓7th **S11.014 Puncture wound with foreign body of larynx** MCC
  - ✓7th **S11.015 Open bite of larynx** MCC
    - Bite of larynx NOS
  - ✓7th **S11.019 Unspecified open wound of larynx** MCC
- ✓6th **S11.02 Open wound of trachea**
  - Open wound of cervical trachea
  - Open wound of trachea NOS
  - EXCLUDES 2 *open wound of thoracic trachea (S27.5-)*
  - ✓7th **S11.021 Laceration without foreign body of trachea** MCC
  - ✓7th **S11.022 Laceration with foreign body of trachea** MCC
  - ✓7th **S11.023 Puncture wound without foreign body of trachea** MCC
  - ✓7th **S11.024 Puncture wound with foreign body of trachea** MCC
  - ✓7th **S11.025 Open bite of trachea** MCC
    - Bite of trachea NOS
  - ✓7th **S11.029 Unspecified open wound of trachea** MCC
- ✓6th **S11.03 Open wound of vocal cord**
  - ✓7th **S11.031 Laceration without foreign body of vocal cord** MCC
  - ✓7th **S11.032 Laceration with foreign body of vocal cord** MCC
  - ✓7th **S11.033 Puncture wound without foreign body of vocal cord** MCC
  - ✓7th **S11.034 Puncture wound with foreign body of vocal cord** MCC
  - ✓7th **S11.035 Open bite of vocal cord** MCC
    - Bite of vocal cord NOS
  - ✓7th **S11.039 Unspecified open wound of vocal cord** MCC

✓5th **S11.1 Open wound of thyroid gland**
- ✓x7th **S11.10 Unspecified open wound of thyroid gland** CC
- ✓x7th **S11.11 Laceration without foreign body of thyroid gland** CC
- ✓x7th **S11.12 Laceration with foreign body of thyroid gland** CC
- ✓x7th **S11.13 Puncture wound without foreign body of thyroid gland** CC
- ✓x7th **S11.14 Puncture wound with foreign body of thyroid gland** CC
- ✓x7th **S11.15 Open bite of thyroid gland** CC
  - Bite of thyroid gland NOS

✓5th **S11.2 Open wound of pharynx and cervical esophagus**
- EXCLUDES 1 *open wound of esophagus NOS (S27.8-)*
- ✓x7th **S11.20 Unspecified open wound of pharynx and cervical esophagus** CC
- ✓x7th **S11.21 Laceration without foreign body of pharynx and cervical esophagus** CC
- ✓x7th **S11.22 Laceration with foreign body of pharynx and cervical esophagus** CC
- ✓x7th **S11.23 Puncture wound without foreign body of pharynx and cervical esophagus** CC
- ✓x7th **S11.24 Puncture wound with foreign body of pharynx and cervical esophagus** CC
- ✓x7th **S11.25 Open bite of pharynx and cervical esophagus** CC
  - Bite of pharynx and cervical esophagus NOS

✓5th **S11.8 Open wound of other specified parts of neck**
- ✓x7th **S11.80 Unspecified open wound of other specified part of neck**
- ✓x7th **S11.81 Laceration without foreign body of other specified part of neck**
- ✓x7th **S11.82 Laceration with foreign body of other specified part of neck**
- ✓x7th **S11.83 Puncture wound without foreign body of other specified part of neck**
- ✓x7th **S11.84 Puncture wound with foreign body of other specified part of neck**
- ✓x7th **S11.85 Open bite of other specified part of neck**
  - Bite of other specified part of neck NOS
  - EXCLUDES 1 *superficial bite of other specified part of neck (S10.87)*
- ✓x7th **S11.89 Other open wound of other specified part of neck**

✓5th **S11.9 Open wound of unspecified part of neck**
- ✓x7th **S11.90 Unspecified open wound of unspecified part of neck**
- ✓x7th **S11.91 Laceration without foreign body of unspecified part of neck**
- ✓x7th **S11.92 Laceration with foreign body of unspecified part of neck**
- ✓x7th **S11.93 Puncture wound without foreign body of unspecified part of neck**
- ✓x7th **S11.94 Puncture wound with foreign body of unspecified part of neck**
- ✓x7th **S11.95 Open bite of unspecified part of neck**
  - Bite of neck NOS
  - EXCLUDES 1 *superficial bite of neck (S10.97)*

S12 Fracture of cervical vertebra and other parts of neck

NOTE A fracture not indicated as displaced or nondisplaced should be coded to displaced.

A fracture not indicated as open or closed should be coded to closed.

INCLUDES fracture of cervical neural arch
fracture of cervical spine
fracture of cervical spinous process
fracture of cervical transverse process
fracture of cervical vertebral arch
fracture of neck

Code first any associated cervical spinal cord injury (S14.Ø, S14.1-)

AHA: 2021,1Q,6; 2018,2Q,12; 2015,3Q,37-39

The appropriate 7th character is to be added to all codes from subcategories S12.Ø-S12.6.
A initial encounter for closed fracture
B initial encounter for open fracture
D subsequent encounter for fracture with routine healing
G subsequent encounter for fracture with delayed healing
K subsequent encounter for fracture with nonunion
S sequela

S12.Ø Fracture of first cervical vertebra
Atlas

S12.ØØ Unspecified fracture of first cervical vertebra
- **S12.ØØØ Unspecified displaced fracture of first cervical vertebra** MCC CC H5 HCC
- **S12.ØØ1 Unspecified nondisplaced fracture of first cervical vertebra** MCC CC H5 HCC

S12.Ø1 Stable burst fracture of first cervical vertebra MCC CC H5 HCC

S12.Ø2 Unstable burst fracture of first cervical vertebra MCC CC H5 HCC

S12.Ø3 Posterior arch fracture of first cervical vertebra
- **S12.Ø3Ø Displaced posterior arch fracture of first cervical vertebra** MCC CC H5 HCC
- **S12.Ø31 Nondisplaced posterior arch fracture of first cervical vertebra** MCC CC H5 HCC

S12.Ø4 Lateral mass fracture of first cervical vertebra
- **S12.Ø4Ø Displaced lateral mass fracture of first cervical vertebra** MCC CC H5 HCC
- **S12.Ø41 Nondisplaced lateral mass fracture of first cervical vertebra** MCC CC H5 HCC

S12.Ø9 Other fracture of first cervical vertebra
- **S12.Ø9Ø Other displaced fracture of first cervical vertebra** MCC CC H5 HCC
- **S12.Ø91 Other nondisplaced fracture of first cervical vertebra** MCC CC H5 HCC

S12.1 Fracture of second cervical vertebra
Axis

S12.1Ø Unspecified fracture of second cervical vertebra
- **S12.1ØØ Unspecified displaced fracture of second cervical vertebra** MCC CC H5 HCC
- **S12.1Ø1 Unspecified nondisplaced fracture of second cervical vertebra** MCC CC H5 HCC

S12.11 Type II dens fracture
- **S12.11Ø Anterior displaced Type II dens fracture** MCC CC H5 HCC
- **S12.111 Posterior displaced Type II dens fracture** MCC CC H5 HCC
- **S12.112 Nondisplaced Type II dens fracture** MCC CC H5 HCC

S12.12 Other dens fracture
- **S12.12Ø Other displaced dens fracture** MCC CC H5 HCC
- **S12.121 Other nondisplaced dens fracture** MCC CC H5 HCC

S12.13 Unspecified traumatic spondylolisthesis of second cervical vertebra
- **S12.13Ø Unspecified traumatic displaced spondylolisthesis of second cervical vertebra** MCC CC H5 HCC
- **S12.131 Unspecified traumatic nondisplaced spondylolisthesis of second cervical vertebra** MCC CC H5 HCC

S12.14 Type III traumatic spondylolisthesis of second cervical vertebra MCC CC H5 HCC

S12.15 Other traumatic spondylolisthesis of second cervical vertebra
- **S12.15Ø Other traumatic displaced spondylolisthesis of second cervical vertebra** MCC CC H5 HCC
- **S12.151 Other traumatic nondisplaced spondylolisthesis of second cervical vertebra** MCC CC H5 HCC

S12.19 Other fracture of second cervical vertebra
- **S12.19Ø Other displaced fracture of second cervical vertebra** MCC CC H5 HCC
- **S12.191 Other nondisplaced fracture of second cervical vertebra** MCC CC H5 HCC

S12.2 Fracture of third cervical vertebra

S12.2Ø Unspecified fracture of third cervical vertebra
- **S12.2ØØ Unspecified displaced fracture of third cervical vertebra** MCC CC H5 HCC
- **S12.2Ø1 Unspecified nondisplaced fracture of third cervical vertebra** MCC CC H5 HCC

S12.23 Unspecified traumatic spondylolisthesis of third cervical vertebra
- **S12.23Ø Unspecified traumatic displaced spondylolisthesis of third cervical vertebra** MCC CC H5 HCC
- **S12.231 Unspecified traumatic nondisplaced spondylolisthesis of third cervical vertebra** MCC CC H5 HCC

S12.24 Type III traumatic spondylolisthesis of third cervical vertebra MCC CC H5 HCC

S12.25 Other traumatic spondylolisthesis of third cervical vertebra
- **S12.25Ø Other traumatic displaced spondylolisthesis of third cervical vertebra** MCC CC H5 HCC
- **S12.251 Other traumatic nondisplaced spondylolisthesis of third cervical vertebra** MCC CC H5 HCC

S12.29 Other fracture of third cervical vertebra
- **S12.29Ø Other displaced fracture of third cervical vertebra** MCC CC H5 HCC
- **S12.291 Other nondisplaced fracture of third cervical vertebra** MCC CC H5 HCC

S12.3 Fracture of fourth cervical vertebra

S12.3Ø Unspecified fracture of fourth cervical vertebra
- **S12.3ØØ Unspecified displaced fracture of fourth cervical vertebra** MCC CC H5 HCC
- **S12.3Ø1 Unspecified nondisplaced fracture of fourth cervical vertebra** MCC CC H5 HCC

S12.33 Unspecified traumatic spondylolisthesis of fourth cervical vertebra
- **S12.33Ø Unspecified traumatic displaced spondylolisthesis of fourth cervical vertebra** MCC CC H5 HCC
- **S12.331 Unspecified traumatic nondisplaced spondylolisthesis of fourth cervical vertebra** MCC CC H5 HCC

S12.34 Type III traumatic spondylolisthesis of fourth cervical vertebra MCC CC H5 HCC

S12.35 Other traumatic spondylolisthesis of fourth cervical vertebra
- **S12.35Ø Other traumatic displaced spondylolisthesis of fourth cervical vertebra** MCC CC H5 HCC
- **S12.351 Other traumatic nondisplaced spondylolisthesis of fourth cervical vertebra** MCC CC H5 HCC

S12.39 Other fracture of fourth cervical vertebra
- **S12.39Ø Other displaced fracture of fourth cervical vertebra** MCC CC H5 HCC
- **S12.391 Other nondisplaced fracture of fourth cervical vertebra** MCC CC H5 HCC

S12.4 Fracture of fifth cervical vertebra

S12.4Ø Unspecified fracture of fifth cervical vertebra
- **S12.4ØØ Unspecified displaced fracture of fifth cervical vertebra** MCC CC H5 HCC
- **S12.4Ø1 Unspecified nondisplaced fracture of fifth cervical vertebra** MCC CC H5 HCC

√6th **S12.43 Unspecified traumatic spondylolisthesis of fifth cervical vertebra**

√7th **S12.430 Unspecified traumatic displaced spondylolisthesis of fifth cervical vertebra** MCC CC HS HCC

√7th **S12.431 Unspecified traumatic nondisplaced spondylolisthesis of fifth cervical vertebra** MCC CC HS HCC

√x7th **S12.44 Type III traumatic spondylolisthesis of fifth cervical vertebra** MCC CC HS HCC

√6th **S12.45 Other traumatic spondylolisthesis of fifth cervical vertebra**

√7th **S12.450 Other traumatic displaced spondylolisthesis of fifth cervical vertebra** MCC CC HS HCC

√7th **S12.451 Other traumatic nondisplaced spondylolisthesis of fifth cervical vertebra** MCC CC HS HCC

√6th **S12.49 Other fracture of fifth cervical vertebra**

√7th **S12.490 Other displaced fracture of fifth cervical vertebra** MCC CC HS HCC

√7th **S12.491 Other nondisplaced fracture of fifth cervical vertebra** MCC CC HS HCC

√5th **S12.5 Fracture of sixth cervical vertebra**

√6th **S12.50 Unspecified fracture of sixth cervical vertebra**

√7th **S12.500 Unspecified displaced fracture of sixth cervical vertebra** MCC CC HS HCC

√7th **S12.501 Unspecified nondisplaced fracture of sixth cervical vertebra** MCC CC HS HCC

√6th **S12.53 Unspecified traumatic spondylolisthesis of sixth cervical vertebra**

√7th **S12.530 Unspecified traumatic displaced spondylolisthesis of sixth cervical vertebra** MCC CC HS HCC

√7th **S12.531 Unspecified traumatic nondisplaced spondylolisthesis of sixth cervical vertebra** MCC CC HS HCC

√x7th **S12.54 Type III traumatic spondylolisthesis of sixth cervical vertebra** MCC CC HS HCC

√6th **S12.55 Other traumatic spondylolisthesis of sixth cervical vertebra**

√7th **S12.550 Other traumatic displaced spondylolisthesis of sixth cervical vertebra** MCC CC HS HCC

√7th **S12.551 Other traumatic nondisplaced spondylolisthesis of sixth cervical vertebra** MCC CC HS HCC

√6th **S12.59 Other fracture of sixth cervical vertebra**

√7th **S12.590 Other displaced fracture of sixth cervical vertebra** MCC CC HS HCC

√7th **S12.591 Other nondisplaced fracture of sixth cervical vertebra** MCC CC HS HCC

√5th **S12.6 Fracture of seventh cervical vertebra**

√6th **S12.60 Unspecified fracture of seventh cervical vertebra**

√7th **S12.600 Unspecified displaced fracture of seventh cervical vertebra** MCC CC HS HCC

√7th **S12.601 Unspecified nondisplaced fracture of seventh cervical vertebra** MCC CC HS HCC

√6th **S12.63 Unspecified traumatic spondylolisthesis of seventh cervical vertebra**

√7th **S12.630 Unspecified traumatic displaced spondylolisthesis of seventh cervical vertebra** MCC CC HS HCC

√7th **S12.631 Unspecified traumatic nondisplaced spondylolisthesis of seventh cervical vertebra** MCC CC HS HCC

√x7th **S12.64 Type III traumatic spondylolisthesis of seventh cervical vertebra** MCC CC HS HCC

√6th **S12.65 Other traumatic spondylolisthesis of seventh cervical vertebra**

√7th **S12.650 Other traumatic displaced spondylolisthesis of seventh cervical vertebra** MCC CC HS HCC

√7th **S12.651 Other traumatic nondisplaced spondylolisthesis of seventh cervical vertebra** MCC CC HS HCC

√6th **S12.69 Other fracture of seventh cervical vertebra**

√7th **S12.690 Other displaced fracture of seventh cervical vertebra** MCC CC HS HCC

√7th **S12.691 Other nondisplaced fracture of seventh cervical vertebra** MCC CC HS HCC

√x7th **S12.8 Fracture of other parts of neck** MCC HS HCC

Hyoid bone
Larynx
Thyroid cartilage
Trachea

The appropriate 7th character is to be added to code S12.8.
A initial encounter
D subsequent encounter
S sequela

√x7th **S12.9 Fracture of neck, unspecified** CC HS HCC

Fracture of neck NOS
Fracture of cervical spine NOS
Fracture of cervical vertebra NOS

The appropriate 7th character is to be added to code S12.9.
A initial encounter
D subsequent encounter
S sequela

√4th **S13 Dislocation and sprain of joints and ligaments at neck level**

INCLUDES avulsion of joint or ligament at neck level
laceration of cartilage, joint or ligament at neck level
sprain of cartilage, joint or ligament at neck level
traumatic hemarthrosis of joint or ligament at neck level
traumatic rupture of joint or ligament at neck level
traumatic subluxation of joint or ligament at neck level
traumatic tear of joint or ligament at neck level

Code also any associated open wound

EXCLUDES 2 *strain of muscle or tendon at neck level (S16.1)*

The appropriate 7th character is to be added to each code from category S13.
A initial encounter
D subsequent encounter
S sequela

√x7th **S13.0 Traumatic rupture of cervical intervertebral disc** CC HS

EXCLUDES 1 *rupture or displacement (nontraumatic) of cervical intervertebral disc NOS (M50.-)*

√5th **S13.1 Subluxation and dislocation of cervical vertebrae**

Code also any associated:
open wound of neck (S11.-)
spinal cord injury (S14.1-)

EXCLUDES 2 *fracture of cervical vertebrae (S12.0-S12.3-)*

√6th **S13.10 Subluxation and dislocation of unspecified cervical vertebrae**

√7th **S13.100 Subluxation of unspecified cervical vertebrae** CC HS

√7th **S13.101 Dislocation of unspecified cervical vertebrae** CC HS

√6th **S13.11 Subluxation and dislocation of C0/C1 cervical vertebrae**

Subluxation and dislocation of atlantooccipital joint
Subluxation and dislocation of atloidooccipital joint
Subluxation and dislocation of occipitoatloid joint

√7th **S13.110 Subluxation of C0/C1 cervical vertebrae** CC HS

√7th **S13.111 Dislocation of C0/C1 cervical vertebrae** CC HS

√6th **S13.12 Subluxation and dislocation of C1/C2 cervical vertebrae**

Subluxation and dislocation of atlantoaxial joint

√7th **S13.120 Subluxation of C1/C2 cervical vertebrae** CC HS

√7th **S13.121 Dislocation of C1/C2 cervical vertebrae** CC HS

√6th **S13.13 Subluxation and dislocation of C2/C3 cervical vertebrae**

√7th **S13.130 Subluxation of C2/C3 cervical vertebrae** CC HS

√7th **S13.131 Dislocation of C2/C3 cervical vertebrae** CC HS

√6th **S13.14 Subluxation and dislocation of C3/C4 cervical vertebrae**

√7th **S13.140 Subluxation of C3/C4 cervical vertebrae** CC HS

√7th **S13.141 Dislocation of C3/C4 cervical vertebrae** CC HS

S13.15 Subluxation and dislocation of C4/C5 cervical vertebrae
S13.150 Subluxation of C4/C5 cervical vertebrae CC H5
S13.151 Dislocation of C4/C5 cervical vertebrae CC H5
S13.16 Subluxation and dislocation of C5/C6 cervical vertebrae
S13.160 Subluxation of C5/C6 cervical vertebrae CC H5
S13.161 Dislocation of C5/C6 cervical vertebrae CC H5
S13.17 Subluxation and dislocation of C6/C7 cervical vertebrae
S13.170 Subluxation of C6/C7 cervical vertebrae CC H5
S13.171 Dislocation of C6/C7 cervical vertebrae CC H5
S13.18 Subluxation and dislocation of C7/T1 cervical vertebrae
S13.180 Subluxation of C7/T1 cervical vertebrae CC H5
S13.181 Dislocation of C7/T1 cervical vertebrae CC H5
S13.2 Dislocation of other and unspecified parts of neck
S13.20 Dislocation of unspecified parts of neck CC H5
S13.29 Dislocation of other parts of neck CC H5
S13.4 Sprain of ligaments of cervical spine
Sprain of anterior longitudinal (ligament), cervical
Sprain of atlanto-axial (joints)
Sprain of atlanto-occipital (joints)
Whiplash injury of cervical spine
S13.5 Sprain of thyroid region
Sprain of cricoarytenoid (joint) (ligament)
Sprain of cricothyroid (joint) (ligament)
Sprain of thyroid cartilage
S13.8 Sprain of joints and ligaments of other parts of neck
S13.9 Sprain of joints and ligaments of unspecified parts of neck

S14 Injury of nerves and spinal cord at neck level

NOTE Code to highest level of cervical cord injury

Code also any associated:
fracture of cervical vertebra (S12.0- — S12.6.-)
open wound of neck (S11.-)
transient paralysis (R29.5)

The appropriate 7th character is to be added to each code from category S14.
A initial encounter
D subsequent encounter
S sequela

S14.0 Concussion and edema of cervical spinal cord MCC HCC
S14.1 Other and unspecified injuries of cervical spinal cord
S14.10 Unspecified injury of cervical spinal cord
S14.101 Unspecified injury at C1 level of cervical spinal cord MCC H5 HCC
S14.102 Unspecified injury at C2 level of cervical spinal cord MCC H5 HCC
S14.103 Unspecified injury at C3 level of cervical spinal cord MCC H5 HCC
S14.104 Unspecified injury at C4 level of cervical spinal cord MCC H5 HCC
S14.105 Unspecified injury at C5 level of cervical spinal cord MCC H5 HCC
S14.106 Unspecified injury at C6 level of cervical spinal cord MCC H5 HCC
S14.107 Unspecified injury at C7 level of cervical spinal cord MCC H5 HCC
S14.108 Unspecified injury at C8 level of cervical spinal cord MCC HCC
S14.109 Unspecified injury at unspecified level of cervical spinal cord HCC
Injury of cervical spinal cord NOS
S14.11 Complete lesion of cervical spinal cord
S14.111 Complete lesion at C1 level of cervical spinal cord MCC H5 HCC
S14.112 Complete lesion at C2 level of cervical spinal cord MCC H5 HCC
S14.113 Complete lesion at C3 level of cervical spinal cord MCC H5 HCC
S14.114 Complete lesion at C4 level of cervical spinal cord MCC H5 HCC
S14.115 Complete lesion at C5 level of cervical spinal cord MCC H5 HCC
S14.116 Complete lesion at C6 level of cervical spinal cord MCC H5 HCC
S14.117 Complete lesion at C7 level of cervical spinal cord MCC H5 HCC
S14.118 Complete lesion at C8 level of cervical spinal cord MCC HCC
S14.119 Complete lesion at unspecified level of cervical spinal cord HCC
S14.12 Central cord syndrome of cervical spinal cord
S14.121 Central cord syndrome at C1 level of cervical spinal cord MCC H5 HCC
S14.122 Central cord syndrome at C2 level of cervical spinal cord MCC H5 HCC
S14.123 Central cord syndrome at C3 level of cervical spinal cord MCC H5 HCC
S14.124 Central cord syndrome at C4 level of cervical spinal cord MCC H5 HCC
S14.125 Central cord syndrome at C5 level of cervical spinal cord MCC H5 HCC
S14.126 Central cord syndrome at C6 level of cervical spinal cord MCC H5 HCC
S14.127 Central cord syndrome at C7 level of cervical spinal cord MCC H5 HCC
S14.128 Central cord syndrome at C8 level of cervical spinal cord MCC HCC
S14.129 Central cord syndrome at unspecified level of cervical spinal cord HCC
S14.13 Anterior cord syndrome of cervical spinal cord
S14.131 Anterior cord syndrome at C1 level of cervical spinal cord MCC H5 HCC
S14.132 Anterior cord syndrome at C2 level of cervical spinal cord MCC H5 HCC
S14.133 Anterior cord syndrome at C3 level of cervical spinal cord MCC H5 HCC
S14.134 Anterior cord syndrome at C4 level of cervical spinal cord MCC H5 HCC
S14.135 Anterior cord syndrome at C5 level of cervical spinal cord MCC H5 HCC
S14.136 Anterior cord syndrome at C6 level of cervical spinal cord MCC H5 HCC
S14.137 Anterior cord syndrome at C7 level of cervical spinal cord MCC H5 HCC
S14.138 Anterior cord syndrome at C8 level of cervical spinal cord MCC HCC
S14.139 Anterior cord syndrome at unspecified level of cervical spinal cord HCC
S14.14 Brown-Sequard syndrome of cervical spinal cord
S14.141 Brown-Sequard syndrome at C1 level of cervical spinal cord MCC HCC
S14.142 Brown-Sequard syndrome at C2 level of cervical spinal cord MCC HCC
S14.143 Brown-Sequard syndrome at C3 level of cervical spinal cord MCC HCC
S14.144 Brown-Sequard syndrome at C4 level of cervical spinal cord MCC HCC
S14.145 Brown-Sequard syndrome at C5 level of cervical spinal cord MCC HCC
S14.146 Brown-Sequard syndrome at C6 level of cervical spinal cord MCC HCC
S14.147 Brown-Sequard syndrome at C7 level of cervical spinal cord MCC HCC
S14.148 Brown-Sequard syndrome at C8 level of cervical spinal cord MCC HCC
S14.149 Brown-Sequard syndrome at unspecified level of cervical spinal cord HCC
S14.15 Other incomplete lesions of cervical spinal cord
Incomplete lesion of cervical spinal cord NOS
Posterior cord syndrome of cervical spinal cord
S14.151 Other incomplete lesion at C1 level of cervical spinal cord MCC H5 HCC
S14.152 Other incomplete lesion at C2 level of cervical spinal cord MCC H5 HCC
S14.153 Other incomplete lesion at C3 level of cervical spinal cord MCC H5 HCC

√7th **S14.154 Other incomplete lesion at C4 level of cervical spinal cord** MCC H5 HCC

√7th **S14.155 Other incomplete lesion at C5 level of cervical spinal cord** MCC H5 HCC

√7th **S14.156 Other incomplete lesion at C6 level of cervical spinal cord** MCC H5 HCC

√7th **S14.157 Other incomplete lesion at C7 level of cervical spinal cord** MCC H5 HCC

√7th **S14.158 Other incomplete lesion at C8 level of cervical spinal cord** MCC HCC

√7th **S14.159 Other incomplete lesion at unspecified level of cervical spinal cord** HCC

√x7th **S14.2 Injury of nerve root of cervical spine**

√x7th **S14.3 Injury of brachial plexus**

√x7th **S14.4 Injury of peripheral nerves of neck**

√x7th **S14.5 Injury of cervical sympathetic nerves**

√x7th **S14.8 Injury of other specified nerves of neck**

√x7th **S14.9 Injury of unspecified nerves of neck**

√4th **S15 Injury of blood vessels at neck level**

Code also any associated open wound (S11.-)

The appropriate 7th character is to be added to each code from category S15.
A initial encounter
D subsequent encounter
S sequela

√5th **S15.Ø Injury of carotid artery of neck**

Injury of carotid artery (common) (external) (internal, extracranial portion)
Injury of carotid artery NOS

EXCLUDES 1 *injury of internal carotid artery, intracranial portion (SØ6.8)*

√6th **S15.ØØ Unspecified injury of carotid artery**

√7th **S15.ØØ1 Unspecified injury of right carotid artery** CC

√7th **S15.ØØ2 Unspecified injury of left carotid artery** CC

√7th **S15.ØØ9 Unspecified injury of unspecified carotid artery** CC UNS

√6th **S15.Ø1 Minor laceration of carotid artery**

Incomplete transection of carotid artery
Laceration of carotid artery NOS
Superficial laceration of carotid artery

√7th **S15.Ø11 Minor laceration of right carotid artery** CC

√7th **S15.Ø12 Minor laceration of left carotid artery** CC

√7th **S15.Ø19 Minor laceration of unspecified carotid artery** CC UNS

√6th **S15.Ø2 Major laceration of carotid artery**

Complete transection of carotid artery
Traumatic rupture of carotid artery

√7th **S15.Ø21 Major laceration of right carotid artery** CC

√7th **S15.Ø22 Major laceration of left carotid artery** CC

√7th **S15.Ø29 Major laceration of unspecified carotid artery** CC UNS

√6th **S15.Ø9 Other specified injury of carotid artery**

√7th **S15.Ø91 Other specified injury of right carotid artery** CC

√7th **S15.Ø92 Other specified injury of left carotid artery** CC

√7th **S15.Ø99 Other specified injury of unspecified carotid artery** CC UNS

√5th **S15.1 Injury of vertebral artery**

√6th **S15.1Ø Unspecified injury of vertebral artery**

√7th **S15.1Ø1 Unspecified injury of right vertebral artery** CC

√7th **S15.1Ø2 Unspecified injury of left vertebral artery** CC

√7th **S15.1Ø9 Unspecified injury of unspecified vertebral artery** CC UNS

√6th **S15.11 Minor laceration of vertebral artery**

Incomplete transection of vertebral artery
Laceration of vertebral artery NOS
Superficial laceration of vertebral artery

√7th **S15.111 Minor laceration of right vertebral artery** CC

√7th **S15.112 Minor laceration of left vertebral artery** CC

√7th **S15.119 Minor laceration of unspecified vertebral artery** CC UNS

√6th **S15.12 Major laceration of vertebral artery**

Complete transection of vertebral artery
Traumatic rupture of vertebral artery

√7th **S15.121 Major laceration of right vertebral artery** CC

√7th **S15.122 Major laceration of left vertebral artery** CC

√7th **S15.129 Major laceration of unspecified vertebral artery** CC UNS

√6th **S15.19 Other specified injury of vertebral artery**

√7th **S15.191 Other specified injury of right vertebral artery** CC

√7th **S15.192 Other specified injury of left vertebral artery** CC

√7th **S15.199 Other specified injury of unspecified vertebral artery** CC UNS

√5th **S15.2 Injury of external jugular vein**

√6th **S15.2Ø Unspecified injury of external jugular vein**

√7th **S15.2Ø1 Unspecified injury of right external jugular vein** CC

√7th **S15.2Ø2 Unspecified injury of left external jugular vein** CC

√7th **S15.2Ø9 Unspecified injury of unspecified external jugular vein** CC UNS

√6th **S15.21 Minor laceration of external jugular vein**

Incomplete transection of external jugular vein
Laceration of external jugular vein NOS
Superficial laceration of external jugular vein

√7th **S15.211 Minor laceration of right external jugular vein** CC

√7th **S15.212 Minor laceration of left external jugular vein** CC

√7th **S15.219 Minor laceration of unspecified external jugular vein** CC UNS

√6th **S15.22 Major laceration of external jugular vein**

Complete transection of external jugular vein
Traumatic rupture of external jugular vein

√7th **S15.221 Major laceration of right external jugular vein** CC

√7th **S15.222 Major laceration of left external jugular vein** CC

√7th **S15.229 Major laceration of unspecified external jugular vein** CC UNS

√6th **S15.29 Other specified injury of external jugular vein**

√7th **S15.291 Other specified injury of right external jugular vein** CC

√7th **S15.292 Other specified injury of left external jugular vein** CC

√7th **S15.299 Other specified injury of unspecified external jugular vein** CC UNS

√5th **S15.3 Injury of internal jugular vein**

√6th **S15.3Ø Unspecified injury of internal jugular vein**

√7th **S15.3Ø1 Unspecified injury of right internal jugular vein** CC

√7th **S15.3Ø2 Unspecified injury of left internal jugular vein** CC

√7th **S15.3Ø9 Unspecified injury of unspecified internal jugular vein** CC UNS

√6th **S15.31 Minor laceration of internal jugular vein**

Incomplete transection of internal jugular vein
Laceration of internal jugular vein NOS
Superficial laceration of internal jugular vein

√7th **S15.311 Minor laceration of right internal jugular vein** CC

√7th **S15.312 Minor laceration of left internal jugular vein** CC

√7th **S15.319 Minor laceration of unspecified internal jugular vein** CC UNS

S15.32 Major laceration of internal jugular vein
Complete transection of internal jugular vein
Traumatic rupture of internal jugular vein
S15.321 Major laceration of right internal jugular vein CC
S15.322 Major laceration of left internal jugular vein CC
S15.329 Major laceration of unspecified internal jugular vein CC UNS
S15.39 Other specified injury of internal jugular vein
S15.391 Other specified injury of right internal jugular vein CC
S15.392 Other specified injury of left internal jugular vein CC
S15.399 Other specified injury of unspecified internal jugular vein CC UNS
S15.8 Injury of other specified blood vessels at neck level CC
S15.9 Injury of unspecified blood vessel at neck level CC

S16 Injury of muscle, fascia and tendon at neck level
Code also any associated open wound (S11.-)
EXCLUDES 2 *sprain of joint or ligament at neck level (S13.9)*

The appropriate 7th character is to be added to each code from category S16.
A initial encounter
D subsequent encounter
S sequela

S16.1 Strain of muscle, fascia and tendon at neck level
S16.2 Laceration of muscle, fascia and tendon at neck level
S16.8 Other specified injury of muscle, fascia and tendon at neck level
S16.9 Unspecified injury of muscle, fascia and tendon at neck level

S17 Crushing injury of neck
Use additional code for all associated injuries, such as:
injury of blood vessels (S15.-)
open wound of neck (S11.-)
spinal cord injury (S14.Ø, S14.1-)
vertebral fracture (S12.Ø- — S12.3-)

The appropriate 7th character is to be added to each code from category S17.
A initial encounter
D subsequent encounter
S sequela

S17.Ø Crushing injury of larynx and trachea CC H5
S17.8 Crushing injury of other specified parts of neck CC H5
S17.9 Crushing injury of neck, part unspecified CC H5

S19 Other specified and unspecified injuries of neck

The appropriate 7th character is to be added to each code from category S19.
A initial encounter
D subsequent encounter
S sequela

S19.8 Other specified injuries of neck
S19.8Ø Other specified injuries of unspecified part of neck
S19.81 Other specified injuries of larynx
S19.82 Other specified injuries of cervical trachea
EXCLUDES 2 *other specified injury of thoracic trachea (S27.5-)*
S19.83 Other specified injuries of vocal cord
S19.84 Other specified injuries of thyroid gland
S19.85 Other specified injuries of pharynx and cervical esophagus
AHA: 2022,1Q,27
S19.89 Other specified injuries of other specified part of neck
S19.9 Unspecified injury of neck

Injuries to the thorax (S2Ø-S29)

INCLUDES injuries of breast
injuries of chest (wall)
injuries of interscapular area
EXCLUDES 2 *burns and corrosions (T2Ø-T32)*
effects of foreign body in bronchus (T17.5)
effects of foreign body in esophagus (T18.1)
effects of foreign body in lung (T17.8)
effects of foreign body in trachea (T17.4)
frostbite (T33-T34)
injuries of axilla
injuries of clavicle
injuries of scapular region
injuries of shoulder
insect bite or sting, venomous (T63.4)

S2Ø Superficial injury of thorax
AHA: 2020,4Q,39

The appropriate 7th character is to be added to each code from category S2Ø.
A initial encounter
D subsequent encounter
S sequela

S2Ø.Ø Contusion of breast
S2Ø.ØØ Contusion of breast, unspecified breast
S2Ø.Ø1 Contusion of right breast
S2Ø.Ø2 Contusion of left breast
S2Ø.1 Other and unspecified superficial injuries of breast
S2Ø.1Ø Unspecified superficial injuries of breast
S2Ø.1Ø1 Unspecified superficial injuries of breast, right breast
S2Ø.1Ø2 Unspecified superficial injuries of breast, left breast
S2Ø.1Ø9 Unspecified superficial injuries of breast, unspecified breast
S2Ø.11 Abrasion of breast
S2Ø.111 Abrasion of breast, right breast
S2Ø.112 Abrasion of breast, left breast
S2Ø.119 Abrasion of breast, unspecified breast
S2Ø.12 Blister (nonthermal) of breast
S2Ø.121 Blister (nonthermal) of breast, right breast
S2Ø.122 Blister (nonthermal) of breast, left breast
S2Ø.129 Blister (nonthermal) of breast, unspecified breast
S2Ø.14 External constriction of part of breast
S2Ø.141 External constriction of part of breast, right breast
S2Ø.142 External constriction of part of breast, left breast
S2Ø.149 External constriction of part of breast, unspecified breast
S2Ø.15 Superficial foreign body of breast
Splinter in the breast
S2Ø.151 Superficial foreign body of breast, right breast
S2Ø.152 Superficial foreign body of breast, left breast
S2Ø.159 Superficial foreign body of breast, unspecified breast
S2Ø.16 Insect bite (nonvenomous) of breast
S2Ø.161 Insect bite (nonvenomous) of breast, right breast
S2Ø.162 Insect bite (nonvenomous) of breast, left breast
S2Ø.169 Insect bite (nonvenomous) of breast, unspecified breast
S2Ø.17 Other superficial bite of breast
EXCLUDES 1 *open bite of breast (S21.Ø5-)*
S2Ø.171 Other superficial bite of breast, right breast
S2Ø.172 Other superficial bite of breast, left breast
S2Ø.179 Other superficial bite of breast, unspecified breast
S2Ø.2 Contusion of thorax
S2Ø.2Ø Contusion of thorax, unspecified
S2Ø.21 Contusion of front wall of thorax
S2Ø.211 Contusion of right front wall of thorax

- √7th S20.212 Contusion of left front wall of thorax
- √7th S20.213 Contusion of bilateral front wall of thorax
- √7th S20.214 Contusion of middle front wall of thorax
- √7th S20.219 Contusion of unspecified front wall of thorax

√6th S20.22 Contusion of back wall of thorax
- √7th S20.221 Contusion of right back wall of thorax
- √7th S20.222 Contusion of left back wall of thorax
- √7th S20.223 Contusion of bilateral back wall of thorax
- √7th S20.224 Contusion of middle back wall of thorax
- √7th S20.229 Contusion of unspecified back wall of thorax

√5th S20.3 Other and unspecified superficial injuries of front wall of thorax

√6th S20.30 Unspecified superficial injuries of front wall of thorax
- √7th S20.301 Unspecified superficial injuries of right front wall of thorax
- √7th S20.302 Unspecified superficial injuries of left front wall of thorax
- √7th S20.303 Unspecified superficial injuries of bilateral front wall of thorax
- √7th S20.304 Unspecified superficial injuries of middle front wall of thorax
- √7th S20.309 Unspecified superficial injuries of unspecified front wall of thorax

√6th S20.31 Abrasion of front wall of thorax
- √7th S20.311 Abrasion of right front wall of thorax
- √7th S20.312 Abrasion of left front wall of thorax
- √7th S20.313 Abrasion of bilateral front wall of thorax
- √7th S20.314 Abrasion of middle front wall of thorax
- √7th S20.319 Abrasion of unspecified front wall of thorax

√6th S20.32 Blister (nonthermal) of front wall of thorax
- √7th S20.321 Blister (nonthermal) of right front wall of thorax
- √7th S20.322 Blister (nonthermal) of left front wall of thorax
- √7th S20.323 Blister (nonthermal) of bilateral front wall of thorax
- √7th S20.324 Blister (nonthermal) of middle front wall of thorax
- √7th S20.329 Blister (nonthermal) of unspecified front wall of thorax

√6th S20.34 External constriction of front wall of thorax
- √7th S20.341 External constriction of right front wall of thorax
- √7th S20.342 External constriction of left front wall of thorax
- √7th S20.343 External constriction of bilateral front wall of thorax
- √7th S20.344 External constriction of middle front wall of thorax
- √7th S20.349 External constriction of unspecified front wall of thorax

√6th S20.35 Superficial foreign body of front wall of thorax

Splinter in front wall of thorax
- √7th S20.351 Superficial foreign body of right front wall of thorax
- √7th S20.352 Superficial foreign body of left front wall of thorax
- √7th S20.353 Superficial foreign body of bilateral front wall of thorax
- √7th S20.354 Superficial foreign body of middle front wall of thorax
- √7th S20.359 Superficial foreign body of unspecified front wall of thorax

√6th S20.36 Insect bite (nonvenomous) of front wall of thorax
- √7th S20.361 Insect bite (nonvenomous) of right front wall of thorax
- √7th S20.362 Insect bite (nonvenomous) of left front wall of thorax
- √7th S20.363 Insect bite (nonvenomous) of bilateral front wall of thorax
- √7th S20.364 Insect bite (nonvenomous) of middle front wall of thorax
- √7th S20.369 Insect bite (nonvenomous) of unspecified front wall of thorax

√6th S20.37 Other superficial bite of front wall of thorax

EXCLUDES 1 *open bite of front wall of thorax (S21.15)*
- √7th S20.371 Other superficial bite of right front wall of thorax
- √7th S20.372 Other superficial bite of left front wall of thorax
- √7th S20.373 Other superficial bite of bilateral front wall of thorax
- √7th S20.374 Other superficial bite of middle front wall of thorax
- √7th S20.379 Other superficial bite of unspecified front wall of thorax

√5th S20.4 Other and unspecified superficial injuries of back wall of thorax

√6th S20.40 Unspecified superficial injuries of back wall of thorax
- √7th S20.401 Unspecified superficial injuries of right back wall of thorax
- √7th S20.402 Unspecified superficial injuries of left back wall of thorax
- √7th S20.409 Unspecified superficial injuries of unspecified back wall of thorax

√6th S20.41 Abrasion of back wall of thorax
- √7th S20.411 Abrasion of right back wall of thorax
- √7th S20.412 Abrasion of left back wall of thorax
- √7th S20.419 Abrasion of unspecified back wall of thorax

√6th S20.42 Blister (nonthermal) of back wall of thorax
- √7th S20.421 Blister (nonthermal) of right back wall of thorax
- √7th S20.422 Blister (nonthermal) of left back wall of thorax
- √7th S20.429 Blister (nonthermal) of unspecified back wall of thorax

√6th S20.44 External constriction of back wall of thorax
- √7th S20.441 External constriction of right back wall of thorax
- √7th S20.442 External constriction of left back wall of thorax
- √7th S20.449 External constriction of unspecified back wall of thorax

√6th S20.45 Superficial foreign body of back wall of thorax

Splinter of back wall of thorax
- √7th S20.451 Superficial foreign body of right back wall of thorax
- √7th S20.452 Superficial foreign body of left back wall of thorax
- √7th S20.459 Superficial foreign body of unspecified back wall of thorax

√6th S20.46 Insect bite (nonvenomous) of back wall of thorax
- √7th S20.461 Insect bite (nonvenomous) of right back wall of thorax
- √7th S20.462 Insect bite (nonvenomous) of left back wall of thorax
- √7th S20.469 Insect bite (nonvenomous) of unspecified back wall of thorax

√6th S20.47 Other superficial bite of back wall of thorax

EXCLUDES 1 *open bite of back wall of thorax (S21.25)*
- √7th S20.471 Other superficial bite of right back wall of thorax
- √7th S20.472 Other superficial bite of left back wall of thorax
- √7th S20.479 Other superficial bite of unspecified back wall of thorax

√5th S20.9 Superficial injury of unspecified parts of thorax

EXCLUDES 1 *contusion of thorax NOS (S20.20)*
- √x7th S20.90 Unspecified superficial injury of unspecified parts of thorax
  - Superficial injury of thoracic wall NOS
- √x7th S20.91 Abrasion of unspecified parts of thorax
- √x7th S20.92 Blister (nonthermal) of unspecified parts of thorax
- √x7th S20.94 External constriction of unspecified parts of thorax
- √x7th S20.95 Superficial foreign body of unspecified parts of thorax
  - Splinter in thorax NOS
- √x7th S20.96 Insect bite (nonvenomous) of unspecified parts of thorax

S20.97 Other superficial bite of unspecified parts of thorax
EXCLUDES 1 *open bite of thorax NOS (S21.95)*

S21 Open wound of thorax

Code also any associated injury, such as:
- injury of heart (S26.-)
- injury of intrathoracic organs (S27.-)
- rib fracture (S22.3-, S22.4-)
- spinal cord injury (S24.0-, S24.1-)
- traumatic hemopneumothorax (S27.3)
- traumatic hemothorax (S27.1)
- traumatic pneumothorax (S27.0)
- wound infection

EXCLUDES 1 *traumatic amputation (partial) of thorax (S28.1)*

The appropriate 7th character is to be added to each code from category S21.
- A initial encounter
- D subsequent encounter
- S sequela

S21.0 Open wound of breast
- S21.00 Unspecified open wound of breast
  - S21.001 Unspecified open wound of right breast
  - S21.002 Unspecified open wound of left breast
  - S21.009 Unspecified open wound of unspecified breast
- S21.01 Laceration without foreign body of breast
  - S21.011 Laceration without foreign body of right breast
  - S21.012 Laceration without foreign body of left breast
  - S21.019 Laceration without foreign body of unspecified breast
- S21.02 Laceration with foreign body of breast
  - S21.021 Laceration with foreign body of right breast
  - S21.022 Laceration with foreign body of left breast
  - S21.029 Laceration with foreign body of unspecified breast
- S21.03 Puncture wound without foreign body of breast
  - S21.031 Puncture wound without foreign body of right breast
  - S21.032 Puncture wound without foreign body of left breast
  - S21.039 Puncture wound without foreign body of unspecified breast
- S21.04 Puncture wound with foreign body of breast
  - S21.041 Puncture wound with foreign body of right breast
  - S21.042 Puncture wound with foreign body of left breast
  - S21.049 Puncture wound with foreign body of unspecified breast
- S21.05 Open bite of breast
  Bite of breast NOS
  EXCLUDES 1 *superficial bite of breast (S20.17)*
  - S21.051 Open bite of right breast
  - S21.052 Open bite of left breast
  - S21.059 Open bite of unspecified breast

S21.1 Open wound of front wall of thorax without penetration into thoracic cavity
Open wound of chest without penetration into thoracic cavity
- S21.10 Unspecified open wound of front wall of thorax without penetration into thoracic cavity
  - S21.101 Unspecified open wound of right front wall of thorax without penetration into thoracic cavity CC
  - S21.102 Unspecified open wound of left front wall of thorax without penetration into thoracic cavity CC
  - S21.109 Unspecified open wound of unspecified front wall of thorax without penetration into thoracic cavity CC UNS
- S21.11 Laceration without foreign body of front wall of thorax without penetration into thoracic cavity
  - S21.111 Laceration without foreign body of right front wall of thorax without penetration into thoracic cavity CC
  - S21.112 Laceration without foreign body of left front wall of thorax without penetration into thoracic cavity CC
  - S21.119 Laceration without foreign body of unspecified front wall of thorax without penetration into thoracic cavity CC UNS
- S21.12 Laceration with foreign body of front wall of thorax without penetration into thoracic cavity
  - S21.121 Laceration with foreign body of right front wall of thorax without penetration into thoracic cavity CC
  - S21.122 Laceration with foreign body of left front wall of thorax without penetration into thoracic cavity CC
  - S21.129 Laceration with foreign body of unspecified front wall of thorax without penetration into thoracic cavity CC UNS
- S21.13 Puncture wound without foreign body of front wall of thorax without penetration into thoracic cavity
  - S21.131 Puncture wound without foreign body of right front wall of thorax without penetration into thoracic cavity CC
  - S21.132 Puncture wound without foreign body of left front wall of thorax without penetration into thoracic cavity CC
  - S21.139 Puncture wound without foreign body of unspecified front wall of thorax without penetration into thoracic cavity CC UNS
- S21.14 Puncture wound with foreign body of front wall of thorax without penetration into thoracic cavity
  - S21.141 Puncture wound with foreign body of right front wall of thorax without penetration into thoracic cavity CC
  - S21.142 Puncture wound with foreign body of left front wall of thorax without penetration into thoracic cavity CC
  - S21.149 Puncture wound with foreign body of unspecified front wall of thorax without penetration into thoracic cavity CC UNS
- S21.15 Open bite of front wall of thorax without penetration into thoracic cavity
  Bite of front wall of thorax NOS
  EXCLUDES 1 *superficial bite of front wall of thorax (S20.37)*
  - S21.151 Open bite of right front wall of thorax without penetration into thoracic cavity CC
  - S21.152 Open bite of left front wall of thorax without penetration into thoracic cavity CC
  - S21.159 Open bite of unspecified front wall of thorax without penetration into thoracic cavity CC UNS

S21.2 Open wound of back wall of thorax without penetration into thoracic cavity
- S21.20 Unspecified open wound of back wall of thorax without penetration into thoracic cavity
  - S21.201 Unspecified open wound of right back wall of thorax without penetration into thoracic cavity
  - S21.202 Unspecified open wound of left back wall of thorax without penetration into thoracic cavity
  - S21.209 Unspecified open wound of unspecified back wall of thorax without penetration into thoracic cavity
- S21.21 Laceration without foreign body of back wall of thorax without penetration into thoracic cavity
  - S21.211 Laceration without foreign body of right back wall of thorax without penetration into thoracic cavity
  - S21.212 Laceration without foreign body of left back wall of thorax without penetration into thoracic cavity
  - S21.219 Laceration without foreign body of unspecified back wall of thorax without penetration into thoracic cavity

6th S21.22 **Laceration with foreign body** of back wall of thorax without penetration into thoracic cavity
7th S21.221 Laceration with foreign body of **right** back wall of thorax without penetration into thoracic cavity
7th S21.222 Laceration with foreign body of **left** back wall of thorax without penetration into thoracic cavity
7th S21.229 Laceration with foreign body of unspecified back wall of thorax without penetration into thoracic cavity
6th S21.23 **Puncture wound without foreign body** of back wall of thorax without penetration into thoracic cavity
7th S21.231 Puncture wound without foreign body of **right** back wall of thorax without penetration into thoracic cavity
7th S21.232 Puncture wound without foreign body of **left** back wall of thorax without penetration into thoracic cavity
7th S21.239 Puncture wound without foreign body of unspecified back wall of thorax without penetration into thoracic cavity
6th S21.24 **Puncture wound with foreign body** of back wall of thorax without penetration into thoracic cavity
7th S21.241 Puncture wound with foreign body of **right** back wall of thorax without penetration into thoracic cavity
7th S21.242 Puncture wound with foreign body of **left** back wall of thorax without penetration into thoracic cavity
7th S21.249 Puncture wound with foreign body of unspecified back wall of thorax without penetration into thoracic cavity
6th S21.25 **Open bite** of back wall of thorax without penetration into thoracic cavity
Bite of back wall of thorax NOS
EXCLUDES 1 *superficial bite of back wall of thorax (S20.47)*
7th S21.251 Open bite of **right** back wall of thorax without penetration into thoracic cavity
7th S21.252 Open bite of **left** back wall of thorax without penetration into thoracic cavity
7th S21.259 Open bite of unspecified back wall of thorax without penetration into thoracic cavity
5th S21.3 Open wound of **front wall of thorax with penetration** into thoracic cavity
Open wound of chest with penetration into thoracic cavity
6th S21.30 Unspecified open wound of front wall of thorax with penetration into thoracic cavity
7th S21.301 Unspecified open wound of **right** front wall of thorax with penetration into thoracic cavity MCC
7th S21.302 Unspecified open wound of **left** front wall of thorax with penetration into thoracic cavity MCC
7th S21.309 Unspecified open wound of unspecified front wall of thorax with penetration into thoracic cavity MCC UNS
6th S21.31 **Laceration without foreign body** of front wall of thorax with penetration into thoracic cavity
7th S21.311 Laceration without foreign body of **right** front wall of thorax with penetration into thoracic cavity MCC
7th S21.312 Laceration without foreign body of **left** front wall of thorax with penetration into thoracic cavity MCC
7th S21.319 Laceration without foreign body of unspecified front wall of thorax with penetration into thoracic cavity MCC UNS
6th S21.32 **Laceration with foreign body** of front wall of thorax with penetration into thoracic cavity
7th S21.321 Laceration with foreign body of **right** front wall of thorax with penetration into thoracic cavity MCC
7th S21.322 Laceration with foreign body of **left** front wall of thorax with penetration into thoracic cavity MCC
7th S21.329 Laceration with foreign body of unspecified front wall of thorax with penetration into thoracic cavity MCC UNS
6th S21.33 **Puncture wound without foreign body** of front wall of thorax with penetration into thoracic cavity
7th S21.331 Puncture wound without foreign body of **right** front wall of thorax with penetration into thoracic cavity MCC
7th S21.332 Puncture wound without foreign body of **left** front wall of thorax with penetration into thoracic cavity MCC
7th S21.339 Puncture wound without foreign body of unspecified front wall of thorax with penetration into thoracic cavity MCC UNS
6th S21.34 **Puncture wound with foreign body** of front wall of thorax with penetration into thoracic cavity
7th S21.341 Puncture wound with foreign body of **right** front wall of thorax with penetration into thoracic cavity MCC
7th S21.342 Puncture wound with foreign body of **left** front wall of thorax with penetration into thoracic cavity MCC
7th S21.349 Puncture wound with foreign body of unspecified front wall of thorax with penetration into thoracic cavity MCC UNS
6th S21.35 **Open bite** of front wall of thorax with penetration into thoracic cavity
EXCLUDES 1 *superficial bite of front wall of thorax (S20.37)*
7th S21.351 Open bite of **right** front wall of thorax with penetration into thoracic cavity MCC
7th S21.352 Open bite of **left** front wall of thorax with penetration into thoracic cavity MCC
7th S21.359 Open bite of unspecified front wall of thorax with penetration into thoracic cavity MCC UNS
5th S21.4 Open wound of **back wall of thorax with penetration** into thoracic cavity
6th S21.40 Unspecified open wound of back wall of thorax with penetration into thoracic cavity
7th S21.401 Unspecified open wound of **right** back wall of thorax with penetration into thoracic cavity MCC
7th S21.402 Unspecified open wound of **left** back wall of thorax with penetration into thoracic cavity MCC
7th S21.409 Unspecified open wound of unspecified back wall of thorax with penetration into thoracic cavity MCC UNS
6th S21.41 **Laceration without foreign body** of back wall of thorax with penetration into thoracic cavity
7th S21.411 Laceration without foreign body of **right** back wall of thorax with penetration into thoracic cavity MCC
7th S21.412 Laceration without foreign body of **left** back wall of thorax with penetration into thoracic cavity MCC
7th S21.419 Laceration without foreign body of unspecified back wall of thorax with penetration into thoracic cavity MCC UNS
6th S21.42 **Laceration with foreign body** of back wall of thorax with penetration into thoracic cavity
7th S21.421 Laceration with foreign body of **right** back wall of thorax with penetration into thoracic cavity MCC
7th S21.422 Laceration with foreign body of **left** back wall of thorax with penetration into thoracic cavity MCC
7th S21.429 Laceration with foreign body of unspecified back wall of thorax with penetration into thoracic cavity MCC UNS
6th S21.43 **Puncture wound without foreign body** of back wall of thorax with penetration into thoracic cavity
7th S21.431 Puncture wound without foreign body of **right** back wall of thorax with penetration into thoracic cavity MCC
7th S21.432 Puncture wound without foreign body of **left** back wall of thorax with penetration into thoracic cavity MCC

S21.439 Puncture wound without foreign body of unspecified back wall of thorax with penetration into thoracic cavity MCC UNS

S21.44 Puncture wound with foreign body of back wall of thorax with penetration into thoracic cavity

S21.441 Puncture wound with foreign body of right back wall of thorax with penetration into thoracic cavity MCC

S21.442 Puncture wound with foreign body of left back wall of thorax with penetration into thoracic cavity MCC

S21.449 Puncture wound with foreign body of unspecified back wall of thorax with penetration into thoracic cavity MCC UNS

S21.45 Open bite of back wall of thorax with penetration into thoracic cavity

Bite of back wall of thorax NOS

EXCLUDES 1 *superficial bite of back wall of thorax (S20.47)*

S21.451 Open bite of right back wall of thorax with penetration into thoracic cavity MCC

S21.452 Open bite of left back wall of thorax with penetration into thoracic cavity MCC

S21.459 Open bite of unspecified back wall of thorax with penetration into thoracic cavity MCC UNS

S21.9 Open wound of unspecified part of thorax

Open wound of thoracic wall NOS

S21.90 Unspecified open wound of unspecified part of thorax CC UNS

S21.91 Laceration without foreign body of unspecified part of thorax CC UNS

S21.92 Laceration with foreign body of unspecified part of thorax CC UNS

S21.93 Puncture wound without foreign body of unspecified part of thorax CC UNS

S21.94 Puncture wound with foreign body of unspecified part of thorax CC UNS

S21.95 Open bite of unspecified part of thorax CC UNS

EXCLUDES 1 *superficial bite of thorax (S20.97)*

S22 Fracture of rib(s), sternum and thoracic spine

NOTE A fracture not indicated as displaced or nondisplaced should be coded to displaced

A fracture not indicated as open or closed should be coded to closed

INCLUDES fracture of thoracic neural arch
fracture of thoracic spinous process
fracture of thoracic transverse process
fracture of thoracic vertebra
fracture of thoracic vertebral arch

~~Code first any associated:~~
~~injury of intrathoracic organ (S27.-)~~
~~spinal cord injury (S24.0-, S24.1-)~~

▶Code also, if applicable, any associated:◀
▶injury of intrathoracic organ (S27.-)◀
▶spinal cord injury (S24.0-, S24.1-)◀

EXCLUDES 1 *transection of thorax (S28.1)*

EXCLUDES 2 *fracture of clavicle (S42.0-)*
fracture of scapula (S42.1-)

AHA: 2021,1Q,6; 2018,2Q,12; 2015,3Q,37-39

The appropriate 7th character is to be added to each code from category S22.
- A initial encounter for closed fracture
- B initial encounter for open fracture
- D subsequent encounter for fracture with routine healing
- G subsequent encounter for fracture with delayed healing
- K subsequent encounter for fracture with nonunion
- S sequela

S22.0 Fracture of thoracic vertebra

S22.00 Fracture of unspecified thoracic vertebra

S22.000 Wedge compression fracture of unspecified thoracic vertebra MCC CC H5 HCC

S22.001 Stable burst fracture of unspecified thoracic vertebra MCC CC H5 HCC

S22.002 Unstable burst fracture of unspecified thoracic vertebra MCC CC H5 HCC

S22.008 Other fracture of unspecified thoracic vertebra MCC CC H5 HCC

S22.009 Unspecified fracture of unspecified thoracic vertebra MCC CC H5 HCC

S22.01 Fracture of first thoracic vertebra

S22.010 Wedge compression fracture of first thoracic vertebra MCC CC H5 HCC

S22.011 Stable burst fracture of first thoracic vertebra MCC CC H5 HCC

S22.012 Unstable burst fracture of first thoracic vertebra MCC CC H5 HCC

S22.018 Other fracture of first thoracic vertebra MCC CC H5 HCC

S22.019 Unspecified fracture of first thoracic vertebra MCC CC H5 HCC

S22.02 Fracture of second thoracic vertebra

S22.020 Wedge compression fracture of second thoracic vertebra MCC CC H5 HCC

S22.021 Stable burst fracture of second thoracic vertebra MCC CC H5 HCC

S22.022 Unstable burst fracture of second thoracic vertebra MCC CC H5 HCC

S22.028 Other fracture of second thoracic vertebra MCC CC H5 HCC

S22.029 Unspecified fracture of second thoracic vertebra MCC CC H5 HCC

S22.03 Fracture of third thoracic vertebra

S22.030 Wedge compression fracture of third thoracic vertebra MCC CC H5 HCC

S22.031 Stable burst fracture of third thoracic vertebra MCC CC H5 HCC

S22.032 Unstable burst fracture of third thoracic vertebra MCC CC H5 HCC

S22.038 Other fracture of third thoracic vertebra MCC CC H5 HCC

S22.039 Unspecified fracture of third thoracic vertebra MCC CC H5 HCC

S22.04 Fracture of fourth thoracic vertebra

S22.040 Wedge compression fracture of fourth thoracic vertebra MCC CC H5 HCC

S22.041 Stable burst fracture of fourth thoracic vertebra MCC CC H5 HCC

S22.042 Unstable burst fracture of fourth thoracic vertebra MCC CC H5 HCC

S22.048 Other fracture of fourth thoracic vertebra MCC CC H5 HCC

S22.049 Unspecified fracture of fourth thoracic vertebra MCC CC H5 HCC

S22.05 Fracture of T5-T6 vertebra

S22.050 Wedge compression fracture of T5-T6 vertebra MCC CC H5 HCC

S22.051 Stable burst fracture of T5-T6 vertebra MCC CC H5 HCC

S22.052 Unstable burst fracture of T5-T6 vertebra MCC CC H5 HCC

S22.058 Other fracture of T5-T6 vertebra MCC CC H5 HCC

S22.059 Unspecified fracture of T5-T6 vertebra MCC CC H5 HCC

S22.06 Fracture of T7-T8 vertebra

S22.060 Wedge compression fracture of T7-T8 vertebra MCC CC H5 HCC

S22.061 Stable burst fracture of T7-T8 vertebra MCC CC H5 HCC

S22.062 Unstable burst fracture of T7-T8 vertebra MCC CC H5 HCC

S22.068 Other fracture of T7-T8 thoracic vertebra MCC CC H5 HCC

S22.069 Unspecified fracture of T7-T8 vertebra MCC CC H5 HCC

S22.07 Fracture of T9-T10 vertebra

S22.070 Wedge compression fracture of T9-T10 vertebra MCC CC H5 HCC

S22.071 Stable burst fracture of T9-T10 vertebra MCC CC H5 HCC

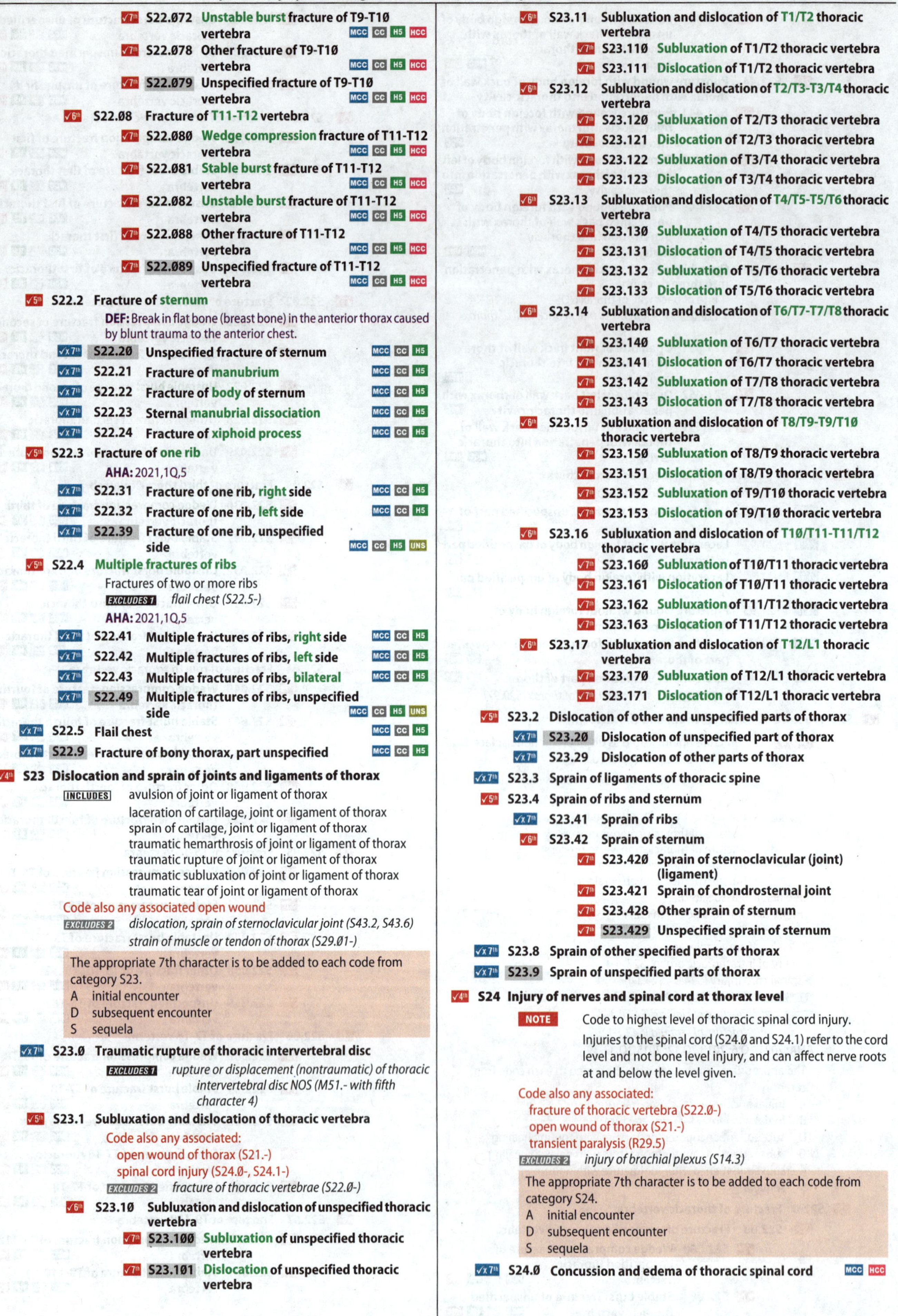

- 7th **S22.072** **Unstable burst** fracture of T9-T10 vertebra MCC CC H5 HCC
- 7th **S22.078** Other fracture of T9-T10 vertebra MCC CC H5 HCC
- 7th **S22.079** Unspecified fracture of T9-T10 vertebra MCC CC H5 HCC
- 6th **S22.08** Fracture of **T11-T12** vertebra
  - 7th **S22.080** **Wedge compression** fracture of T11-T12 vertebra MCC CC H5 HCC
  - 7th **S22.081** **Stable burst** fracture of T11-T12 vertebra MCC CC H5 HCC
  - 7th **S22.082** **Unstable burst** fracture of T11-T12 vertebra MCC CC H5 HCC
  - 7th **S22.088** Other fracture of T11-T12 vertebra MCC CC H5 HCC
  - 7th **S22.089** Unspecified fracture of T11-T12 vertebra MCC CC H5 HCC

5th **S22.2 Fracture of sternum**

DEF: Break in flat bone (breast bone) in the anterior thorax caused by blunt trauma to the anterior chest.

- x7th **S22.20** Unspecified fracture of sternum MCC CC H5
- x7th **S22.21** Fracture of **manubrium** MCC CC H5
- x7th **S22.22** Fracture of **body** of sternum MCC CC H5
- x7th **S22.23** Sternal **manubrial dissociation** MCC CC H5
- x7th **S22.24** Fracture of **xiphoid process** MCC CC H5

5th **S22.3 Fracture of one rib**

AHA: 2021,1Q,5

- x7th **S22.31** Fracture of one rib, **right** side MCC CC H5
- x7th **S22.32** Fracture of one rib, **left** side MCC CC H5
- x7th **S22.39** Fracture of one rib, unspecified side MCC CC H5 UNS

5th **S22.4 Multiple fractures of ribs**

Fractures of two or more ribs

EXCLUDES 1 *flail chest (S22.5-)*

AHA: 2021,1Q,5

- x7th **S22.41** Multiple fractures of ribs, **right** side MCC CC H5
- x7th **S22.42** Multiple fractures of ribs, **left** side MCC CC H5
- x7th **S22.43** Multiple fractures of ribs, **bilateral** MCC CC H5
- x7th **S22.49** Multiple fractures of ribs, unspecified side MCC CC H5 UNS

x7th **S22.5 Flail chest** MCC CC H5

x7th **S22.9 Fracture of bony thorax, part unspecified** MCC CC H5

4th S23 Dislocation and sprain of joints and ligaments of thorax

INCLUDES avulsion of joint or ligament of thorax
laceration of cartilage, joint or ligament of thorax
sprain of cartilage, joint or ligament of thorax
traumatic hemarthrosis of joint or ligament of thorax
traumatic rupture of joint or ligament of thorax
traumatic subluxation of joint or ligament of thorax
traumatic tear of joint or ligament of thorax

Code also any associated open wound

EXCLUDES 2 *dislocation, sprain of sternoclavicular joint (S43.2, S43.6)*
strain of muscle or tendon of thorax (S29.01-)

The appropriate 7th character is to be added to each code from category S23.
A initial encounter
D subsequent encounter
S sequela

x7th **S23.0 Traumatic rupture of thoracic intervertebral disc**

EXCLUDES 1 *rupture or displacement (nontraumatic) of thoracic intervertebral disc NOS (M51.- with fifth character 4)*

5th **S23.1 Subluxation and dislocation of thoracic vertebra**

Code also any associated:
open wound of thorax (S21.-)
spinal cord injury (S24.0-, S24.1-)

EXCLUDES 2 *fracture of thoracic vertebrae (S22.0-)*

- 6th **S23.10** Subluxation and dislocation of unspecified thoracic vertebra
  - 7th **S23.100** **Subluxation** of unspecified thoracic vertebra
  - 7th **S23.101** **Dislocation** of unspecified thoracic vertebra
- 6th **S23.11** Subluxation and dislocation of **T1/T2** thoracic vertebra
  - 7th **S23.110** **Subluxation** of T1/T2 thoracic vertebra
  - 7th **S23.111** **Dislocation** of T1/T2 thoracic vertebra
- 6th **S23.12** Subluxation and dislocation of **T2/T3-T3/T4** thoracic vertebra
  - 7th **S23.120** **Subluxation** of T2/T3 thoracic vertebra
  - 7th **S23.121** **Dislocation** of T2/T3 thoracic vertebra
  - 7th **S23.122** **Subluxation** of T3/T4 thoracic vertebra
  - 7th **S23.123** **Dislocation** of T3/T4 thoracic vertebra
- 6th **S23.13** Subluxation and dislocation of **T4/T5-T5/T6** thoracic vertebra
  - 7th **S23.130** **Subluxation** of T4/T5 thoracic vertebra
  - 7th **S23.131** **Dislocation** of T4/T5 thoracic vertebra
  - 7th **S23.132** **Subluxation** of T5/T6 thoracic vertebra
  - 7th **S23.133** **Dislocation** of T5/T6 thoracic vertebra
- 6th **S23.14** Subluxation and dislocation of **T6/T7-T7/T8** thoracic vertebra
  - 7th **S23.140** **Subluxation** of T6/T7 thoracic vertebra
  - 7th **S23.141** **Dislocation** of T6/T7 thoracic vertebra
  - 7th **S23.142** **Subluxation** of T7/T8 thoracic vertebra
  - 7th **S23.143** **Dislocation** of T7/T8 thoracic vertebra
- 6th **S23.15** Subluxation and dislocation of **T8/T9-T9/T10** thoracic vertebra
  - 7th **S23.150** **Subluxation** of T8/T9 thoracic vertebra
  - 7th **S23.151** **Dislocation** of T8/T9 thoracic vertebra
  - 7th **S23.152** **Subluxation** of T9/T10 thoracic vertebra
  - 7th **S23.153** **Dislocation** of T9/T10 thoracic vertebra
- 6th **S23.16** Subluxation and dislocation of **T10/T11-T11/T12** thoracic vertebra
  - 7th **S23.160** **Subluxation** of T10/T11 thoracic vertebra
  - 7th **S23.161** **Dislocation** of T10/T11 thoracic vertebra
  - 7th **S23.162** **Subluxation** of T11/T12 thoracic vertebra
  - 7th **S23.163** **Dislocation** of T11/T12 thoracic vertebra
- 6th **S23.17** Subluxation and dislocation of **T12/L1** thoracic vertebra
  - 7th **S23.170** **Subluxation** of T12/L1 thoracic vertebra
  - 7th **S23.171** **Dislocation** of T12/L1 thoracic vertebra

5th **S23.2 Dislocation of other and unspecified parts of thorax**

- x7th **S23.20** Dislocation of unspecified part of thorax
- x7th **S23.29** Dislocation of other parts of thorax

x7th **S23.3 Sprain of ligaments of thoracic spine**

5th **S23.4 Sprain of ribs and sternum**

- x7th **S23.41** Sprain of ribs
- 6th **S23.42** Sprain of sternum
  - 7th **S23.420** Sprain of sternoclavicular (joint) (ligament)
  - 7th **S23.421** Sprain of chondrosternal joint
  - 7th **S23.428** Other sprain of sternum
  - 7th **S23.429** Unspecified sprain of sternum

x7th **S23.8 Sprain of other specified parts of thorax**

x7th **S23.9 Sprain of unspecified parts of thorax**

4th S24 Injury of nerves and spinal cord at thorax level

NOTE Code to highest level of thoracic spinal cord injury.
Injuries to the spinal cord (S24.0 and S24.1) refer to the cord level and not bone level injury, and can affect nerve roots at and below the level given.

Code also any associated:
fracture of thoracic vertebra (S22.0-)
open wound of thorax (S21.-)
transient paralysis (R29.5)

EXCLUDES 2 *injury of brachial plexus (S14.3)*

The appropriate 7th character is to be added to each code from category S24.
A initial encounter
D subsequent encounter
S sequela

x7th **S24.0 Concussion and edema of thoracic spinal cord** MCC HCC

S24.1 Other and unspecified injuries of thoracic spinal cord

S24.10 Unspecified injury of thoracic spinal cord

S24.101 Unspecified injury at T1 level of thoracic spinal cord MCC H5 HCC

S24.102 Unspecified injury at T2-T6 level of thoracic spinal cord MCC H5 HCC

S24.103 Unspecified injury at T7-T10 level of thoracic spinal cord MCC H5 HCC

S24.104 Unspecified injury at T11-T12 level of thoracic spinal cord MCC H5 HCC

S24.109 Unspecified injury at unspecified level of thoracic spinal cord HCC

Injury of thoracic spinal cord NOS

S24.11 Complete lesion of thoracic spinal cord

S24.111 Complete lesion at T1 level of thoracic spinal cord MCC H5 HCC

S24.112 Complete lesion at T2-T6 level of thoracic spinal cord MCC H5 HCC

S24.113 Complete lesion at T7-T10 level of thoracic spinal cord MCC H5 HCC

S24.114 Complete lesion at T11-T12 level of thoracic spinal cord MCC H5 HCC

S24.119 Complete lesion at unspecified level of thoracic spinal cord HCC

S24.13 Anterior cord syndrome of thoracic spinal cord

S24.131 Anterior cord syndrome at T1 level of thoracic spinal cord MCC H5 HCC

S24.132 Anterior cord syndrome at T2-T6 level of thoracic spinal cord MCC H5 HCC

S24.133 Anterior cord syndrome at T7-T10 level of thoracic spinal cord MCC H5 HCC

S24.134 Anterior cord syndrome at T11-T12 level of thoracic spinal cord MCC H5 HCC

S24.139 Anterior cord syndrome at unspecified level of thoracic spinal cord HCC

S24.14 Brown-Sequard syndrome of thoracic spinal cord

S24.141 Brown-Sequard syndrome at T1 level of thoracic spinal cord MCC HCC

S24.142 Brown-Sequard syndrome at T2-T6 level of thoracic spinal cord MCC HCC

S24.143 Brown-Sequard syndrome at T7-T10 level of thoracic spinal cord MCC HCC

S24.144 Brown-Sequard syndrome at T11-T12 level of thoracic spinal cord MCC HCC

S24.149 Brown-Sequard syndrome at unspecified level of thoracic spinal cord HCC

S24.15 Other incomplete lesions of thoracic spinal cord

Incomplete lesion of thoracic spinal cord NOS
Posterior cord syndrome of thoracic spinal cord

S24.151 Other incomplete lesion at T1 level of thoracic spinal cord MCC H5 HCC

S24.152 Other incomplete lesion at T2-T6 level of thoracic spinal cord MCC H5 HCC

S24.153 Other incomplete lesion at T7-T10 level of thoracic spinal cord MCC H5 HCC

S24.154 Other incomplete lesion at T11-T12 level of thoracic spinal cord MCC H5 HCC

S24.159 Other incomplete lesion at unspecified level of thoracic spinal cord HCC

S24.2 Injury of nerve root of thoracic spine

S24.3 Injury of peripheral nerves of thorax

S24.4 Injury of thoracic sympathetic nervous system

Injury of cardiac plexus
Injury of esophageal plexus
Injury of pulmonary plexus
Injury of stellate ganglion
Injury of thoracic sympathetic ganglion

S24.8 Injury of other specified nerves of thorax

S24.9 Injury of unspecified nerve of thorax

S25 Injury of blood vessels of thorax

Code also any associated open wound (S21.-)

The appropriate 7th character is to be added to each code from category S25.
A initial encounter
D subsequent encounter
S sequela

S25.0 Injury of thoracic aorta

Injury of aorta NOS

S25.00 Unspecified injury of thoracic aorta MCC

S25.01 Minor laceration of thoracic aorta MCC

Incomplete transection of thoracic aorta
Laceration of thoracic aorta NOS
Superficial laceration of thoracic aorta

S25.02 Major laceration of thoracic aorta MCC

Complete transection of thoracic aorta
Traumatic rupture of thoracic aorta

S25.09 Other specified injury of thoracic aorta MCC

S25.1 Injury of innominate or subclavian artery

S25.10 Unspecified injury of innominate or subclavian artery

S25.101 Unspecified injury of right innominate or subclavian artery MCC

S25.102 Unspecified injury of left innominate or subclavian artery MCC

S25.109 Unspecified injury of unspecified innominate or subclavian artery MCC UNS

S25.11 Minor laceration of innominate or subclavian artery

Incomplete transection of innominate or subclavian artery
Laceration of innominate or subclavian artery NOS
Superficial laceration of innominate or subclavian artery

S25.111 Minor laceration of right innominate or subclavian artery MCC

S25.112 Minor laceration of left innominate or subclavian artery MCC

S25.119 Minor laceration of unspecified innominate or subclavian artery MCC UNS

S25.12 Major laceration of innominate or subclavian artery

Complete transection of innominate or subclavian artery
Traumatic rupture of innominate or subclavian artery

S25.121 Major laceration of right innominate or subclavian artery MCC

S25.122 Major laceration of left innominate or subclavian artery MCC

S25.129 Major laceration of unspecified innominate or subclavian artery MCC UNS

S25.19 Other specified injury of innominate or subclavian artery

S25.191 Other specified injury of right innominate or subclavian artery MCC

S25.192 Other specified injury of left innominate or subclavian artery MCC

S25.199 Other specified injury of unspecified innominate or subclavian artery MCC UNS

S25.2 Injury of superior vena cava

Injury of vena cava NOS

S25.20 Unspecified injury of superior vena cava MCC

S25.21 Minor laceration of superior vena cava MCC

Incomplete transection of superior vena cava
Laceration of superior vena cava NOS
Superficial laceration of superior vena cava

S25.22 Major laceration of superior vena cava MCC

Complete transection of superior vena cava
Traumatic rupture of superior vena cava

S25.29 Other specified injury of superior vena cava MCC

S25.3 Injury of innominate or subclavian vein

S25.30 Unspecified injury of innominate or subclavian vein

S25.301 Unspecified injury of right innominate or subclavian vein MCC

S25.302 Unspecified injury of left innominate or subclavian vein MCC

S25.309 Unspecified injury of unspecified innominate or subclavian vein MCC UNS

S25.31 Minor laceration of innominate or subclavian vein
Incomplete transection of innominate or subclavian vein
Laceration of innominate or subclavian vein NOS
Superficial laceration of innominate or subclavian vein

S25.311 Minor laceration of right innominate or subclavian vein MCC

S25.312 Minor laceration of left innominate or subclavian vein MCC

S25.319 Minor laceration of unspecified innominate or subclavian vein MCC UNS

S25.32 Major laceration of innominate or subclavian vein
Complete transection of innominate or subclavian vein
Traumatic rupture of innominate or subclavian vein

S25.321 Major laceration of right innominate or subclavian vein MCC

S25.322 Major laceration of left innominate or subclavian vein MCC

S25.329 Major laceration of unspecified innominate or subclavian vein MCC UNS

S25.39 Other specified injury of innominate or subclavian vein

S25.391 Other specified injury of right innominate or subclavian vein MCC

S25.392 Other specified injury of left innominate or subclavian vein MCC

S25.399 Other specified injury of unspecified innominate or subclavian vein MCC UNS

S25.4 Injury of pulmonary blood vessels

S25.40 Unspecified injury of pulmonary blood vessels

S25.401 Unspecified injury of right pulmonary blood vessels MCC

S25.402 Unspecified injury of left pulmonary blood vessels MCC

S25.409 Unspecified injury of unspecified pulmonary blood vessels MCC UNS

S25.41 Minor laceration of pulmonary blood vessels
Incomplete transection of pulmonary blood vessels
Laceration of pulmonary blood vessels NOS
Superficial laceration of pulmonary blood vessels

S25.411 Minor laceration of right pulmonary blood vessels MCC

S25.412 Minor laceration of left pulmonary blood vessels MCC

S25.419 Minor laceration of unspecified pulmonary blood vessels MCC UNS

S25.42 Major laceration of pulmonary blood vessels
Complete transection of pulmonary blood vessels
Traumatic rupture of pulmonary blood vessels

S25.421 Major laceration of right pulmonary blood vessels MCC

S25.422 Major laceration of left pulmonary blood vessels MCC

S25.429 Major laceration of unspecified pulmonary blood vessels MCC UNS

S25.49 Other specified injury of pulmonary blood vessels

S25.491 Other specified injury of right pulmonary blood vessels MCC

S25.492 Other specified injury of left pulmonary blood vessels MCC

S25.499 Other specified injury of unspecified pulmonary blood vessels MCC UNS

S25.5 Injury of intercostal blood vessels

S25.50 Unspecified injury of intercostal blood vessels

S25.501 Unspecified injury of intercostal blood vessels, right side CC

S25.502 Unspecified injury of intercostal blood vessels, left side CC

S25.509 Unspecified injury of intercostal blood vessels, unspecified side CC UNS

S25.51 Laceration of intercostal blood vessels

S25.511 Laceration of intercostal blood vessels, right side CC

S25.512 Laceration of intercostal blood vessels, left side CC

S25.519 Laceration of intercostal blood vessels, unspecified side CC UNS

S25.59 Other specified injury of intercostal blood vessels

S25.591 Other specified injury of intercostal blood vessels, right side CC

S25.592 Other specified injury of intercostal blood vessels, left side CC

S25.599 Other specified injury of intercostal blood vessels, unspecified side CC UNS

S25.8 Injury of other blood vessels of thorax
Injury of azygos vein
Injury of mammary artery or vein

S25.80 Unspecified injury of other blood vessels of thorax

S25.801 Unspecified injury of other blood vessels of thorax, right side CC

S25.802 Unspecified injury of other blood vessels of thorax, left side CC

S25.809 Unspecified injury of other blood vessels of thorax, unspecified side CC UNS

S25.81 Laceration of other blood vessels of thorax

S25.811 Laceration of other blood vessels of thorax, right side CC

S25.812 Laceration of other blood vessels of thorax, left side CC

S25.819 Laceration of other blood vessels of thorax, unspecified side CC UNS

S25.89 Other specified injury of other blood vessels of thorax

S25.891 Other specified injury of other blood vessels of thorax, right side CC

S25.892 Other specified injury of other blood vessels of thorax, left side CC

S25.899 Other specified injury of other blood vessels of thorax, unspecified side CC UNS

S25.9 Injury of unspecified blood vessel of thorax

S25.90 Unspecified injury of unspecified blood vessel of thorax CC UNS

S25.91 Laceration of unspecified blood vessel of thorax CC UNS

S25.99 Other specified injury of unspecified blood vessel of thorax CC UNS

S26 Injury of heart

Code also any associated:
open wound of thorax (S21.-)
traumatic hemopneumothorax (S27.2)
traumatic hemothorax (S27.1)
traumatic pneumothorax (S27.0)

The appropriate 7th character is to be added to each code from category S26.
A initial encounter
D subsequent encounter
S sequela

S26.0 Injury of heart with hemopericardium

S26.00 Unspecified injury of heart with hemopericardium CC

S26.01 Contusion of heart with hemopericardium CC

S26.02 Laceration of heart with hemopericardium

S26.020 Mild laceration of heart with hemopericardium MCC
Laceration of heart without penetration of heart chamber

S26.021 Moderate laceration of heart with hemopericardium MCC
Laceration of heart with penetration of heart chamber

√7th S26.022 Major laceration of heart with hemopericardium MCC
Laceration of heart with penetration of multiple heart chambers

√x7th S26.09 Other injury of heart with hemopericardium CC

√5th S26.1 Injury of heart without hemopericardium

√x7th S26.10 Unspecified injury of heart without hemopericardium CC

√x7th S26.11 Contusion of heart without hemopericardium CC

√x7th S26.12 Laceration of heart without hemopericardium MCC

√x7th S26.19 Other injury of heart without hemopericardium CC

√5th S26.9 Injury of heart, unspecified with or without hemopericardium

√x7th S26.90 Unspecified injury of heart, unspecified with or without hemopericardium CC

√x7th S26.91 Contusion of heart, unspecified with or without hemopericardium CC
DEF: Bruising within the heart muscle, with no mention of an open wound, usually caused by blunt chest trauma in motor vehicle accidents, falling from great heights, or receiving CPR.

√x7th S26.92 Laceration of heart, unspecified with or without hemopericardium MCC
Laceration of heart NOS
AHA: 2019,2Q,24

√x7th S26.99 Other injury of heart, unspecified with or without hemopericardium CC

√4th S27 Injury of other and unspecified intrathoracic organs

Code also any associated open wound of thorax (S21.-)

EXCLUDES 2 *injury of cervical esophagus (S10-S19)*
injury of trachea (cervical) (S10-S19)

The appropriate 7th character is to be added to each code from category S27.
A initial encounter
D subsequent encounter
S sequela

√x7th S27.0 Traumatic pneumothorax CC
EXCLUDES 1 *spontaneous pneumothorax (J93.-)*

√x7th S27.1 Traumatic hemothorax MCC

√x7th S27.2 Traumatic hemopneumothorax MCC

√5th S27.3 Other and unspecified injuries of lung

√6th S27.30 Unspecified injury of lung

√7th S27.301 Unspecified injury of lung, unilateral CC

√7th S27.302 Unspecified injury of lung, bilateral CC

√7th S27.309 Unspecified injury of lung, unspecified CC UNS

√6th S27.31 Primary blast injury of lung
Blast injury of lung NOS

√7th S27.311 Primary blast injury of lung, unilateral CC

√7th S27.312 Primary blast injury of lung, bilateral CC

√7th S27.319 Primary blast injury of lung, unspecified CC UNS

√6th S27.32 Contusion of lung
DEF: Bruising of the lung without mention of an open wound.

√7th S27.321 Contusion of lung, unilateral CC

√7th S27.322 Contusion of lung, bilateral CC

√7th S27.329 Contusion of lung, unspecified CC UNS

√6th S27.33 Laceration of lung

√7th S27.331 Laceration of lung, unilateral MCC

√7th S27.332 Laceration of lung, bilateral MCC

√7th S27.339 Laceration of lung, unspecified MCC UNS

√6th S27.39 Other injuries of lung
Secondary blast injury of lung

√7th S27.391 Other injuries of lung, unilateral CC

√7th S27.392 Other injuries of lung, bilateral CC

√7th S27.399 Other injuries of lung, unspecified CC UNS

√5th S27.4 Injury of bronchus

√6th S27.40 Unspecified injury of bronchus

√7th S27.401 Unspecified injury of bronchus, unilateral MCC

√7th S27.402 Unspecified injury of bronchus, bilateral MCC

√7th S27.409 Unspecified injury of bronchus, unspecified MCC UNS

√6th S27.41 Primary blast injury of bronchus
Blast injury of bronchus NOS

√7th S27.411 Primary blast injury of bronchus, unilateral MCC

√7th S27.412 Primary blast injury of bronchus, bilateral MCC

√7th S27.419 Primary blast injury of bronchus, unspecified MCC UNS

√6th S27.42 Contusion of bronchus

√7th S27.421 Contusion of bronchus, unilateral MCC

√7th S27.422 Contusion of bronchus, bilateral MCC

√7th S27.429 Contusion of bronchus, unspecified MCC UNS

√6th S27.43 Laceration of bronchus

√7th S27.431 Laceration of bronchus, unilateral MCC

√7th S27.432 Laceration of bronchus, bilateral MCC

√7th S27.439 Laceration of bronchus, unspecified MCC UNS

√6th S27.49 Other injury of bronchus
Secondary blast injury of bronchus

√7th S27.491 Other injury of bronchus, unilateral MCC

√7th S27.492 Other injury of bronchus, bilateral MCC

√7th S27.499 Other injury of bronchus, unspecified MCC UNS

√5th S27.5 Injury of thoracic trachea

√x7th S27.50 Unspecified injury of thoracic trachea CC

√x7th S27.51 Primary blast injury of thoracic trachea CC
Blast injury of thoracic trachea NOS

√x7th S27.52 Contusion of thoracic trachea CC

√x7th S27.53 Laceration of thoracic trachea CC

√x7th S27.59 Other injury of thoracic trachea CC
Secondary blast injury of thoracic trachea

√5th S27.6 Injury of pleura

√x7th S27.60 Unspecified injury of pleura CC

√x7th S27.63 Laceration of pleura CC

√x7th S27.69 Other injury of pleura CC

√5th S27.8 Injury of other specified intrathoracic organs

√6th S27.80 Injury of diaphragm

√7th S27.802 Contusion of diaphragm CC

√7th S27.803 Laceration of diaphragm CC

√7th S27.808 Other injury of diaphragm CC

√7th S27.809 Unspecified injury of diaphragm CC

√6th S27.81 Injury of esophagus (thoracic part)

√7th S27.812 Contusion of esophagus (thoracic part) MCC

√7th S27.813 Laceration of esophagus (thoracic part) MCC

√7th S27.818 Other injury of esophagus (thoracic part) MCC

√7th S27.819 Unspecified injury of esophagus (thoracic part) MCC

√6th S27.89 Injury of other specified intrathoracic organs
Injury of lymphatic thoracic duct
Injury of thymus gland

√7th S27.892 Contusion of other specified intrathoracic organs CC

√7th S27.893 Laceration of other specified intrathoracic organs CC

√7th S27.898 Other injury of other specified intrathoracic organs CC

√7th S27.899 Unspecified injury of other specified intrathoracic organs CC

√x7th S27.9 Injury of unspecified intrathoracic organ CC

S28 Crushing injury of thorax, and traumatic amputation of part of thorax

The appropriate 7th character is to be added to each code from category S28.
A initial encounter
D subsequent encounter
S sequela

S28.0 Crushed chest
Use additional code for all associated injuries
EXCLUDES 1 *flail chest (S22.5)*

S28.1 Traumatic amputation (partial) of part of thorax, except breast CC

S28.2 Traumatic amputation of breast

S28.21 Complete traumatic amputation of breast
Traumatic amputation of breast NOS

S28.211 Complete traumatic amputation of right breast

S28.212 Complete traumatic amputation of left breast

S28.219 Complete traumatic amputation of unspecified breast

S28.22 Partial traumatic amputation of breast

S28.221 Partial traumatic amputation of right breast

S28.222 Partial traumatic amputation of left breast

S28.229 Partial traumatic amputation of unspecified breast

S29 Other and unspecified injuries of thorax
Code also any associated open wound (S21.-)

The appropriate 7th character is to be added to each code from category S29.
A initial encounter
D subsequent encounter
S sequela

S29.0 Injury of muscle and tendon at thorax level

S29.00 Unspecified injury of muscle and tendon of thorax

S29.001 Unspecified injury of muscle and tendon of front wall of thorax

S29.002 Unspecified injury of muscle and tendon of back wall of thorax

S29.009 Unspecified injury of muscle and tendon of unspecified wall of thorax

S29.01 Strain of muscle and tendon of thorax

S29.011 Strain of muscle and tendon of front wall of thorax

S29.012 Strain of muscle and tendon of back wall of thorax

S29.019 Strain of muscle and tendon of unspecified wall of thorax

S29.02 Laceration of muscle and tendon of thorax

S29.021 Laceration of muscle and tendon of front wall of thorax CC

S29.022 Laceration of muscle and tendon of back wall of thorax

S29.029 Laceration of muscle and tendon of unspecified wall of thorax CC UNS

S29.09 Other injury of muscle and tendon of thorax

S29.091 Other injury of muscle and tendon of front wall of thorax

S29.092 Other injury of muscle and tendon of back wall of thorax

S29.099 Other injury of muscle and tendon of unspecified wall of thorax

S29.8 Other specified injuries of thorax

S29.9 Unspecified injury of thorax

Injuries to the abdomen, lower back, lumbar spine, pelvis and external genitals (S30-S39)

INCLUDES injuries to the abdominal wall
injuries to the anus
injuries to the buttock
injuries to the external genitalia
injuries to the flank
injuries to the groin

EXCLUDES 2 *burns and corrosions (T20-T32)*
effects of foreign body in anus and rectum (T18.5)
effects of foreign body in genitourinary tract (T19.-)
effects of foreign body in stomach, small intestine and colon (T18.2-T18.4)
frostbite (T33-T34)
insect bite or sting, venomous (T63.4)

S30 Superficial injury of abdomen, lower back, pelvis and external genitals
EXCLUDES 2 *superficial injury of hip (S70.-)*

The appropriate 7th character is to be added to each code from category S30.
A initial encounter
D subsequent encounter
S sequela

S30.0 Contusion of lower back and pelvis
Contusion of buttock

S30.1 Contusion of abdominal wall
Contusion of flank
Contusion of groin

S30.2 Contusion of external genital organs

S30.20 Contusion of unspecified external genital organ

S30.201 Contusion of unspecified external genital organ, male ♂

S30.202 Contusion of unspecified external genital organ, female ♀

S30.21 Contusion of penis ♂

S30.22 Contusion of scrotum and testes ♂

S30.23 Contusion of vagina and vulva ♀

S30.3 Contusion of anus

S30.8 Other superficial injuries of abdomen, lower back, pelvis and external genitals

S30.81 Abrasion of abdomen, lower back, pelvis and external genitals

S30.810 Abrasion of lower back and pelvis

S30.811 Abrasion of abdominal wall

S30.812 Abrasion of penis ♂

S30.813 Abrasion of scrotum and testes ♂

S30.814 Abrasion of vagina and vulva ♀

S30.815 Abrasion of unspecified external genital organs, male ♂

S30.816 Abrasion of unspecified external genital organs, female ♀

S30.817 Abrasion of anus

S30.82 Blister (nonthermal) of abdomen, lower back, pelvis and external genitals

S30.820 Blister (nonthermal) of lower back and pelvis

S30.821 Blister (nonthermal) of abdominal wall

S30.822 Blister (nonthermal) of penis ♂

S30.823 Blister (nonthermal) of scrotum and testes ♂

S30.824 Blister (nonthermal) of vagina and vulva ♀

S30.825 Blister (nonthermal) of unspecified external genital organs, male ♂

S30.826 Blister (nonthermal) of unspecified external genital organs, female ♀

S30.827 Blister (nonthermal) of anus

S30.84 External constriction of abdomen, lower back, pelvis and external genitals

S30.840 External constriction of lower back and pelvis

S30.841 External constriction of abdominal wall

S30.842 External constriction of penis ♂
Hair tourniquet syndrome of penis
Use additional cause code to identify the constricting item (W49.0-)

S30.843 External constriction of scrotum and testes ♂
S30.844 External constriction of vagina and vulva ♀
S30.845 External constriction of unspecified external genital organs, male ♂
S30.846 External constriction of unspecified external genital organs, female ♀

S30.85 Superficial foreign body of abdomen, lower back, pelvis and external genitals
Splinter in the abdomen, lower back, pelvis and external genitals
S30.850 Superficial foreign body of lower back and pelvis
S30.851 Superficial foreign body of abdominal wall
S30.852 Superficial foreign body of penis ♂
S30.853 Superficial foreign body of scrotum and testes ♂
S30.854 Superficial foreign body of vagina and vulva ♀
S30.855 Superficial foreign body of unspecified external genital organs, male ♂
S30.856 Superficial foreign body of unspecified external genital organs, female ♀
S30.857 Superficial foreign body of anus

S30.86 Insect bite (nonvenomous) of abdomen, lower back, pelvis and external genitals
S30.860 Insect bite (nonvenomous) of lower back and pelvis
S30.861 Insect bite (nonvenomous) of abdominal wall
S30.862 Insect bite (nonvenomous) of penis ♂
S30.863 Insect bite (nonvenomous) of scrotum and testes ♂
S30.864 Insect bite (nonvenomous) of vagina and vulva ♀
S30.865 Insect bite (nonvenomous) of unspecified external genital organs, male ♂
S30.866 Insect bite (nonvenomous) of unspecified external genital organs, female ♀
S30.867 Insect bite (nonvenomous) of anus

S30.87 Other superficial bite of abdomen, lower back, pelvis and external genitals
EXCLUDES 1 *open bite of abdomen, lower back, pelvis and external genitals (S31.05, S31.15, S31.25, S31.35, S31.45, S31.55)*
S30.870 Other superficial bite of lower back and pelvis
S30.871 Other superficial bite of abdominal wall
S30.872 Other superficial bite of penis ♂
S30.873 Other superficial bite of scrotum and testes ♂
S30.874 Other superficial bite of vagina and vulva ♀
S30.875 Other superficial bite of unspecified external genital organs, male ♂
S30.876 Other superficial bite of unspecified external genital organs, female ♀
S30.877 Other superficial bite of anus

S30.9 Unspecified superficial injury of abdomen, lower back, pelvis and external genitals
S30.91 Unspecified superficial injury of lower back and pelvis
S30.92 Unspecified superficial injury of abdominal wall
S30.93 Unspecified superficial injury of penis ♂
S30.94 Unspecified superficial injury of scrotum and testes ♂
S30.95 Unspecified superficial injury of vagina and vulva ♀
S30.96 Unspecified superficial injury of unspecified external genital organs, male ♂
S30.97 Unspecified superficial injury of unspecified external genital organs, female ♀
S30.98 Unspecified superficial injury of anus

S31 Open wound of abdomen, lower back, pelvis and external genitals

Code also any associated:
spinal cord injury (S24.0, S24.1-, S34.0-, S34.1-)
wound infection

EXCLUDES 1 *traumatic amputation of part of abdomen, lower back and pelvis (S38.2-, S38.3)*
EXCLUDES 2 *open fracture of pelvis (S32.1- - S32.9 with 7th character B)*
open wound of hip (S71.00-S71.02)

The appropriate 7th character is to be added to each code from category S31.
A initial encounter
D subsequent encounter
S sequela

S31.0 Open wound of lower back and pelvis
S31.00 Unspecified open wound of lower back and pelvis
S31.000 Unspecified open wound of lower back and pelvis without penetration into retroperitoneum
Unspecified open wound of lower back and pelvis NOS
S31.001 Unspecified open wound of lower back and pelvis with penetration into retroperitoneum MCC
S31.01 Laceration without foreign body of lower back and pelvis
S31.010 Laceration without foreign body of lower back and pelvis without penetration into retroperitoneum
Laceration without foreign body of lower back and pelvis NOS
S31.011 Laceration without foreign body of lower back and pelvis with penetration into retroperitoneum MCC
S31.02 Laceration with foreign body of lower back and pelvis
S31.020 Laceration with foreign body of lower back and pelvis without penetration into retroperitoneum
Laceration with foreign body of lower back and pelvis NOS
S31.021 Laceration with foreign body of lower back and pelvis with penetration into retroperitoneum MCC
S31.03 Puncture wound without foreign body of lower back and pelvis
S31.030 Puncture wound without foreign body of lower back and pelvis without penetration into retroperitoneum
Puncture wound without foreign body of lower back and pelvis NOS
S31.031 Puncture wound without foreign body of lower back and pelvis with penetration into retroperitoneum MCC
S31.04 Puncture wound with foreign body of lower back and pelvis
S31.040 Puncture wound with foreign body of lower back and pelvis without penetration into retroperitoneum
Puncture wound with foreign body of lower back and pelvis NOS
S31.041 Puncture wound with foreign body of lower back and pelvis with penetration into retroperitoneum MCC
S31.05 Open bite of lower back and pelvis
Bite of lower back and pelvis NOS
EXCLUDES 1 *superficial bite of lower back and pelvis (S30.860, S30.870)*
S31.050 Open bite of lower back and pelvis without penetration into retroperitoneum
Open bite of lower back and pelvis NOS
S31.051 Open bite of lower back and pelvis with penetration into retroperitoneum MCC

√5th **S31.1 Open wound of abdominal wall without penetration into peritoneal cavity**
Open wound of abdominal wall NOS
EXCLUDES 2 *open wound of abdominal wall with penetration into peritoneal cavity (S31.6-)*

√6th **S31.10 Unspecified open wound of abdominal wall without penetration into peritoneal cavity**

√7th **S31.100 Unspecified open wound of abdominal wall, right upper quadrant without penetration into peritoneal cavity**

√7th **S31.101 Unspecified open wound of abdominal wall, left upper quadrant without penetration into peritoneal cavity**

√7th **S31.102 Unspecified open wound of abdominal wall, epigastric region without penetration into peritoneal cavity**

√7th **S31.103 Unspecified open wound of abdominal wall, right lower quadrant without penetration into peritoneal cavity**

√7th **S31.104 Unspecified open wound of abdominal wall, left lower quadrant without penetration into peritoneal cavity**

√7th **S31.105 Unspecified open wound of abdominal wall, periumbilic region without penetration into peritoneal cavity**

√7th **S31.109 Unspecified open wound of abdominal wall, unspecified quadrant without penetration into peritoneal cavity**
Unspecified open wound of abdominal wall NOS

√6th **S31.11 Laceration without foreign body of abdominal wall without penetration into peritoneal cavity**

√7th **S31.110 Laceration without foreign body of abdominal wall, right upper quadrant without penetration into peritoneal cavity**

√7th **S31.111 Laceration without foreign body of abdominal wall, left upper quadrant without penetration into peritoneal cavity**

√7th **S31.112 Laceration without foreign body of abdominal wall, epigastric region without penetration into peritoneal cavity**

√7th **S31.113 Laceration without foreign body of abdominal wall, right lower quadrant without penetration into peritoneal cavity**

√7th **S31.114 Laceration without foreign body of abdominal wall, left lower quadrant without penetration into peritoneal cavity**

√7th **S31.115 Laceration without foreign body of abdominal wall, periumbilic region without penetration into peritoneal cavity**

√7th **S31.119 Laceration without foreign body of abdominal wall, unspecified quadrant without penetration into peritoneal cavity**

√6th **S31.12 Laceration with foreign body of abdominal wall without penetration into peritoneal cavity**

√7th **S31.120 Laceration of abdominal wall with foreign body, right upper quadrant without penetration into peritoneal cavity**

√7th **S31.121 Laceration of abdominal wall with foreign body, left upper quadrant without penetration into peritoneal cavity**

√7th **S31.122 Laceration of abdominal wall with foreign body, epigastric region without penetration into peritoneal cavity**

√7th **S31.123 Laceration of abdominal wall with foreign body, right lower quadrant without penetration into peritoneal cavity**

√7th **S31.124 Laceration of abdominal wall with foreign body, left lower quadrant without penetration into peritoneal cavity**

√7th **S31.125 Laceration of abdominal wall with foreign body, periumbilic region without penetration into peritoneal cavity**

√7th **S31.129 Laceration of abdominal wall with foreign body, unspecified quadrant without penetration into peritoneal cavity**

√6th **S31.13 Puncture wound of abdominal wall without foreign body without penetration into peritoneal cavity**

√7th **S31.130 Puncture wound of abdominal wall without foreign body, right upper quadrant without penetration into peritoneal cavity**

√7th **S31.131 Puncture wound of abdominal wall without foreign body, left upper quadrant without penetration into peritoneal cavity**

√7th **S31.132 Puncture wound of abdominal wall without foreign body, epigastric region without penetration into peritoneal cavity**

√7th **S31.133 Puncture wound of abdominal wall without foreign body, right lower quadrant without penetration into peritoneal cavity**

√7th **S31.134 Puncture wound of abdominal wall without foreign body, left lower quadrant without penetration into peritoneal cavity**

√7th **S31.135 Puncture wound of abdominal wall without foreign body, periumbilic region without penetration into peritoneal cavity**

√7th **S31.139 Puncture wound of abdominal wall without foreign body, unspecified quadrant without penetration into peritoneal cavity**

√6th **S31.14 Puncture wound of abdominal wall with foreign body without penetration into peritoneal cavity**

√7th **S31.140 Puncture wound of abdominal wall with foreign body, right upper quadrant without penetration into peritoneal cavity**

√7th **S31.141 Puncture wound of abdominal wall with foreign body, left upper quadrant without penetration into peritoneal cavity**

√7th **S31.142 Puncture wound of abdominal wall with foreign body, epigastric region without penetration into peritoneal cavity**

√7th **S31.143 Puncture wound of abdominal wall with foreign body, right lower quadrant without penetration into peritoneal cavity**

√7th **S31.144 Puncture wound of abdominal wall with foreign body, left lower quadrant without penetration into peritoneal cavity**

√7th **S31.145 Puncture wound of abdominal wall with foreign body, periumbilic region without penetration into peritoneal cavity**

√7th **S31.149 Puncture wound of abdominal wall with foreign body, unspecified quadrant without penetration into peritoneal cavity**

√6th **S31.15 Open bite of abdominal wall without penetration into peritoneal cavity**
Bite of abdominal wall NOS
EXCLUDES 1 *superficial bite of abdominal wall (S30.871)*

√7th **S31.150 Open bite of abdominal wall, right upper quadrant without penetration into peritoneal cavity**

√7th **S31.151 Open bite of abdominal wall, left upper quadrant without penetration into peritoneal cavity**

√7th **S31.152 Open bite of abdominal wall, epigastric region without penetration into peritoneal cavity**

√7th **S31.153 Open bite of abdominal wall, right lower quadrant without penetration into peritoneal cavity**

√7th **S31.154 Open bite of abdominal wall, left lower quadrant without penetration into peritoneal cavity**

√7th **S31.155 Open bite of abdominal wall, periumbilic region without penetration into peritoneal cavity**

√7th **S31.159 Open bite of abdominal wall, unspecified quadrant without penetration into peritoneal cavity**

√5th **S31.2 Open wound of penis**

√x7th **S31.20 Unspecified open wound of penis** ♂

S31.21 Laceration without foreign body of penis ♂
S31.22 Laceration with foreign body of penis ♂
S31.23 Puncture wound without foreign body of penis ♂
S31.24 Puncture wound with foreign body of penis ♂
S31.25 Open bite of penis ♂
Bite of penis NOS
EXCLUDES 1 *superficial bite of penis (S30.862, S30.872)*

S31.3 Open wound of scrotum and testes
S31.30 Unspecified open wound of scrotum and testes ♂
S31.31 Laceration without foreign body of scrotum and testes ♂
S31.32 Laceration with foreign body of scrotum and testes ♂
S31.33 Puncture wound without foreign body of scrotum and testes ♂
S31.34 Puncture wound with foreign body of scrotum and testes ♂
S31.35 Open bite of scrotum and testes ♂
Bite of scrotum and testes NOS
EXCLUDES 1 *superficial bite of scrotum and testes (S30.863, S30.873)*

S31.4 Open wound of vagina and vulva
EXCLUDES 1 *injury to vagina and vulva during delivery (O70.-, O71.4)*
S31.40 Unspecified open wound of vagina and vulva ♀
S31.41 Laceration without foreign body of vagina and vulva ♀
S31.42 Laceration with foreign body of vagina and vulva ♀
S31.43 Puncture wound without foreign body of vagina and vulva ♀
S31.44 Puncture wound with foreign body of vagina and vulva ♀
S31.45 Open bite of vagina and vulva ♀
Bite of vagina and vulva NOS
EXCLUDES 1 *superficial bite of vagina and vulva (S30.864, S30.874)*

S31.5 Open wound of unspecified external genital organs
EXCLUDES 1 *traumatic amputation of external genital organs (S38.21, S38.22)*
S31.50 Unspecified open wound of unspecified external genital organs
S31.501 Unspecified open wound of unspecified external genital organs, male ♂
S31.502 Unspecified open wound of unspecified external genital organs, female ♀
S31.51 Laceration without foreign body of unspecified external genital organs
S31.511 Laceration without foreign body of unspecified external genital organs, male ♂
S31.512 Laceration without foreign body of unspecified external genital organs, female ♀
S31.52 Laceration with foreign body of unspecified external genital organs
S31.521 Laceration with foreign body of unspecified external genital organs, male ♂
S31.522 Laceration with foreign body of unspecified external genital organs, female ♀
S31.53 Puncture wound without foreign body of unspecified external genital organs
S31.531 Puncture wound without foreign body of unspecified external genital organs, male ♂
S31.532 Puncture wound without foreign body of unspecified external genital organs, female ♀
S31.54 Puncture wound with foreign body of unspecified external genital organs
S31.541 Puncture wound with foreign body of unspecified external genital organs, male ♂
S31.542 Puncture wound with foreign body of unspecified external genital organs, female ♀
S31.55 Open bite of unspecified external genital organs
Bite of unspecified external genital organs NOS
EXCLUDES 1 *superficial bite of unspecified external genital organs (S30.865, S30.866, S30.875, S30.876)*
S31.551 Open bite of unspecified external genital organs, male ♂
S31.552 Open bite of unspecified external genital organs, female ♀

S31.6 Open wound of abdominal wall with penetration into peritoneal cavity
S31.60 Unspecified open wound of abdominal wall with penetration into peritoneal cavity
S31.600 Unspecified open wound of abdominal wall, right upper quadrant with penetration into peritoneal cavity MCC
S31.601 Unspecified open wound of abdominal wall, left upper quadrant with penetration into peritoneal cavity MCC
S31.602 Unspecified open wound of abdominal wall, epigastric region with penetration into peritoneal cavity MCC
S31.603 Unspecified open wound of abdominal wall, right lower quadrant with penetration into peritoneal cavity MCC
S31.604 Unspecified open wound of abdominal wall, left lower quadrant with penetration into peritoneal cavity MCC
S31.605 Unspecified open wound of abdominal wall, periumbilic region with penetration into peritoneal cavity MCC
S31.609 Unspecified open wound of abdominal wall, unspecified quadrant with penetration into peritoneal cavity MCC UNS
S31.61 Laceration without foreign body of abdominal wall with penetration into peritoneal cavity
S31.610 Laceration without foreign body of abdominal wall, right upper quadrant with penetration into peritoneal cavity MCC
S31.611 Laceration without foreign body of abdominal wall, left upper quadrant with penetration into peritoneal cavity MCC
S31.612 Laceration without foreign body of abdominal wall, epigastric region with penetration into peritoneal cavity MCC
S31.613 Laceration without foreign body of abdominal wall, right lower quadrant with penetration into peritoneal cavity MCC
S31.614 Laceration without foreign body of abdominal wall, left lower quadrant with penetration into peritoneal cavity MCC
S31.615 Laceration without foreign body of abdominal wall, periumbilic region with penetration into peritoneal cavity MCC
S31.619 Laceration without foreign body of abdominal wall, unspecified quadrant with penetration into peritoneal cavity MCC UNS
S31.62 Laceration with foreign body of abdominal wall with penetration into peritoneal cavity
S31.620 Laceration with foreign body of abdominal wall, right upper quadrant with penetration into peritoneal cavity MCC
S31.621 Laceration with foreign body of abdominal wall, left upper quadrant with penetration into peritoneal cavity MCC
S31.622 Laceration with foreign body of abdominal wall, epigastric region with penetration into peritoneal cavity MCC
S31.623 Laceration with foreign body of abdominal wall, right lower quadrant with penetration into peritoneal cavity MCC
S31.624 Laceration with foreign body of abdominal wall, left lower quadrant with penetration into peritoneal cavity MCC

7th S31.625 Laceration with foreign body of abdominal wall, periumbilic region with penetration into peritoneal cavity MCC

7th S31.629 Laceration with foreign body of abdominal wall, unspecified quadrant with penetration into peritoneal cavity MCC UNS

6th S31.63 Puncture wound without foreign body of abdominal wall with penetration into peritoneal cavity

7th S31.630 Puncture wound without foreign body of abdominal wall, right upper quadrant with penetration into peritoneal cavity MCC

7th S31.631 Puncture wound without foreign body of abdominal wall, left upper quadrant with penetration into peritoneal cavity MCC

7th S31.632 Puncture wound without foreign body of abdominal wall, epigastric region with penetration into peritoneal cavity MCC

7th S31.633 Puncture wound without foreign body of abdominal wall, right lower quadrant with penetration into peritoneal cavity MCC

7th S31.634 Puncture wound without foreign body of abdominal wall, left lower quadrant with penetration into peritoneal cavity MCC

7th S31.635 Puncture wound without foreign body of abdominal wall, periumbilic region with penetration into peritoneal cavity MCC

7th S31.639 Puncture wound without foreign body of abdominal wall, unspecified quadrant with penetration into peritoneal cavity MCC UNS

6th S31.64 Puncture wound with foreign body of abdominal wall with penetration into peritoneal cavity

7th S31.640 Puncture wound with foreign body of abdominal wall, right upper quadrant with penetration into peritoneal cavity MCC

7th S31.641 Puncture wound with foreign body of abdominal wall, left upper quadrant with penetration into peritoneal cavity MCC

7th S31.642 Puncture wound with foreign body of abdominal wall, epigastric region with penetration into peritoneal cavity MCC

7th S31.643 Puncture wound with foreign body of abdominal wall, right lower quadrant with penetration into peritoneal cavity MCC

7th S31.644 Puncture wound with foreign body of abdominal wall, left lower quadrant with penetration into peritoneal cavity MCC

7th S31.645 Puncture wound with foreign body of abdominal wall, periumbilic region with penetration into peritoneal cavity MCC

7th S31.649 Puncture wound with foreign body of abdominal wall, unspecified quadrant with penetration into peritoneal cavity MCC UNS

6th S31.65 Open bite of abdominal wall with penetration into peritoneal cavity

EXCLUDES 1 *superficial bite of abdominal wall (S30.861, S30.871)*

7th S31.650 Open bite of abdominal wall, right upper quadrant with penetration into peritoneal cavity MCC

7th S31.651 Open bite of abdominal wall, left upper quadrant with penetration into peritoneal cavity MCC

7th S31.652 Open bite of abdominal wall, epigastric region with penetration into peritoneal cavity MCC

7th S31.653 Open bite of abdominal wall, right lower quadrant with penetration into peritoneal cavity MCC

7th S31.654 Open bite of abdominal wall, left lower quadrant with penetration into peritoneal cavity MCC

7th S31.655 Open bite of abdominal wall, periumbilic region with penetration into peritoneal cavity MCC

7th S31.659 Open bite of abdominal wall, unspecified quadrant with penetration into peritoneal cavity MCC UNS

5th S31.8 Open wound of other parts of abdomen, lower back and pelvis

6th S31.80 Open wound of unspecified buttock

7th S31.801 Laceration without foreign body of unspecified buttock

7th S31.802 Laceration with foreign body of unspecified buttock

7th S31.803 Puncture wound without foreign body of unspecified buttock

7th S31.804 Puncture wound with foreign body of unspecified buttock

7th S31.805 Open bite of unspecified buttock

Bite of buttock NOS

EXCLUDES 1 *superficial bite of buttock (S30.870)*

7th S31.809 Unspecified open wound of unspecified buttock

6th S31.81 Open wound of right buttock

7th S31.811 Laceration without foreign body of right buttock

7th S31.812 Laceration with foreign body of right buttock

7th S31.813 Puncture wound without foreign body of right buttock

7th S31.814 Puncture wound with foreign body of right buttock

7th S31.815 Open bite of right buttock

Bite of right buttock NOS

EXCLUDES 1 *superficial bite of buttock (S30.870)*

7th S31.819 Unspecified open wound of right buttock

6th S31.82 Open wound of left buttock

7th S31.821 Laceration without foreign body of left buttock

7th S31.822 Laceration with foreign body of left buttock

7th S31.823 Puncture wound without foreign body of left buttock

7th S31.824 Puncture wound with foreign body of left buttock

7th S31.825 Open bite of left buttock

Bite of left buttock NOS

EXCLUDES 1 *superficial bite of buttock (S30.870)*

7th S31.829 Unspecified open wound of left buttock

6th S31.83 Open wound of anus

7th S31.831 Laceration without foreign body of anus

7th S31.832 Laceration with foreign body of anus

7th S31.833 Puncture wound without foreign body of anus

7th S31.834 Puncture wound with foreign body of anus

7th S31.835 Open bite of anus

Bite of anus NOS

EXCLUDES 1 *superficial bite of anus (S30.877)*

7th S31.839 Unspecified open wound of anus

√4th **S32 Fracture of lumbar spine and pelvis**

NOTE A fracture not indicated as displaced or nondisplaced should be coded to displaced.

A fracture not indicated as opened or closed should be coded to closed.

INCLUDES fracture of lumbosacral neural arch
fracture of lumbosacral spinous process
fracture of lumbosacral transverse process
fracture of lumbosacral vertebra
fracture of lumbosacral vertebral arch

Code first any associated spinal cord and spinal nerve injury (S34.-)

EXCLUDES 1 *transection of abdomen (S38.3)*

EXCLUDES 2 *fracture of hip NOS (S72.Ø-)*

AHA: 2021,1Q,6; 2018,2Q,12; 2015,3Q,37-39; 2012,4Q,93

The appropriate 7th character is to be added to each code from category S32.
A initial encounter for closed fracture
B initial encounter for open fracture
D subsequent encounter for fracture with routine healing
G subsequent encounter for fracture with delayed healing
K subsequent encounter for fracture with nonunion
S sequela

√5th **S32.Ø Fracture of lumbar vertebra**
Fracture of lumbar spine NOS

√6th **S32.ØØ Fracture of unspecified lumbar vertebra**
√7th **S32.ØØØ Wedge compression fracture of unspecified lumbar vertebra** MCC CC H5 HCC
√7th **S32.ØØ1 Stable burst fracture of unspecified lumbar vertebra** MCC CC H5 HCC
√7th **S32.ØØ2 Unstable burst fracture of unspecified lumbar vertebra** MCC CC H5 HCC
√7th **S32.ØØ8 Other fracture of unspecified lumbar vertebra** MCC CC H5 HCC
√7th **S32.ØØ9 Unspecified fracture of unspecified lumbar vertebra** MCC CC H5 HCC

√6th **S32.Ø1 Fracture of first lumbar vertebra**
√7th **S32.Ø1Ø Wedge compression fracture of first lumbar vertebra** MCC CC H5 HCC
√7th **S32.Ø11 Stable burst fracture of first lumbar vertebra** MCC CC H5 HCC
√7th **S32.Ø12 Unstable burst fracture of first lumbar vertebra** MCC CC H5 HCC
√7th **S32.Ø18 Other fracture of first lumbar vertebra** MCC CC H5 HCC
√7th **S32.Ø19 Unspecified fracture of first lumbar vertebra** MCC CC H5 HCC

√6th **S32.Ø2 Fracture of second lumbar vertebra**
√7th **S32.Ø2Ø Wedge compression fracture of second lumbar vertebra** MCC CC H5 HCC
√7th **S32.Ø21 Stable burst fracture of second lumbar vertebra** MCC CC H5 HCC
√7th **S32.Ø22 Unstable burst fracture of second lumbar vertebra** MCC CC H5 HCC
√7th **S32.Ø28 Other fracture of second lumbar vertebra** MCC CC H5 HCC
√7th **S32.Ø29 Unspecified fracture of second lumbar vertebra** MCC CC H5 HCC

√6th **S32.Ø3 Fracture of third lumbar vertebra**
√7th **S32.Ø3Ø Wedge compression fracture of third lumbar vertebra** MCC CC H5 HCC
√7th **S32.Ø31 Stable burst fracture of third lumbar vertebra** MCC CC H5 HCC
√7th **S32.Ø32 Unstable burst fracture of third lumbar vertebra** MCC CC H5 HCC
√7th **S32.Ø38 Other fracture of third lumbar vertebra** MCC CC H5 HCC
√7th **S32.Ø39 Unspecified fracture of third lumbar vertebra** MCC CC H5 HCC

√6th **S32.Ø4 Fracture of fourth lumbar vertebra**
√7th **S32.Ø4Ø Wedge compression fracture of fourth lumbar vertebra** MCC CC H5 HCC
√7th **S32.Ø41 Stable burst fracture of fourth lumbar vertebra** MCC CC H5 HCC
√7th **S32.Ø42 Unstable burst fracture of fourth lumbar vertebra** MCC CC H5 HCC
√7th **S32.Ø48 Other fracture of fourth lumbar vertebra** MCC CC H5 HCC
√7th **S32.Ø49 Unspecified fracture of fourth lumbar vertebra** MCC CC H5 HCC

√6th **S32.Ø5 Fracture of fifth lumbar vertebra**
√7th **S32.Ø5Ø Wedge compression fracture of fifth lumbar vertebra** MCC CC H5 HCC
√7th **S32.Ø51 Stable burst fracture of fifth lumbar vertebra** MCC CC H5 HCC
√7th **S32.Ø52 Unstable burst fracture of fifth lumbar vertebra** MCC CC H5 HCC
√7th **S32.Ø58 Other fracture of fifth lumbar vertebra** MCC CC H5 HCC
√7th **S32.Ø59 Unspecified fracture of fifth lumbar vertebra** MCC CC H5 HCC

√5th **S32.1 Fracture of sacrum**

NOTE For vertical fractures, code to most medial fracture extension

Use two codes if both a vertical and transverse fracture are present

Code also any associated fracture of pelvic ring (S32.8-)

√x 7th **S32.1Ø Unspecified fracture of sacrum** MCC CC H5 HCC

√6th **S32.11 Zone I fracture of sacrum**
Vertical sacral ala fracture of sacrum

Vertical Sacral Fracture Zones

Zones: 1 2 3

√7th **S32.11Ø Nondisplaced Zone I fracture of sacrum** MCC CC H5 HCC
√7th **S32.111 Minimally displaced Zone I fracture of sacrum** MCC CC H5 HCC
√7th **S32.112 Severely displaced Zone I fracture of sacrum** MCC CC H5 HCC
√7th **S32.119 Unspecified Zone I fracture of sacrum** MCC CC H5 HCC

√6th **S32.12 Zone II fracture of sacrum**
Vertical foraminal region fracture of sacrum
√7th **S32.12Ø Nondisplaced Zone II fracture of sacrum** MCC CC H5 HCC
√7th **S32.121 Minimally displaced Zone II fracture of sacrum** MCC CC H5 HCC
√7th **S32.122 Severely displaced Zone II fracture of sacrum** MCC CC H5 HCC
√7th **S32.129 Unspecified Zone II fracture of sacrum** MCC CC H5 HCC

√6th **S32.13 Zone III fracture of sacrum**
Vertical fracture into spinal canal region of sacrum
√7th **S32.13Ø Nondisplaced Zone III fracture of sacrum** MCC CC H5 HCC
√7th **S32.131 Minimally displaced Zone III fracture of sacrum** MCC CC H5 HCC
√7th **S32.132 Severely displaced Zone III fracture of sacrum** MCC CC H5 HCC

7th **S32.139** Unspecified Zone III fracture of sacrum MCC CC H5 HCC

Transverse Sacral Fracture Types

Type 1 Type 2 Type 3 Type 4

x7th **S32.14** Type 1 fracture of sacrum MCC CC H5 HCC
Transverse flexion fracture of sacrum without displacement

x7th **S32.15** Type 2 fracture of sacrum MCC CC H5 HCC
Transverse flexion fracture of sacrum with posterior displacement

x7th **S32.16** Type 3 fracture of sacrum MCC CC H5 HCC
Transverse extension fracture of sacrum with anterior displacement

x7th **S32.17** Type 4 fracture of sacrum MCC CC H5 HCC
Transverse segmental comminution of upper sacrum

x7th **S32.19** Other fracture of sacrum MCC CC H5 HCC

x7th **S32.2** Fracture of coccyx MCC CC H5 HCC

5th **S32.3** Fracture of ilium

EXCLUDES 1 *fracture of ilium with associated disruption of pelvic ring (S32.8-)*

6th **S32.30** Unspecified fracture of ilium

7th **S32.301** Unspecified fracture of right ilium MCC CC H5 HCC

7th **S32.302** Unspecified fracture of left ilium MCC CC H5 HCC

7th **S32.309** Unspecified fracture of unspecified ilium MCC CC H5 UNS HCC

6th **S32.31** Avulsion fracture of ilium

7th **S32.311** Displaced avulsion fracture of right ilium MCC CC H5 HCC

7th **S32.312** Displaced avulsion fracture of left ilium MCC CC H5 HCC

7th **S32.313** Displaced avulsion fracture of unspecified ilium MCC CC H5 UNS HCC

7th **S32.314** Nondisplaced avulsion fracture of right ilium MCC CC H5 HCC

7th **S32.315** Nondisplaced avulsion fracture of left ilium MCC CC H5 HCC

7th **S32.316** Nondisplaced avulsion fracture of unspecified ilium MCC CC H5 UNS HCC

6th **S32.39** Other fracture of ilium

7th **S32.391** Other fracture of right ilium MCC CC H5 HCC

7th **S32.392** Other fracture of left ilium MCC CC H5 HCC

7th **S32.399** Other fracture of unspecified ilium MCC CC H5 UNS HCC

5th **S32.4** Fracture of acetabulum

Code also any associated fracture of pelvic ring (S32.8-)

AHA: 2016,3Q,16

6th **S32.40** Unspecified fracture of acetabulum

7th **S32.401** Unspecified fracture of right acetabulum MCC CC H5 HCC

7th **S32.402** Unspecified fracture of left acetabulum MCC CC H5 HCC

7th **S32.409** Unspecified fracture of unspecified acetabulum MCC CC H5 UNS HCC

6th **S32.41** Fracture of anterior wall of acetabulum

7th **S32.411** Displaced fracture of anterior wall of right acetabulum MCC CC H5 HCC

7th **S32.412** Displaced fracture of anterior wall of left acetabulum MCC CC H5 HCC

7th **S32.413** Displaced fracture of anterior wall of unspecified acetabulum MCC CC H5 UNS HCC

7th **S32.414** Nondisplaced fracture of anterior wall of right acetabulum MCC CC H5 HCC

7th **S32.415** Nondisplaced fracture of anterior wall of left acetabulum MCC CC H5 HCC

7th **S32.416** Nondisplaced fracture of anterior wall of unspecified acetabulum MCC CC H5 UNS HCC

6th **S32.42** Fracture of posterior wall of acetabulum

7th **S32.421** Displaced fracture of posterior wall of right acetabulum MCC CC H5 HCC

7th **S32.422** Displaced fracture of posterior wall of left acetabulum MCC CC H5 HCC

7th **S32.423** Displaced fracture of posterior wall of unspecified acetabulum MCC CC H5 UNS HCC

7th **S32.424** Nondisplaced fracture of posterior wall of right acetabulum MCC CC H5 HCC

7th **S32.425** Nondisplaced fracture of posterior wall of left acetabulum MCC CC H5 HCC

7th **S32.426** Nondisplaced fracture of posterior wall of unspecified acetabulum MCC CC H5 UNS HCC

6th **S32.43** Fracture of anterior column [iliopubic] of acetabulum

7th **S32.431** Displaced fracture of anterior column [iliopubic] of right acetabulum MCC CC H5 HCC

7th **S32.432** Displaced fracture of anterior column [iliopubic] of left acetabulum MCC CC H5 HCC

7th **S32.433** Displaced fracture of anterior column [iliopubic] of unspecified acetabulum MCC CC H5 UNS HCC

7th **S32.434** Nondisplaced fracture of anterior column [iliopubic] of right acetabulum MCC CC H5 HCC

7th **S32.435** Nondisplaced fracture of anterior column [iliopubic] of left acetabulum MCC CC H5 HCC

7th **S32.436** Nondisplaced fracture of anterior column [iliopubic] of unspecified acetabulum MCC CC H5 UNS HCC

6th **S32.44** Fracture of posterior column [ilioischial] of acetabulum

7th **S32.441** Displaced fracture of posterior column [ilioischial] of right acetabulum MCC CC H5 HCC

7th **S32.442** Displaced fracture of posterior column [ilioischial] of left acetabulum MCC CC H5 HCC

7th **S32.443** Displaced fracture of posterior column [ilioischial] of unspecified acetabulum MCC CC H5 UNS HCC

7th **S32.444** Nondisplaced fracture of posterior column [ilioischial] of right acetabulum MCC CC H5 HCC

7th **S32.445** Nondisplaced fracture of posterior column [ilioischial] of left acetabulum MCC CC H5 HCC

7th **S32.446** Nondisplaced fracture of posterior column [ilioischial] of unspecified acetabulum MCC CC H5 UNS HCC

6th **S32.45** Transverse fracture of acetabulum

7th **S32.451** Displaced transverse fracture of right acetabulum MCC CC H5 HCC

7th **S32.452** Displaced transverse fracture of left acetabulum MCC CC H5 HCC

7th **S32.453** Displaced transverse fracture of unspecified acetabulum MCC CC H5 UNS HCC

7th **S32.454** Nondisplaced transverse fracture of right acetabulum MCC CC H5 HCC

7th **S32.455** Nondisplaced transverse fracture of left acetabulum MCC CC H5 HCC

7th **S32.456** Nondisplaced transverse fracture of unspecified acetabulum MCC CC H5 UNS HCC

✓6th **S32.46 Associated transverse-posterior fracture of acetabulum**

✓7th S32.461 Displaced associated transverse-posterior fracture of right acetabulum MCC CC H5 HCC

✓7th S32.462 Displaced associated transverse-posterior fracture of left acetabulum MCC CC H5 HCC

✓7th S32.463 Displaced associated transverse-posterior fracture of unspecified acetabulum MCC CC H5 UNS HCC

✓7th S32.464 Nondisplaced associated transverse-posterior fracture of right acetabulum MCC CC H5 HCC

✓7th S32.465 Nondisplaced associated transverse-posterior fracture of left acetabulum MCC CC H5 HCC

✓7th S32.466 Nondisplaced associated transverse-posterior fracture of unspecified acetabulum MCC CC H5 UNS HCC

✓6th **S32.47 Fracture of medial wall of acetabulum**

✓7th S32.471 Displaced fracture of medial wall of right acetabulum MCC CC H5 HCC

✓7th S32.472 Displaced fracture of medial wall of left acetabulum MCC CC H5 HCC

✓7th S32.473 Displaced fracture of medial wall of unspecified acetabulum MCC CC H5 UNS HCC

✓7th S32.474 Nondisplaced fracture of medial wall of right acetabulum MCC CC H5 HCC

✓7th S32.475 Nondisplaced fracture of medial wall of left acetabulum MCC CC H5 HCC

✓7th S32.476 Nondisplaced fracture of medial wall of unspecified acetabulum MCC CC H5 UNS HCC

✓6th **S32.48 Dome fracture of acetabulum**

✓7th S32.481 Displaced dome fracture of right acetabulum MCC CC H5 HCC

✓7th S32.482 Displaced dome fracture of left acetabulum MCC CC H5 HCC

✓7th S32.483 Displaced dome fracture of unspecified acetabulum MCC CC H5 UNS HCC

✓7th S32.484 Nondisplaced dome fracture of right acetabulum MCC CC H5 HCC

✓7th S32.485 Nondisplaced dome fracture of left acetabulum MCC CC H5 HCC

✓7th S32.486 Nondisplaced dome fracture of unspecified acetabulum MCC CC H5 UNS HCC

✓6th **S32.49 Other specified fracture of acetabulum**

✓7th S32.491 Other specified fracture of right acetabulum MCC CC H5 HCC

✓7th S32.492 Other specified fracture of left acetabulum MCC CC H5 HCC

✓7th S32.499 Other specified fracture of unspecified acetabulum MCC CC H5 UNS HCC

✓5th **S32.5 Fracture of pubis**

EXCLUDES 1 *fracture of pubis with associated disruption of pelvic ring (S32.8-)*

✓6th **S32.50 Unspecified fracture of pubis**

✓7th S32.501 Unspecified fracture of right pubis MCC CC H5 HCC

✓7th S32.502 Unspecified fracture of left pubis MCC CC H5 HCC

✓7th S32.509 Unspecified fracture of unspecified pubis MCC CC H5 UNS HCC

✓6th **S32.51 Fracture of superior rim of pubis**

✓7th S32.511 Fracture of superior rim of right pubis MCC CC H5 HCC

✓7th S32.512 Fracture of superior rim of left pubis MCC CC H5 HCC

✓7th S32.519 Fracture of superior rim of unspecified pubis MCC CC H5 UNS HCC

✓6th **S32.59 Other specified fracture of pubis**

✓7th S32.591 Other specified fracture of right pubis MCC CC H5 HCC

✓7th S32.592 Other specified fracture of left pubis MCC CC H5 HCC

✓7th S32.599 Other specified fracture of unspecified pubis MCC CC H5 UNS HCC

✓5th **S32.6 Fracture of ischium**

EXCLUDES 1 *fracture of ischium with associated disruption of pelvic ring (S32.8-)*

✓6th **S32.60 Unspecified fracture of ischium**

✓7th S32.601 Unspecified fracture of right ischium MCC CC H5 HCC

✓7th S32.602 Unspecified fracture of left ischium MCC CC H5 HCC

✓7th S32.609 Unspecified fracture of unspecified ischium MCC CC H5 UNS HCC

✓6th **S32.61 Avulsion fracture of ischium**

✓7th S32.611 Displaced avulsion fracture of right ischium MCC CC H5 HCC

✓7th S32.612 Displaced avulsion fracture of left ischium MCC CC H5 HCC

✓7th S32.613 Displaced avulsion fracture of unspecified ischium MCC CC H5 UNS HCC

✓7th S32.614 Nondisplaced avulsion fracture of right ischium MCC CC H5 HCC

✓7th S32.615 Nondisplaced avulsion fracture of left ischium MCC CC H5 HCC

✓7th S32.616 Nondisplaced avulsion fracture of unspecified ischium MCC CC H5 UNS HCC

✓6th **S32.69 Other specified fracture of ischium**

✓7th S32.691 Other specified fracture of right ischium MCC CC H5 HCC

✓7th S32.692 Other specified fracture of left ischium MCC CC H5 HCC

✓7th S32.699 Other specified fracture of unspecified ischium MCC CC H5 UNS HCC

✓5th **S32.8 Fracture of other parts of pelvis**

Code also any associated:
fracture of acetabulum (S32.4-)
sacral fracture (S32.1-)

Fractures Disrupting Pelvic Circle

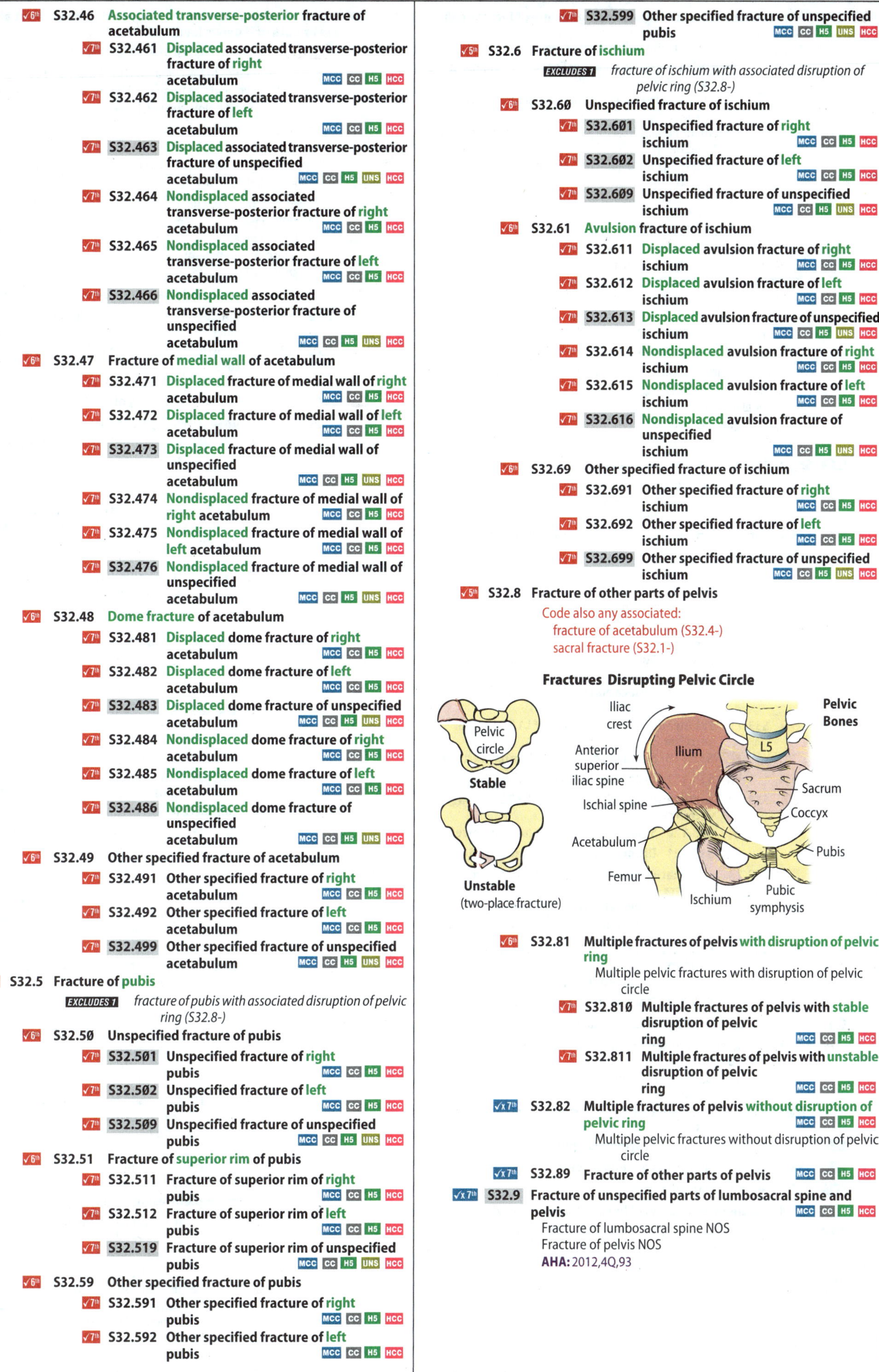

✓6th **S32.81 Multiple fractures of pelvis with disruption of pelvic ring**
Multiple pelvic fractures with disruption of pelvic circle

✓7th S32.810 Multiple fractures of pelvis with stable disruption of pelvic ring MCC CC H5 HCC

✓7th S32.811 Multiple fractures of pelvis with unstable disruption of pelvic ring MCC CC H5 HCC

✓x7th **S32.82 Multiple fractures of pelvis without disruption of pelvic ring** MCC CC H5 HCC
Multiple pelvic fractures without disruption of pelvic circle

✓x7th **S32.89 Fracture of other parts of pelvis** MCC CC H5 HCC

✓x7th **S32.9 Fracture of unspecified parts of lumbosacral spine and pelvis** MCC CC H5 HCC
Fracture of lumbosacral spine NOS
Fracture of pelvis NOS
AHA: 2012,4Q,93

4th **S33 Dislocation and sprain of joints and ligaments of lumbar spine and pelvis**

INCLUDES avulsion of joint or ligament of lumbar spine and pelvis
laceration of cartilage, joint or ligament of lumbar spine and pelvis
sprain of cartilage, joint or ligament of lumbar spine and pelvis
traumatic hemarthrosis of joint or ligament of lumbar spine and pelvis
traumatic rupture of joint or ligament of lumbar spine and pelvis
traumatic subluxation of joint or ligament of lumbar spine and pelvis
traumatic tear of joint or ligament of lumbar spine and pelvis

Code also any associated open wound

EXCLUDES 1 *nontraumatic rupture or displacement of lumbar intervertebral disc NOS (M51.-)*
obstetric damage to pelvic joints and ligaments (O71.6)

EXCLUDES 2 *dislocation and sprain of joints and ligaments of hip (S73.-)*
strain of muscle of lower back and pelvis (S39.01-)

The appropriate 7th character is to be added to each code from category S33.
A initial encounter
D subsequent encounter
S sequela

x7th **S33.0 Traumatic rupture of lumbar intervertebral disc**
EXCLUDES 1 *rupture or displacement (nontraumatic) of lumbar intervertebral disc NOS (M51.- with fifth character 6)*

5th **S33.1 Subluxation and dislocation of lumbar vertebra**
Code also any associated:
open wound of abdomen, lower back and pelvis (S31)
spinal cord injury (S24.0, S24.1-, S34.0-, S34.1-)
EXCLUDES 2 *fracture of lumbar vertebrae (S32.0-)*

6th **S33.10 Subluxation and dislocation of unspecified lumbar vertebra**
7th **S33.100 Subluxation of unspecified lumbar vertebra**
7th **S33.101 Dislocation of unspecified lumbar vertebra**

6th **S33.11 Subluxation and dislocation of L1/L2 lumbar vertebra**
7th **S33.110 Subluxation of L1/L2 lumbar vertebra**
7th **S33.111 Dislocation of L1/L2 lumbar vertebra**

6th **S33.12 Subluxation and dislocation of L2/L3 lumbar vertebra**
7th **S33.120 Subluxation of L2/L3 lumbar vertebra**
7th **S33.121 Dislocation of L2/L3 lumbar vertebra**

6th **S33.13 Subluxation and dislocation of L3/L4 lumbar vertebra**
7th **S33.130 Subluxation of L3/L4 lumbar vertebra**
7th **S33.131 Dislocation of L3/L4 lumbar vertebra**

6th **S33.14 Subluxation and dislocation of L4/L5 lumbar vertebra**
7th **S33.140 Subluxation of L4/L5 lumbar vertebra**
7th **S33.141 Dislocation of L4/L5 lumbar vertebra**

x7th **S33.2 Dislocation of sacroiliac and sacrococcygeal joint**

5th **S33.3 Dislocation of other and unspecified parts of lumbar spine and pelvis**
x7th **S33.30 Dislocation of unspecified parts of lumbar spine and pelvis**
x7th **S33.39 Dislocation of other parts of lumbar spine and pelvis**

x7th **S33.4 Traumatic rupture of symphysis pubis**
x7th **S33.5 Sprain of ligaments of lumbar spine**
x7th **S33.6 Sprain of sacroiliac joint**
x7th **S33.8 Sprain of other parts of lumbar spine and pelvis**
x7th **S33.9 Sprain of unspecified parts of lumbar spine and pelvis**

4th **S34 Injury of lumbar and sacral spinal cord and nerves at abdomen, lower back and pelvis level**

NOTE Code to highest level of lumbar cord injury.
Injuries to the spinal cord (S34.0 and S34.1) refer to the cord level and not bone level injury, and can affect nerve roots at and below the level given.

Code also any associated:
fracture of vertebra (S22.0-, S32.0-)
open wound of abdomen, lower back and pelvis (S31.-)
transient paralysis (R29.5)

The appropriate 7th character is to be added to each code from category S34.
A initial encounter
D subsequent encounter
S sequela

5th **S34.0 Concussion and edema of lumbar and sacral spinal cord**
x7th **S34.01 Concussion and edema of lumbar spinal cord** MCC HCC
x7th **S34.02 Concussion and edema of sacral spinal cord** MCC HCC
Concussion and edema of conus medullaris

5th **S34.1 Other and unspecified injury of lumbar and sacral spinal cord**

6th **S34.10 Unspecified injury to lumbar spinal cord**
7th **S34.101 Unspecified injury to L1 level of lumbar spinal cord** MCC H5 HCC
Unspecified injury to lumbar spinal cord level 1
7th **S34.102 Unspecified injury to L2 level of lumbar spinal cord** MCC H5 HCC
Unspecified injury to lumbar spinal cord level 2
7th **S34.103 Unspecified injury to L3 level of lumbar spinal cord** MCC H5 HCC
Unspecified injury to lumbar spinal cord level 3
7th **S34.104 Unspecified injury to L4 level of lumbar spinal cord** MCC H5 HCC
Unspecified injury to lumbar spinal cord level 4
7th **S34.105 Unspecified injury to L5 level of lumbar spinal cord** MCC H5 HCC
Unspecified injury to lumbar spinal cord level 5
7th **S34.109 Unspecified injury to unspecified level of lumbar spinal cord** MCC H5 HCC

6th **S34.11 Complete lesion of lumbar spinal cord**
7th **S34.111 Complete lesion of L1 level of lumbar spinal cord** MCC H5 HCC
Complete lesion of lumbar spinal cord level 1
7th **S34.112 Complete lesion of L2 level of lumbar spinal cord** MCC H5 HCC
Complete lesion of lumbar spinal cord level 2
7th **S34.113 Complete lesion of L3 level of lumbar spinal cord** MCC H5 HCC
Complete lesion of lumbar spinal cord level 3
7th **S34.114 Complete lesion of L4 level of lumbar spinal cord** MCC H5 HCC
Complete lesion of lumbar spinal cord level 4
7th **S34.115 Complete lesion of L5 level of lumbar spinal cord** MCC H5 HCC
Complete lesion of lumbar spinal cord level 5
7th **S34.119 Complete lesion of unspecified level of lumbar spinal cord** MCC H5 HCC

6th **S34.12 Incomplete lesion of lumbar spinal cord**
7th **S34.121 Incomplete lesion of L1 level of lumbar spinal cord** MCC H5 HCC
Incomplete lesion of lumbar spinal cord level 1
7th **S34.122 Incomplete lesion of L2 level of lumbar spinal cord** MCC H5 HCC
Incomplete lesion of lumbar spinal cord level 2

√7th **S34.123 Incomplete lesion of L3 level of lumbar spinal cord** MCC H5 HCC
Incomplete lesion of lumbar spinal cord level 3

√7th **S34.124 Incomplete lesion of L4 level of lumbar spinal cord** MCC H5 HCC
Incomplete lesion of lumbar spinal cord level 4

√7th **S34.125 Incomplete lesion of L5 level of lumbar spinal cord** MCC H5 HCC
Incomplete lesion of lumbar spinal cord level 5

√7th **S34.129 Incomplete lesion of unspecified level of lumbar spinal cord** MCC H5 HCC

√6th **S34.13 Other and unspecified injury to sacral spinal cord**
Other injury to conus medullaris

√7th **S34.131 Complete lesion of sacral spinal cord** MCC H5 HCC
Complete lesion of conus medullaris

√7th **S34.132 Incomplete lesion of sacral spinal cord** MCC H5 HCC
Incomplete lesion of conus medullaris

√7th **S34.139 Unspecified injury to sacral spinal cord** MCC H5 HCC
Unspecified injury of conus medullaris

√5th **S34.2 Injury of nerve root of lumbar and sacral spine**

√x7th **S34.21 Injury of nerve root of lumbar spine**

√x7th **S34.22 Injury of nerve root of sacral spine**

√x7th **S34.3 Injury of cauda equina** MCC H5 HCC

√x7th **S34.4 Injury of lumbosacral plexus**

√x7th **S34.5 Injury of lumbar, sacral and pelvic sympathetic nerves**
Injury of celiac ganglion or plexus
Injury of hypogastric plexus
Injury of mesenteric plexus (inferior) (superior)
Injury of splanchnic nerve

√x7th **S34.6 Injury of peripheral nerve(s) at abdomen, lower back and pelvis level**

√x7th **S34.8 Injury of other nerves at abdomen, lower back and pelvis level**

√x7th **S34.9 Injury of unspecified nerves at abdomen, lower back and pelvis level**

√4th **S35 Injury of blood vessels at abdomen, lower back and pelvis level**

Code also any associated open wound (S31.-)

The appropriate 7th character is to be added to each code from category S35.
A initial encounter
D subsequent encounter
S sequela

√5th **S35.Ø Injury of abdominal aorta**
EXCLUDES 1 *injury of aorta NOS (S25.Ø)*

√x7th **S35.ØØ Unspecified injury of abdominal aorta** MCC

√x7th **S35.Ø1 Minor laceration of abdominal aorta** MCC
Incomplete transection of abdominal aorta
Laceration of abdominal aorta NOS
Superficial laceration of abdominal aorta

√x7th **S35.Ø2 Major laceration of abdominal aorta** MCC
Complete transection of abdominal aorta
Traumatic rupture of abdominal aorta

√x7th **S35.Ø9 Other injury of abdominal aorta** MCC

√5th **S35.1 Injury of inferior vena cava**
Injury of hepatic vein
EXCLUDES 1 *injury of vena cava NOS (S25.2)*

√x7th **S35.1Ø Unspecified injury of inferior vena cava** MCC

√x7th **S35.11 Minor laceration of inferior vena cava** MCC
Incomplete transection of inferior vena cava
Laceration of inferior vena cava NOS
Superficial laceration of inferior vena cava

√x7th **S35.12 Major laceration of inferior vena cava** MCC
Complete transection of inferior vena cava
Traumatic rupture of inferior vena cava

√x7th **S35.19 Other injury of inferior vena cava** MCC

√5th **S35.2 Injury of celiac or mesenteric artery and branches**

√6th **S35.21 Injury of celiac artery**

√7th **S35.211 Minor laceration of celiac artery** MCC
Incomplete transection of celiac artery
Laceration of celiac artery NOS
Superficial laceration of celiac artery

√7th **S35.212 Major laceration of celiac artery** MCC
Complete transection of celiac artery
Traumatic rupture of celiac artery

√7th **S35.218 Other injury of celiac artery** MCC

√7th **S35.219 Unspecified injury of celiac artery** MCC

√6th **S35.22 Injury of superior mesenteric artery**

√7th **S35.221 Minor laceration of superior mesenteric artery** MCC
Incomplete transection of superior mesenteric artery
Laceration of superior mesenteric artery NOS
Superficial laceration of superior mesenteric artery

√7th **S35.222 Major laceration of superior mesenteric artery** MCC
Complete transection of superior mesenteric artery
Traumatic rupture of superior mesenteric artery

√7th **S35.228 Other injury of superior mesenteric artery** MCC

√7th **S35.229 Unspecified injury of superior mesenteric artery** MCC

√6th **S35.23 Injury of inferior mesenteric artery**

√7th **S35.231 Minor laceration of inferior mesenteric artery** MCC
Incomplete transection of inferior mesenteric artery
Laceration of inferior mesenteric artery NOS
Superficial laceration of inferior mesenteric artery

√7th **S35.232 Major laceration of inferior mesenteric artery** MCC
Complete transection of inferior mesenteric artery
Traumatic rupture of inferior mesenteric artery

√7th **S35.238 Other injury of inferior mesenteric artery** MCC

√7th **S35.239 Unspecified injury of inferior mesenteric artery** MCC

√6th **S35.29 Injury of branches of celiac and mesenteric artery**
Injury of gastric artery
Injury of gastroduodenal artery
Injury of hepatic artery
Injury of splenic artery

√7th **S35.291 Minor laceration of branches of celiac and mesenteric artery** MCC
Incomplete transection of branches of celiac and mesenteric artery
Laceration of branches of celiac and mesenteric artery NOS
Superficial laceration of branches of celiac and mesenteric artery

√7th **S35.292 Major laceration of branches of celiac and mesenteric artery** MCC
Complete transection of branches of celiac and mesenteric artery
Traumatic rupture of branches of celiac and mesenteric artery

√7th **S35.298 Other injury of branches of celiac and mesenteric artery** MCC

√7th **S35.299 Unspecified injury of branches of celiac and mesenteric artery** MCC

√5th **S35.3 Injury of portal or splenic vein and branches**

√6th **S35.31 Injury of portal vein**

√7th **S35.311 Laceration of portal vein** MCC

√7th **S35.318 Other specified injury of portal vein** MCC

√7th **S35.319 Unspecified injury of portal vein** MCC

√6th S35.32 Injury of splenic vein
√7th S35.321 Laceration of splenic vein MCC
√7th S35.328 Other specified injury of splenic vein MCC
√7th S35.329 Unspecified injury of splenic vein MCC
√6th S35.33 Injury of superior mesenteric vein
√7th S35.331 Laceration of superior mesenteric vein MCC
√7th S35.338 Other specified injury of superior mesenteric vein MCC
√7th S35.339 Unspecified injury of superior mesenteric vein MCC
√6th S35.34 Injury of inferior mesenteric vein
√7th S35.341 Laceration of inferior mesenteric vein MCC
√7th S35.348 Other specified injury of inferior mesenteric vein MCC
√7th S35.349 Unspecified injury of inferior mesenteric vein MCC
√5th S35.4 Injury of renal blood vessels
√6th S35.40 Unspecified injury of renal blood vessel
√7th S35.401 Unspecified injury of right renal artery MCC
√7th S35.402 Unspecified injury of left renal artery MCC
√7th S35.403 Unspecified injury of unspecified renal artery MCC UNS
√7th S35.404 Unspecified injury of right renal vein MCC
√7th S35.405 Unspecified injury of left renal vein MCC
√7th S35.406 Unspecified injury of unspecified renal vein MCC UNS
√6th S35.41 Laceration of renal blood vessel
√7th S35.411 Laceration of right renal artery MCC
√7th S35.412 Laceration of left renal artery MCC
√7th S35.413 Laceration of unspecified renal artery MCC UNS
√7th S35.414 Laceration of right renal vein MCC
√7th S35.415 Laceration of left renal vein MCC
√7th S35.416 Laceration of unspecified renal vein MCC UNS
√6th S35.49 Other specified injury of renal blood vessel
√7th S35.491 Other specified injury of right renal artery MCC
√7th S35.492 Other specified injury of left renal artery MCC
√7th S35.493 Other specified injury of unspecified renal artery MCC UNS
√7th S35.494 Other specified injury of right renal vein MCC
√7th S35.495 Other specified injury of left renal vein MCC
√7th S35.496 Other specified injury of unspecified renal vein MCC UNS
√5th S35.5 Injury of iliac blood vessels
√x7th S35.50 Injury of unspecified iliac blood vessel(s) MCC
√6th S35.51 Injury of iliac artery or vein
Injury of hypogastric artery or vein
√7th S35.511 Injury of right iliac artery MCC
√7th S35.512 Injury of left iliac artery MCC
√7th S35.513 Injury of unspecified iliac artery MCC UNS
√7th S35.514 Injury of right iliac vein MCC
√7th S35.515 Injury of left iliac vein MCC
√7th S35.516 Injury of unspecified iliac vein MCC UNS
√6th S35.53 Injury of uterine artery or vein
√7th S35.531 Injury of right uterine artery CC ♀
√7th S35.532 Injury of left uterine artery CC ♀
√7th S35.533 Injury of unspecified uterine artery CC UNS ♀
√7th S35.534 Injury of right uterine vein CC ♀
√7th S35.535 Injury of left uterine vein CC ♀
√7th S35.536 Injury of unspecified uterine vein CC UNS ♀
√x7th S35.59 Injury of other iliac blood vessels MCC
√5th S35.8 Injury of other blood vessels at abdomen, lower back and pelvis level
Injury of ovarian artery or vein
√6th S35.8X Injury of other blood vessels at abdomen, lower back and pelvis level
√7th S35.8X1 Laceration of other blood vessels at abdomen, lower back and pelvis level CC
√7th S35.8X8 Other specified injury of other blood vessels at abdomen, lower back and pelvis level CC
√7th S35.8X9 Unspecified injury of other blood vessels at abdomen, lower back and pelvis level CC
√5th S35.9 Injury of unspecified blood vessel at abdomen, lower back and pelvis level
√x7th S35.90 Unspecified injury of unspecified blood vessel at abdomen, lower back and pelvis level CC
√x7th S35.91 Laceration of unspecified blood vessel at abdomen, lower back and pelvis level CC
√x7th S35.99 Other specified injury of unspecified blood vessel at abdomen, lower back and pelvis level CC

√4th S36 Injury of intra-abdominal organs
Code also any associated open wound (S31.-)

The appropriate 7th character is to be added to each code from category S36.
A initial encounter
D subsequent encounter
S sequela

√5th S36.0 Injury of spleen
AHA: 2015,2Q,36; 2015,1Q,10
√x7th S36.00 Unspecified injury of spleen CC
√6th S36.02 Contusion of spleen
TIP: When both traumatic splenic laceration and contusion are documented in the same encounter, code only the laceration, as contusions are not coded when they occur with a more severe injury in the same body site.
√7th S36.020 Minor contusion of spleen CC
Contusion of spleen less than 2 cm
√7th S36.021 Major contusion of spleen CC
Contusion of spleen greater than 2 cm
√7th S36.029 Unspecified contusion of spleen CC
√6th S36.03 Laceration of spleen
TIP: When both traumatic splenic laceration and contusion are documented in the same encounter, code only the laceration, as contusions are not coded when they occur with a more severe injury in the same body site.
√7th S36.030 Superficial (capsular) laceration of spleen CC
Laceration of spleen less than 1 cm
Minor laceration of spleen
√7th S36.031 Moderate laceration of spleen MCC
Laceration of spleen 1 to 3 cm
√7th S36.032 Major laceration of spleen MCC
Avulsion of spleen
Laceration of spleen greater than 3 cm
Massive laceration of spleen
Multiple moderate lacerations of spleen
Stellate laceration of spleen
√7th S36.039 Unspecified laceration of spleen CC
√x7th S36.09 Other injury of spleen CC
√5th S36.1 Injury of liver and gallbladder and bile duct
√6th S36.11 Injury of liver
√7th S36.112 Contusion of liver CC
√7th S36.113 Laceration of liver, unspecified degree CC
√7th S36.114 Minor laceration of liver CC
Laceration involving capsule only, or, without significant involvement of hepatic parenchyma [i.e., less than 1 cm deep]

S36.115 Moderate laceration of liver MCC
Laceration involving parenchyma but without major disruption of parenchyma [i.e., less than 10 cm long and less than 3 cm deep]

S36.116 Major laceration of liver MCC
Laceration with significant disruption of hepatic parenchyma [i.e., greater than 10 cm long and 3 cm deep]
Multiple moderate lacerations, with or without hematoma
Stellate laceration of liver

S36.118 Other injury of liver CC

S36.119 Unspecified injury of liver CC

S36.12 Injury of gallbladder

S36.122 Contusion of gallbladder CC

S36.123 Laceration of gallbladder CC

S36.128 Other injury of gallbladder CC

S36.129 Unspecified injury of gallbladder CC

S36.13 Injury of bile duct CC

S36.2 Injury of pancreas

S36.20 Unspecified injury of pancreas

S36.200 Unspecified injury of head of pancreas CC

S36.201 Unspecified injury of body of pancreas CC

S36.202 Unspecified injury of tail of pancreas CC

S36.209 Unspecified injury of unspecified part of pancreas CC

S36.22 Contusion of pancreas

S36.220 Contusion of head of pancreas CC

S36.221 Contusion of body of pancreas CC

S36.222 Contusion of tail of pancreas CC

S36.229 Contusion of unspecified part of pancreas CC

S36.23 Laceration of pancreas, unspecified degree

S36.230 Laceration of head of pancreas, unspecified degree CC

S36.231 Laceration of body of pancreas, unspecified degree CC

S36.232 Laceration of tail of pancreas, unspecified degree CC

S36.239 Laceration of unspecified part of pancreas, unspecified degree CC

S36.24 Minor laceration of pancreas

S36.240 Minor laceration of head of pancreas CC

S36.241 Minor laceration of body of pancreas CC

S36.242 Minor laceration of tail of pancreas CC

S36.249 Minor laceration of unspecified part of pancreas CC

S36.25 Moderate laceration of pancreas

S36.250 Moderate laceration of head of pancreas CC

S36.251 Moderate laceration of body of pancreas CC

S36.252 Moderate laceration of tail of pancreas CC

S36.259 Moderate laceration of unspecified part of pancreas CC

S36.26 Major laceration of pancreas

S36.260 Major laceration of head of pancreas CC

S36.261 Major laceration of body of pancreas CC

S36.262 Major laceration of tail of pancreas CC

S36.269 Major laceration of unspecified part of pancreas CC

S36.29 Other injury of pancreas

S36.290 Other injury of head of pancreas CC

S36.291 Other injury of body of pancreas CC

S36.292 Other injury of tail of pancreas CC

S36.299 Other injury of unspecified part of pancreas CC

S36.3 Injury of stomach

S36.30 Unspecified injury of stomach CC

S36.32 Contusion of stomach CC

S36.33 Laceration of stomach CC

S36.39 Other injury of stomach CC

S36.4 Injury of small intestine

S36.40 Unspecified injury of small intestine

S36.400 Unspecified injury of duodenum CC

S36.408 Unspecified injury of other part of small intestine CC

S36.409 Unspecified injury of unspecified part of small intestine CC

S36.41 Primary blast injury of small intestine
Blast injury of small intestine NOS

S36.410 Primary blast injury of duodenum CC

S36.418 Primary blast injury of other part of small intestine CC

S36.419 Primary blast injury of unspecified part of small intestine CC

S36.42 Contusion of small intestine

S36.420 Contusion of duodenum CC

S36.428 Contusion of other part of small intestine CC

S36.429 Contusion of unspecified part of small intestine CC

S36.43 Laceration of small intestine

S36.430 Laceration of duodenum CC

S36.438 Laceration of other part of small intestine CC

S36.439 Laceration of unspecified part of small intestine CC

S36.49 Other injury of small intestine

S36.490 Other injury of duodenum CC

S36.498 Other injury of other part of small intestine CC

S36.499 Other injury of unspecified part of small intestine CC

S36.5 Injury of colon
EXCLUDES 2 *injury of rectum (S36.6-)*

S36.50 Unspecified injury of colon

S36.500 Unspecified injury of ascending [right] colon CC

S36.501 Unspecified injury of transverse colon CC

S36.502 Unspecified injury of descending [left] colon CC

S36.503 Unspecified injury of sigmoid colon CC

S36.508 Unspecified injury of other part of colon CC

S36.509 Unspecified injury of unspecified part of colon CC

S36.51 Primary blast injury of colon
Blast injury of colon NOS

S36.510 Primary blast injury of ascending [right] colon CC

S36.511 Primary blast injury of transverse colon CC

S36.512 Primary blast injury of descending [left] colon CC

S36.513 Primary blast injury of sigmoid colon CC

S36.518 Primary blast injury of other part of colon CC

S36.519 Primary blast injury of unspecified part of colon CC

S36.52 Contusion of colon

S36.520 Contusion of ascending [right] colon CC

S36.521 Contusion of transverse colon CC

S36.522 Contusion of descending [left] colon CC

S36.523 Contusion of sigmoid colon CC

- √7th S36.528 Contusion of other part of colon CC
- √7th S36.529 Contusion of unspecified part of colon CC

√6th S36.53 Laceration of colon
- √7th S36.530 Laceration of ascending [right] colon CC
- √7th S36.531 Laceration of transverse colon CC
- √7th S36.532 Laceration of descending [left] colon CC
- √7th S36.533 Laceration of sigmoid colon CC
- √7th S36.538 Laceration of other part of colon CC
- √7th S36.539 Laceration of unspecified part of colon CC

√6th S36.59 Other injury of colon

Secondary blast injury of colon
- √7th S36.590 Other injury of ascending [right] colon CC
- √7th S36.591 Other injury of transverse colon CC
- √7th S36.592 Other injury of descending [left] colon CC
- √7th S36.593 Other injury of sigmoid colon CC
- √7th S36.598 Other injury of other part of colon CC
- √7th S36.599 Other injury of unspecified part of colon CC

√5th S36.6 Injury of rectum
- √x7th S36.60 Unspecified injury of rectum CC
- √x7th S36.61 Primary blast injury of rectum CC
  Blast injury of rectum NOS
- √x7th S36.62 Contusion of rectum CC
- √x7th S36.63 Laceration of rectum CC
- √x7th S36.69 Other injury of rectum CC
  Secondary blast injury of rectum

√5th S36.8 Injury of other intra-abdominal organs
- √x7th S36.81 Injury of peritoneum CC

√6th S36.89 Injury of other intra-abdominal organs

Injury of retroperitoneum
- √7th S36.892 Contusion of other intra-abdominal organs CC
- √7th S36.893 Laceration of other intra-abdominal organs CC
- √7th S36.898 Other injury of other intra-abdominal organs CC
- √7th S36.899 Unspecified injury of other intra-abdominal organs CC

√5th S36.9 Injury of unspecified intra-abdominal organ
- √x7th S36.90 Unspecified injury of unspecified intra-abdominal organ CC
- √x7th S36.92 Contusion of unspecified intra-abdominal organ CC
- √x7th S36.93 Laceration of unspecified intra-abdominal organ CC
- √x7th S36.99 Other injury of unspecified intra-abdominal organ CC

√4th S37 Injury of urinary and pelvic organs

Code also any associated open wound (S31.-)

EXCLUDES 1 *obstetric trauma to pelvic organs (O71.-)*

EXCLUDES 2 *injury of peritoneum (S36.81)*
injury of retroperitoneum (S36.89-)

The appropriate 7th character is to be added to each code from category S37.
- A initial encounter
- D subsequent encounter
- S sequela

√5th S37.0 Injury of kidney

EXCLUDES 2 *acute kidney injury (nontraumatic) (N17.9)*

√6th S37.00 Unspecified injury of kidney
- √7th S37.001 Unspecified injury of right kidney CC
- √7th S37.002 Unspecified injury of left kidney CC
- √7th S37.009 Unspecified injury of unspecified kidney CC UNS

√6th S37.01 Minor contusion of kidney

Contusion of kidney less than 2 cm
Contusion of kidney NOS
- √7th S37.011 Minor contusion of right kidney CC
- √7th S37.012 Minor contusion of left kidney CC
- √7th S37.019 Minor contusion of unspecified kidney CC UNS

√6th S37.02 Major contusion of kidney

Contusion of kidney greater than 2 cm
- √7th S37.021 Major contusion of right kidney CC
- √7th S37.022 Major contusion of left kidney CC
- √7th S37.029 Major contusion of unspecified kidney CC UNS

√6th S37.03 Laceration of kidney, unspecified degree
- √7th S37.031 Laceration of right kidney, unspecified degree CC
- √7th S37.032 Laceration of left kidney, unspecified degree CC
- √7th S37.039 Laceration of unspecified kidney, unspecified degree CC UNS

√6th S37.04 Minor laceration of kidney

Laceration of kidney less than 1 cm
- √7th S37.041 Minor laceration of right kidney CC
- √7th S37.042 Minor laceration of left kidney CC
- √7th S37.049 Minor laceration of unspecified kidney CC UNS

√6th S37.05 Moderate laceration of kidney

Laceration of kidney 1 to 3 cm
- √7th S37.051 Moderate laceration of right kidney CC
- √7th S37.052 Moderate laceration of left kidney CC
- √7th S37.059 Moderate laceration of unspecified kidney CC UNS

√6th S37.06 Major laceration of kidney

Avulsion of kidney
Laceration of kidney greater than 3 cm
Massive laceration of kidney
Multiple moderate lacerations of kidney
Stellate laceration of kidney
- √7th S37.061 Major laceration of right kidney MCC
- √7th S37.062 Major laceration of left kidney MCC
- √7th S37.069 Major laceration of unspecified kidney MCC UNS

√6th S37.09 Other injury of kidney
- √7th S37.091 Other injury of right kidney MCC
- √7th S37.092 Other injury of left kidney MCC
- √7th S37.099 Other injury of unspecified kidney MCC UNS

√5th S37.1 Injury of ureter
- √x7th S37.10 Unspecified injury of ureter CC
- √x7th S37.12 Contusion of ureter CC
- √x7th S37.13 Laceration of ureter CC
- √x7th S37.19 Other injury of ureter CC

√5th S37.2 Injury of bladder
- √x7th S37.20 Unspecified injury of bladder CC
- √x7th S37.22 Contusion of bladder CC
- √x7th S37.23 Laceration of bladder CC
- √x7th S37.29 Other injury of bladder CC

√5th S37.3 Injury of urethra
- √x7th S37.30 Unspecified injury of urethra CC
- √x7th S37.32 Contusion of urethra CC
- √x7th S37.33 Laceration of urethra CC
- √x7th S37.39 Other injury of urethra CC

√5th S37.4 Injury of ovary

√6th S37.40 Unspecified injury of ovary
- √7th S37.401 Unspecified injury of ovary, unilateral ♀
- √7th S37.402 Unspecified injury of ovary, bilateral ♀
- √7th S37.409 Unspecified injury of ovary, unspecified ♀

N Newborn: 0 P Pediatric: 0-17 M Maternity: 9-64 A Adult: 15-124 UNS Unspecified Site MCC Major Complication/Comorbidity CC Complication/Comorbidity

S37.42 Contusion of ovary
- S37.421 Contusion of ovary, unilateral ♀
- S37.422 Contusion of ovary, bilateral ♀
- S37.429 Contusion of ovary, unspecified ♀

S37.43 Laceration of ovary
- S37.431 Laceration of ovary, unilateral ♀
- S37.432 Laceration of ovary, bilateral ♀
- S37.439 Laceration of ovary, unspecified ♀

S37.49 Other injury of ovary
- S37.491 Other injury of ovary, unilateral ♀
- S37.492 Other injury of ovary, bilateral ♀
- S37.499 Other injury of ovary, unspecified ♀

S37.5 Injury of fallopian tube

S37.50 Unspecified injury of fallopian tube
- S37.501 Unspecified injury of fallopian tube, unilateral ♀
- S37.502 Unspecified injury of fallopian tube, bilateral ♀
- S37.509 Unspecified injury of fallopian tube, unspecified ♀

S37.51 Primary blast injury of fallopian tube

Blast injury of fallopian tube NOS
- S37.511 Primary blast injury of fallopian tube, unilateral ♀
- S37.512 Primary blast injury of fallopian tube, bilateral ♀
- S37.519 Primary blast injury of fallopian tube, unspecified ♀

S37.52 Contusion of fallopian tube
- S37.521 Contusion of fallopian tube, unilateral ♀
- S37.522 Contusion of fallopian tube, bilateral ♀
- S37.529 Contusion of fallopian tube, unspecified ♀

S37.53 Laceration of fallopian tube
- S37.531 Laceration of fallopian tube, unilateral ♀
- S37.532 Laceration of fallopian tube, bilateral ♀
- S37.539 Laceration of fallopian tube, unspecified ♀

S37.59 Other injury of fallopian tube

Secondary blast injury of fallopian tube
- S37.591 Other injury of fallopian tube, unilateral ♀
- S37.592 Other injury of fallopian tube, bilateral ♀
- S37.599 Other injury of fallopian tube, unspecified ♀

S37.6 Injury of uterus

EXCLUDES 1 *injury to gravid uterus (O9A.2-)*
injury to uterus during delivery (O71.-)

- S37.60 Unspecified injury of uterus CC ♀
- S37.62 Contusion of uterus CC ♀
- S37.63 Laceration of uterus CC ♀
- S37.69 Other injury of uterus CC ♀

S37.8 Injury of other urinary and pelvic organs

S37.81 Injury of adrenal gland
- S37.812 Contusion of adrenal gland CC
- S37.813 Laceration of adrenal gland CC
- S37.818 Other injury of adrenal gland CC
- S37.819 Unspecified injury of adrenal gland CC

S37.82 Injury of prostate
- S37.822 Contusion of prostate ♂
- S37.823 Laceration of prostate ♂
- S37.828 Other injury of prostate ♂
- S37.829 Unspecified injury of prostate ♂

S37.89 Injury of other urinary and pelvic organ
- S37.892 Contusion of other urinary and pelvic organ CC
- S37.893 Laceration of other urinary and pelvic organ CC
- S37.898 Other injury of other urinary and pelvic organ CC
- S37.899 Unspecified injury of other urinary and pelvic organ CC

S37.9 Injury of unspecified urinary and pelvic organ
- S37.90 Unspecified injury of unspecified urinary and pelvic organ CC
- S37.92 Contusion of unspecified urinary and pelvic organ CC
- S37.93 Laceration of unspecified urinary and pelvic organ CC
- S37.99 Other injury of unspecified urinary and pelvic organ CC

S38 Crushing injury and traumatic amputation of abdomen, lower back, pelvis and external genitals

NOTE An amputation not identified as partial or complete should be coded to complete

The appropriate 7th character is to be added to each code from category S38.
- A initial encounter
- D subsequent encounter
- S sequela

S38.0 Crushing injury of external genital organs

Use additional code for any associated injuries

S38.00 Crushing injury of unspecified external genital organs
- S38.001 Crushing injury of unspecified external genital organs, male ♂
- S38.002 Crushing injury of unspecified external genital organs, female ♀

- S38.01 Crushing injury of penis ♂
- S38.02 Crushing injury of scrotum and testis ♂
- S38.03 Crushing injury of vulva ♀

S38.1 Crushing injury of abdomen, lower back, and pelvis

Use additional code for all associated injuries, such as:
- fracture of thoracic or lumbar spine and pelvis (S22.0-, S32.-)
- injury to intra-abdominal organs (S36.-)
- injury to urinary and pelvic organs (S37.-)
- open wound of abdominal wall (S31.-)
- spinal cord injury (S34.0, S34.1-)

EXCLUDES 2 *crushing injury of external genital organs (S38.0-)*

S38.2 Traumatic amputation of external genital organs

S38.21 Traumatic amputation of female external genital organs

Traumatic amputation of clitoris
Traumatic amputation of labium (majus) (minus)
Traumatic amputation of vulva
- S38.211 Complete traumatic amputation of female external genital organs ♀
- S38.212 Partial traumatic amputation of female external genital organs ♀

S38.22 Traumatic amputation of penis
- S38.221 Complete traumatic amputation of penis ♂
- S38.222 Partial traumatic amputation of penis ♂

S38.23 Traumatic amputation of scrotum and testis
- S38.231 Complete traumatic amputation of scrotum and testis ♂
- S38.232 Partial traumatic amputation of scrotum and testis ♂

S38.3 Transection (partial) of abdomen

S39 Other and unspecified injuries of abdomen, lower back, pelvis and external genitals

Code also any associated open wound (S31.-)

EXCLUDES 2 *sprain of joints and ligaments of lumbar spine and pelvis (S33.-)*

The appropriate 7th character is to be added to each code from category S39.
A initial encounter
D subsequent encounter
S sequela

S39.0 Injury of muscle, fascia and tendon of abdomen, lower back and pelvis

S39.00 Unspecified injury of muscle, fascia and tendon of abdomen, lower back and pelvis

S39.001 Unspecified injury of muscle, fascia and tendon of abdomen

S39.002 Unspecified injury of muscle, fascia and tendon of lower back

S39.003 Unspecified injury of muscle, fascia and tendon of pelvis

S39.01 Strain of muscle, fascia and tendon of abdomen, lower back and pelvis

S39.011 Strain of muscle, fascia and tendon of abdomen

S39.012 Strain of muscle, fascia and tendon of lower back

S39.013 Strain of muscle, fascia and tendon of pelvis

S39.02 Laceration of muscle, fascia and tendon of abdomen, lower back and pelvis

S39.021 Laceration of muscle, fascia and tendon of abdomen

S39.022 Laceration of muscle, fascia and tendon of lower back

S39.023 Laceration of muscle, fascia and tendon of pelvis

S39.09 Other injury of muscle, fascia and tendon of abdomen, lower back and pelvis

S39.091 Other injury of muscle, fascia and tendon of abdomen

S39.092 Other injury of muscle, fascia and tendon of lower back

S39.093 Other injury of muscle, fascia and tendon of pelvis

S39.8 Other specified injuries of abdomen, lower back, pelvis and external genitals

S39.81 Other specified injuries of abdomen

S39.82 Other specified injuries of lower back

S39.83 Other specified injuries of pelvis

S39.84 Other specified injuries of external genitals

S39.840 Fracture of corpus cavernosum penis ♂

S39.848 Other specified injuries of external genitals

S39.9 Unspecified injury of abdomen, lower back, pelvis and external genitals

S39.91 Unspecified injury of abdomen

S39.92 Unspecified injury of lower back

S39.93 Unspecified injury of pelvis

S39.94 Unspecified injury of external genitals

Injuries to the shoulder and upper arm (S40-S49)

INCLUDES injuries of axilla
injuries of scapular region

EXCLUDES 2 *burns and corrosions (T20-T32)*
frostbite (T33-T34)
injuries of elbow (S50-S59)
insect bite or sting, venomous (T63.4)

S40 Superficial injury of shoulder and upper arm

The appropriate 7th character is to be added to each code from category S40.
A initial encounter
D subsequent encounter
S sequela

S40.0 Contusion of shoulder and upper arm

S40.01 Contusion of shoulder

S40.011 Contusion of right shoulder

S40.012 Contusion of left shoulder

S40.019 Contusion of unspecified shoulder

S40.02 Contusion of upper arm

S40.021 Contusion of right upper arm

S40.022 Contusion of left upper arm

S40.029 Contusion of unspecified upper arm

S40.2 Other superficial injuries of shoulder

S40.21 Abrasion of shoulder

S40.211 Abrasion of right shoulder

S40.212 Abrasion of left shoulder

S40.219 Abrasion of unspecified shoulder

S40.22 Blister (nonthermal) of shoulder

S40.221 Blister (nonthermal) of right shoulder

S40.222 Blister (nonthermal) of left shoulder

S40.229 Blister (nonthermal) of unspecified shoulder

S40.24 External constriction of shoulder

S40.241 External constriction of right shoulder

S40.242 External constriction of left shoulder

S40.249 External constriction of unspecified shoulder

S40.25 Superficial foreign body of shoulder

Splinter in the shoulder

S40.251 Superficial foreign body of right shoulder

S40.252 Superficial foreign body of left shoulder

S40.259 Superficial foreign body of unspecified shoulder

S40.26 Insect bite (nonvenomous) of shoulder

S40.261 Insect bite (nonvenomous) of right shoulder

S40.262 Insect bite (nonvenomous) of left shoulder

S40.269 Insect bite (nonvenomous) of unspecified shoulder

S40.27 Other superficial bite of shoulder

EXCLUDES 1 *open bite of shoulder (S41.05)*

S40.271 Other superficial bite of right shoulder

S40.272 Other superficial bite of left shoulder

S40.279 Other superficial bite of unspecified shoulder

S40.8 Other superficial injuries of upper arm

S40.81 Abrasion of upper arm

S40.811 Abrasion of right upper arm

S40.812 Abrasion of left upper arm

S40.819 Abrasion of unspecified upper arm

S40.82 Blister (nonthermal) of upper arm

S40.821 Blister (nonthermal) of right upper arm

S40.822 Blister (nonthermal) of left upper arm

S40.829 Blister (nonthermal) of unspecified upper arm

S40.84 External constriction of upper arm

S40.841 External constriction of right upper arm

S40.842 External constriction of left upper arm

S40.849 External constriction of unspecified upper arm

S40.85 Superficial foreign body of upper arm

Splinter in the upper arm

S40.851 Superficial foreign body of right upper arm

S40.852 Superficial foreign body of left upper arm

S40.859 Superficial foreign body of unspecified upper arm

S40.86 Insect bite (nonvenomous) of upper arm

S40.861 Insect bite (nonvenomous) of right upper arm

S40.862 Insect bite (nonvenomous) of left upper arm

S40.869 Insect bite (nonvenomous) of unspecified upper arm

S40.87 Other superficial bite of upper arm

EXCLUDES 1 *open bite of upper arm (S41.14)*

EXCLUDES 2 *other superficial bite of shoulder (S40.27-)*

S40.871 Other superficial bite of right upper arm

√7th S4Ø.872 Other superficial bite of left upper arm

√7th S4Ø.879 Other superficial bite of unspecified upper arm

√5th S4Ø.9 Unspecified superficial injury of shoulder and upper arm

√6th S4Ø.91 Unspecified superficial injury of shoulder

√7th S4Ø.911 Unspecified superficial injury of right shoulder

√7th S4Ø.912 Unspecified superficial injury of left shoulder

√7th S4Ø.919 Unspecified superficial injury of unspecified shoulder

√6th S4Ø.92 Unspecified superficial injury of upper arm

√7th S4Ø.921 Unspecified superficial injury of right upper arm

√7th S4Ø.922 Unspecified superficial injury of left upper arm

√7th S4Ø.929 Unspecified superficial injury of unspecified upper arm

√4th S41 Open wound of shoulder and upper arm

Code also any associated wound infection

EXCLUDES 1 *traumatic amputation of shoulder and upper arm (S48.-)*

EXCLUDES 2 *open fracture of shoulder and upper arm (S42.- with 7th character B or C)*

The appropriate 7th character is to be added to each code from category S41.

A initial encounter
D subsequent encounter
S sequela

√5th S41.Ø Open wound of shoulder

√6th S41.ØØ Unspecified open wound of shoulder

√7th S41.ØØ1 Unspecified open wound of right shoulder

√7th S41.ØØ2 Unspecified open wound of left shoulder

√7th S41.ØØ9 Unspecified open wound of unspecified shoulder

√6th S41.Ø1 Laceration without foreign body of shoulder

√7th S41.Ø11 Laceration without foreign body of right shoulder

√7th S41.Ø12 Laceration without foreign body of left shoulder

√7th S41.Ø19 Laceration without foreign body of unspecified shoulder

√6th S41.Ø2 Laceration with foreign body of shoulder

√7th S41.Ø21 Laceration with foreign body of right shoulder

√7th S41.Ø22 Laceration with foreign body of left shoulder

√7th S41.Ø29 Laceration with foreign body of unspecified shoulder

√6th S41.Ø3 Puncture wound without foreign body of shoulder

√7th S41.Ø31 Puncture wound without foreign body of right shoulder

√7th S41.Ø32 Puncture wound without foreign body of left shoulder

√7th S41.Ø39 Puncture wound without foreign body of unspecified shoulder

√6th S41.Ø4 Puncture wound with foreign body of shoulder

√7th S41.Ø41 Puncture wound with foreign body of right shoulder

√7th S41.Ø42 Puncture wound with foreign body of left shoulder

√7th S41.Ø49 Puncture wound with foreign body of unspecified shoulder

√6th S41.Ø5 Open bite of shoulder

Bite of shoulder NOS

EXCLUDES 1 *superficial bite of shoulder (S4Ø.27)*

√7th S41.Ø51 Open bite of right shoulder

√7th S41.Ø52 Open bite of left shoulder

√7th S41.Ø59 Open bite of unspecified shoulder

√5th S41.1 Open wound of upper arm

√6th S41.1Ø Unspecified open wound of upper arm

AHA: 2016,3Q,24

√7th S41.1Ø1 Unspecified open wound of right upper arm

√7th S41.1Ø2 Unspecified open wound of left upper arm

√7th S41.1Ø9 Unspecified open wound of unspecified upper arm

√6th S41.11 Laceration without foreign body of upper arm

√7th S41.111 Laceration without foreign body of right upper arm

√7th S41.112 Laceration without foreign body of left upper arm

√7th S41.119 Laceration without foreign body of unspecified upper arm

√6th S41.12 Laceration with foreign body of upper arm

√7th S41.121 Laceration with foreign body of right upper arm

√7th S41.122 Laceration with foreign body of left upper arm

√7th S41.129 Laceration with foreign body of unspecified upper arm

√6th S41.13 Puncture wound without foreign body of upper arm

AHA: 2016,3Q,24

√7th S41.131 Puncture wound without foreign body of right upper arm

√7th S41.132 Puncture wound without foreign body of left upper arm

√7th S41.139 Puncture wound without foreign body of unspecified upper arm

√6th S41.14 Puncture wound with foreign body of upper arm

AHA: 2016,3Q,24

√7th S41.141 Puncture wound with foreign body of right upper arm

√7th S41.142 Puncture wound with foreign body of left upper arm

√7th S41.149 Puncture wound with foreign body of unspecified upper arm

√6th S41.15 Open bite of upper arm

Bite of upper arm NOS

EXCLUDES 1 *superficial bite of upper arm (S4Ø.87)*

√7th S41.151 Open bite of right upper arm

√7th S41.152 Open bite of left upper arm

√7th S41.159 Open bite of unspecified upper arm

√4th S42 Fracture of shoulder and upper arm

NOTE A fracture not indicated as displaced or nondisplaced should be coded to displaced

A fracture not indicated as open or closed should be coded to closed

EXCLUDES 1 *traumatic amputation of shoulder and upper arm (S48.-)*

EXCLUDES 2 *▶periprosthetic fracture around internal prosthetic shoulder joint (M97.3)◀*

AHA: 2018,2Q,12; 2015,3Q,37-39

DEF: Diaphysis: Central shaft of a long bone.

DEF: Epiphysis: Proximal and distal rounded ends of a long bone, communicates with the joint.

DEF: Metaphysis: Section of a long bone located between the epiphysis and diaphysis at the proximal and distal ends.

DEF: Physis (growth plate): Narrow zone of cartilaginous tissue between the epiphysis and metaphysis at each end of a long bone. In childhood, proliferation of cells in this zone lengthens the bone. As the bone matures, this area thins, ossification eventually fusing into solid bone and growth stops. ***Synonym(s):*** *Epiphyseal plate.*

The appropriate 7th character is to be added to all codes from category S42 [unless otherwise indicated].

A initial encounter for closed fracture
B initial encounter for open fracture
D subsequent encounter for fracture with routine healing
G subsequent encounter for fracture with delayed healing
K subsequent encounter for fracture with nonunion
P subsequent encounter for fracture with malunion
S sequela

√5th S42.Ø Fracture of clavicle

√6th S42.ØØ Fracture of unspecified part of clavicle

√7th S42.ØØ1 Fracture of unspecified part of right clavicle CC H5

√7th S42.ØØ2 Fracture of unspecified part of left clavicle CC H5

√7th S42.ØØ9 Fracture of unspecified part of unspecified clavicle CC H5 UNS

AHA: 2012,4Q,93

- ✓6th S42.01 Fracture of sternal end of clavicle
  - ✓7th S42.011 Anterior displaced fracture of sternal end of right clavicle CC H5
  - ✓7th S42.012 Anterior displaced fracture of sternal end of left clavicle CC H5
  - ✓7th S42.013 Anterior displaced fracture of sternal end of unspecified clavicle CC H5 UNS
    Displaced fracture of sternal end of clavicle NOS
  - ✓7th S42.014 Posterior displaced fracture of sternal end of right clavicle CC H5
  - ✓7th S42.015 Posterior displaced fracture of sternal end of left clavicle CC H5
  - ✓7th S42.016 Posterior displaced fracture of sternal end of unspecified clavicle CC H5 UNS
  - ✓7th S42.017 Nondisplaced fracture of sternal end of right clavicle CC H5
  - ✓7th S42.018 Nondisplaced fracture of sternal end of left clavicle CC H5
  - ✓7th S42.019 Nondisplaced fracture of sternal end of unspecified clavicle CC H5 UNS
- ✓6th S42.02 Fracture of shaft of clavicle
  - ✓7th S42.021 Displaced fracture of shaft of right clavicle CC H5
  - ✓7th S42.022 Displaced fracture of shaft of left clavicle CC H5
  - ✓7th S42.023 Displaced fracture of shaft of unspecified clavicle CC H5 UNS
  - ✓7th S42.024 Nondisplaced fracture of shaft of right clavicle CC H5
  - ✓7th S42.025 Nondisplaced fracture of shaft of left clavicle CC H5
  - ✓7th S42.026 Nondisplaced fracture of shaft of unspecified clavicle CC H5 UNS
- ✓6th S42.03 Fracture of lateral end of clavicle
  Fracture of acromial end of clavicle
  - ✓7th S42.031 Displaced fracture of lateral end of right clavicle CC H5
  - ✓7th S42.032 Displaced fracture of lateral end of left clavicle CC H5
  - ✓7th S42.033 Displaced fracture of lateral end of unspecified clavicle CC H5 UNS
  - ✓7th S42.034 Nondisplaced fracture of lateral end of right clavicle CC H5
  - ✓7th S42.035 Nondisplaced fracture of lateral end of left clavicle CC H5
  - ✓7th S42.036 Nondisplaced fracture of lateral end of unspecified clavicle CC H5 UNS

✓5th S42.1 Fracture of scapula

- ✓6th S42.10 Fracture of unspecified part of scapula
  - ✓7th S42.101 Fracture of unspecified part of scapula, right shoulder CC H5
  - ✓7th S42.102 Fracture of unspecified part of scapula, left shoulder CC H5
  - ✓7th S42.109 Fracture of unspecified part of scapula, unspecified shoulder CC H5 UNS
- ✓6th S42.11 Fracture of body of scapula
  - ✓7th S42.111 Displaced fracture of body of scapula, right shoulder CC H5
  - ✓7th S42.112 Displaced fracture of body of scapula, left shoulder CC H5
  - ✓7th S42.113 Displaced fracture of body of scapula, unspecified shoulder CC H5 UNS
  - ✓7th S42.114 Nondisplaced fracture of body of scapula, right shoulder CC H5
  - ✓7th S42.115 Nondisplaced fracture of body of scapula, left shoulder CC H5
  - ✓7th S42.116 Nondisplaced fracture of body of scapula, unspecified shoulder CC H5 UNS
- ✓6th S42.12 Fracture of acromial process
  - ✓7th S42.121 Displaced fracture of acromial process, right shoulder CC H5
  - ✓7th S42.122 Displaced fracture of acromial process, left shoulder CC H5
  - ✓7th S42.123 Displaced fracture of acromial process, unspecified shoulder CC H5 UNS
  - ✓7th S42.124 Nondisplaced fracture of acromial process, right shoulder CC H5
  - ✓7th S42.125 Nondisplaced fracture of acromial process, left shoulder CC H5
  - ✓7th S42.126 Nondisplaced fracture of acromial process, unspecified shoulder CC H5 UNS
- ✓6th S42.13 Fracture of coracoid process
  - ✓7th S42.131 Displaced fracture of coracoid process, right shoulder CC H5
  - ✓7th S42.132 Displaced fracture of coracoid process, left shoulder CC H5
  - ✓7th S42.133 Displaced fracture of coracoid process, unspecified shoulder CC H5 UNS
  - ✓7th S42.134 Nondisplaced fracture of coracoid process, right shoulder CC H5
  - ✓7th S42.135 Nondisplaced fracture of coracoid process, left shoulder CC H5
  - ✓7th S42.136 Nondisplaced fracture of coracoid process, unspecified shoulder CC H5 UNS
- ✓6th S42.14 Fracture of glenoid cavity of scapula
  - ✓7th S42.141 Displaced fracture of glenoid cavity of scapula, right shoulder CC H5
  - ✓7th S42.142 Displaced fracture of glenoid cavity of scapula, left shoulder CC H5
  - ✓7th S42.143 Displaced fracture of glenoid cavity of scapula, unspecified shoulder CC H5 UNS
  - ✓7th S42.144 Nondisplaced fracture of glenoid cavity of scapula, right shoulder CC H5
  - ✓7th S42.145 Nondisplaced fracture of glenoid cavity of scapula, left shoulder CC H5
  - ✓7th S42.146 Nondisplaced fracture of glenoid cavity of scapula, unspecified shoulder CC H5 UNS
- ✓6th S42.15 Fracture of neck of scapula
  - ✓7th S42.151 Displaced fracture of neck of scapula, right shoulder CC H5
  - ✓7th S42.152 Displaced fracture of neck of scapula, left shoulder CC H5
  - ✓7th S42.153 Displaced fracture of neck of scapula, unspecified shoulder CC H5 UNS
  - ✓7th S42.154 Nondisplaced fracture of neck of scapula, right shoulder CC H5
  - ✓7th S42.155 Nondisplaced fracture of neck of scapula, left shoulder CC H5
  - ✓7th S42.156 Nondisplaced fracture of neck of scapula, unspecified shoulder CC H5 UNS
- ✓6th S42.19 Fracture of other part of scapula
  - ✓7th S42.191 Fracture of other part of scapula, right shoulder CC H5
  - ✓7th S42.192 Fracture of other part of scapula, left shoulder CC H5
  - ✓7th S42.199 Fracture of other part of scapula, unspecified shoulder CC H5 UNS

✓5th S42.2 Fracture of upper end of humerus

Fracture of proximal end of humerus

EXCLUDES 2 *fracture of shaft of humerus (S42.3-)*
physeal fracture of upper end of humerus (S49.0-)

- ✓6th S42.20 Unspecified fracture of upper end of humerus
  - ✓7th S42.201 Unspecified fracture of upper end of right humerus MCC CC H5
  - ✓7th S42.202 Unspecified fracture of upper end of left humerus MCC CC H5
  - ✓7th S42.209 Unspecified fracture of upper end of unspecified humerus MCC CC H5 UNS
- ✓6th S42.21 Unspecified fracture of surgical neck of humerus
  Fracture of neck of humerus NOS
  - ✓7th S42.211 Unspecified displaced fracture of surgical neck of right humerus MCC CC H5
  - ✓7th S42.212 Unspecified displaced fracture of surgical neck of left humerus MCC CC H5
  - ✓7th S42.213 Unspecified displaced fracture of surgical neck of unspecified humerus MCC CC H5 UNS
  - ✓7th S42.214 Unspecified nondisplaced fracture of surgical neck of right humerus MCC CC H5

S42.215 Unspecified nondisplaced fracture of surgical neck of left humerus MCC CC H5
S42.216 Unspecified nondisplaced fracture of surgical neck of unspecified humerus MCC CC H5 UNS

S42.22 2-part fracture of surgical neck of humerus
S42.221 2-part displaced fracture of surgical neck of right humerus MCC CC H5
S42.222 2-part displaced fracture of surgical neck of left humerus MCC CC H5
S42.223 2-part displaced fracture of surgical neck of unspecified humerus MCC CC H5 UNS
S42.224 2-part nondisplaced fracture of surgical neck of right humerus MCC CC H5
S42.225 2-part nondisplaced fracture of surgical neck of left humerus MCC CC H5
S42.226 2-part nondisplaced fracture of surgical neck of unspecified humerus MCC CC H5 UNS

S42.23 3-part fracture of surgical neck of humerus
S42.231 3-part fracture of surgical neck of right humerus MCC CC H5
S42.232 3-part fracture of surgical neck of left humerus MCC CC H5
S42.239 3-part fracture of surgical neck of unspecified humerus MCC CC H5 UNS

S42.24 4-part fracture of surgical neck of humerus
S42.241 4-part fracture of surgical neck of right humerus MCC CC H5
S42.242 4-part fracture of surgical neck of left humerus MCC CC H5
S42.249 4-part fracture of surgical neck of unspecified humerus MCC CC H5 UNS

S42.25 Fracture of greater tuberosity of humerus
S42.251 Displaced fracture of greater tuberosity of right humerus MCC CC H5
S42.252 Displaced fracture of greater tuberosity of left humerus MCC CC H5
S42.253 Displaced fracture of greater tuberosity of unspecified humerus MCC CC H5 UNS
S42.254 Nondisplaced fracture of greater tuberosity of right humerus MCC CC H5
S42.255 Nondisplaced fracture of greater tuberosity of left humerus MCC CC H5
S42.256 Nondisplaced fracture of greater tuberosity of unspecified humerus MCC CC H5 UNS

S42.26 Fracture of lesser tuberosity of humerus
S42.261 Displaced fracture of lesser tuberosity of right humerus MCC CC H5
S42.262 Displaced fracture of lesser tuberosity of left humerus MCC CC H5
S42.263 Displaced fracture of lesser tuberosity of unspecified humerus MCC CC H5 UNS
S42.264 Nondisplaced fracture of lesser tuberosity of right humerus MCC CC H5
S42.265 Nondisplaced fracture of lesser tuberosity of left humerus MCC CC H5
S42.266 Nondisplaced fracture of lesser tuberosity of unspecified humerus MCC CC H5 UNS

S42.27 Torus fracture of upper end of humerus

The appropriate 7th character is to be added to all codes in subcategory S42.27
- A initial encounter for closed fracture
- D subsequent encounter for fracture with routine healing
- G subsequent encounter for fracture with delayed healing
- K subsequent encounter for fracture with nonunion
- P subsequent encounter for fracture with malunion
- S sequela

S42.271 Torus fracture of upper end of right humerus CC H5
S42.272 Torus fracture of upper end of left humerus CC H5
S42.279 Torus fracture of upper end of unspecified humerus CC H5 UNS

S42.29 Other fracture of upper end of humerus
Fracture of anatomical neck of humerus
Fracture of articular head of humerus
AHA: 2019,1Q,18
S42.291 Other displaced fracture of upper end of right humerus MCC CC H5
S42.292 Other displaced fracture of upper end of left humerus MCC CC H5
S42.293 Other displaced fracture of upper end of unspecified humerus MCC CC H5 UNS
S42.294 Other nondisplaced fracture of upper end of right humerus MCC CC H5
S42.295 Other nondisplaced fracture of upper end of left humerus MCC CC H5
S42.296 Other nondisplaced fracture of upper end of unspecified humerus MCC CC H5 UNS

S42.3 Fracture of shaft of humerus
Fracture of humerus NOS
Fracture of upper arm NOS
EXCLUDES 2 *physeal fractures of upper end of humerus (S49.0-)*
physeal fractures of lower end of humerus (S49.1-)

S42.30 Unspecified fracture of shaft of humerus
S42.301 Unspecified fracture of shaft of humerus, right arm MCC CC H5
S42.302 Unspecified fracture of shaft of humerus, left arm MCC CC H5
S42.309 Unspecified fracture of shaft of humerus, unspecified arm MCC CC H5 UNS

S42.31 Greenstick fracture of shaft of humerus

The appropriate 7th character is to be added to all codes in subcategory S42.31
- A initial encounter for closed fracture
- D subsequent encounter for fracture with routine healing
- G subsequent encounter for fracture with delayed healing
- K subsequent encounter for fracture with nonunion
- P subsequent encounter for fracture with malunion
- S sequela

S42.311 Greenstick fracture of shaft of humerus, right arm CC H5
S42.312 Greenstick fracture of shaft of humerus, left arm CC H5
S42.319 Greenstick fracture of shaft of humerus, unspecified arm CC H5 UNS

S42.32 Transverse fracture of shaft of humerus
S42.321 Displaced transverse fracture of shaft of humerus, right arm MCC CC H5
S42.322 Displaced transverse fracture of shaft of humerus, left arm MCC CC H5
S42.323 Displaced transverse fracture of shaft of humerus, unspecified arm MCC CC H5 UNS
S42.324 Nondisplaced transverse fracture of shaft of humerus, right arm MCC CC H5
S42.325 Nondisplaced transverse fracture of shaft of humerus, left arm MCC CC H5
S42.326 Nondisplaced transverse fracture of shaft of humerus, unspecified arm MCC CC H5 UNS

S42.33 Oblique fracture of shaft of humerus
S42.331 Displaced oblique fracture of shaft of humerus, right arm MCC CC H5
S42.332 Displaced oblique fracture of shaft of humerus, left arm MCC CC H5
S42.333 Displaced oblique fracture of shaft of humerus, unspecified arm MCC CC H5 UNS
S42.334 Nondisplaced oblique fracture of shaft of humerus, right arm MCC CC H5
S42.335 Nondisplaced oblique fracture of shaft of humerus, left arm MCC CC H5

7th S42.336 Nondisplaced oblique fracture of shaft of humerus, unspecified arm MCC CC H5 UNS

6th S42.34 Spiral fracture of shaft of humerus

7th S42.341 Displaced spiral fracture of shaft of humerus, right arm MCC CC H5

7th S42.342 Displaced spiral fracture of shaft of humerus, left arm MCC CC H5

7th S42.343 Displaced spiral fracture of shaft of humerus, unspecified arm MCC CC H5 UNS

7th S42.344 Nondisplaced spiral fracture of shaft of humerus, right arm MCC CC H5

7th S42.345 Nondisplaced spiral fracture of shaft of humerus, left arm MCC CC H5

7th S42.346 Nondisplaced spiral fracture of shaft of humerus, unspecified arm MCC CC H5 UNS

6th S42.35 Comminuted fracture of shaft of humerus

7th S42.351 Displaced comminuted fracture of shaft of humerus, right arm MCC CC H5

7th S42.352 Displaced comminuted fracture of shaft of humerus, left arm MCC CC H5

7th S42.353 Displaced comminuted fracture of shaft of humerus, unspecified arm MCC CC H5 UNS

7th S42.354 Nondisplaced comminuted fracture of shaft of humerus, right arm MCC CC H5

7th S42.355 Nondisplaced comminuted fracture of shaft of humerus, left arm MCC CC H5

7th S42.356 Nondisplaced comminuted fracture of shaft of humerus, unspecified arm MCC CC H5 UNS

6th S42.36 Segmental fracture of shaft of humerus

7th S42.361 Displaced segmental fracture of shaft of humerus, right arm MCC CC H5

7th S42.362 Displaced segmental fracture of shaft of humerus, left arm MCC CC H5

7th S42.363 Displaced segmental fracture of shaft of humerus, unspecified arm MCC CC H5 UNS

7th S42.364 Nondisplaced segmental fracture of shaft of humerus, right arm MCC CC H5

7th S42.365 Nondisplaced segmental fracture of shaft of humerus, left arm MCC CC H5

7th S42.366 Nondisplaced segmental fracture of shaft of humerus, unspecified arm MCC CC H5 UNS

6th S42.39 Other fracture of shaft of humerus

7th S42.391 Other fracture of shaft of right humerus MCC CC H5

7th S42.392 Other fracture of shaft of left humerus MCC CC H5

7th S42.399 Other fracture of shaft of unspecified humerus MCC CC H5 UNS

5th S42.4 Fracture of lower end of humerus

Fracture of distal end of humerus

EXCLUDES 2 *fracture of shaft of humerus (S42.3-)*
physeal fracture of lower end of humerus (S49.1-)

6th S42.40 Unspecified fracture of lower end of humerus

Fracture of elbow NOS

7th S42.401 Unspecified fracture of lower end of right humerus MCC CC H5

7th S42.402 Unspecified fracture of lower end of left humerus MCC CC H5

7th S42.409 Unspecified fracture of lower end of unspecified humerus MCC CC H5 UNS

6th S42.41 Simple supracondylar fracture without intercondylar fracture of humerus

7th S42.411 Displaced simple supracondylar fracture without intercondylar fracture of right humerus MCC CC H5

7th S42.412 Displaced simple supracondylar fracture without intercondylar fracture of left humerus MCC CC H5

7th S42.413 Displaced simple supracondylar fracture without intercondylar fracture of unspecified humerus MCC CC H5 UNS

7th S42.414 Nondisplaced simple supracondylar fracture without intercondylar fracture of right humerus MCC CC H5

7th S42.415 Nondisplaced simple supracondylar fracture without intercondylar fracture of left humerus MCC CC H5

7th S42.416 Nondisplaced simple supracondylar fracture without intercondylar fracture of unspecified humerus MCC CC H5 UNS

6th S42.42 Comminuted supracondylar fracture without intercondylar fracture of humerus

7th S42.421 Displaced comminuted supracondylar fracture without intercondylar fracture of right humerus MCC CC H5

7th S42.422 Displaced comminuted supracondylar fracture without intercondylar fracture of left humerus MCC CC H5

7th S42.423 Displaced comminuted supracondylar fracture without intercondylar fracture of unspecified humerus MCC CC H5 UNS

7th S42.424 Nondisplaced comminuted supracondylar fracture without intercondylar fracture of right humerus MCC CC H5

7th S42.425 Nondisplaced comminuted supracondylar fracture without intercondylar fracture of left humerus MCC CC H5

7th S42.426 Nondisplaced comminuted supracondylar fracture without intercondylar fracture of unspecified humerus MCC CC H5 UNS

6th S42.43 Fracture (avulsion) of lateral epicondyle of humerus

7th S42.431 Displaced fracture (avulsion) of lateral epicondyle of right humerus MCC CC H5

7th S42.432 Displaced fracture (avulsion) of lateral epicondyle of left humerus MCC CC H5

7th S42.433 Displaced fracture (avulsion) of lateral epicondyle of unspecified humerus MCC CC H5 UNS

7th S42.434 Nondisplaced fracture (avulsion) of lateral epicondyle of right humerus MCC CC H5

7th S42.435 Nondisplaced fracture (avulsion) of lateral epicondyle of left humerus MCC CC H5

7th S42.436 Nondisplaced fracture (avulsion) of lateral epicondyle of unspecified humerus MCC CC H5 UNS

6th S42.44 Fracture (avulsion) of medial epicondyle of humerus

7th S42.441 Displaced fracture (avulsion) of medial epicondyle of right humerus MCC CC H5

7th S42.442 Displaced fracture (avulsion) of medial epicondyle of left humerus MCC CC H5

7th S42.443 Displaced fracture (avulsion) of medial epicondyle of unspecified humerus MCC CC H5 UNS

7th S42.444 Nondisplaced fracture (avulsion) of medial epicondyle of right humerus MCC CC H5

7th S42.445 Nondisplaced fracture (avulsion) of medial epicondyle of left humerus MCC CC H5

7th S42.446 Nondisplaced fracture (avulsion) of medial epicondyle of unspecified humerus MCC CC H5 UNS

7th S42.447 Incarcerated fracture (avulsion) of medial epicondyle of right humerus MCC CC H5

7th S42.448 Incarcerated fracture (avulsion) of medial epicondyle of left humerus MCC CC H5

7th S42.449 Incarcerated fracture (avulsion) of medial epicondyle of unspecified humerus MCC CC H5 UNS

6th S42.45 Fracture of lateral condyle of humerus

Fracture of capitellum of humerus

7th S42.451 Displaced fracture of lateral condyle of right humerus MCC CC H5

7th S42.452 Displaced fracture of lateral condyle of left humerus MCC CC H5

7th S42.453 Displaced fracture of lateral condyle of unspecified humerus MCC CC H5 UNS

S42.454 Nondisplaced fracture of lateral condyle of right humerus MCC CC H5
S42.455 Nondisplaced fracture of lateral condyle of left humerus MCC CC H5
S42.456 Nondisplaced fracture of lateral condyle of unspecified humerus MCC CC H5 UNS
S42.46 Fracture of medial condyle of humerus
Trochlea fracture of humerus
S42.461 Displaced fracture of medial condyle of right humerus MCC CC H5
S42.462 Displaced fracture of medial condyle of left humerus MCC CC H5
S42.463 Displaced fracture of medial condyle of unspecified humerus MCC CC H5 UNS
S42.464 Nondisplaced fracture of medial condyle of right humerus MCC CC H5
S42.465 Nondisplaced fracture of medial condyle of left humerus MCC CC H5
S42.466 Nondisplaced fracture of medial condyle of unspecified humerus MCC CC H5 UNS
S42.47 Transcondylar fracture of humerus
S42.471 Displaced transcondylar fracture of right humerus MCC CC H5
S42.472 Displaced transcondylar fracture of left humerus MCC CC H5
S42.473 Displaced transcondylar fracture of unspecified humerus MCC CC H5 UNS
S42.474 Nondisplaced transcondylar fracture of right humerus MCC CC H5
S42.475 Nondisplaced transcondylar fracture of left humerus MCC CC H5
S42.476 Nondisplaced transcondylar fracture of unspecified humerus MCC CC H5 UNS
S42.48 Torus fracture of lower end of humerus

The appropriate 7th character is to be added to all codes in subcategory S42.48.
A initial encounter for closed fracture
D subsequent encounter for fracture with routine healing
G subsequent encounter for fracture with delayed healing
K subsequent encounter for fracture with nonunion
P subsequent encounter for fracture with malunion
S sequela

S42.481 Torus fracture of lower end of right humerus CC H5
S42.482 Torus fracture of lower end of left humerus CC H5
S42.489 Torus fracture of lower end of unspecified humerus CC H5 UNS
S42.49 Other fracture of lower end of humerus
S42.491 Other displaced fracture of lower end of right humerus MCC CC H5
S42.492 Other displaced fracture of lower end of left humerus MCC CC H5
S42.493 Other displaced fracture of lower end of unspecified humerus MCC CC H5 UNS
S42.494 Other nondisplaced fracture of lower end of right humerus MCC CC H5
S42.495 Other nondisplaced fracture of lower end of left humerus MCC CC H5
S42.496 Other nondisplaced fracture of lower end of unspecified humerus MCC CC H5 UNS
S42.9 Fracture of shoulder girdle, part unspecified
Fracture of shoulder NOS
S42.90 Fracture of unspecified shoulder girdle, part unspecified MCC CC H5 UNS
S42.91 Fracture of right shoulder girdle, part unspecified MCC CC H5
S42.92 Fracture of left shoulder girdle, part unspecified MCC CC H5

S43 Dislocation and sprain of joints and ligaments of shoulder girdle

INCLUDES avulsion of joint or ligament of shoulder girdle
laceration of cartilage, joint or ligament of shoulder girdle
sprain of cartilage, joint or ligament of shoulder girdle
traumatic hemarthrosis of joint or ligament of shoulder girdle
traumatic rupture of joint or ligament of shoulder girdle
traumatic subluxation of joint or ligament of shoulder girdle
traumatic tear of joint or ligament of shoulder girdle

Code also any associated open wound

EXCLUDES 2 *strain of muscle, fascia and tendon of shoulder and upper arm (S46.-)*

The appropriate 7th character is to be added to each code from category S43.
A initial encounter
D subsequent encounter
S sequela

S43.0 Subluxation and dislocation of shoulder joint
Dislocation of glenohumeral joint
Subluxation of glenohumeral joint
S43.00 Unspecified subluxation and dislocation of shoulder joint
Dislocation of humerus NOS
Subluxation of humerus NOS
S43.001 Unspecified subluxation of right shoulder joint
S43.002 Unspecified subluxation of left shoulder joint
S43.003 Unspecified subluxation of unspecified shoulder joint
S43.004 Unspecified dislocation of right shoulder joint
S43.005 Unspecified dislocation of left shoulder joint
S43.006 Unspecified dislocation of unspecified shoulder joint
S43.01 Anterior subluxation and dislocation of humerus
S43.011 Anterior subluxation of right humerus
S43.012 Anterior subluxation of left humerus
S43.013 Anterior subluxation of unspecified humerus
S43.014 Anterior dislocation of right humerus
S43.015 Anterior dislocation of left humerus
S43.016 Anterior dislocation of unspecified humerus
S43.02 Posterior subluxation and dislocation of humerus
S43.021 Posterior subluxation of right humerus
S43.022 Posterior subluxation of left humerus
S43.023 Posterior subluxation of unspecified humerus
S43.024 Posterior dislocation of right humerus
S43.025 Posterior dislocation of left humerus
S43.026 Posterior dislocation of unspecified humerus
S43.03 Inferior subluxation and dislocation of humerus
S43.031 Inferior subluxation of right humerus
S43.032 Inferior subluxation of left humerus
S43.033 Inferior subluxation of unspecified humerus
S43.034 Inferior dislocation of right humerus
S43.035 Inferior dislocation of left humerus
S43.036 Inferior dislocation of unspecified humerus
S43.08 Other subluxation and dislocation of shoulder joint
S43.081 Other subluxation of right shoulder joint
S43.082 Other subluxation of left shoulder joint
S43.083 Other subluxation of unspecified shoulder joint
S43.084 Other dislocation of right shoulder joint
S43.085 Other dislocation of left shoulder joint
S43.086 Other dislocation of unspecified shoulder joint

5th S43.1 Subluxation and dislocation of acromioclavicular joint
6th S43.10 Unspecified dislocation of acromioclavicular joint
7th S43.101 Unspecified dislocation of right acromioclavicular joint
7th S43.102 Unspecified dislocation of left acromioclavicular joint
7th S43.109 Unspecified dislocation of unspecified acromioclavicular joint
6th S43.11 Subluxation of acromioclavicular joint
7th S43.111 Subluxation of right acromioclavicular joint
7th S43.112 Subluxation of left acromioclavicular joint
7th S43.119 Subluxation of unspecified acromioclavicular joint
6th S43.12 Dislocation of acromioclavicular joint, 100%-200% displacement
7th S43.121 Dislocation of right acromioclavicular joint, 100%-200% displacement
7th S43.122 Dislocation of left acromioclavicular joint, 100%-200% displacement
7th S43.129 Dislocation of unspecified acromioclavicular joint, 100%-200% displacement
6th S43.13 Dislocation of acromioclavicular joint, greater than 200% displacement
7th S43.131 Dislocation of right acromioclavicular joint, greater than 200% displacement
7th S43.132 Dislocation of left acromioclavicular joint, greater than 200% displacement
7th S43.139 Dislocation of unspecified acromioclavicular joint, greater than 200% displacement
6th S43.14 Inferior dislocation of acromioclavicular joint
7th S43.141 Inferior dislocation of right acromioclavicular joint
7th S43.142 Inferior dislocation of left acromioclavicular joint
7th S43.149 Inferior dislocation of unspecified acromioclavicular joint
6th S43.15 Posterior dislocation of acromioclavicular joint
7th S43.151 Posterior dislocation of right acromioclavicular joint
7th S43.152 Posterior dislocation of left acromioclavicular joint
7th S43.159 Posterior dislocation of unspecified acromioclavicular joint
5th S43.2 Subluxation and dislocation of sternoclavicular joint
6th S43.20 Unspecified subluxation and dislocation of sternoclavicular joint
7th S43.201 Unspecified subluxation of right sternoclavicular joint CC H5
7th S43.202 Unspecified subluxation of left sternoclavicular joint CC H5
7th S43.203 Unspecified subluxation of unspecified sternoclavicular joint CC H5 UNS
7th S43.204 Unspecified dislocation of right sternoclavicular joint CC H5
7th S43.205 Unspecified dislocation of left sternoclavicular joint CC H5
7th S43.206 Unspecified dislocation of unspecified sternoclavicular joint CC H5 UNS
6th S43.21 Anterior subluxation and dislocation of sternoclavicular joint
7th S43.211 Anterior subluxation of right sternoclavicular joint CC H5
7th S43.212 Anterior subluxation of left sternoclavicular joint CC H5
7th S43.213 Anterior subluxation of unspecified sternoclavicular joint CC H5 UNS
7th S43.214 Anterior dislocation of right sternoclavicular joint CC H5
7th S43.215 Anterior dislocation of left sternoclavicular joint CC H5
7th S43.216 Anterior dislocation of unspecified sternoclavicular joint CC H5 UNS
6th S43.22 Posterior subluxation and dislocation of sternoclavicular joint
7th S43.221 Posterior subluxation of right sternoclavicular joint CC H5
7th S43.222 Posterior subluxation of left sternoclavicular joint CC H5
7th S43.223 Posterior subluxation of unspecified sternoclavicular joint CC H5 UNS
7th S43.224 Posterior dislocation of right sternoclavicular joint CC H5
7th S43.225 Posterior dislocation of left sternoclavicular joint CC H5
7th S43.226 Posterior dislocation of unspecified sternoclavicular joint CC H5 UNS
5th S43.3 Subluxation and dislocation of other and unspecified parts of shoulder girdle
6th S43.30 Subluxation and dislocation of unspecified parts of shoulder girdle
Dislocation of shoulder girdle NOS
Subluxation of shoulder girdle NOS
7th S43.301 Subluxation of unspecified parts of right shoulder girdle
7th S43.302 Subluxation of unspecified parts of left shoulder girdle
7th S43.303 Subluxation of unspecified parts of unspecified shoulder girdle
7th S43.304 Dislocation of unspecified parts of right shoulder girdle
7th S43.305 Dislocation of unspecified parts of left shoulder girdle
7th S43.306 Dislocation of unspecified parts of unspecified shoulder girdle
6th S43.31 Subluxation and dislocation of scapula
7th S43.311 Subluxation of right scapula
7th S43.312 Subluxation of left scapula
7th S43.313 Subluxation of unspecified scapula
7th S43.314 Dislocation of right scapula
7th S43.315 Dislocation of left scapula
7th S43.316 Dislocation of unspecified scapula
6th S43.39 Subluxation and dislocation of other parts of shoulder girdle
7th S43.391 Subluxation of other parts of right shoulder girdle
7th S43.392 Subluxation of other parts of left shoulder girdle
7th S43.393 Subluxation of other parts of unspecified shoulder girdle
7th S43.394 Dislocation of other parts of right shoulder girdle
7th S43.395 Dislocation of other parts of left shoulder girdle
7th S43.396 Dislocation of other parts of unspecified shoulder girdle
5th S43.4 Sprain of shoulder joint
6th S43.40 Unspecified sprain of shoulder joint
7th S43.401 Unspecified sprain of right shoulder joint
7th S43.402 Unspecified sprain of left shoulder joint
7th S43.409 Unspecified sprain of unspecified shoulder joint
6th S43.41 Sprain of coracohumeral (ligament)
7th S43.411 Sprain of right coracohumeral (ligament)
7th S43.412 Sprain of left coracohumeral (ligament)
7th S43.419 Sprain of unspecified coracohumeral (ligament)
6th S43.42 Sprain of rotator cuff capsule
EXCLUDES 1 *rotator cuff syndrome (complete) (incomplete), not specified as traumatic (M75.1-)*
EXCLUDES 2 *injury of tendon of rotator cuff (S46.0-)*
7th S43.421 Sprain of right rotator cuff capsule
7th S43.422 Sprain of left rotator cuff capsule
7th S43.429 Sprain of unspecified rotator cuff capsule
6th S43.43 Superior glenoid labrum lesion
SLAP lesion
AHA: 2019,2Q,26
DEF: Detachment injury of the superior aspect of the glenoid labrum, which is the ring of fibrocartilage attached to the rim of the glenoid cavity of the scapula.
7th S43.431 Superior glenoid labrum lesion of right shoulder

S43.432 Superior glenoid labrum lesion of left shoulder
S43.439 Superior glenoid labrum lesion of unspecified shoulder
S43.49 Other sprain of shoulder joint
S43.491 Other sprain of right shoulder joint
S43.492 Other sprain of left shoulder joint
S43.499 Other sprain of unspecified shoulder joint
S43.5 Sprain of acromioclavicular joint
Sprain of acromioclavicular ligament
S43.50 Sprain of unspecified acromioclavicular joint
S43.51 Sprain of right acromioclavicular joint
S43.52 Sprain of left acromioclavicular joint
S43.6 Sprain of sternoclavicular joint
S43.60 Sprain of unspecified sternoclavicular joint
S43.61 Sprain of right sternoclavicular joint
S43.62 Sprain of left sternoclavicular joint
S43.8 Sprain of other specified parts of shoulder girdle
S43.80 Sprain of other specified parts of unspecified shoulder girdle
S43.81 Sprain of other specified parts of right shoulder girdle
S43.82 Sprain of other specified parts of left shoulder girdle
S43.9 Sprain of unspecified parts of shoulder girdle
S43.90 Sprain of unspecified parts of unspecified shoulder girdle
Sprain of shoulder girdle NOS
S43.91 Sprain of unspecified parts of right shoulder girdle
S43.92 Sprain of unspecified parts of left shoulder girdle

S44 Injury of nerves at shoulder and upper arm level

Code also any associated open wound (S41.-)

EXCLUDES 2 *injury of brachial plexus (S14.3-)*

The appropriate 7th character is to be added to each code from category S44.
A initial encounter
D subsequent encounter
S sequela

S44.0 Injury of ulnar nerve at upper arm level
EXCLUDES 1 *ulnar nerve NOS (S54.0)*
S44.00 Injury of ulnar nerve at upper arm level, unspecified arm
S44.01 Injury of ulnar nerve at upper arm level, right arm
S44.02 Injury of ulnar nerve at upper arm level, left arm
S44.1 Injury of median nerve at upper arm level
EXCLUDES 1 *median nerve NOS (S54.1)*
S44.10 Injury of median nerve at upper arm level, unspecified arm
S44.11 Injury of median nerve at upper arm level, right arm
S44.12 Injury of median nerve at upper arm level, left arm
S44.2 Injury of radial nerve at upper arm level
EXCLUDES 1 *radial nerve NOS (S54.2)*
S44.20 Injury of radial nerve at upper arm level, unspecified arm
S44.21 Injury of radial nerve at upper arm level, right arm
S44.22 Injury of radial nerve at upper arm level, left arm
S44.3 Injury of axillary nerve
S44.30 Injury of axillary nerve, unspecified arm
S44.31 Injury of axillary nerve, right arm
S44.32 Injury of axillary nerve, left arm
S44.4 Injury of musculocutaneous nerve
S44.40 Injury of musculocutaneous nerve, unspecified arm
S44.41 Injury of musculocutaneous nerve, right arm
S44.42 Injury of musculocutaneous nerve, left arm
S44.5 Injury of cutaneous sensory nerve at shoulder and upper arm level
S44.50 Injury of cutaneous sensory nerve at shoulder and upper arm level, unspecified arm
S44.51 Injury of cutaneous sensory nerve at shoulder and upper arm level, right arm
S44.52 Injury of cutaneous sensory nerve at shoulder and upper arm level, left arm
S44.8 Injury of other nerves at shoulder and upper arm level
S44.8X Injury of other nerves at shoulder and upper arm level
S44.8X1 Injury of other nerves at shoulder and upper arm level, right arm
S44.8X2 Injury of other nerves at shoulder and upper arm level, left arm
S44.8X9 Injury of other nerves at shoulder and upper arm level, unspecified arm
S44.9 Injury of unspecified nerve at shoulder and upper arm level
S44.90 Injury of unspecified nerve at shoulder and upper arm level, unspecified arm
S44.91 Injury of unspecified nerve at shoulder and upper arm level, right arm
S44.92 Injury of unspecified nerve at shoulder and upper arm level, left arm

S45 Injury of blood vessels at shoulder and upper arm level

Code also any associated open wound (S41.-)

EXCLUDES 2 *injury of subclavian artery (S25.1)*
injury of subclavian vein (S25.3)

The appropriate 7th character is to be added to each code from category S45.
A initial encounter
D subsequent encounter
S sequela

S45.0 Injury of axillary artery
S45.00 Unspecified injury of axillary artery
S45.001 Unspecified injury of axillary artery, right side MCC
S45.002 Unspecified injury of axillary artery, left side MCC
S45.009 Unspecified injury of axillary artery, unspecified side MCC UNS
S45.01 Laceration of axillary artery
S45.011 Laceration of axillary artery, right side MCC
S45.012 Laceration of axillary artery, left side MCC
S45.019 Laceration of axillary artery, unspecified side MCC UNS
S45.09 Other specified injury of axillary artery
S45.091 Other specified injury of axillary artery, right side MCC
S45.092 Other specified injury of axillary artery, left side MCC
S45.099 Other specified injury of axillary artery, unspecified side MCC UNS
S45.1 Injury of brachial artery
S45.10 Unspecified injury of brachial artery
S45.101 Unspecified injury of brachial artery, right side CC
S45.102 Unspecified injury of brachial artery, left side CC
S45.109 Unspecified injury of brachial artery, unspecified side CC UNS
S45.11 Laceration of brachial artery
S45.111 Laceration of brachial artery, right side CC
S45.112 Laceration of brachial artery, left side CC
S45.119 Laceration of brachial artery, unspecified side CC UNS
S45.19 Other specified injury of brachial artery
S45.191 Other specified injury of brachial artery, right side CC
S45.192 Other specified injury of brachial artery, left side CC
S45.199 Other specified injury of brachial artery, unspecified side CC UNS
S45.2 Injury of axillary or brachial vein
S45.20 Unspecified injury of axillary or brachial vein
S45.201 Unspecified injury of axillary or brachial vein, right side CC
S45.202 Unspecified injury of axillary or brachial vein, left side CC

√7th **S45.209 Unspecified injury of axillary or brachial vein, unspecified side** CC UNS

√6th **S45.21 Laceration of axillary or brachial vein**

√7th **S45.211 Laceration of axillary or brachial vein, right side** CC

√7th **S45.212 Laceration of axillary or brachial vein, left side** CC

√7th **S45.219 Laceration of axillary or brachial vein, unspecified side** CC UNS

√6th **S45.29 Other specified injury of axillary or brachial vein**

√7th **S45.291 Other specified injury of axillary or brachial vein, right side** CC

√7th **S45.292 Other specified injury of axillary or brachial vein, left side** CC

√7th **S45.299 Other specified injury of axillary or brachial vein, unspecified side** CC UNS

√5th **S45.3 Injury of superficial vein at shoulder and upper arm level**

√6th **S45.30 Unspecified injury of superficial vein at shoulder and upper arm level**

√7th **S45.301 Unspecified injury of superficial vein at shoulder and upper arm level, right arm** CC

√7th **S45.302 Unspecified injury of superficial vein at shoulder and upper arm level, left arm** CC

√7th **S45.309 Unspecified injury of superficial vein at shoulder and upper arm level, unspecified arm** CC UNS

√6th **S45.31 Laceration of superficial vein at shoulder and upper arm level**

√7th **S45.311 Laceration of superficial vein at shoulder and upper arm level, right arm** CC

√7th **S45.312 Laceration of superficial vein at shoulder and upper arm level, left arm** CC

√7th **S45.319 Laceration of superficial vein at shoulder and upper arm level, unspecified arm** CC UNS

√6th **S45.39 Other specified injury of superficial vein at shoulder and upper arm level**

√7th **S45.391 Other specified injury of superficial vein at shoulder and upper arm level, right arm** CC

√7th **S45.392 Other specified injury of superficial vein at shoulder and upper arm level, left arm** CC

√7th **S45.399 Other specified injury of superficial vein at shoulder and upper arm level, unspecified arm** CC UNS

√5th **S45.8 Injury of other specified blood vessels at shoulder and upper arm level**

√6th **S45.80 Unspecified injury of other specified blood vessels at shoulder and upper arm level**

√7th **S45.801 Unspecified injury of other specified blood vessels at shoulder and upper arm level, right arm** CC

√7th **S45.802 Unspecified injury of other specified blood vessels at shoulder and upper arm level, left arm** CC

√7th **S45.809 Unspecified injury of other specified blood vessels at shoulder and upper arm level, unspecified arm** CC UNS

√6th **S45.81 Laceration of other specified blood vessels at shoulder and upper arm level**

√7th **S45.811 Laceration of other specified blood vessels at shoulder and upper arm level, right arm** CC

√7th **S45.812 Laceration of other specified blood vessels at shoulder and upper arm level, left arm** CC

√7th **S45.819 Laceration of other specified blood vessels at shoulder and upper arm level, unspecified arm** CC UNS

√6th **S45.89 Other specified injury of other specified blood vessels at shoulder and upper arm level**

√7th **S45.891 Other specified injury of other specified blood vessels at shoulder and upper arm level, right arm** CC

√7th **S45.892 Other specified injury of other specified blood vessels at shoulder and upper arm level, left arm** CC

√7th **S45.899 Other specified injury of other specified blood vessels at shoulder and upper arm level, unspecified arm** CC UNS

√5th **S45.9 Injury of unspecified blood vessel at shoulder and upper arm level**

√6th **S45.90 Unspecified injury of unspecified blood vessel at shoulder and upper arm level**

√7th **S45.901 Unspecified injury of unspecified blood vessel at shoulder and upper arm level, right arm** CC

√7th **S45.902 Unspecified injury of unspecified blood vessel at shoulder and upper arm level, left arm** CC

√7th **S45.909 Unspecified injury of unspecified blood vessel at shoulder and upper arm level, unspecified arm** CC UNS

√6th **S45.91 Laceration of unspecified blood vessel at shoulder and upper arm level**

√7th **S45.911 Laceration of unspecified blood vessel at shoulder and upper arm level, right arm** CC

√7th **S45.912 Laceration of unspecified blood vessel at shoulder and upper arm level, left arm** CC

√7th **S45.919 Laceration of unspecified blood vessel at shoulder and upper arm level, unspecified arm** CC UNS

√6th **S45.99 Other specified injury of unspecified blood vessel at shoulder and upper arm level**

√7th **S45.991 Other specified injury of unspecified blood vessel at shoulder and upper arm level, right arm** CC

√7th **S45.992 Other specified injury of unspecified blood vessel at shoulder and upper arm level, left arm** CC

√7th **S45.999 Other specified injury of unspecified blood vessel at shoulder and upper arm level, unspecified arm** CC UNS

√4th **S46 Injury of muscle, fascia and tendon at shoulder and upper arm level**

Code also any associated open wound (S41.-)

EXCLUDES 2 *injury of muscle, fascia and tendon at elbow (S56.-)*
sprain of joints and ligaments of shoulder girdle (S43.9)

TIP: Refer to the Muscle/Tendon table at the beginning of this chapter.

The appropriate 7th character is to be added to each code from category S46.
A initial encounter
D subsequent encounter
S sequela

√5th **S46.0 Injury of muscle(s) and tendon(s) of the rotator cuff of shoulder**

√6th **S46.00 Unspecified injury of muscle(s) and tendon(s) of the rotator cuff of shoulder**

√7th **S46.001 Unspecified injury of muscle(s) and tendon(s) of the rotator cuff of right shoulder**

√7th **S46.002 Unspecified injury of muscle(s) and tendon(s) of the rotator cuff of left shoulder**

√7th **S46.009 Unspecified injury of muscle(s) and tendon(s) of the rotator cuff of unspecified shoulder**

√6th **S46.01 Strain of muscle(s) and tendon(s) of the rotator cuff of shoulder**

√7th **S46.011 Strain of muscle(s) and tendon(s) of the rotator cuff of right shoulder**

√7th **S46.012 Strain of muscle(s) and tendon(s) of the rotator cuff of left shoulder**

√7th **S46.019 Strain of muscle(s) and tendon(s) of the rotator cuff of unspecified shoulder**

√6th **S46.02 Laceration of muscle(s) and tendon(s) of the rotator cuff of shoulder**

√7th **S46.021 Laceration of muscle(s) and tendon(s) of the rotator cuff of right shoulder** CC

√7th **S46.022 Laceration of muscle(s) and tendon(s) of the rotator cuff of left shoulder** CC

√7th **S46.029 Laceration of muscle(s) and tendon(s) of the rotator cuff of unspecified shoulder** CC UNS

- 6th S46.09 Other injury of muscle(s) and tendon(s) of the rotator cuff of shoulder
  - 7th S46.091 Other injury of muscle(s) and tendon(s) of the rotator cuff of right shoulder
  - 7th S46.092 Other injury of muscle(s) and tendon(s) of the rotator cuff of left shoulder
  - 7th S46.099 Other injury of muscle(s) and tendon(s) of the rotator cuff of unspecified shoulder

5th S46.1 Injury of muscle, fascia and tendon of long head of biceps

- 6th S46.10 Unspecified injury of muscle, fascia and tendon of long head of biceps
  - 7th S46.101 Unspecified injury of muscle, fascia and tendon of long head of biceps, right arm
  - 7th S46.102 Unspecified injury of muscle, fascia and tendon of long head of biceps, left arm
  - 7th S46.109 Unspecified injury of muscle, fascia and tendon of long head of biceps, unspecified arm
- 6th S46.11 Strain of muscle, fascia and tendon of long head of biceps
  - AHA: 2020,1Q,38; 2019,2Q,27
  - 7th S46.111 Strain of muscle, fascia and tendon of long head of biceps, right arm
  - 7th S46.112 Strain of muscle, fascia and tendon of long head of biceps, left arm
  - 7th S46.119 Strain of muscle, fascia and tendon of long head of biceps, unspecified arm
- 6th S46.12 Laceration of muscle, fascia and tendon of long head of biceps
  - 7th S46.121 Laceration of muscle, fascia and tendon of long head of biceps, right arm CC
  - 7th S46.122 Laceration of muscle, fascia and tendon of long head of biceps, left arm CC
  - 7th S46.129 Laceration of muscle, fascia and tendon of long head of biceps, unspecified arm CC UNS
- 6th S46.19 Other injury of muscle, fascia and tendon of long head of biceps
  - 7th S46.191 Other injury of muscle, fascia and tendon of long head of biceps, right arm
  - 7th S46.192 Other injury of muscle, fascia and tendon of long head of biceps, left arm
  - 7th S46.199 Other injury of muscle, fascia and tendon of long head of biceps, unspecified arm

5th S46.2 Injury of muscle, fascia and tendon of other parts of biceps

- 6th S46.20 Unspecified injury of muscle, fascia and tendon of other parts of biceps
  - 7th S46.201 Unspecified injury of muscle, fascia and tendon of other parts of biceps, right arm
  - 7th S46.202 Unspecified injury of muscle, fascia and tendon of other parts of biceps, left arm
  - 7th S46.209 Unspecified injury of muscle, fascia and tendon of other parts of biceps, unspecified arm
- 6th S46.21 Strain of muscle, fascia and tendon of other parts of biceps
  - 7th S46.211 Strain of muscle, fascia and tendon of other parts of biceps, right arm
  - 7th S46.212 Strain of muscle, fascia and tendon of other parts of biceps, left arm
  - 7th S46.219 Strain of muscle, fascia and tendon of other parts of biceps, unspecified arm
- 6th S46.22 Laceration of muscle, fascia and tendon of other parts of biceps
  - 7th S46.221 Laceration of muscle, fascia and tendon of other parts of biceps, right arm CC
  - 7th S46.222 Laceration of muscle, fascia and tendon of other parts of biceps, left arm CC
  - 7th S46.229 Laceration of muscle, fascia and tendon of other parts of biceps, unspecified arm CC UNS
- 6th S46.29 Other injury of muscle, fascia and tendon of other parts of biceps
  - 7th S46.291 Other injury of muscle, fascia and tendon of other parts of biceps, right arm
  - 7th S46.292 Other injury of muscle, fascia and tendon of other parts of biceps, left arm
  - 7th S46.299 Other injury of muscle, fascia and tendon of other parts of biceps, unspecified arm

5th S46.3 Injury of muscle, fascia and tendon of triceps

- 6th S46.30 Unspecified injury of muscle, fascia and tendon of triceps
  - 7th S46.301 Unspecified injury of muscle, fascia and tendon of triceps, right arm
  - 7th S46.302 Unspecified injury of muscle, fascia and tendon of triceps, left arm
  - 7th S46.309 Unspecified injury of muscle, fascia and tendon of triceps, unspecified arm
- 6th S46.31 Strain of muscle, fascia and tendon of triceps
  - 7th S46.311 Strain of muscle, fascia and tendon of triceps, right arm
  - 7th S46.312 Strain of muscle, fascia and tendon of triceps, left arm
  - 7th S46.319 Strain of muscle, fascia and tendon of triceps, unspecified arm
- 6th S46.32 Laceration of muscle, fascia and tendon of triceps
  - 7th S46.321 Laceration of muscle, fascia and tendon of triceps, right arm CC
  - 7th S46.322 Laceration of muscle, fascia and tendon of triceps, left arm CC
  - 7th S46.329 Laceration of muscle, fascia and tendon of triceps, unspecified arm CC UNS
- 6th S46.39 Other injury of muscle, fascia and tendon of triceps
  - 7th S46.391 Other injury of muscle, fascia and tendon of triceps, right arm
  - 7th S46.392 Other injury of muscle, fascia and tendon of triceps, left arm
  - 7th S46.399 Other injury of muscle, fascia and tendon of triceps, unspecified arm

5th S46.8 Injury of other muscles, fascia and tendons at shoulder and upper arm level

- 6th S46.80 Unspecified injury of other muscles, fascia and tendons at shoulder and upper arm level
  - 7th S46.801 Unspecified injury of other muscles, fascia and tendons at shoulder and upper arm level, right arm
  - 7th S46.802 Unspecified injury of other muscles, fascia and tendons at shoulder and upper arm level, left arm
  - 7th S46.809 Unspecified injury of other muscles, fascia and tendons at shoulder and upper arm level, unspecified arm
- 6th S46.81 Strain of other muscles, fascia and tendons at shoulder and upper arm level
  - 7th S46.811 Strain of other muscles, fascia and tendons at shoulder and upper arm level, right arm
  - 7th S46.812 Strain of other muscles, fascia and tendons at shoulder and upper arm level, left arm
  - 7th S46.819 Strain of other muscles, fascia and tendons at shoulder and upper arm level, unspecified arm
- 6th S46.82 Laceration of other muscles, fascia and tendons at shoulder and upper arm level
  - 7th S46.821 Laceration of other muscles, fascia and tendons at shoulder and upper arm level, right arm CC
  - 7th S46.822 Laceration of other muscles, fascia and tendons at shoulder and upper arm level, left arm CC
  - 7th S46.829 Laceration of other muscles, fascia and tendons at shoulder and upper arm level, unspecified arm CC UNS
- 6th S46.89 Other injury of other muscles, fascia and tendons at shoulder and upper arm level
  - 7th S46.891 Other injury of other muscles, fascia and tendons at shoulder and upper arm level, right arm
  - 7th S46.892 Other injury of other muscles, fascia and tendons at shoulder and upper arm level, left arm
  - 7th S46.899 Other injury of other muscles, fascia and tendons at shoulder and upper arm level, unspecified arm

- S46.9 Injury of unspecified muscle, fascia and tendon at shoulder and upper arm level
  - S46.90 Unspecified injury of unspecified muscle, fascia and tendon at shoulder and upper arm level
    - S46.901 Unspecified injury of unspecified muscle, fascia and tendon at shoulder and upper arm level, right arm
    - S46.902 Unspecified injury of unspecified muscle, fascia and tendon at shoulder and upper arm level, left arm
    - S46.909 Unspecified injury of unspecified muscle, fascia and tendon at shoulder and upper arm level, unspecified arm
  - S46.91 Strain of unspecified muscle, fascia and tendon at shoulder and upper arm level
    - S46.911 Strain of unspecified muscle, fascia and tendon at shoulder and upper arm level, right arm
    - S46.912 Strain of unspecified muscle, fascia and tendon at shoulder and upper arm level, left arm
    - S46.919 Strain of unspecified muscle, fascia and tendon at shoulder and upper arm level, unspecified arm
  - S46.92 Laceration of unspecified muscle, fascia and tendon at shoulder and upper arm level
    - S46.921 Laceration of unspecified muscle, fascia and tendon at shoulder and upper arm level, right arm CC
    - S46.922 Laceration of unspecified muscle, fascia and tendon at shoulder and upper arm level, left arm CC
    - S46.929 Laceration of unspecified muscle, fascia and tendon at shoulder and upper arm level, unspecified arm CC UNS
  - S46.99 Other injury of unspecified muscle, fascia and tendon at shoulder and upper arm level
    - S46.991 Other injury of unspecified muscle, fascia and tendon at shoulder and upper arm level, right arm
    - S46.992 Other injury of unspecified muscle, fascia and tendon at shoulder and upper arm level, left arm
    - S46.999 Other injury of unspecified muscle, fascia and tendon at shoulder and upper arm level, unspecified arm

S47 Crushing injury of shoulder and upper arm

Use additional code for all associated injuries

EXCLUDES 2 *crushing injury of elbow (S57.Ø-)*

The appropriate 7th character is to be added to each code from category S47.
A initial encounter
D subsequent encounter
S sequela

- S47.1 Crushing injury of right shoulder and upper arm
- S47.2 Crushing injury of left shoulder and upper arm
- S47.9 Crushing injury of shoulder and upper arm, unspecified arm

S48 Traumatic amputation of shoulder and upper arm

An amputation not identified as partial or complete should be coded to complete

EXCLUDES 1 *traumatic amputation at elbow level (S58.Ø)*

The appropriate 7th character is to be added to each code from category S48.
A initial encounter
D subsequent encounter
S sequela

- S48.Ø Traumatic amputation at shoulder joint
  - S48.Ø1 Complete traumatic amputation at shoulder joint
    - S48.Ø11 Complete traumatic amputation at right shoulder joint CC HCC
    - S48.Ø12 Complete traumatic amputation at left shoulder joint CC HCC
    - S48.Ø19 Complete traumatic amputation at unspecified shoulder joint CC UNS HCC
  - S48.Ø2 Partial traumatic amputation at shoulder joint
    - S48.Ø21 Partial traumatic amputation at right shoulder joint CC HCC
    - S48.Ø22 Partial traumatic amputation at left shoulder joint CC HCC
    - S48.Ø29 Partial traumatic amputation at unspecified shoulder joint CC UNS HCC
- S48.1 Traumatic amputation at level between shoulder and elbow
  - S48.11 Complete traumatic amputation at level between shoulder and elbow
    - S48.111 Complete traumatic amputation at level between right shoulder and elbow CC HCC
    - S48.112 Complete traumatic amputation at level between left shoulder and elbow CC HCC
    - S48.119 Complete traumatic amputation at level between unspecified shoulder and elbow CC UNS HCC
  - S48.12 Partial traumatic amputation at level between shoulder and elbow
    - S48.121 Partial traumatic amputation at level between right shoulder and elbow CC HCC
    - S48.122 Partial traumatic amputation at level between left shoulder and elbow CC HCC
    - S48.129 Partial traumatic amputation at level between unspecified shoulder and elbow CC UNS HCC
- S48.9 Traumatic amputation of shoulder and upper arm, level unspecified
  - S48.91 Complete traumatic amputation of shoulder and upper arm, level unspecified
    - S48.911 Complete traumatic amputation of right shoulder and upper arm, level unspecified CC HCC
    - S48.912 Complete traumatic amputation of left shoulder and upper arm, level unspecified CC HCC
    - S48.919 Complete traumatic amputation of unspecified shoulder and upper arm, level unspecified CC UNS HCC
  - S48.92 Partial traumatic amputation of shoulder and upper arm, level unspecified
    - S48.921 Partial traumatic amputation of right shoulder and upper arm, level unspecified CC HCC
    - S48.922 Partial traumatic amputation of left shoulder and upper arm, level unspecified CC HCC
    - S48.929 Partial traumatic amputation of unspecified shoulder and upper arm, level unspecified CC UNS HCC

S49 Other and unspecified injuries of shoulder and upper arm

AHA: 2018,2Q,12; 2018,1Q,3

The appropriate 7th character is to be added to each code from subcategories S49.Ø and S49.1.
A initial encounter for closed fracture
D subsequent encounter for fracture with routine healing
G subsequent encounter for fracture with delayed healing
K subsequent encounter for fracture with nonunion
P subsequent encounter for fracture with malunion
S sequela

- S49.Ø Physeal fracture of upper end of humerus
  AHA: 2019,4Q,56
  - S49.ØØ Unspecified physeal fracture of upper end of humerus
    - S49.ØØ1 Unspecified physeal fracture of upper end of humerus, right arm CC H5
    - S49.ØØ2 Unspecified physeal fracture of upper end of humerus, left arm CC H5
    - S49.ØØ9 Unspecified physeal fracture of upper end of humerus, unspecified arm CC H5 UNS
  - S49.Ø1 Salter-Harris Type I physeal fracture of upper end of humerus
    - S49.Ø11 Salter-Harris Type I physeal fracture of upper end of humerus, right arm CC H5
    - S49.Ø12 Salter-Harris Type I physeal fracture of upper end of humerus, left arm CC H5
    - S49.Ø19 Salter-Harris Type I physeal fracture of upper end of humerus, unspecified arm CC H5 UNS

√6th S49.02 Salter-Harris Type II physeal fracture of upper end of humerus
√7th S49.021 Salter-Harris Type II physeal fracture of upper end of humerus, right arm CC H5
√7th S49.022 Salter-Harris Type II physeal fracture of upper end of humerus, left arm CC H5
√7th S49.029 Salter-Harris Type II physeal fracture of upper end of humerus, unspecified arm CC H5 UNS
√6th S49.03 Salter-Harris Type III physeal fracture of upper end of humerus
√7th S49.031 Salter-Harris Type III physeal fracture of upper end of humerus, right arm CC H5
√7th S49.032 Salter-Harris Type III physeal fracture of upper end of humerus, left arm CC H5
√7th S49.039 Salter-Harris Type III physeal fracture of upper end of humerus, unspecified arm CC H5 UNS
√6th S49.04 Salter-Harris Type IV physeal fracture of upper end of humerus
√7th S49.041 Salter-Harris Type IV physeal fracture of upper end of humerus, right arm CC H5
√7th S49.042 Salter-Harris Type IV physeal fracture of upper end of humerus, left arm CC H5
√7th S49.049 Salter-Harris Type IV physeal fracture of upper end of humerus, unspecified arm CC H5 UNS
√6th S49.09 Other physeal fracture of upper end of humerus
√7th S49.091 Other physeal fracture of upper end of humerus, right arm CC H5
√7th S49.092 Other physeal fracture of upper end of humerus, left arm CC H5
√7th S49.099 Other physeal fracture of upper end of humerus, unspecified arm CC H5 UNS
√5th S49.1 Physeal fracture of lower end of humerus
AHA: 2019,4Q,56
√6th S49.10 Unspecified physeal fracture of lower end of humerus
√7th S49.101 Unspecified physeal fracture of lower end of humerus, right arm CC H5
√7th S49.102 Unspecified physeal fracture of lower end of humerus, left arm CC H5
√7th S49.109 Unspecified physeal fracture of lower end of humerus, unspecified arm CC H5 UNS
√6th S49.11 Salter-Harris Type I physeal fracture of lower end of humerus
√7th S49.111 Salter-Harris Type I physeal fracture of lower end of humerus, right arm CC H5
√7th S49.112 Salter-Harris Type I physeal fracture of lower end of humerus, left arm CC H5
√7th S49.119 Salter-Harris Type I physeal fracture of lower end of humerus, unspecified arm CC H5 UNS
√6th S49.12 Salter-Harris Type II physeal fracture of lower end of humerus
√7th S49.121 Salter-Harris Type II physeal fracture of lower end of humerus, right arm CC H5
√7th S49.122 Salter-Harris Type II physeal fracture of lower end of humerus, left arm CC H5
√7th S49.129 Salter-Harris Type II physeal fracture of lower end of humerus, unspecified arm CC H5 UNS
√6th S49.13 Salter-Harris Type III physeal fracture of lower end of humerus
√7th S49.131 Salter-Harris Type III physeal fracture of lower end of humerus, right arm CC H5
√7th S49.132 Salter-Harris Type III physeal fracture of lower end of humerus, left arm CC H5
√7th S49.139 Salter-Harris Type III physeal fracture of lower end of humerus, unspecified arm CC H5 UNS
√6th S49.14 Salter-Harris Type IV physeal fracture of lower end of humerus
√7th S49.141 Salter-Harris Type IV physeal fracture of lower end of humerus, right arm CC H5
√7th S49.142 Salter-Harris Type IV physeal fracture of lower end of humerus, left arm CC H5
√7th S49.149 Salter-Harris Type IV physeal fracture of lower end of humerus, unspecified arm CC H5 UNS
√6th S49.19 Other physeal fracture of lower end of humerus
√7th S49.191 Other physeal fracture of lower end of humerus, right arm CC H5
√7th S49.192 Other physeal fracture of lower end of humerus, left arm CC H5
√7th S49.199 Other physeal fracture of lower end of humerus, unspecified arm CC H5 UNS
√5th S49.8 Other specified injuries of shoulder and upper arm

The appropriate 7th character is to be added to each code in subcategory S49.8.
A initial encounter
D subsequent encounter
S sequela

√x7th S49.80 Other specified injuries of shoulder and upper arm, unspecified arm
√x7th S49.81 Other specified injuries of right shoulder and upper arm
√x7th S49.82 Other specified injuries of left shoulder and upper arm
√5th S49.9 Unspecified injury of shoulder and upper arm

The appropriate 7th character is to be added to each code in subcategory S49.9.
A initial encounter
D subsequent encounter
S sequela

√x7th S49.90 Unspecified injury of shoulder and upper arm, unspecified arm
√x7th S49.91 Unspecified injury of right shoulder and upper arm
√x7th S49.92 Unspecified injury of left shoulder and upper arm

Injuries to the elbow and forearm (S50-S59)

EXCLUDES 2 *burns and corrosions (T20-T32)*
frostbite (T33-T34)
injuries of wrist and hand (S60-S69)
insect bite or sting, venomous (T63.4)

√4th **S50 Superficial injury of elbow and forearm**
EXCLUDES 2 *superficial injury of wrist and hand (S60.-)*

The appropriate 7th character is to be added to each code from category S50.
A initial encounter
D subsequent encounter
S sequela

√5th S50.0 Contusion of elbow
√x7th S50.00 Contusion of unspecified elbow
√x7th S50.01 Contusion of right elbow
√x7th S50.02 Contusion of left elbow
√5th S50.1 Contusion of forearm
√x7th S50.10 Contusion of unspecified forearm
√x7th S50.11 Contusion of right forearm
√x7th S50.12 Contusion of left forearm
√5th S50.3 Other superficial injuries of elbow
√6th S50.31 Abrasion of elbow
√7th S50.311 Abrasion of right elbow
√7th S50.312 Abrasion of left elbow
√7th S50.319 Abrasion of unspecified elbow
√6th S50.32 Blister (nonthermal) of elbow
√7th S50.321 Blister (nonthermal) of right elbow
√7th S50.322 Blister (nonthermal) of left elbow
√7th S50.329 Blister (nonthermal) of unspecified elbow
√6th S50.34 External constriction of elbow
√7th S50.341 External constriction of right elbow
√7th S50.342 External constriction of left elbow

S50.349 External constriction of unspecified elbow

S50.35 Superficial foreign body of elbow
Splinter in the elbow
S50.351 Superficial foreign body of right elbow
S50.352 Superficial foreign body of left elbow
S50.359 Superficial foreign body of unspecified elbow

S50.36 Insect bite (nonvenomous) of elbow
S50.361 Insect bite (nonvenomous) of right elbow
S50.362 Insect bite (nonvenomous) of left elbow
S50.369 Insect bite (nonvenomous) of unspecified elbow

S50.37 Other superficial bite of elbow
EXCLUDES 1 *open bite of elbow (S51.05)*
S50.371 Other superficial bite of right elbow
S50.372 Other superficial bite of left elbow
S50.379 Other superficial bite of unspecified elbow

S50.8 Other superficial injuries of forearm

S50.81 Abrasion of forearm
S50.811 Abrasion of right forearm
S50.812 Abrasion of left forearm
S50.819 Abrasion of unspecified forearm

S50.82 Blister (nonthermal) of forearm
S50.821 Blister (nonthermal) of right forearm
S50.822 Blister (nonthermal) of left forearm
S50.829 Blister (nonthermal) of unspecified forearm

S50.84 External constriction of forearm
S50.841 External constriction of right forearm
S50.842 External constriction of left forearm
S50.849 External constriction of unspecified forearm

S50.85 Superficial foreign body of forearm
Splinter in the forearm
S50.851 Superficial foreign body of right forearm
S50.852 Superficial foreign body of left forearm
S50.859 Superficial foreign body of unspecified forearm

S50.86 Insect bite (nonvenomous) of forearm
S50.861 Insect bite (nonvenomous) of right forearm
S50.862 Insect bite (nonvenomous) of left forearm
S50.869 Insect bite (nonvenomous) of unspecified forearm

S50.87 Other superficial bite of forearm
EXCLUDES 1 *open bite of forearm (S51.85)*
S50.871 Other superficial bite of right forearm
S50.872 Other superficial bite of left forearm
S50.879 Other superficial bite of unspecified forearm

S50.9 Unspecified superficial injury of elbow and forearm

S50.90 Unspecified superficial injury of elbow
S50.901 Unspecified superficial injury of right elbow
S50.902 Unspecified superficial injury of left elbow
S50.909 Unspecified superficial injury of unspecified elbow

S50.91 Unspecified superficial injury of forearm
S50.911 Unspecified superficial injury of right forearm
S50.912 Unspecified superficial injury of left forearm
S50.919 Unspecified superficial injury of unspecified forearm

S51 Open wound of elbow and forearm

Code also any associated wound infection

EXCLUDES 1 *open fracture of elbow and forearm (S52.- with open fracture 7th character)*
traumatic amputation of elbow and forearm (S58.-)

EXCLUDES 2 *open wound of wrist and hand (S61.-)*

The appropriate 7th character is to be added to each code from category S51.
A initial encounter
D subsequent encounter
S sequela

S51.0 Open wound of elbow

S51.00 Unspecified open wound of elbow
S51.001 Unspecified open wound of right elbow
AHA: 2012,4Q,108
S51.002 Unspecified open wound of left elbow
S51.009 Unspecified open wound of unspecified elbow
Open wound of elbow NOS

S51.01 Laceration without foreign body of elbow
S51.011 Laceration without foreign body of right elbow
S51.012 Laceration without foreign body of left elbow
S51.019 Laceration without foreign body of unspecified elbow

S51.02 Laceration with foreign body of elbow
S51.021 Laceration with foreign body of right elbow
S51.022 Laceration with foreign body of left elbow
S51.029 Laceration with foreign body of unspecified elbow

S51.03 Puncture wound without foreign body of elbow
S51.031 Puncture wound without foreign body of right elbow
S51.032 Puncture wound without foreign body of left elbow
S51.039 Puncture wound without foreign body of unspecified elbow

S51.04 Puncture wound with foreign body of elbow
S51.041 Puncture wound with foreign body of right elbow
S51.042 Puncture wound with foreign body of left elbow
S51.049 Puncture wound with foreign body of unspecified elbow

S51.05 Open bite of elbow
Bite of elbow NOS
EXCLUDES 1 *superficial bite of elbow (S50.36, S50.37)*
S51.051 Open bite, right elbow
S51.052 Open bite, left elbow
S51.059 Open bite, unspecified elbow

S51.8 Open wound of forearm
EXCLUDES 2 *open wound of elbow (S51.0-)*

S51.80 Unspecified open wound of forearm
AHA: 2016,3Q,24
S51.801 Unspecified open wound of right forearm
S51.802 Unspecified open wound of left forearm
S51.809 Unspecified open wound of unspecified forearm
Open wound of forearm NOS

S51.81 Laceration without foreign body of forearm
S51.811 Laceration without foreign body of right forearm
S51.812 Laceration without foreign body of left forearm
S51.819 Laceration without foreign body of unspecified forearm

S51.82 Laceration with foreign body of forearm
S51.821 Laceration with foreign body of right forearm
S51.822 Laceration with foreign body of left forearm
S51.829 Laceration with foreign body of unspecified forearm

S51.83 Puncture wound without foreign body of forearm
AHA: 2016,3Q,24
S51.831 Puncture wound without foreign body of right forearm
S51.832 Puncture wound without foreign body of left forearm
S51.839 Puncture wound without foreign body of unspecified forearm
S51.84 Puncture wound with foreign body of forearm
AHA: 2016,3Q,24
S51.841 Puncture wound with foreign body of right forearm
S51.842 Puncture wound with foreign body of left forearm
S51.849 Puncture wound with foreign body of unspecified forearm
S51.85 Open bite of forearm
Bite of forearm NOS
EXCLUDES 1 *superficial bite of forearm (S50.86, S50.87)*
S51.851 Open bite of right forearm
S51.852 Open bite of left forearm
S51.859 Open bite of unspecified forearm

S52 Fracture of forearm

NOTE A fracture not indicated as displaced or nondisplaced should be coded to displaced.
A fracture not indicated as open or closed should be coded to closed.
The open fracture designations are based on the Gustilo open fracture classification.

EXCLUDES 1 *traumatic amputation of forearm (S58.-)*
EXCLUDES 2 *fracture at wrist and hand level (S62.-)*
▶*periprosthetic fracture around internal prosthetic elbow joint (M97.4)*◀

AHA: 2018,2Q,12; 2016,1Q,33; 2015,3Q,37-39
DEF: Diaphysis: Central shaft of a long bone.
DEF: Epiphysis: Proximal and distal rounded ends of a long bone, communicates with the joint.
DEF: Metaphysis: Section of a long bone located between the epiphysis and diaphysis at the proximal and distal ends.
DEF: Physis (growth plate): Narrow zone of cartilaginous tissue between the epiphysis and metaphysis at each end of a long bone. In childhood, proliferation of cells in this zone lengthens the bone. As the bone matures, this area thins, ossification eventually fusing into solid bone and growth stops. *Synonym(s): Epiphyseal plate.*

The appropriate 7th character is to be added to all codes from category S52 [unless otherwise indicated].
A initial encounter for closed fracture
B initial encounter for open fracture type I or II
initial encounter for open fracture NOS
C initial encounter for open fracture type IIIA, IIIB, or IIIC
D subsequent encounter for closed fracture with routine healing
E subsequent encounter for open fracture type I or II with routine healing
F subsequent encounter for open fracture type IIIA, IIIB, or IIIC with routine healing
G subsequent encounter for closed fracture with delayed healing
H subsequent encounter for open fracture type I or II with delayed healing
J subsequent encounter for open fracture type IIIA, IIIB, or IIIC with delayed healing
K subsequent encounter for closed fracture with nonunion
M subsequent encounter for open fracture type I or II with nonunion
N subsequent encounter for open fracture type IIIA, IIIB, or IIIC with nonunion
P subsequent encounter for closed fracture with malunion
Q subsequent encounter for open fracture type I or II with malunion
R subsequent encounter for open fracture type IIIA, IIIB, or IIIC with malunion
S sequela

S52.0 Fracture of upper end of ulna
Fracture of proximal end of ulna
EXCLUDES 2 *fracture of elbow NOS (S42.40-)*
fractures of shaft of ulna (S52.2-)
S52.00 Unspecified fracture of upper end of ulna
S52.001 Unspecified fracture of upper end of right ulna MCC CC H5
S52.002 Unspecified fracture of upper end of left ulna MCC CC H5
S52.009 Unspecified fracture of upper end of unspecified ulna MCC CC H5 UNS
S52.01 Torus fracture of upper end of ulna

The appropriate 7th character is to be added to all codes in subcategory S52.01
A initial encounter for closed fracture
D subsequent encounter for fracture with routine healing
G subsequent encounter for fracture with delayed healing
K subsequent encounter for fracture with nonunion
P subsequent encounter for fracture with malunion
S sequela

S52.011 Torus fracture of upper end of right ulna CC H5
S52.012 Torus fracture of upper end of left ulna CC H5
S52.019 Torus fracture of upper end of unspecified ulna CC H5 UNS
S52.02 Fracture of olecranon process without intraarticular extension of ulna
S52.021 Displaced fracture of olecranon process without intraarticular extension of right ulna MCC CC H5
S52.022 Displaced fracture of olecranon process without intraarticular extension of left ulna MCC CC H5
S52.023 Displaced fracture of olecranon process without intraarticular extension of unspecified ulna MCC CC H5 UNS
S52.024 Nondisplaced fracture of olecranon process without intraarticular extension of right ulna MCC CC H5
S52.025 Nondisplaced fracture of olecranon process without intraarticular extension of left ulna MCC CC H5
S52.026 Nondisplaced fracture of olecranon process without intraarticular extension of unspecified ulna MCC CC H5 UNS
S52.03 Fracture of olecranon process with intraarticular extension of ulna
S52.031 Displaced fracture of olecranon process with intraarticular extension of right ulna MCC CC H5
S52.032 Displaced fracture of olecranon process with intraarticular extension of left ulna MCC CC H5
S52.033 Displaced fracture of olecranon process with intraarticular extension of unspecified ulna MCC CC H5 UNS
S52.034 Nondisplaced fracture of olecranon process with intraarticular extension of right ulna MCC CC H5
S52.035 Nondisplaced fracture of olecranon process with intraarticular extension of left ulna MCC CC H5
S52.036 Nondisplaced fracture of olecranon process with intraarticular extension of unspecified ulna MCC CC H5 UNS
S52.04 Fracture of coronoid process of ulna
S52.041 Displaced fracture of coronoid process of right ulna MCC CC H5
S52.042 Displaced fracture of coronoid process of left ulna MCC CC H5
S52.043 Displaced fracture of coronoid process of unspecified ulna MCC CC H5 UNS
S52.044 Nondisplaced fracture of coronoid process of right ulna MCC CC H5
S52.045 Nondisplaced fracture of coronoid process of left ulna MCC CC H5
S52.046 Nondisplaced fracture of coronoid process of unspecified ulna MCC CC H5 UNS
S52.09 Other fracture of upper end of ulna
S52.091 Other fracture of upper end of right ulna MCC CC H5

7th **S52.092 Other fracture of upper end of left ulna** MCC CC HS

7th **S52.099 Other fracture of upper end of unspecified ulna** MCC CC HS UNS

5th **S52.1 Fracture of upper end of radius**

Fracture of proximal end of radius

EXCLUDES 2 *fracture of shaft of radius (S52.3-)*

physeal fractures of upper end of radius (S59.2-)

6th **S52.10 Unspecified fracture of upper end of radius**

7th **S52.101 Unspecified fracture of upper end of right radius** MCC CC HS

7th **S52.102 Unspecified fracture of upper end of left radius** MCC CC HS

7th **S52.109 Unspecified fracture of upper end of unspecified radius** MCC CC HS UNS

6th **S52.11 Torus fracture of upper end of radius**

The appropriate 7th character is to be added to all codes in subcategory S52.11

A initial encounter for closed fracture

D subsequent encounter for fracture with routine healing

G subsequent encounter for fracture with delayed healing

K subsequent encounter for fracture with nonunion

P subsequent encounter for fracture with malunion

S sequela

7th **S52.111 Torus fracture of upper end of right radius** CC HS

7th **S52.112 Torus fracture of upper end of left radius** CC HS

7th **S52.119 Torus fracture of upper end of unspecified radius** CC HS UNS

6th **S52.12 Fracture of head of radius**

7th **S52.121 Displaced fracture of head of right radius** MCC CC HS

7th **S52.122 Displaced fracture of head of left radius** MCC CC HS

7th **S52.123 Displaced fracture of head of unspecified radius** MCC CC HS UNS

7th **S52.124 Nondisplaced fracture of head of right radius** MCC CC HS

7th **S52.125 Nondisplaced fracture of head of left radius** MCC CC HS

7th **S52.126 Nondisplaced fracture of head of unspecified radius** MCC CC HS UNS

6th **S52.13 Fracture of neck of radius**

7th **S52.131 Displaced fracture of neck of right radius** MCC CC HS

7th **S52.132 Displaced fracture of neck of left radius** MCC CC HS

7th **S52.133 Displaced fracture of neck of unspecified radius** MCC CC HS UNS

7th **S52.134 Nondisplaced fracture of neck of right radius** MCC CC HS

7th **S52.135 Nondisplaced fracture of neck of left radius** MCC CC HS

7th **S52.136 Nondisplaced fracture of neck of unspecified radius** MCC CC HS UNS

6th **S52.18 Other fracture of upper end of radius**

7th **S52.181 Other fracture of upper end of right radius** MCC CC HS

7th **S52.182 Other fracture of upper end of left radius** MCC CC HS

7th **S52.189 Other fracture of upper end of unspecified radius** MCC CC HS UNS

5th **S52.2 Fracture of shaft of ulna**

6th **S52.20 Unspecified fracture of shaft of ulna**

Fracture of ulna NOS

7th **S52.201 Unspecified fracture of shaft of right ulna** MCC CC HS

7th **S52.202 Unspecified fracture of shaft of left ulna** MCC CC HS

7th **S52.209 Unspecified fracture of shaft of unspecified ulna** MCC CC HS UNS

6th **S52.21 Greenstick fracture of shaft of ulna**

The appropriate 7th character is to be added to all codes in subcategory S52.21

A initial encounter for closed fracture

D subsequent encounter for fracture with routine healing

G subsequent encounter for fracture with delayed healing

K subsequent encounter for fracture with nonunion

P subsequent encounter for fracture with malunion

S sequela

7th **S52.211 Greenstick fracture of shaft of right ulna** CC HS

7th **S52.212 Greenstick fracture of shaft of left ulna** CC HS

7th **S52.219 Greenstick fracture of shaft of unspecified ulna** CC HS UNS

6th **S52.22 Transverse fracture of shaft of ulna**

7th **S52.221 Displaced transverse fracture of shaft of right ulna** MCC CC HS

7th **S52.222 Displaced transverse fracture of shaft of left ulna** MCC CC HS

7th **S52.223 Displaced transverse fracture of shaft of unspecified ulna** MCC CC HS UNS

7th **S52.224 Nondisplaced transverse fracture of shaft of right ulna** MCC CC HS

7th **S52.225 Nondisplaced transverse fracture of shaft of left ulna** MCC CC HS

7th **S52.226 Nondisplaced transverse fracture of shaft of unspecified ulna** MCC CC HS UNS

6th **S52.23 Oblique fracture of shaft of ulna**

7th **S52.231 Displaced oblique fracture of shaft of right ulna** MCC CC HS

7th **S52.232 Displaced oblique fracture of shaft of left ulna** MCC CC HS

7th **S52.233 Displaced oblique fracture of shaft of unspecified ulna** MCC CC HS UNS

7th **S52.234 Nondisplaced oblique fracture of shaft of right ulna** MCC CC HS

7th **S52.235 Nondisplaced oblique fracture of shaft of left ulna** MCC CC HS

7th **S52.236 Nondisplaced oblique fracture of shaft of unspecified ulna** MCC CC HS UNS

6th **S52.24 Spiral fracture of shaft of ulna**

7th **S52.241 Displaced spiral fracture of shaft of ulna, right arm** MCC CC HS

7th **S52.242 Displaced spiral fracture of shaft of ulna, left arm** MCC CC HS

7th **S52.243 Displaced spiral fracture of shaft of ulna, unspecified arm** MCC CC HS UNS

7th **S52.244 Nondisplaced spiral fracture of shaft of ulna, right arm** MCC CC HS

7th **S52.245 Nondisplaced spiral fracture of shaft of ulna, left arm** MCC CC HS

7th **S52.246 Nondisplaced spiral fracture of shaft of ulna, unspecified arm** MCC CC HS UNS

6th **S52.25 Comminuted fracture of shaft of ulna**

7th **S52.251 Displaced comminuted fracture of shaft of ulna, right arm** MCC CC HS

7th **S52.252 Displaced comminuted fracture of shaft of ulna, left arm** MCC CC HS

7th **S52.253 Displaced comminuted fracture of shaft of ulna, unspecified arm** MCC CC HS UNS

7th **S52.254 Nondisplaced comminuted fracture of shaft of ulna, right arm** MCC CC HS

7th **S52.255 Nondisplaced comminuted fracture of shaft of ulna, left arm** MCC CC HS

7th **S52.256 Nondisplaced comminuted fracture of shaft of ulna, unspecified arm** MCC CC HS UNS

6th **S52.26 Segmental fracture of shaft of ulna**

7th **S52.261 Displaced segmental fracture of shaft of ulna, right arm** MCC CC HS

7th **S52.262 Displaced segmental fracture of shaft of ulna, left arm** MCC CC HS

S52.263 Displaced segmental fracture of shaft of ulna, unspecified arm MCC CC H5 UNS
S52.264 Nondisplaced segmental fracture of shaft of ulna, right arm MCC CC H5
S52.265 Nondisplaced segmental fracture of shaft of ulna, left arm MCC CC H5
S52.266 Nondisplaced segmental fracture of shaft of ulna, unspecified arm MCC CC H5 UNS

S52.27 Monteggia's fracture of ulna
Fracture of upper shaft of ulna with dislocation of radial head
S52.271 Monteggia's fracture of right ulna MCC CC H5
S52.272 Monteggia's fracture of left ulna MCC CC H5
S52.279 Monteggia's fracture of unspecified ulna MCC CC H5 UNS

S52.28 Bent bone of ulna
S52.281 Bent bone of right ulna MCC CC H5
S52.282 Bent bone of left ulna MCC CC H5
S52.283 Bent bone of unspecified ulna MCC CC H5 UNS

S52.29 Other fracture of shaft of ulna
S52.291 Other fracture of shaft of right ulna MCC CC H5
S52.292 Other fracture of shaft of left ulna MCC CC H5
S52.299 Other fracture of shaft of unspecified ulna MCC CC H5 UNS

S52.3 Fracture of shaft of radius

S52.30 Unspecified fracture of shaft of radius
S52.301 Unspecified fracture of shaft of right radius MCC CC H5
S52.302 Unspecified fracture of shaft of left radius MCC CC H5
S52.309 Unspecified fracture of shaft of unspecified radius MCC CC H5 UNS

S52.31 Greenstick fracture of shaft of radius

The appropriate 7th character is to be added to all codes in subcategory S52.31.
- A initial encounter for closed fracture
- D subsequent encounter for fracture with routine healing
- G subsequent encounter for fracture with delayed healing
- K subsequent encounter for fracture with nonunion
- P subsequent encounter for fracture with malunion
- S sequela

S52.311 Greenstick fracture of shaft of radius, right arm CC H5
S52.312 Greenstick fracture of shaft of radius, left arm CC H5
S52.319 Greenstick fracture of shaft of radius, unspecified arm CC H5 UNS

S52.32 Transverse fracture of shaft of radius
S52.321 Displaced transverse fracture of shaft of right radius MCC CC H5
S52.322 Displaced transverse fracture of shaft of left radius MCC CC H5
S52.323 Displaced transverse fracture of shaft of unspecified radius MCC CC H5 UNS
S52.324 Nondisplaced transverse fracture of shaft of right radius MCC CC H5
S52.325 Nondisplaced transverse fracture of shaft of left radius MCC CC H5
S52.326 Nondisplaced transverse fracture of shaft of unspecified radius MCC CC H5 UNS

S52.33 Oblique fracture of shaft of radius
S52.331 Displaced oblique fracture of shaft of right radius MCC CC H5
S52.332 Displaced oblique fracture of shaft of left radius MCC CC H5
S52.333 Displaced oblique fracture of shaft of unspecified radius MCC CC H5 UNS
S52.334 Nondisplaced oblique fracture of shaft of right radius MCC CC H5
S52.335 Nondisplaced oblique fracture of shaft of left radius MCC CC H5
S52.336 Nondisplaced oblique fracture of shaft of unspecified radius MCC CC H5 UNS

S52.34 Spiral fracture of shaft of radius
S52.341 Displaced spiral fracture of shaft of radius, right arm MCC CC H5
S52.342 Displaced spiral fracture of shaft of radius, left arm MCC CC H5
S52.343 Displaced spiral fracture of shaft of radius, unspecified arm MCC CC H5 UNS
S52.344 Nondisplaced spiral fracture of shaft of radius, right arm MCC CC H5
S52.345 Nondisplaced spiral fracture of shaft of radius, left arm MCC CC H5
S52.346 Nondisplaced spiral fracture of shaft of radius, unspecified arm MCC CC H5 UNS

S52.35 Comminuted fracture of shaft of radius
S52.351 Displaced comminuted fracture of shaft of radius, right arm MCC CC H5
S52.352 Displaced comminuted fracture of shaft of radius, left arm MCC CC H5
S52.353 Displaced comminuted fracture of shaft of radius, unspecified arm MCC CC H5 UNS
S52.354 Nondisplaced comminuted fracture of shaft of radius, right arm MCC CC H5
S52.355 Nondisplaced comminuted fracture of shaft of radius, left arm MCC CC H5
S52.356 Nondisplaced comminuted fracture of shaft of radius, unspecified arm MCC CC H5 UNS

S52.36 Segmental fracture of shaft of radius
S52.361 Displaced segmental fracture of shaft of radius, right arm MCC CC H5
S52.362 Displaced segmental fracture of shaft of radius, left arm MCC CC H5
S52.363 Displaced segmental fracture of shaft of radius, unspecified arm MCC CC H5 UNS
S52.364 Nondisplaced segmental fracture of shaft of radius, right arm MCC CC H5
S52.365 Nondisplaced segmental fracture of shaft of radius, left arm MCC CC H5
S52.366 Nondisplaced segmental fracture of shaft of radius, unspecified arm MCC CC H5 UNS

S52.37 Galeazzi's fracture
Fracture of lower shaft of radius with radioulnar joint dislocation
S52.371 Galeazzi's fracture of right radius MCC CC H5
S52.372 Galeazzi's fracture of left radius MCC CC H5
S52.379 Galeazzi's fracture of unspecified radius MCC CC H5 UNS

S52.38 Bent bone of radius
S52.381 Bent bone of right radius MCC CC H5
S52.382 Bent bone of left radius MCC CC H5
S52.389 Bent bone of unspecified radius MCC CC H5 UNS

S52.39 Other fracture of shaft of radius
S52.391 Other fracture of shaft of radius, right arm MCC CC H5
S52.392 Other fracture of shaft of radius, left arm MCC CC H5
S52.399 Other fracture of shaft of radius, unspecified arm MCC CC H5 UNS

S52.5 Fracture of lower end of radius
Fracture of distal end of radius
EXCLUDES 2 *physeal fractures of lower end of radius (S59.2-)*
DEF: Fracture of the distal end of the radius above the wrist, most commonly caused by a fall onto an outstretched hand.

S52.50 Unspecified fracture of the lower end of radius
S52.501 Unspecified fracture of the lower end of right radius MCC CC H5

√7th S52.502 Unspecified fracture of the lower end of left radius MCC CC H5

√7th S52.509 Unspecified fracture of the lower end of unspecified radius MCC CC H5 UNS

√6th S52.51 Fracture of radial styloid process

√7th S52.511 Displaced fracture of right radial styloid process MCC CC H5

√7th S52.512 Displaced fracture of left radial styloid process MCC CC H5

√7th S52.513 Displaced fracture of unspecified radial styloid process MCC CC H5 UNS

√7th S52.514 Nondisplaced fracture of right radial styloid process MCC CC H5

√7th S52.515 Nondisplaced fracture of left radial styloid process MCC CC H5

√7th S52.516 Nondisplaced fracture of unspecified radial styloid process MCC CC H5 UNS

√6th S52.52 Torus fracture of lower end of radius

The appropriate 7th character is to be added to all codes in subcategory S52.52.
A initial encounter for closed fracture
D subsequent encounter for fracture with routine healing
G subsequent encounter for fracture with delayed healing
K subsequent encounter for fracture with nonunion
P subsequent encounter for fracture with malunion
S sequela

√7th S52.521 Torus fracture of lower end of right radius CC H5

√7th S52.522 Torus fracture of lower end of left radius CC H5

√7th S52.529 Torus fracture of lower end of unspecified radius CC H5 UNS

√6th S52.53 Colles' fracture

AHA: 2016,2Q,4

DEF: Fracture of the radius at the wrist in which the distal fragment is pushed posteriorly. The dorsal angulation of the fragment results in the wrist cocking up.

√7th S52.531 Colles' fracture of right radius MCC CC H5

√7th S52.532 Colles' fracture of left radius MCC CC H5

√7th S52.539 Colles' fracture of unspecified radius MCC CC H5 UNS

√6th S52.54 Smith's fracture

√7th S52.541 Smith's fracture of right radius MCC CC H5

√7th S52.542 Smith's fracture of left radius MCC CC H5

√7th S52.549 Smith's fracture of unspecified radius MCC CC H5 UNS

√6th S52.55 Other extraarticular fracture of lower end of radius

√7th S52.551 Other extraarticular fracture of lower end of right radius MCC CC H5

√7th S52.552 Other extraarticular fracture of lower end of left radius MCC CC H5

√7th S52.559 Other extraarticular fracture of lower end of unspecified radius MCC CC H5 UNS

√6th S52.56 Barton's fracture

√7th S52.561 Barton's fracture of right radius MCC CC H5

√7th S52.562 Barton's fracture of left radius MCC CC H5

√7th S52.569 Barton's fracture of unspecified radius MCC CC H5 UNS

√6th S52.57 Other intraarticular fracture of lower end of radius

√7th S52.571 Other intraarticular fracture of lower end of right radius MCC CC H5

√7th S52.572 Other intraarticular fracture of lower end of left radius MCC CC H5

√7th S52.579 Other intraarticular fracture of lower end of unspecified radius MCC CC H5 UNS

√6th S52.59 Other fractures of lower end of radius

AHA: 2019,3Q,9

√7th S52.591 Other fractures of lower end of right radius MCC CC H5

√7th S52.592 Other fractures of lower end of left radius MCC CC H5

√7th S52.599 Other fractures of lower end of unspecified radius MCC CC H5 UNS

√5th S52.6 Fracture of lower end of ulna

√6th S52.60 Unspecified fracture of lower end of ulna

√7th S52.601 Unspecified fracture of lower end of right ulna MCC CC H5

√7th S52.602 Unspecified fracture of lower end of left ulna MCC CC H5

√7th S52.609 Unspecified fracture of lower end of unspecified ulna MCC CC H5 UNS

√6th S52.61 Fracture of ulna styloid process

√7th S52.611 Displaced fracture of right ulna styloid process MCC CC H5

√7th S52.612 Displaced fracture of left ulna styloid process MCC CC H5

√7th S52.613 Displaced fracture of unspecified ulna styloid process MCC CC H5 UNS

√7th S52.614 Nondisplaced fracture of right ulna styloid process MCC CC H5

√7th S52.615 Nondisplaced fracture of left ulna styloid process MCC CC H5

√7th S52.616 Nondisplaced fracture of unspecified ulna styloid process MCC CC H5 UNS

√6th S52.62 Torus fracture of lower end of ulna

The appropriate 7th character is to be added to all codes in subcategory S52.62.
A initial encounter for closed fracture
D subsequent encounter for fracture with routine healing
G subsequent encounter for fracture with delayed healing
K subsequent encounter for fracture with nonunion
P subsequent encounter for fracture with malunion
S sequela

√7th S52.621 Torus fracture of lower end of right ulna CC H5

√7th S52.622 Torus fracture of lower end of left ulna CC H5

√7th S52.629 Torus fracture of lower end of unspecified ulna CC H5 UNS

√6th S52.69 Other fracture of lower end of ulna

AHA: 2019,3Q,9

√7th S52.691 Other fracture of lower end of right ulna MCC CC H5

√7th S52.692 Other fracture of lower end of left ulna MCC CC H5

√7th S52.699 Other fracture of lower end of unspecified ulna MCC CC H5 UNS

√5th S52.9 Unspecified fracture of forearm

√x7th S52.90 Unspecified fracture of unspecified forearm MCC CC H5 UNS

√x7th S52.91 Unspecified fracture of right forearm MCC CC H5

√x7th S52.92 Unspecified fracture of left forearm MCC CC H5

S53 Dislocation and sprain of joints and ligaments of elbow

INCLUDES avulsion of joint or ligament of elbow
laceration of cartilage, joint or ligament of elbow
sprain of cartilage, joint or ligament of elbow
traumatic hemarthrosis of joint or ligament of elbow
traumatic rupture of joint or ligament of elbow
traumatic subluxation of joint or ligament of elbow
traumatic tear of joint or ligament of elbow

Code also any associated open wound

EXCLUDES 2 *strain of muscle, fascia and tendon at forearm level (S56.-)*

The appropriate 7th character is to be added to each code from category S53.
A initial encounter
D subsequent encounter
S sequela

S53.0 Subluxation and dislocation of radial head
Dislocation of radiohumeral joint
Subluxation of radiohumeral joint
EXCLUDES 1 *Monteggia's fracture-dislocation (S52.27-)*

S53.00 Unspecified subluxation and dislocation of radial head
- **S53.001 Unspecified subluxation of right radial head**
- **S53.002 Unspecified subluxation of left radial head**
- **S53.003 Unspecified subluxation of unspecified radial head**
- **S53.004 Unspecified dislocation of right radial head**
- **S53.005 Unspecified dislocation of left radial head**
- **S53.006 Unspecified dislocation of unspecified radial head**

S53.01 Anterior subluxation and dislocation of radial head
Anteriomedial subluxation and dislocation of radial head
- **S53.011 Anterior subluxation of right radial head**
- **S53.012 Anterior subluxation of left radial head**
- **S53.013 Anterior subluxation of unspecified radial head**
- **S53.014 Anterior dislocation of right radial head**
- **S53.015 Anterior dislocation of left radial head**
- **S53.016 Anterior dislocation of unspecified radial head**

S53.02 Posterior subluxation and dislocation of radial head
Posteriolateral subluxation and dislocation of radial head
- **S53.021 Posterior subluxation of right radial head**
- **S53.022 Posterior subluxation of left radial head**
- **S53.023 Posterior subluxation of unspecified radial head**
- **S53.024 Posterior dislocation of right radial head**
- **S53.025 Posterior dislocation of left radial head**
- **S53.026 Posterior dislocation of unspecified radial head**

S53.03 Nursemaid's elbow
- **S53.031 Nursemaid's elbow, right elbow**
- **S53.032 Nursemaid's elbow, left elbow**
- **S53.033 Nursemaid's elbow, unspecified elbow**

S53.09 Other subluxation and dislocation of radial head
- **S53.091 Other subluxation of right radial head**
- **S53.092 Other subluxation of left radial head**
- **S53.093 Other subluxation of unspecified radial head**
- **S53.094 Other dislocation of right radial head**
- **S53.095 Other dislocation of left radial head**
- **S53.096 Other dislocation of unspecified radial head**

S53.1 Subluxation and dislocation of ulnohumeral joint
Subluxation and dislocation of elbow NOS
EXCLUDES 1 *dislocation of radial head alone (S53.0-)*

S53.10 Unspecified subluxation and dislocation of ulnohumeral joint
- **S53.101 Unspecified subluxation of right ulnohumeral joint**
- **S53.102 Unspecified subluxation of left ulnohumeral joint**
- **S53.103 Unspecified subluxation of unspecified ulnohumeral joint**
- **S53.104 Unspecified dislocation of right ulnohumeral joint**
- **S53.105 Unspecified dislocation of left ulnohumeral joint**
- **S53.106 Unspecified dislocation of unspecified ulnohumeral joint**

S53.11 Anterior subluxation and dislocation of ulnohumeral joint
- **S53.111 Anterior subluxation of right ulnohumeral joint**
- **S53.112 Anterior subluxation of left ulnohumeral joint**
- **S53.113 Anterior subluxation of unspecified ulnohumeral joint**
- **S53.114 Anterior dislocation of right ulnohumeral joint**
  AHA: 2012,4Q,108
- **S53.115 Anterior dislocation of left ulnohumeral joint**
- **S53.116 Anterior dislocation of unspecified ulnohumeral joint**

S53.12 Posterior subluxation and dislocation of ulnohumeral joint
- **S53.121 Posterior subluxation of right ulnohumeral joint**
- **S53.122 Posterior subluxation of left ulnohumeral joint**
- **S53.123 Posterior subluxation of unspecified ulnohumeral joint**
- **S53.124 Posterior dislocation of right ulnohumeral joint**
- **S53.125 Posterior dislocation of left ulnohumeral joint**
- **S53.126 Posterior dislocation of unspecified ulnohumeral joint**

S53.13 Medial subluxation and dislocation of ulnohumeral joint
- **S53.131 Medial subluxation of right ulnohumeral joint**
- **S53.132 Medial subluxation of left ulnohumeral joint**
- **S53.133 Medial subluxation of unspecified ulnohumeral joint**
- **S53.134 Medial dislocation of right ulnohumeral joint**
- **S53.135 Medial dislocation of left ulnohumeral joint**
- **S53.136 Medial dislocation of unspecified ulnohumeral joint**

S53.14 Lateral subluxation and dislocation of ulnohumeral joint
- **S53.141 Lateral subluxation of right ulnohumeral joint**
- **S53.142 Lateral subluxation of left ulnohumeral joint**
- **S53.143 Lateral subluxation of unspecified ulnohumeral joint**
- **S53.144 Lateral dislocation of right ulnohumeral joint**
- **S53.145 Lateral dislocation of left ulnohumeral joint**
- **S53.146 Lateral dislocation of unspecified ulnohumeral joint**

S53.19 Other subluxation and dislocation of ulnohumeral joint
- **S53.191 Other subluxation of right ulnohumeral joint**
- **S53.192 Other subluxation of left ulnohumeral joint**
- **S53.193 Other subluxation of unspecified ulnohumeral joint**
- **S53.194 Other dislocation of right ulnohumeral joint**
- **S53.195 Other dislocation of left ulnohumeral joint**
- **S53.196 Other dislocation of unspecified ulnohumeral joint**

S53.2 Traumatic rupture of radial collateral ligament
EXCLUDES 1 *sprain of radial collateral ligament NOS (S53.43-)*

- **S53.20 Traumatic rupture of unspecified radial collateral ligament**

Chapter 19. Injury, Poisoning and Certain Other Consequences of External Causes

√x7th **S53.21 Traumatic rupture of right radial collateral ligament**

√x7th **S53.22 Traumatic rupture of left radial collateral ligament**

√5th **S53.3 Traumatic rupture of ulnar collateral ligament**

EXCLUDES 1 *sprain of ulnar collateral ligament (S53.44-)*

√x7th **S53.30 Traumatic rupture of unspecified ulnar collateral ligament**

√x7th **S53.31 Traumatic rupture of right ulnar collateral ligament**

√x7th **S53.32 Traumatic rupture of left ulnar collateral ligament**

√5th **S53.4 Sprain of elbow**

EXCLUDES 2 *traumatic rupture of radial collateral ligament (S53.2-)*
traumatic rupture of ulnar collateral ligament (S53.3-)

√6th **S53.40 Unspecified sprain of elbow**

√7th **S53.401 Unspecified sprain of right elbow**

√7th **S53.402 Unspecified sprain of left elbow**

√7th **S53.409 Unspecified sprain of unspecified elbow**
Sprain of elbow NOS

√6th **S53.41 Radiohumeral (joint) sprain**

√7th **S53.411 Radiohumeral (joint) sprain of right elbow**

√7th **S53.412 Radiohumeral (joint) sprain of left elbow**

√7th **S53.419 Radiohumeral (joint) sprain of unspecified elbow**

√6th **S53.42 Ulnohumeral (joint) sprain**

√7th **S53.421 Ulnohumeral (joint) sprain of right elbow**

√7th **S53.422 Ulnohumeral (joint) sprain of left elbow**

√7th **S53.429 Ulnohumeral (joint) sprain of unspecified elbow**

√6th **S53.43 Radial collateral ligament sprain**

√7th **S53.431 Radial collateral ligament sprain of right elbow**

√7th **S53.432 Radial collateral ligament sprain of left elbow**

√7th **S53.439 Radial collateral ligament sprain of unspecified elbow**

√6th **S53.44 Ulnar collateral ligament sprain**

√7th **S53.441 Ulnar collateral ligament sprain of right elbow**

√7th **S53.442 Ulnar collateral ligament sprain of left elbow**

√7th **S53.449 Ulnar collateral ligament sprain of unspecified elbow**

√6th **S53.49 Other sprain of elbow**

√7th **S53.491 Other sprain of right elbow**

√7th **S53.492 Other sprain of left elbow**

√7th **S53.499 Other sprain of unspecified elbow**

√4th **S54 Injury of nerves at forearm level**

Code also any associated open wound (S51.-)

EXCLUDES 2 *injury of nerves at wrist and hand level (S64.-)*

The appropriate 7th character is to be added to each code from category S54.
A initial encounter
D subsequent encounter
S sequela

√5th **S54.0 Injury of ulnar nerve at forearm level**
Injury of ulnar nerve NOS

√x7th **S54.00 Injury of ulnar nerve at forearm level, unspecified arm**

√x7th **S54.01 Injury of ulnar nerve at forearm level, right arm**

√x7th **S54.02 Injury of ulnar nerve at forearm level, left arm**

√5th **S54.1 Injury of median nerve at forearm level**
Injury of median nerve NOS

√x7th **S54.10 Injury of median nerve at forearm level, unspecified arm**

√x7th **S54.11 Injury of median nerve at forearm level, right arm**

√x7th **S54.12 Injury of median nerve at forearm level, left arm**

√5th **S54.2 Injury of radial nerve at forearm level**
Injury of radial nerve NOS

√x7th **S54.20 Injury of radial nerve at forearm level, unspecified arm**

√x7th **S54.21 Injury of radial nerve at forearm level, right arm**

√x7th **S54.22 Injury of radial nerve at forearm level, left arm**

√5th **S54.3 Injury of cutaneous sensory nerve at forearm level**

√x7th **S54.30 Injury of cutaneous sensory nerve at forearm level, unspecified arm**

√x7th **S54.31 Injury of cutaneous sensory nerve at forearm level, right arm**

√x7th **S54.32 Injury of cutaneous sensory nerve at forearm level, left arm**

√5th **S54.8 Injury of other nerves at forearm level**

√6th **S54.8X Injury of other nerves at forearm level**

√7th **S54.8X1 Injury of other nerves at forearm level, right arm**

√7th **S54.8X2 Injury of other nerves at forearm level, left arm**

√7th **S54.8X9 Injury of other nerves at forearm level, unspecified arm**

√5th **S54.9 Injury of unspecified nerve at forearm level**

√x7th **S54.90 Injury of unspecified nerve at forearm level, unspecified arm**

√x7th **S54.91 Injury of unspecified nerve at forearm level, right arm**

√x7th **S54.92 Injury of unspecified nerve at forearm level, left arm**

√4th **S55 Injury of blood vessels at forearm level**

Code also any associated open wound (S51.-)

EXCLUDES 2 *injury of blood vessels at wrist and hand level (S65.-)*
injury of brachial vessels (S45.1-S45.2)

The appropriate 7th character is to be added to each code from category S55.
A initial encounter
D subsequent encounter
S sequela

√5th **S55.0 Injury of ulnar artery at forearm level**

√6th **S55.00 Unspecified injury of ulnar artery at forearm level**

√7th **S55.001 Unspecified injury of ulnar artery at forearm level, right arm** CC

√7th **S55.002 Unspecified injury of ulnar artery at forearm level, left arm** CC

√7th **S55.009 Unspecified injury of ulnar artery at forearm level, unspecified arm** CC UNS

√6th **S55.01 Laceration of ulnar artery at forearm level**

√7th **S55.011 Laceration of ulnar artery at forearm level, right arm** CC

√7th **S55.012 Laceration of ulnar artery at forearm level, left arm** CC

√7th **S55.019 Laceration of ulnar artery at forearm level, unspecified arm** CC UNS

√6th **S55.09 Other specified injury of ulnar artery at forearm level**

√7th **S55.091 Other specified injury of ulnar artery at forearm level, right arm** CC

√7th **S55.092 Other specified injury of ulnar artery at forearm level, left arm** CC

√7th **S55.099 Other specified injury of ulnar artery at forearm level, unspecified arm** CC UNS

√5th **S55.1 Injury of radial artery at forearm level**

√6th **S55.10 Unspecified injury of radial artery at forearm level**

√7th **S55.101 Unspecified injury of radial artery at forearm level, right arm** CC

√7th **S55.102 Unspecified injury of radial artery at forearm level, left arm** CC

√7th **S55.109 Unspecified injury of radial artery at forearm level, unspecified arm** CC UNS

√6th **S55.11 Laceration of radial artery at forearm level**

√7th **S55.111 Laceration of radial artery at forearm level, right arm** CC

√7th **S55.112 Laceration of radial artery at forearm level, left arm** CC

√7th **S55.119 Laceration of radial artery at forearm level, unspecified arm** CC UNS

√6th **S55.19 Other specified injury of radial artery at forearm level**

√7th **S55.191 Other specified injury of radial artery at forearm level, right arm** CC

√7th **S55.192 Other specified injury of radial artery at forearm level, left arm** CC

√7th **S55.199 Other specified injury of radial artery at forearm level, unspecified arm** CC UNS

√5th S55.2 Injury of vein at forearm level
√6th S55.20 Unspecified injury of vein at forearm level
√7th S55.201 Unspecified injury of vein at forearm level, right arm CC
√7th S55.202 Unspecified injury of vein at forearm level, left arm CC
√7th S55.209 Unspecified injury of vein at forearm level, unspecified arm CC UNS
√6th S55.21 Laceration of vein at forearm level
√7th S55.211 Laceration of vein at forearm level, right arm CC
√7th S55.212 Laceration of vein at forearm level, left arm CC
√7th S55.219 Laceration of vein at forearm level, unspecified arm CC UNS
√6th S55.29 Other specified injury of vein at forearm level
√7th S55.291 Other specified injury of vein at forearm level, right arm CC
√7th S55.292 Other specified injury of vein at forearm level, left arm CC
√7th S55.299 Other specified injury of vein at forearm level, unspecified arm CC UNS
√5th S55.8 Injury of other blood vessels at forearm level
√6th S55.80 Unspecified injury of other blood vessels at forearm level
√7th S55.801 Unspecified injury of other blood vessels at forearm level, right arm CC
√7th S55.802 Unspecified injury of other blood vessels at forearm level, left arm CC
√7th S55.809 Unspecified injury of other blood vessels at forearm level, unspecified arm CC UNS
√6th S55.81 Laceration of other blood vessels at forearm level
√7th S55.811 Laceration of other blood vessels at forearm level, right arm CC
√7th S55.812 Laceration of other blood vessels at forearm level, left arm CC
√7th S55.819 Laceration of other blood vessels at forearm level, unspecified arm CC UNS
√6th S55.89 Other specified injury of other blood vessels at forearm level
√7th S55.891 Other specified injury of other blood vessels at forearm level, right arm CC
√7th S55.892 Other specified injury of other blood vessels at forearm level, left arm CC
√7th S55.899 Other specified injury of other blood vessels at forearm level, unspecified arm CC UNS
√5th S55.9 Injury of unspecified blood vessel at forearm level
√6th S55.90 Unspecified injury of unspecified blood vessel at forearm level
√7th S55.901 Unspecified injury of unspecified blood vessel at forearm level, right arm CC
√7th S55.902 Unspecified injury of unspecified blood vessel at forearm level, left arm CC
√7th S55.909 Unspecified injury of unspecified blood vessel at forearm level, unspecified arm CC UNS
√6th S55.91 Laceration of unspecified blood vessel at forearm level
√7th S55.911 Laceration of unspecified blood vessel at forearm level, right arm CC
√7th S55.912 Laceration of unspecified blood vessel at forearm level, left arm CC
√7th S55.919 Laceration of unspecified blood vessel at forearm level, unspecified arm CC UNS
√6th S55.99 Other specified injury of unspecified blood vessel at forearm level
√7th S55.991 Other specified injury of unspecified blood vessel at forearm level, right arm CC
√7th S55.992 Other specified injury of unspecified blood vessel at forearm level, left arm CC
√7th S55.999 Other specified injury of unspecified blood vessel at forearm level, unspecified arm CC UNS

√4th **S56 Injury of muscle, fascia and tendon at forearm level**
Code also any associated open wound (S51.-)
EXCLUDES 2 *injury of muscle, fascia and tendon at or below wrist (S66.-)*
sprain of joints and ligaments of elbow (S53.4-)
TIP: Refer to the Muscle/Tendon table at the beginning of this chapter

The appropriate 7th character is to be added to each code from category S56.
A initial encounter
D subsequent encounter
S sequela

√5th S56.0 Injury of flexor muscle, fascia and tendon of thumb at forearm level
√6th S56.00 Unspecified injury of flexor muscle, fascia and tendon of thumb at forearm level
√7th S56.001 Unspecified injury of flexor muscle, fascia and tendon of right thumb at forearm level
√7th S56.002 Unspecified injury of flexor muscle, fascia and tendon of left thumb at forearm level
√7th S56.009 Unspecified injury of flexor muscle, fascia and tendon of unspecified thumb at forearm level
√6th S56.01 Strain of flexor muscle, fascia and tendon of thumb at forearm level
√7th S56.011 Strain of flexor muscle, fascia and tendon of right thumb at forearm level
√7th S56.012 Strain of flexor muscle, fascia and tendon of left thumb at forearm level
√7th S56.019 Strain of flexor muscle, fascia and tendon of unspecified thumb at forearm level
√6th S56.02 Laceration of flexor muscle, fascia and tendon of thumb at forearm level
√7th S56.021 Laceration of flexor muscle, fascia and tendon of right thumb at forearm level CC
√7th S56.022 Laceration of flexor muscle, fascia and tendon of left thumb at forearm level CC
√7th S56.029 Laceration of flexor muscle, fascia and tendon of unspecified thumb at forearm level CC
√6th S56.09 Other injury of flexor muscle, fascia and tendon of thumb at forearm level
√7th S56.091 Other injury of flexor muscle, fascia and tendon of right thumb at forearm level
√7th S56.092 Other injury of flexor muscle, fascia and tendon of left thumb at forearm level
√7th S56.099 Other injury of flexor muscle, fascia and tendon of unspecified thumb at forearm level
√5th S56.1 Injury of flexor muscle, fascia and tendon of other and unspecified finger at forearm level
√6th S56.10 Unspecified injury of flexor muscle, fascia and tendon of other and unspecified finger at forearm level
√7th S56.101 Unspecified injury of flexor muscle, fascia and tendon of right index finger at forearm level
√7th S56.102 Unspecified injury of flexor muscle, fascia and tendon of left index finger at forearm level
√7th S56.103 Unspecified injury of flexor muscle, fascia and tendon of right middle finger at forearm level
√7th S56.104 Unspecified injury of flexor muscle, fascia and tendon of left middle finger at forearm level
√7th S56.105 Unspecified injury of flexor muscle, fascia and tendon of right ring finger at forearm level
√7th S56.106 Unspecified injury of flexor muscle, fascia and tendon of left ring finger at forearm level
√7th S56.107 Unspecified injury of flexor muscle, fascia and tendon of right little finger at forearm level
√7th S56.108 Unspecified injury of flexor muscle, fascia and tendon of left little finger at forearm level
√7th S56.109 Unspecified injury of flexor muscle, fascia and tendon of unspecified finger at forearm level

Chapter 19. Injury, Poisoning and Certain Other Consequences of External Causes
S55.2–S56.109

✓6th **S56.11** Strain of flexor muscle, fascia and tendon of other and unspecified finger at forearm level

✓7th **S56.111** Strain of flexor muscle, fascia and tendon of right index finger at forearm level

✓7th **S56.112** Strain of flexor muscle, fascia and tendon of left index finger at forearm level

✓7th **S56.113** Strain of flexor muscle, fascia and tendon of right middle finger at forearm level

✓7th **S56.114** Strain of flexor muscle, fascia and tendon of left middle finger at forearm level

✓7th **S56.115** Strain of flexor muscle, fascia and tendon of right ring finger at forearm level

✓7th **S56.116** Strain of flexor muscle, fascia and tendon of left ring finger at forearm level

✓7th **S56.117** Strain of flexor muscle, fascia and tendon of right little finger at forearm level

✓7th **S56.118** Strain of flexor muscle, fascia and tendon of left little finger at forearm level

✓7th **S56.119** Strain of flexor muscle, fascia and tendon of finger of unspecified finger at forearm level

✓6th **S56.12** Laceration of flexor muscle, fascia and tendon of other and unspecified finger at forearm level

✓7th **S56.121** Laceration of flexor muscle, fascia and tendon of right index finger at forearm level CC

✓7th **S56.122** Laceration of flexor muscle, fascia and tendon of left index finger at forearm level CC

✓7th **S56.123** Laceration of flexor muscle, fascia and tendon of right middle finger at forearm level CC

✓7th **S56.124** Laceration of flexor muscle, fascia and tendon of left middle finger at forearm level CC

✓7th **S56.125** Laceration of flexor muscle, fascia and tendon of right ring finger at forearm level CC

✓7th **S56.126** Laceration of flexor muscle, fascia and tendon of left ring finger at forearm level CC

✓7th **S56.127** Laceration of flexor muscle, fascia and tendon of right little finger at forearm level CC

✓7th **S56.128** Laceration of flexor muscle, fascia and tendon of left little finger at forearm level CC

✓7th **S56.129** Laceration of flexor muscle, fascia and tendon of unspecified finger at forearm level CC UNS

✓6th **S56.19** Other injury of flexor muscle, fascia and tendon of other and unspecified finger at forearm level

✓7th **S56.191** Other injury of flexor muscle, fascia and tendon of right index finger at forearm level

✓7th **S56.192** Other injury of flexor muscle, fascia and tendon of left index finger at forearm level

✓7th **S56.193** Other injury of flexor muscle, fascia and tendon of right middle finger at forearm level

✓7th **S56.194** Other injury of flexor muscle, fascia and tendon of left middle finger at forearm level

✓7th **S56.195** Other injury of flexor muscle, fascia and tendon of right ring finger at forearm level

✓7th **S56.196** Other injury of flexor muscle, fascia and tendon of left ring finger at forearm level

✓7th **S56.197** Other injury of flexor muscle, fascia and tendon of right little finger at forearm level

✓7th **S56.198** Other injury of flexor muscle, fascia and tendon of left little finger at forearm level

✓7th **S56.199** Other injury of flexor muscle, fascia and tendon of unspecified finger at forearm level

✓5th **S56.2** Injury of other flexor muscle, fascia and tendon at forearm level

✓6th **S56.20** Unspecified injury of other flexor muscle, fascia and tendon at forearm level

✓7th **S56.201** Unspecified injury of other flexor muscle, fascia and tendon at forearm level, right arm

✓7th **S56.202** Unspecified injury of other flexor muscle, fascia and tendon at forearm level, left arm

✓7th **S56.209** Unspecified injury of other flexor muscle, fascia and tendon at forearm level, unspecified arm

✓6th **S56.21** Strain of other flexor muscle, fascia and tendon at forearm level

✓7th **S56.211** Strain of other flexor muscle, fascia and tendon at forearm level, right arm

✓7th **S56.212** Strain of other flexor muscle, fascia and tendon at forearm level, left arm

✓7th **S56.219** Strain of other flexor muscle, fascia and tendon at forearm level, unspecified arm

✓6th **S56.22** Laceration of other flexor muscle, fascia and tendon at forearm level

✓7th **S56.221** Laceration of other flexor muscle, fascia and tendon at forearm level, right arm CC

✓7th **S56.222** Laceration of other flexor muscle, fascia and tendon at forearm level, left arm CC

✓7th **S56.229** Laceration of other flexor muscle, fascia and tendon at forearm level, unspecified arm CC UNS

✓6th **S56.29** Other injury of other flexor muscle, fascia and tendon at forearm level

✓7th **S56.291** Other injury of other flexor muscle, fascia and tendon at forearm level, right arm

✓7th **S56.292** Other injury of other flexor muscle, fascia and tendon at forearm level, left arm

✓7th **S56.299** Other injury of other flexor muscle, fascia and tendon at forearm level, unspecified arm

✓5th **S56.3** Injury of extensor or abductor muscles, fascia and tendons of thumb at forearm level

✓6th **S56.30** Unspecified injury of extensor or abductor muscles, fascia and tendons of thumb at forearm level

✓7th **S56.301** Unspecified injury of extensor or abductor muscles, fascia and tendons of right thumb at forearm level

✓7th **S56.302** Unspecified injury of extensor or abductor muscles, fascia and tendons of left thumb at forearm level

✓7th **S56.309** Unspecified injury of extensor or abductor muscles, fascia and tendons of unspecified thumb at forearm level

✓6th **S56.31** Strain of extensor or abductor muscles, fascia and tendons of thumb at forearm level

✓7th **S56.311** Strain of extensor or abductor muscles, fascia and tendons of right thumb at forearm level

✓7th **S56.312** Strain of extensor or abductor muscles, fascia and tendons of left thumb at forearm level

✓7th **S56.319** Strain of extensor or abductor muscles, fascia and tendons of unspecified thumb at forearm level

✓6th **S56.32** Laceration of extensor or abductor muscles, fascia and tendons of thumb at forearm level

✓7th **S56.321** Laceration of extensor or abductor muscles, fascia and tendons of right thumb at forearm level CC

✓7th **S56.322** Laceration of extensor or abductor muscles, fascia and tendons of left thumb at forearm level CC

✓7th **S56.329** Laceration of extensor or abductor muscles, fascia and tendons of unspecified thumb at forearm level CC

✓6th **S56.39** Other injury of extensor or abductor muscles, fascia and tendons of thumb at forearm level

✓7th **S56.391** Other injury of extensor or abductor muscles, fascia and tendons of right thumb at forearm level

✓7th **S56.392** Other injury of extensor or abductor muscles, fascia and tendons of left thumb at forearm level

✓7th **S56.399** Other injury of extensor or abductor muscles, fascia and tendons of unspecified thumb at forearm level

√5th S56.4 Injury of extensor muscle, fascia and tendon of other and unspecified finger at forearm level

√6th S56.40 Unspecified injury of extensor muscle, fascia and tendon of other and unspecified finger at forearm level

√7th S56.401 Unspecified injury of extensor muscle, fascia and tendon of right index finger at forearm level

√7th S56.402 Unspecified injury of extensor muscle, fascia and tendon of left index finger at forearm level

√7th S56.403 Unspecified injury of extensor muscle, fascia and tendon of right middle finger at forearm level

√7th S56.404 Unspecified injury of extensor muscle, fascia and tendon of left middle finger at forearm level

√7th S56.405 Unspecified injury of extensor muscle, fascia and tendon of right ring finger at forearm level

√7th S56.406 Unspecified injury of extensor muscle, fascia and tendon of left ring finger at forearm level

√7th S56.407 Unspecified injury of extensor muscle, fascia and tendon of right little finger at forearm level

√7th S56.408 Unspecified injury of extensor muscle, fascia and tendon of left little finger at forearm level

√7th S56.409 Unspecified injury of extensor muscle, fascia and tendon of unspecified finger at forearm level

√6th S56.41 Strain of extensor muscle, fascia and tendon of other and unspecified finger at forearm level

√7th S56.411 Strain of extensor muscle, fascia and tendon of right index finger at forearm level

√7th S56.412 Strain of extensor muscle, fascia and tendon of left index finger at forearm level

√7th S56.413 Strain of extensor muscle, fascia and tendon of right middle finger at forearm level

√7th S56.414 Strain of extensor muscle, fascia and tendon of left middle finger at forearm level

√7th S56.415 Strain of extensor muscle, fascia and tendon of right ring finger at forearm level

√7th S56.416 Strain of extensor muscle, fascia and tendon of left ring finger at forearm level

√7th S56.417 Strain of extensor muscle, fascia and tendon of right little finger at forearm level

√7th S56.418 Strain of extensor muscle, fascia and tendon of left little finger at forearm level

√7th S56.419 Strain of extensor muscle, fascia and tendon of finger, unspecified finger at forearm level

√6th S56.42 Laceration of extensor muscle, fascia and tendon of other and unspecified finger at forearm level

√7th S56.421 Laceration of extensor muscle, fascia and tendon of right index finger at forearm level CC

√7th S56.422 Laceration of extensor muscle, fascia and tendon of left index finger at forearm level CC

√7th S56.423 Laceration of extensor muscle, fascia and tendon of right middle finger at forearm level CC

√7th S56.424 Laceration of extensor muscle, fascia and tendon of left middle finger at forearm level CC

√7th S56.425 Laceration of extensor muscle, fascia and tendon of right ring finger at forearm level CC

√7th S56.426 Laceration of extensor muscle, fascia and tendon of left ring finger at forearm level CC

√7th S56.427 Laceration of extensor muscle, fascia and tendon of right little finger at forearm level CC

√7th S56.428 Laceration of extensor muscle, fascia and tendon of left little finger at forearm level CC

√7th S56.429 Laceration of extensor muscle, fascia and tendon of unspecified finger at forearm level CC UNS

√6th S56.49 Other injury of extensor muscle, fascia and tendon of other and unspecified finger at forearm level

√7th S56.491 Other injury of extensor muscle, fascia and tendon of right index finger at forearm level

√7th S56.492 Other injury of extensor muscle, fascia and tendon of left index finger at forearm level

√7th S56.493 Other injury of extensor muscle, fascia and tendon of right middle finger at forearm level

√7th S56.494 Other injury of extensor muscle, fascia and tendon of left middle finger at forearm level

√7th S56.495 Other injury of extensor muscle, fascia and tendon of right ring finger at forearm level

√7th S56.496 Other injury of extensor muscle, fascia and tendon of left ring finger at forearm level

√7th S56.497 Other injury of extensor muscle, fascia and tendon of right little finger at forearm level

√7th S56.498 Other injury of extensor muscle, fascia and tendon of left little finger at forearm level

√7th S56.499 Other injury of extensor muscle, fascia and tendon of unspecified finger at forearm level

√5th S56.5 Injury of other extensor muscle, fascia and tendon at forearm level

√6th S56.50 Unspecified injury of other extensor muscle, fascia and tendon at forearm level

√7th S56.501 Unspecified injury of other extensor muscle, fascia and tendon at forearm level, right arm

√7th S56.502 Unspecified injury of other extensor muscle, fascia and tendon at forearm level, left arm

√7th S56.509 Unspecified injury of other extensor muscle, fascia and tendon at forearm level, unspecified arm

√6th S56.51 Strain of other extensor muscle, fascia and tendon at forearm level

√7th S56.511 Strain of other extensor muscle, fascia and tendon at forearm level, right arm

√7th S56.512 Strain of other extensor muscle, fascia and tendon at forearm level, left arm

√7th S56.519 Strain of other extensor muscle, fascia and tendon at forearm level, unspecified arm

√6th S56.52 Laceration of other extensor muscle, fascia and tendon at forearm level

√7th S56.521 Laceration of other extensor muscle, fascia and tendon at forearm level, right arm CC

√7th S56.522 Laceration of other extensor muscle, fascia and tendon at forearm level, left arm CC

√7th S56.529 Laceration of other extensor muscle, fascia and tendon at forearm level, unspecified arm CC UNS

√6th S56.59 Other injury of other extensor muscle, fascia and tendon at forearm level

√7th S56.591 Other injury of other extensor muscle, fascia and tendon at forearm level, right arm

√7th S56.592 Other injury of other extensor muscle, fascia and tendon at forearm level, left arm

√7th S56.599 Other injury of other extensor muscle, fascia and tendon at forearm level, unspecified arm

√5th S56.8 Injury of other muscles, fascia and tendons at forearm level

√6th S56.80 Unspecified injury of other muscles, fascia and tendons at forearm level

√7th S56.801 Unspecified injury of other muscles, fascia and tendons at forearm level, right arm

√7th S56.802 Unspecified injury of other muscles, fascia and tendons at forearm level, left arm

✓7th **S56.809 Unspecified injury of other muscles, fascia and tendons at forearm level, unspecified arm**

✓6th **S56.81 Strain of other muscles, fascia and tendons at forearm level**

✓7th **S56.811 Strain of other muscles, fascia and tendons at forearm level, right arm**

✓7th **S56.812 Strain of other muscles, fascia and tendons at forearm level, left arm**

✓7th **S56.819 Strain of other muscles, fascia and tendons at forearm level, unspecified arm**

✓6th **S56.82 Laceration of other muscles, fascia and tendons at forearm level**

✓7th **S56.821 Laceration of other muscles, fascia and tendons at forearm level, right arm** CC

✓7th **S56.822 Laceration of other muscles, fascia and tendons at forearm level, left arm** CC

✓7th **S56.829 Laceration of other muscles, fascia and tendons at forearm level, unspecified arm** CC UNS

✓6th **S56.89 Other injury of other muscles, fascia and tendons at forearm level**

✓7th **S56.891 Other injury of other muscles, fascia and tendons at forearm level, right arm**

✓7th **S56.892 Other injury of other muscles, fascia and tendons at forearm level, left arm**

✓7th **S56.899 Other injury of other muscles, fascia and tendons at forearm level, unspecified arm**

✓5th **S56.9 Injury of unspecified muscles, fascia and tendons at forearm level**

✓6th **S56.90 Unspecified injury of unspecified muscles, fascia and tendons at forearm level**

✓7th **S56.901 Unspecified injury of unspecified muscles, fascia and tendons at forearm level, right arm**

✓7th **S56.902 Unspecified injury of unspecified muscles, fascia and tendons at forearm level, left arm**

✓7th **S56.909 Unspecified injury of unspecified muscles, fascia and tendons at forearm level, unspecified arm**

✓6th **S56.91 Strain of unspecified muscles, fascia and tendons at forearm level**

✓7th **S56.911 Strain of unspecified muscles, fascia and tendons at forearm level, right arm**

✓7th **S56.912 Strain of unspecified muscles, fascia and tendons at forearm level, left arm**

✓7th **S56.919 Strain of unspecified muscles, fascia and tendons at forearm level, unspecified arm**

✓6th **S56.92 Laceration of unspecified muscles, fascia and tendons at forearm level**

✓7th **S56.921 Laceration of unspecified muscles, fascia and tendons at forearm level, right arm** CC

✓7th **S56.922 Laceration of unspecified muscles, fascia and tendons at forearm level, left arm** CC

✓7th **S56.929 Laceration of unspecified muscles, fascia and tendons at forearm level, unspecified arm** CC UNS

✓6th **S56.99 Other injury of unspecified muscles, fascia and tendons at forearm level**

✓7th **S56.991 Other injury of unspecified muscles, fascia and tendons at forearm level, right arm**

✓7th **S56.992 Other injury of unspecified muscles, fascia and tendons at forearm level, left arm**

✓7th **S56.999 Other injury of unspecified muscles, fascia and tendons at forearm level, unspecified arm**

✓4th **S57 Crushing injury of elbow and forearm**

Use additional code(s) for all associated injuries

EXCLUDES 2 *crushing injury of wrist and hand (S67.-)*

The appropriate 7th character is to be added to each code from category S57.
A initial encounter
D subsequent encounter
S sequela

✓5th **S57.0 Crushing injury of elbow**

✓x7th **S57.00 Crushing injury of unspecified elbow**

✓x7th **S57.01 Crushing injury of right elbow**

✓x7th **S57.02 Crushing injury of left elbow**

✓5th **S57.8 Crushing injury of forearm**

✓x7th **S57.80 Crushing injury of unspecified forearm**

✓x7th **S57.81 Crushing injury of right forearm**

✓x7th **S57.82 Crushing injury of left forearm**

✓4th **S58 Traumatic amputation of elbow and forearm**

An amputation not identified as partial or complete should be coded to complete

EXCLUDES 1 *traumatic amputation of wrist and hand (S68.-)*

The appropriate 7th character is to be added to each code from category S58.
A initial encounter
D subsequent encounter
S sequela

✓5th **S58.0 Traumatic amputation at elbow level**

✓6th **S58.01 Complete traumatic amputation at elbow level**

✓7th **S58.011 Complete traumatic amputation at elbow level, right arm** CC HCC

✓7th **S58.012 Complete traumatic amputation at elbow level, left arm** CC HCC

✓7th **S58.019 Complete traumatic amputation at elbow level, unspecified arm** CC UNS HCC

✓6th **S58.02 Partial traumatic amputation at elbow level**

✓7th **S58.021 Partial traumatic amputation at elbow level, right arm** CC HCC

✓7th **S58.022 Partial traumatic amputation at elbow level, left arm** CC HCC

✓7th **S58.029 Partial traumatic amputation at elbow level, unspecified arm** CC UNS HCC

✓5th **S58.1 Traumatic amputation at level between elbow and wrist**

✓6th **S58.11 Complete traumatic amputation at level between elbow and wrist**

✓7th **S58.111 Complete traumatic amputation at level between elbow and wrist, right arm** CC HCC

✓7th **S58.112 Complete traumatic amputation at level between elbow and wrist, left arm** CC HCC

✓7th **S58.119 Complete traumatic amputation at level between elbow and wrist, unspecified arm** CC UNS HCC

✓6th **S58.12 Partial traumatic amputation at level between elbow and wrist**

✓7th **S58.121 Partial traumatic amputation at level between elbow and wrist, right arm** CC HCC

✓7th **S58.122 Partial traumatic amputation at level between elbow and wrist, left arm** CC HCC

✓7th **S58.129 Partial traumatic amputation at level between elbow and wrist, unspecified arm** CC UNS HCC

✓5th **S58.9 Traumatic amputation of forearm, level unspecified**

EXCLUDES 1 *traumatic amputation of wrist (S68.-)*

✓6th **S58.91 Complete traumatic amputation of forearm, level unspecified**

✓7th **S58.911 Complete traumatic amputation of right forearm, level unspecified** CC HCC

✓7th **S58.912 Complete traumatic amputation of left forearm, level unspecified** CC HCC

✓7th **S58.919 Complete traumatic amputation of unspecified forearm, level unspecified** CC UNS HCC

✓6th **S58.92 Partial traumatic amputation of forearm, level unspecified**

✓7th **S58.921 Partial traumatic amputation of right forearm, level unspecified** CC HCC

✓7th **S58.922 Partial traumatic amputation of left forearm, level unspecified** CC HCC

✓7th **S58.929 Partial traumatic amputation of unspecified forearm, level unspecified** CC UNS HCC

S59 Other and unspecified injuries of elbow and forearm

EXCLUDES 2 *other and unspecified injuries of wrist and hand (S69.-)*

AHA: 2018,2Q,12; 2018,1Q,3; 2015,3Q,37-39

The appropriate 7th character is to be added to each code from subcategories S59.Ø, S59.1, and S59.2.
- A initial encounter for closed fracture
- D subsequent encounter for fracture with routine healing
- G subsequent encounter for fracture with delayed healing
- K subsequent encounter for fracture with nonunion
- P subsequent encounter for fracture with malunion
- S sequela

S59.Ø Physeal fracture of lower end of ulna

AHA: 2019,4Q,56

S59.ØØ Unspecified physeal fracture of lower end of ulna
- S59.ØØ1 Unspecified physeal fracture of lower end of ulna, right arm CC H5
- S59.ØØ2 Unspecified physeal fracture of lower end of ulna, left arm CC H5
- S59.ØØ9 Unspecified physeal fracture of lower end of ulna, unspecified arm CC H5 UNS

S59.Ø1 Salter-Harris Type I physeal fracture of lower end of ulna
- S59.Ø11 Salter-Harris Type I physeal fracture of lower end of ulna, right arm CC H5
- S59.Ø12 Salter-Harris Type I physeal fracture of lower end of ulna, left arm CC H5
- S59.Ø19 Salter-Harris Type I physeal fracture of lower end of ulna, unspecified arm CC H5 UNS

S59.Ø2 Salter-Harris Type II physeal fracture of lower end of ulna
- S59.Ø21 Salter-Harris Type II physeal fracture of lower end of ulna, right arm CC H5
- S59.Ø22 Salter-Harris Type II physeal fracture of lower end of ulna, left arm CC H5
- S59.Ø29 Salter-Harris Type II physeal fracture of lower end of ulna, unspecified arm CC H5 UNS

S59.Ø3 Salter-Harris Type III physeal fracture of lower end of ulna
- S59.Ø31 Salter-Harris Type III physeal fracture of lower end of ulna, right arm CC H5
- S59.Ø32 Salter-Harris Type III physeal fracture of lower end of ulna, left arm CC H5
- S59.Ø39 Salter-Harris Type III physeal fracture of lower end of ulna, unspecified arm CC H5 UNS

S59.Ø4 Salter-Harris Type IV physeal fracture of lower end of ulna
- S59.Ø41 Salter-Harris Type IV physeal fracture of lower end of ulna, right arm CC H5
- S59.Ø42 Salter-Harris Type IV physeal fracture of lower end of ulna, left arm CC H5
- S59.Ø49 Salter-Harris Type IV physeal fracture of lower end of ulna, unspecified arm CC H5 UNS

S59.Ø9 Other physeal fracture of lower end of ulna
- S59.Ø91 Other physeal fracture of lower end of ulna, right arm CC H5
- S59.Ø92 Other physeal fracture of lower end of ulna, left arm CC H5
- S59.Ø99 Other physeal fracture of lower end of ulna, unspecified arm CC H5 UNS

S59.1 Physeal fracture of upper end of radius

AHA: 2019,4Q,56

S59.1Ø Unspecified physeal fracture of upper end of radius
- S59.1Ø1 Unspecified physeal fracture of upper end of radius, right arm CC
- S59.1Ø2 Unspecified physeal fracture of upper end of radius, left arm CC
- S59.1Ø9 Unspecified physeal fracture of upper end of radius, unspecified arm CC UNS

S59.11 Salter-Harris Type I physeal fracture of upper end of radius
- S59.111 Salter-Harris Type I physeal fracture of upper end of radius, right arm CC
- S59.112 Salter-Harris Type I physeal fracture of upper end of radius, left arm CC
- S59.119 Salter-Harris Type I physeal fracture of upper end of radius, unspecified arm CC UNS

S59.12 Salter-Harris Type II physeal fracture of upper end of radius
- S59.121 Salter-Harris Type II physeal fracture of upper end of radius, right arm CC
- S59.122 Salter-Harris Type II physeal fracture of upper end of radius, left arm CC
- S59.129 Salter-Harris Type II physeal fracture of upper end of radius, unspecified arm CC UNS

S59.13 Salter-Harris Type III physeal fracture of upper end of radius
- S59.131 Salter-Harris Type III physeal fracture of upper end of radius, right arm CC
- S59.132 Salter-Harris Type III physeal fracture of upper end of radius, left arm CC
- S59.139 Salter-Harris Type III physeal fracture of upper end of radius, unspecified arm CC UNS

S59.14 Salter-Harris Type IV physeal fracture of upper end of radius
- S59.141 Salter-Harris Type IV physeal fracture of upper end of radius, right arm CC
- S59.142 Salter-Harris Type IV physeal fracture of upper end of radius, left arm CC
- S59.149 Salter-Harris Type IV physeal fracture of upper end of radius, unspecified arm CC UNS

S59.19 Other physeal fracture of upper end of radius
- S59.191 Other physeal fracture of upper end of radius, right arm CC
- S59.192 Other physeal fracture of upper end of radius, left arm CC
- S59.199 Other physeal fracture of upper end of radius, unspecified arm CC UNS

S59.2 Physeal fracture of lower end of radius

AHA: 2019,4Q,56

S59.2Ø Unspecified physeal fracture of lower end of radius
- S59.2Ø1 Unspecified physeal fracture of lower end of radius, right arm CC H5
- S59.2Ø2 Unspecified physeal fracture of lower end of radius, left arm CC H5
- S59.2Ø9 Unspecified physeal fracture of lower end of radius, unspecified arm CC H5 UNS

S59.21 Salter-Harris Type I physeal fracture of lower end of radius
- S59.211 Salter-Harris Type I physeal fracture of lower end of radius, right arm CC H5
- S59.212 Salter-Harris Type I physeal fracture of lower end of radius, left arm CC H5
- S59.219 Salter-Harris Type I physeal fracture of lower end of radius, unspecified arm CC H5 UNS

S59.22 Salter-Harris Type II physeal fracture of lower end of radius
- S59.221 Salter-Harris Type II physeal fracture of lower end of radius, right arm CC H5
- S59.222 Salter-Harris Type II physeal fracture of lower end of radius, left arm CC H5
- S59.229 Salter-Harris Type II physeal fracture of lower end of radius, unspecified arm CC H5 UNS

S59.23 Salter-Harris Type III physeal fracture of lower end of radius
- S59.231 Salter-Harris Type III physeal fracture of lower end of radius, right arm CC H5
- S59.232 Salter-Harris Type III physeal fracture of lower end of radius, left arm CC H5
- S59.239 Salter-Harris Type III physeal fracture of lower end of radius, unspecified arm CC H5 UNS

S59.24 Salter-Harris Type IV physeal fracture of lower end of radius
- S59.241 Salter-Harris Type IV physeal fracture of lower end of radius, right arm CC H5
- S59.242 Salter-Harris Type IV physeal fracture of lower end of radius, left arm CC H5

✓7th **S59.249 Salter-Harris Type IV physeal fracture of lower end of radius, unspecified arm** CC H5 UNS

✓6th **S59.29 Other physeal fracture of lower end of radius**

✓7th **S59.291 Other physeal fracture of lower end of radius, right arm** CC H5

✓7th **S59.292 Other physeal fracture of lower end of radius, left arm** CC H5

✓7th **S59.299 Other physeal fracture of lower end of radius, unspecified arm** CC H5 UNS

✓5th **S59.8 Other specified injuries of elbow and forearm**

The appropriate 7th character is to be added to each code in subcategory S59.8.
A initial encounter
D subsequent encounter
S sequela

✓6th **S59.80 Other specified injuries of elbow**

✓7th **S59.801 Other specified injuries of right elbow**

✓7th **S59.802 Other specified injuries of left elbow**

✓7th **S59.809 Other specified injuries of unspecified elbow**

✓6th **S59.81 Other specified injuries of forearm**

✓7th **S59.811 Other specified injuries right forearm**

✓7th **S59.812 Other specified injuries left forearm**

✓7th **S59.819 Other specified injuries unspecified forearm**

✓5th **S59.9 Unspecified injury of elbow and forearm**

The appropriate 7th character is to be added to each code in subcategory S59.9.
A initial encounter
D subsequent encounter
S sequela

✓6th **S59.90 Unspecified injury of elbow**

✓7th **S59.901 Unspecified injury of right elbow**

✓7th **S59.902 Unspecified injury of left elbow**

✓7th **S59.909 Unspecified injury of unspecified elbow**

✓6th **S59.91 Unspecified injury of forearm**

✓7th **S59.911 Unspecified injury of right forearm**

✓7th **S59.912 Unspecified injury of left forearm**

✓7th **S59.919 Unspecified injury of unspecified forearm**

Injuries to the wrist, hand and fingers (S60-S69)

EXCLUDES 2 *burns and corrosions (T20-T32)*
frostbite (T33-T34)
insect bite or sting, venomous (T63.4)

✓4th **S60 Superficial injury of wrist, hand and fingers**

The appropriate 7th character is to be added to each code from category S60.
A initial encounter
D subsequent encounter
S sequela

✓5th **S60.0 Contusion of finger without damage to nail**

EXCLUDES 1 *contusion involving nail (matrix) (S60.1)*

✓x7th **S60.00 Contusion of unspecified finger without damage to nail**
Contusion of finger(s) NOS

✓6th **S60.01 Contusion of thumb without damage to nail**

✓7th **S60.011 Contusion of right thumb without damage to nail**

✓7th **S60.012 Contusion of left thumb without damage to nail**

✓7th **S60.019 Contusion of unspecified thumb without damage to nail**

✓6th **S60.02 Contusion of index finger without damage to nail**

✓7th **S60.021 Contusion of right index finger without damage to nail**

✓7th **S60.022 Contusion of left index finger without damage to nail**

✓7th **S60.029 Contusion of unspecified index finger without damage to nail**

✓6th **S60.03 Contusion of middle finger without damage to nail**

✓7th **S60.031 Contusion of right middle finger without damage to nail**

✓7th **S60.032 Contusion of left middle finger without damage to nail**

✓7th **S60.039 Contusion of unspecified middle finger without damage to nail**

✓6th **S60.04 Contusion of ring finger without damage to nail**

✓7th **S60.041 Contusion of right ring finger without damage to nail**

✓7th **S60.042 Contusion of left ring finger without damage to nail**

✓7th **S60.049 Contusion of unspecified ring finger without damage to nail**

✓6th **S60.05 Contusion of little finger without damage to nail**

✓7th **S60.051 Contusion of right little finger without damage to nail**

✓7th **S60.052 Contusion of left little finger without damage to nail**

✓7th **S60.059 Contusion of unspecified little finger without damage to nail**

✓5th **S60.1 Contusion of finger with damage to nail**

✓x7th **S60.10 Contusion of unspecified finger with damage to nail**

✓6th **S60.11 Contusion of thumb with damage to nail**

✓7th **S60.111 Contusion of right thumb with damage to nail**

✓7th **S60.112 Contusion of left thumb with damage to nail**

✓7th **S60.119 Contusion of unspecified thumb with damage to nail**

✓6th **S60.12 Contusion of index finger with damage to nail**

✓7th **S60.121 Contusion of right index finger with damage to nail**

✓7th **S60.122 Contusion of left index finger with damage to nail**

✓7th **S60.129 Contusion of unspecified index finger with damage to nail**

✓6th **S60.13 Contusion of middle finger with damage to nail**

✓7th **S60.131 Contusion of right middle finger with damage to nail**

✓7th **S60.132 Contusion of left middle finger with damage to nail**

✓7th **S60.139 Contusion of unspecified middle finger with damage to nail**

✓6th **S60.14 Contusion of ring finger with damage to nail**

✓7th **S60.141 Contusion of right ring finger with damage to nail**

✓7th **S60.142 Contusion of left ring finger with damage to nail**

✓7th **S60.149 Contusion of unspecified ring finger with damage to nail**

✓6th **S60.15 Contusion of little finger with damage to nail**

✓7th **S60.151 Contusion of right little finger with damage to nail**

✓7th **S60.152 Contusion of left little finger with damage to nail**

✓7th **S60.159 Contusion of unspecified little finger with damage to nail**

✓5th **S60.2 Contusion of wrist and hand**

EXCLUDES 2 *contusion of fingers (S60.0-, S60.1-)*

✓6th **S60.21 Contusion of wrist**

✓7th **S60.211 Contusion of right wrist**

✓7th **S60.212 Contusion of left wrist**

✓7th **S60.219 Contusion of unspecified wrist**

✓6th **S60.22 Contusion of hand**

✓7th **S60.221 Contusion of right hand**

✓7th **S60.222 Contusion of left hand**

✓7th **S60.229 Contusion of unspecified hand**

✓5th **S60.3 Other superficial injuries of thumb**

✓6th **S60.31 Abrasion of thumb**

✓7th **S60.311 Abrasion of right thumb**

✓7th **S60.312 Abrasion of left thumb**

✓7th **S60.319 Abrasion of unspecified thumb**

✓6th **S60.32 Blister (nonthermal) of thumb**

✓7th **S60.321 Blister (nonthermal) of right thumb**

✓7th **S60.322 Blister (nonthermal) of left thumb**

✓7th **S60.329 Blister (nonthermal) of unspecified thumb**

√6th **S60.34 External constriction of thumb**
Hair tourniquet syndrome of thumb
Use additional cause code to identify the constricting item (W49.0-)
√7th **S60.341 External constriction of right thumb**
√7th **S60.342 External constriction of left thumb**
√7th **S60.349 External constriction of unspecified thumb**
√6th **S60.35 Superficial foreign body of thumb**
Splinter in the thumb
√7th **S60.351 Superficial foreign body of right thumb**
√7th **S60.352 Superficial foreign body of left thumb**
√7th **S60.359 Superficial foreign body of unspecified thumb**
√6th **S60.36 Insect bite (nonvenomous) of thumb**
√7th **S60.361 Insect bite (nonvenomous) of right thumb**
√7th **S60.362 Insect bite (nonvenomous) of left thumb**
√7th **S60.369 Insect bite (nonvenomous) of unspecified thumb**
√6th **S60.37 Other superficial bite of thumb**
EXCLUDES 1 *open bite of thumb (S61.05-, S61.15-)*
√7th **S60.371 Other superficial bite of right thumb**
√7th **S60.372 Other superficial bite of left thumb**
√7th **S60.379 Other superficial bite of unspecified thumb**
√6th **S60.39 Other superficial injuries of thumb**
√7th **S60.391 Other superficial injuries of right thumb**
√7th **S60.392 Other superficial injuries of left thumb**
√7th **S60.399 Other superficial injuries of unspecified thumb**
√5th **S60.4 Other superficial injuries of other fingers**
√6th **S60.41 Abrasion of fingers**
√7th **S60.410 Abrasion of right index finger**
√7th **S60.411 Abrasion of left index finger**
√7th **S60.412 Abrasion of right middle finger**
√7th **S60.413 Abrasion of left middle finger**
√7th **S60.414 Abrasion of right ring finger**
√7th **S60.415 Abrasion of left ring finger**
√7th **S60.416 Abrasion of right little finger**
√7th **S60.417 Abrasion of left little finger**
√7th **S60.418 Abrasion of other finger**
Abrasion of specified finger with unspecified laterality
√7th **S60.419 Abrasion of unspecified finger**
√6th **S60.42 Blister (nonthermal) of fingers**
√7th **S60.420 Blister (nonthermal) of right index finger**
√7th **S60.421 Blister (nonthermal) of left index finger**
√7th **S60.422 Blister (nonthermal) of right middle finger**
√7th **S60.423 Blister (nonthermal) of left middle finger**
√7th **S60.424 Blister (nonthermal) of right ring finger**
√7th **S60.425 Blister (nonthermal) of left ring finger**
√7th **S60.426 Blister (nonthermal) of right little finger**
√7th **S60.427 Blister (nonthermal) of left little finger**
√7th **S60.428 Blister (nonthermal) of other finger**
Blister (nonthermal) of specified finger with unspecified laterality
√7th **S60.429 Blister (nonthermal) of unspecified finger**
√6th **S60.44 External constriction of fingers**
Hair tourniquet syndrome of finger
Use additional cause code to identify the constricting item (W49.0-)
√7th **S60.440 External constriction of right index finger**
√7th **S60.441 External constriction of left index finger**
√7th **S60.442 External constriction of right middle finger**
√7th **S60.443 External constriction of left middle finger**
√7th **S60.444 External constriction of right ring finger**
√7th **S60.445 External constriction of left ring finger**
√7th **S60.446 External constriction of right little finger**
√7th **S60.447 External constriction of left little finger**
√7th **S60.448 External constriction of other finger**
External constriction of specified finger with unspecified laterality
√7th **S60.449 External constriction of unspecified finger**
√6th **S60.45 Superficial foreign body of fingers**
Splinter in the finger(s)
√7th **S60.450 Superficial foreign body of right index finger**
√7th **S60.451 Superficial foreign body of left index finger**
√7th **S60.452 Superficial foreign body of right middle finger**
√7th **S60.453 Superficial foreign body of left middle finger**
√7th **S60.454 Superficial foreign body of right ring finger**
√7th **S60.455 Superficial foreign body of left ring finger**
√7th **S60.456 Superficial foreign body of right little finger**
√7th **S60.457 Superficial foreign body of left little finger**
√7th **S60.458 Superficial foreign body of other finger**
Superficial foreign body of specified finger with unspecified laterality
√7th **S60.459 Superficial foreign body of unspecified finger**
√6th **S60.46 Insect bite (nonvenomous) of fingers**
√7th **S60.460 Insect bite (nonvenomous) of right index finger**
√7th **S60.461 Insect bite (nonvenomous) of left index finger**
√7th **S60.462 Insect bite (nonvenomous) of right middle finger**
√7th **S60.463 Insect bite (nonvenomous) of left middle finger**
√7th **S60.464 Insect bite (nonvenomous) of right ring finger**
√7th **S60.465 Insect bite (nonvenomous) of left ring finger**
√7th **S60.466 Insect bite (nonvenomous) of right little finger**
√7th **S60.467 Insect bite (nonvenomous) of left little finger**
√7th **S60.468 Insect bite (nonvenomous) of other finger**
Insect bite (nonvenomous) of specified finger with unspecified laterality
√7th **S60.469 Insect bite (nonvenomous) of unspecified finger**
√6th **S60.47 Other superficial bite of fingers**
EXCLUDES 1 *open bite of fingers (S61.25-, S61.35-)*
√7th **S60.470 Other superficial bite of right index finger**
√7th **S60.471 Other superficial bite of left index finger**
√7th **S60.472 Other superficial bite of right middle finger**
√7th **S60.473 Other superficial bite of left middle finger**
√7th **S60.474 Other superficial bite of right ring finger**
√7th **S60.475 Other superficial bite of left ring finger**
√7th **S60.476 Other superficial bite of right little finger**
√7th **S60.477 Other superficial bite of left little finger**
√7th **S60.478 Other superficial bite of other finger**
Other superficial bite of specified finger with unspecified laterality
√7th **S60.479 Other superficial bite of unspecified finger**
√5th **S60.5 Other superficial injuries of hand**
EXCLUDES 2 *superficial injuries of fingers (S60.3-, S60.4-)*
√6th **S60.51 Abrasion of hand**
√7th **S60.511 Abrasion of right hand**
√7th **S60.512 Abrasion of left hand**
√7th **S60.519 Abrasion of unspecified hand**
√6th **S60.52 Blister (nonthermal) of hand**
√7th **S60.521 Blister (nonthermal) of right hand**
√7th **S60.522 Blister (nonthermal) of left hand**
√7th **S60.529 Blister (nonthermal) of unspecified hand**
√6th **S60.54 External constriction of hand**
√7th **S60.541 External constriction of right hand**

7th **S60.542** External constriction of left hand
7th **S60.549** External constriction of unspecified hand
6th **S60.55** Superficial foreign body of hand
Splinter in the hand
7th **S60.551** Superficial foreign body of right hand
7th **S60.552** Superficial foreign body of left hand
7th **S60.559** Superficial foreign body of unspecified hand
6th **S60.56** Insect bite (nonvenomous) of hand
7th **S60.561** Insect bite (nonvenomous) of right hand
7th **S60.562** Insect bite (nonvenomous) of left hand
7th **S60.569** Insect bite (nonvenomous) of unspecified hand
6th **S60.57** Other superficial bite of hand
EXCLUDES 1 *open bite of hand (S61.45-)*
7th **S60.571** Other superficial bite of hand of right hand
7th **S60.572** Other superficial bite of hand of left hand
7th **S60.579** Other superficial bite of hand of unspecified hand
5th **S60.8** Other superficial injuries of wrist
6th **S60.81** Abrasion of wrist
7th **S60.811** Abrasion of right wrist
7th **S60.812** Abrasion of left wrist
7th **S60.819** Abrasion of unspecified wrist
6th **S60.82** Blister (nonthermal) of wrist
7th **S60.821** Blister (nonthermal) of right wrist
7th **S60.822** Blister (nonthermal) of left wrist
7th **S60.829** Blister (nonthermal) of unspecified wrist
6th **S60.84** External constriction of wrist
7th **S60.841** External constriction of right wrist
7th **S60.842** External constriction of left wrist
7th **S60.849** External constriction of unspecified wrist
6th **S60.85** Superficial foreign body of wrist
Splinter in the wrist
7th **S60.851** Superficial foreign body of right wrist
7th **S60.852** Superficial foreign body of left wrist
7th **S60.859** Superficial foreign body of unspecified wrist
6th **S60.86** Insect bite (nonvenomous) of wrist
7th **S60.861** Insect bite (nonvenomous) of right wrist
7th **S60.862** Insect bite (nonvenomous) of left wrist
7th **S60.869** Insect bite (nonvenomous) of unspecified wrist
6th **S60.87** Other superficial bite of wrist
EXCLUDES 1 *open bite of wrist (S61.55)*
7th **S60.871** Other superficial bite of right wrist
7th **S60.872** Other superficial bite of left wrist
7th **S60.879** Other superficial bite of unspecified wrist
5th **S60.9** Unspecified superficial injury of wrist, hand and fingers
6th **S60.91** Unspecified superficial injury of wrist
7th **S60.911** Unspecified superficial injury of right wrist
7th **S60.912** Unspecified superficial injury of left wrist
7th **S60.919** Unspecified superficial injury of unspecified wrist
6th **S60.92** Unspecified superficial injury of hand
7th **S60.921** Unspecified superficial injury of right hand
7th **S60.922** Unspecified superficial injury of left hand
7th **S60.929** Unspecified superficial injury of unspecified hand
6th **S60.93** Unspecified superficial injury of thumb
7th **S60.931** Unspecified superficial injury of right thumb
7th **S60.932** Unspecified superficial injury of left thumb
7th **S60.939** Unspecified superficial injury of unspecified thumb
6th **S60.94** Unspecified superficial injury of other fingers
7th **S60.940** Unspecified superficial injury of right index finger
7th **S60.941** Unspecified superficial injury of left index finger
7th **S60.942** Unspecified superficial injury of right middle finger
7th **S60.943** Unspecified superficial injury of left middle finger
7th **S60.944** Unspecified superficial injury of right ring finger
7th **S60.945** Unspecified superficial injury of left ring finger
7th **S60.946** Unspecified superficial injury of right little finger
7th **S60.947** Unspecified superficial injury of left little finger
7th **S60.948** Unspecified superficial injury of other finger
Unspecified superficial injury of specified finger with unspecified laterality
7th **S60.949** Unspecified superficial injury of unspecified finger

4th **S61 Open wound of wrist, hand and fingers**
Code also any associated wound infection
EXCLUDES 1 *open fracture of wrist, hand and finger (S62.- with 7th character B)*
traumatic amputation of wrist and hand (S68.-)

The appropriate 7th character is to be added to each code from category S61.
A initial encounter
D subsequent encounter
S sequela

5th **S61.0** Open wound of thumb without damage to nail
EXCLUDES 1 *open wound of thumb with damage to nail (S61.1-)*
6th **S61.00** Unspecified open wound of thumb without damage to nail
7th **S61.001** Unspecified open wound of right thumb without damage to nail
7th **S61.002** Unspecified open wound of left thumb without damage to nail
7th **S61.009** Unspecified open wound of unspecified thumb without damage to nail
6th **S61.01** Laceration without foreign body of thumb without damage to nail
7th **S61.011** Laceration without foreign body of right thumb without damage to nail
7th **S61.012** Laceration without foreign body of left thumb without damage to nail
7th **S61.019** Laceration without foreign body of unspecified thumb without damage to nail
6th **S61.02** Laceration with foreign body of thumb without damage to nail
7th **S61.021** Laceration with foreign body of right thumb without damage to nail
7th **S61.022** Laceration with foreign body of left thumb without damage to nail
7th **S61.029** Laceration with foreign body of unspecified thumb without damage to nail
6th **S61.03** Puncture wound without foreign body of thumb without damage to nail
7th **S61.031** Puncture wound without foreign body of right thumb without damage to nail
7th **S61.032** Puncture wound without foreign body of left thumb without damage to nail
7th **S61.039** Puncture wound without foreign body of unspecified thumb without damage to nail
6th **S61.04** Puncture wound with foreign body of thumb without damage to nail
7th **S61.041** Puncture wound with foreign body of right thumb without damage to nail
7th **S61.042** Puncture wound with foreign body of left thumb without damage to nail
7th **S61.049** Puncture wound with foreign body of unspecified thumb without damage to nail
6th **S61.05** Open bite of thumb without damage to nail
Bite of thumb NOS
EXCLUDES 1 *superficial bite of thumb (S60.36-, S60.37-)*
7th **S61.051** Open bite of right thumb without damage to nail

√7th S61.052 Open bite of left thumb without damage to nail

√7th S61.059 Open bite of unspecified thumb without damage to nail

√5th S61.1 Open wound of thumb with damage to nail

√6th S61.10 Unspecified open wound of thumb with damage to nail

√7th S61.101 Unspecified open wound of right thumb with damage to nail

√7th S61.102 Unspecified open wound of left thumb with damage to nail

√7th S61.109 Unspecified open wound of unspecified thumb with damage to nail

√6th S61.11 Laceration without foreign body of thumb with damage to nail

√7th S61.111 Laceration without foreign body of right thumb with damage to nail

√7th S61.112 Laceration without foreign body of left thumb with damage to nail

√7th S61.119 Laceration without foreign body of unspecified thumb with damage to nail

√6th S61.12 Laceration with foreign body of thumb with damage to nail

√7th S61.121 Laceration with foreign body of right thumb with damage to nail

√7th S61.122 Laceration with foreign body of left thumb with damage to nail

√7th S61.129 Laceration with foreign body of unspecified thumb with damage to nail

√6th S61.13 Puncture wound without foreign body of thumb with damage to nail

√7th S61.131 Puncture wound without foreign body of right thumb with damage to nail

√7th S61.132 Puncture wound without foreign body of left thumb with damage to nail

√7th S61.139 Puncture wound without foreign body of unspecified thumb with damage to nail

√6th S61.14 Puncture wound with foreign body of thumb with damage to nail

√7th S61.141 Puncture wound with foreign body of right thumb with damage to nail

√7th S61.142 Puncture wound with foreign body of left thumb with damage to nail

√7th S61.149 Puncture wound with foreign body of unspecified thumb with damage to nail

√6th S61.15 Open bite of thumb with damage to nail

Bite of thumb with damage to nail NOS

EXCLUDES 1 *superficial bite of thumb (S60.36-, S60.37-)*

√7th S61.151 Open bite of right thumb with damage to nail

√7th S61.152 Open bite of left thumb with damage to nail

√7th S61.159 Open bite of unspecified thumb with damage to nail

√5th S61.2 Open wound of other finger without damage to nail

EXCLUDES 1 *open wound of finger involving nail (matrix) (S61.3-)*

EXCLUDES 2 *open wound of thumb without damage to nail (S61.0-)*

√6th S61.20 Unspecified open wound of other finger without damage to nail

√7th S61.200 Unspecified open wound of right index finger without damage to nail

√7th S61.201 Unspecified open wound of left index finger without damage to nail

√7th S61.202 Unspecified open wound of right middle finger without damage to nail

√7th S61.203 Unspecified open wound of left middle finger without damage to nail

√7th S61.204 Unspecified open wound of right ring finger without damage to nail

√7th S61.205 Unspecified open wound of left ring finger without damage to nail

√7th S61.206 Unspecified open wound of right little finger without damage to nail

√7th S61.207 Unspecified open wound of left little finger without damage to nail

√7th S61.208 Unspecified open wound of other finger without damage to nail

Unspecified open wound of specified finger with unspecified laterality without damage to nail

√7th S61.209 Unspecified open wound of unspecified finger without damage to nail

√6th S61.21 Laceration without foreign body of finger without damage to nail

√7th S61.210 Laceration without foreign body of right index finger without damage to nail

√7th S61.211 Laceration without foreign body of left index finger without damage to nail

√7th S61.212 Laceration without foreign body of right middle finger without damage to nail

√7th S61.213 Laceration without foreign body of left middle finger without damage to nail

√7th S61.214 Laceration without foreign body of right ring finger without damage to nail

√7th S61.215 Laceration without foreign body of left ring finger without damage to nail

√7th S61.216 Laceration without foreign body of right little finger without damage to nail

√7th S61.217 Laceration without foreign body of left little finger without damage to nail

√7th S61.218 Laceration without foreign body of other finger without damage to nail

Laceration without foreign body of specified finger with unspecified laterality without damage to nail

√7th S61.219 Laceration without foreign body of unspecified finger without damage to nail

√6th S61.22 Laceration with foreign body of finger without damage to nail

√7th S61.220 Laceration with foreign body of right index finger without damage to nail

√7th S61.221 Laceration with foreign body of left index finger without damage to nail

√7th S61.222 Laceration with foreign body of right middle finger without damage to nail

√7th S61.223 Laceration with foreign body of left middle finger without damage to nail

√7th S61.224 Laceration with foreign body of right ring finger without damage to nail

√7th S61.225 Laceration with foreign body of left ring finger without damage to nail

√7th S61.226 Laceration with foreign body of right little finger without damage to nail

√7th S61.227 Laceration with foreign body of left little finger without damage to nail

√7th S61.228 Laceration with foreign body of other finger without damage to nail

Laceration with foreign body of specified finger with unspecified laterality without damage to nail

√7th S61.229 Laceration with foreign body of unspecified finger without damage to nail

√6th S61.23 Puncture wound without foreign body of finger without damage to nail

√7th S61.230 Puncture wound without foreign body of right index finger without damage to nail

√7th S61.231 Puncture wound without foreign body of left index finger without damage to nail

√7th S61.232 Puncture wound without foreign body of right middle finger without damage to nail

√7th S61.233 Puncture wound without foreign body of left middle finger without damage to nail

√7th S61.234 Puncture wound without foreign body of right ring finger without damage to nail

√7th S61.235 Puncture wound without foreign body of left ring finger without damage to nail

√7th S61.236 Puncture wound without foreign body of right little finger without damage to nail

√7th S61.237 Puncture wound without foreign body of left little finger without damage to nail

√7th S61.238 Puncture wound without foreign body of other finger without damage to nail

Puncture wound without foreign body of specified finger with unspecified laterality without damage to nail

√7th S61.239 Puncture wound without foreign body of unspecified finger without damage to nail

6th **S61.24 Puncture wound with foreign body of finger without damage to nail**
- 7th **S61.240 Puncture wound with foreign body of right index finger without damage to nail**
- 7th **S61.241 Puncture wound with foreign body of left index finger without damage to nail**
- 7th **S61.242 Puncture wound with foreign body of right middle finger without damage to nail**
- 7th **S61.243 Puncture wound with foreign body of left middle finger without damage to nail**
- 7th **S61.244 Puncture wound with foreign body of right ring finger without damage to nail**
- 7th **S61.245 Puncture wound with foreign body of left ring finger without damage to nail**
- 7th **S61.246 Puncture wound with foreign body of right little finger without damage to nail**
- 7th **S61.247 Puncture wound with foreign body of left little finger without damage to nail**
- 7th **S61.248 Puncture wound with foreign body of other finger without damage to nail**
  Puncture wound with foreign body of specified finger with unspecified laterality without damage to nail
- 7th **S61.249 Puncture wound with foreign body of unspecified finger without damage to nail**

6th **S61.25 Open bite of finger without damage to nail**
Bite of finger without damage to nail NOS
EXCLUDES 1 *superficial bite of finger (S60.46-, S60.47-)*
- 7th **S61.250 Open bite of right index finger without damage to nail**
- 7th **S61.251 Open bite of left index finger without damage to nail**
- 7th **S61.252 Open bite of right middle finger without damage to nail**
- 7th **S61.253 Open bite of left middle finger without damage to nail**
- 7th **S61.254 Open bite of right ring finger without damage to nail**
- 7th **S61.255 Open bite of left ring finger without damage to nail**
- 7th **S61.256 Open bite of right little finger without damage to nail**
- 7th **S61.257 Open bite of left little finger without damage to nail**
- 7th **S61.258 Open bite of other finger without damage to nail**
  Open bite of specified finger with unspecified laterality without damage to nail
- 7th **S61.259 Open bite of unspecified finger without damage to nail**

5th **S61.3 Open wound of other finger with damage to nail**

6th **S61.30 Unspecified open wound of finger with damage to nail**
- 7th **S61.300 Unspecified open wound of right index finger with damage to nail**
- 7th **S61.301 Unspecified open wound of left index finger with damage to nail**
- 7th **S61.302 Unspecified open wound of right middle finger with damage to nail**
- 7th **S61.303 Unspecified open wound of left middle finger with damage to nail**
- 7th **S61.304 Unspecified open wound of right ring finger with damage to nail**
- 7th **S61.305 Unspecified open wound of left ring finger with damage to nail**
- 7th **S61.306 Unspecified open wound of right little finger with damage to nail**
- 7th **S61.307 Unspecified open wound of left little finger with damage to nail**
- 7th **S61.308 Unspecified open wound of other finger with damage to nail**
  Unspecified open wound of specified finger with unspecified laterality with damage to nail
- 7th **S61.309 Unspecified open wound of unspecified finger with damage to nail**

6th **S61.31 Laceration without foreign body of finger with damage to nail**
- 7th **S61.310 Laceration without foreign body of right index finger with damage to nail**
- 7th **S61.311 Laceration without foreign body of left index finger with damage to nail**
- 7th **S61.312 Laceration without foreign body of right middle finger with damage to nail**
- 7th **S61.313 Laceration without foreign body of left middle finger with damage to nail**
- 7th **S61.314 Laceration without foreign body of right ring finger with damage to nail**
- 7th **S61.315 Laceration without foreign body of left ring finger with damage to nail**
- 7th **S61.316 Laceration without foreign body of right little finger with damage to nail**
- 7th **S61.317 Laceration without foreign body of left little finger with damage to nail**
- 7th **S61.318 Laceration without foreign body of other finger with damage to nail**
  Laceration without foreign body of specified finger with unspecified laterality with damage to nail
- 7th **S61.319 Laceration without foreign body of unspecified finger with damage to nail**

6th **S61.32 Laceration with foreign body of finger with damage to nail**
- 7th **S61.320 Laceration with foreign body of right index finger with damage to nail**
- 7th **S61.321 Laceration with foreign body of left index finger with damage to nail**
- 7th **S61.322 Laceration with foreign body of right middle finger with damage to nail**
- 7th **S61.323 Laceration with foreign body of left middle finger with damage to nail**
- 7th **S61.324 Laceration with foreign body of right ring finger with damage to nail**
- 7th **S61.325 Laceration with foreign body of left ring finger with damage to nail**
- 7th **S61.326 Laceration with foreign body of right little finger with damage to nail**
- 7th **S61.327 Laceration with foreign body of left little finger with damage to nail**
- 7th **S61.328 Laceration with foreign body of other finger with damage to nail**
  Laceration with foreign body of specified finger with unspecified laterality with damage to nail
- 7th **S61.329 Laceration with foreign body of unspecified finger with damage to nail**

6th **S61.33 Puncture wound without foreign body of finger with damage to nail**
- 7th **S61.330 Puncture wound without foreign body of right index finger with damage to nail**
- 7th **S61.331 Puncture wound without foreign body of left index finger with damage to nail**
- 7th **S61.332 Puncture wound without foreign body of right middle finger with damage to nail**
- 7th **S61.333 Puncture wound without foreign body of left middle finger with damage to nail**
- 7th **S61.334 Puncture wound without foreign body of right ring finger with damage to nail**
- 7th **S61.335 Puncture wound without foreign body of left ring finger with damage to nail**
- 7th **S61.336 Puncture wound without foreign body of right little finger with damage to nail**
- 7th **S61.337 Puncture wound without foreign body of left little finger with damage to nail**
- 7th **S61.338 Puncture wound without foreign body of other finger with damage to nail**
  Puncture wound without foreign body of specified finger with unspecified laterality with damage to nail
- 7th **S61.339 Puncture wound without foreign body of unspecified finger with damage to nail**

6th **S61.34 Puncture wound with foreign body of finger with damage to nail**
- 7th **S61.340 Puncture wound with foreign body of right index finger with damage to nail**
- 7th **S61.341 Puncture wound with foreign body of left index finger with damage to nail**
- 7th **S61.342 Puncture wound with foreign body of right middle finger with damage to nail**
- 7th **S61.343 Puncture wound with foreign body of left middle finger with damage to nail**
- 7th **S61.344 Puncture wound with foreign body of right ring finger with damage to nail**

S61.345 Puncture wound with foreign body of left ring finger with damage to nail
S61.346 Puncture wound with foreign body of right little finger with damage to nail
S61.347 Puncture wound with foreign body of left little finger with damage to nail
S61.348 Puncture wound with foreign body of other finger with damage to nail
Puncture wound with foreign body of specified finger with unspecified laterality with damage to nail
S61.349 Puncture wound with foreign body of unspecified finger with damage to nail

S61.35 Open bite of finger with damage to nail
Bite of finger with damage to nail NOS
EXCLUDES 1 *superficial bite of finger (S60.46-, S60.47-)*
S61.350 Open bite of right index finger with damage to nail
S61.351 Open bite of left index finger with damage to nail
S61.352 Open bite of right middle finger with damage to nail
S61.353 Open bite of left middle finger with damage to nail
S61.354 Open bite of right ring finger with damage to nail
S61.355 Open bite of left ring finger with damage to nail
S61.356 Open bite of right little finger with damage to nail
S61.357 Open bite of left little finger with damage to nail
S61.358 Open bite of other finger with damage to nail
Open bite of specified finger with unspecified laterality with damage to nail
S61.359 Open bite of unspecified finger with damage to nail

S61.4 Open wound of hand
S61.40 Unspecified open wound of hand
S61.401 Unspecified open wound of right hand
S61.402 Unspecified open wound of left hand
S61.409 Unspecified open wound of unspecified hand
S61.41 Laceration without foreign body of hand
S61.411 Laceration without foreign body of right hand
S61.412 Laceration without foreign body of left hand
S61.419 Laceration without foreign body of unspecified hand
S61.42 Laceration with foreign body of hand
S61.421 Laceration with foreign body of right hand
S61.422 Laceration with foreign body of left hand
S61.429 Laceration with foreign body of unspecified hand
S61.43 Puncture wound without foreign body of hand
S61.431 Puncture wound without foreign body of right hand
S61.432 Puncture wound without foreign body of left hand
S61.439 Puncture wound without foreign body of unspecified hand
S61.44 Puncture wound with foreign body of hand
S61.441 Puncture wound with foreign body of right hand
S61.442 Puncture wound with foreign body of left hand
S61.449 Puncture wound with foreign body of unspecified hand
S61.45 Open bite of hand
Bite of hand NOS
EXCLUDES 1 *superficial bite of hand (S60.56-, S60.57-)*
S61.451 Open bite of right hand
S61.452 Open bite of left hand
S61.459 Open bite of unspecified hand

S61.5 Open wound of wrist
S61.50 Unspecified open wound of wrist
S61.501 Unspecified open wound of right wrist
S61.502 Unspecified open wound of left wrist
S61.509 Unspecified open wound of unspecified wrist
S61.51 Laceration without foreign body of wrist
S61.511 Laceration without foreign body of right wrist
S61.512 Laceration without foreign body of left wrist
S61.519 Laceration without foreign body of unspecified wrist
S61.52 Laceration with foreign body of wrist
S61.521 Laceration with foreign body of right wrist
S61.522 Laceration with foreign body of left wrist
S61.529 Laceration with foreign body of unspecified wrist
S61.53 Puncture wound without foreign body of wrist
S61.531 Puncture wound without foreign body of right wrist
S61.532 Puncture wound without foreign body of left wrist
S61.539 Puncture wound without foreign body of unspecified wrist
S61.54 Puncture wound with foreign body of wrist
S61.541 Puncture wound with foreign body of right wrist
S61.542 Puncture wound with foreign body of left wrist
S61.549 Puncture wound with foreign body of unspecified wrist
S61.55 Open bite of wrist
Bite of wrist NOS
EXCLUDES 1 *superficial bite of wrist (S60.86-, S60.87-)*
S61.551 Open bite of right wrist
S61.552 Open bite of left wrist
S61.559 Open bite of unspecified wrist

S62 Fracture at wrist and hand level

NOTE A fracture not indicated as displaced or nondisplaced should be coded to displaced

A fracture not indicated as open or closed should be coded to closed

EXCLUDES 1 *traumatic amputation of wrist and hand (S68.-)*
EXCLUDES 2 *fracture of distal parts of ulna and radius (S52.-)*

AHA: 2018,2Q,12; 2015,3Q,37-39

The appropriate 7th character is to be added to each code from category S62.
A initial encounter for closed fracture
B initial encounter for open fracture
D subsequent encounter for fracture with routine healing
G subsequent encounter for fracture with delayed healing
K subsequent encounter for fracture with nonunion
P subsequent encounter for fracture with malunion
S sequela

S62.0 Fracture of navicular [scaphoid] bone of wrist
S62.00 Unspecified fracture of navicular [scaphoid] bone of wrist
S62.001 Unspecified fracture of navicular [scaphoid] bone of right wrist CC H5
S62.002 Unspecified fracture of navicular [scaphoid] bone of left wrist CC H5
AHA: 2012,4Q,106
S62.009 Unspecified fracture of navicular [scaphoid] bone of unspecified wrist CC H5 UNS
S62.01 Fracture of distal pole of navicular [scaphoid] bone of wrist
Fracture of volar tuberosity of navicular [scaphoid] bone of wrist
S62.011 Displaced fracture of distal pole of navicular [scaphoid] bone of right wrist CC H5

√7th S62.012 Displaced fracture of distal pole of navicular [scaphoid] bone of left wrist CC HS

√7th S62.013 Displaced fracture of distal pole of navicular [scaphoid] bone of unspecified wrist CC HS UNS

√7th S62.014 Nondisplaced fracture of distal pole of navicular [scaphoid] bone of right wrist CC HS

√7th S62.015 Nondisplaced fracture of distal pole of navicular [scaphoid] bone of left wrist CC HS

√7th S62.016 Nondisplaced fracture of distal pole of navicular [scaphoid] bone of unspecified wrist CC HS UNS

√6th S62.02 Fracture of middle third of navicular [scaphoid] bone of wrist

√7th S62.021 Displaced fracture of middle third of navicular [scaphoid] bone of right wrist CC HS

√7th S62.022 Displaced fracture of middle third of navicular [scaphoid] bone of left wrist CC HS

√7th S62.023 Displaced fracture of middle third of navicular [scaphoid] bone of unspecified wrist CC HS UNS

√7th S62.024 Nondisplaced fracture of middle third of navicular [scaphoid] bone of right wrist CC HS

√7th S62.025 Nondisplaced fracture of middle third of navicular [scaphoid] bone of left wrist CC HS

√7th S62.026 Nondisplaced fracture of middle third of navicular [scaphoid] bone of unspecified wrist CC HS UNS

√6th S62.03 Fracture of proximal third of navicular [scaphoid] bone of wrist

√7th S62.031 Displaced fracture of proximal third of navicular [scaphoid] bone of right wrist CC HS

√7th S62.032 Displaced fracture of proximal third of navicular [scaphoid] bone of left wrist CC HS

√7th S62.033 Displaced fracture of proximal third of navicular [scaphoid] bone of unspecified wrist CC HS UNS

√7th S62.034 Nondisplaced fracture of proximal third of navicular [scaphoid] bone of right wrist CC HS

√7th S62.035 Nondisplaced fracture of proximal third of navicular [scaphoid] bone of left wrist CC HS

√7th S62.036 Nondisplaced fracture of proximal third of navicular [scaphoid] bone of unspecified wrist CC HS UNS

√5th S62.1 Fracture of other and unspecified carpal bone(s)

EXCLUDES 2 *fracture of scaphoid of wrist (S62.0-)*

√6th S62.10 Fracture of unspecified carpal bone

Fracture of wrist NOS

√7th S62.101 Fracture of unspecified carpal bone, right wrist CC HS

√7th S62.102 Fracture of unspecified carpal bone, left wrist CC HS

AHA: 2012,4Q,95

√7th S62.109 Fracture of unspecified carpal bone, unspecified wrist CC HS UNS

√6th S62.11 Fracture of triquetrum [cuneiform] bone of wrist

√7th S62.111 Displaced fracture of triquetrum [cuneiform] bone, right wrist CC HS

√7th S62.112 Displaced fracture of triquetrum [cuneiform] bone, left wrist CC HS

√7th S62.113 Displaced fracture of triquetrum [cuneiform] bone, unspecified wrist CC HS UNS

√7th S62.114 Nondisplaced fracture of triquetrum [cuneiform] bone, right wrist CC HS

√7th S62.115 Nondisplaced fracture of triquetrum [cuneiform] bone, left wrist CC HS

√7th S62.116 Nondisplaced fracture of triquetrum [cuneiform] bone, unspecified wrist CC HS UNS

√6th S62.12 Fracture of lunate [semilunar]

√7th S62.121 Displaced fracture of lunate [semilunar], right wrist CC HS

√7th S62.122 Displaced fracture of lunate [semilunar], left wrist CC HS

√7th S62.123 Displaced fracture of lunate [semilunar], unspecified wrist CC HS UNS

√7th S62.124 Nondisplaced fracture of lunate [semilunar], right wrist CC HS

√7th S62.125 Nondisplaced fracture of lunate [semilunar], left wrist CC HS

√7th S62.126 Nondisplaced fracture of lunate [semilunar], unspecified wrist CC HS UNS

√6th S62.13 Fracture of capitate [os magnum] bone

√7th S62.131 Displaced fracture of capitate [os magnum] bone, right wrist CC HS

√7th S62.132 Displaced fracture of capitate [os magnum] bone, left wrist CC HS

√7th S62.133 Displaced fracture of capitate [os magnum] bone, unspecified wrist CC HS UNS

√7th S62.134 Nondisplaced fracture of capitate [os magnum] bone, right wrist CC HS

√7th S62.135 Nondisplaced fracture of capitate [os magnum] bone, left wrist CC HS

√7th S62.136 Nondisplaced fracture of capitate [os magnum] bone, unspecified wrist CC HS UNS

√6th S62.14 Fracture of body of hamate [unciform] bone

Fracture of hamate [unciform] bone NOS

√7th S62.141 Displaced fracture of body of hamate [unciform] bone, right wrist CC HS

√7th S62.142 Displaced fracture of body of hamate [unciform] bone, left wrist CC HS

√7th S62.143 Displaced fracture of body of hamate [unciform] bone, unspecified wrist CC HS UNS

√7th S62.144 Nondisplaced fracture of body of hamate [unciform] bone, right wrist CC HS

√7th S62.145 Nondisplaced fracture of body of hamate [unciform] bone, left wrist CC HS

√7th S62.146 Nondisplaced fracture of body of hamate [unciform] bone, unspecified wrist CC HS UNS

√6th S62.15 Fracture of hook process of hamate [unciform] bone

Fracture of unciform process of hamate [unciform] bone

√7th S62.151 Displaced fracture of hook process of hamate [unciform] bone, right wrist CC HS

√7th S62.152 Displaced fracture of hook process of hamate [unciform] bone, left wrist CC HS

√7th S62.153 Displaced fracture of hook process of hamate [unciform] bone, unspecified wrist CC HS UNS

√7th S62.154 Nondisplaced fracture of hook process of hamate [unciform] bone, right wrist CC HS

√7th S62.155 Nondisplaced fracture of hook process of hamate [unciform] bone, left wrist CC HS

√7th S62.156 Nondisplaced fracture of hook process of hamate [unciform] bone, unspecified wrist CC HS UNS

√6th S62.16 Fracture of pisiform

√7th S62.161 Displaced fracture of pisiform, right wrist CC HS

√7th S62.162 Displaced fracture of pisiform, left wrist CC HS

√7th S62.163 Displaced fracture of pisiform, unspecified wrist CC HS UNS

√7th S62.164 Nondisplaced fracture of pisiform, right wrist CC HS

√7th S62.165 Nondisplaced fracture of pisiform, left wrist CC HS

√7th S62.166 Nondisplaced fracture of pisiform, unspecified wrist CC HS UNS

S62.17 Fracture of trapezium [larger multangular]
S62.171 Displaced fracture of trapezium [larger multangular], right wrist CC H5
S62.172 Displaced fracture of trapezium [larger multangular], left wrist CC H5
S62.173 Displaced fracture of trapezium [larger multangular], unspecified wrist CC H5 UNS
S62.174 Nondisplaced fracture of trapezium [larger multangular], right wrist CC H5
S62.175 Nondisplaced fracture of trapezium [larger multangular], left wrist CC H5
S62.176 Nondisplaced fracture of trapezium [larger multangular], unspecified wrist CC H5 UNS
S62.18 Fracture of trapezoid [smaller multangular]
S62.181 Displaced fracture of trapezoid [smaller multangular], right wrist CC H5
S62.182 Displaced fracture of trapezoid [smaller multangular], left wrist CC H5
S62.183 Displaced fracture of trapezoid [smaller multangular], unspecified wrist CC H5 UNS
S62.184 Nondisplaced fracture of trapezoid [smaller multangular], right wrist CC H5
S62.185 Nondisplaced fracture of trapezoid [smaller multangular], left wrist CC H5
S62.186 Nondisplaced fracture of trapezoid [smaller multangular], unspecified wrist CC H5 UNS
S62.2 Fracture of first metacarpal bone
S62.20 Unspecified fracture of first metacarpal bone
S62.201 Unspecified fracture of first metacarpal bone, right hand CC H5
S62.202 Unspecified fracture of first metacarpal bone, left hand CC H5
S62.209 Unspecified fracture of first metacarpal bone, unspecified hand CC H5 UNS
S62.21 Bennett's fracture
DEF: Intra-articular, two-part fracture at the base of the first metacarpal bone (thumb) on the ulnar side at the carpometacarpal (CMC) joint.
S62.211 Bennett's fracture, right hand CC H5
S62.212 Bennett's fracture, left hand CC H5
S62.213 Bennett's fracture, unspecified hand CC H5 UNS
S62.22 Rolando's fracture
DEF: Comminuted, three part intra-articular fracture at the base of the thumb metacarpal.
S62.221 Displaced Rolando's fracture, right hand CC H5
S62.222 Displaced Rolando's fracture, left hand CC H5
S62.223 Displaced Rolando's fracture, unspecified hand CC H5 UNS
S62.224 Nondisplaced Rolando's fracture, right hand CC H5
S62.225 Nondisplaced Rolando's fracture, left hand CC H5
S62.226 Nondisplaced Rolando's fracture, unspecified hand CC H5 UNS
S62.23 Other fracture of base of first metacarpal bone
S62.231 Other displaced fracture of base of first metacarpal bone, right hand CC H5
S62.232 Other displaced fracture of base of first metacarpal bone, left hand CC H5
S62.233 Other displaced fracture of base of first metacarpal bone, unspecified hand CC H5 UNS
S62.234 Other nondisplaced fracture of base of first metacarpal bone, right hand CC H5
S62.235 Other nondisplaced fracture of base of first metacarpal bone, left hand CC H5
S62.236 Other nondisplaced fracture of base of first metacarpal bone, unspecified hand CC H5 UNS
S62.24 Fracture of shaft of first metacarpal bone
S62.241 Displaced fracture of shaft of first metacarpal bone, right hand CC H5
S62.242 Displaced fracture of shaft of first metacarpal bone, left hand CC H5
S62.243 Displaced fracture of shaft of first metacarpal bone, unspecified hand CC H5 UNS
S62.244 Nondisplaced fracture of shaft of first metacarpal bone, right hand CC H5
S62.245 Nondisplaced fracture of shaft of first metacarpal bone, left hand CC H5
S62.246 Nondisplaced fracture of shaft of first metacarpal bone, unspecified hand CC H5 UNS
S62.25 Fracture of neck of first metacarpal bone
S62.251 Displaced fracture of neck of first metacarpal bone, right hand CC H5
S62.252 Displaced fracture of neck of first metacarpal bone, left hand CC H5
S62.253 Displaced fracture of neck of first metacarpal bone, unspecified hand CC H5 UNS
S62.254 Nondisplaced fracture of neck of first metacarpal bone, right hand CC H5
S62.255 Nondisplaced fracture of neck of first metacarpal bone, left hand CC H5
S62.256 Nondisplaced fracture of neck of first metacarpal bone, unspecified hand CC H5 UNS
S62.29 Other fracture of first metacarpal bone
S62.291 Other fracture of first metacarpal bone, right hand CC H5
S62.292 Other fracture of first metacarpal bone, left hand CC H5
S62.299 Other fracture of first metacarpal bone, unspecified hand CC H5 UNS
S62.3 Fracture of other and unspecified metacarpal bone
EXCLUDES 2 *fracture of first metacarpal bone (S62.2-)*
S62.30 Unspecified fracture of other metacarpal bone
S62.300 Unspecified fracture of second metacarpal bone, right hand CC H5
S62.301 Unspecified fracture of second metacarpal bone, left hand CC H5
S62.302 Unspecified fracture of third metacarpal bone, right hand CC H5
S62.303 Unspecified fracture of third metacarpal bone, left hand CC H5
S62.304 Unspecified fracture of fourth metacarpal bone, right hand CC H5
S62.305 Unspecified fracture of fourth metacarpal bone, left hand CC H5
S62.306 Unspecified fracture of fifth metacarpal bone, right hand CC H5
S62.307 Unspecified fracture of fifth metacarpal bone, left hand CC H5
S62.308 Unspecified fracture of other metacarpal bone CC H5
Unspecified fracture of specified metacarpal bone with unspecified laterality
S62.309 Unspecified fracture of unspecified metacarpal bone CC H5 UNS
S62.31 Displaced fracture of base of other metacarpal bone
S62.310 Displaced fracture of base of second metacarpal bone, right hand CC H5
S62.311 Displaced fracture of base of second metacarpal bone, left hand CC H5
S62.312 Displaced fracture of base of third metacarpal bone, right hand CC H5
S62.313 Displaced fracture of base of third metacarpal bone, left hand CC H5
S62.314 Displaced fracture of base of fourth metacarpal bone, right hand CC H5
S62.315 Displaced fracture of base of fourth metacarpal bone, left hand CC H5
S62.316 Displaced fracture of base of fifth metacarpal bone, right hand CC H5

7th S62.317 Displaced fracture of base of fifth metacarpal bone, left hand CC H5
7th S62.318 Displaced fracture of base of other metacarpal bone CC H5
Displaced fracture of base of specified metacarpal bone with unspecified laterality
7th S62.319 Displaced fracture of base of unspecified metacarpal bone CC H5 UNS
6th S62.32 Displaced fracture of shaft of other metacarpal bone
7th S62.320 Displaced fracture of shaft of second metacarpal bone, right hand CC H5
7th S62.321 Displaced fracture of shaft of second metacarpal bone, left hand CC H5
7th S62.322 Displaced fracture of shaft of third metacarpal bone, right hand CC H5
7th S62.323 Displaced fracture of shaft of third metacarpal bone, left hand CC H5
7th S62.324 Displaced fracture of shaft of fourth metacarpal bone, right hand CC H5
7th S62.325 Displaced fracture of shaft of fourth metacarpal bone, left hand CC H5
7th S62.326 Displaced fracture of shaft of fifth metacarpal bone, right hand CC H5
7th S62.327 Displaced fracture of shaft of fifth metacarpal bone, left hand CC H5
7th S62.328 Displaced fracture of shaft of other metacarpal bone CC H5
Displaced fracture of shaft of specified metacarpal bone with unspecified laterality
7th S62.329 Displaced fracture of shaft of unspecified metacarpal bone CC H5 UNS
6th S62.33 Displaced fracture of neck of other metacarpal bone
7th S62.330 Displaced fracture of neck of second metacarpal bone, right hand CC H5
7th S62.331 Displaced fracture of neck of second metacarpal bone, left hand CC H5
7th S62.332 Displaced fracture of neck of third metacarpal bone, right hand CC H5
7th S62.333 Displaced fracture of neck of third metacarpal bone, left hand CC H5
7th S62.334 Displaced fracture of neck of fourth metacarpal bone, right hand CC H5
7th S62.335 Displaced fracture of neck of fourth metacarpal bone, left hand CC H5
7th S62.336 Displaced fracture of neck of fifth metacarpal bone, right hand CC H5
7th S62.337 Displaced fracture of neck of fifth metacarpal bone, left hand CC H5
7th S62.338 Displaced fracture of neck of other metacarpal bone CC H5
Displaced fracture of neck of specified metacarpal bone with unspecified laterality
7th S62.339 Displaced fracture of neck of unspecified metacarpal bone CC H5 UNS
6th S62.34 Nondisplaced fracture of base of other metacarpal bone
7th S62.340 Nondisplaced fracture of base of second metacarpal bone, right hand CC H5
7th S62.341 Nondisplaced fracture of base of second metacarpal bone, left hand CC H5
7th S62.342 Nondisplaced fracture of base of third metacarpal bone, right hand CC H5
7th S62.343 Nondisplaced fracture of base of third metacarpal bone, left hand CC H5
7th S62.344 Nondisplaced fracture of base of fourth metacarpal bone, right hand CC H5
7th S62.345 Nondisplaced fracture of base of fourth metacarpal bone, left hand CC H5
7th S62.346 Nondisplaced fracture of base of fifth metacarpal bone, right hand CC H5
7th S62.347 Nondisplaced fracture of base of fifth metacarpal bone, left hand CC H5
7th S62.348 Nondisplaced fracture of base of other metacarpal bone CC H5
Nondisplaced fracture of base of specified metacarpal bone with unspecified laterality
7th S62.349 Nondisplaced fracture of base of unspecified metacarpal bone CC H5 UNS
6th S62.35 Nondisplaced fracture of shaft of other metacarpal bone
7th S62.350 Nondisplaced fracture of shaft of second metacarpal bone, right hand CC H5
7th S62.351 Nondisplaced fracture of shaft of second metacarpal bone, left hand CC H5
7th S62.352 Nondisplaced fracture of shaft of third metacarpal bone, right hand CC H5
7th S62.353 Nondisplaced fracture of shaft of third metacarpal bone, left hand CC H5
7th S62.354 Nondisplaced fracture of shaft of fourth metacarpal bone, right hand CC H5
7th S62.355 Nondisplaced fracture of shaft of fourth metacarpal bone, left hand CC H5
7th S62.356 Nondisplaced fracture of shaft of fifth metacarpal bone, right hand CC H5
7th S62.357 Nondisplaced fracture of shaft of fifth metacarpal bone, left hand CC H5
7th S62.358 Nondisplaced fracture of shaft of other metacarpal bone CC H5
Nondisplaced fracture of shaft of specified metacarpal bone with unspecified laterality
7th S62.359 Nondisplaced fracture of shaft of unspecified metacarpal bone CC H5 UNS
6th S62.36 Nondisplaced fracture of neck of other metacarpal bone
7th S62.360 Nondisplaced fracture of neck of second metacarpal bone, right hand CC H5
7th S62.361 Nondisplaced fracture of neck of second metacarpal bone, left hand CC H5
7th S62.362 Nondisplaced fracture of neck of third metacarpal bone, right hand CC H5
7th S62.363 Nondisplaced fracture of neck of third metacarpal bone, left hand CC H5
7th S62.364 Nondisplaced fracture of neck of fourth metacarpal bone, right hand CC H5
7th S62.365 Nondisplaced fracture of neck of fourth metacarpal bone, left hand CC H5
7th S62.366 Nondisplaced fracture of neck of fifth metacarpal bone, right hand CC H5
7th S62.367 Nondisplaced fracture of neck of fifth metacarpal bone, left hand CC H5
7th S62.368 Nondisplaced fracture of neck of other metacarpal bone CC H5
Nondisplaced fracture of neck of specified metacarpal bone with unspecified laterality
7th S62.369 Nondisplaced fracture of neck of unspecified metacarpal bone CC H5 UNS
6th S62.39 Other fracture of other metacarpal bone
7th S62.390 Other fracture of second metacarpal bone, right hand CC H5
7th S62.391 Other fracture of second metacarpal bone, left hand CC H5
7th S62.392 Other fracture of third metacarpal bone, right hand CC H5
7th S62.393 Other fracture of third metacarpal bone, left hand CC H5
7th S62.394 Other fracture of fourth metacarpal bone, right hand CC H5
7th S62.395 Other fracture of fourth metacarpal bone, left hand CC H5
7th S62.396 Other fracture of fifth metacarpal bone, right hand CC H5
7th S62.397 Other fracture of fifth metacarpal bone, left hand CC H5

S62.398 Other fracture of other metacarpal bone CC H5
Other fracture of specified metacarpal bone with unspecified laterality

S62.399 Other fracture of unspecified metacarpal bone CC H5 UNS

S62.5 Fracture of thumb

S62.50 Fracture of unspecified phalanx of thumb

S62.501 Fracture of unspecified phalanx of right thumb CC H5

S62.502 Fracture of unspecified phalanx of left thumb CC H5

S62.509 Fracture of unspecified phalanx of unspecified thumb CC H5 UNS

S62.51 Fracture of proximal phalanx of thumb

S62.511 Displaced fracture of proximal phalanx of right thumb CC H5

S62.512 Displaced fracture of proximal phalanx of left thumb CC H5

S62.513 Displaced fracture of proximal phalanx of unspecified thumb CC H5 UNS

S62.514 Nondisplaced fracture of proximal phalanx of right thumb CC H5

S62.515 Nondisplaced fracture of proximal phalanx of left thumb CC H5

S62.516 Nondisplaced fracture of proximal phalanx of unspecified thumb CC H5

S62.52 Fracture of distal phalanx of thumb

S62.521 Displaced fracture of distal phalanx of right thumb CC H5

S62.522 Displaced fracture of distal phalanx of left thumb CC H5

S62.523 Displaced fracture of distal phalanx of unspecified thumb CC H5 UNS

S62.524 Nondisplaced fracture of distal phalanx of right thumb CC H5

S62.525 Nondisplaced fracture of distal phalanx of left thumb CC H5

S62.526 Nondisplaced fracture of distal phalanx of unspecified thumb CC H5 UNS

S62.6 Fracture of other and unspecified finger(s)

EXCLUDES 2 *fracture of thumb (S62.5-)*

S62.60 Fracture of unspecified phalanx of finger

S62.600 Fracture of unspecified phalanx of right index finger CC H5

S62.601 Fracture of unspecified phalanx of left index finger CC H5

S62.602 Fracture of unspecified phalanx of right middle finger CC H5

S62.603 Fracture of unspecified phalanx of left middle finger CC H5

S62.604 Fracture of unspecified phalanx of right ring finger CC H5

S62.605 Fracture of unspecified phalanx of left ring finger CC H5

S62.606 Fracture of unspecified phalanx of right little finger CC H5

S62.607 Fracture of unspecified phalanx of left little finger CC H5

S62.608 Fracture of unspecified phalanx of other finger CC H5
Fracture of unspecified phalanx of specified finger with unspecified laterality

S62.609 Fracture of unspecified phalanx of unspecified finger CC H5 UNS

S62.61 Displaced fracture of proximal phalanx of finger

S62.610 Displaced fracture of proximal phalanx of right index finger CC H5

S62.611 Displaced fracture of proximal phalanx of left index finger CC H5

S62.612 Displaced fracture of proximal phalanx of right middle finger CC H5

S62.613 Displaced fracture of proximal phalanx of left middle finger CC H5

S62.614 Displaced fracture of proximal phalanx of right ring finger CC H5

S62.615 Displaced fracture of proximal phalanx of left ring finger CC H5

S62.616 Displaced fracture of proximal phalanx of right little finger CC H5

S62.617 Displaced fracture of proximal phalanx of left little finger CC H5

S62.618 Displaced fracture of proximal phalanx of other finger CC H5
Displaced fracture of proximal phalanx of specified finger with unspecified laterality

S62.619 Displaced fracture of proximal phalanx of unspecified finger CC H5 UNS

S62.62 Displaced fracture of middle phalanx of finger

S62.620 Displaced fracture of middle phalanx of right index finger CC H5

S62.621 Displaced fracture of middle phalanx of left index finger CC H5

S62.622 Displaced fracture of middle phalanx of right middle finger CC H5

S62.623 Displaced fracture of middle phalanx of left middle finger CC H5

S62.624 Displaced fracture of middle phalanx of right ring finger CC H5

S62.625 Displaced fracture of middle phalanx of left ring finger CC H5

S62.626 Displaced fracture of middle phalanx of right little finger CC H5

S62.627 Displaced fracture of middle phalanx of left little finger CC H5

S62.628 Displaced fracture of middle phalanx of other finger CC H5
Displaced fracture of middle phalanx of specified finger with unspecified laterality

S62.629 Displaced fracture of middle phalanx of unspecified finger CC H5 UNS

S62.63 Displaced fracture of distal phalanx of finger

S62.630 Displaced fracture of distal phalanx of right index finger CC H5

S62.631 Displaced fracture of distal phalanx of left index finger CC H5

S62.632 Displaced fracture of distal phalanx of right middle finger CC H5

S62.633 Displaced fracture of distal phalanx of left middle finger CC H5

S62.634 Displaced fracture of distal phalanx of right ring finger CC H5

S62.635 Displaced fracture of distal phalanx of left ring finger CC H5

S62.636 Displaced fracture of distal phalanx of right little finger CC H5

S62.637 Displaced fracture of distal phalanx of left little finger CC H5

S62.638 Displaced fracture of distal phalanx of other finger CC H5
Displaced fracture of distal phalanx of specified finger with unspecified laterality

S62.639 Displaced fracture of distal phalanx of unspecified finger CC H5 UNS

S62.64 Nondisplaced fracture of proximal phalanx of finger

S62.640 Nondisplaced fracture of proximal phalanx of right index finger CC H5

S62.641 Nondisplaced fracture of proximal phalanx of left index finger CC H5

S62.642 Nondisplaced fracture of proximal phalanx of right middle finger CC H5

S62.643 Nondisplaced fracture of proximal phalanx of left middle finger CC H5

S62.644 Nondisplaced fracture of proximal phalanx of right ring finger CC H5

S62.645 Nondisplaced fracture of proximal phalanx of left ring finger CC H5

S62.646 Nondisplaced fracture of proximal phalanx of right little finger CC H5

S62.647 Nondisplaced fracture of proximal phalanx of left little finger CC H5

√7th **S62.648 Nondisplaced fracture of proximal phalanx of other finger** CC H5
Nondisplaced fracture of proximal phalanx of specified finger with unspecified laterality

√7th **S62.649 Nondisplaced fracture of proximal phalanx of unspecified finger** CC H5 UNS

√6th **S62.65 Nondisplaced fracture of middle phalanx of finger**

√7th **S62.650 Nondisplaced fracture of middle phalanx of right index finger** CC H5

√7th **S62.651 Nondisplaced fracture of middle phalanx of left index finger** CC H5

√7th **S62.652 Nondisplaced fracture of middle phalanx of right middle finger** CC H5

√7th **S62.653 Nondisplaced fracture of middle phalanx of left middle finger** CC H5

√7th **S62.654 Nondisplaced fracture of middle phalanx of right ring finger** CC H5

√7th **S62.655 Nondisplaced fracture of middle phalanx of left ring finger** CC H5

√7th **S62.656 Nondisplaced fracture of middle phalanx of right little finger** CC H5

√7th **S62.657 Nondisplaced fracture of middle phalanx of left little finger** CC H5

√7th **S62.658 Nondisplaced fracture of middle phalanx of other finger** CC H5
Nondisplaced fracture of middle phalanx of specified finger with unspecified laterality

√7th **S62.659 Nondisplaced fracture of middle phalanx of unspecified finger** CC H5 UNS

√6th **S62.66 Nondisplaced fracture of distal phalanx of finger**

√7th **S62.660 Nondisplaced fracture of distal phalanx of right index finger** CC H5

√7th **S62.661 Nondisplaced fracture of distal phalanx of left index finger** CC H5

√7th **S62.662 Nondisplaced fracture of distal phalanx of right middle finger** CC H5

√7th **S62.663 Nondisplaced fracture of distal phalanx of left middle finger** CC H5

√7th **S62.664 Nondisplaced fracture of distal phalanx of right ring finger** CC H5

√7th **S62.665 Nondisplaced fracture of distal phalanx of left ring finger** CC H5

√7th **S62.666 Nondisplaced fracture of distal phalanx of right little finger** CC H5

√7th **S62.667 Nondisplaced fracture of distal phalanx of left little finger** CC H5

√7th **S62.668 Nondisplaced fracture of distal phalanx of other finger** CC H5
Nondisplaced fracture of distal phalanx of specified finger with unspecified laterality

√7th **S62.669 Nondisplaced fracture of distal phalanx of unspecified finger** CC H5 UNS

√5th **S62.9 Unspecified fracture of wrist and hand**

√x7th **S62.90 Unspecified fracture of unspecified wrist and hand** CC H5 UNS

√x7th **S62.91 Unspecified fracture of right wrist and hand** CC H5

√x7th **S62.92 Unspecified fracture of left wrist and hand** CC H5

√4th **S63 Dislocation and sprain of joints and ligaments at wrist and hand level**

INCLUDES avulsion of joint or ligament at wrist and hand level
laceration of cartilage, joint or ligament at wrist and hand level
sprain of cartilage, joint or ligament at wrist and hand level
traumatic hemarthrosis of joint or ligament at wrist and hand level
traumatic rupture of joint or ligament at wrist and hand level
traumatic subluxation of joint or ligament at wrist and hand level
traumatic tear of joint or ligament at wrist and hand level

Code also any associated open wound

EXCLUDES 2 *strain of muscle, fascia and tendon of wrist and hand (S66.-)*

The appropriate 7th character is to be added to each code from category S63.
A initial encounter
D subsequent encounter
S sequela

√5th **S63.0 Subluxation and dislocation of wrist and hand joints**

√6th **S63.00 Unspecified subluxation and dislocation of wrist and hand**
Dislocation of carpal bone NOS
Dislocation of distal end of radius NOS
Subluxation of carpal bone NOS
Subluxation of distal end of radius NOS

√7th **S63.001 Unspecified subluxation of right wrist and hand**

√7th **S63.002 Unspecified subluxation of left wrist and hand**

√7th **S63.003 Unspecified subluxation of unspecified wrist and hand**

√7th **S63.004 Unspecified dislocation of right wrist and hand**

√7th **S63.005 Unspecified dislocation of left wrist and hand**

√7th **S63.006 Unspecified dislocation of unspecified wrist and hand**

√6th **S63.01 Subluxation and dislocation of distal radioulnar joint**

√7th **S63.011 Subluxation of distal radioulnar joint of right wrist**

√7th **S63.012 Subluxation of distal radioulnar joint of left wrist**

√7th **S63.013 Subluxation of distal radioulnar joint of unspecified wrist**

√7th **S63.014 Dislocation of distal radioulnar joint of right wrist**

√7th **S63.015 Dislocation of distal radioulnar joint of left wrist**

√7th **S63.016 Dislocation of distal radioulnar joint of unspecified wrist**

√6th **S63.02 Subluxation and dislocation of radiocarpal joint**

√7th **S63.021 Subluxation of radiocarpal joint of right wrist**

√7th **S63.022 Subluxation of radiocarpal joint of left wrist**

√7th **S63.023 Subluxation of radiocarpal joint of unspecified wrist**

√7th **S63.024 Dislocation of radiocarpal joint of right wrist**

√7th **S63.025 Dislocation of radiocarpal joint of left wrist**

√7th **S63.026 Dislocation of radiocarpal joint of unspecified wrist**

√6th **S63.03 Subluxation and dislocation of midcarpal joint**

√7th **S63.031 Subluxation of midcarpal joint of right wrist**

√7th **S63.032 Subluxation of midcarpal joint of left wrist**

√7th **S63.033 Subluxation of midcarpal joint of unspecified wrist**

√7th **S63.034 Dislocation of midcarpal joint of right wrist**

√7th **S63.035 Dislocation of midcarpal joint of left wrist**

√7th **S63.036 Dislocation of midcarpal joint of unspecified wrist**

✓6th S63.04 Subluxation and dislocation of carpometacarpal joint of thumb
EXCLUDES 2 interphalangeal subluxation and dislocation of thumb (S63.1-)
✓7th S63.041 Subluxation of carpometacarpal joint of right thumb
✓7th S63.042 Subluxation of carpometacarpal joint of left thumb
✓7th S63.043 Subluxation of carpometacarpal joint of unspecified thumb
✓7th S63.044 Dislocation of carpometacarpal joint of right thumb
✓7th S63.045 Dislocation of carpometacarpal joint of left thumb
✓7th S63.046 Dislocation of carpometacarpal joint of unspecified thumb
✓6th S63.05 Subluxation and dislocation of other carpometacarpal joint
EXCLUDES 2 subluxation and dislocation of carpometacarpal joint of thumb (S63.04-)
✓7th S63.051 Subluxation of other carpometacarpal joint of right hand
✓7th S63.052 Subluxation of other carpometacarpal joint of left hand
✓7th S63.053 Subluxation of other carpometacarpal joint of unspecified hand
✓7th S63.054 Dislocation of other carpometacarpal joint of right hand
✓7th S63.055 Dislocation of other carpometacarpal joint of left hand
✓7th S63.056 Dislocation of other carpometacarpal joint of unspecified hand
✓6th S63.06 Subluxation and dislocation of metacarpal (bone), proximal end
✓7th S63.061 Subluxation of metacarpal (bone), proximal end of right hand
✓7th S63.062 Subluxation of metacarpal (bone), proximal end of left hand
✓7th S63.063 Subluxation of metacarpal (bone), proximal end of unspecified hand
✓7th S63.064 Dislocation of metacarpal (bone), proximal end of right hand
✓7th S63.065 Dislocation of metacarpal (bone), proximal end of left hand
✓7th S63.066 Dislocation of metacarpal (bone), proximal end of unspecified hand
✓6th S63.07 Subluxation and dislocation of distal end of ulna
✓7th S63.071 Subluxation of distal end of right ulna
✓7th S63.072 Subluxation of distal end of left ulna
✓7th S63.073 Subluxation of distal end of unspecified ulna
✓7th S63.074 Dislocation of distal end of right ulna
✓7th S63.075 Dislocation of distal end of left ulna
✓7th S63.076 Dislocation of distal end of unspecified ulna
✓6th S63.09 Other subluxation and dislocation of wrist and hand
✓7th S63.091 Other subluxation of right wrist and hand
✓7th S63.092 Other subluxation of left wrist and hand
✓7th S63.093 Other subluxation of unspecified wrist and hand
✓7th S63.094 Other dislocation of right wrist and hand
✓7th S63.095 Other dislocation of left wrist and hand
✓7th S63.096 Other dislocation of unspecified wrist and hand
✓5th S63.1 Subluxation and dislocation of thumb
✓6th S63.10 Unspecified subluxation and dislocation of thumb
✓7th S63.101 Unspecified subluxation of right thumb
✓7th S63.102 Unspecified subluxation of left thumb
✓7th S63.103 Unspecified subluxation of unspecified thumb
✓7th S63.104 Unspecified dislocation of right thumb
✓7th S63.105 Unspecified dislocation of left thumb
✓7th S63.106 Unspecified dislocation of unspecified thumb
✓6th S63.11 Subluxation and dislocation of metacarpophalangeal joint of thumb
✓7th S63.111 Subluxation of metacarpophalangeal joint of right thumb
✓7th S63.112 Subluxation of metacarpophalangeal joint of left thumb
✓7th S63.113 Subluxation of metacarpophalangeal joint of unspecified thumb
✓7th S63.114 Dislocation of metacarpophalangeal joint of right thumb
✓7th S63.115 Dislocation of metacarpophalangeal joint of left thumb
✓7th S63.116 Dislocation of metacarpophalangeal joint of unspecified thumb
✓6th S63.12 Subluxation and dislocation of interphalangeal joint of thumb
✓7th S63.121 Subluxation of interphalangeal joint of right thumb
✓7th S63.122 Subluxation of interphalangeal joint of left thumb
✓7th S63.123 Subluxation of interphalangeal joint of unspecified thumb
✓7th S63.124 Dislocation of interphalangeal joint of right thumb
✓7th S63.125 Dislocation of interphalangeal joint of left thumb
✓7th S63.126 Dislocation of interphalangeal joint of unspecified thumb
✓5th S63.2 Subluxation and dislocation of other finger(s)
EXCLUDES 2 subluxation and dislocation of thumb (S63.1-)
✓6th S63.20 Unspecified subluxation of other finger
✓7th S63.200 Unspecified subluxation of right index finger
✓7th S63.201 Unspecified subluxation of left index finger
✓7th S63.202 Unspecified subluxation of right middle finger
✓7th S63.203 Unspecified subluxation of left middle finger
✓7th S63.204 Unspecified subluxation of right ring finger
✓7th S63.205 Unspecified subluxation of left ring finger
✓7th S63.206 Unspecified subluxation of right little finger
✓7th S63.207 Unspecified subluxation of left little finger
✓7th S63.208 Unspecified subluxation of other finger
Unspecified subluxation of specified finger with unspecified laterality
✓7th S63.209 Unspecified subluxation of unspecified finger
✓6th S63.21 Subluxation of metacarpophalangeal joint of finger
✓7th S63.210 Subluxation of metacarpophalangeal joint of right index finger
✓7th S63.211 Subluxation of metacarpophalangeal joint of left index finger
✓7th S63.212 Subluxation of metacarpophalangeal joint of right middle finger
✓7th S63.213 Subluxation of metacarpophalangeal joint of left middle finger
✓7th S63.214 Subluxation of metacarpophalangeal joint of right ring finger
✓7th S63.215 Subluxation of metacarpophalangeal joint of left ring finger
✓7th S63.216 Subluxation of metacarpophalangeal joint of right little finger
✓7th S63.217 Subluxation of metacarpophalangeal joint of left little finger
✓7th S63.218 Subluxation of metacarpophalangeal joint of other finger
Subluxation of metacarpophalangeal joint of specified finger with unspecified laterality
✓7th S63.219 Subluxation of metacarpophalangeal joint of unspecified finger
✓6th S63.22 Subluxation of unspecified interphalangeal joint of finger
✓7th S63.220 Subluxation of unspecified interphalangeal joint of right index finger
✓7th S63.221 Subluxation of unspecified interphalangeal joint of left index finger
✓7th S63.222 Subluxation of unspecified interphalangeal joint of right middle finger
✓7th S63.223 Subluxation of unspecified interphalangeal joint of left middle finger

√7th **S63.224 Subluxation of unspecified interphalangeal joint of right ring finger**

√7th **S63.225 Subluxation of unspecified interphalangeal joint of left ring finger**

√7th **S63.226 Subluxation of unspecified interphalangeal joint of right little finger**

√7th **S63.227 Subluxation of unspecified interphalangeal joint of left little finger**

√7th **S63.228 Subluxation of unspecified interphalangeal joint of other finger**

Subluxation of unspecified interphalangeal joint of specified finger with unspecified laterality

√7th **S63.229 Subluxation of unspecified interphalangeal joint of unspecified finger**

√6th **S63.23 Subluxation of proximal interphalangeal joint of finger**

√7th **S63.230 Subluxation of proximal interphalangeal joint of right index finger**

√7th **S63.231 Subluxation of proximal interphalangeal joint of left index finger**

√7th **S63.232 Subluxation of proximal interphalangeal joint of right middle finger**

√7th **S63.233 Subluxation of proximal interphalangeal joint of left middle finger**

√7th **S63.234 Subluxation of proximal interphalangeal joint of right ring finger**

√7th **S63.235 Subluxation of proximal interphalangeal joint of left ring finger**

√7th **S63.236 Subluxation of proximal interphalangeal joint of right little finger**

√7th **S63.237 Subluxation of proximal interphalangeal joint of left little finger**

√7th **S63.238 Subluxation of proximal interphalangeal joint of other finger**

Subluxation of proximal interphalangeal joint of specified finger with unspecified laterality

√7th **S63.239 Subluxation of proximal interphalangeal joint of unspecified finger**

√6th **S63.24 Subluxation of distal interphalangeal joint of finger**

√7th **S63.240 Subluxation of distal interphalangeal joint of right index finger**

√7th **S63.241 Subluxation of distal interphalangeal joint of left index finger**

√7th **S63.242 Subluxation of distal interphalangeal joint of right middle finger**

√7th **S63.243 Subluxation of distal interphalangeal joint of left middle finger**

√7th **S63.244 Subluxation of distal interphalangeal joint of right ring finger**

√7th **S63.245 Subluxation of distal interphalangeal joint of left ring finger**

√7th **S63.246 Subluxation of distal interphalangeal joint of right little finger**

√7th **S63.247 Subluxation of distal interphalangeal joint of left little finger**

√7th **S63.248 Subluxation of distal interphalangeal joint of other finger**

Subluxation of distal interphalangeal joint of specified finger with unspecified laterality

√7th **S63.249 Subluxation of distal interphalangeal joint of unspecified finger**

√6th **S63.25 Unspecified dislocation of other finger**

√7th **S63.250 Unspecified dislocation of right index finger**

√7th **S63.251 Unspecified dislocation of left index finger**

√7th **S63.252 Unspecified dislocation of right middle finger**

√7th **S63.253 Unspecified dislocation of left middle finger**

√7th **S63.254 Unspecified dislocation of right ring finger**

√7th **S63.255 Unspecified dislocation of left ring finger**

√7th **S63.256 Unspecified dislocation of right little finger**

√7th **S63.257 Unspecified dislocation of left little finger**

√7th **S63.258 Unspecified dislocation of other finger**

Unspecified dislocation of specified finger with unspecified laterality

√7th **S63.259 Unspecified dislocation of unspecified finger**

Unspecified dislocation of unspecified finger with unspecified laterality

√6th **S63.26 Dislocation of metacarpophalangeal joint of finger**

√7th **S63.260 Dislocation of metacarpophalangeal joint of right index finger**

√7th **S63.261 Dislocation of metacarpophalangeal joint of left index finger**

√7th **S63.262 Dislocation of metacarpophalangeal joint of right middle finger**

√7th **S63.263 Dislocation of metacarpophalangeal joint of left middle finger**

√7th **S63.264 Dislocation of metacarpophalangeal joint of right ring finger**

√7th **S63.265 Dislocation of metacarpophalangeal joint of left ring finger**

√7th **S63.266 Dislocation of metacarpophalangeal joint of right little finger**

√7th **S63.267 Dislocation of metacarpophalangeal joint of left little finger**

√7th **S63.268 Dislocation of metacarpophalangeal joint of other finger**

Dislocation of metacarpophalangeal joint of specified finger with unspecified laterality

√7th **S63.269 Dislocation of metacarpophalangeal joint of unspecified finger**

√6th **S63.27 Dislocation of unspecified interphalangeal joint of finger**

√7th **S63.270 Dislocation of unspecified interphalangeal joint of right index finger**

√7th **S63.271 Dislocation of unspecified interphalangeal joint of left index finger**

√7th **S63.272 Dislocation of unspecified interphalangeal joint of right middle finger**

√7th **S63.273 Dislocation of unspecified interphalangeal joint of left middle finger**

√7th **S63.274 Dislocation of unspecified interphalangeal joint of right ring finger**

√7th **S63.275 Dislocation of unspecified interphalangeal joint of left ring finger**

√7th **S63.276 Dislocation of unspecified interphalangeal joint of right little finger**

√7th **S63.277 Dislocation of unspecified interphalangeal joint of left little finger**

√7th **S63.278 Dislocation of unspecified interphalangeal joint of other finger**

Dislocation of unspecified interphalangeal joint of specified finger with unspecified laterality

√7th **S63.279 Dislocation of unspecified interphalangeal joint of unspecified finger**

Dislocation of unspecified interphalangeal joint of unspecified finger without specified laterality

√6th **S63.28 Dislocation of proximal interphalangeal joint of finger**

√7th **S63.280 Dislocation of proximal interphalangeal joint of right index finger**

√7th **S63.281 Dislocation of proximal interphalangeal joint of left index finger**

√7th **S63.282 Dislocation of proximal interphalangeal joint of right middle finger**

√7th **S63.283 Dislocation of proximal interphalangeal joint of left middle finger**

√7th **S63.284 Dislocation of proximal interphalangeal joint of right ring finger**

√7th **S63.285 Dislocation of proximal interphalangeal joint of left ring finger**

√7th **S63.286 Dislocation of proximal interphalangeal joint of right little finger**

√7th **S63.287 Dislocation of proximal interphalangeal joint of left little finger**

- S63.288 **Dislocation of proximal interphalangeal joint of other finger**
  Dislocation of proximal interphalangeal joint of specified finger with unspecified laterality
- S63.289 **Dislocation of proximal interphalangeal joint of unspecified finger**

S63.29 **Dislocation of distal interphalangeal joint of finger**
- S63.290 **Dislocation of distal interphalangeal joint of right index finger**
- S63.291 **Dislocation of distal interphalangeal joint of left index finger**
- S63.292 **Dislocation of distal interphalangeal joint of right middle finger**
- S63.293 **Dislocation of distal interphalangeal joint of left middle finger**
- S63.294 **Dislocation of distal interphalangeal joint of right ring finger**
- S63.295 **Dislocation of distal interphalangeal joint of left ring finger**
- S63.296 **Dislocation of distal interphalangeal joint of right little finger**
- S63.297 **Dislocation of distal interphalangeal joint of left little finger**
- S63.298 **Dislocation of distal interphalangeal joint of other finger**
  Dislocation of distal interphalangeal joint of specified finger with unspecified laterality
- S63.299 **Dislocation of distal interphalangeal joint of unspecified finger**

S63.3 **Traumatic rupture of ligament of wrist**

S63.30 **Traumatic rupture of unspecified ligament of wrist**
- S63.301 **Traumatic rupture of unspecified ligament of right wrist**
- S63.302 **Traumatic rupture of unspecified ligament of left wrist**
- S63.309 **Traumatic rupture of unspecified ligament of unspecified wrist**

S63.31 **Traumatic rupture of collateral ligament of wrist**
- S63.311 **Traumatic rupture of collateral ligament of right wrist**
- S63.312 **Traumatic rupture of collateral ligament of left wrist**
- S63.319 **Traumatic rupture of collateral ligament of unspecified wrist**

S63.32 **Traumatic rupture of radiocarpal ligament**
- S63.321 **Traumatic rupture of right radiocarpal ligament**
- S63.322 **Traumatic rupture of left radiocarpal ligament**
- S63.329 **Traumatic rupture of unspecified radiocarpal ligament**

S63.33 **Traumatic rupture of ulnocarpal (palmar) ligament**
- S63.331 **Traumatic rupture of right ulnocarpal (palmar) ligament**
- S63.332 **Traumatic rupture of left ulnocarpal (palmar) ligament**
- S63.339 **Traumatic rupture of unspecified ulnocarpal (palmar) ligament**

S63.39 **Traumatic rupture of other ligament of wrist**
- S63.391 **Traumatic rupture of other ligament of right wrist**
- S63.392 **Traumatic rupture of other ligament of left wrist**
- S63.399 **Traumatic rupture of other ligament of unspecified wrist**

S63.4 **Traumatic rupture of ligament of finger at metacarpophalangeal and interphalangeal joint(s)**

S63.40 **Traumatic rupture of unspecified ligament of finger at metacarpophalangeal and interphalangeal joint**
- S63.400 **Traumatic rupture of unspecified ligament of right index finger at metacarpophalangeal and interphalangeal joint**
- S63.401 **Traumatic rupture of unspecified ligament of left index finger at metacarpophalangeal and interphalangeal joint**
- S63.402 **Traumatic rupture of unspecified ligament of right middle finger at metacarpophalangeal and interphalangeal joint**
- S63.403 **Traumatic rupture of unspecified ligament of left middle finger at metacarpophalangeal and interphalangeal joint**
- S63.404 **Traumatic rupture of unspecified ligament of right ring finger at metacarpophalangeal and interphalangeal joint**
- S63.405 **Traumatic rupture of unspecified ligament of left ring finger at metacarpophalangeal and interphalangeal joint**
- S63.406 **Traumatic rupture of unspecified ligament of right little finger at metacarpophalangeal and interphalangeal joint**
- S63.407 **Traumatic rupture of unspecified ligament of left little finger at metacarpophalangeal and interphalangeal joint**
- S63.408 **Traumatic rupture of unspecified ligament of other finger at metacarpophalangeal and interphalangeal joint**
  Traumatic rupture of unspecified ligament of specified finger with unspecified laterality at metacarpophalangeal and interphalangeal joint
- S63.409 **Traumatic rupture of unspecified ligament of unspecified finger at metacarpophalangeal and interphalangeal joint**

S63.41 **Traumatic rupture of collateral ligament of finger at metacarpophalangeal and interphalangeal joint**
- S63.410 **Traumatic rupture of collateral ligament of right index finger at metacarpophalangeal and interphalangeal joint**
- S63.411 **Traumatic rupture of collateral ligament of left index finger at metacarpophalangeal and interphalangeal joint**
- S63.412 **Traumatic rupture of collateral ligament of right middle finger at metacarpophalangeal and interphalangeal joint**
- S63.413 **Traumatic rupture of collateral ligament of left middle finger at metacarpophalangeal and interphalangeal joint**
- S63.414 **Traumatic rupture of collateral ligament of right ring finger at metacarpophalangeal and interphalangeal joint**
- S63.415 **Traumatic rupture of collateral ligament of left ring finger at metacarpophalangeal and interphalangeal joint**
- S63.416 **Traumatic rupture of collateral ligament of right little finger at metacarpophalangeal and interphalangeal joint**
- S63.417 **Traumatic rupture of collateral ligament of left little finger at metacarpophalangeal and interphalangeal joint**
- S63.418 **Traumatic rupture of collateral ligament of other finger at metacarpophalangeal and interphalangeal joint**
  Traumatic rupture of collateral ligament of specified finger with unspecified laterality at metacarpophalangeal and interphalangeal joint
- S63.419 **Traumatic rupture of collateral ligament of unspecified finger at metacarpophalangeal and interphalangeal joint**

6th S63.42 Traumatic rupture of palmar ligament of finger at metacarpophalangeal and interphalangeal joint

7th S63.420 Traumatic rupture of palmar ligament of right index finger at metacarpophalangeal and interphalangeal joint

7th S63.421 Traumatic rupture of palmar ligament of left index finger at metacarpophalangeal and interphalangeal joint

7th S63.422 Traumatic rupture of palmar ligament of right middle finger at metacarpophalangeal and interphalangeal joint

7th S63.423 Traumatic rupture of palmar ligament of left middle finger at metacarpophalangeal and interphalangeal joint

7th S63.424 Traumatic rupture of palmar ligament of right ring finger at metacarpophalangeal and interphalangeal joint

7th S63.425 Traumatic rupture of palmar ligament of left ring finger at metacarpophalangeal and interphalangeal joint

7th S63.426 Traumatic rupture of palmar ligament of right little finger at metacarpophalangeal and interphalangeal joint

7th S63.427 Traumatic rupture of palmar ligament of left little finger at metacarpophalangeal and interphalangeal joint

7th S63.428 Traumatic rupture of palmar ligament of other finger at metacarpophalangeal and interphalangeal joint
Traumatic rupture of palmar ligament of specified finger with unspecified laterality at metacarpophalangeal and interphalangeal joint

7th S63.429 Traumatic rupture of palmar ligament of unspecified finger at metacarpophalangeal and interphalangeal joint

6th S63.43 Traumatic rupture of volar plate of finger at metacarpophalangeal and interphalangeal joint

7th S63.430 Traumatic rupture of volar plate of right index finger at metacarpophalangeal and interphalangeal joint

7th S63.431 Traumatic rupture of volar plate of left index finger at metacarpophalangeal and interphalangeal joint

7th S63.432 Traumatic rupture of volar plate of right middle finger at metacarpophalangeal and interphalangeal joint

7th S63.433 Traumatic rupture of volar plate of left middle finger at metacarpophalangeal and interphalangeal joint

7th S63.434 Traumatic rupture of volar plate of right ring finger at metacarpophalangeal and interphalangeal joint

7th S63.435 Traumatic rupture of volar plate of left ring finger at metacarpophalangeal and interphalangeal joint

7th S63.436 Traumatic rupture of volar plate of right little finger at metacarpophalangeal and interphalangeal joint

7th S63.437 Traumatic rupture of volar plate of left little finger at metacarpophalangeal and interphalangeal joint

7th S63.438 Traumatic rupture of volar plate of other finger at metacarpophalangeal and interphalangeal joint
Traumatic rupture of volar plate of specified finger with unspecified laterality at metacarpophalangeal and interphalangeal joint

7th S63.439 Traumatic rupture of volar plate of unspecified finger at metacarpophalangeal and interphalangeal joint

6th S63.49 Traumatic rupture of other ligament of finger at metacarpophalangeal and interphalangeal joint

7th S63.490 Traumatic rupture of other ligament of right index finger at metacarpophalangeal and interphalangeal joint

7th S63.491 Traumatic rupture of other ligament of left index finger at metacarpophalangeal and interphalangeal joint

7th S63.492 Traumatic rupture of other ligament of right middle finger at metacarpophalangeal and interphalangeal joint

7th S63.493 Traumatic rupture of other ligament of left middle finger at metacarpophalangeal and interphalangeal joint

7th S63.494 Traumatic rupture of other ligament of right ring finger at metacarpophalangeal and interphalangeal joint

7th S63.495 Traumatic rupture of other ligament of left ring finger at metacarpophalangeal and interphalangeal joint

7th S63.496 Traumatic rupture of other ligament of right little finger at metacarpophalangeal and interphalangeal joint

7th S63.497 Traumatic rupture of other ligament of left little finger at metacarpophalangeal and interphalangeal joint

7th S63.498 Traumatic rupture of other ligament of other finger at metacarpophalangeal and interphalangeal joint
Traumatic rupture of ligament of specified finger with unspecified laterality at metacarpophalangeal and interphalangeal joint

7th S63.499 Traumatic rupture of other ligament of unspecified finger at metacarpophalangeal and interphalangeal joint

5th S63.5 Other and unspecified sprain of wrist

6th S63.50 Unspecified sprain of wrist

7th S63.501 Unspecified sprain of right wrist

7th S63.502 Unspecified sprain of left wrist

7th S63.509 Unspecified sprain of unspecified wrist

6th S63.51 Sprain of carpal (joint)

7th S63.511 Sprain of carpal joint of right wrist

7th S63.512 Sprain of carpal joint of left wrist

7th S63.519 Sprain of carpal joint of unspecified wrist

6th S63.52 Sprain of radiocarpal joint

EXCLUDES 1 *traumatic rupture of radiocarpal ligament (S63.32-)*

7th S63.521 Sprain of radiocarpal joint of right wrist

7th S63.522 Sprain of radiocarpal joint of left wrist

7th S63.529 Sprain of radiocarpal joint of unspecified wrist

6th S63.59 Other specified sprain of wrist

7th S63.591 Other specified sprain of right wrist

7th S63.592 Other specified sprain of left wrist

7th S63.599 Other specified sprain of unspecified wrist

5th S63.6 Other and unspecified sprain of finger(s)

EXCLUDES 1 *traumatic rupture of ligament of finger at metacarpophalangeal and interphalangeal joint(s) (S63.4-)*

6th S63.60 Unspecified sprain of thumb

7th S63.601 Unspecified sprain of right thumb

7th S63.602 Unspecified sprain of left thumb

7th S63.609 Unspecified sprain of unspecified thumb

6th S63.61 Unspecified sprain of other and unspecified finger(s)

7th S63.610 Unspecified sprain of right index finger

7th S63.611 Unspecified sprain of left index finger

7th S63.612 Unspecified sprain of right middle finger

7th S63.613 Unspecified sprain of left middle finger

7th S63.614 Unspecified sprain of right ring finger

7th S63.615 Unspecified sprain of left ring finger

7th S63.616 Unspecified sprain of right little finger

7th S63.617 Unspecified sprain of left little finger

S63.618 Unspecified sprain of other finger
Unspecified sprain of specified finger with unspecified laterality

S63.619 Unspecified sprain of unspecified finger

S63.62 Sprain of interphalangeal joint of thumb

S63.621 Sprain of interphalangeal joint of right thumb

S63.622 Sprain of interphalangeal joint of left thumb

S63.629 Sprain of interphalangeal joint of unspecified thumb

S63.63 Sprain of interphalangeal joint of other and unspecified finger(s)

S63.630 Sprain of interphalangeal joint of right index finger

S63.631 Sprain of interphalangeal joint of left index finger

S63.632 Sprain of interphalangeal joint of right middle finger

S63.633 Sprain of interphalangeal joint of left middle finger

S63.634 Sprain of interphalangeal joint of right ring finger

S63.635 Sprain of interphalangeal joint of left ring finger

S63.636 Sprain of interphalangeal joint of right little finger

S63.637 Sprain of interphalangeal joint of left little finger

S63.638 Sprain of interphalangeal joint of other finger

S63.639 Sprain of interphalangeal joint of unspecified finger

S63.64 Sprain of metacarpophalangeal joint of thumb

S63.641 Sprain of metacarpophalangeal joint of right thumb

S63.642 Sprain of metacarpophalangeal joint of left thumb

S63.649 Sprain of metacarpophalangeal joint of unspecified thumb

S63.65 Sprain of metacarpophalangeal joint of other and unspecified finger(s)

S63.650 Sprain of metacarpophalangeal joint of right index finger

S63.651 Sprain of metacarpophalangeal joint of left index finger

S63.652 Sprain of metacarpophalangeal joint of right middle finger

S63.653 Sprain of metacarpophalangeal joint of left middle finger

S63.654 Sprain of metacarpophalangeal joint of right ring finger

S63.655 Sprain of metacarpophalangeal joint of left ring finger

S63.656 Sprain of metacarpophalangeal joint of right little finger

S63.657 Sprain of metacarpophalangeal joint of left little finger

S63.658 Sprain of metacarpophalangeal joint of other finger
Sprain of metacarpophalangeal joint of specified finger with unspecified laterality

S63.659 Sprain of metacarpophalangeal joint of unspecified finger

S63.68 Other sprain of thumb

S63.681 Other sprain of right thumb

S63.682 Other sprain of left thumb

S63.689 Other sprain of unspecified thumb

S63.69 Other sprain of other and unspecified finger(s)

S63.690 Other sprain of right index finger

S63.691 Other sprain of left index finger

S63.692 Other sprain of right middle finger

S63.693 Other sprain of left middle finger

S63.694 Other sprain of right ring finger

S63.695 Other sprain of left ring finger

S63.696 Other sprain of right little finger

S63.697 Other sprain of left little finger

S63.698 Other sprain of other finger
Other sprain of specified finger with unspecified laterality

S63.699 Other sprain of unspecified finger

S63.8 Sprain of other part of wrist and hand

S63.8X Sprain of other part of wrist and hand

S63.8X1 Sprain of other part of right wrist and hand

S63.8X2 Sprain of other part of left wrist and hand

S63.8X9 Sprain of other part of unspecified wrist and hand

S63.9 Sprain of unspecified part of wrist and hand

S63.90 Sprain of unspecified part of unspecified wrist and hand

S63.91 Sprain of unspecified part of right wrist and hand

S63.92 Sprain of unspecified part of left wrist and hand

S64 Injury of nerves at wrist and hand level

Code also any associated open wound (S61.-)

The appropriate 7th character is to be added to each code from category S64.
A initial encounter
D subsequent encounter
S sequela

S64.0 Injury of ulnar nerve at wrist and hand level

S64.00 Injury of ulnar nerve at wrist and hand level of unspecified arm

S64.01 Injury of ulnar nerve at wrist and hand level of right arm

S64.02 Injury of ulnar nerve at wrist and hand level of left arm

S64.1 Injury of median nerve at wrist and hand level

S64.10 Injury of median nerve at wrist and hand level of unspecified arm

S64.11 Injury of median nerve at wrist and hand level of right arm

S64.12 Injury of median nerve at wrist and hand level of left arm

S64.2 Injury of radial nerve at wrist and hand level

S64.20 Injury of radial nerve at wrist and hand level of unspecified arm

S64.21 Injury of radial nerve at wrist and hand level of right arm

S64.22 Injury of radial nerve at wrist and hand level of left arm

S64.3 Injury of digital nerve of thumb

S64.30 Injury of digital nerve of unspecified thumb

S64.31 Injury of digital nerve of right thumb

S64.32 Injury of digital nerve of left thumb

S64.4 Injury of digital nerve of other and unspecified finger

S64.40 Injury of digital nerve of unspecified finger

S64.49 Injury of digital nerve of other finger

S64.490 Injury of digital nerve of right index finger

S64.491 Injury of digital nerve of left index finger

S64.492 Injury of digital nerve of right middle finger

S64.493 Injury of digital nerve of left middle finger

S64.494 Injury of digital nerve of right ring finger

S64.495 Injury of digital nerve of left ring finger

S64.496 Injury of digital nerve of right little finger

S64.497 Injury of digital nerve of left little finger

S64.498 Injury of digital nerve of other finger
Injury of digital nerve of specified finger with unspecified laterality

S64.8 Injury of other nerves at wrist and hand level

S64.8X Injury of other nerves at wrist and hand level

S64.8X1 Injury of other nerves at wrist and hand level of right arm

S64.8X2 Injury of other nerves at wrist and hand level of left arm

S64.8X9 Injury of other nerves at wrist and hand level of unspecified arm

- 5th S64.9 Injury of unspecified nerve at wrist and hand level
  - x7th S64.90 Injury of unspecified nerve at wrist and hand level of unspecified arm
  - x7th S64.91 Injury of unspecified nerve at wrist and hand level of right arm
  - x7th S64.92 Injury of unspecified nerve at wrist and hand level of left arm

4th S65 Injury of blood vessels at wrist and hand level

Code also any associated open wound (S61.-)

The appropriate 7th character is to be added to each code from category S65.
A initial encounter
D subsequent encounter
S sequela

- 5th S65.0 Injury of ulnar artery at wrist and hand level
  - 6th S65.00 Unspecified injury of ulnar artery at wrist and hand level
    - 7th S65.001 Unspecified injury of ulnar artery at wrist and hand level of right arm CC
    - 7th S65.002 Unspecified injury of ulnar artery at wrist and hand level of left arm CC
    - 7th S65.009 Unspecified injury of ulnar artery at wrist and hand level of unspecified arm CC UNS
  - 6th S65.01 Laceration of ulnar artery at wrist and hand level
    - 7th S65.011 Laceration of ulnar artery at wrist and hand level of right arm CC
    - 7th S65.012 Laceration of ulnar artery at wrist and hand level of left arm CC
    - 7th S65.019 Laceration of ulnar artery at wrist and hand level of unspecified arm CC UNS
  - 6th S65.09 Other specified injury of ulnar artery at wrist and hand level
    - 7th S65.091 Other specified injury of ulnar artery at wrist and hand level of right arm CC
    - 7th S65.092 Other specified injury of ulnar artery at wrist and hand level of left arm CC
    - 7th S65.099 Other specified injury of ulnar artery at wrist and hand level of unspecified arm CC UNS
- 5th S65.1 Injury of radial artery at wrist and hand level
  - 6th S65.10 Unspecified injury of radial artery at wrist and hand level
    - 7th S65.101 Unspecified injury of radial artery at wrist and hand level of right arm CC
    - 7th S65.102 Unspecified injury of radial artery at wrist and hand level of left arm CC
    - 7th S65.109 Unspecified injury of radial artery at wrist and hand level of unspecified arm CC UNS
  - 6th S65.11 Laceration of radial artery at wrist and hand level
    - 7th S65.111 Laceration of radial artery at wrist and hand level of right arm CC
    - 7th S65.112 Laceration of radial artery at wrist and hand level of left arm CC
    - 7th S65.119 Laceration of radial artery at wrist and hand level of unspecified arm CC UNS
  - 6th S65.19 Other specified injury of radial artery at wrist and hand level
    - 7th S65.191 Other specified injury of radial artery at wrist and hand level of right arm CC
    - 7th S65.192 Other specified injury of radial artery at wrist and hand level of left arm CC
    - 7th S65.199 Other specified injury of radial artery at wrist and hand level of unspecified arm CC UNS
- 5th S65.2 Injury of superficial palmar arch
  - 6th S65.20 Unspecified injury of superficial palmar arch
    - 7th S65.201 Unspecified injury of superficial palmar arch of right hand CC
    - 7th S65.202 Unspecified injury of superficial palmar arch of left hand CC
    - 7th S65.209 Unspecified injury of superficial palmar arch of unspecified hand CC UNS
  - 6th S65.21 Laceration of superficial palmar arch
    - 7th S65.211 Laceration of superficial palmar arch of right hand CC
    - 7th S65.212 Laceration of superficial palmar arch of left hand CC
    - 7th S65.219 Laceration of superficial palmar arch of unspecified hand CC UNS
  - 6th S65.29 Other specified injury of superficial palmar arch
    - 7th S65.291 Other specified injury of superficial palmar arch of right hand CC
    - 7th S65.292 Other specified injury of superficial palmar arch of left hand CC
    - 7th S65.299 Other specified injury of superficial palmar arch of unspecified hand CC UNS
- 5th S65.3 Injury of deep palmar arch
  - 6th S65.30 Unspecified injury of deep palmar arch
    - 7th S65.301 Unspecified injury of deep palmar arch of right hand CC
    - 7th S65.302 Unspecified injury of deep palmar arch of left hand CC
    - 7th S65.309 Unspecified injury of deep palmar arch of unspecified hand CC UNS
  - 6th S65.31 Laceration of deep palmar arch
    - 7th S65.311 Laceration of deep palmar arch of right hand CC
    - 7th S65.312 Laceration of deep palmar arch of left hand CC
    - 7th S65.319 Laceration of deep palmar arch of unspecified hand CC UNS
  - 6th S65.39 Other specified injury of deep palmar arch
    - 7th S65.391 Other specified injury of deep palmar arch of right hand CC
    - 7th S65.392 Other specified injury of deep palmar arch of left hand CC
    - 7th S65.399 Other specified injury of deep palmar arch of unspecified hand CC UNS
- 5th S65.4 Injury of blood vessel of thumb
  - 6th S65.40 Unspecified injury of blood vessel of thumb
    - 7th S65.401 Unspecified injury of blood vessel of right thumb CC
    - 7th S65.402 Unspecified injury of blood vessel of left thumb CC
    - 7th S65.409 Unspecified injury of blood vessel of unspecified thumb CC UNS
  - 6th S65.41 Laceration of blood vessel of thumb
    - 7th S65.411 Laceration of blood vessel of right thumb CC
    - 7th S65.412 Laceration of blood vessel of left thumb CC
    - 7th S65.419 Laceration of blood vessel of unspecified thumb CC UNS
  - 6th S65.49 Other specified injury of blood vessel of thumb
    - 7th S65.491 Other specified injury of blood vessel of right thumb CC
    - 7th S65.492 Other specified injury of blood vessel of left thumb CC
    - 7th S65.499 Other specified injury of blood vessel of unspecified thumb CC UNS
- 5th S65.5 Injury of blood vessel of other and unspecified finger
  - 6th S65.50 Unspecified injury of blood vessel of other and unspecified finger
    - 7th S65.500 Unspecified injury of blood vessel of right index finger CC
    - 7th S65.501 Unspecified injury of blood vessel of left index finger CC
    - 7th S65.502 Unspecified injury of blood vessel of right middle finger CC
    - 7th S65.503 Unspecified injury of blood vessel of left middle finger CC
    - 7th S65.504 Unspecified injury of blood vessel of right ring finger CC
    - 7th S65.505 Unspecified injury of blood vessel of left ring finger CC
    - 7th S65.506 Unspecified injury of blood vessel of right little finger CC
    - 7th S65.507 Unspecified injury of blood vessel of left little finger CC

√7th **S65.5Ø8 Unspecified injury of blood vessel of other finger** CC UNS
Unspecified injury of blood vessel of specified finger with unspecified laterality

√7th **S65.5Ø9 Unspecified injury of blood vessel of unspecified finger** CC UNS

√6th **S65.51 Laceration of blood vessel of other and unspecified finger**

√7th **S65.51Ø Laceration of blood vessel of right index finger** CC

√7th **S65.511 Laceration of blood vessel of left index finger** CC

√7th **S65.512 Laceration of blood vessel of right middle finger** CC

√7th **S65.513 Laceration of blood vessel of left middle finger** CC

√7th **S65.514 Laceration of blood vessel of right ring finger** CC

√7th **S65.515 Laceration of blood vessel of left ring finger** CC

√7th **S65.516 Laceration of blood vessel of right little finger** CC

√7th **S65.517 Laceration of blood vessel of left little finger** CC

√7th **S65.518 Laceration of blood vessel of other finger** CC
Laceration of blood vessel of specified finger with unspecified laterality

√7th **S65.519 Laceration of blood vessel of unspecified finger** CC UNS

√6th **S65.59 Other specified injury of blood vessel of other and unspecified finger**

√7th **S65.59Ø Other specified injury of blood vessel of right index finger** CC

√7th **S65.591 Other specified injury of blood vessel of left index finger** CC

√7th **S65.592 Other specified injury of blood vessel of right middle finger** CC

√7th **S65.593 Other specified injury of blood vessel of left middle finger** CC

√7th **S65.594 Other specified injury of blood vessel of right ring finger** CC

√7th **S65.595 Other specified injury of blood vessel of left ring finger** CC

√7th **S65.596 Other specified injury of blood vessel of right little finger** CC

√7th **S65.597 Other specified injury of blood vessel of left little finger** CC

√7th **S65.598 Other specified injury of blood vessel of other finger** CC
Other specified injury of blood vessel of specified finger with unspecified laterality

√7th **S65.599 Other specified injury of blood vessel of unspecified finger** CC UNS

√5th **S65.8 Injury of other blood vessels at wrist and hand level**

√6th **S65.8Ø Unspecified injury of other blood vessels at wrist and hand level**

√7th **S65.8Ø1 Unspecified injury of other blood vessels at wrist and hand level of right arm** CC

√7th **S65.8Ø2 Unspecified injury of other blood vessels at wrist and hand level of left arm** CC

√7th **S65.8Ø9 Unspecified injury of other blood vessels at wrist and hand level of unspecified arm** CC UNS

√6th **S65.81 Laceration of other blood vessels at wrist and hand level**

√7th **S65.811 Laceration of other blood vessels at wrist and hand level of right arm** CC

√7th **S65.812 Laceration of other blood vessels at wrist and hand level of left arm** CC

√7th **S65.819 Laceration of other blood vessels at wrist and hand level of unspecified arm** CC UNS

√6th **S65.89 Other specified injury of other blood vessels at wrist and hand level**

√7th **S65.891 Other specified injury of other blood vessels at wrist and hand level of right arm** CC

√7th **S65.892 Other specified injury of other blood vessels at wrist and hand level of left arm** CC

√7th **S65.899 Other specified injury of other blood vessels at wrist and hand level of unspecified arm** CC UNS

√5th **S65.9 Injury of unspecified blood vessel at wrist and hand level**

√6th **S65.9Ø Unspecified injury of unspecified blood vessel at wrist and hand level**

√7th **S65.9Ø1 Unspecified injury of unspecified blood vessel at wrist and hand level of right arm** CC

√7th **S65.9Ø2 Unspecified injury of unspecified blood vessel at wrist and hand level of left arm** CC

√7th **S65.9Ø9 Unspecified injury of unspecified blood vessel at wrist and hand level of unspecified arm** CC UNS

√6th **S65.91 Laceration of unspecified blood vessel at wrist and hand level**

√7th **S65.911 Laceration of unspecified blood vessel at wrist and hand level of right arm** CC

√7th **S65.912 Laceration of unspecified blood vessel at wrist and hand level of left arm** CC

√7th **S65.919 Laceration of unspecified blood vessel at wrist and hand level of unspecified arm** CC UNS

√6th **S65.99 Other specified injury of unspecified blood vessel at wrist and hand level**

√7th **S65.991 Other specified injury of unspecified blood vessel at wrist and hand of right arm** CC

√7th **S65.992 Other specified injury of unspecified blood vessel at wrist and hand of left arm** CC

√7th **S65.999 Other specified injury of unspecified blood vessel at wrist and hand of unspecified arm** CC UNS

√4th **S66 Injury of muscle, fascia and tendon at wrist and hand level**

Code also any associated open wound (S61.-)

EXCLUDES 2 *sprain of joints and ligaments of wrist and hand (S63.-)*

TIP: Refer to the Muscle/Tendon table at the beginning of this chapter.

The appropriate 7th character is to be added to each code from category S66.
A initial encounter
D subsequent encounter
S sequela

√5th **S66.Ø Injury of long flexor muscle, fascia and tendon of thumb at wrist and hand level**

√6th **S66.ØØ Unspecified injury of long flexor muscle, fascia and tendon of thumb at wrist and hand level**

√7th **S66.ØØ1 Unspecified injury of long flexor muscle, fascia and tendon of right thumb at wrist and hand level**

√7th **S66.ØØ2 Unspecified injury of long flexor muscle, fascia and tendon of left thumb at wrist and hand level**

√7th **S66.ØØ9 Unspecified injury of long flexor muscle, fascia and tendon of unspecified thumb at wrist and hand level**

√6th **S66.Ø1 Strain of long flexor muscle, fascia and tendon of thumb at wrist and hand level**

√7th **S66.Ø11 Strain of long flexor muscle, fascia and tendon of right thumb at wrist and hand level**

√7th **S66.Ø12 Strain of long flexor muscle, fascia and tendon of left thumb at wrist and hand level**

√7th **S66.Ø19 Strain of long flexor muscle, fascia and tendon of unspecified thumb at wrist and hand level**

√6th **S66.Ø2 Laceration of long flexor muscle, fascia and tendon of thumb at wrist and hand level**

√7th **S66.Ø21 Laceration of long flexor muscle, fascia and tendon of right thumb at wrist and hand level** CC

√7th **S66.Ø22 Laceration of long flexor muscle, fascia and tendon of left thumb at wrist and hand level** CC

√7th **S66.Ø29 Laceration of long flexor muscle, fascia and tendon of unspecified thumb at wrist and hand level** CC

6th **S66.09 Other specified injury of long flexor muscle, fascia and tendon of thumb at wrist and hand level**

7th **S66.091 Other specified injury of long flexor muscle, fascia and tendon of right thumb at wrist and hand level**

7th **S66.092 Other specified injury of long flexor muscle, fascia and tendon of left thumb at wrist and hand level**

7th **S66.099 Other specified injury of long flexor muscle, fascia and tendon of unspecified thumb at wrist and hand level**

5th **S66.1 Injury of flexor muscle, fascia and tendon of other and unspecified finger at wrist and hand level**

EXCLUDES 2 *injury of long flexor muscle, fascia and tendon of thumb at wrist and hand level (S66.0-)*

6th **S66.10 Unspecified injury of flexor muscle, fascia and tendon of other and unspecified finger at wrist and hand level**

7th **S66.100 Unspecified injury of flexor muscle, fascia and tendon of right index finger at wrist and hand level**

7th **S66.101 Unspecified injury of flexor muscle, fascia and tendon of left index finger at wrist and hand level**

7th **S66.102 Unspecified injury of flexor muscle, fascia and tendon of right middle finger at wrist and hand level**

7th **S66.103 Unspecified injury of flexor muscle, fascia and tendon of left middle finger at wrist and hand level**

7th **S66.104 Unspecified injury of flexor muscle, fascia and tendon of right ring finger at wrist and hand level**

7th **S66.105 Unspecified injury of flexor muscle, fascia and tendon of left ring finger at wrist and hand level**

7th **S66.106 Unspecified injury of flexor muscle, fascia and tendon of right little finger at wrist and hand level**

7th **S66.107 Unspecified injury of flexor muscle, fascia and tendon of left little finger at wrist and hand level**

7th **S66.108 Unspecified injury of flexor muscle, fascia and tendon of other finger at wrist and hand level**

Unspecified injury of flexor muscle, fascia and tendon of specified finger with unspecified laterality at wrist and hand level

7th **S66.109 Unspecified injury of flexor muscle, fascia and tendon of unspecified finger at wrist and hand level**

6th **S66.11 Strain of flexor muscle, fascia and tendon of other and unspecified finger at wrist and hand level**

7th **S66.110 Strain of flexor muscle, fascia and tendon of right index finger at wrist and hand level**

7th **S66.111 Strain of flexor muscle, fascia and tendon of left index finger at wrist and hand level**

7th **S66.112 Strain of flexor muscle, fascia and tendon of right middle finger at wrist and hand level**

7th **S66.113 Strain of flexor muscle, fascia and tendon of left middle finger at wrist and hand level**

7th **S66.114 Strain of flexor muscle, fascia and tendon of right ring finger at wrist and hand level**

7th **S66.115 Strain of flexor muscle, fascia and tendon of left ring finger at wrist and hand level**

7th **S66.116 Strain of flexor muscle, fascia and tendon of right little finger at wrist and hand level**

7th **S66.117 Strain of flexor muscle, fascia and tendon of left little finger at wrist and hand level**

7th **S66.118 Strain of flexor muscle, fascia and tendon of other finger at wrist and hand level**

Strain of flexor muscle, fascia and tendon of specified finger with unspecified laterality at wrist and hand level

7th **S66.119 Strain of flexor muscle, fascia and tendon of unspecified finger at wrist and hand level**

6th **S66.12 Laceration of flexor muscle, fascia and tendon of other and unspecified finger at wrist and hand level**

7th **S66.120 Laceration of flexor muscle, fascia and tendon of right index finger at wrist and hand level** CC

7th **S66.121 Laceration of flexor muscle, fascia and tendon of left index finger at wrist and hand level** CC

7th **S66.122 Laceration of flexor muscle, fascia and tendon of right middle finger at wrist and hand level** CC

7th **S66.123 Laceration of flexor muscle, fascia and tendon of left middle finger at wrist and hand level** CC

7th **S66.124 Laceration of flexor muscle, fascia and tendon of right ring finger at wrist and hand level** CC

7th **S66.125 Laceration of flexor muscle, fascia and tendon of left ring finger at wrist and hand level** CC

7th **S66.126 Laceration of flexor muscle, fascia and tendon of right little finger at wrist and hand level** CC

7th **S66.127 Laceration of flexor muscle, fascia and tendon of left little finger at wrist and hand level** CC

7th **S66.128 Laceration of flexor muscle, fascia and tendon of other finger at wrist and hand level** CC

Laceration of flexor muscle, fascia and tendon of specified finger with unspecified laterality at wrist and hand level

7th **S66.129 Laceration of flexor muscle, fascia and tendon of unspecified finger at wrist and hand level** CC UNS

6th **S66.19 Other injury of flexor muscle, fascia and tendon of other and unspecified finger at wrist and hand level**

7th **S66.190 Other injury of flexor muscle, fascia and tendon of right index finger at wrist and hand level**

7th **S66.191 Other injury of flexor muscle, fascia and tendon of left index finger at wrist and hand level**

7th **S66.192 Other injury of flexor muscle, fascia and tendon of right middle finger at wrist and hand level**

7th **S66.193 Other injury of flexor muscle, fascia and tendon of left middle finger at wrist and hand level**

7th **S66.194 Other injury of flexor muscle, fascia and tendon of right ring finger at wrist and hand level**

7th **S66.195 Other injury of flexor muscle, fascia and tendon of left ring finger at wrist and hand level**

7th **S66.196 Other injury of flexor muscle, fascia and tendon of right little finger at wrist and hand level**

7th **S66.197 Other injury of flexor muscle, fascia and tendon of left little finger at wrist and hand level**

7th **S66.198 Other injury of flexor muscle, fascia and tendon of other finger at wrist and hand level**

Other injury of flexor muscle, fascia and tendon of specified finger with unspecified laterality at wrist and hand level

7th **S66.199 Other injury of flexor muscle, fascia and tendon of unspecified finger at wrist and hand level**

5th **S66.2 Injury of extensor muscle, fascia and tendon of thumb at wrist and hand level**

6th **S66.20 Unspecified injury of extensor muscle, fascia and tendon of thumb at wrist and hand level**

7th **S66.201 Unspecified injury of extensor muscle, fascia and tendon of right thumb at wrist and hand level**

7th **S66.202 Unspecified injury of extensor muscle, fascia and tendon of left thumb at wrist and hand level**

√7th S66.209 Unspecified injury of extensor muscle, fascia and tendon of unspecified thumb at wrist and hand level

√6th S66.21 Strain of extensor muscle, fascia and tendon of thumb at wrist and hand level

√7th S66.211 Strain of extensor muscle, fascia and tendon of right thumb at wrist and hand level

√7th S66.212 Strain of extensor muscle, fascia and tendon of left thumb at wrist and hand level

√7th S66.219 Strain of extensor muscle, fascia and tendon of unspecified thumb at wrist and hand level

√6th S66.22 Laceration of extensor muscle, fascia and tendon of thumb at wrist and hand level

√7th S66.221 Laceration of extensor muscle, fascia and tendon of right thumb at wrist and hand level CC

√7th S66.222 Laceration of extensor muscle, fascia and tendon of left thumb at wrist and hand level CC

√7th S66.229 Laceration of extensor muscle, fascia and tendon of unspecified thumb at wrist and hand level CC

√6th S66.29 Other specified injury of extensor muscle, fascia and tendon of thumb at wrist and hand level

√7th S66.291 Other specified injury of extensor muscle, fascia and tendon of right thumb at wrist and hand level

√7th S66.292 Other specified injury of extensor muscle, fascia and tendon of left thumb at wrist and hand level

√7th S66.299 Other specified injury of extensor muscle, fascia and tendon of unspecified thumb at wrist and hand level

√5th S66.3 Injury of extensor muscle, fascia and tendon of other and unspecified finger at wrist and hand level

EXCLUDES 2 *injury of extensor muscle, fascia and tendon of thumb at wrist and hand level (S66.2-)*

√6th S66.30 Unspecified injury of extensor muscle, fascia and tendon of other and unspecified finger at wrist and hand level

√7th S66.300 Unspecified injury of extensor muscle, fascia and tendon of right index finger at wrist and hand level

√7th S66.301 Unspecified injury of extensor muscle, fascia and tendon of left index finger at wrist and hand level

√7th S66.302 Unspecified injury of extensor muscle, fascia and tendon of right middle finger at wrist and hand level

√7th S66.303 Unspecified injury of extensor muscle, fascia and tendon of left middle finger at wrist and hand level

√7th S66.304 Unspecified injury of extensor muscle, fascia and tendon of right ring finger at wrist and hand level

√7th S66.305 Unspecified injury of extensor muscle, fascia and tendon of left ring finger at wrist and hand level

√7th S66.306 Unspecified injury of extensor muscle, fascia and tendon of right little finger at wrist and hand level

√7th S66.307 Unspecified injury of extensor muscle, fascia and tendon of left little finger at wrist and hand level

√7th S66.308 Unspecified injury of extensor muscle, fascia and tendon of other finger at wrist and hand level

Unspecified injury of extensor muscle, fascia and tendon of specified finger with unspecified laterality at wrist and hand level

√7th S66.309 Unspecified injury of extensor muscle, fascia and tendon of unspecified finger at wrist and hand level

√6th S66.31 Strain of extensor muscle, fascia and tendon of other and unspecified finger at wrist and hand level

√7th S66.310 Strain of extensor muscle, fascia and tendon of right index finger at wrist and hand level

√7th S66.311 Strain of extensor muscle, fascia and tendon of left index finger at wrist and hand level

√7th S66.312 Strain of extensor muscle, fascia and tendon of right middle finger at wrist and hand level

√7th S66.313 Strain of extensor muscle, fascia and tendon of left middle finger at wrist and hand level

√7th S66.314 Strain of extensor muscle, fascia and tendon of right ring finger at wrist and hand level

√7th S66.315 Strain of extensor muscle, fascia and tendon of left ring finger at wrist and hand level

√7th S66.316 Strain of extensor muscle, fascia and tendon of right little finger at wrist and hand level

√7th S66.317 Strain of extensor muscle, fascia and tendon of left little finger at wrist and hand level

√7th S66.318 Strain of extensor muscle, fascia and tendon of other finger at wrist and hand level

Strain of extensor muscle, fascia and tendon of specified finger with unspecified laterality at wrist and hand level

√7th S66.319 Strain of extensor muscle, fascia and tendon of unspecified finger at wrist and hand level

√6th S66.32 Laceration of extensor muscle, fascia and tendon of other and unspecified finger at wrist and hand level

√7th S66.320 Laceration of extensor muscle, fascia and tendon of right index finger at wrist and hand level CC

√7th S66.321 Laceration of extensor muscle, fascia and tendon of left index finger at wrist and hand level CC

√7th S66.322 Laceration of extensor muscle, fascia and tendon of right middle finger at wrist and hand level CC

√7th S66.323 Laceration of extensor muscle, fascia and tendon of left middle finger at wrist and hand level CC

√7th S66.324 Laceration of extensor muscle, fascia and tendon of right ring finger at wrist and hand level CC

√7th S66.325 Laceration of extensor muscle, fascia and tendon of left ring finger at wrist and hand level CC

√7th S66.326 Laceration of extensor muscle, fascia and tendon of right little finger at wrist and hand level CC

√7th S66.327 Laceration of extensor muscle, fascia and tendon of left little finger at wrist and hand level CC

√7th S66.328 Laceration of extensor muscle, fascia and tendon of other finger at wrist and hand level CC

Laceration of extensor muscle, fascia and tendon of specified finger with unspecified laterality at wrist and hand level

√7th S66.329 Laceration of extensor muscle, fascia and tendon of unspecified finger at wrist and hand level CC UNS

√6th S66.39 Other injury of extensor muscle, fascia and tendon of other and unspecified finger at wrist and hand level

√7th S66.390 Other injury of extensor muscle, fascia and tendon of right index finger at wrist and hand level

√7th S66.391 Other injury of extensor muscle, fascia and tendon of left index finger at wrist and hand level

√7th S66.392 Other injury of extensor muscle, fascia and tendon of right middle finger at wrist and hand level

√7th S66.393 Other injury of extensor muscle, fascia and tendon of left middle finger at wrist and hand level

√7th S66.394 Other injury of extensor muscle, fascia and tendon of right ring finger at wrist and hand level

7th **S66.395 Other injury of extensor muscle, fascia and tendon of left ring finger at wrist and hand level**

7th **S66.396 Other injury of extensor muscle, fascia and tendon of right little finger at wrist and hand level**

7th **S66.397 Other injury of extensor muscle, fascia and tendon of left little finger at wrist and hand level**

7th **S66.398 Other injury of extensor muscle, fascia and tendon of other finger at wrist and hand level**

Other injury of extensor muscle, fascia and tendon of specified finger with unspecified laterality at wrist and hand level

7th **S66.399 Other injury of extensor muscle, fascia and tendon of unspecified finger at wrist and hand level**

5th **S66.4 Injury of intrinsic muscle, fascia and tendon of thumb at wrist and hand level**

6th **S66.40 Unspecified injury of intrinsic muscle, fascia and tendon of thumb at wrist and hand level**

7th **S66.401 Unspecified injury of intrinsic muscle, fascia and tendon of right thumb at wrist and hand level**

7th **S66.402 Unspecified injury of intrinsic muscle, fascia and tendon of left thumb at wrist and hand level**

7th **S66.409 Unspecified injury of intrinsic muscle, fascia and tendon of unspecified thumb at wrist and hand level**

6th **S66.41 Strain of intrinsic muscle, fascia and tendon of thumb at wrist and hand level**

7th **S66.411 Strain of intrinsic muscle, fascia and tendon of right thumb at wrist and hand level**

7th **S66.412 Strain of intrinsic muscle, fascia and tendon of left thumb at wrist and hand level**

7th **S66.419 Strain of intrinsic muscle, fascia and tendon of unspecified thumb at wrist and hand level**

6th **S66.42 Laceration of intrinsic muscle, fascia and tendon of thumb at wrist and hand level**

7th **S66.421 Laceration of intrinsic muscle, fascia and tendon of right thumb at wrist and hand level** CC

7th **S66.422 Laceration of intrinsic muscle, fascia and tendon of left thumb at wrist and hand level** CC

7th **S66.429 Laceration of intrinsic muscle, fascia and tendon of unspecified thumb at wrist and hand level** CC

6th **S66.49 Other specified injury of intrinsic muscle, fascia and tendon of thumb at wrist and hand level**

7th **S66.491 Other specified injury of intrinsic muscle, fascia and tendon of right thumb at wrist and hand level**

7th **S66.492 Other specified injury of intrinsic muscle, fascia and tendon of left thumb at wrist and hand level**

7th **S66.499 Other specified injury of intrinsic muscle, fascia and tendon of unspecified thumb at wrist and hand level**

5th **S66.5 Injury of intrinsic muscle, fascia and tendon of other and unspecified finger at wrist and hand level**

EXCLUDES 2 *injury of intrinsic muscle, fascia and tendon of thumb at wrist and hand level (S66.4-)*

6th **S66.50 Unspecified injury of intrinsic muscle, fascia and tendon of other and unspecified finger at wrist and hand level**

7th **S66.500 Unspecified injury of intrinsic muscle, fascia and tendon of right index finger at wrist and hand level**

7th **S66.501 Unspecified injury of intrinsic muscle, fascia and tendon of left index finger at wrist and hand level**

7th **S66.502 Unspecified injury of intrinsic muscle, fascia and tendon of right middle finger at wrist and hand level**

7th **S66.503 Unspecified injury of intrinsic muscle, fascia and tendon of left middle finger at wrist and hand level**

7th **S66.504 Unspecified injury of intrinsic muscle, fascia and tendon of right ring finger at wrist and hand level**

7th **S66.505 Unspecified injury of intrinsic muscle, fascia and tendon of left ring finger at wrist and hand level**

7th **S66.506 Unspecified injury of intrinsic muscle, fascia and tendon of right little finger at wrist and hand level**

7th **S66.507 Unspecified injury of intrinsic muscle, fascia and tendon of left little finger at wrist and hand level**

7th **S66.508 Unspecified injury of intrinsic muscle, fascia and tendon of other finger at wrist and hand level**

Unspecified injury of intrinsic muscle, fascia and tendon of specified finger with unspecified laterality at wrist and hand level

7th **S66.509 Unspecified injury of intrinsic muscle, fascia and tendon of unspecified finger at wrist and hand level**

6th **S66.51 Strain of intrinsic muscle, fascia and tendon of other and unspecified finger at wrist and hand level**

7th **S66.510 Strain of intrinsic muscle, fascia and tendon of right index finger at wrist and hand level**

7th **S66.511 Strain of intrinsic muscle, fascia and tendon of left index finger at wrist and hand level**

7th **S66.512 Strain of intrinsic muscle, fascia and tendon of right middle finger at wrist and hand level**

7th **S66.513 Strain of intrinsic muscle, fascia and tendon of left middle finger at wrist and hand level**

7th **S66.514 Strain of intrinsic muscle, fascia and tendon of right ring finger at wrist and hand level**

7th **S66.515 Strain of intrinsic muscle, fascia and tendon of left ring finger at wrist and hand level**

7th **S66.516 Strain of intrinsic muscle, fascia and tendon of right little finger at wrist and hand level**

7th **S66.517 Strain of intrinsic muscle, fascia and tendon of left little finger at wrist and hand level**

7th **S66.518 Strain of intrinsic muscle, fascia and tendon of other finger at wrist and hand level**

Strain of intrinsic muscle, fascia and tendon of specified finger with unspecified laterality at wrist and hand level

7th **S66.519 Strain of intrinsic muscle, fascia and tendon of unspecified finger at wrist and hand level**

6th **S66.52 Laceration of intrinsic muscle, fascia and tendon of other and unspecified finger at wrist and hand level**

7th **S66.520 Laceration of intrinsic muscle, fascia and tendon of right index finger at wrist and hand level** CC

7th **S66.521 Laceration of intrinsic muscle, fascia and tendon of left index finger at wrist and hand level** CC

7th **S66.522 Laceration of intrinsic muscle, fascia and tendon of right middle finger at wrist and hand level** CC

7th **S66.523 Laceration of intrinsic muscle, fascia and tendon of left middle finger at wrist and hand level** CC

7th **S66.524 Laceration of intrinsic muscle, fascia and tendon of right ring finger at wrist and hand level** CC

7th **S66.525 Laceration of intrinsic muscle, fascia and tendon of left ring finger at wrist and hand level** CC

7th **S66.526 Laceration of intrinsic muscle, fascia and tendon of right little finger at wrist and hand level** CC

7th **S66.527 Laceration of intrinsic muscle, fascia and tendon of left little finger at wrist and hand level** CC

S66.528 Laceration of intrinsic muscle, fascia and tendon of other finger at wrist and hand level CC
Laceration of intrinsic muscle, fascia and tendon of specified finger with unspecified laterality at wrist and hand level

S66.529 Laceration of intrinsic muscle, fascia and tendon of unspecified finger at wrist and hand level CC UNS

S66.59 Other injury of intrinsic muscle, fascia and tendon of other and unspecified finger at wrist and hand level

S66.590 Other injury of intrinsic muscle, fascia and tendon of right index finger at wrist and hand level

S66.591 Other injury of intrinsic muscle, fascia and tendon of left index finger at wrist and hand level

S66.592 Other injury of intrinsic muscle, fascia and tendon of right middle finger at wrist and hand level

S66.593 Other injury of intrinsic muscle, fascia and tendon of left middle finger at wrist and hand level

S66.594 Other injury of intrinsic muscle, fascia and tendon of right ring finger at wrist and hand level

S66.595 Other injury of intrinsic muscle, fascia and tendon of left ring finger at wrist and hand level

S66.596 Other injury of intrinsic muscle, fascia and tendon of right little finger at wrist and hand level

S66.597 Other injury of intrinsic muscle, fascia and tendon of left little finger at wrist and hand level

S66.598 Other injury of intrinsic muscle, fascia and tendon of other finger at wrist and hand level
Other injury of intrinsic muscle, fascia and tendon of specified finger with unspecified laterality at wrist and hand level

S66.599 Other injury of intrinsic muscle, fascia and tendon of unspecified finger at wrist and hand level

S66.8 Injury of other specified muscles, fascia and tendons at wrist and hand level

S66.80 Unspecified injury of other specified muscles, fascia and tendons at wrist and hand level

S66.801 Unspecified injury of other specified muscles, fascia and tendons at wrist and hand level, right hand

S66.802 Unspecified injury of other specified muscles, fascia and tendons at wrist and hand level, left hand

S66.809 Unspecified injury of other specified muscles, fascia and tendons at wrist and hand level, unspecified hand

S66.81 Strain of other specified muscles, fascia and tendons at wrist and hand level

S66.811 Strain of other specified muscles, fascia and tendons at wrist and hand level, right hand

S66.812 Strain of other specified muscles, fascia and tendons at wrist and hand level, left hand

S66.819 Strain of other specified muscles, fascia and tendons at wrist and hand level, unspecified hand

S66.82 Laceration of other specified muscles, fascia and tendons at wrist and hand level

S66.821 Laceration of other specified muscles, fascia and tendons at wrist and hand level, right hand CC

S66.822 Laceration of other specified muscles, fascia and tendons at wrist and hand level, left hand CC

S66.829 Laceration of other specified muscles, fascia and tendons at wrist and hand level, unspecified hand CC UNS

S66.89 Other injury of other specified muscles, fascia and tendons at wrist and hand level

S66.891 Other injury of other specified muscles, fascia and tendons at wrist and hand level, right hand

S66.892 Other injury of other specified muscles, fascia and tendons at wrist and hand level, left hand

S66.899 Other injury of other specified muscles, fascia and tendons at wrist and hand level, unspecified hand

S66.9 Injury of unspecified muscle, fascia and tendon at wrist and hand level

S66.90 Unspecified injury of unspecified muscle, fascia and tendon at wrist and hand level

S66.901 Unspecified injury of unspecified muscle, fascia and tendon at wrist and hand level, right hand

S66.902 Unspecified injury of unspecified muscle, fascia and tendon at wrist and hand level, left hand

S66.909 Unspecified injury of unspecified muscle, fascia and tendon at wrist and hand level, unspecified hand

S66.91 Strain of unspecified muscle, fascia and tendon at wrist and hand level

S66.911 Strain of unspecified muscle, fascia and tendon at wrist and hand level, right hand

S66.912 Strain of unspecified muscle, fascia and tendon at wrist and hand level, left hand

S66.919 Strain of unspecified muscle, fascia and tendon at wrist and hand level, unspecified hand

S66.92 Laceration of unspecified muscle, fascia and tendon at wrist and hand level

S66.921 Laceration of unspecified muscle, fascia and tendon at wrist and hand level, right hand CC

S66.922 Laceration of unspecified muscle, fascia and tendon at wrist and hand level, left hand CC

S66.929 Laceration of unspecified muscle, fascia and tendon at wrist and hand level, unspecified hand CC UNS

S66.99 Other injury of unspecified muscle, fascia and tendon at wrist and hand level

S66.991 Other injury of unspecified muscle, fascia and tendon at wrist and hand level, right hand

S66.992 Other injury of unspecified muscle, fascia and tendon at wrist and hand level, left hand

S66.999 Other injury of unspecified muscle, fascia and tendon at wrist and hand level, unspecified hand

S67 Crushing injury of wrist, hand and fingers

Use additional code for all associated injuries, such as:
fracture of wrist and hand (S62.-)
open wound of wrist and hand (S61.-)

The appropriate 7th character is to be added to each code from category S67.
A initial encounter
D subsequent encounter
S sequela

S67.0 Crushing injury of thumb

S67.00 Crushing injury of unspecified thumb

S67.01 Crushing injury of right thumb

S67.02 Crushing injury of left thumb

S67.1 Crushing injury of other and unspecified finger(s)
EXCLUDES 2 *crushing injury of thumb (S67.0-)*

S67.10 Crushing injury of unspecified finger(s)

S67.19 Crushing injury of other finger(s)

S67.190 Crushing injury of right index finger

S67.191 Crushing injury of left index finger

S67.192 Crushing injury of right middle finger

S67.193 Crushing injury of left middle finger

S67.194 Crushing injury of right ring finger

S67.195 Crushing injury of left ring finger

✓7th **S67.196 Crushing injury of right little finger**

✓7th **S67.197 Crushing injury of left little finger**

✓7th **S67.198 Crushing injury of other finger**

Crushing injury of specified finger with unspecified laterality

✓5th **S67.2 Crushing injury of hand**

EXCLUDES 2 *crushing injury of fingers (S67.1-)*

crushing injury of thumb (S67.0-)

✓x7th **S67.20 Crushing injury of unspecified hand**

✓x7th **S67.21 Crushing injury of right hand**

✓x7th **S67.22 Crushing injury of left hand**

✓5th **S67.3 Crushing injury of wrist**

✓x7th **S67.30 Crushing injury of unspecified wrist**

✓x7th **S67.31 Crushing injury of right wrist**

✓x7th **S67.32 Crushing injury of left wrist**

✓5th **S67.4 Crushing injury of wrist and hand**

EXCLUDES 1 *crushing injury of hand alone (S67.2-)*

crushing injury of wrist alone (S67.3-)

EXCLUDES 2 *crushing injury of fingers (S67.1-)*

crushing injury of thumb (S67.0-)

✓x7th **S67.40 Crushing injury of unspecified wrist and hand**

✓x7th **S67.41 Crushing injury of right wrist and hand**

✓x7th **S67.42 Crushing injury of left wrist and hand**

✓5th **S67.9 Crushing injury of unspecified part(s) of wrist, hand and fingers**

✓x7th **S67.90 Crushing injury of unspecified part(s) of unspecified wrist, hand and fingers**

✓x7th **S67.91 Crushing injury of unspecified part(s) of right wrist, hand and fingers**

✓x7th **S67.92 Crushing injury of unspecified part(s) of left wrist, hand and fingers**

✓4th **S68 Traumatic amputation of wrist, hand and fingers**

An amputation not identified as partial or complete should be coded to complete.

The appropriate 7th character is to be added to each code from category S68.
A initial encounter
D subsequent encounter
S sequela

✓5th **S68.0 Traumatic metacarpophalangeal amputation of thumb**

Traumatic amputation of thumb NOS

✓6th **S68.01 Complete traumatic metacarpophalangeal amputation of thumb**

✓7th **S68.011 Complete traumatic metacarpophalangeal amputation of right thumb** HCC

✓7th **S68.012 Complete traumatic metacarpophalangeal amputation of left thumb** HCC

✓7th **S68.019 Complete traumatic metacarpophalangeal amputation of unspecified thumb** HCC

✓6th **S68.02 Partial traumatic metacarpophalangeal amputation of thumb**

✓7th **S68.021 Partial traumatic metacarpophalangeal amputation of right thumb** HCC

✓7th **S68.022 Partial traumatic metacarpophalangeal amputation of left thumb** HCC

✓7th **S68.029 Partial traumatic metacarpophalangeal amputation of unspecified thumb** HCC

✓5th **S68.1 Traumatic metacarpophalangeal amputation of other and unspecified finger**

Traumatic amputation of finger NOS

EXCLUDES 2 *traumatic metacarpophalangeal amputation of thumb (S68.0-)*

✓6th **S68.11 Complete traumatic metacarpophalangeal amputation of other and unspecified finger**

✓7th **S68.110 Complete traumatic metacarpophalangeal amputation of right index finger** HCC

✓7th **S68.111 Complete traumatic metacarpophalangeal amputation of left index finger** HCC

✓7th **S68.112 Complete traumatic metacarpophalangeal amputation of right middle finger** HCC

✓7th **S68.113 Complete traumatic metacarpophalangeal amputation of left middle finger** HCC

✓7th **S68.114 Complete traumatic metacarpophalangeal amputation of right ring finger** HCC

✓7th **S68.115 Complete traumatic metacarpophalangeal amputation of left ring finger** HCC

✓7th **S68.116 Complete traumatic metacarpophalangeal amputation of right little finger** HCC

✓7th **S68.117 Complete traumatic metacarpophalangeal amputation of left little finger** HCC

✓7th **S68.118 Complete traumatic metacarpophalangeal amputation of other finger** HCC

Complete traumatic metacarpophalangeal amputation of specified finger with unspecified laterality

✓7th **S68.119 Complete traumatic metacarpophalangeal amputation of unspecified finger** HCC

✓6th **S68.12 Partial traumatic metacarpophalangeal amputation of other and unspecified finger**

✓7th **S68.120 Partial traumatic metacarpophalangeal amputation of right index finger** HCC

✓7th **S68.121 Partial traumatic metacarpophalangeal amputation of left index finger** HCC

✓7th **S68.122 Partial traumatic metacarpophalangeal amputation of right middle finger** HCC

✓7th **S68.123 Partial traumatic metacarpophalangeal amputation of left middle finger** HCC

✓7th **S68.124 Partial traumatic metacarpophalangeal amputation of right ring finger** HCC

✓7th **S68.125 Partial traumatic metacarpophalangeal amputation of left ring finger** HCC

✓7th **S68.126 Partial traumatic metacarpophalangeal amputation of right little finger** HCC

✓7th **S68.127 Partial traumatic metacarpophalangeal amputation of left little finger** HCC

✓7th **S68.128 Partial traumatic metacarpophalangeal amputation of other finger** HCC

Partial traumatic metacarpophalangeal amputation of specified finger with unspecified laterality

✓7th **S68.129 Partial traumatic metacarpophalangeal amputation of unspecified finger** HCC

✓5th **S68.4 Traumatic amputation of hand at wrist level**

Traumatic amputation of hand NOS

Traumatic amputation of wrist

✓6th **S68.41 Complete traumatic amputation of hand at wrist level**

✓7th **S68.411 Complete traumatic amputation of right hand at wrist level** CC HCC

✓7th **S68.412 Complete traumatic amputation of left hand at wrist level** CC HCC

✓7th **S68.419 Complete traumatic amputation of unspecified hand at wrist level** CC UNS HCC

✓6th **S68.42 Partial traumatic amputation of hand at wrist level**

✓7th **S68.421 Partial traumatic amputation of right hand at wrist level** CC HCC

✓7th **S68.422 Partial traumatic amputation of left hand at wrist level** CC HCC

✓7th **S68.429 Partial traumatic amputation of unspecified hand at wrist level** CC UNS HCC

✓5th **S68.5 Traumatic transphalangeal amputation of thumb**

Traumatic interphalangeal joint amputation of thumb

✓6th **S68.51 Complete traumatic transphalangeal amputation of thumb**

✓7th **S68.511 Complete traumatic transphalangeal amputation of right thumb** HCC

✓7th **S68.512 Complete traumatic transphalangeal amputation of left thumb** HCC

✓7th **S68.519 Complete traumatic transphalangeal amputation of unspecified thumb** HCC

S68.52 Partial traumatic transphalangeal amputation of thumb
S68.521 Partial traumatic transphalangeal amputation of right thumb HCC
S68.522 Partial traumatic transphalangeal amputation of left thumb HCC
S68.529 Partial traumatic transphalangeal amputation of unspecified thumb HCC
S68.6 Traumatic transphalangeal amputation of other and unspecified finger
S68.61 Complete traumatic transphalangeal amputation of other and unspecified finger(s)
S68.610 Complete traumatic transphalangeal amputation of right index finger HCC
S68.611 Complete traumatic transphalangeal amputation of left index finger HCC
S68.612 Complete traumatic transphalangeal amputation of right middle finger HCC
S68.613 Complete traumatic transphalangeal amputation of left middle finger HCC
S68.614 Complete traumatic transphalangeal amputation of right ring finger HCC
S68.615 Complete traumatic transphalangeal amputation of left ring finger HCC
S68.616 Complete traumatic transphalangeal amputation of right little finger HCC
S68.617 Complete traumatic transphalangeal amputation of left little finger HCC
S68.618 Complete traumatic transphalangeal amputation of other finger HCC
Complete traumatic transphalangeal amputation of specified finger with unspecified laterality
S68.619 Complete traumatic transphalangeal amputation of unspecified finger HCC
S68.62 Partial traumatic transphalangeal amputation of other and unspecified finger
S68.620 Partial traumatic transphalangeal amputation of right index finger HCC
S68.621 Partial traumatic transphalangeal amputation of left index finger HCC
S68.622 Partial traumatic transphalangeal amputation of right middle finger HCC
S68.623 Partial traumatic transphalangeal amputation of left middle finger HCC
S68.624 Partial traumatic transphalangeal amputation of right ring finger HCC
S68.625 Partial traumatic transphalangeal amputation of left ring finger HCC
S68.626 Partial traumatic transphalangeal amputation of right little finger HCC
S68.627 Partial traumatic transphalangeal amputation of left little finger HCC
S68.628 Partial traumatic transphalangeal amputation of other finger HCC
Partial traumatic transphalangeal amputation of specified finger with unspecified laterality
S68.629 Partial traumatic transphalangeal amputation of unspecified finger HCC
S68.7 Traumatic transmetacarpal amputation of hand
S68.71 Complete traumatic transmetacarpal amputation of hand
S68.711 Complete traumatic transmetacarpal amputation of right hand CC HCC
S68.712 Complete traumatic transmetacarpal amputation of left hand CC HCC
S68.719 Complete traumatic transmetacarpal amputation of unspecified hand CC UNS HCC
S68.72 Partial traumatic transmetacarpal amputation of hand
S68.721 Partial traumatic transmetacarpal amputation of right hand CC HCC
S68.722 Partial traumatic transmetacarpal amputation of left hand CC HCC
S68.729 Partial traumatic transmetacarpal amputation of unspecified hand CC UNS HCC

S69 Other and unspecified injuries of wrist, hand and finger(s)

The appropriate 7th character is to be added to each code from category S69.
A initial encounter
D subsequent encounter
S sequela

S69.8 Other specified injuries of wrist, hand and finger(s)
S69.80 Other specified injuries of unspecified wrist, hand and finger(s)
S69.81 Other specified injuries of right wrist, hand and finger(s)
S69.82 Other specified injuries of left wrist, hand and finger(s)
S69.9 Unspecified injury of wrist, hand and finger(s)
S69.90 Unspecified injury of unspecified wrist, hand and finger(s)
S69.91 Unspecified injury of right wrist, hand and finger(s)
S69.92 Unspecified injury of left wrist, hand and finger(s)

Injuries to the hip and thigh (S70-S79)

EXCLUDES 2 *burns and corrosions (T20-T32)*
frostbite (T33-T34)
snake bite (T63.0-)
venomous insect bite or sting (T63.4-)

S70 Superficial injury of hip and thigh

The appropriate 7th character is to be added to each code from category S70.
A initial encounter
D subsequent encounter
S sequela

S70.0 Contusion of hip
S70.00 Contusion of unspecified hip
S70.01 Contusion of right hip
S70.02 Contusion of left hip
S70.1 Contusion of thigh
S70.10 Contusion of unspecified thigh
S70.11 Contusion of right thigh
S70.12 Contusion of left thigh
S70.2 Other superficial injuries of hip
S70.21 Abrasion of hip
S70.211 Abrasion, right hip
S70.212 Abrasion, left hip
S70.219 Abrasion, unspecified hip
S70.22 Blister (nonthermal) of hip
S70.221 Blister (nonthermal), right hip
S70.222 Blister (nonthermal), left hip
S70.229 Blister (nonthermal), unspecified hip
S70.24 External constriction of hip
S70.241 External constriction, right hip
S70.242 External constriction, left hip
S70.249 External constriction, unspecified hip
S70.25 Superficial foreign body of hip
Splinter in the hip
S70.251 Superficial foreign body, right hip
S70.252 Superficial foreign body, left hip
S70.259 Superficial foreign body, unspecified hip
S70.26 Insect bite (nonvenomous) of hip
S70.261 Insect bite (nonvenomous), right hip
S70.262 Insect bite (nonvenomous), left hip
S70.269 Insect bite (nonvenomous), unspecified hip
S70.27 Other superficial bite of hip
EXCLUDES 1 *open bite of hip (S71.05-)*
S70.271 Other superficial bite of hip, right hip
S70.272 Other superficial bite of hip, left hip
S70.279 Other superficial bite of hip, unspecified hip
S70.3 Other superficial injuries of thigh
S70.31 Abrasion of thigh
S70.311 Abrasion, right thigh

7th S70.312 Abrasion, left thigh
7th S70.319 Abrasion, unspecified thigh
6th S70.32 Blister (nonthermal) of thigh
7th S70.321 Blister (nonthermal), right thigh
7th S70.322 Blister (nonthermal), left thigh
7th S70.329 Blister (nonthermal), unspecified thigh
6th S70.34 External constriction of thigh
7th S70.341 External constriction, right thigh
7th S70.342 External constriction, left thigh
7th S70.349 External constriction, unspecified thigh
6th S70.35 Superficial foreign body of thigh
Splinter in the thigh
7th S70.351 Superficial foreign body, right thigh
7th S70.352 Superficial foreign body, left thigh
7th S70.359 Superficial foreign body, unspecified thigh
6th S70.36 Insect bite (nonvenomous) of thigh
7th S70.361 Insect bite (nonvenomous), right thigh
7th S70.362 Insect bite (nonvenomous), left thigh
7th S70.369 Insect bite (nonvenomous), unspecified thigh
6th S70.37 Other superficial bite of thigh
EXCLUDES 1 *open bite of thigh (S71.15)*
7th S70.371 Other superficial bite of right thigh
7th S70.372 Other superficial bite of left thigh
7th S70.379 Other superficial bite of unspecified thigh
5th S70.9 Unspecified superficial injury of hip and thigh
6th S70.91 Unspecified superficial injury of hip
7th S70.911 Unspecified superficial injury of right hip
7th S70.912 Unspecified superficial injury of left hip
7th S70.919 Unspecified superficial injury of unspecified hip
6th S70.92 Unspecified superficial injury of thigh
7th S70.921 Unspecified superficial injury of right thigh
7th S70.922 Unspecified superficial injury of left thigh
7th S70.929 Unspecified superficial injury of unspecified thigh

4th **S71 Open wound of hip and thigh**
Code also any associated wound infection
EXCLUDES 1 *open fracture of hip and thigh (S72.-)*
traumatic amputation of hip and thigh (S78.-)
EXCLUDES 2 *bite of venomous animal (T63.-)*
open wound of ankle, foot and toes (S91.-)
open wound of knee and lower leg (S81.-)

The appropriate 7th character is to be added to each code from category S71.
A initial encounter
D subsequent encounter
S sequela

5th S71.0 Open wound of hip
6th S71.00 Unspecified open wound of hip
7th S71.001 Unspecified open wound, right hip
7th S71.002 Unspecified open wound, left hip
7th S71.009 Unspecified open wound, unspecified hip
6th S71.01 Laceration without foreign body of hip
7th S71.011 Laceration without foreign body, right hip
7th S71.012 Laceration without foreign body, left hip
7th S71.019 Laceration without foreign body, unspecified hip
6th S71.02 Laceration with foreign body of hip
7th S71.021 Laceration with foreign body, right hip
7th S71.022 Laceration with foreign body, left hip
7th S71.029 Laceration with foreign body, unspecified hip
6th S71.03 Puncture wound without foreign body of hip
7th S71.031 Puncture wound without foreign body, right hip
7th S71.032 Puncture wound without foreign body, left hip
7th S71.039 Puncture wound without foreign body, unspecified hip
6th S71.04 Puncture wound with foreign body of hip
7th S71.041 Puncture wound with foreign body, right hip
7th S71.042 Puncture wound with foreign body, left hip
7th S71.049 Puncture wound with foreign body, unspecified hip
6th S71.05 Open bite of hip
Bite of hip NOS
EXCLUDES 1 *superficial bite of hip (S70.26, S70.27)*
7th S71.051 Open bite, right hip
7th S71.052 Open bite, left hip
7th S71.059 Open bite, unspecified hip
5th S71.1 Open wound of thigh
6th S71.10 Unspecified open wound of thigh
AHA: 2016,3Q,24
7th S71.101 Unspecified open wound, right thigh
7th S71.102 Unspecified open wound, left thigh
7th S71.109 Unspecified open wound, unspecified thigh
6th S71.11 Laceration without foreign body of thigh
7th S71.111 Laceration without foreign body, right thigh
7th S71.112 Laceration without foreign body, left thigh
7th S71.119 Laceration without foreign body, unspecified thigh
6th S71.12 Laceration with foreign body of thigh
7th S71.121 Laceration with foreign body, right thigh
7th S71.122 Laceration with foreign body, left thigh
7th S71.129 Laceration with foreign body, unspecified thigh
6th S71.13 Puncture wound without foreign body of thigh
AHA: 2016,3Q,24
7th S71.131 Puncture wound without foreign body, right thigh
7th S71.132 Puncture wound without foreign body, left thigh
7th S71.139 Puncture wound without foreign body, unspecified thigh
6th S71.14 Puncture wound with foreign body of thigh
AHA: 2016,3Q,24
7th S71.141 Puncture wound with foreign body, right thigh
7th S71.142 Puncture wound with foreign body, left thigh
7th S71.149 Puncture wound with foreign body, unspecified thigh
6th S71.15 Open bite of thigh
Bite of thigh NOS
EXCLUDES 1 *superficial bite of thigh (S70.37-)*
7th S71.151 Open bite, right thigh
7th S71.152 Open bite, left thigh
7th S71.159 Open bite, unspecified thigh

S72 Fracture of femur

NOTE A fracture not indicated as displaced or nondisplaced should be coded to displaced.

A fracture not indicated as open or closed should be coded to closed.

The open fracture designations are based on the Gustilo open fracture classification.

EXCLUDES 1 *traumatic amputation of hip and thigh (S78.-)*

EXCLUDES 2 *fracture of foot (S92.-)*
fracture of lower leg and ankle (S82.-)
periprosthetic fracture of prosthetic implant of hip (M97.0-)

AHA: 2018,2Q,12; 2016,1Q,33; 2015,3Q,37-39; 2015,1Q,17; 2013,4Q,128

DEF: Diaphysis: Central shaft of a long bone.

DEF: Epiphysis: Proximal and distal rounded ends of a long bone communicates with the joint.

DEF: Metaphysis: Section of a long bone located between the epiphysis and diaphysis at the proximal and distal ends.

DEF: Physis (growth plate): Narrow zone of cartilaginous tissue between the epiphysis and metaphysis at each end of a long bone. In childhood, proliferation of cells in this zone lengthens the bone. As the bone matures, this area thins, ossification eventually fusing into solid bone and growth stops. ***Synonym(s):*** *Epiphyseal plate.*

The appropriate 7th character is to be added to all codes from category S72 [unless otherwise indicated].

- A initial encounter for closed fracture
- B initial encounter for open fracture type I or II
  initial encounter for open fracture NOS
- C initial encounter for open fracture type IIIA, IIIB, or IIIC
- D subsequent encounter for closed fracture with routine healing
- E subsequent encounter for open fracture type I or II with routine healing
- F subsequent encounter for open fracture type IIIA, IIIB, or IIIC with routine healing
- G subsequent encounter for closed fracture with delayed healing
- H subsequent encounter for open fracture type I or II with delayed healing
- J subsequent encounter for open fracture type IIIA, IIIB, or IIIC with delayed healing
- K subsequent encounter for closed fracture with nonunion
- M subsequent encounter for open fracture type I or II with nonunion
- N subsequent encounter for open fracture type IIIA, IIIB, or IIIC with nonunion
- P subsequent encounter for closed fracture with malunion
- Q subsequent encounter for open fracture type I or II with malunion
- R subsequent encounter for open fracture type IIIA, IIIB, or IIIC with malunion
- S sequela

5th S72.0 Fracture of head and neck of femur

EXCLUDES 2 *►physeal fracture of lower end of femur (S79.1-)◄*
physeal fracture of upper end of femur (S79.0-)

AHA: 2016,3Q,16

6th S72.00 Fracture of unspecified part of neck of femur

Fracture of hip NOS
Fracture of neck of femur NOS

7th S72.001 Fracture of unspecified part of neck of right femur MCC CC H5 HCC

7th S72.002 Fracture of unspecified part of neck of left femur MCC CC H5 HCC

7th S72.009 Fracture of unspecified part of neck of unspecified femur MCC CC H5 UNS HCC

6th S72.01 Unspecified intracapsular fracture of femur

Subcapital fracture of femur

7th S72.011 Unspecified intracapsular fracture of right femur MCC CC H5 HCC

7th S72.012 Unspecified intracapsular fracture of left femur MCC CC H5 HCC

7th S72.019 Unspecified intracapsular fracture of unspecified femur MCC CC H5 UNS HCC

6th S72.02 Fracture of epiphysis (separation) (upper) of femur

Transepiphyseal fracture of femur

EXCLUDES 1 *capital femoral epiphyseal fracture (pediatric) of femur (S79.01-)*
Salter-Harris Type I physeal fracture of upper end of femur (S79.01-)

7th S72.021 Displaced fracture of epiphysis (separation) (upper) of right femur MCC CC H5 HCC

7th S72.022 Displaced fracture of epiphysis (separation) (upper) of left femur MCC CC H5 HCC

7th S72.023 Displaced fracture of epiphysis (separation) (upper) of unspecified femur MCC CC H5 UNS HCC

7th S72.024 Nondisplaced fracture of epiphysis (separation) (upper) of right femur MCC CC H5 HCC

7th S72.025 Nondisplaced fracture of epiphysis (separation) (upper) of left femur MCC CC H5 HCC

7th S72.026 Nondisplaced fracture of epiphysis (separation) (upper) of unspecified femur MCC CC H5 UNS HCC

6th S72.03 Midcervical fracture of femur

Transcervical fracture of femur NOS

7th S72.031 Displaced midcervical fracture of right femur MCC CC H5 HCC

7th S72.032 Displaced midcervical fracture of left femur MCC CC H5 HCC

7th S72.033 Displaced midcervical fracture of unspecified femur MCC CC H5 UNS HCC

7th S72.034 Nondisplaced midcervical fracture of right femur MCC CC H5 HCC

7th S72.035 Nondisplaced midcervical fracture of left femur MCC CC H5 HCC

7th S72.036 Nondisplaced midcervical fracture of unspecified femur MCC CC H5 UNS HCC

6th S72.04 Fracture of base of neck of femur

Cervicotrochanteric fracture of femur

7th S72.041 Displaced fracture of base of neck of right femur MCC CC H5 HCC

7th S72.042 Displaced fracture of base of neck of left femur MCC CC H5 HCC

7th S72.043 Displaced fracture of base of neck of unspecified femur MCC CC H5 UNS HCC

7th S72.044 Nondisplaced fracture of base of neck of right femur MCC CC H5 HCC

7th S72.045 Nondisplaced fracture of base of neck of left femur MCC CC H5 HCC

7th S72.046 Nondisplaced fracture of base of neck of unspecified femur MCC CC H5 UNS HCC

6th S72.05 Unspecified fracture of head of femur

Fracture of head of femur NOS

7th S72.051 Unspecified fracture of head of right femur MCC CC H5 HCC

7th S72.052 Unspecified fracture of head of left femur MCC CC H5 HCC

7th S72.059 Unspecified fracture of head of unspecified femur MCC CC H5 UNS HCC

6th S72.06 Articular fracture of head of femur

7th S72.061 Displaced articular fracture of head of right femur MCC CC H5 HCC

7th S72.062 Displaced articular fracture of head of left femur MCC CC H5 HCC

7th S72.063 Displaced articular fracture of head of unspecified femur MCC CC H5 UNS HCC

7th S72.064 Nondisplaced articular fracture of head of right femur MCC CC H5 HCC

7th S72.065 Nondisplaced articular fracture of head of left femur MCC CC H5 HCC

7th S72.066 Nondisplaced articular fracture of head of unspecified femur MCC CC H5 UNS HCC

6th S72.09 Other fracture of head and neck of femur

7th S72.091 Other fracture of head and neck of right femur MCC CC H5 HCC

7th S72.092 Other fracture of head and neck of left femur MCC CC H5 HCC

7th S72.099 Other fracture of head and neck of unspecified femur MCC CC H5 UNS HCC

5th S72.1 Pertrochanteric fracture

AHA: 2016,3Q,16

6th S72.10 Unspecified trochanteric fracture of femur

Fracture of trochanter NOS

7th S72.101 Unspecified trochanteric fracture of right femur MCC CC H5 HCC

√7th **S72.102** Unspecified trochanteric fracture of left femur MCC CC HS HCC

√7th **S72.109** Unspecified trochanteric fracture of unspecified femur MCC CC HS UNS HCC

√6th **S72.11** Fracture of greater trochanter of femur

√7th **S72.111** Displaced fracture of greater trochanter of right femur MCC CC HS HCC

√7th **S72.112** Displaced fracture of greater trochanter of left femur MCC CC HS HCC

√7th **S72.113** Displaced fracture of greater trochanter of unspecified femur MCC CC HS UNS HCC

√7th **S72.114** Nondisplaced fracture of greater trochanter of right femur MCC CC HS HCC

√7th **S72.115** Nondisplaced fracture of greater trochanter of left femur MCC CC HS HCC

√7th **S72.116** Nondisplaced fracture of greater trochanter of unspecified femur MCC CC HS UNS HCC

√6th **S72.12** Fracture of lesser trochanter of femur

√7th **S72.121** Displaced fracture of lesser trochanter of right femur MCC CC HS HCC

√7th **S72.122** Displaced fracture of lesser trochanter of left femur MCC CC HS HCC

√7th **S72.123** Displaced fracture of lesser trochanter of unspecified femur MCC CC HS UNS HCC

√7th **S72.124** Nondisplaced fracture of lesser trochanter of right femur MCC CC HS HCC

√7th **S72.125** Nondisplaced fracture of lesser trochanter of left femur MCC CC HS HCC

√7th **S72.126** Nondisplaced fracture of lesser trochanter of unspecified femur MCC CC HS UNS HCC

√6th **S72.13** Apophyseal fracture of femur

EXCLUDES 1 *chronic (nontraumatic) slipped upper femoral epiphysis (M93.0-)*

√7th **S72.131** Displaced apophyseal fracture of right femur MCC CC HS HCC

√7th **S72.132** Displaced apophyseal fracture of left femur MCC CC HS HCC

√7th **S72.133** Displaced apophyseal fracture of unspecified femur MCC CC HS UNS HCC

√7th **S72.134** Nondisplaced apophyseal fracture of right femur MCC CC HS HCC

√7th **S72.135** Nondisplaced apophyseal fracture of left femur MCC CC HS HCC

√7th **S72.136** Nondisplaced apophyseal fracture of unspecified femur MCC CC HS UNS HCC

√6th **S72.14** Intertrochanteric fracture of femur

√7th **S72.141** Displaced intertrochanteric fracture of right femur MCC CC HS HCC

√7th **S72.142** Displaced intertrochanteric fracture of left femur MCC CC HS HCC

√7th **S72.143** Displaced intertrochanteric fracture of unspecified femur MCC CC HS UNS HCC

√7th **S72.144** Nondisplaced intertrochanteric fracture of right femur MCC CC HS HCC

√7th **S72.145** Nondisplaced intertrochanteric fracture of left femur MCC CC HS HCC

√7th **S72.146** Nondisplaced intertrochanteric fracture of unspecified femur MCC CC HS UNS HCC

√5th **S72.2** Subtrochanteric fracture of femur

√x7th **S72.21** Displaced subtrochanteric fracture of right femur MCC CC HS HCC

√x7th **S72.22** Displaced subtrochanteric fracture of left femur MCC CC HS HCC

√x7th **S72.23** Displaced subtrochanteric fracture of unspecified femur MCC CC HS UNS HCC

√x7th **S72.24** Nondisplaced subtrochanteric fracture of right femur MCC CC HS HCC

√x7th **S72.25** Nondisplaced subtrochanteric fracture of left femur MCC CC HS HCC

√x7th **S72.26** Nondisplaced subtrochanteric fracture of unspecified femur MCC CC HS UNS HCC

√5th **S72.3** Fracture of shaft of femur

√6th **S72.30** Unspecified fracture of shaft of femur

√7th **S72.301** Unspecified fracture of shaft of right femur MCC CC HS HCC

√7th **S72.302** Unspecified fracture of shaft of left femur MCC CC HS HCC

√7th **S72.309** Unspecified fracture of shaft of unspecified femur MCC CC HS UNS HCC

√6th **S72.32** Transverse fracture of shaft of femur

√7th **S72.321** Displaced transverse fracture of shaft of right femur MCC CC HS HCC

√7th **S72.322** Displaced transverse fracture of shaft of left femur MCC CC HS HCC

√7th **S72.323** Displaced transverse fracture of shaft of unspecified femur MCC CC HS UNS HCC

√7th **S72.324** Nondisplaced transverse fracture of shaft of right femur MCC CC HS HCC

√7th **S72.325** Nondisplaced transverse fracture of shaft of left femur MCC CC HS HCC

√7th **S72.326** Nondisplaced transverse fracture of shaft of unspecified femur MCC CC HS UNS HCC

√6th **S72.33** Oblique fracture of shaft of femur

√7th **S72.331** Displaced oblique fracture of shaft of right femur MCC CC HS HCC

√7th **S72.332** Displaced oblique fracture of shaft of left femur MCC CC HS HCC

√7th **S72.333** Displaced oblique fracture of shaft of unspecified femur MCC CC HS UNS HCC

√7th **S72.334** Nondisplaced oblique fracture of shaft of right femur MCC CC HS HCC

√7th **S72.335** Nondisplaced oblique fracture of shaft of left femur MCC CC HS HCC

√7th **S72.336** Nondisplaced oblique fracture of shaft of unspecified femur MCC CC HS UNS HCC

√6th **S72.34** Spiral fracture of shaft of femur

√7th **S72.341** Displaced spiral fracture of shaft of right femur MCC CC HS HCC

√7th **S72.342** Displaced spiral fracture of shaft of left femur MCC CC HS HCC

√7th **S72.343** Displaced spiral fracture of shaft of unspecified femur MCC CC HS UNS HCC

√7th **S72.344** Nondisplaced spiral fracture of shaft of right femur MCC CC HS HCC

√7th **S72.345** Nondisplaced spiral fracture of shaft of left femur MCC CC HS HCC

√7th **S72.346** Nondisplaced spiral fracture of shaft of unspecified femur MCC CC HS UNS HCC

√6th **S72.35** Comminuted fracture of shaft of femur

√7th **S72.351** Displaced comminuted fracture of shaft of right femur MCC CC HS HCC

√7th **S72.352** Displaced comminuted fracture of shaft of left femur MCC CC HS HCC

√7th **S72.353** Displaced comminuted fracture of shaft of unspecified femur MCC CC HS UNS HCC

√7th **S72.354** Nondisplaced comminuted fracture of shaft of right femur MCC CC HS HCC

√7th **S72.355** Nondisplaced comminuted fracture of shaft of left femur MCC CC HS HCC

√7th **S72.356** Nondisplaced comminuted fracture of shaft of unspecified femur MCC CC HS UNS HCC

√6th **S72.36** Segmental fracture of shaft of femur

√7th **S72.361** Displaced segmental fracture of shaft of right femur MCC CC HS HCC

√7th **S72.362** Displaced segmental fracture of shaft of left femur MCC CC HS HCC

√7th **S72.363** Displaced segmental fracture of shaft of unspecified femur MCC CC HS UNS HCC

√7th **S72.364** Nondisplaced segmental fracture of shaft of right femur MCC CC HS HCC

√7th **S72.365** Nondisplaced segmental fracture of shaft of left femur MCC CC HS HCC

√7th **S72.366** Nondisplaced segmental fracture of shaft of unspecified femur MCC CC HS UNS HCC

✓6th S72.39 Other fracture of shaft of femur
✓7th S72.391 Other fracture of shaft of right femur MCC CC H5 HCC
✓7th S72.392 Other fracture of shaft of left femur MCC CC H5 HCC
✓7th S72.399 Other fracture of shaft of unspecified femur MCC CC H5 UNS HCC
✓5th S72.4 Fracture of lower end of femur
Fracture of distal end of femur
EXCLUDES 2 fracture of shaft of femur (S72.3-)
physeal fracture of lower end of femur (S79.1-)
AHA: 2016,4Q,42
✓6th S72.40 Unspecified fracture of lower end of femur
AHA: 2018,1Q,21; 2016,4Q,42
✓7th S72.401 Unspecified fracture of lower end of right femur MCC CC H5 HCC
✓7th S72.402 Unspecified fracture of lower end of left femur MCC CC H5 HCC
✓7th S72.409 Unspecified fracture of lower end of unspecified femur MCC CC H5 UNS HCC
✓6th S72.41 Unspecified condyle fracture of lower end of femur
Condyle fracture of femur NOS
✓7th S72.411 Displaced unspecified condyle fracture of lower end of right femur MCC CC H5 HCC
✓7th S72.412 Displaced unspecified condyle fracture of lower end of left femur MCC CC H5 HCC
✓7th S72.413 Displaced unspecified condyle fracture of lower end of unspecified femur MCC CC H5 UNS HCC
✓7th S72.414 Nondisplaced unspecified condyle fracture of lower end of right femur MCC CC H5 HCC
✓7th S72.415 Nondisplaced unspecified condyle fracture of lower end of left femur MCC CC H5 HCC
✓7th S72.416 Nondisplaced unspecified condyle fracture of lower end of unspecified femur MCC CC H5 UNS HCC
✓6th S72.42 Fracture of lateral condyle of femur
✓7th S72.421 Displaced fracture of lateral condyle of right femur MCC CC H5 HCC
✓7th S72.422 Displaced fracture of lateral condyle of left femur MCC CC H5 HCC
✓7th S72.423 Displaced fracture of lateral condyle of unspecified femur MCC CC H5 UNS HCC
✓7th S72.424 Nondisplaced fracture of lateral condyle of right femur MCC CC H5 HCC
✓7th S72.425 Nondisplaced fracture of lateral condyle of left femur MCC CC H5 HCC
✓7th S72.426 Nondisplaced fracture of lateral condyle of unspecified femur MCC CC H5 UNS HCC
✓6th S72.43 Fracture of medial condyle of femur
✓7th S72.431 Displaced fracture of medial condyle of right femur MCC CC H5 HCC
✓7th S72.432 Displaced fracture of medial condyle of left femur MCC CC H5 HCC
✓7th S72.433 Displaced fracture of medial condyle of unspecified femur MCC CC H5 UNS HCC
✓7th S72.434 Nondisplaced fracture of medial condyle of right femur MCC CC H5 HCC
✓7th S72.435 Nondisplaced fracture of medial condyle of left femur MCC CC H5 HCC
✓7th S72.436 Nondisplaced fracture of medial condyle of unspecified femur MCC CC H5 UNS HCC
✓6th S72.44 Fracture of lower epiphysis (separation) of femur
EXCLUDES 1 Salter-Harris Type I physeal fracture of lower end of femur (S79.11-)
✓7th S72.441 Displaced fracture of lower epiphysis (separation) of right femur MCC CC H5 HCC
✓7th S72.442 Displaced fracture of lower epiphysis (separation) of left femur MCC CC H5 HCC
✓7th S72.443 Displaced fracture of lower epiphysis (separation) of unspecified femur MCC CC H5 UNS HCC
✓7th S72.444 Nondisplaced fracture of lower epiphysis (separation) of right femur MCC CC H5 HCC
✓7th S72.445 Nondisplaced fracture of lower epiphysis (separation) of left femur MCC CC H5 HCC
✓7th S72.446 Nondisplaced fracture of lower epiphysis (separation) of unspecified femur MCC CC H5 UNS HCC
✓6th S72.45 Supracondylar fracture without intracondylar extension of lower end of femur
Supracondylar fracture of lower end of femur NOS
EXCLUDES 1 supracondylar fracture with intracondylar extension of lower end of femur (S72.46-)
✓7th S72.451 Displaced supracondylar fracture without intracondylar extension of lower end of right femur MCC CC H5 HCC
✓7th S72.452 Displaced supracondylar fracture without intracondylar extension of lower end of left femur MCC CC H5 HCC
✓7th S72.453 Displaced supracondylar fracture without intracondylar extension of lower end of unspecified femur MCC CC H5 UNS HCC
✓7th S72.454 Nondisplaced supracondylar fracture without intracondylar extension of lower end of right femur MCC CC H5 HCC
✓7th S72.455 Nondisplaced supracondylar fracture without intracondylar extension of lower end of left femur MCC CC H5 HCC
✓7th S72.456 Nondisplaced supracondylar fracture without intracondylar extension of lower end of unspecified femur MCC CC H5 UNS HCC
✓6th S72.46 Supracondylar fracture with intracondylar extension of lower end of femur
EXCLUDES 1 supracondylar fracture without intracondylar extension of lower end of femur (S72.45-)
✓7th S72.461 Displaced supracondylar fracture with intracondylar extension of lower end of right femur MCC CC H5 HCC
✓7th S72.462 Displaced supracondylar fracture with intracondylar extension of lower end of left femur MCC CC H5 HCC
✓7th S72.463 Displaced supracondylar fracture with intracondylar extension of lower end of unspecified femur MCC CC H5 UNS HCC
✓7th S72.464 Nondisplaced supracondylar fracture with intracondylar extension of lower end of right femur MCC CC H5 HCC
✓7th S72.465 Nondisplaced supracondylar fracture with intracondylar extension of lower end of left femur MCC CC H5 HCC
✓7th S72.466 Nondisplaced supracondylar fracture with intracondylar extension of lower end of unspecified femur MCC CC H5 UNS HCC
✓6th S72.47 Torus fracture of lower end of femur

The appropriate 7th character is to be added to all codes in subcategory S72.47.
A initial encounter for closed fracture
D subsequent encounter for fracture with routine healing
G subsequent encounter for fracture with delayed healing
K subsequent encounter for fracture with nonunion
P subsequent encounter for fracture with malunion
S sequela

✓7th S72.471 Torus fracture of lower end of right femur CC H5 HCC
✓7th S72.472 Torus fracture of lower end of left femur CC H5 HCC
✓7th S72.479 Torus fracture of lower end of unspecified femur CC H5 UNS HCC

✓6th **S72.49 Other fracture of lower end of femur**
- ✓7th **S72.491 Other fracture of lower end of right femur** MCC CC HS HCC
- ✓7th **S72.492 Other fracture of lower end of left femur** MCC CC HS HCC
- ✓7th **S72.499 Other fracture of lower end of unspecified femur** MCC CC HS UNS HCC

✓5th **S72.8 Other fracture of femur**

✓6th **S72.8X Other fracture of femur**
- ✓7th **S72.8X1 Other fracture of right femur** MCC CC HS HCC
- ✓7th **S72.8X2 Other fracture of left femur** MCC CC HS HCC
- ✓7th **S72.8X9 Other fracture of unspecified femur** MCC CC HS UNS HCC

✓5th **S72.9 Unspecified fracture of femur**

Fracture of thigh NOS
Fracture of upper leg NOS

EXCLUDES 1 *fracture of hip NOS (S72.ØØ-, S72.Ø1-)*

- ✓x7th **S72.9Ø Unspecified fracture of unspecified femur** MCC CC HS UNS HCC
  AHA: 2012,4Q,93
- ✓x7th **S72.91 Unspecified fracture of right femur** MCC CC HS HCC
- ✓x7th **S72.92 Unspecified fracture of left femur** MCC CC HS HCC

✓4th **S73 Dislocation and sprain of joint and ligaments of hip**

INCLUDES avulsion of joint or ligament of hip
laceration of cartilage, joint or ligament of hip
sprain of cartilage, joint or ligament of hip
traumatic hemarthrosis of joint or ligament of hip
traumatic rupture of joint or ligament of hip
traumatic subluxation of joint or ligament of hip
traumatic tear of joint or ligament of hip

Code also any associated open wound

EXCLUDES 2 *strain of muscle, fascia and tendon of hip and thigh (S76.-)*

The appropriate 7th character is to be added to each code from category S73.
A initial encounter
D subsequent encounter
S sequela

✓5th **S73.Ø Subluxation and dislocation of hip**

EXCLUDES 2 *dislocation and subluxation of hip prosthesis (T84.Ø2Ø, T84.Ø21)*

✓6th **S73.ØØ Unspecified subluxation and dislocation of hip**

Dislocation of hip NOS
Subluxation of hip NOS

- ✓7th **S73.ØØ1 Unspecified subluxation of right hip** CC HS HCC
- ✓7th **S73.ØØ2 Unspecified subluxation of left hip** CC HS HCC
- ✓7th **S73.ØØ3 Unspecified subluxation of unspecified hip** CC HS UNS HCC
- ✓7th **S73.ØØ4 Unspecified dislocation of right hip** CC HS HCC
- ✓7th **S73.ØØ5 Unspecified dislocation of left hip** CC HS HCC
- ✓7th **S73.ØØ6 Unspecified dislocation of unspecified hip** CC HS UNS HCC

✓6th **S73.Ø1 Posterior subluxation and dislocation of hip**
- ✓7th **S73.Ø11 Posterior subluxation of right hip** CC HS HCC
- ✓7th **S73.Ø12 Posterior subluxation of left hip** CC HS HCC
- ✓7th **S73.Ø13 Posterior subluxation of unspecified hip** CC HS UNS HCC
- ✓7th **S73.Ø14 Posterior dislocation of right hip** CC HS HCC
- ✓7th **S73.Ø15 Posterior dislocation of left hip** CC HS HCC
- ✓7th **S73.Ø16 Posterior dislocation of unspecified hip** CC HS UNS HCC

✓6th **S73.Ø2 Obturator subluxation and dislocation of hip**
- ✓7th **S73.Ø21 Obturator subluxation of right hip** CC HS HCC
- ✓7th **S73.Ø22 Obturator subluxation of left hip** CC HS HCC
- ✓7th **S73.Ø23 Obturator subluxation of unspecified hip** CC HS UNS HCC
- ✓7th **S73.Ø24 Obturator dislocation of right hip** CC HS HCC
- ✓7th **S73.Ø25 Obturator dislocation of left hip** CC HS HCC
- ✓7th **S73.Ø26 Obturator dislocation of unspecified hip** CC HS UNS HCC

✓6th **S73.Ø3 Other anterior subluxation and dislocation of hip**
- ✓7th **S73.Ø31 Other anterior subluxation of right hip** CC HS HCC
- ✓7th **S73.Ø32 Other anterior subluxation of left hip** CC HS HCC
- ✓7th **S73.Ø33 Other anterior subluxation of unspecified hip** CC HS UNS HCC
- ✓7th **S73.Ø34 Other anterior dislocation of right hip** CC HS HCC
- ✓7th **S73.Ø35 Other anterior dislocation of left hip** CC HS HCC
- ✓7th **S73.Ø36 Other anterior dislocation of unspecified hip** CC HS UNS HCC

✓6th **S73.Ø4 Central subluxation and dislocation of hip**
- ✓7th **S73.Ø41 Central subluxation of right hip** CC HS HCC
- ✓7th **S73.Ø42 Central subluxation of left hip** CC HS HCC
- ✓7th **S73.Ø43 Central subluxation of unspecified hip** CC HS UNS HCC
- ✓7th **S73.Ø44 Central dislocation of right hip** CC HS HCC
- ✓7th **S73.Ø45 Central dislocation of left hip** CC HS HCC
- ✓7th **S73.Ø46 Central dislocation of unspecified hip** CC HS UNS HCC

✓5th **S73.1 Sprain of hip**

AHA: 2014,4Q,25

✓6th **S73.1Ø Unspecified sprain of hip**
- ✓7th **S73.1Ø1 Unspecified sprain of right hip**
- ✓7th **S73.1Ø2 Unspecified sprain of left hip**
- ✓7th **S73.1Ø9 Unspecified sprain of unspecified hip**

✓6th **S73.11 Iliofemoral ligament sprain of hip**
- ✓7th **S73.111 Iliofemoral ligament sprain of right hip**
- ✓7th **S73.112 Iliofemoral ligament sprain of left hip**
- ✓7th **S73.119 Iliofemoral ligament sprain of unspecified hip**

✓6th **S73.12 Ischiocapsular (ligament) sprain of hip**
- ✓7th **S73.121 Ischiocapsular ligament sprain of right hip**
- ✓7th **S73.122 Ischiocapsular ligament sprain of left hip**
- ✓7th **S73.129 Ischiocapsular ligament sprain of unspecified hip**

✓6th **S73.19 Other sprain of hip**
- ✓7th **S73.191 Other sprain of right hip**
- ✓7th **S73.192 Other sprain of left hip**
- ✓7th **S73.199 Other sprain of unspecified hip**

✓4th **S74 Injury of nerves at hip and thigh level**

Code also any associated open wound (S71.-)

EXCLUDES 2 *injury of nerves at ankle and foot level (S94.-)*
injury of nerves at lower leg level (S84.-)

The appropriate 7th character is to be added to each code from category S74.
A initial encounter
D subsequent encounter
S sequela

✓5th **S74.Ø Injury of sciatic nerve at hip and thigh level**
- ✓x7th **S74.ØØ Injury of sciatic nerve at hip and thigh level, unspecified leg**
- ✓x7th **S74.Ø1 Injury of sciatic nerve at hip and thigh level, right leg**
- ✓x7th **S74.Ø2 Injury of sciatic nerve at hip and thigh level, left leg**

✓5th **S74.1 Injury of femoral nerve at hip and thigh level**
- ✓x7th **S74.1Ø Injury of femoral nerve at hip and thigh level, unspecified leg**
- ✓x7th **S74.11 Injury of femoral nerve at hip and thigh level, right leg**

√x7th S74.12 Injury of femoral nerve at hip and thigh level, left leg

√5th S74.2 Injury of cutaneous sensory nerve at hip and thigh level

√x7th S74.20 Injury of cutaneous sensory nerve at hip and thigh level, unspecified leg

√x7th S74.21 Injury of cutaneous sensory nerve at hip and high level, right leg

√x7th S74.22 Injury of cutaneous sensory nerve at hip and thigh level, left leg

√5th S74.8 Injury of other nerves at hip and thigh level

√6th S74.8X Injury of other nerves at hip and thigh level

√7th S74.8X1 Injury of other nerves at hip and thigh level, right leg

√7th S74.8X2 Injury of other nerves at hip and thigh level, left leg

√7th S74.8X9 Injury of other nerves at hip and thigh level, unspecified leg

√5th S74.9 Injury of unspecified nerve at hip and thigh level

√x7th S74.90 Injury of unspecified nerve at hip and thigh level, unspecified leg

√x7th S74.91 Injury of unspecified nerve at hip and thigh level, right leg

√x7th S74.92 Injury of unspecified nerve at hip and thigh level, left leg

√4th **S75 Injury of blood vessels at hip and thigh level**

Code also any associated open wound (S71.-)

EXCLUDES 2 *injury of blood vessels at lower leg level (S85.-)*
injury of popliteal artery (S85.Ø)

The appropriate 7th character is to be added to each code from category S75.
A initial encounter
D subsequent encounter
S sequela

√5th S75.Ø Injury of femoral artery

√6th S75.ØØ Unspecified injury of femoral artery

√7th S75.ØØ1 Unspecified injury of femoral artery, right leg MCC

√7th S75.ØØ2 Unspecified injury of femoral artery, left leg MCC

√7th S75.ØØ9 Unspecified injury of femoral artery, unspecified leg MCC UNS

√6th S75.Ø1 Minor laceration of femoral artery
Incomplete transection of femoral artery
Laceration of femoral artery NOS
Superficial laceration of femoral artery

√7th S75.Ø11 Minor laceration of femoral artery, right leg MCC

√7th S75.Ø12 Minor laceration of femoral artery, left leg MCC

√7th S75.Ø19 Minor laceration of femoral artery, unspecified leg MCC UNS

√6th S75.Ø2 Major laceration of femoral artery
Complete transection of femoral artery
Traumatic rupture of femoral artery

√7th S75.Ø21 Major laceration of femoral artery, right leg MCC

√7th S75.Ø22 Major laceration of femoral artery, left leg MCC

√7th S75.Ø29 Major laceration of femoral artery, unspecified leg MCC UNS

√6th S75.Ø9 Other specified injury of femoral artery

√7th S75.Ø91 Other specified injury of femoral artery, right leg MCC

√7th S75.Ø92 Other specified injury of femoral artery, left leg MCC

√7th S75.Ø99 Other specified injury of femoral artery, unspecified leg MCC UNS

√5th S75.1 Injury of femoral vein at hip and thigh level

√6th S75.1Ø Unspecified injury of femoral vein at hip and thigh level

√7th S75.1Ø1 Unspecified injury of femoral vein at hip and thigh level, right leg MCC

√7th S75.1Ø2 Unspecified injury of femoral vein at hip and thigh level, left leg MCC

√7th S75.1Ø9 Unspecified injury of femoral vein at hip and thigh level, unspecified leg MCC UNS

√6th S75.11 Minor laceration of femoral vein at hip and thigh level
Incomplete transection of femoral vein at hip and thigh level
Laceration of femoral vein at hip and thigh level NOS
Superficial laceration of femoral vein at hip and thigh level

√7th S75.111 Minor laceration of femoral vein at hip and thigh level, right leg MCC

√7th S75.112 Minor laceration of femoral vein at hip and thigh level, left leg MCC

√7th S75.119 Minor laceration of femoral vein at hip and thigh level, unspecified leg MCC UNS

√6th S75.12 Major laceration of femoral vein at hip and thigh level
Complete transection of femoral vein at hip and thigh level
Traumatic rupture of femoral vein at hip and thigh level

√7th S75.121 Major laceration of femoral vein at hip and thigh level, right leg MCC

√7th S75.122 Major laceration of femoral vein at hip and thigh level, left leg MCC

√7th S75.129 Major laceration of femoral vein at hip and thigh level, unspecified leg MCC UNS

√6th S75.19 Other specified injury of femoral vein at hip and thigh level

√7th S75.191 Other specified injury of femoral vein at hip and thigh level, right leg MCC

√7th S75.192 Other specified injury of femoral vein at hip and thigh level, left leg MCC

√7th S75.199 Other specified injury of femoral vein at hip and thigh level, unspecified leg MCC UNS

√5th S75.2 Injury of greater saphenous vein at hip and thigh level

EXCLUDES 1 *greater saphenous vein NOS (S85.3)*

√6th S75.2Ø Unspecified injury of greater saphenous vein at hip and thigh level

√7th S75.2Ø1 Unspecified injury of greater saphenous vein at hip and thigh level, right leg CC

√7th S75.2Ø2 Unspecified injury of greater saphenous vein at hip and thigh level, left leg CC

√7th S75.2Ø9 Unspecified injury of greater saphenous vein at hip and thigh level, unspecified leg CC UNS

√6th S75.21 Minor laceration of greater saphenous vein at hip and thigh level
Incomplete transection of greater saphenous vein at hip and thigh level
Laceration of greater saphenous vein at hip and thigh level NOS
Superficial laceration of greater saphenous vein at hip and thigh level

√7th S75.211 Minor laceration of greater saphenous vein at hip and thigh level, right leg CC

√7th S75.212 Minor laceration of greater saphenous vein at hip and thigh level, left leg CC

√7th S75.219 Minor laceration of greater saphenous vein at hip and thigh level, unspecified leg CC UNS

√6th S75.22 Major laceration of greater saphenous vein at hip and thigh level
Complete transection of greater saphenous vein at hip and thigh level
Traumatic rupture of greater saphenous vein at hip and thigh level

√7th S75.221 Major laceration of greater saphenous vein at hip and thigh level, right leg CC

√7th S75.222 Major laceration of greater saphenous vein at hip and thigh level, left leg CC

√7th S75.229 Major laceration of greater saphenous vein at hip and thigh level, unspecified leg CC UNS

S75.29 Other specified injury of greater saphenous vein at hip and thigh level
- **S75.291** Other specified injury of greater saphenous vein at hip and thigh level, right leg CC
- **S75.292** Other specified injury of greater saphenous vein at hip and thigh level, left leg CC
- **S75.299** Other specified injury of greater saphenous vein at hip and thigh level, unspecified leg CC UNS

S75.8 Injury of other blood vessels at hip and thigh level

S75.80 Unspecified injury of other blood vessels at hip and thigh level
- **S75.801** Unspecified injury of other blood vessels at hip and thigh level, right leg CC
- **S75.802** Unspecified injury of other blood vessels at hip and thigh level, left leg CC
- **S75.809** Unspecified injury of other blood vessels at hip and thigh level, unspecified leg CC UNS

S75.81 Laceration of other blood vessels at hip and thigh level
- **S75.811** Laceration of other blood vessels at hip and thigh level, right leg CC
- **S75.812** Laceration of other blood vessels at hip and thigh level, left leg CC
- **S75.819** Laceration of other blood vessels at hip and thigh level, unspecified leg CC UNS

S75.89 Other specified injury of other blood vessels at hip and thigh level
- **S75.891** Other specified injury of other blood vessels at hip and thigh level, right leg CC
- **S75.892** Other specified injury of other blood vessels at hip and thigh level, left leg CC
- **S75.899** Other specified injury of other blood vessels at hip and thigh level, unspecified leg CC UNS

S75.9 Injury of unspecified blood vessel at hip and thigh level

S75.90 Unspecified injury of unspecified blood vessel at hip and thigh level
- **S75.901** Unspecified injury of unspecified blood vessel at hip and thigh level, right leg CC
- **S75.902** Unspecified injury of unspecified blood vessel at hip and thigh level, left leg CC
- **S75.909** Unspecified injury of unspecified blood vessel at hip and thigh level, unspecified leg CC UNS

S75.91 Laceration of unspecified blood vessel at hip and thigh level
- **S75.911** Laceration of unspecified blood vessel at hip and thigh level, right leg CC
- **S75.912** Laceration of unspecified blood vessel at hip and thigh level, left leg CC
- **S75.919** Laceration of unspecified blood vessel at hip and thigh level, unspecified leg CC UNS

S75.99 Other specified injury of unspecified blood vessel at hip and thigh level
- **S75.991** Other specified injury of unspecified blood vessel at hip and thigh level, right leg CC
- **S75.992** Other specified injury of unspecified blood vessel at hip and thigh level, left leg CC
- **S75.999** Other specified injury of unspecified blood vessel at hip and thigh level, unspecified leg CC UNS

S76 Injury of muscle, fascia and tendon at hip and thigh level

Code also any associated open wound (S71.-)

EXCLUDES 2 *injury of muscle, fascia and tendon at lower leg level (S86)*
sprain of joint and ligament of hip (S73.1)

TIP: Refer to the Muscle/Tendon table at the beginning of this chapter.

The appropriate 7th character is to be added to each code from category S76.
- A initial encounter
- D subsequent encounter
- S sequela

S76.0 Injury of muscle, fascia and tendon of hip

S76.00 Unspecified injury of muscle, fascia and tendon of hip
- **S76.001** Unspecified injury of muscle, fascia and tendon of right hip
- **S76.002** Unspecified injury of muscle, fascia and tendon of left hip
- **S76.009** Unspecified injury of muscle, fascia and tendon of unspecified hip

S76.01 Strain of muscle, fascia and tendon of hip
- **S76.011** Strain of muscle, fascia and tendon of right hip
- **S76.012** Strain of muscle, fascia and tendon of left hip
- **S76.019** Strain of muscle, fascia and tendon of unspecified hip

S76.02 Laceration of muscle, fascia and tendon of hip
- **S76.021** Laceration of muscle, fascia and tendon of right hip CC
- **S76.022** Laceration of muscle, fascia and tendon of left hip CC
- **S76.029** Laceration of muscle, fascia and tendon of unspecified hip CC UNS

S76.09 Other specified injury of muscle, fascia and tendon of hip
- **S76.091** Other specified injury of muscle, fascia and tendon of right hip
- **S76.092** Other specified injury of muscle, fascia and tendon of left hip
- **S76.099** Other specified injury of muscle, fascia and tendon of unspecified hip

S76.1 Injury of quadriceps muscle, fascia and tendon

Injury of patellar ligament (tendon)

S76.10 Unspecified injury of quadriceps muscle, fascia and tendon
- **S76.101** Unspecified injury of right quadriceps muscle, fascia and tendon
- **S76.102** Unspecified injury of left quadriceps muscle, fascia and tendon
- **S76.109** Unspecified injury of unspecified quadriceps muscle, fascia and tendon

S76.11 Strain of quadriceps muscle, fascia and tendon
- **S76.111** Strain of right quadriceps muscle, fascia and tendon
- **S76.112** Strain of left quadriceps muscle, fascia and tendon
- **S76.119** Strain of unspecified quadriceps muscle, fascia and tendon

S76.12 Laceration of quadriceps muscle, fascia and tendon
- **S76.121** Laceration of right quadriceps muscle, fascia and tendon CC
- **S76.122** Laceration of left quadriceps muscle, fascia and tendon CC
- **S76.129** Laceration of unspecified quadriceps muscle, fascia and tendon CC UNS

S76.19 Other specified injury of quadriceps muscle, fascia and tendon
- **S76.191** Other specified injury of right quadriceps muscle, fascia and tendon
- **S76.192** Other specified injury of left quadriceps muscle, fascia and tendon
- **S76.199** Other specified injury of unspecified quadriceps muscle, fascia and tendon

S76.2 Injury of adductor muscle, fascia and tendon of thigh

S76.20 Unspecified injury of adductor muscle, fascia and tendon of thigh
- **S76.201** Unspecified injury of adductor muscle, fascia and tendon of right thigh
- **S76.202** Unspecified injury of adductor muscle, fascia and tendon of left thigh

S76.209 Unspecified injury of adductor muscle, fascia and tendon of unspecified thigh

S76.21 Strain of adductor muscle, fascia and tendon of thigh

S76.211 Strain of adductor muscle, fascia and tendon of right thigh

S76.212 Strain of adductor muscle, fascia and tendon of left thigh

S76.219 Strain of adductor muscle, fascia and tendon of unspecified thigh

S76.22 Laceration of adductor muscle, fascia and tendon of thigh

S76.221 Laceration of adductor muscle, fascia and tendon of right thigh CC

S76.222 Laceration of adductor muscle, fascia and tendon of left thigh CC

S76.229 Laceration of adductor muscle, fascia and tendon of unspecified thigh CC UNS

S76.29 Other injury of adductor muscle, fascia and tendon of thigh

S76.291 Other injury of adductor muscle, fascia and tendon of right thigh

S76.292 Other injury of adductor muscle, fascia and tendon of left thigh

S76.299 Other injury of adductor muscle, fascia and tendon of unspecified thigh

S76.3 Injury of muscle, fascia and tendon of the posterior muscle group at thigh level

S76.30 Unspecified injury of muscle, fascia and tendon of the posterior muscle group at thigh level

S76.301 Unspecified injury of muscle, fascia and tendon of the posterior muscle group at thigh level, right thigh

S76.302 Unspecified injury of muscle, fascia and tendon of the posterior muscle group at thigh level, left thigh

S76.309 Unspecified injury of muscle, fascia and tendon of the posterior muscle group at thigh level, unspecified thigh

S76.31 Strain of muscle, fascia and tendon of the posterior muscle group at thigh level

S76.311 Strain of muscle, fascia and tendon of the posterior muscle group at thigh level, right thigh

S76.312 Strain of muscle, fascia and tendon of the posterior muscle group at thigh level, left thigh

S76.319 Strain of muscle, fascia and tendon of the posterior muscle group at thigh level, unspecified thigh

S76.32 Laceration of muscle, fascia and tendon of the posterior muscle group at thigh level

S76.321 Laceration of muscle, fascia and tendon of the posterior muscle group at thigh level, right thigh CC

S76.322 Laceration of muscle, fascia and tendon of the posterior muscle group at thigh level, left thigh CC

S76.329 Laceration of muscle, fascia and tendon of the posterior muscle group at thigh level, unspecified thigh CC UNS

S76.39 Other specified injury of muscle, fascia and tendon of the posterior muscle group at thigh level

S76.391 Other specified injury of muscle, fascia and tendon of the posterior muscle group at thigh level, right thigh

S76.392 Other specified injury of muscle, fascia and tendon of the posterior muscle group at thigh level, left thigh

S76.399 Other specified injury of muscle, fascia and tendon of the posterior muscle group at thigh level, unspecified thigh

S76.8 Injury of other specified muscles, fascia and tendons at thigh level

S76.80 Unspecified injury of other specified muscles, fascia and tendons at thigh level

S76.801 Unspecified injury of other specified muscles, fascia and tendons at thigh level, right thigh

S76.802 Unspecified injury of other specified muscles, fascia and tendons at thigh level, left thigh

S76.809 Unspecified injury of other specified muscles, fascia and tendons at thigh level, unspecified thigh

S76.81 Strain of other specified muscles, fascia and tendons at thigh level

S76.811 Strain of other specified muscles, fascia and tendons at thigh level, right thigh

S76.812 Strain of other specified muscles, fascia and tendons at thigh level, left thigh

S76.819 Strain of other specified muscles, fascia and tendons at thigh level, unspecified thigh

S76.82 Laceration of other specified muscles, fascia and tendons at thigh level

S76.821 Laceration of other specified muscles, fascia and tendons at thigh level, right thigh CC

S76.822 Laceration of other specified muscles, fascia and tendons at thigh level, left thigh CC

S76.829 Laceration of other specified muscles, fascia and tendons at thigh level, unspecified thigh CC UNS

S76.89 Other injury of other specified muscles, fascia and tendons at thigh level

S76.891 Other injury of other specified muscles, fascia and tendons at thigh level, right thigh

S76.892 Other injury of other specified muscles, fascia and tendons at thigh level, left thigh

S76.899 Other injury of other specified muscles, fascia and tendons at thigh level, unspecified thigh

S76.9 Injury of unspecified muscles, fascia and tendons at thigh level

S76.90 Unspecified injury of unspecified muscles, fascia and tendons at thigh level

S76.901 Unspecified injury of unspecified muscles, fascia and tendons at thigh level, right thigh

S76.902 Unspecified injury of unspecified muscles, fascia and tendons at thigh level, left thigh

S76.909 Unspecified injury of unspecified muscles, fascia and tendons at thigh level, unspecified thigh

S76.91 Strain of unspecified muscles, fascia and tendons at thigh level

S76.911 Strain of unspecified muscles, fascia and tendons at thigh level, right thigh

S76.912 Strain of unspecified muscles, fascia and tendons at thigh level, left thigh

S76.919 Strain of unspecified muscles, fascia and tendons at thigh level, unspecified thigh

S76.92 Laceration of unspecified muscles, fascia and tendons at thigh level

S76.921 Laceration of unspecified muscles, fascia and tendons at thigh level, right thigh CC

S76.922 Laceration of unspecified muscles, fascia and tendons at thigh level, left thigh CC

S76.929 Laceration of unspecified muscles, fascia and tendons at thigh level, unspecified thigh CC UNS

S76.99 Other specified injury of unspecified muscles, fascia and tendons at thigh level

S76.991 Other specified injury of unspecified muscles, fascia and tendons at thigh level, right thigh

S76.992 Other specified injury of unspecified muscles, fascia and tendons at thigh level, left thigh

S76.999 Other specified injury of unspecified muscles, fascia and tendons at thigh level, unspecified thigh

4th S77 Crushing injury of hip and thigh
Use additional code(s) for all associated injuries
EXCLUDES 2 *crushing injury of ankle and foot (S97.-)*
crushing injury of lower leg (S87.-)

The appropriate 7th character is to be added to each code from category S77.
A initial encounter
D subsequent encounter
S sequela

5th **S77.Ø Crushing injury of hip**
x7th **S77.ØØ Crushing injury of unspecified hip** CC H5 UNS
x7th **S77.Ø1 Crushing injury of right hip** CC H5
x7th **S77.Ø2 Crushing injury of left hip** CC H5
5th **S77.1 Crushing injury of thigh**
x7th **S77.1Ø Crushing injury of unspecified thigh** CC H5 UNS
x7th **S77.11 Crushing injury of right thigh** CC H5
x7th **S77.12 Crushing injury of left thigh** CC H5
5th **S77.2 Crushing injury of hip with thigh**
x7th **S77.2Ø Crushing injury of unspecified hip with thigh**
x7th **S77.21 Crushing injury of right hip with thigh**
x7th **S77.22 Crushing injury of left hip with thigh**

4th S78 Traumatic amputation of hip and thigh
An amputation not identified as partial or complete should be coded to complete
EXCLUDES 1 *traumatic amputation of knee (S88.Ø-)*

The appropriate 7th character is to be added to each code from category S78.
A initial encounter
D subsequent encounter
S sequela

5th **S78.Ø Traumatic amputation at hip joint**
6th **S78.Ø1 Complete traumatic amputation at hip joint**
7th **S78.Ø11 Complete traumatic amputation at right hip joint** CC HCC
7th **S78.Ø12 Complete traumatic amputation at left hip joint** CC HCC
7th **S78.Ø19 Complete traumatic amputation at unspecified hip joint** CC UNS HCC
6th **S78.Ø2 Partial traumatic amputation at hip joint**
7th **S78.Ø21 Partial traumatic amputation at right hip joint** CC HCC
7th **S78.Ø22 Partial traumatic amputation at left hip joint** CC HCC
7th **S78.Ø29 Partial traumatic amputation at unspecified hip joint** CC UNS HCC
5th **S78.1 Traumatic amputation at level between hip and knee**
EXCLUDES 1 *traumatic amputation of knee (S88.Ø-)*
6th **S78.11 Complete traumatic amputation at level between hip and knee**
7th **S78.111 Complete traumatic amputation at level between right hip and knee** CC HCC
7th **S78.112 Complete traumatic amputation at level between left hip and knee** CC HCC
7th **S78.119 Complete traumatic amputation at level between unspecified hip and knee** CC UNS HCC
6th **S78.12 Partial traumatic amputation at level between hip and knee**
7th **S78.121 Partial traumatic amputation at level between right hip and knee** CC HCC
7th **S78.122 Partial traumatic amputation at level between left hip and knee** CC HCC
7th **S78.129 Partial traumatic amputation at level between unspecified hip and knee** CC UNS HCC
5th **S78.9 Traumatic amputation of hip and thigh, level unspecified**
6th **S78.91 Complete traumatic amputation of hip and thigh, level unspecified**
7th **S78.911 Complete traumatic amputation of right hip and thigh, level unspecified** CC HCC
7th **S78.912 Complete traumatic amputation of left hip and thigh, level unspecified** CC HCC
7th **S78.919 Complete traumatic amputation of unspecified hip and thigh, level unspecified** CC UNS HCC
6th **S78.92 Partial traumatic amputation of hip and thigh, level unspecified**
7th **S78.921 Partial traumatic amputation of right hip and thigh, level unspecified** CC HCC
7th **S78.922 Partial traumatic amputation of left hip and thigh, level unspecified** CC HCC
7th **S78.929 Partial traumatic amputation of unspecified hip and thigh, level unspecified** CC UNS HCC

4th S79 Other and unspecified injuries of hip and thigh
NOTE A fracture not indicated as open or closed should be coded to closed
AHA: 2018,2Q,12; 2018,1Q,3; 2015,3Q,37-39

The appropriate 7th character is to be added to each code from subcategories S79.Ø and S79.1.
A initial encounter for closed fracture
D subsequent encounter for fracture with routine healing
G subsequent encounter for fracture with delayed healing
K subsequent encounter for fracture with nonunion
P subsequent encounter for fracture with malunion
S sequela

5th **S79.Ø Physeal fracture of upper end of femur**
EXCLUDES 1 *apophyseal fracture of upper end of femur (S72.13-)*
nontraumatic slipped upper femoral epiphysis (M93.Ø-)
AHA: 2019,4Q,56
6th **S79.ØØ Unspecified physeal fracture of upper end of femur**
7th **S79.ØØ1 Unspecified physeal fracture of upper end of right femur** MCC CC H5 HCC
7th **S79.ØØ2 Unspecified physeal fracture of upper end of left femur** MCC CC H5 HCC
7th **S79.ØØ9 Unspecified physeal fracture of upper end of unspecified femur** MCC CC H5 UNS HCC
6th **S79.Ø1 Salter-Harris Type I physeal fracture of upper end of femur**
Acute on chronic slipped capital femoral epiphysis (traumatic)
Acute slipped capital femoral epiphysis (traumatic)
Capital femoral epiphyseal fracture
EXCLUDES 1 *chronic slipped upper femoral epiphysis (nontraumatic) (M93.Ø2-)*
7th **S79.Ø11 Salter-Harris Type I physeal fracture of upper end of right femur** MCC CC H5 HCC
7th **S79.Ø12 Salter-Harris Type I physeal fracture of upper end of left femur** MCC CC H5 HCC
7th **S79.Ø19 Salter-Harris Type I physeal fracture of upper end of unspecified femur** MCC CC H5 UNS HCC
6th **S79.Ø9 Other physeal fracture of upper end of femur**
7th **S79.Ø91 Other physeal fracture of upper end of right femur** MCC CC H5 HCC
7th **S79.Ø92 Other physeal fracture of upper end of left femur** MCC CC H5 HCC
7th **S79.Ø99 Other physeal fracture of upper end of unspecified femur** MCC CC H5 UNS HCC
5th **S79.1 Physeal fracture of lower end of femur**
AHA: 2019,4Q,56
6th **S79.1Ø Unspecified physeal fracture of lower end of femur**
7th **S79.1Ø1 Unspecified physeal fracture of lower end of right femur** CC H5 HCC
7th **S79.1Ø2 Unspecified physeal fracture of lower end of left femur** CC H5 HCC
7th **S79.1Ø9 Unspecified physeal fracture of lower end of unspecified femur** CC H5 UNS HCC
6th **S79.11 Salter-Harris Type I physeal fracture of lower end of femur**
7th **S79.111 Salter-Harris Type I physeal fracture of lower end of right femur** CC H5 HCC
7th **S79.112 Salter-Harris Type I physeal fracture of lower end of left femur** CC H5 HCC
7th **S79.119 Salter-Harris Type I physeal fracture of lower end of unspecified femur** CC H5 UNS HCC

N Newborn: 0 P Pediatric: 0-17 M Maternity: 9-64 A Adult: 15-124 UNS Unspecified Site MCC Major Complication/Comorbidity CC Complication/Comorbidity

- S79.12 Salter-Harris Type II physeal fracture of lower end of femur
  - S79.121 Salter-Harris Type II physeal fracture of lower end of right femur CC H5 HCC
  - S79.122 Salter-Harris Type II physeal fracture of lower end of left femur CC H5 HCC
  - S79.129 Salter-Harris Type II physeal fracture of lower end of unspecified femur CC H5 UNS HCC
- S79.13 Salter-Harris Type III physeal fracture of lower end of femur
  - S79.131 Salter-Harris Type III physeal fracture of lower end of right femur CC H5 HCC
  - S79.132 Salter-Harris Type III physeal fracture of lower end of left femur CC H5 HCC
  - S79.139 Salter-Harris Type III physeal fracture of lower end of unspecified femur CC H5 UNS HCC
- S79.14 Salter-Harris Type IV physeal fracture of lower end of femur
  - S79.141 Salter-Harris Type IV physeal fracture of lower end of right femur CC H5 HCC
  - S79.142 Salter-Harris Type IV physeal fracture of lower end of left femur CC H5 HCC
  - S79.149 Salter-Harris Type IV physeal fracture of lower end of unspecified femur CC H5 UNS HCC
- S79.19 Other physeal fracture of lower end of femur
  - S79.191 Other physeal fracture of lower end of right femur CC H5 HCC
  - S79.192 Other physeal fracture of lower end of left femur CC H5 HCC
  - S79.199 Other physeal fracture of lower end of unspecified femur CC H5 UNS HCC

S79.8 Other specified injuries of hip and thigh

> The appropriate 7th character is to be added to each code in subcategory S79.8.
> A initial encounter
> D subsequent encounter
> S sequela

- S79.81 Other specified injuries of hip
  - S79.811 Other specified injuries of right hip
  - S79.812 Other specified injuries of left hip
  - S79.819 Other specified injuries of unspecified hip
- S79.82 Other specified injuries of thigh
  - S79.821 Other specified injuries of right thigh
  - S79.822 Other specified injuries of left thigh
  - S79.829 Other specified injuries of unspecified thigh

S79.9 Unspecified injury of hip and thigh

> The appropriate 7th character is to be added to each code in subcategory S79.9.
> A initial encounter
> D subsequent encounter
> S sequela

- S79.91 Unspecified injury of hip
  - S79.911 Unspecified injury of right hip
  - S79.912 Unspecified injury of left hip
  - S79.919 Unspecified injury of unspecified hip
- S79.92 Unspecified injury of thigh
  - S79.921 Unspecified injury of right thigh
  - S79.922 Unspecified injury of left thigh
  - S79.929 Unspecified injury of unspecified thigh

Injuries to the knee and lower leg (S80-S89)

EXCLUDES 2 *burns and corrosions (T20-T32)*
frostbite (T33-T34)
injuries of ankle and foot, except fracture of ankle and malleolus (S90-S99)
insect bite or sting, venomous (T63.4)

S80 Superficial injury of knee and lower leg

EXCLUDES 2 *superficial injury of ankle and foot (S90.-)*

> The appropriate 7th character is to be added to each code from category S80.
> A initial encounter
> D subsequent encounter
> S sequela

S80.0 Contusion of knee
- S80.00 Contusion of unspecified knee
- S80.01 Contusion of right knee
- S80.02 Contusion of left knee

S80.1 Contusion of lower leg
- S80.10 Contusion of unspecified lower leg
- S80.11 Contusion of right lower leg
- S80.12 Contusion of left lower leg

S80.2 Other superficial injuries of knee
- S80.21 Abrasion of knee
  - S80.211 Abrasion, right knee
  - S80.212 Abrasion, left knee
  - S80.219 Abrasion, unspecified knee
- S80.22 Blister (nonthermal) of knee
  - S80.221 Blister (nonthermal), right knee
  - S80.222 Blister (nonthermal), left knee
  - S80.229 Blister (nonthermal), unspecified knee
- S80.24 External constriction of knee
  - S80.241 External constriction, right knee
  - S80.242 External constriction, left knee
  - S80.249 External constriction, unspecified knee
- S80.25 Superficial foreign body of knee
  Splinter in the knee
  - S80.251 Superficial foreign body, right knee
  - S80.252 Superficial foreign body, left knee
  - S80.259 Superficial foreign body, unspecified knee
- S80.26 Insect bite (nonvenomous) of knee
  - S80.261 Insect bite (nonvenomous), right knee
  - S80.262 Insect bite (nonvenomous), left knee
  - S80.269 Insect bite (nonvenomous), unspecified knee
- S80.27 Other superficial bite of knee
  EXCLUDES 1 *open bite of knee (S81.05-)*
  - S80.271 Other superficial bite of right knee
  - S80.272 Other superficial bite of left knee
  - S80.279 Other superficial bite of unspecified knee

S80.8 Other superficial injuries of lower leg
- S80.81 Abrasion of lower leg
  - S80.811 Abrasion, right lower leg
  - S80.812 Abrasion, left lower leg
  - S80.819 Abrasion, unspecified lower leg
- S80.82 Blister (nonthermal) of lower leg
  - S80.821 Blister (nonthermal), right lower leg
  - S80.822 Blister (nonthermal), left lower leg
  - S80.829 Blister (nonthermal), unspecified lower leg
- S80.84 External constriction of lower leg
  - S80.841 External constriction, right lower leg
  - S80.842 External constriction, left lower leg
  - S80.849 External constriction, unspecified lower leg
- S80.85 Superficial foreign body of lower leg
  Splinter in the lower leg
  - S80.851 Superficial foreign body, right lower leg

7th S8Ø.852 Superficial foreign body, left lower leg
7th S8Ø.859 Superficial foreign body, unspecified lower leg
6th S8Ø.86 Insect bite (nonvenomous) of lower leg
7th S8Ø.861 Insect bite (nonvenomous), right lower leg
7th S8Ø.862 Insect bite (nonvenomous), left lower leg
7th S8Ø.869 Insect bite (nonvenomous), unspecified lower leg
6th S8Ø.87 Other superficial bite of lower leg
EXCLUDES 1 *open bite of lower leg (S81.85-)*
7th S8Ø.871 Other superficial bite, right lower leg
7th S8Ø.872 Other superficial bite, left lower leg
7th S8Ø.879 Other superficial bite, unspecified lower leg
5th S8Ø.9 Unspecified superficial injury of knee and lower leg
6th S8Ø.91 Unspecified superficial injury of knee
7th S8Ø.911 Unspecified superficial injury of right knee
7th S8Ø.912 Unspecified superficial injury of left knee
7th S8Ø.919 Unspecified superficial injury of unspecified knee
6th S8Ø.92 Unspecified superficial injury of lower leg
7th S8Ø.921 Unspecified superficial injury of right lower leg
7th S8Ø.922 Unspecified superficial injury of left lower leg
7th S8Ø.929 Unspecified superficial injury of unspecified lower leg

4th S81 Open wound of knee and lower leg
Code also any associated wound infection
EXCLUDES 1 *open fracture of knee and lower leg (S82.-)*
traumatic amputation of lower leg (S88.-)
EXCLUDES 2 *open wound of ankle and foot (S91.-)*

The appropriate 7th character is to be added to each code from category S81.
A initial encounter
D subsequent encounter
S sequela

5th S81.Ø Open wound of knee
6th S81.ØØ Unspecified open wound of knee
7th S81.ØØ1 Unspecified open wound, right knee
7th S81.ØØ2 Unspecified open wound, left knee
7th S81.ØØ9 Unspecified open wound, unspecified knee
6th S81.Ø1 Laceration without foreign body of knee
7th S81.Ø11 Laceration without foreign body, right knee
7th S81.Ø12 Laceration without foreign body, left knee
7th S81.Ø19 Laceration without foreign body, unspecified knee
6th S81.Ø2 Laceration with foreign body of knee
7th S81.Ø21 Laceration with foreign body, right knee
7th S81.Ø22 Laceration with foreign body, left knee
7th S81.Ø29 Laceration with foreign body, unspecified knee
6th S81.Ø3 Puncture wound without foreign body of knee
7th S81.Ø31 Puncture wound without foreign body, right knee
7th S81.Ø32 Puncture wound without foreign body, left knee
7th S81.Ø39 Puncture wound without foreign body, unspecified knee
6th S81.Ø4 Puncture wound with foreign body of knee
7th S81.Ø41 Puncture wound with foreign body, right knee
7th S81.Ø42 Puncture wound with foreign body, left knee
7th S81.Ø49 Puncture wound with foreign body, unspecified knee
6th S81.Ø5 Open bite of knee
Bite of knee NOS
EXCLUDES 1 *superficial bite of knee (S8Ø.27-)*
7th S81.Ø51 Open bite, right knee
7th S81.Ø52 Open bite, left knee
7th S81.Ø59 Open bite, unspecified knee
5th S81.8 Open wound of lower leg
6th S81.8Ø Unspecified open wound of lower leg
AHA: 2016,3Q,24
7th S81.8Ø1 Unspecified open wound, right lower leg
7th S81.8Ø2 Unspecified open wound, left lower leg
7th S81.8Ø9 Unspecified open wound, unspecified lower leg
6th S81.81 Laceration without foreign body of lower leg
7th S81.811 Laceration without foreign body, right lower leg
7th S81.812 Laceration without foreign body, left lower leg
7th S81.819 Laceration without foreign body, unspecified lower leg
6th S81.82 Laceration with foreign body of lower leg
7th S81.821 Laceration with foreign body, right lower leg
7th S81.822 Laceration with foreign body, left lower leg
7th S81.829 Laceration with foreign body, unspecified lower leg
6th S81.83 Puncture wound without foreign body of lower leg
AHA: 2016,3Q,24
7th S81.831 Puncture wound without foreign body, right lower leg
7th S81.832 Puncture wound without foreign body, left lower leg
7th S81.839 Puncture wound without foreign body, unspecified lower leg
6th S81.84 Puncture wound with foreign body of lower leg
AHA: 2016,3Q,24
7th S81.841 Puncture wound with foreign body, right lower leg
7th S81.842 Puncture wound with foreign body, left lower leg
7th S81.849 Puncture wound with foreign body, unspecified lower leg
6th S81.85 Open bite of lower leg
Bite of lower leg NOS
EXCLUDES 1 *superficial bite of lower leg (S8Ø.86-, S8Ø.87-)*
7th S81.851 Open bite, right lower leg
7th S81.852 Open bite, left lower leg
7th S81.859 Open bite, unspecified lower leg

S82 Fracture of lower leg, including ankle

NOTE A fracture not indicated as displaced or nondisplaced should be coded to displaced

A fracture not indicated as open or closed should be coded to closed

The open fracture designations are based on the Gustilo open fracture classification.

INCLUDES fracture of malleolus

EXCLUDES 1 *traumatic amputation of lower leg (S88.-)*

EXCLUDES 2 *fracture of foot, except ankle (S92.-)*

▶*periprosthetic fracture around internal prosthetic ankle joint (M97.2)*◀

periprosthetic fracture around internal prosthetic implant of knee joint (M97.1-)

AHA: 2018,2Q,12; 2016,1Q,33; 2015,3Q,37-39

DEF: Diaphysis: Central shaft of a long bone.

DEF: Epiphysis: Proximal and distal rounded ends of a long bone, communicates with the joint.

DEF: Metaphysis: Section of a long bone located between the epiphysis and diaphysis at the proximal and distal ends.

DEF: Physis (growth plate): Narrow zone of cartilaginous tissue between the epiphysis and metaphysis at each end of a long bone. In childhood, proliferation of cells in this zone lengthens the bone. As the bone matures, this area thins, ossification eventually fusing into solid bone and growth stops. ***Synonym(s):*** *Epiphyseal plate.*

The appropriate 7th character is to be added to all codes from category S82 [unless otherwise indicated].

- A initial encounter for closed fracture
- B initial encounter for open fracture type I or II
  initial encounter for open fracture NOS
- C initial encounter for open fracture type IIIA, IIIB, or IIIC
- D subsequent encounter for closed fracture with routine healing
- E subsequent encounter for open fracture type I or II with routine healing
- F subsequent encounter for open fracture type IIIA, IIIB, or IIIC with routine healing
- G subsequent encounter for closed fracture with delayed healing
- H subsequent encounter for open fracture type I or II with delayed healing
- J subsequent encounter for open fracture type IIIA, IIIB, or IIIC with delayed healing
- K subsequent encounter for closed fracture with nonunion
- M subsequent encounter for open fracture type I or II with nonunion
- N subsequent encounter for open fracture type IIIA, IIIB, or IIIC with nonunion
- P subsequent encounter for closed fracture with malunion
- Q subsequent encounter for open fracture type I or II with malunion
- R subsequent encounter for open fracture type IIIA, IIIB, or IIIC with malunion
- S sequela

S82.Ø Fracture of patella
Knee cap

S82.ØØ Unspecified fracture of patella
- **S82.ØØ1** Unspecified fracture of right patella CC H5
- **S82.ØØ2** Unspecified fracture of left patella CC H5
- **S82.ØØ9** Unspecified fracture of unspecified patella CC H5 UNS

S82.Ø1 Osteochondral fracture of patella
- **S82.Ø11** Displaced osteochondral fracture of right patella CC H5
- **S82.Ø12** Displaced osteochondral fracture of left patella CC H5
- **S82.Ø13** Displaced osteochondral fracture of unspecified patella CC H5 UNS
- **S82.Ø14** Nondisplaced osteochondral fracture of right patella CC H5
- **S82.Ø15** Nondisplaced osteochondral fracture of left patella CC H5
- **S82.Ø16** Nondisplaced osteochondral fracture of unspecified patella CC H5 UNS

S82.Ø2 Longitudinal fracture of patella
- **S82.Ø21** Displaced longitudinal fracture of right patella CC H5
- **S82.Ø22** Displaced longitudinal fracture of left patella CC H5
- **S82.Ø23** Displaced longitudinal fracture of unspecified patella CC H5 UNS
- **S82.Ø24** Nondisplaced longitudinal fracture of right patella CC H5
- **S82.Ø25** Nondisplaced longitudinal fracture of left patella CC H5
- **S82.Ø26** Nondisplaced longitudinal fracture of unspecified patella CC H5 UNS

S82.Ø3 Transverse fracture of patella
- **S82.Ø31** Displaced transverse fracture of right patella CC H5
- **S82.Ø32** Displaced transverse fracture of left patella CC H5
- **S82.Ø33** Displaced transverse fracture of unspecified patella CC H5 UNS
- **S82.Ø34** Nondisplaced transverse fracture of right patella CC H5
- **S82.Ø35** Nondisplaced transverse fracture of left patella CC H5
- **S82.Ø36** Nondisplaced transverse fracture of unspecified patella CC H5 UNS

S82.Ø4 Comminuted fracture of patella
- **S82.Ø41** Displaced comminuted fracture of right patella CC H5
- **S82.Ø42** Displaced comminuted fracture of left patella CC H5
- **S82.Ø43** Displaced comminuted fracture of unspecified patella CC H5 UNS
- **S82.Ø44** Nondisplaced comminuted fracture of right patella CC H5
- **S82.Ø45** Nondisplaced comminuted fracture of left patella CC H5
- **S82.Ø46** Nondisplaced comminuted fracture of unspecified patella CC H5 UNS

S82.Ø9 Other fracture of patella
- **S82.Ø91** Other fracture of right patella CC H5
- **S82.Ø92** Other fracture of left patella CC H5
- **S82.Ø99** Other fracture of unspecified patella CC H5 UNS

S82.1 Fracture of upper end of tibia
Fracture of proximal end of tibia

EXCLUDES 2 *fracture of shaft of tibia (S82.2-)*
physeal fracture of upper end of tibia (S89.Ø-)

S82.1Ø Unspecified fracture of upper end of tibia
- **S82.1Ø1** Unspecified fracture of upper end of right tibia MCC CC H5
- **S82.1Ø2** Unspecified fracture of upper end of left tibia MCC CC H5
- **S82.1Ø9** Unspecified fracture of upper end of unspecified tibia MCC CC H5 UNS

S82.11 Fracture of tibial spine
- **S82.111** Displaced fracture of right tibial spine MCC CC H5
- **S82.112** Displaced fracture of left tibial spine MCC CC H5
- **S82.113** Displaced fracture of unspecified tibial spine MCC CC H5 UNS
- **S82.114** Nondisplaced fracture of right tibial spine MCC CC H5
- **S82.115** Nondisplaced fracture of left tibial spine MCC CC H5
- **S82.116** Nondisplaced fracture of unspecified tibial spine MCC CC H5 UNS

S82.12 Fracture of lateral condyle of tibia
- **S82.121** Displaced fracture of lateral condyle of right tibia MCC CC H5
- **S82.122** Displaced fracture of lateral condyle of left tibia MCC CC H5
- **S82.123** Displaced fracture of lateral condyle of unspecified tibia MCC CC H5 UNS
- **S82.124** Nondisplaced fracture of lateral condyle of right tibia MCC CC H5
- **S82.125** Nondisplaced fracture of lateral condyle of left tibia MCC CC H5
- **S82.126** Nondisplaced fracture of lateral condyle of unspecified tibia MCC CC H5 UNS

6th S82.13 Fracture of medial condyle of tibia
7th S82.131 Displaced fracture of medial condyle of right tibia MCC CC H5
7th S82.132 Displaced fracture of medial condyle of left tibia MCC CC H5
7th S82.133 Displaced fracture of medial condyle of unspecified tibia MCC CC H5 UNS
7th S82.134 Nondisplaced fracture of medial condyle of right tibia MCC CC H5
7th S82.135 Nondisplaced fracture of medial condyle of left tibia MCC CC H5
7th S82.136 Nondisplaced fracture of medial condyle of unspecified tibia MCC CC H5 UNS
6th S82.14 Bicondylar fracture of tibia
Fracture of tibial plateau NOS
7th S82.141 Displaced bicondylar fracture of right tibia MCC CC H5
7th S82.142 Displaced bicondylar fracture of left tibia MCC CC H5
7th S82.143 Displaced bicondylar fracture of unspecified tibia MCC CC H5 UNS
7th S82.144 Nondisplaced bicondylar fracture of right tibia MCC CC H5
7th S82.145 Nondisplaced bicondylar fracture of left tibia MCC CC H5
7th S82.146 Nondisplaced bicondylar fracture of unspecified tibia MCC CC H5 UNS
6th S82.15 Fracture of tibial tuberosity
7th S82.151 Displaced fracture of right tibial tuberosity MCC CC H5
7th S82.152 Displaced fracture of left tibial tuberosity MCC CC H5
7th S82.153 Displaced fracture of unspecified tibial tuberosity MCC CC H5 UNS
7th S82.154 Nondisplaced fracture of right tibial tuberosity MCC CC H5
7th S82.155 Nondisplaced fracture of left tibial tuberosity MCC CC H5
7th S82.156 Nondisplaced fracture of unspecified tibial tuberosity MCC CC H5 UNS
6th S82.16 Torus fracture of upper end of tibia

The appropriate 7th character is to be added to all codes in subcategory S82.16.
A initial encounter for closed fracture
D subsequent encounter for fracture with routine healing
G subsequent encounter for fracture with delayed healing
K subsequent encounter for fracture with nonunion
P subsequent encounter for fracture with malunion
S sequela

7th S82.161 Torus fracture of upper end of right tibia CC H5
7th S82.162 Torus fracture of upper end of left tibia CC H5
7th S82.169 Torus fracture of upper end of unspecified tibia CC H5 UNS
6th S82.19 Other fracture of upper end of tibia
7th S82.191 Other fracture of upper end of right tibia MCC CC H5
7th S82.192 Other fracture of upper end of left tibia MCC CC H5
7th S82.199 Other fracture of upper end of unspecified tibia MCC CC H5 UNS
5th S82.2 Fracture of shaft of tibia
6th S82.20 Unspecified fracture of shaft of tibia
Fracture of tibia NOS
7th S82.201 Unspecified fracture of shaft of right tibia MCC CC H5
7th S82.202 Unspecified fracture of shaft of left tibia MCC CC H5
7th S82.209 Unspecified fracture of shaft of unspecified tibia MCC CC H5 UNS
6th S82.22 Transverse fracture of shaft of tibia
7th S82.221 Displaced transverse fracture of shaft of right tibia MCC CC H5
7th S82.222 Displaced transverse fracture of shaft of left tibia MCC CC H5
7th S82.223 Displaced transverse fracture of shaft of unspecified tibia MCC CC H5 UNS
7th S82.224 Nondisplaced transverse fracture of shaft of right tibia MCC CC H5
7th S82.225 Nondisplaced transverse fracture of shaft of left tibia MCC CC H5
7th S82.226 Nondisplaced transverse fracture of shaft of unspecified tibia MCC CC H5 UNS
6th S82.23 Oblique fracture of shaft of tibia
7th S82.231 Displaced oblique fracture of shaft of right tibia MCC CC H5
7th S82.232 Displaced oblique fracture of shaft of left tibia MCC CC H5
7th S82.233 Displaced oblique fracture of shaft of unspecified tibia MCC CC H5 UNS
7th S82.234 Nondisplaced oblique fracture of shaft of right tibia MCC CC H5
7th S82.235 Nondisplaced oblique fracture of shaft of left tibia MCC CC H5
7th S82.236 Nondisplaced oblique fracture of shaft of unspecified tibia MCC CC H5 UNS
6th S82.24 Spiral fracture of shaft of tibia
Toddler fracture
7th S82.241 Displaced spiral fracture of shaft of right tibia MCC CC H5
7th S82.242 Displaced spiral fracture of shaft of left tibia MCC CC H5
7th S82.243 Displaced spiral fracture of shaft of unspecified tibia MCC CC H5 UNS
7th S82.244 Nondisplaced spiral fracture of shaft of right tibia MCC CC H5
7th S82.245 Nondisplaced spiral fracture of shaft of left tibia MCC CC H5
7th S82.246 Nondisplaced spiral fracture of shaft of unspecified tibia MCC CC H5 UNS
6th S82.25 Comminuted fracture of shaft of tibia
7th S82.251 Displaced comminuted fracture of shaft of right tibia MCC CC H5
7th S82.252 Displaced comminuted fracture of shaft of left tibia MCC CC H5
7th S82.253 Displaced comminuted fracture of shaft of unspecified tibia MCC CC H5 UNS
7th S82.254 Nondisplaced comminuted fracture of shaft of right tibia MCC CC H5
7th S82.255 Nondisplaced comminuted fracture of shaft of left tibia MCC CC H5
7th S82.256 Nondisplaced comminuted fracture of shaft of unspecified tibia MCC CC H5 UNS
6th S82.26 Segmental fracture of shaft of tibia
7th S82.261 Displaced segmental fracture of shaft of right tibia MCC CC H5
7th S82.262 Displaced segmental fracture of shaft of left tibia MCC CC H5
7th S82.263 Displaced segmental fracture of shaft of unspecified tibia MCC CC H5 UNS
7th S82.264 Nondisplaced segmental fracture of shaft of right tibia MCC CC H5
7th S82.265 Nondisplaced segmental fracture of shaft of left tibia MCC CC H5
7th S82.266 Nondisplaced segmental fracture of shaft of unspecified tibia MCC CC H5 UNS
6th S82.29 Other fracture of shaft of tibia
7th S82.291 Other fracture of shaft of right tibia MCC CC H5
7th S82.292 Other fracture of shaft of left tibia MCC CC H5
7th S82.299 Other fracture of shaft of unspecified tibia MCC CC H5 UNS

√5th S82.3 Fracture of lower end of tibia

EXCLUDES 1 *bimalleolar fracture of lower leg (S82.84-)*
fracture of medial malleolus alone (S82.5-)
Maisonneuve's fracture (S82.86-)
pilon fracture of distal tibia (S82.87-)
trimalleolar fractures of lower leg (S82.85-)

√6th S82.30 Unspecified fracture of lower end of tibia

√7th S82.301 Unspecified fracture of lower end of right tibia CC H5

√7th S82.302 Unspecified fracture of lower end of left tibia CC H5

√7th S82.309 Unspecified fracture of lower end of unspecified tibia CC H5 UNS

√6th S82.31 Torus fracture of lower end of tibia

The appropriate 7th character is to be added to all codes in subcategory S82.31.
A initial encounter for closed fracture
D subsequent encounter for fracture with routine healing
G subsequent encounter for fracture with delayed healing
K subsequent encounter for fracture with nonunion
P subsequent encounter for fracture with malunion
S sequela

√7th S82.311 Torus fracture of lower end of right tibia CC H5

√7th S82.312 Torus fracture of lower end of left tibia CC H5

√7th S82.319 Torus fracture of lower end of unspecified tibia CC H5 UNS

√6th S82.39 Other fracture of lower end of tibia

AHA: 2015,1Q,25

√7th S82.391 Other fracture of lower end of right tibia CC H5

√7th S82.392 Other fracture of lower end of left tibia CC H5

√7th S82.399 Other fracture of lower end of unspecified tibia CC H5 UNS

√5th S82.4 Fracture of shaft of fibula

EXCLUDES 2 *fracture of lateral malleolus alone (S82.6-)*

√6th S82.40 Unspecified fracture of shaft of fibula

√7th S82.401 Unspecified fracture of shaft of right fibula MCC CC H5

√7th S82.402 Unspecified fracture of shaft of left fibula MCC CC H5

√7th S82.409 Unspecified fracture of shaft of unspecified fibula MCC CC H5 UNS

√6th S82.42 Transverse fracture of shaft of fibula

√7th S82.421 Displaced transverse fracture of shaft of right fibula MCC CC H5

√7th S82.422 Displaced transverse fracture of shaft of left fibula MCC CC H5

√7th S82.423 Displaced transverse fracture of shaft of unspecified fibula MCC CC H5 UNS

√7th S82.424 Nondisplaced transverse fracture of shaft of right fibula MCC CC H5

√7th S82.425 Nondisplaced transverse fracture of shaft of left fibula MCC CC H5

√7th S82.426 Nondisplaced transverse fracture of shaft of unspecified fibula MCC CC H5 UNS

√6th S82.43 Oblique fracture of shaft of fibula

√7th S82.431 Displaced oblique fracture of shaft of right fibula MCC CC H5

√7th S82.432 Displaced oblique fracture of shaft of left fibula MCC CC H5

√7th S82.433 Displaced oblique fracture of shaft of unspecified fibula MCC CC H5 UNS

√7th S82.434 Nondisplaced oblique fracture of shaft of right fibula MCC CC H5

√7th S82.435 Nondisplaced oblique fracture of shaft of left fibula MCC CC H5

√7th S82.436 Nondisplaced oblique fracture of shaft of unspecified fibula MCC CC H5 UNS

√6th S82.44 Spiral fracture of shaft of fibula

√7th S82.441 Displaced spiral fracture of shaft of right fibula MCC CC H5

√7th S82.442 Displaced spiral fracture of shaft of left fibula MCC CC H5

√7th S82.443 Displaced spiral fracture of shaft of unspecified fibula MCC CC H5 UNS

√7th S82.444 Nondisplaced spiral fracture of shaft of right fibula MCC CC H5

√7th S82.445 Nondisplaced spiral fracture of shaft of left fibula MCC CC H5

√7th S82.446 Nondisplaced spiral fracture of shaft of unspecified fibula MCC CC H5 UNS

√6th S82.45 Comminuted fracture of shaft of fibula

√7th S82.451 Displaced comminuted fracture of shaft of right fibula MCC CC H5

√7th S82.452 Displaced comminuted fracture of shaft of left fibula MCC CC H5

√7th S82.453 Displaced comminuted fracture of shaft of unspecified fibula MCC CC H5 UNS

√7th S82.454 Nondisplaced comminuted fracture of shaft of right fibula MCC CC H5

√7th S82.455 Nondisplaced comminuted fracture of shaft of left fibula MCC CC H5

√7th S82.456 Nondisplaced comminuted fracture of shaft of unspecified fibula MCC CC H5 UNS

√6th S82.46 Segmental fracture of shaft of fibula

√7th S82.461 Displaced segmental fracture of shaft of right fibula MCC CC H5

√7th S82.462 Displaced segmental fracture of shaft of left fibula MCC CC H5

√7th S82.463 Displaced segmental fracture of shaft of unspecified fibula MCC CC H5 UNS

√7th S82.464 Nondisplaced segmental fracture of shaft of right fibula MCC CC H5

√7th S82.465 Nondisplaced segmental fracture of shaft of left fibula MCC CC H5

√7th S82.466 Nondisplaced segmental fracture of shaft of unspecified fibula MCC CC H5 UNS

√6th S82.49 Other fracture of shaft of fibula

√7th S82.491 Other fracture of shaft of right fibula MCC CC H5

√7th S82.492 Other fracture of shaft of left fibula MCC CC H5

√7th S82.499 Other fracture of shaft of unspecified fibula MCC CC H5 UNS

√5th S82.5 Fracture of medial malleolus

EXCLUDES 1 *pilon fracture of distal tibia (S82.87-)*
Salter-Harris type III of lower end of tibia (S89.13-)
Salter-Harris type IV of lower end of tibia (S89.14-)

√x7th S82.51 Displaced fracture of medial malleolus of right tibia CC H5

√x7th S82.52 Displaced fracture of medial malleolus of left tibia CC H5

√x7th S82.53 Displaced fracture of medial malleolus of unspecified tibia CC H5 UNS

√x7th S82.54 Nondisplaced fracture of medial malleolus of right tibia CC H5

√x7th S82.55 Nondisplaced fracture of medial malleolus of left tibia CC H5

√x7th S82.56 Nondisplaced fracture of medial malleolus of unspecified tibia CC H5 UNS

√5th S82.6 Fracture of lateral malleolus

EXCLUDES 1 *pilon fracture of distal tibia (S82.87-)*

√x7th S82.61 Displaced fracture of lateral malleolus of right fibula CC H5

√x7th S82.62 Displaced fracture of lateral malleolus of left fibula CC H5

√x7th S82.63 Displaced fracture of lateral malleolus of unspecified fibula CC H5 UNS

√x7th S82.64 Nondisplaced fracture of lateral malleolus of right fibula CC H5

√x7th S82.65 Nondisplaced fracture of lateral malleolus of left fibula CC H5

√x7th S82.66 Nondisplaced fracture of lateral malleolus of unspecified fibula CC H5 UNS

✓5th **S82.8 Other fractures of lower leg**

✓6th **S82.81 Torus fracture of upper end of fibula**

The appropriate 7th character is to be added to all codes in subcategory S82.81
- A initial encounter for closed fracture
- D subsequent encounter for fracture with routine healing
- G subsequent encounter for fracture with delayed healing
- K subsequent encounter for fracture with nonunion
- P subsequent encounter for fracture with malunion
- S sequela

✓7th **S82.811 Torus fracture of upper end of right fibula** CC

✓7th **S82.812 Torus fracture of upper end of left fibula** CC

✓7th **S82.819 Torus fracture of upper end of unspecified fibula** CC UNS

✓6th **S82.82 Torus fracture of lower end of fibula**

The appropriate 7th character is to be added to all codes in subcategory S82.82.
- A initial encounter for closed fracture
- D subsequent encounter for fracture with routine healing
- G subsequent encounter for fracture with delayed healing
- K subsequent encounter for fracture with nonunion
- P subsequent encounter for fracture with malunion
- S sequela

✓7th **S82.821 Torus fracture of lower end of right fibula** CC

✓7th **S82.822 Torus fracture of lower end of left fibula** CC

✓7th **S82.829 Torus fracture of lower end of unspecified fibula** CC UNS

✓6th **S82.83 Other fracture of upper and lower end of fibula**

AHA: 2015,1Q,25

✓7th **S82.831 Other fracture of upper and lower end of right fibula** MCC CC H5

✓7th **S82.832 Other fracture of upper and lower end of left fibula** MCC CC H5

✓7th **S82.839 Other fracture of upper and lower end of unspecified fibula** MCC CC H5 UNS

✓6th **S82.84 Bimalleolar fracture of lower leg**

Right Bimalleolar Fracture

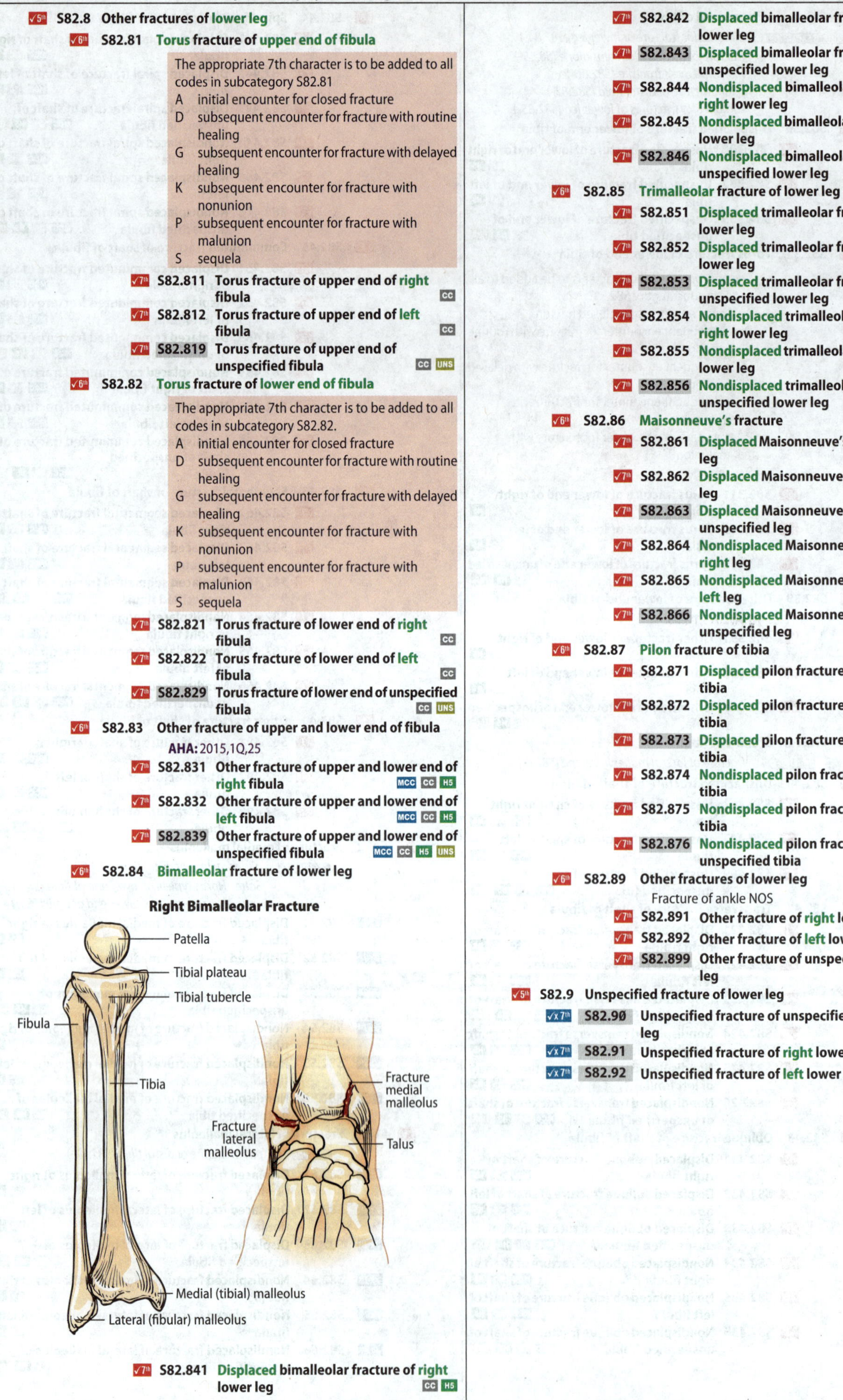

✓7th **S82.841 Displaced bimalleolar fracture of right lower leg** CC H5

✓7th **S82.842 Displaced bimalleolar fracture of left lower leg** CC H5

✓7th **S82.843 Displaced bimalleolar fracture of unspecified lower leg** CC H5 UNS

✓7th **S82.844 Nondisplaced bimalleolar fracture of right lower leg** CC H5

✓7th **S82.845 Nondisplaced bimalleolar fracture of left lower leg** CC H5

✓7th **S82.846 Nondisplaced bimalleolar fracture of unspecified lower leg** CC H5 UNS

✓6th **S82.85 Trimalleolar fracture of lower leg**

✓7th **S82.851 Displaced trimalleolar fracture of right lower leg** CC H5

✓7th **S82.852 Displaced trimalleolar fracture of left lower leg** CC H5

✓7th **S82.853 Displaced trimalleolar fracture of unspecified lower leg** CC H5 UNS

✓7th **S82.854 Nondisplaced trimalleolar fracture of right lower leg** CC H5

✓7th **S82.855 Nondisplaced trimalleolar fracture of left lower leg** CC H5

✓7th **S82.856 Nondisplaced trimalleolar fracture of unspecified lower leg** CC H5 UNS

✓6th **S82.86 Maisonneuve's fracture**

✓7th **S82.861 Displaced Maisonneuve's fracture of right leg** MCC CC H5

✓7th **S82.862 Displaced Maisonneuve's fracture of left leg** MCC CC H5

✓7th **S82.863 Displaced Maisonneuve's fracture of unspecified leg** MCC CC H5 UNS

✓7th **S82.864 Nondisplaced Maisonneuve's fracture of right leg** MCC CC H5

✓7th **S82.865 Nondisplaced Maisonneuve's fracture of left leg** MCC CC H5

✓7th **S82.866 Nondisplaced Maisonneuve's fracture of unspecified leg** MCC CC H5 UNS

✓6th **S82.87 Pilon fracture of tibia**

✓7th **S82.871 Displaced pilon fracture of right tibia** CC H5

✓7th **S82.872 Displaced pilon fracture of left tibia** CC H5

✓7th **S82.873 Displaced pilon fracture of unspecified tibia** CC H5 UNS

✓7th **S82.874 Nondisplaced pilon fracture of right tibia** CC H5

✓7th **S82.875 Nondisplaced pilon fracture of left tibia** CC H5

✓7th **S82.876 Nondisplaced pilon fracture of unspecified tibia** CC H5 UNS

✓6th **S82.89 Other fractures of lower leg**

Fracture of ankle NOS

✓7th **S82.891 Other fracture of right lower leg** CC H5

✓7th **S82.892 Other fracture of left lower leg** CC H5

✓7th **S82.899 Other fracture of unspecified lower leg** CC H5 UNS

✓5th **S82.9 Unspecified fracture of lower leg**

✓x7th **S82.90 Unspecified fracture of unspecified lower leg** CC H5 UNS

✓x7th **S82.91 Unspecified fracture of right lower leg** CC H5

✓x7th **S82.92 Unspecified fracture of left lower leg** CC H5

S83 Dislocation and sprain of joints and ligaments of knee

INCLUDES avulsion of joint or ligament of knee
laceration of cartilage, joint or ligament of knee
sprain of cartilage, joint or ligament of knee
traumatic hemarthrosis of joint or ligament of knee
traumatic rupture of joint or ligament of knee
traumatic subluxation of joint or ligament of knee
traumatic tear of joint or ligament of knee

Code also any associated open wound

EXCLUDES 2 *derangement of patella (M22.Ø-M22.3)*
injury of patellar ligament (tendon) (S76.1-)
internal derangement of knee (M23.-)
old dislocation of knee (M24.36)
pathological dislocation of knee (M24.36)
recurrent dislocation of knee (M22.Ø)
strain of muscle, fascia and tendon of lower leg (S86.-)

The appropriate 7th character is to be added to each code from category S83.
A initial encounter
D subsequent encounter
S sequela

S83.Ø Subluxation and dislocation of patella
S83.ØØ Unspecified subluxation and dislocation of patella
S83.ØØ1 Unspecified subluxation of right patella
S83.ØØ2 Unspecified subluxation of left patella
S83.ØØ3 Unspecified subluxation of unspecified patella
S83.ØØ4 Unspecified dislocation of right patella
S83.ØØ5 Unspecified dislocation of left patella
S83.ØØ6 Unspecified dislocation of unspecified patella
S83.Ø1 Lateral subluxation and dislocation of patella
S83.Ø11 Lateral subluxation of right patella
S83.Ø12 Lateral subluxation of left patella
S83.Ø13 Lateral subluxation of unspecified patella
S83.Ø14 Lateral dislocation of right patella
S83.Ø15 Lateral dislocation of left patella
S83.Ø16 Lateral dislocation of unspecified patella
S83.Ø9 Other subluxation and dislocation of patella
S83.Ø91 Other subluxation of right patella
S83.Ø92 Other subluxation of left patella
S83.Ø93 Other subluxation of unspecified patella
S83.Ø94 Other dislocation of right patella
S83.Ø95 Other dislocation of left patella
S83.Ø96 Other dislocation of unspecified patella
S83.1 Subluxation and dislocation of knee
EXCLUDES 2 *instability of knee prosthesis (T84.Ø22, T84.Ø23)*
S83.1Ø Unspecified subluxation and dislocation of knee
S83.1Ø1 Unspecified subluxation of right knee
S83.1Ø2 Unspecified subluxation of left knee
S83.1Ø3 Unspecified subluxation of unspecified knee
S83.1Ø4 Unspecified dislocation of right knee
S83.1Ø5 Unspecified dislocation of left knee
S83.1Ø6 Unspecified dislocation of unspecified knee
S83.11 Anterior subluxation and dislocation of proximal end of tibia
Posterior subluxation and dislocation of distal end of femur
S83.111 Anterior subluxation of proximal end of tibia, right knee
S83.112 Anterior subluxation of proximal end of tibia, left knee
S83.113 Anterior subluxation of proximal end of tibia, unspecified knee
S83.114 Anterior dislocation of proximal end of tibia, right knee
S83.115 Anterior dislocation of proximal end of tibia, left knee
S83.116 Anterior dislocation of proximal end of tibia, unspecified knee
S83.12 Posterior subluxation and dislocation of proximal end of tibia
Anterior dislocation of distal end of femur
S83.121 Posterior subluxation of proximal end of tibia, right knee
S83.122 Posterior subluxation of proximal end of tibia, left knee
S83.123 Posterior subluxation of proximal end of tibia, unspecified knee
S83.124 Posterior dislocation of proximal end of tibia, right knee
S83.125 Posterior dislocation of proximal end of tibia, left knee
S83.126 Posterior dislocation of proximal end of tibia, unspecified knee
S83.13 Medial subluxation and dislocation of proximal end of tibia
S83.131 Medial subluxation of proximal end of tibia, right knee
S83.132 Medial subluxation of proximal end of tibia, left knee
S83.133 Medial subluxation of proximal end of tibia, unspecified knee
S83.134 Medial dislocation of proximal end of tibia, right knee
S83.135 Medial dislocation of proximal end of tibia, left knee
S83.136 Medial dislocation of proximal end of tibia, unspecified knee
S83.14 Lateral subluxation and dislocation of proximal end of tibia
S83.141 Lateral subluxation of proximal end of tibia, right knee
S83.142 Lateral subluxation of proximal end of tibia, left knee
S83.143 Lateral subluxation of proximal end of tibia, unspecified knee
S83.144 Lateral dislocation of proximal end of tibia, right knee
S83.145 Lateral dislocation of proximal end of tibia, left knee
S83.146 Lateral dislocation of proximal end of tibia, unspecified knee
S83.19 Other subluxation and dislocation of knee
S83.191 Other subluxation of right knee
S83.192 Other subluxation of left knee
S83.193 Other subluxation of unspecified knee
S83.194 Other dislocation of right knee
S83.195 Other dislocation of left knee
S83.196 Other dislocation of unspecified knee
S83.2 Tear of meniscus, current injury
EXCLUDES 1 *old bucket-handle tear (M23.2)*
AHA: 2019,2Q,26
S83.2Ø Tear of unspecified meniscus, current injury
Tear of meniscus of knee NOS
S83.2ØØ Bucket-handle tear of unspecified meniscus, current injury, right knee
S83.2Ø1 Bucket-handle tear of unspecified meniscus, current injury, left knee
S83.2Ø2 Bucket-handle tear of unspecified meniscus, current injury, unspecified knee
S83.2Ø3 Other tear of unspecified meniscus, current injury, right knee
S83.2Ø4 Other tear of unspecified meniscus, current injury, left knee
S83.2Ø5 Other tear of unspecified meniscus, current injury, unspecified knee
S83.2Ø6 Unspecified tear of unspecified meniscus, current injury, right knee
S83.2Ø7 Unspecified tear of unspecified meniscus, current injury, left knee
S83.2Ø9 Unspecified tear of unspecified meniscus, current injury, unspecified knee
S83.21 Bucket-handle tear of medial meniscus, current injury
S83.211 Bucket-handle tear of medial meniscus, current injury, right knee
S83.212 Bucket-handle tear of medial meniscus, current injury, left knee

✓7th S83.219 Bucket-handle tear of medial meniscus, current injury, unspecified knee

✓6th S83.22 Peripheral tear of medial meniscus, current injury

✓7th S83.221 Peripheral tear of medial meniscus, current injury, right knee

✓7th S83.222 Peripheral tear of medial meniscus, current injury, left knee

✓7th S83.229 Peripheral tear of medial meniscus, current injury, unspecified knee

✓6th S83.23 Complex tear of medial meniscus, current injury

✓7th S83.231 Complex tear of medial meniscus, current injury, right knee

✓7th S83.232 Complex tear of medial meniscus, current injury, left knee

✓7th S83.239 Complex tear of medial meniscus, current injury, unspecified knee

✓6th S83.24 Other tear of medial meniscus, current injury

✓7th S83.241 Other tear of medial meniscus, current injury, right knee

✓7th S83.242 Other tear of medial meniscus, current injury, left knee

✓7th S83.249 Other tear of medial meniscus, current injury, unspecified knee

✓6th S83.25 Bucket-handle tear of lateral meniscus, current injury

✓7th S83.251 Bucket-handle tear of lateral meniscus, current injury, right knee

✓7th S83.252 Bucket-handle tear of lateral meniscus, current injury, left knee

✓7th S83.259 Bucket-handle tear of lateral meniscus, current injury, unspecified knee

✓6th S83.26 Peripheral tear of lateral meniscus, current injury

✓7th S83.261 Peripheral tear of lateral meniscus, current injury, right knee

✓7th S83.262 Peripheral tear of lateral meniscus, current injury, left knee

✓7th S83.269 Peripheral tear of lateral meniscus, current injury, unspecified knee

✓6th S83.27 Complex tear of lateral meniscus, current injury

✓7th S83.271 Complex tear of lateral meniscus, current injury, right knee

✓7th S83.272 Complex tear of lateral meniscus, current injury, left knee

✓7th S83.279 Complex tear of lateral meniscus, current injury, unspecified knee

✓6th S83.28 Other tear of lateral meniscus, current injury

✓7th S83.281 Other tear of lateral meniscus, current injury, right knee

✓7th S83.282 Other tear of lateral meniscus, current injury, left knee

✓7th S83.289 Other tear of lateral meniscus, current injury, unspecified knee

✓5th S83.3 Tear of articular cartilage of knee, current

✓x7th S83.30 Tear of articular cartilage of unspecified knee, current

✓x7th S83.31 Tear of articular cartilage of right knee, current

✓x7th S83.32 Tear of articular cartilage of left knee, current

✓5th S83.4 Sprain of collateral ligament of knee

✓6th S83.40 Sprain of unspecified collateral ligament of knee

✓7th S83.401 Sprain of unspecified collateral ligament of right knee

✓7th S83.402 Sprain of unspecified collateral ligament of left knee

✓7th S83.409 Sprain of unspecified collateral ligament of unspecified knee

✓6th S83.41 Sprain of medial collateral ligament of knee

Sprain of tibial collateral ligament

✓7th S83.411 Sprain of medial collateral ligament of right knee

✓7th S83.412 Sprain of medial collateral ligament of left knee

✓7th S83.419 Sprain of medial collateral ligament of unspecified knee

✓6th S83.42 Sprain of lateral collateral ligament of knee

Sprain of fibular collateral ligament

✓7th S83.421 Sprain of lateral collateral ligament of right knee

✓7th S83.422 Sprain of lateral collateral ligament of left knee

✓7th S83.429 Sprain of lateral collateral ligament of unspecified knee

✓5th S83.5 Sprain of cruciate ligament of knee

AHA: 2016,2Q,3

✓6th S83.50 Sprain of unspecified cruciate ligament of knee

✓7th S83.501 Sprain of unspecified cruciate ligament of right knee

✓7th S83.502 Sprain of unspecified cruciate ligament of left knee

✓7th S83.509 Sprain of unspecified cruciate ligament of unspecified knee

✓6th S83.51 Sprain of anterior cruciate ligament of knee

✓7th S83.511 Sprain of anterior cruciate ligament of right knee

✓7th S83.512 Sprain of anterior cruciate ligament of left knee

✓7th S83.519 Sprain of anterior cruciate ligament of unspecified knee

✓6th S83.52 Sprain of posterior cruciate ligament of knee

✓7th S83.521 Sprain of posterior cruciate ligament of right knee

✓7th S83.522 Sprain of posterior cruciate ligament of left knee

✓7th S83.529 Sprain of posterior cruciate ligament of unspecified knee

✓5th S83.6 Sprain of the superior tibiofibular joint and ligament

✓x7th S83.60 Sprain of the superior tibiofibular joint and ligament, unspecified knee

✓x7th S83.61 Sprain of the superior tibiofibular joint and ligament, right knee

✓x7th S83.62 Sprain of the superior tibiofibular joint and ligament, left knee

✓5th S83.8 Sprain of other specified parts of knee

✓6th S83.8X Sprain of other specified parts of knee

✓7th S83.8X1 Sprain of other specified parts of right knee

✓7th S83.8X2 Sprain of other specified parts of left knee

✓7th S83.8X9 Sprain of other specified parts of unspecified knee

✓5th S83.9 Sprain of unspecified site of knee

✓x7th S83.90 Sprain of unspecified site of unspecified knee

✓x7th S83.91 Sprain of unspecified site of right knee

✓x7th S83.92 Sprain of unspecified site of left knee

✓4th S84 Injury of nerves at lower leg level

Code also any associated open wound (S81.-)

EXCLUDES 2 *injury of nerves at ankle and foot level (S94.-)*

The appropriate 7th character is to be added to each code from category S84.
A initial encounter
D subsequent encounter
S sequela

✓5th S84.0 Injury of tibial nerve at lower leg level

✓x7th S84.00 Injury of tibial nerve at lower leg level, unspecified leg

✓x7th S84.01 Injury of tibial nerve at lower leg level, right leg

✓x7th S84.02 Injury of tibial nerve at lower leg level, left leg

✓5th S84.1 Injury of peroneal nerve at lower leg level

✓x7th S84.10 Injury of peroneal nerve at lower leg level, unspecified leg

✓x7th S84.11 Injury of peroneal nerve at lower leg level, right leg

✓x7th S84.12 Injury of peroneal nerve at lower leg level, left leg

✓5th S84.2 Injury of cutaneous sensory nerve at lower leg level

✓x7th S84.20 Injury of cutaneous sensory nerve at lower leg level, unspecified leg

✓x7th S84.21 Injury of cutaneous sensory nerve at lower leg level, right leg

✓x7th S84.22 Injury of cutaneous sensory nerve at lower leg level, left leg

✓5th S84.8 Injury of other nerves at lower leg level

✓6th S84.80 Injury of other nerves at lower leg level

✓7th S84.801 Injury of other nerves at lower leg level, right leg

✓7th S84.802 Injury of other nerves at lower leg level, left leg

√7th **S84.809** Injury of other nerves at lower leg level, unspecified leg

√5th **S84.9** Injury of unspecified nerve at lower leg level

√x7th **S84.90** Injury of unspecified nerve at lower leg level, unspecified leg

√x7th **S84.91** Injury of unspecified nerve at lower leg level, right leg

√x7th **S84.92** Injury of unspecified nerve at lower leg level, left leg

√4th **S85 Injury of blood vessels at lower leg level**

Code also any associated open wound (S81.-)

EXCLUDES 2 *injury of blood vessels at ankle and foot level (S95.-)*

The appropriate 7th character is to be added to each code from category S85.
A initial encounter
D subsequent encounter
S sequela

√5th **S85.0** Injury of popliteal artery

√6th **S85.00** Unspecified injury of popliteal artery

√7th **S85.001** Unspecified injury of popliteal artery, right leg MCC

√7th **S85.002** Unspecified injury of popliteal artery, left leg MCC

√7th **S85.009** Unspecified injury of popliteal artery, unspecified leg MCC UNS

√6th **S85.01** Laceration of popliteal artery

√7th **S85.011** Laceration of popliteal artery, right leg MCC

√7th **S85.012** Laceration of popliteal artery, left leg MCC

√7th **S85.019** Laceration of popliteal artery, unspecified leg MCC UNS

√6th **S85.09** Other specified injury of popliteal artery

√7th **S85.091** Other specified injury of popliteal artery, right leg MCC

√7th **S85.092** Other specified injury of popliteal artery, left leg MCC

√7th **S85.099** Other specified injury of popliteal artery, unspecified leg MCC UNS

√5th **S85.1** Injury of tibial artery

√6th **S85.10** Unspecified injury of unspecified tibial artery

Injury of tibial artery NOS

√7th **S85.101** Unspecified injury of unspecified tibial artery, right leg CC

√7th **S85.102** Unspecified injury of unspecified tibial artery, left leg CC

√7th **S85.109** Unspecified injury of unspecified tibial artery, unspecified leg CC UNS

√6th **S85.11** Laceration of unspecified tibial artery

√7th **S85.111** Laceration of unspecified tibial artery, right leg CC

√7th **S85.112** Laceration of unspecified tibial artery, left leg CC

√7th **S85.119** Laceration of unspecified tibial artery, unspecified leg CC UNS

√6th **S85.12** Other specified injury of unspecified tibial artery

√7th **S85.121** Other specified injury of unspecified tibial artery, right leg CC

√7th **S85.122** Other specified injury of unspecified tibial artery, left leg CC

√7th **S85.129** Other specified injury of unspecified tibial artery, unspecified leg CC UNS

√6th **S85.13** Unspecified injury of anterior tibial artery

√7th **S85.131** Unspecified injury of anterior tibial artery, right leg CC

√7th **S85.132** Unspecified injury of anterior tibial artery, left leg CC

√7th **S85.139** Unspecified injury of anterior tibial artery, unspecified leg CC UNS

√6th **S85.14** Laceration of anterior tibial artery

√7th **S85.141** Laceration of anterior tibial artery, right leg CC

√7th **S85.142** Laceration of anterior tibial artery, left leg CC

√7th **S85.149** Laceration of anterior tibial artery, unspecified leg CC UNS

√6th **S85.15** Other specified injury of anterior tibial artery

√7th **S85.151** Other specified injury of anterior tibial artery, right leg CC

√7th **S85.152** Other specified injury of anterior tibial artery, left leg CC

√7th **S85.159** Other specified injury of anterior tibial artery, unspecified leg CC UNS

√6th **S85.16** Unspecified injury of posterior tibial artery

√7th **S85.161** Unspecified injury of posterior tibial artery, right leg CC

√7th **S85.162** Unspecified injury of posterior tibial artery, left leg CC

√7th **S85.169** Unspecified injury of posterior tibial artery, unspecified leg CC UNS

√6th **S85.17** Laceration of posterior tibial artery

√7th **S85.171** Laceration of posterior tibial artery, right leg CC

√7th **S85.172** Laceration of posterior tibial artery, left leg CC

√7th **S85.179** Laceration of posterior tibial artery, unspecified leg CC UNS

√6th **S85.18** Other specified injury of posterior tibial artery

√7th **S85.181** Other specified injury of posterior tibial artery, right leg CC

√7th **S85.182** Other specified injury of posterior tibial artery, left leg CC

√7th **S85.189** Other specified injury of posterior tibial artery, unspecified leg CC UNS

√5th **S85.2** Injury of peroneal artery

√6th **S85.20** Unspecified injury of peroneal artery

√7th **S85.201** Unspecified injury of peroneal artery, right leg CC

√7th **S85.202** Unspecified injury of peroneal artery, left leg CC

√7th **S85.209** Unspecified injury of peroneal artery, unspecified leg CC UNS

√6th **S85.21** Laceration of peroneal artery

√7th **S85.211** Laceration of peroneal artery, right leg CC

√7th **S85.212** Laceration of peroneal artery, left leg CC

√7th **S85.219** Laceration of peroneal artery, unspecified leg CC UNS

√6th **S85.29** Other specified injury of peroneal artery

√7th **S85.291** Other specified injury of peroneal artery, right leg CC

√7th **S85.292** Other specified injury of peroneal artery, left leg CC

√7th **S85.299** Other specified injury of peroneal artery, unspecified leg CC UNS

√5th **S85.3** Injury of greater saphenous vein at lower leg level

Injury of greater saphenous vein NOS
Injury of saphenous vein NOS

√6th **S85.30** Unspecified injury of greater saphenous vein at lower leg level

√7th **S85.301** Unspecified injury of greater saphenous vein at lower leg level, right leg CC

√7th **S85.302** Unspecified injury of greater saphenous vein at lower leg level, left leg CC

√7th **S85.309** Unspecified injury of greater saphenous vein at lower leg level, unspecified leg CC UNS

√6th **S85.31** Laceration of greater saphenous vein at lower leg level

√7th **S85.311** Laceration of greater saphenous vein at lower leg level, right leg CC

√7th **S85.312** Laceration of greater saphenous vein at lower leg level, left leg CC

√7th **S85.319** Laceration of greater saphenous vein at lower leg level, unspecified leg CC UNS

√6th **S85.39** Other specified injury of greater saphenous vein at lower leg level

√7th **S85.391** Other specified injury of greater saphenous vein at lower leg level, right leg CC

√7th **S85.392** Other specified injury of greater saphenous vein at lower leg level, left leg CC

7th **S85.399** Other specified injury of greater saphenous vein at lower leg level, unspecified leg CC UNS

5th **S85.4** Injury of lesser saphenous vein at lower leg level

6th **S85.40** Unspecified injury of lesser saphenous vein at lower leg level

7th **S85.401** Unspecified injury of lesser saphenous vein at lower leg level, right leg CC

7th **S85.402** Unspecified injury of lesser saphenous vein at lower leg level, left leg CC

7th **S85.409** Unspecified injury of lesser saphenous vein at lower leg level, unspecified leg CC UNS

6th **S85.41** Laceration of lesser saphenous vein at lower leg level

7th **S85.411** Laceration of lesser saphenous vein at lower leg level, right leg CC

7th **S85.412** Laceration of lesser saphenous vein at lower leg level, left leg CC

7th **S85.419** Laceration of lesser saphenous vein at lower leg level, unspecified leg CC UNS

6th **S85.49** Other specified injury of lesser saphenous vein at lower leg level

7th **S85.491** Other specified injury of lesser saphenous vein at lower leg level, right leg CC

7th **S85.492** Other specified injury of lesser saphenous vein at lower leg level, left leg CC

7th **S85.499** Other specified injury of lesser saphenous vein at lower leg level, unspecified leg CC UNS

5th **S85.5** Injury of popliteal vein

6th **S85.50** Unspecified injury of popliteal vein

7th **S85.501** Unspecified injury of popliteal vein, right leg MCC

7th **S85.502** Unspecified injury of popliteal vein, left leg MCC

7th **S85.509** Unspecified injury of popliteal vein, unspecified leg MCC UNS

6th **S85.51** Laceration of popliteal vein

7th **S85.511** Laceration of popliteal vein, right leg MCC

7th **S85.512** Laceration of popliteal vein, left leg MCC

7th **S85.519** Laceration of popliteal vein, unspecified leg MCC UNS

6th **S85.59** Other specified injury of popliteal vein

7th **S85.591** Other specified injury of popliteal vein, right leg MCC

7th **S85.592** Other specified injury of popliteal vein, left leg MCC

7th **S85.599** Other specified injury of popliteal vein, unspecified leg MCC UNS

5th **S85.8** Injury of other blood vessels at lower leg level

6th **S85.80** Unspecified injury of other blood vessels at lower leg level

7th **S85.801** Unspecified injury of other blood vessels at lower leg level, right leg CC

7th **S85.802** Unspecified injury of other blood vessels at lower leg level, left leg CC

7th **S85.809** Unspecified injury of other blood vessels at lower leg level, unspecified leg CC UNS

6th **S85.81** Laceration of other blood vessels at lower leg level

7th **S85.811** Laceration of other blood vessels at lower leg level, right leg CC

7th **S85.812** Laceration of other blood vessels at lower leg level, left leg CC

7th **S85.819** Laceration of other blood vessels at lower leg level, unspecified leg CC UNS

6th **S85.89** Other specified injury of other blood vessels at lower leg level

7th **S85.891** Other specified injury of other blood vessels at lower leg level, right leg CC

7th **S85.892** Other specified injury of other blood vessels at lower leg level, left leg CC

7th **S85.899** Other specified injury of other blood vessels at lower leg level, unspecified leg CC UNS

5th **S85.9** Injury of unspecified blood vessel at lower leg level

6th **S85.90** Unspecified injury of unspecified blood vessel at lower leg level

7th **S85.901** Unspecified injury of unspecified blood vessel at lower leg level, right leg CC

7th **S85.902** Unspecified injury of unspecified blood vessel at lower leg level, left leg CC

7th **S85.909** Unspecified injury of unspecified blood vessel at lower leg level, unspecified leg CC UNS

6th **S85.91** Laceration of unspecified blood vessel at lower leg level

7th **S85.911** Laceration of unspecified blood vessel at lower leg level, right leg CC

7th **S85.912** Laceration of unspecified blood vessel at lower leg level, left leg CC

7th **S85.919** Laceration of unspecified blood vessel at lower leg level, unspecified leg CC UNS

6th **S85.99** Other specified injury of unspecified blood vessel at lower leg level

7th **S85.991** Other specified injury of unspecified blood vessel at lower leg level, right leg CC

7th **S85.992** Other specified injury of unspecified blood vessel at lower leg level, left leg CC

7th **S85.999** Other specified injury of unspecified blood vessel at lower leg level, unspecified leg CC UNS

4th **S86 Injury of muscle, fascia and tendon at lower leg level**

Code also any associated open wound (S81.-)

EXCLUDES 2 *injury of muscle, fascia and tendon at ankle (S96.-)*
injury of patellar ligament (tendon) (S76.1-)
sprain of joints and ligaments of knee (S83.-)

TIP: Refer to the Muscle/Tendon table at the beginning of this chapter.

The appropriate 7th character is to be added to each code from category S86.
A initial encounter
D subsequent encounter
S sequela

5th **S86.0** Injury of Achilles tendon

6th **S86.00** Unspecified injury of Achilles tendon

7th **S86.001** Unspecified injury of right Achilles tendon

7th **S86.002** Unspecified injury of left Achilles tendon

7th **S86.009** Unspecified injury of unspecified Achilles tendon

6th **S86.01** Strain of Achilles tendon

7th **S86.011** Strain of right Achilles tendon

7th **S86.012** Strain of left Achilles tendon

7th **S86.019** Strain of unspecified Achilles tendon

6th **S86.02** Laceration of Achilles tendon

7th **S86.021** Laceration of right Achilles tendon CC

7th **S86.022** Laceration of left Achilles tendon CC

7th **S86.029** Laceration of unspecified Achilles tendon CC UNS

6th **S86.09** Other specified injury of Achilles tendon

7th **S86.091** Other specified injury of right Achilles tendon

7th **S86.092** Other specified injury of left Achilles tendon

7th **S86.099** Other specified injury of unspecified Achilles tendon

5th **S86.1** Injury of other muscle(s) and tendon(s) of posterior muscle group at lower leg level

6th **S86.10** Unspecified injury of other muscle(s) and tendon(s) of posterior muscle group at lower leg level

7th **S86.101** Unspecified injury of other muscle(s) and tendon(s) of posterior muscle group at lower leg level, right leg

7th **S86.102** Unspecified injury of other muscle(s) and tendon(s) of posterior muscle group at lower leg level, left leg

7th **S86.109** Unspecified injury of other muscle(s) and tendon(s) of posterior muscle group at lower leg level, unspecified leg

6th S86.11 Strain of other muscle(s) and tendon(s) of posterior muscle group at lower leg level
- 7th S86.111 Strain of other muscle(s) and tendon(s) of posterior muscle group at lower leg level, right leg
- 7th S86.112 Strain of other muscle(s) and tendon(s) of posterior muscle group at lower leg level, left leg
- 7th S86.119 Strain of other muscle(s) and tendon(s) of posterior muscle group at lower leg level, unspecified leg

6th S86.12 Laceration of other muscle(s) and tendon(s) of posterior muscle group at lower leg level
- 7th S86.121 Laceration of other muscle(s) and tendon(s) of posterior muscle group at lower leg level, right leg CC
- 7th S86.122 Laceration of other muscle(s) and tendon(s) of posterior muscle group at lower leg level, left leg CC
- 7th S86.129 Laceration of other muscle(s) and tendon(s) of posterior muscle group at lower leg level, unspecified leg CC UNS

6th S86.19 Other injury of other muscle(s) and tendon(s) of posterior muscle group at lower leg level
- 7th S86.191 Other injury of other muscle(s) and tendon(s) of posterior muscle group at lower leg level, right leg
- 7th S86.192 Other injury of other muscle(s) and tendon(s) of posterior muscle group at lower leg level, left leg
- 7th S86.199 Other injury of other muscle(s) and tendon(s) of posterior muscle group at lower leg level, unspecified leg

5th S86.2 Injury of muscle(s) and tendon(s) of anterior muscle group at lower leg level

6th S86.20 Unspecified injury of muscle(s) and tendon(s) of anterior muscle group at lower leg level
- 7th S86.201 Unspecified injury of muscle(s) and tendon(s) of anterior muscle group at lower leg level, right leg
- 7th S86.202 Unspecified injury of muscle(s) and tendon(s) of anterior muscle group at lower leg level, left leg
- 7th S86.209 Unspecified injury of muscle(s) and tendon(s) of anterior muscle group at lower leg level, unspecified leg

6th S86.21 Strain of muscle(s) and tendon(s) of anterior muscle group at lower leg level
- 7th S86.211 Strain of muscle(s) and tendon(s) of anterior muscle group at lower leg level, right leg
- 7th S86.212 Strain of muscle(s) and tendon(s) of anterior muscle group at lower leg level, left leg
- 7th S86.219 Strain of muscle(s) and tendon(s) of anterior muscle group at lower leg level, unspecified leg

6th S86.22 Laceration of muscle(s) and tendon(s) of anterior muscle group at lower leg level
- 7th S86.221 Laceration of muscle(s) and tendon(s) of anterior muscle group at lower leg level, right leg CC
- 7th S86.222 Laceration of muscle(s) and tendon(s) of anterior muscle group at lower leg level, left leg CC
- 7th S86.229 Laceration of muscle(s) and tendon(s) of anterior muscle group at lower leg level, unspecified leg CC UNS

6th S86.29 Other injury of muscle(s) and tendon(s) of anterior muscle group at lower leg level
- 7th S86.291 Other injury of muscle(s) and tendon(s) of anterior muscle group at lower leg level, right leg
- 7th S86.292 Other injury of muscle(s) and tendon(s) of anterior muscle group at lower leg level, left leg
- 7th S86.299 Other injury of muscle(s) and tendon(s) of anterior muscle group at lower leg level, unspecified leg

5th S86.3 Injury of muscle(s) and tendon(s) of peroneal muscle group at lower leg level

6th S86.30 Unspecified injury of muscle(s) and tendon(s) of peroneal muscle group at lower leg level
- 7th S86.301 Unspecified injury of muscle(s) and tendon(s) of peroneal muscle group at lower leg level, right leg
- 7th S86.302 Unspecified injury of muscle(s) and tendon(s) of peroneal muscle group at lower leg level, left leg
- 7th S86.309 Unspecified injury of muscle(s) and tendon(s) of peroneal muscle group at lower leg level, unspecified leg

6th S86.31 Strain of muscle(s) and tendon(s) of peroneal muscle group at lower leg level
- 7th S86.311 Strain of muscle(s) and tendon(s) of peroneal muscle group at lower leg level, right leg
- 7th S86.312 Strain of muscle(s) and tendon(s) of peroneal muscle group at lower leg level, left leg
- 7th S86.319 Strain of muscle(s) and tendon(s) of peroneal muscle group at lower leg level, unspecified leg

6th S86.32 Laceration of muscle(s) and tendon(s) of peroneal muscle group at lower leg level
- 7th S86.321 Laceration of muscle(s) and tendon(s) of peroneal muscle group at lower leg level, right leg CC
- 7th S86.322 Laceration of muscle(s) and tendon(s) of peroneal muscle group at lower leg level, left leg CC
- 7th S86.329 Laceration of muscle(s) and tendon(s) of peroneal muscle group at lower leg level, unspecified leg CC UNS

6th S86.39 Other injury of muscle(s) and tendon(s) of peroneal muscle group at lower leg level
- 7th S86.391 Other injury of muscle(s) and tendon(s) of peroneal muscle group at lower leg level, right leg
- 7th S86.392 Other injury of muscle(s) and tendon(s) of peroneal muscle group at lower leg level, left leg
- 7th S86.399 Other injury of muscle(s) and tendon(s) of peroneal muscle group at lower leg level, unspecified leg

5th S86.8 Injury of other muscles and tendons at lower leg level

6th S86.80 Unspecified injury of other muscles and tendons at lower leg level
- 7th S86.801 Unspecified injury of other muscle(s) and tendon(s) at lower leg level, right leg
- 7th S86.802 Unspecified injury of other muscle(s) and tendon(s) at lower leg level, left leg
- 7th S86.809 Unspecified injury of other muscle(s) and tendon(s) at lower leg level, unspecified leg

6th S86.81 Strain of other muscles and tendons at lower leg level
- 7th S86.811 Strain of other muscle(s) and tendon(s) at lower leg level, right leg
- 7th S86.812 Strain of other muscle(s) and tendon(s) at lower leg level, left leg
- 7th S86.819 Strain of other muscle(s) and tendon(s) at lower leg level, unspecified leg

6th S86.82 Laceration of other muscles and tendons at lower leg level
- 7th S86.821 Laceration of other muscle(s) and tendon(s) at lower leg level, right leg CC
- 7th S86.822 Laceration of other muscle(s) and tendon(s) at lower leg level, left leg CC
- 7th S86.829 Laceration of other muscle(s) and tendon(s) at lower leg level, unspecified leg CC UNS

6th S86.89 Other injury of other muscles and tendons at lower leg level
- 7th S86.891 Other injury of other muscle(s) and tendon(s) at lower leg level, right leg
- 7th S86.892 Other injury of other muscle(s) and tendon(s) at lower leg level, left leg
- 7th S86.899 Other injury of other muscle(s) and tendon(s) at lower leg level, unspecified leg

√5th **S86.9 Injury of unspecified muscle and tendon at lower leg level**
- √6th **S86.90 Unspecified injury of unspecified muscle and tendon at lower leg level**
  - √7th **S86.901 Unspecified injury of unspecified muscle(s) and tendon(s) at lower leg level, right leg**
  - √7th **S86.902 Unspecified injury of unspecified muscle(s) and tendon(s) at lower leg level, left leg**
  - √7th **S86.909 Unspecified injury of unspecified muscle(s) and tendon(s) at lower leg level, unspecified leg**
- √6th **S86.91 Strain of unspecified muscle and tendon at lower leg level**
  - √7th **S86.911 Strain of unspecified muscle(s) and tendon(s) at lower leg level, right leg**
  - √7th **S86.912 Strain of unspecified muscle(s) and tendon(s) at lower leg level, left leg**
  - √7th **S86.919 Strain of unspecified muscle(s) and tendon(s) at lower leg level, unspecified leg**
- √6th **S86.92 Laceration of unspecified muscle and tendon at lower leg level**
  - √7th **S86.921 Laceration of unspecified muscle(s) and tendon(s) at lower leg level, right leg** CC
  - √7th **S86.922 Laceration of unspecified muscle(s) and tendon(s) at lower leg level, left leg** CC
  - √7th **S86.929 Laceration of unspecified muscle(s) and tendon(s) at lower leg level, unspecified leg** CC UNS
- √6th **S86.99 Other injury of unspecified muscle and tendon at lower leg level**
  - √7th **S86.991 Other injury of unspecified muscle(s) and tendon(s) at lower leg level, right leg**
  - √7th **S86.992 Other injury of unspecified muscle(s) and tendon(s) at lower leg level, left leg**
  - √7th **S86.999 Other injury of unspecified muscle(s) and tendon(s) at lower leg level, unspecified leg**

√4th **S87 Crushing injury of lower leg**

Use additional code(s) for all associated injuries

EXCLUDES 2 *crushing injury of ankle and foot (S97.-)*

The appropriate 7th character is to be added to each code from category S87.
- A initial encounter
- D subsequent encounter
- S sequela

√5th **S87.0 Crushing injury of knee**
- √x7th **S87.00 Crushing injury of unspecified knee**
- √x7th **S87.01 Crushing injury of right knee**
- √x7th **S87.02 Crushing injury of left knee**

√5th **S87.8 Crushing injury of lower leg**
- √x7th **S87.80 Crushing injury of unspecified lower leg**
- √x7th **S87.81 Crushing injury of right lower leg**
- √x7th **S87.82 Crushing injury of left lower leg**

√4th **S88 Traumatic amputation of lower leg**

An amputation not identified as partial or complete should be coded to complete

EXCLUDES 1 *traumatic amputation of ankle and foot (S98.-)*

The appropriate 7th character is to be added to each code from category S88.
- A initial encounter
- D subsequent encounter
- S sequela

√5th **S88.0 Traumatic amputation at knee level**
- √6th **S88.01 Complete traumatic amputation at knee level**
  - AHA: 2023,1Q,27,29
  - √7th **S88.011 Complete traumatic amputation at knee level, right lower leg** CC HCC
  - √7th **S88.012 Complete traumatic amputation at knee level, left lower leg** CC HCC
  - √7th **S88.019 Complete traumatic amputation at knee level, unspecified lower leg** CC UNS HCC
- √6th **S88.02 Partial traumatic amputation at knee level**
  - √7th **S88.021 Partial traumatic amputation at knee level, right lower leg** CC HCC
  - √7th **S88.022 Partial traumatic amputation at knee level, left lower leg** CC HCC
  - √7th **S88.029 Partial traumatic amputation at knee level, unspecified lower leg** CC UNS HCC

√5th **S88.1 Traumatic amputation at level between knee and ankle**
- √6th **S88.11 Complete traumatic amputation at level between knee and ankle**
  - √7th **S88.111 Complete traumatic amputation at level between knee and ankle, right lower leg** CC HCC
  - √7th **S88.112 Complete traumatic amputation at level between knee and ankle, left lower leg** CC HCC
  - √7th **S88.119 Complete traumatic amputation at level between knee and ankle, unspecified lower leg** CC UNS HCC
- √6th **S88.12 Partial traumatic amputation at level between knee and ankle**
  - √7th **S88.121 Partial traumatic amputation at level between knee and ankle, right lower leg** CC HCC
  - √7th **S88.122 Partial traumatic amputation at level between knee and ankle, left lower leg** CC HCC
  - √7th **S88.129 Partial traumatic amputation at level between knee and ankle, unspecified lower leg** CC UNS HCC

√5th **S88.9 Traumatic amputation of lower leg, level unspecified**
- √6th **S88.91 Complete traumatic amputation of lower leg, level unspecified**
  - √7th **S88.911 Complete traumatic amputation of right lower leg, level unspecified** CC HCC
  - √7th **S88.912 Complete traumatic amputation of left lower leg, level unspecified** CC HCC
  - √7th **S88.919 Complete traumatic amputation of unspecified lower leg, level unspecified** CC HCC
- √6th **S88.92 Partial traumatic amputation of lower leg, level unspecified**
  - √7th **S88.921 Partial traumatic amputation of right lower leg, level unspecified** CC HCC
  - √7th **S88.922 Partial traumatic amputation of left lower leg, level unspecified** CC HCC
  - √7th **S88.929 Partial traumatic amputation of unspecified lower leg, level unspecified** CC UNS HCC

√4th **S89 Other and unspecified injuries of lower leg**

NOTE A fracture not indicated as open or closed should be coded to closed.

EXCLUDES 2 *other and unspecified injuries of ankle and foot (S99.-)*

AHA: 2018,2Q,12; 2018,1Q,3; 2015,3Q,37-39

The appropriate 7th character is to be added to each code from subcategories S89.0, S89.1, S89.2, and S89.3.
- A initial encounter for closed fracture
- D subsequent encounter for fracture with routine healing
- G subsequent encounter for fracture with delayed healing
- K subsequent encounter for fracture with nonunion
- P subsequent encounter for fracture with malunion
- S sequela

√5th **S89.0 Physeal fracture of upper end of tibia**

AHA: 2019,4Q,56
- √6th **S89.00 Unspecified physeal fracture of upper end of tibia**
  - √7th **S89.001 Unspecified physeal fracture of upper end of right tibia** CC H5
  - √7th **S89.002 Unspecified physeal fracture of upper end of left tibia** CC H5
  - √7th **S89.009 Unspecified physeal fracture of upper end of unspecified tibia** CC H5 UNS
- √6th **S89.01 Salter-Harris Type I physeal fracture of upper end of tibia**
  - √7th **S89.011 Salter-Harris Type I physeal fracture of upper end of right tibia** CC H5
  - √7th **S89.012 Salter-Harris Type I physeal fracture of upper end of left tibia** CC H5

S89.019 Salter-Harris Type I physeal fracture of upper end of unspecified tibia CC H5 UNS

S89.02 Salter-Harris Type II physeal fracture of upper end of tibia

S89.021 Salter-Harris Type II physeal fracture of upper end of right tibia CC H5

S89.022 Salter-Harris Type II physeal fracture of upper end of left tibia CC H5

S89.029 Salter-Harris Type II physeal fracture of upper end of unspecified tibia CC H5 UNS

S89.03 Salter-Harris Type III physeal fracture of upper end of tibia

S89.031 Salter-Harris Type III physeal fracture of upper end of right tibia CC H5

S89.032 Salter-Harris Type III physeal fracture of upper end of left tibia CC H5

S89.039 Salter-Harris Type III physeal fracture of upper end of unspecified tibia CC H5 UNS

S89.04 Salter-Harris Type IV physeal fracture of upper end of tibia

S89.041 Salter-Harris Type IV physeal fracture of upper end of right tibia CC H5

S89.042 Salter-Harris Type IV physeal fracture of upper end of left tibia CC H5

S89.049 Salter-Harris Type IV physeal fracture of upper end of unspecified tibia CC H5 UNS

S89.09 Other physeal fracture of upper end of tibia

S89.091 Other physeal fracture of upper end of right tibia CC H5

S89.092 Other physeal fracture of upper end of left tibia CC H5

S89.099 Other physeal fracture of upper end of unspecified tibia CC H5 UNS

S89.1 Physeal fracture of lower end of tibia

AHA: 2019,4Q,56

S89.10 Unspecified physeal fracture of lower end of tibia

S89.101 Unspecified physeal fracture of lower end of right tibia CC

S89.102 Unspecified physeal fracture of lower end of left tibia CC

S89.109 Unspecified physeal fracture of lower end of unspecified tibia CC UNS

S89.11 Salter-Harris Type I physeal fracture of lower end of tibia

S89.111 Salter-Harris Type I physeal fracture of lower end of right tibia CC

S89.112 Salter-Harris Type I physeal fracture of lower end of left tibia CC

S89.119 Salter-Harris Type I physeal fracture of lower end of unspecified tibia CC UNS

S89.12 Salter-Harris Type II physeal fracture of lower end of tibia

S89.121 Salter-Harris Type II physeal fracture of lower end of right tibia CC

S89.122 Salter-Harris Type II physeal fracture of lower end of left tibia CC

S89.129 Salter-Harris Type II physeal fracture of lower end of unspecified tibia CC UNS

S89.13 Salter-Harris Type III physeal fracture of lower end of tibia

EXCLUDES 1 *fracture of medial malleolus (adult) (S82.5-)*

S89.131 Salter-Harris Type III physeal fracture of lower end of right tibia CC

S89.132 Salter-Harris Type III physeal fracture of lower end of left tibia CC

S89.139 Salter-Harris Type III physeal fracture of lower end of unspecified tibia CC UNS

S89.14 Salter-Harris Type IV physeal fracture of lower end of tibia

EXCLUDES 1 *fracture of medial malleolus (adult) (S82.5-)*

S89.141 Salter-Harris Type IV physeal fracture of lower end of right tibia CC

S89.142 Salter-Harris Type IV physeal fracture of lower end of left tibia CC

S89.149 Salter-Harris Type IV physeal fracture of lower end of unspecified tibia CC UNS

S89.19 Other physeal fracture of lower end of tibia

S89.191 Other physeal fracture of lower end of right tibia CC

S89.192 Other physeal fracture of lower end of left tibia CC

S89.199 Other physeal fracture of lower end of unspecified tibia CC UNS

S89.2 Physeal fracture of upper end of fibula

AHA: 2019,4Q,56

S89.20 Unspecified physeal fracture of upper end of fibula

S89.201 Unspecified physeal fracture of upper end of right fibula CC

S89.202 Unspecified physeal fracture of upper end of left fibula CC

S89.209 Unspecified physeal fracture of upper end of unspecified fibula CC UNS

S89.21 Salter-Harris Type I physeal fracture of upper end of fibula

S89.211 Salter-Harris Type I physeal fracture of upper end of right fibula CC

S89.212 Salter-Harris Type I physeal fracture of upper end of left fibula CC

S89.219 Salter-Harris Type I physeal fracture of upper end of unspecified fibula CC UNS

S89.22 Salter-Harris Type II physeal fracture of upper end of fibula

S89.221 Salter-Harris Type II physeal fracture of upper end of right fibula CC

S89.222 Salter-Harris Type II physeal fracture of upper end of left fibula CC

S89.229 Salter-Harris Type II physeal fracture of upper end of unspecified fibula CC UNS

S89.29 Other physeal fracture of upper end of fibula

S89.291 Other physeal fracture of upper end of right fibula CC

S89.292 Other physeal fracture of upper end of left fibula CC

S89.299 Other physeal fracture of upper end of unspecified fibula CC UNS

S89.3 Physeal fracture of lower end of fibula

AHA: 2019,4Q,56

S89.30 Unspecified physeal fracture of lower end of fibula

S89.301 Unspecified physeal fracture of lower end of right fibula CC

S89.302 Unspecified physeal fracture of lower end of left fibula CC

S89.309 Unspecified physeal fracture of lower end of unspecified fibula CC UNS

S89.31 Salter-Harris Type I physeal fracture of lower end of fibula

S89.311 Salter-Harris Type I physeal fracture of lower end of right fibula CC

S89.312 Salter-Harris Type I physeal fracture of lower end of left fibula CC

S89.319 Salter-Harris Type I physeal fracture of lower end of unspecified fibula CC UNS

S89.32 Salter-Harris Type II physeal fracture of lower end of fibula

S89.321 Salter-Harris Type II physeal fracture of lower end of right fibula CC

S89.322 Salter-Harris Type II physeal fracture of lower end of left fibula CC

S89.329 Salter-Harris Type II physeal fracture of lower end of unspecified fibula CC UNS

S89.39 Other physeal fracture of lower end of fibula

S89.391 Other physeal fracture of lower end of right fibula CC

S89.392 Other physeal fracture of lower end of left fibula CC

S89.399 Other physeal fracture of lower end of unspecified fibula CC UNS

S89.8 Other specified injuries of lower leg

The appropriate 7th character is to be added to each code in subcategory S89.8.
A initial encounter
D subsequent encounter
S sequela

S89.80 Other specified injuries of unspecified lower leg
S89.81 Other specified injuries of right lower leg
S89.82 Other specified injuries of left lower leg

S89.9 Unspecified injury of lower leg

The appropriate 7th character is to be added to each code in subcategory S89.9.
A initial encounter
D subsequent encounter
S sequela

S89.90 Unspecified injury of unspecified lower leg
S89.91 Unspecified injury of right lower leg
S89.92 Unspecified injury of left lower leg

Injuries to the ankle and foot (S90-S99)

EXCLUDES 2 *burns and corrosions (T20-T32)*
fracture of ankle and malleolus (S82.-)
frostbite (T33-T34)
insect bite or sting, venomous (T63.4)

S90 Superficial injury of ankle, foot and toes

The appropriate 7th character is to be added to each code from category S90.
A initial encounter
D subsequent encounter
S sequela

S90.0 Contusion of ankle
S90.00 Contusion of unspecified ankle
S90.01 Contusion of right ankle
S90.02 Contusion of left ankle

S90.1 Contusion of toe without damage to nail
S90.11 Contusion of great toe without damage to nail
S90.111 Contusion of right great toe without damage to nail
S90.112 Contusion of left great toe without damage to nail
S90.119 Contusion of unspecified great toe without damage to nail
S90.12 Contusion of lesser toe without damage to nail
S90.121 Contusion of right lesser toe(s) without damage to nail
S90.122 Contusion of left lesser toe(s) without damage to nail
S90.129 Contusion of unspecified lesser toe(s) without damage to nail
Contusion of toe NOS

S90.2 Contusion of toe with damage to nail
S90.21 Contusion of great toe with damage to nail
S90.211 Contusion of right great toe with damage to nail
S90.212 Contusion of left great toe with damage to nail
S90.219 Contusion of unspecified great toe with damage to nail
S90.22 Contusion of lesser toe with damage to nail
S90.221 Contusion of right lesser toe(s) with damage to nail
S90.222 Contusion of left lesser toe(s) with damage to nail
S90.229 Contusion of unspecified lesser toe(s) with damage to nail

S90.3 Contusion of foot
EXCLUDES 2 *contusion of toes (S90.1-, S90.2-)*
S90.30 Contusion of unspecified foot
Contusion of foot NOS
S90.31 Contusion of right foot
S90.32 Contusion of left foot

S90.4 Other superficial injuries of toe
S90.41 Abrasion of toe
S90.411 Abrasion, right great toe
S90.412 Abrasion, left great toe
S90.413 Abrasion, unspecified great toe
S90.414 Abrasion, right lesser toe(s)
S90.415 Abrasion, left lesser toe(s)
S90.416 Abrasion, unspecified lesser toe(s)
S90.42 Blister (nonthermal) of toe
S90.421 Blister (nonthermal), right great toe
S90.422 Blister (nonthermal), left great toe
S90.423 Blister (nonthermal), unspecified great toe
S90.424 Blister (nonthermal), right lesser toe(s)
S90.425 Blister (nonthermal), left lesser toe(s)
S90.426 Blister (nonthermal), unspecified lesser toe(s)
S90.44 External constriction of toe
Hair tourniquet syndrome of toe
S90.441 External constriction, right great toe
S90.442 External constriction, left great toe
S90.443 External constriction, unspecified great toe
S90.444 External constriction, right lesser toe(s)
S90.445 External constriction, left lesser toe(s)
S90.446 External constriction, unspecified lesser toe(s)
S90.45 Superficial foreign body of toe
Splinter in the toe
S90.451 Superficial foreign body, right great toe
S90.452 Superficial foreign body, left great toe
S90.453 Superficial foreign body, unspecified great toe
S90.454 Superficial foreign body, right lesser toe(s)
S90.455 Superficial foreign body, left lesser toe(s)
S90.456 Superficial foreign body, unspecified lesser toe(s)
S90.46 Insect bite (nonvenomous) of toe
S90.461 Insect bite (nonvenomous), right great toe
S90.462 Insect bite (nonvenomous), left great toe
S90.463 Insect bite (nonvenomous), unspecified great toe
S90.464 Insect bite (nonvenomous), right lesser toe(s)
S90.465 Insect bite (nonvenomous), left lesser toe(s)
S90.466 Insect bite (nonvenomous), unspecified lesser toe(s)
S90.47 Other superficial bite of toe
EXCLUDES 1 *open bite of toe (S91.15-, S91.25-)*
S90.471 Other superficial bite of right great toe
S90.472 Other superficial bite of left great toe
S90.473 Other superficial bite of unspecified great toe
S90.474 Other superficial bite of right lesser toe(s)
S90.475 Other superficial bite of left lesser toe(s)
S90.476 Other superficial bite of unspecified lesser toe(s)

S90.5 Other superficial injuries of ankle
S90.51 Abrasion of ankle
S90.511 Abrasion, right ankle
S90.512 Abrasion, left ankle
S90.519 Abrasion, unspecified ankle
S90.52 Blister (nonthermal) of ankle
S90.521 Blister (nonthermal), right ankle
S90.522 Blister (nonthermal), left ankle
S90.529 Blister (nonthermal), unspecified ankle
S90.54 External constriction of ankle
S90.541 External constriction, right ankle
S90.542 External constriction, left ankle

N Newborn: 0 P Pediatric: 0-17 M Maternity: 9-64 A Adult: 15-124 UNS Unspecified Site MCC Major Complication/Comorbidity CC Complication/Comorbidity

S90.549 External constriction, unspecified ankle

S90.55 Superficial foreign body of ankle

Splinter in the ankle

S90.551 Superficial foreign body, right ankle

S90.552 Superficial foreign body, left ankle

S90.559 Superficial foreign body, unspecified ankle

S90.56 Insect bite (nonvenomous) of ankle

S90.561 Insect bite (nonvenomous), right ankle

S90.562 Insect bite (nonvenomous), left ankle

S90.569 Insect bite (nonvenomous), unspecified ankle

S90.57 Other superficial bite of ankle

EXCLUDES 1 *open bite of ankle (S91.05-)*

S90.571 Other superficial bite of ankle, right ankle

S90.572 Other superficial bite of ankle, left ankle

S90.579 Other superficial bite of ankle, unspecified ankle

S90.8 Other superficial injuries of foot

S90.81 Abrasion of foot

S90.811 Abrasion, right foot

S90.812 Abrasion, left foot

S90.819 Abrasion, unspecified foot

S90.82 Blister (nonthermal) of foot

S90.821 Blister (nonthermal), right foot

S90.822 Blister (nonthermal), left foot

S90.829 Blister (nonthermal), unspecified foot

S90.84 External constriction of foot

S90.841 External constriction, right foot

S90.842 External constriction, left foot

S90.849 External constriction, unspecified foot

S90.85 Superficial foreign body of foot

Splinter in the foot

S90.851 Superficial foreign body, right foot

S90.852 Superficial foreign body, left foot

S90.859 Superficial foreign body, unspecified foot

S90.86 Insect bite (nonvenomous) of foot

S90.861 Insect bite (nonvenomous), right foot

S90.862 Insect bite (nonvenomous), left foot

S90.869 Insect bite (nonvenomous), unspecified foot

S90.87 Other superficial bite of foot

EXCLUDES 1 *open bite of foot (S91.35-)*

S90.871 Other superficial bite of right foot

S90.872 Other superficial bite of left foot

S90.879 Other superficial bite of unspecified foot

S90.9 Unspecified superficial injury of ankle, foot and toe

S90.91 Unspecified superficial injury of ankle

S90.911 Unspecified superficial injury of right ankle

S90.912 Unspecified superficial injury of left ankle

S90.919 Unspecified superficial injury of unspecified ankle

S90.92 Unspecified superficial injury of foot

S90.921 Unspecified superficial injury of right foot

S90.922 Unspecified superficial injury of left foot

S90.929 Unspecified superficial injury of unspecified foot

S90.93 Unspecified superficial injury of toes

S90.931 Unspecified superficial injury of right great toe

S90.932 Unspecified superficial injury of left great toe

S90.933 Unspecified superficial injury of unspecified great toe

S90.934 Unspecified superficial injury of right lesser toe(s)

S90.935 Unspecified superficial injury of left lesser toe(s)

S90.936 Unspecified superficial injury of unspecified lesser toe(s)

S91 Open wound of ankle, foot and toes

Code also any associated wound infection

EXCLUDES 1 *open fracture of ankle, foot and toes (S92.- with 7th character B)*
traumatic amputation of ankle and foot (S98.-)

AHA: 2021,1Q,7

The appropriate 7th character is to be added to each code from category S91.
A initial encounter
D subsequent encounter
S sequela

S91.0 Open wound of ankle

S91.00 Unspecified open wound of ankle

S91.001 Unspecified open wound, right ankle

S91.002 Unspecified open wound, left ankle

S91.009 Unspecified open wound, unspecified ankle

S91.01 Laceration without foreign body of ankle

S91.011 Laceration without foreign body, right ankle

S91.012 Laceration without foreign body, left ankle

S91.019 Laceration without foreign body, unspecified ankle

S91.02 Laceration with foreign body of ankle

S91.021 Laceration with foreign body, right ankle

S91.022 Laceration with foreign body, left ankle

S91.029 Laceration with foreign body, unspecified ankle

S91.03 Puncture wound without foreign body of ankle

S91.031 Puncture wound without foreign body, right ankle

S91.032 Puncture wound without foreign body, left ankle

S91.039 Puncture wound without foreign body, unspecified ankle

S91.04 Puncture wound with foreign body of ankle

S91.041 Puncture wound with foreign body, right ankle

S91.042 Puncture wound with foreign body, left ankle

S91.049 Puncture wound with foreign body, unspecified ankle

S91.05 Open bite of ankle

EXCLUDES 1 *superficial bite of ankle (S90.56-, S90.57-)*

S91.051 Open bite, right ankle

S91.052 Open bite, left ankle

S91.059 Open bite, unspecified ankle

S91.1 Open wound of toe without damage to nail

S91.10 Unspecified open wound of toe without damage to nail

S91.101 Unspecified open wound of right great toe without damage to nail

S91.102 Unspecified open wound of left great toe without damage to nail

S91.103 Unspecified open wound of unspecified great toe without damage to nail

S91.104 Unspecified open wound of right lesser toe(s) without damage to nail

S91.105 Unspecified open wound of left lesser toe(s) without damage to nail

S91.106 Unspecified open wound of unspecified lesser toe(s) without damage to nail

S91.109 Unspecified open wound of unspecified toe(s) without damage to nail

S91.11 Laceration without foreign body of toe without damage to nail

S91.111 Laceration without foreign body of right great toe without damage to nail

S91.112 Laceration without foreign body of left great toe without damage to nail

S91.113 Laceration without foreign body of unspecified great toe without damage to nail

S91.114 Laceration without foreign body of right lesser toe(s) without damage to nail

S91.115 Laceration without foreign body of left lesser toe(s) without damage to nail

7th **S91.116** **Laceration without foreign body of unspecified lesser toe(s) without damage to nail**

7th **S91.119** **Laceration without foreign body of unspecified toe without damage to nail**

6th **S91.12** **Laceration with foreign body of toe without damage to nail**

7th **S91.121** **Laceration with foreign body of right great toe without damage to nail**

7th **S91.122** **Laceration with foreign body of left great toe without damage to nail**

7th **S91.123** **Laceration with foreign body of unspecified great toe without damage to nail**

7th **S91.124** **Laceration with foreign body of right lesser toe(s) without damage to nail**

7th **S91.125** **Laceration with foreign body of left lesser toe(s) without damage to nail**

7th **S91.126** **Laceration with foreign body of unspecified lesser toe(s) without damage to nail**

7th **S91.129** **Laceration with foreign body of unspecified toe(s) without damage to nail**

6th **S91.13** **Puncture wound without foreign body of toe without damage to nail**

7th **S91.131** **Puncture wound without foreign body of right great toe without damage to nail**

7th **S91.132** **Puncture wound without foreign body of left great toe without damage to nail**

7th **S91.133** **Puncture wound without foreign body of unspecified great toe without damage to nail**

7th **S91.134** **Puncture wound without foreign body of right lesser toe(s) without damage to nail**

7th **S91.135** **Puncture wound without foreign body of left lesser toe(s) without damage to nail**

7th **S91.136** **Puncture wound without foreign body of unspecified lesser toe(s) without damage to nail**

7th **S91.139** **Puncture wound without foreign body of unspecified toe(s) without damage to nail**

6th **S91.14** **Puncture wound with foreign body of toe without damage to nail**

7th **S91.141** **Puncture wound with foreign body of right great toe without damage to nail**

7th **S91.142** **Puncture wound with foreign body of left great toe without damage to nail**

7th **S91.143** **Puncture wound with foreign body of unspecified great toe without damage to nail**

7th **S91.144** **Puncture wound with foreign body of right lesser toe(s) without damage to nail**

7th **S91.145** **Puncture wound with foreign body of left lesser toe(s) without damage to nail**

7th **S91.146** **Puncture wound with foreign body of unspecified lesser toe(s) without damage to nail**

7th **S91.149** **Puncture wound with foreign body of unspecified toe(s) without damage to nail**

6th **S91.15** **Open bite of toe without damage to nail**

Bite of toe NOS

EXCLUDES 1 *superficial bite of toe (S90.46-, S90.47-)*

7th **S91.151** **Open bite of right great toe without damage to nail**

7th **S91.152** **Open bite of left great toe without damage to nail**

7th **S91.153** **Open bite of unspecified great toe without damage to nail**

7th **S91.154** **Open bite of right lesser toe(s) without damage to nail**

7th **S91.155** **Open bite of left lesser toe(s) without damage to nail**

7th **S91.156** **Open bite of unspecified lesser toe(s) without damage to nail**

7th **S91.159** **Open bite of unspecified toe(s) without damage to nail**

5th **S91.2** **Open wound of toe with damage to nail**

6th **S91.20** **Unspecified open wound of toe with damage to nail**

7th **S91.201** **Unspecified open wound of right great toe with damage to nail**

7th **S91.202** **Unspecified open wound of left great toe with damage to nail**

7th **S91.203** **Unspecified open wound of unspecified great toe with damage to nail**

7th **S91.204** **Unspecified open wound of right lesser toe(s) with damage to nail**

7th **S91.205** **Unspecified open wound of left lesser toe(s) with damage to nail**

7th **S91.206** **Unspecified open wound of unspecified lesser toe(s) with damage to nail**

7th **S91.209** **Unspecified open wound of unspecified toe(s) with damage to nail**

6th **S91.21** **Laceration without foreign body of toe with damage to nail**

7th **S91.211** **Laceration without foreign body of right great toe with damage to nail**

7th **S91.212** **Laceration without foreign body of left great toe with damage to nail**

7th **S91.213** **Laceration without foreign body of unspecified great toe with damage to nail**

7th **S91.214** **Laceration without foreign body of right lesser toe(s) with damage to nail**

7th **S91.215** **Laceration without foreign body of left lesser toe(s) with damage to nail**

7th **S91.216** **Laceration without foreign body of unspecified lesser toe(s) with damage to nail**

7th **S91.219** **Laceration without foreign body of unspecified toe(s) with damage to nail**

6th **S91.22** **Laceration with foreign body of toe with damage to nail**

7th **S91.221** **Laceration with foreign body of right great toe with damage to nail**

7th **S91.222** **Laceration with foreign body of left great toe with damage to nail**

7th **S91.223** **Laceration with foreign body of unspecified great toe with damage to nail**

7th **S91.224** **Laceration with foreign body of right lesser toe(s) with damage to nail**

7th **S91.225** **Laceration with foreign body of left lesser toe(s) with damage to nail**

7th **S91.226** **Laceration with foreign body of unspecified lesser toe(s) with damage to nail**

7th **S91.229** **Laceration with foreign body of unspecified toe(s) with damage to nail**

6th **S91.23** **Puncture wound without foreign body of toe with damage to nail**

7th **S91.231** **Puncture wound without foreign body of right great toe with damage to nail**

7th **S91.232** **Puncture wound without foreign body of left great toe with damage to nail**

7th **S91.233** **Puncture wound without foreign body of unspecified great toe with damage to nail**

7th **S91.234** **Puncture wound without foreign body of right lesser toe(s) with damage to nail**

7th **S91.235** **Puncture wound without foreign body of left lesser toe(s) with damage to nail**

7th **S91.236** **Puncture wound without foreign body of unspecified lesser toe(s) with damage to nail**

7th **S91.239** **Puncture wound without foreign body of unspecified toe(s) with damage to nail**

6th **S91.24** **Puncture wound with foreign body of toe with damage to nail**

7th **S91.241** **Puncture wound with foreign body of right great toe with damage to nail**

7th **S91.242** **Puncture wound with foreign body of left great toe with damage to nail**

7th **S91.243** **Puncture wound with foreign body of unspecified great toe with damage to nail**

7th **S91.244** **Puncture wound with foreign body of right lesser toe(s) with damage to nail**

7th **S91.245** **Puncture wound with foreign body of left lesser toe(s) with damage to nail**

7th **S91.246** **Puncture wound with foreign body of unspecified lesser toe(s) with damage to nail**

7th **S91.249** **Puncture wound with foreign body of unspecified toe(s) with damage to nail**

6th **S91.25** **Open bite of toe with damage to nail**

Bite of toe with damage to nail NOS

EXCLUDES 1 *superficial bite of toe (S90.46-, S90.47-)*

7th **S91.251** **Open bite of right great toe with damage to nail**

S91.252 Open bite of left great toe with damage to nail
S91.253 Open bite of unspecified great toe with damage to nail
S91.254 Open bite of right lesser toe(s) with damage to nail
S91.255 Open bite of left lesser toe(s) with damage to nail
S91.256 Open bite of unspecified lesser toe(s) with damage to nail
S91.259 Open bite of unspecified toe(s) with damage to nail

S91.3 Open wound of foot

S91.30 Unspecified open wound of foot
S91.301 Unspecified open wound, right foot
S91.302 Unspecified open wound, left foot
S91.309 Unspecified open wound, unspecified foot

S91.31 Laceration without foreign body of foot
S91.311 Laceration without foreign body, right foot
S91.312 Laceration without foreign body, left foot
S91.319 Laceration without foreign body, unspecified foot

S91.32 Laceration with foreign body of foot
S91.321 Laceration with foreign body, right foot
S91.322 Laceration with foreign body, left foot
S91.329 Laceration with foreign body, unspecified foot

S91.33 Puncture wound without foreign body of foot
S91.331 Puncture wound without foreign body, right foot
S91.332 Puncture wound without foreign body, left foot
S91.339 Puncture wound without foreign body, unspecified foot

S91.34 Puncture wound with foreign body of foot
S91.341 Puncture wound with foreign body, right foot
S91.342 Puncture wound with foreign body, left foot
S91.349 Puncture wound with foreign body, unspecified foot

S91.35 Open bite of foot
EXCLUDES 1 *superficial bite of foot (S90.86-, S90.87-)*
S91.351 Open bite, right foot
S91.352 Open bite, left foot
S91.359 Open bite, unspecified foot

S92 Fracture of foot and toe, except ankle

NOTE A fracture not indicated as displaced or nondisplaced should be coded to displaced

A fracture not indicated as open or closed should be coded to closed.

EXCLUDES 2 *fracture of ankle (S82.-)*
fracture of malleolus (S82.-)
traumatic amputation of ankle and foot (S98.-)

AHA: 2018,2Q,12; 2015,3Q,37-39

The appropriate 7th character is to be added to each code from category S92.
A initial encounter for closed fracture
B initial encounter for open fracture
D subsequent encounter for fracture with routine healing
G subsequent encounter for fracture with delayed healing
K subsequent encounter for fracture with nonunion
P subsequent encounter for fracture with malunion
S sequela

S92.0 Fracture of calcaneus
Heel bone
Os calcis
EXCLUDES 2 *physeal fracture of calcaneus (S99.0-)*

S92.00 Unspecified fracture of calcaneus
S92.001 Unspecified fracture of right calcaneus CC H5
S92.002 Unspecified fracture of left calcaneus CC H5
S92.009 Unspecified fracture of unspecified calcaneus CC H5 UNS

S92.01 Fracture of body of calcaneus
S92.011 Displaced fracture of body of right calcaneus CC H5
S92.012 Displaced fracture of body of left calcaneus CC H5
S92.013 Displaced fracture of body of unspecified calcaneus CC H5 UNS
S92.014 Nondisplaced fracture of body of right calcaneus CC H5
S92.015 Nondisplaced fracture of body of left calcaneus CC H5
S92.016 Nondisplaced fracture of body of unspecified calcaneus CC H5 UNS

S92.02 Fracture of anterior process of calcaneus
S92.021 Displaced fracture of anterior process of right calcaneus CC H5
S92.022 Displaced fracture of anterior process of left calcaneus CC H5
S92.023 Displaced fracture of anterior process of unspecified calcaneus CC H5 UNS
S92.024 Nondisplaced fracture of anterior process of right calcaneus CC H5
S92.025 Nondisplaced fracture of anterior process of left calcaneus CC H5
S92.026 Nondisplaced fracture of anterior process of unspecified calcaneus CC H5 UNS

S92.03 Avulsion fracture of tuberosity of calcaneus
S92.031 Displaced avulsion fracture of tuberosity of right calcaneus CC H5
S92.032 Displaced avulsion fracture of tuberosity of left calcaneus CC H5
S92.033 Displaced avulsion fracture of tuberosity of unspecified calcaneus CC H5 UNS
S92.034 Nondisplaced avulsion fracture of tuberosity of right calcaneus CC H5
S92.035 Nondisplaced avulsion fracture of tuberosity of left calcaneus CC H5
S92.036 Nondisplaced avulsion fracture of tuberosity of unspecified calcaneus CC H5 UNS

S92.04 Other fracture of tuberosity of calcaneus
S92.041 Displaced other fracture of tuberosity of right calcaneus CC H5
S92.042 Displaced other fracture of tuberosity of left calcaneus CC H5
S92.043 Displaced other fracture of tuberosity of unspecified calcaneus CC H5 UNS
S92.044 Nondisplaced other fracture of tuberosity of right calcaneus CC H5
S92.045 Nondisplaced other fracture of tuberosity of left calcaneus CC H5
S92.046 Nondisplaced other fracture of tuberosity of unspecified calcaneus CC H5 UNS

S92.05 Other extraarticular fracture of calcaneus
S92.051 Displaced other extraarticular fracture of right calcaneus CC H5
S92.052 Displaced other extraarticular fracture of left calcaneus CC H5
S92.053 Displaced other extraarticular fracture of unspecified calcaneus CC H5 UNS
S92.054 Nondisplaced other extraarticular fracture of right calcaneus CC H5
S92.055 Nondisplaced other extraarticular fracture of left calcaneus CC H5
S92.056 Nondisplaced other extraarticular fracture of unspecified calcaneus CC H5 UNS

S92.06 Intraarticular fracture of calcaneus
S92.061 Displaced intraarticular fracture of right calcaneus CC H5
S92.062 Displaced intraarticular fracture of left calcaneus CC H5
S92.063 Displaced intraarticular fracture of unspecified calcaneus CC H5 UNS
S92.064 Nondisplaced intraarticular fracture of right calcaneus CC H5

7th S92.065 Nondisplaced intraarticular fracture of left calcaneus CC H5
7th S92.066 Nondisplaced intraarticular fracture of unspecified calcaneus CC H5 UNS

5th S92.1 Fracture of talus
Astragalus

6th S92.10 Unspecified fracture of talus
7th S92.101 Unspecified fracture of right talus CC H5
7th S92.102 Unspecified fracture of left talus CC H5
7th S92.109 Unspecified fracture of unspecified talus CC H5 UNS

6th S92.11 Fracture of neck of talus
7th S92.111 Displaced fracture of neck of right talus CC H5
7th S92.112 Displaced fracture of neck of left talus CC H5
7th S92.113 Displaced fracture of neck of unspecified talus CC H5 UNS
7th S92.114 Nondisplaced fracture of neck of right talus CC H5
7th S92.115 Nondisplaced fracture of neck of left talus CC H5
7th S92.116 Nondisplaced fracture of neck of unspecified talus CC H5 UNS

6th S92.12 Fracture of body of talus
7th S92.121 Displaced fracture of body of right talus CC H5
7th S92.122 Displaced fracture of body of left talus CC H5
7th S92.123 Displaced fracture of body of unspecified talus CC H5 UNS
7th S92.124 Nondisplaced fracture of body of right talus CC H5
7th S92.125 Nondisplaced fracture of body of left talus CC H5
7th S92.126 Nondisplaced fracture of body of unspecified talus CC H5 UNS

6th S92.13 Fracture of posterior process of talus
7th S92.131 Displaced fracture of posterior process of right talus CC H5
7th S92.132 Displaced fracture of posterior process of left talus CC H5
7th S92.133 Displaced fracture of posterior process of unspecified talus CC H5 UNS
7th S92.134 Nondisplaced fracture of posterior process of right talus CC H5
7th S92.135 Nondisplaced fracture of posterior process of left talus CC H5
7th S92.136 Nondisplaced fracture of posterior process of unspecified talus CC H5 UNS

6th S92.14 Dome fracture of talus
EXCLUDES 1 *osteochondritis dissecans (M93.2)*
7th S92.141 Displaced dome fracture of right talus CC H5
7th S92.142 Displaced dome fracture of left talus CC H5
7th S92.143 Displaced dome fracture of unspecified talus CC H5 UNS
7th S92.144 Nondisplaced dome fracture of right talus CC H5
7th S92.145 Nondisplaced dome fracture of left talus CC H5
7th S92.146 Nondisplaced dome fracture of unspecified talus CC H5 UNS

6th S92.15 Avulsion fracture (chip fracture) of talus
7th S92.151 Displaced avulsion fracture (chip fracture) of right talus CC H5
7th S92.152 Displaced avulsion fracture (chip fracture) of left talus CC H5
7th S92.153 Displaced avulsion fracture (chip fracture) of unspecified talus CC H5 UNS
7th S92.154 Nondisplaced avulsion fracture (chip fracture) of right talus CC H5
7th S92.155 Nondisplaced avulsion fracture (chip fracture) of left talus CC H5
7th S92.156 Nondisplaced avulsion fracture (chip fracture) of unspecified talus CC H5 UNS

6th S92.19 Other fracture of talus
7th S92.191 Other fracture of right talus CC H5
7th S92.192 Other fracture of left talus CC H5
7th S92.199 Other fracture of unspecified talus CC H5 UNS

5th S92.2 Fracture of other and unspecified tarsal bone(s)

6th S92.20 Fracture of unspecified tarsal bone(s)
7th S92.201 Fracture of unspecified tarsal bone(s) of right foot CC H5
7th S92.202 Fracture of unspecified tarsal bone(s) of left foot CC H5
7th S92.209 Fracture of unspecified tarsal bone(s) of unspecified foot CC H5 UNS

6th S92.21 Fracture of cuboid bone
7th S92.211 Displaced fracture of cuboid bone of right foot CC H5
7th S92.212 Displaced fracture of cuboid bone of left foot CC H5
7th S92.213 Displaced fracture of cuboid bone of unspecified foot CC H5 UNS
7th S92.214 Nondisplaced fracture of cuboid bone of right foot CC H5
7th S92.215 Nondisplaced fracture of cuboid bone of left foot CC H5
7th S92.216 Nondisplaced fracture of cuboid bone of unspecified foot CC H5 UNS

6th S92.22 Fracture of lateral cuneiform
7th S92.221 Displaced fracture of lateral cuneiform of right foot CC H5
7th S92.222 Displaced fracture of lateral cuneiform of left foot CC H5
7th S92.223 Displaced fracture of lateral cuneiform of unspecified foot CC H5 UNS
7th S92.224 Nondisplaced fracture of lateral cuneiform of right foot CC H5
7th S92.225 Nondisplaced fracture of lateral cuneiform of left foot CC H5
7th S92.226 Nondisplaced fracture of lateral cuneiform of unspecified foot CC H5 UNS

6th S92.23 Fracture of intermediate cuneiform
7th S92.231 Displaced fracture of intermediate cuneiform of right foot CC H5
7th S92.232 Displaced fracture of intermediate cuneiform of left foot CC H5
7th S92.233 Displaced fracture of intermediate cuneiform of unspecified foot CC H5 UNS
7th S92.234 Nondisplaced fracture of intermediate cuneiform of right foot CC H5
7th S92.235 Nondisplaced fracture of intermediate cuneiform of left foot CC H5
7th S92.236 Nondisplaced fracture of intermediate cuneiform of unspecified foot CC H5 UNS

6th S92.24 Fracture of medial cuneiform
7th S92.241 Displaced fracture of medial cuneiform of right foot CC H5
7th S92.242 Displaced fracture of medial cuneiform of left foot CC H5
7th S92.243 Displaced fracture of medial cuneiform of unspecified foot CC H5 UNS
7th S92.244 Nondisplaced fracture of medial cuneiform of right foot CC H5
7th S92.245 Nondisplaced fracture of medial cuneiform of left foot CC H5
7th S92.246 Nondisplaced fracture of medial cuneiform of unspecified foot CC H5 UNS

6th S92.25 Fracture of navicular [scaphoid] of foot
7th S92.251 Displaced fracture of navicular [scaphoid] of right foot CC H5
7th S92.252 Displaced fracture of navicular [scaphoid] of left foot CC H5

S92.253 Displaced fracture of navicular [scaphoid] of unspecified foot CC H5 UNS
S92.254 Nondisplaced fracture of navicular [scaphoid] of right foot CC H5
S92.255 Nondisplaced fracture of navicular [scaphoid] of left foot CC H5
S92.256 Nondisplaced fracture of navicular [scaphoid] of unspecified foot CC H5 UNS

S92.3 Fracture of metatarsal bone(s)
EXCLUDES 2 *physeal fracture of metatarsal (S99.1-)*
AHA: 2018,1Q,3

S92.30 Fracture of unspecified metatarsal bone(s)
S92.301 Fracture of unspecified metatarsal bone(s), right foot CC H5
S92.302 Fracture of unspecified metatarsal bone(s), left foot CC H5
S92.309 Fracture of unspecified metatarsal bone(s), unspecified foot CC H5 UNS

S92.31 Fracture of first metatarsal bone
S92.311 Displaced fracture of first metatarsal bone, right foot CC H5
S92.312 Displaced fracture of first metatarsal bone, left foot CC H5
S92.313 Displaced fracture of first metatarsal bone, unspecified foot CC H5 UNS
S92.314 Nondisplaced fracture of first metatarsal bone, right foot CC H5
S92.315 Nondisplaced fracture of first metatarsal bone, left foot CC H5
S92.316 Nondisplaced fracture of first metatarsal bone, unspecified foot CC H5 UNS

S92.32 Fracture of second metatarsal bone
S92.321 Displaced fracture of second metatarsal bone, right foot CC H5
S92.322 Displaced fracture of second metatarsal bone, left foot CC H5
S92.323 Displaced fracture of second metatarsal bone, unspecified foot CC H5 UNS
S92.324 Nondisplaced fracture of second metatarsal bone, right foot CC H5
S92.325 Nondisplaced fracture of second metatarsal bone, left foot CC H5
S92.326 Nondisplaced fracture of second metatarsal bone, unspecified foot CC H5 UNS

S92.33 Fracture of third metatarsal bone
S92.331 Displaced fracture of third metatarsal bone, right foot CC H5
S92.332 Displaced fracture of third metatarsal bone, left foot CC H5
S92.333 Displaced fracture of third metatarsal bone, unspecified foot CC H5 UNS
S92.334 Nondisplaced fracture of third metatarsal bone, right foot CC H5
S92.335 Nondisplaced fracture of third metatarsal bone, left foot CC H5
S92.336 Nondisplaced fracture of third metatarsal bone, unspecified foot CC H5 UNS

S92.34 Fracture of fourth metatarsal bone
S92.341 Displaced fracture of fourth metatarsal bone, right foot CC H5
S92.342 Displaced fracture of fourth metatarsal bone, left foot CC H5
S92.343 Displaced fracture of fourth metatarsal bone, unspecified foot CC H5 UNS
S92.344 Nondisplaced fracture of fourth metatarsal bone, right foot CC H5
S92.345 Nondisplaced fracture of fourth metatarsal bone, left foot CC H5
S92.346 Nondisplaced fracture of fourth metatarsal bone, unspecified foot CC H5 UNS

S92.35 Fracture of fifth metatarsal bone
S92.351 Displaced fracture of fifth metatarsal bone, right foot CC H5
S92.352 Displaced fracture of fifth metatarsal bone, left foot CC H5
S92.353 Displaced fracture of fifth metatarsal bone, unspecified foot CC H5 UNS
S92.354 Nondisplaced fracture of fifth metatarsal bone, right foot CC H5
S92.355 Nondisplaced fracture of fifth metatarsal bone, left foot CC H5
S92.356 Nondisplaced fracture of fifth metatarsal bone, unspecified foot CC H5 UNS

S92.4 Fracture of great toe
EXCLUDES 2 *physeal fracture of phalanx of toe (S99.2-)*

S92.40 Unspecified fracture of great toe
S92.401 Displaced unspecified fracture of right great toe CC
S92.402 Displaced unspecified fracture of left great toe CC
S92.403 Displaced unspecified fracture of unspecified great toe CC UNS
S92.404 Nondisplaced unspecified fracture of right great toe CC
S92.405 Nondisplaced unspecified fracture of left great toe CC
S92.406 Nondisplaced unspecified fracture of unspecified great toe CC UNS

S92.41 Fracture of proximal phalanx of great toe
S92.411 Displaced fracture of proximal phalanx of right great toe CC
S92.412 Displaced fracture of proximal phalanx of left great toe CC
S92.413 Displaced fracture of proximal phalanx of unspecified great toe CC UNS
S92.414 Nondisplaced fracture of proximal phalanx of right great toe CC
S92.415 Nondisplaced fracture of proximal phalanx of left great toe CC
S92.416 Nondisplaced fracture of proximal phalanx of unspecified great toe CC UNS

S92.42 Fracture of distal phalanx of great toe
S92.421 Displaced fracture of distal phalanx of right great toe CC
S92.422 Displaced fracture of distal phalanx of left great toe CC
S92.423 Displaced fracture of distal phalanx of unspecified great toe CC UNS
S92.424 Nondisplaced fracture of distal phalanx of right great toe CC
S92.425 Nondisplaced fracture of distal phalanx of left great toe CC
S92.426 Nondisplaced fracture of distal phalanx of unspecified great toe CC UNS

S92.49 Other fracture of great toe
S92.491 Other fracture of right great toe CC
S92.492 Other fracture of left great toe CC
S92.499 Other fracture of unspecified great toe CC UNS

S92.5 Fracture of lesser toe(s)
EXCLUDES 2 *physeal fracture of phalanx of toe (S99.2-)*

S92.50 Unspecified fracture of lesser toe(s)
S92.501 Displaced unspecified fracture of right lesser toe(s) CC
S92.502 Displaced unspecified fracture of left lesser toe(s) CC
S92.503 Displaced unspecified fracture of unspecified lesser toe(s) CC UNS
S92.504 Nondisplaced unspecified fracture of right lesser toe(s) CC
S92.505 Nondisplaced unspecified fracture of left lesser toe(s) CC
S92.506 Nondisplaced unspecified fracture of unspecified lesser toe(s) CC UNS

S92.51 Fracture of proximal phalanx of lesser toe(s)
S92.511 Displaced fracture of proximal phalanx of right lesser toe(s) CC
S92.512 Displaced fracture of proximal phalanx of left lesser toe(s) CC
S92.513 Displaced fracture of proximal phalanx of unspecified lesser toe(s) CC UNS

√7th S92.514 Nondisplaced fracture of proximal phalanx of right lesser toe(s) CC

√7th S92.515 Nondisplaced fracture of proximal phalanx of left lesser toe(s) CC

√7th S92.516 Nondisplaced fracture of proximal phalanx of unspecified lesser toe(s) CC UNS

√6th S92.52 Fracture of middle phalanx of lesser toe(s)

√7th S92.521 Displaced fracture of middle phalanx of right lesser toe(s) CC

√7th S92.522 Displaced fracture of middle phalanx of left lesser toe(s) CC

√7th S92.523 Displaced fracture of middle phalanx of unspecified lesser toe(s) CC UNS

√7th S92.524 Nondisplaced fracture of middle phalanx of right lesser toe(s) CC

√7th S92.525 Nondisplaced fracture of middle phalanx of left lesser toe(s) CC

√7th S92.526 Nondisplaced fracture of middle phalanx of unspecified lesser toe(s) CC UNS

√6th S92.53 Fracture of distal phalanx of lesser toe(s)

√7th S92.531 Displaced fracture of distal phalanx of right lesser toe(s) CC

√7th S92.532 Displaced fracture of distal phalanx of left lesser toe(s) CC

√7th S92.533 Displaced fracture of distal phalanx of unspecified lesser toe(s) CC UNS

√7th S92.534 Nondisplaced fracture of distal phalanx of right lesser toe(s) CC

√7th S92.535 Nondisplaced fracture of distal phalanx of left lesser toe(s) CC

√7th S92.536 Nondisplaced fracture of distal phalanx of unspecified lesser toe(s) CC UNS

√6th S92.59 Other fracture of lesser toe(s)

√7th S92.591 Other fracture of right lesser toe(s) CC

√7th S92.592 Other fracture of left lesser toe(s) CC

√7th S92.599 Other fracture of unspecified lesser toe(s) CC UNS

√5th S92.8 Other fracture of foot, except ankle

√6th S92.81 Other fracture of foot

Sesamoid fracture of foot

AHA: 2016,4Q,68

√7th S92.811 Other fracture of right foot CC H5

√7th S92.812 Other fracture of left foot CC H5

√7th S92.819 Other fracture of unspecified foot CC H5 UNS

√5th S92.9 Unspecified fracture of foot and toe

√6th S92.90 Unspecified fracture of foot

√7th S92.901 Unspecified fracture of right foot CC H5

√7th S92.902 Unspecified fracture of left foot CC H5

√7th S92.909 Unspecified fracture of unspecified foot CC H5 UNS

√6th S92.91 Unspecified fracture of toe

√7th S92.911 Unspecified fracture of right toe(s) CC

√7th S92.912 Unspecified fracture of left toe(s) CC

√7th S92.919 Unspecified fracture of unspecified toe(s) CC UNS

√4th S93 Dislocation and sprain of joints and ligaments at ankle, foot and toe level

INCLUDES avulsion of joint or ligament of ankle, foot and toe
laceration of cartilage, joint or ligament of ankle, foot and toe
sprain of cartilage, joint or ligament of ankle, foot and toe
traumatic hemarthrosis of joint or ligament of ankle, foot and toe
traumatic rupture of joint or ligament of ankle, foot and toe
traumatic subluxation of joint or ligament of ankle, foot and toe
traumatic tear of joint or ligament of ankle, foot and toe

Code also any associated open wound

EXCLUDES 2 *strain of muscle and tendon of ankle and foot (S96.-)*

The appropriate 7th character is to be added to each code from category S93.
A initial encounter
D subsequent encounter
S sequela

√5th S93.0 Subluxation and dislocation of ankle joint

Subluxation and dislocation of astragalus
Subluxation and dislocation of fibula, lower end
Subluxation and dislocation of talus
Subluxation and dislocation of tibia, lower end

√x7th S93.01 Subluxation of right ankle joint

√x7th S93.02 Subluxation of left ankle joint

√x7th S93.03 Subluxation of unspecified ankle joint

√x7th S93.04 Dislocation of right ankle joint

√x7th S93.05 Dislocation of left ankle joint

√x7th S93.06 Dislocation of unspecified ankle joint

√5th S93.1 Subluxation and dislocation of toe

√6th S93.10 Unspecified subluxation and dislocation of toe

Dislocation of toe NOS
Subluxation of toe NOS

√7th S93.101 Unspecified subluxation of right toe(s)

√7th S93.102 Unspecified subluxation of left toe(s)

√7th S93.103 Unspecified subluxation of unspecified toe(s)

√7th S93.104 Unspecified dislocation of right toe(s)

√7th S93.105 Unspecified dislocation of left toe(s)

√7th S93.106 Unspecified dislocation of unspecified toe(s)

√6th S93.11 Dislocation of interphalangeal joint

√7th S93.111 Dislocation of interphalangeal joint of right great toe

√7th S93.112 Dislocation of interphalangeal joint of left great toe

√7th S93.113 Dislocation of interphalangeal joint of unspecified great toe

√7th S93.114 Dislocation of interphalangeal joint of right lesser toe(s)

√7th S93.115 Dislocation of interphalangeal joint of left lesser toe(s)

√7th S93.116 Dislocation of interphalangeal joint of unspecified lesser toe(s)

√7th S93.119 Dislocation of interphalangeal joint of unspecified toe(s)

√6th S93.12 Dislocation of metatarsophalangeal joint

√7th S93.121 Dislocation of metatarsophalangeal joint of right great toe

√7th S93.122 Dislocation of metatarsophalangeal joint of left great toe

√7th S93.123 Dislocation of metatarsophalangeal joint of unspecified great toe

√7th S93.124 Dislocation of metatarsophalangeal joint of right lesser toe(s)

√7th S93.125 Dislocation of metatarsophalangeal joint of left lesser toe(s)

√7th S93.126 Dislocation of metatarsophalangeal joint of unspecified lesser toe(s)

√7th S93.129 Dislocation of metatarsophalangeal joint of unspecified toe(s)

√6th S93.13 Subluxation of interphalangeal joint

√7th S93.131 Subluxation of interphalangeal joint of right great toe

√7th S93.132 Subluxation of interphalangeal joint of left great toe

S93.133 Subluxation of interphalangeal joint of unspecified great toe
S93.134 Subluxation of interphalangeal joint of right lesser toe(s)
S93.135 Subluxation of interphalangeal joint of left lesser toe(s)
S93.136 Subluxation of interphalangeal joint of unspecified lesser toe(s)
S93.139 Subluxation of interphalangeal joint of unspecified toe(s)

S93.14 Subluxation of metatarsophalangeal joint
S93.141 Subluxation of metatarsophalangeal joint of right great toe
S93.142 Subluxation of metatarsophalangeal joint of left great toe
S93.143 Subluxation of metatarsophalangeal joint of unspecified great toe
S93.144 Subluxation of metatarsophalangeal joint of right lesser toe(s)
S93.145 Subluxation of metatarsophalangeal joint of left lesser toe(s)
S93.146 Subluxation of metatarsophalangeal joint of unspecified lesser toe(s)
S93.149 Subluxation of metatarsophalangeal joint of unspecified toe(s)

S93.3 Subluxation and dislocation of foot

EXCLUDES 2 *dislocation of toe (S93.1-)*

S93.30 Unspecified subluxation and dislocation of foot
Dislocation of foot NOS
Subluxation of foot NOS
S93.301 Unspecified subluxation of right foot
S93.302 Unspecified subluxation of left foot
S93.303 Unspecified subluxation of unspecified foot
S93.304 Unspecified dislocation of right foot
S93.305 Unspecified dislocation of left foot
S93.306 Unspecified dislocation of unspecified foot

S93.31 Subluxation and dislocation of tarsal joint
S93.311 Subluxation of tarsal joint of right foot
S93.312 Subluxation of tarsal joint of left foot
S93.313 Subluxation of tarsal joint of unspecified foot
S93.314 Dislocation of tarsal joint of right foot
S93.315 Dislocation of tarsal joint of left foot
S93.316 Dislocation of tarsal joint of unspecified foot

S93.32 Subluxation and dislocation of tarsometatarsal joint
S93.321 Subluxation of tarsometatarsal joint of right foot
S93.322 Subluxation of tarsometatarsal joint of left foot
S93.323 Subluxation of tarsometatarsal joint of unspecified foot
S93.324 Dislocation of tarsometatarsal joint of right foot
S93.325 Dislocation of tarsometatarsal joint of left foot
S93.326 Dislocation of tarsometatarsal joint of unspecified foot

S93.33 Other subluxation and dislocation of foot
S93.331 Other subluxation of right foot
S93.332 Other subluxation of left foot
S93.333 Other subluxation of unspecified foot
S93.334 Other dislocation of right foot
S93.335 Other dislocation of left foot
S93.336 Other dislocation of unspecified foot

S93.4 Sprain of ankle

EXCLUDES 2 *injury of Achilles tendon (S86.0-)*

S93.40 Sprain of unspecified ligament of ankle
Sprain of ankle NOS
Sprained ankle NOS
S93.401 Sprain of unspecified ligament of right ankle
S93.402 Sprain of unspecified ligament of left ankle
S93.409 Sprain of unspecified ligament of unspecified ankle

S93.41 Sprain of calcaneofibular ligament
S93.411 Sprain of calcaneofibular ligament of right ankle
S93.412 Sprain of calcaneofibular ligament of left ankle
S93.419 Sprain of calcaneofibular ligament of unspecified ankle

S93.42 Sprain of deltoid ligament
S93.421 Sprain of deltoid ligament of right ankle
S93.422 Sprain of deltoid ligament of left ankle
S93.429 Sprain of deltoid ligament of unspecified ankle

S93.43 Sprain of tibiofibular ligament
S93.431 Sprain of tibiofibular ligament of right ankle
S93.432 Sprain of tibiofibular ligament of left ankle
S93.439 Sprain of tibiofibular ligament of unspecified ankle

S93.49 Sprain of other ligament of ankle
Sprain of internal collateral ligament
Sprain of talofibular ligament
S93.491 Sprain of other ligament of right ankle
S93.492 Sprain of other ligament of left ankle
S93.499 Sprain of other ligament of unspecified ankle

S93.5 Sprain of toe

S93.50 Unspecified sprain of toe
S93.501 Unspecified sprain of right great toe
S93.502 Unspecified sprain of left great toe
S93.503 Unspecified sprain of unspecified great toe
S93.504 Unspecified sprain of right lesser toe(s)
S93.505 Unspecified sprain of left lesser toe(s)
S93.506 Unspecified sprain of unspecified lesser toe(s)
S93.509 Unspecified sprain of unspecified toe(s)

S93.51 Sprain of interphalangeal joint of toe
S93.511 Sprain of interphalangeal joint of right great toe
S93.512 Sprain of interphalangeal joint of left great toe
S93.513 Sprain of interphalangeal joint of unspecified great toe
S93.514 Sprain of interphalangeal joint of right lesser toe(s)
S93.515 Sprain of interphalangeal joint of left lesser toe(s)
S93.516 Sprain of interphalangeal joint of unspecified lesser toe(s)
S93.519 Sprain of interphalangeal joint of unspecified toe(s)

S93.52 Sprain of metatarsophalangeal joint of toe
S93.521 Sprain of metatarsophalangeal joint of right great toe
S93.522 Sprain of metatarsophalangeal joint of left great toe
S93.523 Sprain of metatarsophalangeal joint of unspecified great toe
S93.524 Sprain of metatarsophalangeal joint of right lesser toe(s)
S93.525 Sprain of metatarsophalangeal joint of left lesser toe(s)
S93.526 Sprain of metatarsophalangeal joint of unspecified lesser toe(s)
S93.529 Sprain of metatarsophalangeal joint of unspecified toe(s)

S93.6 Sprain of foot

EXCLUDES 2 *sprain of metatarsophalangeal joint of toe (S93.52-)*
sprain of toe (S93.5-)

S93.60 Unspecified sprain of foot
S93.601 Unspecified sprain of right foot
S93.602 Unspecified sprain of left foot
S93.609 Unspecified sprain of unspecified foot

✓6th **S93.61 Sprain of tarsal ligament of foot**
- ✓7th **S93.611** Sprain of tarsal ligament of right foot
- ✓7th **S93.612** Sprain of tarsal ligament of left foot
- ✓7th **S93.619** Sprain of tarsal ligament of unspecified foot

✓6th **S93.62 Sprain of tarsometatarsal ligament of foot**
- ✓7th **S93.621** Sprain of tarsometatarsal ligament of right foot
- ✓7th **S93.622** Sprain of tarsometatarsal ligament of left foot
- ✓7th **S93.629** Sprain of tarsometatarsal ligament of unspecified foot

✓6th **S93.69 Other sprain of foot**
- ✓7th **S93.691** Other sprain of right foot
- ✓7th **S93.692** Other sprain of left foot
- ✓7th **S93.699** Other sprain of unspecified foot

✓4th S94 Injury of nerves at ankle and foot level

Code also any associated open wound (S91.-)

The appropriate 7th character is to be added to each code from category S94.
- A initial encounter
- D subsequent encounter
- S sequela

✓5th **S94.0 Injury of lateral plantar nerve**
- ✓x7th **S94.00** Injury of lateral plantar nerve, unspecified leg
- ✓x7th **S94.01** Injury of lateral plantar nerve, right leg
- ✓x7th **S94.02** Injury of lateral plantar nerve, left leg

✓5th **S94.1 Injury of medial plantar nerve**
- ✓x7th **S94.10** Injury of medial plantar nerve, unspecified leg
- ✓x7th **S94.11** Injury of medial plantar nerve, right leg
- ✓x7th **S94.12** Injury of medial plantar nerve, left leg

✓5th **S94.2 Injury of deep peroneal nerve at ankle and foot level**

Injury of terminal, lateral branch of deep peroneal nerve
- ✓x7th **S94.20** Injury of deep peroneal nerve at ankle and foot level, unspecified leg
- ✓x7th **S94.21** Injury of deep peroneal nerve at ankle and foot level, right leg
- ✓x7th **S94.22** Injury of deep peroneal nerve at ankle and foot level, left leg

✓5th **S94.3 Injury of cutaneous sensory nerve at ankle and foot level**
- ✓x7th **S94.30** Injury of cutaneous sensory nerve at ankle and foot level, unspecified leg
- ✓x7th **S94.31** Injury of cutaneous sensory nerve at ankle and foot level, right leg
- ✓x7th **S94.32** Injury of cutaneous sensory nerve at ankle and foot level, left leg

✓5th **S94.8 Injury of other nerves at ankle and foot level**

✓6th **S94.8X Injury of other nerves at ankle and foot level**
- ✓7th **S94.8X1** Injury of other nerves at ankle and foot level, right leg
- ✓7th **S94.8X2** Injury of other nerves at ankle and foot level, left leg
- ✓7th **S94.8X9** Injury of other nerves at ankle and foot level, unspecified leg

✓5th **S94.9 Injury of unspecified nerve at ankle and foot level**
- ✓x7th **S94.90** Injury of unspecified nerve at ankle and foot level, unspecified leg
- ✓x7th **S94.91** Injury of unspecified nerve at ankle and foot level, right leg
- ✓x7th **S94.92** Injury of unspecified nerve at ankle and foot level, left leg

✓4th S95 Injury of blood vessels at ankle and foot level

Code also any associated open wound (S91.-)

EXCLUDES 2 *injury of posterior tibial artery and vein (S85.1-, S85.8-)*

The appropriate 7th character is to be added to each code from category S95.
- A initial encounter
- D subsequent encounter
- S sequela

✓5th **S95.0 Injury of dorsal artery of foot**

✓6th **S95.00 Unspecified injury of dorsal artery of foot**
- ✓7th **S95.001** Unspecified injury of dorsal artery of right foot CC
- ✓7th **S95.002** Unspecified injury of dorsal artery of left foot CC
- ✓7th **S95.009** Unspecified injury of dorsal artery of unspecified foot CC UNS

✓6th **S95.01 Laceration of dorsal artery of foot**
- ✓7th **S95.011** Laceration of dorsal artery of right foot CC
- ✓7th **S95.012** Laceration of dorsal artery of left foot CC
- ✓7th **S95.019** Laceration of dorsal artery of unspecified foot CC UNS

✓6th **S95.09 Other specified injury of dorsal artery of foot**
- ✓7th **S95.091** Other specified injury of dorsal artery of right foot CC
- ✓7th **S95.092** Other specified injury of dorsal artery of left foot CC
- ✓7th **S95.099** Other specified injury of dorsal artery of unspecified foot CC UNS

✓5th **S95.1 Injury of plantar artery of foot**

✓6th **S95.10 Unspecified injury of plantar artery of foot**
- ✓7th **S95.101** Unspecified injury of plantar artery of right foot CC
- ✓7th **S95.102** Unspecified injury of plantar artery of left foot CC
- ✓7th **S95.109** Unspecified injury of plantar artery of unspecified foot CC UNS

✓6th **S95.11 Laceration of plantar artery of foot**
- ✓7th **S95.111** Laceration of plantar artery of right foot CC
- ✓7th **S95.112** Laceration of plantar artery of left foot CC
- ✓7th **S95.119** Laceration of plantar artery of unspecified foot CC UNS

✓6th **S95.19 Other specified injury of plantar artery of foot**
- ✓7th **S95.191** Other specified injury of plantar artery of right foot CC
- ✓7th **S95.192** Other specified injury of plantar artery of left foot CC
- ✓7th **S95.199** Other specified injury of plantar artery of unspecified foot CC UNS

✓5th **S95.2 Injury of dorsal vein of foot**

✓6th **S95.20 Unspecified injury of dorsal vein of foot**
- ✓7th **S95.201** Unspecified injury of dorsal vein of right foot CC
- ✓7th **S95.202** Unspecified injury of dorsal vein of left foot CC
- ✓7th **S95.209** Unspecified injury of dorsal vein of unspecified foot CC UNS

✓6th **S95.21 Laceration of dorsal vein of foot**
- ✓7th **S95.211** Laceration of dorsal vein of right foot CC
- ✓7th **S95.212** Laceration of dorsal vein of left foot CC
- ✓7th **S95.219** Laceration of dorsal vein of unspecified foot CC UNS

✓6th **S95.29 Other specified injury of dorsal vein of foot**
- ✓7th **S95.291** Other specified injury of dorsal vein of right foot CC
- ✓7th **S95.292** Other specified injury of dorsal vein of left foot CC
- ✓7th **S95.299** Other specified injury of dorsal vein of unspecified foot CC UNS

✓5th **S95.8 Injury of other blood vessels at ankle and foot level**

✓6th **S95.80 Unspecified injury of other blood vessels at ankle and foot level**
- ✓7th **S95.801** Unspecified injury of other blood vessels at ankle and foot level, right leg CC
- ✓7th **S95.802** Unspecified injury of other blood vessels at ankle and foot level, left leg CC
- ✓7th **S95.809** Unspecified injury of other blood vessels at ankle and foot level, unspecified leg CC UNS

✓6th **S95.81 Laceration of other blood vessels at ankle and foot level**
- ✓7th **S95.811** Laceration of other blood vessels at ankle and foot level, right leg CC
- ✓7th **S95.812** Laceration of other blood vessels at ankle and foot level, left leg CC

√7th **S95.819** Laceration of other blood vessels at ankle and foot level, unspecified leg CC UNS

√6th **S95.89** Other specified injury of other blood vessels at ankle and foot level

√7th **S95.891** Other specified injury of other blood vessels at ankle and foot level, right leg CC

√7th **S95.892** Other specified injury of other blood vessels at ankle and foot level, left leg CC

√7th **S95.899** Other specified injury of other blood vessels at ankle and foot level, unspecified leg CC UNS

√5th **S95.9** Injury of unspecified blood vessel at ankle and foot level

√6th **S95.90** Unspecified injury of unspecified blood vessel at ankle and foot level

√7th **S95.901** Unspecified injury of unspecified blood vessel at ankle and foot level, right leg CC

√7th **S95.902** Unspecified injury of unspecified blood vessel at ankle and foot level, left leg CC

√7th **S95.909** Unspecified injury of unspecified blood vessel at ankle and foot level, unspecified leg CC UNS

√6th **S95.91** Laceration of unspecified blood vessel at ankle and foot level

√7th **S95.911** Laceration of unspecified blood vessel at ankle and foot level, right leg CC

√7th **S95.912** Laceration of unspecified blood vessel at ankle and foot level, left leg CC

√7th **S95.919** Laceration of unspecified blood vessel at ankle and foot level, unspecified leg CC UNS

√6th **S95.99** Other specified injury of unspecified blood vessel at ankle and foot level

√7th **S95.991** Other specified injury of unspecified blood vessel at ankle and foot level, right leg CC

√7th **S95.992** Other specified injury of unspecified blood vessel at ankle and foot level, left leg CC

√7th **S95.999** Other specified injury of unspecified blood vessel at ankle and foot level, unspecified leg CC UNS

√4th S96 Injury of muscle and tendon at ankle and foot level

Code also any associated open wound (S91.-)

EXCLUDES 2 *injury of Achilles tendon (S86.0-)*
sprain of joints and ligaments of ankle and foot (S93.-)

TIP: Refer to the Muscle/Tendon table at the beginning of this chapter.

The appropriate 7th character is to be added to each code from category S96.
A initial encounter
D subsequent encounter
S sequela

√5th **S96.0** Injury of muscle and tendon of long flexor muscle of toe at ankle and foot level

√6th **S96.00** Unspecified injury of muscle and tendon of long flexor muscle of toe at ankle and foot level

√7th **S96.001** Unspecified injury of muscle and tendon of long flexor muscle of toe at ankle and foot level, right foot

√7th **S96.002** Unspecified injury of muscle and tendon of long flexor muscle of toe at ankle and foot level, left foot

√7th **S96.009** Unspecified injury of muscle and tendon of long flexor muscle of toe at ankle and foot level, unspecified foot

√6th **S96.01** Strain of muscle and tendon of long flexor muscle of toe at ankle and foot level

√7th **S96.011** Strain of muscle and tendon of long flexor muscle of toe at ankle and foot level, right foot

√7th **S96.012** Strain of muscle and tendon of long flexor muscle of toe at ankle and foot level, left foot

√7th **S96.019** Strain of muscle and tendon of long flexor muscle of toe at ankle and foot level, unspecified foot

√6th **S96.02** Laceration of muscle and tendon of long flexor muscle of toe at ankle and foot level

√7th **S96.021** Laceration of muscle and tendon of long flexor muscle of toe at ankle and foot level, right foot CC

√7th **S96.022** Laceration of muscle and tendon of long flexor muscle of toe at ankle and foot level, left foot CC

√7th **S96.029** Laceration of muscle and tendon of long flexor muscle of toe at ankle and foot level, unspecified foot CC UNS

√6th **S96.09** Other injury of muscle and tendon of long flexor muscle of toe at ankle and foot level

√7th **S96.091** Other injury of muscle and tendon of long flexor muscle of toe at ankle and foot level, right foot

√7th **S96.092** Other injury of muscle and tendon of long flexor muscle of toe at ankle and foot level, left foot

√7th **S96.099** Other injury of muscle and tendon of long flexor muscle of toe at ankle and foot level, unspecified foot

√5th **S96.1** Injury of muscle and tendon of long extensor muscle of toe at ankle and foot level

√6th **S96.10** Unspecified injury of muscle and tendon of long extensor muscle of toe at ankle and foot level

√7th **S96.101** Unspecified injury of muscle and tendon of long extensor muscle of toe at ankle and foot level, right foot

√7th **S96.102** Unspecified injury of muscle and tendon of long extensor muscle of toe at ankle and foot level, left foot

√7th **S96.109** Unspecified injury of muscle and tendon of long extensor muscle of toe at ankle and foot level, unspecified foot

√6th **S96.11** Strain of muscle and tendon of long extensor muscle of toe at ankle and foot level

√7th **S96.111** Strain of muscle and tendon of long extensor muscle of toe at ankle and foot level, right foot

√7th **S96.112** Strain of muscle and tendon of long extensor muscle of toe at ankle and foot level, left foot

√7th **S96.119** Strain of muscle and tendon of long extensor muscle of toe at ankle and foot level, unspecified foot

√6th **S96.12** Laceration of muscle and tendon of long extensor muscle of toe at ankle and foot level

√7th **S96.121** Laceration of muscle and tendon of long extensor muscle of toe at ankle and foot level, right foot CC

√7th **S96.122** Laceration of muscle and tendon of long extensor muscle of toe at ankle and foot level, left foot CC

√7th **S96.129** Laceration of muscle and tendon of long extensor muscle of toe at ankle and foot level, unspecified foot CC UNS

√6th **S96.19** Other specified injury of muscle and tendon of long extensor muscle of toe at ankle and foot level

√7th **S96.191** Other specified injury of muscle and tendon of long extensor muscle of toe at ankle and foot level, right foot

√7th **S96.192** Other specified injury of muscle and tendon of long extensor muscle of toe at ankle and foot level, left foot

√7th **S96.199** Other specified injury of muscle and tendon of long extensor muscle of toe at ankle and foot level, unspecified foot

√5th **S96.2** Injury of intrinsic muscle and tendon at ankle and foot level

√6th **S96.20** Unspecified injury of intrinsic muscle and tendon at ankle and foot level

√7th **S96.201** Unspecified injury of intrinsic muscle and tendon at ankle and foot level, right foot

√7th **S96.202** Unspecified injury of intrinsic muscle and tendon at ankle and foot level, left foot

√7th **S96.209** Unspecified injury of intrinsic muscle and tendon at ankle and foot level, unspecified foot

√6th **S96.21** Strain of intrinsic muscle and tendon at ankle and foot level

√7th **S96.211** Strain of intrinsic muscle and tendon at ankle and foot level, right foot

√7th **S96.212** Strain of intrinsic muscle and tendon at ankle and foot level, left foot

- 7th **S96.219** **Strain of intrinsic muscle and tendon at ankle and foot level, unspecified foot**
- 6th **S96.22** **Laceration of intrinsic muscle and tendon at ankle and foot level**
  - 7th **S96.221** **Laceration of intrinsic muscle and tendon at ankle and foot level, right foot** CC
  - 7th **S96.222** **Laceration of intrinsic muscle and tendon at ankle and foot level, left foot** CC
  - 7th **S96.229** **Laceration of intrinsic muscle and tendon at ankle and foot level, unspecified foot** CC UNS
- 6th **S96.29** **Other specified injury of intrinsic muscle and tendon at ankle and foot level**
  - 7th **S96.291** **Other specified injury of intrinsic muscle and tendon at ankle and foot level, right foot**
  - 7th **S96.292** **Other specified injury of intrinsic muscle and tendon at ankle and foot level, left foot**
  - 7th **S96.299** **Other specified injury of intrinsic muscle and tendon at ankle and foot level, unspecified foot**
- 5th **S96.8** **Injury of other specified muscles and tendons at ankle and foot level**
- 6th **S96.80** **Unspecified injury of other specified muscles and tendons at ankle and foot level**
  - 7th **S96.801** **Unspecified injury of other specified muscles and tendons at ankle and foot level, right foot**
  - 7th **S96.802** **Unspecified injury of other specified muscles and tendons at ankle and foot level, left foot**
  - 7th **S96.809** **Unspecified injury of other specified muscles and tendons at ankle and foot level, unspecified foot**
- 6th **S96.81** **Strain of other specified muscles and tendons at ankle and foot level**
  - 7th **S96.811** **Strain of other specified muscles and tendons at ankle and foot level, right foot**
  - 7th **S96.812** **Strain of other specified muscles and tendons at ankle and foot level, left foot**
  - 7th **S96.819** **Strain of other specified muscles and tendons at ankle and foot level, unspecified foot**
- 6th **S96.82** **Laceration of other specified muscles and tendons at ankle and foot level**
  - 7th **S96.821** **Laceration of other specified muscles and tendons at ankle and foot level, right foot** CC
  - 7th **S96.822** **Laceration of other specified muscles and tendons at ankle and foot level, left foot** CC
  - 7th **S96.829** **Laceration of other specified muscles and tendons at ankle and foot level, unspecified foot** CC UNS
- 6th **S96.89** **Other specified injury of other specified muscles and tendons at ankle and foot level**
  - 7th **S96.891** **Other specified injury of other specified muscles and tendons at ankle and foot level, right foot**
  - 7th **S96.892** **Other specified injury of other specified muscles and tendons at ankle and foot level, left foot**
  - 7th **S96.899** **Other specified injury of other specified muscles and tendons at ankle and foot level, unspecified foot**
- 5th **S96.9** **Injury of unspecified muscle and tendon at ankle and foot level**
- 6th **S96.90** **Unspecified injury of unspecified muscle and tendon at ankle and foot level**
  - 7th **S96.901** **Unspecified injury of unspecified muscle and tendon at ankle and foot level, right foot**
  - 7th **S96.902** **Unspecified injury of unspecified muscle and tendon at ankle and foot level, left foot**
  - 7th **S96.909** **Unspecified injury of unspecified muscle and tendon at ankle and foot level, unspecified foot**
- 6th **S96.91** **Strain of unspecified muscle and tendon at ankle and foot level**
  - 7th **S96.911** **Strain of unspecified muscle and tendon at ankle and foot level, right foot**
  - 7th **S96.912** **Strain of unspecified muscle and tendon at ankle and foot level, left foot**
  - 7th **S96.919** **Strain of unspecified muscle and tendon at ankle and foot level, unspecified foot**
- 6th **S96.92** **Laceration of unspecified muscle and tendon at ankle and foot level**
  - 7th **S96.921** **Laceration of unspecified muscle and tendon at ankle and foot level, right foot** CC
  - 7th **S96.922** **Laceration of unspecified muscle and tendon at ankle and foot level, left foot** CC
  - 7th **S96.929** **Laceration of unspecified muscle and tendon at ankle and foot level, unspecified foot** CC UNS
- 6th **S96.99** **Other specified injury of unspecified muscle and tendon at ankle and foot level**
  - 7th **S96.991** **Other specified injury of unspecified muscle and tendon at ankle and foot level, right foot**
  - 7th **S96.992** **Other specified injury of unspecified muscle and tendon at ankle and foot level, left foot**
  - 7th **S96.999** **Other specified injury of unspecified muscle and tendon at ankle and foot level, unspecified foot**

4th **S97** **Crushing injury of ankle and foot**

Use additional code(s) for all associated injuries

The appropriate 7th character is to be added to each code from category S97.
A initial encounter
D subsequent encounter
S sequela

- 5th **S97.0** **Crushing injury of ankle**
  - x7th **S97.00** **Crushing injury of unspecified ankle**
  - x7th **S97.01** **Crushing injury of right ankle**
  - x7th **S97.02** **Crushing injury of left ankle**
- 5th **S97.1** **Crushing injury of toe**
- 6th **S97.10** **Crushing injury of unspecified toe(s)**
  - 7th **S97.101** **Crushing injury of unspecified right toe(s)**
  - 7th **S97.102** **Crushing injury of unspecified left toe(s)**
  - 7th **S97.109** **Crushing injury of unspecified toe(s)**
    Crushing injury of toe NOS
- 6th **S97.11** **Crushing injury of great toe**
  - 7th **S97.111** **Crushing injury of right great toe**
  - 7th **S97.112** **Crushing injury of left great toe**
  - 7th **S97.119** **Crushing injury of unspecified great toe**
- 6th **S97.12** **Crushing injury of lesser toe(s)**
  - 7th **S97.121** **Crushing injury of right lesser toe(s)**
  - 7th **S97.122** **Crushing injury of left lesser toe(s)**
  - 7th **S97.129** **Crushing injury of unspecified lesser toe(s)**
- 5th **S97.8** **Crushing injury of foot**
  - x7th **S97.80** **Crushing injury of unspecified foot**
    Crushing injury of foot NOS
  - x7th **S97.81** **Crushing injury of right foot**
  - x7th **S97.82** **Crushing injury of left foot**

4th **S98** **Traumatic amputation of ankle and foot**

An amputation not identified as partial or complete should be coded to complete

The appropriate 7th character is to be added to each code from category S98.
A initial encounter
D subsequent encounter
S sequela

- 5th **S98.0** **Traumatic amputation of foot at ankle level**
- 6th **S98.01** **Complete traumatic amputation of foot at ankle level**
  - 7th **S98.011** **Complete traumatic amputation of right foot at ankle level** CC HCC
  - 7th **S98.012** **Complete traumatic amputation of left foot at ankle level** CC HCC
  - 7th **S98.019** **Complete traumatic amputation of unspecified foot at ankle level** CC UNS HCC

S98.02 Partial traumatic amputation of foot at ankle level
- S98.021 Partial traumatic amputation of right foot at ankle level CC HCC
- S98.022 Partial traumatic amputation of left foot at ankle level CC HCC
- S98.029 Partial traumatic amputation of unspecified foot at ankle level CC UNS HCC

S98.1 Traumatic amputation of one toe

S98.11 Complete traumatic amputation of great toe
- S98.111 Complete traumatic amputation of right great toe HCC
- S98.112 Complete traumatic amputation of left great toe HCC
- S98.119 Complete traumatic amputation of unspecified great toe HCC

S98.12 Partial traumatic amputation of great toe
- S98.121 Partial traumatic amputation of right great toe HCC
- S98.122 Partial traumatic amputation of left great toe HCC
- S98.129 Partial traumatic amputation of unspecified great toe HCC

S98.13 Complete traumatic amputation of one lesser toe

Traumatic amputation of toe NOS
- S98.131 Complete traumatic amputation of one right lesser toe HCC
- S98.132 Complete traumatic amputation of one left lesser toe HCC
- S98.139 Complete traumatic amputation of one unspecified lesser toe HCC

S98.14 Partial traumatic amputation of one lesser toe
- S98.141 Partial traumatic amputation of one right lesser toe HCC
- S98.142 Partial traumatic amputation of one left lesser toe HCC
- S98.149 Partial traumatic amputation of one unspecified lesser toe HCC

S98.2 Traumatic amputation of two or more lesser toes

S98.21 Complete traumatic amputation of two or more lesser toes
- S98.211 Complete traumatic amputation of two or more right lesser toes HCC
- S98.212 Complete traumatic amputation of two or more left lesser toes HCC
- S98.219 Complete traumatic amputation of two or more unspecified lesser toes HCC

S98.22 Partial traumatic amputation of two or more lesser toes
- S98.221 Partial traumatic amputation of two or more right lesser toes HCC
- S98.222 Partial traumatic amputation of two or more left lesser toes HCC
- S98.229 Partial traumatic amputation of two or more unspecified lesser toes HCC

S98.3 Traumatic amputation of midfoot

S98.31 Complete traumatic amputation of midfoot
- S98.311 Complete traumatic amputation of right midfoot CC HCC
- S98.312 Complete traumatic amputation of left midfoot CC HCC
- S98.319 Complete traumatic amputation of unspecified midfoot CC UNS HCC

S98.32 Partial traumatic amputation of midfoot
- S98.321 Partial traumatic amputation of right midfoot CC HCC
- S98.322 Partial traumatic amputation of left midfoot CC HCC
- S98.329 Partial traumatic amputation of unspecified midfoot CC UNS HCC

S98.9 Traumatic amputation of foot, level unspecified

S98.91 Complete traumatic amputation of foot, level unspecified
- S98.911 Complete traumatic amputation of right foot, level unspecified CC HCC
- S98.912 Complete traumatic amputation of left foot, level unspecified CC HCC
- S98.919 Complete traumatic amputation of unspecified foot, level unspecified CC UNS HCC

S98.92 Partial traumatic amputation of foot, level unspecified
- S98.921 Partial traumatic amputation of right foot, level unspecified CC HCC
- S98.922 Partial traumatic amputation of left foot, level unspecified CC HCC
- S98.929 Partial traumatic amputation of unspecified foot, level unspecified CC UNS HCC

S99 Other and unspecified injuries of ankle and foot

AHA: 2018,2Q,12; 2018,1Q,3; 2016,4Q,68-69

S99.0 Physeal fracture of calcaneus

AHA: 2019,4Q,56

The appropriate 7th character is to be added to each code from subcategory S99.Ø.
- A initial encounter for closed fracture
- B initial encounter for open fracture
- D subsequent encounter for fracture with routine healing
- G subsequent encounter for fracture with delayed healing
- K subsequent encounter for fracture with nonunion
- P subsequent encounter for fracture with malunion
- S sequela

S99.ØØ Unspecified physeal fracture of calcaneus
- S99.ØØ1 Unspecified physeal fracture of right calcaneus
- S99.ØØ2 Unspecified physeal fracture of left calcaneus
- S99.ØØ9 Unspecified physeal fracture of unspecified calcaneus

S99.Ø1 Salter-Harris Type I physeal fracture of calcaneus
- S99.Ø11 Salter-Harris Type I physeal fracture of right calcaneus
- S99.Ø12 Salter-Harris Type I physeal fracture of left calcaneus
- S99.Ø19 Salter-Harris Type I physeal fracture of unspecified calcaneus

S99.Ø2 Salter-Harris Type II physeal fracture of calcaneus
- S99.Ø21 Salter-Harris Type II physeal fracture of right calcaneus
- S99.Ø22 Salter-Harris Type II physeal fracture of left calcaneus
- S99.Ø29 Salter-Harris Type II physeal fracture of unspecified calcaneus

S99.Ø3 Salter-Harris Type III physeal fracture of calcaneus
- S99.Ø31 Salter-Harris Type III physeal fracture of right calcaneus
- S99.Ø32 Salter-Harris Type III physeal fracture of left calcaneus
- S99.Ø39 Salter-Harris Type III physeal fracture of unspecified calcaneus

S99.Ø4 Salter-Harris Type IV physeal fracture of calcaneus
- S99.Ø41 Salter-Harris Type IV physeal fracture of right calcaneus
- S99.Ø42 Salter-Harris Type IV physeal fracture of left calcaneus
- S99.Ø49 Salter-Harris Type IV physeal fracture of unspecified calcaneus

S99.Ø9 Other physeal fracture of calcaneus
- S99.Ø91 Other physeal fracture of right calcaneus
- S99.Ø92 Other physeal fracture of left calcaneus
- S99.Ø99 Other physeal fracture of unspecified calcaneus

5th S99.1 Physeal fracture of metatarsal

AHA: 2019,4Q,56

The appropriate 7th character is to be added to each code from subcategory S99.1
- A initial encounter for closed fracture
- B initial encounter for open fracture
- D subsequent encounter for fracture with routine healing
- G subsequent encounter for fracture with delayed healing
- K subsequent encounter for fracture with nonunion
- P subsequent encounter for fracture with malunion
- S sequela

6th S99.10 Unspecified physeal fracture of metatarsal
- 7th S99.101 Unspecified physeal fracture of right metatarsal
- 7th S99.102 Unspecified physeal fracture of left metatarsal
- 7th S99.109 Unspecified physeal fracture of unspecified metatarsal

6th S99.11 Salter-Harris Type I physeal fracture of metatarsal
- 7th S99.111 Salter-Harris Type I physeal fracture of right metatarsal
- 7th S99.112 Salter-Harris Type I physeal fracture of left metatarsal
- 7th S99.119 Salter-Harris Type I physeal fracture of unspecified metatarsal

6th S99.12 Salter-Harris Type II physeal fracture of metatarsal
- 7th S99.121 Salter-Harris Type II physeal fracture of right metatarsal
- 7th S99.122 Salter-Harris Type II physeal fracture of left metatarsal
- 7th S99.129 Salter-Harris Type II physeal fracture of unspecified metatarsal

6th S99.13 Salter-Harris Type III physeal fracture of metatarsal
- 7th S99.131 Salter-Harris Type III physeal fracture of right metatarsal
- 7th S99.132 Salter-Harris Type III physeal fracture of left metatarsal
- 7th S99.139 Salter-Harris Type III physeal fracture of unspecified metatarsal

6th S99.14 Salter-Harris Type IV physeal fracture of metatarsal
- 7th S99.141 Salter-Harris Type IV physeal fracture of right metatarsal
- 7th S99.142 Salter-Harris Type IV physeal fracture of left metatarsal
- 7th S99.149 Salter-Harris Type IV physeal fracture of unspecified metatarsal

6th S99.19 Other physeal fracture of metatarsal
- 7th S99.191 Other physeal fracture of right metatarsal
- 7th S99.192 Other physeal fracture of left metatarsal
- 7th S99.199 Other physeal fracture of unspecified metatarsal

5th S99.2 Physeal fracture of phalanx of toe

AHA: 2019,4Q,56

The appropriate 7th character is to be added to each code from subcategories S99.2.
- A initial encounter for closed fracture
- B initial encounter for open fracture
- D subsequent encounter for fracture with routine healing
- G subsequent encounter for fracture with delayed healing
- K subsequent encounter for fracture with nonunion
- P subsequent encounter for fracture with malunion
- S sequela

6th S99.20 Unspecified physeal fracture of phalanx of toe
- 7th S99.201 Unspecified physeal fracture of phalanx of right toe
- 7th S99.202 Unspecified physeal fracture of phalanx of left toe
- 7th S99.209 Unspecified physeal fracture of phalanx of unspecified toe

6th S99.21 Salter-Harris Type I physeal fracture of phalanx of toe
- 7th S99.211 Salter-Harris Type I physeal fracture of phalanx of right toe
- 7th S99.212 Salter-Harris Type I physeal fracture of phalanx of left toe
- 7th S99.219 Salter-Harris Type I physeal fracture of phalanx of unspecified toe

6th S99.22 Salter-Harris Type II physeal fracture of phalanx of toe
- 7th S99.221 Salter-Harris Type II physeal fracture of phalanx of right toe
- 7th S99.222 Salter-Harris Type II physeal fracture of phalanx of left toe
- 7th S99.229 Salter-Harris Type II physeal fracture of phalanx of unspecified toe

6th S99.23 Salter-Harris Type III physeal fracture of phalanx of toe
- 7th S99.231 Salter-Harris Type III physeal fracture of phalanx of right toe
- 7th S99.232 Salter-Harris Type III physeal fracture of phalanx of left toe
- 7th S99.239 Salter-Harris Type III physeal fracture of phalanx of unspecified toe

6th S99.24 Salter-Harris Type IV physeal fracture of phalanx of toe
- 7th S99.241 Salter-Harris Type IV physeal fracture of phalanx of right toe
- 7th S99.242 Salter-Harris Type IV physeal fracture of phalanx of left toe
- 7th S99.249 Salter-Harris Type IV physeal fracture of phalanx of unspecified toe

6th S99.29 Other physeal fracture of phalanx of toe
- 7th S99.291 Other physeal fracture of phalanx of right toe
- 7th S99.292 Other physeal fracture of phalanx of left toe
- 7th S99.299 Other physeal fracture of phalanx of unspecified toe

5th S99.8 Other specified injuries of ankle and foot

The appropriate 7th character is to be added to each code from subcategory S99.8.
- A initial encounter
- D subsequent encounter
- S sequela

6th S99.81 Other specified injuries of ankle
- 7th S99.811 Other specified injuries of right ankle
- 7th S99.812 Other specified injuries of left ankle
- 7th S99.819 Other specified injuries of unspecified ankle

6th S99.82 Other specified injuries of foot
- 7th S99.821 Other specified injuries of right foot
- 7th S99.822 Other specified injuries of left foot
- 7th S99.829 Other specified injuries of unspecified foot

5th S99.9 Unspecified injury of ankle and foot

The appropriate 7th character is to be added to each code from subcategory S99.9.
- A initial encounter
- D subsequent encounter
- S sequela

6th S99.91 Unspecified injury of ankle
- 7th S99.911 Unspecified injury of right ankle
- 7th S99.912 Unspecified injury of left ankle
- 7th S99.919 Unspecified injury of unspecified ankle

6th S99.92 Unspecified injury of foot
- 7th S99.921 Unspecified injury of right foot
- 7th S99.922 Unspecified injury of left foot
- 7th S99.929 Unspecified injury of unspecified foot

INJURY, POISONING AND CERTAIN OTHER CONSEQUENCES OF EXTERNAL CAUSES (T07-T88)

Injuries involving multiple body regions (T07)

EXCLUDES 1 *burns and corrosions (T20-T32)*
frostbite (T33-T34)
insect bite or sting, venomous (T63.4)
sunburn (L55.-)

T07 Unspecified multiple injuries
EXCLUDES 1 *injury NOS (T14.90)*
AHA: 2017,4Q,26

The appropriate 7th character is to be added to code T07.
A initial encounter
D subsequent encounter
S sequela

Injury of unspecified body region (T14)

T14 Injury of unspecified body region
EXCLUDES 1 *multiple unspecified injuries (T07)*
AHA: 2017,4Q,26

The appropriate 7th character is to be added to each code from category T14.
A initial encounter
D subsequent encounter
S sequela

T14.8 Other injury of unspecified body region
Abrasion NOS
Contusion NOS
Crush injury NOS
Fracture NOS
Skin injury NOS
Vascular injury NOS
Wound NOS

T14.9 Unspecified injury
T14.90 Injury, unspecified
Injury NOS
T14.91 Suicide attempt HCC
Attempted suicide NOS

Effects of foreign body entering through natural orifice (T15-T19)

▶Use additional code, if known, for foreign body entering into or through a natural orifice (W44.-)◀

EXCLUDES 2 *foreign body accidentally left in operation wound (T81.5-)*
foreign body in penetrating wound - see open wound by body region
residual foreign body in soft tissue (M79.5)
splinter, without open wound - see superficial injury by body region

T15 Foreign body on external eye
EXCLUDES 2 *foreign body in penetrating wound of orbit and eye ball (S05.4-, S05.5-)*
open wound of eyelid and periocular area (S01.1-)
retained foreign body in eyelid (H02.8-)
retained (old) foreign body in penetrating wound of orbit and eye ball (H05.5-, H44.6-, H44.7-)
superficial foreign body of eyelid and periocular area (S00.25-)

The appropriate 7th character is to be added to each code from category T15.
A initial encounter
D subsequent encounter
S sequela

T15.0 Foreign body in cornea
T15.00 Foreign body in cornea, unspecified eye
T15.01 Foreign body in cornea, right eye
T15.02 Foreign body in cornea, left eye

T15.1 Foreign body in conjunctival sac
T15.10 Foreign body in conjunctival sac, unspecified eye
T15.11 Foreign body in conjunctival sac, right eye
T15.12 Foreign body in conjunctival sac, left eye

T15.8 Foreign body in other and multiple parts of external eye
Foreign body in lacrimal punctum
T15.80 Foreign body in other and multiple parts of external eye, unspecified eye
T15.81 Foreign body in other and multiple parts of external eye, right eye
T15.82 Foreign body in other and multiple parts of external eye, left eye

T15.9 Foreign body on external eye, part unspecified
T15.90 Foreign body on external eye, part unspecified, unspecified eye
T15.91 Foreign body on external eye, part unspecified, right eye
T15.92 Foreign body on external eye, part unspecified, left eye

T16 Foreign body in ear
INCLUDES foreign body in auditory canal

The appropriate 7th character is to be added to each code from category T16.
A initial encounter
D subsequent encounter
S sequela

T16.1 Foreign body in right ear
T16.2 Foreign body in left ear
T16.9 Foreign body in ear, unspecified ear

T17 Foreign body in respiratory tract

The appropriate 7th character is to be added to each code from category T17.
A initial encounter
D subsequent encounter
S sequela

T17.0 Foreign body in nasal sinus
T17.1 Foreign body in nostril
Foreign body in nose NOS

T17.2 Foreign body in pharynx
Foreign body in nasopharynx
Foreign body in throat NOS

T17.20 Unspecified foreign body in pharynx
T17.200 Unspecified foreign body in pharynx causing asphyxiation
T17.208 Unspecified foreign body in pharynx causing other injury

T17.21 Gastric contents in pharynx
Aspiration of gastric contents into pharynx
Vomitus in pharynx
T17.210 Gastric contents in pharynx causing asphyxiation
T17.218 Gastric contents in pharynx causing other injury

T17.22 Food in pharynx
Bones in pharynx
Seeds in pharynx
T17.220 Food in pharynx causing asphyxiation
T17.228 Food in pharynx causing other injury

T17.29 Other foreign object in pharynx
T17.290 Other foreign object in pharynx causing asphyxiation
T17.298 Other foreign object in pharynx causing other injury

T17.3 Foreign body in larynx
T17.30 Unspecified foreign body in larynx
T17.300 Unspecified foreign body in larynx causing asphyxiation
T17.308 Unspecified foreign body in larynx causing other injury

T17.31 Gastric contents in larynx
Aspiration of gastric contents into larynx
Vomitus in larynx
T17.310 Gastric contents in larynx causing asphyxiation
T17.318 Gastric contents in larynx causing other injury

T17.32 Food in larynx
Bones in larynx
Seeds in larynx
T17.320 Food in larynx causing asphyxiation
T17.328 Food in larynx causing other injury

✓6th T17.39 Other foreign object in larynx
✓7th T17.390 Other foreign object in larynx causing asphyxiation
✓7th T17.398 Other foreign object in larynx causing other injury

✓5th T17.4 Foreign body in trachea
✓6th T17.40 Unspecified foreign body in trachea
✓7th T17.400 Unspecified foreign body in trachea causing asphyxiation CC
✓7th T17.408 Unspecified foreign body in trachea causing other injury CC

✓6th T17.41 Gastric contents in trachea
Aspiration of gastric contents into trachea
Vomitus in trachea
✓7th T17.410 Gastric contents in trachea causing asphyxiation CC
✓7th T17.418 Gastric contents in trachea causing other injury CC

✓6th T17.42 Food in trachea
Bones in trachea
Seeds in trachea
✓7th T17.420 Food in trachea causing asphyxiation CC
✓7th T17.428 Food in trachea causing other injury CC

✓6th T17.49 Other foreign object in trachea
✓7th T17.490 Other foreign object in trachea causing asphyxiation CC
✓7th T17.498 Other foreign object in trachea causing other injury CC

✓5th T17.5 Foreign body in bronchus
✓6th T17.50 Unspecified foreign body in bronchus
✓7th T17.500 Unspecified foreign body in bronchus causing asphyxiation CC
✓7th T17.508 Unspecified foreign body in bronchus causing other injury CC

✓6th T17.51 Gastric contents in bronchus
Aspiration of gastric contents into bronchus
Vomitus in bronchus
✓7th T17.510 Gastric contents in bronchus causing asphyxiation CC
✓7th T17.518 Gastric contents in bronchus causing other injury CC

✓6th T17.52 Food in bronchus
Bones in bronchus
Seeds in bronchus
✓7th T17.520 Food in bronchus causing asphyxiation CC
✓7th T17.528 Food in bronchus causing other injury CC

✓6th T17.59 Other foreign object in bronchus
✓7th T17.590 Other foreign object in bronchus causing asphyxiation CC
✓7th T17.598 Other foreign object in bronchus causing other injury CC

✓5th T17.8 Foreign body in other parts of respiratory tract
Foreign body in bronchioles
Foreign body in lung
✓6th T17.80 Unspecified foreign body in other parts of respiratory tract
✓7th T17.800 Unspecified foreign body in other parts of respiratory tract causing asphyxiation CC
✓7th T17.808 Unspecified foreign body in other parts of respiratory tract causing other injury CC

✓6th T17.81 Gastric contents in other parts of respiratory tract
Aspiration of gastric contents into other parts of respiratory tract
Vomitus in other parts of respiratory tract
✓7th T17.810 Gastric contents in other parts of respiratory tract causing asphyxiation CC
✓7th T17.818 Gastric contents in other parts of respiratory tract causing other injury CC

✓6th T17.82 Food in other parts of respiratory tract
Bones in other parts of respiratory tract
Seeds in other parts of respiratory tract
✓7th T17.820 Food in other parts of respiratory tract causing asphyxiation CC
✓7th T17.828 Food in other parts of respiratory tract causing other injury CC

✓6th T17.89 Other foreign object in other parts of respiratory tract
✓7th T17.890 Other foreign object in other parts of respiratory tract causing asphyxiation CC
✓7th T17.898 Other foreign object in other parts of respiratory tract causing other injury CC

✓5th T17.9 Foreign body in respiratory tract, part unspecified
✓6th T17.90 Unspecified foreign body in respiratory tract, part unspecified
✓7th T17.900 Unspecified foreign body in respiratory tract, part unspecified causing asphyxiation
✓7th T17.908 Unspecified foreign body in respiratory tract, part unspecified causing other injury

✓6th T17.91 Gastric contents in respiratory tract, part unspecified
Aspiration of gastric contents into respiratory tract, part unspecified
Vomitus in trachea respiratory tract, part unspecified
✓7th T17.910 Gastric contents in respiratory tract, part unspecified causing asphyxiation
✓7th T17.918 Gastric contents in respiratory tract, part unspecified causing other injury

✓6th T17.92 Food in respiratory tract, part unspecified
Bones in respiratory tract, part unspecified
Seeds in respiratory tract, part unspecified
✓7th T17.920 Food in respiratory tract, part unspecified causing asphyxiation
✓7th T17.928 Food in respiratory tract, part unspecified causing other injury

✓6th T17.99 Other foreign object in respiratory tract, part unspecified
✓7th T17.990 Other foreign object in respiratory tract, part unspecified in causing asphyxiation
AHA: 2019,3Q,15
✓7th T17.998 Other foreign object in respiratory tract, part unspecified causing other injury

✓4th **T18 Foreign body in alimentary tract**
EXCLUDES 2 *foreign body in pharynx (T17.2-)*

The appropriate 7th character is to be added to each code from category T18.
A initial encounter
D subsequent encounter
S sequela

✓x 7th T18.0 Foreign body in mouth
✓5th T18.1 Foreign body in esophagus
EXCLUDES 2 *foreign body in respiratory tract (T17.-)*
✓6th T18.10 Unspecified foreign body in esophagus
✓7th T18.100 Unspecified foreign body in esophagus causing compression of trachea
Unspecified foreign body in esophagus causing obstruction of respiration
✓7th T18.108 Unspecified foreign body in esophagus causing other injury

✓6th T18.11 Gastric contents in esophagus
Vomitus in esophagus
✓7th T18.110 Gastric contents in esophagus causing compression of trachea
Gastric contents in esophagus causing obstruction of respiration
✓7th T18.118 Gastric contents in esophagus causing other injury

T18.12 **Food in esophagus**
Bones in esophagus
Seeds in esophagus
T18.120 **Food in esophagus causing compression of trachea**
Food in esophagus causing obstruction of respiration
T18.128 **Food in esophagus causing other injury**
T18.19 **Other foreign object in esophagus**
AHA: 2022,1Q,27; 2015,1Q,23
T18.190 **Other foreign object in esophagus causing compression of trachea**
Other foreign body in esophagus causing obstruction of respiration
TIP: Any foreign object lodged in the esophagus requires immediate treatment and is considered an injury. Assign this code when there is respiratory compromise or compression. If no respiratory compromise or compression is documented, assign code T18.198-.
T18.198 **Other foreign object in esophagus causing other injury**
TIP: Any foreign object lodged in the esophagus requires immediate treatment and is considered an injury. Assign this code when there is no respiratory compromise or compression. If respiratory compromise or compression is documented, assign code T18.190-.
T18.2 **Foreign body in stomach**
T18.3 **Foreign body in small intestine**
T18.4 **Foreign body in colon**
T18.5 **Foreign body in anus and rectum**
Foreign body in rectosigmoid (junction)
T18.8 **Foreign body in other parts of alimentary tract**
T18.9 **Foreign body of alimentary tract, part unspecified**
Foreign body in digestive system NOS
Swallowed foreign body NOS

T19 **Foreign body in genitourinary tract**
EXCLUDES 2 *complications due to implanted mesh (T83.7-)*
mechanical complications of contraceptive device (intrauterine) (vaginal) (T83.3-)
presence of contraceptive device (intrauterine) (vaginal) (Z97.5)

The appropriate 7th character is to be added to each code from category T19.
A initial encounter
D subsequent encounter
S sequela

T19.0 **Foreign body in urethra**
T19.1 **Foreign body in bladder**
T19.2 **Foreign body in vulva and vagina** ♀
T19.3 **Foreign body in uterus** ♀
T19.4 **Foreign body in penis** ♂
T19.8 **Foreign body in other parts of genitourinary tract**
T19.9 **Foreign body in genitourinary tract, part unspecified**

BURNS AND CORROSIONS (T20-T32)

INCLUDES burns (thermal) from electrical heating appliances
burns (thermal) from electricity
burns (thermal) from flame
burns (thermal) from friction
burns (thermal) from hot air and hot gases
burns (thermal) from hot objects
burns (thermal) from lightning
burns (thermal) from radiation
chemical burn [corrosion] (external) (internal)
scalds
EXCLUDES 2 *erythema [dermatitis] ab igne (L59.0)*
radiation-related disorders of the skin and subcutaneous tissue (L55-L59)
sunburn (L55.-)
AHA: 2016,2Q,4

Burns and corrosions of external body surface, specified by site (T20-T25)

INCLUDES burns and corrosions of first degree [erythema]
burns and corrosions of second degree [blisters] [epidermal loss]
burns and corrosions of third degree [deep necrosis of underlying tissue] [full-thickness skin loss]
Use additional code from category T31 or T32 to identify extent of body surface involved

T20 **Burn and corrosion of head, face, and neck**
EXCLUDES 2 *burn and corrosion of ear drum (T28.41, T28.91)*
burn and corrosion of eye and adnexa (T26.-)
burn and corrosion of mouth and pharynx (T28.0)
AHA: 2015,1Q,18-19

The appropriate 7th character is to be added to each code from category T20.
A initial encounter
D subsequent encounter
S sequela

T20.0 **Burn of unspecified degree of head, face, and neck**
Use additional external cause code to identify the source, place and intent of the burn (X00-X19, X75-X77, X96-X98, Y92)
T20.00 **Burn of unspecified degree of head, face, and neck, unspecified site**
T20.01 **Burn of unspecified degree of ear [any part, except ear drum]**
EXCLUDES 2 *burn of ear drum (T28.41-)*
T20.011 **Burn of unspecified degree of right ear [any part, except ear drum]**
T20.012 **Burn of unspecified degree of left ear [any part, except ear drum]**
T20.019 **Burn of unspecified degree of unspecified ear [any part, except ear drum]**
T20.02 **Burn of unspecified degree of lip(s)**
T20.03 **Burn of unspecified degree of chin**
T20.04 **Burn of unspecified degree of nose (septum)**
T20.05 **Burn of unspecified degree of scalp [any part]**
T20.06 **Burn of unspecified degree of forehead and cheek**
T20.07 **Burn of unspecified degree of neck**
T20.09 **Burn of unspecified degree of multiple sites of head, face, and neck**
T20.1 **Burn of first degree of head, face, and neck**
Use additional external cause code to identify the source, place and intent of the burn (X00-X19, X75-X77, X96-X98, Y92)
T20.10 **Burn of first degree of head, face, and neck, unspecified site**
T20.11 **Burn of first degree of ear [any part, except ear drum]**
EXCLUDES 2 *burn of ear drum (T28.41-)*
T20.111 **Burn of first degree of right ear [any part, except ear drum]**
T20.112 **Burn of first degree of left ear [any part, except ear drum]**
T20.119 **Burn of first degree of unspecified ear [any part, except ear drum]**
T20.12 **Burn of first degree of lip(s)**
T20.13 **Burn of first degree of chin**
T20.14 **Burn of first degree of nose (septum)**
T20.15 **Burn of first degree of scalp [any part]**
T20.16 **Burn of first degree of forehead and cheek**
T20.17 **Burn of first degree of neck**

√x7th T20.19 Burn of first degree of multiple sites of head, face, and neck

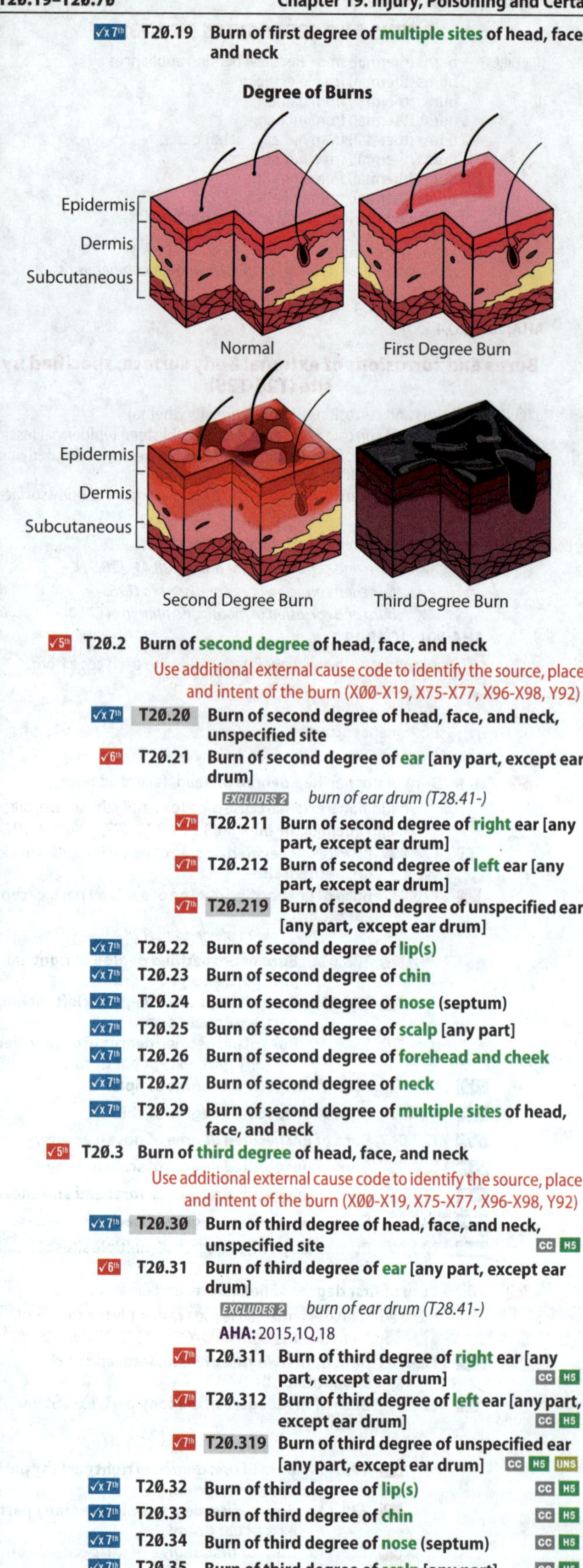

√5th T20.2 Burn of second degree of head, face, and neck
Use additional external cause code to identify the source, place and intent of the burn (X00-X19, X75-X77, X96-X98, Y92)
√x7th T20.20 Burn of second degree of head, face, and neck, unspecified site
√6th T20.21 Burn of second degree of ear [any part, except ear drum]
EXCLUDES 2 *burn of ear drum (T28.41-)*
√7th T20.211 Burn of second degree of right ear [any part, except ear drum]
√7th T20.212 Burn of second degree of left ear [any part, except ear drum]
√7th T20.219 Burn of second degree of unspecified ear [any part, except ear drum]
√x7th T20.22 Burn of second degree of lip(s)
√x7th T20.23 Burn of second degree of chin
√x7th T20.24 Burn of second degree of nose (septum)
√x7th T20.25 Burn of second degree of scalp [any part]
√x7th T20.26 Burn of second degree of forehead and cheek
√x7th T20.27 Burn of second degree of neck
√x7th T20.29 Burn of second degree of multiple sites of head, face, and neck
√5th T20.3 Burn of third degree of head, face, and neck
Use additional external cause code to identify the source, place and intent of the burn (X00-X19, X75-X77, X96-X98, Y92)
√x7th T20.30 Burn of third degree of head, face, and neck, unspecified site CC H5
√6th T20.31 Burn of third degree of ear [any part, except ear drum]
EXCLUDES 2 *burn of ear drum (T28.41-)*
AHA: 2015,1Q,18
√7th T20.311 Burn of third degree of right ear [any part, except ear drum] CC H5
√7th T20.312 Burn of third degree of left ear [any part, except ear drum] CC H5
√7th T20.319 Burn of third degree of unspecified ear [any part, except ear drum] CC H5 UNS
√x7th T20.32 Burn of third degree of lip(s) CC H5
√x7th T20.33 Burn of third degree of chin CC H5
√x7th T20.34 Burn of third degree of nose (septum) CC H5
√x7th T20.35 Burn of third degree of scalp [any part] CC H5
√x7th T20.36 Burn of third degree of forehead and cheek CC H5
√x7th T20.37 Burn of third degree of neck CC H5
√x7th T20.39 Burn of third degree of multiple sites of head, face, and neck CC H5

√5th T20.4 Corrosion of unspecified degree of head, face, and neck
Code first (T51-T65) to identify chemical and intent
Use additional external cause code to identify place (Y92)
√x7th T20.40 Corrosion of unspecified degree of head, face, and neck, unspecified site
√6th T20.41 Corrosion of unspecified degree of ear [any part, except ear drum]
EXCLUDES 2 *corrosion of ear drum (T28.91-)*
√7th T20.411 Corrosion of unspecified degree of right ear [any part, except ear drum]
√7th T20.412 Corrosion of unspecified degree of left ear [any part, except ear drum]
√7th T20.419 Corrosion of unspecified degree of unspecified ear [any part, except ear drum]
√x7th T20.42 Corrosion of unspecified degree of lip(s)
√x7th T20.43 Corrosion of unspecified degree of chin
√x7th T20.44 Corrosion of unspecified degree of nose (septum)
√x7th T20.45 Corrosion of unspecified degree of scalp [any part]
√x7th T20.46 Corrosion of unspecified degree of forehead and cheek
√x7th T20.47 Corrosion of unspecified degree of neck
√x7th T20.49 Corrosion of unspecified degree of multiple sites of head, face, and neck
√5th T20.5 Corrosion of first degree of head, face, and neck
Code first (T51-T65) to identify chemical and intent
Use additional external cause code to identify place (Y92)
√x7th T20.50 Corrosion of first degree of head, face, and neck, unspecified site
√6th T20.51 Corrosion of first degree of ear [any part, except ear drum]
EXCLUDES 2 *corrosion of ear drum (T28.91-)*
√7th T20.511 Corrosion of first degree of right ear [any part, except ear drum]
√7th T20.512 Corrosion of first degree of left ear [any part, except ear drum]
√7th T20.519 Corrosion of first degree of unspecified ear [any part, except ear drum]
√x7th T20.52 Corrosion of first degree of lip(s)
√x7th T20.53 Corrosion of first degree of chin
√x7th T20.54 Corrosion of first degree of nose (septum)
√x7th T20.55 Corrosion of first degree of scalp [any part]
√x7th T20.56 Corrosion of first degree of forehead and cheek
√x7th T20.57 Corrosion of first degree of neck
√x7th T20.59 Corrosion of first degree of multiple sites of head, face, and neck
√5th T20.6 Corrosion of second degree of head, face, and neck
Code first (T51-T65) to identify chemical and intent
Use additional external cause code to identify place (Y92)
√x7th T20.60 Corrosion of second degree of head, face, and neck, unspecified site
√6th T20.61 Corrosion of second degree of ear [any part, except ear drum]
EXCLUDES 2 *corrosion of ear drum (T28.91-)*
√7th T20.611 Corrosion of second degree of right ear [any part, except ear drum]
√7th T20.612 Corrosion of second degree of left ear [any part, except ear drum]
√7th T20.619 Corrosion of second degree of unspecified ear [any part, except ear drum]
√x7th T20.62 Corrosion of second degree of lip(s)
√x7th T20.63 Corrosion of second degree of chin
√x7th T20.64 Corrosion of second degree of nose (septum)
√x7th T20.65 Corrosion of second degree of scalp [any part]
√x7th T20.66 Corrosion of second degree of forehead and cheek
√x7th T20.67 Corrosion of second degree of neck
√x7th T20.69 Corrosion of second degree of multiple sites of head, face, and neck
√5th T20.7 Corrosion of third degree of head, face, and neck
Code first (T51-T65) to identify chemical and intent
Use additional external cause code to identify place (Y92)
√x7th T20.70 Corrosion of third degree of head, face, and neck, unspecified site CC H5

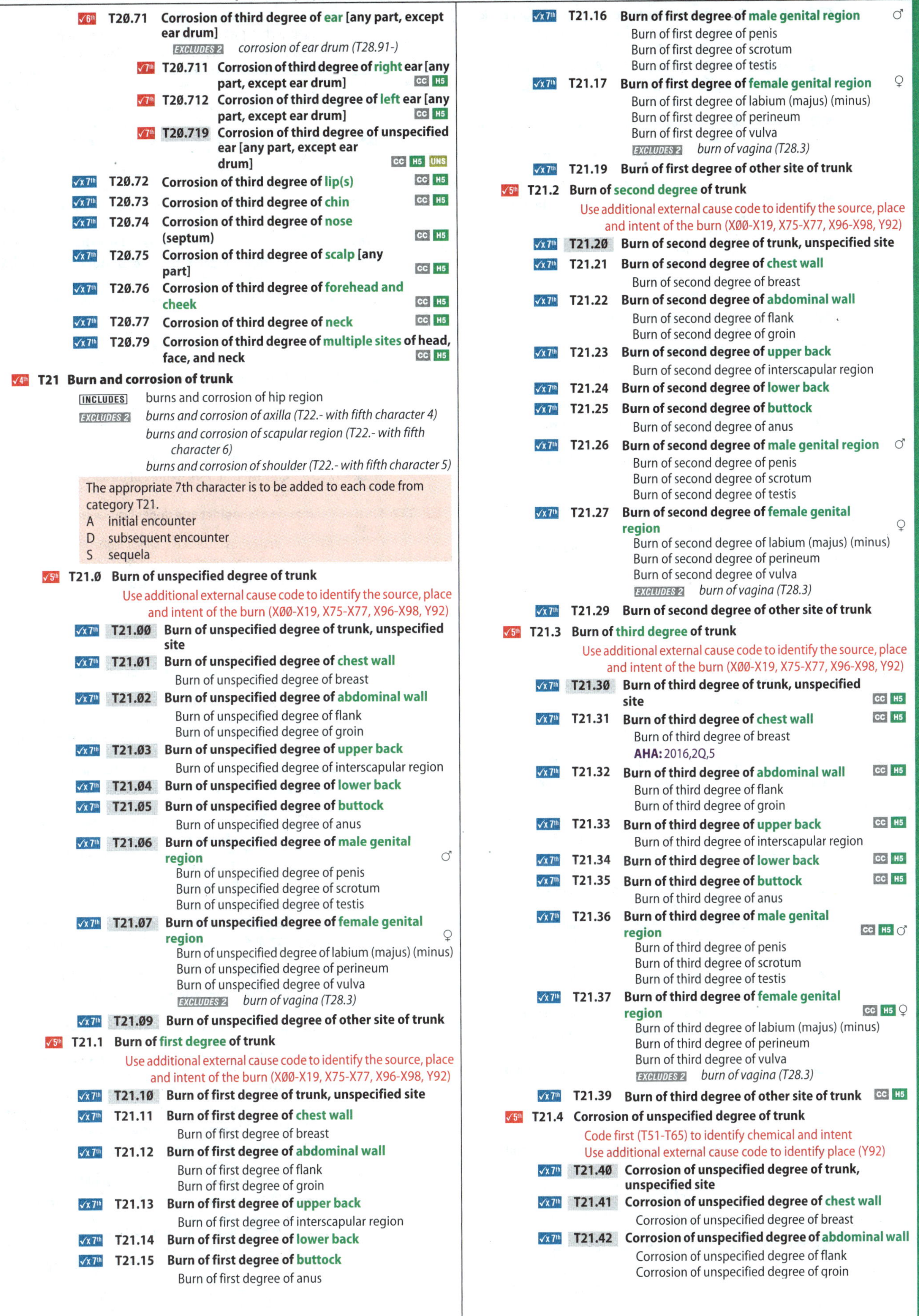

√6th **T20.71 Corrosion of third degree of ear [any part, except ear drum]**
EXCLUDES 2 *corrosion of ear drum (T28.91-)*

√7th **T20.711 Corrosion of third degree of right ear [any part, except ear drum]** CC H5
√7th **T20.712 Corrosion of third degree of left ear [any part, except ear drum]** CC H5
√7th **T20.719 Corrosion of third degree of unspecified ear [any part, except ear drum]** CC H5 UNS

√x7th **T20.72 Corrosion of third degree of lip(s)** CC H5
√x7th **T20.73 Corrosion of third degree of chin** CC H5
√x7th **T20.74 Corrosion of third degree of nose (septum)** CC H5
√x7th **T20.75 Corrosion of third degree of scalp [any part]** CC H5
√x7th **T20.76 Corrosion of third degree of forehead and cheek** CC H5
√x7th **T20.77 Corrosion of third degree of neck** CC H5
√x7th **T20.79 Corrosion of third degree of multiple sites of head, face, and neck** CC H5

√4th **T21 Burn and corrosion of trunk**
INCLUDES burns and corrosion of hip region
EXCLUDES 2 *burns and corrosion of axilla (T22.- with fifth character 4)*
burns and corrosion of scapular region (T22.- with fifth character 6)
burns and corrosion of shoulder (T22.- with fifth character 5)

The appropriate 7th character is to be added to each code from category T21.
A initial encounter
D subsequent encounter
S sequela

√5th **T21.0 Burn of unspecified degree of trunk**
Use additional external cause code to identify the source, place and intent of the burn (X00-X19, X75-X77, X96-X98, Y92)

√x7th **T21.00 Burn of unspecified degree of trunk, unspecified site**
√x7th **T21.01 Burn of unspecified degree of chest wall**
Burn of unspecified degree of breast
√x7th **T21.02 Burn of unspecified degree of abdominal wall**
Burn of unspecified degree of flank
Burn of unspecified degree of groin
√x7th **T21.03 Burn of unspecified degree of upper back**
Burn of unspecified degree of interscapular region
√x7th **T21.04 Burn of unspecified degree of lower back**
√x7th **T21.05 Burn of unspecified degree of buttock**
Burn of unspecified degree of anus
√x7th **T21.06 Burn of unspecified degree of male genital region** ♂
Burn of unspecified degree of penis
Burn of unspecified degree of scrotum
Burn of unspecified degree of testis
√x7th **T21.07 Burn of unspecified degree of female genital region** ♀
Burn of unspecified degree of labium (majus) (minus)
Burn of unspecified degree of perineum
Burn of unspecified degree of vulva
EXCLUDES 2 *burn of vagina (T28.3)*
√x7th **T21.09 Burn of unspecified degree of other site of trunk**

√5th **T21.1 Burn of first degree of trunk**
Use additional external cause code to identify the source, place and intent of the burn (X00-X19, X75-X77, X96-X98, Y92)

√x7th **T21.10 Burn of first degree of trunk, unspecified site**
√x7th **T21.11 Burn of first degree of chest wall**
Burn of first degree of breast
√x7th **T21.12 Burn of first degree of abdominal wall**
Burn of first degree of flank
Burn of first degree of groin
√x7th **T21.13 Burn of first degree of upper back**
Burn of first degree of interscapular region
√x7th **T21.14 Burn of first degree of lower back**
√x7th **T21.15 Burn of first degree of buttock**
Burn of first degree of anus
√x7th **T21.16 Burn of first degree of male genital region** ♂
Burn of first degree of penis
Burn of first degree of scrotum
Burn of first degree of testis
√x7th **T21.17 Burn of first degree of female genital region** ♀
Burn of first degree of labium (majus) (minus)
Burn of first degree of perineum
Burn of first degree of vulva
EXCLUDES 2 *burn of vagina (T28.3)*
√x7th **T21.19 Burn of first degree of other site of trunk**

√5th **T21.2 Burn of second degree of trunk**
Use additional external cause code to identify the source, place and intent of the burn (X00-X19, X75-X77, X96-X98, Y92)

√x7th **T21.20 Burn of second degree of trunk, unspecified site**
√x7th **T21.21 Burn of second degree of chest wall**
Burn of second degree of breast
√x7th **T21.22 Burn of second degree of abdominal wall**
Burn of second degree of flank
Burn of second degree of groin
√x7th **T21.23 Burn of second degree of upper back**
Burn of second degree of interscapular region
√x7th **T21.24 Burn of second degree of lower back**
√x7th **T21.25 Burn of second degree of buttock**
Burn of second degree of anus
√x7th **T21.26 Burn of second degree of male genital region** ♂
Burn of second degree of penis
Burn of second degree of scrotum
Burn of second degree of testis
√x7th **T21.27 Burn of second degree of female genital region** ♀
Burn of second degree of labium (majus) (minus)
Burn of second degree of perineum
Burn of second degree of vulva
EXCLUDES 2 *burn of vagina (T28.3)*
√x7th **T21.29 Burn of second degree of other site of trunk**

√5th **T21.3 Burn of third degree of trunk**
Use additional external cause code to identify the source, place and intent of the burn (X00-X19, X75-X77, X96-X98, Y92)

√x7th **T21.30 Burn of third degree of trunk, unspecified site** CC H5
√x7th **T21.31 Burn of third degree of chest wall** CC H5
Burn of third degree of breast
AHA: 2016,2Q,5
√x7th **T21.32 Burn of third degree of abdominal wall** CC H5
Burn of third degree of flank
Burn of third degree of groin
√x7th **T21.33 Burn of third degree of upper back** CC H5
Burn of third degree of interscapular region
√x7th **T21.34 Burn of third degree of lower back** CC H5
√x7th **T21.35 Burn of third degree of buttock** CC H5
Burn of third degree of anus
√x7th **T21.36 Burn of third degree of male genital region** CC H5 ♂
Burn of third degree of penis
Burn of third degree of scrotum
Burn of third degree of testis
√x7th **T21.37 Burn of third degree of female genital region** CC H5 ♀
Burn of third degree of labium (majus) (minus)
Burn of third degree of perineum
Burn of third degree of vulva
EXCLUDES 2 *burn of vagina (T28.3)*
√x7th **T21.39 Burn of third degree of other site of trunk** CC H5

√5th **T21.4 Corrosion of unspecified degree of trunk**
Code first (T51-T65) to identify chemical and intent
Use additional external cause code to identify place (Y92)

√x7th **T21.40 Corrosion of unspecified degree of trunk, unspecified site**
√x7th **T21.41 Corrosion of unspecified degree of chest wall**
Corrosion of unspecified degree of breast
√x7th **T21.42 Corrosion of unspecified degree of abdominal wall**
Corrosion of unspecified degree of flank
Corrosion of unspecified degree of groin

√x7th **T21.43 Corrosion of unspecified degree of upper back**
Corrosion of unspecified degree of interscapular region

√x7th **T21.44 Corrosion of unspecified degree of lower back**

√x7th **T21.45 Corrosion of unspecified degree of buttock**
Corrosion of unspecified degree of anus

√x7th **T21.46 Corrosion of unspecified degree of male genital region** ♂
Corrosion of unspecified degree of penis
Corrosion of unspecified degree of scrotum
Corrosion of unspecified degree of testis

√x7th **T21.47 Corrosion of unspecified degree of female genital region** ♀
Corrosion of unspecified degree of labium (majus) (minus)
Corrosion of unspecified degree of perineum
Corrosion of unspecified degree of vulva
EXCLUDES 2 *corrosion of vagina (T28.8)*

√x7th **T21.49 Corrosion of unspecified degree of other site of trunk**

√5th **T21.5 Corrosion of first degree of trunk**
Code first (T51-T65) to identify chemical and intent
Use additional external cause code to identify place (Y92)

√x7th **T21.5Ø Corrosion of first degree of trunk, unspecified site**

√x7th **T21.51 Corrosion of first degree of chest wall**
Corrosion of first degree of breast

√x7th **T21.52 Corrosion of first degree of abdominal wall**
Corrosion of first degree of flank
Corrosion of first degree of groin

√x7th **T21.53 Corrosion of first degree of upper back**
Corrosion of first degree of interscapular region

√x7th **T21.54 Corrosion of first degree of lower back**

√x7th **T21.55 Corrosion of first degree of buttock**
Corrosion of first degree of anus

√x7th **T21.56 Corrosion of first degree of male genital region** ♂
Corrosion of first degree of penis
Corrosion of first degree of scrotum
Corrosion of first degree of testis

√x7th **T21.57 Corrosion of first degree of female genital region** ♀
Corrosion of first degree of labium (majus) (minus)
Corrosion of first degree of perineum
Corrosion of first degree of vulva
EXCLUDES 2 *corrosion of vagina (T28.8)*

√x7th **T21.59 Corrosion of first degree of other site of trunk**

√5th **T21.6 Corrosion of second degree of trunk**
Code first (T51-T65) to identify chemical and intent
Use additional external cause code to identify place (Y92)

√x7th **T21.6Ø Corrosion of second degree of trunk, unspecified site**

√x7th **T21.61 Corrosion of second degree of chest wall**
Corrosion of second degree of breast

√x7th **T21.62 Corrosion of second degree of abdominal wall**
Corrosion of second degree of flank
Corrosion of second degree of groin

√x7th **T21.63 Corrosion of second degree of upper back**
Corrosion of second degree of interscapular region

√x7th **T21.64 Corrosion of second degree of lower back**

√x7th **T21.65 Corrosion of second degree of buttock**
Corrosion of second degree of anus

√x7th **T21.66 Corrosion of second degree of male genital region** ♂
Corrosion of second degree of penis
Corrosion of second degree of scrotum
Corrosion of second degree of testis

√x7th **T21.67 Corrosion of second degree of female genital region** ♀
Corrosion of second degree of labium (majus) (minus)
Corrosion of second degree of perineum
Corrosion of second degree of vulva
EXCLUDES 2 *corrosion of vagina (T28.8)*

√x7th **T21.69 Corrosion of second degree of other site of trunk**

√5th **T21.7 Corrosion of third degree of trunk**
Code first (T51-T65) to identify chemical and intent
Use additional external cause code to identify place (Y92)

√x7th **T21.7Ø Corrosion of third degree of trunk, unspecified site** CC HS

√x7th **T21.71 Corrosion of third degree of chest wall** CC HS
Corrosion of third degree of breast

√x7th **T21.72 Corrosion of third degree of abdominal wall** CC HS
Corrosion of third degree of flank
Corrosion of third degree of groin

√x7th **T21.73 Corrosion of third degree of upper back** CC HS
Corrosion of third degree of interscapular region

√x7th **T21.74 Corrosion of third degree of lower back** CC HS

√x7th **T21.75 Corrosion of third degree of buttock** CC HS
Corrosion of third degree of anus

√x7th **T21.76 Corrosion of third degree of male genital region** CC HS ♂
Corrosion of third degree of penis
Corrosion of third degree of scrotum
Corrosion of third degree of testis

√x7th **T21.77 Corrosion of third degree of female genital region** CC HS ♀
Corrosion of third degree of labium (majus) (minus)
Corrosion of third degree of perineum
Corrosion of third degree of vulva
EXCLUDES 2 *corrosion of vagina (T28.8)*

√x7th **T21.79 Corrosion of third degree of other site of trunk** CC HS

√4th **T22 Burn and corrosion of shoulder and upper limb, except wrist and hand**
EXCLUDES 2 *burn and corrosion of interscapular region (T21.-)*
burn and corrosion of wrist and hand (T23.-)

The appropriate 7th character is to be added to each code from category T22.
A initial encounter
D subsequent encounter
S sequela

√5th **T22.Ø Burn of unspecified degree of shoulder and upper limb, except wrist and hand**
Use additional external cause code to identify the source, place and intent of the burn (XØØ-X19, X75-X77, X96-X98, Y92)

√x7th **T22.ØØ Burn of unspecified degree of shoulder and upper limb, except wrist and hand, unspecified site**

√6th **T22.Ø1 Burn of unspecified degree of forearm**

√7th **T22.Ø11 Burn of unspecified degree of right forearm**

√7th **T22.Ø12 Burn of unspecified degree of left forearm**

√7th **T22.Ø19 Burn of unspecified degree of unspecified forearm**

√6th **T22.Ø2 Burn of unspecified degree of elbow**

√7th **T22.Ø21 Burn of unspecified degree of right elbow**

√7th **T22.Ø22 Burn of unspecified degree of left elbow**

√7th **T22.Ø29 Burn of unspecified degree of unspecified elbow**

√6th **T22.Ø3 Burn of unspecified degree of upper arm**

√7th **T22.Ø31 Burn of unspecified degree of right upper arm**

√7th **T22.Ø32 Burn of unspecified degree of left upper arm**

√7th **T22.Ø39 Burn of unspecified degree of unspecified upper arm**

√6th **T22.Ø4 Burn of unspecified degree of axilla**

√7th **T22.Ø41 Burn of unspecified degree of right axilla**

√7th **T22.Ø42 Burn of unspecified degree of left axilla**

√7th **T22.Ø49 Burn of unspecified degree of unspecified axilla**

√6th **T22.Ø5 Burn of unspecified degree of shoulder**

√7th **T22.Ø51 Burn of unspecified degree of right shoulder**

√7th **T22.Ø52 Burn of unspecified degree of left shoulder**

√7th **T22.Ø59 Burn of unspecified degree of unspecified shoulder**

√6th T22.06 Burn of unspecified degree of scapular region
√7th T22.061 Burn of unspecified degree of right scapular region
√7th T22.062 Burn of unspecified degree of left scapular region
√7th T22.069 Burn of unspecified degree of unspecified scapular region

√6th T22.09 Burn of unspecified degree of multiple sites of shoulder and upper limb, except wrist and hand
√7th T22.091 Burn of unspecified degree of multiple sites of right shoulder and upper limb, except wrist and hand
√7th T22.092 Burn of unspecified degree of multiple sites of left shoulder and upper limb, except wrist and hand
√7th T22.099 Burn of unspecified degree of multiple sites of unspecified shoulder and upper limb, except wrist and hand

√5th T22.1 Burn of first degree of shoulder and upper limb, except wrist and hand
Use additional external cause code to identify the source, place and intent of the burn (X00-X19, X75-X77, X96-X98, Y92)
√x7th T22.10 Burn of first degree of shoulder and upper limb, except wrist and hand, unspecified site

√6th T22.11 Burn of first degree of forearm
√7th T22.111 Burn of first degree of right forearm
√7th T22.112 Burn of first degree of left forearm
√7th T22.119 Burn of first degree of unspecified forearm

√6th T22.12 Burn of first degree of elbow
√7th T22.121 Burn of first degree of right elbow
√7th T22.122 Burn of first degree of left elbow
√7th T22.129 Burn of first degree of unspecified elbow

√6th T22.13 Burn of first degree of upper arm
√7th T22.131 Burn of first degree of right upper arm
√7th T22.132 Burn of first degree of left upper arm
√7th T22.139 Burn of first degree of unspecified upper arm

√6th T22.14 Burn of first degree of axilla
√7th T22.141 Burn of first degree of right axilla
√7th T22.142 Burn of first degree of left axilla
√7th T22.149 Burn of first degree of unspecified axilla

√6th T22.15 Burn of first degree of shoulder
√7th T22.151 Burn of first degree of right shoulder
√7th T22.152 Burn of first degree of left shoulder
√7th T22.159 Burn of first degree of unspecified shoulder

√6th T22.16 Burn of first degree of scapular region
√7th T22.161 Burn of first degree of right scapular region
√7th T22.162 Burn of first degree of left scapular region
√7th T22.169 Burn of first degree of unspecified scapular region

√6th T22.19 Burn of first degree of multiple sites of shoulder and upper limb, except wrist and hand
√7th T22.191 Burn of first degree of multiple sites of right shoulder and upper limb, except wrist and hand
√7th T22.192 Burn of first degree of multiple sites of left shoulder and upper limb, except wrist and hand
√7th T22.199 Burn of first degree of multiple sites of unspecified shoulder and upper limb, except wrist and hand

√5th T22.2 Burn of second degree of shoulder and upper limb, except wrist and hand
Use additional external cause code to identify the source, place and intent of the burn (X00-X19, X75-X77, X96-X98, Y92)
√x7th T22.20 Burn of second degree of shoulder and upper limb, except wrist and hand, unspecified site

√6th T22.21 Burn of second degree of forearm
√7th T22.211 Burn of second degree of right forearm
√7th T22.212 Burn of second degree of left forearm
√7th T22.219 Burn of second degree of unspecified forearm

√6th T22.22 Burn of second degree of elbow
√7th T22.221 Burn of second degree of right elbow
√7th T22.222 Burn of second degree of left elbow
√7th T22.229 Burn of second degree of unspecified elbow

√6th T22.23 Burn of second degree of upper arm
√7th T22.231 Burn of second degree of right upper arm
√7th T22.232 Burn of second degree of left upper arm
√7th T22.239 Burn of second degree of unspecified upper arm

√6th T22.24 Burn of second degree of axilla
√7th T22.241 Burn of second degree of right axilla
√7th T22.242 Burn of second degree of left axilla
√7th T22.249 Burn of second degree of unspecified axilla

√6th T22.25 Burn of second degree of shoulder
√7th T22.251 Burn of second degree of right shoulder
√7th T22.252 Burn of second degree of left shoulder
√7th T22.259 Burn of second degree of unspecified shoulder

√6th T22.26 Burn of second degree of scapular region
√7th T22.261 Burn of second degree of right scapular region
√7th T22.262 Burn of second degree of left scapular region
√7th T22.269 Burn of second degree of unspecified scapular region

√6th T22.29 Burn of second degree of multiple sites of shoulder and upper limb, except wrist and hand
√7th T22.291 Burn of second degree of multiple sites of right shoulder and upper limb, except wrist and hand
√7th T22.292 Burn of second degree of multiple sites of left shoulder and upper limb, except wrist and hand
√7th T22.299 Burn of second degree of multiple sites of unspecified shoulder and upper limb, except wrist and hand

√5th T22.3 Burn of third degree of shoulder and upper limb, except wrist and hand
Use additional external cause code to identify the source, place and intent of the burn (X00-X19, X75-X77, X96-X98, Y92)
√x7th T22.30 Burn of third degree of shoulder and upper limb, except wrist and hand, unspecified site CC H5 UNS

√6th T22.31 Burn of third degree of forearm
√7th T22.311 Burn of third degree of right forearm CC H5
√7th T22.312 Burn of third degree of left forearm CC H5
√7th T22.319 Burn of third degree of unspecified forearm CC H5 UNS

√6th T22.32 Burn of third degree of elbow
√7th T22.321 Burn of third degree of right elbow CC H5
√7th T22.322 Burn of third degree of left elbow CC H5
√7th T22.329 Burn of third degree of unspecified elbow CC H5 UNS

√6th T22.33 Burn of third degree of upper arm
√7th T22.331 Burn of third degree of right upper arm CC H5
√7th T22.332 Burn of third degree of left upper arm CC H5
√7th T22.339 Burn of third degree of unspecified upper arm CC H5 UNS

√6th T22.34 Burn of third degree of axilla
√7th T22.341 Burn of third degree of right axilla CC H5
√7th T22.342 Burn of third degree of left axilla CC H5
√7th T22.349 Burn of third degree of unspecified axilla CC H5 UNS

√6th T22.35 Burn of third degree of shoulder
√7th T22.351 Burn of third degree of right shoulder CC H5

Chapter 19. Injury, Poisoning and Certain Other Consequences of External Causes

7th T22.352 Burn of third degree of left shoulder CC H5
7th T22.359 Burn of third degree of unspecified shoulder CC H5 UNS
6th T22.36 Burn of third degree of scapular region
7th T22.361 Burn of third degree of right scapular region CC H5
7th T22.362 Burn of third degree of left scapular region CC H5
7th T22.369 Burn of third degree of unspecified scapular region CC H5 UNS
6th T22.39 Burn of third degree of multiple sites of shoulder and upper limb, except wrist and hand
7th T22.391 Burn of third degree of multiple sites of right shoulder and upper limb, except wrist and hand CC H5
7th T22.392 Burn of third degree of multiple sites of left shoulder and upper limb, except wrist and hand CC H5
7th T22.399 Burn of third degree of multiple sites of unspecified shoulder and upper limb, except wrist and hand CC H5

5th T22.4 Corrosion of unspecified degree of shoulder and upper limb, except wrist and hand
Code first (T51-T65) to identify chemical and intent
Use additional external cause code to identify place (Y92)
x7th T22.40 Corrosion of unspecified degree of shoulder and upper limb, except wrist and hand, unspecified site
6th T22.41 Corrosion of unspecified degree of forearm
7th T22.411 Corrosion of unspecified degree of right forearm
7th T22.412 Corrosion of unspecified degree of left forearm
7th T22.419 Corrosion of unspecified degree of unspecified forearm
6th T22.42 Corrosion of unspecified degree of elbow
7th T22.421 Corrosion of unspecified degree of right elbow
7th T22.422 Corrosion of unspecified degree of left elbow
7th T22.429 Corrosion of unspecified degree of unspecified elbow
6th T22.43 Corrosion of unspecified degree of upper arm
7th T22.431 Corrosion of unspecified degree of right upper arm
7th T22.432 Corrosion of unspecified degree of left upper arm
7th T22.439 Corrosion of unspecified degree of unspecified upper arm
6th T22.44 Corrosion of unspecified degree of axilla
7th T22.441 Corrosion of unspecified degree of right axilla
7th T22.442 Corrosion of unspecified degree of left axilla
7th T22.449 Corrosion of unspecified degree of unspecified axilla
6th T22.45 Corrosion of unspecified degree of shoulder
7th T22.451 Corrosion of unspecified degree of right shoulder
7th T22.452 Corrosion of unspecified degree of left shoulder
7th T22.459 Corrosion of unspecified degree of unspecified shoulder
6th T22.46 Corrosion of unspecified degree of scapular region
7th T22.461 Corrosion of unspecified degree of right scapular region
7th T22.462 Corrosion of unspecified degree of left scapular region
7th T22.469 Corrosion of unspecified degree of unspecified scapular region
6th T22.49 Corrosion of unspecified degree of multiple sites of shoulder and upper limb, except wrist and hand
7th T22.491 Corrosion of unspecified degree of multiple sites of right shoulder and upper limb, except wrist and hand
7th T22.492 Corrosion of unspecified degree of multiple sites of left shoulder and upper limb, except wrist and hand
7th T22.499 Corrosion of unspecified degree of multiple sites of unspecified shoulder and upper limb, except wrist and hand

5th T22.5 Corrosion of first degree of shoulder and upper limb, except wrist and hand
Code first (T51-T65) to identify chemical and intent
Use additional external cause code to identify place (Y92)
x7th T22.50 Corrosion of first degree of shoulder and upper limb, except wrist and hand unspecified site
6th T22.51 Corrosion of first degree of forearm
7th T22.511 Corrosion of first degree of right forearm
7th T22.512 Corrosion of first degree of left forearm
7th T22.519 Corrosion of first degree of unspecified forearm
6th T22.52 Corrosion of first degree of elbow
7th T22.521 Corrosion of first degree of right elbow
7th T22.522 Corrosion of first degree of left elbow
7th T22.529 Corrosion of first degree of unspecified elbow
6th T22.53 Corrosion of first degree of upper arm
7th T22.531 Corrosion of first degree of right upper arm
7th T22.532 Corrosion of first degree of left upper arm
7th T22.539 Corrosion of first degree of unspecified upper arm
6th T22.54 Corrosion of first degree of axilla
7th T22.541 Corrosion of first degree of right axilla
7th T22.542 Corrosion of first degree of left axilla
7th T22.549 Corrosion of first degree of unspecified axilla
6th T22.55 Corrosion of first degree of shoulder
7th T22.551 Corrosion of first degree of right shoulder
7th T22.552 Corrosion of first degree of left shoulder
7th T22.559 Corrosion of first degree of unspecified shoulder
6th T22.56 Corrosion of first degree of scapular region
7th T22.561 Corrosion of first degree of right scapular region
7th T22.562 Corrosion of first degree of left scapular region
7th T22.569 Corrosion of first degree of unspecified scapular region
6th T22.59 Corrosion of first degree of multiple sites of shoulder and upper limb, except wrist and hand
7th T22.591 Corrosion of first degree of multiple sites of right shoulder and upper limb, except wrist and hand
7th T22.592 Corrosion of first degree of multiple sites of left shoulder and upper limb, except wrist and hand
7th T22.599 Corrosion of first degree of multiple sites of unspecified shoulder and upper limb, except wrist and hand

5th T22.6 Corrosion of second degree of shoulder and upper limb, except wrist and hand
Code first (T51-T65) to identify chemical and intent
Use additional external cause code to identify place (Y92)
x7th T22.60 Corrosion of second degree of shoulder and upper limb, except wrist and hand, unspecified site
6th T22.61 Corrosion of second degree of forearm
7th T22.611 Corrosion of second degree of right forearm
7th T22.612 Corrosion of second degree of left forearm
7th T22.619 Corrosion of second degree of unspecified forearm
6th T22.62 Corrosion of second degree of elbow
7th T22.621 Corrosion of second degree of right elbow
7th T22.622 Corrosion of second degree of left elbow
7th T22.629 Corrosion of second degree of unspecified elbow
6th T22.63 Corrosion of second degree of upper arm
7th T22.631 Corrosion of second degree of right upper arm
7th T22.632 Corrosion of second degree of left upper arm
7th T22.639 Corrosion of second degree of unspecified upper arm
6th T22.64 Corrosion of second degree of axilla
7th T22.641 Corrosion of second degree of right axilla

T22.642 Corrosion of second degree of left axilla
T22.649 Corrosion of second degree of unspecified axilla
T22.65 Corrosion of second degree of shoulder
T22.651 Corrosion of second degree of right shoulder
T22.652 Corrosion of second degree of left shoulder
T22.659 Corrosion of second degree of unspecified shoulder
T22.66 Corrosion of second degree of scapular region
T22.661 Corrosion of second degree of right scapular region
T22.662 Corrosion of second degree of left scapular region
T22.669 Corrosion of second degree of unspecified scapular region
T22.69 Corrosion of second degree of multiple sites of shoulder and upper limb, except wrist and hand
T22.691 Corrosion of second degree of multiple sites of right shoulder and upper limb, except wrist and hand
T22.692 Corrosion of second degree of multiple sites of left shoulder and upper limb, except wrist and hand
T22.699 Corrosion of second degree of multiple sites of unspecified shoulder and upper limb, except wrist and hand
T22.7 Corrosion of third degree of shoulder and upper limb, except wrist and hand
Code first (T51-T65) to identify chemical and intent
Use additional external cause code to identify place (Y92)
T22.70 Corrosion of third degree of shoulder and upper limb, except wrist and hand, unspecified site CC H5 UNS
T22.71 Corrosion of third degree of forearm
T22.711 Corrosion of third degree of right forearm CC H5
T22.712 Corrosion of third degree of left forearm CC H5
T22.719 Corrosion of third degree of unspecified forearm CC H5 UNS
T22.72 Corrosion of third degree of elbow
T22.721 Corrosion of third degree of right elbow CC H5
T22.722 Corrosion of third degree of left elbow CC H5
T22.729 Corrosion of third degree of unspecified elbow CC H5 UNS
T22.73 Corrosion of third degree of upper arm
T22.731 Corrosion of third degree of right upper arm CC H5
T22.732 Corrosion of third degree of left upper arm CC H5
T22.739 Corrosion of third degree of unspecified upper arm CC H5 UNS
T22.74 Corrosion of third degree of axilla
T22.741 Corrosion of third degree of right axilla CC H5
T22.742 Corrosion of third degree of left axilla CC H5
T22.749 Corrosion of third degree of unspecified axilla CC H5 UNS
T22.75 Corrosion of third degree of shoulder
T22.751 Corrosion of third degree of right shoulder CC H5
T22.752 Corrosion of third degree of left shoulder CC H5
T22.759 Corrosion of third degree of unspecified shoulder CC H5 UNS
T22.76 Corrosion of third degree of scapular region
T22.761 Corrosion of third degree of right scapular region CC H5
T22.762 Corrosion of third degree of left scapular region CC H5
T22.769 Corrosion of third degree of unspecified scapular region CC H5 UNS
T22.79 Corrosion of third degree of multiple sites of shoulder and upper limb, except wrist and hand
T22.791 Corrosion of third degree of multiple sites of right shoulder and upper limb, except wrist and hand CC H5
T22.792 Corrosion of third degree of multiple sites of left shoulder and upper limb, except wrist and hand CC H5
T22.799 Corrosion of third degree of multiple sites of unspecified shoulder and upper limb, except wrist and hand CC H5

T23 Burn and corrosion of wrist and hand

AHA: 2015,1Q,19

The appropriate 7th character is to be added to each code from category T23.
A initial encounter
D subsequent encounter
S sequela

T23.0 Burn of unspecified degree of wrist and hand
Use additional external cause code to identify the source, place and intent of the burn (X00-X19, X75-X77, X96-X98, Y92)
T23.00 Burn of unspecified degree of hand, unspecified site
T23.001 Burn of unspecified degree of right hand, unspecified site
T23.002 Burn of unspecified degree of left hand, unspecified site
T23.009 Burn of unspecified degree of unspecified hand, unspecified site
T23.01 Burn of unspecified degree of thumb (nail)
T23.011 Burn of unspecified degree of right thumb (nail)
T23.012 Burn of unspecified degree of left thumb (nail)
T23.019 Burn of unspecified degree of unspecified thumb (nail)
T23.02 Burn of unspecified degree of single finger (nail) except thumb
T23.021 Burn of unspecified degree of single right finger (nail) except thumb
T23.022 Burn of unspecified degree of single left finger (nail) except thumb
T23.029 Burn of unspecified degree of unspecified single finger (nail) except thumb
T23.03 Burn of unspecified degree of multiple fingers (nail), not including thumb
T23.031 Burn of unspecified degree of multiple right fingers (nail), not including thumb
T23.032 Burn of unspecified degree of multiple left fingers (nail), not including thumb
T23.039 Burn of unspecified degree of unspecified multiple fingers (nail), not including thumb
T23.04 Burn of unspecified degree of multiple fingers (nail), including thumb
T23.041 Burn of unspecified degree of multiple right fingers (nail), including thumb
T23.042 Burn of unspecified degree of multiple left fingers (nail), including thumb
T23.049 Burn of unspecified degree of unspecified multiple fingers (nail), including thumb
T23.05 Burn of unspecified degree of palm
T23.051 Burn of unspecified degree of right palm
T23.052 Burn of unspecified degree of left palm
T23.059 Burn of unspecified degree of unspecified palm
T23.06 Burn of unspecified degree of back of hand
T23.061 Burn of unspecified degree of back of right hand
T23.062 Burn of unspecified degree of back of left hand
T23.069 Burn of unspecified degree of back of unspecified hand
T23.07 Burn of unspecified degree of wrist
T23.071 Burn of unspecified degree of right wrist
T23.072 Burn of unspecified degree of left wrist
T23.079 Burn of unspecified degree of unspecified wrist

6th **T23.09** Burn of unspecified degree of multiple sites of wrist and hand
- 7th **T23.091** Burn of unspecified degree of multiple sites of right wrist and hand
- 7th **T23.092** Burn of unspecified degree of multiple sites of left wrist and hand
- 7th **T23.099** Burn of unspecified degree of multiple sites of unspecified wrist and hand

5th **T23.1** Burn of first degree of wrist and hand

Use additional external cause code to identify the source, place and intent of the burn (X00-X19, X75-X77, X96-X98, Y92)

6th **T23.10** Burn of first degree of hand, unspecified site
- 7th **T23.101** Burn of first degree of right hand, unspecified site
- 7th **T23.102** Burn of first degree of left hand, unspecified site
- 7th **T23.109** Burn of first degree of unspecified hand, unspecified site

6th **T23.11** Burn of first degree of thumb (nail)
- 7th **T23.111** Burn of first degree of right thumb (nail)
- 7th **T23.112** Burn of first degree of left thumb (nail)
- 7th **T23.119** Burn of first degree of unspecified thumb (nail)

6th **T23.12** Burn of first degree of single finger (nail) except thumb
- 7th **T23.121** Burn of first degree of single right finger (nail) except thumb
- 7th **T23.122** Burn of first degree of single left finger (nail) except thumb
- 7th **T23.129** Burn of first degree of unspecified single finger (nail) except thumb

6th **T23.13** Burn of first degree of multiple fingers (nail), not including thumb
- 7th **T23.131** Burn of first degree of multiple right fingers (nail), not including thumb
- 7th **T23.132** Burn of first degree of multiple left fingers (nail), not including thumb
- 7th **T23.139** Burn of first degree of unspecified multiple fingers (nail), not including thumb

6th **T23.14** Burn of first degree of multiple fingers (nail), including thumb
- 7th **T23.141** Burn of first degree of multiple right fingers (nail), including thumb
- 7th **T23.142** Burn of first degree of multiple left fingers (nail), including thumb
- 7th **T23.149** Burn of first degree of unspecified multiple fingers (nail), including thumb

6th **T23.15** Burn of first degree of palm
- 7th **T23.151** Burn of first degree of right palm
- 7th **T23.152** Burn of first degree of left palm
- 7th **T23.159** Burn of first degree of unspecified palm

6th **T23.16** Burn of first degree of back of hand
- 7th **T23.161** Burn of first degree of back of right hand
- 7th **T23.162** Burn of first degree of back of left hand
- 7th **T23.169** Burn of first degree of back of unspecified hand

6th **T23.17** Burn of first degree of wrist
- 7th **T23.171** Burn of first degree of right wrist
- 7th **T23.172** Burn of first degree of left wrist
- 7th **T23.179** Burn of first degree of unspecified wrist

6th **T23.19** Burn of first degree of multiple sites of wrist and hand
- 7th **T23.191** Burn of first degree of multiple sites of right wrist and hand
- 7th **T23.192** Burn of first degree of multiple sites of left wrist and hand
- 7th **T23.199** Burn of first degree of multiple sites of unspecified wrist and hand

5th **T23.2** Burn of second degree of wrist and hand

Use additional external cause code to identify the source, place and intent of the burn (X00-X19, X75-X77, X96-X98, Y92)

6th **T23.20** Burn of second degree of hand, unspecified site
- 7th **T23.201** Burn of second degree of right hand, unspecified site
- 7th **T23.202** Burn of second degree of left hand, unspecified site
- 7th **T23.209** Burn of second degree of unspecified hand, unspecified site

6th **T23.21** Burn of second degree of thumb (nail)
- 7th **T23.211** Burn of second degree of right thumb (nail)
- 7th **T23.212** Burn of second degree of left thumb (nail)
- 7th **T23.219** Burn of second degree of unspecified thumb (nail)

6th **T23.22** Burn of second degree of single finger (nail) except thumb
- 7th **T23.221** Burn of second degree of single right finger (nail) except thumb
- 7th **T23.222** Burn of second degree of single left finger (nail) except thumb
- 7th **T23.229** Burn of second degree of unspecified single finger (nail) except thumb

6th **T23.23** Burn of second degree of multiple fingers (nail), not including thumb
- 7th **T23.231** Burn of second degree of multiple right fingers (nail), not including thumb
- 7th **T23.232** Burn of second degree of multiple left fingers (nail), not including thumb
- 7th **T23.239** Burn of second degree of unspecified multiple fingers (nail), not including thumb

6th **T23.24** Burn of second degree of multiple fingers (nail), including thumb
- 7th **T23.241** Burn of second degree of multiple right fingers (nail), including thumb
- 7th **T23.242** Burn of second degree of multiple left fingers (nail), including thumb
- 7th **T23.249** Burn of second degree of unspecified multiple fingers (nail), including thumb

6th **T23.25** Burn of second degree of palm
- 7th **T23.251** Burn of second degree of right palm
- 7th **T23.252** Burn of second degree of left palm
- 7th **T23.259** Burn of second degree of unspecified palm

6th **T23.26** Burn of second degree of back of hand
- 7th **T23.261** Burn of second degree of back of right hand
- 7th **T23.262** Burn of second degree of back of left hand
- 7th **T23.269** Burn of second degree of back of unspecified hand

6th **T23.27** Burn of second degree of wrist
- 7th **T23.271** Burn of second degree of right wrist
- 7th **T23.272** Burn of second degree of left wrist
- 7th **T23.279** Burn of second degree of unspecified wrist

6th **T23.29** Burn of second degree of multiple sites of wrist and hand
- 7th **T23.291** Burn of second degree of multiple sites of right wrist and hand
- 7th **T23.292** Burn of second degree of multiple sites of left wrist and hand
- 7th **T23.299** Burn of second degree of multiple sites of unspecified wrist and hand

5th **T23.3** Burn of third degree of wrist and hand

Use additional external cause code to identify the source, place and intent of the burn (X00-X19, X75-X77, X96-X98, Y92)

6th **T23.30** Burn of third degree of hand, unspecified site

AHA: 2016,2Q,5

- 7th **T23.301** Burn of third degree of right hand, unspecified site CC H5
- 7th **T23.302** Burn of third degree of left hand, unspecified site CC H5
- 7th **T23.309** Burn of third degree of unspecified hand, unspecified site CC H5 UNS

6th **T23.31** Burn of third degree of thumb (nail)
- 7th **T23.311** Burn of third degree of right thumb (nail) CC H5
- 7th **T23.312** Burn of third degree of left thumb (nail) CC H5
- 7th **T23.319** Burn of third degree of unspecified thumb (nail) CC H5 UNS

T23.32 Burn of third degree of single finger (nail) except thumb
T23.321 Burn of third degree of single right finger (nail) except thumb CC H5
T23.322 Burn of third degree of single left finger (nail) except thumb CC H5
T23.329 Burn of third degree of unspecified single finger (nail) except thumb CC H5 UNS
T23.33 Burn of third degree of multiple fingers (nail), not including thumb
T23.331 Burn of third degree of multiple right fingers (nail), not including thumb CC H5
T23.332 Burn of third degree of multiple left fingers (nail), not including thumb CC H5
T23.339 Burn of third degree of unspecified multiple fingers (nail), not including thumb CC H5 UNS
T23.34 Burn of third degree of multiple fingers (nail), including thumb
T23.341 Burn of third degree of multiple right fingers (nail), including thumb CC H5
T23.342 Burn of third degree of multiple left fingers (nail), including thumb CC H5
T23.349 Burn of third degree of unspecified multiple fingers (nail), including thumb CC H5 UNS
T23.35 Burn of third degree of palm
T23.351 Burn of third degree of right palm CC H5
T23.352 Burn of third degree of left palm CC H5
T23.359 Burn of third degree of unspecified palm CC H5 UNS
T23.36 Burn of third degree of back of hand
T23.361 Burn of third degree of back of right hand CC H5
T23.362 Burn of third degree of back of left hand CC H5
T23.369 Burn of third degree of back of unspecified hand CC H5 UNS
T23.37 Burn of third degree of wrist
T23.371 Burn of third degree of right wrist CC H5
T23.372 Burn of third degree of left wrist CC H5
T23.379 Burn of third degree of unspecified wrist CC H5 UNS
T23.39 Burn of third degree of multiple sites of wrist and hand
T23.391 Burn of third degree of multiple sites of right wrist and hand CC H5
T23.392 Burn of third degree of multiple sites of left wrist and hand CC H5
T23.399 Burn of third degree of multiple sites of unspecified wrist and hand CC H5 UNS
T23.4 Corrosion of unspecified degree of wrist and hand
Code first (T51-T65) to identify chemical and intent
Use additional external cause code to identify place (Y92)
T23.40 Corrosion of unspecified degree of hand, unspecified site
T23.401 Corrosion of unspecified degree of right hand, unspecified site
T23.402 Corrosion of unspecified degree of left hand, unspecified site
T23.409 Corrosion of unspecified degree of unspecified hand, unspecified site
T23.41 Corrosion of unspecified degree of thumb (nail)
T23.411 Corrosion of unspecified degree of right thumb (nail)
T23.412 Corrosion of unspecified degree of left thumb (nail)
T23.419 Corrosion of unspecified degree of unspecified thumb (nail)
T23.42 Corrosion of unspecified degree of single finger (nail) except thumb
T23.421 Corrosion of unspecified degree of single right finger (nail) except thumb
T23.422 Corrosion of unspecified degree of single left finger (nail) except thumb
T23.429 Corrosion of unspecified degree of unspecified single finger (nail) except thumb
T23.43 Corrosion of unspecified degree of multiple fingers (nail), not including thumb
T23.431 Corrosion of unspecified degree of multiple right fingers (nail), not including thumb
T23.432 Corrosion of unspecified degree of multiple left fingers (nail), not including thumb
T23.439 Corrosion of unspecified degree of unspecified multiple fingers (nail), not including thumb
T23.44 Corrosion of unspecified degree of multiple fingers (nail), including thumb
T23.441 Corrosion of unspecified degree of multiple right fingers (nail), including thumb
T23.442 Corrosion of unspecified degree of multiple left fingers (nail), including thumb
T23.449 Corrosion of unspecified degree of unspecified multiple fingers (nail), including thumb
T23.45 Corrosion of unspecified degree of palm
T23.451 Corrosion of unspecified degree of right palm
T23.452 Corrosion of unspecified degree of left palm
T23.459 Corrosion of unspecified degree of unspecified palm
T23.46 Corrosion of unspecified degree of back of hand
T23.461 Corrosion of unspecified degree of back of right hand
T23.462 Corrosion of unspecified degree of back of left hand
T23.469 Corrosion of unspecified degree of back of unspecified hand
T23.47 Corrosion of unspecified degree of wrist
T23.471 Corrosion of unspecified degree of right wrist
T23.472 Corrosion of unspecified degree of left wrist
T23.479 Corrosion of unspecified degree of unspecified wrist
T23.49 Corrosion of unspecified degree of multiple sites of wrist and hand
T23.491 Corrosion of unspecified degree of multiple sites of right wrist and hand
T23.492 Corrosion of unspecified degree of multiple sites of left wrist and hand
T23.499 Corrosion of unspecified degree of multiple sites of unspecified wrist and hand
T23.5 Corrosion of first degree of wrist and hand
Code first (T51-T65) to identify chemical and intent
Use additional external cause code to identify place (Y92)
T23.50 Corrosion of first degree of hand, unspecified site
T23.501 Corrosion of first degree of right hand, unspecified site
T23.502 Corrosion of first degree of left hand, unspecified site
T23.509 Corrosion of first degree of unspecified hand, unspecified site
T23.51 Corrosion of first degree of thumb (nail)
T23.511 Corrosion of first degree of right thumb (nail)
T23.512 Corrosion of first degree of left thumb (nail)
T23.519 Corrosion of first degree of unspecified thumb (nail)
T23.52 Corrosion of first degree of single finger (nail) except thumb
T23.521 Corrosion of first degree of single right finger (nail) except thumb
T23.522 Corrosion of first degree of single left finger (nail) except thumb
T23.529 Corrosion of first degree of unspecified single finger (nail) except thumb

6th T23.53 Corrosion of first degree of multiple fingers (nail), not including thumb
7th T23.531 Corrosion of first degree of multiple right fingers (nail), not including thumb
7th T23.532 Corrosion of first degree of multiple left fingers (nail), not including thumb
7th T23.539 Corrosion of first degree of unspecified multiple fingers (nail), not including thumb
6th T23.54 Corrosion of first degree of multiple fingers (nail), including thumb
7th T23.541 Corrosion of first degree of multiple right fingers (nail), including thumb
7th T23.542 Corrosion of first degree of multiple left fingers (nail), including thumb
7th T23.549 Corrosion of first degree of unspecified multiple fingers (nail), including thumb
6th T23.55 Corrosion of first degree of palm
7th T23.551 Corrosion of first degree of right palm
7th T23.552 Corrosion of first degree of left palm
7th T23.559 Corrosion of first degree of unspecified palm
6th T23.56 Corrosion of first degree of back of hand
7th T23.561 Corrosion of first degree of back of right hand
7th T23.562 Corrosion of first degree of back of left hand
7th T23.569 Corrosion of first degree of back of unspecified hand
6th T23.57 Corrosion of first degree of wrist
7th T23.571 Corrosion of first degree of right wrist
7th T23.572 Corrosion of first degree of left wrist
7th T23.579 Corrosion of first degree of unspecified wrist
6th T23.59 Corrosion of first degree of multiple sites of wrist and hand
7th T23.591 Corrosion of first degree of multiple sites of right wrist and hand
7th T23.592 Corrosion of first degree of multiple sites of left wrist and hand
7th T23.599 Corrosion of first degree of multiple sites of unspecified wrist and hand
5th T23.6 Corrosion of second degree of wrist and hand
Code first (T51-T65) to identify chemical and intent
Use additional external cause code to identify place (Y92)
6th T23.60 Corrosion of second degree of hand, unspecified site
7th T23.601 Corrosion of second degree of right hand, unspecified site
7th T23.602 Corrosion of second degree of left hand, unspecified site
7th T23.609 Corrosion of second degree of unspecified hand, unspecified site
6th T23.61 Corrosion of second degree of thumb (nail)
7th T23.611 Corrosion of second degree of right thumb (nail)
7th T23.612 Corrosion of second degree of left thumb (nail)
7th T23.619 Corrosion of second degree of unspecified thumb (nail)
6th T23.62 Corrosion of second degree of single finger (nail) except thumb
7th T23.621 Corrosion of second degree of single right finger (nail) except thumb
7th T23.622 Corrosion of second degree of single left finger (nail) except thumb
7th T23.629 Corrosion of second degree of unspecified single finger (nail) except thumb
6th T23.63 Corrosion of second degree of multiple fingers (nail), not including thumb
7th T23.631 Corrosion of second degree of multiple right fingers (nail), not including thumb
7th T23.632 Corrosion of second degree of multiple left fingers (nail), not including thumb
7th T23.639 Corrosion of second degree of unspecified multiple fingers (nail), not including thumb
6th T23.64 Corrosion of second degree of multiple fingers (nail), including thumb
7th T23.641 Corrosion of second degree of multiple right fingers (nail), including thumb
7th T23.642 Corrosion of second degree of multiple left fingers (nail), including thumb
7th T23.649 Corrosion of second degree of unspecified multiple fingers (nail), including thumb
6th T23.65 Corrosion of second degree of palm
7th T23.651 Corrosion of second degree of right palm
7th T23.652 Corrosion of second degree of left palm
7th T23.659 Corrosion of second degree of unspecified palm
6th T23.66 Corrosion of second degree of back of hand
7th T23.661 Corrosion of second degree back of right hand
7th T23.662 Corrosion of second degree back of left hand
7th T23.669 Corrosion of second degree back of unspecified hand
6th T23.67 Corrosion of second degree of wrist
7th T23.671 Corrosion of second degree of right wrist
7th T23.672 Corrosion of second degree of left wrist
7th T23.679 Corrosion of second degree of unspecified wrist
6th T23.69 Corrosion of second degree of multiple sites of wrist and hand
7th T23.691 Corrosion of second degree of multiple sites of right wrist and hand
7th T23.692 Corrosion of second degree of multiple sites of left wrist and hand
7th T23.699 Corrosion of second degree of multiple sites of unspecified wrist and hand
5th T23.7 Corrosion of third degree of wrist and hand
Code first (T51-T65) to identify chemical and intent
Use additional external cause code to identify place (Y92)
6th T23.70 Corrosion of third degree of hand, unspecified site
7th T23.701 Corrosion of third degree of right hand, unspecified site CC HS
7th T23.702 Corrosion of third degree of left hand, unspecified site CC HS
7th T23.709 Corrosion of third degree of unspecified hand, unspecified site CC HS UNS
6th T23.71 Corrosion of third degree of thumb (nail)
7th T23.711 Corrosion of third degree of right thumb (nail) CC HS
7th T23.712 Corrosion of third degree of left thumb (nail) CC HS
7th T23.719 Corrosion of third degree of unspecified thumb (nail) CC HS UNS
6th T23.72 Corrosion of third degree of single finger (nail) except thumb
7th T23.721 Corrosion of third degree of single right finger (nail) except thumb CC HS
7th T23.722 Corrosion of third degree of single left finger (nail) except thumb CC HS
7th T23.729 Corrosion of third degree of unspecified single finger (nail) except thumb CC HS UNS
6th T23.73 Corrosion of third degree of multiple fingers (nail), not including thumb
7th T23.731 Corrosion of third degree of multiple right fingers (nail), not including thumb CC HS
7th T23.732 Corrosion of third degree of multiple left fingers (nail), not including thumb CC HS
7th T23.739 Corrosion of third degree of unspecified multiple fingers (nail), not including thumb CC HS UNS
6th T23.74 Corrosion of third degree of multiple fingers (nail), including thumb
7th T23.741 Corrosion of third degree of multiple right fingers (nail), including thumb CC HS
7th T23.742 Corrosion of third degree of multiple left fingers (nail), including thumb CC HS
7th T23.749 Corrosion of third degree of unspecified multiple fingers (nail), including thumb CC HS UNS
6th T23.75 Corrosion of third degree of palm
7th T23.751 Corrosion of third degree of right palm CC HS

T23.752 Corrosion of third degree of left palm CC H5

T23.759 Corrosion of third degree of unspecified palm CC H5 UNS

T23.76 Corrosion of third degree of back of hand

T23.761 Corrosion of third degree of back of right hand CC H5

T23.762 Corrosion of third degree of back of left hand CC H5

T23.769 Corrosion of third degree back of unspecified hand CC H5 UNS

T23.77 Corrosion of third degree of wrist

T23.771 Corrosion of third degree of right wrist CC H5

T23.772 Corrosion of third degree of left wrist CC H5

T23.779 Corrosion of third degree of unspecified wrist CC H5 UNS

T23.79 Corrosion of third degree of multiple sites of wrist and hand

T23.791 Corrosion of third degree of multiple sites of right wrist and hand CC H5

T23.792 Corrosion of third degree of multiple sites of left wrist and hand CC H5

T23.799 Corrosion of third degree of multiple sites of unspecified wrist and hand CC H5 UNS

T24 Burn and corrosion of lower limb, except ankle and foot

EXCLUDES 2 *burn and corrosion of ankle and foot (T25.-)*

burn and corrosion of hip region (T21.-)

The appropriate 7th character is to be added to each code from category T24.
A initial encounter
D subsequent encounter
S sequela

T24.Ø Burn of unspecified degree of lower limb, except ankle and foot

Use additional external cause code to identify the source, place and intent of the burn (XØØ-X19, X75-X77, X96-X98, Y92)

T24.ØØ Burn of unspecified degree of unspecified site of lower limb, except ankle and foot

T24.ØØ1 Burn of unspecified degree of unspecified site of right lower limb, except ankle and foot

T24.ØØ2 Burn of unspecified degree of unspecified site of left lower limb, except ankle and foot

T24.ØØ9 Burn of unspecified degree of unspecified site of unspecified lower limb, except ankle and foot

T24.Ø1 Burn of unspecified degree of thigh

T24.Ø11 Burn of unspecified degree of right thigh

T24.Ø12 Burn of unspecified degree of left thigh

T24.Ø19 Burn of unspecified degree of unspecified thigh

T24.Ø2 Burn of unspecified degree of knee

T24.Ø21 Burn of unspecified degree of right knee

T24.Ø22 Burn of unspecified degree of left knee

T24.Ø29 Burn of unspecified degree of unspecified knee

T24.Ø3 Burn of unspecified degree of lower leg

T24.Ø31 Burn of unspecified degree of right lower leg

T24.Ø32 Burn of unspecified degree of left lower leg

T24.Ø39 Burn of unspecified degree of unspecified lower leg

T24.Ø9 Burn of unspecified degree of multiple sites of lower limb, except ankle and foot

T24.Ø91 Burn of unspecified degree of multiple sites of right lower limb, except ankle and foot

T24.Ø92 Burn of unspecified degree of multiple sites of left lower limb, except ankle and foot

T24.Ø99 Burn of unspecified degree of multiple sites of unspecified lower limb, except ankle and foot

T24.1 Burn of first degree of lower limb, except ankle and foot

Use additional external cause code to identify the source, place and intent of the burn (XØØ-X19, X75-X77, X96-X98, Y92)

T24.1Ø Burn of first degree of unspecified site of lower limb, except ankle and foot

T24.1Ø1 Burn of first degree of unspecified site of right lower limb, except ankle and foot

T24.1Ø2 Burn of first degree of unspecified site of left lower limb, except ankle and foot

T24.1Ø9 Burn of first degree of unspecified site of unspecified lower limb, except ankle and foot

T24.11 Burn of first degree of thigh

T24.111 Burn of first degree of right thigh

T24.112 Burn of first degree of left thigh

T24.119 Burn of first degree of unspecified thigh

T24.12 Burn of first degree of knee

T24.121 Burn of first degree of right knee

T24.122 Burn of first degree of left knee

T24.129 Burn of first degree of unspecified knee

T24.13 Burn of first degree of lower leg

T24.131 Burn of first degree of right lower leg

T24.132 Burn of first degree of left lower leg

T24.139 Burn of first degree of unspecified lower leg

T24.19 Burn of first degree of multiple sites of lower limb, except ankle and foot

T24.191 Burn of first degree of multiple sites of right lower limb, except ankle and foot

T24.192 Burn of first degree of multiple sites of left lower limb, except ankle and foot

T24.199 Burn of first degree of multiple sites of unspecified lower limb, except ankle and foot

T24.2 Burn of second degree of lower limb, except ankle and foot

Use additional external cause code to identify the source, place and intent of the burn (XØØ-X19, X75-X77, X96-X98, Y92)

T24.2Ø Burn of second degree of unspecified site of lower limb, except ankle and foot

T24.2Ø1 Burn of second degree of unspecified site of right lower limb, except ankle and foot

T24.2Ø2 Burn of second degree of unspecified site of left lower limb, except ankle and foot

T24.2Ø9 Burn of second degree of unspecified site of unspecified lower limb, except ankle and foot

T24.21 Burn of second degree of thigh

T24.211 Burn of second degree of right thigh

T24.212 Burn of second degree of left thigh

T24.219 Burn of second degree of unspecified thigh

T24.22 Burn of second degree of knee

T24.221 Burn of second degree of right knee

T24.222 Burn of second degree of left knee

T24.229 Burn of second degree of unspecified knee

T24.23 Burn of second degree of lower leg

T24.231 Burn of second degree of right lower leg

T24.232 Burn of second degree of left lower leg

T24.239 Burn of second degree of unspecified lower leg

T24.29 Burn of second degree of multiple sites of lower limb, except ankle and foot

T24.291 Burn of second degree of multiple sites of right lower limb, except ankle and foot

T24.292 Burn of second degree of multiple sites of left lower limb, except ankle and foot

T24.299 Burn of second degree of multiple sites of unspecified lower limb, except ankle and foot

5th **T24.3 Burn of third degree of lower limb, except ankle and foot**
Use additional external cause code to identify the source, place and intent of the burn (X00-X19, X75-X77, X96-X98, Y92)

6th **T24.30 Burn of third degree of unspecified site of lower limb, except ankle and foot**
7th **T24.301 Burn of third degree of unspecified site of right lower limb, except ankle and foot** CC HS
7th **T24.302 Burn of third degree of unspecified site of left lower limb, except ankle and foot** CC HS
7th **T24.309 Burn of third degree of unspecified site of unspecified lower limb, except ankle and foot** CC HS UNS

6th **T24.31 Burn of third degree of thigh**
7th **T24.311 Burn of third degree of right thigh** CC HS
7th **T24.312 Burn of third degree of left thigh** CC HS
7th **T24.319 Burn of third degree of unspecified thigh** CC HS UNS

6th **T24.32 Burn of third degree of knee**
7th **T24.321 Burn of third degree of right knee** CC HS
7th **T24.322 Burn of third degree of left knee** CC HS
7th **T24.329 Burn of third degree of unspecified knee** CC HS UNS

6th **T24.33 Burn of third degree of lower leg**
7th **T24.331 Burn of third degree of right lower leg** CC HS
7th **T24.332 Burn of third degree of left lower leg** CC HS
7th **T24.339 Burn of third degree of unspecified lower leg** CC HS UNS

6th **T24.39 Burn of third degree of multiple sites of lower limb, except ankle and foot**
AHA: 2016,2Q,4
7th **T24.391 Burn of third degree of multiple sites of right lower limb, except ankle and foot** CC HS
7th **T24.392 Burn of third degree of multiple sites of left lower limb, except ankle and foot** CC HS
7th **T24.399 Burn of third degree of multiple sites of unspecified lower limb, except ankle and foot** CC HS UNS

5th **T24.4 Corrosion of unspecified degree of lower limb, except ankle and foot**
Code first (T51-T65) to identify chemical and intent
Use additional external cause code to identify place (Y92)

6th **T24.40 Corrosion of unspecified degree of unspecified site of lower limb, except ankle and foot**
7th **T24.401 Corrosion of unspecified degree of unspecified site of right lower limb, except ankle and foot**
7th **T24.402 Corrosion of unspecified degree of unspecified site of left lower limb, except ankle and foot**
7th **T24.409 Corrosion of unspecified degree of unspecified site of unspecified lower limb, except ankle and foot**

6th **T24.41 Corrosion of unspecified degree of thigh**
7th **T24.411 Corrosion of unspecified degree of right thigh**
7th **T24.412 Corrosion of unspecified degree of left thigh**
7th **T24.419 Corrosion of unspecified degree of unspecified thigh**

6th **T24.42 Corrosion of unspecified degree of knee**
7th **T24.421 Corrosion of unspecified degree of right knee**
7th **T24.422 Corrosion of unspecified degree of left knee**
7th **T24.429 Corrosion of unspecified degree of unspecified knee**

6th **T24.43 Corrosion of unspecified degree of lower leg**
7th **T24.431 Corrosion of unspecified degree of right lower leg**
7th **T24.432 Corrosion of unspecified degree of left lower leg**
7th **T24.439 Corrosion of unspecified degree of unspecified lower leg**

6th **T24.49 Corrosion of unspecified degree of multiple sites of lower limb, except ankle and foot**
7th **T24.491 Corrosion of unspecified degree of multiple sites of right lower limb, except ankle and foot**
7th **T24.492 Corrosion of unspecified degree of multiple sites of left lower limb, except ankle and foot**
7th **T24.499 Corrosion of unspecified degree of multiple sites of unspecified lower limb, except ankle and foot**

5th **T24.5 Corrosion of first degree of lower limb, except ankle and foot**
Code first (T51-T65) to identify chemical and intent
Use additional external cause code to identify place (Y92)

6th **T24.50 Corrosion of first degree of unspecified site of lower limb, except ankle and foot**
7th **T24.501 Corrosion of first degree of unspecified site of right lower limb, except ankle and foot**
7th **T24.502 Corrosion of first degree of unspecified site of left lower limb, except ankle and foot**
7th **T24.509 Corrosion of first degree of unspecified site of unspecified lower limb, except ankle and foot**

6th **T24.51 Corrosion of first degree of thigh**
7th **T24.511 Corrosion of first degree of right thigh**
7th **T24.512 Corrosion of first degree of left thigh**
7th **T24.519 Corrosion of first degree of unspecified thigh**

6th **T24.52 Corrosion of first degree of knee**
7th **T24.521 Corrosion of first degree of right knee**
7th **T24.522 Corrosion of first degree of left knee**
7th **T24.529 Corrosion of first degree of unspecified knee**

6th **T24.53 Corrosion of first degree of lower leg**
7th **T24.531 Corrosion of first degree of right lower leg**
7th **T24.532 Corrosion of first degree of left lower leg**
7th **T24.539 Corrosion of first degree of unspecified lower leg**

6th **T24.59 Corrosion of first degree of multiple sites of lower limb, except ankle and foot**
7th **T24.591 Corrosion of first degree of multiple sites of right lower limb, except ankle and foot**
7th **T24.592 Corrosion of first degree of multiple sites of left lower limb, except ankle and foot**
7th **T24.599 Corrosion of first degree of multiple sites of unspecified lower limb, except ankle and foot**

5th **T24.6 Corrosion of second degree of lower limb, except ankle and foot**
Code first (T51-T65) to identify chemical and intent
Use additional external cause code to identify place (Y92)

6th **T24.60 Corrosion of second degree of unspecified site of lower limb, except ankle and foot**
7th **T24.601 Corrosion of second degree of unspecified site of right lower limb, except ankle and foot**
7th **T24.602 Corrosion of second degree of unspecified site of left lower limb, except ankle and foot**
7th **T24.609 Corrosion of second degree of unspecified site of unspecified lower limb, except ankle and foot**

6th **T24.61 Corrosion of second degree of thigh**
7th **T24.611 Corrosion of second degree of right thigh**
7th **T24.612 Corrosion of second degree of left thigh**
7th **T24.619 Corrosion of second degree of unspecified thigh**

6th **T24.62 Corrosion of second degree of knee**
7th **T24.621 Corrosion of second degree of right knee**
7th **T24.622 Corrosion of second degree of left knee**
7th **T24.629 Corrosion of second degree of unspecified knee**

T24.63 Corrosion of second degree of lower leg
T24.631 Corrosion of second degree of right lower leg
T24.632 Corrosion of second degree of left lower leg
T24.639 Corrosion of second degree of unspecified lower leg
T24.69 Corrosion of second degree of multiple sites of lower limb, except ankle and foot
T24.691 Corrosion of second degree of multiple sites of right lower limb, except ankle and foot
T24.692 Corrosion of second degree of multiple sites of left lower limb, except ankle and foot
T24.699 Corrosion of second degree of multiple sites of unspecified lower limb, except ankle and foot
T24.7 Corrosion of third degree of lower limb, except ankle and foot
Code first (T51-T65) to identify chemical and intent
Use additional external cause code to identify place (Y92)
T24.70 Corrosion of third degree of unspecified site of lower limb, except ankle and foot
T24.701 Corrosion of third degree of unspecified site of right lower limb, except ankle and foot CC H5
T24.702 Corrosion of third degree of unspecified site of left lower limb, except ankle and foot CC H5
T24.709 Corrosion of third degree of unspecified site of unspecified lower limb, except ankle and foot CC H5 UNS
T24.71 Corrosion of third degree of thigh
T24.711 Corrosion of third degree of right thigh CC H5
T24.712 Corrosion of third degree of left thigh CC H5
T24.719 Corrosion of third degree of unspecified thigh CC H5 UNS
T24.72 Corrosion of third degree of knee
T24.721 Corrosion of third degree of right knee CC H5
T24.722 Corrosion of third degree of left knee CC H5
T24.729 Corrosion of third degree of unspecified knee CC H5 UNS
T24.73 Corrosion of third degree of lower leg
T24.731 Corrosion of third degree of right lower leg CC H5
T24.732 Corrosion of third degree of left lower leg CC H5
T24.739 Corrosion of third degree of unspecified lower leg CC H5 UNS
T24.79 Corrosion of third degree of multiple sites of lower limb, except ankle and foot
T24.791 Corrosion of third degree of multiple sites of right lower limb, except ankle and foot CC H5
T24.792 Corrosion of third degree of multiple sites of left lower limb, except ankle and foot CC H5
T24.799 Corrosion of third degree of multiple sites of unspecified lower limb, except ankle and foot CC H5 UNS

T25 Burn and corrosion of ankle and foot

The appropriate 7th character is to be added to each code from category T25.
A initial encounter
D subsequent encounter
S sequela

T25.0 Burn of unspecified degree of ankle and foot
Use additional external cause code to identify the source, place and intent of the burn (X00-X19, X75-X77, X96-X98, Y92)
T25.01 Burn of unspecified degree of ankle
T25.011 Burn of unspecified degree of right ankle
T25.012 Burn of unspecified degree of left ankle
T25.019 Burn of unspecified degree of unspecified ankle
T25.02 Burn of unspecified degree of foot
EXCLUDES 2 *burn of unspecified degree of toe(s) (nail) (T25.03-)*
T25.021 Burn of unspecified degree of right foot
T25.022 Burn of unspecified degree of left foot
T25.029 Burn of unspecified degree of unspecified foot
T25.03 Burn of unspecified degree of toe(s) (nail)
T25.031 Burn of unspecified degree of right toe(s) (nail)
T25.032 Burn of unspecified degree of left toe(s) (nail)
T25.039 Burn of unspecified degree of unspecified toe(s) (nail)
T25.09 Burn of unspecified degree of multiple sites of ankle and foot
T25.091 Burn of unspecified degree of multiple sites of right ankle and foot
T25.092 Burn of unspecified degree of multiple sites of left ankle and foot
T25.099 Burn of unspecified degree of multiple sites of unspecified ankle and foot
T25.1 Burn of first degree of ankle and foot
Use additional external cause code to identify the source, place and intent of the burn (X00-X19, X75-X77, X96-X98, Y92)
T25.11 Burn of first degree of ankle
T25.111 Burn of first degree of right ankle
T25.112 Burn of first degree of left ankle
T25.119 Burn of first degree of unspecified ankle
T25.12 Burn of first degree of foot
EXCLUDES 2 *burn of first degree of toe(s) (nail) (T25.13-)*
T25.121 Burn of first degree of right foot
T25.122 Burn of first degree of left foot
T25.129 Burn of first degree of unspecified foot
T25.13 Burn of first degree of toe(s) (nail)
T25.131 Burn of first degree of right toe(s) (nail)
T25.132 Burn of first degree of left toe(s) (nail)
T25.139 Burn of first degree of unspecified toe(s) (nail)
T25.19 Burn of first degree of multiple sites of ankle and foot
T25.191 Burn of first degree of multiple sites of right ankle and foot
T25.192 Burn of first degree of multiple sites of left ankle and foot
T25.199 Burn of first degree of multiple sites of unspecified ankle and foot
T25.2 Burn of second degree of ankle and foot
Use additional external cause code to identify the source, place and intent of the burn (X00-X19, X75-X77, X96-X98, Y92)
T25.21 Burn of second degree of ankle
T25.211 Burn of second degree of right ankle
T25.212 Burn of second degree of left ankle
T25.219 Burn of second degree of unspecified ankle
T25.22 Burn of second degree of foot
EXCLUDES 2 *burn of second degree of toe(s) (nail) (T25.23-)*
T25.221 Burn of second degree of right foot
T25.222 Burn of second degree of left foot
T25.229 Burn of second degree of unspecified foot
T25.23 Burn of second degree of toe(s) (nail)
T25.231 Burn of second degree of right toe(s) (nail)
T25.232 Burn of second degree of left toe(s) (nail)
T25.239 Burn of second degree of unspecified toe(s) (nail)
T25.29 Burn of second degree of multiple sites of ankle and foot
T25.291 Burn of second degree of multiple sites of right ankle and foot
T25.292 Burn of second degree of multiple sites of left ankle and foot
T25.299 Burn of second degree of multiple sites of unspecified ankle and foot

Chapter 19. Injury, Poisoning and Certain Other Consequences of External Causes
T24.63–T25.299

T25.3 Burn of third degree of ankle and foot
Use additional external cause code to identify the source, place and intent of the burn (X00-X19, X75-X77, X96-X98, Y92)
- **T25.31** Burn of third degree of ankle
  - **T25.311** Burn of third degree of right ankle CC HS
  - **T25.312** Burn of third degree of left ankle CC HS
  - **T25.319** Burn of third degree of unspecified ankle CC HS UNS
- **T25.32** Burn of third degree of foot
  EXCLUDES 2 *burn of third degree of toe(s) (nail) (T25.33-)*
  - **T25.321** Burn of third degree of right foot CC HS
  - **T25.322** Burn of third degree of left foot CC HS
  - **T25.329** Burn of third degree of unspecified foot CC HS UNS
- **T25.33** Burn of third degree of toe(s) (nail)
  - **T25.331** Burn of third degree of right toe(s) (nail) CC HS
  - **T25.332** Burn of third degree of left toe(s) (nail) CC HS
  - **T25.339** Burn of third degree of unspecified toe(s) (nail) CC HS UNS
- **T25.39** Burn of third degree of multiple sites of ankle and foot
  - **T25.391** Burn of third degree of multiple sites of right ankle and foot CC HS
  - **T25.392** Burn of third degree of multiple sites of left ankle and foot CC HS
  - **T25.399** Burn of third degree of multiple sites of unspecified ankle and foot CC HS UNS

T25.4 Corrosion of unspecified degree of ankle and foot
Code first (T51-T65) to identify chemical and intent
Use additional external cause code to identify place (Y92)
- **T25.41** Corrosion of unspecified degree of ankle
  - **T25.411** Corrosion of unspecified degree of right ankle
  - **T25.412** Corrosion of unspecified degree of left ankle
  - **T25.419** Corrosion of unspecified degree of unspecified ankle
- **T25.42** Corrosion of unspecified degree of foot
  EXCLUDES 2 *corrosion of unspecified degree of toe(s) (nail) (T25.43-)*
  - **T25.421** Corrosion of unspecified degree of right foot
  - **T25.422** Corrosion of unspecified degree of left foot
  - **T25.429** Corrosion of unspecified degree of unspecified foot
- **T25.43** Corrosion of unspecified degree of toe(s) (nail)
  - **T25.431** Corrosion of unspecified degree of right toe(s) (nail)
  - **T25.432** Corrosion of unspecified degree of left toe(s) (nail)
  - **T25.439** Corrosion of unspecified degree of unspecified toe(s) (nail)
- **T25.49** Corrosion of unspecified degree of multiple sites of ankle and foot
  - **T25.491** Corrosion of unspecified degree of multiple sites of right ankle and foot
  - **T25.492** Corrosion of unspecified degree of multiple sites of left ankle and foot
  - **T25.499** Corrosion of unspecified degree of multiple sites of unspecified ankle and foot

T25.5 Corrosion of first degree of ankle and foot
Code first (T51-T65) to identify chemical and intent
Use additional external cause code to identify place (Y92)
- **T25.51** Corrosion of first degree of ankle
  - **T25.511** Corrosion of first degree of right ankle
  - **T25.512** Corrosion of first degree of left ankle
  - **T25.519** Corrosion of first degree of unspecified ankle
- **T25.52** Corrosion of first degree of foot
  EXCLUDES 2 *corrosion of first degree of toe(s) (nail) (T25.53-)*
  - **T25.521** Corrosion of first degree of right foot
  - **T25.522** Corrosion of first degree of left foot
  - **T25.529** Corrosion of first degree of unspecified foot
- **T25.53** Corrosion of first degree of toe(s) (nail)
  - **T25.531** Corrosion of first degree of right toe(s) (nail)
  - **T25.532** Corrosion of first degree of left toe(s) (nail)
  - **T25.539** Corrosion of first degree of unspecified toe(s) (nail)
- **T25.59** Corrosion of first degree of multiple sites of ankle and foot
  - **T25.591** Corrosion of first degree of multiple sites of right ankle and foot
  - **T25.592** Corrosion of first degree of multiple sites of left ankle and foot
  - **T25.599** Corrosion of first degree of multiple sites of unspecified ankle and foot

T25.6 Corrosion of second degree of ankle and foot
Code first (T51-T65) to identify chemical and intent
Use additional external cause code to identify place (Y92)
- **T25.61** Corrosion of second degree of ankle
  - **T25.611** Corrosion of second degree of right ankle
  - **T25.612** Corrosion of second degree of left ankle
  - **T25.619** Corrosion of second degree of unspecified ankle
- **T25.62** Corrosion of second degree of foot
  EXCLUDES 2 *corrosion of second degree of toe(s) (nail) (T25.63-)*
  - **T25.621** Corrosion of second degree of right foot
  - **T25.622** Corrosion of second degree of left foot
  - **T25.629** Corrosion of second degree of unspecified foot
- **T25.63** Corrosion of second degree of toe(s) (nail)
  - **T25.631** Corrosion of second degree of right toe(s) (nail)
  - **T25.632** Corrosion of second degree of left toe(s) (nail)
  - **T25.639** Corrosion of second degree of unspecified toe(s) (nail)
- **T25.69** Corrosion of second degree of multiple sites of ankle and foot
  - **T25.691** Corrosion of second degree of right ankle and foot
  - **T25.692** Corrosion of second degree of left ankle and foot
  - **T25.699** Corrosion of second degree of unspecified ankle and foot

T25.7 Corrosion of third degree of ankle and foot
Code first (T51-T65) to identify chemical and intent
Use additional external cause code to identify place (Y92)
- **T25.71** Corrosion of third degree of ankle
  - **T25.711** Corrosion of third degree of right ankle CC HS
  - **T25.712** Corrosion of third degree of left ankle CC HS
  - **T25.719** Corrosion of third degree of unspecified ankle CC HS UNS
- **T25.72** Corrosion of third degree of foot
  EXCLUDES 2 *corrosion of third degree of toe(s) (nail) (T25.73-)*
  - **T25.721** Corrosion of third degree of right foot CC HS
  - **T25.722** Corrosion of third degree of left foot CC HS
  - **T25.729** Corrosion of third degree of unspecified foot CC HS UNS
- **T25.73** Corrosion of third degree of toe(s) (nail)
  - **T25.731** Corrosion of third degree of right toe(s) (nail) CC HS
  - **T25.732** Corrosion of third degree of left toe(s) (nail) CC HS
  - **T25.739** Corrosion of third degree of unspecified toe(s) (nail) CC HS UNS

- T25.79 Corrosion of third degree of multiple sites of ankle and foot
  - T25.791 Corrosion of third degree of multiple sites of right ankle and foot CC H5
  - T25.792 Corrosion of third degree of multiple sites of left ankle and foot CC H5
  - T25.799 Corrosion of third degree of multiple sites of unspecified ankle and foot CC H5 UNS

Burns and corrosions confined to eye and internal organs (T26-T28)

T26 Burn and corrosion confined to eye and adnexa

The appropriate 7th character is to be added to each code from category T26.
A initial encounter
D subsequent encounter
S sequela

- T26.Ø Burn of eyelid and periocular area
  Use additional external cause code to identify the source, place and intent of the burn (XØØ-X19, X75-X77, X96-X98, Y92)
  - T26.ØØ Burn of unspecified eyelid and periocular area
  - T26.Ø1 Burn of right eyelid and periocular area
  - T26.Ø2 Burn of left eyelid and periocular area
- T26.1 Burn of cornea and conjunctival sac
  Use additional external cause code to identify the source, place and intent of the burn (XØØ-X19, X75-X77, X96-X98, Y92)
  - T26.1Ø Burn of cornea and conjunctival sac, unspecified eye
  - T26.11 Burn of cornea and conjunctival sac, right eye
  - T26.12 Burn of cornea and conjunctival sac, left eye
- T26.2 Burn with resulting rupture and destruction of eyeball
  Use additional external cause code to identify the source, place and intent of the burn (XØØ-X19, X75-X77, X96-X98, Y92)
  - T26.2Ø Burn with resulting rupture and destruction of unspecified eyeball CC H5 UNS
  - T26.21 Burn with resulting rupture and destruction of right eyeball CC H5
  - T26.22 Burn with resulting rupture and destruction of left eyeball CC H5
- T26.3 Burns of other specified parts of eye and adnexa
  Use additional external cause code to identify the source, place and intent of the burn (XØØ-X19, X75-X77, X96-X98, Y92)
  - T26.3Ø Burns of other specified parts of unspecified eye and adnexa
  - T26.31 Burns of other specified parts of right eye and adnexa
  - T26.32 Burns of other specified parts of left eye and adnexa
- T26.4 Burn of eye and adnexa, part unspecified
  Use additional external cause code to identify the source, place and intent of the burn (XØØ-X19, X75-X77, X96-X98, Y92)
  - T26.4Ø Burn of unspecified eye and adnexa, part unspecified
  - T26.41 Burn of right eye and adnexa, part unspecified
  - T26.42 Burn of left eye and adnexa, part unspecified
- T26.5 Corrosion of eyelid and periocular area
  Code first (T51-T65) to identify chemical and intent
  Use additional external cause code to identify place (Y92)
  - T26.5Ø Corrosion of unspecified eyelid and periocular area
  - T26.51 Corrosion of right eyelid and periocular area
  - T26.52 Corrosion of left eyelid and periocular area
- T26.6 Corrosion of cornea and conjunctival sac
  Code first (T51-T65) to identify chemical and intent
  Use additional external cause code to identify place (Y92)
  - T26.6Ø Corrosion of cornea and conjunctival sac, unspecified eye
  - T26.61 Corrosion of cornea and conjunctival sac, right eye
  - T26.62 Corrosion of cornea and conjunctival sac, left eye
- T26.7 Corrosion with resulting rupture and destruction of eyeball
  Code first (T51-T65) to identify chemical and intent
  Use additional external cause code to identify place (Y92)
  - T26.7Ø Corrosion with resulting rupture and destruction of unspecified eyeball CC H5 UNS
  - T26.71 Corrosion with resulting rupture and destruction of right eyeball CC H5
  - T26.72 Corrosion with resulting rupture and destruction of left eyeball CC H5
- T26.8 Corrosions of other specified parts of eye and adnexa
  Code first (T51-T65) to identify chemical and intent
  Use additional external cause code to identify place (Y92)
  - T26.8Ø Corrosions of other specified parts of unspecified eye and adnexa
  - T26.81 Corrosions of other specified parts of right eye and adnexa
  - T26.82 Corrosions of other specified parts of left eye and adnexa
- T26.9 Corrosion of eye and adnexa, part unspecified
  Code first (T51-T65) to identify chemical and intent
  Use additional external cause code to identify place (Y92)
  - T26.9Ø Corrosion of unspecified eye and adnexa, part unspecified
  - T26.91 Corrosion of right eye and adnexa, part unspecified
  - T26.92 Corrosion of left eye and adnexa, part unspecified

T27 Burn and corrosion of respiratory tract

Use additional external cause code to identify the source and intent of the burn (XØØ-X19, X75-X77, X96-X98)
Use additional external cause code to identify place (Y92)

The appropriate 7th character is to be added to each code from category T27.
A initial encounter
D subsequent encounter
S sequela

- T27.Ø Burn of larynx and trachea CC H5
- T27.1 Burn involving larynx and trachea with lung CC H5
- T27.2 Burn of other parts of respiratory tract CC H5
  Burn of thoracic cavity
- T27.3 Burn of respiratory tract, part unspecified CC H5
- T27.4 Corrosion of larynx and trachea CC H5
  Code first (T51-T65) to identify chemical and intent
- T27.5 Corrosion involving larynx and trachea with lung CC H5
  Code first (T51-T65) to identify chemical and intent
- T27.6 Corrosion of other parts of respiratory tract CC H5
  Code first (T51-T65) to identify chemical and intent
- T27.7 Corrosion of respiratory tract, part unspecified CC H5
  Code first (T51-T65) to identify chemical and intent

T28 Burn and corrosion of other internal organs

Use additional external cause code to identify the source and intent of the burn (XØØ-X19, X75-X77, X96-X98)
Use additional external cause code to identify place (Y92)

The appropriate 7th character is to be added to each code from category T28.
A initial encounter
D subsequent encounter
S sequela

- T28.Ø Burn of mouth and pharynx
- T28.1 Burn of esophagus CC H5
- T28.2 Burn of other parts of alimentary tract CC H5
- T28.3 Burn of internal genitourinary organs
- T28.4 Burns of other and unspecified internal organs
  - T28.4Ø Burn of unspecified internal organ
  - T28.41 Burn of ear drum
    - T28.411 Burn of right ear drum
    - T28.412 Burn of left ear drum
    - T28.419 Burn of unspecified ear drum
  - T28.49 Burn of other internal organ
- T28.5 Corrosion of mouth and pharynx
  Code first (T51-T65) to identify chemical and intent
- T28.6 Corrosion of esophagus CC H5
  Code first (T51-T65) to identify chemical and intent
- T28.7 Corrosion of other parts of alimentary tract CC H5
  Code first (T51-T65) to identify chemical and intent
- T28.8 Corrosion of internal genitourinary organs
  Code first (T51-T65) to identify chemical and intent

✓5th **T28.9** **Corrosions of other and unspecified internal organs**
Code first (T51-T65) to identify chemical and intent

✓x7th **T28.9Ø** **Corrosions of unspecified internal organs**

✓6th **T28.91** **Corrosions of ear drum**

✓7th **T28.911** **Corrosions of right ear drum**

✓7th **T28.912** **Corrosions of left ear drum**

✓7th **T28.919** **Corrosions of unspecified ear drum**

✓x7th **T28.99** **Corrosions of other internal organs**

Burns and corrosions of multiple and unspecified body regions (T3Ø-T32)

✓4th **T3Ø Burn and corrosion, body region unspecified**

T3Ø.Ø Burn of unspecified body region, unspecified degree
This code is not for inpatient use. Code to specified site and degree of burns
Burn NOS
Multiple burns NOS

T3Ø.4 Corrosion of unspecified body region, unspecified degree
This code is not for inpatient use. Code to specified site and degree of corrosion
Corrosion NOS
Multiple corrosion NOS

✓4th **T31 Burns classified according to extent of body surface involved**

NOTE This category is to be used as the primary code only when the site of the burn is unspecified. It should be used as a supplementary code with categories T2Ø-T25 when the site is specified.

T31.Ø Burns involving less than 1Ø% of body surface

✓5th **T31.1 Burns involving 1Ø-19% of body surface**

T31.1Ø Burns involving 1Ø-19% of body surface with Ø% to 9% third degree burns CC H5
Burns involving 1Ø-19% of body surface NOS

T31.11 Burns involving 1Ø-19% of body surface with 1Ø-19% third degree burns CC H5 HCC

✓5th **T31.2 Burns involving 2Ø-29% of body surface**

T31.2Ø Burns involving 2Ø-29% of body surface with Ø% to 9% third degree burns CC H5
Burns involving 2Ø-29% of body surface NOS

T31.21 Burns involving 2Ø-29% of body surface with 1Ø-19% third degree burns MCC H5 HCC

T31.22 Burns involving 2Ø-29% of body surface with 2Ø-29% third degree burns MCC H5 HCC

✓5th **T31.3 Burns involving 3Ø-39% of body surface**

T31.3Ø Burns involving 3Ø-39% of body surface with Ø% to 9% third degree burns CC H5
Burns involving 3Ø-39% of body surface NOS

T31.31 Burns involving 3Ø-39% of body surface with 1Ø-19% third degree burns MCC H5 HCC

T31.32 Burns involving 3Ø-39% of body surface with 2Ø-29% third degree burns MCC H5 HCC

T31.33 Burns involving 3Ø-39% of body surface with 3Ø-39% third degree burns MCC H5 HCC

✓5th **T31.4 Burns involving 4Ø-49% of body surface**

T31.4Ø Burns involving 4Ø-49% of body surface with Ø% to 9% third degree burns CC H5
Burns involving 4Ø-49% of body surface NOS

T31.41 Burns involving 4Ø-49% of body surface with 1Ø-19% third degree burns MCC H5 HCC

T31.42 Burns involving 4Ø-49% of body surface with 2Ø-29% third degree burns MCC H5 HCC

T31.43 Burns involving 4Ø-49% of body surface with 3Ø-39% third degree burns MCC H5 HCC

T31.44 Burns involving 4Ø-49% of body surface with 4Ø-49% third degree burns MCC H5 HCC

✓5th **T31.5 Burns involving 5Ø-59% of body surface**

T31.5Ø Burns involving 5Ø-59% of body surface with Ø% to 9% third degree burns CC H5
Burns involving 5Ø-59% of body surface NOS

T31.51 Burns involving 5Ø-59% of body surface with 1Ø-19% third degree burns MCC H5 HCC

T31.52 Burns involving 5Ø-59% of body surface with 2Ø-29% third degree burns MCC H5 HCC

T31.53 Burns involving 5Ø-59% of body surface with 3Ø-39% third degree burns MCC H5 HCC

T31.54 Burns involving 5Ø-59% of body surface with 4Ø-49% third degree burns MCC H5 HCC

T31.55 Burns involving 5Ø-59% of body surface with 5Ø-59% third degree burns MCC H5 HCC

✓5th **T31.6 Burns involving 6Ø-69% of body surface**

T31.6Ø Burns involving 6Ø-69% of body surface with Ø% to 9% third degree burns CC H5
Burns involving 6Ø-69% of body surface NOS

T31.61 Burns involving 6Ø-69% of body surface with 1Ø-19% third degree burns MCC H5 HCC

T31.62 Burns involving 6Ø-69% of body surface with 2Ø-29% third degree burns MCC H5 HCC

T31.63 Burns involving 6Ø-69% of body surface with 3Ø-39% third degree burns MCC H5 HCC

T31.64 Burns involving 6Ø-69% of body surface with 4Ø-49% third degree burns MCC H5 HCC

T31.65 Burns involving 6Ø-69% of body surface with 5Ø-59% third degree burns MCC H5 HCC

T31.66 Burns involving 6Ø-69% of body surface with 6Ø-69% third degree burns MCC H5 HCC

✓5th **T31.7 Burns involving 7Ø-79% of body surface**

T31.7Ø Burns involving 7Ø-79% of body surface with Ø% to 9% third degree burns CC H5
Burns involving 7Ø-79% of body surface NOS

T31.71 Burns involving 7Ø-79% of body surface with 1Ø-19% third degree burns MCC H5 HCC

T31.72 Burns involving 7Ø-79% of body surface with 2Ø-29% third degree burns MCC H5 HCC

T31.73 Burns involving 7Ø-79% of body surface with 3Ø-39% third degree burns MCC H5 HCC

T31.74 Burns involving 7Ø-79% of body surface with 4Ø-49% third degree burns MCC H5 HCC

T31.75 Burns involving 7Ø-79% of body surface with 5Ø-59% third degree burns MCC H5 HCC

T31.76 Burns involving 7Ø-79% of body surface with 6Ø-69% third degree burns MCC H5 HCC

T31.77 Burns involving 7Ø-79% of body surface with 7Ø-79% third degree burns MCC H5 HCC

✓5th **T31.8 Burns involving 8Ø-89% of body surface**

T31.8Ø Burns involving 8Ø-89% of body surface with Ø% to 9% third degree burns CC H5
Burns involving 8Ø-89% of body surface NOS

T31.81 Burns involving 8Ø-89% of body surface with 1Ø-19% third degree burns MCC H5 HCC

T31.82 Burns involving 8Ø-89% of body surface with 2Ø-29% third degree burns MCC H5 HCC

T31.83 Burns involving 8Ø-89% of body surface with 3Ø-39% third degree burns MCC H5 HCC

T31.84 Burns involving 8Ø-89% of body surface with 4Ø-49% third degree burns MCC H5 HCC

T31.85 Burns involving 8Ø-89% of body surface with 5Ø-59% third degree burns MCC H5 HCC

T31.86 Burns involving 8Ø-89% of body surface with 6Ø-69% third degree burns MCC H5 HCC

T31.87 Burns involving 8Ø-89% of body surface with 7Ø-79% third degree burns MCC H5 HCC

T31.88 Burns involving 8Ø-89% of body surface with 8Ø-89% third degree burns MCC H5 HCC

✓5th **T31.9 Burns involving 9Ø% or more of body surface**

T31.9Ø Burns involving 9Ø% or more of body surface with Ø% to 9% third degree burns CC H5
Burns involving 9Ø% or more of body surface NOS

T31.91 Burns involving 9Ø% or more of body surface with 1Ø-19% third degree burns MCC H5 HCC

T31.92 Burns involving 9Ø% or more of body surface with 2Ø-29% third degree burns MCC H5 HCC

T31.93 Burns involving 9Ø% or more of body surface with 3Ø-39% third degree burns MCC H5 HCC

T31.94 Burns involving 9Ø% or more of body surface with 4Ø-49% third degree burns MCC H5 HCC

T31.95 Burns involving 9Ø% or more of body surface with 5Ø-59% third degree burns MCC H5 HCC

T31.96 Burns involving 9Ø% or more of body surface with 6Ø-69% third degree burns MCC H5 HCC

T31.97 Burns involving 9Ø% or more of body surface with 7Ø-79% third degree burns MCC H5 HCC

T31.98 Burns involving 9Ø% or more of body surface with 8Ø-89% third degree burns MCC H5 HCC

T31.99 Burns involving 90% or more of body surface with 90% or more third degree burns MCC H5 HCC

Rule of Nines Estimation of Total Body Surface Burned

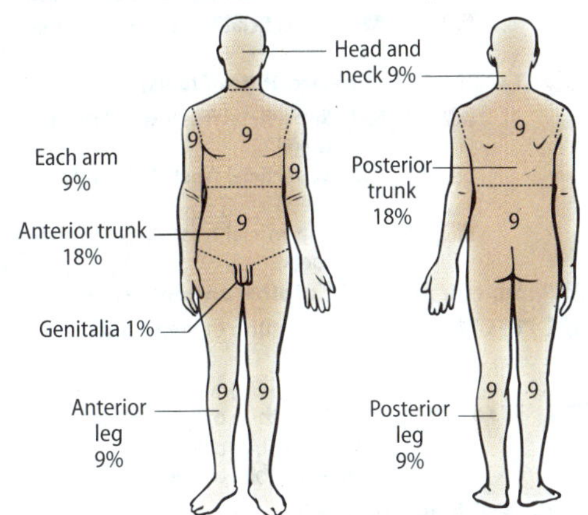

T32 Corrosions classified according to extent of body surface involved

NOTE This category is to be used as the primary code only when the site of the corrosion is unspecified. It may be used as a supplementary code with categories T20-T25 when the site is specified.

T32.0 Corrosions involving less than 10% of body surface

T32.1 Corrosions involving 10-19% of body surface

T32.10 Corrosions involving 10-19% of body surface with 0% to 9% third degree corrosion CC H5
Corrosions involving 10-19% of body surface NOS

T32.11 Corrosions involving 10-19% of body surface with 10-19% third degree corrosion CC H5 HCC

T32.2 Corrosions involving 20-29% of body surface

T32.20 Corrosions involving 20-29% of body surface with 0% to 9% third degree corrosion CC H5

T32.21 Corrosions involving 20-29% of body surface with 10-19% third degree corrosion MCC H5 HCC

T32.22 Corrosions involving 20-29% of body surface with 20-29% third degree corrosion MCC H5 HCC

T32.3 Corrosions involving 30-39% of body surface

T32.30 Corrosions involving 30-39% of body surface with 0% to 9% third degree corrosion CC H5

T32.31 Corrosions involving 30-39% of body surface with 10-19% third degree corrosion MCC H5 HCC

T32.32 Corrosions involving 30-39% of body surface with 20-29% third degree corrosion MCC H5 HCC

T32.33 Corrosions involving 30-39% of body surface with 30-39% third degree corrosion MCC H5 HCC

T32.4 Corrosions involving 40-49% of body surface

T32.40 Corrosions involving 40-49% of body surface with 0% to 9% third degree corrosion CC H5

T32.41 Corrosions involving 40-49% of body surface with 10-19% third degree corrosion MCC H5 HCC

T32.42 Corrosions involving 40-49% of body surface with 20-29% third degree corrosion MCC H5 HCC

T32.43 Corrosions involving 40-49% of body surface with 30-39% third degree corrosion MCC H5 HCC

T32.44 Corrosions involving 40-49% of body surface with 40-49% third degree corrosion MCC H5 HCC

T32.5 Corrosions involving 50-59% of body surface

T32.50 Corrosions involving 50-59% of body surface with 0% to 9% third degree corrosion CC H5

T32.51 Corrosions involving 50-59% of body surface with 10-19% third degree corrosion MCC H5 HCC

T32.52 Corrosions involving 50-59% of body surface with 20-29% third degree corrosion MCC H5 HCC

T32.53 Corrosions involving 50-59% of body surface with 30-39% third degree corrosion MCC H5 HCC

T32.54 Corrosions involving 50-59% of body surface with 40-49% third degree corrosion MCC H5 HCC

T32.55 Corrosions involving 50-59% of body surface with 50-59% third degree corrosion MCC H5 HCC

T32.6 Corrosions involving 60-69% of body surface

T32.60 Corrosions involving 60-69% of body surface with 0% to 9% third degree corrosion CC H5

T32.61 Corrosions involving 60-69% of body surface with 10-19% third degree corrosion MCC H5 HCC

T32.62 Corrosions involving 60-69% of body surface with 20-29% third degree corrosion MCC H5 HCC

T32.63 Corrosions involving 60-69% of body surface with 30-39% third degree corrosion MCC H5 HCC

T32.64 Corrosions involving 60-69% of body surface with 40-49% third degree corrosion MCC H5 HCC

T32.65 Corrosions involving 60-69% of body surface with 50-59% third degree corrosion MCC H5 HCC

T32.66 Corrosions involving 60-69% of body surface with 60-69% third degree corrosion MCC H5 HCC

T32.7 Corrosions involving 70-79% of body surface

T32.70 Corrosions involving 70-79% of body surface with 0% to 9% third degree corrosion CC H5

T32.71 Corrosions involving 70-79% of body surface with 10-19% third degree corrosion MCC H5 HCC

T32.72 Corrosions involving 70-79% of body surface with 20-29% third degree corrosion MCC H5 HCC

T32.73 Corrosions involving 70-79% of body surface with 30-39% third degree corrosion MCC H5 HCC

T32.74 Corrosions involving 70-79% of body surface with 40-49% third degree corrosion MCC H5 HCC

T32.75 Corrosions involving 70-79% of body surface with 50-59% third degree corrosion MCC H5 HCC

T32.76 Corrosions involving 70-79% of body surface with 60-69% third degree corrosion MCC H5 HCC

T32.77 Corrosions involving 70-79% of body surface with 70-79% third degree corrosion MCC H5 HCC

T32.8 Corrosions involving 80-89% of body surface

T32.80 Corrosions involving 80-89% of body surface with 0% to 9% third degree corrosion CC H5

T32.81 Corrosions involving 80-89% of body surface with 10-19% third degree corrosion MCC H5 HCC

T32.82 Corrosions involving 80-89% of body surface with 20-29% third degree corrosion MCC H5 HCC

T32.83 Corrosions involving 80-89% of body surface with 30-39% third degree corrosion MCC H5 HCC

T32.84 Corrosions involving 80-89% of body surface with 40-49% third degree corrosion MCC H5 HCC

T32.85 Corrosions involving 80-89% of body surface with 50-59% third degree corrosion MCC H5 HCC

T32.86 Corrosions involving 80-89% of body surface with 60-69% third degree corrosion MCC H5 HCC

T32.87 Corrosions involving 80-89% of body surface with 70-79% third degree corrosion MCC H5 HCC

T32.88 Corrosions involving 80-89% of body surface with 80-89% third degree corrosion MCC H5 HCC

T32.9 Corrosions involving 90% or more of body surface

T32.90 Corrosions involving 90% or more of body surface with 0% to 9% third degree corrosion CC H5

T32.91 Corrosions involving 90% or more of body surface with 10-19% third degree corrosion MCC H5 HCC

T32.92 Corrosions involving 90% or more of body surface with 20-29% third degree corrosion MCC H5 HCC

T32.93 Corrosions involving 90% or more of body surface with 30-39% third degree corrosion MCC H5 HCC

T32.94 Corrosions involving 90% or more of body surface with 40-49% third degree corrosion MCC H5 HCC

T32.95 Corrosions involving 90% or more of body surface with 50-59% third degree corrosion MCC H5 HCC

T32.96 Corrosions involving 90% or more of body surface with 60-69% third degree corrosion MCC H5 HCC

T32.97 Corrosions involving 90% or more of body surface with 70-79% third degree corrosion MCC H5 HCC

T32.98 Corrosions involving 90% or more of body surface with 80-89% third degree corrosion MCC H5 HCC

T32.99 Corrosions involving 90% or more of body surface with 90% or more third degree corrosion MCC H5 HCC

Frostbite (T33-T34)

EXCLUDES 2 *hypothermia and other effects of reduced temperature (T68, T69.-)*

T33 Superficial frostbite

INCLUDES frostbite with partial thickness skin loss

The appropriate 7th character is to be added to each code from category T33.
A initial encounter
D subsequent encounter
S sequela

T33.0 Superficial frostbite of head

T33.01 Superficial frostbite of ear

T33.011 Superficial frostbite of right ear CC HS

T33.012 Superficial frostbite of left ear CC HS

T33.019 Superficial frostbite of unspecified ear CC HS UNS

T33.02 Superficial frostbite of nose CC HS

T33.09 Superficial frostbite of other part of head CC HS

T33.1 Superficial frostbite of neck CC HS

T33.2 Superficial frostbite of thorax CC HS

T33.3 Superficial frostbite of abdominal wall, lower back and pelvis CC HS

T33.4 Superficial frostbite of arm

EXCLUDES 2 *superficial frostbite of wrist and hand (T33.5-)*

T33.40 Superficial frostbite of unspecified arm CC HS UNS

T33.41 Superficial frostbite of right arm CC HS

T33.42 Superficial frostbite of left arm CC HS

T33.5 Superficial frostbite of wrist, hand, and fingers

T33.51 Superficial frostbite of wrist

T33.511 Superficial frostbite of right wrist CC HS

T33.512 Superficial frostbite of left wrist CC HS

T33.519 Superficial frostbite of unspecified wrist CC HS UNS

T33.52 Superficial frostbite of hand

EXCLUDES 2 *superficial frostbite of fingers (T33.53-)*

T33.521 Superficial frostbite of right hand CC HS

T33.522 Superficial frostbite of left hand CC HS

T33.529 Superficial frostbite of unspecified hand CC HS UNS

T33.53 Superficial frostbite of finger(s)

T33.531 Superficial frostbite of right finger(s) CC HS

T33.532 Superficial frostbite of left finger(s) CC HS

T33.539 Superficial frostbite of unspecified finger(s) CC HS UNS

T33.6 Superficial frostbite of hip and thigh

T33.60 Superficial frostbite of unspecified hip and thigh CC HS UNS

T33.61 Superficial frostbite of right hip and thigh CC HS

T33.62 Superficial frostbite of left hip and thigh CC HS

T33.7 Superficial frostbite of knee and lower leg

EXCLUDES 2 *superficial frostbite of ankle and foot (T33.8-)*

T33.70 Superficial frostbite of unspecified knee and lower leg CC HS UNS

T33.71 Superficial frostbite of right knee and lower leg CC HS

T33.72 Superficial frostbite of left knee and lower leg CC HS

T33.8 Superficial frostbite of ankle, foot, and toe(s)

T33.81 Superficial frostbite of ankle

T33.811 Superficial frostbite of right ankle CC HS

T33.812 Superficial frostbite of left ankle CC HS

T33.819 Superficial frostbite of unspecified ankle CC HS UNS

T33.82 Superficial frostbite of foot

T33.821 Superficial frostbite of right foot CC HS

T33.822 Superficial frostbite of left foot CC HS

T33.829 Superficial frostbite of unspecified foot CC HS UNS

T33.83 Superficial frostbite of toe(s)

T33.831 Superficial frostbite of right toe(s) CC HS

T33.832 Superficial frostbite of left toe(s) CC HS

T33.839 Superficial frostbite of unspecified toe(s) CC HS UNS

T33.9 Superficial frostbite of other and unspecified sites

T33.90 Superficial frostbite of unspecified sites CC HS UNS
Superficial frostbite NOS

T33.99 Superficial frostbite of other sites CC HS
Superficial frostbite of leg NOS
Superficial frostbite of trunk NOS

T34 Frostbite with tissue necrosis

The appropriate 7th character is to be added to each code from category T34.
A initial encounter
D subsequent encounter
S sequela

T34.0 Frostbite with tissue necrosis of head

T34.01 Frostbite with tissue necrosis of ear

T34.011 Frostbite with tissue necrosis of right ear CC HS

T34.012 Frostbite with tissue necrosis of left ear CC HS

T34.019 Frostbite with tissue necrosis of unspecified ear CC HS UNS

T34.02 Frostbite with tissue necrosis of nose CC HS

T34.09 Frostbite with tissue necrosis of other part of head CC HS

T34.1 Frostbite with tissue necrosis of neck CC HS

T34.2 Frostbite with tissue necrosis of thorax CC HS

T34.3 Frostbite with tissue necrosis of abdominal wall, lower back and pelvis CC HS

T34.4 Frostbite with tissue necrosis of arm

EXCLUDES 2 *frostbite with tissue necrosis of wrist and hand (T34.5-)*

T34.40 Frostbite with tissue necrosis of unspecified arm CC HS UNS

T34.41 Frostbite with tissue necrosis of right arm CC HS

T34.42 Frostbite with tissue necrosis of left arm CC HS

T34.5 Frostbite with tissue necrosis of wrist, hand, and finger(s)

T34.51 Frostbite with tissue necrosis of wrist

T34.511 Frostbite with tissue necrosis of right wrist CC HS

T34.512 Frostbite with tissue necrosis of left wrist CC HS

T34.519 Frostbite with tissue necrosis of unspecified wrist CC HS UNS

T34.52 Frostbite with tissue necrosis of hand

EXCLUDES 2 *frostbite with tissue necrosis of finger(s) (T34.53-)*

T34.521 Frostbite with tissue necrosis of right hand CC HS

T34.522 Frostbite with tissue necrosis of left hand CC HS

T34.529 Frostbite with tissue necrosis of unspecified hand CC HS UNS

T34.53 Frostbite with tissue necrosis of finger(s)

T34.531 Frostbite with tissue necrosis of right finger(s) CC HS

T34.532 Frostbite with tissue necrosis of left finger(s) CC HS

T34.539 Frostbite with tissue necrosis of unspecified finger(s) CC HS UNS

T34.6 Frostbite with tissue necrosis of hip and thigh

T34.60 Frostbite with tissue necrosis of unspecified hip and thigh CC HS UNS

T34.61 Frostbite with tissue necrosis of right hip and thigh CC H5

T34.62 Frostbite with tissue necrosis of left hip and thigh CC H5

T34.7 Frostbite with tissue necrosis of knee and lower leg

EXCLUDES 2 *frostbite with tissue necrosis of ankle and foot (T34.8-)*

T34.70 Frostbite with tissue necrosis of unspecified knee and lower leg CC H5 UNS

T34.71 Frostbite with tissue necrosis of right knee and lower leg CC H5

T34.72 Frostbite with tissue necrosis of left knee and lower leg CC H5

T34.8 Frostbite with tissue necrosis of ankle, foot, and toe(s)

T34.81 Frostbite with tissue necrosis of ankle

T34.811 Frostbite with tissue necrosis of right ankle CC H5

T34.812 Frostbite with tissue necrosis of left ankle CC H5

T34.819 Frostbite with tissue necrosis of unspecified ankle CC H5 UNS

T34.82 Frostbite with tissue necrosis of foot

T34.821 Frostbite with tissue necrosis of right foot CC H5

T34.822 Frostbite with tissue necrosis of left foot CC H5

T34.829 Frostbite with tissue necrosis of unspecified foot CC H5 UNS

T34.83 Frostbite with tissue necrosis of toe(s)

T34.831 Frostbite with tissue necrosis of right toe(s) CC H5

T34.832 Frostbite with tissue necrosis of left toe(s) CC H5

T34.839 Frostbite with tissue necrosis of unspecified toe(s) CC H5 UNS

T34.9 Frostbite with tissue necrosis of other and unspecified sites

T34.90 Frostbite with tissue necrosis of unspecified sites CC H5 UNS

Frostbite with tissue necrosis NOS

T34.99 Frostbite with tissue necrosis of other sites CC H5

Frostbite with tissue necrosis of leg NOS

Frostbite with tissue necrosis of trunk NOS

Poisoning by, adverse effects of and underdosing of drugs, medicaments and biological substances (T36-T5Ø)

INCLUDES adverse effect of correct substance properly administered
poisoning by overdose of substance
poisoning by wrong substance given or taken in error
underdosing by (inadvertently) (deliberately) taking less substance than prescribed or instructed

Code first, for adverse effects, the nature of the adverse effect, such as:
- adverse effect NOS (T88.7)
- aspirin gastritis (K29.-)
- blood disorders (D56-D76)
- contact dermatitis (L23-L25)
- dermatitis due to substances taken internally (L27.-)
- nephropathy (N14.Ø-N14.2)

NOTE The drug giving rise to the adverse effect should be identified by use of codes from categories T36-T5Ø with fifth or sixth character 5.

Use additional code(s) to specify:
- manifestations of poisoning
- underdosing or failure in dosage during medical and surgical care (Y63.6, Y63.8-Y63.9)
- underdosing of medication regimen (Z91.12-, Z91.13-)

EXCLUDES 1 *toxic reaction to local anesthesia in pregnancy (O29.3-)*

EXCLUDES 2 *abuse and dependence of psychoactive substances (F1Ø-F19)*
abuse of non-dependence-producing substances (F55.-)
drug reaction and poisoning affecting newborn (PØØ-P96)
immunodeficiency due to drugs (D84.821)
pathological drug intoxication (inebriation) (F1Ø-F19)

AHA: 2018,4Q,71; 2016,2Q,8; 2015,3Q,22

T36 Poisoning by, adverse effect of and underdosing of systemic antibiotics

EXCLUDES 1 *antineoplastic antibiotics (T45.1-)*
locally applied antibiotic NEC (T49.Ø)
topically used antibiotic for ear, nose and throat (T49.6)
topically used antibiotic for eye (T49.5)

The appropriate 7th character is to be added to each code from category T36.
- A initial encounter
- D subsequent encounter
- S sequela

T36.Ø Poisoning by, adverse effect of and underdosing of penicillins

T36.ØX Poisoning by, adverse effect of and underdosing of penicillins

T36.ØX1 Poisoning by penicillins, accidental (unintentional)

Poisoning by penicillins NOS

T36.ØX2 Poisoning by penicillins, intentional self-harm HCC

T36.ØX3 Poisoning by penicillins, assault

T36.ØX4 Poisoning by penicillins, undetermined

T36.ØX5 Adverse effect of penicillins UPD

T36.ØX6 Underdosing of penicillins UPD

T36.1 Poisoning by, adverse effect of and underdosing of cephalosporins and other beta-lactam antibiotics

T36.1X Poisoning by, adverse effect of and underdosing of cephalosporins and other beta-lactam antibiotics

T36.1X1 Poisoning by cephalosporins and other beta-lactam antibiotics, accidental (unintentional)

Poisoning by cephalosporins and other beta-lactam antibiotics NOS

T36.1X2 Poisoning by cephalosporins and other beta-lactam antibiotics, intentional self-harm HCC

T36.1X3 Poisoning by cephalosporins and other beta-lactam antibiotics, assault

T36.1X4 Poisoning by cephalosporins and other beta-lactam antibiotics, undetermined

T36.1X5 Adverse effect of cephalosporins and other beta-lactam antibiotics UPD

T36.1X6 Underdosing of cephalosporins and other beta-lactam antibiotics UPD

T36.2 Poisoning by, adverse effect of and underdosing of chloramphenicol group

T36.2X Poisoning by, adverse effect of and underdosing of chloramphenicol group

T36.2X1 Poisoning by chloramphenicol group, accidental (unintentional)

Poisoning by chloramphenicol group NOS

T36.2X2 Poisoning by chloramphenicol group, intentional self-harm HCC

7th T36.2X3 **Poisoning by chloramphenicol group, assault**

7th T36.2X4 **Poisoning by chloramphenicol group, undetermined**

7th T36.2X5 **Adverse effect of chloramphenicol group** UPD

7th T36.2X6 **Underdosing of chloramphenicol group** UPD

5th **T36.3 Poisoning by, adverse effect of and underdosing of macrolides**

6th **T36.3X Poisoning by, adverse effect of and underdosing of macrolides**

7th T36.3X1 **Poisoning by macrolides, accidental (unintentional)**
Poisoning by macrolides NOS

7th T36.3X2 **Poisoning by macrolides, intentional self-harm** HCC

7th T36.3X3 **Poisoning by macrolides, assault**

7th T36.3X4 **Poisoning by macrolides, undetermined**

7th T36.3X5 **Adverse effect of macrolides** UPD

7th T36.3X6 **Underdosing of macrolides** UPD

5th **T36.4 Poisoning by, adverse effect of and underdosing of tetracyclines**

6th **T36.4X Poisoning by, adverse effect of and underdosing of tetracyclines**

7th T36.4X1 **Poisoning by tetracyclines, accidental (unintentional)**
Poisoning by tetracyclines NOS

7th T36.4X2 **Poisoning by tetracyclines, intentional self-harm** HCC

7th T36.4X3 **Poisoning by tetracyclines, assault**

7th T36.4X4 **Poisoning by tetracyclines, undetermined**

7th T36.4X5 **Adverse effect of tetracyclines** UPD

7th T36.4X6 **Underdosing of tetracyclines** UPD

5th **T36.5 Poisoning by, adverse effect of and underdosing of aminoglycosides**
Poisoning by, adverse effect of and underdosing of streptomycin

6th **T36.5X Poisoning by, adverse effect of and underdosing of aminoglycosides**

7th T36.5X1 **Poisoning by aminoglycosides, accidental (unintentional)**
Poisoning by aminoglycosides NOS

7th T36.5X2 **Poisoning by aminoglycosides, intentional self-harm** HCC

7th T36.5X3 **Poisoning by aminoglycosides, assault**

7th T36.5X4 **Poisoning by aminoglycosides, undetermined**

7th T36.5X5 **Adverse effect of aminoglycosides** UPD

7th T36.5X6 **Underdosing of aminoglycosides** UPD

5th **T36.6 Poisoning by, adverse effect of and underdosing of rifampicins**

6th **T36.6X Poisoning by, adverse effect of and underdosing of rifampicins**

7th T36.6X1 **Poisoning by rifampicins, accidental (unintentional)**
Poisoning by rifampicins NOS

7th T36.6X2 **Poisoning by rifampicins, intentional self-harm** HCC

7th T36.6X3 **Poisoning by rifampicins, assault**

7th T36.6X4 **Poisoning by rifampicins, undetermined**

7th T36.6X5 **Adverse effect of rifampicins** UPD

7th T36.6X6 **Underdosing of rifampicins** UPD

5th **T36.7 Poisoning by, adverse effect of and underdosing of antifungal antibiotics, systemically used**

6th **T36.7X Poisoning by, adverse effect of and underdosing of antifungal antibiotics, systemically used**

7th T36.7X1 **Poisoning by antifungal antibiotics, systemically used, accidental (unintentional)**
Poisoning by antifungal antibiotics, systemically used NOS

7th T36.7X2 **Poisoning by antifungal antibiotics, systemically used, intentional self-harm** HCC

7th T36.7X3 **Poisoning by antifungal antibiotics, systemically used, assault**

7th T36.7X4 **Poisoning by antifungal antibiotics, systemically used, undetermined**

7th T36.7X5 **Adverse effect of antifungal antibiotics, systemically used** UPD

7th T36.7X6 **Underdosing of antifungal antibiotics, systemically used** UPD

5th **T36.8 Poisoning by, adverse effect of and underdosing of other systemic antibiotics**

6th **T36.8X Poisoning by, adverse effect of and underdosing of other systemic antibiotics**
AHA: 2017,1Q,39

7th T36.8X1 **Poisoning by other systemic antibiotics, accidental (unintentional)**
Poisoning by other systemic antibiotics NOS

7th T36.8X2 **Poisoning by other systemic antibiotics, intentional self-harm** HCC

7th T36.8X3 **Poisoning by other systemic antibiotics, assault**

7th T36.8X4 **Poisoning by other systemic antibiotics, undetermined**

7th T36.8X5 **Adverse effect of other systemic antibiotics** UPD

7th T36.8X6 **Underdosing of other systemic antibiotics** UPD

5th **T36.9 Poisoning by, adverse effect of and underdosing of unspecified systemic antibiotic**

x7th T36.91 **Poisoning by unspecified systemic antibiotic, accidental (unintentional)**
Poisoning by systemic antibiotic NOS

x7th T36.92 **Poisoning by unspecified systemic antibiotic, intentional self-harm** HCC

x7th T36.93 **Poisoning by unspecified systemic antibiotic, assault**

x7th T36.94 **Poisoning by unspecified systemic antibiotic, undetermined**

x7th T36.95 **Adverse effect of unspecified systemic antibiotic** UPD

x7th T36.96 **Underdosing of unspecified systemic antibiotic** UPD

4th **T37 Poisoning by, adverse effect of and underdosing of other systemic anti-infectives and antiparasitics**

EXCLUDES 1 *anti-infectives topically used for ear, nose and throat (T49.6-)*
anti-infectives topically used for eye (T49.5-)
locally applied anti-infectives NEC (T49.0-)

The appropriate 7th character is to be added to each code from category T37.
A initial encounter
D subsequent encounter
S sequela

5th **T37.0 Poisoning by, adverse effect of and underdosing of sulfonamides**

6th **T37.0X Poisoning by, adverse effect of and underdosing of sulfonamides**

7th T37.0X1 **Poisoning by sulfonamides, accidental (unintentional)**
Poisoning by sulfonamides NOS

7th T37.0X2 **Poisoning by sulfonamides, intentional self-harm** HCC

7th T37.0X3 **Poisoning by sulfonamides, assault**

7th T37.0X4 **Poisoning by sulfonamides, undetermined**

7th T37.0X5 **Adverse effect of sulfonamides** UPD

7th T37.0X6 **Underdosing of sulfonamides** UPD

5th **T37.1 Poisoning by, adverse effect of and underdosing of antimycobacterial drugs**

EXCLUDES 1 *rifampicins (T36.6-)*
streptomycin (T36.5-)

6th **T37.1X Poisoning by, adverse effect of and underdosing of antimycobacterial drugs**

7th T37.1X1 **Poisoning by antimycobacterial drugs, accidental (unintentional)**
Poisoning by antimycobacterial drugs NOS

7th T37.1X2 **Poisoning by antimycobacterial drugs, intentional self-harm** HCC

7th T37.1X3 **Poisoning by antimycobacterial drugs, assault**

7th T37.1X4 **Poisoning by antimycobacterial drugs, undetermined**

7th T37.1X5 **Adverse effect of antimycobacterial drugs** UPD

T37.1X6 Underdosing of antimycobacterial drugs UPD

T37.2 Poisoning by, adverse effect of and underdosing of antimalarials and drugs acting on other blood protozoa
EXCLUDES 1 *hydroxyquinoline derivatives (T37.8-)*

T37.2X Poisoning by, adverse effect of and underdosing of antimalarials and drugs acting on other blood protozoa

T37.2X1 Poisoning by antimalarials and drugs acting on other blood protozoa, accidental (unintentional)
Poisoning by antimalarials and drugs acting on other blood protozoa NOS

T37.2X2 Poisoning by antimalarials and drugs acting on other blood protozoa, intentional self-harm HCC

T37.2X3 Poisoning by antimalarials and drugs acting on other blood protozoa, assault

T37.2X4 Poisoning by antimalarials and drugs acting on other blood protozoa, undetermined

T37.2X5 Adverse effect of antimalarials and drugs acting on other blood protozoa UPD

T37.2X6 Underdosing of antimalarials and drugs acting on other blood protozoa UPD

T37.3 Poisoning by, adverse effect of and underdosing of other antiprotozoal drugs

T37.3X Poisoning by, adverse effect of and underdosing of other antiprotozoal drugs

T37.3X1 Poisoning by other antiprotozoal drugs, accidental (unintentional)
Poisoning by other antiprotozoal drugs NOS

T37.3X2 Poisoning by other antiprotozoal drugs, intentional self-harm HCC

T37.3X3 Poisoning by other antiprotozoal drugs, assault

T37.3X4 Poisoning by other antiprotozoal drugs, undetermined

T37.3X5 Adverse effect of other antiprotozoal drugs UPD

T37.3X6 Underdosing of other antiprotozoal drugs UPD

T37.4 Poisoning by, adverse effect of and underdosing of anthelminthics

T37.4X Poisoning by, adverse effect of and underdosing of anthelminthics

T37.4X1 Poisoning by anthelminthics, accidental (unintentional)
Poisoning by anthelminthics NOS

T37.4X2 Poisoning by anthelminthics, intentional self-harm HCC

T37.4X3 Poisoning by anthelminthics, assault

T37.4X4 Poisoning by anthelminthics, undetermined

T37.4X5 Adverse effect of anthelminthics UPD

T37.4X6 Underdosing of anthelminthics UPD

T37.5 Poisoning by, adverse effect of and underdosing of antiviral drugs
EXCLUDES 1 *amantadine (T42.8-)*
cytarabine (T45.1-)

T37.5X Poisoning by, adverse effect of and underdosing of antiviral drugs

T37.5X1 Poisoning by antiviral drugs, accidental (unintentional)
Poisoning by antiviral drugs NOS

T37.5X2 Poisoning by antiviral drugs, intentional self-harm HCC

T37.5X3 Poisoning by antiviral drugs, assault

T37.5X4 Poisoning by antiviral drugs, undetermined

T37.5X5 Adverse effect of antiviral drugs UPD

T37.5X6 Underdosing of antiviral drugs UPD

T37.8 Poisoning by, adverse effect of and underdosing of other specified systemic anti-infectives and antiparasitics
Poisoning by, adverse effect of and underdosing of hydroxyquinoline derivatives
EXCLUDES 1 *antimalarial drugs (T37.2-)*

T37.8X Poisoning by, adverse effect of and underdosing of other specified systemic anti-infectives and antiparasitics

T37.8X1 Poisoning by other specified systemic anti-infectives and antiparasitics, accidental (unintentional)
Poisoning by other specified systemic anti-infectives and antiparasitics NOS

T37.8X2 Poisoning by other specified systemic anti-infectives and antiparasitics, intentional self-harm HCC

T37.8X3 Poisoning by other specified systemic anti-infectives and antiparasitics, assault

T37.8X4 Poisoning by other specified systemic anti-infectives and antiparasitics, undetermined

T37.8X5 Adverse effect of other specified systemic anti-infectives and antiparasitics UPD

T37.8X6 Underdosing of other specified systemic anti-infectives and antiparasitics UPD

T37.9 Poisoning by, adverse effect of and underdosing of unspecified systemic anti-infective and antiparasitics

T37.91 Poisoning by unspecified systemic anti-infective and antiparasitics, accidental (unintentional)
Poisoning by, adverse effect of and underdosing of systemic anti-infective and antiparasitics NOS

T37.92 Poisoning by unspecified systemic anti-infective and antiparasitics, intentional self-harm HCC

T37.93 Poisoning by unspecified systemic anti-infective and antiparasitics, assault

T37.94 Poisoning by unspecified systemic anti-infective and antiparasitics, undetermined

T37.95 Adverse effect of unspecified systemic anti-infective and antiparasitic UPD

T37.96 Underdosing of unspecified systemic anti-infectives and antiparasitics UPD

T38 Poisoning by, adverse effect of and underdosing of hormones and their synthetic substitutes and antagonists, not elsewhere classified

EXCLUDES 1 *mineralocorticoids and their antagonists (T50.Ø-)*
oxytocic hormones (T48.Ø-)
parathyroid hormones and derivatives (T5Ø.9-)

The appropriate 7th character is to be added to each code from category T38.
A initial encounter
D subsequent encounter
S sequela

T38.Ø Poisoning by, adverse effect of and underdosing of glucocorticoids and synthetic analogues
EXCLUDES 1 *glucocorticoids, topically used (T49.-)*

T38.ØX Poisoning by, adverse effect of and underdosing of glucocorticoids and synthetic analogues

T38.ØX1 Poisoning by glucocorticoids and synthetic analogues, accidental (unintentional)
Poisoning by glucocorticoids and synthetic analogues NOS

T38.ØX2 Poisoning by glucocorticoids and synthetic analogues, intentional self-harm HCC

T38.ØX3 Poisoning by glucocorticoids and synthetic analogues, assault

T38.ØX4 Poisoning by glucocorticoids and synthetic analogues, undetermined

T38.ØX5 Adverse effect of glucocorticoids and synthetic analogues UPD

T38.ØX6 Underdosing of glucocorticoids and synthetic analogues UPD

√5th **T38.1 Poisoning by, adverse effect of and underdosing of thyroid hormones and substitutes**

√6th **T38.1X Poisoning by, adverse effect of and underdosing of thyroid hormones and substitutes**

√7th **T38.1X1 Poisoning by thyroid hormones and substitutes, accidental (unintentional)**
Poisoning by thyroid hormones and substitutes NOS

√7th **T38.1X2 Poisoning by thyroid hormones and substitutes, intentional self-harm** HCC

√7th **T38.1X3 Poisoning by thyroid hormones and substitutes, assault**

√7th **T38.1X4 Poisoning by thyroid hormones and substitutes, undetermined**

√7th **T38.1X5 Adverse effect of thyroid hormones and substitutes** UPD

√7th **T38.1X6 Underdosing of thyroid hormones and substitutes** UPD

√5th **T38.2 Poisoning by, adverse effect of and underdosing of antithyroid drugs**

√6th **T38.2X Poisoning by, adverse effect of and underdosing of antithyroid drugs**

√7th **T38.2X1 Poisoning by antithyroid drugs, accidental (unintentional)**
Poisoning by antithyroid drugs NOS

√7th **T38.2X2 Poisoning by antithyroid drugs, intentional self-harm** HCC

√7th **T38.2X3 Poisoning by antithyroid drugs, assault**

√7th **T38.2X4 Poisoning by antithyroid drugs, undetermined**

√7th **T38.2X5 Adverse effect of antithyroid drugs** UPD

√7th **T38.2X6 Underdosing of antithyroid drugs** UPD

√5th **T38.3 Poisoning by, adverse effect of and underdosing of insulin and oral hypoglycemic [antidiabetic] drugs**

√6th **T38.3X Poisoning by, adverse effect of and underdosing of insulin and oral hypoglycemic [antidiabetic] drugs**

√7th **T38.3X1 Poisoning by insulin and oral hypoglycemic [antidiabetic] drugs, accidental (unintentional)**
Poisoning by insulin and oral hypoglycemic [antidiabetic] drugs NOS

√7th **T38.3X2 Poisoning by insulin and oral hypoglycemic [antidiabetic] drugs, intentional self-harm** HCC

√7th **T38.3X3 Poisoning by insulin and oral hypoglycemic [antidiabetic] drugs, assault**

√7th **T38.3X4 Poisoning by insulin and oral hypoglycemic [antidiabetic] drugs, undetermined**

√7th **T38.3X5 Adverse effect of insulin and oral hypoglycemic [antidiabetic] drugs** UPD

√7th **T38.3X6 Underdosing of insulin and oral hypoglycemic [antidiabetic] drugs** UPD

√5th **T38.4 Poisoning by, adverse effect of and underdosing of oral contraceptives**
Poisoning by, adverse effect of and underdosing of multiple- and single-ingredient oral contraceptive preparations

√6th **T38.4X Poisoning by, adverse effect of and underdosing of oral contraceptives**

√7th **T38.4X1 Poisoning by oral contraceptives, accidental (unintentional)**
Poisoning by oral contraceptives NOS

√7th **T38.4X2 Poisoning by oral contraceptives, intentional self-harm** HCC

√7th **T38.4X3 Poisoning by oral contraceptives, assault**

√7th **T38.4X4 Poisoning by oral contraceptives, undetermined**

√7th **T38.4X5 Adverse effect of oral contraceptives** UPD

√7th **T38.4X6 Underdosing of oral contraceptives** UPD

√5th **T38.5 Poisoning by, adverse effect of and underdosing of other estrogens and progestogens**
Poisoning by, adverse effect of and underdosing of estrogens and progestogens mixtures and substitutes

√6th **T38.5X Poisoning by, adverse effect of and underdosing of other estrogens and progestogens**

√7th **T38.5X1 Poisoning by other estrogens and progestogens, accidental (unintentional)**
Poisoning by other estrogens and progestogens NOS

√7th **T38.5X2 Poisoning by other estrogens and progestogens, intentional self-harm** HCC

√7th **T38.5X3 Poisoning by other estrogens and progestogens, assault**

√7th **T38.5X4 Poisoning by other estrogens and progestogens, undetermined**

√7th **T38.5X5 Adverse effect of other estrogens and progestogens** UPD

√7th **T38.5X6 Underdosing of other estrogens and progestogens** UPD

√5th **T38.6 Poisoning by, adverse effect of and underdosing of antigonadotrophins, antiestrogens, antiandrogens, not elsewhere classified**
Poisoning by, adverse effect of and underdosing of tamoxifen

√6th **T38.6X Poisoning by, adverse effect of and underdosing of antigonadotrophins, antiestrogens, antiandrogens, not elsewhere classified**

√7th **T38.6X1 Poisoning by antigonadotrophins, antiestrogens, antiandrogens, not elsewhere classified, accidental (unintentional)**
Poisoning by antigonadotrophins, antiestrogens, antiandrogens, not elsewhere classified NOS

√7th **T38.6X2 Poisoning by antigonadotrophins, antiestrogens, antiandrogens, not elsewhere classified, intentional self-harm** HCC

√7th **T38.6X3 Poisoning by antigonadotrophins, antiestrogens, antiandrogens, not elsewhere classified, assault**

√7th **T38.6X4 Poisoning by antigonadotrophins, antiestrogens, antiandrogens, not elsewhere classified, undetermined**

√7th **T38.6X5 Adverse effect of antigonadotrophins, antiestrogens, antiandrogens, not elsewhere classified** UPD

√7th **T38.6X6 Underdosing of antigonadotrophins, antiestrogens, antiandrogens, not elsewhere classified** UPD

√5th **T38.7 Poisoning by, adverse effect of and underdosing of androgens and anabolic congeners**

√6th **T38.7X Poisoning by, adverse effect of and underdosing of androgens and anabolic congeners**

√7th **T38.7X1 Poisoning by androgens and anabolic congeners, accidental (unintentional)**
Poisoning by androgens and anabolic congeners NOS

√7th **T38.7X2 Poisoning by androgens and anabolic congeners, intentional self-harm** HCC

√7th **T38.7X3 Poisoning by androgens and anabolic congeners, assault**

√7th **T38.7X4 Poisoning by androgens and anabolic congeners, undetermined**

√7th **T38.7X5 Adverse effect of androgens and anabolic congeners** UPD

√7th **T38.7X6 Underdosing of androgens and anabolic congeners** UPD

√5th **T38.8 Poisoning by, adverse effect of and underdosing of other and unspecified hormones and synthetic substitutes**

√6th **T38.8Ø Poisoning by, adverse effect of and underdosing of unspecified hormones and synthetic substitutes**

√7th **T38.8Ø1 Poisoning by unspecified hormones and synthetic substitutes, accidental (unintentional)**
Poisoning by unspecified hormones and synthetic substitutes NOS

√7th **T38.8Ø2 Poisoning by unspecified hormones and synthetic substitutes, intentional self-harm** HCC

√7th **T38.8Ø3 Poisoning by unspecified hormones and synthetic substitutes, assault**

T38.804 Poisoning by unspecified hormones and synthetic substitutes, undetermined

T38.805 Adverse effect of unspecified hormones and synthetic substitutes UPD

T38.806 Underdosing of unspecified hormones and synthetic substitutes UPD

T38.81 Poisoning by, adverse effect of and underdosing of anterior pituitary [adenohypophyseal] hormones

T38.811 Poisoning by anterior pituitary [adenohypophyseal] hormones, accidental (unintentional)
Poisoning by anterior pituitary [adenohypophyseal] hormones NOS

T38.812 Poisoning by anterior pituitary [adenohypophyseal] hormones, intentional self-harm HCC

T38.813 Poisoning by anterior pituitary [adenohypophyseal] hormones, assault

T38.814 Poisoning by anterior pituitary [adenohypophyseal] hormones, undetermined

T38.815 Adverse effect of anterior pituitary [adenohypophyseal] hormones UPD

T38.816 Underdosing of anterior pituitary [adenohypophyseal] hormones UPD

T38.89 Poisoning by, adverse effect of and underdosing of other hormones and synthetic substitutes

T38.891 Poisoning by other hormones and synthetic substitutes, accidental (unintentional)
Poisoning by other hormones and synthetic substitutes NOS

T38.892 Poisoning by other hormones and synthetic substitutes, intentional self-harm HCC

T38.893 Poisoning by other hormones and synthetic substitutes, assault

T38.894 Poisoning by other hormones and synthetic substitutes, undetermined

T38.895 Adverse effect of other hormones and synthetic substitutes UPD

T38.896 Underdosing of other hormones and synthetic substitutes UPD

T38.9 Poisoning by, adverse effect of and underdosing of other and unspecified hormone antagonists

T38.90 Poisoning by, adverse effect of and underdosing of unspecified hormone antagonists

T38.901 Poisoning by unspecified hormone antagonists, accidental (unintentional)
Poisoning by unspecified hormone antagonists NOS

T38.902 Poisoning by unspecified hormone antagonists, intentional self-harm HCC

T38.903 Poisoning by unspecified hormone antagonists, assault

T38.904 Poisoning by unspecified hormone antagonists, undetermined

T38.905 Adverse effect of unspecified hormone antagonists UPD

T38.906 Underdosing of unspecified hormone antagonists UPD

T38.99 Poisoning by, adverse effect of and underdosing of other hormone antagonists

T38.991 Poisoning by other hormone antagonists, accidental (unintentional)
Poisoning by other hormone antagonists NOS

T38.992 Poisoning by other hormone antagonists, intentional self-harm HCC

T38.993 Poisoning by other hormone antagonists, assault

T38.994 Poisoning by other hormone antagonists, undetermined

T38.995 Adverse effect of other hormone antagonists UPD

T38.996 Underdosing of other hormone antagonists UPD

T39 Poisoning by, adverse effect of and underdosing of nonopioid analgesics, antipyretics and antirheumatics

The appropriate 7th character is to be added to each code from category T39.
A initial encounter
D subsequent encounter
S sequela

T39.0 Poisoning by, adverse effect of and underdosing of salicylates

T39.01 Poisoning by, adverse effect of and underdosing of aspirin
Poisoning by, adverse effect of and underdosing of acetylsalicylic acid

T39.011 Poisoning by aspirin, accidental (unintentional)

T39.012 Poisoning by aspirin, intentional self-harm HCC

T39.013 Poisoning by aspirin, assault

T39.014 Poisoning by aspirin, undetermined

T39.015 Adverse effect of aspirin UPD
AHA: 2016,1Q,15

T39.016 Underdosing of aspirin UPD

T39.09 Poisoning by, adverse effect of and underdosing of other salicylates

T39.091 Poisoning by salicylates, accidental (unintentional)
Poisoning by salicylates NOS

T39.092 Poisoning by salicylates, intentional self-harm HCC

T39.093 Poisoning by salicylates, assault

T39.094 Poisoning by salicylates, undetermined

T39.095 Adverse effect of salicylates UPD

T39.096 Underdosing of salicylates UPD

T39.1 Poisoning by, adverse effect of and underdosing of 4-Aminophenol derivatives

T39.1X Poisoning by, adverse effect of and underdosing of 4-Aminophenol derivatives

T39.1X1 Poisoning by 4-Aminophenol derivatives, accidental (unintentional)
Poisoning by 4-Aminophenol derivatives NOS

T39.1X2 Poisoning by 4-Aminophenol derivatives, intentional self-harm HCC

T39.1X3 Poisoning by 4-Aminophenol derivatives, assault

T39.1X4 Poisoning by 4-Aminophenol derivatives, undetermined

T39.1X5 Adverse effect of 4-Aminophenol derivatives UPD

T39.1X6 Underdosing of 4-Aminophenol derivatives UPD

T39.2 Poisoning by, adverse effect of and underdosing of pyrazolone derivatives

T39.2X Poisoning by, adverse effect of and underdosing of pyrazolone derivatives

T39.2X1 Poisoning by pyrazolone derivatives, accidental (unintentional)
Poisoning by pyrazolone derivatives NOS

T39.2X2 Poisoning by pyrazolone derivatives, intentional self-harm HCC

T39.2X3 Poisoning by pyrazolone derivatives, assault

T39.2X4 Poisoning by pyrazolone derivatives, undetermined

T39.2X5 Adverse effect of pyrazolone derivatives UPD

T39.2X6 Underdosing of pyrazolone derivatives UPD

T39.3 Poisoning by, adverse effect of and underdosing of other nonsteroidal anti-inflammatory drugs [NSAID]

T39.31 Poisoning by, adverse effect of and underdosing of propionic acid derivatives

Poisoning by, adverse effect of and underdosing of fenoprofen

Poisoning by, adverse effect of and underdosing of flurbiprofen

Poisoning by, adverse effect of and underdosing of ibuprofen

Poisoning by, adverse effect of and underdosing of ketoprofen

Poisoning by, adverse effect of and underdosing of naproxen

Poisoning by, adverse effect of and underdosing of oxaprozin

T39.311 Poisoning by propionic acid derivatives, accidental (unintentional)

T39.312 Poisoning by propionic acid derivatives, intentional self-harm HCC

T39.313 Poisoning by propionic acid derivatives, assault

T39.314 Poisoning by propionic acid derivatives, undetermined

T39.315 Adverse effect of propionic acid derivatives UPD

T39.316 Underdosing of propionic acid derivatives UPD

T39.39 Poisoning by, adverse effect of and underdosing of other nonsteroidal anti-inflammatory drugs [NSAID]

T39.391 Poisoning by other nonsteroidal anti-inflammatory drugs [NSAID], accidental (unintentional)

Poisoning by other nonsteroidal anti-inflammatory drugs NOS

T39.392 Poisoning by other nonsteroidal anti-inflammatory drugs [NSAID], intentional self-harm HCC

T39.393 Poisoning by other nonsteroidal anti-inflammatory drugs [NSAID], assault

T39.394 Poisoning by other nonsteroidal anti-inflammatory drugs [NSAID], undetermined

T39.395 Adverse effect of other nonsteroidal anti-inflammatory drugs [NSAID] UPD

T39.396 Underdosing of other nonsteroidal anti-inflammatory drugs [NSAID] UPD

T39.4 Poisoning by, adverse effect of and underdosing of antirheumatics, not elsewhere classified

EXCLUDES 1 *poisoning by, adverse effect of and underdosing of glucocorticoids (T38.0-)*

poisoning by, adverse effect of and underdosing of salicylates (T39.0-)

T39.4X Poisoning by, adverse effect of and underdosing of antirheumatics, not elsewhere classified

T39.4X1 Poisoning by antirheumatics, not elsewhere classified, accidental (unintentional)

Poisoning by antirheumatics, not elsewhere classified NOS

T39.4X2 Poisoning by antirheumatics, not elsewhere classified, intentional self-harm HCC

T39.4X3 Poisoning by antirheumatics, not elsewhere classified, assault

T39.4X4 Poisoning by antirheumatics, not elsewhere classified, undetermined

T39.4X5 Adverse effect of antirheumatics, not elsewhere classified UPD

T39.4X6 Underdosing of antirheumatics, not elsewhere classified UPD

T39.8 Poisoning by, adverse effect of and underdosing of other nonopioid analgesics and antipyretics, not elsewhere classified

T39.8X Poisoning by, adverse effect of and underdosing of other nonopioid analgesics and antipyretics, not elsewhere classified

T39.8X1 Poisoning by other nonopioid analgesics and antipyretics, not elsewhere classified, accidental (unintentional)

Poisoning by other nonopioid analgesics and antipyretics, not elsewhere classified NOS

T39.8X2 Poisoning by other nonopioid analgesics and antipyretics, not elsewhere classified, intentional self-harm HCC

T39.8X3 Poisoning by other nonopioid analgesics and antipyretics, not elsewhere classified, assault

T39.8X4 Poisoning by other nonopioid analgesics and antipyretics, not elsewhere classified, undetermined

T39.8X5 Adverse effect of other nonopioid analgesics and antipyretics, not elsewhere classified UPD

T39.8X6 Underdosing of other nonopioid analgesics and antipyretics, not elsewhere classified UPD

T39.9 Poisoning by, adverse effect of and underdosing of unspecified nonopioid analgesic, antipyretic and antirheumatic

T39.91 Poisoning by unspecified nonopioid analgesic, antipyretic and antirheumatic, accidental (unintentional)

Poisoning by nonopioid analgesic, antipyretic and antirheumatic NOS

T39.92 Poisoning by unspecified nonopioid analgesic, antipyretic and antirheumatic, intentional self-harm HCC

T39.93 Poisoning by unspecified nonopioid analgesic, antipyretic and antirheumatic, assault

T39.94 Poisoning by unspecified nonopioid analgesic, antipyretic and antirheumatic, undetermined

T39.95 Adverse effect of unspecified nonopioid analgesic, antipyretic and antirheumatic UPD

T39.96 Underdosing of unspecified nonopioid analgesic, antipyretic and antirheumatic UPD

T40 Poisoning by, adverse effect of and underdosing of narcotics and psychodysleptics [hallucinogens]

EXCLUDES 2 *drug dependence and related mental and behavioral disorders due to psychoactive substance use (F10.-F19.-)*

The appropriate 7th character is to be added to each code from category T40.

A initial encounter
D subsequent encounter
S sequela

T40.0 Poisoning by, adverse effect of and underdosing of opium

T40.0X Poisoning by, adverse effect of and underdosing of opium

T40.0X1 Poisoning by opium, accidental (unintentional) HCC

Poisoning by opium NOS

T40.0X2 Poisoning by opium, intentional self-harm HCC

T40.0X3 Poisoning by opium, assault

T40.0X4 Poisoning by opium, undetermined HCC

T40.0X5 Adverse effect of opium UPD

T40.0X6 Underdosing of opium UPD

T40.1 Poisoning by and adverse effect of heroin

T40.1X Poisoning by and adverse effect of heroin

T40.1X1 Poisoning by heroin, accidental (unintentional) HCC

Poisoning by heroin NOS

T40.1X2 Poisoning by heroin, intentional self-harm HCC

T40.1X3 Poisoning by heroin, assault

T40.1X4 Poisoning by heroin, undetermined HCC

T40.2 Poisoning by, adverse effect of and underdosing of other opioids
- **T40.2X Poisoning by, adverse effect of and underdosing of other opioids**
  - **T40.2X1 Poisoning by other opioids, accidental (unintentional)** HCC
    - Poisoning by other opioids NOS
  - **T40.2X2 Poisoning by other opioids, intentional self-harm** HCC
  - **T40.2X3 Poisoning by other opioids, assault**
  - **T40.2X4 Poisoning by other opioids, undetermined** HCC
  - **T40.2X5 Adverse effect of other opioids** UPD
    - AHA: 2020,2Q,24
  - **T40.2X6 Underdosing of other opioids** UPD

T40.3 Poisoning by, adverse effect of and underdosing of methadone
- **T40.3X Poisoning by, adverse effect of and underdosing of methadone**
  - **T40.3X1 Poisoning by methadone, accidental (unintentional)** HCC
    - Poisoning by methadone NOS
  - **T40.3X2 Poisoning by methadone, intentional self-harm** HCC
  - **T40.3X3 Poisoning by methadone, assault**
  - **T40.3X4 Poisoning by methadone, undetermined** HCC
  - **T40.3X5 Adverse effect of methadone** UPD
  - **T40.3X6 Underdosing of methadone** UPD

T40.4 Poisoning by, adverse effect of and underdosing of other synthetic narcotics
- AHA: 2020,4Q,40
- **T40.41 Poisoning by, adverse effect of and underdosing of fentanyl or fentanyl analogs**
  - **T40.411 Poisoning by fentanyl or fentanyl analogs, accidental (unintentional)** HCC
  - **T40.412 Poisoning by fentanyl or fentanyl analogs, intentional self-harm** HCC
  - **T40.413 Poisoning by fentanyl or fentanyl analogs, assault**
  - **T40.414 Poisoning by fentanyl or fentanyl analogs, undetermined** HCC
  - **T40.415 Adverse effect of fentanyl or fentanyl analogs** UPD
  - **T40.416 Underdosing of fentanyl or fentanyl analogs** UPD
- **T40.42 Poisoning by, adverse effect of and underdosing of tramadol**
  - **T40.421 Poisoning by tramadol, accidental (unintentional)** HCC
  - **T40.422 Poisoning by tramadol, intentional self-harm** HCC
  - **T40.423 Poisoning by tramadol, assault**
  - **T40.424 Poisoning by tramadol, undetermined** HCC
  - **T40.425 Adverse effect of tramadol** UPD
  - **T40.426 Underdosing of tramadol** UPD
- **T40.49 Poisoning by, adverse effect of and underdosing of other synthetic narcotics**
  - **T40.491 Poisoning by other synthetic narcotics, accidental (unintentional)** HCC
  - **T40.492 Poisoning by other synthetic narcotics, intentional self-harm** HCC
  - **T40.493 Poisoning by other synthetic narcotics, assault**
  - **T40.494 Poisoning by other synthetic narcotics, undetermined** HCC
  - **T40.495 Adverse effect of other synthetic narcotics** UPD
  - **T40.496 Underdosing of other synthetic narcotics** UPD

T40.5 Poisoning by, adverse effect of and underdosing of cocaine
- **T40.5X Poisoning by, adverse effect of and underdosing of cocaine**
  - **T40.5X1 Poisoning by cocaine, accidental (unintentional)** HCC
    - Poisoning by cocaine NOS
    - AHA: 2016,2Q,8
  - **T40.5X2 Poisoning by cocaine, intentional self-harm** HCC
  - **T40.5X3 Poisoning by cocaine, assault**
  - **T40.5X4 Poisoning by cocaine, undetermined** HCC
  - **T40.5X5 Adverse effect of cocaine** UPD
  - **T40.5X6 Underdosing of cocaine** UPD

T40.6 Poisoning by, adverse effect of and underdosing of other and unspecified narcotics
- **T40.60 Poisoning by, adverse effect of and underdosing of unspecified narcotics**
  - **T40.601 Poisoning by unspecified narcotics, accidental (unintentional)** HCC
    - Poisoning by narcotics NOS
  - **T40.602 Poisoning by unspecified narcotics, intentional self-harm** HCC
  - **T40.603 Poisoning by unspecified narcotics, assault**
  - **T40.604 Poisoning by unspecified narcotics, undetermined** HCC
  - **T40.605 Adverse effect of unspecified narcotics** UPD
  - **T40.606 Underdosing of unspecified narcotics** UPD
- **T40.69 Poisoning by, adverse effect of and underdosing of other narcotics**
  - **T40.691 Poisoning by other narcotics, accidental (unintentional)** HCC
    - Poisoning by other narcotics NOS
  - **T40.692 Poisoning by other narcotics, intentional self-harm** HCC
  - **T40.693 Poisoning by other narcotics, assault**
  - **T40.694 Poisoning by other narcotics, undetermined** HCC
  - **T40.695 Adverse effect of other narcotics** UPD
  - **T40.696 Underdosing of other narcotics** UPD

T40.7 Poisoning by, adverse effect of and underdosing of cannabis (derivatives)
- **T40.71 Poisoning by, adverse effect of and underdosing of cannabis (derivatives)**
  - AHA: 2021,4Q,30
  - **T40.711 Poisoning by cannabis, accidental (unintentional)**
  - **T40.712 Poisoning by cannabis, intentional self-harm** HCC
  - **T40.713 Poisoning by cannabis, assault**
  - **T40.714 Poisoning by cannabis, undetermined**
  - **T40.715 Adverse effect of cannabis** UPD
  - **T40.716 Underdosing of cannabis** UPD
- **T40.72 Poisoning by, adverse effect of and underdosing of synthetic cannabinoids**
  - AHA: 2021,4Q,30
  - **T40.721 Poisoning by synthetic cannabinoids, accidental (unintentional)**
  - **T40.722 Poisoning by synthetic cannabinoids, intentional self-harm** HCC
  - **T40.723 Poisoning by synthetic cannabinoids, assault**
  - **T40.724 Poisoning by synthetic cannabinoids, undetermined**
  - **T40.725 Adverse effect of synthetic cannabinoids** UPD
  - **T40.726 Underdosing of synthetic cannabinoids** UPD

T40.8 Poisoning by and adverse effect of lysergide [LSD]
- **T40.8X Poisoning by and adverse effect of lysergide [LSD]**
  - **T40.8X1 Poisoning by lysergide [LSD], accidental (unintentional)** HCC
    - Poisoning by lysergide [LSD] NOS
  - **T40.8X2 Poisoning by lysergide [LSD], intentional self-harm** HCC

√7th T40.8X3 Poisoning by lysergide [LSD], assault
√7th T40.8X4 Poisoning by lysergide [LSD], undetermined HCC

√5th T40.9 Poisoning by, adverse effect of and underdosing of other and unspecified psychodysleptics [hallucinogens]

√6th T40.90 Poisoning by, adverse effect of and underdosing of unspecified psychodysleptics [hallucinogens]

√7th T40.901 Poisoning by unspecified psychodysleptics [hallucinogens], accidental (unintentional) HCC
√7th T40.902 Poisoning by unspecified psychodysleptics [hallucinogens], intentional self-harm HCC
√7th T40.903 Poisoning by unspecified psychodysleptics [hallucinogens], assault
√7th T40.904 Poisoning by unspecified psychodysleptics [hallucinogens], undetermined HCC
√7th T40.905 Adverse effect of unspecified psychodysleptics [hallucinogens] UPD
√7th T40.906 Underdosing of unspecified psychodysleptics [hallucinogens] UPD

√6th T40.99 Poisoning by, adverse effect of and underdosing of other psychodysleptics [hallucinogens]

√7th T40.991 Poisoning by other psychodysleptics [hallucinogens], accidental (unintentional) HCC
Poisoning by other psychodysleptics [hallucinogens] NOS
√7th T40.992 Poisoning by other psychodysleptics [hallucinogens], intentional self-harm HCC
√7th T40.993 Poisoning by other psychodysleptics [hallucinogens], assault
√7th T40.994 Poisoning by other psychodysleptics [hallucinogens], undetermined HCC
√7th T40.995 Adverse effect of other psychodysleptics [hallucinogens] UPD
√7th T40.996 Underdosing of other psychodysleptics [hallucinogens] UPD

√4th T41 Poisoning by, adverse effect of and underdosing of anesthetics and therapeutic gases

EXCLUDES 1 benzodiazepines (T42.4-)
cocaine (T40.5-)
complications of anesthesia during labor and delivery (O74.-)
complications of anesthesia during pregnancy (O29.-)
complications of anesthesia during the puerperium (O89.-)
opioids (T40.0-T40.2-)

The appropriate 7th character is to be added to each code from category T41.
A initial encounter
D subsequent encounter
S sequela

√5th T41.0 Poisoning by, adverse effect of and underdosing of inhaled anesthetics

EXCLUDES 1 oxygen (T41.5-)

√6th T41.0X Poisoning by, adverse effect of and underdosing of inhaled anesthetics

√7th T41.0X1 Poisoning by inhaled anesthetics, accidental (unintentional)
Poisoning by inhaled anesthetics NOS
√7th T41.0X2 Poisoning by inhaled anesthetics, intentional self-harm HCC
√7th T41.0X3 Poisoning by inhaled anesthetics, assault
√7th T41.0X4 Poisoning by inhaled anesthetics, undetermined
√7th T41.0X5 Adverse effect of inhaled anesthetics UPD
√7th T41.0X6 Underdosing of inhaled anesthetics UPD

√5th T41.1 Poisoning by, adverse effect of and underdosing of intravenous anesthetics
Poisoning by, adverse effect of and underdosing of thiobarbiturates

√6th T41.1X Poisoning by, adverse effect of and underdosing of intravenous anesthetics

√7th T41.1X1 Poisoning by intravenous anesthetics, accidental (unintentional)
Poisoning by intravenous anesthetics NOS
√7th T41.1X2 Poisoning by intravenous anesthetics, intentional self-harm HCC
√7th T41.1X3 Poisoning by intravenous anesthetics, assault
√7th T41.1X4 Poisoning by intravenous anesthetics, undetermined
√7th T41.1X5 Adverse effect of intravenous anesthetics UPD
√7th T41.1X6 Underdosing of intravenous anesthetics UPD

√5th T41.2 Poisoning by, adverse effect of and underdosing of other and unspecified general anesthetics

√6th T41.20 Poisoning by, adverse effect of and underdosing of unspecified general anesthetics

√7th T41.201 Poisoning by unspecified general anesthetics, accidental (unintentional)
Poisoning by general anesthetics NOS
√7th T41.202 Poisoning by unspecified general anesthetics, intentional self-harm HCC
√7th T41.203 Poisoning by unspecified general anesthetics, assault
√7th T41.204 Poisoning by unspecified general anesthetics, undetermined
√7th T41.205 Adverse effect of unspecified general anesthetics UPD
AHA: 2016,4Q,73
√7th T41.206 Underdosing of unspecified general anesthetics UPD

√6th T41.29 Poisoning by, adverse effect of and underdosing of other general anesthetics

√7th T41.291 Poisoning by other general anesthetics, accidental (unintentional)
Poisoning by other general anesthetics NOS
√7th T41.292 Poisoning by other general anesthetics, intentional self-harm HCC
√7th T41.293 Poisoning by other general anesthetics, assault
√7th T41.294 Poisoning by other general anesthetics, undetermined
√7th T41.295 Adverse effect of other general anesthetics UPD
√7th T41.296 Underdosing of other general anesthetics UPD

√5th T41.3 Poisoning by, adverse effect of and underdosing of local anesthetics
Cocaine (topical)

EXCLUDES 2 poisoning by cocaine used as a central nervous system stimulant (T40.5X1-T40.5X4)

√6th T41.3X Poisoning by, adverse effect of and underdosing of local anesthetics

√7th T41.3X1 Poisoning by local anesthetics, accidental (unintentional)
Poisoning by local anesthetics NOS
√7th T41.3X2 Poisoning by local anesthetics, intentional self-harm HCC
√7th T41.3X3 Poisoning by local anesthetics, assault
√7th T41.3X4 Poisoning by local anesthetics, undetermined
√7th T41.3X5 Adverse effect of local anesthetics UPD
√7th T41.3X6 Underdosing of local anesthetics UPD

√5th T41.4 Poisoning by, adverse effect of and underdosing of unspecified anesthetic

√x7th T41.41 Poisoning by unspecified anesthetic, accidental (unintentional)
Poisoning by anesthetic NOS
√x7th T41.42 Poisoning by unspecified anesthetic, intentional self-harm HCC
√x7th T41.43 Poisoning by unspecified anesthetic, assault
√x7th T41.44 Poisoning by unspecified anesthetic, undetermined
√x7th T41.45 Adverse effect of unspecified anesthetic UPD
√x7th T41.46 Underdosing of unspecified anesthetics UPD

√5th T41.5 Poisoning by, adverse effect of and underdosing of therapeutic gases

√6th T41.5X Poisoning by, adverse effect of and underdosing of therapeutic gases

√7th T41.5X1 Poisoning by therapeutic gases, accidental (unintentional)
Poisoning by therapeutic gases NOS

T41.5X2 Poisoning by therapeutic gases, intentional self-harm HCC
T41.5X3 Poisoning by therapeutic gases, assault
T41.5X4 Poisoning by therapeutic gases, undetermined
T41.5X5 Adverse effect of therapeutic gases UPD
T41.5X6 Underdosing of therapeutic gases UPD

T42 Poisoning by, adverse effect of and underdosing of antiepileptic, sedative- hypnotic and antiparkinsonism drugs

EXCLUDES 2 *drug dependence and related mental and behavioral disorders due to psychoactive substance use (F1Ø.- - F19.-)*

The appropriate 7th character is to be added to each code from category T42.
A initial encounter
D subsequent encounter
S sequela

T42.Ø Poisoning by, adverse effect of and underdosing of hydantoin derivatives
T42.ØX Poisoning by, adverse effect of and underdosing of hydantoin derivatives
T42.ØX1 Poisoning by hydantoin derivatives, accidental (unintentional)
Poisoning by hydantoin derivatives NOS
T42.ØX2 Poisoning by hydantoin derivatives, intentional self-harm HCC
T42.ØX3 Poisoning by hydantoin derivatives, assault
T42.ØX4 Poisoning by hydantoin derivatives, undetermined
T42.ØX5 Adverse effect of hydantoin derivatives UPD
T42.ØX6 Underdosing of hydantoin derivatives UPD

T42.1 Poisoning by, adverse effect of and underdosing of iminostilbenes
Poisoning by, adverse effect of and underdosing of carbamazepine
T42.1X Poisoning by, adverse effect of and underdosing of iminostilbenes
T42.1X1 Poisoning by iminostilbenes, accidental (unintentional)
Poisoning by iminostilbenes NOS
T42.1X2 Poisoning by iminostilbenes, intentional self-harm HCC
T42.1X3 Poisoning by iminostilbenes, assault
T42.1X4 Poisoning by iminostilbenes, undetermined
T42.1X5 Adverse effect of iminostilbenes UPD
T42.1X6 Underdosing of iminostilbenes UPD

T42.2 Poisoning by, adverse effect of and underdosing of succinimides and oxazolidinediones
T42.2X Poisoning by, adverse effect of and underdosing of succinimides and oxazolidinediones
T42.2X1 Poisoning by succinimides and oxazolidinediones, accidental (unintentional)
Poisoning by succinimides and oxazolidinediones NOS
T42.2X2 Poisoning by succinimides and oxazolidinediones, intentional self-harm HCC
T42.2X3 Poisoning by succinimides and oxazolidinediones, assault
T42.2X4 Poisoning by succinimides and oxazolidinediones, undetermined
T42.2X5 Adverse effect of succinimides and oxazolidinediones UPD
T42.2X6 Underdosing of succinimides and oxazolidinediones UPD

T42.3 Poisoning by, adverse effect of and underdosing of barbiturates
EXCLUDES 1 *poisoning by, adverse effect of and underdosing of thiobarbiturates (T41.1-)*
T42.3X Poisoning by, adverse effect of and underdosing of barbiturates
T42.3X1 Poisoning by barbiturates, accidental (unintentional)
Poisoning by barbiturates NOS
T42.3X2 Poisoning by barbiturates, intentional self-harm HCC
T42.3X3 Poisoning by barbiturates, assault
T42.3X4 Poisoning by barbiturates, undetermined
T42.3X5 Adverse effect of barbiturates UPD
T42.3X6 Underdosing of barbiturates UPD

T42.4 Poisoning by, adverse effect of and underdosing of benzodiazepines
T42.4X Poisoning by, adverse effect of and underdosing of benzodiazepines
T42.4X1 Poisoning by benzodiazepines, accidental (unintentional)
Poisoning by benzodiazepines NOS
T42.4X2 Poisoning by benzodiazepines, intentional self-harm HCC
T42.4X3 Poisoning by benzodiazepines, assault
T42.4X4 Poisoning by benzodiazepines, undetermined
T42.4X5 Adverse effect of benzodiazepines UPD
T42.4X6 Underdosing of benzodiazepines UPD

T42.5 Poisoning by, adverse effect of and underdosing of mixed antiepileptics
T42.5X Poisoning by, adverse effect of and underdosing of antiepileptics
T42.5X1 Poisoning by mixed antiepileptics, accidental (unintentional)
Poisoning by mixed antiepileptics NOS
T42.5X2 Poisoning by mixed antiepileptics, intentional self-harm HCC
T42.5X3 Poisoning by mixed antiepileptics, assault
T42.5X4 Poisoning by mixed antiepileptics, undetermined
T42.5X5 Adverse effect of mixed antiepileptics UPD
T42.5X6 Underdosing of mixed antiepileptics UPD

T42.6 Poisoning by, adverse effect of and underdosing of other antiepileptic and sedative-hypnotic drugs
Poisoning by, adverse effect of and underdosing of methaqualone
Poisoning by, adverse effect of and underdosing of valproic acid
EXCLUDES 1 *poisoning by, adverse effect of and underdosing of carbamazepine (T42.1-)*
T42.6X Poisoning by, adverse effect of and underdosing of other antiepileptic and sedative-hypnotic drugs
T42.6X1 Poisoning by other antiepileptic and sedative-hypnotic drugs, accidental (unintentional)
Poisoning by other antiepileptic and sedative-hypnotic drugs NOS
T42.6X2 Poisoning by other antiepileptic and sedative-hypnotic drugs, intentional self-harm HCC
T42.6X3 Poisoning by other antiepileptic and sedative-hypnotic drugs, assault
T42.6X4 Poisoning by other antiepileptic and sedative-hypnotic drugs, undetermined
T42.6X5 Adverse effect of other antiepileptic and sedative-hypnotic drugs UPD
T42.6X6 Underdosing of other antiepileptic and sedative-hypnotic drugs UPD

T42.7 Poisoning by, adverse effect of and underdosing of unspecified antiepileptic and sedative-hypnotic drugs
T42.71 Poisoning by unspecified antiepileptic and sedative-hypnotic drugs, accidental (unintentional)
Poisoning by antiepileptic and sedative-hypnotic drugs NOS
T42.72 Poisoning by unspecified antiepileptic and sedative-hypnotic drugs, intentional self-harm HCC
T42.73 Poisoning by unspecified antiepileptic and sedative-hypnotic drugs, assault
T42.74 Poisoning by unspecified antiepileptic and sedative-hypnotic drugs, undetermined
T42.75 Adverse effect of unspecified antiepileptic and sedative-hypnotic drugs UPD
T42.76 Underdosing of unspecified antiepileptic and sedative-hypnotic drugs UPD

5th T42.8 Poisoning by, adverse effect of and underdosing of antiparkinsonism drugs and other central muscle-tone depressants
Poisoning by, adverse effect of and underdosing of amantadine

6th T42.8X Poisoning by, adverse effect of and underdosing of antiparkinsonism drugs and other central muscle-tone depressants

7th T42.8X1 Poisoning by antiparkinsonism drugs and other central muscle-tone depressants, accidental (unintentional)
Poisoning by antiparkinsonism drugs and other central muscle-tone depressants NOS

7th T42.8X2 Poisoning by antiparkinsonism drugs and other central muscle-tone depressants, intentional self-harm HCC

7th T42.8X3 Poisoning by antiparkinsonism drugs and other central muscle-tone depressants, assault

7th T42.8X4 Poisoning by antiparkinsonism drugs and other central muscle-tone depressants, undetermined

7th T42.8X5 Adverse effect of antiparkinsonism drugs and other central muscle-tone depressants UPD

7th T42.8X6 Underdosing of antiparkinsonism drugs and other central muscle-tone depressants UPD

4th T43 Poisoning by, adverse effect of and underdosing of psychotropic drugs, not elsewhere classified

EXCLUDES 1 *appetite depressants (T50.5-)*
barbiturates (T42.3-)
benzodiazepines (T42.4-)
methaqualone (T42.6-)
psychodysleptics [hallucinogens] (T40.7-T40.9-)

EXCLUDES 2 *drug dependence and related mental and behavioral disorders due to psychoactive substance use (F10.- – F19.-)*

The appropriate 7th character is to be added to each code from category T43.
A initial encounter
D subsequent encounter
S sequela

5th T43.0 Poisoning by, adverse effect of and underdosing of tricyclic and tetracyclic antidepressants

6th T43.01 Poisoning by, adverse effect of and underdosing of tricyclic antidepressants

7th T43.011 Poisoning by tricyclic antidepressants, accidental (unintentional)
Poisoning by tricyclic antidepressants NOS

7th T43.012 Poisoning by tricyclic antidepressants, intentional self-harm HCC

7th T43.013 Poisoning by tricyclic antidepressants, assault

7th T43.014 Poisoning by tricyclic antidepressants, undetermined

7th T43.015 Adverse effect of tricyclic antidepressants UPD

7th T43.016 Underdosing of tricyclic antidepressants UPD

6th T43.02 Poisoning by, adverse effect of and underdosing of tetracyclic antidepressants

7th T43.021 Poisoning by tetracyclic antidepressants, accidental (unintentional)
Poisoning by tetracyclic antidepressants NOS

7th T43.022 Poisoning by tetracyclic antidepressants, intentional self-harm HCC

7th T43.023 Poisoning by tetracyclic antidepressants, assault

7th T43.024 Poisoning by tetracyclic antidepressants, undetermined

7th T43.025 Adverse effect of tetracyclic antidepressants UPD

7th T43.026 Underdosing of tetracyclic antidepressants UPD

5th T43.1 Poisoning by, adverse effect of and underdosing of monoamine-oxidase-inhibitor antidepressants

6th T43.1X Poisoning by, adverse effect of and underdosing of monoamine-oxidase-inhibitor antidepressants

7th T43.1X1 Poisoning by monoamine-oxidase-inhibitor antidepressants, accidental (unintentional)
Poisoning by monoamine-oxidase-inhibitor antidepressants NOS

7th T43.1X2 Poisoning by monoamine-oxidase-inhibitor antidepressants, intentional self-harm HCC

7th T43.1X3 Poisoning by monoamine-oxidase-inhibitor antidepressants, assault

7th T43.1X4 Poisoning by monoamine-oxidase-inhibitor antidepressants, undetermined

7th T43.1X5 Adverse effect of monoamine-oxidase-inhibitor antidepressants UPD

7th T43.1X6 Underdosing of monoamine-oxidase-inhibitor antidepressants UPD

5th T43.2 Poisoning by, adverse effect of and underdosing of other and unspecified antidepressants

6th T43.20 Poisoning by, adverse effect of and underdosing of unspecified antidepressants

7th T43.201 Poisoning by unspecified antidepressants, accidental (unintentional)
Poisoning by antidepressants NOS

7th T43.202 Poisoning by unspecified antidepressants, intentional self-harm HCC

7th T43.203 Poisoning by unspecified antidepressants, assault

7th T43.204 Poisoning by unspecified antidepressants, undetermined

7th T43.205 Adverse effect of unspecified antidepressants UPD
Antidepressant discontinuation syndrome

7th T43.206 Underdosing of unspecified antidepressants UPD

6th T43.21 Poisoning by, adverse effect of and underdosing of selective serotonin and norepinephrine reuptake inhibitors
Poisoning by, adverse effect of and underdosing of SSNRI antidepressants

7th T43.211 Poisoning by selective serotonin and norepinephrine reuptake inhibitors, accidental (unintentional)

7th T43.212 Poisoning by selective serotonin and norepinephrine reuptake inhibitors, intentional self-harm HCC

7th T43.213 Poisoning by selective serotonin and norepinephrine reuptake inhibitors, assault

7th T43.214 Poisoning by selective serotonin and norepinephrine reuptake inhibitors, undetermined

7th T43.215 Adverse effect of selective serotonin and norepinephrine reuptake inhibitors UPD

7th T43.216 Underdosing of selective serotonin and norepinephrine reuptake inhibitors UPD

6th T43.22 Poisoning by, adverse effect of and underdosing of selective serotonin reuptake inhibitors
Poisoning by, adverse effect of and underdosing of SSRI antidepressants

7th T43.221 Poisoning by selective serotonin reuptake inhibitors, accidental (unintentional)

7th T43.222 Poisoning by selective serotonin reuptake inhibitors, intentional self-harm HCC

7th T43.223 Poisoning by selective serotonin reuptake inhibitors, assault

7th T43.224 Poisoning by selective serotonin reuptake inhibitors, undetermined

T43.225 Adverse effect of selective serotonin reuptake inhibitors UPD
AHA: 2022,2Q,11

T43.226 Underdosing of selective serotonin reuptake inhibitors UPD

T43.29 Poisoning by, adverse effect of and underdosing of other antidepressants

T43.291 Poisoning by other antidepressants, accidental (unintentional)
Poisoning by other antidepressants NOS

T43.292 Poisoning by other antidepressants, intentional self-harm HCC

T43.293 Poisoning by other antidepressants, assault

T43.294 Poisoning by other antidepressants, undetermined

T43.295 Adverse effect of other antidepressants UPD

T43.296 Underdosing of other antidepressants UPD

T43.3 Poisoning by, adverse effect of and underdosing of phenothiazine antipsychotics and neuroleptics

T43.3X Poisoning by, adverse effect of and underdosing of phenothiazine antipsychotics and neuroleptics

T43.3X1 Poisoning by phenothiazine antipsychotics and neuroleptics, accidental (unintentional)
Poisoning by phenothiazine antipsychotics and neuroleptics NOS

T43.3X2 Poisoning by phenothiazine antipsychotics and neuroleptics, intentional self-harm HCC

T43.3X3 Poisoning by phenothiazine antipsychotics and neuroleptics, assault

T43.3X4 Poisoning by phenothiazine antipsychotics and neuroleptics, undetermined

T43.3X5 Adverse effect of phenothiazine antipsychotics and neuroleptics UPD

T43.3X6 Underdosing of phenothiazine antipsychotics and neuroleptics UPD

T43.4 Poisoning by, adverse effect of and underdosing of butyrophenone and thiothixene neuroleptics

T43.4X Poisoning by, adverse effect of and underdosing of butyrophenone and thiothixene neuroleptics

T43.4X1 Poisoning by butyrophenone and thiothixene neuroleptics, accidental (unintentional)
Poisoning by butyrophenone and thiothixene neuroleptics NOS

T43.4X2 Poisoning by butyrophenone and thiothixene neuroleptics, intentional self-harm HCC

T43.4X3 Poisoning by butyrophenone and thiothixene neuroleptics, assault

T43.4X4 Poisoning by butyrophenone and thiothixene neuroleptics, undetermined

T43.4X5 Adverse effect of butyrophenone and thiothixene neuroleptics UPD

T43.4X6 Underdosing of butyrophenone and thiothixene neuroleptics UPD

T43.5 Poisoning by, adverse effect of and underdosing of other and unspecified antipsychotics and neuroleptics
EXCLUDES 1 *poisoning by, adverse effect of and underdosing of rauwolfia (T46.5-)*

T43.50 Poisoning by, adverse effect of and underdosing of unspecified antipsychotics and neuroleptics

T43.501 Poisoning by unspecified antipsychotics and neuroleptics, accidental (unintentional)
Poisoning by antipsychotics and neuroleptics NOS

T43.502 Poisoning by unspecified antipsychotics and neuroleptics, intentional self-harm HCC

T43.503 Poisoning by unspecified antipsychotics and neuroleptics, assault

T43.504 Poisoning by unspecified antipsychotics and neuroleptics, undetermined

T43.505 Adverse effect of unspecified antipsychotics and neuroleptics UPD
AHA: 2022,4Q,24

T43.506 Underdosing of unspecified antipsychotics and neuroleptics UPD

T43.59 Poisoning by, adverse effect of and underdosing of other antipsychotics and neuroleptics
AHA: 2017,1Q,40

T43.591 Poisoning by other antipsychotics and neuroleptics, accidental (unintentional)
Poisoning by other antipsychotics and neuroleptics NOS

T43.592 Poisoning by other antipsychotics and neuroleptics, intentional self-harm HCC

T43.593 Poisoning by other antipsychotics and neuroleptics, assault

T43.594 Poisoning by other antipsychotics and neuroleptics, undetermined

T43.595 Adverse effect of other antipsychotics and neuroleptics UPD
AHA: 2022,2Q,11

T43.596 Underdosing of other antipsychotics and neuroleptics UPD

T43.6 Poisoning by, adverse effect of and underdosing of psychostimulants
EXCLUDES 1 *poisoning by, adverse effect of and underdosing of cocaine (T40.5-)*

T43.60 Poisoning by, adverse effect of and underdosing of unspecified psychostimulant

T43.601 Poisoning by unspecified psychostimulants, accidental (unintentional) HCC
Poisoning by psychostimulants NOS

T43.602 Poisoning by unspecified psychostimulants, intentional self-harm HCC

T43.603 Poisoning by unspecified psychostimulants, assault

T43.604 Poisoning by unspecified psychostimulants, undetermined HCC

T43.605 Adverse effect of unspecified psychostimulants UPD

T43.606 Underdosing of unspecified psychostimulants UPD

T43.61 Poisoning by, adverse effect of and underdosing of caffeine

T43.611 Poisoning by caffeine, accidental (unintentional) HCC
Poisoning by caffeine NOS

T43.612 Poisoning by caffeine, intentional self-harm HCC

T43.613 Poisoning by caffeine, assault

T43.614 Poisoning by caffeine, undetermined HCC

T43.615 Adverse effect of caffeine UPD

T43.616 Underdosing of caffeine UPD

T43.62 Poisoning by, adverse effect of and underdosing of amphetamines

T43.621 Poisoning by amphetamines, accidental (unintentional) HCC
Poisoning by amphetamines NOS
AHA: 2021,3Q,8

T43.622 Poisoning by amphetamines, intentional self-harm HCC

T43.623 Poisoning by amphetamines, assault

T43.624 Poisoning by amphetamines, undetermined HCC

T43.625 Adverse effect of amphetamines UPD

T43.626 Underdosing of amphetamines UPD

T43.63 Poisoning by, adverse effect of and underdosing of methylphenidate

T43.631 Poisoning by methylphenidate, accidental (unintentional) HCC
Poisoning by methylphenidate NOS

T43.632 Poisoning by methylphenidate, intentional self-harm HCC

T43.633 Poisoning by methylphenidate, assault

T43.634 Poisoning by methylphenidate, undetermined HCC

T43.635 Adverse effect of methylphenidate UPD

T43.636 Underdosing of methylphenidate UPD

T43.64 Poisoning by ecstasy
Poisoning by MDMA
Poisoning by 3,4-methylenedioxymethamphetamine
AHA: 2018,4Q,30-31

T43.641 Poisoning by ecstasy, accidental (unintentional) HCC
Poisoning by ecstasy NOS

T43.642 Poisoning by ecstasy, intentional self-harm HCC

T43.643 Poisoning by ecstasy, assault

T43.644 Poisoning by ecstasy, undetermined HCC

T43.65 Poisoning by, adverse effect of and underdosing of methamphetamines
AHA: 2022,4Q,45-47

T43.651 Poisoning by methamphetamines accidental (unintentional) HCC
Poisoning by methamphetamines NOS
AHA: 2022,4Q,46

T43.652 Poisoning by methamphetamines intentional self-harm HCC

T43.653 Poisoning by methamphetamines, assault

T43.654 Poisoning by methamphetamines, undetermined HCC

T43.655 Adverse effect of methamphetamines UPD
AHA: 2022,4Q,46

T43.656 Underdosing of methamphetamines UPD

T43.69 Poisoning by, adverse effect of and underdosing of other psychostimulants

T43.691 Poisoning by other psychostimulants, accidental (unintentional) HCC
Poisoning by other psychostimulants NOS

T43.692 Poisoning by other psychostimulants, intentional self-harm HCC

T43.693 Poisoning by other psychostimulants, assault

T43.694 Poisoning by other psychostimulants, undetermined HCC

T43.695 Adverse effect of other psychostimulants UPD

T43.696 Underdosing of other psychostimulants UPD

T43.8 Poisoning by, adverse effect of and underdosing of other psychotropic drugs

T43.8X Poisoning by, adverse effect of and underdosing of other psychotropic drugs

T43.8X1 Poisoning by other psychotropic drugs, accidental (unintentional)
Poisoning by other psychotropic drugs NOS

T43.8X2 Poisoning by other psychotropic drugs, intentional self-harm HCC

T43.8X3 Poisoning by other psychotropic drugs, assault

T43.8X4 Poisoning by other psychotropic drugs, undetermined

T43.8X5 Adverse effect of other psychotropic drugs UPD

T43.8X6 Underdosing of other psychotropic drugs UPD

T43.9 Poisoning by, adverse effect of and underdosing of unspecified psychotropic drug

T43.91 Poisoning by unspecified psychotropic drug, accidental (unintentional)
Poisoning by psychotropic drug NOS

T43.92 Poisoning by unspecified psychotropic drug, intentional self-harm HCC

T43.93 Poisoning by unspecified psychotropic drug, assault

T43.94 Poisoning by unspecified psychotropic drug, undetermined

T43.95 Adverse effect of unspecified psychotropic drug UPD

T43.96 Underdosing of unspecified psychotropic drug UPD

T44 Poisoning by, adverse effect of and underdosing of drugs primarily affecting the autonomic nervous system

The appropriate 7th character is to be added to each code from category T44.
A initial encounter
D subsequent encounter
S sequela

T44.Ø Poisoning by, adverse effect of and underdosing of anticholinesterase agents

T44.ØX Poisoning by, adverse effect of and underdosing of anticholinesterase agents

T44.ØX1 Poisoning by anticholinesterase agents, accidental (unintentional)
Poisoning by anticholinesterase agents NOS

T44.ØX2 Poisoning by anticholinesterase agents, intentional self-harm HCC

T44.ØX3 Poisoning by anticholinesterase agents, assault

T44.ØX4 Poisoning by anticholinesterase agents, undetermined

T44.ØX5 Adverse effect of anticholinesterase agents UPD

T44.ØX6 Underdosing of anticholinesterase agents UPD

T44.1 Poisoning by, adverse effect of and underdosing of other parasympathomimetics [cholinergics]

T44.1X Poisoning by, adverse effect of and underdosing of other parasympathomimetics [cholinergics]

T44.1X1 Poisoning by other parasympathomimetics [cholinergics], accidental (unintentional)
Poisoning by other parasympathomimetics [cholinergics] NOS

T44.1X2 Poisoning by other parasympathomimetics [cholinergics], intentional self-harm HCC

T44.1X3 Poisoning by other parasympathomimetics [cholinergics], assault

T44.1X4 Poisoning by other parasympathomimetics [cholinergics], undetermined

T44.1X5 Adverse effect of other parasympathomimetics [cholinergics] UPD

T44.1X6 Underdosing of other parasympathomimetics [cholinergics] UPD

T44.2 Poisoning by, adverse effect of and underdosing of ganglionic blocking drugs

T44.2X Poisoning by, adverse effect of and underdosing of ganglionic blocking drugs

T44.2X1 Poisoning by ganglionic blocking drugs, accidental (unintentional)
Poisoning by ganglionic blocking drugs NOS

T44.2X2 Poisoning by ganglionic blocking drugs, intentional self-harm HCC

T44.2X3 Poisoning by ganglionic blocking drugs, assault

T44.2X4 Poisoning by ganglionic blocking drugs, undetermined

T44.2X5 Adverse effect of ganglionic blocking drugs UPD

T44.2X6 Underdosing of ganglionic blocking drugs UPD

T44.3 Poisoning by, adverse effect of and underdosing of other parasympatholytics [anticholinergics and antimuscarinics] and spasmolytics
Poisoning by, adverse effect of and underdosing of papaverine

T44.3X Poisoning by, adverse effect of and underdosing of other parasympatholytics [anticholinergics and antimuscarinics] and spasmolytics

T44.3X1 Poisoning by other parasympatholytics [anticholinergics and antimuscarinics] and spasmolytics, accidental (unintentional)
Poisoning by other parasympatholytics [anticholinergics and antimuscarinics] and spasmolytics NOS

T44.3X2 Poisoning by other parasympatholytics [anticholinergics and antimuscarinics] and spasmolytics, intentional self-harm HCC

T44.3X3 Poisoning by other parasympatholytics [anticholinergics and antimuscarinics] and spasmolytics, assault

T44.3X4 Poisoning by other parasympatholytics [anticholinergics and antimuscarinics] and spasmolytics, undetermined

T44.3X5 Adverse effect of other parasympatholytics [anticholinergics and antimuscarinics] and spasmolytics UPD

T44.3X6 Underdosing of other parasympatholytics [anticholinergics and antimuscarinics] and spasmolytics UPD

T44.4 Poisoning by, adverse effect of and underdosing of predominantly alpha-adrenoreceptor agonists
Poisoning by, adverse effect of and underdosing of metaraminol

T44.4X Poisoning by, adverse effect of and underdosing of predominantly alpha-adrenoreceptor agonists

T44.4X1 Poisoning by predominantly alpha-adrenoreceptor agonists, accidental (unintentional)
Poisoning by predominantly alpha-adrenoreceptor agonists NOS

T44.4X2 Poisoning by predominantly alpha-adrenoreceptor agonists, intentional self-harm HCC

T44.4X3 Poisoning by predominantly alpha-adrenoreceptor agonists, assault

T44.4X4 Poisoning by predominantly alpha-adrenoreceptor agonists, undetermined

T44.4X5 Adverse effect of predominantly alpha-adrenoreceptor agonists UPD

T44.4X6 Underdosing of predominantly alpha-adrenoreceptor agonists UPD

T44.5 Poisoning by, adverse effect of and underdosing of predominantly beta-adrenoreceptor agonists
EXCLUDES 1 *poisoning by, adverse effect of and underdosing of beta-adrenoreceptor agonists used in asthma therapy (T48.6-)*

T44.5X Poisoning by, adverse effect of and underdosing of predominantly beta-adrenoreceptor agonists

T44.5X1 Poisoning by predominantly beta-adrenoreceptor agonists, accidental (unintentional)
Poisoning by predominantly beta-adrenoreceptor agonists NOS

T44.5X2 Poisoning by predominantly beta-adrenoreceptor agonists, intentional self-harm HCC

T44.5X3 Poisoning by predominantly beta-adrenoreceptor agonists, assault

T44.5X4 Poisoning by predominantly beta-adrenoreceptor agonists, undetermined

T44.5X5 Adverse effect of predominantly beta-adrenoreceptor agonists UPD

T44.5X6 Underdosing of predominantly beta-adrenoreceptor agonists UPD

T44.6 Poisoning by, adverse effect of and underdosing of alpha-adrenoreceptor antagonists
EXCLUDES 1 *poisoning by, adverse effect of and underdosing of ergot alkaloids (T48.Ø)*

T44.6X Poisoning by, adverse effect of and underdosing of alpha-adrenoreceptor antagonists

T44.6X1 Poisoning by alpha-adrenoreceptor antagonists, accidental (unintentional)
Poisoning by alpha-adrenoreceptor antagonists NOS

T44.6X2 Poisoning by alpha-adrenoreceptor antagonists, intentional self-harm HCC

T44.6X3 Poisoning by alpha-adrenoreceptor antagonists, assault

T44.6X4 Poisoning by alpha-adrenoreceptor antagonists, undetermined

T44.6X5 Adverse effect of alpha-adrenoreceptor antagonists UPD

T44.6X6 Underdosing of alpha-adrenoreceptor antagonists UPD

T44.7 Poisoning by, adverse effect of and underdosing of beta-adrenoreceptor antagonists

T44.7X Poisoning by, adverse effect of and underdosing of beta-adrenoreceptor antagonists

T44.7X1 Poisoning by beta-adrenoreceptor antagonists, accidental (unintentional)
Poisoning by beta-adrenoreceptor antagonists NOS

T44.7X2 Poisoning by beta-adrenoreceptor antagonists, intentional self-harm HCC

T44.7X3 Poisoning by beta-adrenoreceptor antagonists, assault

T44.7X4 Poisoning by beta-adrenoreceptor antagonists, undetermined

T44.7X5 Adverse effect of beta-adrenoreceptor antagonists UPD

T44.7X6 Underdosing of beta-adrenoreceptor antagonists UPD

T44.8 Poisoning by, adverse effect of and underdosing of centrally-acting and adrenergic-neuron- blocking agents
EXCLUDES 2 *poisoning by, adverse effect of and underdosing of clonidine (T46.5)*
poisoning by, adverse effect of and underdosing of guanethidine (T46.5)

T44.8X Poisoning by, adverse effect of and underdosing of centrally-acting and adrenergic- neuron-blocking agents

T44.8X1 Poisoning by centrally-acting and adrenergic-neuron-blocking agents, accidental (unintentional)
Poisoning by centrally-acting and adrenergic-neuron-blocking agents NOS

T44.8X2 Poisoning by centrally-acting and adrenergic-neuron-blocking agents, intentional self-harm HCC

T44.8X3 Poisoning by centrally-acting and adrenergic-neuron-blocking agents, assault

T44.8X4 Poisoning by centrally-acting and adrenergic-neuron-blocking agents, undetermined

T44.8X5 Adverse effect of centrally-acting and adrenergic-neuron-blocking agents UPD

T44.8X6 Underdosing of centrally-acting and adrenergic-neuron-blocking agents UPD

T44.9 Poisoning by, adverse effect of and underdosing of other and unspecified drugs primarily affecting the autonomic nervous system
Poisoning by, adverse effect of and underdosing of drug stimulating both alpha and beta-adrenoreceptors

T44.9Ø Poisoning by, adverse effect of and underdosing of unspecified drugs primarily affecting the autonomic nervous system

T44.9Ø1 Poisoning by unspecified drugs primarily affecting the autonomic nervous system, accidental (unintentional)
Poisoning by unspecified drugs primarily affecting the autonomic nervous system NOS

T44.9Ø2 Poisoning by unspecified drugs primarily affecting the autonomic nervous system, intentional self-harm HCC

T44.9Ø3 Poisoning by unspecified drugs primarily affecting the autonomic nervous system, assault

T44.9Ø4 Poisoning by unspecified drugs primarily affecting the autonomic nervous system, undetermined

T44.9Ø5 Adverse effect of unspecified drugs primarily affecting the autonomic nervous system UPD

T44.9Ø6 Underdosing of unspecified drugs primarily affecting the autonomic nervous system UPD

6th **T44.99 Poisoning by, adverse effect of and underdosing of other drugs primarily affecting the autonomic nervous system**

7th **T44.991 Poisoning by other drug primarily affecting the autonomic nervous system, accidental (unintentional)**

Poisoning by other drugs primarily affecting the autonomic nervous system NOS

7th **T44.992 Poisoning by other drug primarily affecting the autonomic nervous system, intentional self-harm** HCC

7th **T44.993 Poisoning by other drug primarily affecting the autonomic nervous system, assault**

7th **T44.994 Poisoning by other drug primarily affecting the autonomic nervous system, undetermined**

7th **T44.995 Adverse effect of other drug primarily affecting the autonomic nervous system** UPD

7th **T44.996 Underdosing of other drug primarily affecting the autonomic nervous system** UPD

4th **T45 Poisoning by, adverse effect of and underdosing of primarily systemic and hematological agents, not elsewhere classified**

The appropriate 7th character is to be added to each code from category T45.
A initial encounter
D subsequent encounter
S sequela

5th **T45.Ø Poisoning by, adverse effect of and underdosing of antiallergic and antiemetic drugs**

EXCLUDES 1 *poisoning by, adverse effect of and underdosing of phenothiazine-based neuroleptics (T43.3)*

6th **T45.ØX Poisoning by, adverse effect of and underdosing of antiallergic and antiemetic drugs**

7th **T45.ØX1 Poisoning by antiallergic and antiemetic drugs, accidental (unintentional)**

Poisoning by antiallergic and antiemetic drugs NOS

7th **T45.ØX2 Poisoning by antiallergic and antiemetic drugs, intentional self-harm** HCC

7th **T45.ØX3 Poisoning by antiallergic and antiemetic drugs, assault**

7th **T45.ØX4 Poisoning by antiallergic and antiemetic drugs, undetermined**

7th **T45.ØX5 Adverse effect of antiallergic and antiemetic drugs** UPD

7th **T45.ØX6 Underdosing of antiallergic and antiemetic drugs** UPD

5th **T45.1 Poisoning by, adverse effect of and underdosing of antineoplastic and immunosuppressive drugs**

EXCLUDES 1 *poisoning by, adverse effect of and underdosing of tamoxifen (T38.6)*

AHA: 2019,1Q,17,20; 2014,4Q,22

6th **T45.1X Poisoning by, adverse effect of and underdosing of antineoplastic and immunosuppressive drugs**

7th **T45.1X1 Poisoning by antineoplastic and immunosuppressive drugs, accidental (unintentional)**

Poisoning by antineoplastic and immunosuppressive drugs NOS

7th **T45.1X2 Poisoning by antineoplastic and immunosuppressive drugs, intentional self-harm** HCC

7th **T45.1X3 Poisoning by antineoplastic and immunosuppressive drugs, assault**

7th **T45.1X4 Poisoning by antineoplastic and immunosuppressive drugs, undetermined**

7th **T45.1X5 Adverse effect of antineoplastic and immunosuppressive drugs** UPD

AHA: 2023,2Q,10; 2021,3Q,4; 2020,4Q,11; 2020,3Q,22; 2019,2Q,24,28

7th **T45.1X6 Underdosing of antineoplastic and immunosuppressive drugs** UPD

5th **T45.2 Poisoning by, adverse effect of and underdosing of vitamins**

EXCLUDES 2 *poisoning by, adverse effect of and underdosing of iron (T45.4)*
poisoning by, adverse effect of and underdosing of nicotinic acid (derivatives) (T46.7)
poisoning by, adverse effect of and underdosing of vitamin K (T45.7)

6th **T45.2X Poisoning by, adverse effect of and underdosing of vitamins**

7th **T45.2X1 Poisoning by vitamins, accidental (unintentional)**

Poisoning by vitamins NOS

7th **T45.2X2 Poisoning by vitamins, intentional self-harm** HCC

7th **T45.2X3 Poisoning by vitamins, assault**

7th **T45.2X4 Poisoning by vitamins, undetermined**

7th **T45.2X5 Adverse effect of vitamins** UPD

7th **T45.2X6 Underdosing of vitamins** UPD

EXCLUDES 1 *vitamin deficiencies (E5Ø-E56)*

5th **T45.3 Poisoning by, adverse effect of and underdosing of enzymes**

6th **T45.3X Poisoning by, adverse effect of and underdosing of enzymes**

7th **T45.3X1 Poisoning by enzymes, accidental (unintentional)**

Poisoning by enzymes NOS

7th **T45.3X2 Poisoning by enzymes, intentional self-harm** HCC

7th **T45.3X3 Poisoning by enzymes, assault**

7th **T45.3X4 Poisoning by enzymes, undetermined**

7th **T45.3X5 Adverse effect of enzymes** UPD

7th **T45.3X6 Underdosing of enzymes** UPD

5th **T45.4 Poisoning by, adverse effect of and underdosing of iron and its compounds**

6th **T45.4X Poisoning by, adverse effect of and underdosing of iron and its compounds**

7th **T45.4X1 Poisoning by iron and its compounds, accidental (unintentional)**

Poisoning by iron and its compounds NOS

7th **T45.4X2 Poisoning by iron and its compounds, intentional self-harm** HCC

7th **T45.4X3 Poisoning by iron and its compounds, assault**

7th **T45.4X4 Poisoning by iron and its compounds, undetermined**

7th **T45.4X5 Adverse effect of iron and its compounds** UPD

7th **T45.4X6 Underdosing of iron and its compounds** UPD

EXCLUDES 1 *iron deficiency (E61.1)*

5th **T45.5 Poisoning by, adverse effect of and underdosing of anticoagulants and antithrombotic drugs**

6th **T45.51 Poisoning by, adverse effect of and underdosing of anticoagulants**

7th **T45.511 Poisoning by anticoagulants, accidental (unintentional)**

Poisoning by anticoagulants NOS

7th **T45.512 Poisoning by anticoagulants, intentional self-harm** HCC

7th **T45.513 Poisoning by anticoagulants, assault**

7th **T45.514 Poisoning by anticoagulants, undetermined**

7th **T45.515 Adverse effect of anticoagulants** UPD

AHA: 2021,1Q,4; 2016,1Q,14; 2013,2Q,34

7th **T45.516 Underdosing of anticoagulants** UPD

6th **T45.52 Poisoning by, adverse effect of and underdosing of antithrombotic drugs**

Poisoning by, adverse effect of and underdosing of antiplatelet drugs

EXCLUDES 2 *poisoning by, adverse effect of and underdosing of acetylsalicylic acid (T39.Ø1-)*
poisoning by, adverse effect of and underdosing of aspirin (T39.Ø1-)

7th **T45.521 Poisoning by antithrombotic drugs, accidental (unintentional)**

Poisoning by antithrombotic drug NOS

7th **T45.522 Poisoning by antithrombotic drugs, intentional self-harm** HCC

T45.523 Poisoning by antithrombotic drugs, assault

T45.524 Poisoning by antithrombotic drugs, undetermined

T45.525 Adverse effect of antithrombotic drugs UPD
AHA: 2016,1Q,15

T45.526 Underdosing of antithrombotic drugs UPD

T45.6 Poisoning by, adverse effect of and underdosing of fibrinolysis-affecting drugs

T45.60 Poisoning by, adverse effect of and underdosing of unspecified fibrinolysis-affecting drugs

T45.601 Poisoning by unspecified fibrinolysis-affecting drugs, accidental (unintentional)
Poisoning by fibrinolysis-affecting drug NOS

T45.602 Poisoning by unspecified fibrinolysis-affecting drugs, intentional self-harm HCC

T45.603 Poisoning by unspecified fibrinolysis-affecting drugs, assault

T45.604 Poisoning by unspecified fibrinolysis-affecting drugs, undetermined

T45.605 Adverse effect of unspecified fibrinolysis-affecting drugs UPD

T45.606 Underdosing of unspecified fibrinolysis-affecting drugs UPD

T45.61 Poisoning by, adverse effect of and underdosing of thrombolytic drugs

T45.611 Poisoning by thrombolytic drug, accidental (unintentional)
Poisoning by thrombolytic drug NOS

T45.612 Poisoning by thrombolytic drug, intentional self-harm HCC

T45.613 Poisoning by thrombolytic drug, assault

T45.614 Poisoning by thrombolytic drug, undetermined

T45.615 Adverse effect of thrombolytic drugs UPD
AHA: 2017,2Q,9

T45.616 Underdosing of thrombolytic drugs UPD

T45.62 Poisoning by, adverse effect of and underdosing of hemostatic drugs

T45.621 Poisoning by hemostatic drug, accidental (unintentional)
Poisoning by hemostatic drug NOS

T45.622 Poisoning by hemostatic drug, intentional self-harm HCC

T45.623 Poisoning by hemostatic drug, assault

T45.624 Poisoning by hemostatic drug, undetermined

T45.625 Adverse effect of hemostatic drug UPD

T45.626 Underdosing of hemostatic drugs UPD

T45.69 Poisoning by, adverse effect of and underdosing of other fibrinolysis-affecting drugs

T45.691 Poisoning by other fibrinolysis-affecting drugs, accidental (unintentional)
Poisoning by other fibrinolysis-affecting drug NOS

T45.692 Poisoning by other fibrinolysis-affecting drugs, intentional self-harm HCC

T45.693 Poisoning by other fibrinolysis-affecting drugs, assault

T45.694 Poisoning by other fibrinolysis-affecting drugs, undetermined

T45.695 Adverse effect of other fibrinolysis-affecting drugs UPD

T45.696 Underdosing of other fibrinolysis-affecting drugs UPD

T45.7 Poisoning by, adverse effect of and underdosing of anticoagulant antagonists, vitamin K and other coagulants

T45.7X Poisoning by, adverse effect of and underdosing of anticoagulant antagonists, vitamin K and other coagulants

T45.7X1 Poisoning by anticoagulant antagonists, vitamin K and other coagulants, accidental (unintentional)
Poisoning by anticoagulant antagonists, vitamin K and other coagulants NOS

T45.7X2 Poisoning by anticoagulant antagonists, vitamin K and other coagulants, intentional self-harm HCC

T45.7X3 Poisoning by anticoagulant antagonists, vitamin K and other coagulants, assault

T45.7X4 Poisoning by anticoagulant antagonists, vitamin K and other coagulants, undetermined

T45.7X5 Adverse effect of anticoagulant antagonists, vitamin K and other coagulants UPD

T45.7X6 Underdosing of anticoagulant antagonist, vitamin K and other coagulants UPD
EXCLUDES 1 *vitamin K deficiency (E56.1)*

T45.8 Poisoning by, adverse effect of and underdosing of other primarily systemic and hematological agents
Poisoning by, adverse effect of and underdosing of liver preparations and other antianemic agents
Poisoning by, adverse effect of and underdosing of natural blood and blood products
Poisoning by, adverse effect of and underdosing of plasma substitute
EXCLUDES 2 *poisoning by, adverse effect of and underdosing of immunoglobulin (T5Ø.Z1)*
poisoning by, adverse effect of and underdosing of iron (T45.4)
transfusion reactions (T8Ø.-)

T45.8X Poisoning by, adverse effect of and underdosing of other primarily systemic and hematological agents

T45.8X1 Poisoning by other primarily systemic and hematological agents, accidental (unintentional)
Poisoning by other primarily systemic and hematological agents NOS

T45.8X2 Poisoning by other primarily systemic and hematological agents, intentional self-harm HCC

T45.8X3 Poisoning by other primarily systemic and hematological agents, assault

T45.8X4 Poisoning by other primarily systemic and hematological agents, undetermined

T45.8X5 Adverse effect of other primarily systemic and hematological agents UPD
AHA: 2016,4Q,42

T45.8X6 Underdosing of other primarily systemic and hematological agents UPD

T45.9 Poisoning by, adverse effect of and underdosing of unspecified primarily systemic and hematological agent

T45.91 Poisoning by unspecified primarily systemic and hematological agent, accidental (unintentional)
Poisoning by primarily systemic and hematological agent NOS

T45.92 Poisoning by unspecified primarily systemic and hematological agent, intentional self-harm HCC

T45.93 Poisoning by unspecified primarily systemic and hematological agent, assault

T45.94 Poisoning by unspecified primarily systemic and hematological agent, undetermined

T45.95 Adverse effect of unspecified primarily systemic and hematological agent UPD

T45.96 Underdosing of unspecified primarily systemic and hematological agent UPD

4th T46 Poisoning by, adverse effect of and underdosing of agents primarily affecting the cardiovascular system

EXCLUDES 1 *poisoning by, adverse effect of and underdosing of metaraminol (T44.4)*

The appropriate 7th character is to be added to each code from category T46.
A initial encounter
D subsequent encounter
S sequela

5th T46.Ø Poisoning by, adverse effect of and underdosing of cardiac-stimulant glycosides and drugs of similar action

6th T46.ØX Poisoning by, adverse effect of and underdosing of cardiac-stimulant glycosides and drugs of similar action

7th T46.ØX1 Poisoning by cardiac-stimulant glycosides and drugs of similar action, accidental (unintentional)
Poisoning by cardiac-stimulant glycosides and drugs of similar action NOS

7th T46.ØX2 Poisoning by cardiac-stimulant glycosides and drugs of similar action, intentional self-harm HCC

7th T46.ØX3 Poisoning by cardiac-stimulant glycosides and drugs of similar action, assault

7th T46.ØX4 Poisoning by cardiac-stimulant glycosides and drugs of similar action, undetermined

7th T46.ØX5 Adverse effect of cardiac-stimulant glycosides and drugs of similar action UPD

7th T46.ØX6 Underdosing of cardiac-stimulant glycosides and drugs of similar action UPD

5th T46.1 Poisoning by, adverse effect of and underdosing of calcium-channel blockers

6th T46.1X Poisoning by, adverse effect of and underdosing of calcium-channel blockers

7th T46.1X1 Poisoning by calcium-channel blockers, accidental (unintentional)
Poisoning by calcium-channel blockers NOS

7th T46.1X2 Poisoning by calcium-channel blockers, intentional self-harm HCC

7th T46.1X3 Poisoning by calcium-channel blockers, assault

7th T46.1X4 Poisoning by calcium-channel blockers, undetermined

7th T46.1X5 Adverse effect of calcium-channel blockers UPD

7th T46.1X6 Underdosing of calcium-channel blockers UPD
AHA: 2023,1Q,39

5th T46.2 Poisoning by, adverse effect of and underdosing of other antidysrhythmic drugs, not elsewhere classified

EXCLUDES 1 *poisoning by, adverse effect of and underdosing of beta-adrenoreceptor antagonists (T44.7-)*

6th T46.2X Poisoning by, adverse effect of and underdosing of other antidysrhythmic drugs

7th T46.2X1 Poisoning by other antidysrhythmic drugs, accidental (unintentional)
Poisoning by other antidysrhythmic drugs NOS

7th T46.2X2 Poisoning by other antidysrhythmic drugs, intentional self-harm HCC

7th T46.2X3 Poisoning by other antidysrhythmic drugs, assault

7th T46.2X4 Poisoning by other antidysrhythmic drugs, undetermined

7th T46.2X5 Adverse effect of other antidysrhythmic drugs UPD

7th T46.2X6 Underdosing of other antidysrhythmic drugs UPD

5th T46.3 Poisoning by, adverse effect of and underdosing of coronary vasodilators
Poisoning by, adverse effect of and underdosing of dipyridamole

EXCLUDES 1 *poisoning by, adverse effect of and underdosing of calcium-channel blockers (T46.1)*

6th T46.3X Poisoning by, adverse effect of and underdosing of coronary vasodilators

7th T46.3X1 Poisoning by coronary vasodilators, accidental (unintentional)
Poisoning by coronary vasodilators NOS

7th T46.3X2 Poisoning by coronary vasodilators, intentional self-harm HCC

7th T46.3X3 Poisoning by coronary vasodilators, assault

7th T46.3X4 Poisoning by coronary vasodilators, undetermined

7th T46.3X5 Adverse effect of coronary vasodilators UPD

7th T46.3X6 Underdosing of coronary vasodilators UPD

5th T46.4 Poisoning by, adverse effect of and underdosing of angiotensin-converting-enzyme inhibitors

6th T46.4X Poisoning by, adverse effect of and underdosing of angiotensin-converting-enzyme inhibitors

7th T46.4X1 Poisoning by angiotensin-converting-enzyme inhibitors, accidental (unintentional)
Poisoning by angiotensin-converting-enzyme inhibitors NOS

7th T46.4X2 Poisoning by angiotensin-converting-enzyme inhibitors, intentional self-harm HCC

7th T46.4X3 Poisoning by angiotensin-converting-enzyme inhibitors, assault

7th T46.4X4 Poisoning by angiotensin-converting-enzyme inhibitors, undetermined

7th T46.4X5 Adverse effect of angiotensin-converting-enzyme inhibitors UPD

7th T46.4X6 Underdosing of angiotensin-converting-enzyme inhibitors UPD

5th T46.5 Poisoning by, adverse effect of and underdosing of other antihypertensive drugs

EXCLUDES 2 *poisoning by, adverse effect of and underdosing of beta-adrenoreceptor antagonists (T44.7)*
poisoning by, adverse effect of and underdosing of calcium-channel blockers (T46.1)
poisoning by, adverse effect of and underdosing of diuretics (T5Ø.Ø-T5Ø.2)

6th T46.5X Poisoning by, adverse effect of and underdosing of other antihypertensive drugs

7th T46.5X1 Poisoning by other antihypertensive drugs, accidental (unintentional)
Poisoning by other antihypertensive drugs NOS

7th T46.5X2 Poisoning by other antihypertensive drugs, intentional self-harm HCC

7th T46.5X3 Poisoning by other antihypertensive drugs, assault

7th T46.5X4 Poisoning by other antihypertensive drugs, undetermined

7th T46.5X5 Adverse effect of other antihypertensive drugs UPD

7th T46.5X6 Underdosing of other antihypertensive drugs UPD
AHA: 2023,1Q,39; 2022,1Q,36

5th T46.6 Poisoning by, adverse effect of and underdosing of antihyperlipidemic and antiarteriosclerotic drugs

6th T46.6X Poisoning by, adverse effect of and underdosing of antihyperlipidemic and antiarteriosclerotic drugs

7th T46.6X1 Poisoning by antihyperlipidemic and antiarteriosclerotic drugs, accidental (unintentional)
Poisoning by antihyperlipidemic and antiarteriosclerotic drugs NOS

7th T46.6X2 Poisoning by antihyperlipidemic and antiarteriosclerotic drugs, intentional self-harm HCC

✓7th T46.6X3 Poisoning by antihyperlipidemic and antiarteriosclerotic drugs, assault

✓7th T46.6X4 Poisoning by antihyperlipidemic and antiarteriosclerotic drugs, undetermined

✓7th T46.6X5 Adverse effect of antihyperlipidemic and antiarteriosclerotic drugs UPD

✓7th T46.6X6 Underdosing of antihyperlipidemic and antiarteriosclerotic drugs UPD

✓5th T46.7 Poisoning by, adverse effect of and underdosing of peripheral vasodilators

Poisoning by, adverse effect of and underdosing of nicotinic acid (derivatives)

EXCLUDES 1 *poisoning by, adverse effect of and underdosing of papaverine (T44.3)*

✓6th T46.7X Poisoning by, adverse effect of and underdosing of peripheral vasodilators

✓7th T46.7X1 Poisoning by peripheral vasodilators, accidental (unintentional)

Poisoning by peripheral vasodilators NOS

✓7th T46.7X2 Poisoning by peripheral vasodilators, intentional self-harm HCC

✓7th T46.7X3 Poisoning by peripheral vasodilators, assault

✓7th T46.7X4 Poisoning by peripheral vasodilators, undetermined

✓7th T46.7X5 Adverse effect of peripheral vasodilators UPD

✓7th T46.7X6 Underdosing of peripheral vasodilators UPD

✓5th T46.8 Poisoning by, adverse effect of and underdosing of antivaricose drugs, including sclerosing agents

✓6th T46.8X Poisoning by, adverse effect of and underdosing of antivaricose drugs, including sclerosing agents

✓7th T46.8X1 Poisoning by antivaricose drugs, including sclerosing agents, accidental (unintentional)

Poisoning by antivaricose drugs, including sclerosing agents NOS

✓7th T46.8X2 Poisoning by antivaricose drugs, including sclerosing agents, intentional self-harm HCC

✓7th T46.8X3 Poisoning by antivaricose drugs, including sclerosing agents, assault

✓7th T46.8X4 Poisoning by antivaricose drugs, including sclerosing agents, undetermined

✓7th T46.8X5 Adverse effect of antivaricose drugs, including sclerosing agents UPD

✓7th T46.8X6 Underdosing of antivaricose drugs, including sclerosing agents UPD

✓5th T46.9 Poisoning by, adverse effect of and underdosing of other and unspecified agents primarily affecting the cardiovascular system

✓6th T46.90 Poisoning by, adverse effect of and underdosing of unspecified agents primarily affecting the cardiovascular system

✓7th T46.901 Poisoning by unspecified agents primarily affecting the cardiovascular system, accidental (unintentional)

✓7th T46.902 Poisoning by unspecified agents primarily affecting the cardiovascular system, intentional self-harm HCC

✓7th T46.903 Poisoning by unspecified agents primarily affecting the cardiovascular system, assault

✓7th T46.904 Poisoning by unspecified agents primarily affecting the cardiovascular system, undetermined

✓7th T46.905 Adverse effect of unspecified agents primarily affecting the cardiovascular system UPD

✓7th T46.906 Underdosing of unspecified agents primarily affecting the cardiovascular system UPD

✓6th T46.99 Poisoning by, adverse effect of and underdosing of other agents primarily affecting the cardiovascular system

✓7th T46.991 Poisoning by other agents primarily affecting the cardiovascular system, accidental (unintentional)

✓7th T46.992 Poisoning by other agents primarily affecting the cardiovascular system, intentional self-harm HCC

✓7th T46.993 Poisoning by other agents primarily affecting the cardiovascular system, assault

✓7th T46.994 Poisoning by other agents primarily affecting the cardiovascular system, undetermined

✓7th T46.995 Adverse effect of other agents primarily affecting the cardiovascular system UPD

✓7th T46.996 Underdosing of other agents primarily affecting the cardiovascular system UPD

✓4th T47 Poisoning by, adverse effect of and underdosing of agents primarily affecting the gastrointestinal system

The appropriate 7th character is to be added to each code from category T47.
A initial encounter
D subsequent encounter
S sequela

✓5th T47.0 Poisoning by, adverse effect of and underdosing of histamine H2-receptor blockers

✓6th T47.0X Poisoning by, adverse effect of and underdosing of histamine H2-receptor blockers

✓7th T47.0X1 Poisoning by histamine H2-receptor blockers, accidental (unintentional)

Poisoning by histamine H2-receptor blockers NOS

✓7th T47.0X2 Poisoning by histamine H2-receptor blockers, intentional self-harm HCC

✓7th T47.0X3 Poisoning by histamine H2-receptor blockers, assault

✓7th T47.0X4 Poisoning by histamine H2-receptor blockers, undetermined

✓7th T47.0X5 Adverse effect of histamine H2-receptor blockers UPD

✓7th T47.0X6 Underdosing of histamine H2-receptor blockers UPD

✓5th T47.1 Poisoning by, adverse effect of and underdosing of other antacids and anti-gastric-secretion drugs

✓6th T47.1X Poisoning by, adverse effect of and underdosing of other antacids and anti-gastric-secretion drugs

✓7th T47.1X1 Poisoning by other antacids and anti-gastric-secretion drugs, accidental (unintentional)

Poisoning by other antacids and anti-gastric-secretion drugs NOS

✓7th T47.1X2 Poisoning by other antacids and anti-gastric-secretion drugs, intentional self-harm HCC

✓7th T47.1X3 Poisoning by other antacids and anti-gastric-secretion drugs, assault

✓7th T47.1X4 Poisoning by other antacids and anti-gastric-secretion drugs, undetermined

✓7th T47.1X5 Adverse effect of other antacids and anti-gastric-secretion drugs UPD

✓7th T47.1X6 Underdosing of other antacids and anti-gastric-secretion drugs UPD

✓5th T47.2 Poisoning by, adverse effect of and underdosing of stimulant laxatives

✓6th T47.2X Poisoning by, adverse effect of and underdosing of stimulant laxatives

✓7th T47.2X1 Poisoning by stimulant laxatives, accidental (unintentional)

Poisoning by stimulant laxatives NOS

✓7th T47.2X2 Poisoning by stimulant laxatives, intentional self-harm HCC

✓7th T47.2X3 Poisoning by stimulant laxatives, assault

✓7th T47.2X4 Poisoning by stimulant laxatives, undetermined

✓7th T47.2X5 Adverse effect of stimulant laxatives UPD

✓7th T47.2X6 Underdosing of stimulant laxatives UPD

T47.3 Poisoning by, adverse effect of and underdosing of saline and osmotic laxatives

T47.3X Poisoning by and adverse effect of saline and osmotic laxatives

T47.3X1 Poisoning by saline and osmotic laxatives, accidental (unintentional)
Poisoning by saline and osmotic laxatives NOS

T47.3X2 Poisoning by saline and osmotic laxatives, intentional self-harm HCC

T47.3X3 Poisoning by saline and osmotic laxatives, assault

T47.3X4 Poisoning by saline and osmotic laxatives, undetermined

T47.3X5 Adverse effect of saline and osmotic laxatives UPD

T47.3X6 Underdosing of saline and osmotic laxatives UPD

T47.4 Poisoning by, adverse effect of and underdosing of other laxatives

T47.4X Poisoning by, adverse effect of and underdosing of other laxatives

T47.4X1 Poisoning by other laxatives, accidental (unintentional)
Poisoning by other laxatives NOS

T47.4X2 Poisoning by other laxatives, intentional self-harm HCC

T47.4X3 Poisoning by other laxatives, assault

T47.4X4 Poisoning by other laxatives, undetermined

T47.4X5 Adverse effect of other laxatives UPD

T47.4X6 Underdosing of other laxatives UPD

T47.5 Poisoning by, adverse effect of and underdosing of digestants

T47.5X Poisoning by, adverse effect of and underdosing of digestants

T47.5X1 Poisoning by digestants, accidental (unintentional)
Poisoning by digestants NOS

T47.5X2 Poisoning by digestants, intentional self-harm HCC

T47.5X3 Poisoning by digestants, assault

T47.5X4 Poisoning by digestants, undetermined

T47.5X5 Adverse effect of digestants UPD

T47.5X6 Underdosing of digestants UPD

T47.6 Poisoning by, adverse effect of and underdosing of antidiarrheal drugs

EXCLUDES 2 *poisoning by, adverse effect of and underdosing of systemic antibiotics and other anti-infectives (T36-T37)*

T47.6X Poisoning by, adverse effect of and underdosing of antidiarrheal drugs

T47.6X1 Poisoning by antidiarrheal drugs, accidental (unintentional)
Poisoning by antidiarrheal drugs NOS

T47.6X2 Poisoning by antidiarrheal drugs, intentional self-harm HCC

T47.6X3 Poisoning by antidiarrheal drugs, assault

T47.6X4 Poisoning by antidiarrheal drugs, undetermined

T47.6X5 Adverse effect of antidiarrheal drugs UPD

T47.6X6 Underdosing of antidiarrheal drugs UPD

T47.7 Poisoning by, adverse effect of and underdosing of emetics

T47.7X Poisoning by, adverse effect of and underdosing of emetics

T47.7X1 Poisoning by emetics, accidental (unintentional)
Poisoning by emetics NOS

T47.7X2 Poisoning by emetics, intentional self-harm HCC

T47.7X3 Poisoning by emetics, assault

T47.7X4 Poisoning by emetics, undetermined

T47.7X5 Adverse effect of emetics UPD

T47.7X6 Underdosing of emetics UPD

T47.8 Poisoning by, adverse effect of and underdosing of other agents primarily affecting gastrointestinal system

T47.8X Poisoning by, adverse effect of and underdosing of other agents primarily affecting gastrointestinal system

T47.8X1 Poisoning by other agents primarily affecting gastrointestinal system, accidental (unintentional)
Poisoning by other agents primarily affecting gastrointestinal system NOS

T47.8X2 Poisoning by other agents primarily affecting gastrointestinal system, intentional self-harm HCC

T47.8X3 Poisoning by other agents primarily affecting gastrointestinal system, assault

T47.8X4 Poisoning by other agents primarily affecting gastrointestinal system, undetermined

T47.8X5 Adverse effect of other agents primarily affecting gastrointestinal system UPD

T47.8X6 Underdosing of other agents primarily affecting gastrointestinal system UPD

T47.9 Poisoning by, adverse effect of and underdosing of unspecified agents primarily affecting the gastrointestinal system

T47.91 Poisoning by unspecified agents primarily affecting the gastrointestinal system, accidental (unintentional)
Poisoning by agents primarily affecting the gastrointestinal system NOS

T47.92 Poisoning by unspecified agents primarily affecting the gastrointestinal system, intentional self-harm HCC

T47.93 Poisoning by unspecified agents primarily affecting the gastrointestinal system, assault

T47.94 Poisoning by unspecified agents primarily affecting the gastrointestinal system, undetermined

T47.95 Adverse effect of unspecified agents primarily affecting the gastrointestinal system UPD

T47.96 Underdosing of unspecified agents primarily affecting the gastrointestinal system UPD

T48 Poisoning by, adverse effect of and underdosing of agents primarily acting on smooth and skeletal muscles and the respiratory system

The appropriate 7th character is to be added to each code from category T48.
A initial encounter
D subsequent encounter
S sequela

T48.Ø Poisoning by, adverse effect of and underdosing of oxytocic drugs

EXCLUDES 1 *poisoning by, adverse effect of and underdosing of estrogens, progestogens and antagonists (T38.4-T38.6)*

T48.ØX Poisoning by, adverse effect of and underdosing of oxytocic drugs

T48.ØX1 Poisoning by oxytocic drugs, accidental (unintentional)
Poisoning by oxytocic drugs NOS

T48.ØX2 Poisoning by oxytocic drugs, intentional self-harm HCC

T48.ØX3 Poisoning by oxytocic drugs, assault

T48.ØX4 Poisoning by oxytocic drugs, undetermined

T48.ØX5 Adverse effect of oxytocic drugs UPD

T48.ØX6 Underdosing of oxytocic drugs UPD

T48.1 Poisoning by, adverse effect of and underdosing of skeletal muscle relaxants [neuromuscular blocking agents]

T48.1X Poisoning by, adverse effect of and underdosing of skeletal muscle relaxants [neuromuscular blocking agents]

T48.1X1 Poisoning by skeletal muscle relaxants [neuromuscular blocking agents], accidental (unintentional)
Poisoning by skeletal muscle relaxants [neuromuscular blocking agents] NOS

T48.1X2 Poisoning by skeletal muscle relaxants [neuromuscular blocking agents], intentional self-harm HCC

T48.1X3 Poisoning by skeletal muscle relaxants [neuromuscular blocking agents], assault

T48.1X4 **Poisoning by skeletal muscle relaxants [neuromuscular blocking agents], undetermined**

T48.1X5 **Adverse effect of skeletal muscle relaxants [neuromuscular blocking agents]** UPD

T48.1X6 **Underdosing of skeletal muscle relaxants [neuromuscular blocking agents]** UPD

T48.2 **Poisoning by, adverse effect of and underdosing of other and unspecified drugs acting on muscles**

T48.20 **Poisoning by, adverse effect of and underdosing of unspecified drugs acting on muscles**

T48.201 **Poisoning by unspecified drugs acting on muscles, accidental (unintentional)**
Poisoning by unspecified drugs acting on muscles NOS

T48.202 **Poisoning by unspecified drugs acting on muscles, intentional self-harm** HCC

T48.203 **Poisoning by unspecified drugs acting on muscles, assault**

T48.204 **Poisoning by unspecified drugs acting on muscles, undetermined**

T48.205 **Adverse effect of unspecified drugs acting on muscles** UPD

T48.206 **Underdosing of unspecified drugs acting on muscles** UPD

T48.29 **Poisoning by, adverse effect of and underdosing of other drugs acting on muscles**

T48.291 **Poisoning by other drugs acting on muscles, accidental (unintentional)**
Poisoning by other drugs acting on muscles NOS

T48.292 **Poisoning by other drugs acting on muscles, intentional self-harm** HCC

T48.293 **Poisoning by other drugs acting on muscles, assault**

T48.294 **Poisoning by other drugs acting on muscles, undetermined**

T48.295 **Adverse effect of other drugs acting on muscles** UPD

T48.296 **Underdosing of other drugs acting on muscles** UPD

T48.3 **Poisoning by, adverse effect of and underdosing of antitussives**

T48.3X **Poisoning by, adverse effect of and underdosing of antitussives**

T48.3X1 **Poisoning by antitussives, accidental (unintentional)**
Poisoning by antitussives NOS

T48.3X2 **Poisoning by antitussives, intentional self-harm** HCC

T48.3X3 **Poisoning by antitussives, assault**

T48.3X4 **Poisoning by antitussives, undetermined**

T48.3X5 **Adverse effect of antitussives** UPD

T48.3X6 **Underdosing of antitussives** UPD

T48.4 **Poisoning by, adverse effect of and underdosing of expectorants**

T48.4X **Poisoning by, adverse effect of and underdosing of expectorants**

T48.4X1 **Poisoning by expectorants, accidental (unintentional)**
Poisoning by expectorants NOS

T48.4X2 **Poisoning by expectorants, intentional self-harm** HCC

T48.4X3 **Poisoning by expectorants, assault**

T48.4X4 **Poisoning by expectorants, undetermined**

T48.4X5 **Adverse effect of expectorants** UPD

T48.4X6 **Underdosing of expectorants** UPD

T48.5 **Poisoning by, adverse effect of and underdosing of other anti-common-cold drugs**
Poisoning by, adverse effect of and underdosing of decongestants
EXCLUDES 2 *poisoning by, adverse effect of and underdosing of antipyretics, NEC (T39.9-)*
poisoning by, adverse effect of and underdosing of non-steroidal antiinflammatory drugs (T39.3-)
poisoning by, adverse effect of and underdosing of salicylates (T39.Ø-)

T48.5X **Poisoning by, adverse effect of and underdosing of other anti-common-cold drugs**

T48.5X1 **Poisoning by other anti-common-cold drugs, accidental (unintentional)**
Poisoning by other anti-common-cold drugs NOS

T48.5X2 **Poisoning by other anti-common-cold drugs, intentional self-harm** HCC

T48.5X3 **Poisoning by other anti-common-cold drugs, assault**

T48.5X4 **Poisoning by other anti-common-cold drugs, undetermined**

T48.5X5 **Adverse effect of other anti-common-cold drugs** UPD

T48.5X6 **Underdosing of other anti-common-cold drugs** UPD

T48.6 **Poisoning by, adverse effect of and underdosing of antiasthmatics, not elsewhere classified**
Poisoning by, adverse effect of and underdosing of beta-adrenoreceptor agonists used in asthma therapy
EXCLUDES 1 *poisoning by, adverse effect of and underdosing of anterior pituitary [adenohypophyseal] hormones (T38.8)*
poisoning by, adverse effect of and underdosing of beta-adrenoreceptor agonists not used in asthma therapy (T44.5)

T48.6X **Poisoning by, adverse effect of and underdosing of antiasthmatics**

T48.6X1 **Poisoning by antiasthmatics, accidental (unintentional)**
Poisoning by antiasthmatics NOS

T48.6X2 **Poisoning by antiasthmatics, intentional self-harm** HCC

T48.6X3 **Poisoning by antiasthmatics, assault**

T48.6X4 **Poisoning by antiasthmatics, undetermined**

T48.6X5 **Adverse effect of antiasthmatics** UPD

T48.6X6 **Underdosing of antiasthmatics** UPD

T48.9 **Poisoning by, adverse effect of and underdosing of other and unspecified agents primarily acting on the respiratory system**

T48.9Ø **Poisoning by, adverse effect of and underdosing of unspecified agents primarily acting on the respiratory system**

T48.9Ø1 **Poisoning by unspecified agents primarily acting on the respiratory system, accidental (unintentional)**

T48.9Ø2 **Poisoning by unspecified agents primarily acting on the respiratory system, intentional self-harm** HCC

T48.9Ø3 **Poisoning by unspecified agents primarily acting on the respiratory system, assault**

T48.9Ø4 **Poisoning by unspecified agents primarily acting on the respiratory system, undetermined**

T48.9Ø5 **Adverse effect of unspecified agents primarily acting on the respiratory system** UPD

T48.9Ø6 **Underdosing of unspecified agents primarily acting on the respiratory system** UPD

T48.99 **Poisoning by, adverse effect of and underdosing of other agents primarily acting on the respiratory system**

T48.991 **Poisoning by other agents primarily acting on the respiratory system, accidental (unintentional)**

T48.992 **Poisoning by other agents primarily acting on the respiratory system, intentional self-harm** HCC

7th T48.993 Poisoning by other agents primarily acting on the respiratory system, assault

7th T48.994 Poisoning by other agents primarily acting on the respiratory system, undetermined

7th T48.995 Adverse effect of other agents primarily acting on the respiratory system UPD

7th T48.996 Underdosing of other agents primarily acting on the respiratory system UPD

4th **T49 Poisoning by, adverse effect of and underdosing of topical agents primarily affecting skin and mucous membrane and by ophthalmological, otorhinolaryngological and dental drugs**

INCLUDES poisoning by, adverse effect of and underdosing of glucocorticoids, topically used

The appropriate 7th character is to be added to each code from category T49.
A initial encounter
D subsequent encounter
S sequela

5th **T49.Ø Poisoning by, adverse effect of and underdosing of local antifungal, anti-infective and anti-inflammatory drugs**

6th T49.ØX Poisoning by, adverse effect of and underdosing of local antifungal, anti-infective and anti-inflammatory drugs

7th T49.ØX1 Poisoning by local antifungal, anti-infective and anti-inflammatory drugs, accidental (unintentional)
Poisoning by local antifungal, anti-infective and anti-inflammatory drugs NOS

7th T49.ØX2 Poisoning by local antifungal, anti-infective and anti-inflammatory drugs, intentional self-harm HCC

7th T49.ØX3 Poisoning by local antifungal, anti-infective and anti-inflammatory drugs, assault

7th T49.ØX4 Poisoning by local antifungal, anti-infective and anti-inflammatory drugs, undetermined

7th T49.ØX5 Adverse effect of local antifungal, anti-infective and anti-inflammatory drugs UPD

7th T49.ØX6 Underdosing of local antifungal, anti-infective and anti-inflammatory drugs UPD

5th **T49.1 Poisoning by, adverse effect of and underdosing of antipruritics**

6th T49.1X Poisoning by, adverse effect of and underdosing of antipruritics

7th T49.1X1 Poisoning by antipruritics, accidental (unintentional)
Poisoning by antipruritics NOS

7th T49.1X2 Poisoning by antipruritics, intentional self-harm HCC

7th T49.1X3 Poisoning by antipruritics, assault

7th T49.1X4 Poisoning by antipruritics, undetermined

7th T49.1X5 Adverse effect of antipruritics UPD

7th T49.1X6 Underdosing of antipruritics UPD

5th **T49.2 Poisoning by, adverse effect of and underdosing of local astringents and local detergents**

6th T49.2X Poisoning by, adverse effect of and underdosing of local astringents and local detergents

7th T49.2X1 Poisoning by local astringents and local detergents, accidental (unintentional)
Poisoning by local astringents and local detergents NOS

7th T49.2X2 Poisoning by local astringents and local detergents, intentional self-harm HCC

7th T49.2X3 Poisoning by local astringents and local detergents, assault

7th T49.2X4 Poisoning by local astringents and local detergents, undetermined

7th T49.2X5 Adverse effect of local astringents and local detergents UPD

7th T49.2X6 Underdosing of local astringents and local detergents UPD

5th **T49.3 Poisoning by, adverse effect of and underdosing of emollients, demulcents and protectants**

6th T49.3X Poisoning by, adverse effect of and underdosing of emollients, demulcents and protectants

7th T49.3X1 Poisoning by emollients, demulcents and protectants, accidental (unintentional)
Poisoning by emollients, demulcents and protectants NOS

7th T49.3X2 Poisoning by emollients, demulcents and protectants, intentional self-harm HCC

7th T49.3X3 Poisoning by emollients, demulcents and protectants, assault

7th T49.3X4 Poisoning by emollients, demulcents and protectants, undetermined

7th T49.3X5 Adverse effect of emollients, demulcents and protectants UPD

7th T49.3X6 Underdosing of emollients, demulcents and protectants UPD

5th **T49.4 Poisoning by, adverse effect of and underdosing of keratolytics, keratoplastics, and other hair treatment drugs and preparations**

6th T49.4X Poisoning by, adverse effect of and underdosing of keratolytics, keratoplastics, and other hair treatment drugs and preparations

7th T49.4X1 Poisoning by keratolytics, keratoplastics, and other hair treatment drugs and preparations, accidental (unintentional)
Poisoning by keratolytics, keratoplastics, and other hair treatment drugs and preparations NOS

7th T49.4X2 Poisoning by keratolytics, keratoplastics, and other hair treatment drugs and preparations, intentional self-harm HCC

7th T49.4X3 Poisoning by keratolytics, keratoplastics, and other hair treatment drugs and preparations, assault

7th T49.4X4 Poisoning by keratolytics, keratoplastics, and other hair treatment drugs and preparations, undetermined

7th T49.4X5 Adverse effect of keratolytics, keratoplastics, and other hair treatment drugs and preparations UPD

7th T49.4X6 Underdosing of keratolytics, keratoplastics, and other hair treatment drugs and preparations UPD

5th **T49.5 Poisoning by, adverse effect of and underdosing of ophthalmological drugs and preparations**

6th T49.5X Poisoning by, adverse effect of and underdosing of ophthalmological drugs and preparations

7th T49.5X1 Poisoning by ophthalmological drugs and preparations, accidental (unintentional)
Poisoning by ophthalmological drugs and preparations NOS

7th T49.5X2 Poisoning by ophthalmological drugs and preparations, intentional self-harm HCC

7th T49.5X3 Poisoning by ophthalmological drugs and preparations, assault

7th T49.5X4 Poisoning by ophthalmological drugs and preparations, undetermined

7th T49.5X5 Adverse effect of ophthalmological drugs and preparations UPD

7th T49.5X6 Underdosing of ophthalmological drugs and preparations UPD

5th **T49.6 Poisoning by, adverse effect of and underdosing of otorhinolaryngological drugs and preparations**

6th T49.6X Poisoning by, adverse effect of and underdosing of otorhinolaryngological drugs and preparations

7th T49.6X1 Poisoning by otorhinolaryngological drugs and preparations, accidental (unintentional)
Poisoning by otorhinolaryngological drugs and preparations NOS

7th T49.6X2 Poisoning by otorhinolaryngological drugs and preparations, intentional self-harm HCC

7th T49.6X3 Poisoning by otorhinolaryngological drugs and preparations, assault

7th T49.6X4 Poisoning by otorhinolaryngological drugs and preparations, undetermined

7th T49.6X5 Adverse effect of otorhinolaryngological drugs and preparations UPD

- T49.6X6 Underdosing of otorhinolaryngological drugs and preparations UPD

T49.7 Poisoning by, adverse effect of and underdosing of dental drugs, topically applied

T49.7X Poisoning by, adverse effect of and underdosing of dental drugs, topically applied

- T49.7X1 Poisoning by dental drugs, topically applied, accidental (unintentional)
  - Poisoning by dental drugs, topically applied NOS
- T49.7X2 Poisoning by dental drugs, topically applied, intentional self-harm HCC
- T49.7X3 Poisoning by dental drugs, topically applied, assault
- T49.7X4 Poisoning by dental drugs, topically applied, undetermined
- T49.7X5 Adverse effect of dental drugs, topically applied UPD
- T49.7X6 Underdosing of dental drugs, topically applied UPD

T49.8 Poisoning by, adverse effect of and underdosing of other topical agents

Poisoning by, adverse effect of and underdosing of spermicides

T49.8X Poisoning by, adverse effect of and underdosing of other topical agents

- T49.8X1 Poisoning by other topical agents, accidental (unintentional)
  - Poisoning by other topical agents NOS
- T49.8X2 Poisoning by other topical agents, intentional self-harm HCC
- T49.8X3 Poisoning by other topical agents, assault
- T49.8X4 Poisoning by other topical agents, undetermined
- T49.8X5 Adverse effect of other topical agents UPD
- T49.8X6 Underdosing of other topical agents UPD

T49.9 Poisoning by, adverse effect of and underdosing of unspecified topical agent

- T49.91 Poisoning by unspecified topical agent, accidental (unintentional)
- T49.92 Poisoning by unspecified topical agent, intentional self-harm HCC
- T49.93 Poisoning by unspecified topical agent, assault
- T49.94 Poisoning by unspecified topical agent, undetermined
- T49.95 Adverse effect of unspecified topical agent UPD
- T49.96 Underdosing of unspecified topical agent UPD

T50 Poisoning by, adverse effect of and underdosing of diuretics and other and unspecified drugs, medicaments and biological substances

The appropriate 7th character is to be added to each code from category T50.

A initial encounter
D subsequent encounter
S sequela

T50.0 Poisoning by, adverse effect of and underdosing of mineralocorticoids and their antagonists

T50.0X Poisoning by, adverse effect of and underdosing of mineralocorticoids and their antagonists

- T50.0X1 Poisoning by mineralocorticoids and their antagonists, accidental (unintentional)
  - Poisoning by mineralocorticoids and their antagonists NOS
- T50.0X2 Poisoning by mineralocorticoids and their antagonists, intentional self-harm HCC
- T50.0X3 Poisoning by mineralocorticoids and their antagonists, assault
- T50.0X4 Poisoning by mineralocorticoids and their antagonists, undetermined
- T50.0X5 Adverse effect of mineralocorticoids and their antagonists UPD
- T50.0X6 Underdosing of mineralocorticoids and their antagonists UPD

T50.1 Poisoning by, adverse effect of and underdosing of loop [high-ceiling] diuretics

T50.1X Poisoning by, adverse effect of and underdosing of loop [high-ceiling] diuretics

- T50.1X1 Poisoning by loop [high-ceiling] diuretics, accidental (unintentional)
  - Poisoning by loop [high-ceiling] diuretics NOS
- T50.1X2 Poisoning by loop [high-ceiling] diuretics, intentional self-harm HCC
- T50.1X3 Poisoning by loop [high-ceiling] diuretics, assault
- T50.1X4 Poisoning by loop [high-ceiling] diuretics, undetermined
- T50.1X5 Adverse effect of loop [high-ceiling] diuretics UPD
- T50.1X6 Underdosing of loop [high-ceiling] diuretics UPD

T50.2 Poisoning by, adverse effect of and underdosing of carbonic-anhydrase inhibitors, benzothiadiazides and other diuretics

Poisoning by, adverse effect of and underdosing of acetazolamide

T50.2X Poisoning by, adverse effect of and underdosing of carbonic-anhydrase inhibitors, benzothiadiazides and other diuretics

- T50.2X1 Poisoning by carbonic-anhydrase inhibitors, benzothiadiazides and other diuretics, accidental (unintentional)
  - Poisoning by carbonic-anhydrase inhibitors, benzothiadiazides and other diuretics NOS
- T50.2X2 Poisoning by carbonic-anhydrase inhibitors, benzothiadiazides and other diuretics, intentional self-harm HCC
- T50.2X3 Poisoning by carbonic-anhydrase inhibitors, benzothiadiazides and other diuretics, assault
- T50.2X4 Poisoning by carbonic-anhydrase inhibitors, benzothiadiazides and other diuretics, undetermined
- T50.2X5 Adverse effect of carbonic-anhydrase inhibitors, benzothiadiazides and other diuretics UPD
- T50.2X6 Underdosing of carbonic-anhydrase inhibitors, benzothiadiazides and other diuretics UPD

T50.3 Poisoning by, adverse effect of and underdosing of electrolytic, caloric and water-balance agents

Poisoning by, adverse effect of and underdosing of oral rehydration salts

T50.3X Poisoning by, adverse effect of and underdosing of electrolytic, caloric and water-balance agents

- T50.3X1 Poisoning by electrolytic, caloric and water-balance agents, accidental (unintentional)
  - Poisoning by electrolytic, caloric and water-balance agents NOS
- T50.3X2 Poisoning by electrolytic, caloric and water-balance agents, intentional self-harm HCC
- T50.3X3 Poisoning by electrolytic, caloric and water-balance agents, assault
- T50.3X4 Poisoning by electrolytic, caloric and water-balance agents, undetermined
- T50.3X5 Adverse effect of electrolytic, caloric and water-balance agents UPD
  - AHA: 2022,2Q,10
- T50.3X6 Underdosing of electrolytic, caloric and water-balance agents UPD

T50.4 Poisoning by, adverse effect of and underdosing of drugs affecting uric acid metabolism

T50.4X Poisoning by, adverse effect of and underdosing of drugs affecting uric acid metabolism

- T50.4X1 Poisoning by drugs affecting uric acid metabolism, accidental (unintentional)
  - Poisoning by drugs affecting uric acid metabolism NOS
- T50.4X2 Poisoning by drugs affecting uric acid metabolism, intentional self-harm HCC
- T50.4X3 Poisoning by drugs affecting uric acid metabolism, assault

√7th **T50.4X4 Poisoning by drugs affecting uric acid metabolism, undetermined**

√7th **T50.4X5 Adverse effect of drugs affecting uric acid metabolism** UPD

√7th **T50.4X6 Underdosing of drugs affecting uric acid metabolism** UPD

√5th **T50.5 Poisoning by, adverse effect of and underdosing of appetite depressants**

√6th **T50.5X Poisoning by, adverse effect of and underdosing of appetite depressants**

√7th **T50.5X1 Poisoning by appetite depressants, accidental (unintentional)**
Poisoning by appetite depressants NOS

√7th **T50.5X2 Poisoning by appetite depressants, intentional self-harm** HCC

√7th **T50.5X3 Poisoning by appetite depressants, assault**

√7th **T50.5X4 Poisoning by appetite depressants, undetermined**

√7th **T50.5X5 Adverse effect of appetite depressants** UPD

√7th **T50.5X6 Underdosing of appetite depressants** UPD

√5th **T50.6 Poisoning by, adverse effect of and underdosing of antidotes and chelating agents**
Poisoning by, adverse effect of and underdosing of alcohol deterrents

√6th **T50.6X Poisoning by, adverse effect of and underdosing of antidotes and chelating agents**

√7th **T50.6X1 Poisoning by antidotes and chelating agents, accidental (unintentional)**
Poisoning by antidotes and chelating agents NOS

√7th **T50.6X2 Poisoning by antidotes and chelating agents, intentional self-harm** HCC

√7th **T50.6X3 Poisoning by antidotes and chelating agents, assault**

√7th **T50.6X4 Poisoning by antidotes and chelating agents, undetermined**

√7th **T50.6X5 Adverse effect of antidotes and chelating agents** UPD

√7th **T50.6X6 Underdosing of antidotes and chelating agents** UPD

√5th **T50.7 Poisoning by, adverse effect of and underdosing of analeptics and opioid receptor antagonists**

√6th **T50.7X Poisoning by, adverse effect of and underdosing of analeptics and opioid receptor antagonists**

√7th **T50.7X1 Poisoning by analeptics and opioid receptor antagonists, accidental (unintentional)**
Poisoning by analeptics and opioid receptor antagonists NOS

√7th **T50.7X2 Poisoning by analeptics and opioid receptor antagonists, intentional self-harm** HCC

√7th **T50.7X3 Poisoning by analeptics and opioid receptor antagonists, assault**

√7th **T50.7X4 Poisoning by analeptics and opioid receptor antagonists, undetermined**

√7th **T50.7X5 Adverse effect of analeptics and opioid receptor antagonists** UPD

√7th **T50.7X6 Underdosing of analeptics and opioid receptor antagonists** UPD

√5th **T50.8 Poisoning by, adverse effect of and underdosing of diagnostic agents**

√6th **T50.8X Poisoning by, adverse effect of and underdosing of diagnostic agents**

√7th **T50.8X1 Poisoning by diagnostic agents, accidental (unintentional)**
Poisoning by diagnostic agents NOS

√7th **T50.8X2 Poisoning by diagnostic agents, intentional self-harm** HCC

√7th **T50.8X3 Poisoning by diagnostic agents, assault**

√7th **T50.8X4 Poisoning by diagnostic agents, undetermined**

√7th **T50.8X5 Adverse effect of diagnostic agents** UPD
AHA: 2022,4Q,33; 2021,3Q,9-10

√7th **T50.8X6 Underdosing of diagnostic agents** UPD

√5th **T50.A Poisoning by, adverse effect of and underdosing of bacterial vaccines**

√6th **T50.A1 Poisoning by, adverse effect of and underdosing of pertussis vaccine, including combinations with a pertussis component**

√7th **T50.A11 Poisoning by pertussis vaccine, including combinations with a pertussis component, accidental (unintentional)**

√7th **T50.A12 Poisoning by pertussis vaccine, including combinations with a pertussis component, intentional self-harm** HCC

√7th **T50.A13 Poisoning by pertussis vaccine, including combinations with a pertussis component, assault**

√7th **T50.A14 Poisoning by pertussis vaccine, including combinations with a pertussis component, undetermined**

√7th **T50.A15 Adverse effect of pertussis vaccine, including combinations with a pertussis component** UPD

√7th **T50.A16 Underdosing of pertussis vaccine, including combinations with a pertussis component** UPD

√6th **T50.A2 Poisoning by, adverse effect of and underdosing of mixed bacterial vaccines without a pertussis component**

√7th **T50.A21 Poisoning by mixed bacterial vaccines without a pertussis component, accidental (unintentional)**

√7th **T50.A22 Poisoning by mixed bacterial vaccines without a pertussis component, intentional self-harm** HCC

√7th **T50.A23 Poisoning by mixed bacterial vaccines without a pertussis component, assault**

√7th **T50.A24 Poisoning by mixed bacterial vaccines without a pertussis component, undetermined**

√7th **T50.A25 Adverse effect of mixed bacterial vaccines without a pertussis component** UPD

√7th **T50.A26 Underdosing of mixed bacterial vaccines without a pertussis component** UPD

√6th **T50.A9 Poisoning by, adverse effect of and underdosing of other bacterial vaccines**

√7th **T50.A91 Poisoning by other bacterial vaccines, accidental (unintentional)**

√7th **T50.A92 Poisoning by other bacterial vaccines, intentional self-harm** HCC

√7th **T50.A93 Poisoning by other bacterial vaccines, assault**

√7th **T50.A94 Poisoning by other bacterial vaccines, undetermined**

√7th **T50.A95 Adverse effect of other bacterial vaccines** UPD

√7th **T50.A96 Underdosing of other bacterial vaccines** UPD

√5th **T50.B Poisoning by, adverse effect of and underdosing of viral vaccines**

√6th **T50.B1 Poisoning by, adverse effect of and underdosing of smallpox vaccines**

√7th **T50.B11 Poisoning by smallpox vaccines, accidental (unintentional)**

√7th **T50.B12 Poisoning by smallpox vaccines, intentional self-harm** HCC

√7th **T50.B13 Poisoning by smallpox vaccines, assault**

√7th **T50.B14 Poisoning by smallpox vaccines, undetermined**

√7th **T50.B15 Adverse effect of smallpox vaccines** UPD

√7th **T50.B16 Underdosing of smallpox vaccines** UPD

√6th **T50.B9 Poisoning by, adverse effect of and underdosing of other viral vaccines**

√7th **T50.B91 Poisoning by other viral vaccines, accidental (unintentional)**

√7th **T50.B92 Poisoning by other viral vaccines, intentional self-harm** HCC

√7th **T50.B93 Poisoning by other viral vaccines, assault**

√7th **T50.B94 Poisoning by other viral vaccines, undetermined**

√7th **T50.B95 Adverse effect of other viral vaccines** UPD
AHA: 2021,1Q,43

T5Ø.B96 Underdosing of other viral vaccines UPD

T5Ø.Z Poisoning by, adverse effect of and underdosing of other vaccines and biological substances

T5Ø.Z1 Poisoning by, adverse effect of and underdosing of immunoglobulin

T5Ø.Z11 Poisoning by immunoglobulin, accidental (unintentional)

T5Ø.Z12 Poisoning by immunoglobulin, intentional self-harm HCC

T5Ø.Z13 Poisoning by immunoglobulin, assault

T5Ø.Z14 Poisoning by immunoglobulin, undetermined

T5Ø.Z15 Adverse effect of immunoglobulin UPD

T5Ø.Z16 Underdosing of immunoglobulin UPD

T5Ø.Z9 Poisoning by, adverse effect of and underdosing of other vaccines and biological substances

T5Ø.Z91 Poisoning by other vaccines and biological substances, accidental (unintentional)

T5Ø.Z92 Poisoning by other vaccines and biological substances, intentional self-harm HCC

T5Ø.Z93 Poisoning by other vaccines and biological substances, assault

T5Ø.Z94 Poisoning by other vaccines and biological substances, undetermined

T5Ø.Z95 Adverse effect of other vaccines and biological substances UPD

AHA: 2020,1Q,18

T5Ø.Z96 Underdosing of other vaccines and biological substances UPD

T5Ø.9 Poisoning by, adverse effect of and underdosing of other and unspecified drugs, medicaments and biological substances

T5Ø.9Ø Poisoning by, adverse effect of and underdosing of unspecified drugs, medicaments and biological substances

T5Ø.9Ø1 Poisoning by unspecified drugs, medicaments and biological substances, accidental (unintentional)

T5Ø.9Ø2 Poisoning by unspecified drugs, medicaments and biological substances, intentional self-harm HCC

T5Ø.9Ø3 Poisoning by unspecified drugs, medicaments and biological substances, assault

T5Ø.9Ø4 Poisoning by unspecified drugs, medicaments and biological substances, undetermined

T5Ø.9Ø5 Adverse effect of unspecified drugs, medicaments and biological substances

T5Ø.9Ø6 Underdosing of unspecified drugs, medicaments and biological substances

T5Ø.91 Poisoning by, adverse effect of and underdosing of multiple unspecified drugs, medicaments and biological substances

Multiple drug ingestion NOS

Code also any specific drugs, medicaments and biological substances

T5Ø.911 Poisoning by multiple unspecified drugs, medicaments and biological substances, accidental (unintentional)

T5Ø.912 Poisoning by multiple unspecified drugs, medicaments and biological substances, intentional self-harm HCC

T5Ø.913 Poisoning by multiple unspecified drugs, medicaments and biological substances, assault

T5Ø.914 Poisoning by multiple unspecified drugs, medicaments and biological substances, undetermined

T5Ø.915 Adverse effect of multiple unspecified drugs, medicaments and biological substances UPD

T5Ø.916 Underdosing of multiple unspecified drugs, medicaments and biological substances UPD

T5Ø.99 Poisoning by, adverse effect of and underdosing of other drugs, medicaments and biological substances

T5Ø.991 Poisoning by other drugs, medicaments and biological substances, accidental (unintentional)

T5Ø.992 Poisoning by other drugs, medicaments and biological substances, intentional self-harm HCC

T5Ø.993 Poisoning by other drugs, medicaments and biological substances, assault

T5Ø.994 Poisoning by other drugs, medicaments and biological substances, undetermined

T5Ø.995 Adverse effect of other drugs, medicaments and biological substances

T5Ø.996 Underdosing of other drugs, medicaments and biological substances

Toxic effects of substances chiefly nonmedicinal as to source (T51-T65)

NOTE When no intent is indicated code to accidental. Undetermined intent is only for use when there is specific documentation in the record that the intent of the toxic effect cannot be determined.

Use additional code(s) for all associated manifestations of toxic effect, such as:
personal history of foreign body fully removed (Z87.821)
respiratory conditions due to external agents (J6Ø-J7Ø)
to identify any retained foreign body, if applicable (Z18.-)

EXCLUDES 1 *contact with and (suspected) exposure to toxic substances (Z77.-)*

AHA: 2017,1Q,39-40

T51 Toxic effect of alcohol

The appropriate 7th character is to be added to each code from category T51.
A initial encounter
D subsequent encounter
S sequela

T51.Ø Toxic effect of ethanol

Toxic effect of ethyl alcohol

EXCLUDES 2 *acute alcohol intoxication or "hangover" effects (F1Ø.129, F1Ø.229, F1Ø.929)*
drunkenness (F1Ø.129, F1Ø.229, F1Ø.929)
pathological alcohol intoxication (F1Ø.129, F1Ø.229, F1Ø.929)

T51.ØX Toxic effect of ethanol

T51.ØX1 Toxic effect of ethanol, accidental (unintentional) HCC

Toxic effect of ethanol NOS

T51.ØX2 Toxic effect of ethanol, intentional self-harm HCC

T51.ØX3 Toxic effect of ethanol, assault

T51.ØX4 Toxic effect of ethanol, undetermined HCC

T51.1 Toxic effect of methanol

Toxic effect of methyl alcohol

T51.1X Toxic effect of methanol

T51.1X1 Toxic effect of methanol, accidental (unintentional)

Toxic effect of methanol NOS

T51.1X2 Toxic effect of methanol, intentional self-harm HCC

T51.1X3 Toxic effect of methanol, assault

T51.1X4 Toxic effect of methanol, undetermined

T51.2 Toxic effect of 2-Propanol

Toxic effect of isopropyl alcohol

T51.2X Toxic effect of 2-Propanol

T51.2X1 Toxic effect of 2-Propanol, accidental (unintentional)

Toxic effect of 2-Propanol NOS

T51.2X2 Toxic effect of 2-Propanol, intentional self-harm HCC

T51.2X3 Toxic effect of 2-Propanol, assault

T51.2X4 Toxic effect of 2-Propanol, undetermined

√5th **T51.3 Toxic effect of fusel oil**
Toxic effect of amyl alcohol
Toxic effect of butyl [1-butanol] alcohol
Toxic effect of propyl [1-propanol] alcohol

√6th **T51.3X Toxic effect of fusel oil**

√7th **T51.3X1 Toxic effect of fusel oil, accidental (unintentional)**
Toxic effect of fusel oil NOS

√7th **T51.3X2 Toxic effect of fusel oil, intentional self-harm** HCC

√7th **T51.3X3 Toxic effect of fusel oil, assault**

√7th **T51.3X4 Toxic effect of fusel oil, undetermined**

√5th **T51.8 Toxic effect of other alcohols**

√6th **T51.8X Toxic effect of other alcohols**

√7th **T51.8X1 Toxic effect of other alcohols, accidental (unintentional)**
Toxic effect of other alcohols NOS

√7th **T51.8X2 Toxic effect of other alcohols, intentional self-harm** HCC

√7th **T51.8X3 Toxic effect of other alcohols, assault**

√7th **T51.8X4 Toxic effect of other alcohols, undetermined**

√5th **T51.9 Toxic effect of unspecified alcohol**

√x7th **T51.91 Toxic effect of unspecified alcohol, accidental (unintentional)**

√x7th **T51.92 Toxic effect of unspecified alcohol, intentional self-harm** HCC

√x7th **T51.93 Toxic effect of unspecified alcohol, assault**

√x7th **T51.94 Toxic effect of unspecified alcohol, undetermined**

√4th **T52 Toxic effect of organic solvents**

EXCLUDES 1 *halogen derivatives of aliphatic and aromatic hydrocarbons (T53.-)*

The appropriate 7th character is to be added to each code from category T52.
A initial encounter
D subsequent encounter
S sequela

√5th **T52.Ø Toxic effects of petroleum products**
Toxic effects of ether petroleum
Toxic effects of gasoline [petrol]
Toxic effects of kerosene [paraffin oil]
Toxic effects of naphtha petroleum
Toxic effects of paraffin wax
Toxic effects of spirit petroleum

√6th **T52.ØX Toxic effects of petroleum products**

√7th **T52.ØX1 Toxic effect of petroleum products, accidental (unintentional)**
Toxic effects of petroleum products NOS

√7th **T52.ØX2 Toxic effect of petroleum products, intentional self-harm** HCC

√7th **T52.ØX3 Toxic effect of petroleum products, assault**

√7th **T52.ØX4 Toxic effect of petroleum products, undetermined**

√5th **T52.1 Toxic effects of benzene**

EXCLUDES 1 *homologues of benzene (T52.2)*
nitroderivatives and aminoderivatives of benzene and its homologues (T65.3)

√6th **T52.1X Toxic effects of benzene**

√7th **T52.1X1 Toxic effect of benzene, accidental (unintentional)**
Toxic effects of benzene NOS

√7th **T52.1X2 Toxic effect of benzene, intentional self-harm** HCC

√7th **T52.1X3 Toxic effect of benzene, assault**

√7th **T52.1X4 Toxic effect of benzene, undetermined**

√5th **T52.2 Toxic effects of homologues of benzene**
Toxic effects of toluene [methylbenzene]
Toxic effects of xylene [dimethylbenzene]

√6th **T52.2X Toxic effects of homologues of benzene**

√7th **T52.2X1 Toxic effect of homologues of benzene, accidental (unintentional)**
Toxic effects of homologues of benzene NOS

√7th **T52.2X2 Toxic effect of homologues of benzene, intentional self-harm** HCC

√7th **T52.2X3 Toxic effect of homologues of benzene, assault**

√7th **T52.2X4 Toxic effect of homologues of benzene, undetermined**

√5th **T52.3 Toxic effects of glycols**

√6th **T52.3X Toxic effects of glycols**

√7th **T52.3X1 Toxic effect of glycols, accidental (unintentional)**
Toxic effects of glycols NOS

√7th **T52.3X2 Toxic effect of glycols, intentional self-harm** HCC

√7th **T52.3X3 Toxic effect of glycols, assault**

√7th **T52.3X4 Toxic effect of glycols, undetermined**

√5th **T52.4 Toxic effects of ketones**

√6th **T52.4X Toxic effects of ketones**

√7th **T52.4X1 Toxic effect of ketones, accidental (unintentional)**
Toxic effects of ketones NOS

√7th **T52.4X2 Toxic effect of ketones, intentional self-harm** HCC

√7th **T52.4X3 Toxic effect of ketones, assault**

√7th **T52.4X4 Toxic effect of ketones, undetermined**

√5th **T52.8 Toxic effects of other organic solvents**

√6th **T52.8X Toxic effects of other organic solvents**

√7th **T52.8X1 Toxic effect of other organic solvents, accidental (unintentional)**
Toxic effects of other organic solvents NOS

√7th **T52.8X2 Toxic effect of other organic solvents, intentional self-harm** HCC

√7th **T52.8X3 Toxic effect of other organic solvents, assault**

√7th **T52.8X4 Toxic effect of other organic solvents, undetermined**

√5th **T52.9 Toxic effects of unspecified organic solvent**

√x7th **T52.91 Toxic effect of unspecified organic solvent, accidental (unintentional)**

√x7th **T52.92 Toxic effect of unspecified organic solvent, intentional self-harm** HCC

√x7th **T52.93 Toxic effect of unspecified organic solvent, assault**

√x7th **T52.94 Toxic effect of unspecified organic solvent, undetermined**

√4th **T53 Toxic effect of halogen derivatives of aliphatic and aromatic hydrocarbons**

The appropriate 7th character is to be added to each code from category T53.
A initial encounter
D subsequent encounter
S sequela

√5th **T53.Ø Toxic effects of carbon tetrachloride**
Toxic effects of tetrachloromethane

√6th **T53.ØX Toxic effects of carbon tetrachloride**

√7th **T53.ØX1 Toxic effect of carbon tetrachloride, accidental (unintentional)**
Toxic effects of carbon tetrachloride NOS

√7th **T53.ØX2 Toxic effect of carbon tetrachloride, intentional self-harm** HCC

√7th **T53.ØX3 Toxic effect of carbon tetrachloride, assault**

√7th **T53.ØX4 Toxic effect of carbon tetrachloride, undetermined**

√5th **T53.1 Toxic effects of chloroform**
Toxic effects of trichloromethane

√6th **T53.1X Toxic effects of chloroform**

√7th **T53.1X1 Toxic effect of chloroform, accidental (unintentional)**
Toxic effects of chloroform NOS

√7th **T53.1X2 Toxic effect of chloroform, intentional self-harm** HCC

√7th **T53.1X3 Toxic effect of chloroform, assault**

√7th **T53.1X4 Toxic effect of chloroform, undetermined**

T53.2 Toxic effects of trichloroethylene
Toxic effects of trichloroethene
T53.2X Toxic effects of trichloroethylene
T53.2X1 Toxic effect of trichloroethylene, accidental (unintentional)
Toxic effects of trichloroethylene NOS
T53.2X2 Toxic effect of trichloroethylene, intentional self-harm HCC
T53.2X3 Toxic effect of trichloroethylene, assault
T53.2X4 Toxic effect of trichloroethylene, undetermined

T53.3 Toxic effects of tetrachloroethylene
Toxic effects of perchloroethylene
Toxic effect of tetrachloroethene
T53.3X Toxic effects of tetrachloroethylene
T53.3X1 Toxic effect of tetrachloroethylene, accidental (unintentional)
Toxic effects of tetrachloroethylene NOS
T53.3X2 Toxic effect of tetrachloroethylene, intentional self-harm HCC
T53.3X3 Toxic effect of tetrachloroethylene, assault
T53.3X4 Toxic effect of tetrachloroethylene, undetermined

T53.4 Toxic effects of dichloromethane
Toxic effects of methylene chloride
T53.4X Toxic effects of dichloromethane
T53.4X1 Toxic effect of dichloromethane, accidental (unintentional)
Toxic effects of dichloromethane NOS
T53.4X2 Toxic effect of dichloromethane, intentional self-harm HCC
T53.4X3 Toxic effect of dichloromethane, assault
T53.4X4 Toxic effect of dichloromethane, undetermined

T53.5 Toxic effects of chlorofluorocarbons
T53.5X Toxic effects of chlorofluorocarbons
T53.5X1 Toxic effect of chlorofluorocarbons, accidental (unintentional)
Toxic effects of chlorofluorocarbons NOS
T53.5X2 Toxic effect of chlorofluorocarbons, intentional self-harm HCC
T53.5X3 Toxic effect of chlorofluorocarbons, assault
T53.5X4 Toxic effect of chlorofluorocarbons, undetermined

T53.6 Toxic effects of other halogen derivatives of aliphatic hydrocarbons
T53.6X Toxic effects of other halogen derivatives of aliphatic hydrocarbons
T53.6X1 Toxic effect of other halogen derivatives of aliphatic hydrocarbons, accidental (unintentional)
Toxic effects of other halogen derivatives of aliphatic hydrocarbons NOS
T53.6X2 Toxic effect of other halogen derivatives of aliphatic hydrocarbons, intentional self-harm HCC
T53.6X3 Toxic effect of other halogen derivatives of aliphatic hydrocarbons, assault
T53.6X4 Toxic effect of other halogen derivatives of aliphatic hydrocarbons, undetermined

T53.7 Toxic effects of other halogen derivatives of aromatic hydrocarbons
T53.7X Toxic effects of other halogen derivatives of aromatic hydrocarbons
T53.7X1 Toxic effect of other halogen derivatives of aromatic hydrocarbons, accidental (unintentional)
Toxic effects of other halogen derivatives of aromatic hydrocarbons NOS
T53.7X2 Toxic effect of other halogen derivatives of aromatic hydrocarbons, intentional self-harm HCC
T53.7X3 Toxic effect of other halogen derivatives of aromatic hydrocarbons, assault
T53.7X4 Toxic effect of other halogen derivatives of aromatic hydrocarbons, undetermined

T53.9 Toxic effects of unspecified halogen derivatives of aliphatic and aromatic hydrocarbons
T53.91 Toxic effect of unspecified halogen derivatives of aliphatic and aromatic hydrocarbons, accidental (unintentional)
T53.92 Toxic effect of unspecified halogen derivatives of aliphatic and aromatic hydrocarbons, intentional self-harm HCC
T53.93 Toxic effect of unspecified halogen derivatives of aliphatic and aromatic hydrocarbons, assault
T53.94 Toxic effect of unspecified halogen derivatives of aliphatic and aromatic hydrocarbons, undetermined

T54 Toxic effect of corrosive substances

The appropriate 7th character is to be added to each code from category T54.
A initial encounter
D subsequent encounter
S sequela

T54.Ø Toxic effects of phenol and phenol homologues
T54.ØX Toxic effects of phenol and phenol homologues
T54.ØX1 Toxic effect of phenol and phenol homologues, accidental (unintentional)
Toxic effects of phenol and phenol homologues NOS
T54.ØX2 Toxic effect of phenol and phenol homologues, intentional self-harm HCC
T54.ØX3 Toxic effect of phenol and phenol homologues, assault
T54.ØX4 Toxic effect of phenol and phenol homologues, undetermined

T54.1 Toxic effects of other corrosive organic compounds
T54.1X Toxic effects of other corrosive organic compounds
T54.1X1 Toxic effect of other corrosive organic compounds, accidental (unintentional)
Toxic effects of other corrosive organic compounds NOS
T54.1X2 Toxic effect of other corrosive organic compounds, intentional self-harm HCC
T54.1X3 Toxic effect of other corrosive organic compounds, assault
T54.1X4 Toxic effect of other corrosive organic compounds, undetermined

T54.2 Toxic effects of corrosive acids and acid-like substances
Toxic effects of hydrochloric acid
Toxic effects of sulfuric acid
T54.2X Toxic effects of corrosive acids and acid-like substances
T54.2X1 Toxic effect of corrosive acids and acid-like substances, accidental (unintentional)
Toxic effects of corrosive acids and acid-like substances NOS
T54.2X2 Toxic effect of corrosive acids and acid-like substances, intentional self-harm HCC
T54.2X3 Toxic effect of corrosive acids and acid-like substances, assault
T54.2X4 Toxic effect of corrosive acids and acid-like substances, undetermined

T54.3 Toxic effects of corrosive alkalis and alkali-like substances
Toxic effects of potassium hydroxide
Toxic effects of sodium hydroxide
T54.3X Toxic effects of corrosive alkalis and alkali-like substances
T54.3X1 Toxic effect of corrosive alkalis and alkali-like substances, accidental (unintentional)
Toxic effects of corrosive alkalis and alkali-like substances NOS
T54.3X2 Toxic effect of corrosive alkalis and alkali-like substances, intentional self-harm HCC
T54.3X3 Toxic effect of corrosive alkalis and alkali-like substances, assault
T54.3X4 Toxic effect of corrosive alkalis and alkali-like substances, undetermined

T54.9 Toxic effects of unspecified corrosive substance
- **T54.91 Toxic effect of unspecified corrosive substance, accidental (unintentional)**
- **T54.92 Toxic effect of unspecified corrosive substance, intentional self-harm** HCC
- **T54.93 Toxic effect of unspecified corrosive substance, assault**
- **T54.94 Toxic effect of unspecified corrosive substance, undetermined**

T55 Toxic effect of soaps and detergents

The appropriate 7th character is to be added to each code from category T55.
A initial encounter
D subsequent encounter
S sequela

T55.Ø Toxic effect of soaps
- **T55.ØX Toxic effect of soaps**
  - **T55.ØX1 Toxic effect of soaps, accidental (unintentional)**
    Toxic effect of soaps NOS
  - **T55.ØX2 Toxic effect of soaps, intentional self-harm** HCC
  - **T55.ØX3 Toxic effect of soaps, assault**
  - **T55.ØX4 Toxic effect of soaps, undetermined**

T55.1 Toxic effect of detergents
- **T55.1X Toxic effect of detergents**
  - **T55.1X1 Toxic effect of detergents, accidental (unintentional)**
    Toxic effect of detergents NOS
  - **T55.1X2 Toxic effect of detergents, intentional self-harm** HCC
  - **T55.1X3 Toxic effect of detergents, assault**
  - **T55.1X4 Toxic effect of detergents, undetermined**

T56 Toxic effect of metals

INCLUDES toxic effects of fumes and vapors of metals
toxic effects of metals from all sources, except medicinal substances

Use additional code to identify any retained metal foreign body, if applicable (Z18.Ø-, T18.1-)

EXCLUDES 1 *arsenic and its compounds (T57.Ø)*
manganese and its compounds (T57.2)

The appropriate 7th character is to be added to each code from category T56.
A initial encounter
D subsequent encounter
S sequela

T56.Ø Toxic effects of lead and its compounds
- **T56.ØX Toxic effects of lead and its compounds**
  - **T56.ØX1 Toxic effect of lead and its compounds, accidental (unintentional)**
    Toxic effects of lead and its compounds NOS
  - **T56.ØX2 Toxic effect of lead and its compounds, intentional self-harm** HCC
  - **T56.ØX3 Toxic effect of lead and its compounds, assault**
  - **T56.ØX4 Toxic effect of lead and its compounds, undetermined**

T56.1 Toxic effects of mercury and its compounds
- **T56.1X Toxic effects of mercury and its compounds**
  - **T56.1X1 Toxic effect of mercury and its compounds, accidental (unintentional)**
    Toxic effects of mercury and its compounds NOS
  - **T56.1X2 Toxic effect of mercury and its compounds, intentional self-harm** HCC
  - **T56.1X3 Toxic effect of mercury and its compounds, assault**
  - **T56.1X4 Toxic effect of mercury and its compounds, undetermined**

T56.2 Toxic effects of chromium and its compounds
- **T56.2X Toxic effects of chromium and its compounds**
  - **T56.2X1 Toxic effect of chromium and its compounds, accidental (unintentional)**
    Toxic effects of chromium and its compounds NOS
  - **T56.2X2 Toxic effect of chromium and its compounds, intentional self-harm** HCC
  - **T56.2X3 Toxic effect of chromium and its compounds, assault**
  - **T56.2X4 Toxic effect of chromium and its compounds, undetermined**

T56.3 Toxic effects of cadmium and its compounds
- **T56.3X Toxic effects of cadmium and its compounds**
  - **T56.3X1 Toxic effect of cadmium and its compounds, accidental (unintentional)**
    Toxic effects of cadmium and its compounds NOS
  - **T56.3X2 Toxic effect of cadmium and its compounds, intentional self-harm** HCC
  - **T56.3X3 Toxic effect of cadmium and its compounds, assault**
  - **T56.3X4 Toxic effect of cadmium and its compounds, undetermined**

T56.4 Toxic effects of copper and its compounds
- **T56.4X Toxic effects of copper and its compounds**
  - **T56.4X1 Toxic effect of copper and its compounds, accidental (unintentional)**
    Toxic effects of copper and its compounds NOS
  - **T56.4X2 Toxic effect of copper and its compounds, intentional self-harm** HCC
  - **T56.4X3 Toxic effect of copper and its compounds, assault**
  - **T56.4X4 Toxic effect of copper and its compounds, undetermined**

T56.5 Toxic effects of zinc and its compounds
- **T56.5X Toxic effects of zinc and its compounds**
  - **T56.5X1 Toxic effect of zinc and its compounds, accidental (unintentional)**
    Toxic effects of zinc and its compounds NOS
  - **T56.5X2 Toxic effect of zinc and its compounds, intentional self-harm** HCC
  - **T56.5X3 Toxic effect of zinc and its compounds, assault**
  - **T56.5X4 Toxic effect of zinc and its compounds, undetermined**

T56.6 Toxic effects of tin and its compounds
- **T56.6X Toxic effects of tin and its compounds**
  - **T56.6X1 Toxic effect of tin and its compounds, accidental (unintentional)**
    Toxic effects of tin and its compounds NOS
  - **T56.6X2 Toxic effect of tin and its compounds, intentional self-harm** HCC
  - **T56.6X3 Toxic effect of tin and its compounds, assault**
  - **T56.6X4 Toxic effect of tin and its compounds, undetermined**

T56.7 Toxic effects of beryllium and its compounds
- **T56.7X Toxic effects of beryllium and its compounds**
  - **T56.7X1 Toxic effect of beryllium and its compounds, accidental (unintentional)**
    Toxic effects of beryllium and its compounds NOS
  - **T56.7X2 Toxic effect of beryllium and its compounds, intentional self-harm** HCC
  - **T56.7X3 Toxic effect of beryllium and its compounds, assault**
  - **T56.7X4 Toxic effect of beryllium and its compounds, undetermined**

T56.8 Toxic effects of other metals
- **T56.81 Toxic effect of thallium**
  - **T56.811 Toxic effect of thallium, accidental (unintentional)**
    Toxic effect of thallium NOS
  - **T56.812 Toxic effect of thallium, intentional self-harm** HCC
  - **T56.813 Toxic effect of thallium, assault**

T56.814 Toxic effect of thallium, undetermined

● T56.82 Toxic effect of gadolinium

EXCLUDES 1 *adverse effect of diagnostic agents (T50.8X5-)*

● T56.821 Toxic effect of gadolinium, accidental (unintentional)
Toxic effect of gadolinium NOS

● T56.822 Toxic effect of gadolinium, intentional self-harm

● T56.823 Toxic effect of gadolinium, assault

● T56.824 Toxic effect of gadolinium, undetermined

T56.89 Toxic effects of other metals

T56.891 Toxic effect of other metals, accidental (unintentional)
Toxic effects of other metals NOS

T56.892 Toxic effect of other metals, intentional self-harm HCC

T56.893 Toxic effect of other metals, assault

T56.894 Toxic effect of other metals, undetermined

T56.9 Toxic effects of unspecified metal

T56.91 Toxic effect of unspecified metal, accidental (unintentional)

T56.92 Toxic effect of unspecified metal, intentional self-harm HCC

T56.93 Toxic effect of unspecified metal, assault

T56.94 Toxic effect of unspecified metal, undetermined

T57 Toxic effect of other inorganic substances

The appropriate 7th character is to be added to each code from category T57.
A initial encounter
D subsequent encounter
S sequela

T57.0 Toxic effect of arsenic and its compounds

T57.0X Toxic effect of arsenic and its compounds

T57.0X1 Toxic effect of arsenic and its compounds, accidental (unintentional)
Toxic effect of arsenic and its compounds NOS

T57.0X2 Toxic effect of arsenic and its compounds, intentional self-harm HCC

T57.0X3 Toxic effect of arsenic and its compounds, assault

T57.0X4 Toxic effect of arsenic and its compounds, undetermined

T57.1 Toxic effect of phosphorus and its compounds

EXCLUDES 1 *organophosphate insecticides (T60.0)*

T57.1X Toxic effect of phosphorus and its compounds

T57.1X1 Toxic effect of phosphorus and its compounds, accidental (unintentional)
Toxic effect of phosphorus and its compounds NOS

T57.1X2 Toxic effect of phosphorus and its compounds, intentional self-harm HCC

T57.1X3 Toxic effect of phosphorus and its compounds, assault

T57.1X4 Toxic effect of phosphorus and its compounds, undetermined

T57.2 Toxic effect of manganese and its compounds

T57.2X Toxic effect of manganese and its compounds

T57.2X1 Toxic effect of manganese and its compounds, accidental (unintentional)
Toxic effect of manganese and its compounds NOS

T57.2X2 Toxic effect of manganese and its compounds, intentional self-harm HCC

T57.2X3 Toxic effect of manganese and its compounds, assault

T57.2X4 Toxic effect of manganese and its compounds, undetermined

T57.3 Toxic effect of hydrogen cyanide

T57.3X Toxic effect of hydrogen cyanide

T57.3X1 Toxic effect of hydrogen cyanide, accidental (unintentional)
Toxic effect of hydrogen cyanide NOS

T57.3X2 Toxic effect of hydrogen cyanide, intentional self-harm HCC

T57.3X3 Toxic effect of hydrogen cyanide, assault

T57.3X4 Toxic effect of hydrogen cyanide, undetermined

T57.8 Toxic effect of other specified inorganic substances

T57.8X Toxic effect of other specified inorganic substances

T57.8X1 Toxic effect of other specified inorganic substances, accidental (unintentional)
Toxic effect of other specified inorganic substances NOS

T57.8X2 Toxic effect of other specified inorganic substances, intentional self-harm HCC

T57.8X3 Toxic effect of other specified inorganic substances, assault

T57.8X4 Toxic effect of other specified inorganic substances, undetermined

T57.9 Toxic effect of unspecified inorganic substance

T57.91 Toxic effect of unspecified inorganic substance, accidental (unintentional)

T57.92 Toxic effect of unspecified inorganic substance, intentional self-harm HCC

T57.93 Toxic effect of unspecified inorganic substance, assault

T57.94 Toxic effect of unspecified inorganic substance, undetermined

T58 Toxic effect of carbon monoxide

INCLUDES asphyxiation from carbon monoxide
toxic effect of carbon monoxide from all sources

The appropriate 7th character is to be added to each code from category T58.
A initial encounter
D subsequent encounter
S sequela

T58.0 Toxic effect of carbon monoxide from motor vehicle exhaust
Toxic effect of exhaust gas from gas engine
Toxic effect of exhaust gas from motor pump

T58.01 Toxic effect of carbon monoxide from motor vehicle exhaust, accidental (unintentional)

T58.02 Toxic effect of carbon monoxide from motor vehicle exhaust, intentional self-harm HCC

T58.03 Toxic effect of carbon monoxide from motor vehicle exhaust, assault

T58.04 Toxic effect of carbon monoxide from motor vehicle exhaust, undetermined

T58.1 Toxic effect of carbon monoxide from utility gas
Toxic effect of acetylene
Toxic effect of gas NOS used for lighting, heating, cooking
Toxic effect of water gas

T58.11 Toxic effect of carbon monoxide from utility gas, accidental (unintentional)

T58.12 Toxic effect of carbon monoxide from utility gas, intentional self-harm HCC

T58.13 Toxic effect of carbon monoxide from utility gas, assault

T58.14 Toxic effect of carbon monoxide from utility gas, undetermined

T58.2 Toxic effect of carbon monoxide from incomplete combustion of other domestic fuels
Toxic effect of carbon monoxide from incomplete combustion of coal, coke, kerosene, wood

T58.2X Toxic effect of carbon monoxide from incomplete combustion of other domestic fuels

T58.2X1 Toxic effect of carbon monoxide from incomplete combustion of other domestic fuels, accidental (unintentional)

T58.2X2 Toxic effect of carbon monoxide from incomplete combustion of other domestic fuels, intentional self-harm HCC

T58.2X3 Toxic effect of carbon monoxide from incomplete combustion of other domestic fuels, assault

T58.2X4 Toxic effect of carbon monoxide from incomplete combustion of other domestic fuels, undetermined

5th T58.8 Toxic effect of carbon monoxide from other source

Toxic effect of carbon monoxide from blast furnace gas
Toxic effect of carbon monoxide from fuels in industrial use
Toxic effect of carbon monoxide from kiln vapor

6th T58.8X Toxic effect of carbon monoxide from other source

7th T58.8X1 Toxic effect of carbon monoxide from other source, accidental (unintentional)

7th T58.8X2 Toxic effect of carbon monoxide from other source, intentional self-harm HCC

7th T58.8X3 Toxic effect of carbon monoxide from other source, assault

7th T58.8X4 Toxic effect of carbon monoxide from other source, undetermined

5th T58.9 Toxic effect of carbon monoxide from unspecified source

x7th T58.91 Toxic effect of carbon monoxide from unspecified source, accidental (unintentional)

x7th T58.92 Toxic effect of carbon monoxide from unspecified source, intentional self-harm HCC

x7th T58.93 Toxic effect of carbon monoxide from unspecified source, assault

x7th T58.94 Toxic effect of carbon monoxide from unspecified source, undetermined

4th T59 Toxic effect of other gases, fumes and vapors

INCLUDES aerosol propellants

EXCLUDES 1 *chlorofluorocarbons (T53.5)*

The appropriate 7th character is to be added to each code from category T59.
A initial encounter
D subsequent encounter
S sequela

5th T59.Ø Toxic effect of nitrogen oxides

6th T59.ØX Toxic effect of nitrogen oxides

7th T59.ØX1 Toxic effect of nitrogen oxides, accidental (unintentional)

Toxic effect of nitrogen oxides NOS

7th T59.ØX2 Toxic effect of nitrogen oxides, intentional self-harm HCC

7th T59.ØX3 Toxic effect of nitrogen oxides, assault

7th T59.ØX4 Toxic effect of nitrogen oxides, undetermined

5th T59.1 Toxic effect of sulfur dioxide

6th T59.1X Toxic effect of sulfur dioxide

7th T59.1X1 Toxic effect of sulfur dioxide, accidental (unintentional)

Toxic effect of sulfur dioxide NOS

7th T59.1X2 Toxic effect of sulfur dioxide, intentional self-harm HCC

7th T59.1X3 Toxic effect of sulfur dioxide, assault

7th T59.1X4 Toxic effect of sulfur dioxide, undetermined

5th T59.2 Toxic effect of formaldehyde

6th T59.2X Toxic effect of formaldehyde

7th T59.2X1 Toxic effect of formaldehyde, accidental (unintentional)

Toxic effect of formaldehyde NOS

7th T59.2X2 Toxic effect of formaldehyde, intentional self-harm HCC

7th T59.2X3 Toxic effect of formaldehyde, assault

7th T59.2X4 Toxic effect of formaldehyde, undetermined

5th T59.3 Toxic effect of lacrimogenic gas

Toxic effect of tear gas

6th T59.3X Toxic effect of lacrimogenic gas

7th T59.3X1 Toxic effect of lacrimogenic gas, accidental (unintentional)

Toxic effect of lacrimogenic gas NOS

7th T59.3X2 Toxic effect of lacrimogenic gas, intentional self-harm HCC

7th T59.3X3 Toxic effect of lacrimogenic gas, assault

7th T59.3X4 Toxic effect of lacrimogenic gas, undetermined

5th T59.4 Toxic effect of chlorine gas

6th T59.4X Toxic effect of chlorine gas

7th T59.4X1 Toxic effect of chlorine gas, accidental (unintentional)

Toxic effect of chlorine gas NOS

7th T59.4X2 Toxic effect of chlorine gas, intentional self-harm HCC

7th T59.4X3 Toxic effect of chlorine gas, assault

7th T59.4X4 Toxic effect of chlorine gas, undetermined

5th T59.5 Toxic effect of fluorine gas and hydrogen fluoride

6th T59.5X Toxic effect of fluorine gas and hydrogen fluoride

7th T59.5X1 Toxic effect of fluorine gas and hydrogen fluoride, accidental (unintentional)

Toxic effect of fluorine gas and hydrogen fluoride NOS

7th T59.5X2 Toxic effect of fluorine gas and hydrogen fluoride, intentional self-harm HCC

7th T59.5X3 Toxic effect of fluorine gas and hydrogen fluoride, assault

7th T59.5X4 Toxic effect of fluorine gas and hydrogen fluoride, undetermined

5th T59.6 Toxic effect of hydrogen sulfide

6th T59.6X Toxic effect of hydrogen sulfide

7th T59.6X1 Toxic effect of hydrogen sulfide, accidental (unintentional)

Toxic effect of hydrogen sulfide NOS

7th T59.6X2 Toxic effect of hydrogen sulfide, intentional self-harm HCC

7th T59.6X3 Toxic effect of hydrogen sulfide, assault

7th T59.6X4 Toxic effect of hydrogen sulfide, undetermined

5th T59.7 Toxic effect of carbon dioxide

6th T59.7X Toxic effect of carbon dioxide

7th T59.7X1 Toxic effect of carbon dioxide, accidental (unintentional)

Toxic effect of carbon dioxide NOS

7th T59.7X2 Toxic effect of carbon dioxide, intentional self-harm HCC

7th T59.7X3 Toxic effect of carbon dioxide, assault

7th T59.7X4 Toxic effect of carbon dioxide, undetermined

5th T59.8 Toxic effect of other specified gases, fumes and vapors

6th T59.81 Toxic effect of smoke

Smoke inhalation

EXCLUDES 2 *toxic effect of cigarette (tobacco) smoke (T65.22-)*

7th T59.811 Toxic effect of smoke, accidental (unintentional)

Toxic effect of smoke NOS

AHA: 2013,4Q,121

7th T59.812 Toxic effect of smoke, intentional self-harm HCC

7th T59.813 Toxic effect of smoke, assault

7th T59.814 Toxic effect of smoke, undetermined

6th T59.89 Toxic effect of other specified gases, fumes and vapors

7th T59.891 Toxic effect of other specified gases, fumes and vapors, accidental (unintentional)

7th T59.892 Toxic effect of other specified gases, fumes and vapors, intentional self-harm HCC

7th T59.893 Toxic effect of other specified gases, fumes and vapors, assault

7th T59.894 Toxic effect of other specified gases, fumes and vapors, undetermined

5th T59.9 Toxic effect of unspecified gases, fumes and vapors

x7th T59.91 Toxic effect of unspecified gases, fumes and vapors, accidental (unintentional)

x7th T59.92 Toxic effect of unspecified gases, fumes and vapors, intentional self-harm HCC

x7th T59.93 Toxic effect of unspecified gases, fumes and vapors, assault

x7th T59.94 Toxic effect of unspecified gases, fumes and vapors, undetermined

T60 Toxic effect of pesticides

INCLUDES toxic effect of wood preservatives

The appropriate 7th character is to be added to each code from category T60.
A initial encounter
D subsequent encounter
S sequela

T60.0 Toxic effect of organophosphate and carbamate insecticides

T60.0X Toxic effect of organophosphate and carbamate insecticides

T60.0X1 Toxic effect of organophosphate and carbamate insecticides, accidental (unintentional)
Toxic effect of organophosphate and carbamate insecticides NOS

T60.0X2 Toxic effect of organophosphate and carbamate insecticides, intentional self-harm HCC

T60.0X3 Toxic effect of organophosphate and carbamate insecticides, assault

T60.0X4 Toxic effect of organophosphate and carbamate insecticides, undetermined

T60.1 Toxic effect of halogenated insecticides

EXCLUDES 1 *chlorinated hydrocarbon (T53.-)*

T60.1X Toxic effect of halogenated insecticides

T60.1X1 Toxic effect of halogenated insecticides, accidental (unintentional)
Toxic effect of halogenated insecticides NOS

T60.1X2 Toxic effect of halogenated insecticides, intentional self-harm HCC

T60.1X3 Toxic effect of halogenated insecticides, assault

T60.1X4 Toxic effect of halogenated insecticides, undetermined

T60.2 Toxic effect of other insecticides

T60.2X Toxic effect of other insecticides

T60.2X1 Toxic effect of other insecticides, accidental (unintentional)
Toxic effect of other insecticides NOS

T60.2X2 Toxic effect of other insecticides, intentional self-harm HCC

T60.2X3 Toxic effect of other insecticides, assault

T60.2X4 Toxic effect of other insecticides, undetermined

T60.3 Toxic effect of herbicides and fungicides

T60.3X Toxic effect of herbicides and fungicides

T60.3X1 Toxic effect of herbicides and fungicides, accidental (unintentional)
Toxic effect of herbicides and fungicides NOS

T60.3X2 Toxic effect of herbicides and fungicides, intentional self-harm HCC

T60.3X3 Toxic effect of herbicides and fungicides, assault

T60.3X4 Toxic effect of herbicides and fungicides, undetermined

T60.4 Toxic effect of rodenticides

EXCLUDES 1 *strychnine and its salts (T65.1)*
thallium (T56.81-)

T60.4X Toxic effect of rodenticides

T60.4X1 Toxic effect of rodenticides, accidental (unintentional)
Toxic effect of rodenticides NOS

T60.4X2 Toxic effect of rodenticides, intentional self-harm HCC

T60.4X3 Toxic effect of rodenticides, assault

T60.4X4 Toxic effect of rodenticides, undetermined

T60.8 Toxic effect of other pesticides

T60.8X Toxic effect of other pesticides

T60.8X1 Toxic effect of other pesticides, accidental (unintentional)
Toxic effect of other pesticides NOS

T60.8X2 Toxic effect of other pesticides, intentional self-harm HCC

T60.8X3 Toxic effect of other pesticides, assault

T60.8X4 Toxic effect of other pesticides, undetermined

T60.9 Toxic effect of unspecified pesticide

T60.91 Toxic effect of unspecified pesticide, accidental (unintentional)

T60.92 Toxic effect of unspecified pesticide, intentional self-harm HCC

T60.93 Toxic effect of unspecified pesticide, assault

T60.94 Toxic effect of unspecified pesticide, undetermined

T61 Toxic effect of noxious substances eaten as seafood

EXCLUDES 1 *allergic reaction to food, such as:*
anaphylactic reaction or shock due to adverse food reaction (T78.0-)
bacterial foodborne intoxications (A05.-)
dermatitis (L23.6, L25.4, L27.2)
food protein-induced enterocolitis syndrome (K52.21)
food protein-induced enteropathy (K52.22)
gastroenteritis (noninfective) (K52.29)
toxic effect of aflatoxin and other mycotoxins (T64)
toxic effect of cyanides (T65.0-)
toxic effect of harmful algae bloom (T65.82-)
toxic effect of hydrogen cyanide (T57.3-)
toxic effect of mercury (T56.1-)
toxic effect of red tide (T65.82-)

The appropriate 7th character is to be added to each code from category T61.
A initial encounter
D subsequent encounter
S sequela

T61.0 Ciguatera fish poisoning

T61.01 Ciguatera fish poisoning, accidental (unintentional)

T61.02 Ciguatera fish poisoning, intentional self-harm HCC

T61.03 Ciguatera fish poisoning, assault

T61.04 Ciguatera fish poisoning, undetermined

T61.1 Scombroid fish poisoning
Histamine-like syndrome

T61.11 Scombroid fish poisoning, accidental (unintentional)

T61.12 Scombroid fish poisoning, intentional self-harm HCC

T61.13 Scombroid fish poisoning, assault

T61.14 Scombroid fish poisoning, undetermined

T61.7 Other fish and shellfish poisoning

T61.77 Other fish poisoning

T61.771 Other fish poisoning, accidental (unintentional)

T61.772 Other fish poisoning, intentional self-harm HCC

T61.773 Other fish poisoning, assault

T61.774 Other fish poisoning, undetermined

T61.78 Other shellfish poisoning

T61.781 Other shellfish poisoning, accidental (unintentional)

T61.782 Other shellfish poisoning, intentional self-harm HCC

T61.783 Other shellfish poisoning, assault

T61.784 Other shellfish poisoning, undetermined

T61.8 Toxic effect of other seafood

T61.8X Toxic effect of other seafood

T61.8X1 Toxic effect of other seafood, accidental (unintentional)

T61.8X2 Toxic effect of other seafood, intentional self-harm HCC

T61.8X3 Toxic effect of other seafood, assault

T61.8X4 Toxic effect of other seafood, undetermined

T61.9 Toxic effect of unspecified seafood

T61.91 Toxic effect of unspecified seafood, accidental (unintentional)

T61.92 Toxic effect of unspecified seafood, intentional self-harm HCC

T61.93 Toxic effect of unspecified seafood, assault

T61.94 Toxic effect of unspecified seafood, undetermined

✓4th T62 Toxic effect of other noxious substances eaten as food

EXCLUDES 1 *allergic reaction to food, such as:*
anaphylactic shock (reaction) due to adverse food reaction (T78.Ø-)
bacterial food borne intoxications (AØ5.-)
dermatitis (L23.6, L25.4, L27.2)
food protein-induced enterocolitis syndrome (K52.21)
food protein-induced enteropathy (K52.22)
gastroenteritis (noninfective) (K52.29)
toxic effect of aflatoxin and other mycotoxins (T64)
toxic effect of cyanides (T65.Ø-)
toxic effect of hydrogen cyanide (T57.3-)
toxic effect of mercury (T56.1-)

The appropriate 7th character is to be added to each code from category T62.
A initial encounter
D subsequent encounter
S sequela

✓5th T62.Ø Toxic effect of ingested mushrooms
✓6th T62.ØX Toxic effect of ingested mushrooms
✓7th T62.ØX1 Toxic effect of ingested mushrooms, accidental (unintentional)
Toxic effect of ingested mushrooms NOS
✓7th T62.ØX2 Toxic effect of ingested mushrooms, intentional self-harm HCC
✓7th T62.ØX3 Toxic effect of ingested mushrooms, assault
✓7th T62.ØX4 Toxic effect of ingested mushrooms, undetermined

✓5th T62.1 Toxic effect of ingested berries
✓6th T62.1X Toxic effect of ingested berries
✓7th T62.1X1 Toxic effect of ingested berries, accidental (unintentional)
Toxic effect of ingested berries NOS
✓7th T62.1X2 Toxic effect of ingested berries, intentional self-harm HCC
✓7th T62.1X3 Toxic effect of ingested berries, assault
✓7th T62.1X4 Toxic effect of ingested berries, undetermined

✓5th T62.2 Toxic effect of other ingested (parts of) plant(s)
✓6th T62.2X Toxic effect of other ingested (parts of) plant(s)
✓7th T62.2X1 Toxic effect of other ingested (parts of) plant(s), accidental (unintentional)
Toxic effect of other ingested (parts of) plant(s) NOS
✓7th T62.2X2 Toxic effect of other ingested (parts of) plant(s), intentional self-harm HCC
✓7th T62.2X3 Toxic effect of other ingested (parts of) plant(s), assault
✓7th T62.2X4 Toxic effect of other ingested (parts of) plant(s), undetermined

✓5th T62.8 Toxic effect of other specified noxious substances eaten as food
✓6th T62.8X Toxic effect of other specified noxious substances eaten as food
✓7th T62.8X1 Toxic effect of other specified noxious substances eaten as food, accidental (unintentional)
Toxic effect of other specified noxious substances eaten as food NOS
✓7th T62.8X2 Toxic effect of other specified noxious substances eaten as food, intentional self-harm HCC
✓7th T62.8X3 Toxic effect of other specified noxious substances eaten as food, assault
✓7th T62.8X4 Toxic effect of other specified noxious substances eaten as food, undetermined

✓5th T62.9 Toxic effect of unspecified noxious substance eaten as food
✓x7th T62.91 Toxic effect of unspecified noxious substance eaten as food, accidental (unintentional)
Toxic effect of unspecified noxious substance eaten as food NOS
✓x7th T62.92 Toxic effect of unspecified noxious substance eaten as food, intentional self-harm HCC
✓x7th T62.93 Toxic effect of unspecified noxious substance eaten as food, assault
✓x7th T62.94 Toxic effect of unspecified noxious substance eaten as food, undetermined

✓4th T63 Toxic effect of contact with venomous animals and plants

INCLUDES bite or touch of venomous animal
pricked or stuck by thorn or leaf

EXCLUDES 2 *ingestion of toxic animal or plant (T61.-, T62.-)*

The appropriate 7th character is to be added to each code from category T63.
A initial encounter
D subsequent encounter
S sequela

✓5th T63.Ø Toxic effect of snake venom
✓6th T63.ØØ Toxic effect of unspecified snake venom
✓7th T63.ØØ1 Toxic effect of unspecified snake venom, accidental (unintentional)
Toxic effect of unspecified snake venom NOS
✓7th T63.ØØ2 Toxic effect of unspecified snake venom, intentional self-harm HCC
✓7th T63.ØØ3 Toxic effect of unspecified snake venom, assault
✓7th T63.ØØ4 Toxic effect of unspecified snake venom, undetermined
✓6th T63.Ø1 Toxic effect of rattlesnake venom
✓7th T63.Ø11 Toxic effect of rattlesnake venom, accidental (unintentional)
Toxic effect of rattlesnake venom NOS
✓7th T63.Ø12 Toxic effect of rattlesnake venom, intentional self-harm HCC
✓7th T63.Ø13 Toxic effect of rattlesnake venom, assault
✓7th T63.Ø14 Toxic effect of rattlesnake venom, undetermined
✓6th T63.Ø2 Toxic effect of coral snake venom
✓7th T63.Ø21 Toxic effect of coral snake venom, accidental (unintentional)
Toxic effect of coral snake venom NOS
✓7th T63.Ø22 Toxic effect of coral snake venom, intentional self-harm HCC
✓7th T63.Ø23 Toxic effect of coral snake venom, assault
✓7th T63.Ø24 Toxic effect of coral snake venom, undetermined
✓6th T63.Ø3 Toxic effect of taipan venom
✓7th T63.Ø31 Toxic effect of taipan venom, accidental (unintentional)
Toxic effect of taipan venom NOS
✓7th T63.Ø32 Toxic effect of taipan venom, intentional self-harm HCC
✓7th T63.Ø33 Toxic effect of taipan venom, assault
✓7th T63.Ø34 Toxic effect of taipan venom, undetermined
✓6th T63.Ø4 Toxic effect of cobra venom
✓7th T63.Ø41 Toxic effect of cobra venom, accidental (unintentional)
Toxic effect of cobra venom NOS
✓7th T63.Ø42 Toxic effect of cobra venom, intentional self-harm HCC
✓7th T63.Ø43 Toxic effect of cobra venom, assault
✓7th T63.Ø44 Toxic effect of cobra venom, undetermined
✓6th T63.Ø6 Toxic effect of venom of other North and South American snake
✓7th T63.Ø61 Toxic effect of venom of other North and South American snake, accidental (unintentional)
Toxic effect of venom of other North and South American snake NOS
✓7th T63.Ø62 Toxic effect of venom of other North and South American snake, intentional self-harm HCC
✓7th T63.Ø63 Toxic effect of venom of other North and South American snake, assault
✓7th T63.Ø64 Toxic effect of venom of other North and South American snake, undetermined
✓6th T63.Ø7 Toxic effect of venom of other Australian snake
✓7th T63.Ø71 Toxic effect of venom of other Australian snake, accidental (unintentional)
Toxic effect of venom of other Australian snake NOS
✓7th T63.Ø72 Toxic effect of venom of other Australian snake, intentional self-harm HCC

- T63.Ø73 Toxic effect of venom of other Australian snake, assault
- T63.Ø74 Toxic effect of venom of other Australian snake, undetermined

T63.Ø8 Toxic effect of venom of other African and Asian snake
- T63.Ø81 Toxic effect of venom of other African and Asian snake, accidental (unintentional)
  Toxic effect of venom of other African and Asian snake NOS
- T63.Ø82 Toxic effect of venom of other African and Asian snake, intentional self-harm HCC
- T63.Ø83 Toxic effect of venom of other African and Asian snake, assault
- T63.Ø84 Toxic effect of venom of other African and Asian snake, undetermined

T63.Ø9 Toxic effect of venom of other snake
- T63.Ø91 Toxic effect of venom of other snake, accidental (unintentional)
  Toxic effect of venom of other snake NOS
- T63.Ø92 Toxic effect of venom of other snake, intentional self-harm HCC
- T63.Ø93 Toxic effect of venom of other snake, assault
- T63.Ø94 Toxic effect of venom of other snake, undetermined

T63.1 Toxic effect of venom of other reptiles

T63.11 Toxic effect of venom of gila monster
- T63.111 Toxic effect of venom of gila monster, accidental (unintentional)
  Toxic effect of venom of gila monster NOS
- T63.112 Toxic effect of venom of gila monster, intentional self-harm HCC
- T63.113 Toxic effect of venom of gila monster, assault
- T63.114 Toxic effect of venom of gila monster, undetermined

T63.12 Toxic effect of venom of other venomous lizard
- T63.121 Toxic effect of venom of other venomous lizard, accidental (unintentional)
  Toxic effect of venom of other venomous lizard NOS
- T63.122 Toxic effect of venom of other venomous lizard, intentional self-harm HCC
- T63.123 Toxic effect of venom of other venomous lizard, assault
- T63.124 Toxic effect of venom of other venomous lizard, undetermined

T63.19 Toxic effect of venom of other reptiles
- T63.191 Toxic effect of venom of other reptiles, accidental (unintentional)
  Toxic effect of venom of other reptiles NOS
- T63.192 Toxic effect of venom of other reptiles, intentional self-harm HCC
- T63.193 Toxic effect of venom of other reptiles, assault
- T63.194 Toxic effect of venom of other reptiles, undetermined

T63.2 Toxic effect of venom of scorpion

T63.2X Toxic effect of venom of scorpion
- T63.2X1 Toxic effect of venom of scorpion, accidental (unintentional)
  Toxic effect of venom of scorpion NOS
- T63.2X2 Toxic effect of venom of scorpion, intentional self-harm HCC
- T63.2X3 Toxic effect of venom of scorpion, assault
- T63.2X4 Toxic effect of venom of scorpion, undetermined

T63.3 Toxic effect of venom of spider

T63.3Ø Toxic effect of unspecified spider venom
- T63.3Ø1 Toxic effect of unspecified spider venom, accidental (unintentional)
- T63.3Ø2 Toxic effect of unspecified spider venom, intentional self-harm HCC
- T63.3Ø3 Toxic effect of unspecified spider venom, assault
- T63.3Ø4 Toxic effect of unspecified spider venom, undetermined

T63.31 Toxic effect of venom of black widow spider
- T63.311 Toxic effect of venom of black widow spider, accidental (unintentional)
- T63.312 Toxic effect of venom of black widow spider, intentional self-harm HCC
- T63.313 Toxic effect of venom of black widow spider, assault
- T63.314 Toxic effect of venom of black widow spider, undetermined

T63.32 Toxic effect of venom of tarantula
- T63.321 Toxic effect of venom of tarantula, accidental (unintentional)
- T63.322 Toxic effect of venom of tarantula, intentional self-harm HCC
- T63.323 Toxic effect of venom of tarantula, assault
- T63.324 Toxic effect of venom of tarantula, undetermined

T63.33 Toxic effect of venom of brown recluse spider
- T63.331 Toxic effect of venom of brown recluse spider, accidental (unintentional)
- T63.332 Toxic effect of venom of brown recluse spider, intentional self-harm HCC
- T63.333 Toxic effect of venom of brown recluse spider, assault
- T63.334 Toxic effect of venom of brown recluse spider, undetermined

T63.39 Toxic effect of venom of other spider
- T63.391 Toxic effect of venom of other spider, accidental (unintentional)
- T63.392 Toxic effect of venom of other spider, intentional self-harm HCC
- T63.393 Toxic effect of venom of other spider, assault
- T63.394 Toxic effect of venom of other spider, undetermined

T63.4 Toxic effect of venom of other arthropods

T63.41 Toxic effect of venom of centipedes and venomous millipedes
- T63.411 Toxic effect of venom of centipedes and venomous millipedes, accidental (unintentional)
- T63.412 Toxic effect of venom of centipedes and venomous millipedes, intentional self-harm HCC
- T63.413 Toxic effect of venom of centipedes and venomous millipedes, assault
- T63.414 Toxic effect of venom of centipedes and venomous millipedes, undetermined

T63.42 Toxic effect of venom of ants
- T63.421 Toxic effect of venom of ants, accidental (unintentional)
- T63.422 Toxic effect of venom of ants, intentional self-harm HCC
- T63.423 Toxic effect of venom of ants, assault
- T63.424 Toxic effect of venom of ants, undetermined

T63.43 Toxic effect of venom of caterpillars
- T63.431 Toxic effect of venom of caterpillars, accidental (unintentional)
- T63.432 Toxic effect of venom of caterpillars, intentional self-harm HCC
- T63.433 Toxic effect of venom of caterpillars, assault
- T63.434 Toxic effect of venom of caterpillars, undetermined

T63.44 Toxic effect of venom of bees
- T63.441 Toxic effect of venom of bees, accidental (unintentional)
- T63.442 Toxic effect of venom of bees, intentional self-harm HCC
- T63.443 Toxic effect of venom of bees, assault
- T63.444 Toxic effect of venom of bees, undetermined

T63.45 Toxic effect of venom of hornets
- T63.451 Toxic effect of venom of hornets, accidental (unintentional)
- T63.452 Toxic effect of venom of hornets, intentional self-harm HCC
- T63.453 Toxic effect of venom of hornets, assault

√7th T63.454 Toxic effect of venom of hornets, undetermined

√6th T63.46 Toxic effect of venom of wasps

Toxic effect of yellow jacket

√7th T63.461 Toxic effect of venom of wasps, accidental (unintentional)

√7th T63.462 Toxic effect of venom of wasps, intentional self-harm HCC

√7th T63.463 Toxic effect of venom of wasps, assault

√7th T63.464 Toxic effect of venom of wasps, undetermined

√6th T63.48 Toxic effect of venom of other arthropod

√7th T63.481 Toxic effect of venom of other arthropod, accidental (unintentional)

√7th T63.482 Toxic effect of venom of other arthropod, intentional self-harm HCC

√7th T63.483 Toxic effect of venom of other arthropod, assault

√7th T63.484 Toxic effect of venom of other arthropod, undetermined

√5th T63.5 Toxic effect of contact with venomous fish

EXCLUDES 2 *poisoning by ingestion of fish (T61.-)*

√6th T63.51 Toxic effect of contact with stingray

√7th T63.511 Toxic effect of contact with stingray, accidental (unintentional)

√7th T63.512 Toxic effect of contact with stingray, intentional self-harm HCC

√7th T63.513 Toxic effect of contact with stingray, assault

√7th T63.514 Toxic effect of contact with stingray, undetermined

√6th T63.59 Toxic effect of contact with other venomous fish

√7th T63.591 Toxic effect of contact with other venomous fish, accidental (unintentional)

√7th T63.592 Toxic effect of contact with other venomous fish, intentional self-harm HCC

√7th T63.593 Toxic effect of contact with other venomous fish, assault

√7th T63.594 Toxic effect of contact with other venomous fish, undetermined

√5th T63.6 Toxic effect of contact with other venomous marine animals

EXCLUDES 1 *sea-snake venom (T63.09)*

EXCLUDES 2 *poisoning by ingestion of shellfish (T61.78-)*

√6th T63.61 Toxic effect of contact with Portuguese Man-o-war

Toxic effect of contact with bluebottle

√7th T63.611 Toxic effect of contact with Portuguese Man-o-war, accidental (unintentional)

√7th T63.612 Toxic effect of contact with Portuguese Man-o-war, intentional self-harm HCC

√7th T63.613 Toxic effect of contact with Portuguese Man-o-war, assault

√7th T63.614 Toxic effect of contact with Portuguese Man-o-war, undetermined

√6th T63.62 Toxic effect of contact with other jellyfish

√7th T63.621 Toxic effect of contact with other jellyfish, accidental (unintentional)

√7th T63.622 Toxic effect of contact with other jellyfish, intentional self-harm HCC

√7th T63.623 Toxic effect of contact with other jellyfish, assault

√7th T63.624 Toxic effect of contact with other jellyfish, undetermined

√6th T63.63 Toxic effect of contact with sea anemone

√7th T63.631 Toxic effect of contact with sea anemone, accidental (unintentional)

√7th T63.632 Toxic effect of contact with sea anemone, intentional self-harm HCC

√7th T63.633 Toxic effect of contact with sea anemone, assault

√7th T63.634 Toxic effect of contact with sea anemone, undetermined

√6th T63.69 Toxic effect of contact with other venomous marine animals

√7th T63.691 Toxic effect of contact with other venomous marine animals, accidental (unintentional)

√7th T63.692 Toxic effect of contact with other venomous marine animals, intentional self-harm HCC

√7th T63.693 Toxic effect of contact with other venomous marine animals, assault

√7th T63.694 Toxic effect of contact with other venomous marine animals, undetermined

√5th T63.7 Toxic effect of contact with venomous plant

√6th T63.71 Toxic effect of contact with venomous marine plant

√7th T63.711 Toxic effect of contact with venomous marine plant, accidental (unintentional)

√7th T63.712 Toxic effect of contact with venomous marine plant, intentional self-harm HCC

√7th T63.713 Toxic effect of contact with venomous marine plant, assault

√7th T63.714 Toxic effect of contact with venomous marine plant, undetermined

√6th T63.79 Toxic effect of contact with other venomous plant

√7th T63.791 Toxic effect of contact with other venomous plant, accidental (unintentional)

√7th T63.792 Toxic effect of contact with other venomous plant, intentional self-harm HCC

√7th T63.793 Toxic effect of contact with other venomous plant, assault

√7th T63.794 Toxic effect of contact with other venomous plant, undetermined

√5th T63.8 Toxic effect of contact with other venomous animals

√6th T63.81 Toxic effect of contact with venomous frog

EXCLUDES 1 *contact with nonvenomous frog (W62.0)*

√7th T63.811 Toxic effect of contact with venomous frog, accidental (unintentional)

√7th T63.812 Toxic effect of contact with venomous frog, intentional self-harm HCC

√7th T63.813 Toxic effect of contact with venomous frog, assault

√7th T63.814 Toxic effect of contact with venomous frog, undetermined

√6th T63.82 Toxic effect of contact with venomous toad

EXCLUDES 1 *contact with nonvenomous toad (W62.1)*

√7th T63.821 Toxic effect of contact with venomous toad, accidental (unintentional)

√7th T63.822 Toxic effect of contact with venomous toad, intentional self-harm HCC

√7th T63.823 Toxic effect of contact with venomous toad, assault

√7th T63.824 Toxic effect of contact with venomous toad, undetermined

√6th T63.83 Toxic effect of contact with other venomous amphibian

EXCLUDES 1 *contact with nonvenomous amphibian (W62.9)*

√7th T63.831 Toxic effect of contact with other venomous amphibian, accidental (unintentional)

√7th T63.832 Toxic effect of contact with other venomous amphibian, intentional self-harm HCC

√7th T63.833 Toxic effect of contact with other venomous amphibian, assault

√7th T63.834 Toxic effect of contact with other venomous amphibian, undetermined

√6th T63.89 Toxic effect of contact with other venomous animals

√7th T63.891 Toxic effect of contact with other venomous animals, accidental (unintentional)

√7th T63.892 Toxic effect of contact with other venomous animals, intentional self-harm HCC

√7th T63.893 Toxic effect of contact with other venomous animals, assault

√7th T63.894 Toxic effect of contact with other venomous animals, undetermined

√5th T63.9 Toxic effect of contact with unspecified venomous animal

√x7th T63.91 Toxic effect of contact with unspecified venomous animal, accidental (unintentional)

√x7th T63.92 Toxic effect of contact with unspecified venomous animal, intentional self-harm HCC

√x7th T63.93 Toxic effect of contact with unspecified venomous animal, assault

√x7th T63.94 Toxic effect of contact with unspecified venomous animal, undetermined

T64 Toxic effect of aflatoxin and other mycotoxin food contaminants

The appropriate 7th character is to be added to each code from category T64.
A initial encounter
D subsequent encounter
S sequela

T64.Ø Toxic effect of aflatoxin

T64.Ø1 Toxic effect of aflatoxin, accidental (unintentional)

T64.Ø2 Toxic effect of aflatoxin, intentional self-harm HCC

T64.Ø3 Toxic effect of aflatoxin, assault

T64.Ø4 Toxic effect of aflatoxin, undetermined

T64.8 Toxic effect of other mycotoxin food contaminants

T64.81 Toxic effect of other mycotoxin food contaminants, accidental (unintentional)

T64.82 Toxic effect of other mycotoxin food contaminants, intentional self-harm HCC

T64.83 Toxic effect of other mycotoxin food contaminants, assault

T64.84 Toxic effect of other mycotoxin food contaminants, undetermined

T65 Toxic effect of other and unspecified substances

The appropriate 7th character is to be added to each code from category T65.
A initial encounter
D subsequent encounter
S sequela

T65.Ø Toxic effect of cyanides

EXCLUDES 1 *hydrogen cyanide (T57.3-)*

T65.ØX Toxic effect of cyanides

T65.ØX1 Toxic effect of cyanides, accidental (unintentional)
Toxic effect of cyanides NOS

T65.ØX2 Toxic effect of cyanides, intentional self-harm HCC

T65.ØX3 Toxic effect of cyanides, assault

T65.ØX4 Toxic effect of cyanides, undetermined

T65.1 Toxic effect of strychnine and its salts

T65.1X Toxic effect of strychnine and its salts

T65.1X1 Toxic effect of strychnine and its salts, accidental (unintentional)
Toxic effect of strychnine and its salts NOS

T65.1X2 Toxic effect of strychnine and its salts, intentional self-harm HCC

T65.1X3 Toxic effect of strychnine and its salts, assault

T65.1X4 Toxic effect of strychnine and its salts, undetermined

T65.2 Toxic effect of tobacco and nicotine

EXCLUDES 2 *nicotine dependence (F17.-)*

T65.21 Toxic effect of chewing tobacco

T65.211 Toxic effect of chewing tobacco, accidental (unintentional)
Toxic effect of chewing tobacco NOS

T65.212 Toxic effect of chewing tobacco, intentional self-harm HCC

T65.213 Toxic effect of chewing tobacco, assault

T65.214 Toxic effect of chewing tobacco, undetermined

T65.22 Toxic effect of tobacco cigarettes
Toxic effect of tobacco smoke
Use additional code for exposure to second hand tobacco smoke (Z57.31, Z77.22)

T65.221 Toxic effect of tobacco cigarettes, accidental (unintentional)
Toxic effect of tobacco cigarettes NOS

T65.222 Toxic effect of tobacco cigarettes, intentional self-harm HCC

T65.223 Toxic effect of tobacco cigarettes, assault

T65.224 Toxic effect of tobacco cigarettes, undetermined

T65.29 Toxic effect of other tobacco and nicotine

T65.291 Toxic effect of other tobacco and nicotine, accidental (unintentional)
Toxic effect of other tobacco and nicotine NOS

T65.292 Toxic effect of other tobacco and nicotine, intentional self-harm HCC

T65.293 Toxic effect of other tobacco and nicotine, assault

T65.294 Toxic effect of other tobacco and nicotine, undetermined

T65.3 Toxic effect of nitroderivatives and aminoderivatives of benzene and its homologues
Toxic effect of anilin [benzenamine]
Toxic effect of nitrobenzene
Toxic effect of trinitrotoluene

T65.3X Toxic effect of nitroderivatives and aminoderivatives of benzene and its homologues

T65.3X1 Toxic effect of nitroderivatives and aminoderivatives of benzene and its homologues, accidental (unintentional)
Toxic effect of nitroderivatives and aminoderivatives of benzene and its homologues NOS

T65.3X2 Toxic effect of nitroderivatives and aminoderivatives of benzene and its homologues, intentional self-harm HCC

T65.3X3 Toxic effect of nitroderivatives and aminoderivatives of benzene and its homologues, assault

T65.3X4 Toxic effect of nitroderivatives and aminoderivatives of benzene and its homologues, undetermined

T65.4 Toxic effect of carbon disulfide

T65.4X Toxic effect of carbon disulfide

T65.4X1 Toxic effect of carbon disulfide, accidental (unintentional)
Toxic effect of carbon disulfide NOS

T65.4X2 Toxic effect of carbon disulfide, intentional self-harm HCC

T65.4X3 Toxic effect of carbon disulfide, assault

T65.4X4 Toxic effect of carbon disulfide, undetermined

T65.5 Toxic effect of nitroglycerin and other nitric acids and esters
Toxic effect of 1,2,3-Propanetriol trinitrate

T65.5X Toxic effect of nitroglycerin and other nitric acids and esters

T65.5X1 Toxic effect of nitroglycerin and other nitric acids and esters, accidental (unintentional)
Toxic effect of nitroglycerin and other nitric acids and esters NOS

T65.5X2 Toxic effect of nitroglycerin and other nitric acids and esters, intentional self-harm HCC

T65.5X3 Toxic effect of nitroglycerin and other nitric acids and esters, assault

T65.5X4 Toxic effect of nitroglycerin and other nitric acids and esters, undetermined

T65.6 Toxic effect of paints and dyes, not elsewhere classified

T65.6X Toxic effect of paints and dyes, not elsewhere classified

T65.6X1 Toxic effect of paints and dyes, not elsewhere classified, accidental (unintentional)
Toxic effect of paints and dyes NOS

T65.6X2 Toxic effect of paints and dyes, not elsewhere classified, intentional self-harm HCC

T65.6X3 Toxic effect of paints and dyes, not elsewhere classified, assault

T65.6X4 Toxic effect of paints and dyes, not elsewhere classified, undetermined

T65.8 Toxic effect of other specified substances

T65.81 Toxic effect of latex

T65.811 Toxic effect of latex, accidental (unintentional)
Toxic effect of latex NOS

T65.812 Toxic effect of latex, intentional self-harm HCC

√7th T65.813 Toxic effect of latex, assault
√7th T65.814 Toxic effect of latex, undetermined
√6th T65.82 Toxic effect of harmful algae and algae toxins
Toxic effect of (harmful) algae bloom NOS
Toxic effect of blue-green algae bloom
Toxic effect of brown tide
Toxic effect of cyanobacteria bloom
Toxic effect of Florida red tide
Toxic effect of pfiesteria piscicida
Toxic effect of red tide
√7th T65.821 Toxic effect of harmful algae and algae toxins, accidental (unintentional)
Toxic effect of harmful algae and algae toxins NOS
√7th T65.822 Toxic effect of harmful algae and algae toxins, intentional self-harm HCC
√7th T65.823 Toxic effect of harmful algae and algae toxins, assault
√7th T65.824 Toxic effect of harmful algae and algae toxins, undetermined
√6th T65.83 Toxic effect of fiberglass
√7th T65.831 Toxic effect of fiberglass, accidental (unintentional)
Toxic effect of fiberglass NOS
√7th T65.832 Toxic effect of fiberglass, intentional self-harm HCC
√7th T65.833 Toxic effect of fiberglass, assault
√7th T65.834 Toxic effect of fiberglass, undetermined
√6th T65.89 Toxic effect of other specified substances
√7th T65.891 Toxic effect of other specified substances, accidental (unintentional)
Toxic effect of other specified substances NOS
AHA: 2018,1Q,5
√7th T65.892 Toxic effect of other specified substances, intentional self-harm HCC
√7th T65.893 Toxic effect of other specified substances, assault
√7th T65.894 Toxic effect of other specified substances, undetermined
√5th T65.9 Toxic effect of unspecified substance
√x7th T65.91 Toxic effect of unspecified substance, accidental (unintentional)
Poisoning NOS
√x7th T65.92 Toxic effect of unspecified substance, intentional self-harm HCC
√x7th T65.93 Toxic effect of unspecified substance, assault
√x7th T65.94 Toxic effect of unspecified substance, undetermined

Other and unspecified effects of external causes (T66-T78)

√x7th **T66 Radiation sickness, unspecified**
EXCLUDES 1 *specified adverse effects of radiation, such as:*
burns (T20-T31)
leukemia (C91-C95)
radiation gastroenteritis and colitis (K52.0)
radiation pneumonitis (J70.0)
radiation related disorders of the skin and subcutaneous tissue (L55-L59)
radiation sunburn (L55.-)

The appropriate 7th character is to be added to code T66.
A initial encounter
D subsequent encounter
S sequela

√4th **T67 Effects of heat and light**
EXCLUDES 1 *erythema [dermatitis] ab igne (L59.0)*
malignant hyperpyrexia due to anesthesia (T88.3)
radiation-related disorders of the skin and subcutaneous tissue (L55-L59)
EXCLUDES 2 *burns (T20-T31)*
sunburn (L55.-)
sweat disorder due to heat (L74-L75)

The appropriate 7th character is to be added to each code from category T67.
A initial encounter
D subsequent encounter
S sequela

√5th T67.0 Heatstroke and sunstroke
Use additional code(s) to identify any associated complications of heatstroke, such as:
coma and stupor (R40.-)
rhabdomyolysis (M62.82)
systemic inflammatory response syndrome (R65.1-)
AHA: 2019,4Q,17-18
DEF: Headache, vertigo, cramps, and elevated body temperature due to prolonged exposure to high environmental temperatures that requires emergency intervention.
√x7th T67.01 Heatstroke and sunstroke CC HS
Heat apoplexy
Heat pyrexia
Siriasis
Thermoplegia
√x7th T67.02 Exertional heatstroke CC HS
√x7th T67.09 Other heatstroke and sunstroke CC HS
√x7th T67.1 Heat syncope
Heat collapse
√x7th T67.2 Heat cramp
√x7th T67.3 Heat exhaustion, anhydrotic
Heat prostration due to water depletion
EXCLUDES 1 *heat exhaustion due to salt depletion (T67.4)*
√x7th T67.4 Heat exhaustion due to salt depletion
Heat prostration due to salt (and water) depletion
√x7th T67.5 Heat exhaustion, unspecified
Heat prostration NOS
√x7th T67.6 Heat fatigue, transient
√x7th T67.7 Heat edema
√x7th T67.8 Other effects of heat and light
√x7th T67.9 Effect of heat and light, unspecified

√x7th **T68 Hypothermia**
Accidental hypothermia
Hypothermia NOS
Use additional code to identify source of exposure:
exposure to excessive cold of man-made origin (W93)
exposure to excessive cold of natural origin (X31)
EXCLUDES 1 *hypothermia following anesthesia (T88.51)*
hypothermia not associated with low environmental temperature (R68.0)
hypothermia of newborn (P80.-)
EXCLUDES 2 *frostbite (T33-T34)*

The appropriate 7th character is to be added to code T68.
A initial encounter
D subsequent encounter
S sequela

√4th **T69 Other effects of reduced temperature**
Use additional code to identify source of exposure:
exposure to excessive cold of man-made origin (W93)
exposure to excessive cold of natural origin (X31)
EXCLUDES 2 *frostbite (T33-T34)*

The appropriate 7th character is to be added to each code from category T69.
A initial encounter
D subsequent encounter
S sequela

√5th T69.0 Immersion hand and foot
√6th T69.01 Immersion hand
√7th T69.011 Immersion hand, right hand

T69.Ø12 **Immersion hand, left hand**

T69.Ø19 **Immersion hand, unspecified hand**

T69.Ø2 **Immersion foot**

Trench foot

T69.Ø21 **Immersion foot, right foot** CC H5

T69.Ø22 **Immersion foot, left foot** CC H5

T69.Ø29 **Immersion foot, unspecified foot** CC H5 UNS

T69.1 **Chilblains**

DEF: Red, swollen, itchy skin primarily affecting the fingers and toes, nose and ears, and legs. Chilblains follows damp-cold exposure, and can also be associated with pruritus and a burning feeling.

T69.8 **Other specified effects of reduced temperature**

T69.9 **Effect of reduced temperature, unspecified**

T7Ø Effects of air pressure and water pressure

The appropriate 7th character is to be added to each code from category T7Ø.
A initial encounter
D subsequent encounter
S sequela

T7Ø.Ø **Otitic barotrauma**

Aero-otitis media
Effects of change in ambient atmospheric pressure or water pressure on ears

T7Ø.1 **Sinus barotrauma**

Aerosinusitis
Effects of change in ambient atmospheric pressure on sinuses

T7Ø.2 **Other and unspecified effects of high altitude**

EXCLUDES 2 *polycythemia due to high altitude (D75.1)*

T7Ø.2Ø **Unspecified effects of high altitude**

T7Ø.29 **Other effects of high altitude**

Alpine sickness
Anoxia due to high altitude
Barotrauma NOS
Hypobaropathy
Mountain sickness

T7Ø.3 **Caisson disease [decompression sickness]** CC H5

Compressed-air disease
Diver's palsy or paralysis
DEF: Rapid reduction in air pressure while breathing compressed air. Symptoms include skin lesions, joint pains, and respiratory and neurological problems.

T7Ø.4 **Effects of high-pressure fluids**

Hydraulic jet injection (industrial)
Pneumatic jet injection (industrial)
Traumatic jet injection (industrial)

T7Ø.8 **Other effects of air pressure and water pressure**

T7Ø.9 **Effect of air pressure and water pressure, unspecified**

T71 Asphyxiation

Mechanical suffocation
Traumatic suffocation

EXCLUDES 1 *acute respiratory distress (syndrome) (J8Ø)*
anoxia due to high altitude (T7Ø.2)
asphyxia NOS (RØ9.Ø1)
asphyxia from carbon monoxide (T58.-)
asphyxia from inhalation of food or foreign body (T17.-)
asphyxia from other gases, fumes and vapors (T59.-)
respiratory distress (syndrome) in newborn (P22.-)

The appropriate 7th character is to be added to each code from category T71.
A initial encounter
D subsequent encounter
S sequela

T71.1 **Asphyxiation due to mechanical threat to breathing**

Suffocation due to mechanical threat to breathing

T71.11 **Asphyxiation due to smothering under pillow**

T71.111 **Asphyxiation due to smothering under pillow, accidental** CC H5

Asphyxiation due to smothering under pillow NOS

T71.112 **Asphyxiation due to smothering under pillow, intentional self-harm** CC H5 HCC

T71.113 **Asphyxiation due to smothering under pillow, assault** CC H5

T71.114 **Asphyxiation due to smothering under pillow, undetermined** CC H5

T71.12 **Asphyxiation due to plastic bag**

T71.121 **Asphyxiation due to plastic bag, accidental** CC H5

Asphyxiation due to plastic bag NOS

T71.122 **Asphyxiation due to plastic bag, intentional self-harm** CC H5 HCC

T71.123 **Asphyxiation due to plastic bag, assault** CC H5

T71.124 **Asphyxiation due to plastic bag, undetermined** CC H5

T71.13 **Asphyxiation due to being trapped in bed linens**

T71.131 **Asphyxiation due to being trapped in bed linens, accidental** CC H5

Asphyxiation due to being trapped in bed linens NOS

T71.132 **Asphyxiation due to being trapped in bed linens, intentional self-harm** CC H5 HCC

T71.133 **Asphyxiation due to being trapped in bed linens, assault** CC H5

T71.134 **Asphyxiation due to being trapped in bed linens, undetermined** CC H5

T71.14 **Asphyxiation due to smothering under another person's body (in bed)**

T71.141 **Asphyxiation due to smothering under another person's body (in bed), accidental** CC H5

Asphyxiation due to smothering under another person's body (in bed) NOS

T71.143 **Asphyxiation due to smothering under another person's body (in bed), assault** CC H5

T71.144 **Asphyxiation due to smothering under another person's body (in bed), undetermined** CC H5

T71.15 **Asphyxiation due to smothering in furniture**

T71.151 **Asphyxiation due to smothering in furniture, accidental** CC H5

Asphyxiation due to smothering in furniture NOS

T71.152 **Asphyxiation due to smothering in furniture, intentional self-harm** CC H5 HCC

T71.153 **Asphyxiation due to smothering in furniture, assault** CC H5

T71.154 **Asphyxiation due to smothering in furniture, undetermined** CC H5

T71.16 **Asphyxiation due to hanging**

Hanging by window shade cord
Use additional code for any associated injuries, such as:
crushing injury of neck (S17.-)
fracture of cervical vertebrae (S12.Ø-S12.2-)
open wound of neck (S11.-)

T71.161 **Asphyxiation due to hanging, accidental** CC H5

Asphyxiation due to hanging NOS
Hanging NOS

T71.162 **Asphyxiation due to hanging, intentional self-harm** CC H5 HCC

T71.163 **Asphyxiation due to hanging, assault** CC H5

T71.164 **Asphyxiation due to hanging, undetermined** CC H5

T71.19 **Asphyxiation due to mechanical threat to breathing due to other causes**

T71.191 **Asphyxiation due to mechanical threat to breathing due to other causes, accidental** CC H5

Asphyxiation due to other causes NOS

T71.192 **Asphyxiation due to mechanical threat to breathing due to other causes, intentional self-harm** CC H5 HCC

T71.193 **Asphyxiation due to mechanical threat to breathing due to other causes, assault** CC H5

T71.194 Asphyxiation due to mechanical threat to breathing due to other causes, undetermined CC HS

T71.2 Asphyxiation due to systemic oxygen deficiency due to low oxygen content in ambient air
Suffocation due to systemic oxygen deficiency due to low oxygen content in ambient air

T71.20 Asphyxiation due to systemic oxygen deficiency due to low oxygen content in ambient air due to unspecified cause CC HS

T71.21 Asphyxiation due to cave-in or falling earth CC HS
Use additional code for any associated cataclysm (X34-X38)

T71.22 Asphyxiation due to being trapped in a car trunk

T71.221 Asphyxiation due to being trapped in a car trunk, accidental CC

T71.222 Asphyxiation due to being trapped in a car trunk, intentional self-harm CC HCC

T71.223 Asphyxiation due to being trapped in a car trunk, assault CC

T71.224 Asphyxiation due to being trapped in a car trunk, undetermined CC

T71.23 Asphyxiation due to being trapped in a (discarded) refrigerator

T71.231 Asphyxiation due to being trapped in a (discarded) refrigerator, accidental CC

T71.232 Asphyxiation due to being trapped in a (discarded) refrigerator, intentional self-harm CC HCC

T71.233 Asphyxiation due to being trapped in a (discarded) refrigerator, assault CC

T71.234 Asphyxiation due to being trapped in a (discarded) refrigerator, undetermined CC

T71.29 Asphyxiation due to being trapped in other low oxygen environment CC HS

T71.9 Asphyxiation due to unspecified cause CC HS
Suffocation (by strangulation) due to unspecified cause
Suffocation NOS
Systemic oxygen deficiency due to low oxygen content in ambient air due to unspecified cause
Systemic oxygen deficiency due to mechanical threat to breathing due to unspecified cause
Traumatic asphyxia NOS

T73 Effects of other deprivation

The appropriate 7th character is to be added to each code from category T73.
A initial encounter
D subsequent encounter
S sequela

T73.0 Starvation
Deprivation of food

T73.1 Deprivation of water

T73.2 Exhaustion due to exposure

T73.3 Exhaustion due to excessive exertion
Exhaustion due to overexertion

T73.8 Other effects of deprivation

T73.9 Effect of deprivation, unspecified

T74 Adult and child abuse, neglect and other maltreatment, confirmed
Use additional code, if applicable, to identify any associated current injury
Use additional external cause code to identify perpetrator, if known (Y07.-)
EXCLUDES 1 *abuse and maltreatment in pregnancy (O9A.3-, O9A.4-, O9A.5-)*
adult and child maltreatment, suspected (T76.-)

The appropriate 7th character is to be added to each code from category T74.
A initial encounter
D subsequent encounter
S sequela

T74.0 Neglect or abandonment, confirmed

T74.01 Adult neglect or abandonment, confirmed CC A

T74.02 Child neglect or abandonment, confirmed CC P

T74.1 Physical abuse, confirmed
EXCLUDES 2 *sexual abuse (T74.2-)*

T74.11 Adult physical abuse, confirmed CC A

T74.12 Child physical abuse, confirmed CC P
EXCLUDES 2 *shaken infant syndrome (T74.4)*

T74.2 Sexual abuse, confirmed
Rape, confirmed
Sexual assault, confirmed

T74.21 Adult sexual abuse, confirmed CC A

T74.22 Child sexual abuse, confirmed CC P

T74.3 Psychological abuse, confirmed
Bullying and intimidation, confirmed
Intimidation through social media, confirmed
▶Target of threatened harm, confirmed◀
▶Target of threatened physical violence, confirmed◀
▶Target of threatened sexual abuse, confirmed◀

T74.31 Adult psychological abuse, confirmed A

T74.32 Child psychological abuse, confirmed CC P

T74.4 Shaken infant syndrome CC P

T74.5 Forced sexual exploitation, confirmed
AHA: 2018,4Q,32-33,65

T74.51 Adult forced sexual exploitation, confirmed CC A

T74.52 Child sexual exploitation, confirmed CC P

T74.6 Forced labor exploitation, confirmed
AHA: 2018,4Q,32-33,65

T74.61 Adult forced labor exploitation, confirmed CC A

T74.62 Child forced labor exploitation, confirmed CC P

T74.9 Unspecified maltreatment, confirmed

T74.91 Unspecified adult maltreatment, confirmed CC A

T74.92 Unspecified child maltreatment, confirmed CC P

● **T74.A Financial abuse, confirmed**
AHA: 2023,1Q,4

● **T74.A1 Adult financial abuse, confirmed** A

● **T74.A2 Child financial abuse, confirmed** P

T75 Other and unspecified effects of other external causes
EXCLUDES 1 *adverse effects NEC (T78.-)*
EXCLUDES 2 *burns (electric) (T20-T31)*

The appropriate 7th character is to be added to each code from category T75.
A initial encounter
D subsequent encounter
S sequela

T75.0 Effects of lightning
Struck by lightning

T75.00 Unspecified effects of lightning
Struck by lightning NOS

T75.01 Shock due to being struck by lightning

T75.09 Other effects of lightning
Use additional code for other effects of lightning

T75.1 Unspecified effects of drowning and nonfatal submersion CC HS
Immersion
EXCLUDES 1 *specified effects of drowning - code to effects*
AHA: 2023,1Q,25

T75.2 Effects of vibration

T75.20 Unspecified effects of vibration

T75.21 Pneumatic hammer syndrome

T75.22 Traumatic vasospastic syndrome

T75.23 Vertigo from infrasound
EXCLUDES 1 *vertigo NOS (R42)*

T75.29 Other effects of vibration

T75.3 Motion sickness
Airsickness
Seasickness
Travel sickness
Use additional external cause code to identify vehicle or type of motion ▶(Y92.81-)◀

T75.4 Electrocution
Shock from electric current
Shock from electroshock gun (taser)

T75.8 Other specified effects of external causes

T75.81 Effects of abnormal gravitation [G] forces

T75.82 Effects of weightlessness

T75.89 Other specified effects of external causes

T76 Adult and child abuse, neglect and other maltreatment, suspected

Use additional code, if applicable, to identify any associated current injury

EXCLUDES 1 *adult and child maltreatment, confirmed (T74.-)*
suspected abuse and maltreatment in pregnancy (O9A.3-, O9A.4-, O9A.5-)
suspected adult physical abuse, ruled out (ZØ4.71)
suspected adult sexual abuse, ruled out (ZØ4.41)
suspected child physical abuse, ruled out (ZØ4.72)
suspected child sexual abuse, ruled out (ZØ4.42)

AHA: 2018,4Q,72

The appropriate 7th character is to be added to each code from category T76.
A initial encounter
D subsequent encounter
S sequela

T76.Ø Neglect or abandonment, suspected

T76.Ø1 Adult neglect or abandonment, suspected CC A

T76.Ø2 Child neglect or abandonment, suspected CC P

T76.1 Physical abuse, suspected

T76.11 Adult physical abuse, suspected CC A

T76.12 Child physical abuse, suspected CC P
AHA: 2019,2Q,12

T76.2 Sexual abuse, suspected
Rape, suspected
EXCLUDES 1 *alleged abuse, ruled out (ZØ4.7)*

T76.21 Adult sexual abuse, suspected CC A

T76.22 Child sexual abuse, suspected CC P

T76.3 Psychological abuse, suspected
Bullying and intimidation, suspected
Intimidation through social media, suspected
▶Target of threatened harm, suspected◀
▶Target of threatened physical violence, suspected◀
▶Target of threatened sexual abuse, suspected◀

T76.31 Adult psychological abuse, suspected A

T76.32 Child psychological abuse, suspected CC P

T76.5 Forced sexual exploitation, suspected
AHA: 2018,4Q,32-33,65

T76.51 Adult forced sexual exploitation, suspected CC A

T76.52 Child sexual exploitation, suspected CC P

T76.6 Forced labor exploitation, suspected
AHA: 2018,4Q,32-33,65

T76.61 Adult forced labor exploitation, suspected CC A

T76.62 Child forced labor exploitation, suspected CC P

T76.9 Unspecified maltreatment, suspected

T76.91 Unspecified adult maltreatment, suspected CC A

T76.92 Unspecified child maltreatment, suspected CC P

● **T76.A Financial abuse, suspected**
AHA: 2023,1Q,4

● **T76.A1 Adult financial abuse, suspected** A

● **T76.A2 Child financial abuse, suspected** P

T78 Adverse effects, not elsewhere classified

EXCLUDES 2 *complications of surgical and medical care NEC (T8Ø-T88)*

The appropriate 7th character is to be added to each code from category T78.
A initial encounter
D subsequent encounter
S sequela

T78.Ø Anaphylactic reaction due to food
Anaphylactic reaction due to adverse food reaction
Anaphylactic shock or reaction due to nonpoisonous foods
Anaphylactoid reaction due to food

T78.ØØ Anaphylactic reaction due to unspecified food CC

T78.Ø1 Anaphylactic reaction due to peanuts CC

T78.Ø2 Anaphylactic reaction due to shellfish (crustaceans) CC

T78.Ø3 Anaphylactic reaction due to other fish CC

T78.Ø4 Anaphylactic reaction due to fruits and vegetables CC

T78.Ø5 Anaphylactic reaction due to tree nuts and seeds CC
EXCLUDES 2 *anaphylactic reaction due to peanuts (T78.Ø1)*

T78.Ø6 Anaphylactic reaction due to food additives CC

T78.Ø7 Anaphylactic reaction due to milk and dairy products CC

T78.Ø8 Anaphylactic reaction due to eggs CC

T78.Ø9 Anaphylactic reaction due to other food products CC

T78.1 Other adverse food reactions, not elsewhere classified
Use additional code to identify the type of reaction, if applicable
EXCLUDES 1 *anaphylactic reaction or shock due to adverse food reaction (T78.Ø-)*
anaphylactic reaction due to food (T78.Ø-)
bacterial food borne intoxications (AØ5.-)
EXCLUDES 2 *allergic and dietetic gastroenteritis and colitis (K52.29)*
allergic rhinitis due to food (J3Ø.5)
dermatitis due to food in contact with skin (L23.6, L24.6, L25.4)
dermatitis due to ingested food (L27.2)
food protein-induced enterocolitis syndrome (K52.21)
food protein-induced enteropathy (K52.22)

T78.2 Anaphylactic shock, unspecified CC
Allergic shock
Anaphylactic reaction
Anaphylaxis
EXCLUDES 1 *anaphylactic reaction or shock due to adverse effect of correct medicinal substance properly administered (T88.6)*
anaphylactic reaction or shock due to adverse food reaction (T78.Ø-)
anaphylactic reaction or shock due to serum (T8Ø.5-)

T78.3 Angioneurotic edema
Allergic angioedema
Giant urticaria
Quincke's edema
EXCLUDES 1 *serum urticaria (T8Ø.6-)*
urticaria (L5Ø.-)

T78.4 Other and unspecified allergy
EXCLUDES 1 *specified types of allergic reaction such as:*
allergic diarrhea (K52.29)
allergic gastroenteritis and colitis (K52.29)
dermatitis (L23-L25, L27.-)
food protein-induced enterocolitis syndrome (K52.21)
food protein-induced enteropathy (K52.22)
hay fever (J3Ø.1)

T78.4Ø Allergy, unspecified
Allergic reaction NOS
Hypersensitivity NOS

T78.41 Arthus phenomenon
Arthus reaction

T78.49 Other allergy
AHA: 2021,1Q,42

T78.8 Other adverse effects, not elsewhere classified

Certain early complications of trauma (T79)

T79 Certain early complications of trauma, not elsewhere classified

EXCLUDES 2 *acute respiratory distress syndrome (J80)*
complications occurring during or following medical procedures (T80-T88)
complications of surgical and medical care NEC (T80-T88)
newborn respiratory distress syndrome (P22.0)

The appropriate 7th character is to be added to each code from category T79.
A initial encounter
D subsequent encounter
S sequela

T79.0 Air embolism (traumatic) MCC HCC
EXCLUDES 1 *air embolism complicating abortion or ectopic or molar pregnancy (O00-O07, O08.2)*
air embolism complicating pregnancy, childbirth and the puerperium (O88.0)
air embolism following infusion, transfusion, and therapeutic injection (T80.0)
air embolism following procedure NEC (T81.7-)
DEF: Arterial or venous obstruction due to the introduction of air bubbles into the blood vessels following surgery or trauma.

T79.1 Fat embolism (traumatic) MCC HCC
EXCLUDES 1 *fat embolism complicating:*
abortion or ectopic or molar pregnancy (O00-O07, O08.2)
pregnancy, childbirth and the puerperium (O88.8)
DEF: Arterial blockage due to the entrance of fat into the circulatory system after a fracture of the large bones or administration of corticosteroids.

T79.2 Traumatic secondary and recurrent hemorrhage and seroma CC HCC

T79.4 Traumatic shock MCC HCC
Shock (immediate) (delayed) following injury
EXCLUDES 1 *anaphylactic shock due to adverse food reaction (T78.0-)*
anaphylactic shock due to correct medicinal substance properly administered (T88.6)
anaphylactic shock due to serum (T80.5-)
anaphylactic shock NOS (T78.2)
electric shock (T75.4)
nontraumatic shock NEC (R57.-)
obstetric shock (O75.1)
postprocedural shock (T81.1-)
septic shock (R65.21)
shock complicating abortion or ectopic or molar pregnancy (O00-O07, O08.3)
shock due to anesthesia (T88.2)
shock due to lightning (T75.01)
shock NOS (R57.9)

T79.5 Traumatic anuria MCC HCC
Crush syndrome
Renal failure following crushing

T79.6 Traumatic ischemia of muscle HCC
Traumatic rhabdomyolysis
Volkmann's ischemic contracture
EXCLUDES 2 *anterior tibial syndrome (M76.8)*
compartment syndrome (traumatic) (T79.A-)
nontraumatic ischemia of muscle (M62.2-)
AHA: 2019,2Q,12

T79.7 Traumatic subcutaneous emphysema CC HCC
EXCLUDES 2 *emphysema NOS (J43)*
emphysema (subcutaneous) resulting from a procedure (T81.82)

T79.A Traumatic compartment syndrome
EXCLUDES 1 *fibromyalgia (M79.7)*
nontraumatic compartment syndrome (M79.A-)
EXCLUDES 2 *traumatic ischemic infarction of muscle (T79.6)*
DEF: Compression of nerves and blood vessels within an enclosed muscle space due to previous trauma, which leads to impaired blood flow and muscle and nerve damage.

T79.A0 Compartment syndrome, unspecified CC HCC
Compartment syndrome NOS

T79.A1 Traumatic compartment syndrome of upper extremity
Traumatic compartment syndrome of shoulder, arm, forearm, wrist, hand, and fingers

T79.A11 Traumatic compartment syndrome of right upper extremity CC HCC

T79.A12 Traumatic compartment syndrome of left upper extremity CC HCC

T79.A19 Traumatic compartment syndrome of unspecified upper extremity CC UNS HCC

T79.A2 Traumatic compartment syndrome of lower extremity
Traumatic compartment syndrome of hip, buttock, thigh, leg, foot, and toes

T79.A21 Traumatic compartment syndrome of right lower extremity CC HCC

T79.A22 Traumatic compartment syndrome of left lower extremity CC HCC

T79.A29 Traumatic compartment syndrome of unspecified lower extremity CC UNS HCC

T79.A3 Traumatic compartment syndrome of abdomen CC HCC

T79.A9 Traumatic compartment syndrome of other sites CC HCC

T79.8 Other early complications of trauma HCC

T79.9 Unspecified early complication of trauma HCC

Complications of surgical and medical care, not elsewhere classified (T80-T88)

Use additional code for adverse effect, if applicable, to identify drug (T36-T50 with fifth or sixth character 5)
Use additional code(s) to identify the specified condition resulting from the complication
Use additional code to identify devices involved and details of circumstances (Y62-Y82)

EXCLUDES 2 *any encounters with medical care for postprocedural conditions in which no complications are present, such as:*
artificial opening status (Z93.-)
closure of external stoma (Z43.-)
fitting and adjustment of external prosthetic device (Z44.-)
burns and corrosions from local applications and irradiation (T20-T32)
complications of surgical procedures during pregnancy, childbirth and the puerperium (O00-O9A)
mechanical complication of respirator [ventilator] (J95.850)
poisoning and toxic effects of drugs and chemicals (T36-T65 with fifth or sixth character 1-4 or 6)
postprocedural fever (R50.82)
specified complications classified elsewhere, such as:
cerebrospinal fluid leak from spinal puncture (G97.0)
colostomy malfunction (K94.0-)
disorders of fluid and electrolyte imbalance (E86-E87)
functional disturbances following cardiac surgery (I97.0-I97.1)
intraoperative and postprocedural complications of specified body systems (D78.-, E36.-, E89.-, G97.3-, G97.4, H59.3-, H59.-, H95.2-, H95.3, I97.4-, I97.5, J95.6-, J95.7, K91.6-, L76.-, M96.-, N99.-)
ostomy complications (J95.0-, K94.-, N99.5-)
postgastric surgery syndromes (K91.1)
postlaminectomy syndrome NEC (M96.1)
postmastectomy lymphedema syndrome (I97.2)
postsurgical blind-loop syndrome (K91.2)
ventilator associated pneumonia (J95.851)
AHA: 2015,1Q,15

T80 Complications following infusion, transfusion and therapeutic injection
INCLUDES complications following perfusion
EXCLUDES 2 *bone marrow transplant rejection (T86.01)*
febrile nonhemolytic transfusion reaction (R50.84)
fluid overload due to transfusion (E87.71)
posttransfusion purpura (D69.51)
transfusion associated circulatory overload (TACO) (E87.71)
transfusion (red blood cell) associated hemochromatosis (E83.111)
transfusion related acute lung injury (TRALI) (J95.84)

The appropriate 7th character is to be added to each code from category T80.
A initial encounter
D subsequent encounter
S sequela

T80.0 Air embolism following infusion, transfusion and therapeutic injection MCC H2

√x7th **T80.1 Vascular complications following infusion, transfusion and therapeutic injection** CC

Use additional code to identify the vascular complication

EXCLUDES 2 *extravasation of vesicant agent (T80.81-)*
infiltration of vesicant agent (T80.81-)
postprocedural vascular complications (T81.7-)
vascular complications specified as due to prosthetic devices, implants and grafts (T82.8-, T83.8-, T84.8-, T85.8-)

√5th **T80.2 Infections following infusion, transfusion and therapeutic injection**

Use additional code to identify the specific infection, such as: sepsis (A41.9)

Use additional code (R65.2-) to identify severe sepsis, if applicable

EXCLUDES 2 *infections specified as due to prosthetic devices, implants and grafts (T82.6-T82.7, T83.5-T83.6, T84.5-T84.7, T85.7)*
postprocedural infections (T81.4-)

AHA: 2018,4Q,62

√6th **T80.21 Infection due to central venous catheter**

Infection due to pulmonary artery catheter (Swan-Ganz catheter)

AHA: 2019,1Q,13-14

DEF: Central venous catheter: Catheter positioned in the superior vena cava or right atrium and introduced through a large vein, such as the jugular or subclavian, and used to measure venous pressure or administer fluids or medication.

TIP: Code assignment is based on the location of the catheter and not how the catheter is being used; for example, for hemodialysis. Infections resulting from catheters that are not central lines should be coded to T82.7-.

√7th **T80.211 Bloodstream infection due to central venous catheter** CC H7

Catheter-related bloodstream infection (CRBSI) NOS
Central line-associated bloodstream infection (CLABSI)
Bloodstream infection due to Hickman catheter
Bloodstream infection due to peripherally inserted central catheter (PICC)
Bloodstream infection due to portacath (port-a-cath)
Bloodstream infection due to pulmonary artery catheter
Bloodstream infection due to triple lumen catheter
Bloodstream infection due to umbilical venous catheter

AHA: 2019,1Q,13,14; 2018,4Q,89

√7th **T80.212 Local infection due to central venous catheter** CC H7

Exit or insertion site infection
Local infection due to Hickman catheter
Local infection due to peripherally inserted central catheter (PICC)
Local infection due to portacath (port-a-cath)
Local infection due to pulmonary artery catheter
Local infection due to triple lumen catheter
Local infection due to umbilical venous catheter
Port or reservoir infection
Tunnel infection

√7th **T80.218 Other infection due to central venous catheter** CC H7

Other central line-associated infection
Other infection due to Hickman catheter
Other infection due to peripherally inserted central catheter (PICC)
Other infection due to portacath (port-a-cath)
Other infection due to pulmonary artery catheter
Other infection due to triple lumen catheter
Other infection due to umbilical venous catheter

√7th **T80.219 Unspecified infection due to central venous catheter** CC H7

Central line-associated infection NOS
Unspecified infection due to Hickman catheter
Unspecified infection due to peripherally inserted central catheter (PICC)
Unspecified infection due to portacath (port-a-cath)
Unspecified infection due to pulmonary artery catheter
Unspecified infection due to triple lumen catheter
Unspecified infection due to umbilical venous catheter

√x7th **T80.22 Acute infection following transfusion, infusion, or injection of blood and blood products** CC

√x7th **T80.29 Infection following other infusion, transfusion and therapeutic injection** CC

√5th **T80.3 ABO incompatibility reaction due to transfusion of blood or blood products**

EXCLUDES 1 *minor blood group antigens reactions (Duffy) (E) (K) (Kell) (Kidd) (Lewis) (M) (N) (P) (S) (T80.A-)*

√x7th **T80.30 ABO incompatibility reaction due to transfusion of blood or blood products, unspecified** CC H3

ABO incompatibility blood transfusion NOS
Reaction to ABO incompatibility from transfusion NOS

√6th **T80.31 ABO incompatibility with hemolytic transfusion reaction**

√7th **T80.310 ABO incompatibility with acute hemolytic transfusion reaction** CC H3

ABO incompatibility with hemolytic transfusion reaction less than 24 hours after transfusion
Acute hemolytic transfusion reaction (AHTR) due to ABO incompatibility

√7th **T80.311 ABO incompatibility with delayed hemolytic transfusion reaction** CC H3

ABO incompatibility with hemolytic transfusion reaction 24 hours or more after transfusion
Delayed hemolytic transfusion reaction (DHTR) due to ABO incompatibility

√7th **T80.319 ABO incompatibility with hemolytic transfusion reaction, unspecified** CC H3

ABO incompatibility with hemolytic transfusion reaction at unspecified time after transfusion
Hemolytic transfusion reaction (HTR) due to ABO incompatibility NOS

√x7th **T80.39 Other ABO incompatibility reaction due to transfusion of blood or blood products** CC H3

Delayed serologic transfusion reaction (DSTR) from ABO incompatibility
Other ABO incompatible blood transfusion
Other reaction to ABO incompatible blood transfusion

√5th **T80.4 Rh incompatibility reaction due to transfusion of blood or blood products**

Reaction due to incompatibility of Rh antigens (C) (c) (D) (E) (e)

√x7th **T80.40 Rh incompatibility reaction due to transfusion of blood or blood products, unspecified** CC

Reaction due to Rh factor in transfusion NOS
Rh incompatible blood transfusion NOS

√6th **T80.41 Rh incompatibility with hemolytic transfusion reaction**

√7th **T80.410 Rh incompatibility with acute hemolytic transfusion reaction** CC
Acute hemolytic transfusion reaction (AHTR) due to Rh incompatibility
Rh incompatibility with hemolytic transfusion reaction less than 24 hours after transfusion

√7th **T80.411 Rh incompatibility with delayed hemolytic transfusion reaction** CC
Delayed hemolytic transfusion reaction (DHTR) due to Rh incompatibility
Rh incompatibility with hemolytic transfusion reaction 24 hours or more after transfusion

√7th **T80.419 Rh incompatibility with hemolytic transfusion reaction, unspecified** CC
Rh incompatibility with hemolytic transfusion reaction at unspecified time after transfusion
Hemolytic transfusion reaction (HTR) due to Rh incompatibility NOS

√x7th **T80.49 Other Rh incompatibility reaction due to transfusion of blood or blood products** CC
Delayed serologic transfusion reaction (DSTR) from Rh incompatibility
Other reaction to Rh incompatible blood transfusion

√5th **T80.A Non-ABO incompatibility reaction due to transfusion of blood or blood products**
Reaction due to incompatibility of minor antigens (Duffy) (Kell) (Kidd) (Lewis) (M) (N) (P) (S)

√x7th **T80.A0 Non-ABO incompatibility reaction due to transfusion of blood or blood products, unspecified** CC
Non-ABO antigen incompatibility reaction from transfusion NOS

√6th **T80.A1 Non-ABO incompatibility with hemolytic transfusion reaction**

√7th **T80.A10 Non-ABO incompatibility with acute hemolytic transfusion reaction** CC
Acute hemolytic transfusion reaction (AHTR) due to non-ABO incompatibility
Non-ABO incompatibility with hemolytic transfusion reaction less than 24 hours after transfusion

√7th **T80.A11 Non-ABO incompatibility with delayed hemolytic transfusion reaction** CC
Delayed hemolytic transfusion reaction (DHTR) due to non-ABO incompatibility
Non-ABO incompatibility with hemolytic transfusion reaction 24 or more hours after transfusion

√7th **T80.A19 Non-ABO incompatibility with hemolytic transfusion reaction, unspecified** CC
Hemolytic transfusion reaction (HTR) due to non-ABO incompatibility NOS
Non-ABO incompatibility with hemolytic transfusion reaction at unspecified time after transfusion

√x7th **T80.A9 Other non-ABO incompatibility reaction due to transfusion of blood or blood products** CC
Delayed serologic transfusion reaction (DSTR) from non-ABO incompatibility
Other reaction to non-ABO incompatible blood transfusion

√5th **T80.5 Anaphylactic reaction due to serum**
Allergic shock due to serum
Anaphylactic shock due to serum
Anaphylactoid reaction due to serum
Anaphylaxis due to serum
EXCLUDES 1 *ABO incompatibility reaction due to transfusion of blood or blood products (T80.3-)*
allergic reaction or shock NOS (T78.2)
anaphylactic reaction or shock NOS (T78.2)
anaphylactic reaction or shock due to adverse effect of correct medicinal substance properly administered (T88.6)
other serum reaction (T80.6-)

DEF: Life-threatening hypersensitivity to a foreign serum causing respiratory distress, vascular collapse, and shock.

√x7th **T80.51 Anaphylactic reaction due to administration of blood and blood products** CC

√x7th **T80.52 Anaphylactic reaction due to vaccination** CC
AHA: 2021,1Q,43

√x7th **T80.59 Anaphylactic reaction due to other serum** CC

√5th **T80.6 Other serum reactions**
Intoxication by serum
Protein sickness
Serum rash
Serum sickness
Serum urticaria
EXCLUDES 2 *serum hepatitis (B16-B19)*

DEF: Serum sickness: Hypersensitivity to a foreign serum that causes fever, hives, swelling, and lymphadenopathy.

√x7th **T80.61 Other serum reaction due to administration of blood and blood products** CC

√x7th **T80.62 Other serum reaction due to vaccination** CC
AHA: 2021,1Q,42

√x7th **T80.69 Other serum reaction due to other serum** CC
Code also, if applicable, arthropathy in hypersensitivity reactions classified elsewhere (M36.4)

√5th **T80.8 Other complications following infusion, transfusion and therapeutic injection**

√6th **T80.81 Extravasation of vesicant agent**
Infiltration of vesicant agent

√7th **T80.810 Extravasation of vesicant antineoplastic chemotherapy** CC
Infiltration of vesicant antineoplastic chemotherapy

√7th **T80.818 Extravasation of other vesicant agent** CC
Infiltration of other vesicant agent

√x7th **T80.82 Complication of immune effector cellular therapy**
Complication of chimeric antigen receptor (CAR-T) cell therapy
Complication of IEC therapy
Use additional code to identify the specific complication, such as:
cytokine release syndrome (D89.83-)
immune effector cell-associated neurotoxicity syndrome (G92.0-)
EXCLUDES 2 *complication of bone marrow transplant (T86.0)*
complication of stem cell transplant (T86.5)
AHA: 2021,4Q,31

√x7th **T80.89 Other complications following infusion, transfusion and therapeutic injection**
Delayed serologic transfusion reaction (DSTR), unspecified incompatibility
Use additional code to identify graft-versus-host reaction, if applicable, (D89.81-)
AHA: 2020,4Q,14

√5th **T80.9 Unspecified complication following infusion, transfusion and therapeutic injection**

√x7th **T80.90 Unspecified complication following infusion and therapeutic injection**

T80.91 Hemolytic transfusion reaction, unspecified incompatibility

EXCLUDES 1 *ABO incompatibility with hemolytic transfusion reaction (T80.31-)*
non-ABO incompatibility with hemolytic transfusion reaction (T80.A1-)
Rh incompatibility with hemolytic transfusion reaction (T80.41-)

T80.910 Acute hemolytic transfusion reaction, unspecified incompatibility CC

T80.911 Delayed hemolytic transfusion reaction, unspecified incompatibility CC

T80.919 Hemolytic transfusion reaction, unspecified incompatibility, unspecified as acute or delayed CC

Hemolytic transfusion reaction NOS

T80.92 Unspecified transfusion reaction

Transfusion reaction NOS

T81 Complications of procedures, not elsewhere classified

Use additional code for adverse effect, if applicable, to identify drug (T36-T50 with fifth or sixth character 5)

EXCLUDES 2 *complications following immunization (T88.0-T88.1)*
complications following infusion, transfusion and therapeutic injection (T80.-)
complications of transplanted organs and tissue (T86.-)
specified complications classified elsewhere, such as:
complication of prosthetic devices, implants and grafts (T82-T85)
dermatitis due to drugs and medicaments (L23.3, L24.4, L25.1, L27.0-L27.1)
endosseous dental implant failure (M27.6-)
floppy iris syndrome (IFIS) (intraoperative) (H21.81)
intraoperative and postprocedural complications of specific body system (D78.-, E36.-, E89.-, G97.3-, G97.4, H59.3-, H59.-, H95.2-, H95.3, I97.4-, I97.5, J95, K91.-, L76.-, M96.-, N99.-)
ostomy complications (J95.0-, K94.-, N99.5-)
plateau iris syndrome (post-iridectomy) (postprocedural) H21.82
poisoning and toxic effects of drugs and chemicals ▶(T36-T65 with fifth or sixth character 1-4)◀

AHA: 2019,2Q,21

The appropriate 7th character is to be added to each code from category T81.
A initial encounter
D subsequent encounter
S sequela

T81.1 Postprocedural shock

Shock during or resulting from a procedure, not elsewhere classified

EXCLUDES 1 *anaphylactic shock NOS (T78.2)*
anaphylactic shock due to correct substance properly administered (T88.6)
anaphylactic shock due to serum (T80.5-)
electric shock (T75.4)
obstetric shock (O75.1)
~~septic shock (R65.21)~~
shock due to anesthesia (T88.2)
shock following abortion or ectopic or molar pregnancy (O00-O07, O08.3)
traumatic shock (T79.4)

AHA: 2021,1Q,13

T81.10 Postprocedural shock unspecified CC

Collapse NOS during or resulting from a procedure, not elsewhere classified
Postprocedural failure of peripheral circulation
Postprocedural shock NOS

T81.11 Postprocedural cardiogenic shock MCC HCC

T81.12 Postprocedural septic shock MCC UPD HCC

Postprocedural endotoxic shock resulting from a procedure, not elsewhere classified
Postprocedural gram-negative shock resulting from a procedure, not elsewhere classified
Code first underlying infection
Use additional code, to identify any associated acute organ dysfunction, if applicable

AHA: 2018,4Q,63

T81.19 Other postprocedural shock MCC

Postprocedural hypovolemic shock

T81.3 Disruption of wound, not elsewhere classified

Disruption of any suture materials or other closure methods

EXCLUDES 1 *breakdown (mechanical) of permanent sutures (T85.612)*
displacement of permanent sutures (T85.622)
disruption of cesarean delivery wound (O90.0)
disruption of perineal obstetric wound (O90.1)
mechanical complication of permanent sutures NEC (T85.692)

AHA: 2014,1Q,23

T81.30 Disruption of wound, unspecified CC

Disruption of wound NOS

T81.31 Disruption of external operation (surgical) wound, not elsewhere classified CC

Dehiscence of operation wound NOS
Disruption of operation wound NOS
Disruption or dehiscence of closure of cornea
Disruption or dehiscence of closure of mucosa
Disruption or dehiscence of closure of skin and subcutaneous tissue
Full-thickness skin disruption or dehiscence
Superficial disruption or dehiscence of operation wound

EXCLUDES 1 *dehiscence of amputation stump (T87.81)*

T81.32 Disruption of internal operation (surgical) wound, not elsewhere classified CC

Deep disruption or dehiscence of operation wound NOS
Disruption or dehiscence of closure of internal organ or other internal tissue
Disruption or dehiscence of closure of muscle or muscle flap
Disruption or dehiscence of closure of ribs or rib cage
Disruption or dehiscence of closure of skull or craniotomy
Disruption or dehiscence of closure of sternum or sternotomy
Disruption or dehiscence of closure of tendon or ligament
Disruption or dehiscence of closure of superficial or muscular fascia

AHA: 2020,2Q,22; 2017,3Q,4

T81.33 Disruption of traumatic injury wound repair CC

Disruption or dehiscence of closure of traumatic laceration (external) (internal)

T81.4 Infection following a procedure

Wound abscess following a procedure
Use additional code to identify infection
Use additional code (R65.2-) to identify severe sepsis, if applicable

EXCLUDES 2 *bleb associated endophthalmitis (H59.4-)*
infection due to infusion, transfusion and therapeutic injection (T80.2-)
infection due to prosthetic devices, implants and grafts (T82.6-T82.7, T83.5-T83.6, T84.5-T84.7, T85.7)
obstetric surgical wound infection (O86.0-)
postprocedural fever NOS (R50.82)
postprocedural retroperitoneal abscess (K68.11)

AHA: 2018,4Q,33-34,62; 2014,1Q,23

T81.40 Infection following a procedure, unspecified CC H11 H12 H13

T81.41 Infection following a procedure, superficial incisional surgical site CC H11 H12 H13

Subcutaneous abscess following a procedure
Stitch abscess following a procedure

T81.42 Infection following a procedure, deep incisional surgical site CC H11 H12 H13

Intra-muscular abscess following a procedure

T81.43 Infection following a procedure, organ and space surgical site CC H11 H12 H13

Intra-abdominal abscess following a procedure
Subphrenic abscess following a procedure

T81.44 Sepsis following a procedure CC H11 H12 H13 HCC

Use additional code to identify the sepsis

T81.49 Infection following a procedure, other surgical site CC H11 H12 H13

√5th **T81.5 Complications of foreign body accidentally left in body following procedure**
AHA: 2014,4Q,24

√6th **T81.50 Unspecified complication of foreign body accidentally left in body following procedure**

√7th **T81.500 Unspecified complication of foreign body accidentally left in body following surgical operation** CC H1

√7th **T81.501 Unspecified complication of foreign body accidentally left in body following infusion or transfusion** CC H1

√7th **T81.502 Unspecified complication of foreign body accidentally left in body following kidney dialysis** CC H1 HCC

√7th **T81.503 Unspecified complication of foreign body accidentally left in body following injection or immunization** CC H1

√7th **T81.504 Unspecified complication of foreign body accidentally left in body following endoscopic examination** CC H1

√7th **T81.505 Unspecified complication of foreign body accidentally left in body following heart catheterization** CC H1

√7th **T81.506 Unspecified complication of foreign body accidentally left in body following aspiration, puncture or other catheterization** CC H1

√7th **T81.507 Unspecified complication of foreign body accidentally left in body following removal of catheter or packing** CC H1

√7th **T81.508 Unspecified complication of foreign body accidentally left in body following other procedure** CC H1

√7th **T81.509 Unspecified complication of foreign body accidentally left in body following unspecified procedure** CC H1

√6th **T81.51 Adhesions due to foreign body accidentally left in body following procedure**

√7th **T81.510 Adhesions due to foreign body accidentally left in body following surgical operation** CC H1

√7th **T81.511 Adhesions due to foreign body accidentally left in body following infusion or transfusion** CC H1

√7th **T81.512 Adhesions due to foreign body accidentally left in body following kidney dialysis** CC H1 HCC

√7th **T81.513 Adhesions due to foreign body accidentally left in body following injection or immunization** CC H1

√7th **T81.514 Adhesions due to foreign body accidentally left in body following endoscopic examination** CC H1

√7th **T81.515 Adhesions due to foreign body accidentally left in body following heart catheterization** CC H1

√7th **T81.516 Adhesions due to foreign body accidentally left in body following aspiration, puncture or other catheterization** CC H1

√7th **T81.517 Adhesions due to foreign body accidentally left in body following removal of catheter or packing** CC H1

√7th **T81.518 Adhesions due to foreign body accidentally left in body following other procedure** CC H1

√7th **T81.519 Adhesions due to foreign body accidentally left in body following unspecified procedure** CC H1

√6th **T81.52 Obstruction due to foreign body accidentally left in body following procedure**

√7th **T81.520 Obstruction due to foreign body accidentally left in body following surgical operation** CC H1

√7th **T81.521 Obstruction due to foreign body accidentally left in body following infusion or transfusion** CC H1

√7th **T81.522 Obstruction due to foreign body accidentally left in body following kidney dialysis** CC H1 HCC

√7th **T81.523 Obstruction due to foreign body accidentally left in body following injection or immunization** CC H1

√7th **T81.524 Obstruction due to foreign body accidentally left in body following endoscopic examination** CC H1

√7th **T81.525 Obstruction due to foreign body accidentally left in body following heart catheterization** CC H1

√7th **T81.526 Obstruction due to foreign body accidentally left in body following aspiration, puncture or other catheterization** CC H1

√7th **T81.527 Obstruction due to foreign body accidentally left in body following removal of catheter or packing** CC H1

√7th **T81.528 Obstruction due to foreign body accidentally left in body following other procedure** CC H1

√7th **T81.529 Obstruction due to foreign body accidentally left in body following unspecified procedure** CC H1

√6th **T81.53 Perforation due to foreign body accidentally left in body following procedure**

√7th **T81.530 Perforation due to foreign body accidentally left in body following surgical operation** CC H1

√7th **T81.531 Perforation due to foreign body accidentally left in body following infusion or transfusion** CC H1

√7th **T81.532 Perforation due to foreign body accidentally left in body following kidney dialysis** CC H1 HCC

√7th **T81.533 Perforation due to foreign body accidentally left in body following injection or immunization** CC H1

√7th **T81.534 Perforation due to foreign body accidentally left in body following endoscopic examination** CC H1

√7th **T81.535 Perforation due to foreign body accidentally left in body following heart catheterization** CC H1

√7th **T81.536 Perforation due to foreign body accidentally left in body following aspiration, puncture or other catheterization** CC H1

√7th **T81.537 Perforation due to foreign body accidentally left in body following removal of catheter or packing** CC H1

√7th **T81.538 Perforation due to foreign body accidentally left in body following other procedure** CC H1

√7th **T81.539 Perforation due to foreign body accidentally left in body following unspecified procedure** CC H1

√6th **T81.59 Other complications of foreign body accidentally left in body following procedure**

EXCLUDES 2 *obstruction or perforation due to prosthetic devices and implants intentionally left in body (T82.0-T82.5, T83.0-T83.4, T83.7, T84.0-T84.4, T85.0-T85.6)*

√7th **T81.590 Other complications of foreign body accidentally left in body following surgical operation** CC H1

√7th **T81.591 Other complications of foreign body accidentally left in body following infusion or transfusion** CC H1

√7th **T81.592 Other complications of foreign body accidentally left in body following kidney dialysis** CC H1 HCC

√7th **T81.593 Other complications of foreign body accidentally left in body following injection or immunization** CC H1

√7th **T81.594 Other complications of foreign body accidentally left in body following endoscopic examination** CC H1

√7th **T81.595 Other complications of foreign body accidentally left in body following heart catheterization** CC H1

√7th **T81.596 Other complications of foreign body accidentally left in body following aspiration, puncture or other catheterization** CC H1

T81.597 Other complications of foreign body accidentally left in body following removal of catheter or packing CC H1

T81.598 Other complications of foreign body accidentally left in body following other procedure CC H1

T81.599 Other complications of foreign body accidentally left in body following unspecified procedure CC H1

T81.6 Acute reaction to foreign substance accidentally left during a procedure

EXCLUDES 2 *complications of foreign body accidentally left in body cavity or operation wound following procedure (T81.5-)*

T81.60 Unspecified acute reaction to foreign substance accidentally left during a procedure CC H1

T81.61 Aseptic peritonitis due to foreign substance accidentally left during a procedure CC H1

Chemical peritonitis

T81.69 Other acute reaction to foreign substance accidentally left during a procedure CC H1

T81.7 Vascular complications following a procedure, not elsewhere classified

Air embolism following procedure NEC

Phlebitis or thrombophlebitis resulting from a procedure

EXCLUDES 1 *embolism complicating abortion or ectopic or molar pregnancy (O00-O07, O08.2)*

embolism complicating pregnancy, childbirth and the puerperium (O88.-)

traumatic embolism (T79.0)

EXCLUDES 2 *embolism due to prosthetic devices, implants and grafts (T82.8-, T83.81, T84.8-, T85.81-)*

embolism following infusion, transfusion and therapeutic injection (T80.0)

AHA: 2019,2Q,22

T81.71 Complication of artery following a procedure, not elsewhere classified

T81.710 Complication of mesenteric artery following a procedure, not elsewhere classified CC

T81.711 Complication of renal artery following a procedure, not elsewhere classified CC

T81.718 Complication of other artery following a procedure, not elsewhere classified CC

AHA: 2019,2Q,21-22

T81.719 Complication of unspecified artery following a procedure, not elsewhere classified CC

T81.72 Complication of vein following a procedure, not elsewhere classified CC

T81.8 Other complications of procedures, not elsewhere classified

EXCLUDES 2 *hypothermia following anesthesia (T88.51)*

malignant hyperpyrexia due to anesthesia (T88.3)

T81.81 Complication of inhalation therapy

T81.82 Emphysema (subcutaneous) resulting from a procedure

T81.83 Persistent postprocedural fistula CC

▶Use additional code, if known, for site of fistula such as:◀

▶anal fistula (K60.3)◀

▶anorectal fistula (K60.5)◀

▶bladder fistula (N32.2)◀

▶other female intestinal-genital tract fistulae (N82.4)◀

AHA: 2023,1Q,30; 2017,3Q,3-4

T81.89 Other complications of procedures, not elsewhere classified

Use additional code to specify complication, such as: postprocedural delirium (F05)

AHA: 2014,1Q,23

T81.9 Unspecified complication of procedure

T82 Complications of cardiac and vascular prosthetic devices, implants and grafts

EXCLUDES 2 *failure and rejection of transplanted organs and tissue (T86.-)*

AHA: 2020,3Q,36-37

The appropriate 7th character is to be added to each code from category T82.

A initial encounter

D subsequent encounter

S sequela

T82.0 Mechanical complication of heart valve prosthesis

Mechanical complication of artificial heart valve

EXCLUDES 1 *mechanical complication of biological heart valve graft (T82.22-)*

T82.01 Breakdown (mechanical) of heart valve prosthesis CC

T82.02 Displacement of heart valve prosthesis CC

Malposition of heart valve prosthesis

T82.03 Leakage of heart valve prosthesis CC

T82.09 Other mechanical complication of heart valve prosthesis CC

Obstruction (mechanical) of heart valve prosthesis

Perforation of heart valve prosthesis

Protrusion of heart valve prosthesis

T82.1 Mechanical complication of cardiac electronic device

T82.11 Breakdown (mechanical) of cardiac electronic device

T82.110 Breakdown (mechanical) of cardiac electrode CC

T82.111 Breakdown (mechanical) of cardiac pulse generator (battery) CC

T82.118 Breakdown (mechanical) of other cardiac electronic device CC

T82.119 Breakdown (mechanical) of unspecified cardiac electronic device CC

T82.12 Displacement of cardiac electronic device

Malposition of cardiac electronic device

T82.120 Displacement of cardiac electrode CC

T82.121 Displacement of cardiac pulse generator (battery) CC

T82.128 Displacement of other cardiac electronic device CC

T82.129 Displacement of unspecified cardiac electronic device CC

T82.19 Other mechanical complication of cardiac electronic device

Leakage of cardiac electronic device

Obstruction of cardiac electronic device

Perforation of cardiac electronic device

Protrusion of cardiac electronic device

T82.190 Other mechanical complication of cardiac electrode CC

T82.191 Other mechanical complication of cardiac pulse generator (battery) CC

T82.198 Other mechanical complication of other cardiac electronic device CC

T82.199 Other mechanical complication of unspecified cardiac device CC

T82.2 Mechanical complication of coronary artery bypass graft and biological heart valve graft

EXCLUDES 1 *mechanical complication of artificial heart valve prosthesis (T82.0-)*

T82.21 Mechanical complication of coronary artery bypass graft

T82.211 Breakdown (mechanical) of coronary artery bypass graft CC

T82.212 Displacement of coronary artery bypass graft CC

Malposition of coronary artery bypass graft

T82.213 Leakage of coronary artery bypass graft CC

T82.218 Other mechanical complication of coronary artery bypass graft CC

Obstruction, mechanical of coronary artery bypass graft

Perforation of coronary artery bypass graft

Protrusion of coronary artery bypass graft

√6th T82.22 **Mechanical complication of biological heart valve graft**
- √7th T82.221 **Breakdown (mechanical) of biological heart valve graft** CC
- √7th T82.222 **Displacement of biological heart valve graft** CC
  Malposition of biological heart valve graft
- √7th T82.223 **Leakage of biological heart valve graft** CC
- √7th T82.228 **Other mechanical complication of biological heart valve graft** CC
  Obstruction of biological heart valve graft
  Perforation of biological heart valve graft
  Protrusion of biological heart valve graft

√5th T82.3 **Mechanical complication of other vascular grafts**

√6th T82.31 **Breakdown (mechanical) of other vascular grafts**
- √7th T82.310 **Breakdown (mechanical) of aortic (bifurcation) graft (replacement)** CC HCC
  AHA: 2020,3Q,3-8
- √7th T82.311 **Breakdown (mechanical) of carotid arterial graft (bypass)** CC HCC
- √7th T82.312 **Breakdown (mechanical) of femoral arterial graft (bypass)** CC HCC
- √7th T82.318 **Breakdown (mechanical) of other vascular grafts** CC HCC
- √7th T82.319 **Breakdown (mechanical) of unspecified vascular grafts** CC HCC

√6th T82.32 **Displacement of other vascular grafts**
Malposition of other vascular grafts
- √7th T82.320 **Displacement of aortic (bifurcation) graft (replacement)** CC HCC
- √7th T82.321 **Displacement of carotid arterial graft (bypass)** CC HCC
- √7th T82.322 **Displacement of femoral arterial graft (bypass)** CC HCC
- √7th T82.328 **Displacement of other vascular grafts** CC HCC
- √7th T82.329 **Displacement of unspecified vascular grafts** CC HCC

√6th T82.33 **Leakage of other vascular grafts**
- √7th T82.330 **Leakage of aortic (bifurcation) graft (replacement)** CC HCC
  AHA: 2020,3Q,3-8
- √7th T82.331 **Leakage of carotid arterial graft (bypass)** CC HCC
- √7th T82.332 **Leakage of femoral arterial graft (bypass)** CC HCC
- √7th T82.338 **Leakage of other vascular grafts** CC HCC
- √7th T82.339 **Leakage of unspecified vascular graft** CC HCC

√6th T82.39 **Other mechanical complication of other vascular grafts**
Obstruction (mechanical) of other vascular grafts
Perforation of other vascular grafts
Protrusion of other vascular grafts
- √7th T82.390 **Other mechanical complication of aortic (bifurcation) graft (replacement)** CC HCC
  AHA: 2020,3Q,3-5
- √7th T82.391 **Other mechanical complication of carotid arterial graft (bypass)** CC HCC
- √7th T82.392 **Other mechanical complication of femoral arterial graft (bypass)** CC HCC
- √7th T82.398 **Other mechanical complication of other vascular grafts** CC HCC
- √7th T82.399 **Other mechanical complication of unspecified vascular grafts** CC HCC

√5th T82.4 **Mechanical complication of vascular dialysis catheter**
Mechanical complication of hemodialysis catheter
EXCLUDES 1 *mechanical complication of intraperitoneal dialysis catheter (T85.62)*

√x7th T82.41 **Breakdown (mechanical) of vascular dialysis catheter** CC HCC

√x7th T82.42 **Displacement of vascular dialysis catheter** CC HCC
Malposition of vascular dialysis catheter

√x7th T82.43 **Leakage of vascular dialysis catheter** CC HCC

√x7th T82.49 **Other complication of vascular dialysis catheter** CC HCC
Obstruction (mechanical) of vascular dialysis catheter
Perforation of vascular dialysis catheter
Protrusion of vascular dialysis catheter

√5th T82.5 **Mechanical complication of other cardiac and vascular devices and implants**
EXCLUDES 2 *mechanical complication of epidural and subdural infusion catheter (T85.61)*

√6th T82.51 **Breakdown (mechanical) of other cardiac and vascular devices and implants**
- √7th T82.510 **Breakdown (mechanical) of surgically created arteriovenous fistula** CC HCC
  AHA: 2020,3Q,36
- √7th T82.511 **Breakdown (mechanical) of surgically created arteriovenous shunt** CC HCC
  AHA: 2020,3Q,37
- √7th T82.512 **Breakdown (mechanical) of artificial heart** CC
- √7th T82.513 **Breakdown (mechanical) of balloon (counterpulsation) device** CC HCC
- √7th T82.514 **Breakdown (mechanical) of infusion catheter** CC HCC
- √7th T82.515 **Breakdown (mechanical) of umbrella device** CC HCC
- √7th T82.518 **Breakdown (mechanical) of other cardiac and vascular devices and implants** CC HCC
- √7th T82.519 **Breakdown (mechanical) of unspecified cardiac and vascular devices and implants** CC

√6th T82.52 **Displacement of other cardiac and vascular devices and implants**
Malposition of other cardiac and vascular devices and implants
- √7th T82.520 **Displacement of surgically created arteriovenous fistula** CC HCC
  AHA: 2020,3Q,36
- √7th T82.521 **Displacement of surgically created arteriovenous shunt** CC HCC
- √7th T82.522 **Displacement of artificial heart** CC
- √7th T82.523 **Displacement of balloon (counterpulsation) device** CC HCC
- √7th T82.524 **Displacement of infusion catheter** CC HCC
  AHA: 2020,2Q,21; 2019,3Q,15
- √7th T82.525 **Displacement of umbrella device** CC HCC
- √7th T82.528 **Displacement of other cardiac and vascular devices and implants** CC HCC
- √7th T82.529 **Displacement of unspecified cardiac and vascular devices and implants** CC

√6th T82.53 **Leakage of other cardiac and vascular devices and implants**
- √7th T82.530 **Leakage of surgically created arteriovenous fistula** CC HCC
  AHA: 2020,3Q,36
- √7th T82.531 **Leakage of surgically created arteriovenous shunt** CC HCC
- √7th T82.532 **Leakage of artificial heart** CC
- √7th T82.533 **Leakage of balloon (counterpulsation) device** CC HCC
- √7th T82.534 **Leakage of infusion catheter** CC HCC
- √7th T82.535 **Leakage of umbrella device** CC HCC
- √7th T82.538 **Leakage of other cardiac and vascular devices and implants** CC HCC
- √7th T82.539 **Leakage of unspecified cardiac and vascular devices and implants** CC

√6th **T82.59 Other mechanical complication of other cardiac and vascular devices and implants**
Obstruction (mechanical) of other cardiac and vascular devices and implants
Perforation of other cardiac and vascular devices and implants
Protrusion of other cardiac and vascular devices and implants

√7th **T82.59Ø Other mechanical complication of surgically created arteriovenous fistula** CC HCC
AHA: 2020,3Q,36

√7th **T82.591 Other mechanical complication of surgically created arteriovenous shunt** CC HCC

√7th **T82.592 Other mechanical complication of artificial heart** CC

√7th **T82.593 Other mechanical complication of balloon (counterpulsation) device** CC HCC

√7th **T82.594 Other mechanical complication of infusion catheter** CC HCC

√7th **T82.595 Other mechanical complication of umbrella device** CC HCC

√7th **T82.598 Other mechanical complication of other cardiac and vascular devices and implants** CC HCC

√7th **T82.599 Other mechanical complication of unspecified cardiac and vascular devices and implants** CC

√x7th **T82.6 Infection and inflammatory reaction due to cardiac valve prosthesis** CC HCC
Use additional code to identify infection

√x7th **T82.7 Infection and inflammatory reaction due to other cardiac and vascular devices, implants and grafts** CC H13 HCC
Use additional code to identify infection
AHA: 2019,1Q,13-14
DEF: Midline catheter: Long peripheral catheter introduced via the cephalic, basilic, brachial, or median cubital veins in the upper arm and positioned so that the tip is level or near the level of the axilla and distal to the shoulder. Midline catheters are typically used for IV access, fluid replacement, and medication administration.
TIP: Assign this code for infections and/or cellulitis resulting from catheters that are not centrally placed (e.g., midline catheters).

√5th **T82.8 Other specified complications of cardiac and vascular prosthetic devices, implants and grafts**
AHA: 2016,4Q,70

√6th **T82.81 Embolism due to cardiac and vascular prosthetic devices, implants and grafts**

√7th **T82.817 Embolism due to cardiac prosthetic devices, implants and grafts** CC

√7th **T82.818 Embolism due to vascular prosthetic devices, implants and grafts** CC HCC

√6th **T82.82 Fibrosis due to cardiac and vascular prosthetic devices, implants and grafts**

√7th **T82.827 Fibrosis due to cardiac prosthetic devices, implants and grafts** CC

√7th **T82.828 Fibrosis due vascular prosthetic devices, implants and grafts** CC HCC

√6th **T82.83 Hemorrhage due to cardiac and vascular prosthetic devices, implants and grafts**

√7th **T82.837 Hemorrhage due to cardiac prosthetic devices, implants and grafts** CC

√7th **T82.838 Hemorrhage due to vascular prosthetic devices, implants and grafts** CC HCC
AHA: 2020,3Q,36-37

√6th **T82.84 Pain due to cardiac and vascular prosthetic devices, implants and grafts**

√7th **T82.847 Pain due to cardiac prosthetic devices, implants and grafts** CC

√7th **T82.848 Pain due to vascular prosthetic devices, implants and grafts** CC HCC

√6th **T82.85 Stenosis due to cardiac and vascular prosthetic devices, implants and grafts**

√7th **T82.855 Stenosis of coronary artery stent** CC
In-stent stenosis (restenosis) of coronary artery stent
Restenosis of coronary artery stent
AHA: 2021,3Q,6-7

√7th **T82.856 Stenosis of peripheral vascular stent** CC HCC
In-stent stenosis (restenosis) of peripheral vascular stent
Restenosis of peripheral vascular stent

√7th **T82.857 Stenosis of other cardiac prosthetic devices, implants and grafts** CC

√7th **T82.858 Stenosis of other vascular prosthetic devices, implants and grafts** CC HCC

√6th **T82.86 Thrombosis of cardiac and vascular prosthetic devices, implants and grafts**
AHA: 2023,2Q,7

√7th **T82.867 Thrombosis due to cardiac prosthetic devices, implants and grafts** CC

√7th **T82.868 Thrombosis due to vascular prosthetic devices, implants and grafts** CC HCC

√6th **T82.89 Other specified complication of cardiac and vascular prosthetic devices, implants and grafts**

√7th **T82.897 Other specified complication of cardiac prosthetic devices, implants and grafts** CC
AHA: 2019,2Q,33

√7th **T82.898 Other specified complication of vascular prosthetic devices, implants and grafts** CC HCC
AHA: 2020,3Q,3-5

√x7th **T82.9 Unspecified complication of cardiac and vascular prosthetic device, implant and graft** CC

√4th **T83 Complications of genitourinary prosthetic devices, implants and grafts**
EXCLUDES 2 *failure and rejection of transplanted organs and tissue (T86.-)*
AHA: 2016,4Q,70-71

The appropriate 7th character is to be added to each code from category T83.
A initial encounter
D subsequent encounter
S sequela

√5th **T83.Ø Mechanical complication of urinary catheter**
EXCLUDES 2 *complications of stoma of urinary tract (N99.5-)*

√6th **T83.Ø1 Breakdown (mechanical) of urinary catheter**

√7th **T83.Ø1Ø Breakdown (mechanical) of cystostomy catheter** CC HCC

√7th **T83.Ø11 Breakdown (mechanical) of indwelling urethral catheter** HCC

√7th **T83.Ø12 Breakdown (mechanical) of nephrostomy catheter** HCC

√7th **T83.Ø18 Breakdown (mechanical) of other urinary catheter** HCC
Breakdown (mechanical) of Hopkins catheter
Breakdown (mechanical) of ileostomy catheter
Breakdown (mechanical) urostomy catheter

√6th **T83.Ø2 Displacement of urinary catheter**
Malposition of urinary catheter

√7th **T83.Ø2Ø Displacement of cystostomy catheter** CC HCC

√7th **T83.Ø21 Displacement of indwelling urethral catheter** HCC

√7th **T83.Ø22 Displacement of nephrostomy catheter** HCC

√7th **T83.Ø28 Displacement of other urinary catheter** HCC
Displacement of Hopkins catheter
Displacement of ileostomy catheter
Displacement of urostomy catheter

√6th **T83.Ø3 Leakage of urinary catheter**

√7th **T83.Ø3Ø Leakage of cystostomy catheter** CC HCC
AHA: 2021,4Q,18

√7th **T83.Ø31 Leakage of indwelling urethral catheter** HCC

√7th **T83.Ø32 Leakage of nephrostomy catheter** HCC

√7th **T83.Ø38 Leakage of other urinary catheter** HCC
Leakage of Hopkins catheter
Leakage of ileostomy catheter
Leakage of urostomy catheter

√6th **T83.09 Other mechanical complication of urinary catheter**
Obstruction (mechanical) of urinary catheter
Perforation of urinary catheter
Protrusion of urinary catheter

√7th **T83.090 Other mechanical complication of cystostomy catheter** CC HCC

√7th **T83.091 Other mechanical complication of indwelling urethral catheter** HCC

√7th **T83.092 Other mechanical complication of nephrostomy catheter** HCC

√7th **T83.098 Other mechanical complication of other urinary catheter** HCC
Other mechanical complication of Hopkins catheter
Other mechanical complication of ileostomy catheter
Other mechanical complication of urostomy catheter

√5th **T83.1 Mechanical complication of other urinary devices and implants**

√6th **T83.11 Breakdown (mechanical) of other urinary devices and implants**

√7th **T83.110 Breakdown (mechanical) of urinary electronic stimulator device** CC HCC
EXCLUDES 2 *breakdown (mechanical) of electrode (lead) for sacral nerve neurostimulator (T85.111)*
breakdown (mechanical) of implanted electronic sacral neurostimulator, pulse generator or receiver (T85.113)

√7th **T83.111 Breakdown (mechanical) of implanted urinary sphincter** CC HCC

√7th **T83.112 Breakdown (mechanical) of indwelling ureteral stent** CC HCC

√7th **T83.113 Breakdown (mechanical) of other urinary stents** CC HCC
Breakdown (mechanical) of ileal conduit stent
Breakdown (mechanical) of nephroureteral stent

√7th **T83.118 Breakdown (mechanical) of other urinary devices and implants** CC HCC

√6th **T83.12 Displacement of other urinary devices and implants**
Malposition of other urinary devices and implants

√7th **T83.120 Displacement of urinary electronic stimulator device** CC HCC
EXCLUDES 2 *displacement of electrode (lead) for sacral nerve neurostimulator (T85.121)*
displacement of implanted electronic sacral neurostimulator, pulse generator or receiver (T85.123)

√7th **T83.121 Displacement of implanted urinary sphincter** CC HCC

√7th **T83.122 Displacement of indwelling ureteral stent** CC HCC

√7th **T83.123 Displacement of other urinary stents** CC HCC
Displacement of ileal conduit stent
Displacement of nephroureteral stent

√7th **T83.128 Displacement of other urinary devices and implants** CC HCC

√6th **T83.19 Other mechanical complication of other urinary devices and implants**
Leakage of other urinary devices and implants
Obstruction (mechanical) of other urinary devices and implants
Perforation of other urinary devices and implants
Protrusion of other urinary devices and implants

√7th **T83.190 Other mechanical complication of urinary electronic stimulator device** CC HCC
EXCLUDES 2 *other mechanical complication of electrode (lead) for sacral nerve neurostimulator (T85.191)*
other mechanical complication of implanted electronic sacral neurostimulator, pulse generator or receiver (T85.193)

√7th **T83.191 Other mechanical complication of implanted urinary sphincter** CC HCC

√7th **T83.192 Other mechanical complication of indwelling ureteral stent** CC HCC

√7th **T83.193 Other mechanical complication of other urinary stent** CC HCC
Other mechanical complication of ileal conduit stent
Other mechanical complication of nephroureteral stent

√7th **T83.198 Other mechanical complication of other urinary devices and implants** CC HCC

√5th **T83.2 Mechanical complication of graft of urinary organ**

√x7th **T83.21 Breakdown (mechanical) of graft of urinary organ** CC HCC

√x7th **T83.22 Displacement of graft of urinary organ** CC HCC
Malposition of graft of urinary organ

√x7th **T83.23 Leakage of graft of urinary organ** CC HCC

√x7th **T83.24 Erosion of graft of urinary organ** CC HCC

√x7th **T83.25 Exposure of graft of urinary organ** CC HCC

√x7th **T83.29 Other mechanical complication of graft of urinary organ** CC HCC
Obstruction (mechanical) of graft of urinary organ
Perforation of graft of urinary organ
Protrusion of graft of urinary organ

√5th **T83.3 Mechanical complication of intrauterine contraceptive device**

√x7th **T83.31 Breakdown (mechanical) of intrauterine contraceptive device** ♀

√x7th **T83.32 Displacement of intrauterine contraceptive device** ♀
Malposition of intrauterine contraceptive device
Missing string of intrauterine contraceptive device
AHA: 2018,1Q,5

√x7th **T83.39 Other mechanical complication of intrauterine contraceptive device** ♀
Leakage of intrauterine contraceptive device
Obstruction (mechanical) of intrauterine contraceptive device
Perforation of intrauterine contraceptive device
Protrusion of intrauterine contraceptive device

√5th **T83.4 Mechanical complication of other prosthetic devices, implants and grafts of genital tract**

√6th **T83.41 Breakdown (mechanical) of other prosthetic devices, implants and grafts of genital tract**

√7th **T83.410 Breakdown (mechanical) of implanted penile prosthesis** CC HCC ♂
Breakdown (mechanical) of penile prosthesis cylinder
Breakdown (mechanical) of penile prosthesis pump
Breakdown (mechanical) of penile prosthesis reservoir

√7th **T83.411 Breakdown (mechanical) of implanted testicular prosthesis** CC HCC

√7th **T83.418 Breakdown (mechanical) of other prosthetic devices, implants and grafts of genital tract** CC HCC

√6th **T83.42 Displacement of other prosthetic devices, implants and grafts of genital tract**
Malposition of other prosthetic devices, implants and grafts of genital tract

√7th **T83.420 Displacement of implanted penile prosthesis** CC HCC ♂
Displacement of penile prosthesis cylinder
Displacement of penile prosthesis pump
Displacement of penile prosthesis reservoir

√7th **T83.421 Displacement of implanted testicular prosthesis** CC HCC

√7th **T83.428 Displacement of other prosthetic devices, implants and grafts of genital tract** CC HCC
AHA: 2018,1Q,5

√6th **T83.49 Other mechanical complication of other prosthetic devices, implants and grafts of genital tract**
Leakage of other prosthetic devices, implants and grafts of genital tract
Obstruction, mechanical of other prosthetic devices, implants and grafts of genital tract
Perforation of other prosthetic devices, implants and grafts of genital tract
Protrusion of other prosthetic devices, implants and grafts of genital tract

√7th **T83.490 Other mechanical complication of implanted penile prosthesis** CC HCC ♂
Other mechanical complication of penile prosthesis cylinder
Other mechanical complication of penile prosthesis pump
Other mechanical complication of penile prosthesis reservoir

√7th **T83.491 Other mechanical complication of implanted testicular prosthesis** CC HCC

√7th **T83.498 Other mechanical complication of other prosthetic devices, implants and grafts of genital tract** CC HCC

√5th **T83.5 Infection and inflammatory reaction due to prosthetic device, implant and graft in urinary system**
Use additional code to identify infection

√6th **T83.51 Infection and inflammatory reaction due to urinary catheter**
EXCLUDES 2 *complications of stoma of urinary tract (N99.5-)*
AHA: 2019,3Q,17

√7th **T83.510 Infection and inflammatory reaction due to cystostomy catheter** CC HCC

√7th **T83.511 Infection and inflammatory reaction due to indwelling urethral catheter** CC H6 HCC
AHA: 2022,2Q,7

√7th **T83.512 Infection and inflammatory reaction due to nephrostomy catheter** CC HCC

√7th **T83.518 Infection and inflammatory reaction due to other urinary catheter** CC H6 HCC
Infection and inflammatory reaction due to Hopkins catheter
Infection and inflammatory reaction due to ileostomy catheter
Infection and inflammatory reaction due to urostomy catheter

√6th **T83.59 Infection and inflammatory reaction due to prosthetic device, implant and graft in urinary system**

√7th **T83.590 Infection and inflammatory reaction due to implanted urinary neurostimulation device** CC HCC
EXCLUDES 2 *infection and inflammatory reaction due to electrode lead of sacral nerve neurostimulator (T85.732)*
infection and inflammatory reaction due to pulse generator or receiver of sacral nerve neurostimulator (T85.734)

√7th **T83.591 Infection and inflammatory reaction due to implanted urinary sphincter** CC HCC

√7th **T83.592 Infection and inflammatory reaction due to indwelling ureteral stent** CC HCC

√7th **T83.593 Infection and inflammatory reaction due to other urinary stents** CC HCC
Infection and inflammatory reaction due to ileal conduit stents
Infection and inflammatory reaction due to nephroureteral stent

√7th **T83.598 Infection and inflammatory reaction due to other prosthetic device, implant and graft in urinary system** CC HCC
AHA: 2020,3Q,25

√5th **T83.6 Infection and inflammatory reaction due to prosthetic device, implant and graft in genital tract**
Use additional code to identify infection

√x7th **T83.61 Infection and inflammatory reaction due to implanted penile prosthesis** CC HCC
Infection and inflammatory reaction due to penile prosthesis cylinder
Infection and inflammatory reaction due to penile prosthesis pump
Infection and inflammatory reaction due to penile prosthesis reservoir

√x7th **T83.62 Infection and inflammatory reaction due to implanted testicular prosthesis** CC HCC

√x7th **T83.69 Infection and inflammatory reaction due to other prosthetic device, implant and graft in genital tract** CC HCC

√5th **T83.7 Complications due to implanted mesh and other prosthetic materials**

√6th **T83.71 Erosion of implanted mesh and other prosthetic materials**

√7th **T83.711 Erosion of implanted vaginal mesh to surrounding organ or tissue** HCC ♀
Erosion of implanted vaginal mesh into pelvic floor muscles

√7th **T83.712 Erosion of implanted urethral mesh to surrounding organ or tissue** CC HCC
Erosion of implanted female urethral sling
Erosion of implanted male urethral sling
Erosion of implanted urethral mesh into pelvic floor muscles

√7th **T83.713 Erosion of implanted urethral bulking agent to surrounding organ or tissue** CC HCC

√7th **T83.714 Erosion of implanted ureteral bulking agent to surrounding organ or tissue** CC HCC

√7th **T83.718 Erosion of other implanted mesh to organ or tissue** CC HCC

√7th **T83.719 Erosion of other prosthetic materials to surrounding organ or tissue** CC HCC

√6th **T83.72 Exposure of implanted mesh and other prosthetic materials into surrounding organ or tissue**
Extrusion of implanted mesh

√7th **T83.721 Exposure of implanted vaginal mesh into vagina** HCC ♀
Exposure of implanted vaginal mesh through vaginal wall

√7th **T83.722 Exposure of implanted urethral mesh into urethra** CC HCC
Exposure of implanted female urethral sling
Exposure of implanted male urethral sling
Exposure of implanted urethral mesh through urethral wall

√7th **T83.723 Exposure of implanted urethral bulking agent into urethra** CC HCC

√7th **T83.724 Exposure of implanted ureteral bulking agent into ureter** CC HCC

√7th **T83.728 Exposure of other implanted mesh into organ or tissue** CC HCC

√7th **T83.729 Exposure of other prosthetic materials into organ or tissue** CC HCC

√x7th **T83.79 Other specified complications due to other genitourinary prosthetic materials** CC HCC

√5th **T83.8 Other specified complications of genitourinary prosthetic devices, implants and grafts**

√x7th **T83.81 Embolism due to genitourinary prosthetic devices, implants and grafts** CC HCC

√x7th **T83.82 Fibrosis due to genitourinary prosthetic devices, implants and grafts** CC HCC

√x7th **T83.83 Hemorrhage due to genitourinary prosthetic devices, implants and grafts** CC HCC

√x7th **T83.84 Pain due to genitourinary prosthetic devices, implants and grafts** CC HCC

√x7th **T83.85 Stenosis due to genitourinary prosthetic devices, implants and grafts** CC HCC

√x7th **T83.86 Thrombosis due to genitourinary prosthetic devices, implants and grafts** CC HCC

√x7th **T83.89 Other specified complication of genitourinary prosthetic devices, implants and grafts** CC HCC

AHA: 2022,3Q,13; 2016,1Q,19

√x7th **T83.9 Unspecified complication of genitourinary prosthetic device, implant and graft** CC HCC

√4th **T84 Complications of internal orthopedic prosthetic devices, implants and grafts**

EXCLUDES 2 *failure and rejection of transplanted organs and tissues (T86.-)*
fracture of bone following insertion of orthopedic implant, joint prosthesis or bone plate (M96.6)

The appropriate 7th character is to be added to each code from category T84.
A initial encounter
D subsequent encounter
S sequela

√5th **T84.Ø Mechanical complication of internal joint prosthesis**

√6th **T84.Ø1 Broken internal joint prosthesis**

Breakage (fracture) of prosthetic joint
Broken prosthetic joint implant

EXCLUDES 1 *periprosthetic joint implant fracture (M97.-)*

AHA: 2016,4Q,42

√7th **T84.Ø1Ø Broken internal right hip prosthesis** CC HCC

√7th **T84.Ø11 Broken internal left hip prosthesis** CC HCC

√7th **T84.Ø12 Broken internal right knee prosthesis** CC HCC

√7th **T84.Ø13 Broken internal left knee prosthesis** CC HCC

√7th **T84.Ø18 Broken internal joint prosthesis, other site** CC HCC

Use additional code to identify the joint (Z96.6-)

√7th **T84.Ø19 Broken internal joint prosthesis, unspecified site** CC UNS HCC

√6th **T84.Ø2 Dislocation of internal joint prosthesis**

Instability of internal joint prosthesis
Subluxation of internal joint prosthesis

AHA: 2019,2Q,27

√7th **T84.Ø2Ø Dislocation of internal right hip prosthesis** CC HCC

√7th **T84.Ø21 Dislocation of internal left hip prosthesis** CC HCC

√7th **T84.Ø22 Instability of internal right knee prosthesis** CC HCC

√7th **T84.Ø23 Instability of internal left knee prosthesis** CC HCC

√7th **T84.Ø28 Dislocation of other internal joint prosthesis** CC HCC

Use additional code to identify the joint (Z96.6-)

√7th **T84.Ø29 Dislocation of unspecified internal joint prosthesis** CC UNS HCC

√6th **T84.Ø3 Mechanical loosening of internal prosthetic joint**

Aseptic loosening of prosthetic joint

√7th **T84.Ø3Ø Mechanical loosening of internal right hip prosthetic joint** CC HCC

√7th **T84.Ø31 Mechanical loosening of internal left hip prosthetic joint** CC HCC

√7th **T84.Ø32 Mechanical loosening of internal right knee prosthetic joint** CC HCC

√7th **T84.Ø33 Mechanical loosening of internal left knee prosthetic joint** CC HCC

√7th **T84.Ø38 Mechanical loosening of other internal prosthetic joint** CC HCC

Use additional code to identify the joint (Z96.6-)

√7th **T84.Ø39 Mechanical loosening of unspecified internal prosthetic joint** CC UNS HCC

√6th **T84.Ø5 Periprosthetic osteolysis of internal prosthetic joint**

Use additional code to identify major osseous defect, if applicable (M89.7-)

√7th **T84.Ø5Ø Periprosthetic osteolysis of internal prosthetic right hip joint** CC HCC

√7th **T84.Ø51 Periprosthetic osteolysis of internal prosthetic left hip joint** CC HCC

√7th **T84.Ø52 Periprosthetic osteolysis of internal prosthetic right knee joint** CC HCC

√7th **T84.Ø53 Periprosthetic osteolysis of internal prosthetic left knee joint** CC HCC

√7th **T84.Ø58 Periprosthetic osteolysis of other internal prosthetic joint** CC HCC

Use additional code to identify the joint (Z96.6-)

√7th **T84.Ø59 Periprosthetic osteolysis of unspecified internal prosthetic joint** CC UNS HCC

√6th **T84.Ø6 Wear of articular bearing surface of internal prosthetic joint**

√7th **T84.Ø6Ø Wear of articular bearing surface of internal prosthetic right hip joint** CC HCC

√7th **T84.Ø61 Wear of articular bearing surface of internal prosthetic left hip joint** CC HCC

√7th **T84.Ø62 Wear of articular bearing surface of internal prosthetic right knee joint** CC HCC

√7th **T84.Ø63 Wear of articular bearing surface of internal prosthetic left knee joint** CC HCC

√7th **T84.Ø68 Wear of articular bearing surface of other internal prosthetic joint** CC HCC

Use additional code to identify the joint (Z96.6-)

√7th **T84.Ø69 Wear of articular bearing surface of unspecified internal prosthetic joint** CC UNS HCC

√6th **T84.Ø9 Other mechanical complication of internal joint prosthesis**

Prosthetic joint implant failure NOS

AHA: 2019,1Q,20

√7th **T84.Ø9Ø Other mechanical complication of internal right hip prosthesis** CC HCC

√7th **T84.Ø91 Other mechanical complication of internal left hip prosthesis** CC HCC

√7th **T84.Ø92 Other mechanical complication of internal right knee prosthesis** CC HCC

√7th **T84.Ø93 Other mechanical complication of internal left knee prosthesis** CC HCC

√7th **T84.Ø98 Other mechanical complication of other internal joint prosthesis** CC HCC

Use additional code to identify the joint (Z96.6-)

√7th **T84.Ø99 Other mechanical complication of unspecified internal joint prosthesis** CC UNS HCC

√5th **T84.1 Mechanical complication of internal fixation device of bones of limb**

EXCLUDES 2 *mechanical complication of internal fixation device of bones of feet (T84.2-)*
mechanical complication of internal fixation device of bones of fingers (T84.2-)
mechanical complication of internal fixation device of bones of hands (T84.2-)
mechanical complication of internal fixation device of bones of toes (T84.2-)

√6th **T84.11 Breakdown (mechanical) of internal fixation device of bones of limb**

√7th **T84.11Ø Breakdown (mechanical) of internal fixation device of right humerus** CC HCC

√7th **T84.111 Breakdown (mechanical) of internal fixation device of left humerus** CC HCC

√7th **T84.112 Breakdown (mechanical) of internal fixation device of bone of right forearm** CC HCC

√7th **T84.113 Breakdown (mechanical) of internal fixation device of bone of left forearm** CC HCC

T84.114 Breakdown (mechanical) of internal fixation device of right femur CC HCC
T84.115 Breakdown (mechanical) of internal fixation device of left femur CC HCC
T84.116 Breakdown (mechanical) of internal fixation device of bone of right lower leg CC HCC
T84.117 Breakdown (mechanical) of internal fixation device of bone of left lower leg CC HCC
T84.119 Breakdown (mechanical) of internal fixation device of unspecified bone of limb CC UNS HCC

T84.12 Displacement of internal fixation device of bones of limb
Malposition of internal fixation device of bones of limb
T84.120 Displacement of internal fixation device of right humerus CC HCC
T84.121 Displacement of internal fixation device of left humerus CC HCC
T84.122 Displacement of internal fixation device of bone of right forearm CC HCC
T84.123 Displacement of internal fixation device of bone of left forearm CC HCC
T84.124 Displacement of internal fixation device of right femur CC HCC
T84.125 Displacement of internal fixation device of left femur CC HCC
T84.126 Displacement of internal fixation device of bone of right lower leg CC HCC
T84.127 Displacement of internal fixation device of bone of left lower leg CC HCC
T84.129 Displacement of internal fixation device of unspecified bone of limb CC UNS HCC

T84.19 Other mechanical complication of internal fixation device of bones of limb
Obstruction (mechanical) of internal fixation device of bones of limb
Perforation of internal fixation device of bones of limb
Protrusion of internal fixation device of bones of limb
T84.190 Other mechanical complication of internal fixation device of right humerus CC HCC
T84.191 Other mechanical complication of internal fixation device of left humerus CC HCC
T84.192 Other mechanical complication of internal fixation device of bone of right forearm CC HCC
T84.193 Other mechanical complication of internal fixation device of bone of left forearm CC HCC
T84.194 Other mechanical complication of internal fixation device of right femur CC HCC
T84.195 Other mechanical complication of internal fixation device of left femur CC HCC
T84.196 Other mechanical complication of internal fixation device of bone of right lower leg CC HCC
T84.197 Other mechanical complication of internal fixation device of bone of left lower leg CC HCC
T84.199 Other mechanical complication of internal fixation device of unspecified bone of limb CC UNS HCC

T84.2 Mechanical complication of internal fixation device of other bones

T84.21 Breakdown (mechanical) of internal fixation device of other bones
T84.210 Breakdown (mechanical) of internal fixation device of bones of hand and fingers CC HCC
T84.213 Breakdown (mechanical) of internal fixation device of bones of foot and toes CC HCC
T84.216 Breakdown (mechanical) of internal fixation device of vertebrae CC HCC
T84.218 Breakdown (mechanical) of internal fixation device of other bones CC HCC

T84.22 Displacement of internal fixation device of other bones
Malposition of internal fixation device of other bones
T84.220 Displacement of internal fixation device of bones of hand and fingers CC HCC
T84.223 Displacement of internal fixation device of bones of foot and toes CC HCC
T84.226 Displacement of internal fixation device of vertebrae CC HCC
T84.228 Displacement of internal fixation device of other bones CC HCC

T84.29 Other mechanical complication of internal fixation device of other bones
Obstruction (mechanical) of internal fixation device of other bones
Perforation of internal fixation device of other bones
Protrusion of internal fixation device of other bones
T84.290 Other mechanical complication of internal fixation device of bones of hand and fingers CC HCC
T84.293 Other mechanical complication of internal fixation device of bones of foot and toes CC HCC
T84.296 Other mechanical complication of internal fixation device of vertebrae CC HCC
T84.298 Other mechanical complication of internal fixation device of other bones CC HCC

T84.3 Mechanical complication of other bone devices, implants and grafts
EXCLUDES 2 *other complications of bone graft (T86.83-)*

T84.31 Breakdown (mechanical) of other bone devices, implants and grafts
T84.310 Breakdown (mechanical) of electronic bone stimulator CC HCC
T84.318 Breakdown (mechanical) of other bone devices, implants and grafts CC HCC

T84.32 Displacement of other bone devices, implants and grafts
Malposition of other bone devices, implants and grafts
T84.320 Displacement of electronic bone stimulator CC HCC
T84.328 Displacement of other bone devices, implants and grafts CC HCC
AHA: 2014,4Q,28

T84.39 Other mechanical complication of other bone devices, implants and grafts
Obstruction (mechanical) of other bone devices, implants and grafts
Perforation of other bone devices, implants and grafts
Protrusion of other bone devices, implants and grafts
T84.390 Other mechanical complication of electronic bone stimulator CC HCC
T84.398 Other mechanical complication of other bone devices, implants and grafts CC HCC

T84.4 Mechanical complication of other internal orthopedic devices, implants and grafts

T84.41 Breakdown (mechanical) of other internal orthopedic devices, implants and grafts
T84.410 Breakdown (mechanical) of muscle and tendon graft CC HCC
T84.418 Breakdown (mechanical) of other internal orthopedic devices, implants and grafts CC HCC

T84.42 Displacement of other internal orthopedic devices, implants and grafts
Malposition of other internal orthopedic devices, implants and grafts
T84.420 Displacement of muscle and tendon graft CC HCC
T84.428 Displacement of other internal orthopedic devices, implants and grafts CC HCC

√6th **T84.49 Other mechanical complication of other internal orthopedic devices, implants and grafts**
Mechanical complication of other internal orthopedic devices, implants and grafts NOS
Obstruction (mechanical) of other internal orthopedic devices, implants and grafts
Perforation of other internal orthopedic devices, implants and grafts
Protrusion of other internal orthopedic devices, implants and grafts

√7th **T84.490 Other mechanical complication of muscle and tendon graft** CC HCC

√7th **T84.498 Other mechanical complication of other internal orthopedic devices, implants and grafts** CC HCC

√5th **T84.5 Infection and inflammatory reaction due to internal joint prosthesis**
Use additional code to identify infection
AHA: 2019,3Q,16; 2015,1Q,16

√x7th **T84.50 Infection and inflammatory reaction due to unspecified internal joint prosthesis** CC UNS HCC

√x7th **T84.51 Infection and inflammatory reaction due to internal right hip prosthesis** CC HCC

√x7th **T84.52 Infection and inflammatory reaction due to internal left hip prosthesis** CC HCC

√x7th **T84.53 Infection and inflammatory reaction due to internal right knee prosthesis** CC HCC

√x7th **T84.54 Infection and inflammatory reaction due to internal left knee prosthesis** CC HCC

√x7th **T84.59 Infection and inflammatory reaction due to other internal joint prosthesis** CC HCC

√5th **T84.6 Infection and inflammatory reaction due to internal fixation device**
Use additional code to identify infection

√x7th **T84.60 Infection and inflammatory reaction due to internal fixation device of unspecified site** CC H12 UNS HCC

√6th **T84.61 Infection and inflammatory reaction due to internal fixation device of arm**

√7th **T84.610 Infection and inflammatory reaction due to internal fixation device of right humerus** CC H12 HCC

√7th **T84.611 Infection and inflammatory reaction due to internal fixation device of left humerus** CC H12 HCC

√7th **T84.612 Infection and inflammatory reaction due to internal fixation device of right radius** CC H12 HCC

√7th **T84.613 Infection and inflammatory reaction due to internal fixation device of left radius** CC H12 HCC

√7th **T84.614 Infection and inflammatory reaction due to internal fixation device of right ulna** CC H12 HCC

√7th **T84.615 Infection and inflammatory reaction due to internal fixation device of left ulna** CC H12 HCC

√7th **T84.619 Infection and inflammatory reaction due to internal fixation device of unspecified bone of arm** CC H12 UNS HCC

√6th **T84.62 Infection and inflammatory reaction due to internal fixation device of leg**

√7th **T84.620 Infection and inflammatory reaction due to internal fixation device of right femur** CC HCC

√7th **T84.621 Infection and inflammatory reaction due to internal fixation device of left femur** CC HCC

√7th **T84.622 Infection and inflammatory reaction due to internal fixation device of right tibia** CC HCC

√7th **T84.623 Infection and inflammatory reaction due to internal fixation device of left tibia** CC HCC

√7th **T84.624 Infection and inflammatory reaction due to internal fixation device of right fibula** CC HCC

√7th **T84.625 Infection and inflammatory reaction due to internal fixation device of left fibula** CC HCC

√7th **T84.629 Infection and inflammatory reaction due to internal fixation device of unspecified bone of leg** CC UNS HCC

√x7th **T84.63 Infection and inflammatory reaction due to internal fixation device of spine** CC H12 HCC

√x7th **T84.69 Infection and inflammatory reaction due to internal fixation device of other site** CC H12 HCC

√x7th **T84.7 Infection and inflammatory reaction due to other internal orthopedic prosthetic devices, implants and grafts** CC H12 HCC
Use additional code to identify infection

√5th **T84.8 Other specified complications of internal orthopedic prosthetic devices, implants and grafts**

√x7th **T84.81 Embolism due to internal orthopedic prosthetic devices, implants and grafts** CC HCC

√x7th **T84.82 Fibrosis due to internal orthopedic prosthetic devices, implants and grafts** CC HCC

√x7th **T84.83 Hemorrhage due to internal orthopedic prosthetic devices, implants and grafts** CC HCC

√x7th **T84.84 Pain due to internal orthopedic prosthetic devices, implants and grafts** CC HCC

√x7th **T84.85 Stenosis due to internal orthopedic prosthetic devices, implants and grafts** CC HCC

√x7th **T84.86 Thrombosis due to internal orthopedic prosthetic devices, implants and grafts** CC HCC

√x7th **T84.89 Other specified complication of internal orthopedic prosthetic devices, implants and grafts** CC HCC

√x7th **T84.9 Unspecified complication of internal orthopedic prosthetic device, implant and graft** CC HCC

√4th **T85 Complications of other internal prosthetic devices, implants and grafts**
EXCLUDES 2 *failure and rejection of transplanted organs and tissue (T86.-)*
AHA: 2023,2Q,7; 2016,4Q,71-72

The appropriate 7th character is to be added to each code from category T85.
A initial encounter
D subsequent encounter
S sequela

√5th **T85.0 Mechanical complication of ventricular intracranial (communicating) shunt**

√x7th **T85.01 Breakdown (mechanical) of ventricular intracranial (communicating) shunt** CC HCC

√x7th **T85.02 Displacement of ventricular intracranial (communicating) shunt** CC HCC
Malposition of ventricular intracranial (communicating) shunt

√x7th **T85.03 Leakage of ventricular intracranial (communicating) shunt** CC HCC

√x7th **T85.09 Other mechanical complication of ventricular intracranial (communicating) shunt** CC HCC
Obstruction (mechanical) of ventricular intracranial (communicating) shunt
Perforation of ventricular intracranial (communicating) shunt
Protrusion of ventricular intracranial (communicating) shunt

√5th **T85.1 Mechanical complication of implanted electronic stimulator of nervous system**

√6th **T85.11 Breakdown (mechanical) of implanted electronic stimulator of nervous system**

√7th **T85.110 Breakdown (mechanical) of implanted electronic neurostimulator of brain electrode (lead)** CC HCC

√7th **T85.111 Breakdown (mechanical) of implanted electronic neurostimulator of peripheral nerve electrode (lead)** CC HCC
Breakdown of electrode (lead) for cranial nerve neurostimulators
Breakdown of electrode (lead) for gastric neurostimulator
Breakdown of electrode (lead) for sacral nerve neurostimulator
Breakdown of electrode (lead) for vagal nerve neurostimulators

√7th **T85.112 Breakdown (mechanical) of implanted electronic neurostimulator of spinal cord electrode (lead)** CC HCC

T85.113 **Breakdown (mechanical) of implanted electronic neurostimulator, generator** CC HCC
Breakdown (mechanical) of implanted electronic neurostimulator generator, brain, peripheral, gastric, spinal
Breakdown (mechanical) of implanted electronic sacral neurostimulator, pulse generator or receiver

T85.118 **Breakdown (mechanical) of other implanted electronic stimulator of nervous system** CC HCC

T85.12 **Displacement of implanted electronic stimulator of nervous system**
Malposition of implanted electronic stimulator of nervous system

T85.120 **Displacement of implanted electronic neurostimulator of brain electrode (lead)** CC HCC

T85.121 **Displacement of implanted electronic neurostimulator of peripheral nerve electrode (lead)** CC HCC
Displacement of electrode (lead) for cranial nerve neurostimulators
Displacement of electrode (lead) for gastric neurostimulator
Displacement of electrode (lead) for sacral nerve neurostimulator
Displacement of electrode (lead) for vagal nerve neurostimulators

T85.122 **Displacement of implanted electronic neurostimulator of spinal cord electrode (lead)** CC HCC

T85.123 **Displacement of implanted electronic neurostimulator, generator** CC HCC
Displacement of implanted electronic neurostimulator generator, brain, peripheral, gastric, spinal
Displacement of implanted electronic sacral neurostimulator, pulse generator or receiver

T85.128 **Displacement of other implanted electronic stimulator of nervous system** CC HCC

T85.19 **Other mechanical complication of implanted electronic stimulator of nervous system**
Leakage of implanted electronic stimulator of nervous system
Obstruction (mechanical) of implanted electronic stimulator of nervous system
Perforation of implanted electronic stimulator of nervous system
Protrusion of implanted electronic stimulator of nervous system

T85.190 **Other mechanical complication of implanted electronic neurostimulator of brain electrode (lead)** CC HCC

T85.191 **Other mechanical complication of implanted electronic neurostimulator of peripheral nerve electrode (lead)** CC HCC
Other mechanical complication of electrode (lead) for cranial nerve neurostimulators
Other mechanical complication of electrode (lead) for gastric neurostimulator
Other mechanical complication of electrode (lead) for sacral nerve neurostimulator
Other mechanical complication of electrode (lead) for vagal nerve neurostimulators

T85.192 **Other mechanical complication of implanted electronic neurostimulator of spinal cord electrode (lead)** CC HCC

T85.193 **Other mechanical complication of implanted electronic neurostimulator, generator** CC HCC
Other mechanical complication of implanted electronic neurostimulator generator, brain, peripheral, gastric, spinal
Other mechanical complication of implanted electronic sacral neurostimulator, pulse generator or receiver

T85.199 **Other mechanical complication of other implanted electronic stimulator of nervous system** CC HCC

T85.2 **Mechanical complication of intraocular lens**

T85.21 **Breakdown (mechanical) of intraocular lens** CC

T85.22 **Displacement of intraocular lens** CC
Malposition of intraocular lens

T85.29 **Other mechanical complication of intraocular lens** CC
Obstruction (mechanical) of intraocular lens
Perforation of intraocular lens
Protrusion of intraocular lens

T85.3 **Mechanical complication of other ocular prosthetic devices, implants and grafts**
EXCLUDES 2 *other complications of corneal graft (T86.84-)*

T85.31 **Breakdown (mechanical) of other ocular prosthetic devices, implants and grafts**

T85.310 **Breakdown (mechanical) of prosthetic orbit of right eye** CC

T85.311 **Breakdown (mechanical) of prosthetic orbit of left eye** CC

T85.318 **Breakdown (mechanical) of other ocular prosthetic devices, implants and grafts**

T85.32 **Displacement of other ocular prosthetic devices, implants and grafts**
Malposition of other ocular prosthetic devices, implants and grafts

T85.320 **Displacement of prosthetic orbit of right eye** CC

T85.321 **Displacement of prosthetic orbit of left eye** CC

T85.328 **Displacement of other ocular prosthetic devices, implants and grafts**

T85.39 **Other mechanical complication of other ocular prosthetic devices, implants and grafts**
Obstruction (mechanical) of other ocular prosthetic devices, implants and grafts
Perforation of other ocular prosthetic devices, implants and grafts
Protrusion of other ocular prosthetic devices, implants and grafts

T85.390 **Other mechanical complication of prosthetic orbit of right eye** CC

T85.391 **Other mechanical complication of prosthetic orbit of left eye** CC

T85.398 **Other mechanical complication of other ocular prosthetic devices, implants and grafts**

T85.4 **Mechanical complication of breast prosthesis and implant**

T85.41 **Breakdown (mechanical) of breast prosthesis and implant** CC

T85.42 **Displacement of breast prosthesis and implant** CC
Malposition of breast prosthesis and implant

T85.43 **Leakage of breast prosthesis and implant** CC

T85.44 **Capsular contracture of breast implant** CC

T85.49 **Other mechanical complication of breast prosthesis and implant** CC
Obstruction (mechanical) of breast prosthesis and implant
Perforation of breast prosthesis and implant
Protrusion of breast prosthesis and implant

T85.5 **Mechanical complication of gastrointestinal prosthetic devices, implants and grafts**

T85.51 **Breakdown (mechanical) of gastrointestinal prosthetic devices, implants and grafts**

T85.510 **Breakdown (mechanical) of bile duct prosthesis** CC

✓7th **T85.511 Breakdown (mechanical) of esophageal anti-reflux device** CC

✓7th **T85.518 Breakdown (mechanical) of other gastrointestinal prosthetic devices, implants and grafts** CC

✓6th **T85.52 Displacement of gastrointestinal prosthetic devices, implants and grafts**
Malposition of gastrointestinal prosthetic devices, implants and grafts

✓7th **T85.520 Displacement of bile duct prosthesis** CC

✓7th **T85.521 Displacement of esophageal anti-reflux device** CC

✓7th **T85.528 Displacement of other gastrointestinal prosthetic devices, implants and grafts** CC

✓6th **T85.59 Other mechanical complication of gastrointestinal prosthetic devices, implants and**
Obstruction, mechanical of gastrointestinal prosthetic devices, implants and grafts
Perforation of gastrointestinal prosthetic devices, implants and grafts
Protrusion of gastrointestinal prosthetic devices, implants and grafts

✓7th **T85.590 Other mechanical complication of bile duct prosthesis** CC

✓7th **T85.591 Other mechanical complication of esophageal anti-reflux device** CC

✓7th **T85.598 Other mechanical complication of other gastrointestinal prosthetic devices, implants and grafts** CC

✓5th **T85.6 Mechanical complication of other specified internal and external prosthetic devices, implants and grafts**

✓6th **T85.61 Breakdown (mechanical) of other specified internal prosthetic devices, implants and grafts**

✓7th **T85.610 Breakdown (mechanical) of cranial or spinal infusion catheter** CC
Breakdown (mechanical) of epidural infusion catheter
Breakdown (mechanical) of intrathecal infusion catheter
Breakdown (mechanical) of subarachnoid infusion catheter
Breakdown (mechanical) of subdural infusion catheter

✓7th **T85.611 Breakdown (mechanical) of intraperitoneal dialysis catheter** CC HCC
EXCLUDES 1 *mechanical complication of vascular dialysis catheter (T82.4-)*

✓7th **T85.612 Breakdown (mechanical) of permanent sutures** CC
EXCLUDES 1 *mechanical complication of permanent (wire) suture used in bone repair (T84.1-T84.2)*

✓7th **T85.613 Breakdown (mechanical) of artificial skin graft and decellularized allodermis** CC
Failure of artificial skin graft and decellularized allodermis
Non-adherence of artificial skin graft and decellularized allodermis
Poor incorporation of artificial skin graft and decellularized allodermis
Shearing of artificial skin graft and decellularized allodermis

✓7th **T85.614 Breakdown (mechanical) of insulin pump** CC

✓7th **T85.615 Breakdown (mechanical) of other nervous system device, implant or graft** CC HCC
Breakdown (mechanical) of intrathecal infusion pump

✓7th **T85.618 Breakdown (mechanical) of other specified internal prosthetic devices, implants and grafts** CC

✓6th **T85.62 Displacement of other specified internal prosthetic devices, implants and grafts**
Malposition of other specified internal prosthetic devices, implants and grafts

✓7th **T85.620 Displacement of cranial or spinal infusion catheter** CC
Displacement of epidural infusion catheter
Displacement of intrathecal infusion catheter
Displacement of subarachnoid infusion catheter
Displacement of subdural infusion catheter

✓7th **T85.621 Displacement of intraperitoneal dialysis catheter** CC HCC
EXCLUDES 1 *mechanical complication of vascular dialysis catheter (T82.4-)*

✓7th **T85.622 Displacement of permanent sutures** CC
EXCLUDES 1 *mechanical complication of permanent (wire) suture used in bone repair (T84.1-T84.2)*

✓7th **T85.623 Displacement of artificial skin graft and decellularized allodermis** CC
Dislodgement of artificial skin graft and decellularized allodermis

✓7th **T85.624 Displacement of insulin pump** CC

✓7th **T85.625 Displacement of other nervous system device, implant or graft** CC HCC
Displacement of intrathecal infusion pump

✓7th **T85.628 Displacement of other specified internal prosthetic devices, implants and grafts** CC

✓6th **T85.63 Leakage of other specified internal prosthetic devices, implants and grafts**

✓7th **T85.630 Leakage of cranial or spinal infusion catheter** CC
Leakage of epidural infusion catheter
Leakage of intrathecal infusion catheter infusion catheter
Leakage of subarachnoid infusion catheter
Leakage of subdural infusion catheter
AHA: 2022,3Q,24

✓7th **T85.631 Leakage of intraperitoneal dialysis catheter** CC HCC
EXCLUDES 1 *mechanical complication of vascular dialysis catheter (T82.4)*

✓7th **T85.633 Leakage of insulin pump** CC

✓7th **T85.635 Leakage of other nervous system device, implant or graft** CC HCC
Leakage of intrathecal infusion pump

✓7th **T85.638 Leakage of other specified internal prosthetic devices, implants and grafts** CC

✓6th **T85.69 Other mechanical complication of other specified internal prosthetic devices, implants and grafts**
Obstruction, mechanical of other specified internal prosthetic devices, implants and grafts
Perforation of other specified internal prosthetic devices, implants and grafts
Protrusion of other specified internal prosthetic devices, implants and grafts

✓7th **T85.690 Other mechanical complication of cranial or spinal infusion catheter** CC
Other mechanical complication of epidural infusion catheter
Other mechanical complication of intrathecal infusion catheter
Other mechanical complication of subarachnoid infusion catheter
Other mechanical complication of subdural infusion catheter

✓7th **T85.691 Other mechanical complication of intraperitoneal dialysis catheter** CC HCC
EXCLUDES 1 *mechanical complication of vascular dialysis catheter (T82.4)*

√7th **T85.692 Other mechanical complication of permanent sutures** CC
EXCLUDES 1 *mechanical complication of permanent (wire) suture used in bone repair (T84.1-T84.2)*

√7th **T85.693 Other mechanical complication of artificial skin graft and decellularized allodermis** CC

√7th **T85.694 Other mechanical complication of insulin pump** CC

√7th **T85.695 Other mechanical complication of other nervous system device, implant or graft** CC HCC
Other mechanical complication of intrathecal infusion pump

√7th **T85.698 Other mechanical complication of other specified internal prosthetic devices, implants and grafts** CC
Mechanical complication of nonabsorbable surgical material NOS

√5th **T85.7 Infection and inflammatory reaction due to other internal prosthetic devices, implants and grafts**
Use additional code to identify infection

√x7th **T85.71 Infection and inflammatory reaction due to peritoneal dialysis catheter** CC HCC

√x7th **T85.72 Infection and inflammatory reaction due to insulin pump** CC HCC

√6th **T85.73 Infection and inflammatory reaction due to nervous system devices, implants and graft**

√7th **T85.730 Infection and inflammatory reaction due to ventricular intracranial (communicating) shunt** CC HCC

√7th **T85.731 Infection and inflammatory reaction due to implanted electronic neurostimulator of brain, electrode (lead)** CC HCC

√7th **T85.732 Infection and inflammatory reaction due to implanted electronic neurostimulator of peripheral nerve, electrode (lead)** CC HCC
Infection and inflammatory reaction due to electrode (lead) for cranial nerve neurostimulators
Infection and inflammatory reaction due to electrode (lead) for gastric neurostimulator
Infection and inflammatory reaction due to electrode (lead) for sacral nerve neurostimulator
Infection and inflammatory reaction due to electrode (lead) for vagal nerve neurostimulators

√7th **T85.733 Infection and inflammatory reaction due to implanted electronic neurostimulator of spinal cord, electrode (lead)** CC HCC

√7th **T85.734 Infection and inflammatory reaction due to implanted electronic neurostimulator, generator** CC HCC
Generator pocket infection

√7th **T85.735 Infection and inflammatory reaction due to cranial or spinal infusion catheter** CC HCC
Infection and inflammatory reaction due to epidural catheter
Infection and inflammatory reaction due to intrathecal infusion catheter
Infection and inflammatory reaction due to subarachnoid catheter
Infection and inflammatory reaction due to subdural catheter

√7th **T85.738 Infection and inflammatory reaction due to other nervous system device, implant or graft** CC HCC
Infection and inflammatory reaction due to intrathecal infusion pump

√x7th **T85.79 Infection and inflammatory reaction due to other internal prosthetic devices, implants and grafts** CC HCC
AHA: 2023,2Q,27; 2022,2Q,7

√5th **T85.8 Other specified complications of internal prosthetic devices, implants and grafts, not elsewhere classified**

√6th **T85.81 Embolism due to internal prosthetic devices, implants and grafts, not elsewhere classified**

√7th **T85.810 Embolism due to nervous system prosthetic devices, implants and grafts** CC HCC

√7th **T85.818 Embolism due to other internal prosthetic devices, implants and grafts**

√6th **T85.82 Fibrosis due to internal prosthetic devices, implants and grafts, not elsewhere classified**

√7th **T85.820 Fibrosis due to nervous system prosthetic devices, implants and grafts** CC HCC

√7th **T85.828 Fibrosis due to other internal prosthetic devices, implants and grafts**

√6th **T85.83 Hemorrhage due to internal prosthetic devices, implants and grafts, not elsewhere classified**

√7th **T85.830 Hemorrhage due to nervous system prosthetic devices, implants and grafts** CC HCC

√7th **T85.838 Hemorrhage due to other internal prosthetic devices, implants and grafts**

√6th **T85.84 Pain due to internal prosthetic devices, implants and grafts, not elsewhere classified**

√7th **T85.840 Pain due to nervous system prosthetic devices, implants and grafts** CC HCC

√7th **T85.848 Pain due to other internal prosthetic devices, implants and grafts**

√6th **T85.85 Stenosis due to internal prosthetic devices, implants and grafts, not elsewhere classified**

√7th **T85.850 Stenosis due to nervous system prosthetic devices, implants and grafts** CC HCC

√7th **T85.858 Stenosis due to other internal prosthetic devices, implants and grafts**

√6th **T85.86 Thrombosis due to internal prosthetic devices, implants and grafts, not elsewhere classified**

√7th **T85.860 Thrombosis due to nervous system prosthetic devices, implants and grafts** CC HCC

√7th **T85.868 Thrombosis due to other internal prosthetic devices, implants and grafts**

√6th **T85.89 Other specified complication of internal prosthetic devices, implants and grafts, not elsewhere classified**
Erosion or breakdown of subcutaneous device pocket

√7th **T85.890 Other specified complication of nervous system prosthetic devices, implants and grafts** CC HCC

√7th **T85.898 Other specified complication of other internal prosthetic devices, implants and grafts**

√x7th **T85.9 Unspecified complication of internal prosthetic device, implant and graft**
Complication of internal prosthetic device, implant and graft NOS

√4th **T86 Complications of transplanted organs and tissue**
Use additional code to identify other transplant complications, such as:
graft-versus-host disease (D89.81-)
malignancy associated with organ transplant (C80.2)
post-transplant lymphoproliferative disorders (PTLD) (D47.Z1)
AHA: 2020,1Q,18

√5th **T86.0 Complications of bone marrow transplant**

T86.00 Unspecified complication of bone marrow transplant CC HCC

T86.01 Bone marrow transplant rejection CC HCC

T86.02 Bone marrow transplant failure CC HCC

T86.03 Bone marrow transplant infection CC HCC

T86.09 Other complications of bone marrow transplant CC HCC

√5th **T86.1 Complications of kidney transplant**

T86.10 Unspecified complication of kidney transplant CC

T86.11 Kidney transplant rejection CC

T86.12 Kidney transplant failure CC
AHA: 2013,1Q,24

T86.13 Kidney transplant infection CC
Use additional code to specify infection

T86.19 Other complication of kidney transplant CC
AHA: 2019,2Q,7

✓5th **T86.2 Complications of heart transplant**
EXCLUDES 1 *complication of:*
artificial heart device (T82.5-)
heart-lung transplant (T86.3-)

T86.20 Unspecified complication of heart transplant CC HCC
T86.21 Heart transplant rejection CC HCC
T86.22 Heart transplant failure CC HCC
T86.23 Heart transplant infection CC HCC
Use additional code to specify infection

✓6th **T86.29 Other complications of heart transplant**
T86.290 Cardiac allograft vasculopathy CC HCC
EXCLUDES 1 *atherosclerosis of coronary arteries (I25.75-, I25.76-, I25.81-)*
T86.298 Other complications of heart transplant CC HCC

✓5th **T86.3 Complications of heart-lung transplant**
T86.30 Unspecified complication of heart-lung transplant CC HCC
T86.31 Heart-lung transplant rejection CC HCC
T86.32 Heart-lung transplant failure CC HCC
T86.33 Heart-lung transplant infection CC HCC
Use additional code to specify infection
T86.39 Other complications of heart-lung transplant CC HCC

✓5th **T86.4 Complications of liver transplant**
T86.40 Unspecified complication of liver transplant CC HCC
T86.41 Liver transplant rejection CC HCC
T86.42 Liver transplant failure CC HCC
T86.43 Liver transplant infection CC HCC
Use additional code to identify infection, such as: cytomegalovirus (CMV) infection (B25.-)
T86.49 Other complications of liver transplant CC HCC

T86.5 Complications of stem cell transplant CC HCC
Complications from stem cells from peripheral blood
Complications from stem cells from umbilical cord
AHA: 2020,4Q,14

✓5th **T86.8 Complications of other transplanted organs and tissues**
✓6th **T86.81 Complications of lung transplant**
EXCLUDES 1 *complication of heart-lung transplant (T86.3-)*
T86.810 Lung transplant rejection CC HCC
T86.811 Lung transplant failure CC HCC
T86.812 Lung transplant infection CC HCC
Use additional code to specify infection
T86.818 Other complications of lung transplant CC HCC
AHA: 2019,2Q,6
T86.819 Unspecified complication of lung transplant CC HCC

✓6th **T86.82 Complications of skin graft (allograft) (autograft)**
EXCLUDES 2 *complication of artificial skin graft (T85.693)*
T86.820 Skin graft (allograft) rejection CC
T86.821 Skin graft (allograft) (autograft) failure CC
T86.822 Skin graft (allograft) (autograft) infection CC
Use additional code to specify infection
T86.828 Other complications of skin graft (allograft) (autograft) CC
T86.829 Unspecified complication of skin graft (allograft) (autograft) CC

✓6th **T86.83 Complications of bone graft**
EXCLUDES 2 *mechanical complications of bone graft (T84.3-)*
T86.830 Bone graft rejection CC
T86.831 Bone graft failure CC
T86.832 Bone graft infection CC
Use additional code to specify infection
T86.838 Other complications of bone graft CC
AHA: 2023,1Q,30
T86.839 Unspecified complication of bone graft CC

✓6th **T86.84 Complications of corneal transplant**
EXCLUDES 2 *mechanical complications of corneal graft (T85.3-)*
AHA: 2020,4Q,40

✓7th **T86.840 Corneal transplant rejection**
T86.8401 Corneal transplant rejection, right eye CC
T86.8402 Corneal transplant rejection, left eye CC
T86.8403 Corneal transplant rejection, bilateral CC
T86.8409 Corneal transplant rejection, unspecified eye CC UNS

✓7th **T86.841 Corneal transplant failure**
T86.8411 Corneal transplant failure, right eye CC
T86.8412 Corneal transplant failure, left eye CC
T86.8413 Corneal transplant failure, bilateral CC
T86.8419 Corneal transplant failure, unspecified eye CC UNS

✓7th **T86.842 Corneal transplant infection**
Use additional code to specify infection
T86.8421 Corneal transplant infection, right eye CC HCC
T86.8422 Corneal transplant infection, left eye CC HCC
T86.8423 Corneal transplant infection, bilateral CC HCC
T86.8429 Corneal transplant infection, unspecified eye CC UNS HCC

✓7th **T86.848 Other complications of corneal transplant**
T86.8481 Other complications of corneal transplant, right eye CC
T86.8482 Other complications of corneal transplant, left eye CC
T86.8483 Other complications of corneal transplant, bilateral CC
T86.8489 Other complications of corneal transplant, unspecified eye CC UNS

✓7th **T86.849 Unspecified complication of corneal transplant**
T86.8491 Unspecified complication of corneal transplant, right eye CC
T86.8492 Unspecified complication of corneal transplant, left eye CC
T86.8493 Unspecified complication of corneal transplant, bilateral CC
T86.8499 Unspecified complication of corneal transplant, unspecified eye CC UNS

✓6th **T86.85 Complication of intestine transplant**
T86.850 Intestine transplant rejection CC HCC
T86.851 Intestine transplant failure CC HCC
T86.852 Intestine transplant infection CC HCC
Use additional code to specify infection
T86.858 Other complications of intestine transplant CC HCC
T86.859 Unspecified complication of intestine transplant CC HCC

✓6th **T86.89 Complications of other transplanted tissue**
Transplant failure or rejection of pancreas
AHA: 2020,1Q,18
T86.890 Other transplanted tissue rejection CC
T86.891 Other transplanted tissue failure CC
T86.892 Other transplanted tissue infection CC
Use additional code to specify infection
T86.898 Other complications of other transplanted tissue CC

T86.899 Unspecified complication of other transplanted tissue CC

T86.9 Complication of unspecified transplanted organ and tissue

T86.90 Unspecified complication of unspecified transplanted organ and tissue CC

T86.91 Unspecified transplanted organ and tissue rejection CC

T86.92 Unspecified transplanted organ and tissue failure CC

T86.93 Unspecified transplanted organ and tissue infection CC

Use additional code to specify infection

T86.99 Other complications of unspecified transplanted organ and tissue CC

T87 Complications peculiar to reattachment and amputation

T87.0 Complications of reattached (part of) upper extremity

T87.0X Complications of reattached (part of) upper extremity

T87.0X1 Complications of reattached (part of) right upper extremity CC HCC

T87.0X2 Complications of reattached (part of) left upper extremity CC HCC

T87.0X9 Complications of reattached (part of) unspecified upper extremity CC UNS HCC

T87.1 Complications of reattached (part of) lower extremity

T87.1X Complications of reattached (part of) lower extremity

T87.1X1 Complications of reattached (part of) right lower extremity CC HCC

T87.1X2 Complications of reattached (part of) left lower extremity CC HCC

T87.1X9 Complications of reattached (part of) unspecified lower extremity CC UNS HCC

T87.2 Complications of other reattached body part CC HCC

T87.3 Neuroma of amputation stump

DEF: Non-neoplastic tumor generated at the proximal end of severed, partially transected, or injured nerve following amputation.

T87.30 Neuroma of amputation stump, unspecified extremity HCC

T87.31 Neuroma of amputation stump, right upper extremity HCC

T87.32 Neuroma of amputation stump, left upper extremity HCC

T87.33 Neuroma of amputation stump, right lower extremity HCC

T87.34 Neuroma of amputation stump, left lower extremity HCC

T87.4 Infection of amputation stump

T87.40 Infection of amputation stump, unspecified extremity CC UNS HCC

T87.41 Infection of amputation stump, right upper extremity CC HCC

T87.42 Infection of amputation stump, left upper extremity CC HCC

T87.43 Infection of amputation stump, right lower extremity CC HCC

T87.44 Infection of amputation stump, left lower extremity CC HCC

T87.5 Necrosis of amputation stump

T87.50 Necrosis of amputation stump, unspecified extremity HCC

T87.51 Necrosis of amputation stump, right upper extremity HCC

T87.52 Necrosis of amputation stump, left upper extremity HCC

T87.53 Necrosis of amputation stump, right lower extremity HCC

T87.54 Necrosis of amputation stump, left lower extremity HCC

T87.8 Other complications of amputation stump

T87.81 Dehiscence of amputation stump HCC

T87.89 Other complications of amputation stump HCC

Amputation stump contracture

Amputation stump contracture of next proximal joint

Amputation stump edema

Amputation stump flexion

Amputation stump hematoma

EXCLUDES 2 *phantom limb syndrome (G54.6-G54.7)*

AHA: 2022,3Q,11

T87.9 Unspecified complications of amputation stump HCC

T88 Other complications of surgical and medical care, not elsewhere classified

EXCLUDES 2 *complication following infusion, transfusion and therapeutic injection (T80.-)*
complication following procedure NEC (T81.-)
complications of anesthesia in labor and delivery (O74.-)
complications of anesthesia in pregnancy (O29.-)
complications of anesthesia in puerperium (O89.-)
complications of devices, implants and grafts (T82-T85)
complications of obstetric surgery and procedure (O75.4)
dermatitis due to drugs and medicaments (L23.3, L24.4, L25.1, L27.0-L27.1)
poisoning and toxic effects of drugs and chemicals ▶(T36-T65 with fifth or sixth character 1-4)◀
specified complications classified elsewhere

The appropriate 7th character is to be added to each code from category T88.
A initial encounter
D subsequent encounter
S sequela

T88.0 Infection following immunization CC

Sepsis following immunization

AHA: 2018,4Q,62-63

T88.1 Other complications following immunization, not elsewhere classified CC

Generalized vaccinia

Rash following immunization

EXCLUDES 1 *vaccinia not from vaccine (B08.011)*

EXCLUDES 2 *anaphylactic shock due to serum (T80.5-)*
other serum reactions (T80.6-)
postimmunization arthropathy (M02.2)
postimmunization encephalitis (G04.02)
postimmunization fever (R50.83)

T88.2 Shock due to anesthesia CC

Use additional code for adverse effect, if applicable, to identify drug (T41.- with fifth or sixth character 5)

EXCLUDES 1 *complications of anesthesia (in):*
labor and delivery (O74.-)
postprocedural shock NOS (T81.1-)
pregnancy (O29.-)
puerperium (O89.-)

T88.3 Malignant hyperthermia due to anesthesia CC

Use additional code for adverse effect, if applicable, to identify drug (T41.- with fifth or sixth character 5)

T88.4 Failed or difficult intubation

T88.5 Other complications of anesthesia

Use additional code for adverse effect, if applicable, to identify drug (T41.- with fifth or sixth character 5)

T88.51 Hypothermia following anesthesia

T88.52 Failed moderate sedation during procedure

Failed conscious sedation during procedure

EXCLUDES 2 *personal history of failed moderate sedation (Z92.83)*

T88.53 Unintended awareness under general anesthesia during procedure

EXCLUDES 2 *personal history of unintended awareness under general anesthesia (Z92.84)*

AHA: 2016,4Q,72-73

T88.59 Other complications of anesthesia

√x7th **T88.6 Anaphylactic reaction due to adverse effect of correct drug or medicament properly administered** CC

Anaphylactic shock due to adverse effect of correct drug or medicament properly administered

Anaphylactoid reaction NOS

Use additional code for adverse effect, if applicable, to identify drug (T36-T5Ø with fifth or sixth character 5)

EXCLUDES 1 *anaphylactic reaction due to serum (T8Ø.5-)*

anaphylactic shock or reaction due to adverse food reaction (T78.Ø-)

AHA: 2020,1Q,18

√x7th **T88.7 Unspecified adverse effect of drug or medicament**

Drug hypersensitivity NOS

Drug reaction NOS

Use additional code for adverse effect, if applicable, to identify drug (T36-T5Ø with fifth or sixth character 5)

EXCLUDES 1 *specified adverse effects of drugs and medicaments (AØØ-R94 and T8Ø-T88.6, T88.8)*

√x7th **T88.8 Other specified complications of surgical and medical care, not elsewhere classified**

Use additional code to identify the complication

AHA: 2022,2Q,7

√x7th **T88.9 Complication of surgical and medical care, unspecified**

Chapter 20. External Causes of Morbidity (VØØ–Y99)

Chapter-specific Guidelines with Coding Examples

The chapter-specific guidelines from the ICD-10-CM Official Guidelines for Coding and Reporting have been provided below. Along with these guidelines are coding examples, contained in the shaded boxes, that have been developed to help illustrate the coding and/or sequencing guidance found in these guidelines.

The external causes of morbidity codes should never be sequenced as the first-listed or principal diagnosis.

External cause codes are intended to provide data for injury research and evaluation of injury prevention strategies. These codes capture how the injury or health condition happened (cause), the intent (unintentional or accidental; or intentional, such as suicide or assault), the place where the event occurred the activity of the patient at the time of the event, and the person's status (e.g., civilian, military).

There is no national requirement for mandatory ICD-10-CM external cause code reporting. Unless a provider is subject to a state-based external cause code reporting mandate or these codes are required by a particular payer, reporting of ICD-10-CM codes in Chapter 20, External Causes of Morbidity, is not required. In the absence of a mandatory reporting requirement, providers are encouraged to voluntarily report external cause codes, as they provide valuable data for injury research and evaluation of injury prevention strategies.

a. General external cause coding guidelines

1) Used with any code in the range of AØØ.Ø–T88.9, ZØØ–Z99

An external cause code may be used with any code in the range of AØØ.Ø–T88.9, ZØØ–Z99, classification that represents a health condition due to an external cause. Though they are most applicable to injuries, they are also valid for use with such things as infections or diseases due to an external source, and other health conditions, such as a heart attack that occurs during strenuous physical activity.

Actinic reticuloid due to tanning bed use

L57.1	**Actinic reticuloid**
W89.1XXA	**Exposure to tanning bed, initial encounter**

Explanation: An external cause code may be used with any code in the range of AØØ.Ø–T88.9, ZØØ–Z99, classifications that describe health conditions due to an external cause. Code W89.1 Exposure to tanning bed requires a seventh character of A to report this initial encounter, with a placeholder X for the fifth and sixth characters.

2) External cause code used for length of treatment

Assign the external cause code, with the appropriate 7th character (initial encounter, subsequent encounter or sequela) for each encounter for which the injury or condition is being treated.

Most categories in chapter 20 have a 7th character requirement for each applicable code. Most categories in this chapter have three 7th character values: A, initial encounter, D, subsequent encounter and S, sequela. While the patient may be seen by a new or different provider over the course of treatment for an injury or condition, assignment of the 7th character for external cause should match the 7th character of the code assigned for the associated injury or condition for the encounter.

3) Use the full range of external cause codes

Use the full range of external cause codes to completely describe the cause, the intent, the place of occurrence, and if applicable, the activity of the patient at the time of the event, and the patient's status, for all injuries, and other health conditions due to an external cause.

4) Assign as many external cause codes as necessary

Assign as many external cause codes as necessary to fully explain each cause. If only one external code can be recorded, assign the code most related to the principal diagnosis.

5) The selection of the appropriate external cause code

The selection of the appropriate external cause code is guided by the Alphabetic Index of External Causes and by Inclusion and Exclusion notes in the Tabular List.

6) External cause code can never be a principal diagnosis

An external cause code can never be a principal (first-listed) diagnosis.

7) Combination external cause codes

Certain of the external cause codes are combination codes that identify sequential events that result in an injury, such as a fall which results in striking against an object. The injury may be due to either event or both. The combination external cause code used should correspond to the sequence of events regardless of which caused the most serious injury.

Toddler tripped and fell while walking and struck his head on an end table, sustaining a scalp contusion

SØØ.Ø3XA	**Contusion of scalp, initial encounter**
WØ1.19ØA	**Fall on same level from slipping, tripping and stumbling with subsequent striking against furniture, initial encounter**

Explanation: Combination external cause codes identify sequential events that result in an injury, such as a fall resulting in striking against an object. The injury may be due to either or both events.

8) No external cause code needed in certain circumstances

No external cause code from Chapter 20 is needed if the external cause and intent are included in a code from another chapter (e.g., T36.ØX1-, Poisoning by penicillins, accidental (unintentional)).

b. Place of occurrence guideline

Codes from category Y92, Place of occurrence of the external cause, are secondary codes for use after other external cause codes to identify the location of the patient at the time of injury or other condition.

Generally, a place of occurrence code is assigned only once, at the initial encounter for treatment. However, in the rare instance that a new injury occurs during hospitalization, an additional place of occurrence code may be assigned. No 7th characters are used for Y92.

Do not use place of occurrence code Y92.9 if the place is not stated or is not applicable.

A farmer was working in his barn and sustained a foot contusion when the horse stepped on his left foot

S9Ø.32XA	**Contusion of left foot, initial encounter**
W55.19XA	**Other contact with horse, initial encounter**
Y92.71	**Barn as the place of occurrence of the external cause**

Explanation: A place-of-occurrence code from category Y92 is assigned at the initial encounter to identify the location of the patient at the time the injury occurred.

c. Activity code

Assign a code from category Y93, Activity code, to describe the activity of the patient at the time the injury or other health condition occurred.

An activity code is used only once, at the initial encounter for treatment. Only one code from Y93 should be recorded on a medical record.

The activity codes are not applicable to poisonings, adverse effects, misadventures or sequela.

Do not assign Y93.9, Unspecified activity, if the activity is not stated.

A code from category Y93 is appropriate for use with external cause and intent codes if identifying the activity provides additional information about the event.

Ranch hand who was grooming a horse sustained a foot contusion when the horse stepped on his left foot

S9Ø.32XA	**Contusion of left foot, initial encounter**
W55.19XA	**Other contact with horse, initial encounter**
Y93.K3	**Activity, grooming and shearing an animal**

Explanation: One activity code from category Y93 is assigned at the initial encounter only to describe the activity of the patient at the time the injury occurred.

d. Place of occurrence, activity, and status codes used with other external cause code

When applicable, place of occurrence, activity, and external cause status codes are sequenced after the main external cause code(s). Regardless of the number of external cause codes assigned, generally there should be only one place of occurrence code, one activity code, and one external cause status code assigned to an encounter. However, in the rare instance that a new injury occurs during hospitalization, an additional place of occurrence code may be assigned.

e. If the reporting format limits the number of external cause codes

If the reporting format limits the number of external cause codes that can be used in reporting clinical data, report the code for the cause/intent most related to the principal diagnosis. If the format permits capture of additional external cause codes, the cause/intent, including medical misadventures, of the additional events should be reported rather than the codes for place, activity, or external status.

f. Multiple external cause coding guidelines

More than one external cause code is required to fully describe the external cause of an illness or injury. The assignment of external cause codes should be sequenced in the following priority:

If two or more events cause separate injuries, an external cause code should be assigned for each cause. The first-listed external cause code will be selected in the following order:

External codes for child and adult abuse take priority over all other external cause codes.

See Section I.C.19., Child and Adult abuse guidelines.

External cause codes for terrorism events take priority over all other external cause codes except child and adult abuse.

External cause codes for cataclysmic events take priority over all other external cause codes except child and adult abuse and terrorism.

External cause codes for transport accidents take priority over all other external cause codes except cataclysmic events, child and adult abuse and terrorism.

Activity and external cause status codes are assigned following all causal (intent) external cause codes.

The first-listed external cause code should correspond to the cause of the most serious diagnosis due to an assault, accident, or self-harm, following the order of hierarchy listed above..

30-year-old man accidentally discharged his hunting rifle, sustaining an open gunshot wound to the right thigh, which caused him to fall down the stairs, resulting in closed displaced comminuted fracture of his left radial shaft

S71.131A	**Puncture wound without foreign body, right thigh, initial encounter**
W33.Ø2XA	**Accidental discharge of hunting rifle, initial encounter**
S52.352A	**Displaced comminuted fracture of shaft of radius, left arm, initial encounter for closed fracture**
W1Ø.9XXA	**Fall (on) (from) unspecified stairs and steps, initial encounter**

Explanation: If two or more events cause separate injuries, an external cause code should be assigned for each cause.

g. Child and adult abuse guideline

Adult and child abuse, neglect and maltreatment are classified as assault. Any of the assault codes may be used to indicate the external cause of any injury resulting from the confirmed abuse.

For confirmed cases of abuse, neglect and maltreatment, when the perpetrator is known, a code from YØ7, Perpetrator of maltreatment and neglect, should accompany any other assault codes.

See Section I.C.19. Adult and child abuse, neglect and other maltreatment

h. Unknown or undetermined intent guideline

If the intent (accident, self-harm, assault) of the cause of an injury or other condition is unknown or unspecified, code the intent as accidental intent. All transport accident categories assume accidental intent.

1) Use of undetermined intent

External cause codes for events of undetermined intent are only for use if the documentation in the record specifies that the intent cannot be determined.

i. Sequelae (late effects) of external cause guidelines

1) Sequelae external cause codes

Sequela are reported using the external cause code with the 7th character "S" for sequela. These codes should be used with any report of a late effect or sequela resulting from a previous injury.

See Section I.B.10. Sequela (Late Effects)

2) Sequela external cause code with a related current injury

A sequela external cause code should never be used with a related current nature of injury code.

3) Use of sequela external cause codes for subsequent visits

Use a late effect external cause code for subsequent visits when a late effect of the initial injury is being treated. Do not use a late effect external cause code for subsequent visits for follow-up care (e.g., to assess healing, to receive rehabilitative therapy) of the injury when no late effect of the injury has been documented.

j. Terrorism guidelines

1) Cause of injury identified by the Federal Government (FBI) as terrorism

When the cause of an injury is identified by the Federal Government (FBI) as terrorism, the first-listed external cause code should be a code from category Y38, Terrorism. The definition of terrorism employed by the FBI is found at the inclusion note at the beginning of category Y38. Use additional code for place of occurrence (Y92.-). More than one Y38 code may be assigned if the injury is the result of more than one mechanism of terrorism.

2) Cause of an injury is suspected to be the result of terrorism

When the cause of an injury is suspected to be the result of terrorism a code from category Y38 should not be assigned. Suspected cases should be classified as assault.

3) Code Y38.9, Terrorism, secondary effects

Assign code Y38.9, Terrorism, secondary effects, for conditions occurring subsequent to the terrorist event. This code should not be assigned for conditions that are due to the initial terrorist act.

It is acceptable to assign code Y38.9 with another code from Y38 if there is an injury due to the initial terrorist event and an injury that is a subsequent result of the terrorist event.

k. External cause status

A code from category Y99, External cause status, should be assigned whenever any other external cause code is assigned for an encounter, including an Activity code, except for the events noted below. Assign a code from category Y99, External cause status, to indicate the work status of the person at the time the event occurred. The status code indicates whether the event occurred during military activity, whether a non-military person was at work, whether an individual including a student or volunteer was involved in a non-work activity at the time of the causal event.

A code from Y99, External cause status, should be assigned, when applicable, with other external cause codes, such as transport accidents and falls. The external cause status codes are not applicable to poisonings, adverse effects, misadventures or late effects.

Do not assign a code from category Y99 if no other external cause codes (cause, activity) are applicable for the encounter.

An external cause status code is used only once, at the initial encounter for treatment. Only one code from Y99 should be recorded on a medical record.

Do not assign code Y99.9, Unspecified external cause status, if the status is not stated.

Chapter 20. External Causes of Morbidity (VØØ-Y99)

NOTE This chapter permits the classification of environmental events and circumstances as the cause of injury, and other adverse effects. Where a code from this section is applicable, it is intended that it shall be used secondary to a code from another chapter of the Classification indicating the nature of the condition. Most often, the condition will be classifiable to Chapter 19, Injury, poisoning and certain other consequences of external causes (SØØ-T88). Other conditions that may be stated to be due to external causes are classified in Chapters I to XVIII. For these conditions, codes from Chapter 2Ø should be used to provide additional information as to the cause of the condition.

AHA: 2018,4Q,58-60

This chapter contains the following blocks:

VØØ-X58 Accidents
VØØ-V99 Transport accidents
VØØ-VØ9 Pedestrian injured in transport accident
V1Ø-V19 Pedal cycle rider injured in transport accident
V2Ø-V29 Motorcycle rider injured in transport accident
V3Ø-V39 Occupant of three-wheeled motor vehicle injured in transport accident
V4Ø-V49 Car occupant injured in transport accident
V5Ø-V59 Occupant of pick-up truck or van injured in transport accident
V6Ø-V69 Occupant of heavy transport vehicle injured in transport accident
V7Ø-V79 Bus occupant injured in transport accident
V8Ø-V89 Other land transport accidents
V9Ø-V94 Water transport accidents
V95-V97 Air and space transport accidents
V98-V99 Other and unspecified transport accidents
WØØ-X58 Other external causes of accidental injury
WØØ-W19 Slipping, tripping, stumbling and falls
W2Ø-W49 Exposure to inanimate mechanical forces
W5Ø-W64 Exposure to animate mechanical forces
W65-W74 Accidental non-transport drowning and submersion
W85-W99 Exposure to electric current, radiation and extreme ambient air temperature and pressure
XØØ-XØ8 Exposure to smoke, fire and flames
X1Ø-X19 Contact with heat and hot substances
X3Ø-X39 Exposure to forces of nature
X5Ø Overexertion and strenuous or repetitive movements
X52-X58 Accidental exposure to other specified factors
X71-X83 Intentional self-harm
X92-YØ9 Assault
Y21-Y33 Event of undetermined intent
Y35-Y38 Legal intervention, operations of war, military operations, and terrorism
Y62-Y84 Complications of medical and surgical care
Y62-Y69 Misadventures to patients during surgical and medical care
Y7Ø-Y82 Medical devices associated with adverse incidents in diagnostic and therapeutic use
Y83-Y84 Surgical and other medical procedures as the cause of abnormal reaction of the patient, or of later complication, without mention of misadventure at the time of the procedure
Y9Ø-Y99 Supplementary factors related to causes of morbidity classified elsewhere

ACCIDENTS (VØØ-X58)

AHA: 2018,2Q,7-8

Transport accidents (VØØ-V99)

NOTE This section is structured in 12 groups. Those relating to land transport accidents (VØØ-V89) reflect the victim's mode of transport and are subdivided to identify the victim's 'counterpart' or the type of event. The vehicle of which the injured person is an occupant is identified in the first two characters since it is seen as the most important factor to identify for prevention purposes. A transport accident is one in which the vehicle involved must be moving or running or in use for transport purposes at the time of the accident.

Use additional code to identify:
airbag injury (W22.1)
type of street or road (Y92.4-)
use of cellular telephone and other electronic equipment at the time of the transport accident (Y93.C-)

EXCLUDES 1 *agricultural vehicles in stationary use or maintenance (W31.-)*
assault by crashing of motor vehicle (YØ3.-)
automobile or motor cycle in stationary use or maintenance - code to type of accident
crashing of motor vehicle, undetermined intent (Y32)
intentional self-harm by crashing of motor vehicle (X82)

EXCLUDES 2 *transport accidents due to cataclysm (X34-X38)*

NOTE Definitions related to transport accidents:

(a) A transport accident (VØØ-V99) is any accident involving a device designed primarily for, or used at the time primarily for, conveying persons or good from one place to another.

(b) A public highway [trafficway] or street is the entire width between property lines (or other boundary lines) of land open to the public as a matter of right or custom for purposes of moving persons or property from one place to another. A roadway is that part of the public highway designed, improved and customarily used for vehicular traffic.

(c) A traffic accident is any vehicle accident occurring on the public highway [i.e. originating on, terminating on, or involving a vehicle partially on the highway]. A vehicle accident is assumed to have occurred on the public highway unless another place is specified, except in the case of accidents involving only off-road motor vehicles, which are classified as nontraffic accidents unless the contrary is stated.

(d) A nontraffic accident is any vehicle accident that occurs entirely in any place other than a public highway.

(e) A pedestrian is any person involved in an accident who was not at the time of the accident riding in or on a motor vehicle, railway train, streetcar or animal-drawn or other vehicle, or on a pedal cycle or animal. This includes, a person changing a tire, working on a parked car, or a person on foot. It also includes the user of a pedestrian conveyance such as a baby stroller, ice-skates, skis, sled, roller skates, a skateboard, nonmotorized or motorized wheelchair, motorized mobility scooter, or nonmotorized scooter.

(f) A driver is an occupant of a transport vehicle who is operating or intending to operate it.

(g) A passenger is any occupant of a transport vehicle other than the driver, except a person traveling on the outside of the vehicle.

(h) A person on the outside of a vehicle is any person being transported by a vehicle but not occupying the space normally reserved for the driver or passengers, or the space intended for the transport of property. This includes a person travelling on the bodywork, bumper, fender, roof, running board or step of a vehicle, as well as, hanging on the outside of the vehicle.

(i) A pedal cycle is any land transport vehicle operated solely by nonmotorized pedals including a bicycle or tricycle.

(j) A pedal cyclist is any person riding a pedal cycle or in a sidecar or trailer attached to a pedal cycle.

(k) A motorcycle is a two-wheeled motor vehicle with one or two riding saddles and sometimes with a third wheel for the support of a sidecar. The sidecar is considered part of the motorcycle. This includes a moped, motor scooter, or motorized bicycle.

(l) A motorcycle rider is any person riding a motorcycle or in a sidecar or trailer attached to the motorcycle.

(m) A three-wheeled motor vehicle is a motorized tricycle designed primarily for on-road use. This includes a motor-driven tricycle, a motorized rickshaw, or a three-wheeled motor car.

(n) A car [automobile] is a four-wheeled motor vehicle designed primarily for carrying up to 7 persons. A trailer being towed by the car is considered part of the car. It does not include a van or minivan — see definition (o).

(o) A pick-up truck or van is a four or six-wheeled motor vehicle designed for carrying passengers as well as property or cargo weighing less than the local limit for classification as a heavy goods vehicle, and not requiring a special driver's license. This includes a minivan and a sport-utility vehicle (SUV).

(p) A heavy transport vehicle is a motor vehicle designed primarily for carrying property, meeting local criteria for classification as a heavy goods vehicle in terms of weight and requiring a special driver's license.

(q) A bus (coach) is a motor vehicle designed or adapted primarily for carrying more than 1Ø passengers, and requiring a special driver's license.

(r) A railway train or railway vehicle is any device, with or without freight or passenger cars couple to it, designed for traffic on a railway track. This includes subterranean (subways) or elevated trains.

(s) A streetcar, is a device designed and used primarily for transporting passengers within a municipality, running on rails, usually subject to normal traffic control signals, and operated principally on a right-of-way that forms part of the roadway. This includes a tram or trolley that runs on rails. A trailer being towed by a streetcar is considered part of the streetcar.

(t) A special vehicle mainly used on industrial premises is a motor vehicle designed primarily for use within the buildings and premises of industrial or commercial establishments. This includes battery-powered airport passenger vehicles or baggage/mail trucks, forklifts, coal-cars in a coal mine, logging cars and trucks used in mines or quarries.

(u) A special vehicle mainly used in agriculture is a motor vehicle designed specifically for use in farming and agriculture (horticulture), to work the land, tend and harvest crops and transport materials on the farm. This includes harvesters, farm machinery and tractor and trailers.

(v) A special construction vehicle is a motor vehicle designed specifically for use on construction and demolition sites. This includes bulldozers, diggers, earth levellers, dump trucks. backhoes, front-end loaders, pavers, and mechanical shovels.

(w) A special all-terrain vehicle is a motor vehicle of special design to enable it to negotiate over rough or soft terrain, snow or sand. Examples of special design are high construction, special wheels and tires, tracks, and support on a cushion of air. This includes snow mobiles, All-terrain vehicles (ATV), and dune buggies. It does not include passenger vehicle designated as Sport Utility Vehicles. (SUV)

(x) A watercraft is any device designed for transporting passengers or goods on water. This includes motor or sailboats, ships, and hovercraft.

(y) An aircraft is any device for transporting passengers or goods in the air. This includes hot-air balloons, gliders, helicopters and airplanes.

(z) A military vehicle is any motorized vehicle operating on a public roadway owned by the military and being operated by a member of the military.

Pedestrian injured in transport accident (V00-V09)

INCLUDES person changing tire on transport vehicle
person examining engine of vehicle broken down in (on side of) road

EXCLUDES 1 *fall due to non-transport collision with other person (W03)*
pedestrian on foot falling (slipping) on ice and snow (W00.-)
struck or bumped by another person (W51)

The appropriate 7th character is to be added to each code from categories V00-V09.
A initial encounter
D subsequent encounter
S sequela

✓4th **V00 Pedestrian conveyance accident**

Use additional place of occurrence and activity external cause codes, if known (Y92.-, Y93.-)

EXCLUDES 1 *collision with another person without fall (W51)*
fall due to person on foot colliding with another person on foot (W03)
fall from non-moving wheelchair, nonmotorized scooter and motorized mobility scooter without collision (W05.-)
pedestrian (conveyance) collision with other land transport vehicle (V01-V09)
pedestrian on foot falling (slipping) on ice and snow (W00.-)

✓5th **V00.0 Pedestrian on foot injured in collision with pedestrian conveyance**

✓x7th **V00.01 Pedestrian on foot injured in collision with roller-skater**

✓x7th **V00.02 Pedestrian on foot injured in collision with skateboarder**

✓6th **V00.03 Pedestrian on foot injured in collision with standing micro-mobility pedestrian conveyance**

✓7th **V00.031 Pedestrian on foot injured in collision with rider of standing electric scooter**

✓7th **V00.038 Pedestrian on foot injured in collision with rider of other standing micro-mobility pedestrian conveyance**
Pedestrian on foot injured in collision with rider of hoverboard
Pedestrian on foot injured in collision with rider of segway

✓x7th **V00.09 Pedestrian on foot injured in collision with other pedestrian conveyance**

✓5th **V00.1 Rolling-type pedestrian conveyance accident**

EXCLUDES 1 *accident with baby stroller (V00.82-)*
accident with motorized mobility scooter (V00.83-)
accident with wheelchair (powered) (V00.81-)

✓6th **V00.11 In-line roller-skate accident**

✓7th **V00.111 Fall from in-line roller-skates**

✓7th **V00.112 In-line roller-skater colliding with stationary object**

✓7th **V00.118 Other in-line roller-skate accident**

EXCLUDES 1 *roller-skater collision with other land transport vehicle (V01-V09 with 5th character 1)*

✓6th **V00.12 Non-in-line roller-skate accident**

✓7th **V00.121 Fall from non-in-line roller-skates**

✓7th **V00.122 Non-in-line roller-skater colliding with stationary object**

✓7th **V00.128 Other non-in-line roller-skating accident**

EXCLUDES 1 *roller-skater collision with other land transport vehicle (V01-V09 with 5th character 1)*

✓6th **V00.13 Skateboard accident**

✓7th **V00.131 Fall from skateboard**

✓7th **V00.132 Skateboarder colliding with stationary object**

✓7th **V00.138 Other skateboard accident**

EXCLUDES 1 *skateboarder collision with other land transport vehicle (V01-V09 with 5th character 2)*

✓6th **V00.14 Scooter (nonmotorized) accident**

EXCLUDES 1 *motor scooter accident (V20-V29)*

✓7th **V00.141 Fall from scooter (nonmotorized)**

✓7th **V00.142 Scooter (nonmotorized) colliding with stationary object**

✓7th **V00.148 Other scooter (nonmotorized) accident**

EXCLUDES 1 *scooter (nonmotorized) collision with other land transport vehicle (V01-V09 with fifth character 9)*

✓6th **V00.15 Heelies accident**
Rolling shoe
Wheeled shoe
Wheelies accident

✓7th **V00.151 Fall from heelies**

✓7th **V00.152 Heelies colliding with stationary object**

✓7th **V00.158 Other heelies accident**

✓6th **V00.18 Accident on other rolling-type pedestrian conveyance**

✓7th **V00.181 Fall from other rolling-type pedestrian conveyance**

✓7th **V00.182 Pedestrian on other rolling-type pedestrian conveyance colliding with stationary object**

✓7th **V00.188 Other accident on other rolling-type pedestrian conveyance**

✓5th **V00.2 Gliding-type pedestrian conveyance accident**

✓6th **V00.21 Ice-skates accident**

✓7th **V00.211 Fall from ice-skates**

✓7th **V00.212 Ice-skater colliding with stationary object**

✓7th **V00.218 Other ice-skates accident**

EXCLUDES 1 *ice-skater collision with other land transport vehicle (V01-V09 with 5th character 9)*

✓6th **V00.22 Sled accident**

✓7th **V00.221 Fall from sled**

✓7th **V00.222 Sledder colliding with stationary object**

✓7th **V00.228 Other sled accident**

EXCLUDES 1 *sled collision with other land transport vehicle (V01-V09 with 5th character 9)*

✓6th **V00.28 Other gliding-type pedestrian conveyance accident**

✓7th **V00.281 Fall from other gliding-type pedestrian conveyance**

✓7th **V00.282 Pedestrian on other gliding-type pedestrian conveyance colliding with stationary object**

✓7th **V00.288 Other accident on other gliding-type pedestrian conveyance**

EXCLUDES 1 *gliding-type pedestrian conveyance collision with other land transport vehicle (V01-V09 with 5th character 9)*

✓5th **V00.3 Flat-bottomed pedestrian conveyance accident**

✓6th **V00.31 Snowboard accident**

✓7th **V00.311 Fall from snowboard**

√7th **V00.312 Snowboarder colliding with stationary object**

√7th **V00.318 Other snowboard accident**

EXCLUDES 1 *snowboarder collision with other land transport vehicle (V01-V09 with 5th character 9)*

√6th **V00.32 Snow-ski accident**

√7th **V00.321 Fall from snow-skis**

√7th **V00.322 Snow-skier colliding with stationary object**

√7th **V00.328 Other snow-ski accident**

EXCLUDES 1 *snow-skier collision with other land transport vehicle (V01-V09 with 5th character 9)*

√6th **V00.38 Other flat-bottomed pedestrian conveyance accident**

√7th **V00.381 Fall from other flat-bottomed pedestrian conveyance**

√7th **V00.382 Pedestrian on other flat-bottomed pedestrian conveyance colliding with stationary object**

√7th **V00.388 Other accident on other flat-bottomed pedestrian conveyance**

√5th **V00.8 Accident on other pedestrian conveyance**

√6th **V00.81 Accident with wheelchair (powered)**

√7th **V00.811 Fall from moving wheelchair (powered)**

EXCLUDES 1 *fall from non-moving wheelchair (W05.0)*

√7th **V00.812 Wheelchair (powered) colliding with stationary object**

√7th **V00.818 Other accident with wheelchair (powered)**

√6th **V00.82 Accident with baby stroller**

√7th **V00.821 Fall from baby stroller**

√7th **V00.822 Baby stroller colliding with stationary object**

√7th **V00.828 Other accident with baby stroller**

√6th **V00.83 Accident with motorized mobility scooter**

√7th **V00.831 Fall from motorized mobility scooter**

EXCLUDES 1 *fall from non-moving motorized mobility scooter (W05.2)*

√7th **V00.832 Motorized mobility scooter colliding with stationary object**

√7th **V00.838 Other accident with motorized mobility scooter**

√6th **V00.84 Accident with standing micro-mobility pedestrian conveyance**

√7th **V00.841 Fall from standing electric scooter**

√7th **V00.842 Pedestrian on standing electric scooter colliding with stationary object**

√7th **V00.848 Other accident with standing micro-mobility pedestrian conveyance**

Accident with hoverboard

Accident with segway

√6th **V00.89 Accident on other pedestrian conveyance**

√7th **V00.891 Fall from other pedestrian conveyance**

√7th **V00.892 Pedestrian on other pedestrian conveyance colliding with stationary object**

√7th **V00.898 Other accident on other pedestrian conveyance**

EXCLUDES 1 *other pedestrian (conveyance) collision with other land transport vehicle (V01-V09 with 5th character 9)*

√4th **V01 Pedestrian injured in collision with pedal cycle**

√5th **V01.0 Pedestrian injured in collision with pedal cycle in nontraffic accident**

√x7th **V01.00 Pedestrian on foot injured in collision with pedal cycle in nontraffic accident**

Pedestrian NOS injured in collision with pedal cycle in nontraffic accident

√x7th **V01.01 Pedestrian on roller-skates injured in collision with pedal cycle in nontraffic accident**

√x7th **V01.02 Pedestrian on skateboard injured in collision with pedal cycle in nontraffic accident**

√6th **V01.03 Pedestrian on standing micro-mobility pedestrian conveyance injured in collision with pedal cycle in nontraffic accident**

√7th **V01.031 Pedestrian on standing electric scooter injured in collision with pedal cycle in nontraffic accident**

√7th **V01.038 Pedestrian on other standing micro-mobility pedestrian conveyance injured in collision with pedal cycle in nontraffic accident**

Pedestrian on hoverboard injured in collision with pedal cycle in nontraffic accident

Pedestrian on segway injured in collision with pedal cycle in nontraffic accident

√x7th **V01.09 Pedestrian with other conveyance injured in collision with pedal cycle in nontraffic accident**

Pedestrian with baby stroller injured in collision with pedal cycle in nontraffic accident

Pedestrian on ice-skates injured in collision with pedal cycle in nontraffic accident

Pedestrian in motorized mobility scooter injured in collision with pedal cycle in nontraffic accident

Pedestrian on nonmotorized scooter injured in collision with pedal cycle in nontraffic accident

Pedestrian on sled injured in collision with pedal cycle in nontraffic accident

Pedestrian on snowboard injured in collision with pedal cycle in nontraffic accident

Pedestrian on snow-skis injured in collision with pedal cycle in nontraffic accident

Pedestrian in wheelchair (powered) injured in collision with pedal cycle in nontraffic accident

√5th **V01.1 Pedestrian injured in collision with pedal cycle in traffic accident**

√x7th **V01.10 Pedestrian on foot injured in collision with pedal cycle in traffic accident**

Pedestrian NOS injured in collision with pedal cycle in traffic accident

√x7th **V01.11 Pedestrian on roller-skates injured in collision with pedal cycle in traffic accident**

√x7th **V01.12 Pedestrian on skateboard injured in collision with pedal cycle in traffic accident**

√6th **V01.13 Pedestrian on standing micro-mobility pedestrian conveyance injured in collision with pedal cycle in traffic accident**

√7th **V01.131 Pedestrian on standing electric scooter injured in collision with pedal cycle in traffic accident**

√7th **V01.138 Pedestrian on other standing micro-mobility pedestrian conveyance injured in collision with pedal cycle in traffic accident**

Pedestrian on hoverboard injured in collision with pedal cycle in traffic accident

Pedestrian on segway injured in collision with pedal cycle in traffic accident

√x7th **V01.19 Pedestrian with other conveyance injured in collision with pedal cycle in traffic accident**

Pedestrian with baby stroller injured in collision with pedal cycle in traffic accident

Pedestrian on ice-skates injured in collision with pedal cycle in traffic accident

Pedestrian in motorized mobility scooter injured in collision with pedal cycle in traffic accident

Pedestrian on nonmotorized scooter injured in collision with pedal cycle in traffic accident

Pedestrian on sled injured in collision with pedal cycle in traffic accident

Pedestrian on snowboard injured in collision with pedal cycle in traffic accident

Pedestrian on snow-skis injured in collision with pedal cycle in traffic accident

Pedestrian in wheelchair (powered) injured in collision with pedal cycle in traffic accident

5th **V01.9 Pedestrian injured in collision with pedal cycle, unspecified whether traffic or nontraffic accident**

√x7th **V01.90 Pedestrian on foot injured in collision with pedal cycle, unspecified whether traffic or nontraffic accident**

Pedestrian NOS injured in collision with pedal cycle, unspecified whether traffic or nontraffic accident

√x7th **V01.91 Pedestrian on roller-skates injured in collision with pedal cycle, unspecified whether traffic or nontraffic accident**

√x7th **V01.92 Pedestrian on skateboard injured in collision with pedal cycle, unspecified whether traffic or nontraffic accident**

6th **V01.93 Pedestrian on standing micro-mobility pedestrian conveyance injured in collision with pedal cycle, unspecified whether traffic or nontraffic accident**

7th **V01.931 Pedestrian on standing electric scooter injured in collision with pedal cycle, unspecified whether traffic or nontraffic accident**

7th **V01.938 Pedestrian on other standing micro-mobility pedestrian conveyance injured in collision with pedal cycle, unspecified whether traffic or nontraffic accident**

Pedestrian on hoverboard injured in collision with pedal cycle, unspecified whether traffic or nontraffic accident

Pedestrian on segway injured in collision with pedal cycle, unspecified whether traffic or nontraffic accident

√x7th **V01.99 Pedestrian with other conveyance injured in collision with pedal cycle, unspecified whether traffic or nontraffic accident**

Pedestrian with baby stroller injured in collision with pedal cycle, unspecified whether traffic or nontraffic accident

Pedestrian on ice-skates injured in collision with pedal cycle unspecified, whether traffic or nontraffic accident

Pedestrian in motorized mobility scooter injured in collision with pedal cycle, unspecified whether traffic or nontraffic accident

Pedestrian on nonmotorized scooter injured in collision with pedal cycle, unspecified whether traffic or nontraffic accident

Pedestrian on sled injured in collision with pedal cycle unspecified, whether traffic or nontraffic accident

Pedestrian on snowboard injured in collision with pedal cycle, unspecified whether traffic or nontraffic accident

Pedestrian on snow-skis injured in collision with pedal cycle, unspecified whether traffic or nontraffic accident

Pedestrian in wheelchair (powered) injured in collision with pedal cycle, unspecified whether traffic or nontraffic accident

4th **V02 Pedestrian injured in collision with two- or three-wheeled motor vehicle**

5th **V02.0 Pedestrian injured in collision with two- or three-wheeled motor vehicle in nontraffic accident**

√x7th **V02.00 Pedestrian on foot injured in collision with two- or three-wheeled motor vehicle in nontraffic accident**

Pedestrian NOS injured in collision with two- or three-wheeled motor vehicle in nontraffic accident

√x7th **V02.01 Pedestrian on roller-skates injured in collision with two- or three-wheeled motor vehicle in nontraffic accident**

√x7th **V02.02 Pedestrian on skateboard injured in collision with two- or three-wheeled motor vehicle in nontraffic accident**

6th **V02.03 Pedestrian on standing micro-mobility pedestrian conveyance injured in collision with two- or three-wheeled motor vehicle in nontraffic accident**

7th **V02.031 Pedestrian on standing electric scooter injured in collision with two- or three-wheeled motor vehicle in nontraffic accident**

7th **V02.038 Pedestrian on other standing micro-mobility pedestrian conveyance injured in collision with two- or three-wheeled motor vehicle in nontraffic accident**

Pedestrian on hoverboard injured in collision with two-or three wheeled motor vehicle in nontraffic accident

Pedestrian on segway injured in collision with two- or three-wheeled motor vehicle in nontraffic accident

√x7th **V02.09 Pedestrian with other conveyance injured in collision with two- or three-wheeled motor vehicle in nontraffic accident**

Pedestrian with baby stroller injured in collision with two- or three-wheeled motor vehicle in nontraffic accident

Pedestrian on ice-skates injured in collision with two- or three-wheeled motor vehicle in nontraffic accident

Pedestrian in motorized mobility scooter injured in collision with two- or three-wheeled motor vehicle in nontraffic accident

Pedestrian on nonmotorized scooter injured in collision with two- or three-wheeled motor vehicle in nontraffic accident

Pedestrian on sled injured in collision with two- or three-wheeled motor vehicle in nontraffic accident

Pedestrian on snowboard injured in collision with two- or three-wheeled motor vehicle in nontraffic accident

Pedestrian on snow-skis injured in collision with two- or three-wheeled motor vehicle in nontraffic accident

Pedestrian in wheelchair (powered) injured in collision with two- or three-wheeled motor vehicle in nontraffic accident

5th **V02.1 Pedestrian injured in collision with two- or three-wheeled motor vehicle in traffic accident**

√x7th **V02.10 Pedestrian on foot injured in collision with two- or three-wheeled motor vehicle in traffic accident**

Pedestrian NOS injured in collision with two- or three-wheeled motor vehicle in traffic accident

√x7th **V02.11 Pedestrian on roller-skates injured in collision with two- or three-wheeled motor vehicle in traffic accident**

√x7th **V02.12 Pedestrian on skateboard injured in collision with two- or three-wheeled motor vehicle in traffic accident**

6th **V02.13 Pedestrian on standing micro-mobility pedestrian conveyance injured in collision with two- or three-wheeled motor vehicle in traffic accident**

7th **V02.131 Pedestrian on standing electric scooter injured in collision with two- or three-wheeled motor vehicle in traffic accident**

7th **V02.138 Pedestrian on other standing micro-mobility pedestrian conveyance injured in collision with two- or three-wheeled motor vehicle in traffic accident**

Pedestrian on hoverboard injured in collision with two-or three wheeled motor vehicle in traffic accident

Pedestrian on segway injured in collision with two- or three-wheeled motor vehicle in traffic accident

✓x7th **V02.19 Pedestrian with other conveyance injured in collision with two- or three-wheeled motor vehicle in traffic accident**

Pedestrian with baby stroller injured in collision with two- or three-wheeled motor vehicle in traffic accident

Pedestrian on ice-skates injured in collision with two- or three-wheeled motor vehicle in traffic accident

Pedestrian in motorized mobility scooter injured in collision with two- or three-wheeled motor vehicle in traffic accident

Pedestrian on nonmotorized scooter injured in collision with two- or three-wheeled motor vehicle in traffic accident

Pedestrian on sled injured in collision with two- or three-wheeled motor vehicle in traffic accident

Pedestrian on snowboard injured in collision with two- or three-wheeled motor vehicle in traffic accident

Pedestrian on snow-skis injured in collision with two- or three-wheeled motor vehicle in traffic accident

Pedestrian in wheelchair (powered) injured in collision with two- or three-wheeled motor vehicle in traffic accident

✓5th **V02.9 Pedestrian injured in collision with two- or three-wheeled motor vehicle, unspecified whether traffic or nontraffic accident**

✓x7th **V02.90 Pedestrian on foot injured in collision with two- or three-wheeled motor vehicle, unspecified whether traffic or nontraffic accident**

Pedestrian NOS injured in collision with two- or three-wheeled motor vehicle, unspecified whether traffic or nontraffic accident

✓x7th **V02.91 Pedestrian on roller-skates injured in collision with two- or three-wheeled motor vehicle, unspecified whether traffic or nontraffic accident**

✓x7th **V02.92 Pedestrian on skateboard injured in collision with two- or three-wheeled motor vehicle, unspecified whether traffic or nontraffic accident**

✓6th **V02.93 Pedestrian on standing micro-mobility pedestrian conveyance injured in collision with two- or three-wheeled motor vehicle, unspecified whether traffic or nontraffic accident**

✓7th **V02.931 Pedestrian on standing electric scooter injured in collision with two- or three wheeled motor vehicle, unspecified whether traffic or nontraffic accident**

✓7th **V02.938 Pedestrian on other standing micro-mobility pedestrian conveyance injured in collision with two- or three wheeled motor vehicle, unspecified whether traffic or nontraffic accident**

Pedestrian on hoverboard injured in collision with two-three-wheeled motor vehicle, unspecified whether traffic or nontraffic accident

Pedestrian on segway injured in collision with two- or three wheeled motor vehicle, unspecified whether traffic or nontraffic accident

✓x7th **V02.99 Pedestrian with other conveyance injured in collision with two- or three-wheeled motor vehicle, unspecified whether traffic or nontraffic accident**

Pedestrian with baby stroller injured in collision with two- or three-wheeled motor vehicle, unspecified whether traffic or nontraffic accident

Pedestrian on ice-skates injured in collision with two- or three-wheeled motor vehicle, unspecified whether traffic or nontraffic accident

Pedestrian on nonmotorized scooter injured in collision with two- or three-wheeled motor vehicle, unspecified whether traffic or nontraffic accident

Pedestrian on sled injured in collision with two- or three-wheeled motor vehicle, unspecified whether traffic or nontraffic accident

Pedestrian on snowboard injured in collision with two- or three-wheeled motor vehicle, unspecified whether traffic or nontraffic accident

Pedestrian on snow-skis injured in collision with two- or three-wheeled motor vehicle, unspecified whether traffic or nontraffic accident

Pedestrian in wheelchair (powered) injured in collision with two- or three-wheeled motor vehicle, unspecified whether traffic or nontraffic accident

Pedestrian in motorized mobility scooter injured in collision with two- or three wheeled motor vehicle, unspecified whether traffic or nontraffic accident

✓4th **V03 Pedestrian injured in collision with car, pick-up truck or van**

✓5th **V03.0 Pedestrian injured in collision with car, pick-up truck or van in nontraffic accident**

✓x7th **V03.00 Pedestrian on foot injured in collision with car, pick-up truck or van in nontraffic accident**

Pedestrian NOS injured in collision with car, pick-up truck or van in nontraffic accident

✓x7th **V03.01 Pedestrian on roller-skates injured in collision with car, pick-up truck or van in nontraffic accident**

✓x7th **V03.02 Pedestrian on skateboard injured in collision with car, pick-up truck or van in nontraffic accident**

✓6th **V03.03 Pedestrian on standing micro-mobility pedestrian conveyance injured in collision with car, pick-up or van in nontraffic accident**

✓7th **V03.031 Pedestrian on standing electric scooter injured in collision with car, pick-up or van in nontraffic accident**

✓7th **V03.038 Pedestrian on other standing micro-mobility pedestrian conveyance injured in collision with car, pick-up or van in nontraffic accident**

Pedestrian on hoverboard injured in collision with car, pick-up or van in nontraffic accident

Pedestrian on segway injured in collision with car, pick-up or van in nontraffic accident

✓x7th **V03.09 Pedestrian with other conveyance injured in collision with car, pick-up truck or van in nontraffic accident**

Pedestrian with baby stroller injured in collision with car, pick-up truck or van in nontraffic accident

Pedestrian on ice-skates injured in collision with car, pick-up truck or van in nontraffic accident

Pedestrian in motorized mobility scooter injured in collision with car, pick-up truck or van in nontraffic accident

Pedestrian on nonmotorized scooter injured in collision with car, pick-up truck or van in nontraffic accident

Pedestrian on sled injured in collision with car, pick-up truck or van in nontraffic accident

Pedestrian on snowboard injured in collision with car, pick-up truck or van in nontraffic accident

Pedestrian on snow-skis injured in collision with car, pick-up truck or van in nontraffic accident

Pedestrian in wheelchair (powered) injured in collision with car, pick-up truck or van in nontraffic accident

V03.1 Pedestrian injured in collision with car, pick-up truck or van in traffic accident

V03.10 Pedestrian on foot injured in collision with car, pick-up truck or van in traffic accident
Pedestrian NOS injured in collision with car, pick-up truck or van in traffic accident

V03.11 Pedestrian on roller-skates injured in collision with car, pick-up truck or van in traffic accident

V03.12 Pedestrian on skateboard injured in collision with car, pick-up truck or van in traffic accident

V03.13 Pedestrian on standing micro-mobility pedestrian conveyance injured in collision with car, pick-up or van in traffic accident

V03.131 Pedestrian on standing electric scooter injured in collision with car, pick-up or van in traffic accident

V03.138 Pedestrian on other standing micro-mobility pedestrian conveyance injured in collision with car, pick-up or van in traffic accident
Pedestrian on hoverboard injured in collision with car, pick-up or van in traffic accident
Pedestrian on segway injured in collision with car, pick-up or van in traffic accident

V03.19 Pedestrian with other conveyance injured in collision with car, pick-up truck or van in traffic accident
Pedestrian with baby stroller injured in collision with car, pick-up truck or van in traffic accident
Pedestrian on ice-skates injured in collision with car, pick-up truck or van in traffic accident
Pedestrian in motorized mobility scooter injured in collision with car, pick-up truck or van in nontraffic accident
Pedestrian on nonmotorized scooter injured in collision with car, pick-up truck or van in nontraffic accident
Pedestrian on sled injured in collision with car, pick-up truck or van in traffic accident
Pedestrian on snowboard injured in collision with car, pick-up truck or van in traffic accident
Pedestrian on snow-skis injured in collision with car, pick-up truck or van in traffic accident
Pedestrian in wheelchair (powered) injured in collision with car, pick-up truck or van in traffic accident

V03.9 Pedestrian injured in collision with car, pick-up truck or van, unspecified whether traffic or nontraffic accident

V03.90 Pedestrian on foot injured in collision with car, pick-up truck or van, unspecified whether traffic or nontraffic accident
Pedestrian NOS injured in collision with car, pick-up truck or van, unspecified whether traffic or nontraffic accident

V03.91 Pedestrian on roller-skates injured in collision with car, pick-up truck or van, unspecified whether traffic or nontraffic accident

V03.92 Pedestrian on skateboard injured in collision with car, pick-up truck or van, unspecified whether traffic or nontraffic accident

V03.93 Pedestrian on standing micro-mobility pedestrian conveyance injured in collision with car, pick-up or van, unspecified whether traffic or nontraffic accident

V03.931 Pedestrian on standing electric scooter injured in collision with car, pick-up or van, unspecified whether traffic or nontraffic accident

V03.938 Pedestrian on other standing micro-mobility pedestrian conveyance injured in collision with car, pick-up or van, unspecified whether traffic or nontraffic accident
Pedestrian on hoverboard injured in collision with car, pick-up or van, unspecified whether traffic or nontraffic accident
Pedestrian on segway injured in collision with car, pick-up or van, unspecified whether traffic or nontraffic accident

V03.99 Pedestrian with other conveyance injured in collision with car, pick-up truck or van, unspecified whether traffic or nontraffic accident
Pedestrian with baby stroller injured in collision with car, pick-up truck or van, unspecified whether traffic or nontraffic accident
Pedestrian on ice-skates injured in collision with car, pick-up truck or van, unspecified whether traffic or nontraffic accident
Pedestrian in motorized mobility scooter injured in collision with car, pick-up truck or van, unspecified whether traffic or nontraffic accident
Pedestrian on nonmotorized scooter injured in collision with car, pick-up truck or van, unspecified whether traffic or nontraffic accident
Pedestrian on sled injured in collision with car, pick-up truck or van in nontraffic accident
Pedestrian on snowboard injured in collision with car, pick-up truck or van, unspecified whether traffic or nontraffic accident
Pedestrian on snow-skis injured in collision with car, pick-up truck or van, unspecified whether traffic or nontraffic accident
Pedestrian in wheelchair (powered) injured in collision with car, pick-up truck or van, unspecified whether traffic or nontraffic accident

V04 Pedestrian injured in collision with heavy transport vehicle or bus

EXCLUDES 1 *pedestrian injured in collision with military vehicle (V09.01, V09.21)*

V04.0 Pedestrian injured in collision with heavy transport vehicle or bus in nontraffic accident

V04.00 Pedestrian on foot injured in collision with heavy transport vehicle or bus in nontraffic accident
Pedestrian NOS injured in collision with heavy transport vehicle or bus in nontraffic accident

V04.01 Pedestrian on roller-skates injured in collision with heavy transport vehicle or bus in nontraffic accident

V04.02 Pedestrian on skateboard injured in collision with heavy transport vehicle or bus in nontraffic accident

V04.03 Pedestrian on standing micro-mobility pedestrian conveyance injured in collision with heavy transport vehicle or bus in nontraffic accident

V04.031 Pedestrian on standing electric scooter injured in collision with heavy transport vehicle or bus in nontraffic accident

V04.038 Pedestrian on other standing micro-mobility pedestrian conveyance injured in collision with heavy transport vehicle or bus in nontraffic accident
Pedestrian on hoverboard injured in collision with heavy transport vehicle or bus in nontraffic accident
Pedestrian on segway injured in collision with heavy transport vehicle or bus in nontraffic accident

V04.09 Pedestrian with other conveyance injured in collision with heavy transport vehicle or bus in nontraffic accident
Pedestrian with baby stroller injured in collision with heavy transport vehicle or bus in nontraffic accident
Pedestrian on ice-skates injured in collision with heavy transport vehicle or bus in nontraffic accident
Pedestrian in motorized mobility scooter injured in collision with heavy transport vehicle or bus in nontraffic accident
Pedestrian on nonmotorized scooter injured in collision with heavy transport vehicle or bus in nontraffic accident
Pedestrian on sled injured in collision with heavy transport vehicle or bus in nontraffic accident
Pedestrian on snowboard injured in collision with heavy transport vehicle or bus in nontraffic accident
Pedestrian on snow-skis injured in collision with heavy transport vehicle or bus in nontraffic accident
Pedestrian in wheelchair (powered) injured in collision with heavy transport vehicle or bus in nontraffic accident

V04.1 Pedestrian injured in collision with heavy transport vehicle or bus in traffic accident

V04.10 Pedestrian on foot injured in collision with heavy transport vehicle or bus in traffic accident
Pedestrian NOS injured in collision with heavy transport vehicle or bus in traffic accident

V04.11 Pedestrian on roller-skates injured in collision with heavy transport vehicle or bus in traffic accident

V04.12 Pedestrian on skateboard injured in collision with heavy transport vehicle or bus in traffic accident

V04.13 Pedestrian on standing micro-mobility pedestrian conveyance injured in collision with heavy transport vehicle or bus in traffic accident

V04.131 Pedestrian on standing electric scooter injured in collision with heavy transport vehicle or bus in traffic accident

V04.138 Pedestrian on other standing micro-mobility pedestrian conveyance injured in collision with heavy transport vehicle or bus in traffic accident
Pedestrian on hoverboard injured in collision with heavy transport vehicle or bus in traffic accident
Pedestrian on segway injured in collision with heavy transport vehicle or bus in traffic accident

V04.19 Pedestrian with other conveyance injured in collision with heavy transport vehicle or bus in traffic accident
Pedestrian with baby stroller injured in collision with heavy transport vehicle or bus in traffic accident
Pedestrian on ice-skates injured in collision with heavy transport vehicle or bus in traffic accident
Pedestrian in motorized mobility scooter injured in collision with heavy transport vehicle or bus in traffic accident
Pedestrian on nonmotorized scooter injured in collision with heavy transport vehicle or bus in traffic accident
Pedestrian on sled injured in collision with heavy transport vehicle or bus in traffic accident
Pedestrian on snowboard injured in collision with heavy transport vehicle or bus in traffic accident
Pedestrian on snow-skis injured in collision with heavy transport vehicle or bus in traffic accident
Pedestrian in wheelchair (powered) injured in collision with heavy transport vehicle or bus in traffic accident

V04.9 Pedestrian injured in collision with heavy transport vehicle or bus, unspecified whether traffic or nontraffic accident

V04.90 Pedestrian on foot injured in collision with heavy transport vehicle or bus, unspecified whether traffic or nontraffic accident
Pedestrian NOS injured in collision with heavy transport vehicle or bus, unspecified whether traffic or nontraffic accident

V04.91 Pedestrian on roller-skates injured in collision with heavy transport vehicle or bus, unspecified whether traffic or nontraffic accident

V04.92 Pedestrian on skateboard injured in collision with heavy transport vehicle or bus, unspecified whether traffic or nontraffic accident

V04.93 Pedestrian on standing micro-mobility pedestrian conveyance injured in collision with heavy transport vehicle or bus, unspecified whether traffic or nontraffic accident

V04.931 Pedestrian on standing electric scooter injured in collision with heavy transport vehicle or bus, unspecified whether traffic or nontraffic accident

V04.938 Pedestrian on other standing micro-mobility pedestrian conveyance injured in collision with heavy transport vehicle or bus, unspecified whether traffic or nontraffic accident
Pedestrian on hoverboard injured in collision with heavy transport vehicle or bus, unspecified whether traffic or nontraffic accident
Pedestrian on segway injured in collision with heavy transport vehicle or bus, unspecified whether traffic or nontraffic accident

V04.99 Pedestrian with other conveyance injured in collision with heavy transport vehicle or bus, unspecified whether traffic or nontraffic accident
Pedestrian with baby stroller injured in collision with heavy transport vehicle or bus, unspecified whether traffic or nontraffic accident
Pedestrian on ice-skates injured in collision with heavy transport vehicle or bus, unspecified whether traffic or nontraffic accident
Pedestrian in motorized mobility scooter injured in collision with heavy transport vehicle or bus, unspecified whether traffic or nontraffic accident
Pedestrian on nonmotorized scooter injured in collision with heavy transport vehicle or bus, unspecified whether traffic or nontraffic accident
Pedestrian on sled injured in collision with heavy transport vehicle or bus, unspecified whether traffic or nontraffic accident
Pedestrian on snowboard injured in collision with heavy transport vehicle or bus, unspecified whether traffic or nontraffic accident
Pedestrian on snow-skis injured in collision with heavy transport vehicle or bus, unspecified whether traffic or nontraffic accident
Pedestrian in wheelchair (powered) injured in collision with heavy transport vehicle or bus, unspecified whether traffic or nontraffic accident

V05 Pedestrian injured in collision with railway train or railway vehicle

V05.0 Pedestrian injured in collision with railway train or railway vehicle in nontraffic accident

V05.00 Pedestrian on foot injured in collision with railway train or railway vehicle in nontraffic accident
Pedestrian NOS injured in collision with railway train or railway vehicle in nontraffic accident

V05.01 Pedestrian on roller-skates injured in collision with railway train or railway vehicle in nontraffic accident

V05.02 Pedestrian on skateboard injured in collision with railway train or railway vehicle in nontraffic accident

V05.03 Pedestrian on standing micro-mobility pedestrian conveyance injured in collision with railway train or railway vehicle in nontraffic accident

V05.031 Pedestrian on standing electric scooter injured in collision with railway train or railway vehicle in nontraffic accident

V05.038 Pedestrian on other standing micro-mobility pedestrian conveyance injured in collision with railway train or railway vehicle in nontraffic accident
Pedestrian on hoverboard injured in collision with railway train or railway vehicle in nontraffic accident
Pedestrian on segway injured in collision with railway train or railway vehicle in nontraffic accident

V05.09 Pedestrian with other conveyance injured in collision with railway train or railway vehicle in nontraffic accident
Pedestrian with baby stroller injured in collision with railway train or railway vehicle in nontraffic accident
Pedestrian on ice-skates injured in collision with railway train or railway vehicle in nontraffic accident
Pedestrian in motorized mobility scooter injured in collision with railway train or railway vehicle in nontraffic accident
Pedestrian on nonmotorized scooter injured in collision with railway train or railway vehicle in nontraffic accident
Pedestrian on sled injured in collision with railway train or railway vehicle in nontraffic accident
Pedestrian on snowboard injured in collision with railway train or railway vehicle in nontraffic accident
Pedestrian on snow-skis injured in collision with railway train or railway vehicle in nontraffic accident
Pedestrian in wheelchair (powered) injured in collision with railway train or railway vehicle in nontraffic accident

5th VØ5.1 Pedestrian injured in collision with railway train or railway vehicle in traffic accident

x7th VØ5.1Ø Pedestrian on foot injured in collision with railway train or railway vehicle in traffic accident
Pedestrian NOS injured in collision with railway train or railway vehicle in traffic accident

x7th VØ5.11 Pedestrian on roller-skates injured in collision with railway train or railway vehicle in traffic accident

x7th VØ5.12 Pedestrian on skateboard injured in collision with railway train or railway vehicle in traffic accident

6th VØ5.13 Pedestrian on standing micro-mobility pedestrian conveyance injured in collision with railway train or railway vehicle in traffic accident

7th VØ5.131 Pedestrian on standing electric scooter injured in collision with railway train or railway vehicle in traffic accident

7th VØ5.138 Pedestrian on other standing micro-mobility pedestrian conveyance injured in collision with railway train or railway vehicle in traffic accident
Pedestrian on hoverboard injured in collision with railway train or railway vehicle in traffic accident
Pedestrian on segway injured in collision with railway train or railway vehicle in traffic accident

x7th VØ5.19 Pedestrian with other conveyance injured in collision with railway train or railway vehicle in traffic accident
Pedestrian with baby stroller injured in collision with railway train or railway vehicle in traffic accident
Pedestrian on ice-skates injured in collision with railway train or railway vehicle in traffic accident
Pedestrian in motorized mobility scooter injured in collision with railway train or railway vehicle in traffic accident
Pedestrian on nonmotorized scooter injured in collision with railway train or railway vehicle in traffic accident
Pedestrian on sled injured in collision with railway train or railway vehicle in traffic accident
Pedestrian on snowboard injured in collision with railway train or railway vehicle in traffic accident
Pedestrian on snow-skis injured in collision with railway train or railway vehicle in traffic accident
Pedestrian in wheelchair (powered) injured in collision with railway train or railway vehicle in traffic accident

5th VØ5.9 Pedestrian injured in collision with railway train or railway vehicle, unspecified whether traffic or nontraffic accident

x7th VØ5.9Ø Pedestrian on foot injured in collision with railway train or railway vehicle, unspecified whether traffic or nontraffic accident
Pedestrian NOS injured in collision with railway train or railway vehicle, unspecified whether traffic or nontraffic accident

x7th VØ5.91 Pedestrian on roller-skates injured in collision with railway train or railway vehicle, unspecified whether traffic or nontraffic accident

x7th VØ5.92 Pedestrian on skateboard injured in collision with railway train or railway vehicle, unspecified whether traffic or nontraffic accident

6th VØ5.93 Pedestrian on standing micro-mobility pedestrian conveyance injured in collision with railway train or railway vehicle, unspecified whether traffic or nontraffic accident

7th VØ5.931 Pedestrian on standing electric scooter injured in collision with railway train or railway vehicle, unspecified whether traffic or nontraffic accident

7th VØ5.938 Pedestrian on other standing micro-mobility pedestrian conveyance injured in collision with railway train or railway vehicle, unspecified whether traffic or nontraffic accident
Pedestrian on hoverboard injured in collision with railway train or railway vehicle, unspecified whether traffic or nontraffic accident
Pedestrian on segway injured in collision with railway train or railway vehicle, unspecified whether traffic or nontraffic accident

x7th VØ5.99 Pedestrian with other conveyance injured in collision with railway train or railway vehicle, unspecified whether traffic or nontraffic accident
Pedestrian with baby stroller injured in collision with railway train or railway vehicle, unspecified whether traffic or nontraffic
Pedestrian on ice-skates injured in collision with railway train or railway vehicle, unspecified whether traffic or nontraffic
Pedestrian on nonmotorized scooter injured in collision with railway train or railway vehicle, unspecified whether traffic or nontraffic
Pedestrian on sled injured in collision with railway train or railway vehicle, unspecified whether traffic or nontraffic
Pedestrian on snowboard injured in collision with railway train or railway vehicle, unspecified whether traffic or nontraffic
Pedestrian on snow-skis injured in collision with railway train or railway vehicle, unspecified whether traffic or nontraffic
Pedestrian in wheelchair (powered) injured in collision with railway train or railway vehicle, unspecified whether traffic or nontraffic
Pedestrian in motorized mobility scooter injured in collision with railway train or railway vehicle, unspecified whether traffic or nontraffic

4th VØ6 Pedestrian injured in collision with other nonmotor vehicle
INCLUDES collision with animal-drawn vehicle, animal being ridden, nonpowered streetcar
EXCLUDES 1 *pedestrian injured in collision with pedestrian conveyance (VØØ.Ø-)*

5th VØ6.Ø Pedestrian injured in collision with other nonmotor vehicle in nontraffic accident

x7th VØ6.ØØ Pedestrian on foot injured in collision with other nonmotor vehicle in nontraffic accident
Pedestrian NOS injured in collision with other nonmotor vehicle in nontraffic accident

x7th VØ6.Ø1 Pedestrian on roller-skates injured in collision with other nonmotor vehicle in nontraffic accident

x7th VØ6.Ø2 Pedestrian on skateboard injured in collision with other nonmotor vehicle in nontraffic accident

6th VØ6.Ø3 Pedestrian on standing micro-mobility pedestrian conveyance injured in collision with other nonmotor vehicle in nontraffic accident

7th VØ6.Ø31 Pedestrian on standing electric scooter injured in collision with other nonmotor vehicle in nontraffic accident

7th VØ6.Ø38 Pedestrian on other standing micro-mobility pedestrian conveyance injured in collision with other nonmotor vehicle in nontraffic accident
Pedestrian on hoverboard injured in collision with other nonmotor vehicle in nontraffic accident
Pedestrian on segway injured in collision with other nonmotor vehicle in nontraffic accident

x7th VØ6.Ø9 Pedestrian with other conveyance injured in collision with other nonmotor vehicle in nontraffic accident
Pedestrian with baby stroller injured in collision with other nonmotor vehicle in nontraffic accident
Pedestrian on ice-skates injured in collision with other nonmotor vehicle in nontraffic accident
Pedestrian in motorized mobility scooter injured in collision with other nonmotor vehicle in nontraffic accident
Pedestrian on nonmotorized scooter injured in collision with other nonmotor vehicle in nontraffic accident
Pedestrian on sled injured in collision with other nonmotor vehicle in nontraffic accident
Pedestrian on snowboard injured in collision with other nonmotor vehicle in nontraffic accident
Pedestrian on snow-skis injured in collision with other nonmotor vehicle in nontraffic accident
Pedestrian in wheelchair (powered) injured in collision with other nonmotor vehicle in nontraffic accident

V06.1 **Pedestrian injured in collision with other nonmotor vehicle in traffic accident**

V06.10 **Pedestrian on foot injured in collision with other nonmotor vehicle in traffic accident**
Pedestrian NOS injured in collision with other nonmotor vehicle in traffic accident

V06.11 **Pedestrian on roller-skates injured in collision with other nonmotor vehicle in traffic accident**

V06.12 **Pedestrian on skateboard injured in collision with other nonmotor vehicle in traffic accident**

V06.13 **Pedestrian on standing micro-mobility pedestrian conveyance injured in collision with other nonmotor vehicle in traffic accident**

V06.131 **Pedestrian on standing electric scooter injured in collision with other nonmotor vehicle in traffic accident**

V06.138 **Pedestrian on other standing micro-mobility pedestrian conveyance injured in collision with other nonmotor vehicle in traffic accident**
Pedestrian on hoverboard injured in collision with other nonmotor vehicle in traffic accident
Pedestrian on segway injured in collision with other nonmotor vehicle in traffic accident

V06.19 **Pedestrian with other conveyance injured in collision with other nonmotor vehicle in traffic accident**
Pedestrian with baby stroller injured in collision with other nonmotor vehicle in nontraffic accident
Pedestrian on ice-skates injured in collision with other nonmotor vehicle in traffic accident
Pedestrian in motorized mobility scooter injured in collision with other nonmotor vehicle in traffic accident
Pedestrian on nonmotorized scooter injured in collision with other nonmotor vehicle in traffic accident
Pedestrian on sled injured in collision with other nonmotor vehicle in traffic accident
Pedestrian on snowboard injured in collision with other nonmotor vehicle in traffic accident
Pedestrian on snow-skis injured in collision with other nonmotor vehicle in traffic accident
Pedestrian in wheelchair (powered) injured in collision with other nonmotor vehicle in traffic accident

V06.9 **Pedestrian injured in collision with other nonmotor vehicle, unspecified whether traffic or nontraffic accident**

V06.90 **Pedestrian on foot injured in collision with other nonmotor vehicle, unspecified whether traffic or nontraffic accident**
Pedestrian NOS injured in collision with other nonmotor vehicle, unspecified whether traffic or nontraffic accident

V06.91 **Pedestrian on roller-skates injured in collision with other nonmotor vehicle, unspecified whether traffic or nontraffic accident**

V06.92 **Pedestrian on skateboard injured in collision with other nonmotor vehicle, unspecified whether traffic or nontraffic accident**

V06.93 **Pedestrian on standing micro-mobility pedestrian conveyance injured in collision with other nonmotor vehicle, unspecified whether traffic or nontraffic accident**

V06.931 **Pedestrian on standing electric scooter injured in collision with other nonmotor vehicle, unspecified whether traffic or nontraffic accident**

V06.938 **Pedestrian on other standing micro-mobility pedestrian conveyance injured in collision with other nonmotor vehicle, unspecified whether traffic or nontraffic accident**
Pedestrian on hoverboard injured in collision with other nonmotor, unspecified whether traffic or nontraffic accident
Pedestrian on segway injured in collision with other nonmotor vehicle, unspecified whether traffic or nontraffic accident

V06.99 **Pedestrian with other conveyance injured in collision with other nonmotor vehicle, unspecified whether traffic or nontraffic accident**
Pedestrian with baby stroller injured in collision with other nonmotor vehicle, unspecified whether traffic or nontraffic accident
Pedestrian on ice-skates injured in collision with other nonmotor vehicle, unspecified whether traffic or nontraffic accident
Pedestrian in motorized mobility scooter injured in collision with other nonmotorized vehicle, unspecified whether traffic or nontraffic accident
Pedestrian on nonmotorized scooter injured in collision with other nonmotor vehicle, unspecified whether traffic or nontraffic accident
Pedestrian on sled injured in collision with other nonmotor vehicle, unspecified whether traffic or nontraffic accident
Pedestrian on snowboard injured in collision with other nonmotor vehicle, unspecified whether traffic or nontraffic accident
Pedestrian on snow-skis injured in collision with other nonmotor vehicle, unspecified whether traffic or nontraffic accident
Pedestrian in wheelchair (powered) injured in collision with other nonmotor vehicle, unspecified whether traffic or nontraffic accident

V09 **Pedestrian injured in other and unspecified transport accidents**

V09.0 **Pedestrian injured in nontraffic accident involving other and unspecified motor vehicles**

V09.00 **Pedestrian injured in nontraffic accident involving unspecified motor vehicles**

V09.01 **Pedestrian injured in nontraffic accident involving military vehicle**

V09.09 **Pedestrian injured in nontraffic accident involving other motor vehicles**
Pedestrian injured in nontraffic accident by special vehicle

V09.1 **Pedestrian injured in unspecified nontraffic accident**

V09.2 **Pedestrian injured in traffic accident involving other and unspecified motor vehicles**

V09.20 **Pedestrian injured in traffic accident involving unspecified motor vehicles**

V09.21 **Pedestrian injured in traffic accident involving military vehicle**

V09.29 **Pedestrian injured in traffic accident involving other motor vehicles**

V09.3 **Pedestrian injured in unspecified traffic accident**

V09.9 **Pedestrian injured in unspecified transport accident**

Pedal cycle rider injured in transport accident (V10-V19)

INCLUDES any non-motorized vehicle, excluding an animal-drawn vehicle, or a sidecar or trailer attached to the pedal cycle

EXCLUDES 2 *rupture of pedal cycle tire (W37.0)*

The appropriate 7th character is to be added to each code from categories V10-V19.
A initial encounter
D subsequent encounter
S sequela

V10 **Pedal cycle rider injured in collision with pedestrian or animal**

EXCLUDES 1 *pedal cycle rider collision with animal-drawn vehicle or animal being ridden (V16.-)*

V10.0 **Pedal cycle driver injured in collision with pedestrian or animal in nontraffic accident**

V10.1 **Pedal cycle passenger injured in collision with pedestrian or animal in nontraffic accident**

V10.2 **Unspecified pedal cyclist injured in collision with pedestrian or animal in nontraffic accident**

V10.3 **Person boarding or alighting a pedal cycle injured in collision with pedestrian or animal**

V10.4 **Pedal cycle driver injured in collision with pedestrian or animal in traffic accident**

V10.5 **Pedal cycle passenger injured in collision with pedestrian or animal in traffic accident**

V10.9 **Unspecified pedal cyclist injured in collision with pedestrian or animal in traffic accident**

V11 **Pedal cycle rider injured in collision with other pedal cycle**

V11.0 **Pedal cycle driver injured in collision with other pedal cycle in nontraffic accident**

√x7th V11.1 **Pedal cycle passenger injured in collision with other pedal cycle in nontraffic accident**

√x7th V11.2 **Unspecified pedal cyclist injured in collision with other pedal cycle in nontraffic accident**

√x7th V11.3 **Person boarding or alighting a pedal cycle injured in collision with other pedal cycle**

√x7th V11.4 **Pedal cycle driver injured in collision with other pedal cycle in traffic accident**

√x7th V11.5 **Pedal cycle passenger injured in collision with other pedal cycle in traffic accident**

√x7th V11.9 **Unspecified pedal cyclist injured in collision with other pedal cycle in traffic accident**

√4th **V12 Pedal cycle rider injured in collision with two- or three-wheeled motor vehicle**

√x7th V12.0 **Pedal cycle driver injured in collision with two- or three-wheeled motor vehicle in nontraffic accident**

√x7th V12.1 **Pedal cycle passenger injured in collision with two- or three-wheeled motor vehicle in nontraffic accident**

√x7th V12.2 **Unspecified pedal cyclist injured in collision with two- or three-wheeled motor vehicle in nontraffic accident**

√x7th V12.3 **Person boarding or alighting a pedal cycle injured in collision with two- or three-wheeled motor vehicle**

√x7th V12.4 **Pedal cycle driver injured in collision with two- or three-wheeled motor vehicle in traffic accident**

√x7th V12.5 **Pedal cycle passenger injured in collision with two- or three-wheeled motor vehicle in traffic accident**

√x7th V12.9 **Unspecified pedal cyclist injured in collision with two- or three-wheeled motor vehicle in traffic accident**

√4th **V13 Pedal cycle rider injured in collision with car, pick-up truck or van**

√x7th V13.0 **Pedal cycle driver injured in collision with car, pick-up truck or van in nontraffic accident**

√x7th V13.1 **Pedal cycle passenger injured in collision with car, pick-up truck or van in nontraffic accident**

√x7th V13.2 **Unspecified pedal cyclist injured in collision with car, pick-up truck or van in nontraffic accident**

√x7th V13.3 **Person boarding or alighting a pedal cycle injured in collision with car, pick-up truck or van**

√x7th V13.4 **Pedal cycle driver injured in collision with car, pick-up truck or van in traffic accident**

√x7th V13.5 **Pedal cycle passenger injured in collision with car, pick-up truck or van in traffic accident**

√x7th V13.9 **Unspecified pedal cyclist injured in collision with car, pick-up truck or van in traffic accident**

√4th **V14 Pedal cycle rider injured in collision with heavy transport vehicle or bus**

EXCLUDES 1 *pedal cycle rider injured in collision with military vehicle (V19.81)*

√x7th V14.0 **Pedal cycle driver injured in collision with heavy transport vehicle or bus in nontraffic accident**

√x7th V14.1 **Pedal cycle passenger injured in collision with heavy transport vehicle or bus in nontraffic accident**

√x7th V14.2 **Unspecified pedal cyclist injured in collision with heavy transport vehicle or bus in nontraffic accident**

√x7th V14.3 **Person boarding or alighting a pedal cycle injured in collision with heavy transport vehicle or bus**

√x7th V14.4 **Pedal cycle driver injured in collision with heavy transport vehicle or bus in traffic accident**

√x7th V14.5 **Pedal cycle passenger injured in collision with heavy transport vehicle or bus in traffic accident**

√x7th V14.9 **Unspecified pedal cyclist injured in collision with heavy transport vehicle or bus in traffic accident**

√4th **V15 Pedal cycle rider injured in collision with railway train or railway vehicle**

√x7th V15.0 **Pedal cycle driver injured in collision with railway train or railway vehicle in nontraffic accident**

√x7th V15.1 **Pedal cycle passenger injured in collision with railway train or railway vehicle in nontraffic accident**

√x7th V15.2 **Unspecified pedal cyclist injured in collision with railway train or railway vehicle in nontraffic accident**

√x7th V15.3 **Person boarding or alighting a pedal cycle injured in collision with railway train or railway vehicle**

√x7th V15.4 **Pedal cycle driver injured in collision with railway train or railway vehicle in traffic accident**

√x7th V15.5 **Pedal cycle passenger injured in collision with railway train or railway vehicle in traffic accident**

√x7th V15.9 **Unspecified pedal cyclist injured in collision with railway train or railway vehicle in traffic accident**

√4th **V16 Pedal cycle rider injured in collision with other nonmotor vehicle**

INCLUDES collision with animal-drawn vehicle, animal being ridden, streetcar

√x7th V16.0 **Pedal cycle driver injured in collision with other nonmotor vehicle in nontraffic accident**

√x7th V16.1 **Pedal cycle passenger injured in collision with other nonmotor vehicle in nontraffic accident**

√x7th V16.2 **Unspecified pedal cyclist injured in collision with other nonmotor vehicle in nontraffic accident**

√x7th V16.3 **Person boarding or alighting a pedal cycle injured in collision with other nonmotor vehicle in nontraffic accident**

√x7th V16.4 **Pedal cycle driver injured in collision with other nonmotor vehicle in traffic accident**

√x7th V16.5 **Pedal cycle passenger injured in collision with other nonmotor vehicle in traffic accident**

√x7th V16.9 **Unspecified pedal cyclist injured in collision with other nonmotor vehicle in traffic accident**

√4th **V17 Pedal cycle rider injured in collision with fixed or stationary object**

√x7th V17.0 **Pedal cycle driver injured in collision with fixed or stationary object in nontraffic accident**

√x7th V17.1 **Pedal cycle passenger injured in collision with fixed or stationary object in nontraffic accident**

√x7th V17.2 **Unspecified pedal cyclist injured in collision with fixed or stationary object in nontraffic accident**

√x7th V17.3 **Person boarding or alighting a pedal cycle injured in collision with fixed or stationary object**

√x7th V17.4 **Pedal cycle driver injured in collision with fixed or stationary object in traffic accident**

√x7th V17.5 **Pedal cycle passenger injured in collision with fixed or stationary object in traffic accident**

√x7th V17.9 **Unspecified pedal cyclist injured in collision with fixed or stationary object in traffic accident**

√4th **V18 Pedal cycle rider injured in noncollision transport accident**

INCLUDES fall or thrown from pedal cycle (without antecedent collision)
overturning pedal cycle NOS
overturning pedal cycle without collision

√x7th V18.0 **Pedal cycle driver injured in noncollision transport accident in nontraffic accident**

√x7th V18.1 **Pedal cycle passenger injured in noncollision transport accident in nontraffic accident**

√x7th V18.2 **Unspecified pedal cyclist injured in noncollision transport accident in nontraffic accident**

√x7th V18.3 **Person boarding or alighting a pedal cycle injured in noncollision transport accident**

√x7th V18.4 **Pedal cycle driver injured in noncollision transport accident in traffic accident**

√x7th V18.5 **Pedal cycle passenger injured in noncollision transport accident in traffic accident**

√x7th V18.9 **Unspecified pedal cyclist injured in noncollision transport accident in traffic accident**

√4th **V19 Pedal cycle rider injured in other and unspecified transport accidents**

√5th V19.0 **Pedal cycle driver injured in collision with other and unspecified motor vehicles in nontraffic accident**

√x7th V19.00 **Pedal cycle driver injured in collision with unspecified motor vehicles in nontraffic accident**

√x7th V19.09 **Pedal cycle driver injured in collision with other motor vehicles in nontraffic accident**

√5th V19.1 **Pedal cycle passenger injured in collision with other and unspecified motor vehicles in nontraffic accident**

√x7th V19.10 **Pedal cycle passenger injured in collision with unspecified motor vehicles in nontraffic accident**

√x7th V19.19 **Pedal cycle passenger injured in collision with other motor vehicles in nontraffic accident**

√5th V19.2 **Unspecified pedal cyclist injured in collision with other and unspecified motor vehicles in nontraffic accident**

√x7th V19.20 **Unspecified pedal cyclist injured in collision with unspecified motor vehicles in nontraffic accident**
Pedal cycle collision NOS, nontraffic

√x7th V19.29 **Unspecified pedal cyclist injured in collision with other motor vehicles in nontraffic accident**

√x7th V19.3 **Pedal cyclist (driver) (passenger) injured in unspecified nontraffic accident**
Pedal cycle accident NOS, nontraffic
Pedal cyclist injured in nontraffic accident NOS

√5th V19.4 **Pedal cycle driver injured in collision with other and unspecified motor vehicles in traffic accident**

√x7th V19.40 **Pedal cycle driver injured in collision with unspecified motor vehicles in traffic accident**

V19.49 Pedal cycle driver injured in collision with other motor vehicles in traffic accident

V19.5 Pedal cycle passenger injured in collision with other and unspecified motor vehicles in traffic accident

V19.50 Pedal cycle passenger injured in collision with unspecified motor vehicles in traffic accident

V19.59 Pedal cycle passenger injured in collision with other motor vehicles in traffic accident

V19.6 Unspecified pedal cyclist injured in collision with other and unspecified motor vehicles in traffic accident

V19.60 Unspecified pedal cyclist injured in collision with unspecified motor vehicles in traffic accident
Pedal cycle collision NOS (traffic)

V19.69 Unspecified pedal cyclist injured in collision with other motor vehicles in traffic accident

V19.8 Pedal cyclist (driver) (passenger) injured in other specified transport accidents

V19.81 Pedal cyclist (driver) (passenger) injured in transport accident with military vehicle

V19.88 Pedal cyclist (driver) (passenger) injured in other specified transport accidents

V19.9 Pedal cyclist (driver) (passenger) injured in unspecified traffic accident
Pedal cycle accident NOS

Motorcycle rider injured in transport accident (V20-V29)

INCLUDES electric bicycle
e-bike
e-bicycle
moped
motorcycle with sidecar
motorized bicycle
motor scooter

EXCLUDES 1 *three-wheeled motor vehicle (V30-V39)*

AHA: 2022,4Q,47

The appropriate 7th character is to be added to each code from categories V20-V29.
A initial encounter
D subsequent encounter
S sequela

V20 Motorcycle rider injured in collision with pedestrian or animal

EXCLUDES 1 *motorcycle rider collision with animal-drawn vehicle or animal being ridden (V26.-)*

V20.0 Motorcycle driver injured in collision with pedestrian or animal in nontraffic accident

V20.01 Electric (assisted) bicycle driver injured in collision with pedestrian or animal in nontraffic accident

V20.09 Other motorcycle driver injured in collision with pedestrian or animal in nontraffic accident

V20.1 Motorcycle passenger injured in collision with pedestrian or animal in nontraffic accident

V20.11 Electric (assisted) bicycle passenger injured in collision with pedestrian or animal in nontraffic accident

V20.19 Other motorcycle passenger injured in collision with pedestrian or animal in nontraffic accident

V20.2 Unspecified motorcycle rider injured in collision with pedestrian or animal in nontraffic accident

V20.21 Unspecified electric (assisted) bicycle rider injured in collision with pedestrian or animal in nontraffic accident

V20.29 Unspecified rider of other motorcycle injured in collision with pedestrian or animal in nontraffic accident

V20.3 Person boarding or alighting a motorcycle injured in collision with pedestrian or animal

V20.31 Person boarding or alighting an electric (assisted) bicycle injured in collision with pedestrian or animal

V20.39 Person boarding or alighting other motorcycle injured in collision with pedestrian or animal

V20.4 Motorcycle driver injured in collision with pedestrian or animal in traffic accident

V20.41 Electric (assisted) bicycle driver injured in collision with pedestrian or animal in traffic accident

V20.49 Other motorcycle driver injured in collision with pedestrian or animal in traffic accident

V20.5 Motorcycle passenger injured in collision with pedestrian or animal in traffic accident

V20.51 Electric (assisted) bicycle passenger injured in collision with pedestrian or animal in traffic accident

V20.59 Other motorcycle passenger injured in collision with pedestrian or animal in traffic accident

V20.9 Unspecified motorcycle rider injured in collision with pedestrian or animal in traffic accident

V20.91 Unspecified electric (assisted) bicycle rider injured in collision with pedestrian or animal in traffic accident

V20.99 Unspecified rider of other motorcycle injured in collision with pedestrian or animal in traffic accident

V21 Motorcycle rider injured in collision with pedal cycle

V21.0 Motorcycle driver injured in collision with pedal cycle in nontraffic accident

V21.01 Electric (assisted) bicycle driver injured in collision with pedal cycle in nontraffic accident

V21.09 Other motorcycle driver injured in collision with pedal cycle in nontraffic accident

V21.1 Motorcycle passenger injured in collision with pedal cycle in nontraffic accident

V21.11 Electric (assisted) bicycle passenger injured in collision with pedal cycle in nontraffic accident

V21.19 Other motorcycle passenger injured in collision with pedal cycle in nontraffic accident

V21.2 Unspecified motorcycle rider injured in collision with pedal cycle in nontraffic accident

V21.21 Unspecified electric (assisted) bicycle rider injured in collision with pedal cycle in nontraffic accident

V21.29 Unspecified rider of other motorcycle injured in collision with pedal cycle in nontraffic accident

V21.3 Person boarding or alighting a motorcycle injured in collision with pedal cycle

V21.31 Person boarding or alighting an electric (assisted) bicycle injured in collision with pedal cycle

V21.39 Person boarding or alighting other motorcycle injured in collision with pedal cycle

V21.4 Motorcycle driver injured in collision with pedal cycle in traffic accident

V21.41 Electric (assisted) bicycle driver injured in collision with pedal cycle in traffic accident

V21.49 Other motorcycle driver injured in collision with pedal cycle in traffic accident

V21.5 Motorcycle passenger injured in collision with pedal cycle in traffic accident

V21.51 Electric (assisted) bicycle passenger injured in collision with pedal cycle in traffic accident

V21.59 Other motorcycle passenger injured in collision with pedal cycle in traffic accident

V21.9 Unspecified motorcycle rider injured in collision with pedal cycle in traffic accident

V21.91 Unspecified electric (assisted) bicycle rider injured in collision with pedal cycle in traffic accident

V21.99 Unspecified rider of other motorcycle injured in collision with pedal cycle in traffic accident

V22 Motorcycle rider injured in collision with two- or three-wheeled motor vehicle

V22.0 Motorcycle driver injured in collision with two- or three-wheeled motor vehicle in nontraffic accident

V22.01 Electric (assisted) bicycle driver injured in collision with two- or three-wheeled motor vehicle in nontraffic accident

V22.09 Other motorcycle driver injured in collision with two- or three-wheeled motor vehicle in nontraffic accident

V22.1 Motorcycle passenger injured in collision with two- or three-wheeled motor vehicle in nontraffic accident

V22.11 Electric (assisted) bicycle passenger injured in collision with two- or three-wheeled motor vehicle in nontraffic accident

V22.19 Other motorcycle passenger injured in collision with two- or three-wheeled motor vehicle in nontraffic accident

V22.2 Unspecified motorcycle rider injured in collision with two- or three-wheeled motor vehicle in nontraffic accident

V22.21 Unspecified electric (assisted) bicycle rider injured in collision with two- or three-wheeled motor vehicle in nontraffic accident

V22.29 Unspecified rider of other motorcycle injured in collision with two- or three-wheeled motor vehicle in nontraffic accident

V22.3 Person boarding or alighting a motorcycle injured in collision with two- or three-wheeled motor vehicle

V22.31 Person boarding or alighting an electric (assisted) bicycle injured in collision with two- or three-wheeled motor vehicle

√x7th **V22.39** Person boarding or alighting other motorcycle injured in collision with two- or three-wheeled motor vehicle

√5th **V22.4** Motorcycle driver injured in collision with two- or three-wheeled motor vehicle in traffic accident

√x7th **V22.41** Electric (assisted) bicycle driver injured in collision with two- or three-wheeled motor vehicle in traffic accident

√x7th **V22.49** Other motorcycle driver injured in collision with two- or three-wheeled motor vehicle in traffic accident

√5th **V22.5** Motorcycle passenger injured in collision with two- or three-wheeled motor vehicle in traffic accident

√x7th **V22.51** Electric (assisted) bicycle passenger injured in collision with two- or three-wheeled motor vehicle in traffic accident

√x7th **V22.59** Other motorcycle passenger injured in collision with two- or three-wheeled motor vehicle in traffic accident

√5th **V22.9** Unspecified motorcycle rider injured in collision with two- or three-wheeled motor vehicle in traffic accident

√x7th **V22.91** Unspecified electric (assisted) bicycle rider injured in collision with two- or three-wheeled motor vehicle in traffic accident

√x7th **V22.99** Unspecified rider of other motorcycle injured in collision with two- or three-wheeled motor vehicle in traffic accident

√4th **V23 Motorcycle rider injured in collision with car, pick-up truck or van**

√5th **V23.Ø** Motorcycle driver injured in collision with car, pick-up truck or van in nontraffic accident

√x7th **V23.Ø1** Electric (assisted) bicycle driver injured in collision with car, pick-up truck or van in nontraffic accident

√x7th **V23.Ø9** Other motorcycle driver injured in collision with car, pick-up truck or van in nontraffic accident

√5th **V23.1** Motorcycle passenger injured in collision with car, pick-up truck or van in nontraffic accident

√x7th **V23.11** Electric (assisted) bicycle passenger injured in collision with car, pick-up truck or van in nontraffic accident

√x7th **V23.19** Other motorcycle passenger injured in collision with car, pick-up truck or van in nontraffic accident

√5th **V23.2** Unspecified motorcycle rider injured in collision with car, pick-up truck or van in nontraffic accident

√x7th **V23.21** Unspecified electric (assisted) bicycle rider injured in collision with car, pick-up truck or van in nontraffic accident

√x7th **V23.29** Unspecified rider of other motorcycle injured in collision with car, pick-up truck or van in nontraffic accident

√5th **V23.3** Person boarding or alighting a motorcycle injured in collision with car, pick-up truck or van

√x7th **V23.31** Person boarding or alighting an electric (assisted) bicycle injured in collision with car, pick-up truck or van

√x7th **V23.39** Person boarding or alighting other motorcycle injured in collision with car, pick-up truck or van

√5th **V23.4** Motorcycle driver injured in collision with car, pick-up truck or van in traffic accident

√x7th **V23.41** Electric (assisted) bicycle driver injured in collision with car, pick-up truck or van in traffic accident

√x7th **V23.49** Other motorcycle driver injured in collision with car, pick-up truck or van in traffic accident

√5th **V23.5** Motorcycle passenger injured in collision with car, pick-up truck or van in traffic accident

√x7th **V23.51** Electric (assisted) bicycle passenger injured in collision with car, pick-up truck or van in traffic accident

√x7th **V23.59** Other motorcycle passenger injured in collision with car, pick-up truck or van in traffic accident

√5th **V23.9** Unspecified motorcycle rider injured in collision with car, pick-up truck or van in traffic accident

√x7th **V23.91** Unspecified electric (assisted) bicycle rider injured in collision with car, pick-up truck or van in traffic accident

√x7th **V23.99** Unspecified rider of other motorcycle injured in collision with car, pick-up truck or van in traffic accident

√4th **V24 Motorcycle rider injured in collision with heavy transport vehicle or bus**

EXCLUDES 1 *motorcycle rider injured in collision with military vehicle (V29.818)*

√5th **V24.Ø** Motorcycle driver injured in collision with heavy transport vehicle or bus in nontraffic accident

√x7th **V24.Ø1** Electric (assisted) bicycle driver injured in collision with heavy transport vehicle or bus in nontraffic accident

√x7th **V24.Ø9** Other motorcycle driver injured in collision with heavy transport vehicle or bus in nontraffic accident

√5th **V24.1** Motorcycle passenger injured in collision with heavy transport vehicle or bus in nontraffic accident

√x7th **V24.11** Electric (assisted) bicycle passenger injured in collision with heavy transport vehicle or bus in nontraffic accident

√x7th **V24.19** Other motorcycle passenger injured in collision with heavy transport vehicle or bus in nontraffic accident

√5th **V24.2** Unspecified motorcycle rider injured in collision with heavy transport vehicle or bus in nontraffic accident

√x7th **V24.21** Unspecified electric (assisted) bicycle rider injured in collision with heavy transport vehicle or bus in nontraffic accident

√x7th **V24.29** Unspecified rider of other motorcycle injured in collision with heavy transport vehicle or bus in nontraffic accident

√5th **V24.3** Person boarding or alighting a motorcycle injured in collision with heavy transport vehicle or bus

√x7th **V24.31** Person boarding or alighting an electric (assisted) bicycle injured in collision with heavy transport vehicle or bus

√x7th **V24.39** Person boarding or alighting other motorcycle injured in collision with heavy transport vehicle or bus

√5th **V24.4** Motorcycle driver injured in collision with heavy transport vehicle or bus in traffic accident

√x7th **V24.41** Electric (assisted) bicycle driver injured in collision with heavy transport vehicle or bus in traffic accident

√x7th **V24.49** Other motorcycle driver injured in collision with heavy transport vehicle or bus in traffic accident

√5th **V24.5** Motorcycle passenger injured in collision with heavy transport vehicle or bus in traffic accident

√x7th **V24.51** Electric (assisted) bicycle passenger injured in collision with heavy transport vehicle or bus in traffic accident

√x7th **V24.59** Other motorcycle passenger injured in collision with heavy transport vehicle or bus in traffic accident

√5th **V24.9** Unspecified motorcycle rider injured in collision with heavy transport vehicle or bus in traffic accident

√x7th **V24.91** Unspecified electric (assisted) bicycle rider injured in collision with heavy transport vehicle or bus in traffic accident

√x7th **V24.99** Unspecified rider of other motorcycle injured in collision with heavy transport vehicle or bus in traffic accident

√4th **V25 Motorcycle rider injured in collision with railway train or railway vehicle**

√5th **V25.Ø** Motorcycle driver injured in collision with railway train or railway vehicle in nontraffic accident

√x7th **V25.Ø1** Electric (assisted) bicycle driver injured in collision with railway train or railway vehicle in nontraffic accident

√x7th **V25.Ø9** Other motorcycle driver injured in collision with railway train or railway vehicle in nontraffic accident

√5th **V25.1** Motorcycle passenger injured in collision with railway train or railway vehicle in nontraffic accident

√x7th **V25.11** Electric (assisted) bicycle passenger injured in collision with railway train or railway vehicle in nontraffic accident

√x7th **V25.19** Other motorcycle passenger injured in collision with railway train or railway vehicle in nontraffic accident

√5th **V25.2** Unspecified motorcycle rider injured in collision with railway train or railway vehicle in nontraffic accident

√x7th **V25.21** Unspecified electric (assisted) bicycle rider injured in collision with railway train or railway vehicle in nontraffic accident

V25.29 Unspecified rider of other motorcycle injured in collision with railway train or railway vehicle in nontraffic accident

V25.3 Person boarding or alighting a motorcycle injured in collision with railway train or railway vehicle

V25.31 Person boarding or alighting an electric (assisted) bicycle injured in collision with railway train or railway vehicle

V25.39 Person boarding or alighting other motorcycle injured in collision with railway train or railway vehicle

V25.4 Motorcycle driver injured in collision with railway train or railway vehicle in traffic accident

V25.41 Electric (assisted) bicycle driver injured in collision with railway train or railway vehicle in traffic accident

V25.49 Other motorcycle driver injured in collision with railway train or railway vehicle in traffic accident

V25.5 Motorcycle passenger injured in collision with railway train or railway vehicle in traffic accident

V25.51 Electric (assisted) bicycle passenger injured in collision with railway train or railway vehicle in traffic accident

V25.59 Other motorcycle passenger injured in collision with railway train or railway vehicle in traffic accident

V25.9 Unspecified motorcycle rider injured in collision with railway train or railway vehicle in traffic accident

V25.91 Unspecified electric (assisted) bicycle rider injured in collision with railway train or railway vehicle in traffic accident

V25.99 Unspecified rider of other motorcycle injured in collision with railway train or railway vehicle in traffic accident

V26 Motorcycle rider injured in collision with other nonmotor vehicle

INCLUDES collision with animal-drawn vehicle, animal being ridden, streetcar

V26.0 Motorcycle driver injured in collision with other nonmotor vehicle in nontraffic accident

V26.01 Electric (assisted) bicycle driver injured in collision with other nonmotor vehicle in nontraffic accident

V26.09 Other motorcycle driver injured in collision with other nonmotor vehicle in nontraffic accident

V26.1 Motorcycle passenger injured in collision with other nonmotor vehicle in nontraffic accident

V26.11 Electric (assisted) bicycle passenger injured in collision with other nonmotor vehicle in nontraffic accident

V26.19 Other motorcycle passenger injured in collision with other nonmotor vehicle in nontraffic accident

V26.2 Unspecified motorcycle rider injured in collision with other nonmotor vehicle in nontraffic accident

V26.21 Unspecified electric (assisted) bicycle rider injured in collision with other nonmotor vehicle in nontraffic accident

V26.29 Unspecified rider of other motorcycle injured in collision with other nonmotor vehicle in nontraffic accident

V26.3 Person boarding or alighting a motorcycle injured in collision with other nonmotor vehicle

V26.31 Person boarding or alighting an electric (assisted) bicycle injured in collision with other nonmotor vehicle

V26.39 Person boarding or alighting other motorcycle injured in collision with other nonmotor vehicle

V26.4 Motorcycle driver injured in collision with other nonmotor vehicle in traffic accident

V26.41 Electric (assisted) bicycle driver injured in collision with other nonmotor vehicle in traffic accident

V26.49 Other motorcycle driver injured in collision with other nonmotor vehicle in traffic accident

V26.5 Motorcycle passenger injured in collision with other nonmotor vehicle in traffic accident

V26.51 Electric (assisted) bicycle passenger injured in collision with other nonmotor vehicle in traffic accident

V26.59 Other motorcycle passenger injured in collision with other nonmotor vehicle in traffic accident

V26.9 Unspecified motorcycle rider injured in collision with other nonmotor vehicle in traffic accident

V26.91 Unspecified electric (assisted) bicycle rider injured in collision with other nonmotor vehicle in traffic accident

V26.99 Unspecified rider of other motorcycle injured in collision with other nonmotor vehicle in traffic accident

V27 Motorcycle rider injured in collision with fixed or stationary object

V27.0 Motorcycle driver injured in collision with fixed or stationary object in nontraffic accident

V27.01 Electric (assisted) bicycle driver injured in collision with fixed or stationary object in nontraffic accident

V27.09 Other motorcycle driver injured in collision with fixed or stationary object in nontraffic accident

V27.1 Motorcycle passenger injured in collision with fixed or stationary object in nontraffic accident

V27.11 Electric (assisted) bicycle passenger injured in collision with fixed or stationary object in nontraffic accident

V27.19 Other motorcycle passenger injured in collision with fixed or stationary object in nontraffic accident

V27.2 Unspecified motorcycle rider injured in collision with fixed or stationary object in nontraffic accident

V27.21 Unspecified electric (assisted) bicycle rider injured in collision with fixed or stationary object in nontraffic accident

V27.29 Unspecified rider of other motorcycle injured in collision with fixed or stationary object in nontraffic accident

V27.3 Person boarding or alighting a motorcycle injured in collision with fixed or stationary object

V27.31 Person boarding or alighting an electric (assisted) bicycle injured in collision with fixed or stationary object

V27.39 Person boarding or alighting other motorcycle injured in collision with fixed or stationary object

V27.4 Motorcycle driver injured in collision with fixed or stationary object in traffic accident

V27.41 Electric (assisted) bicycle driver injured in collision with fixed or stationary object in traffic accident

V27.49 Other motorcycle driver injured in collision with fixed or stationary object in traffic accident

V27.5 Motorcycle passenger injured in collision with fixed or stationary object in traffic accident

V27.51 Electric (assisted) bicycle passenger injured in collision with fixed or stationary object in traffic accident

V27.59 Other motorcycle passenger injured in collision with fixed or stationary object in traffic accident

V27.9 Unspecified motorcycle rider injured in collision with fixed or stationary object in traffic accident

V27.91 Unspecified electric (assisted) bicycle rider injured in collision with fixed or stationary object in traffic accident

V27.99 Unspecified rider of other motorcycle injured in collision with fixed or stationary object in traffic accident

V28 Motorcycle rider injured in noncollision transport accident

INCLUDES fall or thrown from motorcycle (without antecedent collision)
overturning motorcycle NOS
overturning motorcycle without collision

V28.0 Motorcycle driver injured in noncollision transport accident in nontraffic accident

V28.01 Electric (assisted) bicycle driver injured in noncollision transport accident in nontraffic accident

V28.09 Other motorcycle driver injured in noncollision transport accident in nontraffic accident

V28.1 Motorcycle passenger injured in noncollision transport accident in nontraffic accident

V28.11 Electric (assisted) bicycle passenger injured in noncollision transport accident in nontraffic accident

V28.19 Other motorcycle passenger injured in noncollision transport accident in nontraffic accident

V28.2 Unspecified motorcycle rider injured in noncollision transport accident in nontraffic accident

V28.21 Unspecified electric (assisted) bicycle rider injured in noncollision transport accident in nontraffic accident

V28.29 Unspecified rider of other motorcycle injured in noncollision transport accident in nontraffic accident

5th **V28.3** **Person boarding or alighting a motorcycle injured in noncollision transport accident**
- √x7th **V28.31** **Person boarding or alighting an electric (assisted) bicycle injured in noncollision transport accident**
- √x7th **V28.39** **Person boarding or alighting other motorcycle injured in noncollision transport accident**

5th **V28.4** **Motorcycle driver injured in noncollision transport accident in traffic accident**
- √x7th **V28.41** **Electric (assisted) bicycle driver injured in noncollision transport accident in traffic accident**
- √x7th **V28.49** **Other motorcycle driver injured in noncollision transport accident in traffic accident**

5th **V28.5** **Motorcycle passenger injured in noncollision transport accident in traffic accident**
- √x7th **V28.51** **Electric (assisted) bicycle passenger injured in noncollision transport accident in traffic accident**
- √x7th **V28.59** **Other motorcycle passenger injured in noncollision transport accident in traffic accident**

5th **V28.9** **Unspecified motorcycle rider injured in noncollision transport accident in traffic accident**
- √x7th **V28.91** **Unspecified electric (assisted) bicycle rider injured in noncollision transport accident in traffic accident**
- √x7th **V28.99** **Unspecified rider of other motorcycle injured in noncollision transport accident in traffic accident**

4th **V29** **Motorcycle rider injured in other and unspecified transport accidents**

5th **V29.0** **Motorcycle driver injured in collision with other and unspecified motor vehicles in nontraffic accident**
- 6th **V29.00** **Motorcycle driver injured in collision with unspecified motor vehicles in nontraffic accident**
  - 7th **V29.001** **Electric (assisted) bicycle driver injured in collision with unspecified motor vehicles in nontraffic accident**
  - 7th **V29.008** **Other motorcycle driver injured in collision with unspecified motor vehicles in nontraffic accident**
- 6th **V29.09** **Motorcycle driver injured in collision with other motor vehicles in nontraffic accident**
  - 7th **V29.091** **Electric (assisted) bicycle driver injured in collision with other motor vehicles in nontraffic accident**
  - 7th **V29.098** **Other motorcycle driver injured in collision with other motor vehicles in nontraffic accident**

5th **V29.1** **Motorcycle passenger injured in collision with other and unspecified motor vehicles in nontraffic accident**
- 6th **V29.10** **Motorcycle passenger injured in collision with unspecified motor vehicles in nontraffic accident**
  - 7th **V29.101** **Electric (assisted) bicycle passenger injured in collision with unspecified motor vehicles in nontraffic accident**
  - 7th **V29.108** **Other motorcycle passenger injured in collision with unspecified motor vehicles in nontraffic accident**
- 6th **V29.19** **Motorcycle passenger injured in collision with other motor vehicles in nontraffic accident**
  - 7th **V29.191** **Electric (assisted) bicycle passenger injured in collision with other motor vehicles in nontraffic accident**
  - 7th **V29.198** **Other motorcycle passenger injured in collision with other motor vehicles in nontraffic accident**

5th **V29.2** **Unspecified motorcycle rider injured in collision with other and unspecified motor vehicles in nontraffic accident**
- 6th **V29.20** **Unspecified motorcycle rider injured in collision with unspecified motor vehicles in nontraffic accident**
  - 7th **V29.201** **Unspecified electric (assisted) bicycle rider injured in collision with unspecified motor vehicles in nontraffic accident**
  - 7th **V29.208** **Unspecified rider of other motorcycle injured in collision with unspecified motor vehicles in nontraffic accident**
    Motorcycle collision NOS, nontraffic
- 6th **V29.29** **Unspecified motorcycle rider injured in collision with other motor vehicles in nontraffic accident**
  - 7th **V29.291** **Unspecified electric (assisted) bicycle rider injured in collision with other motor vehicles in nontraffic accident**
  - 7th **V29.298** **Unspecified rider of other motorcycle injured in collision with other motor vehicles in nontraffic accident**

5th **V29.3** **Motorcycle rider (driver) (passenger) injured in unspecified nontraffic accident**
- √x7th **V29.31** **Electric (assisted) bicycle (driver) (passenger) injured in unspecified nontraffic accident**
- √x7th **V29.39** **Other motorcycle (driver) (passenger) injured in unspecified nontraffic accident**
  Motorcycle accident NOS, nontraffic
  Motorcycle rider injured in nontraffic accident NOS

5th **V29.4** **Motorcycle driver injured in collision with other and unspecified motor vehicles in traffic accident**
- 6th **V29.40** **Motorcycle driver injured in collision with unspecified motor vehicles in traffic accident**
  - 7th **V29.401** **Electric (assisted) bicycle driver injured in collision with unspecified motor vehicles in traffic accident**
  - 7th **V29.408** **Other motorcycle driver injured in collision with unspecified motor vehicles in traffic accident**
- 6th **V29.49** **Motorcycle driver injured in collision with other motor vehicles in traffic accident**
  - 7th **V29.491** **Electric (assisted) bicycle driver injured in collision with other motor vehicles in traffic accident**
  - 7th **V29.498** **Other motorcycle driver injured in collision with other motor vehicles in traffic accident**

5th **V29.5** **Motorcycle passenger injured in collision with other and unspecified motor vehicles in traffic accident**
- 6th **V29.50** **Motorcycle passenger injured in collision with unspecified motor vehicles in traffic accident**
  - 7th **V29.501** **Electric (assisted) bicycle passenger injured in collision with unspecified motor vehicles in traffic accident**
  - 7th **V29.508** **Other motorcycle passenger injured in collision with unspecified motor vehicles in traffic accident**
- 6th **V29.59** **Motorcycle passenger injured in collision with other motor vehicles in traffic accident**
  - 7th **V29.591** **Electric (assisted) bicycle passenger injured in collision with other motor vehicles in traffic accident**
  - 7th **V29.598** **Other motorcycle passenger injured in collision with other motor vehicles in traffic accident**

5th **V29.6** **Unspecified motorcycle rider injured in collision with other and unspecified motor vehicles in traffic accident**
- 6th **V29.60** **Unspecified motorcycle rider injured in collision with unspecified motor vehicles in traffic accident**
  - 7th **V29.601** **Unspecified electric (assisted) bicycle rider injured in collision with unspecified motor vehicles in traffic accident**
  - 7th **V29.608** **Unspecified rider of other motorcycle injured in collision with unspecified motor vehicles in traffic accident**
    Motorcycle collision NOS (traffic)
- 6th **V29.69** **Unspecified motorcycle rider injured in collision with other motor vehicles in traffic accident**
  - 7th **V29.691** **Unspecified electric (assisted) bicycle rider injured in collision with other motor vehicles in traffic accident**
  - 7th **V29.698** **Unspecified rider of other motorcycle injured in collision with other motor vehicles in traffic accident**

5th **V29.8** **Motorcycle rider (driver) (passenger) injured in other specified transport accidents**
- 6th **V29.81** **Motorcycle rider (driver) (passenger) injured in transport accident with military vehicle**
  - 7th **V29.811** **Electric (assisted) bicycle rider (driver) (passenger) injured in transport accident with military vehicle**
  - 7th **V29.818** **Rider (driver) (passenger) of other motorcycle injured in transport accident with military vehicle**
- 6th **V29.88** **Motorcycle rider (driver) (passenger) injured in other specified transport accidents**
  - 7th **V29.881** **Electric (assisted) bicycle rider (driver) (passenger) injured in other specified transport accidents**
  - 7th **V29.888** **Rider (driver) (passenger) of other motorcycle injured in other specified transport accidents**

5th **V29.9 Motorcycle rider (driver) (passenger) injured in unspecified traffic accident**

x7th **V29.91 Electric (assisted) bicycle rider (driver) (passenger) injured in unspecified traffic accident**

x7th **V29.99 Rider (driver) (passenger) of other motorcycle injured in unspecified traffic accident**
Motorcycle accident NOS

Occupant of three-wheeled motor vehicle injured in transport accident (V30-V39)

INCLUDES motorized tricycle
motorized rickshaw
three-wheeled motor car

EXCLUDES 1 *all-terrain vehicles (V86.-)*
motorcycle with sidecar (V20-V29)
vehicle designed primarily for off-road use (V86.-)

The appropriate 7th character is to be added to each code from categories V30-V39.
A initial encounter
D subsequent encounter
S sequela

4th **V30 Occupant of three-wheeled motor vehicle injured in collision with pedestrian or animal**
EXCLUDES 1 *three-wheeled motor vehicle collision with animal-drawn vehicle or animal being ridden (V36.-)*

x7th **V30.0 Driver of three-wheeled motor vehicle injured in collision with pedestrian or animal in nontraffic accident**

x7th **V30.1 Passenger in three-wheeled motor vehicle injured in collision with pedestrian or animal in nontraffic accident**

x7th **V30.2 Person on outside of three-wheeled motor vehicle injured in collision with pedestrian or animal in nontraffic accident**

x7th **V30.3 Unspecified occupant of three-wheeled motor vehicle injured in collision with pedestrian or animal in nontraffic accident**

x7th **V30.4 Person boarding or alighting a three-wheeled motor vehicle injured in collision with pedestrian or animal**

x7th **V30.5 Driver of three-wheeled motor vehicle injured in collision with pedestrian or animal in traffic accident**

x7th **V30.6 Passenger in three-wheeled motor vehicle injured in collision with pedestrian or animal in traffic accident**

x7th **V30.7 Person on outside of three-wheeled motor vehicle injured in collision with pedestrian or animal in traffic accident**

x7th **V30.9 Unspecified occupant of three-wheeled motor vehicle injured in collision with pedestrian or animal in traffic accident**

4th **V31 Occupant of three-wheeled motor vehicle injured in collision with pedal cycle**

x7th **V31.0 Driver of three-wheeled motor vehicle injured in collision with pedal cycle in nontraffic accident**

x7th **V31.1 Passenger in three-wheeled motor vehicle injured in collision with pedal cycle in nontraffic accident**

x7th **V31.2 Person on outside of three-wheeled motor vehicle injured in collision with pedal cycle in nontraffic accident**

x7th **V31.3 Unspecified occupant of three-wheeled motor vehicle injured in collision with pedal cycle in nontraffic accident**

x7th **V31.4 Person boarding or alighting a three-wheeled motor vehicle injured in collision with pedal cycle**

x7th **V31.5 Driver of three-wheeled motor vehicle injured in collision with pedal cycle in traffic accident**

x7th **V31.6 Passenger in three-wheeled motor vehicle injured in collision with pedal cycle in traffic accident**

x7th **V31.7 Person on outside of three-wheeled motor vehicle injured in collision with pedal cycle in traffic accident**

x7th **V31.9 Unspecified occupant of three-wheeled motor vehicle injured in collision with pedal cycle in traffic accident**

4th **V32 Occupant of three-wheeled motor vehicle injured in collision with two- or three-wheeled motor vehicle**

x7th **V32.0 Driver of three-wheeled motor vehicle injured in collision with two- or three-wheeled motor vehicle in nontraffic accident**

x7th **V32.1 Passenger in three-wheeled motor vehicle injured in collision with two- or three-wheeled motor vehicle in nontraffic accident**

x7th **V32.2 Person on outside of three-wheeled motor vehicle injured in collision with two- or three-wheeled motor vehicle in nontraffic accident**

x7th **V32.3 Unspecified occupant of three-wheeled motor vehicle injured in collision with two- or three-wheeled motor vehicle in nontraffic accident**

x7th **V32.4 Person boarding or alighting a three-wheeled motor vehicle injured in collision with two- or three-wheeled motor vehicle**

x7th **V32.5 Driver of three-wheeled motor vehicle injured in collision with two- or three-wheeled motor vehicle in traffic accident**

x7th **V32.6 Passenger in three-wheeled motor vehicle injured in collision with two- or three-wheeled motor vehicle in traffic accident**

x7th **V32.7 Person on outside of three-wheeled motor vehicle injured in collision with two- or three-wheeled motor vehicle in traffic accident**

x7th **V32.9 Unspecified occupant of three-wheeled motor vehicle injured in collision with two- or three-wheeled motor vehicle in traffic accident**

4th **V33 Occupant of three-wheeled motor vehicle injured in collision with car, pick-up truck or van**

x7th **V33.0 Driver of three-wheeled motor vehicle injured in collision with car, pick-up truck or van in nontraffic accident**

x7th **V33.1 Passenger in three-wheeled motor vehicle injured in collision with car, pick-up truck or van in nontraffic accident**

x7th **V33.2 Person on outside of three-wheeled motor vehicle injured in collision with car, pick-up truck or van in nontraffic accident**

x7th **V33.3 Unspecified occupant of three-wheeled motor vehicle injured in collision with car, pick-up truck or van in nontraffic accident**

x7th **V33.4 Person boarding or alighting a three-wheeled motor vehicle injured in collision with car, pick-up truck or van**

x7th **V33.5 Driver of three-wheeled motor vehicle injured in collision with car, pick-up truck or van in traffic accident**

x7th **V33.6 Passenger in three-wheeled motor vehicle injured in collision with car, pick-up truck or van in traffic accident**

x7th **V33.7 Person on outside of three-wheeled motor vehicle injured in collision with car, pick-up truck or van in traffic accident**

x7th **V33.9 Unspecified occupant of three-wheeled motor vehicle injured in collision with car, pick-up truck or van in traffic accident**

4th **V34 Occupant of three-wheeled motor vehicle injured in collision with heavy transport vehicle or bus**
EXCLUDES 1 *occupant of three-wheeled motor vehicle injured in collision with military vehicle (V39.81)*

x7th **V34.0 Driver of three-wheeled motor vehicle injured in collision with heavy transport vehicle or bus in nontraffic accident**

x7th **V34.1 Passenger in three-wheeled motor vehicle injured in collision with heavy transport vehicle or bus in nontraffic accident**

x7th **V34.2 Person on outside of three-wheeled motor vehicle injured in collision with heavy transport vehicle or bus in nontraffic accident**

x7th **V34.3 Unspecified occupant of three-wheeled motor vehicle injured in collision with heavy transport vehicle or bus in nontraffic accident**

x7th **V34.4 Person boarding or alighting a three-wheeled motor vehicle injured in collision with heavy transport vehicle or bus**

x7th **V34.5 Driver of three-wheeled motor vehicle injured in collision with heavy transport vehicle or bus in traffic accident**

x7th **V34.6 Passenger in three-wheeled motor vehicle injured in collision with heavy transport vehicle or bus in traffic accident**

x7th **V34.7 Person on outside of three-wheeled motor vehicle injured in collision with heavy transport vehicle or bus in traffic accident**

x7th **V34.9 Unspecified occupant of three-wheeled motor vehicle injured in collision with heavy transport vehicle or bus in traffic accident**

4th **V35 Occupant of three-wheeled motor vehicle injured in collision with railway train or railway vehicle**

x7th **V35.0 Driver of three-wheeled motor vehicle injured in collision with railway train or railway vehicle in nontraffic accident**

x7th **V35.1 Passenger in three-wheeled motor vehicle injured in collision with railway train or railway vehicle in nontraffic accident**

x7th **V35.2 Person on outside of three-wheeled motor vehicle injured in collision with railway train or railway vehicle in nontraffic accident**

x7th **V35.3 Unspecified occupant of three-wheeled motor vehicle injured in collision with railway train or railway vehicle in nontraffic accident**

x7th **V35.4 Person boarding or alighting a three-wheeled motor vehicle injured in collision with railway train or railway vehicle**

x7th **V35.5 Driver of three-wheeled motor vehicle injured in collision with railway train or railway vehicle in traffic accident**

x7th **V35.6 Passenger in three-wheeled motor vehicle injured in collision with railway train or railway vehicle in traffic accident**

x7th **V35.7 Person on outside of three-wheeled motor vehicle injured in collision with railway train or railway vehicle in traffic accident**

x7th **V35.9 Unspecified occupant of three-wheeled motor vehicle injured in collision with railway train or railway vehicle in traffic accident**

V36 Occupant of three-wheeled motor vehicle injured in collision with other nonmotor vehicle

INCLUDES collision with animal-drawn vehicle, animal being ridden, streetcar

V36.0 Driver of three-wheeled motor vehicle injured in collision with other nonmotor vehicle in nontraffic accident

V36.1 Passenger in three-wheeled motor vehicle injured in collision with other nonmotor vehicle in nontraffic accident

V36.2 Person on outside of three-wheeled motor vehicle injured in collision with other nonmotor vehicle in nontraffic accident

V36.3 Unspecified occupant of three-wheeled motor vehicle injured in collision with other nonmotor vehicle in nontraffic accident

V36.4 Person boarding or alighting a three-wheeled motor vehicle injured in collision with other nonmotor vehicle

V36.5 Driver of three-wheeled motor vehicle injured in collision with other nonmotor vehicle in traffic accident

V36.6 Passenger in three-wheeled motor vehicle injured in collision with other nonmotor vehicle in traffic accident

V36.7 Person on outside of three-wheeled motor vehicle injured in collision with other nonmotor vehicle in traffic accident

V36.9 Unspecified occupant of three-wheeled motor vehicle injured in collision with other nonmotor vehicle in traffic accident

V37 Occupant of three-wheeled motor vehicle injured in collision with fixed or stationary object

V37.0 Driver of three-wheeled motor vehicle injured in collision with fixed or stationary object in nontraffic accident

V37.1 Passenger in three-wheeled motor vehicle injured in collision with fixed or stationary object in nontraffic accident

V37.2 Person on outside of three-wheeled motor vehicle injured in collision with fixed or stationary object in nontraffic accident

V37.3 Unspecified occupant of three-wheeled motor vehicle injured in collision with fixed or stationary object in nontraffic accident

V37.4 Person boarding or alighting a three-wheeled motor vehicle injured in collision with fixed or stationary object

V37.5 Driver of three-wheeled motor vehicle injured in collision with fixed or stationary object in traffic accident

V37.6 Passenger in three-wheeled motor vehicle injured in collision with fixed or stationary object in traffic accident

V37.7 Person on outside of three-wheeled motor vehicle injured in collision with fixed or stationary object in traffic accident

V37.9 Unspecified occupant of three-wheeled motor vehicle injured in collision with fixed or stationary object in traffic accident

V38 Occupant of three-wheeled motor vehicle injured in noncollision transport accident

INCLUDES fall or thrown from three-wheeled motor vehicle
overturning of three-wheeled motor vehicle NOS
overturning of three-wheeled motor vehicle without collision

V38.0 Driver of three-wheeled motor vehicle injured in noncollision transport accident in nontraffic accident

V38.1 Passenger in three-wheeled motor vehicle injured in noncollision transport accident in nontraffic accident

V38.2 Person on outside of three-wheeled motor vehicle injured in noncollision transport accident in nontraffic accident

V38.3 Unspecified occupant of three-wheeled motor vehicle injured in noncollision transport accident in nontraffic accident

V38.4 Person boarding or alighting a three-wheeled motor vehicle injured in noncollision transport accident

V38.5 Driver of three-wheeled motor vehicle injured in noncollision transport accident in traffic accident

V38.6 Passenger in three-wheeled motor vehicle injured in noncollision transport accident in traffic accident

V38.7 Person on outside of three-wheeled motor vehicle injured in noncollision transport accident in traffic accident

V38.9 Unspecified occupant of three-wheeled motor vehicle injured in noncollision transport accident in traffic accident

V39 Occupant of three-wheeled motor vehicle injured in other and unspecified transport accidents

V39.0 Driver of three-wheeled motor vehicle injured in collision with other and unspecified motor vehicles in nontraffic accident

V39.00 Driver of three-wheeled motor vehicle injured in collision with unspecified motor vehicles in nontraffic accident

V39.09 Driver of three-wheeled motor vehicle injured in collision with other motor vehicles in nontraffic accident

V39.1 Passenger in three-wheeled motor vehicle injured in collision with other and unspecified motor vehicles in nontraffic accident

V39.10 Passenger in three-wheeled motor vehicle injured in collision with unspecified motor vehicles in nontraffic accident

V39.19 Passenger in three-wheeled motor vehicle injured in collision with other motor vehicles in nontraffic accident

V39.2 Unspecified occupant of three-wheeled motor vehicle injured in collision with other and unspecified motor vehicles in nontraffic accident

V39.20 Unspecified occupant of three-wheeled motor vehicle injured in collision with unspecified motor vehicles in nontraffic accident

Collision NOS involving three-wheeled motor vehicle, nontraffic

V39.29 Unspecified occupant of three-wheeled motor vehicle injured in collision with other motor vehicles in nontraffic accident

V39.3 Occupant (driver) (passenger) of three-wheeled motor vehicle injured in unspecified nontraffic accident

Accident NOS involving three-wheeled motor vehicle, nontraffic
Occupant of three-wheeled motor vehicle injured in nontraffic accident NOS

V39.4 Driver of three-wheeled motor vehicle injured in collision with other and unspecified motor vehicles in traffic accident

V39.40 Driver of three-wheeled motor vehicle injured in collision with unspecified motor vehicles in traffic accident

V39.49 Driver of three-wheeled motor vehicle injured in collision with other motor vehicles in traffic accident

V39.5 Passenger in three-wheeled motor vehicle injured in collision with other and unspecified motor vehicles in traffic accident

V39.50 Passenger in three-wheeled motor vehicle injured in collision with unspecified motor vehicles in traffic accident

V39.59 Passenger in three-wheeled motor vehicle injured in collision with other motor vehicles in traffic accident

V39.6 Unspecified occupant of three-wheeled motor vehicle injured in collision with other and unspecified motor vehicles in traffic accident

V39.60 Unspecified occupant of three-wheeled motor vehicle injured in collision with unspecified motor vehicles in traffic accident

Collision NOS involving three-wheeled motor vehicle (traffic)

V39.69 Unspecified occupant of three-wheeled motor vehicle injured in collision with other motor vehicles in traffic accident

V39.8 Occupant (driver) (passenger) of three-wheeled motor vehicle injured in other specified transport accidents

V39.81 Occupant (driver) (passenger) of three-wheeled motor vehicle injured in transport accident with military vehicle

V39.89 Occupant (driver) (passenger) of three-wheeled motor vehicle injured in other specified transport accidents

V39.9 Occupant (driver) (passenger) of three-wheeled motor vehicle injured in unspecified traffic accident

Accident NOS involving three-wheeled motor vehicle

Car occupant injured in transport accident (V40-V49)

INCLUDES a four-wheeled motor vehicle designed primarily for carrying passengers
automobile (pulling a trailer or camper)

EXCLUDES1 *bus (V50-V59)*
minibus (V50-V59)
minivan (V50-V59)
motorcoach (V70-V79)
pick-up truck (V50-V59)
sport utility vehicle (SUV) (V50-V59)

The appropriate 7th character is to be added to each code from categories V40-V49.
A initial encounter
D subsequent encounter
S sequela

V40 Car occupant injured in collision with pedestrian or animal

EXCLUDES1 *car collision with animal-drawn vehicle or animal being ridden (V46.-)*

V40.0 Car driver injured in collision with pedestrian or animal in nontraffic accident

V40.1 Car passenger injured in collision with pedestrian or animal in nontraffic accident
V40.2 Person on outside of car injured in collision with pedestrian or animal in nontraffic accident
V40.3 Unspecified car occupant injured in collision with pedestrian or animal in nontraffic accident
V40.4 Person boarding or alighting a car injured in collision with pedestrian or animal
V40.5 Car driver injured in collision with pedestrian or animal in traffic accident
V40.6 Car passenger injured in collision with pedestrian or animal in traffic accident
V40.7 Person on outside of car injured in collision with pedestrian or animal in traffic accident
V40.9 Unspecified car occupant injured in collision with pedestrian or animal in traffic accident

V41 Car occupant injured in collision with pedal cycle

V41.0 Car driver injured in collision with pedal cycle in nontraffic accident
V41.1 Car passenger injured in collision with pedal cycle in nontraffic accident
V41.2 Person on outside of car injured in collision with pedal cycle in nontraffic accident
V41.3 Unspecified car occupant injured in collision with pedal cycle in nontraffic accident
V41.4 Person boarding or alighting a car injured in collision with pedal cycle
V41.5 Car driver injured in collision with pedal cycle in traffic accident
V41.6 Car passenger injured in collision with pedal cycle in traffic accident
V41.7 Person on outside of car injured in collision with pedal cycle in traffic accident
V41.9 Unspecified car occupant injured in collision with pedal cycle in traffic accident

V42 Car occupant injured in collision with two- or three-wheeled motor vehicle

V42.0 Car driver injured in collision with two- or three-wheeled motor vehicle in nontraffic accident
V42.1 Car passenger injured in collision with two- or three-wheeled motor vehicle in nontraffic accident
V42.2 Person on outside of car injured in collision with two- or three-wheeled motor vehicle in nontraffic accident
V42.3 Unspecified car occupant injured in collision with two- or three-wheeled motor vehicle in nontraffic accident
V42.4 Person boarding or alighting a car injured in collision with two- or three-wheeled motor vehicle
V42.5 Car driver injured in collision with two- or three-wheeled motor vehicle in traffic accident
V42.6 Car passenger injured in collision with two- or three-wheeled motor vehicle in traffic accident
V42.7 Person on outside of car injured in collision with two- or three-wheeled motor vehicle in traffic accident
V42.9 Unspecified car occupant injured in collision with two- or three-wheeled motor vehicle in traffic accident

V43 Car occupant injured in collision with car, pick-up truck or van

V43.0 Car driver injured in collision with car, pick-up truck or van in nontraffic accident
- V43.01 Car driver injured in collision with sport utility vehicle in nontraffic accident
- V43.02 Car driver injured in collision with other type car in nontraffic accident
- V43.03 Car driver injured in collision with pick-up truck in nontraffic accident
- V43.04 Car driver injured in collision with van in nontraffic accident

V43.1 Car passenger injured in collision with car, pick-up truck or van in nontraffic accident
- V43.11 Car passenger injured in collision with sport utility vehicle in nontraffic accident
- V43.12 Car passenger injured in collision with other type car in nontraffic accident
- V43.13 Car passenger injured in collision with pick-up truck in nontraffic accident
- V43.14 Car passenger injured in collision with van in nontraffic accident

V43.2 Person on outside of car injured in collision with car, pick-up truck or van in nontraffic accident
- V43.21 Person on outside of car injured in collision with sport utility vehicle in nontraffic accident
- V43.22 Person on outside of car injured in collision with other type car in nontraffic accident
- V43.23 Person on outside of car injured in collision with pick-up truck in nontraffic accident
- V43.24 Person on outside of car injured in collision with van in nontraffic accident

V43.3 Unspecified car occupant injured in collision with car, pick-up truck or van in nontraffic accident
- V43.31 Unspecified car occupant injured in collision with sport utility vehicle in nontraffic accident
- V43.32 Unspecified car occupant injured in collision with other type car in nontraffic accident
- V43.33 Unspecified car occupant injured in collision with pick-up truck in nontraffic accident
- V43.34 Unspecified car occupant injured in collision with van in nontraffic accident

V43.4 Person boarding or alighting a car injured in collision with car, pick-up truck or van
- V43.41 Person boarding or alighting a car injured in collision with sport utility vehicle
- V43.42 Person boarding or alighting a car injured in collision with other type car
- V43.43 Person boarding or alighting a car injured in collision with pick-up truck
- V43.44 Person boarding or alighting a car injured in collision with van

V43.5 Car driver injured in collision with car, pick-up truck or van in traffic accident
- V43.51 Car driver injured in collision with sport utility vehicle in traffic accident
- V43.52 Car driver injured in collision with other type car in traffic accident
- V43.53 Car driver injured in collision with pick-up truck in traffic accident
- V43.54 Car driver injured in collision with van in traffic accident

V43.6 Car passenger injured in collision with car, pick-up truck or van in traffic accident
- V43.61 Car passenger injured in collision with sport utility vehicle in traffic accident
- V43.62 Car passenger injured in collision with other type car in traffic accident
- V43.63 Car passenger injured in collision with pick-up truck in traffic accident
- V43.64 Car passenger injured in collision with van in traffic accident

V43.7 Person on outside of car injured in collision with car, pick-up truck or van in traffic accident
- V43.71 Person on outside of car injured in collision with sport utility vehicle in traffic accident
- V43.72 Person on outside of car injured in collision with other type car in traffic accident
- V43.73 Person on outside of car injured in collision with pick-up truck in traffic accident
- V43.74 Person on outside of car injured in collision with van in traffic accident

V43.9 Unspecified car occupant injured in collision with car, pick-up truck or van in traffic accident
- V43.91 Unspecified car occupant injured in collision with sport utility vehicle in traffic accident
- V43.92 Unspecified car occupant injured in collision with other type car in traffic accident
- V43.93 Unspecified car occupant injured in collision with pick-up truck in traffic accident
- V43.94 Unspecified car occupant injured in collision with van in traffic accident

V44 Car occupant injured in collision with heavy transport vehicle or bus

EXCLUDES 1 *car occupant injured in collision with military vehicle (V49.81)*

V44.0 Car driver injured in collision with heavy transport vehicle or bus in nontraffic accident
V44.1 Car passenger injured in collision with heavy transport vehicle or bus in nontraffic accident
V44.2 Person on outside of car injured in collision with heavy transport vehicle or bus in nontraffic accident
V44.3 Unspecified car occupant injured in collision with heavy transport vehicle or bus in nontraffic accident
V44.4 Person boarding or alighting a car injured in collision with heavy transport vehicle or bus
V44.5 Car driver injured in collision with heavy transport vehicle or bus in traffic accident

√x7th V44.6 Car passenger injured in collision with heavy transport vehicle or bus in traffic accident

√x7th V44.7 Person on outside of car injured in collision with heavy transport vehicle or bus in traffic accident

√x7th V44.9 Unspecified car occupant injured in collision with heavy transport vehicle or bus in traffic accident

√4th **V45 Car occupant injured in collision with railway train or railway vehicle**

√x7th V45.0 Car driver injured in collision with railway train or railway vehicle in nontraffic accident

√x7th V45.1 Car passenger injured in collision with railway train or railway vehicle in nontraffic accident

√x7th V45.2 Person on outside of car injured in collision with railway train or railway vehicle in nontraffic accident

√x7th V45.3 Unspecified car occupant injured in collision with railway train or railway vehicle in nontraffic accident

√x7th V45.4 Person boarding or alighting a car injured in collision with railway train or railway vehicle

√x7th V45.5 Car driver injured in collision with railway train or railway vehicle in traffic accident

√x7th V45.6 Car passenger injured in collision with railway train or railway vehicle in traffic accident

√x7th V45.7 Person on outside of car injured in collision with railway train or railway vehicle in traffic accident

√x7th V45.9 Unspecified car occupant injured in collision with railway train or railway vehicle in traffic accident

√4th **V46 Car occupant injured in collision with other nonmotor vehicle**

INCLUDES collision with animal-drawn vehicle, animal being ridden, streetcar

√x7th V46.0 Car driver injured in collision with other nonmotor vehicle in nontraffic accident

√x7th V46.1 Car passenger injured in collision with other nonmotor vehicle in nontraffic accident

√x7th V46.2 Person on outside of car injured in collision with other nonmotor vehicle in nontraffic accident

√x7th V46.3 Unspecified car occupant injured in collision with other nonmotor vehicle in nontraffic accident

√x7th V46.4 Person boarding or alighting a car injured in collision with other nonmotor vehicle

√x7th V46.5 Car driver injured in collision with other nonmotor vehicle in traffic accident

√x7th V46.6 Car passenger injured in collision with other nonmotor vehicle in traffic accident

√x7th V46.7 Person on outside of car injured in collision with other nonmotor vehicle in traffic accident

√x7th V46.9 Unspecified car occupant injured in collision with other nonmotor vehicle in traffic accident

√4th **V47 Car occupant injured in collision with fixed or stationary object**

AHA: 2016,4Q,73

√x7th V47.0 Car driver injured in collision with fixed or stationary object in nontraffic accident

√x7th V47.1 Car passenger injured in collision with fixed or stationary object in nontraffic accident

√x7th V47.2 Person on outside of car injured in collision with fixed or stationary object in nontraffic accident

√x7th V47.3 Unspecified car occupant injured in collision with fixed or stationary object in nontraffic accident

√x7th V47.4 Person boarding or alighting a car injured in collision with fixed or stationary object

√x7th V47.5 Car driver injured in collision with fixed or stationary object in traffic accident

√x7th V47.6 Car passenger injured in collision with fixed or stationary object in traffic accident

√x7th V47.7 Person on outside of car injured in collision with fixed or stationary object in traffic accident

√x7th V47.9 Unspecified car occupant injured in collision with fixed or stationary object in traffic accident

√4th **V48 Car occupant injured in noncollision transport accident**

INCLUDES overturning car NOS
overturning car without collision

√x7th V48.0 Car driver injured in noncollision transport accident in nontraffic accident

√x7th V48.1 Car passenger injured in noncollision transport accident in nontraffic accident

√x7th V48.2 Person on outside of car injured in noncollision transport accident in nontraffic accident

√x7th V48.3 Unspecified car occupant injured in noncollision transport accident in nontraffic accident

√x7th V48.4 Person boarding or alighting a car injured in noncollision transport accident

√x7th V48.5 Car driver injured in noncollision transport accident in traffic accident

√x7th V48.6 Car passenger injured in noncollision transport accident in traffic accident

√x7th V48.7 Person on outside of car injured in noncollision transport accident in traffic accident

√x7th V48.9 Unspecified car occupant injured in noncollision transport accident in traffic accident

√4th **V49 Car occupant injured in other and unspecified transport accidents**

√5th V49.0 Driver injured in collision with other and unspecified motor vehicles in nontraffic accident

√x7th V49.00 Driver injured in collision with unspecified motor vehicles in nontraffic accident

√x7th V49.09 Driver injured in collision with other motor vehicles in nontraffic accident

√5th V49.1 Passenger injured in collision with other and unspecified motor vehicles in nontraffic accident

√x7th V49.10 Passenger injured in collision with unspecified motor vehicles in nontraffic accident

√x7th V49.19 Passenger injured in collision with other motor vehicles in nontraffic accident

√5th V49.2 Unspecified car occupant injured in collision with other and unspecified motor vehicles in nontraffic accident

√x7th V49.20 Unspecified car occupant injured in collision with unspecified motor vehicles in nontraffic accident
Car collision NOS, nontraffic

√x7th V49.29 Unspecified car occupant injured in collision with other motor vehicles in nontraffic accident

√x7th V49.3 Car occupant (driver) (passenger) injured in unspecified nontraffic accident
Car accident NOS, nontraffic
Car occupant injured in nontraffic accident NOS

√5th V49.4 Driver injured in collision with other and unspecified motor vehicles in traffic accident

√x7th V49.40 Driver injured in collision with unspecified motor vehicles in traffic accident

√x7th V49.49 Driver injured in collision with other motor vehicles in traffic accident

√5th V49.5 Passenger injured in collision with other and unspecified motor vehicles in traffic accident

√x7th V49.50 Passenger injured in collision with unspecified motor vehicles in traffic accident

√x7th V49.59 Passenger injured in collision with other motor vehicles in traffic accident

√5th V49.6 Unspecified car occupant injured in collision with other and unspecified motor vehicles in traffic accident

√x7th V49.60 Unspecified car occupant injured in collision with unspecified motor vehicles in traffic accident
Car collision NOS (traffic)

√x7th V49.69 Unspecified car occupant injured in collision with other motor vehicles in traffic accident

√5th V49.8 Car occupant (driver) (passenger) injured in other specified transport accidents

√x7th V49.81 Car occupant (driver) (passenger) injured in transport accident with military vehicle

√x7th V49.88 Car occupant (driver) (passenger) injured in other specified transport accidents

√x7th V49.9 Car occupant (driver) (passenger) injured in unspecified traffic accident
Car accident NOS

Occupant of pick-up truck or van injured in transport accident (V50-V59)

INCLUDES a four or six wheel motor vehicle designed primarily for carrying passengers and property but weighing less than the local limit for classification as a heavy goods vehicle
minibus
minivan
sport utility vehicle (SUV)
truck
van

EXCLUDES 1 *heavy transport vehicle (V60-V69)*

The appropriate 7th character is to be added to each code from categories V50-V59.
A initial encounter
D subsequent encounter
S sequela

V50 Occupant of pick-up truck or van injured in collision with pedestrian or animal
EXCLUDES 1 *pick-up truck or van collision with animal-drawn vehicle or animal being ridden (V56.-)*
- V50.0 Driver of pick-up truck or van injured in collision with pedestrian or animal in nontraffic accident
- V50.1 Passenger in pick-up truck or van injured in collision with pedestrian or animal in nontraffic accident
- V50.2 Person on outside of pick-up truck or van injured in collision with pedestrian or animal in nontraffic accident
- V50.3 Unspecified occupant of pick-up truck or van injured in collision with pedestrian or animal in nontraffic accident
- V50.4 Person boarding or alighting a pick-up truck or van injured in collision with pedestrian or animal
- V50.5 Driver of pick-up truck or van injured in collision with pedestrian or animal in traffic accident
- V50.6 Passenger in pick-up truck or van injured in collision with pedestrian or animal in traffic accident
- V50.7 Person on outside of pick-up truck or van injured in collision with pedestrian or animal in traffic accident
- V50.9 Unspecified occupant of pick-up truck or van injured in collision with pedestrian or animal in traffic accident

V51 Occupant of pick-up truck or van injured in collision with pedal cycle
- V51.0 Driver of pick-up truck or van injured in collision with pedal cycle in nontraffic accident
- V51.1 Passenger in pick-up truck or van injured in collision with pedal cycle in nontraffic accident
- V51.2 Person on outside of pick-up truck or van injured in collision with pedal cycle in nontraffic accident
- V51.3 Unspecified occupant of pick-up truck or van injured in collision with pedal cycle in nontraffic accident
- V51.4 Person boarding or alighting a pick-up truck or van injured in collision with pedal cycle
- V51.5 Driver of pick-up truck or van injured in collision with pedal cycle in traffic accident
- V51.6 Passenger in pick-up truck or van injured in collision with pedal cycle in traffic accident
- V51.7 Person on outside of pick-up truck or van injured in collision with pedal cycle in traffic accident
- V51.9 Unspecified occupant of pick-up truck or van injured in collision with pedal cycle in traffic accident

V52 Occupant of pick-up truck or van injured in collision with two- or three-wheeled motor vehicle
- V52.0 Driver of pick-up truck or van injured in collision with two- or three-wheeled motor vehicle in nontraffic accident
- V52.1 Passenger in pick-up truck or van injured in collision with two- or three-wheeled motor vehicle in nontraffic accident
- V52.2 Person on outside of pick-up truck or van injured in collision with two- or three-wheeled motor vehicle in nontraffic accident
- V52.3 Unspecified occupant of pick-up truck or van injured in collision with two- or three-wheeled motor vehicle in nontraffic accident
- V52.4 Person boarding or alighting a pick-up truck or van injured in collision with two- or three-wheeled motor vehicle
- V52.5 Driver of pick-up truck or van injured in collision with two- or three-wheeled motor vehicle in traffic accident
- V52.6 Passenger in pick-up truck or van injured in collision with two- or three-wheeled motor vehicle in traffic accident
- V52.7 Person on outside of pick-up truck or van injured in collision with two- or three-wheeled motor vehicle in traffic accident
- V52.9 Unspecified occupant of pick-up truck or van injured in collision with two- or three-wheeled motor vehicle in traffic accident

V53 Occupant of pick-up truck or van injured in collision with car, pick-up truck or van
- V53.0 Driver of pick-up truck or van injured in collision with car, pick-up truck or van in nontraffic accident
- V53.1 Passenger in pick-up truck or van injured in collision with car, pick-up truck or van in nontraffic accident
- V53.2 Person on outside of pick-up truck or van injured in collision with car, pick-up truck or van in nontraffic accident
- V53.3 Unspecified occupant of pick-up truck or van injured in collision with car, pick-up truck or van in nontraffic accident
- V53.4 Person boarding or alighting a pick-up truck or van injured in collision with car, pick-up truck or van
- V53.5 Driver of pick-up truck or van injured in collision with car, pick-up truck or van in traffic accident
- V53.6 Passenger in pick-up truck or van injured in collision with car, pick-up truck or van in traffic accident
- V53.7 Person on outside of pick-up truck or van injured in collision with car, pick-up truck or van in traffic accident
- V53.9 Unspecified occupant of pick-up truck or van injured in collision with car, pick-up truck or van in traffic accident

V54 Occupant of pick-up truck or van injured in collision with heavy transport vehicle or bus
EXCLUDES 1 *occupant of pick-up truck or van injured in collision with military vehicle (V59.81)*
- V54.0 Driver of pick-up truck or van injured in collision with heavy transport vehicle or bus in nontraffic accident
- V54.1 Passenger in pick-up truck or van injured in collision with heavy transport vehicle or bus in nontraffic accident
- V54.2 Person on outside of pick-up truck or van injured in collision with heavy transport vehicle or bus in nontraffic accident
- V54.3 Unspecified occupant of pick-up truck or van injured in collision with heavy transport vehicle or bus in nontraffic accident
- V54.4 Person boarding or alighting a pick-up truck or van injured in collision with heavy transport vehicle or bus
- V54.5 Driver of pick-up truck or van injured in collision with heavy transport vehicle or bus in traffic accident
- V54.6 Passenger in pick-up truck or van injured in collision with heavy transport vehicle or bus in traffic accident
- V54.7 Person on outside of pick-up truck or van injured in collision with heavy transport vehicle or bus in traffic accident
- V54.9 Unspecified occupant of pick-up truck or van injured in collision with heavy transport vehicle or bus in traffic accident

V55 Occupant of pick-up truck or van injured in collision with railway train or railway vehicle
- V55.0 Driver of pick-up truck or van injured in collision with railway train or railway vehicle in nontraffic accident
- V55.1 Passenger in pick-up truck or van injured in collision with railway train or railway vehicle in nontraffic accident
- V55.2 Person on outside of pick-up truck or van injured in collision with railway train or railway vehicle in nontraffic accident
- V55.3 Unspecified occupant of pick-up truck or van injured in collision with railway train or railway vehicle in nontraffic accident
- V55.4 Person boarding or alighting a pick-up truck or van injured in collision with railway train or railway vehicle
- V55.5 Driver of pick-up truck or van injured in collision with railway train or railway vehicle in traffic accident
- V55.6 Passenger in pick-up truck or van injured in collision with railway train or railway vehicle in traffic accident
- V55.7 Person on outside of pick-up truck or van injured in collision with railway train or railway vehicle in traffic accident
- V55.9 Unspecified occupant of pick-up truck or van injured in collision with railway train or railway vehicle in traffic accident

V56 Occupant of pick-up truck or van injured in collision with other nonmotor vehicle
INCLUDES collision with animal-drawn vehicle, animal being ridden, streetcar
- V56.0 Driver of pick-up truck or van injured in collision with other nonmotor vehicle in nontraffic accident
- V56.1 Passenger in pick-up truck or van injured in collision with other nonmotor vehicle in nontraffic accident
- V56.2 Person on outside of pick-up truck or van injured in collision with other nonmotor vehicle in nontraffic accident
- V56.3 Unspecified occupant of pick-up truck or van injured in collision with other nonmotor vehicle in nontraffic accident
- V56.4 Person boarding or alighting a pick-up truck or van injured in collision with other nonmotor vehicle

- **V56.5** Driver of pick-up truck or van injured in collision with other nonmotor vehicle in traffic accident
- **V56.6** Passenger in pick-up truck or van injured in collision with other nonmotor vehicle in traffic accident
- **V56.7** Person on outside of pick-up truck or van injured in collision with other nonmotor vehicle in traffic accident
- **V56.9** Unspecified occupant of pick-up truck or van injured in collision with other nonmotor vehicle in traffic accident

V57 Occupant of pick-up truck or van injured in collision with fixed or stationary object

- **V57.0** Driver of pick-up truck or van injured in collision with fixed or stationary object in nontraffic accident
- **V57.1** Passenger in pick-up truck or van injured in collision with fixed or stationary object in nontraffic accident
- **V57.2** Person on outside of pick-up truck or van injured in collision with fixed or stationary object in nontraffic accident
- **V57.3** Unspecified occupant of pick-up truck or van injured in collision with fixed or stationary object in nontraffic accident
- **V57.4** Person boarding or alighting a pick-up truck or van injured in collision with fixed or stationary object
- **V57.5** Driver of pick-up truck or van injured in collision with fixed or stationary object in traffic accident
- **V57.6** Passenger in pick-up truck or van injured in collision with fixed or stationary object in traffic accident
- **V57.7** Person on outside of pick-up truck or van injured in collision with fixed or stationary object in traffic accident
- **V57.9** Unspecified occupant of pick-up truck or van injured in collision with fixed or stationary object in traffic accident

V58 Occupant of pick-up truck or van injured in noncollision transport accident

INCLUDES overturning pick-up truck or van NOS
overturning pick-up truck or van without collision

- **V58.0** Driver of pick-up truck or van injured in noncollision transport accident in nontraffic accident
- **V58.1** Passenger in pick-up truck or van injured in noncollision transport accident in nontraffic accident
- **V58.2** Person on outside of pick-up truck or van injured in noncollision transport accident in nontraffic accident
- **V58.3** Unspecified occupant of pick-up truck or van injured in noncollision transport accident in nontraffic accident
- **V58.4** Person boarding or alighting a pick-up truck or van injured in noncollision transport accident
- **V58.5** Driver of pick-up truck or van injured in noncollision transport accident in traffic accident
- **V58.6** Passenger in pick-up truck or van injured in noncollision transport accident in traffic accident
- **V58.7** Person on outside of pick-up truck or van injured in noncollision transport accident in traffic accident
- **V58.9** Unspecified occupant of pick-up truck or van injured in noncollision transport accident in traffic accident

V59 Occupant of pick-up truck or van injured in other and unspecified transport accidents

- **V59.0** Driver of pick-up truck or van injured in collision with other and unspecified motor vehicles in nontraffic accident
  - **V59.00** Driver of pick-up truck or van injured in collision with unspecified motor vehicles in nontraffic accident
  - **V59.09** Driver of pick-up truck or van injured in collision with other motor vehicles in nontraffic accident
- **V59.1** Passenger in pick-up truck or van injured in collision with other and unspecified motor vehicles in nontraffic accident
  - **V59.10** Passenger in pick-up truck or van injured in collision with unspecified motor vehicles in nontraffic accident
  - **V59.19** Passenger in pick-up truck or van injured in collision with other motor vehicles in nontraffic accident
- **V59.2** Unspecified occupant of pick-up truck or van injured in collision with other and unspecified motor vehicles in nontraffic accident
  - **V59.20** Unspecified occupant of pick-up truck or van injured in collision with unspecified motor vehicles in nontraffic accident
    Collision NOS involving pick-up truck or van, nontraffic
  - **V59.29** Unspecified occupant of pick-up truck or van injured in collision with other motor vehicles in nontraffic accident
- **V59.3** Occupant (driver) (passenger) of pick-up truck or van injured in unspecified nontraffic accident
  Accident NOS involving pick-up truck or van, nontraffic
  Occupant of pick-up truck or van injured in nontraffic accident NOS
- **V59.4** Driver of pick-up truck or van injured in collision with other and unspecified motor vehicles in traffic accident
  - **V59.40** Driver of pick-up truck or van injured in collision with unspecified motor vehicles in traffic accident
  - **V59.49** Driver of pick-up truck or van injured in collision with other motor vehicles in traffic accident
- **V59.5** Passenger in pick-up truck or van injured in collision with other and unspecified motor vehicles in traffic accident
  - **V59.50** Passenger in pick-up truck or van injured in collision with unspecified motor vehicles in traffic accident
  - **V59.59** Passenger in pick-up truck or van injured in collision with other motor vehicles in traffic accident
- **V59.6** Unspecified occupant of pick-up truck or van injured in collision with other and unspecified motor vehicles in traffic accident
  - **V59.60** Unspecified occupant of pick-up truck or van injured in collision with unspecified motor vehicles in traffic accident
    Collision NOS involving pick-up truck or van (traffic)
  - **V59.69** Unspecified occupant of pick-up truck or van injured in collision with other motor vehicles in traffic accident
- **V59.8** Occupant (driver) (passenger) of pick-up truck or van injured in other specified transport accidents
  - **V59.81** Occupant (driver) (passenger) of pick-up truck or van injured in transport accident with military vehicle
  - **V59.88** Occupant (driver) (passenger) of pick-up truck or van injured in other specified transport accidents
- **V59.9** Occupant (driver) (passenger) of pick-up truck or van injured in unspecified traffic accident
  Accident NOS involving pick-up truck or van

Occupant of heavy transport vehicle injured in transport accident (V60-V69)

INCLUDES 18 wheeler
armored car
panel truck

EXCLUDES 1 *bus*
motorcoach

The appropriate 7th character is to be added to each code from categories V60-V69.
A initial encounter
D subsequent encounter
S sequela

V60 Occupant of heavy transport vehicle injured in collision with pedestrian or animal

EXCLUDES 1 *heavy transport vehicle collision with animal-drawn vehicle or animal being ridden (V66.-)*

- **V60.0** Driver of heavy transport vehicle injured in collision with pedestrian or animal in nontraffic accident
- **V60.1** Passenger in heavy transport vehicle injured in collision with pedestrian or animal in nontraffic accident
- **V60.2** Person on outside of heavy transport vehicle injured in collision with pedestrian or animal in nontraffic accident
- **V60.3** Unspecified occupant of heavy transport vehicle injured in collision with pedestrian or animal in nontraffic accident
- **V60.4** Person boarding or alighting a heavy transport vehicle injured in collision with pedestrian or animal
- **V60.5** Driver of heavy transport vehicle injured in collision with pedestrian or animal in traffic accident
- **V60.6** Passenger in heavy transport vehicle injured in collision with pedestrian or animal in traffic accident
- **V60.7** Person on outside of heavy transport vehicle injured in collision with pedestrian or animal in traffic accident
- **V60.9** Unspecified occupant of heavy transport vehicle injured in collision with pedestrian or animal in traffic accident

V61 Occupant of heavy transport vehicle injured in collision with pedal cycle

- **V61.0** Driver of heavy transport vehicle injured in collision with pedal cycle in nontraffic accident
- **V61.1** Passenger in heavy transport vehicle injured in collision with pedal cycle in nontraffic accident
- **V61.2** Person on outside of heavy transport vehicle injured in collision with pedal cycle in nontraffic accident
- **V61.3** Unspecified occupant of heavy transport vehicle injured in collision with pedal cycle in nontraffic accident

✓x7th V61.4 Person boarding or alighting a heavy transport vehicle injured in collision with pedal cycle while boarding or alighting

✓x7th V61.5 Driver of heavy transport vehicle injured in collision with pedal cycle in traffic accident

✓x7th V61.6 Passenger in heavy transport vehicle injured in collision with pedal cycle in traffic accident

✓x7th V61.7 Person on outside of heavy transport vehicle injured in collision with pedal cycle in traffic accident

✓x7th V61.9 Unspecified occupant of heavy transport vehicle injured in collision with pedal cycle in traffic accident

✓4th **V62 Occupant of heavy transport vehicle injured in collision with two- or three-wheeled motor vehicle**

✓x7th V62.Ø Driver of heavy transport vehicle injured in collision with two- or three-wheeled motor vehicle in nontraffic accident

✓x7th V62.1 Passenger in heavy transport vehicle injured in collision with two- or three-wheeled motor vehicle in nontraffic accident

✓x7th V62.2 Person on outside of heavy transport vehicle injured in collision with two- or three-wheeled motor vehicle in nontraffic accident

✓x7th V62.3 Unspecified occupant of heavy transport vehicle injured in collision with two- or three-wheeled motor vehicle in nontraffic accident

✓x7th V62.4 Person boarding or alighting a heavy transport vehicle injured in collision with two- or three-wheeled motor vehicle

✓x7th V62.5 Driver of heavy transport vehicle injured in collision with two- or three-wheeled motor vehicle in traffic accident

✓x7th V62.6 Passenger in heavy transport vehicle injured in collision with two- or three-wheeled motor vehicle in traffic accident

✓x7th V62.7 Person on outside of heavy transport vehicle injured in collision with two- or three-wheeled motor vehicle in traffic accident

✓x7th V62.9 Unspecified occupant of heavy transport vehicle injured in collision with two- or three-wheeled motor vehicle in traffic accident

✓4th **V63 Occupant of heavy transport vehicle injured in collision with car, pick-up truck or van**

✓x7th V63.Ø Driver of heavy transport vehicle injured in collision with car, pick-up truck or van in nontraffic accident

✓x7th V63.1 Passenger in heavy transport vehicle injured in collision with car, pick-up truck or van in nontraffic accident

✓x7th V63.2 Person on outside of heavy transport vehicle injured in collision with car, pick-up truck or van in nontraffic accident

✓x7th V63.3 Unspecified occupant of heavy transport vehicle injured in collision with car, pick-up truck or van in nontraffic accident

✓x7th V63.4 Person boarding or alighting a heavy transport vehicle injured in collision with car, pick-up truck or van

✓x7th V63.5 Driver of heavy transport vehicle injured in collision with car, pick-up truck or van in traffic accident

✓x7th V63.6 Passenger in heavy transport vehicle injured in collision with car, pick-up truck or van in traffic accident

✓x7th V63.7 Person on outside of heavy transport vehicle injured in collision with car, pick-up truck or van in traffic accident

✓x7th V63.9 Unspecified occupant of heavy transport vehicle injured in collision with car, pick-up truck or van in traffic accident

✓4th **V64 Occupant of heavy transport vehicle injured in collision with heavy transport vehicle or bus**

EXCLUDES 1 *occupant of heavy transport vehicle injured in collision with military vehicle (V69.81)*

✓x7th V64.Ø Driver of heavy transport vehicle injured in collision with heavy transport vehicle or bus in nontraffic accident

✓x7th V64.1 Passenger in heavy transport vehicle injured in collision with heavy transport vehicle or bus in nontraffic accident

✓x7th V64.2 Person on outside of heavy transport vehicle injured in collision with heavy transport vehicle or bus in nontraffic accident

✓x7th V64.3 Unspecified occupant of heavy transport vehicle injured in collision with heavy transport vehicle or bus in nontraffic accident

✓x7th V64.4 Person boarding or alighting a heavy transport vehicle injured in collision with heavy transport vehicle or bus while boarding or alighting

✓x7th V64.5 Driver of heavy transport vehicle injured in collision with heavy transport vehicle or bus in traffic accident

✓x7th V64.6 Passenger in heavy transport vehicle injured in collision with heavy transport vehicle or bus in traffic accident

✓x7th V64.7 Person on outside of heavy transport vehicle injured in collision with heavy transport vehicle or bus in traffic accident

✓x7th V64.9 Unspecified occupant of heavy transport vehicle injured in collision with heavy transport vehicle or bus in traffic accident

✓4th **V65 Occupant of heavy transport vehicle injured in collision with railway train or railway vehicle**

✓x7th V65.Ø Driver of heavy transport vehicle injured in collision with railway train or railway vehicle in nontraffic accident

✓x7th V65.1 Passenger in heavy transport vehicle injured in collision with railway train or railway vehicle in nontraffic accident

✓x7th V65.2 Person on outside of heavy transport vehicle injured in collision with railway train or railway vehicle in nontraffic accident

✓x7th V65.3 Unspecified occupant of heavy transport vehicle injured in collision with railway train or railway vehicle in nontraffic accident

✓x7th V65.4 Person boarding or alighting a heavy transport vehicle injured in collision with railway train or railway vehicle

✓x7th V65.5 Driver of heavy transport vehicle injured in collision with railway train or railway vehicle in traffic accident

✓x7th V65.6 Passenger in heavy transport vehicle injured in collision with railway train or railway vehicle in traffic accident

✓x7th V65.7 Person on outside of heavy transport vehicle injured in collision with railway train or railway vehicle in traffic accident

✓x7th V65.9 Unspecified occupant of heavy transport vehicle injured in collision with railway train or railway vehicle in traffic accident

✓4th **V66 Occupant of heavy transport vehicle injured in collision with other nonmotor vehicle**

INCLUDES collision with animal-drawn vehicle, animal being ridden, streetcar

✓x7th V66.Ø Driver of heavy transport vehicle injured in collision with other nonmotor vehicle in nontraffic accident

✓x7th V66.1 Passenger in heavy transport vehicle injured in collision with other nonmotor vehicle in nontraffic accident

✓x7th V66.2 Person on outside of heavy transport vehicle injured in collision with other nonmotor vehicle in nontraffic accident

✓x7th V66.3 Unspecified occupant of heavy transport vehicle injured in collision with other nonmotor vehicle in nontraffic accident

✓x7th V66.4 Person boarding or alighting a heavy transport vehicle injured in collision with other nonmotor vehicle

✓x7th V66.5 Driver of heavy transport vehicle injured in collision with other nonmotor vehicle in traffic accident

✓x7th V66.6 Passenger in heavy transport vehicle injured in collision with other nonmotor vehicle in traffic accident

✓x7th V66.7 Person on outside of heavy transport vehicle injured in collision with other nonmotor vehicle in traffic accident

✓x7th V66.9 Unspecified occupant of heavy transport vehicle injured in collision with other nonmotor vehicle in traffic accident

✓4th **V67 Occupant of heavy transport vehicle injured in collision with fixed or stationary object**

✓x7th V67.Ø Driver of heavy transport vehicle injured in collision with fixed or stationary object in nontraffic accident

✓x7th V67.1 Passenger in heavy transport vehicle injured in collision with fixed or stationary object in nontraffic accident

✓x7th V67.2 Person on outside of heavy transport vehicle injured in collision with fixed or stationary object in nontraffic accident

✓x7th V67.3 Unspecified occupant of heavy transport vehicle injured in collision with fixed or stationary object in nontraffic accident

✓x7th V67.4 Person boarding or alighting a heavy transport vehicle injured in collision with fixed or stationary object

✓x7th V67.5 Driver of heavy transport vehicle injured in collision with fixed or stationary object in traffic accident

✓x7th V67.6 Passenger in heavy transport vehicle injured in collision with fixed or stationary object in traffic accident

✓x7th V67.7 Person on outside of heavy transport vehicle injured in collision with fixed or stationary object in traffic accident

✓x7th V67.9 Unspecified occupant of heavy transport vehicle injured in collision with fixed or stationary object in traffic accident

✓4th **V68 Occupant of heavy transport vehicle injured in noncollision transport accident**

INCLUDES overturning heavy transport vehicle NOS
overturning heavy transport vehicle without collision

✓x7th V68.Ø Driver of heavy transport vehicle injured in noncollision transport accident in nontraffic accident

✓x7th V68.1 Passenger in heavy transport vehicle injured in noncollision transport accident in nontraffic accident

✓x7th V68.2 Person on outside of heavy transport vehicle injured in noncollision transport accident in nontraffic accident

✓x7th V68.3 Unspecified occupant of heavy transport vehicle injured in noncollision transport accident in nontraffic accident

√x7th V68.4 Person boarding or alighting a heavy transport vehicle injured in noncollision transport accident

√x7th V68.5 Driver of heavy transport vehicle injured in noncollision transport accident in traffic accident

√x7th V68.6 Passenger in heavy transport vehicle injured in noncollision transport accident in traffic accident

√x7th V68.7 Person on outside of heavy transport vehicle injured in noncollision transport accident in traffic accident

√x7th V68.9 Unspecified occupant of heavy transport vehicle injured in noncollision transport accident in traffic accident

√4th **V69 Occupant of heavy transport vehicle injured in other and unspecified transport accidents**

√5th V69.0 Driver of heavy transport vehicle injured in collision with other and unspecified motor vehicles in nontraffic accident

√x7th V69.00 Driver of heavy transport vehicle injured in collision with unspecified motor vehicles in nontraffic accident

√x7th V69.09 Driver of heavy transport vehicle injured in collision with other motor vehicles in nontraffic accident

√5th V69.1 Passenger in heavy transport vehicle injured in collision with other and unspecified motor vehicles in nontraffic accident

√x7th V69.10 Passenger in heavy transport vehicle injured in collision with unspecified motor vehicles in nontraffic accident

√x7th V69.19 Passenger in heavy transport vehicle injured in collision with other motor vehicles in nontraffic accident

√5th V69.2 Unspecified occupant of heavy transport vehicle injured in collision with other and unspecified motor vehicles in nontraffic accident

√x7th V69.20 Unspecified occupant of heavy transport vehicle injured in collision with unspecified motor vehicles in nontraffic accident

Collision NOS involving heavy transport vehicle, nontraffic

√x7th V69.29 Unspecified occupant of heavy transport vehicle injured in collision with other motor vehicles in nontraffic accident

√x7th V69.3 Occupant (driver) (passenger) of heavy transport vehicle injured in unspecified nontraffic accident

Accident NOS involving heavy transport vehicle, nontraffic

Occupant of heavy transport vehicle injured in nontraffic accident NOS

√5th V69.4 Driver of heavy transport vehicle injured in collision with other and unspecified motor vehicles in traffic accident

√x7th V69.40 Driver of heavy transport vehicle injured in collision with unspecified motor vehicles in traffic accident

√x7th V69.49 Driver of heavy transport vehicle injured in collision with other motor vehicles in traffic accident

√5th V69.5 Passenger in heavy transport vehicle injured in collision with other and unspecified motor vehicles in traffic accident

√x7th V69.50 Passenger in heavy transport vehicle injured in collision with unspecified motor vehicles in traffic accident

√x7th V69.59 Passenger in heavy transport vehicle injured in collision with other motor vehicles in traffic accident

√5th V69.6 Unspecified occupant of heavy transport vehicle injured in collision with other and unspecified motor vehicles in traffic accident

√x7th V69.60 Unspecified occupant of heavy transport vehicle injured in collision with unspecified motor vehicles in traffic accident

Collision NOS involving heavy transport vehicle (traffic)

√x7th V69.69 Unspecified occupant of heavy transport vehicle injured in collision with other motor vehicles in traffic accident

√5th V69.8 Occupant (driver) (passenger) of heavy transport vehicle injured in other specified transport accidents

√x7th V69.81 Occupant (driver) (passenger) of heavy transport vehicle injured in transport accidents with military vehicle

√x7th V69.88 Occupant (driver) (passenger) of heavy transport vehicle injured in other specified transport accidents

√x7th V69.9 Occupant (driver) (passenger) of heavy transport vehicle injured in unspecified traffic accident

Accident NOS involving heavy transport vehicle

Bus occupant injured in transport accident (V70-V79)

INCLUDES motorcoach

EXCLUDES 1 *minibus (V50-V59)*

The appropriate 7th character is to be added to each code from categories V70-V79.
A initial encounter
D subsequent encounter
S sequela

√4th **V70 Bus occupant injured in collision with pedestrian or animal**

EXCLUDES 1 *bus collision with animal-drawn vehicle or animal being ridden (V76.-)*

√x7th V70.0 Driver of bus injured in collision with pedestrian or animal in nontraffic accident

√x7th V70.1 Passenger on bus injured in collision with pedestrian or animal in nontraffic accident

√x7th V70.2 Person on outside of bus injured in collision with pedestrian or animal in nontraffic accident

√x7th V70.3 Unspecified occupant of bus injured in collision with pedestrian or animal in nontraffic accident

√x7th V70.4 Person boarding or alighting from bus injured in collision with pedestrian or animal

√x7th V70.5 Driver of bus injured in collision with pedestrian or animal in traffic accident

√x7th V70.6 Passenger on bus injured in collision with pedestrian or animal in traffic accident

√x7th V70.7 Person on outside of bus injured in collision with pedestrian or animal in traffic accident

√x7th V70.9 Unspecified occupant of bus injured in collision with pedestrian or animal in traffic accident

√4th **V71 Bus occupant injured in collision with pedal cycle**

√x7th V71.0 Driver of bus injured in collision with pedal cycle in nontraffic accident

√x7th V71.1 Passenger on bus injured in collision with pedal cycle in nontraffic accident

√x7th V71.2 Person on outside of bus injured in collision with pedal cycle in nontraffic accident

√x7th V71.3 Unspecified occupant of bus injured in collision with pedal cycle in nontraffic accident

√x7th V71.4 Person boarding or alighting from bus injured in collision with pedal cycle

√x7th V71.5 Driver of bus injured in collision with pedal cycle in traffic accident

√x7th V71.6 Passenger on bus injured in collision with pedal cycle in traffic accident

√x7th V71.7 Person on outside of bus injured in collision with pedal cycle in traffic accident

√x7th V71.9 Unspecified occupant of bus injured in collision with pedal cycle in traffic accident

√4th **V72 Bus occupant injured in collision with two- or three-wheeled motor vehicle**

√x7th V72.0 Driver of bus injured in collision with two- or three-wheeled motor vehicle in nontraffic accident

√x7th V72.1 Passenger on bus injured in collision with two- or three-wheeled motor vehicle in nontraffic accident

√x7th V72.2 Person on outside of bus injured in collision with two- or three-wheeled motor vehicle in nontraffic accident

√x7th V72.3 Unspecified occupant of bus injured in collision with two- or three-wheeled motor vehicle in nontraffic accident

√x7th V72.4 Person boarding or alighting from bus injured in collision with two- or three-wheeled motor vehicle

√x7th V72.5 Driver of bus injured in collision with two- or three-wheeled motor vehicle in traffic accident

√x7th V72.6 Passenger on bus injured in collision with two- or three-wheeled motor vehicle in traffic accident

√x7th V72.7 Person on outside of bus injured in collision with two- or three-wheeled motor vehicle in traffic accident

√x7th V72.9 Unspecified occupant of bus injured in collision with two- or three-wheeled motor vehicle in traffic accident

√4th **V73 Bus occupant injured in collision with car, pick-up truck or van**

√x7th V73.0 Driver of bus injured in collision with car, pick-up truck or van in nontraffic accident

√x7th V73.1 Passenger on bus injured in collision with car, pick-up truck or van in nontraffic accident

√x7th V73.2 Person on outside of bus injured in collision with car, pick-up truck or van in nontraffic accident

√x7th V73.3 Unspecified occupant of bus injured in collision with car, pick-up truck or van in nontraffic accident

V73.4 Person boarding or alighting from bus injured in collision with car, pick-up truck or van
V73.5 Driver of bus injured in collision with car, pick-up truck or van in traffic accident
V73.6 Passenger on bus injured in collision with car, pick-up truck or van in traffic accident
V73.7 Person on outside of bus injured in collision with car, pick-up truck or van in traffic accident
V73.9 Unspecified occupant of bus injured in collision with car, pick-up truck or van in traffic accident

V74 Bus occupant injured in collision with heavy transport vehicle or bus
EXCLUDES 1 *bus occupant injured in collision with military vehicle (V79.81)*
V74.0 Driver of bus injured in collision with heavy transport vehicle or bus in nontraffic accident
V74.1 Passenger on bus injured in collision with heavy transport vehicle or bus in nontraffic accident
V74.2 Person on outside of bus injured in collision with heavy transport vehicle or bus in nontraffic accident
V74.3 Unspecified occupant of bus injured in collision with heavy transport vehicle or bus in nontraffic accident
V74.4 Person boarding or alighting from bus injured in collision with heavy transport vehicle or bus
V74.5 Driver of bus injured in collision with heavy transport vehicle or bus in traffic accident
V74.6 Passenger on bus injured in collision with heavy transport vehicle or bus in traffic accident
V74.7 Person on outside of bus injured in collision with heavy transport vehicle or bus in traffic accident
V74.9 Unspecified occupant of bus injured in collision with heavy transport vehicle or bus in traffic accident

V75 Bus occupant injured in collision with railway train or railway vehicle
V75.0 Driver of bus injured in collision with railway train or railway vehicle in nontraffic accident
V75.1 Passenger on bus injured in collision with railway train or railway vehicle in nontraffic accident
V75.2 Person on outside of bus injured in collision with railway train or railway vehicle in nontraffic accident
V75.3 Unspecified occupant of bus injured in collision with railway train or railway vehicle in nontraffic accident
V75.4 Person boarding or alighting from bus injured in collision with railway train or railway vehicle
V75.5 Driver of bus injured in collision with railway train or railway vehicle in traffic accident
V75.6 Passenger on bus injured in collision with railway train or railway vehicle in traffic accident
V75.7 Person on outside of bus injured in collision with railway train or railway vehicle in traffic accident
V75.9 Unspecified occupant of bus injured in collision with railway train or railway vehicle in traffic accident

V76 Bus occupant injured in collision with other nonmotor vehicle
INCLUDES collision with animal-drawn vehicle, animal being ridden, streetcar
V76.0 Driver of bus injured in collision with other nonmotor vehicle in nontraffic accident
V76.1 Passenger on bus injured in collision with other nonmotor vehicle in nontraffic accident
V76.2 Person on outside of bus injured in collision with other nonmotor vehicle in nontraffic accident
V76.3 Unspecified occupant of bus injured in collision with other nonmotor vehicle in nontraffic accident
V76.4 Person boarding or alighting from bus injured in collision with other nonmotor vehicle
V76.5 Driver of bus injured in collision with other nonmotor vehicle in traffic accident
V76.6 Passenger on bus injured in collision with other nonmotor vehicle in traffic accident
V76.7 Person on outside of bus injured in collision with other nonmotor vehicle in traffic accident
V76.9 Unspecified occupant of bus injured in collision with other nonmotor vehicle in traffic accident

V77 Bus occupant injured in collision with fixed or stationary object
V77.0 Driver of bus injured in collision with fixed or stationary object in nontraffic accident
V77.1 Passenger on bus injured in collision with fixed or stationary object in nontraffic accident
V77.2 Person on outside of bus injured in collision with fixed or stationary object in nontraffic accident
V77.3 Unspecified occupant of bus injured in collision with fixed or stationary object in nontraffic accident
V77.4 Person boarding or alighting from bus injured in collision with fixed or stationary object
V77.5 Driver of bus injured in collision with fixed or stationary object in traffic accident
V77.6 Passenger on bus injured in collision with fixed or stationary object in traffic accident
V77.7 Person on outside of bus injured in collision with fixed or stationary object in traffic accident
V77.9 Unspecified occupant of bus injured in collision with fixed or stationary object in traffic accident

V78 Bus occupant injured in noncollision transport accident
INCLUDES overturning bus NOS
overturning bus without collision
V78.0 Driver of bus injured in noncollision transport accident in nontraffic accident
V78.1 Passenger on bus injured in noncollision transport accident in nontraffic accident
V78.2 Person on outside of bus injured in noncollision transport accident in nontraffic accident
V78.3 Unspecified occupant of bus injured in noncollision transport accident in nontraffic accident
V78.4 Person boarding or alighting from bus injured in noncollision transport accident
V78.5 Driver of bus injured in noncollision transport accident in traffic accident
V78.6 Passenger on bus injured in noncollision transport accident in traffic accident
V78.7 Person on outside of bus injured in noncollision transport accident in traffic accident
V78.9 Unspecified occupant of bus injured in noncollision transport accident in traffic accident

V79 Bus occupant injured in other and unspecified transport accidents
V79.0 Driver of bus injured in collision with other and unspecified motor vehicles in nontraffic accident
V79.00 Driver of bus injured in collision with unspecified motor vehicles in nontraffic accident
V79.09 Driver of bus injured in collision with other motor vehicles in nontraffic accident
V79.1 Passenger on bus injured in collision with other and unspecified motor vehicles in nontraffic accident
V79.10 Passenger on bus injured in collision with unspecified motor vehicles in nontraffic accident
V79.19 Passenger on bus injured in collision with other motor vehicles in nontraffic accident
V79.2 Unspecified bus occupant injured in collision with other and unspecified motor vehicles in nontraffic accident
V79.20 Unspecified bus occupant injured in collision with unspecified motor vehicles in nontraffic accident
Bus collision NOS, nontraffic
V79.29 Unspecified bus occupant injured in collision with other motor vehicles in nontraffic accident
V79.3 Bus occupant (driver) (passenger) injured in unspecified nontraffic accident
Bus accident NOS, nontraffic
Bus occupant injured in nontraffic accident NOS
V79.4 Driver of bus injured in collision with other and unspecified motor vehicles in traffic accident
V79.40 Driver of bus injured in collision with unspecified motor vehicles in traffic accident
V79.49 Driver of bus injured in collision with other motor vehicles in traffic accident
V79.5 Passenger on bus injured in collision with other and unspecified motor vehicles in traffic accident
V79.50 Passenger on bus injured in collision with unspecified motor vehicles in traffic accident
V79.59 Passenger on bus injured in collision with other motor vehicles in traffic accident
V79.6 Unspecified bus occupant injured in collision with other and unspecified motor vehicles in traffic accident
V79.60 Unspecified bus occupant injured in collision with unspecified motor vehicles in traffic accident
Bus collision NOS (traffic)
V79.69 Unspecified bus occupant injured in collision with other motor vehicles in traffic accident
V79.8 Bus occupant (driver) (passenger) injured in other specified transport accidents
V79.81 Bus occupant (driver) (passenger) injured in transport accidents with military vehicle

√x7th V79.88 **Bus occupant (driver) (passenger) injured in other specified transport accidents**

√x7th V79.9 **Bus occupant (driver) (passenger) injured in unspecified traffic accident**
Bus accident NOS

Other land transport accidents (V80-V89)

The appropriate 7th character is to be added to each code from categories V80-V89.
A initial encounter
D subsequent encounter
S sequela

√4th **V80 Animal-rider or occupant of animal-drawn vehicle injured in transport accident**

√5th **V80.0 Animal-rider or occupant of animal drawn vehicle injured by fall from or being thrown from animal or animal-drawn vehicle in noncollision accident**

√6th **V80.01 Animal-rider injured by fall from or being thrown from animal in noncollision accident**

√7th **V80.010 Animal-rider injured by fall from or being thrown from horse in noncollision accident**

√7th **V80.018 Animal-rider injured by fall from or being thrown from other animal in noncollision accident**

√x7th **V80.02 Occupant of animal-drawn vehicle injured by fall from or being thrown from animal-drawn vehicle in noncollision accident**
Overturning animal-drawn vehicle NOS
Overturning animal-drawn vehicle without collision

√5th **V80.1 Animal-rider or occupant of animal-drawn vehicle injured in collision with pedestrian or animal**
EXCLUDES 1 *animal-rider or animal-drawn vehicle collision with animal-drawn vehicle or animal being ridden (V80.7)*

√x7th **V80.11 Animal-rider injured in collision with pedestrian or animal**

√x7th **V80.12 Occupant of animal-drawn vehicle injured in collision with pedestrian or animal**

√5th **V80.2 Animal-rider or occupant of animal-drawn vehicle injured in collision with pedal cycle**

√x7th **V80.21 Animal-rider injured in collision with pedal cycle**

√x7th **V80.22 Occupant of animal-drawn vehicle injured in collision with pedal cycle**

√5th **V80.3 Animal-rider or occupant of animal-drawn vehicle injured in collision with two- or three-wheeled motor vehicle**

√x7th **V80.31 Animal-rider injured in collision with two- or three-wheeled motor vehicle**

√x7th **V80.32 Occupant of animal-drawn vehicle injured in collision with two- or three-wheeled motor vehicle**

√5th **V80.4 Animal-rider or occupant of animal-drawn vehicle injured in collision with car, pick-up truck, van, heavy transport vehicle or bus**
EXCLUDES 1 *animal-rider injured in collision with military vehicle (V80.910)*
occupant of animal-drawn vehicle injured in collision with military vehicle (V80.920)

√x7th **V80.41 Animal-rider injured in collision with car, pick-up truck, van, heavy transport vehicle or bus**

√x7th **V80.42 Occupant of animal-drawn vehicle injured in collision with car, pick-up truck, van, heavy transport vehicle or bus**

√5th **V80.5 Animal-rider or occupant of animal-drawn vehicle injured in collision with other specified motor vehicle**

√x7th **V80.51 Animal-rider injured in collision with other specified motor vehicle**

√x7th **V80.52 Occupant of animal-drawn vehicle injured in collision with other specified motor vehicle**

√5th **V80.6 Animal-rider or occupant of animal-drawn vehicle injured in collision with railway train or railway vehicle**

√x7th **V80.61 Animal-rider injured in collision with railway train or railway vehicle**

√x7th **V80.62 Occupant of animal-drawn vehicle injured in collision with railway train or railway vehicle**

√5th **V80.7 Animal-rider or occupant of animal-drawn vehicle injured in collision with other nonmotor vehicles**

√6th **V80.71 Animal-rider or occupant of animal-drawn vehicle injured in collision with animal being ridden**

√7th **V80.710 Animal-rider injured in collision with other animal being ridden**

√7th **V80.711 Occupant of animal-drawn vehicle injured in collision with animal being ridden**

√6th **V80.72 Animal-rider or occupant of animal-drawn vehicle injured in collision with other animal-drawn vehicle**

√7th **V80.720 Animal-rider injured in collision with animal-drawn vehicle**

√7th **V80.721 Occupant of animal-drawn vehicle injured in collision with other animal-drawn vehicle**

√6th **V80.73 Animal-rider or occupant of animal-drawn vehicle injured in collision with streetcar**

√7th **V80.730 Animal-rider injured in collision with streetcar**

√7th **V80.731 Occupant of animal-drawn vehicle injured in collision with streetcar**

√6th **V80.79 Animal-rider or occupant of animal-drawn vehicle injured in collision with other nonmotor vehicles**

√7th **V80.790 Animal-rider injured in collision with other nonmotor vehicles**

√7th **V80.791 Occupant of animal-drawn vehicle injured in collision with other nonmotor vehicles**

√5th **V80.8 Animal-rider or occupant of animal-drawn vehicle injured in collision with fixed or stationary object**

√x7th **V80.81 Animal-rider injured in collision with fixed or stationary object**

√x7th **V80.82 Occupant of animal-drawn vehicle injured in collision with fixed or stationary object**

√5th **V80.9 Animal-rider or occupant of animal-drawn vehicle injured in other and unspecified transport accidents**

√6th **V80.91 Animal-rider injured in other and unspecified transport accidents**

√7th **V80.910 Animal-rider injured in transport accident with military vehicle**

√7th **V80.918 Animal-rider injured in other transport accident**

√7th **V80.919 Animal-rider injured in unspecified transport accident**
Animal rider accident NOS

√6th **V80.92 Occupant of animal-drawn vehicle injured in other and unspecified transport accidents**

√7th **V80.920 Occupant of animal-drawn vehicle injured in transport accident with military vehicle**

√7th **V80.928 Occupant of animal-drawn vehicle injured in other transport accident**

√7th **V80.929 Occupant of animal-drawn vehicle injured in unspecified transport accident**
Animal-drawn vehicle accident NOS

√4th **V81 Occupant of railway train or railway vehicle injured in transport accident**
INCLUDES derailment of railway train or railway vehicle
person on outside of train
EXCLUDES 1 *streetcar (V82.-)*

√x7th **V81.0 Occupant of railway train or railway vehicle injured in collision with motor vehicle in nontraffic accident**
EXCLUDES 1 *occupant of railway train or railway vehicle injured due to collision with military vehicle (V81.83)*

√x7th **V81.1 Occupant of railway train or railway vehicle injured in collision with motor vehicle in traffic accident**
EXCLUDES 1 *occupant of railway train or railway vehicle injured due to collision with military vehicle (V81.83)*

√x7th **V81.2 Occupant of railway train or railway vehicle injured in collision with or hit by rolling stock**

√x7th **V81.3 Occupant of railway train or railway vehicle injured in collision with other object**
Railway collision NOS

√x7th **V81.4 Person injured while boarding or alighting from railway train or railway vehicle**

√x7th **V81.5 Occupant of railway train or railway vehicle injured by fall in railway train or railway vehicle**

√x7th **V81.6 Occupant of railway train or railway vehicle injured by fall from railway train or railway vehicle**

√x7th **V81.7 Occupant of railway train or railway vehicle injured in derailment without antecedent collision**

√5th **V81.8 Occupant of railway train or railway vehicle injured in other specified railway accidents**

√x7th **V81.81 Occupant of railway train or railway vehicle injured due to explosion or fire on train**

V81.82 Occupant of railway train or railway vehicle injured due to object falling onto train
Occupant of railway train or railway vehicle injured due to falling earth onto train
Occupant of railway train or railway vehicle injured due to falling rocks onto train
Occupant of railway train or railway vehicle injured due to falling snow onto train
Occupant of railway train or railway vehicle injured due to falling trees onto train

V81.83 Occupant of railway train or railway vehicle injured due to collision with military vehicle

V81.89 Occupant of railway train or railway vehicle injured due to other specified railway accident

V81.9 Occupant of railway train or railway vehicle injured in unspecified railway accident
Railway accident NOS

V82 Occupant of powered streetcar injured in transport accident

INCLUDES interurban electric car
person on outside of streetcar
tram (car)
trolley (car)

EXCLUDES 1 *bus (V7Ø-V79)*
motorcoach (V7Ø-V79)
nonpowered streetcar (V76.-)
train (V81.-)

V82.Ø Occupant of streetcar injured in collision with motor vehicle in nontraffic accident

V82.1 Occupant of streetcar injured in collision with motor vehicle in traffic accident

V82.2 Occupant of streetcar injured in collision with or hit by rolling stock

V82.3 Occupant of streetcar injured in collision with other object
EXCLUDES 1 *collision with animal-drawn vehicle or animal being ridden (V82.8)*

V82.4 Person injured while boarding or alighting from streetcar

V82.5 Occupant of streetcar injured by fall in streetcar
EXCLUDES 1 *fall in streetcar:*
while boarding or alighting (V82.4)
with antecedent collision (V82.Ø-V82.3)

V82.6 Occupant of streetcar injured by fall from streetcar
EXCLUDES 1 *fall from streetcar:*
while boarding or alighting (V82.4)
with antecedent collision (V82.Ø-V82.3)

V82.7 Occupant of streetcar injured in derailment without antecedent collision
EXCLUDES 1 *occupant of streetcar injured in derailment with antecedent collision (V82.Ø-V82.3)*

V82.8 Occupant of streetcar injured in other specified transport accidents
Streetcar collision with military vehicle
Streetcar collision with train or nonmotor vehicles

V82.9 Occupant of streetcar injured in unspecified traffic accident
Streetcar accident NOS

V83 Occupant of special vehicle mainly used on industrial premises injured in transport accident

INCLUDES battery-powered airport passenger vehicle
battery-powered truck (baggage) (mail)
coal-car in mine
forklift (truck)
logging car
self-propelled industrial truck
station baggage truck (powered)
tram, truck, or tub (powered) in mine or quarry

EXCLUDES 1 *special construction vehicles (V85.-)*
special industrial vehicle in stationary use or maintenance (W31.-)

V83.Ø Driver of special industrial vehicle injured in traffic accident

V83.1 Passenger of special industrial vehicle injured in traffic accident

V83.2 Person on outside of special industrial vehicle injured in traffic accident

V83.3 Unspecified occupant of special industrial vehicle injured in traffic accident

V83.4 Person injured while boarding or alighting from special industrial vehicle

V83.5 Driver of special industrial vehicle injured in nontraffic accident

V83.6 Passenger of special industrial vehicle injured in nontraffic accident

V83.7 Person on outside of special industrial vehicle injured in nontraffic accident

V83.9 Unspecified occupant of special industrial vehicle injured in nontraffic accident
Special-industrial-vehicle accident NOS

V84 Occupant of special vehicle mainly used in agriculture injured in transport accident

INCLUDES self-propelled farm machinery
tractor (and trailer)

EXCLUDES 1 *animal-powered farm machinery accident (W3Ø.8-)*
contact with combine harvester (W3Ø.Ø)
special agricultural vehicle in stationary use or maintenance (W3Ø.-)

V84.Ø Driver of special agricultural vehicle injured in traffic accident

V84.1 Passenger of special agricultural vehicle injured in traffic accident

V84.2 Person on outside of special agricultural vehicle injured in traffic accident

V84.3 Unspecified occupant of special agricultural vehicle injured in traffic accident

V84.4 Person injured while boarding or alighting from special agricultural vehicle

V84.5 Driver of special agricultural vehicle injured in nontraffic accident

V84.6 Passenger of special agricultural vehicle injured in nontraffic accident

V84.7 Person on outside of special agricultural vehicle injured in nontraffic accident

V84.9 Unspecified occupant of special agricultural vehicle injured in nontraffic accident
Special-agricultural vehicle accident NOS

V85 Occupant of special construction vehicle injured in transport accident

INCLUDES bulldozer
digger
dump truck
earth-leveller
mechanical shovel
road-roller

EXCLUDES 1 *special construction vehicle in stationary use or maintenance (W31.-)*
special industrial vehicle (V83.-)

V85.Ø Driver of special construction vehicle injured in traffic accident

V85.1 Passenger of special construction vehicle injured in traffic accident

V85.2 Person on outside of special construction vehicle injured in traffic accident

V85.3 Unspecified occupant of special construction vehicle injured in traffic accident

V85.4 Person injured while boarding or alighting from special construction vehicle

V85.5 Driver of special construction vehicle injured in nontraffic accident

V85.6 Passenger of special construction vehicle injured in nontraffic accident

V85.7 Person on outside of special construction vehicle injured in nontraffic accident

V85.9 Unspecified occupant of special construction vehicle injured in nontraffic accident
Special-construction-vehicle accident NOS

V86 Occupant of special all-terrain or other off-road motor vehicle, injured in transport accident

EXCLUDES 1 *special all-terrain vehicle in stationary use or maintenance (W31.-)*
sport-utility vehicle (V5Ø-V59)
three-wheeled motor vehicle designed for on-road use (V3Ø-V39)

AHA: 2017,4Q,26

V86.Ø Driver of special all-terrain or other off-road motor vehicle injured in traffic accident

V86.Ø1 Driver of ambulance or fire engine injured in traffic accident

V86.Ø2 Driver of snowmobile injured in traffic accident

V86.Ø3 Driver of dune buggy injured in traffic accident

V86.Ø4 Driver of military vehicle injured in traffic accident

√x7th **V86.05 Driver of 3- or 4- wheeled all-terrain vehicle (ATV) injured in traffic accident**

√x7th **V86.06 Driver of dirt bike or motor/cross bike injured in traffic accident**

√x7th **V86.09 Driver of other special all-terrain or other off-road motor vehicle injured in traffic accident**
Driver of go cart injured in traffic accident
Driver of golf cart injured in traffic accident

√5th **V86.1 Passenger of special all-terrain or other off-road motor vehicle injured in traffic accident**

√x7th **V86.11 Passenger of ambulance or fire engine injured in traffic accident**

√x7th **V86.12 Passenger of snowmobile injured in traffic accident**

√x7th **V86.13 Passenger of dune buggy injured in traffic accident**

√x7th **V86.14 Passenger of military vehicle injured in traffic accident**

√x7th **V86.15 Passenger of 3- or 4- wheeled all-terrain vehicle (ATV) injured in traffic accident**

√x7th **V86.16 Passenger of dirt bike or motor/cross bike injured in traffic accident**

√x7th **V86.19 Passenger of other special all-terrain or other off-road motor vehicle injured in traffic accident**
Passenger of go cart injured in traffic accident
Passenger of golf cart injured in traffic accident

√5th **V86.2 Person on outside of special all-terrain or other off-road motor vehicle injured in traffic accident**

√x7th **V86.21 Person on outside of ambulance or fire engine injured in traffic accident**

√x7th **V86.22 Person on outside of snowmobile injured in traffic accident**

√x7th **V86.23 Person on outside of dune buggy injured in traffic accident**

√x7th **V86.24 Person on outside of military vehicle injured in traffic accident**

√x7th **V86.25 Person on outside of 3- or 4- wheeled all-terrain vehicle (ATV) injured in traffic accident**

√x7th **V86.26 Person on outside of dirt bike or motor/cross bike injured in traffic accident**

√x7th **V86.29 Person on outside of other special all-terrain or other off-road motor vehicle injured in traffic accident**
Person on outside of go cart in traffic accident
Person on outside of golf cart injured in traffic accident

√5th **V86.3 Unspecified occupant of special all-terrain or other off-road motor vehicle injured in traffic accident**

√x7th **V86.31 Unspecified occupant of ambulance or fire engine injured in traffic accident**

√x7th **V86.32 Unspecified occupant of snowmobile injured in traffic accident**

√x7th **V86.33 Unspecified occupant of dune buggy injured in traffic accident**

√x7th **V86.34 Unspecified occupant of military vehicle injured in traffic accident**

√x7th **V86.35 Unspecified occupant of 3- or 4- wheeled all-terrain vehicle (ATV) injured in traffic accident**

√x7th **V86.36 Unspecified occupant of dirt bike or motor/cross bike injured in traffic accident**

√x7th **V86.39 Unspecified occupant of other special all-terrain or other off-road motor vehicle injured in traffic accident**
Unspecified occupant of go cart injured in traffic accident
Unspecified occupant of golf cart injured in traffic accident

√5th **V86.4 Person injured while boarding or alighting from special all-terrain or other off-road motor vehicle**

√x7th **V86.41 Person injured while boarding or alighting from ambulance or fire engine**

√x7th **V86.42 Person injured while boarding or alighting from snowmobile**

√x7th **V86.43 Person injured while boarding or alighting from dune buggy**

√x7th **V86.44 Person injured while boarding or alighting from military vehicle**

√x7th **V86.45 Person injured while boarding or alighting from a 3- or 4- wheeled all-terrain vehicle (ATV)**

√x7th **V86.46 Person injured while boarding or alighting from a dirt bike or motor/cross bike**

√x7th **V86.49 Person injured while boarding or alighting from other special all-terrain or other off-road motor vehicle**
Person injured while boarding or alighting from go cart
Person injured while boarding or alighting from golf cart

√5th **V86.5 Driver of special all-terrain or other off-road motor vehicle injured in nontraffic accident**

√x7th **V86.51 Driver of ambulance or fire engine injured in nontraffic accident**

√x7th **V86.52 Driver of snowmobile injured in nontraffic accident**

√x7th **V86.53 Driver of dune buggy injured in nontraffic accident**

√x7th **V86.54 Driver of military vehicle injured in nontraffic accident**

√x7th **V86.55 Driver of 3- or 4- wheeled all-terrain vehicle (ATV) injured in nontraffic accident**

√x7th **V86.56 Driver of dirt bike or motor/cross bike injured in nontraffic accident**

√x7th **V86.59 Driver of other special all-terrain or other off-road motor vehicle injured in nontraffic accident**
Driver of go cart injured in nontraffic accident
Driver of golf cart injured in nontraffic accident

√5th **V86.6 Passenger of special all-terrain or other off-road motor vehicle injured in nontraffic accident**

√x7th **V86.61 Passenger of ambulance or fire engine injured in nontraffic accident**

√x7th **V86.62 Passenger of snowmobile injured in nontraffic accident**

√x7th **V86.63 Passenger of dune buggy injured in nontraffic accident**

√x7th **V86.64 Passenger of military vehicle injured in nontraffic accident**

√x7th **V86.65 Passenger of 3- or 4- wheeled all-terrain vehicle (ATV) injured in nontraffic accident**

√x7th **V86.66 Passenger of dirt bike or motor/cross bike injured in nontraffic accident**

√x7th **V86.69 Passenger of other special all-terrain or other off-road motor vehicle injured in nontraffic accident**
Passenger of go cart injured in nontraffic accident
Passenger of golf cart injured in nontraffic accident

√5th **V86.7 Person on outside of special all-terrain or other off-road motor vehicle injured in nontraffic accident**

√x7th **V86.71 Person on outside of ambulance or fire engine injured in nontraffic accident**

√x7th **V86.72 Person on outside of snowmobile injured in nontraffic accident**

√x7th **V86.73 Person on outside of dune buggy injured in nontraffic accident**

√x7th **V86.74 Person on outside of military vehicle injured in nontraffic accident**

√x7th **V86.75 Person on outside of 3- or 4- wheeled all-terrain vehicle (ATV) injured in nontraffic accident**

√x7th **V86.76 Person on outside of dirt bike or motor/cross bike injured in nontraffic accident**

√x7th **V86.79 Person on outside of other special all-terrain or other off-road motor vehicles injured in nontraffic accident**
Person on outside of go cart injured in nontraffic accident
Person on outside of golf cart injured in nontraffic accident

√5th **V86.9 Unspecified occupant of special all-terrain or other off-road motor vehicle injured in nontraffic accident**

√x7th **V86.91 Unspecified occupant of ambulance or fire engine injured in nontraffic accident**

√x7th **V86.92 Unspecified occupant of snowmobile injured in nontraffic accident**

√x7th **V86.93 Unspecified occupant of dune buggy injured in nontraffic accident**

√x7th **V86.94 Unspecified occupant of military vehicle injured in nontraffic accident**

√x7th **V86.95 Unspecified occupant of 3- or 4- wheeled all-terrain vehicle (ATV) injured in nontraffic accident**

√x7th **V86.96 Unspecified occupant of dirt bike or motor/cross bike injured in nontraffic accident**

✓x7th **V86.99 Unspecified occupant of other special all-terrain or other off-road motor vehicle injured in nontraffic accident**
Off-road motor-vehicle accident NOS
Other motor-vehicle accident NOS
Unspecified occupant of go cart injured in nontraffic accident
Unspecified occupant of golf cart injured in nontraffic accident

✓4th **V87 Traffic accident of specified type but victim's mode of transport unknown**
EXCLUDES 1 *collision involving:*
pedal cycle (V10-V19)
pedestrian (V01-V09)

✓x7th **V87.0 Person injured in collision between car and two- or three-wheeled powered vehicle (traffic)**
✓x7th **V87.1 Person injured in collision between other motor vehicle and two- or three-wheeled motor vehicle (traffic)**
✓x7th **V87.2 Person injured in collision between car and pick-up truck or van (traffic)**
✓x7th **V87.3 Person injured in collision between car and bus (traffic)**
✓x7th **V87.4 Person injured in collision between car and heavy transport vehicle (traffic)**
✓x7th **V87.5 Person injured in collision between heavy transport vehicle and bus (traffic)**
✓x7th **V87.6 Person injured in collision between railway train or railway vehicle and car (traffic)**
✓x7th **V87.7 Person injured in collision between other specified motor vehicles (traffic)**
✓x7th **V87.8 Person injured in other specified noncollision transport accidents involving motor vehicle (traffic)**
✓x7th **V87.9 Person injured in other specified (collision)(noncollision) transport accidents involving nonmotor vehicle (traffic)**

✓4th **V88 Nontraffic accident of specified type but victim's mode of transport unknown**
EXCLUDES 1 *collision involving:*
pedal cycle (V10-V19)
pedestrian (V01-V09)

✓x7th **V88.0 Person injured in collision between car and two- or three-wheeled motor vehicle, nontraffic**
✓x7th **V88.1 Person injured in collision between other motor vehicle and two- or three-wheeled motor vehicle, nontraffic**
✓x7th **V88.2 Person injured in collision between car and pick-up truck or van, nontraffic**
✓x7th **V88.3 Person injured in collision between car and bus, nontraffic**
✓x7th **V88.4 Person injured in collision between car and heavy transport vehicle, nontraffic**
✓x7th **V88.5 Person injured in collision between heavy transport vehicle and bus, nontraffic**
✓x7th **V88.6 Person injured in collision between railway train or railway vehicle and car, nontraffic**
✓x7th **V88.7 Person injured in collision between other specified motor vehicle, nontraffic**
✓x7th **V88.8 Person injured in other specified noncollision transport accidents involving motor vehicle, nontraffic**
✓x7th **V88.9 Person injured in other specified (collision)(noncollision) transport accidents involving nonmotor vehicle, nontraffic**

✓4th **V89 Motor- or nonmotor-vehicle accident, type of vehicle unspecified**

✓x7th **V89.0 Person injured in unspecified motor-vehicle accident, nontraffic**
Motor-vehicle accident NOS, nontraffic
✓x7th **V89.1 Person injured in unspecified nonmotor-vehicle accident, nontraffic**
Nonmotor-vehicle accident NOS (nontraffic)
✓x7th **V89.2 Person injured in unspecified motor-vehicle accident, traffic**
Motor-vehicle accident [MVA] NOS
Road (traffic) accident [RTA] NOS
✓x7th **V89.3 Person injured in unspecified nonmotor-vehicle accident, traffic**
Nonmotor-vehicle traffic accident NOS
✓x7th **V89.9 Person injured in unspecified vehicle accident**
Collision NOS

Water transport accidents (V90-V94)

The appropriate 7th character is to be added to each code from categories V90-V94.
A initial encounter
D subsequent encounter
S sequela

✓4th **V90 Drowning and submersion due to accident to watercraft**
EXCLUDES 1 *civilian water transport accident involving military watercraft (V94.81-)*
fall into water not from watercraft (W16.-)
military watercraft accident in military or war operations (Y36.0-, Y37.0-)
water-transport-related drowning or submersion without accident to watercraft (V92.-)

✓5th **V90.0 Drowning and submersion due to watercraft overturning**
✓x7th **V90.00 Drowning and submersion due to merchant ship overturning**
✓x7th **V90.01 Drowning and submersion due to passenger ship overturning**
Drowning and submersion due to Ferry-boat overturning
Drowning and submersion due to Liner overturning
✓x7th **V90.02 Drowning and submersion due to fishing boat overturning**
✓x7th **V90.03 Drowning and submersion due to other powered watercraft overturning**
Drowning and submersion due to Hovercraft (on open water) overturning
Drowning and submersion due to Jet ski overturning
✓x7th **V90.04 Drowning and submersion due to sailboat overturning**
✓x7th **V90.05 Drowning and submersion due to canoe or kayak overturning**
✓x7th **V90.06 Drowning and submersion due to (nonpowered) inflatable craft overturning**
✓x7th **V90.08 Drowning and submersion due to other unpowered watercraft overturning**
Drowning and submersion due to windsurfer overturning
✓x7th **V90.09 Drowning and submersion due to unspecified watercraft overturning**
Drowning and submersion due to boat NOS overturning
Drowning and submersion due to ship NOS overturning
Drowning and submersion due to watercraft NOS overturning

✓5th **V90.1 Drowning and submersion due to watercraft sinking**
✓x7th **V90.10 Drowning and submersion due to merchant ship sinking**
✓x7th **V90.11 Drowning and submersion due to passenger ship sinking**
Drowning and submersion due to Ferry-boat sinking
Drowning and submersion due to Liner sinking
✓x7th **V90.12 Drowning and submersion due to fishing boat sinking**
✓x7th **V90.13 Drowning and submersion due to other powered watercraft sinking**
Drowning and submersion due to Hovercraft (on open water) sinking
Drowning and submersion due to Jet ski sinking
✓x7th **V90.14 Drowning and submersion due to sailboat sinking**
✓x7th **V90.15 Drowning and submersion due to canoe or kayak sinking**
✓x7th **V90.16 Drowning and submersion due to (nonpowered) inflatable craft sinking**
✓x7th **V90.18 Drowning and submersion due to other unpowered watercraft sinking**
✓x7th **V90.19 Drowning and submersion due to unspecified watercraft sinking**
Drowning and submersion due to boat NOS sinking
Drowning and submersion due to ship NOS sinking
Drowning and submersion due to watercraft NOS sinking

✓5th **V90.2 Drowning and submersion due to falling or jumping from burning watercraft**
✓x7th **V90.20 Drowning and submersion due to falling or jumping from burning merchant ship**

√x7th **V90.21 Drowning and submersion due to falling or jumping from burning passenger ship**
Drowning and submersion due to falling or jumping from burning Ferry-boat
Drowning and submersion due to falling or jumping from burning Liner

√x7th **V90.22 Drowning and submersion due to falling or jumping from burning fishing boat**

√x7th **V90.23 Drowning and submersion due to falling or jumping from other burning powered watercraft**
Drowning and submersion due to falling and jumping from burning Hovercraft (on open water)
Drowning and submersion due to falling and jumping from burning Jet ski

√x7th **V90.24 Drowning and submersion due to falling or jumping from burning sailboat**

√x7th **V90.25 Drowning and submersion due to falling or jumping from burning canoe or kayak**

√x7th **V90.26 Drowning and submersion due to falling or jumping from burning (nonpowered) inflatable craft**

√x7th **V90.27 Drowning and submersion due to falling or jumping from burning water-skis**

√x7th **V90.28 Drowning and submersion due to falling or jumping from other burning unpowered watercraft**
Drowning and submersion due to falling and jumping from burning surf-board
Drowning and submersion due to falling and jumping from burning windsurfer

√x7th **V90.29 Drowning and submersion due to falling or jumping from unspecified burning watercraft**
Drowning and submersion due to falling or jumping from burning boat NOS
Drowning and submersion due to falling or jumping from burning ship NOS
Drowning and submersion due to falling or jumping from burning watercraft NOS

√5th **V90.3 Drowning and submersion due to falling or jumping from crushed watercraft**

√x7th **V90.30 Drowning and submersion due to falling or jumping from crushed merchant ship**

√x7th **V90.31 Drowning and submersion due to falling or jumping from crushed passenger ship**
Drowning and submersion due to falling and jumping from crushed Ferry boat
Drowning and submersion due to falling and jumping from crushed Liner

√x7th **V90.32 Drowning and submersion due to falling or jumping from crushed fishing boat**

√x7th **V90.33 Drowning and submersion due to falling or jumping from other crushed powered watercraft**
Drowning and submersion due to falling and jumping from crushed Hovercraft
Drowning and submersion due to falling and jumping from crushed Jet ski

√x7th **V90.34 Drowning and submersion due to falling or jumping from crushed sailboat**

√x7th **V90.35 Drowning and submersion due to falling or jumping from crushed canoe or kayak**

√x7th **V90.36 Drowning and submersion due to falling or jumping from crushed (nonpowered) inflatable craft**

√x7th **V90.37 Drowning and submersion due to falling or jumping from crushed water-skis**

√x7th **V90.38 Drowning and submersion due to falling or jumping from other crushed unpowered watercraft**
Drowning and submersion due to falling and jumping from crushed surf-board
Drowning and submersion due to falling and jumping from crushed windsurfer

√x7th **V90.39 Drowning and submersion due to falling or jumping from crushed unspecified watercraft**
Drowning and submersion due to falling and jumping from crushed boat NOS
Drowning and submersion due to falling and jumping from crushed ship NOS
Drowning and submersion due to falling and jumping from crushed watercraft NOS

√5th **V90.8 Drowning and submersion due to other accident to watercraft**

√x7th **V90.80 Drowning and submersion due to other accident to merchant ship**

√x7th **V90.81 Drowning and submersion due to other accident to passenger ship**
Drowning and submersion due to other accident to Ferry-boat
Drowning and submersion due to other accident to Liner

√x7th **V90.82 Drowning and submersion due to other accident to fishing boat**

√x7th **V90.83 Drowning and submersion due to other accident to other powered watercraft**
Drowning and submersion due to other accident to Hovercraft (on open water)
Drowning and submersion due to other accident to Jet ski

√x7th **V90.84 Drowning and submersion due to other accident to sailboat**

√x7th **V90.85 Drowning and submersion due to other accident to canoe or kayak**

√x7th **V90.86 Drowning and submersion due to other accident to (nonpowered) inflatable craft**

√x7th **V90.87 Drowning and submersion due to other accident to water-skis**

√x7th **V90.88 Drowning and submersion due to other accident to other unpowered watercraft**
Drowning and submersion due to other accident to surf-board
Drowning and submersion due to other accident to windsurfer

√x7th **V90.89 Drowning and submersion due to other accident to unspecified watercraft**
Drowning and submersion due to other accident to boat NOS
Drowning and submersion due to other accident to ship NOS
Drowning and submersion due to other accident to watercraft NOS

√4th **V91 Other injury due to accident to watercraft**

INCLUDES any injury except drowning and submersion as a result of an accident to watercraft

EXCLUDES 1 *civilian water transport accident involving military watercraft (V94.81-)*
military watercraft accident in military or war operations (Y36, Y37.-)

EXCLUDES 2 *drowning and submersion due to accident to watercraft (V90.-)*

√5th **V91.0 Burn due to watercraft on fire**

EXCLUDES 1 *burn from localized fire or explosion on board ship without accident to watercraft (V93.-)*

√x7th **V91.00 Burn due to merchant ship on fire**

√x7th **V91.01 Burn due to passenger ship on fire**
Burn due to Ferry-boat on fire
Burn due to Liner on fire

√x7th **V91.02 Burn due to fishing boat on fire**

√x7th **V91.03 Burn due to other powered watercraft on fire**
Burn due to Hovercraft (on open water) on fire
Burn due to Jet ski on fire

√x7th **V91.04 Burn due to sailboat on fire**

√x7th **V91.05 Burn due to canoe or kayak on fire**

√x7th **V91.06 Burn due to (nonpowered) inflatable craft on fire**

√x7th **V91.07 Burn due to water-skis on fire**

√x7th **V91.08 Burn due to other unpowered watercraft on fire**

√x7th **V91.09 Burn due to unspecified watercraft on fire**
Burn due to boat NOS on fire
Burn due to ship NOS on fire
Burn due to watercraft NOS on fire

√5th **V91.1 Crushed between watercraft and other watercraft or other object due to collision**
Crushed by lifeboat after abandoning ship in a collision

NOTE Select the specified type of watercraft that the victim was on at the time of the collision

√x7th **V91.10 Crushed between merchant ship and other watercraft or other object due to collision**

√x7th **V91.11 Crushed between passenger ship and other watercraft or other object due to collision**
Crushed between Ferry-boat and other watercraft or other object due to collision
Crushed between Liner and other watercraft or other object due to collision

√x7th **V91.12 Crushed between fishing boat and other watercraft or other object due to collision**

√x7th **V91.13 Crushed between other powered watercraft and other watercraft or other object due to collision**
Crushed between Hovercraft (on open water) and other watercraft or other object due to collision
Crushed between Jet ski and other watercraft or other object due to collision

√x7th **V91.14 Crushed between sailboat and other watercraft or other object due to collision**

√x7th **V91.15 Crushed between canoe or kayak and other watercraft or other object due to collision**

√x7th **V91.16 Crushed between (nonpowered) inflatable craft and other watercraft or other object due to collision**

√x7th **V91.18 Crushed between other unpowered watercraft and other watercraft or other object due to collision**
Crushed between surfboard and other watercraft or other object due to collision
Crushed between windsurfer and other watercraft or other object due to collision

√x7th **V91.19 Crushed between unspecified watercraft and other watercraft or other object due to collision**
Crushed between boat NOS and other watercraft or other object due to collision
Crushed between ship NOS and other watercraft or other object due to collision
Crushed between watercraft NOS and other watercraft or other object due to collision

√5th **V91.2 Fall due to collision between watercraft and other watercraft or other object**
Fall while remaining on watercraft after collision

NOTE Select the specified type of watercraft that the victim was on at the time of the collision

EXCLUDES 1 *crushed between watercraft and other watercraft and other object due to collision (V91.1-)*
drowning and submersion due to falling from crushed watercraft (V90.3-)

√x7th **V91.20 Fall due to collision between merchant ship and other watercraft or other object**

√x7th **V91.21 Fall due to collision between passenger ship and other watercraft or other object**
Fall due to collision between Ferry-boat and other watercraft or other object
Fall due to collision between Liner and other watercraft or other object

√x7th **V91.22 Fall due to collision between fishing boat and other watercraft or other object**

√x7th **V91.23 Fall due to collision between other powered watercraft and other watercraft or other object**
Fall due to collision between Hovercraft (on open water) and other watercraft or other object
Fall due to collision between Jet ski and other watercraft or other object

√x7th **V91.24 Fall due to collision between sailboat and other watercraft or other object**

√x7th **V91.25 Fall due to collision between canoe or kayak and other watercraft or other object**

√x7th **V91.26 Fall due to collision between (nonpowered) inflatable craft and other watercraft or other object**

√x7th **V91.29 Fall due to collision between unspecified watercraft and other watercraft or other object**
Fall due to collision between boat NOS and other watercraft or other object
Fall due to collision between ship NOS and other watercraft or other object
Fall due to collision between watercraft NOS and other watercraft or other object

√5th **V91.3 Hit or struck by falling object due to accident to watercraft**
Hit or struck by falling object (part of damaged watercraft or other object) after falling or jumping from damaged watercraft

EXCLUDES 2 *drowning or submersion due to fall or jumping from damaged watercraft (V90.2-, V90.3-)*

√x7th **V91.30 Hit or struck by falling object due to accident to merchant ship**

√x7th **V91.31 Hit or struck by falling object due to accident to passenger ship**
Hit or struck by falling object due to accident to Ferry-boat
Hit or struck by falling object due to accident to Liner

√x7th **V91.32 Hit or struck by falling object due to accident to fishing boat**

√x7th **V91.33 Hit or struck by falling object due to accident to other powered watercraft**
Hit or struck by falling object due to accident to Hovercraft (on open water)
Hit or struck by falling object due to accident to Jet ski

√x7th **V91.34 Hit or struck by falling object due to accident to sailboat**

√x7th **V91.35 Hit or struck by falling object due to accident to canoe or kayak**

√x7th **V91.36 Hit or struck by falling object due to accident to (nonpowered) inflatable craft**

√x7th **V91.37 Hit or struck by falling object due to accident to water-skis**
Hit by water-skis after jumping off of waterskis

√x7th **V91.38 Hit or struck by falling object due to accident to other unpowered watercraft**
Hit or struck by surf-board after falling off damaged surf-board
Hit or struck by object after falling off damaged windsurfer

√x7th **V91.39 Hit or struck by falling object due to accident to unspecified watercraft**
Hit or struck by falling object due to accident to boat NOS
Hit or struck by falling object due to accident to ship NOS
Hit or struck by falling object due to accident to watercraft NOS

√5th **V91.8 Other injury due to other accident to watercraft**

√x7th **V91.80 Other injury due to other accident to merchant ship**

√x7th **V91.81 Other injury due to other accident to passenger ship**
Other injury due to other accident to Ferry-boat
Other injury due to other accident to Liner

√x7th **V91.82 Other injury due to other accident to fishing boat**

√x7th **V91.83 Other injury due to other accident to other powered watercraft**
Other injury due to other accident to Hovercraft (on open water)
Other injury due to other accident to Jet ski

√x7th **V91.84 Other injury due to other accident to sailboat**

√x7th **V91.85 Other injury due to other accident to canoe or kayak**

√x7th **V91.86 Other injury due to other accident to (nonpowered) inflatable craft**

√x7th **V91.87 Other injury due to other accident to water-skis**

√x7th **V91.88 Other injury due to other accident to other unpowered watercraft**
Other injury due to other accident to surf-board
Other injury due to other accident to windsurfer

√x7th **V91.89 Other injury due to other accident to unspecified watercraft**
Other injury due to other accident to boat NOS
Other injury due to other accident to ship NOS
Other injury due to other accident to watercraft NOS

√4th **V92 Drowning and submersion due to accident on board watercraft, without accident to watercraft**

EXCLUDES 1 *civilian water transport accident involving military watercraft (V94.81-)*
drowning or submersion due to accident to watercraft (VØØ-V91)
drowning or submersion of diver who voluntarily jumps from boat not involved in an accident (W16.711, W16.721)
fall into water without watercraft (W16.-)
military watercraft accident in military or war operations (Y36, Y37)

√5th **V92.Ø Drowning and submersion due to fall off watercraft**
Drowning and submersion due to fall from gangplank of watercraft
Drowning and submersion due to fall overboard watercraft
EXCLUDES 2 *hitting head on object or bottom of body of water due to fall from watercraft (V94.Ø-)*

√x7th **V92.ØØ Drowning and submersion due to fall off merchant ship**

√x7th **V92.Ø1 Drowning and submersion due to fall off passenger ship**
Drowning and submersion due to fall off Ferry-boat
Drowning and submersion due to fall off Liner

√x7th **V92.Ø2 Drowning and submersion due to fall off fishing boat**

√x7th **V92.Ø3 Drowning and submersion due to fall off other powered watercraft**
Drowning and submersion due to fall off Hovercraft (on open water)
Drowning and submersion due to fall off Jet ski

√x7th **V92.Ø4 Drowning and submersion due to fall off sailboat**

√x7th **V92.Ø5 Drowning and submersion due to fall off canoe or kayak**

√x7th **V92.Ø6 Drowning and submersion due to fall off (nonpowered) inflatable craft**

√x7th **V92.Ø7 Drowning and submersion due to fall off water-skis**
EXCLUDES 1 *drowning and submersion due to falling off burning water-skis (V9Ø.27)*
drowning and submersion due to falling off crushed water-skis (V9Ø.37)
hit by boat while water-skiing NOS ▶(V94.-)◀

√x7th **V92.Ø8 Drowning and submersion due to fall off other unpowered watercraft**
Drowning and submersion due to fall off surf-board
Drowning and submersion due to fall off windsurfer
EXCLUDES 1 *drowning and submersion due to fall off burning unpowered watercraft (V9Ø.28)*
drowning and submersion due to fall off crushed unpowered watercraft (V9Ø.38)
drowning and submersion due to fall off damaged unpowered watercraft (V9Ø.88)
drowning and submersion due to rider of nonpowered watercraft being hit by other watercraft (V94.-)
other injury due to rider of nonpowered watercraft being hit by other watercraft (V94.-)

√x7th **V92.Ø9 Drowning and submersion due to fall off unspecified watercraft**
Drowning and submersion due to fall off boat NOS
Drowning and submersion due to fall off ship
Drowning and submersion due to fall off watercraft NOS

√5th **V92.1 Drowning and submersion due to being thrown overboard by motion of watercraft**
EXCLUDES 1 *drowning and submersion due to fall off surf-board (V92.Ø8)*
drowning and submersion due to fall off water-skis (V92.Ø7)
drowning and submersion due to fall off windsurfer (V92.Ø8)

√x7th **V92.1Ø Drowning and submersion due to being thrown overboard by motion of merchant ship**

√x7th **V92.11 Drowning and submersion due to being thrown overboard by motion of passenger ship**
Drowning and submersion due to being thrown overboard by motion of Ferry-boat
Drowning and submersion due to being thrown overboard by motion of Liner

√x7th **V92.12 Drowning and submersion due to being thrown overboard by motion of fishing boat**

√x7th **V92.13 Drowning and submersion due to being thrown overboard by motion of other powered watercraft**
Drowning and submersion due to being thrown overboard by motion of Hovercraft

√x7th **V92.14 Drowning and submersion due to being thrown overboard by motion of sailboat**

√x7th **V92.15 Drowning and submersion due to being thrown overboard by motion of canoe or kayak**

√x7th **V92.16 Drowning and submersion due to being thrown overboard by motion of (nonpowered) inflatable craft**

√x7th **V92.19 Drowning and submersion due to being thrown overboard by motion of unspecified watercraft**
Drowning and submersion due to being thrown overboard by motion of boat NOS
Drowning and submersion due to being thrown overboard by motion of ship NOS
Drowning and submersion due to being thrown overboard by motion of watercraft NOS

√5th **V92.2 Drowning and submersion due to being washed overboard from watercraft**
Code first any associated cataclysm (X37.Ø-)

√x7th **V92.2Ø Drowning and submersion due to being washed overboard from merchant ship**

√x7th **V92.21 Drowning and submersion due to being washed overboard from passenger ship**
Drowning and submersion due to being washed overboard from Ferry-boat
Drowning and submersion due to being washed overboard from Liner

√x7th **V92.22 Drowning and submersion due to being washed overboard from fishing boat**

√x7th **V92.23 Drowning and submersion due to being washed overboard from other powered watercraft**
Drowning and submersion due to being washed overboard from Hovercraft (on open water)
Drowning and submersion due to being washed overboard from Jet ski

√x7th **V92.24 Drowning and submersion due to being washed overboard from sailboat**

√x7th **V92.25 Drowning and submersion due to being washed overboard from canoe or kayak**

√x7th **V92.26 Drowning and submersion due to being washed overboard from (nonpowered) inflatable craft**

√x7th **V92.27 Drowning and submersion due to being washed overboard from water-skis**
EXCLUDES 1 *drowning and submersion due to fall off water-skis (V92.Ø7)*

√x7th **V92.28 Drowning and submersion due to being washed overboard from other unpowered watercraft**
Drowning and submersion due to being washed overboard from surf-board
Drowning and submersion due to being washed overboard from windsurfer

√x7th **V92.29 Drowning and submersion due to being washed overboard from unspecified watercraft**
Drowning and submersion due to being washed overboard from boat NOS
Drowning and submersion due to being washed overboard from ship NOS
Drowning and submersion due to being washed overboard from watercraft NOS

√4th **V93 Other injury due to accident on board watercraft, without accident to watercraft**
EXCLUDES 1 *civilian water transport accident involving military watercraft (V94.81-)*
military watercraft accident in military or war operations (Y36, Y37.-)
other injury due to accident to watercraft (V91.-)
EXCLUDES 2 *drowning and submersion due to accident on board watercraft, without accident to watercraft (V92.-)*

√5th **V93.Ø Burn due to localized fire on board watercraft**
EXCLUDES 1 *burn due to watercraft on fire (V91.Ø-)*

√x7th **V93.ØØ Burn due to localized fire on board merchant vessel**

√x7th **V93.01 Burn due to localized fire on board passenger vessel**
Burn due to localized fire on board Ferry-boat
Burn due to localized fire on board Liner

√x7th **V93.02 Burn due to localized fire on board fishing boat**

√x7th **V93.03 Burn due to localized fire on board other powered watercraft**
Burn due to localized fire on board Hovercraft
Burn due to localized fire on board Jet ski

√x7th **V93.04 Burn due to localized fire on board sailboat**

√x7th **V93.09 Burn due to localized fire on board unspecified watercraft**
Burn due to localized fire on board boat NOS
Burn due to localized fire on board ship NOS
Burn due to localized fire on board watercraft NOS

√5th **V93.1 Other burn on board watercraft**
Burn due to source other than fire on board watercraft
EXCLUDES 1 *burn due to watercraft on fire (V91.0-)*

√x7th **V93.10 Other burn on board merchant vessel**

√x7th **V93.11 Other burn on board passenger vessel**
Other burn on board Ferry-boat
Other burn on board Liner

√x7th **V93.12 Other burn on board fishing boat**

√x7th **V93.13 Other burn on board other powered watercraft**
Other burn on board Hovercraft
Other burn on board Jet ski

√x7th **V93.14 Other burn on board sailboat**

√x7th **V93.19 Other burn on board unspecified watercraft**
Other burn on board boat NOS
Other burn on board ship NOS
Other burn on board watercraft NOS

√5th **V93.2 Heat exposure on board watercraft**
EXCLUDES 1 *exposure to man-made heat not aboard watercraft (W92)*
exposure to natural heat while on board watercraft (X30)
exposure to sunlight while on board watercraft (X32)
EXCLUDES 2 *burn due to fire on board watercraft (V93.0-)*

√x7th **V93.20 Heat exposure on board merchant ship**

√x7th **V93.21 Heat exposure on board passenger ship**
Heat exposure on board Ferry-boat
Heat exposure on board Liner

√x7th **V93.22 Heat exposure on board fishing boat**

√x7th **V93.23 Heat exposure on board other powered watercraft**
Heat exposure on board hovercraft

√x7th **V93.24 Heat exposure on board sailboat**

√x7th **V93.29 Heat exposure on board unspecified watercraft**
Heat exposure on board boat NOS
Heat exposure on board ship NOS
Heat exposure on board watercraft NOS

√5th **V93.3 Fall on board watercraft**
EXCLUDES 1 *fall due to collision of watercraft (V91.2-)*

√x7th **V93.30 Fall on board merchant ship**

√x7th **V93.31 Fall on board passenger ship**
Fall on board Ferry-boat
Fall on board Liner

√x7th **V93.32 Fall on board fishing boat**

√x7th **V93.33 Fall on board other powered watercraft**
Fall on board Hovercraft (on open water)
Fall on board Jet ski

√x7th **V93.34 Fall on board sailboat**

√x7th **V93.35 Fall on board canoe or kayak**

√x7th **V93.36 Fall on board (nonpowered) inflatable craft**

√x7th **V93.38 Fall on board other unpowered watercraft**

√x7th **V93.39 Fall on board unspecified watercraft**
Fall on board boat NOS
Fall on board ship NOS
Fall on board watercraft NOS

√5th **V93.4 Struck by falling object on board watercraft**
Hit by falling object on board watercraft
EXCLUDES 1 *struck by falling object due to accident to watercraft (V91.3)*

√x7th **V93.40 Struck by falling object on merchant ship**

√x7th **V93.41 Struck by falling object on passenger ship**
Struck by falling object on Ferry-boat
Struck by falling object on Liner

√x7th **V93.42 Struck by falling object on fishing boat**

√x7th **V93.43 Struck by falling object on other powered watercraft**
Struck by falling object on Hovercraft

√x7th **V93.44 Struck by falling object on sailboat**

√x7th **V93.48 Struck by falling object on other unpowered watercraft**

√x7th **V93.49 Struck by falling object on unspecified watercraft**

√5th **V93.5 Explosion on board watercraft**
Boiler explosion on steamship
EXCLUDES 2 *fire on board watercraft (V93.0-)*

√x7th **V93.50 Explosion on board merchant ship**

√x7th **V93.51 Explosion on board passenger ship**
Explosion on board Ferry-boat
Explosion on board Liner

√x7th **V93.52 Explosion on board fishing boat**

√x7th **V93.53 Explosion on board other powered watercraft**
Explosion on board Hovercraft
Explosion on board Jet ski

√x7th **V93.54 Explosion on board sailboat**

√x7th **V93.59 Explosion on board unspecified watercraft**
Explosion on board boat NOS
Explosion on board ship NOS
Explosion on board watercraft NOS

√5th **V93.6 Machinery accident on board watercraft**
EXCLUDES 1 *machinery explosion on board watercraft (V93.4-)*
machinery fire on board watercraft (V93.0-)

√x7th **V93.60 Machinery accident on board merchant ship**

√x7th **V93.61 Machinery accident on board passenger ship**
Machinery accident on board Ferry-boat
Machinery accident on board Liner

√x7th **V93.62 Machinery accident on board fishing boat**

√x7th **V93.63 Machinery accident on board other powered watercraft**
Machinery accident on board Hovercraft

√x7th **V93.64 Machinery accident on board sailboat**

√x7th **V93.69 Machinery accident on board unspecified watercraft**
Machinery accident on board boat NOS
Machinery accident on board ship NOS
Machinery accident on board watercraft NOS

√5th **V93.8 Other injury due to other accident on board watercraft**
Accidental poisoning by gases or fumes on watercraft

√x7th **V93.80 Other injury due to other accident on board merchant ship**

√x7th **V93.81 Other injury due to other accident on board passenger ship**
Other injury due to other accident on board Ferry-boat
Other injury due to other accident on board Liner

√x7th **V93.82 Other injury due to other accident on board fishing boat**

√x7th **V93.83 Other injury due to other accident on board other powered watercraft**
Other injury due to other accident on board Hovercraft
Other injury due to other accident on board Jet ski

√x7th **V93.84 Other injury due to other accident on board sailboat**

√x7th **V93.85 Other injury due to other accident on board canoe or kayak**

√x7th **V93.86 Other injury due to other accident on board (nonpowered) inflatable craft**

√x7th **V93.87 Other injury due to other accident on board water-skis**
Hit or struck by object while waterskiing

√x7th **V93.88 Other injury due to other accident on board other unpowered watercraft**
Hit or struck by object while surfing
Hit or struck by object while on board windsurfer

√x7th **V93.89 Other injury due to other accident on board unspecified watercraft**
Other injury due to other accident on board boat NOS
Other injury due to other accident on board ship NOS
Other injury due to other accident on board watercraft NOS

√4th **V94 Other and unspecified water transport accidents**
EXCLUDES 1 *military watercraft accidents in military or war operations (Y36, Y37)*

√x7th **V94.Ø Hitting object or bottom of body of water due to fall from watercraft**
EXCLUDES 2 *drowning and submersion due to fall from watercraft (V92.Ø-)*

√5th **V94.1 Bather struck by watercraft**
Swimmer hit by watercraft

√x7th **V94.11 Bather struck by powered watercraft**

√x7th **V94.12 Bather struck by nonpowered watercraft**

√5th **V94.2 Rider of nonpowered watercraft struck by other watercraft**

√x7th **V94.21 Rider of nonpowered watercraft struck by other nonpowered watercraft**
Canoer hit by other nonpowered watercraft
Surfer hit by other nonpowered watercraft
Windsurfer hit by other nonpowered watercraft

√x7th **V94.22 Rider of nonpowered watercraft struck by powered watercraft**
Canoer hit by motorboat
Surfer hit by motorboat
Windsurfer hit by motorboat

√5th **V94.3 Injury to rider of (inflatable) watercraft being pulled behind other watercraft**

√x7th **V94.31 Injury to rider of (inflatable) recreational watercraft being pulled behind other watercraft**
Injury to rider of inner-tube pulled behind motor boat

√x7th **V94.32 Injury to rider of non-recreational watercraft being pulled behind other watercraft**
Injury to occupant of dingy being pulled behind boat or ship
Injury to occupant of life-raft being pulled behind boat or ship

√x7th **V94.4 Injury to barefoot water-skier**
Injury to person being pulled behind boat or ship

√5th **V94.8 Other water transport accident**

√6th **V94.81 Water transport accident involving military watercraft**

√7th **V94.81Ø Civilian watercraft involved in water transport accident with military watercraft**
Passenger on civilian watercraft injured due to accident with military watercraft

√7th **V94.811 Civilian in water injured by military watercraft**

√7th **V94.818 Other water transport accident involving military watercraft**

√x7th **V94.89 Other water transport accident**

√x7th **V94.9 Unspecified water transport accident**
Water transport accident NOS

Air and space transport accidents (V95-V97)

EXCLUDES 1 *military aircraft accidents in military or war operations (Y36, Y37)*

The appropriate 7th character is to be added to each code from categories V95-V97.
A initial encounter
D subsequent encounter
S sequela

√4th **V95 Accident to powered aircraft causing injury to occupant**

√5th **V95.Ø Helicopter accident injuring occupant**

√x7th **V95.ØØ Unspecified helicopter accident injuring occupant**

√x7th **V95.Ø1 Helicopter crash injuring occupant**

√x7th **V95.Ø2 Forced landing of helicopter injuring occupant**

√x7th **V95.Ø3 Helicopter collision injuring occupant**
Helicopter collision with any object, fixed, movable or moving

√x7th **V95.Ø4 Helicopter fire injuring occupant**

√x7th **V95.Ø5 Helicopter explosion injuring occupant**

√x7th **V95.Ø9 Other helicopter accident injuring occupant**

√5th **V95.1 Ultralight, microlight or powered-glider accident injuring occupant**

√x7th **V95.1Ø Unspecified ultralight, microlight or powered-glider accident injuring occupant**

√x7th **V95.11 Ultralight, microlight or powered-glider crash injuring occupant**

√x7th **V95.12 Forced landing of ultralight, microlight or powered-glider injuring occupant**

√x7th **V95.13 Ultralight, microlight or powered-glider collision injuring occupant**
Ultralight, microlight or powered-glider collision with any object, fixed, movable or moving

√x7th **V95.14 Ultralight, microlight or powered-glider fire injuring occupant**

√x7th **V95.15 Ultralight, microlight or powered-glider explosion injuring occupant**

√x7th **V95.19 Other ultralight, microlight or powered-glider accident injuring occupant**

√5th **V95.2 Other private fixed-wing aircraft accident injuring occupant**

√x7th **V95.2Ø Unspecified accident to other private fixed-wing aircraft, injuring occupant**

√x7th **V95.21 Other private fixed-wing aircraft crash injuring occupant**

√x7th **V95.22 Forced landing of other private fixed-wing aircraft injuring occupant**

√x7th **V95.23 Other private fixed-wing aircraft collision injuring occupant**
Other private fixed-wing aircraft collision with any object, fixed, movable or moving

√x7th **V95.24 Other private fixed-wing aircraft fire injuring occupant**

√x7th **V95.25 Other private fixed-wing aircraft explosion injuring occupant**

√x7th **V95.29 Other accident to other private fixed-wing aircraft injuring occupant**

√5th **V95.3 Commercial fixed-wing aircraft accident injuring occupant**

√x7th **V95.3Ø Unspecified accident to commercial fixed-wing aircraft injuring occupant**

√x7th **V95.31 Commercial fixed-wing aircraft crash injuring occupant**

√x7th **V95.32 Forced landing of commercial fixed-wing aircraft injuring occupant**

√x7th **V95.33 Commercial fixed-wing aircraft collision injuring occupant**
Commercial fixed-wing aircraft collision with any object, fixed, movable or moving

√x7th **V95.34 Commercial fixed-wing aircraft fire injuring occupant**

√x7th **V95.35 Commercial fixed-wing aircraft explosion injuring occupant**

√x7th **V95.39 Other accident to commercial fixed-wing aircraft injuring occupant**

√5th **V95.4 Spacecraft accident injuring occupant**

√x7th **V95.4Ø Unspecified spacecraft accident injuring occupant**

√x7th **V95.41 Spacecraft crash injuring occupant**

√x7th **V95.42 Forced landing of spacecraft injuring occupant**

√x7th **V95.43 Spacecraft collision injuring occupant**
Spacecraft collision with any object, fixed, moveable or moving

√x7th **V95.44 Spacecraft fire injuring occupant**

√x7th **V95.45 Spacecraft explosion injuring occupant**

√x7th **V95.49 Other spacecraft accident injuring occupant**

√x7th **V95.8 Other powered aircraft accidents injuring occupant**

√x7th **V95.9 Unspecified aircraft accident injuring occupant**
Aircraft accident NOS
Air transport accident NOS

√4th **V96 Accident to nonpowered aircraft causing injury to occupant**

√5th **V96.Ø Balloon accident injuring occupant**

√x7th **V96.ØØ Unspecified balloon accident injuring occupant**

√x7th **V96.Ø1 Balloon crash injuring occupant**

√x7th **V96.Ø2 Forced landing of balloon injuring occupant**

√x7th **V96.Ø3 Balloon collision injuring occupant**
Balloon collision with any object, fixed, moveable or moving

√x7th **V96.Ø4 Balloon fire injuring occupant**

√x7th **V96.Ø5 Balloon explosion injuring occupant**

V96.09 Other balloon accident injuring occupant

V96.1 Hang-glider accident injuring occupant

V96.10 Unspecified hang-glider accident injuring occupant

V96.11 Hang-glider crash injuring occupant

V96.12 Forced landing of hang-glider injuring occupant

V96.13 Hang-glider collision injuring occupant
Hang-glider collision with any object, fixed, moveable or moving

V96.14 Hang-glider fire injuring occupant

V96.15 Hang-glider explosion injuring occupant

V96.19 Other hang-glider accident injuring occupant

V96.2 Glider (nonpowered) accident injuring occupant

V96.20 Unspecified glider (nonpowered) accident injuring occupant

V96.21 Glider (nonpowered) crash injuring occupant

V96.22 Forced landing of glider (nonpowered) injuring occupant

V96.23 Glider (nonpowered) collision injuring occupant
Glider (nonpowered) collision with any object, fixed, moveable or moving

V96.24 Glider (nonpowered) fire injuring occupant

V96.25 Glider (nonpowered) explosion injuring occupant

V96.29 Other glider (nonpowered) accident injuring occupant

V96.8 Other nonpowered-aircraft accidents injuring occupant
Kite carrying a person accident injuring occupant

V96.9 Unspecified nonpowered-aircraft accident injuring occupant
Nonpowered-aircraft accident NOS

V97 Other specified air transport accidents

V97.0 Occupant of aircraft injured in other specified air transport accidents
Fall in, on or from aircraft in air transport accident
EXCLUDES 1 *accident while boarding or alighting aircraft (V97.1)*

V97.1 Person injured while boarding or alighting from aircraft

V97.2 Parachutist accident

V97.21 Parachutist entangled in object
Parachutist landing in tree

V97.22 Parachutist injured on landing

V97.29 Other parachutist accident

V97.3 Person on ground injured in air transport accident

V97.31 Hit by object falling from aircraft
Hit by crashing aircraft
Injured by aircraft hitting house
Injured by aircraft hitting car

V97.32 Injured by rotating propeller

V97.33 Sucked into jet engine

V97.39 Other injury to person on ground due to air transport accident

V97.8 Other air transport accidents, not elsewhere classified
EXCLUDES 1 *aircraft accident NOS (V95.9)*
exposure to changes in air pressure during ascent or descent (W94.-)

V97.81 Air transport accident involving military aircraft

V97.810 Civilian aircraft involved in air transport accident with military aircraft
Passenger in civilian aircraft injured due to accident with military aircraft

V97.811 Civilian injured by military aircraft

V97.818 Other air transport accident involving military aircraft

V97.89 Other air transport accidents, not elsewhere classified
Injury from machinery on aircraft

Other and unspecified transport accidents (V98-V99)

EXCLUDES 1 *vehicle accident, type of vehicle unspecified (V89.-)*

The appropriate 7th character is to be added to each code from categories V98-V99.
A initial encounter
D subsequent encounter
S sequela

V98 Other specified transport accidents

V98.0 Accident to, on or involving cable-car, not on rails
Caught or dragged by cable-car, not on rails
Fall or jump from cable-car, not on rails
Object thrown from or in cable-car, not on rails

V98.1 Accident to, on or involving land-yacht

V98.2 Accident to, on or involving ice yacht

V98.3 Accident to, on or involving ski lift
Accident to, on or involving ski chair-lift
Accident to, on or involving ski-lift with gondola

V98.8 Other specified transport accidents

V99 Unspecified transport accident

OTHER EXTERNAL CAUSES OF ACCIDENTAL INJURY (W00-X58)

Slipping, tripping, stumbling and falls (W00-W19)

EXCLUDES 1 *assault involving a fall (Y01-Y02)*
fall from animal (V80.-)
fall (in) (from) machinery (in operation) (W28-W31)
fall (in) (from) transport vehicle (V01-V99)
intentional self-harm involving a fall (X80-X81)
EXCLUDES 2 *at risk for fall (history of fall) Z91.81*
fall (in) (from) burning building (X00.-)
fall into fire (X00-X04, X08)

The appropriate 7th character is to be added to each code from categories W00-W19.
A initial encounter
D subsequent encounter
S sequela

W00 Fall due to ice and snow
INCLUDES pedestrian on foot falling (slipping) on ice and snow
EXCLUDES 1 *fall on (from) ice and snow involving pedestrian conveyance (V00.-)*
fall from stairs and steps not due to ice and snow (W10.-)
AHA: 2016,2Q,4

W00.0 Fall on same level due to ice and snow

W00.1 Fall from stairs and steps due to ice and snow

W00.2 Other fall from one level to another due to ice and snow

W00.9 Unspecified fall due to ice and snow

W01 Fall on same level from slipping, tripping and stumbling
INCLUDES fall on moving sidewalk
EXCLUDES 1 *fall due to bumping (striking) against object (W18.0-)*
fall in shower or bathtub (W18.2-)
fall on same level NOS (W18.30)
fall on same level from slipping, tripping and stumbling due to ice or snow (W00.0)
fall off or from toilet (W18.1-)
slipping, tripping and stumbling NOS (W18.40)
slipping, tripping and stumbling without falling (W18.4-)

W01.0 Fall on same level from slipping, tripping and stumbling without subsequent striking against object
Falling over animal

W01.1 Fall on same level from slipping, tripping and stumbling with subsequent striking against object

W01.10 Fall on same level from slipping, tripping and stumbling with subsequent striking against unspecified object

W01.11 Fall on same level from slipping, tripping and stumbling with subsequent striking against sharp object

W01.110 Fall on same level from slipping, tripping and stumbling with subsequent striking against sharp glass

W01.111 Fall on same level from slipping, tripping and stumbling with subsequent striking against power tool or machine

W01.118 Fall on same level from slipping, tripping and stumbling with subsequent striking against other sharp object

√7th **W01.119 Fall on same level from slipping, tripping and stumbling with subsequent striking against unspecified sharp object**

√6th **W01.19 Fall on same level from slipping, tripping and stumbling with subsequent striking against other object**

√7th **W01.190 Fall on same level from slipping, tripping and stumbling with subsequent striking against furniture**

√7th **W01.198 Fall on same level from slipping, tripping and stumbling with subsequent striking against other object**

√x7th **W03 Other fall on same level due to collision with another person**

Fall due to non-transport collision with other person

EXCLUDES 1 *collision with another person without fall (W51)*
crushed or pushed by a crowd or human stampede (W52)
fall due to ice or snow (W00)
fall involving pedestrian conveyance (V00-V09)
fall on same level NOS (W18.30)

AHA: 2012,4Q,108

√x7th **W04 Fall while being carried or supported by other persons**

Accidentally dropped while being carried

√4th **W05 Fall from non-moving wheelchair, nonmotorized scooter and motorized mobility scooter**

EXCLUDES 1 *fall from moving motorized mobility scooter (V00.831)*
fall from moving wheelchair (powered) (V00.811)
fall from nonmotorized scooter (V00.141)

√x7th **W05.0 Fall from non-moving wheelchair**

AHA: 2019,2Q,27

√x7th **W05.1 Fall from non-moving nonmotorized scooter**

√x7th **W05.2 Fall from non-moving motorized mobility scooter**

√x7th **W06 Fall from bed**

√x7th **W07 Fall from chair**

√x7th **W08 Fall from other furniture**

Fall from stool

√4th **W09 Fall on and from playground equipment**

EXCLUDES 1 *fall involving recreational machinery (W31)*

√x7th **W09.0 Fall on or from playground slide**

√x7th **W09.1 Fall from playground swing**

√x7th **W09.2 Fall on or from jungle gym**

√x7th **W09.8 Fall on or from other playground equipment**

√4th **W10 Fall on and from stairs and steps**

EXCLUDES 1 *Fall from stairs and steps due to ice and snow (W00.1)*

√x7th **W10.0 Fall (on)(from) escalator**

√x7th **W10.1 Fall (on)(from) sidewalk curb**

√x7th **W10.2 Fall (on)(from) incline**

Fall (on) (from) ramp

√x7th **W10.8 Fall (on) (from) other stairs and steps**

√x7th **W10.9 Fall (on) (from) unspecified stairs and steps**

√x7th **W11 Fall on and from ladder**

√x7th **W12 Fall on and from scaffolding**

√4th **W13 Fall from, out of or through building or structure**

√x7th **W13.0 Fall from, out of or through balcony**

Fall from, out of or through railing

√x7th **W13.1 Fall from, out of or through bridge**

√x7th **W13.2 Fall from, out of or through roof**

√x7th **W13.3 Fall through floor**

√x7th **W13.4 Fall from, out of or through window**

EXCLUDES 2 *fall with subsequent striking against sharp glass (W01.110-)*

√x7th **W13.8 Fall from, out of or through other building or structure**

Fall from, out of or through viaduct
Fall from, out of or through wall
Fall from, out of or through flag-pole

√x7th **W13.9 Fall from, out of or through building, not otherwise specified**

EXCLUDES 1 *collapse of a building or structure (W20.-)*
fall or jump from burning building or structure (X00.-)

√x7th **W14 Fall from tree**

√x7th **W15 Fall from cliff**

√4th **W16 Fall, jump or diving into water**

EXCLUDES 1 *accidental non-watercraft drowning and submersion not involving fall (W65-W74)*
effects of air pressure from diving (W94.-)
fall into water from watercraft (V90-V94)
hitting an object or against bottom when falling from watercraft (V94.0)

EXCLUDES 2 *striking or hitting diving board (W21.4)*

√5th **W16.0 Fall into swimming pool**

Fall into swimming pool NOS

EXCLUDES 1 *fall into empty swimming pool (W17.3)*

√6th **W16.01 Fall into swimming pool striking water surface**

√7th **W16.011 Fall into swimming pool striking water surface causing drowning and submersion**

EXCLUDES 1 *drowning and submersion while in swimming pool without fall (W67)*

√7th **W16.012 Fall into swimming pool striking water surface causing other injury**

√6th **W16.02 Fall into swimming pool striking bottom**

√7th **W16.021 Fall into swimming pool striking bottom causing drowning and submersion**

EXCLUDES 1 *drowning and submersion while in swimming pool without fall (W67)*

√7th **W16.022 Fall into swimming pool striking bottom causing other injury**

√6th **W16.03 Fall into swimming pool striking wall**

√7th **W16.031 Fall into swimming pool striking wall causing drowning and submersion**

EXCLUDES 1 *drowning and submersion while in swimming pool without fall (W67)*

√7th **W16.032 Fall into swimming pool striking wall causing other injury**

√5th **W16.1 Fall into natural body of water**

Fall into lake
Fall into open sea
Fall into river
Fall into stream

√6th **W16.11 Fall into natural body of water striking water surface**

√7th **W16.111 Fall into natural body of water striking water surface causing drowning and submersion**

EXCLUDES 1 *drowning and submersion while in natural body of water without fall (W69)*

√7th **W16.112 Fall into natural body of water striking water surface causing other injury**

√6th **W16.12 Fall into natural body of water striking bottom**

√7th **W16.121 Fall into natural body of water striking bottom causing drowning and submersion**

EXCLUDES 1 *drowning and submersion while in natural body of water without fall (W69)*

√7th **W16.122 Fall into natural body of water striking bottom causing other injury**

√6th **W16.13 Fall into natural body of water striking side**

√7th **W16.131 Fall into natural body of water striking side causing drowning and submersion**

EXCLUDES 1 *drowning and submersion while in natural body of water without fall (W69)*

√7th **W16.132 Fall into natural body of water striking side causing other injury**

√5th **W16.2 Fall in (into) filled bathtub or bucket of water**

√6th **W16.21 Fall in (into) filled bathtub**

EXCLUDES 1 *fall into empty bathtub (W18.2)*

√7th **W16.211 Fall in (into) filled bathtub causing drowning and submersion**

EXCLUDES 1 *drowning and submersion while in filled bathtub without fall (W65)*

√7th **W16.212 Fall in (into) filled bathtub causing other injury**

✓6th **W16.22 Fall in (into) bucket of water**

✓7th **W16.221 Fall in (into) bucket of water causing drowning and submersion**

✓7th **W16.222 Fall in (into) bucket of water causing other injury**

✓5th **W16.3 Fall into other water**

Fall into fountain
Fall into reservoir

✓6th **W16.31 Fall into other water striking water surface**

✓7th **W16.311 Fall into other water striking water surface causing drowning and submersion**

EXCLUDES 1 *drowning and submersion while in other water without fall (W73)*

✓7th **W16.312 Fall into other water striking water surface causing other injury**

✓6th **W16.32 Fall into other water striking bottom**

✓7th **W16.321 Fall into other water striking bottom causing drowning and submersion**

EXCLUDES 1 *drowning and submersion while in other water without fall (W73)*

✓7th **W16.322 Fall into other water striking bottom causing other injury**

✓6th **W16.33 Fall into other water striking wall**

✓7th **W16.331 Fall into other water striking wall causing drowning and submersion**

EXCLUDES 1 *drowning and submersion while in other water without fall (W73)*

✓7th **W16.332 Fall into other water striking wall causing other injury**

✓5th **W16.4 Fall into unspecified water**

✓x7th **W16.41 Fall into unspecified water causing drowning and submersion**

✓x7th **W16.42 Fall into unspecified water causing other injury**

✓5th **W16.5 Jumping or diving into swimming pool**

✓6th **W16.51 Jumping or diving into swimming pool striking water surface**

✓7th **W16.511 Jumping or diving into swimming pool striking water surface causing drowning and submersion**

EXCLUDES 1 *drowning and submersion while in swimming pool without jumping or diving (W67)*

✓7th **W16.512 Jumping or diving into swimming pool striking water surface causing other injury**

✓6th **W16.52 Jumping or diving into swimming pool striking bottom**

✓7th **W16.521 Jumping or diving into swimming pool striking bottom causing drowning and submersion**

EXCLUDES 1 *drowning and submersion while in swimming pool without jumping or diving (W67)*

✓7th **W16.522 Jumping or diving into swimming pool striking bottom causing other injury**

✓6th **W16.53 Jumping or diving into swimming pool striking wall**

✓7th **W16.531 Jumping or diving into swimming pool striking wall causing drowning and submersion**

EXCLUDES 1 *drowning and submersion while in swimming pool without jumping or diving (W67)*

✓7th **W16.532 Jumping or diving into swimming pool striking wall causing other injury**

✓5th **W16.6 Jumping or diving into natural body of water**

Jumping or diving into lake
Jumping or diving into open sea
Jumping or diving into river
Jumping or diving into stream

✓6th **W16.61 Jumping or diving into natural body of water striking water surface**

✓7th **W16.611 Jumping or diving into natural body of water striking water surface causing drowning and submersion**

EXCLUDES 1 *drowning and submersion while in natural body of water without jumping or diving (W69)*

✓7th **W16.612 Jumping or diving into natural body of water striking water surface causing other injury**

✓6th **W16.62 Jumping or diving into natural body of water striking bottom**

✓7th **W16.621 Jumping or diving into natural body of water striking bottom causing drowning and submersion**

EXCLUDES 1 *drowning and submersion while in natural body of water without jumping or diving (W69)*

✓7th **W16.622 Jumping or diving into natural body of water striking bottom causing other injury**

✓5th **W16.7 Jumping or diving from boat**

EXCLUDES 1 *fall from boat into water - see watercraft accident (V90-V94)*

✓6th **W16.71 Jumping or diving from boat striking water surface**

✓7th **W16.711 Jumping or diving from boat striking water surface causing drowning and submersion**

✓7th **W16.712 Jumping or diving from boat striking water surface causing other injury**

✓6th **W16.72 Jumping or diving from boat striking bottom**

✓7th **W16.721 Jumping or diving from boat striking bottom causing drowning and submersion**

✓7th **W16.722 Jumping or diving from boat striking bottom causing other injury**

✓5th **W16.8 Jumping or diving into other water**

Jumping or diving into fountain
Jumping or diving into reservoir

✓6th **W16.81 Jumping or diving into other water striking water surface**

✓7th **W16.811 Jumping or diving into other water striking water surface causing drowning and submersion**

EXCLUDES 1 *drowning and submersion while in other water without jumping or diving (W73)*

✓7th **W16.812 Jumping or diving into other water striking water surface causing other injury**

✓6th **W16.82 Jumping or diving into other water striking bottom**

✓7th **W16.821 Jumping or diving into other water striking bottom causing drowning and submersion**

EXCLUDES 1 *drowning and submersion while in other water without jumping or diving (W73)*

✓7th **W16.822 Jumping or diving into other water striking bottom causing other injury**

✓6th **W16.83 Jumping or diving into other water striking wall**

✓7th **W16.831 Jumping or diving into other water striking wall causing drowning and submersion**

EXCLUDES 1 *drowning and submersion while in other water without jumping or diving (W73)*

✓7th **W16.832 Jumping or diving into other water striking wall causing other injury**

W16.9 Jumping or diving into unspecified water

W16.91 Jumping or diving into unspecified water causing drowning and submersion

W16.92 Jumping or diving into unspecified water causing other injury

W17 Other fall from one level to another

W17.Ø Fall into well

W17.1 Fall into storm drain or manhole

W17.2 Fall into hole

Fall into pit

W17.3 Fall into empty swimming pool

EXCLUDES 1 *fall into filled swimming pool (W16.Ø-)*

W17.4 Fall from dock

W17.8 Other fall from one level to another

W17.81 Fall down embankment (hill)

W17.82 Fall from (out of) grocery cart

Fall due to grocery cart tipping over

W17.89 Other fall from one level to another

Fall from cherry picker
Fall from lifting device
Fall from mobile elevated work platform [MEWP]
Fall from sky lift

AHA: 2015,2Q,6

W18 Other slipping, tripping and stumbling and falls

W18.Ø Fall due to bumping against object

Striking against object with subsequent fall

EXCLUDES 1 *fall on same level due to slipping, tripping, or stumbling with subsequent striking against object (WØ1.1-)*

W18.ØØ Striking against unspecified object with subsequent fall

W18.Ø1 Striking against sports equipment with subsequent fall

W18.Ø2 Striking against glass with subsequent fall

W18.Ø9 Striking against other object with subsequent fall

W18.1 Fall from or off toilet

W18.11 Fall from or off toilet without subsequent striking against object

Fall from (off) toilet NOS

W18.12 Fall from or off toilet with subsequent striking against object

W18.2 Fall in (into) shower or empty bathtub

EXCLUDES 1 *fall in full bathtub causing drowning or submersion (W16.21-)*

W18.3 Other and unspecified fall on same level

W18.3Ø Fall on same level, unspecified

W18.31 Fall on same level due to stepping on an object

Fall on same level due to stepping on an animal

EXCLUDES 1 *slipping, tripping and stumbling without fall due to stepping on animal (W18.41)*

W18.39 Other fall on same level

W18.4 Slipping, tripping and stumbling without falling

EXCLUDES 1 *collision with another person without fall (W51)*

W18.4Ø Slipping, tripping and stumbling without falling, unspecified

W18.41 Slipping, tripping and stumbling without falling due to stepping on object

Slipping, tripping and stumbling without falling due to stepping on animal

EXCLUDES 1 *slipping, tripping and stumbling with fall due to stepping on animal (W18.31)*

W18.42 Slipping, tripping and stumbling without falling due to stepping into hole or opening

W18.43 Slipping, tripping and stumbling without falling due to stepping from one level to another

W18.49 Other slipping, tripping and stumbling without falling

W19 Unspecified fall

Accidental fall NOS

AHA: 2012,4Q,95

Exposure to inanimate mechanical forces (W2Ø-W49)

EXCLUDES 1 *assault (X92-YØ9)*
contact or collision with animals or persons (W5Ø-W64)
exposure to inanimate mechanical forces involving military or war operations (Y36.-, Y37.-)
intentional self-harm (X71-X83)

The appropriate 7th character is to be added to each code from categories W2Ø-W49.
A initial encounter
D subsequent encounter
S sequela

W2Ø Struck by thrown, projected or falling object

Code first any associated:
cataclysm (X34-X39)
lightning strike (T75.ØØ)

EXCLUDES 1 *falling object in machinery accident (W24, W28-W31)*
falling object in transport accident (VØ1-V99)
object set in motion by explosion (W35-W4Ø)
object set in motion by firearm (W32-W34)
struck by thrown sports equipment (W21.-)

W2Ø.Ø Struck by falling object in cave-in

EXCLUDES 2 *asphyxiation due to cave-in (T71.21)*

W2Ø.1 Struck by object due to collapse of building

EXCLUDES 1 *struck by object due to collapse of burning building (XØØ.2, XØ2.2)*

W2Ø.8 Other cause of strike by thrown, projected or falling object

EXCLUDES 1 *struck by thrown sports equipment (W21.-)*

W21 Striking against or struck by sports equipment

EXCLUDES 1 *assault with sports equipment (YØ8.Ø-)*
striking against or struck by sports equipment with subsequent fall (W18.Ø1)

W21.Ø Struck by hit or thrown ball

W21.ØØ Struck by hit or thrown ball, unspecified type

W21.Ø1 Struck by football

W21.Ø2 Struck by soccer ball

W21.Ø3 Struck by baseball

W21.Ø4 Struck by golf ball

W21.Ø5 Struck by basketball

W21.Ø6 Struck by volleyball

W21.Ø7 Struck by softball

W21.Ø9 Struck by other hit or thrown ball

W21.1 Struck by bat, racquet or club

W21.11 Struck by baseball bat

W21.12 Struck by tennis racquet

W21.13 Struck by golf club

W21.19 Struck by other bat, racquet or club

W21.2 Struck by hockey stick or puck

W21.21 Struck by hockey stick

W21.21Ø Struck by ice hockey stick

W21.211 Struck by field hockey stick

W21.22 Struck by hockey puck

W21.22Ø Struck by ice hockey puck

W21.221 Struck by field hockey puck

W21.3 Struck by sports foot wear

W21.31 Struck by shoe cleats

Stepped on by shoe cleats

W21.32 Struck by skate blades

Skated over by skate blades

W21.39 Struck by other sports foot wear

W21.4 Striking against diving board

Use additional code for subsequent falling into water, if applicable (W16.-)

W21.8 Striking against or struck by other sports equipment

W21.81 Striking against or struck by football helmet

W21.89 Striking against or struck by other sports equipment

W21.9 Striking against or struck by unspecified sports equipment

W22 Striking against or struck by other objects

EXCLUDES 1 *striking against or struck by object with subsequent fall (W18.09)*

W22.0 Striking against stationary object

EXCLUDES 1 *striking against stationary sports equipment (W21.8)*

W22.01 Walked into wall

W22.02 Walked into lamppost

W22.03 Walked into furniture

W22.04 Striking against wall of swimming pool

W22.041 Striking against wall of swimming pool causing drowning and submersion

EXCLUDES 1 *drowning and submersion while swimming without striking against wall (W67)*

W22.042 Striking against wall of swimming pool causing other injury

W22.09 Striking against other stationary object

W22.1 Striking against or struck by automobile airbag

W22.10 Striking against or struck by unspecified automobile airbag

W22.11 Striking against or struck by driver side automobile airbag

W22.12 Striking against or struck by front passenger side automobile airbag

W22.19 Striking against or struck by other automobile airbag

W22.8 Striking against or struck by other objects

Striking against or struck by object NOS

EXCLUDES 1 *struck by thrown, projected or falling object (W20.-)*

W23 Caught, crushed, jammed or pinched in or between objects

EXCLUDES 1 *injury caused by cutting or piercing instruments (W25-W27)*
injury caused by firearms malfunction (W32.1, W33.1-, W34.1-)
injury caused by lifting and transmission devices (W24.-)
injury caused by machinery (W28-W31)
injury caused by nonpowered hand tools (W27.-)
injury caused by struck by thrown, projected or falling object (W20.-)
injury caused by transport vehicle being used as a means of transportation (V01-V99)

W23.0 Caught, crushed, jammed, or pinched between moving objects

W23.1 Caught, crushed, jammed, or pinched between stationary objects

W23.2 Caught, crushed, jammed or pinched between a moving and stationary object

AHA: 2022,4Q,48

W24 Contact with lifting and transmission devices, not elsewhere classified

EXCLUDES 1 *transport accidents (V01-V99)*

W24.0 Contact with lifting devices, not elsewhere classified

Contact with chain hoist
Contact with drive belt
Contact with pulley (block)

W24.1 Contact with transmission devices, not elsewhere classified

Contact with transmission belt or cable

W25 Contact with sharp glass

Code first any associated:
injury due to flying glass from explosion or firearm discharge (W32-W40)
transport accident (V00-V99)

EXCLUDES 1 *fall on same level due to slipping, tripping and stumbling with subsequent striking against sharp glass (W01.110-)*
striking against sharp glass with subsequent fall (W18.02-)

EXCLUDES 2 *glass embedded in skin (W45.-)*

W26 Contact with other sharp objects

EXCLUDES 2 *sharp object(s) embedded in skin (W45.-)*

AHA: 2016,4Q,73

W26.0 Contact with knife

EXCLUDES 1 *contact with electric knife (W29.1)*

W26.1 Contact with sword or dagger

W26.2 Contact with edge of stiff paper

Paper cut

W26.8 Contact with other sharp object(s), not elsewhere classified

Contact with tin can lid

W26.9 Contact with unspecified sharp object(s)

W27 Contact with nonpowered hand tool

W27.0 Contact with workbench tool

Contact with auger
Contact with axe
Contact with chisel
Contact with handsaw
Contact with screwdriver

W27.1 Contact with garden tool

Contact with hoe
Contact with nonpowered lawn mower
Contact with pitchfork
Contact with rake

W27.2 Contact with scissors

W27.3 Contact with needle (sewing)

EXCLUDES 1 *contact with hypodermic needle (W46.-)*

W27.4 Contact with kitchen utensil

Contact with fork
Contact with ice-pick
Contact with can-opener NOS

W27.5 Contact with paper-cutter

W27.8 Contact with other nonpowered hand tool

Contact with nonpowered sewing machine
Contact with shovel

W28 Contact with powered lawn mower

Powered lawn mower (commercial) (residential)

EXCLUDES 1 *contact with nonpowered lawn mower (W27.1)*

EXCLUDES 2 *exposure to electric current (W86.-)*

W29 Contact with other powered hand tools and household machinery

EXCLUDES 1 *contact with commercial machinery (W31.82)*
contact with hot household appliance (X15)
contact with nonpowered hand tool (W27.-)
exposure to electric current (W86)

W29.0 Contact with powered kitchen appliance

Contact with blender
Contact with can-opener
Contact with garbage disposal
Contact with mixer

W29.1 Contact with electric knife

W29.2 Contact with other powered household machinery

Contact with electric fan
Contact with powered dryer (clothes) (powered) (spin)
Contact with sewing machine
Contact with washing-machine

W29.3 Contact with powered garden and outdoor hand tools and machinery

Contact with chainsaw
Contact with edger
Contact with garden cultivator (tiller)
Contact with hedge trimmer
Contact with other powered garden tool

EXCLUDES 1 *contact with powered lawn mower (W28)*

W29.4 Contact with nail gun

W29.8 Contact with other powered hand tools and household machinery

Contact with do-it-yourself tool NOS

W30 Contact with agricultural machinery

INCLUDES animal-powered farm machine

EXCLUDES 1 *agricultural transport vehicle accident (V01-V99)*
explosion of grain store (W40.8)
exposure to electric current (W86.-)

W30.0 Contact with combine harvester

Contact with reaper
Contact with thresher

W30.1 Contact with power take-off devices (PTO)

W30.2 Contact with hay derrick

W30.3 Contact with grain storage elevator

EXCLUDES 1 *explosion of grain store (W40.8)*

Chapter 20. External Causes of Morbidity

W22–W30.3

√5th **W30.8 Contact with other specified agricultural machinery**

√x7th **W30.81 Contact with agricultural transport vehicle in stationary use**

Contact with agricultural transport vehicle under repair, not on public roadway

EXCLUDES 1 *agricultural transport vehicle accident (V01-V99)*

√x7th **W30.89 Contact with other specified agricultural machinery**

√x7th **W30.9 Contact with unspecified agricultural machinery**

Contact with farm machinery NOS

√4th **W31 Contact with other and unspecified machinery**

EXCLUDES 1 *contact with agricultural machinery (W30.-)*
contact with machinery in transport under own power or being towed by a vehicle (V01-V99)
exposure to electric current (W86)

√x7th **W31.0 Contact with mining and earth-drilling machinery**

Contact with bore or drill (land) (seabed)
Contact with shaft hoist
Contact with shaft lift
Contact with undercutter

√x7th **W31.1 Contact with metalworking machines**

Contact with abrasive wheel
Contact with forging machine
Contact with lathe
Contact with mechanical shears
Contact with metal drilling machine
Contact with milling machine
Contact with power press
Contact with rolling-mill
Contact with metal sawing machine

√x7th **W31.2 Contact with powered woodworking and forming machines**

Contact with band saw
Contact with bench saw
Contact with circular saw
Contact with molding machine
Contact with overhead plane
Contact with powered saw
Contact with radial saw
Contact with sander

EXCLUDES 1 *nonpowered woodworking tools (W27.0)*

√x7th **W31.3 Contact with prime movers**

Contact with gas turbine
Contact with internal combustion engine
Contact with steam engine
Contact with water driven turbine

√5th **W31.8 Contact with other specified machinery**

√x7th **W31.81 Contact with recreational machinery**

Contact with roller coaster

√x7th **W31.82 Contact with other commercial machinery**

Contact with commercial electric fan
Contact with commercial kitchen appliances
Contact with commercial powered dryer (clothes) (powered) (spin)
Contact with commercial sewing machine
Contact with commercial washing-machine

EXCLUDES 1 *contact with household machinery (W29.-)*
contact with powered lawn mower (W28)

√x7th **W31.83 Contact with special construction vehicle in stationary use**

Contact with special construction vehicle under repair, not on public roadway

EXCLUDES 1 *special construction vehicle accident (V01-V99)*

√x7th **W31.89 Contact with other specified machinery**

√x7th **W31.9 Contact with unspecified machinery**

Contact with machinery NOS

√4th **W32 Accidental handgun discharge and malfunction**

INCLUDES accidental discharge and malfunction of gun for single hand use
accidental discharge and malfunction of pistol
accidental discharge and malfunction of revolver
handgun discharge and malfunction NOS

EXCLUDES 1 *accidental airgun discharge and malfunction (W34.010, W34.110)*
accidental BB gun discharge and malfunction (W34.010, W34.110)
accidental pellet gun discharge and malfunction (W34.010, W34.110)
accidental shotgun discharge and malfunction (W33.01, W33.11)
assault by handgun discharge (X93)
handgun discharge involving legal intervention (Y35.0-)
handgun discharge involving military or war operations (Y36.4-)
intentional self-harm by handgun discharge (X72)
Very pistol discharge and malfunction (W34.09, W34.19)

√x7th **W32.0 Accidental handgun discharge**

√x7th **W32.1 Accidental handgun malfunction**

Injury due to explosion of handgun (parts)
Injury due to malfunction of mechanism or component of handgun
Injury due to recoil of handgun
Powder burn from handgun

√4th **W33 Accidental rifle, shotgun and larger firearm discharge and malfunction**

INCLUDES rifle, shotgun and larger firearm discharge and malfunction NOS

EXCLUDES 1 *accidental airgun discharge and malfunction (W34.010, W34.110)*
accidental BB gun discharge and malfunction (W34.010, W34.110)
accidental handgun discharge and malfunction (W32.-)
accidental pellet gun discharge and malfunction (W34.010, W34.110)
assault by rifle, shotgun and larger firearm discharge (X94)
firearm discharge involving legal intervention (Y35.0-)
firearm discharge involving military or war operations (Y36.4-)
intentional self-harm by rifle, shotgun and larger firearm discharge (X73)

√5th **W33.0 Accidental rifle, shotgun and larger firearm discharge**

√x7th **W33.00 Accidental discharge of unspecified larger firearm**

Discharge of unspecified larger firearm NOS

√x7th **W33.01 Accidental discharge of shotgun**

Discharge of shotgun NOS

√x7th **W33.02 Accidental discharge of hunting rifle**

Discharge of hunting rifle NOS

√x7th **W33.03 Accidental discharge of machine gun**

Discharge of machine gun NOS

√x7th **W33.09 Accidental discharge of other larger firearm**

Discharge of other larger firearm NOS

√5th **W33.1 Accidental rifle, shotgun and larger firearm malfunction**

Injury due to explosion of rifle, shotgun and larger firearm (parts)
Injury due to malfunction of mechanism or component of rifle, shotgun and larger firearm
Injury due to piercing, cutting, crushing or pinching due to (by) slide trigger mechanism, scope or other gun part
Injury due to recoil of rifle, shotgun and larger firearm
Powder burn from rifle, shotgun and larger firearm

√x7th **W33.10 Accidental malfunction of unspecified larger firearm**

Malfunction of unspecified larger firearm NOS

√x7th **W33.11 Accidental malfunction of shotgun**

Malfunction of shotgun NOS

√x7th **W33.12 Accidental malfunction of hunting rifle**

Malfunction of hunting rifle NOS

√x7th **W33.13 Accidental malfunction of machine gun**

Malfunction of machine gun NOS

√x7th **W33.19 Accidental malfunction of other larger firearm**

Malfunction of other larger firearm NOS

W34 Accidental discharge and malfunction from other and unspecified firearms and guns

W34.0 Accidental discharge from other and unspecified firearms and guns

W34.00 Accidental discharge from unspecified firearms or gun
Discharge from firearm NOS
Gunshot wound NOS
Shot NOS

W34.01 Accidental discharge of gas, air or spring-operated guns

W34.010 Accidental discharge of airgun
Accidental discharge of BB gun
Accidental discharge of pellet gun

W34.011 Accidental discharge of paintball gun
Accidental injury due to paintball discharge

W34.018 Accidental discharge of other gas, air or spring-operated gun

W34.09 Accidental discharge from other specified firearms
Accidental discharge from Very pistol [flare]

W34.1 Accidental malfunction from other and unspecified firearms and guns

W34.10 Accidental malfunction from unspecified firearms or gun
Firearm malfunction NOS

W34.11 Accidental malfunction of gas, air or spring-operated guns

W34.110 Accidental malfunction of airgun
Accidental malfunction of BB gun
Accidental malfunction of pellet gun

W34.111 Accidental malfunction of paintball gun
Accidental injury due to paintball gun malfunction

W34.118 Accidental malfunction of other gas, air or spring-operated gun

W34.19 Accidental malfunction from other specified firearms
Accidental malfunction from Very pistol [flare]

W35 Explosion and rupture of boiler
EXCLUDES 1 *explosion and rupture of boiler on watercraft (V93.4)*

W36 Explosion and rupture of gas cylinder

W36.1 Explosion and rupture of aerosol can

W36.2 Explosion and rupture of air tank

W36.3 Explosion and rupture of pressurized-gas tank

W36.8 Explosion and rupture of other gas cylinder

W36.9 Explosion and rupture of unspecified gas cylinder

W37 Explosion and rupture of pressurized tire, pipe or hose

W37.0 Explosion of bicycle tire

W37.8 Explosion and rupture of other pressurized tire, pipe or hose

W38 Explosion and rupture of other specified pressurized devices

W39 Discharge of firework

W40 Explosion of other materials
EXCLUDES 1 *assault by explosive material (X96)*
explosion involving legal intervention (Y35.1-)
explosion involving military or war operations (Y36.0-, Y36.2-)
intentional self-harm by explosive material (X75)

W40.0 Explosion of blasting material
Explosion of blasting cap
Explosion of detonator
Explosion of dynamite
Explosion of explosive (any) used in blasting operations

W40.1 Explosion of explosive gases
Explosion of acetylene
Explosion of butane
Explosion of coal gas
Explosion in mine NOS
Explosion of explosive gas
Explosion of fire damp
Explosion of gasoline fumes
Explosion of methane
Explosion of propane

W40.8 Explosion of other specified explosive materials
Explosion in dump NOS
Explosion in factory NOS
Explosion in grain store
Explosion in munitions
EXCLUDES 1 *explosion involving legal intervention (Y35.1-)*
explosion involving military or war operations (Y36.0-, Y36.2-)

W40.9 Explosion of unspecified explosive materials
Explosion NOS

W42 Exposure to noise

W42.0 Exposure to supersonic waves

W42.9 Exposure to other noise
Exposure to sound waves NOS

● **W44 Foreign body entering into or through a natural orifice**
EXCLUDES 2 *contact with other sharp objects (W26)*
contact with sharp glass (W25)
foreign body or object entering through skin (W45)

● **W44.A Battery entering into or through a natural orifice**

● **W44.A0 Battery unspecified, entering into or through a natural orifice**

● **W44.A1 Button battery entering into or through a natural orifice**

● **W44.A9 Other batteries entering into or through a natural orifice**
Cylindrical battery

● **W44.B Plastic entering into or through a natural orifice**

● **W44.B0 Plastic object unspecified, entering into or through a natural orifice**

● **W44.B1 Plastic bead entering into or through a natural orifice**
EXCLUDES 2 *plastic jewelry entering into or through a natural orifice (W44.B4)*

● **W44.B2 Plastic coin entering into or through a natural orifice**

● **W44.B3 Plastic toy and toy part entering into or through a natural orifice**

● **W44.B4 Plastic jewelry entering into or through a natural orifice**
EXCLUDES 2 *plastic bead entering into or through a natural orifice (W44.B1)*

● **W44.B5 Plastic bottle entering into or through a natural orifice**

● **W44.B9 Other plastic object entering into or through a natural orifice**

● **W44.C Glass entering into or through a natural orifice**

● **W44.C0 Glass unspecified, entering into or through a natural orifice**

● **W44.C1 Sharp glass entering into or through a natural orifice**
Glass shard entering into or through a natural orifice

● **W44.C2 Intact glass entering into or through a natural orifice**
Intact glass bottle entering into or through a natural orifice

● **W44.D Magnetic metal entering into or through a natural orifice**

● **W44.D0 Magnetic metal object unspecified, entering into or through a natural orifice**

● **W44.D1 Magnetic metal bead entering into or through a natural orifice**

● **W44.D2 Magnetic metal coin entering into or through a natural orifice**

● **W44.D3 Magnetic metal toy entering into or through a natural orifice**

● **W44.D4 Magnetic metal jewelry entering into or through a natural orifice**

● **W44.D9 Other magnetic metal objects entering into or through a natural orifice**

● **W44.E Non-magnetic metal entering into or through a natural orifice**

● **W44.E0 Non-magnetic metal object unspecified, entering into or through a natural orifice**

● **W44.E1 Non-magnetic metal bead entering into or through a natural orifice**

● **W44.E2 Non-magnetic metal coin entering into or through a natural orifice**

● **W44.E3 Non-magnetic metal toy entering into or through a natural orifice**

- ● ✓x7th **W44.E4 Non-magnetic metal jewelry entering into or through a natural orifice**
- ● ✓x7th **W44.E9 Other non-magnetic metal objects entering into or through a natural orifice**
  - Bottle cap entering into or through a natural orifice
  - Can lid entering into or through a natural orifice
  - Pull tab entering into or through a natural orifice
- ● ✓5th **W44.F Objects of natural or organic material entering into or through a natural orifice**
- ● ✓x7th **W44.FØ Objects of natural or organic material unspecified, entering into or through a natural orifice**
- ● ✓x7th **W44.F1 Bezoar entering into or through a natural orifice**
- ● ✓x7th **W44.F2 Rubber band entering into or through a natural orifice**
- ● ✓x7th **W44.F3 Food entering into or through a natural orifice**
- ● ✓x7th **W44.F4 Insect entering into or through a natural orifice**
- ● ✓x7th **W44.F9 Other object of natural or organic material, entering into or through a natural orifice**
- ● ✓5th **W44.G Other non-organic objects entering into or through a natural orifice**
- ● ✓x7th **W44.GØ Other non-organic objects unspecified, entering into or through a natural orifice**
- ● ✓x7th **W44.G1 Audio device entering into or through a natural orifice**
  - Ear buds
  - Hearing aids
- ● ✓x7th **W44.G2 Combination metal and plastic toy and toy part entering into or through natural orifice**
- ● ✓x7th **W44.G3 Combination metal and plastic jewelry entering into or through a natural orifice**
- ● ✓x7th **W44.G9 Other non-organic objects entering into or through a natural orifice**
- ● ✓5th **W44.H Other sharp object entering into or through a natural orifice**
- ● ✓x7th **W44.HØ Other sharp object unspecified, entering into or through a natural orifice**
- ● ✓x7th **W44.H1 Needle entering into or through a natural orifice**
  - Dart entering into or through a natural orifice
  - Hypodermic needle entering into or through a natural orifice
  - Safety pin entering into or through a natural orifice
  - Sewing needle entering into or through a natural orifice
- ● ✓x7th **W44.H2 Knife, sword or dagger entering into or through a natural orifice**
- ● ✓x7th **W44.8 Other foreign body entering into or through a natural orifice**
- ● ✓x7th **W44.9 Unspecified foreign body entering into or through a natural orifice**
  - Foreign body NOS entering into or through a natural orifice

✓4th **W45 Foreign body or object entering through skin**

INCLUDES foreign body or object embedded in skin
nail embedded in skin

EXCLUDES 2 *contact with hand tools (nonpowered) (powered) (W27-W29)*
contact with other sharp objects (W26.-)
contact with sharp glass (W25.-)
struck by objects (W2Ø-W22)

- ✓x7th **W45.Ø Nail entering through skin**
- ✓x7th **W45.8 Other foreign body or object entering through skin**
  - Splinter in skin NOS

✓4th **W46 Contact with hypodermic needle**

- ✓x7th **W46.Ø Contact with hypodermic needle**
  - Hypodermic needle stick NOS
- ✓x7th **W46.1 Contact with contaminated hypodermic needle**

✓4th **W49 Exposure to other inanimate mechanical forces**

INCLUDES exposure to abnormal gravitational [G] forces
exposure to inanimate mechanical forces NEC

EXCLUDES 1 *exposure to inanimate mechanical forces involving military or war operations (Y36.-, Y37.-)*

- ✓5th **W49.Ø Item causing external constriction**
  - ✓x7th **W49.Ø1 Hair causing external constriction**
  - ✓x7th **W49.Ø2 String or thread causing external constriction**
  - ✓x7th **W49.Ø3 Rubber band causing external constriction**
  - ✓x7th **W49.Ø4 Ring or other jewelry causing external constriction**
  - ✓x7th **W49.Ø9 Other specified item causing external constriction**
- ✓x7th **W49.9 Exposure to other inanimate mechanical forces**

Exposure to animate mechanical forces (W5Ø-W64)

EXCLUDES 1 *toxic effect of contact with venomous animals and plants (T63.-)*

The appropriate 7th character is to be added to each code from categories W5Ø-W64.
A initial encounter
D subsequent encounter
S sequela

✓4th **W5Ø Accidental hit, strike, kick, twist, bite or scratch by another person**

INCLUDES hit, strike, kick, twist, bite, or scratch by another person NOS

EXCLUDES 1 *assault by bodily force (YØ4)*
struck by objects (W2Ø-W22)

- ✓x7th **W5Ø.Ø Accidental hit or strike by another person**
  - Hit or strike by another person NOS
- ✓x7th **W5Ø.1 Accidental kick by another person**
  - Kick by another person NOS
- ✓x7th **W5Ø.2 Accidental twist by another person**
  - Twist by another person NOS
- ✓x7th **W5Ø.3 Accidental bite by another person**
  - Human bite
  - Bite by another person NOS
- ✓x7th **W5Ø.4 Accidental scratch by another person**
  - Scratch by another person NOS

✓x7th **W51 Accidental striking against or bumped into by another person**

EXCLUDES 1 *assault by striking against or bumping into by another person (YØ4.2)*
fall due to collision with another person (WØ3)

✓x7th **W52 Crushed, pushed or stepped on by crowd or human stampede**

Crushed, pushed or stepped on by crowd or human stampede with or without fall

✓4th **W53 Contact with rodent**

INCLUDES contact with saliva, feces or urine of rodent

- ✓5th **W53.Ø Contact with mouse**
  - ✓x7th **W53.Ø1 Bitten by mouse**
  - ✓x7th **W53.Ø9 Other contact with mouse**
- ✓5th **W53.1 Contact with rat**
  - ✓x7th **W53.11 Bitten by rat**
  - ✓x7th **W53.19 Other contact with rat**
- ✓5th **W53.2 Contact with squirrel**
  - ✓x7th **W53.21 Bitten by squirrel**
  - ✓x7th **W53.29 Other contact with squirrel**
- ✓5th **W53.8 Contact with other rodent**
  - ✓x7th **W53.81 Bitten by other rodent**
  - ✓x7th **W53.89 Other contact with other rodent**

✓4th **W54 Contact with dog**

INCLUDES contact with saliva, feces or urine of dog

- ✓x7th **W54.Ø Bitten by dog**
- ✓x7th **W54.1 Struck by dog**
  - Knocked over by dog
- ✓x7th **W54.8 Other contact with dog**

✓4th **W55 Contact with other mammals**

INCLUDES contact with saliva, feces or urine of mammal

EXCLUDES 1 *animal being ridden - see transport accidents*
bitten or struck by dog (W54)
bitten or struck by rodent (W53.-)
contact with marine mammals (W56.-)

- ✓5th **W55.Ø Contact with cat**
  - ✓x7th **W55.Ø1 Bitten by cat**
  - ✓x7th **W55.Ø3 Scratched by cat**
  - ✓x7th **W55.Ø9 Other contact with cat**
- ✓5th **W55.1 Contact with horse**
  - ✓x7th **W55.11 Bitten by horse**
  - ✓x7th **W55.12 Struck by horse**
  - ✓x7th **W55.19 Other contact with horse**
- ✓5th **W55.2 Contact with cow**
  - Contact with bull
  - ✓x7th **W55.21 Bitten by cow**

W55.22 Struck by cow
Gored by bull
W55.29 Other contact with cow
W55.3 Contact with other hoof stock
Contact with goats
Contact with sheep
W55.31 Bitten by other hoof stock
W55.32 Struck by other hoof stock
Gored by goat
Gored by ram
W55.39 Other contact with other hoof stock
W55.4 Contact with pig
W55.41 Bitten by pig
W55.42 Struck by pig
W55.49 Other contact with pig
W55.5 Contact with raccoon
W55.51 Bitten by raccoon
W55.52 Struck by raccoon
W55.59 Other contact with raccoon
W55.8 Contact with other mammals
W55.81 Bitten by other mammals
W55.82 Struck by other mammals
W55.89 Other contact with other mammals

W56 Contact with nonvenomous marine animal
EXCLUDES 1 *contact with venomous marine animal (T63.-)*
W56.Ø Contact with dolphin
W56.Ø1 Bitten by dolphin
W56.Ø2 Struck by dolphin
W56.Ø9 Other contact with dolphin
W56.1 Contact with sea lion
W56.11 Bitten by sea lion
W56.12 Struck by sea lion
W56.19 Other contact with sea lion
W56.2 Contact with orca
Contact with killer whale
W56.21 Bitten by orca
W56.22 Struck by orca
W56.29 Other contact with orca
W56.3 Contact with other marine mammals
W56.31 Bitten by other marine mammals
W56.32 Struck by other marine mammals
W56.39 Other contact with other marine mammals
W56.4 Contact with shark
W56.41 Bitten by shark
W56.42 Struck by shark
W56.49 Other contact with shark
W56.5 Contact with other fish
W56.51 Bitten by other fish
W56.52 Struck by other fish
W56.59 Other contact with other fish
W56.8 Contact with other nonvenomous marine animals
W56.81 Bitten by other nonvenomous marine animals
W56.82 Struck by other nonvenomous marine animals
W56.89 Other contact with other nonvenomous marine animals

W57 Bitten or stung by nonvenomous insect and other nonvenomous arthropods
EXCLUDES 1 *contact with venomous insects and arthropods (T63.2-, T63.3-, T63.4-)*

W58 Contact with crocodile or alligator
W58.Ø Contact with alligator
W58.Ø1 Bitten by alligator
W58.Ø2 Struck by alligator
W58.Ø3 Crushed by alligator
W58.Ø9 Other contact with alligator
W58.1 Contact with crocodile
W58.11 Bitten by crocodile
W58.12 Struck by crocodile
W58.13 Crushed by crocodile
W58.19 Other contact with crocodile

W59 Contact with other nonvenomous reptiles
EXCLUDES 1 *contact with venomous reptile (T63.Ø-, T63.1-)*
W59.Ø Contact with nonvenomous lizards
W59.Ø1 Bitten by nonvenomous lizards
W59.Ø2 Struck by nonvenomous lizards
W59.Ø9 Other contact with nonvenomous lizards
Exposure to nonvenomous lizards
W59.1 Contact with nonvenomous snakes
W59.11 Bitten by nonvenomous snake
W59.12 Struck by nonvenomous snake
W59.13 Crushed by nonvenomous snake
W59.19 Other contact with nonvenomous snake
W59.2 Contact with turtles
EXCLUDES 1 *contact with tortoises (W59.8-)*
W59.21 Bitten by turtle
W59.22 Struck by turtle
W59.29 Other contact with turtle
Exposure to turtles
W59.8 Contact with other nonvenomous reptiles
W59.81 Bitten by other nonvenomous reptiles
W59.82 Struck by other nonvenomous reptiles
W59.83 Crushed by other nonvenomous reptiles
W59.89 Other contact with other nonvenomous reptiles

W6Ø Contact with nonvenomous plant thorns and spines and sharp leaves
EXCLUDES 1 *contact with venomous plants (T63.7-)*

W61 Contact with birds (domestic) (wild)
INCLUDES contact with excreta of birds
W61.Ø Contact with parrot
W61.Ø1 Bitten by parrot
W61.Ø2 Struck by parrot
W61.Ø9 Other contact with parrot
Exposure to parrots
W61.1 Contact with macaw
W61.11 Bitten by macaw
W61.12 Struck by macaw
W61.19 Other contact with macaw
Exposure to macaws
W61.2 Contact with other psittacines
W61.21 Bitten by other psittacines
W61.22 Struck by other psittacines
W61.29 Other contact with other psittacines
Exposure to other psittacines
W61.3 Contact with chicken
W61.32 Struck by chicken
W61.33 Pecked by chicken
W61.39 Other contact with chicken
Exposure to chickens
W61.4 Contact with turkey
W61.42 Struck by turkey
W61.43 Pecked by turkey
W61.49 Other contact with turkey
W61.5 Contact with goose
W61.51 Bitten by goose
W61.52 Struck by goose
W61.59 Other contact with goose
W61.6 Contact with duck
W61.61 Bitten by duck
W61.62 Struck by duck
W61.69 Other contact with duck

√5th **W61.9 Contact with other birds**

√x7th **W61.91 Bitten by other birds**

√x7th **W61.92 Struck by other birds**

√x7th **W61.99 Other contact with other birds**

Contact with bird NOS

√4th **W62 Contact with nonvenomous amphibians**

EXCLUDES 1 *contact with venomous amphibians ▶(T63.81-T63.83)◀*

√x7th **W62.0 Contact with nonvenomous frogs**

√x7th **W62.1 Contact with nonvenomous toads**

√x7th **W62.9 Contact with other nonvenomous amphibians**

√x7th **W64 Exposure to other animate mechanical forces**

INCLUDES exposure to nonvenomous animal NOS

EXCLUDES 1 *contact with venomous animal (T63.-)*

Accidental non-transport drowning and submersion (W65-W74)

EXCLUDES 1 *accidental drowning and submersion due to fall into water (W16.-)*
accidental drowning and submersion due to water transport accident (V90.-, V92.-)

EXCLUDES 2 *accidental drowning and submersion due to cataclysm (X34-X39)*

The appropriate 7th character is to be added to each code from categories W65-W74.
A initial encounter
D subsequent encounter
S sequela

√x7th **W65 Accidental drowning and submersion while in bath-tub**

EXCLUDES 1 *accidental drowning and submersion due to fall in (into) bathtub (W16.211)*

√x7th **W67 Accidental drowning and submersion while in swimming-pool**

EXCLUDES 1 *accidental drowning and submersion due to fall into swimming pool (W16.011, W16.021, W16.031)*
accidental drowning and submersion due to striking into wall of swimming pool (W22.041)

AHA: 2023,1Q,25

√x7th **W69 Accidental drowning and submersion while in natural water**

Accidental drowning and submersion while in lake
Accidental drowning and submersion while in open sea
Accidental drowning and submersion while in river
Accidental drowning and submersion while in stream

EXCLUDES 1 *accidental drowning and submersion due to fall into natural body of water (W16.111, W16.121, W16.131)*

√x7th **W73 Other specified cause of accidental non-transport drowning and submersion**

Accidental drowning and submersion while in quenching tank
Accidental drowning and submersion while in reservoir

EXCLUDES 1 *accidental drowning and submersion due to fall into other water (W16.311, W16.321, W16.331)*

√x7th **W74 Unspecified cause of accidental drowning and submersion**

Drowning NOS

Exposure to electric current, radiation and extreme ambient air temperature and pressure (W85-W99)

EXCLUDES 1 *exposure to:*
failure in dosage of radiation or temperature during surgical and medical care (Y63.2-Y63.5)
lightning (T75.0-)
natural cold (X31)
natural heat (X30)
natural radiation NOS (X39)
radiological procedure and radiotherapy (Y84.2)
sunlight (X32)

AHA: 2018,2Q,7-8

The appropriate 7th character is to be added to each code from categories W85-W99.
A initial encounter
D subsequent encounter
S sequela

√x7th **W85 Exposure to electric transmission lines**

Broken power line

√4th **W86 Exposure to other specified electric current**

√x7th **W86.0 Exposure to domestic wiring and appliances**

√x7th **W86.1 Exposure to industrial wiring, appliances and electrical machinery**

Exposure to conductors
Exposure to control apparatus
Exposure to electrical equipment and machinery
Exposure to transformers

√x7th **W86.8 Exposure to other electric current**

Exposure to wiring and appliances in or on farm (not farmhouse)
Exposure to wiring and appliances outdoors
Exposure to wiring and appliances in or on public building
Exposure to wiring and appliances in or on residential institutions
Exposure to wiring and appliances in or on schools

√4th **W88 Exposure to ionizing radiation**

EXCLUDES 1 *exposure to sunlight (X32)*

√x7th **W88.0 Exposure to X-rays**

√x7th **W88.1 Exposure to radioactive isotopes**

√x7th **W88.8 Exposure to other ionizing radiation**

√4th **W89 Exposure to man-made visible and ultraviolet light**

INCLUDES exposure to welding light (arc)

EXCLUDES 2 *exposure to sunlight (X32)*

√x7th **W89.0 Exposure to welding light (arc)**

√x7th **W89.1 Exposure to tanning bed**

√x7th **W89.8 Exposure to other man-made visible and ultraviolet light**

√x7th **W89.9 Exposure to unspecified man-made visible and ultraviolet light**

√4th **W90 Exposure to other nonionizing radiation**

EXCLUDES 2 *exposure to sunlight (X32)*

AHA: 2019,1Q,21

√x7th **W90.0 Exposure to radiofrequency**

√x7th **W90.1 Exposure to infrared radiation**

√x7th **W90.2 Exposure to laser radiation**

√x7th **W90.8 Exposure to other nonionizing radiation**

√x7th **W92 Exposure to excessive heat of man-made origin**

√4th **W93 Exposure to excessive cold of man-made origin**

√5th **W93.0 Contact with or inhalation of dry ice**

√x7th **W93.01 Contact with dry ice**

√x7th **W93.02 Inhalation of dry ice**

√5th **W93.1 Contact with or inhalation of liquid air**

√x7th **W93.11 Contact with liquid air**

Contact with liquid hydrogen
Contact with liquid nitrogen

√x7th **W93.12 Inhalation of liquid air**

Inhalation of liquid hydrogen
Inhalation of liquid nitrogen

√x7th **W93.2 Prolonged exposure in deep freeze unit or refrigerator**

√x7th **W93.8 Exposure to other excessive cold of man-made origin**

√4th **W94 Exposure to high and low air pressure and changes in air pressure**

√x7th **W94.0 Exposure to prolonged high air pressure**

√5th **W94.1 Exposure to prolonged low air pressure**

√x7th **W94.11 Exposure to residence or prolonged visit at high altitude**

√x7th **W94.12 Exposure to other prolonged low air pressure**

√5th **W94.2 Exposure to rapid changes in air pressure during ascent**

√x7th **W94.21 Exposure to reduction in atmospheric pressure while surfacing from deep-water diving**

√x7th **W94.22 Exposure to reduction in atmospheric pressure while surfacing from underground**

√x7th **W94.23 Exposure to sudden change in air pressure in aircraft during ascent**

√x7th **W94.29 Exposure to other rapid changes in air pressure during ascent**

√5th **W94.3 Exposure to rapid changes in air pressure during descent**

√x7th **W94.31 Exposure to sudden change in air pressure in aircraft during descent**

√x7th **W94.32 Exposure to high air pressure from rapid descent in water**

√x7th **W94.39 Exposure to other rapid changes in air pressure during descent**

√x7th **W99 Exposure to other man-made environmental factors**

Exposure to smoke, fire and flames (X00-X08)

EXCLUDES 1 *arson (X97)*
EXCLUDES 2 *explosions (W35-W40)*
lightning (T75.0-)
transport accident (V01-V99)

AHA: 2018,2Q,7-8

The appropriate 7th character is to be added to each code from categories X00-X08.
A initial encounter
D subsequent encounter
S sequela

X00 Exposure to uncontrolled fire in building or structure
INCLUDES conflagration in building or structure
Code first any associated cataclysm
EXCLUDES 2 *exposure to ignition or melting of nightwear (X05)*
exposure to ignition or melting of other clothing and apparel (X06.-)
exposure to other specified smoke, fire and flames (X08.-)
AHA: 2016,2Q,5

- **X00.0 Exposure to flames in uncontrolled fire in building or structure**
- **X00.1 Exposure to smoke in uncontrolled fire in building or structure**
- **X00.2 Injury due to collapse of burning building or structure in uncontrolled fire**
  EXCLUDES 1 *injury due to collapse of building not on fire (W20.1)*
- **X00.3 Fall from burning building or structure in uncontrolled fire**
- **X00.4 Hit by object from burning building or structure in uncontrolled fire**
  AHA: 2016,2Q,4
- **X00.5 Jump from burning building or structure in uncontrolled fire**
- **X00.8 Other exposure to uncontrolled fire in building or structure**

X01 Exposure to uncontrolled fire, not in building or structure
INCLUDES exposure to forest fire

- **X01.0 Exposure to flames in uncontrolled fire, not in building or structure**
- **X01.1 Exposure to smoke in uncontrolled fire, not in building or structure**
- **X01.3 Fall due to uncontrolled fire, not in building or structure**
- **X01.4 Hit by object due to uncontrolled fire, not in building or structure**
- **X01.8 Other exposure to uncontrolled fire, not in building or structure**

X02 Exposure to controlled fire in building or structure
INCLUDES exposure to fire in fireplace
exposure to fire in stove

- **X02.0 Exposure to flames in controlled fire in building or structure**
- **X02.1 Exposure to smoke in controlled fire in building or structure**
- **X02.2 Injury due to collapse of burning building or structure in controlled fire**
  EXCLUDES 1 *injury due to collapse of building not on fire (W20.1)*
- **X02.3 Fall from burning building or structure in controlled fire**
- **X02.4 Hit by object from burning building or structure in controlled fire**
- **X02.5 Jump from burning building or structure in controlled fire**
- **X02.8 Other exposure to controlled fire in building or structure**

X03 Exposure to controlled fire, not in building or structure
INCLUDES exposure to bon fire
exposure to camp-fire
exposure to trash fire

- **X03.0 Exposure to flames in controlled fire, not in building or structure**
- **X03.1 Exposure to smoke in controlled fire, not in building or structure**
- **X03.3 Fall due to controlled fire, not in building or structure**
- **X03.4 Hit by object due to controlled fire, not in building or structure**
- **X03.8 Other exposure to controlled fire, not in building or structure**

X04 Exposure to ignition of highly flammable material
Exposure to ignition of gasoline
Exposure to ignition of kerosene
Exposure to ignition of petrol
EXCLUDES 2 *exposure to ignition or melting of nightwear (X05)*
exposure to ignition or melting of other clothing and apparel (X06)
AHA: 2016,2Q,4

X05 Exposure to ignition or melting of nightwear
EXCLUDES 2 *exposure to uncontrolled fire in building or structure (X00.-)*
exposure to uncontrolled fire, not in building or structure (X01.-)
exposure to controlled fire in building or structure (X02.-)
exposure to controlled fire, not in building or structure (X03.-)
exposure to ignition of highly flammable materials (X04.-)

X06 Exposure to ignition or melting of other clothing and apparel
EXCLUDES 2 *exposure to uncontrolled fire in building or structure (X00.-)*
exposure to uncontrolled fire, not in building or structure (X01.-)
exposure to controlled fire in building or structure (X02.-)
exposure to controlled fire, not in building or structure (X03.-)
exposure to ignition of highly flammable materials (X04.-)

- **X06.0 Exposure to ignition of plastic jewelry**
- **X06.1 Exposure to melting of plastic jewelry**
- **X06.2 Exposure to ignition of other clothing and apparel**
- **X06.3 Exposure to melting of other clothing and apparel**

X08 Exposure to other specified smoke, fire and flames

- **X08.0 Exposure to bed fire**
  Exposure to mattress fire
  - **X08.00 Exposure to bed fire due to unspecified burning material**
  - **X08.01 Exposure to bed fire due to burning cigarette**
  - **X08.09 Exposure to bed fire due to other burning material**
- **X08.1 Exposure to sofa fire**
  - **X08.10 Exposure to sofa fire due to unspecified burning material**
  - **X08.11 Exposure to sofa fire due to burning cigarette**
  - **X08.19 Exposure to sofa fire due to other burning material**
- **X08.2 Exposure to other furniture fire**
  - **X08.20 Exposure to other furniture fire due to unspecified burning material**
  - **X08.21 Exposure to other furniture fire due to burning cigarette**
  - **X08.29 Exposure to other furniture fire due to other burning material**
- **X08.8 Exposure to other specified smoke, fire and flames**

Contact with heat and hot substances (X10-X19)

EXCLUDES 1 *exposure to excessive natural heat (X30)*
exposure to fire and flames (X00-X08)

AHA: 2018,2Q,7-8

The appropriate 7th character is to be added to each code from categories X10-X19.
A initial encounter
D subsequent encounter
S sequela

X10 Contact with hot drinks, food, fats and cooking oils

- **X10.0 Contact with hot drinks**
- **X10.1 Contact with hot food**
- **X10.2 Contact with fats and cooking oils**

X11 Contact with hot tap-water
INCLUDES contact with boiling tap-water
contact with boiling water NOS
EXCLUDES 1 *contact with water heated on stove (X12)*

- **X11.0 Contact with hot water in bath or tub**
  EXCLUDES 1 *contact with running hot water in bath or tub (X11.1)*
- **X11.1 Contact with running hot water**
  Contact with hot water running out of hose
  Contact with hot water running out of tap

Chapter 20. External Causes of Morbidity

√x 7th **X11.8 Contact with other hot tap-water**
Contact with hot water in bucket
Contact with hot tap-water NOS

√x 7th **X12 Contact with other hot fluids**
Contact with water heated on stove
EXCLUDES 1 *hot (liquid) metals (X18)*

√4th **X13 Contact with steam and other hot vapors**
√x 7th **X13.0 Inhalation of steam and other hot vapors**
√x 7th **X13.1 Other contact with steam and other hot vapors**

√4th **X14 Contact with hot air and other hot gases**
√x 7th **X14.0 Inhalation of hot air and gases**
√x 7th **X14.1 Other contact with hot air and other hot gases**

√4th **X15 Contact with hot household appliances**
EXCLUDES 1 *contact with heating appliances (X16)*
contact with powered household appliances (W29.-)
exposure to controlled fire in building or structure due to household appliance (X02.8)
exposure to household appliances electrical current (W86.0)
√x 7th **X15.0 Contact with hot stove (kitchen)**
√x 7th **X15.1 Contact with hot toaster**
√x 7th **X15.2 Contact with hotplate**
√x 7th **X15.3 Contact with hot saucepan or skillet**
Contact with hot cooking pan
Contact with hot cooking pot
√x 7th **X15.8 Contact with other hot household appliances**
Contact with cooker
Contact with kettle
Contact with light bulbs

√x 7th **X16 Contact with hot heating appliances, radiators and pipes**
EXCLUDES 1 *contact with powered appliances (W29.-)*
exposure to controlled fire in building or structure due to appliance (X02.8)
exposure to industrial appliances electrical current (W86.1)

√x 7th **X17 Contact with hot engines, machinery and tools**
EXCLUDES 1 *contact with hot heating appliances, radiators and pipes (X16)*
contact with hot household appliances (X15)

√x 7th **X18 Contact with other hot metals**
Contact with liquid metal

√x 7th **X19 Contact with other heat and hot substances**
EXCLUDES 1 *objects that are not normally hot, e.g., an object made hot by a house fire (X00-X08)*

Exposure to forces of nature (X30-X39)

AHA: 2018,2Q,7-8

The appropriate 7th character is to be added to each code from categories X30-X39.
A initial encounter
D subsequent encounter
S sequela

√x 7th **X30 Exposure to excessive natural heat**
Exposure to excessive heat as the cause of sunstroke
Exposure to heat NOS
EXCLUDES 1 *excessive heat of man-made origin (W92)*
exposure to man-made radiation (W89)
exposure to sunlight (X32)
exposure to tanning bed (W89)

√x 7th **X31 Exposure to excessive natural cold**
Excessive cold as the cause of chilblains NOS
Excessive cold as the cause of immersion foot or hand
Exposure to cold NOS
Exposure to weather conditions
EXCLUDES 1 *cold of man-made origin (W93.-)*
contact with or inhalation of dry ice (W93.-)
contact with or inhalation of liquefied gas (W93.-)

√x 7th **X32 Exposure to sunlight**
EXCLUDES 1 *man-made radiation (tanning bed) (W89)*
EXCLUDES 2 *radiation-related disorders of the skin and subcutaneous tissue (L55-L59)*

√x 7th **X34 Earthquake**
EXCLUDES 2 *tidal wave (tsunami) due to earthquake (X37.41)*

√x 7th **X35 Volcanic eruption**
EXCLUDES 2 *tidal wave (tsunami) due to volcanic eruption (X37.41)*

√4th **X36 Avalanche, landslide and other earth movements**
INCLUDES victim of mudslide of cataclysmic nature
EXCLUDES 1 *earthquake (X34)*
EXCLUDES 2 *transport accident involving collision with avalanche or landslide not in motion (V01-V99)*
√x 7th **X36.0 Collapse of dam or man-made structure causing earth movement**
√x 7th **X36.1 Avalanche, landslide, or mudslide**

√4th **X37 Cataclysmic storm**
√x 7th **X37.0 Hurricane**
Storm surge
Typhoon
√x 7th **X37.1 Tornado**
Cyclone
Twister
√x 7th **X37.2 Blizzard (snow)(ice)**
√x 7th **X37.3 Dust storm**
√5th **X37.4 Tidalwave**
√x 7th **X37.41 Tidal wave due to earthquake or volcanic eruption**
Tidal wave NOS
Tsunami
√x 7th **X37.42 Tidal wave due to storm**
√x 7th **X37.43 Tidal wave due to landslide**
√x 7th **X37.8 Other cataclysmic storms**
Cloudburst
Torrential rain
EXCLUDES 2 *flood (X38)*
√x 7th **X37.9 Unspecified cataclysmic storm**
Storm NOS
EXCLUDES 1 *collapse of dam or man-made structure causing earth movement (X36.0)*

√x 7th **X38 Flood**
Flood arising from remote storm
Flood of cataclysmic nature arising from melting snow
Flood resulting directly from storm
EXCLUDES 1 *collapse of dam or man-made structure causing earth movement (X36.0)*
tidal wave NOS (X37.41)
tidal wave caused by storm (X37.42)

√4th **X39 Exposure to other forces of nature**
√5th **X39.0 Exposure to natural radiation**
EXCLUDES 1 *contact with and (suspected) exposure to radon and other naturally occurring radiation (Z77.123)*
exposure to man-made radiation (W88-W90)
exposure to sunlight (X32)
√x 7th **X39.01 Exposure to radon**
√x 7th **X39.08 Exposure to other natural radiation**
√x 7th **X39.8 Other exposure to forces of nature**

Overexertion and strenuous or repetitive movements (X50)

√4th **X50 Overexertion and strenuous or repetitive movements**
AHA: 2018,2Q,7-8; 2016,4Q,73-74

The appropriate 7th character is to be added to each code from category X50.
A initial encounter
D subsequent encounter
S sequela

√x 7th **X50.0 Overexertion from strenuous movement or load**
Lifting heavy objects
Lifting weights

√x7th **X50.1 Overexertion from prolonged static or awkward postures**
Prolonged bending
Prolonged kneeling
Prolonged reaching
Prolonged sitting
Prolonged standing
Prolonged twisting
Static bending
Static kneeling
Static reaching
Static sitting
Static standing
Static twisting

√x7th **X50.3 Overexertion from repetitive movements**
Use of hand as hammer
EXCLUDES 2 *overuse from prolonged static or awkward postures (X50.1)*

√x7th **X50.9 Other and unspecified overexertion or strenuous movements or postures**
Contact pressure
Contact stress

Accidental exposure to other specified factors (X52-X58)

AHA: 2018,2Q,7-8

The appropriate 7th character is to be added to each code from categories X52-X58.
A initial encounter
D subsequent encounter
S sequela

√x7th **X52 Prolonged stay in weightless environment**
Weightlessness in spacecraft (simulator)

√x7th **X58 Exposure to other specified factors**
Accident NOS
Exposure NOS

Intentional self-harm (X71-X83)

Purposely self-inflicted injury
Suicide (attempted)

The appropriate 7th character is to be added to each code from categories X71-X83.
A initial encounter
D subsequent encounter
S sequela

√4th **X71 Intentional self-harm by drowning and submersion**

√x7th **X71.0 Intentional self-harm by drowning and submersion while in bathtub** HCC

√x7th **X71.1 Intentional self-harm by drowning and submersion while in swimming pool** HCC

√x7th **X71.2 Intentional self-harm by drowning and submersion after jump into swimming pool** HCC

√x7th **X71.3 Intentional self-harm by drowning and submersion in natural water** HCC

√x7th **X71.8 Other intentional self-harm by drowning and submersion** HCC

√x7th **X71.9 Intentional self-harm by drowning and submersion, unspecified** HCC

√x7th **X72 Intentional self-harm by handgun discharge** HCC
Intentional self-harm by gun for single hand use
Intentional self-harm by pistol
Intentional self-harm by revolver
EXCLUDES 1 *Very pistol (X74.8)*

√4th **X73 Intentional self-harm by rifle, shotgun and larger firearm discharge**
EXCLUDES 1 *airgun (X74.01)*

√x7th **X73.0 Intentional self-harm by shotgun discharge** HCC

√x7th **X73.1 Intentional self-harm by hunting rifle discharge** HCC

√x7th **X73.2 Intentional self-harm by machine gun discharge** HCC

√x7th **X73.8 Intentional self-harm by other larger firearm discharge** HCC

√x7th **X73.9 Intentional self-harm by unspecified larger firearm discharge** HCC

√4th **X74 Intentional self-harm by other and unspecified firearm and gun discharge**

√5th **X74.0 Intentional self-harm by gas, air or spring-operated guns**

√x7th **X74.01 Intentional self-harm by airgun** HCC
Intentional self-harm by BB gun discharge
Intentional self-harm by pellet gun discharge

√x7th **X74.02 Intentional self-harm by paintball gun** HCC

√x7th **X74.09 Intentional self-harm by other gas, air or spring-operated gun** HCC

√x7th **X74.8 Intentional self-harm by other firearm discharge** HCC
Intentional self-harm by Very pistol [flare] discharge

√x7th **X74.9 Intentional self-harm by unspecified firearm discharge** HCC

√x7th **X75 Intentional self-harm by explosive material** HCC

√x7th **X76 Intentional self-harm by smoke, fire and flames** HCC

√4th **X77 Intentional self-harm by steam, hot vapors and hot objects**

√x7th **X77.0 Intentional self-harm by steam or hot vapors** HCC

√x7th **X77.1 Intentional self-harm by hot tap water** HCC

√x7th **X77.2 Intentional self-harm by other hot fluids** HCC

√x7th **X77.3 Intentional self-harm by hot household appliances** HCC

√x7th **X77.8 Intentional self-harm by other hot objects** HCC

√x7th **X77.9 Intentional self-harm by unspecified hot objects** HCC

√4th **X78 Intentional self-harm by sharp object**

√x7th **X78.0 Intentional self-harm by sharp glass** HCC

√x7th **X78.1 Intentional self-harm by knife** HCC

√x7th **X78.2 Intentional self-harm by sword or dagger** HCC

√x7th **X78.8 Intentional self-harm by other sharp object** HCC
AHA: 2022,1Q,27

√x7th **X78.9 Intentional self-harm by unspecified sharp object** HCC

√x7th **X79 Intentional self-harm by blunt object** HCC

√x7th **X80 Intentional self-harm by jumping from a high place** HCC
Intentional fall from one level to another

√4th **X81 Intentional self-harm by jumping or lying in front of moving object**

√x7th **X81.0 Intentional self-harm by jumping or lying in front of motor vehicle** HCC

√x7th **X81.1 Intentional self-harm by jumping or lying in front of (subway) train** HCC

√x7th **X81.8 Intentional self-harm by jumping or lying in front of other moving object** HCC

√4th **X82 Intentional self-harm by crashing of motor vehicle**

√x7th **X82.0 Intentional collision of motor vehicle with other motor vehicle** HCC

√x7th **X82.1 Intentional collision of motor vehicle with train** HCC

√x7th **X82.2 Intentional collision of motor vehicle with tree** HCC

√x7th **X82.8 Other intentional self-harm by crashing of motor vehicle** HCC

√4th **X83 Intentional self-harm by other specified means**
EXCLUDES 1 *intentional self-harm by poisoning or contact with toxic substance - see Table of Drugs and Chemicals*

√x7th **X83.0 Intentional self-harm by crashing of aircraft** HCC

√x7th **X83.1 Intentional self-harm by electrocution** HCC

√x7th **X83.2 Intentional self-harm by exposure to extremes of cold** HCC

√x7th **X83.8 Intentional self-harm by other specified means** HCC

Assault (X92-Y09)

INCLUDES homicide
injuries inflicted by another person with intent to injure or kill, by any means

EXCLUDES 1 *injuries due to legal intervention (Y35.-)*
injuries due to operations of war (Y36.-)
injuries due to terrorism (Y38.-)

The appropriate 7th character is to be added to each code from categories X92-Y04 and Y08.
A initial encounter
D subsequent encounter
S sequela

√4th **X92 Assault by drowning and submersion**

√x7th **X92.0 Assault by drowning and submersion while in bathtub**

√x7th **X92.1 Assault by drowning and submersion while in swimming pool**

X92.2 Assault by drowning and submersion after push into swimming pool

X92.3 Assault by drowning and submersion in natural water

X92.8 Other assault by drowning and submersion

X92.9 Assault by drowning and submersion, unspecified

X93 Assault by handgun discharge

Assault by discharge of gun for single hand use
Assault by discharge of pistol
Assault by discharge of revolver

EXCLUDES 1 *Very pistol (X95.8)*

X94 Assault by rifle, shotgun and larger firearm discharge

EXCLUDES 1 *airgun (X95.01)*

X94.0 Assault by shotgun

X94.1 Assault by hunting rifle

X94.2 Assault by machine gun

X94.8 Assault by other larger firearm discharge

X94.9 Assault by unspecified larger firearm discharge

X95 Assault by other and unspecified firearm and gun discharge

X95.0 Assault by gas, air or spring-operated guns

X95.01 Assault by airgun discharge
Assault by BB gun discharge
Assault by pellet gun discharge

X95.02 Assault by paintball gun discharge

X95.09 Assault by other gas, air or spring-operated gun

X95.8 Assault by other firearm discharge
Assault by Very pistol [flare] discharge

X95.9 Assault by unspecified firearm discharge

X96 Assault by explosive material

EXCLUDES 1 *incendiary device (X97)*
terrorism involving explosive material (Y38.2-)

X96.0 Assault by antipersonnel bomb

EXCLUDES 1 *antipersonnel bomb use in military or war (Y36.2-)*

X96.1 Assault by gasoline bomb

X96.2 Assault by letter bomb

X96.3 Assault by fertilizer bomb

X96.4 Assault by pipe bomb

X96.8 Assault by other specified explosive

X96.9 Assault by unspecified explosive

X97 Assault by smoke, fire and flames

Assault by arson
Assault by cigarettes
Assault by incendiary device

X98 Assault by steam, hot vapors and hot objects

X98.0 Assault by steam or hot vapors

X98.1 Assault by hot tap water

X98.2 Assault by hot fluids

X98.3 Assault by hot household appliances

X98.8 Assault by other hot objects

X98.9 Assault by unspecified hot objects

X99 Assault by sharp object

EXCLUDES 1 *assault by strike by sports equipment (Y08.0-)*

X99.0 Assault by sharp glass

X99.1 Assault by knife

X99.2 Assault by sword or dagger

X99.8 Assault by other sharp object

X99.9 Assault by unspecified sharp object
Assault by stabbing NOS

Y00 Assault by blunt object

EXCLUDES 1 *assault by strike by sports equipment (Y08.0-)*

Y01 Assault by pushing from high place

Y02 Assault by pushing or placing victim in front of moving object

Y02.0 Assault by pushing or placing victim in front of motor vehicle

Y02.1 Assault by pushing or placing victim in front of (subway) train

Y02.8 Assault by pushing or placing victim in front of other moving object

Y03 Assault by crashing of motor vehicle

Y03.0 Assault by being hit or run over by motor vehicle

Y03.8 Other assault by crashing of motor vehicle

Y04 Assault by bodily force

EXCLUDES 1 *assault by:*
submersion (X92.-)
use of weapon (X93-X95, X99, Y00)

Y04.0 Assault by unarmed brawl or fight

Y04.1 Assault by human bite

Y04.2 Assault by strike against or bumped into by another person

Y04.8 Assault by other bodily force
Assault by bodily force NOS

Y07 Perpetrator of assault, maltreatment and neglect

NOTE Codes from this category are for use only in cases of confirmed abuse (T74.-)
Selection of the correct perpetrator code is based on the relationship between the perpetrator and the victim

INCLUDES perpetrator of abandonment
perpetrator of emotional neglect
perpetrator of mental cruelty
perpetrator of physical abuse
perpetrator of physical neglect
perpetrator of sexual abuse
perpetrator of torture
▶perpetrator of verbal abuse◀

Y07.0 Spouse or partner, perpetrator of maltreatment and neglect
Spouse or partner, perpetrator of maltreatment and neglect against spouse or partner
AHA: 2023,1Q,5

Y07.01 Husband, perpetrator of maltreatment and neglect

Y07.010 Husband, current, perpetrator of maltreatment and neglect

Y07.011 Husband, former, perpetrator of maltreatment and neglect

Y07.02 Wife, perpetrator of maltreatment and neglect

Y07.020 Wife, current, perpetrator of maltreatment and neglect

Y07.021 Wife, former, perpetrator of maltreatment and neglect

Y07.03 Male partner, perpetrator of maltreatment and neglect
▶Male intimate or dating partner, perpetrator of maltreatment and neglect◀

Y07.030 Male partner, current, perpetrator of maltreatment and neglect

Y07.031 Male partner, former, perpetrator of maltreatment and neglect

Y07.04 Female partner, perpetrator of maltreatment and neglect
▶Female intimate or dating partner, perpetrator of maltreatment and neglect◀

Y07.040 Female partner, current, perpetrator of maltreatment and neglect

Y07.041 Female partner, former, perpetrator of maltreatment and neglect

Y07.05 Non-binary partner, perpetrator of maltreatment and neglect
Gender non-conforming partner, perpetrator of maltreatment and neglect

Y07.050 Non-binary partner, current, perpetrator of maltreatment and neglect

Y07.051 Non-binary partner, former, perpetrator of maltreatment and neglect

Y07.1 Parent (adoptive) (biological), perpetrator of maltreatment and neglect

Y07.11 Biological father, perpetrator of maltreatment and neglect

Y07.12 Biological mother, perpetrator of maltreatment and neglect

Y07.13 Adoptive father, perpetrator of maltreatment and neglect

Y07.14 Adoptive mother, perpetrator of maltreatment and neglect

Y07.4 Other family member, perpetrator of maltreatment and neglect
AHA: 2023,1Q,5

Y07.41 Sibling, perpetrator of maltreatment and neglect
EXCLUDES 1 stepsibling, perpetrator of maltreatment and neglect (Y07.435, Y07.436)

Y07.410 Brother, perpetrator of maltreatment and neglect

Y07.411 Sister, perpetrator of maltreatment and neglect

Y07.42 Foster parent, perpetrator of maltreatment and neglect

Y07.420 Foster father, perpetrator of maltreatment and neglect

Y07.421 Foster mother, perpetrator of maltreatment and neglect

Y07.43 Stepparent or stepsibling, perpetrator of maltreatment and neglect

Y07.430 Stepfather, perpetrator of maltreatment and neglect

Y07.432 Male friend of parent (co-residing in household), perpetrator of maltreatment and neglect

Y07.433 Stepmother, perpetrator of maltreatment and neglect

Y07.434 Female friend of parent (co-residing in household), perpetrator of maltreatment and neglect

Y07.435 Stepbrother, perpetrator or maltreatment and neglect

Y07.436 Stepsister, perpetrator of maltreatment and neglect

Y07.44 Child, perpetrator of maltreatment and neglect
Adopted child, perpetrator of maltreatment and neglect
Biological child, perpetrator of maltreatment and neglect
Daughter, perpetrator of maltreatment and neglect
Foster child, perpetrator of maltreatment and neglect
In-law child, perpetrator of maltreatment and neglect
Non-binary child, perpetrator of maltreatment and neglect
Son, perpetrator of maltreatment and neglect
Stepchild, perpetrator of maltreatment and neglect

Y07.45 Grandchild, perpetrator of maltreatment and neglect
Adopted grandchild, perpetrator of maltreatment and neglect
Biological grandchild, perpetrator of maltreatment and neglect
Foster grandchild, perpetrator of maltreatment and neglect
Granddaughter, perpetrator of maltreatment and neglect
Grandson, perpetrator of maltreatment and neglect
In-law grandchild, perpetrator of maltreatment and neglect
Non-binary grandchild, perpetrator of maltreatment and neglect
Step grandchild, perpetrator of maltreatment and neglect

Y07.46 Grandparent, perpetrator of maltreatment and neglect
Grandfather, perpetrator of maltreatment and neglect
Grandmother, perpetrator of maltreatment and neglect
Non-binary grandparent, perpetrator of maltreatment and neglect

Y07.47 Parental sibling, perpetrator of maltreatment and neglect
Aunt, perpetrator of maltreatment and neglect
Non-binary parental sibling, perpetrator of maltreatment and neglect
Uncle, perpetrator of maltreatment and neglect

Y07.49 Other family member, perpetrator of maltreatment and neglect

Y07.490 Male cousin, perpetrator of maltreatment and neglect

Y07.491 Female cousin, perpetrator of maltreatment and neglect

Y07.499 Other family member, perpetrator of maltreatment and neglect

Y07.5 Non-family member, perpetrator of maltreatment and neglect
AHA: 2023,1Q,5

Y07.50 Unspecified non-family member, perpetrator of maltreatment and neglect

Y07.51 Daycare provider, perpetrator of maltreatment and neglect

Y07.510 At-home childcare provider, perpetrator of maltreatment and neglect

Y07.511 Daycare center childcare provider, perpetrator of maltreatment and neglect

Y07.512 At-home adultcare provider, perpetrator of maltreatment and neglect

Y07.513 Adultcare center provider, perpetrator of maltreatment and neglect

Y07.519 Unspecified daycare provider, perpetrator of maltreatment and neglect

Y07.52 Healthcare provider, perpetrator of maltreatment and neglect

Y07.521 Mental health provider, perpetrator of maltreatment and neglect

Y07.528 Other therapist or healthcare provider, perpetrator of maltreatment and neglect
Nurse perpetrator of maltreatment and neglect
Occupational therapist perpetrator of maltreatment and neglect
Physical therapist perpetrator of maltreatment and neglect
Speech therapist perpetrator of maltreatment and neglect

Y07.529 Unspecified healthcare provider, perpetrator of maltreatment and neglect

Y07.53 Teacher or instructor, perpetrator of maltreatment and neglect
Coach, perpetrator of maltreatment and neglect

Y07.54 Acquaintance or friend, perpetrator of maltreatment and neglect

Y07.59 Other non-family member, perpetrator of maltreatment and neglect

Y07.6 Multiple perpetrators of maltreatment and neglect
AHA: 2018,4Q,32

Y07.9 Unspecified perpetrator of maltreatment and neglect

Y08 Assault by other specified means

Y08.0 Assault by strike by sport equipment

Y08.01 Assault by strike by hockey stick

Y08.02 Assault by strike by baseball bat

Y08.09 Assault by strike by other specified type of sport equipment

Y08.8 Assault by other specified means

Y08.81 Assault by crashing of aircraft

Y08.89 Assault by other specified means

Y09 Assault by unspecified means
Assassination (attempted) NOS
Homicide (attempted) NOS
Manslaughter (attempted) NOS
Murder (attempted) NOS

Event of undetermined intent (Y21-Y33)

Undetermined intent is only for use when there is specific documentation in the record that the intent of the injury cannot be determined. If no such documentation is present, code to accidental (unintentional).

The appropriate 7th character is to be added to each code from categories Y21-Y33.
A initial encounter
D subsequent encounter
S sequela

Y21 Drowning and submersion, undetermined intent

Y21.0 Drowning and submersion while in bathtub, undetermined intent

Y21.1 Drowning and submersion after fall into bathtub, undetermined intent

Y21.2 Drowning and submersion while in swimming pool, undetermined intent

Y21.3 Drowning and submersion after fall into swimming pool, undetermined intent

Y21.4 Drowning and submersion in natural water, undetermined intent

Y21.8 Other drowning and submersion, undetermined intent

Y21.9 Unspecified drowning and submersion, undetermined intent

Y22 Handgun discharge, undetermined intent
Discharge of gun for single hand use, undetermined intent
Discharge of pistol, undetermined intent
Discharge of revolver, undetermined intent
EXCLUDES 2 Very pistol (Y24.8)

Y23 Rifle, shotgun and larger firearm discharge, undetermined intent
EXCLUDES 2 airgun (Y24.0)

Y23.0 Shotgun discharge, undetermined intent
Y23.1 Hunting rifle discharge, undetermined intent
Y23.2 Military firearm discharge, undetermined intent
Y23.3 Machine gun discharge, undetermined intent
Y23.8 Other larger firearm discharge, undetermined intent
Y23.9 Unspecified larger firearm discharge, undetermined intent

Y24 Other and unspecified firearm discharge, undetermined intent

Y24.0 Airgun discharge, undetermined intent
BB gun discharge, undetermined intent
Pellet gun discharge, undetermined intent
Y24.8 Other firearm discharge, undetermined intent
Paintball gun discharge, undetermined intent
Very pistol [flare] discharge, undetermined intent
Y24.9 Unspecified firearm discharge, undetermined intent

Y25 Contact with explosive material, undetermined intent

Y26 Exposure to smoke, fire and flames, undetermined intent

Y27 Contact with steam, hot vapors and hot objects, undetermined intent

Y27.0 Contact with steam and hot vapors, undetermined intent
Y27.1 Contact with hot tap water, undetermined intent
Y27.2 Contact with hot fluids, undetermined intent
Y27.3 Contact with hot household appliance, undetermined intent
Y27.8 Contact with other hot objects, undetermined intent
Y27.9 Contact with unspecified hot objects, undetermined intent

Y28 Contact with sharp object, undetermined intent

Y28.0 Contact with sharp glass, undetermined intent
Y28.1 Contact with knife, undetermined intent
Y28.2 Contact with sword or dagger, undetermined intent
Y28.8 Contact with other sharp object, undetermined intent
Y28.9 Contact with unspecified sharp object, undetermined intent

Y29 Contact with blunt object, undetermined intent

Y30 Falling, jumping or pushed from a high place, undetermined intent
Victim falling from one level to another, undetermined intent

Y31 Falling, lying or running before or into moving object, undetermined intent

Y32 Crashing of motor vehicle, undetermined intent

Y33 Other specified events, undetermined intent

Legal intervention, operations of war, military operations, and terrorism (Y35-Y38)

The appropriate 7th character is to be added to each code from categories Y35-Y38.
A initial encounter
D subsequent encounter
S sequela

Y35 Legal intervention
INCLUDES any injury sustained as a result of an encounter with any law enforcement official, serving in any capacity at the time of the encounter, whether on-duty or off-duty. Includes injury to law enforcement official, suspect and bystander
AHA: 2019,4Q,18-19

Y35.0 Legal intervention involving firearm discharge
Y35.00 Legal intervention involving unspecified firearm discharge
Legal intervention involving gunshot wound
Legal intervention involving shot NOS
Y35.001 Legal intervention involving unspecified firearm discharge, law enforcement official injured
Y35.002 Legal intervention involving unspecified firearm discharge, bystander injured
Y35.003 Legal intervention involving unspecified firearm discharge, suspect injured
Y35.009 Legal intervention involving unspecified firearm discharge, unspecified person injured
Y35.01 Legal intervention involving injury by machine gun
Y35.011 Legal intervention involving injury by machine gun, law enforcement official injured
Y35.012 Legal intervention involving injury by machine gun, bystander injured
Y35.013 Legal intervention involving injury by machine gun, suspect injured
Y35.019 Legal intervention involving injury by machine gun, unspecified person injured
Y35.02 Legal intervention involving injury by handgun
Y35.021 Legal intervention involving injury by handgun, law enforcement official injured
Y35.022 Legal intervention involving injury by handgun, bystander injured
Y35.023 Legal intervention involving injury by handgun, suspect injured
Y35.029 Legal intervention involving injury by handgun, unspecified person injured
Y35.03 Legal intervention involving injury by rifle pellet
Y35.031 Legal intervention involving injury by rifle pellet, law enforcement official injured
Y35.032 Legal intervention involving injury by rifle pellet, bystander injured
Y35.033 Legal intervention involving injury by rifle pellet, suspect injured
Y35.039 Legal intervention involving injury by rifle pellet, unspecified person injured
Y35.04 Legal intervention involving injury by rubber bullet
Y35.041 Legal intervention involving injury by rubber bullet, law enforcement official injured
Y35.042 Legal intervention involving injury by rubber bullet, bystander injured
Y35.043 Legal intervention involving injury by rubber bullet, suspect injured
Y35.049 Legal intervention involving injury by rubber bullet, unspecified person injured
Y35.09 Legal intervention involving other firearm discharge
Y35.091 Legal intervention involving other firearm discharge, law enforcement official injured
Y35.092 Legal intervention involving other firearm discharge, bystander injured
Y35.093 Legal intervention involving other firearm discharge, suspect injured
Y35.099 Legal intervention involving other firearm discharge, unspecified person injured
Y35.1 Legal intervention involving explosives
Y35.10 Legal intervention involving unspecified explosives
Y35.101 Legal intervention involving unspecified explosives, law enforcement official injured
Y35.102 Legal intervention involving unspecified explosives, bystander injured
Y35.103 Legal intervention involving unspecified explosives, suspect injured
Y35.109 Legal intervention involving unspecified explosives, unspecified person injured
Y35.11 Legal intervention involving injury by dynamite
Y35.111 Legal intervention involving injury by dynamite, law enforcement official injured
Y35.112 Legal intervention involving injury by dynamite, bystander injured
Y35.113 Legal intervention involving injury by dynamite, suspect injured
Y35.119 Legal intervention involving injury by dynamite, unspecified person injured

N Newborn: 0 P Pediatric: 0-17 M Maternity: 9-64 A Adult: 15-124 UNS Unspecified Site MCC Major Complication/Comorbidity CC Complication/Comorbidity

Y35.12 Legal intervention involving injury by explosive shell
Y35.121 Legal intervention involving injury by explosive shell, law enforcement official injured
Y35.122 Legal intervention involving injury by explosive shell, bystander injured
Y35.123 Legal intervention involving injury by explosive shell, suspect injured
Y35.129 Legal intervention involving injury by explosive shell, unspecified person injured
Y35.19 Legal intervention involving other explosives
Legal intervention involving injury by grenade
Legal intervention involving injury by mortar bomb
Y35.191 Legal intervention involving other explosives, law enforcement official injured
Y35.192 Legal intervention involving other explosives, bystander injured
Y35.193 Legal intervention involving other explosives, suspect injured
Y35.199 Legal intervention involving other explosives, unspecified person injured
Y35.2 Legal intervention involving gas
Legal intervention involving asphyxiation by gas
Legal intervention involving poisoning by gas
Y35.20 Legal intervention involving unspecified gas
Y35.201 Legal intervention involving unspecified gas, law enforcement official injured
Y35.202 Legal intervention involving unspecified gas, bystander injured
Y35.203 Legal intervention involving unspecified gas, suspect injured
Y35.209 Legal intervention involving unspecified gas, unspecified person injured
Y35.21 Legal intervention involving injury by tear gas
Y35.211 Legal intervention involving injury by tear gas, law enforcement official injured
Y35.212 Legal intervention involving injury by tear gas, bystander injured
Y35.213 Legal intervention involving injury by tear gas, suspect injured
Y35.219 Legal intervention involving injury by tear gas, unspecified person injured
Y35.29 Legal intervention involving other gas
Y35.291 Legal intervention involving other gas, law enforcement official injured
Y35.292 Legal intervention involving other gas, bystander injured
Y35.293 Legal intervention involving other gas, suspect injured
Y35.299 Legal intervention involving other gas, unspecified person injured
Y35.3 Legal intervention involving blunt objects
Legal intervention involving being hit or struck by blunt object
Y35.30 Legal intervention involving unspecified blunt objects
Y35.301 Legal intervention involving unspecified blunt objects, law enforcement official injured
Y35.302 Legal intervention involving unspecified blunt objects, bystander injured
Y35.303 Legal intervention involving unspecified blunt objects, suspect injured
Y35.309 Legal intervention involving unspecified blunt objects, unspecified person injured
Y35.31 Legal intervention involving baton
Y35.311 Legal intervention involving baton, law enforcement official injured
Y35.312 Legal intervention involving baton, bystander injured
Y35.313 Legal intervention involving baton, suspect injured
Y35.319 Legal intervention involving baton, unspecified person injured
Y35.39 Legal intervention involving other blunt objects
Y35.391 Legal intervention involving other blunt objects, law enforcement official injured
Y35.392 Legal intervention involving other blunt objects, bystander injured
Y35.393 Legal intervention involving other blunt objects, suspect injured
Y35.399 Legal intervention involving other blunt objects, unspecified person injured
Y35.4 Legal intervention involving sharp objects
Legal intervention involving being cut by sharp objects
Legal intervention involving being stabbed by sharp objects
Y35.40 Legal intervention involving unspecified sharp objects
Y35.401 Legal intervention involving unspecified sharp objects, law enforcement official injured
Y35.402 Legal intervention involving unspecified sharp objects, bystander injured
Y35.403 Legal intervention involving unspecified sharp objects, suspect injured
Y35.409 Legal intervention involving unspecified sharp objects, unspecified person injured
Y35.41 Legal intervention involving bayonet
Y35.411 Legal intervention involving bayonet, law enforcement official injured
Y35.412 Legal intervention involving bayonet, bystander injured
Y35.413 Legal intervention involving bayonet, suspect injured
Y35.419 Legal intervention involving bayonet, unspecified person injured
Y35.49 Legal intervention involving other sharp objects
Y35.491 Legal intervention involving other sharp objects, law enforcement official injured
Y35.492 Legal intervention involving other sharp objects, bystander injured
Y35.493 Legal intervention involving other sharp objects, suspect injured
Y35.499 Legal intervention involving other sharp objects, unspecified person injured
Y35.8 Legal intervention involving other specified means
AHA: 2019,4Q,19
Y35.81 Legal intervention involving manhandling
Y35.811 Legal intervention involving manhandling, law enforcement official injured
Y35.812 Legal intervention involving manhandling, bystander injured
Y35.813 Legal intervention involving manhandling, suspect injured
Y35.819 Legal intervention involving manhandling, unspecified person injured
Y35.83 Legal intervention involving a conducted energy device
Electroshock device (taser)
Stun gun
Y35.831 Legal intervention involving a conducted energy device, law enforcement official injured
Y35.832 Legal intervention involving a conducted energy device, bystander injured
Y35.833 Legal intervention involving a conducted energy device, suspect injured
Y35.839 Legal intervention involving a conducted energy device, unspecified person injured
Y35.89 Legal intervention involving other specified means
Y35.891 Legal intervention involving other specified means, law enforcement official injured
Y35.892 Legal intervention involving other specified means, bystander injured
Y35.893 Legal intervention involving other specified means, suspect injured
AHA: 2018,1Q,5
Y35.899 Legal intervention involving other specified means, unspecified person injured
Y35.9 Legal intervention, means unspecified
Y35.91 Legal intervention, means unspecified, law enforcement official injured
Y35.92 Legal intervention, means unspecified, bystander injured
Y35.93 Legal intervention, means unspecified, suspect injured

Y35.99 Legal intervention, means unspecified, unspecified person injured

Y36 Operations of war

INCLUDES injuries to military personnel and civilians caused by war, civil insurrection, and peacekeeping missions

EXCLUDES 1 *injury to military personnel occurring during peacetime military operations (Y37.-)*
military vehicles involved in transport accidents with non-military vehicle during peacetime (V09.01, V09.21, V19.81, V29.818, V39.81, V49.81, V59.81, V69.81, V79.81)

AHA: 2014,3Q,4

Y36.0 War operations involving explosion of marine weapons

Y36.00 War operations involving explosion of unspecified marine weapon
War operations involving underwater blast NOS

Y36.000 War operations involving explosion of unspecified marine weapon, military personnel

Y36.001 War operations involving explosion of unspecified marine weapon, civilian

Y36.01 War operations involving explosion of depth-charge

Y36.010 War operations involving explosion of depth-charge, military personnel

Y36.011 War operations involving explosion of depth-charge, civilian

Y36.02 War operations involving explosion of marine mine
War operations involving explosion of marine mine, at sea or in harbor

Y36.020 War operations involving explosion of marine mine, military personnel

Y36.021 War operations involving explosion of marine mine, civilian

Y36.03 War operations involving explosion of sea-based artillery shell

Y36.030 War operations involving explosion of sea-based artillery shell, military personnel

Y36.031 War operations involving explosion of sea-based artillery shell, civilian

Y36.04 War operations involving explosion of torpedo

Y36.040 War operations involving explosion of torpedo, military personnel

Y36.041 War operations involving explosion of torpedo, civilian

Y36.05 War operations involving accidental detonation of onboard marine weapons

Y36.050 War operations involving accidental detonation of onboard marine weapons, military personnel

Y36.051 War operations involving accidental detonation of onboard marine weapons, civilian

Y36.09 War operations involving explosion of other marine weapons

Y36.090 War operations involving explosion of other marine weapons, military personnel

Y36.091 War operations involving explosion of other marine weapons, civilian

Y36.1 War operations involving destruction of aircraft

Y36.10 War operations involving unspecified destruction of aircraft

Y36.100 War operations involving unspecified destruction of aircraft, military personnel

Y36.101 War operations involving unspecified destruction of aircraft, civilian

Y36.11 War operations involving destruction of aircraft due to enemy fire or explosives
War operations involving destruction of aircraft due to air to air missile
War operations involving destruction of aircraft due to explosive placed on aircraft
War operations involving destruction of aircraft due to rocket propelled grenade [RPG]
War operations involving destruction of aircraft due to small arms fire
War operations involving destruction of aircraft due to surface to air missile

Y36.110 War operations involving destruction of aircraft due to enemy fire or explosives, military personnel

Y36.111 War operations involving destruction of aircraft due to enemy fire or explosives, civilian

Y36.12 War operations involving destruction of aircraft due to collision with other aircraft

Y36.120 War operations involving destruction of aircraft due to collision with other aircraft, military personnel

Y36.121 War operations involving destruction of aircraft due to collision with other aircraft, civilian

Y36.13 War operations involving destruction of aircraft due to onboard fire

Y36.130 War operations involving destruction of aircraft due to onboard fire, military personnel

Y36.131 War operations involving destruction of aircraft due to onboard fire, civilian

Y36.14 War operations involving destruction of aircraft due to accidental detonation of onboard munitions and explosives

Y36.140 War operations involving destruction of aircraft due to accidental detonation of onboard munitions and explosives, military personnel

Y36.141 War operations involving destruction of aircraft due to accidental detonation of onboard munitions and explosives, civilian

Y36.19 War operations involving other destruction of aircraft

Y36.190 War operations involving other destruction of aircraft, military personnel

Y36.191 War operations involving other destruction of aircraft, civilian

Y36.2 War operations involving other explosions and fragments

EXCLUDES 1 *war operations involving explosion of aircraft (Y36.1-)*
war operations involving explosion of marine weapons (Y36.0-)
war operations involving explosion of nuclear weapons (Y36.5-)
war operations involving explosion occurring after cessation of hostilities (Y36.8-)

Y36.20 War operations involving unspecified explosion and fragments
War operations involving air blast NOS
War operations involving blast NOS
War operations involving blast fragments NOS
War operations involving blast wave NOS
War operations involving blast wind NOS
War operations involving explosion NOS
War operations involving explosion of bomb NOS

Y36.200 War operations involving unspecified explosion and fragments, military personnel

Y36.201 War operations involving unspecified explosion and fragments, civilian

Y36.21 War operations involving explosion of aerial bomb

Y36.210 War operations involving explosion of aerial bomb, military personnel

Y36.211 War operations involving explosion of aerial bomb, civilian

Y36.22 War operations involving explosion of guided missile

Y36.220 War operations involving explosion of guided missile, military personnel

Y36.221 War operations involving explosion of guided missile, civilian

Y36.23 War operations involving explosion of improvised explosive device [IED]
War operations involving explosion of person-borne improvised explosive device [IED]
War operations involving explosion of vehicle-borne improvised explosive device [IED]
War operations involving explosion of roadside improvised explosive device [IED]

Y36.230 War operations involving explosion of improvised explosive device [IED], military personnel

Y36.231 War operations involving explosion of improvised explosive device [IED], civilian

✓6th Y36.24 **War operations involving explosion due to accidental detonation and discharge of own munitions or munitions launch device**

✓7th Y36.240 **War operations involving explosion due to accidental detonation and discharge of own munitions or munitions launch device, military personnel**

✓7th Y36.241 **War operations involving explosion due to accidental detonation and discharge of own munitions or munitions launch device, civilian**

✓6th Y36.25 **War operations involving fragments from munitions**

✓7th Y36.250 **War operations involving fragments from munitions, military personnel**

✓7th Y36.251 **War operations involving fragments from munitions, civilian**

✓6th Y36.26 **War operations involving fragments of improvised explosive device [IED]**

War operations involving fragments of person-borne improvised explosive device [IED]

War operations involving fragments of roadside improvised explosive device [IED]

War operations involving fragments of vehicle-borne improvised explosive device [IED]

✓7th Y36.260 **War operations involving fragments of improvised explosive device [IED], military personnel**

✓7th Y36.261 **War operations involving fragments of improvised explosive device [IED], civilian**

✓6th Y36.27 **War operations involving fragments from weapons**

✓7th Y36.270 **War operations involving fragments from weapons, military personnel**

✓7th Y36.271 **War operations involving fragments from weapons, civilian**

✓6th Y36.29 **War operations involving other explosions and fragments**

War operations involving explosion of grenade

War operations involving explosions of land mine

War operations involving shrapnel NOS

✓7th Y36.290 **War operations involving other explosions and fragments, military personnel**

✓7th Y36.291 **War operations involving other explosions and fragments, civilian**

✓5th Y36.3 **War operations involving fires, conflagrations and hot substances**

War operations involving smoke, fumes, and heat from fires, conflagrations and hot substances

EXCLUDES 1 *war operations involving fires and conflagrations aboard military aircraft (Y36.1-)*

war operations involving fires and conflagrations aboard military watercraft (Y36.0-)

war operations involving fires and conflagrations caused indirectly by conventional weapons (Y36.2-)

war operations involving fires and thermal effects of nuclear weapons (Y36.53-)

✓6th Y36.30 **War operations involving unspecified fire, conflagration and hot substance**

✓7th Y36.300 **War operations involving unspecified fire, conflagration and hot substance, military personnel**

✓7th Y36.301 **War operations involving unspecified fire, conflagration and hot substance, civilian**

✓6th Y36.31 **War operations involving gasoline bomb**

War operations involving incendiary bomb

War operations involving petrol bomb

✓7th Y36.310 **War operations involving gasoline bomb, military personnel**

✓7th Y36.311 **War operations involving gasoline bomb, civilian**

✓6th Y36.32 **War operations involving incendiary bullet**

✓7th Y36.320 **War operations involving incendiary bullet, military personnel**

✓7th Y36.321 **War operations involving incendiary bullet, civilian**

✓6th Y36.33 **War operations involving flamethrower**

✓7th Y36.330 **War operations involving flamethrower, military personnel**

✓7th Y36.331 **War operations involving flamethrower, civilian**

✓6th Y36.39 **War operations involving other fires, conflagrations and hot substances**

✓7th Y36.390 **War operations involving other fires, conflagrations and hot substances, military personnel**

✓7th Y36.391 **War operations involving other fires, conflagrations and hot substances, civilian**

✓5th Y36.4 **War operations involving firearm discharge and other forms of conventional warfare**

✓6th Y36.41 **War operations involving rubber bullets**

✓7th Y36.410 **War operations involving rubber bullets, military personnel**

✓7th Y36.411 **War operations involving rubber bullets, civilian**

✓6th Y36.42 **War operations involving firearms pellets**

✓7th Y36.420 **War operations involving firearms pellets, military personnel**

✓7th Y36.421 **War operations involving firearms pellets, civilian**

✓6th Y36.43 **War operations involving other firearms discharge**

War operations involving bullets NOS

EXCLUDES 1 *war operations involving munitions fragments (Y36.25-)*

war operations involving incendiary bullets (Y36.32-)

✓7th Y36.430 **War operations involving other firearms discharge, military personnel**

✓7th Y36.431 **War operations involving other firearms discharge, civilian**

✓6th Y36.44 **War operations involving unarmed hand to hand combat**

EXCLUDES 1 *war operations involving combat using blunt or piercing object (Y36.45-)*

war operations involving intentional restriction of air and airway (Y36.46-)

war operations involving unintentional restriction of air and airway (Y36.47-)

✓7th Y36.440 **War operations involving unarmed hand to hand combat, military personnel**

✓7th Y36.441 **War operations involving unarmed hand to hand combat, civilian**

✓6th Y36.45 **War operations involving combat using blunt or piercing object**

✓7th Y36.450 **War operations involving combat using blunt or piercing object, military personnel**

✓7th Y36.451 **War operations involving combat using blunt or piercing object, civilian**

✓6th Y36.46 **War operations involving intentional restriction of air and airway**

✓7th Y36.460 **War operations involving intentional restriction of air and airway, military personnel**

✓7th Y36.461 **War operations involving intentional restriction of air and airway, civilian**

✓6th Y36.47 **War operations involving unintentional restriction of air and airway**

✓7th Y36.470 **War operations involving unintentional restriction of air and airway, military personnel**

✓7th Y36.471 **War operations involving unintentional restriction of air and airway, civilian**

✓6th Y36.49 **War operations involving other forms of conventional warfare**

✓7th Y36.490 **War operations involving other forms of conventional warfare, military personnel**

✓7th Y36.491 **War operations involving other forms of conventional warfare, civilian**

✓5th Y36.5 **War operations involving nuclear weapons**

War operations involving dirty bomb NOS

✓6th Y36.50 **War operations involving unspecified effect of nuclear weapon**

✓7th Y36.500 **War operations involving unspecified effect of nuclear weapon, military personnel**

✓7th Y36.501 **War operations involving unspecified effect of nuclear weapon, civilian**

- **Y36.51 War operations involving direct blast effect of nuclear weapon**
  - War operations involving blast pressure of nuclear weapon
  - **Y36.510 War operations involving direct blast effect of nuclear weapon, military personnel**
  - **Y36.511 War operations involving direct blast effect of nuclear weapon, civilian**
- **Y36.52 War operations involving indirect blast effect of nuclear weapon**
  - War operations involving being thrown by blast of nuclear weapon
  - War operations involving being struck or crushed by blast debris of nuclear weapon
  - **Y36.520 War operations involving indirect blast effect of nuclear weapon, military personnel**
  - **Y36.521 War operations involving indirect blast effect of nuclear weapon, civilian**
- **Y36.53 War operations involving thermal radiation effect of nuclear weapon**
  - War operations involving direct heat from nuclear weapon
  - War operation involving fireball effects from nuclear weapon
  - **Y36.530 War operations involving thermal radiation effect of nuclear weapon, military personnel**
  - **Y36.531 War operations involving thermal radiation effect of nuclear weapon, civilian**
- **Y36.54 War operation involving nuclear radiation effects of nuclear weapon**
  - War operation involving acute radiation exposure from nuclear weapon
  - War operation involving exposure to immediate ionizing radiation from nuclear weapon
  - War operation involving fallout exposure from nuclear weapon
  - War operation involving secondary effects of nuclear weapons
  - **Y36.540 War operation involving nuclear radiation effects of nuclear weapon, military personnel**
  - **Y36.541 War operation involving nuclear radiation effects of nuclear weapon, civilian**
- **Y36.59 War operation involving other effects of nuclear weapons**
  - **Y36.590 War operation involving other effects of nuclear weapons, military personnel**
  - **Y36.591 War operation involving other effects of nuclear weapons, civilian**

Y36.6 War operations involving biological weapons

- **Y36.6X War operations involving biological weapons**
  - **Y36.6X0 War operations involving biological weapons, military personnel**
  - **Y36.6X1 War operations involving biological weapons, civilian**

Y36.7 War operations involving chemical weapons and other forms of unconventional warfare

EXCLUDES 1 *war operations involving incendiary devices (Y36.3-, Y36.5-)*

- **Y36.7X War operations involving chemical weapons and other forms of unconventional warfare**
  - **Y36.7X0 War operations involving chemical weapons and other forms of unconventional warfare, military personnel**
  - **Y36.7X1 War operations involving chemical weapons and other forms of unconventional warfare, civilian**

Y36.8 War operations occurring after cessation of hostilities

War operations classifiable to categories Y36.0-Y36.8 but occurring after cessation of hostilities

- **Y36.81 Explosion of mine placed during war operations but exploding after cessation of hostilities**
  - **Y36.810 Explosion of mine placed during war operations but exploding after cessation of hostilities, military personnel**
  - **Y36.811 Explosion of mine placed during war operations but exploding after cessation of hostilities, civilian**
- **Y36.82 Explosion of bomb placed during war operations but exploding after cessation of hostilities**
  - **Y36.820 Explosion of bomb placed during war operations but exploding after cessation of hostilities, military personnel**
  - **Y36.821 Explosion of bomb placed during war operations but exploding after cessation of hostilities, civilian**
- **Y36.88 Other war operations occurring after cessation of hostilities**
  - **Y36.880 Other war operations occurring after cessation of hostilities, military personnel**
  - **Y36.881 Other war operations occurring after cessation of hostilities, civilian**
- **Y36.89 Unspecified war operations occurring after cessation of hostilities**
  - **Y36.890 Unspecified war operations occurring after cessation of hostilities, military personnel**
  - **Y36.891 Unspecified war operations occurring after cessation of hostilities, civilian**

Y36.9 Other and unspecified war operations

- **Y36.90 War operations, unspecified**
- **Y36.91 War operations involving unspecified weapon of mass destruction [WMD]**
- **Y36.92 War operations involving friendly fire**

Y37 Military operations

INCLUDES injuries to military personnel and civilians occurring during peacetime on military property and during routine military exercises and operations

EXCLUDES 1 *military aircraft involved in aircraft accident with civilian aircraft (V97.81-)*
military vehicles involved in transport accident with civilian vehicle (V09.01, V09.21, V19.81, V29.818, V39.81, V49.81, V59.81, V69.81, V79.81)
military watercraft involved in water transport accident with civilian watercraft (V94.81-)
war operations (Y36.-)

Y37.0 Military operations involving explosion of marine weapons

- **Y37.00 Military operations involving explosion of unspecified marine weapon**
  - Military operations involving underwater blast NOS
  - **Y37.000 Military operations involving explosion of unspecified marine weapon, military personnel**
  - **Y37.001 Military operations involving explosion of unspecified marine weapon, civilian**
- **Y37.01 Military operations involving explosion of depth-charge**
  - **Y37.010 Military operations involving explosion of depth-charge, military personnel**
  - **Y37.011 Military operations involving explosion of depth-charge, civilian**
- **Y37.02 Military operations involving explosion of marine mine**
  - Military operations involving explosion of marine mine, at sea or in harbor
  - **Y37.020 Military operations involving explosion of marine mine, military personnel**
  - **Y37.021 Military operations involving explosion of marine mine, civilian**
- **Y37.03 Military operations involving explosion of sea-based artillery shell**
  - **Y37.030 Military operations involving explosion of sea-based artillery shell, military personnel**
  - **Y37.031 Military operations involving explosion of sea-based artillery shell, civilian**
- **Y37.04 Military operations involving explosion of torpedo**
  - **Y37.040 Military operations involving explosion of torpedo, military personnel**
  - **Y37.041 Military operations involving explosion of torpedo, civilian**
- **Y37.05 Military operations involving accidental detonation of onboard marine weapons**
  - **Y37.050 Military operations involving accidental detonation of onboard marine weapons, military personnel**

7th Y37.051 **Military operations involving accidental detonation of onboard marine weapons, civilian**

6th Y37.09 **Military operations involving explosion of other marine weapons**

7th Y37.090 **Military operations involving explosion of other marine weapons, military personnel**

7th Y37.091 **Military operations involving explosion of other marine weapons, civilian**

5th Y37.1 **Military operations involving destruction of aircraft**

6th Y37.10 **Military operations involving unspecified destruction of aircraft**

7th Y37.100 **Military operations involving unspecified destruction of aircraft, military personnel**

7th Y37.101 **Military operations involving unspecified destruction of aircraft, civilian**

6th Y37.11 **Military operations involving destruction of aircraft due to enemy fire or explosives**

Military operations involving destruction of aircraft due to air to air missile
Military operations involving destruction of aircraft due to explosive placed on aircraft
Military operations involving destruction of aircraft due to rocket propelled grenade [RPG]
Military operations involving destruction of aircraft due to small arms fire
Military operations involving destruction of aircraft due to surface to air missile

7th Y37.110 **Military operations involving destruction of aircraft due to enemy fire or explosives, military personnel**

7th Y37.111 **Military operations involving destruction of aircraft due to enemy fire or explosives, civilian**

6th Y37.12 **Military operations involving destruction of aircraft due to collision with other aircraft**

7th Y37.120 **Military operations involving destruction of aircraft due to collision with other aircraft, military personnel**

7th Y37.121 **Military operations involving destruction of aircraft due to collision with other aircraft, civilian**

6th Y37.13 **Military operations involving destruction of aircraft due to onboard fire**

7th Y37.130 **Military operations involving destruction of aircraft due to onboard fire, military personnel**

7th Y37.131 **Military operations involving destruction of aircraft due to onboard fire, civilian**

6th Y37.14 **Military operations involving destruction of aircraft due to accidental detonation of onboard munitions and explosives**

7th Y37.140 **Military operations involving destruction of aircraft due to accidental detonation of onboard munitions and explosives, military personnel**

7th Y37.141 **Military operations involving destruction of aircraft due to accidental detonation of onboard munitions and explosives, civilian**

6th Y37.19 **Military operations involving other destruction of aircraft**

7th Y37.190 **Military operations involving other destruction of aircraft, military personnel**

7th Y37.191 **Military operations involving other destruction of aircraft, civilian**

5th Y37.2 **Military operations involving other explosions and fragments**

EXCLUDES 1 *military operations involving explosion of aircraft (Y37.1-)*
military operations involving explosion of marine weapons (Y37.0-)
military operations involving explosion of nuclear weapons (Y37.5-)

6th Y37.20 **Military operations involving unspecified explosion and fragments**

Military operations involving air blast NOS
Military operations involving blast NOS
Military operations involving blast fragments NOS
Military operations involving blast wave NOS
Military operations involving blast wind NOS
Military operations involving explosion NOS
Military operations involving explosion of bomb NOS

7th Y37.200 **Military operations involving unspecified explosion and fragments, military personnel**

7th Y37.201 **Military operations involving unspecified explosion and fragments, civilian**

6th Y37.21 **Military operations involving explosion of aerial bomb**

7th Y37.210 **Military operations involving explosion of aerial bomb, military personnel**

7th Y37.211 **Military operations involving explosion of aerial bomb, civilian**

6th Y37.22 **Military operations involving explosion of guided missile**

7th Y37.220 **Military operations involving explosion of guided missile, military personnel**

7th Y37.221 **Military operations involving explosion of guided missile, civilian**

6th Y37.23 **Military operations involving explosion of improvised explosive device [IED]**

Military operations involving explosion of person-borne improvised explosive device [IED]
Military operations involving explosion of vehicle-borne improvised explosive device [IED]
Military operations involving explosion of roadside improvised explosive device [IED]

7th Y37.230 **Military operations involving explosion of improvised explosive device [IED], military personnel**

7th Y37.231 **Military operations involving explosion of improvised explosive device [IED], civilian**

6th Y37.24 **Military operations involving explosion due to accidental detonation and discharge of own munitions or munitions launch device**

7th Y37.240 **Military operations involving explosion due to accidental detonation and discharge of own munitions or munitions launch device, military personnel**

7th Y37.241 **Military operations involving explosion due to accidental detonation and discharge of own munitions or munitions launch device, civilian**

6th Y37.25 **Military operations involving fragments from munitions**

7th Y37.250 **Military operations involving fragments from munitions, military personnel**

7th Y37.251 **Military operations involving fragments from munitions, civilian**

6th Y37.26 **Military operations involving fragments of improvised explosive device [IED]**

Military operations involving fragments of person-borne improvised explosive device [IED]
Military operations involving fragments of vehicle-borne improvised explosive device [IED]
Military operations involving fragments of roadside improvised explosive device [IED]

7th Y37.260 **Military operations involving fragments of improvised explosive device [IED], military personnel**

7th Y37.261 **Military operations involving fragments of improvised explosive device [IED], civilian**

6th Y37.27 **Military operations involving fragments from weapons**

7th Y37.270 **Military operations involving fragments from weapons, military personnel**

✓7th **Y37.271 Military operations involving fragments from weapons, civilian**

✓6th **Y37.29 Military operations involving other explosions and fragments**

Military operations involving explosion of grenade
Military operations involving explosions of land mine
Military operations involving shrapnel NOS

✓7th **Y37.290 Military operations involving other explosions and fragments, military personnel**

✓7th **Y37.291 Military operations involving other explosions and fragments, civilian**

✓5th **Y37.3 Military operations involving fires, conflagrations and hot substances**

Military operations involving smoke, fumes, and heat from fires, conflagrations and hot substances

EXCLUDES 1 *military operations involving fires and conflagrations aboard military aircraft (Y37.1-)*
military operations involving fires and conflagrations aboard military watercraft (Y37.0-)
military operations involving fires and conflagrations caused indirectly by conventional weapons (Y37.2-)
military operations involving fires and thermal effects of nuclear weapons (Y36.53-)

✓6th **Y37.30 Military operations involving unspecified fire, conflagration and hot substance**

✓7th **Y37.300 Military operations involving unspecified fire, conflagration and hot substance, military personnel**

✓7th **Y37.301 Military operations involving unspecified fire, conflagration and hot substance, civilian**

✓6th **Y37.31 Military operations involving gasoline bomb**

Military operations involving incendiary bomb
Military operations involving petrol bomb

✓7th **Y37.310 Military operations involving gasoline bomb, military personnel**

✓7th **Y37.311 Military operations involving gasoline bomb, civilian**

✓6th **Y37.32 Military operations involving incendiary bullet**

✓7th **Y37.320 Military operations involving incendiary bullet, military personnel**

✓7th **Y37.321 Military operations involving incendiary bullet, civilian**

✓6th **Y37.33 Military operations involving flamethrower**

✓7th **Y37.330 Military operations involving flamethrower, military personnel**

✓7th **Y37.331 Military operations involving flamethrower, civilian**

✓6th **Y37.39 Military operations involving other fires, conflagrations and hot substances**

✓7th **Y37.390 Military operations involving other fires, conflagrations and hot substances, military personnel**

✓7th **Y37.391 Military operations involving other fires, conflagrations and hot substances, civilian**

✓5th **Y37.4 Military operations involving firearm discharge and other forms of conventional warfare**

✓6th **Y37.41 Military operations involving rubber bullets**

✓7th **Y37.410 Military operations involving rubber bullets, military personnel**

✓7th **Y37.411 Military operations involving rubber bullets, civilian**

✓6th **Y37.42 Military operations involving firearms pellets**

✓7th **Y37.420 Military operations involving firearms pellets, military personnel**

✓7th **Y37.421 Military operations involving firearms pellets, civilian**

✓6th **Y37.43 Military operations involving other firearms discharge**

Military operations involving bullets NOS

EXCLUDES 1 *military operations involving munitions fragments (Y37.25-)*
military operations involving incendiary bullets (Y37.32-)

✓7th **Y37.430 Military operations involving other firearms discharge, military personnel**

✓7th **Y37.431 Military operations involving other firearms discharge, civilian**

✓6th **Y37.44 Military operations involving unarmed hand to hand combat**

EXCLUDES 1 *military operations involving combat using blunt or piercing object (Y37.45-)*
military operations involving intentional restriction of air and airway (Y37.46-)
military operations involving unintentional restriction of air and airway (Y37.47-)

✓7th **Y37.440 Military operations involving unarmed hand to hand combat, military personnel**

✓7th **Y37.441 Military operations involving unarmed hand to hand combat, civilian**

✓6th **Y37.45 Military operations involving combat using blunt or piercing object**

✓7th **Y37.450 Military operations involving combat using blunt or piercing object, military personnel**

✓7th **Y37.451 Military operations involving combat using blunt or piercing object, civilian**

✓6th **Y37.46 Military operations involving intentional restriction of air and airway**

✓7th **Y37.460 Military operations involving intentional restriction of air and airway, military personnel**

✓7th **Y37.461 Military operations involving intentional restriction of air and airway, civilian**

✓6th **Y37.47 Military operations involving unintentional restriction of air and airway**

✓7th **Y37.470 Military operations involving unintentional restriction of air and airway, military personnel**

✓7th **Y37.471 Military operations involving unintentional restriction of air and airway, civilian**

✓6th **Y37.49 Military operations involving other forms of conventional warfare**

✓7th **Y37.490 Military operations involving other forms of conventional warfare, military personnel**

✓7th **Y37.491 Military operations involving other forms of conventional warfare, civilian**

✓5th **Y37.5 Military operations involving nuclear weapons**

Military operation involving dirty bomb NOS

✓6th **Y37.50 Military operations involving unspecified effect of nuclear weapon**

✓7th **Y37.500 Military operations involving unspecified effect of nuclear weapon, military personnel**

✓7th **Y37.501 Military operations involving unspecified effect of nuclear weapon, civilian**

✓6th **Y37.51 Military operations involving direct blast effect of nuclear weapon**

Military operations involving blast pressure of nuclear weapon

✓7th **Y37.510 Military operations involving direct blast effect of nuclear weapon, military personnel**

✓7th **Y37.511 Military operations involving direct blast effect of nuclear weapon, civilian**

✓6th **Y37.52 Military operations involving indirect blast effect of nuclear weapon**

Military operations involving being thrown by blast of nuclear weapon
Military operations involving being struck or crushed by blast debris of nuclear weapon

✓7th **Y37.520 Military operations involving indirect blast effect of nuclear weapon, military personnel**

✓7th **Y37.521 Military operations involving indirect blast effect of nuclear weapon, civilian**

✓6th **Y37.53 Military operations involving thermal radiation effect of nuclear weapon**

Military operations involving direct heat from nuclear weapon
Military operation involving fireball effects from nuclear weapon

✓7th **Y37.530 Military operations involving thermal radiation effect of nuclear weapon, military personnel**

✓7th **Y37.531 Military operations involving thermal radiation effect of nuclear weapon, civilian**

Y37.54 **Military operation involving nuclear radiation effects of nuclear weapon**
Military operation involving acute radiation exposure from nuclear weapon
Military operation involving exposure to immediate ionizing radiation from nuclear weapon
Military operation involving fallout exposure from nuclear weapon
Military operation involving secondary effects of nuclear weapons

Y37.540 **Military operation involving nuclear radiation effects of nuclear weapon, military personnel**

Y37.541 **Military operation involving nuclear radiation effects of nuclear weapon, civilian**

Y37.59 **Military operation involving other effects of nuclear weapons**

Y37.590 **Military operation involving other effects of nuclear weapons, military personnel**

Y37.591 **Military operation involving other effects of nuclear weapons, civilian**

Y37.6 **Military operations involving biological weapons**

Y37.6X **Military operations involving biological weapons**

Y37.6X0 **Military operations involving biological weapons, military personnel**

Y37.6X1 **Military operations involving biological weapons, civilian**

Y37.7 **Military operations involving chemical weapons and other forms of unconventional warfare**
EXCLUDES 1 *military operations involving incendiary devices (Y36.3-, Y36.5-)*

Y37.7X **Military operations involving chemical weapons and other forms of unconventional warfare**

Y37.7X0 **Military operations involving chemical weapons and other forms of unconventional warfare, military personnel**

Y37.7X1 **Military operations involving chemical weapons and other forms of unconventional warfare, civilian**

Y37.9 **Other and unspecified military operations**

Y37.90 **Military operations, unspecified**

Y37.91 **Military operations involving unspecified weapon of mass destruction [WMD]**

Y37.92 **Military operations involving friendly fire**

Y38 Terrorism

NOTE These codes are for use to identify injuries resulting from the unlawful use of force or violence against persons or property to intimidate or coerce a Government, the civilian population, or any segment thereof, in furtherance of political or social objective

Use additional code for place of occurrence (Y92.-)

Y38.0 **Terrorism involving explosion of marine weapons**
Terrorism involving depth-charge
Terrorism involving marine mine
Terrorism involving mine NOS, at sea or in harbor
Terrorism involving sea-based artillery shell
Terrorism involving torpedo
Terrorism involving underwater blast

Y38.0X **Terrorism involving explosion of marine weapons**

Y38.0X1 **Terrorism involving explosion of marine weapons, public safety official injured**

Y38.0X2 **Terrorism involving explosion of marine weapons, civilian injured**

Y38.0X3 **Terrorism involving explosion of marine weapons, terrorist injured**

Y38.1 **Terrorism involving destruction of aircraft**
Terrorism involving aircraft burned
Terrorism involving aircraft exploded
Terrorism involving aircraft being shot down
Terrorism involving aircraft used as a weapon

Y38.1X **Terrorism involving destruction of aircraft**

Y38.1X1 **Terrorism involving destruction of aircraft, public safety official injured**

Y38.1X2 **Terrorism involving destruction of aircraft, civilian injured**

Y38.1X3 **Terrorism involving destruction of aircraft, terrorist injured**

Y38.2 **Terrorism involving other explosions and fragments**
Terrorism involving antipersonnel (fragments) bomb
Terrorism involving blast NOS
Terrorism involving explosion NOS
Terrorism involving explosion of breech block
Terrorism involving explosion of cannon block
Terrorism involving explosion (fragments) of artillery shell
Terrorism involving explosion (fragments) of bomb
Terrorism involving explosion (fragments) of grenade
Terrorism involving explosion (fragments) of guided missile
Terrorism involving explosion (fragments) of land mine
Terrorism involving explosion of mortar bomb
Terrorism involving explosion of munitions
Terrorism involving explosion (fragments) of rocket
Terrorism involving explosion (fragments) of shell
Terrorism involving shrapnel
Terrorism involving mine NOS, on land
EXCLUDES 1 *terrorism involving explosion of nuclear weapon (Y38.5)*
terrorism involving suicide bomber (Y38.81)

Y38.2X **Terrorism involving other explosions and fragments**

Y38.2X1 **Terrorism involving other explosions and fragments, public safety official injured**

Y38.2X2 **Terrorism involving other explosions and fragments, civilian injured**

Y38.2X3 **Terrorism involving other explosions and fragments, terrorist injured**

Y38.3 **Terrorism involving fires, conflagration and hot substances**
Terrorism involving conflagration NOS
Terrorism involving fire NOS
Terrorism involving petrol bomb
EXCLUDES 1 *terrorism involving fire or heat of nuclear weapon (Y38.5)*

Y38.3X **Terrorism involving fires, conflagration and hot substances**

Y38.3X1 **Terrorism involving fires, conflagration and hot substances, public safety official injured**

Y38.3X2 **Terrorism involving fires, conflagration and hot substances, civilian injured**

Y38.3X3 **Terrorism involving fires, conflagration and hot substances, terrorist injured**

Y38.4 **Terrorism involving firearms**
Terrorism involving carbine bullet
Terrorism involving machine gun bullet
Terrorism involving pellets (shotgun)
Terrorism involving pistol bullet
Terrorism involving rifle bullet
Terrorism involving rubber (rifle) bullet

Y38.4X **Terrorism involving firearms**

Y38.4X1 **Terrorism involving firearms, public safety official injured**

Y38.4X2 **Terrorism involving firearms, civilian injured**

Y38.4X3 **Terrorism involving firearms, terrorist injured**

Y38.5 **Terrorism involving nuclear weapons**
Terrorism involving blast effects of nuclear weapon
Terrorism involving exposure to ionizing radiation from nuclear weapon
Terrorism involving fireball effect of nuclear weapon
Terrorism involving heat from nuclear weapon

Y38.5X **Terrorism involving nuclear weapons**

Y38.5X1 **Terrorism involving nuclear weapons, public safety official injured**

Y38.5X2 **Terrorism involving nuclear weapons, civilian injured**

Y38.5X3 **Terrorism involving nuclear weapons, terrorist injured**

Y38.6 **Terrorism involving biological weapons**
Terrorism involving anthrax
Terrorism involving cholera
Terrorism involving smallpox

Y38.6X **Terrorism involving biological weapons**

Y38.6X1 **Terrorism involving biological weapons, public safety official injured**

Y38.6X2 **Terrorism involving biological weapons, civilian injured**

Y38.6X3 **Terrorism involving biological weapons, terrorist injured**

√5th **Y38.7 Terrorism involving chemical weapons**
Terrorism involving gases, fumes, chemicals
Terrorism involving hydrogen cyanide
Terrorism involving phosgene
Terrorism involving sarin

√6th **Y38.7X Terrorism involving chemical weapons**

√7th **Y38.7X1 Terrorism involving chemical weapons, public safety official injured**

√7th **Y38.7X2 Terrorism involving chemical weapons, civilian injured**

√7th **Y38.7X3 Terrorism involving chemical weapons, terrorist injured**

√5th **Y38.8 Terrorism involving other and unspecified means**

√x7th **Y38.80 Terrorism involving unspecified means**
Terrorism NOS

√6th **Y38.81 Terrorism involving suicide bomber**

√7th **Y38.811 Terrorism involving suicide bomber, public safety official injured**

√7th **Y38.812 Terrorism involving suicide bomber, civilian injured**

√6th **Y38.89 Terrorism involving other means**
Terrorism involving drowning and submersion
Terrorism involving lasers
Terrorism involving piercing or stabbing instruments

√7th **Y38.891 Terrorism involving other means, public safety official injured**

√7th **Y38.892 Terrorism involving other means, civilian injured**

√7th **Y38.893 Terrorism involving other means, terrorist injured**

√5th **Y38.9 Terrorism, secondary effects**

NOTE This code is for use to identify conditions occurring subsequent to a terrorist attack not those that are due to the initial terrorist attack

√6th **Y38.9X Terrorism, secondary effects**

√7th **Y38.9X1 Terrorism, secondary effects, public safety official injured**

√7th **Y38.9X2 Terrorism, secondary effects, civilian injured**

COMPLICATIONS OF MEDICAL AND SURGICAL CARE (Y62-Y84)

INCLUDES complications of medical devices
surgical and medical procedures as the cause of abnormal reaction of the patient, or of later complication, without mention of misadventure at the time of the procedure

Misadventures to patients during surgical and medical care (Y62-Y69)

EXCLUDES 1 *surgical and medical procedures as the cause of abnormal reaction of the patient, without mention of misadventure at the time of the procedure (Y83-Y84)*

EXCLUDES 2 *breakdown or malfunctioning of medical device (during procedure) (after implantation) (ongoing use) (Y70-Y82)*

√4th **Y62 Failure of sterile precautions during surgical and medical care**

Y62.0 Failure of sterile precautions during surgical operation
Y62.1 Failure of sterile precautions during infusion or transfusion
Y62.2 Failure of sterile precautions during kidney dialysis and other perfusion HCC
Y62.3 Failure of sterile precautions during injection or immunization
Y62.4 Failure of sterile precautions during endoscopic examination
Y62.5 Failure of sterile precautions during heart catheterization
Y62.6 Failure of sterile precautions during aspiration, puncture and other catheterization
Y62.8 Failure of sterile precautions during other surgical and medical care
Y62.9 Failure of sterile precautions during unspecified surgical and medical care

√4th **Y63 Failure in dosage during surgical and medical care**

EXCLUDES 2 *accidental overdose of drug or wrong drug given in error (T36-T50)*

Y63.0 Excessive amount of blood or other fluid given during transfusion or infusion
Y63.1 Incorrect dilution of fluid used during infusion
Y63.2 Overdose of radiation given during therapy
Y63.3 Inadvertent exposure of patient to radiation during medical care
Y63.4 Failure in dosage in electroshock or insulin-shock therapy
Y63.5 Inappropriate temperature in local application and packing
Y63.6 Underdosing and nonadministration of necessary drug, medicament or biological substance
AHA: 2018,4Q,72
Y63.8 Failure in dosage during other surgical and medical care
AHA: 2018,4Q,72
Y63.9 Failure in dosage during unspecified surgical and medical care
AHA: 2018,4Q,72

√4th **Y64 Contaminated medical or biological substances**

Y64.0 Contaminated medical or biological substance, transfused or infused
Y64.1 Contaminated medical or biological substance, injected or used for immunization
Y64.8 Contaminated medical or biological substance administered by other means
Y64.9 Contaminated medical or biological substance administered by unspecified means
Administered contaminated medical or biological substance NOS

√4th **Y65 Other misadventures during surgical and medical care**

Y65.0 Mismatched blood in transfusion
Y65.1 Wrong fluid used in infusion
Y65.2 Failure in suture or ligature during surgical operation
Y65.3 Endotracheal tube wrongly placed during anesthetic procedure
Y65.4 Failure to introduce or to remove other tube or instrument

√5th **Y65.5 Performance of wrong procedure (operation)**

Y65.51 Performance of wrong procedure (operation) on correct patient
Wrong device implanted into correct surgical site
EXCLUDES 1 *performance of correct procedure (operation) on wrong side or body part (Y65.53)*

Y65.52 Performance of procedure (operation) on patient not scheduled for surgery
Performance of procedure (operation) intended for another patient
Performance of procedure (operation) on wrong patient

Y65.53 Performance of correct procedure (operation) on wrong side or body part
Performance of correct procedure (operation) on wrong side
Performance of correct procedure (operation) on wrong site

Y65.8 Other specified misadventures during surgical and medical care
AHA: 2022,1Q,22; 2019,2Q,23-24

Y66 Nonadministration of surgical and medical care
Premature cessation of surgical and medical care
EXCLUDES 1 *DNR status (Z66)*
palliative care (Z51.5)

Y69 Unspecified misadventure during surgical and medical care

Medical devices associated with adverse incidents in diagnostic and therapeutic use (Y70-Y82)

INCLUDES breakdown or malfunction of medical devices (during use) (after implantation) (ongoing use)

EXCLUDES 2 *later complications following use of medical devices without breakdown or malfunctioning of device (Y83-Y84)*
misadventure to patients during surgical and medical care, classifiable to (Y62-Y69)
surgical and other medical procedures as the cause of abnormal reaction of the patient, or of later complication, without mention of misadventure at the time of the procedure (Y83-Y84)

√4th **Y70 Anesthesiology devices associated with adverse incidents**

Y70.0 Diagnostic and monitoring anesthesiology devices associated with adverse incidents
Y70.1 Therapeutic (nonsurgical) and rehabilitative anesthesiology devices associated with adverse incidents
Y70.2 Prosthetic and other implants, materials and accessory anesthesiology devices associated with adverse incidents
Y70.3 Surgical instruments, materials and anesthesiology devices (including sutures) associated with adverse incidents
Y70.8 Miscellaneous anesthesiology devices associated with adverse incidents, not elsewhere classified

√4th **Y71 Cardiovascular devices associated with adverse incidents**

Y71.0 Diagnostic and monitoring cardiovascular devices associated with adverse incidents
Y71.1 Therapeutic (nonsurgical) and rehabilitative cardiovascular devices associated with adverse incidents

Y71.2 Prosthetic and other implants, materials and accessory cardiovascular devices associated with adverse incidents

Y71.3 Surgical instruments, materials and cardiovascular devices (including sutures) associated with adverse incidents

Y71.8 Miscellaneous cardiovascular devices associated with adverse incidents, not elsewhere classified

Y72 Otorhinolaryngological devices associated with adverse incidents

Y72.Ø Diagnostic and monitoring otorhinolaryngological devices associated with adverse incidents

Y72.1 Therapeutic (nonsurgical) and rehabilitative otorhinolaryngological devices associated with adverse incidents

Y72.2 Prosthetic and other implants, materials and accessory otorhinolaryngological devices associated with adverse incidents

Y72.3 Surgical instruments, materials and otorhinolaryngological devices (including sutures) associated with adverse incidents

Y72.8 Miscellaneous otorhinolaryngological devices associated with adverse incidents, not elsewhere classified

Y73 Gastroenterology and urology devices associated with adverse incidents

Y73.Ø Diagnostic and monitoring gastroenterology and urology devices associated with adverse incidents

Y73.1 Therapeutic (nonsurgical) and rehabilitative gastroenterology and urology devices associated with adverse incidents

Y73.2 Prosthetic and other implants, materials and accessory gastroenterology and urology devices associated with adverse incidents

Y73.3 Surgical instruments, materials and gastroenterology and urology devices (including sutures) associated with adverse incidents

Y73.8 Miscellaneous gastroenterology and urology devices associated with adverse incidents, not elsewhere classified

Y74 General hospital and personal-use devices associated with adverse incidents

Y74.Ø Diagnostic and monitoring general hospital and personal-use devices associated with adverse incidents

Y74.1 Therapeutic (nonsurgical) and rehabilitative general hospital and personal-use devices associated with adverse incidents

Y74.2 Prosthetic and other implants, materials and accessory general hospital and personal-use devices associated with adverse incidents

Y74.3 Surgical instruments, materials and general hospital and personal-use devices (including sutures) associated with adverse incidents

Y74.8 Miscellaneous general hospital and personal-use devices associated with adverse incidents, not elsewhere classified

Y75 Neurological devices associated with adverse incidents

Y75.Ø Diagnostic and monitoring neurological devices associated with adverse incidents

Y75.1 Therapeutic (nonsurgical) and rehabilitative neurological devices associated with adverse incidents

Y75.2 Prosthetic and other implants, materials and neurological devices associated with adverse incidents

Y75.3 Surgical instruments, materials and neurological devices (including sutures) associated with adverse incidents

Y75.8 Miscellaneous neurological devices associated with adverse incidents, not elsewhere classified

Y76 Obstetric and gynecological devices associated with adverse incidents

Y76.Ø Diagnostic and monitoring obstetric and gynecological devices associated with adverse incidents ♀

Y76.1 Therapeutic (nonsurgical) and rehabilitative obstetric and gynecological devices associated with adverse incidents ♀

Y76.2 Prosthetic and other implants, materials and accessory obstetric and gynecological devices associated with adverse incidents ♀

Y76.3 Surgical instruments, materials and obstetric and gynecological devices (including sutures) associated with adverse incidents ♀

Y76.8 Miscellaneous obstetric and gynecological devices associated with adverse incidents, not elsewhere classified ♀

Y77 Ophthalmic devices associated with adverse incidents

Y77.Ø Diagnostic and monitoring ophthalmic devices associated with adverse incidents

Y77.1 Therapeutic (nonsurgical) and rehabilitative ophthalmic devices associated with adverse incidents

AHA: 2020,4Q,41

Y77.11 Contact lens associated with adverse incidents

Rigid gas permeable contact lens associated with adverse incidents

Soft (hydrophilic) contact lens associated with adverse incidents

Y77.19 Other therapeutic (nonsurgical) and rehabilitative ophthalmic devices associated with adverse incidents

Y77.2 Prosthetic and other implants, materials and accessory ophthalmic devices associated with adverse incidents

Y77.3 Surgical instruments, materials and ophthalmic devices (including sutures) associated with adverse incidents

Y77.8 Miscellaneous ophthalmic devices associated with adverse incidents, not elsewhere classified

Y78 Radiological devices associated with adverse incidents

Y78.Ø Diagnostic and monitoring radiological devices associated with adverse incidents

Y78.1 Therapeutic (nonsurgical) and rehabilitative radiological devices associated with adverse incidents

Y78.2 Prosthetic and other implants, materials and accessory radiological devices associated with adverse incidents

Y78.3 Surgical instruments, materials and radiological devices (including sutures) associated with adverse incidents

Y78.8 Miscellaneous radiological devices associated with adverse incidents, not elsewhere classified

Y79 Orthopedic devices associated with adverse incidents

Y79.Ø Diagnostic and monitoring orthopedic devices associated with adverse incidents

Y79.1 Therapeutic (nonsurgical) and rehabilitative orthopedic devices associated with adverse incidents

Y79.2 Prosthetic and other implants, materials and accessory orthopedic devices associated with adverse incidents

Y79.3 Surgical instruments, materials and orthopedic devices (including sutures) associated with adverse incidents

Y79.8 Miscellaneous orthopedic devices associated with adverse incidents, not elsewhere classified

Y8Ø Physical medicine devices associated with adverse incidents

Y8Ø.Ø Diagnostic and monitoring physical medicine devices associated with adverse incidents

Y8Ø.1 Therapeutic (nonsurgical) and rehabilitative physical medicine devices associated with adverse incidents

Y8Ø.2 Prosthetic and other implants, materials and accessory physical medicine devices associated with adverse incidents

Y8Ø.3 Surgical instruments, materials and physical medicine devices (including sutures) associated with adverse incidents

Y8Ø.8 Miscellaneous physical medicine devices associated with adverse incidents, not elsewhere classified

Y81 General- and plastic-surgery devices associated with adverse incidents

Y81.Ø Diagnostic and monitoring general- and plastic-surgery devices associated with adverse incidents

Y81.1 Therapeutic (nonsurgical) and rehabilitative general- and plastic-surgery devices associated with adverse incidents

Y81.2 Prosthetic and other implants, materials and accessory general- and plastic-surgery devices associated with adverse incidents

Y81.3 Surgical instruments, materials and general- and plastic-surgery devices (including sutures) associated with adverse incidents

Y81.8 Miscellaneous general- and plastic-surgery devices associated with adverse incidents, not elsewhere classified

Y82 Other and unspecified medical devices associated with adverse incidents

Y82.8 Other medical devices associated with adverse incidents

Y82.9 Unspecified medical devices associated with adverse incidents

Surgical and other medical procedures as the cause of abnormal reaction of the patient, or of later complication, without mention of misadventure at the time of the procedure (Y83-Y84)

EXCLUDES 1 *misadventures to patients during surgical and medical care, classifiable to (Y62-Y69)*

EXCLUDES 2 *breakdown or malfunctioning of medical device (during procedure) (after implantation) (ongoing use) (Y7Ø-Y82)*

4th Y83 Surgical operation and other surgical procedures as the cause of abnormal reaction of the patient, or of later complication, without mention of misadventure at the time of the procedure

Y83.Ø Surgical operation with transplant of whole organ as the cause of abnormal reaction of the patient, or of later complication, without mention of misadventure at the time of the procedure

Y83.1 Surgical operation with implant of artificial internal device as the cause of abnormal reaction of the patient, or of later complication, without mention of misadventure at the time of the procedure

Y83.2 Surgical operation with anastomosis, bypass or graft as the cause of abnormal reaction of the patient, or of later complication, without mention of misadventure at the time of the procedure

Y83.3 Surgical operation with formation of external stoma as the cause of abnormal reaction of the patient, or of later complication, without mention of misadventure at the time of the procedure

Y83.4 Other reconstructive surgery as the cause of abnormal reaction of the patient, or of later complication, without mention of misadventure at the time of the procedure

Y83.5 Amputation of limb(s) as the cause of abnormal reaction of the patient, or of later complication, without mention of misadventure at the time of the procedure

Y83.6 Removal of other organ (partial) (total) as the cause of abnormal reaction of the patient, or of later complication, without mention of misadventure at the time of the procedure

Y83.8 Other surgical procedures as the cause of abnormal reaction of the patient, or of later complication, without mention of misadventure at the time of the procedure

AHA: 2023,2Q,14

Y83.9 Surgical procedure, unspecified as the cause of abnormal reaction of the patient, or of later complication, without mention of misadventure at the time of the procedure

4th Y84 Other medical procedures as the cause of abnormal reaction of the patient, or of later complication, without mention of misadventure at the time of the procedure

Y84.Ø Cardiac catheterization as the cause of abnormal reaction of the patient, or of later complication, without mention of misadventure at the time of the procedure

Y84.1 Kidney dialysis as the cause of abnormal reaction of the patient, or of later complication, without mention of misadventure at the time of the procedure

Y84.2 Radiological procedure and radiotherapy as the cause of abnormal reaction of the patient, or of later complication, without mention of misadventure at the time of the procedure

AHA: 2019,1Q,21; 2017,1Q,33

Y84.3 Shock therapy as the cause of abnormal reaction of the patient, or of later complication, without mention of misadventure at the time of the procedure

Y84.4 Aspiration of fluid as the cause of abnormal reaction of the patient, or of later complication, without mention of misadventure at the time of the procedure

Y84.5 Insertion of gastric or duodenal sound as the cause of abnormal reaction of the patient, or of later complication, without mention of misadventure at the time of the procedure

Y84.6 Urinary catheterization as the cause of abnormal reaction of the patient, or of later complication, without mention of misadventure at the time of the procedure

Y84.7 Blood-sampling as the cause of abnormal reaction of the patient, or of later complication, without mention of misadventure at the time of the procedure

Y84.8 Other medical procedures as the cause of abnormal reaction of the patient, or of later complication, without mention of misadventure at the time of the procedure

AHA: 2023,2Q,28; 2021,1Q,5; 2014,4Q,24

Y84.9 Medical procedure, unspecified as the cause of abnormal reaction of the patient, or of later complication, without mention of misadventure at the time of the procedure

Supplementary factors related to causes of morbidity classified elsewhere (Y9Ø-Y99)

NOTE These categories may be used to provide supplementary information concerning causes of morbidity. They are not to be used for single-condition coding.

4th Y9Ø Evidence of alcohol involvement determined by blood alcohol level

Code first any associated alcohol related disorders (F1Ø)

Y9Ø.Ø Blood alcohol level of less than 2Ø mg/1ØØ ml

Y9Ø.1 Blood alcohol level of 2Ø-39 mg/1ØØ ml

Y9Ø.2 Blood alcohol level of 4Ø-59 mg/1ØØ ml

Y9Ø.3 Blood alcohol level of 6Ø-79 mg/1ØØ ml

Y9Ø.4 Blood alcohol level of 8Ø-99 mg/1ØØ ml

Y9Ø.5 Blood alcohol level of 1ØØ-119 mg/1ØØ ml

Y9Ø.6 Blood alcohol level of 12Ø-199 mg/1ØØ ml

Y9Ø.7 Blood alcohol level of 2ØØ-239 mg/1ØØ ml

Y9Ø.8 Blood alcohol level of 24Ø mg/1ØØ ml or more

Y9Ø.9 Presence of alcohol in blood, level not specified

4th Y92 Place of occurrence of the external cause

The following category is for use, when relevant, to identify the place of occurrence of the external cause. Use in conjunction with an activity code.

Place of occurrence should be recorded only at the initial encounter for treatment

5th Y92.Ø Non-institutional (private) residence as the place of occurrence of the external cause

EXCLUDES 1 *abandoned or derelict house (Y92.89)*
home under construction but not yet occupied (Y92.6-)
institutional place of residence (Y92.1-)

6th Y92.ØØ Unspecified non-institutional (private) residence as the place of occurrence of the external cause

Y92.ØØØ Kitchen of unspecified non-institutional (private) residence as the place of occurrence of the external cause

Y92.ØØ1 Dining room of unspecified non-institutional (private) residence as the place of occurrence of the external cause

Y92.ØØ2 Bathroom of unspecified non-institutional (private) residence as the place of occurrence of the external cause

Y92.ØØ3 Bedroom of unspecified non-institutional (private) residence as the place of occurrence of the external cause

Y92.ØØ7 Garden or yard of unspecified non-institutional (private) residence as the place of occurrence of the external cause

Y92.ØØ8 Other place in unspecified non-institutional (private) residence as the place of occurrence of the external cause

Y92.ØØ9 Unspecified place in unspecified non-institutional (private) residence as the place of occurrence of the external cause

Home (NOS) as the place of occurrence of the external cause

6th Y92.Ø1 Single-family non-institutional (private) house as the place of occurrence of the external cause

Farmhouse as the place of occurrence of the external cause

EXCLUDES 1 *barn (Y92.71)*
chicken coop or hen house (Y92.72)
farm field (Y92.73)
orchard (Y92.74)
single family mobile home or trailer (Y92.Ø2-)
slaughter house (Y92.86)

Y92.Ø1Ø Kitchen of single-family (private) house as the place of occurrence of the external cause

Y92.Ø11 Dining room of single-family (private) house as the place of occurrence of the external cause

Y92.Ø12 Bathroom of single-family (private) house as the place of occurrence of the external cause

Y92.Ø13 Bedroom of single-family (private) house as the place of occurrence of the external cause
Y92.Ø14 Private driveway to single-family (private) house as the place of occurrence of the external cause
Y92.Ø15 Private garage of single-family (private) house as the place of occurrence of the external cause
Y92.Ø16 Swimming-pool in single-family (private) house or garden as the place of occurrence of the external cause
AHA: 2023,1Q,25
Y92.Ø17 Garden or yard in single-family (private) house as the place of occurrence of the external cause
Y92.Ø18 Other place in single-family (private) house as the place of occurrence of the external cause
Y92.Ø19 Unspecified place in single-family (private) house as the place of occurrence of the external cause

Y92.Ø2 Mobile home as the place of occurrence of the external cause
Y92.Ø2Ø Kitchen in mobile home as the place of occurrence of the external cause
Y92.Ø21 Dining room in mobile home as the place of occurrence of the external cause
Y92.Ø22 Bathroom in mobile home as the place of occurrence of the external cause
Y92.Ø23 Bedroom in mobile home as the place of occurrence of the external cause
Y92.Ø24 Driveway of mobile home as the place of occurrence of the external cause
Y92.Ø25 Garage of mobile home as the place of occurrence of the external cause
Y92.Ø26 Swimming-pool of mobile home as the place of occurrence of the external cause
Y92.Ø27 Garden or yard of mobile home as the place of occurrence of the external cause
Y92.Ø28 Other place in mobile home as the place of occurrence of the external cause
Y92.Ø29 Unspecified place in mobile home as the place of occurrence of the external cause

Y92.Ø3 Apartment as the place of occurrence of the external cause
Condominium as the place of occurrence of the external cause
Co-op apartment as the place of occurrence of the external cause
Y92.Ø3Ø Kitchen in apartment as the place of occurrence of the external cause
Y92.Ø31 Bathroom in apartment as the place of occurrence of the external cause
Y92.Ø32 Bedroom in apartment as the place of occurrence of the external cause
Y92.Ø38 Other place in apartment as the place of occurrence of the external cause
Y92.Ø39 Unspecified place in apartment as the place of occurrence of the external cause

Y92.Ø4 Boarding-house as the place of occurrence of the external cause
Y92.Ø4Ø Kitchen in boarding-house as the place of occurrence of the external cause
Y92.Ø41 Bathroom in boarding-house as the place of occurrence of the external cause
Y92.Ø42 Bedroom in boarding-house as the place of occurrence of the external cause
Y92.Ø43 Driveway of boarding-house as the place of occurrence of the external cause
Y92.Ø44 Garage of boarding-house as the place of occurrence of the external cause
Y92.Ø45 Swimming-pool of boarding-house as the place of occurrence of the external cause
Y92.Ø46 Garden or yard of boarding-house as the place of occurrence of the external cause
Y92.Ø48 Other place in boarding-house as the place of occurrence of the external cause
Y92.Ø49 Unspecified place in boarding-house as the place of occurrence of the external cause

Y92.Ø9 Other non-institutional residence as the place of occurrence of the external cause
AHA: 2017,2Q,10
Y92.Ø9Ø Kitchen in other non-institutional residence as the place of occurrence of the external cause
Y92.Ø91 Bathroom in other non-institutional residence as the place of occurrence of the external cause
Y92.Ø92 Bedroom in other non-institutional residence as the place of occurrence of the external cause
Y92.Ø93 Driveway of other non-institutional residence as the place of occurrence of the external cause
Y92.Ø94 Garage of other non-institutional residence as the place of occurrence of the external cause
Y92.Ø95 Swimming-pool of other non-institutional residence as the place of occurrence of the external cause
Y92.Ø96 Garden or yard of other non-institutional residence as the place of occurrence of the external cause
Y92.Ø98 Other place in other non-institutional residence as the place of occurrence of the external cause
Y92.Ø99 Unspecified place in other non-institutional residence as the place of occurrence of the external cause

Y92.1 Institutional (nonprivate) residence as the place of occurrence of the external cause
Y92.1Ø Unspecified residential institution as the place of occurrence of the external cause

Y92.11 Children's home and orphanage as the place of occurrence of the external cause
Y92.11Ø Kitchen in children's home and orphanage as the place of occurrence of the external cause
Y92.111 Bathroom in children's home and orphanage as the place of occurrence of the external cause
Y92.112 Bedroom in children's home and orphanage as the place of occurrence of the external cause
Y92.113 Driveway of children's home and orphanage as the place of occurrence of the external cause
Y92.114 Garage of children's home and orphanage as the place of occurrence of the external cause
Y92.115 Swimming-pool of children's home and orphanage as the place of occurrence of the external cause
Y92.116 Garden or yard of children's home and orphanage as the place of occurrence of the external cause
Y92.118 Other place in children's home and orphanage as the place of occurrence of the external cause
Y92.119 Unspecified place in children's home and orphanage as the place of occurrence of the external cause

Y92.12 Nursing home as the place of occurrence of the external cause
Home for the sick as the place of occurrence of the external cause
Hospice as the place of occurrence of the external cause
AHA: 2017,2Q,10
Y92.12Ø Kitchen in nursing home as the place of occurrence of the external cause
Y92.121 Bathroom in nursing home as the place of occurrence of the external cause
Y92.122 Bedroom in nursing home as the place of occurrence of the external cause
Y92.123 Driveway of nursing home as the place of occurrence of the external cause
Y92.124 Garage of nursing home as the place of occurrence of the external cause
Y92.125 Swimming-pool of nursing home as the place of occurrence of the external cause
Y92.126 Garden or yard of nursing home as the place of occurrence of the external cause

Y92.128 **Other place in nursing home as the place of occurrence of the external cause**

Y92.129 **Unspecified place in nursing home as the place of occurrence of the external cause**

6th **Y92.13** **Military base as the place of occurrence of the external cause**

EXCLUDES 1 *military training grounds (Y92.84)*

Y92.130 **Kitchen on military base as the place of occurrence of the external cause**

Y92.131 **Mess hall on military base as the place of occurrence of the external cause**

Y92.133 **Barracks on military base as the place of occurrence of the external cause**

Y92.135 **Garage on military base as the place of occurrence of the external cause**

Y92.136 **Swimming-pool on military base as the place of occurrence of the external cause**

Y92.137 **Garden or yard on military base as the place of occurrence of the external cause**

Y92.138 **Other place on military base as the place of occurrence of the external cause**

Y92.139 **Unspecified place military base as the place of occurrence of the external cause**

6th **Y92.14** **Prison as the place of occurrence of the external cause**

Y92.140 **Kitchen in prison as the place of occurrence of the external cause**

Y92.141 **Dining room in prison as the place of occurrence of the external cause**

Y92.142 **Bathroom in prison as the place of occurrence of the external cause**

Y92.143 **Cell of prison as the place of occurrence of the external cause**

Y92.146 **Swimming-pool of prison as the place of occurrence of the external cause**

Y92.147 **Courtyard of prison as the place of occurrence of the external cause**

Y92.148 **Other place in prison as the place of occurrence of the external cause**

Y92.149 **Unspecified place in prison as the place of occurrence of the external cause**

6th **Y92.15** **Reform school as the place of occurrence of the external cause**

Y92.150 **Kitchen in reform school as the place of occurrence of the external cause**

Y92.151 **Dining room in reform school as the place of occurrence of the external cause**

Y92.152 **Bathroom in reform school as the place of occurrence of the external cause**

Y92.153 **Bedroom in reform school as the place of occurrence of the external cause**

Y92.154 **Driveway of reform school as the place of occurrence of the external cause**

Y92.155 **Garage of reform school as the place of occurrence of the external cause**

Y92.156 **Swimming-pool of reform school as the place of occurrence of the external cause**

Y92.157 **Garden or yard of reform school as the place of occurrence of the external cause**

Y92.158 **Other place in reform school as the place of occurrence of the external cause**

Y92.159 **Unspecified place in reform school as the place of occurrence of the external cause**

6th **Y92.16** **School dormitory as the place of occurrence of the external cause**

EXCLUDES 1 *reform school as the place of occurrence of the external cause (Y92.15-)*
school buildings and grounds as the place of occurrence of the external cause (Y92.2-)
school sports and athletic areas as the place of occurrence of the external cause (Y92.3-)

Y92.160 **Kitchen in school dormitory as the place of occurrence of the external cause**

Y92.161 **Dining room in school dormitory as the place of occurrence of the external cause**

Y92.162 **Bathroom in school dormitory as the place of occurrence of the external cause**

Y92.163 **Bedroom in school dormitory as the place of occurrence of the external cause**

Y92.168 **Other place in school dormitory as the place of occurrence of the external cause**

Y92.169 **Unspecified place in school dormitory as the place of occurrence of the external cause**

6th **Y92.19** **Other specified residential institution as the place of occurrence of the external cause**

AHA: 2017,2Q,10

Y92.190 **Kitchen in other specified residential institution as the place of occurrence of the external cause**

Y92.191 **Dining room in other specified residential institution as the place of occurrence of the external cause**

Y92.192 **Bathroom in other specified residential institution as the place of occurrence of the external cause**

Y92.193 **Bedroom in other specified residential institution as the place of occurrence of the external cause**

Y92.194 **Driveway of other specified residential institution as the place of occurrence of the external cause**

Y92.195 **Garage of other specified residential institution as the place of occurrence of the external cause**

Y92.196 **Pool of other specified residential institution as the place of occurrence of the external cause**

Y92.197 **Garden or yard of other specified residential institution as the place of occurrence of the external cause**

Y92.198 **Other place in other specified residential institution as the place of occurrence of the external cause**

Y92.199 **Unspecified place in other specified residential institution as the place of occurrence of the external cause**

5th **Y92.2** **School, other institution and public administrative area as the place of occurrence of the external cause**

Building and adjacent grounds used by the general public or by a particular group of the public

EXCLUDES 1 *building under construction as the place of occurrence of the external cause (Y92.6)*
residential institution as the place of occurrence of the external cause (Y92.1)
school dormitory as the place of occurrence of the external cause (Y92.16-)
sports and athletics area of schools as the place of occurrence of the external cause (Y92.3-)

6th **Y92.21** **School (private) (public) (state) as the place of occurrence of the external cause**

Y92.210 **Daycare center as the place of occurrence of the external cause**

Y92.211 **Elementary school as the place of occurrence of the external cause**

Kindergarten as the place of occurrence of the external cause

Y92.212 **Middle school as the place of occurrence of the external cause**

Y92.213 **High school as the place of occurrence of the external cause**

AHA: 2012,4Q,108

Y92.214 **College as the place of occurrence of the external cause**

University as the place of occurrence of the external cause

Y92.215 **Trade school as the place of occurrence of the external cause**

Y92.218 **Other school as the place of occurrence of the external cause**

Y92.219 **Unspecified school as the place of occurrence of the external cause**

Y92.22 **Religious institution as the place of occurrence of the external cause**

Church as the place of occurrence of the external cause

Mosque as the place of occurrence of the external cause

Synagogue as the place of occurrence of the external cause

✓6th **Y92.23 Hospital as the place of occurrence of the external cause**
EXCLUDES 1 *ambulatory (outpatient) health services establishments (Y92.53-)*
home for the sick as the place of occurrence of the external cause (Y92.12-)
hospice as the place of occurrence of the external cause (Y92.12-)
nursing home as the place of occurrence of the external cause (Y92.12-)

Y92.230 Patient room in hospital as the place of occurrence of the external cause
Y92.231 Patient bathroom in hospital as the place of occurrence of the external cause
Y92.232 Corridor of hospital as the place of occurrence of the external cause
Y92.233 Cafeteria of hospital as the place of occurrence of the external cause
Y92.234 Operating room of hospital as the place of occurrence of the external cause
Y92.238 Other place in hospital as the place of occurrence of the external cause
Y92.239 Unspecified place in hospital as the place of occurrence of the external cause

✓6th **Y92.24 Public administrative building as the place of occurrence of the external cause**
Y92.240 Courthouse as the place of occurrence of the external cause
Y92.241 Library as the place of occurrence of the external cause
Y92.242 Post office as the place of occurrence of the external cause
Y92.243 City hall as the place of occurrence of the external cause
Y92.248 Other public administrative building as the place of occurrence of the external cause

✓6th **Y92.25 Cultural building as the place of occurrence of the external cause**
Y92.250 Art Gallery as the place of occurrence of the external cause
Y92.251 Museum as the place of occurrence of the external cause
Y92.252 Music hall as the place of occurrence of the external cause
Y92.253 Opera house as the place of occurrence of the external cause
Y92.254 Theater (live) as the place of occurrence of the external cause
Y92.258 Other cultural public building as the place of occurrence of the external cause

Y92.26 Movie house or cinema as the place of occurrence of the external cause

Y92.29 Other specified public building as the place of occurrence of the external cause
Assembly hall as the place of occurrence of the external cause
Clubhouse as the place of occurrence of the external cause

✓5th **Y92.3 Sports and athletics area as the place of occurrence of the external cause**

✓6th **Y92.31 Athletic court as the place of occurrence of the external cause**
EXCLUDES 1 *tennis court in private home or garden (Y92.09)*

Y92.310 Basketball court as the place of occurrence of the external cause
Y92.311 Squash court as the place of occurrence of the external cause
Y92.312 Tennis court as the place of occurrence of the external cause
Y92.318 Other athletic court as the place of occurrence of the external cause

✓6th **Y92.32 Athletic field as the place of occurrence of the external cause**
Y92.320 Baseball field as the place of occurrence of the external cause
Y92.321 Football field as the place of occurrence of the external cause
Y92.322 Soccer field as the place of occurrence of the external cause
Y92.328 Other athletic field as the place of occurrence of the external cause
Cricket field as the place of occurrence of the external cause
Hockey field as the place of occurrence of the external cause

✓6th **Y92.33 Skating rink as the place of occurrence of the external cause**
Y92.330 Ice skating rink (indoor) (outdoor) as the place of occurrence of the external cause
Y92.331 Roller skating rink as the place of occurrence of the external cause

Y92.34 Swimming pool (public) as the place of occurrence of the external cause
EXCLUDES 1 *swimming pool in private home or garden (Y92.016)*

Y92.39 Other specified sports and athletic area as the place of occurrence of the external cause
Golf-course as the place of occurrence of the external cause
Gymnasium as the place of occurrence of the external cause
Riding-school as the place of occurrence of the external cause
Stadium as the place of occurrence of the external cause

✓5th **Y92.4 Street, highway and other paved roadways as the place of occurrence of the external cause**
EXCLUDES 1 *private driveway of residence (Y92.014, Y92.024, Y92.043, Y92.093, Y92.113, Y92.123, Y92.154, Y92.194)*

✓6th **Y92.41 Street and highway as the place of occurrence of the external cause**
Y92.410 Unspecified street and highway as the place of occurrence of the external cause
Road NOS as the place of occurrence of the external cause
Y92.411 Interstate highway as the place of occurrence of the external cause
Freeway as the place of occurrence of the external cause
Motorway as the place of occurrence of the external cause
Y92.412 Parkway as the place of occurrence of the external cause
Y92.413 State road as the place of occurrence of the external cause
Y92.414 Local residential or business street as the place of occurrence of the external cause
Y92.415 Exit ramp or entrance ramp of street or highway as the place of occurrence of the external cause

✓6th **Y92.48 Other paved roadways as the place of occurrence of the external cause**
Y92.480 Sidewalk as the place of occurrence of the external cause
Y92.481 Parking lot as the place of occurrence of the external cause
Y92.482 Bike path as the place of occurrence of the external cause
Y92.488 Other paved roadways as the place of occurrence of the external cause

✓5th **Y92.5 Trade and service area as the place of occurrence of the external cause**
EXCLUDES 1 *garage in private home (Y92.015)*
schools and other public administration buildings (Y92.2-)

✓6th **Y92.51 Private commercial establishments as the place of occurrence of the external cause**
Y92.510 Bank as the place of occurrence of the external cause
Y92.511 Restaurant or cafe as the place of occurrence of the external cause
Y92.512 Supermarket, store or market as the place of occurrence of the external cause
Y92.513 Shop (commercial) as the place of occurrence of the external cause

✓6th **Y92.52 Service areas as the place of occurrence of the external cause**
Y92.520 Airport as the place of occurrence of the external cause
Y92.521 Bus station as the place of occurrence of the external cause

Y92.522 Railway station as the place of occurrence of the external cause

Y92.523 Highway rest stop as the place of occurrence of the external cause

Y92.524 Gas station as the place of occurrence of the external cause

Petroleum station as the place of occurrence of the external cause

Service station as the place of occurrence of the external cause

√6th **Y92.53 Ambulatory health services establishments as the place of occurrence of the external cause**

Y92.530 Ambulatory surgery center as the place of occurrence of the external cause

Outpatient surgery center, including that connected with a hospital as the place of occurrence of the external cause

Same day surgery center, including that connected with a hospital as the place of occurrence of the external cause

Y92.531 Health care provider office as the place of occurrence of the external cause

Physician office as the place of occurrence of the external cause

Y92.532 Urgent care center as the place of occurrence of the external cause

Y92.538 Other ambulatory health services establishments as the place of occurrence of the external cause

AHA: 2019,1Q,21

Y92.59 Other trade areas as the place of occurrence of the external cause

Office building as the place of occurrence of the external cause

Casino as the place of occurrence of the external cause

Garage (commercial) as the place of occurrence of the external cause

Hotel as the place of occurrence of the external cause

Radio or television station as the place of occurrence of the external cause

Shopping mall as the place of occurrence of the external cause

Warehouse as the place of occurrence of the external cause

√5th **Y92.6 Industrial and construction area as the place of occurrence of the external cause**

Y92.61 Building [any] under construction as the place of occurrence of the external cause

Y92.62 Dock or shipyard as the place of occurrence of the external cause

Dockyard as the place of occurrence of the external cause

Dry dock as the place of occurrence of the external cause

Shipyard as the place of occurrence of the external cause

Y92.63 Factory as the place of occurrence of the external cause

Factory building as the place of occurrence of the external cause

Factory premises as the place of occurrence of the external cause

Industrial yard as the place of occurrence of the external cause

Y92.64 Mine or pit as the place of occurrence of the external cause

Mine as the place of occurrence of the external cause

Y92.65 Oil rig as the place of occurrence of the external cause

Pit (coal) (gravel) (sand) as the place of occurrence of the external cause

Y92.69 Other specified industrial and construction area as the place of occurrence of the external cause

Gasworks as the place of occurrence of the external cause

Power-station (coal) (nuclear) (oil) as the place of occurrence of the external cause

Tunnel under construction as the place of occurrence of the external cause

Workshop as the place of occurrence of the external cause

√5th **Y92.7 Farm as the place of occurrence of the external cause**

Ranch as the place of occurrence of the external cause

EXCLUDES 1 *farmhouse and home premises of farm (Y92.01-)*

Y92.71 Barn as the place of occurrence of the external cause

Y92.72 Chicken coop as the place of occurrence of the external cause

Hen house as the place of occurrence of the external cause

Y92.73 Farm field as the place of occurrence of the external cause

Y92.74 Orchard as the place of occurrence of the external cause

Y92.79 Other farm location as the place of occurrence of the external cause

√5th **Y92.8 Other places as the place of occurrence of the external cause**

√6th **Y92.81 Transport vehicle as the place of occurrence of the external cause**

EXCLUDES 1 *transport accidents (V00-V99)*

Y92.810 Car as the place of occurrence of the external cause

Y92.811 Bus as the place of occurrence of the external cause

Y92.812 Truck as the place of occurrence of the external cause

Y92.813 Airplane as the place of occurrence of the external cause

Y92.814 Boat as the place of occurrence of the external cause

Y92.815 Train as the place of occurrence of the external cause

Y92.816 Subway car as the place of occurrence of the external cause

Y92.818 Other transport vehicle as the place of occurrence of the external cause

√6th **Y92.82 Wilderness area**

Y92.820 Desert as the place of occurrence of the external cause

Y92.821 Forest as the place of occurrence of the external cause

Y92.828 Other wilderness area as the place of occurrence of the external cause

Swamp as the place of occurrence of the external cause

Mountain as the place of occurrence of the external cause

Marsh as the place of occurrence of the external cause

Prairie as the place of occurrence of the external cause

√6th **Y92.83 Recreation area as the place of occurrence of the external cause**

Y92.830 Public park as the place of occurrence of the external cause

Y92.831 Amusement park as the place of occurrence of the external cause

Y92.832 Beach as the place of occurrence of the external cause

Seashore as the place of occurrence of the external cause

Y92.833 Campsite as the place of occurrence of the external cause

Y92.834 Zoological garden (Zoo) as the place of occurrence of the external cause

Y92.838 Other recreation area as the place of occurrence of the external cause

Y92.84 Military training ground as the place of occurrence of the external cause

Y92.85 Railroad track as the place of occurrence of the external cause

Y92.86 Slaughter house as the place of occurrence of the external cause

Y92.89 Other specified places as the place of occurrence of the external cause

Derelict house as the place of occurrence of the external cause

Y92.9 Unspecified place or not applicable

Y93 Activity codes

NOTE Category Y93 is provided for use to indicate the activity of the person seeking healthcare for an injury or health condition, such as a heart attack while shoveling snow, which resulted from, or was contributed to, by the activity. These codes are appropriate for use for both acute injuries, such as those from chapter 19, and conditions that are due to the long-term, cumulative effects of an activity, such as those from chapter 13. They are also appropriate for use with external cause codes for cause and intent if identifying the activity provides additional information on the event. These codes should be used in conjunction with codes for external cause status (Y99) and place of occurrence (Y92).

This section contains the following broad activity categories:

Y93.Ø Activities involving walking and running
Y93.1 Activities involving water and water craft
Y93.2 Activities involving ice and snow
Y93.3 Activities involving climbing, rappelling, and jumping off
Y93.4 Activities involving dancing and other rhythmic movement
Y93.5 Activities involving other sports and athletics played individually
Y93.6 Activities involving other sports and athletics played as a team or group
Y93.7 Activities involving other specified sports and athletics
Y93.A Activities involving other cardiorespiratory exercise
Y93.B Activities involving other muscle strengthening exercises
Y93.C Activities involving computer technology and electronic devices
Y93.D Activities involving arts and handcrafts
Y93.E Activities involving personal hygiene and interior property and clothing maintenance
Y93.F Activities involving caregiving
Y93.G Activities involving food preparation, cooking and grilling
Y93.H Activities involving exterior property and land maintenance, building and construction
Y93.I Activities involving roller coasters and other types of external motion
Y93.J Activities involving playing musical instrument
Y93.K Activities involving animal care
Y93.8 Activities, other specified
Y93.9 Activity, unspecified

Y93.Ø Activities involving walking and running

EXCLUDES 1 *activity, walking an animal (Y93.K1)*
activity, walking or running on a treadmill (Y93.A1)

Y93.Ø1 Activity, walking, marching and hiking
Activity, walking, marching and hiking on level or elevated terrain
EXCLUDES 1 *activity, mountain climbing (Y93.31)*

Y93.Ø2 Activity, running

Y93.1 Activities involving water and water craft

EXCLUDES 1 *activities involving ice (Y93.2-)*

Y93.11 Activity, swimming
Y93.12 Activity, springboard and platform diving
Y93.13 Activity, water polo
Y93.14 Activity, water aerobics and water exercise
Y93.15 Activity, underwater diving and snorkeling
Activity, SCUBA diving
Y93.16 Activity, rowing, canoeing, kayaking, rafting and tubing
Activity, canoeing, kayaking, rafting and tubing in calm and turbulent water
Y93.17 Activity, water skiing and wake boarding
Y93.18 Activity, surfing, windsurfing and boogie boarding
Activity, water sliding
Y93.19 Activity, other involving water and watercraft
Activity involving water NOS
Activity, parasailing
Activity, water survival training and testing

Y93.2 Activities involving ice and snow

EXCLUDES 1 *activity, shoveling ice and snow (Y93.H1)*

Y93.21 Activity, ice skating
Activity, figure skating (singles) (pairs)
Activity, ice dancing
EXCLUDES 1 *activity, ice hockey (Y93.22)*
Y93.22 Activity, ice hockey
Y93.23 Activity, snow (alpine) (downhill) skiing, snowboarding, sledding, tobogganing and snow tubing
EXCLUDES 1 *activity, cross country skiing (Y93.24)*
Y93.24 Activity, cross country skiing
Activity, nordic skiing
Y93.29 Activity, other involving ice and snow
Activity involving ice and snow NOS

Y93.3 Activities involving climbing, rappelling and jumping off

EXCLUDES 1 *activity, hiking on level or elevated terrain (Y93.Ø1)*
activity, jumping rope (Y93.56)
activity, trampoline jumping (Y93.44)

Y93.31 Activity, mountain climbing, rock climbing and wall climbing
Y93.32 Activity, rappelling
Y93.33 Activity, BASE jumping
Activity, Building, Antenna, Span, Earth jumping
Y93.34 Activity, bungee jumping
Y93.35 Activity, hang gliding
Y93.39 Activity, other involving climbing, rappelling and jumping off

Y93.4 Activities involving dancing and other rhythmic movement

EXCLUDES 1 *activity, martial arts (Y93.75)*

Y93.41 Activity, dancing
AHA: 2012,4Q,108
Y93.42 Activity, yoga
Y93.43 Activity, gymnastics
Activity, rhythmic gymnastics
EXCLUDES 1 *activity, trampolining (Y93.44)*
Y93.44 Activity, trampolining
Y93.45 Activity, cheerleading
Y93.49 Activity, other involving dancing and other rhythmic movements

Y93.5 Activities involving other sports and athletics played individually

EXCLUDES 1 *activity, dancing (Y93.41)*
activity, gymnastic (Y93.43)
activity, trampolining (Y93.44)
activity, yoga (Y93.42)

Y93.51 Activity, roller skating (inline) and skateboarding
Y93.52 Activity, horseback riding
Y93.53 Activity, golf
Y93.54 Activity, bowling
Y93.55 Activity, bike riding
Y93.56 Activity, jumping rope
Y93.57 Activity, non-running track and field events
EXCLUDES 1 *activity, running (any form) (Y93.Ø2)*
Y93.59 Activity, other involving other sports and athletics played individually
EXCLUDES 1 *activities involving climbing, rappelling, and jumping (Y93.3-)*
activities involving ice and snow (Y93.2-)
activities involving walking and running (Y93.Ø-)
activities involving water and watercraft (Y93.1-)

Y93.6 Activities involving other sports and athletics played as a team or group

EXCLUDES 1 *activity, ice hockey (Y93.22)*
activity, water polo (Y93.13)

Y93.61 Activity, American tackle football
Activity, football NOS
Y93.62 Activity, American flag or touch football
Y93.63 Activity, rugby
Y93.64 Activity, baseball
Activity, softball
Y93.65 Activity, lacrosse and field hockey
Y93.66 Activity, soccer
Y93.67 Activity, basketball
Y93.68 Activity, volleyball (beach) (court)

Y93.6A Activity, physical games generally associated with school recess, summer camp and children
Activity, capture the flag
Activity, dodge ball
Activity, four square
Activity, kickball

Y93.69 Activity, other involving other sports and athletics played as a team or group
Activity, cricket

5th **Y93.7 Activities involving other specified sports and athletics**

Y93.71 Activity, boxing

Y93.72 Activity, wrestling

Y93.73 Activity, racquet and hand sports
Activity, handball
Activity, racquetball
Activity, squash
Activity, tennis

Y93.74 Activity, frisbee
Activity, ultimate frisbee

Y93.75 Activity, martial arts
Activity, combatives

Y93.79 Activity, other specified sports and athletics
EXCLUDES 1 *sports and athletics activities specified in categories Y93.Ø-Y93.6*

5th **Y93.A Activities involving other cardiorespiratory exercise**
Activities involving physical training

Y93.A1 Activity, exercise machines primarily for cardiorespiratory conditioning
Activity, elliptical and stepper machines
Activity, stationary bike
Activity, treadmill

Y93.A2 Activity, calisthenics
Activity, jumping jacks
Activity, warm up and cool down

Y93.A3 Activity, aerobic and step exercise

Y93.A4 Activity, circuit training

Y93.A5 Activity, obstacle course
Activity, challenge course
Activity, confidence course

Y93.A6 Activity, grass drills
Activity, guerilla drills

Y93.A9 Activity, other involving cardiorespiratory exercise
EXCLUDES 1 *activities involving cardiorespiratory exercise specified in categories Y93.Ø-Y93.7*

5th **Y93.B Activities involving other muscle strengthening exercises**

Y93.B1 Activity, exercise machines primarily for muscle strengthening

Y93.B2 Activity, push-ups, pull-ups, sit-ups

Y93.B3 Activity, free weights
Activity, barbells
Activity, dumbbells

Y93.B4 Activity, pilates

Y93.B9 Activity, other involving muscle strengthening exercises
EXCLUDES 1 *activities involving muscle strengthening specified in categories Y93.Ø-Y93.A*

5th **Y93.C Activities involving computer technology and electronic devices**
EXCLUDES 1 *activity, electronic musical keyboard or instruments (Y93.J-)*

Y93.C1 Activity, computer keyboarding
Activity, electronic game playing using keyboard or other stationary device

Y93.C2 Activity, hand held interactive electronic device
Activity, cellular telephone and communication device
Activity, electronic game playing using interactive device
EXCLUDES 1 *activity, electronic game playing using keyboard or other stationary device (Y93.C1)*

Y93.C9 Activity, other involving computer technology and electronic devices

5th **Y93.D Activities involving arts and handcrafts**
EXCLUDES 1 *activities involving playing musical instrument (Y93.J-)*

Y93.D1 Activity, knitting and crocheting

Y93.D2 Activity, sewing

Y93.D3 Activity, furniture building and finishing
Activity, furniture repair

Y93.D9 Activity, other involving arts and handcrafts

5th **Y93.E Activities involving personal hygiene and interior property and clothing maintenance**
EXCLUDES 1 *activities involving cooking and grilling (Y93.G-)*
activities involving exterior property and land maintenance, building and construction (Y93.H-)
activities involving caregiving (Y93.F-)
activity, dishwashing (Y93.G1)
activity, food preparation (Y93.G1)
activity, gardening (Y93.H2)

Y93.E1 Activity, personal bathing and showering

Y93.E2 Activity, laundry

Y93.E3 Activity, vacuuming

Y93.E4 Activity, ironing

Y93.E5 Activity, floor mopping and cleaning

Y93.E6 Activity, residential relocation
Activity, packing up and unpacking involved in moving to a new residence

Y93.E8 Activity, other personal hygiene

Y93.E9 Activity, other interior property and clothing maintenance

5th **Y93.F Activities involving caregiving**
Activity involving the provider of caregiving

Y93.F1 Activity, caregiving, bathing

Y93.F2 Activity, caregiving, lifting

Y93.F9 Activity, other caregiving

5th **Y93.G Activities involving food preparation, cooking and grilling**

Y93.G1 Activity, food preparation and clean up
Activity, dishwashing

Y93.G2 Activity, grilling and smoking food

Y93.G3 Activity, cooking and baking
Activity, use of stove, oven and microwave oven

Y93.G9 Activity, other involving cooking and grilling

5th **Y93.H Activities involving exterior property and land maintenance, building and construction**

Y93.H1 Activity, digging, shoveling and raking
Activity, dirt digging
Activity, raking leaves
Activity, snow shoveling

Y93.H2 Activity, gardening and landscaping
Activity, pruning, trimming shrubs, weeding

Y93.H3 Activity, building and construction

Y93.H9 Activity, other involving exterior property and land maintenance, building and construction

5th **Y93.I Activities involving roller coasters and other types of external motion**

Y93.I1 Activity, rollercoaster riding

Y93.I9 Activity, other involving external motion

5th **Y93.J Activities involving playing musical instrument**
Activity involving playing electric musical instrument

Y93.J1 Activity, piano playing
Activity, musical keyboard (electronic) playing

Y93.J2 Activity, drum and other percussion instrument playing

Y93.J3 Activity, string instrument playing

Y93.J4 Activity, winds and brass instrument playing

5th **Y93.K Activities involving animal care**
EXCLUDES 1 *activity, horseback riding (Y93.52)*

Y93.K1 Activity, walking an animal

Y93.K2 Activity, milking an animal

Y93.K3 Activity, grooming and shearing an animal

Y93.K9 Activity, other involving animal care

5th **Y93.8 Activities, other specified**

Y93.81 Activity, refereeing a sports activity

Y93.82 Activity, spectator at an event

Y93.83 Activity, rough housing and horseplay

Y93.84 Activity, sleeping

Y93.85 Activity, choking game
Activity, blackout game
Activity, fainting game
Activity, pass out game
AHA: 2016,4Q,74-76

Y93.89 Activity, other specified

Y93.9 Activity, unspecified

Y95 Nosocomial condition
AHA: 2013,4Q,119

✓4th **Y99 External cause status**

NOTE A single code from category Y99 should be used in conjunction with the external cause code(s) assigned to a record to indicate the status of the person at the time the event occurred.

Y99.Ø Civilian activity done for income or pay
Civilian activity done for financial or other compensation
EXCLUDES 1 *military activity (Y99.1)*
volunteer activity (Y99.2)

Y99.1 Military activity
EXCLUDES 1 *activity of off duty military personnel (Y99.8)*

Y99.2 Volunteer activity
EXCLUDES 1 *activity of child or other family member assisting in compensated work of other family member (Y99.8)*

Y99.8 Other external cause status
Activity NEC
Activity of child or other family member assisting in compensated work of other family member
Hobby not done for income
Leisure activity
Off-duty activity of military personnel
Recreation or sport not for income or while a student
Student activity
EXCLUDES 1 *civilian activity done for income or compensation (Y99.Ø)*
military activity (Y99.1)
AHA: 2012,4Q,108

Y99.9 Unspecified external cause status

Chapter 21. Factors Influencing Health Status and Contact with Health Services (Z00–Z99)

Chapter-specific Guidelines with Coding Examples

The chapter-specific guidelines from the ICD-10-CM Official Guidelines for Coding and Reporting have been provided below. Along with these guidelines are coding examples, contained in the shaded boxes, that have been developed to help illustrate the coding and/or sequencing guidance found in these guidelines.

Note: The chapter-specific guidelines provide additional information about the use of Z codes for specified encounters.

a. Use of Z Codes in any healthcare setting

Z codes are for use in any healthcare setting. Z codes may be used as either a first-listed (principal diagnosis code in the inpatient setting) or secondary code, depending on the circumstances of the encounter. Certain Z codes may only be used as first-listed or principal diagnosis.

Patient with middle lobe lung cancer admitted for initiation of chemotherapy

Z51.11 Encounter for antineoplastic chemotherapy

C34.2 Malignant neoplasm of middle lobe, bronchus or lung

Explanation: A Z code can be used as first-listed in this situation based on guidelines in this chapter as well as chapter 2, "Neoplasms."

b. Z Codes indicate a reason for an encounter or provide additional information about a patient encounter

Z codes are not procedure codes. A corresponding procedure code must accompany a Z code to describe any procedure performed.

c. Categories of Z Codes

1) Contact/exposure

Category Z20 indicates contact with, and suspected exposure to, communicable diseases. These codes are for patients who are suspected to have been exposed to a disease by close personal contact with an infected individual or are in an area where a disease is epidemic.

Category Z77, Other contact with and (suspected) exposures hazardous to health, indicates contact with and suspected exposures hazardous to health.

Contact/exposure codes may be used as a first-listed code to explain an encounter for testing, or, more commonly, as a secondary code to identify a potential risk.

2) Inoculations and vaccinations

Code Z23 is for encounters for inoculations and vaccinations. It indicates that a patient is being seen to receive a prophylactic inoculation against a disease. Procedure codes are required to identify the actual administration of the injection and the type(s) of immunizations given. Code Z23 may be used as a secondary code if the inoculation is given as a routine part of preventive health care, such as a well-baby visit.

3) Status

Status codes indicate that a patient is either a carrier of a disease or has the sequelae or residual of a past disease or condition. This includes such things as the presence of prosthetic or mechanical devices resulting from past treatment. A status code is informative, because the status may affect the course of treatment and its outcome. A status code is distinct from a history code. The history code indicates that the patient no longer has the condition.

A status code should not be used with a diagnosis code from one of the body system chapters, if the diagnosis code includes the information provided by the status code. For example, code Z94.1, Heart transplant status, should not be used with a code from subcategory T86.2, Complications of heart transplant. The status code does not provide additional information. The complication code indicates that the patient is a heart transplant patient.

For encounters for weaning from a mechanical ventilator, assign a code from subcategory J96.1, Chronic respiratory failure, followed by code Z99.11, Dependence on respirator [ventilator] status.

The status Z codes/categories are:

Z14 Genetic carrier

Genetic carrier status indicates that a person carries a gene, associated with a particular disease, which may be passed to offspring who may develop that disease. The person does not have the disease and is not at risk of developing the disease.

Z15 Genetic susceptibility to disease

Genetic susceptibility indicates that a person has a gene that increases the risk of that person developing the disease.

Codes from category Z15 should not be used as principal or first-listed codes. If the patient has the condition to which he/she is susceptible, and that condition is the reason for the encounter, the code for the current condition should be sequenced first. If the patient is being seen for follow-up after completed treatment for this condition, and the condition no longer exists, a follow-up code should be sequenced first, followed by the appropriate personal history and genetic susceptibility codes. If the purpose of the encounter is genetic counseling associated with procreative management, code Z31.5, Encounter for genetic counseling, should be assigned as the first-listed code, followed by a code from category Z15. Additional codes should be assigned for any applicable family or personal history.

Z16 Resistance to antimicrobial drugs

This code indicates that a patient has a condition that is resistant to antimicrobial drug treatment. Sequence the infection code first.

Penicillin resistant streptococcus pneumoniae meningitis

G00.1 Pneumococcal meningitis

Z16.11 Resistance to penicillins

Explanation: The status Z code is used to describe the presence of a drug-resistant organism that most likely altered how the meningitis was treated.

Z17 Estrogen receptor status

Z18 Retained foreign body fragments

Z19 Hormone sensitivity malignancy status

Z21 Asymptomatic HIV infection status

This code indicates that a patient has tested positive for HIV but has manifested no signs or symptoms of the disease.

Z22 Carrier of infectious disease

Carrier status indicates that a person harbors the specific organisms of a disease without manifest symptoms and is capable of transmitting the infection.

Z28.3 Underimmunization status

See Section I.B.14. for underimmunization documentation by clinicians other than the patient's provider.

Z33.1 Pregnant state, incidental

This code is a secondary code only for use when the pregnancy is in no way complicating the reason for visit. Otherwise, a code from the obstetric chapter is required.

Z66 Do not resuscitate

This code may be used when it is documented by the provider that a patient is on do not resuscitate status at any time during the stay.

Z67 Blood type

Z68 Body mass index (BMI)

BMI codes should only be assigned when there is an associated, reportable diagnosis (such as obesity). Do not assign BMI codes during pregnancy.

See Section I.B.14. for BMI documentation by clinicians other than the patient's provider.

Z74.01 Bed confinement status

Z76.82 Awaiting organ transplant status

Z78 Other specified health status

Code Z78.1, Physical restraint status, may be used when it is documented by the provider that a patient has been put in restraints during the current encounter. Please note that this code should not be reported when it is documented by the provider that a patient is temporarily restrained during a procedure.

Z79 Long-term (current) drug therapy

Codes from this category indicate a patient's continuous use of a prescribed drug (including such things as aspirin therapy) for the long-term treatment of a condition or for prophylactic use.

It is not for use for patients who have addictions to drugs. This subcategory is not for use of medications for detoxification or maintenance programs to prevent withdrawal symptoms (e.g., methadone maintenance for opiate dependence). Assign the appropriate code for the drug use, abuse, or dependence instead.

Assign a code from Z79 if the patient is receiving a medication for an extended period as a prophylactic measure (such as for the prevention of deep vein thrombosis) or as treatment of a chronic condition (such as arthritis) or a disease requiring a lengthy course of treatment (such as cancer). Do not assign a code from category Z79 for medication being administered for a brief period of time to treat an acute illness or injury (such as a course of antibiotics to treat acute bronchitis).

Z88 Allergy status to drugs, medicaments and biological substances

Except: Z88.9, Allergy status to unspecified drugs, medicaments and biological substances status

Z89 Acquired absence of limb

Z9Ø Acquired absence of organs, not elsewhere classified

Z91.Ø- Allergy status, other than to drugs and biological substances

Z92.82 Status post administration of tPA (rtPA) in a different facility within the last 24 hours prior to admission to a current facility

Assign code Z92.82, Status post administration of tPA (rtPA) in a different facility within the last 24 hours prior to admission to current facility, as a secondary diagnosis when a patient is received by transfer into a facility and documentation indicates they were administered tissue plasminogen activator (tPA) within the last 24 hours prior to admission to the current facility.

This guideline applies even if the patient is still receiving the tPA at the time they are received into the current facility.

The appropriate code for the condition for which the tPA was administered (such as cerebrovascular disease or myocardial infarction) should be assigned first.

Code Z92.82 is only applicable to the receiving facility record and not to the transferring facility record.

Z93 Artificial opening status

Z94 Transplanted organ and tissue status

Z95 Presence of cardiac and vascular implants and grafts

Z96 Presence of other functional implants

Z97 Presence of other devices

Z98 Other postprocedural states

Assign code Z98.85, Transplanted organ removal status, to indicate that a transplanted organ has been previously removed. This code should not be assigned for the encounter in which the transplanted organ is removed. The complication necessitating removal of the transplant organ should be assigned for that encounter.

See section I.C.19. for information on the coding of organ transplant complications.

Z99 Dependence on enabling machines and devices, not elsewhere classified

Note: Categories Z89–Z9Ø and Z93–Z99 are for use only if there are no complications or malfunctions of the organ or tissue replaced, the amputation site or the equipment on which the patient is dependent.

4) History (of)

There are two types of history Z codes, personal and family. Personal history codes explain a patient's past medical condition that no longer exists and is not receiving any treatment, but that has the potential for recurrence, and therefore may require continued monitoring.

Family history codes are for use when a patient has a family member(s) who has had a particular disease that causes the patient to be at higher risk of also contracting the disease.

Personal history codes may be used in conjunction with follow-up codes and family history codes may be used in conjunction with screening codes to explain the need for a test or procedure. History codes are also acceptable on any medical record regardless of the reason for visit. A history of an illness, even if no longer present, is important information that may alter the type of treatment ordered.

The reason for the encounter (for example, screening or counseling) should be sequenced first and the appropriate personal and/or family history code(s) should be assigned as additional diagnos(es).

The history Z code categories are:

Z8Ø Family history of primary malignant neoplasm

Z81 Family history of mental and behavioral disorders

Z82 Family history of certain disabilities and chronic diseases (leading to disablement)

Z83 Family history of other specific disorders

Z84 Family history of other conditions

Z85 Personal history of malignant neoplasm

Z86 Personal history of certain other diseases

Z87 Personal history of other diseases and conditions

Z91.4- Personal history of psychological trauma, not elsewhere classified

Z91.5- Personal history of self-harm

Z91.81 History of falling

Z91.82 Personal history of military deployment

Z91.85 Personal history of military service

Z92 Personal history of medical treatment

Except: Z92.Ø, Personal history of contraception

Except: Z92.82, Status post administration of tPA (rtPA) in a different facility within the last 24 hours prior to admission to a current facility

Patient has chronic lymphocytic leukemia for which the patient had previous chemotherapy and is now in remission

C91.11 Chronic lymphocytic leukemia of B-cell type in remission

Z92.21 Personal history of antineoplastic chemotherapy

Explanation: The personal history Z code is used to describe a secondary (supplementary) diagnosis to identify that this patient has had chemotherapy in the past.

5) Screening

Screening is the testing for disease or disease precursors in seemingly well individuals so that early detection and treatment can be provided for those who test positive for the disease (e.g., screening mammogram).

The testing of a person to rule out or confirm a suspected diagnosis because the patient has some sign or symptom is a diagnostic examination, not a screening. In these cases, the sign or symptom is used to explain the reason for the test.

A screening code may be a first-listed code if the reason for the visit is specifically the screening exam. It may also be used as an additional code if the screening is done during an office visit for other health problems. A screening code is not necessary if the screening is inherent to a routine examination, such as a pap smear done during a routine pelvic examination.

Should a condition be discovered during the screening then the code for the condition may be assigned as an additional diagnosis.

The Z code indicates that a screening exam is planned. A procedure code is required to confirm that the screening was performed.

The screening Z codes/categories:

Z11 Encounter for screening for infectious and parasitic diseases

Z12 Encounter for screening for malignant neoplasms

Z13 Encounter for screening for other diseases and disorders

Except: Z13.9, Encounter for screening, unspecified

Z36 Encounter for antenatal screening for mother

6) Observation

There are three observation Z code categories. They are for use in very limited circumstances when a person is being observed for a suspected condition that is ruled out. The observation codes are not for use if an injury or illness or any signs or symptoms related to the suspected condition are present. In such cases the diagnosis/symptom code is used with the corresponding external cause code.

The observation codes are primarily to be used as a principal/first-listed diagnosis. An observation code may be assigned as a secondary diagnosis code when the patient is being observed for a condition that is ruled out and is unrelated to the principal/first-listed diagnosis Also, when the principal diagnosis is required to be a code from category Z38, Liveborn infants according to place of birth and type of delivery, then a code from category ZØ5, Encounter for observation and evaluation of newborn for suspected diseases and conditions ruled out, is sequenced after the Z38 code. Additional codes may be used in addition to the observation code, but only if they are unrelated to the suspected condition being observed.

Codes from subcategory ZØ3.7, Encounter for suspected maternal and fetal conditions ruled out, may either be used as a first-listed or as an additional code assignment depending on the case. They are for use in very limited circumstances on a maternal record when an encounter is for a suspected maternal or fetal condition that is ruled out during that encounter (for example, a maternal or fetal condition may be suspected due to an abnormal test result). These codes should not be used when the condition is confirmed. In those cases, the confirmed condition should be coded. In addition, these codes are not for use if an illness or any signs or symptoms related to the suspected condition or problem are present. In such cases the diagnosis/symptom code is used.

Additional codes may be used in addition to the code from subcategory Z03.7, but only if they are unrelated to the suspected condition being evaluated.

Codes from subcategory Z03.7 may not be used for encounters for antenatal screening of mother. *See Section I.C.21. Screening.*

For encounters for suspected fetal condition that are inconclusive following testing and evaluation, assign the appropriate code from category O35, O36, O40 or O41.

The observation Z code categories:

- Z03 Encounter for medical observation for suspected diseases and conditions ruled out
- Z04 Encounter for examination and observation for other reasons
  Except: Z04.9, Encounter for examination and observation for unspecified reason
- Z05 Encounter for observation and evaluation of newborn for suspected diseases and conditions ruled out

Upon initial examination, a heart murmur was heard in a newborn infant delivered vaginally in the hospital; however, after further observation, any serious cardiac conditions were ruled out.

Z38.00 Single liveborn infant, delivered vaginally

Z05.0 Observation and evaluation of newborn for suspected cardiac condition ruled out

Explanation: Normally an observation code is used as the principal diagnosis except when the patient is a newborn. A code from category Z38 Liveborn infants according to place of birth and type of delivery code would be sequenced first, followed by the encounter for observation and evaluation of newborn for suspected diseases and conditions ruled out.

7) Aftercare

Aftercare visit codes cover situations when the initial treatment of a disease has been performed and the patient requires continued care during the healing or recovery phase, or for the long-term consequences of the disease. The aftercare Z code should not be used if treatment is directed at a current, acute disease. The diagnosis code is to be used in these cases. Exceptions to this rule are codes Z51.0, Encounter for antineoplastic radiation therapy, and codes from subcategory Z51.1, Encounter for antineoplastic chemotherapy and immunotherapy. These codes are to be first listed, followed by the diagnosis code when a patient's encounter is solely to receive radiation therapy, chemotherapy, or immunotherapy for the treatment of a neoplasm. If the reason for the encounter is more than one type of antineoplastic therapy, code Z51.0 and a code from subcategory Z51.1 may be assigned together, in which case one of these codes would be reported as a secondary diagnosis.

The aftercare Z codes should also not be used for aftercare for injuries. For aftercare of an injury, assign the acute injury code with the appropriate 7th character (for subsequent encounter).

The aftercare codes are generally first listed to explain the specific reason for the encounter. An aftercare code may be used as an additional code when some type of aftercare is provided in addition to the reason for admission and no diagnosis code is applicable. An example of this would be the closure of a colostomy during an encounter for treatment of another condition.

Aftercare codes should be used in conjunction with other aftercare codes or diagnosis codes to provide better detail on the specifics of an aftercare encounter visit, unless otherwise directed by the classification. The sequencing of multiple aftercare codes depends on the circumstances of the encounter.

Certain aftercare Z code categories need a secondary diagnosis code to describe the resolving condition or sequelae. For others, the condition is included in the code title.

Additional Z code aftercare category terms include fitting and adjustment, and attention to artificial openings.

Status Z codes may be used with aftercare Z codes to indicate the nature of the aftercare. For example code Z95.1, Presence of aortocoronary bypass graft, may be used with code Z48.812, Encounter for surgical aftercare following surgery on the circulatory system, to indicate the surgery for which the aftercare is being performed. A status code should not be used when the aftercare code indicates the type of status, such as using Z43.0, Encounter for attention to tracheostomy, with Z93.0, Tracheostomy status.

The aftercare Z category/codes:

- Z42 Encounter for plastic and reconstructive surgery following medical procedure or healed injury
- Z43 Encounter for attention to artificial openings
- Z44 Encounter for fitting and adjustment of external prosthetic device
- Z45 Encounter for adjustment and management of implanted device
- Z46 Encounter for fitting and adjustment of other devices
- Z47 Orthopedic aftercare
- Z48 Encounter for other postprocedural aftercare
- Z49 Encounter for care involving renal dialysis
- Z51 Encounter for other aftercare and medical care

8) Follow-up

The follow-up codes are used to explain continuing surveillance following completed treatment of a disease, condition, or injury. They imply that the condition has been fully treated and no longer exists. They should not be confused with aftercare codes, or injury codes with a 7th character for subsequent encounter, that explain ongoing care of a healing condition or its sequelae. Follow-up codes may be used in conjunction with history codes to provide the full picture of the healed condition and its treatment. The follow-up code is sequenced first, followed by the history code.

A follow-up code may be used to explain multiple visits. Should a condition be found to have recurred on the follow-up visit, then the diagnosis code for the condition should be assigned in place of the follow-up code.

The follow-up **Z codes/categories**:

- Z08 Encounter for follow-up examination after completed treatment for malignant neoplasm
- Z09 Encounter for follow-up examination after completed treatment for conditions other than malignant neoplasm

Codes Z08, Encounter for follow-up examination after completed treatment for malignant neoplasm, and Z09, Encounter for follow up examination after completed treatment for conditions other than malignant neoplasm, may be assigned following any type of completed treatment modality (including both medical and surgical treatments).

- Z39 Encounter for maternal postpartum care and examination

9) Donor

Codes in category Z52, Donors of organs and tissues, are used for living individuals who are donating blood or other body tissue. These codes are for individuals donating for others, as well as for self-donations. They are not used to identify cadaveric donations.

10)Counseling

Counseling Z codes are used when a patient or family member receives assistance in the aftermath of an illness or injury, or when support is required in coping with family or social problems.

The counseling Z codes/categories:

- Z30.0- Encounter for general counseling and advice on contraception
- Z31.5 Encounter for procreative genetic counseling
- Z31.6- Encounter for general counseling and advice on procreation
- Z32.2 Encounter for childbirth instruction
- Z32.3 Encounter for childcare instruction
- Z69 Encounter for mental health services for victim and perpetrator of abuse
- Z70 Counseling related to sexual attitude, behavior and orientation
- Z71 Persons encountering health services for other counseling and medical advice, not elsewhere classified
  Note: Code Z71.84, Encounter for health counseling related to travel, is to be used for health risk and safety counseling for future travel purposes.
  Code Z71.85, Encounter for immunization safety counseling, is to be used for counseling of the patient or caregiver regarding the safety of a vaccine. This code should not be used for the provision of general information regarding risks and potential side effects during routine encounters for the administration of vaccines.
  Code Z71.87, Encounter for pediatric-to-adult transition counseling, should be assigned when pediatric-to-adult transition counseling is the sole reason for the encounter or when this counseling is provided In addition to other services, such as treatment of a chronic condition. If both transition

counseling and treatment of a medical condition are provided during the same encounter, the code(s) for the medical condition(s) treated and code Z71.87 should be assigned, with sequencing depending on the circumstances of the encounter.

Z76.81 Expectant mother prebirth pediatrician visit

11)Encounters for obstetrical and reproductive services

See Section I.C.15. Pregnancy, Childbirth, and the Puerperium, for further instruction on the use of these codes.

Z codes for pregnancy are for use in those circumstances when none of the problems or complications included in the codes from the Obstetrics chapter exist (a routine prenatal visit or postpartum care). Codes in category Z34, Encounter for supervision of normal pregnancy, are always first listed and are not to be used with any other code from the OB chapter.

Codes in category Z3A, Weeks of gestation, may be assigned to provide additional information about the pregnancy. Category Z3A codes should not be assigned for pregnancies with abortive outcomes (categories O00–O08), elective termination of pregnancy (code Z33.2), nor for postpartum conditions, as category Z3A is not applicable to these conditions. The date of the admission should be used to determine weeks of gestation for inpatient admissions that encompass more than one gestational week.

The outcome of delivery, category Z37, should be included on all maternal delivery records. It is always a secondary code.

Codes in category Z37 should not be used on the newborn record.

Z codes for family planning (contraceptive) or procreative management and counseling should be included on an obstetric record either during the pregnancy or the postpartum stage, if applicable.

Z codes/categories for obstetrical and reproductive services:

Z30	Encounter for contraceptive management
Z31	Encounter for procreative management
Z32.2	Encounter for childbirth instruction
Z32.3	Encounter for childcare instruction
Z33	Pregnant state
Z34	Encounter for supervision of normal pregnancy
Z36	Encounter for antenatal screening of mother
Z3A	Weeks of gestation
Z37	Outcome of delivery
Z39	Encounter for maternal postpartum care and examination
Z76.81	Expectant mother prebirth pediatrician visit

12)Newborns and infants

See Section I.C.16. Newborn (Perinatal) Guidelines, for further instruction on the use of these codes.

Newborn Z codes/categories:

Z76.1	Encounter for health supervision and care of foundling
Z00.1-	Encounter for routine child health examination
Z38	Liveborn infants according to place of birth and type of delivery

13)Routine and administrative examinations

The Z codes allow for the description of encounters for routine examinations, such as, a general check-up, or, examinations for administrative purposes, such as, a pre-employment physical. The codes are not to be used if the examination is for diagnosis of a suspected condition or for treatment purposes. In such cases the diagnosis code is used. During a routine exam, should a diagnosis or condition be discovered, it should be coded as an additional code. Pre-existing and chronic conditions and history codes may also be included as additional codes as long as the examination is for administrative purposes and not focused on any particular condition.

Some of the codes for routine health examinations distinguish between "with" and "without" abnormal findings. Code assignment depends on the information that is known at the time the encounter is being coded. For example, if no abnormal findings were found during the examination, but the encounter is being coded before test results are back, it is acceptable to assign the code for "without abnormal findings." When assigning a code for "with abnormal findings," additional code(s) should be assigned to identify the specific abnormal finding(s).

Pre-operative examination and pre-procedural laboratory examination Z codes are for use only in those situations when a patient is being cleared for a procedure or surgery and no treatment is given.

The Z codes/categories for routine and administrative examinations:

Z00	Encounter for general examination without complaint, suspected or reported diagnosis
Z01	Encounter for other special examination without complaint, suspected or reported diagnosis
Z02	Encounter for administrative examination Except: Z02.9, Encounter for administrative examinations, unspecified
Z32.0-	Encounter for pregnancy test

14)Miscellaneous Z codes

The miscellaneous Z codes capture a number of other health care encounters that do not fall into one of the other categories. Some of these codes identify the reason for the encounter; others are for use as additional codes that provide useful information on circumstances that may affect a patient's care and treatment.

Prophylactic organ removal

For encounters specifically for prophylactic removal of an organ (such as prophylactic removal of breasts due to a genetic susceptibility to cancer or a family history of cancer), the principal or first-listed code should be a code from category Z40, Encounter for prophylactic surgery, followed by the appropriate codes to identify the associated risk factor (such as genetic susceptibility or family history).

If the patient has a malignancy of one site and is having prophylactic removal at another site to prevent either a new primary malignancy or metastatic disease, a code for the malignancy should also be assigned in addition to a code from subcategory Z40.0, Encounter for prophylactic surgery for risk factors related to malignant neoplasms. A Z40.0 code should not be assigned if the patient is having organ removal for treatment of a malignancy, such as the removal of the testes for the treatment of prostate cancer.

Female patient with cancer in lower inner quadrant of right breast and positive BRCA 1 noted on testing is admitted for mastectomy of right breast and prophylactic removal of left breast

C50.311	**Malignant neoplasm of lower-inner quadrant of right female breast**
Z40.01	**Encounter for prophylactic removal of breast**
Z15.01	**Genetic susceptibility to malignant neoplasm of breast**

Explanation: Removal of the current neoplastic disease in the right breast was the focus of treatment for this admission and is sequenced first. The removal of the left breast was not required to treat a current disease process but as a means of prevention. The two Z codes are informational; they capture the reason behind the removal of what is currently a healthy left breast.

Miscellaneous Z codes/categories:

Z28	Immunization not carried out Except: Z28.3-, Underimmunization status
Z29	Encounter for other prophylactic measures
Z40	Encounter for prophylactic surgery
Z41	Encounter for procedures for purposes other than remedying health state Except: Z41.9, Encounter for procedure for purposes other than remedying health state, unspecified
Z53	Persons encountering health services for specific procedures and treatment, not carried out
Z72	Problems related to lifestyle Note: These codes should be assigned only when the documentation specifies that the patient has an associated problem
Z73	Problems related to life management difficulty Note: These codes should be assigned only when the documentation specifies that the patient has an associated problem.
Z74	Problems related to care provider dependency Except: Z74.01, Bed confinement status
Z75	Problems related to medical facilities and other health care
Z76.0	Encounter for issue of repeat prescription
Z76.3	Healthy person accompanying sick person
Z76.4	Other boarder to healthcare facility
Z76.5	Malingerer [conscious simulation]
Z91.1-	Patient's noncompliance with medical treatment and regimen
Z91.A-	**Caregiver's noncompliance with patient's medical treatment and regimen**
Z91.83	Wandering in diseases classified elsewhere

Z91.84- Oral health risk factors

Z91.89 Other specified personal risk factors, not elsewhere classified

See Section I.B.14. for Z55–Z65 Persons with potential health hazards related to socioeconomic and psychosocial circumstances, documentation by clinicians other than the patient's provider

15) Nonspecific Z codes

Certain Z codes are so non-specific, or potentially redundant with other codes in the classification, that there can be little justification for their use in the inpatient setting. Their use in the outpatient setting should be limited to those instances when there is no further documentation to permit more precise coding. Otherwise, any sign or symptom or any other reason for visit that is captured in another code should be used.

Nonspecific Z codes/categories:

Z02.9	Encounter for administrative examinations, unspecified
Z04.9	Encounter for examination and observation for unspecified reason
Z13.9	Encounter for screening, unspecified
Z41.9	Encounter for procedure for purposes other than remedying health state, unspecified
Z52.9	Donor of unspecified organ or tissue
Z86.59	Personal history of other mental and behavioral disorders
Z88.9	Allergy status to unspecified drugs, medicaments and biological substances status
Z92.0	Personal history of contraception

16) Z codes that may only be principal/first-listed diagnosis

The following Z codes/categories may only be reported as the principal/first-listed diagnosis, except when there are multiple encounters on the same day and the medical records for the encounters are combined:

Z00	Encounter for general examination without complaint, suspected or reported diagnosis Except: Z00.6
Z01	Encounter for other special examination without complaint, suspected or reported diagnosis
Z02	Encounter for administrative examination
Z04	Encounter for examination and observation for other reasons
Z33.2	Encounter for elective termination of pregnancy
Z31.81	Encounter for male factor infertility in female patient
Z31.83	Encounter for assisted reproductive fertility procedure cycle
Z31.84	Encounter for fertility preservation procedure
Z34	Encounter for supervision of normal pregnancy
Z39	Encounter for maternal postpartum care and examination
Z38	Liveborn infants according to place of birth and type of delivery
Z40	Encounter for prophylactic surgery
Z42	Encounter for plastic and reconstructive surgery following medical procedure or healed injury
Z51.0	Encounter for antineoplastic radiation therapy
Z51.1-	Encounter for antineoplastic chemotherapy and immunotherapy
Z52	Donors of organs and tissues Except: Z52.9, Donor of unspecified organ or tissue
Z76.1	Encounter for health supervision and care of foundling
Z76.2	Encounter for health supervision and care of other healthy infant and child
Z99.12	Encounter for respirator [ventilator] dependence during power failure

17) Social Determinants of Health

Social determinants of health (SDOH) codes describing social problems, conditions, or risk factors that influence a patient's health should be assigned when this information is documented in the patient's medical record. Assign as many SDOH codes as are necessary to describe all of the social problems, conditions, or risk factors documented during the current episode of care. For example, a patient who lives alone may suffer an acute injury temporarily impacting their ability to perform routine activities of daily living. When documented as such, this would support assignment of code Z60.2, Problems related to living alone. However, merely living alone, without documentation of a risk or unmet need for assistance at home, would not support assignment of code Z60.2. Documentation by a clinician (or patient-reported information that is signed off by a clinician) that the patient expressed concerns with access and availability of food would support assignment of code Z59.41, Food insecurity. Similarly, medical record documentation indicating the patient is homeless would support assignment of a code from subcategory Z59.0-, Homelessness.

For social determinants of health **classified to chapter 21**, such as information found in categories Z55-Z65, Persons with potential health hazards related to socioeconomic and psychosocial circumstances, code assignment may be based on medical record documentation from clinicians involved in the care of the patient who are not the patient's provider since this information represents social information, rather than medical diagnoses. For example, coding professionals may utilize documentation of social information from social workers, community health workers, case managers, or nurses, if their documentation is included in the official medical record.

Patient self-reported documentation may be used to assign codes for social determinants of health, as long as the patient self-reported information is signed-off by and incorporated into the medical record by either a clinician or provider.

Social determinants of health codes are located primarily in these Z code categories:

Z55	Problems related to education and literacy
Z56	Problems related to employment and unemployment
Z57	Occupational exposure to risk factors
Z58	Problems related to physical environment
Z59	Problems related to housing and economic circumstances
Z60	Problems related to social environment
Z62	Problems related to upbringing
Z63	Other problems related to primary support group, including family circumstances
Z64	Problems related to certain psychosocial circumstances
Z65	Problems related to other psychosocial circumstances

See Section I.B.14. Documentation by Clinicians Other than the Patient's Provider.

Chapter 21. Factors Influencing Health Status and Contact With Health Services (Z00-Z99)

NOTE Z codes represent reasons for encounters. A corresponding procedure code must accompany a Z code if a procedure is performed. Categories Z00-Z99 are provided for occasions when circumstances other than a disease, injury or external cause classifiable to categories A00-Y89 are recorded as "diagnoses" or "problems." This can arise in two main ways:

(a) When a person who may or may not be sick encounters the health services for some specific purpose, such as to receive limited care or service for a current condition, to donate an organ or tissue, to receive prophylactic vaccination (immunization), or to discuss a problem which is in itself not a disease or injury.

(b) When some circumstance or problem is present which influences the person's health status but is not in itself a current illness or injury.

AHA: 2018,4Q,60-61

This chapter contains the following blocks:

Z00-Z13	Persons encountering health services for examinations
Z14-Z15	Genetic carrier and genetic susceptibility to disease
Z16	Resistance to antimicrobial drugs
Z17	Estrogen receptor status
Z18	Retained foreign body fragments
Z19	Hormone sensitivity malignancy status
Z20-Z29	Persons with potential health hazards related to communicable diseases
Z30-Z39	Persons encountering health services in circumstances related to reproduction
Z40-Z53	Encounters for other specific health care
Z55-Z65	Persons with potential health hazards related to socioeconomic and psychosocial circumstances
Z66	Do not resuscitate status
Z67	Blood type
Z68	Body mass index (BMI)
Z69-Z76	Persons encountering health services in other circumstances
Z77-Z99	Persons with potential health hazards related to family and personal history and certain conditions influencing health status

Persons encountering health services for examinations (Z00-Z13)

NOTE Nonspecific abnormal findings disclosed at the time of these examinations are classified to categories R70-R94.

EXCLUDES 1 *examinations related to pregnancy and reproduction (Z30-Z36, Z39.-)*

✓4th **Z00 Encounter for general examination without complaint, suspected or reported diagnosis**

EXCLUDES 1 *encounter for examination for administrative purposes (Z02.-)*

EXCLUDES 2 *encounter for pre-procedural examinations (Z01.81-)*

special screening examinations (Z11-Z13)

AHA: 2017,4Q,95

✓5th **Z00.0 Encounter for general adult medical examination**

Encounter for adult periodic examination (annual) (physical) and any associated laboratory and radiologic examinations

EXCLUDES 1 *encounter for examination of sign or symptom - code to sign or symptom*

general health check-up of infant or child (Z00.12.-)

Z00.00 Encounter for general adult medical examination without abnormal findings UPD A

Encounter for adult health check-up NOS

AHA: 2016,1Q,36

Z00.01 Encounter for general adult medical examination with abnormal findings UPD A

Use additional code to identify abnormal findings

AHA: 2016,1Q,35-36

✓5th **Z00.1 Encounter for newborn, infant and child health examinations**

✓6th **Z00.11 Newborn health examination**

Health check for child under 29 days old

Use additional code to identify any abnormal findings

EXCLUDES 1 *health check for child over 28 days old (Z00.12-)*

Z00.110 Health examination for newborn under 8 days old UPD N

Health check for newborn under 8 days old

Z00.111 Health examination for newborn 8 to 28 days old UPD N

Health check for newborn 8 to 28 days old

Newborn weight check

✓6th **Z00.12 Encounter for routine child health examination**

Health check (routine) for child over 28 days old

Immunizations appropriate for age

Routine developmental screening of infant or child

Routine vison and hearing testing

EXCLUDES 1 *health check for child under 29 days old (Z00.11-)*

health supervision of foundling or other healthy infant or child (Z76.1-Z76.2)

newborn health examination (Z00.11-)

AHA: 2018,4Q,36

Z00.121 Encounter for routine child health examination with abnormal findings UPD P

Use additional code to identify abnormal findings

AHA: 2016,1Q,34-35

Z00.129 Encounter for routine child health examination without abnormal findings UPD P

Encounter for routine child health examination NOS

AHA: 2016,1Q,34

Z00.2 Encounter for examination for period of rapid growth in childhood UPD P

Z00.3 Encounter for examination for adolescent development state UPD P

Encounter for puberty development state

Z00.5 Encounter for examination of potential donor of organ and tissue UPD

Z00.6 Encounter for examination for normal comparison and control in clinical research program

Examination of participant or control in clinical research program

✓5th **Z00.7 Encounter for examination for period of delayed growth in childhood**

Z00.70 Encounter for examination for period of delayed growth in childhood without abnormal findings UPD P

Z00.71 Encounter for examination for period of delayed growth in childhood with abnormal findings UPD P

Use additional code to identify abnormal findings

Z00.8 Encounter for other general examination UPD

Encounter for health examination in population surveys

✓4th **Z01 Encounter for other special examination without complaint, suspected or reported diagnosis**

INCLUDES routine examination of specific system

NOTE Codes from category Z01 represent the reason for the encounter. A separate procedure code is required to identify any examinations or procedures performed

EXCLUDES 1 *encounter for examination for administrative purposes (Z02.-)*

encounter for examination for suspected conditions, proven not to exist (Z03.-)

encounter for laboratory and radiologic examinations as a component of general medical examinations (Z00.0-)

encounter for laboratory, radiologic and imaging examinations for sign(s) and symptom(s) - code to the sign(s) or symptom(s)

EXCLUDES 2 *screening examinations (Z11-Z13)*

✓5th **Z01.0 Encounter for examination of eyes and vision**

EXCLUDES 1 *examination for driving license (Z02.4)*

Z01.00 Encounter for examination of eyes and vision without abnormal findings

Encounter for examination of eyes and vision NOS

Z01.01 Encounter for examination of eyes and vision with abnormal findings

Use additional code to identify abnormal findings

AHA: 2016,4Q,21

✓6th **Z01.02 Encounter for examination of eyes and vision following failed vision screening**

EXCLUDES 1 *encounter for examination of eyes and vision with abnormal findings (Z01.01)*
encounter for examination of eyes and vision without abnormal findings (Z01.00)

AHA: 2019,4Q,20

Z01.020 Encounter for examination of eyes and vision following failed vision screening without abnormal findings

Z01.021 Encounter for examination of eyes and vision following failed vision screening with abnormal findings
Use additional code to identify abnormal findings

✓5th **Z01.1 Encounter for examination of ears and hearing**

Z01.10 Encounter for examination of ears and hearing without abnormal findings UPD
Encounter for examination of ears and hearing NOS
AHA: 2016,4Q,24

✓6th **Z01.11 Encounter for examination of ears and hearing with abnormal findings**
AHA: 2016,3Q,17-18

Z01.110 Encounter for hearing examination following failed hearing screening UPD

Z01.118 Encounter for examination of ears and hearing with other abnormal findings UPD
Use additional code to identify abnormal findings

Z01.12 Encounter for hearing conservation and treatment UPD

✓5th **Z01.2 Encounter for dental examination and cleaning**

Z01.20 Encounter for dental examination and cleaning without abnormal findings UPD
Encounter for dental examination and cleaning NOS

Z01.21 Encounter for dental examination and cleaning with abnormal findings UPD
Use additional code to identify abnormal findings

✓5th **Z01.3 Encounter for examination of blood pressure**

Z01.30 Encounter for examination of blood pressure without abnormal findings UPD
Encounter for examination of blood pressure NOS

Z01.31 Encounter for examination of blood pressure with abnormal findings UPD
Use additional code to identify abnormal findings

✓5th **Z01.4 Encounter for gynecological examination**

EXCLUDES 2 *pregnancy examination or test (Z32.0-)*
routine examination for contraceptive maintenance (Z30.4-)

✓6th **Z01.41 Encounter for routine gynecological examination**
Encounter for general gynecological examination with or without cervical smear
Encounter for gynecological examination (general) (routine) NOS
Encounter for pelvic examination (annual) (periodic)
Use additional code:
for screening for human papillomavirus, if applicable, (Z11.51)
for screening vaginal pap smear, if applicable (Z12.72)
to identify acquired absence of uterus, if applicable (Z90.71-)

EXCLUDES 1 *gynecologic examination status-post hysterectomy for malignant condition (Z08)*
screening cervical pap smear not a part of a routine gynecological examination (Z12.4)

Z01.411 Encounter for gynecological examination (general) (routine) with abnormal findings ♀
Use additional code to identify abnormal findings

Z01.419 Encounter for gynecological examination (general) (routine) without abnormal findings ♀

Z01.42 Encounter for cervical smear to confirm findings of recent normal smear following initial abnormal smear ♀

✓5th **Z01.8 Encounter for other specified special examinations**

✓6th **Z01.81 Encounter for preprocedural examinations**
Encounter for preoperative examinations
Encounter for radiological and imaging examinations as part of preprocedural examination

Z01.810 Encounter for preprocedural cardiovascular examination

Z01.811 Encounter for preprocedural respiratory examination

Z01.812 Encounter for preprocedural laboratory examination UPD
Blood and urine tests prior to treatment or procedure
AHA: 2023,2Q,3; 2020,3Q,14

Z01.818 Encounter for other preprocedural examination UPD
Encounter for preprocedural examination NOS
Encounter for examinations prior to antineoplastic chemotherapy

Z01.82 Encounter for allergy testing UPD
EXCLUDES 1 *encounter for antibody response examination (Z01.84)*

Z01.83 Encounter for blood typing UPD
Encounter for Rh typing

Z01.84 Encounter for antibody response examination UPD
Encounter for immunity status testing
EXCLUDES 1 *encounter for allergy testing (Z01.82)*
AHA: 2020,2Q,11

Z01.89 Encounter for other specified special examinations UPD

✓4th **Z02 Encounter for administrative examination**

Z02.0 Encounter for examination for admission to educational institution UPD
Encounter for examination for admission to preschool (education)
Encounter for examination for re-admission to school following illness or medical treatment

Z02.1 Encounter for pre-employment examination

Z02.2 Encounter for examination for admission to residential institution UPD
EXCLUDES 1 *examination for admission to prison (Z02.89)*

Z02.3 Encounter for examination for recruitment to armed forces

Z02.4 Encounter for examination for driving license UPD

Z02.5 Encounter for examination for participation in sport UPD
EXCLUDES 1 *blood-alcohol and blood-drug test (Z02.83)*

Z02.6 Encounter for examination for insurance purposes UPD

✓5th **Z02.7 Encounter for issue of medical certificate**
EXCLUDES 1 *encounter for general medical examination (Z00-Z01, Z02.0-Z02.6, Z02.8-Z02.9)*

Z02.71 Encounter for disability determination UPD
Encounter for issue of medical certificate of incapacity
Encounter for issue of medical certificate of invalidity

Z02.79 Encounter for issue of other medical certificate UPD

✓5th **Z02.8 Encounter for other administrative examinations**

Z02.81 Encounter for paternity testing

Z02.82 Encounter for adoption services UPD

Z02.83 Encounter for blood-alcohol and blood-drug test
Use additional code for findings of alcohol or drugs in blood (R78.-)

● **Z02.84 Encounter for child welfare exam**
Encounter for child welfare screening exam
EXCLUDES 2 *encounter for examination and observation for alleged child physical abuse (Z04.72)*
encounter for examination and observation for alleged child rape (Z04.42)

Z02.89 **Encounter for other administrative examinations** UPD
Encounter for examination for admission to prison
Encounter for examination for admission to summer camp
Encounter for immigration examination
Encounter for naturalization examination
Encounter for premarital examination
EXCLUDES 1 *health supervision of foundling or other healthy infant or child (Z76.1-Z76.2)*

Z02.9 **Encounter for administrative examinations, unspecified** UPD

✓4th Z03 **Encounter for medical observation for suspected diseases and conditions ruled out**
This category is to be used when a person without a diagnosis is suspected of having an abnormal condition, without signs or symptoms, which requires study, but after examination and observation, is ruled out. This category is also for use for administrative and legal observation status.
EXCLUDES 1 *contact with and (suspected) exposures hazardous to health (Z77.-)*
encounter for observation and evaluation of newborn for suspected diseases and conditions ruled out (Z05.-)
person with feared complaint in whom no diagnosis is made (Z71.1)
signs or symptoms under study - code to signs or symptoms
AHA: 2020,2Q,8; 2018,2Q,7-8; 2017,4Q,27

Z03.6 **Encounter for observation for suspected toxic effect from ingested substance ruled out**
Encounter for observation for suspected adverse effect from drug
Encounter for observation for suspected poisoning

✓5th Z03.7 **Encounter for suspected maternal and fetal conditions ruled out**
Encounter for suspected maternal and fetal conditions not found
EXCLUDES 1 *known or suspected fetal anomalies affecting management of mother, not ruled out (O26.-, O35.-, O36.-, O40.-, O41.-)*

Z03.71 **Encounter for suspected problem with amniotic cavity and membrane ruled out** UPD M ♀
Encounter for suspected oligohydramnios ruled out
Encounter for suspected polyhydramnios ruled out

Z03.72 **Encounter for suspected placental problem ruled out** UPD M ♀

Z03.73 **Encounter for suspected fetal anomaly ruled out** UPD M ♀

Z03.74 **Encounter for suspected problem with fetal growth ruled out** UPD M ♀

Z03.75 **Encounter for suspected cervical shortening ruled out** UPD M ♀

Z03.79 **Encounter for other suspected maternal and fetal conditions ruled out** UPD M ♀

✓5th Z03.8 **Encounter for observation for other suspected diseases and conditions ruled out**

✓6th Z03.81 **Encounter for observation for suspected exposure to biological agents ruled out**

Z03.810 **Encounter for observation for suspected exposure to anthrax ruled out**

Z03.818 **Encounter for observation for suspected exposure to other biological agents ruled out**
AHA: 2020,2Q,8; 2020,1Q,34-36
TIP: During the COVID-19 pandemic, possible exposure to COVID-19 should be coded using Z20.822 Contact with and (suspected) exposure to COVID-19, even when the COVID-19 infection has been ruled out.

✓6th Z03.82 **Encounter for observation for suspected foreign body ruled out**
EXCLUDES 1 *retained foreign body (Z18.-)*
retained foreign body in eyelid (H02.81)
residual foreign body in soft tissue (M79.5)
EXCLUDES 2 *confirmed foreign body ingestion or aspiration including:*
foreign body in alimentary tract (T18)
foreign body in ear (T16)
foreign body on external eye (T15)
foreign body in respiratory tract (T17)
AHA: 2020,4Q,42

Z03.821 **Encounter for observation for suspected ingested foreign body ruled out** UPD

Z03.822 **Encounter for observation for suspected aspirated (inhaled) foreign body ruled out** UPD

Z03.823 **Encounter for observation for suspected inserted (injected) foreign body ruled out** UPD
Encounter for observation for suspected inserted (injected) foreign body in eye ruled out
Encounter for observation for suspected inserted (injected) foreign body in orifice ruled out
Encounter for observation for suspected inserted (injected) foreign body in skin ruled out

Z03.83 **Encounter for observation for suspected conditions related to home physiologic monitoring device ruled out** UPD
Encounter for observation for apnea alarm without findings
Encounter for observation for bradycardia alarm without findings
Encounter for observation for malfunction of home cardiorespiratory monitor
Encounter for observation for non-specific findings home physiologic monitoring device
Encounter for observation for pulse oximeter alarm without findings
EXCLUDES 1 *apnea NOS (R06.81)*
neonatal bradycardia (P29.12)
newborn apnea (P28.4-)
primary sleep apnea of newborn (P28.3-)
sleep apnea (G47.3-)
AHA: 2022,4Q,51

Z03.89 **Encounter for observation for other suspected diseases and conditions ruled out**

✓4th Z04 **Encounter for examination and observation for other reasons**
INCLUDES encounter for examination for medicolegal reasons
This category is to be used when a person without a diagnosis is suspected of having an abnormal condition, without signs or symptoms, which requires study, but after examination and observation, is ruled-out. This category is also for use for administrative and legal observation status.
AHA: 2018,2Q,7-8

Z04.1 **Encounter for examination and observation following transport accident**
EXCLUDES 1 *encounter for examination and observation following work accident (Z04.2)*
AHA: 2019,2Q,11; 2018,2Q,8

Z04.2 **Encounter for examination and observation following work accident**

Z04.3 **Encounter for examination and observation following other accident**

✓5th Z04.4 **Encounter for examination and observation following alleged rape**
Encounter for examination and observation of victim following alleged rape
Encounter for examination and observation of victim following alleged sexual abuse

Z04.41 **Encounter for examination and observation following alleged adult rape** A
Suspected adult rape, ruled out
Suspected adult sexual abuse, ruled out

Z04.42 Encounter for examination and observation following alleged child rape P
Suspected child rape, ruled out
Suspected child sexual abuse, ruled out

Z04.6 Encounter for general psychiatric examination, requested by authority

✓5th **Z04.7 Encounter for examination and observation following alleged physical abuse**

Z04.71 Encounter for examination and observation following alleged adult physical abuse A
Suspected adult physical abuse, ruled out
EXCLUDES 1 *confirmed case of adult physical abuse (T74.-)*
encounter for examination and observation following alleged adult sexual abuse (Z04.41)
suspected case of adult physical abuse, not ruled out (T76.-)

Z04.72 Encounter for examination and observation following alleged child physical abuse P
Suspected child physical abuse, ruled out
EXCLUDES 1 *confirmed case of child physical abuse (T74.-)*
encounter for examination and observation following alleged child sexual abuse (Z04.42)
suspected case of child physical abuse, not ruled out (T76.-)

✓5th **Z04.8 Encounter for examination and observation for other specified reasons**
Encounter for examination and observation for request for expert evidence
AHA: 2018,4Q,32,35,72

Z04.81 Encounter for examination and observation of victim following forced sexual exploitation

Z04.82 Encounter for examination and observation of victim following forced labor exploitation

Z04.89 Encounter for examination and observation for other specified reasons

Z04.9 Encounter for examination and observation for unspecified reason UPD
Encounter for observation NOS

✓4th **Z05 Encounter for observation and evaluation of newborn for suspected diseases and conditions ruled out**
This category is to be used for newborns, within the neonatal period (the first 28 days of life), who are suspected of having an abnormal condition, but without signs or symptoms, and which, after examination and observation, is ruled out.
AHA: 2022,1Q,17-18; 2017,4Q,27; 2016,4Q,77

Z05.0 Observation and evaluation of newborn for suspected cardiac condition ruled out N

Z05.1 Observation and evaluation of newborn for suspected infectious condition ruled out N
AHA: 2019,2Q,10

Z05.2 Observation and evaluation of newborn for suspected neurological condition ruled out N

Z05.3 Observation and evaluation of newborn for suspected respiratory condition ruled out N

✓5th **Z05.4 Observation and evaluation of newborn for suspected genetic, metabolic or immunologic condition ruled out**

Z05.41 Observation and evaluation of newborn for suspected genetic condition ruled out N
AHA: 2016,4Q,55

Z05.42 Observation and evaluation of newborn for suspected metabolic condition ruled out N

Z05.43 Observation and evaluation of newborn for suspected immunologic condition ruled out N

Z05.5 Observation and evaluation of newborn for suspected gastrointestinal condition ruled out N

Z05.6 Observation and evaluation of newborn for suspected genitourinary condition ruled out N

✓5th **Z05.7 Observation and evaluation of newborn for suspected skin, subcutaneous, musculoskeletal and connective tissue condition ruled out**

Z05.71 Observation and evaluation of newborn for suspected skin and subcutaneous tissue condition ruled out N

Z05.72 Observation and evaluation of newborn for suspected musculoskeletal condition ruled out N

Z05.73 Observation and evaluation of newborn for suspected connective tissue condition ruled out N

▲ ✓5th **Z05.8 Observation and evaluation of newborn for other specified suspected condition ruled out**
AHA: 2022,1Q,17-18

● **Z05.81 Observation and evaluation of newborn for suspected condition related to home physiologic monitoring device ruled out**
Encounter for observation of newborn for apnea alarm without findings
Encounter for observation of newborn for bradycardia alarm without findings
Encounter for observation of newborn for malfunction of home cardiorespiratory monitor
Encounter for observation of newborn for non-specific findings home physiologic monitoring device
Encounter for observation of newborn for pulse oximeter alarm without findings
EXCLUDES 1 *encounter for observation for suspected conditions related to home physiologic monitoring device ruled out (Z03.83)*
neonatal bradycardia (P29.12)
other newborn apnea (P28.4-)
primary sleep apnea of newborn (P28.3-)

● **Z05.89 Observation and evaluation of newborn for other specified suspected condition ruled out**

Z05.9 Observation and evaluation of newborn for unspecified suspected condition ruled out N

Z08 Encounter for follow-up examination after completed treatment for malignant neoplasm UPD
Medical surveillance following completed treatment
Use additional code to identify any acquired absence of organs (Z90.-)
Use additional code to identify the personal history of malignant neoplasm (Z85.-)
EXCLUDES 1 *aftercare following medical care (Z43-Z49, Z51)*
AHA: 2020,3Q,30

Z09 Encounter for follow-up examination after completed treatment for conditions other than malignant neoplasm UPD
Medical surveillance following completed treatment
Use additional code to identify any applicable history of disease code (Z86.-, Z87.-)
EXCLUDES 1 *aftercare following medical care (Z43-Z49, Z51)*
surveillance of contraception (Z30.4-)
surveillance of prosthetic and other medical devices (Z44-Z46)
AHA: 2022,3Q,4; 2021,1Q,33; 2020,2Q,10; 2017,1Q,9; 2015,1Q,8

✓4th **Z11 Encounter for screening for infectious and parasitic diseases**
Screening is the testing for disease or disease precursors in asymptomatic individuals so that early detection and treatment can be provided for those who test positive for the disease.
EXCLUDES 1 *encounter for diagnostic examination - code to sign or symptom*

Z11.0 Encounter for screening for intestinal infectious diseases UPD

Z11.1 Encounter for screening for respiratory tuberculosis UPD
Encounter for screening for active tuberculosis disease

Z11.2 Encounter for screening for other bacterial diseases UPD

Z11.3 Encounter for screening for infections with a predominantly sexual mode of transmission UPD
EXCLUDES 2 *encounter for screening for human immunodeficiency virus [HIV] (Z11.4)*
encounter for screening for human papillomavirus (Z11.51)

Z11.4 Encounter for screening for human immunodeficiency virus [HIV] UPD

✓5th **Z11.5 Encounter for screening for other viral diseases**
EXCLUDES 2 *encounter for screening for viral intestinal disease (Z11.0)*

Z11.51 Encounter for screening for human papillomavirus (HPV) UPD

Z11.52 Encounter for screening for COVID-19 UPD
AHA: 2023,2Q,3; 2021,1Q,27,37,41

Z11.59 Encounter for screening for other viral diseases UPD
AHA: 2020,3Q,14

Z11.6 Encounter for screening for other protozoal diseases and helminthiases UPD
EXCLUDES 2 *encounter for screening for protozoal intestinal disease (Z11.Ø)*

Z11.7 Encounter for testing for latent tuberculosis infection UPD
AHA: 2019,4Q,20

Z11.8 Encounter for screening for other infectious and parasitic diseases UPD
Encounter for screening for chlamydia
Encounter for screening for rickettsial
Encounter for screening for spirochetal
Encounter for screening for mycoses

Z11.9 Encounter for screening for infectious and parasitic diseases, unspecified UPD

✓4th **Z12 Encounter for screening for malignant neoplasms**
Screening is the testing for disease or disease precursors in asymptomatic individuals so that early detection and treatment can be provided for those who test positive for the disease.
Use additional code to identify any family history of malignant neoplasm (Z8Ø.-)
EXCLUDES 1 *encounter for diagnostic examination - code to sign or symptom*

Z12.Ø Encounter for screening for malignant neoplasm of stomach UPD

✓5th **Z12.1 Encounter for screening for malignant neoplasm of intestinal tract**
AHA: 2017,1Q,8,9

Z12.1Ø Encounter for screening for malignant neoplasm of intestinal tract, unspecified UPD

Z12.11 Encounter for screening for malignant neoplasm of colon UPD
Encounter for screening colonoscopy NOS
AHA: 2019,1Q,32-33; 2018,1Q,6

Z12.12 Encounter for screening for malignant neoplasm of rectum UPD
AHA: 2018,1Q,6

Z12.13 Encounter for screening for malignant neoplasm of small intestine UPD

Z12.2 Encounter for screening for malignant neoplasm of respiratory organs UPD

✓5th **Z12.3 Encounter for screening for malignant neoplasm of breast**

Z12.31 Encounter for screening mammogram for malignant neoplasm of breast UPD
EXCLUDES 1 *inconclusive mammogram (R92.2)*
AHA: 2015,1Q,24

Z12.39 Encounter for other screening for malignant neoplasm of breast UPD

Z12.4 Encounter for screening for malignant neoplasm of cervix UPD ♀
Encounter for screening pap smear for malignant neoplasm of cervix
EXCLUDES 1 *when screening is part of general gynecological examination (ZØ1.4-)*
EXCLUDES 2 *encounter for screening for human papillomavirus (Z11.51)*

Z12.5 Encounter for screening for malignant neoplasm of prostate ♂

Z12.6 Encounter for screening for malignant neoplasm of bladder UPD

✓5th **Z12.7 Encounter for screening for malignant neoplasm of other genitourinary organs**

Z12.71 Encounter for screening for malignant neoplasm of testis UPD ♂

Z12.72 Encounter for screening for malignant neoplasm of vagina UPD ♀
Vaginal pap smear status-post hysterectomy for non-malignant condition
Use additional code to identify acquired absence of uterus (Z9Ø.71-)
EXCLUDES 1 *vaginal pap smear status-post hysterectomy for malignant conditions (ZØ8)*

Z12.73 Encounter for screening for malignant neoplasm of ovary UPD ♀

Z12.79 Encounter for screening for malignant neoplasm of other genitourinary organs UPD

✓5th **Z12.8 Encounter for screening for malignant neoplasm of other sites**

Z12.81 Encounter for screening for malignant neoplasm of oral cavity UPD

Z12.82 Encounter for screening for malignant neoplasm of nervous system UPD

Z12.83 Encounter for screening for malignant neoplasm of skin UPD

Z12.89 Encounter for screening for malignant neoplasm of other sites UPD
AHA: 2021,1Q,14

Z12.9 Encounter for screening for malignant neoplasm, site unspecified UPD

✓4th **Z13 Encounter for screening for other diseases and disorders**
Screening is the testing for disease or disease precursors in asymptomatic individuals so that early detection and treatment can be provided for those who test positive for the disease.
EXCLUDES 1 *encounter for diagnostic examination - code to sign or symptom*

Z13.Ø Encounter for screening for diseases of the blood and blood-forming organs and certain disorders involving the immune mechanism UPD

Z13.1 Encounter for screening for diabetes mellitus UPD

✓5th **Z13.2 Encounter for screening for nutritional, metabolic and other endocrine disorders**

Z13.21 Encounter for screening for nutritional disorder UPD

✓6th **Z13.22 Encounter for screening for metabolic disorder**

Z13.22Ø Encounter for screening for lipoid disorders UPD
Encounter for screening for cholesterol level
Encounter for screening for hypercholesterolemia
Encounter for screening for hyperlipidemia

Z13.228 Encounter for screening for other metabolic disorders UPD

Z13.29 Encounter for screening for other suspected endocrine disorder UPD
EXCLUDES 2 *encounter for screening for diabetes mellitus (Z13.1)*

✓5th **Z13.3 Encounter for screening examination for mental health and behavioral disorders**
AHA: 2018,4Q,35-36

Z13.3Ø Encounter for screening examination for mental health and behavioral disorders, unspecified UPD

Z13.31 Encounter for screening for depression UPD
Encounter for screening for depression, adult
Encounter for screening for depression for child or adolescent

Z13.32 Encounter for screening for maternal depression UPD ♀
Encounter for screening for perinatal depression

Z13.39 Encounter for screening examination for other mental health and behavioral disorders UPD
Encounter for screening for alcoholism
Encounter for screening for intellectual disabilities

✓5th **Z13.4 Encounter for screening for certain developmental disorders in childhood**
Encounter for development testing of infant or child
Encounter for screening for developmental handicaps in early childhood
EXCLUDES 2 *encounter for routine child health examination (ZØØ.12-)*
AHA: 2018,4Q,36

Z13.4Ø Encounter for screening for unspecified developmental delays UPD

Z13.41 Encounter for autism screening UPD

Z13.42 Encounter for screening for global developmental delays (milestones) UPD
Encounter for screening for developmental handicaps in early childhood

Z13.49 Encounter for screening for other developmental delays UPD

Z13.5 Encounter for screening for eye and ear disorders UPD
EXCLUDES 2 *encounter for general hearing examination (ZØ1.1-)*
encounter for general vision examination (ZØ1.Ø-)
AHA: 2016,3Q,17

Z13.6 Encounter for screening for cardiovascular disorders UPD

Z13.7 Encounter for screening for genetic and chromosomal anomalies
EXCLUDES 1 *genetic testing for procreative management (Z31.4-)*
Z13.71 Encounter for nonprocreative screening for genetic disease carrier status UPD
Z13.79 Encounter for other screening for genetic and chromosomal anomalies UPD

Z13.8 Encounter for screening for other specified diseases and disorders
EXCLUDES 2 *screening for malignant neoplasms (Z12.-)*
Z13.81 Encounter for screening for digestive system disorders
Z13.810 Encounter for screening for upper gastrointestinal disorder UPD
Z13.811 Encounter for screening for lower gastrointestinal disorder UPD
EXCLUDES 1 *encounter for screening for intestinal infectious disease (Z11.0)*
Z13.818 Encounter for screening for other digestive system disorders UPD
Z13.82 Encounter for screening for musculoskeletal disorder
Z13.820 Encounter for screening for osteoporosis UPD
Z13.828 Encounter for screening for other musculoskeletal disorder UPD
Z13.83 Encounter for screening for respiratory disorder NEC UPD
EXCLUDES 1 *encounter for screening for respiratory tuberculosis (Z11.1)*
Z13.84 Encounter for screening for dental disorders UPD
Z13.85 Encounter for screening for nervous system disorders
Z13.850 Encounter for screening for traumatic brain injury UPD
Z13.858 Encounter for screening for other nervous system disorders UPD
Z13.88 Encounter for screening for disorder due to exposure to contaminants UPD
EXCLUDES 1 *those exposed to contaminants without suspected disorders (Z57.-, Z77.-)*
Z13.89 Encounter for screening for other disorder UPD
Encounter for screening for genitourinary disorders
Z13.9 Encounter for screening, unspecified UPD

Genetic carrier and genetic susceptibility to disease (Z14-Z15)

Z14 Genetic carrier
DEF: Individuals carrying a gene mutation associated with a certain disease that typically do not develop the disease but are able to pass the mutated genes to offspring.
Z14.0 Hemophilia A carrier
Z14.01 Asymptomatic hemophilia A carrier UPD
Z14.02 Symptomatic hemophilia A carrier UPD
Z14.1 Cystic fibrosis carrier UPD
Z14.8 Genetic carrier of other disease UPD

Z15 Genetic susceptibility to disease
INCLUDES confirmed abnormal gene
Use additional code, if applicable, for any associated family history of the disease (Z80-Z84)
EXCLUDES 1 *chromosomal anomalies (Q90-Q99)*
Z15.0 Genetic susceptibility to malignant neoplasm
Code first, if applicable, any current malignant neoplasm (C00-C75, C81-C96)
Use additional code, if applicable, for any personal history of malignant neoplasm (Z85.-)
Z15.01 Genetic susceptibility to malignant neoplasm of breast UPD
Z15.02 Genetic susceptibility to malignant neoplasm of ovary UPD ♀
Z15.03 Genetic susceptibility to malignant neoplasm of prostate UPD ♂
Z15.04 Genetic susceptibility to malignant neoplasm of endometrium UPD ♀
Z15.09 Genetic susceptibility to other malignant neoplasm UPD
AHA: 2021,1Q,14
Z15.8 Genetic susceptibility to other disease
Z15.81 Genetic susceptibility to multiple endocrine neoplasia [MEN] UPD
EXCLUDES 1 *multiple endocrine neoplasia [MEN] syndromes (E31.2-)*
DEF: Group of conditions in which several endocrine glands grow excessively (such as in adenomatous hyperplasia) and/or develop benign or malignant tumors. Tumors and hyperplasia associated with MEN often produce excess hormones, which impede normal physiology. There is no comprehensive cure known for MEN syndrome. Treatment is directed at the hyperplasia or tumors in each individual gland. Tumors are usually surgically removed and oral medications or hormonal injections are used to correct hormone imbalances.
Z15.89 Genetic susceptibility to other disease UPD

Resistance to antimicrobial drugs (Z16)

Z16 Resistance to antimicrobial drugs
NOTE The codes in this category are provided for use as additional codes to identify the resistance and non-responsiveness of a condition to antimicrobial drugs.
Code first the infection
EXCLUDES 1 *Methicillin resistant Staphylococcus aureus infection (A49.02)*
Methicillin resistant Staphylococcus aureus pneumonia (J15.212)
sepsis due to Methicillin resistant Staphylococcus aureus (A41.02)
Z16.1 Resistance to beta lactam antibiotics
Z16.10 Resistance to unspecified beta lactam antibiotics CC UPD
Z16.11 Resistance to penicillins CC UPD
Resistance to amoxicillin
Resistance to ampicillin
Z16.12 Extended spectrum beta lactamase (ESBL) resistance CC UPD
EXCLUDES 2 *Methicillin resistant Staphylococcus aureus infection in diseases classified elsewhere (B95.62)*
• **Z16.13 Resistance to carbapenem** CC
Z16.19 Resistance to other specified beta lactam antibiotics CC UPD
Resistance to cephalosporins
Z16.2 Resistance to other antibiotics
Z16.20 Resistance to unspecified antibiotic CC UPD
Resistance to antibiotics NOS
Z16.21 Resistance to vancomycin CC UPD
Z16.22 Resistance to vancomycin related antibiotics CC UPD
Z16.23 Resistance to quinolones and fluoroquinolones CC UPD
Z16.24 Resistance to multiple antibiotics CC UPD
Z16.29 Resistance to other single specified antibiotic CC UPD
Resistance to aminoglycosides
Resistance to macrolides
Resistance to sulfonamides
Resistance to tetracyclines
Z16.3 Resistance to other antimicrobial drugs
EXCLUDES 1 *resistance to antibiotics (Z16.1-, Z16.2-)*
Z16.30 Resistance to unspecified antimicrobial drugs CC UPD
Drug resistance NOS
Z16.31 Resistance to antiparasitic drug(s) CC UPD
Resistance to quinine and related compounds
Z16.32 Resistance to antifungal drug(s) CC UPD
Z16.33 Resistance to antiviral drug(s) CC UPD
Z16.34 Resistance to antimycobacterial drug(s)
Resistance to tuberculostatics
Z16.341 Resistance to single antimycobacterial drug CC UPD
Resistance to antimycobacterial drug NOS
Z16.342 Resistance to multiple antimycobacterial drugs CC UPD

Z16.35 Resistance to multiple antimicrobial drugs CC UPD
EXCLUDES 1 *resistance to multiple antibiotics only (Z16.24)*

Z16.39 Resistance to other specified antimicrobial drug CC UPD

Estrogen receptor status (Z17)

✓4th **Z17 Estrogen receptor status**
Code first malignant neoplasm of breast (C50.-)
AHA: 2022,3Q,14
DEF: Receptor status of breast cancer cells for the hormone estrogen that is used to help determine treatment and evaluate prognosis. ER+ breast cancer responds to hormone therapies while ER- breast cancer does not.

Z17.0 Estrogen receptor positive status [ER+] UPD
Z17.1 Estrogen receptor negative status [ER-] UPD

Retained foreign body fragments (Z18)

✓4th **Z18 Retained foreign body fragments**
INCLUDES embedded fragment (status)
embedded splinter (status)
retained foreign body status
EXCLUDES 1 *artificial joint prosthesis status (Z96.6-)*
foreign body accidentally left during a procedure (T81.5-)
foreign body entering through orifice (T15-T19)
in situ cardiac device (Z95.-)
organ or tissue replaced by means other than transplant (Z96.-, Z97.-)
organ or tissue replaced by transplant (Z94.-)
personal history of retained foreign body fully removed Z87.821
superficial foreign body (non-embedded splinter) - code to superficial foreign body, by site
AHA: 2023,2Q,27
DEF: Embedded or retained fragment, splinter, or foreign body, natural or synthetic that can cause infection.

✓5th **Z18.0 Retained radioactive fragments**
Z18.01 Retained depleted uranium fragments UPD
Z18.09 Other retained radioactive fragments UPD
Other retained depleted isotope fragments
Retained nontherapeutic radioactive fragments

✓5th **Z18.1 Retained metal fragments**
EXCLUDES 1 *retained radioactive metal fragments (Z18.01-Z18.09)*
Z18.10 Retained metal fragments, unspecified UPD
Retained metal fragment NOS
Z18.11 Retained magnetic metal fragments UPD
Z18.12 Retained nonmagnetic metal fragments UPD

Z18.2 Retained plastic fragments UPD
Acrylics fragments
Diethylhexyl phthalates fragments
Isocyanate fragments

✓5th **Z18.3 Retained organic fragments**
Z18.31 Retained animal quills or spines UPD
Z18.32 Retained tooth UPD
Z18.33 Retained wood fragments UPD
Z18.39 Other retained organic fragments UPD

✓5th **Z18.8 Other specified retained foreign body**
Z18.81 Retained glass fragments UPD
Z18.83 Retained stone or crystalline fragments UPD
Retained concrete or cement fragments
Z18.89 Other specified retained foreign body fragments UPD

Z18.9 Retained foreign body fragments, unspecified material UPD

Hormone sensitivity malignancy status (Z19)

✓4th **Z19 Hormone sensitivity malignancy status**
Code first malignant neoplasm — see Table of Neoplasms, by site, malignant
AHA: 2016,4Q,76

Z19.1 Hormone sensitive malignancy status UPD
Z19.2 Hormone resistant malignancy status UPD
Castrate resistant prostate malignancy status

Persons with potential health hazards related to communicable diseases (Z20-Z29)

✓4th **Z20 Contact with and (suspected) exposure to communicable diseases**
EXCLUDES 1 *carrier of infectious disease (Z22.-)*
diagnosed current infectious or parasitic disease - see Alphabetic Index
EXCLUDES 2 *personal history of infectious and parasitic diseases (Z86.1-)*

✓5th **Z20.0 Contact with and (suspected) exposure to intestinal infectious diseases**
Z20.01 Contact with and (suspected) exposure to intestinal infectious diseases due to Escherichia coli (E. coli)
Z20.09 Contact with and (suspected) exposure to other intestinal infectious diseases UPD

Z20.1 Contact with and (suspected) exposure to tuberculosis UPD
Z20.2 Contact with and (suspected) exposure to infections with a predominantly sexual mode of transmission UPD
Z20.3 Contact with and (suspected) exposure to rabies UPD
Z20.4 Contact with and (suspected) exposure to rubella UPD
Z20.5 Contact with and (suspected) exposure to viral hepatitis
Z20.6 Contact with and (suspected) exposure to human immunodeficiency virus [HIV]
EXCLUDES 1 *asymptomatic human immunodeficiency virus [HIV] HIV infection status (Z21)*
Z20.7 Contact with and (suspected) exposure to pediculosis, acariasis and other infestations UPD

✓5th **Z20.8 Contact with and (suspected) exposure to other communicable diseases**
✓6th **Z20.81 Contact with and (suspected) exposure to other bacterial communicable diseases**
Z20.810 Contact with and (suspected) exposure to anthrax UPD
Z20.811 Contact with and (suspected) exposure to meningococcus
Z20.818 Contact with and (suspected) exposure to other bacterial communicable diseases UPD
AHA: 2019,2Q,10

✓6th **Z20.82 Contact with and (suspected) exposure to other viral communicable diseases**
Z20.820 Contact with and (suspected) exposure to varicella
Z20.821 Contact with and (suspected) exposure to Zika virus UPD
AHA: 2018,4Q,35,64
Z20.822 Contact with and (suspected) exposure to COVID-19 UPD
Contact with and (suspected) exposure to SARS-CoV-2
AHA: 2023,2Q,3; 2022,2Q,28-29; 2021,4Q,109; 2021,1Q,27-29,37-38,41
Z20.828 Contact with and (suspected) exposure to other viral communicable diseases
AHA: 2022,3Q,4; 2021,1Q,37-38; 2020,4Q,99; 2020,3Q,14-15; 2020,2Q,4,8; 2020,1Q,34-36

Z20.89 Contact with and (suspected) exposure to other communicable diseases UPD

Z20.9 Contact with and (suspected) exposure to unspecified communicable disease UPD

Z21 Asymptomatic human immunodeficiency virus [HIV] infection status HCC
HIV positive NOS
Code first human immunodeficiency virus [HIV] disease complicating pregnancy, childbirth and the puerperium, if applicable (O98.7-)
EXCLUDES 1 *acquired immunodeficiency syndrome (B20)*
contact with human immunodeficiency virus [HIV] (Z20.6)
exposure to human immunodeficiency virus [HIV] (Z20.6)
human immunodeficiency virus [HIV] disease (B20)
inconclusive laboratory evidence of human immunodeficiency virus [HIV] (R75)
AHA: 2022,1Q,36; 2019,1Q,8-11
DEF: Phase of human immunodeficiency virus (HIV) infection with no clinical symptoms. This phase may last for 10 years or more.

Z22 Carrier of infectious disease
INCLUDES colonization status
suspected carrier
EXCLUDES 2 *carrier of viral hepatitis (B18.-)*

Z22.0 Carrier of typhoid UPD
Z22.1 Carrier of other intestinal infectious diseases UPD
Z22.2 Carrier of diphtheria UPD
Z22.3 Carrier of other specified bacterial diseases
Z22.31 Carrier of bacterial disease due to meningococci UPD
Z22.32 Carrier of bacterial disease due to staphylococci
Z22.321 Carrier or suspected carrier of Methicillin susceptible Staphylococcus aureus UPD
MSSA colonization
Z22.322 Carrier or suspected carrier of Methicillin resistant Staphylococcus aureus UPD
MRSA colonization
DEF: Carriers (colonization) of methicillin resistant *Staphylococcus aureus* (MRSA) have MRSA on their skin or in their body but do not exhibit signs of infection. These individuals are able to pass MRSA on to others who may develop an infection.
Z22.33 Carrier of bacterial disease due to streptococci
Z22.330 Carrier of Group B streptococcus UPD
EXCLUDES 1 *carrier of streptococcus group B (GBS) complicating pregnancy, childbirth and the puerperium (O99.82-)*
Z22.338 Carrier of other streptococcus UPD
● **Z22.34 Carrier of Acinetobacter baumannii**
● **Z22.340 Carrier of carbapenem-resistant Acinetobacter baumannii**
● **Z22.341 Carrier of carbapenem-sensitive Acinetobacter baumannii**
● **Z22.349 Carrier of Acinetobacter baumannii, unspecified**
● **Z22.35 Carrier of Enterobacterales**
Carrier of E. coli
Carrier of K. pneumoniae
● **Z22.350 Carrier of carbapenem-resistant Enterobacterales**
● **Z22.358 Carrier of other Enterobacterales**
Carrier of carbapenem-sensitive Enterobacterales
Carrier of ESBL-producing Enterobacterales
Carrier of extended-spectrum beta-lactamase producing Enterobacterales
● **Z22.359 Carrier of Enterobacterales, unspecified**
Z22.39 Carrier of other specified bacterial diseases UPD
Z22.4 Carrier of infections with a predominantly sexual mode of transmission UPD
Z22.6 Carrier of human T-lymphotropic virus type-1 [HTLV-1] infection UPD
Z22.7 Latent tuberculosis UPD
Latent tuberculosis infection (LTBI)
EXCLUDES 1 *nonspecific reaction to cell mediated immunity measurement of gamma interferon antigen response without active tuberculosis (R76.12)*
nonspecific reaction to tuberculin skin test without active tuberculosis (R76.11)
AHA: 2019,4Q,19
Z22.8 Carrier of other infectious diseases UPD
Z22.9 Carrier of infectious disease, unspecified UPD

Z23 Encounter for immunization UPD
NOTE Procedure codes are required to identify the types of immunizations given
Code first any routine childhood examination
Code also, if applicable, encounter for immunization safety counseling (Z71.85)

Z28 Immunization not carried out and underimmunization status
INCLUDES vaccination not carried out
Code also, if applicable, encounter for immunization safety counseling (Z71.85)

Z28.0 Immunization not carried out because of contraindication
DEF: Contraindication: Situation where a drug, surgery, or other procedure may negatively affect or cause harm to a patient.
Z28.01 Immunization not carried out because of acute illness of patient UPD
Z28.02 Immunization not carried out because of chronic illness or condition of patient UPD
Z28.03 Immunization not carried out because of immune compromised state of patient UPD
Z28.04 Immunization not carried out because of patient allergy to vaccine or component UPD
Z28.09 Immunization not carried out because of other contraindication UPD
Z28.1 Immunization not carried out because of patient decision for reasons of belief or group pressure UPD
Immunization not carried out because of religious belief
Z28.2 Immunization not carried out because of patient decision for other and unspecified reason
Z28.20 Immunization not carried out because of patient decision for unspecified reason UPD
Z28.21 Immunization not carried out because of patient refusal UPD
Z28.29 Immunization not carried out because of patient decision for other reason UPD
Z28.3 Underimmunization status
Use additional code, if applicable, to identify:
immunization not carried out because of contraindication (Z28.0-)
immunization not carried out because of patient decision for other and unspecified reason (Z28.2-)
immunization not carried out because of patient decision for reasons of belief or group pressure (Z28.1)
immunization not carried out for other reason (Z28.8-)
AHA: 2022,1Q,4-5
Z28.31 Underimmunization for COVID-19 status
NOTE These codes should not be used for individuals who are not eligible for the COVID-19 vaccines, as determined by the healthcare provider.
Z28.310 Unvaccinated for COVID-19 UPD
Z28.311 Partially vaccinated for COVID-19 UPD
Z28.39 Other underimmunization status UPD
Delinquent immunization status
Lapsed immunization schedule status
Z28.8 Immunization not carried out for other reason
Z28.81 Immunization not carried out due to patient having had the disease UPD
Z28.82 Immunization not carried out because of caregiver refusal UPD
Immunization not carried out because of guardian refusal
Immunization not carried out because of parent refusal
EXCLUDES 1 *immunization not carried out because of caregiver refusal because of religious belief (Z28.1)*
Z28.83 Immunization not carried out due to unavailability of vaccine UPD
Delay in delivery of vaccine
Lack of availability of vaccine
Manufacturer delay of vaccine
AHA: 2018,4Q,36
Z28.89 Immunization not carried out for other reason UPD
Z28.9 Immunization not carried out for unspecified reason UPD

Z29 Encounter for other prophylactic measures
EXCLUDES 1 *desensitization to allergens (Z51.6)*
prophylactic surgery (Z40.-)
AHA: 2016,4Q,78-79
Z29.1 Encounter for prophylactic immunotherapy
Encounter for administration of immunoglobulin
Z29.11 Encounter for prophylactic immunotherapy for respiratory syncytial virus (RSV) UPD

Z29.12 Encounter for prophylactic antivenin UPD

Z29.13 Encounter for prophylactic Rho(D) immune globulin UPD
AHA: 2019,3Q,5

Z29.14 Encounter for prophylactic rabies immune globulin UPD

Z29.3 Encounter for prophylactic fluoride administration UPD

▲ ✓5th Z29.8 Encounter for other specified prophylactic measures
AHA: 2022,2Q,27

● Z29.81 Encounter for HIV pre-exposure prophylaxis
Code also, if applicable, risk factors for HIV, such as:
contact with and (suspected) exposure to human immunodeficiency virus [HIV] (Z20.6)
high risk sexual behavior (Z72.5-)

● Z29.89 Encounter for other specified prophylactic measures

Z29.9 Encounter for prophylactic measures, unspecified UPD

Persons encountering health services in circumstances related to reproduction (Z30-Z39)

✓4th **Z30 Encounter for contraceptive management**
AHA: 2016,4Q,78
DEF: Contraceptive management to prevent pregnancy. Methods include oral medications, intrauterine devices, and surgical procedures for males and females (sterilization).

✓5th Z30.0 Encounter for general counseling and advice on contraception

✓6th Z30.01 Encounter for initial prescription of contraceptives
EXCLUDES 1 *encounter for surveillance of contraceptives (Z30.4-)*

Z30.011 Encounter for initial prescription of contraceptive pills UPD ♀

Z30.012 Encounter for prescription of emergency contraception UPD ♀
Encounter for postcoital contraception

Z30.013 Encounter for initial prescription of injectable contraceptive UPD ♀

Z30.014 Encounter for initial prescription of intrauterine contraceptive device UPD ♀
EXCLUDES 1 *encounter for insertion of intrauterine contraceptive device (Z30.430, Z30.432)*

Z30.015 Encounter for initial prescription of vaginal ring hormonal contraceptive UPD ♀

Z30.016 Encounter for initial prescription of transdermal patch hormonal contraceptive device UPD

Z30.017 Encounter for initial prescription of implantable subdermal contraceptive UPD

Z30.018 Encounter for initial prescription of other contraceptives UPD ♀
Encounter for initial prescription of barrier contraception
Encounter for initial prescription of diaphragm

Z30.019 Encounter for initial prescription of contraceptives, unspecified UPD ♀

Z30.02 Counseling and instruction in natural family planning to avoid pregnancy UPD

Z30.09 Encounter for other general counseling and advice on contraception UPD
Encounter for family planning advice NOS

Z30.2 Encounter for sterilization
AHA: 2021,3Q,13

✓5th Z30.4 Encounter for surveillance of contraceptives

Z30.40 Encounter for surveillance of contraceptives, unspecified UPD

Z30.41 Encounter for surveillance of contraceptive pills UPD ♀
Encounter for repeat prescription for contraceptive pill

Z30.42 Encounter for surveillance of injectable contraceptive UPD ♀

✓6th Z30.43 Encounter for surveillance of intrauterine contraceptive device

Z30.430 Encounter for insertion of intrauterine contraceptive device UPD ♀

Z30.431 Encounter for routine checking of intrauterine contraceptive device UPD ♀

Z30.432 Encounter for removal of intrauterine contraceptive device UPD ♀

Z30.433 Encounter for removal and reinsertion of intrauterine contraceptive device UPD ♀
Encounter for replacement of intrauterine contraceptive device

Z30.44 Encounter for surveillance of vaginal ring hormonal contraceptive device UPD ♀

Z30.45 Encounter for surveillance of transdermal patch hormonal contraceptive device UPD ♀

Z30.46 Encounter for surveillance of implantable subdermal contraceptive UPD ♀
Encounter for checking, reinsertion or removal of implantable subdermal contraceptive

Z30.49 Encounter for surveillance of other contraceptives UPD ♀
Encounter for surveillance of barrier contraception
Encounter for surveillance of diaphragm

Z30.8 Encounter for other contraceptive management UPD
Encounter for postvasectomy sperm count
Encounter for routine examination for contraceptive maintenance
EXCLUDES 1 *sperm count following sterilization reversal (Z31.42)*
sperm count for fertility testing (Z31.41)

Z30.9 Encounter for contraceptive management, unspecified UPD

✓4th **Z31 Encounter for procreative management**
EXCLUDES 2 *complications associated with artificial fertilization (N98.-)*
female infertility (N97.-)
male infertility (N46.-)

Z31.0 Encounter for reversal of previous sterilization

✓5th Z31.4 Encounter for procreative investigation and testing
EXCLUDES 1 *postvasectomy sperm count (Z30.8)*

Z31.41 Encounter for fertility testing UPD
Encounter for fallopian tube patency testing
Encounter for sperm count for fertility testing

Z31.42 Aftercare following sterilization reversal UPD
Sperm count following sterilization reversal

✓6th Z31.43 Encounter for genetic testing of female for procreative management
Use additional code for recurrent pregnancy loss, if applicable (N96, O26.2-)
EXCLUDES 1 *nonprocreative genetic testing (Z13.7-)*

Z31.430 Encounter of female for testing for genetic disease carrier status for procreative management UPD ♀

Z31.438 Encounter for other genetic testing of female for procreative management UPD ♀

✓6th Z31.44 Encounter for genetic testing of male for procreative management
EXCLUDES 1 *nonprocreative genetic testing (Z13.7-)*

Z31.440 Encounter of male for testing for genetic disease carrier status for procreative management UPD ♂

Z31.441 Encounter for testing of male partner of patient with recurrent pregnancy loss UPD A ♂

Z31.448 Encounter for other genetic testing of male for procreative management UPD A ♂

Z31.49 Encounter for other procreative investigation and testing UPD

Z31.5 Encounter for procreative genetic counseling UPD
AHA: 2017,4Q,27

✓5th Z31.6 Encounter for general counseling and advice on procreation

Z31.61 Procreative counseling and advice using natural family planning UPD

Z31.62 Encounter for fertility preservation counseling UPD
Encounter for fertility preservation counseling prior to cancer therapy
Encounter for fertility preservation counseling prior to surgical removal of gonads

Z31.69 Encounter for other general counseling and advice on procreation UPD

Z31.7 Encounter for procreative management and counseling for gestational carrier UPD ♀
EXCLUDES 1 *pregnant state, gestational carrier (Z33.3)*
AHA: 2016,4Q,78

✓5th **Z31.8 Encounter for other procreative management**

Z31.81 Encounter for male factor infertility in female patient UPD ♀

Z31.82 Encounter for Rh incompatibility status UPD ♀
AHA: 2015,3Q,40; 2014,4Q,17

Z31.83 Encounter for assisted reproductive fertility procedure cycle UPD ♀
Patient undergoing in vitro fertilization cycle
Use additional code to identify the type of infertility
EXCLUDES 1 *pre-cycle diagnosis and testing - code to reason for encounter*
AHA: 2022,2Q,15-16

Z31.84 Encounter for fertility preservation procedure UPD
Encounter for fertility preservation procedure prior to cancer therapy
Encounter for fertility preservation procedure prior to surgical removal of gonads

Z31.89 Encounter for other procreative management UPD

Z31.9 Encounter for procreative management, unspecified UPD

✓4th **Z32 Encounter for pregnancy test and childbirth and childcare instruction**

✓5th **Z32.0 Encounter for pregnancy test**

Z32.00 Encounter for pregnancy test, result unknown ♀
Encounter for pregnancy test NOS

Z32.01 Encounter for pregnancy test, result positive M ♀

Z32.02 Encounter for pregnancy test, result negative ♀

Z32.2 Encounter for childbirth instruction UPD

Z32.3 Encounter for childcare instruction UPD
Encounter for prenatal or postpartum childcare instruction

✓4th **Z33 Pregnant state**

Z33.1 Pregnant state, incidental UPD M ♀
Pregnancy NOS
Pregnant state NOS
EXCLUDES 1 *complications of pregnancy (O00-O9A)*
pregnant state, gestational carrier (Z33.3)

Z33.2 Encounter for elective termination of pregnancy M ♀
EXCLUDES 1 *early fetal death with retention of dead fetus (O02.1)*
late fetal death (O36.4)
spontaneous abortion (O03)
AHA: 2023,2Q,15; 2022,1Q,20
TIP: Do not assign a code from category Z3A with this code.

Z33.3 Pregnant state, gestational carrier UPD M ♀
EXCLUDES 1 *encounter for procreative management and counseling for gestational carrier (Z31.7)*
AHA: 2016,4Q,78

✓4th **Z34 Encounter for supervision of normal pregnancy**
EXCLUDES 1 *any complication of pregnancy (O00-O9A)*
encounter for pregnancy test (Z32.0-)
encounter for supervision of high risk pregnancy (O09.-)
AHA: 2019,3Q,5; 2014,4Q,17

✓5th **Z34.0 Encounter for supervision of normal first pregnancy**

Z34.00 Encounter for supervision of normal first pregnancy, unspecified trimester UPD M ♀

Z34.01 Encounter for supervision of normal first pregnancy, first trimester UPD M ♀

Z34.02 Encounter for supervision of normal first pregnancy, second trimester UPD M ♀

Z34.03 Encounter for supervision of normal first pregnancy, third trimester UPD M ♀

✓5th **Z34.8 Encounter for supervision of other normal pregnancy**

Z34.80 Encounter for supervision of other normal pregnancy, unspecified trimester UPD M ♀

Z34.81 Encounter for supervision of other normal pregnancy, first trimester UPD M ♀

Z34.82 Encounter for supervision of other normal pregnancy, second trimester UPD M ♀

Z34.83 Encounter for supervision of other normal pregnancy, third trimester UPD M ♀

✓5th **Z34.9 Encounter for supervision of normal pregnancy, unspecified**

Z34.90 Encounter for supervision of normal pregnancy, unspecified, unspecified trimester UPD M ♀

Z34.91 Encounter for supervision of normal pregnancy, unspecified, first trimester UPD M ♀

Z34.92 Encounter for supervision of normal pregnancy, unspecified, second trimester UPD M ♀

Z34.93 Encounter for supervision of normal pregnancy, unspecified, third trimester UPD M ♀

✓4th **Z36 Encounter for antenatal screening of mother**
INCLUDES encounter for placental sample (taken vaginally)
screening is the testing for disease or disease precursors in asymptomatic individuals so that early detection and treatment can be provided for those who test positive for the disease.
EXCLUDES 1 *diagnostic examination - code to sign or symptom*
encounter for suspected maternal and fetal conditions ruled out (Z03.7-)
suspected fetal condition affecting management of pregnancy - code to condition in Chapter 15
EXCLUDES 2 *abnormal findings on antenatal screening of mother (O28.-)*
genetic counseling and testing (Z31.43-, Z31.5)
routine prenatal care (Z34)
AHA: 2017,4Q,28

Z36.0 Encounter for antenatal screening for chromosomal anomalies M ♀

Z36.1 Encounter for antenatal screening for raised alphafetoprotein level M ♀
Encounter for antenatal screening for elevated maternal serum alphafetoprotein level
DEF: High levels of alpha-fetoprotein (AFP) that may indicate a possibility of spina bifida and other neural tube defects, anencephaly, or omphalocele in the fetus.

Z36.2 Encounter for other antenatal screening follow-up M ♀
Non-visualized anatomy on a previous scan

Z36.3 Encounter for antenatal screening for malformations M ♀
Screening for a suspected anomaly

Z36.4 Encounter for antenatal screening for fetal growth retardation M ♀
Intrauterine growth restriction (IUGR)/small-for-dates

Z36.5 Encounter for antenatal screening for isoimmunization M ♀

✓5th **Z36.8 Encounter for other antenatal screening**

Z36.81 Encounter for antenatal screening for hydrops fetalis M ♀
DEF: Hydrops fetalis: Abnormal accumulation of fluid in two or more parts of the fetus, such as ascites, effusion of the pleural or pericardial tissues, or edema.

Z36.82 Encounter for antenatal screening for nuchal translucency M ♀

Z36.83 Encounter for fetal screening for congenital cardiac abnormalities M ♀

Z36.84 Encounter for antenatal screening for fetal lung maturity M ♀

Z36.85 Encounter for antenatal screening for Streptococcus B M ♀

Z36.86 Encounter for antenatal screening for cervical length M ♀
Screening for risk of pre-term labor

Z36.87 Encounter for antenatal screening for uncertain dates M ♀

Z36.88 Encounter for antenatal screening for fetal macrosomia M ♀
Screening for large-for-dates

Z36.89 Encounter for other specified antenatal screening M ♀

Z36.8A Encounter for antenatal screening for other genetic defects M ♀

Z36.9 Encounter for antenatal screening, unspecified M ♀

Z3A Weeks of gestation

NOTE Codes from category Z3A are for use, only on the maternal record, to indicate the weeks of gestation of the pregnancy, if known.

Code first obstetric condition or encounter for delivery (O09-O60, O80-O82)

AHA: 2022,2Q,3; 2019,2Q,11; 2016,2Q,34; 2014,3Q,17; 2014,2Q,9; 2013,2Q,33

TIP: Do not assign a code from this category with codes from categories O00-O08 or code Z33.2.

Z3A.0 Weeks of gestation of pregnancy, unspecified or less than 10 weeks

- **Z3A.00 Weeks of gestation of pregnancy not specified** UPD M ♀
- **Z3A.01 Less than 8 weeks gestation of pregnancy** UPD M ♀
- **Z3A.08 8 weeks gestation of pregnancy** UPD M ♀
- **Z3A.09 9 weeks gestation of pregnancy** UPD M ♀

Z3A.1 Weeks of gestation of pregnancy, weeks 10-19

- **Z3A.10 10 weeks gestation of pregnancy** UPD M ♀
- **Z3A.11 11 weeks gestation of pregnancy** UPD M ♀
- **Z3A.12 12 weeks gestation of pregnancy** UPD M ♀
- **Z3A.13 13 weeks gestation of pregnancy** UPD M ♀
- **Z3A.14 14 weeks gestation of pregnancy** UPD M ♀
- **Z3A.15 15 weeks gestation of pregnancy** UPD M ♀
- **Z3A.16 16 weeks gestation of pregnancy** UPD M ♀
- **Z3A.17 17 weeks gestation of pregnancy** UPD M ♀
- **Z3A.18 18 weeks gestation of pregnancy** UPD M ♀
- **Z3A.19 19 weeks gestation of pregnancy** UPD M ♀

Z3A.2 Weeks of gestation of pregnancy, weeks 20-29

- **Z3A.20 20 weeks gestation of pregnancy** UPD M ♀
- **Z3A.21 21 weeks gestation of pregnancy** UPD M ♀
- **Z3A.22 22 weeks gestation of pregnancy** UPD M ♀
- **Z3A.23 23 weeks gestation of pregnancy** UPD M ♀
- **Z3A.24 24 weeks gestation of pregnancy** UPD M ♀
- **Z3A.25 25 weeks gestation of pregnancy** UPD M ♀
- **Z3A.26 26 weeks gestation of pregnancy** UPD M ♀
- **Z3A.27 27 weeks gestation of pregnancy** UPD M ♀
- **Z3A.28 28 weeks gestation of pregnancy** UPD M ♀
- **Z3A.29 29 weeks gestation of pregnancy** UPD M ♀

Z3A.3 Weeks of gestation of pregnancy, weeks 30-39

- **Z3A.30 30 weeks gestation of pregnancy** UPD M ♀
- **Z3A.31 31 weeks gestation of pregnancy** UPD M ♀
- **Z3A.32 32 weeks gestation of pregnancy** UPD M ♀
- **Z3A.33 33 weeks gestation of pregnancy** UPD M ♀
- **Z3A.34 34 weeks gestation of pregnancy** UPD M ♀
- **Z3A.35 35 weeks gestation of pregnancy** UPD M ♀
- **Z3A.36 36 weeks gestation of pregnancy** UPD M ♀
- **Z3A.37 37 weeks gestation of pregnancy** UPD M ♀
- **Z3A.38 38 weeks gestation of pregnancy** UPD M ♀
- **Z3A.39 39 weeks gestation of pregnancy** UPD M ♀

Z3A.4 Weeks of gestation of pregnancy, weeks 40 or greater

AHA: 2014,4Q,23

- **Z3A.40 40 weeks gestation of pregnancy** UPD M ♀
- **Z3A.41 41 weeks gestation of pregnancy** UPD M ♀
- **Z3A.42 42 weeks gestation of pregnancy** UPD M ♀
- **Z3A.49 Greater than 42 weeks gestation of pregnancy** UPD M ♀

Z37 Outcome of delivery

This category is intended for use as an additional code to identify the outcome of delivery on the mother's record. It is not for use on the newborn record.

EXCLUDES 1 *stillbirth (P95)*

- **Z37.0 Single live birth** UPD M ♀
  AHA: 2016,2Q,34; 2014,2Q,9
- **Z37.1 Single stillbirth** UPD M ♀
- **Z37.2 Twins, both liveborn** UPD M ♀
- **Z37.3 Twins, one liveborn and one stillborn** UPD M ♀
- **Z37.4 Twins, both stillborn** UPD M ♀

Z37.5 Other multiple births, all liveborn

- **Z37.50 Multiple births, unspecified, all liveborn** UPD M ♀
- **Z37.51 Triplets, all liveborn** UPD M ♀
- **Z37.52 Quadruplets, all liveborn** UPD M ♀
- **Z37.53 Quintuplets, all liveborn** UPD M ♀
- **Z37.54 Sextuplets, all liveborn** UPD M ♀
- **Z37.59 Other multiple births, all liveborn** UPD M ♀

Z37.6 Other multiple births, some liveborn

- **Z37.60 Multiple births, unspecified, some liveborn** UPD M ♀
- **Z37.61 Triplets, some liveborn** UPD M ♀
- **Z37.62 Quadruplets, some liveborn** UPD M ♀
- **Z37.63 Quintuplets, some liveborn** UPD M ♀
- **Z37.64 Sextuplets, some liveborn** UPD M ♀
- **Z37.69 Other multiple births, some liveborn** UPD M ♀

- **Z37.7 Other multiple births, all stillborn** UPD M ♀
- **Z37.9 Outcome of delivery, unspecified** UPD M ♀
  Multiple birth NOS
  Single birth NOS

Z38 Liveborn infants according to place of birth and type of delivery

This category is for use as the principal code on the initial record of a newborn baby. It is to be used for the initial birth record only. It is not to be used on the mother's record.

AHA: 2020,2Q,13; 2017,2Q,5-7; 2016,3Q,18; 2015,2Q,15

Z38.0 Single liveborn infant, born in hospital

Single liveborn infant, born in birthing center or other health care facility

- **Z38.00 Single liveborn infant, delivered vaginally** N
- **Z38.01 Single liveborn infant, delivered by cesarean** N

- **Z38.1 Single liveborn infant, born outside hospital** N
- **Z38.2 Single liveborn infant, unspecified as to place of birth** N
  Single liveborn infant NOS

Z38.3 Twin liveborn infant, born in hospital

- **Z38.30 Twin liveborn infant, delivered vaginally** N
- **Z38.31 Twin liveborn infant, delivered by cesarean** N

- **Z38.4 Twin liveborn infant, born outside hospital** N
- **Z38.5 Twin liveborn infant, unspecified as to place of birth** N

Z38.6 Other multiple liveborn infant, born in hospital

- **Z38.61 Triplet liveborn infant, delivered vaginally** N
- **Z38.62 Triplet liveborn infant, delivered by cesarean** N
- **Z38.63 Quadruplet liveborn infant, delivered vaginally** N
- **Z38.64 Quadruplet liveborn infant, delivered by cesarean** N
- **Z38.65 Quintuplet liveborn infant, delivered vaginally** N
- **Z38.66 Quintuplet liveborn infant, delivered by cesarean** N
- **Z38.68 Other multiple liveborn infant, delivered vaginally** N
- **Z38.69 Other multiple liveborn infant, delivered by cesarean** N

- **Z38.7 Other multiple liveborn infant, born outside hospital** N
- **Z38.8 Other multiple liveborn infant, unspecified as to place of birth** N

Z39 Encounter for maternal postpartum care and examination

- **Z39.0 Encounter for care and examination of mother immediately after delivery** M ♀
  Care and observation in uncomplicated cases when the delivery occurs outside a healthcare facility
  EXCLUDES 1 *care for postpartum complication - see Alphabetic Index*
  AHA: 2021,3Q,13
- **Z39.1 Encounter for care and examination of lactating mother** UPD M ♀
  Encounter for supervision of lactation
  EXCLUDES 1 *disorders of lactation (O92.-)*
- **Z39.2 Encounter for routine postpartum follow-up** UPD M ♀

Encounters for other specific health care (Z40-Z53)

Categories Z40-Z53 are intended for use to indicate a reason for care. They may be used for patients who have already been treated for a disease or injury, but who are receiving aftercare or prophylactic care, or care to consolidate the treatment, or to deal with a residual state

EXCLUDES 2 *follow-up examination for medical surveillance after treatment (Z08-Z09)*

Z40 Encounter for prophylactic surgery

EXCLUDES 1 *organ donations (Z52.-)*
therapeutic organ removal - code to condition

DEF: Treatment measure intended to prevent or ward off a disease or condition.

Z40.0 Encounter for prophylactic surgery for risk factors related to malignant neoplasms
Admission for prophylactic organ removal
Use additional code to identify risk factor
AHA: 2017,4Q,28-29

Z40.00 Encounter for prophylactic removal of unspecified organ
Z40.01 Encounter for prophylactic removal of breast
Z40.02 Encounter for prophylactic removal of ovary(s) ♀
Encounter for prophylactic removal of ovary(s) and fallopian tube(s)
Z40.03 Encounter for prophylactic removal of fallopian tube(s) ♀
Z40.09 Encounter for prophylactic removal of other organ

Z40.8 Encounter for other prophylactic surgery UPD
Z40.9 Encounter for prophylactic surgery, unspecified UPD

Z41 Encounter for procedures for purposes other than remedying health state

Z41.1 Encounter for cosmetic surgery
Encounter for cosmetic breast implant
Encounter for cosmetic procedure
EXCLUDES 1 *encounter for plastic and reconstructive surgery following medical procedure or healed injury (Z42.-)*
encounter for post-mastectomy breast implantation (Z42.1)

Z41.2 Encounter for routine and ritual male circumcision ♂
AHA: 2018,3Q,15
TIP: Do not report this code when circumcision is performed during the birth admission.

Z41.3 Encounter for ear piercing UPD
Z41.8 Encounter for other procedures for purposes other than remedying health state
Z41.9 Encounter for procedure for purposes other than remedying health state, unspecified UPD

Z42 Encounter for plastic and reconstructive surgery following medical procedure or healed injury

EXCLUDES 1 *encounter for cosmetic plastic surgery (Z41.1)*
encounter for plastic surgery for treatment of current injury - code to relevent injury

Z42.1 Encounter for breast reconstruction following mastectomy A
EXCLUDES 1 *deformity and disproportion of reconstructed breast (N65.1-)*

Z42.8 Encounter for other plastic and reconstructive surgery following medical procedure or healed injury
AHA: 2017,1Q,42

Z43 Encounter for attention to artificial openings

INCLUDES closure of artificial openings
passage of sounds or bougies through artificial openings
reforming artificial openings
removal of catheter from artificial openings
toilet or cleansing of artificial openings

EXCLUDES 1 *complications of external stoma (J95.0-, K94.-, N99.5-)*
EXCLUDES 2 *fitting and adjustment of prosthetic and other devices (Z44-Z46)*

AHA: 2019,2Q,33

Z43.0 Encounter for attention to tracheostomy HCC
Z43.1 Encounter for attention to gastrostomy CC HCC
EXCLUDES 2 *artificial opening status only, without need for care (Z93.-)*
Z43.2 Encounter for attention to ileostomy HCC
Z43.3 Encounter for attention to colostomy HCC
Z43.4 Encounter for attention to other artificial openings of digestive tract HCC
Z43.5 Encounter for attention to cystostomy HCC
Z43.6 Encounter for attention to other artificial openings of urinary tract HCC
Encounter for attention to nephrostomy
Encounter for attention to ureterostomy
Encounter for attention to urethrostomy
Z43.7 Encounter for attention to artificial vagina
Z43.8 Encounter for attention to other artificial openings HCC
Z43.9 Encounter for attention to unspecified artificial opening UPD HCC

Z44 Encounter for fitting and adjustment of external prosthetic device

INCLUDES removal or replacement of external prosthetic device
EXCLUDES 1 *malfunction or other complications of device - see Alphabetical Index*
presence of prosthetic device (Z97.-)

Z44.0 Encounter for fitting and adjustment of artificial arm

Z44.00 Encounter for fitting and adjustment of unspecified artificial arm
Z44.001 Encounter for fitting and adjustment of unspecified right artificial arm
Z44.002 Encounter for fitting and adjustment of unspecified left artificial arm
Z44.009 Encounter for fitting and adjustment of unspecified artificial arm, unspecified arm

Z44.01 Encounter for fitting and adjustment of complete artificial arm
Z44.011 Encounter for fitting and adjustment of complete right artificial arm
Z44.012 Encounter for fitting and adjustment of complete left artificial arm
Z44.019 Encounter for fitting and adjustment of complete artificial arm, unspecified arm

Z44.02 Encounter for fitting and adjustment of partial artificial arm
Z44.021 Encounter for fitting and adjustment of partial artificial right arm
Z44.022 Encounter for fitting and adjustment of partial artificial left arm
Z44.029 Encounter for fitting and adjustment of partial artificial arm, unspecified arm

Z44.1 Encounter for fitting and adjustment of artificial leg

Z44.10 Encounter for fitting and adjustment of unspecified artificial leg
Z44.101 Encounter for fitting and adjustment of unspecified right artificial leg HCC
Z44.102 Encounter for fitting and adjustment of unspecified left artificial leg HCC
Z44.109 Encounter for fitting and adjustment of unspecified artificial leg, unspecified leg HCC

Z44.11 Encounter for fitting and adjustment of complete artificial leg
Z44.111 Encounter for fitting and adjustment of complete right artificial leg HCC
Z44.112 Encounter for fitting and adjustment of complete left artificial leg HCC
Z44.119 Encounter for fitting and adjustment of complete artificial leg, unspecified leg HCC

Z44.12 Encounter for fitting and adjustment of partial artificial leg
Z44.121 Encounter for fitting and adjustment of partial artificial right leg HCC
Z44.122 Encounter for fitting and adjustment of partial artificial left leg HCC
Z44.129 Encounter for fitting and adjustment of partial artificial leg, unspecified leg HCC

Z44.2 Encounter for fitting and adjustment of artificial eye
EXCLUDES 1 *mechanical complication of ocular prosthesis (T85.3)*

Z44.20 Encounter for fitting and adjustment of artificial eye, unspecified
Z44.21 Encounter for fitting and adjustment of artificial right eye
Z44.22 Encounter for fitting and adjustment of artificial left eye

5th **Z44.3 Encounter for fitting and adjustment of external breast prosthesis**
EXCLUDES 1 *complications of breast implant (T85.4-)*
encounter for adjustment or removal of breast implant (Z45.81-)
encounter for initial breast implant insertion for cosmetic breast augmentation (Z41.1)
encounter for breast reconstruction following mastectomy (Z42.1)

Z44.30 Encounter for fitting and adjustment of external breast prosthesis, unspecified breast

Z44.31 Encounter for fitting and adjustment of external right breast prosthesis

Z44.32 Encounter for fitting and adjustment of external left breast prosthesis

Z44.8 Encounter for fitting and adjustment of other external prosthetic devices

Z44.9 Encounter for fitting and adjustment of unspecified external prosthetic device UPD

4th **Z45 Encounter for adjustment and management of implanted device**
INCLUDES removal or replacement of implanted device
EXCLUDES 1 *malfunction or other complications of device - see Alphabetical Index*
EXCLUDES 2 *encounter for fitting and adjustment of non-implanted device (Z46.-)*

5th **Z45.0 Encounter for adjustment and management of cardiac device**
TIP: Assign an additional code for the associated condition if that condition requires constant intervention from the device, as in cases of sick sinus syndrome. For conditions that do not require constant intervention from the device, as in cases of ventricular fibrillation, an additional code for the associated condition should be assigned only if the patient is experiencing the condition and the device is firing during the current admission.

6th **Z45.01 Encounter for adjustment and management of cardiac pacemaker**
Encounter for adjustment and management of cardiac resynchronization therapy pacemaker (CRT-P)
EXCLUDES 1 *encounter for adjustment and management of automatic implantable cardiac defibrillator with synchronous cardiac pacemaker (Z45.02)*

Z45.010 Encounter for checking and testing of cardiac pacemaker pulse generator [battery]
Encounter for replacing cardiac pacemaker pulse generator [battery]

Z45.018 Encounter for adjustment and management of other part of cardiac pacemaker
EXCLUDES 1 *presence of other part of cardiac pacemaker (Z95.0)*
EXCLUDES 2 *presence of prosthetic and other devices (Z95.1-Z95.5, Z95.811-Z97)*

Z45.02 Encounter for adjustment and management of automatic implantable cardiac defibrillator
Encounter for adjustment and management of automatic implantable cardiac defibrillator with synchronous cardiac pacemaker
Encounter for adjustment and management of cardiac resynchronization therapy defibrillator (CRT-D)

Z45.09 Encounter for adjustment and management of other cardiac device

Z45.1 Encounter for adjustment and management of infusion pump

Z45.2 Encounter for adjustment and management of vascular access device
Encounter for adjustment and management of vascular catheters
EXCLUDES 1 *encounter for adjustment and management of renal dialysis catheter (Z49.01)*
AHA: 2020,2Q,21; 2018,3Q,20

5th **Z45.3 Encounter for adjustment and management of implanted devices of the special senses**

Z45.31 Encounter for adjustment and management of implanted visual substitution device

6th **Z45.32 Encounter for adjustment and management of implanted hearing device**
EXCLUDES 1 *encounter for fitting and adjustment of hearing aide (Z46.1)*

Z45.320 Encounter for adjustment and management of bone conduction device

Z45.321 Encounter for adjustment and management of cochlear device

Z45.328 Encounter for adjustment and management of other implanted hearing device

5th **Z45.4 Encounter for adjustment and management of implanted nervous system device**

Z45.41 Encounter for adjustment and management of cerebrospinal fluid drainage device
Encounter for adjustment and management of cerebral ventricular (communicating) shunt

Z45.42 Encounter for adjustment and management of neurostimulator
Encounter for adjustment and management of brain neurostimulator
Encounter for adjustment and management of gastric neurostimulator
Encounter for adjustment and management of peripheral nerve neurostimulator
Encounter for adjustment and management of sacral nerve neurostimulator
Encounter for adjustment and management of spinal cord neurostimulator
Encounter for adjustment and management of vagus nerve neurostimulator

Z45.49 Encounter for adjustment and management of other implanted nervous system device
AHA: 2014,3Q,19

5th **Z45.8 Encounter for adjustment and management of other implanted devices**

6th **Z45.81 Encounter for adjustment or removal of breast implant**
Encounter for elective implant exchange (different material) (different size)
Encounter for removal of tissue expander with or without synchronous insertion of permanent implant
EXCLUDES 1 *complications of breast implant (T85.4-)*
encounter for initial breast implant insertion for cosmetic breast augmentation (Z41.1)
encounter for breast reconstruction following mastectomy (Z42.1)

Z45.811 Encounter for adjustment or removal of right breast implant

Z45.812 Encounter for adjustment or removal of left breast implant

Z45.819 Encounter for adjustment or removal of unspecified breast implant

Z45.82 Encounter for adjustment or removal of myringotomy device (stent) (tube) UPD

Z45.89 Encounter for adjustment and management of other implanted devices UPD
AHA: 2014,4Q,26-28

Z45.9 Encounter for adjustment and management of unspecified implanted device UPD

4th **Z46 Encounter for fitting and adjustment of other devices**
INCLUDES removal or replacement of other device
EXCLUDES 1 *malfunction or other complications of device - see Alphabetical Index*
EXCLUDES 2 *encounter for fitting and management of implanted devices (Z45.-)*
issue of repeat prescription only (Z76.0)
presence of prosthetic and other devices (Z95-Z97)

Z46.0 Encounter for fitting and adjustment of spectacles and contact lenses UPD

Z46.1 Encounter for fitting and adjustment of hearing aid UPD
EXCLUDES 1 *encounter for adjustment and management of implanted hearing device (Z45.32-)*

Z46.2 Encounter for fitting and adjustment of other devices related to nervous system and special senses
EXCLUDES 2 *encounter for adjustment and management of implanted nervous system device (Z45.4-)*
encounter for adjustment and management of implanted visual substitution device (Z45.31)

Z46.3 Encounter for fitting and adjustment of dental prosthetic device
Encounter for fitting and adjustment of dentures

Z46.4 Encounter for fitting and adjustment of orthodontic device UPD

✓5th **Z46.5 Encounter for fitting and adjustment of other gastrointestinal appliance and device**
EXCLUDES 1 *encounter for attention to artificial openings of digestive tract (Z43.1-Z43.4)*

Z46.51 Encounter for fitting and adjustment of gastric lap band UPD

Z46.59 Encounter for fitting and adjustment of other gastrointestinal appliance and device UPD

Z46.6 Encounter for fitting and adjustment of urinary device UPD
EXCLUDES 2 *attention to artificial openings of urinary tract (Z43.5, Z43.6)*

✓5th **Z46.8 Encounter for fitting and adjustment of other specified devices**

Z46.81 Encounter for fitting and adjustment of insulin pump UPD
Encounter for insulin pump instruction and training
Encounter for insulin pump titration

Z46.82 Encounter for fitting and adjustment of non-vascular catheter

Z46.89 Encounter for fitting and adjustment of other specified devices UPD
Encounter for fitting and adjustment of wheelchair

Z46.9 Encounter for fitting and adjustment of unspecified device UPD

✓4th **Z47 Orthopedic aftercare**
EXCLUDES 1 *aftercare for healing fracture - code to fracture with 7th character D*

Z47.1 Aftercare following joint replacement surgery
Use additional code to identify the joint (Z96.6-)
AHA: 2020,1Q,23

Z47.2 Encounter for removal of internal fixation device
EXCLUDES 1 *encounter for adjustment of internal fixation device for fracture treatment - code to fracture with appropriate 7th character*
encounter for removal of external fixation device - code to fracture with 7th character D
infection or inflammatory reaction to internal fixation device (T84.6-)
mechanical complication of internal fixation device (T84.1-)

✓5th **Z47.3 Aftercare following explantation of joint prosthesis**
Aftercare following explantation of joint prosthesis, staged procedure
Encounter for joint prosthesis insertion following prior explantation of joint prosthesis
AHA: 2020,1Q,23; 2015,1Q,16
TIP: For staged removal of elbow joint prosthesis, assign code Z47.1.

Z47.31 Aftercare following explantation of shoulder joint prosthesis
EXCLUDES 1 *acquired absence of shoulder joint following prior explantation of shoulder joint prosthesis (Z89.23-)*
shoulder joint prosthesis explantation status (Z89.23-)

Z47.32 Aftercare following explantation of hip joint prosthesis
EXCLUDES 1 *acquired absence of hip joint following prior explantation of hip joint prosthesis (Z89.62-)*
hip joint prosthesis explantation status (Z89.62-)

Z47.33 Aftercare following explantation of knee joint prosthesis
EXCLUDES 1 *acquired absence of knee joint following prior explantation of knee prosthesis (Z89.52-)*
knee joint prosthesis explantation status (Z89.52-)

✓5th **Z47.8 Encounter for other orthopedic aftercare**

Z47.81 Encounter for orthopedic aftercare following surgical amputation
Use additional code to identify the limb amputated (Z89.-)

Z47.82 Encounter for orthopedic aftercare following scoliosis surgery

Z47.89 Encounter for other orthopedic aftercare
AHA: 2015,1Q,8

✓4th **Z48 Encounter for other postprocedural aftercare**
EXCLUDES 1 *encounter for aftercare following injury - code to Injury, by site, with appropriate 7th character for subsequent encounter*
encounter for follow-up examination after completed treatment (Z08-Z09)
EXCLUDES 2 *encounter for attention to artificial openings (Z43.-)*
encounter for fitting and adjustment of prosthetic and other devices (Z44-Z46)
AHA: 2015,4Q,38; 2015,1Q,6-7

✓5th **Z48.0 Encounter for attention to dressings, sutures and drains**
EXCLUDES 1 *encounter for planned postprocedural wound closure (Z48.1)*

Z48.00 Encounter for change or removal of nonsurgical wound dressing UPD
Encounter for change or removal of wound dressing NOS

Z48.01 Encounter for change or removal of surgical wound dressing UPD
AHA: 2019,2Q,33

Z48.02 Encounter for removal of sutures UPD
Encounter for removal of staples

Z48.03 Encounter for change or removal of drains
AHA: 2019,2Q,33

Z48.1 Encounter for planned postprocedural wound closure
EXCLUDES 1 *encounter for attention to dressings and sutures (Z48.0-)*

✓5th **Z48.2 Encounter for aftercare following organ transplant**

Z48.21 Encounter for aftercare following heart transplant CC HCC

Z48.22 Encounter for aftercare following kidney transplant CC

Z48.23 Encounter for aftercare following liver transplant CC HCC

Z48.24 Encounter for aftercare following lung transplant CC HCC

✓6th **Z48.28 Encounter for aftercare following multiple organ transplant**

Z48.280 Encounter for aftercare following heart-lung transplant CC HCC

Z48.288 Encounter for aftercare following multiple organ transplant

✓6th **Z48.29 Encounter for aftercare following other organ transplant**

Z48.290 Encounter for aftercare following bone marrow transplant CC HCC

Z48.298 Encounter for aftercare following other organ transplant

Z48.3 Aftercare following surgery for neoplasm
Use additional code to identify the neoplasm

5th **Z48.8 Encounter for other specified postprocedural aftercare**

6th **Z48.81 Encounter for surgical aftercare following surgery on specified body systems**

These codes identify the body system requiring aftercare. They are for use in conjunction with other aftercare codes to fully explain the aftercare encounter. The condition treated should also be coded if still present.

EXCLUDES 1 *aftercare for injury - code the injury with 7th character D*

aftercare following surgery for neoplasm (Z48.3)

EXCLUDES 2 *aftercare following organ transplant (Z48.2-)*

orthopedic aftercare (Z47.-)

AHA: 2015,4Q,38

Z48.810 Encounter for surgical aftercare following surgery on the sense organs

Z48.811 Encounter for surgical aftercare following surgery on the nervous system

EXCLUDES 2 *encounter for surgical aftercare following surgery on the sense organs (Z48.810)*

Z48.812 Encounter for surgical aftercare following surgery on the circulatory system

AHA: 2012,4Q,96

Z48.813 Encounter for surgical aftercare following surgery on the respiratory system

AHA: 2019,2Q,33

Z48.814 Encounter for surgical aftercare following surgery on the teeth or oral cavity

Z48.815 Encounter for surgical aftercare following surgery on the digestive system

Z48.816 Encounter for surgical aftercare following surgery on the genitourinary system

EXCLUDES 1 *encounter for aftercare following sterilization reversal (Z31.42)*

Z48.817 Encounter for surgical aftercare following surgery on the skin and subcutaneous tissue

Z48.89 Encounter for other specified surgical aftercare

4th **Z49 Encounter for care involving renal dialysis**

Code also associated end stage renal disease (N18.6)

5th **Z49.0 Preparatory care for renal dialysis**

Encounter for dialysis instruction and training

Z49.01 Encounter for fitting and adjustment of extracorporeal dialysis catheter UPD HCC

Removal or replacement of renal dialysis catheter

Toilet or cleansing of renal dialysis catheter

Z49.02 Encounter for fitting and adjustment of peritoneal dialysis catheter UPD HCC

5th **Z49.3 Encounter for adequacy testing for dialysis**

Z49.31 Encounter for adequacy testing for hemodialysis UPD HCC

Z49.32 Encounter for adequacy testing for peritoneal dialysis UPD HCC

Encounter for peritoneal equilibration test

4th **Z51 Encounter for other aftercare and medical care**

Code also condition requiring care

EXCLUDES 1 *follow-up examination after treatment (Z08-Z09)*

Z51.0 Encounter for antineoplastic radiation therapy

AHA: 2017,4Q,103

TIP: Do not assign when admission is for insertion/implantation of radioactive elements. Assign a code for the malignancy instead. Any complications related to the radioactive elements should be assigned as secondary diagnoses.

5th **Z51.1 Encounter for antineoplastic chemotherapy and immunotherapy**

EXCLUDES 2 *encounter for chemotherapy and immunotherapy for nonneoplastic condition - code to condition*

Z51.11 Encounter for antineoplastic chemotherapy

AHA: 2022,1Q,16; 2015,3Q,19

Z51.12 Encounter for antineoplastic immunotherapy

Z51.5 Encounter for palliative care

AHA: 2022,1Q,18; 2020,4Q,98; 2017,1Q,48

Z51.6 Encounter for desensitization to allergens UPD

AHA: 2016,4Q,77

5th **Z51.8 Encounter for other specified aftercare**

EXCLUDES 1 *holiday relief care (Z75.5)*

Z51.81 Encounter for therapeutic drug level monitoring

Code also any long-term (current) drug therapy (Z79.-)

EXCLUDES 1 *encounter for blood-drug test for administrative or medicolegal reasons (Z02.83)*

DEF: Drug monitoring: Measurement of the level of a specific drug in the body or measurement of a specific function to assess effectiveness of a drug.

Z51.89 Encounter for other specified aftercare UPD

AHA: 2012,4Q,95-97

4th **Z52 Donors of organs and tissues**

INCLUDES autologous and other living donors

EXCLUDES 1 *cadaveric donor - omit code*

examination of potential donor (Z00.5)

AHA: 2012,4Q,99

5th **Z52.0 Blood donor**

6th **Z52.00 Unspecified blood donor**

Z52.000 Unspecified donor, whole blood UPD

Z52.001 Unspecified donor, stem cells UPD

Z52.008 Unspecified donor, other blood UPD

6th **Z52.01 Autologous blood donor**

Z52.010 Autologous donor, whole blood UPD

Z52.011 Autologous donor, stem cells UPD

Z52.018 Autologous donor, other blood UPD

6th **Z52.09 Other blood donor**

Volunteer donor

Z52.090 Other blood donor, whole blood UPD

Z52.091 Other blood donor, stem cells UPD

Z52.098 Other blood donor, other blood UPD

5th **Z52.1 Skin donor**

Z52.10 Skin donor, unspecified

Z52.11 Skin donor, autologous

Z52.19 Skin donor, other

5th **Z52.2 Bone donor**

Z52.20 Bone donor, unspecified

Z52.21 Bone donor, autologous

Z52.29 Bone donor, other

Z52.3 Bone marrow donor

Z52.4 Kidney donor

Z52.5 Cornea donor

Z52.6 Liver donor

5th **Z52.8 Donor of other specified organs or tissues**

6th **Z52.81 Egg (Oocyte) donor**

Z52.810 Egg (Oocyte) donor under age 35, anonymous recipient UPD ♀

Egg donor under age 35 NOS

Z52.811 Egg (Oocyte) donor under age 35, designated recipient UPD ♀

Z52.812 Egg (Oocyte) donor age 35 and over, anonymous recipient UPD ♀

Egg donor age 35 and over NOS

Z52.813 Egg (Oocyte) donor age 35 and over, designated recipient UPD ♀

Z52.819 Egg (Oocyte) donor, unspecified UPD ♀

Z52.89 Donor of other specified organs or tissues

Z52.9 Donor of unspecified organ or tissue

Donor NOS

4th **Z53 Persons encountering health services for specific procedures and treatment, not carried out**

5th **Z53.0 Procedure and treatment not carried out because of contraindication**

Z53.01 Procedure and treatment not carried out due to patient smoking UPD

Z53.09 Procedure and treatment not carried out because of other contraindication UPD

Z53.1 Procedure and treatment not carried out because of patient's decision for reasons of belief and group pressure UPD

5th **Z53.2 Procedure and treatment not carried out because of patient's decision for other and unspecified reasons**

Z53.20 Procedure and treatment not carried out because of patient's decision for unspecified reasons UPD

Z53.21 Procedure and treatment not carried out due to patient leaving prior to being seen by health care provider UPD

Z53.29 Procedure and treatment not carried out because of patient's decision for other reasons UPD

Z53.3 Procedure converted to open procedure
AHA: 2016,4Q,79

Z53.31 Laparoscopic surgical procedure converted to open procedure UPD

Z53.32 Thoracoscopic surgical procedure converted to open procedure UPD

Z53.33 Arthroscopic surgical procedure converted to open procedure UPD

Z53.39 Other specified procedure converted to open procedure UPD

Z53.8 Procedure and treatment not carried out for other reasons UPD

Z53.9 Procedure and treatment not carried out, unspecified reason UPD

Persons with potential health hazards related to socioeconomic and psychosocial circumstances (Z55-Z65)

AHA: 2021,4Q,34-37; 2019,4Q,66; 2018,4Q,58,73; 2018,1Q,18

DEF: Social determinants of health: Socioeconomic factors that can affect a person's health, including both environmental and societal conditions such as education and literacy, employment, health behaviors, housing, lack of adequate food or water, occupational exposure to risk factors, social support, transportation, and violence. Tracking social needs that impact patients allows providers to identify population health trends and to promote the personalized care that addresses the medical and social needs of individual patients. ***Synonym(s):*** *SDOH.*

TIP: Because codes in these categories represent social information rather than medical diagnoses, they can be assigned based on documentation by nonphysician clinicians involved in the care of these patients as well as self-reported documentation from the patient, as long as the information is approved and incorporated into the medical record by a clinician or provider.

Z55 Problems related to education and literacy
EXCLUDES 1 *disorders of psychological development (F80-F89)*

Z55.0 Illiteracy and low-level literacy UPD

Z55.1 Schooling unavailable and unattainable UPD

Z55.2 Failed school examinations UPD

Z55.3 Underachievement in school UPD

Z55.4 Educational maladjustment and discord with teachers and classmates UPD

Z55.5 Less than a high school diploma UPD
No general equivalence degree (GED)

Z55.6 Problems related to health literacy UPD
Difficulty understanding health related information
Difficulty understanding medication instructions
Problem completing medical forms
AHA: 2023,1Q,6

Z55.8 Other problems related to education and literacy UPD
Problems related to inadequate teaching

Z55.9 Problems related to education and literacy, unspecified UPD
Academic problems NOS

Z56 Problems related to employment and unemployment
EXCLUDES 2 *occupational exposure to risk factors (Z57.-)*
problems related to housing and economic circumstances (Z59.-)

Z56.0 Unemployment, unspecified UPD

Z56.1 Change of job UPD A

Z56.2 Threat of job loss UPD

Z56.3 Stressful work schedule UPD

Z56.4 Discord with boss and workmates UPD

Z56.5 Uncongenial work environment UPD
Difficult conditions at work

Z56.6 Other physical and mental strain related to work UPD

Z56.8 Other problems related to employment

Z56.81 Sexual harassment on the job UPD

Z56.82 Military deployment status UPD
Individual (civilian or military) currently deployed in theater or in support of military war, peacekeeping and humanitarian operations

Z56.89 Other problems related to employment UPD

Z56.9 Unspecified problems related to employment UPD
Occupational problems NOS

Z57 Occupational exposure to risk factors

Z57.0 Occupational exposure to noise UPD

Z57.1 Occupational exposure to radiation UPD

Z57.2 Occupational exposure to dust UPD

Z57.3 Occupational exposure to other air contaminants

Z57.31 Occupational exposure to environmental tobacco smoke UPD
EXCLUDES 2 *exposure to environmental tobacco smoke (Z77.22)*

Z57.39 Occupational exposure to other air contaminants UPD

Z57.4 Occupational exposure to toxic agents in agriculture UPD
Occupational exposure to solids, liquids, gases or vapors in agriculture

Z57.5 Occupational exposure to toxic agents in other industries UPD
Occupational exposure to solids, liquids, gases or vapors in other industries

Z57.6 Occupational exposure to extreme temperature UPD

Z57.7 Occupational exposure to vibration UPD

Z57.8 Occupational exposure to other risk factors UPD

Z57.9 Occupational exposure to unspecified risk factor UPD

Z58 Problems related to physical environment
EXCLUDES 2 *occupational exposure (Z57.-)*

Z58.6 Inadequate drinking-water supply UPD
Lack of safe drinking water
EXCLUDES 2 *deprivation of water (T73.1)*

Z58.8 Other problems related to physical environment
AHA: 2023,1Q,6

Z58.81 Basic services unavailable in physical environment UPD
Unable to obtain internet service, due to unavailability in geographic area
Unable to obtain telephone service, due to unavailability in geographic area
Unable to obtain utilities, due to inadequate physical environment

Z58.89 Other problems related to physical environment UPD

Z59 Problems related to housing and economic circumstances
EXCLUDES 2 *problems related to upbringing (Z62.-)*

Z59.0 Homelessness

Z59.00 Homelessness unspecified CC UPD

Z59.01 Sheltered homelessness CC UPD
Doubled up
Living in a shelter such as: motel, scattered site housing, temporary or transitional living situation

Z59.02 Unsheltered homelessness CC UPD
Residing in place not meant for human habitation such as: abandoned buildings, cars, parks, sidewalk
Residing on the street

Z59.1 Inadequate housing
~~Lack of heating~~
~~Restriction of space~~
~~Technical defects in home preventing adequate care~~
~~Unsatisfactory surroundings~~
EXCLUDES 1 *problems related to the natural and physical environment (Z77.1-)*
AHA: 2023,1Q,6

Z59.10 Inadequate housing, unspecified UPD
Inadequate housing NOS

Z59.11 Inadequate housing environmental temperature UPD
Lack of air conditioning
Lack of heating

Z59.12 Inadequate housing utilities UPD
Lack of electricity services
Lack of gas services
Lack of oil services
Lack of water services
EXCLUDES 2 *basic services unavailable in physical environment (Z58.81)*
lack of adequate food (Z59.4-)
other problems related to housing and economic circumstances (Z59.8-)

● Z59.19 **Other inadequate housing** UPD
Pest infestation
Restriction of space
Technical defects in home preventing adequate care
Unsatisfactory surroundings

Z59.2 **Discord with neighbors, lodgers and landlord** UPD

Z59.3 **Problems related to living in residential institution** UPD
Boarding-school resident
EXCLUDES 1 *institutional upbringing ▶(Z62.22)◀*

✓5th Z59.4 **Lack of adequate food**
EXCLUDES 2 *deprivation of food (T73.Ø)*
effects of hunger (T73.Ø)
inappropriate diet or eating habits (Z72.4)
malnutrition (E4Ø-E46)

Z59.41 **Food insecurity** UPD

Z59.48 **Other specified lack of adequate food** UPD
Inadequate food
Lack of food

Z59.5 **Extreme poverty** UPD

Z59.6 **Low income** UPD

Z59.7 **Insufficient social insurance and welfare support** UPD

✓5th Z59.8 **Other problems related to housing and economic circumstances**
AHA: 2022,4Q,52

✓6th Z59.81 **Housing instability, housed**
Foreclosure on home loan
Past due on rent or mortgage
Unwanted multiple moves in the last 12 months

Z59.811 **Housing instability, housed, with risk of homelessness** UPD
Imminent risk of homelessness

Z59.812 **Housing instability, housed, homelessness in past 12 months** UPD

Z59.819 **Housing instability, housed unspecified** UPD
EXCLUDES 2 ▶*extreme poverty (Z59.5)*◀
▶*financial insecurity (Z59.86)*◀
▶*low income (Z59.6)*◀
▶*material hardship due to limited financial resources, not elsewhere classified (Z59.87)*◀

Z59.82 **Transportation insecurity** UPD
Excessive transportation time
Inaccessible transportation
Inadequate transportation
Lack of transportation
Unaffordable transportation
Unreliable transportation
Unsafe transportation
EXCLUDES 2 ▶*unavailability and inaccessibility of healthcare facilities (Z75.3)*◀

Z59.86 **Financial insecurity** UPD
Bankruptcy
Burdensome debt
Economic strain
Financial strain
Money problems
Running out of money
Unable to make ends meet
EXCLUDES 2 *extreme poverty (Z59.5)*
low income (Z59.6)
material hardship, not elsewhere classified (Z59.87)

▲ Z59.87 **Material hardship due to limited financial resources, not elsewhere classified** UPD
▶Material deprivation due to limited financial resources◀
▶Unable to obtain adequate childcare due to limited financial resources◀
▶Unable to obtain adequate clothing due to limited financial resources◀
▶Unable to obtain adequate utilities due to limited financial resources◀
▶Unable to obtain basic needs due to limited financial resources◀
EXCLUDES 2 *extreme poverty (Z59.5)*
financial insecurity, not elsewhere classified (Z59.86)
low income (Z59.6)

Z59.89 **Other problems related to housing and economic circumstances** UPD
Foreclosure on loan
Isolated dwelling
Problems with creditors

Z59.9 **Problem related to housing and economic circumstances, unspecified** UPD

✓4th **Z6Ø Problems related to social environment**

Z6Ø.Ø **Problems of adjustment to life-cycle transitions** UPD
Empty nest syndrome
Phase of life problem
Problem with adjustment to retirement [pension]

Z6Ø.2 **Problems related to living alone** UPD

Z6Ø.3 **Acculturation difficulty** UPD
Problem with migration
Problem with social transplantation
DEF: Problem adapting to a different culture or environment not based on any coexisting mental disorder.

Z6Ø.4 **Social exclusion and rejection** UPD
Exclusion and rejection on the basis of personal characteristics, such as unusual physical appearance, illness or behavior.
▶Social isolation◀
EXCLUDES 1 *target of adverse discrimination such as for racial or religious reasons (Z6Ø.5)*

Z6Ø.5 **Target of (perceived) adverse discrimination and persecution** UPD
EXCLUDES 1 *social exclusion and rejection (Z6Ø.4)*

Z6Ø.8 **Other problems related to social environment** UPD
▶Inadequate social support◀
▶Lack of emotional support◀

Z6Ø.9 **Problem related to social environment, unspecified** UPD

✓4th **Z62 Problems related to upbringing**
INCLUDES current and past negative life events in childhood
current and past problems of a child related to upbringing
EXCLUDES 2 *maltreatment syndrome (T74.-)*
problems related to housing and economic circumstances (Z59.-)

Z62.Ø **Inadequate parental supervision and control** UPD

Z62.1 **Parental overprotection** UPD

✓5th Z62.2 **Upbringing away from parents**
EXCLUDES 1 *problems with boarding school (Z59.3)*

Z62.21 **Child in welfare custody** UPD P
~~Child in care of non-parental family member~~
Child in foster care
▶Child in welfare guardianship◀
EXCLUDES 2 ~~*problem for parent due to child in welfare custody (Z63.5)*~~

Z62.22 **Institutional upbringing** UPD
▶Child living in group home◀
▶Child living in orphanage◀
▶Code also, if applicable, child in welfare custody (Z62.21)◀

● Z62.23 **Child in custody of non-parental relative**
Child in care of non-parental family member
Child in custody of grandparent
Child in kinship care
Guardianship by non-parental relative
Code also, if applicable, child in welfare custody (Z62.21)

Z62.24 Child in custody of non-relative guardian
Code also, if applicable, child in welfare custody (Z62.21)
Z62.29 Other upbringing away from parents UPD
Z62.3 Hostility towards and scapegoating of child UPD P
Z62.6 Inappropriate (excessive) parental pressure UPD
Z62.8 Other specified problems related to upbringing
Code also, if applicable:
- absence of family member (Z63.3-)
- disappearance and death of family member (Z63.4)
- disruption of family by separation and divorce (Z63.5)
- other specified problems related to primary support group (Z63.8)
- other stressful life events affecting family and household (Z63.7-)

Z62.81 Personal history of abuse in childhood
Personal history of abuse in adolescence
AHA: 2023,1Q,6
Z62.810 Personal history of physical and sexual abuse in childhood UPD
EXCLUDES 1 *current child physical abuse (T74.12, T76.12)*
current child sexual abuse (T74.22, T76.22)
Z62.811 Personal history of psychological abuse in childhood UPD
EXCLUDES 1 *current child psychological abuse (T74.32, T76.32)*
Z62.812 Personal history of neglect in childhood UPD
EXCLUDES 1 *current child neglect (T74.02, T76.02)*
Z62.813 Personal history of forced labor or sexual exploitation in childhood UPD
AHA: 2018,4Q,32,35
Z62.814 Personal history of child financial abuse UPD
EXCLUDES 1 *current child financial abuse (T74.A2)*
Z62.815 Personal history of intimate partner abuse in childhood UPD
EXCLUDES 2 *adult and child abuse, neglect and other maltreatment, confirmed (T74.-)*
Z62.819 Personal history of unspecified abuse in childhood UPD
EXCLUDES 1 *current child abuse NOS (T74.92, T76.92)*
Z62.82 Parent-child conflict
Z62.820 Parent-biological child conflict UPD
Parent-child problem NOS
Z62.821 Parent-adopted child conflict UPD
Z62.822 Parent-foster child conflict UPD
Z62.823 Parent-step child conflict
Z62.83 Non-parental relative or guardian-child conflict
Z62.831 Non-parental relative-child conflict
Grandparent-child conflict
Kinship-care child conflict
Non-parental relative legal guardian-child conflict
Other relative-child conflict
EXCLUDES 1 *group home staff-child conflict (Z62.833)*
Z62.832 Non-relative guardian-child conflict
EXCLUDES 1 *group home staff-child conflict (Z62.833)*
Z62.833 Group home staff-child conflict
Z62.89 Other specified problems related to upbringing
Z62.890 Parent-child estrangement NEC UPD
Z62.891 Sibling rivalry UPD
Z62.892 Runaway [from current living environment]
Child leaving living situation without permission
Z62.898 Other specified problems related to upbringing UPD
Z62.9 Problem related to upbringing, unspecified UPD

Z63 Other problems related to primary support group, including family circumstances
EXCLUDES 2 *maltreatment syndrome (T74.-, T76)*
parent-child problems (Z62.-)
problems related to negative life events in childhood (Z62.-)
problems related to upbringing (Z62.-)
Z63.0 Problems in relationship with spouse or partner UPD
Relationship distress with spouse or intimate partner
EXCLUDES 1 *counseling for spousal or partner abuse problems (Z69.1)*
counseling related to sexual attitude, behavior, and orientation (Z70.-)
Z63.1 Problems in relationship with in-laws UPD
Z63.3 Absence of family member
EXCLUDES 1 *absence of family member due to disappearance and death (Z63.4)*
absence of family member due to separation and divorce (Z63.5)
Z63.31 Absence of family member due to military deployment UPD
Individual or family affected by other family member being on military deployment
EXCLUDES 1 *family disruption due to return of family member from military deployment (Z63.71)*
Z63.32 Other absence of family member UPD
Z63.4 Disappearance and death of family member UPD
Assumed death of family member
Bereavement
AHA: 2014,1Q,25
Z63.5 Disruption of family by separation and divorce UPD
Marital estrangement
Z63.6 Dependent relative needing care at home UPD
Z63.7 Other stressful life events affecting family and household
Z63.71 Stress on family due to return of family member from military deployment UPD
Individual or family affected by family member having returned from military deployment (current or past conflict)
Z63.72 Alcoholism and drug addiction in family UPD
Z63.79 Other stressful life events affecting family and household UPD
Anxiety (normal) about sick person in family
Health problems within family
Ill or disturbed family member
Isolated family
Z63.8 Other specified problems related to primary support group UPD
Family discord NOS
Family estrangement NOS
High expressed emotional level within family
Inadequate family support NOS
Inadequate or distorted communication within family
Z63.9 Problem related to primary support group, unspecified UPD
Relationship disorder NOS

Z64 Problems related to certain psychosocial circumstances
Z64.0 Problems related to unwanted pregnancy UPD ♀
Z64.1 Problems related to multiparity UPD ♀
Z64.4 Discord with counselors UPD
Discord with probation officer
Discord with social worker

Z65 Problems related to other psychosocial circumstances
Z65.0 Conviction in civil and criminal proceedings without imprisonment UPD
Z65.1 Imprisonment and other incarceration UPD
Z65.2 Problems related to release from prison UPD
Z65.3 Problems related to other legal circumstances UPD
Arrest
Child custody or support proceedings
Litigation
Prosecution
Z65.4 Victim of crime and terrorism UPD
Victim of torture
Z65.5 Exposure to disaster, war and other hostilities UPD
EXCLUDES 1 *target of perceived discrimination or persecution (Z60.5)*

Z65.8 Other specified problems related to psychosocial circumstances UPD
▶At risk for feeling loneliness◀
Religious or spiritual problem

Z65.9 Problem related to unspecified psychosocial circumstances UPD

Do not resuscitate status (Z66)

Z66 Do not resuscitate UPD
DNR status
DEF: Medical order written by a physician that instructs others not to perform cardiopulmonary resuscitation (CPR), intubation, or advanced cardiac life support (ACLS). It prevents unnecessary invasive treatment to prolong life should breathing stop or cardiac arrest occur.

Blood type (Z67)

✓4th **Z67 Blood type**
AHA: 2015,3Q,40

✓5th **Z67.1 Type A blood**
- **Z67.10 Type A blood, Rh positive** UPD
- **Z67.11 Type A blood, Rh negative** UPD

✓5th **Z67.2 Type B blood**
- **Z67.20 Type B blood, Rh positive** UPD
- **Z67.21 Type B blood, Rh negative** UPD

✓5th **Z67.3 Type AB blood**
- **Z67.30 Type AB blood, Rh positive** UPD
- **Z67.31 Type AB blood, Rh negative** UPD

✓5th **Z67.4 Type O blood**
- **Z67.40 Type O blood, Rh positive** UPD
- **Z67.41 Type O blood, Rh negative** UPD

✓5th **Z67.9 Unspecified blood type**
- **Z67.90 Unspecified blood type, Rh positive** UPD
- **Z67.91 Unspecified blood type, Rh negative** UPD

Body mass index [BMI] (Z68)

✓4th **Z68 Body mass index [BMI]**
Kilograms per meters squared

NOTE BMI adult codes are for use for persons 20 years of age or older

BMI pediatric codes are for use for persons 2-19 years of age.

These percentiles are based on the growth charts published by the Centers for Disease Control and Prevention (CDC)

AHA: 2022,3Q,6; 2019,4Q,19,57; 2018,4Q,73,77-83; 2017,1Q,39
DEF: Index used to help determine whether an individual is underweight, a healthy weight, overweight, or obese.
TIP: A BMI code may be assigned to support an associated condition based on medical record documentation from clinicians who are not the patient's provider.
TIP: Do not assign when used in association with fluctuations in body fluid during an encounter, such as fluid overload or fluid retention, or during pregnancy.
TIP: In order to assign a BMI code, the associated condition must meet the definition of a reportable diagnosis for nonoutpatient encounters, per section III of the *ICD-10-CM Official Guidelines for Coding and Reporting*.

Z68.1 Body mass index [BMI] 19.9 or less, adult CC UPD A

✓5th **Z68.2 Body mass index [BMI] 20-29, adult**
- **Z68.20 Body mass index [BMI] 20.0-20.9, adult** UPD A
- **Z68.21 Body mass index [BMI] 21.0-21.9, adult** UPD A
- **Z68.22 Body mass index [BMI] 22.0-22.9, adult** UPD A
- **Z68.23 Body mass index [BMI] 23.0-23.9, adult** UPD A
- **Z68.24 Body mass index [BMI] 24.0-24.9, adult** UPD A
- **Z68.25 Body mass index [BMI] 25.0-25.9, adult** UPD A
- **Z68.26 Body mass index [BMI] 26.0-26.9, adult** UPD A
- **Z68.27 Body mass index [BMI] 27.0-27.9, adult** UPD A
- **Z68.28 Body mass index [BMI] 28.0-28.9, adult** UPD A
- **Z68.29 Body mass index [BMI] 29.0-29.9, adult** UPD A

✓5th **Z68.3 Body mass index [BMI] 30-39, adult**
- **Z68.30 Body mass index [BMI] 30.0-30.9, adult** UPD A
- **Z68.31 Body mass index [BMI] 31.0-31.9, adult** UPD A
- **Z68.32 Body mass index [BMI] 32.0-32.9, adult** UPD A
- **Z68.33 Body mass index [BMI] 33.0-33.9, adult** UPD A
- **Z68.34 Body mass index [BMI] 34.0-34.9, adult** UPD A
- **Z68.35 Body mass index [BMI] 35.0-35.9, adult** UPD A
- **Z68.36 Body mass index [BMI] 36.0-36.9, adult** UPD A
- **Z68.37 Body mass index [BMI] 37.0-37.9, adult** UPD A
- **Z68.38 Body mass index [BMI] 38.0-38.9, adult** UPD A
- **Z68.39 Body mass index [BMI] 39.0-39.9, adult** UPD A

✓5th **Z68.4 Body mass index [BMI] 40 or greater, adult**
- **Z68.41 Body mass index [BMI] 40.0-44.9, adult** CC UPD HCC A
- **Z68.42 Body mass index [BMI] 45.0-49.9, adult** CC UPD HCC A
- **Z68.43 Body mass index [BMI] 50.0-59.9, adult** CC UPD HCC A
- **Z68.44 Body mass index [BMI] 60.0-69.9, adult** CC UPD HCC A
- **Z68.45 Body mass index [BMI] 70 or greater, adult** CC UPD HCC A

✓5th **Z68.5 Body mass index [BMI] pediatric**
AHA: 2018,4Q,81-82
- **Z68.51 Body mass index [BMI] pediatric, less than 5th percentile for age** UPD
- **Z68.52 Body mass index [BMI] pediatric, 5th percentile to less than 85th percentile for age** UPD
- **Z68.53 Body mass index [BMI] pediatric, 85th percentile to less than 95th percentile for age** UPD
- **Z68.54 Body mass index [BMI] pediatric, greater than or equal to 95th percentile for age** UPD

Persons encountering health services in other circumstances (Z69-Z76)

✓4th **Z69 Encounter for mental health services for victim and perpetrator of abuse**
INCLUDES counseling for victims and perpetrators of abuse

✓5th **Z69.0 Encounter for mental health services for child abuse problems**

✓6th **Z69.01 Encounter for mental health services for parental child abuse**

Z69.010 Encounter for mental health services for victim of parental child abuse P
Encounter for mental health services for victim of child abuse by parent
Encounter for mental health services for victim of child neglect by parent
Encounter for mental health services for victim of child psychological abuse by parent
Encounter for mental health services for victim of child sexual abuse by parent

Z69.011 Encounter for mental health services for perpetrator of parental child abuse UPD
Encounter for mental health services for perpetrator of parental child neglect
Encounter for mental health services for perpetrator of parental child psychological abuse
Encounter for mental health services for perpetrator of parental child sexual abuse
EXCLUDES 1 *encounter for mental health services for non-parental child abuse (Z69.02-)*

✓6th **Z69.02 Encounter for mental health services for non-parental child abuse**

Z69.020 Encounter for mental health services for victim of non-parental child abuse P
Encounter for mental health services for victim of non-parental child neglect
Encounter for mental health services for victim of non-parental child psychological abuse
Encounter for mental health services for victim of non-parental child sexual abuse

Z69.021 Encounter for mental health services for perpetrator of non-parental child abuse UPD
Encounter for mental health services for perpetrator of non-parental child neglect
Encounter for mental health services for perpetrator of non-parental child psychological abuse
Encounter for mental health services for perpetrator of non-parental child sexual abuse

✓5th **Z69.1 Encounter for mental health services for spousal or partner abuse problems**

Z69.11 Encounter for mental health services for victim of spousal or partner abuse UPD
Encounter for mental health services for victim of spouse or partner neglect
Encounter for mental health services for victim of spouse or partner psychological abuse
Encounter for mental health services for victim of spouse or partner violence, physical

Z69.12 Encounter for mental health services for perpetrator of spousal or partner abuse UPD
Encounter for mental health services for perpetrator of spouse or partner neglect
Encounter for mental health services for perpetrator of spouse or partner psychological abuse
Encounter for mental health services for perpetrator of spouse or partner violence, physical
Encounter for mental health services for perpetrator of spouse or partner violence, sexual

✓5th **Z69.8 Encounter for mental health services for victim or perpetrator of other abuse**

Z69.81 Encounter for mental health services for victim of other abuse UPD
Encounter for mental health services for victim of non-spousal adult abuse
Encounter for mental health services for victim of spouse or partner violence, sexual
Encounter for rape victim counseling

Z69.82 Encounter for mental health services for perpetrator of other abuse UPD
Encounter for mental health services for perpetrator of non-spousal adult abuse

✓4th **Z70 Counseling related to sexual attitude, behavior and orientation**

INCLUDES encounter for mental health services for sexual attitude, behavior and orientation

EXCLUDES 2 *contraceptive or procreative counseling (Z30-Z31)*

Z70.0 Counseling related to sexual attitude UPD

Z70.1 Counseling related to patient's sexual behavior and orientation UPD
Patient concerned regarding impotence
Patient concerned regarding non-responsiveness
Patient concerned regarding promiscuity
Patient concerned regarding sexual orientation

Z70.2 Counseling related to sexual behavior and orientation of third party UPD
Advice sought regarding sexual behavior and orientation of child
Advice sought regarding sexual behavior and orientation of partner
Advice sought regarding sexual behavior and orientation of spouse

Z70.3 Counseling related to combined concerns regarding sexual attitude, behavior and orientation UPD

Z70.8 Other sex counseling UPD
Encounter for sex education

Z70.9 Sex counseling, unspecified UPD

✓4th **Z71 Persons encountering health services for other counseling and medical advice, not elsewhere classified**

EXCLUDES 2 *contraceptive or procreation counseling (Z30-Z31)*
sex counseling (Z70.-)

Z71.0 Person encountering health services to consult on behalf of another person UPD
Person encountering health services to seek advice or treatment for non-attending third party
EXCLUDES 2 *anxiety (normal) about sick person in family (Z63.7)*
expectant (adoptive) parent(s) pre-birth pediatrician visit (Z76.81)

Z71.1 Person with feared health complaint in whom no diagnosis is made UPD
Person encountering health services with feared condition which was not demonstrated
Person encountering health services in which problem was normal state
"Worried well"
EXCLUDES 1 *medical observation for suspected diseases and conditions proven not to exist (Z03.-)*

Z71.2 Person consulting for explanation of examination or test findings UPD

Z71.3 Dietary counseling and surveillance UPD
Use additional code for any associated underlying medical condition
Use additional code to identify body mass index (BMI), if known (Z68.-)

✓5th **Z71.4 Alcohol abuse counseling and surveillance**
Use additional code for alcohol abuse or dependence (F10.-)

Z71.41 Alcohol abuse counseling and surveillance of alcoholic UPD

Z71.42 Counseling for family member of alcoholic UPD
Counseling for significant other, partner, or friend of alcoholic

✓5th **Z71.5 Drug abuse counseling and surveillance**
Use additional code for drug abuse or dependence (F11-F16, F18-F19)

Z71.51 Drug abuse counseling and surveillance of drug abuser UPD

Z71.52 Counseling for family member of drug abuser UPD
Counseling for significant other, partner, or friend of drug abuser

Z71.6 Tobacco abuse counseling UPD
Use additional code for nicotine dependence (F17.-)

Z71.7 Human immunodeficiency virus [HIV] counseling UPD

✓5th **Z71.8 Other specified counseling**
EXCLUDES 2 *counseling for contraception (Z30.0-)*
AHA: 2017,4Q,27

Z71.81 Spiritual or religious counseling UPD

Z71.82 Exercise counseling UPD

Z71.83 Encounter for nonprocreative genetic counseling
EXCLUDES 1 *counseling for procreative genetics (Z31.5)*
counseling for procreative management (Z31.6)

Z71.84 Encounter for health counseling related to travel UPD
Encounter for health risk and safety counseling for (international) travel
Code also, if applicable, encounter for immunization (Z23)
EXCLUDES 2 *encounter for administrative examination (Z02.-)*
encounter for other special examination without complaint, suspected or reported diagnosis (Z01.-)
AHA: 2019,4Q,20,57

Z71.85 Encounter for immunization safety counseling UPD
Encounter for vaccine product safety counseling
Code also, if applicable, encounter for immunization (Z23)
Code also, if applicable, immunization not carried out (Z28.-)
EXCLUDES 1 *encounter for health counseling related to travel (Z71.84)*
AHA: 2021,4Q,34

Z71.87 Encounter for pediatric-to-adult transition counseling UPD
Code also chronic condition, if applicable, such as:
autism spectrum disorder (F84.0)
congenital malformations of the circulatory system (Q20-Q28)
cystic fibrosis (E84-)
sickle-cell disorder (D57-)
AHA: 2022,4Q,51

Z71.88 Encounter for counseling for socioeconomic factors UPD
AHA: 2022,4Q,51

Z71.89 Other specified counseling UPD

Z71.9 Counseling, unspecified UPD
Encounter for medical advice NOS

Z72 Problems related to lifestyle
EXCLUDES 2 *problems related to life-management difficulty (Z73*
problems related to socioeconomic and psychosoc
circumstances (Z55-Z65)

Z72.0 Tobacco use UPD
Tobacco use NOS
EXCLUDES 1 *history of tobacco dependence (Z87.891)*
nicotine dependence (F17.2-)
tobacco dependence (F17.2-)
tobacco use during pregnancy (O99.33-)

Z72.3 Lack of physical exercise UPD

Z72.4 Inappropriate diet and eating habits UPD
EXCLUDES 1 *behavioral eating disorders of infancy or childhood (F98.2-F98.3)*
eating disorders (F50.-)
lack of adequate food (Z59.48)
malnutrition and other nutritional deficiencies (E40-E64)

Z72.5 High risk sexual behavior
Promiscuity
EXCLUDES 1 *paraphilias (F65)*

Z72.51 High risk heterosexual behavior UPD
Z72.52 High risk homosexual behavior UPD
Z72.53 High risk bisexual behavior UPD

Z72.6 Gambling and betting UPD
EXCLUDES 1 *compulsive or pathological gambling (F63.0)*

Z72.8 Other problems related to lifestyle

Z72.81 Antisocial behavior
EXCLUDES 1 *conduct disorders (F91.-)*

Z72.810 Child and adolescent antisocial behavior P
Antisocial behavior (child) (adolescent) without manifest psychiatric disorder
Delinquency NOS
Group delinquency
Offenses in the context of gang membership
Stealing in company with others
Truancy from school

Z72.811 Adult antisocial behavior A
Adult antisocial behavior without manifest psychiatric disorder

Z72.82 Problems related to sleep

Z72.820 Sleep deprivation
Lack of adequate sleep
EXCLUDES 1 *insomnia (G47.0-)*

Z72.821 Inadequate sleep hygiene UPD
Bad sleep habits
Irregular sleep habits
Unhealthy sleep wake schedule
EXCLUDES 1 *insomnia (F51.0-, G47.0-)*

Z72.823 Risk of suffocation (smothering) under another while sleeping UPD
Child-caregiver co-sleeping
Infant bed-sharing
AHA: 2022,4Q,51

Z72.89 Other problems related to lifestyle UPD
Self-damaging behavior

Z72.9 Problem related to lifestyle, unspecified UPD

Z73 Problems related to life management difficulty
EXCLUDES 2 *problems related to socioeconomic and psychosocial circumstances (Z55-Z65)*
DEF: State of emotional, mental, and physical exhaustion causing difficulties in managing personal, school, or work circumstances. It is usually due to prolonged stress or poor interpersonal relationship skills or parenting skills.

Z73.0 Burn-out UPD
Z73.1 Type A behavior pattern UPD
Z73.2 Lack of relaxation and leisure UPD
Z73.3 Stress, not elsewhere classified UPD
Physical and mental strain NOS
EXCLUDES 1 *stress related to employment or unemployment (Z56.-)*
Z73.4 Inadequate social skills, not elsewhere classified UPD
Z73.5 Social role conflict, not elsewhere classified UPD
Z73.6 Limitation of activities due to disability UPD
EXCLUDES 1 *care-provider dependency (Z74.-)*

Z73.8 Other problems related to life management difficulty

Z73.81 Behavioral insomnia of childhood
DEF: Behaviors on the part of the child or caregivers that cause negative compliance with a child's sleep schedule resulting in lack of adequate sleep.

Z73.810 Behavioral insomnia of childhood, sleep-onset association type UPD P
Z73.811 Behavioral insomnia of childhood, limit setting type UPD P
Z73.812 Behavioral insomnia of childhood, combined type UPD P
Z73.819 Behavioral insomnia of childhood, unspecified type UPD P

Z73.82 Dual sensory impairment UPD
Z73.89 Other problems related to life management difficulty UPD

Z73.9 Problem related to life management difficulty, unspecified UPD

Z74 Problems related to care provider dependency
EXCLUDES 2 *dependence on enabling machines or devices NEC (Z99.-)*

Z74.0 Reduced mobility

Z74.01 Bed confinement status UPD
Bedridden

Z74.09 Other reduced mobility UPD
Chair ridden
Reduced mobility NOS
EXCLUDES 2 *wheelchair dependence (Z99.3)*

Z74.1 Need for assistance with personal care UPD
Z74.2 Need for assistance at home and no other household member able to render care UPD
Z74.3 Need for continuous supervision UPD
Z74.8 Other problems related to care provider dependency UPD
Z74.9 Problem related to care provider dependency, unspecified UPD

Z75 Problems related to medical facilities and other health care

Z75.0 Medical services not available in home UPD
EXCLUDES 1 *no other household member able to render care (Z74.2)*
Z75.1 Person awaiting admission to adequate facility elsewhere UPD
Z75.2 Other waiting period for investigation and treatment UPD
Z75.3 Unavailability and inaccessibility of health-care facilities UPD
EXCLUDES 1 *bed unavailable (Z75.1)*
Z75.4 Unavailability and inaccessibility of other helping agencies UPD
Z75.5 Holiday relief care UPD
Z75.8 Other problems related to medical facilities and other health care UPD
Z75.9 Unspecified problem related to medical facilities and other health care UPD

Z76 Persons encountering health services in other circumstances

Z76.Ø Encounter for issue of repeat prescription UPD
Encounter for issue of repeat prescription for appliance
Encounter for issue of repeat prescription for medicaments
Encounter for issue of repeat prescription for spectacles
EXCLUDES 2 *issue of medical certificate (ZØ2.7)*
repeat prescription for contraceptive (Z3Ø.4-)

Z76.1 Encounter for health supervision and care of foundling

Z76.2 Encounter for health supervision and care of other healthy infant and child UPD P
Encounter for medical or nursing care or supervision of healthy infant under circumstances such as adverse socioeconomic conditions at home
Encounter for medical or nursing care or supervision of healthy infant under circumstances such as awaiting foster or adoptive placement
Encounter for medical or nursing care or supervision of healthy infant under circumstances such as maternal illness
Encounter for medical or nursing care or supervision of healthy infant under circumstances such as number of children at home preventing or interfering with normal care

Z76.3 Healthy person accompanying sick person

Z76.4 Other boarder to healthcare facility
EXCLUDES 1 *homelessness (Z59.Ø-)*

Z76.5 Malingerer [conscious simulation]
Person feigning illness (with obvious motivation)
EXCLUDES 1 *factitious disorder (F68.1-, F68.A)*
peregrinating patient (F68.1-)
DEF: Act of intentionally exaggerating an illness or disability in order to receive personal gain or to avoid punishment or responsibility.

Z76.8 Persons encountering health services in other specified circumstances

Z76.81 Expectant parent(s) prebirth pediatrician visit UPD
Pre-adoption pediatrician visit for adoptive parent(s)

Z76.82 Awaiting organ transplant status UPD
Patient waiting for organ availability

Z76.89 Persons encountering health services in other specified circumstances UPD
Persons encountering health services NOS
AHA: 2014,2Q,10

Persons with potential health hazards related to family and personal history and certain conditions influencing health status (Z77-Z99)

Code also any follow-up examination (ZØ8-ZØ9)

Z77 Other contact with and (suspected) exposures hazardous to health
INCLUDES contact with and (suspected) exposures to potential hazards to health
EXCLUDES 2 *contact with and (suspected) exposure to communicable diseases (Z2Ø.-)*
exposure to (parental) (environmental) tobacco smoke in the perinatal period (P96.81)
newborn affected by noxious substances transmitted via placenta or breast milk (PØ4.-)
occupational exposure to risk factors (Z57.-)
retained foreign body (Z18.-)
retained foreign body fully removed (Z87.821)
toxic effects of substances chiefly nonmedicinal as to source (T51-T65)

Z77.Ø Contact with and (suspected) exposure to hazardous, chiefly nonmedicinal, chemicals

Z77.Ø1 Contact with and (suspected) exposure to hazardous metals

Z77.Ø1Ø Contact with and (suspected) exposure to arsenic UPD

Z77.Ø11 Contact with and (suspected) exposure to lead UPD

Z77.Ø12 Contact with and (suspected) exposure to uranium UPD
EXCLUDES 1 *retained depleted uranium fragments (Z18.Ø1)*

Z77.Ø18 Contact with and (suspected) exposure to other hazardous metals UPD
Contact with and (suspected) exposure to chromium compounds
Contact with and (suspected) exposure to nickel dust

Z77.Ø2 Contact with and (suspected) exposure to hazardous aromatic compounds

Z77.Ø2Ø Contact with and (suspected) exposure to aromatic amines UPD

Z77.Ø21 Contact with and (suspected) exposure to benzene UPD

Z77.Ø28 Contact with and (suspected) exposure to other hazardous aromatic compounds UPD
Aromatic dyes NOS
Polycyclic aromatic hydrocarbons

Z77.Ø9 Contact with and (suspected) exposure to other hazardous, chiefly nonmedicinal, chemicals

Z77.Ø9Ø Contact with and (suspected) exposure to asbestos UPD

Z77.Ø98 Contact with and (suspected) exposure to other hazardous, chiefly nonmedicinal, chemicals UPD
Dyes NOS

Z77.1 Contact with and (suspected) exposure to environmental pollution and hazards in the physical environment

Z77.11 Contact with and (suspected) exposure to environmental pollution

Z77.11Ø Contact with and (suspected) exposure to air pollution UPD

Z77.111 Contact with and (suspected) exposure to water pollution UPD

Z77.112 Contact with and (suspected) exposure to soil pollution UPD

Z77.118 Contact with and (suspected) exposure to other environmental pollution UPD

Z77.12 Contact with and (suspected) exposure to hazards in the physical environment

Z77.12Ø Contact with and (suspected) exposure to mold (toxic) UPD

Z77.121 Contact with and (suspected) exposure to harmful algae and algae toxins UPD
Contact with and (suspected) exposure to (harmful) algae bloom NOS
Contact with and (suspected) exposure to blue-green algae bloom
Contact with and (suspected) exposure to brown tide
Contact with and (suspected) exposure to cyanobacteria bloom
Contact with and (suspected) exposure to Florida red tide
Contact with and (suspected) exposure to pfiesteria piscicida
Contact with and (suspected) exposure to red tide

Z77.122 Contact with and (suspected) exposure to noise UPD

Z77.123 Contact with and (suspected) exposure to radon and other naturally occurring radiation UPD
EXCLUDES 2 *radiation exposure as the cause of a confirmed condition (W88-W9Ø, X39.Ø-)*
radiation sickness NOS (T66)

Z77.128 Contact with and (suspected) exposure to other hazards in the physical environment UPD

Z77.2 Contact with and (suspected) exposure to other hazardous substances

Z77.21 Contact with and (suspected) exposure to potentially hazardous body fluids UPD

Z77.22 Contact with and (suspected) exposure to environmental tobacco smoke (acute) (chronic) UPD
Exposure to second hand tobacco smoke (acute) (chronic)
Passive smoking (acute) (chronic)
EXCLUDES 1 *nicotine dependence (F17.-)*
tobacco use (Z72.Ø)
EXCLUDES 2 *occupational exposure to environmental tobacco smoke (Z57.31)*

Z77.29 Contact with and (suspected) exposure to other hazardous substances UPD
AHA: 2016,2Q,33

Z77.9 Other contact with and (suspected) exposures hazardous to health UPD

Z78 Other specified health status
EXCLUDES 2 *asymptomatic human immunodeficiency virus [HIV] infection status (Z21)*
postprocedural status (Z93-Z99)
sex reassignment status (Z87.89Ø)

Z78.Ø Asymptomatic menopausal state UPD A ♀
Menopausal state NOS
Postmenopausal status NOS
EXCLUDES 2 *symptomatic menopausal state (N95.1)*

Z78.1 Physical restraint status UPD
EXCLUDES 1 *physical restraint due to a procedure - omit code*
DEF: Application of mechanical restraining devices or manual restraints to limit physical mobility of a patient.

Z78.9 Other specified health status UPD

Z79 Long term (current) drug therapy
INCLUDES long term (current) drug use for prophylactic purposes
Code also any therapeutic drug level monitoring (Z51.81)
EXCLUDES 2 *drug abuse and dependence (F11-F19)*
drug use complicating pregnancy, childbirth, and the puerperium (O99.32-)
AHA: 2021,1Q,12

Z79.Ø Long term (current) use of anticoagulants and antithrombotics/antiplatelets
EXCLUDES 2 *long term (current) use of aspirin (Z79.82)*

Z79.Ø1 Long term (current) use of anticoagulants
AHA: 2023,2Q,28; 2022,2Q,17; 2021,1Q,4; 2020,2Q,20

Z79.Ø2 Long term (current) use of antithrombotics/antiplatelets UPD

Z79.1 Long term (current) use of non-steroidal anti-inflammatories (NSAID) UPD
EXCLUDES 2 *long term (current) use of aspirin (Z79.82)*

Z79.2 Long term (current) use of antibiotics UPD

Z79.3 Long term (current) use of hormonal contraceptives
Long term (current) use of birth control pill or patch

Z79.4 Long term (current) use of insulin HCC
EXCLUDES 2 *long-term (current) use of injectable non-insulin antidiabetic drugs (Z79.85)*
long term (current) use of oral antidiabetic drugs (Z79.84)
long term (current) use of oral hypoglycemic drugs (Z79.84)
AHA: 2020,3Q,31

Z79.5 Long term (current) use of steroids

Z79.51 Long term (current) use of inhaled steroids UPD

Z79.52 Long term (current) use of systemic steroids UPD

Z79.6 Long term (current) use of immunomodulators and immunosuppressants
EXCLUDES 2 *long term (current) use of steroids (Z79.5-)*
long term (current) use of agents affecting estrogen receptors and estrogen levels (Z79.81-)
AHA: 2022,4Q,50

Z79.6Ø Long term (current) use of unspecified immunomodulators and immunosuppressants UPD

Z79.61 Long term (current) use of immunomodulator UPD
Long term (current) use of apremilast
Long term (current) use of immunomodulatory imide drug
Long term (current) use of lenalidomide
Long term (current) use of pomalidomide

Z79.62 Long term (current) use of immunosuppressant

Z79.62Ø Long term (current) use of immunosuppressive biologic UPD
Long term (current) use of adalimumab
Long term (current) use of etanercept
Long term (current) use of infliximab
Long term (current) use of monoclonal antibodies

Z79.621 Long term (current) use of calcineurin inhibitor UPD
Long term (current) use of cyclosporine
Long term (current) use of tacrolimus

Z79.622 Long term (current) use of Janus kinase inhibitor UPD
Long term (current) use of tofacitinib

Z79.623 Long term (current) use of mammalian target of rapamycin (mTOR) inhibitor UPD
Long term (current) use of sirolimus

Z79.624 Long term (current) use of inhibitors of nucleotide synthesis UPD
Long term (current) use of azathioprine
Long term (current) use omycophenolate
Long term (current) use of purine synthesis (IMDH) inhibitors

Z79.63 Long term (current) use of chemotherapeutic agent

Z79.63Ø Long term (current) use of alkylating agent UPD
Long term (current) use of chlorambucil
Long term (current) use of cisplatin
Long term (current) use of cyclophosphamide

Z79.631 Long term (current) use of antimetabolite agent UPD
Long term (current) use of 5-fluorouracil
Long term (current) use of 6-mercaptopurine
Long term (current) use of cytarabine
Long term (current) use of methotrexate

Z79.632 Long term (current) use of antitumor antibiotic UPD
Long term (current) use of bleomycin
Long term (current) use of doxorubicin
Long term (current) use of mitomycin C

Z79.633 Long term (current) use of mitotic inhibitor UPD
Long term (current) use of paclitaxel
Long term (current) use of plant alkaloids
Long term (current) use of vinblastine
Long term (current) use of vincristine

Z79.634 Long term (current) use of topoisomerase inhibitor UPD
Long term (current) use of etoposide
Long term (current) use of irinotecan
Long term (current) use of topotecan

Z79.64 Long term (current) use of myelosuppressive agent UPD
Long term (current) use of hydroxyurea

Z79.69 Long term (current) use of other immunomodulators and immunosuppressants UPD

Z79.8 Other long term (current) drug therapy

Z79.81 Long term (current) use of agents affecting estrogen receptors and estrogen levels

Code first, if applicable:
- malignant neoplasm of breast (C5Ø.-)
- malignant neoplasm of prostate (C61)

Use additional code, if applicable, to identify:
- estrogen receptor positive status (Z17.Ø)
- family history of breast cancer (Z8Ø.3)
- genetic susceptibility to malignant neoplasm (cancer) (Z15.Ø-)
- personal history of breast cancer (Z85.3)
- personal history of prostate cancer (Z85.46)
- postmenopausal status (Z78.Ø)

EXCLUDES 1 *hormone replacement therapy (Z79.89Ø)*

AHA: 2022,3Q,14

Z79.81Ø Long term (current) use of selective estrogen receptor modulators (SERMs) UPD
- Long term (current) use of raloxifene (Evista)
- Long term (current) use of tamoxifen (Nolvadex)
- Long term (current) use of toremifene (Fareston)

Z79.811 Long term (current) use of aromatase inhibitors UPD
- Long term (current) use of anastrozole (Arimidex)
- Long term (current) use of exemestane (Aromasin)
- Long term (current) use of letrozole (Femara)

Z79.818 Long term (current) use of other agents affecting estrogen receptors and estrogen levels UPD
- Long term (current) use of estrogen receptor downregulators
- Long term (current) use of fulvestrant (Faslodex)
- Long term (current) use of gonadotropin-releasing hormone (GnRH) agonist
- Long term (current) use of goserelin acetate (Zoladex)
- Long term (current) use of leuprolide acetate (leuprorelin) (Lupron)
- Long term (current) use of megestrol acetate (Megace)

Z79.82 Long term (current) use of aspirin

Z79.83 Long term (current) use of bisphosphonates UPD

AHA: 2016,4Q,42

Z79.84 Long term (current) use of oral hypoglycemic drugs UPD

Long term (current) use of oral antidiabetic drugs

EXCLUDES 2 *long-term (current) use of injectable non-insulin antidiabetic drugs (Z79.85)*
long term (current) use of insulin (Z79.4)

AHA: 2020,3Q,31; 2016,4Q,76

Z79.85 Long-term (current) use of injectable non-insulin antidiabetic drugs UPD

EXCLUDES 2 *long term (current) use of insulin (Z79.4)*
long term (current) use of oral hypoglycemic drugs (Z79.84)

AHA: 2022,4Q,50

Z79.89 Other long term (current) drug therapy

Z79.89Ø Hormone replacement therapy UPD

Z79.891 Long term (current) use of opiate analgesic

Long term (current) use of methadone for pain management

EXCLUDES 1 *methadone use NOS (F11.9-)*
use of methodone for treatment of heroin addiction (F11.2-)

Z79.899 Other long term (current) drug therapy

AHA: 2020,4Q,11; 2020,3Q,31; 2020,2Q,14; 2015,4Q,34; 2015,3Q,21

Z8Ø Family history of primary malignant neoplasm

Z8Ø.Ø Family history of malignant neoplasm of digestive organs UPD

Conditions classifiable to C15-C26

AHA: 2018,1Q,6

Z8Ø.1 Family history of malignant neoplasm of trachea, bronchus and lung UPD

Conditions classifiable to C33-C34

Z8Ø.2 Family history of malignant neoplasm of other respiratory and intrathoracic organs UPD

Conditions classifiable to C3Ø-C32, C37-C39

Z8Ø.3 Family history of malignant neoplasm of breast UPD

Conditions classifiable to C5Ø.-

Z8Ø.4 Family history of malignant neoplasm of genital organs

Conditions classifiable to C51-C63

Z8Ø.41 Family history of malignant neoplasm of ovary UPD

Z8Ø.42 Family history of malignant neoplasm of prostate UPD

Z8Ø.43 Family history of malignant neoplasm of testis UPD

Z8Ø.49 Family history of malignant neoplasm of other genital organs UPD

Z8Ø.5 Family history of malignant neoplasm of urinary tract

Conditions classifiable to C64-C68

Z8Ø.51 Family history of malignant neoplasm of kidney UPD

Z8Ø.52 Family history of malignant neoplasm of bladder UPD

Z8Ø.59 Family history of malignant neoplasm of other urinary tract organ UPD

Z8Ø.6 Family history of leukemia UPD

Conditions classifiable to C91-C95

Z8Ø.7 Family history of other malignant neoplasms of lymphoid, hematopoietic and related tissues UPD

Conditions classifiable to C81-C9Ø, C96.-

Z8Ø.8 Family history of malignant neoplasm of other organs or systems UPD

Conditions classifiable to CØØ-C14, C4Ø-C49, C69-C79

Z8Ø.9 Family history of malignant neoplasm, unspecified UPD

Conditions classifiable to C8Ø.1

Z81 Family history of mental and behavioral disorders

Z81.Ø Family history of intellectual disabilities UPD

Conditions classifiable to F7Ø-F79

Z81.1 Family history of alcohol abuse and dependence UPD

Conditions classifiable to F1Ø.-

Z81.2 Family history of tobacco abuse and dependence UPD

Conditions classifiable to F17.-

Z81.3 Family history of other psychoactive substance abuse and dependence UPD

Conditions classifiable to F11-F16, F18-F19

Z81.4 Family history of other substance abuse and dependence UPD

Conditions classifiable to F55

Z81.8 Family history of other mental and behavioral disorders UPD

Conditions classifiable elsewhere in FØ1-F99

Z82 Family history of certain disabilities and chronic diseases (leading to disablement)

Z82.Ø Family history of epilepsy and other diseases of the nervous system UPD

Conditions classifiable to GØØ-G99

Z82.1 Family history of blindness and visual loss UPD

Conditions classifiable to H54.-

Z82.2 Family history of deafness and hearing loss UPD

Conditions classifiable to H9Ø-H91

Z82.3 Family history of stroke UPD

Conditions classifiable to I6Ø-I64

Z82.4 Family history of ischemic heart disease and other diseases of the circulatory system

Conditions classifiable to IØØ-I5A, I65-I99

Z82.41 Family history of sudden cardiac death UPD

Z82.49 Family history of ischemic heart disease and other diseases of the circulatory system UPD

Z82.5 **Family history of asthma and other chronic lower respiratory diseases** UPD
Conditions classifiable to J40-J47
EXCLUDES 2 *family history of other diseases of the respiratory system (Z83.6)*

✓5th Z82.6 **Family history of arthritis and other diseases of the musculoskeletal system and connective tissue**
Conditions classifiable to M00-M99

Z82.61 **Family history of arthritis** UPD

Z82.62 **Family history of osteoporosis** UPD

Z82.69 **Family history of other diseases of the musculoskeletal system and connective tissue** UPD

✓5th Z82.7 **Family history of congenital malformations, deformations and chromosomal abnormalities**
Conditions classifiable to Q00-Q99

Z82.71 **Family history of polycystic kidney** UPD

Z82.79 **Family history of other congenital malformations, deformations and chromosomal abnormalities** UPD

Z82.8 **Family history of other disabilities and chronic diseases leading to disablement, not elsewhere classified** UPD

✓4th **Z83 Family history of other specific disorders**
EXCLUDES 2 *contact with and (suspected) exposure to communicable disease in the family (Z20.-)*

Z83.0 **Family history of human immunodeficiency virus [HIV] disease** UPD
Conditions classifiable to B20

Z83.1 **Family history of other infectious and parasitic diseases** UPD
Conditions classifiable to A00-B19, B25-B94, B99

Z83.2 **Family history of diseases of the blood and blood-forming organs and certain disorders involving the immune mechanism** UPD
Conditions classifiable to D50-D89

Z83.3 **Family history of diabetes mellitus** UPD
Conditions classifiable to E08-E13

✓5th Z83.4 **Family history of other endocrine, nutritional and metabolic diseases**
Conditions classifiable to E00-E07, E15-E88

Z83.41 **Family history of multiple endocrine neoplasia [MEN] syndrome** UPD

Z83.42 **Family history of familial hypercholesterolemia** UPD
AHA: 2016,4Q,77

✓6th Z83.43 **Family history of other disorder of lipoprotein metabolism and other lipidemias**
AHA: 2018,4Q,6,35

Z83.430 **Family history of elevated lipoprotein(a)** UPD
Family history of elevated Lp(a)

Z83.438 **Family history of other disorder of lipoprotein metabolism and other lipidemia** UPD
Family history of familial combined hyperlipidemia

Z83.49 **Family history of other endocrine, nutritional and metabolic diseases** UPD

✓5th Z83.5 **Family history of eye and ear disorders**

✓6th Z83.51 **Family history of eye disorders**
Conditions classifiable to H00-H53, H55-H59
EXCLUDES 2 *family history of blindness and visual loss (Z82.1)*

Z83.511 **Family history of glaucoma** UPD

Z83.518 **Family history of other specified eye disorder** UPD

Z83.52 **Family history of ear disorders** UPD
Conditions classifiable to H60-H83, H92-H95
EXCLUDES 2 *family history of deafness and hearing loss (Z82.2)*

Z83.6 **Family history of other diseases of the respiratory system** UPD
Conditions classifiable to J00-J39, J60-J99
EXCLUDES 2 *family history of asthma and other chronic lower respiratory diseases (Z82.5)*

✓5th Z83.7 **Family history of diseases of the digestive system**
Conditions classifiable to ▶D12, K00-K93◀

▲ ✓6th Z83.71 **Family history of colonic polyps**
EXCLUDES 2 *family history of malignant neoplasm of digestive organs (Z80.0)*
AHA: 2021,1Q,14

● Z83.710 **Family history of adenomatous and serrated polyps**
Conditions classifiable to D12.-
Family history of tubular adenoma polyps
Family history of tubulovillous adenoma polyps
Family history of villous adenoma polyps

● Z83.711 **Family history of hyperplastic colon polyps**

● Z83.718 **Other family history of colon polyps**
Family history of inflammatory colon polyps

● Z83.719 **Family history of colon polyps, unspecified**
Family history of colon polyps NOS

Z83.79 **Family history of other diseases of the digestive system** UPD

✓4th **Z84 Family history of other conditions**

Z84.0 **Family history of diseases of the skin and subcutaneous tissue** UPD
Conditions classifiable to L00-L99

Z84.1 **Family history of disorders of kidney and ureter** UPD
Conditions classifiable to N00-N29

Z84.2 **Family history of other diseases of the genitourinary system** UPD
Conditions classifiable to N30-N99

Z84.3 **Family history of consanguinity** UPD

✓5th Z84.8 **Family history of other specified conditions**

Z84.81 **Family history of carrier of genetic disease** UPD
AHA: 2021,1Q,14

Z84.82 **Family history of sudden infant death syndrome** UPD
Family history of SIDS
AHA: 2016,4Q,77

Z84.89 **Family history of other specified conditions** UPD

✓4th **Z85 Personal history of malignant neoplasm**
Code first any follow-up examination after treatment of malignant neoplasm (Z08)
Use additional code to identify:
alcohol use and dependence (F10.-)
exposure to environmental tobacco smoke (Z77.22)
history of tobacco dependence (Z87.891)
occupational exposure to environmental tobacco smoke (Z57.31)
tobacco dependence (F17.-)
tobacco use (Z72.0)
EXCLUDES 2 *personal history of benign neoplasm (Z86.01-)*
personal history of carcinoma-in-situ (Z86.00-)
AHA: 2022,3Q,28; 2020,3Q,30; 2018,4Q,64

✓5th Z85.0 **Personal history of malignant neoplasm of digestive organs**
AHA: 2017,1Q,9

Z85.00 **Personal history of malignant neoplasm of unspecified digestive organ** UPD

Z85.01 **Personal history of malignant neoplasm of esophagus** UPD
Conditions classifiable to C15

✓6th Z85.02 **Personal history of malignant neoplasm of stomach**

Z85.020 **Personal history of malignant carcinoid tumor of stomach** UPD
Conditions classifiable to C7A.092

Z85.028 **Personal history of other malignant neoplasm of stomach** UPD
Conditions classifiable to C16

✓6th Z85.03 **Personal history of malignant neoplasm of large intestine**

Z85.030 **Personal history of malignant carcinoid tumor of large intestine** UPD
Conditions classifiable to C7A.022-C7A.025, C7A.029

Z85.038 **Personal history of other malignant neoplasm of large intestine** UPD
Conditions classifiable to C18

Z85.04 Personal history of malignant neoplasm of rectum, rectosigmoid junction, and anus

Z85.040 Personal history of malignant carcinoid tumor of rectum UPD
Conditions classifiable to C7A.026

Z85.048 Personal history of other malignant neoplasm of rectum, rectosigmoid junction, and anus UPD
Conditions classifiable to C19-C21

Z85.05 Personal history of malignant neoplasm of liver UPD
Conditions classifiable to C22

Z85.06 Personal history of malignant neoplasm of small intestine

Z85.060 Personal history of malignant carcinoid tumor of small intestine UPD
Conditions classifiable to C7A.01-

Z85.068 Personal history of other malignant neoplasm of small intestine UPD
Conditions classifiable to C17

Z85.07 Personal history of malignant neoplasm of pancreas UPD
Conditions classifiable to C25

Z85.09 Personal history of malignant neoplasm of other digestive organs UPD

Z85.1 Personal history of malignant neoplasm of trachea, bronchus and lung

Z85.11 Personal history of malignant neoplasm of bronchus and lung

Z85.110 Personal history of malignant carcinoid tumor of bronchus and lung UPD
Conditions classifiable to C7A.090

Z85.118 Personal history of other malignant neoplasm of bronchus and lung UPD
Conditions classifiable to C34

Z85.12 Personal history of malignant neoplasm of trachea UPD
Conditions classifiable to C33

Z85.2 Personal history of malignant neoplasm of other respiratory and intrathoracic organs

Z85.20 Personal history of malignant neoplasm of unspecified respiratory organ UPD

Z85.21 Personal history of malignant neoplasm of larynx UPD
Conditions classifiable to C32

Z85.22 Personal history of malignant neoplasm of nasal cavities, middle ear, and accessory sinuses UPD
Conditions classifiable to C30-C31

Z85.23 Personal history of malignant neoplasm of thymus

Z85.230 Personal history of malignant carcinoid tumor of thymus UPD
Conditions classifiable to C7A.091

Z85.238 Personal history of other malignant neoplasm of thymus UPD
Conditions classifiable to C37

Z85.29 Personal history of malignant neoplasm of other respiratory and intrathoracic organs UPD

Z85.3 Personal history of malignant neoplasm of breast UPD
Conditions classifiable to C50.-

Z85.4 Personal history of malignant neoplasm of genital organs
Conditions classifiable to C51-C63

Z85.40 Personal history of malignant neoplasm of unspecified female genital organ UPD ♀

Z85.41 Personal history of malignant neoplasm of cervix uteri UPD ♀

Z85.42 Personal history of malignant neoplasm of other parts of uterus UPD ♀

Z85.43 Personal history of malignant neoplasm of ovary UPD ♀

Z85.44 Personal history of malignant neoplasm of other female genital organs UPD ♀

Z85.45 Personal history of malignant neoplasm of unspecified male genital organ UPD ♂

Z85.46 Personal history of malignant neoplasm of prostate UPD ♂
AHA: 2023,2Q,5

Z85.47 Personal history of malignant neoplasm of testis UPD ♂

Z85.48 Personal history of malignant neoplasm of epididymis UPD ♂

Z85.49 Personal history of malignant neoplasm of other male genital organs UPD ♂

Z85.5 Personal history of malignant neoplasm of urinary tract
Conditions classifiable to C64-C68

Z85.50 Personal history of malignant neoplasm of unspecified urinary tract organ UPD

Z85.51 Personal history of malignant neoplasm of bladder UPD

Z85.52 Personal history of malignant neoplasm of kidney
EXCLUDES 1 *personal history of malignant neoplasm of renal pelvis (Z85.53)*

Z85.520 Personal history of malignant carcinoid tumor of kidney UPD
Conditions classifiable to C7A.093

Z85.528 Personal history of other malignant neoplasm of kidney UPD
Conditions classifiable to C64

Z85.53 Personal history of malignant neoplasm of renal pelvis UPD

Z85.54 Personal history of malignant neoplasm of ureter UPD

Z85.59 Personal history of malignant neoplasm of other urinary tract organ UPD

Z85.6 Personal history of leukemia UPD
Conditions classifiable to C91-C95
EXCLUDES 1 *leukemia in remission C91.0-C95.9 with 5th character 1*

Z85.7 Personal history of other malignant neoplasms of lymphoid, hematopoietic and related tissues

Z85.71 Personal history of Hodgkin lymphoma UPD
Conditions classifiable to C81

Z85.72 Personal history of non-Hodgkin lymphomas UPD
Conditions classifiable to C82-C85
AHA: 2022,3Q,28

Z85.79 Personal history of other malignant neoplasms of lymphoid, hematopoietic and related tissues UPD
Conditions classifiable to C88-C90, C96
EXCLUDES 1 *multiple myeloma in remission (C90.01)*
plasma cell leukemia in remission (C90.11)
plasmacytoma in remission (C90.21)

Z85.8 Personal history of malignant neoplasms of other organs and systems
Conditions classifiable to C00-C14, C40-C49, C69-C75, C7A.098, C76-C79

Z85.81 Personal history of malignant neoplasm of lip, oral cavity, and pharynx
Conditions classifiable to C00-C14

Z85.810 Personal history of malignant neoplasm of tongue UPD

Z85.818 Personal history of malignant neoplasm of other sites of lip, oral cavity, and pharynx UPD

Z85.819 Personal history of malignant neoplasm of unspecified site of lip, oral cavity, and pharynx UPD

Z85.82 Personal history of malignant neoplasm of skin

Z85.820 Personal history of malignant melanoma of skin UPD
Conditions classifiable to C43
AHA: 2022,3Q,9

Z85.821 Personal history of Merkel cell carcinoma UPD
Conditions classifiable to C4A

Z85.828 Personal history of other malignant neoplasm of skin UPD
Conditions classifiable to C44

Z85.83 Personal history of malignant neoplasm of bone and soft tissue
Conditions classifiable to C40-C41; C45-C49

Z85.830 Personal history of malignant neoplasm of bone UPD

Z85.831 Personal history of malignant neoplasm of soft tissue UPD
EXCLUDES 2 *personal history of malignant neoplasm of skin (Z85.82-)*

✓6th **Z85.84 Personal history of malignant neoplasm of eye and nervous tissue**
Conditions classifiable to C69-C72
Z85.840 Personal history of malignant neoplasm of eye UPD
Z85.841 Personal history of malignant neoplasm of brain UPD
Z85.848 Personal history of malignant neoplasm of other parts of nervous tissue UPD

✓6th **Z85.85 Personal history of malignant neoplasm of endocrine glands**
Conditions classifiable to C73-C75
Z85.850 Personal history of malignant neoplasm of thyroid UPD
Z85.858 Personal history of malignant neoplasm of other endocrine glands UPD

Z85.89 Personal history of malignant neoplasm of other organs and systems UPD
Conditions classifiable to C7A.098, C76, C77-C79

Z85.9 Personal history of malignant neoplasm, unspecified UPD
Conditions classifiable to C7A.00, C80.1

✓4th **Z86 Personal history of certain other diseases**
Code first any follow-up examination after treatment (Z09)

✓5th **Z86.0 Personal history of in-situ and benign neoplasms and neoplasms of uncertain behavior**
EXCLUDES 2 *personal history of malignant neoplasms (Z85.-)*
AHA: 2017,1Q,9

✓6th **Z86.00 Personal history of in-situ neoplasm**
Conditions classifiable to D00-D09
AHA: 2019,4Q,20
Z86.000 Personal history of in-situ neoplasm of breast UPD
Conditions classifiable to D05
Z86.001 Personal history of in-situ neoplasm of cervix uteri UPD ♀
Conditions classifiable to D06
Personal history of cervical intraepithelial neoplasia III [CIN III]
Z86.002 Personal history of in-situ neoplasm of other and unspecified genital organs UPD
Conditions classifiable to D07
Personal history of high-grade prostatic intraepithelial neoplasia III [HGPIN III]
Personal history of vaginal intraepithelial neoplasia III [VAIN III]
Personal history of vulvar intraepithelial neoplasia III [VIN III]
Z86.003 Personal history of in-situ neoplasm of oral cavity, esophagus and stomach UPD
Conditions classifiable to D00
Z86.004 Personal history of in-situ neoplasm of other and unspecified digestive organs UPD
Conditions classifiable to D01
Personal history of anal intraepithelial neoplasia (AIN III)
Z86.005 Personal history of in-situ neoplasm of middle ear and respiratory system UPD
Conditions classifiable to D02
Z86.006 Personal history of melanoma in-situ UPD
Conditions classifiable to D03
EXCLUDES 2 *sites other than skin - code to personal history of in-situ neoplasm of the site*
Z86.007 Personal history of in-situ neoplasm of skin UPD
Conditions classifiable to D04
Personal history of carcinoma in situ of skin
Z86.008 Personal history of in-situ neoplasm of other site UPD
Conditions classifiable to D09

✓6th **Z86.01 Personal history of benign neoplasm**
Z86.010 Personal history of colonic polyps UPD
AHA: 2021,1Q,14; 2017,1Q,14
Z86.011 Personal history of benign neoplasm of the brain UPD
Z86.012 Personal history of benign carcinoid tumor UPD
Z86.018 Personal history of other benign neoplasm UPD
AHA: 2017,1Q,14

Z86.03 Personal history of neoplasm of uncertain behavior UPD

✓5th **Z86.1 Personal history of infectious and parasitic diseases**
Conditions classifiable to A00-B89, B99
EXCLUDES 1 *personal history of infectious diseases specific to a body system*
sequelae of infectious and parasitic diseases (B90-B94)
Z86.11 Personal history of tuberculosis UPD
Z86.12 Personal history of poliomyelitis UPD
Z86.13 Personal history of malaria UPD
Z86.14 Personal history of Methicillin resistant Staphylococcus aureus infection UPD
Personal history of MRSA infection
Z86.15 Personal history of latent tuberculosis infection UPD
Z86.16 Personal history of COVID-19 UPD
EXCLUDES 1 *post COVID-19 condition (U09.9)*
AHA: 2021,4Q,107-108; 2021,1Q,28-29,33-35,40-41,44-45
Z86.19 Personal history of other infectious and parasitic diseases UPD
AHA: 2022,3Q,4; 2021,1Q,33-34,40; 2020,3Q,13; 2020,2Q,10,12

Z86.2 Personal history of diseases of the blood and blood-forming organs and certain disorders involving the immune mechanism UPD
Conditions classifiable to D50-D89

✓5th **Z86.3 Personal history of endocrine, nutritional and metabolic diseases**
Conditions classifiable to E00-E88
Z86.31 Personal history of diabetic foot ulcer UPD
EXCLUDES 2 *current diabetic foot ulcer (E08.621, E09.621, E10.621, E11.621, E13.621)*
Z86.32 Personal history of gestational diabetes UPD ♀
Personal history of conditions classifiable to O24.4-
EXCLUDES 1 *gestational diabetes mellitus in current pregnancy (O24.4-)*
Z86.39 Personal history of other endocrine, nutritional and metabolic disease UPD
AHA: 2020,1Q,12

✓5th **Z86.5 Personal history of mental and behavioral disorders**
Conditions classifiable to F40-F59
Z86.51 Personal history of combat and operational stress reaction UPD A
Z86.59 Personal history of other mental and behavioral disorders UPD

✓5th **Z86.6 Personal history of diseases of the nervous system and sense organs**
Conditions classifiable to G00-G99, H00-H95
Z86.61 Personal history of infections of the central nervous system UPD
Personal history of encephalitis
Personal history of meningitis
Z86.69 Personal history of other diseases of the nervous system and sense organs UPD
AHA: 2016,4Q,24

✓5th **Z86.7 Personal history of diseases of the circulatory system**
Conditions classifiable to I00-I99
EXCLUDES 2 *old myocardial infarction (I25.2)*
personal history of anaphylactic shock (Z87.892)
postmyocardial infarction syndrome (I24.1)

✓6th **Z86.71 Personal history of venous thrombosis and embolism**
Z86.711 Personal history of pulmonary embolism UPD
Z86.718 Personal history of other venous thrombosis and embolism UPD
AHA: 2020,2Q,20

Z86.72 Personal history of thrombophlebitis UPD

Z86.73 Personal history of transient ischemic attack (TIA), and cerebral infarction without residual deficits UPD

Personal history of prolonged reversible ischemic neurological deficit (PRIND)

Personal history of stroke NOS without residual deficits

EXCLUDES 1 *personal history of traumatic brain injury (Z87.820)*

sequelae of cerebrovascular disease (I69.-)

AHA: 2023,1Q,37; 2012,4Q,92

Z86.74 Personal history of sudden cardiac arrest UPD

Personal history of sudden cardiac death successfully resuscitated

Z86.79 Personal history of other diseases of the circulatory system UPD

AHA: 2022,2Q,14; 2020,1Q,12

√4th **Z87 Personal history of other diseases and conditions**

Code first any follow-up examination after treatment (Z09)

AHA: 2022,4Q,50-51

√5th **Z87.0 Personal history of diseases of the respiratory system**

Conditions classifiable to J00-J99

Z87.01 Personal history of pneumonia (recurrent) UPD

Z87.09 Personal history of other diseases of the respiratory system UPD

√5th **Z87.1 Personal history of diseases of the digestive system**

Conditions classifiable to K00-K93

Z87.11 Personal history of peptic ulcer disease UPD

Z87.19 Personal history of other diseases of the digestive system UPD

AHA: 2017,1Q,14

Z87.2 Personal history of diseases of the skin and subcutaneous tissue UPD

Conditions classifiable to L00-L99

EXCLUDES 2 *personal history of diabetic foot ulcer (Z86.31)*

√5th **Z87.3 Personal history of diseases of the musculoskeletal system and connective tissue**

Conditions classifiable to M00-M99

EXCLUDES 2 *personal history of (healed) traumatic fracture (Z87.81)*

√6th **Z87.31 Personal history of (healed) nontraumatic fracture**

Z87.310 Personal history of (healed) osteoporosis fracture UPD

Personal history of (healed) fragility fracture

Personal history of (healed) collapsed vertebra due to osteoporosis

TIP: Assign for history of osteoporosis fractures that have resolved, even when a code from category M80 indicating current osteoporosis fracture is also reported.

Z87.311 Personal history of (healed) other pathological fracture UPD

Personal history of (healed) collapsed vertebra NOS

EXCLUDES 2 *personal history of osteoporosis fracture (Z87.310)*

Z87.312 Personal history of (healed) stress fracture UPD

Personal history of (healed) fatigue fracture

Z87.39 Personal history of other diseases of the musculoskeletal system and connective tissue UPD

√5th **Z87.4 Personal history of diseases of the genitourinary system**

Conditions classifiable to N00-N99

√6th **Z87.41 Personal history of dysplasia of the female genital tract**

EXCLUDES 1 *personal history of intraepithelial neoplasia III of female genital tract (Z86.001, Z86.008)*

personal history of malignant neoplasm of female genital tract (Z85.40-Z85.44)

Z87.410 Personal history of cervical dysplasia UPD ♀

Z87.411 Personal history of vaginal dysplasia UPD ♀

Z87.412 Personal history of vulvar dysplasia UPD ♀

Z87.42 Personal history of other diseases of the female genital tract UPD ♀

√6th **Z87.43 Personal history of diseases of the male genital organs**

Z87.430 Personal history of prostatic dysplasia UPD ♂

EXCLUDES 1 *personal history of malignant neoplasm of prostate (Z85.46)*

Z87.438 Personal history of other diseases of male genital organs UPD ♂

√6th **Z87.44 Personal history of diseases of the urinary system**

EXCLUDES 1 *personal history of malignant neoplasm of cervix uteri (Z85.41)*

Z87.440 Personal history of urinary (tract) infections UPD

Z87.441 Personal history of nephrotic syndrome UPD

Z87.442 Personal history of urinary calculi UPD

Personal history of kidney stones

Z87.448 Personal history of other diseases of urinary system UPD

√5th **Z87.5 Personal history of complications of pregnancy, childbirth and the puerperium**

Conditions classifiable to O00-O9A

EXCLUDES 2 *recurrent pregnancy loss (N96)*

Z87.51 Personal history of pre-term labor UPD ♀

EXCLUDES 1 *current pregnancy with history of pre-term labor (O09.21-)*

Z87.59 Personal history of other complications of pregnancy, childbirth and the puerperium UPD ♀

Personal history of trophoblastic disease

√5th **Z87.6 Personal history of certain (corrected) conditions arising in the perinatal period**

Conditions classifiable to P00-P96

EXCLUDES 1 *personal history of (corrected) congenital malformations (Z87.7-)*

Z87.61 Personal history of (corrected) necrotizing enterocolitis of newborn UPD

Z87.68 Personal history of other (corrected) conditions arising in the perinatal period UPD

√5th **Z87.7 Personal history of (corrected) congenital malformations**

Conditions classifiable to Q00-Q89 that have been repaired or corrected

EXCLUDES 2 *congenital malformations that have been partially corrected or repaired but which still require medical treatment - code to condition*

other postprocedural states (Z98.-)

personal history of medical treatment (Z92.-)

presence of cardiac and vascular implants and grafts (Z95.-)

presence of other devices (Z97.-)

presence of other functional implants (Z96.-)

transplanted organ and tissue status (Z94.-)

√6th **Z87.71 Personal history of (corrected) congenital malformations of genitourinary system**

Z87.710 Personal history of (corrected) hypospadias UPD ♂

Z87.718 Personal history of other specified (corrected) congenital malformations of genitourinary system UPD

√6th **Z87.72 Personal history of (corrected) congenital malformations of nervous system and sense organs**

Z87.720 Personal history of (corrected) congenital malformations of eye UPD

Z87.721 Personal history of (corrected) congenital malformations of ear UPD

Z87.728 Personal history of other specified (corrected) congenital malformations of nervous system and sense organs UPD

√6th **Z87.73 Personal history of (corrected) congenital malformations of digestive system**

Z87.730 Personal history of (corrected) cleft lip and palate UPD

Z87.731 Personal history of (corrected) tracheoesophageal fistula or atresia UPD

Z87.732 Personal history of (corrected) persistent cloaca or cloacal malformations UPD

Z87.738 Personal history of other specified (corrected) congenital malformations of digestive system UPD

Z87.74 Personal history of (corrected) congenital malformations of heart and circulatory system UPD

Z87.75 Personal history of (corrected) congenital malformations of respiratory system UPD

√6th Z87.76 Personal history of (corrected) congenital malformations of integument, limbs and musculoskeletal system

Z87.760 Personal history of (corrected) congenital diaphragmatic hernia or other congenital diaphragm malformations UPD

Z87.761 Personal history of (corrected) gastroschisis UPD

Z87.762 Personal history of (corrected) prune belly malformation UPD

Z87.763 Personal history of other (corrected) congenital abdominal wall malformations UPD

Z87.768 Personal history of other specified (corrected) congenital malformations of integument, limbs and musculoskeletal system UPD

√6th Z87.79 Personal history of other (corrected) congenital malformations

Z87.790 Personal history of (corrected) congenital malformations of face and neck UPD

Z87.798 Personal history of other (corrected) congenital malformations UPD

√5th Z87.8 Personal history of other specified conditions

EXCLUDES 2 *personal history of self harm (Z91.5-)*

Z87.81 Personal history of (healed) traumatic fracture UPD

EXCLUDES 2 *personal history of (healed) nontraumatic fracture (Z87.31-)*

√6th Z87.82 Personal history of other (healed) physical injury and trauma

Conditions classifiable to SØØ-T88, except traumatic fractures

Z87.820 Personal history of traumatic brain injury UPD

EXCLUDES 1 *personal history of transient ischemic attack (TIA), and cerebral infarction without residual deficits (Z86.73)*

Z87.821 Personal history of retained foreign body fully removed UPD

Z87.828 Personal history of other (healed) physical injury and trauma UPD

√6th Z87.89 Personal history of other specified conditions

Z87.890 Personal history of sex reassignment

Z87.891 Personal history of nicotine dependence UPD

EXCLUDES 1 *current nicotine dependence (F17.2-)*

AHA: 2017,2Q,27

Z87.892 Personal history of anaphylaxis UPD

Code also allergy status such as:
allergy status to drugs, medicaments and biological substances (Z88.-)
allergy status, other than to drugs and biological substances (Z91.Ø-)

Z87.898 Personal history of other specified conditions UPD

AHA: 2013,1Q,21

√4th Z88 Allergy status to drugs, medicaments and biological substances

EXCLUDES 2 *allergy status, other than to drugs and biological substances (Z91.Ø-)*

AHA: 2015,3Q,23

Z88.Ø Allergy status to penicillin UPD

Z88.1 Allergy status to other antibiotic agents UPD

Z88.2 Allergy status to sulfonamides UPD

Z88.3 Allergy status to other anti-infective agents UPD

Z88.4 Allergy status to anesthetic agent UPD

Z88.5 Allergy status to narcotic agent UPD

Z88.6 Allergy status to analgesic agent UPD

Z88.7 Allergy status to serum and vaccine UPD

Z88.8 Allergy status to other drugs, medicaments and biological substances UPD

Z88.9 Allergy status to unspecified drugs, medicaments and biological substances UPD

√4th Z89 Acquired absence of limb

INCLUDES amputation status
postprocedural loss of limb
post-traumatic loss of limb

EXCLUDES 1 *acquired deformities of limbs (M2Ø-M21)*
congenital absence of limbs (Q71-Q73)

√5th Z89.Ø Acquired absence of thumb and other finger(s)

√6th Z89.Ø1 Acquired absence of thumb

Z89.Ø11 Acquired absence of right thumb UPD

Z89.Ø12 Acquired absence of left thumb UPD

Z89.Ø19 Acquired absence of unspecified thumb UPD

√6th Z89.Ø2 Acquired absence of other finger(s)

EXCLUDES 2 *acquired absence of thumb (Z89.Ø1-)*

Z89.Ø21 Acquired absence of right finger(s) UPD

Z89.Ø22 Acquired absence of left finger(s) UPD

Z89.Ø29 Acquired absence of unspecified finger(s) UPD

√5th Z89.1 Acquired absence of hand and wrist

√6th Z89.11 Acquired absence of hand

Z89.111 Acquired absence of right hand UPD

Z89.112 Acquired absence of left hand UPD

Z89.119 Acquired absence of unspecified hand UPD

√6th Z89.12 Acquired absence of wrist

Disarticulation at wrist

Z89.121 Acquired absence of right wrist UPD

Z89.122 Acquired absence of left wrist UPD

Z89.129 Acquired absence of unspecified wrist UPD

√5th Z89.2 Acquired absence of upper limb above wrist

√6th Z89.2Ø Acquired absence of upper limb, unspecified level

Z89.2Ø1 Acquired absence of right upper limb, unspecified level UPD

Z89.2Ø2 Acquired absence of left upper limb, unspecified level UPD

Z89.2Ø9 Acquired absence of unspecified upper limb, unspecified level UPD

Acquired absence of arm NOS

√6th Z89.21 Acquired absence of upper limb below elbow

Z89.211 Acquired absence of right upper limb below elbow UPD

Z89.212 Acquired absence of left upper limb below elbow UPD

Z89.219 Acquired absence of unspecified upper limb below elbow UPD

√6th Z89.22 Acquired absence of upper limb above elbow

Disarticulation at elbow

Z89.221 Acquired absence of right upper limb above elbow UPD

Z89.222 Acquired absence of left upper limb above elbow UPD

Z89.229 Acquired absence of unspecified upper limb above elbow UPD

√6th Z89.23 Acquired absence of shoulder

Acquired absence of shoulder joint following explantation of shoulder joint prosthesis, with or without presence of antibiotic-impregnated cement spacer

Z89.231 Acquired absence of right shoulder UPD

Z89.232 Acquired absence of left shoulder UPD

Z89.239 Acquired absence of unspecified shoulder UPD

√5th Z89.4 Acquired absence of toe(s), foot, and ankle

√6th Z89.41 Acquired absence of great toe

Z89.411 Acquired absence of right great toe UPD HCC

Z89.412 Acquired absence of left great toe UPD HCC

Z89.419 Acquired absence of unspecified great toe UPD HCC

✓6th Z89.42 Acquired absence of other toe(s)
EXCLUDES 2 *acquired absence of great toe (Z89.41-)*
Z89.421 Acquired absence of other right toe(s) UPD HCC
Z89.422 Acquired absence of other left toe(s) UPD HCC
Z89.429 Acquired absence of other toe(s), unspecified side UPD HCC

✓6th Z89.43 Acquired absence of foot
Z89.431 Acquired absence of right foot UPD HCC
Z89.432 Acquired absence of left foot UPD HCC
Z89.439 Acquired absence of unspecified foot UPD HCC

✓6th Z89.44 Acquired absence of ankle
Disarticulation of ankle
Z89.441 Acquired absence of right ankle UPD HCC
Z89.442 Acquired absence of left ankle UPD HCC
Z89.449 Acquired absence of unspecified ankle UPD HCC

✓5th Z89.5 Acquired absence of leg below knee

✓6th Z89.51 Acquired absence of leg below knee
Z89.511 Acquired absence of right leg below knee UPD HCC
Z89.512 Acquired absence of left leg below knee UPD HCC
Z89.519 Acquired absence of unspecified leg below knee UPD HCC

✓6th Z89.52 Acquired absence of knee
Acquired absence of knee joint following explantation of knee joint prosthesis, with or without presence of antibiotic-impregnated cement spacer
Z89.521 Acquired absence of right knee UPD
Z89.522 Acquired absence of left knee UPD
Z89.529 Acquired absence of unspecified knee UPD

✓5th Z89.6 Acquired absence of leg above knee

✓6th Z89.61 Acquired absence of leg above knee
Acquired absence of leg NOS
Disarticulation at knee
Z89.611 Acquired absence of right leg above knee UPD HCC
Z89.612 Acquired absence of left leg above knee UPD HCC
Z89.619 Acquired absence of unspecified leg above knee UPD HCC

✓6th Z89.62 Acquired absence of hip
Acquired absence of hip joint following explantation of hip joint prosthesis, with or without presence of antibiotic-impregnated cement spacer
Disarticulation at hip
Z89.621 Acquired absence of right hip joint UPD
Z89.622 Acquired absence of left hip joint UPD
Z89.629 Acquired absence of unspecified hip joint UPD

Z89.9 Acquired absence of limb, unspecified UPD

✓4th Z90 Acquired absence of organs, not elsewhere classified
INCLUDES postprocedural or post-traumatic loss of body part NEC
EXCLUDES 1 *congenital absence - see Alphabetical Index*
EXCLUDES 2 *postprocedural absence of endocrine glands (E89.-)*

✓5th Z90.0 Acquired absence of part of head and neck
Z90.01 Acquired absence of eye UPD
Z90.02 Acquired absence of larynx UPD
Z90.09 Acquired absence of other part of head and neck UPD
Acquired absence of nose
EXCLUDES 2 *teeth (K08.1)*

✓5th Z90.1 Acquired absence of breast and nipple
AHA: 2022,3Q,8
Z90.10 Acquired absence of unspecified breast and nipple
Z90.11 Acquired absence of right breast and nipple
Z90.12 Acquired absence of left breast and nipple
Z90.13 Acquired absence of bilateral breasts and nipples

Z90.2 Acquired absence of lung [part of] UPD
Z90.3 Acquired absence of stomach [part of] UPD

✓5th Z90.4 Acquired absence of other specified parts of digestive tract

✓6th Z90.41 Acquired absence of pancreas
Code also exocrine pancreatic insufficiency (K86.81)
Use additional code to identify any associated:
diabetes mellitus, postpancreatectomy (E13.-)
insulin use (Z79.4)
Z90.410 Acquired total absence of pancreas UPD
Acquired absence of pancreas NOS
Z90.411 Acquired partial absence of pancreas UPD

Z90.49 Acquired absence of other specified parts of digestive tract UPD

Z90.5 Acquired absence of kidney UPD
Z90.6 Acquired absence of other parts of urinary tract UPD
Acquired absence of bladder

✓5th Z90.7 Acquired absence of genital organ(s)
EXCLUDES 1 *personal history of sex reassignment (Z87.890)*
EXCLUDES 2 *female genital mutilation status (N90.81-)*

✓6th Z90.71 Acquired absence of cervix and uterus
Z90.710 Acquired absence of both cervix and uterus UPD ♀
Acquired absence of uterus NOS
Status post total hysterectomy
Z90.711 Acquired absence of uterus with remaining cervical stump UPD ♀
Status post partial hysterectomy with remaining cervical stump
Z90.712 Acquired absence of cervix with remaining uterus UPD ♀

✓6th Z90.72 Acquired absence of ovaries
Z90.721 Acquired absence of ovaries, unilateral UPD ♀
Z90.722 Acquired absence of ovaries, bilateral UPD ♀

Z90.79 Acquired absence of other genital organ(s) UPD
AHA: 2023,2Q,5

✓5th Z90.8 Acquired absence of other organs
Z90.81 Acquired absence of spleen UPD
Z90.89 Acquired absence of other organs UPD

✓4th Z91 Personal risk factors, not elsewhere classified
EXCLUDES 2 *contact with and (suspected) exposures hazardous to health (Z77.-)*
exposure to pollution and other problems related to physical environment (Z77.1-)
female genital mutilation status (N90.81-)
occupational exposure to risk factors (Z57.-)
personal history of physical injury and trauma (Z87.81, Z87.82-)

✓5th Z91.0 Allergy status, other than to drugs and biological substances
EXCLUDES 2 *allergy status to drugs, medicaments, and biological substances (Z88.-)*

✓6th Z91.01 Food allergy status
EXCLUDES 2 *food additives allergy status (Z91.02)*
Z91.010 Allergy to peanuts UPD
Z91.011 Allergy to milk products UPD
EXCLUDES 1 *lactose intolerance (E73.-)*
Z91.012 Allergy to eggs UPD
Z91.013 Allergy to seafood UPD
Allergy to octopus or squid ink
Allergy to shellfish
Z91.014 Allergy to mammalian meats UPD
Allergy to beef
Allergy to lamb
Allergy to pork
Allergy to red meats
AHA: 2021,4Q,33
Z91.018 Allergy to other foods UPD
Allergy to nuts other than peanuts

Z91.02 Food additives allergy status UPD

✓6th Z91.03 Insect allergy status
Z91.030 Bee allergy status UPD
Z91.038 Other insect allergy status UPD

Z91.04 Nonmedicinal substance allergy status

Z91.040 Latex allergy status UPD
Latex sensitivity status

Z91.041 Radiographic dye allergy status UPD
Allergy status to contrast media used for diagnostic X-ray procedure

Z91.048 Other nonmedicinal substance allergy status UPD

Z91.09 Other allergy status, other than to drugs and biological substances UPD

Z91.1 Patient's noncompliance with medical treatment and regimen
▶Code also, if applicable, to identify underdosing of specific drug (T36-T50 with final character 6)◀
EXCLUDES 2 *caregiver noncompliance with patient's medical treatment and regimen (Z91.A-)*
AHA: 2022,4Q,49

Z91.11 Patient's noncompliance with dietary regimen
Code also, if applicable, food insecurity (Z59.4-)

Z91.110 Patient's noncompliance with dietary regimen due to financial hardship UPD

Z91.118 Patient's noncompliance with dietary regimen for other reason UPD
Inability to comply with dietary regimen

Z91.119 Patient's noncompliance with dietary regimen due to unspecified reason UPD

Z91.12 Patient's intentional underdosing of medication regimen
Code first underdosing of medication (T36-T50) with fifth or sixth character 6
EXCLUDES 1 *adverse effect of prescribed drug taken as directed - code to adverse effect*
poisoning (overdose) - code to poisoning
AHA: 2018,4Q,72

Z91.120 Patient's intentional underdosing of medication regimen due to financial hardship UPD

Z91.128 Patient's intentional underdosing of medication regimen for other reason UPD

Z91.13 Patient's unintentional underdosing of medication regimen
Code first underdosing of medication (T36-T50) with fifth or sixth character 6
EXCLUDES 1 *adverse effect of prescribed drug taken as directed - code to adverse effect*
poisoning (overdose) - code to poisoning
AHA: 2018,4Q,72

Z91.130 Patient's unintentional underdosing of medication regimen due to age-related debility UPD

Z91.138 Patient's unintentional underdosing of medication regimen for other reason UPD

▲ **Z91.14 Patient's other noncompliance with medication regimen**
Patient's underdosing of medication NOS
AHA: 2023,1Q,7; 2022,1Q,36; 2018,4Q,72

● **Z91.141 Patient's other noncompliance with medication regimen due to financial hardship** UPD

● **Z91.148 Patient's other noncompliance with medication regimen for other reason** UPD

▲ **Z91.15 Patient's noncompliance with renal dialysis**
AHA: 2023,1Q,7

● **Z91.151 Patient's noncompliance with renal dialysis due to financial hardship** UPD

● **Z91.158 Patient's noncompliance with renal dialysis for other reason** UPD

Z91.19 Patient's noncompliance with other medical treatment and regimen
Patient's nonadherence to medical treatment

Z91.190 Patient's noncompliance with other medical treatment and regimen due to financial hardship UPD

Z91.198 Patient's noncompliance with other medical treatment and regimen for other reason UPD

Z91.199 Patient's noncompliance with other medical treatment and regimen due to unspecified reason UPD

Z91.A Caregiver's noncompliance with patient's medical treatment and regimen
AHA: 2022,4Q,49

Z91.A1 Caregiver's noncompliance with patient's dietary regimen
Caregiver's inability to comply with patient's dietary regimen
Code also, if applicable, food insecurity (Z59.4-)

Z91.A10 Caregiver's noncompliance with patient's dietary regimen due to financial hardship UPD

Z91.A18 Caregiver's noncompliance with patient's dietary regimen for other reason UPD

Z91.A2 Caregiver's intentional underdosing of patient's medication regimen
Code first underdosing of medication (T36-T50) with fifth or sixth character 6

Z91.A20 Caregiver's intentional underdosing of patient's medication regimen due to financial hardship UPD

Z91.A28 Caregiver's intentional underdosing of medication regimen for other reason UPD

Z91.A3 Caregiver's unintentional underdosing of patient's medication regimen UPD
Code first underdosing of medication (T36-T50) with fifth or sixth character 6

▲ **Z91.A4 Caregiver's other noncompliance with patient's medication regimen**
Caregiver's underdosing of patient's medication NOS
▶Caregiver's underdosing with patient's medication NOS◀

● **Z91.A41 Caregiver's other noncompliance with patient's medication regimen due to financial hardship**

● **Z91.A48 Caregiver's other noncompliance with patient's medication regimen for other reason**

▲ **Z91.A5 Caregiver's noncompliance with patient's renal dialysis**

● **Z91.A51 Caregiver's noncompliance with patient's renal dialysis due to financial hardship**

● **Z91.A58 Caregiver's noncompliance with patient's renal dialysis for other reason**

▲ **Z91.A9 Caregiver's noncompliance with patient's other medical treatment and regimen**
Caregiver's nonadherence to patient's medical treatment

● **Z91.A91 Caregiver's noncompliance with patient's other medical treatment and regimen due to financial hardship**

● **Z91.A98 Caregiver's noncompliance with patient's other medical treatment and regimen for other reason**

Z91.4 Personal history of psychological trauma, not elsewhere classified
AHA: 2023,1Q,7

Z91.41 Personal history of adult abuse
EXCLUDES 2 *personal history of abuse in childhood (Z62.81-)*

Z91.410 Personal history of adult physical and sexual abuse UPD A
EXCLUDES 1 *current adult physical abuse (T74.11, T76.11)*
current adult sexual abuse (T74.21, T76.11)

Z91.411 Personal history of adult psychological abuse UPD A

Z91.412 Personal history of adult neglect UPD A
EXCLUDES 1 *current adult neglect (T74.01, T76.01)*

● **Z91.413 Personal history of adult financial abuse** UPD

● **Z91.414 Personal history of adult intimate partner abuse** UPD

Z91.419 Personal history of unspecified adult abuse UPD A

Z91.42 Personal history of forced labor or sexual exploitation UPD
AHA: 2018,4Q,32,35

Z91.49 Other personal history of psychological trauma, not elsewhere classified UPD

✓5th **Z91.5 Personal history of self-harm**
Code also mental health disorder, if known
AHA: 2021,4Q,33

Z91.51 Personal history of suicidal behavior UPD
Personal history of parasuicide
Personal history of self-poisoning
Personal history of suicide attempt

Z91.52 Personal history of nonsuicidal self-harm UPD
Personal history of nonsuicidal self-injury
Personal history of self-inflicted injury without suicidal intent
Personal history of self-mutilation

✓5th **Z91.8 Other specified personal risk factors, not elsewhere classified**

Z91.81 History of falling UPD
At risk for falling

Z91.82 Personal history of military deployment UPD A
Individual (civilian or military) with past history of military war, peacekeeping and humanitarian deployment (current or past conflict)
Returned from military deployment
EXCLUDES 2 ▶*personal history of military service (Z91.85)*◀

Z91.83 Wandering in diseases classified elsewhere
Code first underlying disorder such as:
Alzheimer's disease (G30.-)
autism or pervasive developmental disorder (F84.-)
intellectual disabilities (F70-F79)
unspecified dementia with behavioral disturbance (F03.9-, F03.A-, F03.B-, F03.C-)

✓6th **Z91.84 Oral health risk factors**
AHA: 2017,4Q,29

Z91.841 Risk for dental caries, low UPD
Z91.842 Risk for dental caries, moderate UPD
Z91.843 Risk for dental caries, high UPD
Z91.849 Unspecified risk for dental caries UPD

● **Z91.85 Personal history of military service**
Personal history of serving in the armed forces
Personal history of veteran
EXCLUDES 2 *personal history of military deployment (Z91.82)*

Z91.89 Other specified personal risk factors, not elsewhere classified UPD
▶Increased risk for social isolation◀
AHA: 2017,1Q,45

✓4th **Z92 Personal history of medical treatment**
EXCLUDES 2 *postprocedural states (Z98.-)*

Z92.0 Personal history of contraception UPD
EXCLUDES 1 *counseling or management of current contraceptive practices (Z30.-)*
long term (current) use of contraception (Z79.3)
presence of (intrauterine) contraceptive device (Z97.5)

✓5th **Z92.2 Personal history of drug therapy**
EXCLUDES 2 *long term (current) drug therapy (Z79.-)*

Z92.21 Personal history of antineoplastic chemotherapy UPD
Z92.22 Personal history of monoclonal drug therapy UPD
Z92.23 Personal history of estrogen therapy UPD

✓6th **Z92.24 Personal history of steroid therapy**

Z92.240 Personal history of inhaled steroid therapy UPD
Z92.241 Personal history of systemic steroid therapy UPD
Personal history of steroid therapy NOS

Z92.25 Personal history of immunosuppression therapy UPD
EXCLUDES 2 *personal history of steroid therapy (Z92.24)*

Z92.29 Personal history of other drug therapy UPD

Z92.3 Personal history of irradiation UPD
Personal history of exposure to therapeutic radiation
EXCLUDES 1 *exposure to radiation in the physical environment (Z77.12)*
occupational exposure to radiation (Z57.1)

✓5th **Z92.8 Personal history of other medical treatment**

Z92.81 Personal history of extracorporeal membrane oxygenation (ECMO) UPD

Z92.82 Status post administration of tPA (rtPA) in a different facility within the last 24 hours prior to admission to current facility UPD
Code first condition requiring tPA administration, such as:
acute cerebral infarction (I63.-)
acute myocardial infarction (I21.-, I22.-)
AHA: 2013,4Q,124

Z92.83 Personal history of failed moderate sedation UPD
Personal history of failed conscious sedation
EXCLUDES 2 *failed moderate sedation during procedure (T88.52)*

Z92.84 Personal history of unintended awareness under general anesthesia UPD
EXCLUDES 2 *unintended awareness under general anesthesia during procedure (T88.53)*
AHA: 2016,4Q,72-73,77

✓6th **Z92.85 Personal history of cellular therapy**
AHA: 2021,4Q,33-34

Z92.850 Personal history of Chimeric Antigen Receptor T-cell therapy UPD
Personal history of CAR T-cell therapy
Z92.858 Personal history of other cellular therapy UPD
Z92.859 Personal history of cellular therapy, unspecified UPD

Z92.86 Personal history of gene therapy UPD
AHA: 2021,4Q,33-34

Z92.89 Personal history of other medical treatment UPD
AHA: 2020,1Q,18

✓4th **Z93 Artificial opening status**
EXCLUDES 1 *artificial openings requiring attention or management (Z43.-)*
complications of external stoma (J95.0-, K94.-, N99.5-)

Z93.0 Tracheostomy status UPD HCC
AHA: 2013,4Q,129
Z93.1 Gastrostomy status UPD HCC
Z93.2 Ileostomy status UPD HCC
Z93.3 Colostomy status UPD HCC
Z93.4 Other artificial openings of gastrointestinal tract status UPD HCC

✓5th **Z93.5 Cystostomy status**
Z93.50 Unspecified cystostomy status UPD HCC
Z93.51 Cutaneous-vesicostomy status UPD HCC
Z93.52 Appendico-vesicostomy status UPD HCC
Z93.59 Other cystostomy status UPD HCC

Z93.6 Other artificial openings of urinary tract status UPD HCC
Nephrostomy status
Ureterostomy status
Urethrostomy status
Z93.8 Other artificial opening status UPD HCC
Z93.9 Artificial opening status, unspecified UPD HCC

✓4th **Z94 Transplanted organ and tissue status**
INCLUDES organ or tissue replaced by heterogenous or homogenous transplant
EXCLUDES 1 *complications of transplanted organ or tissue - see Alphabetical Index*
EXCLUDES 2 *presence of vascular grafts (Z95.-)*

Z94.0 Kidney transplant status CC UPD
Z94.1 Heart transplant status CC UPD HCC
EXCLUDES 1 *artificial heart status (Z95.812)*
heart-valve replacement status (Z95.2-Z95.4)
Z94.2 Lung transplant status CC UPD HCC
Z94.3 Heart and lungs transplant status CC UPD HCC
Z94.4 Liver transplant status CC UPD HCC
Z94.5 Skin transplant status UPD
Autogenous skin transplant status
Z94.6 Bone transplant status UPD
Z94.7 Corneal transplant status UPD

√5th **Z94.8 Other transplanted organ and tissue status**

Z94.81 Bone marrow transplant status CC UPD HCC

Z94.82 Intestine transplant status CC UPD HCC

Z94.83 Pancreas transplant status CC UPD HCC

Z94.84 Stem cells transplant status CC UPD HCC

Z94.89 Other transplanted organ and tissue status UPD

Z94.9 Transplanted organ and tissue status, unspecified UPD

√4th **Z95 Presence of cardiac and vascular implants and grafts**

EXCLUDES 2 *complications of cardiac and vascular devices, implants and grafts (T82.-)*

Z95.Ø Presence of cardiac pacemaker UPD

Presence of cardiac resynchronization therapy (CRT-P) pacemaker

EXCLUDES 1 *adjustment or management of cardiac device (Z45.Ø-)*

adjustment or management of cardiac pacemaker (Z45.Ø)

presence of automatic (implantable) cardiac defibrillator with synchronous cardiac pacemaker (Z95.81Ø)

AHA: 2022,2Q,14; 2019,1Q,33

TIP: Assign an additional code for the associated condition if that condition requires constant intervention from the device, as in cases of sick sinus syndrome. For conditions that do not require constant intervention from the device, as in cases of ventricular fibrillation, an additional code for the associated condition should be assigned only if the patient is experiencing the condition and the device is firing during the current admission.

Z95.1 Presence of aortocoronary bypass graft UPD

Presence of coronary artery bypass graft

Z95.2 Presence of prosthetic heart valve UPD

Presence of heart valve NOS

Z95.3 Presence of xenogenic heart valve UPD

Z95.4 Presence of other heart-valve replacement UPD

Z95.5 Presence of coronary angioplasty implant and graft UPD

EXCLUDES 1 *coronary angioplasty status without implant and graft (Z98.61)*

√5th **Z95.8 Presence of other cardiac and vascular implants and grafts**

√6th **Z95.81 Presence of other cardiac implants and grafts**

Z95.81Ø Presence of automatic (implantable) cardiac defibrillator UPD

Presence of automatic (implantable) cardiac defibrillator with synchronous cardiac pacemaker

Presence of cardiac resynchronization therapy defibrillator (CRT-D)

Presence of cardioverter-defibrillator (ICD)

AHA: 2022,2Q,14; 2019,1Q,33

TIP: Assign an additional code for the associated condition if that condition requires constant intervention from the device, as in cases of sick sinus syndrome. For conditions that do not require constant intervention from the device, as in cases of ventricular fibrillation, an additional code for the associated condition should be assigned only if the patient is experiencing the condition and the device is firing during the current admission.

Z95.811 Presence of heart assist device CC UPD HCC

Z95.812 Presence of fully implantable artificial heart CC UPD HCC

Z95.818 Presence of other cardiac implants and grafts UPD

√6th **Z95.82 Presence of other vascular implants and grafts**

Z95.82Ø Peripheral vascular angioplasty status with implants and grafts UPD

EXCLUDES 1 *peripheral vascular angioplasty without implant and graft (Z98.62)*

Z95.828 Presence of other vascular implants and grafts UPD

Presence of intravascular prosthesis NEC

Z95.9 Presence of cardiac and vascular implant and graft, unspecified UPD

√4th **Z96 Presence of other functional implants**

EXCLUDES 2 *complications of internal prosthetic devices, implants and grafts (T82-T85)*

fitting and adjustment of prosthetic and other devices (Z44-Z46)

Z96.Ø Presence of urogenital implants UPD

Z96.1 Presence of intraocular lens UPD

Presence of pseudophakia

√5th **Z96.2 Presence of otological and audiological implants**

Z96.2Ø Presence of otological and audiological implant, unspecified UPD

Z96.21 Cochlear implant status UPD

Z96.22 Myringotomy tube(s) status UPD

Z96.29 Presence of other otological and audiological implants UPD

Presence of bone-conduction hearing device

Presence of eustachian tube stent

Stapes replacement

Z96.3 Presence of artificial larynx UPD

√5th **Z96.4 Presence of endocrine implants**

Z96.41 Presence of insulin pump (external) (internal) UPD

Z96.49 Presence of other endocrine implants UPD

Z96.5 Presence of tooth-root and mandibular implants UPD

√5th **Z96.6 Presence of orthopedic joint implants**

AHA: 2019,3Q,16

Z96.6Ø Presence of unspecified orthopedic joint implant UPD

√6th **Z96.61 Presence of artificial shoulder joint**

Z96.611 Presence of right artificial shoulder joint UPD

Z96.612 Presence of left artificial shoulder joint UPD

Z96.619 Presence of unspecified artificial shoulder joint UPD

√6th **Z96.62 Presence of artificial elbow joint**

Z96.621 Presence of right artificial elbow joint UPD

Z96.622 Presence of left artificial elbow joint UPD

Z96.629 Presence of unspecified artificial elbow joint UPD

√6th **Z96.63 Presence of artificial wrist joint**

Z96.631 Presence of right artificial wrist joint UPD

Z96.632 Presence of left artificial wrist joint UPD

Z96.639 Presence of unspecified artificial wrist joint UPD

√6th **Z96.64 Presence of artificial hip joint**

Hip-joint replacement (partial) (total)

Z96.641 Presence of right artificial hip joint UPD

Z96.642 Presence of left artificial hip joint UPD

Z96.643 Presence of artificial hip joint, bilateral UPD

Z96.649 Presence of unspecified artificial hip joint UPD

√6th **Z96.65 Presence of artificial knee joint**

Z96.651 Presence of right artificial knee joint UPD

Z96.652 Presence of left artificial knee joint UPD

Z96.653 Presence of artificial knee joint, bilateral UPD

Z96.659 Presence of unspecified artificial knee joint UPD

√6th **Z96.66 Presence of artificial ankle joint**

Z96.661 Presence of right artificial ankle joint UPD

Z96.662 Presence of left artificial ankle joint UPD

Z96.669 Presence of unspecified artificial ankle joint UPD

√6th **Z96.69 Presence of other orthopedic joint implants**

Z96.691 Finger-joint replacement of right hand UPD

Z96.692 **Finger-joint replacement of left hand** UPD

Z96.693 **Finger-joint replacement, bilateral** UPD

Z96.698 **Presence of other orthopedic joint implants** UPD

Z96.7 **Presence of other bone and tendon implants** UPD
Presence of skull plate

Z96.8 **Presence of other specified functional implants**

Z96.81 **Presence of artificial skin** UPD

Z96.82 **Presence of neurostimulator** UPD
Presence of brain neurostimulator
Presence of gastric neurostimulator
Presence of peripheral nerve neurostimulator
Presence of sacral nerve neurostimulator
Presence of spinal cord neurostimulator
Presence of vagus nerve neurostimulator
AHA: 2019,4Q,19

Z96.89 **Presence of other specified functional implants** UPD

Z96.9 **Presence of functional implant, unspecified** UPD

Z97 Presence of other devices
EXCLUDES 1 *complications of internal prosthetic devices, implants and grafts (T82-T85)*
EXCLUDES 2 *fitting and adjustment of prosthetic and other devices (Z44-Z46)*
presence of cerebrospinal fluid drainage device (Z98.2)

Z97.Ø **Presence of artificial eye** UPD

Z97.1 **Presence of artificial limb (complete) (partial)**

Z97.1Ø **Presence of artificial limb (complete) (partial), unspecified** UPD

Z97.11 **Presence of artificial right arm (complete) (partial)** UPD

Z97.12 **Presence of artificial left arm (complete) (partial)** UPD

Z97.13 **Presence of artificial right leg (complete) (partial)** UPD

Z97.14 **Presence of artificial left leg (complete) (partial)** UPD

Z97.15 **Presence of artificial arms, bilateral (complete) (partial)** UPD

Z97.16 **Presence of artificial legs, bilateral (complete) (partial)** UPD

Z97.2 **Presence of dental prosthetic device (complete) (partial)** UPD
Presence of dentures (complete) (partial)

Z97.3 **Presence of spectacles and contact lenses** UPD

Z97.4 **Presence of external hearing-aid** UPD

Z97.5 **Presence of (intrauterine) contraceptive device** UPD ♀
EXCLUDES 1 *checking, reinsertion or removal of implantable subdermal contraceptive (Z3Ø.46)*
checking, reinsertion or removal of intrauterine contraceptive device (Z3Ø.43-)

Z97.8 **Presence of other specified devices** UPD

Z98 Other postprocedural states
EXCLUDES 2 *aftercare (Z43-Z49, Z51)*
follow-up medical care (ZØ8-ZØ9)
postprocedural complication - see Alphabetical Index

Z98.Ø **Intestinal bypass and anastomosis status** UPD
EXCLUDES 2 *bariatric surgery status (Z98.84)*
gastric bypass status (Z98.84)
obesity surgery status (Z98.84)

Z98.1 **Arthrodesis status** UPD

Z98.2 **Presence of cerebrospinal fluid drainage device** UPD
Presence of CSF shunt

Z98.3 **Post therapeutic collapse of lung status** UPD
Code first underlying disease

Z98.4 **Cataract extraction status**
Use additional code to identify intraocular lens implant status (Z96.1)
EXCLUDES 1 *aphakia (H27.Ø)*

Z98.41 **Cataract extraction status, right eye** UPD

Z98.42 **Cataract extraction status, left eye** UPD

Z98.49 **Cataract extraction status, unspecified eye** UPD

Z98.5 **Sterilization status**
EXCLUDES 1 *female infertility (N97.-)*
male infertility (N46.-)

Z98.51 **Tubal ligation status** UPD ♀

Z98.52 **Vasectomy status** UPD A ♂

Z98.6 **Angioplasty status**

Z98.61 **Coronary angioplasty status** UPD
EXCLUDES 1 *coronary angioplasty status with implant and graft (Z95.5)*

Z98.62 **Peripheral vascular angioplasty status** UPD
EXCLUDES 1 *peripheral vascular angioplasty status with implant and graft (Z95.82Ø)*

Z98.8 **Other specified postprocedural states**

Z98.81 **Dental procedure status**

Z98.81Ø **Dental sealant status** UPD

Z98.811 **Dental restoration status** UPD
Dental crown status
Dental fillings status

Z98.818 **Other dental procedure status** UPD

Z98.82 **Breast implant status** UPD
EXCLUDES 1 *breast implant removal status (Z98.86)*
AHA: 2022,3Q,8

Z98.83 **Filtering (vitreous) bleb after glaucoma surgery status** UPD
EXCLUDES 1 *inflammation (infection) of postprocedural bleb (H59.4-)*
AHA: 2020,3Q,29

Z98.84 **Bariatric surgery status** UPD
Gastric banding status
Gastric bypass status for obesity
Obesity surgery status
EXCLUDES 1 *bariatric surgery status complicating pregnancy, childbirth, or the puerperium (O99.84)*
EXCLUDES 2 *intestinal bypass and anastomosis status (Z98.Ø)*
AHA: 2020,1Q,12

Z98.85 **Transplanted organ removal status** UPD
Transplanted organ previously removed due to complication, failure, rejection or infection
EXCLUDES 1 *encounter for removal of transplanted organ - code to complication of transplanted organ (T86.-)*

Z98.86 **Personal history of breast implant removal** UPD

Z98.87 **Personal history of in utero procedure**

Z98.87Ø **Personal history of in utero procedure during pregnancy** UPD ♀
EXCLUDES 2 *complications from in utero procedure for current pregnancy (O35.7)*
supervision of current pregnancy with history of in utero procedure during previous pregnancy (OØ9.82-)

Z98.871 **Personal history of in utero procedure while a fetus** UPD

Z98.89 **Other specified postprocedural states**

Z98.89Ø **Other specified postprocedural states** UPD
Personal history of surgery, not elsewhere classified

Z98.891 **History of uterine scar from previous surgery** UPD ♀
EXCLUDES 1 *maternal care due to uterine scar from previous surgery (O34.2-)*
AHA: 2016,4Q,51-52,76

Z99 Dependence on enabling machines and devices, not elsewhere classified
AHA: 2020,1Q,11

Z99.Ø **Dependence on aspirator** UPD

Z99.1 **Dependence on respirator**
Dependence on ventilator

Z99.11 **Dependence on respirator [ventilator] status** CC HCC
AHA: 2015,1Q,21

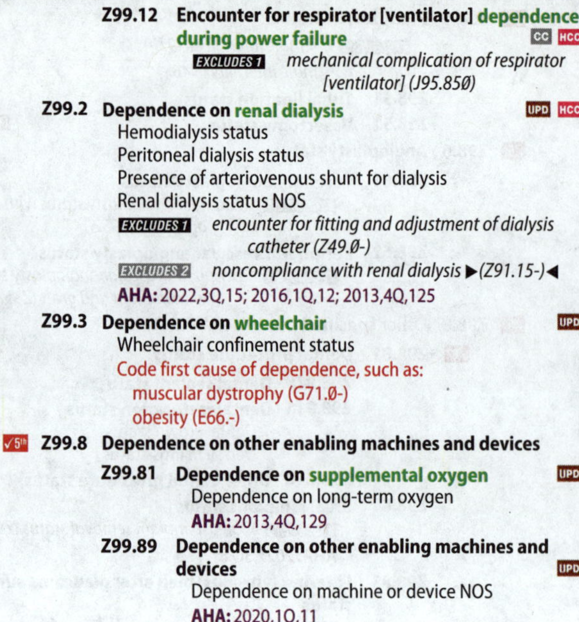

Z99.12 Encounter for respirator [ventilator] dependence during power failure CC HCC

EXCLUDES 1 *mechanical complication of respirator [ventilator] (J95.85Ø)*

Z99.2 Dependence on renal dialysis UPD HCC

Hemodialysis status
Peritoneal dialysis status
Presence of arteriovenous shunt for dialysis
Renal dialysis status NOS

EXCLUDES 1 *encounter for fitting and adjustment of dialysis catheter (Z49.Ø-)*

EXCLUDES 2 *noncompliance with renal dialysis ▶(Z91.15-)◀*

AHA: 2022,3Q,15; 2016,1Q,12; 2013,4Q,125

Z99.3 Dependence on wheelchair UPD

Wheelchair confinement status

Code first cause of dependence, such as:
muscular dystrophy (G71.Ø-)
obesity (E66.-)

√5th **Z99.8 Dependence on other enabling machines and devices**

Z99.81 Dependence on supplemental oxygen UPD

Dependence on long-term oxygen

AHA: 2013,4Q,129

Z99.89 Dependence on other enabling machines and devices UPD

Dependence on machine or device NOS

AHA: 2020,1Q,11

Chapter 22. Codes for Special Purposes (UØØ–U85)

Chapter-specific Guidelines

UØ7.Ø Vaping-related disorder (see Section I.C.10.e., Vaping-related disorders)

UØ7.1 COVID-19 (see Section I.C.1.g.1., COVID-19 infection)

UØ9.9 Post COVID-19 condition, unspecified (see Section I.C.1.g.1.m.)

Chapter 22. Codes for Special Purposes (UØØ-U85)

This chapter contains the following blocks:

UØØ-U49 Provisional assignment of new diseases of uncertain etiology or emergency use

Provisional assignment of new diseases of uncertain etiology or emergency use (UØØ-U49)

UØ7 Emergency use of UØ7

UØ7.Ø Vaping-related disorder

Dabbing related lung damage
Dabbing related lung injury
E-cigarette, or vaping, product use associated lung injury [EVALI]
Electronic cigarette related lung damage
Electronic cigarette related lung injury

Use additional code, to identify manifestations, such as:
- abdominal pain (R1Ø.84)
- acute respiratory distress syndrome (J8Ø)
- diarrhea (R19.7)
- drug-induced interstitial lung disorder (J7Ø.4)
- lipoid pneumonia (J69.1)
- weight loss (R63.4)

DEF: Respiratory illness or injury caused by harmful aerosolized substances and chemicals produced by electronic cigarettes, vapes, e-pipes, and other battery-powered vaping devices. Symptoms may include shortness of breath and fever, while some patients experience severe, sometimes fatal, lung damage. ***Synonym(s):*** *e-cigarette and vaping product use-associated lung injury, EVALI.*

UØ7.1 COVID-19 HIV MCC

Use additional code to identify pneumonia or other manifestations, such as:
- pneumonia due to COVID-19 (J12.82)

▶Use additional code, if applicable, for associated conditions such as:◀
- ▶COVID-19 associated coagulopathy (D68.8)◀
- ▶disseminated intravascular coagulation (D65)◀
- ▶hypercoagulable states (D68.69)◀
- ▶thrombophilia (D68.69)◀

EXCLUDES 2 *coronavirus as the cause of diseases classified elsewhere (B97.2-)*
~~*coronavirus infection, unspecified (B34.2)*~~
pneumonia due to SARS-associated coronavirus (J12.81)

AHA: 2022,2Q,28; 2021,4Q,101,107-108; 2021,1Q,25-30,31-49; 2020,4Q,14,99; 2020,3Q,9-16; 2020,2Q,3-13

DEF: First diagnosed in December 2019 in China, coronavirus disease 2019 (COVID-19) is a respiratory infection caused by a newly identified (novel) virus not previously seen in humans, known as severe acute respiratory syndrome coronavirus 2 (SARS-CoV-2). Symptoms of this lower respiratory illness include fever, dry cough, and tiredness that may progress to include difficulty breathing. Older patients and those with high blood pressure, heart problems, and diabetes are more likely to develop serious symptoms of the illness. ***Synonym(s):*** *SARS-CoV-2, coronavirus disease 2019.*

TIP: Only a confirmed diagnosis of COVID-19, either through a positive test result documented in the medical record or documentation by the provider, can be coded to U07.1.

TIP: Assign for asymptomatic individuals who test positive for COVID-19. Even though asymptomatic, the individual is considered to have the COVID-19 infection due to the positive test result.

TIP: Assign appropriate codes for presenting signs/symptoms associated with COVID-19 (cough, fever, shortness of breath), instead of U07.1, if a definitive diagnosis has not been established.

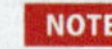 **UØ9 Post COVID-19 condition**

UØ9.9 Post COVID-19 condition, unspecified

NOTE This code enables establishment of a link with COVID-19.

This code is not to be used in cases that are still presenting with active COVID-19. However, an exception is made in cases of re-infection with COVID-19, occurring with a condition related to prior COVID-19.

Post-acute sequela of COVID-19

Code first the specific condition related to COVID-19 if known, such as:
- chronic respiratory failure (J96.1-)
- loss of smell (R43.8)
- loss of taste (R43.8)
- multisystem inflammatory syndrome (M35.81)
- pulmonary embolism (I26.-)
- pulmonary fibrosis (J84.1Ø)

AHA: 2021,4Q,31-32,102-106

Chapter 3. Diseases of the Blood and Blood-forming Organs and Certain Disorders Involving the Immune Mechanism (D5Ø–D89)

Red Blood Cells

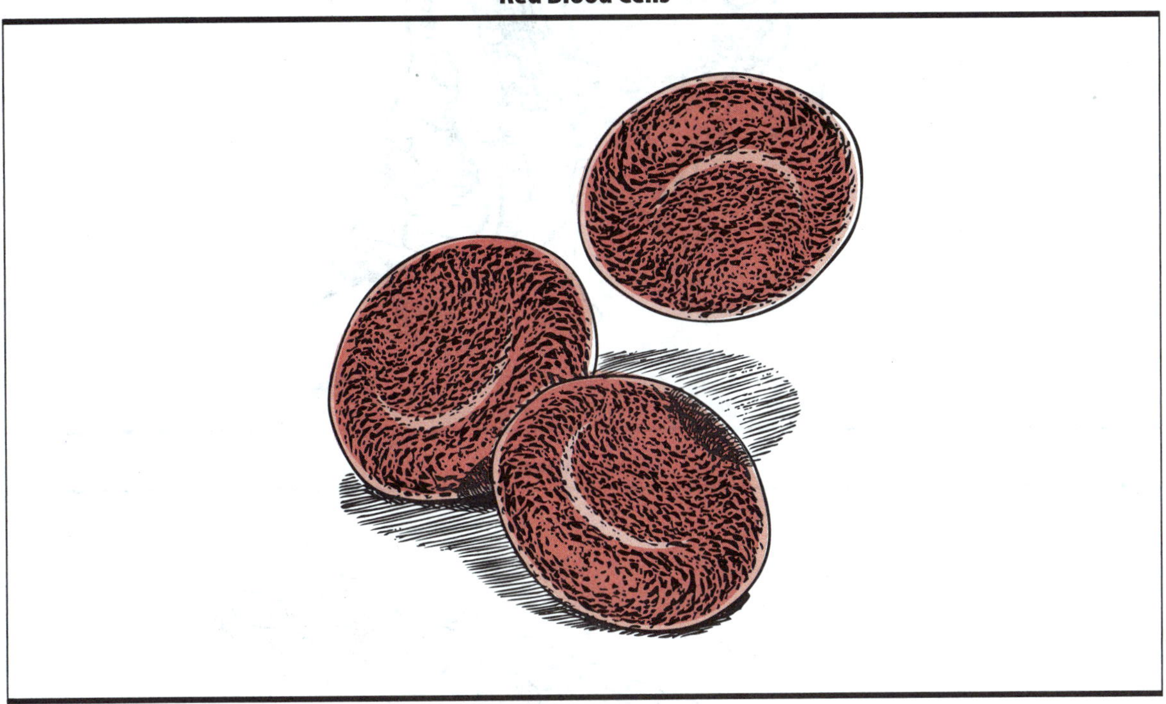

White Blood Cell

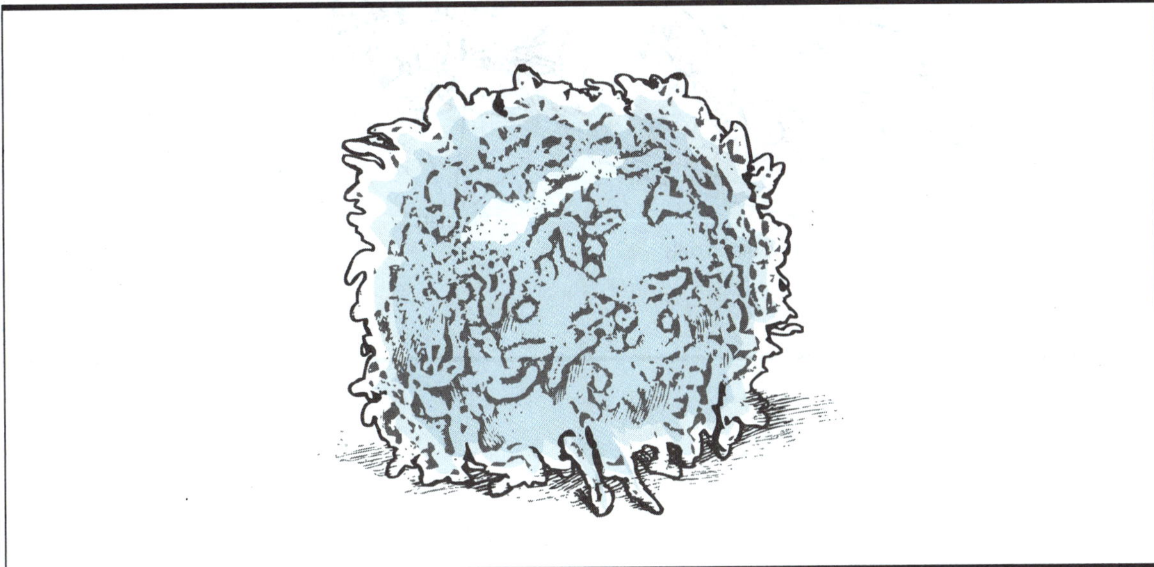

Platelet

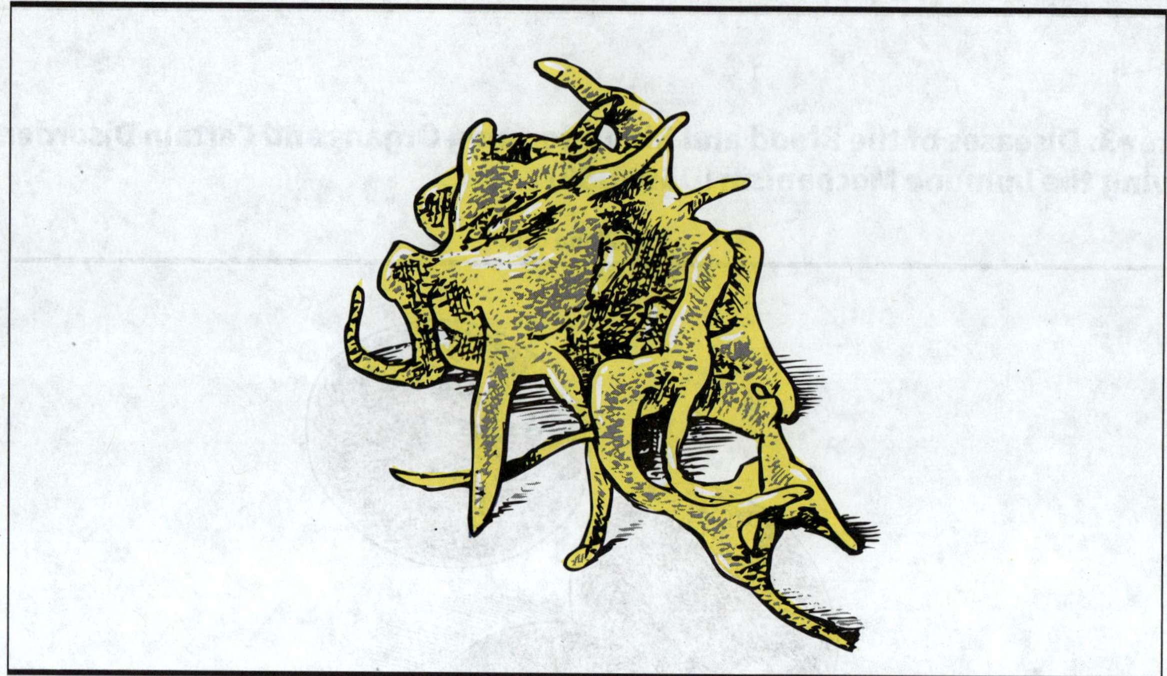

Coagulation

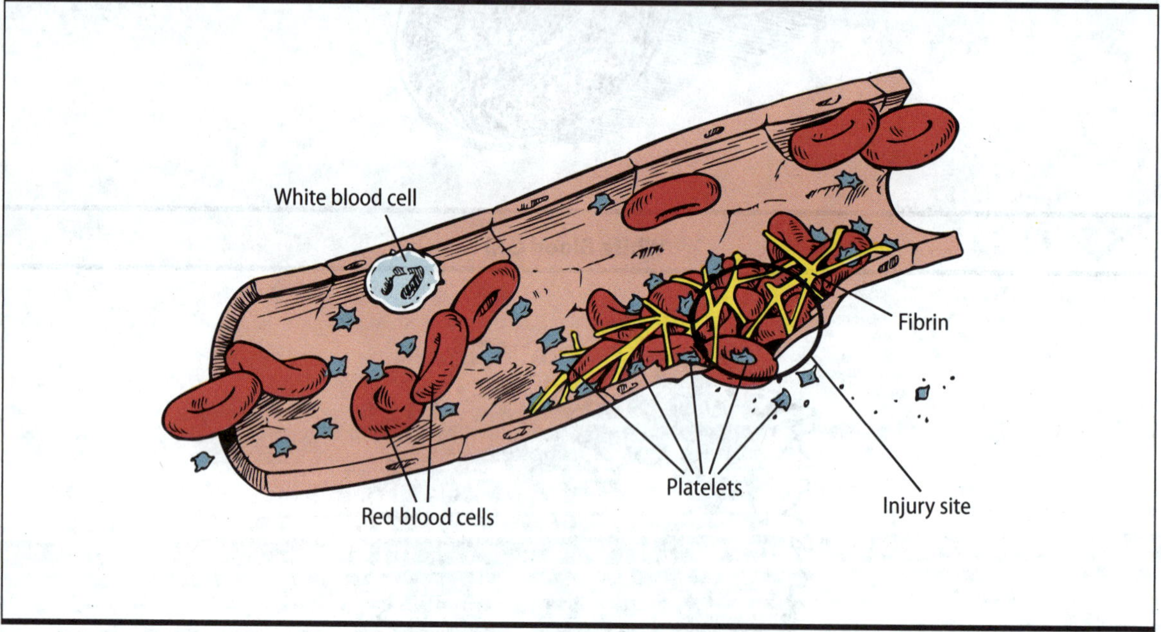

Spleen Anatomical Location and External Structures

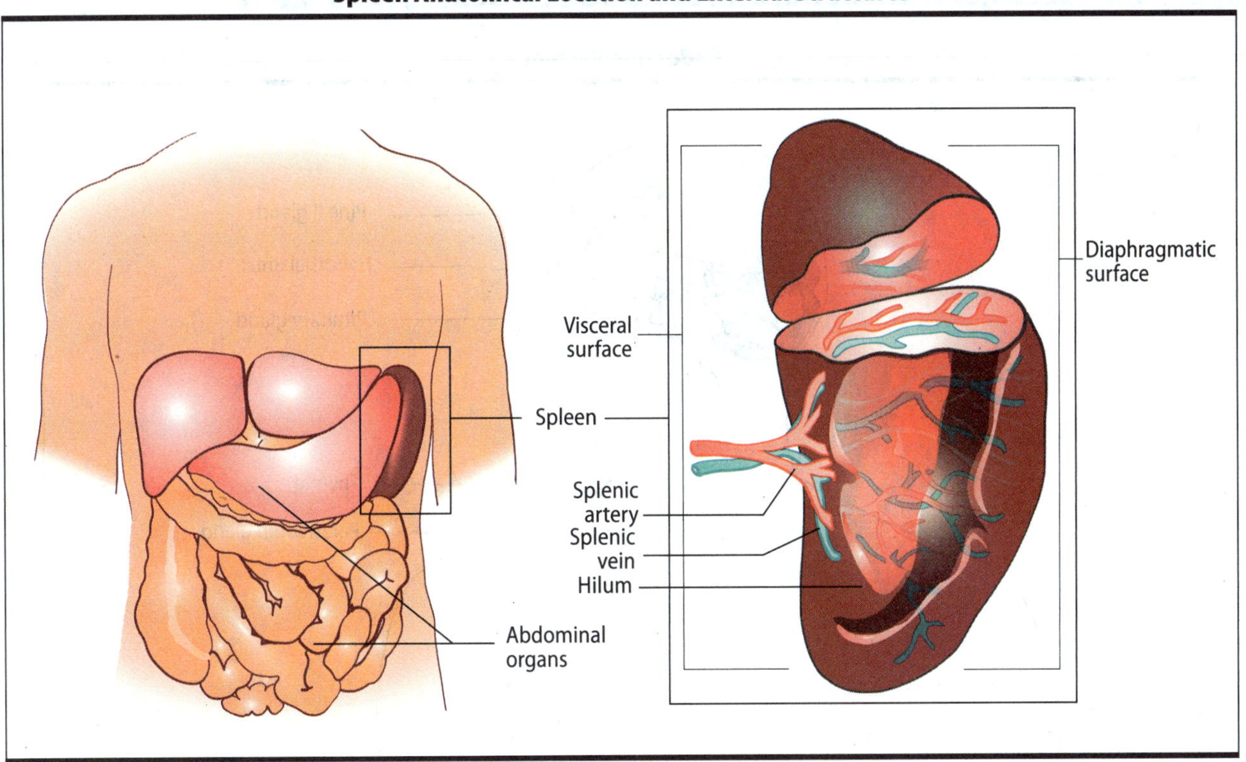

Spleen Interior Structures

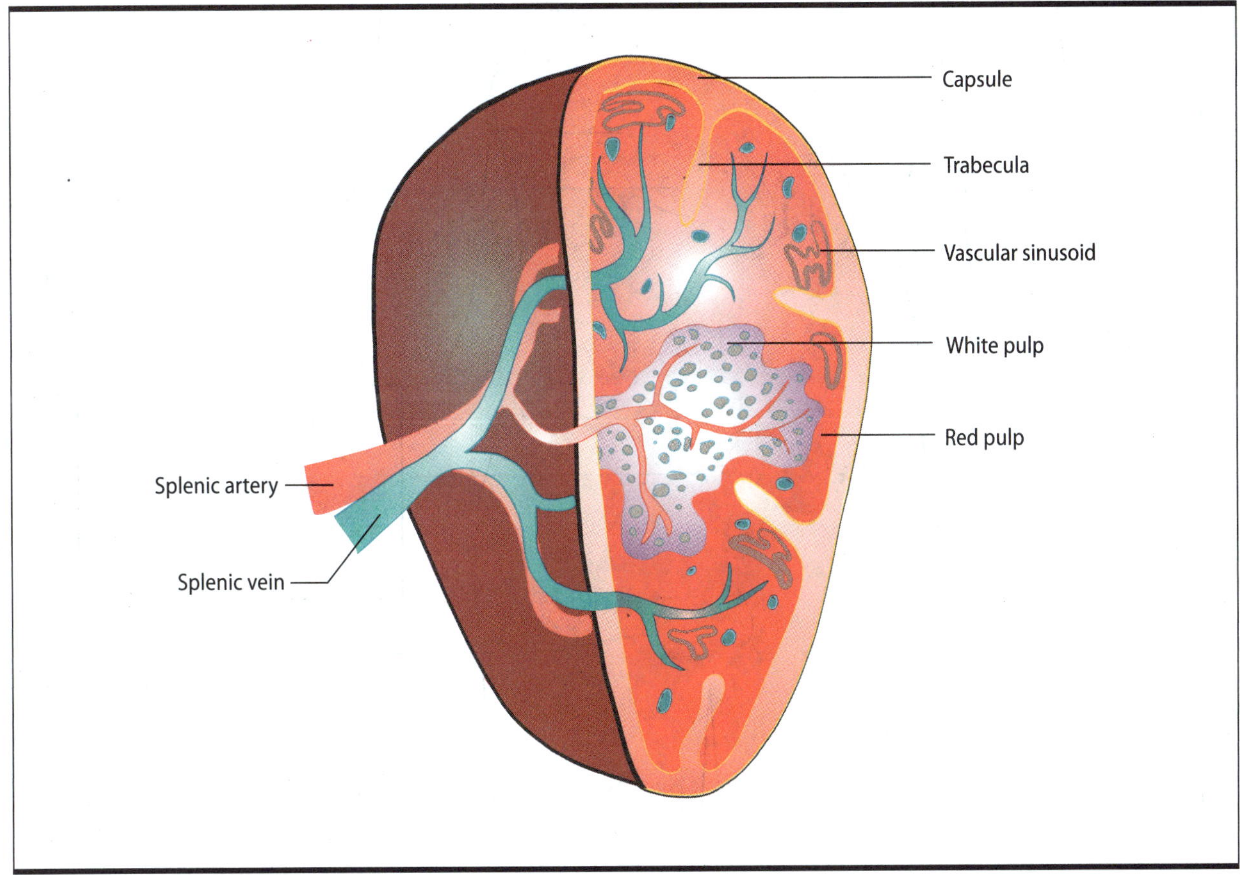

Chapter 4. Endocrine, Nutritional and Metabolic Diseases (EØØ–E89)

Endocrine System

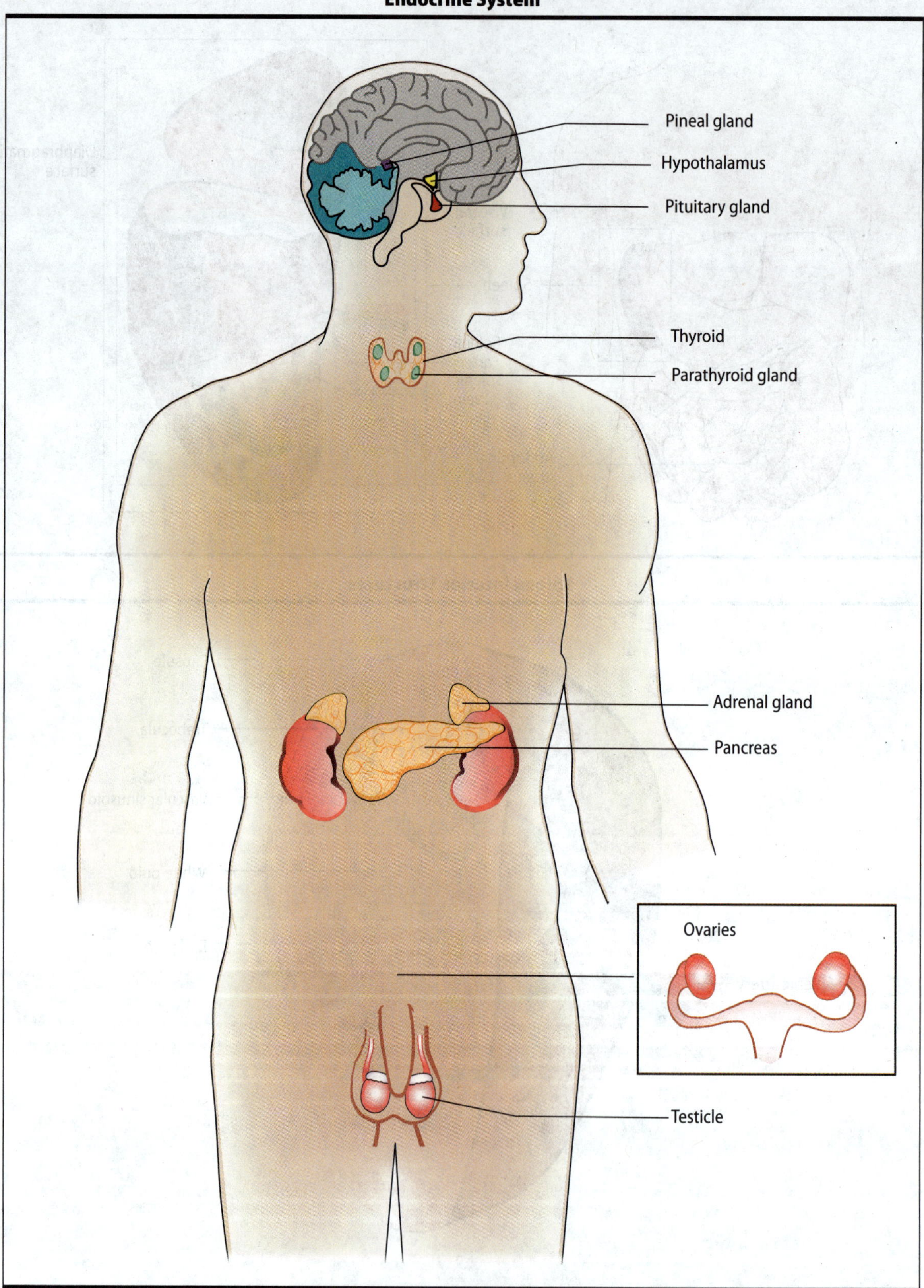

Thyroid

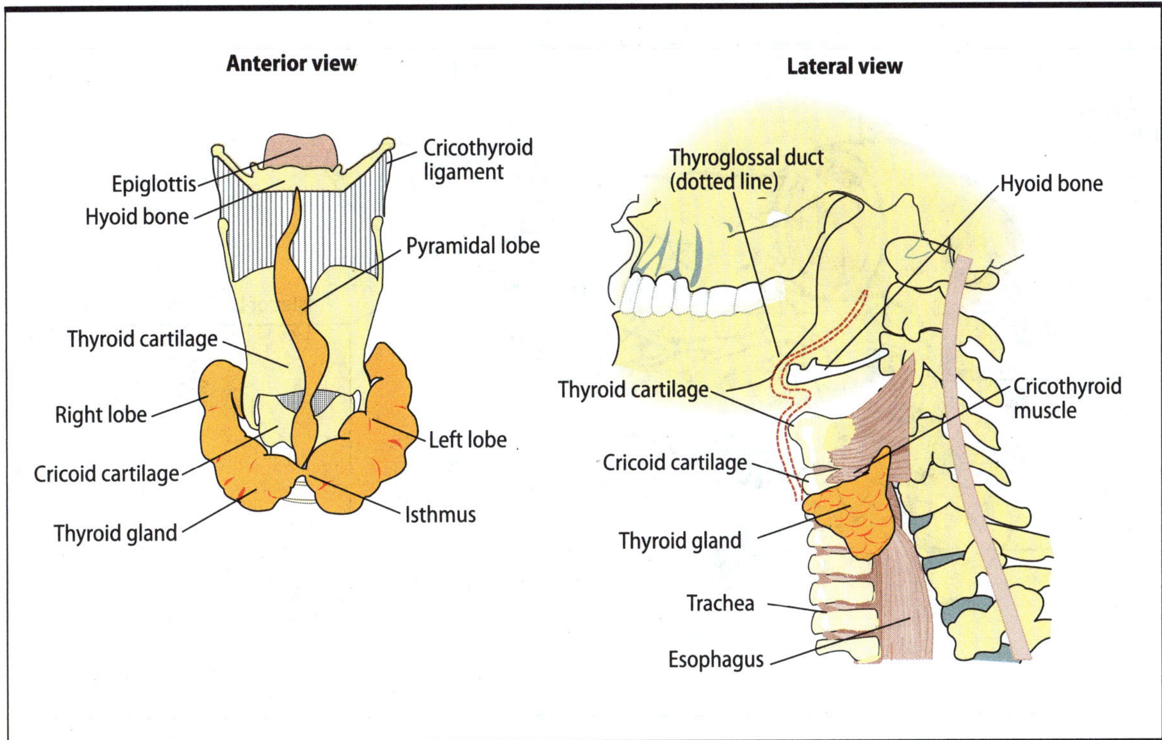

Thyroid and Parathyroid Glands

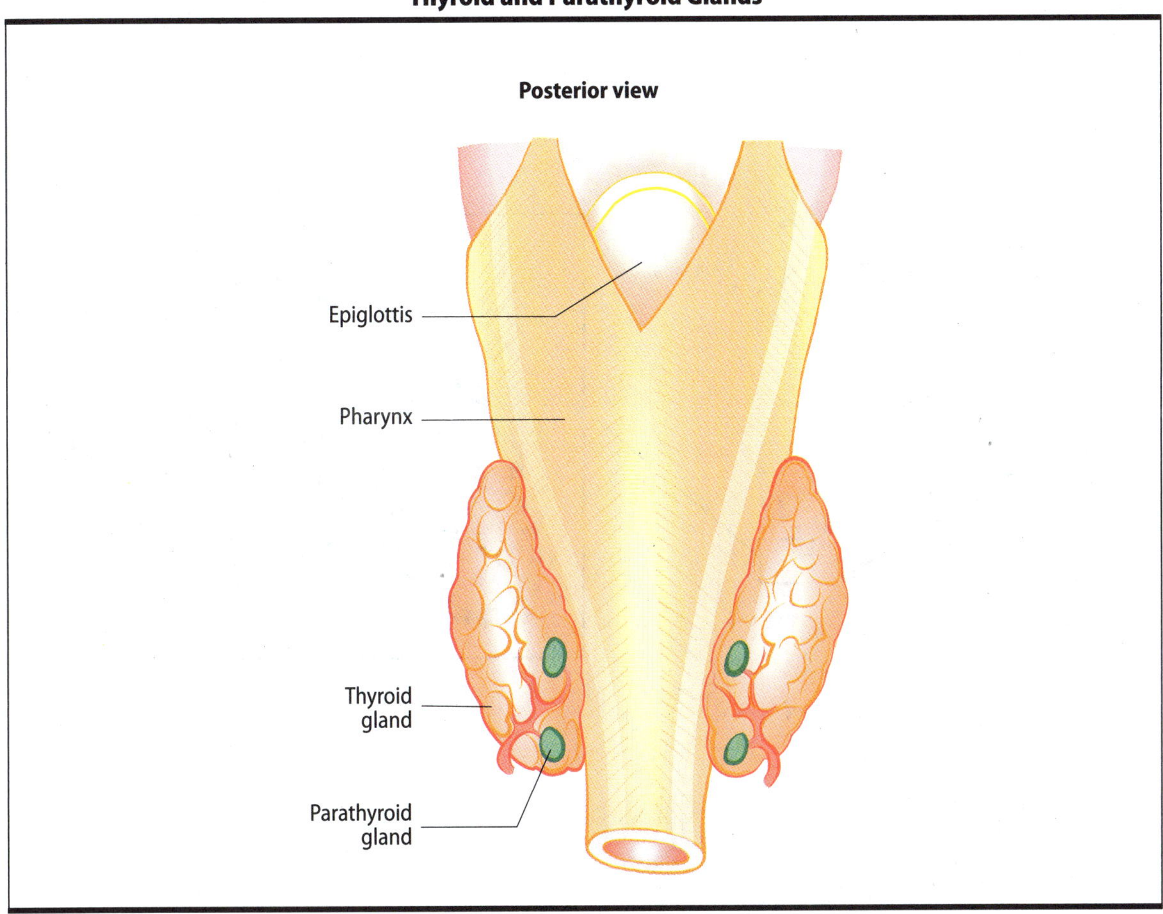

Pancreas

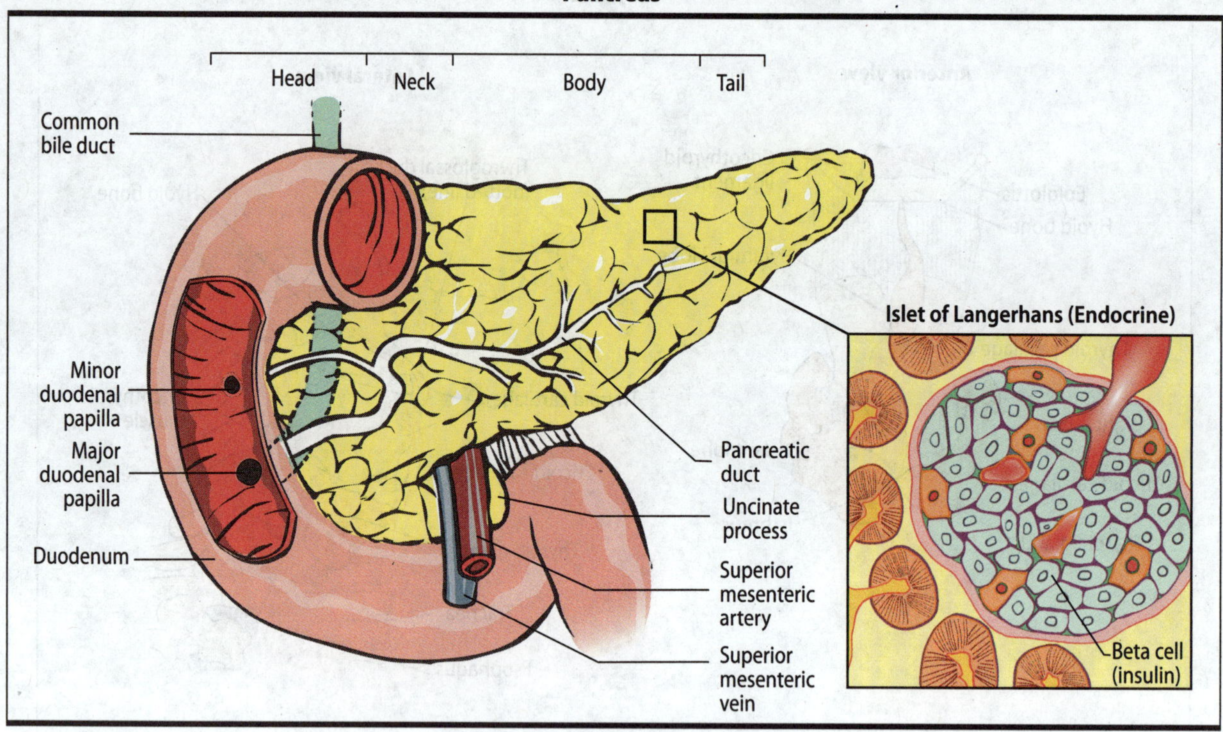

Anatomy of the Adrenal Gland

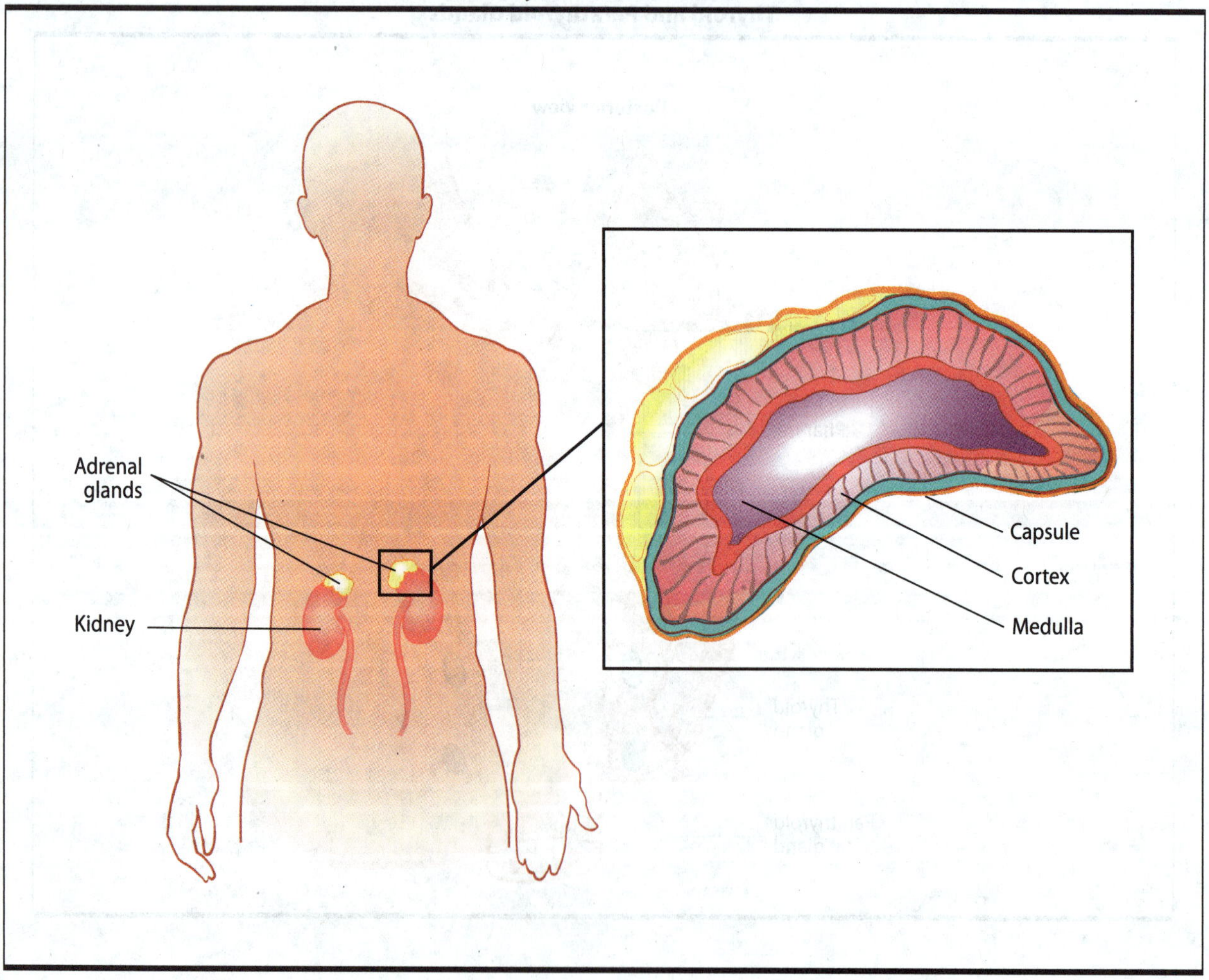

Adrenal glands

Kidney

Capsule

Cortex

Medulla

Structure of an Ovary

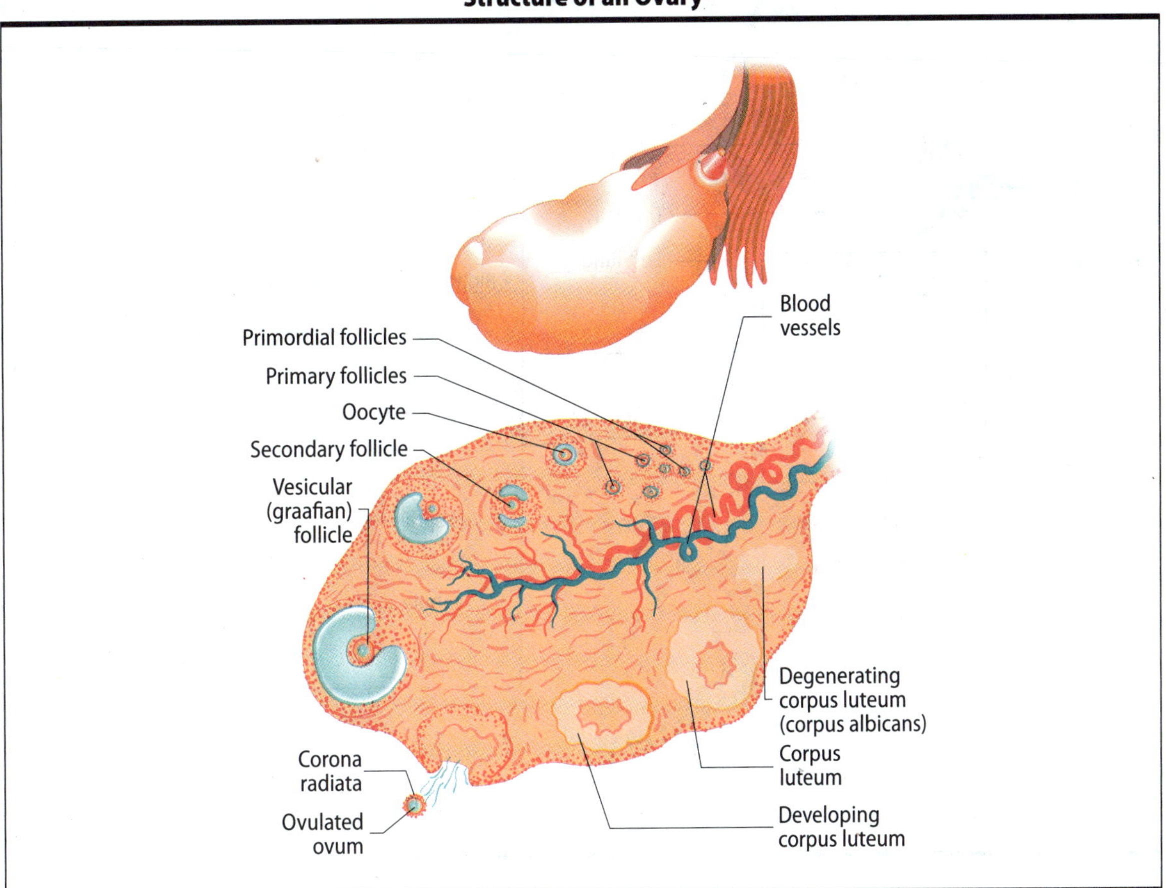

Testis and Associated Structures

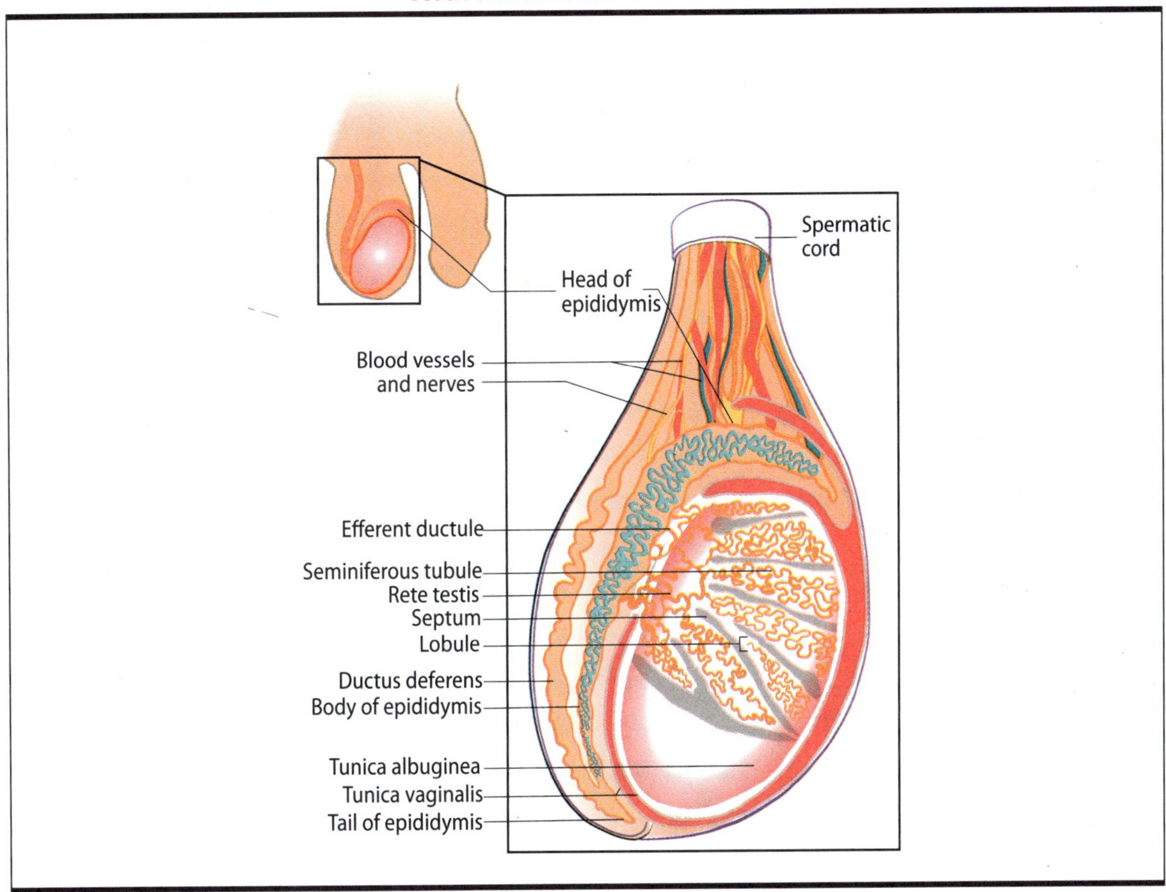

Thymus

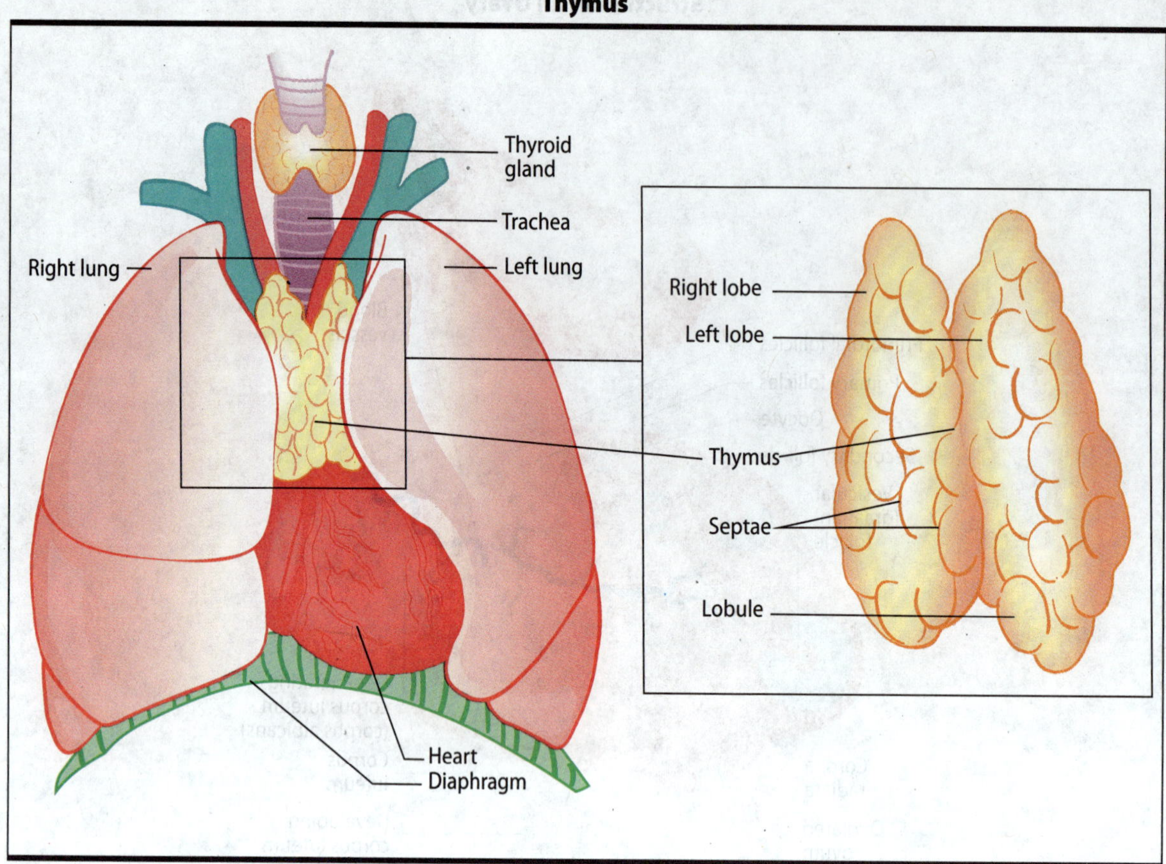

Thyroid gland
Trachea
Right lung
Left lung
Right lobe
Left lobe
Thymus
Septae
Lobule
Heart
Diaphragm

Chapter 6. Diseases of the Nervous System (GØØ–G99)

Brain

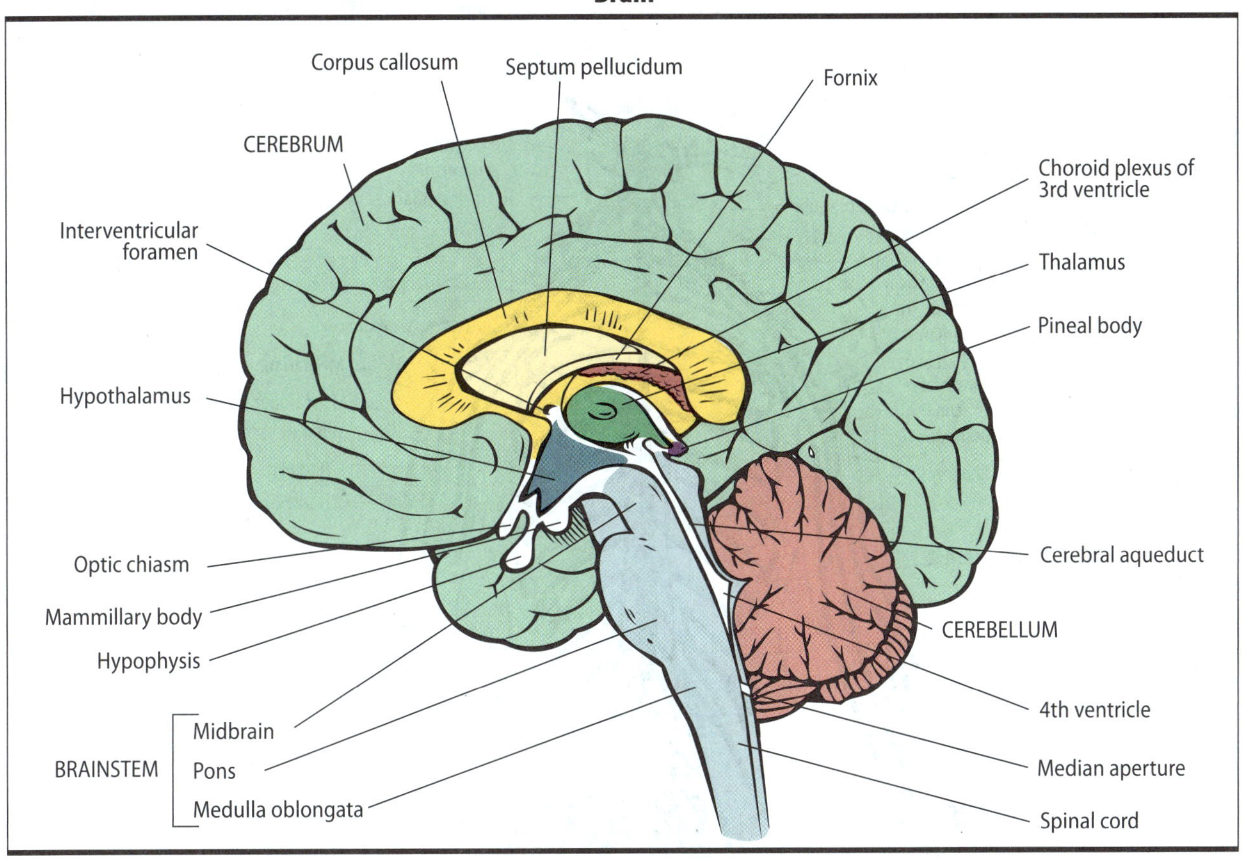

Cranial Nerves

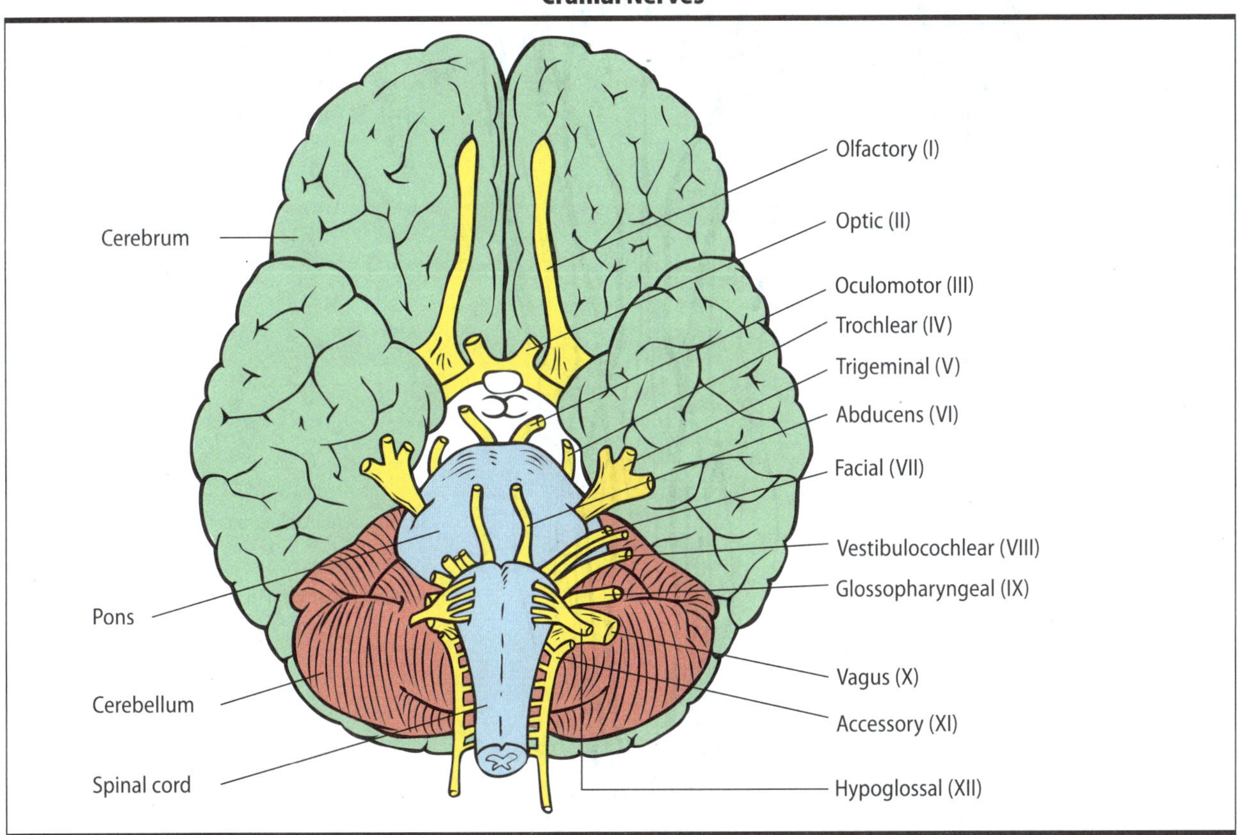

Peripheral Nervous System

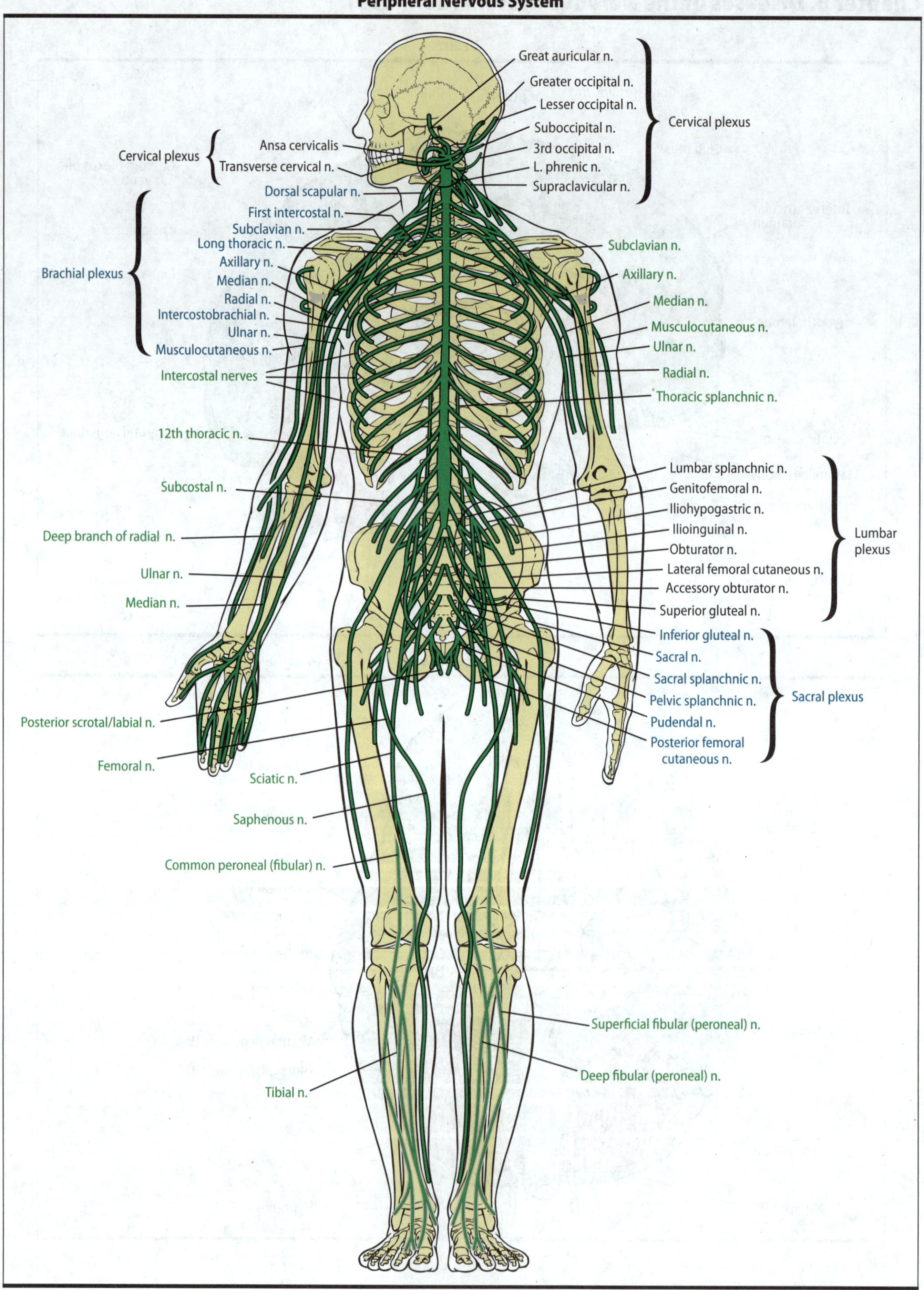

Spinal Cord and Spinal Nerves

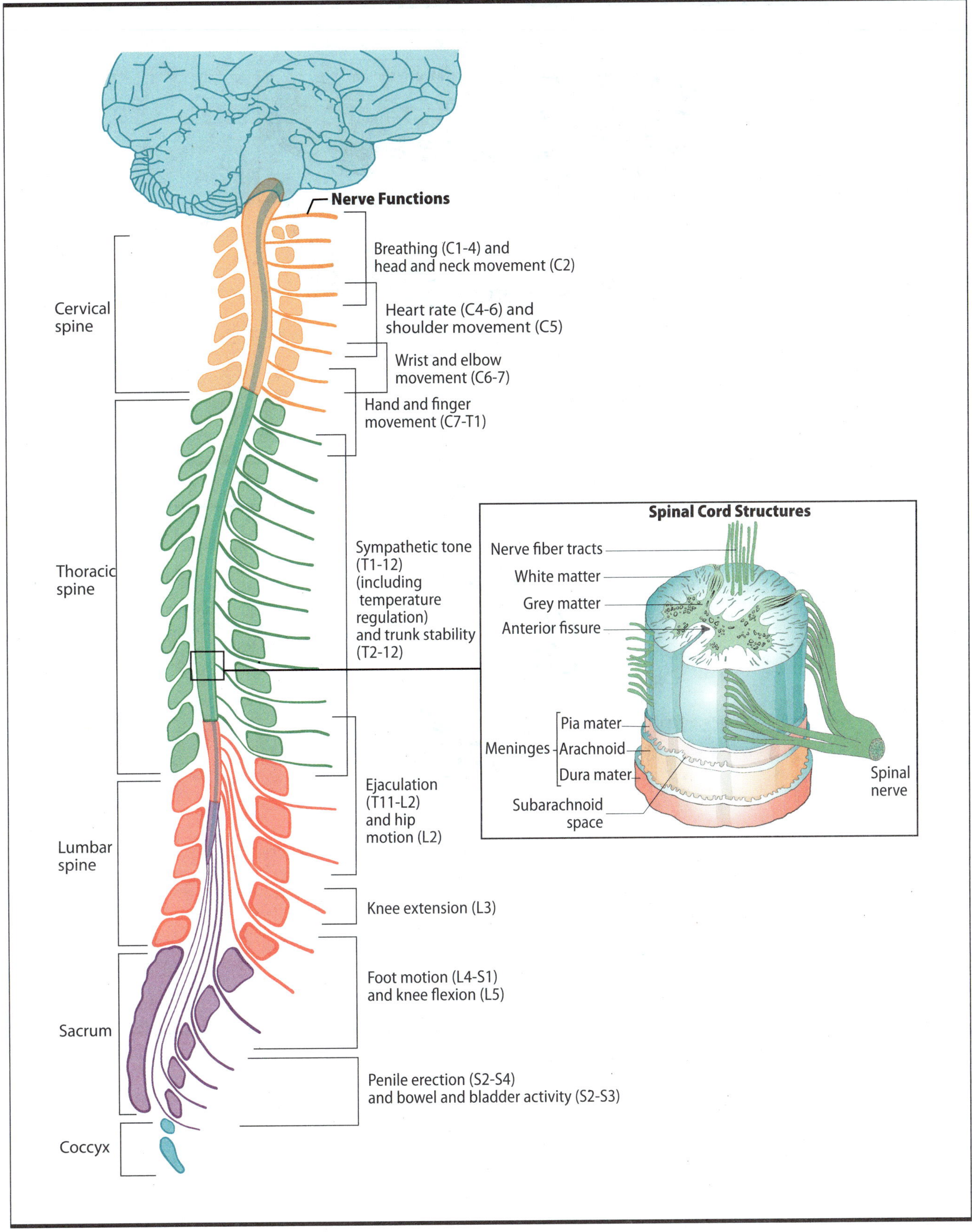

Nerve Cell

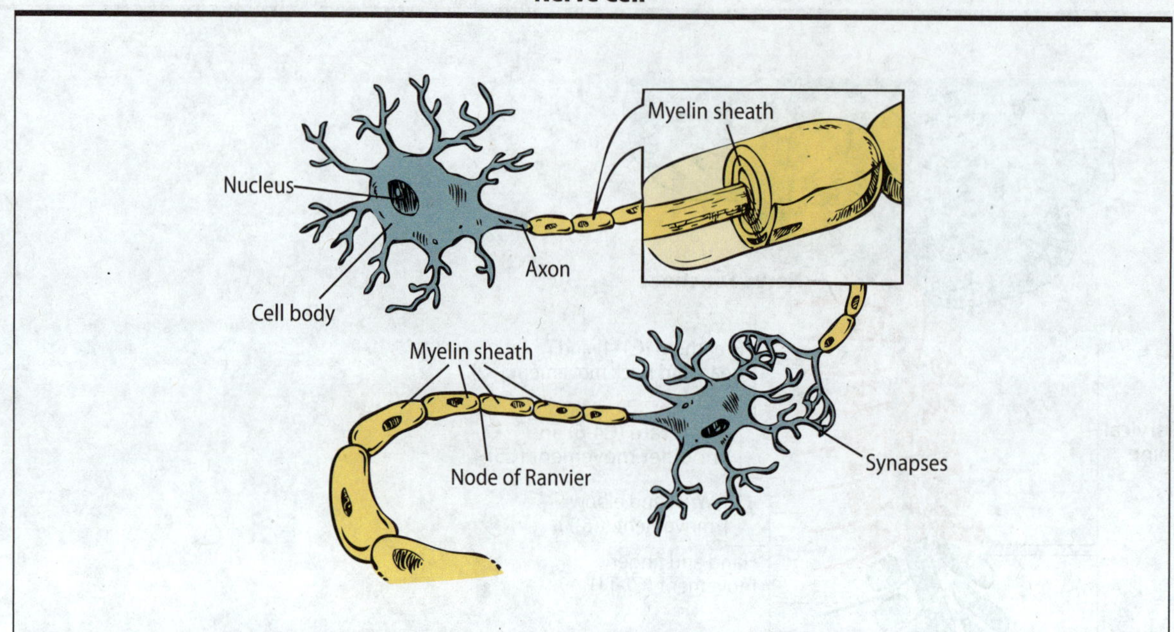

Trigeminal and Facial Nerve Branches

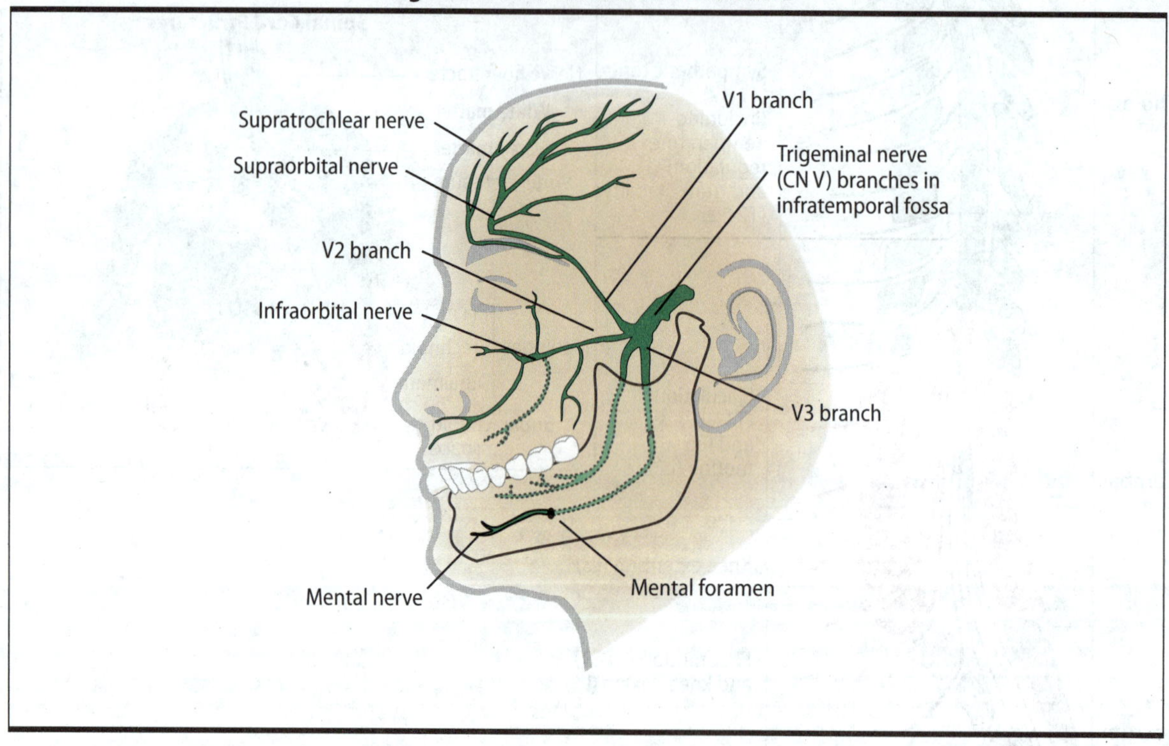

Chapter 7. Diseases of the Eye and Adnexa (HØØ–H59)

Eye

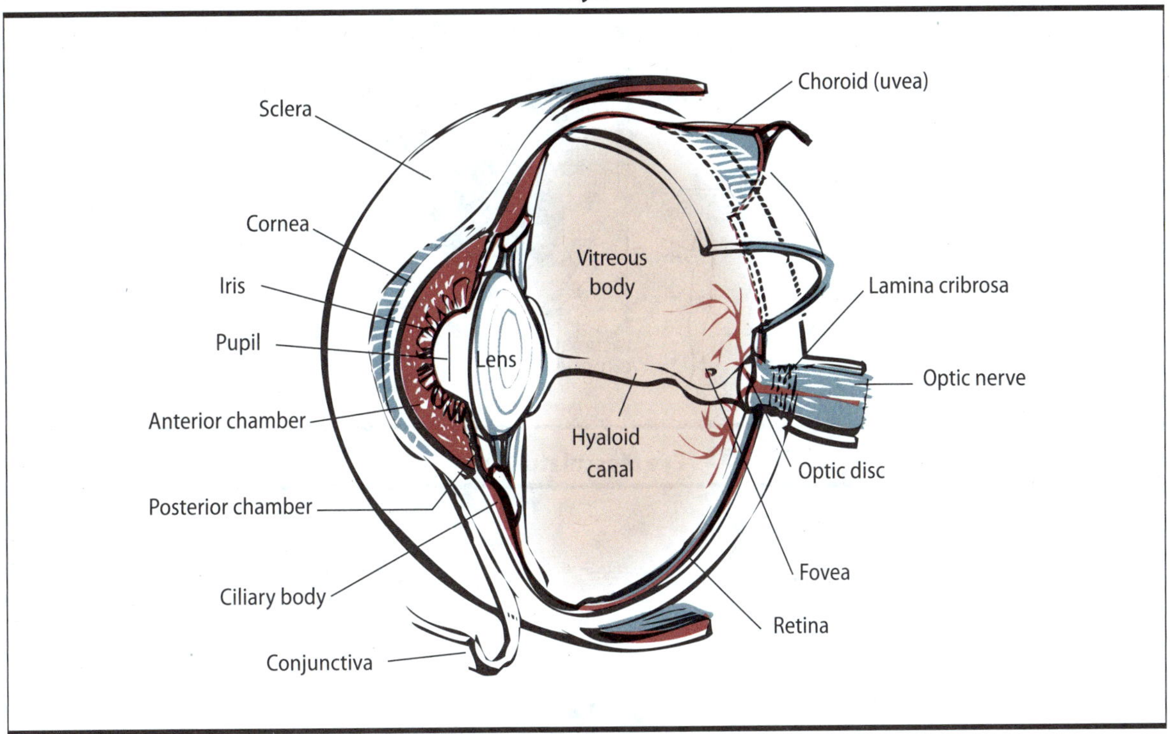

Posterior Pole of Globe/Flow of Aqueous Humor

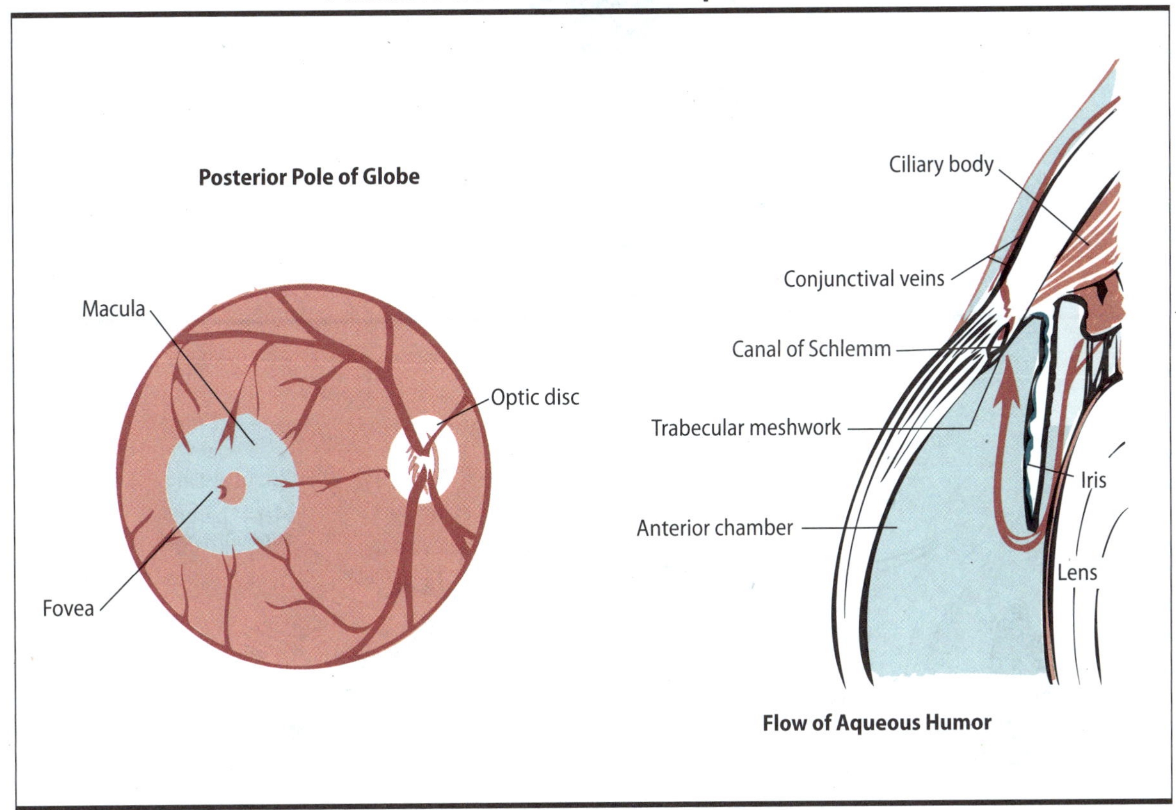

Lacrimal System

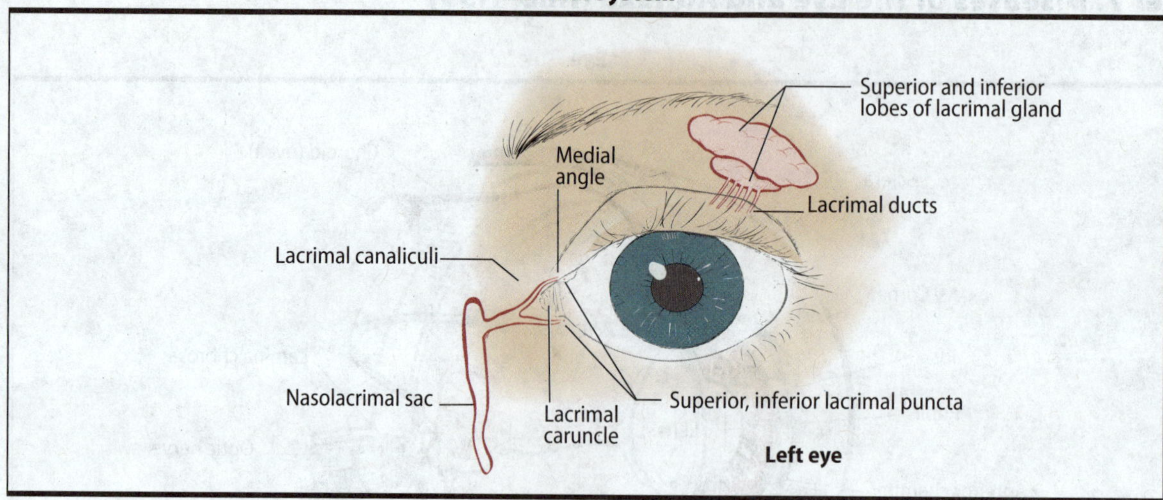

Eye Musculature

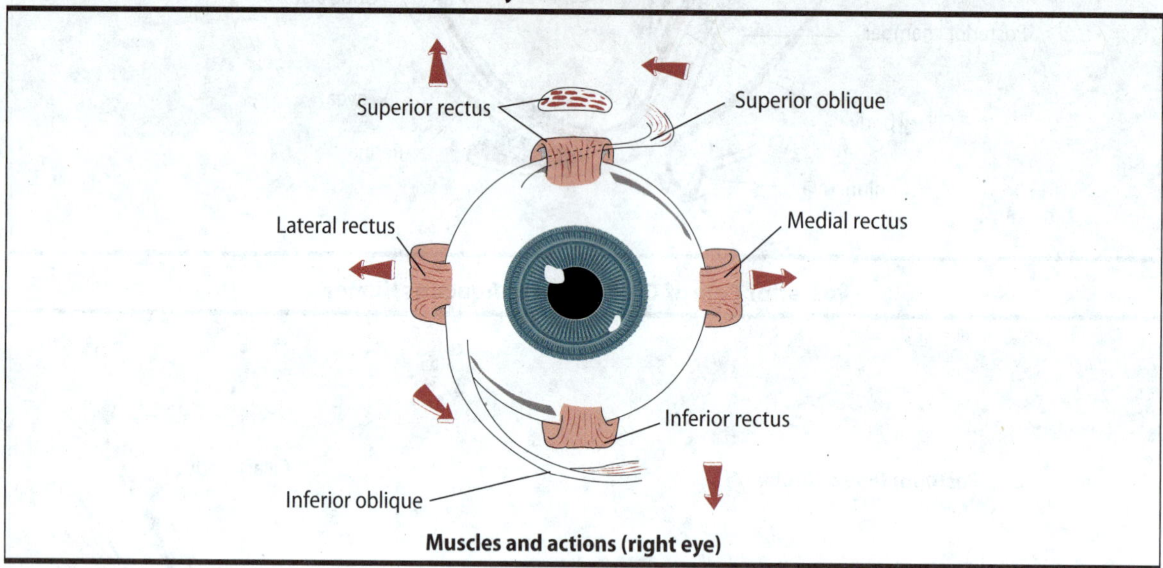

Muscles and actions (right eye)

Eyelid Structures

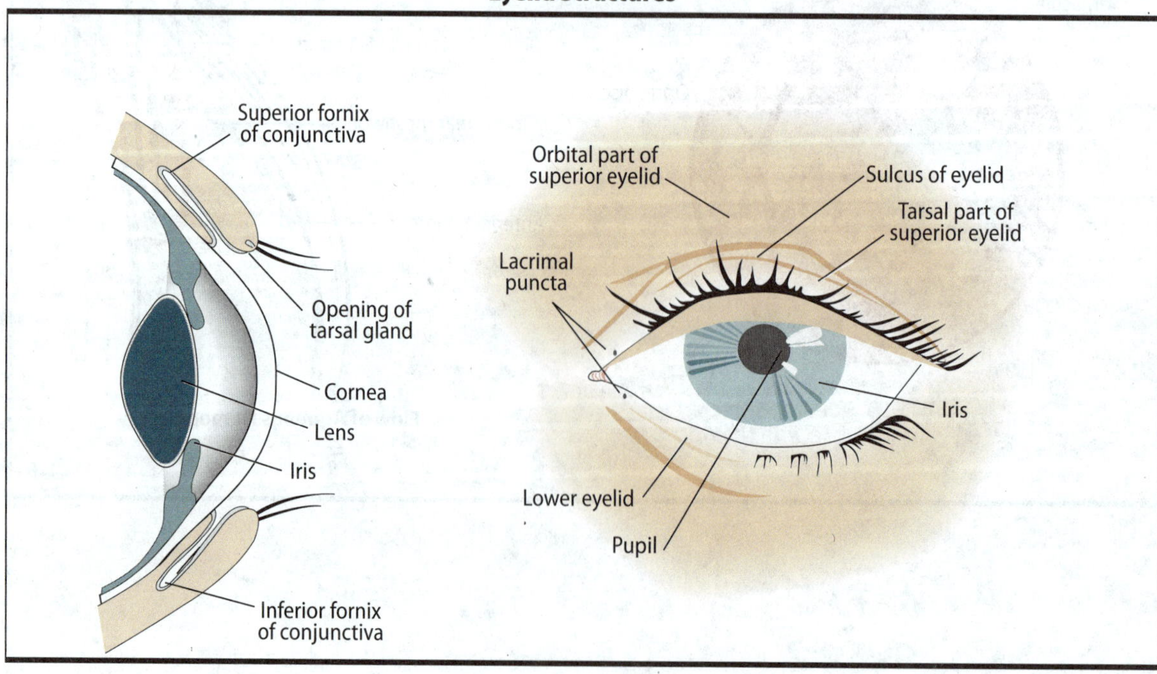

Chapter 8. Diseases of the Ear and Mastoid Process (H6Ø–H95)

Ear Anatomy

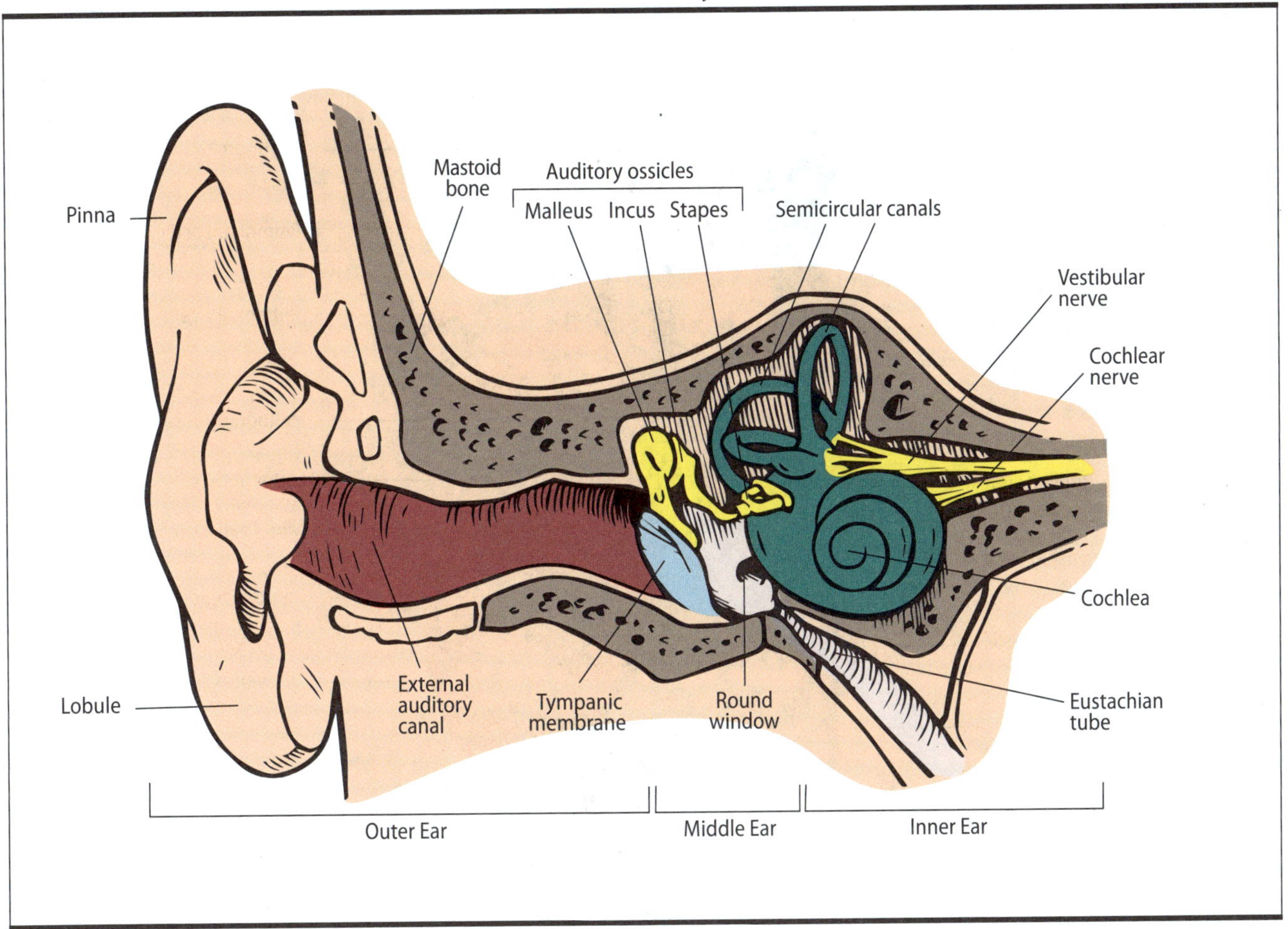

Chapter 9. Diseases of the Circulatory System (I00–I99)

Anatomy of the Heart

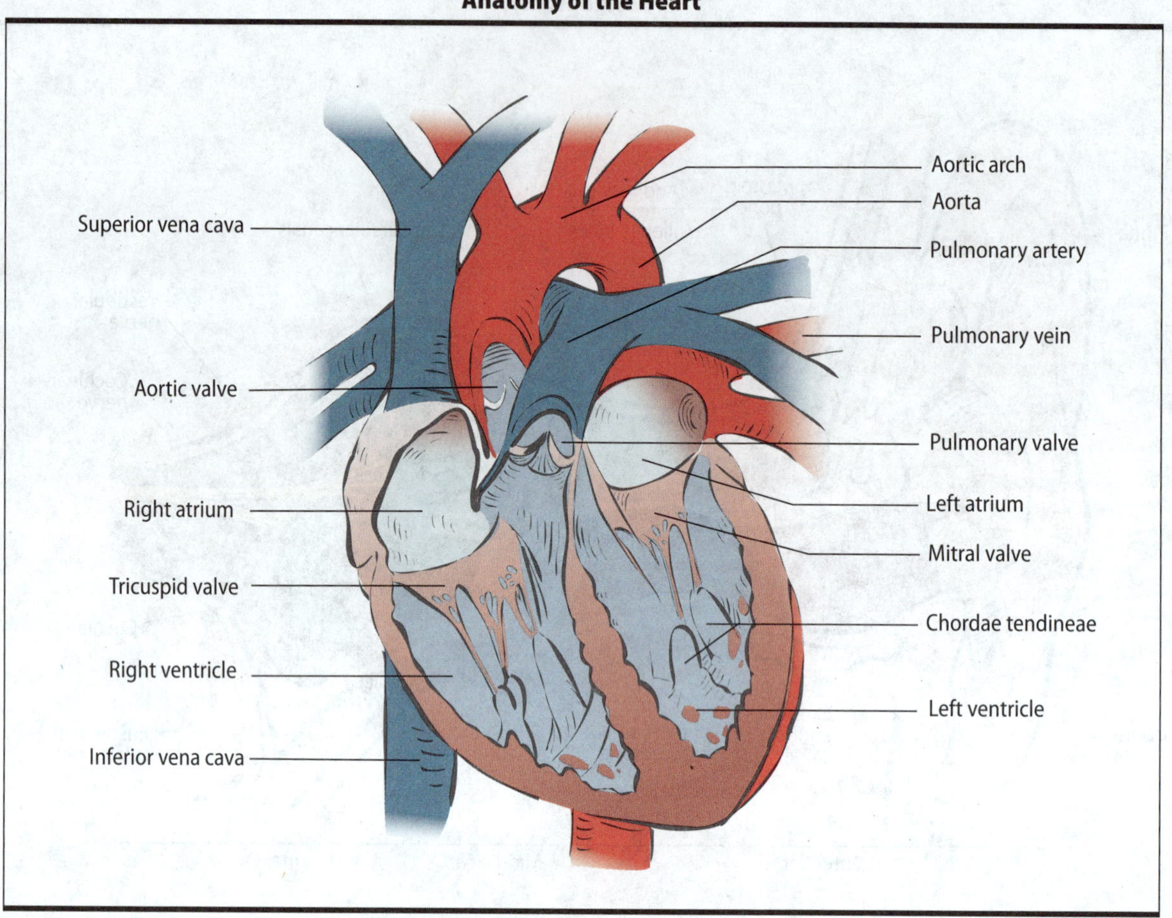

Heart Cross Section

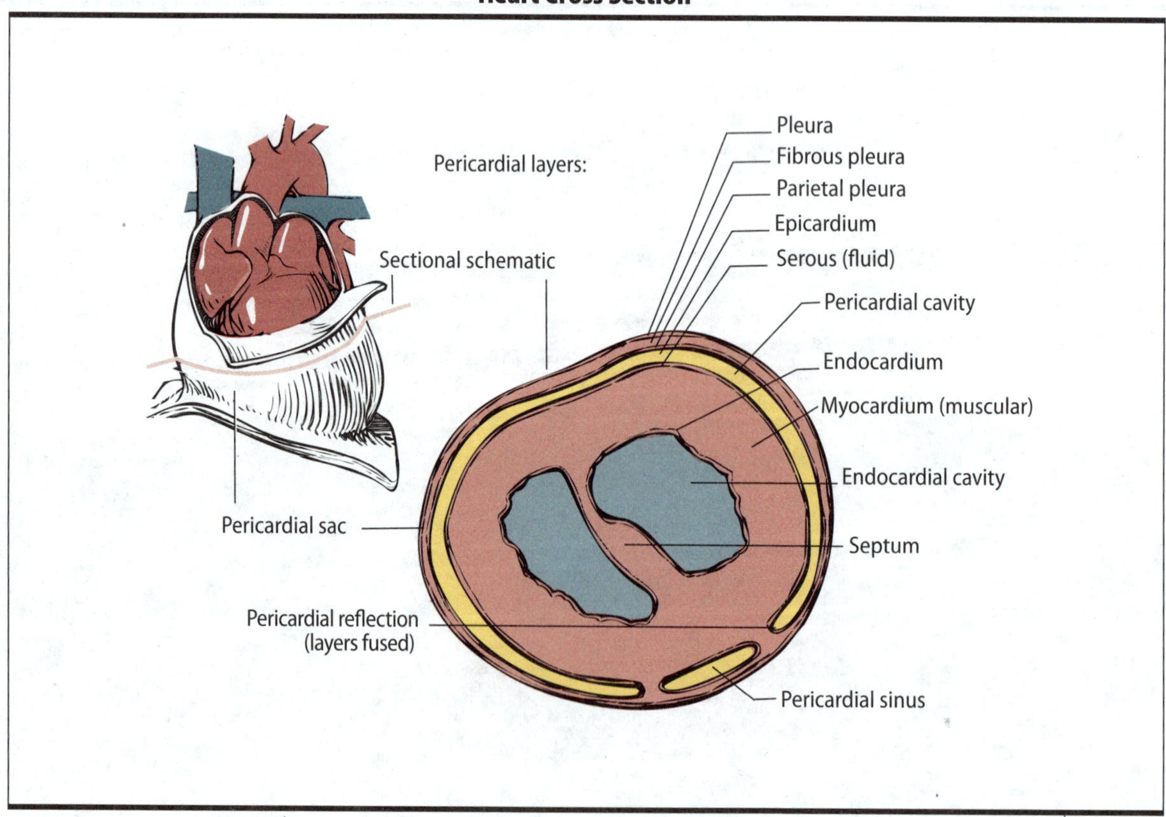

Heart Valves

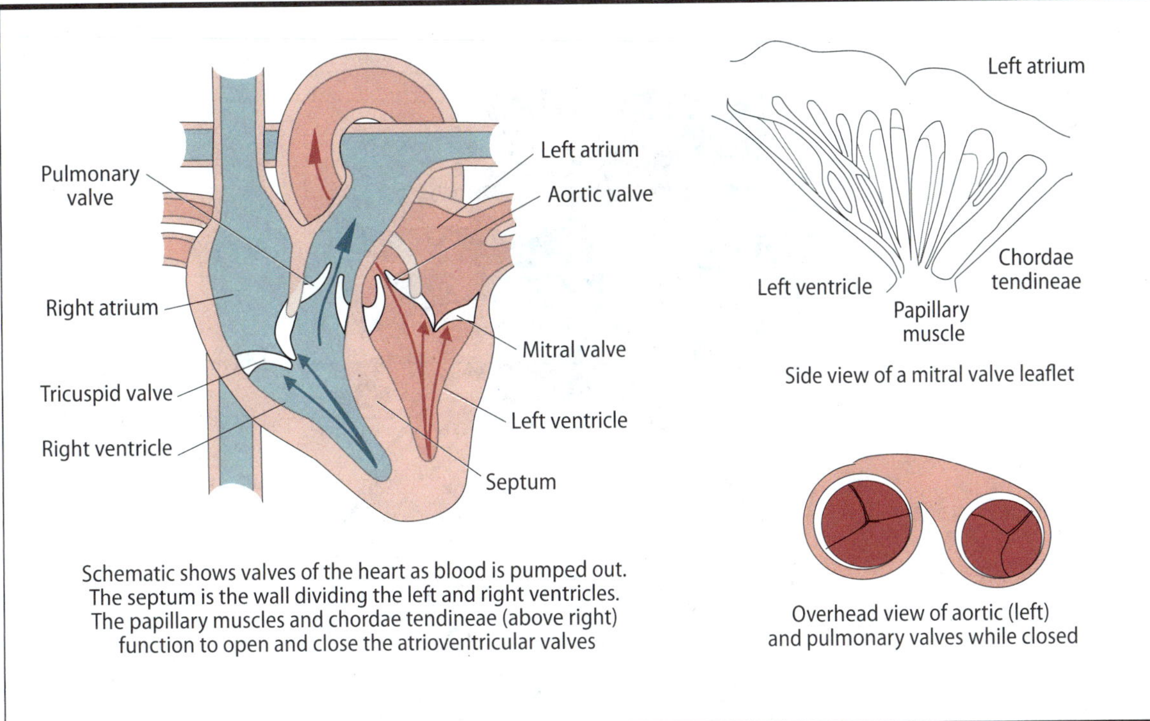

Schematic shows valves of the heart as blood is pumped out. The septum is the wall dividing the left and right ventricles. The papillary muscles and chordae tendineae (above right) function to open and close the atrioventricular valves

Side view of a mitral valve leaflet

Overhead view of aortic (left) and pulmonary valves while closed

Heart Conduction System

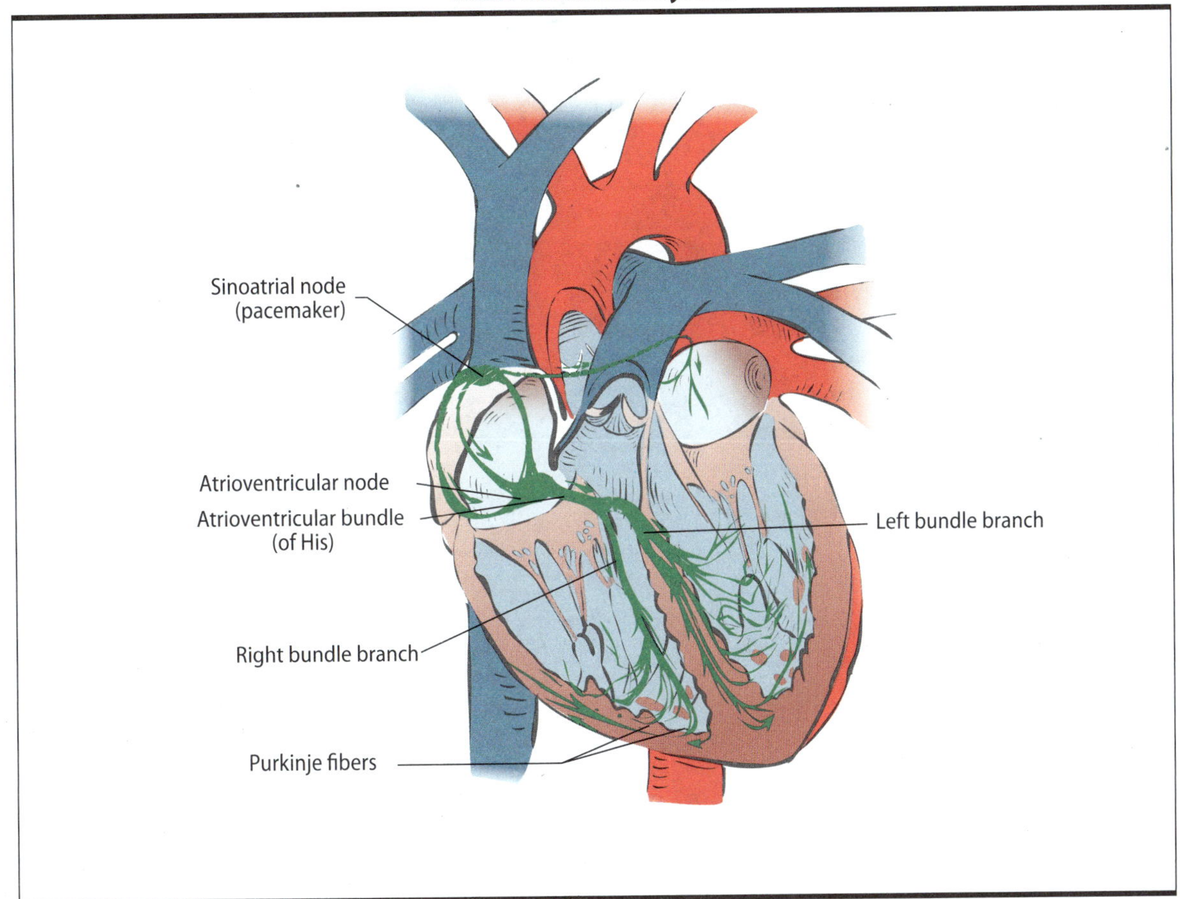

Coronary Arteries

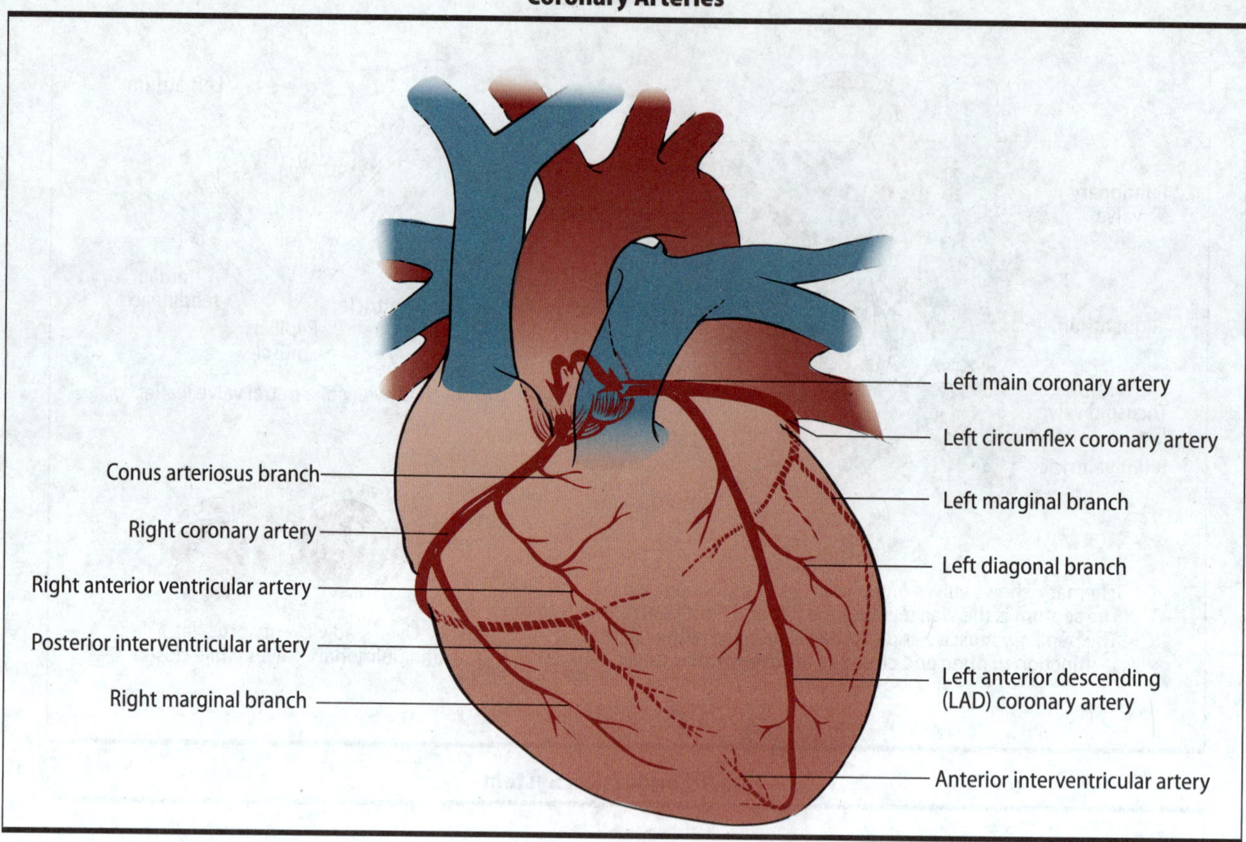

Arteries

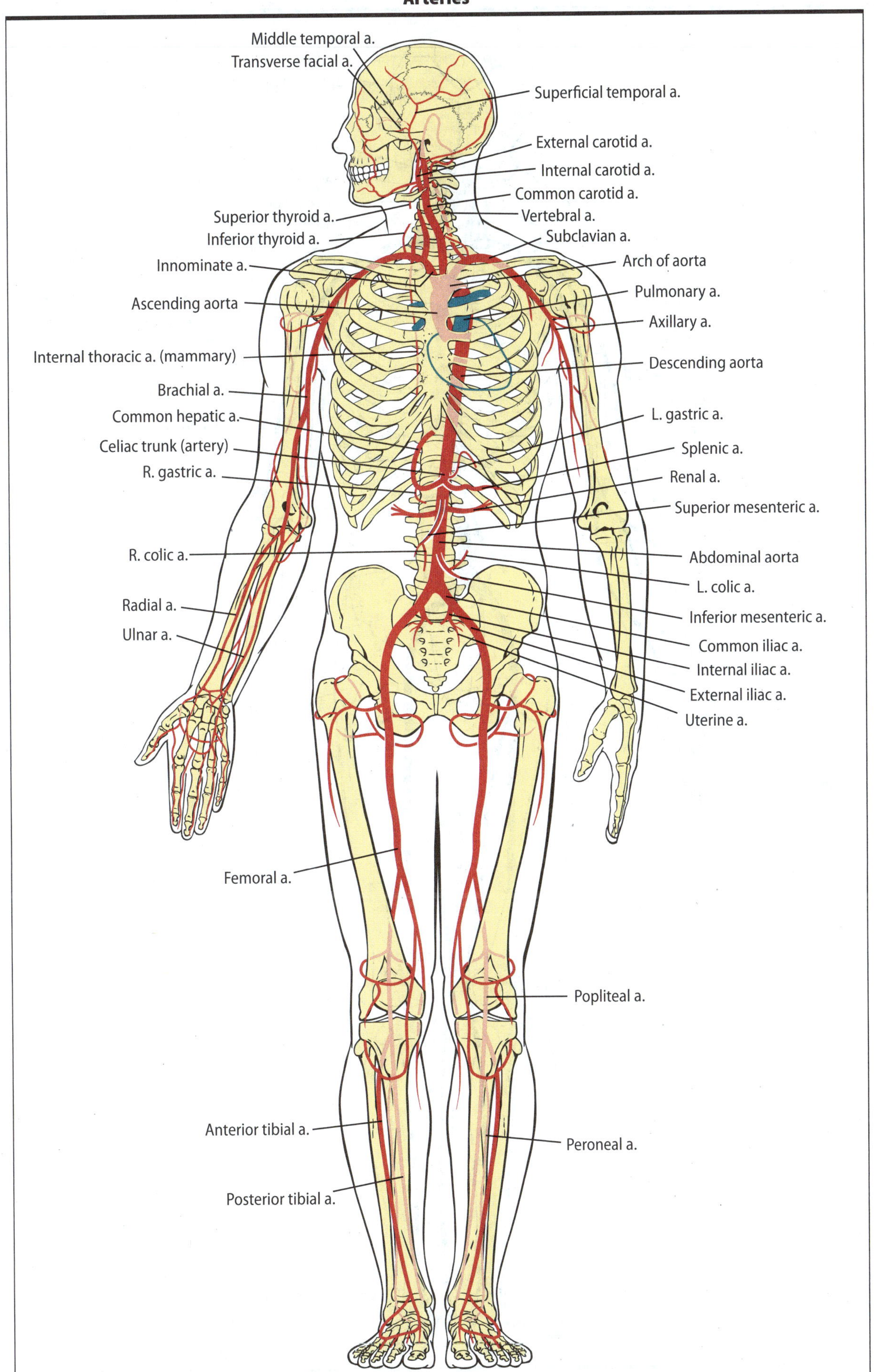

Middle temporal a.
Transverse facial a.
Superficial temporal a.
External carotid a.
Internal carotid a.
Common carotid a.
Superior thyroid a.
Vertebral a.
Inferior thyroid a.
Subclavian a.
Arch of aorta
Innominate a.
Pulmonary a.
Ascending aorta
Axillary a.
Internal thoracic a. (mammary)
Descending aorta
Brachial a.
Common hepatic a.
L. gastric a.
Celiac trunk (artery)
Splenic a.
R. gastric a.
Renal a.
Superior mesenteric a.
R. colic a.
Abdominal aorta
L. colic a.
Radial a.
Inferior mesenteric a.
Ulnar a.
Common iliac a.
Internal iliac a.
External iliac a.
Uterine a.
Femoral a.
Popliteal a.
Anterior tibial a.
Peroneal a.
Posterior tibial a.

Veins

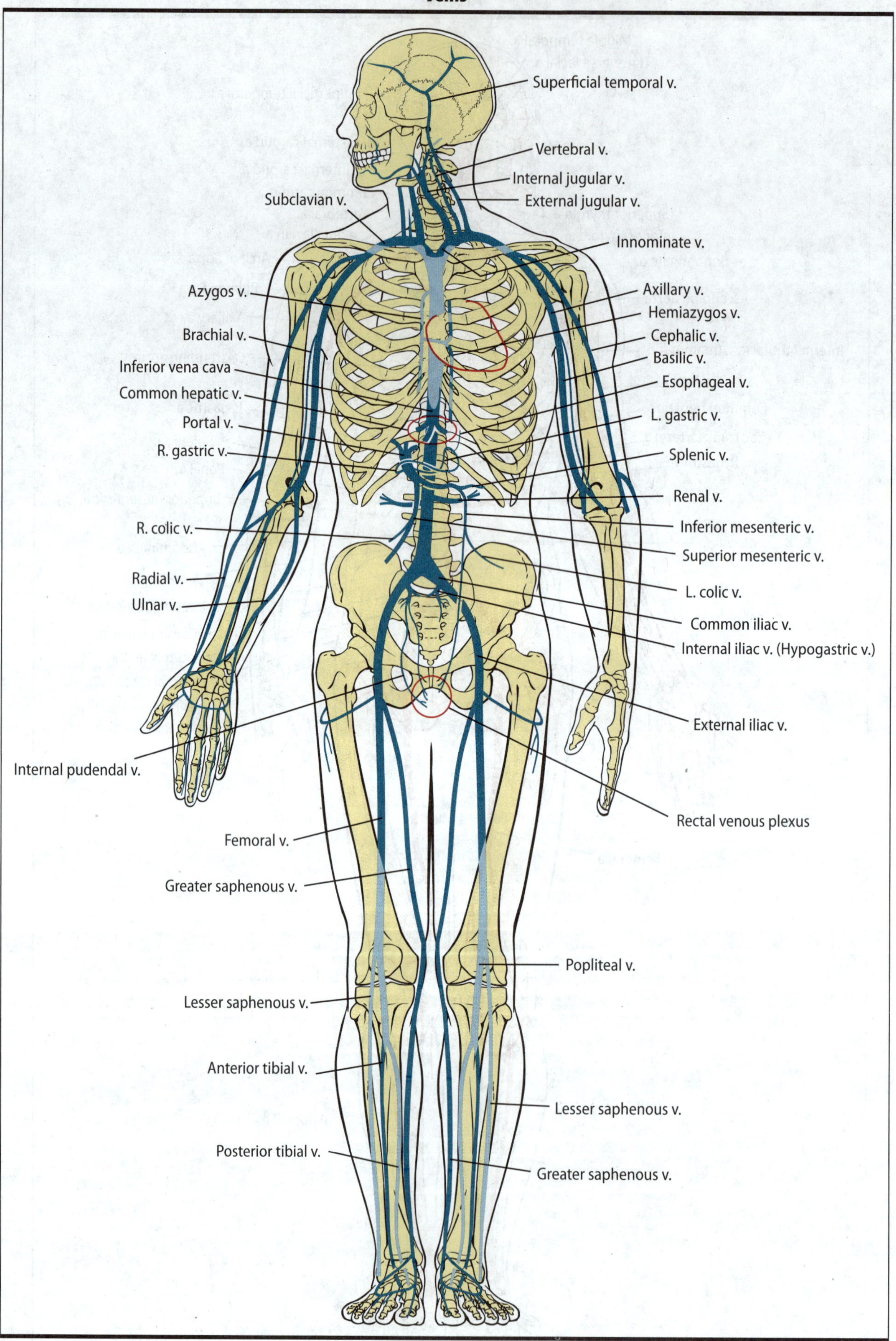

Superficial temporal v.
Vertebral v.
Internal jugular v.
External jugular v.
Subclavian v.
Innominate v.
Azygos v.
Axillary v.
Hemiazygos v.
Brachial v.
Cephalic v.
Basilic v.
Inferior vena cava
Esophageal v.
Common hepatic v.
L. gastric v.
Portal v.
R. gastric v.
Splenic v.
Renal v.
Inferior mesenteric v.
R. colic v.
Superior mesenteric v.
Radial v.
L. colic v.
Ulnar v.
Common iliac v.
Internal iliac v. (Hypogastric v.)
External iliac v.
Internal pudendal v.
Rectal venous plexus
Femoral v.
Greater saphenous v.
Popliteal v.
Lesser saphenous v.
Anterior tibial v.
Lesser saphenous v.
Posterior tibial v.
Greater saphenous v.

Internal Carotid and Vertebral Arteries and Branches

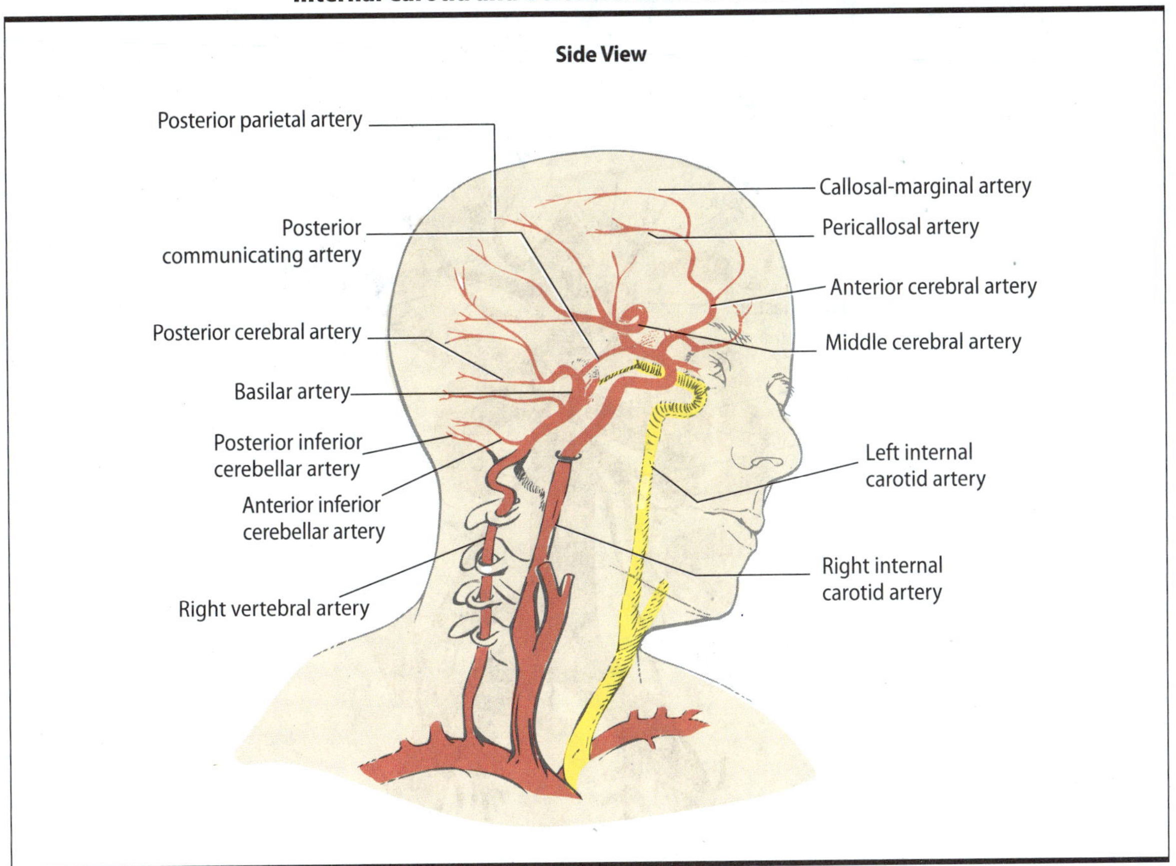

External Carotid Artery and Branches

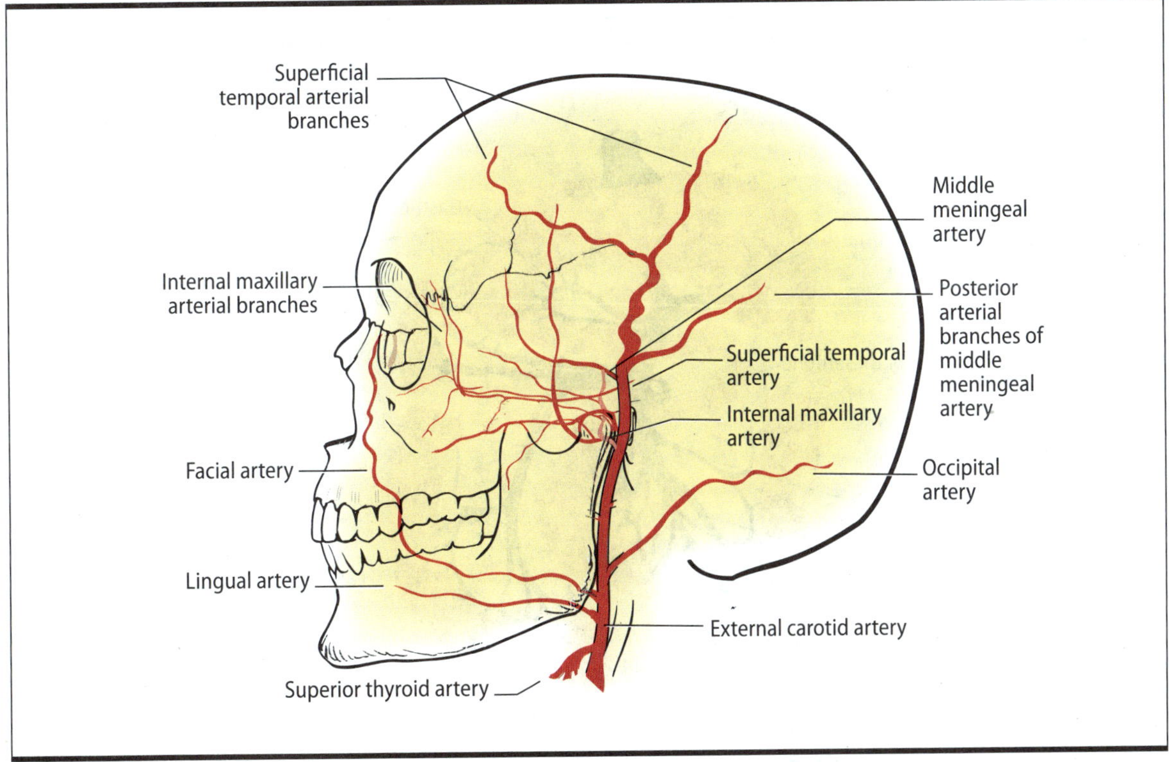

Branches of Abdominal Aorta

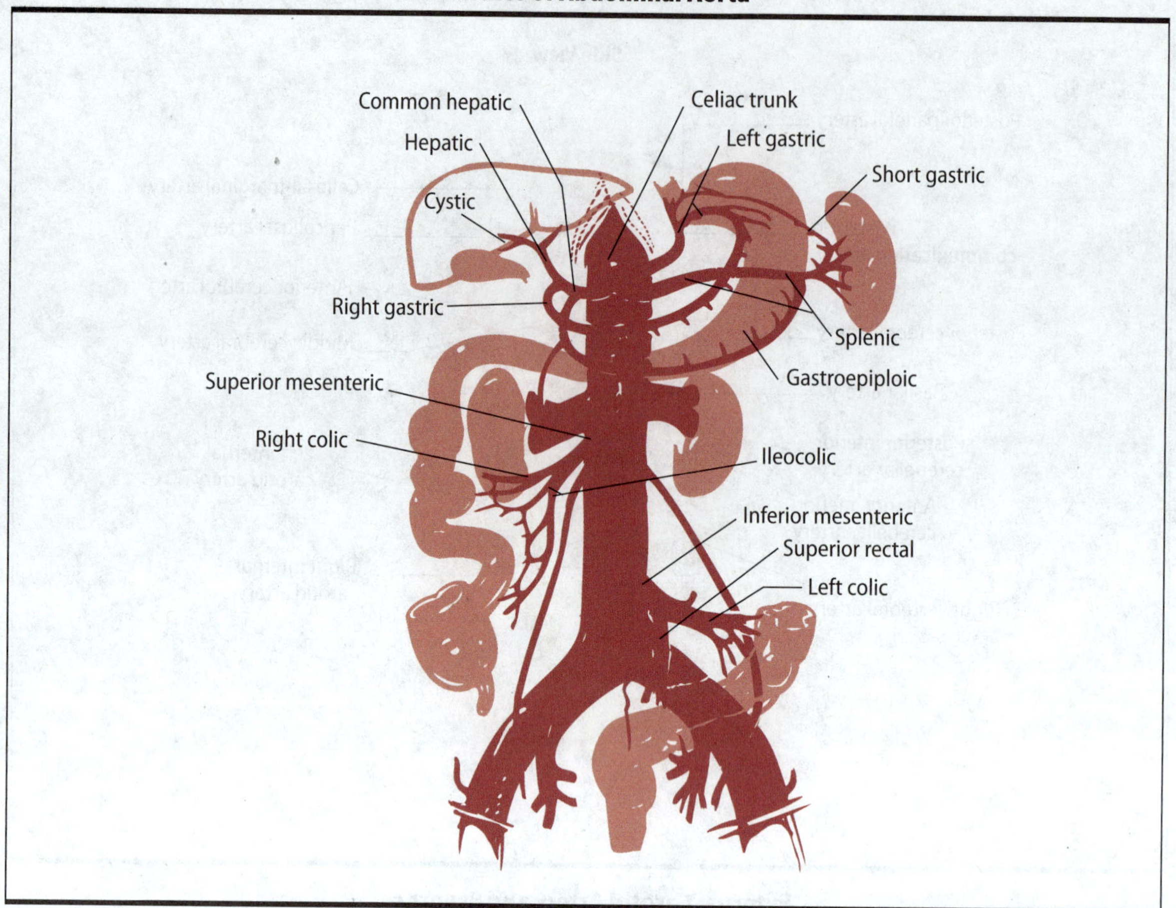

Portal Venous Circulation

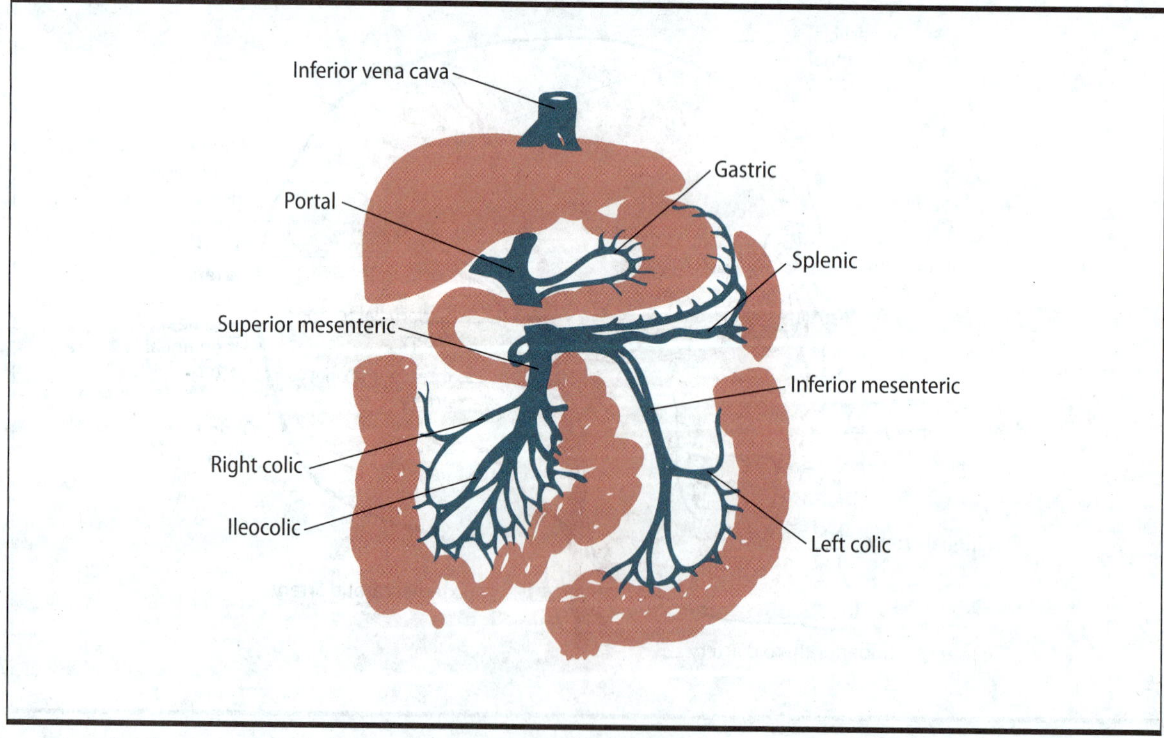

Lymphatic System

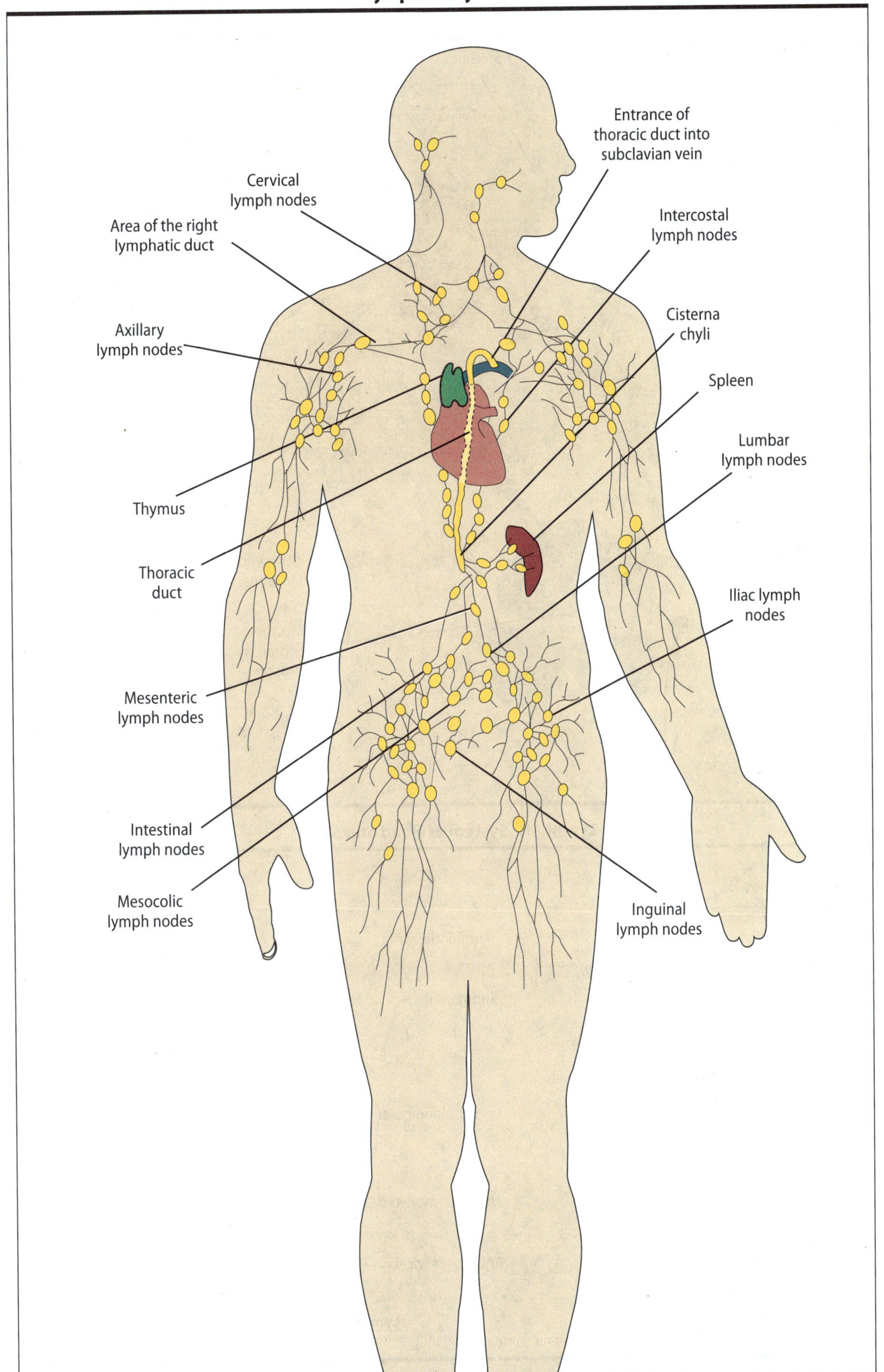

Axillary Lymph Nodes

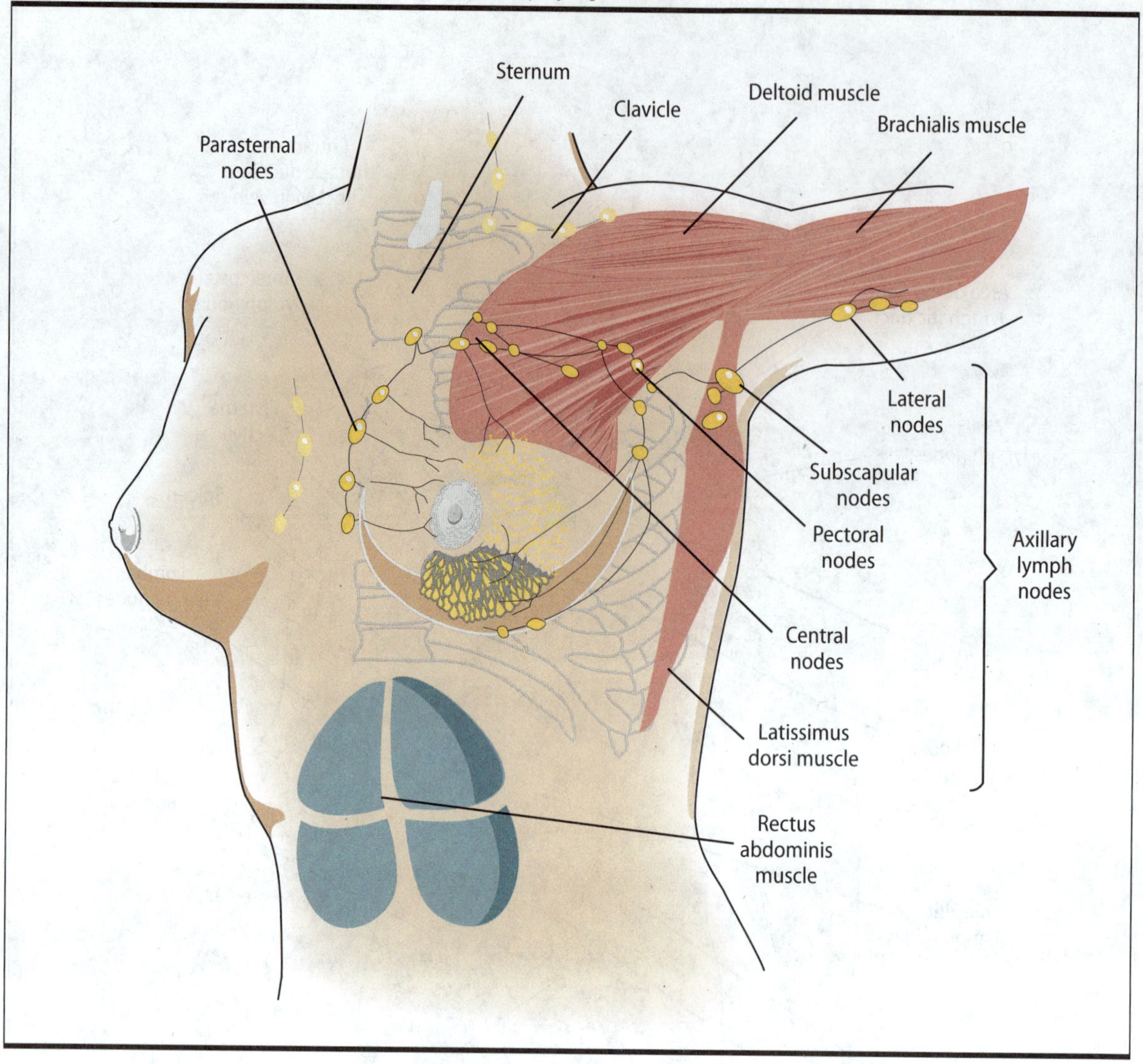

Sternum
Clavicle
Deltoid muscle
Brachialis muscle
Parasternal nodes
Lateral nodes
Subscapular nodes
Pectoral nodes
Axillary lymph nodes
Central nodes
Latissimus dorsi muscle
Rectus abdominis muscle

Lymphatic System of Head and Neck

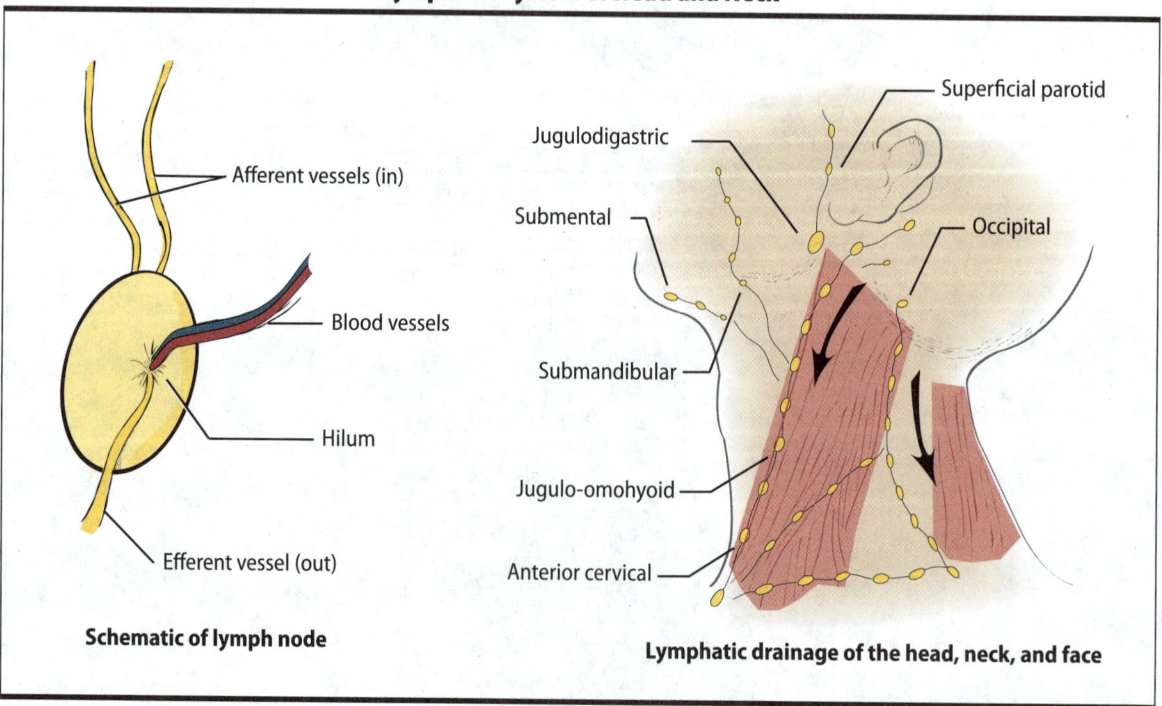

Schematic of lymph node

Lymphatic drainage of the head, neck, and face

Lymphatic Capillaries

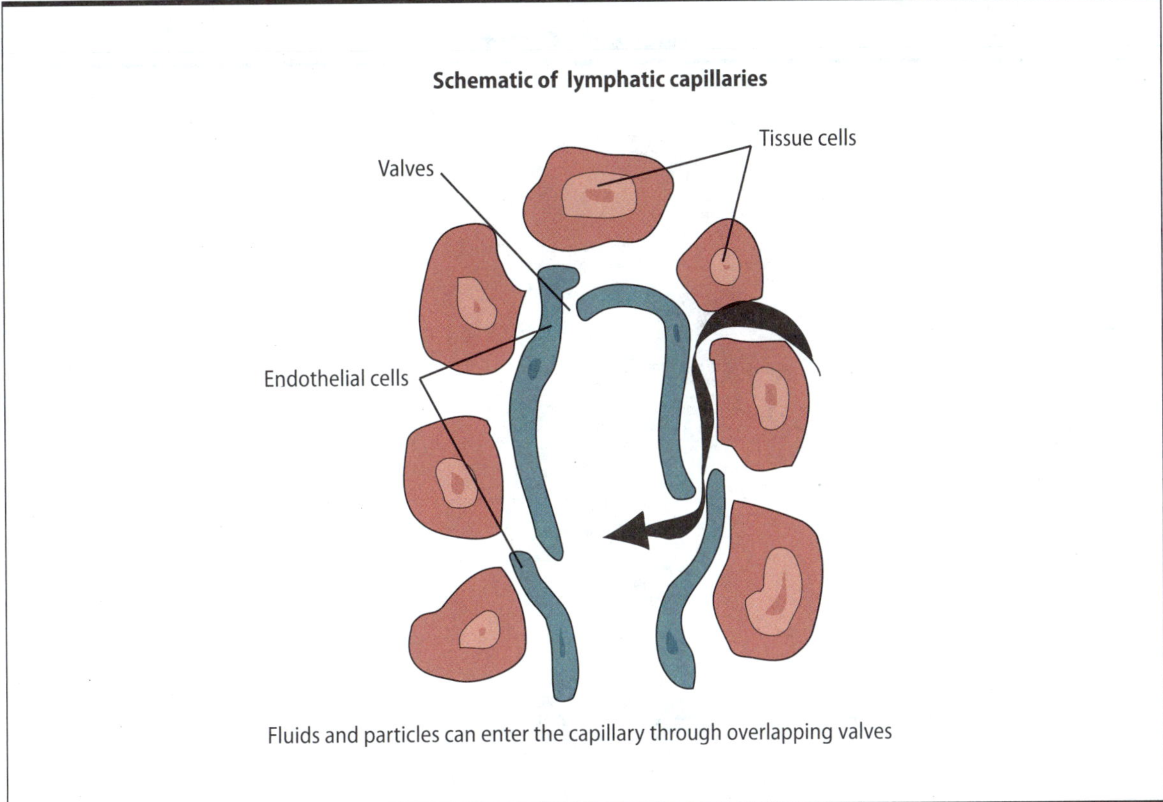

Fluids and particles can enter the capillary through overlapping valves

Lymphatic Drainage

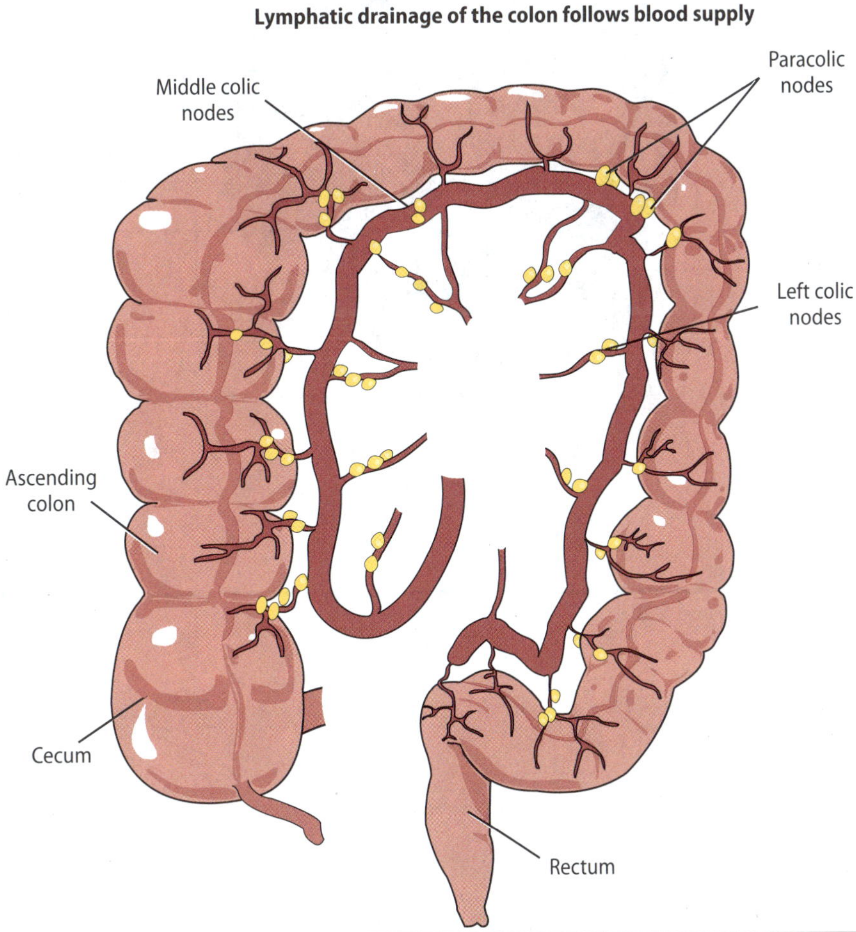

Lymphatic drainage of the colon follows blood supply

Middle colic nodes

Paracolic nodes

Left colic nodes

Ascending colon

Cecum

Rectum

Chapter 10. Diseases of the Respiratory System (JØØ–J99)

Respiratory System

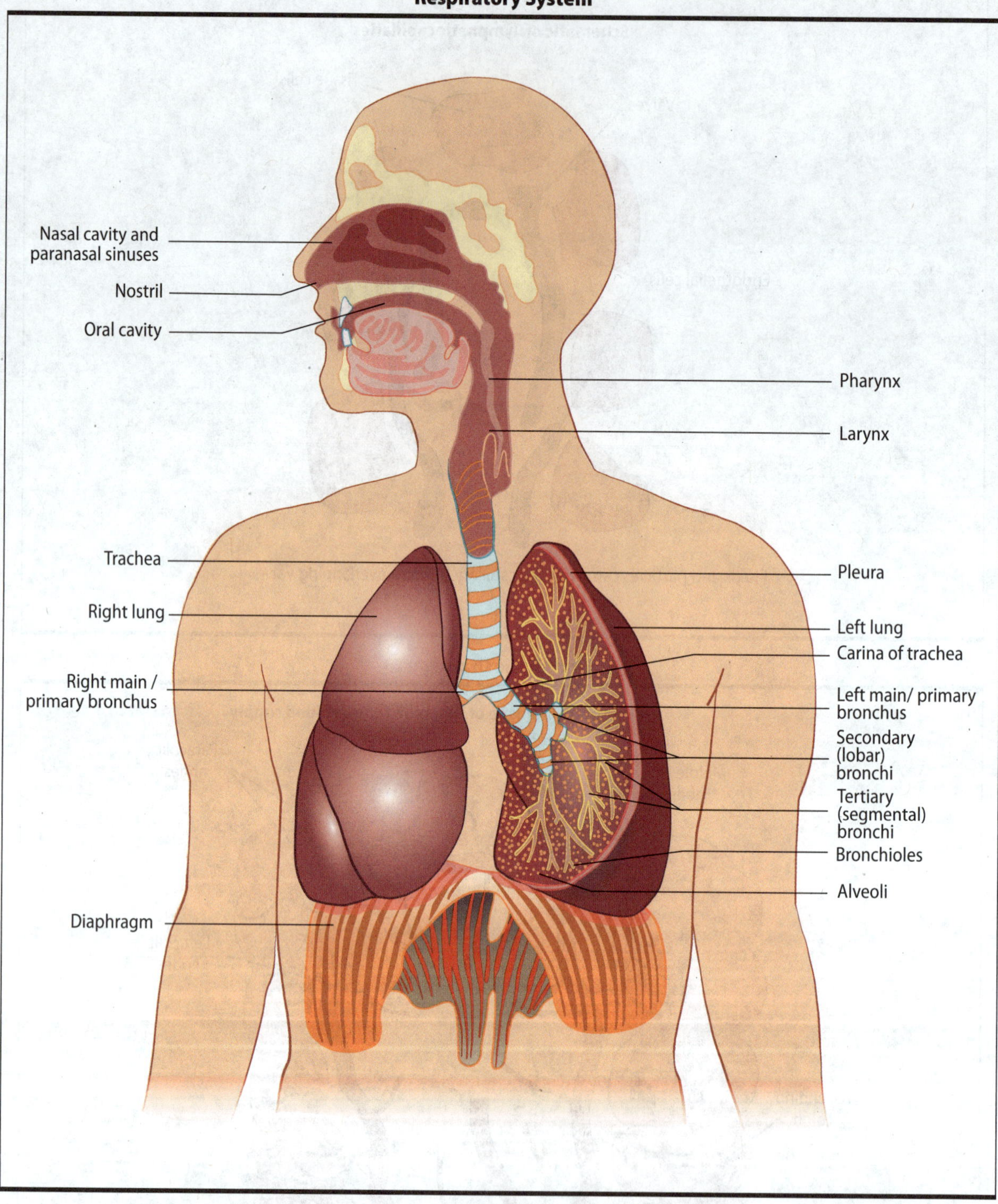

Upper Respiratory System

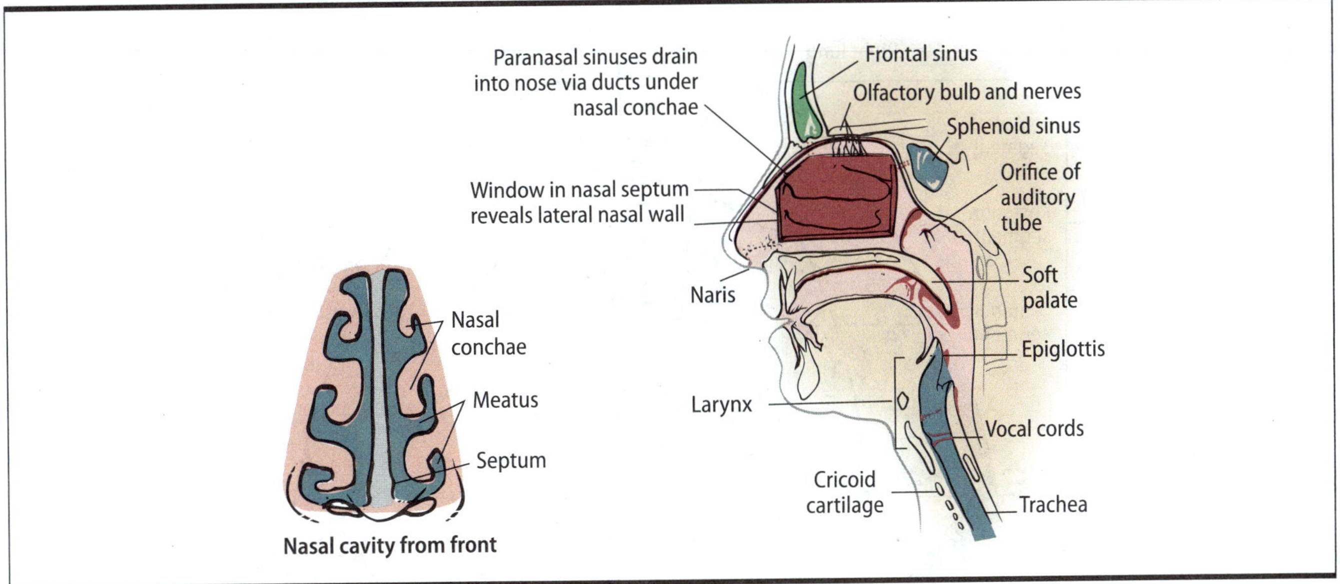

Nasal cavity from front

Lower Respiratory System

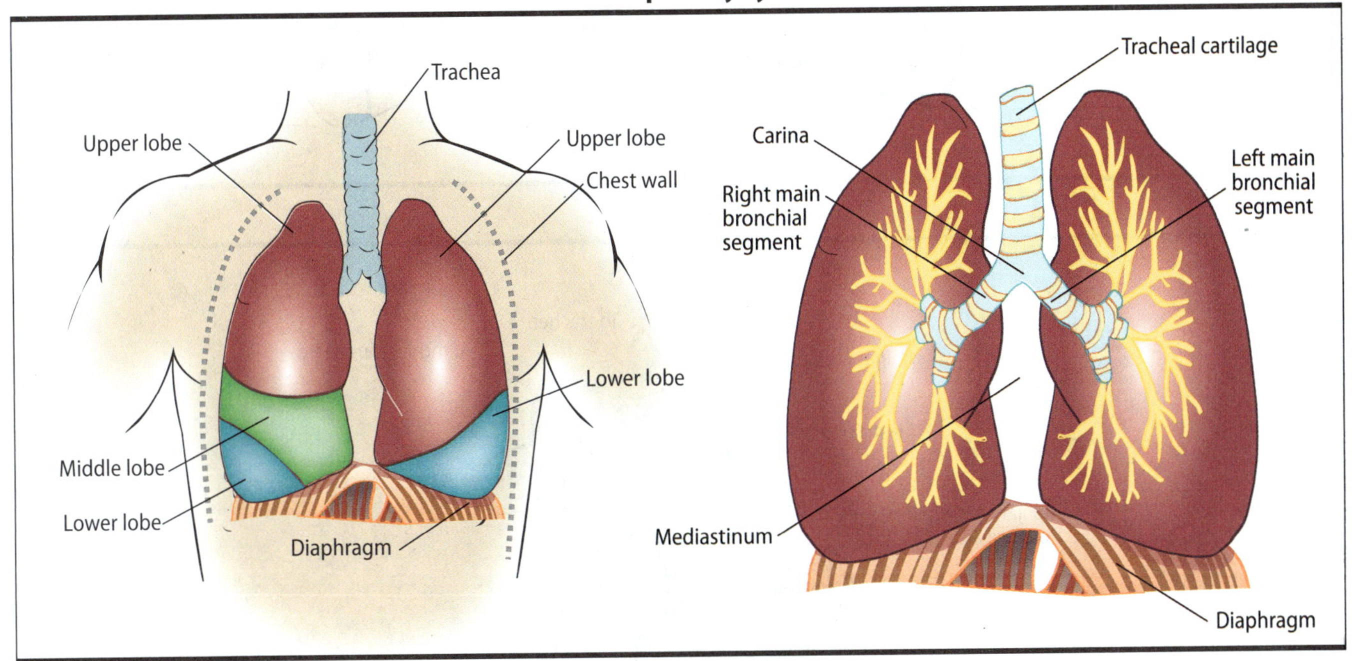

Paranasal Sinuses

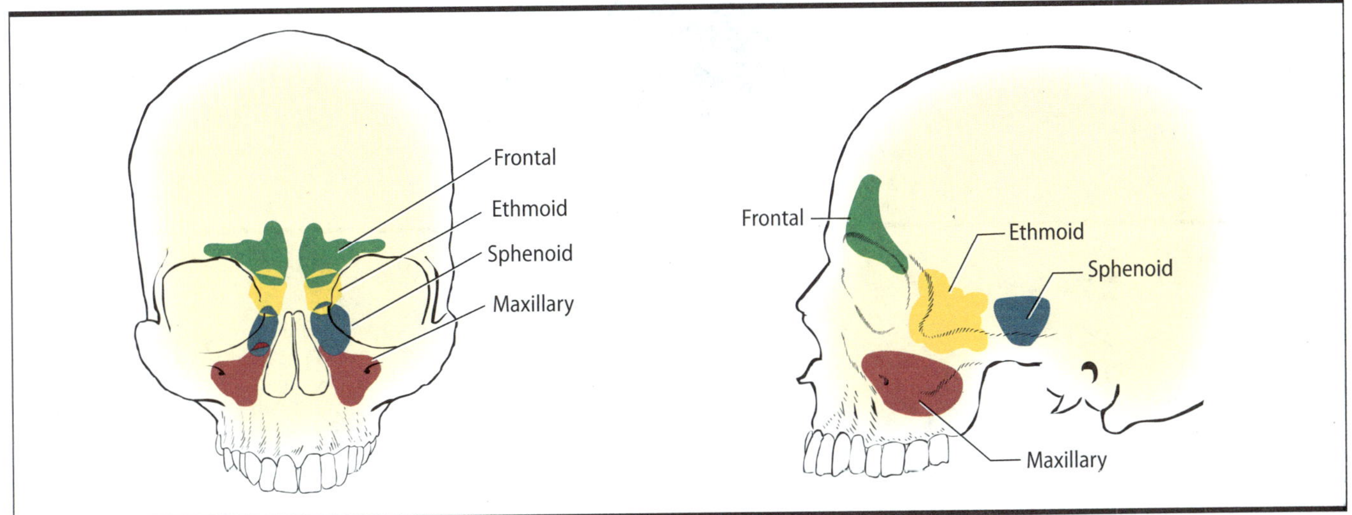

Lung Segments

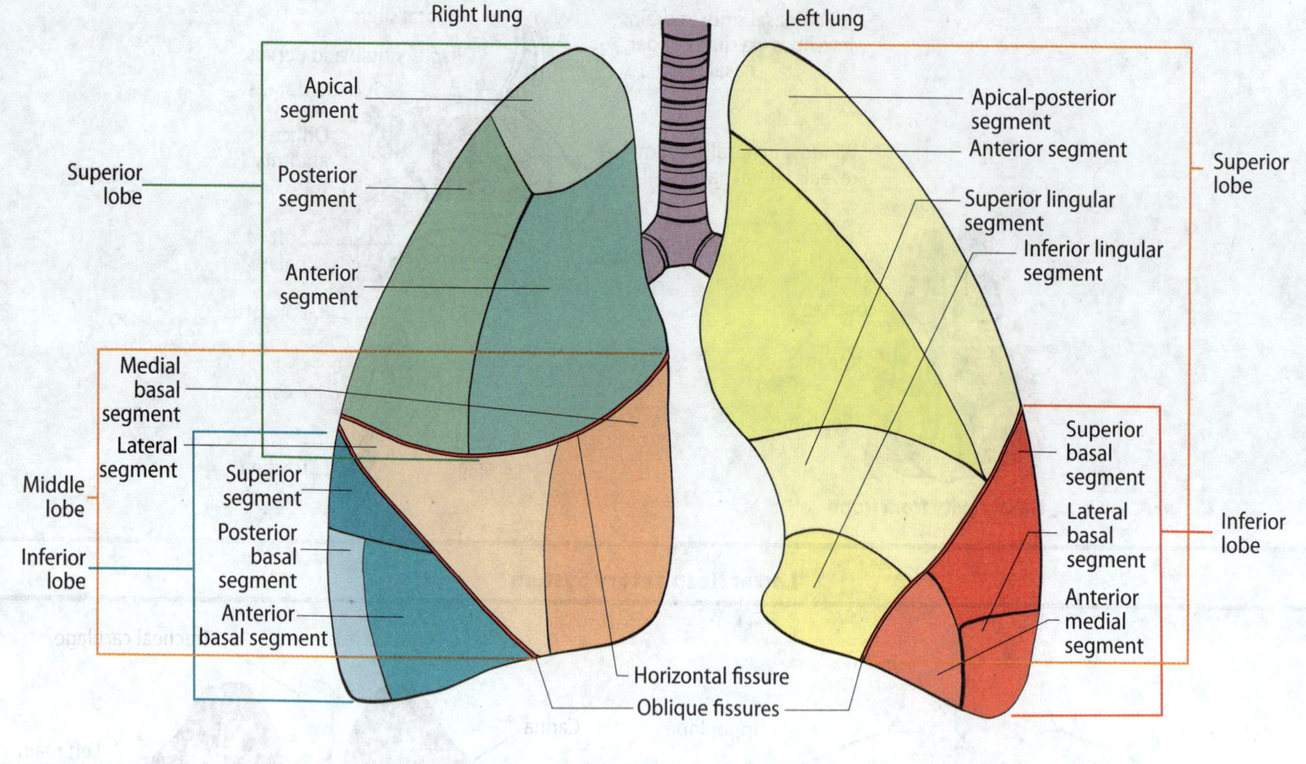

Right lung
Left lung
Superior lobe
Apical segment
Posterior segment
Anterior segment
Medial basal segment
Lateral segment
Middle lobe
Inferior lobe
Superior segment
Posterior basal segment
Anterior basal segment
Horizontal fissure
Oblique fissures
Apical-posterior segment
Anterior segment
Superior lingular segment
Inferior lingular segment
Superior lobe
Superior basal segment
Lateral basal segment
Anterior medial segment
Inferior lobe

Alveoli

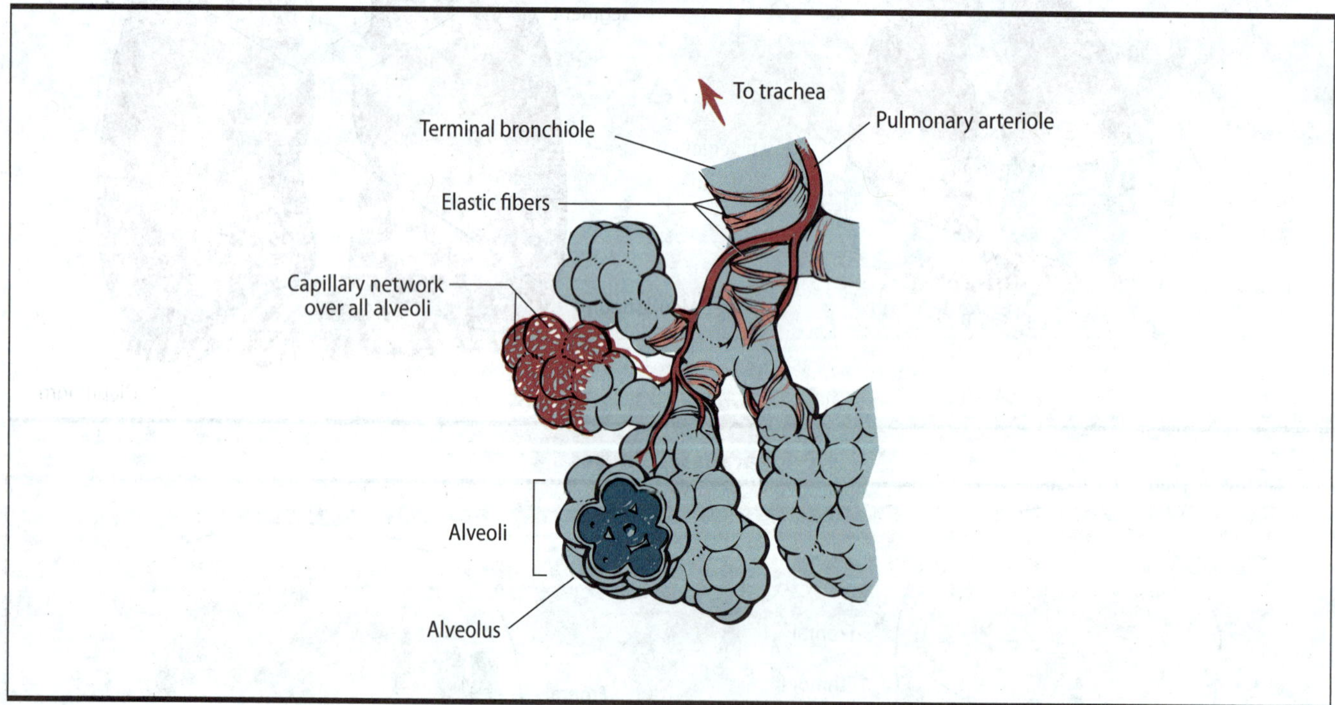

Chapter 11. Diseases of the Digestive System (KØØ–K95)

Digestive System

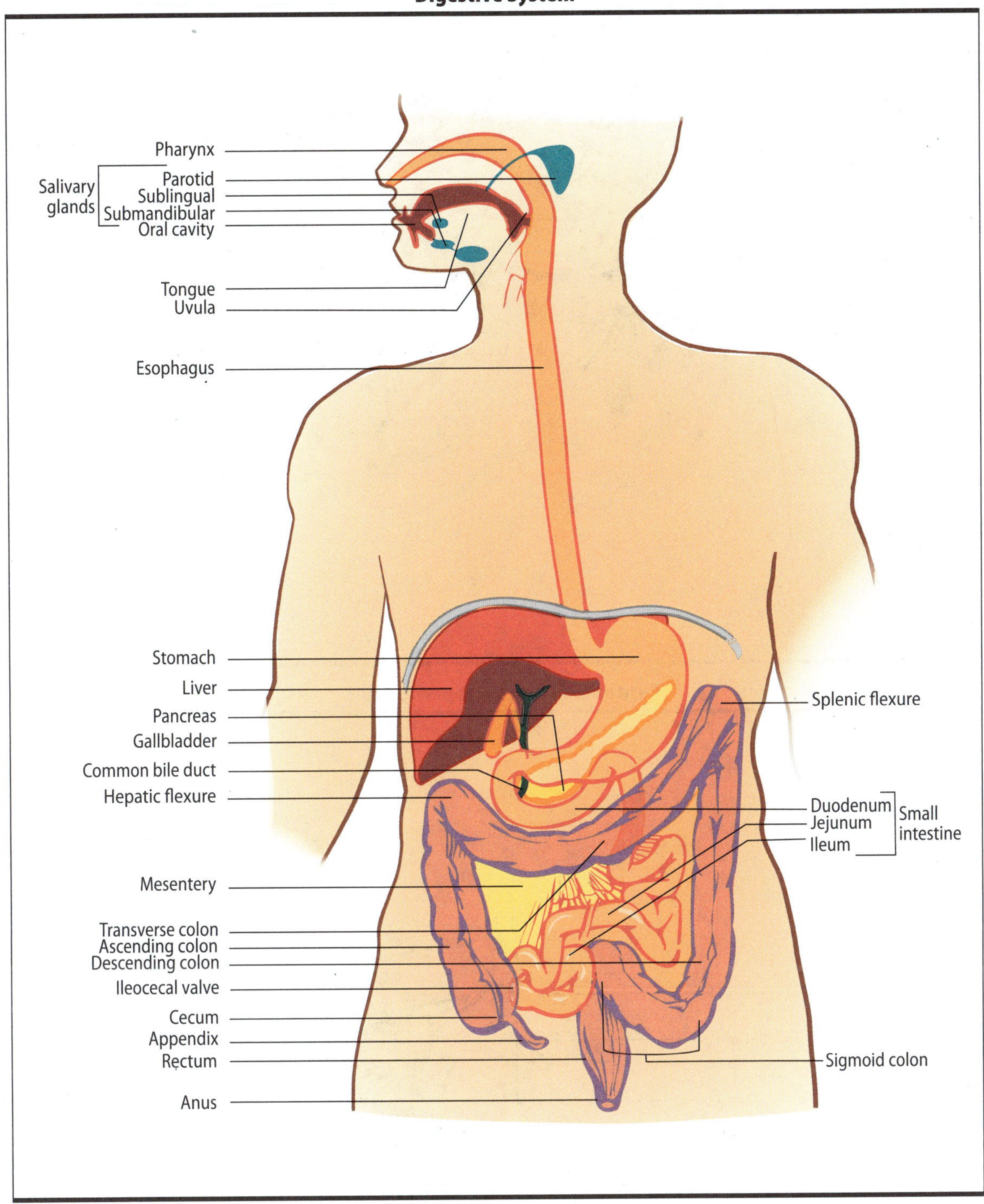

Omentum and Mesentery

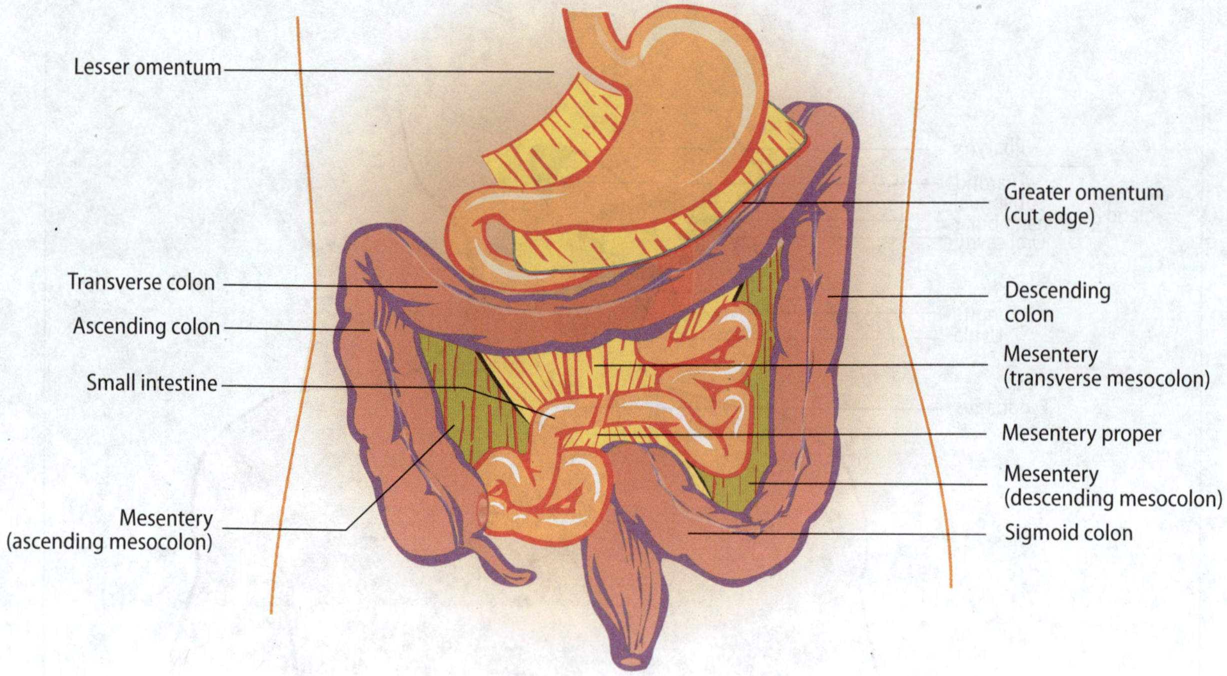

Peritoneum and Retroperitoneum

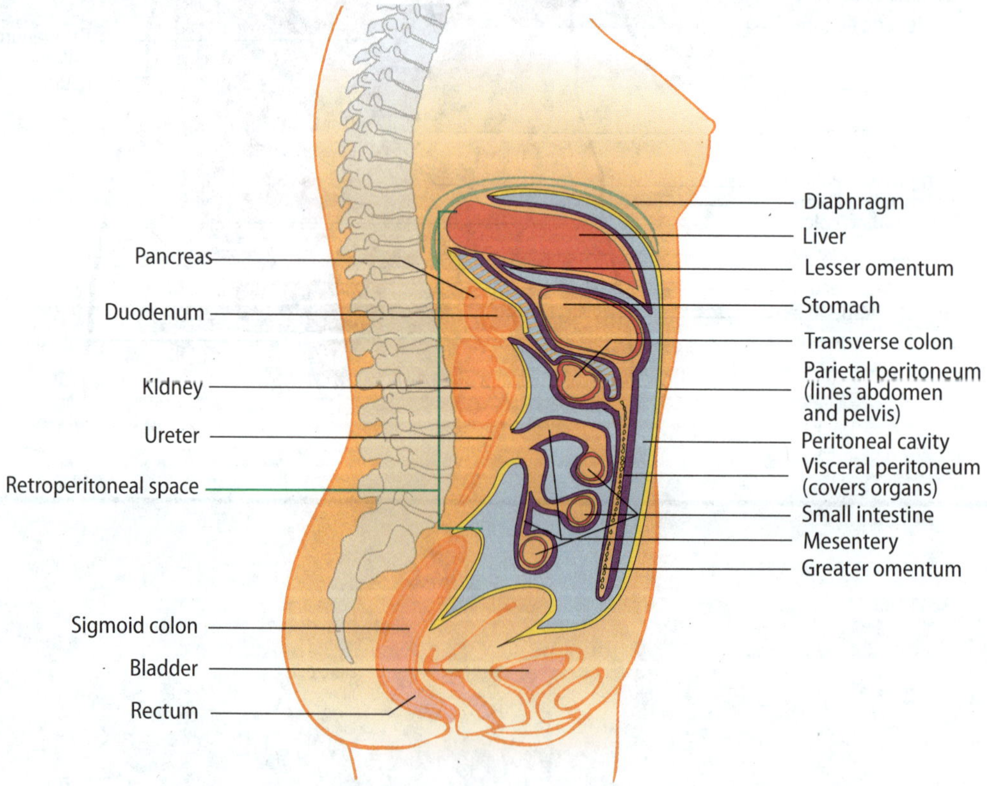

Chapter 12. Diseases of the Skin and Subcutaneous Tissue (LØØ–L99)

Nail Anatomy

Hyponychium
Cuticle
Nail plate
Nail fold
Nail bed
Nail root
Hyponychium
Matrix
Skin
Distal phalanx bone

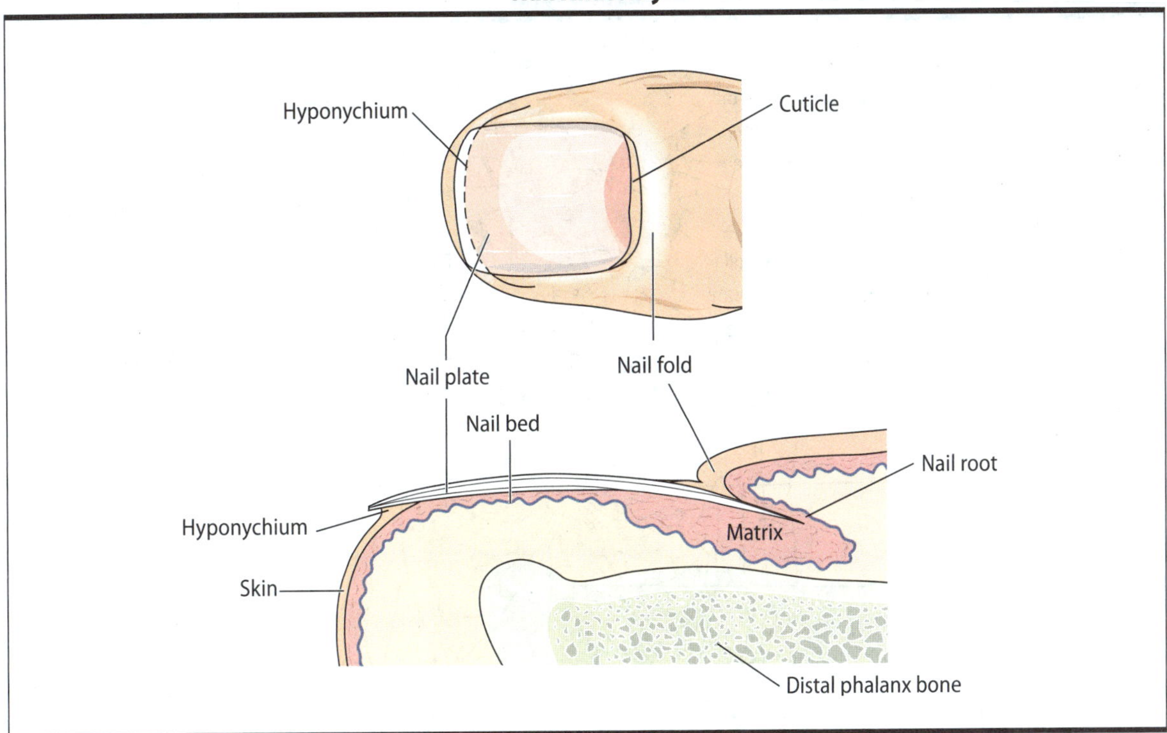

Skin and Subcutaneous Tissue

Hair
Basal layer
Corneal layer (corneum)
Epidermis
Hair shaft
Dermis
Sebaceous gland
Bulb
Hypodermis
(subcutaneous layer)
Hair follicles
Sweat (eccrine gland)
Sensory nerve
Adipose tissue
Blood vessels

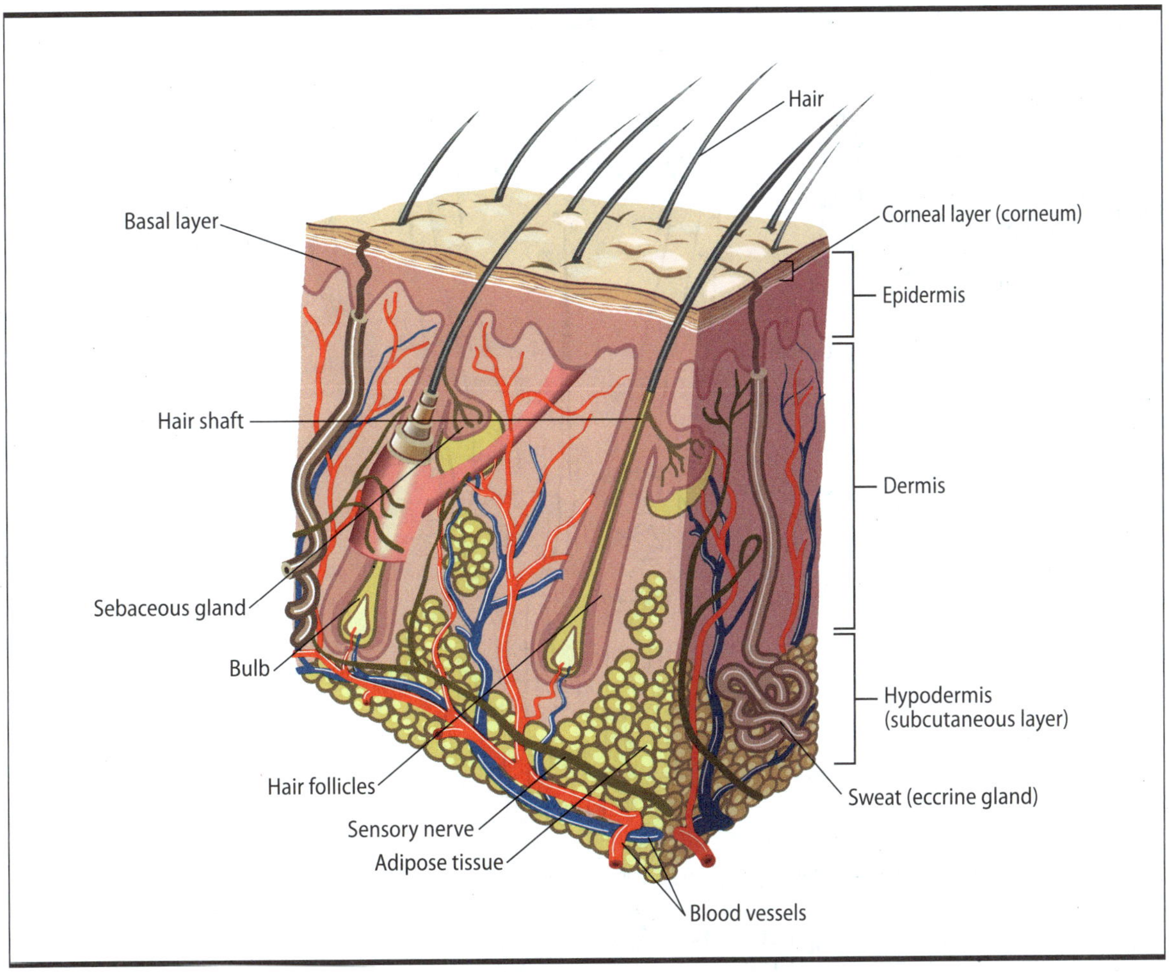

Chapter 13. Diseases of the Musculoskeletal System and Connective Tissue (MØØ–M99)

Bones and Joints

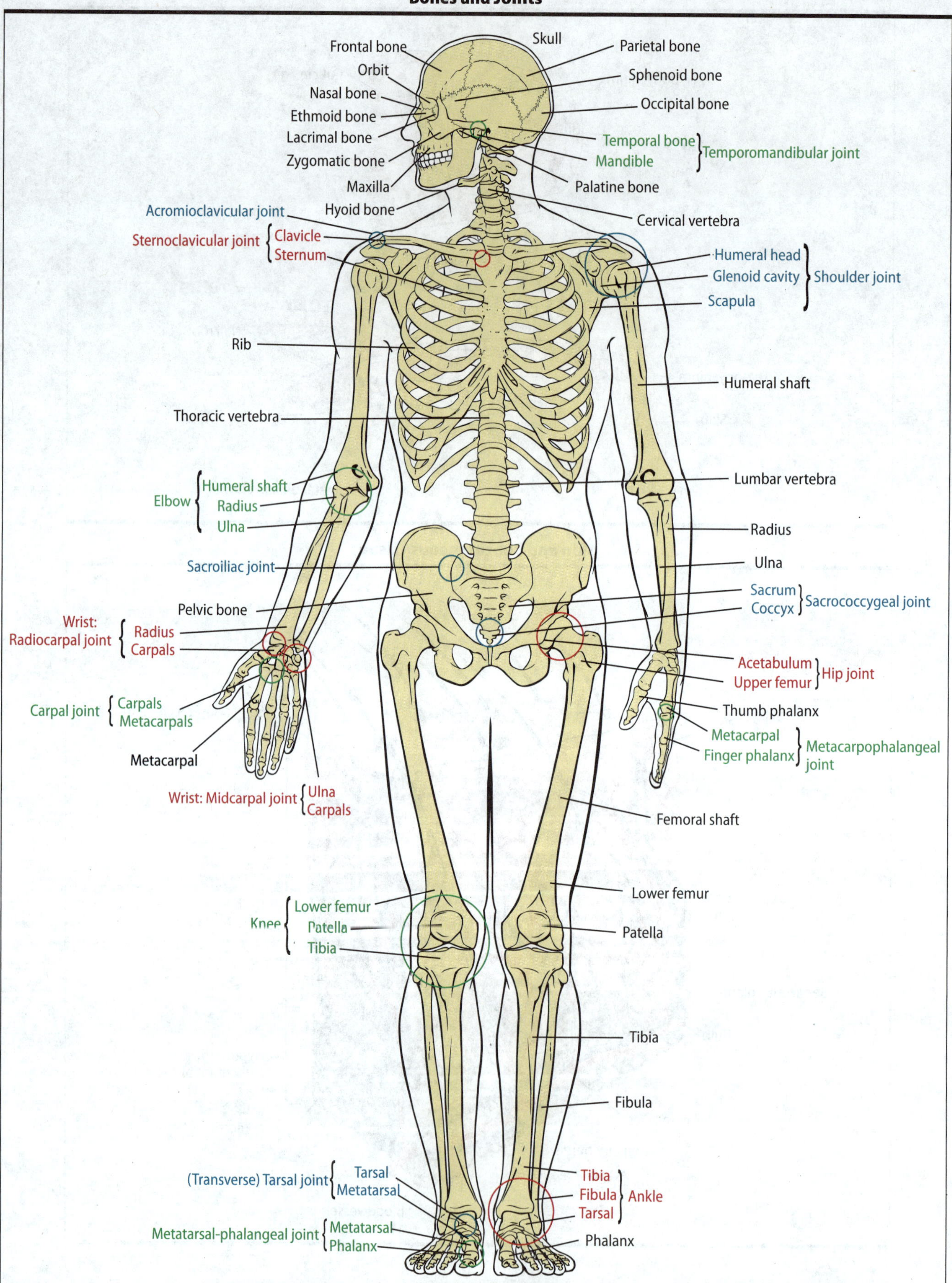

Shoulder Anterior View

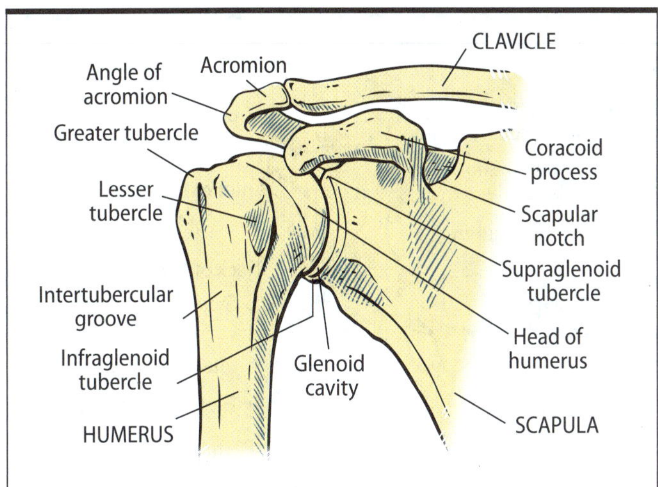

Shoulder Posterior View

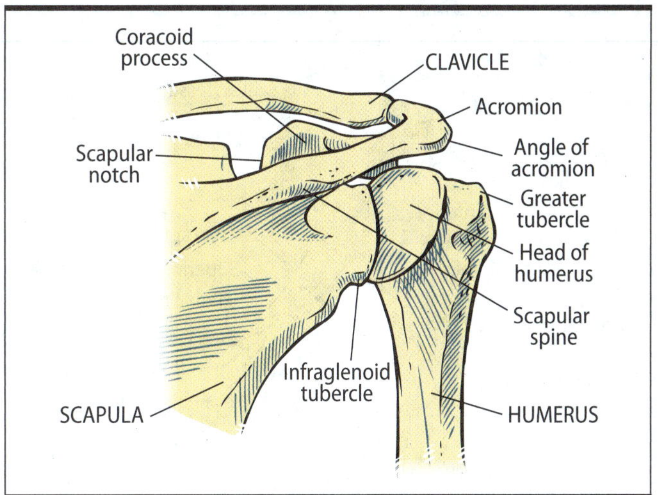

Elbow Anterior View

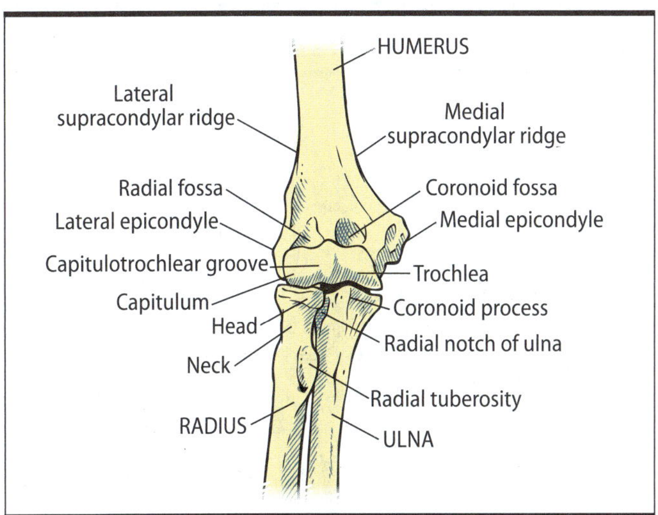

Elbow Posterior View

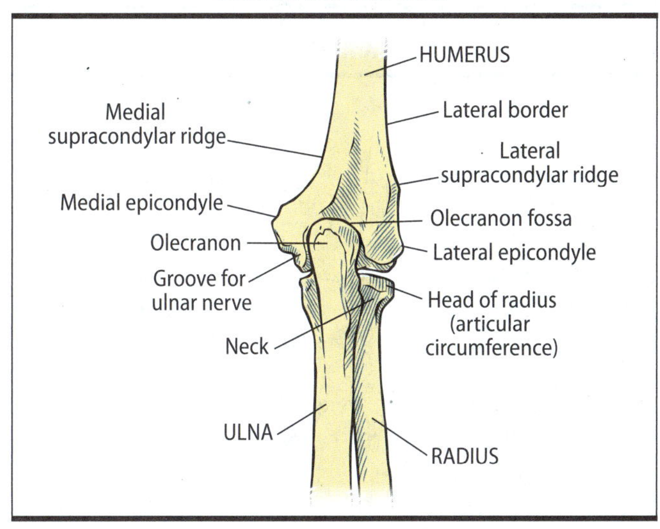

Hand

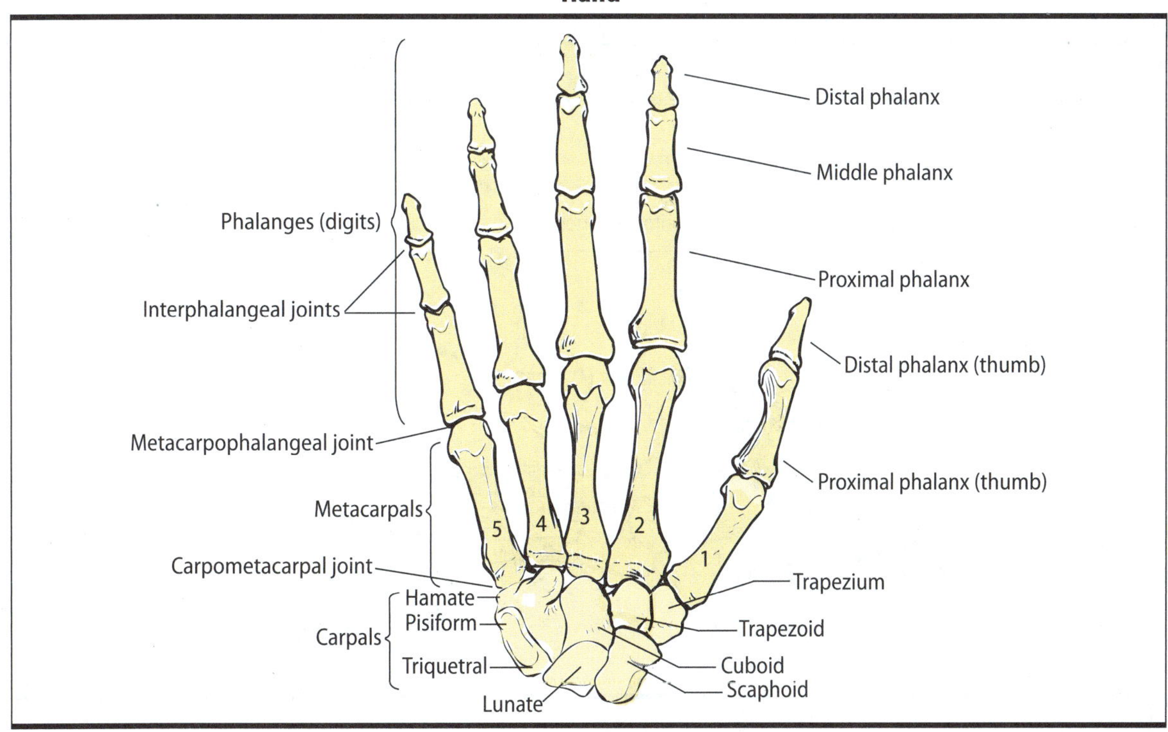

Hip Anterior View

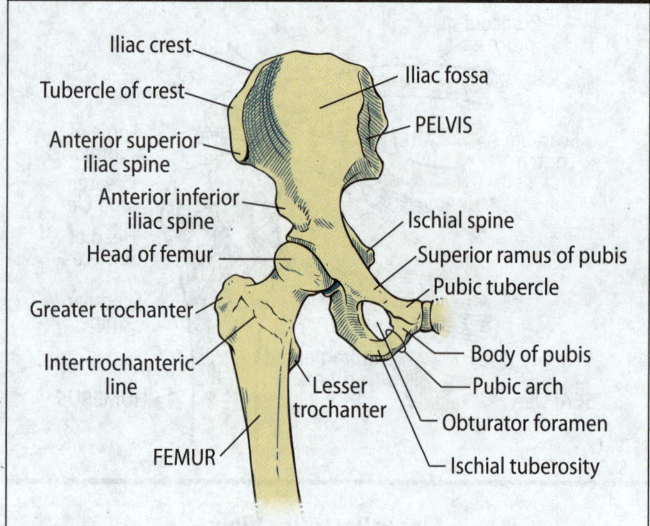

Hip Posterior View

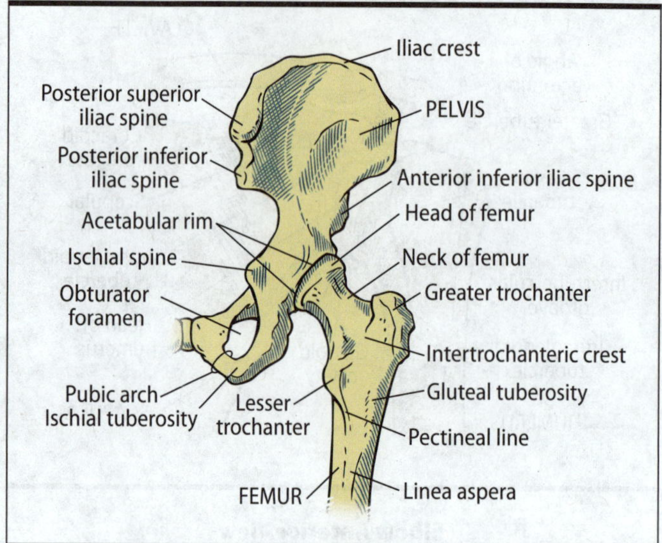

Knee Anterior View

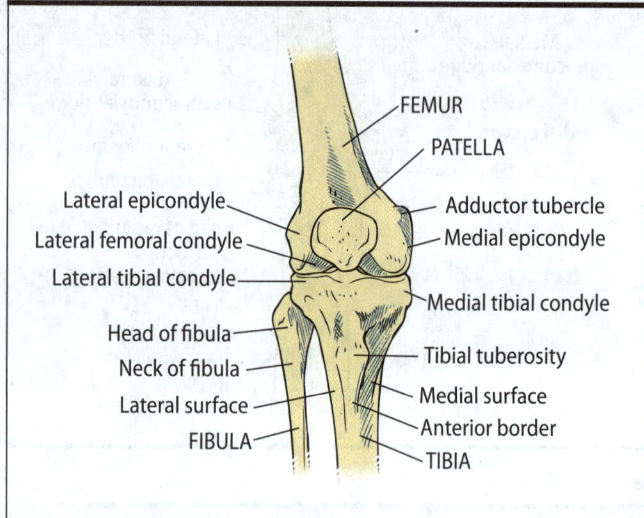

Knee Posterior View

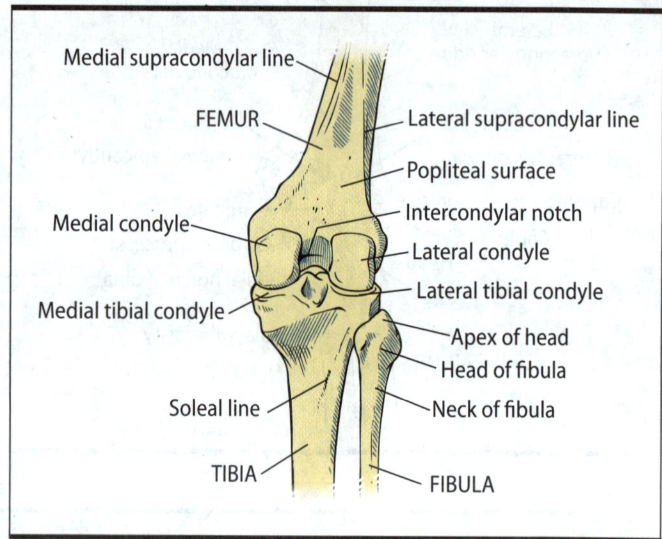

Foot

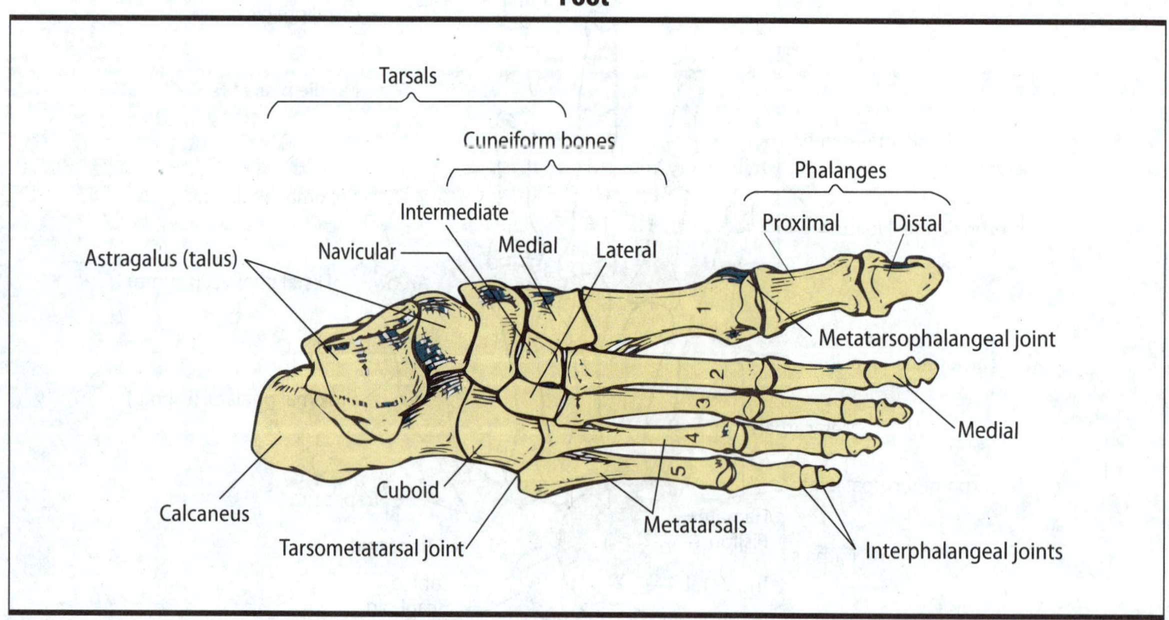

Muscles

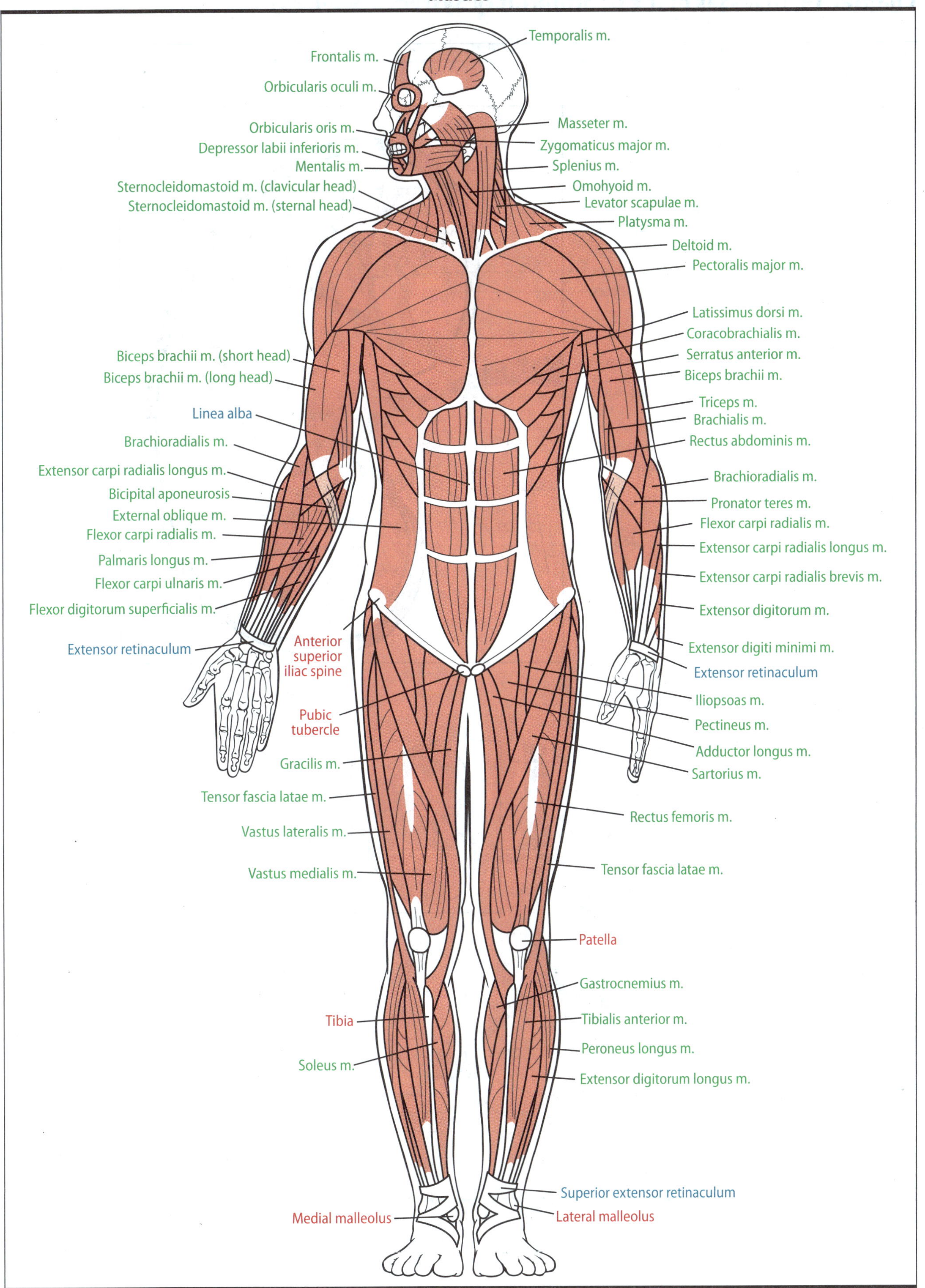

Temporalis m.
Frontalis m.
Orbicularis oculi m.
Orbicularis oris m.
Depressor labii inferioris m.
Mentalis m.
Sternocleidomastoid m. (clavicular head)
Sternocleidomastoid m. (sternal head)
Masseter m.
Zygomaticus major m.
Splenius m.
Omohyoid m.
Levator scapulae m.
Platysma m.
Deltoid m.
Pectoralis major m.
Latissimus dorsi m.
Coracobrachialis m.
Serratus anterior m.
Biceps brachii m.
Biceps brachii m. (short head)
Biceps brachii m. (long head)
Triceps m.
Brachialis m.
Linea alba
Rectus abdominis m.
Brachioradialis m.
Extensor carpi radialis longus m.
Bicipital aponeurosis
External oblique m.
Flexor carpi radialis m.
Palmaris longus m.
Flexor carpi ulnaris m.
Flexor digitorum superficialis m.
Brachioradialis m.
Pronator teres m.
Flexor carpi radialis m.
Extensor carpi radialis longus m.
Extensor carpi radialis brevis m.
Extensor digitorum m.
Extensor digiti minimi m.
Extensor retinaculum
Extensor retinaculum
Anterior superior iliac spine
Pubic tubercle
Iliopsoas m.
Pectineus m.
Adductor longus m.
Sartorius m.
Gracilis m.
Tensor fascia latae m.
Vastus lateralis m.
Vastus medialis m.
Rectus femoris m.
Tensor fascia latae m.
Patella
Gastrocnemius m.
Tibia
Tibialis anterior m.
Peroneus longus m.
Soleus m.
Extensor digitorum longus m.
Superior extensor retinaculum
Medial malleolus
Lateral malleolus

Chapter 14. Diseases of the Genitourinary System (NØØ–N99)

Urinary System

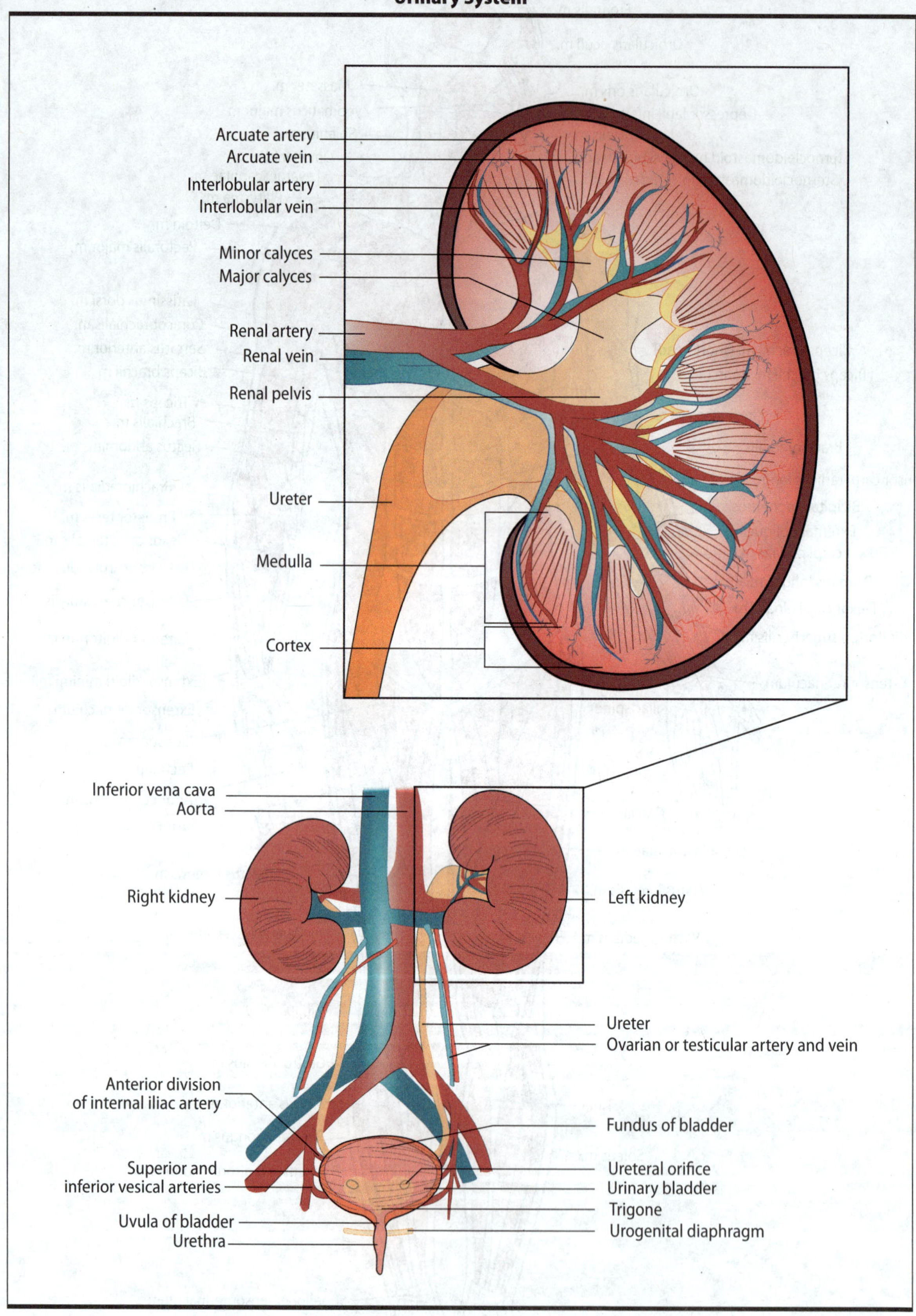

Male Genitourinary System

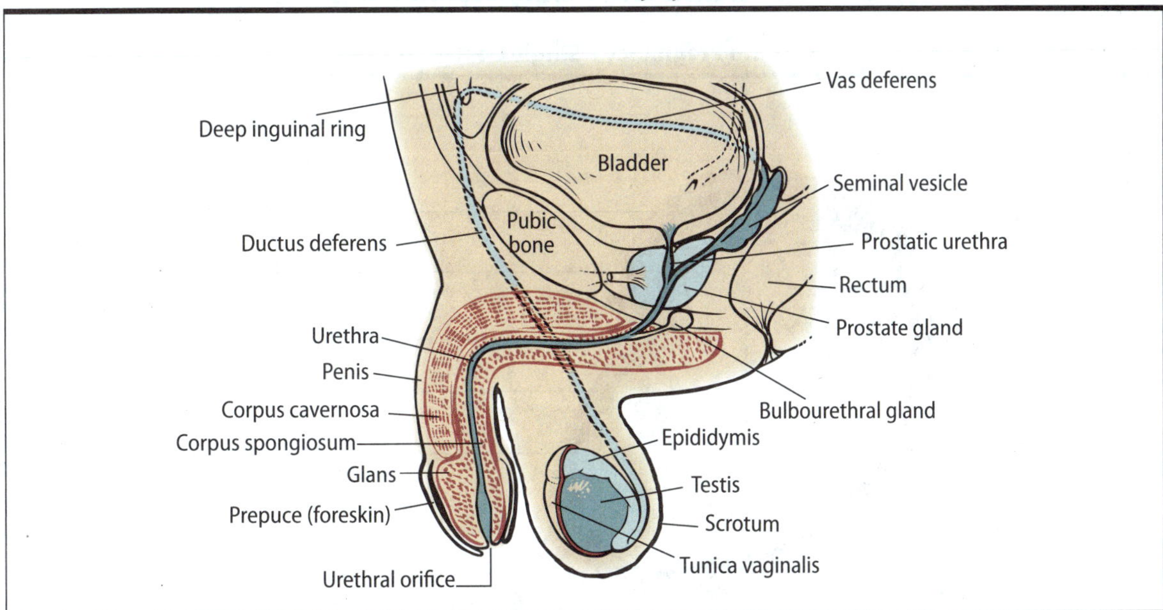

Female Internal Genitalia

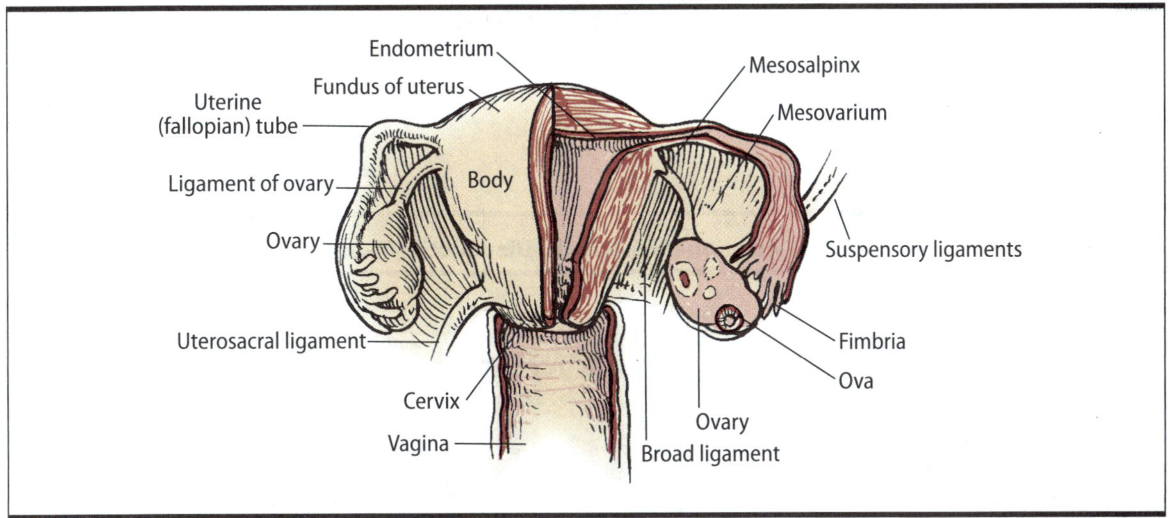

Female Genitourinary Tract Lateral View

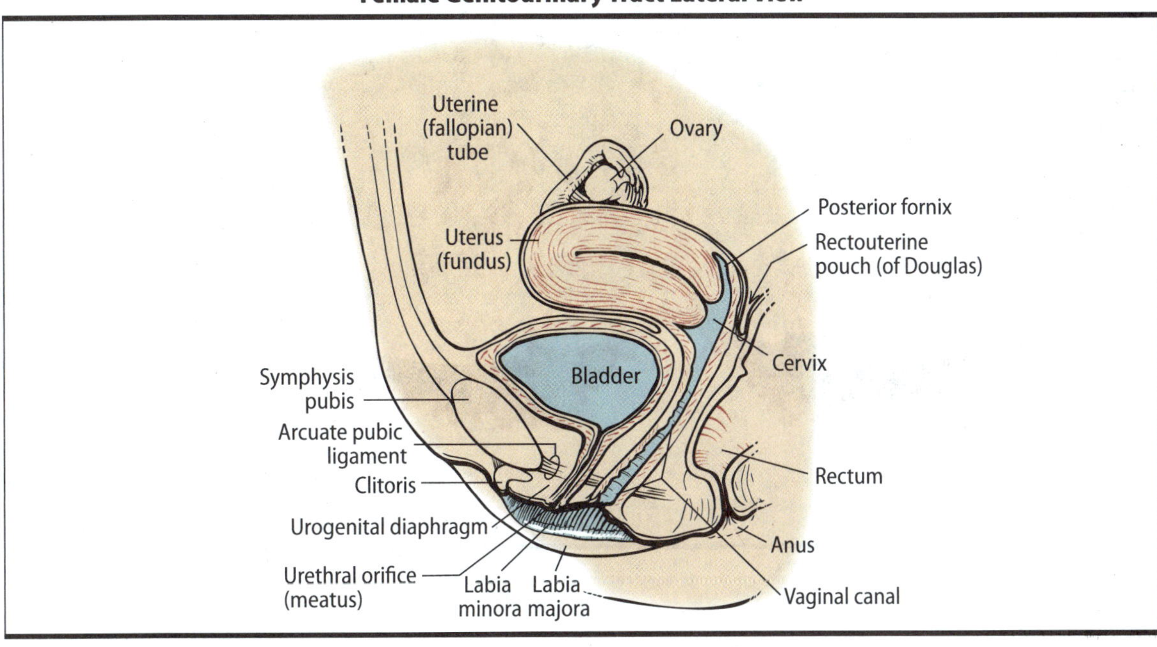

Chapter 15. Pregnancy, Childbirth and the Puerperium (O00–O9A)

Term Pregnancy – Single Gestation

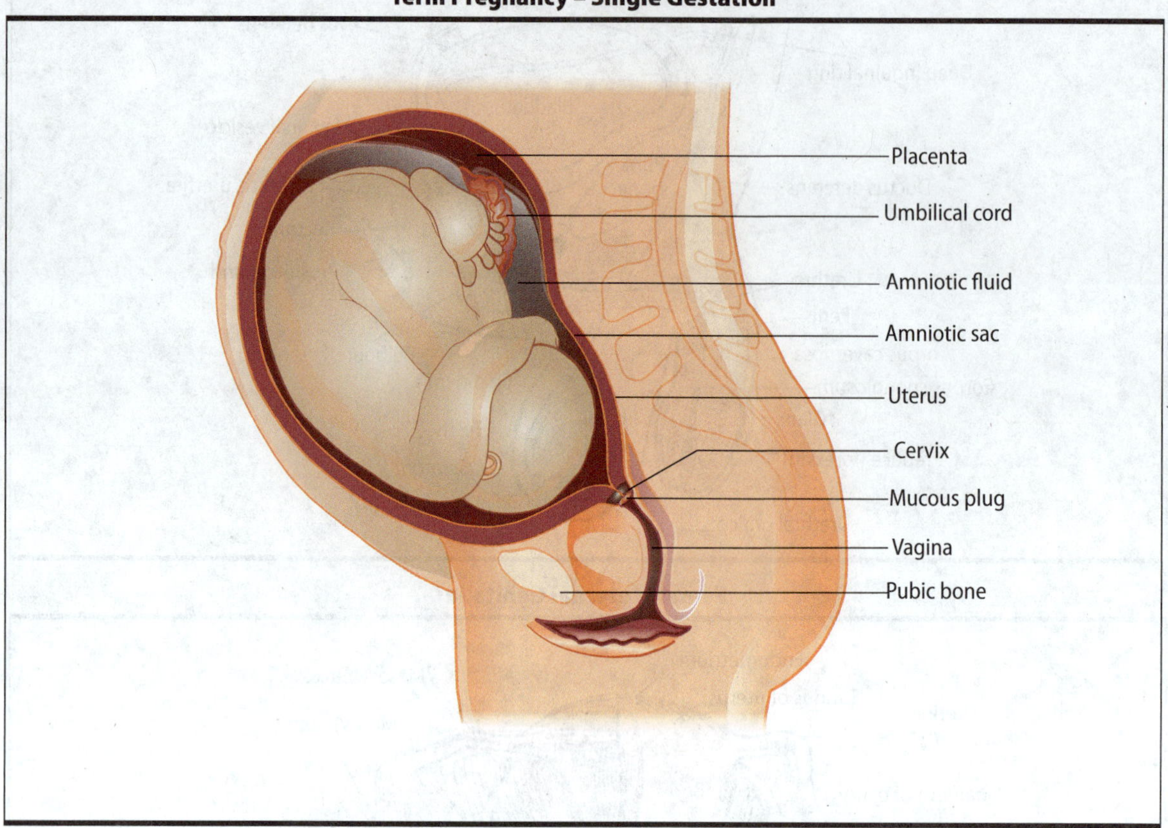

Twin Gestation–Dichorionic–Diamniotic (DI-DI)

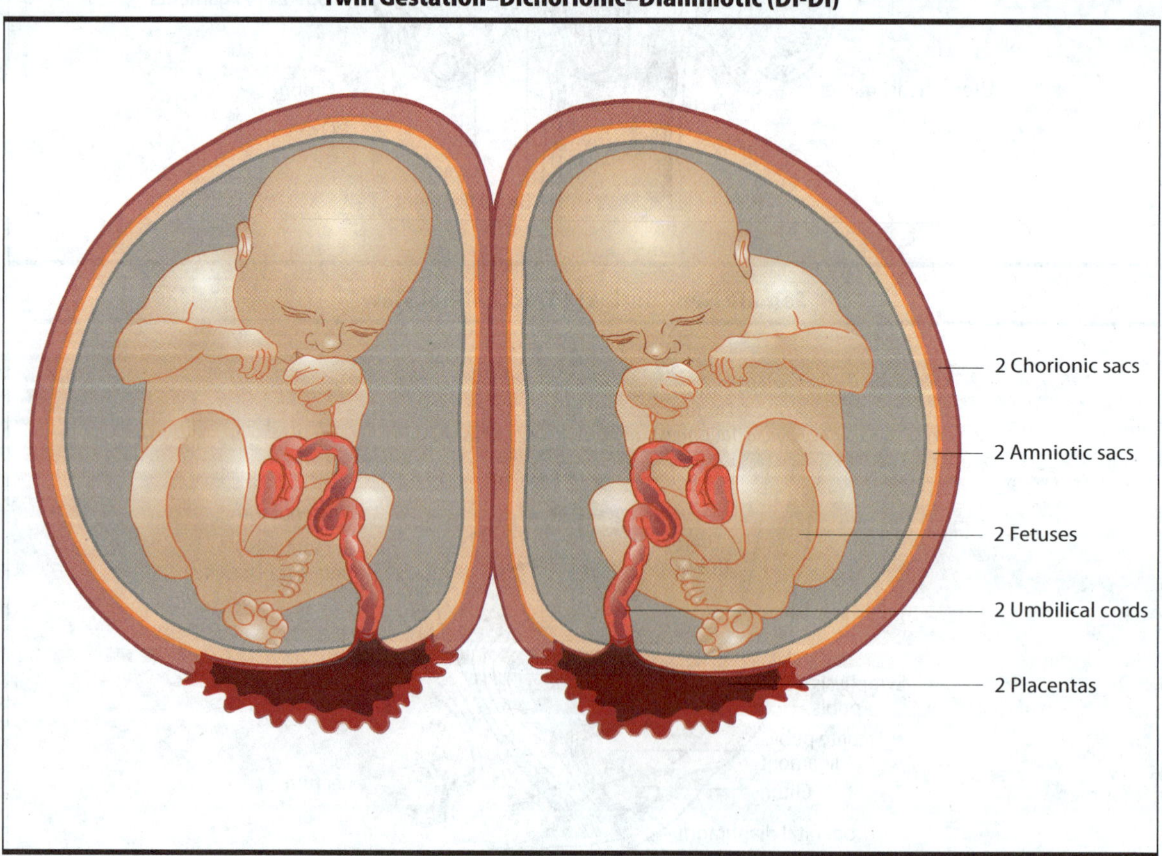

Twin Gestation–Monochorionic–Diamniotic (MO-DI)

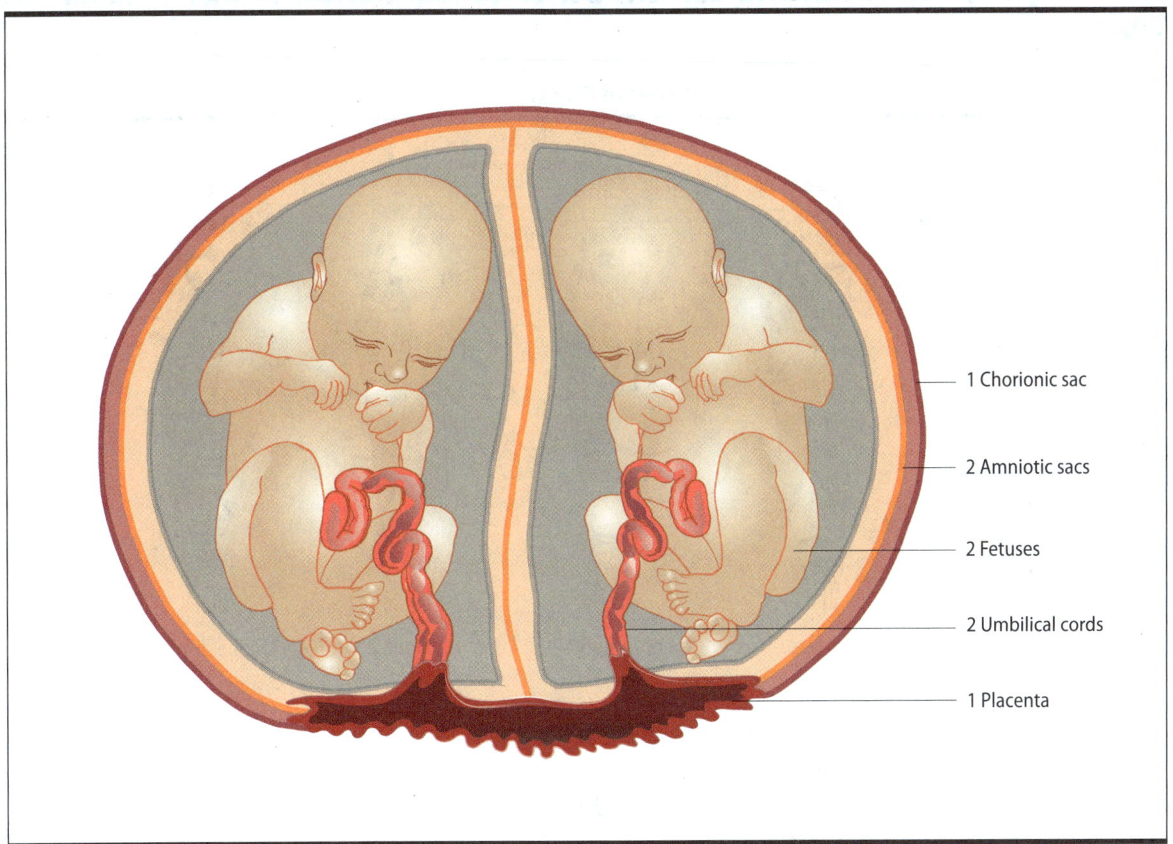

Twin Gestation–Monochorionic–Monoamniotic (MO-MO)

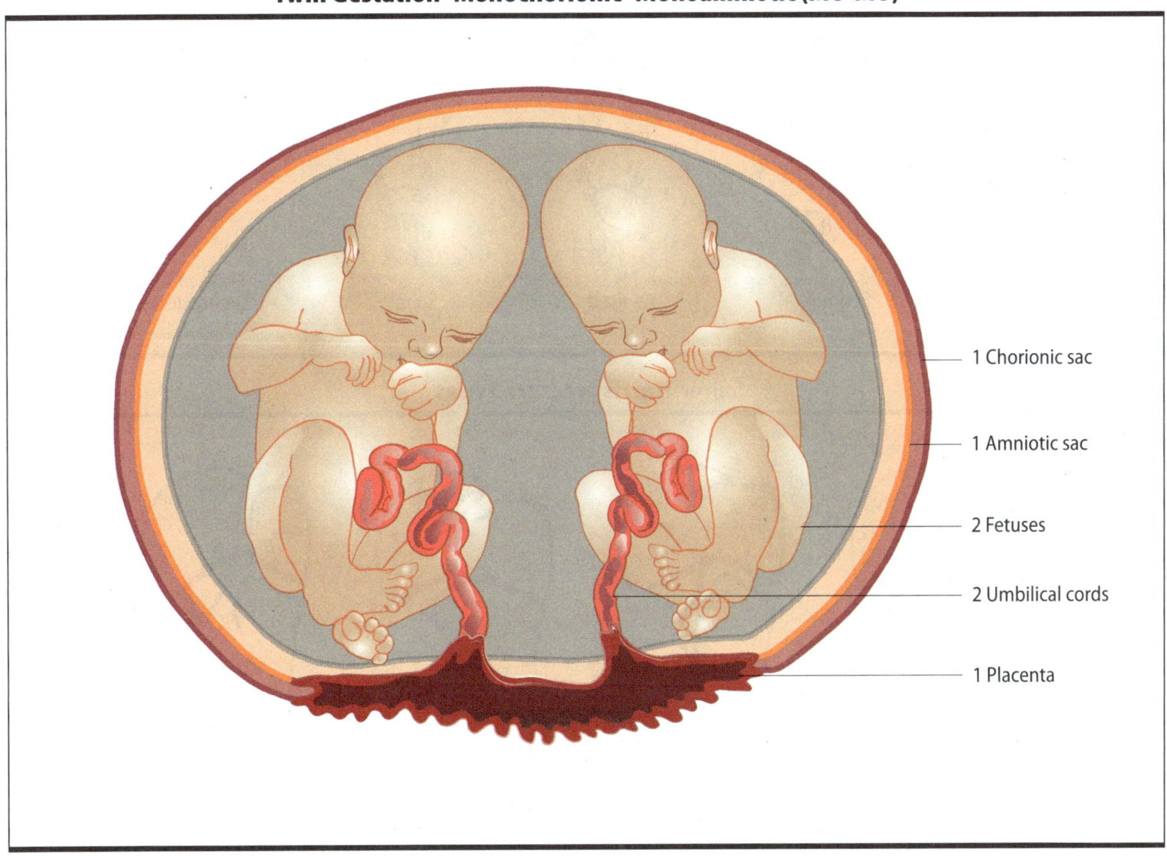

Chapter 19. Injury, Poisoning and Certain Other Consequences of External Causes (SØØ–T88)

Types of Fractures

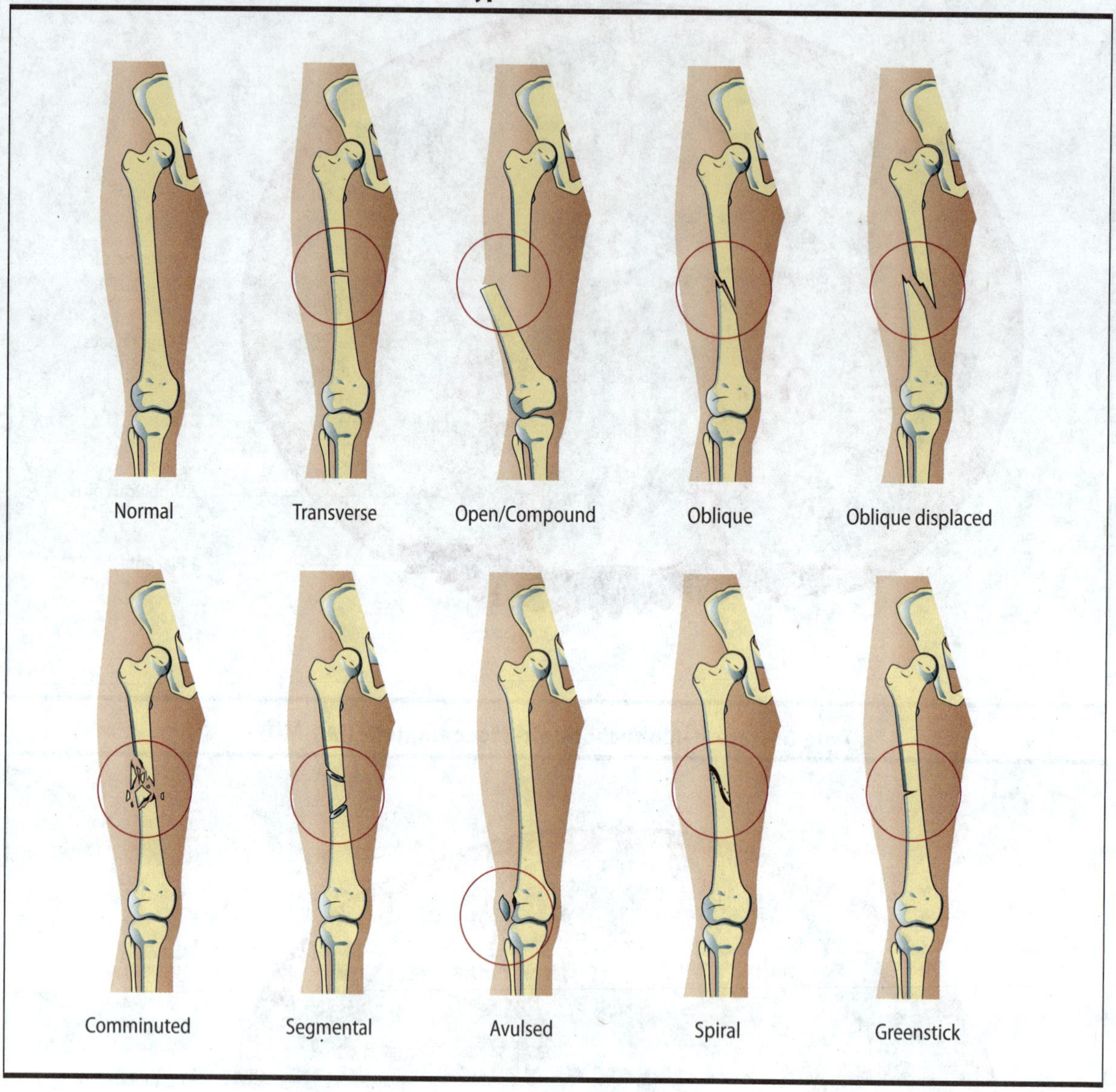

Normal
Transverse
Open/Compound
Oblique
Oblique displaced
Comminuted
Segmental
Avulsed
Spiral
Greenstick

Salter-Harris Fracture Types

Type I
Type II
Type III
Type IV

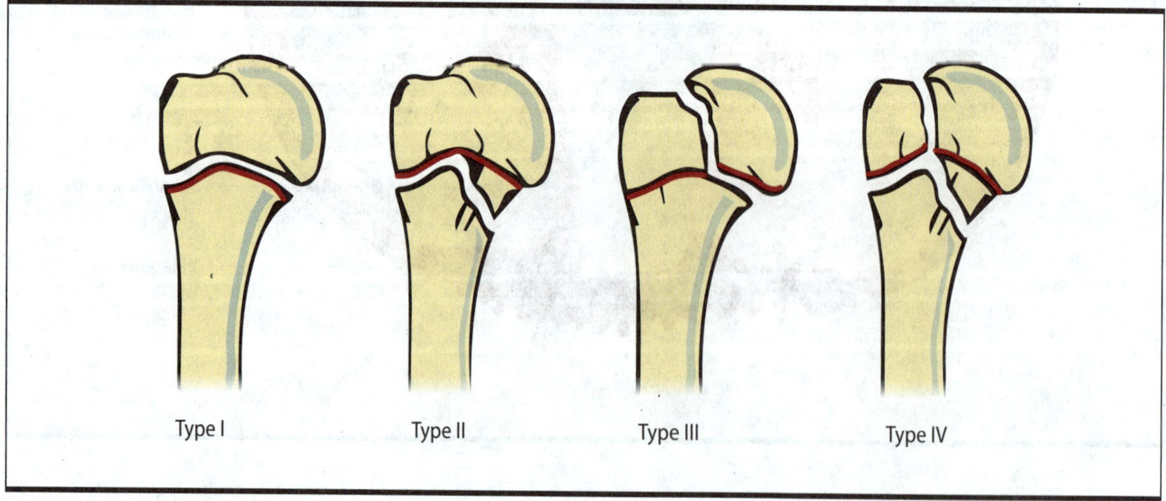